CURRENT SURGICAL THERAPY

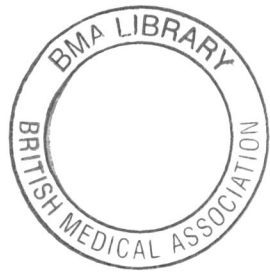

CURRENT SURGICAL THERAPY

11th EDITION

JOHN L. CAMERON
MD, FACS, FRCS (Eng) (hon), FRCS (Ed) (hon), FRCSI (hon)

The Alfred Blalock Distinguished Service Professor
Department of Surgery
The Johns Hopkins Medical Institutions
Baltimore, Maryland

ANDREW M. CAMERON
MD, PhD, FACS

Associate Professor of Surgery
Surgical Director of Liver Transplantation
Department of Surgery
The Johns Hopkins Medical Institutions
Baltimore, Maryland

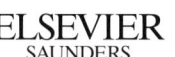

ELSEVIER
SAUNDERS

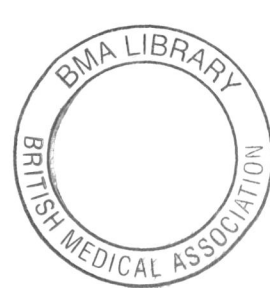

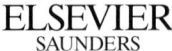

ELSEVIER
SAUNDERS

1600 John F. Kennedy Blvd.
Ste 1800
Philadelphia, PA 19103-2899

CURRENT SURGICAL THERAPY, ELEVENTH EDITION   ISBN: 978-1-4557-4007-9

Notices

Knowledge and best practice in this field are constantly changing. As new research and experience broaden our understanding, changes in research methods, professional practices, or medical treatment may become necessary.

Practitioners and researchers must always rely on their own experience and knowledge in evaluating and using any information, methods, compounds, or experiments described herein. In using such information or methods they should be mindful of their own safety and the safety of others, including parties for whom they have a professional responsibility.

With respect to any drug or pharmaceutical products identified, readers are advised to check the most current information provided (i) on procedures featured or (ii) by the manufacturer of each product to be administered, to verify the recommended dose or formula, the method and duration of administration, and contraindications. It is the responsibility of practitioners, relying on their own experience and knowledge of their patients, to make diagnoses, to determine dosages and the best treatment for each individual patient, and to take all appropriate safety precautions.

To the fullest extent of the law, neither the Publisher nor the authors, contributors, or editors, assume any liability for any injury and/or damage to persons or property as a matter of products liability, negligence or otherwise, or from any use or operation of any methods, products, instructions, or ideas contained in the material herein.

ISBN: 978-1-4557-4007-9

Publishing Manager: Michael Houston
Managing Editor: Kathryn DeFrancesco
Publishing Services Manager: Catherine Jackson
Senior Project Manager: Mary Pohlman
Design Direction: Steven Stave

Printed in the U.S.A.

Last digit is the print number: 9   8   7   6   5   4   3   2   1

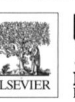

Working together
to grow libraries in
developing countries

www.elsevier.com • www.bookaid.org

LIST OF CONTRIBUTORS

Herand Abcarian, MD
Professor of Surgery
University of Illinois at Chicago
Chicago, Illinois

HEMORRHOIDS

THE MANAGEMENT OF RECTOVAGINAL FISTULA

Raafat Z. Abdel-Misih, MD, FRCS Edin, FRCS Eng, FACS
Department of Surgery
Christiana Care Health System
Newark, Delaware

THE MANAGEMENT OF BENIGN GASTRIC ULCER

Sherif R. Abdel-Misih, MD
Assistant Professor of Surgery
Wexner Medical Center at The Ohio State
  University
Arthur G James Cancer Hospital
Columbus, Ohio

THE MANAGEMENT OF BENIGN GASTRIC ULCER

Fizan Abdullah, MD, PhD
Johns Hopkins University
Baltimore, Maryland

REPAIR OF PECTUS EXCAVATUM

Christopher J. Abularrage, MD, FACS
Director, Multidisiplinary Diabetic Foot &
  Wound Clinic
Assistant Professor of Surgery
Division of Vascular Surgery and
  Endovascular Therapy
The Johns Hopkins Hospital
Baltimore, Maryland

CAROTID ENDARTERECTOMY

David B. Adams, MD, FACS
Professor of Surgery
Head, Section of General and
  Gastrointestinal Surgery
Medical University of South Carolina
Charleston, South Carolina

THE MANAGEMENT OF PANCREATIC PSEUDOCYST

Reid B. Adams, MD
Claude A. Jessup Professor of Surgery
Chief, Division of Surgical Oncology
Chief, Hepatobiliary and Pancreatic
  Surgery
Director, Gastrointestinal Oncology
  Program
Department of Surgery
University of Virginia Health System
Charlottesville, Virginia

GALLBLADDER CANCER

Suresh Mitu Agarwal, MD
Associate Professor of Surgery
Section Chief, Trauma, Acute Care Surgery,
  Burn, and Surgical Critical Care
Department of Surgery
University of Wisconsin School of Medicine
  and Public Health
Madison, Wisconsin

TRACHEOSTOMY

Rizwan Ahmed, MD
Division of Surgery
Johns Hopkins Bayview Medical Center
Baltimore, Maryland

THE MANAGEMENT OF COMMON BILE DUCT STONES

Steven A. Ahrendt, MD
Associate Professor of Surgery
University of Pittsburgh
Pittsburgh, Pennsylvania

PRIMARY SCLEROSING CHOLANGITIS

Nita Ahuja, MD
The Johns Hopkins Hospital
Baltimore, Maryland

THE MANAGEMENT OF ADRENAL CORTICAL TUMORS

Gilbert Aidinian, MD, FACS, RPVI
Chief, Vascular and Endovascular Surgery
William Beaumont Army Medical Center
El Paso, Texas;
Assistant Professor of Surgery
The Norman M. Rich Department of
  Surgery
The Uniformed Services University of the
  Health Sciences
Bethesda, Maryland

THE DIABETIC FOOT

Daniel S. Alam, MD, FACS
Cleveland Clinic
Cleveland, Ohio

FACIAL TRAUMA: EVALUATION AND MANAGEMENT

Scott P. Albert, MD
Surgical Oncology Fellow
The Ohio State University
Columbus, Ohio

THE MANAGEMENT OF PANCREATIC ISLET CELL TUMORS EXCLUDING GASTRINOMAS

Marco Ettore Allaix, MD
Department of Surgery
University of Chicago Medical Center
Chicago, Illinois;
Department of Surgical Sciences
University of Torino
Torino, Italy

TUMORS OF THE ANAL CANAL

Benjamin O. Anderson, MD
Surgical Oncology Section, Division of
  General Surgery
Department of Surgery
University of Washington
Seattle, Washington

BREAST RECONSTRUCTION FOLLOWING MASTECTOMY: INDICATIONS, TECHNIQUES, AND RESULTS

Mark P. Androes, MD
Division of Vascular Surgery
Greenville Hospital System Clinical
  University
University of South Carolina School of
  Medicine
Greenville, South Carolina

PROFUNDA FEMORIS RECONSTRUCTION

George Apostolides, MD, FACS, FASCRS
Program Director
Greater Baltimore Medical Center
Baltimore, Maryland

HEREDITARY POLYPOSIS SYNDROMES

George J. Arnaoutakis, MD
Senior Resident, Department of Surgery
The Johns Hopkins University School of
   Medicine
Baltimore, Maryland

*THE MANAGEMENT OF PRIMARY CHEST
WALL TUMORS*

Kengo Asai, MD, PhD
Hepatobiliary Surgery Fellow
Department of Surgery
Mayo Clinic
Rochester, Minnesota

*THE MANAGEMENT OF ASYMPTOMATIC
(SILENT) GALLSTONES*

Stanley W. Ashley, MD
Chief Medical Officer
Senior Vice President for Medical Affairs
Brigham and Women's Hospital
Boston, Massachusetts

*THE MANAGEMENT OF GALLSTONE
PANCREATITIS*

Malachy E. Asuku, MBBS, FWACS
Johns Hopkins Burn Center
Michael D. Hendrix Burn Research Center
The Johns Hopkins University School of
   Medicine
Baltimore, Maryland

BURN WOUND MANAGEMENT

Hugh G. Auchincloss, MD, MPH
Massachusetts General Hospital
Boston, Massachusetts

*COMPARATIVE EFFECTIVENESS RESEARCH
IN SURGERY*

Edward D. Auyang, MD, MS
Assistant Professor
Department of Surgery
University of New Mexico
Albuquerque, New Mexico

*LAPAROSCOPIC TREATMENT OF
ESOPHAGEAL MOTILITY DISORDERS*

Oluwafunmi O. Awonuga, MD
General Surgery Resident
University of Alabama Birmingham
Birmingham, Alabama

MOLECULAR TARGETS IN BREAST CANCER

Ezana M. Azene, MD, PhD
Vascular and Interventional Radiologist
Gundersen Health System
La Crosse, Wisconsin

*TRANSJUGULAR INTRAHEPATIC
PORTOSYSTEMIC SHUNT*

Ellen Hunter Bailey, MD
Resident in General Surgery
Department of Surgery
Vanderbilt University Medical Center
Nashville, Tennessee

GALLSTONE ILEUS

Matthew J. Bak, MD
Department of Otolaryngology-Head and
   Neck Surgery
Eastern Virginia Medical School
Norfolk, Virginia

*THE MANAGEMENT OF THYROID
NODULES*

Megan K. Baker, MD
Department of Surgery
Medical University of South Carolina
Charleston, South Carolina

*BREAST CANCER: SURGICAL
MANAGEMENT*

Anthony J. Baldea, Jr., MD
University of California Davis Medical
   Center
Sacramento, California

*CENTRAL LINE–ASSOCIATED BLOODSTREAM
INFECTIONS*

Douglas Ball, MD
The Johns Hopkins Hospital
Baltimore, Maryland

*THE MANAGEMENT OF ADRENAL
CORTICAL TUMORS*

Keki R. Balsara, MD
Resident
Division of Cardiac Surgery
The Johns Hopkins Hospital
Baltimore, Maryland

BLUNT CARDIAC INJURY

Pablo A. Baltodano, MD
Postdoctoral Research Fellow, Department
   of Plastic and Reconstructive Surgery
The Johns Hopkins Hospital
Baltimore, Maryland

NERVE INJURY AND REPAIR

Adrian Barbul, MD, FACS
Vice-Chair, Department of Surgery
Surgical Director, Operating Rooms
Washington Hospital Center
Washington, DC

*IS A NASOGASTRIC TUBE NECESSARY AFTER
ALIMENTARY TRACT SURGERY?*

**Philip S. Barie, MD, MBA, FIDSA,
FCCM, FACS**
Departments of Surgery and Public Health
Weill Cornell Medical College
NewYork-Presbyterian Hospital/Weill
   Cornell Medical Center
New York, New York

ANTIBIOTICS FOR CRITICALLY ILL PATIENTS

Neal R. Barshes, MD, MPH
Assistant Professor of Surgery
Division of Vascular Surgery and
   Endovascular Therapy
Baylor College of Medicine
Operative Care Line, Michael E. DeBakey
   Veterans Affairs Medical Center
Houston, Texas

THE TREATMENT OF CLAUDICATION

Rolf N. Barth, MD
University of Maryland Medical Ceneter
Baltimore, Maryland

*LAPAROENDOSCOPIC SINGLE-SITE SURGERY
AS AN EVOLVING SURGICAL APPROACH*

John G. Bartlett, MD
The Johns Hopkins Hospital
Baltimore, Maryland

*OCCUPATIONAL EXPOSURE TO HUMAN
IMMUNODEFICIENCY VIRUS AND OTHER
BLOODBORNE PATHOGENS*

Todd W. Bauer, MD
Associate Professor of Surgery
Director, High Risk Pancreatic Cancer
   Program
Department of Surgery
University of Virginia Health System
Charlottesville, Virginia

GALLBLADDER CANCER

Robert J. Beaulieu, MD
Resident
The Johns Hopkins School of Medicine
Baltimore, Maryland

*THE MANAGEMENT OF DUODENAL
ULCERS*

CAROTID ENDARTERECTOMY

David E. Beck, MD, FACS, FASCRS
Professor and Chairman
Department of Colon and Rectal Surgery
Ochsner Clinic Foundation
New Orleans, Louisiana

*LAPAROSCOPIC REPAIR OF PARISTOMAL
HERNIAS*

Matthew V. Benns, MD
University of Louisville
Louisville, Kentucky

EMERGENCY DEPARTMENT THORACOTOMY

David L. Berger, MD
Director, Colo-Rectal Group
Visiting Surgeon
Massachusetts General Hospital
Associate Professor
Harvard Medical School
Boston, Massachusetts

LARGE BOWEL OBSTRUCTION

Nikhil Bhagat, MD
Assistant Professor of Radiology and
    Surgery
The Johns Hopkins University School of
    Medicine
Baltimore, Maryland

*TRANSARTERIAL CHEMOEMBOLIZATION
FOR LIVER METASTASES*

Anton J. Bilchik, MD, PhD
Gastrointestinal Research Program
John Wayne Cancer Institute at Saint John's
    Health Center
Santa Monica, California;
California Oncology Research Institute
Los Angeles, California

*RADIOFREQUENCY ABLATION OF HEPATIC
METASTASES FROM COLORECTAL CANCER*

Danielle A. Bischof, MD
Clinical Fellow
Surgical Oncology
The Johns Hopkins Hospital
Baltimore, Maryland

*THE MANAGEMENT OF ADRENAL
CORTICAL TUMORS*

James H. Black III, MD
The Bertram M. Bernheim MD Associate
    Professor of Surgery
Division of Vascular and Endovasular
    Surgery
Johns Hopkins University
Baltimore, Maryland

*OPEN REPAIR OF ABDOMINAL AORTIC
ANEURYSMS*

Kirby Bland, MD
University of Alabama at Birmingham
Birmingham, Alabama

MOLECULAR TARGETS IN BREAST CANCER

Mark Bloomston, MD
Associate Professor of Surgery
Division of Surgical Oncology
The Ohio State University
Columbus, Ohio

*THE MANAGEMENT OF PANCREATIC ISLET
CELL TUMORS EXCLUDING GASTRINOMAS*

Jennifer Blumetti, MD, FACS
Attending Surgeon
Division of Colon and Rectal Surgery
Stroger Hospital of Cook County
Clinical Assistant Professor
Division of Colon and Rectal Surgery
University of Illinois at Chicago
Chicago, Illinois

ANORECTAL ABSCESS AND FISTULA

Liliana Bordeianou, MD, MPH
Department of Surgery
Massachusetts General Hospital Digestive
    Healthcare Center
Harvard Medical School
Boston, Massachusetts

*SURGICAL TREATMENT OF FECAL
INCONTINENCE*

Joseph E. Bornstein, MD, MBA
Resident
Department of Surgery
Massachusetts General Hospital
Boston, Massachusetts

LARGE BOWEL OBSTRUCTION

Judy C. Boughey, MD
Department of Surgery
Mayo Clinic
Rochester, Minnesota

*THE MANAGEMENT OF RECURRENT AND
DISSEMINATED BREAST CANCER*

Mantaj S. Brar, MD, FRCSC
Colorectal Surgery Fellow
University of Calgary
Calgary, Alberta, Canada

THE MANAGEMENT OF PRURITUS ANI

Stacy A. Brethauer, MD
Cleveland Clinic Foundation
Cleveland, Ohio

*GLYCEMIC CONTROL AND
CARDIOVASCULAR DISEASE RISK
REDUCTION AFTER BARIATRIC SURGERY*

Benjamin N. Breyer, MD, MAS
Assistant Professor
Department of Urology
University of California, San Francisco
Interim Chief of Urology, San Francisco
    General Hospital
Director, UCSF Male Genitourinary
    Reconstruction and Trama Surgery
    Fellowship
San Francisco, California

*RETROPERITONEAL INJURIES: KIDNEY AND
URETER*

Kristine E. W. Breyer, MD
University of California, San Francisco
San Francisco, California

*PREOPERATIVE PREPARATION OF THE
SURGICAL PATIENT*

Alexandra Briggs, MD
Clinical Fellow in Surgery
Department of Surgery
Brigham and Women's Hospital
Boston, Massachusetts

*THE MANAGEMENT OF GALLSTONE
PANCREATITIS*

Nelya Brindzei, MD
Memorial Sloan-Kettering Cancer Center
New York, New York

*THE USE OF POSITRON EMISSION
TOMOGRAPHIC SCANNING IN THE
MANAGEMENT OF COLORECTAL CANCER*

**LD Britt, MD, MPH, D.Sc (Hon),
FACS, FCCM, FRCSEng (Hon),
FRCSEd (Hon), FWACS (Hon),
FRCSI (Hon), FCS(SA) (Hon)**
Brickhouse Professor and Chairman
Department of Surgery
Eastern Virginia Medical School
Norfolk, Virginia

ABDOMINAL TRAUMA

Malcolm V. Brock, MD
Associate Professor of Surgery
Associate Professor of Oncology
Director of Clinical and Translational
    Research in Thoracic Surgery
Department of Surgery
The Johns Hopkins Hospital
Baltimore, Maryland

*THE MANAGEMENT OF BARRETT'S
ESOPHAGUS*

PARAESOPHAGEAL HERNIA

L. Michael Brunt, MD
Professor of Surgery
Section of Minimally Invasive Surgery
Washington University School of Medicine
St. Louis, Missouri

LAPAROSCOPIC CHOLECYSTECTOMY

**Timothy G. Buchman, PhD, MD,
FACS, FCCP, MCCM**
Director, Emory Center for Critical Care
Professor of Surgery and of Anesthesiology
Emory University
Atlanta, Georgia

*INITIAL ASSESSMENT AND RESUSCITATION
OF THE TRAUMA PATIENT*

Ronald W. Busuttil, MD, PhD
Professor and Executive Chairman
Department of Surgery
University of California, Los Angeles
Los Angeles, California

*PORTAL HYPERTENSION: THE ROLE OF
SHUNTING PROCEDURES*

Richard P. Cambria, MD
Massachusetts General Hospital
Boston, Massachusetts

*THE MANAGEMENT OF THORACIC
AND THORACOABDOMINAL AORTIC
ANEURYSMS*

Andrew M. Cameron, MD, PhD, FACS
Associate Professor of Surgery
Surgical Director of Liver Transplantation
The Johns Hopkins Hospital
Baltimore, Maryland

*TREATMENT FOR HEPATOCELLULAR
CARCINOMA: RESECTION VERSUS
TRANSPLANTATION*

*VASCULAR RECONSTRUCTION DURING THE
WHIPPLE OPERATION*

Melissa S. Camp, MD, MPH
The Johns Hopkins Hospital
Baltimore, Maryland

*LYMPHATIC MAPPING AND SENTINEL
LYMPHADENECTOMY*

Kurtis A. Campbell, MD, FACS
Associate Professor of Surgery
The Johns Hopkins University School of
 Medicine
Attending Surgeon
Mercy Medical Center and The Johns
 Hopkins Hospital
Baltimore, Maryland

ABDOMINAL WALL RECONSTRUCTION

Michael J. Campbell, MD
Assistant Professor of Surgery
University of California, Davis
Sacramento, California

*PERSISTENT AND RECURRENT
HYPERPARATHYROIDISM*

Rebecca R. Cannom, MD, MS
Clinical Assistant Professor of Surgery,
 University of Southern California
Attending Surgeon, Kaiser Permanente
Los Angeles, California

*THE MANAGEMENT OF COLORECTAL
POLYPS*

Francis J. Caputo, MD
Cooper University Physician
Department of Vascular and Endovascular
 Surgery
Cooper University Health Care
Camden, New Jersey

ATHEROSCLEROTIC RENAL ARTERY DISEASE

Diana Caragacianu, MD
Department of Neurosurgery
Brigham and Women's Hospital
Harvard Medical School
Boston, Massachusetts

SURGICAL APPROACH TO THYROID CANCER

Philip W. Carrott, Jr., MD
Division of Thoracic and Cardiovascular
 Surgery
University of Virginia Health System
Charlottesville, Virginia

ESOPHAGEAL FUNCTION TESTING

Joseph Caruso, MD
Department of General Surgery
Walter Reed National Military Medical
 Center
Bethesda, Maryland

GANGRENE OF THE FOOT

John Y. Cha, MD
Assistant Professor of Surgery
Division of Acute Care Surgery
University of South Florida
Tampa, Florida

THE MANAGEMENT OF RECTAL INJURIES

Elliot L. Chaikof, MD, PhD
Johnson and Johnson Professor of Surgery
Harvard Medical School
Surgeon-in-Chief
Beth Israel Deaconess Medical Center
Boston, Massachusetts

RAYNAUD'S SYNDROME

**Bipan Chand, MD, FACS, FASMBS,
FASGE**
Associate Professor of Surgery
Chief, Division of GI/Minimally Invasive
 Surgery
Loyola University Medical Center
Stritch School of Medicine
Maywood, Illinois

*LAPAROSCOPIC COMMON BILE DUCT
EXPLORATION*

Michael C. Chang, MD, FACS
Professor of Surgery
Department of Surgery
Wake Forest University School of Medicine
Winston-Salem, North Carolina

*ABDOMINAL COMPARTMENT SYNDROME
AND MANAGEMENT OF THE OPEN
ABDOMEN*

Philip H. Chang, MD
Instructor in Surgery
Harvard Medical School
Sumner Redstone Burn Center
Massachusetts General Hospital
Shriners Hospital for Children-Boston
Boston, Massachusetts

*COLD INJURY, FROSTBITE, AND
HYPOTHERMIA*

Vivek Chaudhry, MD, FACS, FASCRS
Section Head, Surgical Endoscopy
Director, Research Division of Colon and
 Rectal Surgery
John H. Stroger Hospital of Cook County
Interim Chief, Colon And Rectal Surgery
Clinical Assistant Professor, University of
 Illinois at Chicago
Instructor, Rush University
Chicago, Illinois

HEMORRHOIDS

Zulfiqar Cheema, MD
Department of Surgery
University of Texas Medical Branch at
 Galveston
Galveston, Texas

ACUTE MESENTERIC ISCHEMIA

Herbert Chen, MD, FACS
Chairman, General Surgery
Layton F. Rikkers, M.D. Chair in Surgical
 Leadership
Vice-Chair for Research
Professor of Surgery
Department of Surgery
University of Wisconsin
Madison, Wisconsin

ZOLLINGER-ELLISON SYNDROME

Charlie C. Cheng, MD
Department of Surgery
University of Texas Medical Branch at
 Galveston
Galveston, Texas

ACUTE MESENTERIC ISCHEMIA

Elaine Y. Cheng, MD
Fellow in Abdominal Transplant Surgery
Department of Surgery
University of California–Los Angeles
Los Angeles, California

*PORTAL HYPERTENSION: THE ROLE OF
SHUNTING PROCEDURES*

Albert Chi, MD
The Johns Hopkins Hospital
Baltimore, Maryland

FLUIDS AND ELECTROLYTES

John J. Chi, MD
Washington University School of Medicine
St. Louis, Missouri

*FACIAL TRAUMA: EVALUATION AND
MANAGEMENT*

Lorraine Choi, MD
Department of Surgery
University of Texas Medical Branch at
 Galveston
Galveston, Texas

ACUTE MESENTERIC ISCHEMIA

Michael A. Choti, MD, MBA, FACS
The Hall and Mary Lucille Shannon
 Distinguished Professor of Surgery
Chair of the Department of Surgery and
 Surgeon-in-Chief
University of Texas Southwestern Medical
 Center
Dallas, Texas

CAVERNOUS HEPATIC HEMANGIOMA

David P. Ciceri, MD
Assistant Professor of Anesthesiology
Director, Cardiovascular Anesthesiology
Director, Surgical Trauma Intensive
  Care Unit
Scott and White Memorial Hospital
Department of Anesthesiology
Texas A & M Health Science Center, College
  of Medicine
Temple, Texas

CARDIOVASCULAR PHARMACOLOGY

David J. Ciesla, MD
Professor of Surgery
Division of Acute Care Surgery
University of South Florida;
Director
Regional Trauma Program
Tampa General Hospital
Tampa, Florida

THE MANAGEMENT OF RECTAL INJURIES

Jose R. Cintron, MD, FACS
Attending Surgeon
Division of Colon and Rectal Surgery
Stroger Hospital of Cook County;
Associate Professor
Division of Colon and Rectal Surgery
University of Illinois at Chicago
Chicago, Illinois

ANORECTAL ABSCESS AND FISTULA

William G. Cioffi, Jr., MD
Professor and Chair
Department of Surgery
Brown Medical School
Providence, Rhode Island

THE SEPTIC RESPONSE

John Clarke, MD
Assistant Professor of Medicine
Director of Esophageal Motility
The Johns Hopkins Hospital
Baltimore, Maryland

*MOTILITY DISORDERS OF THE STOMACH
AND SMALL BOWEL*

**Christine S. Cocanour, MD, FACS,
FCCM**
University of California Davis Medical
  Center
Sacramento, California

INJURY TO THE SPLEEN

*CENTRAL LINE–ASSOCIATED BLOODSTREAM
INFECTIONS*

Raul Coimbra, MD, PhD, FACS
The Monroe E. Trout Professor of Surgery
Executive Vice-Chairman Department of
  Surgery
Chief, Division of Trauma, Surgical Critical
  Care, and Burns
University of California San Diego Health
  Sciences
San Diego, California

ISCHEMIC COLITIS

*CHEST WALL TRAUMA, HEMOTHORAX, AND
PNEUMOTHORAX*

Shannon Colohan, MD
Division of Plastic Surgery, Department of
  Surgery
University of Washington
Seattle, Washington

*BREAST RECONSTRUCTION FOLLOWING
MASTECTOMY: INDICATIONS, TECHNIQUES,
AND RESULTS*

**Paul Colombani, MD, MBA, FACS,
FAAP**
Professor of Surgery
Pediatrics and Oncology
Vice-Chairman
Department of Surgery
Chief
Division of Pediatric Surgery
The Johns Hopkins Hospital
Baltimore, Maryland

REPAIR OF PECTUS EXCAVATUM

Michael D. Connolly, MD
Assistant Professor
Department of Surgery
Brown Medical School
Providence, Rhode Island

THE SEPTIC RESPONSE

Claudius Conrad, MD, PhD
Assistant in Surgery, Massachusetts General
  Hospital
Instructor, Harvard Medical School
Boston, Massachusetts

*PALLIATIVE THERAPY FOR PANCREATIC
CANCER*

Michael S. Conte, MD
Division of Vascular and Endovascular
  Surgery
University of California
San Francisco, California

AORTOILIAC OCCLUSIVE DISEASE

Patrick R. Cook, DO, FACS, RPVI
Chief, Department of Anesthesia and
  Operative Services
William Beaumont Army Medical Center
El Paso, Texas;
Vascular Surgery Consultant to the Office
  of the Surgeon General
Assistant Professor of Surgery
The Norman M. Rich Department of
  Surgery
The Uniformed Services University of the
  Health Sciences
Bethesda, Maryland

THE DIABETIC FOOT

Robert N. Cooney, MD
Department of Surgery
SUNY Upstate Medical Center
Syracuse, New York

*METABOLIC CHANGES FOLLOWING
BARIATRIC SURGERY*

**Edward E. Cornwell, III, MD, FACS,
FCCM**
LaSalle D. Leffall, Jr., MD Professor and
  Chairman of Surgery
Howard University College of Medicine
Surgeon-in-Chief
Howard University Hospital
Washington, DC

*INJURIES TO THE SMALL AND LARGE
BOWEL*

David Cosgrove, MBBCh
Assistant Professor of Oncology
Johns Hopkins Sidney Kimmel
  Comprehensive Cancer Center
Baltimore, Maryland

*THE USE OF NEOADJUVANT AND
ADJUVANT TREATMENT FOR COLORECTAL
CANCER*

Bard C. Cosman, MD, MPH
Halasz General Surgery Section, Surgical
  Service
VA San Diego Healthcare System
Department of Surgery
University of California San Diego School
  of Medicine
San Diego, California

ANORECTAL STRICTURE

Todd W. Costantini, MD
Assistant Professor of Surgery
Division of Trauma, Surgical Critical Care,
  and Burns
Department of Surgery
University of California San Diego Health
  Sciences
San Diego, California

ISCHEMIC COLITIS

Charles Cox, MD
Tampa Bay Breast Care Specialists
Department of Surgery
University of South Florida, Morsani
   College of Medicine
Tampa, Florida

*ABLATIVE THERAPIES IN BENIGN AND
MALIGNANT BREAST DISEASE*

John Cox, MD
Tampa Bay Breast Care Specialists
Tampa, Florida

*ABLATIVE THERAPIES IN BENIGN AND
MALIGNANT BREAST DISEASE*

Martin A. Croce, MD, FACS
Professor of Surgery
University of Tennessee Health Science
   Center
Memphis, Tennessee

THE MANAGEMENT OF LIVER INJURIES

David M. Cromwell, MD
Assistant Professor of Medicine
Johns Hopkins University
Baltimore, Maryland

*ACUTE COLONIC PSEUDO-OBSTRUCTION
(OGILVIE'S SYNDROME)*

Paul G. Curcillo II, MD, FACS
Associate Professor, Surgical Oncology
Section Chief, Minimally Invasive Surgery
Director, Minimally Invasive Surgical
   Initiatives and Development
Fox Chase Cancer Center
Philadelphia, Pennsylvania

*INCISIONAL, EPIGASTRIC, AND UMBILICAL
HERNIAS*

James C. Cusack, Jr., MD
Associate Professor of Surgery
Division of Surgical Oncology
Harvard Medical School
Department of Surgery
Massachusetts General Hospital
Boston, Massachusetts

*THE MANAGEMENT OF
PHEOCHROMOCYTOMA*

Alan P. B. Dackiw, MD, PhD
Department of Surgery
The Johns Hopkins Hospital
The Johns Hopkins University School of
   Medicine
Baltimore, Maryland

ADRENAL INCIDENTALOMA

Phong T. Dargon, MD
Oregon Health & Science University
Portland, Oregon

*PSEUDOANEURYSMS AND ARTERIOVENOUS
FISTULAS*

Benjamin W. Dart IV, MD, FACS
Associate Professor of Surgery
Department of Surgery
University of Tennessee College of Medicine
Chattanooga, Tennessee

*THE MANAGEMENT OF CLOSTRIDIUM
DIFFICILE COLITIS*

S. Scott Davis, Jr., MD, FACS
Associate Professor of Surgery
Associate Program Director, Emory
   Endosurgery Fellowship
Division of General and GI Surgery
Department of Surgery
Emory University School of Medicine
Atlanta, Georgia

*LAPAROSCOPIC 360-DEGREE
FUNDOPLICATION*

Ana De Jesus-Acosta, MD
Gastrointestinal Medical Oncology
Sidney Kimmel Comprehensive Cancer
   Center at Johns Hopkins
Baltimore, Maryland

*NEOADJUVANT AND ADJUVANT THERAPY
OF PANCREATIC CANCER*

Christopher J. Dente, MD
Department of Surgery
Emory University School of Medicine
Atlanta, Georgia

*THE SURGEON'S USE OF ULTRASOUND IN
THORACOABDOMINAL TRAUMA*

Marcello Deraco, MD
Surgical Oncologist
Department of Surgery
National Cancer Institute
Milan, Italy

*THE MANAGEMENT OF PERITONEAL
SURFACE MALIGNANCY*

Niraj M. Desai, MD
Director of the Kidney and Pancreas
   Transplant Program
The Johns Hopkins Hospital
Transplant Surgery Division, Department of
   Surgery
Johns Hopkins University
Baltimore, Maryland

TRANSPLANTATION OF THE PANCREAS

**Ashwin L. deSouza, MS, MRCSEd,
DNB, FCPS, MNAMS**
Fellow, Minimally Invasive and
   Laparoscopic Colon and Rectal Surgery
University of Illinois at Chicago
Chicago, Illinois

*THE MANAGEMENT OF RECTOVAGINAL
FISTULA*

Karen Deveney, MD
Professor of Surgery
Vice Chair of Education and Program
   Director
Department of Surgery
Oregon Health & Science University
Portland, Oregon

*THE MANAGEMENT OF COLONIC
VOLVULUS*

Gerard M. Doherty, MD, FACS
Utley Professor and Chair of Surgery
Professor of Medicine
Boston University
Surgeon-in-Chief
Boston Medical Center
Boston, Massachusetts

NONTOXIC GOITER

Timothy R. Donahue, MD
Assistant Professor of Surgery, and
   Molecular and Medical Pharmacology
University of California, Los Angeles
Los Angeles, California

*THE MANAGEMENT OF CHRONIC
PANCREATITIS*

Graham W. Donald, MD
Department of Surgery
David Geffen School of Medicine at UCLA
Los Angeles, California

*PANCREATIC DUCTAL DISRUPTIONS
LEADING TO PANCREATIC FISTULA,
PANCREATIC ASCITES, OR PANCREATIC
PLEURAL EFFUSION*

**Juan Carlos Duchesne, MD, FACS,
FCCP, FCCM**
Trauma Medical Director
North Oaks Shock/Trauma Center
Hammond, Louisiana;
Associate Professor of Surgery
Tulane University
Chairman
Louisiana Committee of Trauma
New Orleans, Louisiana

*PANCREATIC AND DUODENAL INJURIES
AND CURRENT SURGICAL THERAPIES*

Quan-Yang Duh, MD
Professor of Surgery
University of California, San Francisco
San Francisco, California

*PERSISTENT AND RECURRENT
HYPERPARATHYROIDISM*

William S. Duke, MD
Assistant Professor
Department of Otolaryngology-Head and
   Neck Surgery
Georgia Regents University
Augusta, Georgia

HYPERTHYROIDISM

Casey Boyd Duncan, MD, MS
Department of Surgery
The University of Texas Medical Branch
Galveston, Texas

UNUSUAL PANCREATIC TUMORS

Mark D. Duncan, MD
Associate Professor, Surgery
Chief, Surgical Oncology
Johns Hopkins Bayview Medical Center,
    Division of Surgery
Baltimore, Maryland

*THE MANAGEMENT OF COMMON BILE
DUCT STONES*

Geoffrey P. Dunn, MD, FACS
Department of Surgery and Palliative Care
    Consultation Service
UPMC Hamot Medical Center
Erie, Pennsylvania

SURGICAL PALLIATIVE CARE

Francisco Antonio Durazo, MD, FACP
Associate Professor of Medicine and
    Surgery
David Geffen UCLA School of Medicine
Division of Gastrointestinal and Liver
    Diseases
Medical Director, Dumont-UCLA Liver
    Transplant Center
Los Angeles, CA

*ENDOSCOPIC THERAPY FOR ESOPHAGEAL
VARICEAL HEMORRHAGE*

Frederic E. Eckhauser, MD, FACS
Professor of Surgery
Director of Clinical Operation
The Johns Hopkins Hospital
Baltimore, Maryland

*THE MANAGEMENT OF DUODENAL
ULCERS*

Barish H. Edil, MD
Associate Professor of Surgery
University of Colorado
Denver, Colorado

CYSTIC DISORDERS OF THE BILE DUCTS

PERIAMPULLARY CARCINOMA

Jonathan E. Efron, MD
Associate Professor of Surgery
Chief of Ravitch Service
The Mark M. Ravitch, MD Endowed
    Professorship in Gastrointestinal Surgery
Johns Hopkins University
Baltimore, Maryland

*THE MANAGEMENT OF CHRONIC
ULCERATIVE COLITIS*

Dominique Elias, MD, PhD
Department of Surgical Oncology
Gustave Roussy Institute
Villejuif, Paris, France

*THE MANAGEMENT OF PERITONEAL
SURFACE MALIGNANCY*

E. Christopher Ellison, MD
Professor of Surgery
The Ohio State University
Columbus, Ohio

*THE MANAGEMENT OF PANCREATIC ISLET
CELL TUMORS EXCLUDING GASTRINOMAS*

Nassrene Elmadhun, MD
PGY 3 Resident, Department of Surgery
Beth Israel Deaconess Medical Center
Boston, Massachusetts

*ENDOSCOPIC TREATMENT OF BARRETT'S
ESOPHAGUS*

James K. Elsey, MD, FACS
Gwinnett Surgical Associates
Lawrenceville, Georgia

ACUTE CHOLECYSTITIS

Timothy C. Fabian, MD
Harwell Wilson Alumni Professor &
    Chairman, Department of Surgery
University of Tennessee Health Science
    Center
Memphis, Tennessee

THE ABDOMEN THAT WILL NOT CLOSE

Sandy H. Fang, MD
Assistant Professor of Surgery
Department of Surgery
Johns Hopkins University
Baltimore, Maryland

*THE MANAGEMENT OF CHRONIC
ULCERATIVE COLITIS*

Alik Farber, MD, FACS
Chief of Vascular and Endovascular Surgery
Boston University Medical Center
Associate Professor of Surgery and
    Radiology
Boston University School of Medicine
Boston, Massachusetts

*THE MANAGEMENT OF PERIPHERAL
ARTERIAL EMBOLI*

Mark B. Faries, MD
Melanoma Research Program, John Wayne
    Cancer Institute at Saint John's Health
    Center
Santa Monica, California

*THE MANAGEMENT OF CUTANEOUS
MELANOMA*

Russell Farmer, MD
Fellow, Colorectal Surgery
PGY5, General Surgery
Department of Surgery
School of Medicine
University of Louisville
Louisville, Kentucky

CROHN'S COLITIS

Amir H. Fathi, MD
Case Comprehensive Hernia Center
Department of Surgery
University Hospitals Case Medical Center
Cleveland, Ohio

*LAPAROSCOPIC REPAIR OF RECURRENT
INGUINAL HERNIAS*

David V. Feliciano, MD
Battersby Professor and Chief, Division of
    General Surgery
Attending Surgeon, Indiana University and
    IU Methodist Hospitals
Indiana University Medical Center
Indianapolis, Indiana

DIAPHRAGMATIC INJURIES

Charles M. Ferguson, MD
Surgeon/Clinical Medical Staff
Emory Clark-Holder Clinic
LaGrange, Georgia

ESOPHAGEAL PERFORATION

Carlos Fernandez-del Castillo, MD
Department of Surgery
Massachusetts General Hospital
Harvard Medical School
Boston, Massachusetts

*INTRADUCTAL PAPILLARY MUCINOUS
NEOPLASMS OF THE PANCREAS*

Paula Ferrada, MD, FACS
Division of Trauma, Critical Care &
    Emergency Surgery
Department of Surgery
Virginia Commonwealth University
Richmond, Virginia

*THE MANAGEMENT OF DIVERTICULAR
DISEASE OF THE COLON*

Cristina R. Ferrone, MD
Surgeon, General and Gastrointestinal
    Surgery
Department of Surgery
Massachusetts General Hospital
Assistant Professor, Department of Surgery
Harvard Medical School
Dana-Farber/Harvard Cancer Center
Boston, Massachusetts

CYSTIC DISEASE OF THE LIVER

**Alessandro Fichera, MD, FACS,
FASCRS**
Professor
Department of Surgery
University of Washington
Seattle, Washington

TUMORS OF THE ANAL CANAL

*LAPAROSCOPIC MANAGEMENT OF CROHN'S
DISEASE*

Christina Finlayson, MD
Professor, Surgery
Director, Diane O'Connor Thompson
  Breast Center
University of Colorado School of
  Medicine
Aurora, Colorado

*ADVANCES IN NEOADJUVANT AND
ADJUVANT THERAPY FOR BREAST CANCER*

Jordan E. Fishman, MD, MPH
Surgical House Officer
New Jersey Medical School—Rutgers
  University
Newark, New Jersey

*IS A NASOGASTRIC TUBE NECESSARY AFTER
ALIMENTARY TRACT SURGERY?*

**Mark E. Fleming, DO, MC(FS/FMF),
USN**
Orthopedic Trauma Surgeon
Assistant Deputy Commander for
  Surgery
Walter Reed National Military Medical
  Center
Assistant Professor of Surgery
Uniformed Services University of the
  Health Sciences
Bethesda, Maryland

GANGRENE OF THE FOOT

**James W. Fleshman, MD, FACS,
FASCRS**
Chief of Surgery
Baylor University Medical Center
Dallas, Texas

*THE MANAGEMENT OF TOXIC
MEGACOLON*

*LAPAROSCOPIC COLON AND RECTAL
SURGERY*

Yuman Fong, MD
Murray F. Brennan Chair in Surgery
Memorial Sloan-Kettering Cancer Center
New York, New York

*THE MANAGEMENT OF MALIGNANT LIVER
TUMORS*

Christopher L. Forthman, MD
Consultant, Curtis National Hand Center
Union Memorial Hospital
Baltimore, Maryland

HAND INFECTIONS

Adam D. Fox, DPM, DO, FACS
Assistant Professor of Surgery
Division of Trauma Surgery and Critical
  Care
Rutgers—New Jersey Medical School
Newark, New Jersey

*THE MANAGEMENT OF INTRAABDOMINAL
INFECTIONS*

Julie A. Freischlag, MD
The William Stewart Halsted Professor
Chair, Department of Surgery
Surgeon-in-Chief
The Johns Hopkins Hospital
Baltimore, Maryland

THORACIC OUTLET SYNDROMES

Randall S. Friese, MD
Division of Trauma and Critical Care
University of Arizona
Tucson, Arizona

ELECTROLYTE DISORDERS

Robert Gabordi, MD
Department of Surgery
University of South Florida
Morsani College of Medicine
Tampa, Florida

*ABLATIVE THERAPIES IN BENIGN AND
MALIGNANT BREAST DISEASE*

Michele A. Gadd, MD
Massachusetts General Hospital
Division of Surgical Oncology
Boston, Massachusetts

SCREENING FOR BREAST CANCER

Csaba Gajdos, MD
Assistant Professor of Surgery
University of Colorado
Aurora, Colorado

PERIAMPULLARY CARCIMOMA

Susan Galandiuk, MD
Professor of Surgery
Section of Colon and Rectal Surgery
Director, Price Institute of Surgical Research
Department of Surgery
University of Louisville
Louisville, Kentucky

CROHN'S COLITIS

Samuel M. Galvagno, Jr., DO, PhD
Assistant Professor
Divisions of Trauma, Anesthesiology, and
  Critical Care Medicine
Department of Anesthesiology and the
  Program in Trauma
Shock Trauma Center
University of Maryland School of Medicine
Baltimore, Maryland

*AIRWAY MANAGEMENT IN THE TRAUMA
PATIENT*

Julio Garcia-Aguilar, MD, PhD
Chief, Colorectal Service
Department of Surgery
Memorial Sloan-Kettering Cancer Center
New York, New York

*THE USE OF POSITRON EMISSION
TOMOGRAPHIC SCANNING IN THE
MANAGEMENT OF COLORECTAL CANCER*

Alan D. Garely, MD, FACOG, FACS
Chair of Obstetrics and Gynecology
Director of Urogynecology and Pelvic
  Reconstructive Surgery
South Nassau Communities Hospital
Clinical Associate Professor
Mount Sinai School of Medicine
New York, New York

RECTAL PROLAPSE

**Susan L. Gearhart, MD, FACS,
FASCAS**
Assistant Professor of Colorectal Surgery
Johns Hopkins University
Baltimore, Maryland

*THE MANAGEMENT OF CROHN'S DISEASE
OF THE SMALL BOWEL*

ANAL FISSURES

**Christos S. Georgiades, MD, PhD,
FSIR**
Director
Vascular and Interventional Radiology
American Medical Center
Nicosia, Cyprus

VENA CAVA FILTERS

Jean-Francois H. (Jeff) Geschwind, MD
Professor of Radiology, Surgery and
  Oncology
The Johns Hopkins University School of
  Medicine
Baltimore, Maryland

*THE TRANSARTERIAL
CHEMOEMBOLIZATION FOR LIVER
METASTASES*

Bruce L. Gewertz, MD
Department of Surgery
Cedars-Sinai Medical Center
Los Angeles, California

*BUERGER'S DISEASE (THROMBOANGIITIS
OBLITERANS)*

**Armando E. Giuliano, MD, FACS,
FRCSEd**
Executive Vice Chair, Surgery
Chief, Surgical Oncology
Cedars-Sinai Medical Center
Los Angeles, California

*THE MANAGEMENT OF THE AXILLA IN
BREAST CANCER*

Natalia O. Glebova, MD, PhD
Fellow in Vascular Surgery
Johns Hopkins Medicical Institutions
Baltimore, Maryland

*THE MANAGEMENT OF RUPTURED
ABDOMINAL AORTIC ANEURYSM*

FEMOROPOPLITEAL OCCLUSIVE DISEASE

LYMPHEDEMA

Olivier Glehen, MD, PhD
Professor of Surgery
Surgical Oncology Department
Centre Hospitalo-Universitaire Lyon Sud
Pierre Benite, France

*THE MANAGEMENT OF PERITONEAL
SURFACE MALIGNANCY*

Catherine Go
Fourth Year Medical Student
University of Pittsburgh School of Medicine
Pittsburgh, Pennsylvania

ESOPHAGEAL STENTS

Jason S. Gold, MD
Departments of Surgery
VA Boston Healthcare System
Brigham and Women's Hospital
Harvard Medical School
Boston, Massachusetts

ACUTE CHOLANGITIS

Steven B. Goldin, MD, PhD
Professor of Surgery
Chief of Hepatobiliary and Pancreatic
    Surgery
Vice Chairman of Surgical Education
Medical Student Clerkship Director
University of South Florida
Tampa, Florida

*PANCREAS DIVISUM AND OTHER VARIANTS
OF DOMINANT DORSAL DUCT ANATOMY*

Seth Goldstein, MD
Johns Hopkins University
Baltimore, Maryland

CYSTIC DISORDERS OF THE BILE DUCTS

FLUIDS AND ELECTROLYTES

**Jerry Goldstone, MD, FACS, FRCSEd
(Hon)**
Division of Vascular Surgery and
    Endovascular Therapy
University Hospital Case Medical Center
Case Western Reserve University School of
    Medicine
Cleveland, Ohio

*THE MANAGEMENT OF ANEURYSMS OF
THE EXTRACRANIAL CAROTID AND
VERTEBRAL ARTERIES*

Alexandra June Gordon
Medical Student
University of Illinois, College of Medicine
Chicago, Illinois

*THE ROLE OF STEREOTACTIC BREAST
BIOPSY IN THE MANAGEMENT OF BREAST
DISEASE*

Jay A. Graham, MD
Department of Surgery
Georgetown University Hospital
Washington, DC

LAPAROSCOPIC LIVER RESECTION

Caprice C. Greenberg, MD, MPH
Associate Professor of Surgery
WARF Professor of Surgical Research
Director, Wisconsin Surgical Outcomes
    Research (WiSOR)
Department of Surgery
University of Wisconsin
Madison, Wisconsin

MEASURING OUTCOMES IN SURGERY

Alessandro Gronchi, MD
Department of Surgery, Sarcoma Service
Fondazione IRCCS Istituto Nazionale dei
    Tumori
Milan, Italy

*THE MANAGEMENT OF SOFT TISSUE
SARCOMA*

Michael A. Gropper, MD, PhD
Professor and Executive Vice Chair
Department of Anesthesia and
    Perioperative Care
Director, Critical Care Medicine
Investigator, Cardiovascular Research
    Institute
University of California, San Francisco
San Francisco, California

*PREOPERATIVE PREPARATION OF THE
SURGICAL PATIENT*

Ahmet Gurakar, MD
Associate Professor of Medicine
Section of Gastroenterology and
    Hepatology
Medical Director, Liver Transplantation
The Johns Hopkins Hospital
Baltimore, Maryland

*THE MANAGEMENT OF REFRACTORY
ASCITES*

James L. Guzzo, MD
Division of Vascular & Endovascular
    Surgery
Department of Surgery
Lehigh Valley Hospital
Allentown, Pennsylvania

*FEMORAL AND POPLITEAL ARTERY
ANEURYSMS*

Adil Haider, MD, MPH, FACS
Department of Surgery
The Johns Hopkins Hospital
Baltimore, Maryland

DAMAGE CONTROL OPERATION

Yarah M. Haidar, MD
Department of Surgery
University of California, San Diego School
    of Medicine
San Diego, California

ANORECTAL STRICTURE

James P. Hamilton, MD
Assistant Professor of Medicine
The Johns Hopkins Hospital
Baltimore, Maryland

*THE MANAGEMENT OF BUDD-CHIARI
SYNDROME*

John B. Hanks, MD
C. Bruce Morton Professor and Chief
Division of General Surgery
Department of Surgery
University of Virginia
Charlottesville, Virginia

EVALUATION OF THE ISOLATED NECK MASS

Tod M. Hanover, MD
Division of Vascular Surgery
Greenville Hospital System Clinical
    University
University of South Carolina School of
    Medicine
Greenville, South Carolina

PROFUNDA FEMORIS RECONSTRUCTION

Nora Hansen, MD
Feinberg School of Medicine
Northwestern University
Chicago, Illinois

*THE ROLE OF STEREOTACTIC BREAST
BIOPSY IN THE MANAGEMENT OF BREAST
DISEASE*

Rosemarie Hardin, MD
Wheeling Hospital
Wheeling, West Virginia

*THE MANAGEMENT OF BENIGN BREAST
DISEASE*

INFLAMMATORY BREAST CARCINOMA

MALE BREAST CANCER

Elliott R. Haut, MD, FACS
Associate Professor of Surgery,
    Anesthesiology / Critical Care Medicine
    (ACCM) and Emergency Medicine
Division of Acute Care Surgery,
    Department of Surgery
The Johns Hopkins University School of
    Medicine
Core faculty, The Armstrong Institute for
    Patient Safety & Quality, John Hopkins
    Medicine
Director, Trama/Acute Care Surgery
    Fellowship, The John Hopkins Hospital
Baltimore, Maryland

*VENOUS THROMBOEMBOLISM:
PREVENTION, DIAGNOSIS, AND TREATMENT*

William G. Hawkins, MD
Section of Hepatobiliary-Pancreatic Surgery,
  Department of Surgery
Washington University
St. Louis, Missouri

BENIGN BILIARY STRICTURES

Elizabeth Hechenbleikner, MD
Research: Colorectal
The John Hopkins Hospital
Baltimore, Maryland;
Research Resident, MedStar Georgetown
  University Hospital
Washington, DC

COLON CANCER

Robert Evans Heithaus, Jr., MD
Baylor University Medical Center
Dallas, Texas

*PANCREAS DIVISUM AND OTHER VARIANTS
OF DOMINANT DORSAL DUCT ANATOMY*

Richard F. Heitmiller, MD, FACS
J.M.T. Finney Chairman of Surgery
Union Memorial Hospital
Baltimore, Maryland

*THE MANAGEMENT OF PHARYNGEAL
ESOPHAGEAL (ZENKER'S) DIVERTICULA*

Jennifer Heller, MD
Department of Surgery
Bayview Medical Center
Baltimore, Maryland

LYMPHEDEMA

C. William Helm, MB.BChir
Department of Obstetrics, Gynecology and
  Women's Health
Saint Louis University
St. Louis, Missouri

*THE MANAGEMENT OF PERITONEAL
SURFACE MALIGNANCY*

Sharon Henry, MD
Professor of Surgery
Anne Scalea Professor in Trauma
Director, Division of Wound Healing and
  Metabolism
R Adams Cowley Shock Trauma Center
University of Maryland School of Medicine
Baltimore, Maryland

EXTREMITY GAS GANGRENE

Joseph M. Herman, MD, MS
Associate Professor, Radiation Oncology
The Johns Hopkins Kimmel Cancer Center
Baltimore, Maryland

*RADIATION INJURY TO THE SMALL AND
LARGE BOWEL*

Jonathan R. Hiatt, MD
Professor of Surgery
Vice Dean for Faculty
Department of Surgery
University of California–Los Angeles
Los Angeles, California

*PORTAL HYPERTENSION: THE ROLE OF
SHUNTING PROCEDURES*

Caitlin W. Hicks, MD, MS
Department of Surgery
The Johns Hopkins Hospital
Baltimore, Maryland

DAMAGE CONTROL OPERATION

O. Joseph Hines, MD
Department of Surgery
David Geffen School of Medicine
  at UCLA
Los Angeles, California

*PANCREATIC DUCTAL DISRUPTIONS
LEADING TO PANCREATIC FISTULA,
PANCREATIC ASCITES, OR PANCREATIC
PLEURAL EFFUSION*

Kenzo Hirose, MD
Assistant Professor
Department of Surgery
Division of Surgical Oncology
Johns Hopkins University
Baltimore, Maryland

*THE MANAGEMENT OF BENIGN LIVER
LESIONS*

Vanessa P. Ho, MD, MPH
Department of Surgery
University of Medicine and Dentistry of
  New Jersey-New Jersey Medical School
Newark, New Jersey

ANTIBIOTICS FOR CRITICALLY ILL PATIENTS

Richard Hodin, MD
Chief, Endocrine Surgery
Surgical Director, MGH Center for
  Inflammatory Bowel Disease
Massachusetts General Hospital
Boston, Massachusetts

*THE MANAGEMENT OF SMALL BOWEL
TUMORS*

Tammy M. Holm, MD, PhD
Department of General Surgery
Brigham and Women's Hospital
Harvard Medical School
Boston, Massachusetts

SURGICAL APPROACH TO THYROID CANCER

Johnny C. Hong, MD, FACS
Associate Professor of Surgery
The Mark B. Adams Chair in Surgery
Division of Transplant Surgery, Department
  of Surgery
Medical College of Wisconsin
Director, Solid Organ Transplantation Joint
  Program
Medical College of Wisconsin-Froedtert
  Health-Children's Hospital of Wisconsin-
  Blood Center of Wisconsin
Milwaukee, Wisconsin

THE MANAGEMENT OF HEPATIC ABSCESS

Kelvin Hong, MD
Clinical Director
Fellowship Program Director
Vascular and Interventional Radiology
Johns Hopkins Medical Institutions
Baltimore, Maryland

*TRANSJUGULAR INTRAHEPATIC
PORTOSYSTEMIC SHUNT*

Karen D. Horvath, MD, FACS
Professor of Surgery
Director, Residency Program in General
  Surgery
Associate Chair for Education
Department of Surgery
University of Washington
Seattle, Washington

*LAPAROSCOPIC MANAGEMENT OF
PANCREATIC PSEUDOCYST*

Isaac Howley, MD
Department of Surgery
The Johns Hopkins Hospital
Baltimore, Maryland

*THE MANAGEMENT OF CROHN'S DISEASE
OF THE SMALL BOWEL*

David B. Hoyt, MD, FACS
Executive Director
American College of Surgeons
Chicago, Illinois;
Professor of Surgery—Emeritus
Department of Surgery
University of California, Irvine
Irvine, California

*CHEST WALL TRAUMA, HEMOTHORAX, AND
PNEUMOTHORAX*

Michal Hubka, MD
Department of General and Thoracic
  Surgery
Virginia Mason Medical Center
Seattle, Washington

PRIMARY TUMORS OF THE THYMUS

Matthew M. Hutter, MD, MPH
Massachusetts General Hospital
Boston, Massachusetts

*COMPARATIVE EFFECTIVENESS RESEARCH
IN SURGERY*

Andre Ilbawi, MD
Department of Surgery
University of Washington Medical Center
Seattle, Washington

*LAPAROSCOPIC MANAGEMENT OF
PANCREATIC PSEUDOCYST*

Kamal M.F. Itani, MD, FACS
Department of Surgery
Boston Veteran's Administration Health
    Care System
Boston University School of Medicine
Harvard University School of Medicine
Boston, Massachusetts

*NECROTIZING SKIN AND SOFT TISSUE
INFECTIONS*

Rao R. Ivatury, MD, FACS
Division of Trauma, Critical Care &
    Emergency Surgery
Department of Surgery
Virginia Commonwealth University
Richmond, Virginia

*THE MANAGEMENT OF DIVERTICULAR
DISEASE OF THE COLON*

Lisa Jacobs, MD
Department of Surgery
The Johns Hopkins Hospital
Baltimore, Maryland

*THE MANAGEMENT OF BENIGN BREAST
DISEASE*

Tom Jaksic, MD, PhD
W. Hardy Hendren Professor of Surgery
Harvard Medical School
Surgical Director, Center for Advanced
    Intestinal Rehabilitation
Boston Children's Hospital
Boston, Massachusetts

*THE MANAGEMENT OF SHORT BOWEL
SYNDROME*

Nagamallika Jasti, MD
MedStar Harbor Hospital
Baltimore, Maryland

*COAGULOPATHY IN THE CRITICALLY ILL
PATIENT*

Sara H. Javid, MD
Surgical Oncology Section
Division of General Surgery
Department of Surgery
University of Washington
Seattle, Washington

*BREAST RECONSTRUCTION FOLLOWING
MASTECTOMY: INDICATIONS, TECHNIQUES,
AND RESULTS*

Lynt B. Johnson, MD, MBA, FACS
Robert J. Coffey Professor & Chairman
Department of Surgery
Georgetown University Hospital
Washington, DC

LAPAROSCOPIC LIVER RESECTION

Bellal Joseph, MD
University of Arizona Medical Center
Tucson, Arizona

FLUIDS AND ELECTROLYTES

Nora Eve Joseph, MD
Gastrointestinal and Liver Pathology Fellow
Department of Pathology
University of Chicago Medical Center
Chicago, Illinois

TUMORS OF THE ANAL CANAL

Gregory J. Jurkovich, MD
Director, Surgery Trauma
Denver Health Medical Center
University of Colorado School of Medicine
Denver, Colorado

PENETRATING ABDOMINAL TRAUMA

Fady Michael Kaldas, MD
Assistant Professor of Surgery
Associate Director, Multi-Organ
    Transplantation & Hepatobiliary Surgery
    Fellowship Program
Director, Liver Transplantation Service
The Pfleger Liver Institute
The Dumont-UCLA Transplant Center
Department of Surgery, David Geffen
    School of Medicine-UCLA
Los Angeles, California

THE MANAGEMENT OF HEPATIC ABSCESS

Anthony N. Kalloo, MD
The Moses and Helen Golden Paulson
    Professor of Gastroenterology
Director, Division of Gastroenterology &
    Hepatology
The Johns Hopkins Hospital
Baltimore, Maryland

NOTES: WHAT IS CURRENTLY POSSIBLE?

Daniel W. Karakla, MD
Department of Otolaryngology-Head and
    Neck Surgery
Eastern Virginia Medical School
Norfolk, Virginia

THE MANAGEMENT OF THYROID NODULES

Jeffry L. Kashuk, MD, FACS
Director of Surgical Research and Academic
    Development
EmCare-Acute Care Surgery
Dallas, Texas

*COAGULATION ISSUES AND THE TRAUMA
PATIENT*

Vikram S. Kashyap, MD, FACS
Professor of Surgery, Case Western Reserve
    University School of Medicine
Chief, Division of Vascular Surgery and
    Endovascular Therapy
Co-Director, Harrington Heart and
    Vascular Institute
University Hospitals Case Medical Center
Cleveland, Ohio

*UPPER EXTREMITY ARTERIAL OCCLUSIVE
DISEASE*

Dierdre C. Kelleher, MD
Resident Physician, Department of Surgery
Weill Cornell Medical Center
New York, New York;
Research Fellow, Section of Colon and
    Rectal Surgery
Department of Surgery
MedStar Washington Hospital Center
Washington, DC

*THE MANAGEMENT OF SOLITARY RECTAL
ULCER SYNDROME*

Michael Kent, MD
Department of Surgery
Beth Israel Deaconess Medical Center
Boston, Massachusetts

*ENDOSCOPIC TREATMENT OF BARRETT'S
ESOPHAGUS*

Heung Bae Kim, MD
Associate Professor of Surgery
Harvard Medical School
Director, Pediatric Transplant Center
Boston Children's Hospital
Boston, Massachusetts

*THE MANAGEMENT OF SHORT BOWEL
SYNDROME*

Karen M. Kim, MD
Fellow in Cardiothoracic Surgery
Hospital of the University of Pennsylvania
Philadelphia, Pennsylvania

*THE MANAGEMENT OF ACUTE AORTIC
DISSECTIONS*

Lisa M. Kodadek, MD
Resident in General Surgery
The Johns Hopkins Hospital
Baltimore, Maryland

SMALL BOWEL OBSTRUCTION

Ayman A. Koteish, MD
The Johns Hopkins Hospital
Baltimore, Maryland

*THE MANAGEMENT OF HEPATIC
ENCEPHALOPATHY*

Nicole Kounalakis, MD
Assistant Professor of Surgery
University of Colorado School of Medicine
Denver, Colorado

*ADVANCES IN NEOADJUVANT AND
ADJUVANT THERAPY FOR BREAST CANCER*

**Benjamin D. Kozower, MD, MPH,
FACS**
Division of Thoracic and Cardiovascular
    Surgery
University of Virginia Health System
Charlottesville, Virginia

ESOPHAGEAL FUNCTION TESTING

Beth R. Krieger, MD
General and Colorectal Surgery
Fox Valley Surgical Associates
Appleton, Wisconsin
RECTAL PROLAPSE

Helen Krontiras, MD
Associate Professor
Co-Director, UAB Breast Health Center
Co-Director, Lynne Cohen Prevention
   Program for Women's Cancer
University of Alabama, Birmingham
Birmingham, Alabama
MOLECULAR TARGETS IN BREAST CANCER

Anjali S. Kumar, MD, MPH
Director, Research and Education
Section of Colon and Rectal Surgery
Department of Surgery
MedStar Washington Hospital Center
Assistant Professor of Surgery
Georgetown University
Washington, DC
*THE MANAGEMENT OF SOLITARY RECTAL
ULCER SYNDROME*

Hari Kumar, MD
Vascular Surgery Fellow
Northwestern Univeristy School of
   Medicine
Chicago, Illinois
*TIBIOPERONEAL ARTERIAL OCCLUSIVE
DISEASE*

Rachit Kumar, MD
Resident, The Johns Hopkins Hospital
Department of Radiation Oncology and
   Molecular Radiation Sciences
Baltimore, Maryland
*RADIATION INJURY TO THE SMALL AND
LARGE BOWEL*

Hiroko Kunitake, MD
Assistant Professor, Department of Surgery
Boston University School of Medicine
Boston, Massachusetts
*THE MANAGEMENT OF SMALL BOWEL
TUMORS*

Christopher J. Kwolek, MD
Division of Vascular and Endovascular
   Surgery
Massachusetts General Hospital
Boston, Massachusetts
*ENDOVASCULAR TREATMENT OF
ABDOMINAL AORTIC ANEURYSM*

Sebastianus Kwon, MBBS, FRACS
Visiting Surgical Fellow
Seoul National University Hospital
Seoul, South Korea
LAPAROSCOPIC GASTRIC SURGERY

Alex J. Ky, MD
Associate Professor
Department of Surgery
The Mount Sinai Hospital
New York, New York
RECTAL PROLAPSE

Michal J. Lada, MD
General Surgery Resident
University of Rochester Medical Center
Rochester, New York
*THE MANAGEMENT OF ESOPHAGEAL
CARCINOMA*

Dan Laheru, MD
Department of Oncology
The Johns Hopkins Hospital
Baltimore, Maryland
*NEOADJUVANT AND ADJUVANT THERAPY
OF PANCREATIC CANCER*

John C. LaMattina, MD
Assistant Professor of Surgery
University of Maryland Medical Center
Baltimore, Maryland
*LAPAROENDOSCOPIC SINGLE-SITE SURGERY
AS AN EVOLVING SURGICAL APPROACH*

Katherine Graw Lamond, MD, MS
Assistant Professor of Surgery
Division of General and Oncologic Surgery
UM Center for Weight Management and
   Wellness
University of Maryland School of Medicine
Baltimore, Maryland
MORBID OBESITY

R. Todd Lancaster, MD
Instructor in Surgery
Massachusetts General Hospital
Boston, Massachusetts
*THE MANAGEMENT OF THORACIC AND
THORACOABDOMINAL AORTIC ANEURYSMS*

Gregory J. Landry, MD
Associate Professor of Surgery
Knight Cardiovascular Institute
Oregon Health & Science University
Portland, Oregon
*ACUTE PERIPHERAL ARTERIAL AND BYPASS
GRAFT OCCLUSION: THROMBOLYTIC
THERAPY*

Julie R. Lange, MD, ScM
Department of Surgery
Johns Hopkins Medical Institutions
Baltimore, Maryland
INFLAMMATORY BREAST CARCINOMA

James D. Larson, MD
General Surgery Resident
Christiana Care Health System
Newark, Delaware
*THE MANAGEMENT OF BENIGN GASTRIC
ULCER*

Nyan L. Latt, MD
Fellow at Gastroenterology and Hepatology
Kaiser Permanente Los Angeles Medical
   Center
Los Angeles, California
*THE MANAGEMENT OF REFRACTORY
ASCITES*

Joanna K. Law, MD, MA (Ed)
Fellow in Therapeutic Endoscopy
Johns Hopkins Medical Institutions
Baltimore, Maryland
COLONIC STENTING

Anna M. Ledgerwood, MD
Department of Surgery
Wayne State University
Detroit, Michigan
*THE MANAGEMENT OF EXTREMITY
COMPARTMENT SYNDROME*

Andy M. Lee, MD
Department of Surgery
Beth Israel Deaconess Medical Center
Harvard Medical School
Boston, Massachusetts
RAYNAUD'S SYNDROME

Michael J. Lee, MD
Department of Surgery
Cedars-Sinai Medical Center
Los Angeles, California
LAPAROSCOPIC SPLENECTOMY

Anna M. Leung, MD
Gastrointestinal Research Program
Melanoma Research Program
John Wayne Cancer Institute at Saint John's
   Health Center
Santa Monica, California
*RADIOFREQUENCY ABLATION OF HEPATIC
METASTASES FROM COLORECTAL CANCER*
*THE MANAGEMENT OF CUTANEOUS
MELANOMA*

Louis Lewandowski, MD
Department of Orthopaedic Surgery
Walter Reed National Military Medical
   Center
Norman M. Rich Department of Surgery
Uniformed Services University of Health
   Sciences
Bethesda, Maryland
GANGRENE OF THE FOOT

Meghan Lewis, MD
Staff Surgeon
Naval Hospital Camp Pendleton
Newport Beach, California

GLUCOSE CONTROL IN THE POSTOPERATIVE PERIOD

Zhiping Li, MD
The Johns Hopkins University
Baltimore, Maryland

OBSTRUCTIVE JAUNDICE: ENDOSCOPIC THERAPY

Anne O. Lidor, MD, MPH
Associate Professor of Surgery
The Johns Hopkins University School of Medicine
Baltimore, Maryland

MORBID OBESITY

Keith D. Lillemoe, MD
Chief of Surgery
Surgeon-in-Chief
Massachusetts General Hospital
W. Gerald Austen Professor
Harvard Medical School
Boston, Massachusetts

PALLIATIVE THERAPY FOR PANCREATIC CANCER

Jennifer H. Lin, MD
Attending Surgeon
Breast Service, Department of Surgery
Kaiser Permanente Los Angeles Medical Center
Los Angeles, California

THE MANAGEMENT OF THE AXILLA IN BREAST CANCER

Peter H. Lin, MD
Professor of Surgery, Chief of Division of Vascular Surgery & Endovascular Therapy
Michael E. DeBakey Department of Surgery
Baylor College of Medicine
Houston, Texas

DEEP VENOUS THROMBOSIS

Pamela A. Lipsett, MD, MHPE, FACS, FCCM
Warfield M. Firor Endowed Professorship in Surgery
Professor of Surgery
Departments of Surgery, Anesthesiology, Critical Care Medicine, and Nursing
The Johns Hopkins University Schools of Medicine and Nursing
Baltimore, Maryland

PREOPERATIVE BOWEL PREPARATION: IS IT REALLY NECESSARY?

Evan C. Lipsitz, MD
Associate Professor of Surgery
Chief, Division of Vascular and Endovascular Surgery
Montefiore Medical Center and the Albert Einstein College of Medicine
Bronx, New York

AXILLOFEMORAL BYPASS

David H. Livingston, MD, FACS
Wesley J. Howe Professor of Surgery
Chief, Division of Trauma and Critical Care
Rutgers-New Jersey Medical School
Newark, New Jersey

THE MANAGEMENT OF INTRAABDOMINAL INFECTIONS

Jayme E. Locke, MD, MPH
Assistant Professor of Surgery
The University of Alabama, Birmingham
Birmingham, Alabama

TREATMENT FOR HEPATOCELLULAR CARCINOMA: RESECTION VERSUS TRANSPLANTATION

Laurie Anne Loiacono, MD, FCCP
Chief, Surgical Critical Care
Director, Hyperbaric Medicine
Saint Francis Hospital and Medical Center
Hartford, Connecticut

ELECTRICAL AND LIGHTNING INJURY

Joseph V. Lombardi, MD, FACS
Head, Division of Vascular and Endovascular Surgery
Associate Professor of Surgery
Cooper Medical School of Rowan University
Program Director, Vascular and Endovascular Surgery Fellowship
Cooper University Health Care
Camden, New Jersey

ENDOVASCULAR MANAGEMENT OF ARTERIAL INJURY

Bonnie E. Lonze, MD, PhD
Clinical Fellow in Transplant Surgery
Department of Surgery
The Johns Hopkins University School of Medicine
Baltimore, Maryland

HEMODIALYSIS ACCESS SURGERY

Otway Louie, MD
Division of Plastic Surgery
Department of Surgery
University of Washington
Seattle, Washington

BREAST RECONSTRUCTION FOLLOWING MASTECTOMY: INDICATIONS, TECHNIQUES, AND RESULTS

Donald E. Low, MD
Head of Department of Thoracic Surgery
Virginia Mason Medical Center
Seattle, Washington

THE MANAGEMENT OF ACHALASIA OF THE ESOPHAGUS

Charles E. Lucas, MD
Department of Surgery
Wayne State University
Detroit, Michigan

THE MANAGEMENT OF EXTREMITY COMPARTMENT SYNDROME

James D. Luketich, MD
Henry T. Bahnson Professor of Cardiothoracic Surgery
Chief of the Division of Thoracic and Foregut Surgery
Director of the Heart, Lung, and Esophageal Institute
University of Pittsburgh Medical Center
Pittsburgh, Pennsylvania

ESOPHAGEAL STENTS

Ying Wei Lum, MD
Assistant Professor
Division of Vascular Surgery & Endovascular Therapy
Department of Surgery
The Johns Hopkins Hospital
Baltimore, Maryland;
Section Director for Anatomy
Perdana University Graduate School of Medicine
Serdang, Malaysia

FEMORAL AND POPLITEAL ARTERY ANEURYSMS

Kimberly M. Lumpkins, MD
University of Maryland Medical Center
Baltimore, Maryland

REPAIR OF PECTUS EXCAVATUM

Sean P. Lyden, MD
Associate Professor
Vascular Surgery
Cleveland Clinic Foundation
Cleveland, Ohio

THE PREVENTION OF VENOUS THROMBOEMBOLISM

Thomas E. MacGillivary, MD
Co-Director, Thoracic Aortic Center of Cardiac Surgery
Massachusetts General Hospital
Boston, Massachusetts

THE MANAGEMENT OF ACUTE AORTIC DISSECTIONS

Anthony R. MacLean, MD, FRCSC, FACS
Clinical Associate Professor of Surgery
University of Calgary
Colorectal Surgeon
Department of Surgery
Foothills Medical Center
Calgary, Alberta, Canada

THE MANAGEMENT OF PRURITUS ANI

Leon Maggiori, MD
Department of Surgery
New York-Presbyterian Hospital
Weill Cornell Medical College
New York, New York

STRICTUREPLASTY IN CROHN'S DISEASE

Thomas Magnuson, MD
Chief of General Surgery
Johns Hopkins Bayview Medical Center
Baltimore, Maryland

LAPAROSCOPIC SURGERY FOR MORBID OBESITY

George J. Magovern, MD
Professor and Chairman
Department of Thoracic and
    Cardiovascular Surgery
Allegheny General Hospital
Pittsburgh, Pennsylvania

EXTRACORPOREAL MEMBRANE OXYGENATION FOR RESPIRATORY FAILURE IN ADULTS

Ronald V. Maier, MD, FACS
Jane and Donald D. Trunkey Professor and
    Vice Chair of Surgery
University of Washington
Surgeon-in-Chief
Department of Surgery
Harborview Medical Center
Seattle, Washington

PENETRATING NECK TRAUMA

Martin A. Makary, MD, MPH
Associate Professor of Surgery and Health
    Policy & Management
Director, Surgical Quality and Safety
The Johns Hopkins Hospital
Baltimore, Maryland

SMALL BOWEL OBSTRUCTION

LAPAROSCOPIC PANCREAS SURGERY

Junaid Makel, MD
Vascular Surgeon
The Rhode Island Hospital
The Miriam Hospital
Providence, Rhode Island

ABDOMINAL AORTIC ANEURYSM AND UNEXPECTED ABDOMINAL PATHOLOGY

Mahmoud B. Malas, MD, MHS, FACS
Associate Professor of Surgery
Director of Endovascular Surgery
Director of The Vascular and Endovascular
    Clinical Research Center
Johns Hopkins Bayview Medical Center
Baltimore, Maryland

THE MANAGEMENT OF RUPTURED ABDOMINAL AORTIC ANEURYSM

James A. Mann, MD
Division of Gastroenterology and
    Hepatology
University of Virginia Health System
Charlottesville, Virginia

ESOPHAGEAL FUNCTION TESTING

Lindsey L. Manos, MPAS, PA-C
Department of Surgery
The Johns Hopkins Hospital
Baltimore, Maryland

THE MANAGEMENT OF ENTEROCUTANEOUS FISTULAS

Paul N. Manson, MD
Professor of Plastic Surgery
Johns Hopkins Medical Institutions
Baltimore, Maryland

NONMELANOMA SKIN CANCERS

David A. Margolin, MD
Colon and Rectal Research Director
Ochsner Medical Center
New Orleans, Louisiana

THE MANAGEMENT OF CONDYLOMA ACUMINATA

Sheraz R. Markar, MD
Department of Thoracic Surgery
Virginia Mason Medical Center
Seattle, Washington

THE MANAGEMENT OF ACHALASIA OF THE ESOPHAGUS

James F. Markmann, MD, PhD
Claude E. Welch Professor of Surgery
Harvard Medical School
Chief, Division of Transplant Surgery
Massachusetts General Hospital
Boston, Massachusetts

TRANSPLANTATION OF THE PANCREAS

Deborah Lane Marquardt, MD
Trauma / Surgical Critical Care Fellow
Department of Surgery
Harborview Medical Center
Seattle, Washington

PENETRATING NECK TRAUMA

Kieren A. Marr, MD
The Johns Hopkins Hospital
Baltimore, Maryland

ANTIFUNGAL THERAPY IN THE SURGICAL PATIENT

Derek L. Masden, MD
Fellow, Curtis National Hand Center
Union Memorial Hospital
Baltimore, Maryland

HAND INFECTIONS

David W. Mathes, MD
Division of Plastic Surgery, Department of
    Surgery
University of Washington
Seattle, Washington

BREAST RECONSTRUCTION FOLLOWING MASTECTOMY: INDICATIONS, TECHNIQUES, AND RESULTS

Douglas Mathisen, MD
Massachusetts General Hospital
Boston, Massachusetts

MEDIASTINAL MASSES

Jeffrey B. Matthews, MD, FACS
Dallas B. Phemister Professor and
    Chairman
Department of Surgery
The University of Chicago
Chicago, Illinois

PANCREATIC NECROSIS

Haggi Mazeh, MD
Assistant Professor
Section of Endocrine Surgery
Department of Surgery
Hadassah-Hebrew University Medical
    Center
Jerusalem, Israel

ZOLLINGER-ELLISON SYNDROME

Mara McAdams-DeMarco, PhD
Assistant Professor of Surgery and
    Epidemiology
Johns Hopkins University
Johns Hopkins Bloomberg School of Public
    Health
Baltimore, Maryland

PREOPERATIVE ASSESSMENT OF THE OLDER PATIENT: FRAILTY

Jack W. McAninch, MD, FACS
Professor and Vice Chair of Urology
University of California, San Francisco
Chief of Urology
San Francisco General Hospital
San Francisco, California

RETROPERITONEAL INJURIES: KIDNEY AND URETER

Martin McCarter, MD
Professor and Director of Endocrine
    Surgery
University of Colorado
Aurora, Colorado

PERIAMPULLARY CARCINOMA

David W. McFadden, MD
Professor and Chairman
Department of Surgery
University of Connecticut School of
Medicine
Farmington, Connecticut

MALLORY-WEISS SYNDROME

Thomas McIntyre, MD
Assistant Professor of Surgery
SUNY Downstate School of Medicine
Brooklyn, New York

*CYSTS, TUMORS, AND ABSCESSES OF THE
SPLEEN*

**Elisabeth C. McLemore, MD, FACS,
FASCRS**
Associate Professor of Surgery
University of California, San Diego Health
System
San Diego, California

*STAGING LAPAROSCROPY FOR
GASTROINTESTINAL CANCER*

Norman McSwain, Jr., MD, FACS
Professor of Surgery, Tulane University
School of Medicine
Trauma Director, Charity Hospital
Police Surgeon, NOPD
New Orleans, Louisiana

*PANCREATIC AND DUODENAL INJURIES
AND CURRENT SURGICAL THERAPIES*

Rachel L. Medbery, MD
General Surgery Resident
Department of Surgery
Emory University School of Medicine
Atlanta, Georgia

*LAPAROSCOPIC 360-DEGREE
FUNDOPLICATION*

Laleh G. Melstrom, MD, MS
Assistant Professor of Surgery
Rutgers Cancer Institute of New Jersey
New Brunswick, New Jersey

*THE MANAGEMENT OF MALIGNANT LIVER
TUMORS*

Genevieve B. Melton, MD, MA
Associate Professor, Department of Surgery
Faculty Fellow, Institute for Health
Informatics
University of Minnesota
Minneapolis, Minnesota

*THE MANAGEMENT OF COLORECTAL
POLYPS*

W. Scott Melvin, MD
Department of Surgery
The Ohio State University Wexner Medical
Center
Columbus, Ohio

*ENDOLUMINAL APPROACHES TO
GASTROESOPHAGEAL REFLUX DISEASE*

Avedis Meneshian, MD
Assistant Professor, Department of Surgery
The Johns Hopkins University School of
Medicine
Baltimore, Maryland;
Division of Thoracic Surgery
Anne Arundel Medical Center
Annapolis, Maryland

*THE MANAGEMENT OF PRIMARY CHEST
WALL TUMORS*

J. Wayne Meredith, MD, FACS
Professor and Chair
Department of Surgery
Wake Forest University School of Medicine
Winston-Salem, North Carolina

*ABDOMINAL COMPARTMENT SYNDROME
AND MANAGEMENT OF THE OPEN
ABDOMEN*

Fabrizio Michelassi, MD
Department of Surgery
New York-Presbyterian Hospital
Weill Cornell Medical College
New York, New York

STRICTUREPLASTY IN CROHN'S DISEASE

Kresimira Milas, MD, FACS
Professor and Director of Endocrine
Surgery
Department of Surgery and the Thyroid
and Parathyroid Center
Oregon Health & Sciences University
Portland, Oregon

ENDOCRINE CHANGES IN CRITICAL ILLNESS

Zvonimir Milas, MD, FACS
Associate Professor of Surgery
Department of Surgical Oncology and the
Levine Cancer Institute
Carolinas Medical Center
Charlotte, North Carolina

ENDOCRINE CHANGES IN CRITICAL ILLNESS

Preston R. Miller, MD, FACS
Associate Professor of Surgery
Department of Surgery
Wake Forest University School of Medicine
Winston-Salem, North Carolina

*ABDOMINAL COMPARTMENT SYNDROME
AND MANAGEMENT OF THE OPEN
ABDOMEN*

**Stephen M. Milner, MBBS, BDS, DSc
(Hon), FRCS (Ed), FACS**
Professor of Plastic Surgery
Director, Johns Hopkins Burn Center
Surgical Director, Johns Hopkins Wound
Healing Center
Director, Michael D. Hendrix Burn
Research Center
The Johns Hopkins University School of
Medicine
Baltimore, Maryland

BURN WOUND MANAGEMENT

Issa Mirmehdi, MD
Halifax Health-Hernia Institute
Daytona Beach, Florida

ATHLETIC PUBALGIA: THE "SPORTS HERNIA"

Erica L. Mitchell, MD
Associate Professor of Surgery
Division of Vascular Surgery
Oregon Health & Science University
Portland, Oregon

*PSEUDOANEURYSMS AND ARTERIOVENOUS
FISTULAS*

Robert Moesinger, MD
Intermountain Healthcare
Adjunct Assistant Professor
Department of Surgery
Director Rural Surgery Fellowship
University of Utah
Ogden, Utah

RECURRENT INGUINAL HERNIA

Jahan Mohebali, MD
Cardiac Surgery Research Fellow
Brigham and Women's Hospital
General Surgery Resident
Massachusetts General Hospital
Boston, Massachusetts

*THE MANAGEMENT OF ACQUIRED
ESOPHAGEAL RESPIRATORY TRACT FISTULA*

Daniela Molena, MD
Department of Surgery
Assistant Professor of Surgery
Director, Robotic and Minimally Invasive
Thoracic Surgery
Director of Thoracic Surgery, Johns
Hopkins Bayview Medical Center
The Johns Hopkins Hospital
Baltimore, Maryland

PARAESOPHAGEAL HERNIA

VIDEO-ASSISTED THORACIC SURGERY

Robert J. Moraca, MD
Assistant Professor of Surgery
Chief, Section of Arrhythmia and Thoracic
Aortic Surgery
Department of Thoracic and
Cardiovascular Surgery
Allegheny General Hospital
Pittsburgh, Pennsylvania

*EXTRACORPOREAL MEMBRANE
OXYGENATION FOR RESPIRATORY FAILURE
IN ADULTS*

Katherine A. Morgan, MD
Medical University of South Carolina
Charleston, South Carolina

*THE MANAGEMENT OF PANCREATIC
PSEUDOCYST*

Christopher R. Morse, MD
Department of Surgery
Massachusetts General Hospital
Boston, Massachusetts

*THE MANAGEMENT OF ACQUIRED
ESOPHAGEAL RESPIRATORY TRACT FISTULA*

MINIMALLY INVASIVE ESOPHAGECTOMY

Donald L. Morton, MD
Melanoma Research Program
John Wayne Cancer Institute at Saint John's
Health Center
Santa Monica, California

*THE MANAGEMENT OF CUTANEOUS
MELANOMA*

Anne C. Mosenthal, MD, FACS
Professor and Chair
Department of Surgery
Rutgers New Jersey Medical School
Newark, New Jersey

*THE MULTIPLE ORGAN DYSFUNCTION AND
FAILURE*

Raghu Motaganahalli, MD, FACS
Associate Professor of Surgery
Residency Program Director, Vascular and
Endovascular Surgery
Indiana University School of Medicine
Indianapolis, Indiana

*TIBIOPERONEAL ARTERIAL OCCLUSIVE
DISEASE*

**Fady Moustarah, MD, MPH, FRCS(C)
General Surgery**
Associate Professor, Department of Surgery
Laval University
Institut Universitaire de Cardiologie et de
Pneumologie de Québec (IUCPQ)
Research Co-Chair in Bariatric & Metabolic
Surgery
Centre de Recherche de l'IUCPQ, Université
Laval
Québec, QC, Canada

*GLYCEMIC CONTROL AND
CARDIOVASCULAR DISEASE RISK
REDUCTION AFTER BARIATRIC SURGERY*

Nathan T. Mowery, MD, FACS
Assistant Professor
Department of Surgery
Wake Forest University School of Medicine
Winston-Salem, North Carolina

*ABDOMINAL COMPARTMENT SYNDROME
AND MANAGEMENT OF THE OPEN
ABDOMEN*

Benedetto Mungo, MD
Post Doctoral Fellow
Department of Surgery
The Johns Hopkins Hospital
Baltimore, Maryland

PARAESOPHAGEAL HERNIA

VIDEO-ASSISTED THORACIC SURGERY

Ashok Muniappan, MD
Division of Thoracic Surgery
Department of Surgery
Massachusetts General Hospital
Boston, Massachusetts

MEDIASTINAL MASSES

Michael Patrick Murphy, MD
Associate Professor of Surgery and Cellular
& Integrative Physiology
Chief, Vascular and Endovascular Surgery
Richard Roudebush VAMC
Indiana University School of Medicine
Indianapolis, Indiana

*TIBIOPERONEAL ARTERIAL OCCLUSIVE
DISEASE*

Peter Muscarella, MD
Department of Surgery
Ohio State University
Columbus, Ohio

*LAPAROSCOPIC BYPASS FOR PANCREATIC
CANCER*

**Lena M. Napolitano, MD, FACS, FCCP,
FCCM**
Professor of Surgery
University of Michigan School of Medicine
Division Chief, Acute Care Surgery
[Trauma, Burn, Surgical Critical Care,
Emergency Surgery]
Associate Chair, Department of Surgery
Director, Trauma and Surgical Critical Care
University of Michigan Medical System
Ann Arbor, Michigan

POSTOPERATIVE RESPIRATORY FAILURE

Peter Nau, MD, MS
Department of Surgery
The University of Iowa
Iowa City, Iowa

*LAPAROSCOPIC BYPASS FOR PANCREATIC
CANCER*

**Douglas F. Naylor, Jr., MD,
FACS, FCCM**
Departments of General Anesthesia/Critical
Care Medicine and General Surgery
Cleveland Clinic
Cleveland, Ohio

ENDOCRINE CHANGES IN CRITICAL ILLNESS

Susanna Nazarian, MD, PhD
Department of Surgery
The Johns Hopkins Hospital
Baltimore, Maryland

*THE ROLE OF LIVER TRANSPLANTATION IN
PORTAL HYPERTENSION*

Matthew D. Neal, MD
University of Pittsburgh Medical Center
Pittsburgh, Pennsylvania

*NUTRITIONAL SUPPORT IN THE CRITICALLY
ILL*

Peter C. Neligan, MD
Division of Plastic Surgery, Department of
Surgery
University of Washington
Seattle, Washington

*BREAST RECONSTRUCTION FOLLOWING
MASTECTOMY: INDICATIONS, TECHNIQUES,
AND RESULTS*

Leigh Neumayer, MD, MS
Huntsman Cancer Hospital
University of Utah
Salt Lake City, Utah

INGUINAL HERNIA

Hien T. Nguyen, MD, FACS
Director, Comprehensive Hernia Center
Assistant Professor of Surgery, School of
Medicine
Associate Medical Director, Center for
Bioengineering Innovation and Design
(CBID) School of Engineering
Johns Hopkins University
Baltimore, Maryland

LAPAROSCOPIC INGUINAL HERNIORRHAPHY

Ninh T. Nguyen, MD, FACS
Department of Surgery
University of California, Irvine Medical
Center
Orange, California

LAPAROSCOPIC APPENDECTOMY

Raminder Nirula, MD
Surgical Critical Care Fellowship Director
Co-Director, Surgical ICU
Trauma Medical Director, University of
Utah
Salt Lake City, Utah

*GLUCOSE CONTROL IN THE POSTOPERATIVE
PERIOD*

Yuri W. Novitsky, MD
Associate Professor of Surgery
Case Western Reserve University
Co-Director, Case Comprehensive Hernia
Center
Director, Surgical Research
Department of Surgery
University Hospitals Case Medical Center
Cleveland, Ohio

*LAPAROSCOPIC REPAIR OF RECURRENT
INGUINAL HERNIAS*

Terence O'Keeffe, MD, FACS
University of Arizona
Tucson, Arizona

BLOOD TRANSFUSION THERAPY IN TRAUMA

Patrick I. Okolo III, MD, MPH, FASGE
Chief, Gastrointestinal Endoscopy
Associate Professor of Medicine
Johns Hopkins University
Baltimore, Maryland

COLONIC STENTING

Charles S. O'Mara, MD, MBA
Professor of Surgery
University of Mississippi Medical Center
Jackson, Mississippi

*BALLOON ANGIOPLASTY AND STENTS IN
CAROTID ARTERY OCCLUSIVE DISEASE*

Patrick B. O'Neal, MD
Department of Surgery
Boston Veteran's Administration Health
   Care System
Boston University School of Medicine
Boston, Massachusetts

*NECROTIZING SKIN AND SOFT TISSUE
INFECTIONS*

Edwin O. Onkendi, MB, ChB
Department of Surgery
Mayo Clinic
Rochester, Minnesota

*THE MANAGEMENT OF RECURRENT AND
DISSEMINATED BREAST CANCER*

Babak J. Orandi, MD, MSc
The Johns Hopkins Hospital
Baltimore, Maryland

*OPEN REPAIR OF ABDOMINAL AORTIC
ANEURYSMS*

C. Keith Ozaki, MD, FACS
Vascular and Endovascular Surgery
Brigham and Women's Hospital
Boston, Massachusetts

THE TREATMENT OF CLAUDICATION

John Paige, MD, FACS
Associate Professor of Clinical Surgery
Department of Surgery
LSU Health New Orleans School of
   Medicine
New Orleans, Louisiana

*THE MANAGEMENT OF SEMILUNAR LINE,
LUMBAR, AND OBTURATOR HERNIATION*

Theodore N. Pappas, MD
Distinguished Professor of Surgical
   Innovation
Interim Chair, Department of Surgery
Chief, General and Advanced
   Gastrointestinal Surgery
Vice Dean for Medical Affairs
Duke University Medical Center
Durham, North Carolina

*MANAGEMENT OF
CHOLANGIOCARCINOMA*

**Adrian Park, MD, FRCSC, FACS,
FCS (ECSA)**
Chair, Department of Surgery
Anne Arundel Medical Center
Annapolis, Maryland

*HEMATOLOGIC INDICATIONS FOR
SPLENECTOMY*

Do Joong Park, MD, PhD
Department of Surgery
Seoul National University College of
   Medicine
Seoul, Korea

GASTRIC ADENOCARCINOMA

Charles Parker, MD
University of Cincinnati
Cincinnati, Ohio

THE MANAGEMENT OF THYROIDITIS

Nishant D. Patel, MD
Resident, Department of Surgery
The Johns Hopkins Hospital
Baltimore, Maryland

PRIMARY HYPERPARATHYROIDISM

Supriya S. Patel, MD
Resident in Surgery
Department of General Surgery
University of Southern California Medical
   Center
Los Angeles, California

*SURGICAL MANAGEMENT OF
CONSTIPATION*

Timothy M. Pawlik, MD, MPH, PhD
Professor of Surgery and Oncology
Chief, Division of Surgical Oncology
John L. Cameron M.D. Professor of
   Alimentary Tract Diseases
The Johns Hopkins Hospital
Baltimore, MD

GASTROINTESTINAL STROMAL TUMORS

Gregory J. Pearl, MD
Professor of Surgery
Texas A & M Health Sciences Center
Chief, Division of Vascular Surgery
Baylor University Medical Center
Dallas, Texas

BRACHIOCEPHALIC RECONSTRUCTION

Gregory Peck, DO
Trauma and Critical Care Fellow
Emory University
Atlanta, Georgia

*INITIAL ASSESSMENT AND RESUSCITATION
OF THE TRAUMA PATIENT*

**Carlos A. Pellegrini, MD, FACS,
FRCSI (Hon)**
Henry N. Harkins Professor and Chair
Department of Surgery
University of Washington
Seattle, Washington

*LAPAROSCOPIC TREATMENT OF
ESOPHAGEAL MOTILITY DISORDERS*

Peter D. Peng, MD
Department of Surgery
Kaiser Foundation Hospital
Oakland, California

*THE MANAGEMENT OF ADRENAL
CORTICAL TUMORS*

Bruce A. Perler, MD, MBA
Julius H. Jacobson, II Professor of Surgery
The Johns Hopkins University School of
   Medicine
Chief, Division of Vascular Surgery and
   Endovascular Therpay
The John Hopkins Hospital
Baltimore, Maryland

*THE MANAGEMENT OF RECURRENT
CAROTID ARTERY STENOSIS*

Jeffrey H. Peters, MD
Professor of Surgery
Chair of the Department of Surgery
University of Rochester Medical Center
Rochester, New York

*THE MANAGEMENT OF ESOPHAGEAL
CARCINOMA*

Ho Phan, MD
UC Davis Medical Center
Sacramento, California

INJURY TO THE SPLEEN

K. Shad Pharaon, MD
Department of Surgery
Oregon Health & Science University
Portland, Oregon

*THE MANAGEMENT OF VASCULAR
INJURIES*

Edward H. Phillips, MD, FACS
Department of Surgery
Cedars-Sinai Medical Center
Los Angeles, California

LAPAROSCOPIC SPLENECTOMY

Roy Phitayakorn, MD, MHPE (MEd)
Instructor of Surgery
Harvard Medical School
General and Endocrine Surgery
Director of Surgical Education Research
Boston, Massachusetts

*THE MANAGEMENT OF
PHEOCHROMOCYTOMA*

Fredric M. Pieracci, MD, MPH
Staff Surgeon
Denver Health Medical Center
Assistant Professor of Surgery
University of Colorado School of Medicine
Denver, Colorado

PENETRATING ABDOMINAL TRAUMA

Henry A. Pitt, MD
Chief Quality Officer
Temple University Health System
Philadelphia, Pennsylvania

*THE MANAGEMENT OF ECHINOCOCCAL
CYST DISEASE OF THE LIVER*

Susan C. Pitt, MD
Department of Surgery
Washington University
St. Louis, Missouri

*THE MANAGEMENT OF ECHINOCOCCAL
CYST DISEASE OF THE LIVER*

Mun Jye Poi, MD
Assistant Professor of Surgery, Division of
   Vascular Surgery & Endovascular
   Therapy
Michael E. DeBakey Department of Surgery
Baylor College of Medicine
Houston, Texas

DEEP VENOUS THROMBOSIS

Jason D. Prescott, MD, PhD
Massachusetts General Hospital
Boston, Massachusetts

*SECONDARY AND TERTIARY
HYPERPARATHYROIDISM*

Jennifer C. Price, MD
Fellow in Advanced Hepatology
The Johns Hopkins Hospital
Baltimore, Maryland

*THE MANAGEMENT OF BUDD CHIARI
SYNDROME*

Leigh Ann Price, MD
Assistant Professor of Plastic and
   Reconstructive Surgery
Director, Burn Fellowship Program
The Johns Hopkins University School of
   Medicine
Baltimore, Maryland

ELECTRICAL AND LIGHTNING INJURY

Brandon W. Propper, MD
The Johns Hopkins Hospital
Baltimore, Maryland

THORACIC OUTLET SYNDROMES

Reuven Rabinovici, MD, FACS
Professor of Surgery
Tufts University School of Medicine
Chief
Division of Trauma and Acute Care Surgery
Tufts Medical Center
Boston, Massachusetts

*COAGULATION ISSUES AND THE TRAUMA
PATIENT*

Philip T. Ramsay, MD
Attending Surgeon and Director of General
   Surgery Residency
Atlanta Medical Center
Atlanta, Georgia

DIAPHRAGMATIC INJURIES

Bruce Ramshaw, MD, FACS
Halifax Health-Hernia Institute
Daytona Beach, Florida

ATHLETIC PUBALGIA: THE "SPORTS HERNIA"

Gregory W. Randolph, MD
Department of Otolaryngology—Head and
   Neck Surgery
Massachusetts Eye and Ear Infirmary
Department of Otology and Laryngology
Harvard Medical School
Boston, Massachusetts

SURGICAL APPROACH TO THYROID CANCER

Todd E. Rasmussen, MD, FACS
Deputy Commander
The U.S. Army Institute of Surgical
   Research
Fort Sam Houston, Texas;
Professor of Surgery
The Norman M. Rich Department of
   Surgery
The Uniformed Services University of the
   Health Sciences
Bethesda, Maryland

THE DIABETIC FOOT

David W. Rattner, MD
Chief, Division of Gastrointestinal and
   General Surgery
Massachusetts General Hospital
Professor of Surgery
Harvard Medical School
Boston, Massachusetts

GASTROESOPHAGEAL REFLUX DISEASE

Chandrajit P. Raut, MS, MSc
Associate Professor
Department of Surgery
Brigham & Women's Hospital
Center for Sarcoma and Bone Oncology
Dana-Farber Cancer Institute
Harvard Medical School
Boston, Massachusetts

GASTROINTESTINAL STROMAL TUMORS

*THE MANAGEMENT OF SOFT TISSUE
SARCOMA*

Howard A. Reber, MD
Professor and Chief
Division of Gastrointestinal Surgery
Director, UCLA Center for Pancreatic
   Diseases
Department of Surgery
David Geffen School of Medicine at UCLA
Los Angeles, California

*THE MANAGEMENT OF CHRONIC
PANCREATITIS*

Thomas Reifsnyder, MD, FACS
Department of Surgery
Bayview Medical Center
The Johns Hopkins University School of
   Medicine
Baltimore, Maryland

FEMOROPOPLITEAL OCCLUSIVE DISEASE

HEMODIALYSIS ACCESS SURGERY

Linda M. Reilly, MD
Professor of Surgery
University of California, San Francisco
San Francisco, California

*THE MANAGEMENT OF CHRONIC
MESENTERIC ISCHEMIA*

Justin A. Reynolds, MD
Division of Digestive Diseases
Department of Medicine
David Geffen School of Medicine at UCLA
Los Angeles, California

*ENDOSCOPIC THERAPY FOR ESOPHAGEAL
VARICEAL HEMORRHAGE*

Peter Rhee, MD, MPH, FACS, FCCM
Chief, Division of Trauma, Critical Care
   and Emergency Surgery
Professor of Surgery
Medical Director, UMC Trauma Center
Co-Medical Director, Pediatric ICU
Program Director, Acute Care Surgery
   Fellowship
Program Director, Critical Care Fellowship
Vice Chair, Clinical Affairs
Martin Gluck Endowed Chair in Trauma,
   Critical Care and Emergency Surgery
The University of Arizona
Tucson, Arizona

BLOOD TRANSFUSION THERAPY IN TRAUMA

Taylor S. Riall, MD, PhD
Associate Professor
John Sealy Distinguished Chair in Clinical
   Research
Department of Surgery
University of Texas Medical Branch
Galveston, Texas

UNUSUAL PANCREATIC TUMORS

J. David Richardson, MD
University of Louisville
Louisville, Kentucky

EMERGENCY DEPARTMENT THORACOTOMY

Nabil P. Rizk, MD
General Thoracic Surgeon
Memorial Sloan-Kettering Cancer Center
New York, New York

*NEOADJUVANT AND ADJUVANT THERAPY
OF ESOPHAGEAL CANCER*

**Miguel A. Rodriguez-Bigas, MD, FACS,
FASCRS**
Professor, Department of Surgical Oncology
Division of Surgery
The University of Texas MD Anderson
   Cancer Center
Houston, Texas

THE MANAGEMENT OF RECTAL CANCER

Michael J. Rosen, MD, FACS
Professor of Surgery
Chief, Division of GI and General Surgery
Director, Case Comprehensive Hernia
   Center
Co-Director, Case Acute Intestinal Failure
   Unit
University Hospitals Case Medical Center
Cleveland, Ohio
LAPAROSCOPIC VENTRAL HERNIA REPAIR

Laura H. Rosenberger, MD, MS
Resident, Department of Surgery
University of Virginia School of Medicine
Charlottesville, Virginia
SURGICAL SITE INFECTIONS

Robert E. Roses, MD
Assistant Professor
Department of Surgery
Hospital of the University of Pennsylvania
University of Pennsylvania School of
   Medicine
Philadelphia, Pennsylvania
THE MANAGEMENT OF RECTAL CANCER

Gedge D. Rosson, MD
Associate Professor, Department of Plastic
   and Reconstructive Surgery
The Johns Hopkins Hospital
Baltimore, Maryland
NERVE INJURY AND REPAIR

Grace S. Rozycki, MD, MBA
Willis D. Gatch Professor of Surgery
Executive Vice-Chair
Department of Surgery
Director, Indiana Injury Institute
Indiana University
Indianapolis, Indiana
*THE SURGEON'S USE OF ULTRASOUND IN
THORACOABDOMINAL TRAUMA*

Amy Rushing, MD
Assistant Professor of Surgery
Division of Acute Care Surgery, Trauma,
   and Surgical Critical Care
The Johns Hopkins Hospital
Baltimore, Maryland
VENTILATOR-ASSOCIATED PNEUMONIA

Colleen M. Ryan, MD
Associate Professor of Surgery
Harvard Medical School
Sumner Redstone Burn Center
Massachusetts General Hospital
Shriners Hospital for Children-Boston
Boston, Massachusetts
*COLD INJURY, FROSTBITE, AND
HYPOTHERMIA*

Shirin Sabbaghian, MD
Fellow, Surgical Oncology
University of Pittsburgh
Pittsburgh, Pennsylvania
PRIMARY SCLEROSING CHOLANGITIS

Teviah E. Sachs, MD, MPH
Department of Surgery
The Johns Hopkins School of Medicine
Baltimore, Maryland
CAVERNOUS HEPATIC HEMANGIOMA

Bashar Safar, MBBS
Department of Surgery
The Johns Hopkins School of Medicine
Baltimore, Maryland
*THE MANAGEMENT OF TOXIC
MEGACOLON*

Klaus Sahora, MD
Department of Surgery
Massachusetts General Hospital
Harvard Medical School
Boston, Massachusetts
*INTRADUCTAL PAPILLARY MUCINOUS
NEOPLASMS OF THE PANCREAS*

Hakim K. Said, MD, FACS
Director, Microvascular Reconstructive
   Surgery Fellowship
Associate Professor, Surgery
Division of Plastic Surgery
University of Washington
Seattle, Washington
*BREAST RECONSTRUCTION FOLLOWING
MASTECTOMY: INDICATIONS, TECHNIQUES,
AND RESULTS*

Bulent Salman, MD
Associate Professor of Surgery
Gazi University School of Medicine
Ankara, Turkey
CYSTIC DISORDERS OF THE BILE DUCTS

Michael G. Sarr, MD
James C. Mason Professor of Surgery
Mayo Clinic
Rochester, Minnesota
*THE MANAGEMENT OF ASYMPTOMATIC
(SILENT) GALLSTONES*

Stephanie A. Savage, MD, MS, FACS
Assistant Professor of Surgery
University of Tennessee Health Science
   Center
Memphis, Tennessee
THE MANAGEMENT OF LIVER INJURIES

Robert G. Sawyer, MD
University of Virginia
Charlottesville, Virginia
SURGICAL SITE INFECTIONS

Thomas M. Scalea, MD
Francis X. Kelly Professorship in Trauma
   Surgery
Director, Program in Trauma
Physician-in-Chief, R Adams Cowley Shock
   Trauma Center
University of Maryland School of Medicine
Baltimore, Maryland
*AIRWAY MANAGEMENT IN THE TRAUMA
PATIENT*

Philip R. Schauer, MD
Cleveland Clinic Foundation
Cleveland, Ohio
*GLYCEMIC CONTROL AND
CARDIOVASCULAR DISEASE RISK
REDUCTION AFTER BARIATRIC SURGERY*

Todd Schlachter, MD
Vascular & Interventional Radiology
Johns Hopkins University
Baltimore, Maryland
VENA CAVA FILTERS

David R. Schmidt, MD, FACS
Gwinnett Surgical Associates
Lawrenceville, Georgia
ACUTE CHOLECYSTITIS

Matthew J. Schuchert, MD
Assistant Professor of Surgery
Department of Cardiothoracic Surgery
University of Pittsburgh Medical Center
Pittsburgh, Pennsylvania
ESOPHAGEAL STENTS

Richard D. Schulick, MD
The Aragon/Gonzalez-Giusti Professor and
   Chair of Surgery
University of Colorado
Aurora, Colorado
PERIAMPULLARY CARCINOMA

Michael A. Schweitzer, MD
Assistant Professor of Surgery
The Johns Hopkins University School of
   Medicine
Director of Minimally Invasive Bariatric
   Surgery
Department of Surgery
Johns Hopkins Bayview Medical Center
Baltimore, Maryland
*LAPAROSCOPIC SURGERY FOR MORBID
OBESITY*

Christopher M. Sciortino, MD, PhD
Assistant Professor of Surgery
Division of Cardiac Surgery
The Johns Hopkins Hospital
Baltimore, Maryland
DISORDERS OF ESOPHAGEAL MOTILITY

VIDEO-ASSISTED THORACIC SURGERY

Dorry Segev, MD, PhD
Associate Professor of Surgery and
    Epidemiology
Johns Hopkins University
Johns Hopkins Bloomberg School of Public
    Health
Baltimore, Maryland
*PREOPERATIVE ASSESSMENT OF THE OLDER
PATIENT: FRAILTY*
LAPAROSCOPIC DONOR NEPHRECTOMY

**Anthony J. Senagore, MD, MS, MBA,
FACS, FASCRS**
Professor and Division Chief
Charles W. and Carolyn Costello Chair for
    Colorectal Diseases
Department of Surgery
Division of Colorectal Surgery
Keck School of Medicine of University of
    Southern California
Los Angeles, California
*SURGICAL MANAGEMENT OF
CONSTIPATION*

Ashish Shah, MD
Associate Professor of Surgery
Division of Cardiac Surgery
The Johns Hopkins Hospital
Baltimore, Maryland
BLUNT CARDIAC INJURY

Jay G. Shake, MD, MS, FACS
Division of Cardiothoracic Surgery
Assistant Professor of Surgery
Director, Cardiothoracic Intensive Care
    Unit
Scott and White Memorial Hospital
Texas A & M Health Science Center, College
    of Medicine
Temple, Texas
CARDIOVASCULAR PHARMACOLOGY

Brian D. Shames, MD
Associate Professor of Surgery, Department
    of Surgery
Chief, Division of General Surgery
University of Connecticut School of
    Medicine
Farmington, Connecticut
MALLORY-WEISS SYNDROME

Skandan Shanmugan, MD
Resident in Colon and Rectal Surgery
University Hospitals, Case Medical Center
Cleveland, Ohio
LOWER GASTROINTESTINAL BLEEDING

Reem Zeyad Sharaiha, MD, MSc
Weill Cornell Medical Center
New York, New York
*OBSTRUCTIVE JAUNDICE: ENDOSCOPIC
THERAPY*

Gaurav Sharma, MD, MS
Surgical Resident
Brigham and Women's Hospital
Boston, Massachusetts
ACUTE CHOLANGITIS

Kenneth W. Sharp, MD
Professor of Surgery
Vice-Chair, Department of General Surgery
Vanderbilt University Medical Center
Nashville, Tennessee
GALLSTONE ILEUS

Robert Sheridan, MD
Massachusetts General Hospital
Shriners Hospital for Children
Boston, Massachusetts
*PRACTICAL MANAGEMENT OF THE BURN
PATIENT*

Shmuel Shoham, MD
The Johns Hopkins Hospital
Baltimore, Maryland
*ANTIFUNGAL THERAPY IN THE SURGICAL
PATIENT*

Fahad Shuja, MD
Department of Surgery
Massachusetts General Hospital
Boston, Massachusetts
*ENDOVASCULAR TREATMENT OF
ABDOMINAL AORTIC ANEURYSM*

Gregorio A. Sicard, MD
Vice-Chairman
Eugene M. Bricker Professor of Surgery
Section of Vascular Surgery
Department of Surgery
Washington University, School of Medicine
St. Louis, Missouri
ATHEROSCLEROTIC RENAL ARTERY DISEASE

Michael B. Silva, Jr., MD
Department of Surgery
University of Texas Medical Branch at
    Galveston
Galveston, Texas
ACUTE MESENTERIC ISCHEMIA

Eric R. Simms, MD
Resident, Department of Surgery
Tulane University School of Medicine
New Orleans, Louisiana
*PANCREATIC AND DUODENAL INJURIES
AND CURRENT SURGICAL THERAPIES*

Andrew Singer, MD, PhD
Assistant Professor of Surgery
Surgical Director of Kidney Transplantation
The Johns Hopkins Hospital
Baltimore, Maryland
*THE ROLE OF LIVER TRANSPLANTATION IN
PORTAL HYPERTENSION*

Smrita Sinha, MD
Gastroenterology Fellow
Johns Hopkins University
Baltimore, Maryland
*ACUTE COLONIC PSEUDO-OBSTRUCTION
(OGILVIE'S SYNDROME)*

Barbara L. Smith, MD, PhD
Massachusetts General Hospital
Boston, Massachusetts
*LYMPHATIC MAPPING AND SENTINEL
LYMPHADENECTOMY*

Brian R. Smith, MD, FACS
Department of Surgery
University of California, Irvine Medical
    Center
Orange, California
LAPAROSCOPIC APPENDECTOMY

Lee E. Smith, MD
Emeritus Faculty, Section of Colon and
    Rectal Surgery
Department of Surgery
MedStar Washington Hospital Center
Professor of Surgery, Georgetown
    University
Washington, DC
*THE MANAGEMENT OF SOLITARY RECTAL
ULCER SYNDROME*

Philip W. Smith, MD
Assistant Professor of Surgery
University of Virginia
Charlottesville, Virginia
*EVALUATION OF THE ISOLATED
NECK MASS*

Julie Ann Sosa, MD, MA, FACS
Professor of Surgery and Medicine
Chief, Section of Endocrine Surgery
Director of Health Services Research
Department of Surgery
Duke University School of Medicine
Leader, Endocrine Neoplasia Diseases
    Group
Duke Cancer Institute and Duke Clinical
    Research Institute
Durham, North Carolina
MINIMALLY INVASIVE PARATHYROIDECTOMY

Jason L. Sperry, MD
University of Pittsburgh Medical Center
Pittsburgh, Pennsylvania
*NUTRITIONAL SUPPORT IN THE
CRITICALLY ILL*

Jennifer A. Stableford, MD
Assistant Professor of Surgery
Montefiore Medical Center and the Albert
　Einstein College of Medicine
Bronx, New York

AXILLOFEMORAL BYPASS

J. Daniel Stanley, MD, FACS, FASCRS
Associate Professor of Surgery
Department of Surgery
University of Tennessee College of Medicine
Chattanooga, Tennessee

*THE MANAGEMENT OF CLOSTRIDIUM
DIFFICILE COLITIS*

Sharon L. Stein, MD
Assistant Professor of Surgery
University Hospitals, Case Medical Center
Cleveland, Ohio

LOWER GASTROINTESTINAL BLEEDING

Antonia Stephen, MD
Assistant Professor of Surgery
Massachusetts General Hospital
Boston, Massachusetts

*SECONDARY AND TERTIARY
HYPERPARATHYROIDISM*

Jordan R. Stern, MD
Senior Resident in Surgery
The University of Chicago
Chicago, Illinois

PANCREATIC NECROSIS

**Jeffrey A. Sternberg, MD, FACS,
FASCRS**
Surgical Director, Center For Inflammatory
　Diseases
California Pacific Medical Center
Clinical Assistant Professor of Surgery
University of California San Francisco
San Francisco, California

THE MANAGEMENT OF PILONIDAL DISEASE

Kent A. Stevens, MD, MPH
Assistant Professor of Surgery
Department of Surgery
Johns Hopkins Medical Institutions
Baltimore, Maryland

*SPLENIC SALVAGE PROCEDURES:
THERAPEUTIC OPTIONS*

David Steward, MD
University of Cincinnati
Cincinnati, Ohio

THE MANAGEMENT OF THYROIDITIS

Dylan Stewart, MD
Assistant Professor of Surgery
Director of Pediatric Trauma Program
Division of Pediatric Surgery
Johns Hopkins Children Center
The Johns Hopkins Hospital
Baltimore, Maryland

*THE MANAGEMENT OF ACUTE
APPENDICITIS*

Tiffany Stoddard, MD
Department of Surgery
Anne Arundel Medical Center
Annapolis, Maryland

*HEMATOLOGIC INDICATIONS FOR
SPLENECTOMY*

Steven M. Strasberg, MD
Section of Hepatobiliary-Pancreatic Surgery
　Department of Surgery
Washington University
St. Louis, Missouri

BENIGN BILIARY STRICTURES

Michael B. Streiff, MD
Associate Professor of Medicine and
　Pathology
Johns Hopkins Medical Institutions
Baltimore, Maryland

*COAGULOPATHY IN THE CRITICALLY ILL
PATIENT*

Paul H. Sugarbaker, MD, FACS, FRCS
Medical Director, Center for
　Gastrointestinal Malignancies
MedStar Washington Hospital Center
Washington, DC

*THE MANAGEMENT OF PERITONEAL
SURFACE MALIGNANCY*

Lee L. Swanstrom, MD, FACS
Clinical Professor of Surgery
Oregon Health & Sciences University
Division of GI and MIS Surgery
The Oregon Clinic
Portland, Oregon;
Chief Innovations Officer, Institute
　l'Hopital Univeritaire
Strasbourg, Strasbourg, France

LAPAROSCOPIC ADRENALECTOMY

Tze-Woei Tan, MD
Smithwick Vascular Surgery Fellow
Boston University Medical Center
Boston University School of Medicine
Boston, Massachusetts

*THE MANAGEMENT OF PERIPHERAL
ARTERIAL EMBOLI*

Luis F. Tapias, MD
Department of Surgery
Massachusetts General Hospital
Boston, Massachusetts

MINIMALLY INVASIVE ESOPHAGECTOMY

John L. Tarpley, MD
Professor of Surgery and Anesthesiology
Department of Surgery
Vanderbilt University School of Medicine
Associate Chief, Surgical Service
Nashville VA
Nashville, Tennessee

*THE MANAGEMENT OF DIVERTICULOSIS OF
THE SMALL BOWEL*

Ali Tavakkoli, MD
Department of Surgery
Brigham and Women's Hospital
Boston, Massachusetts

*METABOLIC CHANGES FOLLOWING
BARIATRIC SURGERY*

Nyali Taylor, MD
Albert Einstein Medical Center
Philadelphia, Pennsylvania

*ENDOVASCULAR MANAGEMENT OF
ARTERIAL INJURY*

Spence M. Taylor, MD
Division of Vascular Surgery
Greenville Hospital System Clinical
　University
University of South Carolina School of
　Medicine
Greenville, South Carolina

PROFUNDA FEMORIS RECONSTRUCTION

Dana A. Telem, MD
Assistant Professor of Surgery
Department of General Surgery
Stony Brook University Medical Center
Stony Brook, New York

GASTROESOPHAGEAL REFLUX DISEASE

Mario D. Terán, MD
Division of Thoracic Surgery
Johns Hopkins University
Baltimore, Maryland

*THE MANAGEMENT OF BARRETT'S
ESOPHAGUS*

Kyla P. Terhune, MD
Assistant Professor of Surgery and
　Anesthesiology
Department of Surgery
Vanderbilt University School of Medicine
Nashville, Tennessee

*THE MANAGEMENT OF DIVERTICULOSIS OF
THE SMALL BOWEL*

David J. Terris, MD
Surgical Director, GRU Thyroid and
　Parathyroid Center
Porubsky Professor and Chairman
Department of Otolaryngology-Head and
　Neck Surgery
Georgia Regents University
Augusta, Georgia

HYPERTHYROIDISM

Sarah P. Thayer, MD, PhD
Associate Professor
Department of Surgery
Andrew L. Warshaw, MD, Institute for
　Pancreatic Cancer Research
W. Gerald Austen Scholar in Academic
　Surgery
Masachusetts General Hospital and
Harvard Medical School
Boston, Massachusetts

*THE MANAGEMENT OF ACUTE
PANCREATITIS*

William D. Tobler, Jr., MD
Neurological Surgeon
The Mayfield Clinic
Cincinnati, Ohio
TRACHEOSTOMY

Paul Toomey, MD
Department of Surgery
University of South Florida, Morsani
    College of Medicine
Tampa, Florida
*ABLATIVE THERAPIES IN BENIGN AND
MALIGNANT BREAST DISEASE*

Shirin Towfigh, MD
Cedars Sinai Medical Center
Los Angeles, California
INGUINAL HERNIA

Donald D. Trunkey, MD
Department of Surgery
Oregon Health & Science University
Portland, Oregon
THE MANAGEMENT OF VASCULAR INJURIES

Theodore Tsangaris, MD
Director, Breast Surgery
Jefferson University Hospitals
Philadelphia, Pennsylvania
MALE BREAST CANCER

Anthony P. Tufaro, DDS, MD, FACS
Associate Professor of Plastic Surgery &
    Oncology
Johns Hopkins University School of
    Medicine
The Johns Hopkins Outpatient Center
Baltimore, Maryland
ABDOMINAL WALL RECONSTRUCTION

Evan Tummel, MD
Department of Surgery
University of South Florida
Morsani College of Medicine
Tampa, Florida
*ABLATIVE THERAPIES IN BENIGN AND
MALIGNANT BREAST DISEASE*

Eric J. Turney, MD
Staff Surgeon
Vascular Surgery
Mike O'Callaghan Federal Medical Center
Las Vegas, Nevada
*THE PREVENTION OF VENOUS
THROMBOEMBOLISM*

Konstantin Umanskiy, MD, FACS
Assistant Professor
Department of Surgery
University of Chicago
Chicago, Illinois
*LAPAROSCOPIC MANAGEMENT OF CROHN'S
DISEASE*

Marshall M. Urist, MD
University of Alabama at Birmingham
Birmingham, Alabama
*DUCTAL AND LOBULAR CARCINOMA IN
SITU OF THE BREAST*

Nakul Valsangkar, MD
Department of Surgery
Andrew L. Warshaw, M.D., Institute for
    Pancreatic Cancer Research
Massachusetts General Hospital and
    Harvard Medical School
Boston, Massachusetts
ACUTE PANCREATITIS

Shant M. Vartanian, MD
Division of Vascular and Endovascular
    Surgery
University of California, San Francisco
San Francisco, California
AORTOILIAC OCCLUSIVE DISEASE

Catherine G. Velopulos, MD, MHS
Assistant Professor of Surgery
Anesthesiology/Critical Care Medicine and
    Emergency Medicine
Division of Acute Care Surgery
Department of Surgery
The Johns Hopkins University School of
    Medicine
Baltimore, Maryland
*VENOUS THROMBOEMBOLISM:
PREVENTION, DIAGNOSIS, AND TREATMENT*

David Victor, MD
The Johns Hopkins Hospital
Baltimore, Maryland
*THE MANAGEMENT OF HEPATIC
ENCEPHALOPATHY*

Carl Magnus Wahlgren, MD, PhD
Consultant Vascular Surgeon
Associate Professor
Department of Vascular Surgery
Karolinska University Hospital
171 76 Stockholm, Sweden
*BUERGER'S DISEASE (THROMBOANGIITIS
OBLITERANS)*

Thomas N. Wang, MD, PhD
University of Alabama at Birmingham
Birmingham, Alabama
*DUCTAL AND LOBULAR CARCINOMA IN
SITU OF THE BREAST*

Tracy S. Wang, MD, MPH
Associate Professor
Department of Surgery
Medical College of Wisconsin
Milwaukee, Wisconsin
MINIMALLY INVASIVE PARATHYROIDECTOMY

Michael T. Watkins, MD
Division of Vascular and Endovascular
    Surgery
Department of Surgery
Massachusetts General Hospital
Boston, Massachusetts
*ABDOMINAL AORTIC ANEURYSM AND
UNEXPECTED ABDOMINAL PATHOLOGY*

Kenneth Waxman, MD, FACS
Santa Barbara Cottage Hospital
Santa Barbara, California
ACUTE KIDNEY FAILURE

Jordan A. Weinberg, MD
Associate Professor, Department of Surgery
University of Tennessee Health Science
    Center
Memphis, Tennessee
THE ABDOMEN THAT WILL NOT CLOSE

Jon David Weingart, MD
The Johns Hopkins Hospital
Baltimore, Maryland
*THE MANAGEMENT OF TRAUMATIC BRAIN
INJURY*

Mark R. Wendling, MD
General Surgery Resident
The Ohio State University Wexner Medical
    Center
Columbus, Ohio
*ENDOLUMINAL APPROACHES TO
GASTROESOPHAGEAL REFLUX DISEASE*

Hunter Wessells, MD, FACS
Professor and Nelson Chair in Urology
University of Washington, School of
    Medicine
Attending Urologist, Harborview Medical
    Center
Affiliate Member, Harborview Injury
    Prevention Research Center
Seattle, Washington
*UROLOGIC COMPLICATIONS OF PELVIC
FRACTURE*

Hadley K.H. Wesson, MD, MPH
Department of General Surgery
Virginia Commonwealth University Medical
    Center
Richmond, Virginia
*SPLENIC SALVAGE PROCEDURES:
THERAPEUTIC OPTIONS*

Russell N. Wesson, MBChB
Resident in General Surgery
The Johns Hopkins Hospital
Baltimore, Maryland
*VASCULAR RECONSTRUCTION DURING THE
WHIPPLE OPERATION*

Steven D. Wexner, MD, PhD (Hon), FASCRS, FRCS (Ed)
Director, Digestive Disease Center
Chairman, Department of Colorectal
    Surgery
Cleveland Clinic Foundation, Weston
Weston, Florida

STAGING LAPAROSCROPY FOR GASTROINTESTINAL CANCER

Edward E. Whang, MD
Departments of Surgery
VA Boston Healthcare System and Brigham
    and Women's Hospital
Harvard Medical School
Boston, Massachusetts

ACUTE CHOLANGITIS

Charles B. Whitlow, MD
Program Director, Colon & Rectal Surgery
    Fellowship Program
Board Member, American Board of Colon
    and Rectal Surgery
Residency Review Committee for Colon
    and Rectal Surgery
Vice-President, Program Directors
    Association for Colon and Rectal Surgery
Ochsner Medical Center
New Orleans, Louisiana

THE MANAGEMENT OF CONDYLOMA ACUMINATA

Glen Whitman, MD
The Johns Hopkins Hospital
Baltimore, Maryland

ACID-BASE PROBLEMS

Elizabeth Wick, MD, FACS
Assistant Professor
Department of Surgery
John Hopkins University
Baltimore, Maryland

COLON CANCER

Timothy K. Williams, MD
Assistant Clinical Professor
Department of Surgery
The University of California Davis
Sacramento, California

THE MANAGEMENT OF RECURRENT CAROTID ARTERY STENOSIS

Christopher L. Wolfgang, MD, PhD
Assistant Professor of Surgery
The Johns Hopkins University School of
    Medicine
Attending Surgeon
The Johns Hopkins Hospital
Baltimore, Maryland

The MANAGEMENT OF ENTEROCUTANEOUS FISTULAS

Virginia L. Wong, MD, FACS
Assistant Professor of Surgery, Case Western
    Reserve University
Division of Vascular Surgery and
    Endovascular Therapy
University Hospitals Case Medical Center
Director of Vascular Services
University Hospitals Richmond Medical
    Center
Cleveland, Ohio

THE MANAGEMENT OF ANEURYSMS OF THE EXTRACRANIAL CAROTID AND VERTEBRAL ARTERIES

UPPER EXTREMITY ARTERIAL OCCLUSIVE DISEASE

Yee Wong, MD
General Surgery Resident
Loyola University Medical Center
Maywood, Illinois

LAPAROSCOPIC COMMON BILE DUCT EXPLORATION

Douglas E. Wood, MD
University of Washington
Seattle, Washington

PRIMARY TUMORS OF THE THYMUS

Cameron D. Wright, MD
Professor of Surgery
Harvard Medical School
Division of Thoracic Surgery
Massachusetts General Hospital
Boston, Massachusetts

THE MANAGEMENT OF TRACHEAL STENOSIS

Han-Kwang Yang, MD, PhD, FACS
Department of Surgery
Seoul National University Hospital
Seoul, South Korea

LAPAROSCOPIC GASTRIC SURGERY

Stephen C. Yang, MD
The Arthur B. and Patricia B. Modell
    Professor in Thoracic Surgery
Chief of Thoracic Surgery
Director, Thoracic Oncology Program
Surgical Curriculum and Clerkship Director
The Johns Hopkins School of Medicine
Baltimore, Maryland

DISORDERS OF ESOPHAGEAL MOTILITY

Sam S. Yoon, MD
Department of Surgery
Memorial Sloan-Kettering Cancer Center
New York, New York

GASTRIC ADENOCARCINOMA

Syed Nabeel Zafar, MB, BS, MPH
Resident, General Surgery
Department of Surgery
Howard University Hospital
Washington, DC

INJURIES TO THE SMALL AND LARGE BOWEL

Sabino Zani, Jr., MD
Duke University Medical Center
Durham, North Carolina

MANAGEMENT OF CHOLANGIOCARCINOMA

Victor Zaydfudim, MD, MPH
Hepatobiliary Surgery Fellow
Department of Surgery
Mayo Clinic
Rochester, Minnesota

THE MANAGEMENT OF ASYMPTOMATIC (SILENT) GALLSTONES

Martha A. Zeiger, MD
The Johns Hopkins Hospital
Baltimore, Maryland

PRIMARY HYPERPARATHYROIDISM

Michael E. Zenilman, MD
Professor of Surgery
The Johns Hopkins School of Medicine
Baltimore, Maryland;
Professor Emeritus
SUNY Downstate
Brooklyn, New York

CYSTS, TUMORS, AND ABSCESSES OF THE SPLEEN

Faming Zhang, MD, PhD
Johns Hopkins Medical Institutions
Baltimore, Maryland

NOTES: WHAT IS CURRENTLY POSSIBLE?

Kashif A. Zuberi, MD
Sanford Health
Bemidji, Minnesota

LAPAROSCOPIC SURGERY FOR MORBID OBESITY

PREFACE

The first edition of *Current Surgical Therapy* was published in 1984. The text has thus been in existence for 30 years, and this represents the eleventh edition. We have updated the material to reflect the continuing evolution of minimally invasive surgery, critical care, and vascular surgery. The text continues to be perhaps the most popular surgical book in the country, and as long as it fulfills a need, we plan to continue the publication every three years. In addition, it is a special privilege and honor for the two editors to be able to review contributions from surgeons around the country, and indeed from around the world, on what they believe is current surgical therapy for virtually all general surgical topics. It is an enjoyable task and keeps two surgeons, who care for surgical patients and operate daily, current on all general surgical topics.

The eleventh edition contains more than 270 chapters. This is twice the number of chapters in the first edition of *Current Surgical Therapy*. The length, however, has been held constant through the last few editions in an effort to keep the text at a manageable size. As with prior editions, nearly every chapter is new, and has been written by a new author. All authors have contributed their specific and personal thoughts on the current surgical therapy of the disease about which they are experts. Thus, to obtain a broad view of the topic, the reader should review the contributions of other experts in the last two or three editions of *Current Surgical Therapy*.

As with the past editions, disease presentation, pathophysiology, and diagnosis are discussed only briefly, with the emphasis being on current surgical therapy. When an operative procedure is discussed, an effort has been made to contain brief and concise descriptions, with figures and diagrams when possible. *Current Surgical Therapy* is written for surgical residents, fellows, and fully trained surgeons in private practice or an academic setting. Many have told us that it is an excellent text to review prior to taking the general surgical boards or recertifying. In addition, medical students have given us feedback that they believe the text is of value to them. However, *Current Surgical Therapy* is not written principally for medical students. We believe a more classic surgical textbook with substantial sections on disease presentation, diagnosis, and pathophysiology is more appropriate for medical students.

We remain grateful to the many surgeons throughout the country, as well as the international surgeons, who participated in creating this textbook. Most of the potential authors that we solicit respond enthusiastically to the opportunity to present their expert views. Their efforts obviously are what make this textbook a success. In addition, Andrew and I could not have compiled this textbook without the herculean efforts of Ms. Irma Silkworth, who has been involved with virtually all of these editions.

Both editors continue to enjoy and thrive in our chosen profession of general surgery. In recruiting medical students into our specialty over the last 40 years, I have used the statement, "If you pick a profession you love, you never have to work the rest of your life." In our view, that profession is surgery.

Finally, we would like to dedicate this edition, as with the others, to the surgical house staff at The Johns Hopkins Hospital, who are "the best of the best."

Andrew M. Cameron, MD
John L. Cameron, MD

CONTENTS

SKIN AND SOFT TISSUE

CHEST WALL, MEDIASTINUM, TRACHEA

VASCULAR SURGERY

TRAUMA AND EMERGENCY CARE

PREOPERATIVE AND POSTOPERATIVE CARE

SURGICAL CRITICAL CARE

MINIMALLY INVASIVE SURGERY

INDEX

THE ESOPHAGUS

ESOPHAGEAL FUNCTION TESTING

Philip W. Carrott, Jr., MD, James A. Mann, MD, and
Benjamin D. Kozower, MD, MPH, FACS

The function of the esophagus is to facilitate the passage of food and drink to the stomach and to ensure that they stay there. Disorders of this function are complex and are caused by a variety of anatomic or intrinsic issues that can be measured and diagnosed with esophageal function tests. Esophageal dysfunction can be present at any level of the esophagus, although most patients evaluated by surgeons have issues with lower esophageal sphincter (LES) function. Common symptoms such as dysphagia, regurgitation, reflux, and pain prompt a diagnostic work up workup, and esophageal function tests are essential for optimal surgical intervention. A detailed history from patients with dysphagia is imperative; many patients suffer unnecessarily because physicians are unfamiliar with this topic.

This chapter provides a brief overview of commonly encountered esophageal function disorders and a review of the primary esophageal function tests used in their diagnosis.

DISORDERS OF ESOPHAGEAL FUNCTION

Gastroesophageal Reflux

Gastroesophageal reflux disease (GERD) is a common disorder that often brings patients to medical attention for acid-suppressing medication. Chronic reflux, Barrett's esophagus, stricture and regurgitation of stomach contents into the mouth or pharynx are common symptoms that lead to surgical referral. The etiology with aspiration of the reflux or regurgitation can be complex and may be related to the amount and type of dietary consumption or to an anatomic problem, usually a hiatal hernia that alters the geometry of the gastroesophageal junction (GEJ). A mechanically defective LES is diagnosed when one of the anatomic components is abnormal (pressure, <6 mm Hg; total length, <2 cm; abdominal length, <1 cm). As one expects, the chance of GERD increases with the increasing number of defective components and is more than 90% when all three LES components are abnormal. The etiology and severity of reflux varies with every patient and can be investigated with pH studies, impedance testing, and motility or manometry studies. Newer technologies can combine these tests into one catheter.

Achalasia

Achalasia is the most common esophageal motility disorder and is defined as relaxation failure or incomplete relaxation of the LES accompanied by an absence of peristalsis in the esophageal body. The LES is hypertensive in about 50% and almost always shows a failure of normal relaxation of patients with achalasia. Patients need to know that although swallowing is improved after surgery or pneumatic dilation of the LES, it is never normal because of the abnormal peristalsis. The cause of achalasia remains unknown, but a decreased number of inhibitory ganglion cells is seen on pathologic review. An esophagram is a good screening test for a patient with dysphagia; the classic findings are a dilated esophagus with smooth tapering at the GEJ, to the classic "bird's beak" appearance (Figure 1). The diagnosis of achalasia should always rule out pseudoachalasia, any condition that can masquerade as achalasia, such as a malignant disease. Endoscopic examination is an imperative part of this evaluation and usually shows some resistance at the GEJ, with a classic "popping" feeling as the scope passes into the stomach. Endoscopy can also include the placement of a wire to facilitate the passage of a manometric catheter, where blind passage proves difficult. Manometry is the gold standard for confirmation of the diagnosis and classically shows aperistalsis and incomplete relaxation of the LES after a swallow (Figure 2). Medical therapy can include calcium channel blockers, nitrates, and sildenafil. However, these are minimally effective. Endoscopic therapies include botulinum toxin and pneumatic dilation. Botulinum toxin is effective but only works for 3 to 6 months. Pneumatic dilation is slightly less effective than surgery, and many radiologists and gastroenterologists no longer are comfortable performing this procedure. Importantly, pneumatic dilation makes surgery considerably more difficult. Surgery involves a myotomy of the LES, which can usually be performed laparoscopically, from the stomach, across the LES, and well on to the esophagus. Some patients with end-stage achalasia and a dilated nonfunctional esophagus may need an esophagectomy.

Hypertensive Lower Esophageal Sphincter

Hypertensive LES is diagnosed when a patient has an LES pressure above the 95th percentile of normal and has symptoms of dysphagia or noncardiac chest pain. The exact value differs according to the method used for measurement, but this condition can only be diagnosed with manometry. In hypertensive LES, relaxation of the LES and peristalsis are present, unlike in achalasia.

Diffuse Esophageal Spasm

Diffuse esophageal spasm (DES) is an uncommon condition that accounts for less than 10% of esophageal motility abnormalities. DES is characterized by uncoordinated contractions of the esophagus that

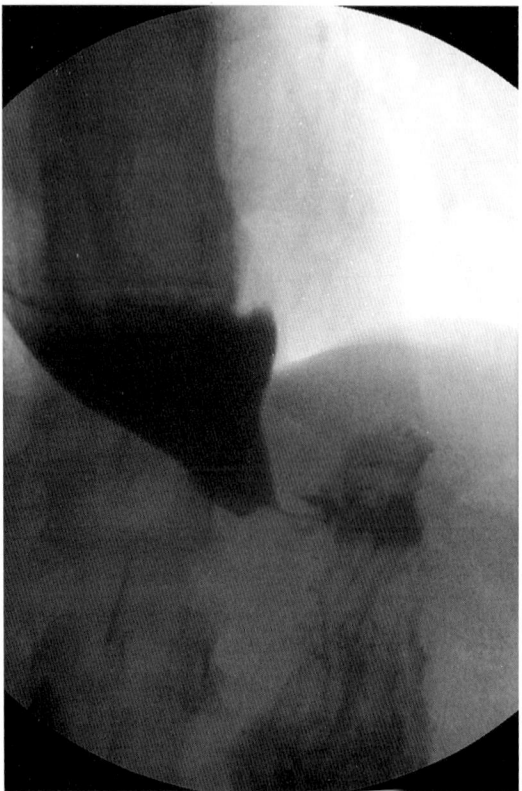

FIGURE 1   Classic bird's-beak appearance of achalasia on upper gastrointestinal series.

typically result in symptoms of chest pain, dysphagia, or both. The esophagram may be abnormal, but manometry is usually necessary for the diagnosis. Manometric findings, however, may not correlate with symptoms. DES is usually characterized by disordered rather than high pressure esophageal contractions.

Medical treatment options include nitrates and sildenafil and tricyclic antidepressants, which help with noncardiac chest pain. Valium and Ativan are also frequently effective if both the drugs fail to control symptoms. Use of proton pump inhibitors (PPIs) for treatment of concomitant GERD may also be helpful. A long myotomy can be effective in many patients with refractory DES but has a very high morbidity rate.

Hypercontractile "Nutcracker" Esophagus

Hypercontractile, or "nutcracker," esophagus is a manometric diagnosis defined by high pressure (>180 mm Hg) or long duration of swallow responses (>7 seconds) in patients who have either chest pain or dysphagia (Figures 3 and 4). The peristaltic contractions propagate normally, and the LES relaxes appropriately. Diltiazem has been shown to lower distal peristaltic pressures and may reduce chest pain; however, these results are not reliably reproducible. As in DES, nitrates, sildenafil, PPIs, and tricyclic antidepressants may be useful in the treatment of noncardiac chest pain.

Ineffective Esophageal Motility

Ineffective esophageal motility is characterized by decreased distal esophageal peristaltic wave pressures (amplitudes <30 mm Hg) or an absence of esophageal contractions in more than 30% of wet swallows. A distinguishing feature between ineffective esophageal motility and achalasia is that resting LES pressure is typically decreased in ineffective esophageal motility. Systemic conditions, such as scleroderma, can be associated with ineffective esophageal motility. Unfortunately, no standard treatment options exist, besides PPIs and lifestyle modifications. Patients are advised to eat small meals, remain upright after eating, chew food well, and take acid-suppressing medication.

Nonspecific Esophageal Motility

Nonspecific esophageal motility disorder refers to an esophageal motility disorder that does not have features of a named motility disorder. These abnormalities are often not associated with dysphagia and are nonspecific. Examples of frequently encountered nonspecific esophageal motility disorders are triple-peaked and retrograde contractions. Systemic diseases such as diabetes mellitus, hypothyroidism, eosinophilic esophagitis, and amyloidosis can be associated with nonspecific esophageal motor abnormalities. These abnormalities may also be seen in patients with paraesophageal hernia who have a shortened esophagus.

Hiatal Hernia

The presence of a hiatal hernia alters the usual location and structure of the LES, displacing it into the negatively pressured thorax and disrupting the reinforcement offered by the diaphragmatic crura. The manometric profile often shows the LES and the crura and intra-abdominal stomach as having increased pressure, a "double hump." High resolution manometry makes the diagnosis of hiatal hernia by manometry relatively easy. Manometry in paraesophageal hernias can be unpredictable depending on the anatomy of the hernia and the stomach because the esophagus may be shortened or of normal length. Manometry guides surgeons in repair of the hiatal hernia and helps them to choose the type of fundoplication to perform. Although a paucity of evidence is found, most esophageal surgeons avoid a complete wrap for patients with abnormal peristalsis and perform a partial, 180-degree or 270-degree, fundoplication to prevent postoperative dysphagia.

DIAGNOSTIC TESTS FOR ESOPHAGEAL DISEASES

Radiographic Imaging

Radiographic tests of the esophagus include the fluoroscopic esophagram and cross-sectional imaging. An esophagram, or barium swallow, is often performed as a biphasic examination in which double or single contrast techniques are used and should always have a solid bolus administered as a 13 mm barium tablet. Liquid and solid contrast agents are used in most diagnostic tests for dysphagia. Because the act of swallowing is a dynamic process, the inclusion of video or cine recording is imperative for better assessment of oropharyngeal function and esophageal motility.

A properly conducted videoesophagram allows the physician to comment on oropharyngeal function, morphology of the esophagus, esophageal motility, appearance of the mucosal surface, evaluation of the GEJ, presence and degree of reflux, and efficiency of secondary wave clearance. A videoesophagram is sensitive for detection of certain motility disorders, such as achalasia (94%) and scleroderma (100%); however, it is relatively insensitive for detection of most other motility disorders. The decision of whether to obtain radiographic imaging before endoscopic examination or to proceed directly to esophagogastroduodenoscopy (EGD) can be difficult. The authors recommend a videoesophagram as the initial diagnostic test in conditions such as a suspected cricopharyngeal bar, esophageal

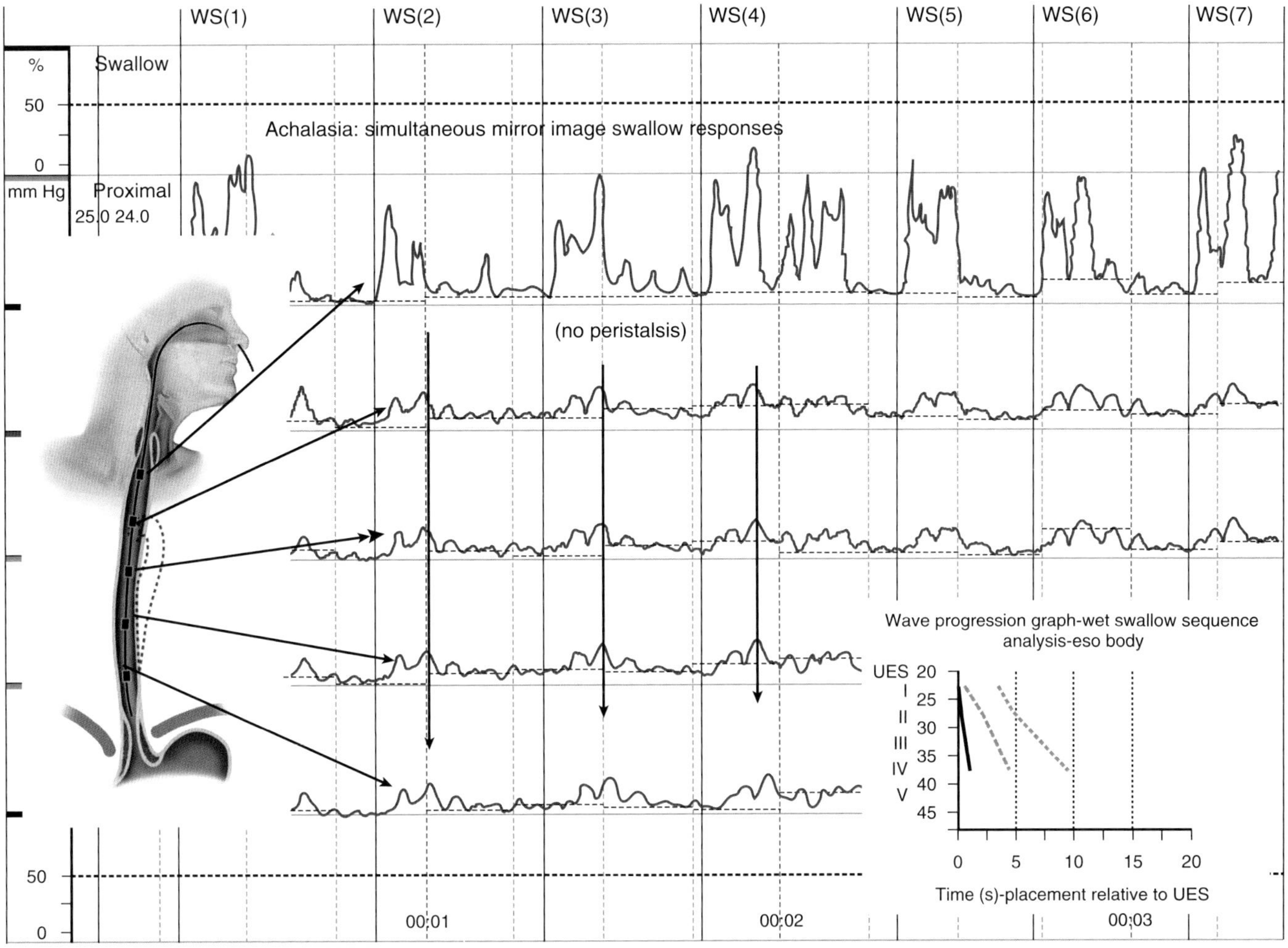

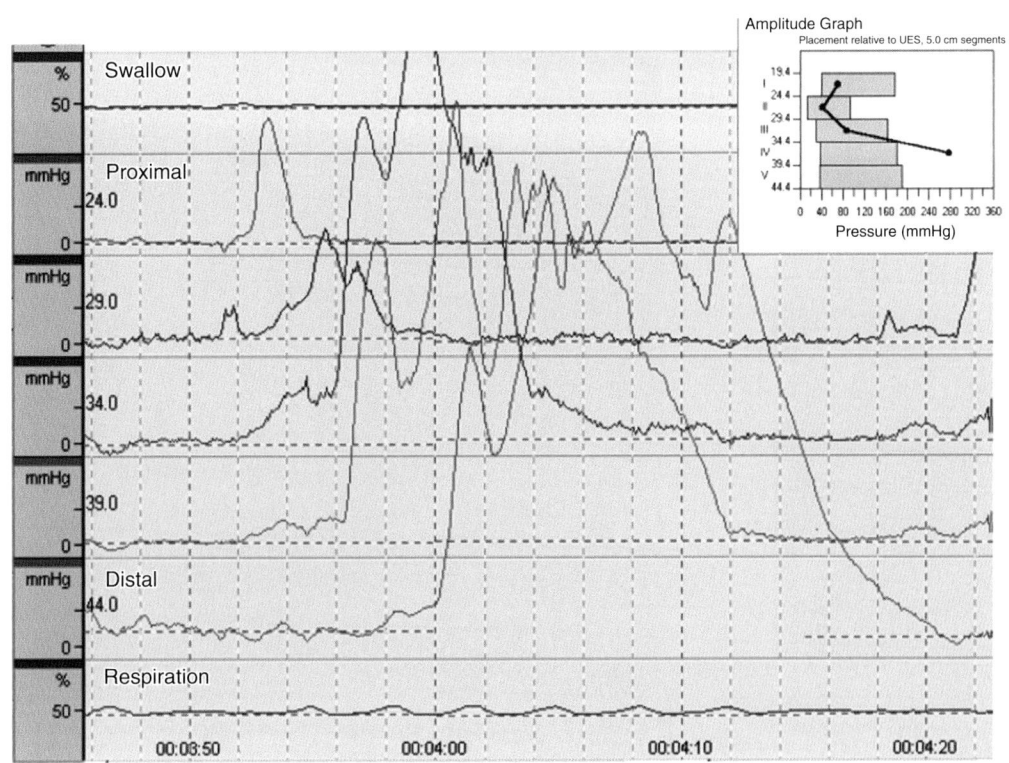

FIGURE 2 Manometry tracing of achalasia. The swallow study shows mirror-image swallow responses in the esophageal body.

FIGURE 3 Manometry showing hypercontractile esophageal body with pressures more than 180 mm Hg, which is designated as a "nutcracker" esophagus with these high pressures and symptoms of chest pain or dysphagia.

web, diverticulum, Schatzki's ring, early achalasia, or complex stricture, where an esophagram may provide the endoscopist a "road map."

Cross-sectional imaging with computed tomographic (CT) scan is helpful for evaluation of extraluminal esophageal disease, including staging for esophageal cancer and evaluation of esophageal trauma. However, the videoesophagram is still the gold standard in evaluation for esophageal leak. CT scan is used in evaluation of esophageal changes of the wall, such as thickening, but is not accurate in the evaluation of esophageal mucosal disease or motility disorders. Magnetic resonance imaging can produce high-quality multiplanar images without use of ionizing radiation but has limited utility for most esophageal diseases because of motion artifact and long imaging times.

Endoscopy

Although not strictly an esophageal function test, endoscopic examination is often necessary for evaluation or treatment for esophageal disorders. The authors routinely perform an on-table endoscopy before esophageal surgery because the surgeon is ultimately responsible for the diagnosis and treatment option selected. For example,

endoscopic evaluation in achalasia rules out pseudoachalasia and can confirm the diagnosis with the characteristic "pop" on passing through the LES. For hiatal hernia surgery, it can identify Barrett's esophagus, rule out early malignant disease of the stomach or esophagus that has been missed, and help identify the presence of a short esophagus that may need an esophageal lengthening procedure as part of the hernia repair.

Endoscopic evaluation for esophageal disorders begins with a good view of the vocal cords and aryepiglottic folds, which can appear inflamed in patients with chronic GERD. The upper esophageal sphincter (UES) consists of the cricopharyngeal muscle and is best seen on the final withdrawal of the endoscope. As the esophagus is entered, the mucosa can be carefully inspected for signs of mucosal inflammation or luminal irregularities, such as esophageal webs, rings, strictures, or esophagitis. Evaluation of the esophagus for distension or tonicity is also important because an atonic or patulous appearance may indicate the presence of a motility disorder.

At the level of the aortic arch, the striated muscle of the upper esophagus transitions to smooth muscle in the distal half of the esophagus. Patients with dysphagia should have random biopsies sampled from the distal and proximal esophagus for evaluation for eosinophilic esophagitis, particularly if the endoscopic examination shows the corrugated "feline" esophagus, with multiple concentric rings and linear furrows (Figure 5). In patients with longstanding GERD, the squamocolumnar junction proximal to the LES should be carefully inspected for signs of Barrett's esophagus (Figure 6), which appears as intestinal mucosa, with a pinker or salmon-colored appearance. The length of the Barrett's mucosa should be quantified, and multiple biopsies should be taken for assessment for dysplasia or malignancy.

The LES should really be called the LES complex because it is not one discrete muscle but rather a combination of esophageal muscle, phrenoesophageal ligament, and diaphragm. On endoscopy, it appears as a flap valve. Once the endoscope has entered the stomach, the endoscopist notes whether the gastric wall is poorly distensible and uses retroflex to examine the cardia and GEJ. The flap valve of the GEJ may be seen and assessed for competence under air pressure or for whether a hiatal hernia has expanded this area and allowed reflux and regurgitation.

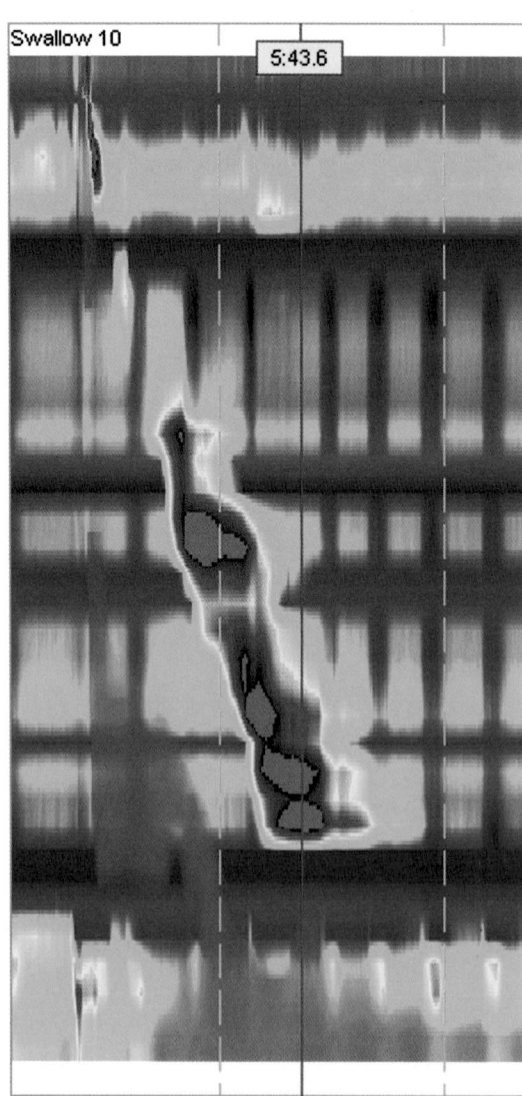

FIGURE 4   High-resolution manometry showing "nutcracker" esophagus and relaxation after the swallow.

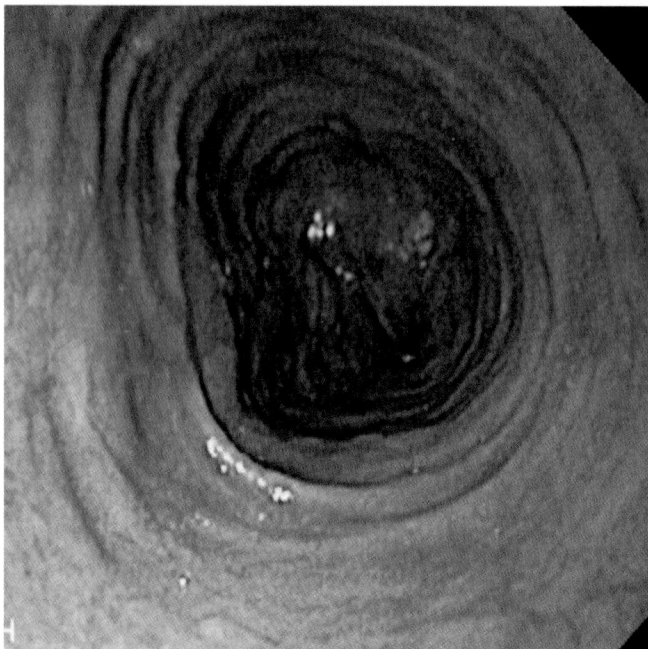

FIGURE 5   Eosinophilic esophagitis. Mucosal rings consistent with "trachealization" of the esophagus.

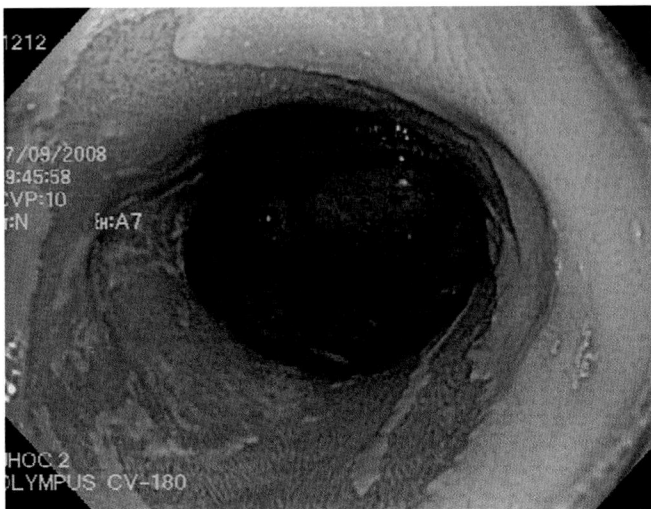

FIGURE 6 Salmon-colored mucosal changes seen in Barrett's esophagus.

BOX 1: Indications for esophageal manometry

1. Dysphagia: For the assessment of functional disorders after structural causes have been ruled out.
2. Noncardiac chest pain: For assessment for esophageal dysmotility as a cause of symptoms.
3. Diagnosis or confirmation of a suspected motility disorder.
4. Preoperative assessment of esophageal motility before planned esophageal surgery.
5. Postoperative assessment: For detection of response to surgery or confirmation of response to treatment or for assessment of the cause of persistent symptoms after surgery.

Endoscopy offers multiple therapeutic maneuvers, from dilation to biopsy to botulinum toxin injection. Mucosal ablative techniques are also used for Barrett's esophagus, and endoscopic ultrasound scan (EUS) has become the gold standard for the local and regional lymph node staging of esophageal cancer.

Esophageal Manometry

Esophageal manometry is the gold standard for assessment of esophageal motor function. It is the only modality that can define the pressure profile of peristalsis and measure LES pressure. Conventional manometry uses eight sensors, placed at various points of the esophagus, typically four in the esophageal body and four at the level of the GEJ. High-resolution manometry, specifically the Manoscan (Sierra Scientific Instruments, LLC, Los Angeles, Calif), is vastly superior and will replace older manometry equipment. High-resolution manometry provides a much clearer picture of esophageal pressure changes during swallowing and includes pressure monitors every centimeter along the catheter. This new technology offers the ability to simplify the procedural setup, eliminate motion artifact, simplify the ability to interpret data, and allow for a more sophisticated interpretation of esophageal motility. Indications for esophageal manometry are summarized in Box 1.

Technical Considerations

For conventional manometry, a solid-state or water-perfused catheter is used. The manometry catheter is swallowed until all of the sensors are in the stomach, and the catheter is then pulled back in increments of 0.5 to 1 cm for measurement of the resting pressure of the LES, esophageal body, and UES (Figure 7). Once the resting pressures have been calibrated, the catheter is positioned across the entire esophagus for recording of pressure changes during swallowing. The contraction and relaxation of the UES, the body of the esophagus, and the LES are recorded with 10 consecutive swallows of a 5-mL bolus of water. These pressure values are compared with standardized normal values (Figure 8; Table 1). Plotting of the pressure values with the passage of the water bolus down the esophagus allows for the detection of abnormal peristalsis and sphincter dysfunction. These patterns form the basis of esophageal dysmotility conditions.

The high-resolution manometry catheters have sensors every 1 cm. These catheters are able to span from the pharynx to the stomach, which obviates the need to retract the catheter to measure resting pressures. Pressure measurements are recorded both in the resting phase and for 10 swallows in a similar fashion to the older equipment. However, these pressure measurements are displayed as a topographic pressure reading over time. A typical scan of a high-resolution swallow in achalasia is shown in Figure 9. This figure also shows impedance in magenta, as the catheter used included impedance monitoring. Figures 4 and 9 are also examples of high-resolution manometry.

Diagnostic Tests for Gastroesophageal Reflux

A surgeon performing a procedure for GERD should order four principal tests before performing a fundoplication or hiatal hernia repair. First, an acid exposure test is used to document the presence of reflux because many patients with heartburn do not actually have GERD. Second, manometry is essential to ensure that esophageal dysmotility is not contributing to reflux as patients with dysmotility may not be able to clear physiologic reflux. Surgeons need to be careful when operating on patients with documented GERD and impaired motility because postoperative dysphagia can be a significant problem. A partial fundoplication or a floppy complete fundoplication may prevent dysphagia in these patients. Third, a barium swallow helps with identification of the presence and size of a hiatal hernia and may alert the surgeon to the presence of a short esophagus. A tension-free intra-abdominal GEJ at the end of the procedure is imperative, and a variety of esophageal lengthening procedures can be used if necessary. Finally, an EGD should be performed to rule out malignant disease and to identify Barrett's esophagus in patients with severe GERD. The authors typically perform the EGD in the operating room at the same setting as the procedure.

Acid exposure in the esophagus is measured with an intraluminal pH probe with one of two methods: either an intraluminal tube with a nasopharyngeal catheter or a wireless Bravo pH probe (Medtronic, Minneapolis, Minn). Both methods provide the physician with similar data, particularly relating to the amount of time the esophagus is exposed to acid reflux. When the information is correlated with a symptom log, determination is possible of whether the patient's symptoms are related to acid exposure within the esophagus. This information is commonly expressed with use of six standard parameters (Box 2) to calculate a DeMeester score, or a composite pH score. A score of less than 14.72 (95th percentile of normal) is considered physiologic reflux, whereas a score greater than 14.72 is considered abnormal. Acid exposure in the esophagus may be physiologic, and it is recorded according to the position of the patient (supine or upright) and the relation of acid exposure to meals. pH monitoring may also be used while the patient is on acid-suppressing therapy to determine whether there is adequate acid suppression with the current medication regimen. The data collected from each

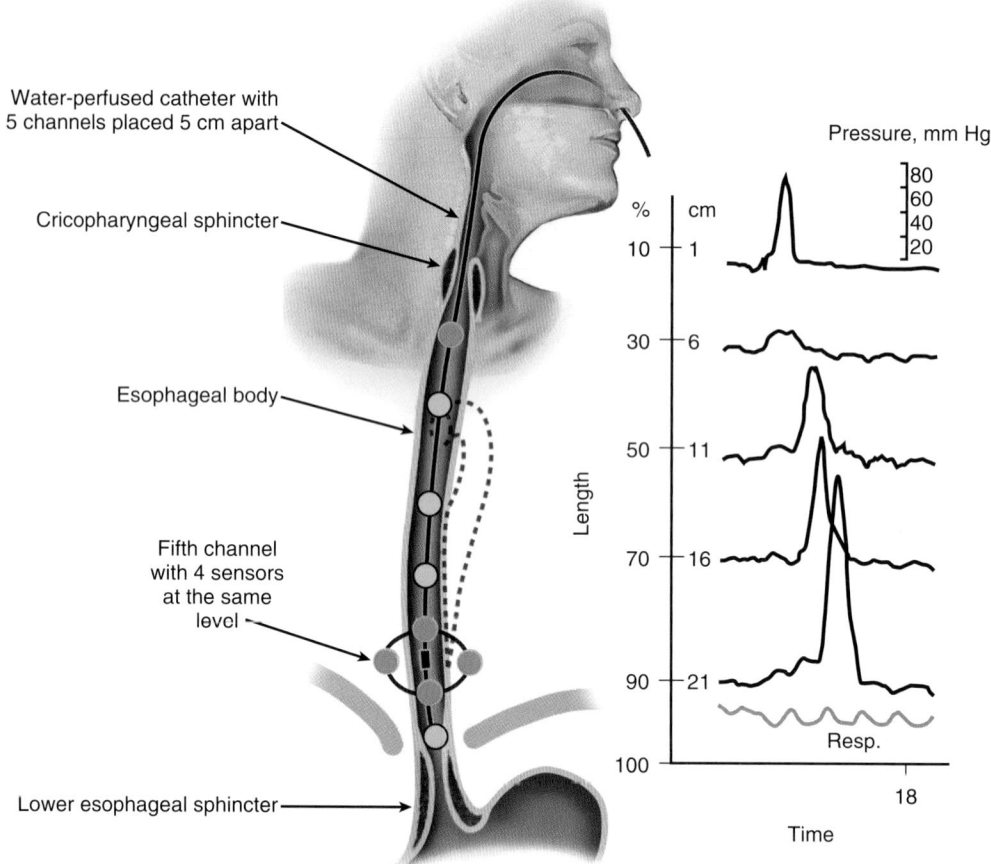

FIGURE 7 Esophageal manometry. A water-perfused or solid-state catheter is positioned in the esophagus. The sensors here are 5 cm apart, and the manometry shows normal wave propagation. Newer catheters that have sensors every 1 cm are termed high-resolution manometry.

TABLE 1: Normal LES parameters in 50 healthy volunteers

LES measurements	Mean	SD	Median	Maximum	Minimum	Percentile 2.5	Percentile 5
Pressure (mm Hg)	14.87	5.14	13.8	25.6	5.2	6.1	8
Abdominal length (cm)	2.18	0.72	2.2	5	0.8	0.89	1.1
Overall length (cm)	3.65	0.68	3.5	5.5	2.4	2.4	2.6

LES, Lower esophageal sphincter; *SD*, standard deviation.
Zaninotto G, DeMeester TR, Schwizer W, et al: The lower esophageal sphincter in health and disease, Am J Surg, 155:104-111, 1988.

individual's tests are compared with normal values derived from data from healthy volunteers. The Bravo probe is often preferred by patients for pH monitoring because it is placed at the time of upper endoscopy and does not require an extended time with a nasopharyngeal catheter. The Bravo probe is placed 5 cm above the LES and wirelessly transmits data to a recorder worn by the patient. It measures ph for 48 hours while a wired probe is worn for 24 hours which gives a larger sampling of ph changes in the esophagus and is more accurate.

Esophageal Impedance

Impedance monitoring measures bolus transport by measuring the resistance to electrical conductivity of the esophagus and its contents.

Impedance testing is an important adjunct to traditional pH testing because it can be useful for patients taking PPIs and for evaluation of bile (nonacid) reflux. Impedance measurement works by using low AC voltage to apply an electrical potential between two electrodes on a catheter separated by an isolator. The circuit is then closed by the surrounding material spanning the electrodes. Because air, liquid, and esophageal mucosa have unique impedance characteristics, identification of the material that is bridging the electrodes is easy. Air is resistant to current flow and has a high impedance; liquid has a low impedance value. Esophageal tissue has an indeterminate range and is used as a baseline during monitoring. With multiple electrodes along a catheter system, identification of changes in impedance makes possible determination of the direction of bolus transport within the esophagus and identification of reflux of a bolus that has cleared the esophagus but comes back up from the stomach (Figure 10).

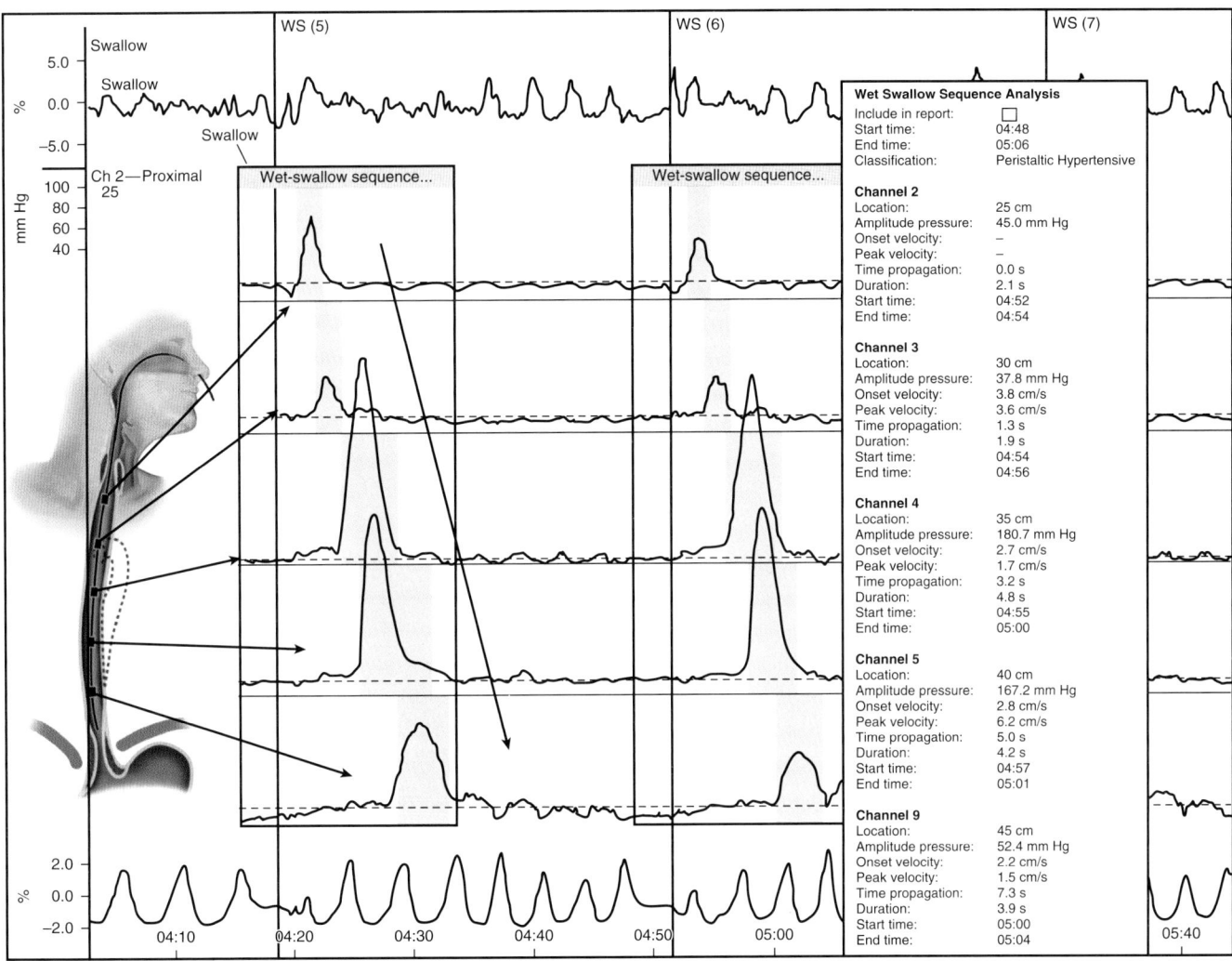

FIGURE 8   Normal esophageal body study. The channels are positioned at 5-cm intervals. The values shown are calculated for each wet swallow.

Multichannel intraluminal impedance (MII) is a new technology that incorporates impedance transducers for pressure measurement and a pH probe in one catheter. As a result, MII is used for the same indications as esophageal manometry and for detection and measurement of acid and nonacid reflux.

SUMMARY

The diagnosis of esophageal function disorders can be made from a careful history and the use of appropriate diagnostic testing. Several tests are frequently needed for the thorough evaluation of these disorders. Surgeons must understand the utility of these tests to evaluate whether a patient is a good surgical candidate for intervention and to determine the best treatment for a particular patient. A surgeon who is not familiar with these tests is not able to achieve optimal outcomes in the management of complex esophageal disorders. The authors also stress the importance of close collaboration between the radiologist, gastroenterologist, and surgeon in evaluating and treating this complicated group of patients.

BOX 2:   Measured parameters during 24-hour esophageal pH monitoring

1. Percent total time pH <4
2. Percent upright time pH <4
3. Percent supine time pH <4
4. Number of reflux episodes
5. Number of reflux episodes ≥5 minutes
6. Longest reflux episode (in minutes)

Acknowledgment

The authors recognize Vinay Chandrasekhara, MD, and Sanjay Jagannath, MD, the authors of this chapter in the 10th edition, as they have revised and updated their excellent work.

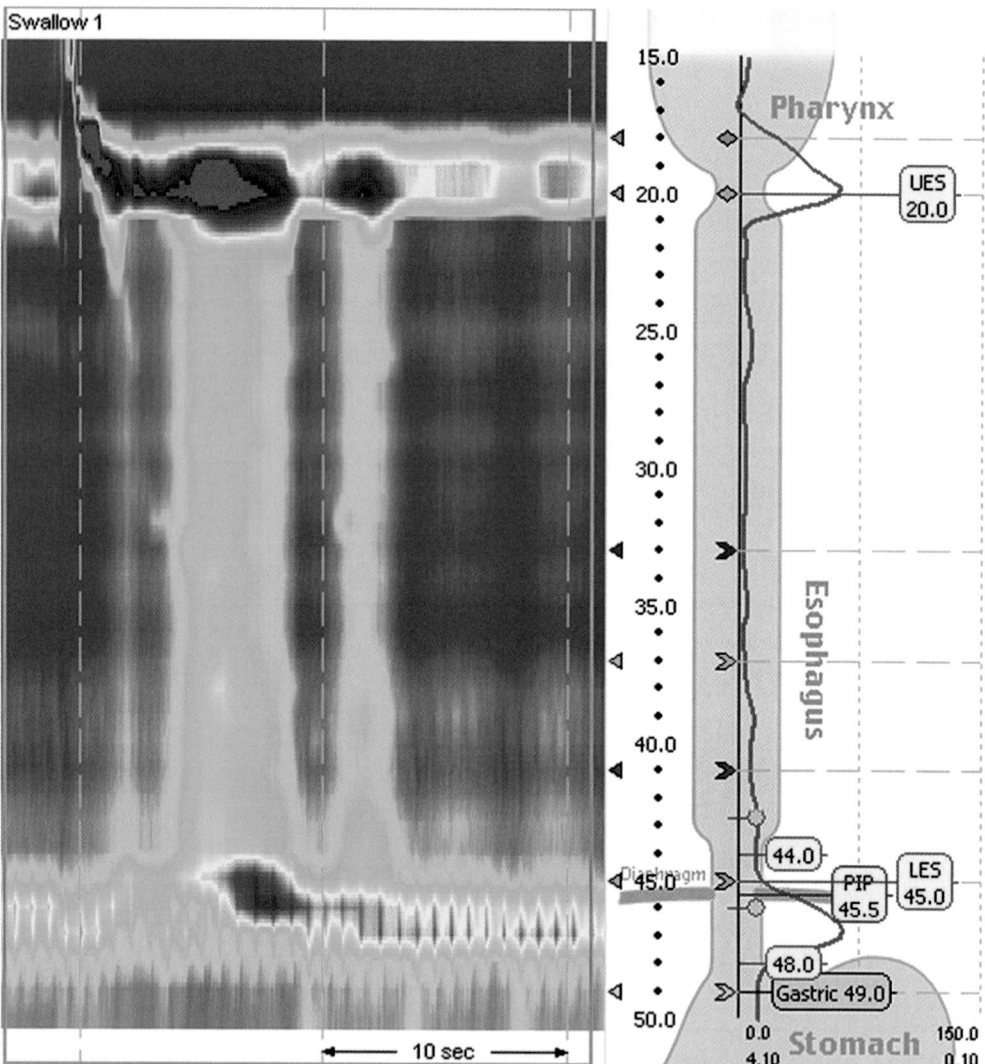

FIGURE 9 High-resolution manometry in a patient with achalasia. Note the simultaneous contractions and lack of swallow propagation. The lower esophageal sphincter is not hypertensive, but complete relaxation is not seen.

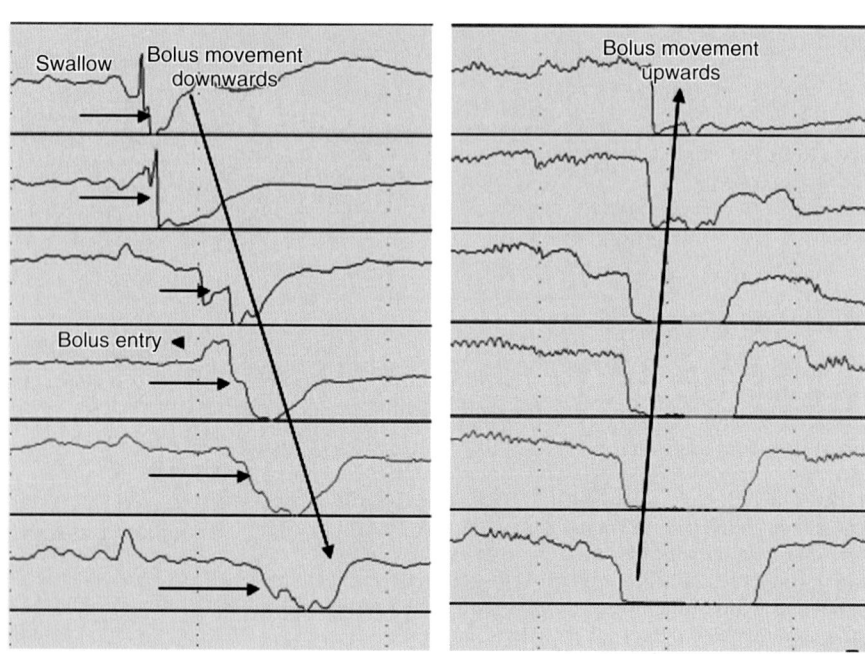

FIGURE 10 Impedance study showing antegrade and retrograde movements of a swallowed bolus.

SUGGESTED READING

Kuo P, Holloway RH, Nguyen NQ: Current and future techniques in the evaluation of dysphagia, *J Gastroenterol Hepatol* 27(5):873–881, 2012.

Lacy BE, Weiser K, Chertoff J, et al: The diagnosis of gastroesophageal reflux disease, *Am J Med* 123(7):583–592, 2010.

Stein HJ, Barlow AP, DeMeester TR, et al: Complications of gastroesophageal reflux disease: role of the lower esophageal sphincter, esophageal acid and acid/alkaline exposure and duodenogastric reflux, *Ann Surg* 216:35–45, 1992.

Stein HK, DeMeester TR: Indications, technique and clinical use of ambulatory 24-hour esophageal motility monitoring in a surgical practice, *Ann Surg* 217:128–137, 1993.

GASTROESOPHAGEAL REFLUX DISEASE

Dana A. Telem, MD, and David W. Rattner, MD

INTRODUCTION

Gastroesophageal reflux disease (GERD) is caused by incompetence of antireflux barriers at the gastroesophageal junction (GEJ) that results in acid or alkaline substances refluxing into the esophagus. In the past decade, the prevalence of GERD has steadily increased. Although most patients with GERD experience intermittent symptoms, an estimated 20% of adults experience symptoms weekly and 7% to 10% have daily symptoms. Treatment of GERD involves a stepwise approach. Initial treatment focuses on lifestyle modifications and medical therapy directed at neutralizing acid. Goals of treatment center on symptom control, resolution of esophagitis when present, and prevention of disease complications. Surgical therapy for GERD has evolved a great deal since the first antireflux procedures were described more than half a century ago. Despite improved surgical techniques, debate comparing the benefit of surgical intervention with optimal medical therapy continues. The outcome of surgical treatment for gastroesophageal reflux depends on key preoperative patient factors and adherence to proper surgical technique. Thus, surgeons who treat GERD must be familiar with the tenets of proper patient selection and with the principles of operative therapy.

OPERATIVE INDICATIONS

Proper patient selection is essential both to obtain optimal surgical outcomes and to manage postoperative patient expectations. The most frequent indication for surgery has traditionally been reflux symptoms refractory to pharmacologic therapy. However, in the era of powerful acid suppressive medications (i.e., proton pump inhibitors [PPIs]), the outcomes after fundoplication in this subset of patients are suboptimal. Multiple studies show worse outcomes with regards to resolution of reflux symptoms in patients whose conditions do not respond to antisecretory medications. Although GERD refractory to pharmacologic therapy should remain an operative indication, physiologic testing must show that pathologic acid reflux exists and that when reflux occurs that it correlates with the patient's symptoms.

Ideal candidates for an antireflux operation are patients who show a response to medical therapy but are either unwilling or unable to take daily medications. As more data become available detailing the risks associated with long-term PPI use, such as osteoporosis, this operative indication may represent a larger portion of antireflux operations performed. Additional operative indications for an antireflux procedure include noncompliance with medical therapy, complications of GERD, and atypical symptoms of GERD, such as chest pain, asthma, chronic cough, hoarseness, dental erosions, idiopathic pulmonary fibrosis, recurrent pneumonia, aspiration, and chronic bronchitis (Box 1).

Absolute contraindications to an anti-reflux procedure are few but most importantly include patients with esophageal cancer or those with Barrett's mucosa with untreated high-grade dysplasia. Although multiple relative contraindications exist, obesity is perhaps the most significant. Obesity is a well-established risk factor for the development of GERD, and symptoms typically improve with weight loss. Furthermore, obesity has been shown to adversely impact the durability of an antireflux operation. As such, patients with body mass index (BMI) greater than 35 kg/m^2 are more likely to benefit from a weight loss procedure, such as Roux-en-Y gastric bypass, than fundoplication and should be referred accordingly (see Box 1).

PREOPERATIVE EVALUATION

A systematic evaluation is necessary before consideration of an antireflux procedure. Initial evaluation of all patients should include a thorough history and physical examination. Patient reflux history is predictive of operative success and should center on duration, pattern, and type of reflux symptoms. Patients with typical symptoms of GERD, such as heartburn and regurgitation, tend to have a better response to fundoplication than those with atypical symptoms. Evidence also suggests that patients who experience worse symptoms in a supine rather than upright position have better outcomes after fundoplication. A thorough history of previous and current medical therapies attempted, and compliance with therapy, must also be obtained. A good response to antisecretory medications is generally predictive of a good surgical outcome. After a thorough initial evaluation, all patients deemed candidates for an antireflux procedure should undergo a preoperative evaluation that includes the following studies: endoscopy, upper gastrointestinal (UGI) series, manometry, and ambulatory pH monitoring (Box 2).

Endoscopy

Endoscopy has a high specificity for diagnosing of GERD. Visual or histopathologic changes of the esophageal mucosa that are present on endoscopy are diagnostic of GERD, with specificity upwards of 95%. Biopsy of the mucosa is an essential procedure in evaluation of patients with reflux or dysphagia. Although Barrett's esophagus (BE) often has a characteristic salmon color, visual inspection alone is inadequate for this diagnosis. Endoscopic findings are very specific for GERD, but endoscopy lacks sensitivity. Approximately 50% of patients with GERD have normal endoscopic findings and are thus classified as having nonerosive reflux disease (NERD) or uncomplicated GERD. Perhaps more important than diagnosis is the ability of endoscopy to detect complications of gastroesophageal reflux. Such complications include erosive esophagitis, peptic stricture, BE, esophageal cancer, gastric outlet obstruction, and other potentially significant UGI findings that impact operative management.

Upper Gastrointestinal Series

Although not all surgeons find a UGI series useful, the authors obtain it fairly liberally. The benefit of a UGI series pertains more to the diagnosis and characterization of a potential hiatal hernia and to the opportunity to observe esophageal motility fluoroscopically. A close association between reflux and presence of hiatal hernia has been found. A hiatal hernia results in reflux both by affecting the competence of the lower esophageal sphincter (LES) and by compromising esophageal acid clearance once reflux has occurred. Thus, presence of a hiatal hernia necessitates repair during an antireflux procedure. A UGI provides valuable information regarding gastric morphology, size and type of hiatal hernia, presence of gastric volvulus, and other anatomic abnormalities, such as a "short" esophagus, that are useful for preoperative planning. Although a UGI has some utility in showing reflux and motility abnormalities in patients with atypical symptoms of GERD or in those with NERD, it cannot be used to determine the presence of pathologic reflux.

Esophageal Manometry

Data that show that the best predictor of postoperative dysphagia is the presence of preoperative dysphagia have led some surgeons to abandon this test as part of the preoperative evaluation. However, the authors routinely obtain esophageal manometry before recommending a fundoplication. Manometry occasionally provides an alternative diagnosis, such as achalasia, for which antireflux surgery may be contraindicated. In addition, manometric findings may lead to a modification of the surgical approach. In patients with markedly disordered peristalsis or very low amplitude contractions, a partial fundoplication or nonsurgical management should be considered. Ineffective clearance of small amounts of reflux can significantly contribute to symptoms in these patients. Although it reduces reflux, a complete fundoplication in this setting can also make esophageal clearance more difficult, which is one of the reasons a partial rather than complete fundoplication in the presence of esophageal dysmotility is controversial. Level II evidence suggests that patients with nonspecific esophageal motility disorders may be at increased risk for postoperative heartburn, regurgitation, and dysphagia after a complete fundoplication.

Ambulatory pH Monitoring

Ambulatory pH monitoring is the gold standard for confirmation of pathologic acid reflux and, even more importantly, of correlation with the patient's symptoms. A 24-hour pH test should be performed in patients with typical reflux symptoms who do not have evidence of mucosal damage on endoscopy and in all patients who have atypical symptoms. The only patients that do not need a 24-hour pH study are those who have typical symptoms of reflux, histologic evidence of esophagitis, and a good response to PPIs. Several key points are crucial in ensuring the validity of this study. First, the esophageal probe must be positioned correctly in the distal esophagus. The pH probe should be placed 5 cm above the manometrically determined upper limit of the LES. This distance is standardized and was chosen to avoid possible displacement of the probe within the stomach during swallowing. Confirmation of the LES is crucial because incorrect placement of the probe compromises the sensitivity of the test. Manometric placement is preferred; other methods of LES detection have been proven inaccurate and inferior in determination of LES position. In evaluation of patients for surgery, this test is most useful if patients discontinue use of antisecretory medications at least 1 week before the study. If the test is performed while patient's acid production is suppressed with medication, the test may not answer the question the surgeon should be asking—that is, is pathologic acid reflux causing the patient's symptoms? Patients who cannot discontinue their acid suppressive medications should be evaluated with esophageal impedance testing. Impedance testing has the ability to distinguish between acidic and nonacidic reflux but still captures all reflux events irrespective of pH.

SURGICAL TREATMENT OPTIONS

Once a patient has met the requirements for antireflux surgery and has undergone the appropriate preoperative evaluation, surgical options may then be discussed. The probability of an antireflux operation relieving a patient's symptoms is directly related to how well the patient's symptoms have been correlated to the physiology. When a solid cause and effect relationship is established, good outcomes are routine. A variety of operative techniques and approaches to antireflux surgery have been described (Box 3). A laparoscopic transabdominal approach is the preferred approach for most patients undergoing a primary antireflux operation. Transthoracic and open abdominal approaches are typically reserved for patients who need revisional antireflux operations, those who have had multiple previous abdominal operations, and those with other contraindications to laparoscopic surgery. The benefits of a laparoscopic approach include shorter recovery time, decreased pain, decreased rate of hernia formation and other wound complications, and perhaps most importantly, improved visualization of hiatal structures. In the United States, a 360-degree fundoplication is the most common operation performed. In Europe, however, surgeons are more inclined to perform partial fundoplication. Several recent randomized controlled studies have showed comparable efficacy between 360-degree and 270-degree fundoplication. Nonetheless, proponents of the full 360-degree fundoplication argue that durability of the Nissen fundoplication is superior to that of partial fundoplication. Advocates of partial fundoplication argue that the ability of their patients to vomit and a lower incidence rate of bloating symptoms make partial fundoplication the procedure of choice. Regardless of the specific fundoplication performed, the principles of the operation remain the same. The purpose of the antireflux operation is to restore the functional and mechanical competence of the LES, reconstruct the diaphragmatic hiatus, and repair any hiatal hernia if present.

MINIMALLY INVASIVE SURGICAL TECHNIQUE

Proper operative instruments, port placement, and patient positioning are key factors to consider for the operation. The patient is placed in the supine position with the surgeon standing on the patient's right side and the assistant at the patient's left side. Laparoscopic monitors are placed at eye level at each side of the patient. Five trocars, two 10-mm and three 5-mm, are used for the operation. A Veress needle is placed in the left upper quadrant and is used to establish pneumoperitoneum. Once the abdomen has been insufflated to 15 mm Hg, a 10-mm supraumbilical trocar is placed off of the midline towards the patient's left side. This trocar serves as the camera port and is placed in this position to improve visualization of the hiatus and not interfere with working ports. A 5-mm port is then placed laterally in the right upper quadrant for a flexible arm liver retractor. After placement of the liver retractor, a 5-mm port for the surgeon's left hand is placed just below the right subcostal margin in the midclavicular line, and a 10-mm port for the surgeon's right

hand is placed along the left subcostal margin at the midclavicular line. A 5-mm assistant port is also placed laterally in the left upper quadrant. A 30-degree laparoscope is preferred for this procedure. Correct port placement is critical to ensuring proper visualization of hiatal structures and optimizing ergonomics for hiatal dissection and laparoscopic suturing (Figure 1).

With the patient in reverse Trendelenburg's position, the dissection is initiated with division of the gastrohepatic ligament. Care must be taken at this point to identify a completely replaced left hepatic artery. Oftentimes, an accessory hepatic artery is encountered. If present, one may attempt to preserve this vessel; however, if it impedes exposure or positioning of the fundoplication, division is recommended and typically inconsequential. If the vessel is large and concern exists that the vessel provides most of the arterial supply to the left lobe of the liver, it should be temporarily occluded and the liver observed for ischemia. Once the gastrohepatic ligament has been divided, the right crus is identified and the phrenoesophageal ligament opened. Care must be taken during this portion of the procedure to ensure that only the peritoneum is opened because deeper dissection may result in injury to the anterior vagus nerve or esophagus. Once the phrenoesophageal ligament is opened, the right crus is mobilized from the esophagus with careful blunt dissection. This dissection is carried anteriorly and circumferentially to the left crus. The anterior vagus nerve must be identified during this dissection to prevent inadvertent injury. Visualization for the caudal dissection onto the left crus can be hindered by fat, particularly in an obese patient. When this caudal dissection becomes challenging, division of the short gastric vessels usually provides improved exposure to the caudal portion of the left crus. Caution must be taken during this portion of the operation to ensure that the vessels are taken without any thermal injury to the stomach.

Once the left crus has been completely cleared, attention is then turned to creation of a posterior window behind the esophagus. This maneuver should be approached delicately, and the dissection should proceed easily to the other side. The posterior vagus nerve must be identified at this time. Once a window has been created, a vessel loop is placed around the esophagus to facilitate retraction. With the esophagus retracted upwards, attention can now be turned to crural closure. The crura are then closed starting caudally and moving in a cephalad direction with interrupted pledgeted nonabsorbable suture (Figure 2). Crural closure should be performed at low-pressure pneumoperitoneum (8–mm Hg to 9–mm Hg) to reduce diaphragmatic stretch and to more accurately approximate anatomy that will exist when the pneumoperitoneum is released. Crural closure should leave

BOX 3: Options for fundoplication

Complete Fundoplication
Nissen: 360-degree wrap

Partial Fundoplication
Toupet: Posterior 270-degree wrap
Anterior fundoplication: 180-degree or 90-degree
Hill Repair: Recreation of Angle of His and posterior gastropexy
Belsey Mark IV: Transthoracic 240-degree wrap

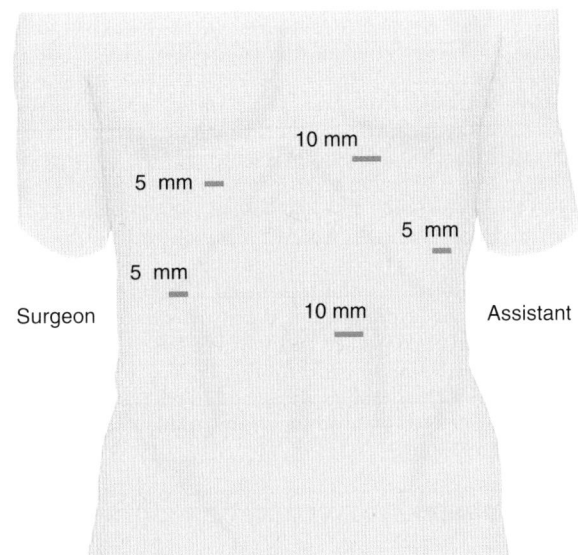

FIGURE 1   Port positioning for fundoplication.

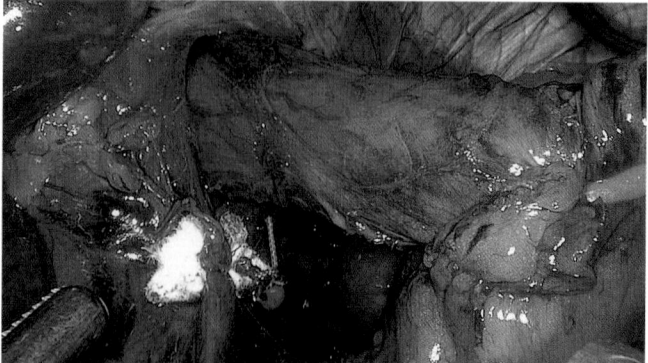

FIGURE 2 Closure of the diaphragmatic hiatus.

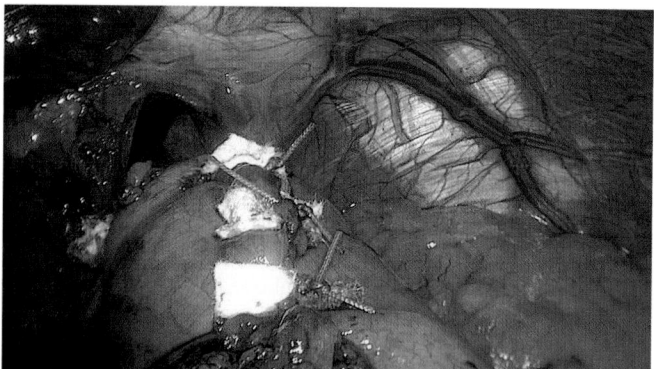

FIGURE 3 Completed 360-degree fundoplication.

approximately 1.5 cm of free space in the hiatus. An overzealous crural closure can lead to dysphagia that is unresponsive to esophageal dilation.

Once the crura have been reapproximated, the fundoplication is performed. The fundus of the stomach is grasped and brought underneath the esophagus. A "shoeshine" maneuver is then performed in which both sides of the fundus are grasped and pulled back and forth behind the esophagus to assess for proper orientation and tension. The remnants of the short gastric vessels should line up if the fundus has been delivered without twisting it. Once the fundus is pulled underneath the esophagus, it should remain in place after the grasper is released. If the fundus retracts back under the esophagus, further dissection to eliminate tension is necessary. A 56F bougie is then passed by either the surgeon or an experienced team member. Once the bougie is in place, a complete, 360-degree fundoplication is performed. A minimum of 2.5 cm of intra-abdominal esophageal length is necessary for an adequate wrap, and the fundoplication must be performed over the distal esophagus. Three nonabsorbable pledgeted sutures are used to create the wrap, all incorporating esophageal wall (Figure 3). At the conclusion of the operation, an endoscopy may be performed to assess the adequacy of the fundoplication. This is particularly useful in difficult cases or reoperations (Figure 4).

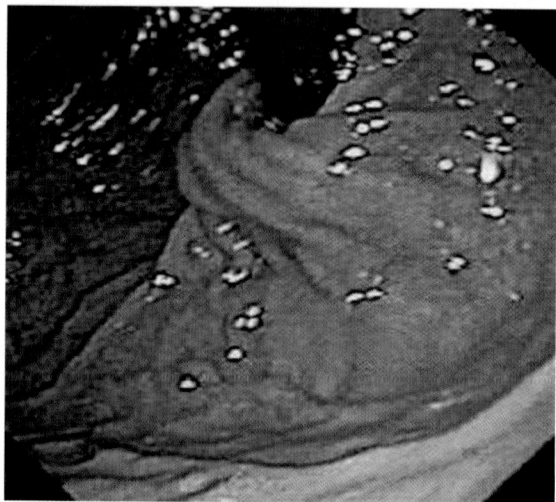

FIGURE 4 Normal endoscopic appearance of a 360-degree fundoplication.

POTENTIAL OPERATIVE PITFALLS

Bleeding

When dissection is performed in proper anatomic planes, significant bleeding is unusual. Bleeding during dissection of the right crus and GEJ usually originates from branches of the left gastric vessels and usually means the surgeon has dissected too close to the lesser curvature vessels. Care should be taken when energy devices are used for hemostasis in the GEJ region because these can easily cause a thermal injury to the vagus nerve. In some patients, the fundus and upper pole of the spleen appear fused and make division of the highest short gastric vessels difficult. This can be managed by carefully opening the peritoneum in this region and working layer by layer to isolate these vessels before dividing them. When bleeding occurs in this region, it can be controlled by applying pressure while the team sets up to make a definitive effort to stop the bleeding. The surgeon should have a low threshold to add an additional port so that exposure can be maintained or an additional instrument used to help get control of the bleeding.

Short Esophagus

The incidence rate of a "short" esophagus is estimated to be up to 10% in patients undergoing an antireflux procedure. A

short esophagus is the result of chronic reflux disease that involves recurring cycles of inflammation and healing, with subsequent fibrosis. This entity can pose a unique challenge for the surgeon because sufficient intra-abdominal esophageal length is a key tenet to performance of a fundoplication. Failure to recognize and correct a short esophagus results in a higher potential for a "slipped" fundoplication, mediastinal herniation, and suboptimal operative outcome. In most patients, this entity can be managed with more extensive mediastinal mobilization of the esophagus and complete reduction of a hiatal hernia, if present. However, gaining more than 2 cm of esophageal length is difficult even if one mobilizes the esophagus all the way up to the aortic arch. Therefore, some patients need an esophageal lengthening procedure, such as a Collis gastroplasty. Attempts at full mobilization should be performed before any lengthening procedure, and intraabdominal esophageal length should be assessed after the crural closure is completed. Closure of the crura from a caudal to cephalad direction displaces the hiatal opening in an anterior and cephalad direction. In patients with moderate sized hiatal hernias, this maneuver can often gain several centimeters of intraabdominal length.

Esophageal or Gastric Perforation

A dreaded complication of an antireflux operation is an unrecognized intraoperative gastric or esophageal perforation. Injuries typically result from either thermal damage during dissection or excessive traction on the stomach or esophagus. At the end of the operation, the stomach and distal esophagus should be thoroughly inspected for any evidence of compromise. An endoscopy may also help in identification of a perforation. If an injury is identified during surgery, depending on surgeon comfort level and skill set, it may be managed laparoscopically with oversewing of the defect. Larger defects may be excised and stapled closed. If any question as to the adequacy of repair exists, conversion to open surgery is necessary.

POSTOPERATIVE CARE

After the operation, patients are admitted to a regular hospital room. Neither a nasogastric tube nor a Foley catheter is placed in these patients. Use of narcotics is kept at a minimum, and standing ketorolac tromethamine is given routinely to reduce narcotic use. Patients are started on a clear liquid diet the next morning. Patients are discharged on postoperative day 1 and kept on a full liquid diet for 1 week, at which time a soft diet is introduced. A postoperative UGI study is not routinely obtained unless clinically indicated. Patients with chest pain, retching, or unexplained tachycardia should undergo immediate imaging to exclude the possibility of a herniated wrap.

COMMON POSTOPERATIVE PROBLEMS

Dysphagia

Most patients have some degree of dysphagia after fundoplication, which is why they are maintained on a liquid diet for 1 week after surgery with slow introduction of soft solids after that time. As long as the patient is able to take liquids and remain hydrated, they may be managed expectantly as an outpatient. Over time, the dysphagia should improve and eventually resolve. Dysphagia that persists more than 12 weeks is concerning and should be evaluated. Initial evaluation consists of an UGI to evaluate the anatomic position and tightness of the wrap. In patients with a tight wrap, serial endoscopic dilation can be attempted with good results. If dysphagia persists or an anatomic cause of dysphagia is identified, revision of the fundoplication is likely necessary.

Gas Bloat Syndrome

Gas bloat syndrome refers to recurrent abdominal pain and distention caused by air trapping in the stomach. Before modification of Nissen's original operation, this occurred in up to 40% of patients. However, with the adoption of the short and floppy wrap that is performed by most contemporary surgeons, the incidence rate of true gas bloat syndrome has decreased substantially. Although patients commonly experience some bloating and increased flatulence in the first several months after surgery, severe gas bloat syndrome is now uncommon. The diagnosis is made by obtaining a plain abdominal x-ray while the patient is symptomatic (Figure 5). If the stomach is gas filled and distended in the absence of bowel distention, then the diagnosis is secure. Confirmation can be achieved if placement of an nasogastric tube promptly relieves the patient's symptoms. Gas bloat syndrome can be exacerbated by dietary habits, such as drinking carbonated beverages, and behavioral habits, such as aerophagia. Initial treatment centers on dietary modification and use of prokinetic agents. These interventions are occasionally effective; however, most patients with true gas bloat syndrome need conversion of the full fundoplication to a partial wrap.

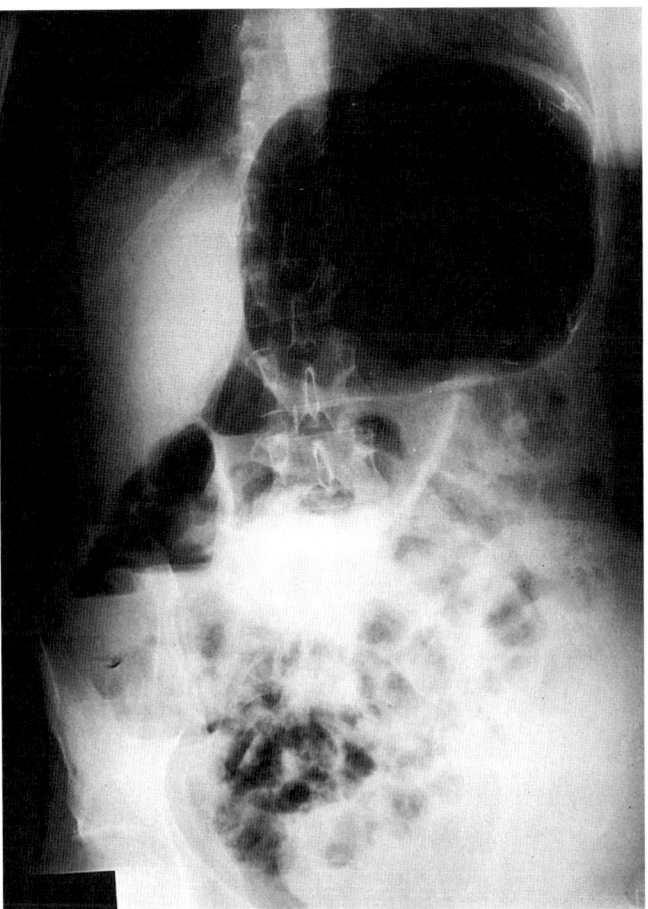

FIGURE 5 Abdominal x-ray showing distended stomach as seen in gas bloat syndrome.

REOPERATIVE FUNDOPLICATION

Failure rate of flowing fundoplication is estimated to be between 5% and 30%, depending on the series. Not every patient with a failed fundoplication needs reoperation. Candidates for reoperative surgery should have evidence of failure based on physiologic studies or an anatomic abnormality that can be surgically corrected. The most common indication for reoperation is recurrent symptoms from either a "slipped" fundoplication or herniation of the fundoplication into the mediastinum. Regardless of indication, the key principle of reoperative fundoplication is complete restoration of normal anatomy before any revision. Revisional surgery may be attempted laparoscopically; however, a low threshold for open conversion should be maintained. In patients in whom the revision cannot be completed laparoscopically because of dense adhesions or other anatomic abnormality, a transthoracic or thoracoabdominal approach may be beneficial.

EMERGING SURGICAL THERAPIES FOR GASTROESOPHAGEAL REFLUX DISEASE

Many innovative endoscopic therapies for GERD have been described. Although multiple devices have been developed for the endoscopic treatment of GERD, very few have had much long-term success. Several new endoluminal devices that create partial fundoplication with robust fixation mechanisms are currently undergoing clinical trials. Another novel approach being introduced is augmentation of the LES with a ring of laparoscopically placed magnetic beads. More data are needed before the efficacy of these devices can be adequately evaluated. Given the high incidence of GERD and its impact on lifestyle, emerging therapies for GERD remain an area of intense activity for the foreseeable future.

SUGGESTED READINGS

Broeders JA, Roks DJ, Jamieson GG, et al: Five-year outcome after laparoscopic anterior partial versus Nissen fundoplication: four randomized trials, Ann Surg 255(4):637–642, 2012.

Galmiche JP, Hatlebakk J, Attwood S, et al: Laparoscopic antireflux surgery vs esomeprazole treatment for chronic GERD: the LOTUS randomized clinical trial, JAMA 305(19):1969–1977, 2011.

Gee DW, Andreoli MT, Rattner DW: Measuring the effectiveness of laparoscopic antireflux surgery: long-term results, Arch Surg 143(5):482–487, 2008.

Nijjar RS, Watson DI, Jamieson GG, et al: Five-year follow-up of a multicenter, double-blind randomized clinical trial of laparoscopic Nissen vs anterior 90 degrees partial fundoplication, Arch Surg 145(6):552–557, 2010.

Stefanidis D, Hope WW, Kohn GP, et al: Guidelines for surgical treatment of gastroesophageal reflux disease, Surg Endosc 24(11):2647–2669, 2010.

ENDOLUMINAL APPROACHES TO GASTROESOPHAGEAL REFLUX DISEASE

Mark R. Wendling, MD, and W. Scott Melvin, MD

INTRODUCTION

Gastroesophageal reflux disease (GERD) is a prevalent disease that greatly influences the quality of life of those it afflicts. Surgical fundoplication has become the gold standard treatment when medical therapy is no longer effective or desired. However, the side effect profile of traditional antireflux surgery leaves some patients and referring physicians hesitant, and the desire for endoluminal therapies has become evident.

In 2000, the EndoCinch (Bard Endoscopic Technologies, Billerica, Mass) was the first modern endoluminal therapy to gain U.S. Food and Drug Administration (FDA) approval. Since that time, numerous other devices have used myriad techniques in the attempt to achieve symptom and disease control. Some techniques, such as injection of bulking agents and partial-thickness gastric plication, are no longer available because of respective safety concerns and ineffectiveness. Currently, two treatments, the Stretta system (Mederi Therapeutics, Greenwich, Conn) and EsophyX (EndoGastric Solutions, Redmond, Wash), essentially constitute the landscape of FDA-approved devices commercially available today, with more techniques in various stages of development.

PREOPERATIVE CONSIDERATIONS

Indications for endoluminal therapy may be similar to those for Nissen fundoplication. However, with the reduction of side effects and decrease in invasiveness of endoluminal approaches, the indications could be expanded to those patients with less severe symptoms. Patients who wish to control GERD symptoms without medication or those in whom medication is no longer effective are candidates. Although the presence of a large hiatal hernia (>2 cm) and

complications of reflux, such as severe esophagitis, stricture, and mucosal ulceration, represent indications for Nissen fundoplication, these are contraindications to endoluminal therapies. Other contraindications include Barrett's esophagus, portal hypertension, and motility disorders of the esophagus. In some studies, body mass index (BMI) of more than 35 is listed as a contraindication because symptoms are likely to improve with weight-reduction surgery. However, this is inconsistently applied, and a uniform cutoff has not been established.

Preoperative workup before endoluminal treatment first requires confirmation of the GERD diagnosis with 24-hour pH monitoring. Diagnostic upper endoscopy is also necessary to evaluate esophageal anatomy and rule out complications of GERD, which may represent contraindications to treatment. Because endoluminal treatments are limited to patients without esophageal motility disorders, manometry is also used.

OUTCOMES ASSESSMENT

Little agreement exists on what outcomes are most important in evaluation of endoluminal therapies for GERD. Treatment of GERD is based on the presence of clinically significant symptoms. Therefore, one could argue that the goal of therapy should be subjective improvement of these symptoms, which has traditionally been measured through surveys such as the GERD–health-related quality of life (GERD-HRQL) survey, the reflux symptom index (RSI) survey, successful discontinuation of proton pump inhibitor (PPI) therapy, and patient satisfaction metrics. However, any treatment that does not correct the underlying pathologic process and achieve disease control is seen as unacceptable to some. Normalization of objective indices, such as mean esophageal acid exposure time, quantification of reflux episodes, and DeMeester score, are customarily used as outcomes to assess for disease control. Currently, no endoluminal therapy has been able to show consistent normalization of pH metrics or healing of esophagitis. For this reason, Barrett's esophagus remains a contraindication to treatment.

Another topic of debate is whether these therapies should be compared with medical or surgical therapy when determining their efficacy. If endoluminal therapies are to be an addition to our treatment armamentarium of the spectrum of disease between the medical and surgical extremes, then direct comparison may not be applicable. The more important task is identifying the correct patient population for these therapies. When this population is determined, then useful comparisons can be made. However, if we do not identify this population, then any assessment will surely show endoluminal treatment to be inferior.

Controversy exists in regards to which outcomes to measure, what patient population to study, and what current therapies to compare them with. This creates quite a challenge in evaluating the merit of endoluminal therapies.

STRETTA

Background

The Stretta system (Figure 1) is the only device to use radiofrequency energy as a treatment for GERD. The system has been approved by the FDA since 2000 and consists of a flexible catheter with a 30F bougie tip and a balloon basket assembly with four 22-gauge, 5.5-mm–long, nickel-plated, radially placed electrodes. The catheter has two channels: a suction channel and another for cool water irrigation to keep mucosal temperature regulated. Stretta's mechanism remains unclear but could be induction of thermal injury to the lower esophageal sphincter (LES), which results in scarring and collagen deposition at the gastroesophageal junction (GEJ). This scarring decreases the compliance of the LES and may reduce transient LES relaxation. Another rational explanation is that fewer transient LES relaxations occur as a result of ablation of vagal afferent fibers.

Technique

The procedure is performed with conscious sedation with the patient in the left lateral decubitus position. First, upper endoscopy is performed. The esophageal and gastric anatomy is evaluated for any unexpected abnormality, and the distance from the incisors to the Z-line is measured. After a guidewire is placed through the working port, the endoscope is withdrawn. The radiofrequency delivery catheter is introduced orally over the guidewire into the stomach with fluoroscopic guidance. The device is withdrawn to approximately 2 cm proximal to the Z-line, and the balloon is inflated to 2.5 psi. This maneuver deploys the electrode needles into the muscular layer of the esophagus, and radiofrequency energy is delivered for 90 seconds. Tissue temperature is monitored with a built-in feedback thermostat to maintain muscular temperature at less than 85°C and mucosal temperatures at less than 50°C. After the application of energy, the needles are withdrawn and the balloon is deflated. The catheter is then rotated 45 degrees and the process is repeated, creating eight radial lesions at a given level. Radiofrequency energy is applied every 0.5cm, covering an area 2cm above and 1.5cm below the Z-line (Figure 2). The procedure is then completed with upper endoscopy to ensure the application of energy in the desired location and to evaluate for complications. The Stretta procedure takes approximately 40 minutes to complete.

Postoperative Care

The Stretta procedure is commonly performed as an outpatient procedure. Patients are kept on a liquid diet the day of the procedure and may resume a normal diet thereafter. Because the benefit of Stretta relies on scarring and collagen deposition for their effect, PPI therapy is continued and reevaluated at follow-up examination.

Outcomes

As the Stretta system has been available for more than a decade, a plethora of data has been published regarding its safety and efficacy. The procedure appears to be quite safe; most complications are minor and need no further intervention. A recently published systematic review found that, other than postprocedure pain, the most common complications were mucosal tears (4%), esophageal ulceration (4%), and dysphagia (3%). Esophageal perforation is exceedingly rare, and only one death has been reported from aspiration pneumonia.

At short-term follow-up examination, the Stretta procedure has shown to be reasonably effective. A randomized, double-blinded, sham-controlled, multicenter clinical trial evaluated 64 patients at 6-month and 12-month follow-up periods. No difference was seen in regards to PPI use or esophageal acid exposure times at 6 months. However, heartburn symptoms and GERD-HRQL scores were significantly better for the treatment group compared with those who underwent a sham procedure; this symptom improvement persisted at the 12-month follow-up period. Similar results were seen in another study of 94 patients with follow-up at 1 year. Again, mean heartburn scores (4 to 1; $P = 0.0001$), GERD-HRQL scores (27 to 9; $P = 0.0001$), and patient satisfaction were significantly improved. But unlike the previous study, PPI use decreased from 88% before the procedure to 30% after the procedure; esophageal acid exposure time was also significantly improved.

Long-term efficacy of the Stretta procedure has been less conclusive. In a study of the 4-year follow-up period, significant improvements in both heartburn and GERD-HRQL scores were reported. Also, 72.3% of patients were no longer taking PPIs. However, in

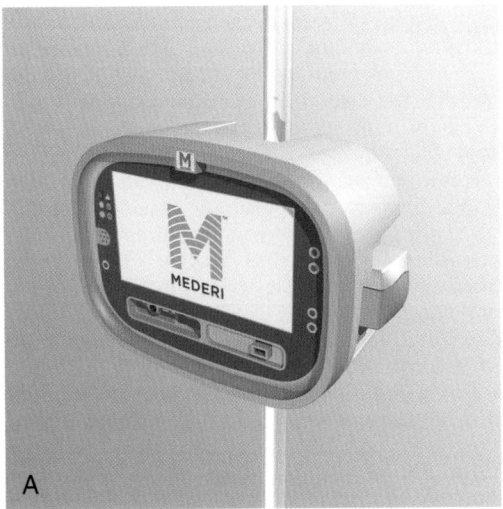

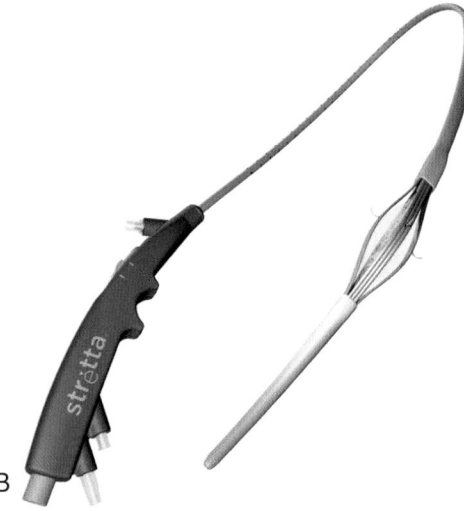

FIGURE 1 The Stretta system: **A,** radiofrequency generator; **B,** catheter. *(Courtesy of Mederi Therapeutics, Greenwich, Conn.)*

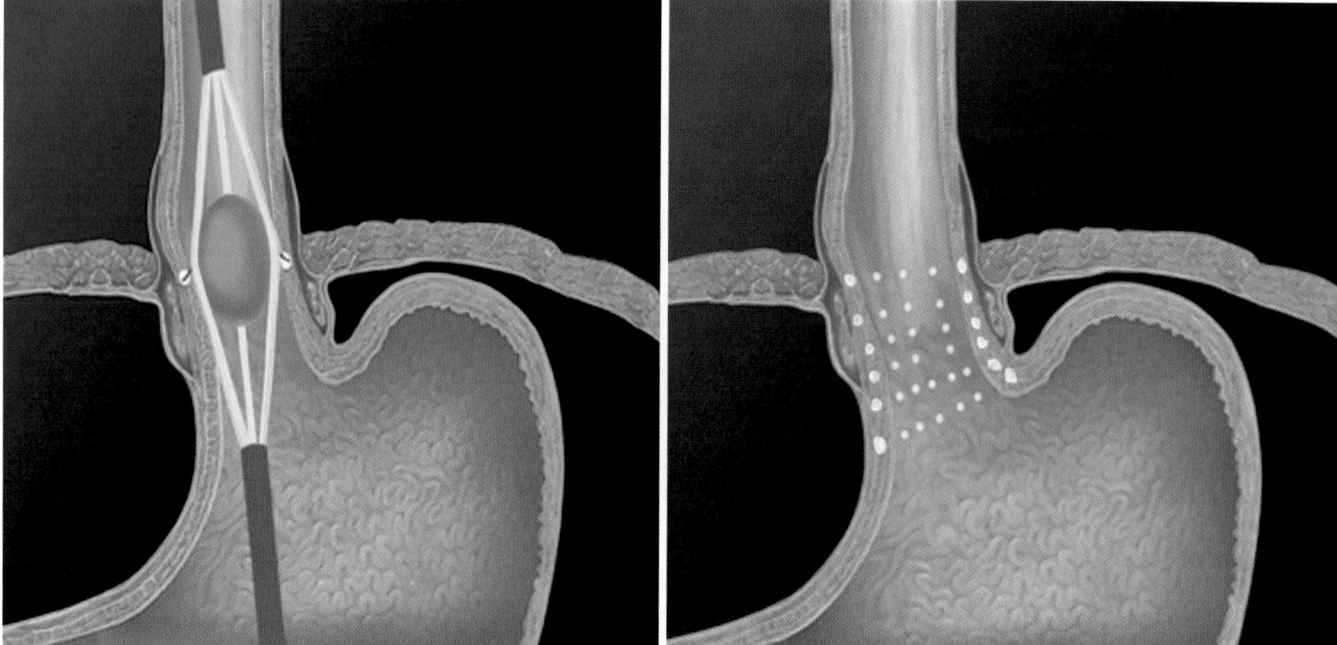

FIGURE 2   Serial application of radiofrequency energy at multiple levels along the lower esophageal sphincter with the Stretta system.

another study with a minimum of a 3-year follow-up period, 19 of 32 patients had been deemed treatment failures and went on to need a traditional antireflux operation. These differences were possibly the result of patient selection because findings showed that those whose conditions responded to the Stretta procedure had significantly lower preprocedure heartburn scores than those whose conditions did not respond.

Overall, a recent meta-analysis of the published literature from 2000 to 2010 identified 18 studies with a total of 1441 patients who underwent the Stretta procedure for treatment of GERD. Significant improvements in heartburn and patient satisfaction scores were found. GERD-HRQL scores also significantly improved and were on average normalized (26.11 vs 9.25; $P = 0.0001$) at a mean 19.8-month follow-up period. Esophageal acid exposure time (10.29 vs 6.51; $P = 0.0003$) and DeMeester score (44.37 vs 28.53; $P = 0.0074$) also improved significantly; however, they failed to normalize. LES pressure (mm Hg; 16.5 vs 20.24; $P = 0.0302$) also improved significantly. These data suggest that Stretta indeed produces significant improvement in reflux symptoms and improvement in objective GERD indices beyond the short-term follow-up period.

ESOPHYX

Background

The EsophyX device (Figure 3) consists of a disposable element that fits over a standard forward viewing endoscope and is used to perform transoral incisionless fundoplication (TIF). It is the most recent attempt in the use of endoluminal plication for the treatment of GERD. As previously mentioned, the EndoCinch device began this trend with the creation of a partial-thickness gastric plication, but it is no longer sold by Bard. Later, the NDO Full-Thickness Plicator (NDO Medical, Mansfield, Mass) gained FDA approval in 2004; as its name implies, it used full-thickness gastric plication for the treatment of GERD. The company has since ceased operations, and this product is off the market. EsophyX continues to evolve the technique

of endoscopic plication with the creation of esophagogastric plication with rotational and longitudinal elements to reconstruct the gastroesophageal valve.

Technique

Transoral incisionless fundoplication is performed with the patient in the left lateral decubitus position with general anesthesia and nasotracheal intubation. Deep venous thrombosis prophylaxis is administered as a standard component of care for those undergoing general anesthesia. Because the plication is full thickness, preoperative antibiotics are administered.

Two physicians are needed to perform the procedure. The first operates the endoscope while the other operates the EsophyX device. Initial upper endoscopy is performed to assess for unexpected pathology. The endoscope is withdrawn and placed through the EsophyX device, and both are introduced into the esophagus to the stomach. The authors' practice is to dilate the esophagus with a 56F bougie before this introduction to ensure ease of passing the EsophyX device.

The device contains a vacuum invaginator, which is used to reduce small hiatal hernias by returning the squamocolumnar junction to a position below the diaphragm. A helical retractor is then deployed at the GEJ at the lesser curve to draw tissue into the device, creating a tissue fold with esophageal epithelium against the body of the device, gastric epithelium facing outwards and serosa in between. The helical retractor is used to manipulate the tissue to mold an omega-shaped valve with serial placement of polypropylene H fasteners full thickness across the tissue, thus creating a full-thickness, esophagogastric plication (Figure 4). The device is rotated both anteriorly and posteriorly to create multiple plication sets with H fasteners deployed at different distances from the GEJ. The authors strive to create an omega-shaped valve of at least 270 degrees in circumference and 3 cm in length and typically use an entire cartridge of H fasteners (20 fasteners) during the procedure. The device is then withdrawn, and the endoscope is reintroduced to evaluate the newly created valve and ensure hemostasis. The procedure commonly takes less than 90 minutes to complete.

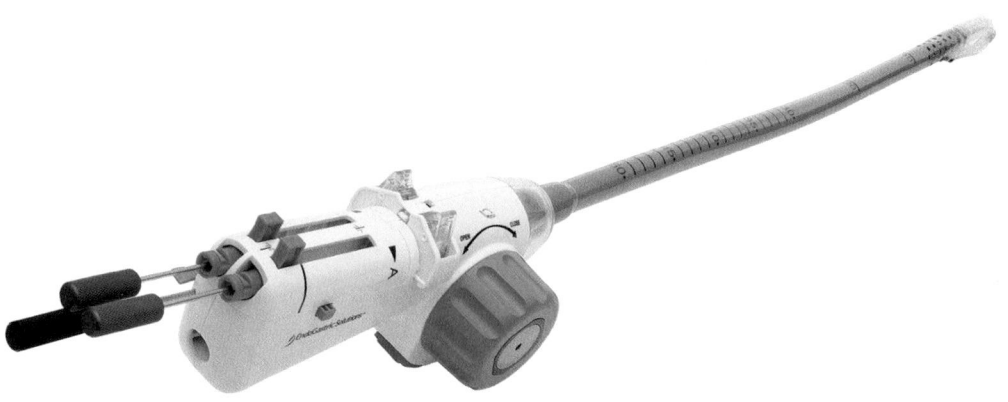

FIGURE 3 The EsophyX device with magnification on the working end. *(Courtesy of EndoGastric Solutions, Redmond, Wash.)*

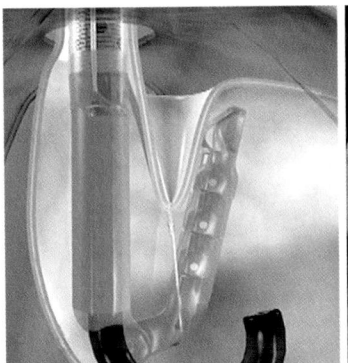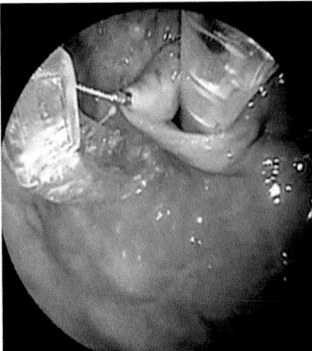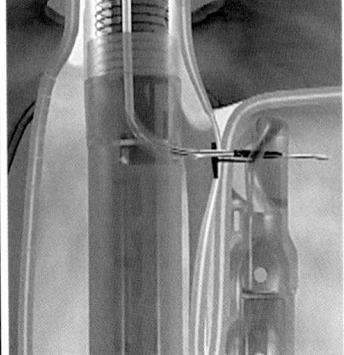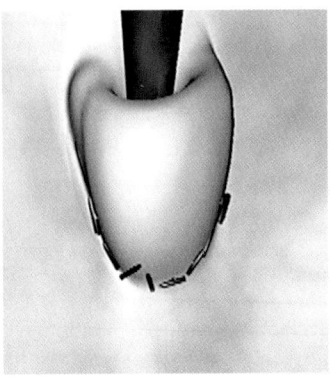

FIGURE 4 The EsophyX device drawing the gastroesophageal junction down into the jaws of the device, with full-thickness polypropylene H fasteners placed to mold an omega-shaped valve.

TABLE 1: Summary of outcome measures after transoral incisionless fundoplication

Outcome measure	Weighted mean	Number of studies measuring outcome	Mean follow-up period across studies (months)
Decrease in GERD-HRQL score	16.0	10	9.8
Decrease in RSI score	19.1	4	7.6
Patient satisfaction	72%	11	8.5
PPI discontinuation	67%	14	8.3

GERD-HRQL, Gastroesophageal reflux disease health-related quality of life; *PPI,* proton pump inhibitor; *RSI,* reflux symptom index.

Postoperative Care

Patients are observed overnight and discharged the next day. They remain on a liquid diet for up to 1 week and a soft diet until 2 to 3 weeks at follow-up examination. The authors' practice is to stop acid-reducing medications at the time of the procedure.

Outcomes

Because TIF is a relatively new procedure, the available data are immature. Currently, no randomized control trials compare TIF with either antireflux or PPI therapy. Many of the observational studies that have been performed have relatively small patient numbers. Also, the results of these studies have had significant variability.

Among the initial reports of TIF was a multicenter study of 86 patients. At the 12-month follow-up period, all hiatal hernias remained reduced. Median GERD-HRQL scores improved from 24 before TIF to 7 after TIF (*P* = 0.0001). PPIs were discontinued by 68% of the study population, and patient satisfaction was 65%. Another study of 37 consecutive patients at a single center found that atypical symptoms improved after TIF as measured with the RSI survey. Improvement from a mean score of 22.8 to 12.9 (*P* = 0.003) after TIF was shown. A statistically significant decrease in regurgitation scores was also seen (11.2 vs 4.3; *P* = 0.006). In a global assessment of the 24 patients who underwent pH testing off PPIs both before surgery and at follow-up examination, 54% were found to be in complete remission, needed no PPIs, and had normalized pH studies.

The authors recently conducted a systematic review of the published literature on TIF. A summary of the results can be found in Table 1. The 15 studies included reported on more than 550 procedures. Weighted means were calculated across the studies. Both GERD-HRQL scores (21.9 vs 5.9; *P* <0.0001) and RSI scores (24.5 vs

5.4; $P = <0.0001$) were significantly reduced after TIF. Overall patient satisfaction was found to be 72% after the procedure. The overall rate of PPI discontinuation was 67% across all studies. TIF appears to be safe; the major complication rate was 3.2%. The most common complication reported was hemorrhage that necessitated transfusion. Four cases of esophageal perforation were reported across all studies. The total failure rate was 8.1% (patients subsequently needed either Nissen fundoplication or redo-TIF). Currently, no studies have been able to show consistent normalization of pH metrics.

Multiple prospective clinical trials are currently underway. The Randomized EsophyX Versus Sham/Placebo Controlled TIF Trial (RESPECT study) is a multicenter randomized sham-controlled trial of 120 patients to evaluate the safety and effectiveness of TIF. The TIF versus Medical PPI Management of Refractory GERD Symptoms (TEMPO) trial is a multicenter randomized trial that will compare TIF directly with PPI therapy in 42 patients. Other sham-controlled trials are taking place in Europe as well. When these data become available, we will have a much better picture of whether EsophyX will live up to it promising potential.

FUTURE METHODS

In 2012, the SRS flexible endoscope (Medigus Ltd, Omer, Israel) gained FDA approval for endoluminal treatment of GERD. The SRS endoscope combines a miniaturized video camera, a surgical stapler, and ultrasonic sights for alignment in a single instrument (Figure 5). The SRS is designed to allow one to perform a true endoscopic 180-degree anterior fundoplication by stapling the stomach to the esophagus in two or three locations with a quintuplet of standard B-shaped, 4.8-mm titanium staples in each location. The safety and efficacy is currently being evaluated by an industry-sponsored multicenter clinical trial. Other significant endoluminal devices are under development for the reconstruction of the GEJ and may eventually allow more patients whose conditions are managed with medical therapy to be treated surgically.

SUMMARY

Development of an effective endoluminal treatment for GERD has proven as difficult as it is enticing. Most attempts have resulted in products that are off the market. Multiple factors are responsible for the demise of previous therapies, and product development remains a high-risk proposition. Payers have not consistently been willing to cover these procedures because of high costs and lack of conclusive evidence of long-term benefit beyond standard medical and surgical therapy. Still, the proliferation of devices continues. Matching current treatments with severity of disease, a niche exists between PPI use for mild symptoms and surgical intervention for severe disease. Filling this gap with endoluminal therapies seems logical and guarantees further effort on this front.

The current systems of Stretta and EsophyX have shown promising short-term results like many endoluminal therapies before them. Some positive data for Stretta exist in long-term follow-up periods,

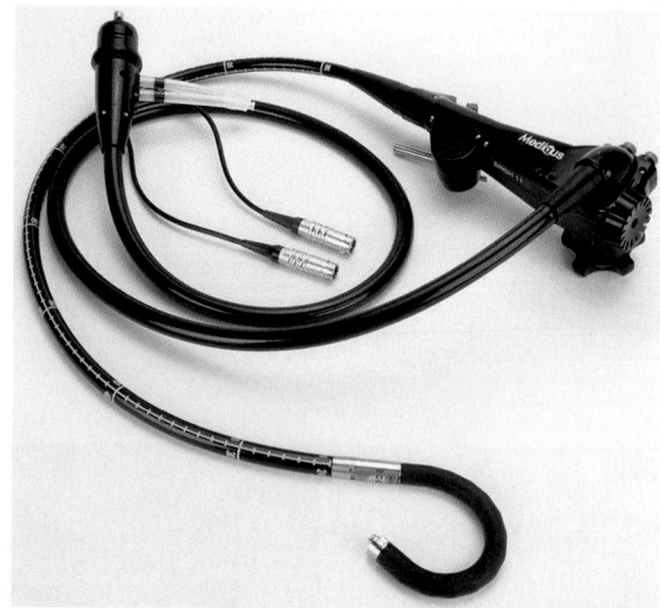

FIGURE 5 The SRS endoscope.

but the results are far from conclusive. Data on long-term efficacy of EsophyX are not yet available but may be promising based on favorable mid-term results. The greatest challenge may be identification of the correct patient population for these procedures. Currently, most patients being offered endoluminal treatments are at the severe end to the spectrum of disease. Well-designed clinical trials are needed not only to further describe efficacy but also to identify optimal candidates for these procedures.

SUGGESTED READINGS

Bell RC, Cadière GB: Transoral rotational esophagogastric fundoplication: technical, anatomical, and safety considerations, *Surg Endosc* 25(7):2387–2399, 2011.

Cadière GB, Buset M, Muls V, et al: Antireflux transoral incisionless fundoplication using Esophyx: 12-month results of a prospective multicenter study, *World J Surg* 32(8):1676–1688, 2008.

Chen D, Barber C, McLoughlin P, et al: Systematic review of endoscopic treatments for gastro-oesophageal reflux disease, *Br J Surg* 96(2):128–136, 2009.

Corley DA, Katz P, Wo JM, et al: Improvement of gastroesophageal reflux symptoms after radiofrequency energy: a randomized sham-controlled trial, *Gastroenterology* 125(3):668–676, 2003.

Dundon JM, Davis SS, Hazey JW, et al: Radiofrequency energy delivery to the lower esophageal sphincter (Stretta procedure) does not provide long-term symptom control, *Surg Innov* 15(4):297–301, 2008.

Hoppo T, Immanuel A, Schechert M, et al: Transoral incisionless fundoplication 2.0 procedure using EsophyX for gastroesophageal reflux disease, *J Gastrointest Surg* 14:1895–1901, 2010.

THE MANAGEMENT OF BARRETT'S ESOPHAGUS

Mario D. Terán, MD, and Malcolm V. Brock, MD

INTRODUCTION

The understanding of Barrett's esophagus (BE) has changed dramatically since 1950, when Norman Barrett first described his finding of a distal esophageal ulcer associated with esophagitis and columnar epithelium. Since Dr. Barrett's initial observation, the condition that bears his name has received multiple descriptions, formal definitions, and clinical associations. Today, BE is defined as the pathologic replacement of the esophagus' normal stratified squamous epithelium with an intestinal-like columnar epithelium. This replacement, also known as *intestinal metaplasia,* is a clear abnormality and is induced by chronic esophageal injury and inflammation caused by gastroesophageal reflux disease (GERD). It is conservatively estimated that 6% to 15% of American patients with GERD develop BE.

CLINICAL IMPACT

By far the greatest clinical concern with BE is that it is the most identifiable risk factor for the progression to esophageal adenocarcinoma (EAC), a malignancy with one of the fastest rising incidence rates worldwide. Multiple studies have shown that the presence of BE can confer at least a fortyfold increase in risk for the development of EAC. However, despite the increased cancer risk, most patients with BE do not progress to EAC; the overall annual rate of neoplastic transformation is approximately 0.5%. However, because of the aggressive and lethal nature of EAC (overall 5-year survival <17%), diagnosis, surveillance, and treatment of BE are sought by both patients and physicians alike.

The natural progression of BE to carcinoma develops over time; prospective studies have demonstrated the transformation of non-dysplastic columnar epithelium to dysplasia and eventually to invasive carcinoma. The transition through the dysplastic phase is further characterized as low- or high-grade dysplasia. Low-grade dysplasia (LGD) is distinguished from high-grade dysplasia (HGD) according to the degree of architectural and cytologic aberrations of the cells (Figure 1). However, the characterization of dysplasia is largely subjective, inasmuch as studies have shown poor interobserver agreement among experienced pathologists in diagnosing LGD (<50% interobserver agreement) and HGD (85% interobserver agreement). The difficulty in determining the severity of dysplasia with reproducible accuracy has led to controversy in quantifying the risk of progression through the dysplastic phase. As a result, the annual rates of dysplasia-to-cancer progression estimated in published studies vary from 0.9% to 13.5%. In addition, although biomarkers of dysplastic progression remain an active area of research, no biologic markers of progression that distinguish LGD from HGD have been clinically defined. Currently, HGD is regarded as the most reliable predictor for the development of invasive malignancy. A meta-analysis demonstrated that the overall risk of progression from HGD to EAC is 6% per patient per year.

Despite controversies surrounding the dysplastic progression and risk stratification of BE, there is overwhelming consensus on the primary cause: chronic mucosal injury induced by GERD. Exposure to both the acidic and alkali (unconjugated bile acids) substances, through reflux, has been shown, in multiple in vitro and in vivo

studies, to activate inflammatory pathways, promote cellular proliferation, and induce genetic alterations. These latter aberrations have even been shown to be correlated with increasing severity of gastrointestinal reflux exposure. In clinical studies of patients with GERD in which patients with and without BE were compared, findings have corroborated with wet-laboratory results, inasmuch as patients with BE have a greater severity of reflux symptoms, significantly higher esophageal acid exposure, and increased frequencies of erosive esophagitis, stricture formation, and ulceration than do patients without BE. Thus the presence of BE alone is an indication of severe GERD and necessitates treatment. These investigations have also revealed additional clinical risk factors for BE, such as age higher than 50 years, male gender, white race, presence of hiatal hernia, elevated body mass index, and a high distribution of intraabdominal body fat.

CLINICAL FEATURES

As the definition of BE has evolved considerably since its inception, so has its clinical characterization. Historically, BE was diagnosed and classified on the basis of (1) the length of visible columnar epithelium-lined esophageal mucosa present above the gastroesophageal junction (GEJ) and (2) the identification of intestinal metaplasia on histologic study (i.e., goblet cells; Figures 2 and 3). Hence, classic "long-segment" BE was defined endoscopically as columnar epithelium-lined esophageal mucosa extending more than 3 cm above the GEJ; "short-segment" BE, as columnar epithelium-lined esophageal mucosa within 3 cm of the GEJ. However, this classification did not account for the identification of gastric cardia-type intestinal metaplasia on biopsy when no obvious columnar epithelium was seen endoscopically. This latter entity was later defined as "ultra–short-segment" BE, or *cardia intestinal metaplasia,* and its significance has been extremely controversial. Currently, BE is diagnosed according to two criteria: when any length of columnar epithelia is visualized endoscopically and then confirmed histologically as present in the esophagus above the GEJ. Any intestinal-type epithelium in the esophagus is thus a clear abnormality and predisposes to cancer. Moreover, there is still clinical value in recording and measuring the extent of BE in the esophagus during endoscopic examination because cancer risk has been shown to be correlated with the extent of metaplastic lining. However, historical subjective classifications—such as the terms "long," "short," and "ultra-short"—have been replaced by the systematic recording of the circumferential extent and maximal length of BE. Known as the *Prague C and M criteria,* the circumferential extent (C) and the maximal extent (M) of BE above the GEJ are now used as a grading system to document and characterize BE.

TREATMENT OF NONDYSPLASTIC BARRETT'S ESOPHAGUS

Medical Management and Treatment

One of the principal treatment goals for any patient with BE is to control the GERD effectively. Medical therapy, consisting primarily of proton-pump inhibitors (PPIs), are a first-line therapy of any patient with BE and symptomatic GERD. Overall, PPIs are generally well tolerated and have been effective in controlling GERD symptoms and healing erosive esophagitis. However, the rate at which PPIs reduce EAC is unknown because it would be unethical to perform any prospective study of the incidence rates of EAC in patients with GERD taking PPIs versus a placebo. However, studies such as A Phase III, Randomized Study of Aspirin and Esomeprazole Chemoprevention in Barrett's Metaplasia (AspECT trial) in the United Kingdom

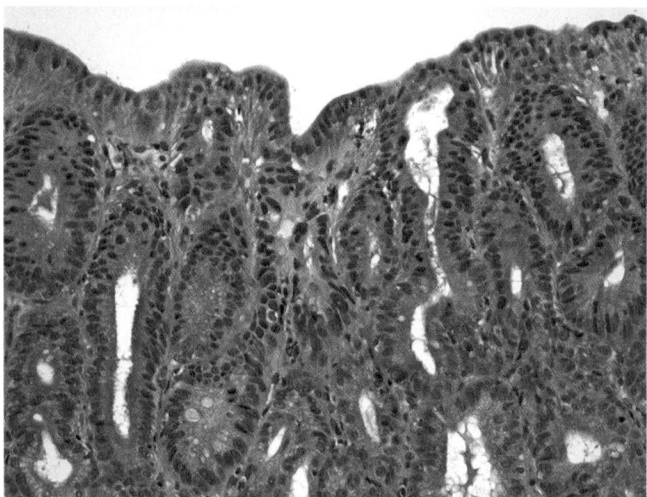

FIGURE 1   Barrett's esophagus (BE): intestinal metaplasia (IM) with high-grade dysplasia (HGD).

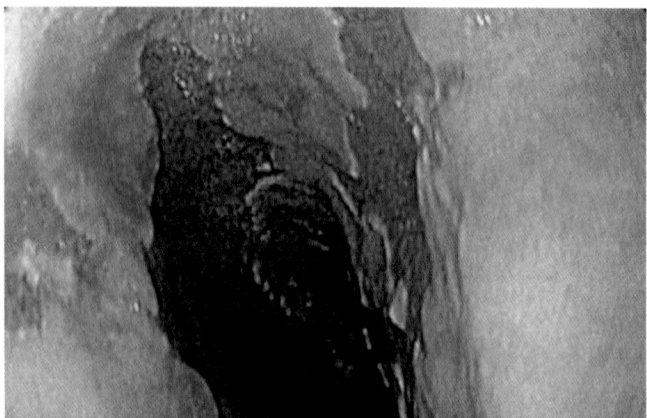

FIGURE 2   Long-segment Barrett's esophagus.

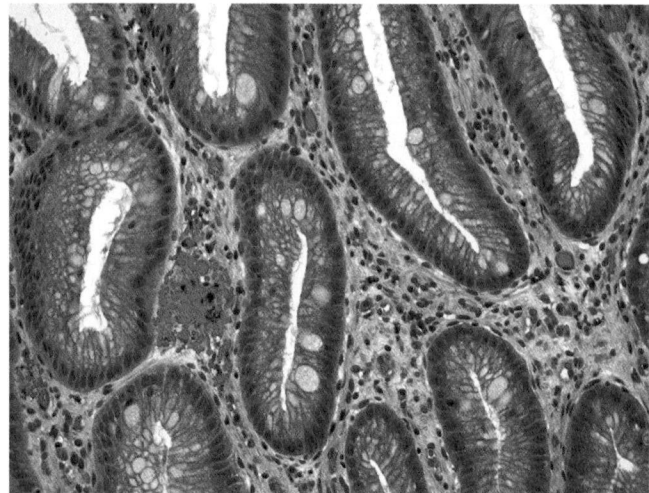

FIGURE 3   Barrett's esophagus/intestinal metaplasia (BE/IM) with goblet cells.

are attempts to investigate the prophylactic effects of PPIs in preventing esophageal cancer. In the AspECT trial, 5000 patients with BE were randomly assigned to receive either low-dose or high-dose PPIs; the primary outcome measure was progression of BE to HGD or EAC (completion of trial expected in 2019).

The long-term safety of PPI use has come into question. In 2010, the U.S. Food and Drug Administration (FDA) issued warnings regarding the potential for spine, hip, and wrist fractures among long-term PPI users. In addition, by increasing gastric pH levels, PPIs may also encourage the overgrowth of gut microflora, thereby increasing the susceptibility to bacterial infection. In a systematic review published in 2011, PPI users were found to have increased susceptibility for *Salmonella, Campylobacter,* and *Clostridium. difficile* infections. *C. difficile* infection had the strongest correlation with PPI use. Of 27 studies, 17 demonstrated a positive association (relative risk = 1.2 to 5.0). As with any medication, the potential adverse effects must be weighed against the potential benefits in each patient.

In addition to PPIs, nonsteroidal antiinflammatory drugs (NSAIDs), specifically cyclooxygenase-2 inhibitors, have also been identified as possibly chemopreventive agents in the progression of BE to cancer and as therapeutic agents in EAC. In in vitro studies, NSAIDs have been shown to decrease the proliferation of BE cells. Furthermore, in 2005, Vaughan and associates showed in a prospective study that these agents seemed to decrease the neoplastic progression of BE to EAC; the 5-year cumulative incidence was 14.3% among patients not taking NSAIDs, in contrast to 6.6% of patients taking NSAIDs. The AspECT trial is intended to evaluate the chemopreventive effects of PPIs, as well as aspirin, in two conditions. Despite available evidence suggesting a prophylactic effect of NSAIDs against EAC, it is not yet clear whether this outweighs the long-term risks of these medications. Therefore, initiating NSAID treatment in a patient with BE for the sole purpose of EAC chemoprevention is currently not recommended.

Antireflux Surgery

Antireflux surgery has been shown to be an effective treatment strategy for most patients with GERD and BE. Long-term results are equal or superior to those of medical therapy. In a study with a 12-year follow-up period, patients randomly assigned to undergo fundoplication had significantly higher remission rates of GERD than did those treated with omeprazole (53% vs 45%; *P* = 0.02). According to a 2010 Cochrane review of four controlled randomized trials with more than 1200 patients randomly assigned to undergo either surgery or medical management, GERD-specific quality of life was significantly higher with surgery than with medical management. In addition, symptoms of heartburn, reflux, and bloating were much better after surgery than after medical therapy.

Antireflux surgery has also produced higher rates of BE regression than has medical therapy. In a 2006 study, Rossi and associates compared the effects of medical therapy and Nissen fundoplication on LGD regression and, in a multivariate analysis, determined that Nissen fundoplication was the only factor significantly associated with the regression of LGD in nondysplastic BE (odds ratio = 15.33; *P* = 0.033). In a systematic review, Chang and colleagues in 2007 reached a similar conclusion. In this review, the probability of regression to lower grades of dysplasia, nondysplastic BE, or nonmetaplastic tissue was 15.4% in surgically treated patients but only 1.9% in patients receiving medical therapy (*P* = 0.004). The long-term effects of antireflux surgery in the prevention of EAC, however, remain controversial. In the same review, Chang and colleagues found among controlled studies no significant difference in EAC incidence rates between surgically and medically treated patients (6.5 vs 4.8 per 1000 patient-years; *P* = 0.32).

Endoscopic Therapies

Endoscopic therapies for the management and treatment of GERD and nondysplastic BE are constantly evolving. Methods have included radiofrequency augmentation of the lower esophageal sphincter, endoscopic suturing of the lower esophageal sphincter, and transoral incisionless fundoplication. However, none of these methods has demonstrated long-term improvement in pH levels or cessation of the need for antireflux medications. A 2012 study showed that at 36 months, the majority of patients who underwent transoral incisionless fundoplication had required additional medical therapy or a surgical revision of the fundoplication. Sphincter augmentation by means of a system of titanium beads (the LINX Reflux Management System) has shown promise in the long-term control of GERD. After 4 years, patients with this device were found consistently to have symptom relief and pH control. However, more data are required before widespread routine use can be recommended.

Other treatment modalities such as radiofrequency ablation (RFA) and photodynamic therapy (PDT) have been shown to eradicate BE cells and promote reversion of the mucosa in BE to normal squamous epithelium. RFA has successfully achieved reversion in 97% of patients with nondysplastic BE by means of a balloon-based device (HALO[360] System). Of importance, however, is that no data from controlled trials in nondysplastic BE have shown that endoscopic ablative therapies are more effective at reducing cancer risk or are more cost effective than periodic long-term endoscopic surveillance.

TREATMENT OF DYSPLASTIC BARRETT'S ESOPHAGUS

Despite the controversies in factors for risk progression and overall risk, dysplastic formation remains a significant neoplastic progression and warrants frequent surveillance and consideration of eradication treatment modalities. In patients with dysplastic BE, endoscopic surveillance varies with the severity of dysplasia. Surveillance is recommended every 6 to 12 months for patients with LGD and every 3 months for patients with HGD who have not undergone ablative therapy. During a surveillance examination, four-quadrant biopsy specimens should be taken at 2-cm intervals in patients without dysplasia and at 1-cm intervals in patients with established dysplasia. Any additional mucosal irregularities should also be sampled. Submitted biopsy specimens should be reviewed by two pathologists, with preferably one with expertise in gastrointestinal pathology, because disparities in intraobserver agreement are often reported.

Endoscopic Ablative Treatments

Current endoscopic ablative treatments include RFA, PDT, argon plasma coagulation, and cryoablation (Figures 4 through 6). RFA and PDT are very effective in the treatment of dysplastic BE. RFA has been shown to lead to reversion to normal squamous epithelium in more than 90% of patients with LGD. In 2009, researchers in a large sham-controlled U.S. trial reported that RFA therapy in HGD reduced the progression to EAC. In that study, 127 patients with dysplastic BE were assigned to receive either RFA therapy or a sham procedure. Of the patients with HGD who received RFA, 2.4% developed EAC, whereas of those who received sham therapy, 19% developed EAC ($P <0.001$). Overall, 9.3% of patients who received sham therapy, in comparison with 1.2% who received RFA, progressed to cancer ($P = 0.45$).

Like RFA, PDT also leads to the destruction of BE cells. After systemic administration of a photosensitizer such as porfimer sodium that accumulates in HGD and neoplastic cells, endoscopic delivery of a low-energy, nonthermal laser beam activates the photosensitizer, enabling singlet oxygen formation and subsequent cell destruction. In 2005, Overholt and colleagues published the results of a multicenter, prospective, randomized controlled trial in which PDT plus omeprazole was compared with omeprazole alone in patients with HGD. They found that HGD was eliminated in 77% of patients

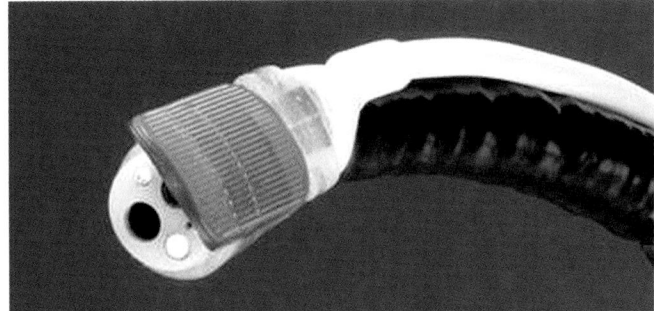

FIGURE 4   HALO[90] device. *(Courtesy Covidien LP d/b/a BÂRRX Medical, Sunnyvale, CA.)*

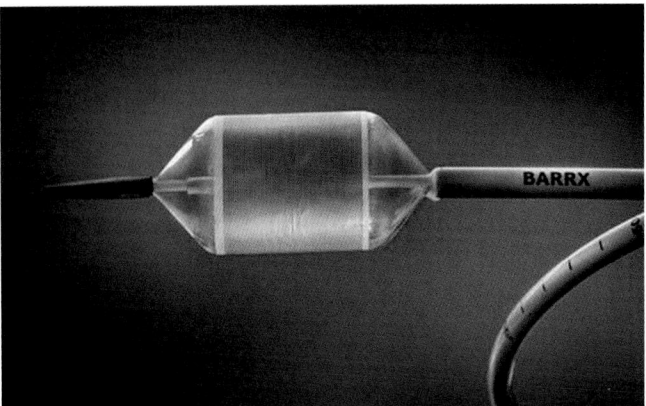

FIGURE 5   HALO[360] device. *(Courtesy Covidien LP d/b/a BÂRRX Medical, Sunnyvale, CA.)*

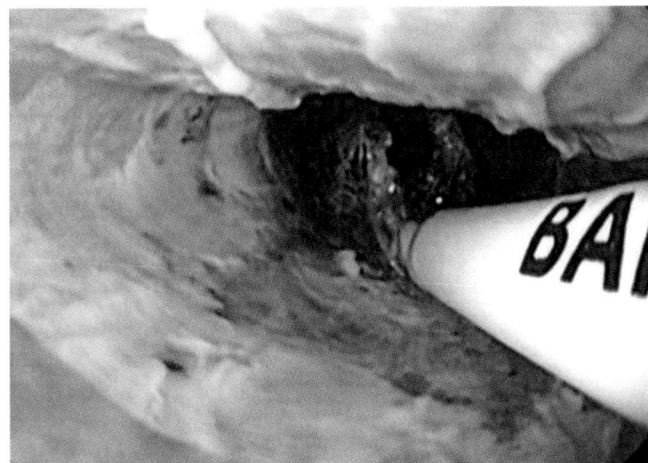

FIGURE 6   Metaplastic esophageal mucosa treated with a radiofrequency ablation HALO[360] device. *(Courtesy Covidien LP d/b/a BÂRRX Medical, Sunnyvale, CA.)*

receiving PDT plus omeprazole but in only 39% of patients who received only omeprazole ($P <0.0001$). In addition, invasive cancer developed in only 13% of patients who received PDT plus omeprazole, in comparison with 28% of patients treated with omeprazole alone ($P = 0.006$). These effects remained durable inasmuch as after 5 years, cancer had developed in only 15% of patients who received PDT plus omeprazole, in comparison with 29% of those receiving only omeprazole ($P = 0.027$).

No controlled trials have been performed to compare the effectiveness of RFA with that of PDT. Both methods have been shown to have low complication rates and are well tolerated by patients. PDT does produce a greater depth of ablation than does RFA, although with higher complication rates. Both modalities have limited usefulness in assessing the depth of HGD, as well as in detecting foci of unsuspected EAC. It has been estimated that EAC can be found in 25% to 75% of patients with HGD undergoing esophagectomy; more recent data favor the lower end of this estimate.

Endoscopic Mucosal Resection

Endoscopic mucosal resection (EMR) is another important modality in the treatment of HGD and intramucosal carcinomas (Figures 7 through 11). EMR is now offered as a curative treatment for HGD or early EAC, with or without conjunctive ablative therapies (i.e., RFA or PDT). In addition, a major advantage of EMR over ablative treatments is the ability to obtain a large specimen in biopsy that is both lateral and deep to irregular dysplastic lesions. A single-institution study of the efficacy of EMR treatment on HGD or mucosal adenocarcinoma showed that after a mean follow-up of 63.6 months, complete response was seen in 96.6% of patients, and the 5-year survival rate was 84%. Eligibility criteria for the use of EMR as a definitive therapy include focal HGD or stage T1a intramucosal lesion smaller than 2 cm in diameter, no evidence of lymph node involvement or systemic disease, flat or polypoid lesions without ulceration, and lesions without lymphovascular invasion.

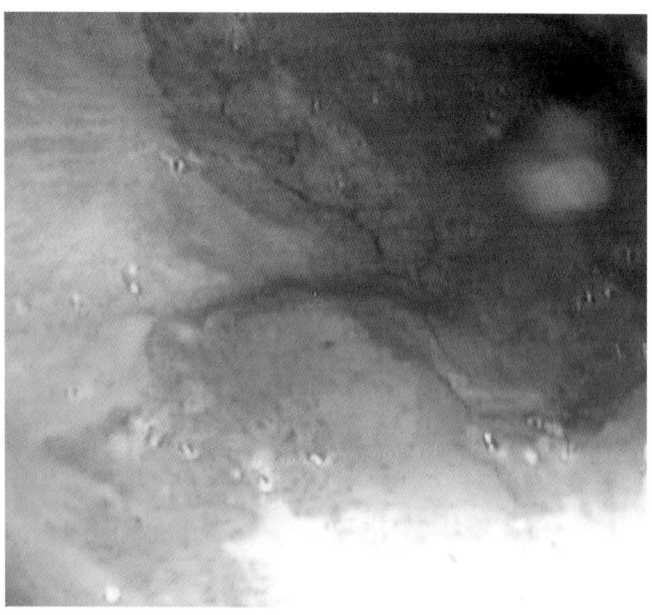

FIGURE 7   Lesion visible on endoscopy.

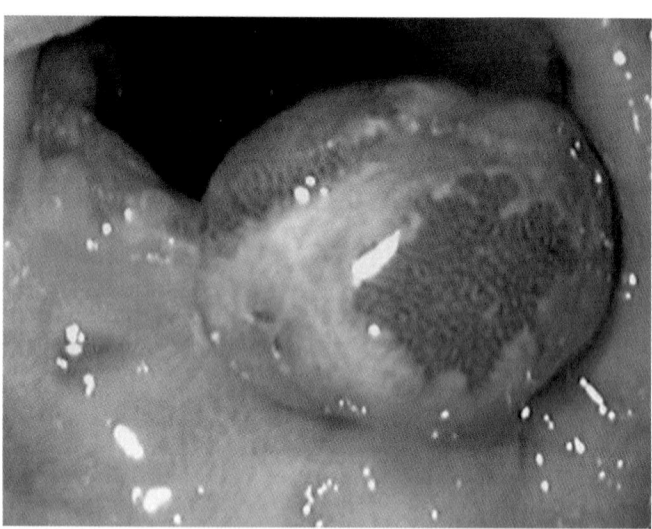

FIGURE 9   Pseudopolyp of visible lesion created with suction cap and rubber band.

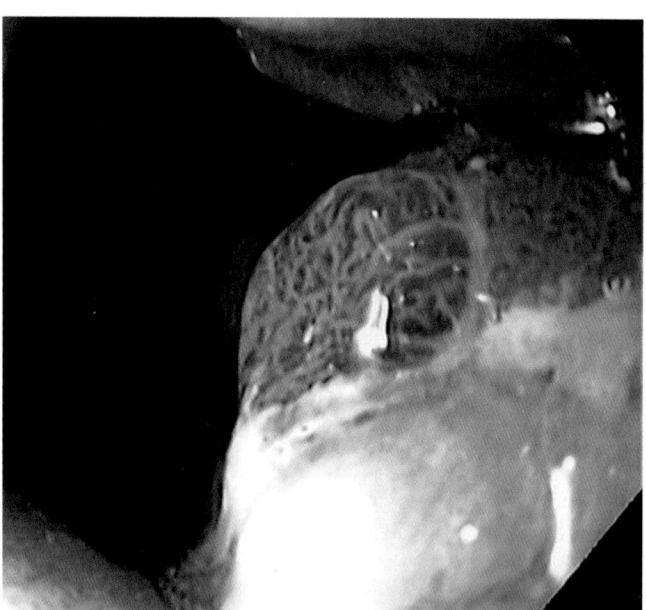

FIGURE 8   Lesion visible on endoscopy (view augmented with narrow-band imaging).

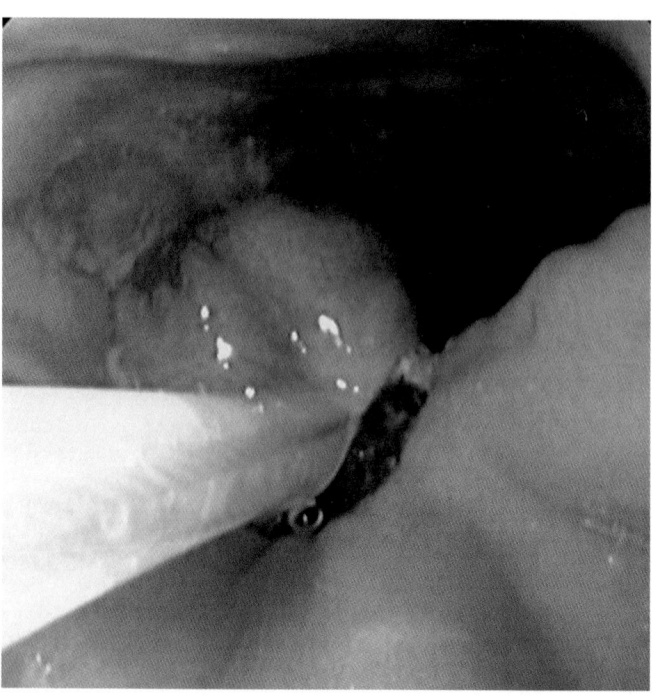

FIGURE 10   Snaring of the pseudopolyp.

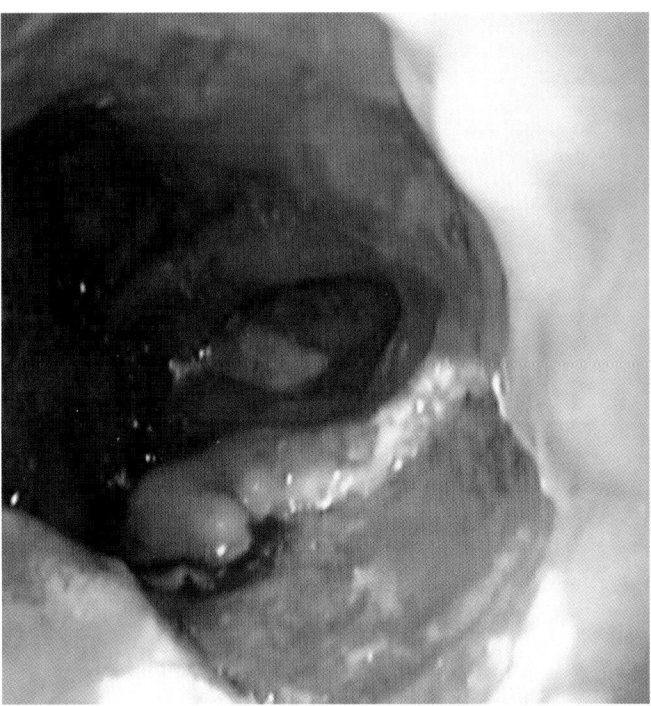

FIGURE 11   Excised lesion.

Esophagectomy

Historically, an esophagectomy was the "gold standard" in the treatment of HGD. Currently, 70% to 80% of patients with HGD are successfully treated instead with endoscopic eradication therapies. A common argument opposing the use of esophagectomy has been the magnitude of the procedure, as well as the rates of associated morbidity and mortality. However, because no molecular markers have been developed and validated to identify occult EAC, esophagectomy not only cures HGD in patients with undiagnosed carcinomas but also serves as an effective prophylaxis. Studies have also shown that the historical concern over high reported mortality rates with esophagectomies may be inflated. In 2007, Williams and colleagues reviewed 22 published reports on the outcomes of esophagectomy for patients with HGD. They found the overall perioperative mortality rate to be 0.94%, and in 17 of the reviewed reports, the mortality rate was 0.

Longitudinal studies have demonstrated that the quality of life after an esophagectomy is good to excellent and can return to preoperative levels. Despite an initial and prolonged adjustment period, patients who underwent esophagectomy for HGD have demonstrated quality-of-life scores similar to national norms by 5 years later. The new techniques of vagal-sparing esophagectomies and minimally invasive esophagectomies may further improve the quality of life for these patients.

SUMMARY

The diagnosis, risk assessment, and management of BE have been highly dynamic since their inception. However, with the rising incidence rate of EAC and its poor associated outcomes, the management and early treatment of BE has the potential to affect public health greatly. Control of a patient's underlying GERD has to be the initial step of BE management. Once BE is diagnosed, patients should undergo endoscopic surveillance, with the frequency determined according to the severity of their dysplasia. Although the therapeutic armamentarium for BE has expanded, judicious evaluation, good judgment, and thorough patient discussions are still needed to evaluate the best therapeutic options for each individual. Much still remains to be learned concerning the management and treatment of BE, and clinicians must be able to adapt and implement new information as it becomes available to achieve the best possible outcomes.

SELECTED READINGS

American Gastroenterological Association Institute Medical Panel: American Gastroenterological Association medical position statement on the management of Barrett's esophagus, *Gastroenterology* 140:1084–1091, 2011.

Atwood SE, Lundell L, Hatlback JG, et al: Medical or surgical management of GERD patients with Barrett's esophagus: the LOTUS trial 3-year experience, *J Gastrointest Surg* 12(10):1646–1654, 2008.

Fernando HC, Murthy SC, Hofstetter W, et al: The Society of Thoracic Surgeons practice guideline series: guidelines for the management of Barrett's esophagus with high-grade dysplasia, *Ann Thorac Surg* 87: 1993–2002, 2009.

Shaheen N, Sharma P, Overholt BF, et al, Radiofrequency ablation in Barrett's esophagus with dysplasia, *N Engl J Med* 360(22):2353–2355, 2009.

ENDOSCOPIC TREATMENT OF BARRETT'S ESOPHAGUS

Nassrene Elmadhun, MD, and Michael Kent, MD

INTRODUCTION

Barrett's esophagus (BE) is an acquired condition in which the normal squamous epithelial lining of the esophagus is replaced with columnar epithelium and characteristic goblet cells, also known as intestinal metaplasia. BE develops as a result of long-standing gastroesophageal reflux disease and occurs in 10% to 15% of patients undergoing upper gastrointestinal endoscopy for reflux symptoms. BE increases the risk of development of esophageal adenocarcinoma (EAC) by 30 to 125 times. In the United States, the prevalence rate of BE is estimated to be 5.6%, and the annual risk of EAC is 0.5% per year. Esophageal carcinogenesis involves the progression of intestinal metaplasia to dysplasia and finally to adenocarcinoma. In a randomized control trial of patients with BE followed endoscopically over the course of 1 year, 22.7% of patients with low-grade dysplasia (LGD) and 19% of patients with high-grade dysplasia (HGD) had complete regression of dysplasia without treatment. However, 19% of patients with HGD had disease progression to EAC. Given that EAC is one of the fastest rising solid cancers in the Western world, with a dismal 5-year survival rate of 12%, there is increased public health interest for targeted therapies to treat individuals at high risk.

HISTOLOGIC FEATURES OF BARRETT'S ESOPHAGUS

Barrett's esophagus classically appears on endoscopy as salmon-colored "tongues" or extensions of mucosa that stretch into the tubular esophagus from the esophagogastric junction. The American Gastroenterological Association recommends standardized four-quadrant biopsies at intervals of every other centimeter of suspected BE and specific biopsy of any mucosal irregularities (such as nodules and ulcers). Histologic classification of BE dysplasia is as follows:

1. Negative for dysplasia: This classification indicates benign BE with intestinal metaplasia and columnar epithelium. All cells have normal morphology.
2. Indefinite for dysplasia: These biopsy results show mucosal injury and regenerative changes as a result of long-standing reflux disease. Distinguishing between regeneration and dysplasia is difficult. In this case, providers may repeat the endoscopy after a course of treatment with a secretory inhibitor to reduce the acid reflux–induced cellular injury.
3. Low-grade dysplasia: This classification designates atypical epithelium with increased mitosis and nuclear-to-cytoplasmic ratio, but the crypt architecture is preserved.
4. High-grade dysplasia: This classification designates abnormal columnar epithelium with loss of cell polarity, atypical mitotic activity, loss of goblet cells, and distortion of the crypt architecture.
5. Intramucosal adenocarcinoma: This classification is defined by dysplasia that penetrates the basement membrane and infiltrates into the lamina propria but not into the submucosa. Lesions that penetrate past the lamina propria or muscularis mucosa are designated as T1b invasive EAC.

An important note is that these histologic changes and degree of dysplasia occur on a continuum, and pathologists may find difficulty in distinguishing LGD from HGD. In fact, significant interobserver variability occurs even among experienced gastrointestinal pathologists. As a result, the American Gastroenterological Association recommends that all dysplasia diagnoses are confirmed by at least one other experienced gastrointestinal pathologist given the implications of a dysplasia diagnosis on treatment and management.

SURVEILLANCE ALGORITHM FOR BARRETT'S ESOPHAGUS

In patients with BE without dysplasia, endoscopy is recommended in 3-year to 5-year intervals. Patients with BE and LGD should undergo surveillance endoscopy every 6 to 12 months. Although endoscopic surveillance for patients with BE and no dysplasia or LGD is the standard of care, little evidence supports the assumption that surveillance reduces the number of deaths from BE. Treatment of patients with nondysplastic BE or with LGD is also controversial. In a randomized prospective study conducted by Parrilla and colleagues, 101 patients with nondysplastic BE or LGD were randomized to antireflux surgery and medical therapy. After a mean follow-up period of 5 years, HGD developed in 5% of the medical arm and 3% of the surgical arm, which was not statistically different. This result was corroborated by a meta-analysis published by Chang and colleagues in 2007 that showed no difference in EAC incidence rate between antireflux surgery and antisecretory medical therapy. Given the lack of data on the benefit of antireflux medical or surgical therapy, treatment of nondysplastic BE with the intention to prevent EAC is cost ineffective.

In patients with HGD, surveillance endoscopy should be conducted every 3 months in the absence of endoscopic eradication or surgical therapy. HGD is of particular importance because these patients are at high risk for development of EAC. In a study of 30 patients with HGD who were undergoing prophylactic esophagectomy, 43% had occult adenocarcinoma on pathology. Certain features of HGD confer a higher risk of development of EAC, including multifocal HGD or an endoscopically visible lesion, such as ulceration or a discrete nodule. Patients with these concerning features have an estimated risk of concurrent EAC of 60% to 78%, but patients with unifocal, flat HGD have a 17% risk of concurrent EAC. Patients with HGD and low-risk features should be treated endoscopically with the intention to eradicate BE and prevent neoplastic progression. Although most patients with HGD can be treated endoscopically, major medical societies recommend that patients with high-risk features or intramucosal EAC are evaluated for esophagectomy in a high-volume center by an experienced esophageal surgeon. However, patients who refuse esophagectomy or have conditions that are unfit for surgery should undergo endoscopic ablation as an alternative to surgery.

ENDOSCOPIC ABLATION THERAPIES

Several endoscopic ablation therapies have been described to manage BE with HGD and include thermal ablation (including multipolar electrocoagulation [MPEC] and argon beam plasma coagulation [ABPC]), chemical ablation (photodynamic therapy [PDT]), cryotherapy, and radiofrequency ablation (RFA). The goal for all ablation therapies is to eradicate BE and repopulation with normal squamous cells. Ideally, ablation should extend through the muscularis mucosa. Ablation, however, should not extend to the submucosa because that can increase the risk of stricture (Figure 1).

Thermal Ablation

Multipolar electrocoagulation involves passing a current between electrodes, which are in direct contact with the tissue. ABPC transfers monopolar electrocautery to the tissue via the flow of ionized argon gas plasma. ABPC distributes the ablation more evenly than MPEC, and the ablation depth can be better controlled. These techniques are falling out of favor because they require multiple treatment sessions and the depth of ablation is not well controlled, which results in complications such as stricture and perforation. Also, reports of

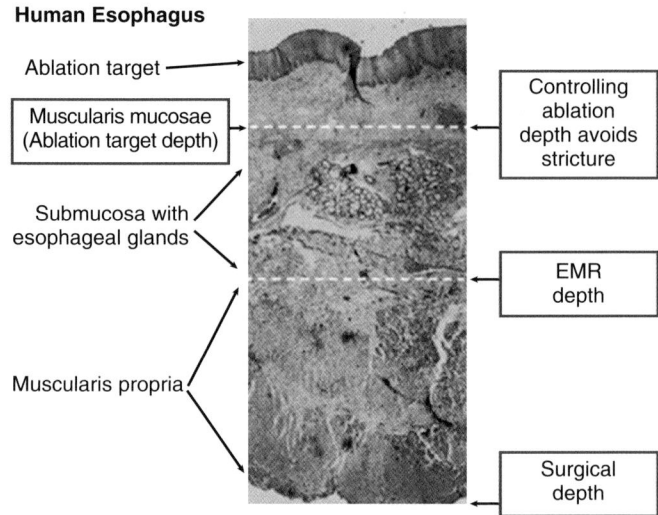

Human Esophagus

Ablation target
Muscularis mucosae (Ablation target depth)
Submucosa with esophageal glands
Muscularis propria

Controlling ablation depth avoids stricture

EMR depth

Surgical depth

FIGURE 1 Histology of the normal layers of the esophagus. Appropriate ablation and resection depths are noted for the varying endoscopic treatments of Barrett's esophagus. *EMR,* Endoscopic mucosal resection.

buried BE have been documented after MPEC and ABPC, in which islands of intestinal metaplasia are found under normal-appearing regenerated squamous mucosa that may progress to occult EAC.

Photodynamic Therapy

Photodynamic therapy involves the administration of an inactive photosensitizing agent before endoscopy, which accumulates preferentially in diseased esophageal mucosa. The photosensitizing agent is then activated by a wavelength-specific light during endoscopy, which triggers the formation of oxygen radicals and eradication of BE. PDT is also falling out of favor because of skin photosensitivity that can last for weeks to months, symptomatic strictures in 36% of patients, high cost, and buried BE in 58% of patients.

Cryospray Ablation

Cryospray ablation (CSA) is a noncontact method that uses endoscopically applied low-pressure liquid nitrogen and carbon dioxide spray to eradicate BE. The rapid tissue freeze-thaw cycle results in destruction of diseased epithelium followed by the regeneration of normal squamous epithelium. The depth is limited to 2 mm and requires repeat CSA sessions every 4 to 6 weeks until BE is completely eradicated. Early results reported that 79% to 87% of patients with HGD had no evidence of dysplasia after CSA and that 46% to 78% of patients had complete eradication of BE. Side effects of CSA are generally mild and consist mainly of noncardiac/acid reflux–like chest pain that lasts a few days after treatment. One case of gastric perforation was reported in a patient with Marfan syndrome. As a result, the stomach must be decompressed because the carbon insufflates the stomach.

Cryospray Ablation Technique

With moderate sedation, a surveillance endoscopy is performed. An orogastric tube is then advanced to the stomach and connected to continuous suction to allow for decompression of the stomach and esophagus. The cryotherapy catheter is passed through the working port of the endoscope and extended beyond the tip of the endoscope. With direct visualization, liquid nitrogen is sprayed through the catheter for 10-second intervals for four cycles to freeze the mucosa. Between cycles, the tissue is given 45 seconds to thaw. This process is repeated until all abnormal esophageal tissue is treated. The patients are discharged home the same day.

Radiofrequency Ablation

Radiofrequency ablation delivers bipolar energy via direct contact with esophageal mucosa in a controlled duration and intensity for reliable tissue penetration without submucosal injury. The initial treatment uses a sizing balloon catheter to deliver circumferential treatment (Figure 2, A). Subsequent treatments for focal disease deliver RFA through a targeted ablation catheter that is mounted to the tip of an endoscope (Figure 2, B). Unlike PDT, CSA, or other thermal ablation techniques, RFA is precisely programmed through the energy generator to deliver high power with a controlled energy density, while the balloon catheter allows for uniform mucosa electrode contact, which results in controlled ablation depth. However, the target lesions must be flat to ensure adequate ablation.

Multiple prospective trials have shown that RFA is a safe, effective, and reliable ablation tool to eradicate BE and dysplasia. Fleischer and colleagues conducted the Ablation of Intestinal Metaplasia (AIMII) trials, a prospective multicenter trial to evaluate the use of RFA to eradicate BE in patients without dysplasia after a 2.5-year and 5-year follow-up period. They found that at 12 months, 70% of patients

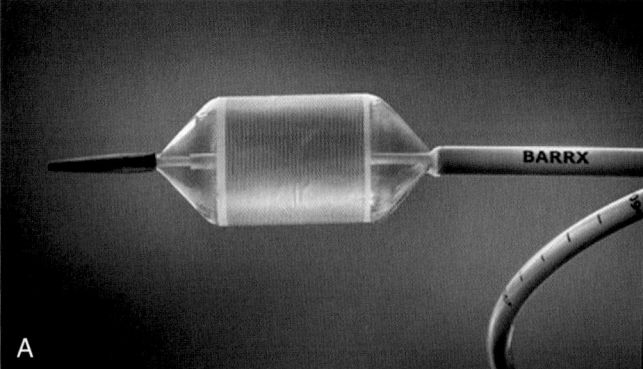
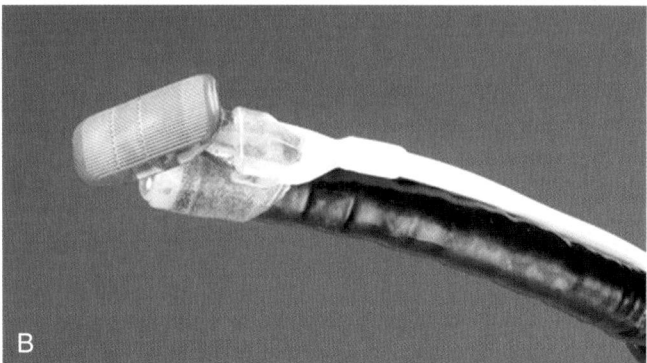

FIGURE 2 Radiofrequency ablation catheters. **A,** Balloon catheter used for initial circumferential ablation of Barrett's esophagus. **B,** Focal treatment catheter used in subsequent treatments to ablate small residual areas of disease.

with nondysplastic BE who had one treatment session of RFA had complete eradication of BE. After a 2.5-year follow-up period and repeat focal treatment for the remaining 30% with residual disease, 98.4% of patients had complete eradication of BE. After 5 years, 92% had complete eradication of BE. Although patients with BE and HGD clearly should undergo treatment, the current literature does not support routine treatment for nondysplastic BE. Nevertheless, this study established the safety and efficacy of RFA; AIMII reported no buried glands in the 2396 specimens analyzed and no strictures or serious complications.

Shaheen and colleagues published the first multicenter sham-controlled trial of 127 patients with LGD and HGD randomized to RFA or sham procedure. At 12 months, 90% of patients with LGD and 81% of patients with HGD had complete eradication of dysplasia. Patients who underwent RFA had less disease progression and less EAC (3.6% and 1.2%, respectively) compared with the control group (16.3% and 9.3%, respectively). The authors noted that the decreased incidence rate of cancer in this study should be viewed with caution as a shift of a single incidence of cancer would have resulted in a loss of statistical significance. They also reported one case of upper gastrointestinal bleeding, a 6% rate of esophageal stricture, and a 5.1% rate of buried BE. In comparison, these complication rates are lower than those reported in the literature for PDT and other ablation therapies. Therefore, RFA has supplanted many of the other ablative technique as a safe and effective ablation tool.

Radiofrequency Ablation Technique

With moderate sedation, an endoscope is passed into the esophagus and the esophageal mucosa is sprayed with 1% acetylcysteine and flushed with water to remove esophageal mucus. The inner diameter of the esophagus is then measured with a sizing catheter passed over a guidewire through the endoscope working port. The sizing catheter is removed, and an appropriately sized treatment balloon catheter is then passed into the esophagus. The balloon is deployed 1 cm above the proximal margin of BE. The energy generator delivers approximately 300 W in a density of 12 to 15 J/cm^2 in less than 300 ms. The delivered treatment is circumferential and is 3 cm in length. The balloon is then repositioned, moving distally down the esophagus with a small amount of overlap. After the treatment, the esophagus is inspected to ensure that all the BE is adequately treated. Patients are generally discharged the same day, with a follow-up endoscopy in 3 months. If residual BE is seen on follow-up endoscopy, ablation is carried out with either a balloon catheter (for large areas of BE) or a focal ablation catheter (for smaller lesions; Figure 2,*B*). The focal ablation catheter is mounted to the tip of the endoscope, so the operator must be careful when advancing the endoscope from the oropharynx through the upper esophageal sphincter to avoid injury.

ENDOSCOPIC MUCOSAL RESECTION

Endoscopic mucosal resection (EMR) involves the resection of mucosa and submucosal layer down to the muscularis propria. EMR has emerged as a safe and effective treatment of BE with HGD or intramucosal EAC. Although esophagectomy is the most conservative therapy for patients who are good surgical candidates with HGD or intramucosal EAC, it also carries a 1% mortality rate in high-volume centers and can be as high as 10% or more in low-volume centers. Therefore, although esophagectomy is an established therapy for BE with HGD, EMR is increasing in popularity as an esophageal-sparing procedure for patients with low risk for nodal spread.

Endoscopic ultrasound scan (EUS) should be performed in all patients with BE and focal nodules or ulcers to evaluate the depth of invasion and periesophageal lymphadenopathy. Although EUS is a useful tool for EAC staging, providers need to be cautious because EUS is often not sensitive enough to differentiate superficial tumors. In a blinded trial of 100 patients with suspicion of early esophageal cancer, patients underwent endoscopy and EUS followed by esophagectomy. Although EUS was 90% sensitive for mucosal involvement, the sensitivity for submucosal invasion was only 48%.

After appropriate staging including EUS and preliminary endoscopy with standard BE biopsies, EMR can be considered if the HGD or intramucosal EAC is considered low risk for nodal disease. Indications for EMR include:

1. Small lesions (<2 cm).
2. Nonulcerated lesions.
3. Lesions without submucosal invasion.
4. Lesions without lymphovascular invasion.
5. Well-differentiated or moderately differentiated lesions.

Ell and colleagues have published several prospective studies investigating the efficacy and safety of EMR in patients with HGD and intramucosal EAC. In the study published in 2000, they found that 97% of patients with HGD had complete remission at 1 year. In 2007, the same group found that 88% of patients with low-risk intramucosal EAC had complete remission at 36 months after EMR treatment. After a 5-year follow-up period, 96% of patients with HGD and intramucosal EAC had complete remission and 3.7% needed curative esophagectomy. In these studies, patients followed a rigorous follow-up schedule with endoscopies at 1, 2, 3, 6, 9, and 12 months and then every 6 months for an additional 5 years. Every other follow-up examination also included EUS, computed tomographic (CT) scan, and abdominal ultrasound scan. Such a vigorous follow-up routine is certainly not feasible outside of a research study setting.

The most commonly reported complications are bleeding and stenosis. The risk of stenosis increases particularly after multiple or circumferential treatments. Although arterial bleeding is uncommon, venous bleeding is not and can usually be managed endoscopically with injection. Stenosis can take months to develop and can be

managed with serial dilations. Esophageal perforation has also been reported at a rate of 0.06% to 5%.

Endoscopic Mucosal Resection Technique

Many EMR techniques have been described in the literature. In general, moderate sedation is used and an endoscope is passed into the esophagus for initial surveillance.

Snare Technique

If the lesion is polypoid and small, no submucosal injection is necessary to elevate the lesion. A diathermy snare is advanced through the working port of the endoscope and positioned around the base of the lesion. The snare is then tightened securely around the lesion and resected with electrocautery.

If the lesion is small and flat, a 1:100,000 dilution of epinephrine in saline solution is injected in the submucosa to elevate the target lesion, creating a pseudopolyp. The snare is introduced and used to capture and ligate the lesion. A double-channeled endoscope can be useful in the snare technique, with one port used to pass the snare and the other port used to pass a grasping forceps to aid in pulling the lesion into the snare. The double-channeled endoscope can be too bulky to carry out technically difficult resections in the esophagus, especially if the esophagus is tortuous or if the lesion is at the esophagogastric junction.

"Suck and Cut" Technique

Ligation Technique

A variceal ligation device is used to suction the target lesion into the cylinder of the ligation device. A rubber band is released around the lesion, creating a pseudopolyp. A diathermy snare is then looped around the pseudopolyp to resect the lesion.

Cap Technique

The target lesion should first be marked with electrocautery because the lesion can be difficult to identify after submucosal injection. The submucosa is injected with a saline-epinephrine solution. A special transparent cap is then affixed to the end of the endoscope (Figure 3). A diathermy snare is advanced through the working port, and the lesion is sucked into the cap and resected with the diathermy snare. A prospective randomized trial that compared the cap technique with the ligation technique in 100 consecutive EMRs for early EAC did not find any differences in the incidence of bleeding, diameter of the resected specimen, or the resection area. Therefore, these two techniques can safely be used interchangeably according to operator preference.

ENDOSCOPIC SUBMUCOSAL DISSECTION

Endoscopic submucosal dissection (ESD) is an endoscopic resection technique that was developed in Japan to resect large (>2 cm), flat, or ulcerated esophageal tumors and the surrounding mucosa in an en bloc fashion. Ulcerated lesions and large lesions (>2 cm) cannot be resected en bloc with negative lateral margins with standard EMR techniques. Ulcerated lesions are often fixed to the submucosa and muscularis propria and therefore cannot be elevated with a submucosal injection. Large lesions can only be resected in a piecemeal fashion with EMR, which increases the risk of recurrence from residual dysplastic tissue. Therefore, ESD was developed for the treatment of early esophageal cancer limited to the epithelium or lamina

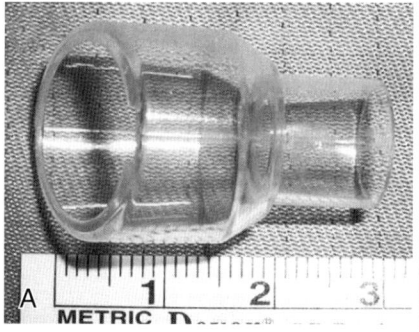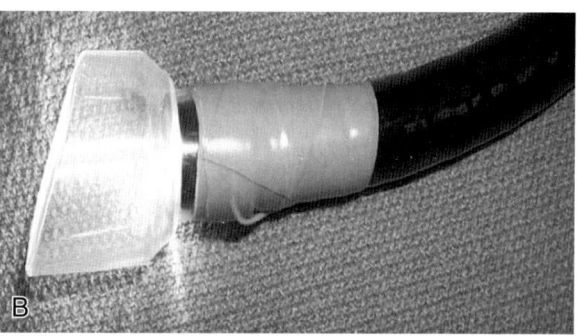

FIGURE 3 Endoscopic mucosal resection cap technique instruments. **A,** Olympus cap. **B,** Cap affixed to the end of a standard flexible endoscope. *(From Watson TJ: Endoscopic resection for Barrett's esophagus with high-grade dysplasia or early esophageal adenocarcinoma, Semin Thorac Cardiovasc Surg 20(4):310–319, 2008, Figure 2).*

propria for patients who are poor surgical candidates or who refuse esophagectomy. Although ESD is one of the gold standards for treatment of early esophageal cancer in Japan, it is not widely available in the United States. Notably, the predominant esophageal neoplasm in Japan is squamous cell carcinoma, whereas the predominant esophageal carcinoma in the United States is adenocarcinoma. All of the reports out of Japan describe ESD for squamous cell carcinoma. Unlike adenocarcinoma, squamous cell carcinoma does not arise from BE and tends to arise in the middle third of the esophagus where the esophagus is tubular and technically more amenable to a complex dissection compared with the esophagogastric junction.

In a prospective study of 102 patients with early squamous cell carcinoma by Oyama and colleagues, ESD was technically successful in resecting the tumor en bloc in 95% of patients with a 6% rate of pneumomediastinum. In 2007, the Japanese Gastroenterological Endoscopy Society reported an impressive 3-year survival rate of 95% for early esophageal squamous cell carcinoma resected with ESD. However, ESD carries a perforation rate as high as 10% compared with 0.6% to 0.5% with EMR. Bleeding and stricture have also been reported with ESD, and it is a time-consuming, technically challenging procedure with a steep learning curve. Also, unlike EMR, which can be performed in an outpatient setting, ESD requires hospitalization after the procedure so the patient can be closely monitored for complications, such as bleeding and perforation, and to slowly advance the diet in a controlled manner.

Endoscopic Submucosal Resection Technique

After surveillance esophagoscopy, the margins of the lesions are marked with electrocautery and the submucosa is injected with 1% hyaluronic acid solution to create a submucosal cushion to lift the lesion. Specialized ESD electrocautery instruments are used to make a circumferential incision around the lesion. The lesion is then carefully dissected from the connective tissue of the submucosa underlying the lesion. Follow-up endoscopy is usually performed after 2 months to assess the healing and to evaluate for recurrence.

SUMMARY

Endoscopic techniques including ablation and EMR have emerged as useful tools for treatment of dysplastic BE. In patients with BE and LGD, screening endoscopy is adequate and no further treatment is necessary. In patients with BE and HGD, RFA, cryotherapy, and EMR are reasonable esophageal-sparing therapies. However, patients with HGD who refuse esophagectomy or have significant comorbidities that preclude surgery must be committed to multiple endoscopies because many of these therapies require several repeat treatment sessions and follow-up examinations. Management of patients with dysplastic BE should be individualized and in collaboration with providers experienced in endoscopy and esophageal surgery.

SUGGESTED READINGS

Fernando HC, Murthy SC, Hofstetter W, et al: The society of thoracic surgeons practice guideline series: guidelines for the management of Barrett's esophagus with high-grade dysplasia, *Ann Thorac Surg* 87:1993–2002, 2009.

Pech O, Behrens A, May A, et al: Long-term results and risk factor analysis for recurrence after curative endoscopic therapy in 349 patients with high-grade intraepithelial neoplasia and mucosal adenocarcinoma in Barrett's oesophagus, *Gut* 57:1200–1206, 2008.

Shaheen NJ, Sharma P, Overholt BF, et al: Radiofrequency ablation in Barrett's esophagus with dysplasia, *N Engl J Med* 360:2277–2288, 2009.

Spechler SJ, Sharma P, Souza RF, et al: American gastroenterological association medical position statement on the management of Barrett's esophagus, *Gastroenterology* 140:1084–1091, 2011.

PARAESOPHAGEAL HERNIA

Benedetto Mungo, MD, Daniela Molena, MD, and Malcolm V. Brock, MD

DEFINITION

The first description of a paraesophageal hernia (PEH) may be attributed to Henry Ingersoll Bowditch. He reported, in 1853, some "dilatation of the esophageal opening" in postmortem assessments, observing that the "esophagus presented a very abrupt change of its course. In all, it descended through the diaphragm as usual but turned back toward the left to enter the abnormal aperture caused by the hernia and to join the stomach in the chest."

It is estimated that the prevalence of hiatal hernias in the population ranges from 10% to 60%, in relation to age.

Sliding hiatal hernias represent more than 95% of all hiatal hernias, while PEHs account for the remaining 5%.

Late-middle-aged and older individuals are more affected by large hiatal hernias compared with younger people (occurrence before age 50 is infrequent); hence, the need for PEH surgery is increasing in the West as the population progressively becomes older.

Hiatal hernias are usually classified into four types.

- Type I, or sliding hiatal hernias, are characterized by the migration of the gastroesophageal junction (GEJ) above the diaphragm, allowed by laxity of the phrenoesophageal ligament, with the contextual creation of a peritoneal sac (Figure 1). This condition results in the typical distortion of the physiologic anatomy of the GEJ, represented by the absence of an adequate portion of intraabdominal esophagus, along with an increasing opening of the angle of His. These hernias can be observed in cases of increased intraabdominal pressure that occurs, for example, in obese or pregnant patients and in patients with constipation.
- True PEHs, or Type II, are the rarest of all hiatal hernias. These are characterized by the intrathoracic migration of the fundus of the stomach alongside the esophagus, while the GEJ remains in the abdomen, below the diaphragm. The combination of anterior weakness in the phrenoesophageal ligament, contextual weakening of the pleuroperitoneal membrane, and enlargement of the esophageal diaphragmatic hiatus may permit the herniation of the fundus and the body of the stomach into the thorax. At the same time, the GEJ stays in its usual intraabdominal location, held in place by the posterolateral attachments of the phrenoesophageal ligaments, which are not altered.
- Type III hiatal hernias represent a combination of sliding hernias and type II hernias and account for the majority of PEHs (Figure 2). In this condition, both the GEJ and the cranial portion of the stomach migrate across the esophageal hiatus of the diaphragm, and the gastric fundus takes its place alongside the esophagus, above the intrathoracic GEJ.
- Type IV PEH occurs when another abdominal organ, such as the spleen, the small intestine, or, more frequently, the colon herniates and joins the stomach in the intrathoracic sac. This is the result of an increased intraabdominal pressure in the presence of a large hiatal defect and abnormal laxity of the gastrosplenic and gastrocolic ligaments (Figure 3). Type IV PEH may or, less frequently, may not be associated with an abnormal location of the GEJ.

The term *giant paraesophageal hernia* is used to describe a hiatal hernia in which 30% or more of the stomach is herniated into the thorax.

The intrathoracic stomach, instead, is the condition in which nearly all of the stomach lies within the chest. If the stomach herniates into the thorax through a defect adjacent to the esophageal

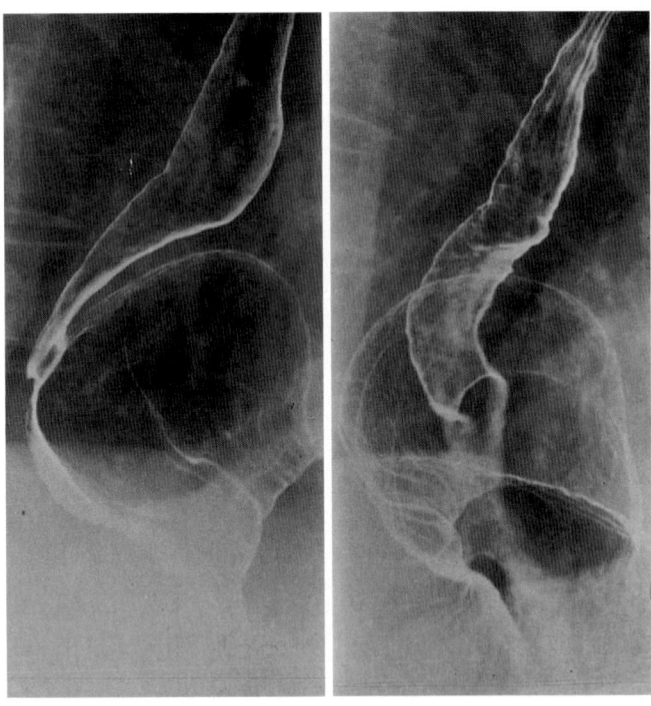

FIGURE 2 Air contrast/barium radiograph showing a type III hiatal hernia. The gastroesophageal junction (GE) has slid above the diaphragm, as in a type I hernia, and the fundus of the stomach is herniated alongside the esophagus above the GEJ, as in a type II hernia.

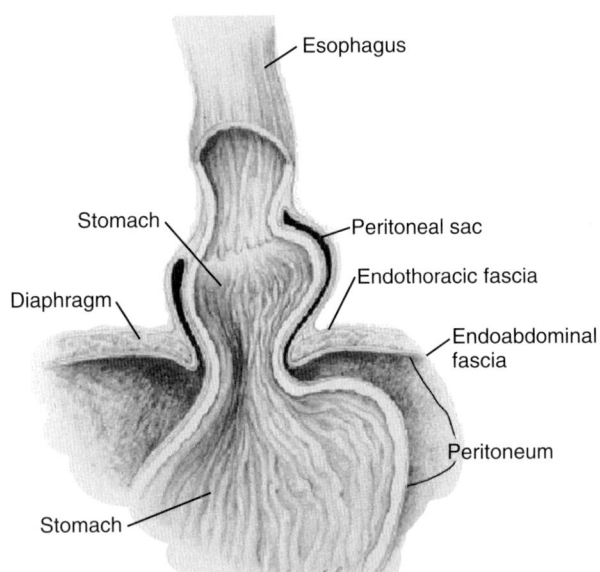

FIGURE 1 Illustration showing a type I. Paraesophageal hernia. *(From Landreneau RF, Del Pino M, Santos R: Management of paraesophageal hernias, Surg Clin North Am 85:411, 2005.)*

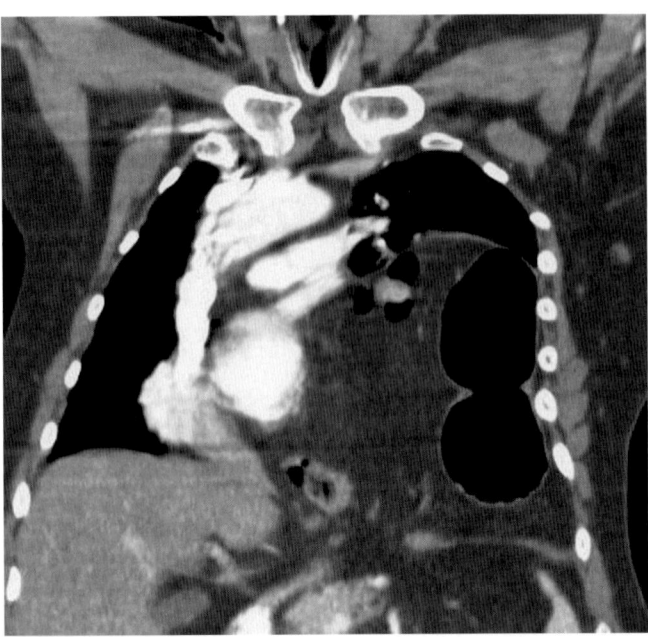

FIGURE 3 Computed tomographic scan showing a type IV giant paraesophageal hernia. The entire stomach and part of the colon and of the small bowel are displaced in the thorax.

hiatus and not through the esophageal hiatus itself, the resulting condition is commonly named *parahiatal hernia* and represents a different and less frequent pathologic entity.

CLINICAL MANIFESTATION

The clinical presentation of a patient with PEH can be heterogeneous. A significant percentage of these patients may be asymptomatic, and the PEH can be an incidental finding in the course of radiographic investigations for another condition.

The patients with PEH may complain of obstructive symptoms, which usually manifest intermittently, related to gastric twisting within the intrathoracic hernia sac. This is due to the upside-down rotational movement that the stomach, attached to the GEJ and the pylorus, is forced to undergo as it ascends into the sac. If the gastric twisting or rotation causes a transient obstruction of the GEJ, the patient experiences acute dysphagia and regurgitation. Obstruction of the distal stomach, on the other hand, may cause gastric distension, which results in nausea, vomiting, palpitation, shortness of breath, dyspnea, chest pain (which often radiates toward the back), and early satiety.

Moreover, after meals, the ingested bolus enters the herniated stomach, causing distension, which results in postprandial fullness and pain that can be confused with angina. The food-related symptoms can cause so much discomfort that the patient may avoid eating altogether; this situation can lead to significant weight loss.

PEH manifests itself not only through obstruction-related symptoms. During the passage of the stomach through the hiatus, the engorged gastric mucosa of the opposing gastric walls may ulcerate, because of repeated friction, and give rise to the so-called Cameron ulcers, which can lead to bleeding and chronic iron-deficiency anemia. This blood loss–related anemia can become symptomatic (pallor, palpitations, exertional dyspnea), but symptoms usually occur in the absence of bleeding, hematemesis, or melena. Type IV PEHs may also show obstructive symptoms that are attributable to other herniated organs, such as the colon or small intestine.

Gastroesophageal reflux disease (GERD) symptoms such as heartburn are sometimes present but are far less common in sliding hernias. In fact, despite the gastric dilation usually found in PEH, the presence of a normal-functioning lower esophageal sphincter prevents reflux and, consequently, esophagitis and esophageal ulceration. If gastric obstruction caused by rotation or twisting fails to resolve, the result is acute gastric volvulus. This represents an emergent condition that can lead to incarceration, strangulation, and gastric ischemia. Occasionally, a gastric volvulus can manifest as conspicuous bleeding, infarction, necrosis, and gastric perforation. A gastric volvulus is a well-known life-threatening complication of PEH, and patients affected by this condition may present with Borchardt's triad, originally described in 1904, which consists of epigastric or chest pain, retching without vomiting, and inability to pass a nasogastric tube (Figure 4).

PATHOPHISIOLOGY

The pathophysiology of hiatal hernias is, to date, not completely understood. There is no dominant pathogenic theory to explain them, and, thus, hiatal hernias are probably caused by a combination of factors such as the following:

- Widening of the esophageal hiatus of the diaphragm due to developmental defects or in response to acquired molecular and cellular changes
- Alterations in collagen metabolism
- Increased intraabdominal pressure and subsequent creation of an abdominal-thoracic pressure gradient
- Esophageal shortening due to fibrosis or excessive vagal nerve stimulation
- Aging-related acquired laxity of the phrenoesophageal membrane

Modifications in the structure of the periesophageal ligaments and of the muscular crura of the diaphragm, due to compromised integrity of muscle fibers and components of the extracellular matrix,

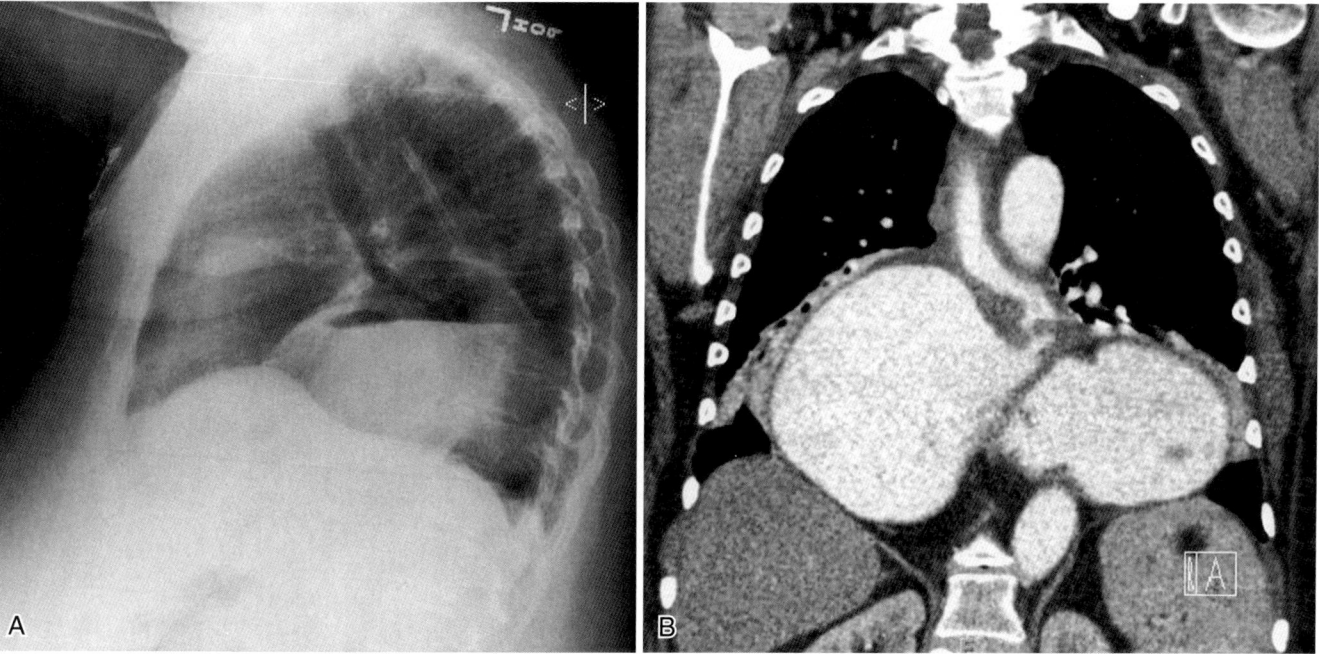

FIGURE 4 Anterolateral chest radiograph **(A)** and computed tomographic (CT) scan **(B)** showing a gastric volvulus in a patient affected by paraesophageal hernia (PEH) with an intrathoracic stomach. A retrocardiac fluid level is evident in the *left* image. The CT scan demonstrates an esophageal tortuosity caused by the thoracic migration of the stomach.

may predispose individuals to the progressive formation of an intrathoracic hernia sac.

Moreover, the increase in intraabdominal pressure promotes the migration of the cranial portions of the stomach into the sac, within the thorax. If the ligaments of the GEJ remain intact, the stomach ascends adjacent to the esophagus through a rotational movement (hence the name "rolling hernia") that creates predisposing conditions for future volvulization. Because of this movement, the stomach may lay upside-down in the mediastinum and exert even further traction on the greater omentum and on other abdominal organs, such as the colon or the spleen. A gastric volvulus is the most common severe complication of PEH and represents one of the most frequent causes of gastric volvulization in the adult population.

There are three ways the stomach can rotate to give rise to a gastric volvulus: organoaxial rotation, mesenteroaxial rotation, and combined rotation. In an organoaxial gastric volvulus, the most frequent type (approximately 60% of cases), the stomach rotates horizontally around an axis passing through the GEJ and the pylorus, while the antrum rotates in an opposite direction to the fundus.

In a mesenteroaxial gastric volvulus, the stomach rotates vertically so that the posterior surface of the stomach progressively brings itself anteriorly (Figure 5). This rotation is less frequent, occurs intermittently, and is usually incomplete. Accordingly, vascular compromise is less frequent compared with organoaxial volvulus. When the stomach rotates both mesenteroaxially and organoaxially, it is called a combined gastric volvulus; this type of stomach rotation is rare.

Diagnosis

Physical examination often provides poor clues to the diagnosis, leaving radiology and flexible endoscopy to play the central role in the diagnostic process. PEHs are sometimes found incidentally on routine chest radiographs, and they appear as a shadow in the posterior mediastinum or as a retrocardiac mass with or without an air-fluid level. The latter is often suggestive of gastric volvulus (see Figure 4). Barium contrast fluoroscopy of the upper gastrointestinal tract is one of the most important diagnostic tools in PEH. Not only can it show the presence of PEH in almost all patients, but it can provide precious information on the anatomy of the hernia, orientation of the stomach (as well as its relationship to the esophagus), and location of the GEJ.

Although it is difficult, except in obvious cases, to diagnose the so-called short esophagus with contrast fluoroscopy, the latter is helpful in identifying patients at risk of having this condition. Finally, barium contrast studies can help to select patients with esophageal motor dysfunction (uncoordinated contractility of the esophageal body and poor esophageal clearance of contrast) who should undergo a manometric study.

Upper endoscopy should also be used in patients with PEH, since it allows assessment of the intrathoracic stomach, the presence of Cameron ulcers, and the ability to evaluate the degree of esophageal mucosal inflammation, gastritis, gastric mucosal venous engorgement, stricture, and other associated pathologies such as Barrett's esophagus and cancer (Figure 6). If esophageal dysmotility is suspected, a preoperatory manometric assessment is recommended.

Esophageal manometry or, if possible, high-resolution manometry (HRM), can provide useful information on intraluminal pressure, lower esophageal sphincter function, and coordinated contractile movements of the esophagus. These findings are important in guiding the surgeon to choose the most suitable antireflux procedure for each patient. In cases of severely impaired peristalsis, a partial fundoplication is preferred to a 360-degree fundoplication, because it reduces the risk of postoperative dysphagia. However, manometric probe placement in PEH patients can be difficult; therefore, the study is not always performed. A 24- to 48-hour pH test is not routinely needed because it does not change the surgical management.

Finally, in selected patients, computed tomographic (CT) scan may be useful as a second-level exam to assess the widening of the esophageal hiatus, PEH size, content and position, and orientation of the herniated stomach.

■ THERAPY

Indications for Surgery

There is unanimous agreement among surgeons that symptomatic hernias require surgery as the mainstay of therapy. On the contrary, the management of asymptomatic or mildly symptomatic patients remains controversial. A well-known probabilistic model, built to evaluate the risks versus benefits of elective repair of asymptomatic large paraesophageal hiatus hernia, determined that the risk of elective repair exceeded any benefits in otherwise asymptomatic patients aged 65 years or older. At the same time, the results of emergent surgery for acute PEH have improved through the years. Therefore, we prefer a conservative approach and suggest "watchful waiting" for asymptomatic, or minimally symptomatic patients. This is especially true for elderly patients with many comorbidities.

FIGURE 5 The two ways that the stomach can rotate when a volvulus occurs.

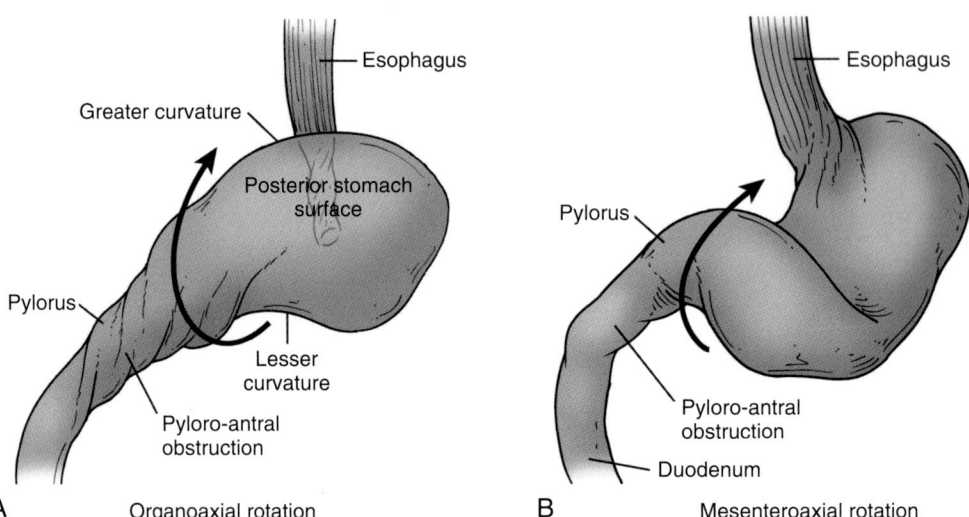

A   Organoaxial rotation

B   Mesenteroaxial rotation

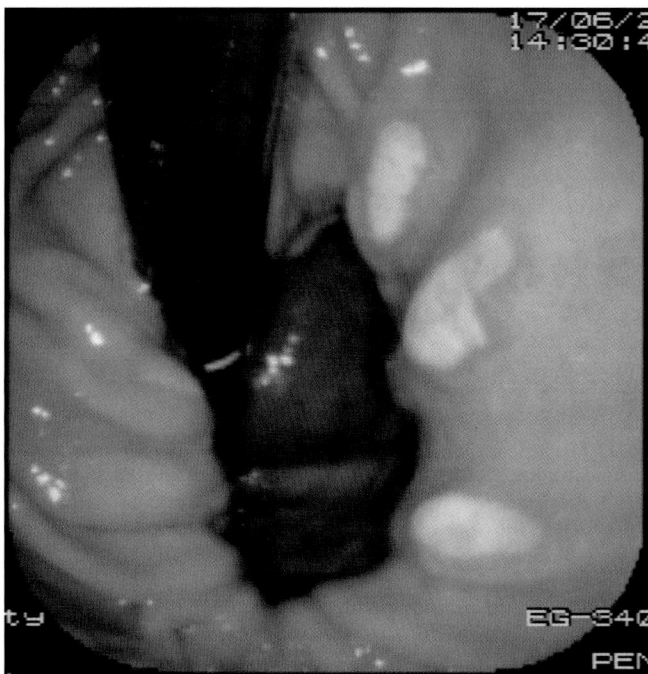

FIGURE 6 Endoscopic view of Cameron ulcers. The endoscopic maneuver of retroversion shows the ascension of the stomach through the esophageal hiatus of the diaphragm. *(From Muller U, Schachschal G, Voderholzer WA: Image of the month. Cameron ulcers,* Gastroenterology *129(1):7, 399, 2005. http://www.ncbi.nlm.nih.gov/pubmed/16012929#.)*

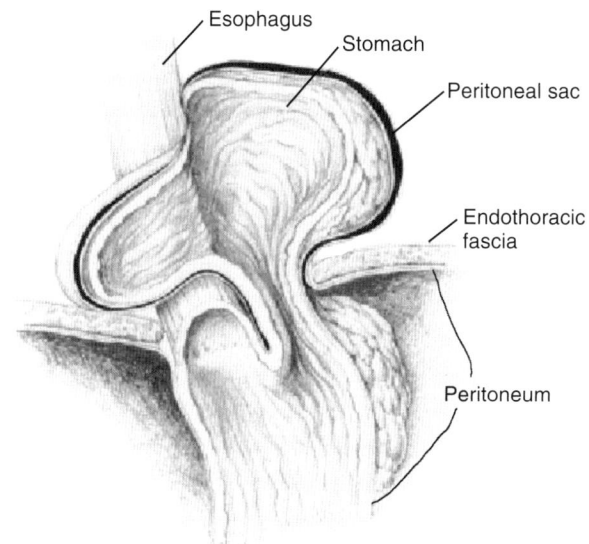

FIGURE 7 View of the gastroesophageal junction (GEJ) region in a type II paraesophageal hernia (PEH). *(From Landreneau RF, Del Pino M, Santos R: Management of paraesophageal hernias,* Surg Clin North Am *85:411, 2005.)*

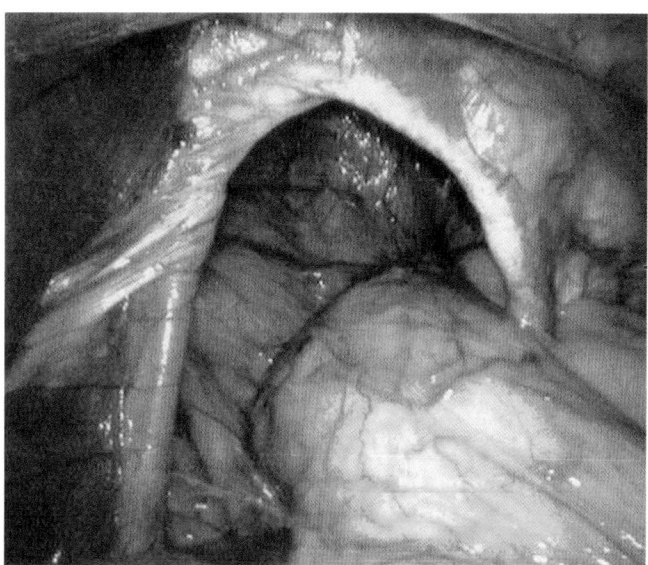

FIGURE 8 A laparoscopic view of an enlarged esophageal hiatus.

Surgical Anatomy

The esophagus enters the abdominal cavity through the diaphragmatic hiatus, whose borders are formed by the arms of the diaphragmatic crura and the median arcuate ligament (Figure 7). The esophageal hiatus is therefore a muscular structure, composed mainly of fibers belonging to the right crus, and its pliability makes it susceptible to visceral herniation. The anterior part of the crura is more tendinous and although anterior crural repair is technically easier and may seem a good choice, this technique leads to kinking of the esophagus that may cause dysphagia.

In the course of surgical repair, particular attention must be paid not to compromise crural integrity during sac dissection, in order to prevent recurrences. When performing surgical procedures on the esophageal hiatus, it is mandatory to recognize and preserve the contiguous structures, which could be accidentally injured. The anterior and posterior vagal trunks cross the hiatus along the esophagus, together with the esophageal branches of the left gastric artery and vein, and some lymphatic vessels.

The thoracic duct, the celiac ganglia, the phrenic artery and vein, the mediastinal pleura, and an inconstant aberrant left hepatic artery lie close to the hiatus and should also be preserved.

The phrenoesophageal ligament, or Laimer's membrane, is an elastic connective tissue membrane that ensures the proximity between the diaphragm and the esophagus, permitting, however, some vertical sliding of the latter.

An anterior weakness in Laimer's membrane, together with a contextual weakening of the pleuroperitoneal membrane and the enlargement of the esophageal diaphragmatic hiatus, may permit the herniation of the fundus and the body of the stomach into the thorax, alongside the esophagus (Figure 8).

There is usually a fat pad surrounding the GEJ, which should be dissected carefully during the course of a PEH repair to enhance visualization and mobilization. One of the anatomic structures that maintains the location of the GEJ is the mesoesophagus, a dense fibrous cellular tissue, included in the posterior gap between the peritoneal leaflets interposed between the esophagus, the aorta, and the diaphragmatic pillars.

The mesoesophagus is prolonged inferiorly by the gastrophrenic ligament, whose dissection is necessary when the gastric fundus is mobilized to strengthen the fundoplication.

Surgical Approach

After an informed consent is obtained, the patient is taken to the operating room, accurately positioned, and given antithrombotic and antibiotic prophylaxis. We usually operate with the patient in reverse Trendelenburg, with the surgeon on the patient's right side and the assistant on the left. We use a 12-mm Visiport trocar (Covidien, Mansfield, Mass) to enter the abdominal cavity with a 0-degree scope, insufflation to a pressure of 15 mm Hg and using a camera angled to 45 degrees. A thorough exploration of the peritoneal cavity is performed. A second 12-mm port is placed in the midline, at about 15 cm from the xyphoid process; this port is used for the camera. A camera holder is used for assistance. A 12-mm trocar and a 5-mm trocar are placed in the right upper quadrant, as showed in Figure 9, and both are used by the surgeon. An additional 5-mm trocar is placed in the left upper quadrant and is used by the assistant. After positioning the patient in steep reversed Trendelenburg, a Nathanson liver retractor is placed through a small subxyphoid incision to hold the liver in place. The important steps of the operation are listed below.

Excision of the Hernia Sac

To begin the dissection of the hernia sac, the displaced organs should be carefully reduced, as far as possible, into the abdominal cavity. It is important that the traction should be placed on the hernia sac and not on the stomach, which could be inadvertently injured. A Penrose drain is used around the stomach or the esophagus to facilitate dissection. The complete reduction of the herniated organs can be achieved only by dissecting the sac off the mediastinum. It is important to remain in the correct avascular plane during the dissection, in order to avoid injury to intrathoracic structures that may have been displaced by the hernia. Once reduced into the abdomen, the sac can be excised, accurately preserving the vagal nerves. The complete sac dissection and excision and respect for the crural integrity are crucial for a successful and long lasting repair. If this procedure is carried out correctly and the surgical handling of the crura is

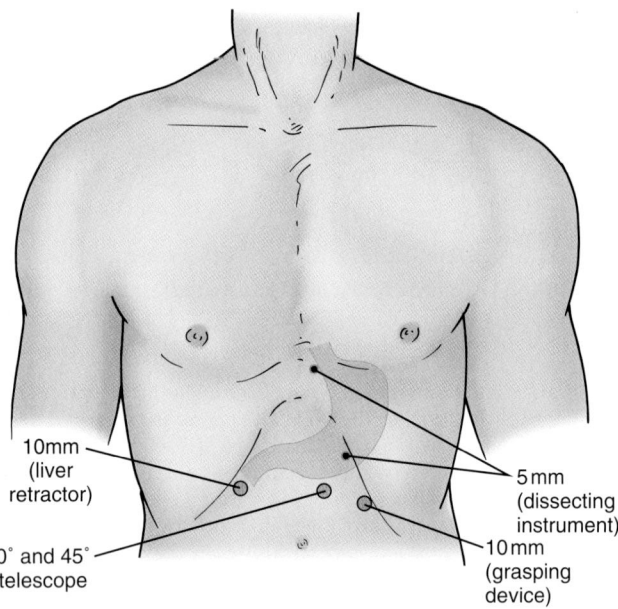

FIGURE 9   Port placement for paraesophageal hernia (PEH) repair. The *red* spot is the camera, the *green* one the liver retractor, and the *blue* spots the operative trocars. *(Modified from Landreneau RF, Del Pino M, Santos R: Management of paraesophageal hernias,* Surg Clin North Am *85:411, 2005.)*

10mm (liver retractor)

0° and 45° telescope

5mm (dissecting instrument)

10mm (grasping device)

minimized, no muscular fibers should be visible, at a glance, on the crural surface.

Assessment of Adequate Intraabdominal Esophageal Length and Management of a Short Esophagus

The preoperative diagnosis of short esophagus is unpredictable and therefore the surgeon must rely on the intraoperative assessment. If at least 2.5 to 3 cm of distal esophagus can be surgically mobilized into the abdomen without tension, no further esophageal lengthening procedures are required. We prefer to dissect the gastric fat pad off the GEJ to enhance visualization of the GEJ and more accurately evaluate the esophageal length by direct visualization of the serosal lining of the cardia. This will also facilitate the creation of a window between the esophagus and the posterior vagus nerve where the stomach will be passed to create the fundoplication. We then divide the short gastric vessels completely to allow full mobilization of the gastric fundus. This will allow constructing a tension-free wrap and, in addition, will provide a useful landmark for keeping the fundoplication correctly oriented. To gain an adequate intraabdominal esophageal length, we perform an extended mediastinal dissection up to the level of the inferior pulmonary veins. A Collis gastroplasty is needed when the esophageal intraabdominal length is not satisfactory despite extensive mobilization. In this case, our preferred technique is a laparoscopic wedge Collis gastroplasty with Endo GIA stapler (Covidien, Mansfield, Mass) over a 52F or 54F bougie (see Collis Gastroplasty in the next section for more details).

Creating the Antireflux Barrier

The esophageal dissection and the disruption of the phrenoesophageal ligament predispose to the onset of GERD symptoms. The creation of a gastric fundoplication protects the esophagus from reflux and, at the same time, represents a method of fixation for the stomach to prevent reherniation.

We usually rely on the results of barium swallow and, occasionally, esophageal manometry to choose the most suitable fundoplication for each patient: in case of severely impaired peristalsis, a partial posterior fundoplication is preferred to a complete wrap. The wrap is created around a 54F or 56F bougie carefully inserted into the esophagus under direct vision. The anterior fundic lip is pulled through the window previously created behind the GEJ, and the surgeon must pay attention to maintain the correct anteroposterior orientation so that the anterior aspect of the stomach would lie against the posterior side of the esophagus. We use three nonabsorbable stitches for a Nissen fundoplication, only the proximal one of them including the esophageal muscle; in a Toupet fundoplication the gastric valves are sutured to each side of the esophagus with one row of three nonabsorbable stitches, the proximal stitch including the diaphragm. If the tension of the wrap has been calibrated correctly, after removal of the bougie, there should be room for a blunt instrument to be inserted easily between the stomach and esophagus.

Repairing the Hiatus

To obtain a tension-free crural closure, we perform a meticulous dissection of all crural attachments with contextual sparing of the crural peritoneal lining and of the pleural reflection. We usually perform a primary tension-free posterior closure of the hiatus with nonabsorbable 0 stitches. In the presence of a very wide hiatal opening, we consider placing additional anterior interrupted stitches, always paying attention not to induce an iatrogenic kinking of the distal esophagus.

We do not routinely buttress the primary closure with a mesh or use pledgeted sutures. In selected cases, in the presence of weak crural muscle or when there is not a tension-free crural reapproximation, we reinforce the hiatal closure by placing a biologic mesh as an onlay to buttress the underlying suture. The mesh is sutured at the corners with 2-0 absorbable stitches and then glued to the crural surface using fibrin glue.

Gastropexy

An anterior gastropexy is routinely performed to decrease recurrence. The pneumoperitoneum is reduced to 8 mm Hg. Two nonabsorbable 0 stitches are placed into the anterior stomach wall and secured to the left anterior abdominal wall with the help of a Carter-Thompson suture passer (Box 1).

INSIGHTS AND CONTROVERSIES IN PARAESOPHAGEAL HERNIA SURGERY

Surgical Management of Acute Paraesophageal Hernia

Acute PEH can present as a potentially life-threatening surgical emergency. Even asymptomatic patients with PEH may be subject to this

---

BOX 1: Technical pearls

- Operate with the patient in the **supine position**, in **reverse Trendelenburg,** to improve visualization and accessibility of the hiatal area.
- Place **traction on the hernia sac** and not on the stomach while trying to reduce the organs into the abdomen.
- Use a **Penrose drain** around the stomach or the esophagus to facilitate dissection.
- Remain in the correct **avascular plane** during the sac dissection.
- Respect the **crural integrity** and the **crural peritoneal** lining during dissection.
- **Dissect the gastric fat pad** and **preserve the vagus nerves.**
- Be sure to **gain** at least **2.5 to 3 cm of tension-free** distal **esophagus** into the abdomen.
- Perform an **extended mediastinal dissection** to lengthen the esophagus and only use Collis gastroplasty as a last resort.
- Create a window between the esophagus and the posterior vagus nerve for the fundoplication.
- Divide the short gastric vessels completely.
- Rely on the results of **barium swallow and esophageal manometry** to choose the most suitable fundoplication.
- Construct the wrap around a **54F or 56F** intraesophageal **bougie.**
- Pay attention to the **correct anteroposterior orientation** of the fundic lip.
- Perform a **primary tension-free posterior closure** of the hiatus with nonabsorbable stitches.
- Use additional anterior interrupted stitches only in the presence of a very wide hiatal opening.
- Use biologic mesh only for selected cases, fixing it with cardinal stitches and glue.
- Add an **anterior gastropexy** to secure the stomach within the abdomen.

---

dreadful condition, usually presenting with sudden chest or abdominal pain, dysphagia, vomiting, retching, severe bleeding due to mucosal venous engorgement, and severe anemia. This may happen when the gastric twisting causing obstruction fails to resolve and, on the contrary, evolves into a gastric volvulus, which can lead to strangulation, gastric ischemia, and gastric rupture. This unfortunate evolution can be so rapid that the patient can present on admission with respiratory failure or systemic sepsis.

In patients presenting with acute symptoms, nasogastric tube decompression of the stomach should always be attempted. If successful, this maneuver, together with appropriate and prompt fluid resuscitation, can preempt emergent surgery and provide time to perform better preoperative studies, allow patient stabilization, and permit more elective laparoscopic repair.

If nasogastric tube decompression fails or if the condition has already evolved to include serious gastric ischemia or gastric perforation, emergent surgery, traditionally performed with an open approach, either through the abdomen or chest, should be considered.

In selected patients, emergent laparoscopic repair of PEH can be safe and feasible.

Laparoscopic Versus Open

Both laparoscopic and laparotomic surgical repair have good symptomatic results and similar recurrence rates. Open surgery for PEH can be performed through an abdominal or a thoracic approach. Similar results have been described with both techniques even if some small differences have emerged. Recurrences are slightly less frequent in transthoracic approaches, but significant postoperative pain and morbidity are less represented with the transabdominal approach. Moreover, the finding of a "short esophagus" is more common in the transthoracic approach (maybe suggesting a technique-related bias); therefore, more esophageal lengthening procedures are carried out with consequent enhanced risk of staple line leak.

There is documented evidence that patients who underwent laparoscopic surgery have better scores in quality-of-life measures. In addition, laparoscopic surgery has the advantage of ensuring reduced morbidity, shorter hospital stay, and faster recovery, particularly in the elderly and patients with comorbidities. Currently, laparoscopic repair of PEHs has reported mortality rates ranging from 0.3% to 0.5%, versus 2% with open surgery. The median length of stay after open PEH repair is 7 to 10 days, and the overall morbidity is reported to be approximately 20%. In comparison, the median length of stay after laparoscopy is 3 days, and postoperative complication rates are reported to range between 0 and 15%.

In addition, technical advantages have been attributed to laparoscopy, such as better visualization of the hiatal region and easier esophageal mobilization in the mediastinum.

These data suggest that laparoscopic repair should be considered, when possible, the first choice for surgical treatment of PEH.

Open surgery for PEH still plays an important role in an emergency context, in cases of contraindications to pneumoperitoneum, and for those patients who have had multiple previous repairs. However, it is not to be forgotten that laparoscopy for PEH is challenging and should be performed by surgeons who are experienced in antireflux surgery and technically skilled in minimally invasive surgical approaches.

A Novel Approach: Robotic-Assisted Surgery

Robotic-assisted surgery (RAS) represents a novel approach to PEH repair that could be advantageous for the surgeon, especially during the most challenging cases. According to a few recent studies, RAS may prove useful in overcoming some well-known pitfalls of traditional laparoscopic PEH repair, such as an unstable video camera platform, physiologic tremor, limited motion of straight laparoscopic instruments, two-dimensional imaging, and poor ergonomics for the surgeon. Some potential advantages of RAS are a better degree of freedom of the robotic instruments, hand-like motions of the instruments, and three-dimensional visualization with depth perception and magnification effect.

In the course of surgery for PEH, the robotic system has proven to be particularly useful in situations when movements are limited by fixed anatomic structures, such as through the narrow hiatus or in the case of an upside-down stomach. Moreover, thanks to the articulated robotic tools, there has been a remarkable improvement in intracorporeal suturing, in tying knots, and in allowing an easier dissection of the fundus. Finally, the intraoperative blood loss is reported to be lower and the learning curve for the surgeon to be shorter than in traditional laparoscopic surgery. However, RAS isn't flawless. The loss of tactile feedback, for example, could make knot tightening with the proper force challenging and increase the risk of damage to nearby structures. Finally, it must be remembered that RAS is very expensive, and this could constitute a limitation to its widespread adaptation.

"To Mesh or Not to Mesh?"

The use of prosthetic mesh for PEH repair is still debated. The most common use of mesh is for reinforcement of the hiatal closure by placing the mesh as an onlay to buttress the underlying suture. In the literature, however, mesh has been used in a bridging fashion to tailor and narrow the esophageal hiatus, especially in the case of a marked crural defect, or to cover a lateral relaxing diaphragmatic incision made to allow a tension-free primary closure of the crura. The prosthesis can be fixed to the crura by means of absorbable or nonabsorbable sutures, tacks, or glue.

Many different types of meshes have been employed for PEH surgery, including the following:

- Synthetic nonabsorbable meshes (polypropylene, Gore-Tex polytetrafluoroethylene [W. L. Gore & Associates, Flagstaff, Ariz], polyester)
- Synthetic absorbable meshes (polyglactin)
- Bioprosthetic meshes (porcine small intestinal submucosa, acellular human dermis)

The claimed advantage to using mesh is the reduction of the recurrence rate as supported by the analysis of numerous published series. Nevertheless, the placement of a prosthesis close to the esophagus unquestionably carries a burden of risks: mesh erosion into the esophageal lumen, fibrosis of the hiatus leading to progressive stenosis and consequent dysphagia, esophageal obstruction, fistulization or perforation, and foreign body reactions.

These complications are not to be underestimated, because they can be life threatening and/or require further drastic measures like esophagogastrectomy or esophagectomy. These consequences have progressively led to the abandonment of permanent meshes for PEH surgery.

Biologic meshes, thanks to their capability of being progressively colonized and replaced by autologous tissue, may help surgeons avoid these dreadful complications and are still considered helpful adjuncts to esophageal hiatus surgery. Animal studies and a wide experience in surgery for abdominal wall defect repair show that biologic meshes may ensure adequate tensile strength and, at the same time, form minimal adhesions. Furthermore, they are more resistant to infections and induce less fibrosis compared with synthetic meshes.

A multicenter prospective randomized study showed that a biologic mesh–buttressed repair significantly decreased recurrence rates at 6 months. However, the long-term 5-year follow-up from the same study showed the recurrence rate to be about 50% for both buttressed and nonbuttressed PEH repairs.

In conclusion, surgeons should knowingly balance the risk of complications and the possible reduction in recurrence rate before making their choice.

Collis Gastroplasty

A shortened esophagus may jeopardize optimal outcome for PEH surgery, increasing the risk of recurrence by placing excessive axial tension on the repair. It is believed that the acquired shortening of the esophagus is caused by repeated acid-related damage against the lower esophageal wall. The subsequent injury and repetitive healing leads to fibrotic remodeling (in particular, affecting the outer longitudinal muscle) that progressively causes contracture and shortening of the esophagus. While a severely shortened esophagus is detectable by contrast fluoroscopy, less obvious shortening is often a subjective intraoperative diagnosis. Predictors of esophageal shortening have been proposed, such as the endoscopic finding of esophageal stricture, but there is no unanimous consensus on how to define a shortened esophagus preoperatively. Moreover, the overall concept of a short esophagus is controversial, and the number of lengthening procedures performed reflects the orientation of each surgical school ranging between 0 and more than 50%.

Collis gastroplasty has been reported to decrease recurrence rates in several published series (Figure 10). However, this procedure is associated with a small but significant risk of staple-line leakage and therefore adds morbidity and mortality to PEH repair. Moreover, the results of Collis gastroplasty have not been studied. Although the procedure is claimed to have similar results to a Nissen

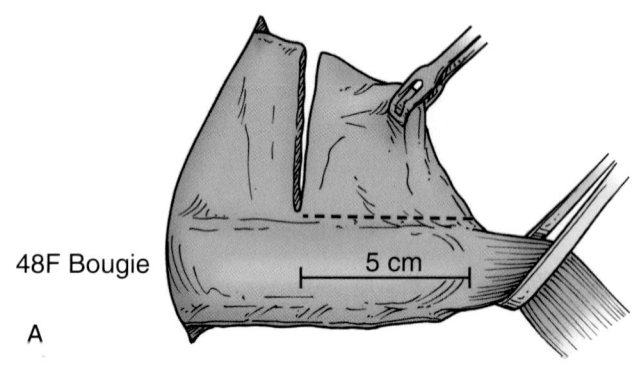

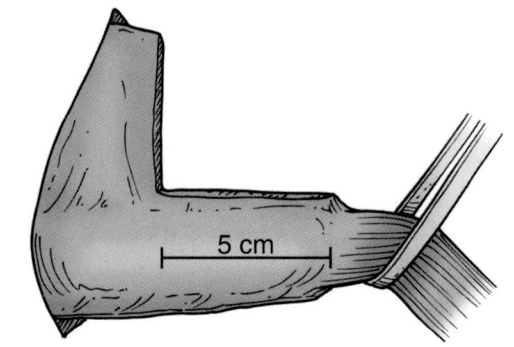

FIGURE 10 A laparoscopic Collis gastroplasty. **A,** The stomach is divided with an Endo GIA from the greater curvature down to a 52F or 54F bougie placed along the lesser curvature and 5 cm from the gastroesophageal junction (GEJ). **B,** A wedge of stomach is removed by dividing the stomach with an Endo GIA along the bougie up to the GEJ. This usually requires that the Endo GIA is placed through the left lateral flank port. The remaining fundus and body of the stomach are advanced cephalad to form the fundoplication around the newly constructed gastroplasty tube.

48F Bougie   5 cm

A

5 cm

B

fundoplication, problems with dysphagia and poor control of GERD have been reported. This is usually because the fundoplication was constructed too inferiorly, often below a portion of aperistaltic stomach or neoesophagus, which maintains its secretory properties. Therefore, balancing the risks and benefits of a Collis should be considered before performing this procedure.

Antireflux Procedure

The choice of adding or not adding an antireflux procedure to the surgical repair of PEH represents another controversial surgical decision. If the majority of surgeons agree that constructing a fundoplication is recommended for those patients with PEH affected by reflux symptoms, the addition of this procedure in absence of such symptoms often remains a subjective choice. Those who always choose to perform a fundoplication advocate that it could be useful to place an intraabdominal buttress, which may help, together with the crural closure, to prevent reherniation of the stomach. Moreover, it could help prevent the future onset of reflux symptoms in patients in which further hiatal surgery would be challenging.

Those who do not routinely perform a fundoplication in asymptomatic or in minimally symptomatic patients assert, on the contrary, that the side effects of a fundoplication overwhelm the possible reduction in recurrence rates.

We prefer to add a fundoplication to our PEH repairs not only to improve gastric fixation below the diaphragm but also to treat GERD, which is often present and underestimated (Figure 11). Furthermore, the extensive esophageal dissection and mobilization during the repair destroys the phrenoesophageal attachments and places patients at a high risk for GERD postoperatively.

The decision about the use of a partial versus a complete wrap is made by carefully evaluating esophageal peristalsis. The first carries a lower risk of postoperative dysphagia but is less effective and less durable against reflux symptoms. The use of a barium swallow evaluation and, in selected cases, esophageal manometry helps the surgeon choose the most suitable antireflux procedure for each patient. In the case of severely impaired peristalsis, a partial fundoplication is preferred to a Nissen procedure to reduce the risk of postoperative dysphagia.

RESULTS

Although PEH repairs are technically challenging, the perioperative morbidity is low and the short- and long-term results are encouraging. Among the most frequent complications, traumatic visceral injury is reported in as many as 4% to 10% of the patients. It is thought to be due to either improper surgical tissue handling or traumatic bougie insertion. However, in many cases, a trained laparoscopist can manage these events intraoperatively, with little impact on the final result of the operation. Delayed perforations, either due to missed intraoperative injury or ischemic necrosis, will almost inevitably require revisional surgery. Other reported complications include vagus nerve injury, which is likely to cause delayed gastric emptying; pneumothorax due to pleural violation during mediastinal dissection; and complications such as pneumonia, respiratory distress, and myocardial infarction, which are more often observed in elderly patients.

The long-term symptomatic outcome of repair of PEH is very good, with reported success rates ranging from 80% to 90%, depending on the series.

Anatomic and radiologic recurrences, detected through videoesophagram or upper endoscopy, are higher than clinically symptomatic recurrences and may occur in more than 50% of PEH surgical repairs. Most radiologic hernia recurrences after PEH repair are asymptomatic or minimally symptomatic and follow a benign course, requiring no further therapy, and only 3% to 5% of patients develop large recurrent PEH with significant symptoms requiring revisional surgery.

It is believed that many factors contribute to a predisposition to recurrence, including tension on the crural repair, short esophagus, large hiatal defects, attenuated crural muscle fibers, inadequate mobilization of the esophagus, and inappropriate diaphragmatic stressors in the early postoperative period, such as vomiting and retching. Recurrences usually occur in the early postoperative period and are

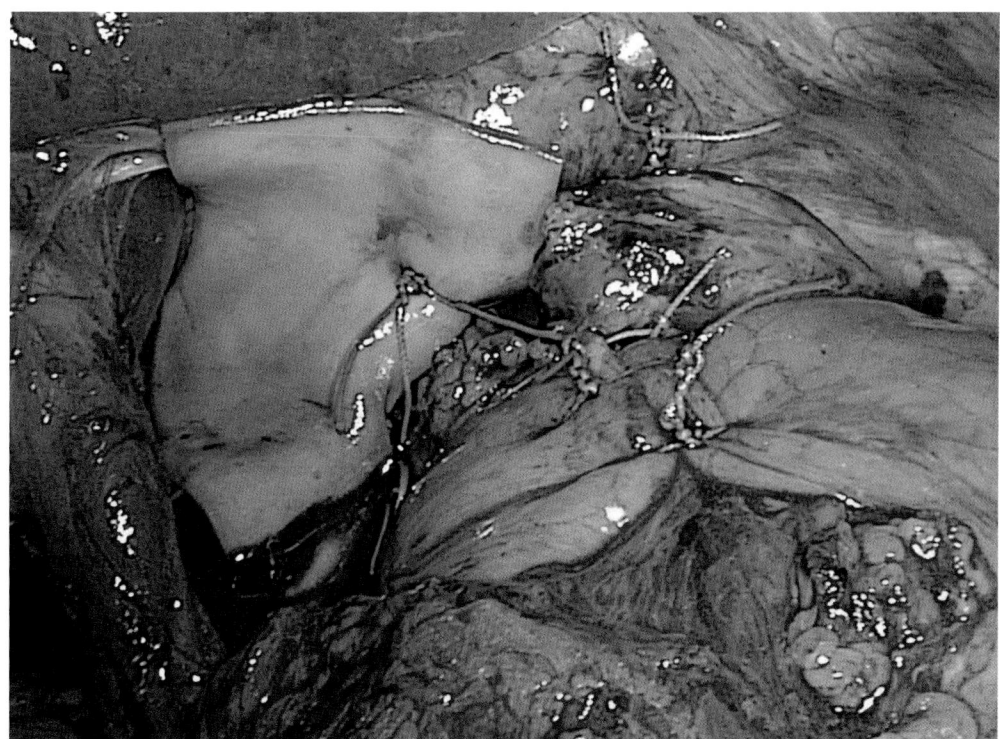

FIGURE 11 A laparoscopic view of a Nissen fundoplication. A biologic mesh–buttressed hiatal closure is visible as well.

often represented by intrathoracic migration of the fundoplication, when present, or wrap disruption with recurrent herniation.

It has been also postulated that recurrent PEHs have a lower risk of evolving into a gastric volvulus. This is probably due to the presence of adhesions in the hiatal area and around the upper stomach that prevent the stomach from rotating and twisting within the new hernia sac.

SUMMARY

PEHs are far less common than type I hiatal hernias, but they can lead to dreadful complications. They are probably caused by a synergic effect of increasing abdominal pressure and weakening of the ligamentous structures of the GEJ region.

Rarely symptomatic, PEHs can commonly manifest through obstruction-related symptoms, GERD-related symptoms or complications, bleeding, or arrhythmias. Evaluation with endoscopy, videoesophagram, and occasionally esophageal manometry should be considered in choosing the correct surgical procedure.

The gold standard treatment for PEH is laparoscopic repair following some key steps:

1. Excision of the hernia sac
2. Assessment of adequate intraabdominal esophageal length and management of a shortened esophagus
3. Repair of the hiatal defect
4. Gastric fixation and antireflux barrier

There are numerous controversies concerning selected topics in PEH repair, and the surgeon should have a deep knowledge of this subject, in order to make the best choice for every patient.

Finally, the results of laparoscopic PEH repair are very good, but laparoscopy for PEH is challenging and should be performed by surgeons who are experienced in antireflux surgery and technically skilled in minimally invasive surgical approaches.

SUGGESTED READINGS

Dean C, Etienne D, Carpentier B, et al: Hiatal hernias, *Surg Radiol Anat* 34(4):291–299, 2012.
Landreneau RJ, Del Pino M, Santos R: Management of paraesophageal hernias, *Surg Clin North Am* 85(3):411–432, 2005.
Nason KS, Luketich JD, Witteman BP, et al: The laparoscopic approach to paraesophageal hernia repair, *J Gastrointest Surg* 16(2):417–426, 2012.
Scott Davis SJ: Current controversies in paraesophageal hernia repair, *Surg Clin North Am* 88:959–978, 2008.
Watson DI: Evolution and development of surgery for large paraesophageal hiatus hernia, *World J Surg* 35:1436–1441, 2011.

THE MANAGEMENT OF PHARYNGEAL ESOPHAGEAL (ZENKER'S) DIVERTICULA

Richard F. Heitmiller, MD, FACS

INTRODUCTION

Pharyngeal esophageal diverticula, more commonly referred to as Zenker's diverticula, are uncommon, benign, easy to diagnose, and safe to treat regardless of patient age. The three types of esophageal diverticula are Zenker's (upper), parabronchial (middle), and epiphrenic (lower). Zenker's is the most common type, accounting for almost two thirds of esophageal diverticula. In addition to anatomic location, diverticula are also classified by their etiology as pulsion (Zenker's and epiphrenic) and traction (parabronchial) types. This classification underscores diverticular etiology and factors into the rationale for specific surgical repair methods.

A Zenker's diverticulum is a posterior, midline outpouching of pharyngeal mucosa, just proximal to the cricopharyngeal muscle through an area of anatomic weakness known as Killian's triangle. It is therefore actually a preesophageal diverticulum. It is also a false diverticulum because only the mucosa herniates, not all layers of the bowel wall. Zenker's diverticula are uncommon, although undoubtedly many result in minimal symptoms and are never discovered. They are diagnosed in patients over a very large age range that spans from 30 years to well above 90 years. They are most prevalent in patients in the 6th decade of life. Zenker's diverticulum is more common in males than in females by a ratio of approximately 3:1 (Table 1).

HISTORY

Historically, symptomatic Zenker's diverticulum was a serious disease process that often resulted in death from malnutrition, aspiration pneumonia, or both. In 1877, Zenker and von Ziemsen described the postmortem findings in 34 patients with pharyngeal esophageal diverticula, proposed their etiology, and correlated the anatomic findings with patient symptoms. It was the correlation of anatomic findings to clinical symptoms that established Zenker's name as the moniker for this disease process. Their detailed findings are as specific and relevant today as they were then. They also are credited with classifying esophageal diverticula into pulsion and traction types. However, the ability to diagnose diverticula preceded the ability to treat them. As Zenker and von Ziemsen wrote, "the radical cure of diverticula by operative procedure from without is at the present time one of our vain wishes . . ." Initial attempts to treat patients by instilling caustic fluids into the diverticulum led to disastrous outcomes, including aspiration pneumonia, leakage with mediastinitis, and death. Early open repairs fared no better. The first successful open surgical repair is credited to Wheeler in Dublin (1885), and the first successful repair in the United States is credited to Mixter in Boston (1895). These early repairs were heroic surgeries with long hospital stays. Currently, surgical repair can be performed quickly and safely with short lengths of stay and excellent results.

ETIOLOGY

A Zenker's diverticulum is a benign, acquired abnormality that is either slow in development or delayed in onset, which leads to patients presenting most commonly between ages 50 and 80 years. A great deal has been published on the pathophysiology of Zenker's. The characteristic mucosal outpouching is thought to develop as a result of an imbalance between pressure developed by posterior pharyngeal muscular contraction and weakness of the mucosa in Killian's triangle. Either hypertensive upper esophageal sphincter (UES), or

TABLE 1: Zenker's diverticulum: Summary

Age (y)	Mean: 68; range, 30-90
Gender (male : female)	3 : 1
Symptoms	Dysphagia Regurgitation Cough Choking episodes Globus sensation
Diagnosis	Contrast esophagogram Video esophagography preferred
Surgical options	Open diverticulectomy with CP myotomy Diverticular suspension with CP myotomy Transoral stapled (vs laser or harmonic scalpel) diverticulectomy
Open surgery results	Mortality: 0 to 2% Complications: 4% to 10% Functional result (good or better): 75% to 99% Recurrence: 3%

CP, Cricopharyngeal.

one that relaxes in a poorly coordinated fashion, have been cited as causes of pharyngeal high pressure. Whether these diverticula arise more from high pressure, intrinsic wall weakness, or a combination is unclear.

Jones states in her comprehensive text that "In our experience, almost all patients with Zenker's diverticulum have esophageal disorders such as gastroesophageal reflux, segmental spasm, acid-induced spasm, hiatal hernia, or Schatzi's ring." Therefore, the data suggest that a Zenker's diverticulum is rarely a truly isolated esophageal disorder.

Documented cases are found of posterior pharyngeal mucosal ulceration or focal injury from an impacted foreign body that subsequently led to diverticular formation as well. Whether these cases would have developed anyway and were initiated by wall weakness or not is unclear.

SYMPTOMS

Dysphagia is the most common symptom. Swallowed food and fluid preferentially fill the diverticulum, which then distends and compresses the adjacent esophagus in the confines of the tight cervical space. Radiographically, this is clearly depicted (Figure 1). The compressed cervical esophagus is often thought to be strictured because of its appearance, but the author has never seen this to be so. Patients report that it is easiest for them to eat in the morning. As the day progresses, they have increasing dysphagia as the diverticulum fills. Diverticular contents have only one way out, which is back into the pharynx, leading to regurgitation, cough, and choking episodes. Choking episodes may wake a patient up at night and, in the worst case, are associated with a history of pneumonia. In addition, patients may have vague reports of a lump in the throat. Many have a characteristic voice, described as a "wet" voice, which sounds as if a person were talking while gargling a small quantity of fluid.

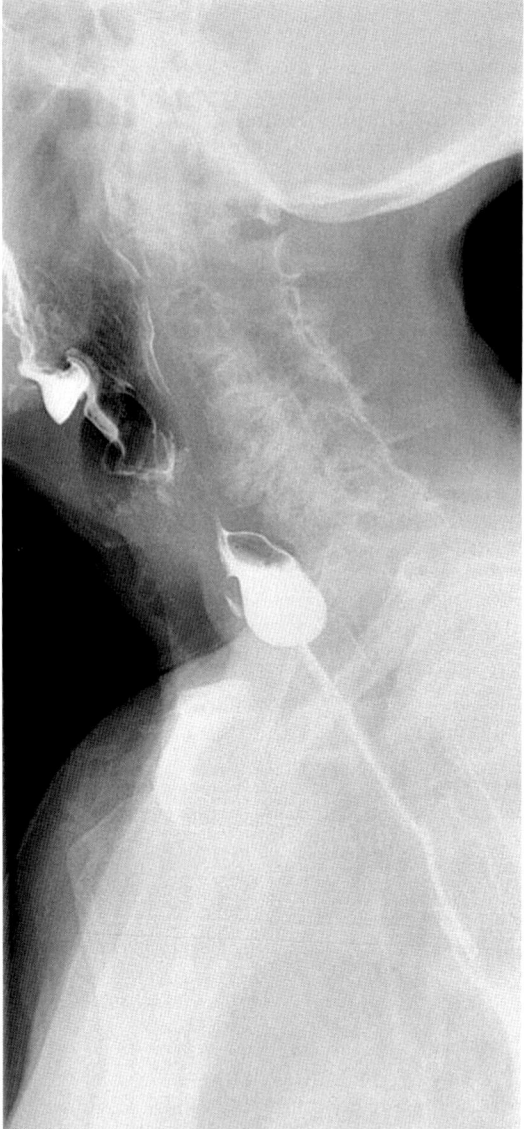

FIGURE 1 Select lateral spot image from contrast esophagogram showing moderate sized Zenker's diverticulum with compression of adjacent cervical esophagus.

DIAGNOSIS

Even in their classic form, the symptoms of Zenker's diverticulum are suggestive, not diagnostic, of the disease. A contrast swallow is the ideal first test. It is readily available and well tolerated by patients. The radiologist should be told that this may be a patient with Zenker's so that precautions against possible aspiration can be taken and appropriate views obtained. Video esophagography is superior to fluoroscopy and spot films in that it can screen for possible pharyngoesophageal motility disorders in addition to defining anatomy. Unless the contrast swallow reveals some unusual esophageal findings, endoscopy is not needed.

INDICATIONS FOR SURGERY

Once the diagnosis is made, the author explains to patients what they have, that it is a benign process, and how it accounts for their symptoms. Patients are followed as long as they are comfortable with their symptoms. Once patients are tired of dealing with the swallowing symptoms, the author has them return for surgery. Prominent respiratory symptoms, such as nighttime choking episodes or history of pneumonia that sounds like aspiration, however, are an indication for surgical repair. Dysphagia with weight loss is another indication for surgery, although significant weight loss is no longer commonly encountered.

OPERATIVE TECHNIQUE

Three operative techniques have been described for management of Zenker's: diverticulectomy with primary repair and cricopharyngeal myotomy, diverticular suspension to the prevertebral fascia and cricopharyngeal myotomy, and transoral endoscopic stapled diverticulectomy. A modification of the last technique uses the harmonic scalpel or laser to create an open channel between the diverticulum into the adjacent esophagus. Only the first, diverticulectomy with primary closure and myotomy, is discussed here. This procedure is simple, safe, and fast and directly corrects the functional (cricopharyngeus muscle) and anatomic (diverticulum) abnormality. A neck incision is well tolerated, and the evolution of stapling devices has made this direct repair even faster. The author has never encountered a patient who was a candidate for any procedure who could not tolerate this form of repair, regardless of age.

For diverticulectomy with primary repair and cricopharyngeal myotomy, patients are at nothing by mouth (NPO) status before surgery. Preoperative prophylactic antibiotics are routine. General endotracheal anesthesia is used, and patients are positioned supine with the neck in extension. Sweet commented that hyperextension of the neck was to be avoided because it narrowed the space between the airway and the spine. The author asks anesthesia colleagues to hold off putting anything into the esophagus at this time because it would preferentially tend to go into the diverticulum. A left neck incision is used because this is most comfortable for right-handed surgeons. The left side could be used if indicated. A modified collar incision is preferred, similar to that used with thyroid surgery except it is slightly higher in the neck and extends asymmetrically to the left side. Use the cricoids cartilage as the landmark to determine the exact location of this incision.

The incision is carried down to the prevertebral space, retracting the sternocleidomastoid muscle laterally, passing medial to the carotid sheath contents, and dividing the omohyoid and superior thyroid vessels as needed. Bluntly develop the posterior esophageal, prevertebral space. Avoid this dissection too far proximally because it tends to adversely affect postoperative pharyngeal function. With the posterior pharynx, left piriform sinus, and distal cervical esophagus exposed, have the anesthesiologist pass an orogastric catheter past the diverticulum into the cervical esophagus. This could be a nasogastric tube passed through the mouth or just an esophageal stethoscope. With this tube in place to help with orientation, dissect posteriorly to identify the diverticulum. The bigger the diverticulum, the easier it is to find. Most of the time, the diverticulum is easy to find. To help with exposure, a small rake or set of retracting hooks can be used to grasp the left posterior edge of the laryngeal cartilage, which rotates the larynx to the right, improving posterior exposure. The recurrent laryngeal nerve is protected in this fashion. Pharyngoscopy may also be used during surgery to help find difficult diverticula or ones in which the anatomy is confusing. Once the diverticulum is identified, take a moment to be sure identification is correct. With the target structure grasped, review its appearance and origin in relation to the cricoid cartilage. The author has seen cases in which the ipsilateral piriform sinus has been mistakenly resected. Once identification is ensured, dissect the diverticulum down to its neck. Generally, there is a good but somewhat vascular plane between the pseudocapsule covering the diverticulum and the mucosa. By doing so, you ensure you have the right structure and that it is completely removed. Either staple the diverticulum flush with the

esophagus and remove it (use the indwelling catheter to ensure the esophagus passes over and past your staple line) or resect the diverticulum and close the mucosal defect primarily in two layers of inverting sutures. No indwelling bougie or spacer is needed. Overtightening of the gastrointestinal tract from this repair is not possible. A 30-mm right angled stapler works well, given its 90-degree configuration that fits into the prevertebral space. However, the newer linear staplers are getting smaller, and the tip articulates so that it can be a good choice as well. The author always closes the adjacent muscle over the stapled closure with interrupted sutures.

Cricopharyngeal myotomy is performed in a different plane from the diverticular suture line closure, usually 90 degrees to the ipsilateral operative side. Use the cricoids cartilage as a landmark and divide the muscle down to the mucosa with scissors. Extend slightly proximal and then distal to the level of the cricoid so that the length of myotomy is approximately 3 cm total.

The wound is irrigated and closed in layers. The author uses a closed suction drain that does not lie adjacent to the suture or stapled line and is removed the next day. Drain use is not imperative. When patients undergo extubation in the operating room at case conclusion, no tubes are left in the esophagus.

POSTOPERATIVE CARE

After surgery, patients are admitted to the hospital. Continued antibiotics are not needed. Patients are kept NPO and hydrated with maintenance intravenous fluids. If a cervical drain is used, it is removed the next day. The wound is left uncovered so it can easily be seen and inspected. Signs of a leak are fevers; tachycardia; increasing neck pain; wound redness, swelling, or drainage; and leukocytosis. Signs are generally not subtle. On postoperative day 3, a contrast swallow is obtained. Radiology should be warned about the possibility of some aspiration. The swallowing study confirms complete diverticular removal and no suture or staple line leak. After successful study, the diet is advanced to soft regular and the patient is discharged home. Observation of patients after surgery during the time of greatest risk for aspiration and leakage is still important. After discharge, patients return to the office in approximately 3 weeks for their first visit.

RESULTS

As mentioned previously, open repair is safe and effective. Overall, the safety of the procedure continues to improve with advancements in anesthesia and patient care. A summary of the open method results show complication rates of approximately 4% to 10%, mortality rates of 0 to 2% (but more recently <1%), good to excellent swallowing achieved in 75% to 99% of patients, and recurrence rates of about 3% or less (see Table 1). Complications include temporary swallowing or speech changes, local wound infections or hematoma, pneumonia, and rarely recurrent laryngeal nerve injury, which should be very uncommon because the repair and retraction is posterior and superior to the nerve path and insertion point.

CONCLUSION

Zenker's diverticulum is an uncommon, benign esophageal disorder that is easy to diagnose and safe to treat with surgery regardless of patient age. Functional results are good, and clinical recurrence rates very low.

SUGGESTED READINGS

Jones B: Common structural lesions. In Jones B, editor: *Normal and abnormal swallowing*, ed 2, New York, 2003, Springer-Verlag, pp 103–118.

Lerut T, Coosemans W, Decker G, et al: Pathophysiology and treatment of Zenker's diverticulum. In Peters JH, editor: *Shakelford's surgery of the alimentary tract*, ed 6, vol 1, Philadelphia, 2007, Saunders Elsevier, pp 391–404.

Meade RH: The surgical treatment of diverticula of the esophagus. In *A history of thoracic surgery*, Springfield, IL, 1961, Charles C Thomas, pp 606–629.

Sweet RH: Thoracic surgery, Philadelphia, 1950, WB Saunders Co, pp 246–250.

Zenker FA, Ziemsen H: Krankheiten des oesophagus. In *Ziemsen's Handbuch der speciellen Pathologie und Therapie*, vol VII, part 1, Leipzig, Germany, 1877, Leipzig Publishers.

THE MANAGEMENT OF ACHALASIA OF THE ESOPHAGUS

Sheraz R. Markar, MD, and Donald E. Low, MD

BACKGROUND

Esophageal achalasia is a rare motility disorder that affects 1 person per 100,000 and is characterized by the failure of the lower esophageal sphincter (LES) to relax appropriately in response to swallowing and the decrease or absence of peristalsis. Findings that have been associated with the diagnosis include myenteric inflammation with associated injury and loss of ganglion cells, along with fibrosis of myenteric nerves, reduced synthesis of nitric oxide, and vasoactive intestinal polypeptide. The exact etiology of achalasia remains unknown; however, autoimmune-mediated destruction of inhibitory neurons is a possible explanation. Common symptoms associated with achalasia include progressive chest pain, odynophagia, dysphagia, regurgitation, and weight loss.

DIAGNOSIS

The diagnostic workup typically includes esophagogastroduodenoscopy (EGD), contrast esophagram, and esophageal manometry.

Esophagogastroduodenoscopy: EGD may show a dilated esophagus with retained saliva, fluid, and food and increased resistance to passage of the scope through the esophagogastric junction. EGD may also be used to assess for the presence of other diagnoses, including pseudoachalasia, esophageal tumors, reflux induced strictures, and eosinophilic esophagitis. Pseudoachalasia is defined as a spectrum of diseases that secondarily impair distal esophageal motility and imperfectly mimic achalasia. Originally described by Oglive in 1947, it is the result of a primary or metastatic submucosal cancer that involves the distal esophagus or esophagogastric junction. If pseudoachalasia is suggested on EGD, further investigations should include computed tomographic (CT) scan or endoscopic ultrasound scan. EGD is often suggestive but is not typically diagnostic of achalasia.

Contrast esophagram: The classic appearance seen with a contrast esophagram is tapering of the lower esophagus, described as a bird's beak (Figure 1). Other features may include a dilated esophageal body with an air-fluid level, the absence of a gastric air bubble, and absent or asynchronous esophageal contractions. Contrast studies have historically been considered diagnostic in approximately two thirds of patients.

Esophageal manometry: This test shows incomplete or absent LES relaxation and the absence of esophageal peristalsis during swallowing and sometimes elevated resting LES pressure. Manometry is considered the gold standard preoperative assessment and is diagnostic of achalasia in 90% of cases. Occasionally, manometric catheters do not pass into the stomach without fluoroscopic or endoscopic guidance.

Treatment for achalasia is not curative; it is primarily aimed at improving esophageal emptying by decreasing the functional obstruction at the level of the gastroesophageal junction, providing symptomatic relief and preventing the long-term development of megaesophagus.

MEDICAL THERAPY

Pharmacologic

Calcium channel blockers and long-acting nitrates that act as smooth muscle relaxants have been shown to be effective in reducing LES pressure and providing temporary relief of dysphagia in a small proportion of patients. However, their use is limited because they do not improve LES relaxation or peristalsis and they have a short duration of action and typically provide incomplete symptom relief. Their role is limited to symptom relief in patients with very early achalasia or those who are at high risk or refuse more aggressive treatments; in patients with severe achalasia, pharmacologic treatments have not been shown to be beneficial.

Botulinum Toxin Injection

Botulinum toxin is a neurotoxin that inhibits acetylcholine release at motor neuron presynaptic terminals and thereby promotes LES relaxation. Botulinum toxin is injected endoscopically with a sclerotherapy needle in four aliquots into each quadrant of the LES, with a total of 100 units. The complication rate associated with botulinum toxin injection is very low, and this method has been shown to provide a good short-term response, with symptomatic reduction in up to 75% of cases. However, beneficial effects decrease over time, with symptoms typically recurring in 1 to 4 months. A recent Cochrane review of four randomized controlled trials suggested that when compared with pneumatic dilation, botulinum toxin injection was less effective in the long-term control of symptoms arising from achalasia, with only 25.6% having symptomatic remission at 1 year compared with 70.2% in the pneumatic dilation group (Table 1). Furthermore, botulinum toxin injections can hypothetically produce submucosal scarring that impacts the dissection of the mucosal plane at myotomy, which some surgeons believe can increase the risk of intraoperative esophageal mucosal injury. Thus, currently botulinum toxin injection should be reserved for patients who do not wish to have other treatments or those who are at too high a risk for more invasive procedures, including pneumatic dilation and surgical myotomy.

Esophageal Pneumatic Dilation

Endoscopic pneumatic dilation is considered the most effective non-surgical treatment for the palliation of dysphagia associated with achalasia. Pneumatic dilation is preferred over standard balloon or bougie dilation because it not only stretches but also produces localized rupture of the LES muscle fibers. Most endoscopists advocate a sequential graded approach to pneumatic dilation, with noncompliant polyethylene balloon diameters currently used being 30, 35, and 40 mm. The most commonly used system is the Microinvasive Rigiflex balloon system (Boston Scientific Corporation, Natick, Mass). The balloon is placed across the LES, and position is confirmed with fluoroscopy with radiopaque markers on the catheter and within the balloon (Figure 2). The pressure necessary is usually 7 to 15 psi, with balloon inflation maintained for 15 to 60 seconds with confirmation of LES waist obliteration with fluoroscopy. Commonly, a multiple treatment regimen is used, based on active surveillance for symptomatic recurrence; this has been shown to be effective in the palliation of dysphagia associated with achalasia. The most severe complication associated with pneumatic dilation is esophageal perforation, which is quoted to occur in 4% to 7% of dilations and which occurred in 4% of patients in a recent randomized controlled trial. Esophageal perforation in this context is a serious complication, requiring urgent surgery, combining primary repair with surgical myotomy. Long-term functional results of perforation when managed by an experienced surgical team can be comparable with primary surgical treatment. Many gastroenterologists perform a postprocedure esophageal contrast swallow to rule out perforation before discharge from

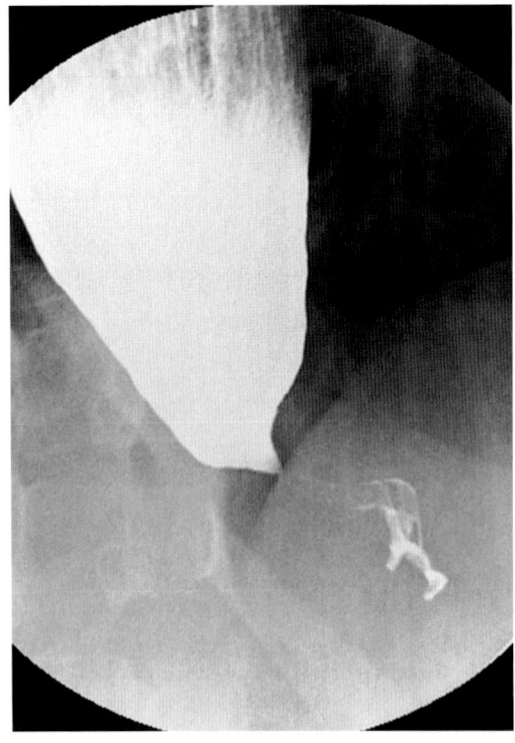

FIGURE 1 Contrast esophagram showing tapering of the lower esophagus with a classic bird's beak appearance.

TABLE 1: Endoscopic pneumatic dilation versus botulinum toxin injection in the management of primary achalasia

Follow-up period	Pneumatic dilation: symptom remission (N = 158)	Botulinum toxin: symptom remission (N = 121)
6 months	76%	26%
12 months	70%	25%

Data from Leyden JE, Moss AC, MacMathuna P: Endoscopic pneumatic dilation versus botulinum toxin injection in the management of primary achalasia. Cochrane Database Sys Rev (4):CD005046, 2006.

FIGURE 2 **A** and **B,** Microinvasive Rigiflex balloon system used for pneumatic dilation.

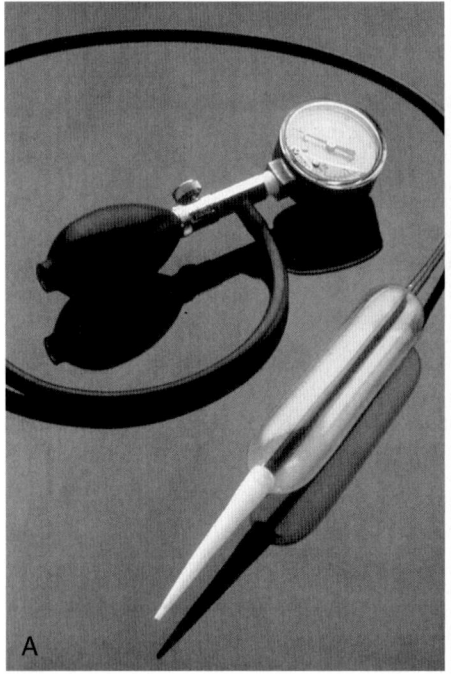
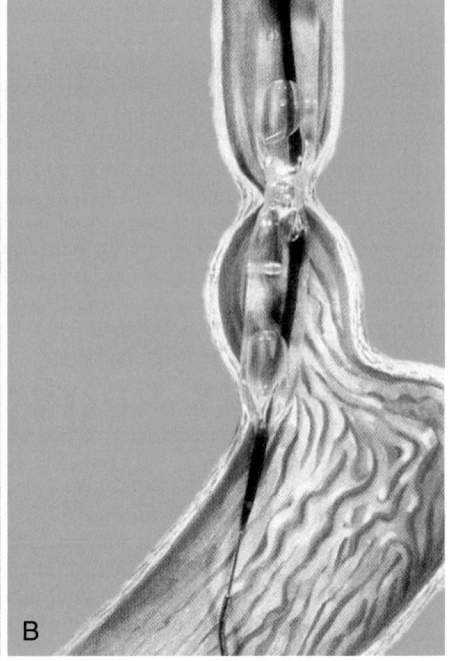

hospital. Furthermore, the long-term effectiveness of pneumatic dilation regimens is questionable, with treatment success rates of 50% at 5 years. A major advantage of pneumatic dilation is that it can be performed in an outpatient setting, enhancing its cost effectiveness in the treatment of esophageal achalasia.

Per-Oral Endoscopic Myotomy

Per-oral endoscopic myotomy (POEM) has been recently introduced as a potential new endoscopic approach to myotomy. Significant variability has been found in the technical approach used in POEM surgery. The most commonly described technique involves submucosal injection of saline solution at the midesophageal level approximately 13 cm from the gastroesophageal junction. A standard endoscope with a cap is introduced into the submucosal layer through a 2-cm longitudinal incision on the mucosal surface. A submucosal tunnel is then created and extended to 3 cm onto the stomach with a triangular tip knife and spray coagulation with direct endoscopic vision, or blunt dissection with the flexible endoscope or standard balloon dilation. Dissection of the circular muscle begins approximately 7 cm from the gastroesophageal junction with spray coagulation and a triangular tip knife. Division of the muscle continues for approximately 2 cm distal to the gastroesophageal junction; narrowing is typically seen endoscopically during passage through the LES. The outer longitudinal muscles are identified at the limit of the dissected area, and after myotomy, smooth passage of the endoscope through the gastroesophageal junction should be seen. The site of entry in the mucosa is then closed with hemostatic clips or fibrin glue. Table 2 discusses the results from clinical POEM studies to date. The attraction of this technique is the minimally invasive nature of the procedure, with no external scarring and less surgical stress, but the creation of a myotomy that replicates what is done surgically. This is an innovative and potentially important addition to the treatment approaches for achalasia. However, currently, insufficient follow-up assessment exists on the long-term success rate or consequences of POEM.

SURGICAL TREATMENT

Myotomy Technique and Outcomes

Surgical myotomy with division of the muscle fibers of the cardia for the treatment of achalasia was first described by Ernst Heller in 1913. Over the years, several technical issues have undergone clinical assessment; transthoracic versus transabdominal, open versus laparoscopic, and extended versus limited myotomy and whether a

concomitant antireflux procedure including Nissen, Toupet, or Dor fundoplication should be done in conjunction with the myotomy. The authors describe the method of esophageal myotomy that is used routinely at their institution and discuss some of the issues regarding modifications of this technique.

Most commonly, the authors use a laparoscopic transabdominal approach to esophageal myotomy. The patient is positioned in a modified lithotomy position in reverse Trendenlenburg's position. A five-port technique is used: one camera port, two ports for retraction, and two working ports. The first incision is made typically one third to one half the distance from the umbilicus to the xiphisternum, to allow placement of a 12-mm Hassan or Optiview port (Johnson & Johnson, Calif). A 12-mm working port is placed in the left upper quadrant adjacent to the costal margin as high as possible but also maximizing triangulation of the right and left working ports. A 5-mm port is placed in the groove between the xiphisternum and the right costal margin to allow insertion of the liver retractor (Nathanson liver retractor, Cook Medical Bloomington, Ind), which is used to retract the liver anteriorly and to the right. Two further 5-mm ports are placed to the left and right of the camera port, the one on the right used for retraction and taking down the short gastric vessels and one on the left to be the other dissection or working port. The left 5-mm port is typically placed through or beneath the falciform ligament. The assistant stands on the left side of the patient, the camera operator to the right, and the operating surgeon between the legs.

Dissection begins with division of the phrenoesophageal membrane and gastrophrenic ligaments, with dissection extending posteriorly to the decussation of the crura. This dissection is continued circumferentially, the right and left crura are freed, and the dissection is carried into the mediastinum to allow adequate circumferential mobilization of the esophagus, which is encircled by a Penrose drain. Esophageal mobilization is continued until there are 4 to 5 cm below the hiatus without tension. This mobilization is done to a greater degree when the distal esophagus is tortuous. The authors divide the short gastric vessels and omental attachments over a distance of 15 cm until the fundus is completely free.

The anterior esophageal fat pad is removed down to the gastric serosa to expose the gastroesophageal junction and increase the ease of doing the myotomy. This dissection is typically started to the left of the anterior vagus nerve and can facilitate the mobilization of the anterior vagus nerve to the right to take it well away from the site of the proposed myotomy. The myotomy is initiated 1 to 2 cm above the esophagogastric junction, typically with hook cautery initially but then with blunt tearing of the last circular muscle fibers. The authors commonly extend the myotomy a minimum of 5 cm in a cephalad direction along the anterior esophagus then across the esophagogastric junction, continuing for a minimum of 2 cm caudally onto the stomach (Figure 3). The change from esophageal to gastric muscle

TABLE 2:   Results from clinical trials of per-oral endoscopic myotomy

Author	No. of patients	Myotomy length (cm)	Follow-up period	Dysphagia score improvement	LES pressure change
Inoue (2010)	17	8.1 (6.1 in esophagus + 2 in stomach)	5 mo (1-16 mo)	10 to 1.3 (0-4)	52.4 to 19.8 (9.3-42.7)
Von Renteln (2011)	16	12 (8-17)	3 mo	94% patients with Eckhard score of ≤3	27.2 to 11.8
Swanstrom (2011)	5	7 (6-12)	2 wk	All patients reported immediate dysphagia relief	No postoperative study
Costamagna (2012)	11	10.2 ± 2.8	1 mo	7.1 to 1.1 (Eckardt score)	45.1 to 16.9

LES, Lower esophageal sphincter.

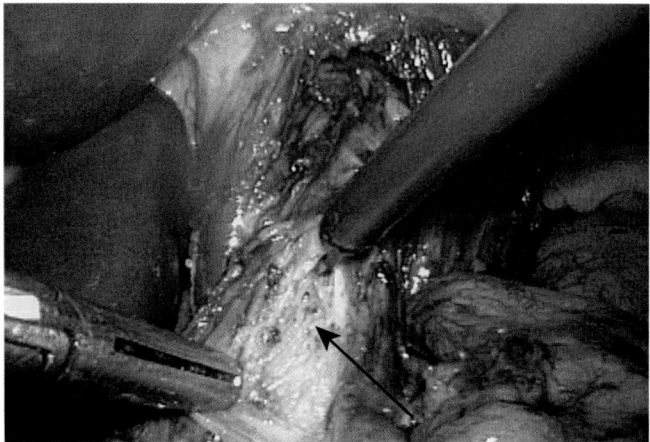

FIGURE 3 Myotomy dissection *(arrow)* extended 5 cm in a cephalad direction along the anterior esophagus and a minimum of 2 cm caudally onto the stomach.

fibers can be seen as they change from a horizontal circular orientation to an oblique direction and are more adherent to mucosa in the region of the LES. Once the myotomy is completed, a 48F to 52F bougie is passed with laparoscopic guidance, which stretches the mucosa and helps to ensure that all muscle fibers are divided. At the end of the myotomy, intraoperative endoscopy is selectively undertaken to confirm an adequate myotomy has been performed, with the easy passage of the endoscope into the stomach, and to transilluminate the mucosa, checking for defects with air insufflations. The crura are loosely opposed posterior to the esophagus with permanent sutures.

After myotomy, the authors typically perform an antireflux procedure, most commonly a Toupet but selectively a Dor fundoplication. For a Toupet fundoplication, the fundus is brought posterior to the esophagus where it should sit in place without any tendency to retract. The right limb of the fundus is then sutured to the right edge of the esophageal myotomy with three interrupted 2-0 Ethibond sutures (Ethicon, Johnson & Johnson, Calif) placed 1 cm apart and careful avoidance of the anterior vagus nerve. The most superior suture includes a bite of the edge of the hiatus and the fundus and esophageal muscular wall. The left limb of the fundus is then sutured in a similar manner to the left side of the esophageal myotomy with interrupted Ethibond sutures placed 1 cm apart to create a 2-cm fundoplication over 270 degrees. The fundus lateral to the fundoplication is tacked to the undersurface of the diaphragm with an additional 2-0 Ethibond suture to accentuate the antireflux valve and remove any residual drag on the repair sutures.

For a Dor fundoplication, the authors use interrupted sutures to fix the posterior wall of the left anterior fundus to the esophagus to the left of the myotomy and to the left crus of the diaphragm. The leading edge of the fundus is then positioned anteriorly to the esophagus overlying the myotomy and is sutured to the right side of the esophagus to the right of the myotomy, with separate sutures placed into the right crus of the diaphragm.

FURTHER DISCUSSION

Transthoracic Versus Transabdominal

Open transthoracic and transabdominal myotomy have similar outcomes in terms of postoperative complications, palliation of dysphagia, and symptom control for the treatment of achalasia. However, transabdominal esophageal myotomy is associated with less physio-

logic impact than a thoracotomy and, when combined with an antireflux procedure, produces less postoperative reflux.

Open Versus Laparoscopic Versus Thoracoscopic

In comparison of laparoscopic and thoracoscopic approaches with myotomy, the outcomes of the laparoscopic approach are superior, particularly with respect to symptomatic improvement. Laparoscopic myotomy has several advantages over an open approach, including reduced postoperative pain, length of hospital stay, and pulmonary dysfunction and shorter return to normal activities. The authors advocate the preferential use of laparoscopic esophageal myotomy with partial fundoplication for the treatment of achalasia, where a contraindication to laparoscopic surgery does not exist.

Length of Myotomy

Palliation of dysphagia remains the most important treatment outcome after surgical myotomy for achalasia; for this reason, a longer myotomy is considered the most appropriate approach in all cases. The acceptable length for myotomy ranges from 4 to 8 cm on the esophageal aspect and from 2 to 3 cm on the stomach. Within this range, symptomatic improvement and lower esophageal resting pressure reduction are equivalent.

Concomitant Antireflux Procedure: Nissen/Toupet/Dor

The authors advocate the use of a partial fundoplication procedure (Toupet or Dor) as a routine addition to the surgical esophageal myotomy for the treatment of achalasia. The rate of dysphagia improvement is not affected; however, the incidence rate of gastroesophageal reflux symptoms is greater when an antireflux procedure is not combined with myotomy. Furthermore, poor long-term outcomes associated with surgical myotomy are commonly the result of severe uncontrolled reflux. The authors preferentially use a Toupet or Dor fundoplication over a 360-degree Nissen fundoplication. Controversy exists as to whether a full 360-degree Nissen fundoplication increases the rate of dysphagia compared with an incomplete fundoplication. Currently, no significant difference in short-term clinical outcomes, including dysphagia control and reflux symptoms, has been shown in comparison of Toupet and Dor fundoplications after esophageal myotomy. Potential benefits of Toupet fundoplication include improved long-term reflux control; however, the benefits of Dor fundoplication include less disruption of hiatal anatomy and fundal coverage of the esophageal mucosa after myotomy. The authors use a Toupet reconstruction in most cases for better visualization during the myotomy and the production of a more robust antireflux gastroesophageal valve. There is a hypothetical advantage of using the two limbs of the fundoplication to hold the edges of the myotomy apart. In cases with concern regarding the integrity of the mucosa after myotomy, the authors use a Dor repair to allow fundal coverage of the esophageal mucosa.

Sigmoid Esophagus or Megaesophagus

Sigmoid esophagus is characterized by a widened (>6-cm diameter) and tortuous esophageal body that results in a sigmoid-shaped appearance and a more advanced stage of achalasia. Surgical treatment for sigmoid achalasia has traditionally been esophagectomy because the suggestion was that the dilated tortuous and aperistaltic esophagus would not empty sufficiently to improve dysphagia after myotomy of the LES. More recently, many surgeons have shown successful outcomes with myotomy and Dor fundoplication as the

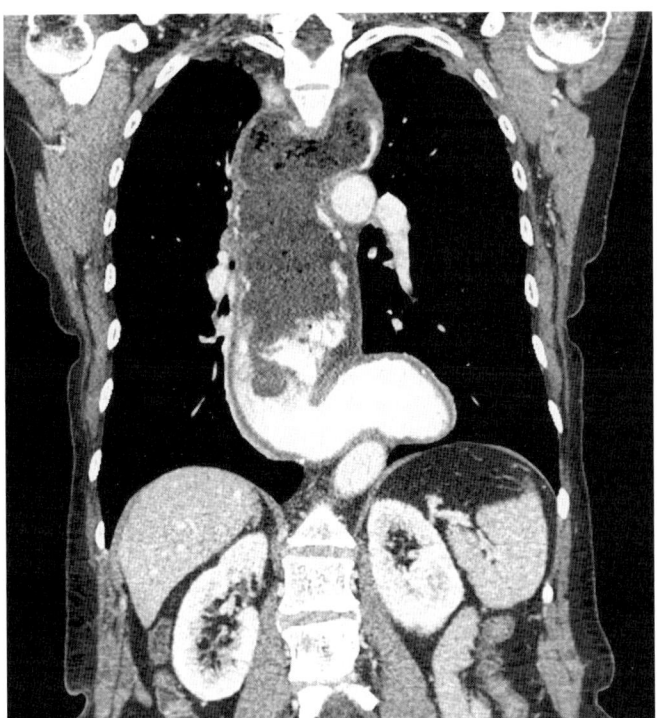

FIGURE 4 Computerized tomographic scan showing severe case of megaesophagus.

treatment of choice, with 92% of patients reporting improvement in dysphagia. The benefits of myotomy in this situation are clear with the avoidance of the morbidity and mortality associated with esophagectomy. However, in certain cases of megaesophagus (Figure 4), myotomy is unlikely to provide adequate relief from dysphagia, and primary esophageal resection is indicated.

Surgical Myotomy Versus Endoscopic Treatment

The debate regarding what is the "best" treatment for achalasia remains unresolved in the current literature. The advantages of endoscopic treatment with pneumatic dilation include a less invasive approach and good short-term relief of dysphagia. Many gastroenterologists find a 5% risk of perforation associated with this procedure unacceptable. There is also the well-documented issue of the need for sequential treatments in many patients.

Surgical myotomy when performed laparoscopically has the benefits of good long-term relief of dysphagia and symptom control. The disadvantages are related to the risks of surgery and include bleeding, infection, reflux symptoms, and esophageal perforation (although in the context of surgery, this is typically recognized and addressed at the time of the myotomy). The most recent multicenter randomized

control trial comparing surgical myotomy with pneumatic dilation showed equivalent rates of success at 2 years. In spite of this trial showing a total perforation rate of 4%, the authors believe that in experienced hands pneumatic dilation should still remain a treatment option for patients. However, at their center, they are currently offering laparoscopic myotomy and antireflux reconstruction as primary treatment for all appropriate patients.

SUMMARY

Esophageal achalasia is a rare disorder, and treatment approach is dependent on several factors, including patient's severity of symptoms, patient's medical comorbidities and physiologic fitness, and the level of experience of the managing gastroenterologist or surgeon. Centers of excellence that are experienced in managing esophageal motility disorders including achalasia allow specialized gastroenterologists and surgeons to work together to provide the best outcomes for patients with esophageal achalasia.

ACKNOWLEDGMENT

This work was supported in part by the Ryan Hill Research Foundation.

SUGGESTED READINGS

Boeckxstaens GE, Annese V, Bruley des Varammes S, et al: Pneumatic dilation versus laparoscopic Heller myotomy for idiopathic achalasia, *N Engl J Med* 364:1807–1816, 2011.
Campos GM, Vittinghoff E, Rabl C, et al: Endoscopic and surgical treatments for achalasia: a systematic review and meta-analysis, *Ann Surg* 249:45–57, 2009.
Ferguson MK, Reeder LB, Olak J: Results of myotomy and partial fundoplication after pneumatic dilation for achalasia, *Ann Thorac Surg* 62:327–330, 1996.
Inoue H, Tianle KM, Ikeda H, et al: Peroral endoscopic myotomy for esophageal achalasia: technique, indication and outcomes, *Thorac Surg Clin* 21:519–525, 2011.
Leyden JE, Moss AC, MacMathuna P: Endoscopic pneumatic dilation versus botulinum toxin injection in the management of primary achalasia, *Cochrane Database Sys Rev* (4):CD005046, 2006.
Patti MG, Fisichella PM, Perretta S, et al: Impact of minimally invasive surgery on the treatment of achalasia: a decade of change, *J Am Coll Surg* 196:698–703, 2003.
Rawlings A, Soper N, Oelschlager B, et al: Laparoscopic Dor versus Toupet fundoplication following Heller myotomy for achalasia: results of a multicenter, prospective randomized-controlled trial, *Surg Endosc* 26:18–26, 2012.
Richter JE, Boeckxstaens GE: Management of achalasia: surgery or pneumatic dilation, *Gut* 60:869–876, 2011.
Stefanidis D, Richardson W, Farrell TM, et al: SAGES guidelines for the surgical treatment of esophageal achalasia, *Surg Endosc* 26:296–311, 2012.
West RL, Hirsch DP, Bartelsman JF, et al: Long term results of pneumatic dilation in achalasia followed for more than 5 years, *Am J Gastroenterol* 97:1346–1351, 2002.

Disorders of Esophageal Motility

Christopher M. Sciortino, MD, PhD, and
Stephen C. Yang, MD

INTRODUCTION

Disorders of esophageal motility can result in major morbidity and decreased quality of life and, in some cases, in an increased risk of cancer and death. Several classes of motility disorders of the esophagus have been described, including primary esophageal motility disorders (Box 1), such as achalasia and the spastic dysmotility disorders (diffuse esophageal spasm), and secondary diseases (Box 2) that affect esophageal motility (scleroderma, diabetes). This chapter describes the types of esophageal motility disorders, their workup, and treatment options. Achalasia will not be discussed, as this disorder is the subject of another chapter in this textbook.

CLASSES OF ESOPHAGEAL MOTILITY DISORDERS

Spastic Dysmotility Disorders

Diffuse Esophageal Spasm

Diffuse esophageal spasm (DES) is a disorder that results from the uncoordinated contraction of the esophagus with subsequent loss of coordinated peristalsis. It is a rare disorder, constituting less than 10% of all motility abnormalities. The etiology is unknown, but similar to achalasia, there may be loss of neuronal activity and secretion of nitric oxide, vasoactive intestinal polypeptide, or both. Familial clustering has been identified in some studies. The most common presenting symptoms of patients with DES are noncardiac chest pain, globus, dysphagia, and modest weight loss. Many patients present after a negative cardiac workup for angina pectoris and thus can be differentiated with nonexertional onset. Dysphagia is usually sporadic, self-limiting, not associated with liquids or solids, and sometimes associated with extreme food temperatures. Although demographic studies are lacking, patients tend to be older (in their 60s or 70s) and may have a significant history of hypertension, anxiety, or psychiatric disorder. Gastroesophageal reflux disease (GERD) is a simultaneous finding in 20% to 50% of patients diagnosed with DES.

DES is diagnosed primarily with esophageal manometry, which demonstrates normal peristalsis with intermittent loss of coordinated contractions primarily in the lower esophagus; the lower esophageal sphincter (LES) functions normally. Some call this *distal* esophageal spasm rather than *diffuse* esophageal spasm. Simultaneous contractions are observed in more than 20% (but less than 100%) of wet swallows. Contractions have normal intensity, and LES tone is typically normal but may be hypertensive in some cases. Because symptoms may occur intermittently, diagnostic tests such as barium swallow may fail to diagnose DES; however, video esophagrams may be diagnostic in up to 50% of cases. Static pictures can depict the typical "corkscrew" or "rosary bead" pattern. Esophagogastroduodenoscopy usually fails to reveal any mucosal or structural abnormalities.

Treatment of DES ranges from reassurance to surgical myotomy. Initial treatment includes workup for possible underlying contributing factors (e.g., GERD, medications, stress). Patients frequently present after extensive cardiac workup. Depending on symptoms at presentation, patients may warrant a workup for GERD, including pH monitoring and endoscopic evaluation. Those patients found to have GERD should be treated and their symptoms tracked for reduction/resolution. Patients with ongoing symptoms may require a trial of medical therapy, including nitrates, calcium channel blockers, antidepressants, or sildenafil. Botulinum toxin as a treatment for DES has been described as having variable results.

Patients refractory to these therapies and who have intolerable symptoms may seek surgical consultation for a long esophageal myotomy. Results are optimal when effective contractions measured by manometry are below 30%. Surgery is aimed at eliminating the functional obstruction caused by the simultaneous muscular contractions, thereby relieving the propulsive contractions. The three issues that dictate the operative intervention include the extent of the myotomy, the need for a fundoplication, and the operative technique (right vs left, open vs minimally invasive). Length of the myotomy is based on manometry results regarding the proximal and distal extent. If it is carried through the esophagogastric junction (EGJ), fundoplication is considered, especially in patients with a history of GERD. Laparoscopic, video-assisted thoracic surgery (VATS), and robotic techniques are currently used to perform the myotomy. The authors prefer to approach it by VATS through the left chest. A synopsis of these variations is outlined in Table 1.

Single lung ventilation with a double-lumen tube or bronchial blocker is needed if the myotomy is done through the chest. The flexible esophagoscope or a Maloney dilator is left in place to help the esophageal myotomy dissection. Three or four port sites are placed along the fifth and eighth intercostal spaces along the anterior and posterior axillary lines. The inferior pulmonary ligament is mobilized. An area on the lateral lower side of the esophagus is picked to begin the site for the myotomy. The hook cautery or scissors is used to begin the dissection through the outer and inner circular muscle fibers until the mucosal layer is reached. Gentle dissection of the mucosa is performed to tease it off the muscle as the cautery is advanced superiorly and inferiorly to divide the muscle layers up to the desired level. The muscle is dissected for 50% of the circumference of the esophagus to prevent recurrence (Figure 1). Care is taken not to injure the vagus nerve. At the end, the esophagus is insufflated with the scope in place to check for violations of the mucosa. On the left side, the myotomy is carried up to the level of the aortic arch and 1 cm short of the hiatus if the EGJ is left intact; on the right, access can be obtained up to the level of the thoracic inlet. If a fundoplication is needed or if the myotomy is carried down across the EGJ (2 cm), then a modified Belsey fundoplication is performed. In this modification (Figure 2), a tongue of the gastric fundus is sutured over the myotomy site for a distance of 4 cm with two lines of sutures in front and in back of the myotomy (as opposed to the traditional three for a Belsey Mark IV fundoplication). After tucking the cardia under the diaphragmatic crura, the top sutures are passed through the diaphragm and tied.

Published results reveal resolution of symptoms and improved quality of life in approximately 70% of patients. Counseling patients about the potential for modest improvement of symptoms after myotomy is important to manage expectations given somewhat modest outcomes. Surgery for DES is somewhat controversial; results are not as good as with myotomy for achalasia.

Hypercontracting Esophagus (Nutcracker Esophagus)

Hypercontracting esophagus, also known as nutcracker esophagus, is a disorder resulting from increased intensity of esophageal contraction rather than disordered contraction. It is less common than DES,

BOX 1: Primary motility disorders of the esophagus

Hypertensive LES
Classic achalasia
Diffuse esophageal spasm
Atypical disorders of LES relaxation
Uncoordinated contraction

Hypercontraction
Hypertensive esophagus (nutcracker esophagus)
Hypertensive LES

Hypocontraction
Ineffective esophageal motility
Hypotensive LES

LES, Lower esophageal motility.

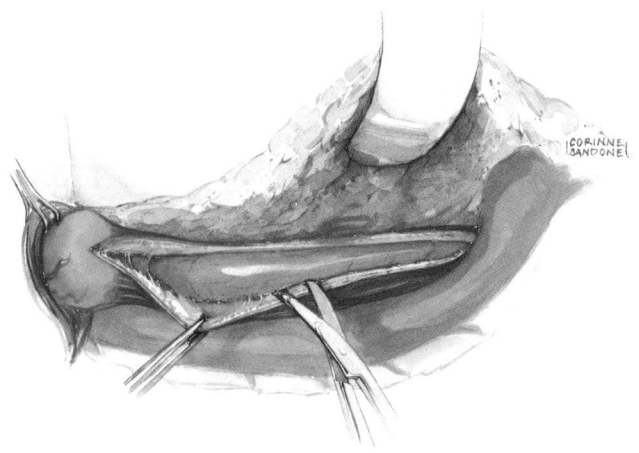

FIGURE 1   Long myotomy for diffuse esophageal spasm. *(Illustration by Corinne Sandone, from Cameron JL:* Atlas of surgery, *vol 2, St. Louis, 1994, Mosby-Year Book. Reprinted with permission.)*

BOX 2: Secondary motility disorders of the esophagus

Malignancy (Pseudoachalasia)
Primary EGJ tumors (adenocarcinoma, squamous, lymphoma)
Remote EGJ tumors (lung, lymphoma, sarcoma, mesothelioma, gastric, liver)

Rheumatologic Disorders
Progressive systemic sclerosis (scleroderma)
Systemic lupus erythematosus
Mixed connective tissue disease
Raynaud's phenomenon
Sjögren's syndrome
Polymyositis

Infectious Diseases
Human immunodeficiency virus
Chagas' disease
Candida
Cytomegalovirus
Herpes simplex virus

Infiltrative Disorders
Amyloidosis
Leiomyomatosis
Eosinophilic esophagitis
Sarcoidosis

Miscellaneous
Congenital diaphragmatic web
Diabetes mellitus
Iatrogenic (postvagotomy, post–gastric banding)
Multiple endocrine neoplasia (type 2B)

EGJ, Esophagogastric junction.

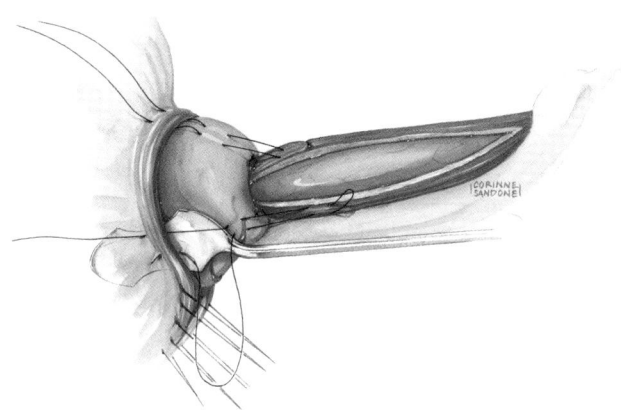

FIGURE 2   Modified Belsey fundoplication for diffuse esophageal spasm. *(Illustration by Corinne Sandone, from Cameron JL:* Atlas of surgery, *vol 2, St. Louis, 1994, Mosby-Year Book. Reprinted with permission.)*

TABLE 1: Operative approaches and techniques for diffuse esophageal spasm

Length of myotomy	Need for fundoplication	Procedure
Aortic arch → hiatus	No	L VATS or open thoracotomy, myotomy
Thoracic inlet → hiatus	No	R VATS or open thoracotomy, myotomy
Through EGJ	Yes	L VATS or open thoracotomy, myotomy with Belsey, or laparoscopic myotomy with partial fundoplication
Thoracic only	Yes	L VATS or open thoracotomy, myotomy with Belsey, or laparoscopic myotomy with partial fundoplication

EGJ, Esophagogastric junction; *L*, left; *R*, right; *VATS*, video-assisted thoracic surgery.

and GERD is less strongly associated with this disorder. The etiology is also unidentified, but like DES, some patients have been found to transition to classic achalasia and thus may be part of the clinical spectrum that eventually leads up to it. Pain is the usual presenting symptom with dysphagia a less common complaint. Compared to the other motility disorders, it has the poorest correlation with symptoms, yet it has the highest correlation with psychological issues. There is significant symptom overlap with irritable bowel syndrome, and up to 30% have a psychiatric illness.

Barium studies are usually normal, and nuclear emptying studies often produce conflicting results. Manometric findings are defined by either high-pressure contractions (>180 mm Hg) or swallow duration of greater than 6 seconds. The diagnosis requires the contraction amplitude to be greater than 2 standard deviations (SD) above normal, with all contractions peristaltic. The peristaltic wave progresses normally, and the LES has normal relaxation characteristics. Risk factor modification and reassurance are again the initial steps in treatment. Patients should be evaluated for GERD and treated if necessary. Medical management is similar to DES, relying primarily on calcium channel blockers. Dilation is not effective. Surgery is rarely used to treat hypercontracting esophagus because the outcomes are inconsistent at best. A long thoracic myotomy (as described for DES), although relieving the pain associated with contractions, may actually worsen the dysphagia.

Hypertensive Lower Esophageal Sphincter

Patients with hypertensive LES typically have symptoms of noncardiac chest pain, dysphagia, globus, and regurgitation. Hypertensive LES can be diagnosed concomitantly with nutcracker esophagus and GERD, but it is dissimilar in character to the reported occasional dysphagia. Manometric findings include normal peristaltic progression and LES pressure greater than the 95th percentile of normal (>45 mm Hg). Unlike achalasia, there is high residual pressure, and 50% have high-amplitude peristaltic contractions in the distal esophagus. Esophageal contrast studies show only a hiatal hernia in half of all patients.

Treatment is primarily aimed at controlling the primary symptoms of GERD with proton pump inhibitors and using interventions directed at the LES, including pharmacologic (e.g., Botox injection), and endoscopic (bougienage or balloon dilatation). Medical treatment with nitrates or calcium channel blockers is typically very effective. Surgery is reserved for patients with refractory symptoms. Those with isolated hypertensive LES should have a myotomy similar to achalasia and partial fundoplication. If GERD is present, then a Nissen fundoplication only should be performed. The approach can be done either by thoracoscopic, laparoscopic, or robotic approach. These techniques are described in other chapters.

Ineffective Motility Disorder

Hypocontracting, or ineffective, esophageal motility is a rare disorder, in which patients experience mild dysphagia or acid reflux but no chest pain. This condition is defined by the manometric findings of either nontransmitted or low-amplitude peristaltic contractions (<30 mm Hg) in more than 30% of wet swallows and a decreased LES tone. Contractions can also be characterized as spontaneous, prolonged duration (>6 seconds), retrograde, or triple-peaked. Peristaltic waves, if detectable, may be unable to clear barium from the esophagus. Some patients have associated GERD, but this is not universal. Prokinetic agents (metoclopramide) and/or GERD treatment may reduce symptoms, and surgery is rarely indicated.

Secondary Esophageal Motility Disorders

There is a wide spectrum of medical diseases that can have secondary consequences on the esophagus; these diseases are outlined in Box 2.

They can be categorized based on associated rheumatologic diseases, infiltrative processes, infectious etiologies, or other, less common entities. Pseudoachalasia will not be covered.

Two connective tissue diseases that have frequent esophageal manifestations are progressive systemic sclerosis (PSS) or scleroderma and systemic lupus erythematosus (SLE). Both are autoimmune diseases that target the distal third of the esophagus. Esophageal symptoms occur in 50% to 90% of patients with PSS and 1% to 25% of patients with SLE, which can coexist with Raynaud's phenomena.

Many patients with PSS will have the complete manifestations of the CREST syndrome (calcinosis, Raynaud's phenomenon, esophageal dysfunction, sclerodactyly, and telangiectasia), and demonstrate dysfunction of the distal esophagus and EGJ. Consequently, dysphagia and reflux are the two most common symptoms. Although the etiology of esophageal dysmotility is not clear, inflammation of esophageal smooth muscle or ischemic vascular changes to Auerbach's plexus have been proposed. Ultimately, all esophageal function studies are used in the evaluation. Video esophagram reveals dilation and marked aperistalsis in the distal one third of the esophagus. Twenty-four-hour pH probe monitoring will document reflux in up to 80% of patients, but not all symptoms will correlate with pathologic reflux. Manometric studies may demonstrate low-amplitude or absent peristalsis and reduced LES tone. Finally, endoscopy may reveal an asymptomatic esophageal stricture, infection (esophageal candidiasis), and/or ulceration, as medications may also contribute to symptoms.

Common to the rest of the miscellaneous diseases, patients with secondary esophageal motility disorders typically have dysphasia and mild pain usually related to the GERD. Management focuses on treatment of the underlying diseases. Infectious etiologies have a wide spectrum of effect on esophageal motility (usually hypocontractions) and on the LES (usually hypertension and incomplete relaxation). Inflammatory diseases such as eosinophilic esophagitis usually result in spasms or hypercontractility of the esophageal body. Neuropathic causes such as in advanced diabetes mellitus result in the obvious consequences of reduced amplitude in the upper and lower esophageal sphincters, slow transit time, and loss of peristaltic waves.

Overall therapy for patients with secondary esophageal motility disorders is directed at the underlying medical cause and conservative management of their swallowing symptoms. Since GERD is usually the root cause for the majority of symptoms, aggressive medical therapies and lifestyle changes are first instituted. Gastroparesis can be addressed pharmacologically. Surgical intervention is rarely indicated and thus is reserved for failure of medical therapies or when patients have end-stage disease, stricture, or perforation when salvage procedures are needed.

Patients who develop GERD should be considered for antireflux surgery to prevent stricture formation. Laparoscopic approaches are clearly the preferred route, given the presence of medical comorbidities, and are described in the Gastroesophageal Reflux Disease chapter. In planning the appropriate operative approach, other variables that should be taken into account include the presence of a distal stricture or shortened esophagus, aperistalsis or dilation of the distal esophagus, delayed gastric emptying, Barrett's metaplasia, and severity of bile reflux. Timing of the procedure is also a critical decision point, for input from a multidisciplinary team of those involved in the patient's care must figure in future interventions such as transplantation for associated organ failure and the use of higher dose immunosuppressive agents.

In deciding the appropriate operative intervention, one must achieve a delicate balance between dysphagia (too tight a wrap) and reflux (too loose). A partial fundoplication (Toupet) is preferred to minimize the risk of postoperative dysphagia secondary to inefficient peristalsis against a complete wrap (Nissen). Surgical results for the former are quite satisfactory, as the lower risk of progressive gastrointestinal symptoms (dysphagia, gas bloat) are balanced by the higher recurrence of reflux with a less than circumferential wrap (e.g., Toupet wrap). Long-term results in patients with PSS have shown a benefit combining an esophageal lengthening procedure (Collis gastroplasty) with fundoplication. However, patients continue to have symptoms of reflux (25%) and dysphagia (40%). Thus, our preference is not to add a gastroplasty because of the associated risk of leaks, given the common presence of steroid use, and to perform only a partial 270-degree wrap. Results of preoperative studies on gastric emptying suggest that pyloromyotomy may be needed. Radical procedures such as biliary diversion and esophagectomy are reserved for palliative situations when carcinoma cannot be excluded, the presence of an untreatable stricture, or acute events such as perforation or bleeding.

SUGGESTED READINGS

Almansa C, Heckman MG, DeVault KR, Bouras E, Achem SR: Esophageal spasm: demographic, clinical, radiographic, and manometric features in 108 patients, *Dis Esophagus* 25:214–221, 2012.
Richter JE: Esophageal motility disorders, *Lancet* 358:823–828, 2001.
Roman S, Kahrilas PJ: Distal esophageal spasm, *Dysphagia* 27:115–123, 2012.
Spechler SJ, Castell DO: Classification of esophageal motility abnormalities, *Gut* 49:145–151, 2001.
Woltman TA, Oelschlager BK, Pellegrini CA: Surgical management of esophageal motility disorders, *J Surg Res* 117:34–43, 2004.

THE MANAGEMENT OF ESOPHAGEAL CARCINOMA

Michal J. Lada, MD, and Jeffrey H. Peters, MD

Over the past several decades, there has been an unprecedented shift in the relative prevalence of the two primary histologic types of esophageal carcinoma. Historically, esophageal squamous cell carcinoma (SCC), largely related to tobacco and alcohol use, has accounted for more than 90% of esophageal malignancies. In the 1970s, the incidence of esophageal adenocarcinoma began rising steadily, at a relative rate unparalleled by any other cancer. Adenocarcinoma now makes up the predominant histologic type in most Western countries. Reasons for this dramatic change are not clear, although the increasing prevalence of both obesity and gastroesophageal reflux disease almost certainly plays a leading role. National Cancer Institute data indicate that 17,460 new cases of tubular esophageal cancer (13,950 male and 3510 female) and 15,070 deaths will occur in the United States in 2012. The prevalence nearly doubles when cancers of the gastric cardia are included.

ASSESSMENT OF THE EXTENT OF DISEASE AND SELECTION OF TREATMENT OPTIONS

Although the majority of patients with esophageal carcinoma have symptoms at the time of presentation, an important minority (15%-25% in most referral centers) are identified via surveillance of a known Barrett's esophagus or endoscopic evaluation for nonspecific symptoms and anemia. These patients form a group that has a high likelihood of intramucosal and early-stage disease and thus are more curable than those who present with dysphagia. In the majority of patients who present with symptoms, dysphagia and weight loss are the two most common presenting complaints. Other less common presenting symptoms include worsening gastroesophageal reflux disease symptoms (heartburn or regurgitation), chest pain, anorexia, and cough. Approximately two thirds of patients present with resectable disease, of which a majority (50%-60%) will have nodal metastases at the time of diagnosis. Metastases most often spread to regional, celiac, and supraclavicular lymph nodes as well as the liver,

lungs, and adrenal glands. A multidisciplinary approach including surgery, gastroenterology, medical oncology, radiation oncology, and pathology is important to optimize stage-specific survival.

Initial staging includes upper endoscopy to assess the location, length, and circumference of the tumor; the extent of gastric cardia involvement, if any; and the suitability of the stomach for reconstruction. This is followed by positron emission tomography combined with a computed tomographic scan (PET-CT), possibly endoscopic ultrasound, and increasingly molecular staging such as HER-2 receptor testing. The seventh edition American Joint Commitee on Cancer (AJCC 2010) TNM classification for esophageal carcinoma is shown in Table 1. Recent data have suggested different outcomes for adenocarcinoma and SCC, which is now reflected in separate AJCC staging systems for each histologic type (Table 2). Other important changes also occurred in the seventh edition staging, including defining gastroesophageal junction tumors as esophageal and changing nodal classification from location to number of nodes.

Endoscopic ultrasound (EUS) may be a useful modality in the assessment of locoregional disease. Its accuracy is better in advanced compared to superficial disease; the latter is better staged with endoscopic mucosal resection (EMR) when possible. Combined with fine-needle aspiration (FNA), EUS provides the most accurate staging modality to prove regional lymph node involvement. T-stage accuracy is approximately 85%. Lymph nodes appear as hypoechoic, well-circumscribed areas greater than 10 mm in the area of the tumor. Lymph node FNA is possible if the needle tract is not obstructed by the tumor itself. For stenotic cancers, it may be difficult to pass the EUS probe distally. Patients with small (<1-1.5 cm) endoscopically visible lesions or identifiable areas should undergo EMR, which allows for accurate histologic distinction between mucosal (T1a) and submucosal (T1b) tumors. The former may be definitively treated with endoscopic methods, while submucosal lesions are best treated via surgical resection. This is due to the fact that esophageal lymphatics are located in the submucosa, leading to a low prevalence of nodal metastases in mucosal lesions. T1b lesions that penetrate the muscularis mucosa carry a potential for metastatic nodes of approximately 30%, rendering them more appropriate for esophagectomy.

An 18F-fluorodeoxyglucose positron emission tomography (PET) scan in combination with a CT scan is the single best systemic staging modality. This combination of PET-CT allows for optimization of the relationship of anatomic abnormalities to hypermetabolic areas (Figure 1). The magnitude of hypermetabolism, measured as the standard uptake value (SUV_{max}) has also been reported to have prognostic significance.

The identification of cancer-related biomarkers is becoming an increasingly important area of esophageal cancer treatment. The

TABLE 1: 2010 AJCC TNM classifications

Primary tumor (T)

TX	Primary tumor cannot be assessed.
T0	No evidence of primary tumor.
Tis	High-grade dysplasia.
T1	Tumor invades lamina propria, muscularis mucosae, or submucosa.
T1a	Tumor invades lamina propria or muscularis mucosae.
T1b	Tumor invades submucosa.
T2	Tumor invades muscularis propria.
T3	Tumor invades adventitia.
T4	Tumor invades adjacent structures.
T4a	Resectable tumor invading pleura, pericardium, or diaphragm.
T4b	Unresectable tumor invading other adjacent structures, such as aorta, vertebral body, trachea, etc.

Regional lymph nodes (N)

NX	Regional lymph nodes cannot be assessed.
N0	No regional lymph node metastasis.
N1	Metastases in 1 or 2 regional lymph nodes.
N2	Metastases in 3 to 6 regional lymph nodes.
N3	Metastases in 7 or more regional lymph nodes. Regional lymph node is defined as any periesophageal lymph node from the cervical lymph nodes to the celiac lymph nodes.

Distant metastasis (M)

M0	No distant metastasis.
M1	Distant metastasis.

Histologic grade

G1	Well differentiated.
G2	Moderately differentiated.
G3	Poorly differentiated.
G4	Undifferentiated.

Cancer location

Upper Thoracic	20-25 cm from the incisors.
Middle Thoracic	>25-30 cm from the incisors.
Lower Thoracic	>30-40 cm from the incisors.
Esophagogastric Junction	Includes cancers whose epicenter is in the distal thoracic esophagus, esophagogastric junction, or the proximal 5 cm of the stomach that extends into the esophagogastric junction or distal thoracic esophagus.

Adapted from 2010 AJCC cancer staging manual, ed 7, American Joint Committee on Cancer, New York, 2010, Springer.

TABLE 2: 2010 AJCC staging of esophageal adenocarcinoma and squamous cell carcinoma

Squamous cell carcinoma

Stage	T	N	M	Grade	Tumor Location
0	Tis (HGD)	N0	M0	1, X	Any
IA	T1	N0	M0	1, X	Any
IB	T1	N0	M0	2-3	Any
	T2-3	N0	M0	1, X	Lower, X
IIA	T2-3	N0	M0	1, X	Upper, middle
	T2-3	N0	M0	2-3	Lower, X
IIB	T2-3	N0	M0	2-3	Upper, middle
	T1-2	N1	M0	Any	Any
IIIA	T1-2	N2	M0	Any	Any
	T3	N1	M0	Any	Any
	T4a	N0	M0	Any	Any
IIIB	T3	N2	M0	Any	Any
IIIC	T4a	N1-2	M0	Any	Any
	T4b	Any	M0	Any	Any
	Any	N3	M0	Any	Any
IV	Any	Any	M1	Any	Any

Adenocarcinoma

Stage	T	N	M	Grade
0	Tis (HGD)	N0	M0	1, X
IA	T1	N0	M0	1-2, X
IB	T1	N0	M0	3
	T2	N0	M0	1-2, X
IIA	T2	N0	M0	3
IIB	T3	N0	M0	Any
	T1-2	N1	M0	Any
IIIA	T1-2	N2	M0	Any
	T3	N1	M0	Any
	T4a	N0	M0	Any
IIIB	T3	N2	M0	Any
IIIC	T4a	N1-2	M0	Any
	T4b	Any	M0	Any
	Any	N3	M0	Any
IV	Any	Any	M1	Any

Adapted from 2010 AJCC cancer staging manual, ed 7, American Joint Committee on Cancer, New York, 2010, Springer.

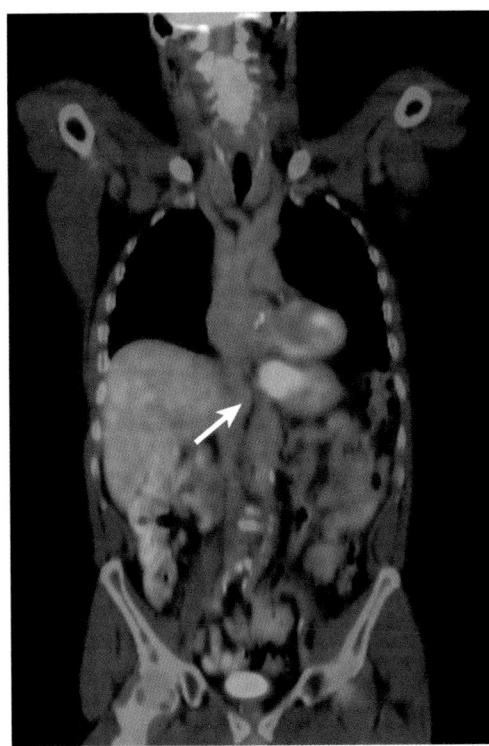

FIGURE 1   PET-CT imaging revealing distal esophageal/gastroesophageal junction (GEJ) hypermetabolic area (increased standardized uptake value [SUV] marked by arrow) in area of confirmed esophageal adenocarcinoma.

Survival according to treatment group

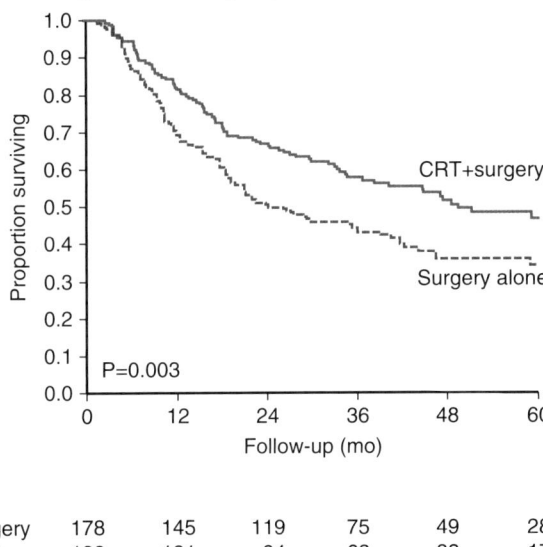

No. at risk						
CRT+surgery	178	145	119	75	49	28
Surgery alone	188	131	94	62	33	17
Total	366	276	213	137	82	45

FIGURE 2   Survival advantage in chemoradiotherapy (CRT) plus surgery compared to surgery alone. *(Data from van Hagen P, et al: Preoperative chemoradiotherapy for esophageal or junctional cancer, N Engl J Med 366(22):2074–2084, 2012.)*

immunohistochemical protein expression profile of markers, including Her2, p53, c-myc, Notch, and EGFR, has been analyzed with respect to esophageal carcinogenesis. Current evidence suggests that Her2 overexpression correlates with cancer progression and may be amenable to therapeutic intervention via medications such as trastuzumab. Although preliminary results are promising, extensive work remains to be done to formulate new treatment regimens or interventions based on a patient's genetic profile.

Despite all available diagnostic modalities—particularly esophagogastroduodenoscopy (EGD), EUS, and PET-CT—the clinical staging of esophageal adenocarcinoma is far from ideal. The TNM staging accuracy and the sensitivity and specificity of any individual modality have been widely reported. It is accepted that combinations of diagnostic modalities offer greater TNM clinical staging accuracy—approximately 80%—compared to the use of any single test. Furthermore, it has been reported that the accuracy of clinical staging significantly increases when the diagnostic tests are performed at a referral center and the results are analyzed by expert radiologists.

Due to the increasing implementation of neoadjuvant therapy in the treatment of esophageal carcinoma in the recent decade, pathologic staging classification has been altered so that it is no longer useful. Current staging systems are based on survival outcomes of patients undergoing esophagectomy alone; therefore, as a result, there is no good staging system as we move forward in 2012.

TREATMENT

Treatment of esophageal cancer, including the type of resection, can and should be individualized. Although far from precise, it is useful clinically to divide patients into those with a high probability of disease limited to the mucosa, those with a high probability of regional disease, and those with likely systemic disease. Among the

most significant treatment advances in recent years are the successful management of intramucosal carcinoma with endoscopic therapeutics and the routine use of neoadjuvant multimodal chemoradiotherapy in patients undergoing surgical resection.

Neoadjuvant Chemotherapy and Chemoradiotherapy

Most patients with carcinoma extending beyond the mucosa will be candidates for neoadjuvant therapy. Although controversy remains regarding its use in patients with clinical T1b (submucosal by EMR) node negative (by EUS) tumors, the probability of nodal metastases (15%-25%) and the false negative rate of EUS (25%-40%) provide rationale for neoadjuvant therapy even in these patients. Several randomized trials and meta-analyses have compared various regimens of neoadjuvant chemotherapy only and combined chemoradiotherapy (CRT). Despite these data, a consensus standard remains to be determined. The most recent, and among the best of these, is the Dutch chemotherapy and radiation in esophageal surgery study (CROSS) trial that compared neoadjuvant CRT and surgery to surgery alone. Patients with resectable (T2-3N0-1, M0) tumors received weekly administrations of paclitaxel and carboplatin for 5 weeks with 41.4 Gy of concurrent radiotherapy. The trial included 368 patients, of which 75% had adenocarcinoma and 23% squamous cell cancer. The R0 resection rate was 92% in the CRT arm versus 69% in the surgery alone arm. Twenty-nine percent (47/161) of those undergoing resection after CRT had a pathologic complete response. Five-year survival (47% vs 34%) was significantly improved in the neoadjuvant group (Figure 2).

Preoperative and postoperative chemotherapy alone (epirubicin, cisplatin, and fluorouracil) was compared to surgery in the medical research council adjuvant gastric infusional chemotherapy (MAGIC) trial, which also showed a benefit of neoadjuvant chemotherapy. This UK-based trial included 503 patients randomized to surgery alone or surgery plus 3 cycles of preoperative and postoperative chemotherapy. Survival was significantly better in the group receiving chemotherapy (5-year: 36% vs 23%). Twenty-six percent of the patients had carcinoma of the lower esophagus or GE junction. Either of these regimens is currently an acceptable option for treatment of patients with resectable esophageal adenocarcinoma, with evidence favoring combined CRT. Neoadjuvant combined chemoradiation utilizing 5-fluorouracil and cisplatin is the current standard for esophageal SCC.

Restaging via upper endoscopy and PET-CT should be performed following neoadjuvant treatment. A significant minority of patients (35%-50%) will achieve a clinical complete response (cCR, defined as endoscopic biopsy and PET-CT negative); therefore, surgical resection is currently recommended because most will have viable tumor identified in the surgical specimen.

Surgical Resection

High Probability of Localized Disease Confined to the Mucosa

Patients with invasive cancer penetrating beyond the basement membrane but limited to the mucosa (not penetrating through the muscularis mucosa; Figure 3), although once rare, currently comprise a significant proportion of patients with esophageal adenocarcinoma. Clinically, intramucosal cancer is characterized by minimal, if any, cancer-related symptoms and known Barrett's esophagus. As such, intramucosal cancer is usually identified via routine surveillance. Endoscopically, the tumors range from flat, nonvisible lesions to small (<1-2 cm), visible nodules. Proof that the neoplasia is confined to the mucosa is best provided by EMR of any and all identifiable areas. Both high-grade dysplasia and intramucosal esophageal adenocarcinoma are amenable to curative treatment via endoscopic intervention, including EMR and radiofrequency mucosal ablation (RFA) (Figure 4). Identifiable lesions are first excised via EMR followed by RFA ablation of the remaining Barrett's esophagus. Although no randomized, controlled trials of EMR versus esophagectomy exist, several case-control studies suggest that most, if not all, patients with intramucosal cancer have similar long-term outcomes with fewer complications following EMR than esophagectomy. Balancing this is the probability of recurrent dysplasia or carcinoma, which has been reported as high as 22%. Endoscopic therapy is often a lifelong process, not a single event. Complications of EMR are infrequent and

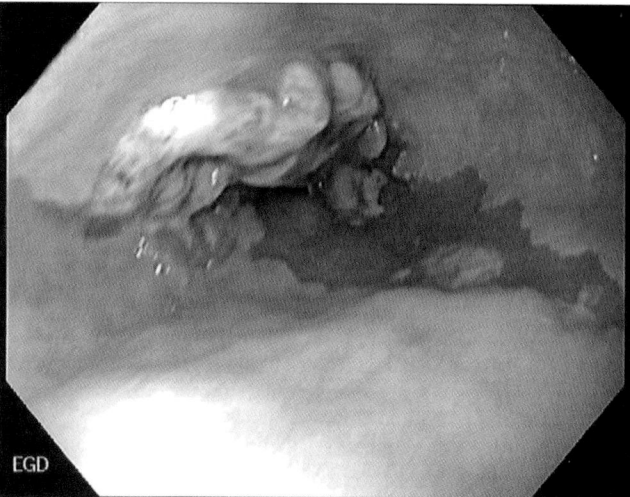

FIGURE 3 Endoscopic appearance of a tumor with a high probability of regional disease. Note a 2-cm to 3-cm 25% circumferential lesion and obvious Barrett's esophagus opposite the tumor. The lesion was identified incidentally via computed tomographic scan.

include bleeding, esophageal perforation, and delayed strictures. The 5-year survival in patients with superficial cancer approaches 90%.

High Probability of Regional Disease

Patients with regional disease are characterized clinically as those with minimal symptoms, including the absence of weight loss or dysphagia, and small (<2-3 cm) partially circumferential tumors identified endoscopically. Although debated, the preponderance of current evidence suggests that surgical resection ideally consists of en bloc esophagectomy with mediastinal and upper abdominal lymphadenectomy.

High Probability of Systemic Disease

Patients with a high probability of systemic disease are characterized clinically as those with systemic symptoms of cancer (weight loss, pain, anorexia), dysphagia, and large (>3 cm), usually circumferential, tumors on endoscopy. Extended lymphadenectomy is less likely to be of benefit in this group, although given the clinical ambiguities of the classifications, overtreatment is preferable to undertreatment, particularly in young, otherwise healthy patients. Patients with extensive locoregional tumor invasion (stage T4b) and PET-positive metastatic disease benefit from a chemoradiation regimen rather than resection.

Options for Esophageal Resection

A variety of options are available for esophageal resection in patients with esophageal cancer. Each has unique and sometimes important characteristics that allow individualization of surgical decision making. They include transhiatal esophagectomy; combined abdominal and right transthoracic esophagectomy with intrathoracic anastomosis (Ivor Lewis), or resection via combined abdominal, right transthoracic and neck incision with cervical anastomosis (McKeown); and left thoracoabdominal resection. The last two can be accompanied by an extended en bloc lymphadenotomy, and all three have been performed with combined laparoscopic and thoracoscopic minimally invasive techniques.

Transhiatal esophagectomy (THE) is performed via an upper midline laparotomy and a left cervical incision. The patient is positioned supine with arms tucked. Via the upper midline laparotomy, the left lateral segment of the liver is mobilized and retracted to the patient's right, and the esophagus is dissected at the hiatus. After entering the lesser sac, the stomach is mobilized and the short gastric vessels are ligated, with attention to preserving the right gastroepiploic artery and vein as the pedicle for the gastric graft. The left gastric artery and vein are dissected, and celiac nodal tissue is taken with the specimen. A Penrose drain is placed around the esophagus for traction and further mobilization. The lower third of the esophagus is dissected under direct vision via retraction of the hiatus. Both vagal nerves are cut, and the proximal two thirds of the esophagus are dissected bluntly via a hand through the hiatus. The posterior and anterior aspects are dissected first, followed by the right and left lateral portions. A 4-cm left-sided cervical incision is made paralleling the anterior border of the sternocleidomastoid muscle (SCM). After the SCM and carotid sheath are retracted laterally, the cervical esophagus is dissected. A Penrose drain is placed around the cervical esophagus to aid in further dissection along the esophageal wall. With traction on both the abdominal and cervical esophageal segments, final dissection of the thoracic esophagus is performed from both directions. The mobilized esophagus is divided, leaving a 3- to 4-cm cervical esophageal remnant, and the specimen is brought out of the laparotomy incision.

The stomach is divided in a vertical fashion via several firings of a 75-mm GIA stapler, taking a generous portion of the lesser curve with the specimen. Maintaining orientation, the gastric conduit is

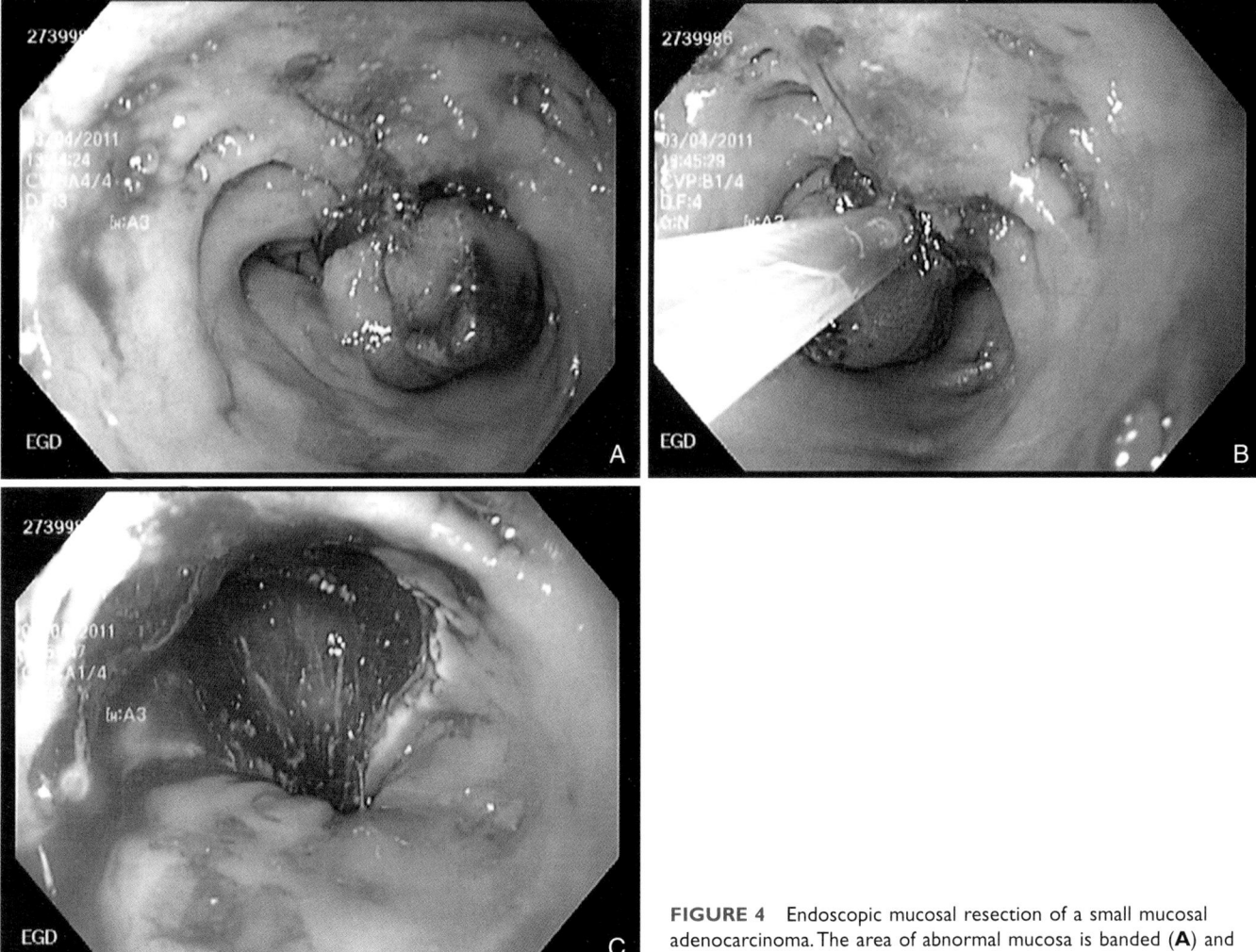

FIGURE 4 Endoscopic mucosal resection of a small mucosal adenocarcinoma. The area of abnormal mucosa is banded (**A**) and resected (**B**). Appearance of esophagus post-EMR (**C**).

sutured to a chest tube and is passed though the thorax to the cervical stump. A stapled or hand-sewn anastomosis is then performed via the cervical approach. A nasogastric tube is placed, and a J-tube is left in place for postoperative nutrition. The limitations of THE include a limited thoracic lymph node dissection and lack of direct visualization in the thoracic cavity. THE is preferable in distal esophageal cancer and is most appropriate in patients with a high likelihood of systemic disease and those with other underlying comorbidities. In patients with transmural tumors above the carina, the authors favor a transthoracic approach.

An Ivor Lewis esophagectomy includes a combined upper midline laparotomy and right thoracotomy and a high intrathoracic anastomosis. After an upper midline laparotomy incision is made, the hiatal dissection and mobilization of the stomach and distal esophagus are performed in the same fashion as in THE. We prefer to divide the stomach prior to pulling it into the chest. Upon completion of the abdominal mobilization, the patient is repositioned and a right posterolateral thoracotomy is made in the fifth intercostal space. The right lung is deflated and retracted, and the distal third of the esophagus is dissected and circled with a Penrose drain. The esophageal dissection can then be taken toward the neck and abdomen. A subcarinal lymphadenectomy is generally performed, and the thoracic duct may be ligated as it enters the thoracic cavity to minimize the risk of a chyle leak. The stomach is pulled into the chest through the hiatus and positioned into the thoracic inlet. An end (esophagus) to side (stomach) anastomosis is performed above the azygous vein. The anastomosis is generally 3 to 5 cm lower when performed through

the chest, which has the advantage of allowing better gastric blood supply at the level of the anastomosis and the disadvantage of a higher incidence of postoperative reflux. Ivor Lewis esophagectomy is preferable in patients with middle or distal esophageal tumors.

A three-incision esophagectomy incorporates characteristics of the previous two approaches. The patient is placed in the left lateral decubitus position, and a right posterolateral thoracotomy is made as in the Ivor Lewis technique. The esophagus is mobilized from the diaphragm to the cervical inlet. A chest tube is left in place, and the thorax is closed. The patient is then placed in the supine position. An upper midline laparotomy is performed, and the hiatus, esophagus, and stomach are mobilized as in the previous two techniques. A left cervical incision is made to mobilize the cervical esophagus where it is divided. The gastric conduit is brought up to the cervical incision, where the anastomosis is fashioned. This technique may be preferable for mid- to upper-esophageal cancers because it allows for visual inspection of the thoracic esophagus.

An en bloc lymphadenectomy can be performed via either of the transthoracic approaches. The aim is to resect the esophagus en bloc with all surrounding lymphatic tissue from the carina to the celiac axis. The thoracic resection field is bound by the carina superiorly, esophageal hiatus inferiorly, hilum of lung and pericardium anteriorly, and the descending aorta and spine posteriorly (Figure 5). The pleura is initially incised along the azygous vein. The dissection proceeds toward the aortic adventitia with identification of the thoracic duct, which is ligated as it enters the chest. The left pleura is incised from the left mainstem bronchus to the diaphragm, and the azygous

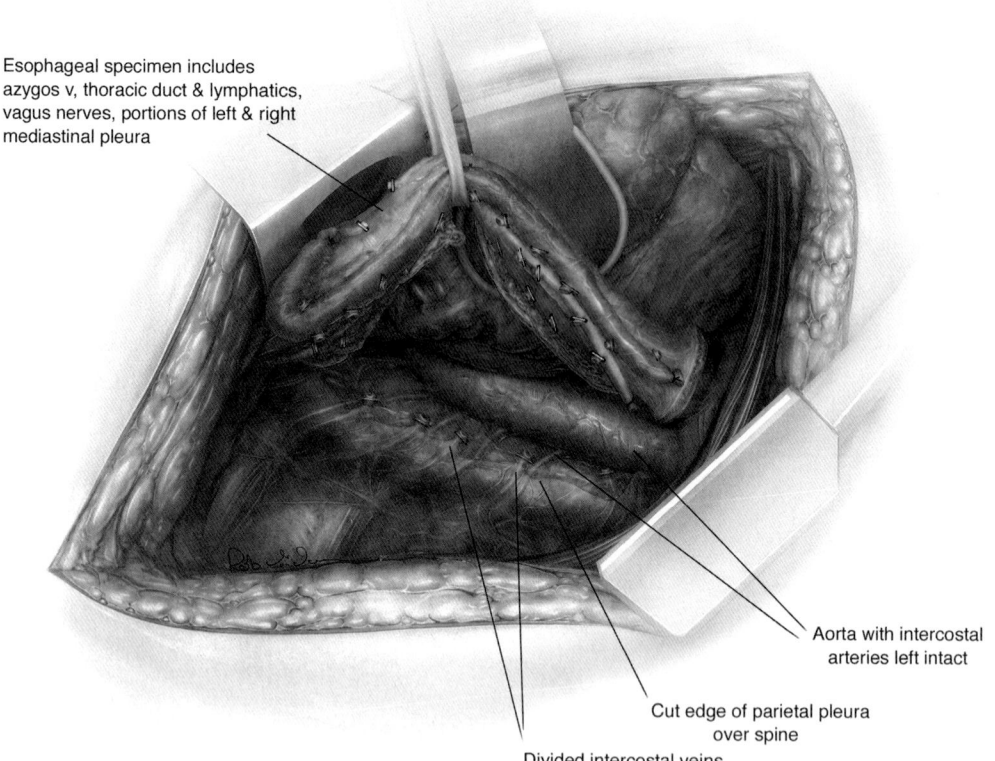

Esophageal specimen includes
azygos v, thoracic duct & lymphatics,
vagus nerves, portions of left & right
mediastinal pleura

Aorta with intercostal
arteries left intact

Cut edge of parietal pleura
over spine

Divided intercostal veins

FIGURE 5 Extent of dissection at completion of mediastinal lymphadenectomy and esophageal mobilization during en bloc esophagectomy. *(From Peters JH: En-bloc esophagectomy,* Operative Techniques in General Surgery Journal *8(3):150–155, 2006.)*

vein is divided at the vena cava. The resection specimen contains the subcarinal lymph node basins. An abdominal incision is then made, and a celiac lymph node dissection is also carried out. The abdominal resection field is bound by the hiatus superiorly, pancreas inferiorly, splenic hilum laterally, and the inferior vena cava and common hepatic artery medially. A gastric conduit is constructed, and a thoracic or cervical anastomosis is constructed.

Minimally invasive esophagectomy (MIE) has been slow to be adopted and currently accounts for approximately 15% of esophagectomies performed. This technique can be performed via combinations of laparoscopy and thoracoscopy with the same basic principles of thoracic and abdominal dissection as in open techniques. The most common version begins with placing the patient in a left lateral decubitus position, after which a four-port entry technique is utilized to dissect the esophagus via the right thoracic cavity. The right lung is deflated and retracted, exposing the posterior mediastinum. The esophageal dissection proceeds in a caudad to cephalad direction, with concurrent dissection of the paraesophageal and subcarinal lymph nodes. The azygous vein is ligated with an endoscopic linear stapler to aid in cephalad dissection into the thoracic inlet. After the esophagus is mobilized from the diaphragm to the thoracic inlet, Penrose drains can be tied around the mobilized esophagus distally and proximally to aid in retrieval during the abdominal and cervical phases, respectively. A chest tube is left in the right pleural cavity, and the incisions are closed. The abdominal phase begins with placing the patient in a supine position and involves the placement of five ports. The dissection involves the hiatus, mobilization of the stomach with preservation of the right gastroepiploic artery, and creation of a gastric conduit with several deployments of a linear endoscopic stapler. A cervical anastomosis can then be fashioned via a hand-sewn or stapled technique through a cervical incision. Although a standardized MIE technique has not yet emerged, MIE may be optimal for patients with small tumors and limited nodal involvement.

Outcomes after MIE compared to open resection have been similar as far as mortality and 30-day morbidity; however, MIE may result in less respiratory complications, albeit with higher rates of reintervention and reoperation. The only randomized controlled trial of MIE versus open esophagectomy concluded that the incidence of pulmonary complications is lower in the MIE group (12% vs 34%). The extent of lymphadenectomy in MIE appears to be comparable to open esophagectomy; however, there are no studies to assess the long-term oncologic outcomes of patients undergoing MIE.

Perioperative Care: Morbidity and Mortality of Esophageal Resection

A 7-day to 14-day hospital stay is common following esophagectomy for cancer. Clinical care plans and standardized protocols have been shown to decrease stay and associated costs. Most surgeons, including the authors, continue to place a nasogastric tube for the first 5 to 7 days postoperatively to allow for decompression of the gastric conduit and to minimize aspiration risk, although its benefit has not been shown in prospective, randomized trials. Most also place a feeding jejunostomy at the time of surgery and begin daily tube feed on postoperative day 2 or 3. This allows not only for early enteral feeding but also for complete nutrition and discharge home in the case of an anastomotic leak and prolonged NPO. A clinical assessment of the integrity of the anastomosis is often helpful 5 to 7 days postoperatively. The authors prefer to do this via routine upper endoscopy. This has several advantages over barium contrast studies, including an accurate assessment of the size and location of any potential anastomotic disruption, an assessment of the mucosal blood supply of the upper gastric conduit, and the avoidance of potential oral contrast leakage and contamination. Furthermore, barium studies have been well documented to have a high prevalence of false negative and occasionally false positive interpretation.

Complications occur in 50% to 75% of patients. Esophagogastric anastomotic leak rates average 15% for a cervical and 5% for an intrathoracic anastomosis. Most patients can and should be managed without the need for transfusion, allowing postoperative hematocrit levels to drift into the low 20s if necessary. Pulmonary complications predominate. Common complications include atrial fibrillation (17%), delirium (13%), pneumonia (9%), urinary infection (6%), ileus (5%), pleural effusion requiring treatment (4%), chyle leak (3%), pulmonary embolism (3%), pneumothorax (3%), and wound infection (2%-3%). Less common are myocardial infarction, deep venous thrombosis, stroke, reoperation for bleeding, recurrent laryngeal nerve paralysis, and sepsis. Esophageal resection is among the surgical procedures in which mortality is significantly affected by both surgeon and hospital volume. In high-volume centers, defined as those performing more than 20 esophagectomies per year, 30-day esophagectomy-related mortality is approximately 2% to 4%. This compares to 15% to 25% mortality in low-volume centers. It is no surprise, however, that many esophagectomies are still being performed in low-volume centers across the United States.

Management of Complications

Optimization of postoperative analgesia and implementation of proper pulmonary toilet are paramount to the prevention of respiratory failure, pneumonia, and reintubation. The interplay of the surgeon, respiratory therapists, and nursing staff is critical in preventing respiratory complications. Should respiratory complications arise, patients are supported with antibiotics and mechanical ventilation, if necessary.

Atrial fibrillation most commonly occurs on postoperative days 2 through 5. Due to the decreased cardiac output and perfusion of the gastric conduit in atrial fibrillation, it is essential to establish rate-control with beta-blockade and amiodarone. In the case of hypotension, occasional cardioversion may be necessary. As a whole, atrial fibrillation usually resolves spontaneously. If medical intervention is utilized, treatment should be maintained for 6 weeks.

An anastomotic leak is usually heralded by new onset fever, tachycardia, and increasing leukocytosis around postoperative days 5 through 7. It is of utmost importance to assess the surgical drains daily and to identify new pleural effusions on chest x-ray. Should a leak arise, it is managed by early broad-spectrum antibiotics (piperacillin/tazobactam plus or minus vancomycin), NPO, and appropriate drainage if there is a collection either via chest tube or by opening the cervical wound. A determination of the size and location of the leak can be established via EGD, and reassessment should be done on a weekly basis. If the leak is large with systemic compromise, the placement of a plastic anastomotic stent may be utilized. Anastomotic leaks that are well managed are not as lethal as in the past, and many can be managed without ICU transfer if anticipated and treated early.

Chyle leaks are most often identified by milky drain output. The management of a chyle leak depends largely on the volume and duration of the leak. As a general rule, drain outputs of less than 500 mL per day that are trending downward can be managed expectantly with NPO status and total parenteral nutrition. Chyle leaks of greater than 1 L per day with continued high output should be addressed surgically with exploration of the thoracic cavity either through a minimally invasive or open approach, with the goal to ligate the thoracic duct at its entrance into the thoracic cavity at the level of the diaphragm.

Survival

Five-year survival after esophagectomy alone is well documented to average 25% to 30%. This can be improved to 40% to 50% with the combination of neoadjuvant therapy and selective use of en bloc lymphadenectomy. Both a higher number of removed nodes and the use of en bloc resection have been shown to be independent predictors of improved survival. Stage-specific survival is shown in Figure 6. Overall, outcomes are better after neoadjuvant chemoradiotherapy, which seems in large part due to increasing R0 resection rates to approximately 95%. Most recurrences occur within 12 to 18 months, and more than 90% by 3 years. Surveillance after treatment should include clinical follow-up every 3 to 4 months for the first 2 years, every 6 months up to 5 years, and then annually. Blood sampling and repeat imaging are utilized as clinically indicated. CT is the preferred imaging modality for detecting recurrence after esophagectomy.

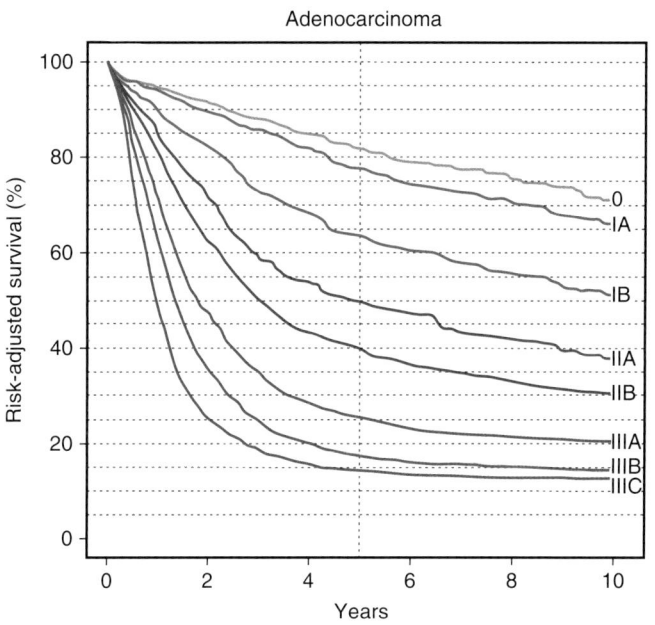

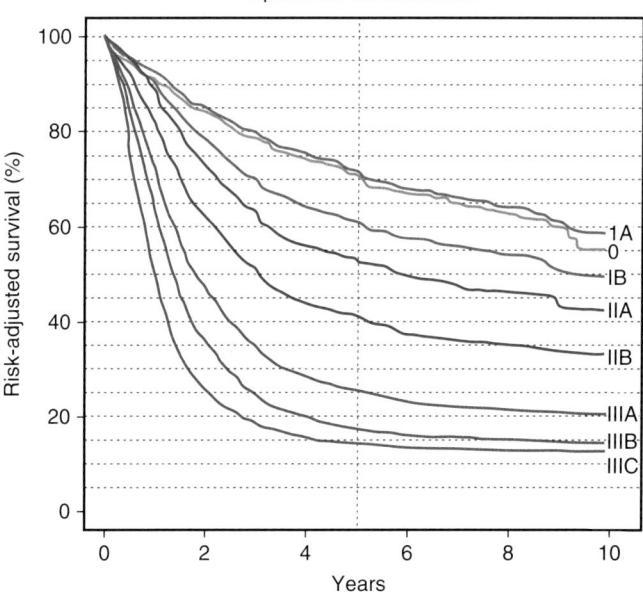

FIGURE 6 Risk-adjusted survival curves for adenocarcinoma and squamous cell carcinoma. *(Adapted from* AJCC cancer staging manual, *ed 7, 2010.)*

Functional Outcomes

Despite a wide range of postsurgical recovery time, functional outcomes after esophagectomy are generally good. Most patients are eventually either asymptomatic or have minor symptoms that do not require intervention. Less than 50% have dysphagia, regurgitation, or other gastrointestinal symptoms that may require intervention. Patients who survive more than 2 years regain their preop quality of life (QOL) within 6 to 9 months. In contrast, most patients who die within 2 years never regain their preop QOL.

CONCLUSIONS

The treatment paradigms of both esophageal adenocarcinoma and SCC currently include multimodal therapy tailored to each patient's specific clinical circumstances. Patients with early-stage adenocarcinoma (T1a, intramucosal) are ideally treated with endoscopic resection rather than traditional esophagectomy. Patients with T1b to T4a disease benefit from combinations of neoadjuvant and adjuvant chemotherapy and CRT in addition to surgical resection. Patients with T4b staging do not benefit from resection and are palliated with systemic chemotherapy often in combination with other procedures such as esophageal stenting. With the increasing incidence of esophageal adenocarcinoma, current and future efforts must be focused on optimizing treatment regimens to optimize survival in patients with this all too lethal disease.

SUGGESTED READINGS

Carrott PW, et al: Accordion severity grading system: assessment of relationship between costs, length of hospital stay, and survival in patients with complications after esophagectomy for cancer, *J Am Coll Surg* 215(3):331–336, 2012.

Li C, et al: An enhanced recovery pathway decreases duration of stay after esophagectomy, *Surgery* 152(4):606–616, 2012.

Portale G, et al: Modern 5-year survival of resectable esophageal adenocarcinoma: single institution experience with 263 patients, *J Am Coll Surg* 202(4):588–596; discussion 596–598, 2006.

Sjoquist KM, et al: Survival after neoadjuvant chemotherapy or chemoradiotherapy for resectable oesophageal carcinoma: an updated meta-analysis, *Lancet Oncol* 12(7):681–692, 2011.

Vallbohmer D, Oh DS, Peters JH: The role of lymphadenectomy in the surgical treatment of esophageal and gastric cancer, *Curr Probl Surg* 49(8):471–515, 2012.

van Hagen P, et al: Preoperative chemoradiotherapy for esophageal or junctional cancer, *N Engl J Med* 366(22):2074–2084, 2012.

NEOADJUVANT AND ADJUVANT THERAPY OF ESOPHAGEAL CANCER

Nabil P. Rizk, MD

INTRODUCTION

A few skeptics still remain regarding the benefits of multimodality therapy in esophageal cancer. However, with recent advances in the understanding of the disease (including a new staging system, better clinical staging capabilities, better algorithms for combined chemotherapy and radiation, and better tolerated therapeutic options) and the culmination of the recent publication of the Chemoradiotherapy for Oesophageal Cancer Followed by Surgery Study (CROSS) Group trial in which many of these new developments are accounted for, most investigators now agree that a subset of patients with esophageal cancer benefits from multimodality therapy. This is a marked departure from a previous era in which evidence cited as support for multimodality therapy was scarce and in which reliance on meta-analyses of flawed data was necessary to support the approach. Our current, more nuanced understanding of the treatment of esophageal cancer incorporates a better appreciation of the different stages of disease and the variable outcomes of the different histology. Consequently, although in the past all esophageal cancers were treated uniformly, current standards of care represent a marked evolution in treatment and outcomes. In the present era, a near consensus exists that early stage esophageal cancers (T1aN0 tumors) are most appropriately treated with either endoscopic means or surgery alone and that the only tumors considered appropriate for multimodality therapy are those which are *local-regionally advanced*. In this chapter, part I provides a summary of the patients whose conditions are appropriate for multimodality therapy; part II discusses various aspects of multimodality therapy, including what is commonly accepted, what remains controversial, and what is unknown.

PART I: DEFINITION OF LOCAL-REGIONAL ADVANCED ESOPHAGEAL CANCER

Patients with local-regional advanced esophageal cancer are candidates for multimodality therapy. Local-regional advanced esophageal cancer includes T2-T4 tumors and tumors with nodal disease (N1-N2) that are M0. In these patients, positron emission tomography (PET scan) is considered to be the gold standard for exclusion of metastatic disease, and endoscopic ultrasound scan (EUS) is considered to be the gold standard for evaluation of depth of disease. Nodal status, both the presence and the number of nodes, is the least predictable of the staging variables.

Clinical T1 Tumors

The recently updated American Joint Committee on Cancer (AJCC) system for esophageal cancer recognizes but does not distinguish between superficial (T1a) and deep (T1b) T1 tumors. T1a tumors by definition invade the mucosa only; T1b tumors invade into the submucosa. Although the depth of invasion in T1 tumors has implications regarding the possibility of successful endoscopic management, an equally important distinction is the potential for nodal metastases; namely, T1a and superficial T1b tumors (<50 of the submucosa invaded) rarely metastasize to regional lymph nodes, and deep T1b tumors (>50% of the submucosa invasion) can metastasize to regional lymph nodes more than 40% of the time. The clinical implication of this early propensity for development of regional nodal disease is that T1b tumors are often understaged clinically, both because EUS is not accurate at distinguishing T1a and superficial T1b tumors from deep T1b tumors and because nodal disease is not accurately detected in T1 tumors with standard EUS and PET techniques. Less commonly used adjuncts to these two studies, EUS fine needle aspiration (FNA) and the PET maximal standard uptake value (SUV-max) of the primary tumor, have both been shown to increase the accuracy of detection of nodal disease. In summary, a reasonable approach to clinical T1 tumors is an attempt of an endoscopic mucosal resection as a possible therapeutic or diagnostic modality; if the deep pathologic margin invades the submucosa, with or without an involved deep margin, the possibility exists that this tumor represents a "deep" T1b tumor with a reasonable potential for regional nodal involvement. In this situation, additional efforts should be made to establish nodal disease, including the use of PET SUV-max and EUS FNA. If nodal disease is confirmed with reasonable certainty, these patients should be considered to have local-regionally advanced disease and should receive multimodality therapy.

Clinical T2 Tumors

Pathologic T2 tumors treated with surgery alone are associated with poor long-term survival and have a high likelihood of nodal disease; therefore, all of these tumors should be considered for multimodality therapy. Clinical establishment of whether a patient has a pathologic T2 tumor remains a challenge, however. Although EUS is the only means of establishing depth of invasion with any accuracy, T2 tumors are commonly overstaged and most frequently pathologically are deep T1b tumors. Less frequently, these tumors are in fact T3 tumors. One clinical correlate that is helpful in deciding whether patients are overstaged or understaged with EUS T2 is the presence of dysphagia; T1b tumors are rarely associated with dysphagia, whereas T2 and T3 tumors frequently are. In summary, if a patient presents with a EUS T2 tumor without dysphagia, then the workup should proceed as for a T1 tumor. If the patient has dysphagia, then multimodality therapy should be considered.

Clinical T3 Tumors

Diagnosis of clinical T3 tumors is most reliably done with EUS with a high level of confidence. Establishing nodal status is less relevant in these tumors because invariably these tumors are also node positive (if an adequate lymphadenectomy is done).

Clinical N1-N2 Tumors

Establishment of nodal disease is most relevant in more superficial tumors because in these tumors the option of a local therapy is available. In patients with EUS T1b tumors and EUS T2 tumors without dysphagia, the nodal status must be established as definitively as possible before resection. EUS appearance is unreliable, especially in superficial tumors. Likewise, visual identification of nodal disease with PET and computed tomographic (CT) scan is unreliable in more superficial esophageal cancers. The most accurate diagnostic tool is EUS-guided FNA. PET SUV-max is also a useful tool when EUS FNA is unavailable or when no nodes are identified. Some studies indicate that a low PET SUV-max of the primary tumor is rarely associated with a nodal disease.

Restaging After Preoperative Therapy

After completion of preoperative therapy, restaging of patients before surgery usually incorporates a CT scan to evaluate the possibility of locally invasive and potentially unresectable disease and a PET scan to exclude metastatic disease. Repeat esophagoscopy should be used to evaluate the endoluminal extent of disease; it is not, however, predictive of the presence of persistent disease. Repeat EUS likewise has minimal utility in restaging of patients.

PART II: MANAGEMENT OF LOCAL-REGIONAL ADVANCED ESOPHAGEAL CANCERS

Near Consensus

Multimodality Therapy

Many previously cited publications that were used to either support or refute the advantages of multimodality therapy or surgery alone for esophageal cancer resulted from multiinstitutional prospective randomized trials. For various reasons, many of these trials have been rendered irrelevant with the current approach to staging and treating the disease. Most of these studies did not have the availability of current standard staging studies, including PET scan, EUS, or even CT scan. Furthermore, these trials often treated an undefined number of patients with early stage disease, with the presence of any non-metastatic disease as the sole trial cancer-related entry criteria (Tables 1 and 2). The potential benefit of adjuvant therapy can only be expected in: (1) patients at risk for metastatic disease, which is unlikely in T1a and in superficial T1b tumors; and (2) patients without overt metastatic disease, which was probably underestimated in a significant number of patients given the limited clinical staging capabilities of the era. Thus, that these older studies did not reliably inform management is not surprising. Another important limitation in these studies includes wide variations in the administration of multimodality therapy. Concurrent chemoradiation is now accepted to be better than sequential chemotherapy and radiation, and some of the newer chemotherapy agents are considered at least equally effective but more tolerable than prior regimens. Because of these many limitations, many of the relevant advances made to the current understanding of multimodality therapy resulted partly from single-institution phase II trials. These trials were able to consistently innovate and evolve as newer technologies and therapies became available. Likewise, over time, large institutional databases became available and were able to validate certain treatment approaches. Ultimately, information from such trials and datasets culminated in several recent prospective clinical trials, which have significantly increased the understanding of the management of local-regional advanced esophageal cancer.

Currently, a near consensus exists that surgery alone for local-regional advanced esophageal cancer is inadequate. Furthermore, although little data directly compare chemotherapy alone before surgery with chemoradiation before surgery, the relevant studies that individually evaluate each approach tend to favor chemoradiation over chemotherapy only; certainly that is the approach most commonly used in the United States.

In addition to the perception of the superiority of preoperative chemoradiation over chemotherapy, squamous cell cancer (SCC) of the esophagus is also increasingly recognized to be significantly more responsive to chemoradiation than adenocarcinoma. One obvious implication of this finding is that predicting a clinical complete response is more reliable in SCC given the underlying higher incidence of the event; but a broader question raised is whether surgery should only be used as salvage therapy in squamous cell cancers after definitive chemoradiotherapy. Lastly, another recognized pathologic feature after chemoradiation is the higher likelihood of uninvolved surgical radial margins when compared with chemotherapy followed by surgery.

TABLE 1: Prospective randomized trials comparing preoperative chemo-radiation to surgery alone

Trial	No. of patients	Tumor type	Clinical stage	Staging workup	Chemotherapy	Radiation	Median survival rate	Significance
Nygaard (1992)	53	Squamous cell	All stages	CT, EGD	Cis, bleomycin	35 Gy	17%, 3-y	NS
	50				None	None	9%, 3-y	
LePrise (1994)	41	Squamous cell	All stages	CXR, ultrasound	Cis, 5-FU	20 Gy*	19.2%, 3-y	NS
	45				None	None	13.8%, 3-y	
Bosset (1997)	143	Squamous cell	All stages	CT, EGD, bronchoscopy	Cis	37 Gy	18.6 mo	NS
	139				None	None	18.6 mo	
Walsh (1996)	58	Adenocarcinoma	All stages	CXR, EGD, ultrasound	Cis, 5-FU	40 Gy	16 mo	P = 0.01
	55				None	None	11 mo	
Urba (2001)	50	Adenocarcinoma (50%)	All stages	CT, bone scan, endoscopy	Cis, 5-FU, vinblastine	45 Gy	16.9 mo	NS
	50	Squamous cell (50%)			None	None	17.6 mo	
Burmeister (2005)	128	Adenocarcinoma (62.9%)	All stages	CT, EGD	Cis, 5-FU	35 Gy	22.2 mo	NS
	128	Squamous cell (37.1%)			None	None	19.3 mo	
Tepper (2008)	30	Adenocarcinoma (75.0%)	All stages	CT, EGD	Cis, 5-FU	50.4 Gy	53.8 mo	P = 0.002
	26	Squamous cell (25.0%)			None	None	21.5 mo	
CROSS (2012)	178	Adenocarcinoma (75.0%)	≥Stage II	CT, EUS, EGD	Carbo, paclitaxel	41.4 Gy	49.4 mo	P = 0.003
	188	Squamous cell (25.0%)			None	None	24.0 mo	

*Sequential.

Carbo, Carboplatin; *Cis,* cisplatin; *CT,* computed tomographic scan of chest and abdomen; *CXR,* chest x-ray; *EGD,* esophagoscopy; *EUS,* endoscopic ultrasound scan; *5-FU,* 5-fluorouracil; *NS,* not significant.

TABLE 2: Prospective randomized trials comparing preoperative chemotherapy to surgery alone

Trial	No. of patients	Tumor type	Clinical stage	Chemotherapy	5-year survival rate	Significance
MRC (2002)	400	Adenocarcinoma (66%)	All stages	Cisplatin, 5-fluorouracil	25.0%	P = 0.004
	402	Squamous cell (31%)		None	15.0%	
RTOG 8911 (1998)	233	Adenocarcinoma (53%)	All stages	Cisplatin, 5-fluorouracil	18%	P = 0.53
	234	Squamous cell (47%)		None	20%	
MAGIC (2006)*	250	Adenocarcinoma	≥Stage II	Epirubicin, cisplatin, 5-fluorouracil	36.3%	P = 0.008
	253			None	23.0%	

*25% Gastroesophageal junction tumors.

MAGIC, Medical Research Council Adjuvant Gastric Infusional Chemotherapy Trial; *MRC,* Medical Research Council; *RTOG,* Radiation Therapy Oncology Group.

Type of Chemotherapy

Before the CROSS trial, data from various studies strongly supported the use of a cisplatin-based two-drug regimen (used in most randomized trials since the 1980s). Over time, the second drug evolved from the more poorly tolerated fluorouracil to several other better-tolerated drugs such as paclitaxel and irinotecan. The CROSS trial used carboplatin and paclitaxel concurrently with 41.40 Gy and showed impressive benefits. Given the ease of administration and relatively lower toxicity, this regimen is rapidly being adopted as the default new standard of care.

Controversial

Definitive Chemoradiation

Although the use of chemoradiation therapy followed by esophagectomy for local-regional advanced esophageal cancers has become accepted by most surgeons as the standard of care, this acceptance is not necessarily true of all physicians; the perception exists among some that definitive chemoradiation is the most appropriate treatment for all esophageal cancers, with surgery relegated to salvage recurrent disease. One reason for this approach stems from a sense of nihilism concerning a cancer with such poor outcomes, and part stems from fear of an operation with historically high morbidity and mortality rates. A major reason for this approach, however, is the presence of conflicting data in the literature regarding the added benefit of surgery in patients after chemoradiotherapy. The most important study that evaluated the marginal benefit of surgery after chemoradiation (Stahl) did not show a survival advantage with the addition of surgery. In this study, patients were randomized to either chemoradiation followed by surgery or to chemoradiation alone. Although this study raises important questions about the added benefit of surgery in this patient population, it is also important to note that the large majority of the patients had squamous cell cancer, the mortality rate of the operative arms was high (11.3%), and the local recurrence rate was higher in the nonsurgical arm. The relevance of these points includes the fact that adenocarcinoma is far more common in the western hemisphere and that it is not possible to extrapolate results from this study given the known differences in treatment response between squamous cell carcinoma and adenocarcinoma.

Selective Definitive Chemoradiation

Selective definitive chemoradiation implies definitive treatment with evaluation of clinical response either during or at the completion of the therapy. Surgery is then offered only to patients with persistent disease after chemoradiation. Supporters of this approach point to the Bedenne trial as evidence that surgery provides no additional benefit in patients whose conditions respond to therapy. Most proponents of this approach reserve it specifically for squamous cell carcinoma. They point to the fact that both Stahl's and Bedenne's trials included predominantly squamous cell carcinomas and that in a subgroup analysis of the CROSS trial and the Burmeister trial, patients with squamous cell cancer seem to benefit relatively more from chemoradiation than those with adenocarcinoma. Further supporting this approach is the significantly higher rates of complete pathologic response in squamous cell carcinoma and the fact that this is the standard approach for cervical esophageal squamous cell carcinomas. Some concerns are raised by this approach, however, and have not been addressed in these trials. Most importantly is the consequence of a local-regional recurrence. How often a salvage esophagectomy is possible in these patients is unclear. What happens when salvage is not possible? And what were the complications when salvage was done? Although conflicting studies are found regarding the risks of salvage esophagectomy, some attribute significantly

increased risks for complications and death. An additional concern is specific regarding squamous cell cancers: these tumors typically arise in the mid esophagus, and when they recur local-regionally, they are frequently unresectable with very few available palliative options. Lastly, the definition of achievement of an adequate clinical response is not yet clear.

Selective Chemoradiation Versus Chemotherapy in Adenocarcinoma

The data supporting the benefits of preoperative chemoradiotherapy are most convincing in squamous cell carcinoma, whereas the data in adenocarcinoma are more tenuous. This differential benefit is best seen in the CROSS and Burmeister trials. One question, which is raised as a result of this difference, is whether adenocarcinoma is better treated with preoperative chemotherapy instead of chemoradiotherapy. Proponents of this selective preoperative approach based on histologic type also extrapolate the results from the Cunningham trial, which included primarily gastric cancer trials but also 25% esophageal and gastroesophageal junction adenocarcinomas. Proponents of the addition of radiation to the management of adenocarcinoma, however, point to the higher likelihood of achieving R0 resections with the addition of radiation, with several studies showing a correlation between R0 resection and survival. No good clinical trials are found to compare these two approaches.

Added Risks to Surgery of Chemoradiation

A persistent concern about the use of preoperative chemoradiation has been the potential of increased postoperative complications. This concern should be addressed as two separate questions: (1) what are the added risks after preoperative chemoradiation? and (2) what are the added risks after definitive chemoradiation and salvage esophagectomy? Most of the data regarding the added risks of preoperative chemoradiation compared with surgery alone, culminating in the CROSS trial, do not support any added risks. The caveat in these data is that the average patient receiving preoperative therapy tends to be younger and healthier than the average esophageal cancer population. In this vein, some good data support increased postoperative morbidity in older patients who received preoperative therapy, defined variably as age greater than 70 years or 80 years. The data regarding increased morbidity after salvage esophagectomy are less consistent, with some studies showing significant added risks and others showing none. One likely reason for these inconsistencies is that these series tend to be in highly skewed populations, typically patients at high risk who were not initially good surgical candidates. The available randomized data do not inform us on this issue.

Optimal Radiation Dose

Concurrent chemoradiation was proven to be superior to radiation alone in an early Radiation Therapy Oncology Group (RTOG) trial (RTOG 85-01). A subsequent RTOG trial (RTOG 94-05) evaluated the optimal radiation dose and compared 50.4 Gy with 64.8 Gy as a definitive concurrent chemoradiation dose. This trial determined that the higher dose was associated with higher complication rates, including fistulae and deaths, without any survival benefit. These data were then extrapolated for use as preoperative therapy in deciding the optimal tolerable preoperative radiation dose. In reality, many of the complications seen in the higher radiation group in the RTOG trial occurred before even reaching the 50.4 Gy dose, so whether higher doses necessarily result in higher complications is unclear. What is more clear is that higher radiation doses can be associated with improved pathologic response rates, and in situations where definitive chemoradiation (such as in squamous cell carcinoma) is being considered, that higher dosing may be worth exploring.

Different Approach to Siewert II and Siewert III Tumors

Although the most recent AJCC staging recommendations have combined all gastroesophageal junction (GEJ) tumors into the same esophageal staging system, this change did not result in a consensus about the best management of GEJ tumors. Because gastric cancer multimodality trials include patients with GEJ tumors, notably Siewert II and III tumors, the tumors are frequently managed as gastric cancers. Alternatively, some make a distinction between Siewert II and III tumors and manage local-regional advanced Siewert III lesions as gastric cancers, typically with either preoperative and postoperative chemotherapy or with postoperative chemoradiation, and local-regional advanced Siewert II lesions with preoperative chemoradiotherapy.

PET-Directed Therapy

There are expanded indications for the use of PET scans to assist in directing multimodality treatment beyond excluding metastatic disease. The indications most supported by evidence stem from the Metabolic response evaluation for individualisation of neoadjuvant chemotherapy in esophageal and esophagogastric adenocarcinoma (MUNCON) trials, which prospectively showed that patients who have evidence of a PET response to induction chemotherapy have a better prognosis and that the lack of PET response might be an indication to alter the planned therapy. Use of PET scan at the completion of chemoradiotherapy to either establish the lack of residual disease or to estimate response to therapy is least supported by clinical data, likely because of the confounding effects of radiation.

Unknown

Very little data are found on what the optimal management is for patients initially managed surgically who subsequently are found to have a more advanced stage of disease for which multimodality therapy is appropriate. Options include observation, adjuvant chemotherapy, or adjuvant chemoradiation. Another area without clear guidelines is the management of patients with involved radial margins, especially in patients who did not receive preoperative radiation. Although radiation is frequently added in this situation, no evidence is found to support any particular treatment approach.

SUMMARY

Multimodality has become the standard of care for the management of local-regional advanced esophageal cancer, with concurrent chemoradiation as the most accepted preoperative therapy. In the future, further attempts will be seen to define which subset of patients are most appropriately treated with definitive chemoradiation, reserving surgery for palliation of either persistent or recurrent disease.

SUGGESTED READINGS

Bedenne L, Michel P, Bouche O, et al: Chemoradiation followed by surgery compared with chemoradiation alone in squamous cancer of the esophagus: FFCD 9102, *J Clin Oncol* 25:1160–1168, 2007.

Burmeister BH, Smithers BM, Gebski V, et al: Surgery alone versus chemoradiotherapy followed by surgery for resectable cancer of the oesophagus: A randomised controlled phase III trial, *Lancet Oncol* 6:659–668, 2005.

Kranzfelder M, Schuster T, Geinitz H, et al: Meta-analysis of neoadjuvant treatment modalities and definitive non-surgical therapy for oesophageal squamous cell cancer, *Br J Surg* 98(6):768–783, 2011.

Kutup A, Link BC, Schurr PG, et al: Quality control of endoscopic ultrasound in preoperative staging of esophageal cancer, *Endoscopy* 39(8):715–719, 2007.

Minsky BD, Pajak TF, Ginsberg RJ, et al: INT 0123 (Radiation Therapy Oncology Group 94-05) phase III trial of combined-modality therapy for esophageal cancer: high-dose versus standard-dose radiation therapy, *J Clin Oncol* 20(5):1167–1174, 2002.

Miyata H, Yamasaki M, Takiguchi S, et al: Salvage esophagectomy after definitive chemoradiotherapy for thoracic esophageal cancer, *J Surg Oncol* 100(6):442–446, 2009.

Pech O, Behrens A, May A, et al: Long-term results and risk factor analysis for recurrence after curative endoscopic therapy in 349 patients with high-grade intraepithelial neoplasia and mucosal adenocarcinoma in Barrett's oesophagus, *Gut* 57(9):1200–1206, 2008.

Stahl M, Stuschke M, Lehmann N, et al: Chemoradiation with and without surgery in patients with locally advanced squamous cell carcinoma of the esophagus, *J Clin Oncol* 23:2310–2317, 2005.

Stiles BM, Mirza F, Coppolino A, et al: Clinical T2-T3N0M0 esophageal cancer: the risk of node positive disease, *Ann Thorac Surg* 92(2):491–498, 2011.

van Hagen P, Hulsho MCCM, van Lanschot JJB, et al: Preoperative chemoradiotherapy for esophageal or junctional cancer, *N Engl J Med* 366:2074–2084, 2012.

van Vliet EP, Heijenbrok-Kal MH, Hunink MG, et al: Staging investigations for oesophageal cancer: a meta-analysis, *Br J Cancer* 98(3):547–557, 2008.

zum Büschenfelde CM, Herrmann K, Schuster T, et al: (18)F-FDG PET-guided salvage neoadjuvant radiochemotherapy of adenocarcinoma of the esophagogastric junction: the MUNICON II trial, *J Nucl Med* 52(8):1189–1196, 2011.

ESOPHAGEAL STENTS

Matthew J. Schuchert, MD, Catherine Go, and James D. Luketich, MD

The primary goals of palliation in patients with unresectable esophageal cancer include the relief of dysphagia, maintenance of oral intake, management of complications, relief of pain, and prevention of reflux, regurgitation, and aspiration, while minimizing the length of hospital stay and maximizing quality of life. Although a variety of treatment options exist (including photodynamic therapy [PDT], chemotherapy, radiation therapy, brachytherapy, and laser ablation), esophageal stenting appears to provide the most immediate and durable results. A combination of modalities can be employed to maximize the palliative effects.

Stenting of the esophagus is the most commonly used first-line modality to palliate dysphagia and prevent malnutrition secondary to esophageal and proximal gastric cancers (Figure 1). The repertoire of available devices includes rigid plastic conduits, self-expanding metal stents, and self-expanding plastic stents. Uncovered stents have the advantage of better purchase on the esophageal wall, thus limiting

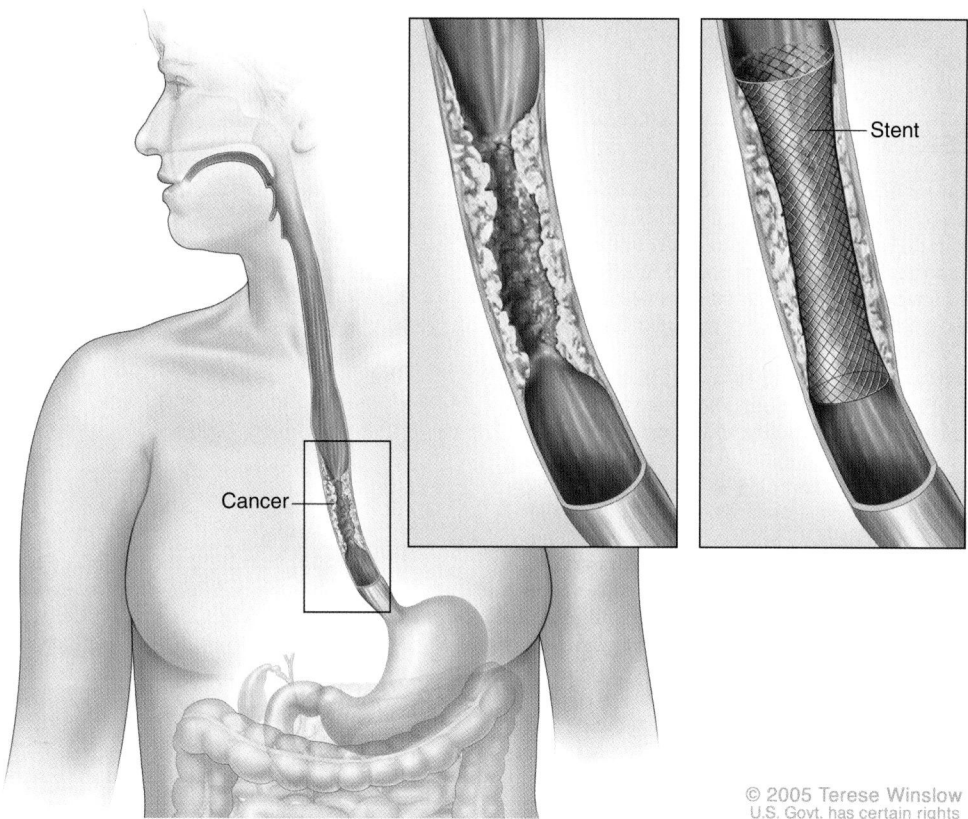

© 2005 Terese Winslow
U.S. Govt. has certain rights

FIGURE I   Esophageal stent insertion for malignant disease. *(© 2005 Terese Winslow, U.S. Government.)*

stent migration. However, they allow (and even stimulate) tumor and granulation tissue ingrowth. Expandable stents may be covered with a plastic coating to retard tissue ingrowth, but they have an increased risk of stent migration. Stent selection is tailored to the individual patient and is dependent on tumor length, bulk, and location. Deployment is achieved under fluoroscopic and/or endoscopic guidance. Stents are highly effective in palliating dysphagia in the setting of esophageal malignancy but can be associated with a substantial complication rate, predominantly due to the patient's poor functional and nutritional status as well as the extent of the underlying esophageal disease. In this chapter, we review the indications, techniques, and outcomes of esophageal stenting.

INDICATIONS

Current indications for stent placement approved by the Food and Drug Administration include the palliation of esophageal obstruction and tracheoesophageal fistulas secondary to malignancy. Other less common applications for esophageal stent placement include dysphagia secondary to external compression by benign neoplasms, benign strictures, and esophageal leak or perforation. Recently, stents have also found a role in management of esophageal varices.

The most common indication for esophageal stent insertion is relief of dysphagia in the setting of unresectable esophageal cancer. The significant majority of newly diagnosed cases have advanced disease at the time of diagnosis, with dismal five-year survival rates of approximately 20%. Palliation of dysphagia, therefore, becomes a paramount component of care. Stents provide safe and expeditious relief of dysphagia, thereby enhancing the patient's nutritional status and quality of life. Dysphagia can also result from obstructing lesions

of the esophagus related to adjacent lung cancer or mediastinal lymphadenopathy due to extrinsic compression. Benign, refractory strictures related to peptic ulcer disease or prior caustic injury can be treated with stent insertion in select cases. Stent placement may be either temporary or permanent, depending on the clinical circumstances. In the setting of malignancy, temporary stents represent useful adjuncts before surgical resection by relieving dysphagia and enhancing nutrition during neoadjuvant therapy (chemotherapy, radiation therapy). Temporary stent placement may also be useful in the management of perforations, leaks, and benign strictures.

HISTORICAL ASPECTS

The first generation of endoluminal stents consisted of rigid plastic or rubber prostheses inserted at the time of rigid esophagoscopy. Dilation to 48F to 54F was commonly required to permit introduction of these devices. The bulky insertion techniques resulted in a higher risk of perioperative complications—perforation in particular. With the advent of flexible endoscopic techniques, a new generation of self-expanding metallic stents (SEMS) was introduced that greatly simplified stent insertion. In a seminal prospective, randomized trial by Knyrim and associates, SEMS were associated with significant reduction of perioperative complications, reduced perioperative 30-day mortality (29% vs 14%), and were found to be cost-effective when compared with rigid prostheses. Numerous studies have established that SEMS are superior to rigid prostheses in the management of patients with malignant esophageal obstruction. Self-expanding esophageal stents are now the most commonly used method of palliation in esophageal cancer. Over the last two decades, there has been a dramatic evolution in stenting technology that has broadened its application in the management of a variety of esophageal conditions.

STENT DESIGN

With the introduction of SEMS, the use of rigid stent prostheses fell out of favor. SEMS are easier to deploy, achieve a wider luminal diameter, and are associated with a reduced periprocedural complication rate (including mortality). Though the cost of SEMS is greater than rigid prostheses, fewer repeat interventions are needed, leading to an overall reduced cost over the limited expected lifetime of a patient with advanced esophageal cancer.

Most SEMS that are currently available today are constructed with Nitinol (a composite of nickel and titanium), which is a highly elastic alloy with intrinsic properties of elasticity and shape memory that allow conformation to varying degrees of stenosis and angulation. The design of these pliable constructs allows the use of a lower-profile delivery system and efficient transmission of adequate radial force upon stent expansion. Initially, all SEMs were uncovered (Figure 2, A). Uncovered stents expand radially and incorporate into the wall of the esophagus with time, which dramatically reduces the potential for stent migration. However, the open spaces within the interstices of the uncovered metallic stent permit the ingrowth of granulation tissue or tumor, leading to recurrent symptoms of dysphagia in 13% to 26% of cases.

To minimize the occurrence of tumor ingrowth and the development of esophageal erosions or tracheoesophageal fistulas, stents were developed that were partially covered with silicone, polyurethane, or other polymers (Figure 2, B). Current designs maintain a 1 to 1.5 cm margin of exposed wire struts on the proximal and distal flanges of the stents that optimize stent purchase and permit integration into the esophageal wall. The use of a covered stents significantly decreases the severity of tumor ingrowth and consequent dysphagia, but it is associated with a slightly higher migration rate.

Completely covered self-expanding plastic stents (SEPS) were introduced into the market in 2001 and expanded the number of applications for stent usage, including benign conditions not readily treatable by SEMS due to their erosive tendencies. SEPS lack the ingrowth properties of metallic stents and are removable. Prospective randomized studies comparing SEMs with SEPS have demonstrated equivalent relief of dysphagia in the setting of esophageal cancer. Plastic stents are limited, however, by increased migration rates due to the mechanical characteristics of the plastic coating and decreased purchase upon the esophageal wall. Plastic stents do exert greater radial force than SEMS, which can lead to migration by "squirting" either proximally or distally with respect to the narrowed segment. The increased radial force can also lead to the subjective sense of discomfort or pain. Some of the plastic stent delivery systems are stiff and bulky, making deployment difficult in severely narrowed segments.

The most recent generation of stents includes fully covered SEMS that are designed to overcome the limitations of partially covered SEMS and SEPS. These stents may promote less granulation tissue and associated stenosis and may be removable after several weeks. However, an increased migration rate still may be expected as a result. Published data on the performance of fully covered stents are awaited.

CLINICAL EVALUATION AND TECHNIQUE

Preoperative assessment of clinical symptoms should be objectively recorded. Dysphagia scores are utilized to gauge the degree of symptomatic esophageal obstruction. The following dysphagia scoring

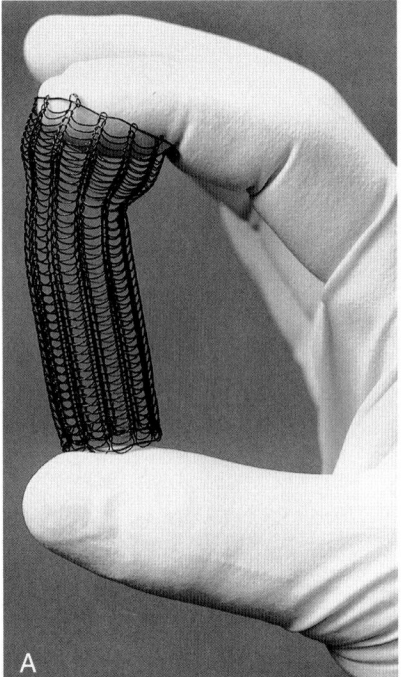

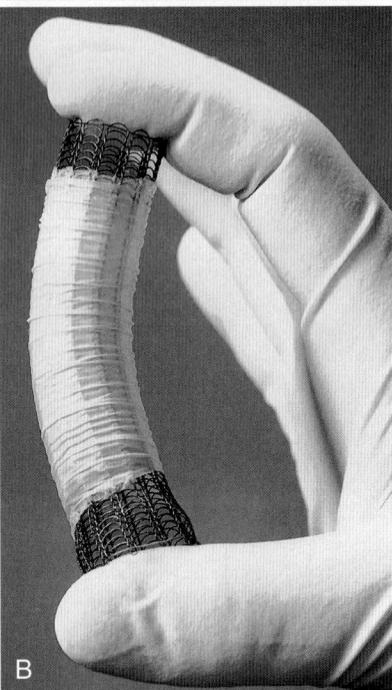

FIGURE 2   Uncovered (**A**) and covered (**B**) expanding metallic stent.

system is commonly employed: 0—Tolerating a regular diet, no dysphagia; 1—Difficulty with solids; 2—Difficulty with soft foods; 3—Difficulty with liquids; 4—Difficulty managing saliva. Careful preoperative radiographic assessment is imperative in planning the optimal approach. Barium esophagography provides a road map of the esophagus and allows assessment of the extent of obstruction, the length of esophageal involvement, and the presence of other anatomic abnormalities such as leak, perforation, or fistula. Computed tomographic (CT) and positron emission tomography (PET) scanning are critical in the setting of malignancy in helping to stage the extent of disease. Esophagogastroduodenoscopy allows confirmation of the underlying pathology and a real-time assessment of the extent of disease and whether the obstruction is intrinsic or extrinsic in nature. Flexible bronchoscopy is a useful adjunct in assessing patients with esophageal cancers of the proximal-mid esophagus and in those with suspected tracheoesophageal fistulas.

Esophageal stents may be inserted using endoscopic or fluoroscopic guidance under conscious sedation or general anesthesia. The authors prefer to employ a general anesthetic in most cases in an effort to minimize the risk of aspiration and to optimize stent positioning. During EGD, the degree of esophageal narrowing, the location and length of esophageal involvement, and the integrity of surrounding esophageal tissues are assessed. On occasion, significant narrowing may prevent the safe passage of the endoscope, and gentle dilation is performed to enable advancement of the scope beyond the distal extent of the lesion. Care should be taken to minimize the extent of dilation if anticipating the need for stent insertion. Over-dilation of a malignant stricture might decrease stent purchase after deployment, leading to a higher risk of stent migration. Alternatively, a smaller-caliber endoscope can be used.

Once the lesion has been assessed, the appropriate length stent is selected—usually 2 cm longer than the lesion—and a guidewire is passed into the esophagus past the distal end of the stricture. The scope is withdrawn and the stent deployment device is passed over the wire, followed by reintubation with the scope. The stent can then be deployed under direct visualization.

Fluoroscopic guidance is the more traditional method of monitoring stent deployment. The proximal and distal extent of the lesion is mapped with radiopaque markers that are placed on the skin of the chest wall (Figure 3). A scope is then advanced into the

duodenum, and a guidewire is inserted. The scope is withdrawn, and the distance between the two external markers is measured and an appropriate stent is selected. The stent delivery system (Figure 4) is then advanced over the wire under fluoroscopic guidance. The stent is identified by radiopaque proximal and distal markers that are aligned with the previously placed skin markers. Once adequate position is confirmed via fluoroscopy, the stent is deployed.

Delivery systems may employ a proximal release or distal release technique. Slight adjustments to stent position can be made during deployment to optimize stent position or after deployment using endoscopic graspers. Following deployment, the delivery system and guidewire are removed, and repeat endoscopy is performed to assess the adequacy of stent position and expansion. Stents should be slightly oversized to permit increased pressure of the stent against the esophageal wall so as to minimize the risk of stent migration. Care should be taken not to select a diameter that is too large, which can lead to incomplete stent expansion with residual infolding of the

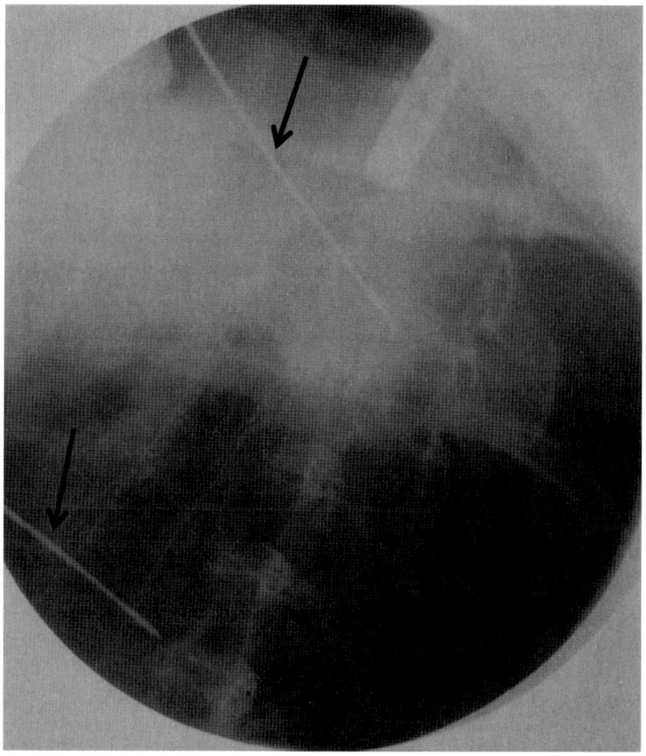

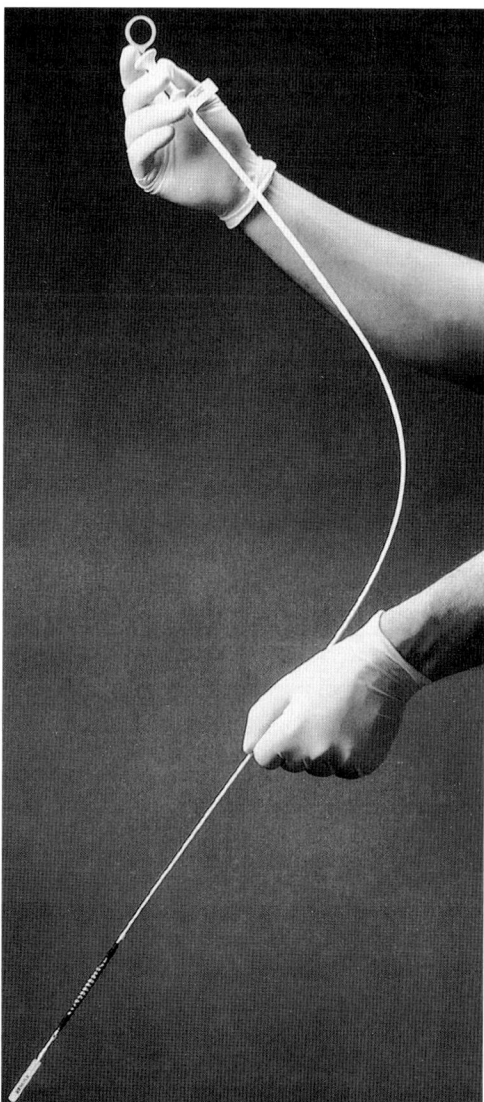

FIGURE 4 Esophageal stent delivery system. The Ultraflex stent is mounted on a plastic delivery vehicle and is advanced over a wire to the desired position. The stent is then deployed by pulling the release string while monitoring stent expansion under fluoroscopic guidance.

FIGURE 3 Deployment of esophageal stent. Note the proximal and distal skin markers that delineate the extent of obstructing tumor *(arrows)*. Fluoroscopy demonstrates good stent position and expansion.

stent that will partially obstruct the stent lumen. Appropriate deployment will result in a stent that is well expanded with good purchase along the esophageal wall. Areas of incomplete expansion can be augmented with the assistance of a balloon dilator. Most stents are equipped with proximal and distal purse strings that permit stent repositioning as required after deployment. Utilizing careful technique, success rates of 90% to 100% for stent deployment can be expected.

COMPLICATIONS

Numerous complications related to stent placement have been documented and range from 30% to 50% in most series (Table 1). The most common complication encountered with SEMS placement is the development of exuberant granulation tissue or tumor ingrowth in the proximal and distal uncovered portions of the stent, which occurs in approximately half of patients within 2 to 3 months of stent placement and can result in recurring dysphagia. Stent migration is another common complication. Proximal stents are associated with a higher rate of airway compromise due to tracheal compression and migration, and distal stents (especially those that span the gastroesophageal junction) can lead to wide open reflux (10%-20%), regurgitation, and even aspiration (1%-2%). Stents can be associated with severe discomfort and/or nausea following placement that may be unremitting in nature and may require stent repositioning, revision, or removal (1%-2%). Procedure-related perforation is rare and has only been reported in 1% to 2% of cases. It has been reported that over half of patients require endoscopic reintervention for complications at a mean interval of 88 days. It is important to note, however, that despite numerous modifications in stent design over time, there has been no significant reduction in postprocedure complications, which is likely due to the generally poor medical and nutritional status of patients experiencing malignant esophageal obstruction.

Following stent insertion, patients should be carefully followed in an outpatient setting to ensure adequate symptomatic palliation and to monitor for any of the above-mentioned complications. Hospital admission is advisable if there are any intraoperative complications. Adequacy of stent position can be assessed with a standard chest x-ray in most cases or via chest CT. Objective assessment of swallowing function can be performed with a barium swallow (Figure 5).

SPECIAL CONSIDERATIONS

Bridge to surgery: Esophageal stents can be utilized as a temporary measure to enhance oral intake in preparation for definitive surgical resection. Uncovered stents are not usually recommended due to increased periesophageal desmoplastic reaction that can obscure tissue planes and make the planned surgery difficult. This is especially notable in the setting of neoadjuvant therapy (chemotherapy, chemoradiation). Fully covered stents can be placed preoperatively and removed before surgery during the course of neoadjuvant therapy to minimize the risk of complications.

Long-term usage: Recent data suggest that long-term placement of stents is safe (13.5 months in one study). Over time, patients should be monitored for signs of recurring dysphagia, which could be due to stent migration or tumor ingrowth.

Proximal esophageal cancer: Esophageal stents can be employed in the proximal esophagus to relieve esophageal obstruction and control fistulae. The use of stents in this setting can be limited due to patient intolerance secondary to pain and globus sensation, as well as airway compression. Stent positioning distal to the cricopharyngeus is critical in minimizing the risk of these symptoms.

Antireflux valves: For tumors involving the GE junction, stent placement can lead to the development of severe reflux symptoms due to compromise of the lower esophageal sphincter valve mechanism. Several stent modifications have been developed in an attempt to create an antireflux valve mechanism. Results from randomized studies, however, are mixed, and as a result, the use of reflux valves has not entered the mainstream during esophageal stenting in the setting of malignancy.

Radioactive stents: Stents covered with iodine-125 have been studied in the setting of malignant dysphagia and have shown some survival benefit, but they are still in nascent stages.

CONCLUSIONS

The use of expandable stents represents a safe and expeditious approach in the palliation of malignant dysphagia. Changes in stent design have simplified stent insertion and have broadened its application to a variety of benign conditions. SEMs have emerged as a superior construct when compared with rigid prostheses in terms of ease of insertion and procedure-related morbidity. Partially covered SEMs are associated with reduced tissue ingrowth and recurrent dysphagia when compared with uncovered stents. Among partially covered SEMS, there are no proven advantages of one design versus another. Although SEPS have demonstrated equivalent relief of dysphagia when compared with SEMS, SEPS have been associated with increased difficulty of insertion and complication rates (migration, hemorrhage, food impaction) in the management of patients with malignant dysphagia. The use of temporary SEMS or SEPS for the management of esophageal perforation and anastomotic leaks is promising but will need to be validated in larger studies with more detailed follow-up. Careful patient selection and postoperative follow-up are required to enhance patient outcomes. As technology improves, and as surgeons gain experience in employing an individualized multimodality approach in the treatment of malignant obstruction of the esophagus (stenting, dilation, laser ablation, photodynamic therapy, radiotherapy, chemotherapy), the palliative benefits of these approaches will be optimized.

TABLE 1: Complications arising from SEMS insertion

Chest pain or odynophagia	13%
Tumor ingrowth/overgrowth	10%
Stent migration	9%
Severe reflux	8%
Food impaction	6%
Nausea or vomiting	6%
Aspiration pneumonia	3%
Esophageal erosion/fistula	0.8%
Perforation	0.4%

Adapted from Battersby NJ, Bonney GK, Subar D, et al: Outcomes following oesophageal stent insertion for palliation of malignant strictures: a large single centre series, J Surg Oncol 105:60–65, 2012.

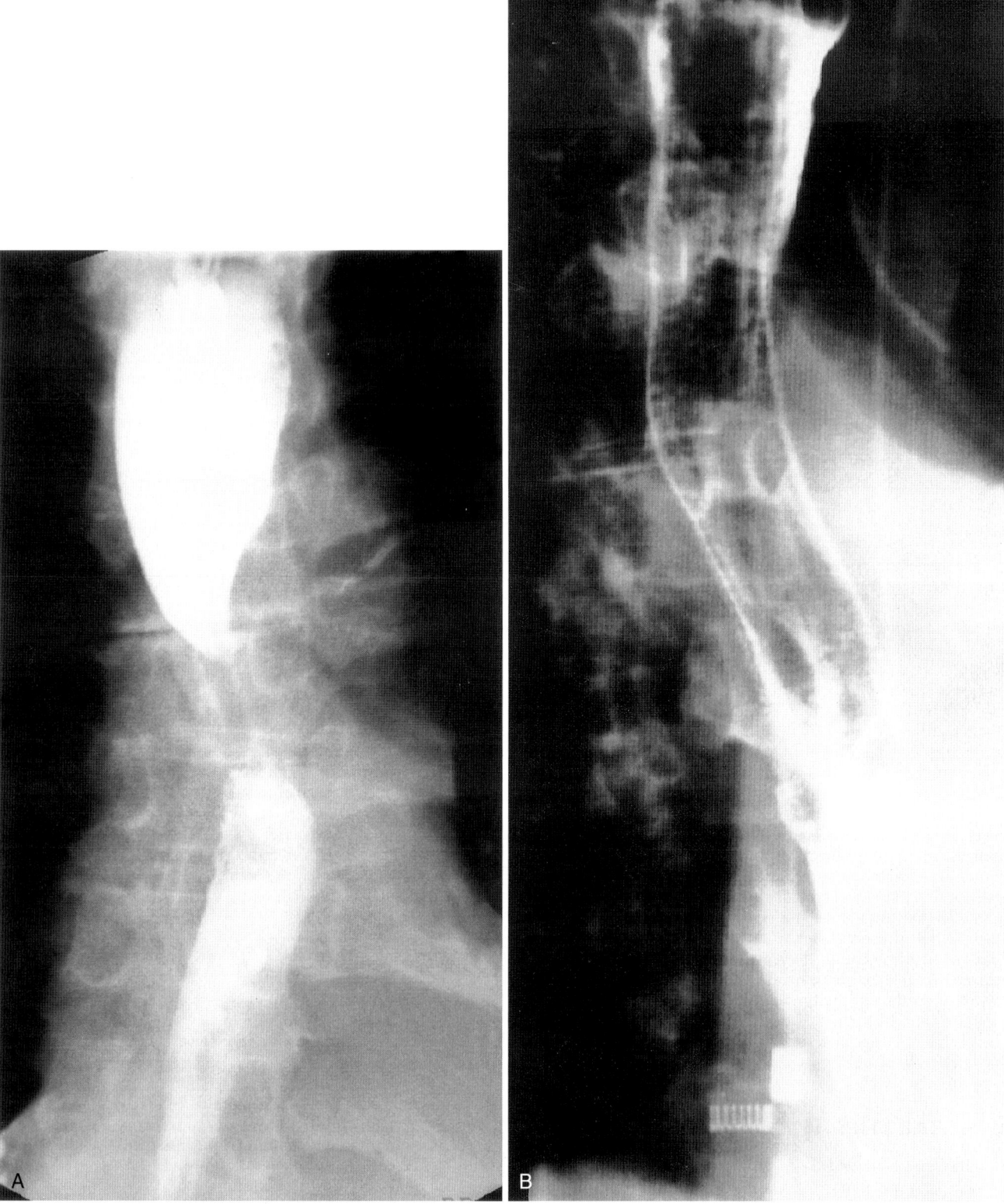

FIGURE 5   Barium esophagram prior to (**A**) and after (**B**) esophageal stent placement for a malignant stricture.

SUGGESTED READINGS

Battersby NJ, Bonney GK, Subar D, et al: Outcomes following oesophageal stent insertion for palliation of malignant strictures: a large single centre series, *J Surg Oncol* 105:60–65, 2012.

Christie NA, Buenaventura PO, Fernando HC, et al: Results of expandable metal stents for malignant esophageal obstruction in 100 patients: short-term and long-term follow-up, *Ann Thorac Surg* 71:1797–1802, 2001.

Ferreira F, Bastos P, Ribeiro A, et al: A comparative study between fluoroscopic and endoscopic guidance in palliative esophageal stent placement, *Diseases of the Esophagus*, 25(76):608–613, 2011.

Pennathur A, Chang AC, McGrath KM, et al: Polyflex expandable stents in the treatment of esophageal disease: initial experience, *Ann Thorac Surg* 85:1968–1972; discussion 73, 2008.

Schoppmann SF, Langer FB, Prager G, et al: Outcome and complications of long-term self-expanding esophageal stenting, *Diseases of the Esophagus*, 26(2):154–158, 2012.

Zhongmin W, Xunbo H, Jun C, et al: Intraluminal radioactive stent compared with covered stent alone for the treatment of malignant esophageal stricture, *Cardiovasc Intervent Radiol* 35:351–358, 2012.

ESOPHAGEAL PERFORATION

Charles M. Ferguson, MD

Esophageal perforation is a life-threatening condition that requires early accurate diagnosis, superb judgment in choice of method of repair, meticulous technique in repair, and conscientious and comprehensive postoperative care to ensure a good result. Thus, a good result in management of esophageal perforation is generally a marker for superb clinical care. The mortality rate for esophageal perforation continues to range from 10% to 40% and is associated with the cause of the perforation, the location of the perforation, the underlying pathology, delay in diagnosis, and the method of treatment of the perforation. Most perforations today follow instrumentation of the esophagus, after esophagoscopy, transesophageal echocardiography, pneumatic dilation, placement of intraesophageal tubes, and traumatic intubation. Spontaneous perforations (Boerhaave's syndrome), foreign body perforations, and caustic ingestion are less common causes, as are postsurgical perforations (from mediastinoscopy, antireflux surgery, anterior spinal surgery, and even thyroidectomy). Finally, both blunt and penetrating trauma may result in esophageal trauma. The key to early diagnosis is suspicion of perforation in any patient with pain, cervical crepitation or swelling, and fever after any of the previously mentioned events (Figure 1). An esophagogram with water-soluble contrast generally reveals the perforation, although barium has greater sensitivity and specificity, despite the risk of local contamination with barium (Figure 2). Computed tomographic (CT) scan is helpful in determination of the presence or absence of a contained perforation, which may change the treatment plan.

INITIAL THERAPY

Once the diagnosis of esophageal perforation is made, therapy must be directed at resuscitation. All patients with esophageal perforation should be started on broad-spectrum antibiotics that cover upper gastrointestinal (UGI) pathogens (the author favors coverage of gram-positive and gram-negative organisms and fungi). A nasogastric (NG) tube should generally be placed just above the perforation at the time of the water-soluble swallow and placed to suction to prevent further contamination. Patients with uncontained intrathoracic or intraabdominal perforations usually have development of an immediate chemical pleuritis or peritonitis with third spacing of fluid and thus should be started on vigorous intravenous (IV) fluid resuscitation with monitoring of urine output. Any significant pleural effusion should be drained via chest tube.

MANAGEMENT DECISIONS

The decision on how to manage an esophageal perforation can be quite difficult, and the wrong decision can be costly and painful to the patient and surgeon. The only easy management decision is the cervical esophagus—if the perforation is large enough to see on the UGI swallow, it should be drained, unless it is well contained and drains back into the esophagus.

Cervical Perforation

The preferred method is a left-sided neck incision at the anterior border of the sternocleidomastoid muscle, retracting it and the carotid sheath laterally (Figure 3). The retroesophageal space is then entered bluntly along the prevertebral fascia, with care taken to preserve the recurrent laryngeal nerve. Blunt dissection should be carried down to the posterior mediastinum to drain all collections, and if the perforation is identified, the defect is closed with absorbable sutures. Oftentimes, the actual defect in the esophagus is not identifiable; if so, simple draining of the space generally results in healing of the defect.

Thoracic Perforations

Patients with uncontained thoracic perforation generally need surgery (operative or endoscopic) to ensure healing; the sooner it is performed, the better the outcome. An algorithm (Figure 4) is helpful in the decision on how to manage thoracic perforations with an otherwise normal esophagus. It should be noted that any underlying pathology may well affect the ability to repair a perforation. Thus, patients with a perforation through a malignancy should undergo resection, and patients with perforation and achalasia need myotomy to ensure the ability of the perforation to heal.

Endoscopic clips and stents seem to be most effective for small perforations, and stents can be particularly useful for anastomotic leaks after esophagogastrectomy, provided the gastric tube conduit has adequate blood supply (this can generally be determined at the time of endoscopy). If the gastric tube is necrotic, then therapy necessitates resection and diversion with cervical esophagostomy, reduction of viable stomach into the abdomen, and feeding jejunostomy

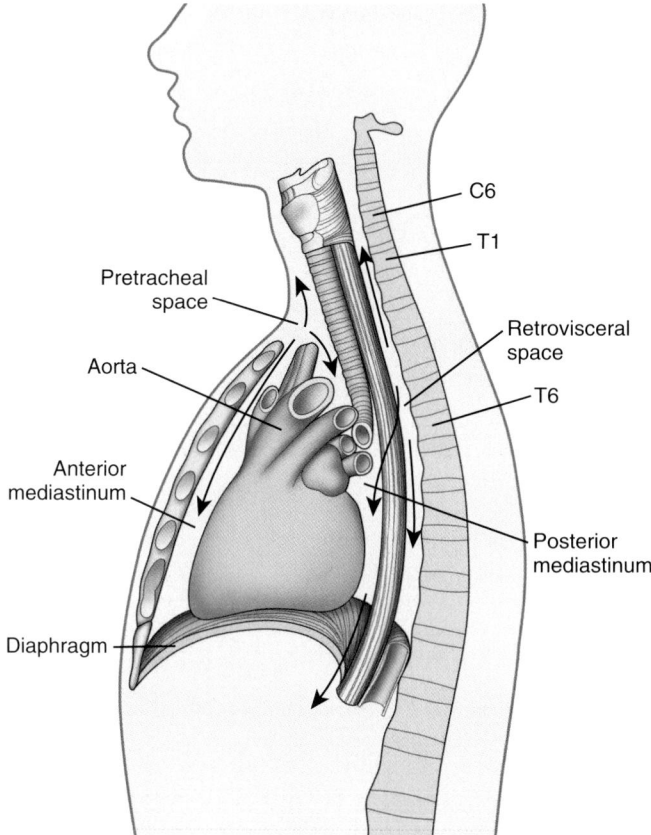

FIGURE 1 Direction of descent of mediastinal infections. *(From Patterson A, Cooper JD, Deslauriers J, et al: Pearson's thoracic and esophageal surgery, ed 3, Philadelphia, 2008, Churchill Livingstone.)*

with plan for later reconstruction with colonic interposition. For patients in whom endoscopic stents are chosen, any associated collections must be adequately drained. This can usually be done via chest tube, although some authors recommend thoracoscopic débridement of the pleura and drain placement.

Perforations of the upper two thirds of the esophagus for which operative therapy are chosen are best approached through a right thoracotomy via the fifth interspace. The pleura is opened in the area of the perforation and the esophagus dissected out such that the perforation can be clearly identified. The edges of the perforation should be débrided, and the mucosa and muscularis closed in layers with absorbable suture material, with a 40F to 48F bougie in place to prevent narrowing (Figures 5 and 6). Surrounding tissue should be used as a buttress over the repair; pleura or pericardial fat pad are described, but the author prefers a vascularized intercostal muscle flap, harvested from the fifth interspace. The wound should be copiously irrigated and drained with large chest tubes adjacent to the injury. If any concern exists about the repair, the patient is generally turned supine at the conclusion of the repair and a feeding tube placed (gastrostomy or jejunostomy). In the rare case with delayed presentation of a perforation, one should consider cervical esophagoscopy and gastrostomy with feeding jejunostomy. The cervical esophagostomy can be performed through an incision along the anterior border of the sternocleidomastoid, with the carotid sheath retracted laterally. The esophagus is easily dissected out bluntly with an index finger. Once it is dissected bluntly from the prevertebral fascia down to the posterior mediastinum, it is brought up to the skin, where a bridge can be placed beneath it, and opened longitudinally as a loop esophagostomy. Alternatively, it can be divided and an end esophagostomy created, but this complicates subsequent reconstruction.

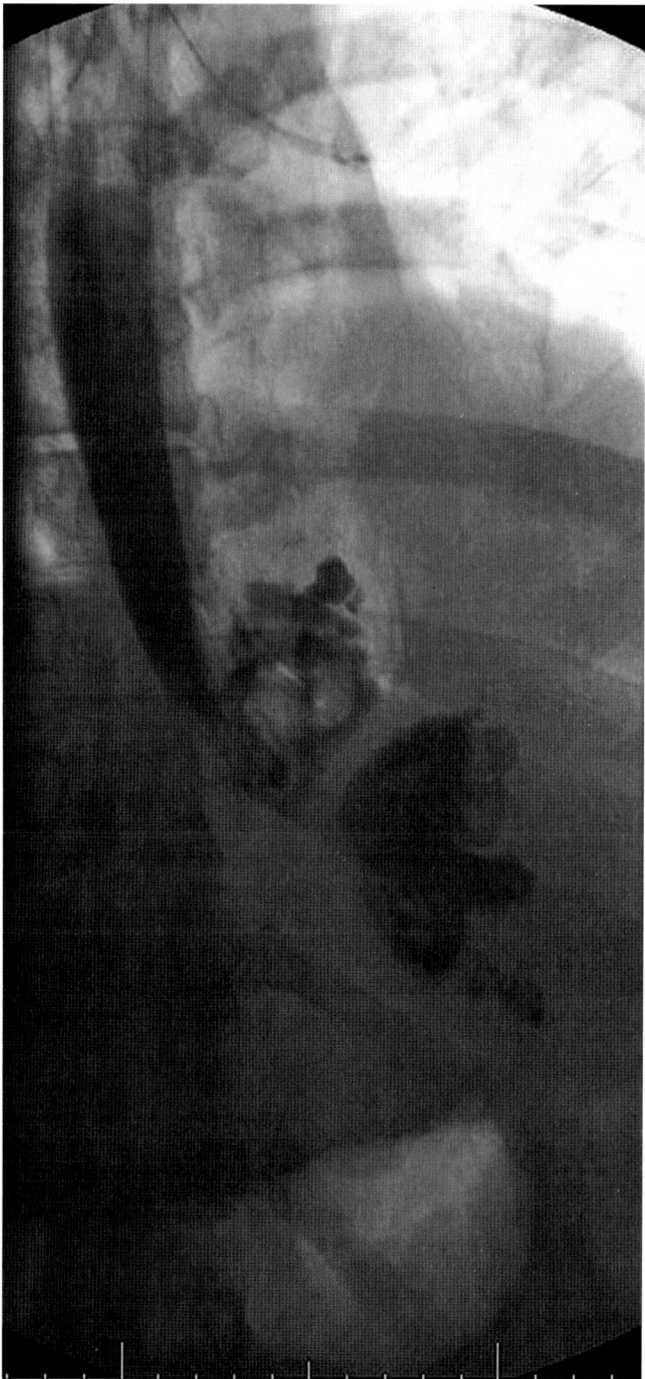

FIGURE 2 Barium swallow showing a lower esophageal perforation.

Perforations of the lower third of the esophagus should be approached through the left seventh interspace. Again, primary repair is preferred and should be buttressed with an intercostal muscle flap.

Abdominal Perforations

Perforations of the abdominal esophagus can usually be approached via an upper midline incision. In the occasional heavy patient with a large hiatus hernia and perforation of the abdominal esophagus, exposure may be better through a low left thoracotomy; this situation is rare. Once exposed and débrided, the perforation should be closed

FIGURE 3 Make an incision over the anterior border of the sternocleidomastoid muscle. If necessary, ligate the middle thyroid vein and inferior thyroid artery. Retract the trachea and thyroid gland medially to help expose the esophagus. *(From Cooke DT, Lau CL: Primary repair of esophageal perforation, Op Tech Thor Cardiovasc Surg 13(2):126–137, 2008.)*

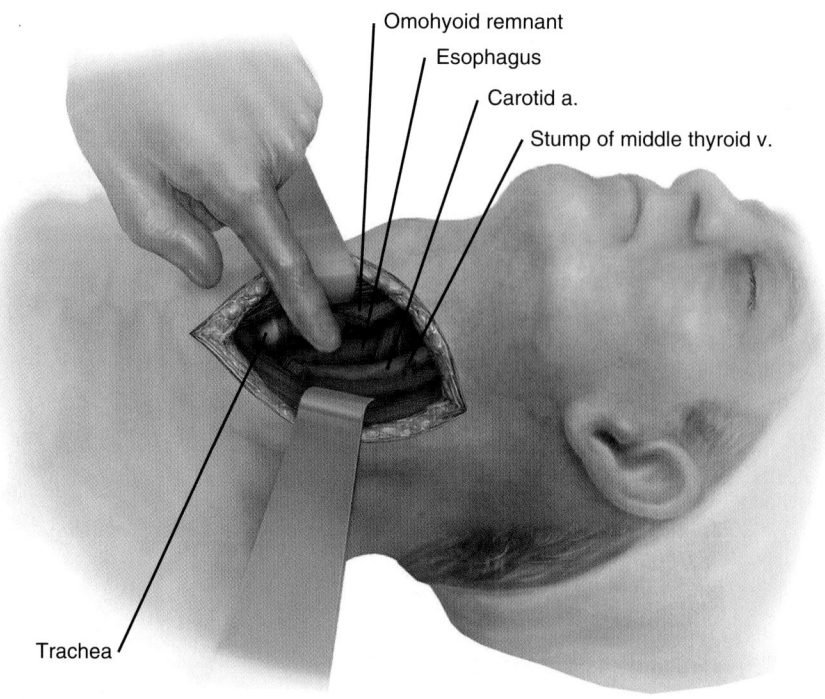

Omohyoid remnant
Esophagus
Carotid a.
Stump of middle thyroid v.

Trachea

FIGURE 4 Algorithm for the management of thoracic perforations.

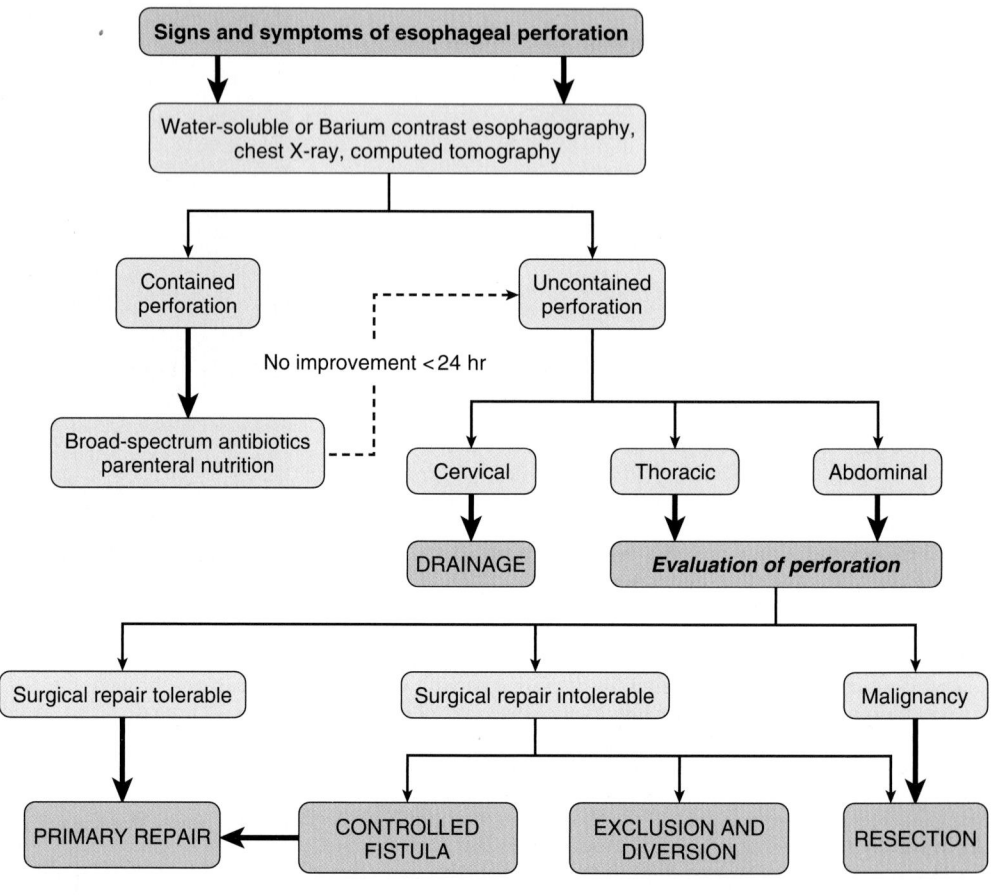

Signs and symptoms of esophageal perforation

Water-soluble or Barium contrast esophagography, chest X-ray, computed tomography

Contained perforation

Uncontained perforation

No improvement < 24 hr

Broad-spectrum antibiotics parenteral nutrition

Cervical

Thoracic

Abdominal

DRAINAGE

Evaluation of perforation

Surgical repair tolerable

Surgical repair intolerable

Malignancy

PRIMARY REPAIR

CONTROLLED FISTULA

EXCLUSION AND DIVERSION

RESECTION

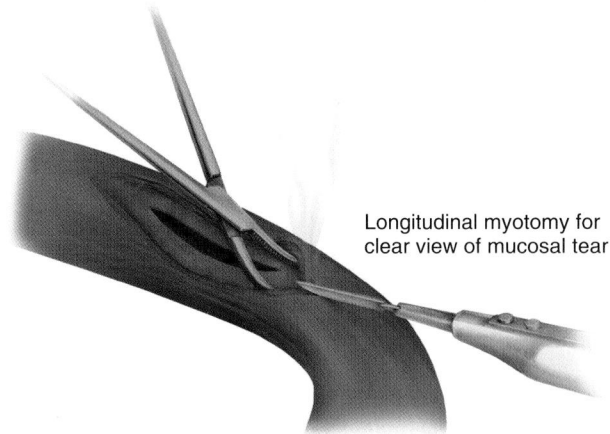

FIGURE 5 Mucosal injury is usually more extensive than the apparent muscular defect. A longitudinal myotomy is performed until the full extent of the mucosal tear is apparent. The mucosa is débrided as necessary to freshen edges. *(From Cooke DT, Lau CL: Primary repair of esophageal perforation,* Op Tech Thor Cardiovasc Surg *13(2):126–137, 2008.)*

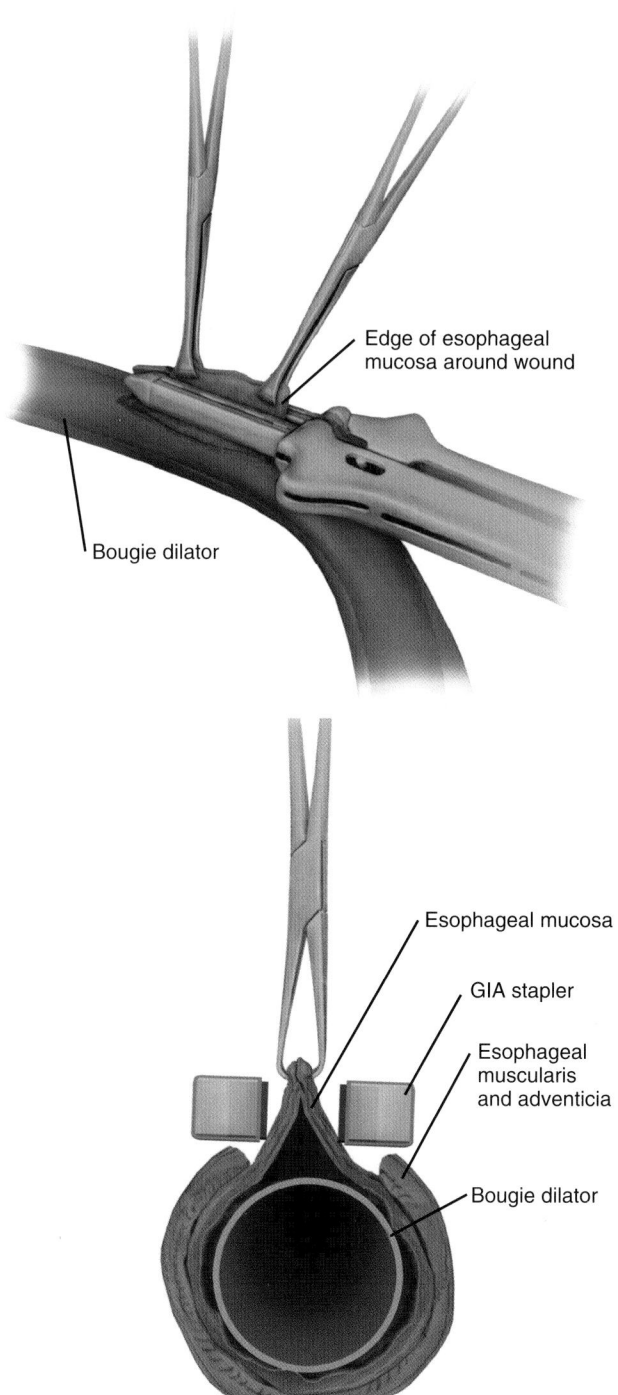

FIGURE 6 A 40F or 46F Maloney bougie is inserted into the lumen, the esophageal mucosal edges are grasped and approximated with Allis clamps or interrupted sutures, and the mucosa is closed with a 3.5-mm load. *GIA,* Gastrointestinal anastomosis. *(From Cooke DT, Lau CL: Primary repair of esophageal perforation,* Op Tech Thor Cardiovasc Surg *13(2):126–137, 2008.)*

as previously mentioned and the repair buttressed. Omentum works well for a buttress, as does the fundus of the stomach as a Nissen or Thal-type fundoplication.

SPECIAL SITUATIONS

Perforation Through a Malignancy

When one is faced with a perforation through a malignancy, the question is whether one can treat both problems. If the contamination can be adequately drained with chest tubes, the better part of valor in this situation is probably to place an endoscopic stent to control contamination and to place chest tubes to control the pleuritis, leaving the oncologic problem for another day. If this is not possible, then resection is necessary. Ideally, a resection and anastomosis appropriate to the site should be performed. However, in the setting of massive contamination, this may not be possible, and resection with cervical esophagostomy and gastrostomy for feeding should be considered. The resection can be performed via a right thoracotomy and then the patient turned supine for the cervical esophagostomy and gastrostomy.

Perforation With Achalasia

When an esophagus with achalasia is perforated (either via pneumatic dilation, at the time of myotomy, or via some other mechanism), the problem is that if the perforation is above the lower esophageal sphincter, the intraluminal esophageal pressure may preclude healing of the repair. Thus, a myotomy must be performed at the time of the repair. Generally, this is best performed through a left thoracotomy through the seventh interspace. The esophagus is bluntly dissected out circumferentially, with care taken to avoid injury to the vagi. The myotomy should be performed on the opposite side of the esophagus from the perforation, and the perforation closed in layers with absorbable suture, buttressed with omentum. A NG tube can be left above the repair to suction for a week.

Perforation of the Esophagus After Nissen Fundoplication

Occasionally, patients present 3 or 4 days after Nissen fundoplication with upper abdominal pain, fever, tachycardia, and leukocytosis and are found on barium swallow or CT scan to have a perforation of the esophagus. These perforations can generally be cured with immediate laparotomy, dismantling of the fundoplication, direct repair of the esophagotomy in layers (with 40F bougie in place to prevent narrowing), and rewrap of the Nissen. Temporary endoscopic stenting is tempting to try in this situation, although no reports are found of this as yet.

Leakage of Esophagogastrostomy After Esophagectomy

Anastomotic leak is a dreaded complication of Ivor Lewis esophagectomy. Management of this leak is dependent on the size of the leak, degree of contamination, and viability of the gastric conduit. In patients with necrosis of the gastric conduit, clearly the anastomosis needs to be dismantled and a cervical esophagostomy and gastrostomy performed. On the other hand, in patients with a viable conduit and contamination that can be handled with chest tube drainage, an endoscopic stent often solves the problem. The author recommends endoscopy in the operating room after stabilization of the patient's condition. If the conduit appears viable at endoscopy, then placement of stent and chest tube drainage or thoracoscopy is recommended, or even thoracotomy and drainage of the pleural and mediastinal spaces. If the gastric conduit appears gangrenous, then a thoracotomy is performed to resect the gangrenous stomach. The gastric remnant is reduced into the abdomen with gastrostomy for feeding, and an esophagostomy is performed as described previously. Once the patient has recovered from this critical illness, one can contemplate reconstruction of the esophagus.

SUGGESTED READINGS

Brinster CJ, Singhai S, Lee L, et al: Evolving options in the management of esophageal perforation, *Ann Thoracic Surg* 77(4):1475–1483, 2009.

Carrott PW, Low DE: Advances in the management of esophageal perforation, *Thoracic Surg Clin* 21(4):541–555, 2011.

David EA, Kim MP, Backman SH: Esophageal salvage with removable covered self-expanding metal stents in the setting of intrathoracic esophageal leakage, *Am J Surg* 202(6):796–811, 2011.

THE STOMACH

THE MANAGEMENT OF BENIGN GASTRIC ULCER

Raafat Z. Abdel-Misih, MD, FRCS Edin, FRCS Eng, FACS,
James D. Larson, MD, and Sherif R. Abdel-Misih, MD

INTRODUCTION

The number of elective operations for benign gastric ulcer disease has decreased dramatically over recent decades. As generations of surgeons with less direct experience encounter this disease, the significance of proper patient selection and appropriate intervention becomes of increasing importance. Overall, the annual incidence rate of peptic ulcer disease (PUD) is 0.1% to 0.3%, resulting in nearly 300,000 new cases diagnosed each year; approximately one third of these are gastric ulcers. The advent of pharmacologic therapy to address acid hypersecretion and treat *Helicobacter pylori* infection is the primary reason for reduction in the need for elective surgical intervention.

ETIOLOGY

The etiology of benign gastric ulceration is multifactorial and is best described in the context of each ulcer type. *H. pylori* infection and nonsteroidal antiinflammatory drug (NSAID) usage contribute to a great majority of cases; thus, nonoperative management of the disease is indicated in nearly all cases, with the exceptions of hemorrhage, perforation, obstruction, and refractory disease. Direct *Helicobacter* treatment and eradication is paramount because complete mucosal healing occurs less than 0.5% of the time with persistent infection. Other notable sources implicated in benign disease include smoking, steroid usage, and Zollinger-Ellison syndrome.

PRESENTATION AND DIAGNOSIS

The hallmark symptom of ulcer disease is epigastric pain. Most often, this pain is relieved with the ingestion of food or antacids and recurs after a short interval. Evaluation of the patient generally involves multiple modalities, given the broad differential diagnosis of epigastric discomfort, but ultimately, the diagnosis rests with endoscopy. Esophagogastroduodenoscopy provides definitive diagnosis, allows for characterization of the lesion's location and extent, and provides tissue for detection of microorganisms and malignant disease.

In the setting of appropriate conservative management, a failure of medical therapy is typically considered persistence of disease beyond 12 weeks. Many patients are given considerably longer periods of time, however, before surgical evaluation. The amount of time given to each patient is dependent on several factors. The treating physician may prefer a longer wait before evaluation by a surgeon, and patients with multiple comorbidities who are generally poor surgical candidates typically receive longer trial periods. Ulcers along the greater curvature tend to prompt earlier intervention given the association of disease in this location with malignancy.

GASTRIC ULCER TYPES AND LOCATION

The location of a gastric ulcer determines the preferred treatment modality, with the classification system proposed by Johnson (Figure 1) typically used to define each type. Type I ulcers, located along the lesser curvature, are the most common. Ulcer types II and III are associated with acid hypersecretion, and thus, vagotomy is recommended when surgical intervention is necessary. Lesions along the lesser curvature near the gastroesophageal junction are type IV. Type V disease is diffuse and associated with NSAID usage. Giant ulcers, often located along the greater curve, have a greater tendency to harbor malignant disease. Only 10% of benign ulcers are located on the greater curvature. The surgical management is described in detail for each ulcer type.

Type I

Located near the incisura on the lesser curvature, type I disease is the most common and comprises approximately 60% of benign gastric ulcers. The etiology of type I ulcers is not fully understood; these lesions are not associated with acid hypersecretion and, in some cases, are noted in the setting of low levels of gastric acid production. *H. pylori* infection can be found in most patients with type I disease, but it also occurs in those whose infections have been eradicated or who have no history of infection. As with other gastric ulcers, most are treated successfully with conservative therapy. For refractory disease, antrectomy and vagotomy with Billroth I reconstruction is the procedure of choice when possible. Despite the lack of definitive association with acid production, the rationale for vagotomy arises from the unclear nature of these ulcers and in general the addition of minimal, if any, morbidity. A Billroth II or Roux-en-Y technique may prove necessary when the anatomy is such that gastroduodenostomy is not feasible; however, this is often possible with good gastric mobilization and wide Kocher's maneuver.

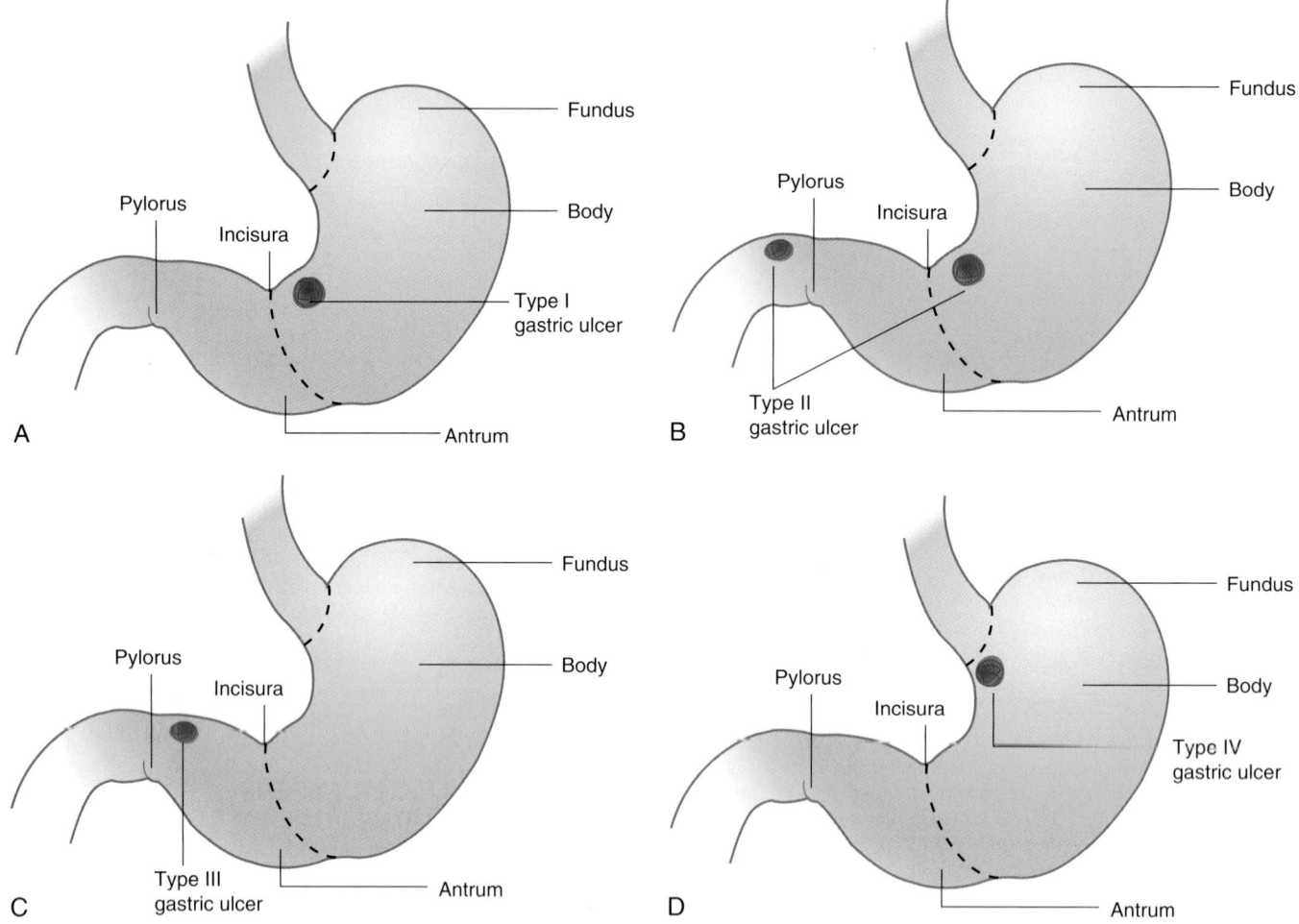

FIGURE 1 **A** to **D,** Johnson classification of gastric ulcers. *(From Townsend CM, Beauchamp RD, Evers BM, Mattox KL: Sabiston textbook of surgery, ed 18, Philadelphia, 2007, Saunders, Fig. 47-10.)*

Types II and III

Type II disease involves concomitant ulcers along the lesser curvature near the incisura and a duodenal ulcer, and type III ulcerations are prepyloric. Distal gastrectomy that includes the ulcer is the preferred surgical resection, again with Billroth I reconstruction when possible. Because of the duodenal involvement in the type II and the distal location of type III ulcers, sufficient mobilization of the duodenum may prove difficult, if not impossible, necessitating Billroth II or Roux-en-Y creation. These ulcers *are* associated with acid hypersecretion; as such, when resection is performed, a vagotomy is recommended because conservative acid reduction therapy has already failed. Depending on the comfort of the surgeon with the various techniques, type III ulcers are occasionally amenable to full-thickness excision combined with highly selective vagotomy; this is not recommended unless the surgeon has considerable experience because the gastrin-secreting tissue is left in place and recurrence rates are higher with incomplete vagotomy.

Type IV

Although type IV ulcers are not related to acid hypersecretion, they do pose a particular surgical challenge because of their proximal location along the lesser curvature near the gastroesophageal junction. Resection is directed at preserving a maximal length of healthy stomach such that a gastroduodenostomy may be possible even after

such a proximal ulcer is removed. The Pauchet's and Csendes' techniques described subsequently (Figure 2) facilitate this goal. A Kelling-Madlener resection, in which total gastrectomy is avoided for very proximal locations with the ulcer left in place and an antrectomy with vagotomy performed, is not recommended given the unclear etiology of these ulcers and lack of association with acid production. In general, total gastrectomy is rarely necessary for gastroesophageal junction ulcers.

Type V

The diffuse nature of type V ulceration makes surgical intervention difficult; fortunately, the need for operation is rare. The use of NSAIDs or steroids is the primary etiology, and resolution is generally facilitated simply with cessation of the offending agent and the addition of a proton pump inhibitor (PPI) or histamine blocker. Bleeding is the most common indication for operation in this setting. Should intervention become necessary, the initial therapy is endoscopic with injection or cautery of significant points of hemorrhage. Unfortunately, because of the diffuse nature of the disease, endoscopic treatment may be inadequate. The localization of bleeding vessels and subsequent coiling or embolization via interventional radiology can be attempted next. Surgical approaches should be reserved for cases refractory to other measures. In that situation, an anterior gastrostomy facilitates inspection of the gastric mucosa with

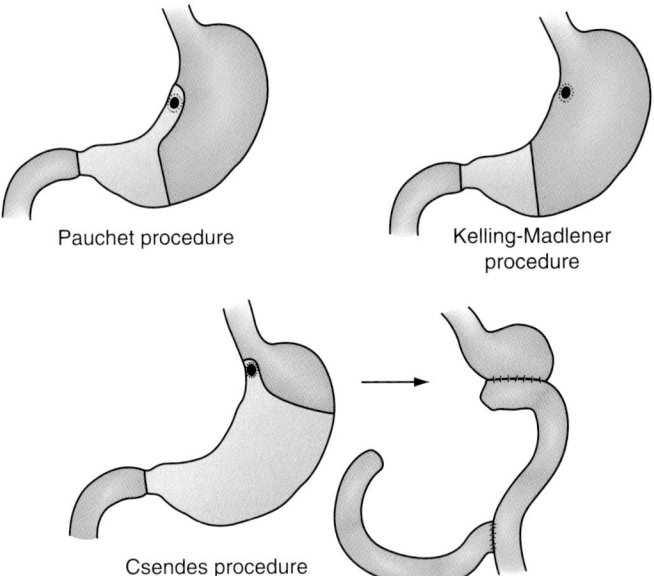

FIGURE 2   Special surgical procedures for gastric ulcers. *(From Townsend CM, Beauchamp RD, Evers BM, Mattox KL: Sabiston textbook of surgery, ed 18, Philadelphia, 2007, Saunders, Fig. 47-16.)*

the goal of oversewing major sites of bleeding. If this is unsuccessful, one should be prepared to perform a total gastrectomy because it may prove to be a life-saving measure. Gastric devascularization has been described in small studies in the past, whereby the major vessels are ligated and the short gastric vessels remain as the primary blood supply. This approach has been virtually replaced with interventional radiology and is uncommon.

Stress-Related Mucosal Disease

Stress-related mucosal disease, or stress gastritis, is generally encountered in the critical care setting and can occur as early as 12 hours after admission. Relative mucosal ischemia appears to play a principal role, with acid secretion likely a secondary association. Many clinical factors are associated with the risk of stress gastritis, including acute respiratory distress syndrome, multiple long bone fractures, transfusion requirements greater than 6 units, sepsis, acute renal failure, and specific associated trauma, such as central nervous system (CNS) injury (Cushing's ulcer) and extensive burns over 35% body surface area (Curling's ulcer). Patients at particular risk of clinically significant hemorrhage seem to be those who need mechanical ventilation for greater than 48 hours or with coagulopathy, defined as a platelet count less than $50,000/mm^3$ or international normalized ratio (INR) of more than 1.5. Prevention of gastritis with addition of pharmaceutical prophylaxis is paramount. However, should further intervention become necessary, then treatment parallels that for type V ulceration; endoscopic and interventional techniques are generally applied first, with surgical involvement reserved for refractory cases.

Cancer Risk After Resection

Data regarding the risk of gastric malignant disease after partial resection are conflicting, in regards to both the time course and the actual (if any) extent of increase. Malignant disease usually appears 15 to 30 years after surgery and may in fact be less common than in the general population during the first 10 years. Significant variability in the literature is also present as to the ultimate risk conferred by resection, anywhere from no additional risk to five times that of normal. On the basis of the largely inconsistent information, no

strong recommendations can be made for routine surveillance of these patients. Rather, a strong suspicion and low threshold for workup of upper gastrointestinal symptoms should be maintained, particularly as time from resection elapses.

Giant Ulcer

Giant ulcers are those that are more than 3 cm in diameter. These ulcers have an increased association with cancer: 30% of those larger than 3 cm harbor malignant disease. Earlier surgical intervention is generally warranted given this association. Endoscopy with multiple biopsies (at least four with jumbo forceps and eight with regular) to include both the ulcer base and edge usually provide sufficient tissue for diagnosis to guide therapy, with treatment of nonmalignant ulcers adhering to guidelines as outlined previously, depending on the location.

Obstruction

Obstruction is the least common complication of gastric ulcer disease. It is not an emergency, and initial management involves nasogastric decompression and fluid and electrolyte replacement. This nonoperative therapy can result in at least temporary resolution of a significant percentage of obstructions, which may be the result of edema or acute inflammation. Subsequent definitive management usually rests with resection and reconstruction, ideally as a Billroth I procedure. If chronic scarring and local derangement of tissues prevents safe resection or a tension-free gastroduodenostomy, then vagotomy and diversion with gastrojejunostomy is appropriate. Endoscopic dilation with or without stenting has yielded some favorable short-term results, but recurrence rates are much higher than with resection. Dilation may be preferable in those patients who are poor surgical candidates.

Perforation

Perforation is the most common complication of gastric ulcers, and the patients tend to be older and have more debilitated conditions than those with perforated duodenal ulcers. Surgical intervention is usually necessary, ideally with a partial gastrectomy to include the ulcer and reconstruction. Rarely, in the setting of a patient with a hemodynamically stable condition without signs of peritonitis, nonoperative treatment may be considered. If the patient cannot tolerate a resection, then full-thickness excision of the ulcer is appropriate, with care to send that tissue as a specimen to rule out malignant disease. Redundancy of the gastric walls generally allows for reapproximation of healthy tissue edges, without the need for an omental patch. In the case of a perforated type II or III ulcer, a vagotomy and drainage procedure can be considered. If before the perforation, however, the patient has never had a period of medical management to include eradication of *H. pylori*, if present, and PPI or H2 antagonist medications, it is reasonable to attempt these first, assuming close follow-up evaluation is possible.

SURGICAL TECHNIQUE

Vagotomy and Drainage

For those patients whose ulcers are associated with acid hypersecretion and are refractory to medical management, a vagotomy is recommended at the time of definitive surgical therapy. Although many variations in description and technique exist, in general, three approaches to vagotomy are recognized (Figure 3); it is important to

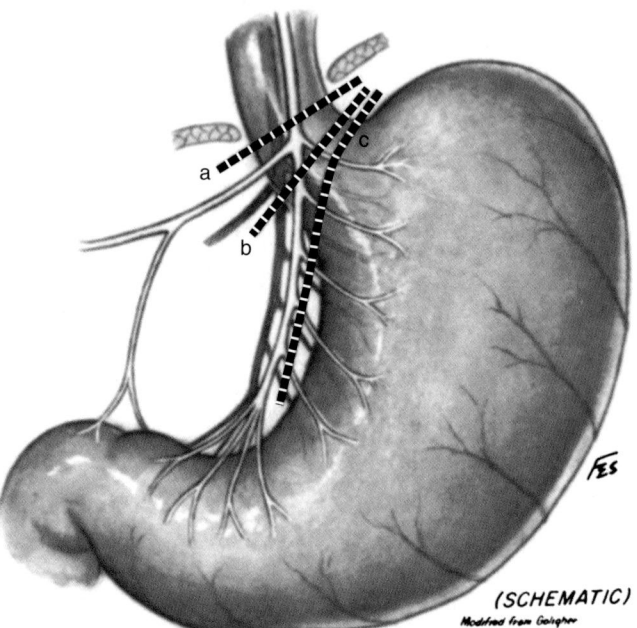

(SCHEMATIC)
Modified from Gallagher

FIGURE 3 Vagotomy: Truncal vagotomy *(a)*; selective vagotomy *(b)*; highly selective vagotomy *(c)*. *(From Zuidema GD, Yeo CJ: Shackelford's surgery of the alimentary tract, ed 5, Philadelphia, 2001, Saunders, Fig. 11-1.)*

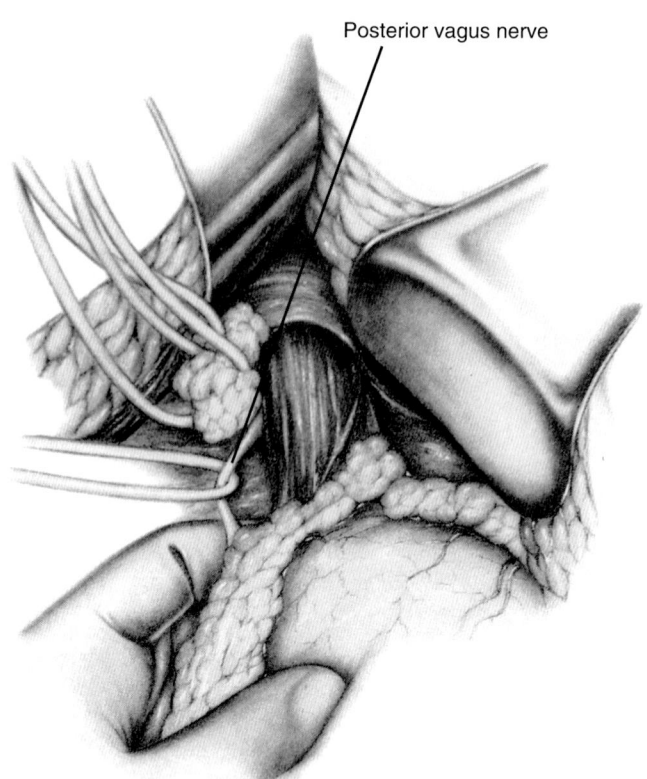

Posterior vagus nerve

FIGURE 4 Exposure of posterior vagus. *(From Malt R: Surgical techniques illustrated: a comparative atlas, Boston, 1985, Saunders.)*

be acquainted with each method and the rationale behind it. Keep in mind that the ultimate goal is parasympathetic denervation of any remaining acid-producing stomach tissue, a feat best accomplished with the technique the operating surgeon is most familiar with and comfortable pursuing.

The first, and usually most straightforward from a technical standpoint, is truncal vagotomy. The anterior and posterior nerves are divided at the level of the distal esophagus, ideally approximately 4 cm proximal to the gastroesophageal junction. At this level, one has the best chance of finding a single trunk for both branches: 90% of anterior and 75% of posterior vagi. This requires mobilization of approximately 5 to 6 cm of the esophagus to provide adequate exposure for complete nerve identification because those that are branching by this point form several smaller cords. Clips are placed proximally and distally on each vagal trunk and then transected, with the segment sent for pathologic confirmation. The so-called "criminal" nerve of Grassi, the first gastric branch of the posterior vagus, is of particular importance because its separation point can be proximal to the celiac division of the posterior nerve. It travels to the posterior fundus, running past the angle of His, and failure to identify and divide it can result in a higher rate of failure; two thirds of cases with ulcer recurrence after an initial antisecretory operation have evidence of incomplete vagotomy.

Several points can be made that facilitate identification of the posterior vagus nerve. Place downward traction by grasping the proximal stomach with the left hand, keeping the gastroesophageal junction between the index and middle fingers. This pull allows the esophageal muscular layers to stretch and puts the posterior nerve under tension such that it can be palpated as an identifiable and relatively isolated cord toward the right side of the esophagus (Figure 4). Unlike the anterior vagus, which is running directly on the esophagus, the posterior nerve is generally located approximately a centimeter away from the wall itself.

A second approach is a selective vagotomy. This method spares the posterior branches that innervate the pancreas and small intestine, and the anterior branches that course to the liver and gallbladder. Preservation of these distal sites of innervation is directed at decreasing the potential morbidity of vagotomy; the incidence of

postoperative diarrhea and dumping has in some cases proven to be less with a properly performed selective versus truncal vagotomy, and the recurrence rate of ulceration is equivalent. Selective vagotomy is performed more frequently for refractory duodenal ulcers in the setting of a concomitant drainage procedure; when used after a gastric resection for benign ulcer disease, its benefit over truncal vagotomy is less clear.

A third approach is a highly selective (parietal cell) vagotomy that seeks to preserve Latarjet's nerves that terminate on, and provide motor function to, the pylorus. This makes it distinct from the other denervation techniques in that no drainage procedure is necessary. Successful completion requires substantial familiarity with the technique; in most cases of refractory benign gastric ulcer, it is unnecessary because a resection of the pylorus is often a part of the procedure. Highly selective vagotomy involves identification of the terminal fronds of both the anterior and the posterior branches; these are located at the junction of the corpus and antrum and have a characteristic "crow's foot" configuration with three divisions. This point is generally 6 cm proximal to the pylorus, and these terminal branches are left intact. The individual neurovascular bundles originating from the vagal trunks and running within the anterior and posterior leaves of the lesser omentum to the stomach are divided up to and including the distal esophagus for approximately 5 cm, with the integrity of the trunks preserved. An alternative method of dealing with the anterior row of vagal fibers is to perform a running anterior seromyotomy at the level of their junction with the stomach; because of its location, this technique is difficult to perform on the posterior row, which is dealt with as described previously.

In those cases in which a truncal or selective vagotomy is executed but no resection is done, usually because of extensive scar tissue or an emergent situation, a procedure to allow drainage through the pylorus is warranted. Most commonly, a pyloroplasty (Figure 5) is performed in the manner described by Heineke-Mikulicz, whereby a longitudinal incision is created through the pylorus and closed

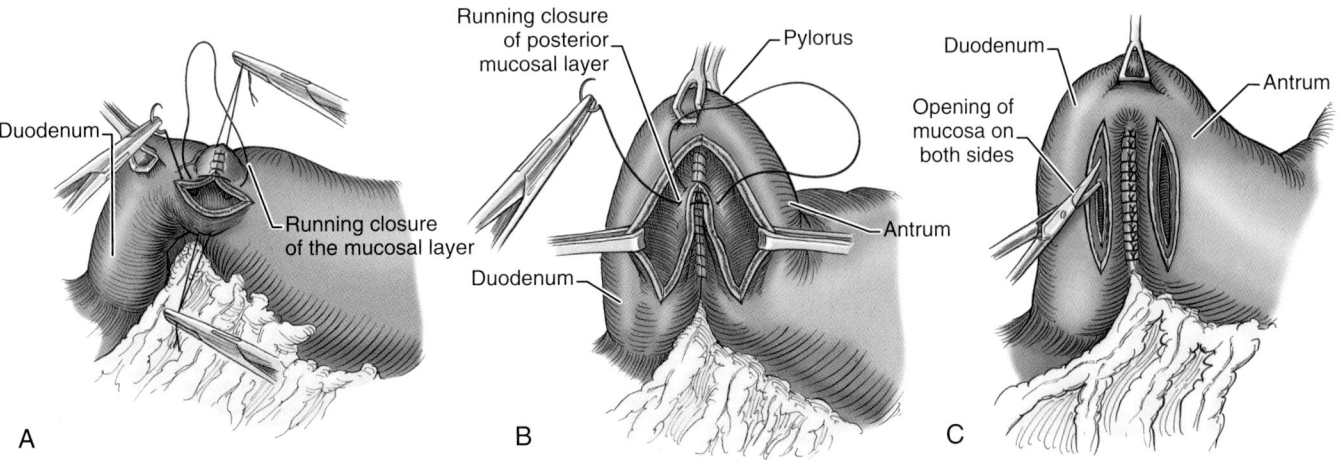

FIGURE 5 **A,** Heineke-Mikulicz pyloroplasty; **B,** Finney pyloroplasty; **C,** Jaboulay gastroduodenostomy. *(From Townsend CM, Evers BM: Atlas of general surgical techniques, ed 1, Philadelphia, 2010, Saunders, Figs. 23-3, 24-3, 25-4.)*

transversely. In cases in which the duodenum is heavily scarred, the Finney and Jaboulay techniques may afford more mobility to allow closure. If a pyloroplasty is not possible via these methods, then a gastrojejunostomy is appropriate.

Extent of Resection

In general, an antrectomy with resection of less than 50% of the stomach is suitable for most benign gastric ulcer disease treatment. Minor variations usually enable the surgeon to remove the ulcer itself and all of the gastrin-secreting tissue without significantly compromising the remaining gastric volume. Although arbitrary, some gross anatomic landmarks help delineate the approximate area of removal. The antrum-body physiologic junction is estimated by a line drawn from 2/5 the distance from pylorus to the cardia on the lesser curvature to 1/8 the same distance on the greater curve. This corresponds to about 7 cm on the lesser curve (2 to 3 cm from the aforementioned crow's foot) and 5 cm on the greater curve, although it becomes more proximal with advancing age. If the resources are available, intraoperative frozen section to determine the presence of antral glands containing G cells in remaining tissue can be obtained, thus directing further resection.

As the ulcer location (or proximal extent of a large ulcer) moves progressively more proximal, principally on the lesser curve, the ability to preserve enough length to create a tension-free gastroduodenostomy becomes challenging. Pauchet's procedure (see Figure 2) addresses this issue by starting proximal to the ulcer on the lesser curve and extending distally to increase the distance along the greater curve. Those ulcers within approximately 2 cm of the esophagus are particularly difficult and may necessitate a subtotal gastrectomy with Roux-en-Y reconstruction, even when saving as much stomach as possible (Csendes' procedure). The need for a total gastrectomy, however, is rare and should be avoided.

The distal extent of resection is usually straightforward with a transection through healthy duodenal tissue just distal to the pylorus. When the local inflammatory reaction of a gastric ulcer or the ulcer itself creates an ill-defined margin, determination of the point at which to stop can be difficult. This is particularly troubling when the ulcer is posterior and involves the surface of the pancreas. It is best to avoid attempting complete resection of the ulcer base; perform the antrectomy as usual, leaving the base in place (Figure 6), and reconstruct overtop the area. With the source of inflammation removed, the area heals without adversely affecting the anastomosis, which generally lies just proximal to the ulcer base.

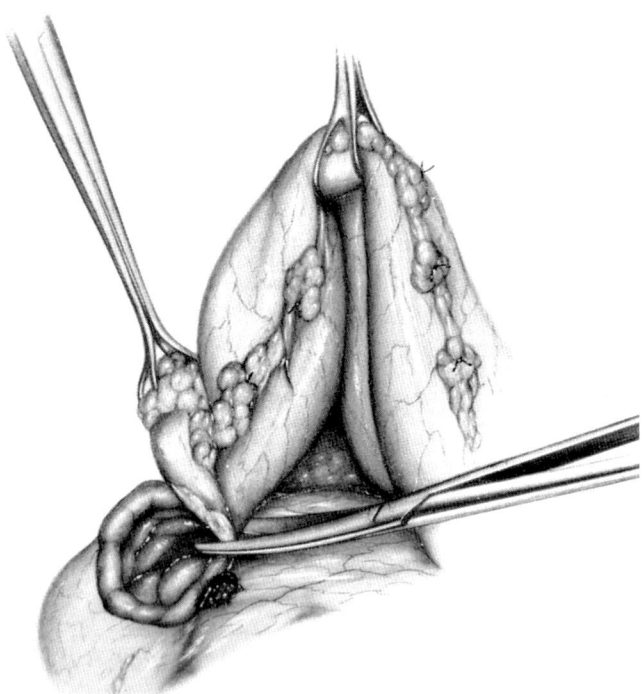

FIGURE 6 In the setting of an ulcer closely associated with the pancreas, the resection is performed while the base is left undisturbed. *(From Malt R: Surgical techniques illustrated: a comparative atlas, Boston, 1985, Saunders.)*

RECONSTRUCTION TECHNIQUES

Billroth I

Gastroduodenostomy has taken many forms since its inception well over a century ago and persists today most commonly as one of the early modifications performed by Billroth (Figure 7). The reconstruction via anastomosis of the end of the duodenum to the distal greater curvature of the stomach is the preferred technique for most benign gastric ulcer disease.

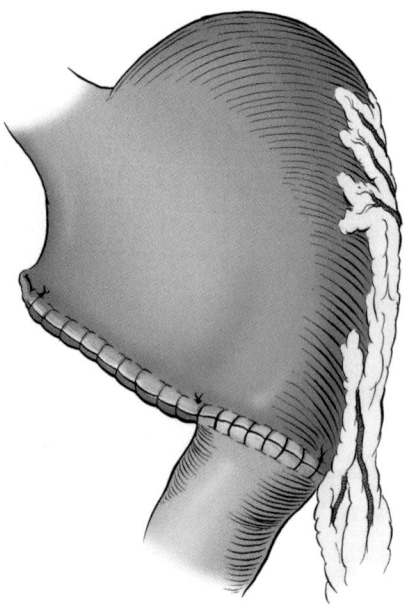

FIGURE 7   Billroth I. *(From Townsend CM, Evers BM:* Atlas of general surgical techniques, *ed 1, Philadelphia, 2010, Saunders, Fig. 26-13.)*

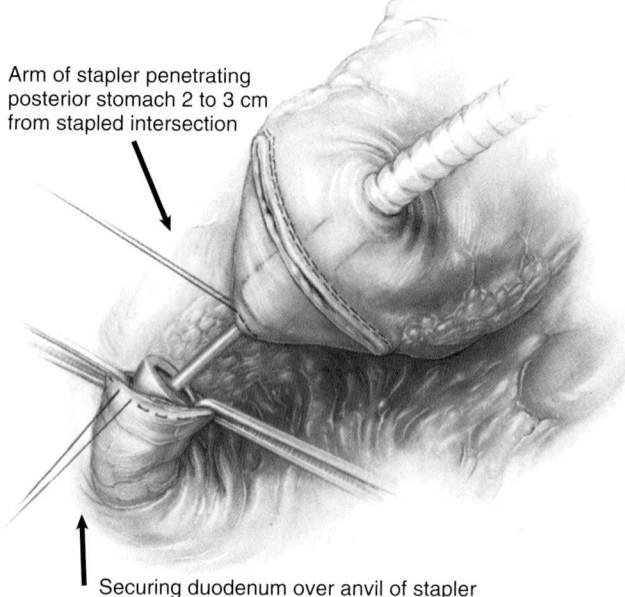

Arm of stapler penetrating posterior stomach 2 to 3 cm from stapled intersection

Securing duodenum over anvil of stapler

FIGURE 8   Stapled Billroth I. *(From Zuidema GD, Yeo CJ:* Shackelford's surgery of the alimentary tract, *ed 5, Philadelphia, 2001, Saunders, Fig. 11-56.)*

The authors perform the anastomosis in a single layer with simple sutures of 3-0 silk. Much attention is given in the literature to the point where the reconstructed lesser curve meets the gastroduodenal suture line (the "angle of sorrow"), with many variations on closing this defect. The authors' practice is to simply place an incorporating u-stitch that involves all three lines—the presence of healthy, well-vascularized tissue and lack of tension are likely of much greater importance than the specific technique used to place this particular suture. Performing Kocher's maneuver does not always prove necessary but can provide added length when the anastomosis is otherwise placed under tension. The use of an end-to-end anastomosis (EEA) stapler placed through an anterior gastrotomy to create the anastomosis is also acceptable (Figure 8). The gastrotomy can then be closed with another staple line or be hand sewn. With the exception of somewhat increased cost, stapling seems to afford equivalent operative experience and outcomes.

After surgery, a nasogastric tube is left in place to monitor for bleeding and is removed on postoperative day 1. A liquid diet is then started and maintained until bowel recovery, at which point the patient is discharged after tolerating a regular diet.

Billroth II

The authors reserve the use of a Billroth II gastroenterostomy for those patients in whom a Billroth I is not feasible, most often because of an inability of the duodenum and greater curvature to approximate without tension. As with gastroduodenostomy, many amendments to this reconstruction exist. A combination of the Reichel-Polya and Hofmeister-Finsterer modifications, first described in the early 20th century, is the preferred technique (Figure 9). Globally, this involves creation of a wide-mouthed gastroenterostomy with extension of the afferent limb along the closed portion of stomach nearest the lesser curve. Many aspects of the variation in this reconstruction have been, and still remain, points of debate with no clear superiority identified. The following are several topics that have generated much discussion and the authors' general approach to them.

- The ideal afferent limb should be as short as possible (no longer than 20 cm and less if the anatomy allows) to decrease the incidence of afferent loop syndrome. Mobilization of the ligament of Treitz can be performed to provide an even shorter limb.
- The authors' preference has been for a one-layered hand-sewn anastomosis, performed with 3-0 silk suture. Stapled techniques appear to be equivalent.
- The gastroenterostomy is performed in a retrocolic position, with the anastomosis placed through and lying below the colonic mesentery. This infracolic location helps prevent kinking of both the afferent and the efferent jejunal limbs and thus their respective obstructive pathologies; placement of sutures from the gastric wall to the transverse colon mesentery is important to maintain this setting.
- Use of a retrogastric location facilitates drainage of the stomach.
- An isoperistaltic orientation takes advantage of the natural course of the small intestine and permits a shorter afferent limb.
- The creation of a Braun's enteroenterostomy distally during the initial operation is acceptable but not routinely necessary.

Management of the duodenal stump with a Billroth II reconstruction is a subject that merits attention because of the potential for great morbidity. As a result of marked advances in intensive care, the mortality of duodenal stump leaks has improved from the historic reports of greater than 50% to around 10%, and in some accounts, even less. Stump leak rates are approximately 1% to 3%; postoperative leaks occur most frequently on postoperative day 6 to 10, but late stump "blow-out" can happen years after the initial surgery. Accordingly, a drain should be used near the stump; it can be removed in the office if the patient has been discharged before passage of the critical early time period.

Closure of the stump can be accomplished in many ways. If the tissue is well vascularized and healthy, it can be stapled or hand-sewn closed in a single layer and no further reinforcement is needed. Dissection of the duodenum away from the pancreas is not necessary,

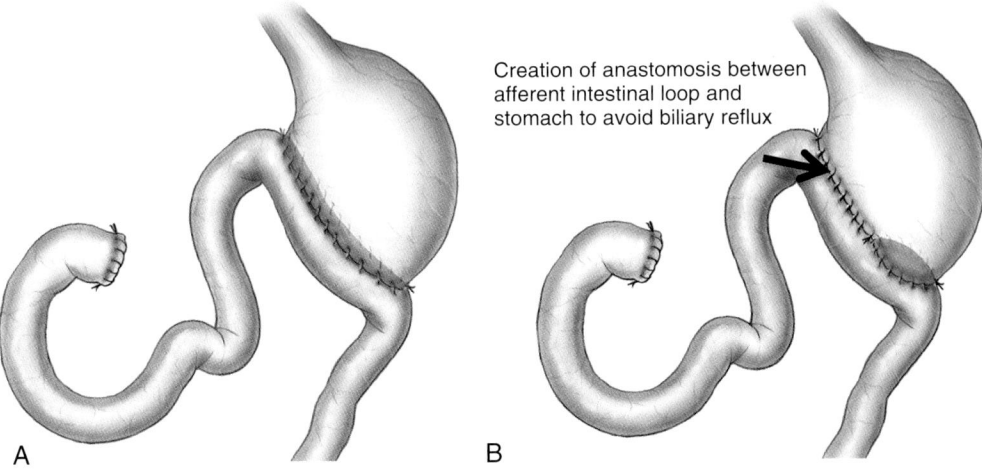

Creation of anastomosis between
afferent intestinal loop and
stomach to avoid biliary reflux

A   B

FIGURE 9   Gastrojejunostomy:
A, Along entire length of gastric
division (Polya); **B,** along part of
the gastric division (Finsterer).
*(From Piessen G: Reconstruction after
gastrectomy: which technique is best,*
J Visceral Surg *147(5):e273–e283,*
2010.)

and in fact, should be avoided, to obtain closure. An extensive review regarding the management of the difficult duodenal stump is beyond the scope of this chapter, but end or lateral stump drains, technically demanding techniques such as those described by Nissen and Bancroft, multiple layer closures, and omental patches are not routinely necessary.

Roux-en-Y

Several aspects appear to be important in creation of a successful Roux-en-Y reconstruction (Figure 10). A Roux limb length of at least 40 cm helps prevent bile reflux. When performed during an open procedure, both retrocolic and antecolic positions for the Roux limb appear to be equivalent in terms of outcome, but more length can generally be gained with the retrocolic version. Variations on the standard reconstruction such as an uncut Roux-en-Y or the creation of a rho-shaped Roux limb are acceptable but likely unnecessary, and both hand-sewn and stapled anastomoses are acceptable. Some comparisons of Roux-en-Y have shown it to be superior to Billroth II in terms of untoward subjective symptoms and objective endoscopic evidence of bile reflux. The choice between the two depends primarily on the operator's experience and comfort with each technique and its potential morbidities.

Minimally Invasive Approach

As previously mentioned, surgical indications for PUD include hemorrhage, obstruction, perforation, and refractory ulcer disease. As minimally invasive surgery has become more pervasive and widely accepted for surgery for both benign and malignant disease, increasing use of laparoscopy for PUD has been seen but still remains uncommon.

Like all minimally invasive approaches, patient selection and surgeon experience are paramount to success. Patient factors such as previous surgery, comorbidities, and body habitus must be considered because they may often make laparoscopy difficult, necessitating conversion to laparotomy. However, more important in the case of PUD is the patient's medical condition. Patients with any degree of hemodynamic instability or long-standing peritonitis are best managed with a traditional open approach, whereas patients with stable conditions may be considered.

Laparoscopic techniques used in foregut operations as in antireflux and bariatric surgery have made many surgeons facile with techniques that can similarly be used for laparoscopic PUD operations. Most commonly, this involves a four-port or five-port technique

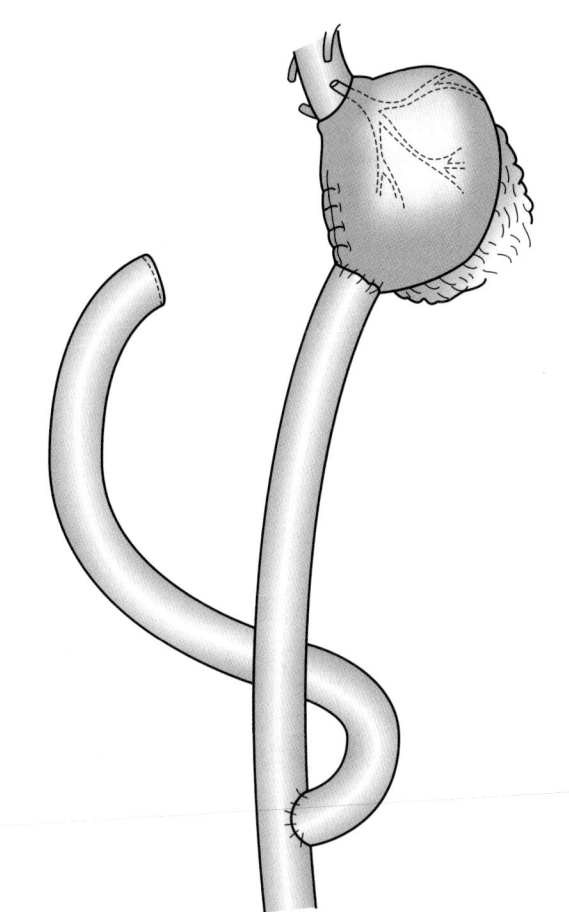

FIGURE 10   Roux-en-Y reconstruction. *(From Cameron JL:* Current surgical therapy, *ed 5, St Louis, 1995, Mosby.)*

(Figure 11), depending on the complexity of the operation, as it is sometimes necessary to have a retractor for the left hepatic lobe or an additional assistant port. As in many minimally invasive foregut operations, patients are positioned with the legs abducted in a split-leg position. Patients need to be well secured for safety because the table is typically placed into a reverse Trendelenburg's position with the surgeon operating between the patient's legs and assistants at the sides.

Port placement

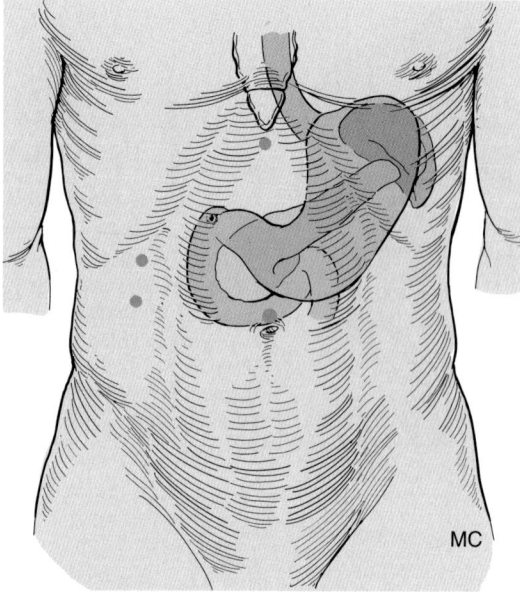

MC

FIGURE 11   Possible port arrangement for laparoscopic approach to foregut surgery, showing port placement in relation to an ulcer. *(From Townsend CM, Evers BM: Atlas of general surgical techniques, ed 1, Philadelphia, 2010, Saunders, Fig. 29-6.)*

With the advent and efficacy of PPIs, current surgical management of perforated peptic ulcers most commonly involves omental patch repair with vigilant pharmacotherapy afterwards. Omental patch repair has been pursued with the use of laparoscopy for some time and has accumulated good data including several randomized controlled clinical trials that support its use and equivalency to traditional open approach.

A minimally invasive approach is not generally advocated for active hemorrhage associated with a peptic ulcer; however, a minimally invasive approach is not unreasonable to pursue for definitive operation when hemorrhage has been temporarily controlled with medical, endoscopic, or interventional radiology management. In those cases of controlled hemorrhage that have a high risk of rebleeding (such as adherent clot, a visible vessel, or active bleeding at the time of endoscopy), definitive surgical intervention may be reasonable to pursue in experienced, skilled hands.

In patients with disease refractory to PPI pharmacotherapy, elective laparoscopic approaches similar to the open approaches previously discussed may be pursued. Again, a surgeon's expertise and experience with laparoscopy may allow for operations like truncal vagotomy, pyloroplasty, gastric resections, and reconstructions.

Robotic surgery continues to evolve within all fields of surgery, including general surgery, although its role and benefits remain somewhat uncertain. The robotic system offers high-definition, three-dimensional visual quality with the enhanced range of motion and dexterity that may be useful in more complex operations as in selective vagotomies or gastric resections with reconstructions. However, the caveat, as with laparoscopy, is that surgeon experience is of utmost importance in optimization of said benefits and outcomes in these patients.

SUGGESTED READINGS

Jordan PH: Surgery for peptic ulcer disease, *Curr Probl Surg* 28(4):267–330, 1991.

Isuel BJ: Management of the difficult duodenum, *Curr Rev Gastrointest Minimally Invasive Endocr Surg* 61(2):166–171, 2004.

Yeo CJ: Operations for peptic ulcer. In Shackelford's surgery of the alimentary tract, ed 6, Philadelphia, 2006, Saunders.

THE MANAGEMENT OF DUODENAL ULCERS

Robert J. Beaulieu, MD, and
Frederic E. Eckhauser, MD, FACS

INTRODUCTION

With the improvement in medical management of peptic ulcer disease, the incidence of hospitalization for duodenal ulcer (DU) disease has declined dramatically since 1990. The two improvements in care largely responsible for the reduction in surgeries for DU are antisecretory medications, such as proton pump inhibitors (PPIs) and histamine-receptor blockers, and therapy targeting the eradication of *Helicobacter pylori*. However, surgery remains an important element in the care of DUs because of the high rate of morbidity and mortality as a result of associated complications, such as bleeding, perforation, or obstruction.

Approximately 60,000 patients are hospitalized annually for DU disease, with an in-hospital mortality of 3.7%, a rate significantly higher than that of gastric ulceration (2.1%). Of patients hospitalized for duodenal ulceration, 10% will require surgery for progression to complicated ulceration, most commonly hemorrhage, and the overall operatively mortality rate may be as high as 10%. The two most common causes of duodenal ulceration are *H. pylori* infection and recent use of nonsteroidal antiinflammatory drugs (NSAIDs), accounting for more than 90% of cases of DU disease. Other important factors include gastrinoma (Zollinger-Ellison syndrome), smoking, steroid or cocaine use, and, likely, gastroduodenal dysmotility. The underlying pathophysiology involves dysregulation of acid secretion and impaired mucosal defense. Patients with DU disease usually have normal fasting gastrin levels but exhibit a higher acid load secretion when exposed to gastrin stimulus than do healthy patients. Further, duodenal mucosa demonstrates gastric metaplasia as a response to damage, allowing for *H. pylori* colonization and infection. *H. pylori* infection disrupts mucosal integrity and stimulates increased acid secretion through excretion of histamine N-methyltransferase.

Duodenal ulceration is marked by sudden onset epigastric pain that is commonly described as gnawing, burning, or stabbing in nature. Patients particularly complain of onset of pain between midnight and 3:00 AM. Although uncommon, pain of duodenal ulceration may be referred elsewhere, typically the back, if the ulcer has extended into the pancreatic head or free perforation has occurred. More than 90% of ulcers are visualized in the first portion of the duodenum on endoscopic evaluation. Ulceration in the more distal portions should raise concern for gastrinoma, which accounts for only 1% to 2% of patients with newly diagnosed duodenal ulceration. DUs have a characteristic appearance with sharply demarcated, clean edges with exposed submucosa. In the case of recent hemorrhage, an eschar or clot may be adherent to the ulcer bed. If duodenal ulceration is visualized on upper endoscopy, gastric mucosal biopsies should be taken to demonstrate the presence of *H. pylori* as a causative agent.

MEDICAL MANAGEMENT OF DUODENAL ULCERS

The majority of regimens for medical management of DUs are focused on eradication of *H. pylori* infection. After the initial diagnosis of active infection by serology, antral biopsy, and/or breath test with carbon-labeled urea, combined therapy with antibiotics active toward *H. pylori* (clarithromycin and amoxicillin typically) and an antisecretory agent should be initiated (Table 1). In this setting, eradication of *H. pylori* significantly reduces rates of ulcer recurrence and ulcer complications, such as bleeding. NSAIDs or aspirin should be avoided, and smoking cessation is essential. In a large meta-analysis examining eradication therapy compared to none, the number of patients that needed to be treated to avoid recurrence was only two. Patients who have uncomplicated DU disease should take antisecretory drugs such as PPIs for 2 to 4 weeks, whereas patients with complicated DU disease should probably receive indefinite PPI therapy.

SURGICAL MANAGEMENT OF DUODENAL ULCERS

Operative management of DUs is indicated when there are complications such as perforation, hemorrhage, and obstruction. Most surgery is performed emergently for the treatment of bleeding or perforation. Because of the effectiveness of medical management, surgery for intractable disease has become rare. Increasingly, surgical techniques focus on repairing the primary defect as in simple closure and oversewing, with subsequent medical eradication of *H. pylori*. However, in some cases, it may be necessary to induce gastric denervation by highly selective vagotomy (HSV), vagotomy and drainage (pyloroplasty or gastrojejunostomy), or vagotomy and antrectomy.

TABLE 1: Medical management regimens for eradication of *H. pylori*

Agent	Length of treatment
PPI (omeprazole 20 mg OR lansoprazole 30 mg) + Amoxicillin 1000 mg + Clarithromycin 500 mg	Orally, twice daily for 14 days
PPI (omeprazole 20 mg OR lansoprazole 30 mg) + Metronidazole 500 mg + Clarithromycin 500 mg	Orally, twice daily for 14 days
Alternative regimen: Bismuth subsalicylate 525 mg qid + Metronidazole 500 mg tid + Tetracycline 500 mg qid + PPI (omeprazole 20 mg OR lansoprazole 30 mg daily)	Orally, given as indicated for 14 days

PPI, Proton pump inhibitor; *qid,* four times daily; *tid,* three times daily.

Operations tailored toward reduction of acid secretion, either by truncal vagotomy or more selective approaches, must be measured against the effectiveness of medical therapy with antisecretory agents. Truncal vagotomy results in 60% to 70% reduction in acid secretion with liquid meal stimulation when compared with normal subjects but is associated with 10% risk of postoperative dumping, diarrhea, or gastroparesis. Inclusion of an antrectomy may further decrease acid secretion by 85% compared with normal individuals. However, PPI therapy allows for nearly 100% acid reduction at 6 hours after dosing yet falls to 60% to 70% reduction by 24 hours (most are doses on a once-daily schedule). It is no surprise, therefore, that the rates of operation for intractability have fallen dramatically since the introduction of these agents in the 1990s. However, early operative management remains essential for the treatment of bleeding, perforation, and obstruction associated with DUs.

Perforated Duodenal Ulcers

Perforation is the most common fatal complication of DUs. The vast majority of patients (>90%) with perforation of a DU experience sudden onset of severe, diffuse abdominal pain and/or demonstrate pneumoperitoneum on plain radiograph. However, up to 20% of patients do not show free intraperitoneal air on plain radiography and may require computed tomography for diagnosis. Early diagnosis is paramount, as delay beyond 12 hours increases the risk of cardiovascular collapse and subsequent risk for morbidity and mortality. Initial management of a perforated DU consists of insertion of a nasogastric tube, fluid resuscitation, intravenous PPI, and broad-spectrum intravenous antibiotics. The patient should then be taken to the operating room emergently for closure and peritoneal washout.

Most perforations are located on the anterior surface of the first portion of the duodenum, immediately distal to the pylorus, and are less than 5 mm in diameter. In younger patients, patients with pre-existent anemia, and patients whose time-to-operation was less than 24 hours, simple closure and peritoneal irrigation are as effective as more extensive gastric resection. Typically, the peritoneal cavity is washed with 5 to 10 liters of warm saline before repair of perforation is attempted. For perforations larger than 5 mm, a patch of omentum is secured in a tension-free fashion over the defect, with absorbable sutures placed into the seromuscular layer adjacent to the ulcer, provided it appears to be healthy, viable tissue. The integrity of the repair is tested by insufflating air through the nasogastric tube under low pressure. To prevent fluid collections and monitor for ongoing leakage, a Jackson-Pratt drain is left in the hepatorenal recess. The anesthesia team should be made aware that the nasogastric tube should be left in place at the cessation of the procedure.

Postoperatively, repair of perforated DU should be followed by PPI and antibiotic therapy to reduce the risk of recurrence. If the suspected cause of perforation is NSAID use, these agents should be discontinued in the postoperative period. However, in patients who require continued postoperative NSAID use or those unlikely to comply with anti–*H. pylori* and antisecretory regimens, HSV or truncal vagotomy and drainage should be considered instead of patch closure. Patients who have previously failed medical management—namely, those who have developed perforation while on antibiotics and antisecretory drugs—should be considered for acid reduction surgery as well. Patients with ongoing shock, delayed presentation beyond 48 hours, marked comorbid disease, and significant peritoneal contamination are poor candidates for definitive surgery, and patch closure should be used in these patients.

There is growing evidence that laparoscopic approaches, especially the Graham patch or vagotomy, to repair DUs are safe and effective in experienced hands. Patients with ongoing hemodynamic stability, multiple medical comorbidities, or peritonitis lasting longer than 24 hours are best served with an open approach. Patients with radiographic evidence of large duodenal defects or complex locations may preclude use of a laparoscopic approach and should probably be managed openly initially. Multiple trials report improved rates of wound infection and pain control among patients treated laparoscopically. However, there appears to be no difference in the length of hospital stay or rates of postoperative complications between the open and laparoscopic approaches. Therefore, for the stable patient with minimal risk factors, it is reasonable to consider laparoscopic HSV or the Taylor procedure (posterior truncal vagotomy and anterior seromyotomy or anterior parietal cell vagotomy). However, patients with large or complex duodenal perforations are best served with an open surgical approach.

Postoperatively, we perform an upper gastrointestinal (GI) study on every patient on the second or third day. If there is no evidence of leakage and the stomach is emptying appropriately, the patient is started on a clear liquid diet. Perioperative antibiotics are not required unless there was peritoneal purulence noted at time of operation. All patients receive intravenous PPIs, and patients for whom serologic findings showed the presence of *H. pylori* are initiated on appropriate treatment immediately. Drain outputs are collected routinely to observe for bilious drainage to suggest postoperative leakage, especially at the initiation of oral diet. Postoperative leak in the stable patient, without signs of peritonitis or clinical decompensation, can be managed conservatively. On discharge, all patients who did not undergo definitive acid suppression surgery are placed on PPI. A carbon-labeled breath test is scheduled in one month for patients undergoing treatment for *H. pylori* to confirm eradication.

Perforations due to DU are typically small and anteriorly placed. However, large or even "giant" perforations (>2.5 cm) and those that are inconveniently placed may be better treated by definitive surgery such as vagotomy and pyloroplasty or duodenal intubation and serosal jejunal packing. Omental patching may still be successful in the case of large perforation in the emergent setting and may be recommended for the inexperienced technician because of the ease of performance (Figure 1). Total gastrectomy is rarely indicated

because it often creates more technical difficulty in the repair and because omental and serosal patching have such high success rates.

Bleeding Duodenal Ulcers

Bleeding DUs are a common initial presentation for DU disease and carry a significant mortality rate. Approximately 2.5% of patients hospitalized with bleeding ulceration will die of this complication. There is a 15% risk at 5 years for hemorrhage in patients with DUs who have not had surgery and who have not received continuing maintenance therapy. For patients treated with H2 blockers, PPIs, or therapy for *H. pylori*, the risk of hemorrhage has not changed significantly since the introduction of these agents. Patients with history of hemorrhage from duodenal ulceration are at an increased risk of bleeding again, in which the rebleeding rate may be as high as 30% to 40% and the mortality rate 10% to 40%. However, the rates of surgery for bleeding ulcer have steadily declined as endoscopic management has become more popular and has been shown to achieve excellent results in initial management of acute GI bleed. Patients older than age 65 also appear to be at an increased risk of experiencing hemorrhage associated with their DUs than do younger patients.

Patients should be placed on a PPI drip immediately on suspicion of a bleeding DU. Endoscopic management has largely surpassed surgery as the initial approach in acute GI hemorrhage and can correctly identify the source of bleeding in approximately 90% of patients. Clipping, cautery, and epinephrine injection are often employed techniques for endoscopic hemorrhage control and are commonly used in conjunction with one another. There is some evidence that, after successful treatment of bleeding, an endoscopic "second look" procedure the following day may decrease the risk of rebleeding. Endoscopic management is less likely to be successful in patients who experience hemodynamic instability at presentation, who have an ulcer base greater than 2 cm, a deep posterior location of the DU, and a transfusion requirement greater than 4 units in a 24-hour period. Endoscopic management should be performed in tandem with surgical consultation to allow for timely identification of patients for whom surgery is required.

Patients with bleeding DUs are typically referred to surgery if bleeding continues after conservative management or if there is evidence of recurrent bleeding after two attempts at endoscopic therapy. Many of these lesions are in the posterior proximal duodenum. In patients demonstrating hemodynamic instability at the time of evaluation, simple oversewing of the ulcer is the procedure of choice. After a midline or upper midline laparotomy, anterolateral duodenectomy is performed, allowing for visualization of the posterior ulcer. Heavy permanent sutures and a u-stitch are used to oversew any visible bleeding vessel in the ulcer base. If bleeding is vigorous, especially to the point of obstructing the view of the ulcer base, a Kocher maneuver may be performed to mobilize the proximal duodenum and allow for manual compressing of the ulcer between the thumb and finger of the surgeon. Multiple u-stitches may be required and care should be taken to avoid unintentional involvement of the common bile duct in the stitch because of its close approximation with the posterior duodenum. A two-layer closure technique is used to repair the duodenectomy and the operation is completed. Postoperatively, the patient should be maintained on intravenous PPI infusion.

Definitive ulcer management with truncal vagotomy or HSV should be reserved for patients at low risk who are hemodynamically stable. In this case, the initial approach is the same. However, the duodenectomy may then be carried through the pylorus, which will be later closed in a Heineke-Mikulicz or Finney pyloroplasty. Until recently, vagotomy with antrectomy was considered the gold-standard definitive ulcer surgery for patients with recurrent DU bleeding. However, recent studies have placed its position as such in question. Yet, vagotomy with antrectomy and subsequent Billroth II

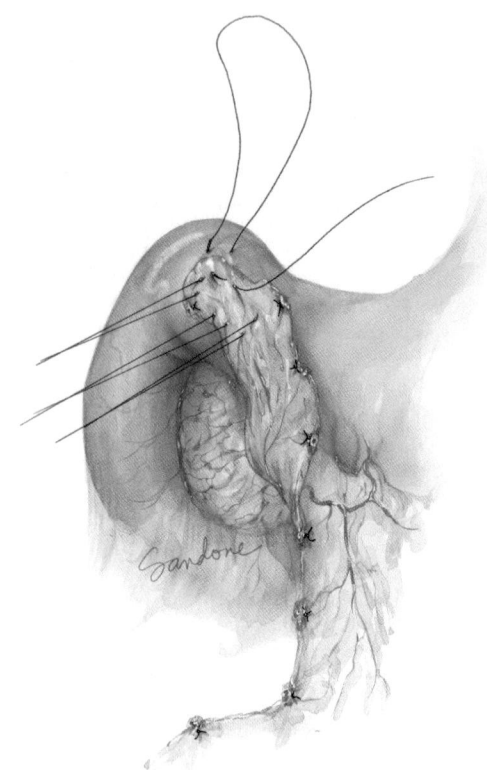

FIGURE 1   Omental patch. *(Illustration by Corinne Sandone, from Cameron JL: Atlas of surgery, vol 2, St. Louis, 1994, Mosby-Year Book. Reprinted with permission.)*

reconstruction is still a reasonable option in stable patients with chronic ulcer diathesis (Figure 2). In patients for whom a partial gastrectomy results in more than 50% of the gastric area removed, reconstruction should be performed using a Roux method. Closure of the DU is essential regardless of the method of reconstruction. The ulcer may be oversewn through an anterior duodenectomy, as previously described, or through the open end of the duodenum. Lesions that are within the proximal duodenum can create difficulty with closure of the duodenum stump and may preclude this method of treatment.

Postoperatively, the patient should be continued on intravenous PPI infusion. If *H. pylori* status was not determined preoperatively, operative biopsy of the gastric mucosa may prove helpful in determining this diagnosis. The role of definitive ulcer therapy, such as truncal vagotomy and antrectomy or HSV, in patients who have not been adequately treated for *H. pylori* has not yet been examined. In such cases, oversewing of the ulcer bed alone with postoperative therapy for *H. pylori* eradication may be reasonable. In patients with sources of duodenal bleeding that are difficult to identify, angiographic embolization may be helpful. Recent series, although small, report high success rates and low risks of recurrent bleeding in patients treated by angiography. Patients who experience recurrent bleeding after definitive surgery may be initially managed by antisecretory agents, but up to 50% require reoperation.

Obstruction Duodenal Ulcers

Acute and chronic gastric outlet obstruction may occur as a result of a large, edematous DU. Patients with untreated duodenal ulceration have a lifetime risk of 10% for pyloric stenosis. Acute obstruction is often successfully managed with conservative treatment involving nasogastric decompression with nasogastric intubation, fluid resuscitation, and intravenous PPI administration. Symptoms of acute disease typically include early satiety, bloating, nausea, and vomiting. Laboratory examinations reveal hypochloremic alkalosis due to the loss of gastric secretions. These patients rarely require operative intervention. Upper endoscopy is indicated to rule out malignancy, a far more common cause of gastric outlet obstruction, and will demonstrate active ulceration with significant edema.

Chronic outlet obstruction due to DU differs from acute in both the length of the settings (typically weeks to months) and the severity of the weight loss. Diagnostic tests, including an upper GI series, will reveal a distended stomach and significant narrowing of the pylorus, secondary to stenosis due to chronic edema and inflammation. The resulting scar and fibrosis may prevent the progression of an endoscope beyond the pylorus. Patients with chronic outlet obstruction do not experience durable relief of symptoms with gastric decompression and PPI infusion. As such, operative intervention is often required (>90% of patients).

After confirmation that the pyloric stenosis and subsequent obstruction are due to duodenal ulceration and not malignancy, relief of the anatomic abnormality is the focus of intervention. Upper endoscopy with balloon dilatation of the pyloric cicatrix is the first-line therapy in most instances. Success rates are high with initial relief achieved in 80% of patients and sustained improvement in 50% to 70% of those treated, but many patients will have to undergo multiple dilatations. Patients who require more than two dilatations should be considered for operative intervention, as they are at a high risk for failure of endoscopic treatment. Yet another consideration for the progression to surgery is the fact that an estimated 67% of patients treated for gastric outlet obstruction due to duodenal ulceration do not have *H. pylori* infection, and early acid-reducing surgery is warranted.

The surgical options for treatment of gastric outlet obstruction are primarily laparoscopic or open HSV with gastrojejunostomy (HSV/GJ) or vagotomy and antrectomy. Although both treatments are equally effective clinically, several other factors are helpful in determining the appropriate therapy. Surgeons adept in laparoscopic techniques may prefer the HSV/GJ because of its minimally invasive nature. However, malignancy is by far the most common cause of gastric outlet obstruction in the adult population, and this may be difficult to diagnose by laparoscopic techniques. Biopsy of the ulcer should be performed when the patient is undergoing laparoscopic repair for gastric outlet obstruction. When HSV is performed, gastrojejunostomy is the preferred drainage procedure compared with pyloroplasty. Some centers recommend the placement of a feeding jejunostomy tube at the time of surgery to minimize the risk of postoperative malnutrition and delayed gastric emptying, which may be complications for 10% to 50% of postoperative patients.

Intractable Duodenal Ulcers

The number of patients affected by intractable DUs has decreased since the advent of PPI therapy. Much of the literature regarding treatment of intractable DUs relies on patients undergoing therapy before the widespread use of antisecretory agents. Therefore, patients afflicted with intractable ulcers today may represent a population different from those previously described, including atypical pathophysiology that is largely as yet unrecognized. Intractable ulcers should also prompt a workup for gastrinoma. A history of noncompliance with medications complicates both the acute and postoperative management of many of these patients. Acid-reducing surgery, particularly HSV, serves as the mainstay of therapy, although the surgeon should strongly judge the ability of large resections to address the underlying etiology, which may be unknown, of the duodenal disease and the likelihood of patient adherence to a strict postoperative regimen. Gastrojejunostomy may also be performed in conjunction with HSV. Prior to either operation, many patients are treated empirically for *H. pylori* infection. Factors that increase the risk of developing duodenal ulceration, including smoking and aspirin or other NSAID use, should be stopped. Postoperatively, the patient should be placed on PPIs indefinitely.

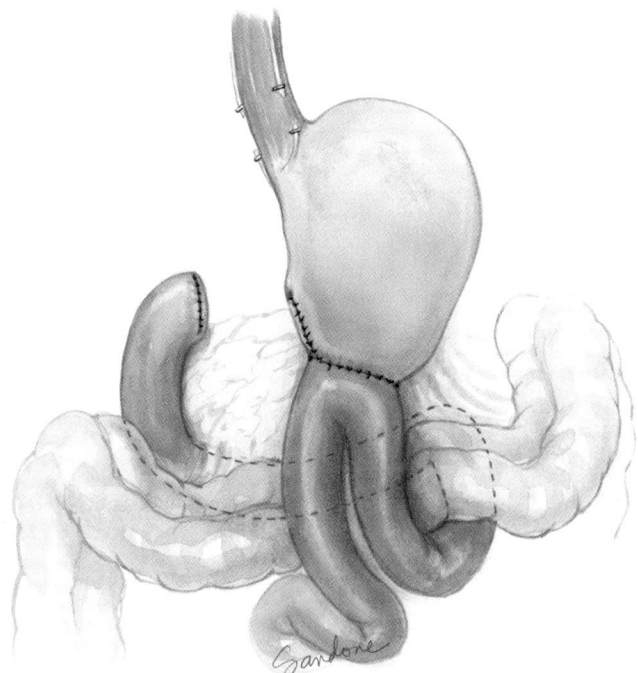

FIGURE 2 Billroth II reconstruction. *(Illustration by Corinne Sandone, from Cameron JL: Atlas of surgery, vol 2, St. Louis, 1994, Mosby-Year Book. Reprinted with permission.)*

Atypical Indications

Giant DUs are those measuring greater than 2 cm. Given their size, they represent a surgical challenge and leakage following repair with typical patch methods is a common complication. No consensus management exists regarding the care of these patients. Patients that present with hemodynamic instability warrant immediate operative intervention with attempted repair or patch of the perforation and identification of any sites of bleeding. In the low risk patient, more definitive ulcer operation may be indicated, including vagotomy and antrectomy. An innovative approach using placement of gastrostomy and jejunostomy tubes at the time of repair, to drain the gastric contents without the use of a nasogastric tube, decompress the duodenum, and allow for early enteral feeding has also been suggested in these patients.

Marginal ulcerations are those that affect the perianastomotic region following a gastrojejunostomy, most commonly seen after gastric bypass operations for morbid obesity. Factors that may affect the risk of marginal ulcer include ischemia, aspirin or other NSAID use, gastrinoma, smoking, and excluded antrum following revisional gastric bypass surgery. In the setting of recurrent marginal ulcer following previous vagotomy or acid-reduction surgery, further differential diagnosis includes incomplete vagotomy, retained antrum, long afferent limb (after Billroth II), and ongoing *H. pylori* infection. Retained or excluded antrum causes the antrum to no longer be exposed to gastric acidification and, therefore, hypergastrinemia results, causing further gastric acid creation. Pancreatic polypeptide levels and gastric acid output after feeding are used to assess completeness of the vagotomy, as they are both mediated through vagal stimulation.

Initial evaluation with upper endoscopy will help to make the diagnosis and allows for control of bleeding from the ulceration site. It is recommended that insufflation during the procedure be kept to a minimum to reduce gastric distention and tension on the anastomosis. Patients with recurrent or persistent *H. pylori* infection should receive an appropriate regimen. For persistent marginal ulcer, operative intervention may be warranted. The goal of the surgeon should be to remove the affected mucosa with reanastomosis and reduction in the acid-secreting capabilities of the stomach. Incomplete truncal vagotomy is often addressed through thoracoscopic truncal vagotomy. Open or laparoscopic approach is performed by resection of the distal gastric remnant, including the gastrojejunostomy, and reanastomosis. Simple conversion of a gastroduodenostomy or gastrojejunostomy to a Roux-en-Y gastrojejunostomy must be done in conjunction with acid reducing surgery.

Duodenal Closure

The posterior location of many DUs increases the complexity of duodenal stump closure following partial gastrectomy and subsequent gastrojejunostomy. The duodenal stump is most easily closed with a GI anastomosis or thoracoabdominal stapler (blue cartridge). Not uncommonly, stapler use is precluded because of grossly friable tissue in the posterior duodenal wall, an already challenging location for closure. In these cases, the anterior wall of the duodenum may be sewn to the most proximal aspect of the distal ulcer lip demonstrating a healthy seromuscular layer. Repair is usually carried out with an absorbable suture in interrupted fashion. An omental patch can be then oversewn to the closure site. Air may be insufflated with a nasogastric tube to allow for inspection of the integrity of the closure. If possible, end duodenostomy, with closure of the duodenal stump around a tube to allow for decompression, should be avoided because of the high likelihood for leakage. Instead, duodenal decompression should be accomplished by a retrograde placed jejunostomy tube. Placement of a gastrostomy and jejunal feeding tube should be considered as at initial intervention.

SUGGESTED READINGS

Lap P, Vindal A, Hadke NS: Controlled tube duodenostomy in the management of fiant duodenal ulcer perforation: a new technique for a surgically challenging condition, *Am J Surg* 198(3):319–323, 2009.

Malfertheiner P, Selgrad M, Bornschein J: Helicobacter pylori: clinical management, *Curr Opin Gastroenterol* 28(6):608–614, 2012.

Millat B, Fingerhut A, Borie F: Surgical treatment of complicated duodenal ulcers: controlled trials, *World J Surg* 24(3):299–306, 2000.

Najm WI: Peptic ulcer disease, *Prim Care* 38(3):383–394, vii.doi:10.1016/j.pop.2011.05.001.Review 2011.

Sachdeva AK, Zaren HA, Sigel B: Surgical treatment of peptic ulcer disease, *Med Clin North Am* 75(4):999–1012, 1991.

ZOLLINGER-ELLISON SYNDROME

Haggi Mazeh, MD, and Herbert Chen, MD, FACS

INTRODUCTION

In 1955, Zollinger and Ellison described a syndrome characterized by ulceration of the upper jejunum, hypersecretion of gastric acid (gastrinoma), and non-beta islet cell tumors of the pancreas. Since their first description, more than 1000 patients have been diagnosed with Zollinger-Ellison syndrome (ZES) and more than 3400 papers have been published on this rare disease. ZES differs from typical peptic ulcer disease in nearly every aspect and therefore requires special consideration. Despite its rarity, surgeons should be aware of the current available diagnostic tools and the different management aspects of ZES because an increasing number of patients are diagnosed with ZES and appropriate management should be tailored to each one. The purpose of this chapter is to review the epidemiology, pathogenesis, presentation, diagnosis, and management of ZES. Management controversies are highlighted.

EPIDEMIOLOGY

Zollinger-Ellison syndrome is a very rare entity, and its incidence rate in the United States is estimated at 1 to 3 per million per year. ZES is also estimated to constitute 0.1% to 1% of all patients with peptic ulcer disease; however, the actual number may be higher because some of the patients with entitled peptic ulcer disease may have undiagnosed ZES. Most ZES cases are sporadic (80%), but 20% are associated with multiple endocrine neoplasia type 1 (MEN 1). Only approximately 25% of the patients with MEN 1 have ZES. The mean age of symptom onset is 41 years, and up to 90% of the patients are diagnosed between ages 20 and 60 years. Nevertheless, patients as young as 7 years and as old as 90 years have been identified. Patients with MEN 1 are more likely to present younger (at the third decade of life). A slight male predominance is seen, with a male:female ratio of 1.5-2:1.

PATHOGENESIS

Gastrinomas are derived from the enteroendocrine cells that are multipotential endodermal stem cells and are found mainly in the pancreas and small intestine. Tumors that arise from these cells are considered neuroendocrine tumors and are entitled gastrinomas when these cells secrete gastrin that results in the typical clinical manifestation. Recent advances identified several genetic mutations that are involved in ZES. These include the oncogenes *c-myc* and *HER-2/neu* and the tumor suppressor genes *MEN-1, p16INK4a,* and *DPC4/Smad.*

The result of excessive gastrin secretion is high gastric acid output. Gastrin has a trophic effect on parietal cells that secrete acid and enterochromaffin-like cells that secrete histamine, a potent acid secretion stimulant.

CLINICAL PRESENTATION

- Peptic ulcers. More than 90% of the patients with ZES have development of peptic ulcers. The ulcers are most commonly solitary and less than 1 cm in diameter. Ulcer location may vary; 75% occur in the first part of the duodenum, 14% in the distal duodenum, and 11% in the jejunum. Ulcers in patients with ZES are more often persistent and tend to recur.
- Diarrhea. More than 70% of the patients with ZES have diarrhea that results from the high rate of acid secretion, inactivation of pancreatic enzymes by low pH, and the inhibition of sodium and water absorption in the small bowel.
- Other symptoms include abdominal pain (90%), heartburn (44%), nausea/emesis (30%), gastrointestinal bleeding (25%), and weight loss (17%).
- Metastatic disease to the liver and bone is present in up to 33% of the patients with ZES and may cause local symptoms.

DIAGNOSIS

The diagnosis of ZES is based on clinical evaluation, laboratory testing, and imaging.

Clinical Evaluation

Despite increased awareness to ZES, the mean delay between symptom onset and correct diagnosis is 5 to 6 years. Correct diagnosis at the time of presentation is made in only 5% of patients with MEN 1 ZES and in only 2% of the patients with sporadic disease. This can partially be explained by the high prevalence of proton pump inhibitor (PPI) usage that may mask symptoms by providing very effective acid secretion suppression. A high index of suspicion should be maintained in patients with: 1, a combination of diarrhea, abdominal pain, and weight loss; 2, refractory or recurrent ulcers; 3, any symptoms of acid hypersecretion that are associated with diarrhea; 4, prominent gastric folds on endoscopy (caused by trophic gastrin effect); and 5, any gastrointestinal symptoms in patients with MEN 1. Family history and pituitary and parathyroid disease should be assessed to evaluate the possibility of MEN 1.

Laboratory Testing

- Fasting serum gastrin. This test should be routinely performed in all patients with suspected ZES. Patients should be off PPIs for 72 hours and fasting for 12 hours. A serum gastrin level greater than 1000 pg/mL (normal limits <110 pg/mL) is virtually diagnostic; however, multiple circumstances may cause gastrin elevation (Table 1). Specifically, achlorhydria with elevated gastric pH should be considered. Up to 60% of patients with ZES have gastrin levels less than 500 pg/mL, and additional testing should be obtained when ZES is suspected.
- Secretin stimulation test. This test can be used to differentiate between patients with ZES and patients with other causes of hypergastrinemia and should be performed routinely. Secretin (intravenous [IV], 0.4 µg/kg) is administered, and gastrin levels are measured at 0, 2, 5, 10, 15, and 30 minutes. Patients with ZES have a dramatic increase in gastrin levels, and an increment greater than 110 pg/mL is considered positive. A rise of 200 pg/mL above baseline has a sensitivity of 83% to 93% and a specificity of 100% for the detection of ZES.
- Ruling out of MEN 1. Serum calcium, parathyroid hormone, prolactin, and fasting insulin levels should be measured. Patients with suspected MEN 1 should undergo genetic testing.
- Other tests. Gastric acid secretion studies have been largely abandoned because of their invasiveness, and serum chromogranin A level is not as specific and sensitive as the previous tests and therefore is not routinely used. Selective arterial stimulation with calcium gluconate (calcium infusion study) followed by venous sampling is another test that is not routinely used because of decreased sensitivity.

Imaging Modalities

As many as 70% of the gastrinomas form in the duodenum, and the remainder arise in the pancreas (20%) and in adjacent lymph nodes (10%). Although up to 80% of the gastrinomas are located in the gastrinoma triangle (Figure 1), 20% may occur at different sites; because of their small size, accurate preoperative localization is of utter importance. Another purpose of the imaging modalities is assessment of local extension and identification of metastatic disease. Such studies include ultrasound scan, computed tomographic (CT) scan, magnetic resonance imaging (MRI), somatostatin receptor scintigraphy (SRS), fluorodeoxyglucose positron emission tomography (FDG-PET), endoscopic ultrasound scan (EUS), and angiography.

Because 80% of the gastrinomas express type 2 somatostatin receptors, SRS is the modality of choice with a sensitivity of 85% and specificity close to 100%. EUS has a sensitivity that reaches 70% and is particularly useful for intrapancreatic primary tumors. The

TABLE 1: Different causes of hypergastrinemia

Hypersecretory	Hyposecretory
Gastrinoma (ZES)	Pernicious anemia
Gastric outlet obstruction	Atrophic gastritis
Retained gastric antrum	Previous vagotomy
Antral hyperplasia	Diabetes mellitus
Helicobacter pylori infection	Renal failure
Pheochromocytoma	Acid-reducing medications
Short gut syndrome	

ZES, Zollinger-Ellison syndrome.

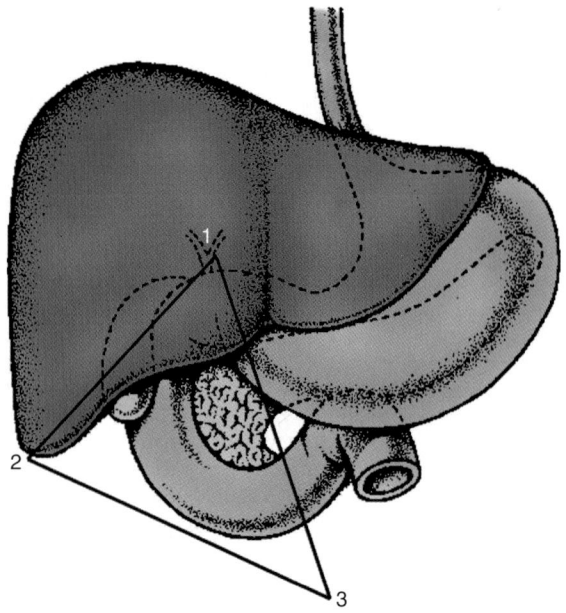

FIGURE I The gastrinoma triangle is composed of: *1*, the confluence of the cystic and common bile duct; *2*, the junction of the second and third portions of the duodenum; and *3*, the junction of the neck and body of the pancreas.

hypervascularity of gastrinomas can be used with contrast CT scan (50% sensitivity), MRI (30% to 50% sensitivity), and angiography (60% sensitivity). Gastrinomas located within the duodenal wall appear to be particularly resistant to detection with these modalities. Intraoperative ultrasound scan may be used to facilitate localization of small lesions that were not readily visible on preoperative studies. Arterial secretin stimulation and gastrin measurement at specific locations may also aid in intraoperative localization.

MANAGEMENT

The management of patients with ZES has evolved over the years. Before the development of effective acid-reducing medications, the morbidity and mortality associated with ZES was mainly the result of hypersecretion complications, and the only effective treatment was total gastrectomy. With the introduction of H2 antagonist and PPI medications, the mortality associated with hypersecretory complications has been, for all intents and purposes, eliminated. Estimates are that 60% to 90% of the gastrinomas are malignant, and therefore current management of ZES includes medical therapy to control the symptoms and complications of gastrin hypersecretion and surgery for selected patients to control the tumor.

Medical Management

Patients with ZES should be started on a high dose of PPIs (omeprazole, 60 mg daily; pantoprazole, 120 mg daily) to control acid secretion. Half the patients without MEN 1 are able to titrate down to a maintenance dose of 20 mg daily. Long-term treatment with PPIs has been generally safe, even in high doses.

Systemic therapy with somatostatin receptor analogs such as octreotide reduces gastrin secretion. Such therapies have been used with variable results and are not considered first-line agents. Systemic chemotherapies such as cisplatin and doxorubicin have also been tried with limited success.

Surgical Management

The effective use of PPIs to control acid secretion has dramatically altered the surgical management of ZES. The current role of surgery is to manage the long-term outcome of patients because of the malignant potential of the primary tumor.

Sporadic Disease

Because gastrinoma resection results in excellent prognosis and because the importance of malignancy control is increasingly appreciated, all patients at good risk with sporadic gastrinoma and no evidence of metastatic spread should be offered resection with curative intent. Such resection may eliminate or decrease the need for PPIs and prevent the morbidity and mortality associated with future metastatic spread. Patient selection and preferably preoperative localization are of utter importance as the medical treatment enables elective surgery that must be performed safely with specific goals and weighed against effective expectant management and excellent long-term prognosis of these patients.

The surgical goal is to detect and resect the primary tumor and to identify local spread to lymph nodes or distant metastasis to the liver. At laparotomy, abdominal exploration to identify peritoneal spread and liver palpation should be performed in every patient. This should be followed by a wide Kocher's mobilization of the duodenum and the pancreas head. The entire pancreas and duodenum should be exposed and mobilized to permit bimanual palpation. Intraoperative ultrasound scan, duodenal transillumination, and duodenotomy are advocated in all patients. For lesions not identifiable with other imaging modalities, palpation may identify 50% to 65% of duodenal gastrinomas, endoscopic transillumination may detect an additional 15% to 20%, and duodenotomy another 15%. Routine duodenotomy resulted in doubling the surgical cure rate from 30% to 60%. The use of intraoperative ultrasound scan may facilitate lesion localization and assess the relation of the tumor to pancreatic duct. Single lesions identified on exploration should be resected, including in the liver. Pancreatic head and neck gastrinomas should be enucleated when possible or resected with pancreaticoduodenectomy (Whipple's procedure) in selected patients. Distal pancreatectomy should be performed for pancreatic tail lesions. If the gastrinoma is not found in surgery, blind distal pancreatectomy should be avoided as different ectopic locations include small bowel mesentery, liver, and ovary. The resection of pancreatic or duodenal gastrinoma should be accompanied by regional lymph node dissection.

Because of the trophic effect of gastrin and excess of gastric parietal cells, gastric secretion may not return to normal after surgical gastrinoma resection. Up to 40% of the patients need long-term PPI treatment as a result of increased acid secretion for a mean of 8 years.

Multiple Endocrine Neoplasia Type 1

In patients with MEN 1 ZES, diagnosis and treatment of hyperparathyroidism before the gastrinoma surgical management is considered is important. The correction of hyperparathyroidism reduces the fasting serum gastrin concentration by eliminating the hypercalcemia as a contributing factor and decreases the basal acid secretion. Total parathyroidectomy with autotransplantation or subtotal parathyroidectomy is generally advocated for patients with hyperparathyroidism and MEN 1.

The surgical management of patients with MEN 1 ZES is challenging, and surgical recommendations are in evolution. Short of pancreaticoduodenectomy, cure is uniformly not possible in MEN 1 ZES because 30% of the patients have more than 20 duodenal tumors and 86% have positive lymph nodes. Biochemical relapse occurs in more than 95% of the patients within 3 to 5 years of surgery, and liver metastases develop rarely and in correlation to tumor size. In contrast, acid secretion can be managed medically in these patients; therefore, current recommendations include surgery only for patients

TABLE 2: Differences between sporadic Zollinger-Ellison syndrome (ZES) and multiple endocrine neoplasia type I (MEN I) ZES

	Sporadic ZES	MEN I ZES
Prevalence rate	80%	20%
Family history	–	+
Other endocrinopathies	–	+
Gastrinoma size	>2 cm	<2 cm
Number of tumors	Single	Multiple
Most common tumor location	Pancreas	Duodenum
Lymph node primary	10%	–
Surgical cure rate	60%	Rare
Malignant potential	High	Low

TABLE 3: Gastrinoma staging and prognosis with or without surgery

Stage	TNM	10-Year survival rate with surgery	10-Year survival rate without surgery
I	T < 2 cm	94%-96%	68%-82%
II	T > 2 cm	86%-91%	40%-55%
III	Any T, any N, M1	65%-90%	7%-50%

TNM, Tumor node metastasis.

with a tumor greater than 2 to 2.5 cm in size. Table 2 summarizes the differences between sporadic and MEN 1 ZES.

Metastatic Disease

Metastatic gastrinoma is currently the most common cause of morbidity and mortality in patients with ZES, but unfortunately, current therapy is limited. Liver resection is indicated in resectable disease and in the absence of compromised liver function and extrahepatic metastasis. The effect of somatostatin analogs (octreotide) in controlling gastrinoma symptoms is not predictable and has shown inconclusive results in metastatic disease. Hepatic artery embolization with or without selective artery chemotherapy infusion is used in patients who are symptomatic but are not surgical candidates with an approximately 50% response rate. Radiofrequency ablation or cryoablation may be used for small liver lesions. Liver transplantation is reserved for patients with isolated metastases to the liver, and most clinicians consider it an investigational approach. Chemotherapy and radiotherapy have limited effect in gastrinomas, which resulted in the development of novel therapeutic approaches that include molecular targeted therapy such as tyrosine kinase and mTOR inhibitors. These therapies are under clinical trials.

Reoperation

Because 70% of the patients with sporadic ZES have persistent or recurrent disease, the role of reoperation is important. Reoperation may prove beneficial in cases where cure can be achieved. Unfortunately, such cure intent cannot be accomplished in most patients; therefore, the increased potential risk should be weighed against the cure odds in every patient.

OUTCOMES AND PROGNOSIS

Surgery results in cure of ZES in 60% of the patients with sporadic disease, but MEN 1 ZES is rarely cured. Benign gastrinomas rarely cause mortality, and the prognosis of patients with ZES largely depends on the presence of malignant disease (60% to 90%) and the extent of disease. The staging of gastrinomas is dictated by tumor size, lymph node involvement, and presence of distant metastases

(tumor node metastasis [TNM]) and is detailed in Table 3. Up to one fourth of the patients have liver metastases at the time of diagnosis, and patients with liver metastases have only a 30% 10-year survival rate as compared with a more than 80% rate in those without. Patients with MEN 1 ZES have as low as a 6% rate of metastases at the time of diagnosis, which translates to an excellent survival rate (100% at 20 years). The 10-year survival rate with or without surgery for patients with sporadic ZES is detailed in Table 3.

Clear association between gastrin level at the time of diagnosis and the prognosis has been shown. Patients with mildly elevated gastrin levels (0 to 499 pg/mL) had 94% and 86% 5-year and 10-year survival rates, respectively. Patients with moderate elevation (500 to 1000 pg/mL) had 92% and 87% 5-year and 10-year survival rates, respectively. Lastly, patients with severe elevations (>1000 pg/mL) had 86% and 73% 5-year and 10-year survival rates, respectively.

POSTOPERATIVE SURVEILLANCE

Current surveillance guidelines include history and physical examination, serum gastrin values, and abdominal imaging (CT scan or MRI) at 3 and 6 months after resection. Thereafter, history, physical examination, and serum gastrin values are recommended every 6 to 12 months for 1 to 3 years and then as clinically indicated. Imaging studies are recommended only as clinically indicated.

AREAS OF CONTROVERSIES

- Vagotomy during laparotomy. Despite effective medical management of acid hypersecretion, parietal cell vagotomy decreases the need for long-term PPIs and avoids the side effects that include achlorhydria that may lead to vitamin B_{12} and iron deficiency. Long-term use of PPIs may also result in the development of gastric carcinoid tumors, and for these reasons, selective vagotomy may be considered when laparotomy is performed for gastrinoma.
- Pancreaticoduodenectomy. Given the good prognosis of patients with ZES, pancreaticoduodenectomy should be carefully weighed against the risks. Whipple's procedure also modifies the anatomy and may affect future interventional methods for liver metastases. Because most gastrinomas in MEN 1 ZES are located in the duodenum, Whipple's procedure may increase the cure rates in these patients; however, this should be offered only to patients in whom gastrin source is localized to the pancreatic head.
- Lymph nodes. Lymph node primary gastrinomas do occur in up to 10% of the cases, and lymph nodes may be involved with tumor from another primary. The extent of lymph node

dissection is controversial and should be tailored to each patient as the routine lymph node removal may increase surgical cure rates.

- Liver metastases resection. Patients with liver metastases who undergo removal of all known disease have a 5-year survival rate of up to 85%. Patients with tumor burden that is unresectable may still benefit from cytoreduction surgery that may affect symptoms that result from tumor endocrine function. Surgical liver metastases resection should probably be offered only to patients in whom at least 90% of the tumor could be removed.
- Laparoscopy. Despite increased technical laparoscopic capabilities and experience, gastrinomas present several challenges. Duodenotomy and palpation of duodenal wall is an essential part of the exploration of all patients with ZES gastrinoma, and the tumors tend to be large and often present with liver metastases. These factors make laparoscopy unappealing for the treatment of gastrinomas.

CONCLUSION

The surgical management of ZES has evolved since its first introduction. At present, gastric acid reducing medications can control symptoms, and the current role of surgery is to manage the long-term outcome of patients because of the malignant potential of the primary tumor. Because of the rarity of this syndrome, areas of controversy exist and future studies with larger cohorts are needed to shed light on the optimal management of these complicated cases.

SUGGESTED READINGS

Chen H, Sippel RS, O'Dorisio MS, et al: The North American Neuroendocrine Tumor Society consensus guideline for the diagnosis and management of neuroendocrine tumors: pheochromocytoma, paraganglioma, and medullary thyroid cancer, *Pancreas* 39:775–783, 2010.

Ellison EC, Johnson JA: The Zollinger-Ellison syndrome: a comprehensive review of historical, scientific, and clinical considerations, *Curr Probl Surg* 46:13–106, 2009.

Libutti SK, Alexander HR Jr: Gastrinoma: sporadic and familial disease, *Surg Oncol Clin North Am* 15:479–496, 2006.

Morrow EH, Norton JA: Surgical management of Zollinger-Ellison syndrome: state of the art, *Surg Clin North Am* 89:1091–1103, 2009.

Norton JA, Jensen RT: Resolved and unresolved controversies in the surgical management of patients with Zollinger-Ellison syndrome, *Ann Surg* 240:757–773, 2004.

MALLORY-WEISS SYNDROME

Brian D. Shames, MD, and David W. McFadden, MD

HISTORY

In 1879, Heinrich Quincke described three cases of gastrointestinal (GI) bleeding caused by ulcers of the esophagus. Subsequently, in 1929, G. Kenneth Mallory and Soma Weiss, described a syndrome of massive upper GI (UGI) hemorrhage from fissure-like lesions of the esophageal mucosa. These lesions developed at the junction of the esophagus and gastric cardia and were caused by alcohol-induced retching or vomiting. For the next 40 years, reports of Mallory-Weiss syndrome were sporadic and numbered less than 250 in total. Treatment was equally divided between supportive observation and surgical hemostasis. The introduction of flexible endoscopy in the early 1970s revolutionized the diagnosis and management of UGI hemorrhage. Mallory-Weiss syndrome has since become a more commonly diagnosed cause of UGI hemorrhage, and a myriad of associated causal factors for the development of Mallory-Weiss tears have been described. The syndrome that bears their names now encompasses all causes of linear mucosal lacerations of the gastroesophageal junction (GEJ) that lead to UGI bleeding. The syndrome should not be confused with Boerhaave's syndrome, which is distal esophageal perforation as a result of vomiting.

INCIDENCE, PATHOPHYSIOLOGY, AND ASSOCIATED CONDITIONS

Although the syndrome was once thought to be a rare cause of UGI bleeding, multiple large studies with flexible endoscopy have shown a 5% to 15% incidence rate of Mallory-Weiss syndrome in patients with acute UGI hemorrhage. Mallory-Weiss tears are the second most common etiology of upper GI nonvariceal bleeding after ulcer disease. How frequently a Mallory-Weiss tear occurs without bleeding cannot be determined with any certainty. It is highly likely that the condition occurs in a less severe form more often than is clinically recognized.

The pathophysiology of Mallory-Weiss tears has not been completely defined. A factor common to most causes of Mallory-Weiss tear is an acute increase in intraabdominal pressure. The most common symptoms before the development of hemorrhage are vomiting and retching. During emesis, the pylorus closes, the abdominal wall and diaphragm contract, the gastric cardia relaxes as the distal stomach contracts, and intragastric contents are forcefully expelled in a cephalad direction. Mucosal tears are thought to be the result of the rapid development of a large gradient between the intragastric pressure and the intrathoracic pressure at the GEJ, which occurs in actions like vomiting and retching. The forceful elevation of the GEJ above the diaphragm leads to the dilation and subsequent tearing of the gastroesophageal mucosa.

Reported risks factors for the development of a Mallory-Weiss tear include hiatal hernia, chronic alcoholism, and increasing age. Mallory-Weiss syndrome usually occurs in the fifth and sixth decades of life. In one report, 44% of cases were associated with alcohol use, but no risk factor was documented in 23%. Any disorder that initiates vomiting or retching may result in the development of a Mallory-Weiss tear. This includes reports of Mallory-Weiss tears associated with hyperemesis gravidarum, pancreatitis-related emesis, eating disorders such as bulimia, cardiopulmonary resuscitation, primal scream therapy, blunt abdominal trauma, chemotherapy-associated emesis, paroxysms of coughing, childbirth, straining for bowel movement, seizures, scuba barotrauma, and endoscopy. In women of childbearing age, the most common cause of these tears is hyperemesis gravidarum, which usually occurs in the first trimester and causes severe persistent nausea and vomiting.

Alcohol use and liver disease have long been associated with Mallory-Weiss syndrome. However, Mallory-Weiss tears represent a cause of UGI bleeding in only 3% to 10% of patients with cirrhosis, which is similar to the prevalence rate of this condition in the general population. The frequency of bleeding from a Mallory-Weiss tear has been reported to be significantly higher in patients with advanced liver disease, especially in patients with Child-Pugh grades B and C. In a second study, 14 of 42 patients (33%) with acute esophageal bleeding related to Mallory-Weiss tears had liver disease. The severity of bleeding was significantly worse in patients with liver disease, but it was not correlated with portal hypertension or Child-Pugh classification.

Hiatal hernia has been found in 40% to 100% of patients with Mallory-Weiss tears and has been considered by some to be a necessary predisposing factor. It has been proposed that, in hiatus hernia, a higher pressure gradient develops in the hernia compared with that in the rest of the stomach during retching, thereby increasing the potential for mucosal laceration. Mallory-Weiss tears may also be more likely to occur when the upper esophageal sphincter does not relax during vomiting. However, the presence of a hiatal hernia is found in a minority of patients with Mallory-Weiss syndrome, which makes its relevance questionable.

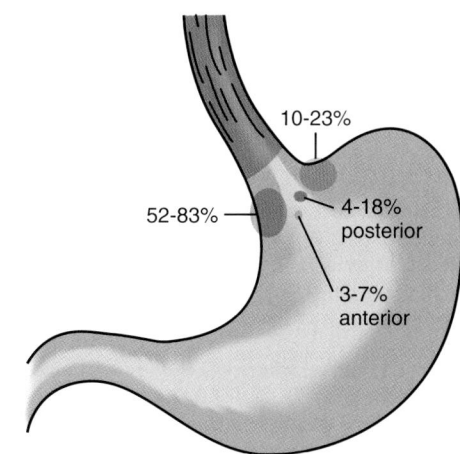

FIGURE 1   Distribution of mucosal tears in Mallory-Weiss syndrome. Data compiled from multiple series.

DIAGNOSES AND OUTCOMES

Hematemesis is the presenting symptom in 80% to 90% of patients with Mallory-Weiss syndrome, although 10% may have melena as the first sign of bleeding. The triad of retching and vomiting followed by hematemesis varies in occurrence, ranging from 30% to 80% of cases. A history of recent alcohol ingestion is common but not invariable. The use of aspirin or nonsteroidal antiinflammatory medications before Mallory-Weiss hemorrhage has been found in up to 30% of cases. Abdominal pain is not a common presenting symptom because most episodes of bleeding from Mallory-Weiss tears are painless. As many as 50% of patients may not have a history of vomiting preceding hematemesis, and 25% may have no identifiable risk factor. Because the history and symptoms of Mallory-Weiss syndrome can be indistinguishable from those of other common causes of UGI bleeding, differentiation of Mallory-Weiss tears from other causes of UGI hemorrhage without invasive diagnostic studies is difficult.

Before diagnostic interventions are undertaken, as with all patients with GI bleeding, the patient needs to have appropriate intravenous access and the severity of the bleeding assessed. Hemodynamic instability and shock are present in up to 10% of patients with Mallory-Weiss tears. Volume resuscitation should consist of crystalloids and blood products when deemed necessary. Initial laboratory studies should include measures of hematocrit, blood type and crossmatch, and coagulation parameters. Any defects in coagulation should be corrected, and this effort should be considered part of the initial resuscitation. Serial assessments of the hematocrit and hemodynamic monitoring should be used to judge the efficacy of resuscitation and any therapeutic maneuvers. Nasogastric tube placement and gastric lavage with 250 mL of room temperature saline solution can be used to assess for the presence of active hemorrhage and to clear the stomach of blood that may obscure subsequent endoscopy. Once resuscitative efforts have been instituted and the patient's condition has been stabilized, diagnostic interventions should be considered.

Flexible endoscopy is the current standard of evaluation of UGI bleeding. A complete evaluation of the esophagus, stomach, and proximal duodenum should be performed. A retroflexion view of the GEJ is essential in the evaluation. Mallory-Weiss tears appear as linear lacerations of the mucosa of the gastric cardia, GEJ, or distal esophagus. Tears that involve only esophageal mucosa are uncommon. Most Mallory-Weiss tears (52% to 83%) occur below the GEJ along the lesser curve of the stomach; 10% to 23% occur along the greater curvature below the GEJ. Anterior and posterior tears range between 3% and 7% and 4% and 18%, respectively (Figure 1). Most tears average 0.5 to 2.5 cm, but they may be up to 5 cm in length. Endoscopy reveals a single tear in 76% to 90% of cases. Two lacerations

have been described in 8% to 15%, and three tears have been found in 1% to 8%. The coexistence of other sources of UGI bleeding, such as esophageal varices, gastritis, duodenitis, and peptic ulcerations has been seen in 32% to 82% of patients.

Bleeding from Mallory-Weiss tears is self limited in 90% of patients, and therapeutic action is not needed. Healing of the tears occurs in 48 to 72 hours. When no active bleeding is seen at the initial endoscopy, which occurs in 50% to 75% of cases, cases can be managed with supportive care only. Recurrent bleeding is unusual but has been described in up to 10% of cases. In one retrospective study of 159 patients with Mallory-Weiss syndrome, 17 patients (10.7%) presented with recurrent bleeding. These patients were compared with 142 patients who had a benign course. The demographics of the patient and initial general physical status were not associated with the risk of recurrent bleeding. In addition, no significant differences were seen in the risk of recurrent bleeding for those patients with comorbid diseases, including diabetes and cardiovascular disease. A history of peptic ulcer or alcohol abuse had no influence on the risk of recurrent bleeding. However, the proportion of patients with comorbid liver cirrhosis was higher (41% vs 18%; $P = 0.028$) in those patients with recurrent bleeding.

Active bleeding, such as spurting or active oozing from the tear, is associated with recurrent bleeding. Active bleeding was seen during endoscopy in 88% of patients (15 of 17) with recurrent bleeding as opposed to 38% of patients (55 of 142) without ($P < 0.001$) in a retrospective study. The risk of recurrent bleeding was not associated with the number and location of the tear, the length of the tear, the presence of hiatal hernia, or waiting time for endoscopy. Additional studies have suggested that an initial hematocrit value less than 30%, the presence of a nonbleeding visible vessel, coagulopathy, or the presence of liver dysfunction predict recurrent bleeding. The presence of any one of these factors requires more aggressive treatment and monitoring.

Reported mortality rates related to Mallory-Weiss syndrome range from a low of 1.5% to a high of 10%. Identified risk factors for mortality in a retrospective study that analyzed 93 patients with Mallory-Weiss syndrome included advanced age, very low hemoglobin levels, elevated aspartate aminotransferase (AST) level, and the presence of the clinical sign of tarry stool. A separate study revealed the following significant risk factors for mortality: the presence of liver cirrhosis or shock, low hemoglobin levels and platelet counts, low blood pressure and a high pulse rate at admission, and an endoscopic finding of active bleeding.

TREATMENT

Endoscopic therapy is the mainstay for treatment of Mallory-Weiss syndrome. The need for surgical or alternative therapies such as angiographic techniques or the use of a Sengstaken-Blakemore tube is increasingly rare given the success of endoscopic techniques. In modern studies, surgery is necessary in less than 1% of patients. Endoscopic hemostasis is accomplished with various techniques, including injection therapy, multipolar electrocoagulation, band ligation, and hemoclipping. Combinations of the various techniques have also been reported. Unfortunately, no definitive randomized trials have been performed to determine which therapy is most effective.

Lessons learned from treatment of other more common causes of GI bleeding have been applied to the treatment of Mallory-Weiss tears. Mechanical hemostasis (hemoclip, banding) has been effectively used in patients with peptic ulcer bleeding or Dieulafoy's-like lesions. The advantages of a mechanical technique include greater patient safety, fewer associated complications, and a less expert technique needed. Endoscopic band ligation is commonly used to treat variceal bleeding and is indicated for nonfibrotic bleeding lesions that can be aspirated into the hood of the ligation device. Band ligation has some advantages, including ease of deployment, even if the bleeding site must be approached tangentially. Furthermore, the hood of the device fixes the bleeding site, which minimizes motion, and the visible vessel is ligated in its deeper aspect. Hemoclips have a similar ease of use and are highly effective. Band ligation and clip application appear to be equivalent treatment for primary hemostasis (100%) and have a similar incidence rate of rebleeding (6% vs 10%).

Endoscopic injection therapy has been shown to be an effective and safe treatment of UGI hemorrhage. Injection therapy has varied from the use of purely vasoconstricting agents like epinephrine to sclerosing agents like polidocanol and dehydrated ethanol or combinations thereof. Epinephrine injection is most commonly used to treat Mallory-Weiss tears; reported rates of primary hemostasis range from 93% to 100%. However, several series have suggested that the use of epinephrine injection alone could lead to an increased risk of recurrent bleeding as compared with mechanical techniques. However, epinephrine injection in combination with hemoclip placement has been used extensively in bleeding peptic ulcer and has also been used with Mallory-Weiss tears in an attempt to decrease recurrent bleeding.

Which endoscopic therapy is best? Although no definitive studies are found, some data from prospective studies, case series, and retrospective studies do exist. In 2004, a prospective, randomized trial compared the effectiveness of endoscopic band ligation with epinephrine injection for actively bleeding Mallory-Weiss tears. Although the study was small (17 patients per group), the authors showed no difference in the efficacy or safety of band ligation versus epinephrine injection for the treatment of actively bleeding Mallory-Weiss tears. No reoccurrence of bleeding was seen in either group. A 2009 retrospective trial compared the efficacy of band ligation (29 patients) with hemoclip placement associated with epinephrine injection (27 patients). This study found that both techniques are safe and effective in primary hemostasis. However, recurrent bleeding occurred significantly more often in patients treated with hemoclip placement and epinephrine injection versus treatment with band ligation (18% vs 0%; $P = 0.02$). One explanation for this finding is that treatment of Mallory-Weiss tears at the GEJ is probably more technically demanding when a hemoclip is used compared with band ligation at this site. Furthermore, clip placement is quite superficial, and esophageal and gastric motility may result in the clip falling off. In contrast, band ligation is much easier to perform, even when the scope is tangential to the lesion, and it results in a much deeper ligation. The authors of this study suggest that the first-line treatment of bleeding Mallory-Weiss tears should be endoscopic band ligation. However, in practice, the choice of endoscopic therapy depends on local expertise.

Angiographic techniques for control of UGI bleeding consist of intraarterial infusion of vasopressin and transcatheter embolization. The use of intraarterial vasopressin at rates of 0.2 to 0.5 U/min over varying lengths of time has yielded rates of hemostasis of 50% to 100% in small studies of Mallory-Weiss syndrome. Selective embolization of the left gastric artery or its branches has also been reported to be effective in the cessation of bleeding from Mallory-Weiss tears. In general, intra-arterial therapy should be reserved for those patients with failed endoscopic therapy and who are poor surgical candidates.

The use of Sengstaken-Blakemore tubes for control of Mallory-Weiss bleeding has been reported with varying degrees of success. Their use is controversial and considered an act of desperation. Concern about their usage in patients with Mallory-Weiss syndrome centers on the risk of extending the mucosal tears into full-thickness tears of the esophagus or stomach. The presence of hiatal hernia is also a contraindication to the use of such tubes because the asymmetric pressure gradient generated by the gastric balloon may lead to necrosis and perforation of the herniated portion of the stomach.

SURGERY

Before the widespread use of flexible fiberoptic endoscopy, surgery was needed to control hemorrhage from Mallory-Weiss tears in approximately half of all cases. Today, surgery for Mallory-Weiss syndrome is uncommon and rare, even at many tertiary referral centers. Surgical rates have declined from a high of 50% in the preendoscopy era to 0 to 3% in the most recent published series. Surgery is usually reserved for those patients with failed endoscopic therapy. In general, if patients have rebleeding after initial endoscopic therapy, a repeat endoscopy is indicated. A suggested treatment algorithm is shown in Figure 2.

Surgical control of bleeding from Malloy-Weiss tears has classically been performed through open surgery with a high anterior longitudinal gastrotomy to gain visualization of the mucosa at the GEJ. Localization of the site of bleeding before laparotomy is important. Subserosal staining of blood near the GEJ is characteristic of Mallory-Weiss bleeding and can be used as a clue to the location of the mucosal tear. This sign, however, is present in only a minority of patients. Simple oversewing of the tear with absorbable sutures suffices. When localization of the site of bleeding has not occurred or when visualization is impaired by ongoing hemorrhage, packing the stomach with laparotomy pads and sequential inspection of all of the gastric mucosa can help in locating the source of bleeding. Intraoperative endoscopy is also a technique that may aide in the identification of the source of bleeding. Inspection for other sources of hemorrhage is wise because 32% to 82% of the Mallory-Weiss tears coexist with other common causes of UGI bleeding.

A combined laparoscopic and endoscopic technique for oversewing Mallory-Weiss tears has been described. Laparoscopy was performed with port placement as is customary for foregut surgery. Endoscopy was then used to localize the site of the tear. Full-thickness absorbable sutures were then placed with endoscopic guidance to occlude the site of hemorrhage. Patients who come to surgery are typically at higher risk for complications and mortality. This is more a reflection of the contribution of comorbid conditions and the sequelae of severe hemorrhage rather than the complexity of surgery.

SUMMARY

Mallory-Weiss tear is a linear mucosal laceration of the GEJ that leads to UGI bleeding. It is caused by any condition associated with forceful vomiting or retching. The bleeding is self limited in 90% of patients, and when treatment is mandated, endoscopic therapy is successful 99% of the time. Surgery, which consists of a simple

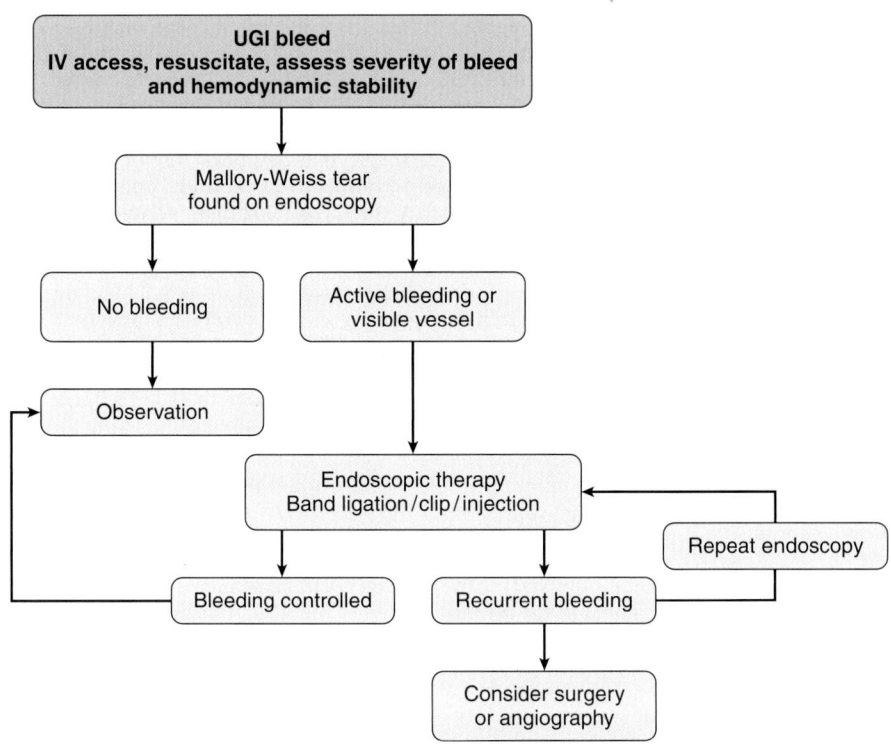

FIGURE 2 Treatment algorithm for Mallory-Weiss syndrome. *IV,* Intravenous; *UGI,* upper gastrointestinal.

oversewing of the bleeding mucosa, is reserved for patients with failed endoscopic therapy.

SUGGESTED READINGS

Akhtar AJ, Padda MS: Natural history of Mallory-Weiss tear in African American and Hispanic patients, *J Natl Med Assoc* 103(5):412–415, 2011.

Cho YS, Chai HS, Kim HK, et al: Endoscopic band ligation and endoscopic hemoclip placement for patients with Mallory-Weiss syndrome and active bleeding, *W J Gastroentrol* 14(3):2080–2084, 2008.

Chung IK, Kim EJ, Hwang KY, et al: Evaluation of endoscopic hemostasis in upper gastrointestinal bleeding related to Mallory-Weiss syndrome, *Endoscopy* 34(6):474–479, 2002.

Grimes OF: Surgical management of massive gastrointestinal hemorrhage from cardioesophageal lacerations, *Am J Surg* 108:285–296, 1964.

Lecleire S, Antoniette M, Wanicki-Caron I, et al: Endoscopic band ligation could decrease recurrent bleeding in Mallory-Weiss syndrome as compared to haemostasis by hemoclips plus epinephrine, *Aliment Pharmacol Ther* 30:399–405, 2009.

Park CH, Min SW, Sohn YH, et al: A prospective, randomized trial of endoscopic band ligation vs. epinephrine injection for actively bleeding Mallory-Weiss syndrome, *Gastrointest Endosc* 60(1):22–27, 2004.

GASTRIC ADENOCARCINOMA

Sam S. Yoon, MD, and Do Joong Park, MD, PhD

INTRODUCTION

Epidemiology and Presentation

More than 1 million cases of gastric cancer are estimated to occur worldwide per year, with more than 700,000 deaths each year. Thus, gastric cancer is the fourth most common cancer and the second leading cause of cancer death. Gastric adenocarcinoma accounts for about 95% of gastric cancer cases. The incidence rate of gastric adenocarcinoma varies tremendously throughout the world and country by country. Nearly three quarters of cases occur in developing countries, and the countries with the highest incidence rates are in Eastern Asia (e.g., Korea, Japan, and China). The incidence rate of gastric cancer in the United States and Western Europe has been steadily declining and is currently only about one sixth that of Eastern Asia. Despite this, the incidence rate of proximal gastric cancer in Western countries is rising. Overall, males are affected twice as frequently as females, and the average age of presentation is between 60 and 70 years old.

Risk factors for gastric adenocarcinoma include *Helicobacter pylori* infection, diets high in smoked or salty foods, pernicious anemia, prior gastric surgery, chronic atrophic gastritis, and intestinal metaplasia. Genetic cancer syndromes that increase the risk of gastric cancer include hereditary nonpolyposis colon cancer (HNPCC), Li-Fraumeni syndrome, Peutz-Jeghers syndrome, and hereditary diffuse gastric cancer (HDGC) syndrome.

Gastric adenocarcinoma is often asymptomatic in its early stages and in later stages causes weight loss, epigastric pain or discomfort, gastrointestinal bleeding, vomiting, and anorexia. In Japan and Korea, high awareness and common endoscopic screening for gastric cancer has led to the proportion of patients with early gastric cancer (i.e., T1 tumors) to reach about 50%. Unfortunately, in other countries, gastric cancer is found most frequently in advanced stages.

Pathology

Gastric adenocarcinoma arises in the inner mucosal lining of the stomach in the epithelial cell layer. As tumors grow deeper into the wall of the stomach (i.e., submucosa and muscularis propria), they can spread via lymphatics to regional lymph nodes and hematogenously to distant sites, most commonly to the liver. For T1b tumors (invading the submucosa), lymph node metastases are found in about 20% of patients. For T2 tumors (invading the muscularis propria), the lymph node metastasis rate increases to more than 50%. Tumors that penetrate the subserosa (T3) or serosa (T4a) of the stomach can progress to invade adjacent structures such as the pancreas, spleen, and colon (T4b) or disseminate via the peritoneal cavity, leading to carcinomatosis.

Several systems have been developed to classify gastric adenocarcinomas by macroscopic or histologic appearance. The most widely used histologic classification is the Lauren classification. The Lauren intestinal type exhibits components of glandular, solid, or intestinal architecture and tubular structures. This type is more common in men and older patients, is associated with environmental exposures such as *H. pylori* infection, and arises often from precancerous areas, such as chronic atrophic gastritis or intestinal metaplasia. The Lauren diffuse type shows single cells or poorly cohesive cells infiltrating the gastric wall, and progressive disease can ultimately lead to linitis plastica (also known as leather bottle stomach). The diffuse type does not typically arise from precancerous areas, is slightly more common in women and in younger patients, and is more associated with familial occurrence, thus suggesting a more genetic etiology. The incidence rate of the intestinal type has been declining, but the incidence rate of the diffuse type has remained either stable or increased.

Signet ring cells are neoplastic cells that contain a large amount of mucin, which pushes the nucleus to the periphery. The general perception is that the presence of these cells is a poor prognostic factor. However, signet ring cells can be found in early T1 tumors and may be associated with *improved* survival compared with T1 tumors without signet ring cells. Furthermore, for T2 or greater tumors, the presence of signet ring cells may not be an independent prognostic factor when patients are stratified by stage.

Preoperative Evaluation

The preoperative evaluation of patients with gastric adenocarcinoma involves establishing the diagnosis, assessing the extent of local disease, ruling out distant metastases, and assessing the patient's general medical condition. All patients should have an upper endoscopy, and information should be obtained as to the location, size, and degree of infiltration of the tumor. If endoscopic ultrasound (EUS) is available, this modality can give additional information, especially regarding T stage. An abdominal computed tomographic (CT) scan should be performed to identify possible regional and distant nodal disease, local extension of tumor to adjacent organs, liver metastases, and peritoneal metastases. The role of chest CT scan to rule out lung metastases or mediastinal nodal disease is controversial because the yield is low in the absence of intraabdominal metastases. Positron emission tomography (PET) or PET/CT scans are not generally obtained for staging given the low yield, but PET scans may be useful in the assessment of response of tumors to neoadjuvant treatment.

Small volume peritoneal carcinomatosis can be missed on abdominal CT scans, and so diagnostic laparoscopy can be performed. Furthermore, patients without overt peritoneal carcinomatosis may have microscopic free peritoneal tumor cells when peritoneal washings are performed. In one study from Memorial Sloan-Kettering Cancer Center, radiologically occult metastatic disease was identified with laparoscopy in 25% of patients who were determined with EUS to have T3-T4 or N+ disease and in only 4% of patient who were determined with EUS to have T1-T2 and N0 disease. The survival of patients without peritoneal carcinomatosis but with free peritoneal tumor cells in peritoneal washings may be similar to that of those with overt peritoneal carcinomatosis, although the increased efficacy of more recent chemotherapy regimens has called this into question.

Staging

The American Joint Committee on Cancer (AJCC) changed T and N definitions and the overall staging classifications of gastric adenocarcinoma in the seventh edition of the AJCC Cancer Staging Manual published in 2010 (Table 1).

SURGERY

Extent of Gastric Resection

For tumors in the middle or distal stomach, several studies have compared distal or subtotal gastrectomy with total gastrectomy. In the French cooperative trial of 169 patients with antrum tumors, 93 patients underwent total gastrectomy, and 76 underwent subtotal gastrectomy. No significant difference was found in perioperative mortality rate, and no difference was seen in 5-year survival rate (48%). In the Italian Gastrointestinal Study group multicenter, randomized trial of 618 patients with tumors of the distal half of stomach, there was also no difference in 5-year survival rate between subtotal and total gastrectomy (65% vs 62%). Thus, for patients with middle or distal tumors, distal or subtotal gastrectomy is adequate and total gastrectomy does not improve survival.

For proximal gastric cancers, few high-quality studies have examined the extent of gastric resection, and thus, the extent of gastric resection is largely governed by the preference of the surgeon. In one nonrandomized Norwegian study of 763 patients, complication and mortality rates were *higher* for patients who underwent proximal gastrectomy (52% and 16%) compared with total gastrectomy (38% and 8%). In another large study from Korea, An and colleagues examined a total of 89 patients who had a proximal gastrectomy and 334 patients who had a total gastrectomy for proximal gastric cancer. Complications were markedly higher in the proximal gastrectomy group, with major differences found in the rate of anastomotic stenosis and reflux esophagitis. Some groups, however, continue to advocate proximal gastrectomies for proximal gastric cancers.

In terms of the surgical incision required to remove a tumor confined to the proximal stomach, a laparotomy incision is usually sufficient. The National Cancer Center (NCC) group in Tokyo randomized 167 patients with proximal gastric tumors to total gastrectomy and D2 lymphadenectomy via a laparotomy or via a left thoracoabdominal incision. Higher morbidity and mortality rates were seen in the left thoracoabdominal incision group, but no difference was found in survival rate. However, for proximal third tumors extending into the gastroesophageal junction (GEJ) or distal esophagus, a left thoracoabdominal or Ivor-Lewis approach may be necessary.

TABLE 1: Seventh American Joint Committee on Cancer staging system for gastric adenocarcinoma

Primary Tumor		
	Tx	Primary tumor cannot be assessed.
	T0	No evidence of primary tumor.
	Tis	Carcinoma in situ: intraepithelial tumor without invasion of the lamina propria.
	T1	Tumor invades lamina propria, muscularis mucosae, or submucosa.
	T1a	Tumor invades lamina propria or muscularis mucosae.
	T1b	Tumor invades submucosa.
	T2	Tumor invades muscularis propria.
	T3	Tumor penetrates subserosal connective tissue without invasion of visceral peritoneum or adjacent structures. T3 tumors also include those extending into the gastrocolic or gastrohepatic ligaments or into the greater or lesser omentum, without perforation of the visceral peritoneum covering these structures.
	T4	Tumor invades serosa (visceral peritoneum) or adjacent structures.
	T4a	Tumor invades serosa (visceral peritoneum).
	T4b	Tumor invades adjacent structures, such as spleen, transverse colon, liver, diaphragm, pancreas, abdominal wall, adrenal gland, kidney, small intestine, and retroperitoneum.
Regional Nodes		
	Nx	Regional lymph node(s) cannot be assessed.
	N0	No regional lymph node metastasis.
	N1	Metastasis in 1 to 2 regional lymph nodes.
	N2	Metastasis in 3 to 6 regional lymph nodes.
	N3	Metastasis in 7 or more regional lymph nodes.
	N3a	Metastasis in 7 to 15 regional lymph nodes.
	N3b	Metastasis in 16 or more regional lymph nodes.
Metastases		
	Mx	Distant metastases cannot be assessed.
	M0	No distant metastases.
	M1	Distant metastases.

Stage Groupings				
0	Tis N0 M0		IIIA	T2 N3 M0
IA	T1 N0 M0			T3 N2 M0
IB	T1 N1 M0			T4a N1 M0
	T2 N0 M0		IIIB	T3 N3 M0
IIA	T1 N2 M0			T4a N2 M0
	T2 N1 M0			T4b N0 or N1 M0
	T3 N0 M0		IIIC	T4a N3 M0
IIB	T1 N3 M0			T4b N2 or N3 M0
	T2 N2 M0		IV	Any T Any N M1
	T3 N1 M0			
	T4a N0 M0			

Adapted from American Joint Committee on Cancer: AJCC cancer staging manual, *ed 7, New York, 2010, Springer, 117–126.*

Gastric Reconstruction

Few good studies are found on the optimal reconstruction after distal or subtotal gastrectomy. In Japan and Korea, the preferred type of reconstruction is generally a Billroth I reconstruction; most United States surgeons prefer a Billroth II reconstruction. Roux-en-Y reconstruction results in less bile reflux into the stomach but can result in a Roux stasis syndrome. One Japanese study randomized 50 patients after distal gastrectomy for cancer to Billroth I or Roux-en-Y reconstruction. Five of 24 patients (21%) in the Roux group had gastrojejunal stasis develop in the early postoperative period, and this group had a longer mean hospital stay, but the Billroth I group had a higher incidence rate of bile reflux gastritis at 6 months after surgery (62% vs 30%).

Reconstruction after total gastrectomy is generally performed with a Roux-en-Y esophagojejunostomy with or without a jejunal pouch. Lehnert and colleagues reviewed 14 small randomized trials of jejunal pouch versus no pouch, each with 20 to 70 patients. The pouch added minimal operative time and did not increase morbidity. Food intake was somewhat improved in the early months, but this advantage decreased with time. Only 2 of 12 trials found a difference is postoperative weight, and only 2 of 9 trials found an improvement in quality of life. More recently, Fein and colleagues randomized 138 patients and found no differences in operative morbidity or mortality rates; short-term and long-term weight loss were similar in both groups. However, quality of life was found to be improved in years 3 to 5 after surgery in the pouch group.

Nodal Station and Lymphadenectomy Definitions

The extent of lymphadenectomy has been a persistent area of controversy in the treatment of gastric adenocarcinoma. Before discussion of lymph node dissections for gastric adenocarcinoma, one must define the terms to be used. The lymph node stations that surround the stomach have been precisely defined by the Japanese Gastric Cancer Association (JGCA) (Figure 1 and Table 2). Table 3 shows the lymph node stations that should be removed for a D1 and D2 lymphadenectomy based on the extent of gastrectomy. The JGCA recommends D2 lymphadenectomy for any tumor T2 or deeper or with clinically positive nodes.

Location of Metastatic Lymph Nodes

For decades, centers in Japan and Korea have performed gastrectomies with extensive lymphadenectomies and then *ex vivo* dissected out and labeled the nodal stations. Pathologists then examine each nodal station separately and document which nodal stations contain metastatic disease. Thus, many excellent studies are found on the location of metastatic lymph nodes from gastric cancer based on tumor location and other tumor and patient factors. With use of a large database of patients treated with D2 or greater lymphadenectomy, Maruyama and colleagues at the NCC calculated the risk of the lymph node metastases in each lymph node station by location of primary tumor (Table 4). In 1989, the NCC database of 3843 cases was used to create the Maruyama computer program. This program estimates the risk of lymph node metastasis for each lymph

node station based on the input of eight variables: gender, age, endoscopic or Bormann classification, depth of invasion, maximal diameter, location (upper, middle, or lower third), position (lesser or greater curvature, anterior or posterior wall, or circumferential), and World Health Organization (WHO) histologic classification. The Maruyama computer program was later expanded to include 4302 cases (WinEstimate 2.5, Springer, Berlin, Germany). By matching input variables to this large database of patients, the program gives a percent likelihood of disease in each of 16 lymph node stations. The applicability and accuracy of the Maruyama computer program have been confirmed in Western patients treated in Germany and in Italy.

Potential Benefits of More Extensive Lymphadenectomy

Lymphadenectomy for cancer can serve three *potential* purposes: staging of disease, prevention of locoregional recurrence, and improvement in overall survival. There is little doubt that more extensive lymphadenectomies for gastric adenocarcinoma lead to better staging of disease. The 2010 7th edition of AJCC Staging

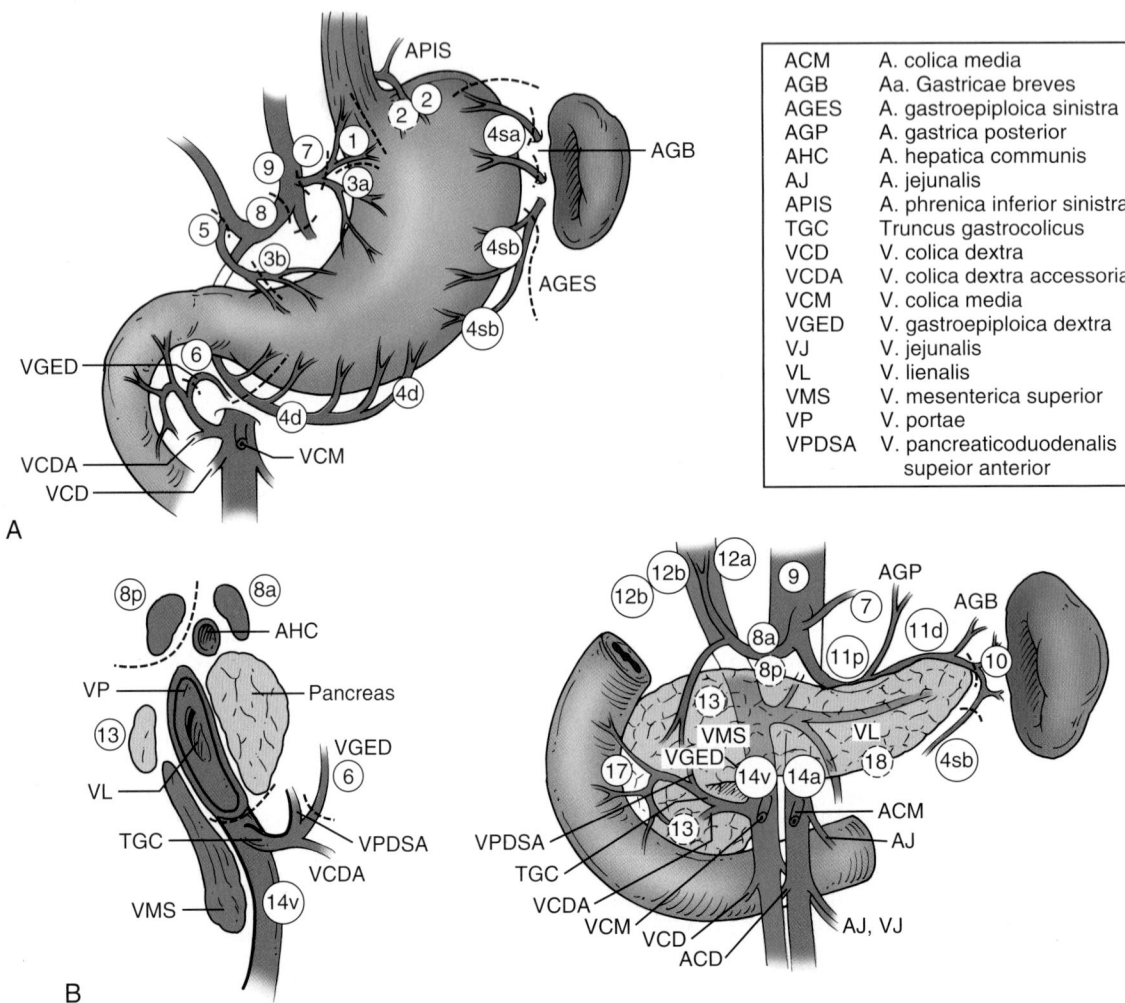

ACM	A. colica media
AGB	Aa. Gastricae breves
AGES	A. gastroepiploica sinistra
AGP	A. gastrica posterior
AHC	A. hepatica communis
AJ	A. jejunalis
APIS	A. phrenica inferior sinistra
TGC	Truncus gastrocolicus
VCD	V. colica dextra
VCDA	V. colica dextra accessoria
VCM	V. colica media
VGED	V. gastroepiploica dextra
VJ	V. jejunalis
VL	V. lienalis
VMS	V. mesenterica superior
VP	V. portae
VPDSA	V. pancreaticoduodenalis supeior anterior

FIGURE I   Locations of lymph node stations. **A,** Lymph node stations 1-9. **B,** Lymph node stations 6-17. *(Adapted from Japanese Gastric Cancer Association: Japanese classification of gastric carcinoma: 3rd English edition,* Gastric Cancer *14:101–112, 2011.)*

TABLE 2: Regional lymph nodes of the stomach

Number	Description
1	Right paracardial
2	Left paracardial
3	Lesser curvature
a	Along branches of left gastric artery
b	Along 2nd branch and distal part of right gastric artery
4	Greater curvature
sa	Along short gastric arteries
sb	Along left gastroepiploic artery
d	Along 2nd branch and distal part of right gastroepiploic artery
5	Suprapyloric along 1st branch and proximal part of right gastric artery
6	Infrapyloric along 1st branch and proximal part of right gastroepiploic artery
7	Left gastric artery
8	Common hepatic artery
a	Anterosuperior group
p	Posterior group
9	Celiac artery
10	Splenic hilum
11	Along splenic artery
p	Along proximal splenic artery
d	Along distal splenic artery
12	Hepatoduodenal ligament
a	Along proper hepatic artery
b	Along bile duct
p	Along portal vein
14	Along superior mesenteric vessels
v	Along superior mesenteric vein
a	Along superior mesenteric artery

Adapted from Japanese Gastric Cancer Association: Japanese classification of gastric carcinoma: 3rd English edition, Gastric Cancer 14:101–112, 2011.

TABLE 3: Extent of lymphadenectomy

Extent of gastrectomy	D1 dissection	D2 dissection
Distal/subtotal gastrectomy	1, 3, 4sb, 4d, 5, 6, 7	D1 + 8a, 9, 11p, 12a
Proximal gastrectomy	1, 2, 3a, 4sa, 4sb, 7	N/A
Total gastrectomy	1-7	D1 + 8a, 9, 10, 11p, 11d, 12a

Adapted from Japanese Gastric Cancer Association: Japanese gastric cancer treatment guidelines 2010 (ver 3), Gastric Cancer 14:113–123, 2011.

Manual for gastric adenocarcinoma recommends that at least 16 lymph nodes be examined for correct assessment of the N category. Despite this, one analysis of the United States Surveillance, Epidemiology and End Results (SEER) database found that only 29% of 10,807 resected gastric cancer patients had 15 or more lymph nodes examined. It is difficult to be confident that a gastric cancer is truly node negative when few lymph nodes are examined, and N1 tumors can be upstaged to N2 or even N3 tumors as more lymph nodes are harvested. Furthermore, it is impossible to be categorized as N3b if less than 16 lymph nodes are harvested. In our analysis of more than 18,000 patients with gastric cancer in the SEER database, we found that more than 50% of patients were misclassified because of inadequate lymph node sampling.

Some evidence shows that more extensive lymphadenectomies result in lower rates of locoregional recurrence. Locoregional recurrence after potentially curative surgery for gastric adenocarcinoma can be quite high. In a 1982 series from the University of Minnesota, 107 patients with gastric adenocarcinoma underwent second look laparotomy, and 80% had a recurrence. Of these recurrences, 88% were locoregional, 54% were peritoneal, and 29% were distant. More recently, in United States Intergroup 0116 trial, 177 of 275 patients (64%) in the surgery-only group had recurrent disease develop. In terms of the site of first relapse, 29% had local recurrence, 72% had regional recurrence, and only 18% had distant recurrence. Rates of locoregional recurrence are generally lower in reports from both Western and Asian institutions that perform more extensive lymphadenectomies.

The effect of more extensive lymphadenectomies on overall survival for gastric cancer is still quite controversial. Most gastric surgeons in Japan and Korea believe that D2 or greater lymphadenectomies improve overall survival and refuse to perform a prospective, randomized trial of D1 versus D2 lymphadenectomy. Maruyama and colleagues determined the 5-year survival rate of patients with positive lymph nodes in each of the nodal stations, and many D2 node stations, when positive for metastases, have a significant percentage of patients surviving 5 years. For example, a lower third tumor has a 25% incidence rate of metastases in the common hepatic artery nodes. When these nodes were positive and resected as part of a D2 lymphadenectomy, the 5-year survival rate was 31%.

Several *retrospective* studies show that more extensive lymphadenectomies are correlated with improved survival. However, these retrospective studies suffer from the confounding issue of stage migration. Dissecting out additional lymph nodes results in patients often being upstaged, which makes subsequent comparisons regarding therapeutic benefit invalid.

Two large prospective randomized trials in the United Kingdom and the Netherlands failed to identify a survival advantage for D2 over D1 lymphadenectomy. However, these two trials had fairly high morbidity (43% to 46%) and mortality (10% to 13%) rates for the D2 lymphadenectomy group. In these trials, the distal pancreas and spleen were often resected during dissection of station 10 and 11 nodes, which significantly increased morbidity. Of note, in the Dutch trial, if patients with hospital mortality are excluded, patients with N2 disease had significant survival advantage when treated with a D2 lymphadenectomy. Several more recent studies now show that D2 lymphadenectomies can be performed without the need for distal pancreatectomy or splenectomy. Furthermore, a recent randomized trial in Taiwan showed an overall survival advantage of more extensive lymphadenectomy over D1 lymphadenectomy, with an overall 5-year survival rate of 59.5% compared with 53.6%, respectively ($P = 0.041$). Fifteen-year follow-up results from the previously described Dutch trial now show decreased locoregional recurrence and gastric cancer–related death in the D2 group. Degiuli and colleagues in Italy have shown that Western surgeons, following extensive training, can perform D2 lymphadenectomies on Western patients with low morbidity and almost no mortality, and survival results from a prospective randomized trial of D1 versus D2 lymphadenectomy from this group are pending.

TABLE 4: Frequency of lymph node metastasis based on location of primary tumor

Lymph node basin	Upper third (% with metastasis)	Middle third (% with metastasis)	Lower third (% with metastasis)
Paracardial (stations 1 and 2)	22	9	4
Lesser or greater curve (stations 3 and 4)	25	36	37
Right gastric artery/suprapyloric (station 5)	2	3	12
Infrapyloric (station 6)	3	15	49
Left gastric artery (station 7)	19	22	23
Common hepatic artery (station 8)	7	11	25
Celiac axis (station 9)	13	8	13
Splenic artery/hilum (stations 10 and 11)	11	3	2
Hepatodudodenal (station 12)	1	2	8
Other	0-5	0-5	0-5

Adapted from Maruyama K, Gunven P, Okabayashi K, et al: Lymph node metastases of gastric cancer. General pattern in 1931 patients. Ann Surg 210:596-602, 1989.

D2 LYMPHADENECTOMY TECHNIQUE FOR SUBTOTAL/DISTAL GASTRECTOMY

Greater Curvature (Station 4sb and 4d) Node Dissection

An upper midline incision is made from the xiphoid to just below the umbilicus. An Omni retractor can be used to provide optimal exposure. The abdomen should be explored to rule out intraabdominal or liver metastases. The primary tumor should be assessed for proximal and distal extent and possible invasion of adjacent structures. A marking suture can be placed on the anterior gastric wall to identify the proximal extent of the tumor. One or two lap pads should be placed behind the spleen to push the spleen forward and prevent capsular tears.

The greater omentum is taken off the transverse colon, beginning from center and moving to the left, widely opening up the lesser sac (Figure 2, A). The dissection is continued such that the greater omentum is taken off the splenic flexure and the inferior aspect of the spleen. This dissection should expose the body and tail of the pancreas, and the left gastroepiploic vessels are divided near their origin from the splenic vessels just anterior to the pancreas (Figure 2, B). The greater curvature of the stomach between the end of the left gastroepiploic arcade and the start of the short gastric vessels should then be identified. This marks the left-most end of the greater omentum dissection. The omentum is divided from peripherally toward the gastric wall. On reaching the gastric wall, ultrasonic coagulating shears can be then used to dissect between the gastric wall and greater omentum from proximal to distal (Figure 2, C).

Infrapyloric (Station 6) Node Dissection

One should now return to where the mid portion of the greater omentum was taken off the transverse colon and continue this dissection toward the hepatic flexure. The infrapyloric lymph nodes are now dissected off the head of the pancreas. Dissection in this area should proceed cautiously to avoid tearing small vessels that lead to troublesome bleeding; use of ultrasonic coagulating shears is often helpful. Dissection should proceed such that all the soft tissue anterior to the pancreas is swept superiorly onto the specimen. The right gastroepiploic vein should be identified at its origin from the inferior pancreaticoduodenal arcade, ligated, and divided (Figure 2, D). The right gastroepiploic artery should also be divided at its origin from the gastroduodenal artery. A tunnel is then created between the first portion of the duodenum and the head of the pancreas.

Hepatoduodenal Ligament Hepatic Artery (Station 12a) and Suprapyloric (Station 5) Node Dissection

The peritoneal covering and soft tissue of the porta hepatis is opened from the mid lesser omentum near the undersurface of the liver toward the superior porta hepatis. One should then dissect on the lateral border of the proper hepatic artery from superior to inferior. The soft tissue between the suprapyloric nodes and proper hepatic artery nodes is then divided. This nodal tissue is then dissected from right to left, completely exposing the common hepatic artery/proper hepatic artery/gastroduodenal artery trifurcation. To the left of the proper hepatic artery, dissection continues posteriorly, exposing the left side of the portal vein. Once this portion of the dissection is completed, the right gastric artery (which usually originates from the proper hepatic artery or the gastroduodenal artery) is divided (Figure 3, A). The right gastric vein that originates from portal vein should also be divided.

The plane between the superior first portion of the duodenum and underlying pancreas is developed until the prior dissection from inferiorly is reached. Small vessels to the first portion of the duodenum are ligated and divided with the harmonic sealing device, thus mobilizing the entire first portion of the duodenum. The duodenum can now be transected distal to the pylorus (Figure 3,B).

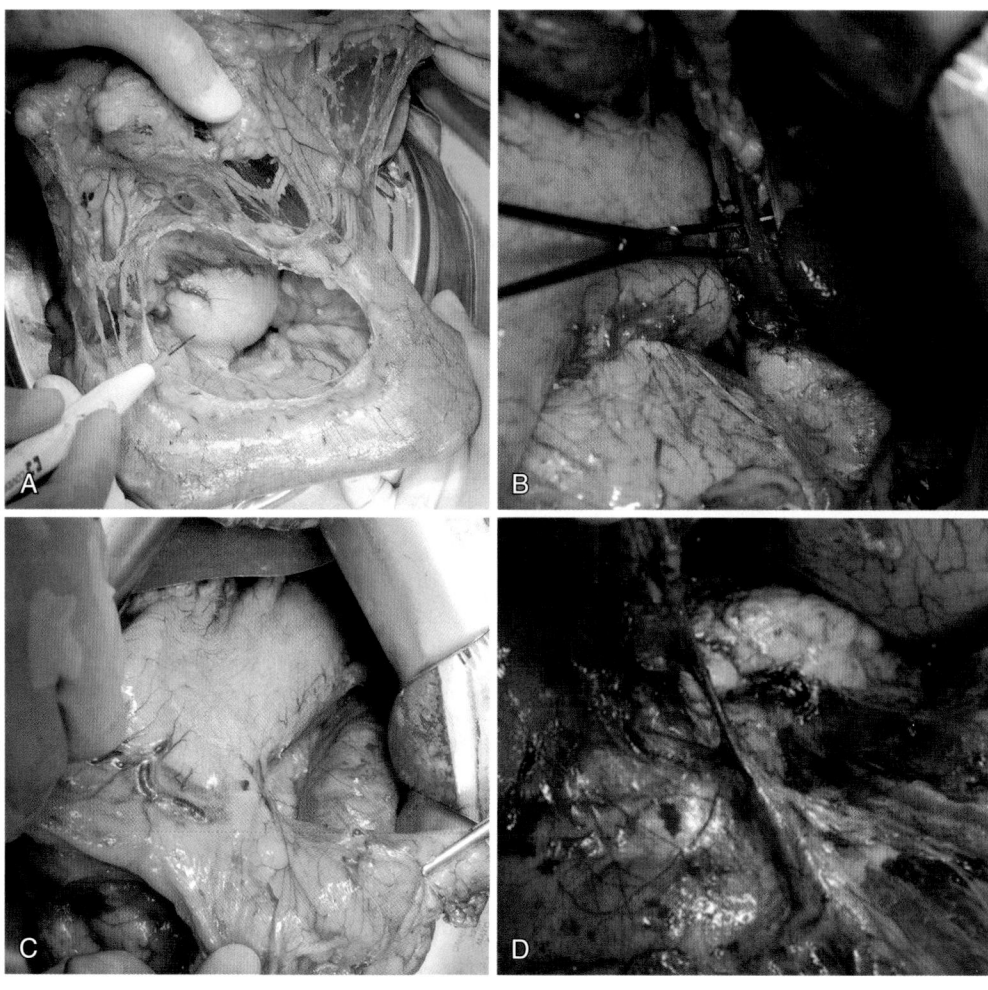

FIGURE 2 Operative photographs show: **A,** dissection of greater omentum off transverse colon; **B,** dissection of left gastroepiploic vessels near their origin from splenic vessels; **C,** dissection of greater curvature nodes; and **D,** dissection of right gastroepiploic vein from inferior pancreaticoduodenal arcade.

Common Hepatic Artery Dissection (Station 8a), Celiac Axis (Station 9), Proximal Splenic Artery (Station 11p), and Left Gastric Artery (Station 7) Lymph Node Dissection

This dissection begins with opening up the peritoneum overlying the superior border of the pancreas from the proximal splenic artery toward the common hepatic artery. Dissection proceeds from left to right and inferiorly to superiorly. All the nodal tissue anterior and superior to the proximal splenic artery should be cleared until retroperitoneal fat is reached. All the nodal tissue medial to the portal vein and anterosuperior to the common hepatic artery should be swept off the retroperitoneum and right crus. Again, this tissue tends to be vascular, and use of the ultrasonic coagulating shears is helpful. The left gastric vein (also known as coronary vein) originates from the portal vein and travels just to the right of the origin of the left gastric artery. This vessel should now be identified and divided. Dissection proceeds from inferior to superior, exposing the left gastric artery, which is taken at its origin. At the end of this dissection, the celiac axis and its branches are skeletonized (Figure 3,*C*).

Lesser Curvature (Station 3) and Right Paracardial (Station 1) Node Dissection

The lesser omentum is divided inferiorly to superiorly near its insertion onto the liver. A replaced/accessory left hepatic artery may be encountered and is generally divided unless the patient has underlying hepatic dysfunction. The lesser omentum dissection is continued to the GEJ, ensuring that the right paracardial nodes are incorporated. To ensure that the lesser curvature lymph nodes are included, all the soft tissue on the lesser curvature is taken off the lesser curvature of the stomach, from the GEJ to beyond where the stomach will be transected (Figure 3,*D*). The soft tissue in this region exists in two leaflets. A finger can be inserted between the leaflets, and soft tissue anterior and posterior to the finger can be divided off the stomach wall with the harmonic sealing device. The stomach can now be transected, and the proximal and distal margins should be sent for frozen section analysis.

Specimen Processing for Pathology

Back table ex vivo dissection of the operative specimen after removal of the specimen can aid the pathologist in identifying lymph nodes. Separate containers with each nodal station optimize the chances of having an adequate number of lymph nodes recovered by the pathologist. On the back table, the proximal and distal gastric staple lines are removed. The stomach is opened longitudinally along the lesser or greater curvature, whichever is away from the tumor. The gross proximal and distal margins are examined. The lymph node stations are then dissected out and sent as separate specimen. During initial cases, it may be best to mark these node stations with tags during the dissection to ensure proper ex vivo nodal dissection.

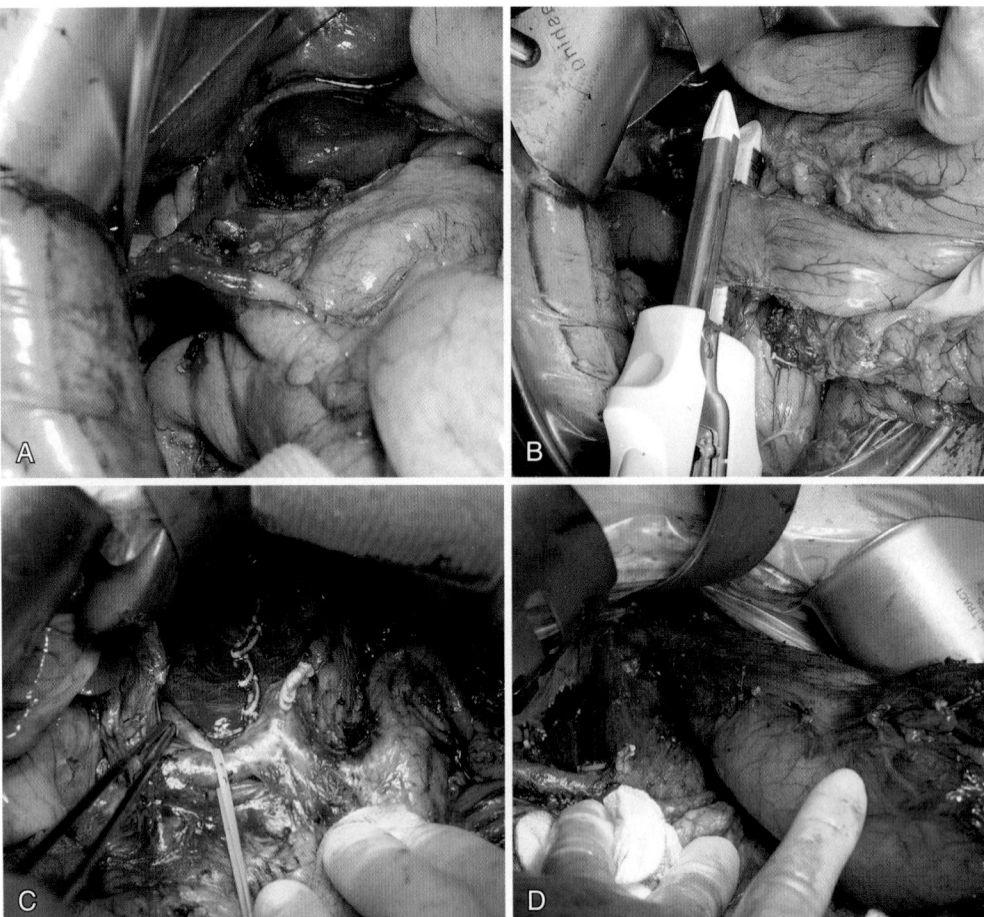

FIGURE 3 Operative photographs show: **A,** dissection of right gastric artery near origin from proper hepatic artery; **B,** transection of duodenum; **C,** completed dissection of proximal splenic artery, celiac axis, common hepatic artery, and divided left gastric artery; and **D,** dissection of right paracardial nodes off the gastroesophageal junction and lesser curvature.

D2 LYMPHADENECTOMY TECHNIQUE FOR TOTAL GASTRECTOMY

Compared with a distal gastrectomy, the only additional nodal stations that require dissection for a total gastrectomy are the greater curvature nodes along the short gastric vessels (station 4sa), left paracardial nodes (station 2), distal splenic artery nodes (station 11d), and splenic hilum nodes (station 10).

The station 4sa nodes can be taken early on after dividing the left gastroepiploic vessels near their origin. One can then continue the greater curvature dissection superiorly toward the GEJ, dividing the short gastric vessels near the medial border of the spleen. On reaching the GEJ, the left paracardial nodes can be dissected by dividing the phrenoesophageal ligament and sweeping all nodal tissue toward the GEJ.

Dissection of the distal splenic artery nodes should be performed after dissection off the proximal splenic artery nodes. Nodal tissue anterior and superior to the splenic artery is dissected of the retroperitoneal fat (Figure 4, A). To facilitate dissection of the splenic hilum nodes, the spleen and tail of pancreas can be mobilized anterior and to the left. The splenic artery forms several segmental branches, and all the nodal tissue anterior to these branches is dissected (Figure 4, B).

Reconstruction is generally performed with a Roux-en-Y method. The use of an end-to-end anastomosis (EEA) circular stapler may result in anastomotic stricture, which requires dilation. The authors now generally perform the side-to-side stapled technique, which is a modification of a technique described by Orringer. The esophagus is transected with endoscopic linear staples (3.5-mm staple size; Figure 4,C). The jejunal limb is brought posterior to the transected

esophagus. A small enterotomy is made in the jejunal limb, 6 to 7 cm proximal to the transected end, and the mid portion of the esophageal staple line is removed. An endoscopic linear stapler (3.5-mm staple size, 45 mm in length) is used to create a side-to-side anastomosis (Figure 4,D), and the holes are closed with interrupted 3-0 silk sutures.

NEOADJUVANT AND ADJUVANT THERAPY

The risks of locoregional and distant recurrence are high for all T2 or more or node-positive gastric cancers even with surgical resection, thus providing rationale for the delivery of neoadjuvant and adjuvant therapies. The United States Intergroup 0116 trial was the first prospective randomized trial to show a survival benefit of 5-fluorouracil (5-FU) chemoradiation after surgery over surgery alone. Three-year overall survival rate was increased from 41% to 50% with chemoradiation ($P = 0.005$). In this trial, 54% of patients received less than a D1 lymphadenectomy and only 10% of patients received a D2 lymphadenectomy, and the chemoradiation appeared to primarily reduce logoregional recurrence. Thus, some have argued that the chemoradiation likely improved survival by making up for inadequate surgery. Of note, an observational study from Samsung Medical Center (Seoul, Korea) of 990 patients who underwent surgical resection along with D2 lymphadenectomy found that median survival rate was significantly increased in the 544 patients who underwent chemoradiation compared with the 446 patients who underwent no adjuvant therapy. More recently, the Adjuvant Chemoradiation Therapy in Stomach Cancer (ARTIST) trial randomized Korean

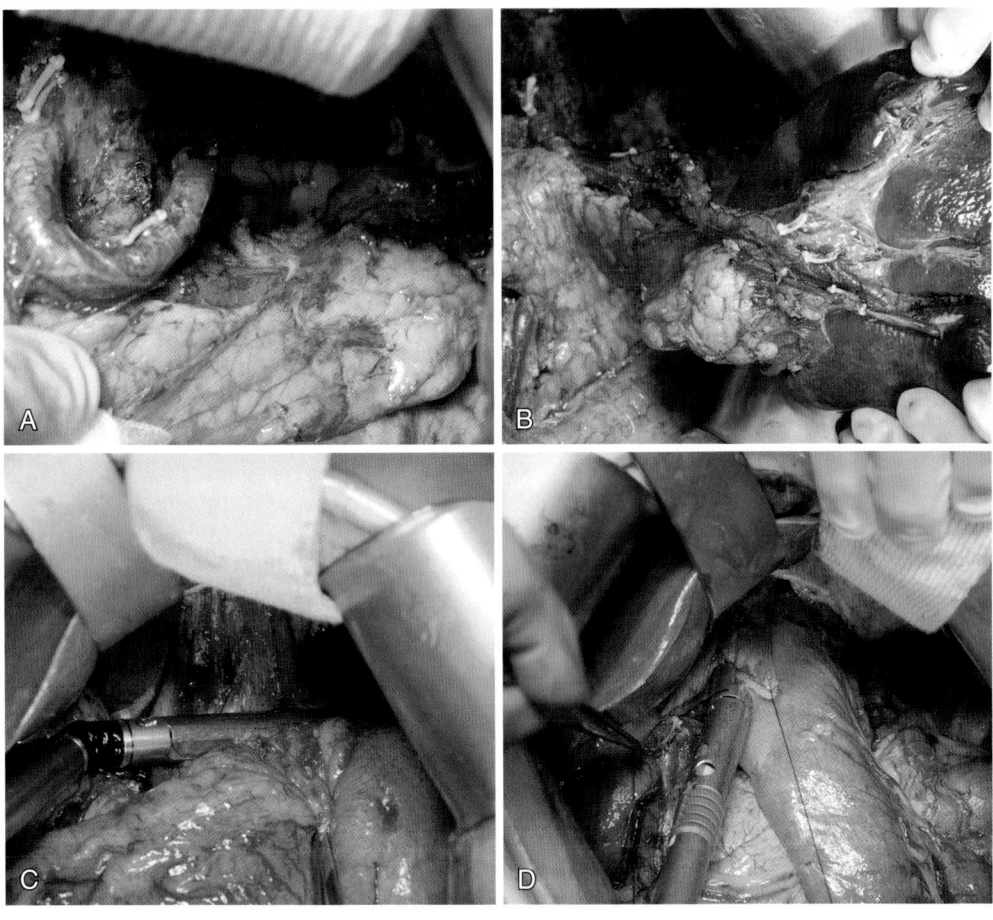

FIGURE 4 Operative photographs show: **A,** dissection of distal splenic artery; **B,** dissection of splenic hilum; **C,** transection of esophagus; and **D,** side-to-side esophagojejunostomy with linear stapler.

patients after gastrectomy to capecitabine and cisplatin (XP) chemotherapy or XP plus radiation and capecitabine. The overall trial results were negative, but disease-free survival rate was improved with chemoradiation in the subgroup of patients with node-positive disease.

Three prospective randomized trials, one from Europe and two from Asia, have shown survival benefits for neoadjuvant or adjuvant chemotherapy without radiation therapy. The European Organisation for Research and Treatment of Cancer (EORTC) Medical research Council Adjuvant Gastric Infusional Chemotherapy (MAGIC) trial randomized patients to three cycles of epirubicin, cisplatin, and 5-FU (ECF) chemotherapy before and after surgery or surgery alone and found a 5-year overall survival rate of 36% in the chemotherapy plus surgery group and 23% in the surgery-alone group (P = 0.009). Sakuramoto and colleagues randomized Japanese patients to surgery plus S-1, a 5-FU prodrug combined with an agent that lowers bowel toxicity and an agent that prevents 5-FU degradation, or surgery alone and found that the 3-year overall survival rate was 80% in the S-1 plus surgery group and 70% in the surgery-alone group (P = 0.002). Most patients in the EORTC MAGIC trial received at least a D1 lymphadenectomy, and most patients in the Japanese trial received a D2 lymphadenectomy, supporting the notion that chemotherapy alone can improve survival in patients with gastric cancer. The Adjuvant Capecitabine and Oxaliplatin for Gastric Cancer after D2 Gastrectomy (CLASSIC) trial randomized Asian patients after D2 gastrectomy to capecitabine and oxaliplatin chemotherapy or no chemotherapy; the 3-year disease-free survival rate was 74% in the chemotherapy group compared with 59% in the no-chemotherapy group (P = 0.0001). The Chemoradiation after Induction Chemotherapy in Cancer of the Stomach (CRITICS) multicenter trial is currently comparing MAGIC-style perioperative

chemotherapy with preoperative chemotherapy followed by postoperative chemoradiation.

FOLLOW-UP

The utility of intensive follow-up of patients with gastric cancer after surgical resection is controversial, and significant differences are found in the recommendations of various groups. The European Society for Medical Oncology (ESMO) clinical recommendations for the follow-up of gastric cancer state, "there is no evidence that regular intensive follow-up improves patient outcomes, [and] symptom-driven visits are recommended for most cases." However, many patients are uncomfortable with minimal or no follow-up. The National Comprehensive Cancer Network practice guidelines for gastric cancer recommend a history and physical examination every 3 to 6 months for 1 to 3 years, every 6 months for 3 to 5 years, and then annually. Complete blood cell count (CBC), chemistry profile, tumor markers (carcinoembryonic antigen [CEA] and carbohydrate antigen 19-9 [CA19-9]), radiologic imaging, and endoscopy are recommended as clinically indicated. Ultimately, the decision regarding the intensiveness of follow-up is left to the treating physician after discussion with the patient.

SUMMARY

The surgical management of patients with gastric adenocarcinoma varies significantly around the world, and much of this is related to the wide range in incidence rates and thus wide range in exposure of surgeons to this disease. Useful diagnostic studies include upper endoscopy, EUS, abdomen and pelvis CT scan, and diagnostic laparoscopy with peritoneal washings. The extent of gastric resection is governed by the location of the tumor. For mid and distal tumors, distal or subtotal gastrectomy can be performed, but for proximal tumors, total gastrectomy is generally performed. The extent of lymphadenectomy is also governed by the location of the tumor, but controversy exists as to whether a D1 or D2 lymphadenectomy is optimal. Unfortunately, more than half of patients in the United States receive less even a D1 lymphadenectomy. Two large randomized studies from Western countries that compared D1 and D2 lymphadenectomy showed no survival benefit for a D2 lymphadenectomy when performed with high morbidity and mortality. Performance of a D2 lymphadenectomy requires surgical training. Experienced surgeons in countries with high incidence rates such as Japan and Korea perform D2 lymphadenectomies for gastric with low morbidity and almost no mortality. Long-term results from the

Dutch randomized trial and a Taiwanese trial suggest there may be a survival benefit for D2 lymphadenectomy. Overall survival results are pending from an Italian prospective randomized trial of D1 versus D2 lymphadenectomy in which the D2 group had low morbidity and mortality.

SUGGESTED READINGS

Japanese gastric cancer treatment guidelines 2010 (ver. 3), *Gastric Cancer* 14:113–123, 2011.
Maduekwe UN, Yoon SS: An evidence-based review of the surgical treatment of gastric adenocarcinoma, *J Gastrointest Surg* 15:730–741, 2011.
Songun I, Putter H, Kranenbarg EM, et al: Surgical treatment of gastric cancer: 15-year follow-up results of the randomised nationwide Dutch D1D2 trial, *Lancet Oncol* 11:439–449, 2010.

GASTROINTESTINAL STROMAL TUMORS

Chandrajit P. Raut, MS, MSc, and
Timothy M. Pawlik, MD, MPH, PhD

INTRODUCTION

Gastrointestinal stromal tumors (GISTs) are rare neoplasms that represent only 0.1% to 3% of all gastrointestinal malignancies. However, they are the most common sarcoma and account for 80% of gastrointestinal mesenchymal neoplasms. In the last 12 years, the understanding and treatment of GIST have witnessed remarkable advances as the result of two key developments: (1) the identification of constitutively active signals (oncogenic mutation of the c-KIT and platelet-derived growth factor alpha [PDGFRA] genes encoding receptor tyrosine kinases); and (2) the development of therapeutic agents that suppress tumor growth by specifically targeting and inhibiting this signal (imatinib mesylate, sunitinib malate). These developments in the management of GIST represent a proof of principle of translational therapeutics in oncology, confirming that specific inhibition of tumor-associated receptor tyrosine kinase activity may be an effective cancer treatment. The advent of effective therapy has dramatically improved outcomes for GIST, and instead of diminishing the role of surgery, it has redefined it. This chapter reviews the biology, treatment, and emerging clinical challenges of these mesenchymal neoplasms.

PATHOLOGIC FEATURES

Historical Background

The term *GIST* was initially proposed in 1983 by Mazur and Clark to describe intra-abdominal nonepithelial neoplasms that lacked

the ultrastructural features of smooth muscle cells and the immunohistochemical characteristics of Schwann cells. A diagnosis of GIST is often suspected histologically because most cases have uniform appearances that fall into one of three categories: spindle cell type, epithelioid type, or mixed type. Interestingly, most gastric GISTs feature an epithelioid phenotype, and small intestinal, anorectal, colonic, and esophageal tumors more often feature spindle cell morphology.

On the basis of their histologic and immunohistochemical features, GISTs are believed to arise from the interstitial cells of Cajal, components of the intestinal autonomic nervous system that serve as potential intestinal pacemakers. Nonetheless, until the late 1990s, no objective criteria existed to classify GISTs. They were frequently misclassified as leiomyomas, leiomyoblastomas, leiomyosarcomas, schwannomas, gastrointestinal autonomic nerve tumors, or other similar soft tissue histologies. Consequently, interpretation of clinical results for reports on GISTs published before 2000 can be challenging.

Receptor Tyrosine Kinase Mutations

In a landmark publication in 1998, Hirota and colleagues reported two critical findings: (1) near-universal expression of the transmembrane receptor tyrosine kinase KIT in GIST; and (2) presence of gain-of-function mutations in the corresponding c-*KIT* proto-oncogene. The KIT receptor is normally activated by binding its cytokine ligand known as steel factor or stem cell factor and plays a critical role in the development and maintenance of components of hematopoiesis, gametogenesis, and intestinal pacemaker cells. Oncogenic *KIT* mutations have been identified in neoplasms corresponding to these functions, including mast cell tumors, myelofibrosis, chronic myelogenous leukemia, germ cell tumors, and GIST. Mutated KIT remains constitutively active even in the absence of ligand binding and results in both unregulated cell growth and malignant transformation.

GISTs are now identified with immunohistochemical staining for the CD117 antigen, part of the KIT receptor, in the appropriate histopathologic context. CD117 expression (KIT positivity) is characteristic of most GISTs but not of other gastrointestinal smooth muscle tumors such as leiomyosarcoma. Application of CD117 staining as a diagnostic criterion for GIST has altered the understanding of the prevalence of this disease.

More than 85% of GISTs have activating *KIT* mutations. These mutations commonly occur in exon 11 (in 57% to 71% of cases), exon 9 (10% to 18%), exon 13 (1% to 4%), and exon 17 (1% to 4%). The presence of CD117 immunoreactivity does not necessarily correlate with a *KIT* gene mutation, and conversely, a *KIT* mutation can exist in the absence of CD117 immunoreactivity. GISTs with *KIT* exon 9 mutations predominantly arise in the small intestine. Approximately 35% of neoplasms that lack *KIT* mutations have activating mutations in a gene encoding a related receptor tyrosine kinase, the platelet-derived growth factor receptor alpha (PDGFRA). *PDGFRA* mutations have been identified in exon 12 (1% to 2% of GISTs), exon 18 (2% to 6%), and exon 14 (<1%). Finally, a few GISTs, the so-called wild-type (WT) GISTs, exhibit no detectable *KIT* or *PDGFRA* mutations and have alternate pathways for pathogenesis. Recently, additional putative mutations in several succinate dehydrogenase (SDH) subunits and *BRAF* and overexpression of insulin-like growth factor–1 receptor have been identified in a small percentage of WT tumors.

DOG1, a monoclonal antibody against a chloride channel protein expressed by GIST, is immunoreactive in 95% of GISTs irrespective of their mutation status. However, DOG1 is not specific to GIST, and uterine retroperitoneal leiomyomas, peritoneal leiomyomatosis, and synovial sarcomas may also be positive for DOG1.

EPIDEMIOLOGY

Age

The median age at diagnosis of GIST is 60 years (range, 40 to 80 years). GISTs are equally common in men and women, and no racial or ethnic predilection is found. GIST does occur rarely in children, often as a familial syndrome or as part of Carney's triad. The clinical presentation is typically different in children, who tend to present with multifocal gastric GISTs, with WT for *KIT* and *PDGFRA*, and have a higher incidence of lymph node metastases.

Hereditary Gastrointestinal Stromal Tumors

The overwhelming majority of GISTs are sporadic. Nevertheless, kindred germline *KIT* or *PDFGRA* mutations have been reported. Individuals with GISTs secondary to germline *KIT* mutations are usually younger than those with sporadic GISTs, manifest multifocal disease at presentation, and only rarely have metastatic disease develop. The phenotype includes skin hyperpigmentation and diffuse hyperplasia of the intestinal myenteric plexus, and cases of melanoma and esophageal and breast cancers have also been reported in individuals with hereditary GIST.

Approximately 7% of individuals with the autosomal dominant disorder Recklinghausen's neurofibromatosis (NF1) have GIST, most commonly multifocal in the small intestine and with a higher incidence in women (1.4:1). In addition to their *NF1* mutations, these individuals express *KIT* and *PDGFRA* point mutations in 8% and 6% of GISTs, respectively. Conversely, *NF1* mutations have not been identified in individuals without NF1 with sporadic GISTs.

Gastric GISTs can be a component of both Carney's triad and Carney-Stratakis syndrome. Described by Carney in 1977, Carney's triad consists of GIST, paraganglioma, and pulmonary chondromas. More recently, esophageal leiomyomas and adrenal cortical adenomas have been added as components of the syndrome. Approximately 85% occur in women, and 80% are diagnosed before the age of 30 years. Patients with Carney's triad do not have somatic *KIT* or *PDGFRA* mutations. The similarly eponymous

Carney-Stratakis syndrome describes familial cases expressing the dyad of gastric GIST and paraganglioma. Mutations in several SDH subunits have been reported in Carney-Stratakis syndrome kindreds. GISTs associated with both syndromes have a chronic yet indolent course.

Incidence

Investigators have attempted to determine the true incidence of GIST with the Surveillance, Epidemiology, and End Results (SEER) database from the National Cancer Institute. However, these data are difficult to interpret because many GISTs were previously misclassified as other gastrointestinal (GI) mesenchymal neoplasms. Although a near doubling of the incidence rate of all GI mesenchymal tumors (more than 80% were GIST) has been reported (0.17/100,000 in 1992 to 0.31/100,000 in 2002), this may be the result of increased recognition or increased screening or a true increased incidence rate. The annual incidence rate in the United States is estimated to be approximately 5000 to 6000 new cases per year (15 to 20 cases per million). European population-based studies identified annual incidence rates ranging from 11 to 15 cases per million population, with an estimated prevalence of approximately 129 per million.

CLINICAL PRESENTATION

GISTs commonly arise in the stomach (50% to 70%), small intestine (25% to 35%), colon and rectum (5% to 10%), mesentery or omentum (7%), and esophagus (<5%). Occasionally, GIST may arise in the duodenal ampulla, appendix, gallbladder, and urinary bladder.

GISTs are generally found as a result of symptoms. In one study, 69% of tumors were symptomatic, 21% were discovered incidentally at surgery, and 10% were discovered at autopsy. GISTs are often highly vascular, soft, and friable, and bleeding is a common presenting symptom. They may cause life-threatening hemorrhage by erosion into the bowel lumen. Alternatively, tumor rupture may cause potentially catastrophic intraperitoneal bleeding or dissemination by peritoneal seeding. Intestinal obstruction may lead to perforation. Smaller tumors may remain asymptomatic and only be incidentally detected on radiographic studies, endoscopy, or laparotomy. Between 15% and approximately 50% of patients with GIST have metastatic disease at diagnosis. Common sites of metastasis include liver, peritoneum, and omentum; metastases to lymph nodes and extra-abdominal structures (lung, bone, subcutaneous tissues, and brain) are rare (<5% of patients).

DIAGNOSIS

Radiographic Studies

The initial imaging study of choice for a suspected or confirmed GIST is a contrast-enhanced computed tomographic (CT) scan of the abdomen and pelvis. Primary GISTs are typically well-circumscribed masses within the walls of hollow viscera. Magnetic resonance imaging (MRI) may help characterize primary rectal disease (Figure 1) or metastatic liver. Although [18F]fluoro-2-deoxy-D-glucose positron emission tomography (FDG-PET) may help characterize masses ambiguous on CT scan, monitor response to therapy, and detect emergence of drug-resistant clones, it is not specific for GIST and thus is not recommended for most patients with suspected primary disease. Much has been written about its utility in patients with metastatic GIST, but in general, PET scans are not necessary in the management of patients with metastatic disease and thus may be used sparingly.

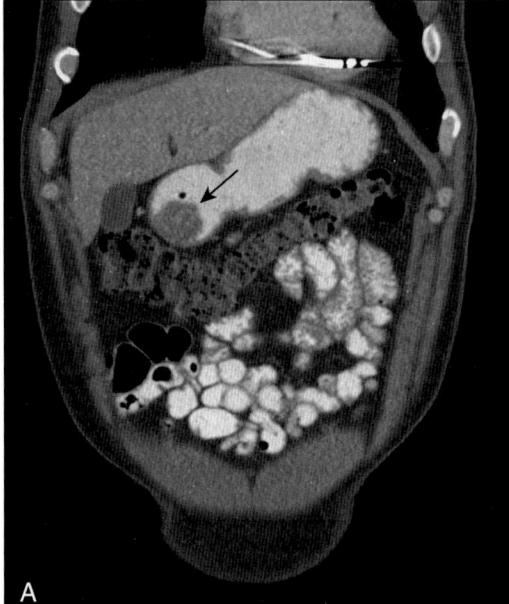

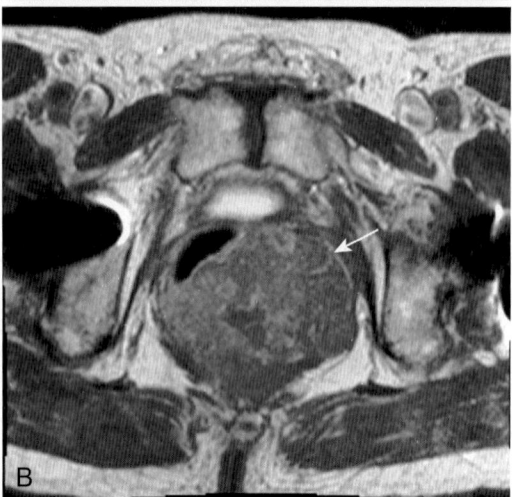

FIGURE 1   Cross-sectional imaging depicts: **A,** a computed tomographic scan image of a distal gastric gastrointestinal stromal tumor *(arrow);* and **B,** a magnetic resonance image of a nearly obstructing rectal gastrointestinal stromal tumor *(arrow).*

Endoscopy, Fine-Needle Aspiration, and Biopsy

Endoscopically, a primary GIST may appear as a submucosal lesion, with or without ulceration, present in the upper or lower GI tract. GISTs are often indistinguishable from other GI tumors of smooth muscle origin, such as leiomyomas. Upper endoscopy with endoscopic biopsy has a low diagnostic yield (17% to 42%). Endoscopic ultrasound scan (EUS) is not necessary to evaluate a confirmed GIST. However, EUS-guided fine-needle aspiration (FNA) may be attempted to establish diagnosis, with a diagnostic yield and sensitivity of approximately 80%. Nevertheless, EUS FNA is not consistently diagnostic. Additional cytologic morphology, immunohistochemistry, and reverse-transcriptase polymerase chain reaction analysis for *KIT* mutations may be necessary to confirm a diagnosis.

A preoperative biopsy is not routinely necessary for a primary, resectable neoplasm suspicious for GIST. In fact, preoperative biopsy may rupture a suspected GIST and increase the risk of dissemination. However, if the differential diagnosis includes entities such as lymphoma that would be treated differently, if neoadjuvant therapy is

under consideration, or if there is metastatic disease, biopsy is appropriate.

PROGNOSTIC FACTORS

Although tumors of less than 1 cm likely have a low risk of recurrence, no tumors can be definitively called benign and most large tumors have malignant potential. The three established prognostic factors are tumor size (single largest dimension), mitotic index, and tumor site of origin, with mitotic count being the most important as the strongest predictor of recurrence (Table 1). Individuals with small bowel GISTs have a higher risk of progression than those with gastric GISTs of comparable size and mitotic count.

More recently, a validated nomogram has been reported (Figure 2). The nomogram assigns points for each of the three known prognostic factors based on a particular patient's presentation and uses the point totals to predict the probability of remaining recurrence-free at 2 and 5 years. Tumors that arise in the small intestine carry more "points" because of their worse prognosis compared with those that arise in the stomach or colon or rectum. Of note, the nomogram bases the probability of recurrence on a cohort of patients diagnosed initially in the therapy era before tyrosine kinase inhibitors (TKIs).

Additional adverse prognostic factors observed in some but not all studies include high cellular proliferation index, aneuploidy, telomerase expression, *KIT* exon 9 mutations, and *KIT* exon 11 deletions that involve amino acid W557 or K558. Point mutations and insertions of *KIT* exon 11 appear to have a favorable prognosis.

THERAPY FOR PRIMARY DISEASE

Surgery

Technique

Surgery remains the standard of care and only potentially curative therapy for patients with primary, resectable, localized GIST. At laparotomy, the abdomen is thoroughly explored to identify and remove any previously undetected peritoneal metastatic deposits. Although primary GISTs may demonstrate inflammatory adhesions to surrounding organs, they do not generally invade other organs beyond the site of origin despite CT scan appearance. The goal of the operation should be a margin negative resection. The ideal margin of resection is unknown. A macroscopically complete resection with negative or positive microscopic margins (R0 or R1 resection, respectively) is associated with a better prognosis than a macroscopically incomplete resection (R2 resection). Post hoc analysis of a randomized trial evaluating the utility of 1 year of adjuvant imatinib mesylate therapy after resection of primary GISTs at least 3 cm in size showed no significant difference in recurrence-free survival (RFS) for patients undergoing an R0 versus R1 resection with or without the use of adjuvant imatinib. However, data on overall survival (OS) rates are unknown. What is clearly known is that tumor rupture or violation of the tumor capsule during surgery is associated with an increased risk of recurrence and therefore should be avoided.

In general, the extent of surgery is usually a wedge or segmental resection of the involved stomach or bowel without the wide margins necessary for adenocarcinoma. In a series of 140 patients with gastric GISTs, wedge resections were performed in 68%, partial gastrectomies in 28%, and total gastrectomies in only 4%. Occasionally, a more extensive resection (total gastrectomy for a large proximal gastric GIST, pancreaticoduodenectomy for a periampullary GIST, or abdominoperineal resection for a low rectal GIST) may be necessary. Several recent multiinstitutional retrospective series have questioned the need for extensive resections such as pancreaticoduodenectomy or abdominoperineal resection in the setting of well-tolerated, orally

TABLE 1: Risk assessment for primary gastrointestinal stromal tumors

Mitotic rate	Tumor size	Percentage of patients with progressive disease/risk classification, based on site of origin			
		Stomach	Duodenum	Jejunum/Ileum	Rectum
≤5 per 50 HPF	≤2 cm	0	0	0	0
	>2, ≤5 cm	1.9/very low	8.3/low	4.3/low	8.5/low
	>5, ≤10 cm	3.6/low	34/high	24/moderate	57/high
	>10 cm	12/moderate	34/high	52/high	57/high
>5 per 50 HPF	≤2 cm	–	–	–	54/high
	>2, ≤5 cm	16/moderate	50/high	73/high	52/high
	>5, ≤10 cm	55/high	86/high	85/high	71/high
	>10 cm	86/high	86/high	90/high	71/high

HPF, High-power field; –, insufficient data.
Adapted from Miettinen and Lasota (with permission). Gastrointestinal stromal tumors: pathology and prognosis at different sites, Semin Diagn Pathol 23(2):70–83, 2010.

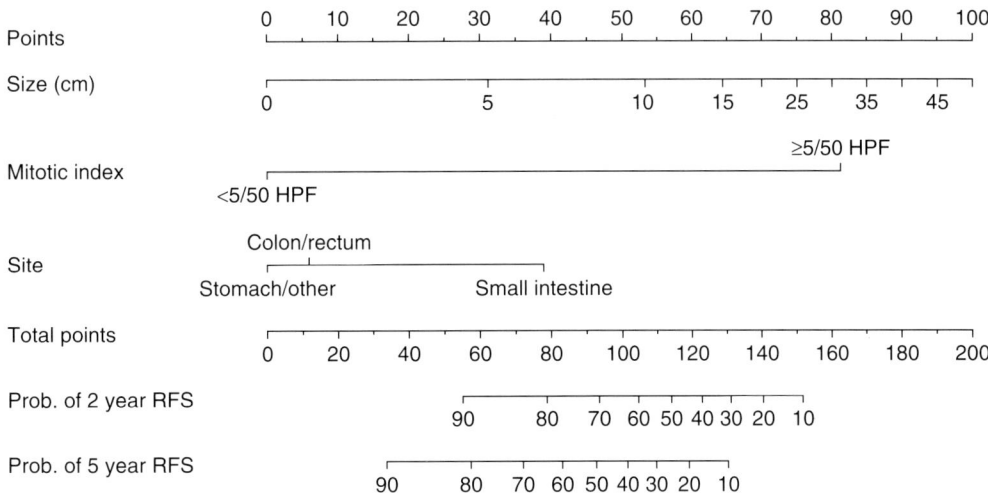

FIGURE 2   Nomogram to predict the probabilities of 2-year and 5-year recurrence-free survival (RFS). Points are assigned for size, mitotic index, and site of origin by drawing a line upward from the corresponding values to the *Points* line. The sum of these three points, plotted on the *Total points* line, corresponds to predictions of 2-year and 5-year RFS. HPF, High-power field. *(Used with permission from Gold JS, Gonen M, Guiterrez A, et al: Development and validation of a prognostic nomogram for recurrence-free survival after complete surgical resection of localised primary gastrointestinal stromal tumour: a retrospective analysis,* Lancet Oncol 10[11]:1045–1052, 2009.)

available targeted therapies. No data indicate that patients who have an R1 resection need reexcision, and in fact, the lack of any difference in RFS between patients undergoing R0 versus R1 resection suggests that reexcision or more radical resections may be avoided. Furthermore, margins may retract after resection, or the pathologist may trim away the staple line (converting a technically negative microscopic margin into a positive one). Therefore, all cases of positive microscopic margins should be carefully reviewed by a multidisciplinary team of surgical oncologists, pathologists, and medical oncologists to assess the need for reexcision. Lymphadenectomy is not required because lymph nodes are rarely involved (in adult patients).

All GISTs 2 cm in size or greater should be resected when possible because none of these can be considered benign. However, the natural history of GISTs less than 2 cm in size is unknown; thus, their management is more debatable. Although the low risk of progression of GISTs less than 2 cm may support a more conservative approach, an accurate mitotic index cannot be determined with biopsy or FNA.

Therefore, observation for GIST 1 to 2 cm is difficult to recommend. As such, resection of GIST measuring 1 to 2 cm should be considered, and the risks and benefits of surgery versus observation should be reviewed with the patient. Given the higher risk of aggressive behavior of small bowel and colon GISTs, any tumor in such locations should be resected irrespective of size. In contrast, most gastric GISTs under 1 cm in size may be followed. Two studies have established that subcentimeter gastric GISTs are relatively common, with detection in 22.5% of autopsies in adults over the age of 50 years in Germany and in 35% of patients undergoing gastrectomy for gastric cancer in Japan. Despite their relative frequency, few of these neoplasms appear to become clinically relevant. Until further data are available, the most appropriate management of such small tumors remains uncertain. Although endoscopic resection of small gastric GISTs has been reported, this cannot be recommended. Unlike early gastric cancers (mucosal malignancies) amenable to endoscopic mucosal resection, GISTs involve the muscularis propria, so attempts at endoscopic resection risk leaving a positive margin and, because of the depth of the lesion, could result in perforation. Regardless of their size, any small GISTs that are symptomatic (e.g., hemorrhage from erosion through the mucosa) or increase in size on serial follow-up examination should be resected.

Laparoscopic or laparoscopy-assisted resection of primary GISTs may be performed following standard oncologic principles. Two early studies confirmed both the safety and the feasibility of a laparoscopic approach. In a series of 35 gastric GISTs (2 to 5 cm) resected laparoscopically, no local or distant recurrences were observed for tumors under 4 cm in size with a median follow-up period of 53 months. In a study of 50 patients with gastric GISTs (1.0 to 8.5 cm) resected laparoscopically or with laparoscopy assistance, 92% of patients were disease-free with a mean follow-up period of 3 years.

Despite a macroscopically complete resection, as many as 50% of individuals may have recurrent disease develop at a median of 24 months after surgery. An R0 or R1 resection is associated with 5-year OS rates of 34% to 63%, whereas R2 resection is associated with 5-year OS rates as low as 8% in the preimatinib era.

Perioperative Therapy for Primary Disease

The identification of two effective, relatively well-tolerated orally available targeted TKIs, imatinib mesylate (STI571, Gleevec, Novartis Pharmaceuticals, Basel, Switzerland) and sunitinib malate (SU11248, Sutent, Pfizer, Inc., New York, NY), revolutionized the treatment of GIST. Imatinib selectively inhibits several tyrosine kinases, including KIT, PDGFRA, and BCR-ABL. Several clinical trials have confirmed that up to 80% of patients with metastatic GIST achieve a complete response or partial response or show stable disease radiographically on imatinib. Although these agents were initially developed for the management of patients with metastatic disease, increasing interest has been seen in using imatinib in the perioperative period given the high incidence rate of recurrence after resection of GIST.

The role of neoadjuvant therapy with imatinib combined with resection has been prospectively studied (Table 2). Specifically, the Radiation Therapy Oncology Group (RTOG) 0312 phase II trial was a multicenter study that evaluated the use of imatinib as a neoadjuvant agent. Patients with resectable primary or recurrent GIST were treated with 600 mg per day of imatinib for 8 to 12 weeks before surgery. Patients without progression underwent surgery and were then maintained on adjuvant imatinib for 2 years. An objective response was shown in 90% of patients with primary GIST, and 92% underwent R0/R1 resections. The 2-year RFS rate was 83%. Although this trial confirmed the safety of imatinib as a neoadjuvant therapy, the optimal length of preoperative therapy is still unclear. Data from trials of advanced GIST have shown that maximal radiographic response to imatinib generally required 6 to 9 months of treatment. Thus, the optimal preoperative imatinib regimen may be 6 months or more as long as continued radiographic response is observed.

In practice, when to use neoadjuvant imatinib is still unclear. In situations where tumor shrinkage may either simplify an operation or potentially allow the scope of an operation to be downstaged (for instance, converting a pancreaticoduodenectomy into a localized resection for a duodenal GIST or converting an abdominoperineal resection into a transanal excision for a rectal GIST), neoadjuvant imatinib may be used. Alternatively, even if the extent of resection is unlikely to change, converting from an open procedure to a laparoscopic one may be another indication for neoadjuvant imatinib.

The role of adjuvant therapy with imatinib combined with resection of primary disease has been explored in numerous prospective trials (see Table 2). These trials examined different durations of adjuvant imatinib of 12 months (American College of Surgeons Oncology Group [ACOSOG] Z9000, ACOSOG Z9001, China Cooperative Group), 24 months (European Organization for the Research and Treatment of Cancer [EORTC] 62024, Korean trial), 12 versus 36 months (Scandinavian Sarcoma Group [SSG] XVIII), or 5 years

(recently completed phase II multiinstitutional trial, PERSIST5). In the phase III ACOSOG Z9011 trial, patients with completely resected primary GIST at least 3 cm in size were randomized to receive either placebo or imatinib postoperatively for 12 months. The trial was halted early after a planned interim analysis of 644 evaluable patients confirmed that the 1-year RFS rate was significantly better in the imatinib arm (97% vs 83%; $P = 0.0000014$). Interestingly, the slopes of the Kaplan-Meier curves representing the two treatment arms, once recurrences were observed, were similar. This suggests that 1 year of adjuvant imatinib may delay recurrence but may not necessarily cure anyone over the short follow-up interval. Furthermore, no difference was seen in OS between the two treatment arms.

In the phase III SSG XVIII trial, patients with high-risk GISTs who underwent a complete resection were randomized to receive either imatinib postoperatively for 12 months versus 36 months. The key entry criteria were: (1) tumor at least 10 cm in size; (2) tumor rupture; (3) mitotic count of more than 10 per 50 high-power field (HPF); (4) tumor greater than 5 cm in size and mitotic count more than 5 per 50 HPF; or (5) primary GIST of any size or mitotic count with synchronous liver or peritoneal metastases (which were also resected). The trial, which included 397 evaluable patients, confirmed that patients treated with 36 months of adjuvant imatinib had longer 5-year RFS rates than those treated with 12 months of adjuvant imatinib (66% vs 48%; $P <0.01$). More importantly, it showed that those treated with longer duration of imatinib had improved 5-year OS rates (92% vs 82%; $P = 0.02$).

The EORTC 62024 trial has completed accrual, but data are not yet available. Data from that trial plus the recently completed PERSIST5 trial will help determine the comparative benefit of 2 and 5 years of imatinib on RFS and time to imatinib failure. Perhaps the most important question is whether administration of imatinib after resection of primary disease or after disease recurrence delays time to second-line therapy (imatinib dose escalation or changing to sunitinib). However, with the recent approval of imatinib for adjuvant use by both the Food and Drug Administration in the United States and the European Medicines Agency in Europe, it seems unlikely that any trial will ever be designed to answer this question. Therefore, at this time, the standard of care is that patients with high-risk GIST should be treated with a minimum of 36 months of adjuvant imatinib.

THERAPY FOR ADVANCED DISEASE

Targeted Therapy

Despite successful resection of the primary tumor, most patients experience tumor recurrence. Recurrences are most commonly in the liver (two thirds) or along the peritoneal surface (half). Before the advent of TKI therapy, median survival time after recurrence was approximately 18 months. Historically, patients with recurrent GIST had limited therapeutic options. More recently, imatinib mesylate and sunitinib malate are now available for the treatment of metastatic GIST. Imatinib is the first-line therapy for advanced (unresectable primary or metastatic) GIST, based on data from international phase I, II, and III trials. Partial responses (PRs) or stable disease (SD) were noted in nearly 85% of patients with advanced GIST treated with imatinib. In the U.S. phase III trial, the median RSF and OS times with imatinib therapy were 18 to 20 months and 51 to 55 months, respectively. The starting dose for imatinib is generally 400 mg once daily. In patients with development of progressive disease on 400 mg, dose escalation up to 400 mg twice daily is effective. However, greater toxicity and more dose reductions are generally required at doses above 400 mg per day. The toxicities of imatinib include edema, nausea, muscle cramps, diarrhea, headache, dermatitis, fatigue, anemia, and neutropenia. Fortunately, most side effects (>70%) are mild to moderate in severity and often resolve with continuing

TABLE 2: Multiinstitutional trials of the use of neoadjuvant or adjuvant imatinib in the perioperative management of resected primary gastrointestinal stromal tumors

Trial	Imatinib therapy	Design	Eligibility	Dose	Primary endpoint	Status
RTOG S0132	Neoadjuvant	Phase II	Any of the following: primary tumor ≥ 5 cm recurrent tumor ≥ 2 cm Potentially resectable	600 mg daily × 8-10 wk before surgery + 600 mg daily × 24 mo after surgery	RFS	Published
ACOSOG Z9000	Adjuvant	Phase II	Any of the following: tumor ≥ 10 cm rupture/hemorrhage multiple tumors (<5) Complete resection	400 mg daily × 12 mo	RFS	Reported
ACOSOG Z9001	Adjuvant	Phase III	Tumor ≥ 3 cm Complete resection	400 mg daily vs placebo × 12 mo	RFS	Published
China Gastrointestinal Cooperative Group	Adjuvant	Phase II	Any of the following: tumor > 5 cm mitotic rate > 5/50 HPF	400 mg daily × 12 mo	RFS	Reported
SSG XVIII	Adjuvant	Phase III	Any of the following: tumor ≥ 10 cm rupture mitotic rate > 10 tumor > 5 cm + mitotic rate > 5 primary tumor + liver/ peritoneal metastases Complete resection	400 mg daily × 12 mo or 36 mo	RFS	Published
EORTC 62024	Adjuvant	Phase III	Any of the following: tumor > 5 cm mitotic rate > 10 tumor < 5 cm + mitotic count 6-10/50 HPF Complete resection	400 mg daily vs no treatment × 24 mo	Time to second-line therapy	Completed
Korea	Adjuvant	Phase II	Any of the following: tumor > 5 cm + mitotic count > 5/50 HPF tumor > 10 cm mitotic count > 10/50 HPF Complete resection	400 mg daily × 24 mo	RFS	Reported
CSIT571BUS282	Adjuvant	Phase II	Any of the following: tumor ≥ 2 cm + mitotic count ≥ 5/50 HPF any nongastric tumor ≥ 5 cm Complete resection	400 mg daily × 5 y	RFS	Completed

ACOSOG, American College of Surgeons Oncology Group; *EORTC,* European Organization for the Research and Treatment of Cancer; *HPF,* high-power field; *RFS,* recurrence-free survival; *RTOG,* Radiation Therapy Oncology Group; *SSG,* Scandinavian Sarcoma Group.

therapy. The location of the *KIT* mutation correlates with response to imatinib therapy. In a 121 patient subset from the U.S.-Finland study, patients whose disease harbored an exon 11 mutation had a response rate of 72%, and only 32% of patients with exon 9 *KIT* mutants and 12% of wild type *KIT* patients responded to imatinib. In a study of 117 patients treated with imatinib for metastatic GIST, the median event-free survival for patients whose tumors had mutations of exon 11 was 22.5 months, compared with 6.6 months for

patients with mutations in exon 9. In a meta-analysis of the two large phase III studies, a slight advantage in progression-free survival (PFS) was noted in patients initially treated with higher dose imatinib, but that advantage was essentially limited to patients with *KIT* exon 9 mutations.

A French randomized imatinib discontinuation study showed that patients with GIST on imatinib who stop imatinib therapy after 1, 3, and 5 years had a much higher rate of disease progression than those who continued on therapy. Interestingly, from the original U.S. phase II trial, approximately 18% of the original cohort remained on imatinib after 9.4 years. As such, imatinib should be continued indefinitely in the setting of advanced disease. If patients continue to progress on higher doses of imatinib or do not tolerate such doses, then second-line sunitinib is started. Sunitinib is a multitargeted TKI whose targets include KIT, PDGFR, vascular endothelial growth factor receptor (VEGFR1, VEGFR2, VEGFR3), the ret proto-oncogene receptor (RET), and Fms-like tyrosine kinase-3 receptor (Flt3). A placebo-controlled phase III trial showed significant improvement in time to progression in patients treated with sunitinib compared with those treated with placebo (27.3 weeks vs 6.4 weeks, respectively), as well as PFS and OS. Initially dosed as 50 mg daily in a 4-week-on/2-week-off cycle, many oncologists now favor a continuous dose regimen of 37.5 mg daily.

When sunitinib resistance develops, protocol-based therapies should be considered. Additional TKIs under investigation include regorafenib (which recently showed benefit as a third-line agent), sorafenib, nilotinib, dasatinib, masitinib, and vatalanib among others. Crenolanib is a novel PDGFR kinase inhibitor undergoing evaluation in patients with GIST whose tumors carry a *PDGFRA* D842V mutation to most other kinases available. Other potential molecules for targeted therapy include heat shock protein–90, mammalian target of rapamycin (mTOR), histone deacetylyase, and insulin-like growth factor type I receptor.

Surgery

Cytoreductive surgery for resectable advanced or metastatic disease is a relatively common practice for disseminated solid tumors that originate in the colon, appendix, ovary, and testicle. With the advent of imatinib and sunitinib therapy, a number of investigators have pursued a similar strategy of aggressive cytoreductive surgery in patients with advanced, metastatic GIST on TKI therapy. Three observations support such an approach. First, most patients experience durable periods of PR or SD on imatinib, lasting months to years. Second, pathologic complete responses are rare, noted in fewer than 5% of patients. Third, response to imatinib is not maintained indefinitely; the median time to progression from the development of secondary resistance to imatinib is 18 to 24 months. Once drug resistance develops, disease progression may be either limited (progression at one site of tumor, with other tumor deposits showing ongoing response to TKI) or generalized (progression at more than one site).

Several single-institution retrospective studies have documented the PFS and OS rates after extensive cytoreductive surgery in patients with advanced GIST treated with TKI therapy. The goal of such operations is to perform a macroscopically complete (R0 or R1) resection when safely possible. However, the disease may frequently be too extensive to be removed completely, in which case progressing lesions are preferentially removed. In the experience at Brigham and Women's Hospital/Dana-Farber Cancer Institute, the best results were generally seen in patients whose disease was still responsive to TKI therapy at the time of surgery. The ability to remove all macroscopic disease was greatest in patients with ongoing response to TKI therapy. After surgery, no evidence was found of any residual disease in 78%, 25%, and 7% of patients with responsive disease, limited progression, and generalized progression, respectively (*P* <0.0001). In contrast, bulky residual disease remained postoperatively in 4%, 16%, and 43% of patients with responsive disease, limited progression, and generalized progression, respectively.

On the basis of the available data, from limited single-institution series, the patients who seemed to derive the most benefit from cytoreductive surgery are the ones still responding to TKI therapy at the time of surgery (PR or SD). Such patients should be considered for surgery on an individual basis. Patients with generalized progression do not appear to derive any benefit from cytoreductive surgery

and are best treated without surgery. Such patients may nevertheless need urgent surgery for palliative or emergency purposes such as obstruction or hemorrhage. Although cytoreductive surgery is feasible in patients with responsive disease, there is still no evidence that outcomes are superior or even equal to those for patients who continue on TKI therapy without surgery. Efforts to answer this question in a randomized controlled trial in the United States, Europe, and China have been unsuccessful because of accrual issues.

SURVEILLANCE

The National Comprehensive Cancer Network (NCCN) consensus panel recommended that patients who have had resection of a primary GIST should undergo a history, physical examination, and abdomen/pelvis CT scans with intravenous contrast every 3 to 6 months during the first 3 to 5 years and then annually thereafter. Given the rarity of pulmonary or other extraabdominal metastases, CT scans of the chest, head, etc, are unnecessary. Routine PET scans for screening are also unnecessary. Because more recurrences occur within the first 5 years after surgery, imaging intervals of 3 to 6 months are standard for patients in the first 5 years of posttreatment follow-up, with annual evaluation thereafter. At present, no specific serum-based markers are used for the detection of recurrent GIST.

CONCLUSION

The principal and only potentially curative treatment for GIST is surgery. However, recurrences are common. In the era before the institution of TKI therapy, survival in the setting of recurrent or metastatic disease was poor. Because of its relatively low toxicity and significant efficacy in the treatment of GIST, TKI therapy has dramatically altered the natural history of this disease. The type and dose of TKI administered may soon be guided by mutational analysis. The role of imatinib has been expanded to patients with primary GIST, where it may be used safely as a neoadjuvant agent and improves RFS as an adjuvant agent after complete macroscopic resection. Ongoing studies will address the issues of optimal length and dose of adjuvant and neoadjuvant imatinib therapy, define the subset of candidates most likely to benefit from such therapy, and determine the long-term impact on OS. Cytoreductive surgery may be considered in a subset of patients with advanced disease, but phase III trial data are necessary to determine whether surgery adds any PFS or OS benefit over continuing imatinib therapy alone. Future studies will focus on the integration of surgery with targeted therapy and the development of new agents for drug-resistant GIST.

SUGGESTED READINGS

NCCN Guidelines

Demetri GD, von Mehren M, Antonescu CR, et al: NCCN Task Force report: update on the management of patients with gastrointestinal stromal tumors, *J Natl Compr Canc Netw* 8(Suppl 2):S1–S44, 2010.

Neoadjuvant Therapy

Eisenberg BL, Harris J, Blanke CD, et al: Phase II trial of neoadjuvant/adjuvant imatinib mesylate (IM) for advanced primary and metastatic/recurrent operable gastrointestinal stromal tumor (GIST): early results of RTOG 0132/ACRIN 6665, *J Surg Oncol* 99(1):42–47, 2009.

Adjuvant Therapy

Dematteo RP, Ballman KV, Antonescu CR, et al: Adjuvant imatinib mesylate after resection of localised, primary gastrointestinal stromal tumour: a randomised, double-blind, placebo-controlled trial, *Lancet* 373(9669): 1097–1104, 2009.

Joensuu H, Eriksson M, Sundby Hall K, et al: One vs three years of adjuvant imatinib for operable gastrointestinal stromal tumor: a randomized trial, *JAMA* 307(12):1265–1272, 2012.

Metastatic GIST: Imatinib Mesylate

Blanke CD, Rankin C, Demetri GD, et al: Phase III randomized, intergroup trial assessing imatinib mesylate at two dose levels in patients with unresectable or metastatic gastrointestinal stromal tumors expressing the kit receptor tyrosine kinase: S0033, *J Clin Oncol* 26(4):626–632, 2008.

Metastatic GIST: Sunitinib Malate

Demetri GD, van Oosterom AT, Garrett CR, et al: Efficacy and safety of sunitinib in patients with advanced gastrointestinal stromal tumour after failure of imatinib: a randomised controlled trial, *Lancet* 368(9544):1329–1338, 2006.

Metastatic Disease: Surgery

Raut CP, Posner M, Desai J, et al: Surgical management of advanced gastrointestinal stromal tumors after treatment with targeted systemic therapy using kinase inhibitors, *J Clin Oncol* 24(15):2325–2331, 2006.

Raut CP, Wang Q, Manola J, et al: Cytoreductive surgery in patients with metastatic gastrointestinal stromal tumor treated with sunitinib, *Ann Surg Oncol* 17(2):407–415, 2010.

Predicting Outcomes

Gold JS, Gonen M, Gutierrez A, et al: Development and validation of a prognostic nomogram for recurrence-free survival after complete surgical resection of localised primary gastrointestinal stromal tumour: a retrospective analysis, *Lancet Oncol* 10(11):1045–1052, 2009.

Hirota S, Isozaki K, Moriyama Y, et al. Gain-of-function mutations of c-kit in human gastrointestinal stromal tumors, *Scienc* 379(5350):577–580, 1998.

Miettinen M, Lasota J: Gastrointestinal stromal tumors: pathology and prognosis at different sites, *Semin Diagn Pathol* 23(2):70–83, 2006.

Background

Hirota S, Isozaki K, Moriyama Y, et al: Gain-of-function mutations of c-kit in human gastrointestinal stromal tumors, *Scienc* 379(5350):577–580, 1998.

MORBID OBESITY

Katherine Graw Lamond, MD, MS, and
Anne O. Lidor, MD, MPH

OVERVIEW

Morbid obesity is becoming increasingly prevalent throughout the United States and other industrialized nations. Body mass index (BMI) is a calculated measurement that takes into account height and weight (BMI = weight [kg]/height [m]).

More than 60% of adults in the United States are considered overweight (BMI ≥25), and more than 33% of Americans are obese (BMI ≥30). Almost one in three children and adolescents in the United States are also overweight (Table 1).

The medical comorbidities of obesity are hazardous and include type 2 diabetes, obstructive sleep apnea, heart disease, and increased risk of stroke, gastroesophageal reflux disease (GERD), osteoarthritis, and liver disease. Medical therapies for weight reduction are largely unsuccessful at maintaining significant weight loss in the severely obese population.

Bariatric surgery continues to be the only durable method to achieve sustained weight loss for many patients. Almost 150,000 bariatric procedures are performed in the United States annually. The two fundamental mechanisms of surgical weight loss are: 1, restrictive; and 2, malabsorptive. Some of the procedures described have components of both. There are multiple theories surrounding the metabolic changes which occur following bariatric surgery. These changes can result in a near instant resolution of diabetes mellitus, as well as a change in set-point of body weight. These alterations may occur by hormonal influences and neuronal feedback loops which are made possible by surgery.

The three most common operations include the laparoscopic Roux-en-Y gastric bypass, laparoscopic adjustable gastric band (LAGB), and vertical sleeve gastrectomy. All of these procedures assist with weight loss by restriction of calorie intake. The Roux-en-Y gastric bypass also causes malabsorption of food, which leads to weight loss.

Duodenal switch with biliopancreatic diversion is a less commonly performed malabsorptive and restrictive procedure.

PATIENT SELECTION

In 1991, the National Institute of Health issued a consensus statement regarding the effectiveness of bariatric surgery based on certain patient criteria. Insurance companies, including Medicare and Medicaid, typically base their reimbursements on these indications. The indications include a BMI of 40 or more, or 35 or more with a significant obesity-related comorbidity. Patients must have documented attempts at weight loss that were unsuccessful, typically for a 6-month period. Finally, patients must also be cleared by a dietician and a mental health profession and have no other medical contraindications for surgery.

The American Society for Metabolic and Bariatric Surgery and the American College of Surgeons have produced guidelines of accreditation for both bariatric programs and hospitals. The policies insist that programs can provide excellent surgical technique and thorough postoperative care, follow-up, and specialty consultants.

A multidisciplinary team approach has been shown to provide the best benefit for the evaluation of potential bariatric surgery cases. This team should include a dietician and a mental health professional familiar with bariatric surgery. Their purpose is to obtain a complete dietary and behavioral eating history, educate the patient on postoperative dietary expectations, examine the social support structure, and ensure that any psychiatric or behavioral disorders are optimally controlled.

At the Johns Hopkins Center for Bariatric Surgery, all patients are required to attend a multidisciplinary preoperative education seminar. Preoperative and postoperative participation in obesity and bariatric support groups is also encouraged.

Age limits for surgery have expanded considerably over the last decade. Select centers, including Johns Hopkins, may offer surgery to adolescent patients and to patients over the age of 70 years.

OPERATIVE PROCEDURES

Most bariatric surgical procedures are now performed laparoscopically, with a hospital stay of 48 hours or less. Open surgery may be necessary and planned for patients who undergo revision surgery,

TABLE 1: Body mass index

Classification	Body mass index (kg/m^2)
Underweight	≤18.49
Normal range	18.5-24.9
Overweight	≥25.0
Obese	≥30.0
Obese class I	30.0-34.9
Obese class II (moderately obese)	35.0-39.9
Obese class III (severely obese)	40.0-49.9
Obese class IV (super obese)	≥50.0

those with prior extensive abdominal operations, or patients with a high BMI (>70).

Before surgery, all patients should receive appropriate antibiotics and subcutaneous unfractionated or low–molecular weight heparin within an hour of incision. Obese patients undergoing laparoscopic surgery have a significant risk of development of potentially life-threatening deep venous thrombosis.

Patient positioning on the operative table is essential for safe placement of the patient in the steep reverse Trendelenburg's position. This placement should include a footboard, secured arms and legs, and a split leg table if possible. Laparoscopic entry in a morbidly obese patient can be difficult. The authors have found that the safest way to enter is in the left upper quadrant with direct vision, with a device that allows visualization of the abdominal wall layers during entry with a 0-degree laparoscope (12-mm Visiport; Covidien, Norwalk, Conn).

Laparoscopic Roux-en-Y Gastric Bypass

Gastric bypass (Figure 1) is the most common bariatric procedure performed in the United States (60% to 70%). Numerous reports have shown achievement of durable long-term weight loss and remission of metabolic disease with a reasonably low complication rate.

The authors perform the procedure with five laparoscopic trocars (three 12-mm and two 5-mm) and a subxiphoid puncture for placement of a Nathanson liver retractor (Cook Medical, Bloomington, Ind).

The jejunojejunal anastomosis is created first. The jejunum is divided approximately 40 cm distal to the ligament of Treitz with a 60-mm white stapler cartridge (Endo-GIA Universal XL; Covidien, Norwalk, Conn). The mesentery is divided with a gray stapler cartridge and ultrasonic shears (AutoSonix XL; Covidien, Norwalk, Conn). The proximal biliopancreatic limb of jejunum is then anastomosed to the distal segment of jejunum 75 to 100 cm distal to the point of division. The authors perform this anastomosis in a side-to-side fashion with a white Endo-GIA stapler cartridge and complete it with a blue or tan tristaple Endo-GIA load and running suture. The mesenteric defect is then closed with a running permanent suture to help minimize the risk of internal hernia.

Next, the patient is placed in steep reverse Trendelenburg's position, and the gastric pouch is created. Dissection is performed at the angle of His, to expose the left crus, and at the gastrohepatic ligament, to gain access to the lesser sac. Division of the neurovascular bundle on the lesser curve side of the stomach, just distal to the left gastric artery and vein, is accomplished with a gray vascular cartridge. Multiple 60-mm blue staple or tan tristaple cartridges are then used to transect the stomach up to the angle of His, creating a vertically oriented, 20-mL proximal gastric pouch. Any bleeding at the staple lines is controlled with clips or suture ligation. Care is taken not to

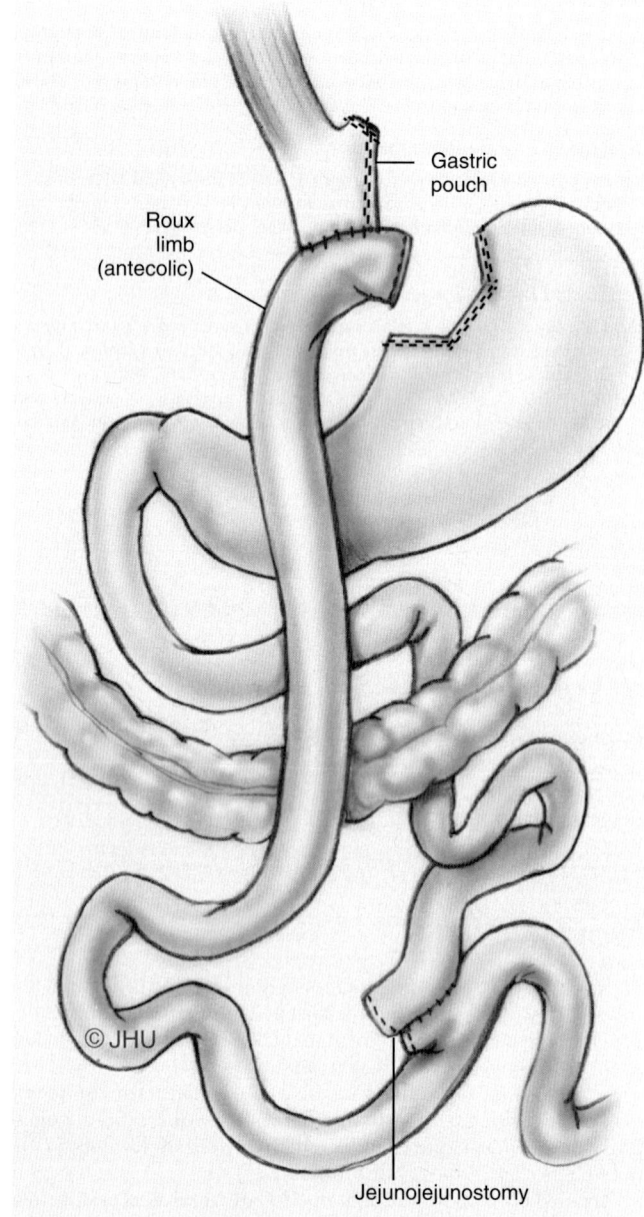

FIGURE 1 Antecolic-antegastric Roux-en-Y gastric bypass. *(Courtesy Corinne Sandone, Johns Hopkins University.)*

place clips in a region that interferes with the gastrojejunal anastomosis.

The authors routinely bring the Roux limb of the jejunum up to the gastric pouch in an antecolic-antegastric orientation. This has been shown to reduce the incidence of internal hernia and is simpler to perform than the retrocolic-retrogastric approach.

The gastrojejunostomy is performed by first suturing the side of the Roux limb to the gastric pouch staple line. A small enterotomy is performed proximal to the end of the Roux limb, and a similarly sized gastrotomy is made in the gastric pouch for insertion of the Endo-GIA blue 45-mm stapler. The stapler is fired with 30-mm of the cartridge to create an appropriately sized anastomosis. A stay suture is then placed on the lesser curve of the opening and is used to retract the anastomosis to expose the posterior staple line. This staple line is reinforced with a running 2-0 suture.

Carefully, a blunt 32F bougie is then passed by the anesthesia or surgical team via the patient's mouth through the gastrojejunal anastomosis and into the Roux limb. The bougie can be seen through the opening formed after the stapler is removed. Another stay suture is placed at the halfway point of this opening. The stay sutures are then elevated, and a 60-mm blue staple or purple tristapler is used to close half of the opening. The remaining small defect is closed with a 2-0 vicryl running suture.

For completion of the gastrojejunostomy, a running 2-0 suture is used to create a second layer across the entire anterior portion of the anastomosis. The resultant ostomy is approximately 12 mm in diameter. A leak test can be performed by clamping the Roux limb distal to the anastomosis and insufflating air via endoscope or orogastric tube, while the anastomosis is submerged in saline solution. Alternatively, a retrograde air leak test can be performed by puncturing the Roux limb with a large bore 14-gauge needle and placing the CO_2 insufflator on low (3 L/min) to provide flow. This can be accomplished via a tool similar to one used for laparoscopic gallbladder drainage. Once the retrograde leak test is performed, a stitch must be placed over the bowel entry point to avoid leakage.

The mesenteric defects between the Roux limb mesentery and the transverse mesocolon (Petersen's defect) is then closed to the level of the transverse colon. If desired, a drain can be placed adjacent to the gastric pouch. If clinically indicated, a Gastrografin swallow study is performed on postoperative day 1 or 2 to check for leakage or obstruction.

Laparoscopic Adjustable Gastric Band

The LAGB received United States Food and Drug Administration approval in 2002. Before this time, the LAGB was widely used in Europe. The band is adjustable via fluid injection into a subcutaneous port to allow for tightening or loosening of the band. Advantages of the band include reversibility, lack of stapling, and ease of placement. The band requires an average of five to six adjustments in the first year after surgery, and its success requires patient compliance with return appointments and a diet and exercise regimen. Relative contraindications for band placement include the super obese (see Table 1), large paraesophageal hernia, prior gastric resection or Nissen fundoplication, and chronic inflammatory changes in the gastroesophageal junction.

The LAGB procedure (Figure 2) is routinely performed via the pars flaccida technique, with two 12-mm trocars, one 5-mm trocar, and a 15-mm trocar for band insertion. The liver is retracted with a Nathanson retractor. Dissection is performed bluntly at the angle of His, freeing up attachments for later insertion of the band. The gastrohepatic ligament adjacent to the lesser curve of the stomach is then divided with electrocautery. The right crus is identified, and the anterior peritoneal tissue is divided. If a hiatal hernia is identified, reinforcement of the hiatus is important, either anteriorly or posteriorly, to discourage further herniation once the band has been placed. Two graspers are used to carefully dissect the plane of tissue posterior to the gastroesophageal junction to provide a tunnel for the LAGB.

An articulating dissector such as the Realize Endoscopic Dissector (RED; Ethicon Endosurgery, Cincinnati, Ohio) is then placed from the right crus toward the angle of His. The RED is then flexed to create a right angle and locked into place. The adjustable band is placed into the abdomen through the 15-mm trocar in the left upper quadrant. The band is secured to the articulating dissector and brought around the stomach while the instrument is withdrawn. The band is then locked into place with approximately a 45-degree angle towards the patient's left shoulder. A minimum of two sutures are then placed from the fundus to the proximal gastric tissue around the band to secure the band into place. This reduces the possibility of band migration or herniation. The authors use two 2-0 vicryl sutures to accomplish this. It is important to ensure that the balloon portion of the band has not been compromised while either placing the band or suturing it into position.

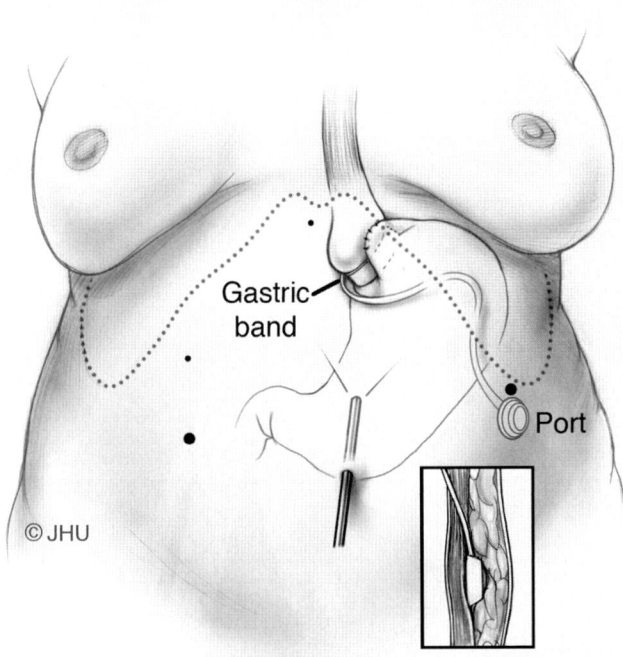

FIGURE 2 Laparoscopic adjustable gastric band. *(Courtesy Corinne Sandone, Johns Hopkins University.)*

The band tubing is brought out through the left upper quadrant port and secured externally to the subcutaneous injection port. Manufacturer's instructions must be followed, so as not to institute fluid or air into the band at this time. When securing the port to the fascia, a sufficient space must be cleared along the rectus sheath. After hemostasis has been achieved in the pocket, the port can be sutured or deployed into position while care is taken to leave the majority of the tubing intraabdominally. Finally, the port can be tested via Huber needle to ensure that the tube and band are functional and not kinked or malpositioned.

The authors do not perform a band fill before 6 weeks after surgery so that the site heals appropriately. If manual palpation of the subcutaneous port is difficult, fluoroscopy can be of assistance to fill the band. In patients with very thick subcutaneous tissue, placement of the band at the costal margin may be advantageous, for better palpation of the port during fills. Bands are typically filled approximately six times during the first year after placement. Each fill volume is 0.5 to 1 mL, depending on the amount of restriction. The patients must be able to swallow liquid without difficulty before leaving the clinic.

Laparoscopic Vertical Sleeve Gastrectomy

Laparoscopic vertical sleeve gastrectomy (LVSG) is the most recently introduced of the bariatric surgery procedures (Figure 3).

As mentioned previously, this procedure is primarily restrictive, as it removes the lateral aspect of the stomach to create a sleeve-like reservoir. The resection may also assist with weight loss by causing hormonally assisted satiety. The fundus produces the proappetite hormone ghrelin, and because the fundus is removed, these hormone levels are reduced after LVSG. Although this bariatric procedure is not reversible, it can be converted into a Roux-en-Y gastric bypass or duodenal switch if greater weight loss is desired.

The LVSG is typically performed with one 5-mm, two 12-mm, and one 15-mm trocar. With the liver retracted with the Nathanson,

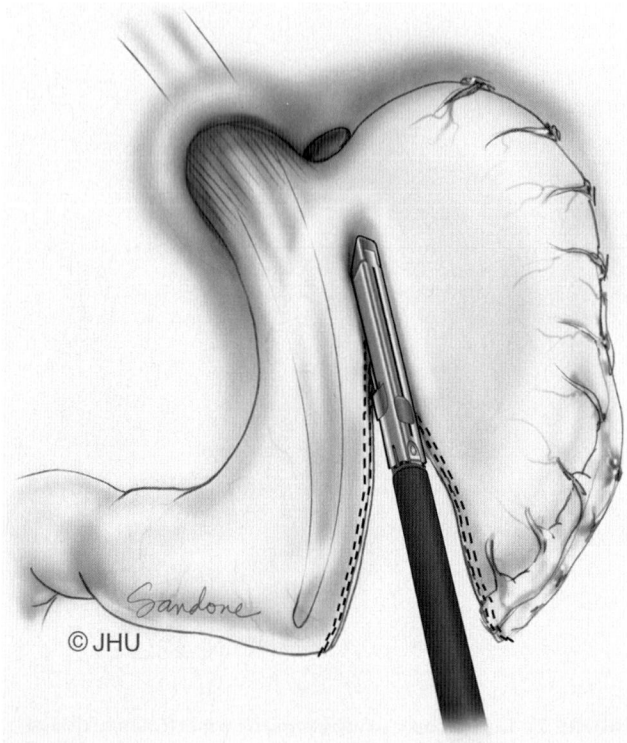

FIGURE 3 Creation of the gastric sleeve. *(Courtesy Corinne Sandone, Johns Hopkins University.)*

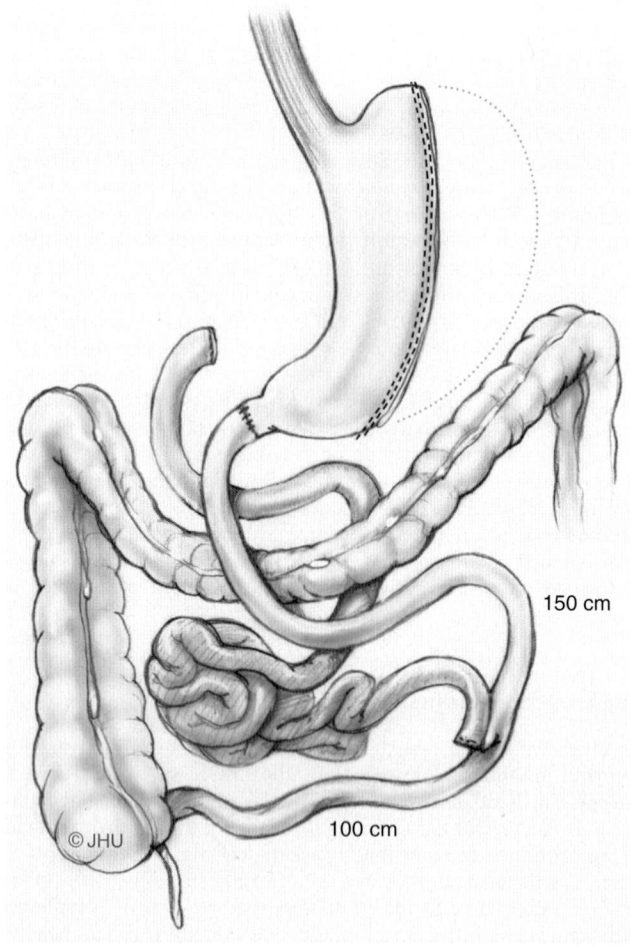

150 cm

100 cm

FIGURE 4 Antecolic duodenal switch with biliopancreatic diversion. *(Courtesy Corinne Sandone, Johns Hopkins University.)*

the short gastric vessels are divided along the greater curve of the stomach. A LigaSure device (Covidien, Norwalk, Conn) is typically used to accomplish this. A 40F blunt tip bougie is placed in the stomach and directed along the lesser curve. The stomach is divided at the greater curvature, beginning 6 cm proximal to the pylorus. Green and blue staple loads are used adjacent to the 40F bougie and extending to the angle of His. The staple line is oversewn or an absorbable buttress material can be used with the staples to assist with hemostasis. To test the anastomosis, an endoscopic air test or liquid dye infused through an orogastric tube can be used.

The partial gastrectomy specimen is removed through the 15-mm trocar site. Care should be taken to repair the fascial opening of this enlarged trocar site to prevent postoperative herniation. The authors typically place a drain in the left upper quadrant that is removed before discharge. As with Roux-en-Y gastric bypass, an UGI study is only performed if clinically indicated.

Laparoscopic Duodenal Switch With Biliopancreatic Diversion

The laparoscopic duodenal switch with biliopancreatic diversion (DS-BPD) is primarily a malabsorptive operation that involves preservation of the pylorus and creation of a short, 100-cm ileal "common channel" (Figure 4). The DS-BPD is the least common bariatric procedure performed because of its surgical complexity and potential for extreme malabsorptive nutritional deficiencies.

This procedure can be performed in a single operation, or in two stages if the patient has a high BMI (>70). The first stage is similar to LVSG. After approximately a 1-year period of weight loss, the patients can be converted to DS-BPD. This is performed by dividing the small bowel 250 cm from the ileocecal valve. The proximal end of bowel is then anastomosed to the distal ileum 100 cm from the cecum.

The patient is then placed in steep reverse Trendelenburg's position and the liver is retracted. If the sleeve gastrectomy portion has not been previously performed, then partial gastrectomy proceeds as described previously. The duodenum is then divided approximately 3 to 4 cm distal to the pylorus with a blue Endo-GIA 60-mm stapler.

The Roux limb is directed in an antecolic fashion, and a side-to-side anastomosis is performed with the duodenum. An air leak or dye test can be performed to check for leaks at the stomach staple line and new duodenal-jejunal anastomosis. Finally, the mesenteric defect is then closed between the Roux limb mesentery and the transverse mesocolon.

OUTCOMES AND COMPLICATIONS

After all bariatric procedures, patients are seen in follow-up at 2 weeks to ensure that they are well hydrated, exercising, and without wound complications. They are then seen at 3, 6, 12, 18, and 24 months and annually thereafter to follow weight loss and nutritional issues. Patients are encouraged to meet with dieticians and remain with their support groups indefinitely.

For 1 month after surgery, patients are all maintained on a high-protein puree consistency diet; they are gradually advanced to solid food. They also receive multivitamins, calcium, and vitamin B_{12} supplements. This is especially important for patients with gastric bypass and DS-BPD who are at higher risk for malabsorption and possible malnutrition. Supplemental iron is always considered for menstruating women.

Weight loss after gastric bypass and DS-BPD occurs primarily in the first 12 to 18 months after surgery and averages approximately 70% and 80% excess weight loss (EWL), respectively. Gastric banding and sleeve gastrectomy typically have less EWL, typically 40% to 50% over a 2-year to 3-year period.

One of the most important outcome measures after bariatric surgery is remission of obesity-related metabolic diseases, such as type 2 diabetes. More than 70% to 80% of patients with diabetes experience complete resolution after undergoing gastric bypass or DS-BPD. The restrictive operations have a 50% remission rate of diabetes. Hypertension, sleep apnea, hyperlipidemia, and fatty liver disease have similar remission rates.

Overall complication rates after bariatric surgery are less than 15% in most reports. Like most surgeries, there are early and late complications for bariatric surgery. Early or perioperative complications include bleeding, anastomotic leaking, and deep venous thrombosis. The mortality rate is less than 1% and is usually attributable to a pulmonary emboli or sepsis from anastomotic leak. Typical symptoms such as anorexia and abdominal pain can be difficult to elicit from morbidly obese patients, so it is important to be prompted by unexplained persistent tachycardia. This should raise suspicion for possible staple line leak or pulmonary embolus and trigger a thorough workup.

Vitamin B_{12}, calcium, iron, vitamin D, and protein deficiencies are long-term complications that can occur within the first year after surgery. Rigorous monitoring of nutrition status is necessary. Vitamin B_1 deficiency can also occur in patients with protracted vomiting after surgery and may present with extremity paresthesias and confusion. Lower extremity weakness and paresthesias can also be seen with vitamin B_{12} deficiency. Anastomotic stenosis and obstruction at the gastrojejunostomy in the first few months after surgery occur in less than 5% of patients after gastric bypass and can usually be managed with endoscopic dilation.

Internal hernias are also a possible complication and can occur at any time after surgery. The symptoms of internal hernia can be similar to an acute bowel obstruction or be chronic in nature and described as postprandial cramping pain. If there is even a slight suspicion of internal hernia, operative intervention is important to avoid bowel ischemia.

In general, the results of weight-loss surgery are excellent, with most patients losing more than 50% of their excess weight and resolving comorbidities. Approximately 10% to 15% of patients either do not achieve significant weight loss or partially regain their weight after 2 to 3 years. Ideally, these patients respond to dietary counseling, although some may need operative revision or conversion to a more malabsorptive procedure, such as the DS-BPD.

Unfortunately, no perfect method exists for choosing the best operation for each individual patient. Certainly, a multidisciplinary team approach is helpful in providing patient support throughout the preoperative and postoperative course. Reducing obesity-related diseases should be the major goal, not merely cosmetic improvement. Patients must understand that bariatric surgery is a tool to assist with weight loss, and it must be combined with drastic changes in dietary, exercise, and lifestyle habits.

SUGGESTED READINGS

ASMBS Clinical Issues Committee: Updated position statement on sleeve gastrectomy as a bariatric procedure, *Surg Obs Relat Dis* 8:e21, 2012.

Adams TD, Gress RE, Smith SC, et al: Long-term mortality after gastric bypass surgery, *N Engl J Med* 357:753, 2007.

Buchwald H, Avidor Y, Braunwald E, et al: Bariatric surgery: a systemic review and meta-analysis, *JAMA* 292:1724, 2004.

Melton, G, Steele K, Schweitzer MA, et al: Suboptimal weight loss after gastric bypass surgery: correlation of demographics, comorbidities, and insurance status with outcomes, *J Gastrointest Surg* 12:250, 2008.

Schweitzer MA, Lidor A, Magnuson TH: 251 consecutive laparoscopic gastric bypass operations using a 2-layer gastrojejunostomy technique with a zero leak rate, *J Laparoendosc Adv Surg Tech* 16:83, 2006.

SMALL BOWEL

SMALL BOWEL OBSTRUCTION

**Lisa M. Kodadek, MD, and
Martin A. Makary, MD, MPH**

OVERVIEW

Although the incidence of mechanical small bowel obstruction (SBO) is decreasing with the advent of laparoscopic surgery, it remains a common surgical problem. Postoperative adhesions are the most common cause and account for nearly 75% of all cases. More than 300,000 patients are hospitalized each year in the United States for an adhesiolysis operation, and SBO represents nearly 20% of surgical admissions for acute abdominal conditions. After some open surgeries, 4% to 30% of patients may develop adhesion-related SBO. Approximately 10% to 30% of patients who undergo adhesiolysis for SBO will develop recurrent SBO and will require an additional operation.

Hernia and neoplasm are other common causes of SBO. Metastatic disease, such as melanoma or ovarian cancer, is more common than primary neoplasm of the small bowel. Less common causes of SBO include Crohn's disease, abscess, intussusception, Meckel's diverticulum, bezoar, gallstone ileus, volvulus, radiation enteritis, traumatic intramural hematoma, congenital abnormalities, and superior mesenteric artery syndrome.

Approximately 25% of all patients with SBO need an operation during the index admission, and those who undergo operative management have fewer recurrent episodes of SBO when compared with those managed without surgery (Foster, 2006). Patients who have not had prior abdominal surgery are far more likely to need surgery than those with a history of abdominal surgery.

Diagnosis of SBO is most often made after a focused history and physical examination. Imaging studies are important adjuncts, and laboratory studies are important to ascertain the degree of metabolic derangement and fluid status. The white blood cell count can help indicate the timing and level of urgency to operate. The etiology of obstruction, the type and location of obstruction, and patient factors including surgical history and comorbidities are important considerations in determining the need for operative intervention. Some patients with regular patterns of recurrent bowel obstruction know themselves best. They often describe a predictable frequency and duration of episodes. In fact, in the absence of leukocytosis or other concerning signs, patients can play an important role in the decision to have surgery versus continue a pattern of nonoperative management, especially in patients at high surgical risk.

Much of the management of SBO surrounds recognition of signs and symptoms concerning for bowel strangulation. For most patients with SBO, bowel strangulation is not present. In these cases, early diagnosis, gastrointestinal decompression, bowel rest, and fluid resuscitation remain the most important strategies. When strangulation is a concern, timely operative intervention is critical to prevent further complications of bowel strangulation, such as perforation, septic shock, and death.

EVALUATION AND DIAGNOSIS

Classic symptoms of SBO include colicky abdominal pain, nausea, emesis, distension, and obstipation. Diarrhea may also be present. Mechanical SBO must be distinguished from nonobstructive motility disorders such as paralytic ileus. Ileus may be associated with abdominal trauma, mesenteric ischemia, or electrolyte disturbances, such as hypokalemia, or most commonly, with open abdominal operations involving bowel manipulation,. The distinction can be subtle and often requires a careful history taking.

The clinical presentation of SBO may vary based on three factors: (1) severity of the obstruction; (2) anatomic site of obstruction; and (3) elapsed time between onset and presentation. Early recognition of SBO severity is critical for proper management. A SBO may be *complete,* meaning the bowel lumen is completely obstructed with no distal passage of stool or air, or only *partial,* meaning the bowel lumen is narrowed and there is some distal passage of bowel contents. An *open-loop* obstruction occurs when proximal decompression is possible via emesis or nasogastric tube (NGT). *Closed-loop* obstruction occurs when both proximal and distal bowel are obstructed; common causes include bowel incarceration in a hernia sac or intestinal torsion. *Simple* obstruction does not compromise blood flow to the bowel; *strangulation* involves compromise of blood flow with inevitable bowel necrosis. Anatomic site of obstruction may be classified as proximal (pylorus to proximal jejunum), intermediate (midjejunum to midileum), or distal (distal ileum to ileocecal valve). The anatomic site of obstruction may also be classified in relation to the intestinal wall as intraluminal (intussusception or bezoar), intramural (neoplasm or Crohn's disease), or extrinsic (adhesions or hernia).

A shorter period of elapsed time is typical between onset of symptoms and presentation for closed-loop obstruction as compared with open-loop obstruction because of the rapid evolution of symptoms in the former. Similarly, a complete obstruction often presents earlier and with more acute findings than partial obstruction. The character of vomitus should be ascertained; feculent vomitus is typically associated with a later presentation and a more established obstruction.

Physical examination findings and signs that portend risk of strangulation include findings consistent with an infection (fever, tachycardia, leukocytosis) and localized abdominal tenderness. Laboratory tests are often advocated for detection of strangulation, but

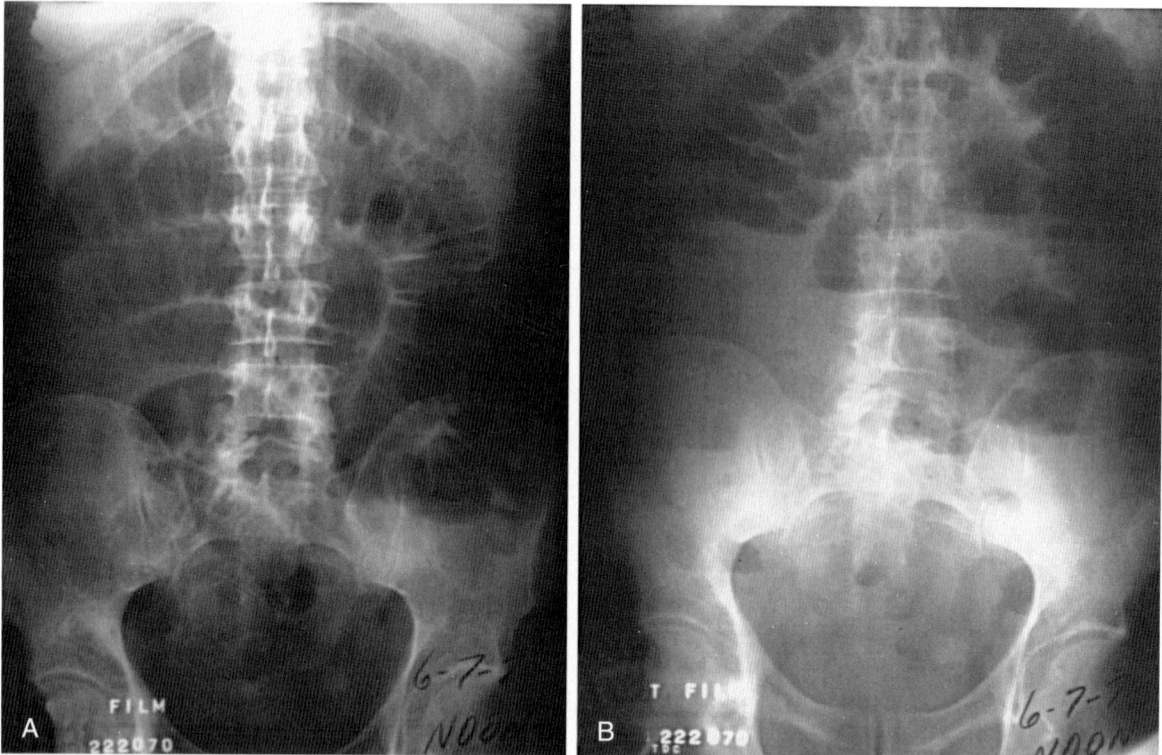

FIGURE 1   Plain abdominal radiographs of a patient with complete small bowel obstruction. **A,** Supine film shows dilated loops of small bowel without evidence of colonic gas. **B,** Upright film shows multiple, short air-fluid levels arranged in a stepwise pattern. *(Courtesy of Melvyn H. Schreiber, MD, The University of Texas Medical Branch, Galveston, Tx.)*

keep in mind that there is no definitive laboratory test to diagnose imminent bowel necrosis and, similarly, there are no laboratory criteria to reliably exclude strangulation. However, increases in serum amylase, serum D-lactate, and intestinal fatty acid binding protein are associated with intestinal ischemia.

Radiographic evaluation often includes an abdominal x-ray series, which includes supine and upright plain radiographs of the abdomen and an upright chest radiograph. The most specific findings for SBO on plain film are dilated loops of small bowel (greater than 3 cm), air-fluid levels, and a paucity of gas in the colon (Figure 1). The chest film is critical to rule out pneumoperitoneum (free air) because this finding in the setting of bowel obstruction may warrant immediate operative exploration (Figure 2). Although an abdominal series may be a reasonable first study, the sensitivity of this test for SBO is poor.

The computed tomographic (CT) scan with intravenous (IV) contrast has become the favored radiographic study for evaluation of SBO. Given the rapid study time, the CT scan has the advantage of more information than an x-ray and evaluation of the passage of contrast when an ileus is also suspected. CT scan also has the advantage of diagnosis of the cause of obstruction such as hernia, mass, inflammatory lesion, or intussusception (Figure 3). CT scan can also be used for assessment of the presence of strangulation with signs such as bowel wall thickening, poor contrast enhancement of the bowel wall, pneumatosis intestinalis, mesenteric vascular engorgement, and mesenteric haziness (Figure 4). CT scan is accurate in distinguishing malignant from benign obstruction in patients with a history of abdominal surgery for malignant disease (Figure 5). Studies have shown that CT scan has an 80% to 90% sensitivity and a 70% to 100% specificity for diagnosis of SBO. One study has shown that helical CT scan has an 84% sensitivity and 90% specificity for diagnosis of the cause of SBO and 100% sensitivity and specificity for diagnosing strangulation (Obuz et al., 2003).

For evaluation of a SBO in the postoperative setting, a study with gastrointestinal contrast can evaluate obstruction. Contrast studies

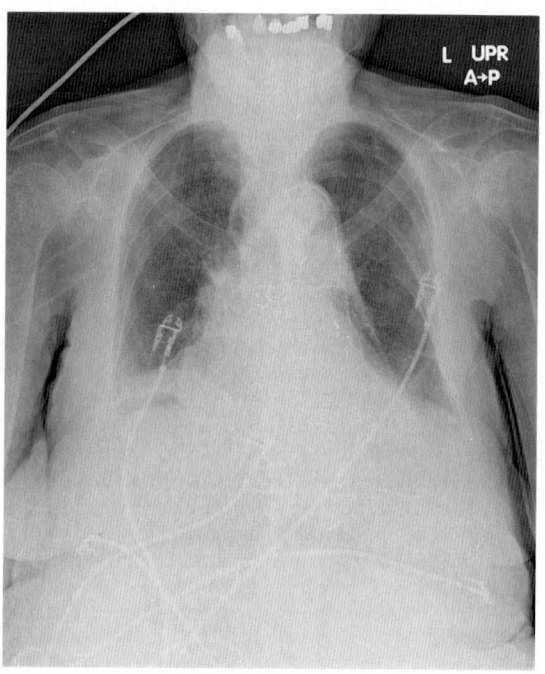

FIGURE 2   Plain upright chest radiograph shows pneumoperitoneum in an individual with bowel perforation. *(Courtesy of Lisa M. Kodadek, MD, The Johns Hopkins Hospital, Baltimore, Md.)*

of the small intestine include CT enterography, enteroclysis, and small bowel series.

CT enterography involves administration of large volumes of oral contrast such as water-methylcellulose solution to achieve intraluminal distension. This study is most often used for patients with Crohn's disease–related strictures and allows excellent imaging of the bowel

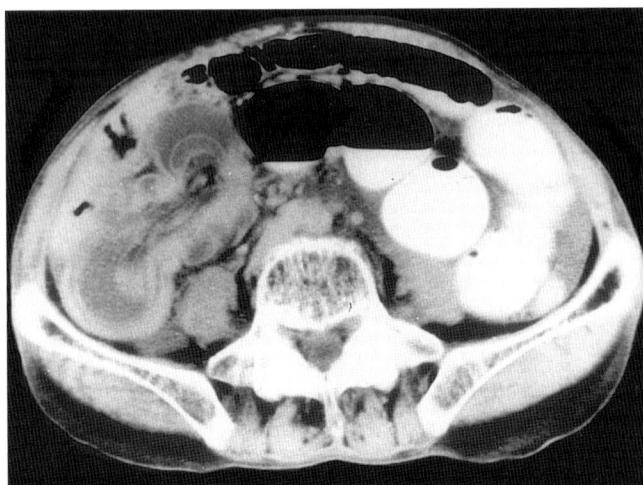

FIGURE 3 Strangulated small bowel obstruction from ileocecal tumor causing intussusception with characteristic "bowel in bowel appearance." *(From Obuz F, Terzi C, Sokmen S, et al: The efficacy of helical CT in the diagnosis of small bowel obstruction,* Eur J Radiol *48(3):299–304, 2003, Fig 5,A.)*

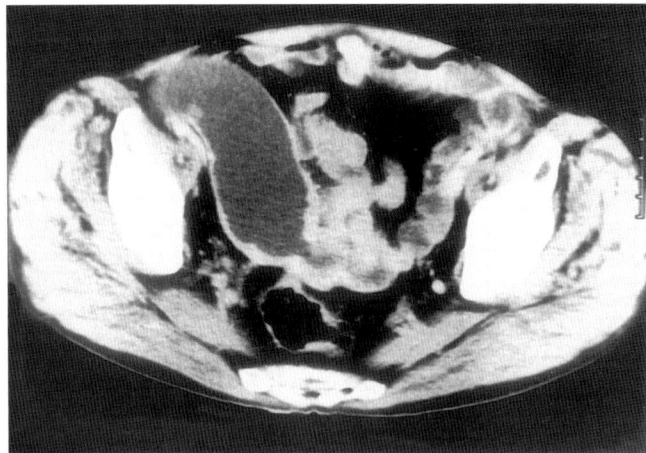

FIGURE 5 Small bowel obstruction from peritoneal carcinomatosis. The patient had a history of total gastrectomy for gastric carcinoma. There is irregularly concentric wall thickness as a result of serosal implants and proximal bowel dilation. *(From Obuz F, Terzi C, Sokmen S, et al: The efficacy of helical CT in the diagnosis of small bowel obstruction,* Eur J Radiol *48(3):299–304, 2003, Fig 2.)*

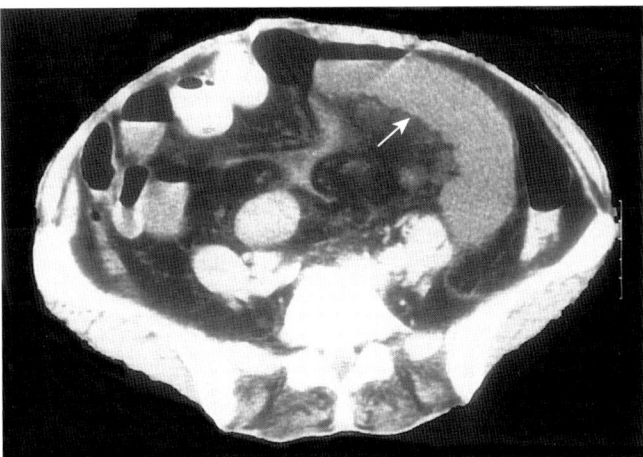

FIGURE 4 Strangulated small bowel obstruction with computed tomographic scan shows poor contrast enhancement of the small bowel wall *(arrow). (From Obuz F, Terzi C, Sokmen S, et al: The efficacy of helical CT in the diagnosis of small bowel obstruction,* Eur J Radiol *48(3):299–304, 2003, Fig 4,A.)*

wall. However, this study is impractical in patients with gastrointestinal distress who are unable to tolerate contrast by mouth. The amount of oral contrast administered and the timing of the oral contrast should be determined based on the purpose of the CT scan.

Enteroclysis, a fluoroscopic study in which the proximal small bowel is instilled with air and contrast, can detect minimal adhesions and mucosal changes. However, this modality has many disadvantages, including the need for nasoenteric intubation and sedation; furthermore, enteroclysis is contraindicated in patients with complete obstruction.

If small bowel series is used, it is important to recognize that barium use may delay CT examination and surgery. Barium should not be used in cases of suspected perforation, strangulation, or a complete or closed loop obstruction. Barium impaction, although rare, is a known complication of this modality and may ultimately worsen a SBO.

An endoscopy procedure is contraindicated for a SBO. The exception to this rule is a gastric outlet obstruction in a patient who is not optimized for surgery (e.g., a malnourished patient). When a narrowing of the distal stomach or duodenum is the cause of a gastric

outlet obstruction (e.g., a periampullary tumor, distal gastric mass, etc.) and endoscopic intervention can dilate or stent the obstruction, endoscopy may be warranted and can be ideal to bridge a patient to surgery at a time when the patient is less sick and better nourished. This interval strategy can lower the complication risk of definitive surgery.

NONOPERATIVE MANAGEMENT

An initial trial of conservative therapy is appropriate for most cases of partial SBO, obstruction in the early postoperative period, obstruction from Crohn's disease, and those patients with history of SBO. Nonoperative management is appropriate provided there is no clinical deterioration and the patient shows some evidence of improvement over the first 12 to 24 hours. Heightened clinical awareness and repeat assessments are critical to ensure that no change in patient status necessitates operative intervention.

Nonoperative management begins with aggressive fluid resuscitation and correction of any electrolyte disorders. Adequate IV access and urinary output monitoring are important. Patients who present after protracted emesis classically have a hypochloremic, hypokalemic metabolic alkalosis with concomitant paradoxical aciduria.

Intraluminal distension can lead to mucosal ischemia. Thus, gastrointestinal decompression and bowel rest is paramount in management of a SBO. A standard NGT provides symptomatic relief, minimizes intraluminal distension with air and fluid, and allows for serial assessment of NGT output as a marker of antegrade small bowel movement. Care should be taken to ensure that nasoenteric tubes are properly functioning because they render the lower and upper esophageal sphincters incompetent and pose a risk for aspiration. A NGT may not be necessary in a patient who does not have gastric dilation.

The use of narcotic pain medication during nonoperative treatment of SBO has been debated because pain medication can mask worsening symptoms that may be diagnostic. Because CT scans are such a tremendous diagnostic tool in management of patients with a SBO, the authors advocate for adequate pain control with a patient-controlled analgesic device or equivalent regimen. Patients with escalating need for pain medication indicate the need for repeat CT scanning.

Many cases of SBO resolve with fluid resuscitation, bowel rest, and gastrointestinal decompression. Over the subsequent days, patients often begin to show improving symptoms, decreased distension, and improving imaging studies. Occasionally, small bowel series or enteroclysis may be helpful for those patients who do not achieve complete resolution, especially in the postoperative period when a prolonged ileus may be high on the differential diagnosis. For those with Crohn's disease, medical therapy (steroids and other immunosuppressive therapy) may help resolve partial SBO from inflammatory lesions. For those with SBO after blunt abdominal trauma, obstruction is typically the result of an intramural hematoma and usually resolves with nonoperative therapy after 2 to 4 weeks. Total parenteral nutrition may be considered for selected patients with SBO to prevent the sequelae of negative nitrogen balance. Patients with Crohn's disease and trauma are two common exceptions to the principle that SBO patients without prior surgery are more likely to need surgery intervention.

A recent systematic review and meta-analysis of 14 prospective studies has shown diagnostic and therapeutic use of water-soluble contrast in patients with adhesive SBO (Branco et al., 2010). The appearance of contrast in the colon within 4 to 24 hours after administration had a sensitivity of 96% and specificity of 98% in predicting resolution of SBO. In cases in which contrast reached the colon, obstruction resolved in 99% without surgery. In cases in which contrast failed to reach the colon, obstruction failed to resolve without surgery in 90% of patients.

OPERATIVE MANAGEMENT

Approximately 25% of inpatients admitted for a SBO need an operation. Patients with a complete or high-grade partial SBO are most likely to need surgery. Patients with evidence of peritonitis, bowel perforation, or strangulation need immediate surgery. Patients with development of fever, tachycardia, or worsening leukocytosis should be considered for operative intervention.

Patients with no history of abdominal surgery are unlikely to have adhesions and are likely to need operative management. Hernia, tumor, or Crohn's disease should be considered in the differential for this group of patients.

Patients with a history of intraabdominal malignancy may be difficult to manage. When a patient has known recurrent disease, nonoperative therapy or surgical palliation may be most appropriate depending on the stage of the malignancy and the patient's goals. However, studies have shown that two thirds of these patients have a lesion amenable to surgical correction such as an adhesive band. Surgical palliation for patients with advanced disease such as carcinomatosis may involve a percutaneous gastrostomy tube placement, a diverting ileostomy, or a limited small bowel resection. Carcinomatosis can be difficult to ascertain with preoperative imaging.

Intussusception is much more common in the pediatric population, but it may present in adults as a SBO. In adults, intussusception is the result of a pathologic nidus such as a polyp or tumor. Whereas most pediatric cases are benign, 50% of adults with intussusception are diagnosed with a malignancy. Radiographic decompression is often successful for pediatric patients, but adults generally need surgery to rule out a malignant lead point.

For patients with a history of recurrent SBO, an initial trial of nonoperative treatment is preferred. However, if the patient does not respond to a course of bowel rest, gastrointestinal decompression, and use of total parenteral nutrition, operative intervention is warranted. These cases can present a significant technical challenge because most patients have undergone multiple prior abdominal operations.

For patients with suspected duodenal intramural hematoma after traumatic injury, surgical intervention is infrequently needed. However, if symptoms of obstruction persist beyond 6 to 8 weeks, consideration of possible progression to fibrosis is important. Surgery should be reserved for those with development of fibrosis; gastrojejunostomy or duodenojejunostomy may be necessary to bypass the area of fibrotic narrowing.

Rare sources of intraluminal obstruction include bezoar, gallstone ileus, and barium impaction. These conditions generally cause complete obstruction and warrant surgery. Patients with gallstone ileus usually have radiographically apparent stones within the intestinal lumen, often in the distal ileum or at the ileocecal valve. Pneumobilia may also be apparent from a biliary-enteric fistula. Operative management involves enterotomy in a region of proximally dilated small bowel with stone extraction. Partial small bowel resection may be required for severely impacted stones. The entire small bowel should be inspected for evidence of remaining stones. Cholecystectomy and biliary-enteric fistula repair should be performed to prevent recurrence of gallstone ileus and cholangitis from reflux of intestinal contents. If the fistula occurs between the distal common bile duct and the duodenum, the definitive repair necessitates closure of the fistula and biliary reconstruction with choledochojejunostomy. The timing of cholecystectomy and fistula repair depends on a patient's overall condition and hemodynamic stability.

Technical Considerations

When small bowel distention does not allow for adequate visualization with laparoscopic insufflation, a laparotomy is performed. In cases in which the bowel is decompressed or the distention is mild, a laparoscopic approach can be attempted, but the initial port site should not involve a previous scar where adhesive disease could risk a bowel perforation on entry. Data from retrospective trials suggest that laparoscopy may have lower mortality and morbidity, faster recovery, and shorter hospital stay than the traditional open approach for SBO. Some series have reported an 80% success rate for resolution of SBO with laparoscopic approach. Surgeon experience likely plays a major factor in successful laparoscopic adhesiolysis.

Once the obstruction has been addressed with appropriate surgical treatment, a diligent and complete determination of bowel viability is critical. The bowel often appears pink and clearly viable; assessment can be rendered with subjective criteria in this situation.

If a large segment of bowel appears threatened, or if bowel viability cannot be clearly established, the surgeon can leave the abdomen open with plans to return to the operating room in 24 to 48 hours for a repeat assessment. If a small segment of bowel appears threatened, resection and closure at the initial operation is usually best.

Luminal decompression may be a helpful maneuver to promote blood flow to bowel that is distended and edematous from obstruction. This maneuver may also help allow closure of the abdomen. Enteric contents may be milked in the retrograde direction to reach the NGT. This should be performed in close communication with the anesthesia team to ensure a properly functioning NGT given the risk for aspiration. Great care should be taken to avoid extensive manipulation and injury. If bowel resection is deemed necessary, decompression can be achieved by inserting a drainage catheter into the proximal segment before completing the anastomosis.

Adhesion Prevention

The overall increased use of laparoscopy in surgery is decreasing the incidence of SBO from adhesions. Laparoscopy when possible results in a lower rate of long-term SBO than laparotomy.

Bioresorbable membrane technology holds promise in adhesion prevention but has not been shown to decrease the rate of SBO. Currently available products include Seprafilm (chemically modified sodium hyaluronate/carboxymethylcellulose; Genzyme, Cambridge, Mass) and Interceed (oxidized regenerated cellulose; Ethicon, Somerville, NJ). These products are supplied as a thin transparent film and may be difficult to handle. SurgiWrap (polyactide; MAST Biosurgery, San Diego, Calif) is also a bioresorbable sheet but may be easier to handle and can be used laparoscopically. Although bioresorbable membrane technology has been shown to decrease adhesion formation and severity, no evidence is found to suggest that these products reduce the rate of SBO or decrease the need for reoperation.

SUGGESTED READINGS

Branco BC, Barmparas G, Schnuriger B, et al: Systematic review and meta-analysis of the diagnostic and therapeutic role of water-soluble contrast agent in adhesive small bowel obstruction, *Br J Surg* 97:470–478, 2010.

Foster NM, McGory ML, Zingmond DS, et al: Small bowel obstruction: a population-based appraisal, *J Am Coll Surg* 203:170–176, 2006.

Landercasper J, Cogbill TH, Merry WH, et al: Long-term outcome after hospitalization for small-bowel obstruction, *Arch Surg* 128:765–770, 1993.

Obuz F, Terzi C, Sokmen S, et al: The efficacy of helical CT in the diagnosis of small bowel obstruction, *Eur J Radiol* 48:299–304, 2003.

Ray NF, Denton WG, Thamer M, et al: Abdominal adhesiolysis: inpatient care and expenditures in the United States in 1994, *J Am Coll Surg* 186:1–9, 1998.

THE MANAGEMENT OF CROHN'S DISEASE OF THE SMALL BOWEL

Isaac Howley, MD, and
Susan L. Gearhart, MD, FACS, FASCAS

OVERVIEW

Crohn's disease (CD), or *regional enteritis,* is a complex, multifactorial disorder that affects the entirety of the gastrointestinal (GI) tract. The hallmark of the disease is a chronic, relapsing, and remitting inflammatory process that may ultimately cause infectious, obstructive, hemorrhagic, or neoplastic complications. The cause of CD is unknown, but there is strong evidence of a genetic predilection; more than 100 genes and loci for inflammatory bowel disease (IBD) have been defined. First-degree relatives of patients with IBD have a five-fold to twentyfold increased risk for developing the disease. The genetic variants of the *NOD2* gene appear to have the greatest association with CD; however, the presence of this gene and others varies among different populations of various descents. Environmental factors, such as intestinal microbes, are also known to influence the development of the disease.

There is currently no known cure for CD. Medical interventions are aimed at control of symptoms and prevention of long-term sequelae, such as disease recurrence and loss of functional intestinal length, which leads to malabsorption. Therefore endpoints of medical therapy are somewhat ambiguous, with no universally accepted mark of efficacy for treatments. Commonly used endpoints include various quality-of-life grading systems, evidence of mucosal healing by endoscopic assessment, and failure of medical therapy, documented by the requirement for surgical intervention. Surgical interventions are aimed at restoring normal gastrointestinal function when medical therapy has not been successful. Approximately 70% of patients with CD eventually require surgery for the disease, and 50% of these require a second operation for disease recurrence.

Patients with CD frequently present with nonspecific symptoms such as abdominal pain, bloating, diarrhea, and anorexia. Unlike acute abdominal processes such as appendicitis, CD may be characterized by progressive, chronic, intermittent GI distress that is localized or diffuse. Many affected patients are malnourished and anemic. Approximately 40% of affected patients have involvement of the terminal ileum, 20% have involvement of the colon, 10% have isolated disease in the jejunum and ileum, and 10% have isolated involvement of the anus. The remaining 20% have disease in multiple locations throughout the GI tract.

The clinical diagnosis of CD is based on an accurate history and physical examination, including anal examination, and a combination of several of the following studies: (1) upper endoscopy to evaluate gastroesophageal and duodenal disease; (2) colonoscopy to characterize colonic or ileal disease; (3) traditional small bowel contrast studies, advanced computed tomographic (CT) enterography, or magnetic resonance enterography to reveal intraluminal manifestations that include strictures and fistulas, and (4) traditional CT scan with oral contrast media to evaluate extraluminal complications such as intraabdominal abscesses or inflammatory masses. The disease is confirmed pathologically when gross features of the disease—including fat wrapping, aphthous ulcers, and transmural inflammation—are seen. Microscopic inspection of gastrointestinal biopsy samples may reveal increased inflammatory features, architectural abnormalities, and epithelial abnormalities.

MEDICAL MANAGEMENT

In the Vienna Classification of CD, age, location, and disease type are the key variables used to predict disease behavior. The most widely quoted variable is disease type, which is based on the following phenotypes; *inflammatory, fibrostenotic,* and *penetrating.* This classification can be problematic at times because there is crossover that occurs between each phenotype, and perianal fistulizing disease does not seem to characterize a specific phenotype. However, CD classification systems may be helpful in guiding therapy and predicting recurrent disease. Recurrent disease commonly occurs with the same phenotypic presentation and in the same anatomic location: for example, ileocolic fibrostenotic disease recurrence at the site of a prior ileocecectomy anastomosis. Furthermore, the inflammatory phenotype in CD is the most common and frequently the most responsive to medical therapy. Fibrostenotic phenotypes tend to be the least responsive to medical therapy.

In the absence of a clear surgical indication, CD is managed with medical therapy. Several classes of medications are used to treat it, including aminosalicylate (5-ASA) derivatives, steroids, antibiotics, immunomodulators, and biologic agents. 5-ASA derivatives, steroids, and immunomodulators have been the mainstay therapy for CD since the 1970s and have well-described side effects. The mechanisms by which these agents exert their effects are uncertain and probably nonspecific. Newer entities, the biologic agents, are intended to target known immune and inflammatory pathways. Although highly specific, biologic agents can cause severe side effects, such as allergic reactions and increased incidence of new or reactivation of old viral infections (meningitis, John Cunningham [JC] virus, progressive multifocal leukoencephalopathy). Furthermore, biologic therapy is expensive. As biologic therapy becomes more widely used, more information regarding its safety and efficacy will become available.

Smoking cessation is among the most effective treatments for Crohn's disease, as well as being inexpensive and free of toxic side effects. Among patients with Crohn's, smoking is associated with a higher incidence of fibrostenotic and penetrating phenotypes. In patients with CD who smoke, perianal disease is worse, rates of surgical therapy are higher, and rates of postsurgical recurrence are higher. Despite its clear benefits, smoking cessation remains a difficult goal for such patients, as it does with other patients. Even in cessation programs targeted at patients with CD, only 12% to 23% of patients have been reported to be successful with abstinence on long-term follow-up.

Traditionally, medications have been prescribed along a "step-up" approach (Figure 1). Therapy begins with the least toxic, least expensive, but least effective drugs, such as 5-ASA derivatives, and proceeds "upwards" with enterally active steroids, antimetabolites, systemic corticosteroids, and biologic drugs. There has been considerable discussion about a "top-down" approach, which starts with powerful biologic therapies for treating medication-naïve disease. This approach to use the most effective therapies initially has not achieved widespread use. Although certain CD types may respond to more aggressive therapy first, a top-down approach involves treating many patients who would be well served by the less expensive and less toxic regimens.

In the following paragraphs, the most commonly used medications in the treatment of CD are discussed (Table 1). Aminosalicylates such as sulfasalazine and mesalamine are antiinflammatory derivatives used orally or rectally to treat and maintain remission in mild to moderate CD with a known 70% response rate. These 5-ASA derivatives are formulated to allow distribution of medication to a specific intestinal location. Mesalamine (Pentasa) 4 g/day, which is released throughout the gastrointestinal tract, has been shown to be effective in the treatment of small bowel and large bowel disease. Derivatives of 5-ASA have not been shown to prevent relapse of CD, are not associated with increased perioperative complications, and can be taken until surgery and restarted immediately afterwards.

Steroids may be used orally, intravenously, or rectally for the treatment of acute moderate to severe disease. In the short term, steroids decrease inflammation in 60% to 92% of affected patients and allow for improved intestinal function, but long-term steroid dependence is associated with significant side effects that include growth retardation, osteopenia, cushingoid features, hypertension, glomerular nephritis, cataracts, necrosis of the femoral head, and adrenal suppression. It has been reported that up to 35% of patients treated with corticosteroids develop either steroid dependence or steroid

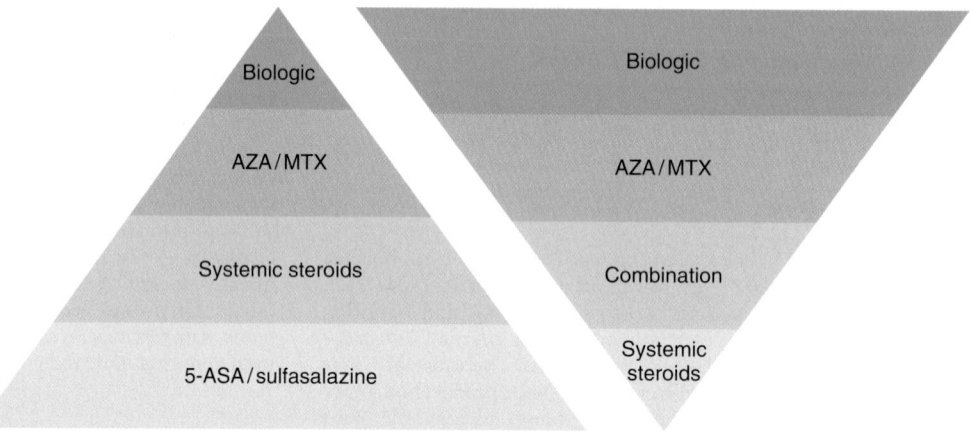

FIGURE 1 Step-up approach versus top-down approach in the medical management of Crohn's disease. *5-ASA, aminosalicylate; AZA, azathioprine; MTX, methotrexate. (Modified from Buchner AM, Blonski W, Lichtenstein GR: Update on the management of Crohn's disease, Curr Gastroenterol Rep 13(5):465-474, 2011.)*

TABLE 1: Indications and risk of perioperative use of commonly used medication for the treatment of Crohn's disease

Medical therapy	Indication	Effect on perioperative risks
Aminosalicylate (5-ASA) derivatives	Mild acute small and large bowel disease	None
Corticosteroids	Mild to moderate ileocecal disease No role in maintenance	Increased infection risk, poor wound healing greatest at ≥40 mg/day For adrenal insufficiency, stress dose needed if steroids have been used in the past 6 mo (no need for stress dose steroids with oral budesonide therapy)
Antibiotics	Perianal disease, in combination for acute intestinal disease	Increased prevalence of *Clostridium difficile* colitis
Immunomodulators	Maintenance therapy for moderate to severe disease	None
Biologic agents	Acute moderate to severe disease	Recommendation to stop therapy 30 days before surgery

resistance. Unless stress-dose steroids are administered, patients receiving long-term steroid therapy are at risk for perioperative adrenal crisis that can result in hemodynamic instability. In addition, long-term use of steroids can result in poor wound healing, increased risk of infectious complications, and other perioperative problems. Long-term use of steroids may complicate diagnosis of abdominal complications such as perforation and abscess by masking signs and symptoms of disease. The side effects of systemic corticosteroids can be avoided by the use of budesonide (Entocort), which has extensive first-pass liver metabolism. Budesonide has been shown to be more effective than placebo for inducing remission in patients with mild to moderate CD of the terminal ileum and proximal colon. However, no data suggest that budesonide alone can reduce the incidence or relapse, and therefore it has no utility in maintenance therapy. Because of the limited systemic effects, the use of budesonide has not been shown to be problematic during the perioperative period.

The rationale for the use of antibiotics in the treatment of CD is the hypothesis that the cause of CD may be related to unidentified bacterial pathogens. A meta-analysis showed that treatment with broad-spectrum antibiotics was more than twice as effective as placebo at inducing clinical improvement. Antibiotics are often used in conjunction with other medications for the treatment of acute inflammation, including perianal fistulas. Fluoroquinolones (e.g., ciprofloxacin), metronidazole, and rifaximin are commonly used. Antibiotics have not been shown to be detrimental when used in the perioperative setting, but they are associated with an increase in the prevalence of *Clostridium difficile* diarrhea in patients with inflammatory bowel disease. This complication may occur even in patients receiving metronidazole, despite this drug's frequent use in the treatment of *C. difficile*.

Immunologic antimetabolites such as azathioprine (AZA) and 6-mercaptopurine (6-MP) work by inhibiting RNA synthesis, having a disproportionate effect on the rapidly proliferating lymphocyte cell lines that mediate CD. These drugs have a slow onset of action (up to 6 months) and are not used in the treatment of acute flares, but they are a mainstay of maintenance therapy for patients in remission. Their use is particularly beneficial in reducing corticosteroid use and the incidence of postoperative recurrence of disease. Studies have shown that in patients who take an immunomodulator postoperatively, the need for recurrent surgery is reduced by 8% and the risk of endoscopic recurrence is reduced by 15% at 1 year. The disadvantage of immunomodulator therapy is the increased rate of adverse events that necessitate withdrawal of the drug in up to 17% of patients in some studies. Side effects include pancreatitis, flu-like symptoms, myelosuppression, and lymphoma. To limit side effects, it is important to evaluate thiopurine methyltransferase (TPMT) activity in each patient before therapy with 6-MP or AZA begins. This enzyme is responsible for the metabolism of these drugs, and up to 11% of patients have abnormal TPMT activity. There is no evidence of higher rates of postoperative complications with these drugs. Methotrexate (MTX), a folic acid antagonist that inhibits purine synthesis, has also been used for remission in the attempt to avoid steroids. A Cochrane meta-analysis showed that low-dose MTX is threefold more effective than placebo in maintaining remission. The side effects of higher dose MTX include myelosuppression and hepatotoxicity.

Biologic agents are the newest, most effective, and most expensive class of medications in the CD armamentarium; response rates are as high as 70%, even in previously difficult-to-treat, penetrating disease. The three biologic agents in use in the United States are infliximab (IFX, Remicade), adalimumab (Humira), and certolizumab pegol (Cimzia). All are directed at tumor necrosis factor (TNF) and reduce T-cell proliferation, thereby decreasing inflammation. These medications are delivered by intravenous infusion or subcutaneous injection and may be used for both acute flares and, on a continuing basis, to maintain remission. Side effects include infusion reactions, increased risk of infections such as tuberculosis and histoplasmosis, and lymphoma. A newer selective adhesion

molecule inhibitor, natalizumab (Tysabri), has been evaluated for use in patients with active moderate to severe CD who do not respond to or tolerate conventional biologic agents. Some research findings suggest an increased risk of postoperative complications in patients receiving biologic therapy, especially intraabdominal sepsis and wound healing. To date, these studies have focused only on infliximab and are limited by small study populations and heterogeneous methods. It is best to avoid operating on patients with therapeutic levels of biologic agents. Unfortunately this is frequently not possible, as patients needing operations are those whom have received maximal medical management without response.

Combination therapy for the treatment of patients with moderate to severe disease has gained favor since the publication of the recent Study of Immunomodulator-Naive Patients in Crohn's Disease (SONIC). In this study, the 508 participants were randomly assigned to receive AZA alone, IFX alone, or AZA plus IFX. The results showed that patients treated with combination therapy (AZA plus IFX) had a nearly twofold increase in steroid-free clinical remission and mucosal healing rates at 26 weeks. Furthermore, immunoreaction to IFX therapy was reduced when the drug was given in combination. No data suggested that combination therapy may be beneficial in the prevention of postoperative recurrence of disease.

Patients with CD may require nutritional supplementation. Absorption may be decreased as a result of inflammation or stricture. Furthermore, bacterial overgrowth in prestenotic dilated intestinal loops may contribute to malabsorption. Absorption of fat-soluble vitamins such as vitamins A, D, E, and K may be reduced as a result of ileal disease or prior resections. Bowel rest with parenteral supplementation may also be used as a treatment for CD, but this has not been supported by results of randomized studies. Furthermore, research continues with regard to the disease-modifying properties of enteral formulas.

A newer modality that is gaining enthusiasm is endoscopic balloon dilatation. Small bowel CD strictures may be endoscopically dilated; however, endoscopic therapy is frequently limited by inaccessibility and fixed strictures. A systematic review of this treatment showed that strictures dilated endoscopically that are 4 cm or smaller were more likely (odds ratio = 4.01) not to necessitate surgery. Furthermore, the reported mean complication rate was 2%.

INDICATIONS FOR SURGICAL MANAGEMENT

Timing of when a patient should go to surgery is important in the management of this disease. Treatment planning is best performed by a multidisciplinary team that includes gastroenterologists, surgeons, radiologists, pathologists, nutritionists, and, when needed, enterostomal therapists and psychologists. As all surgeons know, it is very difficult to promote healing and improve quality of life in a malnourished, immunocompromised patient. In part for this reason, a multicenter trial is currently under way to investigate whether patients should continue with more aggressive therapy (biologic) or undergo laparoscopic surgery for distal ileitis. Further evaluations of the timing of surgery in this population are needed.

The most common indication for surgical intervention is medically refractory CD. Disease symptoms continue or worsen with therapy, or patients are unable to tolerate pharmacologic treatment. Patients may continue to lose weight, have substantial diarrhea, or have recurrent abdominal pain despite optimal therapy, and they may elect to undergo surgery. Growth retardation secondary to chronic disease and use of medications, including steroids, are an indication for surgery in up to 50% of children with CD. Other indications include progression of disease to complete obstruction, abscess, fistulization, presence of neoplasia, toxic megacolon, and GI hemorrhage.

The development of a bowel obstruction in CD frequently results from acute inflammation on top of preexisting fibrostenotic disease.

As with patients without CD, conservative management with nasogastric tube decompression, bowel rest, and IV hydration is frequently appropriate, and medical management may continue if symptoms resolve. Progressive disease is a common feature, and surgery may be required for recurrent obstructions.

Inflammatory masses (phlegmon) and abscesses typically cause abdominal pain and obstruction; in severe cases, they progress to fistulas or become the source of systemic sepsis. They may be palpated on examination or noted on computed tomography (Figure 2). When patients are stable, initial treatment consists of percutaneous drainage of the liquid component under ultrasound or CT guidance. Antibiotics with gram-negative and anaerobic coverage are prescribed until the surrounding inflammation has resolved. A period of initial bowel rest aids in decreasing inflammation and should be maintained while symptoms persist. Surgery may be necessary if the inflammation does not completely resolve with drainage, bowel rest, and antibiotics. If necessary, parenteral nutrition can be used for nutritional supplementation while the abscess resolves and inflammation subsides.

Not all internal fistulas in CD are symptomatic, and some may not require surgical therapy. A large fistula from proximal ileum to the distal sigmoid colon may cause a functional bypass of absorptive intestinal surface and consequent diarrhea or malabsorption, whereas a short fistula from the terminal ileum to the cecum may be tolerated without difficulty. In addition, enterocutaneous or colocutaneous fistulas, fistulas to the vagina after hysterectomy, or fistulas to the bladder are often symptomatic and require surgical resection.

Patients with CD are at increased risk for neoplasia. Colorectal cancer is more prevalent among such patients than in the general population, and small bowel adenocarcinoma is as much as 100 times more likely to occur. In patients without IBD, the incidence of small bowel cancer tends to decrease from proximal to distal small bowel. In CD, the incidence increases along the length of the small bowel and mimics disease distribution. Sporadic small bowel cancers form a mass or growth that is noted on imaging or at the time of resection. In CD, cancers are often not associated with a mass lesion, which complicates diagnosis and screening. Therefore, it is recommended that in patients with long-standing CD, any strictures treated with strictureplasty and not resection should be subjected to biopsy.

Hemorrhage and toxic megacolon are common indications for surgery in ulcerative colitis, but these are much less common in CD. GI hemorrhage can originate from anywhere in the GI tract. Localization techniques—including endoscopy, angiography, and nuclear imaging—can be helpful in preoperative planning or in directing treatment. Intraoperative enteroscopy can be helpful in localizing small bowel hemorrhage. Toxic megacolon occurs in the setting of Crohn's colitis, and significant dilatation of the colon with signs of sepsis such as leukocytosis, fever, or hemodynamic instability is an indication for immediate surgical intervention.

Technical Considerations of Surgical Intervention

Thorough preoperative evaluation is paramount in the success of operative outcomes in patients with CD. Such patients may be dehydrated from chronic diarrhea and may have electrolyte imbalances that should be addressed before surgery. Malnutrition, anemia, and vitamin deficiencies are common and may require preoperative repletion or, on occasion, parenteral supplementation. Knowledge of preoperative medications is necessary. Concern remains about increased infectious complications among patients receiving anti–TNF therapy, and attempts should be made to delay surgery for several weeks after administration when possible. Chronic steroid use causes adrenal insufficiency. Patients maintained on chronic steroids, or recently weaned from steroids, may require perioperative stress dosing, generally with intravenous hydrocortisone or methylprednisolone. Steroid doses should be rapidly tapered over several postoperative days to avoid adrenal insufficiency. Patients who have been appropriately surgically treated for CD should not require continued long-term steroid administration.

Preoperative planning for all but the most urgent indications should involve a careful review of surgical history and thoughtful use of imaging studies. This is particularly true for planning a laparoscopic approach, in which there will be loss of tactile sensation. Reports of previous operations should be obtained and reviewed as part of the preoperative planning process. This information allows estimation of residual small bowel length, an important factor for deciding between resection and strictureplasty. Colonoscopy helps to evaluate the extent of colonic disease. CT or MRI, capsule or push enteroscopy, and upper GI series with small bowel follow-through studies help evaluate small bowel disease, especially abscesses, strictures, and fistulas (see Figure 2). Upper endoscopy is useful in evaluating for gastroesophageal and duodenal disease.

The appropriate preoperative evaluation guides discussions of informed consent, although these discussions should account for the fact that some pathologic processes may not be detectable until operative exploration. It is important to note that up to 50% of fistulas are not detected on preoperative evaluation, and strictures distal to a proximal obstruction may be undetectable before exploration. Consent forms should also address possible additional surgical treatments, including creation of a diverting ostomy. In addition, malabsorption after small bowel resection may occur when insufficient small bowel remains, especially in the absence of an ileocecal valve. Loss of the terminal ileum may lead to deficiencies of fat, fat-soluble vitamins, and bile salts, which cause increased diarrhea. Severe malnutrition and diarrhea may occur, especially when less than 200 cm of small bowel remains.

Any operation on a patient with CD should begin with a thorough intraabdominal examination, with evaluation of both known and possible previously undetected pathologic processes that may be amenable to surgical repair. The small bowel and intraperitoneal colon should be inspected in entirety and their total length measured to assess the potential for the development of the short gut syndrome. Because CD is a lifelong recurring disease, affected patients are at risk for intestinal failure with sequential resections.

All attempts should be made to preserve intestinal length when possible. Only symptomatic and heavily diseased segments should be resected. Findings of mild disease, such as creeping fat, are not an indication for resection. A Foley catheter may be used to grossly evaluate segments for resection or strictureplasty. After gentle insertion of the catheter into the intestinal loop via an enterotomy in the anticipated site of resection or strictureplasty, the balloon is inflated

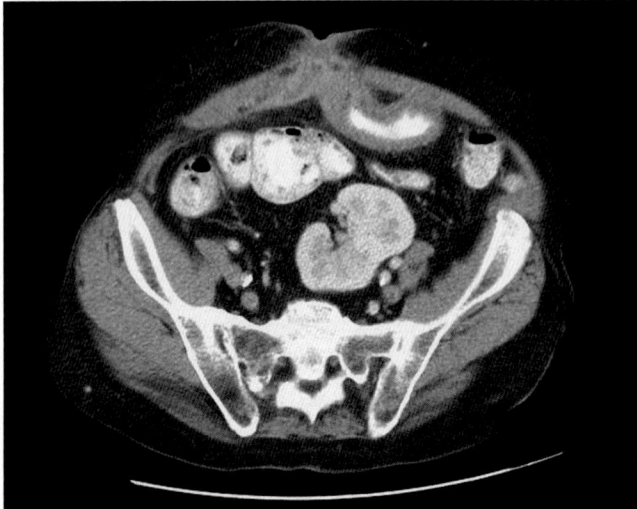

FIGURE 2 Computerized tomographic image of small intestinal stricture with an associated enterocutaneous fistula in Crohn's disease.

to 1 cm and gently pulled through the potentially narrowed bowel. Any site through which the balloon does not easily pass should be carefully evaluated for additional surgical therapy.

Longer segments of small intestine and any segment of large intestine affected with CD are resected with a primary anastomosis. A 2-cm margin of grossly normal-appearing bowel is all that is necessary. Microscopic evaluation of margins is not necessary during resections for benign disease. The authors typically use a GIA stapler to divide the bowel at the proximal and distal resection margins, and create a classic side-to-side, functional end-to-end two-layered hand-sewn anastomosis. Often the bowel may be thicker and less amenable to stapling; however, a stapled anastomosis is an acceptable alternative.

To preserve bowel length, strictureplasty should be considered when technically feasible, especially in patients who have undergone prior resection. Contraindications to strictureplasty, relative and absolute, are listed in Table 2. For short, isolated segments, a 2-layered Heineke-Mikulicz strictureplasty can be used. A Finney strictureplasty is useful for longer segments but has the unwanted side effect of a capacious intestinal side diverticulum. The Michelassi strictureplasty is an option for more extensive disease of the small bowel. In the appropriately selected patient, strictureplasty provides a favorable risk/benefit ratio: Despite longer operative time and slightly increased incidence of postoperative bleeding, recurrence rate is decreased, bowel length is preserved, and function may be restored.

Fistulas are treated with resection of the primary diseased segment and closure of the opening on the target organ, if it is uninvolved with CD. In most cases, fistulas arise from a diseased segment of intestine and drain into an "innocent bystander" loop of bowel. This commonly occurs between two loops of small bowel or between diseased terminal ileum and adjacent sigmoid colon. Recurrent disease of the neoterminal ileum may fistulize to the duodenum, or primary disease from the transverse colon may fistulize to the stomach or fourth portion of the duodenum. When the bystander segment is closed, care should be taken to avoid narrowing the lumen by closing in a transverse direction. If the fistulous opening on the target loop is large, very edematous, or situated on the mesenteric side, a segmental resection with primary anastomosis may be necessary. Fistulas to the bladder may be oversewn with absorbable suture to minimize the risk of stone formation at the site of permanent suture. Vaginal and uterine fistulas often heal spontaneously after resection of the primary diseased intestine. Overlaying the repair with a vascularized tissue pedicle such as omentum can prevent leak or recurrence. Enterocutaneous or colocutaneous fistulas necessitate débridement of the fistulous tract through the aponeurotic and cutaneous planes of the abdominal wall, with complete drainage of intervening abscesses.

Surgery for CD is frequently performed laparoscopically. This holds the potential advantage of reducing not only postoperative pain but also postoperative adhesion formation in a patient population with a high chance of needing further abdominal surgery. Challenges facing the laparoscopic approach include matted loops of bowel, adhesions, fistulas, thickened mesentery, and prior surgical interventions. There are no contraindications to laparoscopy in CD patients, although patients with prior abdominal operations may have longer operative times and potentially higher rates of conversion to open operation. It appears that after age and comorbid conditions are controlled, laparoscopic surgery is associated with significantly fewer complications—including abdominal sepsis, wound complications, and postoperative pneumonia—than is open surgery. In addition, by hastening return of bowel function, laparoscopic surgery reduces length of hospital stay. Laparoscopy should be strongly considered for initial ileocecectomy, but is frequently appropriate for reoperative surgery.

The practice at the author's institution is to obtain abdominal access through the open Hassan technique. As with open surgery, the abdomen should be inspected thoroughly after any necessary adhesiolysis. The small intestine should be inspected for any disease that may not have been visualized on preoperative imaging. When technically possible, we perform exploration and resection laparoscopically and then mobilize the bowel so that it can be extracted through a small laparotomy incision at one of the port sites, and a standard two-layer hand-sewn anastomosis is created.

Recurrence of Disease

Recurrence is a significant concern in patients with Crohn's disease. Up to 50% of patients eventually require a second surgery, often at the site of prior interventions (e.g., ileocolectomy for recurrence at the site of prior ileocecectomy). Smoking cessation reduces the long-term chance of disease recurrence by as much as 50%, but remains a difficult goal for most smokers. Other less well elucidated factors play a role in disease recurrence; phenotype, granulomas, and prior recurrence are risk factors for future surgical interventions. Early postoperative medical therapy has been advocated for CD patients at high risk of recurrence. Patients may be prescribed antibiotics, aminosalicylates, antimetabolites, or biologic agents within 10 days of surgical intervention. Metronidazole has been shown to decrease the rate of endoscopic recurrence when used for 3 months postoperatively, and aminosalicylates have been shows to reduce recurrence rates in postoperative patients by up to 30%. Antimetabolites such as AZA and 6-MP show a decrease in recurrence rates of up to 50%. In patients with severe inflammation who present with abscess that is probably secondary to occult perforations, prolonged bowel rest with parenteral support may be considered. Infliximab has also been shown to prevent recurrence, although to date this has been demonstrated only in very small series. Multidisciplinary management in conjunction with medical gastroenterology consultation should be considered before discharge for all CD patients.

SELECTED READINGS

Ali T, Yun L, Rubin DT: Risk of post-operative complications associated with anti-TNF therapy in inflammatory bowel disease, *World J Gastroenterol* 18(3):197–204, 2012.

Buchner A, Blonski W, Lichtenstein G: Update on the management of Crohn's disease, *Curr Gastroenterol Rep* 13:465–474, 2011.

Hassan C, Zullo A, De Francesco V, et al: Systematic review: endoscopic dilatation in Crohn's disease, *Aliment Pharmacol Ther* 1457–1464, 2007.

Khan KJ, Ullman TA, Ford AC, et al: Antibiotic therapy in inflammatory bowel disease: a systematic review and meta-analysis, *Am J Gastroenterol* 106(5):1014, 2011.

Lee Y, Fleming FJ, Deeb AP, et al: A laparoscopic approach reduces short term complications and length of stay following ileocolic resection in Crohn's disease: an analysis of outcomes from the NSQIP database, *Colorectal Dis* 14(5):572–577, 2012.

Lichtenstein GR, Hanauer SB, Sandborn WJ, et al: Management of Crohn's disease in adults, *Am J Gastroenterol* 104(2):465–483, 2009.

Spurio FF, Aratari A, Margagnoni G, et al: Early treatment in Crohn's disease: do we have enough evidence to reverse the therapeutic pyramid? *J Gastrointest Liver Dis* 21(1):67–73, 2012.

TABLE 2: Relative and absolute contraindications to strictureplasty in Crohn's disease*

Absolute	Relative
Perforation neoplasia	Abscess
Fistula	Long, severely narrowed
Severe malnutrition	segments†

*As techniques improve, contraindications to strictureplasty become fewer.
†In the presence of long, severely narrowed segment of small bowel preceded and followed by a loop with sequential strictures, the middle segment can be resected; the proximal and distal diseased loop may be preserved as part of a side-to-side isoperistaltic strictureplasty.

Strictureplasty in Crohn's Disease

Leon Maggiori, MD, and Fabrizio Michelassi, MD

INTRODUCTION

Crohn's disease (CD) is a chronic inflammatory bowel disease, characterized by transmural bowel inflammation that may occur anywhere in the gastrointestinal tract, from the mouth to the anus. Chronic intestinal inflammation can lead to the development of strictures, septic complications such as abscesses and fistulas, hemorrhage, and malignant transformation. Despite improvements in medical therapy, more than half of all patients with CD need surgical treatment for such complications within 10 years of diagnosis.

Unfortunately, CD is a recurrent disease, and 20% to 60% of patients have postoperative clinical symptoms of recurrence and 15% to 50% need further surgical intervention at some time after the index procedure. With the need for repeated intestinal resections, patients may eventually have intestinal insufficiency and short bowel syndrome develop, leading to the need for total parenteral nutrition support. Surgical treatment of CD should therefore aim to address complications without jeopardizing bowel function.

Bowel-sparing surgical techniques, such as strictureplasty, have been proposed as an alternative to lengthy intestinal resections in the treatment of CD small bowel strictures. This chapter reviews indications, contraindications, technical aspects, and results of strictureplasty techniques.

OVERVIEW

Indications and Contraindications

Strictureplasty is the treatment of choice for patients with symptomatic nonphlegmonous jejuno-ileal CD fibrotic strictures, as highlighted in both American and European guidelines for CD management. Symptoms may vary from postprandial cramped abdominal pain to complete bowel obstruction.

Several studies have also reported excellent results when strictureplasty techniques have been performed for strictures in other gastrointestinal locations, such as in the duodenum or at the site of a strictured ileocolonic anastomosis. Strictureplasty has been reported also in the treatment of isolated colonic strictures: yet, the length and thickness of colonic strictures is usually not conducive to strictureplasty techniques.

Strictureplasty is contraindicated in the presence of local sepsis, such as phlegmon, abscess, or generalized peritonitis. In these situations, strictureplasty is associated with a higher risk of postoperative dehiscence. The presence of enteric fistulae has been hitherto viewed as a contraindication for strictureplasty, but recent reports have suggested that strictureplasty might be performed in the presence of fistulae surrounded by chronic, rather than active, inflammation without increasing postoperative morbidity.

Profoundly impaired nutritional status is also considered as a contraindication to this technique. Suspicion of small bowel adenocarcinoma or dysplasia should lead to intraoperative biopsy and, if confirmed, resection of the bowel loop rather than a bowel-sparing procedure (Box 1). Finally, in the economy of a surgical procedure, if a stricture is located in close proximity of a diseased intestinal segment in need of resection, the resection is usually extended to include the stricture to minimize the length of the overall surgical procedure and the number of suture length.

Preoperative Preparation

As for all elective surgical procedures for CD, a complete assessment of disease extension should be performed with magnetic resonance imaging (MRI) or computed tomographic (CT) scan enterography. MRI is the most sensitive and specific imaging procedure for CD extension assessment: it aids in distinguishing between active inflammatory strictures, which might be medically managed, and fibrotic strictures, which should be surgically treated. The authors also advocate a preoperative total colonoscopy, even in patients with CD apparently strictly limited to small bowel.

Several studies have focused on predictive risk factors of postoperative morbidity in CD surgery. Yamamoto and colleagues identified three independent risk factors: preoperative corticosteroids medication, poor nutritional status, and intraabdominal phlegmon or fistula. Corticosteroid weaning is rarely feasible without a recrudescence of the disease, and abdominal phlegmons are frequently the reason for surgical intervention; by contrast, poor nutritional status should be addressed before surgery with enteric or intravenous nutrition. On the other hand, azathioprine has no impact on postoperative morbidity and can therefore be maintained. Finally, the influence of infliximab on postoperative CD complication is still controversial, although several recent studies have suggested that it has no negative impact on healing of intraabdominal anastomosis.

Intraoperative "Design of a Roadmap"

The authors start all of their small bowel CD cases with examination of the entire small bowel from the ligament of Treitz to the ileocecal valve, with special care paid to recording all CD-related complications (strictures, phlegmonous masses, abscesses, fistulae). This phase of the procedure is called "the design of a roadmap." A strategic approach to the patient's disease is then developed by studying the "roadmap" and includes the use of strictureplasty, intestinal resection, drainage of abscesses, repair of fistulous openings on target intestinal loops or hollow viscera, or a combination of these techniques (Figure 1).

STRICTUREPLASTY TECHNIQUES

Strictureplasty techniques may be divided into three subgroups: short strictureplasty, including the highly common Heineke-Mikulicz technique; intermediate length procedure, including the Finney and Jaboulay procedures; and long enteroenterostomy, like the side-to-side isoperistaltic strictureplasty. The choice among these different techniques should be made according to the number of strictures and length of each one (Table 1).

Short Strictureplasty

The most common strictureplasty technique is the Heineke-Mikulicz technique. This strictureplasty was introduced by Emmanuel Lee for the treatment of CD in 1976 after he became aware of a similar technique on tubercular strictures of the terminal ileum described by Katarya. The technique is similar to a Heineke-Mikulicz pyloroplasty from which it derives its name. The technique is optimal to address short strictures (≤7 cm). This technique is performed by making a longitudinal incision on the antimesenteric side of the bowel,

BOX 1: Absolute contraindications for strictureplasty in Crohn's disease surgical management

Impaired nutritional status
Dysplasia or cancer at the stricture site
Locoregional sepsis:
   Phlegmon
   Abscess
   Peritonitis

TABLE 1: Choice of strictureplasty technique according to disease characteristics

Stricture length	Technique
Short (≤7 cm)	Heineke-Mickulicz
Intermediate (>7 cm and ≤15 cm)	Finney
Multiple short strictures clustered over a lengthy segment	Side-to-side isoperistaltic

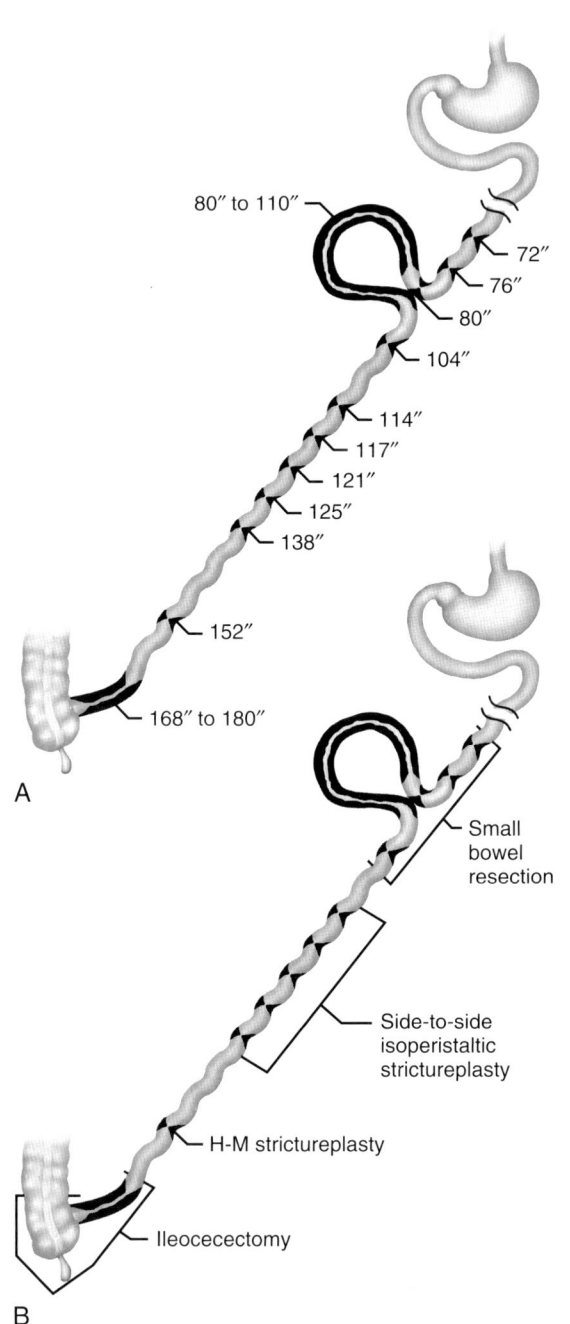

FIGURE 1 Design of a roadmap **(A)** and subsequent surgical plan **(B)** for extensive Crohn's disease. *H-M,* Heineke-Mikulicz.

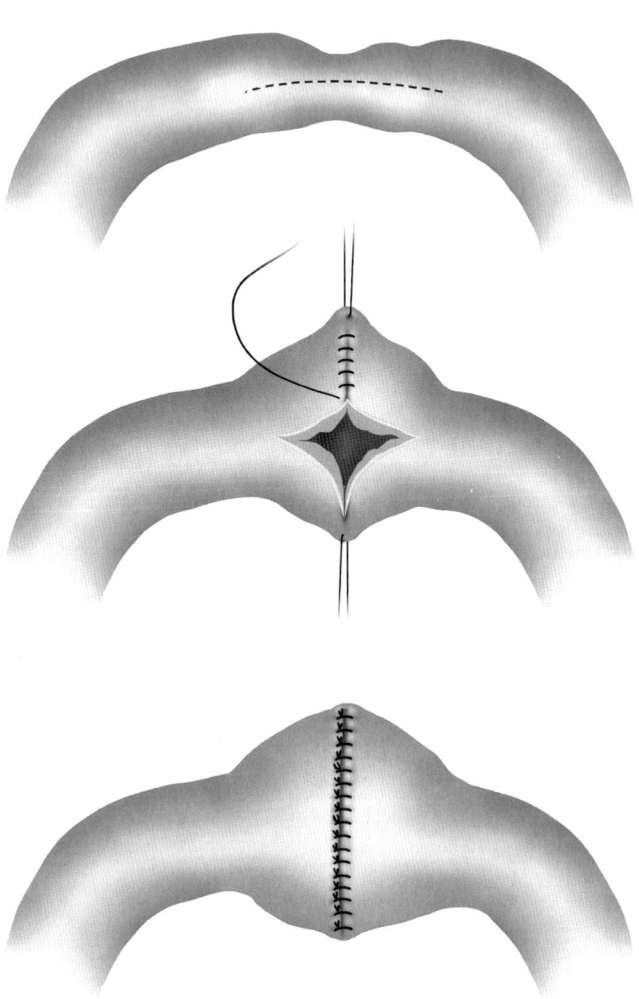

FIGURE 2 Heineke-Mikulicz strictureplasty on an isolated, short, small bowel stricture.

extending from 2 cm proximal to 2 cm distal to the stricture. The enterotomy is then closed in a transverse fashion in one or two layers. The senior author prefers to close this enterotomy in two layers with interrupted Lembert nonabsorbable 3-0 sutures for the outer layer and a running absorbable 3-0 suture for the inner layer (Figure 2).

The Judd strictureplasty is a variation of the Heineke-Mikulicz technique described for the surgical management of short strictures associated with a fistula opening. During this procedure, the longitudinal incision encompasses the fistula opening. The enterotomy is then closed as described in Heineke-Mikulicz technique.

Small bowel stricture can be responsible for a dilation on the proximal loop, leading to a size discrepancy between the proximal and distal loops. In this situation, the Moskel-Walske-Neumayer

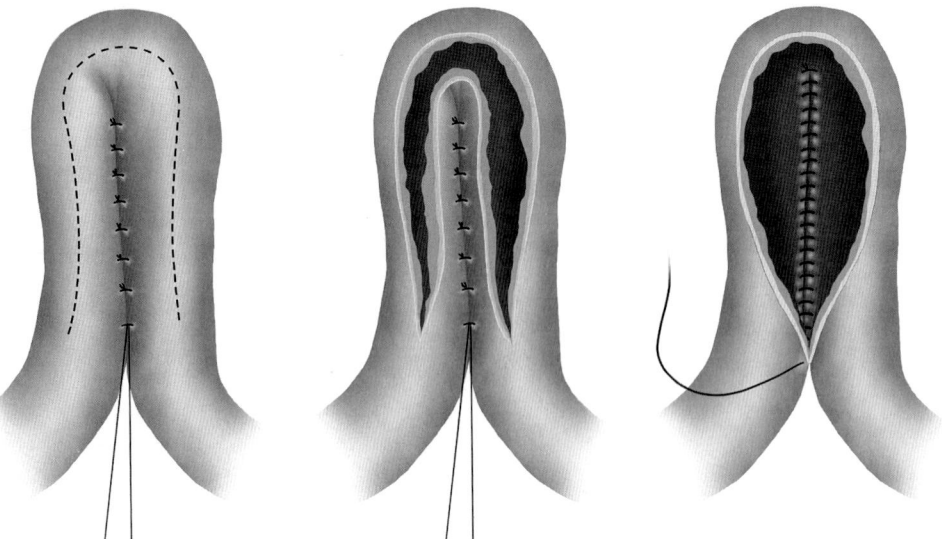

FIGURE 3 Finney strictureplasty on an intermediate small bowel stricture.

strictureplasty compares favorably with the original Heineke-Mikulicz technique. A Y-shaped enterotomy is performed on the stricture, with the Y fork pointing to the dilated loop. The enterotomy is then closed in a transverse fashion in a V shape.

Intermediate Length Procedures

Intermediate length procedures have been described to address longer strictures (>7 cm and ≤15 cm) than those manageable with the Heineke-Mikulicz technique or its variations. In this situation, the most commonly performed procedure is the Finney stricture-plasty, named after the Finney pyloroplasty, first described in 1937. The strictured loop is folded over itself at its midpoint section, forming a U shape. A longitudinal enterotomy is then performed halfway between the mesenteric and the antimesenteric side on the folded loop. The opposed edges of the bowel are sutured together to create a short side-to-side anisoperistaltic enteroenterostomy (Figure 3). The senior author prefers a two-layer closure similar to the one described for the Heineke-Mikulicz strictureplasty. Concerns about long-term complications, such as bacterial overgrowth in the bypassed segment, limit the length of the stricture to be addressed by this strictureplasty to less than 15 cm.

Long Enteroenterostomy

The side-to-side strictureplasty, first described in 1996 by the senior author, is the technique of choice to address multiple short strictures closely clustered over a lengthy small bowel segment (>15 cm).

In this technique, the mesentery of the small bowel loop to undergo the strictureplasty is first divided at its midpoint. The proximal intestinal loop is then moved over the distal one in a side-to-side fashion. Care is taken to ensure that stenotic areas of one loop are placed adjacent to the dilated areas of the other loop. The two loops are then approximated by a layer of interrupted seromuscular Lembert stitches, with nonabsorbable 3-0 sutures (Figure 4, A). A longitudinal enterotomy is performed on both loops, with the intestinal ends tapered to avoid blind stumps (Figure 4, B). Frozen-section biopsies of suspicious areas of disease are obtained to exclude occult malignant disease. Hemostasis is obtained with suture ligatures or electrocautery. The outer suture line is reinforced with an internal row of running full-thickness 3-0 absorbable sutures, continued anteriorly as a running Connell suture (Figure 4, C); this layer is reinforced by an outer layer of interrupted seromuscular Lembert stitches with nonabsorbable 3-0 sutures (Figure 4, D).

Many variations of this side-to-side isoperistaltic strictureplasty technique have been described. These variations fall into four distinct categories: integration of other strictureplasty techniques (e.g., Heineke-Mikulicz or Finney techniques) with the side-to-side isoperistaltic strictureplasty technique, length of bowel selected for strictureplasty, bowel location selected for procedure (jejunum, ileum, or terminal ileum where the side-to-side isoperistaltic strictureplasty is performed between the ileum and the ascending colon), and the condition for which this technique is applied (CD, multiple nonsteroidal antiinflammatory drug [NSAID]–small bowel strictures, and small bowel stricture arising from chronic ischemic enteritis).

RESULTS

Postoperative Short-Term Outcomes

A large number of publications highlighted the safety of strictureplasty for CD. A meta-analysis that included more than 3000 strictureplasties was published in 2007. Short strictureplasties were the most commonly performed (81%), followed by intermediate procedures (10%) and long enteroenterostomies. Overall, mortality was nil, and 13% of patients had postoperative complications, including 4% septic complications (anastomotic leak, fistula, and abscess) and 3% postoperative hemorrhages. This meta-analysis also showed that the strictureplasty technique had no impact on postoperative outcomes.

The short-term results associated with the side-to-side isoperistaltic strictureplasty technique have been reported by one single-center study. This study showed the feasibility and safety of the procedure and the optimal gastrointestinal motility at the level of the side-to-side isoperistaltic strictureplasty.

A recent comparative study has evaluated strictureplasty versus resection in small bowel CD and has established that the postoperative outcomes of strictureplasty compare favorably with those obtained after small bowel resection. In specific regard to functional outcomes, efficacy of strictureplasty has been largely shown, with satisfactory relief of obstructive symptoms, improved food tolerance, and subsequent weight gain.

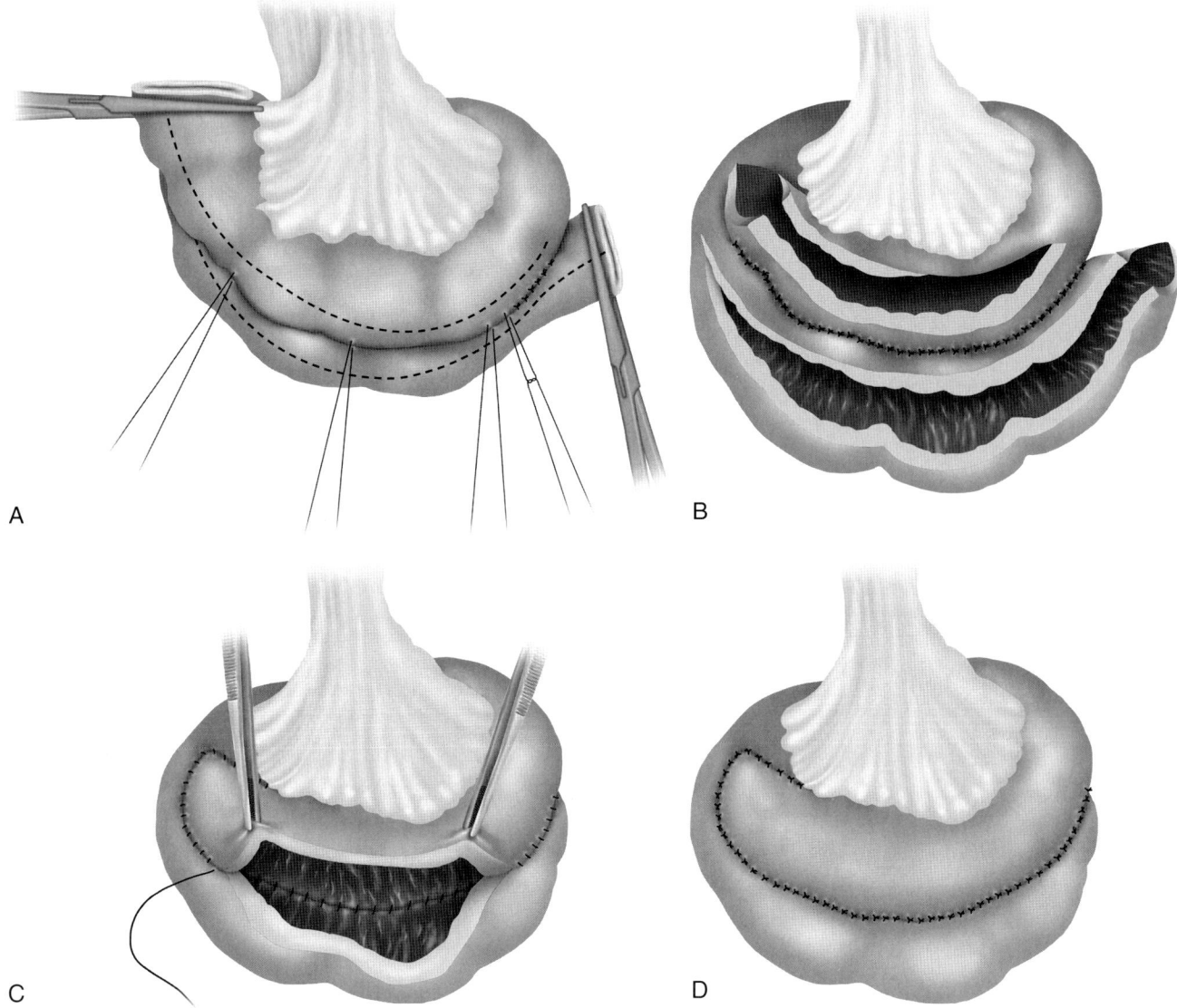

FIGURE 4 **A** to **D,** Side-to-side isoperistaltic strictureplasty. *(Modified from Maggiori L, Michelassi F: How I do it: side-to-side isoperistaltic strictureplasty for extensive Crohn's disease,* J Gastrointest Surg *16:1976-1980, 2012.)*

Long-Term Outcomes

The meta-analysis from 2007 reported an overall symptomatic recurrence rate of 39% with a median follow-up period of 107 months. In this study, recurrence on a previous strictureplasty requiring surgical management occurred in only 10% of cases, which compares favorably with results obtained with small bowel resection. Yamamoto and associates have suggested that strictureplasty may induce a higher recurrence-free survival rate than intestinal resection. Endoscopic, radiologic, and histopathologic evaluations after strictureplasty have indeed highlighted complete CD regression at strictureplasty site in several reports. The mechanism associated with such inflammation regression remains unknown.

Reports of development of small bowel adenocarcinoma arising at the site of strictureplasty have been documented. To date, four cases of such complication have been published, including one reported by the senior author. The risk of neoplastic transformation after strictureplasty is assumed to be low and not sufficient enough to dissuade surgeons from performing those techniques.

Long-term results associated with the side-to-side isoperistaltic strictureplasty technique were reported by a multicenter study in 2007. This study showed that only 14 of 184 total patients needed surgery for recurrent disease at the side-to-side isoperistaltic strictureplasty site, after an average follow-up period of 35 months. Recurrences occurred mostly at the inlet and at the outlet of the side-to-side strictureplasty, leading some authors to suggest the addition of a Heineke-Mikulicz strictureplasty at the inlet and the outlet of the side-to-side strictureplasty during its original construction.

SUMMARY

Crohn's disease is a chronic and recurrent panintestinal inflammatory disorder. Surgical treatment is indicated to address complications of the disease or failure of medical treatment. Symptom alleviation expected from the procedure should be balanced with potential postoperative morbidity and long-term side effects. In this context, strictureplasty for CD-related small bowel stenosis has been shown to be a safe and effective solution, relieving obstructive symptoms without any bowel sacrifice.

Different strictureplasty procedures have been described to address different settings of CD. The choice of strictureplasty techniques should be made based on the length and the number of strictures.

ACKNOWLEDGMENT

Supported in part by the Alice Bohmfalk Charitable Trust.

SUGGESTED READINGS

Ambe R, Campbell L, Cagir B: A comprehensive review of strictureplasty techniques in Crohn's disease: types, indications, comparisons, and safety, *J Gastrointest Surg* 16:209–217, 2012.

Fearnhead NS, Chowdhury R, Box B, et al: Long-term follow-up of strictureplasty for Crohn's disease, *Br J Surg* 93:475–482, 2006.

Fichera A, Lovadina S, Rubin M, et al: Patterns and operative treatment of recurrent Crohn's disease: a prospective longitudinal study, *Surgery* 140:649–654, 2006.

Greenstein AJ, Zhang LP, Miller AT, et al: Relationship of the number of Crohn's strictures and strictureplasties to postoperative recurrence, *J Am Coll Surg* 208:1065–1070, 2009.

Michelassi F, Hurst RD, Melis M, et al: Side-to-side isoperistaltic strictureplasty in extensive Crohn's disease: a prospective longitudinal study, *Ann Surg* 232:401–408, 2000.

Michelassi F, Taschieri A, Tonelli F, et al: An international, multicenter, prospective, observational study of the side-to-side isoperistaltic strictureplasty in Crohn's disease, *Dis Colon Rectum* 50:277–284, 2007.

Roy P, Kumar D: Strictureplasty, *Br J Surg* 91:1428–1437, 2004.

Yamamoto T, Fazio VW, Tekkis PP: Safety and efficacy of strictureplasty for Crohn's disease: a systematic review and meta-analysis, *Dis Colon Rectum* 50:1968–1986, 2007.

THE MANAGEMENT OF SMALL BOWEL TUMORS

Hiroko Kunitake, MD, and Richard Hodin, MD

OVERVIEW

Small bowel mucosa comprises approximately 75% of the length and 90% of the absorptive surface area of the digestive system, yet only 2.8% of new digestive system cancers each year occur in the small intestine. The American Cancer Society estimates that each year, more than 8000 new small bowel malignancies are found, and approximately 1100 people die of their disease.

Several reasons for the low incidence of small bowel tumors have been proposed, including the rapid transit of contents through the small bowel, lower bacterial load, high amount of lymphoid tissue, rapid turnover of epithelial cells, and decreased inflammation owing to the liquidity and alkaline nature of small bowel contents.

Signs and symptoms of these tumors are usually nonspecific and include abdominal pain, weight loss, nausea, vomiting, occult bleeding, and obstruction or perforation. Vague symptoms, limited findings on examination, and failure to obtain or correctly interpret diagnostic tests have all been implicated in delaying the diagnosis of small intestine cancers, and because of this, more than 50% of patients have nodal or distant metastases at the time of presentation.

Diagnosing small bowel tumors has historically been difficult due to limited means of gaining access to distal portions of the small bowel. Common methods have included small bowel follow-through, enteroclysis, computed tomographic (CT) scans, magnetic resonance enterography, upper endoscopy, and push enteroscopy. Wireless capsule endoscopy and double-balloon endoscopy have become increasingly more common. Capsule endoscopy allows painless endoscopic imaging of the whole small bowel, and it has become the standard diagnostic approach for patients with obscure gastrointestinal bleeding, often a presenting symptom of small bowel tumors. However, it is contraindicated for patients with suspected or documented intestinal obstruction, and it does not allow for tissue sampling or interventional therapies in the small bowel. Double-balloon enteroscopy allows for direct inspection of most or all of the small intestine, with better visualization of the duodenum and proximal jejunum compared with capsule endoscopy as well as the option of tissue biopsy and therapeutic intervention. The treatment of small bowel neoplasms has not changed significantly over the past two decades, and surgery continues to be the primary therapy in most cases.

CARCINOID/NEUROENDOCRINE TUMORS

Tumor Characteristics

Gastrointestinal carcinoid tumors, more recently referred to as neuroendocrine tumors, are the most common malignancy of the small bowel. They include a diverse range of slow-growing neoplasms arising from various cells of the neuroendocrine system. Carcinoids can occur anywhere along the gastrointestinal tract; 45% occur in the small intestine, most commonly in the ileum. Up to one third of cases of small bowel carcinoid tumors are multifocal, and more than 50% of patients have nonlocalized disease at the time of diagnosis. Gastrointestinal carcinoid tumors, especially those of the small intestine, are also often associated with other cancers. Synchronous or metachronous noncarcinoid cancers occur in approximately 29% of patients with small intestinal carcinoid tumors. Carcinoid tumors synthesize, store, and release a variety of polypeptides, biogenic amines, and prostaglandins. Most jejunal and ileal carcinoids are serotonin-producing enterochromaffin-cell tumors. The majority of duodenal carcinoids are gastrin-producing G-cell tumors (two thirds) followed by somatostatin-producing D-cell tumors (one fifth). Most small intestine carcinoid tumors occur sporadically, but others may occur in the background of an inherited neoplasia syndrome such as multiple endocrine neoplasia type I (MEN1) or neurofibromatosis type 1 (NF1).

Clinical Presentation

Patients with carcinoid tumors may present with abdominal pain and obstructive symptoms. Carcinoid tumors may act as a lead point for intussusception, and they can also elicit an intense desmoplastic reaction, causing adhesions of intestinal loops and stricturing of the bowel. Fibrosis around mesenteric metastases can cause contraction of the mesentery or fixation of the mesentery to the retroperitoneum, leading to kinking and obstruction via fibrous bands. Encasement of mesenteric vessels by tumor can lead to venous stasis and even ischemia in portions of the small bowel. Duodenal carcinoids (Figure 1) are often identified incidentally or because of symptoms from hormone or peptide production, but they may also arise in the periampullary region and obstruct the ampulla of Vater, causing jaundice.

Approximately 35% of carcinoids of the small intestine are associated with carcinoid syndrome. Carcinoid syndrome is caused by the release of metabolically undegraded vasoactive amines into the systemic circulation. Because vasoactive amines are efficiently metabolized by the liver, carcinoid syndrome rarely occurs in the absence of hepatic metastases. Exceptions include circumstances in which venous blood draining from a tumor enters directly into the systemic circulation (e.g., pelvic or retroperitoneal involvement by metastatic or locally invasive small bowel carcinoids, or extensive bone metastases). Carcinoid syndrome is associated with flushing, abdominal pain and diarrhea, bronchoconstriction, and carcinoid heart disease, manifested by endocardial fibrotic plaques and thickening and fibrosis of the tricuspid and pulmonary valves, and to a lesser extent the mitral and aortic valves.

Diagnosis

Biochemical diagnosis of carcinoid tumors may be achieved by measurement of 5-hydroxyindolacetic acid (5-HIAA) in a 24-hour urine sample or by serum analysis of chromogranin A (CgA), which is believed to be a superior screening test. However, false-positive plasma levels of CgA may occur in patients on proton pump inhibitors. Common imaging studies for localizing carcinoid tumors include abdominal CT, magnetic resonance imaging (MRI), somatostatin receptor scintigraphy (octreotide scan), and positron emission tomography (PET). Octreotide scanning is a useful initial imaging method, with a diagnostic sensitivity estimated to be as high as 90%.

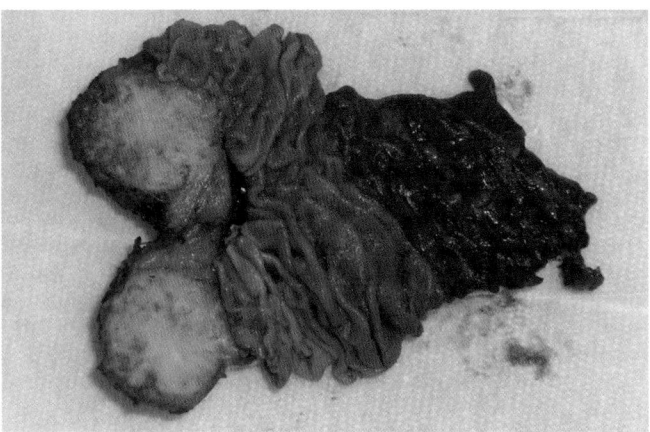

FIGURE 1 Small bowel neuroendocrine tumor.

Treatment

Surgery remains the only potentially curative therapy and is the most effective treatment for averting both local tumor effects, such as obstruction and bleeding, and symptoms caused by the secreted bioactive agents. Because metastatic spread to regional lymph nodes is common, small bowel carcinoids warrant an en bloc resection with extensive lymphadenectomy and wide resection of the mesentery. The abdomen should be carefully inspected for multicentric lesions and liver metastases. If liver metastases are identified, the primary tumor should still be resected to diminish later complications such as obstruction, perforation, and bleeding. Hepatic metastases may be managed with surgical resection, hepatic artery embolization, cryoablation, radiofrequency ablation, or liver transplantation. In the case of duodenal tumors, lesions less than 1 cm may be resected endoscopically, and lesions smaller than 2 cm may be excised locally. Tumors larger than 2 cm should be treated with full-thickness excision and regional lymphadenectomy, even with negative imaging, because of the high rate of lymph node metastases for these tumors. If the tumor is in proximity to the ampulla, a pancreaticoduodenectomy may be necessary to obtain complete resection.

The role of surgery in metastatic disease is not well defined, but resection of bowel, mesenteric tumors, lymph node and hepatic metastases, and fibrotic areas may improve symptoms and quality of life. Extensive resections of metastatic disease may even prolong survival, though it is estimated that 90% of the disease needs to be resected to achieve palliation. Tumor debulking may also improve the efficacy of pharmacologic therapy by reducing the bioactive substances secreted. If future treatment with octreotide is anticipated, a prophylactic cholecystectomy should be considered given the association between the long-term treatment with somatostatin analogs and the development of biliary symptoms and gallstones.

Long-acting and depot formulations of somatostatin analogs have been shown to be highly effective in controlling carcinoid syndrome symptoms, resulting in significant improvement in quality of life with relatively mild adverse effects. Routine preoperative administration can also prevent carcinoid crisis, which is characterized by excessive cutaneous flushing, hyperthermia, shock, arrhythmias, and bronchial obstruction. Aside from octreotide, which is associated with delayed progression of small bowel carcinoid, no treatment has proven antitumor activity. Chemotherapy seems to be of limited value, and the role of interferon is controversial. Peptide receptor radionuclide therapy may have cytoreductive activity in patients with somatostatin (SST) receptor–expressing tumors, but randomized controlled trials are lacking. Various therapies targeting vascular endothelial growth factor (VEGF), platelet-derived growth factor receptor (PDGFR), and mammalian target of rapamycin (mTOR) are now in development.

Overall, the 5- and 10-year survival rates for well-differentiated small bowel carcinoids is 65% and 49% in localized disease; 71% and 46% for regional disease; and 54% and 30% for distant disease, respectively. Age greater than 55 years, male sex, primary tumor size greater than 1 cm, and distant metastases negatively affect outcome.

■ ADENOCARCINOMA

Tumor Characteristics

Adenocarcinoma is the second most common malignancy of the small intestine, comprising approximately 37% of small bowel cancers. It occurs most often in the duodenum and decreases progressively throughout the rest of the small intestine. An exception to the predominantly proximal location is in patients with Crohn's disease. Seventy percent of the adenocarcinomas that arise in Crohn's disease are located in the ileum, the most common site of chronic inflammation. Small bowel adenocarcinoma is also associated with a variety of other diseases and syndromes, including celiac disease, familial adenomatous polyposis, hereditary nonpolyposis colorectal cancer, and Peutz-Jeghers syndrome.

Clinical Presentation

Symptoms of small bowel adenocarcinoma are frequently nonspecific, leading to significant delays in diagnosis. More than 50% of patients are found to have advanced disease (stage III or IV) at presentation, 24% have distant metastases, and approximately 30% have nodal involvement. Patients with ampullary adenocarcinoma often present earlier in their disease course because of symptoms that result from biliary obstruction.

Diagnosis

Periampullary lesions can be diagnosed by upper endoscopy, endoscopic ultrasound, and magnetic resonance cholangiopancreatography. Cancers distal to the ligament of Treitz are more amenable to video capsule endoscopy and double-balloon endoscopy. Advanced adenocarcinomas may appear on barium contrast studies as "apple core" lesions: short, annular, narrowed portions that show evidence of mucosal ulceration and appear rigid and unchanging with compression. CT features of adenocarcinoma are similar to those seen on barium studies; abrupt transitions and irregular shouldered overhanging margins are typical. After intravenous contrast administration, these mucosal-based soft-tissue lesions demonstrate enhancement. CT is advantageous over conventional barium studies for detection of extramucosal spread, lymphadenopathy, and distant metastases. CT enterography and MR enterography are emerging as valuable imaging techniques for accurate diagnosis of small bowel adenocarcinoma (Figure 2).

Treatment

The primary treatment and only potential for cure for small bowel adenocarcinoma continues to be surgical resection. Tumors of the first and second portions of the duodenum require pancreaticoduodenectomy. For tumors arising in the third and fourth portions of

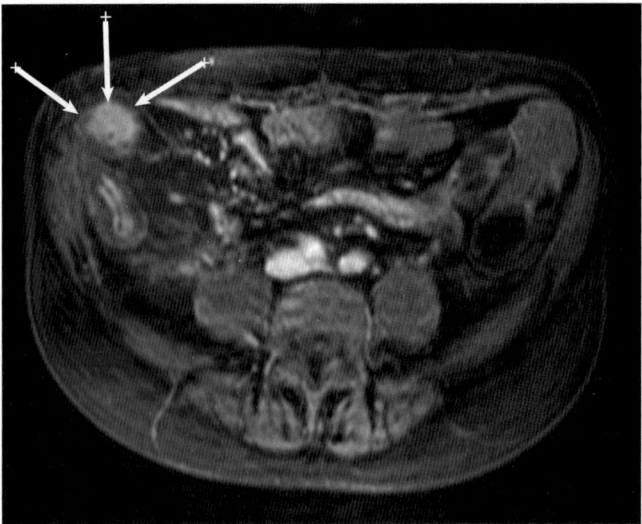

FIGURE 2 MRI showing a small bowel adenocarcinoma *(arrows)* in a Crohn's patient.

the duodenum, segmental resection is preferred over pancreaticoduodenectomy as long as a margin-negative resection can be obtained. Jejunal and ileal tumors require segmental bowel resection with a wide resection of the lymph node–bearing mesentery. An ileocolectomy is indicated for tumors of the distal ileum.

Patients with locally advanced, unresectable, or metastatic small bowel adenocarcinoma may benefit from palliative surgical resection of the primary tumor to prevent bowel obstruction or bleeding. In some advanced cases, intestinal bypass may be needed to relieve obstruction. For tumors in the duodenum, palliation may be achieved by endoscopic placement of an intraluminal duodenal stent. There are no widely accepted criteria for selecting patients for neoadjuvant therapy, nor any standard chemotherapy regimens. However, neoadjuvant therapy is sometimes used in patients with bulky or locally advanced tumors. Similarly, there is a paucity of data demonstrating the benefit of adjuvant chemotherapy, although patients with completely resected, lymph node positive small bowel adenocarcinoma are selectively being offered chemotherapy based on principles established for colorectal cancer. Cytoreductive surgery and intraperitoneal hyperthermic chemotherapy have also been reported to be successful in a handful of highly selected patients with peritoneal carcinomatosis.

A recent SEER registry analysis of 4518 cases from 1988 to 2007 demonstrated that 5-year disease-specific survival was 65% for stage I, 55% for stage II, 40% for stage III, and less than 10% for stage IV disease. However, in the subset of these patients who had 8 or more lymph nodes evaluated, the 5-year disease-specific survival markedly improved to 80% for stage I, 70% for stage II, 45% for stage III, and 10% for stage IV disease. These data suggest that a portion of stage I or II small bowel adenocarcinomas are undergoing inadequate lymph node evaluation and consequently are being understaged (and undertreated). Factors negatively affecting survival for small bowel adenocarcinoma include male sex, age greater than 55 years, tumor location in the duodenum or ileum (compared to jejunum), and the presence of distant metastases.

GASTROINTESTINAL STROMAL TUMORS

Tumor Characteristics

Gastrointestinal stromal tumors (GISTs) are the most common nonepithelial neoplasm of the small bowel. They originate from the interstitial cells of Cajal or their precursors and can occur anywhere along the GI tract. They are most frequently found in the stomach (60%) and the small bowel (30%), and within the small bowel, they are most likely to be located in the jejunum. The majority of GISTs (>90%) express the CD117 antigen, part of the KIT transmembrane receptor tyrosine kinase that is the product of the KIT (also denoted c-kit) protooncogene. Mutation in the KIT gene leads to an abnormally activated KIT protein and enables oncogenic signaling in the cell. A subset of GISTs lacking KIT mutations has activating mutations in the related receptor tyrosine kinase, platelet-derived growth factor receptor alpha (PDGFRA). These findings led to the development of effective systemic therapies in the form of tyrosine kinase inhibitors (TKIs), such as imatinib that block signaling via KIT and PDGFRA and inhibit tumor proliferation.

Most GISTs arise sporadically. Hereditary GIST is a rare, autosomal dominant genetic disorder, with the majority attributable to germline KIT mutations and a small percentage due to germline mutation in PDGFRA. GISTs may also arise in the setting of the autosomal dominant disorder neurofibromatosis type I (NF1) or as part of Carney's triad (GIST, paraganglioma, and pulmonary chondromas) or Carney-Stratakis dyad (GIST and paragangliomas).

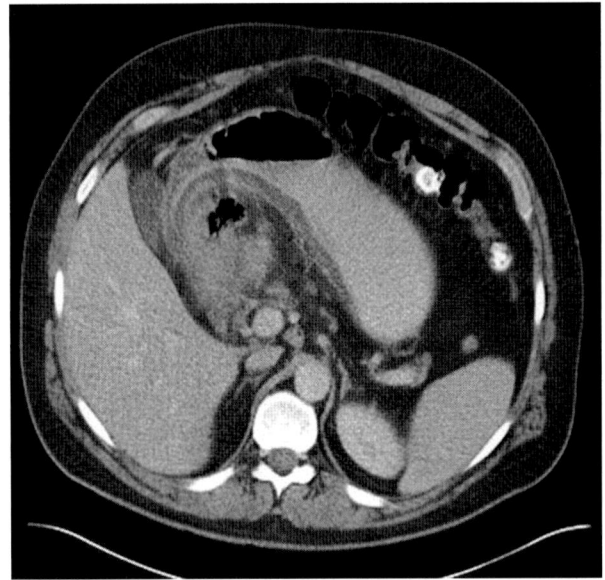

FIGURE 3 Duodenal perforated astrointestinal stromal tumors.

TABLE 1: Risk of aggressive behavior in GISTs

	Size (largest dimension)	Mitotic count
Very low risk	<2 cm	<5/50 HPF
Low risk	2-5 cm	<5/50 HPF
Intermediate risk	<5 cm	6-10/50 HPF
	5-10 cm	<5/50 HPF
High risk	>5 cm	>5/50 HPF
	>10 cm	Any mitotic rate

GISTs, Gastrointestinal stromal tumors; HPF, high-powered field.
Fletcher CD, Berman JJ, Corless C, et al: Diagnosis of gastrointestinal stromal tumors: a consensus approach, Hum Pathol 33(5):459–465, 2002.

GISTs associated with both syndromes have a chronic, yet indolent course.

Clinical Presentation

Presenting complaints include obstructive symptoms, abdominal discomfort, early satiety, and abdominal distension due to the space-occupying nature of these masses. Most GISTs arise within the muscular wall of the GI tract, and they can grow into the mucosa to form solid subserosal, intramural, or polypoid intraluminal masses. Alternatively, they can protrude outward and form external masses attached to the outer aspect of the gut. GISTs may grow to a massive size prior to presentation, with a median tumor size of 7.5 cm. Bleeding can occur when GISTs erode through the bowel wall or result in intraperitoneal rupture (Figure 3).

Diagnosis

On upper endoscopy, GISTs may appear as a submucosal mass with smooth margins with a normal overlying mucosa. Performing preoperative biopsy for tissue diagnosis is generally discouraged, especially if the tumor is easily resectable. GISTs are soft, fragile masses, and biopsies increase the risk of tumor hemorrhage and dissemination. Biopsy may be appropriate when planning neoadjuvant therapy with imatinib, whether for localized, potentially resectable lesions whose surgical morbidity would be improved by tumor size reduction or for unresectable or metastatic lesions.

Radiographic evaluation often includes CT of the abdomen and pelvis with contrast. Attention should be given to the liver and peritoneum, the most common sites of metastases. Chest CT can be performed to assess for rare lung metastases. Staging and determination of surgical resection is generally based on CT findings. The characteristic finding is of a smooth and well-circumscribed mass in the bowel wall that demonstrates exophytic growth. Larger GISTs may demonstrate central necrosis or hemorrhage.

The clinical behavior of GISTs is highly variable. Virtually all GISTs, especially those larger than 1 cm, have malignant potential. Tumor size and mitotic rate are the two major criteria used to define the risk of aggressive behavior (Table 1).

Treatment

Treatment depends on the extent of disease. For localized disease, resection is the primary therapy and should consist of segmental resection of the affected bowel. Periampullary tumors may require pancreaticoduodenectomy. Tumors with adjacent organs adherent to the mass must have all disease resected en bloc. The abdomen should be thoroughly explored for peritoneal and liver metastases. Because GISTs rarely metastasize to lymph nodes, routine lymphadenectomy is not recommended. The goal is complete gross resection with an intact pseudocapsule and negative microscopic margins. Careful handling of these tumors is critical to avoid rupture and tumor dissemination. Some evidence has suggested that patients whose complete resection is complicated by tumor rupture have a shortened survival compared with those who do not have tumor rupture.

Preoperative administration of imatinib should be considered for marginally resectable GISTs in patients whose surgical morbidity would be improved by reducing the size of the tumor preoperatively. Postoperative treatment with imatinib has been shown to prolong recurrence-free survival and is considered a standard approach following complete resection of all small bowel GIST tumors larger than 3 cm. The optimal duration of treatment is still not clear, but it is recommended that patients with intermediate- to high-risk GISTs be treated for a minimum of 36 months. Imatinib should also be given postoperatively to patients with incomplete resection, recurrent disease, and/or metastatic disease.

Patients with unresectable or metastatic GISTs should be treated with imatinib, and because disease progression has been reported to follow the cessation of imatinib therapy, these patients are often treated with tyrosine kinase inhibitor therapy indefinitely, as long as the disease does not progress and patient tolerance permits. The majority of patients treated with imatinib ultimately experience disease progression after an initial response because of the development of delayed imatinib resistance at a median of 18 to 24 months. The oral tyrosine kinase receptor sunitinib malate is generally given to patients who progress on imatinib.

The decision to operate for metastatic or recurrent GIST should be tailored to each patient and limited to patients with stable or shrinking tumors while on tyrosine kinase inhibitor therapy or for limited disease progression, especially for those lesions that appear potentially easy to resect. The 5-year overall observed survival for patients with a small bowel GIST undergoing resection is 40%. Factors that negatively affect prognosis include larger tumor size, high mitotic index per high-powered field, tumor rupture, male gender, age greater than 55 years, metastases, poorly differentiated tumors, and involved margins.

NON-HODGKIN'S LYMPHOMA

Tumor Characteristics

Gastrointestinal lymphomas are the most frequently occurring extranodal lymphomas. Primary lymphomas of the small intestine consist of a variety of non-Hodgkin's lymphoma subtypes that vary significantly in tumor behavior, response to chemotherapy, and prognosis. Most gastrointestinal lymphomas are of B-cell origin, including diffuse large B-cell lymphoma, mantle cell lymphoma, B-cell lymphoma of mucosa-associated lymphoid tissue (MALT) type, follicular lymphoma, Burkitt lymphoma, and immunoproliferative lymphoma. MALT tumors can be associated with *Helicobacter pylori* infection, and primary treatment includes eradication of *H. pylori*, often leading to complete histologic remission. The distribution of lymphoma in the small intestine parallels the distribution of lymphoid follicles, with the lymphoid-rich ileum representing the most common location. Lymphomas are characteristically bulky tumors, and approximately 70% of them are larger than 5 cm in diameter at presentation.

T-cell lymphomas of the small intestine are more common than B-cell lymphomas and are typically associated with celiac disease. Most enteropathy-associated T-cell lymphomas (EATL) are located in the proximal small intestine. The diagnosis of small bowel lymphoma should be entertained in celiac patients who do not improve on a gluten-free diet or who develop recurrent gastrointestinal symptoms, anemia, or weight loss. Finally, patients with human immunodeficiency virus and low CD4 count are at risk for developing B-cell gastrointestinal lymphomas, which often have a high grade of malignancy and a poor prognosis.

Clinical Presentation

The clinical presentation of patients with lymphoma of the small intestine differs according to the histologic tumor type. Abdominal pain is the most frequent symptom of all types, occurring in approximately two thirds of patients. Other symptoms include gastrointestinal (GI) bleeding, intestinal obstruction or perforation, or a palpable abdominal mass. Patients with EATL often present with acute bleeding, obstruction, or perforation.

Diagnosis

Radiographic evaluation may include a CT scan, which characteristically demonstrates multiple, large tumors and bowel wall segments with homogenous thickening and a normal or enlarged lumen (Figure 4). Diagnosis of lymphoma requires a tissue biopsy so that studies including immunohistochemistry, flow cytometry, and cytogenetic and molecular genetic evaluation can be performed. These allow classification of the lymphoma and ultimately determine optimal treatment and prognosis. One of the major reasons to biopsy ulcerating or nodular lesions in the small bowel remains assessment for lymphoma because this may change the management from surgical to medical. Taking multiple endoscopic biopsies provides sufficient material to diagnose lymphoma in nearly all cases.

The Ann Arbor staging system used for most lymphomas is considered to be inadequate for the staging of GI lymphoma since it does not incorporate information on the depth of tumor invasion, that is known to affect prognosis. Several other staging systems have been proposed, and the most widely accepted is the Lugano staging system (Table 2).

Treatment

Optimal treatment of GI lymphoma remains poorly defined. The treatment of nongastric MALT lymphoma depends principally upon the stage of disease at diagnosis. Treatment of small intestinal MALT

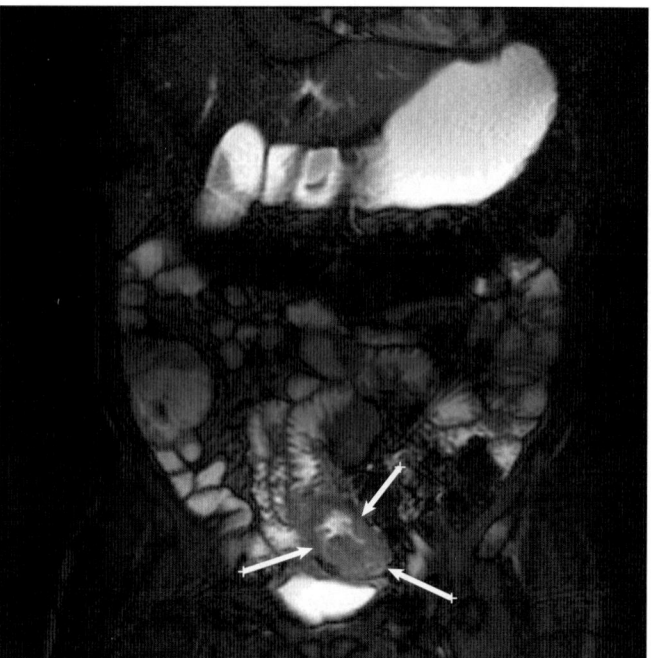

FIGURE 4 Lymphoma involving the ileum.

TABLE 2: Lugano staging system for gastrointestinal lymphomas

Stage I—The tumor is confined to the gastrointestinal tract. It can be a single primary lesion or multiple noncontiguous lesions.

Stage II—The tumor extends into the abdomen. This is further subdivided based upon the location of nodal involvement.

Stage II₁—There is involvement of local nodes (perigastric nodes for gastric lymphoma or paraintestinal nodes for intestinal lymphoma).

Stage II₂—There is involvement of distant nodes (paraaortic, paracaval, pelvic, or inguinal nodes for most tumors; mesenteric nodes in the case of intestinal lymphoma).

Stage IIE—The tumor penetrates the serosa to involve adjacent organs or tissues.

Stage III—There is no stage III disease in this system.

Stage IV—There is disseminated extranodal involvement or concomitant supradiaphragmatic nodal involvement.

Rohatiner A, d'Amore F, Coiffier B, et al: Report on a workshop convened to discuss the pathological and staging classification of gastrointestinal tract lymphoma, Ann Oncol 5:397, 1994.

---

lymphomas diagnosed at an early stage with antibiotics directed against *Campylobacter jejuni* or *H. pylori* may lead to regression. Most patients ultimately relapse and present with an aggressive high-grade histology requiring radiation therapy and/or combination chemotherapy. Most patients with diffuse large B-cell lymphoma are treated with combination chemoimmunotherapy regimens such as R-CHOP with or without radiation therapy. Surgery is reserved for patients with complications such as perforation or obstruction or intractable bleeding.

EATL is almost always of high-grade histology. Prognosis is poor and worse than that of other intestinal lymphomas. Treatment consists of combination chemotherapy that can be followed by autologous hematopoietic cell transplantation. Systemic chemotherapy is the treatment of choice for mantle cell lymphoma. However, if the tumor is localized, chemotherapy followed by radiation may be curative. Chemotherapy is the mainstay of treatment of Burkitt lymphoma, but resection may be an option for isolated lesions or may be required to alleviate symptoms or avoid perforation during chemotherapy.

METASTASES

Secondary neoplastic involvement of the intestine is more common than primary small intestinal neoplasia, most frequently from melanoma, lung cancer, and breast cancer. Metastases to the small bowel can occur via direct invasion, hematogenous or lymphatic spread, and intraperitoneal seeding. The most common presentation of metastasis is small bowel obstruction, although ascites, mesenteric ischemia, perforation, and bleeding can also be seen. Unfortunately, small bowel metastases indicate an advanced stage of the primary neoplasm, so treatment usually is focused on alleviating symptoms. Small bowel obstructions are treated in the standard fashion: with nasogastric decompression, bowel rest, and intravenous hydration. Failure of conservative treatment necessitates surgical intervention, typically resection of obstructed or intussuscepted bowel with primary anastomosis.

Patients with diffuse carcinomatosis are high-risk operative candidates who must be medically optimized prior to undergoing surgery. In those patients whose tumors are so advanced that definitive treatment cannot be performed, placement of a gastrostomy tube or an ostomy for decompression may be considered. Before any surgery, however, it is useful to repeat tumor staging to define the patient's prognosis.

BENIGN TUMORS

Similar to their malignant counterparts, benign small intestine tumors often are undetected. Those patients who are symptomatic most commonly present with abdominal pain and bleeding. Despite their benign nature, endoscopic or surgical resection is usually indicated to obtain adequate tissue for diagnosis and to reduce the risk of subsequent complications, such as bleeding and obstruction.

Adenomas

Three types of small intestine adenomas have been described: simple villous, tubular, and Brunner's gland adenomas. In general, they may develop as single or multiple lesions, both sessile and pedunculated, and are found most commonly in the duodenum. Villous adenomas carry the highest risk of malignant transformation. Malignant cells are found in as many as 42% of duodenal villous adenomas, with an adenoma-carcinoma sequence similar to that of colorectal cancer. Patients with familial adenomatous polyposis have a significantly higher prevalence of duodenal adenomas, as well as a much greater risk of duodenal adenocarcinoma. Tubular adenomas are less likely to undergo malignant transformation. Brunner's gland adenomas exhibit benign proliferation of the Brunner's glands, with scattered ductal and stromal elements.

Ampullary adenomas most commonly present with painless jaundice related to the mass effect on the ampulla and sometimes with pruritus or cholangitis. MRCP and percutaneous transhepatic cholangiography will show findings suggestive of biliary obstruction at the ampullary level, but endoscopic retrograde cholangiopancreatography (ERCP) has the advantage of permitting direct visualization of the ampulla, biliary decompression via an internal stent if necessary, and biopsy of the ampullary mass.

Although endoscopic evaluation is a common and useful means of evaluating these tumors, endoscopic biopsies have been shown to miss malignancies. Treatment of small intestinal adenoma varies by their pathology, and local excision may be appropriate for small tumors. For villous tumors of the duodenum, treatment recommendations vary from local excision to pancreas-sparing duodenectomy to pancreaticoduodenectomy. Patients whose tumor has no features that raise concerns for malignancy, such as ulceration, severe dysplasia on preoperative biopsy, or dilation of pancreatic and common bile duct, may be treated with local excision; if any of the aforementioned worrisome traits are present, pancreaticoduodenectomy should be considered.

Because of the high rate of tumor recurrence with local excision (up to 30% at 5 years) and the potential for recurrence as invasive cancer, regular endoscopic surveillance postoperatively is required. Villous tumors of the duodenum that recur after local excision call for pancreaticoduodenectomy. Patients with familial adenomatous polyposis and duodenal tumors showing high-grade dysplasia should undergo either pancreas-sparing duodenectomy or pancreaticoduodenectomy.

Lipomas

Small intestinal lipomas are benign tumors that arise from the submucosal adipose tissue and expand with compression of the lumen. They are most commonly found in the ileum. Histologic features include collections of mature adipose tissue and fibrous tissue strands. Symptoms, when they do occur, are usually related to obstruction, bleeding, and/or intussusception. Lipomas are seen on CT as a homogenous mass with the density of fat. On barium studies they appear as smooth, radiolucent, well-circumscribed intramural masses whose size and form change with peristalsis and pressure. Small, asymptomatic lipomas can be treated conservatively, whereas symptomatic lipomas or those greater than 2 cm should be resected.

Hamartomas

Hamartomatous polyps consist of a smooth muscle core arising from the muscularis mucosa and extending into the polyp. They usually occur in multiples and in varying sizes and shapes. Hamartomas are characteristic of Peutz-Jeghers syndrome, an autosomal dominant condition. They occur throughout the bowel and in varying number, from solitary polyps to hundreds coating the intestine. The polyps can cause abdominal pain, intussusception, obstruction, and GI bleeding. Endoscopic polypectomy reduces polyp-related complications and the risk of needing future operative polypectomy. If a laparotomy is performed either emergently for obstruction/intussusception, or electively for the removal of large or symptomatic polyps, intraoperative endoscopy and "clean sweep" polypectomy should be undertaken. There are a number of potentially promising agents for reduction of polyp burden in Peutz-Jeghers syndrome, but none of these are in routine clinical use.

Hemangiomas

Vascular tumors account for 7% to 10% of all benign small bowel tumors. They can be solitary or multiple, and in the small intestine, the jejunum is the most common site of involvement. Occult chronic GI bleeding and iron deficiency anemia are the most common forms of presentation. Hemangiomas can be classified as cavernous (most frequent), capillary, or mixed-type, according to the diameter of the involved vessel. Microscopically, they consist of numerous dilated, irregular, blood-filled spaces or sinuses lined by layers of endothelial cells. They can vary in size from a few millimeters to several centimeters. They are usually localized in the submucosa but can be infiltrative and affect the entire thickness of the intestinal wall, as well as the mesentery, retroperitoneum, or pelvis.

Preoperative diagnosis is difficult. MRI and, more recently, capsule endoscopy have been useful means of identifying these lesions. Complete surgical resection is the procedure of choice, particularly when a solitary lesion is found. For appropriately sized and located lesions, endoscopic sclerotherapy or angiographic embolization may also be used.

SUGGESTED READINGS

Bilimoria KY, Bentrem DJ, Wayne JD, et al: Small bowel cancer in the United States: changes in epidemiology, treatment, and survival over the last 20 years, *Ann Surg* 249(1):63–71, 2009.

Grover S, Ashley SW, Raut CP: Small intestine gastrointestinal stromal tumors, *Curr Opin Gastroenterol* 28:113–123, 2012.

Modlin IM, Lye KD, Kidd M: A 5-decade analysis of 13,715 carcinoid tumors, *Cancer* 97:934–959, 2003.

Overman MJ, Hu CY, Kopetz S, et al: A population-based comparison of adenocarcinoma of the large and small intestine: insights into a rare disease, *Ann Surg Oncol* 19(5):1439–1445, 2012.

Pera M, Marquez L, Dedeu J, et al: Solitary cavernous hemangioma of the small intestine as the cause of long-standing iron deficiency anemia, *J Gastrointestinal Surg* 16(12):2288–2290, 2012.

Yao J, Hassan M, Phan A, et al: One hundred years after "carcinoid": epidemiology of and prognostic factors for neuroendocrine tumors in 35,825 cases in the United States, *J Clin Oncol* 26:3063–3072, 2008.

THE MANAGEMENT OF DIVERTICULOSIS OF THE SMALL BOWEL

Kyla P. Terhune, MD, and John L. Tarpley, MD

Diverticulosis of the small bowel is often overlooked because its presentation may be similar but its prevalence pales in comparison with diverticulosis of the large bowel (15% to 40% of those older than 40 years are reported to have colonic diverticula). However, three small bowel diverticula merit particular consideration: duodenal, jejuno-ileal, and Meckel's. These may present acutely or chronically, and management varies depending on location, acuity, and patient age. Descriptions of small bowel diverticula can be categorized by structure or cause: (1) congenital or acquired; (2) true (all three layers) or false (mucosa, submucosa); and (3) location (duodenal or jejuno-ileal). Most duodenal and jejuno-ileal diverticula are false or pseudodiverticula, pulsion phenomena related to increased intraluminal pressure and intestinal dysmotility with consequent herniation of mucosa and submucosa through muscular defects. These occur at the points of entrance or exit of blood vessels, the vasa recta, located on the mesenteric border of the small bowel. Perhaps 5% of adults over 40 years of age harbor duodenal diverticula, with incidence rate increasing with age, but only about 1% has jejunal or ileal pseudodiverticula and about 2% a Meckel's. Although Meckel's diverticula can be described with these descriptors, it is a specific entity unto itself, defined as a congenital true diverticulum that is a result of incomplete closure of the omphalomesenteric or vitelline duct during gestation.

The objective of this chapter is to address the practical approaches to small bowel diverticula, partitioning them by duodenal, jejuno-ileal, or Meckel's. A description of the characteristics of each is followed by proposed guidelines for surgical management: nonoperative or operative, with or without endoscopic or interventional techniques.

DUODENAL DIVERTICULA

Duodenal diverticula are fairly common in adults, and because they are rarely symptomatic, the true incidence and prevalence rates are likely underestimated. Most are detected incidentally on imaging studies, upper endoscopy, occasionally at operation or at postmortem examination. Frequently reported incidence rates are approximately 5% with radiologic contrast studies, 15% with upper endoscopy, and up to 20% in some autopsy reports. The incidence rate rises with increasing age and affects more women than men. Two thirds of cases reside in the periampullary region, located mostly on the medial wall (Figure 1). Duodenal diverticula sometimes are stated to produce symptoms 5% to 10% of the time when present. Symptoms may be the result of inflammation of the diverticulum, perforation, bleeding, or compression of the biliopancreatic ducts. Resist the temptation to "do something" for the asymptomatic, incidentally discovered duodenal diverticulum. As one of the authors says, "Don't poke a skunk."

Occasionally, duodenal diverticula are symptomatic and present with abdominal pain, both acute and chronic. Acute presentations can be the result of diverticulitis, bleeding, pancreatitis, and biliary obstruction. Location of the diverticulum and surrounding structures determines the symptoms from compression. In patients with diverticula immediately adjacent to the ampulla of Vater, the biliopancreatic ducts usually enter the duodenum at the superior margin rather than through the diverticulum. In addition, diverticula on the medial wall of the duodenum are, in reality, embedded in the pancreas. Diverticula in proximity to the ampulla increase in importance during endoscopic procedures, especially endoscopic retrograde cholangiopancreatography (ERCP). The likelihood of an unsuccessful study or, even worse, an iatrogenic injury with duodenal perforation can accompany such efforts when a duodenal diverticulum is present.

Chronic presentations of small bowel diverticular disease can be the result of bleeding or stasis-related steatorrhea with bacterial overgrowth. However, even when symptomatic, diverticula should be addressed operatively only after much reflection given the historically high morbidity and even mortality rates associated with operative management. Patients should instead "earn" their operation, and the physician should be as certain as possible that the diverticulum is causal to the presentation.

When a duodenal diverticulum has been determined to be the source, the least intervention that accomplishes a good outcome is the aim. Nonoperative options in these usually elderly patients include bowel rest, antibiotics, parenteral nutrition, endoscopic treatment, and interventional radiologic (IR) techniques. For patients with a perforation, one can consider IR percutaneous drainage. For patients with bleeding, endoscopic coagulation options or IR angio-embolization are options.

In the past, direct attack on the offending bleeding, inflamed, or perforated diverticulum was the strategy. Now, this is reserved for emergent situations and failure of nonoperative interventions because surgical intervention often comes with significant morbidity and mortality, including high recurrence rates and duodenal fistulae

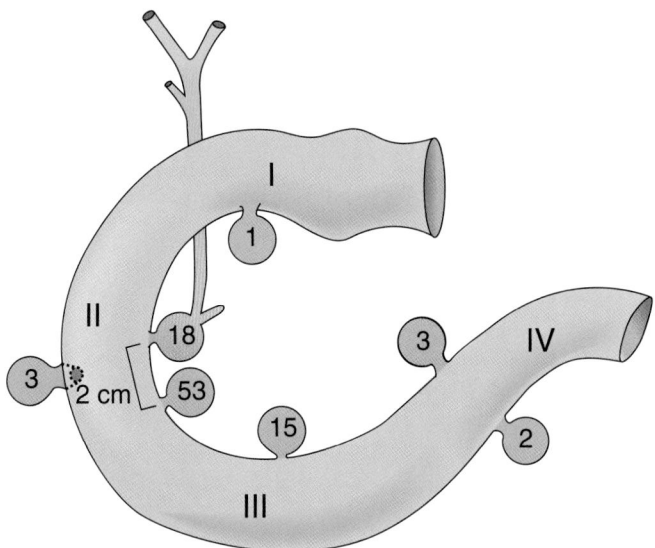

FIGURE 1   Distribution of 95 duodenal diverticula within the four portions of the duodenum. *(From Eggert A, Teichmann W, Wittmann DH: The pathologic implication of duodenal diverticula,* Surg Gynecol Obstet *154:62-64, 1982.)*

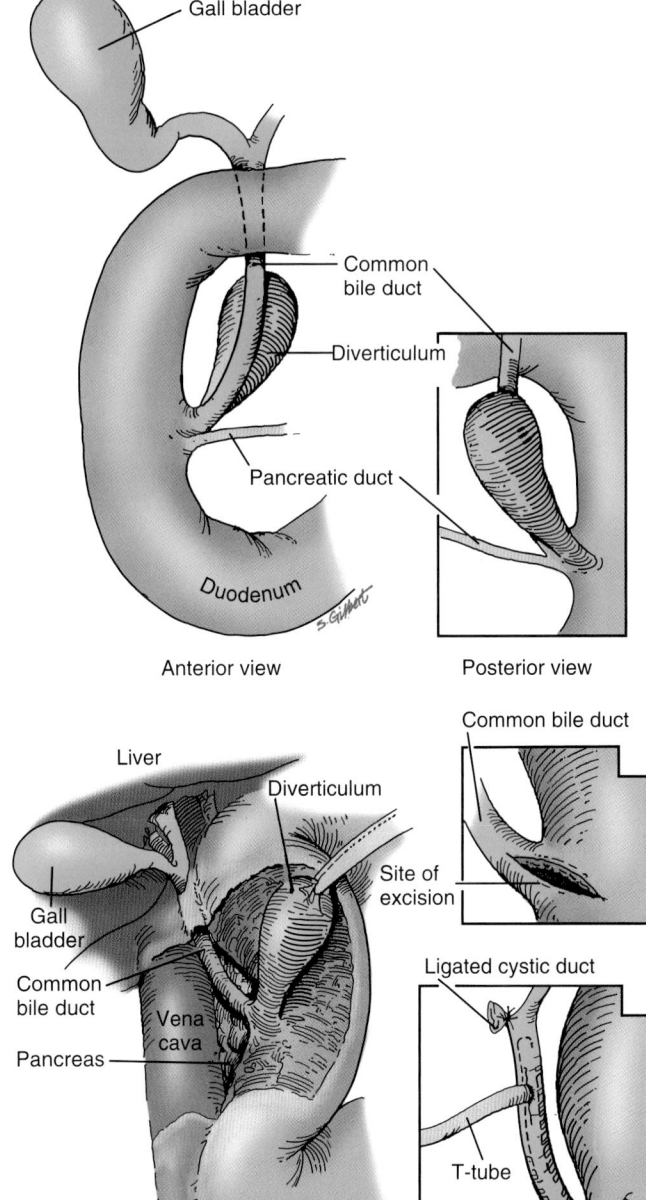

FIGURE 2   Usefulness of the Kocher's maneuver in demonstrating duodenal diverticula. *(From Jones TW, Merendino KA: The perplexing duodenal diverticulum,* Surgery *48:1068, 1960.)*

formation. When operative intervention is necessary, it consists of open laparotomy with generous Kocher's maneuver, followed by diverticulectomy, duodenal resection, inversion, or drainage (Figure 2). Anatomically, most of the diverticula are against and into the head of the pancreas, one of the primary reasons for difficulty and consequent morbidity. It is imperative to know the relationship between the duodenal diverticulum and the biliary system, particularly the ampulla. After the Kocher's maneuver and anterolateral duodenotomy for exposure, one can either place a probe retrograde via the papilla or pass a Fogarty biliary or red rubber catheter anterograde through an opening in the cystic duct or via the common duct to define the anatomy. The challenge is to identify the diverticulum, protect key structures, and then either resect or invert the diverticulum. One then closes the duodenum in two layers with absorbable suture for the inner layer and nonabsorbable sutures for the outer layer, taking care not to compromise the diameter of the bowel. Historically, with a large diverticulum, a serosal patch technique or Roux-en-Y duodenojejunostomy was at times used to thwart narrowing of the lumen. Safer alternatives to resection or inversion of the diverticulum include diversions of the biliary or alimentary stream. These indirect or flanking procedures such as a Roux-en-Y hepaticojejunostomy or a Roux-en-Y duodenojejunostomy as advocated by Silen and more recently Mathews are worthy of consideration and often safer and more effective (Figure 3).

A second type of duodenal diverticulum that is rare but worth describing is a congenital anomaly often referred to as an intraluminal duodenal diverticulum. It can lead to duodenal obstruction, bleeding, and acute pancreatitis. This rarely encountered entity is a variant of an intestinal web, caused by incomplete recanalization of the duodenum, appearing to develop in utero at approximately the 7th week of gestation when a partial duodenal diaphragm forms and elongates, forming a diverticulum. With entrapment of food, peristalsis, and distension, this "diverticulum" increases in size. Radiographically, the region appears as a "windsock" or "thumb of a glove" and resides in the lumen of the duodenum. Other coexistent gastrointestinal congenital abnormalities can be found in up to 40% of patients who also have intraluminal duodenal diverticula. Operative intervention is necessary because the "diverticulum" should be excised; for planning, it is again important to understand the

anatomic relationship of surrounding ductal structures. The common bile duct and pancreatic duct usually empty into the diverticulum near its attachment to the duodenal wall at the proximal extent of the diverticulum. The approach is similar to that described previously, with an anterior duodenotomy and careful preservation of the ampulla of Vater. This is followed by a subtotal resection of the intraluminal diverticulum. Endoscopic approaches have also been reported recently, but currently laparotomy with excision via duodenotomy is recommended.

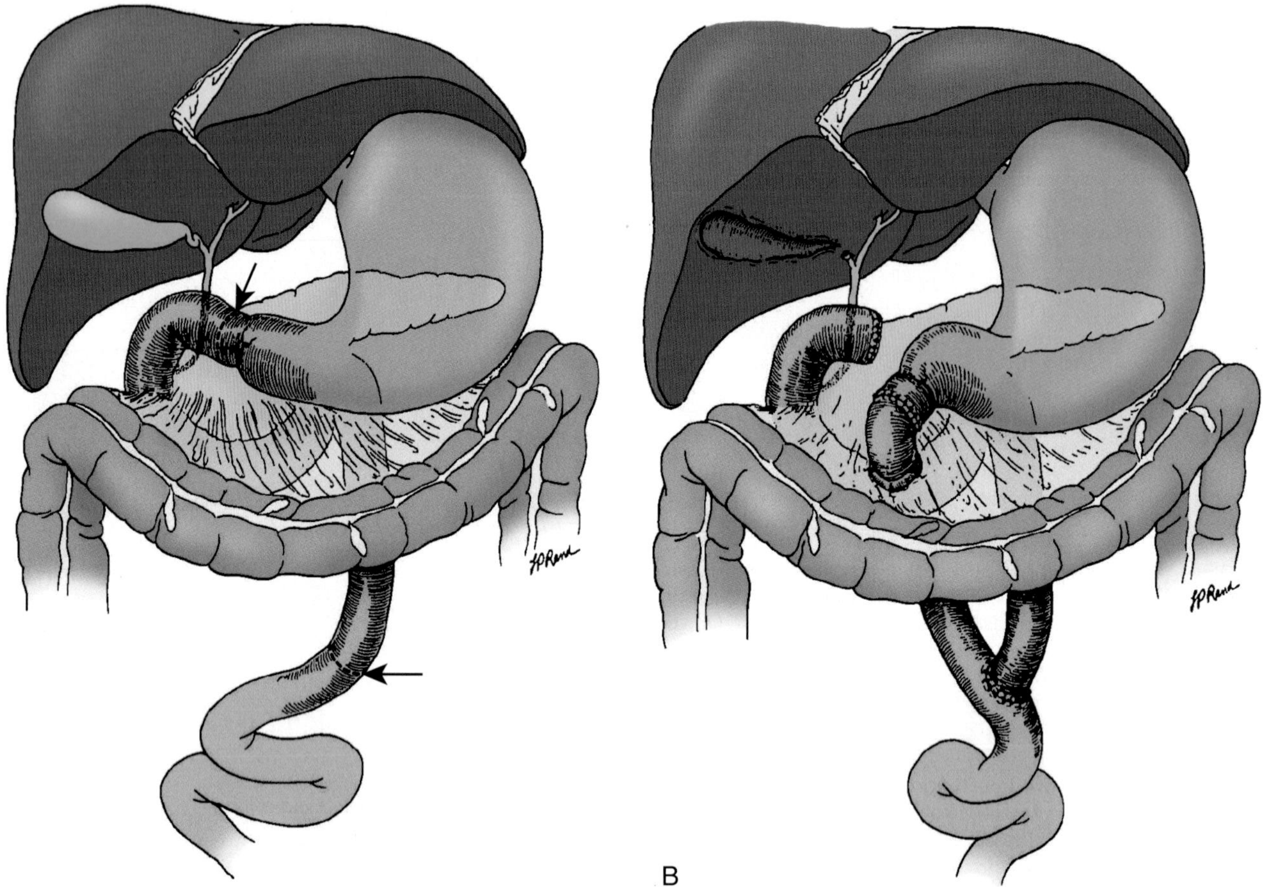

FIGURE 3 Duodenojejunostomy for pancreaticobiliary complications of duodenal diverticulum. **A,** Anatomy before reconstruction. *Arrows* point to dotted lines that indicate proposed sites of division of the intestine. **B,** Anatomy after reconstruction. The gallbladder has been removed. The Roux limb has been brought through the mesocolon, the duodenojejunostomy completed, and the mesentery closed. *(From Critchlow JF, Shapiro ME, Silen W: Duodenojejunostomy for the pancreaticobiliary complications of duodenal diverticulum.* Ann Surg *202:56-58, 1985.)*

JEJUNO-ILEAL DIVERTICULAR DISEASE

Similar to duodenal diverticula but even less frequent, jejuno-ileal diverticula are also false diverticula. Usually in the elderly and multiple in number, diverticula are stated to be seven times more frequent in the jejunum than in the ileum (Figure 4). In the evaluation of patients with chronic symptoms, detection of lesions may be noted with computed tomographic (CT) scan, enteroclysis, push enteroscopy, double-balloon endoscopy, and capsule endoscopy. Jejuno-ileal diverticulitis is an overlooked cause of acute abdominal pain in the elderly and can be confused with colonic diverticulitis, appendicitis, and other entities on the long list of candidates for the differential diagnoses of the acute abdomen. Similarly, patients with a subacute or chronic presentation can be confused as having inflammatory bowel disease, tuberculosis, and even neoplasms. Acute complications from jejuno-ileal diverticula are infrequent but, just as in duodenal disease as described previously, may occur from inflammation, perforation, obstruction, and bleeding. The approach to operative intervention is similar, but because these lesions are not proximately associated with the biliopancreatic tract, the danger of injury to surrounding structures is decreased.

Acute inflammation in the setting of jejuno-ileal diverticulosis can result in uncomplicated diverticulitis, microperforation with phlegmon or abscess formation, and free perforation without containment resulting in generalized peritonitis. The CT scan can prove most helpful in detecting inflammation, stranding, presence of other

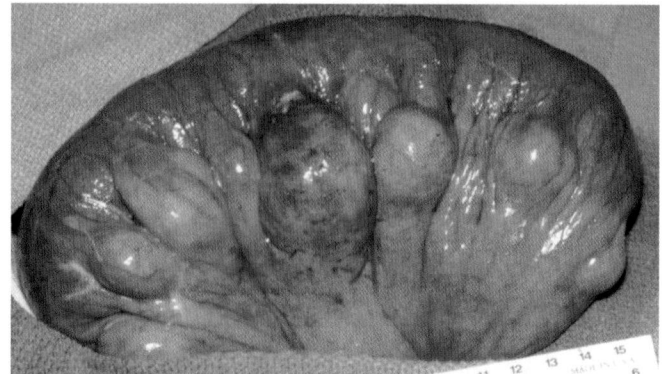

FIGURE 4 Multiple large jejunal diverticula located in the mesentery in an older patient with obstruction from an enterolith. *(From Evers BM, Townsend CM Jr, Thompson JC: Small intestine. In Schwartz SI, editor:* Principles of surgery, *ed 7, New York, 1999, McGraw-Hill, p 1248.)*

diverticula, bowel-wall thickening, microperforations with focal extraluminal air, abscesses, and other features not dissimilar to the more frequent colonic diverticular disease. Symptomatic patients often have an accompanying leukocytosis, although this is sometimes absent in the elderly. Chronic symptoms include abdominal pain, stasis, bacterial overgrowth, and malnutrition. In the symptomatic but nonperitonitic case with a failed trial of nonoperative management with bowel rest, antibiotics, and decompression, the operative treatment is a judicious segmental resection of the involved segment of small bowel with enteroenterostomy. One should not attempt to remove all diverticular disease but instead resect the portion responsible for the current illness.

MECKEL'S DIVERTICULUM

Meckel's diverticulum (Figure 5) is the most common congenital anomaly of the alimentary tract, with a reported prevalence rate of 1% to 4% in the general population. As noted previously, this is the result of incomplete closure of the omphalomesenteric or vitelline duct during gestation. Most Meckel's diverticula remain asymptomatic over the course of a patient's lifetime but may be discovered incidentally at operation or with an imaging study. When symptomatic, it is the result of bleeding, bowel obstruction, diverticulitis, and, very rarely, neoplasia. Meckel's diverticulum is affectionately taught early in medical school as the "Rule of Twos:" it is usually found within 2 feet of the ileocecal valve, in 2% of the population, with two possible heterotopic mucosae (gastric or pancreatic), two times as prevalent in men compared with women, wherein only 2% (0.5 to 2.0%) become symptomatic, usually within the first 2 years of life. When symptomatic in the pediatric population, it is often from bleeding, as secretions from the heterotopic gastric mucosa within the Meckel's diverticulum ulcerate the ileal mucosa on the mesenteric border, opposite the diverticulum. This bleeding may be acute or chronic. If suspected, one can use Meckel's scintigraphy, with technetium-99m pertechnetate, which then is concentrated and secreted by the heterotopic gastric mucosa (Figure 6). Although it has a sensitivity of approximately 85% in children, it shows the presence of gastric mucosa so is less useful in adults where the gastric mucosa may be atrophic.

On rare occasion, IR has a diagnostic role during active bleeding for localization or confirmation. A persistent right vitelline artery arising from the superior mesenteric artery or a nonbranching embryonic ileal artery may be encountered. Treatment for bleeding incited by a Meckel's diverticulum requires a segmental ileal resection so that both the Meckel's diverticulum and the ileal ulceration are removed. When the resection is for symptoms other than bleeding, a simple V-shaped diverticulectomy with transverse closure of the ileum can be performed.

Most children who undergo an operation for a Meckel's diverticulum are under 4 years of age. In a recent national study directed by B.T. Campbell of Hartford, Conn, with an administrative database from 43 freestanding, not-for-profit U.S. children's hospitals, 815 children underwent Meckel's diverticulectomy over a 24-month period. The boy:girl ratio was 2.3:1, and half of the children (53%) needed operation before their 4th birthday. Children less than 2 years of age had the highest incidence rate of Meckel's diverticulectomy. The most common presentations for primary (intentional, directed for the Meckel's diverticulum, not incidental) resection were obstruction (30%), bleeding (27%), and intussusception (19%) in children under 18 years old.

In adults, diverticulitis and obstruction are more likely presentations of a symptomatic Meckel's diverticulum, although both acute and chronic bleeding can occur. The presentation of Meckel's diverticulitis is virtually indistinguishable from acute appendicitis. In fact, it is recommended that when acute appendicitis is suspected but not found operatively, one should run the terminal ileum to exclude Meckel's diverticula. Obstruction can be secondary to a residual fibrous band or cord from the obliterated omphalomesenteric duct with creation of an intestinal volvulus. Other obstructive etiologies include ileo-ileal or an ileo-colic intussusception with the Meckel's diverticulum as a lead point. Rarely, a Meckel's diverticulum becomes incarcerated in an inguinal hernia, known as Littre's hernia.

Resection of the incidentally found Meckel's diverticulum depends on patient age, circumstances of the procedure, and whether the risk of resection is higher or lower than the likelihood of subsequent symptomatology. In the multiinstitutional study from Hartford, 40% of the Meckel's resections in the 815 patients under age 18 years were performed as a secondary procedure after the Meckel's was discovered during an operation for another diagnosis. A study from Seattle by Soltero and Bill in the 1970s argued that the likelihood for

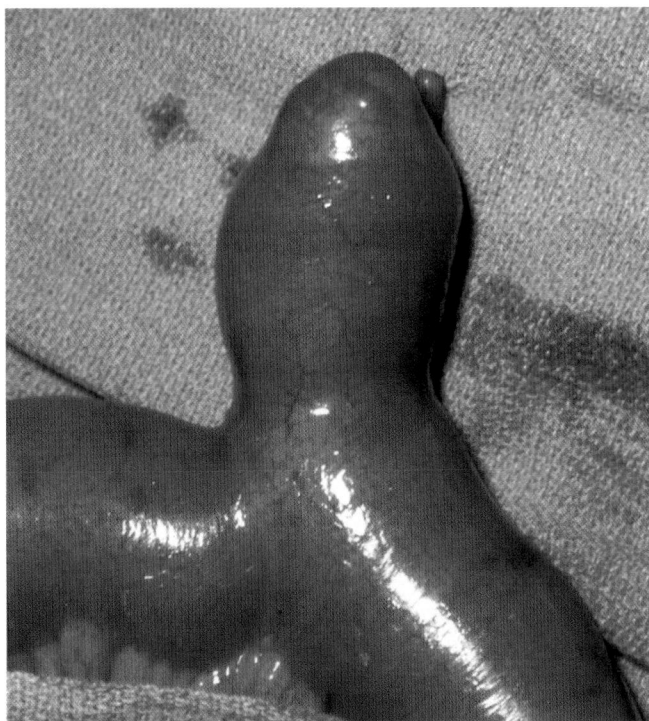

FIGURE 5 Common presentation of a Meckel's diverticulum projecting from the antimesenteric border of the ileum. *(From McKenzie S, Evers BM: Small intestine. In Townsend CM Jr editor: Sabiston textbook of surgery, ed 19, Philadelphia, 2012, Elsevier Saunders.)*

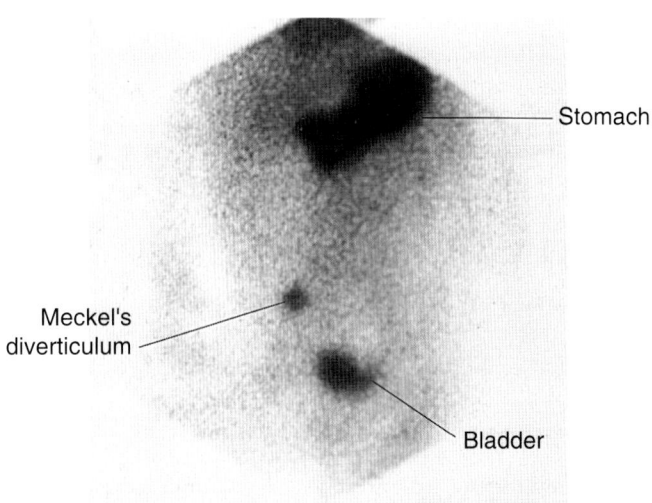

FIGURE 6 ^{99m}Tc-pertchnetate scintigram from a child with a Meckel's diverticulum clearly differentiated from the stomach and bladder. *(From McKenzie S, Evers BM: Small intestine. In Townsend Jr CM editor: Sabiston textbook of surgery, ed 19, Philadelphia, 2012, Elsevier Saunders.)*

a Meckel's becoming symptomatic in an adult was only 2% but the projected morbidity for resection may be as high as 12%. Cullen and associates from the Mayo Clinic in 1994 challenged the practice of ignoring an incidentally found Meckel's and quoted a 6.4% likelihood of symptoms from a Meckel's over a lifetime. Noting a low complication rate from the removal of the Meckel's diverticulum itself as opposed to that of the primary operation, they recommended removal at any age up to 80 years, as long as no additional conditions made removal hazardous. From a meta-analysis of 244 studies, Zani and colleagues reported increased morbidity associated with incidental resection over no treatment and determined that more than 700 patients with incidental Meckel's diverticulum required resection to avoid one Meckel's-related death. Thus, general practice is to resect incidentally found Meckel's diverticulum in children but not in adults.

SUMMARY

In summary, small bowel diverticula are rarely symptomatic, as they are in continuity with the lumen and thus function as a part of the small bowel lumen. On occasion, a diverticulum can become secondarily inflamed, perforate, cause obstruction, or bleed. Bleeding from false diverticula of the duodenum, jejunum, and non-Meckel's ileum arises from blood vessels along their perimeter associated with the vasa recta; bleeding in association with a Meckel's diverticulum results from ulceration secondary to acid secretion from heterotopic gastric mucosa. Asymptomatic diverticula, including incidentally found Meckel's diverticula in the adult, should be left alone. In cases of acute or chronic symptoms associated with the pulsion diverticula, one must ask whether the option for observation and nonoperative management exists. Intraluminal duodenal diverticulum, a congenital anomaly associated with web formation, and symptomatic Meckel's diverticula should be resected. With symptomatic pulsion diverticula (duodenal or jejuno-ileal), operative management is sometimes required. Understanding the anatomic relationship of the diverticulum to surrounding structures, particularly to the biliopancreatic anatomy in the case of the duodenal diverticulum, is imperative. When considering any operation for a patient with a complication from a duodenal diverticulum, be mindful of the counsel of Emperor Augustus: *Festina Lente,* or "Make haste slowly."

SUGGESTED READINGS

Boyd KB, Blondeau B: Bleeding duodenal diverticuli, *Am Surg* 76:232–234, 2010.

Critchlow JF, Shapiro ME, Silen W: Duodenojejunostomy for the pancreaticobiliary complications of duodenal diverticulum, *Ann Surg* 202:56–58, 1985.

Critchlow JF, Shapiro ME, Silen W: Symptomatic duodenal diverticulum, *World J Surg* 20:118, 1996. http://www.ncbi.nlm.nih.gov/pubmed/8588405.

Cullen JJ, Kelly KA, Moir CR, et al: Surgical management of Meckel's diverticulum. An epidemiologic population-based study, *Ann Surg* 220:564–569, 1994.

D'Alessio MJ, Rana A, Martin JA, Moser AJ: Surgical management of intraluminal duodenal diverticulum and coexisting anomalies, *J Am Coll Surg* 201:143–148, 2005.

Jones TW, Merendino KA: The perplexing duodenal diverticulum, *Surgery* 48:1068, 1960.

Mathis KL, Farley DR: Operative management of symptomatic duodenal diverticula, *Am J Surg* 193:305–309, 2007.

Ruscher KA, Fisher JN, Hughes CD, Neff S, Lerer TJ, Hight DW, et al: National trends in the surgical management of Meckel's diverticulum, *J Pediatr Surg* 46:893–896, 2011.

Soltero MJ, Bill AH: The natural history of Meckel's diverticulum and its relation to incidental removal. A study of 202 cases of diseased Meckel's diverticulum found in King County, Washington, over a fifteen year period, *Am J Surg* 132:168–173, 1976.

Teven CM, Grossman E, Roggin KK, Mathews JB: Surgical management of pancreaticobiliary disease associated with juxtapapillary duodenal diverticula: case series and review of the literature, *J Gastrointest Surg* 16:1436–1441, 2012.

Zani A, Eaton S, Rees CM, et al: Incidentally detected Meckel diverticulum: to resect of not resect? *Ann Surg* 247:276–281, 2008.

MOTILITY DISORDERS OF THE STOMACH AND SMALL BOWEL

John Clarke, MD

OVERVIEW

Motility disorders of the gastrointestinal (GI) tract are most commonly encountered by surgeons in two of the following circumstances: either postoperatively or as a consequence of functional or directed denervation. Paralysis of the small intestine commonly manifests in patients undergoing manipulation of the abdominal viscera during laparotomy (especially during colectomy). Primary motility disorders of the GI tract are less commonly encountered in the realm of surgery, but they require a surgeon's evaluation because they are included in the differential diagnosis of surgical conditions and may require surgical intervention. As a rule, most cases of GI motility disorders may require surgical intervention when the symptoms are debilitating and unresponsive to medical management. This chapter is a review of the different motility disorders of the stomach and small bowel, with emphasis on surgical management.

MOTILITY DISORDERS OF THE STOMACH

Gastroparesis

Gastroparesis is a syndrome characterized by delayed gastric emptying in the absence of mechanical obstruction. The hallmark symptoms are nausea, vomiting, abdominal pain, early satiety, and postprandial sense of fullness. Symptom severity can be assessed with the Gastroparesis Cardinal Symptom Index (GCSI), which is a validated scale to assess symptom severity, although symptom severity is not a reliable predictor of the degree of gastric emptying impairment. Other symptoms may include bloating, uncontrolled reflux, post-prandial hypoglycemia, and weight change.

These symptoms can range from mild to severe and can be described within a classification scheme of gastroparesis. Three categories have been proposed: mild (grade 1), compensated (grade 2), and severe (grade 3). In grade 1 gastroparesis, symptoms are easily controlled and nutrition is maintained with a regular diet or with minor modifications. In grade 2 gastroparesis, symptoms are partially controlled by pharmacotherapy, dietary modifications are required, and patients rarely require hospital admission. In grade 3 gastroparesis, symptoms are refractory to medical therapy, oral nutrition intake is compromised, and patients may require frequent hospital admissions.

The incidence and prevalence of gastroparesis are controversial. The best data to date suggest that the age-adjusted incidences of definite gastroparesis are 2.4 for men and 9.8 for women per 100,000 person-years, and the prevalences per 100,000 persons are 9.6 for men and 38 for women. In all subsets of gastroparesis, there is a gender imbalance; women are affected in much greater numbers than are men. Some sources quote a female/male ratio of involvement of as high as 7 : 1.

Gastroparesis is a heterogeneous disease with distinct causes, the most common being idiopathic factors (36% to 49% of cases), diabetes mellitus (25% to 29%), and postsurgical factors (7% to 13%). Idiopathic gastroparesis is currently the most common subset at presentation. A potential autoimmune or postinfectious origin has been a subject of speculation, but the exact cause remains unknown, and active research to better understand involved mechanisms is ongoing.

Although diabetes is classically associated with gastroparesis, diabetic patients represent less than one third of patients with gastroparesis in most series. Approximately 10% to 15% of patients with gastroparesis have upper GI symptoms consistent with potential gastroparesis; however, the true prevalence of gastroparesis in patients with diabetes remains unclear. In tertiary referral centers, a delay is documented in more than 50% of diabetic patients referred for gastric emptying studies; however, this relationship may not exist in community settings. Gastroparesis can affect patients with both type 1 and type 2 diabetes. Usually, symptoms develop after at least 10 years of having documented diabetes, and these patients usually have some other sign of end-organ involvement, such as retinopathy, neuropathy, or nephropathy. Diabetic gastroparesis can cause severe symptoms and hence lead to nutritional compromise, impaired glycemic control, and poor overall quality of life, independent of other confounding factors such as age, smoking, alcohol, or type of diabetes.

The surgical procedure for gastroparesis that may be most commonly encountered in clinical practice and leads to reversible or irreversible vagal injury is fundoplication. Loss of extrinsic vagal stimulation reduces the capacity of the stomach to empty, whether in the fasting or postprandial state, and leads to gastroparesis and possible bezoar formation. Other surgical procedures that are implicated include the Billroth II gastrectomy, botulinum toxin injection for medical treatment of achalasia, variceal sclerotherapy, and lung or heart transplantation. Measuring the plasma pancreatic polypeptide may help establish the diagnosis of vagal injury; however, this is not often required in clinical practice as confirmation of vagal injury may not change management and the diagnosis can usually be established from clinical history. The plasma pancreatic polypeptide level normally increases by at least 25 pg/mL in the first 20 minutes after sham feeding, as a result of cephalic vagal stimulation. In cases of vagal injury, this increase may be blunted or absent.

Medications that have been implicated in gastroparesis include narcotics, α_2-adrenergic agonists (clonidine), tricyclic antidepressants, calcium channel blockers, dopamine agonists, muscarinic anticholinergics, and octreotide. Of interest, intermittent or prolonged use of erythromycin, which is known to accelerate gastric emptying,

may cause vomiting and upper abdominal discomfort, which can mimic symptoms of gastroparesis.

Gastroparesis can also be secondary to other causes, such as connective tissue diseases (typically scleroderma), viral illnesses (Norwalk virus and rotavirus), iatrogenic causes (medications, postsurgical status), infiltrating diseases (amyloidosis), thyroid dysfunction, metabolic abnormalities (hypokalemia, hypomagnesemia, hyperglycemia), and neuromuscular disorders.

In view of the varied causes implicated in gastroparesis, exact predictions regarding prognosis can prove difficult, although it has been suggested that patients with connective tissue disorders and the subset of patients with idiopathic gastroparesis with predominant symptoms of abdominal pain, have a worse prognosis. In addition, it has been noted that emptying of solids is more often compromised than that of liquids. Patients with poor tolerance of a liquid diet have a more unfavorable outcome.

Evaluation of Gastroparesis

Gastroparesis is often suspected from the history and physical examination findings and is subsequently confirmed with the appropriate diagnostic tests. Although no routine laboratory tests aid in the diagnosis, they may be helpful for ruling out secondary causes of gastroparesis. The basic laboratory tests to obtain include measurements of hemoglobin, fasting plasma glucose level, thyroid-stimulating hormone concentration, total serum protein, and albumin to assess the nutritional state of the patient or presence of metabolic abnormalities. If potential rheumatic disease is highly suspected, an antinuclear antibody titer can be measured. A plain radiograph of the abdomen could also reveal any evidence of bowel dilatation.

As symptoms of gastroparesis are nonspecific, upper endoscopy is necessary to rule out mechanical obstruction or significant mucosal disease. Endoscopy also allows for the detection of potential retained food (or bezoar formation). The finding of retained food on endoscopy is more specific for gastroparesis, but sensitivity is lower, and the absence of retained food on endoscopy does not guarantee normal findings of a gastric emptying study. If obstruction is highly suspected, an upper GI series or small bowel follow-through may be performed to rule out a mechanical process.

The "gold standard" for the diagnosis of gastroparesis is the gastric emptying scintigraphy. In the United States, this is the most standardized, simplest, and most widely available technique to document postprandial gastric stasis. In this test, the patient ingests a low-fat egg-white meal labeled with technetium 99 m and sulfur colloid and then undergoes scintigraphy immediately and 1, 2, and 4 hours after ingesting the meal. Many centers may perform studies of shorter duration; however, a 4-hour study has more optimal performance characteristics and is specifically recommended by joint consensus of the American Neurogastroenterology and Motility Society and the Society of Nuclear Medicine. Gastric emptying scintigraphy has 62% sensitivity and 93% specificity when performed 4 hours after meal ingestion. Medications that affect gastric emptying should be discontinued 48 to 72 hours in advance, and the blood glucose level in diabetic patients should be less than 275 mg/dL (and ideally normal) on the day of the test. In clinical practice, abnormal values are higher than 10% retained at 4 hours and higher than 60% retained at 2 hours. Approximately 20% of patients with symptoms suggestive of abnormal gastric emptying and normal 2-hour emptying parameters have abnormal emptying parameters at the 4-hour time point. At some centers, intravenous prokinetic agents may administered after 4 hours to determine whether the patient is a "responder" or "nonresponder," although this is not standard of care at the present time.

Liquids often empty from the stomach normally despite the presence of solid retention, which helps document the presence of gastric stasis, and its severity is most commonly assessed by evaluation of the gastric emptying of solids. Liquid-phase gastric emptying tests can be performed with the use of water labeled with a different isotope, indium 111–diethylenetriaminepentaacetic acid, (^{111}In-DTPA) and technetium 99 m (^{99m}Tc) . This test helps identify the small group of patients who may have altered liquid emptying with a normal solid-phase emptying and persistent nausea, although the clinical significance of this pattern remains unclear.

Other tests that can be used to assist the diagnosis of gastroparesis include the stable isotope breath test, wireless motility capsule (SmartPill), and antroduodenal manometry. The stable isotope breath test is not currently available in the United States, but it is commonly performed in Europe and other parts of the world and has certain potential benefits that will probably lead to more widespread use, including (1) lack of radiation exposure and (2) lower cost. This test is an indirect measure of gastric emptying. The patient ingests a solid meal labeled with carbon 13 (C^{13}) and another substance, such as C^{13} octanoic acid, C^{13} acetate, or C^{13}Spirulina (*Arthrospira platensis,* a plant-based protein source). When the C^{13}–labeled meal is emptied from the stomach, it is rapidly absorbed in the small intestine and metabolized in the liver to $C^{13}O_2$, which is exhaled from the lungs and subsequently detected in the breath test. Breath samples are collected 45, 90, 120, 150, and 180 minutes after meal ingestion. Accuracy and specificity of the stable isotope breath test are comparable with those of scintigraphy; however, the results may be less accurate in cases of malabsorption, liver disease, or lung disease, all of which may hinder the excretion of C^{13}-labeled foods.

The wireless motility capsule provides the opportunity to directly measure gastric emptying time and stomach contractile adequacy. The indigestible capsule has temperature, pressure, and pH sensors and is ingested with a meal or a standardized nutrient bar (e.g., SmartBar). As the capsule traverses the GI tract, it detects changes in pH and measures phasic pressure amplitudes. Gastric emptying time for a nondigestible solid is measured as the characteristic change in pH between the stomach and small intestine. In addition, the pattern and amplitude of contractions immediately before gastric emptying may provide useful information regarding gastric contractile adequacy and potentially may help distinguish patients with heightened gastric contractions from those with a more flaccid stomach. Emptying of the capsule appears to be correlated reasonably well with gastric emptying, as demonstrated by scintigraphy, and this technology has been approved by the U.S. Food and Drug Administration (FDA) as a valid means of evaluating gastric emptying. The wireless motility capsule also has the benefit of enabling clinicians to view whole-gut transit, potentially allowing detection of pan-gastrointestinal motility disorders that may alter therapy; however, at present this technology is expensive and insurance coverage is limited, and although vast amounts of information are derived with regard to gastric and small bowel pressure parameters, normative data to put that information in context are limited.

Antroduodenal manometry is often suggested as an additional modality to assess patients with scintigraphic evidence of gastric stasis and without an identifiable cause. It is an invasive technique that involves insertion of a water-perfused or solid-state multilumen manometry catheter placed through the nose. The proximal catheter port is placed in the distal antrum, and the distal catheter port is placed in the duodenum. This placement can be performed either under fluoroscopic guidance or through endoscopy. Antroduodenal manometry helps differentiate patterns of myopathic origin (low-amplitude contractions), as observed in amyloid deposition and scleroderma, from patterns of neuropathic origin (normal-amplitude contractions with abnormal contractile response), as observed in diabetes mellitus and idiopathic autonomic neuropathy. Although this technology provides helpful diagnostic information, the degree to which this information alters management of patients with gastroparesis remains unclear. For this reason, this study is offered in only select tertiary referral centers and in not widely available.

Management of Gastroparesis

Management of gastroparesis can be divided into four components: supportive measures, including hydration and dietary modifications; optimizing glycemic control in diabetic patients; medical therapy; and surgical therapy.

First-line therapy for these patients remains dietary modification. Usually, fat delays gastric emptying, and nondigestible fibers in fruits and vegetables are emptied poorly because they require effective interdigestive antral motility, which is absent in patients with gastroparesis. For these reasons, patients are usually recommended low-fat diets without nondigestible fibers in small quantities and frequent meals. Because liquid emptying is rarely affected, noncarbonated fluids can be taken throughout the meal, and proper liquid caloric supplementation can be used in lieu of a solid diet. In severe cases in which the patient is severely malnourished (>10% unintentional weight loss in the past 6 months) or is unable to maintain weight by oral intake alone, enteral access via jejunostomy or gastrojejunostomy tube is considered. It is of utmost importance that diabetic patients maintain glycemic control at all times because hyperglycemia results in antral hypomotility and delay in gastric emptying, and it appears to attenuate the efficacy of prokinetic drugs.

Prokinetic and antiemetic medications can be tried when dietary modification alone has not been successful. Antiemetics that can be used include phenothiazines, antihistamines, and 5-HT$_3$ antagonists (granisetron or ondansetron). For outpatients who have difficulty taking oral medications, rectal suppositories (promethazine) or transdermal agents (scopolamine) can be considered, as absorption may be more readily achieved. If patients are hospitalized, intravenous formulations may have more rapid onset and produce a more predictable response.

Prokinetic therapy is often touted as the mainstay of medical therapy for gastroparesis, but evidence to support efficacy is limited. Metoclopramide is the only medication that is endorsed by the FDA for treatment of gastroparesis in the United States; however, it is approved only for short-term use (up to 12 weeks) and has significant potential toxic effects, including tardive dyskinesia in a small percentage of patients who take this drug long term. If metoclopramide is chosen for outpatient use, the liquid formulation may offer more predictable bioavailability, and the dose should be tapered to the smallest amount that controls symptoms. Erythromycin is a macrolide antibiotic that has been shown to significantly increase antral contractions and, for this reason, has been used for treatment of gastroparesis. It may be helpful in a hospital setting for acute use, but long-term use is limited by tachyphylaxis and concern regarding potential toxic effects (including ototoxicity and QT prolongation). Domperidone is not approved in the United States but is frequently used in other countries and works through peripheral dopamine receptors. Comparisons of domperidone with metoclopramide have shown similar efficacy with fewer adverse effects noted in the patients who received domperidone; however, toxicity is not insignificant, and increase in cardiac arrhythmias and QT prolongation have been reported. If the clinician does wish to prescribe this agent in the United States, an Investigational New Drug (IND) application should be obtained from the FDA. Finally, cisapride has the most extensive data with regard to prokinetic use; however, this was withdrawn from the market because of QT prolongation and increased risk of sudden cardiac death. This agent can be obtained on the basis of compassionate use from Janssen Pharmaceuticals (Titusville, N.J.) if desired; however, this is reserved for rare cases in which the potential benefits are believed to outweigh the significant potential cardiac risks.

Neuromodulators have also been used as a potential treatment option for patients with gastroparesis; the rationale is that improvement in visceral sensation may lead to fewer gastroparesis-mediated symptoms. Options available for use include low-dose tricyclic antidepressants (nortriptyline), atypical antidepressants (mirtazapine), or sertraline, which may also have a mild prokinetic effect.

In view of the chronic nature of gastroparesis and the limited medical options available, there has been significant interest in potential alternative and complementary options. Ginger (*Zingiber officinale*) has been shown to accelerate gastric emptying in animals and people and has been used as a treatment for pregnancy-associated nausea, although it has not been studied in gastroparesis per se. Iberogast (an herbal extract) showed efficacy equivalent to that of cisapride for the treatment of patients with functional dyspepsia and gastroparesis in one case series. Acupuncture has been evaluated in idiopathic and postsurgical gastroparesis in small series with good results, although mechanisms remain unclear.

The role of endoscopic therapy at present for gastroparesis is limited. Several large open-label series showed improvement with prepyloric injection of botulinum toxin in approximately 50% of patients with gastroparesis and suspected pylorospasm; however, two small randomized controlled trials showed no difference between the groups that received botulinum toxin as opposed to placebo. Endoscopic placement of a pyloric channel stent has also been reported in a single small pilot study; however, numbers of patients were small, and these data are still very preliminary.

In refractory and severe cases, surgery is often considered after unsuccessful trials of dietary modification and medical therapy. Gastric electric stimulation was given a humanitarian device exemption (HDE) by the FDA for use in patients with gastroparesis and is, at present, the most common surgical procedure performed for these patients. Contrary to expectations, this device involves the use of high-frequency, low-energy settings to modify gastric sensation, but it is not designed to induce gastric contractions or "pace" the stomach. Data with regard to gastric electrical stimulation are controversial. Two randomized controlled trials have been published. Abell and colleagues (2003) showed that high-frequency, low-energy stimulation significantly decreased vomiting frequency and GI symptoms and improved quality of life in patients with gastroparesis. McCallum and colleagues showed that gastric stimulation significantly improved subjective and objective parameters at 1 year, including vomiting frequency, overall quality of life, and 4-hour gastric emptying. However, although both studies showed significant improvement in gastroparesis parameters, neither study demonstrated a convincing difference between the group for which the stimulator was activated and the group for which it was not (although all patients had the device activated at some point in the study and there may have been lingering effects that affected the final measurements). In these studies, as well as several observational series, patients who seemed to derive the most benefit from this procedure were patients with diabetic or postsurgical gastroparesis (as opposed to idiopathic); patients with primary symptoms of nausea, vomiting, or both (as opposed to pain); and patients who were not taking narcotic analgesic drugs.

Gastric electrical stimulation can be performed either laparoscopically or in an open approach. Traditionally, a region 10 cm proximal to the pylorus along the greater curvature is identified, and two leads are placed in the seromuscular layer of the stomach, approximately 1 cm apart. These leads are connected to a separate generator, which is positioned in the subcutaneous layer of the anterior abdominal wall. Intraoperative endoscopy should be performed to ensure that the leads have not perforated the gastric wall. Estimated battery life with the current device (Enterra Neurostimulator; Medtronic, Minneapolis, Minn.) is approximately 7 years, and the generator can be exchanged (without adjustment of the leads) if need be when the battery is depleted. The device can be interrogated and adjusted as needed with a handheld device that is telemetrically connected to the generator.

Other surgical options that have been considered for treatment of refractory gastroparesis include pyloroplasty and complete or subtotal gastrectomy. Although data with regards to pyloroplasty are limited, Swanstrom and colleagues reported 83% clinical improvement in 28 patients who underwent isolated pyloroplasty for treatment of refractory gastroparesis, with significant improvement in symptoms, gastric emptying, and prokinetic use. Completion or subtotal gastrectomy has also been evaluated as a potential option in patients with refractory symptoms in whom other treatment options have failed. Data suggest that patients who do best with this approach are those with continued nausea and vomiting after a prior partial gastrectomy. Symptom improvement has been reported in up to 79% of patients who undergo this procedure; however, other studies have suggested failure rates of more than 50% at 5 years.

Patients unable to maintain adequate caloric intake need aggressive measures for nutritional support, including insertion of an enteral feeding tube (jejunostomy or gastrojejunostomy), and if enteral feeding is not tolerated, total parenteral nutrition is recommended. A venting gastrostomy tube can also be considered, although data supporting its efficacy are limited.

Postgastrectomy Dumping

Rapid transit disorders occur as a consequence of previous gastric and perigastric operative procedures, most commonly any surgery involving a vagotomy. Approximately 25% to 50% of patients undergoing Roux-en-Y gastric bypass, gastrectomy, gastroenterostomy, or vagotomy experience dumping syndrome, but only approximately 5% have symptoms severe enough to require medical or surgical management. Clinically, dumping syndrome can be categorized as early dumping (which affects most patients) and late dumping, although these subgroups may be difficult to distinguish in practice. Early dumping classically manifests with nausea, abdominal pain, diaphoresis, and palpitations approximately 15 to 30 minutes postprandially, followed by diarrhea approximately 30 to 60 minutes later. Late dumping occurs within 1 to 3 hours postprandially secondary to reactive hypoglycemia. After ingestion of a meal, carbohydrates enter the small intestine, inducing the release of glucagon-like peptide–1 (GLP-1), which exaggerates insulin release and thereby leads to hypoglycemia. This results in a surge of catecholamines with subsequent adrenergic symptoms, including lightheadedness, palpitations, diaphoresis, and tremulousness. Late dumping is rare in comparison with early dumping. Patients experiencing dumping syndrome most commonly improve with time and dietary modifications. If the condition is refractory, they might benefit from a trial of subcutaneous octreotide.

Diagnosis of dumping syndrome is made clinically and confirmed by provocation tests. The patient is given 50 g of oral glucose, and several parameters (hematocrit, plasma glucose level, and heart rate) are monitored every 30 minutes for 3 hours. A positive test result shows more than a 3% rise in hematocrit, hypoglycemia (plasma glucose level, <50 mg/dL), or a rise in heart rate of more than 10 beats/min, along with reproduction of the patient's symptoms. Solid-meal scintigraphy assists in documenting rapid gastric emptying. In the ^{13}C–acetic acid and hydrogen breath tests, bacterial fermentation of glucose is a marker for gastric emptying.

The first-line of management remains dietary modification, because symptoms generally improve over time with improvement of dietary habits. Patients are counseled to eat frequent small meals high in protein and fats and with minimal simple carbohydrates. Patients should not drink liquids with solid meals and 2 hours postprandially. It is recommended to add to the diet nonabsorbable polysaccharides such as glucomannan, pectin, and guar gum, which decrease glucose absorption, reduce reactive hypoglycemia, and thus improve dumping symptoms.

In cases in which dumping symptoms persist, medical therapy should be considered. Acarbose (α-glucosidase inhibitor) prevents the digestion of complex polysaccharides and sucrose, which reduces the surge of postprandial plasma glucose. Although acarbose is very efficacious in treating dumping symptoms, it has widely undesirable side effects, including flatulence and diarrhea, because of the fermentation of the unabsorbed carbohydrates. Octreotide (a somatostatin analogue) has been used to slow gastric emptying, inhibit secretion of insulin and enteric peptides, and attenuate the postprandial hemodynamic changes by splanchnic vasoconstriction and hormonal release. Octreotide is typically administered subcutaneously three times a day, 30 min before each meal. Another formulation often preferred by patients is the depot long-acting octreotide (Sandostatin-LAR), administered monthly. Studies have suggested this to be as effective as the intermittent subcutaneous formulation, and it is preferred by patients because it is administered less frequently.

The rare patient with intractable symptoms may be considered for operative therapy with the goal of delaying gastric emptying. Surgery is not always effective, but its goal is usually to prevent rapid delivery of food to the proximal intestine and re-create gastric reservoir function. Although few studies have been conducted to compare different surgical procedures, conversion Roux-en-Y gastrojejunostomy and antiperistaltic jejunal interposition loops provide the most satisfactory results, depending on the initial surgery that resulted in the dumping syndrome. If a patient underwent pyloroplasty, pyloric reconstruction is recommended. Patients who underwent Billroth II or Billroth I gastrectomies should undergo conversion Roux-en-Y gastrojejunostomy. This tends to slow motility by interrupting the migrating motor complexes and introducing a retrograde jejunal contraction. Although ineffective in 25% of patients, the Billroth II gastrectomy can be converted to a Billroth I gastrectomy to restore the physiologic delivery of meal to the duodenum. The surgeon must emphasize to the patient that the outcome may be suboptimal.

Roux Stasis Syndrome

Roux stasis syndrome is usually encountered in patients after Roux-en-Y gastrojejunostomy. It occurs in approximately 25% to 30% of these patients, affecting predominantly women, and usually in cases in which the Roux limb is longer than 40 cm. The motility disorder most commonly occurs in the gastric remnant and in the distal efferent jejunal Roux limb, resulting in symptoms of nausea, vomiting, and early satiety (indistinguishable from gastroparesis). It can also affect the Roux limb alone, but this is generally a late complication, occurring after months or years. The mechanism is related to the transection of the jejunum from the duodenum. This is believed to separate the jejunum from the natural small intestinal pacemaker (in the duodenum), which leads to the development of ectopic pacemakers in the Roux limb with resultant retrograde contractions.

Diagnosis can be made clinically from a thorough history. It can be confirmed with scintigraphy to document delayed gastrojejunal transit, but because of manipulation of the anatomy, interpretation of the results may be difficult. Manometry theoretically can also be used, although in practice this is not commonly performed. Pancreatic polypeptide response to insulin-induced hypoglycemia (pancreatic polypeptide test) can be used to test for vagal function. Pancreatic polypeptide is secreted from the pancreas in response to vagal nerve stimulation in the cephalic phase of digestion. Pancreatic polypeptide can be measured in the blood after sham feeding. However, after vagotomy, this response is lost.

Prokinetics, antiemetics, and minimal narcotics have been used as medical treatment options for patients with Roux stasis syndrome, with approximately 50% improvement. Cisapride may provide long-lasting symptom relief and improved transit in 40% of patients; however, this is not available commercially in the United States and is available only on the basis of compassionate use from Janssen Pharmaceuticals (Titusville, NJ). Intravenous erythromycin and bethanechol have also been used; however, up to 50% of patients continue to have symptoms despite medical therapy and may ultimately require total or near-total gastrectomy. Total gastrectomy has been successful in 43% of patients in improving symptoms; the prognosis is worse in patients receiving total parenteral nutrition, those with endoscopically observed retained food, and those with nausea.

Postvagotomy Diarrhea

Postvagotomy diarrhea occurs in 20% of patients after truncal vagotomy and can be severe in 4% of these patients. If selective vagotomy is performed, especially if the celiac and hepatic branches are preserved, diarrhea is almost nonexistent. It is difficult to distinguish from dumping syndrome, although distinction is important because of the therapeutic and prognostic implications. Patients typically experience approximately 20 watery bowel movements in a 24-hour period, not related to food intake, and this can occur nocturnally. Signs and symptoms similar to dumping syndrome occur, but unlike dumping syndrome, they usually occur 30 to 60 minutes postprandially.

Pathophysiologic features, although unclear, have been described as a combination of impaired gastric relaxation and bile acid malabsorption. With complete vagotomy, gastric motility is, in addition, altered to gastric acidity, favoring bacterial overgrowth, which leads to diarrhea. In addition, in cases of hepatic and celiac branch denervation, gallbladder contraction and coordination are impaired, causing the enterohepatic circulation to be overwhelmed with bile salts, which themselves trigger a secretory and osmotic diarrhea. High bile salt content in the feces can help in the diagnosis of postvagotomy diarrhea, but it does not exclude other causes of diarrhea.

Dietary modification remains the mainstay of treatment. Patients are instructed to avoid carbohydrate-dense foods and to have small, frequent, low-fat meals. Introduction of bulk-forming agents into the diet, such as fibers, psyllium, or pectin, can be helpful. Pharmacologic agents can be used if the diarrhea persists. Codeine phosphate (60 mg, qd) and loperamide (12 to 24 mg, qd) inhibit GI transit time and have proven efficacy as short-term treatments. Bile salt resins, such as cholestyramine, reduce the bile salt load to the gut and alleviate diarrhea, but their unfavorable side effects and their uncertain long-term benefit limit their use. Octreotide, although used in the past to target bile acid malabsorption, has not proven effective for this indication. If diarrhea is persistent, the entire GI tract should be evaluated with endoscopy. In addition, surgery can be tried, although it is rarely beneficial. Procedures, such as Roux-en-Y conversion or using an interposition segment of antiperistaltic jejunum to slow gastric emptying, may be attempted, although data regarding their efficacy are limited.

MOTILITY DISORDERS OF THE SMALL INTESTINE

Ileus of the Small Intestine

Ileus refers to dysmotility in the bowels in the absence of a mechanical obstruction; such dysmotility results in signs and symptoms similar to those of obstruction. These include bloating, diffuse abdominal pain, abdominal distension, obstipation, constipation, nausea, vomiting, and inability to tolerate oral intake. The term *ileus* originated from the Greek word *eileos,* meaning "twisting."

Ileus can be either normal postoperative ileus or paralytic ileus. If symptoms are less severe and last for up to 5 days after the operation, then ileus is considered postoperative. If the symptoms are protracted and prolonged, then it is called *prolonged postoperative ileus.* It is important to distinguish between mechanical bowel obstruction and ileus because management differs. Intense colicky pain, feculent emesis, or acute pain and distension are more suggestive of small bowel obstruction. Emergency surgical intervention is needed when signs and symptoms of shock are suggestive of bowel ischemia or perforation.

Inhibitory neural reflexes are thought to act locally through noxious spinal afferent signals that increase inhibitory sympathetic activity in the GI tract. Blocking these spinal afferents with epidural local anesthetics can improve postoperative paralytic ileus. Intestinal manipulation and trauma during surgery leads to an inflammatory response that contributes to ileus. In addition, neurohumoral peptides (nitric oxide, vasoactive intestinal polypeptide, and substance P) are thought to act as inhibitory neurotransmitters in the gut, which slow gut motility. Use of opioids has an inhibitory effect on the GI tract by increasing the resting tone while decreasing gastric motility and emptying, increasing small intestinal periodic spasm, and decreasing propulsive colonic movements, all of which further contribute to the pathogenesis of ileus.

Risk factors for paralytic ileus include narcotic overuse, peritoneal or retroperitoneal inflammation, sepsis, severe pelvic fractures, and spinal cord injury. Ileus can be prolonged by metabolic disturbances such as hypomagnesemia, hypermagnesemia, hypercalcemia, hyponatremia, hypokalemia, and ketoacidosis. Medications other than opioids are implicated in ileus, including anticholinergics, phenothiazines, calcium channel blockers, and tricyclic antidepressants, which are all notorious for adversely affecting gut motility.

When paralytic or prolonged ileus is suspected, plain radiographs of the abdomen may reveal gas in segments of both the small and large bowel. Differentiating obstruction from ileus can be made by contrast studies, or computed tomographic study, which is usually more useful in a nonacute setting because it helps identify other hidden pathologic processes such as abscesses that might be contributing to ileus.

Prevention measures of paralytic ileus have been attempted when its occurrence is anticipated during surgery. The surgeon assesses intraoperative findings, prolonged handling and packing of the bowels, intensive use of narcotics or other antikinetic agents, presence of peritonitis or sepsis, or extensive blood loss, and accordingly decides on the preventive measures used. Nasogastric suction has been commonly used to prevent accumulation of secreted fluids and swallowed gases in the paralyzed gut. Studies have shown that nasogastric tubes increase the risk of aspiration and may cause additional discomfort for patients, and hence may confer a greater risk than benefit.

When the surgeon elects not to place a nasogastric tube, the patient is allowed nothing by mouth. Oral intake is advanced gradually, beginning with sips of water, then adding a liquid diet, then adding solid food in accordance with evidence of resolution of postoperative ileus, such as positive bowel sounds, the subjective feeling of "rumbling," or passage of flatus. In the meantime, the patient is supported with ample intravenous hydration.

Use of epidural analgesia, whether thoracic or high abdominal, has been beneficial in reducing the duration of postoperative ileus.

For maximal effect, analgesic placement must block nociceptive afferent signals from the surgical site and be used postoperatively for 48 to 72 hours. In addition, correction of metabolic disturbances (whether electrolytes, minerals, or endocrine) and fluid imbalances is of importance in prevention and management of ileus.

Experimental data suggest that the length of the incision may affect GI motility postoperatively. Perhaps for this reason, minimally invasive surgery appears to be associated with decreased incidence of postoperative ileus, although this observation may be confounded by other factors, such as decreased postoperative opiate burden. The development of prolonged ileus after laparoscopy is unusual and should raise concern for potential occult injury.

Finally, several pharmacologic agents have been assessed to treat ileus. Prokinetic agents such as metoclopramide, cisapride (not FDA approved), and erythromycin have been shown to promote gastric emptying after upper GI procedures; however, they did not show benefit for ileus after abdominal or pelvic procedures. Peripherally acting opioid antagonists such as alvimopan and methylnaltrexone have been used in several studies to assess their effect on management of ileus. To date, the FDA has approved alvimopan only in perioperative care after partial large or small bowel resections with primary anastomosis and not for the treatment of protracted ileus.

Surgeons should always keep in mind that gentle handling of tissue, meticulous attention to hemostasis, and abiding by the principles of wound management during laparotomy or laparoscopy provide the best safeguards against ileus development and reduce the risk of a protracted course. Use of minimally invasive surgery (to decrease incision size and reduce the time the intestines are handled), as opposed to open laparotomy, decreases the likelihood of ileus that much more.

SUGGESTED READINGS

Abell T, Lou J, Tabbaa M, et al: Gastric electrical stimulation for gastroparesis improves nutritional parameters at short, intermediate, and long-term follow-up, *JPEN J Parenter Enteral Nutr* 27(4):277–281, 2003

Hibbard ML, Dunst CM, Swanström LL: Laparoscopic and endoscopic pyloroplasty for gastroparesis results in sustained symptom improvement, *J Gastrointest Surg* 15(9):1513–1519, 2011. doi: 10.1007/s11605-011-1607-6. Epub 2011 Jul 1.

McCallum RW, Lin Z, Forster J, et al: Gastric electrical stimulation improves outcomes of patients with gastroparesis for up to 10 years, *Clin Gastroenterol Hepatol* 9(4):314–319, 2011. doi: 10.1016/j.cgh.2010.12.013. Epub 2010 Dec 23.

THE MANAGEMENT OF SHORT BOWEL SYNDROME

Heung Bae Kim, MD, and Tom Jaksic, MD, PhD

INTRODUCTION

Throughout the care of patients with short bowel syndrome (SBS), a multidisciplinary approach to management is essential because no one provider has the expertise to care for these complex cases alone.

The key focus of medical management should be on the meticulous management of parenteral nutrition (PN) to avoid metabolic and hepatotoxic complications of this life-saving treatment. Enteral feedings should be introduced as early as possible and carefully advanced with observation for signs of feeding intolerance. In general, elemental formulas are preferred over more complex formulas because absorption is better and there are less allergic complications. Breast milk is tried before elemental formulas in neonates with SBS. PN may be weaned as tolerated as long as the patient continues to meet growth and weight milestones. Meticulous attention to care of the central venous line is also critical because repeated line sepsis episodes can lead to worsening of liver function and loss of central venous access sites. The authors use ethanol locks for the long-term outpatient management of SBS because several case series have shown a decreased rate of line sepsis with this therapy. The management of PN has evolved significantly over the past 40 years since Dr. Dudrick's first report of the use of total PN to support the growth of animals and infants. Commercially available intravenous amino acids, glucose, lipids, vitamins, and trace minerals are provided through a central line to meet patient-specific nutritional requirements. Studies indicate that the avoidance of overfeeding and parenteral lipid restriction (1 g/kg/d or less) is associated with reduced hyperbilirubinemia. Newer experimental lipid formulas that contain fish oil or a combination of fish oil and olive oil may prove to have additional hepatoprotective properties. Studies of growth factors active on the intestine are also ongoing. Glucagon-like peptide-2 (GLP-2) and its longer acting analogue teduglutide appear to facilitate intestinal adaptation, and in one recent trial, the administration of teduglutide was found to reduce PN requirements. A concern with the protracted application of growth factors is the potential induction of intestinal carcinoma.

INITIAL MANAGEMENT OF THE ABDOMINAL CATASTROPHE THAT LEADS TO SHORT BOWEL SYNDROME

The surgical management of SBS usually begins with treatment of the initial condition that leads to acute intestinal loss. In children, SBS is most commonly caused by gastroschisis, intestinal atresia, or midgut volvulus. In adults, additional conditions include Crohn's disease, tumors, or trauma. During these initial operations, the surgeon must not only consider the short-term goals of survival and recovery but also the long-term goal of preserving as much intestinal mucosal surface area as possible. This may require balancing the risks of early aggressive resection of all questionable intestine versus use of a second look laparotomy to allow for complete demarcation of nonviable bowel. In general, if the patient's condition allows, a second look laparotomy often results in preservation of intestine that otherwise appeared nonviable at the initial operation. Intestinal stomas are often necessary to optimize recovery from the initial insult, but the surgeon must balance this against the additional mandatory loss of a small portion of intestine during the future stoma takedown. In general, bowel-preserving surgery is critical to optimize the long-term outcome for patients with SBS.

Once bowel function has been documented, enteral feedings are generally initiated at 10 mL/kg/d and advanced by 10 mL/kg/d until enteral goals are reached. The authors often use nasogastric or gastrostomy tubes to advance feeds because many infants and children with intestinal failure have an oral aversion or swallowing difficulties related to prematurity. Factors that limit the advancement of enteral feedings include vomiting, increased gastrostomy tube output, stool output of more than 2 mL/kg/h, abdominal distention, or skin breakdown from acidic stool output. Promotility agents, postpyloric tube feeds, or fundoplication may be indicated if vomiting and reflux are a major problem. In cases of increased stool output, infection with *Clostridium difficile* and rotavirus should be ruled out because these commonly occur in children with SBS. Once infectious causes of diarrhea have been ruled out, loperamide can be initiated and titrated to effect.

At some point when the patient is of adequate size and comorbid conditions have been minimized, all ostomies should be closed to maximize the mucosal surface area that is exposed to the enteric stream. This also brings the colon back into the enteric stream, which improves reabsorption of both fluids and electrolytes. In some cases, the increased delivery of incompletely digested enteric contents to the colon may lead to significant diarrhea, abdominal pain, perianal skin breakdown, or metabolic derangements. The authors usually recommend a "poop prep" for children in diapers in which stoma contents are placed on the perianal skin within the diaper for 30 minutes at a time several times a day to prepare the perianal skin for diarrhea before stoma closure. This allows for the skin to adapt and may prevent severe diaper rash after stoma closure.

If full enteral autonomy and appropriate growth and developmental milestones are achieved, there is usually no role for additional surgical procedures to treat SBS. The one instance in which surgical management may be useful is when bacterial overgrowth develops and results in intermittent diarrhea, abdominal pain or distention, and D-lactic acidosis. Initial treatment for this usually involves enteral antibiotics for intestinal decontamination. If this fails to improve symptoms, radiographic studies of the intestine are indicated to determine whether segments of dilated intestine might be the cause of stasis. If present, dilated bowel causing symptomatic bacterial overgrowth may be an indication for surgical treatment despite full enteral autonomy.

Despite optimal early surgical and medical therapy, some patients remain dependent on PN to achieve normal growth and development. When progress halts or the patient's enteral tolerance worsens, surgical procedures may be indicated to improve intestinal function and allow for continuation of weaning from PN.

INDICATIONS FOR SURGICAL MANAGEMENT OF SHORT BOWEL SYNDROME

The initial insult that occurs after massive intestinal resection is a loss of mucosal mass, which leads to an inability to absorb sufficient nutrients to maintain normal growth and development. In response to intestinal loss, the remaining intestine adapts with both microscopic and macroscopic changes that occur within the intestine. Although microscopic changes like increases in villus height and crypt depth and proliferation of enterocytes tend to improve intestinal function, the usual macroscopic adaptive response is intestinal dilation. With mild dilation, the intestinal function may improve, but with ongoing massive dilation, the response becomes maladaptive and results in poor intestinal motility and bacterial overgrowth. This dilated bowel does not have normal peristalsis because the increased diameter prevents proper and complete approximation of the bowel walls. Failure of the bowel edges to fully coapt leads to a sloshing motion of the intraluminal contents and disorganized antegrade peristalsis. The goal of intestinal lengthening and tapering procedures is to correct the two major functional problems of adapted short bowel: namely, poor motility and bacterial overgrowth. Once a patient has reached a plateau in the advancement of enteral nutrition and all medical strategies have been exhausted, surgical intestinal lengthening and tapering procedures should be considered. A contrast study should be performed to give an approximation of the residual intestinal length and to define any areas of dilation or stricturing that may benefit from surgical intervention. In addition to definition of the anatomy, preoperative assessment of liver function and other comorbid conditions is critical. Coagulopathy and decreased hepatic synthetic function may preclude any major abdominal surgery, and in these cases, the patient may benefit from direct referral for liver and small bowel or multivisceral transplantation. Insertion of an enteral access tube and liver biopsy should also be considered during the operation, if not already done. It is our practice to use a preoperative antibiotic and antifungal bowel preparation because many of these patients have significant bacterial or fungal overgrowth at the time of surgery that may result in postoperative sepsis from the significant bowel manipulation during surgery.

A number of procedures to improve intestinal function in patients with SBS have been developed over the past 50 years, but only two are widely used today. The longitudinal intestinal lengthening and tailoring (LILT) and the serial transverse enteroplasty (STEP) procedures are both autologous intestinal reconstruction procedures that combine the benefits of intestinal tapering and lengthening with maximal preservation of enterocyte mass. Although both procedures may be used successfully in select cases with similar outcomes, the STEP procedure has recently gained more widespread popularity among surgeons because of its simplicity and adaptability to bowel that is variably dilated. Both the LILT and the STEP procedures have been shown to improve enteral autonomy in select patients with SBS. With rare exceptions, other procedures, including reversed intestinal segments, intestinal valves, recirculating loops, and isolated bowel segments (Iowa procedure), are of historical interest only and are not discussed further.

LONGITUDINAL INTESTINAL LENGTHENING AND TAILORING

The first paper describing a readily reproducible procedure for intestinal lengthening was reported by Bianchi in 1980. The procedure was initially referred to as intestinal loop lengthening and then later renamed the LILT procedure, although in the modern surgical vernacular, it is commonly referred to as the Bianchi procedure. The initial step of this procedure involves the use of blunt dissection to separate the mesentery into two leaves, each of which supplies blood to half of the intestine. The intestine is then divided longitudinally, with either a surgical stapler or a hand-sewn anastomosis. This

results in two separate loops of intestine, each with half the circumference of the original loop. When these two loops are then anastomosed end to end, the result is a doubling of the length and a tapering of the diameter of the intestine (Figure 1). Since its introduction, LILT has been performed worldwide with variable success. In one report of a 6-year follow-up period in 25 patients who underwent LILT, 17 of 18 survivors were able to be weaned from PN and no intraoperative deaths occurred. In another 5-year follow-up study of 13 children who underwent LILT, bacterial overgrowth was eliminated in 8 of 10 patients who had this documented before surgery. At both 1 and 5 years after surgery, 6 of 13 patients (46%) were on full enteral nutrition. In a more recent series from 2006 of 49 patients who underwent LILT, the reported mortality rate was 18%, and 39% of patients were successfully weaned from PN in a mean of 9 months. Bianchi himself reviewed the worldwide experience with LILT in 2006, with a total of 150 patients from eight published studies. Results were varied, with overall survival rate ranging from 30% to 100% and 28% to 100% of patients achieving full enteral autonomy. The most common causes of death in children who underwent LILT were related to progression of PN-associated liver disease and sepsis. Most of the fatal septic episodes occurred in children with long-term central venous catheters. To date, no intraoperative deaths have been reported. Necrosis of one of the divided limbs necessitating surgical resection of the affected bowel has been reported. Reoperation for

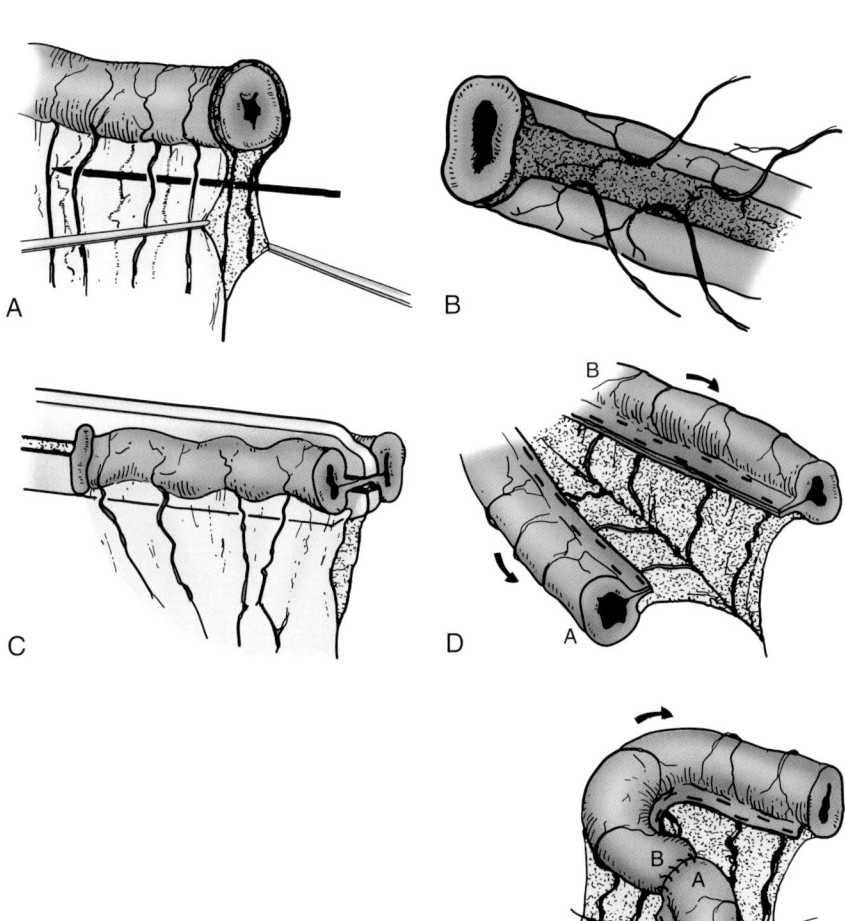

FIGURE 1 Longitudinal intestinal lengthening and tailoring. **A** and **B,** Creation of the mesenteric tunnel. **C** and **D,** Division of the dilated bowel into two hemiloops. **E,** Reanastomosis in an isoperistaltic fashion. *(From Bianchi A: Intestinal loop lengthening: a technique for increasing small intestinal length,* J Pediatr Surg *15(2):145–151, 1980, pp 147, Fig 1.)*

anastomotic strictures, adhesive small bowel obstruction, and inter-loop fistula formation have been noted. Recurrent dilation is common in the lengthened bowel, sometimes requiring reoperation for additional tapering. In patients who are unable to wean from PN after the LILT procedure, small bowel transplantation has been used as a salvage procedure.

The LILT procedure has undergone technical modifications since its original description in 1980. Bianchi reported a change in his preferred method of bowel division in 1984, opting to use bipolar cautery to divide the bowel in half along the mesenteric and antimesenteric borders, rather than the surgical stapler. A hand-sewn suture line was then used to form the divided bowel into the new hemiloops. A surgical nipple valve has been used in some patients with SBS who lack a maladaptive intestinal dilation response to create a partial obstruction and induce bowel dilation so that the LILT procedure can be performed. This technique was used to induce dilation sufficient to perform LILT in six patients at 3 to 9 months after nipple valve construction. The primary criticism of this method is the possibility of creating a complete bowel obstruction. Bianchi's group has also developed a modification of this dilation model for use in patients with jejunal atresia. They reported placing a tube jejunostomy into the proximal dilated small bowel and a separate tube colostomy into the distal bowel. Jejunal contents were then intermittently refed into the distal bowel, and intermittent occlusion of the jejunostomy tube was used to induce proximal bowel dilation. Another modification of the LILT procedure enables the elimination of two of the three intestinal anastomoses usually required for the LILT. In this modification, the stapling device is be applied obliquely at both the proximal and the distal ends of the LILT segment, tapering the diameter down to the size of the native intestine without completely dividing the intestine as originally described. Once the dilated segment has been divided into two equal-sized tubes, a single hand-sewn anastomosis can be fashioned between the two, thus eliminating both the proximal and distal anastomoses as potential sites of leak or stricture.

SERIAL TRANSVERSE ENTEROPLASTY PROCEDURE

In 2003, Kim and colleagues described a novel intestinal lengthening and tapering procedure called the STEP. As in the LILT procedure,

the first description of the STEP procedure was in an animal model of dilated intestine that was obtained with a reversed jejunal segment. Once the intestine was dilated, a stapler was placed on the distal dilated intestine perpendicular to the long axis of the intestine and fired to partially transect the intestine, leaving an approximately 2-cm portion undivided. A second stapler was then applied about 2 cm proximal to this and similarly fired to only partially transect the intestine. This pattern of alternating partial transection of the intestine was carried proximally, maintaining a 2-cm zigzag channel until the length of the staple firings became too short to continue. To accommodate the stapler, a small defect in the mesentery was created at each point of stapler application. The end result was a zigzag pattern to the lengthened and tapered intestine (Figure 2).

These original animal studies showed an immediate 68% increase in the length of intestine after the STEP procedure. Six weeks after the STEP procedure, all animals were noted to have gained weight appropriately and there were no deaths or episodes of bowel obstruction. Subsequent studies in an animal model of SBS showed that the STEP procedure not only increased the length of intestine but also had a beneficial effect on nutrient absorption, bacterial overgrowth, and overall weight gain. In addition, animals that underwent the STEP procedure were found to have higher postoperative levels of serum citrulline, a nonprotein amino acid that is a surrogate for total small intestine enterocyte mass. Though the STEP procedure does not result in an immediate increase in mucosal surface area, the authors hypothesize that by tapering the previously dysfunctional dilated bowel, bacterial overgrowth is reduced and the process of adaptation may be facilitated.

The first human case of the STEP procedure was also reported by Kim and associates in 2003. The patient was a 2-year-old boy who had SBS secondary to gastroschisis with midgut volvulus. He had previously undergone a LILT at age 11 months, which increased his bowel length from 72 to 130 cm, but despite this increase, he remained dependent on PN. At 23 months of age, he returned to the operating room for a STEP procedure. Preoperative imaging had confirmed that the intestine that had undergone the LILT had redilated. Intraoperative measurement revealed 83 cm of dilated intestine that measured approximately 6 cm across. After 26 firings of the stapler, this segment was lengthened to 147 cm, with a channel width of 2 cm. This left the patient with a total small bowel length of approximately 200 cm (Figure 3). Postoperative absorption studies showed a statistically significant increase in serum D-xylose after oral loading. In

FIGURE 2 Serial transverse enteroplasty. The dilated bowel is flattened, and the stapler is applied perpendicular to the long axis of the bowel, from alternating sides. A small defect in the mesentery was created at each point of stapler application. The end result is a zigzag pattern to the lengthened bowel. *(Adapted from Kim HB, Fauza D, Garza J, et al: Serial transverse enteroplasty (STEP): a novel bowel lengthening procedure, J Pediatr Surg 38(3):425–429, 2003, Fig 1.)*

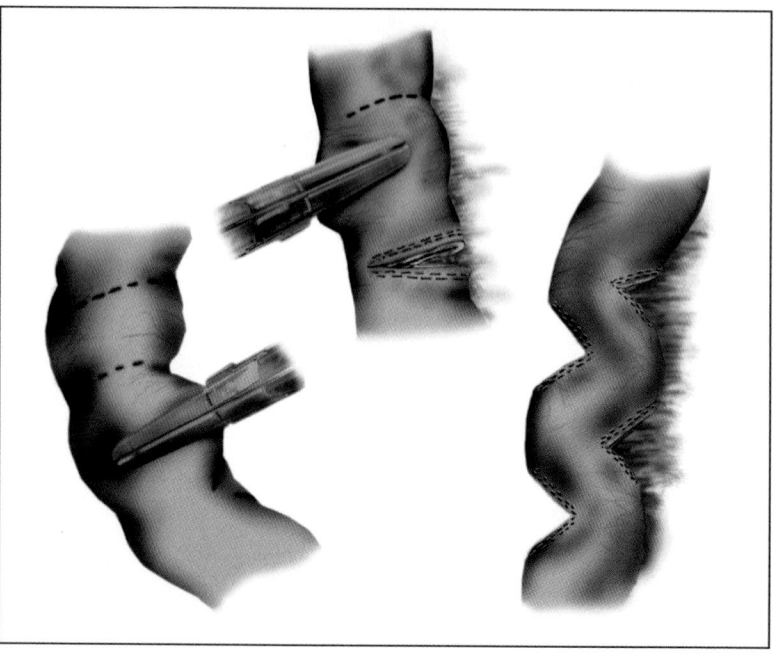

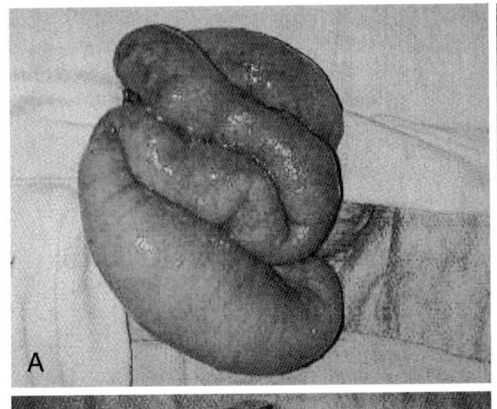

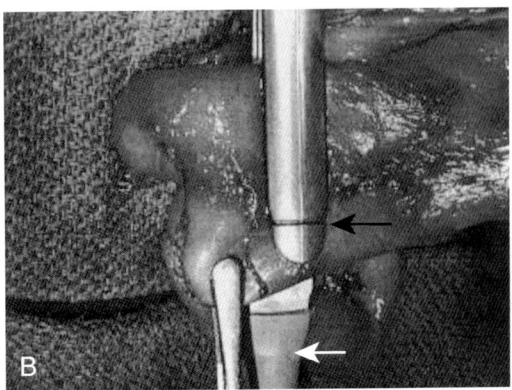

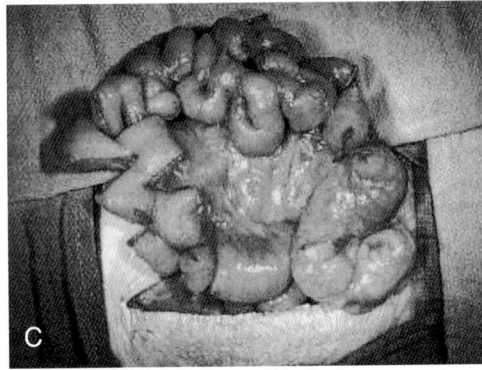

FIGURE 3   A, Appearance of dilated bowel at time of serial transverse enteroplasty. **B,** Stapler being applied with red rubber catheter *(white arrow)* guiding larger end of stapler through mesenteric defect and notch *(black arrow)* on stapler showing where staple line will end. **C,** Bowel after serial transverse enteroplasty procedure is complete. *(From Kim HB, Lee PW, Garza J, et al: Serial transverse enteroplasty for short bowel syndrome: a case report,* J Pediatr Surg 38(6):881–885, 2003, Fig 2.)

addition, 6 months after surgery, the patient had advanced to 50% enteral nutrition.

After these initial reports, the STEP rapidly increased in popularity for the surgical management of patients with SBS who were unable to wean from PN because of dysfunctional dilated intestine. Subsequent reports also described two additional indications for the procedure beyond established SBS with PN dependence. The second published indication for the use of the STEP procedure was to treat newborns with intestinal atresia and marginal bowel length. In these cases, the STEP procedure is used primarily as a mucosa-sparing tapering procedure. When children are born with intestinal atresia, the proximal intestine is very dilated, and when there is a loss of a significant portion of the overall intestinal length, it is critical to save as much of the intestinal mucosa as possible. Rather than performing a standard tapering enteroplasty that results in the removal of a significant portion of the antimesenteric portion of the intestine, the same tapering can be achieved with the STEP, without the need for any intestinal resection. The third published indication for the STEP procedure is for the treatment of recalcitrant D-lactic acidosis that results from bacterial overgrowth. In this report, an 18-year-old woman who previously has SBS from a midgut volvulus developed neurologic impairment from bacterial overgrowth that resulted in elevated serum levels of D-lactic acid. Although she did not need PN, her overall intestine length was marginal and any intestinal resection was undesirable. Preoperative imaging showed a dilated duodenum, which at the time of surgery measured 8 cm in diameter. The STEP procedure was performed on this isolated segment of bowel and resulted in a significant decrease in postoperative episodes of D-lactic acidosis.

Although STEP remains a relatively new procedure, several reported case series with follow-up after STEP have been published and show good short-term and intermediate-term results. To better track STEP outcomes worldwide, a web-based international data registry for patients undergoing the STEP procedure was established at www.stepoperation.org. The first publication from this registry in 2006 summarized the largest experience to date of the STEP procedure, in 38 patients from 19 centers. The indications for STEP included anatomic SBS (n = 29), neonatal jejuno-ileal atresia with marginal intestinal length (n = 3), and bacterial overgrowth (n = 6). In those patients who underwent STEP for SBS, enteral tolerance increased significantly from 31% enteral nutrition before surgery to 67% enteral nutrition after a median follow-up period of 12.9 months after the STEP. Similar to the LILT, all three of the deaths after the STEP procedure were secondary to progressive liver disease and sepsis. Three patients required combined liver-intestine transplant. Complications related to the procedure included ulcer formation along the staple lines and intraoperative leaks from the staple lines. The authors generally recommend that buttress sutures are placed at the apex of each staple line to minimize this risk of leakage. Postoperative small bowel obstructions have also been reported, although most of these have been managed successfully with nasogastric decompression and bowel rest.

After surgery, a nasogastric tube should be left to suction until bowel function has returned. A slow advancement of enteral nutrition then proceeds. Recent data have shown that even after the STEP procedure, enteral advancement may be slow. In a study of 61 patients registered in the International STEP Data Registry who underwent STEP to treat SBS, 31 eventually advanced to full enteral tolerance, but the median time to achieve enteral autonomy was 19 months, with a range of 1 to 44 months.

Similar to LILT, intestinal redilation occurs frequently after the STEP procedure as intestinal adaptation continues. Although repeat LILT is technically not possible after an initial LILT, it has been shown that the STEP procedure may be performed after either the LILT or the STEP, as was clearly shown in the first reported STEP case. The first demonstration of the feasibility of a second STEP procedure was in an animal model; this was quickly followed by the first reported clinical case in 2007. To date, patients have been reported to have had LILT-STEP-STEP, STEP-STEP-STEP, and even STEP-LILT. The limits of repeated procedures have yet to be determined.

CONCLUSION

The last 30 years have seen great advances in the medical and surgical management of children with SBS. The advent of PN has allowed many of these children to survive long enough to develop the bowel adaptation necessary to compensate for their original losses and reach enteral independence. For children who are unable to reach this goal with medical therapy alone, surgical strategies have been devised to both lengthen and taper the remaining intestine. The most commonly performed procedures today are the LILT and STEP. The primary indication for each procedure is to improve the function of dilated poorly functional intestine through intestinal lengthening and tapering in patients who are unable to achieve enteral autonomy despite maximal medical management. Both the LILT and STEP procedures have been reported to increase enteral tolerance, with approximately half of patients achieving enteral autonomy at some point after surgery. However, it must be emphasized that the optimal care for these patient requires a multidisciplinary approach to achieve excellent overall outcomes and that surgical treatment should be limited to select cases in which progression to enteral autonomy is: (1) being hampered by surgically correctable anatomic problems; and (2) not attainable through optimal medical management alone. Application of these surgical techniques without appropriate ongoing evaluation and management may result in poorer than expected outcomes.

SUGGESTED READINGS

Bianchi A: Intestinal loop lengthening: a technique for increasing small intestinal length, *J Pediatr Surg* 15(2):145–151, 1980.

Chang RW, Javid PJ, Oh JT, et al: Serial transverse enteroplasty enhances intestinal function in a model of short bowel syndrome, *Ann Surg* 243(2):223–228, 2006.

Kim HB, Lee PW, Garza J, et al: Serial transverse enteroplasty for short bowel syndrome: a case report, *J Pediatr Surg* 38(6):881–885, 2003.

Kim HB, Fauza D, Garza J, et al: Serial transverse enteroplasty (STEP): a novel bowel lengthening procedure, *J Pediatr Surg* 38(3):425–429, 2003.

Modi BP, Javid PJ, Jaksic T, et al: First report of the international serial transverse enteroplasty data registry: indications, efficacy, and complications, *J Am Coll Surg* 204(3):365–371, 2007.

THE MANAGEMENT OF ENTEROCUTANEOUS FISTULAS

Lindsey L. Manos, MPAS, PA-C, and
Christopher L. Wolfgang, MD, PhD

OVERVIEW

Management of enterocutaneous (EC) fistulas presents a complex problem that falls on the shoulders of general and gastrointestinal surgeons. At the very least, the successful management of an EC fistula is labor-intensive with regards to nutritional support, fluid and electrolyte management, and wound care. Approximately one third of EC fistulas close spontaneously in patients in whom these factors are controlled. In patients whose fistulas do not close with conservative management, operative care becomes necessary. These operations are often complex procedures that involve bowel resection with reconstruction of the abdominal wall. Overall, the mortality rate of EC fistulas remains approximately 15% to 25% and is typically associated with sepsis, malnutrition, and electrolyte imbalance. Expert management of EC fistulas through conservative measures or definitive surgical repair is necessary to reduce morbidity and mortality and ultimately improve the patient's quality of life.

DEFINITION AND ETIOLOGY

A fistula is an abnormal connection between two hollow epithelial-lined organs or between an epithelial-lined organ and the exterior of the body. This differs from a sinus tract, which is a communication between an infected cavity and the surface of the body. An EC fistula occurs when a communication is present between the alimentary tract and the surface of the skin. Often included within this category is the enteroatmospheric (EA) fistula, which is a communication between the alimentary tract and a nonepithelialized granulating wound (Figure 1). This chapter focuses specifically on EC and EA fistulas. Essentially all of the information presented within this chapter pertains to both EC and EA fistulas, and the terminology throughout states EC fistula only for brevity. Unique to EA fistulas is the wound care and drainage control management; this difference is noted where applicable. Postoperative pancreatic and biliary fistulas are unique entities with some differences in management and are discussed elsewhere.

Most EC fistulas develop after an operation that requires an enteric anastomosis, extensive lysis of adhesions, or removal of infected mesh from a prior hernia repair (Table 1). Note that EC fistulas can spontaneously occur in some conditions such as Crohn's disease, malignant disease, or less commonly diverticular disease. Spontaneous formation accounts for a small percentage of EC fistulas and occurs when underlying conditions such as inflammatory bowel disease or malignancy are present. Poor nutrition, prior radiation therapy, and emergency procedures or trauma are associated with postoperative fistula formation.

PRESENTATION

An EC fistula begins with a disruption in the integrity of the bowel wall that results in the leakage of enteric contents either into the abdominal cavity or from the body surface. A typical presentation often begins with fever and a leukocytosis 3 to 5 days after surgery. On physical examination, a wound infection may be encountered and opened at the bedside. This progresses to efflux of enteric fluid through the wound. Another manifestation is that the patient is found to have an intraabdominal abscess on computerized tomographic (CT) scan. This is managed with the placement of a percutaneous drain, which then goes on to drain enteric contents once the

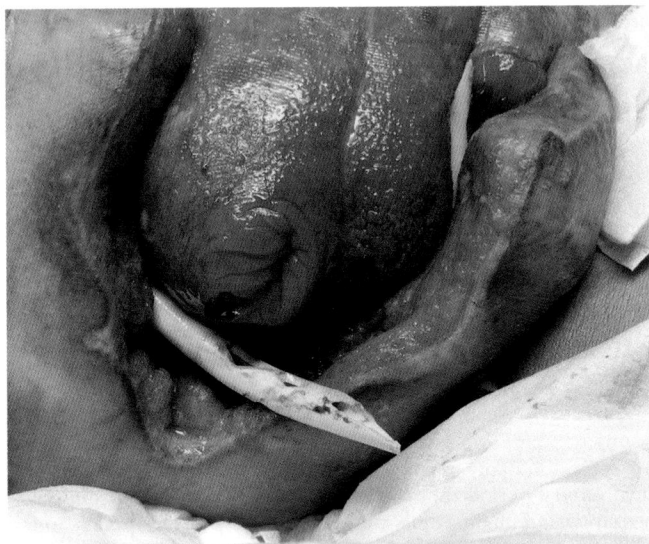

FIGURE 1   Example of enteroatmospheric fistula.

TABLE 1: Common causes of fistula formation

Spontaneous Formation (15% to 25%)

Malignant disease
   Radiation therapy
Inflammatory conditions
   Inflammatory bowel disease (Crohn's disease)
   Bowel obstruction or ischemia
   Complicated diverticular disease
   Complicated appendicitis
   Perforated ulcer disease

Postoperative Formation (75% to 85%)

Oncologic procedures
Bowel resection
Colostomy or ileostomy reversal
Emergent laparotomy (trauma)
Appendectomy
Adhesiolysis

TABLE 2: Enterocutaneous fistula daily output

Classification	mL/d
Low	<200
Moderate	200-500
High	>500

TABLE 3: Stepwise management of enterocutaneous fistulas

1. Sepsis control
   Identification and treatment of source
   Pharmacologic agents
2. Stabilization
   Fluid resuscitation
   Electrolyte homeostasis
3. Nutritional support
   Enteral feeding vs parenteral feeding
4. Effluent management
   Pharmacologic agents
   Wound care
5. Definitive repair
   Spontaneous
   Surgical

initial infected fluid clears. In the case of spontaneous EC fistula formation, the patient presents with fever, leukocytosis, ileus, and abdominal pain or peritonitis. These findings are typical in inflammatory bowel disease. If the abscess is close to the surface, spontaneous drainage may occur or the placement of a percutaneous drain forms a controlled fistula.

PHYSIOLOGIC EFFECT AND COMPLICATIONS

Fluid and electrolyte imbalances, malnutrition, and sepsis are the most common complications associated with EC and EA fistulas. Undrained or incompletely drained collections can be associated with ileus, peritonitis, or even sepsis. Once the infection is cleared through either intentional drainage or spontaneous efflux, the septic complications often resolve and give way to the other long-term problems. For example, the inability to feed through the enteric tract and loss of protein-rich fluid can result in malnutrition if not already present. Fluid loss results in dehydration and electrolyte

abnormalities. The extent of fluid and electrolyte imbalance is directly related to the composition and volume of the fistula output. EC fistulas are characterized as low output (<200 mL/d), moderate output (200 to 500 mL/d), or high output (>500 mL/d; Table 2). Colonic fistulas tend to be low output; small bowel fistulas tend to be moderate to high output and are therefore associated with a higher degree of dehydration. The location also affects the composition of the output and degree of electrolyte imbalances. Proximal fistulas within the duodenum tend to have an output high in bicarbonate and can lead to a metabolic acidosis. Nearly all fistulas have output that is high in potassium, which leads to hypokalemia.

MANAGEMENT

The management of an EC fistula is complex and requires a detailed, stepwise approach to achieve successful closure. The ultimate goal of management is to reestablish the continuity of the patient's alimentary tract while limiting the morbidity and mortality. Approximately one third of EC fistulas close with supportive care and without operative management. The remainder need operative intervention. Achieving metabolic stability and control of sepsis in the first few hours to days of fistula formation is crucial for patient stabilization. Instituting a plan for controlling fistula output and achieving adequate nutritional support is necessary to resuscitate the patient and so that a definitive plan for closure can be developed (Table 3).

Stabilization and Sepsis Control

Sepsis control is imperative in the initial phase of fistula management. The lack of complete source control of the sepsis can lead to rapid multisystem organ failure or even death. In all cases, the principle to eliminate the source of infection is the same. For cases in which the initial abscess spontaneously drains, this may be as simple as débridement of the wound and adequate conduit for egress of the collection. Percutaneous drainage is often necessary for deeper infections. This can be done through image-guided drainage of the abdominal abscess. Antibiotics alone are seldom sufficient in clearing the infection and should only be used as an adjunct to drainage in patients who display sepsis. Unnecessary use of antibiotics creates drug-resistant bacteria and only compounds the complexity of future management. Antibiotic therapy should be maintained for approximately 4 to 7 days or until the sepsis clears. CT scanning should be used liberally with percutaneous drain upsizing used as needed until source control is completed. Operative source control in this phase is often not necessary and may even complicate the problem by creating more enterotomies, completely disrupting an anastomosis, or converting a contained abscess into widespread abdominal sepsis. The exception to this general principle is in the case of a retained foreign body, such as nonabsorbable mesh within the area of the fistula or abscess cavity. When this is present, good source control becomes unlikely, and the foreign body also interferes with subsequent closure of the fistula.

Resuscitation and Nutritional Support

By the time an EC fistula presents, the patient has typically endured multiple stresses, such as a malignant process, inflammatory bowel disease, or a surgical procedure including a complicated postoperative course. On presentation, the patient can be expected to have a decrease in lean muscle mass, anemia, dehydration, and suboptimal nutritional status.

Fluid resuscitation should begin with several liters of isotonic crystalloid solution and transfusion of red blood cells to improve oxygenation in patients who are severely anemic. The type of replacement fluid and electrolyte repletion should be tailored to the type and volume of fistula output as described previously and serum electrolyte status as measured with laboratory assessment. Electrolyte abnormalities of Na, K, Mg, and phosphate are common. These disturbances must be addressed, with special attention paid to relatively rapid correction of hypokalemia and hypophosphatemia, which are important for normal cardiac and respiratory muscle function. Metabolic acidosis may be present in duodenal fistulas and requires replacement of sodium bicarbonate.

Both enteral and parenteral nutrition have a role in the management of EC fistulas and should be used to achieve optimal nutritional support. Baseline nutritional needs are 20 kcal/kg/d of carbohydrate and fat and 0.8 g/kg/d of protein. These requirements can increase to approximately 30 kcal/kg/d and 1.5 to 2.5 g/kg/d in the setting of high-output fistulas. The route for nutrition delivery is based on caloric needs, patient symptoms, and fistula output. Enteral feeding is the physiologically preferred method, and numerous studies performed in the setting of various conditions have shown a benefit to enteral feeding with regards to healing, nutrition, and immune function. Enteral nutrition also supports the intestinal tract with regards to maintaining function while also preserving the integrity of intestinal mucosa. The drawback to this approach is that the initiation of enteral feeds may be associated with increased fistula output or in some cases is simply not tolerated because of ileus or obstruction. In these cases, total parenteral nutrition (TPN) is often necessary in the management of a fistula. Moreover, TPN is often needed in the interim between initiation of enteral support and achievement of caloric goals.

In the authors' practice, all patients start on enteral feeds once the ileus has resolved. If the fistula output does not increase to the level of a high-output fistula, and if it is tolerated, enteral feeds are continued and TPN is discontinued. A bulking agent, such as psyllium, may be added to assist in output control. Antimotility agents and octreotide, a long-acting somatostatin analog, may also help to control output. Although octreotide use has shown no proven benefit, it offers a potential decrease in fistula output by inhibiting secretion of various gastrointestinal hormones. In the authors' experience, some high-output fistulas are converted to medium or low output with the use of octreotide, which makes fluid and electrolyte management easier. If these measures do not work, the authors then revert to TPN to reduce the output.

When a trial of enteral feeds is initiated in a patient who has been on long-term TPN, one must be careful to assess for refeeding syndrome. This condition results in metabolic and fluid abnormalities, especially hypophosphatemia, on reintroducing enteral feeding. Refeeding syndrome typically presents in the first 4 days of renourishment. The chance of refeeding syndrome is reduced through the gradual reinstitution of enteral feeds while weaning the TPN.

Wound Care

Maintenance of skin integrity through control of fistula output and proper wound care is a crucial aspect of successful management. Involvement of skilled nursing staff or an enterostomal therapist can help to ensure that optimal wound care is received, especially in the outpatient setting.

H_2-receptor antagonists, proton pump inhibitors, and sucralfate can suppress acid production to decrease the acidity of the effluent. These medications can potentially limit corrosive effects on skin and assist in acid-base and electrolyte regulation but have shown no benefit with associated wound closure.

Although these pharmacologic agents may assist in controlling the volume of output, the corrosive properties of the effluent are actually most detrimental to skin integrity. Skin barriers (solid wafers, powder, paste, and sealants), adhesives (liquid, aerosol, and double-faced adhesive sheets or discs), dressings, and pouches (one-piece or two-piece appliances) are all useful for protecting the patient's skin and containing effluent.

Vacuum-assisted closure (VAC) dressings are frequently used to manage nonfistula wounds. VAC dressings promote formation of healthy granulation tissue and limit frequent dressing changes. Some studies suggest that applying VAC dressings to EC fistula wounds can assist in effluent management and promote wound healing. However, concerns continue to exist with this method. Effluent confined under VAC dressing sponges can potentially impair wound healing and place the patient at an increased risk of wound infection. Different sponge types are available to prevent this, such as standard VAC GranuFoam, GranuFoam Silver and WhiteFoam (Kinetic Concepts, Inc., San Antonio, Tex). However, VAC dressings are not accepted as standard of care for EC fistula wound management at this time. In the setting of deep EA fistulas, VAC dressings provide constant suction, which reduces contact between the peritoneum and fistula contents. In superficial EA fistulas, split thickness skin grafts can be done around the fistula site and a VAC dressing applied. VAC dressings placed around the fistula site keep effluent away from granulating tissue. When graft healing has progressed, skin barriers and stoma control appliances can replace VAC dressings.

SURGICAL MANAGEMENT

Spontaneous closure of EC fistulas is seen in approximately one third of patients in the first 4 to 6 weeks after formation. In those patients who do not have spontaneous closure, surgical repair is necessary. The operations to repair EC fistulas can be some of the more challenging, unforgiving, and time-consuming operations for the general surgeon. The operation is usually characterized by difficult entry into the abdomen, extensive adhesiolysis, removal of embedded mesh, bowel resection, and complex abdominal wall reconstruction. The tissue encountered is often suboptimal because of malnutrition and chronic inflammation. Not surprisingly, the risk of postoperative wound infection, anastomotic dehiscence, and even reformation of a fistula is not insignificant.

The timing of operation for EC fistula is critical in maximizing the chances of success. First and foremost, electrolyte imbalances need to be corrected and nutrition must be optimized before operation. In general, with the use of aggressive nutritional support, most patients can achieve serum albumin levels of greater than 3 g/dL, which should be the goal before operative intervention. The passage of time itself also plays an important role in preparing the surgical field. With time, the adhesions among bowel loops and other abdominal viscera become soft and filmy, which allows easier dissection and minimizes the chances of inadvertent enterotomy or serosal tear. In addition, the inflammation surrounding a fistula resolves and involves less of the surrounding structures, thus reducing the potential need for resection of adjacent bowel loops. In general, at least 12 weeks should pass from fistula formation to operative intervention. Unless other circumstances, such as uncontrolled sepsis or failure to progress, force an earlier operation, this amount of time should be the minimal wait period. In patients who are doing nutritionally well and have good control of fistula output, waiting an additional 4 to 6 weeks optimizes the chances of a good outcome even further. If a skin graft was placed on a granulation tissue bed, it should pass the "pinch-test" before operation. This test is performed by pinching the skin graft and elevating it off of the underlying tissues. The ability of the graft to elevate from the bowel shows that the surgeon will be able to separate the skin from the viscera at operation.

The operation for fistula takedown is often extensive, and ample preparations should be made. Patients should have appropriate intravenous access to allow resuscitation of the significant insensible fluid loss from the relatively long operative time. A Foley catheter should be placed, and an arterial line should be considered for monitoring hemodynamics and resuscitative effort. In patients who undergo an extensive abdominal operation combined with a complex abdominal wall reconstruction, consideration should also be given to a postoperative intensive care unit (ICU) bed for ongoing resuscitation and monitoring of respiratory function.

The operation should begin with a generous incision away from the EC fistula itself and in virgin tissue if possible. The abdomen should be entered sharply, and care should be taken to avoid injury to the bowel, which is almost always adherent to the previous incision, particularly in the area of the fistula. Once the abdomen is entered, the viscera should be completely freed from each other with extensive adhesiolysis. A thorough inspection of all of the abdominal viscera should be made. In particular, assessment for an obstruction downstream of an EC fistula is important. Often, most of the abdomen is normal appearing, and the area of the fistula is apparent from dense thick adhesions, inflammatory rind, and associated phlegmon. The authors typically separate all structures and leave the fistula attached to the abdominal wall for the very last part of the dissection. In this way, an assessment can be made of the relative location of the fistula on the bowel and any other involved structures before resection. This is important to minimize the length of resected bowel. It is not uncommon that a "single" fistula is often made up of multiple loops of small bowel that are physically close but are separated by a long linear distance. A decision must then be made to resect these enterotomies as a single segment with one anastomosis or multiple segments with several anastomoses, keeping in mind the need to balance the development of short gut syndrome with the added risk of a complication added by each additional anastomosis.

The closure of a fistula almost always involves a bowel resection and anastomosis. Direct suture closure of the dissected fistula tract has been described but is seldom possible in practice. Often the fistula involves a significant portion of the bowel circumference or is surrounded by scarred abnormal bowel and simple closure is not possible. The exceptions to this are fistulas created by a percutaneous drain that inadvertently traverses bowel or a surgically created fistula such as a tube jejunostomy. These can often be dissected and stapled or oversewn.

Once the gastrointestinal portion of the operation is complete, attention must be turned to closure of the abdominal wall. This also carries complex problems not seen with most simple closures. Often the takedown of the fistula requires a full-thickness resection and débridement of scarred and inflamed abdominal wall. The area of resection can be quite large, especially if it includes previously placed mesh. In many cases, the amount of abdominal wall resected precludes a primary closure and an abdominal wall reconstruction must be performed. A few important principles that apply to abdominal closure after EC fistula takedown should be pointed out. At the very least, EC fistula closures are clean-contaminated cases and the use of nonabsorbable meshes such as proline should be avoided. If primary closure cannot be achieved, the midline can often be medialized with a component wall separation. This is often reinforced with an underlay of a biologic material, such as xenograft of bovine or porcine acellular dermis. Further reinforcement can be gained by quilting an overlay of absorbable mesh onto the anterior fascia. Closure of a large defect with these measures is associated with a high risk of subsequent incisional hernia but is superior to the risk of infecting nonabsorbable mesh. With this in mind, a decision should be made on how complex of a closure should be performed at the fistula reversal. A component separation "burns bridges" for future definitive repairs and should not be undertaken if the judgment is that it will not be definitive. The principle of "live to fight another day" applies.

SUMMARY

Enterocutaneous fistulas are a common, complex problem in the surgical patient population. Diligent control of sepsis, electrolyte imbalance, fistula output, and nutrition management can significantly reduce the patient's morbidity and mortality. A patient's course can be optimized through definitive surgical repair when spontaneous closure does not occur.

SUGGESTED READINGS

Evenson AR, Fischer JE: Current management of enterocutaneous fistulas, *J Gastrointest Surg* 10:455–464, 2006.

Martinez JL, Luque-de-Leon E: Factors predictive of recurrence and mortality after surgical repair of enterocutaneous fistula, *J Gastrointest Surg* 16:156–164, 2012.

Polk TM, Schawb, CW: Metabolic and nutritional support of the enterocutaneous fistula patient a three phase approach, *World J Surg* 36:514–533, 2012.

LARGE BOWEL

PREOPERATIVE BOWEL PREPARATION: IS IT REALLY NECESSARY?

Pamela A. Lipsett, MD, MHPE, FACS, FCCM

OVERVIEW

Among elective surgical procedures, elective resection of the colon has the highest rates of surgical site infection (SSI), often at or above 20% when postoperative surveillance is continued for 4 weeks after surgery and strict definitions of infection are applied. No doubt this is related to the fact that the colon contains more than 10^{12} colony-forming units (CFU)/g bacteria that can be released and contaminate the surgical site when the surgical procedure opens the lumen of the bowel. Mechanical bowel preparation (MBP) combined with oral antimicrobial agents was designed to reduce infections after colorectal surgery. However, the routine use of intravenous systemic antibiotics during surgery has brought into question the necessity of preoperative oral antibiotics. Further, evidence-based reviews have routinely called for surgeons to eliminate MBP as lacking evidence to support its usefulness. Moreover, incomplete MBP has been associated with a paradoxical increase in complications, such as intraoperative contamination of the operative field with liquefied bowel contents. Thus, it is reasonable to consider whether MBP should be used in addition to systemic antibiotics, whether MBP should be combined with oral antibiotics, or whether both should be abandoned.

HISTORICAL BACKGROUND

In the 1930s, with mortality rates of 10% to 12% and SSI as high as 80% to 90% after colon resection, it seemed logical to focus on reducing microbial contamination by cleansing of the colon of gross fecal material. Further, some surgeons believe that reduction of the mass of colon contents allows for enhanced manipulation of the colon, ease of stapler use, and palpation of tumors. Edgar Poth noted that MBP reduced the burden of total bacteria in the colon but that it did not reduce the concentration of bacteria. He believed that it was essential to reduce the microbial concentration by MBP for intraluminal antibiotics to have any effect on the mucosal concentration of bacteria. In addition, Nichols and associates similarly concluded that MBP alone had no impact on microbial concentration in the colon. Thus, one can conclude that no clinical or microbiologic evidence

supports MBP alone as a method to reduce SSI rates for elective colon surgery.

MECHANISM OF ACTION OF ORAL ANTIMICROBIAL AGENTS

Magnesium citrate, sodium phosphate, enemas, polyethylene glycol (PEG), and whole-bowel irrigation clear the colon of solid fecal components but do not influence the species or concentration of organisms in residual fluid within the colon at the time of operation. Early experience with oral antimicrobial prophylaxis did not adequately consider the importance of both aerobic and anaerobic bacteria in the colon. However, the combination of an antianaerobic agent with neomycin resulted in a significant reduction of both *Escherichia coli* and *Bacteroides fragilis* species in the colon. In the surgically resected colon, oral antibiotics produce a 4-log to 5-log decrease in the concentrations of both aerobic and anaerobic bacteria. Further, the use of an oral preparation with neomycin and erythromycin base both quantitatively and qualitatively reduces evidence of intraluminal and mucosal wall microflora. No doubt, the reduction in bacterial concentration coupled with a reduction in SSI began the modern era of bowel preparation in elective colorectal surgery.

MECHANICAL BOWEL PREPARATION

Early preparations of MBP used dietary limitations, cathartics, and enemas and lasted 48 to 72 hours. Oral cathartics traditionally use isotonic PEG solution or hyperosmolar insoluble salts that contain magnesium or phosphate. Many studies of various preparations for colonoscopy have concluded that various preparations are effective: 4L PEG, 3L PEG, 2L PEG, or 45-mL and 90-mL preparations of sodium phosphate, However, in several studies, sodium phosphate–based preparations are better tolerated with less patient nausea, emesis, bloating, and cramps. Acute phosphate nephropathy has been rarely reported with the use of some oral sodium phosphate for bowel cleansing (Fleet Phospho-soda or Fleet ACCU-PREP, CB Fleet, Inc., Lynchburg, Va.) but not others (Osmo-Prep, CB Fleet, Inc., Lynchburg, Va.). The use of PEG solutions may be slightly favored for colonoscopy, with perhaps a slight advantage of proximal colon cleansing, but these advantages have not been measured in elective colon surgery.

IS MECHANICAL BOWEL PREPARATION STILL WARRANTED?

If evidence-based reviews, systematic reviews, metaanalyses, and national (Canadian) guidelines for the use of MBP were examined for their recommendations about the use of MBP in elective

147

colorectal surgery, this section would simply say: MBP can be safely omitted. The Cochrane review in 2011 by Guenaga and colleagues examined 5805 patient outcomes and showed that no differences were found in anastomotic leakage rate for low anterior resection (MBP, 8.8% vs 10.3%; odds ratio [OR], 0.88 [0.55,1.40]), colon surgery (MBP, 3.0% vs 3.5%; OR, 0.85 [0.58,1.26]), and SSI (MBP, 9.6% vs 8.5%; OR, 1.15 [0.95,1.42]). Yet, in 2006, a multinational audit of 1082 patients from 295 hospitals in both Europe and the United States revealed that 86% to 97% of patients received preoperative MBP. These surveys indicate that a large gap exists between the evidence surrounding the use of MBP and surgeon practices. Can this gap be explained by lack of awareness of the evidence, or is there more behind the reluctance of surgeons to abandon this practice?

Much of the published evidence suggests that MBP does not reduce SSI or other infectious risks with elective colorectal surgery. Certainly, MBP is unpleasant for patients. Further, in traumatic injury with unprepared bowel, systemic antibiotics alone have complication rates that are considered acceptable. Trials conducted in Europe suggest that when broad-spectrum systemic antibiotics are used, MBP alone provides no advantage in important infectious clinical outcomes. Aside from potential patient concerns and complaints about MBP and dehydration that may be induced with colon cleansing, some adverse effects of MBP have also been identified. First, histologic evidence suggests that cleansing with PEG is associated with depletion of the superficial mucous layer and epithelial cells and severe infiltration of both lymphocytes and neutrophils in the wall of the large bowel. In an interesting report by Wren and colleagues, in which all 304 patients received cathartics and intravenous antibiotics but some patients also received oral antibiotics, *Clostridium difficile* infection was higher in patients who received oral antibiotics (7.4%) versus those who did not (2.6%). Although this single-center report did show an increase in *C. difficile* infection, additional reviews did not support this conclusion.

Despite the lack of efficacy of MBP alone, several authors have suggested that the combined role of MBP and oral antibiotics be reexamined. For example, Lewis showed a reduction in SSI from 17% in the oral placebo group to 5% among those receiving oral neomycin (2 g) and metronidazole (2 g) at 7:00 PM and 11:00 PM the night before surgery. Importantly, the bowel preparation with sodium phosphate was complete by 6:00 PM. Randomized controlled studies with 100 or more patients showed a summary odds reduction with systemic antibiotics, MBP, and oral antibiotics of 0.47 (95% confidence interval [CI], 0.16 to 0.77). Finally, in a naturalistic experiment from the Michigan Surgical Quality Collaborative-Colectomy Best Practices Project, data on MBP and *C. difficile* outcomes were prospectively collected. A total of 49.6% of the 2011 elective colectomies that were performed over 16 months received MBP and no oral antibiotics, and 36.4% received both MBP and oral antibiotics. First, these data show that real-life surgeons still believe in and use MBP. In this report, patients receiving MBP and oral antibiotics were less likely to have any SSI (4.5% vs 11.8%; *P* = 0.0001), to have an organ space infection (1.8% vs 4.2%; *P* = 0.044), or to have a superficial SSI (2.6% vs 7.6%; *P* = 0.001). Patients receiving bowel preparation with oral antibiotics were also less likely to have a prolonged ileus (3.9% vs 8.6%; *P* = 0.011) and had similar rates of *C. difficile* colitis (1.3% vs 1.8%; *P* = 0.58). Although these data are not from a randomized controlled trial, they are real-world experiences that suggest a possible benefit of combining systematic antibiotics with MBP and oral antibiotics.

SUMMARY

Significant controversy remains with respect to the value of MBP and oral antibiotics, alone or in combination. Evidence suggests that MBP does not provide incremental value in the decrease of SSI. However, studies have not examined whether value is provided in colon manipulation, ease of stapler use, and palpation of tumors with MBP. Perhaps the greatest benefit of MBP may well be when used in combination with oral antimicrobial agents. Although the topic of MBP and oral agents may be closed for some, perhaps additional clinical studies to investigate the best agent for MBP in the setting of oral antimicrobials, the timing of MBP and oral agents, and the best oral agents to be used remain valid research questions in providing the best outcomes for our patients after colorectal surgery. However, no additional trials of MBP alone are needed; we know that alone, MBP has no benefit for SSI prevention.

SUGGESTED READINGS

American Society of Colon and Rectal Surgeons (ASCRS), American Society for Gastrointestinal Endoscopy (ASGE), Society of American Gastrointestinal and Endoscopic Surgeons (SAGES), Wexner SD, Beck DE, Baron TH, et al: A consensus document on bowel preparation before colonoscopy: prepared by a Task Force from the American Society of Colon and Rectal Surgeons (ASCRS), the American Society for Gastrointestinal Endoscopy (ASGE), and the Society of American Gastrointestinal and Endoscopic Surgeons (SAGES), *Surg Endosc* 20(7):1161, 2006.

Belsey J, Crosta C, Epstein O, et al: Meta-analysis: the relative efficacy of oral bowel preparations for colonoscopy 1985-2010, *Aliment Pharmacol Ther* 35(2):222–237, 2012; Epub 2011.

Dellinger EP: Re: "Colon preparation and surgical site infection," *Am J Surg* 204(5):804–805, 2012.

Eskicioglu C, Forbes SS, Fenech DS, et al: Best Practice in General Surgery Committee: preoperative bowel preparation for patients undergoing elective colorectal surgery: a clinical practice guideline endorsed by the Canadian Society of Colon and Rectal Surgeons, *Can J Surg* 53(6):385–395, 2010.

Fry DE: Colon preparation and surgical site infection, *Am J Surg* 202(2):225–232, 2011; Epub 2011.

Güenaga KF, Matos D, Wille-Jørgensen P: Mechanical bowel preparation for elective colorectal surgery, *Cochrane Database Syst Rev* (9):CD001544, 2011.

Hayashi MS, Wilson SE: Is there a current role for preoperative non-absorbable oral antimicrobial agents for prophylaxis of infection after colorectal surgery? *Surg Infect (Larchmt)* 10(3):285–288, 2009.

Krapohl GL, Phillips LR, Campbell DA Jr, et al: Bowel preparation for colectomy and risk of Clostridium difficile infection, *Dis Colon Rectum* 54(7):810–817, 2011. Erratum in *Dis Colon Rectum* 54(11):1461, 2011.

Lewis RT: Oral versus systemic antibiotic prophylaxis in elective colon surgery: a randomized study and meta-analysis send a message from the 1990s, *Can J Surg* 45:171–180, 2002.

Slim K, Vicaut E, Launay-Savary MV: Updated systematic review and meta-analysis of randomized clinical trials on the role of mechanical bowel preparation before colorectal surgery, *Ann Surg* 249(2):203–209, 2009.

Van't Sant HP, Weidema WF, Hop WC, et al: The influence of mechanical bowel preparation in elective lower colorectal surgery, *Ann Surg* 251(1):59–63, 2010.

Wren SM, Ahmed N, Jamal A, et al: Preoperative oral antibiotics in colorectal surgery increase the rate of Clostridium difficile colitis, *Arch Surg* 140(8):752–756, 2005.

THE MANAGEMENT OF DIVERTICULAR DISEASE OF THE COLON

Paula Ferrada, MD, FACS, and
Rao R. Ivatury, MD, FACS

Diverticular disease of the colon is very common with advancing age and is higher in prevalence in countries with Western diets. The two important complications of this condition are inflammation and bleeding. In both of these clinical situations, newer concepts of diagnosis and management have emerged in recent years.

DIVERTICULITIS: CLINICAL PRESENTATION

Diverticulitis is defined as inflammation or infection associated with diverticula and is manifested clinically in about one third of patients with diverticula. The process through which a diverticulum becomes inflamed has been linked to obstruction of the diverticula and venous congestion, ultimately leading to perforation. The extent and localization of this perforation determines the clinical behavior of the disease. Small perforations can remain well localized, contained by the pericolic fat and mesentery, leading to small abscesses, and larger perforations result in more extensive abscess formation, remotely in the mesocolon and in the pelvis. Fecal peritonitis results if the perforation is freed into the general peritoneal cavity and may present as life-threatening sepsis (Figure 1).

Hinchey and colleagues described a grading system to reflect the degree of perforation:

- Stage I: Confined pericolic abscess.
- Stage II: Distant abscess (retroperitoneal or pelvic).
- Stage III: Generalized peritonitis caused by rupture of a pericolic or pelvic abscess, noncommunicating with bowel lumen because of obliteration of diverticular neck by inflammation.
- Stage IV: Fecal peritonitis caused by free perforation of a diverticulum (communicating).

MANAGEMENT

Mild cases of diverticulitis, even with the presence of small abscesses (Hinchey I) can be treated conservatively, with antibiotics (aerobic and anaerobic coverage; e.g., combination of ciprofloxacin and metronidazole). Clinical improvement is monitored with serial monitoring of the patient's temperature, abdominal findings, and white blood cell count (WBC). Once these values are normal, patients are progressed on their diet and encouraged to eat a high-fiber diet to avoid recurrent symptoms. Patients with more severe symptoms and those who do not show improvement on outpatient therapy are admitted for intravenous antibiotics and gradual progression of diet. Responders may be discharged after a brief hospital stay.

After resolution of symptoms and signs (diminished tenderness, reduction of leukocytosis), the patient can be treated as an outpatient with oral antibiotics and follow-up. Older patients should be followed with a colonoscopy to rule out malignant lesions in the colon. Larger abscesses (Hinchey II) may be amenable for computed tomographic (CT) scan or ultrasound-guided percutaneous drainage (PCD). However, even after a successful conservatively treated episode, complications such as excessive scaring and strictures or fistulas to hollow organs may still ensue. In the absence of these complications, surgery may be deferred.

Role of Elective Surgery in Acute Uncomplicated Diverticulitis

Elective colectomy was previously recommended after the first bout of diverticulitis. The Standards Task Force of the American Society of Colon and Rectal Surgeons (ACCRS) recommended colectomy after one to two episodes of uncomplicated diverticulitis and after one episode of complicated diverticulitis. More recent studies began to question this recommendation. In a retrospective cohort study from 12 Kaiser Permanente hospitals, among 2551 patients, 185 (7.3%) had elective colectomy and 2366 (92.7%) did not. In a mean follow-up period of 8.9 years, only 13.3% had recurrence after nonoperative treatment. Only advanced age and higher comorbidity was associated with recurrence. Interestingly, percutaneous abscess drainage was not associated with a higher recurrence rate.

Many authorities suggest that younger patients with diverticulitis requiring hospitalization should have an elective colectomy because the disease is more virulent in these patients. In a statistical model that analyzed the probabilities of clinical events and costs from a large cohort, the group from Seattle concluded that performing colectomy after the fourth episode (rather than the second episode) resulted in 1% fewer deaths and 2% fewer colostomies and saved $5429 per patient. The data were similar for older patients as well. Other studies also challenged the concept of an interval sigmoidectomy after diverticulitis, concluding that morbidity and mortality rates are not significantly different between patients with multiple episodes of diverticulitis compared with those with one or two prior attacks. There appears to be a consensus now that elective colectomy after the first episode of diverticulitis should no longer be a routine practice, regardless of age.

Complicated Diverticulitis

Complicated diverticulitis is defined as diverticulitis associated with abscess formation, free perforation, fistula formation, or stenosis. Not all intraabdominal abscesses need drainage. For pericolic and intramesenteric abscesses, initial management with intravenous antibiotics and close observation may be appropriate, reserving PCD for patients with failure to improve rapidly from a clinical standpoint. The threshold for PCD, however, should remain low, if the patient does not show evidence of sepsis control. Once drainage is established, drains may be removed after clinical symptoms improve and output is minimal or ceases. After successful nonoperative management, patients should be referred for colonoscopy to rule out malignant lesions in the colon.

Role of Elective Surgery in Acute Complicated Diverticulitis (Pericolic Abscess, Hinchey I and II)

The necessity for elective interval resection after successful PCD of pericolic abscesses is controversial. Although recommended by most leaders, several smaller series confirm that drainage of smaller mesocolic abscesses can be the definitive treatment without subsequent sigmoid resection.

Role of Elective Surgery in Acute Complicated Diverticulitis After Successful Treatment

The current indications for elective sigmoidectomy after initial successful nonoperative treatment are recurrent episodes of

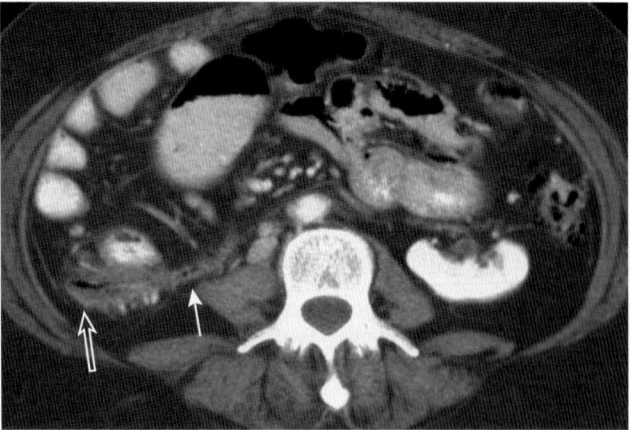

FIGURE 1 Computed tomographic scan of a patient with right lower quadrant abscess *(open arrow)* as a result of perforated sigmoid diverticulitis. The *closed arrow* shows the normal-appearing appendix. *(From Yu J, Fulcher AS, Turner MA, et al: Helical CT evaluation of acute right lower quadrant pain: part II, uncommon mimics of appendicitis,* Am J Roentgenol *184(4):1143–1149, 2005.)*

diverticulitis in patients with immunosuppression or transplant and in those who had pelvic abscess drainage and recovered from it. Diverticular fistulae arise when the inflamed colon erodes into adjacent organs, thus causing a fistulous connection. The most common fistulae are colovesical fistulae, and the presenting symptoms are pneumaturia and fecaluria. The finding of air within the bladder on CT scan is considered pathognomonic. Less commonly fistulas are to other structures within the pelvis: ureter, prostate, fallopian tubes, or uterus. In these patients, preoperative colonoscopy is helpful to rule out malignant lesions. Occasionally, diverticulitis may result in chronic inflammation and stenosis of a segment of sigmoid colon. Such diverticular strictures, if significant and causing increasing constipation, are an indication for surgical resection.

All these patients must have bowel preparation, both mechanical and chemical, before surgery. Concurrent comorbid conditions must be evaluated before surgery and the patients optimized for surgery. The surgical procedure of choice is resection of sigmoid colon up to the level of proximal rectum and colorectal anastomosis.

Current literature strongly supports the superiority of laparoscopic resection and hand-assisted primary anastomosis. In a sigma trial from Europe (a prospective, multicenter, double-blind, parallel-arm, randomized trial), 104 patients were randomized for these two methods. The conversion rate to open operation on initial laparoscopic attempts was 19.2%. Laparoscopic resection took longer ($P = 0.0001$) but caused less blood loss ($P = 0.033$). Mortality rate was 1%. Significantly more major complications were seen in open resection (9.6% vs 25.0%; $P = 0.038$), along with more pain on the visual analog scale, and in systemic analgesia requirement ($P = 0.029$). The short form–36 questionnaire showed significantly better quality of life for the laparoscopy group. At the 6-month follow-up evaluation, no significant differences in morbidity or mortality rates were found. Two patients died of cardiac causes (overall mortality, 3%). Late complications occurred in seven of the laparoscopy group and in 12 of the open group and consisted of three incisional hernias, five small bowel obstructions, four enterocutaneous fistulas, one intraabdominal abscess, one retained gauze, two anastomotic strictures, and three recurrent episodes of diverticulitis. Nine of these patients underwent additional surgical interventions. The total morbidity in these 6 months was significantly less for the laparoscopy group (9 vs 23; $P = 0.003$).

Role of Emergent Surgery in Acute Complicated Diverticulitis

Free Perforation: Purulent and Fecal Peritonitis (Hinchey Stages III and IV)

Peritonitis from free perforation of the diverticula presents with a clinical picture of sepsis, exhibiting signs such as tachycardia, high or very low WBC, hypotension, hyperthermia or hypothermia, peritoneal signs, renal failure, hyperglycemia, and occasionally, frank septic shock. Early, aggressive, goal-directed therapy for sepsis should focus on appropriate oxygen delivery, early initiation of broad coverage antibiotic therapy, and source control with immediate laparotomy, all the time with a careful assessment of the physiologic reserve of the patient.

Critical Care Management and Resuscitation

Starting with the management of an appropriate airway, ensuring adequate ventilation, and continuing with fluid resuscitation are lifesaving measures for these patients in extremis. Placement of a central line, optimization of mixed venous saturation (SvO_2) and central venous pressure (CVP) to guide fluid resuscitation, and early initiation of antibiotics to cover gram-negative and anaerobic organisms are the essential elements of preoperative therapy.

Surgical Management

Emergent operative management is the treatment of choice for patients with perforated diverticulitis. The abdomen is explored with a long midline incision, the intraperitoneal pus and feces are evacuated, and the offending perforation in the sigmoid is controlled with staples, sutures, or clamps. The abdomen is thoroughly irrigated with saline solution, ensuring manual evacuation of stool. Resection of the perforation-bearing segment of the colon (perforectomy) is the preferred procedure in most cases. The safest option in treatment of severe sepsis and generalized purulent or fecal peritonitis is limited resection with colostomy and closure of the distal rectum (Hartmann's procedure) or creation of a mucous fistula. Hartmann's resection is preferred by the authors because it obviates the need for extensive mobilization of the distal colon and avoids violating tissue planes in the pelvis that make the next operation more difficult.

Abbreviated Laparotomy in Unstable Conditions

Massive volume resuscitation and vasopressor therapy is often needed, especially in patients whose conditions are hemodynamically challenged because of severe purulent or fecal peritonitis resulting in acidosis and septic shock. In such cases, the current strategy of abbreviating the laparotomy, rapid perforectomy leaving the colon in discontinuity, abdominal wash out to evacuate pus and feces, and temporary abdominal closure with application of any variation of the vacuum assisted closure (VAC) system constitute the so-called damage-control surgery. The advantages of this approach are the avoidance of continuing operative trauma and resuscitation in the intensive care unit (ICU) with fluids, antibiotics, and, if necessary, vasopressors. Once the goals of correction of acidosis and septic shock are accomplished, usually within 24 to 48 hours, patients are returned for definitive resection, colostomy, and Hartmann's pouch, or in very rare instances, colocolic anastomosis.

Colostomy Versus Colocolostomy

The decision to perform a primary anastomosis with or without an ileostomy or to perform a sigmoid colostomy and Hartmann's pouch hinges on overall stability, the degree and type of peritonitis, and the condition of the colon. In general, Hinchey IV cases with fecal peritonitis are poor candidates for this approach. Patients with hemodynamically stable conditions with purulent peritonitis may be treated with primary anastomosis and a diverting loop ileostomy. Primary anastomosis, in general, is reserved for the most favorable conditions, including a stable condition and well-vascularized ends of colon. Tension on the anastomotic line must be avoided, if necessary with splenic flexure mobilization. Intraoperative colonic lavage may be an adequate substitute for lack of preoperative bowel preparation. Constantinides and associates analyzed 15 recent series with a random effects model and sensitivity analysis to control for heterogeneity of confounding variables. They showed a significantly reduced postoperative mortality rate of 4.9% in resection-anastomosis versus a rate of 15.1% with Hartmann's procedure (odds ratio [OR], 0.41). In emergency operations, matched for severity of peritonitis (Hinchey >II), no difference in mortality rates was seen between these two procedures (14.1% vs 14.4%). Most of the recent literature supports a proximal defunctioning loop ileostomy if there is any doubt about the integrity of the anastomosis, a concept supported by the European Association of Endoscopic Surgeons.

Laparoscopic Irrigation and Drainage for Hinchey II and III

This provocative approach to Hinchey II and III cases is being reported with frequency. In a prospective study reported by Myers and colleagues in 2008, 92 patients with Hinchey grade II pelvic abscess (n = 25) or grade III (n = 67) were treated with laparoscopic irrigation of the peritoneal cavity with 4 L of warm saline solution and the placement of two Penrose drains in the vicinity of perforation along with antibiotic therapy. Eighty-seven had resolution of disease, and only two had recurring pelvic abscesses; one of these had Hartmann's resection. The mortality rate was 3%, 3 of 92 (two from multi-organ failure and one from pulmonary embolism [PE]). The authors noted no recurrence of the disease after a follow-up period of 3 years. Multiple centers are beginning to accumulate experience with this approach that deserves a careful consideration in the future (Table 1).

The optimal strategy for surgical treatment for diverticulitis, whether elective or emergent, depends on a host of factors related to the patient, the disease, the environment, and the surgical team. These are nicely summarized in the graphic described by Bauer (Figure 2).

SUMMARY AND CONCLUSION

The management of diverticulitis appears to have undergone revision in recent years because of a better understanding of the natural history of the disease. Elective sigmoidectomy is deferred in most patients and is reserved for patients with immunocompromise or transplant and for the more severe forms of complicated diverticulitis. Laparoscopic approaches are playing an increasing role both in emergency situations and for elective sigmoid resection.

DIVERTICULAR BLEEDING

Diverticular bleeding is the most common cause of significant lower gastrointestinal (GI) bleeding, defined as bleeding into the bowel lumen from a source that is distal to the ligament of Treitz. Approximately 15% of patients with colonic diverticulosis experience bleeding, which may range from minor to severe and life threatening. Most diverticular hemorrhages stop spontaneously. In general, patients who need more than 4 units of blood in a 24-hour period for hemodynamic stability, who have not stopped bleeding after 72 hours, or who experience rebleeding within 1 week after an initial episode should undergo surgery. Endoscopic treatment may have a role, but large-scale prospective randomized trials are not available.

Diagnosis and Management

1. Resuscitation is performed with ABC (airway, breathing, and circulation) and transfusion as necessary.
2. Upper GI (UGI) bleed must be ruled out with inserting a nasogastric tube and ensuring that there is bile and no blood in the aspirate. Clear fluid is not enough; one has to see bile to be sure that a postpyloric bleed with pylorospasm is not happening. If UGI bleed is not ruled out, an esophagogastroduodenoscopy (EGD) is indicated.
3. Efforts must be made to localize the site of lower GI bleed. The factors that determine the choice of the diagnostic test are the hemodynamic stability of the patient, the bleeding rate, patient comorbidities, therapeutic options, and local expertise available. The various techniques of localization available are colonoscopy; radionuclide scanning, which is highly sensitive (capable of detecting bleeding at rates as slow as 0.1 to 0.4 mL/min); selective mesenteric angiography (less sensitive but offers therapeutic embolization); or, occasionally, a provocative angiography to provoke bleeding with the use of short-acting anticoagulant agents. The recent availability of multidetector CT scan (MDCT), with its increased resolution and faster scanning, allows for identification of extravasation of intraluminal contrast before it is diluted by intestinal contents. MDCT is also noninvasive and can demonstrate acute lower GI bleeding rates as low as 0.2 mL/min. Overall rates of detection and localization range around 50% to 80%. Figure 3 presents an algorithm for the management of lower GI bleeding.

"Blind" subtotal colectomy or resection without localization is associated with a high rebleeding rate of up to 42%. Subtotal colectomy should be reserved for hemodynamically unstable conditions without a localized source of bleeding.

TABLE 1: Reported experience with laparoscopic irrigation and drainage in Hinchey stage II and stage III diverticulitis

Author, year	N	Resolution	Mortality	Morbidity
Taylor CJ, 2006	14	79%	–	3*
Myers E, 2008	92	87%	3%	3 (abscess)
Karoui M, 2009	35	97%	–	1 (Hartmann's)
White SI, 2010	35	77%	–	8†
Afshar S, 2012‡	301	–	0.3%	19%

*Three patients did not show improvement and underwent acute resection.
†Perforated cancer (1), fecal fistula (2), inadequate washout and ongoing sepsis (5).
‡Collected results from 12 studies.

FIGURE 2   Risk assessment and strategies for management after colonic diverticulitis. *CAD,* Coronary artery disease; *DM,* diabetes mellitus; *HP,* Hartmann procedure; *HTN,* hypertension; *MOF,* multi-organ failure; *PRA,* primary resection anastomosis. *(From Bauer VP: Emergency management of diverticulitis,* Clin Colon Rectal Surg 22(3):161–168, 2009.)

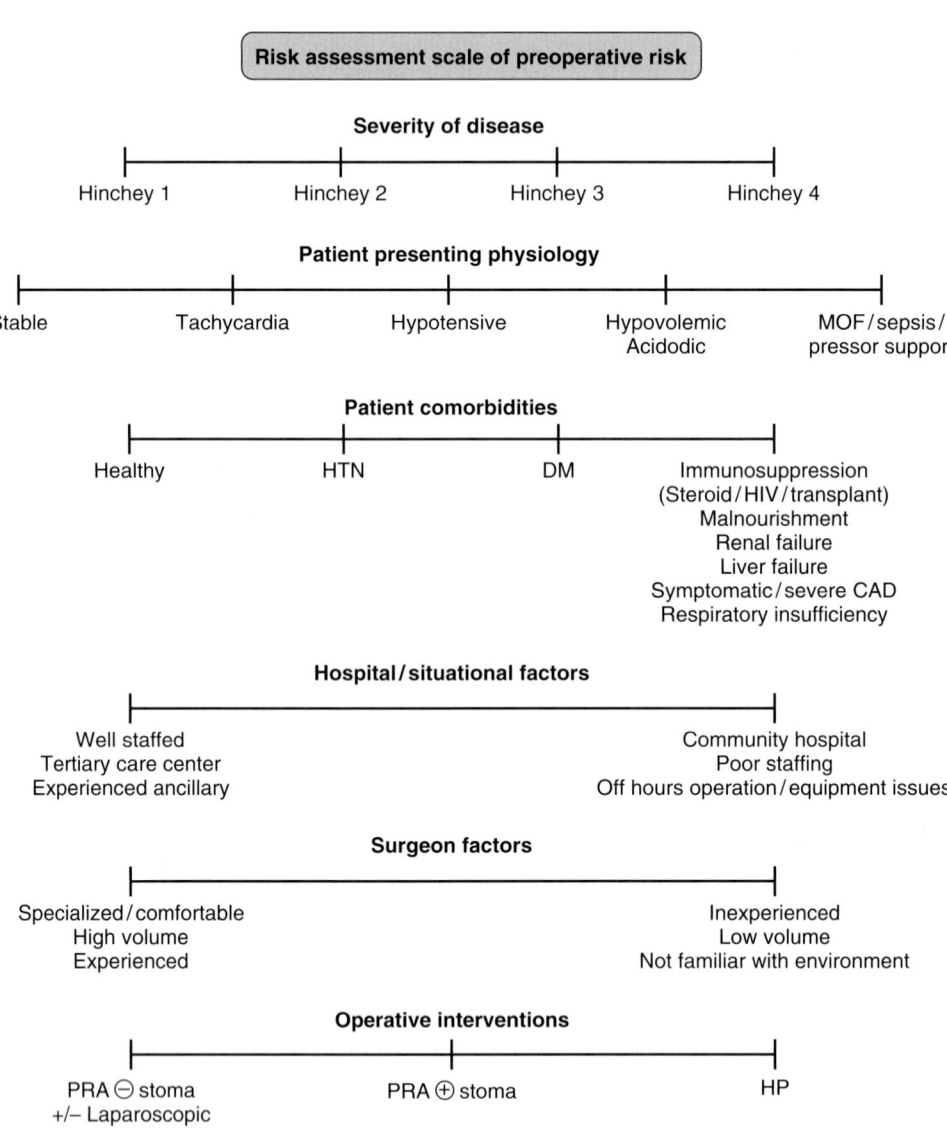

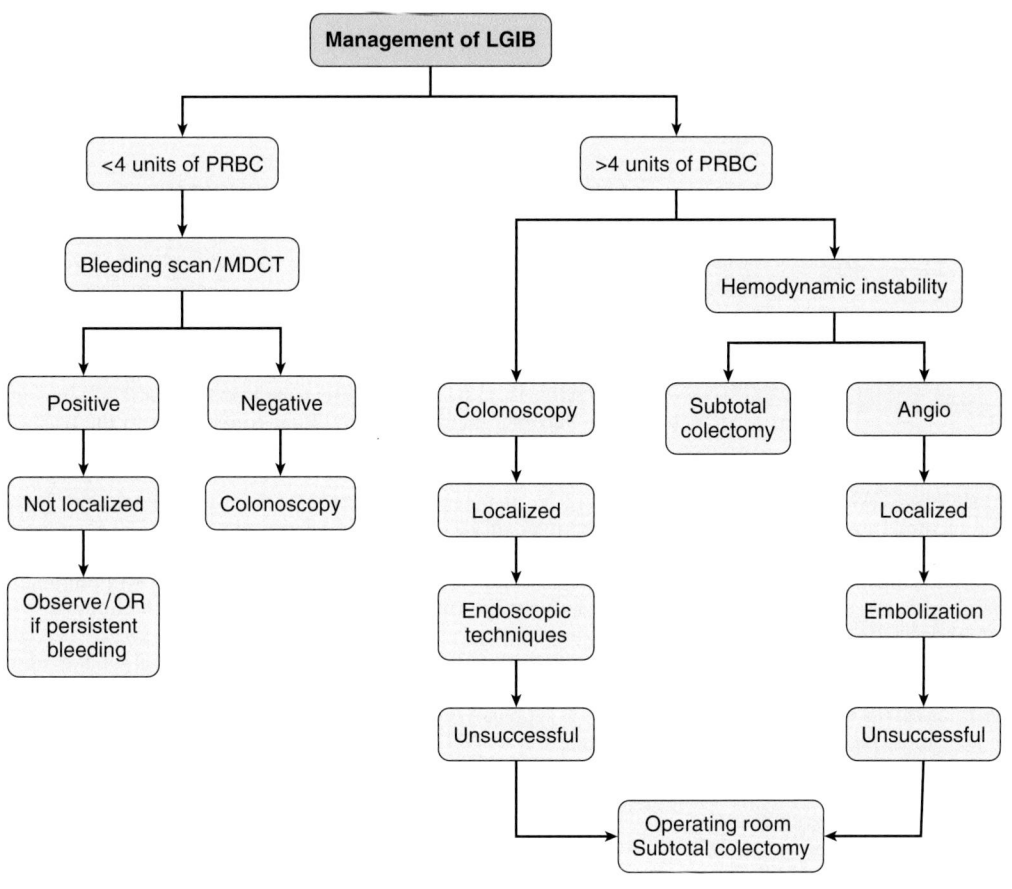

FIGURE 3 Algorithm for management of lower gastrointestinal bleeding (LGIB). *MDCT,* Multi-detector computerized tomography; *OR,* operating room; *PRBC,* packed red blood cells. *(From Lee J, et al: Acute lower GI bleeding for the acute care surgeon: current diagnosis and management,* Scand J Surg *98:135–142, 2009.)*

Suggested Readings

Afshar S, Kurer MA: Laparoscopic peritoneal lavage for perforated sigmoid diverticulitis, *Colorectal Dis* 14(2):135–142, 2012.

Bauer VP: Emergency management of diverticulitis, *Clin Colon Rectal Surg* 22(3):161–168, 2009.

Breitenstein S, Kraus A, Hahnloser D, et al: Emergency left colon resection for acute perforation: primary anastomosis or Hartmann's procedure? A case-matched control study, *World J Surg* 31(11):2117–2124, 2007; Epub 2007.

Broderick-Villa G, Burchette RJ, Collins JC, et al: Hospitalization for acute diverticulitis does not mandate routine elective colectomy, *Arch Surg* 140:576–583, 2005.

Chait MM: Lower gastrointestinal bleeding in the elderly, *World J Gastrointest Endosc* 2(5):147–154, 2010.

Chapman J, Davies M, Wolff B, et al: Complicated diverticulitis: is it time to rethink the rules? *Ann Surg* 242:576–683, 2005.

Chapman JR, Dozois ED, Wolff BG, et al: Diverticulitis; a progressive disease? Do multiple recurrences predict less favorable outcomes? *Ann Surg* 243:876–883, 2006.

Constantinides VA, Heriot A, Remzi F, et al: Operative strategies for diverticular peritonitis: a decision analysis between primary resection and anastomosis versus Hartmann's procedures, *Ann Surg* 245(1):94–103, 2007.

Czymek R, Kempf A, Roblick UJ, et al: Surgical treatment concepts for acute lower gastrointestinal bleeding, *J Gastrointest Surg* 12:2212–2220, 2008.

Hoedema RE, Luchtefeld MA: The management of lower gastrointestinal hemorrhage, *Dis Colon Rectum* 48:2010–2024, 2005.

Karoui M, Champault A, Pautrat K, et al: Laparoscopic peritoneal lavage or primary anastomosis with defunctioning stoma for Hinchey 3 complicated diverticulitis: results of a comparative study, *Dis Colon Rectum* 52(4):609–615, 2009.

Klarenbeek BR, Bergamaschi R, Veenhof AA, et al: Laparoscopic versus open sigmoid resection for diverticular disease: follow-up assessment of the randomized control Sigma trial, *Surg Endosc* 25(4):1121–1126, 2011; Epub 2010.

Lee J, Costantini TW, Coimbra R: Acute lower GI bleeding for the acute care surgeon: current diagnosis and management, *Scand J Surg* 98:135–142, 2009.

Marti M, Artigas JM, Garzon G, et al: Acute lower intestinal bleeding: feasibility and diagnostic performance of CT angiography, *Radiology* 262:109–116, 2012.

Myers E, Hurley M, O'Sullivan GC, et al: Laparoscopic peritoneal lavage for generalized peritonitis due to perforated diverticulitis, *Br J Surg* 95:97–101, 2008.

Salem L, Veenstra DL, Sullivan SD, et al: The timing of elective colectomy in diverticulitis: a decision analysis, *J Am Coll Surg* 199:904–912, 2004.

Stocchi L: Current indications and role of surgery in the management of sigmoid diverticulitis, *World J Gastroenterol* 16(7):804–817, 2010.

Weldon DT, Burke SJ, Sun S, et al: Interventional management of lower gastrointestinal bleeding, *Eur Radiol* 18(5):857–867, 2008; Epub 2008.

White SI, Frenkiel B, Martin PJ: A ten-year audit of perforated sigmoid diverticulitis: highlighting the outcomes of laparoscopic lavage, *Dis Colon Rectum* 53(11):1537–1541, 2010.

THE MANAGEMENT OF CHRONIC ULCERATIVE COLITIS

Sandy H. Fang, MD, and Jonathan E. Efron, MD

INTRODUCTION

Ulcerative colitis (UC) is a chronic mucosal inflammatory bowel disorder (IBD) characterized by remissions and exacerbations. The disease starts with involvement of the rectum (proctitis) and may extend to include the sigmoid colon (proctosigmoiditis) or further contiguous involvement of the colon (proctocolitis). The small intestine is not involved; however, diarrheal stool from severe inflammation in the cecum may cause inflammation in the terminal ileum called backwash ileitis and this may be confused with Crohn's ileitis.

IBD is a multifactorial disorder caused by both genetic and environmental components. A family history of IBD is the most prominent risk factor. UC probands tend to have more relatives diagnosed with UC, and the same holds true for Crohn's disease. Seventy-five percent of patients with UC have perinuclear antineutrophil cytoplasmic antibodies (p-ANCA). Environmental stimuli include increased sugar consumption, low-fiber diet, food allergies, food additives, infectious agents, and shortened breastfeeding time. Cigarette smoking is a protective influence in UC, whereas it is a risk factor for development of Crohn's disease.

Patients usually present with diarrhea and bleeding per rectum. Pain is an uncommon clinical feature except in severe active disease, when inflammation extends to the serosa. After long-term medical therapy, patients may actually present with constipation as opposed to diarrhea.

Diagnosis is made via endoscopy with multiple biopsies. Because inflammation starts in the rectum, proctoscopy or flexible sigmoidoscopy usually provides evidence for the initial diagnosis of UC; however, complete colonoscopy with evaluation of the terminal ileum is necessary to define the extent of disease and to rule out other pathology, such as benign or malignant neoplasia. Colonoscopy is contraindicated in the face of severe inflammation of the colon that may occur during an acute exacerbation, and in these cases, endoscopic evaluation is limited to the rectum and sigmoid colon. Other conditions that cause diarrhea and rectal bleeding must be ruled out, such as infectious etiology (*Clostridium difficile, Campylobacter jejuni, Salmonella enterocolitis, Escherichia coli* 0157:H7, amebiasis), collagenous colitis, and Crohn's colitis. Stool cultures for pathogenic bacteria, ova, and parasites should be sent for analysis.

INDICATIONS FOR SURGICAL THERAPY

Medically Refractory Disease

Medical therapy for UC refers to administration of a variety of immunosuppressive medications, which includes the 5-aminosalicylic acid (5-ASA) compounds, steroids, antipurine or pyrimidine compounds, and antitumor necrosis factor antibodies. However, UC is chronic, often lasting for decades, and patients may see progression to steroid dependence or a disease state that is medically refractory.

Intractability to medical treatment is the most common indication for surgical therapy in patients with UC.

Fulminant Colitis and Toxic Megacolon

Severe colitis affects 5% to 15% of patients with UC and is characterized by bloody diarrhea, weight loss, volume depletion, fever, and severe anemia. Fulminant colitis refers to patients with severe colitis with progressive symptoms of toxicity. Attempts at conservative management with bowel rest, parenteral nutrition, parenteral steroids, and broad spectrum antibiotics are necessary. Progression to toxic colitis is indicated by fevers, leukocytosis, and distention, despite maximal medical therapy. Toxic colitis refers to the triad of fever, tachycardia, and leukocytosis in patients with UC. Toxic megacolon refers to patients who have distention of the transverse colon greater than 8 cm in diameter as seen on abdominal x-ray. Toxic colitis or toxic megacolon should be viewed as a surgical emergency because they indicate impending colonic perforation. Urgent or emergent resection is needed. If a patient's condition with fulminant colitis does not improve or deteriorates within 48 to 96 hours of the initiation of therapy, surgery should be considered. Twenty percent to 30% of patients with fulminant colitis need surgical intervention. If perforation ensues, the mortality rate after surgical intervention may be as high as 57%; therefore, surgery is warranted.

Bleeding

The incidence of massive hemorrhage in UC is low, ranging from 0 to 4.5%. However, it accounts for 10% of all urgent colectomies performed for UC. Although colectomy for bleeding is rare, requirement of blood transfusions is common.

Cancer

Risk factors for malignant disease in patients with UC include extensive involvement of the colon and duration of disease. The risk of development of a malignancy in UC is increased as compared with the general population after the patient's disease duration exceeds 10 years. At 10 years, the risk is 2% above the general population; at 20 years, it is 10%; and after 30 and 40 years, the risk increases to 50% and 75%, respectively. Endoscopic surveillance for dysplasia or cancer must begin 8 to 10 years after onset of symptoms or sooner, depending on age of the patient, and be performed on an annual or biannual basis. If a patient also has primary sclerosing cholangitis (PSC) or has a positive family history of colorectal cancer, surveillance should be performed annually. Ideally, the patient should undergo surveillance colonoscopy while in disease remission to minimize the risk of missing a carcinoma because of inflammation. Because cancer may arise from flat mucosa, random serial four-quadrant biopsies should be obtained every 10 cm for a total of 33 biopsies or more as an adequate sampling for dysplasia or cancer.

If biopsy results are positive for high-grade dysplasia or cancer, a patient should undergo proctocolectomy. The risk of an undetected cancer that is found after colectomy for high-grade dysplasia is 42%. In the setting of low-grade dysplasia, patients are encouraged to undergo elective prophylactic proctocolectomy. Unrecognized synchronous colorectal carcinoma is present in up to 20% of individuals who undergo surgery with the initial diagnosis of low-grade dysplasia. If the patient declines surgery, then close surveillance, every 3 to 6 months, is necessary. Polyps should be biopsied as per routine; however, the surrounding mucosa in four quadrants should also be sampled for dysplasia/carcinoma (non–adenoma-like dysplasia-associated lesion or mass [DALM]). Resection of adenomatous tissue or a polyp is not an absolute indication for proctocolectomy but in conjunction with a DALM lesion is of greater concern. Typically, patients with dysplastic changes have had their colitis for many years and are no longer having inflammatory symptoms. They are having normal bowel movements and therefore are often satisfied with their ileal pouch function. For this reason, patients are often reluctant to undergo surgery.

Stricture formation occurs in 5% to 12% of patients, with 25% of the strictures being malignant. Malignant strictures appear late in the course of disease (61% after 20 years of disease), are usually located proximal to the splenic flexure (86%), and cause large bowel obstructions (100% vs 14% in benign strictures). Thus, proctocolectomy is recommended for stricturing disease in UC.

Extracolonic Manifestations

Hepatobiliary-associated disorders are the most likely to influence surgical management of the colon and rectum in UC. These patients may need orthotopic liver transplantation for primary sclerosing cholangitis. If colectomy is necessitated, formation of a permanent ileostomy is avoided, because of the complications associated with periileostomy varices from portal hypertension. Proctocolectomy for UC is beneficial for erythema nodosum (most responsive), arthritis, and eye diseases (episcleritis, uveitis, iritis, conjunctivitis) but does not affect outcomes for primary sclerosing cholangitis, ankylosing spondylitis, and sacroiliitis.

Growth Failure in Children

Surgery should be considered if children have growth retardation despite maximization of nutritional and medical therapy.

SURGICAL OPTIONS

Many surgical options exist for UC. Each surgical plan is tailored toward the individual patient according to their preoperative comorbidities, functional status, continence, and urgency of the operation. An algorithm to deciding the surgical approach to UC is shown in Figure 1. Patients should have extensive counseling regarding the potential for an ostomy. Several circumstances involve planning for future operations. Patients may need multiple staged procedures because of their disease status or whether they require an emergent operation.

Today, selected patients may be offered a minimally invasive approach. Advocates of the laparoscopic approach cite improved patient comfort, better cosmesis, decreased length of hospital stay, and faster recovery as advantages over the open approach. Studies in minimally invasive ileal pouch–anal anastomosis (IPAA) creation have shown a decrease in adhesion formation and incisional hernias. The many different approaches to minimally invasive proctocolectomy include strict laparoscopy and laparoscopic-assisted, hand-assisted, and single-incision surgery. Specimen extraction or the ileal pouch may be formed through a lower midline incision, Pfannenstiel incision, right lower quadrant incision (the previously marked ileostomy site), or a periumbilical incision. All of the incisions have their benefits. The hand-port incision may also be used for an open approach for the pelvic dissection and pouch creation. Regardless of approach, all patients undergo a standard mechanical bowel preparation, if their condition is stable, and receive perioperative parenteral antibiotics.

INDICATIONS FOR A SUBTOTAL COLECTOMY

A subtotal colectomy with end ileostomy and Hartmann's procedure is the least morbid operation. It is the operation of choice in an emergent situation. It is indicated in moribund patients with fulminant colitis, toxic megacolon, and perforation and in those patients with numerous comorbidities. It is also used for those undergoing a three-stage pouch procedure because they are on high-dose steroids or multiple immunosuppression drugs, are malnourished, or have indeterminate colitis. Patients with indeterminate colitis who the surgeon suspects may have Crohn's disease should undergo the three-stage procedure to allow for complete pathologic evaluation of the colon. For a planned first-stage procedure, it may be an option for those patients wanting to preserve fertility. In men, the risk of damaging the pelvic nerves is reduced by not entering the pelvis with active rectal inflammation. Avoiding the proctectomy in women may prevent pelvic adhesions that may affect fertility.

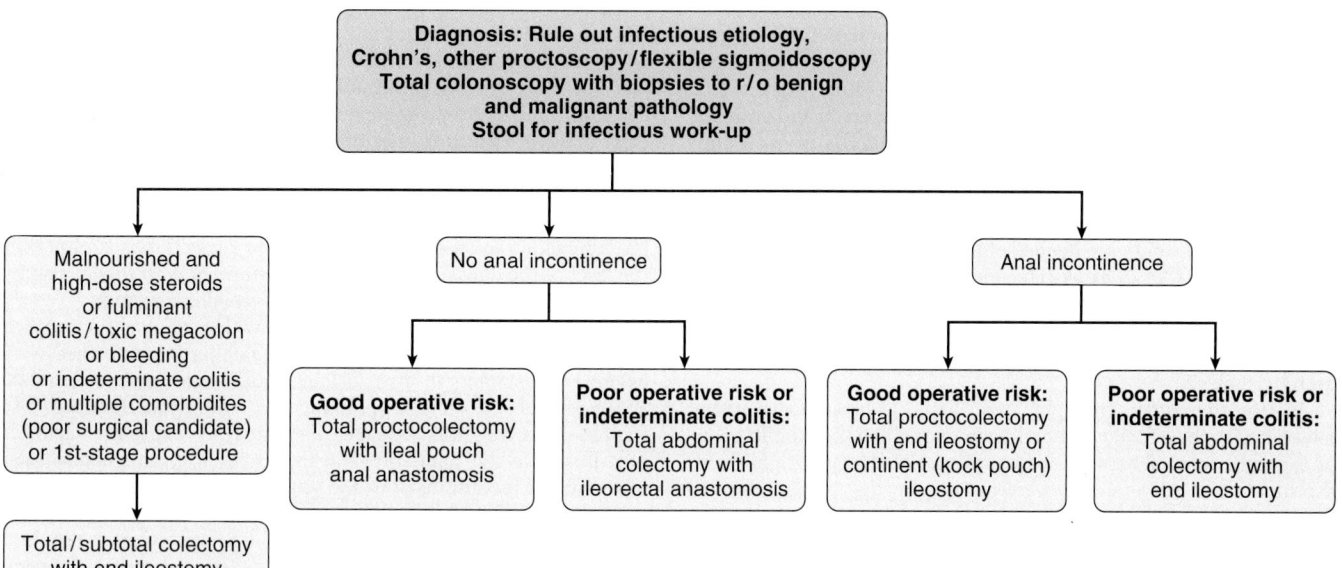

FIGURE 1 Surgical management of chronic ulcerative colitis.

In an emergent situation or when the colon wall is extremely fragile with a high risk of perforation, an open operation should be performed. The lower sigmoid colon is transected with a stapler just above the sacral promontory, leaving a rectal stump. A rectal tube or Foley catheter is left in the rectum to decompress the rectal stump and to prevent perforation of the stump. The Hartmann's pouch may be placed extrafascial, which lowers the risk of pelvic sepsis and subsequently facilitates future pelvic dissection. This is often done by bringing the divided colonic stump up through the most inferior aspect of the midline facial incision and securing the colon in place.

The specimen is submitted for pathologic diagnosis. If the pathology shows UC, a completion proctectomy and IPAA can be planned for a future definitive operation; however, if the pathology shows Crohn's disease and the rectum is without disease, an ileorectal anastomosis may be an option.

A disadvantage of this procedure is that a diseased rectum is left behind. The fate of the retained rectum is not well known. A 10% risk of rectal cancer is believed to exist, so patients need lifelong surveillance of the stump. Other issues include seepage and bleeding. Massive bleeding is rare, but when it occurs, it may require completion proctectomy. Most of these patients proceed on to completion proctectomy with IPAA.

SURGICAL PROCEDURES

Total Colectomy

Laparoscopic

The patient is placed in the modified lithotomy position. Both arms are tucked at the patient's side, and the patient is secured to the operating room table. For the minimally invasive approach, access is secured through an umbilical port with a Hasson technique. All ports are placed under direct visualization, and the right-sided ports include a 12-mm trocar placed 4 fingerbreadths superomedial to the anterior superior iliac spine with a 5-mm port located 4 fingerbreadths cranial in the right upper quadrant and two left-sided 5-mm ports placed to mirror the right-sided ports. As an alternative, a suprapubic port may be placed instead of the more cranial ports.

The omentum is swept above the transverse colon and liver. The small bowel is tucked to the right side of the abdomen. The patient is positioned in steep Trendelenburg position with the right side down. To mobilize the left colon, the surgeon first incises the peritoenum overlying medial aspect of the sigmoid mesentery starting at the sacral promontory and going up toward the inferior mesenteric artery. The mesentery of the sigmoid and descending colon is dissected off the retroperitoneum, identifying the left ureter and gonadal vessels. The base of the inferior mesenteric artery is isolated and divided either with a vessel-sealing device, clips, or an endovascular stapler. The mesentery to the colon is dissected free from Gerota's fascia up to the splenic flexure. The lateral peritoneal attachments, the white line of Toldt, are divided entering the previously dissected plane up to the splenic flexure. The splenic flexure is mobilized entering the lesser sac, and the omentum is freed from the transverse colon with the use of a vessel-sealing device. Shifting the patient into the reverse Trendelenburg's position helps facilitate transverse colon mobilization.

Placing the patient in slight Trendelenburg's position with the table tilted to the left allows the surgeon to perform the mobilization of the right colon. The ileocolic artery is isolated at its origin from the superior mesenteric artery, freeing it from the duodenum and retroperitoneum. The right colon mesentery is mobilized off of the retroperitoneum, identifying the right ureter. The lateral peritoneal attachments are divided entering the previously dissected plane, and the mesentery based on the superior mesenteric artery is completely freed up to the duodenum. The hepatic flexure is mobilized by dividing the colohepatic ligament and omentum with a vessel-sealing device. To prevent bacterial translocation, the colon mesentery is transected last to minimize time that necrotic colon is intracorporeal. The entire colonic mesentery is divided last using a vessel-sealing device or isolating individual vessels such as the right, middle, and left colic vessels with clips or laparoscopic staplers. If an ileal J pouch is performed, the small intestine mesentery must be completely mobilized off of the duodenum to provide maximum reach to the pelvis.

Open

The left colon is mobilized off the white line of Toldt, with care taken to identify and lateralize the left ureter and gonadal vessels. The splenic flexure is mobilized, entering the lesser sac and either dividing the omentum below the gastroepiploic artery, thereby resecting the omentum, or mobilizing the omentum off of the transverse colon in the avascular plane that exists between the two structures.

The right colon is mobilized along the white line of Toldt, identifying the right ureter and gonadal vessels. The hepatic flexure is mobilized by dividing the colohepatic ligament. Complete mobilization of the superior mesenteric artery to its base is necessary, completely exposing the C loop of the duodenum. This is to facilitate reach of an ileal J pouch to the anus. The mesentery to the entire colon is divided down to the sacral promontory. The terminal ileum is divided with a stapler.

Proctectomy

Laparoscopic Approach

The surgeon and the assistant operate on the left and right side of the patient, and a monitor is placed between the patient's legs. The patient is placed in steep Trendelenburg position and in a neutral position with respect to the tilt. In a female patient with a uterus, positioning the uterus to the anterior abdominal wall is often helpful. A suture on a Keith needle is passed into the abdomen, through the abdominal wall just above the pubis. It is passed through the body of the uterus and then back up through the abdominal wall and sutured in place with a bolster. This elevates the uterus and adnexa out of the pelvis and helps facilitate the anterior dissection of the rectum. The rectum is initially retracted superiorly, and the peritoneum is incised over the sacral promontory, with care taken to identify the pelvic nerves and mobilize them off of the mesorectum. The presacral space is entered, and dissection is continued inferiorly in this avascular plane. Rectal mobilization is facilitated by providing adequate traction and counter traction to help identify the correct plane of dissection. Posterior mobilization of the rectum is continued down through Waldeyer's fascia to the levator sling. The lateral avascular plane is identified inferiorly in the previously dissected presacral space. Mobilization is often completed with electrocautery or a vessel-sealing device. Retracting the rectum inferiorly and applying counter pressure with graspers on the vagina or seminal vesicles and prostate allows for the anterior dissection. Dissection is complete at the level of the anorectal ring. This is confirmed with digital examination with cross clamping of the distal mobilized rectum.

At this point, the rectum is divided with a stapler if a J-pouch anastomosis is to be performed. This can either be performed with laparoscopic staplers or a small Pfannenstiel incision may be made above the pubis to facilitate placement of a thoracoabdominal (TA) stapler. Great care must be taken in women to ensure the vagina is kept free from the staple line and that there is approximately 1 cm of mobilized rectum distal to the staple line to allow a safe double-stapled IPAA. The colon and rectum are then removed through either a periumbilical or suprapubic incision. If a mucosectomy is required or the patient is undergoing an intersphincteric dissection, the perineal dissection is initiated after completing the rectal mobilization. In this case, the specimen is often removed via the anus.

Open Proctectomy

The sacral promontory is identified and entered, with care taken to mobilize the hypogastric nerves from the mesorectal fascia. The St. Mark's retractor is then placed in the pelvis, and dissection is continued posteriorly in the avascular plane of the presacral space. Mobilization posteriorly should continue past Waldeyer's fascia to the levator ani muscles. Lateral rectal dissection is facilitated with lateral retraction of the pelvic sidewall with the St. Mark's retractor while the surgeon places medial traction on the rectum and mesorectal fascia. The anterior dissection is completed last, again with the St. Mark's retractor to retract the anterior structures anteriorly while the surgeon applies counter pressure on the rectum. The dissection is complete with the rectum fully mobilized to the levator ani muscles. The level of division is confirmed with digital palpation through the anus while clamping the distal rectum. The rectum should be divided at a level to allow room for stapling of the pouch to the anus, typically 1 to 2 cm above the dentate line. Great care is taken not to incorporate anterior or lateral structures into the staple line. Anterior retraction with the St. Marks retractor helps facilitate rectal division. In women, digital examination of the vagina before firing a TA stapler should be performed to ensure the vagina is not incorporated in to the TA staple line. If a mucosectomy is required or the patient is undergoing an intersphincteric dissection, the perineal dissection is initiated after completing the rectal mobilization.

Perineal Approaches to Remove the Distal Rectum

These dissections are enhanced by the use of a self-retaining retractor to efface the anus. For patients who are undergoing resection with permanent ileostomy, an intersphincteric dissection of the distal rectum and anus is favored. This allows the perineum to be closed with a complete muscular tube and significantly reduces the risk of perineal wound complications. An exception is when the operation is performed in a patient with a low rectal cancer where an abdominoperineal resection is required.

Intersphincteric Proctectomy

A lone star retractor or other self-retaining retractor is sutured to the perineum, and the anus is effaced. A skin incision is created in the intersphincteric groove. The intersphincteric dissection is carried out in the avascular plane, preserving the external sphincter and the levator ani muscles. This avascular plane allows for easy dissection and is initiated in the posterior aspect of the anus extending laterally, reserving the anterior dissection to last. One continues in this plane proximally until the abdominal pelvic dissection is reached and the peritoneal cavity is entered. The entire specimen is removed through the perineum. An omental pedicle flap can be rotated into the pelvis to fill the dead space if it has not been resected with the specimen. Closed suction drains are positioned in the pelvis, and the perineal wound is closed in layers, with all muscular layers closed with absorbable suture. After both abdominal and perineal incisions are closed, a Brooke ileostomy is matured in the right lower quadrant at a previously marked ideal site.

Complications

Postoperative complications include intestinal obstruction, delayed healing of the perineal wound, sexual dysfunction (including postoperative infertility), and issues related to the ileostomy. Patients who present with a chronically draining perineal wound should be investigated for retained mucosa, foreign bodies, and Crohn's disease. Sexual dysfunction after a low pelvic dissection in men consists of impotence, retrograde ejaculation, or both; in women, 30% have dyspareunia. Complications related to the ileostomy include dehydration, skin irritation, stomal stenosis, prolapse, and hernias.

Proctocolectomy with Ileal Pouch–Anal Anastomosis

Proctocolectomy with IPAA (TPC with IPAA) is the procedure of choice for many patients with UC. It eliminates all active disease and eventually leaves the patient stoma free. Patients on average stool six times a day with liquid or pasty stools. This stool consistency requires patients to have normal sphincter tone for continence. Patients who have poor anal continence are not candidates for IPAA and require an end ileostomy.

An ileal pouch performed in patients with middle or distal rectal cancers is controversial. Adjuvant radiation therapy should be performed before pouch creation because postoperative radiotherapy is associated with radiation enteritis and poor pouch function and consequent failure. Finally, in patients with UC with a cecal cancer, a long segment of distal ileum with its associated mesenteric vessel may need to be resected, precluding the formation of a tension-free IPAA.

Typically, the ultimate goal of the TPC with IPAA is accomplished through staged procedures. In a select group of patients, a single-stage procedure may be performed by an experienced surgeon. Most often, patients undergo a two-stage procedure: (1) TPC with IPAA and diverting loop ileostomy; and (2) reversal of the ileostomy. Those who go through a three-stage procedure ([1] subtotal colectomy and end ileostomy; [2] restorative proctectomy with ileoanal pouch anastomosis and diverting loop ileostomy; and [3] reversal of ileostomy) usually are malnourished patients receiving high-dose steroids and are too sick to undergo a total proctocolectomy. Those with fulminant colitis or toxic megacolon have been shown to have a high risk of intraabdominal sepsis; thus, simultaneous IPAA should not be performed at the initial operation because of the high risk of pouch failure.

The patient's positioning and mobilization of the colon and rectum are as described previously. The terminal ileum is transected flush to the cecum, making sure to preserve the ileal branch of the ileocolic vessels. The rectum is transected just above the levator ani muscle. The root of the small bowel mesentery is mobilized to the level of the ligament of Treitz.

J-Pouch Creation

In the laparoscopic technique, the terminal ileum may be exteriorized through the planned diverting loop ileostomy site, a small Pfannenstiel's incision, or a midline incision. Otherwise, the J-pouch is formed through the hand-port or open incision. The J pouch should be 15 to 18 cm in length; the exact length is determined by identifying which point of the antimesenteric edge of ileum provides the maximal reach to the pelvis. Adequate reach for the pouch is confirmed when the distal aspect of the pouch reaches below the pubic symphysis. Sutures are placed to approximate the antimesenteric border of the planned J pouch. A 2-cm curvilinear incision is created at the base of the J. Multiple firings of a linear stapler are used to create the J pouch, usually two or three firings of a stapler 100 cm in length. The tip of the J staple line is oversewn to prevent a leak. The mucosal border of the staple line is inspected to ensure hemostasis and is oversewn if needed (Figure 2).

Ileal Pouch–Anal Anastomosis

A double-stapled pouch–anal anastomosis is thought to provide better postoperative pouch function by maintaining the anal transition zone. It is the preferred method of the authors except in patients with rectal dysplasia or in patients with rectal carcinoma. In those cases, mucosectomy with hand-sewn anastomosis is performed.

Double-Stapled Anastomosis

The curvilinear incision in which the stapler was inserted to create the J pouch is used for the anastomosis. The anvil is inserted into the base of the J pouch and secured with a purse-string suture.

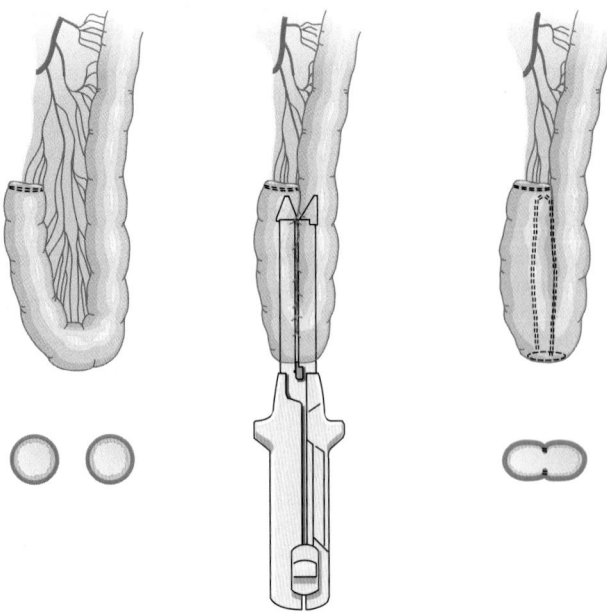

FIGURE 2   Creation of an ileal J pouch with a cutting linear stapler. For replacement of the rectum, a reservoir is created from the distal ileum. The stapler joins two limbs of intestine with staples while dividing the intervening wall. The diameter of the pouch so created is twice as large as the original diameter of the ileum. *(From Townsend CM, Beauchamp RD, Evers BM, Mattox KL, editors: Sabiston textbook of surgery, ed 18, Philadelphia, 2008, Elsevier Saunders, pp 1381, Fig 50-33.)*

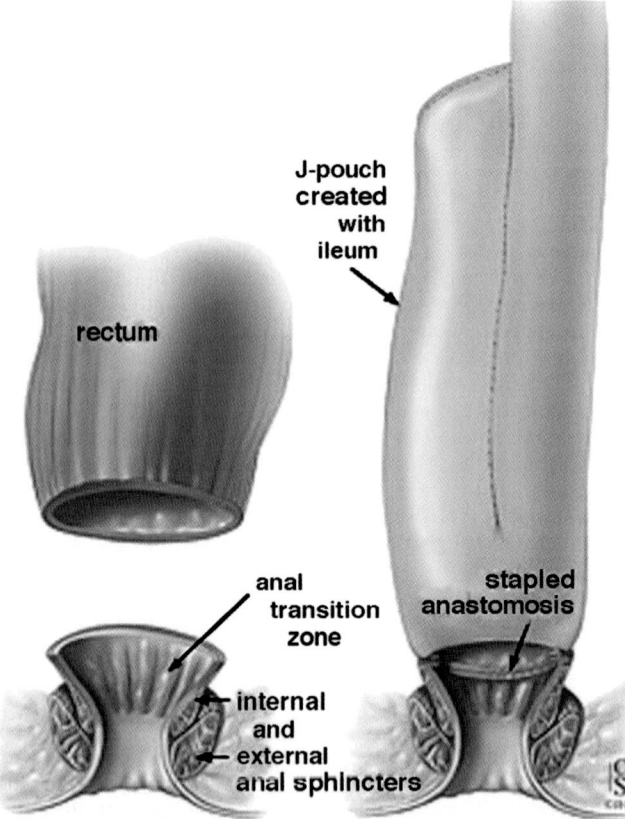

FIGURE 3   Creation of the J pouch. *(From Johns Hopkins Sidney Kimmel Comprehensive Cancer Center website:* http://www.hopkinskimmelcancercenter.org/images/coloncancer/J-pouch2.jpg. *Accessed July 13, 2012.)*

The stapler is inserted transanally, and the pin protruded posterior to the rectal staple line (Figures 3 and 4) Great care must be taken to ensure the pouch is not twisted on its mesenteric pedicle and that anterior structures, most commonly the vagina, are not incorporated into the anterior or lateral staple line. These are key points whether a laparoscopic or open procedure. A loop ileostomy is then formed 40 cm from the ileal pouch at a previously marked location in the right lower quadrant.

Mucosectomy and Hand-Sewn Anastomosis

The mucosa from the anal canal and the distal rectum are removed transanally with the specimen. After the surgeon has completed the abdominal and pelvic dissection, attention is turned towards the anus. A self-retaining retractor is secured to the perineum, and the anus is effaced. Normal saline solution or lidocaine with 1% epinephrine is injected in the submucosal space to help to identify the correct plane of dissection. The mucosa is elevated with electrocautery, generating a circular tube of tissue, and initiating the dissection at the dentate line. The peritoneal cavity is entered posteriorly, dividing the muscularis above the level of the puborectalis sling. The rectum is completely divided, and the specimen is removed. The ileal pouch is brought down to the anus with an empty sponge stick or Babcock clamp. The long instrument is passed through the anus to grasp the pouch, creating a hand-sewn anastomosis. Great care is made to keep the correct orientation of the pouch to avoid twisting the pouch on its vascular pedicle. The pouch is sutured to the anus, anastomosing to the denuded anorectal cuff with interrupted absorbable sutures placed circumferentially. A closed suction drain is placed in the presacral space behind the pouch, and the pouch itself is drained. A loop ileostomy is formed 40 cm from the ileal pouch at a previously marked site in the right lower quadrant.

The risk of the inflammation and dysplasia of the anal transitional zone left behind in a double-stapled technique is low, but present. Similarly, in a mucosectomy procedure, there is a risk of inadvertently leaving small islands of mucosa. For these reasons, long-term annual examinations and biopsies are recommended for all patients with IPAA regardless of the anastomotic technique. These examinations include pouchoscopy and are biannually performed. Biopsies of any retained rectal cuff or suspicious areas in the ileal pouch are required.

Maneuvers to Ensure Reach of the J Pouch

The J pouch should reach comfortably, without tension, to the anorectum. Maneuvers to achieve lengthening of the ileal mesentery include complete mobilization of the superior mesenteric artery off the retroperitoneum and up to the pancreas (including partially Kocher's maneuver of the duodenum). The ileocolic artery may be divided to increase length, with care taken to maintain collateral flow. Backlighting to outline mesenteric vessels is helpful in identifying mesenteric vessels while working on the mesentery. Scoring the mesentery overlying the superior mesenteric artery helps increase the mesenteric length, as does opening mesenteric windows between collateral vessels near the border of the small intestine. These maneuvers are performed before creating the pouch. After formation of the J pouch, the surgeon should wait 15 minutes to reassess viability of the J pouch.

If the J pouch still does not reach, the procedure is aborted by dropping the J pouch into the pelvis and attempting to suture it to a point on the sacrum or coccyx and create a loop ileostomy. Often the pouch mesentery stretches over time, and in 6 months, the patient can be reoperated on and the pouch anal anastomosis completed.

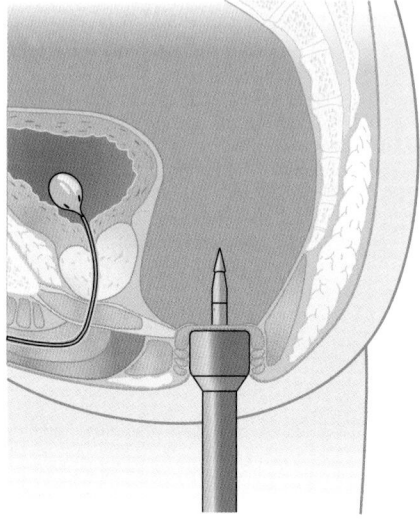
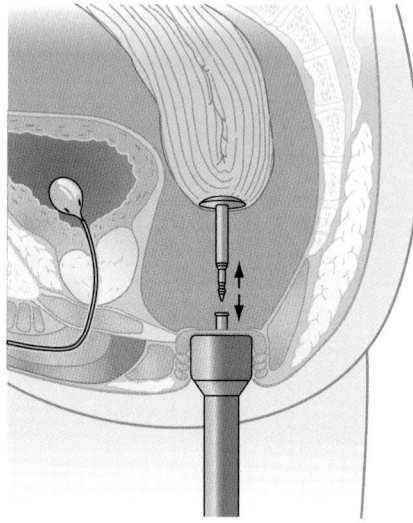

FIGURE 4 Fashioning of stapled ileal pouch–anal anastomosis. *(From Townsend CM, Beauchamp RD, Evers BM, et al, editors: Sabiston textbook of surgery, ed 18, Philadelphia, 2008, Elsevier Saunders, pp 1382, Fig 50-34.)*

Other Types of Pouches

An S pouch has two 10-cm to 12-cm limbs and uses its efferent limb (end of the terminal ileum) as the anastomosis to the anus. Evacuation difficulties are high, so functional results are not as beneficial as with a J pouch. The S pouch does provide extra length and therefore is reserved for cases where the J pouch cannot reach. A lateral isoperistaltic H pouch has a long outlet tract with similar sequelae of pouch distention, stasis, and pouchitis issues as the S Pouch. A four-loop reservoir (W pouch) was developed to increase capacity; however, studies have shown there is no difference in reservoir function in terms of incontinence, urgency, and soiling as compared with the J pouch.

Postoperative Course

Before closure of the ileostomy, the pouch should be studied to ensure healing of the pouch and pouch–anal anastomosis. Nonhealing is often manifested by a fistula or abscess. Digital rectal examination is performed to assess sphincter tone and anastomotic stricture or defects. Endoscopy shows the course of healing of the suture lines. The pouch is studied with Gastrografin (Bracco Diagnostics Inc., Princeton, N.J.) to detect evidence of leak, abscess, fistulas, or sinus tracts. Only after confirmation of no abnormality with the pouch should the ileostomy be closed.

Complications

Small bowel obstruction occurs in 20% of patients who undergo ileal pouch operations. Patients also encounter similar issues with sexual dysfunction (including postoperative infertility) and ileostomy complications after a total proctocolectomy. The literature indicates that 5% of patients have pelvic sepsis develop after an IPAA as a result of anastomotic dehiscence (with early or late manifestations as an abscess or fistula) or an infected pelvic hematoma. This rate may be higher, and patients who have pelvic sepsis have a higher likelihood of subsequent pouch failure. Hence, pelvic sepsis should be treated aggressively with intravenous antibiotics and drainage of the abscess. Some studies have shown that pouch failure rates for patients with development of a leak after a hand-sewn anastomosis to be higher than those who had a stapled anastomosis. The incidence rate of pouch-vaginal fistula ranges from 3% to 16%. It requires surgical correction either through an abdominal or perineal approach. Ileo-anal anastomotic stricture occurrence rates vary from 5% to 38%. Management includes finger dilation or repeated dilations with

anesthesia and, rarely, a transanal approach with excision of the stricture and pouch advancement.

The most frequent long-term complication is pouchitis or nonspecific inflammation of the ileal pouch. Medical management with oral metronidazole or ciprofloxacin and probiotics is usually successful, but those with severe medically refractory pouchitis may need diversion or pouch excision.

Colectomy With Ileorectal Anastomosis

The colectomy with ileorectal anastomosis (IRA) is rarely performed for UC. A select group for patients—those who have indeterminate colitis and those who are young with good anal continence and good rectal compliance, with only mild inflammation of the rectum—are considered. It may be considered in young females who want to preserve fertility and avoid a stoma, but it is rare to have a patient with UC who requires surgery but has minimal rectal inflammation. Moreover, the lack of a pelvic dissection reduces the risk of sexual dysfunction. However, patients tend to have more bowel movements per day. In addition, disease and the potential for malignancy are left behind. The risk of malignant disease of the rectum after IRA is approximately 10%. Twenty-five percent of patients after IRA require a proctectomy as a result of severe proctitis. IRA is contraindicated in patients who have moderate to severe inflammation of the rectum, dysplasia, or cancer of the rectum, perianal disease, and known anal incontinence.

Total Proctocolectomy With Continent Ileostomy (Kock's Pouch)

The continent ileostomy was introduced by Kock for patients who did not want to wear an ostomy appliance for a Brooke end ileostomy. A nipple valve is created with intussusception of a portion of ileum into the planned reservoir. The procedure has essentially been abandoned in the management of UC because of the excellent long-term outcomes with the ileal J pouch and the large complication rate associated with the Kock's pouch. These complications include obstruction and incontinence, usually as a result of nipple valve slippage or dysfunction in 50% of patients. Patients develop difficulty with catheterization of their pouch. Surgical reconstruction is the only option for repair. Twenty-five percent of patients also suffer from pouchitis, 25% from intestinal obstruction, and 10% from pouch fistulas. Most patients with Kock's pouches eventually require resection and formation of an end ileostomy.

CONCLUSION

Many options exist in the surgical management of chronic UC. An approach is tailored according to the individual patient's preferences and their comorbidities and severity of disease.

SUGGESTED READINGS

Biondi A, Zoccali M, Costa S, et al: Surgical treatment of ulcerative colitis in the biologic therapy era, *World J Gastroenterol* 18:1861–1870, 2012.

Cohen JL, Strong SA, Hyman NH, et al: Practice parameters for the surgical treatment of ulcerative colitis, *Dis Colon Rectum* 48:1997–2009, 2005.

Holubar SD, Larson DW, Dozois EJ, et al: Minimally invasive subtotal colectomy and ileal pouch-anal anastomosis for fulminant ulcerative colitis: a reasonable approach? *Dis Colon Rectum* 52:187–192, 2009.

Wick EC, Efron J: Minimally invasive rectal procedures for ulcerative colitis, rectal prolapse, and rectal cancer, *US Gastroenterol Hepatol Rev* 6:85–89, 2010.

THE MANAGEMENT OF TOXIC MEGACOLON

Bashar Safar, MBBS, and
James W. Fleshman, MD, FACS, FASCRS

OVERVIEW

Toxic megacolon (TM) is a serious, life-threatening condition that can result as a complication of ulcerative colitis, Crohn's colitis, and infectious colitides such as pseudomembranous colitis. TM was first described in 1950 by Marschak and colleagues as a complication of colitis, and it is defined as segmental or total colonic distension of 6 cm in the presence of acute colitis and signs of systemic toxicity.

Rapid dilation of the proximal colon produces the radiographic picture. The thickened, severely inflamed distal colon is, however, the segment of colon in which perforation is imminent; moreover, pneumatosis can be seen radiographically. The dilated proximal colon will perforate only if the inflammatory process has weakened the wall of the cecum. Most commonly the point of perforation is the splenic flexure, where a walled-off perforation is found in a phlegmon involving the colon, spleen, and omentum.

Systemic manifestations of toxicity distinguish patients with megacolon from those with colonic dilation due to other causes, such as colonic pseudoobstruction or Hirschsprung disease. Aggressive conservative management is increasingly advocated and may spare some patients an operation. However, prompt recognition of disease severity and surgical intervention may be lifesaving.

INCIDENCE AND ETIOLOGY

TM can result from any disease that causes inflammation of the colon. Although it is most readily recognized as a complication of inflammatory bowel disease (IBD), other causes include pseudomembranous colitis, bacteria (*Salmonella, Shigella, Campylobacter, Entamoeba*), and ischemic colitis (Box 1).

The incidence of the syndrome varies on the basis of the etiology and the study population. The incidence of TM in IBD has been the most extensively reported and has been estimated to range between 1% and 5% of patients with IBD. However, the incidence is believed to be decreasing because of improved medical management of

patients with severe colitis. Conversely, pseudomembranous colitis, which occurs in up to 1% of hospitalized patients, is responsible for an increasing number of patients with TM.

Since 2000 *Clostridium difficile* infections were observed to be more frequent, more severe, more refractory to standard therapy, and more likely to relapse than previously described. These observations have occurred throughout North America and Europe and have been attributed to a new strain (BI/NAP1/027) of *C. difficile*. In a 2008 report of *C. difficile* toxic colitis, only 10% of cases required admission to intensive care, and 2.5% required an emergency colectomy. Other causes of TM are exceedingly rare.

The mechanisms responsible for the toxic dilation of the colon are not fully understood and probably involve a combination of factors, including severe inflammation and local mediator release. Inflammatory damage to colonic mucosa due to severe colitis seems to extend into the smooth muscle layer in TM, resulting in damage and paralysis. Bacterial translocation occurs and results in bacteremia and the toxic/septic response.

Nitric oxide generated by severely inflamed smooth muscle cells in the colonic wall may play an important role in dysmotility and atony, resulting in dilation of the colon proximal to the severely inflamed segment, which in turn leads to the development of TM. In fact, *toxic megacolon* may be a misnomer, because the dilated segment is not the toxic segment, nor is it the cause of the syndrome. In the majority of patients experiencing toxicity from colitis, there is minimal dilation. Thus the terms *severe toxic colitis* and *fulminant colitis* are more accurate.

A number of factors can lead to the induction or exacerbation of colonic dysmotility and dilation. These include hypokalemia, antimotility agents, opiates, anticholinergics, antidepressants, barium enema, and colonoscopy. These, combined with an inflammatory process, can be deadly.

DIAGNOSIS

Patients with IBD are at highest risk of developing TM early on in the disease course. Up to one third of patients with IBD develop colonic dilation within 3 months of their diagnosis, and another two thirds do so within the first 3 years. The mean duration of disease before development of TM has been reported to be between 3 and 5 years.

Toxic megacolon must be suspected in all patients who come in with abdominal distension, diarrhea, and systemic toxicity. In patients with IBD, dilation of the proximal, less inflamed colon frequently complicates severe distal colitis. In such cases the diagnosis

BOX 1: Causes of toxic megacolon

Inflammatory
Ulcerative colitis
Crohn's disease

Infectious
Bacterial
- *Clostridium difficile* pseudomembranous colitis
- *Salmonella* (typhoid and nontyphoid)
- *Shigella*
- *Campylobacter*
- *Yersinia*

Parasitic
- *Entamoeba histolytica*
- *Cryptosporidium*

Viral
- Cytomegalovirus colitis

Other
Ischemia
Kaposi sarcoma

is often preceded or accompanied by severe bloody diarrhea, fever, chills, and abdominal pain. Patients are thought to develop TM when massive colonic distension and functional obstruction ensues and results in worsening signs of systemic disease, including tachycardia and hypotension. The physical examination finding is often remarkable for significant abdominal tenderness, localized or generalized.

The diagnosis of toxic megacolon should be suspected on the basis of physical and radiographic findings, so a thorough history and physical examination are crucial. History of previous bouts of IBD (extent of colonic involvement, previous therapy, extracolonic manifestations), recent use of certain medications (broad-spectrum antibiotics, steroids, antimotility agents, chemotherapy), foreign travel, human immunodeficiency virus (HIV) status, and recent barium enema study must be carefully elicited.

Jalan and colleagues (1969) described the best accepted clinical criteria for diagnosis as any three of the following: fever of 101.5° F (38.6° C) or higher, heart rate of 120 beats/min or higher, white blood cell count greater than 10.5×10^6/L, or anemia. Patients should also have one of the following: dehydration, mental changes, electrolyte disturbances, or hypotension.

A plain abdominal radiograph can aid in making the diagnosis and is crucial in following the disease course. Dilation of the ascending or transverse colon is typical and can vary from 6 cm, which is suggestive of the diagnosis, to as much as 15 cm. The absolute width of the colon is not as important as the rate of expansion along with the overall clinical condition. Small bowel as well as gastric distension may also be present and may be a significant predictor of TM and multiorgan dysfunction in severe ulcerative colitis. Thickening and edema of the wall of the transverse and left colon, with a thin trail of luminal air or none at all, is the typical finding on the left side.

An initial computed tomographic (CT) scan of the abdomen and pelvis can confirm the diagnosis and exclude pneumatosis or colonic perforation. In addition, CT scan may be useful to determine the etiology of the colonic dilation and exclude other causes of colonic distension, such as obstructing colon cancer or a diverticular stricture. Pronounced thickening of the colonic wall is more suggestive of *C. difficile* and IBD as the causative factors.

Laboratory tests should be obtained to both confirm the diagnosis and identify any correctable abnormality. Anemia and leukocytosis are frequently present. Electrolyte abnormalities are common, as a result of the severe inflammation, and they lead to increased fluid loss from the colon; salt and water losses can lead to severe dehydration and hypokalemia. Hypoalbuminemia may herald a poor prognosis. Stool samples should be sent for culture, sensitivity, and *C. difficile* toxin assay. Blood cultures should be considered, as bacteremia occurs in up to 25% of patients with TM.

Limited endoscopy may be useful, but incorrect treatment can result in significant harm to the patient. Endoscopy is especially useful in patients with no previous diagnosis of IBD. Complete colonoscopy should be avoided because of the high risk of perforation, but biopsies can identify inclusion bodies in the case of cytomegalovirus colitis; pseudomembranes in the rectum and sigmoid colon suggest *C. difficile* colitis.

THERAPY

Management of patients with TM and severe acute fulminant colitis necessitates a multidisciplinary approach with early surgical consultation. Communication between the admitting team and the surgical team is crucial. Clear management goals should be defined at the time of diagnosis, and criteria for continuing medical management versus surgical intervention should be set out at the outset and communicated to the patient and the patient's family. An aggressive attempt at medical management is warranted; however, in the absence of measurable improvement or any deterioration, surgical intervention should be instituted early to avoid the high rate of morbidity and mortality associated with colonic perforation.

Medical Therapy

All patients with TM should be admitted to the intensive care unit. Bowel rest and decompression with nasogastric tube is recommended, along with frequent clinical assessment by the nursing and medical staff. Complete blood cell counts, electrolyte measurements, and serial abdominal plain radiographs are reviewed every 12 hours initially and then daily as the patient improves. Anemia, dehydration, and electrolyte deficits, particularly hypokalemia, may aggravate colonic dysmotility and should be treated aggressively. All antimotility agents, opiates, and anticholinergics should be discontinued. Patients should be given prophylaxis for both gastric stress ulcerations and deep venous thrombosis. Broad-spectrum antibiotics are recommended to reduce septic complications. Significant improvement in the intensive care management of these patients has led to a significant decrease in morbidity and mortality.

Management of Patients With Inflammatory Bowel Disease

Patients known to suffer from IBD who show signs and symptoms of TM should be managed as mentioned above with the addition of high-dose intravenous steroids. A typical dose is hydrocortisone 100 mg every 8 hours or an equivalent dose of other intravenous steroids. High-dose steroids have not been shown to result in higher risk of colonic perforation.

Aminosalicylic acid products have no role in the management of TM. They are used in patients with mild to moderate disease, and their clinical efficacy is not proven in severe disease. Other immunosuppressive medication, such as cyclosporin and anti–tumor necrosis factor-alpha (TNF-α) agents, have been successfully used in the management of severe steroid-refractory colitis; however, their use in patients with TM has not been substantiated beyond anecdotal case reports. Their use is not recommended for the management of TM.

Frequent patient repositioning resulting in redistribution of air in the lumen of the colon has been reported to be successful in decompressing colonic distension in patients with TM. The true value of this technique has not been confirmed by randomized trial;

however, the intervention is fairly simple and should be attempted. Medical therapy is reported to be successful in 50% to 75% of patients with TM.

Management of Patients Without Inflammatory Bowel Disease

Management of patients with other diseases follows the same medical principle of aggressive supportive therapy and bowel rest. In addition, depending on the cause, other interventions may also be appropriate.

Clostridium Difficile Colitis

Withdrawal of the offending antibiotics and initiation of oral vancomycin, 500 mg four times daily, taken with intravenous metronidazole, 500 mg three times daily, are effective in the majority of patients. Patients with severe ileus may have the vancomycin delivered through an enema preparation or by colonoscopic spraying of the mucosa. It has been suggested that earlier surgical intervention may be lifesaving. Patients who survived had lower white blood cell counts and less preoperative multisystem organ failure, were less likely to be taking pressors preoperatively, and were more likely to be operated on sooner than patients who did not survive.

In another study, leukocyte counts greater than $50,000/mm^3$ and lactate at concentrations greater than 5 mmol/L were found to predict mortality. Both of these reports suggest that earlier intervention saves lives. Most patients need an aggressive medical management trial with close observation; however, in the presence of any deterioration, delaying surgical intervention may result in higher rates of morbidity and mortality.

The surgical management of patients with TM secondary to *C. difficile* colitis is similar to that in patients with IBD.

Surgical Therapy

Free perforation, massive hemorrhage, and progression of colonic dilation are absolute indications for surgery. Failure to improve within 48 hours is a relative indication. Some authorities suggest continuing medical therapy for up to 7 days in the absence of any signs of deterioration, but proponents of early surgical intervention highlight the high mortality rate once colonic perforation occurs (40% vs 9%). Goligher and colleagues' (1970) popular dictum to "save the patient, not the colon" was based on a study that reduced the rate of perforation from 32.5% to 11.6%, and mortality rate from 20% to 7%, by means of early surgery. The investigators concluded that surgery should be performed shortly after diagnosis. D'Amico and colleagues (2005) confirmed this finding; they suggested that lower mortality rates (13%) can be achieved by surgical intervention at the time of diagnosis with no trial of medical therapy. However, as mentioned previously, medical management can be effective in 50% to 75% of patients and should be instituted without delay. Patients should be observed closely for signs of deterioration, but the length of medical management should be limited to 7 days, provided that the patient is stable clinically or improving.

Subtotal colectomy and end ileostomy is the treatment of choice, once surgery is deemed necessary. Because of the amount of dilation in the colon, laparoscopy should be avoided in patients with TM.

Upon admission of a patient with TM, the enterostomal therapist should be consulted as soon as possible for marking the site of an end ileostomy; a generous midline incision is used to gain access to the abdominal cavity. Mechanical bowel preparation should be avoided.

Once the abdomen is entered, the bowel should be handled with care; the bowel is fragile, and the likelihood of intraoperative perforation is high. The hepatic flexure and splenic flexure should be mobilized and the colonic mesentery divided close to the bowel wall to avoid damage to retroperitoneal structures, including the ureters and nerves. The colon mesentery can be divided with Kelly clamps and ties; alternatively, a hemostatic coagulation device can be employed. The rectum should be divided as low as possible to avoid a rectal stump blowout, and the staple line should be marked with long, permanent sutures for future identification. A large mushroom catheter is left in the rectum, taped to the inside of the thigh to prevent dislodgment, for continued drainage of the rectal stump.

The patient is transported postoperatively back to the intensive care unit, where fluid resuscitation and further support are provided (e.g., ventilatory support, antibiotics, pressure support as needed). The nasogastric tube may be removed and enteric feeds initiated upon resumption of gastric motility. The rectal tube should remain in place for a minimum of 5 days or until the patient is ready to be discharged; perioperative antibiotics should be discontinued within 24 hours, unless a perforation is encountered. Intravenous steroids should be weaned rapidly to the patient's preoperative dose over the course of a few days.

OUTCOMES

The rate of mortality as a consequence of TM has improved markedly since 1980. Jalan and colleagues reported an overall mortality rate of 45% in 1969, but studies with no deaths were being published by the end of the 1970s.

Teeuwen and colleagues (2009) reviewed the literature for colectomy in 1257 patients with colitis who were operated on in an acute setting (urgent or emergency colectomy). Since the 1970s, there has been a shift in incidence: TM has become less common (71.1% from 1975 through 1984 to 21.6% from 1995 through 2005) than severe acute colitis not responding to conservative treatment (16.5% from 1975 through 1984 to 58.1% from 1995 through 2007). Mortality rate decreased from 10.0% to 1.8%, and the review suggests that improvement in medical management of IBD may be responsible for the decreases in incidence of TM and overall mortality.

SUMMARY

TM is a severe, life-threatening emergency that can result from a variety of conditions, but it is most commonly associated with severe ulcerative colitis. Improved medical management has resulted in a decrease in its incidence due to IBD; however, increasing use of broad-spectrum antibiotics has lead to a sharp increase secondary to *C. difficile* colitis. Early recognition and multidisciplinary management are crucial if significant morbidity and mortality are to be avoided.

SUGGESTED READINGS

Ali SO, Welch JP, Dring RJ: Early surgical intervention for fulminant pseudomembranous colitis, *Am Surg* 74:20, 2008.

Ausch C, Madoff RD, Gnant M, et al: Aetiology and surgical management of toxic megacolon, *Colorectal Dis* 8:195, 2006.

D'Amico C, Vitale A, Angriman I, et al: Early surgery for the treatment of toxic megacolon, *Digestion* 72:146–149, 2005.

Gan SI, Beck PL: A new look at toxic megacolon: an update and review of incidence, etiology, pathogenesis, and management, *Am J Gastroenterol* 98:2363, 2003.

Goligher JC, Hoffman DC, DeDombal FT, et al: Surgical treatment of severe attacks of ulcerative colitis, with special reference to the advantages of early operation, *Br Med J* 4:703–706, 1970.

Grieco MB, Bordan DL, Geiss AC, et al: Toxic megacolon complicating Crohn's colitis, *Ann Surg* 191:75–80, 1980.

Jalan K, Sircus W, Card WI, et al: An experience of ulcerative colitis, I. Toxic dilation in 55 cases, *Gastroenterology* 57:68–82, 1969.

Latella G, Vernia P, Viscido A, et al: GI distension in severe ulcerative colitis, *Am J Gastroenterol* 97:1169–1175, 2002.

Pepin J, Valiquette L, Cossette B: Mortality attributable to nosocomial *Clostridium difficile*–associated disease during an epidemic caused by a hypervirulent strain in Quebec, *CMAJ* 173(9):1037–1042, 2005.

Pepin J, Vo TT, Boutros M, et al: Risk factors for mortality following emergency colectomy for fulminant *Clostridium difficile* infection, *Dis Colon Rectum* 52:400–405, 2009.

Sheth SG, LaMont JT: Toxic megacolon, *Lancet* 351:509, 1998.

Strauss RJ, Flint GW, Platt N, et al: The surgical management of toxic dilatation of the colon: a report of 28 cases and a review of the literature, *Ann Surg* 184:682, 1976.

Teeuwen PH, Stommel MW, Bremers AJ, et al: Colectomy in patients with acute colitis: a systematic review, *J Gastrointest Surg* 13:676–686, 2009.

CROHN'S COLITIS

Russell Farmer, MD, and Susan Galandiuk, MD

INTRODUCTION

Originally described as inflammation of the terminal ileum, Crohn's disease (CD) has grown to describe a group of patients with myriad clinical presentations. Colitis is one of the most common of these. CD is seen primarily in the United States and Europe, with an incidence of 2 to 4 patients per 100,000, but there has been a recent increase in Crohn's colitis (CC) in Asian countries as well. Crohn's patients have a bimodal age distribution at the time of presentation (20s-30s or 50s-60s) and with a female predominance. CD is a complex disease whose etiology is still not clear. Both genetic and environmental factors play a role. Whites, especially Ashkenazi Jews, are also more likely to develop CD. Patients with a positive familial history of Crohn's are 20 times more likely to develop CD. Although high-risk variants of the NOD2/CARD 15 gene have been identified in some patients, this has not yet been found a reliable diagnostic clinical utility in practice. The best-studied environmental factor is cigarette smoking. There is increasing recognition that, like ulcerative colitis (UC), patients with CC are at increased colorectal cancer risk (CRC) due to the presence of long-standing chronic inflammation. This is true for many chronic inflammatory conditions, such as inflammatory bowel disease (IBD), Barrett's esophagitis, or hepatitis, where chronic inflammation leads to an increased risk of malignancy. This risk is further increased by the coexistence of sclerosing cholangitis, a family history of CRC, and increasing duration and extent of colonic inflammation. Pertinent clinical factors that should be foremost in the evaluation of CC patients include the anatomic location and distribution of the disease, the acuity of the disease, and the nature of the underlying disease (inflammatory, obstructing, or fistulizing). These will guide both medical and surgical treatment.

CLINICAL FEATURES

Patients with CC have an array of clinical presentations. Frequently, patients will present with vague and intermittent abdominal pain accompanied by diarrhea. Patients may also describe hematochezia; melena is rare. Given the wide differential diagnosis for these symptoms, infectious and parasitic causes should be excluded at initial evaluation. Frequently, patients will present describing symptoms associated with recurrent inflammatory colitis that they experience or recognize as a "Crohn's flare." Advanced colitis may present in the form of major lower gastrointestinal bleeding, colonic perforation, large bowel obstruction, or fulminant colitis. Pancolitis is among the most common manifestations of colonic CD, which makes differentiation from UC difficult. Direct mucosal examination using endoscopy with biopsy as initial evaluation is essential. Only one third of CC patients will display granulomas on biopsy. Frequently, computed tomographic (CT) scanning is used as an adjunct in diagnosis and can potentially elucidate overlooked areas of foregut or midgut disease, thereby establishing a diagnosis of CD versus UC. CT scanning can also indicate the presence of associated intra-abdominal abscesses. Small bowel follow-through with barium is useful in patients with established diagnoses of CD to evaluate for active small bowel disease. The clinical scenario of acuity versus chronicity will often determine the order of diagnostic testing. For example, one should seldom, if ever, plan colonoscopy in the face of an acute abdomen; a CT scan (preferably with contrast) would better suit. Conversely, endoscopy is a good starting point for a patient with chronic complaints. Approximately one quarter of patients with CD will have coexisting perianal CD. This can include anal fissures, anal strictures, and anal and rectovaginal fistula. The presence of such perianal disease simplifies diagnosis.

In order to delineate the potentially nebulous diagnosis of CD, the Working Party of the World Congress of Gastroenterology has produced successive criteria for classifications of CD. While not used as widely as traumatic or oncologic classification schema, this system established in Vienna (1994) and later updated in Montreal (2005) codified the predominant clinical forms of CD (Table 1). A portion of CC patients present with disease that is limited to isolated inflammatory episodes that can be managed medically. Conversely, some will develop significant colonic strictures or colonic perforation and fistula formation, either of which may require operation. Spontaneous sigmoid colon to terminal ileum fistula due to inflammation or obstruction is another common operative finding during operative exploration and should raise the index of suspicion for CD.

DIAGNOSIS

Patients with concomitant extracolonic CD (15%) related to IBD often simplify diagnosis. However, patients will frequently present with isolated colonic disease, making the underlying differentiation between CD and UC difficult. Use of the term *indeterminate colitis* has been employed in patients with acute colitis whose clinical and pathologic diagnoses remain indistinguishable following resection. The imperfection of pathologic examination requires synthetic reasoning by the clinician. Up to one third of patients with the pathologic diagnoses of CD or UC will be in error. Classic findings associated with CD include "skip lesions"—namely segments of intestine that appear thickened and inflamed with intervening normal segments. CC can, however, appear "UC-like" with continuous disease extending from the rectum proximally on endoscopy. External examination of the bowel shows "creeping fat"—mesenteric fat that has begun to encircle the bowel in areas of active disease. When opened, surgical specimens show a characteristic "cobble

TABLE 1: Classification schemes

	Vienna (1994)	Montreal (2005)
Age at Diagnosis	A1: Below 40 y/o A2: Above 40 y/o	A1: Below 16 y/o A2: From 17 to 40 y/o A3: Above 40 y/o
Location	L1: Ileal L2: Colonic L3: Ileocolonic L4: Upper GI tract	L1: Ileal L2: Colonic L3: Ileocolonic L4: Isolated upper disease*
Behavior	B1: Nonstricturing, nonpenetrating B2: Stricturing B3: Penetrating	B1: Nonsticturing, nonpenetrating B2: Stricturing B3: Penetrating p: Perineal disease modifier[†]

GI, Gastrointestinal.

*L4 modifier added to L1-3 when upper GI disease is present.

[†]"p" added to B1-3 when perineal disease is present.

Satsangi J, Silverberg MS, Vermeire S, Colombel J-F: The Montreal classification of inflammatory bowel disease: controversies, consensus, and implications, Gut 55(6):749–753, 2006.

stoning" or "bear claw" pattern with deep linear ulcers, usually along the mesenteric border of the colon (Figure 1). Macroscopically, patients with UC virtually always have some rectal disease with proximal extension, lending to a diagnosis of CD in any patient with a normal rectum and proximal colitis. Frequently, findings at operation and surgeon judgment will prove the definitive means of differential diagnosis between CD and UC.

Histology

In many patients with pancolitis, it is difficult to make an accurate diagnosis, as only one third of patients with colonic CD will display granulomas on biopsy. Other criteria, such as the presence of a transmural lymphoid aggregated in an area not deeply ulcerated, are needed to make a diagnosis of CD. Recently, "indeterminate colitis" has been adopted by pathologists for any biopsy that shows features in common with both CD and UC or for inflammation that is so profound as to preclude diagnosis.

Serology

While serology is readily available and antisaccharomyces cerevisiae IgG and IgA, anti-OmpC IgA, as well as other antibodies, have been described more frequently in patients with CD, this is not foolproof and is only one piece of supporting evidence to make a diagnosis. It is neither 100% specific nor sensitive. Similarly, genetic markers for CD do not yet have proven clinical utility.

TREATMENT

In treating the patient with CC, it is first important to differentiate which anatomic areas are affected and the type of disease (inflammatory, structuring, or fistulizing). With respect to patients with colonic CD, medical therapy will be ineffective in the presence of fibrotic strictures. The most frequently overlooked obstruction of this type that results in failure of medical therapy is the presence of an anal or lower rectal Crohn's stricture. Despite patients being on intensive medical treatment, this is often overlooked or not

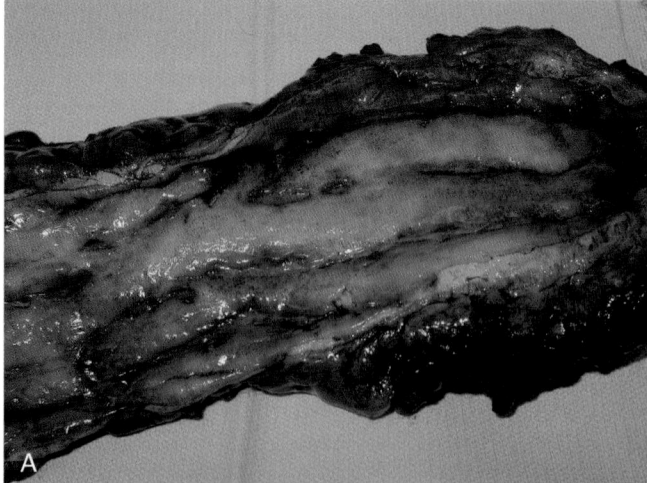
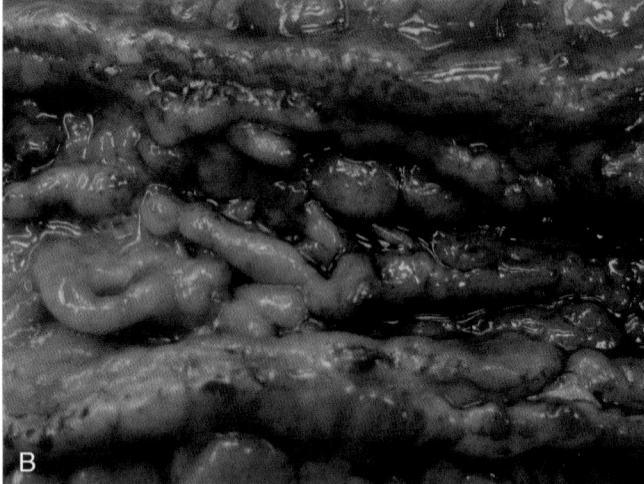

FIGURE 1 **A,** Bear claw or long linear ulcers in the colon of a patient undergoing resection for Crohn's colitis. **B,** Close-up view of colonic mucosa showing "cobblestoning" indicative of severe Crohn's with a combination of linear and transverse ulcerations. The raised areas consist of retained mucosa.

evaluated. If this is not dilated, medical therapy will not likely be effective. The same applies for more proximal colonic strictures if they pose a significant obstruction. Fibrotic strictures are less likely to respond to antiinflammatory medications and more likely to require surgical treatment.

Medical Management

The last 10 years have seen significant changes in the medical treatment of patients with CC. There are two treatment philosophies regarding medical management of CC, as there are for Crohn's treatment in general. One is the *bottom-up* strategy—that is, starting with the safest low-side-effect medications first and then gradually building up toward medications that have more side effects and are stronger (Table 2). The other is the *top-down* strategy, where one starts with more powerful agents with potentially more side effects first (see Table 2). There are pros and cons to both approaches. Advocates of the top-down approach hope to break the cycle of chronic inflammation and scar formation associated with chronic CD and limit permanent architectural damage to tissue. There are, however, cost issues to consider, such as the fact that biologic agents, a mainstay in the therapy of severe CD, are expensive and out of reach of many

TABLE 2: Organization of medical therapy for Crohn's colitis

Systemic effects	Top-down
Fewest	Other: • Antibiotics/metronidazole • Probiotics • 5-ASA and derivatives Steroids: • Intravenous prednisone • Oral prednisone • Oral budesonide Antimetabolites: • Methotrexate • Azathioprine • 6-Mercaptopurine
Most	Biologics: • Imfliximab • Adalimumab • Certulizumab pegol

Systemic effects	Bottom-up
Most	Biologics: • Imfliximab • Adalimumab • Certulizumab pegol Antimetabolites: • Methotrexate • Azathioprine • 6-Mercaptopurine Steroids: • Intravenous prednisone • Oral prednisone • Oral budesonide Other: • Antibiotics/metronidazole • Probiotics • 5-ASA and derivatives

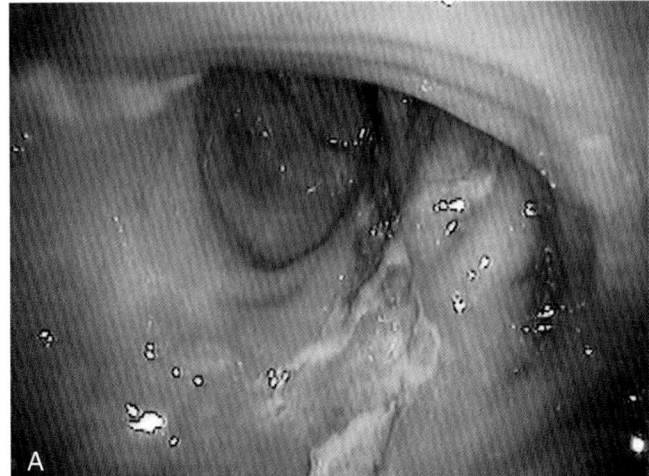
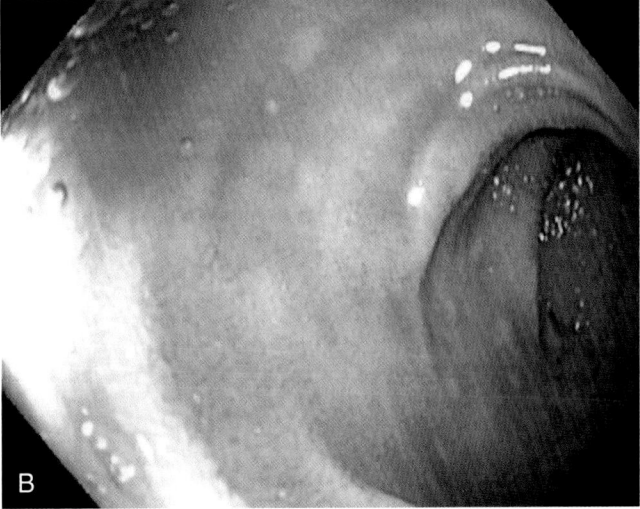

FIGURE 2   A, Colonoscopic view of a patient with severe Crohn's colitis before and **(B)** 1 year after beginning adalimumab therapy.

patients who have no or limited insurance. In addition, many insurance carriers have requirements that patients must have tried other agents prior to proceeding to biologic therapy because of their associated expense.

The safest medications for CD are generally antiinflammatory drugs, which include sulfasalazine and the 5-ASA drugs. The 5-ASA drugs are modifications of sulfasalazine without the sulfapyridine ring. These have been modified into many different forms, which determine their site of drug release. There are many designed for colonic drug delivery, including Asacol, Dipentem, Apriso, and Lialda. Such drugs can also be administered in topical form, such as via suppository (Canasa), which delivers the drug to the rectosigmoid or in small-volume enema form (Rowasa), which delivers the drug to the rectosigmoid and left colon. If the use of these drugs alone is ineffective at inducing disease remission, steroids are frequently utilized in the form of "pulse therapy." Due to the significant side-effect profile of steroids with prolonged use with side effects such as hypertension, increased blood sugar, cataracts, aseptic hip necrosis, striae, Cushingoid appearance, and so on, the goal is to use these agents for a short time but in a fairly potent dose that rapidly deescalates. Typical regimens for severe disease would be to start a patient on 60 mg/day and then taper down by 10 mg every 2 weeks. Budesonide

is a useful oral steroid that can be considered to be a *topical* steroid, since it is nearly completely metabolized as it passes through the enterohepatic circulation. This medication is useful for treating cases of mild to moderate colitis. Although its effect is largely topical, it does have some slight degree of systemic effect, and bone density must be monitored in patients who are on this medication long term. If oral steroids are ineffective, patients are frequently hospitalized for intravenous steroid therapy, or biologic therapy is considered. Intravenous therapy typically would consist of 100 mg of hydrocortisone intravenously every 6 to 8 hours. Clinical improvement should be seen within 48 hours.

There are currently three "biologic" agents that are FDA-approved for the treatment of CD in the United States. *Biologics*, when speaking of IBD, is the commonly used term for monoclonal antibodies directed against tumor necrosis factor alpha. These include Cimzia (Certolizumab pegol), Humira (Adalimumab), and Remicade (Infliximab). The latter is given as an intravenous infusion over 2 hours. The former two are given subcutaneously. Each of these agents requires a loading dose and then is followed by maintenance doses. Side effects of biologic agents include reactivation of tuberculosis or histoplasmosis, as well as an approximately fivefold increased risk of developing non-Hodgkin's lymphoma. In young adults who are also receiving antimetabolite therapy (azathioprine, 6-mercaptopurine), there is a greatly increased risk of fatal hepatosplenic T-cell lymphoma. The introduction of biologic therapy has done much to decrease the frequency with which patients with colonic CD require surgery (Figure 2).

For patients in whom there is a desire to maintain remission, a class of medications known as antimetabolites is frequently used. This comprises both azathioprine, as well as its metabolite 6-mercaptopurine. Both of these medications take approximately 4 months after they are started for their effect to begin, and as such they cannot be used for treatment of flares. The two main side effects with these medications are, as with biologics, an increased risk of non-Hodgkin's lymphoma, as well as an increased risk of leukopenia and pancreatitis. One can, with some reliability, predict individuals at higher risk of developing these latter two side effects by genetic testing to determine which individuals have a lower-efficiency enzyme (thiopurine methyl transferase) for metabolizing this drug. This type of genetic testing is in routine clinical practice.

Surgical Management

The indications and techniques for operation in CC are unique in scope. Determining the short- and long-term goals of surgery cannot be overemphasized prior to any operation for CD. Surgery for CD will only relieve the intestinal complications of the disease; it does not "cure" CD. The surgeon should include the patient's family, gastroenterologist, and likely psychiatrist in face-to-face preoperative consultation to determine what the desired result of surgery will be. Choice of a specific operation must be decided at an individual patient level because there are many factors that go into selection of the most appropriate operation for a given patient. This includes the condition of the anal sphincter, the coexistence of perianal disease, the presence or absence of an anal canal/lower rectal stricture, the presence or absence of small bowel CD, patient age and body habitus, their occupation, and their level of intelligence. The surgeon should pay particular attention to the duration of medical therapy, results of pathologic examinations, previous endoscopy, and previous operations, if any. A careful history of fecal continence should also be taken to avoid an exaggerated colectomy on patients likely to become incontinent. Also, the continence history may elucidate the presence of perineal CD in a patient with progressive difficulty with controlling, initiation, or terminating defecation. Performing an ileorectal anastomosis in such a patient could be devastating to quality of life and exacerbate underlying fluid and electrolyte imbalances from long-term corticosteroid treatment.

With the progression of medical therapy, the majority of patients undergoing operations for CD are now doing so following a prolonged period of treatment with either intravenous steroids or biologic agents. The vigilant surgeon would be traditionally reticent to operate on a patient who is on these medicines for fear of complications. Recent evidence shows, however, that there is little difference in outcomes in patients undergoing colectomy for CD in either the presence or absence of infliximab or steroids (Mascarenhas C, et al., 2012). Similarly, there is no difference in the complication rate for those patients receiving these medicines postoperatively (Regueiro M, et al., 2011). Furthermore, CD medical management with high-dose steroids or biologics that has "failed" is an indication for surgery. "Failed" medical treatment is considered when there is either progression of disease while taking these medicines or having no response to therapy over a 3- to 6- month period. These patients frequently present with stricture or obstruction, or any combination of the following operative indications.

STRICTURE/OBSTRUCTION

A significant majority of CD patients will present with a stricture of the small bowel, terminal ileum, or colon as the initial sign of disease. Nasogastric decompression, correction of electrolyte and fluid imbalance, and nutritional support are standard. Medical management of active CC is possible, but the surgeon must be vigilant to prevent a prolonged period of parenteral nutrition and antiinflammatory agents, which will be a potential setup for operative disaster. CT and water-soluble contrast enema are helpful in outlining the area of active CC resulting in intestinal blockage. Endoscopic dilation of colonic strictures in CD is increasingly performed, but it should be relegated to the hands of expert endoscopists because the risk of perforation is significant. This obviously also applies to stent placement. The risk of malignancy in CC strictures is real. If the affected area is not resected, biopsies should be taken to exclude cancer. Obtaining adequate endoscopic biopsies of strictures may, however, be difficult due to the fibrotic nature of these strictures.

PERFORATION, FISTULAE, AND ABSCESS

A potential first sign of CD is the development of small bowel or colonic perforation and its sequelae. Frequently, patients will present with chronic perforation that has resulted in fistula formation, development of abscess, or the presence of phlegmon. These complications are rendered more difficult to diagnose in a large subset of CD patients given the immunosuppressive nature of many maintenance medications for CD. Steroids, in particular, tend to mask inflammation and chronic leukocytosis. A CT scan is the modality of choice to determine the location of active disease. While a discrete abscess may not be seen, the presence of fatty inflammation on CT often points to the site of ongoing perforation or fistulae.

The preferred method of treatment for pericolonic abscess is bowel rest, nutritional support, parenteral antibiotics, and image-guided percutaneous drainage. An urgent operation is only needed in the case of fecal or purulent peritonitis. If not amenable to percutaneous drainage, colonic resection and abscess drainage are necessary. A classic scenario is the presence of an ileosigmoid fistula resulting from terminal ileitis, the traditional management of which has been to free the inflamed ileum from the sigmoid colon, perform an ileocolic resection, and repair the sigmoid colon primarily. Sigmoid resection may be required if there is significant fibrosis or inability to achieve a safe primary repair. A diverting stoma should be considered for patients whose disease precludes safe anastomosis; that is, there is significant associated malnutrition or pelvic inflammation to warrant concerns regarding postoperative healing.

MASSIVE LOWER GASTROINTESTINAL BLEEDING

CC patients rarely present with lower GI bleeding severe enough to require surgery. Bleeding may be in the form of melena or hematochezia, depending on the site of colonic disease. Initial therapy is medical. Endoscopic control of bleeding is difficult, considering the multifocal or pancolonic nature of CC. It is unusual for CC patients to require significant transfusion for bleeding. The administration of more than 2 units of blood over a 24-hour period, and certainly any sign of hemodynamic abnormality, should prompt surgical therapy. The evaluation of the rectum is essential and repeatable in the operating room using rigid proctoscopy. Rectal resection for severe bleeding is rarely indicated to complement total abdominal colectomy. Anastomosis is not warranted in these critically ill patients, and ileostomy should be performed.

SEVERE COLITIS/FULMINANT COLITIS/TOXIC MEGACOLON

Occasionally, patients with CC will develop progressive colonic disease to the point of systemic inflammatory response. This clinical manifestation of colonic mucosal destruction has been given several different names, but the end or final clinical presentation is the same. Patients develop fever, leukocytosis, tachycardia, and hypoalbuminemia, which are frequently accompanied by hemodynamic instability. Ileus may be present, which may result in colonic dilation seen on plain abdominal film, leading to the moniker of "toxic megacolon." Initial care of these patients is supportive. Standard therapy of euvolemic restoration, antibiotics, gastric decompression, and urine monitoring with a Foley catheter should be supplemented with advanced hemodynamic monitoring in a critical care setting. The use of steroids as adjunctive therapy may be helpful. Operation is indicated for signs of disease progression and nonresponse to conservative treatment. Ideally, surgery should occur prior to bowel perforation. The choice of vasopressors as additional therapy is unwise because it will precipitate ongoing mucosal ischemia and only exacerbate the etiology of the disease. If a patient has progressed to the point of hypotension, colectomy is warranted.

EXTRACOLONIC MANIFESTATIONS OF CROHN'S DISEASE

Many forms of extracolonic CD exist. Commonly, patients will have disease present in the small bowel with similar presentation as in CC: stenosis and stricture, perforation with fistula formation, or perforation with abscess. These are managed largely in the same manner as CC, with the exception of those patients with recurrent small bowel Crohn's being at risk for short-gut syndrome from multiple resections. These patients are best treated with measures designed to preserve absorptive capacity and small intestinal length such as strictureplasty. Other manifestations include perineal Crohn's, cutaneous disease such as pyoderma gangrenosum, Crohn's uveitis, ankylosing spondylitis, primary sclerosing cholangitis (PSC), and growth retardation in children. Many of these improve with surgery; PSC and spondylitis are exceptions to this, however, and are often progressive. Growth retardation in children is of specific concern. Prompt surgery is needed in children with active CC because ongoing inflammation can result in epiphyseal closure and near cessation of growth.

OPERATIONS FOR CROHN'S COLITIS

The extent of surgical resection for CC is defined by the anatomic distribution of disease as well as the nature of the Crohn's inflammation. Patients undergoing surgery for CC require particular perioperative and operative considerations (Box 1). CD patients are often malnourished. Measuring serum albumin and prealbumin prior to operation serves as a means of determining nutrition status. Recognizing occult malnutrition is key, because it is a major operative risk factor. If these nutritional parameters are insufficient, increasing enteral nutrition, if possible, is desired. Patients unable to tolerate a diet may require supplemental parenteral nutrition. Midline incisions are indicated for virtually all operations for CC to preserve all four quadrants for stoma creation, if necessary. Special care must be taken in the creation of these stomas and in the abdominal incisions made because many CD patients will have these stomas for life.

BOX 1: Essential operative considerations

1. Discuss possibility of diversion (+/− temporary)
2. Mark stoma sites prior to operation*
3. Modified lithotomy position*
4. Intraoperative technique:
    a. Work from normal to abnormal tissue
    b. Frequently, fingers better than scissors for dissection of severely inflamed bowel

*Even if not anticipated to need a stoma or special positioning.

Stoma complications can lead to the need for stoma relocation, which can be made more difficult if the original operation was not planned carefully.

In the elective operative patient, antibiotic prophylaxis for the coverage of gram-negative bacteria and anaerobes is appropriate using a single dose of a second-generation cephalosporin (such as cefotetan) within 1 hour of skin incision. This dose is repeated 4 hours following incision in prolonged cases (cases >4 hours). Prevention of deep venous thrombosis and their sequelae are accomplished with a combination of serial compression devices (SCDs) and compression stockings. Perioperative heparin or low-molecular-weight heparin administration can also be used.

EMERGENT OPERATION

Emergent operation for CC is increasingly infrequent. Indications for emergent operation include perforation, abdominal or pelvic sepsis, obstruction, and major bleeding. The operation of choice for emergent treatment of CC is a subtotal colectomy with a long rectal stump. CC will result in severe mesenteric inflammation. This inflamed mesentery cannot be treated the same as that present for normal bowel. It is tempting to use measures to expedite bowel resection in this profoundly ill cohort. While energy devices are appropriate for normal bowel, in some cases of severely indurated, thickened Crohn's mesentery, they work less well. Inflamed mesentery should be divided carefully between clamps and ligated.

Care must be taken to adequately evert the ileostomy to avoid pouching complications. The rectal stump should be brought through the midline incision and tacked to the fascia in the manner of a mucous fistula. If the distal rectal stump dehisces, this is then essentially a complicated wound infection that progresses to a controlled enterocutaneous fistula rather than a pelvic abscess, which would be the case if the stump were left short and within the pelvis. Placement of a rectal drainage tube is a useful adjunct if there is high concern of "blow out" of the rectal stump or if, due to technical reasons, the distal rectosigmoid cannot be incorporated into the fascial closure. Box 1 lists essential operative considerations that are particularly useful in emergent colectomy for CD.

SEGMENTAL COLECTOMY

The use of segmental colectomy in the presence of resectable CC has become increasingly accepted as a means of surgical management. Accomplished by identifying proximal and distal areas of healthy bowel and mesentery suitable for anastomosis, segmental colectomy has become a viable alternative to total colectomy. The use of postoperative adjunctive immune modulating medicines following segmental colectomy is essential because the rate of recurrent colitis is higher than those patients undergoing total abdominal colectomy. However, in patients where preservation of colonic function (water absorption) and delay of stoma are desirable, this recurrence risk is acceptable when compared with the complications and consequences of total colectomy and proctocolectomy. Colonic strictures due to CD should generally be resected, except in the case where a right colon stricture is contiguous with a short stricture of the terminal ileum. In select cases, this can be managed with strictureplasty.

ILEORECTAL ANASTOMOSIS

Primary ileorectal anastomosis (IRA) following subtotal colectomy is a viable option for patients that do not desire an ileostomy. Rectal sparing by the disease process is a prerequisite of this choice for operation. Preoperative evaluation should focus on continence because direct ileum to rectum anastomosis will result in an increase of stool volume and number of bowel movements. This can be severely limiting in a patient with poor resting rectal tone or a nonpliant rectum. Some surgeons have espoused the use of preoperative anorectal manometry to determine if a patient will tolerate this alternative to ileostomy. This is most often done in patients who appear to have questionable tone on digital rectal examination. In fact, if the surgeon is unsure about the ability of the patient to maintain continence after ileorectal anastomosis, manometry will be of little use, and IRA should ordinarily be avoided altogether. The ability of the rectum to stretch on insufflation of air either on rigid proctoscopy or flexible sigmoidoscopy is a good predictor of function. A rectum that does not distend well will result in poor functional results for the patient. Several issues pertaining to IRA make patient selection and preoperative consultation as essential as the operation itself. Patients with IRA will require ongoing surveillance of the rectum to assess for recurrence of CD as well as the possibility of dysplasia and cancer. Recurrence in the remaining rectum is a frequent sequela of IRA. A significant percentage (40%-50%) of patients undergoing IRA will eventually require completion proctectomy with end ileostomy.

TOTAL PROCTOCOLECTOMY WITH END ILEOSTOMY

Total proctocolectomy (TPC) with formation of an end ileostomy is the treatment of choice for several presentations of CD. For patients with pancolitis and perianal Crohn's, patients with dysplasia TPC, and those with multiply recurrent disease, TPC may be the ideal operation. It has the lowest recurrence risk of any operation performed for CD. TPC dissection is performed with the patient in modified lithotomy position so as to allow for access to both the perineum and abdominal cavity. The perineal dissection should be done in the plane between the internal and external anal sphincters. This "intersphincteric proctectomy" minimizes the size of the perineal wound and associated healing complications. The perineal wound is closed in layers with absorbable suture so as to provide coverage for eventual possible breakdown. Roughly 25% of these perineal wounds will ultimately break down and heal by secondary intention. Patients need to be aware of this.

Ileal Pouch Anal Anastomosis

Patients will often present with ileal pouches after having been initially diagnosed with UC or indeterminate colitis, only to later manifest the signs of CD. Pouch surgery is traditionally not performed in patients with CD due to the risk of fistulizing small bowel and perianal CD. In very select CC patients without perianal disease and after a very in-depth discussion of all the potential complications, ileal pouch anal anastomosis may be undertaken. This should only be done by surgeons and centers with significant experience in treating patients with IBD. Once CD is diagnosed in a patient with an ileal pouch, it is generally possible to maintain the pouch with a combination of supportive measures, including frequent examination, endoscopy, and medical therapy.

PROCTECTOMY

Completion proctectomy for CC is often performed following subtotal colectomy for recurrent disease in the rectum. The patient is placed in modified lithotomy position, and after abdominal mobilization of the rectum, the intersphincteric dissection is begun from the perineum. If cancer is present, a conventional abdominoperineal resection is performed with resection of both the internal and external sphincters. Occasionally, patients will have isolated rectal CD, or extracolonic CD, with the rectum as the only site of colonic disease. In that case, proctectomy and end-colostomy may be performed with the understanding of the potential for reoperation should the colonic disease progress.

THE ROLE OF LAPAROSCOPIC AND ROBOTIC SURGERY FOR CROHN'S COLITIS

The role of new surgical techniques for treating CC is still evolving. Clearly, the worst-case scenario is that in which a surgeon moderately skilled in minimal access surgery and with limited clinical familiarity with CD must consider which method to use. In such circumstances, we encourage the use of open or traditional skills but, most of all, organized access to a skilled gastrointestinal pathologist. Given much more ideal circumstances of technical expertise in laparoscopic and robotic surgery, one can then proceed according to the basics of Box 1 as noted above. As is true for most abdominal and alimentary tract operations, the principles are the same, although the issues of incision, pain, herniation, and so on are lessened with minimally invasive approaches. It is especially important for the general surgeon working in a remote area from specialists in gastrointestinal medicine or pathology to have a good communication path with a surgeon experienced in CD, and especially CC. That sort of channel can be arranged through a telephone call and guidance provided on a one-to-one basis in a meaningful way with patient referral as needed. The future of the surgical approach to CD will obviously become progressively less invasive over time, but familiarity with the disease and/or the techniques is essential and both are preferable.

SUGGESTED READINGS

Farmer M, Petras RE, Hunt LE, et al: The importance of diagnostic accuracy in colonic inflammatory bowel disease, *Am J Gastroenterol* 95:3184–3188, 2000.

Galandiuk S, Kimberling J, Al-Mishlag TG, Stromberg AJ: Perianal Crohn's disease: predictors of need for permanent diversion, *Ann Surg* 241:796–802, 2005.

Mascarenhas C, Nunoo R, Asgeirsson T, et al: Outcomes of ileocolic resection and right hemicolectomies for Crohn's patients in comparison with non-Crohn's patients and the impact of perioperative immunosuppressive therapy with biologics and steroids on inpatient complications, *Am J Surg* 203:375–378, 2012.

Regueiro M, El-Hachem S, Kip KE, et al: Postoperative infliximab is not associated with an increase in adverse events in Crohn's disease, *Dig Dis Sci* 56:3610–3615, 2011.

Satsangi J, Silverberg MS, Vermeire S, Colombel J-F: The Montreal classification of inflammatory bowel disease: controversies, consensus, and implications, *Gut* 55:749–753, 2006.

ISCHEMIC COLITIS

Raul Coimbra, MD, PhD, FACS, and
Todd W. Costantini, MD

OVERVIEW

Ischemic colitis is the most common form of intestinal ischemia and is responsible for as many as 1 in every 1000 hospital admissions. The incidence rate of colon ischemia is likely underestimated because patients with transient episodes may not seek medical attention. Ischemic colitis is predominantly a disease of the elderly, with most cases occurring in patients over age 65 years. The numerous potential causes of ischemic colitis (Box 1) result in a diverse clinical presentation that ranges from mild, self-limiting mucosal ischemia to severe transmural infarction and necrosis. Approximately 20% of patients presenting to the hospital with ischemic colitis need surgical intervention; therefore, understanding the pathophysiology of ischemic colitis and the factors associated with the progression of ischemia are necessary to provide appropriate surgical care.

ANATOMIC CONSIDERATIONS

The colon receives its arterial blood supply from the superior mesenteric artery (SMA) and the inferior mesenteric artery (IMA). The SMA gives the blood supply to the right colon via the ileocolic, right colic, and middle colic arteries. The ascending colon is supplied by the ileocolic and right colic arteries, and the transverse colon is supplied predominantly by the middle colic artery. The IMA gives rise to the left colic, sigmoid, and superior rectal arteries, which supply the distal transverse colon through the proximal rectum. The SMA and the IMA communicate through an extensive collateral circulation that limits the risk of ischemia to the colon (Figure 1).

The arch of Riolan, also referred to as the meandering mesenteric artery, is a collateral vessel that connects the proximal SMA with the proximal IMA at the base of the mesentery. This collateral vessel is variable in caliber and may serve a vital role in delivering blood to the colon in the case of either SMA or IMA stenosis or occlusion. The marginal artery of Drummond forms a continuous arterial arcade that runs along the distal mesentery near the colonic wall and serves as another collateral connection between the SMA and the IMA. Despite this collateral circulation, specific areas of the colon are more susceptible to ischemia. These watershed areas of the colon include the right colon, splenic flexure (Griffith's point), and the rectosigmoid junction (Sudek's point).

The right colon is vulnerable to ischemic insults because of low-flow states caused by hypotension resulting from hemorrhage, sepsis, or heart failure. The right colon is also at risk for ischemia from embolic events because the ileocolic artery is the terminal branch of the SMA and susceptible to embolic occlusion based on its straight take-off from the SMA. The splenic flexure is another watershed area because of its location at the distal extent of the arterial supply of the left colic (IMA) and middle colic arteries (SMA). The collateral circulation of the splenic flexure is the most inconsistent amongst individuals and accounts for its predisposition to local ischemia. In some individuals, the marginal artery of Drummond is either diminutive or absent, which limits the collateral circulation and places this segment of colon at risk for ischemic insults. The rectosigmoid junction is also considered a watershed area because it receives its arterial supply from the distal sigmoid artery branches and from the superior hemorrhoidal artery, both distal branches of the IMA. Its anatomic location, the increased incidence of significant IMA stenosis with age from atherosclerosis, and the need for IMA ligation during aortic surgery place the rectosigmoid region at risk for ischemia.

CLINICAL PRESENTATION

The signs and symptoms of ischemic colitis are often nonspecific and require a high index of suspicion to achieve prompt diagnosis. Patients presenting with ischemic colitis frequently experience sudden onset of abdominal pain that is not well localized. This may be associated with nausea and vomiting. Patients may have low-grade fever and leukocytosis. Patients often have mild hematochezia beginning within 24 hours of abdominal pain. Bleeding associated with ischemic colitis is usually minor and does not frequently require blood transfusion.

Medical history is often critical in the diagnosis of ischemic colitis, with specific focus on cardiovascular risk factors, history of hypercoagulability, embolic and thrombotic risk factors, and surgical history (specifically aortic and cardiac surgery). Other factors that have been associated with ischemic colitis include history of vasculitis, cocaine use, oral contraceptive pills, and long-distance running. For patients in whom ischemic colitis develops in the inpatient setting, factors such as heart failure, hypotensive episodes, and recent vasopressor use may favor a diagnosis of ischemic colitis.

DIAGNOSIS

On the basis of the nonspecific clinical presentation of ischemic colitis, patients often undergo an extensive imaging workup for evaluation of abdominal pain. Plain film radiographs of the abdomen may show thumb printing, colonic dilation, or mural thickening. Thumb printing, which is indicative of submucosal edema, is the most common radiographic finding in patients with ischemic colitis; however, it is nonspecific and may be the result of other etiologies causing colonic inflammation. Computed tomographic (CT) scan of the abdomen may localize the site of colitis by demonstrating segmental pericolonic fat stranding and bowel wall thickening. The presence of gas in the colonic wall (pneumatosis) suggests more severe, transmural ischemia. Abdominal free fluid may also be present on the abdominal CT scan and has been shown in one retrospective review to be predictive of the need for surgical intervention in patients with ischemic colitis.

The gold standard for the diagnosis of ischemic colitis is flexible endoscopy. Either colonoscopy or sigmoidoscopy can be used to visualize the mucosa for signs of ulceration or ischemic changes. Endoscopy is usually performed without mechanical bowel preparation to limit the occurrence of further dehydration and potential hypotension, which may exacerbate the ischemic insult. Lower insufflation pressures are advocated during endoscopy to limit the risk of colon perforation. It is also generally recommended that the colonoscope not be advanced beyond the affected area.

Findings on endoscopy that are characteristic of mild ischemic colitis include the presence of pale-appearing mucosa, mucosal edema, erythema, and petechial hemorrhages. Ulceration is also frequently noted on endoscopic examination, with a single longitudinal ulcer called the "single-stripe" sign characteristic of ischemic colitis. More severe ischemia is characterized by the dusky appearance of the tissue, submucosal hemorrhage, and hemorrhagic ulcerations, which progress to frank necrosis in advanced cases. Ischemic colitis is usually segmental in distribution with an abrupt change to normal mucosa in the nonaffected region of the colon. Histologic changes of the bowel during ischemic colitis include inflammatory cell infiltration, mucosal edema and sloughing, altered crypt morphology, and hemorrhage within the lamina propria.

BOX 1: Common causes of ischemic colitis

Hypoperfusion
Hypovolemia
Septic shock
Heart failure
Hemorrhagic shock

Surgery
Aortic repair
Cardiac surgery

Vascular Disease
Atherosclerosis
Systemic lupus erythematosus
Rheumatoid arthritis
Wegener's granulomatosis

Hypercoagulable States
Factor V Leiden
Protein C and S deficiency

Antithrombin III deficiency
Prothrombin G20210A mutation
Antiphospholipid syndrome
Disseminated intravascular coagulation

Drugs
Vasopressors
Oral contraceptive medications
Antihypertensive drugs
Cocaine

Other
Mechanical colon obstruction
Hemodialysis
Cardiac emboli
Cholesterol emboli
Long-distance running

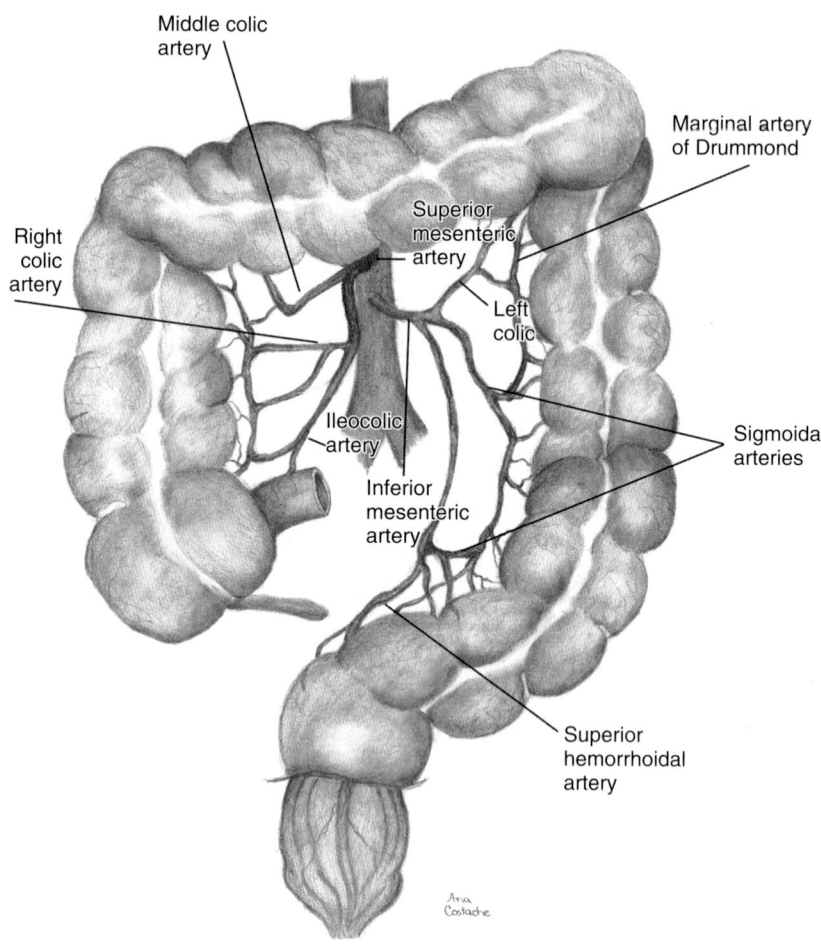

FIGURE 1 Arterial blood supply to the colon.
(Courtesy Ana Costache.)

There is limited role for angiography in the diagnosis of ischemic colitis because the large mesenteric vessels are generally patent in this disease process, with the ischemia present at the arteriolar level. Angiography should be performed to evaluate for acute mesenteric ischemia or acute embolic event. In the past, barium enema was commonly used to diagnose ischemic colitis; however, the utility of this technique is diminished with the improved images obtained with CT scanning. The use of magnetic resonance imaging (MRI) in the diagnosis of ischemic colitis is the subject of ongoing research in animal models and clinical studies.

The differential diagnosis for patients believed to have ischemic colitis includes acute mesenteric ischemia, infectious colitis, inflammatory bowel disease, and colon cancer. It is important to differentiate ischemic colitis from acute mesenteric ischemia, which primarily affects the small intestine and requires urgent intervention. Patients with acute mesenteric ischemia generally present with severe acute-onset abdominal pain, which is out of proportion to their physical examination results. In contrast to patients with ischemic colitis, they generally do not have bloody diarrhea until late in their clinical course. Infectious colitis should also be considered in patients being evaluated for potential ischemic colitis. Invasive bacteria, most commonly *Escherichia coli* O157:H7, *Salmonella,* and *Shigella* should be evaluated for with stool culture studies. Patients with recent hospitalization or recent antibiotic use should be evaluated for *Clostridium difficile* colitis, which may be associated with the presence of pseudomembranes on endoscopic evaluation.

TREATMENT

The initial treatment of the patient with ischemic colitis should focus on determination of the severity of ischemia and whether any indications for urgent surgical intervention are present (Figure 2). Most patients present with mild ischemic colitis that responds to supportive, nonsurgical management. Although less common, some patients present with colonic ischemia causing transmural necrosis that requires urgent operative intervention. Therefore, prompt evaluation of patients with ischemic colitis is needed to evaluate for indications for urgent operative evaluations.

Nonsurgical Management

Nearly 80% of patients with ischemic colitis respond to conservative treatment with resolution of symptoms within a few days. Patients should initially be placed on bowel rest with aggressive fluid rehydration, as needed, if hypovolemia is believed to be a culprit in the development of colon ischemia. Nasogastric tube decompression should be considered in patients with nausea and vomiting or evidence of bowel dilation. The authors do not advocate the routine use of nasogastric tube decompression in all patients. Colon ischemia results in intestinal epithelial barrier failure, which may lead to bacterial translocation and septic complications. For that reason, empiric broad-spectrum antibiotics are recommended when ischemic colitis is suspected, despite the lack of clinical trials supporting their efficacy. Antibiotics against both anaerobic and aerobic coliform bacteria are recommended to cover the normal bacterial flora of the large intestine. Cathartics should be avoided because they may lead to colon perforation. Serial abdominal radiographs may be useful to follow changes in colonic dilation.

In critically ill patients in whom ischemic colitis develops as a complication of another illness, treatment should focus on limiting vasopressor use, if possible, to maximize mesenteric blood flow. Cardiac output should also be optimized with the consideration for use of pulmonary artery catheterization or other noninvasive hemodynamic monitoring tools to guide fluid resuscitation strategies to optimize perfusion to the ischemic colon.

Patient are at increased risk of ischemic colitis after abdominal aortic aneurysm (AAA) repair because of ligation of the IMA in open aortic surgery or coverage of the IMA takeoff during endovascular AAA repair. Patients in whom fever, leukocytosis, bloody diarrhea, abdominal pain, abdominal distention, or unexplained acidosis develops after AAA repair should be evaluated for potential colon ischemia. Supportive measure should be initiated as described previously in addition to an urgent, bedside flexible sigmoidoscopy to

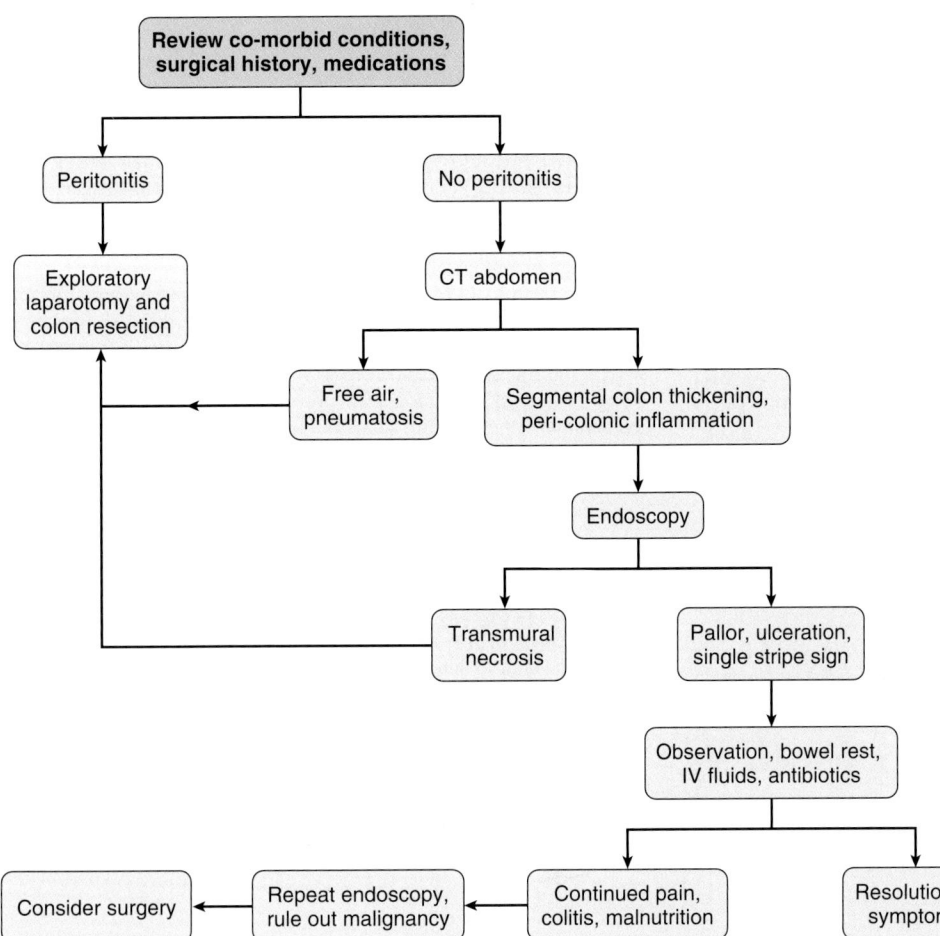

FIGURE 2 Algorithm describing the treatment of ischemic colitis. *CT,* Computed tomographic; *IV,* intravenous.

evaluate for evidence of colon ischemia. In the absence of any indication for urgent exploration, the patient should receive supportive management with consideration for repeat endoscopy to evaluate for signs of worsening ischemia.

Surgical Management

Mortality rate is greater than 50% in patients requiring acute surgical intervention for ischemic colitis. Indications for acute surgical exploration in patients with ischemic colitis include peritonitis, pneumoperitoneum, massive hemorrhage, or signs of transmural necrosis on abdominal imaging including pneumatosis or portal venous gas (Box 2). In addition, those patients with ongoing or worsening abdominal pain, increasing leukocytosis, acidosis, oliguria, or signs of sepsis during treatment with supportive measures should be considered for abdominal exploration. Right-sided colon ischemia tends to be more severe with increased likelihood of operative intervention and increased mortality compared with left-sided colon ischemia.

Surgical intervention for patient with ischemic colitis should include a thorough exploration of the abdomen through a midline incision. The entire small and large intestine should be visualized and evaluated for signs of ischemia. Segmental colon resection should be performed for segments of colon demonstrating ischemia, necrosis, or perforation. It is imperative to ensure that the resection margins are well perfused with no signs of ischemia. Confirmation of normal-appearing serosa at the margins is not adequate to confirm the presence of viable tissue because the underlying mucosa and submucosa may be ischemic despite normal-appearing overlying serosa. The resected bowel should be opened on the back table to confirm healthy, well-perfused mucosa and submucosa at the resection margins. If question exists regarding the viability of the margins, frozen section can be used to confirm the presence of normal mucosa and submucosa; however, visual inspection should be adequate to guide the need for further resection to well-perfused, viable tissue.

Ischemic colitis should be managed operatively with a segmental colon resection with diverting end ileostomy or colostomy in the urgent setting. Creation of an anastomosis is not advised because of the presence of potential tenuous blood flow to the newly created anastomosis and the presence of physiologic derangements that are likely to be present in the patient requiring emergent operation for colon ischemia. The surgeon must remember the etiology of ischemia when planning segmental resection. Because ischemic colitis usually occurs in watershed areas, an anatomic colon resection should be performed such that the remaining colon is supplied by sufficient arterial inflow. In cases of extensive or patchy involvement of the large bowel, a temporary abdominal closure with planned second-look laparotomy in 24 hours may be advisable to determine the need for further resection. In rare cases of ischemia of the entire colon or massive hemorrhage that is not localized, a subtotal colectomy and end ileostomy may be required. In contrast to mesenteric ischemia of the small intestine, interventions aimed at revascularizing the large bowel in patient with ischemic colitis are not indicated.

Patients successfully treated with nonsurgical management at the time of diagnosis of ischemic colitis may have sequelae develop in the subacute and chronic setting that may require operative intervention. Patients with ongoing colitis causing continued abdominal pain, bloody diarrhea, or recurrent sepsis lasting more than 2 weeks from the initial diagnosis should be considered for colon resection. Colonic stricture and chronic colitis may develop as a chronic consequence of ischemic colitis. Patients with chronic colitis experience intermittent bouts of abdominal pain, distention, and bloody diarrhea, which are often self limiting. Patients should undergo repeat colonoscopy with biopsy and culture to evaluate for an infectious cause of colitis. Surgical resection is rarely indicated for chronic colitis caused by ischemia; however, malnutrition or intractable symptoms may prompt the need for elective surgical resection of the affected colon.

Patients with colon stricture from ischemic colitis should undergo repeat colonoscopy and biopsy to rule out malignant disease as the cause of stricture. Once malignancy is ruled out, strictures can be observed as some resolve over time. For strictures causing ongoing symptoms, endoscopic dilation may be considered, but segmental resection with primary anastomosis is the procedure of choice in younger patients with low operative risk. Surgical resection should also be considered for those patients in whom malignant disease cannot be conclusively ruled out.

SUMMARY

Ischemic colitis represents a spectrum of disease that ranges from mild, self-limiting abdominal pain and bloody diarrhea treated with bowel rest and antibiotics to transmural necrosis with peritonitis requiring emergent colon resection. Ischemic colitis is typically a disease of the elderly but should be considered in younger patients with symptoms of colon ischemia. Although most patients present with the mild form of ischemic colitis, nearly 20% have clinical deterioration that necessitates operative intervention, which is associated with a significant increase in morbidity and mortality. Maintaining a high index of suspicion and promptly identifying patients with irreversible ischemic injury is of paramount importance in achieving prompt surgical treatment to correct the physiologic derangements caused by large bowel ischemia.

BOX 2: Indications for surgical intervention in patients with ischemic colitis

Acute
Peritonitis
Bowel perforation
Bowel necrosis
Fulminant colitis
Massive hemorrhage
Sepsis

Chronic
Intractable symptoms lasting >2 weeks
Recurrent sepsis
Chronic colitis
Ischemic stricture
Malnutrition from protein-losing colopathy

SUGGESTED READINGS

Brandt LJ, Boley SJ: AGA technical review on intestinal ischemia, *Gastroenterology* 118:954–968, 2000.

Brandt LJ, Feuerstadt P, Blaszka MC: Anatomic patterns, patient characteristics, and clinical outcomes in ischemic colitis: a study of 313 cases supported by histology, *Am J Gastroenterol* 105:2245–2252, 2010.

Elder K, Lashner BA, Al Solaiman F: Clinical approach to colonic ischemia, *Cleve Clin J Med* 76:401–409, 2009.

Paterno F, McGillicuddy EA, Schuster KM, et al: Ischemic colitis: risk factors for eventual surgery, *Am J Surg* 200:646–650, 2010.

Scharff LR, Longo WE, Vartanian SM, et al: Ischemic colitis: spectrum of disease and outcome. *Surgery* 134:624–629, 2003.

The Management of Clostridium Difficile Colitis

Benjamin W. Dart IV, MD, FACS, and
J. Daniel Stanley, MD, FACS, FASCRS

OVERVIEW

Clostridium difficile is a gram-positive, spore-forming anaerobic bacillus. Currently, the accepted term for colonic and, rarely, small intestinal disease caused by *C. difficile* toxins is *C. difficile* infection (CDI). Approximately 3 million CDI cases occur in the United States each year, with data to suggest that severe CDI is occurring in populations previously thought to be at low risk. The incidence and severity of CDI has increased dramatically over the last decade because of changing patterns of antibiotic use, an aging and more susceptible population, and the emergence of hypervirulent strains. For these reasons, surgical intervention for the treatment of CDI is more frequently required. The surgeon must be familiar with the medical and surgical treatment of the patient with CDI.

Multiple risk factors have been identified for the development of CDI (Box 1). Primary risk factors reflect the most commonly recognized elements of pathogenesis: a source of colonization, a change in intestinal microflora, and host debility or altered immunity. A fourth important factor in CDI pathogenesis is the degree of toxin production related to the emergence of hypervirulent strains of *C. difficile*.

Carrier state prevalence for *C. difficile* varies with age. The carrier state is common in the very young, with a prevalence rate of 25% to 80% in infants, but symptoms rarely develop. In contrast, only approximately 3% of adults are asymptomatic carriers. These individuals and patients with active disease serve as a reservoir for the spread of *C. difficile* via a fecal-oral route.

Control of transmission is difficult in the institutional setting because *C. difficile* spores can survive in the dormant state for weeks to years on inanimate objects and may be carried from patient to patient by caregivers. Colonization rates of 20% to 50% may result after hospitalization of 1 and 4 weeks, respectively.

Progression to an active infection usually requires that the protective effects of an individual's normal intestinal flora have been weakened, as with antibiotic usage. Almost all antibiotics increase the risk of development of CDI. Risk further increases with administration of multiple antibiotics or with prolonged treatment. At this time, the antibiotics most frequently associated with the development of CDI are fluoroquinolones and cephalosporins. Bowel preparation and chemotherapy may also alter the colonic microflora and result in CDI.

The postsurgical patient is particularly susceptible to CDI. In addition to having multiple established risk factors for CDI (routine perioperative antibiotic exposure, aging population, and hospitalization), surgical patient conditions are relatively immunosuppressed in the postoperative period. Not surprisingly, patients who have undergone organ transplantation and those with inflammatory bowel disease are at an increased risk for the development of CDI.

All pathogenic strains of *C. difficile* produce toxins that are responsible for the symptoms of CDI. The most important toxins are toxin A, which is primarily endotoxic, and toxin B, which is primarily cytotoxic. Recently, hypervirulent strains of *C. difficile* have emerged that are capable of producing toxins A and B in quantities sixteenfold to twentyfold higher than less virulent strains. The most often identified hypervirulent strain is known as Bi, NAP1/O27, toxinotype III, or polymerase chain reaction (PCR) ribotype 027.

CLINICAL MANIFESTATIONS

The clinical manifestations of CDI are of variable severity. The most common presentation is a mild antibiotic-associated diarrhea, which typically consists of less than 10 nonbloody stools per day, with abdominal cramping and without systemic symptoms. Classically, the colitis resulting from CDI has been synonymous with pseudomembranous colitis, but this is somewhat of a misnomer because pseudomembranes are not always present.

Surgeons must be keenly aware of worsening symptoms because progression beyond mild disease significantly increases the need for an eventual surgical intervention. Moderate to severe CDI consists of profuse diarrhea, fever, nausea, abdominal pain, leukocytosis, abdominal distention, and varying degrees of abdominal tenderness or peritoneal signs. Fulminant CDI (FCDI), which occurs in 1% to 8% of cases, is characterized by a severe systemic inflammatory response and is associated with mortality rates in the range of 30% to 90%. To further complicate the clinical presentation, as many as 37% of patients with FCDI may present without diarrhea because of an associated ileus.

DIAGNOSIS OF *CLOSTRIDIUM DIFFICILE* INFECTION

The timely diagnosis of CDI is important because evidence shows that the length of time from onset of symptoms to initiation of treatment directly correlates with mortality. Once the clinical suspicion of CDI is entertained, there are a number of options for establishing the diagnosis while assessing the severity of the disease. The most useful diagnostic tests are stool analysis, imaging studies, and occasionally, endoscopic evaluation.

Stool studies for establishing a definitive diagnosis of CDI include: 1, enzyme immunoassay for toxins A and B (ToxA/ToxB EIA); 2, PCR to identify DNA coding for the toxins; 3, stool cell cytotoxicity neutralization assay (CCNA); and 4, an enzyme immunoassay for glutamate dehydrogenase antigen (GDH; Table 1). The surgeon must be familiar with these tests given that they each have certain advantages and limitations. Other laboratory studies that are useful in evaluating and stratifying patients with CDI include white blood cell count (WBC), serum lactate, and albumin. All three have been reported as important in identifying those patients with severe and fulminant CDI. The finding of a WBC in the range of 30,000 to 60,000 may be particularly useful when considering CDI because this degree of leukocytosis is much less common in other types of bacterial infection.

Plain abdominal x-rays may reveal a megacolon, ileus, or colonic wall edema. Abdominal computed tomographic (CT) scan may be particularly sensitive in the patient with a severe or fulminant presentation, with the most common findings being localized or diffuse colonic thickening and ascites (Figure 1).

Endoscopic evaluation may be useful in the presence of colonic pseudomembranes and, in the correct clinical setting, renders an almost certain diagnosis of CDI. Colonoscopy is generally preferred over sigmoidoscopy because colitis is limited to the right colon in approximately one third of cases. It may also be used for decompression and placement of a long colonic tube for vancomycin irrigation.

MEDICAL TREATMENT

Treatment recommendations for CDI depend on the severity of disease. Asymptomatic carriers do not need medical treatment, but some general principles should be applied to both carriers and symptomatic patients. Hospital infection control practices should be implemented in patients with *C. difficile* to limit spread within the institution (Box 2). General contact precautions and hand hygiene with soap and water must be observed. Routine hand cleaning with alcohol-based products is not adequate protection against CDI because spores can be resistant to alcohol.

Patients diagnosed with CDI should have offending antibiotics discontinued if possible. If patients are severely ill with other potential sources of infection, continued administration of offending antibiotics must be weighed against the risk of prolonging the duration of CDI and increasing the chance of recurrence. Likewise, antimotility agents commonly used to treat diarrhea should be avoided because administration may result in progression to more severe disease and toxic megacolon.

Initiation of medical treatment should not be delayed for diagnostic studies in patients when the clinical suspicion for CDI is high. The duration of treatment should be for 10 to 14 days. Consideration should be given to extending the duration of this treatment in patients who need ongoing administration of other antibiotics to treat concomitant infections.

The antibiotics most commonly used to treat CDI are metronidazole and vancomycin.

Oral metronidazole (500 mg three times a day) is almost completely absorbed in the more proximal gastrointestinal (GI) tract, and the therapeutic effect is thought to be a result of both the absorbed and the residual unabsorbed component. Intravenous metronidazole (500 mg every 8 hours) provides effective concentrations within the colon and may be used if the enteral route is not available, as in the case of ileus. In mild cases, oral metronidazole is recommended as first-line therapy.

Oral vancomycin (125 to 500 mg four times a day) is recommended over metronidazole in moderate, severe, or recurrent cases. Vancomycin is not absorbed by the GI tract; therefore, high

---

BOX 1: Risk factors for *Clostridium difficile* infection

Primary Risk Factors
Age greater than 65 years
Antibiotic use within the previous 3 months
Hospitalization

Secondary Risk Factors
Female gender
Double occupancy rooms
Intensive care unit admission
Admission to a long-term care facility within the last year
Postpyloric tube feedings
Chemotherapy
Acid-reducing therapy with proton pump inhibitors or histamine receptor blockers
Gastrointestinal procedures
Renal disorders
Organ transplantation
Human immunodeficiency virus
Autoimmune disease
Hypoalbuminemia
Inflammatory bowel disease

Modified from Stanley JD, Burns RP: Invited commentary: Clostridium difficile and the surgeon, Am Surg 76(3):235–244, 2010.

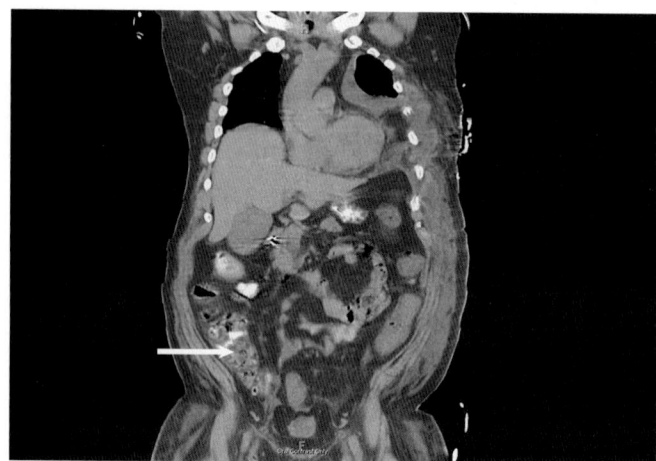

FIGURE 1   Coronal cut from a computed tomographic scan after thoracoabdominal surgery of a patient with fever and elevated white blood cell count. Note the thickened right colon with thumb printing and poor contrast filling *(arrow)*. This patient recovered after treatment with vancomycin and metronidazole.

TABLE 1: Diagnostic tests for *Clostridium difficile* infection

Test	Reported sensitivity	Reported specificity	Comments
Enzyme immunoassay for toxins A and B (ToxA/ToxB EIA)	48% to 96%	94% to 100%	Most commonly used; commercially available; 30-minute turnaround
Common antigen glutamate dehydrogenase	99% to 100%	60%	Excellent as cheap and rapid screening test; negative predictive value close to 100%; confirming test required because of low specificity
Cell cytotoxicity neutralization assay	77%; 92% to 100%	99% to 100%	Typically considered gold standard; long turnaround; requires cell culture
Polymerase chain reaction	87% to 93%	90% to 100%	Emerging as test of choice because of improved sensitivity compared with ToxA/ToxB EIA and rapid turnaround

Modified from Stanley JD, Burns RP: Invited commentary: Clostridium difficile and the surgeon, Am Surg 76(3):235–244, 2010.

BOX 2: Infection control practices to limit the spread of *Clostridium difficile* infection

Avoidance of Inoculation
Minimize intensive care unit stay
Use private rooms
Use gloves
Hand wash with soap or chlorhexidine instead of alcohol-based solutions
Use patient-dedicated stethoscopes and instruments
Wash all nondedicated instruments between patient contacts
Follow isolation precautions

Interventions
Minimize antibiotics
    Follow guidelines for perioperative antibiotics
    Avoid broad-spectrum or multiple antibiotics
    Avoid prolonged courses of antibiotics
Avoid proton pump inhibitors and H2 blockers
Avoid unnecessary bowel preparations
Avoid antidiarrheals
Minimize gastrointestinal intubation for feeding or decompression

Institutional Measures
Consider antibiotic formulary changes in case of institutional epidemic

Modified from Stanley JD, Burns RP: Invited commentary: Clostridium difficile and the surgeon, Am Surg *76(3):235–244, 2010.*

BOX 3: Characteristics of moderate, severe, and fulminant *Clostridium difficile* infection

Moderate Colitis
Pulse, >90 bpm; SBP, >100 mm Hg; temperature, 100°F to 101.5°F; WBC, 12,000 to 15,000
Pseudomembranes on colonoscopy
Colonic thickening on CT scan
Colon, >6 cm
Oliguria responsive to volume
Normal lactate
Mild abdominal tenderness
Mild tachypnea

Severe Colitis
Moderate colitis and the following:
Pulse, >120 bpm; SBP, <100 mm Hg; WBC, >15,000
Renal failure
Respiratory distress or intubation
Albumin, <2.0
Lactate, >2.0
Mental status changes
Moderate abdominal tenderness

Fulminant Colitis
Severe colitis and any of the following:
Condition unimproved after 12 to 24 hours of treatment
Need for vasopressors
Ventilator dependence
Abrupt rise in WBC

CT, Computed tomographic; *SBP,* systolic blood pressure; *WBC,* white blood cell count. *Modified from Stanley JD, Burns RP: Invited commentary: Clostridium difficile and the surgeon,* Am Surg *76(3):235–244, 2010.*

concentrations are achieved in the colon with oral administration. Intravenous vancomycin is not recommended in CDI treatment. In the patient in whom the enteral route is not an option, vancomycin enemas or irrigations through a colonic tube may be of benefit. The typical dose is 500 mg in 100 mL of normal saline solution given as a retention enema or irrigation administered every 6 hours. This may be given in addition to intravenous metronidazole.

Another antimicrobial agent, fidaxomicin, was recently approved by the U.S. Food and Drug Administration (FDA) for treatment of CDI. It is a macrocyclic antibiotic with a narrow therapeutic spectrum. It has been found to be noninferior to vancomycin, with lower recurrence rates. Despite promising results, the widespread adoption of fidaxomicin in the treatment of initial episodes of CDI is limited because of a lack of familiarity and cost.

SURGERY

The surgeon must be involved early in the assessment and treatment of CDI. Increased survival rates have been reported for patients on a surgical service, and earlier surgical intervention may improve survival in patients with severe and fulminant CDI. Surgical intervention is necessary in approximately 20% of patients who are critically ill with CDI. The classic indications for surgery include toxic megacolon or colonic perforation and, less clearly, fulminant disease or failure of medical therapy in 48 to 72 hours with continued signs of toxicity. Toxic megacolon in CDI has been defined as a cecal diameter of greater than 12 cm or a colonic diameter of greater than 6 cm on radiographic imaging. Not uncommonly, patients with CDI with a toxic megacolon may have a conspicuous lack of diarrhea. This finding should not be misinterpreted as an improvement of the disease process. A very low threshold for operative intervention must remain when toxic megacolon exists. The presence of colonic perforation with CDI has an especially poor prognosis, and emergent surgical treatment is the only option for survival.

Standardized definitions of disease severity are not well established. Likewise, failure of medical therapy in patients with severe colitis is a subjective indication of the need for surgery. A severity classification scheme is needed to guide appropriate treatment algorithms that include early surgical intervention. Although several scoring systems have been proposed and appear promising, validated studies are needed before widespread adoption. However, several observations can be made from the collective experience regarding the characteristics of moderate, severe, and fulminant colitis (Box 3). Patients who meet these criteria need close clinical monitoring, typically in an intensive care setting. On the basis of severity of illness and response to aggressive medical management, the authors recommend consideration for surgical intervention as described in Box 4. The presence or absence of a hypervirulent strain (if serotyping is available) may impact decision making.

Once the decision has been made to pursue surgical treatment, the operation must be performed in an expeditious and aggressive manner. Removal of the entire colon with preservation of the rectum and end ileostomy should be performed. A segmental colonic resection should not be performed for CDI regardless of the perceived extent of disease.

An anastomosis is not recommended. Because of the need to perform a rapid colectomy and the critical illness of the patient, a laparoscopic colectomy is also not recommended.

In preparation for surgical intervention, invasive cardiopulmonary monitoring with arterial line placement and central venous access is recommended. Aggressive fluid resuscitation is critical. Marking of a site for a planned ileostomy by an enterostomal specialist is ideal but not always immediately possible. The patient should be placed supine on the operating table. The abdomen is prepped and draped widely. A large midline laparotomy incision should be made. The length of the incision should allow for rapid mobilization of the colon. The gross external appearance of the colon can vary from normal to markedly edematous, ischemic, or frankly necrotic. At this point, the surgeon must resist the temptation to perform a

BOX 4: Guidelines for surgery in *Clostridium difficile* infection

Immediate Surgical Intervention
Peritonitis
Perforation
Fulminant colitis
Recalcitrant severe colitis

Surgery, if no Improvement within 12 Hours of Initial Resuscitation
Severe colitis with megacolon
Severe colitis and history of inflammatory bowel disease
Severe colitis and age >65 years

Surgery if no Improvement within 12 to 24 Hours
Severe colitis

Surgical Consultation for Consideration of Surgery within 48 to 72 Hours if no Improvement with Medical Management
Moderate colitis

Modified from Stanley JD, Burns RP: Invited commentary: Clostridium difficile and the surgeon, Am Surg 76(3):235–244, 2010.

less aggressive operation solely on the basis of the appearance of the colon itself. If the diagnosis of CDI is secure and laparotomy is performed, the surgeon should proceed with a total colectomy and end ileostomy. The distal ileum and the rectum can be quickly divided with linear staplers, and the mesentery can be ligated with a clamp and tie technique. Alternatively, bipolar or ultrasonic tissue sealing and cutting devices can be helpful to quickly divide the mesentery and maintain adequate hemostasis. The omentum can be removed from the colon or divided and resected along with colon, whichever is most expeditious. Once the colon has been removed from the abdomen, the distal ileum is brought through an opening in the rectus muscle and fascia and the stoma matured after closure of the midline wound. Rarely, the patient may remain in extremis or the retroperitoneal and bowel edema may preclude closure. In this event, a damage control philosophy may be used. Delayed maturation of the stoma or use of an open abdomen strategy may be necessary to quickly conclude the operation. Stoma reversal may be considered once the patient has recovered fully. Reversal rates are low, ranging from 20% to 35% with a median interval to closure of 234 days.

The mortality after colectomy for CDI has been reported to be 34% to 57% in most series. Likely contributors to this finding include: delays in the initial diagnosis or surgical consultation, poor patient selection, and difficulty predicting the disease course.

Recognition of unacceptably high perioperative mortality has led many surgeons to reconsider whether total colectomy is the best surgical procedure for CDI. An alternative surgical procedure for the treatment of CDI has recently been proposed. A loop ileostomy is constructed (often laparoscopically). The colon is then irrigated with warmed polyethylene glycol 3350/electrolyte solution via the ileostomy. Postoperative antegrade irrigation of vancomycin solution through the ileostomy is continued for 10 days. Early data show improved mortality and high stoma closure rates. Although intriguing, recommendation of this procedure as first-line surgical treatment is premature.

After an operation for CDI, the patient should be taken to the intensive care unit. Although some patients show almost immediate improvement in their condition after removal of the diseased colon, ongoing critical care is necessary to limit morbidity and mortality. Hemodynamic support including vasopressors and large volume fluid resuscitation may be required. Likewise, aggressive treatment of multisystem organ failure may be necessary in the postoperative period.

RECURRENT INFECTION

Recurrence is a major challenge in the treatment of CDI, with reports of rates between 6% and 47% within the first 2 weeks after completion of initial medical treatment. This risk is further increased with each subsequent recurrence. For patients with a first recurrence of CDI, repeated standard dosing regimens of metronidazole or vancomycin are reasonable. Recurrence does not indicate resistance to the initial choice of antibiotic, and therefore, the specific antibiotic chosen for treatment of recurrent disease does not seem to matter in mild cases of CDI. However, in severe cases of first recurrences, oral vancomycin alone or combination therapy to include intravenous metronidazole is recommended. Subsequent recurrences require consideration of additional treatment options, such as tapering and pulsed antibiotic strategies, donor-directed fecal transplantation, and combination or adjunctive drug regimens. Antibiotic tapering is accomplished by decreasing antibiotic dosage over 4 to 6 weeks. Because the spores of *C. difficile* are resistant to antibiotics, pulsed dosing can be added to the end of a taper to allow for residual *C. difficile* spores to germinate. Although published dose-tapering and pulsed strategies may differ slightly, it is generally believed that vancomycin should be the drug of choice in this setting because prolonged use of metronidazole can lead to peripheral neuropathy.

Donor-directed fecal transplant has also been reported to be effective in the treatment of recurrent and recalcitrant CDI. Patients are given a bowel preparation with a polyethylene glycol solution. Two hundred to 300 g of stool from a healthy donor, screened for pathogenic bacteria or transmissible disease, is suspended in 250 mL of saline solution and administered via retention enema daily for 5 days. Alternatively, colonoscopic and nasoenteric tube infusions have also been described with minimal adverse effects. Cure rates in small series are high.

Other suggested drug regimens include fidaxomicin, rifaximin, tigecycline, rifampin, cholestyramine, and monoclonal antibodies. Unfortunately, no one option has shown superiority. Consequently, treatment for recurrent CDI must be individualized based on the number of recurrences, the severity of disease, comorbidities, and available resources. The role of surgical therapy for recurrent CDI has not been established. One can only speculate that novel, less invasive, surgical techniques may spark interest in operative treatment of recurrent CDI.

CLOSTRIDIUM DIFFICILE INFECTION AND INFLAMMATORY BOWEL DISEASE

C. difficile infection is well established to be increased in patients with inflammatory bowel disease (IBD), especially ulcerative colitis (UC). These patients typically experience an increased hospital length of stay, an increased need for surgical intervention, and higher morbidity and mortality independent of the stress of surgical intervention.

Although steroids, debility, frequent use of antibiotics, and episodic hospitalization contribute to CDI in patients with IBD, to what degree other immunomodulators exacerbate the problem is unclear. A diagnostic dilemma can certainly exist because many of the symptoms of IBD can mimic CDI. Therefore, the clinician must check for CDI in patients with worsening or relapsing IBD.

Treatment of CDI in patients with IBD differs little from that in the general population with few exceptions. Oral vancomycin is recommended as first-line therapy, which may be given in combination with intravenous metronidazole in more severe cases. Minimization of corticosteroids and other immunomodulators and broad-spectrum antibiotics is important. There should be a low threshold for total colectomy with ileostomy in patients with severe, fulminant, and persistent CDI.

CONCLUSION

With the increasing incidence and severity of CDI, surgeons will be called on more frequently to manage these often challenging cases. Mitigation of risk factors, early diagnosis, and aggressive treatment must be realized to improve outcomes. A high index of suspicion in those at risk helps the surgeon identify the patient with an early, atypical, or subtle presentation. CDI must be considered in any patient with a history of recent antibiotic use, unexplained abdominal pain, abdominal distention, fever, or leukocytosis, even in the absence of diarrhea.

The mortality rate of those who need surgical intervention remains high. If mortality rates are to improve, there is current consensus, albeit in the absence of significant prospective data, that early and expeditious surgery is of likely benefit and that patients will ideally receive surgical intervention before reaching a fulminant state. It is clear that when the surgeon encounters a patient with CDI who has peritonitis, perforation, or fulminate colitis, the first consideration after resuscitation is to proceed to operative intervention.

Patients with severe CDI whose conditions fail to promptly respond to nonsurgical therapy should also be strongly considered for surgical intervention even in the face of contributing comorbidities. Although total colectomy with ileostomy is the accepted procedure of choice, laparoscopic ileostomy with vancomycin lavage may emerge as a promising treatment option for severe and fulminant CDI.

SUGGESTED READINGS

Bartlett JG: *Clostridium difficile*: progress and challenges, *Ann N Y Acad Sci* 1213:62–69, 2010.

Efron PA, Mazuski JE: *Clostridium difficile* colitis, *Surg Clin North Am* 89:483–500, 2009.

Neal MD, Alverdy JC, Hall DE, et al: Diverting loop ileostomy and colonic lavage: an alternative to total abdominal colectomy for the treatment of severe, complicated *Clostridium difficile* associated disease, *Ann Surg* 254(3):423–427, 2011.

Stanley JD, Burns RP: Invited commentary: *Clostridium difficile* and the surgeon, *Am Surg* 76(3):235–244, 2010.

LARGE BOWEL
OBSTRUCTION

**Joseph E. Bornstein, MD, MBA, and
David L. Berger, MD**

OVERVIEW

Large bowel obstruction is defined as an intestinal obstruction that begins distal to the ileocecal valve. Surgery is the definitive therapy for most causes of large bowel obstruction. Morbidity and mortality rates can be as high as 46% and 18%, respectively, but vary depending on the etiology and patient characteristics.

Large bowel obstruction may be partial or complete (no passage of stool or flatus). The etiology can be intrinsic or extrinsic to the colon and mechanical or adynamic. These causes can include neoplasms, inflammatory lesions, ischemia, hernias, volvulus, intussusception, endometriosis, pseudoobstruction, and foreign body/fecal impaction. Box 1 provides a list of common causes of large bowel obstruction. The most common mechanical cause of large bowel obstruction is colorectal carcinoma, followed by diverticulitis and volvulus. A common adynamic cause of large bowel obstruction is acute colonic pseudoobstruction (Ogilvie's syndrome). Ogilvie's syndrome is often found in association with a wide variety of medical and surgical illnesses.

Accurate diagnosis and therapeutic planning require a thoughtful collection of the history, the physical examination, and pertinent laboratory and radiologic studies. Epidemiologic factors, surgical history, and the physical examination can often suggest a specific cause. Examination for abdominal wall or inguinal hernias is a must, as is a rectal examination and fecal occult blood test. The exact treatment varies based on the location of the obstruction, the mechanism of obstruction, the viability of the bowel, and goals of care.

Immediate management should include attainment of adequate intravenous (IV) access and IV fluid hydration. Fever, tachycardia, or hypotension may indicate systemic toxicity or hypovolemia. Vital signs and urine output should be monitored for endpoints of resuscitation. A nasogastric tube should be inserted, and in most cases, antibiotics should be started and blood cultures drawn.

The goals of further evaluation are to assess the degree of physiologic derangement and identify characteristics of the obstructing lesion. Useful laboratory tests include a complete blood cell count (CBC) and chemistry panel, which can reveal evidence of inflammation, bleeding, electrolyte disorders, and dehydration. An upright chest x-ray can be obtained to look for free intraperitoneal air. Computed tomographic (CT) scan is the imaging modality of choice for patients with a clinical suspicion of obstruction. CT scans can further demonstrate carcinomatosis, liver metastases, and ascites when advanced malignant disease is present.

OBSTRUCTIONS AS A RESULT OF CANCER

Colorectal cancer is the third most common cancer in the United States, representing 9% of all cancer deaths. Furthermore, 15% of colorectal cancers present as a surgical emergency. The most common symptom of a large bowel obstruction from malignancy is abdominal distention. Additional aspects of the history to obtain include recent weight loss, change in bowel habits, change in stool consistency, recent passage of flatus, nausea, and emesis. Because of the distal focus of obstruction, nausea and vomiting are late findings, especially if the vomit is stercoraceous. Chronic symptoms may represent evidence of a process that has evolved over time, and the patient may report a prolonged history of altered bowel movements. Older patients who present with acute malignant large bowel obstruction often have not had any recent colonoscopic evaluations (Figure 1).

Partial obstruction that does not require urgent surgical intervention may initially be managed with nasogastric decompression and resuscitation. This may allow added surgical planning and staging and allow for a single-stage procedure if possible.

Surgical planning in the event of complete malignant obstruction depends on the viability of bowel, the location of obstruction, the resectability of the tumor, and the goals of care. Patients may either go straight to surgery or pursue nonsurgical, palliative options. Nonsurgical therapy has evolved for malignant obstruction since the introduction of stents in 1991. Stents have been successfully applied for palliation where surgery should be avoided. A stent can also be used as a temporizing measure to allow for preoperative bowel preparation or physiologic correction. The data on the utility of bowel preparation, however, are lacking. Table 1 shows the results of a recent meta-analysis by van Hooft and associates that compares

---

BOX 1: Common causes of large bowel obstruction

- Neoplasm
  - Colorectal origin
  - Local noncolonic origin with tissue invasion or compression
  - Metastatic
- Volvulus: cecal, sigmoid
- Inflammatory-mediated
  - Diverticulitis
  - Acute
  - Chronic: stricture
  - Crohn's disease
  - Radiation
- Hernias
  - Inguinal or abdominal wall
  - Internal
- Intussusception
- Adynamic: Ogilvie's syndrome
- Ischemic stricture
- Foreign body
- Fecal impaction

---

emergency surgery with temporizing colonic stenting followed by resection for acute left-sided obstruction. As shown, no significant difference was seen in the number of adverse events or mortality when used as a bridge to surgery versus proceeding directly to surgery.

The most compelling indication for stenting in colorectal cancer is for palliation. This allows the patient to avoid a colostomy in the presence of unresectable disease or advanced cancer. Stoma creation, however, remains the gold standard. Stents should not be performed in patients who have evidence of peritonitis, perforation, or ischemia. Placement of the stent requires that a catheter can cross the obstructed point. This is successful in greater than 90% of cases by experienced operators with experience greater than 20 cases. Complications from the procedure can include colonic perforation, stent migration, and stent obstruction. The use of stents appears to be safe; however, they confer no advantage to morbidity or mortality and have a lower overall success rate at relieving obstruction, based on a recent Cochrane review. One clear advantage of stents is decreased length of hospital stay and possibly decreased overall cost.

Patients who have a resectable lesion are managed with surgery. Multiple surgical options exist, and considerable advancement has taken place to decrease patient morbidity over the last 30 years. Right-sided lesions have been a matter of little debate and are best managed with a single-stage segmental colectomy. With regard to left-sided lesions, historically, a two-stage or three-stage procedure has been performed; however, when possible, a single-stage procedure is preferable and has shown to be safe and effective. Morbidity and mortality appear equivalent when a single-stage operation is performed when compared with a staged procedure. In fact, single-stage operations appear to be equally successful on both right-sided and left-sided colonic lesions.

The extent of resection has been a matter of debate. For right-sided lesions, segmental resection is appropriate. In the case of left-sided obstruction, segmental resection should be performed unless concern exists for proximal bowel viability or additional areas of colon with lesions of concern. In that event, subtotal colectomy is appropriate. Some have advocated that subtotal colectomy is the preferred operation, arguing that synchronous tumors have been found in up to 11% of patients and that the addition of on-table lavage is onerous. Current data do not support the need to remove additional colon without cause. Concern amongst surgeons about performing primary anastomosis in unprepped bowel led to the use of intraoperative colonic lavage. On-table lavage of the colon is often time consuming and caries additional risk of spillage. Some have

---

FIGURE 1 **A** and **B**, Obstructing sigmoid colon cancer. *(Courtesy of Harisinghani Mukesh, MD, MGH Radiology.)*

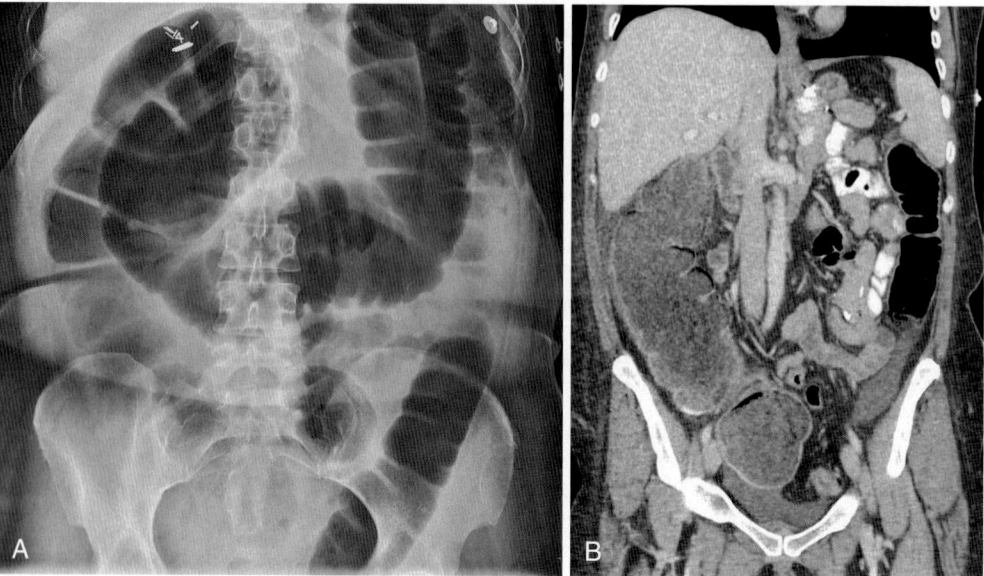

TABLE 1: Colonic stenting versus emergency surgery: morbidity, mortality and stoma rates

	Colonic stenting (N = 47)	Emergency surgery (N = 51)	Absolute risk difference (95% CI)	Relative risk (95% CI)	P value
Mortality					
30-Day mortality	5	5	−0.01 (−0.14-0.12)	0.92 (0.28-2.98)	0.89
Overall mortality	9	9	−0.02 (−0.17-0.14)	0.92 (0.40-2.12)	0.84
Morbidity	25	23	−0.08 (−0.27-0.11)	0.85 (0.57-1.27)	0.43
Stoma Rates					
Directly after initial intervention	24	38	0.23 (0.04-0.40)	1.46 (1.06-2.01)	0.016
At latest follow-up	27	34	0.09 (−0.10-0.27)	1.16 (0.85-1.59)	0.35

CI, Confidence interval.

From van Hooft JE, Bemelman WA, Breumelhof R, et al: Colonic stenting versus emergency surgery for acute left-sided malignant colonic obstruction: a multicentre randomised trial, Lancet Oncol 12(4):344-352, 2011.

omitted this step and use manual decompression with equivalent outcomes. Furthermore, if the patient is in extremis, on-table lavage is not recommended.

After primary anastomosis, some surgeons perform a protective loop ileostomy to decrease the chance of leak at the anastomosis; however, the need for an additional procedure is not without added morbidity and removes some of the benefit of a single-stage operation.

When patients are ill, it may be necessary to perform resection and diversion or even simply divert alone as an initial operation followed by colonic resection at an additional procedure. Principles of damage control hold true in this circumstance and should guide operative planning in the unstable condition.

OBSTRUCTIONS AS A RESULT OF INFLAMMATION

Obstructions from inflammation may be secondary to an active process (acute diverticulitis) or chronic inflammation and fibrosis. The management of inflammatory mediated strictures continues to evolve. Patients with strictures from diverticulitis, Crohn's disease, or radiation colitis or at points of prior anastomoses have been treated both operatively and nonoperatively with colonic stents. Patients with chronic strictures often present with signs and symptoms consistent with a partial obstruction or constipation.

In the case of acute diverticulitis, patients may undergo an attempt at nonoperative management in the absence of hemodynamic instability and purulent or feculent peritonitis. A history of episodes of diverticulitis is highly suggestive of the diagnosis. A CBC may reveal leukocytosis. CT scan shows a transition point in the colon in the area of diverticulitis. A nasogastric tube should be placed, and IV antibiotics started. If the obstruction fails to improve, or the patient's condition begins to deteriorate, a Hartmann's procedure may be necessary. Malignancy must always be a concern, and ideally, colonoscopic biopsies should be taken at a later date if the patient is managed nonoperatively.

When an operation is required, there can be significant inflammation around the sigmoid colon. Surgery can be hazardous because difficult dissection may increase the risk of iatrogenic injury to adjacent structures, such as the ureter. Temporary loop colostomy may be necessary under these circumstances.

Chronic colonic strictures may be sequelae of prior episodes of diverticulitis, pelvic radiation, or prior bowel anastomoses. Generally, these patients present with chronic constipation and partial obstructive symptoms. Under most circumstances, patients should undergo

evaluation to rule out malignancy and subsequently undergo an elective resection. Alternatively, the use of colonic stents for benign colorectal obstructions is increasing. At this time, limited data exist on its long-term efficacy and morbidity; and most studies have a small sample size. The most common benign indications for stenting are anastomotic stricture and diverticular stricture. Patients may benefit from preoperative optimization, and the stent may be used as a bridge to surgery to allow time for inflammation to resolve or physiology to improve. Alternatively, some moderately long-term results have been obtained on select patients who either are unsuitable candidates for operative resection or have refused surgery. Keranen and colleagues reported a success rate of 75% (16 of 21 cases) in clinical relief of obstruction. Unfortunately, 43% of patients experienced a complication. A significant number of the complications were from delayed perforation presenting greater than 4 weeks after stent placement. Complication rates for colonic stenting in benign disease appear higher than their malignant counterpart. The effectiveness in diverticular strictures also appears somewhat limited. Seventy percent of patients in this trial treated for diverticular stricture ultimately underwent surgical therapy. Stenting may play a role as a temporizing solution for elective repair. However, stenting should not be viewed as a definitive or long term solution for patients with benign disease.

OBSTRUCTIONS AS A RESULT OF COLONIC VOLVULUS

Acute colonic volvulus is the third most common cause of mechanical bowel obstruction after cancer and diverticulitis. Volvulus generally involves the cecum or sigmoid colon when the colon twists around its mesenteric blood supply. Sigmoid volvulus is the most common and tends to occur in elderly patients with chronic constipation. In contrast, cecal volvulus generally occurs in younger individuals.

The clinical presentation includes rapid onset of abdominal distention, pain, nausea, and vomiting. Patients may present with significant bowel ischemia that leads to perforation and peritonitis. Plain x-rays are potentially sufficient to make the diagnosis. An abdominal x-ray can show classic findings, such as a "bent inner tube" or "coffee bean sign," which are consistent with sigmoid volvulus. Cecal volvulus shows a twisted cecum in the left upper quadrant of the plain abdominal x-ray. When the diagnosis is in doubt, a CT scan may be obtained and often shows a characteristic "whirl sign," in which the mesentery twists around the vascular supply (Figure 2).

In the absence of peritonitis or perforation, sigmoid volvulus should initially be treated with colonoscopic detorsion and decompression. A rectal tube is subsequently placed for continued rectal decompression. Historically, bowel preparation was performed preoperatively, but it may not be necessary as described for other elective colonic resections. In the event of a successful detorsion, a single-stage resection and primary anastomosis is performed during the same admission. Failure to perform a definitive operation results in a high recurrence rate. In one study, up to 86% of patients treated with decompression alone recurred, which in some cases required emergency surgery. The mortality rate of nonoperative management was significantly higher than for patients treated operatively for all American Society of Anesthesiologists (ASA) classes, suggesting that nonoperative management is inferior.

In the setting of peritonitis, blood per rectum, free intraperitoneal air, signs of sepsis, or failure of endoscopic decompression, the patient should be taken to the operating room for emergency resection. Resection with colostomy may be necessary with peritoneal contamination, ischemic-appearing bowel, or hemodynamic instability. Otherwise, the patient may undergo primary resection and anastomosis. A study comparing patients with uncomplicated sigmoid volvulus who underwent Hartmann's procedure alone, Hartmann's plus colostomy closure, and primary anastomosis of uncomplicated sigmoid volvulus showed no significant difference in morbidity or mortality across the three surgical groups. A 5% rate of stoma complications was observed in addition to the added burden and cost of a second procedure.

The purpose of resection after successful detorsion is therefore to prevent recurrence and more complicated presentation necessitating emergency surgery. Some reports of percutaneous-endoscopic sigmoidopexy have been performed, but long-term studies and large series are lacking at this time.

Unlike sigmoid volvulus, surgery is the immediate definitive therapy for cecal volvulus. The multiple surgical options include resection, detorsion alone, or detorsion with cecopexy. Table 2 details the results of a retrospective review of a large series of patients with cecal volvulus. Simple surgical detorsion with or without cecopexy has been performed with some success but result in a high rate of recurrence. Given improvements in perioperative care since this review, the morbidity of right colectomy with primary ileocolic anastmosis is significantly lessened and offers the best chance of definitive cure from recurrence.

OBSTRUCTIONS AS A RESULT OF INTUSSUSCEPTION

The workup and initial treatment for intussusception is similar to that of other causes of large bowel obstruction. Patients with colonic intussusception present more commonly with melena or guaiac-positive stool and less so with abdominal pain, nausea, and vomiting relative to the small bowel counterpart. In a small proportion of patients, a palpable abdominal mass is evident. CT scan is the most useful diagnostic test, but up to one fourth of cases are diagnosed in the operating room. CT scan often shows a target-shaped area of colon that represents the intussusceptum in the center surrounded by the intussuscipiens (Figure 3).

Unlike the pediatric equivalent, a significant portion of intussusceptions in adults are caused by a malignant focus. Colonic intussusceptions have been found to be malignant in up to 43% of cases. Surgical resection along lymphatic drainage without reduction is the preferred treatment. Right-sided lesions can be repaired with primary anastomosis, whereas left-sided lesions historically have been repaired in two stages with a Hartmann's procedure and subsequent colostomy takedown. A single operation is feasible for left-sided lesions given the outcomes in similar large bowel obstruction cases in the absence of contamination.

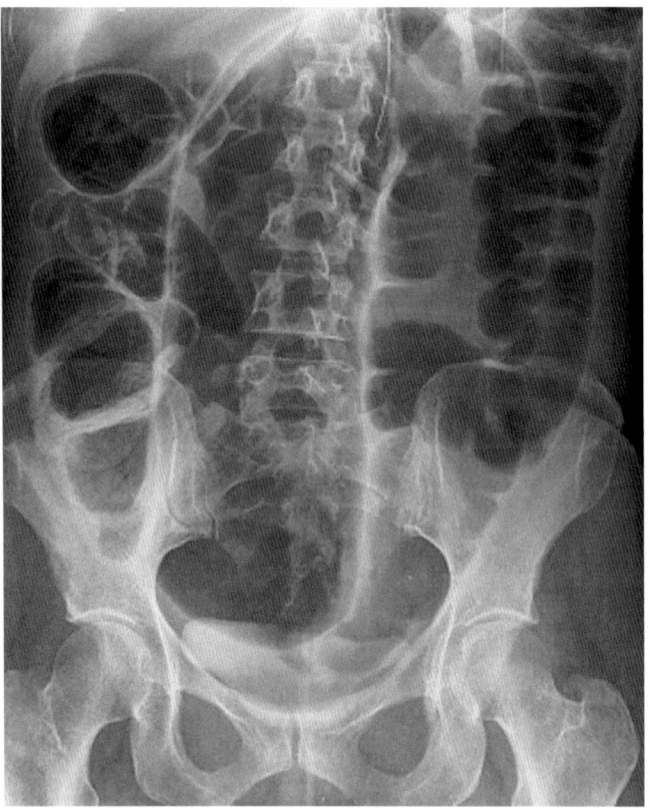

FIGURE 2 Sigmoid volvulus. *(Courtesy of Harisinghani Mukesh, MD, MGH Radiology.)*

TABLE 2: Morbidity and mortality after operation for cecal volvulus

Operation	Percent	Abdominal complications (%)	Wound complications (%)	Mortality (%)	Recurrence (%)
Cecopexy	32	8	7	10	13
Detorsion	25	9	6	13	12
Resection	25	16	13	22	–
Cecostomy	16	25	27	32	14

From Rabinovici, Simansky DA, Kaplan O, et al: Surgical treatment and results in 561 patients with cecal volvulus (1959-1989), Dis Colon Rect 33(9):765-769, 1990.

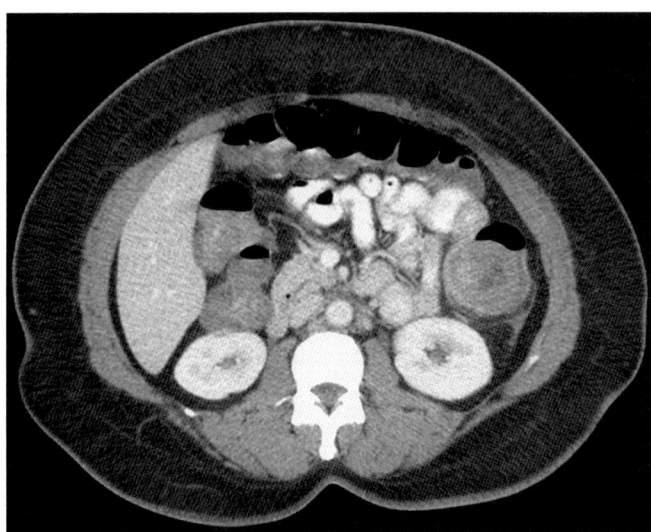

FIGURE 3 Descending colonic intussusceptions.

OBSTRUCTIONS AS A RESULT OF HERNIA

Abdominal wall and inguinal hernias should be sought out on the clinical examination. If an incarcerated hernia is the cause of large bowel obstruction, the patient should be taken to the operating room for reduction, assessment of bowel viability, and possible resection. For an incarcerated inguinal hernia, if the bowel appears viable before surgery, a groin incision may be performed in standard fashion. With signs of perforation or ischemia, a midline laparotomy should be performed in anticipation of resection. Avoidance of non-biologic materials is required when bowel is resected. Internal hernias have been reported in the literature and are diagnosed largely with cross-sectional imaging or at the time of surgery.

OBSTRUCTIONS AS A RESULT OF OGILVIE'S SYNDROME (PSEUDOOBSTRUCTION)

Patients with colonic pseudoobstruction often have a variety of preceding medical conditions, and occurs with increased frequency in the elderly population. The exact mechanism of visceral dilation in pseudoobstruction is not clear. Massive dilation of the large bowel can result in ischemia and perforation, which is an urgent indication for operative intervention. After resuscitative measures have been taken, and potentially offending agents (narcotics, anticholinergics) have been stopped, IV neostigmine has been used with moderate success. Side effects of neostigmine must be carefully observed, including nausea, vomiting, bradycardia, bronchospasm, and hypotension. Atropine should be available, and the patient should be placed on telemetry during administration. Colonoscopic decompression can be performed with significant risk in the unprepped bowel. If these options fail to resolve the obstruction, the patient should undergo definitive operation. Endoscopic stoma placement in either the left or right colon has been performed, but the risks are high. Operative intervention can include a venting stoma if the bowel is viable. Otherwise, segmental or subtotal colectomy may be necessary. If medical therapy is successful, some data suggest that administration of polyethylene glycol helps maintain remission and prevent early recurrence.

CONCLUSION

The principles and treatment of large bowel obstruction have evolved over the last 20 years. Appropriate resuscitation should begin in the emergency department. The specific intervention is dependent on the cause and location of the obstruction in addition to the viability of the bowel. In most cases, when resection is necessary, a single-stage operation is preferable and can be performed safely without added morbidity. In cases of advanced cancer, a loop colostomy may be necessary. In some palliative and benign circumstances, the use of colonic stents is evolving and should be considered where available.

SUGGESTED READINGS

Akcan A, Akyildiz H, Artis T, et al: Feasibility of single-stage resection and primary anastamosis with acute noncomplicated sigmoid volvulus, *Am J Surg* 193:421–426, 2007.
Ansaloni, Andersson RE, Bazzoli F, et al: Guidelines in the management of obstructing cancer of the left colon: Consensus Conference of the World Society of Emergency Surgery and Peritoneum and Surgery Society, *World J Emerg Surg* 5:29, 2010.
Azar T, Berger D: Adult intussusception, *Ann Surg* 226(2):134–138, 1997.
Keranen I, Lepistö A, Udd M, et al: Outcome of patients after endoluminal stent placement for benign colorectal obstruction, *Scand J Gastroenterol* 45:725–731, 2010.
Sagar J: Colorectal stents for the management of malignant colonic obstructions, *Cochrane Database of Systematic Reviews* 2011, Issue 11.

COLONIC STENTING

Patrick I. Okolo III, MD, MPH, FASGE, and Joanna K. Law, MD, MA (Ed)

INTRODUCTION

Colonic obstruction, whether of neoplastic or nonneoplastic origin, can result in significant morbidity, including hypovolemic or septic shock, acute renal or multiorgan failure, perforation, and peritonitis.

Between 10% and 30% of patients with colorectal cancer present with impending or complete obstruction, which is traditionally treated with emergency surgery, which itself is associated with significant rates of perioperative and postoperative morbidity and mortality. Predictors of death include older age, a higher grade obstruction according to the American Society of Anesthesiologist (ASA), metastatic or locally advanced disease, and emergency surgery for obstruction.

In an otherwise healthy patient presenting with acute obstruction, surgical management typically involves colonic resection and primary anastomosis with or without a diverting stoma. In the patient with comorbid conditions, decompression of the obstruction with a diverting colostomy is often the first of a multistaged approach that, when possible, will subsequently include colonic resection and reconnection. With the advent of self-expandable metal stents (SEMS), a minimally invasive alternative to emergency surgery became available to relieve colorectal obstruction. Colorectal stenting has become an effective, nonoperative, immediate means of colonic decompression that, in turn, may allow for patients to proceed to a more elective bowel resection.

At present, there are two major indications for colonic stenting in patients with colorectal cancer: (1) palliation of advanced disease that is otherwise nonoperative and (2) decompression in patients as a "bridge" to surgical resection. In the latter indication, surgical intervention in a patient at high risk can be avoided, and the patient's medical condition can be optimized before either a laparoscopic or open procedure for definitive management.

Although the role of SEMS is very well accepted in the palliative situation, the use of SEMS as a bridge in patients with acute colonic obstruction has been controversial because of the associated costs and possible complications associated with SEMS. However, several studies have demonstrated a cost savings in patients who undergo stenting as a bridge to surgery. Other observed benefits of stenting as a bridge to surgery are (1) the opportunity for patients to undergo a full bowel evaluation to rule out a synchronous lesion either endoscopically or radiologically and (2) enabling some patients to receive systemic chemotherapy and thereby downgrade liver metastases.

Colonic stenting, however, is not without risk. In a multicenter study from the Netherlands, patients with incurable left-sided colorectal cancer were randomly assigned to either a surgical or nonsurgical treatment condition in which the latter was colonic stenting. However, this study closed early because of a high number of serious adverse events in the patients in the nonsurgical condition, with six perforations, of which at least two were directly attributable to the stent. Other complications of colonic stenting include stent migration and occlusion, which may result in recurrent obstruction.

Over the years, as endoscopists have gained experience with colonic stent placement in the malignant setting, its use and indications have expanded to nonneoplastic causes of colonic obstruction, including benign strictures, such as those in diverticulitis, and disturbance of luminal integrity by fistulizing diseases such as inflammatory bowel disease (Box 1). In an institution with endoscopic, radiologic, and surgical support, the use of SEMS for colonic obstruction can be performed safely and with good outcomes for the appropriate indications.

TECHNIQUE

Enteral stents are generally self-expandable, preconstrained tubular meshwork devices usually made of nitinol, and they may be uncovered or covered. In the Unites States, most commercially available stents are uncovered stents. Endoscopic insertion of stents in colorectal obstruction is best accomplished with stents that can be placed "through the scope" (TTS). The most commonly used stents in the United States are available in 60-mm, 90-mm, and 120-mm lengths, with internal diameters of 20 and 22 mm. The TTS stent can be inserted via the accessory channel of a therapeutic endoscope, thus enabling precise placement under endoscopic visualization (Figure 1).

Another delivery mechanism that is too large to enable passage through the working channel of the therapeutic endoscope is one in which the stent is delivered alongside the endoscope or under fluoroscopic visualization. These stents are often made from nitinol and are available in lengths of 57, 87, and 117 mm, with internal diameters in the range of 18 to 25 mm. The advantages of these stents are limited in comparison with the TTS stents, and the decision to use these stents should be driven by the clinical circumstances along with the input of an expert endoscopist.

Preprocedure imaging is very helpful but not an absolute requirement in certain situations in which the clinical acuity may not allow for safe and extensive imaging. When appropriate, a water-soluble contrast enema study or abdominal/pelvic computed tomographic scan with rectal contrast medium should be performed to demonstrate the length, course, and mural complexity of the obstruction and thus facilitate in preprocedural planning (Figure 2). These studies may be particularly useful in ruling out synchronous sites of obstruction proximal to an identified colorectal stricture and may indicate the need for additional or different intervention.

Patient Preparation

Rectal enemas can be used in patients with complete obstruction to clear the field of view. In patients with incomplete obstruction, an

---

BOX 1: Indications for colonic stent placement

Benign Disease
- Treatment of colonic mural integrity in certain colonic fistula
- Treatment of selected refractory benign strictures

Malignant Disease
- Acute decompression of colonic obstruction before surgical resection
- Palliation of colonic obstruction in advanced disease

FIGURE 1   A, Nearly complete obstruction of the proximal rectum by tumor. **B,** After deployment of self-expandable metal stents (SEMS).

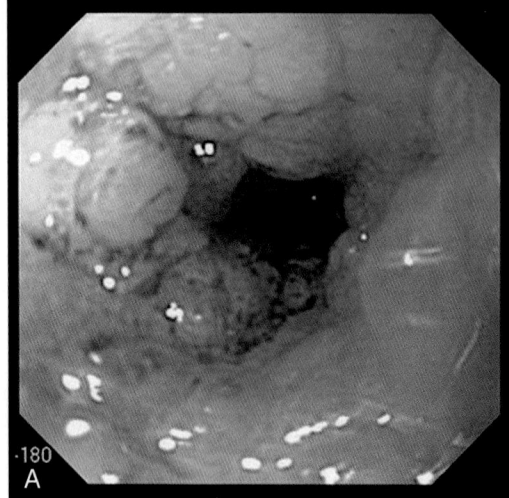
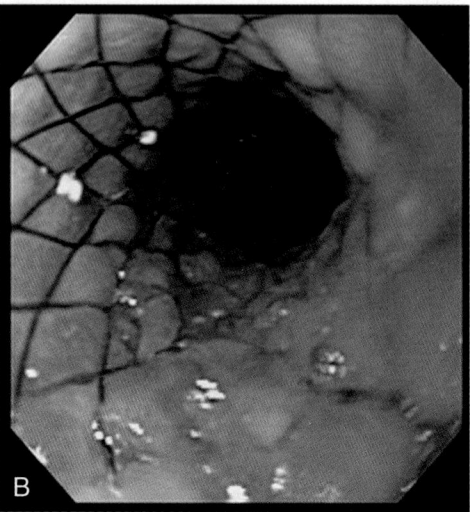

oral electrolyte solution can be used, especially if the lesion is proximal to the splenic flexure. Low-volume polyethylene glycol solutions are favored in this setting. It is prudent to administer antibiotics prophylactically to minimize the entry of procedure-associated bacteremia. When available, carbon dioxide insufflation (rather than air) should be used for these procedures because it reduces the consequences of barotrauma.

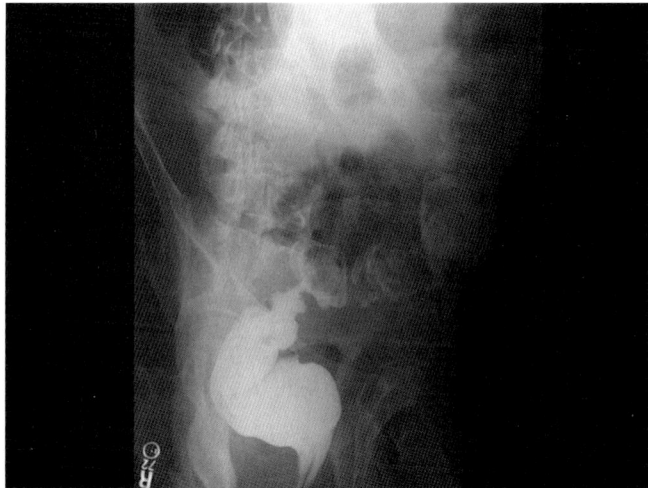

FIGURE 2   Computed tomographic study with water-soluble contrast enema, demonstrating a 4-cm length of narrowing in the distal rectosigmoid colon.

Endoscopic Delivery

A therapeutic endoscope is often used for these procedures and advanced to the point at which the most distal aspect of the lesion is visualized. It is often not necessary or prudent to traverse the lesion with the endoscope. A guidewire is then advanced through the endoscope and traverses the lesion under fluoroscopic or endoscopic visualization, or both. The caliber, length, and course of the obstruction can then be demonstrated with the aid of contrast medium. This step allows the endoscopist to choose the appropriate stent. If the intent is to place a TTS stent, the stent is then passed through the accessory channel of the endoscope over the guidewire; the surgeon must take time to traverse the lesion appropriately. If the intent is to place a stent nonendoscopically, the endoscope is removed, and the guidewire is left in place. The stent is then placed over the guidewire under fluoroscopic or endoscopic guidance (the endoscope is reinserted and passed alongside the guidewire to allow visualization). The stent is then deployed carefully with the intent of positioning the fully deployed stent ideally 2 cm above and below the stricture. The "waist" (narrowest, not fully expanded portion) of the stent should optimally be in the middle of the stent/stent assembly (Figure 3). It may be necessary to use multiple, overlapping stents to achieve this technical goal.

Proximal Lesions and Stent Delivery

The use of colonic stents for the treatment of proximal lesions is less well described, as many patients with these lesions proceed to surgery, and because of concerns about the safety of SEMS in the right side of the colon. In one series of 82 patients, Yao and associates (2011)

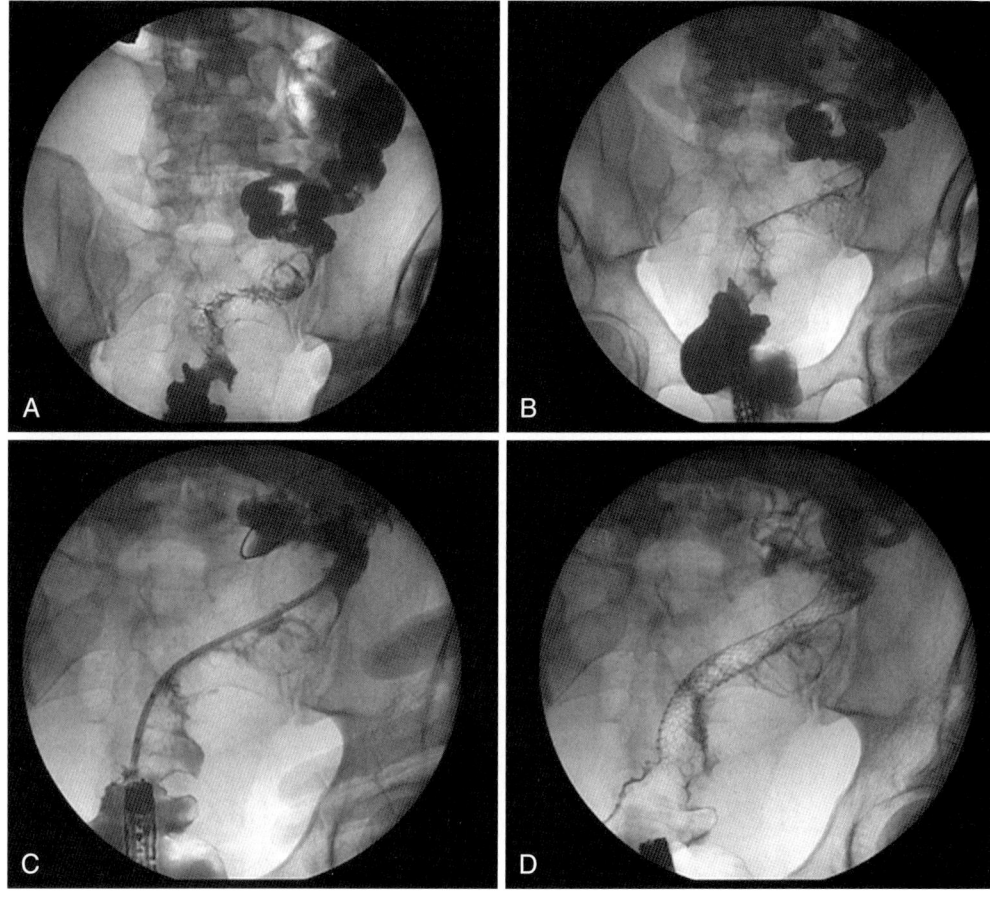

FIGURE 3   **A,** A contrast enema study performed with endoscopic and fluoroscopic visualization. **B,** Advancement of the guidewire traversing the stricture. **C,** "Through the scope" (TTS) stent bridging the stricture. **D,** Deployment of the stent across the stricture; contrast medium is observed flowing from the proximal colon.

described improved immediate outcomes among patients who underwent stent placement for obstructing lesions in the ascending colon, hepatic flexure, and transverse colon. Many patients in this series proceeded to surgical resection after stent decompression, which demonstrates the possibility of a sequential approach to colonic obstruction proximal to the left side of the colon.

Postplacement Care

The prevention of stent impaction by inspissated stool is the major thrust of care after the placement of a colonic stent. Patients should be instructed to avoid high-fiber foods. Polyethylene glycol powder may be used to titrate to a clinical response and is a useful agent in the management of patients to prevent impaction.

COMPLICATIONS

Stent-related perforation and migration are the two most worrisome common complications associated with stenting and are reported at rates of 2% to 5% and 4% to 9%, respectively. Abdominal pain after stent placement is often transient; bleeding occurs infrequently and is usually self-limited unless related to the primary tumor.

Perforations can occur immediately during or after the procedure but can be a delayed occurrence, especially when a large-caliber stent with high radial force is used. Perforations are more likely to occur in the sigmoid colon, where angulation and redundancy make stent deployment technically challenging. Experienced endoscopists are sensitive to the vulnerability of the left side of the colon to this manner of perforation and are able to mitigate these technical issues. In the systematic review by Cirocchi and colleagues (2013), perforation rates for the three included studies were in the range of those reported in previous studies, although two of the randomized controlled trials in this analysis were prematurely discontinued because of high rates of perforation. Several factors have been attributed to higher risks for perforation; patient-related factors include previous radiation therapy and certain types of chemotherapy, and procedure-related factors include predilation with a balloon before stent deployment.

According to anecdotal reports, radiation therapy appears to be a predisposition to stent-related perforation; however, the data to support this suspicion are limited. Use of the angiogenesis inhibitor bevacizumab may be associated with an increased risk of stent-related perforation. In a retrospective study, patients with stents who received bevacizumab appeared to be at higher risk for perforation (odds ratio: 20; 95% confidence interval: 5.9 to 65). Although these data are emerging, it is prudent to use stents with caution in patients receiving bevacizumab or when its use is being contemplated.

Stent migration tends to occur within the first 5 to 7 days after stent placement. Factors that promote migration include suboptimal length of stent/stent assembly, small-caliber stents, and a nonobstructing lesion. Migration may occur after oncologic or debulking therapy. In the study by Vanbiervliet and associates (2013), fully covered SEMS were used for benign strictures. The authors reported a high rate of migration (63%) but, interestingly, did not demonstrate any reduction in the efficacy rate of the stent or the recurrence rate of obstructive symptoms.

Stent failure is defined as the inability of the stent to restore luminal patency and may occur immediately after stent placement or in a delayed manner after tumor recurrence or overgrowth. Immediate stent failure may be related to mismatch between stent length and stricture length, peritoneal carcinomatosis, associated intestinal hypomotility, multifocal strictures, and early stent migration. The rate of immediate stent failure can be as high as 12% of patients in the immediate postprocedure period; the most common reason is a very tight "waist" in the stent that results in no resolution of obstructive symptoms. Pelvic computed tomographic scan with rectal contrast medium or a barium enema is essential for the evaluation of stent failure. Reintervention is often necessary to achieve luminal patency in situations in which the stent is occluded.

Stent occlusion after a period of relief may denote late recurrence of obstruction and may be caused by tumor overgrowth or by luminal compromise through the stent as a result of ingrowth. Endoscopic reintervention often involves placing another stent through the original stent or restoring luminal patency by tissue ablation (usually by argon plasma coagulation and less commonly by laser debulking).

Experienced endoscopists achieve a rate of technical success higher than 90% and a low rate of procedure-associated complications. Caution and procedural modification in patients at higher risk help minimize complications. These risk factors include:

1. The presence of multifocal obstruction
2. Extrinsic compression rather than intraluminal disease
3. Strictures longer than 10 cm
4. Use of certain chemotherapeutic agents (e.g., bevacizumab).

OUTCOMES

The bulk of experience with stents in the colon has been in the relief of left-sided colonic obstruction. Published reports have traversed all levels of evidence, including pooled/systematic analyses. From pooled analysis, these studies demonstrate technical success rates that range from 66% to 100%, with a median of 94%, and clinical success rates that range from 55% to 100%, with a median of 91% in patients undergoing colonic stenting for palliative indication. Ho and colleagues (2012) randomly assigned 39 patients with acute left-sided malignant colonic obstruction to undergo stenting, followed by elective colon resection, or to immediate emergency surgical resection. They noted no differences in mortality; however, there were significantly less stoma formations and postsurgical complications in the group who underwent stenting. The number of days spent in the intensive care unit was also significantly less in the stent recipients. Stent migration occurred in 11% of patients, and approximately 20% of patients required reintervention to reestablish luminal patency. In a systematic review of the 14 studies, Watt and associates (2007), using a survival analysis approach, found that the duration of luminal patency ranged from 68 to 288 days, with a median of 106 days. Perforations occurred in 4% of patients overall, but the rate was greater than 75% in some studies. The wide range of outcomes highlights the heterogeneity of outcomes in these studies.

SUMMARY

Successful stent placement for colonic obstruction relies upon various patient and technical factors. In patients with nonoperative malignant obstruction, more than 75% obtain successful relief of obstruction, although tumor ingrowth, stent migration, and stent-related complications may necessitate endoscopic reintervention. Stenting is favored over surgical intervention in patients presenting with incurable, malignant colonic obstruction caused by intraluminal disease with poor performance status, multiple comorbid conditions, and a colonic stricture of less than 10 cm in length. Conversely, stenting should be used with caution in patients with multifocal or long (>10 cm) strictures or extraluminal compression that results in obstruction. Concomitant or planned use of bevacizumab and possibly radiation treatment should temper the enthusiasm for stents, and full consideration should be given to alternatives so as to optimize palliative outcomes.

Stenting for acute malignant colorectal obstruction is an important option for patients with obstructing colorectal cancer, and its use for patients with nonmalignant obstruction is evolving.

SUGGESTED READINGS

Cennamo V, Fuccio L, Mutri V, et al: Does stent placement for advanced colon cancer increase the risk of perforation during bevacizumab-based therapy? *Clin Gastroenterol Hepatol* 7:1174–1176, 2009.

Cirocchi R, Farinella E, Trastulli S, et al: Safety and efficacy of endoscopic colonic stenting as a bridge to surgery in the management of intestinal obstruction due to left colon and rectal cancer: a systematic review and meta-analysis, *Surg Oncol* 22:14–21, 2013.

Ho KS, Quah HM, Lim JF, et al: Endoscopic stenting and elective surgery versus emergency surgery for left-sided malignant colonic obstruction: a prospective randomized trial, *Int J Colorectal Dis* 27:355–362, 2012.

Leitman IM, Sullivan JD, Brams D, et al: Multivariate analysis of morbidity and mortality from the initial surgical management of obstructing carcinoma of the colon, *Surg Gynecol Obstet* 174:513–518, 1992.

Pirlet IA, Slim K, Kwiatkowski F, et al: Emergency preoperative stenting versus surgery for acute left-sided malignant colonic obstruction: a multicenter randomized controlled trial, *Surg Endosc* 25:1814–1821, 2011.

Targownik LE, Spiegel BM, Sack J, et al: Colonic stent vs. emergency surgery for management of acute left-sided malignant colonic obstruction: a decision analysis, *Gastrointest Endosc* 60:865–874, 2004.

van Hooft JE, Fockens P, Marinelli AW, et al: Early closure of a multicenter randomized clinical trial of endoscopic stenting versus surgery for stage IV left-sided colorectal cancer, *Endoscopy* 40:184–191, 2008.

Vanbiervliet G, Bichard P, Demarquay JF, et al: Fully covered self-expanding metal stents for benign colonic strictures, *Endoscopy* 45:35–41, 2013.

Watt AM, Faragher IG, Griffin TT, et al: Self-expanding metallic stents for relieving malignant colorectal obstruction: a systematic review, *Ann Surg* 246:24–30, 2007.

Yao LQ, Zhong YS, Xu MD, et al: Self-expanding metallic stents drainage for acute proximal colon obstruction, *World J Gastroenterol* 17:3342–3346, 2011.

ACUTE COLONIC PSEUDO-OBSTRUCTION (OGILVIE'S SYNDROME)

Smrita Sinha, MD, and David M. Cromwell, MD

INTRODUCTION

Acute colonic pseudo-obstruction, also known as Ogilvie's syndrome, is a disorder defined by colonic distention in the absence of mechanical obstruction. It was first reported by Sir William Heneage Ogilvie in 1948. Although the exact pathogenesis of acute colonic pseudo-obstruction is unknown, the disruption of normal colonic motility is hypothesized to result in massive distention and symptoms of obstruction. Resulting complications of ischemia or perforation can be associated with mortality rates that exceed 40%.

PRESENTATION AND DIAGNOSIS

The diagnosis of acute colonic pseudo-obstruction is based on clinical presentation combined with abdominal radiographs that confirm colonic distention. Clinical features include abdominal distention, abdominal pain (80%), and nausea or vomiting (60%). Examination reveals a tympanitic abdomen, and bowel sounds are usually present. Marked abdominal pain, fever, and leukocytosis can suggest the development of perforation or ischemia. Acute colonic pseudo-obstruction occurs almost exclusively in hospitalized patients who have a significant underlying medical or surgical comorbidity. In published reviews, most patients have had nonoperative trauma, infection, or cardiac disease. Surgical patients have most commonly undergone obstetric/gynecologic, abdominal, and orthopedic procedures. Abdominal distention occurs on average on postoperative day 4.5.

MANAGEMENT

The management of colonic pseudo-obstruction depends foremost on the patient's clinical status. Fevers, leukocytosis, and peritoneal signs can suggest colonic perforation or ischemia, and these complications should be ruled out immediately. The rate of spontaneous perforation is estimated to be 3% and is generally associated with cecum diameter greater than 12 cm and prolonged distention for more than 6 days. In the absence of suspected ischemia or perforation, initial management includes supportive care and elimination of exacerbating factors (Table 1). Supportive care includes bowel rest, maintenance intravenous fluids, and correction of electrolyte abnormalities, especially potassium, magnesium, and calcium. Underlying conditions such as cardiopulmonary derangements and infections should be treated. Nasogastric tube decompression remains a recommendation even though no published proof of its efficacy has been seen. Some practitioners also use rectal tube decompression. Medications that slow gut transit, especially opiates and those with anticholinergic side effects, should be discontinued. Frequent culprits include: antidiarrheal medications, such as loperamide; tricyclic antidepressants; antipsychotics; calcium channel blockers; and beta-blockers. Laxatives and enemas have been shown to worsen the condition and should be avoided. If air cannot be found in the rectosigmoid on abdominal radiographs, mechanical obstruction should be ruled out with a water-soluble enema. Serial abdominal examinations are recommended. Mortality doubles when the cecum diameter increases from less than 12 cm to greater than 14 cm. Upright and supine abdominal x-rays should be performed every 12 to 24 hours.

Neostigmine

Neostigmine, an acetylcholinesterase inhibitor, should be used if supportive care does not lead to improvement in 24 to 48 hours or if the patient has prolonged distention. Published success rates with neostigmine range from 60% to 100%, with clinical response within 30 minutes. The most common side effects of neostigmine are self-limited abdominal pain, nausea, and excessive salivation. Neostigmine (2 mg intravenously [IV]) should be given with atropine readily

TABLE 1: Supportive treatment for acute colonic pseudo-obstruction

Nothing by mouth
Correct fluid and electrolyte imbalances
Treat systemic illness
Stop exacerbating medications
Consider nasogastric and rectal tubes
Encourage patient to be out of bed if possible

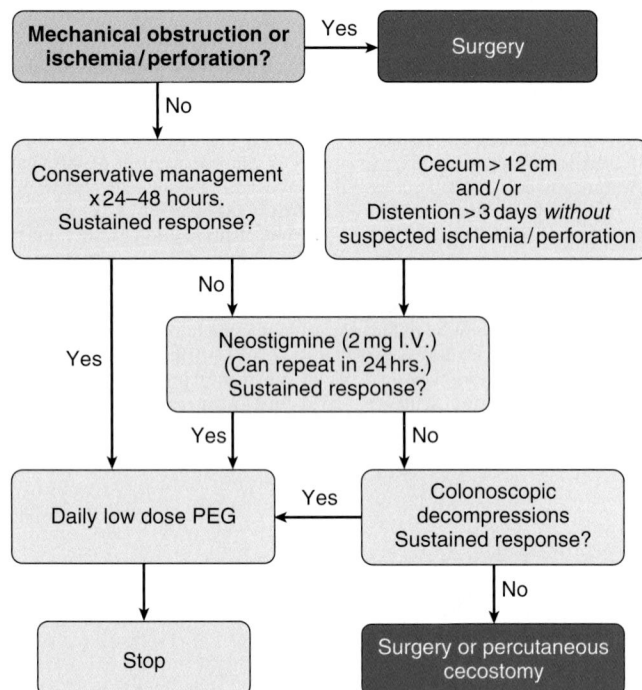

FIGURE 1   Acute colonic distension. *IV,* Intravenous; *PEG,* polyethylene glycol.

available and with continuous cardiac monitoring for 30 minutes because it can cause bradyarrhythmias at a reported incidence rate of 7%. The side effects of neostigmine may be more pronounced in renal failure, so the dose should be adjusted based on creatinine clearance. Neostigmine can also exacerbate bronchoconstriction. Contraindications to its use include: suspected gut ischemia or perforation; ongoing cardiac arrhythmias; active bronchospasm; baseline heart rate of less than 60 beats per minute; systolic blood pressure of less than 90 mm Hg; serum creatinine level of more than 3 mg/dL; and pregnancy. Concomitant use of glycopyrrolate (0.4 mg IV) can mitigate the side effects of neostigmine. Pseudo-obstruction can recur after neostigmine administration. Risks for a failed response include older age, electrolyte disturbances, and use of medications that decrease gut motility. The dose of neostigmine can be repeated. The optimal interval between doses is unknown, but many practitioners repeat the dose once after 24 hours. Overall, neostigmine is an effective and safe option for colonic decompression in those patients with failed conservative management who need more urgent intervention when there are no contraindications to its use.

Very limited data suggest that erythromycin and methylnaltrexone might play a role in addition to or instead of neostigmine. Following initial response of acute pseudo-obstruction to conservative, medical, or endoscopic measures, polyethylene glycol (PEG) has been shown to be effective in preventing recurrence. In this setting, PEG can be administered orally for 7 days. Low doses appropriate for the management of constipation are recommended. The safety and tolerability of PEG make it a reasonable pharmacologic agent to help prevent recurrence of acute colonic pseudo-obstruction.

Colonoscopy

Endoscopic colonic decompression should be considered in patients who do not have improvement after 24 to 48 hours of conservative therapy, have marked cecal distention of significant duration, and have failure of or cannot tolerate initial treatment with neostigmine. Colonoscopy is contraindicated for suspicion of bowel perforation, evidence of peritonitis, or frank mucosal ischemia seen at the start of the procedure. In retrospective studies, sustained response to colonic decompression ranged from 36% to 88%. Colonoscopy with large diameter channels should be used to allow for optimal suctioning of stool and gas. The colon should not be prepped with enemas before the procedure to minimize the risk of perforation. The colonoscopy can be technically difficult in an unprepped colon and should be performed only by a skilled endoscopist. When reaching the cecum is not possible, advancement of the scope to the hepatic flexure may suffice. Anecdotal evidence suggests increased sustained response rates with placement of a decompression tube. The decompression tube should be placed to gravity or to low intermittent suction and flushed every 4 to 6 hours with saline solution to maintain patency. The tube should be removed after 72 hours if it has not already passed spontaneously with restoration of peristalsis. Colonoscopic perforation is reported to occur in approximately 3% of patients with colonic pseudo-obstruction compared with 0.1% to 0.2% in patients undergoing routine colonoscopies. Up to 20% of patients can need two to four colonoscopic decompressions before a sustained clinical response is achieved. Therefore, colonoscopy in patients with acute pseudo-obstruction should be performed carefully and with appropriate delineation of the risks to patients when obtaining consent.

Tube Cecostomy

A percutaneous tube cecostomy can be considered in patients who do not respond to pharmacologic or endoscopic decompression, who have no evidence of ischemia or perforation, and who are poor surgical candidates. A percutaneous cecostomy can be performed with endoscopic, computed tomographic (CT) scan–guided, or laparoscopic techniques. Small case report series with these techniques report some success but cannot accurately reflect on overall safety and efficacy. Risks of the procedure include: peritonitis, wound infection, problems with tube patency, and inadequate decompression. Minimally invasive percutaneous cecostomy should be reserved for patients with failed medical and endoscopic decompression and who cannot tolerate surgery.

Surgery

Surgical intervention for the treatment of acute colonic pseudo-obstruction should only be considered when conservative, pharmacologic, and minimally invasive interventions have been unsuccessful and the patient has prolonged distention lasting more than 6 days. Overall mortality rates in patients with acute colonic pseudo-obstruction undergoing any form of surgical intervention range from 30% to 60%. For surgical tube cecostomy, the morbidity rate approaches 50% and the overall mortality rate is close to 20% to 30%. No published data exist comparing the efficacy of tube cecostomy with more invasive techniques in the management of colonic pseudo-obstruction. In the absence of colonic perforation or ischemia, the surgical procedure of choice may be placement of some form of venting stoma. Stomas have a low immediate morbidity but have been associated with recurrence of pseudo-obstruction and increased long-term morbidity. No published studies compare different types of stoma or stomas versus resection. The high mortality and morbidity with surgical decompression or resection derive from the underlying comorbid conditions in this patient population (Figure 1).

SUMMARY

Acute colonic pseudo-obstruction is a disorder of colonic motility that results in significant colonic distention in the absence of a mechanical obstruction. It occurs almost exclusively in hospitalized patients with comorbid medical and surgical illnesses. Complications such as ischemia and perforation can result in high mortality and make the timely recognition and treatment of acute colonic pseudo-obstruction paramount. Initial management should include supportive care followed by pharmacologic and endoscopic decompression. The presence of significant colonic dilation and the duration of clinical symptoms should prompt earlier attempts at endoscopic or even percutaneous decompression. Surgical intervention should be reserved for patients who do not respond to conservative management or pharmacologic or endoscopic strategies. Surgical decompression and resection are associated with high overall morbidity and mortality.

SUGGESTED READINGS

Benacci JC, Wolff BG: Cecostomy: therapeutic indications and results, *Dis Colon Rectum* 38:530–534, 1995.

De Giorgio R, Knowles CH: Acute colonic pseudo-obstruction, *Br J Surg* 96:229–239, 2009.

Harrison ME, Anderson MA, Appalaneni V, et al: The role of endoscopy in the management of patients with known and suspected colonic obstruction and pseudo-obstruction, *Gastrointest Endosc* 71:669–679, 2010.

Ponec RJ, Saunders MD, Kimmey MB: Neostigmine for the treatment of acute colonic pseudo-obstruction, *N Engl J Med* 341:137–141, 1999.

Saunders MD: Acute colonic pseudo-obstruction, *Best Pract Res Clin Gastroenterol* 21:671–687, 2007.

Sgouros SN, Vlachogiannakos J, Vassiliadis K, et al: Effect of polyethylene glycol electrolyte balanced solution on patients with acute colonic pseudo obstruction after resolution of colonic dilation: a prospective, randomized, placebo controlled trial, *Gut* 55:638–642, 2005.

Vanek VW, Al-Salti M: Acute pseudo-obstruction of the colon (Ogilivie's syndrome): an analysis of 400 cases, *Dis Colon Rectum* 29:203–210, 1986.

THE MANAGEMENT OF COLONIC VOLVULUS

Karen Deveney, MD

OVERVIEW

The term *volvulus* refers to any twisting or turning of the intestine that causes obstruction. Volvulus can occur in either the small or the large intestine. Although colonic volvulus can occur in children as a result of congenital conditions, such as malrotation or Hirschsprung's disease, or infectious disease, such as Chagas' disease, colonic volvulus is most commonly an acquired condition that occurs in adults. Characteristics of the colon that predispose to volvulus include lack of colonic fixation to the retroperitoneum, an elongated mesentery and colon, and a narrow base of origin of the mesentery. Adhesions are not a common cause of volvulus of the colon because they are in the small intestine, and most people with volvulus have not had prior abdominal operations.

Colonic volvulus is estimated to cause 10% to 15% of colonic obstructions. The sigmoid colon is the site of 60% to 80% of all cases of colonic volvulus, with 15% to 30% occurring in the cecum, 2% to 5% in the transverse colon, and about 1% in the splenic flexure. The average age of individuals with development of sigmoid volvulus is older than those with cecal volvulus, and a higher percentage of those with cecal volvulus are women; sigmoid volvulus affects men and women equally. The incidences that occur in the transverse colon or splenic flexure are too small to make accurate generalities about age and gender.

The predominant factors associated with colonic volvulus include anything that results in constipation and thereby leads to lengthening of the colon, such as advanced age, low-fiber diet, psychiatric medications, Parkinson's disease, Chagas' disease, and sedentary lifestyle. The exact pathophysiology of its development is not entirely clear, however, because colonic volvulus is far more common in non-Westernized countries, such as Africa, Asia, the Middle East, Eastern Europe, and South America, where it occurs in a younger age group and where a high-fiber diet has been suggested as a predisposing factor. Volvulus can also occur during pregnancy, which also can cause colonic lengthening.

SIGMOID VOLVULUS

Sigmoid volvulus is much more common worldwide than in North America or Western Europe. In other regions, it occurs more frequently in children than in the United States and is most often associated with congenital abnormalities, such as Hirschsprung's disease, or parasitic diseases, such as Chagas' disease *(Trypanosoma cruzii)*. In Western countries, sigmoid volvulus is predominantly a condition that affects the elderly and those taking psychiatric medications or with neurologic conditions. Because these individuals may not be able to appreciate or report their symptoms, recognition that volvulus has occurred may be delayed and the presentation may be nonspecific.

When the sigmoid colon twists, it usually obstructs the lumen completely but occludes only venous return, not arterial flow. For that reason, symptoms may be gradual and muted rather than abrupt and dramatic. Volvulus usually presents with cramping, vague lower abdominal fullness, and gradual distention of the abdomen. The volvulus may detorse spontaneously and result in explosive, large-volume bowel movements. A history of such past episodes is not uncommon. If the volvulus persists, it eventually results in nausea, anorexia, and more severe pain as the bowel becomes more distended. At that point, the individual may exhibit tachycardia and tachypnea as the elevated diaphragm restricts respiratory excursion.

When the individual comes to medical attention, volvulus has usually been present for several days. On examination, the abdomen is distended and usually only mildly and diffusely tender. Although gangrene and perforation are not common, they can occur in individuals with a tight twist or with longstanding volvulus that has led to extreme colonic distention or venous thrombosis. The perforation may occur in the sigmoid or in the cecum, whose wall is thinner and pressures higher than in the sigmoid. The presence of peritoneal signs on examination, fever, or elevated white blood cell count (WBC) suggests ischemia or perforation.

The diagnosis of sigmoid volvulus can usually be made with abdominal x-rays, which show dilated colon occupying the majority of the abdomen and a colon configuration in the shape of a "bent inner tube" with its point in the left pelvis (Figure 1). An upright or left lateral decubitus film should also be obtained to look for free air. Although a computed tomographic (CT) scan can also be used to make the diagnosis, it is usually not necessary. Barium or water-soluble contrast enemas may also be diagnostic, showing a "bird's beak" appearance in the rectosigmoid, but are usually unnecessary and are unwise if signs of perforation are present.

When sigmoid volvulus has been diagnosed, an attempt at detorsion of the bowel is warranted if the point of torsion looks viable. Although traditionally and somewhat more successfully accomplished with rigid sigmoidoscopy with patients on their hands and knees and buttocks elevated, this position may be difficult for elderly patients to assume and maintain. Current practice most commonly uses flexible sigmoidoscopy with the patient in the left lateral position. Reduction of the volvulus with sigmoidoscopy is achieved in 70% to 80% of patients, but the volvulus recurs in more than half if definitive surgery is not performed. For this reason, a rectal tube is customarily left in place to prevent immediate recurrence and allow colonic decompression while the patient's overall condition is optimized for colonic resection as soon as it can be accomplished. Because these individuals usually are elderly and frail and may have cardiac and respiratory diseases and be on anticoagulant therapy, multidisciplinary teamwork is essential to achieve the most favorable outcome. Recurrence of the volvulus is almost unavoidable without

surgery, so all but those with the most prohibitive anesthetic risk should be offered surgery. A bowel preparation and colonoscopy should ideally be performed before surgery to rule out the presence of malignancy at the site of the volvulus or elsewhere in the colon. If results of a recent colonoscopy are available and show no abnormalities, the need for a bowel preparation before surgery is controversial. Although it has been conventional practice for decades in the United States to perform bowel cleansing before elective colonic surgery, current best evidence suggests lower complications and better outcomes without a bowel preparation. The example from trauma surgery of successful anastomoses and low infection rates in primary colonic repair after penetrating colonic trauma also supports the omission of bowel preparation as safe practice.

If the volvulus was not able to be reduced nonoperatively or the patient's presentation suggests perforation or ischemia, emergency operation is indicated as soon as the patient is rendered normovolemic and the medical condition is optimized.

Although simple pexy of the sigmoid to the sidewall of the lateral abdomen was previously considered a surgical option, the recurrence rate (30% to 50%) is so high after this procedure that it is no longer considered a good choice. If the bowel has signs of gangrene at operation, the affected bowel should be resected without first reducing the volvulus, to avoid the release of toxins into the circulation. If gangrene is not present, the sigmoid can be resected in the usual fashion after reducing the volvulus. To minimize fecal contamination when a bowel preparation is not possible or not performed, the proximal and distal sites of resection can be identified and cleared and the mesentery resected before dividing the bowel. The distal bowel is then divided and bowel contents directed off the field into a bucket, before the proximal site is divided and the specimen passed off the field.

If the patient is hemodynamically stable and nutrition is reasonable, a primary anastomosis is generally preferable to a colostomy with Hartmann's procedure or mucous fistula. If the patient is nutritionally or immunologically compromised (e.g., renal failure, transplant, steroids, severe diabetes), a colostomy should be performed. Impaired fecal continence is another indication for a colostomy.

Series that report outcomes of sigmoid resection for volvulus show lower mortality with primary anastomosis than with colostomy and higher mortality with emergency procedures. However, these studies are all retrospective case series in which the patient's condition likely factored into the decision whether to perform a primary anastomosis or colostomy.

Occasionally, the entire colon may be massively dilated, such as in a patient with Ogilvie's syndrome (colonic pseudo-obstruction). In that case, a subtotal colectomy is indicated with ileostomy or ileoproctostomy, again depending on the patient's overall nutrition and immunocompetence.

A laparoscopic approach has been described for treatment of sigmoid volvulus and is an option if the surgeon is a very skilled laparoscopic surgeon but should probably be avoided in the emergency situation when the bowel has not been reduced because the limited working room in the abdomen makes the laparoscopic approach more difficult. In the patient whose volvulus has been reduced and colon decompressed, the same surgical options are available for a laparoscopic approach as for an open procedure. Colopexy or mesosigmoidopexy can be achieved with low mortality and morbidity and a short procedure time, but the recurrence is much higher than with resection.

An algorithm for treatment of sigmoid volvulus is presented in Figure 2.

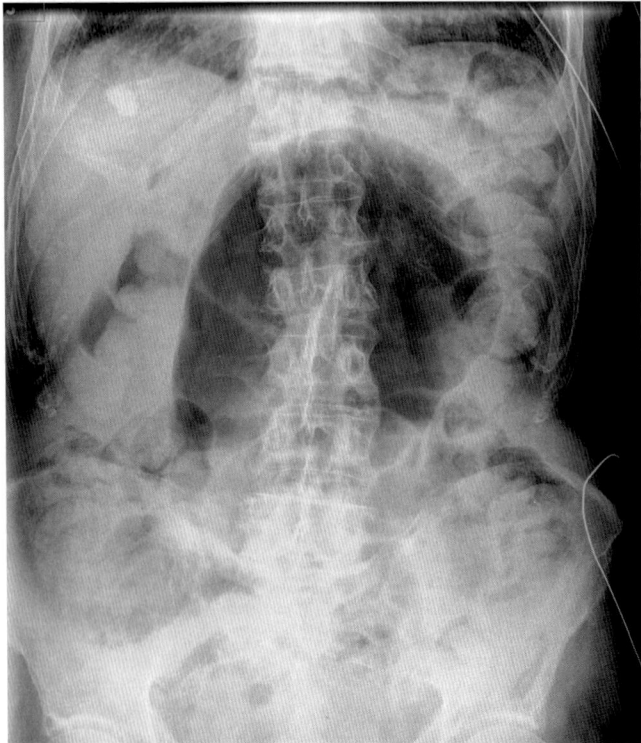

FIGURE 1   Plain abdominal film of an 88-year-old man with sigmoid volvulus, displaying the "bent inner tube" appearance. The volvulus was successfully reduced with rigid sigmoidoscopy.

CECAL VOLVULUS

Cecal volvulus is far less common than sigmoid volvulus, it usually occurs at a younger age (40 to 60 years) than sigmoid volvulus, and it is more frequently seen in women than in men. As in sigmoid

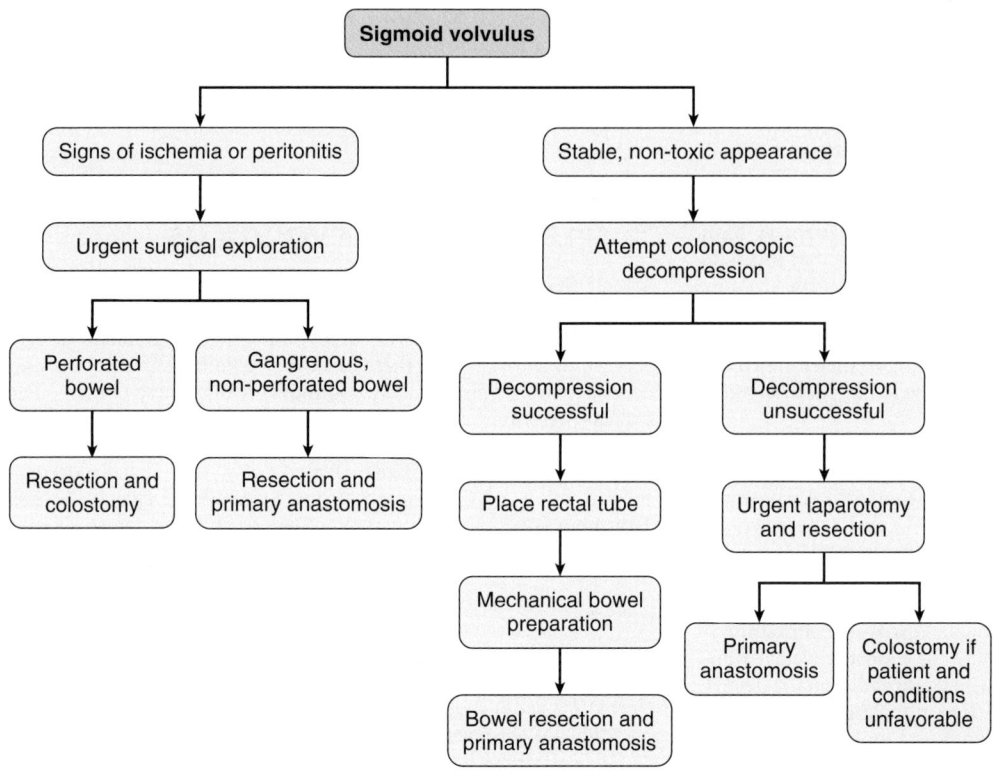

FIGURE 2 Suggested algorithm for management of sigmoid volvulus.

volvulus, the occurrence of cecal volvulus requires an elongated, mobile cecum that is not fixed to the retroperitoneum. Although it is also usually associated with constipation, cecal volvulus is less commonly associated with the elderly, nursing home patients, or those on psychiatric medications than is sigmoid volvulus.

When the entire cecum and terminal ileum rotate on a narrow mesenteric axis, a true ileocecal volvulus occurs. These individuals most commonly note sudden abdominal pain across the mid abdomen and come to medical attention sooner after the onset than patients with sigmoid volvulus. The abdomen is distended and tender; localized peritoneal signs on examination suggest ischemic bowel, and diffuse peritoneal irritation indicates perforation. Although plain abdominal films can show a dilated loop of small and large bowel extending across the abdomen to the left upper quadrant, the appearance of the gas-filled loops is often less definitive and may require CT scan for confirmation (Figure 3). Endoscopic detorsion is less likely to be successful than with sigmoid volvulus, with less than 10% success. Resolution invariably requires operative intervention, either with open or laparoscopic method. Ileocolic resection with primary anastomosis is the procedure with the highest success rate, with a mortality rate of less than 10% and equally low recurrence. If the patient is hemodynamically unstable or has perforation of the bowel with peritonitis, ileostomy may be a safer choice. As in sigmoid volvulus, gangrenous bowel should not be detorsed but resected as it lies to avoid systemic dissemination of toxic substances. Detorsion and cecopexy is an option if the length of procedure must be minimized and the bowel is totally viable, although the recurrence rate of 30% to 40% makes it a less attractive choice in any patient who is clinically stable enough to undergo resection.

A special type of cecal volvulus is cecal bascule, a condition in which the cecum folds up on itself anteriorly. The resultant obstruction may be incomplete and intermittent, making it more difficult to diagnose than a true cecal volvulus. Patients with this condition present with right midabdominal pain that may resolve and recur for several months or years. Plain abdominal films are often not definitive and difficult to interpret correctly. Cross-sectional CT images may also not reveal the abnormality, although it is more easily seen

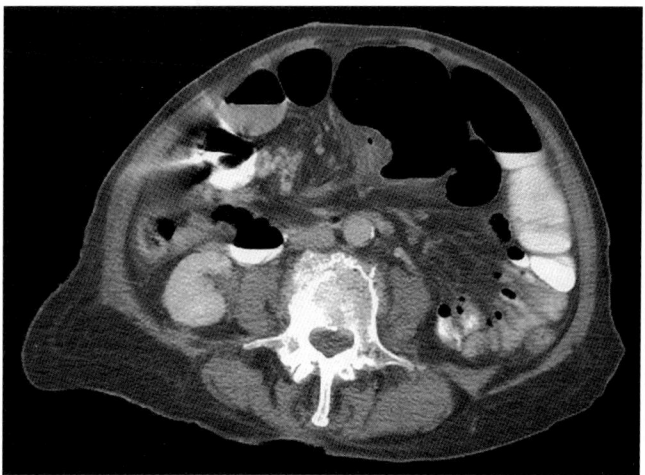

FIGURE 3 A 58-year-old woman with distal ileal and cecal volvulus. The computed tomographic scan shows a dilated cecum and distal ileum in the left upper quadrant, with an abrupt transition point as the right colon crosses the central mesentery.

on the sagittal reconstructions. Operation is necessary for effective treatment, but the best surgical option depends on the operative findings and ranges from cecopexy to cecectomy to ileocolic resection, depending on how much of the cecum and right colon is mobile and nonfixed. Recurrence rates are 10% to 30% and depend on selecting the most appropriate procedure to resolve the hypermobile segment.

TRANSVERSE COLON VOLVULUS

Volvulus of the transverse colon is seen far less frequently than sigmoid or cecal volvulus, with most reports in the literature being case reports or a handful of cases collected over many years. Only 1% to 4% of colonic volvulus involves the transverse colon. Volvulus of the transverse colon is far more common in some geographic areas, including Scandinavia, Eastern Europe, India, and Africa. The most common anatomy of the transverse colon with its short, wide mesentery and its location between the usually fixed hepatic and splenic flexures makes it less inclined to volvulus. Factors that allow the transverse colon to twist on its axis include an abnormally long mesentery, intestinal malrotation with a narrower mesentery than normal, or lack of fixation of the flexures. Conditions that promote elongation of the colon, such as constipation or distal colonic obstruction, can also create a predisposition for the transverse colon to twist around its mesenteric axis. Most likely because of their irregular bowel patterns with subsequent lengthening of the entire colon, the mentally disabled are predisposed to volvulus of the transverse colon and the sigmoid colon.

Patients with transverse colon volvulus present in an acute or subacute fashion. Those with a sudden, more complete volvulus present with epigastric pain, abdominal distention, nausea, vomiting, and abdominal tenderness. They are tachycardic and appear very ill. The more chronic type of transverse colon volvulus, with a less complete twist or intermittent torsion, may be more gradual in onset with less severe symptoms and intermittent cramping pain. A plain abdominal film may be diagnostic, showing distension of the proximal colon and collapsed distal colon. With the almost universal availability and use in patients presenting with acute abdominal pain, CT scanning is usually the diagnostic test used in making the diagnosis. Findings on CT scan include the torsed bowel loop and the "whirl sign" of the mesenteric vessels.

The safest and most practical treatment option for transverse colon volvulus is surgical resection. Clearly, resection is mandatory if any bowel ischemia or perforation is found at exploration. The option of colopexy is less attractive in this form of volvulus because of a lack of convenient structures to which the transverse colon can be safely anchored. Whether to perform an anastomosis or proximal stoma with a mucous fistula or long Hartmann's procedure depends on the condition of the patient and the findings at surgery. The presence of perforation with peritonitis or a malnourished or hemodynamically unstable patient makes anastomosis risky and colostomy a safer option.

SPLENIC FLEXURE VOLVULUS

Splenic flexure volvulus is an extremely rare condition that occurs when the normal fixation of the splenic flexure is absent for congenital reasons or because of prior surgery that renders the splenic flexure more mobile. As with other forms of volvulus, constipation and neuropsychiatric disorders are commonly seen in these patients. The clinical presentation is similar to that of volvulus of the cecum or transverse colon. Radiographic diagnosis can be made either with plain films, showing proximal dilated colon with distally decompressed colon, or CT scan that shows the twisted splenic flexure. Treatment is surgical and can be either resection or detorsion with fixation of the splenic flexure by colopexy, depending on the surgical findings.

SUGGESTED READINGS

Ören D, Atamanalp SS, Aydinli B, et al: An algorithm for the management of sigmoid colon volvulus and the safety of primary resection: experience with 827 cases, *Dis Col Rect* 50:489–497, 2007.

Swenson BR, Kwaan MR, Burkart NE, et al: Colonic volvulus: presentation and management in metropolitan Minnesota, United States, *Dis Colon Rectum* 55:444–449, 2012.

Vandendries C, Julles MC, Boulay-Coletta I, et al: Diagnosis of colonic volvulus: findings on multidetector CT with three-dimensional reconstructions, *Br J Radiol* 83:983–990, 2010.

RECTAL PROLAPSE

Alan D. Garely, MD, FACOG, FACS,
Beth R. Krieger, MD, and Alex J. Ky, MD

Rectal prolapse is a protrusion of the walls of the rectum outside the anus. Full-thickness prolapse refers to prolapse of all layers of the bowel wall; partial prolapse involves only the mucosa. Full-thickness prolapse has a characteristic circular mucosal fold appearance, whereas partial or hemorrhoidal prolapse has radial folds. Internal rectal intussusception is when the rectum folds in on itself, but it usually does not fall outside the anus. The best method for diagnosis of prolapse is with the patient sitting on a commode bearing down to simulate a bowel movement.

ETIOLOGY AND PRESENTATION

The etiology of rectal prolapse is not entirely understood. The two most popular theories are those put forth by Moschowitz and by Broden and Snellman who, respectively, believed that prolapse was the result of a sliding hernia through a defect in the pelvic fascia or an intussusception of the rectum. A variety of anatomic defects occur with rectal prolapse. These include pelvic floor laxity, weak sphincter complex, redundant rectosigmoid, deep pouch of Douglas, pudendal neuropathy, and a lack of rectal fixation.

Most patients with rectal prolapse are women (up to 90%) over the age of 50 years with a history of vaginal childbirth. Men are typically younger, 20 to 40 years of age; the incidence rate decreases with advancing age. An increased incidence rate is also found in nursing home and psychiatric patients. Prolapse may be associated with rectal bleeding, especially after defecation, and frequently has an associated mucoid discharge. Other reported symptoms include a sensation of incomplete evacuation, tenesmus, constipation with straining, and incontinence.

EVALUATION

The evaluation of a patient with rectal prolapse should always start with a history and physical examination. During examination, the prolapse is often reduced. Patients frequently have a patulous anus and diminished resting tone and squeeze pressures on digital rectal examination. The prolapse is best reproduced by having the patient sit on a commode and bear down. Full-thickness prolapse is distinguished from mucosal prolapse by the appearance of concentric folds. This examination may also show a concomitant cystocele or prolapse of the uterus.

Additional workup should include colonoscopy to exclude any other colonic or rectal pathology, especially in patients who are over the age of 50 years. Manometry can help assess any sphincter damage that may result from chronic prolapse. Levatorplasty at the time of surgery may improve the continence in these patients. Patients with a history of constipation should undergo colonic transit studies because this may influence their surgical options. If evidence of slow transit constipation or colonic inertia is found, a sigmoid resection or subtotal colectomy should be considered at the time of operation.

TREATMENT

Surgery is the only definitive form of treatment. Options include narrowing of the anal orifice, obliteration of the pouch of Douglas, restoration of the pelvic floor, bowel resection, suspension/fixation of the rectum to the sacrum, or any combination of these procedures. Surgery is usually divided into abdominal and perineal approaches. Traditionally, the perineal approaches have been reserved for older patients who are not appropriate surgical candidates for a more invasive abdominal operation that requires general anesthesia. Abdominal surgeries are thought to be more effective, with lower rates of recurrence. Because full-thickness rectal prolapse is relatively rare and long-term follow-up studies are limited, there is no clear gold standard surgical approach. Surgery needs to be individualized to each patient for optimization of functional outcomes.

Perineal Procedures

Perineal surgeries are typically reserved for the elderly with significant comorbidities because these surgeries can be done with local anesthesia and are usually well tolerated. Patients usually have minimal pain, earlier return of bowel function, and quicker tolerance of a regular diet and are ambulating much sooner than patients who undergo an abdominal operation. Perineal approaches include anal encirclement, Delorme's procedure, and perineal rectosigmoidectomy.

Thiersch's Procedure

Anal encirclement or the Thiersch's procedure was first described in 1891 with a silver wire. It has since been modified to use any number of products, but the basic principle involves passing a foreign material around the anus to narrow it and act as a physical barrier to prevent further prolapse. The narrowed anus should still allow passage of a 16-mm or 18-mm Hagar dilator. This procedure has largely been abandoned because of its high recurrence rates (33% to 44%) and significant morbidity. Common complications have included fecal impaction, wound infection, and erosion, all of which usually necessitate implant removal. An additional concern is that when prolapse recurs, the rectum may become incarcerated and strangulated.

Mucosal Sleeve Resection (Delorme's Procedure)

Delorme's procedure was first described in 1900 and is considered the treatment of choice for mucosal and short-segment full-thickness prolapse. A circumferential incision is made in the mucosa 1 cm above the dentate line, and the submucosa and mucosal layers are dissected off the muscularis. Injection of local anesthesia with epinephrine in the submucosa facilitates this dissection and aids in hemostasis. The stripped mucosa is excised, and a plicating stitch is then placed from the cut edge of the mucosa to the muscularis and to the mucosa just proximal to the dentate line (Figure 1).

Morbidity and mortality rates have been reported as 4% to 33% and 0 to 2.5%, respectively. Complications associated with the

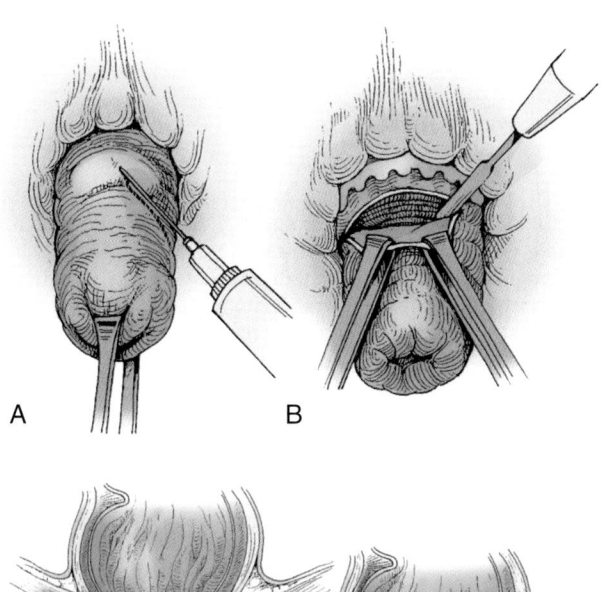
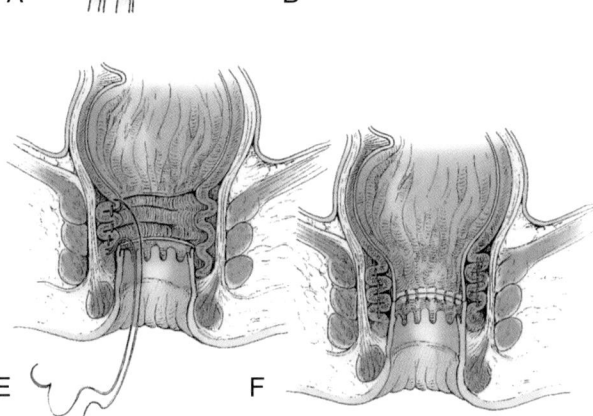
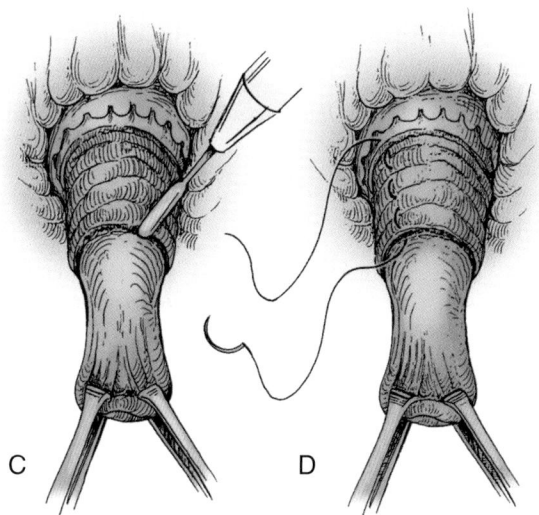

FIGURE 1 Mucosal proctectomy (Delorme's procedure). **A,** Submucosal infiltration with epinephrine solution. **B,** Circumferential mucosal incision. **C,** Dissection of mucosa away from muscular layer. **D** and **E,** Plicating stitch including cut edge of mucosa and muscular wall. **F,** Completed anastomosis. (*From Whitlow CB: Rectal prolapse and intussusceptions. In Beck DE, editor:* Handbook of colorectal surgery, *St Louis, 1997, Quality Medical Publishing, 274–298.*)

procedure include bleeding, anastomotic leak, stricture, and diarrhea. Recurrence rates have been reported to range from 6% to 26%. Up to 50% of patients reported an improvement in incontinence after the procedure and no associated constipation.

One of the largest case series was by Lieberth and colleagues who reported on 76 patients who underwent Delorme's procedure. The median age of the patients was 74 years; they were followed over an average of 36 months. There were no perioperative deaths, and the morbidity rate was 25%. The most common postoperative complication was urinary retention (12%). One patient had a myocardial infarction, and three patients had *Clostridium difficile* colitis develop. Three patients (4%) had development of suture line bleeding, two patients (3%) had an anastomotic leak, and one (1%) an anastomotic stricture. Overall recurrence rate was 14.5%, with a mean time to recurrence of 31 months (range, 1 to 60 months). No predictors of recurrence were identified.

Perineal Rectosigmoidectomy (Altemeier's Procedure)

The perineal rectosigmoidectomy was first performed by Mikulicz in 1889, but it was not until the 1970s that it became popularized by Altemeier. The rectum is prolapsed and then injected with epinephrine-containing local anesthesia. A circumferential incision is made through all layers of the rectal wall 1 to 2 cm above the dentate line. Once the full-thickness incision is complete, the redundant rectum is continually pulled out as the mesorectum is ligated and divided. For this portion of the procedure, the authors use the LigaSure device (Covidien, New Haven, Conn) for both its speed and its hemostatic properties. The anterior peritoneal reflection is opened and allows for a high ligation of the hernia sac. The rectum/sigmoid colon is pulled out through the peritoneal defect until there is no further redundancy. The rectum/colon is then divided, and the end is anastomosed to the anal ring. One modification of this procedure involves plication of the levators, which is thought to decrease recurrence and improve continence (Figures 2 and 3).

Mortality rates associated with this procedure are low (0 to 6%), and most of the morbidity (5% to 24%) stems from the patient's underlying medical problems, but there is a possibility of postoperative bleeding and anastomotic dehiscence. This is where experience comes into play; resecting too much colon and mesentery makes for an anastomosis that is under tension and poorly vascularized, thereby increasing the risk of a leak, whereas not resecting enough can lead to recurrence. Recurrence rates have been reported as 0 to 10% but are believed to increase with longer patient follow-up periods.

In an effort to report long-term data, Altomare and associates performed a retrospective review of 93 patients who had undergone Altemeier's procedure and had at least 1 year of follow-up. Fifteen percent of patients had previously had surgery for prolapse. After an average follow-up period of 41 months, 18% had recurrence of full-thickness prolapse and 6% had mucosal prolapse develop. A previous unsuccessful repair was the only predictor of recurrence (odds ratio [OR], 3.8; $P = 0.042$).

Options for recurrent prolapse after Altemeier's procedure include a repeat Altemeier's procedure or an abdominal approach. Theoretic concern exists that an abdominal resection can devascularize the distal bowel unless a coloanal anastomosis is performed. An abdominal fixation or suspension is considered a reasonable alternative.

Abdominal Procedures

Ripstein's Procedure

This technique was first described by Ripstein and Lanter in 1963. They believed that rectal prolapse was primarily the result of intussusception of the rectum that occurs with loss of the rectal attachments. This belief leads to the design of a surgical technique that affixes the rectum to the sacrum and thus prevents rectal prolapse.

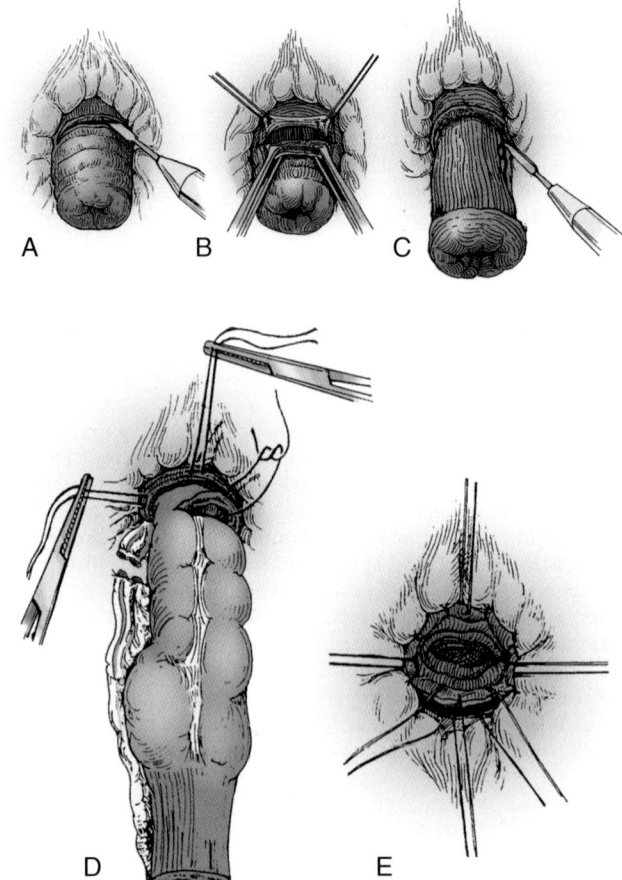

FIGURE 2 Perineal rectosigmoidectomy (Altemeier's procedure). **A** to **C**, Full-thickness excision of the outer cylinder of the prolapse. **D**, Mesenteric vessels ligated; stay sutures placed in distal edge of inner cylinder. **E**, Anastomosis of the distal aspect of the remaining colon to the rectal stump. (*From Whitlow CB: Rectal prolapse and intussusceptions. In Beck DE, editor:* Handbook of colorectal surgery, *St Louis, 1997, Quality Medical Publishing, 274–298.*)

Initially, they used fascia lata to create a sling that they could use to fix the rectum to the sacrum, but they subsequently modified the technique and started using prosthetic mesh.

The procedure involves mobilization of the rectum down to the coccyx with dividing the lateral peritoneal attachments but preserving the lateral ligaments. While the rectum is pulled upward, a 5-cm piece of mesh is wrapped anteriorly around the rectum at the level of the peritoneal reflection and then sutured bilaterally to the presacral fascia approximately 5 cm below the sacral promontory. The sling should allow the passage of one to two fingers between the rectum and fascia because too tight of a wrap can cause obstruction.

Studies have shown that this procedure is best suited for the patient without preexisting constipation. Up to 50% of patients had improvement of incontinence; persistence of constipation occurred in 57%, and new onset constipation developed in 10%. Recurrence and mortality rates after this procedure are relatively low, 0 to 8% and 0 to 1.6%, respectively.

Unfortunately, Ripstein's procedure does have a significant morbidity associated with it; it is not used that frequently anymore. Complication rates are reported from 17% to 33% and are largely related to the placement of the sling. The most common problem was constipation and fecal impaction, but presacral hemorrhage, stricture, small bowel obstruction, impotence, and fistula formation were also notable. One of the more catastrophic complications associated with placement of a mesh is the development of infection or erosion into the bladder. Modifying the procedure to a posterior wrap or substitution of polyvinyl alcohol sponge for the mesh have reduced the complication rates to 20%.

Abdominal Rectopexy and Sigmoid Resection

This technique, originally described in 1955, remains today as one of the commonly used and effective treatment options for full-thickness rectal prolapse. Frykman describes four essential steps to this procedure: (1) complete mobilization of the rectum down to the levator complex, with the lateral ligaments left intact; (2) elevation of the rectum with suture fixation to the presacral fascia just below the sacral promontory; (3) obliteration of the cul-de-sac with suturing the endopelvic fascia anteriorly to the rectum; and (4) resection of the redundant sigmoid colon with an end-to-end anastomosis. The procedure remains essentially the same today, but some surgeons chose to omit the obliteration of the cul-de-sac.

A recent meta-analysis of 418 patients reported a recurrence rate of 0 to 9% and morbidity and mortality rates of 0 to 23% and 0 to 6.7%, respectively. Complications related to the procedure itself included colonic and small bowel obstructions, anastomotic leak, and presacral bleeding. Most patients reported an improvement in bowel habits after the procedure. Huber and colleagues found a reduction in constipation from 44% to 26% and in incontinence from 67% to 23%.

Abdominal Rectopexy

Rectopexy without a sigmoid resection can also be used for the treatment of rectal prolapse. Fixation of the rectum to the sacrum can be accomplished with placement of interrupted nonabsorbable sutures or with use of a mesh (Ripstein's). Recurrence rates also range from 0 to 9%, but the functional outcomes are quite different as compared with a resection rectopexy. Generally speaking, constipation is worsened in these patients and incontinence improved (Table 1).

Management of the Lateral Ligaments

The Cochrane review is a meta-analysis of 12 randomized controlled trials evaluating 380 patients. One of the outcomes assessed in this review was division versus preservation of the lateral ligaments during rectal mobilization in patients undergoing open mesh rectopexy. The three distinct trials examined a total of 64 patients. Division of the ligaments was associated with a decreased recurrence rate (0 vs 19%) but increased rates of constipation (67% vs 43%).

Laparoscopy

Laparoscopy has been used to perform both abdominal rectopexy and resection rextopexy. The rates of recurrence, morbidity, and mortality have been shown to be comparable between the open and laparoscopic techniques. However, laparoscopy is associated with shorter hospital stays and faster patient recovery. A meta-analysis of 467 patients undergoing 275 open and 192 laparoscopic procedures showed no significant difference between recurrence and improvements in constipation or incontinence (Table 2).

Robotics is the next potential step in the treatment of rectal prolapse. Theoretically, one expects to see improved outcomes, particularly in patients undergoing rectopexy, because suturing in the pelvis is more facile with the robot as compared with standard laparoscopy. Because this is a newer technology, studies are small and have short

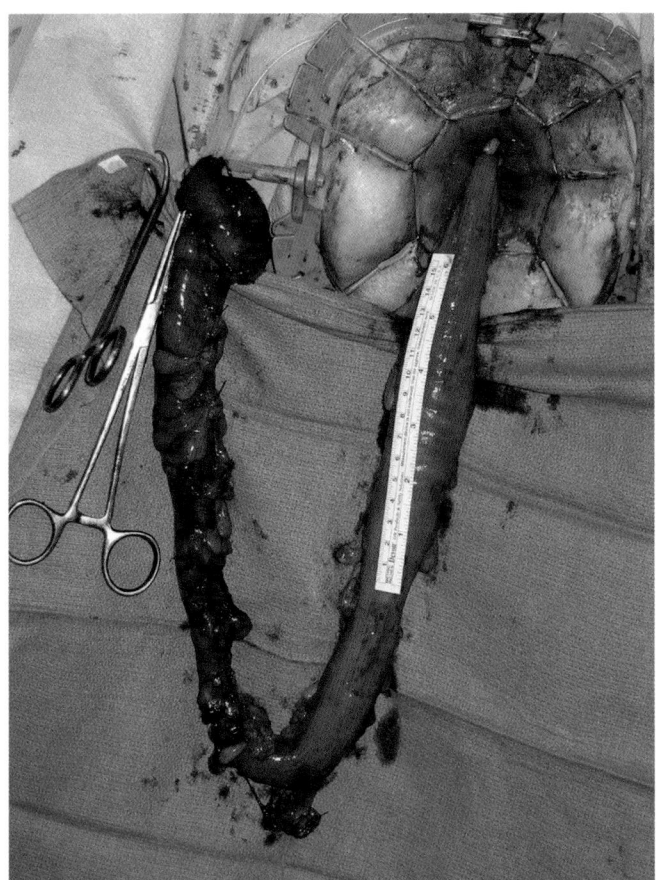

FIGURE 3 An example of how much colon can be resected from an Altemeier's procedure.

TABLE 1: Open abdominal procedures

Procedure	Mortality rates	Morbidity rates	Recurrence rates
Suture rectopexy	0	9.3%-20%	0-9%
Ripstein's procedure	0-2.8%	3.7%-33%	0-12%
Posterior mesh repair	0-1%	15%-28%	0-6%
Resection rectopexy	0-6.7%	7.1%-17.2%	0-5%

TABLE 2: Laparoscopic abdominal procedures

Procedure	Mortality rates	Morbidity rates	Recurrence rates
Suture rectopexy	0	9%-19%	0-7%
Posterior mesh repair	0	8%-14%	0-4%
Resection rectopexy	0	8%-13%	0

follow-up periods. One study of 82 patients found higher recurrence rates with laparoscopy and robotics as compared with open procedures.

Recurrent Prolapse

Because of a significant incidence rate of recurrent rectal prolapse, a discussion of the potential surgical options is important. The most important determinant of subsequent surgery is the remaining blood supply of the bowel. Patients who have previously undergone resection are at risk for development of ischemia to the segment of bowel between the two anastomoses should a second resection be attempted.

The surgeon must know the details of the patient's prior surgery. Patients who have undergone a perineal rectosigmoidectomy are candidates for a repeat perineal rectosigmoidectomy or an abdominal rectopexy without resection. Addition of a sigmoid resection could potentially cause ischemia to the remaining rectal segment. Patients who have undergone a previous abdominal rectopexy can have a redo rectopexy with or without resection or a perineal rectosigmoidectomy. Patients with prior abdominal rectopexy and resection are best treated with a redo abdominal rectopexy with or without resection; perineal rectosigmoidectomy should be avoided.

■ SUMMARY

Rectal prolapse can be a difficult entity to manage. A proper evaluation should be completed so that the surgeon can pick the surgical technique that will minimize morbidity and mortality, prevent recurrence, and improve the functional outcomes of the patient. Generally speaking, perineal procedures have lower rates of morbidity and mortality but higher rates of recurrence. Resection and rectopexy improve constipation, whereas rectopexy alone worsens it. Laparoscopy has similar outcomes as open procedures but reduced length of hospital stay. Patients with recurrent rectal prolapse can undergo additional surgery, but the initial surgical procedure must be taken into account. Robotics have the potential to improve patient outcomes, but larger studies with longer follow-up periods are needed to adequately assess its role in the treatment of rectal prolapse.

SUGGESTED READINGS

Altemeier WA, Culbertson WR, Schowengardt C, et al: Nineteen years experience with the one-stage perineal repair of rectal prolapse, *Ann Surg* 173:993–1006, 1971.

Altomare DF, Binda G, Ganio E, et al: Long-term outcome of Altemeier's procedure for rectal prolapse, *Dis Colon Rectum* 52:698–703, 2009.

Cadeddu F, Sileri P, Grande M, et al: Focus on abdominal rectopexy for full-thickness rectal prolapse: meta-analysis of literature, *Tech Coloproctol* 16:37–53, 2012.

Dulucq JL, Wintringer P, Mahajna A: Clinical and functional outcomes of laparoscopic posterior rextopexy for full thickness rectal prolapse: a prospective study, *Surg Endosc* 21:2226–2230, 2007.

Frykman HM: Abdominal proctopexy and primary sigmoid resection for rectal procidentia, *Am J Surg* 90:780–789, 1955.

Huber FT, Stein H, Siewert JR: Functional results after treatment of rectal prolapse with rectopexy and sigmoid resection, *World J Surg* 19:138–143, 1995.

Kuijpers HC: Treatment of complete rectal prolapse: to narrow, to wrap, to suspend, to fix, to encircle, to plicate or to resect? *World J Surg* 16: 826–830, 1992.

Lieberth M, Kondylis LA, Reilly JC, et al: The Delorme repair for full-thickness rectal prolapse: a retrospective review, *Am J Surg* 197:418–423, 2009.

Madiba TE, Baig MK, Wexner SD: Surgical management of rectal prolapse, *Arch Surg* 140:63–73, 2005.

Prasad ML, Pearl RK, Abcarian H, et al: Perineal proctectomy, posterior rectopexy, and postanal levator repair for the treatment of rectal prolapse, *Dis Colon Rectum* 29:547–552, 1986.

Schultz I, Mellgren A, Dolk A, et al: Long-term results and functional outcome after Ripstein rectopexy, *Dis Colon Rectum* 43:35–43, 2000.

Tou S, Brown SR, Malik AI, et al: Surgery for complete rectal prolapse in adults, *Cochrane Database Sys Rev* (4):CD001758, 2008.

Watkins BP, Landercasper J, Belzer GE, et al: Long-term follow-up of the modified Delorme procedure for rectal prolapse, *Arch Surg* 197:418–423, 2009.

Zbar A, Takashim S, Hasegawa T, et al: Perineal rectosigmoidectomy: a review of physiology, technique and outcome, *Tech Coloproctol* 6:109–116, 2002.

THE MANAGEMENT OF SOLITARY RECTAL ULCER SYNDROME

Anjali S. Kumar, MD, MPH, Deirdre C. Kelleher, MD, and Lee E. Smith, MD

Solitary rectal ulcer syndrome (SRUS) is a relatively new term, introduced in 1964 by M.R. Madigan. The terms *solitary* and *ulcer* may be misnomers, as the condition is a physical sequela of both internal rectal prolapse and outlet obstruction constipation. The physical manifestations may not be solitary in nature, with circumferential involvement occasionally seen. Furthermore, SRUS does not always produce an ulcer, and the ulcers seen are rarely typical. Unlike the lesions seen in ulcerative proctitis, the ulcer may appear as a shallow "punched-out" gray-white lesion with a hyperemic base, caused by ischemic changes from the pressures exerted on the prolapsed tissues during defecation. Other times, a mucosal injury results from the repetitive trauma of chronic digitation or enema use to alleviate symptoms of outlet obstruction constipation. In cases of severe constipation, hard stool may cause this mucosal injury and lead to "ulcerative" damage of the rectum. In other cases, there may be no ulcer at all, but the patient specifically reports bleeding, passage of mucous, straining during defecation, and a sense of incomplete evacuation. For these patients, the only finding on inspection may be rectal erythema. Alternatively, rectal pseudopolyps may develop from repeated inflammation and healing with residual granulation.

Inflamed areas may also fill with mucin, resulting in a cystic-appearing neoplasm termed colitis cystica profunda (CCP). CCP and SRUS are related diagnoses that some clinicians consider interchangeable. SRUS and CCP are seen more commonly in women (3.2 : 1.0 ratio) and in individuals ranging in age from young 20s to late 60s, although SRUS has been reported in pediatric patients as young as 3 years.

CLINICAL FINDINGS

The initial symptom of SRUS is often passage of bright red blood and mucous from the rectum; rarely, massive hemorrhage can occur. Patients more frequently seek medical attention for pain, usually localized to the rectum. On interview, almost all patients report tenesmus and feelings of outlet obstruction. Some may also have incontinence to gas and liquid.

On physical examination, induration may be palpated near the lesion if it is within reach. On sigmoidoscopy, the classic finding is a shallow, well-demarcated ulcer with a red margin and yellow-gray eschar over the base, typically located 10 to 12 cm from the anus. The ulcer is most frequently located anteriorly, as a result of anterior internal intussusception. Valsalva's maneuver during defecation causes strain against a physiologically obstructed outlet and results in anterior rectal wall prolapse with a lead point near the peritoneal reflection or pouch of Douglas. The posterior rectum prolapses less frequently because its sacral attachment provides better support. However, prolapses may be seen in any location in the rectum and occasionally appear circumferential. Other examination findings include a raised ulcer margin and presence of pseudopolyps.

DIAGNOSIS

Clinical suspicion is the key to diagnosis of SRUS. Recognizing the signs and symptoms associated with the syndrome aids in ordering the correct confirmatory diagnostic tests. For visible lesions, biopsy is of the utmost importance to rule out neoplasm and inflammatory bowel disease. In a series of 14 patients with SRUS, nine patients (64%) had an initial diagnosis of rectal cancer that was subsequently corrected to the benign diagnosis after biopsy. Mistaking the benign ulcer for a carcinoma or inflammatory bowel disease (or vice versa) might lead to inappropriate therapy. Because the clinical symptoms of the syndrome can mimic other disorders, the final determination of SRUS must lie with the pathologist.

Other imaging studies are available and may aid in diagnosis of SRUS. Defecography is especially useful but is often only available at specialized centers. For this study, barium paste is introduced into the rectal vault via an enema device, and lateral video fluoroscopy images are obtained during patient defecation of the paste. The resulting film may show intussusception, nonrelaxing puborectalis muscle (resulting in abnormal angulation of the anorectal junction), incomplete or delayed rectal emptying, or a thickened rectal wall. The dynamic results of defecography are more specific than the static films from barium enema, which may only show rectal stricture, mucosal granularity, or thickened rectal folds.

Magnetic resonance (MR) defecography is a newer radiologic option for imaging internal intussusception; it adds a three-dimensional view of the anatomy. Performed at highly specialized radiographic centers, MR defecography involves insertion of a water-soluble agent (such as gel) into the rectum, followed by imaging of the patient during relaxation, straining, and postevacuation phases. In a 19-patient series, MR images were found to be comparable with those of conventional defecography, with no significant differences in detection of sphincter hypotonia, dyssynergia, or rectal prolapse during the evacuation phase. However, in a separate series, MR defecography was found to overdetect incomplete evacuation in 30% of patients. Smaller anorectal angles have also been observed, possibly as a result of the supine or left-lateral positioning of the patient, which removes the effect of gravity and alters the normal pelvic floor anatomy. Patients report difficulty mimicking defecation in this position, and many physicians believe it is less representative of the dynamic forces of defecation than conventional fluoroscopic defecography. Seated MR defecography is currently being developed and may increase the utility of this study.

In patients without defecatory dysfunction, the Valsalva's maneuver should result in pelvic floor relaxation. However, patients with SRUS frequently have nonrelaxing pelvic floor muscles. Electromyographic and dynamic manometry studies can confirm this functional abnormality. However, these tests have not been consistently useful in diagnosis or in prediction of a patient's response to therapy. Other available studies include anal and rectal ultrasound scan, which can show a hypertrophic anal sphincter or rectal wall thickening. Sometimes a shallow ulcer may also be seen with ultrasound scan, most often within the layers of the intact rectal wall. None of these supplementary tests are mandatory for diagnosis of SRUS; however, lesion biopsy is essential.

HISTOLOGIC FINDINGS

The hallmark microscopic findings of SRUS include an obliterated, fibrotic lamina propria that contains excess collagen and disorganized hypertrophy of the smooth muscle fibers from the muscularis mucosae towards the lumen. This appearance has been coined fibromuscular obliteration. Microscopic inspection of the ulcer base reveals local fibrosis and leukocytic exudates, which contribute to its characteristic gray-white color. The presence of collagen infiltration of the lamina propria distinguishes SRUS from other inflammatory, infectious and ischemic colitis. A trichrome stain can accentuate the characteristic fibrosis and collagen deposition. Lack of malignant and adenomatous features is also key to confirmation of the diagnosis of SRUS.

The distinguishing feature of CCP is the presence of mucin-filled cysts lined with columnar epithelium. CCP cysts are typically located deep to the muscularis mucosae. The overlying mucosa may be ulcerated, and the surrounding submucosa may be fibrotic, containing a mixed inflammatory infiltrate. These cysts can appear throughout the intestinal tract but are most frequently found in the colon and rectum. Given the submucosal location of these cysts, a biopsy that includes this layer is critical.

ETIOLOGY

Prolapse of the rectum leads to many of the signs and symptoms of SRUS. Ulcer formation is usually found at the tip of the prolapse. Direct pressure at the point where the prolapse abuts against the pelvic floor, especially at the level of the puborectalis muscle, can lead to blood vessel compromise and ischemia, which contributes to ulcer formation. Anismus, paradoxical contraction of the puborectalis muscle in response to the stimulus of defecation, may also manifest at this demarcation of the rectum and anus, resulting in outlet obstruction constipation. Repeated efforts to defecate against the tense sphincter mechanism contribute to the pressure and trauma on the tip of the prolapse. Because the anus distal to the dentate is quite sensate, the patient may describe a "sliding" in and out sensation with Valsalva's maneuver. This often leads patients to digitally explore the area. On palpation, patients feel the tip of the intussusception and may restore the prolapse to its normal anatomic position. Doing so alters the anorectal angle and allows stool to pass. After a sensation of incomplete evacuation, digitation finally allows some patients to complete defecation. If this becomes a daily practice, the repeated digitation may also lead to ulcer formation on the prolapsed rectum. However, this cannot explain all SRUS lesions, as a number are located beyond the reach of an inserted finger.

TREATMENT

Treatment is typically guided by the severity of symptoms. In patients with minimal symptoms, observation alone or treatment with bulk laxatives, bowel retraining, and reassurance is a reasonable initial management. The use of topical enemas, such as steroids, 5-ASA, sucralfate, or sulfasalazine, may not heal the lesions because they are typically not true ulcers. Products to ease bowel movements are of value in reducing the efforts at defecation; bulking agents, glycerin suppositories, polyethylene glycol (PEG) solutions, or other stool softeners may help with constipation and should be tried as an initial step. Large-volume enemas may help evacuate the contents of the distal colon and rectum and alleviate the need to strain. This being said, some investigators believe that the trauma from enema tips can result in the ulcer that is frequently seen. Unfortunately, conservative therapy frequently does not result in full ulcer healing or symptom resolution. In a series of 23 patients, 16 (70%) had failed nonsurgical therapy.

In patients whose conditions are more symptomatic or unresponsive to conservative therapy, treatment must be aimed at the two features of this rare ulcer: the anismus of the pelvic floor and the intussusception. Biofeedback may be used to treat anismus by helping to promote the normal relaxation reflexes that must occur to open the anal sphincter. In a series of 11 patients, biofeedback resulted in decreased straining effort and stool frequency and improved quality-of-life measures. At least 50% healing of the ulcer was also seen in six patients (54%). Biofeedback alone often fails to treat outlet obstruction, but it may be helpful in teaching patients with incontinence to tighten the sphincter. Long-term improvements in patient quality of life are best ensured by addressing this part of the pathophysiology.

If the ulcer is caused by prolapse, the intussusception must be stopped to treat the condition definitively. Stabilizing the rectum with surgical fixation can be used for this purpose, with a reported 55% to 60% long-term improvement in symptoms. Before the introduction of laparoscopic and robotic techniques, primary fixation procedures involved suture proctopexy to the sacrum, with suture placement at the distal third of the rectum. A low short midline incision allows for good retraction of the rectum and suture placement into the lateral stalks of the rectum. Early experience with laparoscopy resulted in some failures, perhaps as a result of bleeding, operator timidity, or inability to retract the rectum adequately. In the authors' initial experience, the most frequent failures encountered after suture proctopexy for prolapse were after laparoscopic proctopexy referred from outside institutions. However, a recent series of 39 patients reported 70% success rate after laparoscopic rectopexy. As surgeons worldwide become more adept at laparoscopic rectal procedures, laparoscopic failures are expected to be rare, especially if laparoscopic visualization of the puborectalis muscle is achieved circumferentially. Enhanced visualization and articulating instrumentation of robotic surgery may also result in better outcomes with robotic-assisted approaches.

After fixation, occasionally some redundant distal mucosa or hemorrhoids may require an extended hemorrhoidectomy. This is evident 4 to 6 weeks after fixation, when the inflammation related to the initial surgery has resolved.

SUGGESTED READINGS

Chiang JM, Changchien CR, Chen JR: Solitary rectal ulcer syndrome: an endoscopic and histologic presentation and literature review, *Int J Colorectal Dis* 21:348–356, 2006.

Halligan S, Nicholls RJ, Bartram CI: Evacuation proctography in patients with solitary rectal ulcer syndrome: anatomic abnormalities and frequency of impaired emptying and prolapse, *Am J Roentgenol* 164:91, 1995.

Kargar S, Salmanroughani H, Binesh F, et al: Laparoscopic rectopexy in solitary rectal ulcer, *Acta Med Iran* 49:810–813, 2011.

Madigan MR, Morson BC: Solitary ulcer of the rectum, *Gut* 10:871, 1969.

Otto SD, Oesterheld A, Ritz JP, et al: Rectal anatomy after rectopexy: cinedefecography versus MR-defecography, *J Surg Res* 165:52–58, 2011.

Perito ER, Mileti E, Dalal DH, et al: Solitary rectal ulcer syndrome in children and adolescents, *JPGN* 54:266–270, 2012.

Rao SS, Ozturk R, De Ocampo S, et al: Pathophysiology and role of biofeedback therapy in solitary rectal ulcer syndrome, *Am J Gastroenterol* 101:613–618, 2006.

Sitzler PJ, Kamm MA, Nicholls RJ, et al: Long-term clinical outcome of surgery for solitary rectal ulcer syndrome, *Br J Surg* 85:1246–1250, 1998.

Torres C, Khaikin M, Bracho J, et al: Solitary rectal ulcer syndrome: clinical findings, surgical treatment, and outcomes, *Int J Colorectal Dis* 22:1389–1393, 2007.

SURGICAL MANAGEMENT OF CONSTIPATION

Supriya S. Patel, MD, and Anthony J. Senagore, MD, MS, MBA, FACS, FASCRS

Constipation is a common medical condition that accounts for millions of office visits per year and significant resource consumption. Successful management of constipation requires a clear delineation of the scope of the problem. Several definitions and classification schemes have been proposed. One of the most commonly used is the Rome III criteria, which is based on the following symptoms: straining, hard stools, sensation of incomplete evacuation, sensation of outlet obstruction, frequent need for manual evacuation maneuvers, fewer than three defecations per week, and infrequent loose stools without laxative use. To fulfill the Rome III criteria, symptoms must be present for at least 12 weeks, in the 6 months before diagnosis, and irritable bowel syndrome must be excluded. Although these criteria are not entirely comprehensive, they do provide a useful basis for the initial evaluation of patients with the chief symptom of constipation.

ETIOLOGY AND WORKUP

The process of defecation involves a complex interplay between the sphincter complex, the colonic musculature, and the anorectal vault. The sphincter complex is composed of an external, striated muscle under voluntary control and an internal, smooth muscle under autonomic control. In normal situations, the sensation of stool in the anorectum results in relaxation of the pelvic floor and widening of the anorectal angle, thus facilitating stool evacuation with rectal contraction (Figure 1). A disorder in any step of this pathway can lead to impaired defecation.

The vast majority of office visits for constipation can be treated medically. Increased fiber consumption to 25 g/d coupled with increased fluid intake often improves stool frequency. Approximately 10% of patients have significant flatulence develop with psyllium-based products; their condition may be better managed with a cellulose-based fiber supplement. Constipation refractory to increased fiber and water consumption may require additional maneuvers aimed at either increasing luminal fluid content or reducing colonic transit time. Options include polyethylene glycol agents (increase fluid) and combinations of laxatives, suppositories, and prokinetic agents.

A thorough history and physical examination is critical for distinguishing between those cases that can be managed medically and

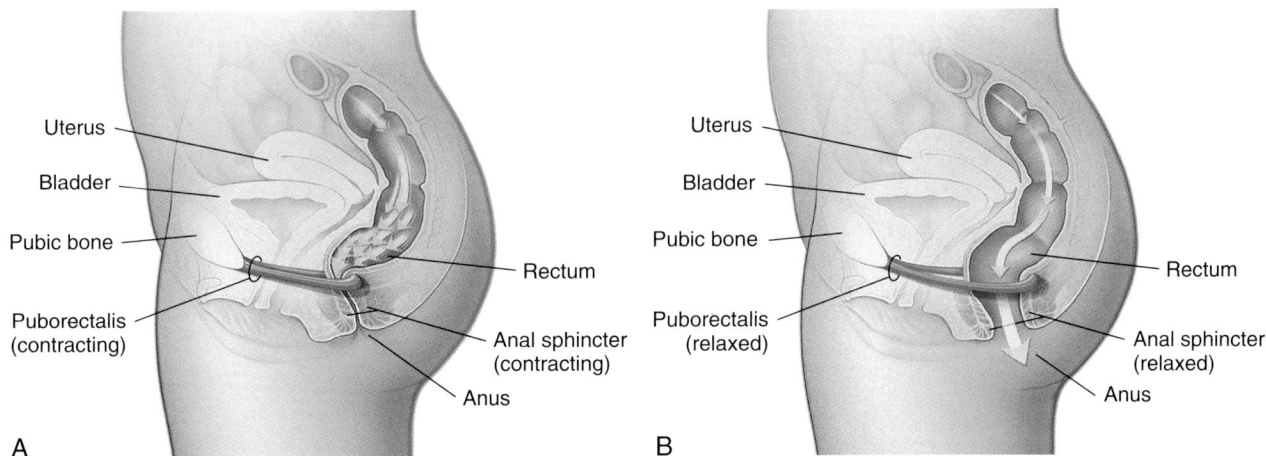

FIGURE 1   Normal anatomy of anorectal complex **(A)** at rest and **(B)** during defecation. During defecation the anorectal angle widens and the sphincter complexe relaxes, enabling evacuation of stool. *(From Bouras EP, Tangalos EG: Chronic constipation in the elderly, Gastroenterol Clin North Am 38(3):463–480, 2009, Fig 2.)*

those that may benefit from surgical intervention (Table 1). Electrolyte abnormalities should be corrected, and comorbidities that may affect gut transit, such as diabetes and hypothyroidism, should be optimized. In addition, medications known to induce constipation, such as opioid analgesics, should be limited when possible. Physical examination should include a rectal examination to rule out a distal obstructing mass and to assess anal sphincter tone. The presence of fecal impaction or impaired perianal sensation may shed insight into the etiology of the problem. Colonoscopy or barium enema should almost always be performed before empiric therapy to exclude colonic obstruction from either malignancy or inflammatory bowel disease.

Constipation can be divided into two main categories based on the underlying pathophysiology: (1) disorders of colonic motility; and (2) disorders of defecation. In terms of motility, constipation is categorized as either normal-transit constipation or slow-transit constipation on the basis of the rate at which stool passes through the colon. Obstructed defecation syndrome (ODS) is typically used to define the various entities associated with impaired defecation.

Patients whose symptoms fail to improve with conservative measures should begin the evaluation process to exclude ODS with anorectal physiologic testing. Anorectal manometry enables detection of sphincter pressures during relaxation and straining. High sphincter pressures may indicate the presence of an anal fissure, anismus, or paradoxic puborectalis syndrome; low pressures may be suggestive of impaired sensation. Distension of the rectum normally results in relaxation of internal anal sphincter, known as the rectoanal inhibitory reflex (RAIR). The presence of this reflex effectively rules out Hirschsprung's disease. The balloon expulsion test is used for assessing ability to evacuate; normal results are indicated with the ability to evacuate a 50-mL rectal balloon in less than 2 minutes. Finally, defecography is the gold standard test for evaluation of defecatory disorders and is especially useful in the setting of suspected anatomic abnormalities. In addition to enabling visualization of perineal descent and measurement of the anorectal angle, instillation of contrast into the small bowel, vagina, and rectum facilitates the diagnosis of enteroceles, sigmoidoceles, rectoceles, and intussusceptions. An often overlooked important finding associated with ODS on defecography is internal intussusception. Classic findings associated with significant rectoceles include size of more than 3 cm and incomplete emptying, both of which are worse with an intussusception. Images can be obtained via traditional x-rays, video fluoroscopy, or magnetic resonance imaging (MRI).

A select group of patients with either ODS or slow transit constipation may benefit from surgical intervention; however, exclusion of the former is essential before colonic resection is offered. Many cases

TABLE 1: Preoperative workup of the patient presenting with chronic constipation

Recommended	Optional
History	Anal manometry
Physical	Cine defecography
Laboratory (hemoglobin, electrolytes, TSH, T_4, etc., if not previously obtained)	Small bowel transit study (breath hydrogen)
	Gastric emptying
Anatomic study (barium enema or colonoscopy)	Small bowel follow through
Transit study	
Balloon expulsion test	

T_4, Thyroxine; *TSH*, thyroid-stimulating hormone.
From Beck DE: Surgical management of constipation, Clin Colon Rectal Surg *18(2):81–84, 2005.*

of ODS can be managed with biofeedback, which avoids the risk of surgery and improves quality of life. If a surgical option is selected, a thorough preoperative discussion is essential to define patient expectations regarding the potential outcomes because success is often relative, rather than complete, with any of the available surgical options.

OBSTRUCTED DEFECATION SYNDROME

ODS is a common cause of symptomatic chronic constipation, characterized by straining and difficulty in evacuation, frequently requiring digitation of the anus or vagina to facilitate defecation. A variety of different scoring systems exists to grade the severity of symptoms; an example is shown in Table 2. The symptoms of ODS have classically been attributed to rectocele; however, better recognition of this syndrome defined by anophysiology evaluation has shown the concomitant occurrence of other abnormalities, such as intussusception, in many of these cases. ODS most frequently occurs in females and may present after an inciting event, such as childbirth or total abdominal hysterectomy. Large nonemptying rectoceles (>3 cm) are often visualized on defecography, but the degree of internal rectal intussusception may be a more important component of ODS and is frequently underappreciated. A rectocele involves a weakening of the rectovaginal septum and anterior prolapse of the rectum into the vagina; an intussusception involves the telescoping of a proximal segment of rectum distally, often as low as the anal canal (Figure 2). Therefore, even small rectoceles with significant degrees of intussusception may be symptomatic. Initial management consists of dietary modification and biofeedback to attempt to improve coordination between anal sphincter relaxation and rectal contraction; surgical management is indicated if these measures fail and symptoms persist.

Classically, rectoceles have been repaired via transvaginal and transanal approaches, with or without mesh placement. The traditional approach to repair is the transvaginal posterior colporrhaphy. In this procedure, the posterior vaginal mucosa is incised and elevated, followed by plication of the entire length of the fibromuscular tissue of the septum and reapproximation of the vaginal mucosa. Anatomic cure is achieved in more than 80% of patients with this technique. More recently, attempts were made to refine the technique by performing site-specific repair of septal defects in hopes of reducing the incidence of dyspareunia associated with longer repairs. Similarly, the use of either biologic or polypropylene mesh has been proposed in hopes of reducing recurrence rates. There has been recent concern regarding the use of permanent mesh because of the risk of infection, pain, and erosion. Conversely, transanal rectocele repair involves the excision of redundant rectal mucosal tissue and suture reenforcement of the rectal muscularis layer as a means of repairing the defect.

STAPLED TRANSANAL RECTAL RESECTION

Stapled transanal rectal resection (STARR) represents a shift in thought as to the underlying mechanism of ODS, with a greater appreciation of the role of dysfunction of the rectal muscular wall. This is manifested by internal intussusception in addition to the typical presence of a rectocele. The goal of the procedure is primarily to separately resect a section of anterior and posterior rectal wall and only secondarily to impact the rectocele. This technique involves the use of two circular staplers to perform separate full-thickness, circumferential rectal resections (Figures 3 and 4). The anal canal is first dilated with lubricated dilators. The anoscope is then introduced and secured to the skin. Several nonabsorbable purse-string sutures, incorporating mucosa, submucosa, and muscularis, are placed along the anterior rectal wall, above the level of the dentate line and tip of the prolapse/intussusception. The first circular stapler is introduced and fired, with care taken not to involve the rectovaginal septum. The procedure is repeated along the posterior rectal wall; purse-string sutures are placed, and the second stapler is introduced and fired. Both staple lines are reenforced with absorbable suture as needed to ensure hemostasis.

Anatomic correction and symptomatic improvement are achieved in most patients. Upwards of 30% of patients report fecal urgency;

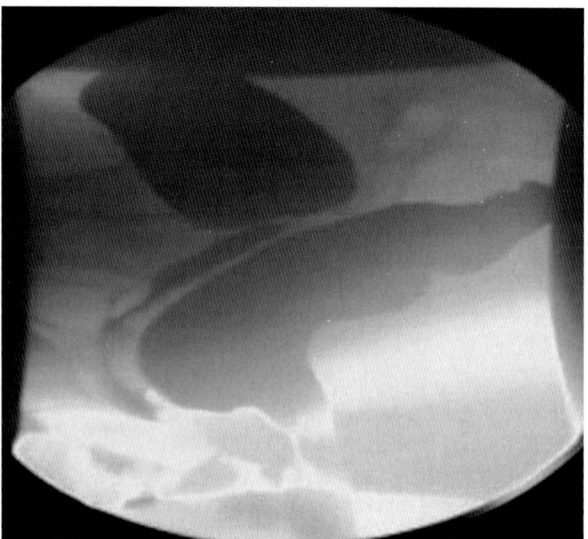

FIGURE 2   Rectocele and rectal intussusception causing impingement of the vaginal wall. *(From Hasan HM: Stapled transanal rectal resection for the surgical treatment of obstructed defecation syndrome associated with rectocele and rectal intussusception,* ISRN Surg 2012:652345, 2012, Fig 1.)

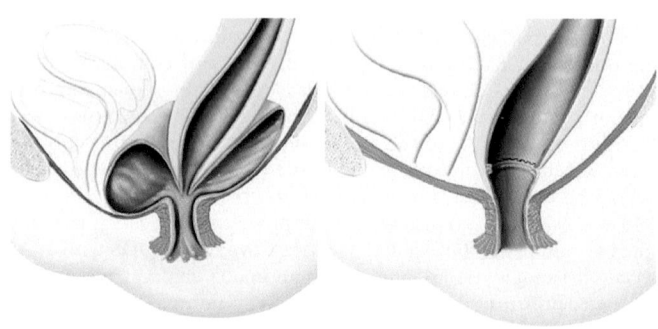

FIGURE 3   Stapled transanal rectal resection procedure. *(From Schwandner O, et al: Decision-making algorithm for the STARR procedure in obstructed defecation syndrome: position statement of the group of STARR Pioneers,* Surg Innovation 15(2):105-109, 2008, Fig 1.)

TABLE 2: Obstructive defecation syndrome: symptom scoring

Symptoms	Never	Rarely	Sometimes	Usually	Always
Excessive straining	0	1	2	3	4
Incomplete rectal evacuation	0	1	2	3	4
Use of enemas/laxative	0	1	2	3	4
Vaginal/perineal digital pressure	0	1	2	3	4
Constipation	0	1	2	3	4

Never, 0 (never); rarely, <1/month; sometimes, <1/week, ≥1/month; usually, <1/day, ≥1/week; always, ≥1/day.
From Hasan HM: Stapled transanal rectal resection for the surgical treatment of obstructed defecation syndrome associated with rectocele and rectal intussusception, ISRN Surg 2012:652345, 2012.

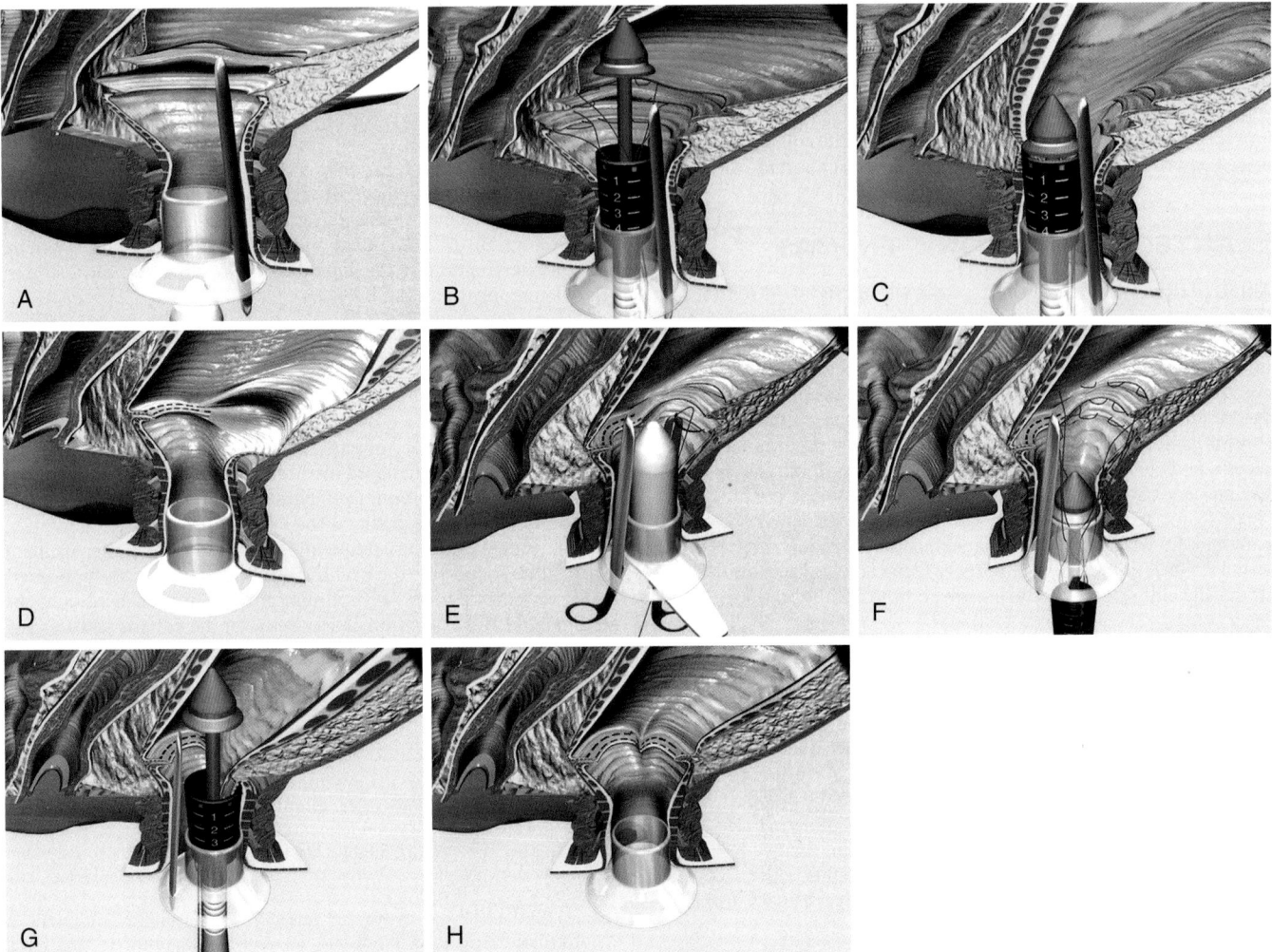

FIGURE 4 A to H, Stapled transanal rectal resection. Anal dilator is introduced, and anterior purse-string sutures are placed into the redundant rectal tissue. A retractor is placed along the posterior rectal wall to protect it during the stapling process. A circular stapler is fired. The procedure is repeated along the posterior rectal wall. *(From Pinto RA, Sands DR: Surgery and sacral nerve stimulation for constipation and fecal incontinence, Gastrointest Endosc Clin North Am 19(1):83–116, vi–vii, 2009, Fig 7.)*

however, the symptoms typically ameliorate over several months. With appropriate procedural training, STARR is generally associated with a low morbidity rate. Nonetheless, serious complications have been reported (i.e., hemorrhage, pelvic sepsis, and rectovaginal fistula).

The stapled transanal prolapsectomy with perineal levatorplasty (STAPL) procedure is a similar technique, in which redundant tissue is excised with a circular stapler and a levator reapproximation is performed via a perineal incision. In addition to the circular stapling techniques, ODS can also be treated via application of linear stapling devices; these procedures generally involve two firings of the linear stapling devices for excision of redundant rectal tissue. Limited comparative data examining the advantages of these approaches are available.

SLOW-TRANSIT CONSTIPATION

The etiology of slow-transit constipation is unknown, but neuronal and muscular factors have both been implicated in the pathogenesis. Patients are most commonly female and frequently present with symptoms of abdominal pain, straining, and bloating. Before surgical intervention, the evaluation should include: (1) anophysiologic evaluation to exclude ODS; (2) a colonic transit study (i.e., Sitzmark's study) to confirm slow transit; and (3) either a barium enema or colonoscopy to exclude luminal disease. Upper gastrointestinal motility studies may also be indicated to rule out pangastrointestinal dysmotility. Correction of concomitant disorders of evacuation before surgery for slow-transit constipation is recommended. In addition, patients with suspected psychiatric disorders should be referred for preoperative counseling, given the high incidence rates of failure and dissatisfaction after surgery observed in this population.

The operative procedure of choice for documented slow-transit constipation is a total abdominal colectomy (TAC) with ileorectal anastomosis. This procedure can be performed open or laparoscopically. The entire colon is mobilized and resected, and the ileum is anastomosed to the rectum. Anastomoses to the distal sigmoid colon have also been performed but are associated with a higher incidence of persistent constipation and are thus generally avoided. The mean stool frequency after TAC with ileorectal anastomosis typically ranges from two to four bowel movements a day. Unfortunately, however, this procedure is associated with a high morbidity rate (especially small bowel obstruction), and greater than 40% of patients experience persistence of their symptoms or a procedure-related complication. A laparoscopic approach may reduce the technical complication rate. Common complications after surgery include diarrhea, incontinence, small bowel obstruction, and recurrent constipation.

Several alternative resection strategies for slow-transit constipation have been described (i.e., subtotal colectomy with cecorectal anastomosis, segmental colectomy). These approaches are based on the concept that minimizing the amount of colon that is resected may reduce the incidence of postoperative diarrhea. However, these limited colonic procedures typically fail to treat the constipation and often require conversion to a TAC with ileorectal anastomosis.

ANTEGRADE COLONIC ENEMAS

Antegrade colonic enemas (ACE) are a viable treatment option for the management of both fecal incontinence and constipation and avoid the risks of colectomy. The procedure involves the administration of enemas directly into the colon to facilitate the controlled evacuation of stool. The traditional Malone's procedure, first described in the 1990s, involves the use of the appendix as the conduit. Since that time, conduit constructions with terminal ileum, cecum, and colon have been described. Advances in minimally invasive surgery have made construction of these stomas possible with laparoscopic techniques. ACE is an especially attractive option in patients who wish to avoid permanent ostomy creation and has been well described in the pediatric surgery literature. Leakage around the stoma site and stomal stricturing are common complications.

SACRAL NERVE STIMULATION

Sacral nerve stimulation (SNS), a U.S. Food and Drug Administration (FDA)–approved method for treatment of fecal incontinence, is gaining increasing attention in the management of chronic constipation. The procedure involves two components. In the first part, a test stimulation is performed with placement of a stimulating electrode, connected to an external pulse generator, into the S3 foramen; peripheral nerve function is then evaluated. Patients with successful responses to the test stimulation proceed to permanent implant placement.

The exact mechanism of action by which SNS regulates bowel function is poorly understood, but it is thought to involve a modulation of neuronal signaling pathways. The subset of patients with chronic constipation who may benefit from this technique has not been clearly defined. Further investigation is required before the routine application of this technique for chronic constipation is implemented.

OSTOMY CREATION

In most cases, ostomy creation is a considered a last-resort measure for patients with refractory chronic constipation. Options include ileostomy and colostomy formation. Stoma marking before surgery is critical, given the high likelihood of the stoma being permanent. Careful construction of the stoma can help avoid common stoma-related complications.

SUMMARY

Chronic constipation is a common and debilitating medical condition with a wide variety of causes. Careful differentiation of those patients who are best managed medically from those who may benefit from surgical intervention, is of paramount importance. Disorders of motility should be distinguished from disorders of defecation because these conditions frequently require different management algorithms. To increase the likelihood of success in the surgical treatment of constipation, a multidisciplinary approach should be adopted and clear communication between the patient and treating physicians established.

SUGGESTED READINGS

Corman ML, Carriero A, et al: Consensus conference on the stapled transanal rectal resection (STARR) for disordered defaecation, *Colorectal Dis* 8(2):98–101, 2006.
Gladman MA, Knowles CH: Surgical treatment of patients with constipation and fecal incontinence, *Gastroenterol Clin North Am* 37(3):605–625, viii, 2008.
Hasan HM: Stapled transanal rectal resection for the surgical treatment of obstructed defecation syndrome associated with rectocele and rectal intussusception, *ISRN Surg* 2012:652345, 2012.
Levitt MA, Mathis KL, et al: Surgical treatment for constipation in children and adults, *Best Pract Res Clin Gastroenterol* 25(1):167–179, 2011.
Ternent CA, Bastawrous AL, et al: Practice parameters for the evaluation and management of constipation, *Dis Colon Rectum* 50(12):2013–2022, 2007.

RADIATION INJURY TO THE SMALL AND LARGE BOWEL

Rachit Kumar, MD, and Joseph M. Herman, MD, MS

OVERVIEW

The treatment of most malignancies in the abdomen and pelvis requires a multimodality approach. The combination of surgery, chemotherapy, and radiation has improved survival in malignancies of the genitourinary tract, gastrointestinal tract, and gynecologic systems. Specifically, not only has the use of radiation led to improvements in local control and disease-free survival in the primary setting, but it is also used frequently in the palliative setting. The small and large intestines are two of the radiation dose-limiting organs in malignancies of the abdomen and pelvis. Modern technologic advances, including three-dimensional (3D) conformal, intensity-modulated, stereotactic, and intraoperative radiation therapy, allow for higher radiation doses to the tumor or tumor bed while limiting dose to the bowel and subsequent toxicity. As such, knowledge of the radiation dose limits, timing of radiation toxicity, and management of subsequent side effects are critical for both general surgeons and surgical oncologists.

Radiation as a treatment modality has advanced significantly over the past two decades. Traditional radiation therapy uses external beam radiation from the anterior-posterior direction (AP-PA) or with additional beams applied laterally (3D or conformal radiation). However, the increased implementation of intensity-modulated radiation therapy (IMRT) has allowed for a higher dose of radiation to a tumor with decreased toxicity to surrounding tissue. IMRT uses several radiation beams (>3) from multiple angles that are modulated (shaped) and converge to conformally cover the tumor volume. Stereotactic body radiation therapy (SBRT) is a form of IMRT that increases the daily dose of radiation applied to each individual radiation beam while decreasing the overall number of treatments (generally one to five treatments total). SBRT allows for a very high (ablative) dose of radiation to the tumor plus a small margin (<5 mm) but can result in an increased risk of damage to adjacent bowel if included in the radiation field. Intraoperative radiation therapy (IORT) can be delivered with x-ray radiation (electrons) and brachytherapy (the application of radiation sources in close approximation to the tumor). IORT allows for increased doses of radiation to the tumor bed with decreased normal tissue toxicity. Because IORT is delivered at the time of surgery, a higher dose of radiation (>10 Gy) can be delivered because the normal bowel has been removed from the treatment area. IORT is often combined with preoperative and postoperative radiation to achieve a dose that is high enough (>60 Gy) to sterilize microscopic residual disease (R1 resection). In general, IORT has been shown to be most effective when used with preoperative and neoadjuvant radiation therapy and when margins are negative (R0). However, emerging data have shown that IORT with high dose rate brachytherapy (HDR-IORT) can sometimes be effective even with R1/R2 resections.

RADIATION DOSE TOLERANCE TO THE SMALL INTESTINE AND RECTUM

A surgeon working with irradiated tissue needs to have a familiarity with the terminology used in describing radiation dose and tissue sensitivity. The small bowel is an organ arranged in a serial configuration (i.e., a relatively small volume of the small bowel receiving a high dose of radiation may lead to severe, irreversible side effects). In contrast, the large bowel and rectum are arranged in a parallel configuration; a single area of the organ may tolerate a very high dose, whereas the whole organ dose should be limited. A landmark paper from Emami and associates published in 1991 evaluated the radiation dose limits of multiple tissues. From this paper, a maximal dose limit to the small intestine was established at 45 to 50 Gy. More recent data from the QUANTEC investigators at the Radiation Therapy Oncology Group has compiled results from multiple studies to improve on Emami's initially identified dose limits. The investigators conclude that the radiation dose limit to the small intestine should be limited to no more than 195 cm³ of small bowel receiving greater than 45 Gy (V45, or volume receiving 45 Gy or more, should be <195 cm³). With SBRT, radiation to the small bowel should be limited to 12.5 Gy in a single fraction (V12.5 <30 cm³), or limited to 30 Gy in a 3 to 5 fraction regimen.

In contrast to the small and large bowels, the rectum has a much higher radiation dose tolerance. As noted previously, radiation toxicity to the rectum is largely based on the volume of the organ receiving a given a dose. From Emami and associates, if the rectum receives more than 60 Gy of radiation, there is only a 5% risk of long-term complications. However, if the bowel receives more than 80 Gy, there is a 50% risk of long-term complications. The risk of complications from radiation can also increase if concurrent chemotherapy is used or if the patient has conditions that may make the bowel more sensitive to radiation, such as Crohn's disease. The QUANTEC investigators refined these dose limits based on their analyses of prostate cancer radiation dose escalation studies. The risk of grade 3 or higher proctitis was determined to be less than 10% with a dose of 79.2 Gy with 1.8 to 2.0 Gy fractions. A more practical model based on dose-volume constraints is that less than 20% of the rectum should receive greater than 70 Gy (V70 <20%). Adhering to these dose limitations helps to ensure that the both the acute and the late complications of radiation are minimized.

PATHOPHYSIOLOGY OF RADIATION TO THE INTESTINAL TRACT

Radiation therapy has both short-term and long-term effects on malignant and healthy tissue. Short-term side effects typically occur

from the end of the first week of therapy and may be seen up to 2 weeks after the completion of radiation. Subacute effects occur between 2 weeks and 3 months. Long-term side effects may occur from 3 months to many years after the radiation therapy is completed. The pathophysiology of these side effects occurs by significantly different mechanisms. A better understanding of these processes assists practitioners in the management of both categories of complications.

Acute radiation to the bowel results in a decline in crypt cell mitosis and mucosal cell necrosis. The combination of these effects leads to villous sloughing. Symptomatically, patients report diarrhea as a consequence of the decreased absorptive surface area. Radiation enteritis often results in nausea and vomiting and in abdominal pain. The high radiosensitivity of the small bowel may result in an ulcer. Late radiation damage to the bowel is a consequence of both submucosal/serosal fibrosis and injury to the microvascular support structure within the intestinal wall. Fibrosis may result in adhesions that lead to kinked bowel loops, potentially resulting in small bowel obstruction. Although this risk is less than 10% in most cases, it is increased in the postoperative setting and should be considered in evaluation of a patient with an emergent abdomen.

Early radiation effects in the rectum generally result in crypt abscesses, decreased mucous production, and eosinophil infiltration. As with the small intestine, this may result in tenesmus, bleeding, pain with defecation, and diarrhea, although this tends to be self limited, with resolution of symptoms shortly after the completion of therapy. Colorectal fibrosis may be seen from 6 months to many years after the completion of radiation, with an incidence similar to that of the small bowel. Damage to the serosal blood vessels is an important mediator of this effect. Radiation proctitis, as manifest by recurrent bleeding years after completion of the radiation, is typically less than 15% and is usually increased in patients with rectal manipulation after radiation.

Certain factors may predispose to radiation enteritis, including pelvic inflammatory disease and endometriosis. A history of abdominopelvic surgery, either before or after radiation, significantly increases the risk of stricture and small bowel obstruction (SBO). As expected, preexisting vascular damage from hypertension, diabetes mellitus, and cardiovascular disease is detrimental on two accounts. First, the patient likely has initial damage to the vascular support structure within the lumen of the vessels. Second, any damage that occurs has more limited repair capacity because of poor nutrient transport. A thorough history of all patients for radiation should always include an assessment for collagen vascular disease, including rheumatoid arthritis, inflammatory bowel disease, and systemic lupus erythematosus, because these conditions often cause a greater acute and delayed response to irradiation. Many of these conditions may be discovered years after the completion of radiation in the setting of delayed radiation toxicity.

The risk of a second malignancy after radiation is extremely small, typically less than 1% in the lifetime of most patients with irradiation. This is an age-dependent value, with most cases of radiation-induced malignancy requiring more than 8 years to develop. Therefore, this is an important consideration in younger patients undergoing radiation and should be discussed with the patient's treating radiation oncologist.

The Radiation Therapy Oncology Group (RTOG) has developed a scoring scale to standardize side effects reported during and after radiation therapy (Table 1).

MANAGEMENT OF RADIATION ENTERITIS

As discussed previously, acute side effects of small intestine irradiation include malabsorption, altered gut mobility, diarrhea, nausea, and vomiting. Later side effects may include mucosal ulceration, eventually developing into perforations, fistulae, bleeding, and

TABLE 1: RTOG acute and late gastrointestinal toxicity scale

	Acute toxicity	Late toxicity
Grade 1	Increased frequency or change in bowel habits not requiring medication; rectal discomfort not requiring analgesics.	Increased frequency of bowel movements or rectal discomfort not requiring medications.
Grade 2	Diarrhea requiring parasympathetic drugs; mucous discharge not necessitating sanitary pads; rectal or abdominal pain requiring analgesics.	Frequent stools requiring parasympatholytic drugs; mucous discharge not requiring pads; pain requiring analgesics.
Grade 3	Diarrhea requiring parenteral support; severe mucous or blood discharge necessitating sanitary pads; abdominal distension.	Diarrhea requiring parenteral support; severe mucus or blood requiring pads; abdominal distension on x-ray.
Grade 4	Obstruction, fistula, or perforation; gastrointestinal bleeding requiring transfusion; abdominal pain or tenesmus requiring tube decompression or bowel diversion.	Acute or subacute obstruction, fistula, or perforation requiring surgical intervention; gastrointestinal bleeding requiring transfusion; abdominal pain or tenesmus requiring tube decompression or bowel diversion.
Grade 5	Death as a consequence of radiation-induced side effects.	Death as a consequence of radiation-related side effects to the intestine.

Radiation Therapy Oncology Group (RTOG) early and late toxicity scale for both genitourinary and gastrointestinal toxicity.
Adapted from Cox JD, Stetz J, Pajak TF: Toxicity criteria of the Radiation Therapy Oncology Group (RTOG) and the European organization for research and treatment of cancer (EORTC), Int J Radiat Oncol Biol Phys 31(5):1341–1346, 1995.

abscesses. The development of fibrosis may cause a stricture and SBO. Chronic malabsorption may lead to severe anemia and hypoalbuminemia. Although many of the acute side effects resolve quickly after radiation, late side effects may be severe, progressive, and irreversible.

Generally, acute radiation enteritis should be managed conservatively. This includes antidiarrheal, antispasmodic, and antiemetic medications as necessary. In patients with ongoing diarrhea despite medical management, a low residue diet should be applied. In some cases, this approach may be used for patients without antidiarrheal medications. Nonetheless, most patients respond to antidiarrheal medications rapidly. Careful observation should be made to a patient's nutritional status in the event that oral intake becomes particularly limited. In cases of severe nausea, total parenteral nutrition may be needed. Given the rapid repair capacity of the small bowel, a short radiation break often leads to functional improvements. Care is required with this approach because the risk of repopulation of the tumor with a more aggressive phenotype has been well recognized.

Small bowel obstruction after irradiation may be a consequence of stricture or adhesions leading to bowel loop entrapment. This surgical emergency should be managed as would any acute abdomen case. Initially, patients should be put on nothing by mouth (NPO) status for bowel rest and allowed to decompress. The site of stricture may be identified with enteroclysis. In certain cases, strictureplasty or dilation of the affected segment may be possible. However, this is not the preferred technique for treatment. Anastomosis with a proximal, nonirradiated segment of bowel has been performed with good results. In cases in which the viability of tissue is of concern, a temporary ileostomy is recommended. Of note, this is generally accepted as the standard of care in patients in whom a low rectal repair is required. The typical time of reversal of the ileostomy is approximately 3 to 6 months once the nutritional status has improved. Adhesiolysis may also be necessary in this patient population and, as expected, is more commonly seen in patients in the postoperative setting. In regards to the appropriate method of incisional approach, emerging data suggest improved outcome with transverse, subumbilical incisions as opposed to standard, vertical incisions. The former allows excellent exposure with fewer postoperative wound complications (Figure 1).

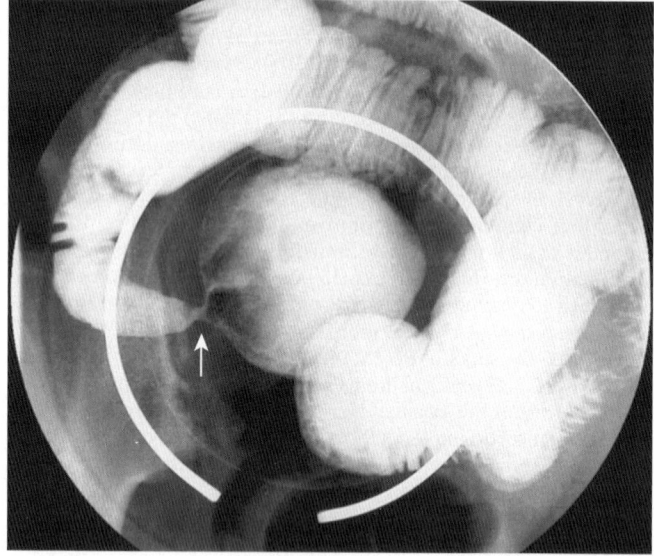

FIGURE 1 Enteroclysis shows a small bowel stricture and obstruction from a postoperative adhesion. The white arrow denotes a stricture with dilated proximal bowel on the right and normal caliber distal bowel on the left. *(From Nicolaou S, et al: Imaging of acute small-bowel obstruction, Am J Roentgen 185(4):1036–1044, 2005, Fig 4.)*

Perforation and fistulae may be caused by radiation but are also a consequence of tumor recurrence. Therefore, the first evaluation must be whether recurrent or residual tumor is the precipitating agent of this effect. If a perforation is noted, the loop of involved segment should be resected and, as with cases of obstruction, an anastomosis between healthy loops of bowel should be performed. Again, a temporary ostomy may be indicated if there is concern regarding the viability of the anastomotic segments. Further, the surgeon should understand the vulnerability of irradiated tissue, including skin, to the risk of wound-healing complications. As noted from a review of patients for irradiation in whom surgery was required for enteric complications, wound healing was the most commonly seen adverse event after surgery (Table 2).

Postradiation fistulae not associated with biopsy-confirmed tumor recurrence should be managed based on the involved segment of bowel and the site of drainage. A water contrast study can help identify the afferent and efferent ends of the fistula if not clinically apparent. Computed tomographic (CT) scans are highly sensitive in identifying the site of a fistula, particularly within the bladder. Fistulae involving the proximal bowel prior to the ileum are typically high output with a significant risk of malnutrition and dehydration. These cases are best managed with resection with anastomosis rather than with diversion or bypass. For lower fistulae, bypass or diversion with an ostomy is an effective way to allow for healing while preserving later continent function. Further, in cases of acute enterocutaneous fistulae, it is sometimes prudent to allow the fistula to mature before closure is attempted. Fistulae involving the bladder and vagina require similar measures as those described previously. Resection and anastomosis are preferred over bypass because of the risk of perforation, bleeding, abscess, and carcinogenesis associated with the remnant bowel. A critical part of the process of anastomosis is to ensure that a section of healthy bowel is identified. An increasingly used technique in preventing anastomotic leak or stricture is via a stapled side-to-side anastomosis. Omental or rectus flaps may occasionally be used to provide a healthy tissue barrier between the anastomosis and the affected organ (Figure 2).

Patients with massive intestinal damage after radiation may need significant surgical resection of affected segments resulting in short bowel syndrome, clinically presenting as severe diarrhea. This is best managed with fasting, total parental nutrition (TPN), and somatostatin.

MANAGEMENT OF RADIATION PROCTITIS

Acute radiation proctitis is generally manifest by tenesmus, bleeding, and diarrhea. Late-term side effects include bleeding, ulcers, strictures, and fistula. Unlike small bowel, malabsorption tends not to be a consequence of radiation to the pelvis. Instead, painless rectal bleeding is the most common long-term side effect.

Similar to radiation enteritis, acute side effects of radiation to the distal colon and rectum should be managed conservatively. The most common side effects reported by patients in the acute setting for rectal and lower genitourinary malignancies are tenesmus and diarrhea. Repeated episodes of rectal urgency are common during definitive radiation for prostate cancer, as the length of treatment for this malignancy lasts up to 8 weeks. Initial management for these symptoms includes antispasmodic medications. A low-fiber, low-residue diet also helps mitigate these symptoms and may reduce pain associated with tenesmus. Nonsteroidal anti-inflammatory medications (NSAIDs) may assist with the initial symptoms of pain associated with defecation. If pain is refractory to NSAIDs, opiates should be added to the patient's medication regimen. Opiate-induced constipation can be a secondary benefit in the patient with both diarrhea and dyschezia.

The treatment of certain long-term side effects, including strictures and fistulae, has been discussed previously. Radiation proctitis,

TABLE 2: Morbidity seen after surgery for chronic radiation enteritis

Complications	No. of events (%)
Overall morbidity*	
Wound complications[†]	21 (15.67)
Intestinal obstruction	5 (3.73)
Anastomotic dehiscence	3 (2.24)
Urinary fistula	3 (2.24)
Intra-abdominal hemorrhage[‡]	1 (0.75)
Disruption of ureteroileal anastomosis	1 (0.75)
Necrotic sigmoidostomy	1 (0.75)
Failure of rectovaginal fistula repair	1 (0.75)
Total	36 (26.87)

*Morbidity seen after surgery for chronic radiation enteritis.
[†]One patient with vertical incision had wound dehiscence and resuture.
[‡]The patient died.
From Zhu W, Gong J, Li Y, et al: A retrospective study of surgical treatment of chronic radiation enteritis. J Surg Oncol 105(7):632–6, 2012.

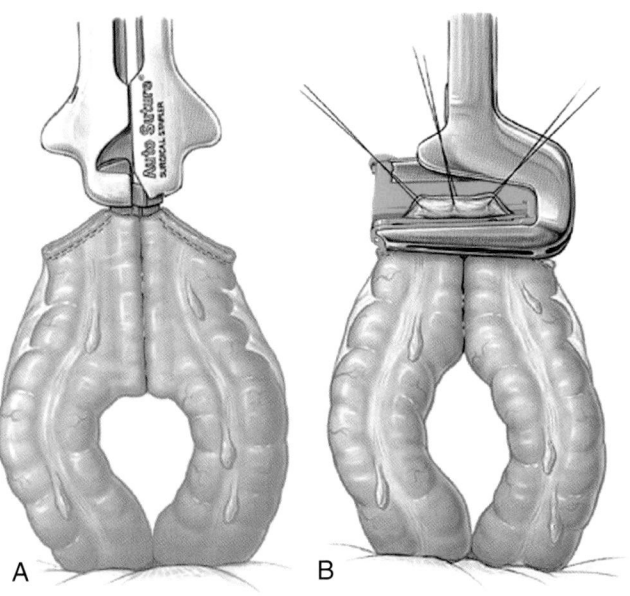

A   B   C

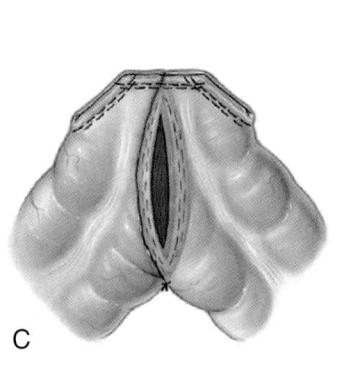

FIGURE 2 Demonstration of a side-to-side anastomosis technique. **A,** Bowel ends aligned and walls compressed, instrument is locked and activated. **B,** The entire circumference of the opening, tissue layers, and staple lines are closed. **C,** Final result. *(Illustrations reprinted with permission from Cine-Med, Inc. Copyright of illustrations are retained by Cine-Med, Inc., Woodbury, Conn.)*

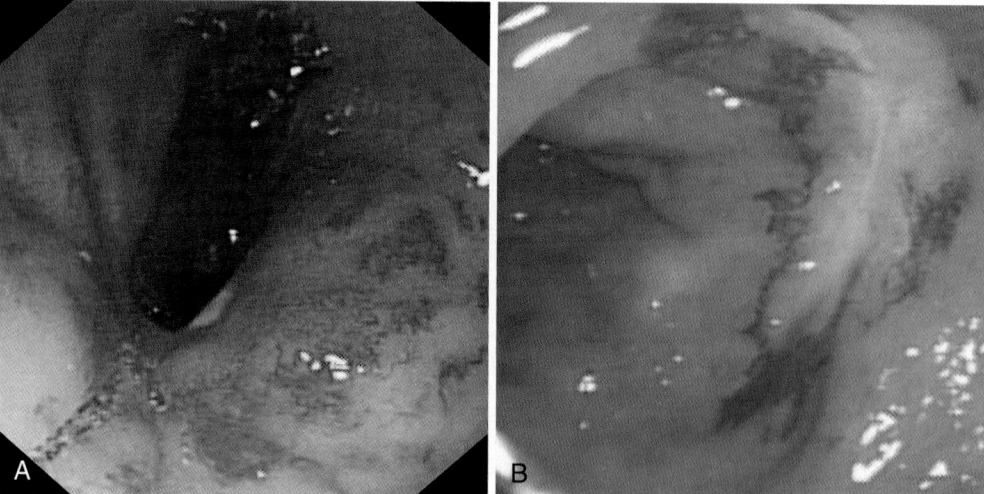

FIGURE 3 **A** and **B,** Tortuous blood vessels consistent with telangiectatic change after radiation therapy for prostate cancer. *(From Leiper K, Morris AI: Treatment of radiation proctitis,* Clin Oncol *19(9):724–729, 2007, Fig 1, A and B.)*

manifested by hematochezia, is established as the most likely complication of rectal irradiation months to years after therapy. In the setting of hematochezia after radiation, a thorough history and physical examination should be performed. Hemorrhoids are not uncommon in this population, and the patient's sexual practices should be determined. Endoscopic evaluation is the gold standard for diagnosis of radiation-induced rectal bleeding. The affected rectum has friable telangiectasia along the mucosa (see Figure 1). Many of these cases resolve spontaneously with time, and unnecessary biopsies of the affected mucosa prolong bleeding and delay healing. The treating physician should notify the performing gastroenterologist regarding a history of radiation therapy to the rectum to avoid a protracted course of hematochezia. The diagnosis of radiation proctitis can be made clinically without a mucosal biopsy (Figure 3).

Patients in whom hematochezia is continuous and progressive may consider a variety of nonsurgical treatment techniques. These include preparations of topical lidocaine, steroid-containing suppositories (prednisone), short chain fatty acid enemas, sucralfate, or steroid enemas (hydrocortisone) concurrently with metronidazole, which have been effective. No consensus regarding medical management procedure exists at this time, but the generally accepted course of therapy is to proceed with a single medication before proceeding to multimodality medication therapy.

Progressive hematochezia despite medical management should prompt consideration for minimally invasive surgical or topical procedures. These options include formalin therapy (chemical cauterization) and thermal coagulation therapy. Formalin therapy produces local chemical cauterization at the site of telangiectatic vessels and ulcers. Typical formalin solutions include 3.6% and 4% formalin, although 10% formalin has been described in the literature. Formalin is applied via either irrigation or direct application of formalin-soaked gauze. Complete response rates vary from 64% to 100%, with a duration of response lasting between 3 and 20 months. Side effects include stricture, anal ulcers, anal pain, incontinence, anal stenosis, and bleeding.

Thermal coagulation is accomplished with bipolar/heater cautery, an argon laser, or a yttrium aluminum garnet (YAG) laser. Bipolar or heater cautery is performed with a probe attached to a standard colonoscope. Multiple treatment sessions are often necessary for complete response. Cautery was found more effective than medical management in the long-term treatment of recurrent bleeding episodes. Further, this form of treatment is relatively rapid, with a response rate of 100% noted in most studies, and no major side effects reported. Both plasma argon therapy and YAG laser show high levels of response, with better response rates noted for plasma argon therapy. Side effects are noted to be potentially significant for this approach and include mucous discharge, prostatitis, rectal stric-

ture, tenesmus, ileus, abdominal pain, rectal ulcers, and rectal strictures.

Hyperbaric oxygen therapy has also been used in subacute and chronic radiation proctitis. Increasing local tissue oxygen tension is thought to promote wound healing by stimulating collagen formation. Despite a number of studies that assessed the results of this method, the quantification of improvement remains vague. Hyperbaric oxygen therapy may require as many as 80 or more treatments for symptom relief. Potential side effects include visual trauma, aural trauma, ear drum perforation, and angina. This therapy can also potentiate tumor growth; therefore, patients with residual disease must be excluded. The benefit of this form of therapy may be limited to patients in whom multiple other therapies have been unsuccessful.

PREVENTION OF RADIATION ENTERITIS AND PROCTITIS

Modern radiation techniques use a variety of methods to help reduce normal tissue radiation dose. Some of these have been mentioned previously and include IMRT, SBRT, IORT, and brachytherapy. Despite the improvements these technologies provide, potential for significant toxicity remains because of very high dose per fraction (SBRT), proximity to healthy tissue (IORT and brachytherapy), and radiation dose inhomogeneity (IMRT/SBRT). Information needed to assist in determination of whether radiation is the cause of specific symptoms includes the radiation plan, dose, fractionation, and treatment delivery. Optimally, the patient should be presented in a multidisciplinary tumor board to determine the best course of management.

Radiation oncologists may implement a variety of methods at the time of CT simulation (also known as the "planning scan") to help reduce side effects at the time of therapy. This includes treating the patient with a rectal balloon in place, and a full bladder and empty rectum to limit the dose to the small bowel and rectum. A rectal balloon helps push the posterior wall of the rectum away from the radiation field and is often used in patients with prostate cancer, especially those treated with high radiation doses per fraction. Placement of a spacer at the time of surgery can limit the volume of bowel in the radiation field; the spacer is often used during surgery in patients undergoing cystectomy or hysterectomy if radiation therapy is expected in the adjuvant setting.

Treatment of the patient in the preoperative setting is routinely done in multiple malignancies, including rectal cancer and sarcoma. The advantage of treating patients in the neoadjuvant setting, in terms of tissue toxicity, is that the organ of interest acts as a tissue spacer: physical space is provided by the organ against the entry of other organs, such as the bowel, as may be seen in the postoperative cases. Neoadjuvant treatment also takes advantage of reoxygenation and reassortment, which may be more effective in sterilization of the tumor. Another benefit of neoadjuvant therapy is the organ of concern is often excised, thereby preventing late side effects from occurring. However, practitioners should understand that this approach entails a higher risk of poor wound healing. A temporary diverting ileostomy should be considered if a low anastomosis is planned after chemoradiation. Optimally, a complete treatment plan, including an explanation of potential toxicity and prevention of long-term side effects, should be discussed with all practitioners at the time of the initial diagnosis and consultation.

Medicinal techniques that have been successfully used in the prevention of acute radiation enteritis include sulfasalazine and a low-residue diet. Although sulfasalazine has been shown to be effective in reducing radiation-induced diarrhea, questions remain regarding its potential radioprotective effects on the tumor. As such, many practitioners recommend a low-residue diet as prophylactic treatment of radiation enteritis.

SUGGESTED READINGS

Denton AS, Andreyev HJ, Forbes A, et al: Systematic review for non-surgical interventions for the management of late radiation proctitis, *Br J Cancer* 87(2):134–143, 2002.

Emami B, Lyman J, Brown A, et al: Tolerance of normal tissue to therapeutic irradiation, *Int J Radiat Oncol Biol Phys* 21(1):109–122, 1991.
Fajardo LF, Berthrong M, Anderson RE: *Radiation pathology*, New York, 2001, Oxford University Press.
Hall EJ, Giaccia AJ: *Radiobiology for the radiologist*, ed 6, Philadelphia, 2006, Lippincott Williams & Wilkins.
Hauer-Jensen M, Wang J, Boerma M, et al: Radiation damage to the gastrointestinal tract: mechanisms, diagnosis, and management, *Curr Opin Support Palliat Care* 1(1):23–29, 2007.
Kavanagh BD, Pan CC, Dawson LA, et al: Radiation dose-volume effects in the stomach and small bowel, *Int J Radiat Oncol Biol Phys* 76(3 Suppl):S101–S107, 2010.
Michalski JM, Gay H, Jackson A, et al: Radiation dose-volume effects in radiation-induced rectal injury, *Int J Radiat Oncol Biol Phys* 76(3 Suppl):S123–S129, 2010.
Nuyttens JJ, Kolkman-Deurloo IK, Vermaas M, et al: High-dose-rate intraoperative radiotherapy for close or positive margins in patients with locally advanced or recurrent rectal cancer, *Int J Radiat Oncol Biol Phys* 58(1):106–112, 2004.
O'Sullivan B, Davis AM, Turcotte R, et al: Preoperative versus postoperative radiotherapy in soft-tissue sarcoma of the limbs: a randomised trial, *Lancet* 359(9325):2235–2241, 2002.
Sauer R, Becker H, Hohenberger W, et al: Preoperative versus postoperative chemoradiotherapy for rectal cancer, *N Engl J Med* 351(17):1731–1740, 2004.
Small W, Woloschak GE: *Radiation toxicity: a practical guide*, New York, 2006, Springer.
Zhu W, Gong J, Li Y, et al: A retrospective study of surgical treatment of chronic radiation enteritis, *J Surg Oncol* 105(7):632–636, 2012.

HEREDITARY POLYPOSIS SYNDROMES

George Apostolides, MD, FACS, FASCRS

INTRODUCTION

Within the realm of gastrointestinal pathology and disease are a number of conditions, aside from polyposis, associated with multiple colorectal polyps. This condition can occur with inflammatory polyps of inflammatory bowel disorder (IBD), intestinal lipomatosis, and neurofibromatosis. Therefore, biopsy is of the utmost importance for proper diagnosis and classification.

In this chapter, the discussion is limited to the true polyposis syndromes, which include:

1. Adenomatous types (familial adenomatous polyposis [FAP], mut y homolog [MYH] polyposis and some of its clinical variants, attenuated FAP, Turcot's syndrome); and
2. Hamartomatous types (Peutz-Jeghers syndrome [PJS], juvenile polyposis [JPS], PTEN hamartomatous polyposis syndromes).

The chapter focuses on the characteristics of the individual polyposis syndromes and their genetics, diagnosis, surgical and medical therapy, and extracolonic manifestations.

ADENOMATOUS POLYPOSIS SYNDROMES

Familial Adenomatous Polyposis

Familial adenomatous polyposis is an autosomal dominant inherited condition caused by a mutation of the APC gene. FAP frequency is 1/10,000 (Table 1). Cardinal elements to meet the criteria for this disease are either greater than 100 adenomas or fewer than 100 with a positive family history. The polyps usually develop in adolescence, with the onset of cancer around 40 years of age. Approximately 25% of patients do not have a family history of FAP. Bleeding is the most common symptom (80%), followed by diarrhea (70%), abdominal pain, and mucous discharge. Mount Sinai Hospital, New York, reported a 27% incidence rate of colorectal cancer at the time of presentation in a series of 115 patients (Table 2).

Congenital hypertrophy of retinal pigment epithelium (CHRPE) is a patchy fundus discoloration. The presence of four or more on examination is a specific phenotypic marker present in two thirds of families with FAP.

Attenuated Familial Adenomatous Polyposis

Unlike classical FAP, attenuated FAP is characterized by patients with fewer than 100 adenomas that develop at a later age (34 to 44 years). Similar to patients with classic FAP, these patients are also at high risk of colorectal cancer. They may exhibit extracolonic manifestations and carry a germ line APC mutation. Cancer onset occurs at a later age than with classic FAP (mean age, 56 years). The polyps are mostly proximal to the splenic flexure, and their numbers vary

TABLE 1: Hereditary colorectal polyposis syndromes

Polyposis syndromes	Phenotypic expression	Genotype
Familial adenomatous polyposis	Attenuated: <100 synchronous adenomas Mild: <1000 synchronous adenomas Severe: >1000 synchronous adenomas	Dominant inheritance of germ-line mutation in APC
Mut y homolog–associated polyposis	Attenuated/mild polyposis	Recessive inheritance: biallelic mutations of yMUTYH
Hyperplastic polyposis	>30 hyperplastic polyps, any size or location >10 hyperplastic polyps, proximal to sigmoid Any number of hyperplastic polyps with a family history of hyperplastic polyposis	Unknown
Hamartomatous polyps Peutz-Jeghers syndrome	Two of the following criteria: Mucocutaneous pigmentation Gastrointestinal Peutz-Jeghers polyps Family history of Peutz-Jeghers polyposis	Dominant inheritance of germ-line mutation in STK11
Juvenile polyposis coli	>4 juvenile polyps in the colorectum Any number of juvenile polyps and a family history of juvenile polyposis	Dominant inheritance of germ-line mutation in SMAD4 or BMPR1
PTEN tumor-hamaroma syndromes		
Cowden's syndrome Bannayan-Riley-Ruvalcaba syndrome Proteus syndrome	International Cowden's consortium criteria	Dominant inheritance of a germ-line mutation in PTEN

TABLE 2: The extracolonic features of familial adenomatous polyposis

Most frequent	Upper GI adenomas	95%
	Osteomas, mainly jaw	80%
	CHRPE	75%
	Epidermoid cysts	50%
	Fundic gland polyps	40%
Less frequent	Unerupted and supernumerary teeth	17%
	Desmoids	15%
	Upper GI cancers	5%
	Adrenocortical adenomas	5%
Rare	Papillary thyroid carcinoma	<1%
	Biliary tract carcinoma	<1%
	Hepatoblastoma	<1%
	Medulloblastoma	<1%

CHRPE, Congenital hypertrophy of retinal pigment epithelium; GI, gastrointestinal.

significantly between family members. The genotype can be one of three groups: germ-line APC mutation, biallelic MYH mutations (30% of patients when APC is normal), and germ-line DNA mismatch repair (MMR) gene mutations. With regards to extracolonic findings, fundic glands and duodenal adenomas are frequent, but CHRPE are not found in this group. Desmoid disease is rare in 5′ mutations but frequent in 3′ mutations.

A full colonoscopy and genetic testing of APC/MYH mutations should be done in patients with 10 or more colonic adenomas, especially with a positive family history of colorectal adenomas or cancers. A full search for extracolonic features of FAP, including upper

gastrointestinal (GI) endoscopy, testing of polyps or tumor for microsatellite instability (MSI), and MMR immunochemistry (IHC), may be helpful to exclude Lynch's syndrome. If the polyps are few and endoscopically controllable, then yearly endoscopy is reasonable. If the adenoma burden is uncontrollable, then colectomy with ileorectal anastomosis (IRA) should be performed.

Mut Y Homolog–Associated Polyposis

Mut y homolog–associated polyposis (MAP) is the autosomal recessive form of FAP caused by a mutation in the MYH gene, not the APC gene. Most affected individuals have fewer than 100 adenomas, but some may have several hundred and thus present as a true FAP case. Most polyps are predominantly right sided. Colonic microadenomas, duodenal adenomas, desmoid tumors, and fundic gland polyps can all be present. MAP can mimic many of the other hereditary forms of colorectal cancer, from sporadic cancer to FAP, and from Lynch's syndrome to hyperplastic polyposis (HPP). Because of its uniquely autosomal recessive inheritance, MAP has major implications for genetic counseling. MAP should be suspected and testing for MYH should be done with the following criteria: no APC mutation is found, the mode of inheritance is not clearly autosomal dominant, or the number of polyps is low.

The genetic mechanism of MAP is a biallelic mutation in MYH. Its protein product functions in the base excision repair pathway to correct base-pair mismatches that result from oxidative damage. Those biallelic carriers have an 80% cumulative lifetime chance of development of colorectal cancer by age 70 years. The locations of the pathogenic human muty homolog (hMUTYH) mutations vary with ethnicity. The most common mutations involve Y179C (associated with a more severe phenotype) and G396D.

The presence of 10 or more synchronous adenomas, or the presence of serrated polyps with multiple adenomas, warrants a genetic counseling and testing referral. Once MAP is confirmed, colonoscopy

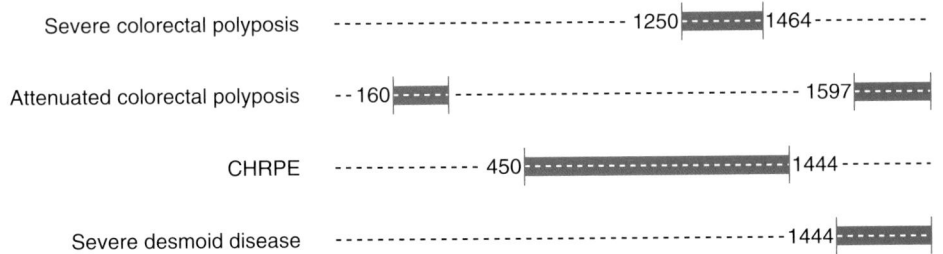

FIGURE 1 Schematic representation of the APC gene showing genotype-phenotype correlations. The *shaded areas* indicate regions of the codon where mutations are mostly found. *CHRPE,* Congenital hypertrophy of retinal pigment epithelium.

and esophagogastroduodenoscopy (EGD) are done, starting between the ages of 25 and 30 years. In rare cases with limited colonic adenomas, endoscopy can control disease and surgery can be avoided. More often than not, surgery is necessary with colectomy and IRA.

Turcot's Syndrome

Turcot's syndrome is the association of colorectal adenomatous polyposis and central nervous system tumors. In two thirds of the families, an APC gene mutation is present and the predominant tumor is a cerebellar medulloblastoma. In the other third of cases, variants of hereditary nonpolyposis colon cancer (HNPCC) are associated with glioblastoma.

GENETICS

The APC gene is a large gene situated on chromosome 5q21. In FAP and most sporadic colorectal cancers (CRC), a mutation of the APC gene is one of the earliest events. It is a key gene in colorectal carcinogenesis and is mutated in a majority of sporadic colorectal cancers. Most mutations are between codons 168 and 1640 (exon 15), with a particular concentration in two hotspot codons 1061 and 1309. More than 820 germ-line APC mutations have been found to cause FAP, and all result in a truncated APC protein product that then fails to act as a tumor suppressor in the *wnt* signaling pathway.

Although the APC protein is expressed in all organs, the messenger RNA is found in particularly high levels in normal colonic mucosa. The 300-kd APC protein is found in the cell cytoplasm and interacts with several other proteins, including β-catenin and the cytoskeleton. It plays a role in the *wnt* signaling pathway, which is involved in the normal development of three-dimensional structures and is abnormally activated in some malignant diseases. APC binds and downregulates cytoplasmic β-catenin, thereby preventing its translocation to the nucleus. In contrast, abnormal APC fails to do this, so that β-catenin is free to enter the nucleus and form a complex that results in a specific transcription of cell cycle, simulating DNA sequences and ultimately cell proliferation.

Genotype-Phenotype Correlation in Familial Adenomatous Polyposis

Several genotype-phenotype correlations have been observed in FAP. Evidence is found of significant correlation between the position of the germ-line APC mutation (genotype) and the various aspects of the phenotype (Figure 1).

SURGICAL THERAPY

Once the molecular genetic diagnosis of FAP is confirmed, and irrespective of whether the patient is symptomatic, prophylactic surgery is recommended. Full colonoscopy is mandatory to evaluate the number and distribution of the polyps. Biopsies are taken to detect any cancer or dysplasia, especially in the rectal and anal mucosa. Close collaboration between the surgeon, gastroenterologist, geneticist, and the patient is needed. Many factors need to be considered in deciding the optimal management and subsequent surgical procedure.

Although the prevention of cancer remains a crucial priority in the management of patients with hereditary colorectal cancer, one should also aim to maintain a good quality of life. This is especially true in the young asymptomatic patient diagnosed with screening. Considering that surgery does not cure FAP, the timing and choice of surgery should be the one with the least impact on social, academic and vocational activities.

Timing of Surgery

Patients with severe polyposis (>1000 colonic or >20 rectal polyps) or symptomatic patients should have surgery as soon as possible. Asymptomatic patients with mild disease (100 to 1000 adenomas, <1 cm size, without severe dysplasia) can have surgery delayed until the patient reaches appropriate physical and intellectual maturity. Another important reason for surgical delay is the concern for the development of desmoid disease, especially in women with a family history of desmoid disease, extracolonic manifestations of Gardner's syndrome, and a 3′ APC mutation. In these cases, annual colonoscopy is advised for monitoring of the polyps. Most patients with classic polyposis have surgery between the ages of 16 and 20 years, well before cancer typically develops.

Choice of Operative Procedure

The most common surgical therapy for FAP includes: (1) total proctocolectomy (TPC) and end ileostomy or Kock's pouch (done in select centers); (2) total abdominal colectomy (TAC) and IRA; and (3) TPC and ileal pouch–anal anastomosis (IPAA), stapled or hand sewn, with or without mucosectomy. Any of these surgeries can be done with equal efficacy and safety, through the conventional open or laparoscopic approach, depending on the expertise of the surgeon (Table 3).

Total Abdominal Colectomy and Ileorectal Anastomosis

Total abdominal colectomy with IRA is a reasonable and safe option in young patients, particularly children and teenagers without 1309 mutation or severe polyposis, especially with fewer than five to 10 rectal polyps. Any polyp of more than 5 mm should be removed, and polyps with high-grade dysplasia are a relative indication for completion proctectomy. The main disadvantage of this surgical technique for FAP is that follow-up studies have shown a 12% to 29% risk of cancer developing in the rectal stump within 20 to 25 years, despite close follow-up observation. Patients with IRA should undergo yearly endoscopic surveillance of the rectum. If severe dysplasia or uncontrolled polyposis develops, completion proctectomy, with or without ileoanal pouch formation, is recommended.

TABLE 3: Indications for prophylactic surgery for patients with familial adenomatous polyposis

Factor	TAC and IRA (leave 15 cm rectum)	TPC and IPAA	PC with Ileostomy (or kock's pouch in select centers)
Indications for surgery	<20 rectal polyps APC	Most of patients with FAP Rectal polyp carpeting Resectable rectal cancer Desmoids in family history	Older patients after IRA Poor sphincter tone Low rectal cancer nonresectable oncologically
Age at surgery	Within 2 years of phenotypic expression and molecular diagnosis	Within 2 years of phenotypic expression and molecular diagnosis	At CRC diagnosis
Mortality rate	Very low	Very low	Very low
Morbidity rate	Low (15%-20%)	High (15%-50%)	Very low
Functional outcome Early Late Follow-up	 Good Good Rectal endoscopy 1×/y	 Average Good Pouch endoscopy 1×/3 y	 Good Good Same as for sporadic CRC Pouch endoscopy 1×/3 y
Disadvantages	Risk of rectal cancer	Complex surgery, often needs stoma, bowel function unpredictable, risk of damage to pelvic nerves and decreased fecundity in women, risk of ATZ adenomas and cancer	Permanent stoma

ATZ, Anal transition zone; *CRC,* colorectal cancers; *FAP,* familial adenomatous polyposis; *IPAA,* ileal pouch–anal anastomosis; *IRA,* ileorectal anastomosis; *PC,* proctocolectomy; *TAC,* total abdominal colectomy; *TPC,* total proctocolectomy.

Patients are at higher risk of development of rectal stump cancer when the polyposis is more severe, with a mutation in exon 15 G, and in codon 1309. The advantage of this approach is the avoidance of risk of damage to erection, ejaculation, and bladder function in men that occurs in about 1% of patients and to fertility in women. This procedure removes the entire colon and leaves about 15 cm of rectum to which the ileum is anastomosed. One should avoid entering the presacral plane to facilitate future pelvic dissection when the prospects of a completion proctectomy and a restorative IPAA become more appropriate.

Restorative Proctocolectomy With Ileal Pouch–Anal Anastomosis, Stapled or With Mucosectomy

This option is favored in cases with severe polyposis or severe rectal disease or in patients predisposed to duodenal or desmoid disease. IPAA is thought to alter bile salt absorption via the enterohepatic circulation with secondary decreased bile acid production and less duodenal exposure to intestinal carcinogens. Reports by Blasco and associates indicate a lower incidence rate of duodenal adenomas after IPAA than after IRA.

In this operation, the colon and rectum down to the level of the dentate line are removed, thereby theoretically eliminating the risk of colorectal cancer. The dissection plane must be close to the rectal wall to avoid injury to the pelvic nerves. If the lower rectum is spared from heavy polyp burden, then a stapled anastomosis is adequate as the bowel function is better than with mucosectomy or hand-sewn anastomosis. When the lower rectum is carpeted with adenomas to the dentate line, then a mucosectomy and hand-sewn anastomosis is recommended. This method does minimize the risk of cancer in the anal transitional zone. The endoanal mucosal stripping can be done either in the prone (the author's preferred method) or lithotomy position. Division of the rectal mucosal dissection is easier in three quadrants through a vertical incision from the dentate line extending proximally about 6 to 8 cm. The dissection is performed with electrocautery, after an infiltration of the submucosa with a diluted solution of 1:100000 epinephrine mixed in normal saline solution; then each mucosal strip is removed separately. The Lone Star retractor (Lone Star Medical, Strafford, Tex) greatly facilitates the exposure during this dissection. Another method is to perform a circular sleeve resection. In both methods, removal of all of the mucosa is imperative. Nevertheless, controversy still remains as to whether a mucosectomy should be done in the absence of dysplasia in the transition zone because it results in more complications and poorer function.

In the case of cancer of the upper or middle rectum, an oncologic dissection can be done with the IPAA by incorporating a total mesorectal dissection. Then, the abdominal colectomy is performed, laparoscopically or open, with a Pfannestiel's or lower vertical midline incision for construction of the ileal pouch and a diverting loop ileostomy. The ileostomy can then be closed 3 months later. A J pouch (most common type, 15-cm to 25-cm limbs) or S-shaped pouch can be constructed with either stapled or hand-sewn anastomosis with similar functional results. In select patients, the obese patient, or tall slender men, there can be difficulties with mesenteric reach. Various maneuvers can be done to lengthen the reach of the pouch. Complete mobilization of the mesentery to the level of the duodenum and near the pancreatic head, transection of the ileum close to the colon, transverse scoring of the peritoneum over the superior mesenteric artery (SMA), and occasionally selective division of mesenteric arcade may be needed for lengthening. In practical terms, the author has found the following simple maneuver to be a good indication of whether the pouch will reach the dentate line. When the apex of the pouch reaches approximately 6 cm beyond the symphysis pubis, then the pouch most likely will reach its target. It may be helpful to anchor the pouch to the pelvic sidewall to prevent twisting or torsion and subsequent ischemia.

Early postoperative complications of this procedure are: pouch leaks in 5% to 7%, small bowel obstruction in 20% to 25%, and pouchitis in 5% (much less than the 20% to 25% seen in ulcerative colitis), for an overall complication rate of 15% to 50%. This is the operation of choice for most patients with FAP. Short-term results are inferior to IRA as far as stool frequency, urgency, day and night-time continence, and need for antidiarrheal medications. In the long term, after 2 years, the results are comparable with IRA.

Ileoanal pouches should also be followed endoscopically because of a high rate of adenoma formation in pouches, with reported rates as high as 50% and even reported cases of cancer formation. Adenomas in the anal transition zone occur twice as commonly with stapled anastomosis compared with the hand-sewn IPAA. These adenomas can be excised individually or the entire anal transitional zone (ATZ) can be stripped. If stripping is to be performed because of the extent of the polyposis, it should be performed in two stages to avoid stenosis. Dysplasia in the ATZ occurs twice as often in the stapled anastomosis (18.5% vs 7.2%) with the mucosectomy method. Needless to say, redo pelvic procedures in patients with FAP are technically demanding as the tissue planes are nonexistent and scarring can be severe. Ureteral stents should be placed before surgery. Recommendations are to refer this kind of secondary revisional surgery to experienced surgeons.

Proctocolectomy With Permanent Terminal Ileostomy (or Kock's Pouch)

Proctocolectomy with permanent terminal ileostomy is rarely indicated except in cases of advanced rectal cancer requiring subsequent pelvic radiation or low rectal cancer, older patients, and poor sphincter function or preclusion of IPAA. It is a simple operation with low morbidity and reoperation rates. It does, however, mean creation of a permanent stoma. The creation of a Kock's pouch to achieve full continence is performed in select centers, but there is a significant complication rate. The most common complication is valve slippage (10% to 20%), which necessitates reoperation and small bowel obstruction (6% to 15%). Although patient satisfaction is high, morbidity and reoperation rates are also high.

Other facts may also dictate the surgical procedure that should be done. These involve the patient's comorbidities, ability to withstand potential complications, baseline sexual and bladder function, and patient's priorities and preferences.

MEDICAL THERAPY

Adenoma Chemoprevention

Both nonsteroidal antiinflammatory drug (NSAID) sulindac and cox-2 inhibitor celecoxib were found to be effective in reducing the number and size of adenomas in the retained rectum. Chemoprevention, however, is not an alternative to prophylactic surgery because no reduction in the rate of cancer was shown. In fact, cases are seen of rectal cancer in patients on sulindac despite reduction in the number and size of polyps.

The circumstances in which the use of chemoprevention is indicated are: unfeasible completion proctectomy because of desmoid disease, delayed surgery, a very high family risk of desmoid disease, or treatment of pouch polyposis.

EXTRACOLONIC DISEASE

Upper Gastrointestinal Polyposis

Upper GI polyposis is a major extracolonic finding in patients with FAP. Fundic gland polyps are seen in the stomach in 80% to 90% of patients with FAP. They are made up of areas of cystic hyperplasia. Usually the condition is benign, but recent reports show a 40% rate of low-grade dysplasia and a 3% rate of high-grade dysplasia. The best clinical practice is to biopsy representative fundie gland polyps (FGPs) during regular surveillance.

Gastric adenomas occur in 10% of patients, usually in the antrum. The incidence rate of gastric cancer in FAP in Japan is seven times that in the West; for Koreans, it is three times the rate.

More than 95% of individuals with FAP have duodenal adenomas. These occur about 15 years later than colonic polyps. Duodenal cancers, although rare (5%), are the second most common cause of death in FAP. Average age at diagnosis is 50 years.

The adenomas are mostly found in the area of the ampulla of Vater. In fact, up to 50% of normal-appearing ampullas are dysplastic on biopsy. Adenomas and even cancer can also occur in the small bowel.

Duodenal surveillance is essential in properly managing FAP. Duodenal adenomas are flat, white mucosal patches. They are completely different from in appearance from colonic adenomas. The Spigelman staging system allows for an objective assessment of the severity of duodenal polyposis in FAP (Table 4).

In Spigelman's original cohort of patients at 10-year follow-up, there was a 2% risk of cancer in stages II or III compared with a 36% risk of invasive duodenal carcinoma in stage IV. Regular endoscopic surveillance of the stomach and duodenum is therefore recommended. The use of forward-viewing and side-viewing scopes starts at age 25 years. The interval of recommended surveillance is outlined in Table 5.

The management of severe duodenal polyposis is difficult, and once invasive carcinoma develops, outcome is poor. Endoscopic mucosal resection is an attractive option but is made difficult by the plaque-like morphology of the polyps and their proximity to the ampulla, as even a simple biopsy of the ampulla can result in acute pancreatitis and repeated diathermy can result in scarring and stricturing. Duodenectomy and open polypectomy carry a 100% recurrence rate at 1 year.

Chemoprevention with sulindac can result in small polyp regression but has no effect on large ones. A randomized trial of cox-2 inhibitor has shown a significant improvement for those with mild to moderate disease.

Duodenectomy is a last resort option. Pancreas-preserving duodenectomy for Spigelman stage IV provides satisfactory control with reasonable low morbidity. If cancer is suspected, a Whipple's procedure is the best choice, although associated with a high rate of complications.

TABLE 4: Polyp scoring system in Spigelman staging for duodenal adenomas

Points	Number of polyps	Size of polyps (mm)	Histology	Dysplasia
1	1-4	1-4	Tubular	Mild
2	5-20	5-10	Tubulovillous	Moderate
3	>20	>10	Villous	Severe

TABLE 5: Derivation of Spigelman stage from scores

Total points	Spigelman stage	Suggested interval to next duodenoscopy (years)
0	0	5
1-4	I	3-5
5-6	II	3
7-8	III	1
9-12	IV	Duodenectomy; if not, rescope in 6 months

TABLE 6: Intra-abdominal desmoid tumor staging

Stage	Description
I	Size <10 cm, not growing, asymptomatic
II	Size <10 cm, mildly symptomatic, slow growing (<50% growth in 6 months)
III	Size 10-20 cm, moderate symptoms (bowel or ureteric obstruction), slow growing
IV	Size >20 cm, severe symptoms (abscess, fistula, hemorrhage) or rapid growth (>50% growth in 6 months)

Desmoid Disease

A desmoid tumor is by far the most troublesome and disabling consequence of FAP. It is a locally invasive, nonmetastasizing clonal proliferation of myofibroblasts. Although rare in the general population, the tumors are found in up to 30% of FAP cases. It is the third most common cause of death in patients with FAP overall (11%), after metastatic colorectal (58%) and duodenal cancer. Desmoids can vary from white sheet-like plaques to large rapidly growing tumors. Intra-abdominal desmoids tend to pucker and distort adjacent tissues, causing obstruction in tubular organs. Peak incidence is around 30 years of age, or 2 to 3 years after surgery. In patients with FAP, desmoids typically occur within the abdomen (50% of cases), especially in the small bowel, and in the abdominal wall in about 45%. Trauma (as in surgery) and estrogens are causative factors. There is also some degree of genotype-phenotype correlation as desmoids have been reported more frequently in patients with 3′ germline APC mutations. Many patients with desmoids also have mutations in the 5′ half of the APC gene. Surgeons should be alert to recent publications mentioning a "desmoid risk factor" score, with the important elements being: female gender, presence of extracolonic manifestations (as in Gardner's syndrome), and, most predictive, a family history of desmoids.

Computed tomographic (CT) scan and magnetic resonance imaging (MRI) are the most useful tools for investigation and follow-up, allowing for visualization and measurements and demonstrating the relationship of the desmoid tumor to other key structures such as ureter and bowel.

The treatment is controversial, often empirical and difficult. The natural history is variable, with about 10% resolving spontaneously, 10% growing rapidly and relentlessly, and the rest showing variable cycles of resolution and growth or remaining stable. Abdominal wall and extraabdominal desmoids are best treated with surgery. Even if recurrences are common (20% to 50%), complications are few.

A staging system for intra-abdominal desmoid tumors has been proposed by Church and Bomann and colleagues and is shown in Table 6.

Intra-abdominal desmoids are much harder to treat. Because most desmoids involve the root of the mesentery, complete resection is often impossible. Even after residual free (R0) resections, recurrence rates are around 50%. Any foolhardy attempt at resection of a desmoid tumor affecting the root of the small bowel mesentery is associated with high mortality from hemorrhage or high morbidity from extensive loss of small bowel. Ureteric obstruction is best treated with stents, and in rare instances, renal autotransplantation has proven effective. Often nonresective surgery is effective to treat the complications, such as careful lysis of adhesions, bypass procedures in the face of bowel obstruction, and occasionally diversion by means of stoma creation.

Clinical Scenarios

If one finds an unexpected desmoid at time of the first surgery, then it is best to do a proctocolectomy and pouch if possible. If the pouch does not reach, then an IRA is the next best choice for mild polyp load, with a proctocolectomy with end ileostomy reserved for severe polyposis.

If a desmoid is found at a completion proctectomy after a previous IRA, the rectum must be removed because it may well be impossible to do a restorative proctectomy.

The third scenario is with a need for prophylactic surgery in a patient with a strong family history of desmoids. Surgery in this case should be delayed as long as it is possible and safe. Yearly colonoscopy and treatment with sulindac are reasonable options for patients in their 20s. Otherwise, IRA or a proctocolectomy and pouch are both adequate options.

Conflicting reports exist regarding the value of radiotherapy. Its use for intra-abdominal desmoids is limited because of the risk of radiation enteritis. Medical treatment may involve NSAIDs, such as sulindac; antiestrogens, such as tamoxifen, raloxifene or toremifene; and cytotoxic chemotherapy in aggressive nonresectable disease, such as doxorubicin, dacarbazine or a combination of vinblastine and methotrexate.

The following algorithm for management of intra-abdominal desmoids may provide useful suggestions in their management (Figure 2).

HAMARTOMATOUS POLYPOSIS TYPES

Peutz-Jeghers Syndrome

Peutz-Jeghers syndrome is an autosomal dominant inherited cancer syndrome with an incidence rate of 1/200,000. It is caused by mutation of LKB1 (or STK11) on chromosome 19. This LKB1 mutation is found in 60% to 70% of cases. A significant number of cases occur de novo. They are hamartomas with a characteristic branching morphology containing smooth muscle in the submucosa.

The presence of two of three of the following characteristics defines this disease: perioral, buccal, or genital melanin pigmentation; gastrointestinal hamartomatous polyposis (PJS); and a family history of PJS. Pigmentation appears in childhood and fades in the late 20s. The polyps occur mostly in the small intestine (78%), stomach (38%), colon (42%), and rectum (28%).

Clinical concerns in PJS are many. Anemia from chronic blood loss and small bowel obstruction are the most common clinical issues. The risk of malignancy increases with age. In one series, by age 57 years, approximately half of patients had died of cancer. The

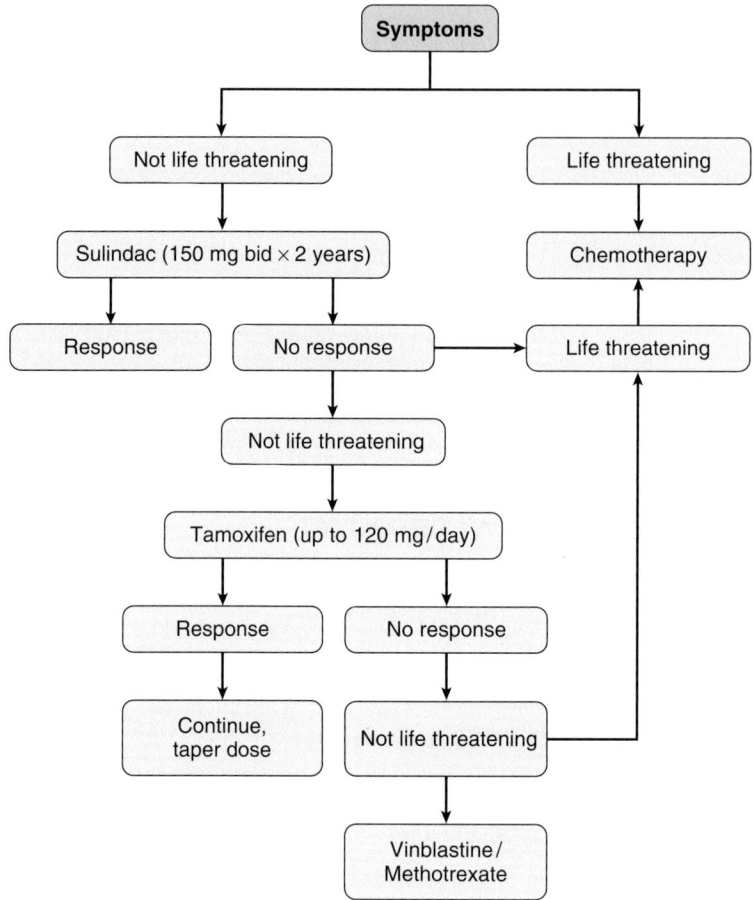

FIGURE 2 Algorithm for management of intra-abdominal desmoids.

cause of death in half of those cases was gastrointestinal related. In a lifetime, 90% of patients have cancer develop: colorectal, 20%; gastric, 5%; breast, pancreas, 30%; ovarian sex cord tumors, pulmonary, and cervical malignancies.

Medical and surgical management of PJS can be complex. Emergency laparotomy may be necessary for intussusception or bleeding. The best technique is the "clean sweep" technique where at the time of laparotomy, endoscopy per anus to the small bowel and per oral into the jejunum are performed. The scope is then withdrawn in a darkened room, and all polyps marked with sutures for later removal through enterotomies with suture ligation at the stalk of the polyps. With this technique, the entire small bowel is cleared of polyps, minimizing the need for future reexploration. Capsule endoscopy is useful for surveillance of asymptomatic patients. Colonic polyps are controlled endoscopically.

Surveillance depends on the number, size, histology, and location of the polyps. An EGD, capsule endoscopy, and colonoscopy should follow a normal examination 2 to 3 years later. Hemoglobin should be checked annually. Any polyps over 1.5 cm should be removed. Extra intestinal surveillance should be done according to national standards for breast and cervical screening and physical examination for testicular tumors in prepubertal boys. Clinicians should be aware of the high cancer risk and maintain a low index of suspicion.

Juvenile Polyposis

Juvenile polyps (JPS) are hamartomas that lack smooth muscle. Juvenile polyposis is defined as the presence of five or more juvenile polyps in the colon, or any number of juvenile polyps associated with a family history of JPS or multiple juvenile polyps in the upper and lower GI tract. The colon is affected 100% of the time, and the stomach and small bowel up to 50%. Most affected patients have between 50 and 200 polyps. It is a rare condition, occurring in 1/100,000. Associated morphologic abnormalities (macrocephaly, cleft lip/palate, congenital heart disease, genitourinary malformations, malrotations) are present in 10% to 20% of patients. Disease presents with rectal bleeding, anemia, and polyp prolapse at around 9 years of age. Adenomatous dysplasia in those hamartomatous polyps can develop in up to 50% of cases, with possibility of progression into adenocarcinoma.

This condition is different from a solitary juvenile polyp, which is the most common colorectal lesion in children (2%) and carries no malignant potential.

Genetic studies have shown JPS to be heterogeneous, as three separate germ-line mutations have been identified. The first mutation is present in SMAD4, a tumor suppressor gene on chromosome 18q21, and occurs in about 40% of patients with JPS in the United States but in only 3% to 28% in Europe. Mutations in a second gene, BMPRIA on 10q22, have been found in 15% of cases. Lastly, mutations in PTEN have been reported in JPS. Mutations in SMAD4 carry a high risk of hereditary hemorrhagic telangiectasia (HHT), manifesting as multiple vascular anomalies in the brain, lungs, mediastinum, and bowel.

In JPS, the cumulative colorectal cancer risk is about 30% to 50%, and upper GI cancer is at about 10% to 20%. Management of first-degree relatives should include a colonoscopy by age 12 years; if the patient is asymptomatic, then 5 years thereafter is appropriate if colonoscopy was normal. Upper GI endoscopy is advised by age 25 years. When the polyp load is minimal, the condition can be controlled endoscopically. When the polyp load is too large, or if the patient is symptomatic with diarrhea, bleeding, or abdominal cramps, a colectomy and IRA or a restorative proctocolectomy may be advisable.

PTEN Tumor Hamartoma Syndromes

PTEN tumor hamartoma syndromes are three very rare dominant inherited conditions involving hamartomatous colorectal polyps and craniofacial, skeletal, and dermatologic phenotypic features. The three syndromes are: Cowden's syndrome, Bannayan-Riley-Ruvalcaba syndrome, and serrated polyposis (SPP). All share common germ-line mutations of PTEN, which is an important tumor suppressor gene.

Cowden's Syndrome

Cowden's syndrome consists of macrocephaly, trichilemmomas (pathognomonic), and benign or malignant tumors of the thyroid, breast, uterus, and skin. Hamartomas occur in the mouth and give a nodular appearance to the buccal mucosa. The colon is affected with various polyps (hamartomas, lipomas, fibromas, neurofibromas adenomas). The colorectal cancer risk in Cowden's syndrome is not yet well defined. Colonoscopy should be done by age 30 years and every 3 years if findings are minimal.

Bannayan-Riley-Ruvalcaba Syndrome

This syndrome involves colorectal hamartomas (50%), characteristic pigmented penile macules, macrocephaly, mental retardation (50%), lipomatosis, and hemangiomas. It is caused by mutations of the same gene. No evidence of increased colorectal cancer risk.

Serrated Polyposis

Initially thought to carry no premalignant potential, the polyps in SPP are now known to be potential premalignant precursors to cancer pathways. These polyps are called serrated because the overcrowded hyperplastic glands are thrown into a saw-toothed or serrated pattern. When patients have multiple lesions, they are at high risk of colorectal cancer, with reported rates up to 50%.

The World Health Organization definition of serrated polyposis is:

At least 30 serrated polyps, any size and location.
More than 10 serrated polyps proximal to the splenic flexure, of which two are larger than 10 mm.
Any number of serrated polyps with a family history of SPP.

No germ-line mutation has been identified yet, and the pattern of inheritance is not clear. The treatment is either endoscopic or surgical. These polyps can be easily missed on colonoscopy; therefore, yearly colonoscopy is advisable to prevent cancer. When the polyp load is too large and not controlled with endoscopy, then colectomy and IRA is advised.

CONCLUSION

The ultimate concern in polyposis syndromes is the potential for malignant transformation and development of colorectal cancers. Each particular syndrome is associated with a certain risk for this outcome. The essence of proper management is to balance the elimination of cancer risk with maintenance and preservation of quality of life. This principle allows for the selection of the most appropriate surgical intervention and proper timing. Understanding the genetic basis of the polyposis syndrome, diagnosis, and surveillance assist in selecting the surgical therapy. A multidisciplinary approach involving genetic counselor, pediatrician, gastroenterologist, and surgeon is crucial to maximizing appropriate medical care.

ACKNOWLEDGMENT

The author acknowledges the previously authored works by James M, Church, MD, Y. Nancy You, MD, Bruce G. Wolff, MD, Claudio Soravia, MD, and Zane Cohen, MD, and also thanks John G. Apostolides, MD, for his help in editing this chapter.

SUGGESTED READINGS

Bianchi LK, Burke CA, Bennett AE, et al: Fundic gland dysplasia is common in familial adenomatous polyposis, *Clin Gastroenterol* 6(2):180–185, 2008.
Church J, Simmang C: Practice parameters for the treatment of patients with dominantly inherited colorectal cancer, *Dis Colon Rectum* 46(8):1001–1012, 2003.
Fazio VW, Church JM, Delaney CP: Current therapy in colon and rectal surgery, ed 2, St. Louis, 2005, Mosby, p 357.
Lathford AR, Sturt NJ, Neale K, et al: A 10 year review of surgery for desmoid disease associated with familial adenomatous polyposis, *Br J Surg* 93:1258–1264, 2006.
Nieuwenhuis MH, Bulow S, Bjork J, et al: Genotype predicting phenotype in familial adenomatous polyposis: a practical application to the choice of surgery, *Dis Colon Rectum* 52(7):1259–1263, 2009.
Parks TG: Extracolonic manifestations associated with familial adenomatous polyposis, *Ann R Coll Surg Engl* 72:181–184, 1990.
Remzi FH, Church JM, Bast J, et al: Mucosectomy vs stapled ileal pouch-anal anastomosis in patients with familial adenomatous polyposis: functional outcome and neoplasia control, *Dis Colon Rectum* 44(11):1590–1596, 2001.
Sieber OM, Lipton L, Crabtree M, et al: Multiple colorectal adenomas, classic adenomatous polyposis and germ-line mutations in MYH, *N Engl J Med* 348:791–799, 2003.
Spigelman AD, Williams CB, Talbot IC, et al: Upper gastrointestinal cancer in patients with familial adenomatous polyposis, *Lancet* 2:783–785, 1989.
Van Lier MD, Wagner A, Mathus-Vliegen EM, et al: High cancer risk in Peutz-Jeghers syndrome: a systematic review and surveillance recommendations, *Am J Gastroenterol* 60:141–147, 2011.

COLON CANCER

Elizabeth Hechenbleikner, MD, and
Elizabeth Wick, MD, FACS

BACKGROUND AND EPIDEMIOLOGY

Colorectal cancer arises from the epithelial lining of the colon or rectum, with roughly 75% of cases occurring in the colon and 25% in the rectum. Colon cancer is one of the most commonly diagnosed cancers and a leading cause of cancer death in the United States. There is considerable geographic variation in colon cancer incidence, both within the United States and across the world, with increased incidence associated with developed and developing countries. Differences in diet, physical activity, and access to healthcare services are some of the proposed reasons for this regional variation. Most colon cancers are sporadic adenocarcinomas diagnosed in adults over the age of 50 years. In the United States, over the past decade, a consistent decline has been seen in colon cancer incidence rate in adults greater than 50 years old; however, in adults under the age of 50 years, the incidence rate has been rising nearly every year since 1992. Colon cancer mortality has also been decreasing in the United States, but disproportionately fewer white patients die from colon cancer as compared with African American patients, regardless of cancer stage. Because screening colonoscopy is not recommended until 50 years of age for individuals at average risk, colon cancers in younger patients generally present later, when symptoms such as abdominal pain or bloating develop. Timely screening colonoscopy is paramount for the early detection and potentially curative treatment for premalignant (adenomatous) and malignant lesions.

SCREENING RECOMMENDATIONS

Colonoscopy is considered the gold standard among colon cancer screening techniques because it is highly sensitive and allows for biopsy of abnormal areas and polyp removal. Overall screening colonoscopy rates are improving but continue to fall short of recommended levels in the United States, with cost and fear of the procedure and bowel preparation the major barriers to widespread adoption. Key goals during colonoscopy are to visualize the entire colon, including adequate cecal inspection, and to identify and remove all polyps. Two common screening tests that are less expensive than colonoscopy are the fecal occult blood test (FOBT) and flexible sigmoidoscopy. FOBT is less sensitive than colonoscopy, and sigmoidoscopy only visualizes the lower one third of the colon; however, decreased colon cancer mortality has been associated with regular use of FOBT and one-time screening sigmoidoscopy in select patients. Another test that has been available since the 1990s is computed tomographic colonography (CTC) or virtual colonoscopy. CTC, which still requires a bowel preparation, has been shown in some settings to be as effective as colonoscopy for detection of tumors 1 cm in size or larger.

Screening recommendations are based on one's lifetime risk of development of colon cancer. Most individuals have no identifiable risk factors and are considered average risk, with a 5% to 6% lifetime risk of colon cancer. In patients at average risk who are 50 years of age or older, the 2008 joint guidelines from the American Cancer Society, the U.S. Multi-Society Task Force on Colorectal Cancer, and the American College of Radiology recommend: (1) annual FOBT; (2) flexible sigmoidoscopy every 5 years; (3) flexible sigmoidoscopy every 5 years with annual FOBT; (4) colonoscopy every 10 years; or (5) double-contrast barium enema every 5 years. In the 2008 joint guidelines, CTC was endorsed as a suitable screening option for those who decline or cannot tolerate colonoscopy, but the timing of repeat examinations is still uncertain. Moreover, a positive finding on FOBT, sigmoidoscopy, double-contrast barium enema, or CTC mandates follow-up colonoscopy.

About 25% of the population is at increased or moderate risk of development of colon cancer because of a personal or family history of colon cancer or adenomatous polyps. In this group, timing of colonoscopy screening examinations varies based on the individual's clinical situation. For example, patients with three to 10 adenomas or one adenoma larger than 1 cm or with high-grade dysplasia should have all lesions removed at initial colonoscopy, with a repeat examination within 3 years. In individuals with first-degree relatives with colon cancer diagnosed before the age of 60 years, colonoscopy should begin either at age 40 years or 10 years before the youngest diagnosed family member, with follow-up colonoscopy every 5 years.

Approximately 6% to 8% of the population is at high risk of development of colon cancer because of a hereditary syndrome like familial adenomatous polyposis (FAP) or hereditary nonpolyposis colon cancer (HNPCC) or a chronic medical condition like inflammatory bowel disease (IBD). Patients with suspected hereditary colon cancer should undergo genetic testing and counseling. Individuals with known or suspected FAP should undergo yearly flexible sigmoidoscopy or colonoscopy starting in childhood (age 10 to 12 years) until prophylactic or therapeutic total colectomy or proctocolectomy is deemed appropriate. Patients with HNPCC should have screening colonoscopies every 1 to 2 years starting in early adulthood (age 20 to 25 years) or 10 years before the youngest immediate family member with colon cancer. Patients with IBD should undergo screening colonoscopies with biopsies for dysplasia every 1 to 2 years after 8 years of pancolitis or 12 to 15 years of left-sided colitis.

PRESENTATION, DIAGNOSIS, AND WORKUP

Early colon cancer typically has no symptoms but may be discovered with a positive FOBT and subsequent colonoscopy. As the primary lesion enlarges, a change in bowel habits may be seen, such as decreasing stool caliber or rectal bleeding. Patients with late or advanced colon cancer often present with fatigue, weight loss, iron-deficiency anemia, or abdominal pain. Presenting symptoms may differ in patients with early or advanced colon cancer based on the location of the tumor. Right-sided tumors have a tendency to present with anemia; left-sided lesions are more likely to cause abdominal pain, obstruction, or rectal bleeding. Interestingly, various studies since the 1980s have reported an increasing percentage of right-sided colon cancers, perhaps in part because of increased colonoscopy utilization and different tumor biology and environmental factors that are currently under investigation.

When a patient is diagnosed with colon cancer, a thorough evaluation is required to establish the proper treatment. Medical comorbidities should be identified as should pertinent family history to rule out hereditary cancer syndromes. Complete colonoscopy with biopsies must be performed to confirm and tattoo the primary lesion along with any synchronous lesions. When a sporadic colon cancer is diagnosed, there is a 6% to 8% chance of having a synchronous lesion. Computerized tomographic (CT) scan of the abdomen and pelvis is done to evaluate the presence of metastases and adjacent organ invasion from the primary tumor. Chest x-rays should also be performed, and abnormal findings usually require chest CT scanning. Approximately 20% of patients in the United States present with metastatic disease, with the liver, lung, and peritoneum as the most common sites. Currently, the National Comprehensive Cancer Network (NCCN) does not recommend positron emission tomography with CT scan for the initial staging of a primary colon cancer intended for surgical resection. Regarding laboratory data, a baseline serum carcinoembryonic antigen (CEA) level should be measured before treatment, particularly surgical resection. After surgical resection, CEA levels that do not normalize or subsequently become elevated indicate inadequate tumor resection, recurrence, or progression of disease and require further evaluation. Serum electrolytes, liver function tests, and a complete blood count are part of a standard workup, along with a proper nutrition assessment, and should be optimized before surgery whenever possible.

SURGICAL RESECTION AND STAGING

Surgical resection is the foundation of curative treatment for localized colon cancer and select patients with limited metastatic disease. Approximately 75% of patients are candidates for potentially curative surgical resection at the time of diagnosis. Ten percent to 25% of patients with isolated liver metastases are operative candidates. The goal of surgery is to achieve an appropriate oncologic resection, ideally an R0 resection, while minimizing complications like infection, hemorrhage, and sexual or urinary dysfunction. The abdomen should be thoroughly explored and any extracolonic tumor spread to the liver, omentum, hemidiaphragm, abdominal wall, or pelvis identified, along with careful palpation of the entire large bowel. The involved colonic segment should be completely removed with a 2-cm to 5-cm margin and en bloc resection of any local structures or organs invaded by the primary tumor. The major vascular pedicle and lymphatic drainage basins of the involved colonic segment should be removed in a curative resection. Per NCCN guidelines, a minimum of 12 lymph nodes are required for accurate assessment of nodal involvement. Bowel continuity should be restored when possible with a well-vascularized, tension-free anastomosis.

Selection of the appropriate surgical procedure is based on the location of the primary tumor and the presence of synchronous lesions or a hereditary cancer syndrome. The vascular supply to the involved colonic segment dictates the extent of resection. Removal of the appropriate vascular supply should ensure adequate lymphadenectomy. A right colectomy is performed for cancers of the cecum, ascending colon, and hepatic flexure. In this procedure, the ileocolic artery is ligated, as is the right colic artery if present, and the terminal ileum is transected roughly 10 to 15 cm proximal to the ileocecal valve (Figure 1). The transverse colon is divided proximal to the right branch of the middle colic artery (MCA), which can be ligated if necessary. An extended right or, in some instances, transverse colectomy can be performed for tumors in the mid transverse colon. For an extended right colectomy, the ileocolic and MCA are ligated at their origin; for a transverse colectomy, only the MCA is ligated. In this case, an anastomosis is created between either the ileum (extended right colectomy) or the ascending (transverse colectomy) and distal transverse colon. A transverse colectomy requires mobilization of both the hepatic and the splenic flexure to allow for adequate reach and a tension-free anastomosis. Splenic flexure tumors can be treated with either a subtotal colectomy or, if adequate mobility is present, a left colectomy. Descending colon cancers and select proximal sigmoid colon cancers are managed with a left colectomy with a descending to sigmoid or rectal anastomosis. With a left colectomy, the inferior mesenteric artery (IMA) should be ligated high near the aorta to allow for a tension-free anastomosis. The inferior mesenteric vein can be ligated just below the duodenum if additional mobility is needed. Sigmoid cancers are treated with a sigmoid colectomy and high ligation of the IMA (see Figure 1). The splenic flexure should be mobilized for left colon resections to ensure creation of a tension-free anastomosis. In the case of patients with synchronous colon cancers or a hereditary cancer syndrome, a total abdominal colectomy with ileorectal anastomosis may be warranted.

The most important prognostic factor after surgical resection is the pathologic stage. The tumor node metastasis (TNM) classification system developed and maintained by the American Joint Committee on Cancer (AJCC) and the Union for International Cancer Control (UICC) is the most universally used staging system for colon and rectal malignant diseases. Table 1 includes the most updated TNM staging for colorectal cancer. Colon cancer is localized to the bowel wall in stage I and II, regionally spread in stage III (i.e., lymph node involvement), and distantly spread or metastatic in stage IV. The 5-year survival rate decreases with stage progression: (1) stage I, 70% to 95%; (2) stage II, 54% to 65%; (3) stage III, 39% to 60%; and (4) stage IV, 0 to 16%. The risk of regional lymph node spread correlates with bowel wall penetration by the primary tumor (T status). Primary tumors limited to the submucosa have a 10% risk of regional spread, whereas those penetrating to the subserosa have a 45% risk. Extent of nodal metastases (N status) is the most important determinant for long-term survival and treatment planning. Inadequate lymphadenectomy is a poor prognostic indicator in localized and regionally spread colon cancers. Lymph node retrieval can be difficult but is facilitated by high ligation of vasculature. Too few lymph nodes can lead to understaging and thus inappropriate adjuvant treatment. Moreover, accurate histologic assessment of lymph nodes can vary markedly based on the pathologist's technique and skill.

OPEN VERSUS LAPAROSCOPIC COLECTOMY

Open colectomies are typically performed through a midline incision with the patient supine for right colon resections and in modified lithotomy position for left colon resections. The right or left colon is mobilized off the retroperitoneum via a lateral-to-medial approach. This approach begins in an avascular plane known as the white line of Toldt (the lateral reflection of parietal peritoneum). Peritoneal attachments at the hepatic or splenic flexure are taken with electrocautery, clipping, or suture ligation with care to avoid undue traction, which can cause avulsion injuries. The transverse colon is mobilized as far as required for an adequate oncologic resection and to facilitate bowel anastomosis, and a portion of the omentum near the tumor is removed with the specimen. The vascular supply is divided and ligated at the base of the mesentery based on tumor location as previously described. A hand-sewn or stapled bowel anastomosis is performed per surgeon preference with no significant difference in complications or outcomes. For transverse colectomy, the greater omentum is removed with the specimen.

Laparoscopic colectomy offers many advantages over traditional open surgery. Postoperative pain and length of hospital stay are significantly reduced, but oncologic outcomes remain similar for localized colon cancer. Correct patient positioning is an integral part of successful laparoscopic colectomy. The patient is secured supine for right colectomies and in the modified lithotomy position with minimal hip flexion and legs in padded stirrups for left colectomies. The patient must be secured to the bed with a strap to prevent the patient from slipping because the bed is frequently repositioned to facilitate laparoscopic dissection. For right colectomy via a lateral-to-medial approach, four basic ports can be placed as follows: an umbilical camera port and three working ports in the left upper quadrant, left lower quadrant, and suprapubic midline (Figure 2, A). Similarly for left colectomy, a four-trocar technique can be set up as follows: an umbilical camera port and three working ports in the right upper quadrant, right lower quadrant, and suprapubic midline (Figure 2, B). Additional ports can be placed to optimize exposure based on surgeon preference.

Passive exposure of the colon is achieved with steep Trendelburg's positioning and rotating the table away from the anatomic location of the tumor. The small bowel and omentum are moved into the upper abdomen. The colon can be mobilized via a lateral-to-medial or medial-to-lateral approach. In the latter, the main vascular pedicles are divided first followed by complete mobilization and transection of the involved colonic segment. The colon can then exteriorized

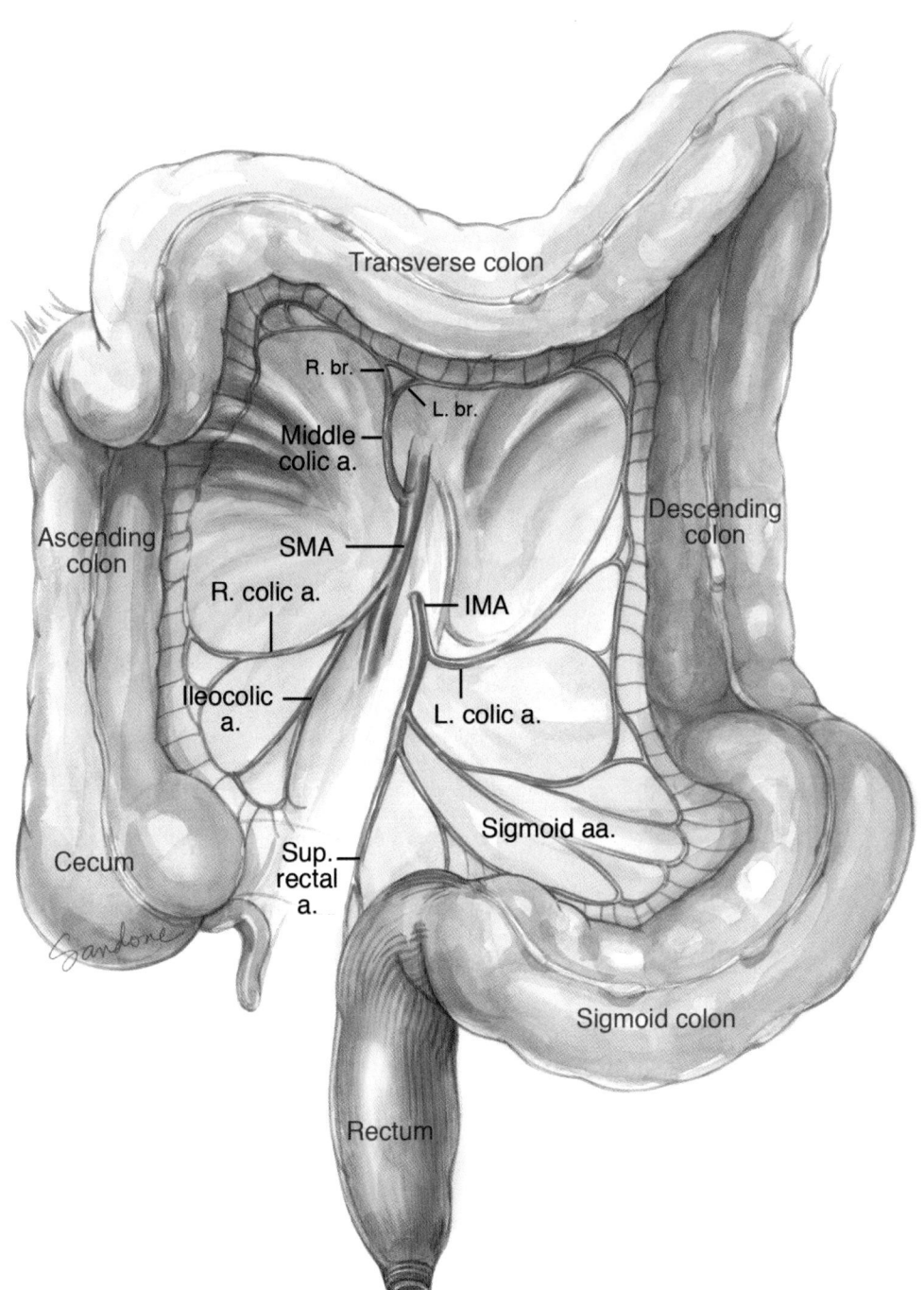

FIGURE 1 Different segments of the colon with the corresponding vascular supply. *a.,* Artery; *aa.,* arteries; *IMA,* inferior mesenteric artery; *L.,* left; *R.,* right; *R. br.,* right branch of middle colic artery; *L. br.,* left branch of middle colic artery; *SMA,* superior mesenteric artery; *Sup. Rectal,* superior rectal. *(Illustration used with permission from Cameron JL, Sandone C: Atlas of gastrointestinal surgery, ed 2, vol II, 2012, Shelton, CT, PMPH-USA.)*

through either an enlarged trocar incision or a separate incision followed by extracorporeal anastomosis. Hand-assist ports can also be used for bulky tumors or difficult patient anatomy. Hallmark anatomic complications include injury to the ureters (right and left colectomy), duodenum (right colectomy), and spleen (left colectomy). When recognized during surgery, all injuries should be repaired immediately with conversion to an open procedure as necessary. Roughly 30% of ureteral injuries involve the distal ureter, and most can be repaired with ureteroneocystostomy and stent placement. Iatrogenic splenic injury is uncommon and usually involves a capsular tear from excessive traction. Splenic salvage should be attempted with packing, topical hemostatic agents, or suture repair. If bleeding persists and is uncontrollable, splenectomy is required.

CHALLENGING AND COMPLICATED CASES

The location of the primary tumor predisposes patients to specific complications like malignant duodenocolic fistula in the setting of transverse colon cancers. If the cancer is localized, surgical management includes a right hemicolectomy and pancreaticoduodenectomy

TABLE 1: Tumor node metastasis (TNM) staging system for colorectal cancer

		Anatomic stage/prognostic groups			
Stage	T	N	M	Dukes*	MAC*
0	Tis	N0	M0	—	—
I	T1	N0	M0	A	A
	T2	N0	M0	A	B1
IIA	T3	N0	M0	B	B2
IIB	T4a	N0	M0	B	B2
IIC	T4b	N0	M0	B	B3
IIIA	T1-T2	N1/N1c	M0	C	C1
	T1	N2a	M0	C	C1
IIIB	T3-T4a	N1/N1c	M0	C	C2
	T2-T3	N2a	M0	C	C1/C2
	T1-T2	N2b	M0	C	C1
IIIC	T4a	N2a	M0	C	C2
	T3-T4	N2b	M0	C	C2
	T4b	N1-N2	M0	C	C3
IVA	Any T	Any N	M1a	—	—
IVB	Any T	Any N	M1b	—	—

Note: cTNM is the clinical classification, and pTNM is the pathologic classification. The y prefix is used for those cancers that are classified after neoadjuvant pretreatment (e.g., ypTNM). Patients who have a complete pathologic response are ypT0N0cM0 that may be similar to stage group 0 or 1. The r prefix is to be used for those cancers that have recurred after a disease-free interval (rTNM).

*Dukes B is a composite of better (T3 N0 M0) and worse (T4 N0 M0) prognostic groups, as is Dukes C (and TN1 M0 and any T N2 M0). MAC is the modified Astler-Coller classification.

Primary tumor (T): T0, no evidence of primary tumor; Tis, carcinoma in situ: intraepithelial or invasion of lamina propria; T1, tumor invades submucosa; T2, tumor invades muscularis propria; T3, tumor invades through muscular propria into pericolorectal tissues; T4a, tumor penetrates to the surface of the visceral peritoneum; T4b, tumor directly invades or is adherent to other organs or structures.

Regional lymph nodes (N): N0, no regional lymph node metastasis; N1, metastasis in one to three regional lymph nodes; N1a, metastasis in one regional lymph node; N1b, metastasis in two to three regional lymph nodes; N1c, tumor deposit(s) in the subserosa, mesentery, or nonperitonealized pericolic or perirectal tissues without regional nodal metastasis; N2, metastasis in four or more regional lymph nodes; N2a, metastasis in four to six regional lymph nodes; N2b, metastasis in seven or more regional lymph nodes.

Distant metastasis (M): M0, no distant metastasis; M1, distant metastasis; M1a, metastasis confined to one organ or site (e.g., liver, lung, ovary, nonregional node); M1b, metastasis in more than one organ/site or the peritoneum.

American Joint Committee on Cancer: AJCC cancer staging manual, ed 7, New York, 2010, Springer.

or segmental duodenectomy (en bloc). Ascending colon cancers invading the right kidney require right hemicolectomy with en bloc partial or total nephrectomy. Malignant colovesical fistulae can occur in the setting of sigmoid colon cancers. Surgical management in this setting is often a sigmoid colectomy or Hartmann's procedure (rectosigmoid colon resection with rectal stump closure and end colostomy) with en bloc partial cystectomy, but total pelvic exenteration may be required for extensive tumors or those involving the prostate. Advanced colon cancers can also involve the ovaries. Oophorectomy is recommended during colon cancer resection if the ovaries look grossly abnormal, are invaded by the primary tumor, or have known metastases. Ovarian metastases develop in less than 15% of women with colon cancer, and prognosis is generally poor. Routine prophylactic oophorectomy is not recommended unless there are pertinent risk factors, such as a history of HNPCC or a breast cancer susceptibility (BRCA) gene mutation.

Although most colon cancer resections are elective, some patients present emergently if there is acute obstruction or perforation. Emergent surgery in this setting is associated with high morbidity and mortality. Surgical management is based on the location of the obstructing lesion. One-stage right hemicolectomy with primary anastomosis is the preferred approach for right-sided lesions. Left-sided colonic obstructions can be challenging to manage, and the optimal approach is somewhat controversial. The historically advocated three-stage approach is as follows: defunctioning colostomy (first stage), primary resection of colon tumor (second stage), and colostomy closure (third stage). Given the morbidity associated with three operations, this approach is now typically reserved for cases where neoadjuvant treatment is needed to facilitate an R0 resection. More recently, a Hartmann's procedure was the operation of choice for patients presenting with colorectal cancer (CRC) and acute obstruction, but now, surgeons favor resection with primary anastomosis with or without a diverting loop ileostomy for patients with hemodynamically stable conditions and acute presentations. Sometimes an on-table, intraoperative colonic lavage can be done to facilitate primary anastomosis in the patient with obstruction. When patients with left-sided colon cancers present with obstruction, the entire colon can be very dilated and the cecum, the area of the colon with the thinnest wall, can even perforate. In this case, a subtotal colectomy may be indicated. Colonic stents have been available since the 1990s and can be used when appropriately skilled endoscopists are available, usually for left-sided cancers. Stents are used for palliation in unresectable cases or as a temporizing measure to allow for proper staging workup so that a definitive treatment plan can be determined.

The role of surgery in metastatic colon cancer continues to evolve. Patients with liver-only metastasis should be offered surgical resection when feasible because this offers the greatest likelihood of cure. Five-year survival rates after surgical resection range from 24% to 58%, with median survival times averaging approximately 35 to 40 months. Resectability is defined as the ability to remove all macroscopic tumor tissue (R0 resection) while maintaining adequate inflow, outflow, and remnant liver parenchyma. High-quality cross-sectional CT imaging with three-dimensional volume rendering is routinely used to determine tumor resectability. When hepatic resection is not feasible, other nonextirpative treatment options include radiofrequency ablation (RFA), hepatic artery infusion (HAI) chemotherapy, transarterial chemoembolization (TACE), and transarterial brachytherapy. The integration of chemotherapy with liver surgery for the treatment of stage IV colon cancer has increased the complexity of patient treatment. Patients with initially resectable liver metastases may be given chemotherapy in the neoadjuvant or adjuvant setting with the goal of improving curability and survival by eliminating occult micrometastatic disease. Patients with initially unresectable liver disease are sometimes given neoadjuvant chemotherapy to convert metastases to resectable lesions. The timing of liver resection in patients with metastases is a controversial issue. A one-stage approach with combined colon and hepatic resection is a reasonable option for patients with low-volume liver metastases who can tolerate simultaneous procedures. Complications with the primary tumor such as perforation or bleeding take priority and delay liver resection until further workup is completed. Bilobar liver metastases or questionably resectable lesions should be managed

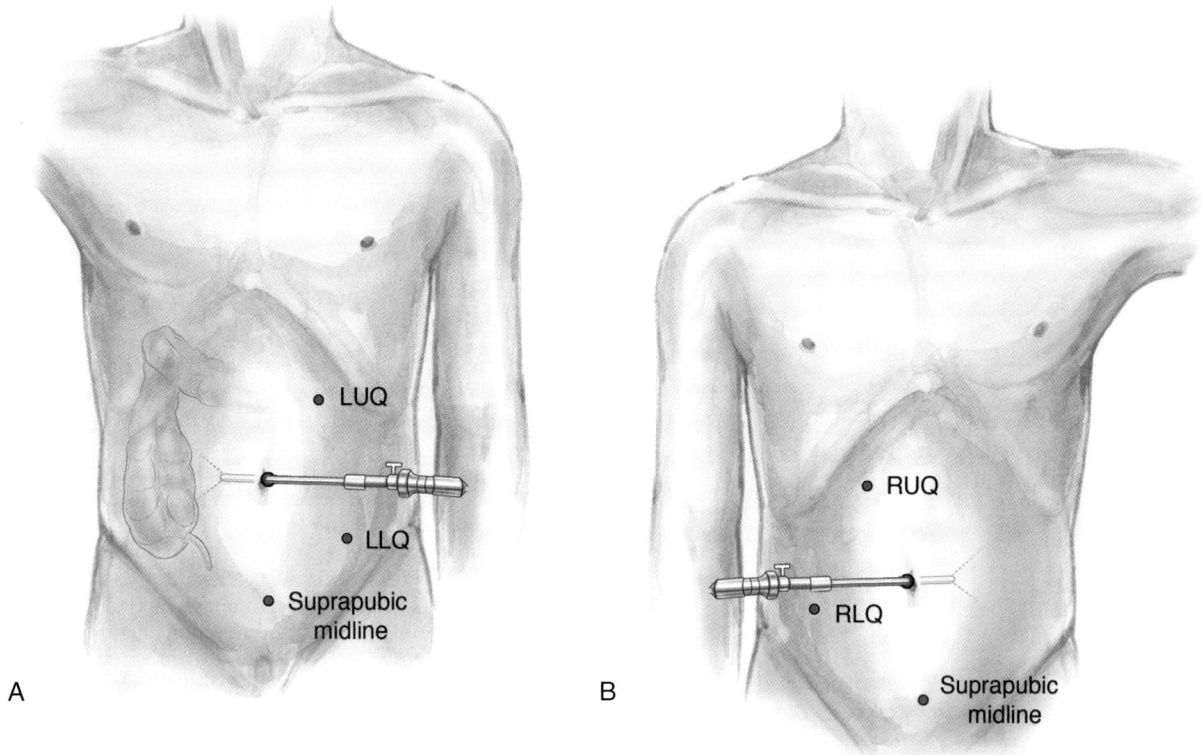

FIGURE 2   Laparoscopic port placement sites for right colectomy **(A)** and left colectomy **(B)**. *LLQ,* Left lower quadrant; *LUQ,* left upper quadrant; *RLQ,* right lower quadrant; *RUQ,* right upper quadrant. *(Illustration used with permission from Cameron JL, Sandone C: Atlas of gastrointestinal surgery, ed 2, vol II, 2012, Shelton, CT, PMPH-USA.)*

with delayed hepatic resection after primary tumor resection and chemotherapy.

ADJUVANT TREATMENT

Multiple options exist for systemic chemotherapy after complete resection of primary colon cancer. In contrast, postoperative radiation therapy is rarely indicated because of the risk of toxicity to the small intestine. Radiation therapy is sometimes used to irradiate the tumor bed in cases where the primary lesion invades local structures and there is an incomplete resection. Since the 1960s, 5-fluorouracil (5-FU) with leucovorin (LV) has been the cornerstone of first-line therapy for stage III colon cancer in the adjuvant setting and has been shown to decrease recurrence rates by 40%. Oxaliplatin combined with 5-FU and LV (FOLFOX) has shown even further benefit and is now standard of care for stage III disease. NCCN guidelines currently recommend 6 months of adjuvant chemotherapy. Certain stage II colon cancers are considered high risk for recurrence because of poor prognostic features like perforation, poor tumor differentiation, or histologic evidence of lymphovascular invasion. Postoperative chemotherapy should be considered in this subset of patients with stage II disease.

Increasing knowledge about the genetic diversity of colon cancers has facilitated the use of targeted adjuvant therapies in select patients. KRAS (v-Ki-ras2 Kirsten rat sarcoma viral homolog) gene molecular testing opened the era for targeted treatments. Only wild-type KRAS tumors respond to anti–epidermal growth factor receptor (EGFR) monoclonal antibodies like cetuximab. Up to 50% of colon cancers harbor a KRAS mutation, which indicates that roughly 50% of patients may benefit from this therapy. For KRAS wild-type tumors, further testing should establish BRAF (v-raf murine sarcoma viral homolog B1) gene mutation status because some data suggest that anti-EGFR agents have limited efficacy in patients with BRAF mutation.

SURVEILLANCE AND FOLLOW-UP

Intensive surveillance is important in the first 2 to 3 years after primary colon cancer resection because most patients have recurrence during this time. The goal is to identify patients with metachronous cancers or recurrent disease early so that appropriate treatment is given. Follow-up colonoscopy is recommended within 1 year of resection. If results are normal, repeat colonoscopies are generally done at 3-year intervals. Any abnormal findings mandate modification to the colonoscopy interval based on appropriate screening guidelines. A history and physical examination with a serum CEA test should be done every 4 months for the first 2 to 3 years, every 6 months for 2 years, and annually thereafter. Per NCCN guidelines, annual CT scan of the chest, abdomen, and pelvis should be considered for the first 3 years in individuals at high risk, such as patients with stage III disease or stage II disease with poor prognostic features.

SUGGESTED READINGS

American Cancer Society: *Colorectal cancer facts & figures 2011-2013,* Atlanta, 2011, American Cancer Society.

Ansaloni L, Andersson RE, Bazzoli F, et al: Guidelines in the management of obstructing cancer of the left colon: consensus conference of the world society of emergency surgery (WSES) and peritoneum and surgery (PnS) society, *World J Emerg Surg* 5(29):1–10, 2010.

Chang GJ, Kaiser AM, Mills S, et al: Practice parameters for the management of colon cancer, *Dis Colon Rectum* 55(8):831–843, 2012.

Choti MA, Sitzmann JV, Tiburi MF, et al: Trends in long-term survival following liver resection for hepatic colorectal metastases, *Ann Surg* 235(6):759–766, 2002.

Landmann RG, Weiser MR: Surgical management of locally advanced and locally recurrent colon cancer, *Clin Colon Rectal Surg* 18(3):182–189, 2005.

Levin B, Lieberman DA, McFarland B, et al: Screening and surveillance for the early detection of colorectal cancer and adenomatous polyps, 2008: a joint guideline from the American Cancer Society, the US Multi-Society Task Force on Colorectal Cancer, and the American College of Radiology, *Gastroenterology* 134(5):1570–1595, 2008.

National Comprehensive Cancer Network: *NCCN clinical practice guidelines in oncology: colon cancer,* version 3.2013, Fort Washington, PA, 2013.

Nelson H, Sargent D, Wieand HS, et al, COST Study Group: A comparison of laparoscopically assisted and open colectomy for colon cancer, *N Engl J Med* 350:2050–2059, 2004.

THE MANAGEMENT OF RECTAL CANCER

Robert E. Roses, MD, and
Miguel A. Rodriguez-Bigas, MD, FACS, FASCRS

INTRODUCTION

Colorectal cancer is the third most common malignancy and cause of cancer death in American men and women. Cancers of the rectum specifically account for approximately one third of these cases. Confinement of the rectum within the bony pelvis and proximity of more distal tumors to the anal sphincter complex make surgical therapy for rectal cancer particularly challenging. Over the last two centuries, a range of surgical approaches, including transperineal, transanal, posterior, and transabdominal, have been applied with variable success. The description of total mesorectal excision (TME) in the early 1980s as well as the emergence of more effective systemic therapies and demonstration of the advantages of preoperative radiotherapy have made a significant impact on the management of rectal cancer over the past two decades. Contemporary treatment paradigms for rectal cancer emphasize TME, sphincter preservation, and multimodality therapy. Defining the role of local excision and the identification of those patients who can forgo radiation or systemic therapy are focuses of ongoing investigations.

DIAGNOSIS

Goals of the initial assessment of the patient with a suspected rectal cancer include confirmation of the diagnosis, accurate pretreatment staging, and an evaluation of comorbidity and baseline bowel function. A complete history should establish baseline bowel function, comorbidities, and physical disability, and should elicit signs and symptoms of advanced disease (e.g., obstructive symptoms, pelvic pain, urinary symptoms, weight loss). A personal or family history of cancer should be sought as well and may alert the clinician to the possibility of a familial colorectal cancer syndrome.

The physical examination is invaluable in localizing the tumor and may alert the clinician to the presence of more advanced disease or unrecognized comorbidity. Low tumors may be appreciable on digital rectal examination (DRE), and fixation of the tumor to the sphincter complex or involvement of adjacent structures (e.g., the vagina or prostate) can often be identified. DRE also allows an assessment of sphincter tone and function. Both rigid and flexible endoscopy are valuable adjuncts to physical examination and can establish the precise location of the tumor and the degree to which the rectal lumen is obscured by the mass.

A complete blood count, basic chemistries, liver function tests, carcinoembryonic antigen (CEA) level, and staging computed tomographic (CT) scan of the chest, abdomen, and pelvis are routinely obtained. Both endorectal ultrasound (ERUS) and orthogonal axial high-resolution T2-weighted magnetic resonance imaging (MRI) can be used to assess pretreatment T and N status. Both modalities have a reported accuracy of up to 90% for both T and N staging, with N staging being slightly less accurate than T staging. MRI allows for an evaluation of involvement of the mesorectal fascia (circumferential margin) and adjacent organs. Figures 1 and 2 illustrate lymphadenopathy in and outside the mesorectum, respectively. The choice of EUS or MRI depends on institution-specific expertise and availability. Positron emission tomography (PET)/CT scan is not used for staging primary rectal cancer. A complete colonoscopy, when feasible, should be performed before the initiation of treatment to exclude the presence of additional colorectal pathology. If complete colonoscopy is not possible (e.g., obstructing tumor), CT colonography can be considered.

TREATMENT APPROACH BY STAGE

Staging based upon a clinical assessment and preoperative imaging forms the basis for the initial treatment strategy (Figure 3). Definitive pathologic staging is only possible after surgical resection. Currently, the TNM classification is preferred (Table 1).

Localized Disease

Radical surgery is the mainstay in the treatment of early-stage (stage I) rectal cancer. The role of local excision continues to evolve. In general, tumors smaller than 4 cm, occupying less than 40% of the circumference of the lumen, and without evidence of lymphadenopathy are amenable to local excision (Box 1). In our experience, transanal excision should only be attempted when the proximal extent of the tumor is palpable on DRE. It also bears emphasis that tumors involving the sphincter complex are no more appropriately removed via a transanal approach than they are with sphincter-sparing proctectomy. Transanal endoscopic microsurgery (TEM) is broadening the indications for local excision, because this approach allows for safer excision of higher lesions and, perhaps, more consistent negative margin excision. Even when strict selection criteria for local excision are utilized, there is a significant local recurrence rate (upwards of 10% for T1 tumors in most series with long-term follow-up). In the Cancer and Leukemia Group B (CALGB) 8984 prospective registration study, at a median follow-up of 7.1 years, rates of local recurrence and distant metastasis after local excision alone for T1 tumors were 8% and 5%, respectively. The 10-year overall survival and disease-free survival rates were 84% with 75%, respectively.

Importantly, local excision does not allow an adequate surgical assessment of lymph node status. Pathologic features associated with a higher rate of nodal positivity include poor differentiation, lymphovascular invasion, and mucin production. These findings should prompt consideration of complete surgical extirpation of the rectum and mesorectum. Additionally, the depth of invasion of the

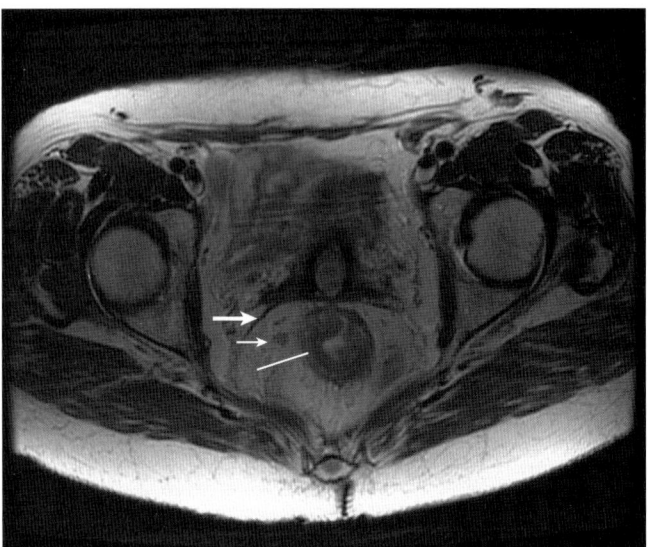

FIGURE 1 Primary rectal tumor with mesorectal lymphadenopathy. *Line,* primary rectal tumor; *large arrow,* mesorectal fascia; *small arrow,* mesorectal lymph node.

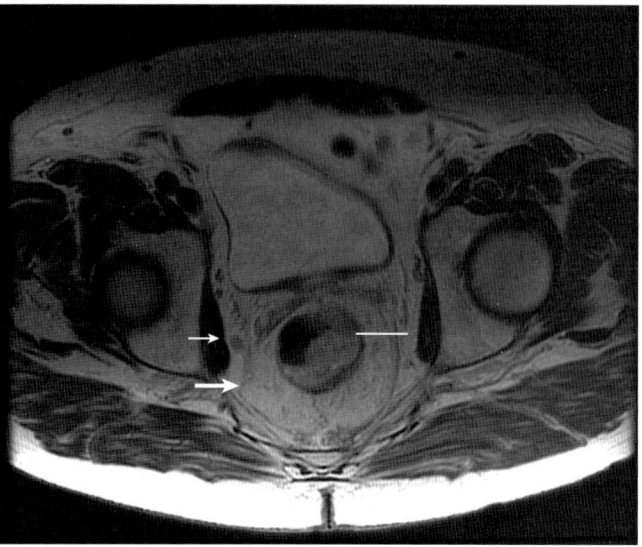

FIGURE 2 MRI with lymphadenopathy outside the mesorectum. *Line,* primary rectal tumor; *large arrow,* mesorectal fascia; *small arrow,* lymph node outside mesorectal fascia.

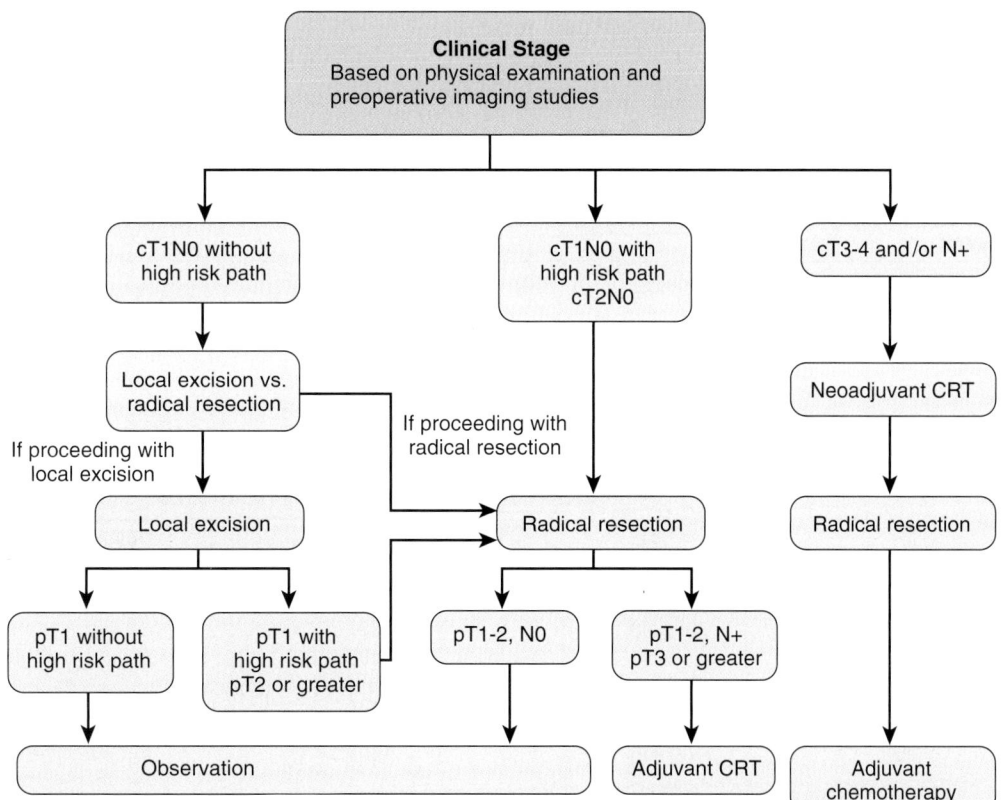

FIGURE 3 Treatment algorithm based on clinical stage of disease for patients with rectal cancer and no evidence of distant metastasis. *C,* clinical stage; *P,* pathologic stage. *High-risk path* refers to (1) poor differentiation, (2) the presence of lymphovascular or perineural invasion, or (3) deep submucosal invasion (sm2 or sm3). Note: Local excision can be considered in patients who have a significant medical contraindication to major abdominal surgery or who make the informed decision to avoid the short-term morbidity, functional consequences, and possible stoma associated with radical surgery with full knowledge that local excision is associated with a significantly higher recurrence rate and may compromise their chances of cure.

TABLE 1: AJCC TNM staging for colon and rectal cancers

Primary tumor (T)

TX	Primary tumor cannot be assessed
T0	No evidence of primary tumor
Tis	Carcinoma in situ: intraepithelial or invasion of lamina propria*
T1	Tumor invades submucosa
T2	Tumor invades muscularis propria
T3	Tumor invades through the muscularis propria into pericolorectal tissue
T4a	Tumor penetrates to the surface of the visceral peritoneum[†]
T4b	Tumor directly invades or is adherent to other organs or structures[†,‡]

Regional lymph nodes (N)

NX	Regional lymph nodes cannot be assessed
N0	No regional lymph node metastasis
N1	Metastasis in one to three regional lymph nodes
N1a	Metastasis in one regional lymph node
N1b	Metastasis in two to three regional lymph nodes
N1c	Tumor deposits in the subserosa, mesentery, or nonperitonealized pericolic or perirectal tissues without regional nodal metastasis
N2	Metastasis in four or more regional lymph nodes
N2a	Metastasis in four to six regional lymph nodes
N2b	Metastasis in seven or more regional lymph nodes

Distant metastasis (M)

M0	No distant metastasis
M1	Distant metastasis
M1a	Metastasis confined to one organ or site (e.g., liver, lung, ovary, nonregional node)
M1b	Metastasis in more than one organ or site or peritoneum

	ANATOMIC STAGE/PROGNOSTIC GROUP				
Stage	**T**	**N**	**M**	**Duke[§]**	**MAC[§]**
0	Tis	N0	M0	—	—
I	T1	N0	M0	A	A
	T2	N0	M0	A	B1
IIA	T3	N0	M0	B	B2
IIB	T4a	N0	M0	B	B2
IIC	T4b	N0	M0	B	B3
IIIA	T1-T2	N1/N1c	M0	C	C1
	T1	N2a	M0	C	C1
IIIB	T3-T4a	N1/N1c	M0	C	C2
	T2-T3	N2a	M0	C	C1/C2
	T1-T2	N2b	M0	C	C1

TABLE 1: AJCC TNM staging for colon and rectal cancers—cont'd

	ANATOMIC STAGE/PROGNOSTIC GROUP				
Stage	**T**	**N**	**M**	**Duke§**	**MAC§**
IIIC	T4a	N2a	M0	C	C2
	T3-T4a	N2b	M0	C	C2
	T4b	N1-N2	M0	C	C3
IVA	Any T	Any N	M1a	—	—
IVB	Any T	Any N	M2a	—	—

Used with the permission of the American Joint Committee on Cancer (AJCC), Chicago, Illinois. The original source for this material is the AJCC Cancer Staging Manual, Seventh Edition (2010) published by Springer New York, Inc.

*This includes cancer cells confined within the glandular basement membrane (intraepithelial) or mucosal lamina propria (intramucosal) with no extension through the muscularis mucosae into the submucosa.

†Direct invasion in T4 includes invasion of other organs or other segments of the colorectum as a result of the direct extension through the serosa, as confirmed on microscopic examination (for example, invasion of the sigmoid colon by a carcinoma of the cecum) or, for cancers in a retroperitoneal or subperitoneal location, direct invasion of other organs or structures by virtue of extension beyond the muscularis propria (i.e., respectively, a tumor on the posterior wall of the descending colon invading the left kidney or lateral abdominal wall; or a mid or distal rectal cancer with invasion of prostate, seminal vesicles, cervix, or vagina).

‡Tumor that is adherent to other organs or structures, grossly, is classified cT4b. However, if no tumor is present in the adhesion, microscopically, the classification should be pT1-4a depending on the anatomical depth of wall invasion. The V and L classifications should be used to identify the presence or absence of vascular or lymphatic invasion whereas the PN site-specific factor should be used for perineural invasion.

§Dukes B is a composite of better (T3 N0 M0) and worse (T4 N0 M0) prognostic groups, as is Dukes C (Any TN1 M0 and Any T N2 M0). MAC is the modified Astler-Coller classification.

Note: cTNM is the clinical classification, pTNM is the pathologic classification. The y prefix is used for those cancers that are classified after neoadjuvant pretreatment (e.g., ypTNM). Patients who have a complete pathologic response are ypT0N0cM0 that may be similar to Stage Group 0 or I. The r prefix is to be used for those cancers that have recurred after a disease-free interval (rTNM).

BOX 1: Criteria for local excision of rectal cancers

Tumor Location and Size
<4 cm and <40% of the circumference of the rectum
<8 cm from the anal verge

Clinical Features
Mobile, nonfixed
T1/N0 or T2/N0* on pretreatment imaging

Histologic Features
Well to moderately differentiated
No lymphovascular or perineural invasion
No mucinous component
T1 or T2 on final histologic examination

*Adjuvant chemoradiation should be administered to patients with T2 lesions (the results of ACOSOG Z6041, which evaluated the role of neoadjuvant chemoradiation followed by local excision, are not yet available).

submucosa has been correlated with the potential for lymph node involvement. Invasion of the upper, middle, and lower thirds of the submucosa have been reported to be associated with a 3%, 8%, and 23% risk of lymph node metastases in T1 lesions, respectively.

Although an increasing utilization of local excision has been reported, local excision alone of T2 tumors is associated with an unacceptably high rate of recurrence (upwards of 20% and as high as 47%) and should only be considered in patients at prohibitive risk for laparotomy. Adjuvant and neoadjuvant chemoradiation have been utilized in addition to local excision for T2 tumors. These approaches have been justified by prospective registration data. In the CALGB 8984 study, the rates of local recurrence and distant metastasis after local excision of T2 tumors followed by chemoradiation were 18% and 12%, respectively. The 10-year overall survival for patients with T2 tumors was reported to be 66%, with a disease-free survival rate of 64%. The use of neoadjuvant chemoradiation for T2 tumors followed by local excision has been evaluated in another prospective multicenter registration study (ACOSOG Z-6041). In this study, 44% of patients with T2 tumors achieved a complete pathologic response after neoadjuvant therapy. Local recurrence rate and overall survival have not yet been reported.

Consideration of these approaches must weigh the risks of local and distant failure against the benefits of avoiding a laparotomy and the risks of TME. Moreover, clinicians must recognize that failure after local excision is frequently unsalvageable. When feasible, salvage often requires multimodality treatment, including multivisceral resection, pelvic irradiation, and chemotherapy, and is associated with potentially lasting treatment-related morbidities and only modest long-term success. Indeed, in an analysis from our institution, the 5-year overall and disease-free survival rates were 59% and 35%, respectively, after salvage for failure after local excision; this is concerning given that most of these patients had relatively favorable disease at the time of initial local excision.

Total mesorectal excision remains the primary treatment for most rectal cancers, including early-stage lesions. When appropriate, every effort is made to preserve sphincter function and reestablish intestinal continuity. For proximal rectal lesions, selective mesorectal excision (at least a 5-cm mesorectal margin) is recommended. For low- and midrectal cancers, TME and a mucosal margin of at least 2 cm is preferred. Lesser mucosal margins may be associated with acceptable outcomes as well and are often necessary if intestinal continuity is to be restored during resection of more distal tumors. If the distal location of the tumor allows resection with a clear margin without violation of the sphincter complex but precludes a stapled anastomosis, a hand-sewn coloanal anastomosis can be performed, albeit with poorer anticipated functional outcomes. Abutment or involvement of the sphincter complex mandates abdominoperineal resection and permanent colostomy.

Locally Advanced Disease

Patients with T3 or T4 tumors or nodal disease are treated with neoadjuvant 5-fluorouracil or capecitabine-based chemoradiation.

This approach is supported by data from randomized control trials that established improved local control with surgery after neoadjuvant radiotherapy compared to surgery alone (Swedish Rectal Cancer Trial and Dutch Colorectal Cancer Group Trial) and with preoperative versus postoperative chemoradiotherapy (German Rectal Cancer Study Group Trial CAO/ARO/AIO-04). To date, only the Swedish trial has demonstrated a survival benefit with preoperative radiotherapy. Both the Swedish and Dutch trials utilized short-course radiation (25 Gy in five fractions over a week), followed shortly thereafter by surgery, whereas the German trial and most long-course chemoradiation trials utilized 50.4 Gy in 28 fractions, followed by a break of 6 to 8 weeks prior to surgery. In the German Trial, at a median follow-up of 134 months, the cumulative incidence of local recurrence was 7.1% in the preoperative treatment group and 10.1% in the postoperative treatment group ($P = 0.048$). There was no difference in the incidence of distant metastases (29.8% vs 29.6%) or overall survival (59.6% vs 59.9%) between groups. Our preferred approach to the management of stage 2 or 3 rectal cancer includes 45 Gy of preoperative radiation delivered in 25 fractions with a boost to the tumor bed of 5.4 Gy in three fractions with concomitant infusional 5-FU or capecitabine. Surgical resection is performed 6 to 8 weeks after the completion of chemoradiotherapy.

A more nuanced approach to the use of preoperative radiation therapy may emerge in the near future. A pooled analysis of prospective adjuvant combined modality trials in rectal cancer in the United States and a more recent report from the Mercury Study Group in Europe suggest that some patients with stage II or III rectal cancer may not need radiation therapy. This hypothesis will be tested in the forthcoming Preoperative Radiation and Evaluation before Chemotherapy and TME (PROSPECT trial sponsored by the Alliance for Clinical Trials in Oncology Foundation). In this study, patients will be randomized to a "Standard Arm" or "Selective Arm." In the latter, preoperative radiation will be omitted in patients with a good response to preoperative chemotherapy.

As with earlier-stage rectal cancers, the cornerstones of surgical therapy are total mesorectal excision and sphincter preservation, when possible. The latter is feasible for the majority of patients, including many with low T3 tumors. Indeed, in a review of our own experience, low anterior resection was possible in 44% of patients with pretreatment T3 tumors within 3 cm of the anal verge following neoadjuvant chemoradiation with a local control rate of 90%. Adjuvant chemotherapy is generally given to patients with stage 2 or 3 disease in accordance with recommendations from the National Comprehensive Cancer Network (NCCN), though randomized data supporting this practice in rectal cancer specifically are lacking. In our experience of 725 cT3-T4 N0-N+ patients treated with neoadjuvant chemoradiation followed by radical surgery, at a median of 65 months, 18.3% developed distant metastases.

The safety of a nonoperative approach in patients who have a good response to neoadjuvant chemotherapy has also been explored in the recent literature. The rate of complete pathologic response following neoadjuvant long-course chemoradiation is reported to be around 17%. A study from Brazil and a recent small trial from the Netherlands both suggest that patients with a *complete clinical response* who are followed very closely do well with low rates of local and distant recurrence. However, in our experience, the applicability of this approach is limited by the inability to reliably identify those patients who have had a *complete pathologic response*.

Disseminated Disease

Patients with metastatic disease represent a highly heterogeneous group. Long-term survival and even clinical cure are possible in patients with limited disease amenable to surgical resection. More challenging still are those patients who present with multiple foci of distant metastatic disease. In this group, systemic therapy is the cornerstone of treatment, and prolonged survival can be achieved in a subset of patients treated with contemporary chemotherapy regimens. The management of these patients must be multidisciplinary,

and in the patient with a symptomatic primary tumor, consideration should be given to diversion or endoscopic stenting prior to initiation of chemotherapy. In our experience, the latter is of limited utility for all but the highest rectal cancers. Stenting of lower lesions is too frequently associated with complications of pain, stent migration, and poor sphincter control, and the creation of a colostomy is usually preferable.

The role of resection of the primary tumor in the setting of stage IV disease remains controversial. Advocates for a more aggressive approach cite the risk of bleeding and perforation in patients receiving systemic therapy. Opponents of a more aggressive surgical approach invoke the risks of delaying systemic therapy. The absolute risk of complications requiring surgical intervention in this cohort has been evaluated in the multiinstitutional prospective National Surgical Adjuvant Breast and Bowel Program (NSABP) Trial C-10. In this study of asymptomatic stage IV patients with intact primary tumors, the rate of major morbidity was 16%, with 11% of patients requiring surgery during treatment with systemic therapy. There were two deaths related to the primary tumor. In other retrospective studies, the rate of primary tumor-related complications in patients treated with systemic therapy has been similar. Features that reliably identify patients who will require, or benefit from, more aggressive surgery remain elusive, and treatment decisions must be individualized.

SURGICAL THERAPY

Transanal Excision

Optimal exposure is mandatory to perform an adequate transanal excision. The patient can be placed in either lithotomy position or in the prone jackknife position. Anterior tumors are sometimes more easily accessed with the patient in prone jackknife position. A self-retaining retractor is placed to efface the anus. Local anesthetic is injected circumferentially in the intersphincteric plane to relax the sphincter. A combination of bivalve and deep curved handheld retractors are then used to expose the lesion.

A traction suture is placed, optimally 2 or more centimeters above the lesion, which aids in drawing the tumor forward into the operating field. The margins of resection are then marked with the electrocautery. A full thickness excision down to the level of the perirectal fat is performed. The defect is usually closed with absorbable sutures, though this is not mandatory. Care must be taken to ensure that the rectal lumen is not compromised during this closure, and if there is any concern for this, proctoscopy should be performed.

Total Mesorectal Excision

The goals of radical surgery for rectal cancer should include (1) resection of the tumor with an adequate distal and circumferential margin, (2) resection of sufficient regional nodal tissue to allow for accurate postoperative staging and good local control, and (3) autonomic nerve preservation. Notions regarding the adequacy of a distal margin continue to evolve. In particular, the implications of a less than 2 cm distal mucosal margin after neoadjuvant chemoradiotherapy are uncertain, although retrospective literature suggests that a negative margin of less than 1 cm is adequate for local control after neoadjuvant chemoradiation and TME in patients undergoing sphincter-preserving surgery (coloanal anastomosis). It appears that in this situation, margin extent likely has less of an impact on outcome than was the case in the preneoadjuvant therapy era. We aim for at least a 2 cm distal mucosal margin unless sphincter preservation requires less. With regards to the radial margin, en bloc resection of adjacent structures (e.g., vagina, bladder, ureter) is justified in appropriately selected patients if R0 resection can be achieved. It cannot be overemphasized that sharp dissection is a must in TME; there is no role for blunt dissection. When the tumor is adherent to other organs, en bloc resection should be performed because local recurrence and survival are compromised if tumor adhesions are violated.

In preparation for TME, the patient is placed in the supine position, with lower extremities in stirrups. The buttocks are positioned so that they extend beyond the edge of the operating table, and a cushion is placed beneath the sacrum to elevate the coccyx. Systemic antibiotics with a sufficiently broad spectrum of activity to cover enteric and skin flora and 5000 units of subcutaneous heparin are administered. In the reoperative setting or in the presence of bulky tumors or inflammatory change in the pelvis, the placement of ureteral stents under cystoscopic guidance aids in the more ready intraoperative identification of the ureters.

A laparotomy incision is made down to the level of the pubic bone. Superiorly, the incision is extended above the umbilicus to a level that allows safe mobilization of the splenic flexure. A thorough exploration of the abdomen is undertaken to exclude the presence of metastatic disease and should include visualization or palpation of the liver and lesser sac and entire small bowel. The sigmoid colon and descending colon are mobilized from the retroperitoneum along the white line of Toldt. The left ureter is identified coursing through the retroperitoneum just lateral to the mesorectum in the intersigmoid fossa and is protected. Full mobilization of the rectosigmoid is achieved by dividing the peritoneum along the right side of the mesorectum. The right ureter is identified as it courses over the right iliac vessels and is protected. The superior rectal artery, the terminal branch of the inferior mesenteric artery, is then identified as it courses inferiorly through the mesocolon and is ligated. The rectosigmoid junction is divided with a linear stapler, and the intervening mesorectum between the divided bowel wall and divided superior rectal artery is transected.

The rectum is retracted anteriorly, and the plane between the fascia propria of the mesorectum and the pelvic fascia is developed sharply. The hypogastric nerves are identified where they descend over the sacral promontory and are preserved. Dissection is carried down to the pelvic floor. Care is taken to avoid injury to the presacral veins during posterior dissection. The correct posterior plane then guides the surgeon to the lateral plane. The nervi erigentes are identified along the pelvic sidewall and are preserved. The middle rectal arteries, if encountered, can usually be cauterized, particularly in the irradiated patient, but they are ligated if troublesome bleeding is encountered. The lateral dissection continues to the level of the levator muscles. Anteriorly, the peritoneum overlying the cul-de-sac is incised. Dissection is continued by sharply dividing the rectovaginal septum or the rectovesical septum under Denonvillier's fascia. In this manner a bloodless anterior plane between the rectum and the vagina or bladder (and prostate in males) is developed and carried down to the levator ani muscles.

Reconstruction

If sphincter preservation is to be attempted, the splenic flexure is mobilized. Undue downward traction on the transverse colon and the omentum are avoided to minimize the risk of splenic injury. If the proximal colon does not readily reach the distal rectal stump, maneuvers to provide greater length include division of the inferior mesenteric artery at its origin (if it has not been previously divided) and division of the inferior mesenteric vein. Provided there is good perfusion through the Arc of Riolan, these maneuvers generally allow for a healthy and tension-free anastomosis. After creation of the anastomosis, the pelvis is filled with saline. The colon above the anastomosis is occluded, and air is insufflated into the distal rectum to confirm the integrity of the staple line.

When the laxity of the proximal colon is sufficient and the pelvis is wide enough, we prefer reconstruction with a colonic J pouch after resection of lower tumors (anastomosis <8 cm from the dentate line). While data from five randomized trials comparing colonic J pouch and straight anastomoses have not conclusively demonstrated improved functional outcomes, a subset of patients likely benefit, particularly in the first 18 months after surgery. In patients who have

undergone preoperative radiation therapy and those with tumors below the peritoneal reflection, we perform a diverting ileostomy.

Abdominoperineal Resection

Lower tumors involving the sphincter complex require abdominoperineal resection. The transabdominal portion of the operation is identical to that described above, excluding the formation of an anastomosis. Additionally, mobilization of the splenic flexure is usually unnecessary prior to creation of a descending colostomy.

Perineal Dissection and Closure

An elliptical skin incision extending from the perineal body to the coccyx that is wide enough to encompass the anal sphincter complex is used. The superficial fascia between the subcutaneous tissue and the ischiorectal fat is divided bilaterally. The coccyx is palpated, and dissection proceeds until the tip of the coccyx is exposed. On the ventral aspect, the anococcygeal ligament is divided, releasing the attachments of the superficial external sphincter muscle. Further dissection in this plane exposes the Waldeyer fascia, which, if it has not been divided from above, is divided transversely, allowing access to the presacral plane of dissection. Blunt dissection without division of the Waldeyer fascia should be avoided because it can result in bleeding from the presacral venous plexus. The anal canal and rectum are retracted anteriorly, and dissection proceeds to the level of the ventral curve of the sacrum, with guidance from the abdominal operator.

Having freed the rectum posteriorly, attention is directed laterally. The ischiorectal adipose tissue is divided on both sides, close to the lateral pelvic walls. As the levator ani are approached, branches of the inferior hemorrhoidal vessels are encountered and divided. The levator ani are divided circumferentially, with the ischial tuberosities defining the lateral extent of the dissection. The rectosigmoid can often be delivered through the perineal defect at this point to facilitate the remaining anterior dissection. The anterior subcutaneous tissues and decussating fibers of the external sphincter are divided, allowing identification of the superficial transverse perineal muscle. Care must be taken to avoid injury to the membranous urethra. The dissection is performed in the plane dorsal to the bulbocavernosus muscle. In males, this is the most difficult portion of the perineal dissection because the anorectum is closely apposed to the membranous urethra, prostate, and seminal vesicles. Intermittent palpation of the urinary catheter assists in keeping the dissection along a safe plane.

Closure of the perineal wound requires particular attention to detail because wound complication rates exceed 30% in multiple series. It bears emphasis that the levator ani muscles cannot be approximated if the proper dissection has been performed. Presacral drainage is accomplished with closed suction catheters brought out through stab wounds to one side of the perineal closure. The subcutaneous tissues and skin are approximated with interrupted sutures in multiple layers. In patients at higher risk for wound failure (e.g., prior irradiation, obesity, diabetes mellitus), closure with a muscle or myocutaneous flap may be justified.

Laparoscopic and Robotic Proctectomy

An increasing body of literature suggests oncologic equivalency of laparoscopic and open proctectomy for rectal cancer. Data demonstrating clear advantages of the laparoscopic approach, however, are lacking. The Conventional versus Laparoscopic Assisted Surgery in Colorectal Cancer (CLASICC) trial from the United Kingdom randomized 794 patients with colorectal cancer (381 of whom had rectal cancer) to laparoscopic assisted or open resection. No differences in 3-year local control or disease-free or overall survival were seen. The outcomes of the Colorectal Cancer Laparoscopic or Open Resection (COLOR II) and ACOSOC Z6051 trials (now sponsored by the Alliance for Clinical Trials in Oncology Foundation) are eagerly awaited. Robotic-assisted approaches are also gaining popularity. Theoretical advantages include the improved visualization and technical control afforded by the robotic instrumentation. Disadvantages include longer operating times and increased cost. Greater experience may allow for the identification of patients who benefit most from these approaches.

SELECTED READINGS

Bedrosian I, Rodriguez-Bigas MA, Feig B: Predicting the node-negative mesorectum after preoperative chemoradiation for locally advanced rectal carcinoma, *J Gastrointest Surg* 8(1):56–62, 2004.

Greenberg JA, Shibata D, Herndon JE II, et al: Local excision of distal rectal cancer: an update of Cancer and Leukemia Group B 8984, *Dis Colon Rectum* 51:1185–1194, 2008.

Kosinski L, Habr-Gama A, Ludwig K, Perez R: Shifting concepts in rectal cancer management: a review of contemporary primary rectal cancer treatment strategies, *CA Cancer J Clin* 62(3):173–202, 2012.

Park IJ, You YN, Agarwal A, et al: Neoadjuvant treatment response as an early response indicator for patients with rectal cancer, *J Clin Oncol* 30(15):1770–1776, 2012.

Sauer R, Liersch T, Merkel S, et al: Preoperative versus postoperative chemoradiotherapy for locally advanced rectal cancer: Results of the German CAO/ARO/AIO-94 randomized phase III trial after a median follow-up of 11 years, *J Clin Oncol* 30(16):1926–1933, 2012.

Silberfein EJ, Kattepogu KM, Hu CY, et al: Long-term survival and recurrence outcomes following surgery for distal rectal cancer, *Ann Surg Oncol* 17(11):2863–2869, 2010.

Taylor FGM, Quirke P, Heald RJ: Preoperative high-resolution magnetic resonance imaging can identify good prognosis stage I, II, and III rectal cancer best managed by surgery alone. A prospective, multicenter, European study, *Ann Surg* 253:711–719, 2011.

You YN, Baxter NN, Stewart A, et al: Is the increasing rate of local excision for stage I rectal cancer in the United States justified? A nationwide cohort study from the National Cancer Database, *Ann Surg* 245:726–733, 2007.

TUMORS OF THE ANAL CANAL

Marco Ettore Allaix, MD, Nora Eve Joseph, MD, and Alessandro Fichera, MD, FACS, FASCRS

GENERAL CONSIDERATIONS

The surgical anal canal extends from the level of the pelvic floor (the anorectal ring or the junction of the puborectalis portion of the levator ani muscle with the external anal sphincter) to the proximal margin of the anal verge. Thus defined, the anal canal corresponds to the extent of the sphincter complex and is approximately 4.0 cm in length. At midpoint is the dentate line, which is defined macroscopically by the anal valves and bases of the anal columns. Microscopically, the anal canal is divided into three zones based on characteristic histologic features. The upper zone lies proximal to the dentate line and is lined by colorectal type glandular mucosa. Extending distally from the dentate line is the mid or anal transition zone (ATZ) defined by a specialized or transitional type epithelium. The third and most distal zone is comprised mostly of non-keratinized and occasionally keratinized squamous mucosa (Figure 1).

The ATZ has been intensively studied for its role in continence and as a potential site for neoplastic degeneration after stapled ileoanal anastomosis in patients with ulcerative colitis. In the literature, this epithelium has been variously classified as transitional, intermediate, or cloacogenic. The ATZ epithelium may also contain mucin-producing cells, endocrine cells, and melanocytes.

The arterial blood supply of the anal canal derives from the superior, middle, and inferior rectal arteries, whose terminal branches reach the anal submucosa. Three main arterial trunks in the right anterior, right posterior, and left lateral positions can be isolated below the dentate line. They originate primarily from the superior rectal artery. The middle rectal veins drain the upper anal canal into the systemic system via the internal iliac veins. The inferior rectal veins drain the lower anal canal, communicating with the pudendal veins and draining into the internal iliac veins.

Lymphatic drainage of the anal canal varies based on the level: below the dentate line drainage is to the inguinal lymph nodes; above, lymphatic drainage goes to the mesorectal, lateral pelvic, and inferior mesenteric nodes.

With focus primarily on anal neoplasms, presenting symptoms are often nonspecific and may include pain, bleeding, discharge, pruritus, and ulceration. Frequently, anal tumors are completely asymptomatic and are diagnosed only incidentally, or because of palpable inguinal lymph nodes.

The macroscopic appearance of an anal lesion may be nonspecific also: it may be flat or raised, and the surface may be verrucous, erythematous, or scaly. An ulcerated mass is usually very suspicious of malignant degeneration.

Diagnosis of anal neoplasm requires a high index of suspicion, particularly in patients with known risk factors who present with new symptoms. For a definitive diagnosis, a biopsy of the suspicious area is often indicated, unless the patient has severe immunocompromise.

Imaging is used for cancer staging. Magnetic resonance imaging of the pelvis and endoanal ultrasound scan define tumor size and invasion and the involvement of local lymph nodes. Distant metastatic spread can be assessed with computed tomographic scan of the chest, abdomen, and pelvis.

The various elements of the anal canal account for the different neoplasms that are described: (1) squamous cell tumors, including condyloma acuminatum, flat squamous dysplasia, Bowen's disease, and invasive squamous cell carcinoma and its variants; (2) adenocarcinoma and its variants, including rectal-type adenocarcinoma, the so-called anal gland adenocarcinoma, fistula-related mucinous adenocarcinoma, and intraepithelial adenocarcinoma (i.e., Paget's disease); (3) neuroendocrine neoplasms, including carcinoid tumor, small cell carcinoma, and non–small cell high-grade neuroendocrine carcinoma; (4) malignant melanoma; (5) mesenchymal tumors; and (6) malignant lymphoma. Although these anal canal tumors as a group account for only about 1.5% of all gastrointestinal neoplasms, their diagnosis and management can be challenging for pathologists and clinicians alike.

SQUAMOUS NEOPLASMS

Condyloma Acuminatum (Anal Wart)

Condyloma acuminatum, or anal wart, is caused by human papilloma virus (HPV). HPV is the most common sexually transmitted infection. Its incidence rate has increased over the past 30 years. In the United States, the prevalence rate of anogenital HPV is estimated to be 15%, equal to 24 million individuals. In addition, 500,000 to 1 million new cases of genital warts are believed to occur annually, resulting in 600,000 healthcare provider visits per year. Currently, more than 100 different HPV types have been sequenced and officially classified, about one third of which have been found to infect the anogenital epithelium.

Although the natural history and the potential for progression to squamous dysplasia and squamous cell carcinoma still needs to be completely elucidated, condyloma acuminatum (anal wart) is generally regarded as a premalignant lesion. The incidence rate of squamous cell carcinoma of the anus in patients with anal condyloma has been reported to be up to 4%. The key histologic features of condyloma acuminatum are a verrucous architecture composed of papillary excrescences and hyperkeratosis as well as the presence of koilocytic changes within a maturing squamous epithelium. Koilocytes are epithelial cells displaying characteristic changes secondary to HPV infection: vacuolated cytoplasm, wrinkled, hyperchromatic nuclei and perinuclear halos. Binucleated and trinucleated epithelial cells are also often present (Figure 2). Koilocytic changes may be absent, however, when the viral infection subsides.

Although many anal condylomata, particularly those of perianal skin, are caused by low-risk HPV (types 6 or 11) and should therefore be regarded as low risk for progression, those lesions in the anal canal are often associated with high-risk HPV (such as 16) and are more likely to progress to an invasive cancer. This is particularly true in patients with immunocompromise.

Several different medical and surgical approaches have been proposed for the treatment of anal condylomata with limited clinical data to support. No consensus has been reached on a gold standard, and whether treatment eliminates infectivity is not even clear, given the fact that both topical and surgical treatments are only aimed at eradication of the visible lesions. Topical treatments include podophyllotoxin, imiquimod cream, and trichloroacetic acid. Invasive therapies include cryotherapy, argon plasma beam treatment, and surgical excision/fulguration. Repeated sessions are needed with cryotherapy that is mainly indicated for small lesions. Surgical excision/fulguration and argon plasma beam treatment are highly effective in the short term. It is mandatory to submit several samples to the pathologists for definitive diagnosis of these lesions that may harbor an invasive component. Skin bridges must be left intact

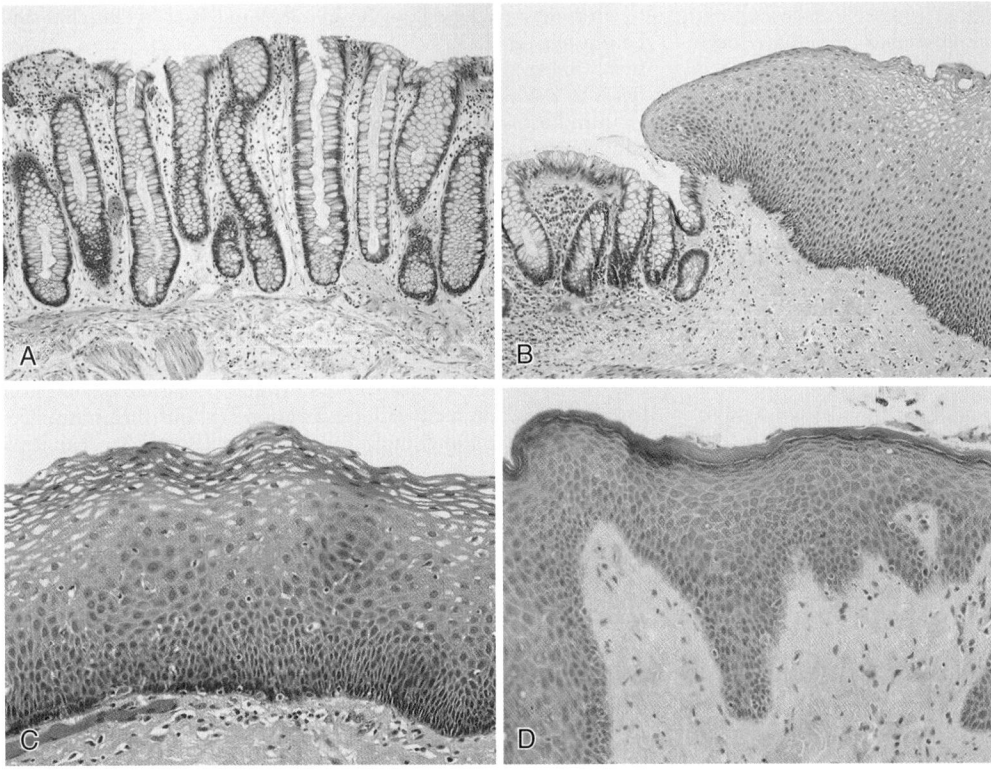

FIGURE 1 A, Normal columnar epithelium lining the upper zone of the anal canal. **B,** Normal mid zone transition from proximal to distal *(left to right)*. **C,** Normal non-keratinized and **D,** keratinized stratified squamous epithelium of the distal anal canal.

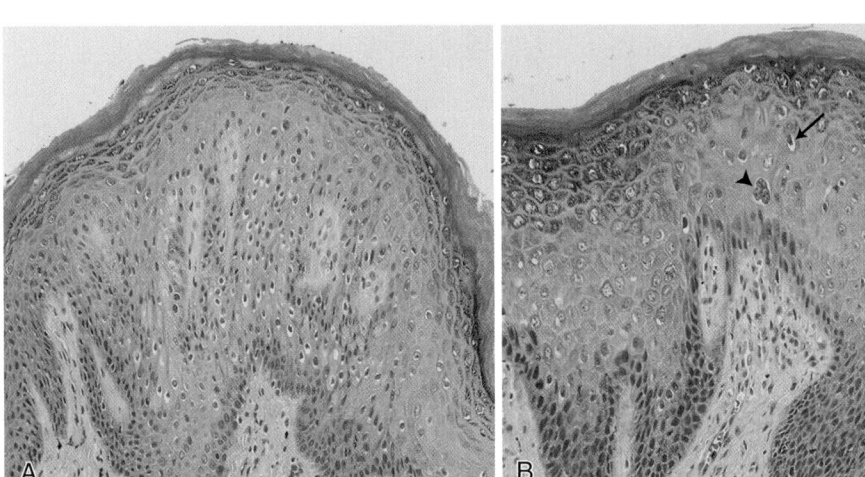

FIGURE 2 A and **B,** Condyloma acuminatum. Papillae of squamous mucosa with features of HPV infection: hyperkeratosis, koilocytic change *(arrow)* and trinucleation *(arrowhead)*.

between wounds to minimize scarring and to avoid anal stenosis (Figure 3).

The many topical treatments have very limited efficacy in the presence of large lesions and are associated with significant side effects. They should be considered only in addition to surgical eradications or in patients with compromised conditions that would not tolerate surgery. Podophyllin has potential oncogenic and teratogenic effects and should not be applied on the cervix and in the anal canal or used during pregnancy. Marrow suppression, hepatic dysfunction, neurologic effects, hallucinations, psychosis, nausea, vomiting, diarrhea, abdominal pain, and genital burns have been rarely described. Trichloroacetic acid may cause an intense burning sensation and ulceration to the dermis and is therefore not recommended for large warts. 5-Fluorouracil has limited use because of its severe local effect and teratogenicity. Conflicting results have been reported with interferon, which is an expensive drug with significant systemic side effects. Imiquimod is not recommended during pregnancy or for internal use. Mild to severe erythema may occur; other side effects include localized erosions, an impetigo-like reaction, and an itching or burning sensation.

Overall recurrence rates between 20% and 50% have been reported irrespective of the treatment approach. Still unclear is whether disease recurrence is the result of recrudescence, reinfection, or other factors such as individual immune response or inadequate treatment. The presence of genital HPV types in plucked pubic and perianal hair suggests that an endogenous reservoir for HPV may play a role in recurrence. Thus, if only the visible lesions are destroyed, latent HPV likely remains in the surrounding tissue. The lack of antiviral activity of most recommended topical therapies supports this hypothesis.

The immune system appears to play a major role in regression of genital HPV disease. In patients with spontaneous regression, significant differences are present in the epidermal and dermal concentration of CD4+ activated memory lymphocytes compared with those without regression. Although there is an association of serum antibodies to HPV proteins with HPV-related diseases, their role is uncertain because their presence does not correlate with wart regression. Evidence suggests that T cells in male and the female genital epithelium secrete protective antibodies against many HPV infections, but the significance of this is unclear. Anal condylomata in patients with immunosuppressed conditions treated with surgery has a higher recurrence rate and recurrence at a faster pace than in patients with a competent immune system. In patients with human immunodeficiency virus (HIV)-seropositive conditions, CD4 counts should be maximized to prevent early recurrence.

Many pharmacologic topical treatments have been proposed to reduce recurrence after surgical treatment. Imiquimod and interferon are the only drugs that exhibit antiviral activity. Both have shown lower recurrence rates compared with other therapies. In particular, adjuvant interferon treatment can reduce recurrence after surgical excision and is more effective in patients with condylomata present for more than 6 months and in the presence of HPV subtype 6 or 11. Further evidence shows that, particularly in patients with immunocompromise, immunostimulation may lead to a reduction in the size of lesions and in recurrence after surgery.

First described by Buschke in 1886, and later by Buschke and Lowenstein in 1925, the "giant condyloma of Buschke and Lowenstein" (or verrucous carcinoma) is a rare form of condyloma that refers to a slow-growing neoplasm that has a tendency to recur and to form abscesses and fistulae. It is an intermediate form between condyloma acuminatum and squamous cell carcinoma. This tumor does not appear to arise from malignant transformation of a condyloma but represents a low-grade form of squamous cell carcinoma. Like conventional condylomata, these lesions are more likely to be associated with low-risk HPV. The histologic appearance on a biopsy specimen may be identical to that seen in common condyloma acuminatum (surface hyperkeratosis, prominent acanthosis and papillomatosis, with orderly arrangement of the epithelial layers). However, excision specimens often demonstrate an endophytic component that is not present in ordinary condylomata. The biology of such lesions is typically that of local invasion without metastasis. The treatment consists of complete wide local excision often requiring

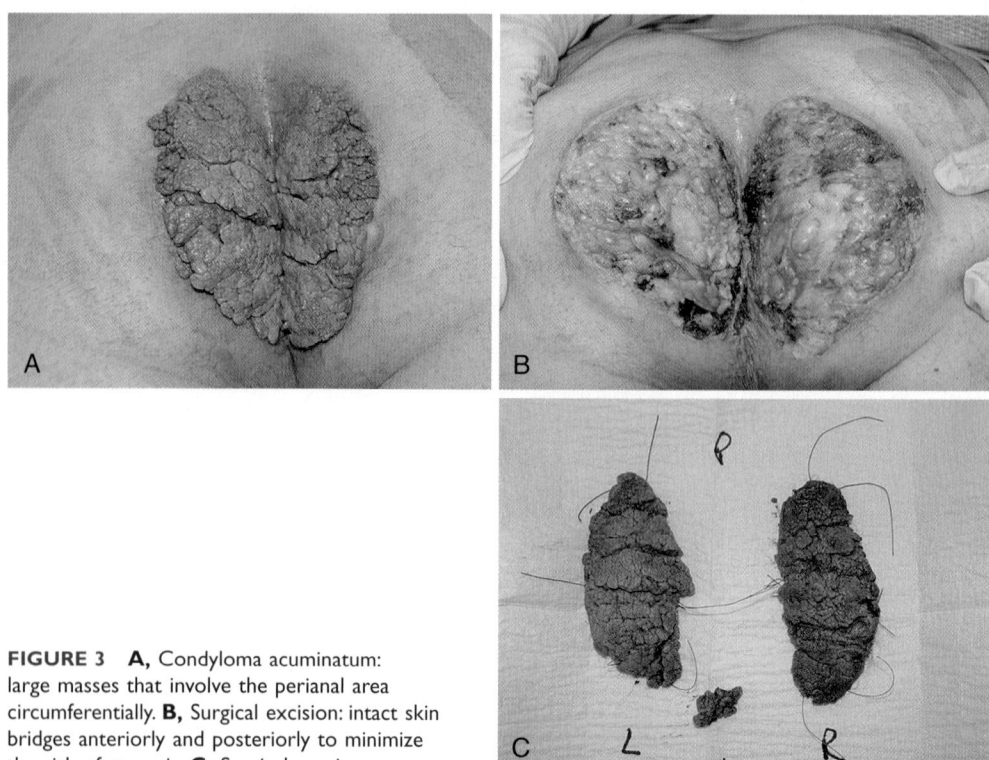

FIGURE 3 A, Condyloma acuminatum: large masses that involve the perianal area circumferentially. **B,** Surgical excision: intact skin bridges anteriorly and posteriorly to minimize the risk of stenosis. **C,** Surgical specimen.

flap closure. An abdominoperineal resection is required in case of deep tissue involvement (Figure 4). The role of chemoradiotherapy is still unclear and seldom indicated.

Anal Intraepithelial Neoplasia

Anal intraepithelial neoplasia (AIN) is often a precursor to invasive squamous anal carcinoma. The disease process may involve both the perianal skin and the anal canal, including the anal transition zone, but anal canal lesions without evidence of perianal involvement are very unusual. It is a multifocal disease process strongly associated with human papillomavirus (usually HPV types 6, 11, 16, and 18). Strong etiologic and clinical similarities are seen between AIN and cervical (CIN) and vulvar (VIN) intraepithelial neoplasia.

AIN is characterized by cellular and nuclear abnormalities within squamous epithelial cells limited to the basement membrane. Histologic features include nuclear atypia such as pleomorphism, enlargement and hyperchromasia as well as increased mitotic activity above an expanded basal layer. The extent of basal layer expansion, or loss of maturing epithelium, is the basis for grading dysplasia in tissue biopsies of anal lesions. AIN I refers to nuclear abnormalities confined to the lower one third of the epithelium and is considered a low-grade dysplastic lesion. AIN II and III are high grade lesions with AIN II limited to the lower two thirds and AIN III involving the full-thickness of the epithelium, or carcinoma in situ (Figure 5). In anal cytology the Bethesda grading system categories dysplastic lesions as low-grade squamous intraepithelial lesions (LSIL) and high-grade intraepithelial lesions (HSIL). LSIL is equivalent to AIN I seen in a tissue biopsy and HSIL encompasses AIN II and III.

The exact prevalence rate of AIN in the general population is unknown, but it is thought to be less than 1%. Identified risk factors for AIN include HPV infection, anal warts, multiple sexual partners, men who have sex with men, anal receptive intercourse, cervical dysplasia or cancer, smoking, and immunosuppression (such as in transplant and HIV).

Although AIN I and II have been known to have the potential to regress, AIN III very rarely regresses. The risk of progression of AIN to invasive anal cancer approximates 10% at 5 years in patients with immunocompetent conditions and up to 50% in patients with immunosuppressed conditions. Those at the highest risk of invasive cancer are those with multifocal disease or immunocompromise.

A high index of suspicion is required for diagnosis of AIN. Around 10% of AIN lesions are diagnosed as an incidental finding after excision of an "innocent" anal tag or condyloma-like lesion. AIN III lesions are usually flat, and their appearance is variable. The presence of ulceration in an AIN lesion suggests invasion. Symptoms include pruritus and anal discharge; other symptoms of pain, bleeding, and tenesmus suggest invasion.

No consensus exists about the best management of AIN. The primary goal is to prevent the development of anal cancer and minimize symptoms. Proposed strategies range from watchful waiting to aggressive surgery.

Conservative strategies are supported by the high recurrence rates seen after aggressive attempts at complete eradication. This is particularly true in patients with HIV and is likely the result of persistent HPV infection. Also, the rate of progression of high-grade AIN to invasive cancer is relatively low with the possibility of detection of invasive disease at an early and still treatable stage.

Ablative therapies used in AIN include CO_2 laser ablation, cryotherapy, and electrocautery fulguration. All the options are burdened by high recurrence rates and significant morbidity.

Excision of small lesions for histologic evaluation is preferred to purely ablative therapy because the latter precludes the possibility of a definitive diagnosis to guide further management. In the authors' practice, for definition of the extent of disease at diagnosis, anal mapping and anal pap smear with excision/ablation of the suspicious areas is performed. This should be done with high-resolution anoscopy (HRA). The advantage of HRA is more accurate identification of the suspicious lesions and minimization of damage to surrounding healthy tissue. In brief, this technique is based on the principle that, with the application of acetic acid, dysplastic tissue exhibits

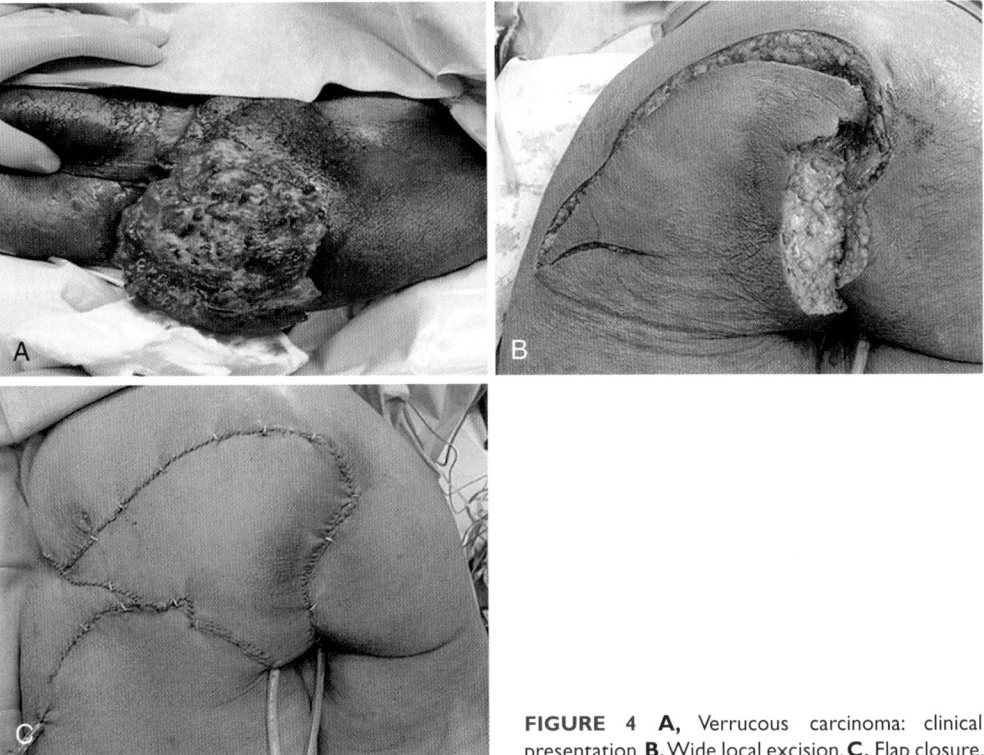

FIGURE 4 A, Verrucous carcinoma: clinical presentation. **B,** Wide local excision. **C,** Flap closure.

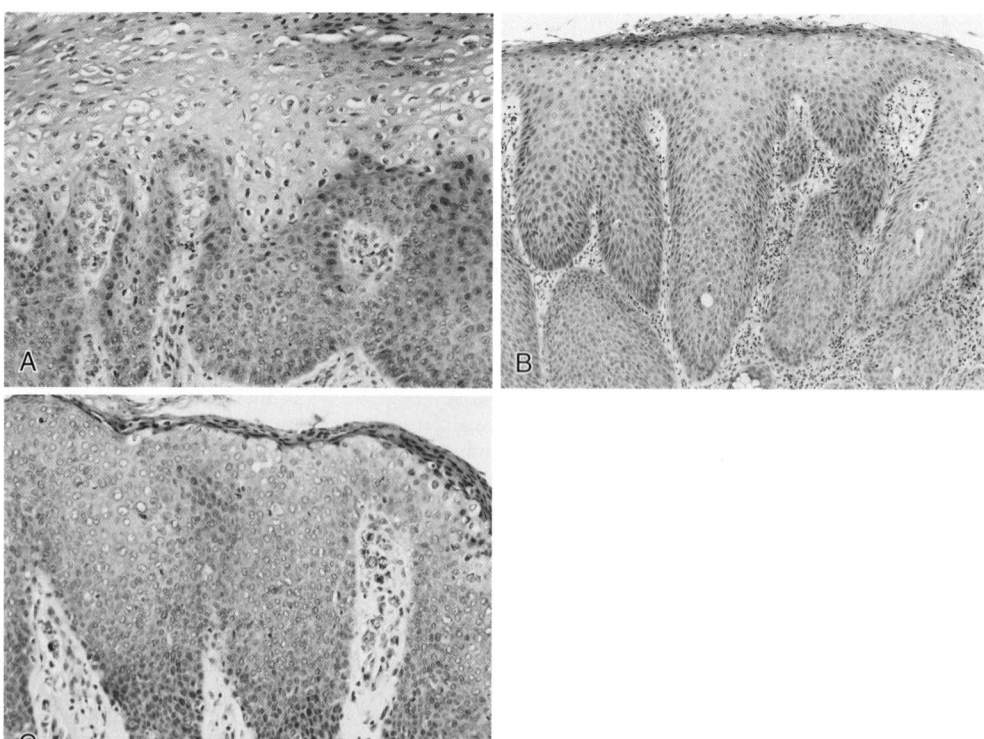

FIGURE 5   **A,** Human papilloma virus (HPV) infected epithelial cells can become dysplastic. The earliest form of dysplasia, or anal intraepithelial neoplasia I (AIN I), is limited to the lower one third of the epithelium. **B,** In AIN II, the grade of dysplasia increases as evidenced by expansion of cellular abnormalities and increased mitotic activity into the lower two thirds of the epithelium. **C,** Dysplastic cells take over the entire epithelium in AIN III, the highest grade of dysplasia. Note the complete loss of an identifiable basal layer with the top of the epithelium identical in appearance to the bottom. Further progression leads to invasive squamous cell carcinoma.

distinct changes and patterns in the anal mucosa. After application of 5% acetic acid to the anal canal and perianal skin, tissues that harbor AIN turn acetowhite. Acetowhitening alone is nonspecific. It sets the background on which the clinicians identify the characteristic vascular changes of low-grade and high-grade dysplastic lesions. Lugol's solution may be applied in areas of diagnostic uncertainty. Areas that do not take up Lugol's solution are considered at high risk for harboring high-grade dysplastic tissue. A biopsy of these areas should be obtained.

After the initial diagnosis is reached and invasive cancer has been ruled out, the authors continue to follow the patients with anal pap smear, excision of the suspicious areas, and fulguration of the less concerning lesions.

Other treatments, such as photodynamic therapy, immunomodulation therapies with imiquimod cream and cidofovir gel, and HPV immunotherapy, have been proposed. Although they are promising, the data are too limited to draw any definitive conclusions regarding their long-term efficacy.

Bowen's Disease

Bowen's disease is synonymous with AIN III. Patients with anal-margin Bowen's disease typically present with minor symptoms, such as burning or pruritus. Up to a third of the patients report a mass or bleeding. Clinically, Bowen's disease presents as erythematous, occasionally brown-red pigmented, noninfiltrating, scaly, or crusted plaques, that sometimes have a moist surface or even nodules (Figure 6). Differential diagnosis is extensive and includes different benign dermatologic conditions like psoriasis, eczema, and leukoplakia. The standard treatment is wide surgical excision. To ensure clear resection margins, a systematic four-quadrant biopsy technique, with intraoperative frozen sections including intraanal biopsies, has been advocated. Despite a wide excision, recurrence rates up to 30% have been reported. The major disadvantage of wide local excision is the difficulty to primarily close the wound; skin flaps may be necessary. Given the multifocality of these lesions, anal mapping is often performed

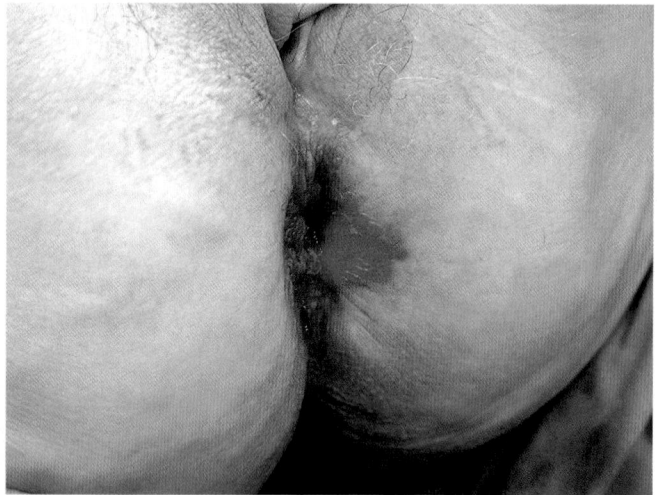

FIGURE 6   Bowen's disease: clinical presentation as brown-red pigmented, noninfiltrating, scaly plaques, with a moist surface and nodules.

in the authors' practice. Four-quadrant biopsies are obtained, starting at the dentate line, at the anal verge, and on the perianal skin (Figure 7). They are sent separately to the pathologist for permanent section.

Squamous Cell Carcinoma

Traditionally squamous cell carcinoma of the anal canal occurs more frequently in women than in men (1.5 vs 1.0/100,000). Epidemiologic studies have shown that most anal cancers are associated with HPV infection, predominately oncogenic types 16 and 18. Anal intercourse is among the presumed mechanisms by which HPV is introduced into the anal canal. Other risk factors include

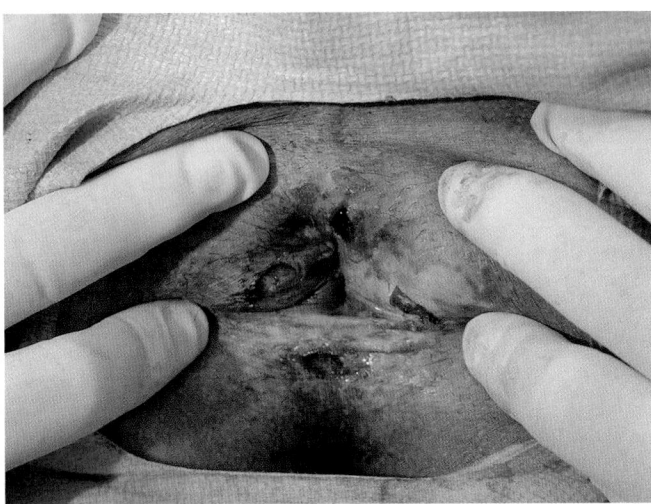

FIGURE 7 Anal mapping for Bowen's disease. Four-quadrant biopsies are obtained, starting at the dentate line, at the anal verge, and on the perianal skin. They are sent separately to the pathologist for permanent section.

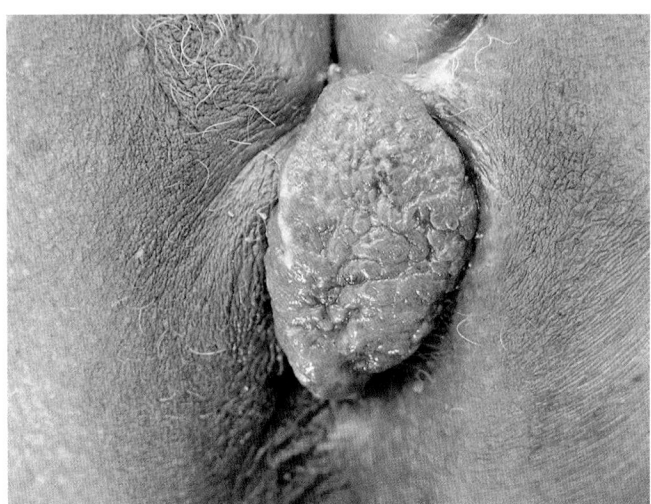

FIGURE 8 Anal squamous cell carcinoma: fungating mass at the anal verge.

immunosuppression (transplant, immune disorders, and HIV infection), an increasing number of sexual partners, a history of anogenital warts, previous lower genital tract dysplasia or carcinoma, and a history of smoking.

The clinical presentation is nonspecific (Figure 8). Anal bleeding appears to be the most common presenting symptom. Squamous cell carcinomas (SCC) are defined histologically by invasion of tumor cells beyond the basement membrane. Upon resection each tumor is given a grade and pathologic stage according to the TMN staging system (Figure 9). Although previous editions of the WHO classified three subtypes of SCC's current guidelines recommend a generic line diagnosis of "squamous cell carcinoma" due to low reproducibility and lack of prognostic relevance. However, the WHO does suggest adding a comment regarding the presence of additional histologic features such as degree of keratinization, cell size, basaloid features and adjacent AIN.

Before 1974, the management of squamous cell carcinoma of the anal canal consisted of primary surgical treatment in the form of an abdominoperineal resection. Since then, Dr Norman Nigro introduced his regimen. In his original description in three patients, radiation was given as a 3000-rad full-pelvis dose calculated to the mid plane of the pelvis, delivered in 15 treatments of 200 rad each in a 3-week period. The day after the start of radiation therapy, patients were given 25 mg/kg body weight of 5-fluorouracil daily continuous infusion for 5 days. Also, on the first day, the patients were given mitomycin-C, 0.5 mg/kg body weight. This protocol has undergone several modifications over the years, but it has completely revolutionized the treatment of squamous cell carcinoma of the anal canal, turning it into a "medical disease," with surgery indicated only as salvage therapy for persistent or recurrent disease. Combined modality therapy is delivered to the primary tumor and the locoregional lymph nodes, achieving complete response and 5-year overall survival rates as high as 92%. The presence of inguinal lymph node metastases at diagnosis reduces 5-year overall survival rates to 58%. Approximately, 10% to 15% of patients eventually have distant metastases develop, most commonly in the liver and lungs, and lymph node metastases occur in 10% to 25% of cases.

Controversy persists about the approach to the inguinal lymph nodes. Some authors favor prophylactic inguinal irradiation, and others reserve inguinal irradiation only for patients with histologically proven inguinal metastases. Inguinal irradiation has a 48% rate of acute and late morbidity. Moreover, in series of patients treated with the "Nigro protocol" avoiding the inguinal fields, inguinal

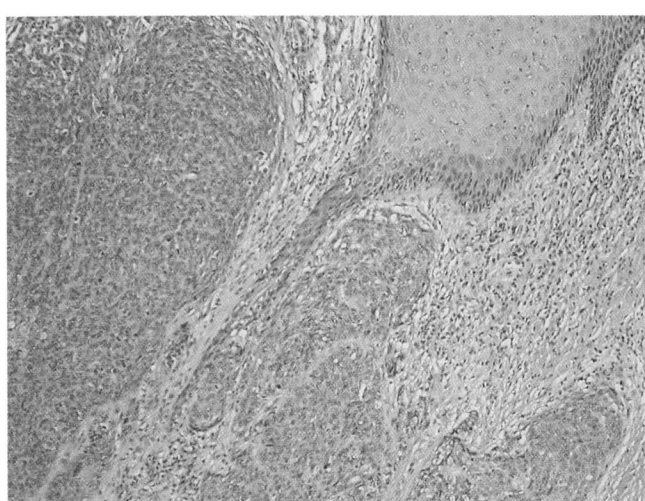

FIGURE 9 Although some residual nonneoplastic epithelium is present in the upper right hand corner, the majority of cells are malignant squamous cells invading through the lamina propria and submucosa (not identified in this image).

metastases were observed in 7% to 8% of patients, with the hypothetical potential risk of overtreating 92% to 93% of patients. Irrespective of the treatment the patient has undergone, surveillance of the inguinal lymphonodal stations remains critically important to detection of early inguinal metastases. Because lymph node size at the imaging studies is not a reliable predictor of metastases, the use of sentinel lymph node biopsy has improved staging of the inguinal status in these patients and is considered the procedure of choice for correct staging.

Inguinal lymph node dissection is associated with high morbidity: an overall wound infection rate of 24%, an incidence rate of moderate to severe infection of 16%, and lower extremity edema in 40% of patients. Superficial groin dissection involves only the inguinal nodes, and a deep groin dissection includes also the iliac and obturator nodes. Through a diagonally oriented skin incision from a point medial to the anterior superior iliac spine down to the apex of the femoral triangle, the fat and lymph nodes are dissected from the femoral triangle, starting medially at the lateral edge of the adductor longus and proceeding laterally. The femoral vessels are preserved, and the saphenous vein is ligated and divided. Finally, the lymph nodes are dissected free from the femoral nerve. The deep groin dissection begins with the division of the inguinal ligament. The deep circumflex iliac vessels are ligated, and the peritoneum is separated from the preperitoneal fat and nodes by means of blunt dissection. Then, the chain of lymph nodes along the external iliac vessels is dissected until the origin of the internal iliac vessels. The dissection incorporates the nodes overlying the obturator foramen. After the lymph nodes have been removed, the inguinal canal is reconstructed to prevent hernias.

Although in the era of improved antiviral therapy, the disease-related outcomes are similar (5-year overall survival rate about 71% to 75%), tolerability of combined modality therapy seems to be worse in patients with HIV-positive conditions in the setting of low CD4 T-cell counts. The "Nigro protocol" has been proven to be very effective, but a small percentage of patients still do not respond to it and an equally small percentage eventually have local recurrence. Interestingly, patients that do not respond have a worse outcome after salvage surgery, typically an abdominoperineal resection, even when an R0 resection is achieved. The 5-year overall survival rate after salvage surgery for persistent disease is 31% to 33%, compared with 51% to 82% after surgery for local recurrence. This is likely the result of more aggressive tumor biology. When to declare a patient a nonresponder is another topic of controversy. The radiation oncology literature clearly shows that the effects of treatment may continue for several months. In the authors' practice, a biopsy is not performed for 6 months to a year after the end of treatment.

Options for patients with metastatic anal cancer are limited and primarily involve combination chemotherapy. A regimen consisting of 5-fluorouracil and cisplatin has been the most frequently studied and results in overall response rates of around 60%, most of which are partial responses. The median survival time is approximately 12 months.

ADENOCARCINOMA

Adenocarcinoma of the anal canal accounts for about 10% of all anal canal cancers. Most of these neoplasms show a colorectal phenotype and originate from the columnar epithelium in the upper portion of the anal canal or from the glandular cells of the ATZ zone (Figure 10). Adenocarcinoma can also arise from anal glands and within established fistulas. The WHO categorizes these entities as extramucosal (perianal) adenocarcinomas.

Although the distinction between these tumors and the truly lower rectal adenocarcinomas directly extending into the anal canal is often very difficult, the difference is purely semantic because the treatment algorithm is the same. For stage II and III lesions, the treatment consists of neoadjuvant 5-fluorouracil–based combined modality therapy, then surgery often as an abdominoperineal resection, finally followed by 5-fluorouracil–based consolidation chemotherapy. For stage I, surgery alone is sufficient, and as in rectal cancer, for small very superficial T1 lesions with favorable histologic features, the role of local excision is currently debated.

Paget's Disease

Perianal Paget's disease is a rare clinical entity with only a few hundred cases reported in the literature. In its early stages symptoms are often limited, therefore, diagnosis and treatment is usually delayed. In addition, the condition can be confused with eczema or dermatitis, thus further delaying treatment. In many patients, the disease is present several years without progressing. Histologically, pale tumor cells with abundant clear cytoplasm and large nuclei are seen infiltrating throughout non neoplastic squamous epithelium

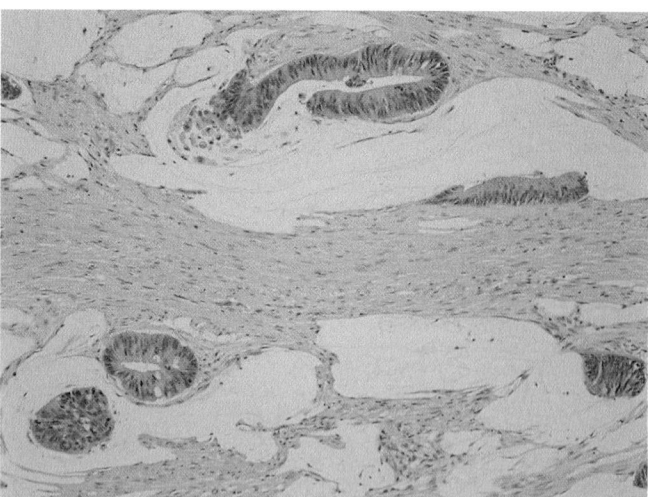

FIGURE 10 Invasive mucinous adenocarcinoma. Note the malignant glands arising from columnar epithelium floating in mucin pools.

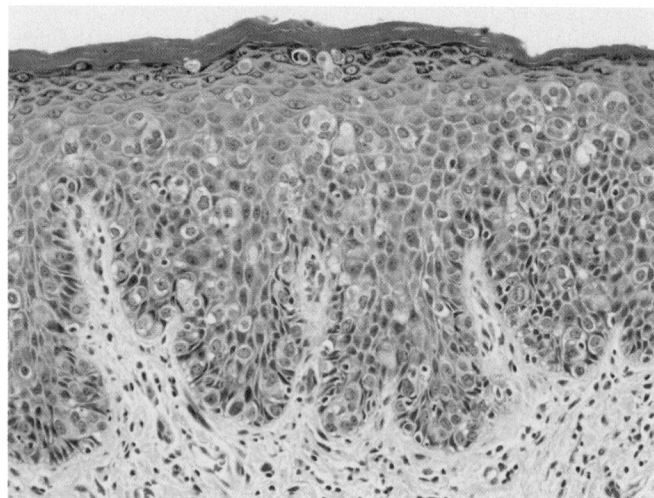

FIGURE 11 Extramammary Paget's disease. Many individual, large, pale cells represent adenocarcinoma in normal external squamous mucosa of the anal skin.

(Figure 11). There are two proposed etiologies. The first is a true primary lesion of apocrine glands exhibiting epidermotropism. These lesions are seen primarily in white women over the age of 50, have a high local recurrence rate and often express markers of apocrine cells. The other lesions are considered synchronous or metachronous lesions in patients with internal malignancies (33% to 86% have colorectal adenocarcinoma, or carcinomas of the Bartholin glands, urethra, bladder, vagina, cervix, endometrium, or prostate).

Staging classification of perianal Paget's disease and stage-appropriate treatment protocols have been proposed. Prognosis remains good for stage I (Paget's cells found in perianal epidermis and adnexa without primary carcinoma), but it progressively worsens for stage II (invasive cutaneous disease penetrating the basement membrane into the underlying stroma or synchronous localized malignancies: i.e., IIa adnexal malignancy, IIb visceral malignancy) and for stages III and IV, where regional involvement and distant metastatic disease are present, respectively.

The treatment of Paget's disease is surgical. However, because Paget's disease typically extends microscopically beyond the visible lesion, it is difficult to obtain a negative margin without sacrificing large skin areas. Consequently, recurrence rates between 30% and 70% after surgery have been reported.

Nonsurgical approaches have been advocated in selected cases, for those patients who are medically unfit for surgery or wish to avoid radical surgery or those who have multifocal widespread disease precluding complete resection.

Radiotherapy can be used as a primary treatment or in the adjuvant setting. Recurrence rates from 0 to 60% have been reported, with no apparent differences between primary treatment and adjuvant therapy.

Systemic chemotherapy is used when surgery is not recommended, in cases of advanced disease, or in a neoadjuvant setting to reduce the tumor mass before surgical excision. Applied in combination with radiotherapy, it appears to improve responses and prevent recurrences, but the use of systemic chemotherapy alone requires further investigation.

Mohs' micrographic surgery has been associated with lower recurrence rates (8% to 28%) and less morbidity compared with standard surgical excision. It is typically performed in steps. A small scalpel is used to cut around the visible tumor. A very small surgical margin is used, usually with 1 to 1.5 mm of "free margin" or uninvolved skin. After each surgical removal of tissue, the specimen is processed, cut on the cryostat and placed on slides, stained with hematoxylin and eosin, and then read by the pathologist who examines the sections for cancerous cells. If cancer is found, its location is marked on the map (drawing of the tissue) and the surgeon removes the indicated cancerous tissue from the patient. This procedure is repeated until no further cancer is found.

Recent series with CO_2 laser treatment have reported recurrence rates similar to surgical excision but with significant post-treatment pain.

MELANOMA

Anal melanomas account for about 4% of anal canal tumors and less than 1% of all melanomas. Frequently it is not pigmented and does not have a macroscopically suspicious appearance. Management of anal melanoma remains a major challenge, and the prognosis is dismal. Despite the fact that most patients present with localized and apparently curable primary tumors, the mean survival time is only 2 years. Surgery is the treatment of choice because anal melanoma does not respond to chemoradiation. The extent of surgical resection (abdominoperineal resection vs local excision) does not seem to significantly impact outcome, as patients often die of distant metastases.

NEUROENDOCRINE TUMORS

Neuroendocrine neoplasms may occasionally occur in the anal canal. Most such tumors probably originate from neuroendocrine cells residing in colorectal type mucosa, although neuroendocrine cells are known to exist in ATZ mucosa as well. Because these lesions are often small, the treatment is typically a local excision.

MESENCHYMAL TUMORS

The most common types of mesenchymal tumors in the anal canal are smooth muscle tumors and gastrointestinal stromal tumors (GISTs). The treatment is typically just a local excision because the vast majority of them are small.

MALIGNANT LYMPHOMA

Primary lymphoma of the anal canal is rare. However, cases of both Hodgkin's disease and non-Hodgkin's lymphomas are reported. Patients with immunocompromise are particularly at risk. In this population, the lymphomas are mainly B-cell type and high grade. The treatment is chemoradiation.

SUGGESTED READINGS

Fichera A, Ragauskaite L, Silvestri MT, et al: Preservation of the anal transition zone in ulcerative colitis. Long-term effects on defecatory function, *J Gastrointest Surg* 11:1647–1652, 2007.

Forcier M, Musacchio N: An overview of human papillomavirus infection for the dermatologist: disease, diagnosis, management, and prevention, *Dermatol Ther* 23:458–476, 2010.

Kanaan Z, Mulhall A, Mahid S, et al: A systematic review of prognosis and therapy of anal malignant melanoma: a plea for more precise reporting of location and thickness, *Am Surg* 78:28–35, 2012.

Kyriazanos ID, Stamos NP, Miliadis L, et al: Extra-mammary Paget's disease of the perianal region: a review of the literature emphasizing the operative management technique, *Surg Oncol* 20:e61–e71, 2011.

Mistrangelo M, Morino M: Sentinel lymph node biopsy in anal cancer: a review, *Gastroenterol Clin Biol* 33:446–450, 2009.

Scholefield JH, Harris D, Radcliffe A: Guidelines from management of anal intraepithelial neoplasia, *Colorectal Dis* 13:S3–S10, 2011.

Shia J: An update of tumors of the anal canal, *Arch Pathol Lab Med* 134:1601–1611, 2010.

Simpson JAD, Scholefield JH: Diagnosis and management of anal intraepithelial neoplasia and anal cancer [review], *BMJ* 343:d6818.doi:10.1136/bmj.d6818, 2011.

The Use of Positron Emission Tomographic Scanning in the Management of Colorectal Cancer

Nelya Brindzei, MD, and
Julio Garcia-Aguilar, MD, PhD

INTRODUCTION

The introduction of positron emission tomography (PET) scanning has been one of the most important advances made in oncology imaging over the last two decades. PET has revolutionized cancer treatment with its ability to identify tumors based on their biologic—metabolic or molecular, rather than anatomic—characteristics. An understanding of the science behind PET imaging is important in order to grasp the current and future clinical applications of this technology. PET and integrated PET/computed tomographic (CT) scan imaging are now used in multiple aspects of colorectal cancer care, including screening, diagnosis, staging, monitoring of response, diagnosis of recurrence, and posttreatment surveillance. In this chapter, we review the evidence supporting applications of PET imaging in the management of colorectal cancer.

BACKGROUND

PET imaging takes advantage of the photons emitted in the process of positron-electron annihilation. The reaction of a positron emitted from a proton-rich unstable isotope, with a nearby electron, leads to the simultaneous emission of two annihilating photons in opposite directions. These photons are identified with two separate detectors in a PET camera, located diametrically opposite one another. Both photons are detected within a short period of time, indicating that an annihilation effect has occurred somewhere in the area between detectors. The data from multiple pairs of opposing detectors is mathematically integrated and reconstructed tomographically, providing the images seen in PET scans.

The positron-emitting radioisotopes used in PET imaging are short-lived, which minimizes the radiation absorbed by the patient and makes it possible to repeat the examination within a short period of time, even on the same day. These radioisotopes combine with tracers that accumulate preferentially or selectively in tumor versus healthy tissue.

The radiotracer most commonly used in oncologic evaluation is $[^{18}F]$-2-fluoro-2-deoxy-D-glucose (FDG), which uses the radionuclide fluorine-18 attached to a glucose analog. FDG takes advantage of the fact that cancer cells preferentially use glycolysis as the source of energy at a much higher rate than healthy cells. This is known as Warburg's effect. FDG competes with normal glucose for transport across the cell membrane, but unlike glucose, FDG cannot be metabolized and accumulates inside the cell. The resultant emission of photons, and therefore the intensity of the PET signal, is proportional to the accumulation of FDG within cells. The relatively higher accumulation of FDG in the more metabolically active cancer cells results in differential intensity signal between the tumor and the adjacent healthy tissue. Tissue activity can be measured at a fixed point and normalized to body surface area, a technique known as standardized uptake value (SUV). These measurements are relatively simple, and the values are reproducible as long as they are taken at the same time point. Tissue activity can also be quantified kinetically with measurement of the constant rate of uptake of tracer by the tumor, a technique known as the Gjedde-Patlak analysis. This measurement is more precise than SUV but requires dynamic data acquisition, which can be influenced by patient movement. In general, there is no significant advantage to the Gjedde-Patlak plot model, and SUV is routinely used in clinical practice.

The use of a radiotracer as a marker of glucose metabolism, which is enhanced in all cancers, has extended the clinical applications of FDG-PET to many different malignancies. However, the targeting of a metabolic process that is enhanced in, but not exclusive to, cancer cells represents the main limitations of its use: low sensitivity and specificity. FDG-PET may provide inadequate differentiation between inflammation and tumor, or between a benign polyp and an invasive cancer. FDG-PET can also provide low signals in slow-growing tumors, or tumors with low cellularity such as mucinous carcinomas. On the other hand, PET imaging may be inaccurate in distinguishing the focal FDG uptake of a tumor from the normal high physiologic background uptake in some metabolically active organs such as bowel or brain. Remember that FDG competes with normal glucose for uptake into the cell and that patients are required to fast for a number of hours before the study. FDG-PET can also provide false-negative results in patients with diabetes with elevated serum glucose levels.

In hopes of overcoming the lack of specificity of FDG-PET, a new generation of radiotracers is under investigation. These tracers are directed against a variety of cellular processes or molecular targets, such as proliferation (fluorothymidine), hypoxia (fluoromisonidazole [FMISO]), angiogenesis (arginine-glycine-aspartate [RGD] peptides), cell surface antigens (*Her2 neu* or carcinoembryonic antigen [CEA]), or cellular receptors (epidermal growth factor receptor [EGFR] or somatostatin), which may be more tumor-specific than glucose metabolism. Some of these new tracers require isotopes with a half-life that matches the kinetics of the compound in which they are embedded, be it a monoclonal antibody (such as ^{89}Zr-Trastuzumab, ^{64}Cu-antiCEA), a small peptide (^{11}C-Erlotinib), or a receptor ligand (^{68}Ga-somatostatin analogues). However, these new PET modalities have not been fully incorporated into clinical practice. FDG-PET is currently the only form of PET used in clinical evaluation of colorectal cancer.

The main advantage of PET imaging—the detection of biologic changes that precede anatomic abnormalities—also represents its main drawback: the lack of anatomic correlation. Since 1999, the biologic information provided by PET scans can be integrated electronically with the detailed anatomic images obtained simultaneously in a CT scan. The recent technologic advances in PET detectors and the CT component, such as contrast enhancement and multidetector scanners, have improved resolution and reduced scanning time. The integration of PET and contrast-enhanced CT scan provides better results than the sum of its parts; therefore, the standalone PET is rarely performed today.

DETECTION OF COLORECTAL CANCER

The colon normally demonstrates a relatively high metabolic background activity, but a focal increase in FDG uptake over background often indicates the presence of relevant neoplasm defined as invasive cancer, polyps with high-grade dysplasia, or polyps greater than 1 cm in diameter. However, FDG-PET is incapable of differentiating adequately between inflammation, benign polyps, or cancer. Because of this, a focal increase in FDG uptake requires subsequent endoscopic examination.

Incidental colorectal focal FDG uptake is observed in 1% to 3% of FDG-PET/CT scans obtained for an unrelated reason, and follow-up colonoscopy detects cancer or polyps in almost half of these patients. A prospective study investigating the clinical significance of an incidental FDG uptake in FDG-PET/CT scans with a colonoscopy performed within 30 days reported that 23% of patients had colorectal cancer and 20% had polyps. In the remaining 56% of cases, the study results were falsely positive. The false-positive rate was higher for FDG uptake found in the right colon, which is probably related to the higher physiologic FDG uptake in the region of the terminal ileum. The maximal SUV (SUV-max) values varied significantly and were unable to discriminate between malignant and nonmalignant lesions. Other studies have reported similar rates of neoplastic lesions among patients with incidental focal colonic FDG uptake on FDG-PET/CT scans. They have also confirmed that a high SUV-max is not a good predictor of malignancy. Although these data support the need for follow-up colonoscopy in patients with incidental FDG uptake in the colon, the true accuracy of FDG-PET/CT in diagnosis of colorectal cancer is unknown because, in most of these series, patients without focal FDG uptake did not undergo colonoscopy. A recent study reported findings of advanced colonic neoplasms in 53% of patients who underwent colonoscopy after incidental focal FDG uptake was noted on PET/CT scans obtained for unrelated reasons. The rate of advanced colorectal neoplasms was only 6% among a subset of patients without focal FDG uptake on PET/CT who underwent colonoscopy for unrelated reasons, most of them for screening purposes. On the basis of these data, the authors concluded that FDG-PET/CT scan has an accuracy of 76% in diagnosis of advanced colonic neoplasia.

SCREENING FOR COLORECTAL CANCER

Conclusive evidence now shows that screening reduces colorectal cancer mortality. Although colonoscopy is the preferred method for colorectal cancer screening, computed tomographic colonography (CTC) has shown excellent diagnostic performance in detection of both cancers and polyps, and is an accepted option for colorectal cancer screening when colonoscopy is incomplete or contraindicated. However, similar to colonoscopy, CTC requires bowel cleansing and distension during the examination. The development of alternatives that could detect clinically relevant lesions, while sparing bowel cleansing, could simplify screening and increase compliance.

FDG-PET/CT scan has been proposed as a potential tool for colorectal cancer screening because it correlates the increased focal FDG uptake characteristic of neoplastic tissue with the anatomic definition of the integrated CT scan. However, CTC is so accurate in detecting colon cancer and polyps that, when the CT component of the FDG-PET/CT scan is performed with cleansed and distended bowel, the added value of the FDG-PET component is negligible. FDG-PET could have a role in screening for colorectal cancer and polyps by adding specificity to a CTC performed in noncleansed, nondistended colon. A recent retrospective study of 84 patients who had PET/CT scan with noncleansed and nondistended bowel, followed by colonoscopy (n = 79) or sigmoidoscopy (n = 5), reported that FDG-PET identified all carcinomas and 83% of all relevant adenomas. The SUV-max in all carcinomas and adenomas with high-grade dysplasia was 5 or more. False-positive FDG uptake occurred in 48 of 107 examinations (45%). Many of the false-positive results had stool as correlate on CT scan, and most of these false-positive results (41 of 48, or 85%) were correctly identified with the CT component. The authors concluded that, with a standardized cut-off value (e.g., SUV-max, ≥5), FDG-PET/CT scan provides promising accuracy in colorectal cancer screening. However, although the adoption of FDG-PET/CT scan for screening may potentially help patients

avoid the discomfort of bowel cleansing and distension, it may increase the proportion of false-positive results and unnecessary colonoscopies compared with CTC. Therefore, in the absence of prospective data, the role of FDG-PET/CT scan in screening for colorectal cancer remains undefined.

TUMOR STAGING AND TREATMENT PLANNING

Surgery is the primary therapy for most patients with colorectal cancer. However, with the development of safer radiotherapy techniques and more effective chemotherapeutic agents, a higher proportion of patients are now being treated primarily by nonsurgical means. Because decisions regarding initial treatment are based primarily on disease stage, the need for accurate clinical staging is increasing. FDG-PET/CT scan is used selectively in specific clinical scenarios, such as detection of occult disease in patients with potentially resectable metastases based on conventional anatomic imaging, and selection of patients with locally advanced rectal cancer for neoadjuvant therapy.

Between 20% and 25% of patients with colorectal cancer have distant metastasis at the time of the initial diagnosis. Until recently, median survival without treatment for patients with stage IV disease was less than 12 months. With the introduction of more effective chemotherapy agents, median survival for patients with metastatic colorectal cancer is now measured in years. A subset of patients with metastasis confined to the liver or lungs, and amenable to complete surgical resection, can now be cured. Detection of disseminated disease in patients with potentially resectable metastasis based on conventional anatomic imaging could help to avoid unnecessary, expensive, and potentially morbid surgery.

Early studies assessing the utility of FDG-PET before hepatic resection for liver metastasis reported that PET diagnosed extrahepatic disease, directly influencing the treatment plan in as many as 25% of patients. Recently, a number of retrospective and prospective studies have compared the performance of FDG-PET/CT scan with conventional imaging modalities in preoperative assessment of patients with metastatic disease. The combined results of these series suggest that FDG-PET/CT scan has greater diagnostic accuracy (sensitivity, 78% to 100%; specificity, 78% to 100%) than contrast-enhanced CT scan (sensitivity, 75% to 98%; specificity, 25% to 100%) when the patient is used as the unit analysis. However, no differences are seen in accuracy between tests when individual lesions are used as the unit analysis. This discrepancy probably reflects the relatively high rates of false-positive lesions on FDG-PET and false-negative lesions on contrast-enhanced CT scan. Similar to FDG-PET, FDG-PET/CT scan impacts management in up to 30% of patients with potentially operable distant metastasis appreciated by conventional anatomic imaging. The results of studies comparing the accuracy of PET-CT with magnetic resonance imaging (MRI) in detection of hepatic and extrahepatic metastasis are mixed: some studies report higher accuracy for MRI, and others report higher patient-level estimate for FDG-PET/CT scan accuracy. However, the results of studies comparing the diagnostic accuracy of these different imaging modalities should be interpreted with caution because these studies are very heterogeneous in terms of patient characteristics, FDG-PET/CT scan equipment and techniques, image interpretation, and reference standards.

In a recent meta-analysis of prospective studies comparing different imaging modalities in patients with known or suspected untreated liver metastasis, the sensitivity estimates on a per-lesion basis were 74.4% for CT scan, 80.3% for MRI, and 81.4% for FDG-PET. These differences were not statistically significant. On a per-patient basis, FDG-PET had a sensitivity of 94.1%, significantly higher than CT scan (83.6%), but not MRI (88.2%). Specificity estimates for all three modalities were similarly high. The number of studies on FDG-PET/CT scan was too small to reach meaningful conclusions. In the subgroup analysis, MRI was more accurate than CT scan in the diagnosis of liver lesions smaller than 1 cm in diameter. The authors concluded that MRI was the preferred first-line modality for imaging of the liver because of its relatively high accuracy, anatomic definition, and ability to detect small lesions. FDG-PET/CT scan was considered a second-line modality in patients requiring additional workup to exclude extrahepatic disease. However, this meta-analysis included few series reporting FDG-PET/CT scan data. It is possible that, with the newer multidetector scanners, FDG-PET/CT scan may be the most accurate and cost-effective imaging technique for evaluation of patients with suspected colorectal liver metastasis.

Patients with locally advanced rectal cancer are now commonly treated with neoadjuvant chemoradiation therapy (nCRT), and selection for neoadjuvant therapy is based on clinical tumor, node, metastasis (TNM) staging. Only patients with tumors that penetrate into the mesorectum (T3) or metastasize to the mesorectal lymph nodes (N+) are candidates for nCRT. In some patients, rectal cancer spreads to pelvic lymph nodes located outside the tissues that are usually removed with total mesorectal excision (TME). Identification of nodal metastasis to the mesorectal and iliac nodes is important, not only in selection of patients for nCRT but in planning of surgical resection. Therefore, accurate local and regional clinical TNM staging is crucial in selecting the optimal therapy for patients with rectal cancer. Because the treatment options for rectal cancer are more diverse than those for colon cancer, identification of distant metastasis in patients with seemingly localized rectal cancer can potentially have a greater treatment impact, compared with patients with colon cancer.

FDG-PET/CT scan, even with contrast enhancement, cannot delineate the different layers of the rectal wall. Thus, similar to CT scan and MRI, FDG-PET/CT scan is not accurate in defining the depth of tumor invasion in the bowel wall, or distinguishing tumors localized to the bowel wall, from those that penetrate into the perirectal fat. FDG-PET/CT scan is also less accurate than MRI for assessing the relationship of the tumor to the fascia propria of the rectum and predicting tumor involvement of the circumferential resection margin. However, FDG uptake correlates well with tumor specimen measurements on pathologic specimens, compared with CT scan or MRI. Preliminary studies suggest that, compared with MRI, FDG-PET/CT scan may reduce interobserver variability in delineating gross tumor volume in patients with rectal cancer, enabling better planning of preoperative radiotherapy.

Although scatter uptake from the primary tumor limits assessment of the perirectal lymph nodes, multiple studies have investigated the contribution of FDG-PET and FDG-PET/CT scan to preoperative staging of rectal cancer with CT scan or MRI. In an early study of 37 patients with rectal cancer initially staged with MRI or endorectal ultrasound and spiral CT scan, FDG-PET/CT scan identified discordant findings in 14 patients (38%). FDG-PET resulted in upstaging seven patients (50%) and downstaging three (21%). The most common discordant findings between the CT scan and FDG-PET/CT scan were lymph node metastasis, for which FDG-PET/CT scan was always accurate. FDG-PET/CT scan changed the treatment plan in 10 patients (27%). These results were confirmed by a later series, which also reported up to 31% change in tumor staging and 12% change in management.

With a qualitative analysis (focal increase in FDG uptake at a location corresponding to regional lymph node chains, compared with surrounding tissues), FDG-PET/CT scan detected nodal metastasis with a sensitivity of 85% at the patient level when compared with histopathology of the resected specimen. However, the specificity was only 42%. Quantitative interpretation of FDG-PET images, and the use of contrast-enhanced CT scan, increased specificity but decreased sensitivity. In a study with an SUV threshold of 1.5-fold, comparing surrounding tissue with diagnosed nodal metastasis, PET/CT scan showed a sensitivity of 53% and specificity of 90% compared with histopathology. As expected, the specificity could be increased to 100% by raising the threshold from 1.5-fold to 3.5-fold

compared with healthy tissue, but the sensitivity dropped even further to 24%. In nodes of more than 1 cm in diameter, PET/CT scan had a sensitivity of 30% and a specificity of 95%. Recent series have reported that FDG -PET/CT scan is as accurate as CT scan, but less accurate than high-resolution pelvic MRI, in nodal staging of rectal cancer. Consequently, FDG-PET/CT scan adds little information to other imaging modalities, such as multidetector, contrast-enhanced CT scan and MRI, in preoperative staging of rectal cancer, except in identifying distant metastasis in patients with high-risk tumors.

ASSESSMENT OF TUMOR RESPONSE

The development of more effective chemotherapeutic drugs and the widespread use of nCRT in rectal cancer have accentuated the importance of assessing tumor response when making therapeutic decisions. FDG-PET is a functional study that can detect metabolic and molecular changes in response to therapy, before volume reduction becomes measurable with conventional anatomic imaging. FDG-PET has been proven very valuable for assessing response to therapy in tumors such as Hodgkin's lymphoma, in which fibrosis cannot be reliably distinguished from residual disease with CT scan. The role of FDG-PET in assessment of colorectal cancer response to therapy, both in the locoregional and metastatic setting, has been studied broadly in recent years.

Some patients with rectal cancer treated with nCRT and TME have no detectable cancer cells in their surgical specimens. Therefore, the nominal value of surgery in these patients has been questioned. If responders could be identified clinically, surgery might be deferred indefinitely, sparing these patients unnecessary morbidity. Unfortunately, the correlation between clinical examination and pathologic analysis is inexact, and some patients with a clinical response have viable cancer cells in their surgical specimens. The discordance between a clinical complete response (cCR) and a pathologic complete response (pCR) is currently the primary limiting factor to an organ preservation approach for patients with rectal cancer who achieve a sustained response to nCRT.

Extensive study of the role of FDG-PET in assessment of rectal cancer response to nCRT has yielded conflicting results. Earlier studies showed a possible correlation between PET parameters and tumor regression, but in most series, PET did not accurately identify patients with a pathologic complete response to chemoradiation therapy (CRT). A recent large prospective series of patients treated with nCRT and TME reported that 70% of patients showing a complete response on FDG-PET had residual tumor on histopathologic examination. For patients with a complete response on CT scan, 50% had residual tumor in the surgical specimen. Conversely, of patients with an incomplete response on PET or CT scan, 16% and 19%, respectively, had pCR in the surgical specimen. It can be concluded that neither FDG-PET nor CT scan are sufficiently accurate in distinguishing between partial and complete rectal cancer response to CRT. Some studies have reported that a decrease in FDG uptake in PET performed early in the course of nCRT is associated with lower risk of tumor recurrence and improved patient survival. However, recent studies have not confirmed these findings.

Changes in SUV, metabolic volume, and lesion glycolysis in post-chemotherapy FDG-PET imaging, compared with baseline, have been correlated with response to chemotherapy in patients treated for colorectal liver metastasis. A number of studies have reported significant differences in one or more of these parameters between responders and nonresponders. However, similar to rectal cancer response to nCRT, FDG-PET/CT scan cannot distinguish with certainty patients with metastasis who achieve a pCR in response to systemic chemotherapy from those with residual disease.

The diagnostic accuracy of most imaging modalities in identification of liver metastasis is lower in patients after chemotherapy, compared with chemo-naive patients. The drop in accuracy after chemotherapy is more significant for FDG-PET and FDG-PET/CT scan compared with other imaging modalities such as MRI or CT scan. A recent meta-analysis of the published series on preoperative imaging of colorectal liver metastasis concluded that MRI appears to be the most appropriate preoperative imaging modality for detection of liver metastasis after chemotherapy. CT scan was the second-best imaging modality. PET-CT scan was not particularly useful in the postchemotherapy setting.

RECURRENT COLORECTAL CANCER

More than one third of patients with colorectal cancer treated with curative intent have recurrence within 5 years of surgery. Most recurrences develop in distant organs, such as the liver or lungs, or locally at the site of the primary tumor. Chemotherapy or radiation can prolong survival and improve quality of life for some of these patients, but surgical resection with negative margins is the only curative treatment for recurrent colorectal cancer. Therefore, identification of patients with isolated resectable recurrences could potentially increase survival in patients with colorectal cancer. A systematic review of several prospective randomized trials concluded that close surveillance improves survival through early detection of recurrences and second primaries in selected patients who are at high risk of recurrence after treatment for primary colorectal cancer. Most professional societies recommend surveillance consisting of periodic clinic visits, measurement of plasma CEA levels, and abdominal CT scans.

The diagnosis of tumor recurrence is often challenging because conventional imaging cannot distinguish between surgical changes or benign incidental lesions and tumor recurrence. FDG-PET/CT scan is especially valuable in diagnosis of tumor recurrence because it combines FDG uptake—a marker of the enhanced glycolytic activity characteristic of cancer cells—and the anatomic definition of the CT scan. In addition, FDG-PET can occasionally detect small foci of increased FDG uptake in structures that appear normal on conventional imaging. Therefore, FDG-PET/CT scan has the potential to impact the treatment of these patients by finding previously undiagnosed recurrences but also by detecting disseminated disease in patients already diagnosed with seemingly localized colorectal cancer recurrences.

A meta-analysis of the literature assessing the use of FDG-PET without CT scan integration in the diagnosis of recurrent colorectal cancer showed an overall sensitivity of 97% and an overall specificity of 76%. These findings changed management in 29% to 40% of patients who had been previously diagnosed with tumor recurrence, based on CT imaging. Furthermore, a decision analysis suggested that FDG-PET was cost-effective in the management of recurrent colorectal cancer. A more recent meta-analysis of a series comparing FDG-PET, FDG-PET/CT scan, CT scan, and MRI for detection of recurrent disease in patients with high suspicion of recurrent colorectal cancer, based on symptoms or rising CEA levels, suggested that FDG-PET and FDG-PET/CT scan had higher diagnostic performance compared with CT scan. PET/CT scan seems to be more accurate than MRI in detection of lymph node recurrences in a lesion level analysis. In patients who had both tests, integrated FDG-PET/CT scan had a higher diagnostic performance compared with FDG-PET alone.

Altered pelvic anatomy and presacral abnormalities are common on CT scan or MRI after TME for rectal cancer, and FDG-PET/CT scan is particularly accurate in distinguishing benign scar from recurrent tumor in these patients. The FDG findings are clinically relevant, as they may change clinical management for many of these patients. However, false-positive results, mainly from FDG uptake in displaced pelvic organs, are not uncommon, and may result in unnecessary treatments.

FDG-PET, particularly when integrated with contrast-enhanced CT scan, is useful for investigating unexplained CEA elevation in patients undergoing surveillance after curative resection for colorectal cancer. The accuracy of FDG-PET/CT scan in detection of tumor recurrence in patients with elevated CEA is independent of the CEA level.

Despite its diagnostic accuracy in patients suspected of colorectal cancer recurrence based on symptoms, rising CEA levels, or conventional imaging, information on the utility of FDG-PET/CT scan for surveillance after curative resection is limited. One study randomized 130 patients who had undergone curative surgery for colon or rectal cancer to conventional surveillance or surveillance with FDG-PET/CT scan. The proportion of patients with recurrence was similar in both groups, but recurrences were detected after a shorter time interval (12.1 vs 15.4; $P = 0.01$) in the FDG-PET cohort. In addition, more patients in the PET group had curative resection. Unfortunately, the study did not provide survival data; thus, the real benefit of routine use of FDG-PET/CT scan in the surveillance of patients after curative treatment of colorectal cancer remains unknown.

SUMMARY

The use of FDG-PET in the management of patients with colorectal cancer is increasing, but its indications are not well defined. At this time, the information available does not support its use for colorectal cancer screening, even in the subset of patients who have a complete colonoscopy, because of the high false-positive rate of the PET component and the lack of advantage shown by the CT component over CTC. The main role of FDG-PET/CT scan in clinical staging is limited to detection of nodal or distant metastasis in patients at high risk.

The greatest impact of FDG-PET/CT scan is in the management of recurrent colorectal cancer, because it can facilitate diagnosis in patients suspected of recurrence based on symptoms, rising CEA, or conventional imaging. In addition, it may be helpful in selecting patients with resectable metastasis for surgical therapy, by identifying those with disseminated disease who will not benefit from surgery. However, at the present time, FDG-PET/CT scan is not cost-effective as a primary tool in routine surveillance after curative resection for colorectal cancer.

FDG-PET and FDG-PET/CT scan measurements, before and after treatment, are able to detect partial tumor response. However, neither modality can predict pathologic complete response with enough accuracy to be considered clinically useful. Therefore, although FDG-PET and FDG-PET/CT scan may be useful in assessing the efficacy of systemic therapy, they cannot be used to select patients for nonoperative management. Future studies should focus on increasing PET resolution, identifying the optimal time to assess tumor response, increasing the rate of tumor response, and using more specific molecular radiotracers.

SUGGESTED READINGS

Brush J, Boyd K, Chappell F, et al: The value of FDG positron emission tomography/computerised tomography (PET/CT) in pre-operative staging of colorectal cancer: a systematic review and economic evaluation, *Health Technol Assess* 15(35):1–192, 2011.

Buijsen J, van den Bogaard J, Janssen MH, et al: FDG-PET provides the best correlation with the tumor specimen compared to MRI and CT in rectal cancer, *Radiother Oncol* 98(2):270–276, 2011.

Guillem JG, Ruby JA, Leibold T, et al: Neither FDG-PET nor CT is able to distinguish between a pathological complete response and an incomplete response after neoadjuvant chemoradiation in locally advanced rectal cancer: a prospective study, *Ann Surg* 2012; epub ahead of print.

Kramer-Marek G, Capala J: The role of nuclear medicine in modern therapy of cancer, *Tumor Biol* 33:629–640, 2012.

Kwak JY, Kim JS, Kim HJ, et al: Diagnostic value of FDG/PET for lymph node metastases of colorectal cancer, *Word J Surg* 36(8):1898–1905, 2012.

Lee C, Koh SJ, Kim JW, et al: Incidental colonic (18)F-Fluorodeoxyglucose uptake: do we need colonoscopy for patients with focal uptake confined to the left-sided colon? *Dig Dis Sci* 58(1):229–235, 2013.

Luboldt W, Volker T, Wiedemann B, et al: Detection of relevant colonic neoplasms with PET/CT: promising accuracy with minimal CT dose and a standardised PET cut-off, *Eur Radiol* 20(9):2274–2285, 2010.

Maas M, Rutten IJ, Nelemans PJ, et al: What is the most accurate whole-body imaging modality for assessment of local and distant recurrent disease in colorectal cancer? A meta-analysis: imaging for recurrent colorectal cancer, *Eur J Nucl Med Mol Imaging* 38(8):1560–1571, 2011.

Niekel MC, Bipat S, Stoker J: Diagnostic imaging of colorectal liver metastases with CT, MR imaging, FDG PET, and/or FDG PET/CT: a meta-analysis of prospective studies including patients who have not previously undergone treatment, *Radiology* 257(3):674–684, 2010.

Ozkan E, Soydal C, Araz M, et al: The role of 18F-FDG PET/CT in detecting colorectal cancer recurrence in patients with elevated CEA levels, *Nucl Med Commun* 33(4):395–402, 2012.

Panagiotidis E, Datseris IE, Exarhos D, et al: High incidence of peritoneal implants in recurrence of intra-abdominal cancer revealed by 18F-FDG PET/CT in patients with increased tumor markers and negative findings on conventional imaging, *Nucl Med Commun* 33(4):431–438, 2012.

Ruby JA, Leibold T, Akhurst TJ, et al: FDG-PET assessment of rectal cancer response to neoadjuvant chemoradiotherapy is not associated with long-term prognosis: a prospective evaluation, *Dis Colon Rectum* 55(4):378–386, 2012.

Sobhani I, Tiret E, Lebtahi R, et al: Early detection of recurrence by 18FDG-PET in the follow-up of patients with colorectal cancer, *Br J Cancer* 98(5):875–880, 2008.

Tateishi U, Maeda T, Morimoto T, et al: Non-enhanced CT versus contrast-enhanced CT in integrated PET/CT studies for nodal staging of rectal cancer, *Eur J Nucl Med Mol Imaging* 34(10):1627–1634, 2007.

Tsunoda Y, Ito M, Fujii H, et al: Preoperative diagnosis of lymph node metastases of colorectal cancer by FDG-PET/CT, *Jpn J Clin Oncol* 38(5):347–353, 2008.

van Lessel CS, Buckens CFM, van den Bosch MAAJ, et al: Preoperative imaging of colorectal liver metastases after neoadjuvant chemotherapy: a meta-analysis, *Ann Surg Oncol* 19:2805–2813, 2012.

THE USE OF NEOADJUVANT AND ADJUVANT TREATMENT FOR COLORECTAL CANCER

David Cosgrove, MBBCh

OVERVIEW

Colorectal cancer (CRC) is a common malignancy and a major public health problem in the United States; an estimated 142,820 new cases are projected to occur in 2013. Although the rate of mortality from CRC has been steadily declining since 1990, there are still more than 50,000 U.S. deaths from the disease each year. Screening for CRC can lead to diagnosis at an earlier stage, potentially curative therapy, and a reduction in cause-specific mortality, but population compliance with screening guidelines remains disappointingly low; only approximately 50% of all eligible adult patients report completion of recommended screening tests.

Surgical resection is the foundation of a curative treatment approach to CRC. Despite appropriate surgical intervention in early-stage disease, the emergence of distant metastatic disease is common. The cause of this recurrence is the presence of micrometastatic spread before or during the surgical intervention, with a tumor burden below the threshold of detection of standard diagnostic tools. The goal of neoadjuvant and adjuvant therapy is to eradicate these micrometastases and enhance the potential for long-term survival. However, the majority of patients undergoing curative-intent surgical resection for this disease do not derive any discernible benefit from adjuvant treatments, either because surgery alone is truly curative (i.e., there are no micrometastatic deposits) or because the disease recurs in spite of additional treatments (i.e., the micrometastatic deposits prove refractory to eradication). Unfortunately, at the time of writing, the ability to predict which patients are more likely to benefit from adjuvant therapy is limited. Physicians still rely on the anatomic tumor stage to assess the recurrence risk, even though the available staging systems consist of broad categories, each of which contains a wide spectrum of actual recurrence risks. Molecular assessment of tumor cells and surrounding stroma has the potential to refine the prognostic armamentarium and could serve to identify individual patients likely to benefit from specific adjuvant therapies, but such assessments are still investigational for the most part and have yet to influence clinical decision making in this arena. Such assessments have a more robust role in clinical decision making for patients with metastatic CRC.

CRC is subdivided into colon cancer and rectal cancer with regard to the specifics of adjuvant treatment options. Because of the unique anatomic challenges to complete surgical clearance posed by lesions in the rectum, radiation therapy has served as a treatment adjunct to reduce local recurrence, whereas it has no role in the adjunctive treatment of true colon lesions. These clinical scenarios are discussed separately in this chapter.

STAGING

Despite the limitations just noted, formal CRC staging remains essential to establish the likely risk of recurrence in an individual patient and to implement appropriate curative-intent treatment. The National Comprehensive Cancer Network® (NCCN®) recommends that the preoperative workup for CRC should include a colonoscopy; complete blood cell counts; liver and kidney function tests; carcinoembryonic antigen (CEA) serum level; computed tomographic (CT) scan of the chest, abdomen, and pelvis; and pathologic assessment of the tumor tissue. Patients presenting with a rectal cancer should additionally undergo rigid proctoscopy and formal pelvic imaging, with either magnetic resonance imaging or endoscopic ultrasonography, to accurately define the depth of tumor invasion and degree of lymph node involvement. Accurate preoperative staging in rectal cancer is of particular importance because radiation therapy will be incorporated in the neoadjuvant setting, which can often lead to an anatomic downstaging of the primary tumor and lymph node metastases before curative resection and final pathologic staging. Positron emission tomography (PET) is not considered standard in the staging workup of localized CRC; however, it may be utilized as a confirmatory test if suspect findings on CT scans suggest the presence of distant metastatic disease.*

CRC is staged on the TNM staging system (T, primary tumor; N, regional lymph nodes; M, distant metastasis), adopted by the American Joint Committee on Cancer (AJCC). The 2010 revision of this staging system is outlined in Table 1. The importance of accurate staging is reflected in Table 2, which outlines the predicted 5-year survival rates among patients with a diagnosis of nonmetastatic CRC. In all patients represented in this table, except those with truly stage I disease, a conversation about the relative risks and benefits of adjuvant therapy is warranted. As discussed in the following sections, the more aggressive the disease biology, or the more widespread its extent, the greater the potential benefit of such therapy.

ADJUVANT THERAPY FOR COLON CANCER

Stage III Colon Cancer

Adjuvant chemotherapy has been an accepted standard of care in stage III colon cancer since 1990, when a survival benefit over surgery alone for such patients was defined in both the National Surgical Adjuvant Breast and Bowel Project (NSABP) C-01 study and the North Central Cancer Treatment Group (NCCTG) trial. The specific

TABLE 1: American Joint Committee on Cancer TNM classification of colon cancer

Primary Tumor (T)

TX	Primary tumor cannot be assessed
T0	No evidence of primary tumor
Tis	Carcinoma in situ: intraepithelial or invasion of lamina propria*
T1	Tumor invades submucosa
T2	Tumor invades muscularis propria
T3	Tumor invades through the muscularis propria into pericolorectal tissues
T4a	Tumor penetrates to the surface of the visceral peritoneum†
T4b	Tumor directly invades or is adherent to other organs or structures†,‡

Regional Lymph Nodes (N)

NX	Regional lymph nodes cannot be assessed
N0	No regional lymph node metastases
N1	Metastasis in one to three regional lymph nodes
N1a	Metastasis in one regional lymph node
N1b	Metastasis in two to three regional lymph nodes
N1c	Tumor deposit(s) in the subserosa, mesentery, or nonperitonealized pericolic or perirectal tissues without regional nodal metastasis
N2	Metastasis in four or more regional lymph nodes
N2a	Metastasis in four to six regional lymph nodes
N2b	Metastasis in seven or more regional lymph nodes

Distant Metastasis (M)

M0	No distant metastasis
M1	Distant metastases
M1a	Metastasis confined to one organ or site (e.g., liver, lung, ovary, nonregional node)
M1b	Metastases in more than one organ/site or the peritoneum

From American Joint Committee on Cancer: AJCC Cancer Staging Manual, 7th ed, New York, 2010, Springer.
*Note: This includes cancer cells confined within the glandular basement membrane (intraepithelial) or mucosal lamina propria (intramucosal) with no extension through the muscularis mucosae in the submucosa.
†Note: Direct invasion in T4 includes invasion of other organs or other segments of the colorectum as a result of direct extension through the serosa, as confirmed on microscopic examination (e.g., invasion of the sigmoid colon by a carcinoma of the cecum) or, for cancers in a retroperitoneal or subperitoneal location, direct invasion of other organs or structures by virtue of extension beyond the muscularis propria (i.e., respectively, a tumor on the posterior wall of the descending colon invading the left kidney or lateral abdominal wall; or a mid or distal rectal cancer with invasion of prostate, seminal vesicles, cervix, or vagina).
‡Note: Tumor that is adherent to other organs or structures, grossly, is classified cT4b. However, if no tumor is present in the adhesion, microscopically, the classification should be pT1-4a, depending on the anatomic depth of wall invasion. The V and L classifications should be used to identify the presence or absence of vascular or lymphatic invasion whereas the PN site-specific factor should be used for perineural invasion.

TABLE 2: TNM classification, staging, and survival

TNM category	% of patients	TNM stage	5-year survival rate (%)
T1 N0	9.9	I	97.4
T2 N0	11.8	I	96.8
T3 N0	36.7	IIA	87.5
T4a N0	4.6	IIB	79.6
T4b N0	2.8	IIC	58.4
T1-T2 N1a	1.7	IIIA	90.7
T1-T2 N1b	1.1	IIIA	83.0
T1 N2a	0.3	IIIA	79.0
T2 N2a		IIIB	
T1-T2 N2b	0.1	IIIB	74.2
T3 N1a	8.0	IIIB	74.2
T3 N1b	8.3	IIIB	65.3
T3 N2a	4.8	IIIB	53.4
T3 N2b	2.9	IIIC	37.3
T4a N1a	1.2	IIIB	67.6
T4b N1a	0.8	IIIC	38.5
T4a N1b	1.3	IIIB	54.0
T4b N1b	0.8	IIIC	31.2
T4a N2a	0.9	IIIC	40.9
T4b N2a	0.7	IIIC	23.3
T4a N2b	0.6	IIIC	21.8
T4b N2b	0.6	IIIC	15.7

Data from American Joint Committee on Cancer: AJCC cancer staging manual, 7th ed, New York, 2010, Springer.
TNM, Tumor, node, metastasis.

chemotherapy combinations used in these studies (semustine, vincristine, and fluorouracil in NSABP C-01; 5-fluorouracil [5-FU] and levimasole in NCCTG) ultimately proved too toxic and were replaced with the fluoropyrimidine 5-fluorouracil and leucovorin (5-FU/LV), a combination that provided an outcome superior to those of the prior agents, when given for a total of 6 months after surgical resection. This regimen was the standard until the early 2000s, when the advent of a number of newer chemotherapeutic agents that produced benefit in patients with metastatic colon cancer drove many researchers in large clinical trials to assess the additional benefit from other combinations.

The original trials in stage III colon cancer had used a strict endpoint of overall survival rate; however, a meta-analysis carried out in follow-up to these studies confirmed that 3-year disease-free survival (DFS) was an acceptable surrogate for 5-year overall survival, and so researchers in subsequent studies of adjuvant colon cancer utilized this endpoint, which has been approved by the U.S. Food and Drug Administration.

One such study demonstrated that the 5-FU prodrug capecitabine was a safe and efficacious alternative to bolus 5-FU/LV in patients with stage III disease. Researchers in three major trials have assessed the efficacy of combining oxaliplatin with a fluoropyrimidine in this group, and researchers in three other trials have assessing the integration of irinotecan into a fluoropyrimidine-based regimen. A number of investigators have attempted to add a monoclonal antibody (so-called targeted therapeutic agents) to cytotoxic chemotherapy in the adjuvant setting, mostly with disappointing results.

The pivotal Multicenter International Study of Oxaliplatin/5-FU/LV in the Adjuvant Treatment of Colon Cancer (MOSAIC) demonstrated that folinic acid and oxaliplatin plus infusional 5-FU/LV (FOLFOX) was superior to 5-FU/LV alone, with improved DFS at 5 years for patients with stage III disease (hazard ratio, 0.78; $P = 0.05$), albeit with an increased risk for peripheral neuropathy, diarrhea, and febrile neutropenia. Certain patients with stage II disease (those presenting with T4 lesions, perforation, obstruction, or undifferentiated tumors) also gleaned a survival benefit with the addition of oxaliplatin, although patients with stage II disease in general experienced no overall improvement in outcome with FOLFOX. The NSABP C-07 study cemented the beneficial role of oxaliplatin-containing regimens as adjuvant therapy for patients with stage III colon cancer. Substituting infusional 5-FU for capecitabine has no detrimental effect on this benefit, as outlined in the Roche No. 16968 ("XELOXA") trial, in which almost 2000 patients were randomly assigned to receive either bolus 5-FU/LV or the XELOX combination of capecitabine (Xeloda) and oxaliplatin (Eloxatin). An incremental increase in 3-year DFS of 4% was noted in the patients who received XELOX, a similar magnitude of benefit to that seen in the prior studies (Table 3).

Although irinotecan-containing and oxaliplatin-containing regimens offer equivalent outcomes in the treatment of metastatic colon cancer, the studies of irinotecan in the adjuvant setting (Pan-European Trials in Alimentary Tract Cancers [PETACC-3] and the Action to Control Cardiovascular Risk in Diabetes [ACCORD] study) have surprisingly failed to demonstrate and survival benefit over 5-FU/LV alone. Similarly, adding the vascular endothelial growth factor (VEGF)–targeted agent bevacizumab (approved in the treatment of metastatic colon cancer) to FOLFOX in the adjuvant setting did not lead to any improvement in DFS or overall survival in two large studies (NSABP C-08 and AVastin adjuvANT [AVANT]). The epithelial growth factor receptor (EGFR)–targeted agent cetuximab, also approved for the treatment of wild-type *KRAS* metastatic colon cancer, had no effect on survival endpoints over chemotherapy alone.

According to the current body of literature, the standard adjuvant protocol for stage III colon cancer is an oxaliplatin-containing regimen (FOLFOX; 5-FU, leucovorin, and oxaliplatin [FLOX]; or XELOX) administered for 6 months after the patient recovers from surgery. Capecitabine or 5-FU/LV alone should be considered in only patients who are not good candidates for oxaliplatin therapy (because of pre-existing neuropathy, borderline performance status). Elderly patients should also not be considered for oxaliplatin regimens, inasmuch as metaanalysis of the MOSAIC and NSABP C-07 findings revealed no DFS or overall survival benefit for patients older than 70 years. Typical practice suggests that physically fit elderly patients should nonetheless be offered oxaliplatin, ideally within the FOLFOX regimen.

Stage II Colon Cancer

Although adjuvant chemotherapy has an established role in treatment of stage III colon cancer, there is much less certainty of that role in treatment of stage II disease. As noted in Table 2, the predicted 5-year survival rate in most patients with fully resected stage II disease is excellent, from 80% to 90%, and so adjuvant chemotherapy would have to have a profoundly beneficial effect to reach a statistically significant improvement in survival endpoints. Because most of the original adjuvant chemotherapy trials (including MOASIC and

TABLE 3: Results of selected phase III adjuvant trials in colon cancer (oxaliplatin regimens)

Trial	Stage (% of patients)	Regimen	3-year outcomes		6-year outcomes	
			Disease-free survival rate (%)	P value, HR	Overall survival rate (%)	P value, HR
Multicenter International Study of Oxaliplatin/5-FU/LV in the Adjuvant Treatment of Colon Cancer (MOSAIC); N = 2246	II/III (40/60)	LV5FU2		$P < 0.001$, HR = 0.77 (95% CI: 0.65-0.90)	76.0	$P = 0.046$, HR = 0.84 (95% CI: 0.71-1.00)
		FOLFOX			78.5	
	II	LV5FU2		HR = 0.82 (95% CI: 0.60-1.13)	86.8	$P = 0.986$, HR = 1.00 (95% CI: 0.70-1.41)
		FOLFOX			86.9	
	III	LV5FU2		HR = 0.75 (95% CI: 0.62-0.89)	68.7	$P = 0.023$, HR = 0.80 (95% CI: 0.65-0.97)
		FOLFOX			72.9	
National Surgical Adjuvant Breast and Bowel Project (NSABP) C-07; N = 2407	II/III (29/71)	RP	71.6	$P < 0.004$, HR = 0.79 (95% CI: 0.67-0.93)	73.5	$P = 0.06$, HR = 0.85 (95% CI: 0.72-1.01)
		FLOX	76.5		78.3	
Roche No. 16968 (XELOXA): N = 1886	III	RP/Mayo	67.0	$P = 0.0045$, HR = 0.80 (95% CI: 0.69-0.93)	NA	
		XELOX	71.0			

Cape, Capecitabine; *CI,* confidence intervals; *FLOX,* bolus 5-FU/LV plus oxaliplatin; *FOLFOX,* bolus/infusional 5-FU/LV plus oxaliplatin; *HR,* hazard ratio; *LV5FU2,* bolus/infusional 5-FU/LV regimen; *Mayo,* Mayo Clinic bolus 5-FU/LV regimen; *NA,* not available; *RP,* Roswell Park bolus 5-FU/LV regimen; *XELOX,* capecitabine plus oxaliplatin.

NSABP C-07) enrolled both patients with stage II and patients with stage III disease, and because the benefits accrued in those trials were clinically and statistically significant only for those with stage III disease, a number of prospective studies dedicated to stage II colon cancer were undertaken. The QUick And Simple And Reliable (QUASAR) trial in the United Kingdom enrolled more than 3000 patients, mostly with stage II disease, and randomly assigned them to receive adjuvant chemotherapy (5-FU/LV with or without levimasole); there was a 3% improvement in 5-year overall survival, although the trend was not statistically significant in patients with stage II disease (hazard ratio, 0.86; 95% confidence interval [CI]: 0.54 to 1.19). The International Multicentre Pooled Analysis of B2 Colon Cancer Trials (IMPACT B2) involved pooled data from more than 1000 patients with T3 N0 disease, assigned to observation or adjuvant 5-FU/LV, and it revealed no difference in 5-year overall survival (80% to 82%). Of the patients enrolled in the MOSAIC trial, as noted previously, 40% had stage II disease. These patients did not glean any additional benefit from adjuvant oxaliplatin therapy; the overall survival rate at 6 years was 87% in both study conditions.

Although most of these studies hint at only a very small benefit from adjuvant chemotherapy in unselected patients with resected stage II disease, there is room for further risk stratification within this group. There are well-established clinicopathologic variables that indicate which patients with stage II disease are at higher risk: namely a T4 primary tumor, bowel obstruction or perforation, poorly differentiated histologic features, inadequate lymph node sampling, perineural or lymphovascular invasion, and markedly elevated CEA level. These are recognized prognostic factors for patients with stage II colon cancer, but data to indicate that adjuvant chemotherapy in these cases will improve outcomes are lacking. Professional society guidelines, including those from the American Society of Clinical Oncology (ASCO) and NCCN®, acknowledge this lack of evidence and stress that medically fit patients with resected stage II colon cancer, who have high-risk features, should be made aware of the risks and benefits of adjuvant chemotherapy in their individual cases.

Advances in the identification of tumor molecular factors have increased the expectation of truly prognostic or predictive biomarker development that can more appropriately risk stratify patients with stage II colon cancer. Research areas with promise include *KRAS* and *BRAF* mutations, 18q deletion, microsatellite instability, hypermethylation, and thymidylate synthase overexpression, and a number of commercial gene assays have been developed (Coloprint, Oncotype DX Colon), but none have thus far provided any predictive utility to guide chemotherapy choices. One subset of patients has been clinically assessed: those with defective mismatch repair (MMR-D) or microsatellite instability (MSI-H), akin to the phenotype of patients with Lynch's syndrome. This subset represents about 15% to 20% of all patients with colon cancer, and they have an excellent prognosis but have exhibited resistance to 5-FU–based chemotherapy. Of note, more modern combination regimens have not been fully explored in this population, and investigations are ongoing.

At this time, unselected patients with resected stage II colon cancer should not routinely be offered adjuvant chemotherapy because the survival benefit is minimal in large studies. It is appropriate to review the risks and benefits of adjuvant therapy with patients, in view of their clinicopathologic characteristics and any available molecular data, and to consider individual cases in the context of comorbid conditions and anticipated life expectancy. This conversation can be facilitated by two web-based tools (Adjuvant! Online and Numeracy), which each provide a visual representation of calculated therapy benefits, although both are informed by somewhat limited datasets and are not necessarily directly applicable to individual patients.

NEOADJUVANT AND ADJUVANT THERAPY FOR RECTAL CANCER

Cancers arising within the rectum, although molecularly similar to other colon cancers, exhibit higher rates of local recurrence after curative intent surgical resection than those arising elsewhere in the colon. The rationale for this increased recurrence risk is thought to be multifactorial, including both tumor-related factors, such as challenging anatomic location and local lymphatic invasion, and surgery-related factors, such as excision of the mesorectum and extent of lymphadenectomy. Total mesorectal excision (TME) is the preferred approach for all but the smallest rectal tumors and requires meticulous sharp dissection and avoidance of disruption of the mesorectum; this should ideally be undertaken at high-volume surgery centers to minimize variation. A number of studies suggest that TME, in combination with appropriate adjunctive therapies, can reduce local recurrence from rectal cancer to below 10%.

The historically high local recurrence rates in rectal cancer, and their rates of associated morbidity and mortality, prompted the study of both preoperative and postoperative radiation therapy for these tumors in recent decades. Two approaches have been predominantly assessed in the preoperative setting: short-term, high-dose radiation delivered immediately before surgical resection, typically delivered in a dose of 5 Gy daily for 5 days, or combined-modality therapy with radiosensitizing chemotherapy doses concomitant with 50.4 Gy total radiation dose over 5 to 6 weeks, with a subsequent 3- to 4-week interval before surgery. Both approaches are associated with decreased locoregional failure, but only the longer duration chemoradiotherapy has resulted in tumor downstaging, tumor shrinkage, and improved sphincter-preservation. The short-course radiation approach has been assessed in two large European trials: a Swedish study randomly assigned more than 1100 patients to receive 5 days of high-dose radiation (total 25 Gy) 1 week before surgery or to undergo surgery alone; in patients who received radiation, the local recurrence rate was reduced (11% vs 27%, $P < 0.001$), and the overall survival advantage at 5 years was higher (58% vs 48%, $P = 0.004$). A subsequent Dutch study assessed similar radiation doses, although this time in conjunction with quality-controlled TME surgery, and once again demonstrated an improved local recurrence rate (2.4% vs 8.4% at 2 years, $P < 0.001$), but there was no overall survival effect. This perhaps highlights the critical importance of adequate surgery in terms of survival in this disease.

Short-course radiation therapy is commonly used in Europe, but longer duration combination therapy is still preferred in the United States. Initial studies demonstrating its effect were undertaken in the adjuvant setting, in which 5-FU–based chemotherapy with concomitant irradiation proved better than irradiation or surgery alone in preventing both local and distant recurrences. Prolonged infusional 5-FU and twice-daily oral capecitabine are considered equivalent in terms of radiosensitization, although no trial data are available to compare the two. The appropriate sequencing of therapy was assessed in a large German study, in which patients were randomly assigned to receive standard, infusional 5-FU plus irradiation either before or after definitive TME. Preoperative combined modality therapy resulted in a lower rate of local recurrence (6% vs 13% at 5 years), a lower toxicity rate (acute and chronic), and a higher rate of sphincter preservation than did postoperative therapy. Preoperative chemoradiotherapy has thus become the standard of care for patients with stages II and III rectal cancer. Studies are ongoing to assess the effect of additional cytotoxic therapy or biologic agents delivered concomitantly with this standard approach or in the adjuvant setting to reduce distant metastases. Current practice in the United States is to deliver adjuvant FOLFOX to all patients with resected rectal cancer, independent of response to preoperative therapy.

Surveillance

As noted previously, therapy for localized colon and rectal cancers is undertaken with curative intent. Despite this, up to 50% of these patients experience relapse with distant (and occasionally local) metastases. Some patients exhibit only solitary or oligometastatic deposits at this relapse and are candidates for salvage surgery, once again with curative intent, especially if the deposits are confined to the liver or lungs. Long-term DFS and even cure remains possible. Because of this, posttreatment surveillance is deemed important,

BOX 1: NCCN Clinical Practice Guidelines In Oncology (NCCN Guidelines®) for Colon Cancer and NCCN Guidelines® for Rectal Cancer : Surveillance After Curative Surgery

- History and physical examination every 3 to 6 months for 2 years, then every 6 months for a total of 5 years
- CEA every 3 to 6 months for 2 years, then every 6 months for a total of 5 years*
- Chest/abdomen/pelvis CT annually for 5 years for patients at high risk for recurrence
- Colonoscopy at 1 year, unless no preoperative colonoscopy due to obstructing lesion, then colonoscopy in 3 to 6 months
  - If advanced adenoma found, repeat in 1 year
  - If no advanced adenoma found, repeat in 3 years, then every 5 years

*For rectal cancer, consider proctoscopy every 6 months for 3 to 5 years for patient post LAR or transanal excision.
CEA, Carcinoembryonic antigen; *CT,* computed tomographic scan.

although data on the effect close surveillance actually has on overall survival are relatively lacking.

Most professional society guidelines mirror those recommended by the NCCN (Box 1), and reflect the reality that recurrence is most common in the first 18 to 24 months after completion of adjuvant therapy: for patients with stage II and III colon cancer and stages I through III rectal cancer, history and physical examination, along with serum CEA if the patient is a candidate for further intervention, every 3 to 6 months for 2 years, then every 6 months for years 3 to 5; colonoscopy within 1 year of resection, unless not completed preoperatively, in which case it should occur within 3 to 6 months, and subsequent colonoscopies dependent on findings at most recent procedure; and chest, abdomen, and pelvis CT annually for 5 years after resection in patients deemed to be at high risk for recurrence (although in practice, the majority of patients undergo this testing). PET-CT is not incorporated into routine surveillance guidelines.

Proctoscopy every 6 months for 3 to 5 years can also be considered for patients with rectal cancer post low anterior resection or transanal excision. The NCCN surveillance recommendations for patients with stage I colon cancer are simply colonoscopy at 1 year after resection and subsequent colonoscopies dependent upon findings.*

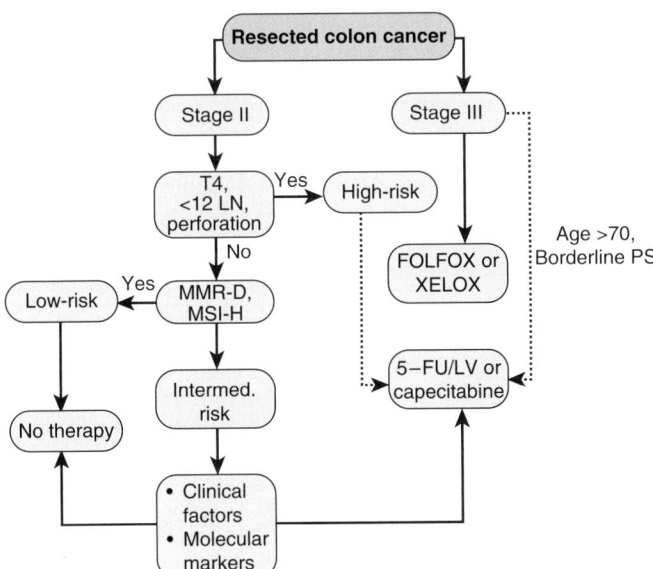

FIGURE 1 Algorithm for use of adjuvant treatment for colorectal cancer. *FOLFOX,* folinic acid, 5-fluorouracil, oxaliplatin; *5-FU/LV,* 5-fluorouracil and leucovorin; *LNs,* lymph nodes; *MMR-D,* defective mismatch repair; *MSI-H,* microsatellite instability; *PS,* performance status; *XELOX,* capecitabine and oxaliplatin.

Recommendations

The magnitude of benefit from adjuvant therapy in these diseases is correlated with the risk of relapse on the basis of pathologic stage, and basic recommendations are outlined algorithmically in Figure 1.

Rectal Cancer. Preoperative chemoradiotherapy is the appropriate treatment; adjuvant chemoradiotherapy is also an option if surgical intervention is urgent, but it is associated with an inferior compliance rate and somewhat increased short- and long-term toxic effects.

Stage III Colon Cancer. Adjuvant chemotherapy for 6 months is the appropriate treatment; FOLFOX and XELOX are considered standards of care in patients fit enough to complete a planned 6-month course.

Stage II Colon Cancer. Adjuvant chemotherapy for 6 months should be discussed as a treatment option and may be recommended for patients with high-risk features. FOLFOX and XELOX are, again, the standard choices in such patients. For patients without these defined high-risk features, other clinical and basic molecular assessments will inform the risk-benefit discussion of adjuvant therapy.

SUGGESTED READINGS

Alberts SR, Sargent DJ, Nair S, et al: Effect of oxaliplatin, fluorouracil, and leucovorin with or without cetuximab on survival among patients with resected stage III colon cancer: a randomized trial, *JAMA* 307(13):1383–1393, 2012.

André T, Boni C, Navarro M, et al: Improved overall survival with oxaliplatin, fluorouracil, and leucovorin as adjuvant treatment in stage II or III colon cancer in the MOSAIC trial, *J Clin Oncol* 27(19):3109–3116, 2009.

Benson AB 3rd, Schrag D, Somerfield MR, et al: American Society of Clinical Oncology recommendations on adjuvant chemotherapy for stage II colon cancer, *J Clin Oncol* 22(16):3408–3419, 2004.

Birgisson H, Påhlman L, Gunnarsson U, et al: Adverse effects of preoperative radiation therapy for rectal cancer: long-term follow-up of the Swedish Rectal Cancer Trial, *J Clin Oncol* 23(34):8697–8705, 2005.

Kapiteijn E, Marijnen CA, Nagtegaal ID, et al: Preoperative radiotherapy combined with total mesorectal excision for resectable rectal cancer, *N Engl J Med* 345(9):638–646, 2001.

Kuebler JP, Wieand HS, O'Connell MJ, et al: Oxaliplatin combined with weekly bolus fluorouracil and leucovorin as surgical adjuvant chemotherapy for stage II and III colon cancer: results from NSABP C-07, *J Clin Oncol* 25(16):2198–2204, 2007.

O'Connor ES, Greenblatt DY, LoConte NK, et al: Adjuvant chemotherapy for stage II colon cancer with poor prognostic features, *J Clin Oncol* 29(25):3381–3388, 2011.

QUASAR Collaborative Group, Gray R, Barnwell J, et al: Adjuvant chemotherapy versus observation in patients with colorectal cancer: a randomised study, *Lancet* 370(9604):2020–2029, 2007.

Referenced with permission from the NCCN Clinical Practice Guidelines in Oncology (NCCN Guidelines®) for Colon Cancer V.1.2014. © National Comprehensive Cancer Network, Inc 2013. All rights reserved. Accessed [April 12, 2010]. To view the most recent and complete version of the guideline, go online to www.nccn.org. NATIONAL COMPREHENSIVE CANCER NETWORK, NCCN, NCCN GUIDELINES, and all other NCCN Content are trademarks owned by the National Comprehensive Cancer Network, Inc.

Referenced with permission from the NCCN Clinical Practice Guidelines in Oncology (NCCN Guidelines®) for Rectal Cancer V.1.2014. © National Comprehensive Cancer Network, Inc 2013. All rights reserved. Accessed [April 12, 2010]. To view the most recent and complete version of the guideline, go online to www.nccn.org. NATIONAL COMPREHENSIVE CANCER NETWORK, NCCN, NCCN GUIDELINES, and all other NCCN Content are trademarks owned by the National Comprehensive Cancer Network, Inc.

Sauer R, Becker H, Hohenberger W, et al: Preoperative versus postoperative chemoradiotherapy for rectal cancer, *N Engl J Med* 351(17):1731–1740, 2004.

THE MANAGEMENT OF COLORECTAL POLYPS

Rebecca R. Cannom, MD, MS, and
Genevieve B. Melton, MD, MA

OVERVIEW

A colorectal polyp is a macroscopically visible lesion or mass that results from pathologic epithelial elevation of the colonic mucosa. A number of other lesions can present as luminal masses, such as lipomas, carcinoid tumors, and leiomyomas. These lesions are covered by normal mucosa and, by definition, are not polyps. Most colonic polyps are asymptomatic; however, these are of clinical concern because of their malignant potential.

The term *polyp* is nonspecific, and the importance of any one colorectal polyp is based on its histopathology, which determines the patient's risk of malignancy and, therefore, further treatment and follow-up. On the basis of clinical information or, in a few cases, genetic testing, colorectal polyps can be classified as either sporadic or hereditary, with the latter comprising a variety of familial syndromes that are potentially malignant conditions. Larger polyps may necessitate prompt treatment for hemorrhage, obstruction, or intussusception. Flexible endoscopy is a safe and highly effective treatment modality for colorectal polyps that in most cases allows for complete excision or histologic evaluation of the polyp.

HISTOPATHOLOGY AND NATURAL HISTORY OF POLYPS

Hyperplastic Polyps and Serrated Adenomas

Hyperplastic polyps are considered nonneoplastic polyps. They contain an increased number of glandular cells in contrast to adenomas, which have decreased numbers of goblet cells. Hyperplastic polyps occur as a result of normal epithelial cells accumulating on the mucosal surface and typically appear pale and sessile. These are the most frequently identified polyp on flexible sigmoidoscopy, with the rectum the most common location. Conflicting data are found as to whether hyperplastic polyps identified on screening endoscopy confer an increased risk of future colorectal neoplasia; however, if a risk exists, it appears to be very small.

Factors associated with hyperplastic polyps and an increased risk of malignant disease are: large size (>1 cm diameter), right colon hyperplastic lesions, mixed adenoma/hyperplastic histology, more than 20 hyperplastic colonic polyps, familial hyperplastic polyposis, and a family history of colorectal cancer. Serrated adenomas, in contrast, were previously classified as hyperplastic; they are now known to have the phenotype of a sporadic adenoma and are associated with an increased risk of colon cancer. Serrated adenomas are less common (0.5% to 4% of colorectal polyps) in comparison with hyperplastic polyps, frequently have a similar endoscopic appearance as hyperplastic polyps, and can be difficult to distinguish from normal mucosa. Serrated adenomas tend to be larger, have a right-sided location and increased incidence in females, and may have a separate oncogenic pathway, which includes *BRAF* genetic mutations and DNA methylation.

Hamartomas

A hamartoma is an outgrowth composed of normal mature cells that originate from below the mucosa. When sporadic, hamartomas are frequently called juvenile polyps because they are relatively common in children. This second histologic category of colorectal polyps is most commonly associated with one of three autosomal-dominant familial syndromes: Peutz-Jeghers syndrome, juvenile polyposis, and Cowden's syndrome. Although sporadic hamartomatous polyps are not considered premalignant, the aforementioned familial syndromes have a significant rate of cancer development, and therefore, patients with these syndromes should undergo regular colonoscopic surveillance.

The typical phenotype of patients with Peutz-Jeghers syndrome includes perioral hyperpigmentation and multiple hamartomatous polyps located in the small or large bowel. These polyps may cause intussusception, bleeding, or obstruction at a young age. After the third decade, patients with Peutz-Jeghers have a 2% to 13% risk of gastrointestinal (GI) cancer and therefore should undergo regular endoscopic surveillance.

Juvenile polyposis is diagnosed when a young patient has 10 or more hamartomatous GI polyps. Lesions may occur anywhere within the GI tract, although they are frequently in the colon. These polyps may twist and auto amputate, causing bleeding. Colon cancer affects up to 50% of those afflicted with juvenile polyposis and may occur in the fourth decade of life.

Cowden's disease, also known as multiple hamartoma syndrome, is characterized by hamartomatous neoplasms of the skin and mucosa, GI tract, bones, central nervous system, eyes, and genitourinary tract. A significant risk exists for skin, thyroid, endometrial, and breast cancer in Cowden's syndrome. Emerging evidence suggests an increased incidence of colorectal cancer as well.

Adenomas

Adenomas are the most common neoplastic polyp identified in patients undergoing colonoscopy, representing 50% to 65% of all colonic polyps. Approximately 10% to 25% of asymptomatic patients at average risk and older than 50 years have an adenomatous polyp. Histology of these adenomas is most commonly tubular (65% to 85%), but they may also be tubulovillous (10% to 25%) or villous (10%). Adenomas differ from hyperplastic polyps in that adenomas have cellular atypia. Therefore, identification of an adenoma on flexible sigmoidoscopy is an indication for a complete colonoscopy. Advanced adenomas are those that are greater than 1 cm or have villous architecture, severe dysplasia, or carcinoma. The prevalence rate of advanced adenomas ranges from 3.5% to 9.5%, depending on gender and age.

The molecular alterations that lead to the development of colorectal polyps, and colorectal cancer, known as the adenoma-carcinoma sequence, are increasingly understood. This relationship is supported by the following data: 1, almost all colon cancers arise within an adenoma; 2, the incidence rate of synchronous adenoma in colon cancer resection specimens is approximately 30%; 3, the risk of colon cancer increases with larger and increasing numbers of adenomatous polyps; 4, the incidence of colorectal cancer in patients with familial adenomatous polyposis is high; and 5, the risk of cancer in unresected polyps is 4% after 5 years and 14% after 10 years.

Most sporadic colorectal cancers (approximately 80%) develop from adenomas. The adenoma-carcinoma sequence, also known as the loss of heterozygosity or chromosomal instability pathway, is a cascade of sequentially accumulated genetic mutations. Our understanding of the genetic alterations leading to colon cancer represents one of the most advanced of all solid malignancies. One of the first mutations leading to sporadic adenomatous polyps is loss of the tumor suppressor adenomatous polyposis coli (APC) gene, the same mutation as in familial adenomatous polyposis (FAP). The next gene thought to be affected in the adenoma-carcinoma sequence is the oncogene *kras*, followed by the loss of deleted in colon cancer (DCC), which likely plays a key role in transitioning to an advanced adenoma. A mutation in the *p53* gene, which regulates the cell cycle that allows for time for either DNA repair or apoptosis, is the final step in development of cancer from an adenoma (Figure 1).

Sessile villous adenomas are frequently found in the rectum and may not be amenable to endoscopic polypectomy because of their size. For lesions in the distal rectum, transanal excision is generally preferred. For adenomas located too proximal for transanal excision, transanal endoscopic microsurgery (TEM) and now transanal minimally invasive surgery (TAMIS) are excellent means for local excision. An anterior resection is indicated in a patient with reasonable surgical risk with a rectal lesion that is not amenable to the aforementioned techniques or with a lesion that has concerning features for invasive malignancy, particularly palpable firmness.

Identification of an adenoma should prompt a complete colonoscopy as a result of the 20% to 40% risk of proximal neoplastic lesions. Recommendations for follow-up colonoscopy are made based on the number, size, and histopathology of the adenomas and other clinical factors such as personal risk factors and family history. Removal of adenomas reduces future colorectal cancer and the development of advanced adenomas.

COLONOSCOPIC POLYPECTOMY

Polypectomy has proven to be an effective means of colon cancer prevention, allowing for identification, removal, and histopathologic evaluation of the polyp. Most colorectal polyps are treated with endoscopic polypectomy, either with biopsy forceps or snare polypectomy, both of which can be either hot with electrocautery or cold. Snare excision typically provides a larger specimen, and the stalk (or base) can be evaluated histopathologically to better define the level of superficial malignancy if present. Large lesions may be removed with a piecemeal excisional technique, which allows for sequential excision of the entire lesion. A submucosal lift with the injection of saline solution (with or without epinephrine or methylene blue) into the submucosa can be helpful to remove larger lesions. This

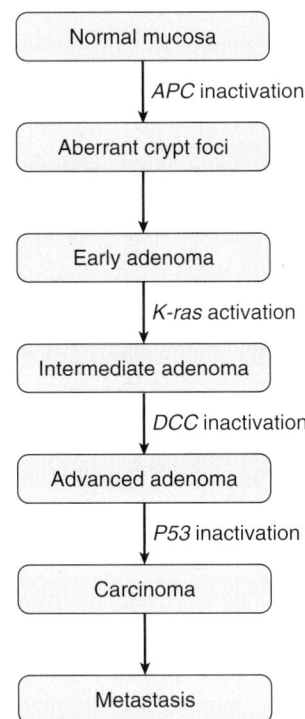

FIGURE 1 Adenoma to carcinoma sequence.

TABLE 1: Current guidelines for colorectal cancer screening after polypectomy

Risk category	Recommended colonoscopy interval
1-2 Small tubular adenomas	5-10 years
3-10 Small adenomas or 1 Adenoma >1 cm or A polyp with villous or High-grade dysplasia	3 years
>10 Adenomas	<3 years
Sessile adenomas removed piecemeal	3-6 months

technique improves the safety of polypectomy by increasing the distance between the mucosa and the muscularis propria. It is critical to tattoo the area with India ink when large or suspicious polyps are removed because typically further endoscopic evaluation or resection is indicated.

Relative contraindications to colonoscopic polypectomy include anticoagulation therapy, bleeding diathesis, acute colitis, and evidence of invasive malignancy, such as central ulceration, a hard or fixed lesion, necrosis, or inability to raise the lesion with submucosal injection.

Complications related to colonoscopic polypectomy are uncommon and typically minor. The risk of death is 1 in 14,000. The most common serious complications are bleeding and perforation. Bleeding occurs in 4.8 in 1000 patients after colonoscopic polypectomy and may occur immediately or days later when clot dissolution occurs. Most postpolypectomy bleeds stop spontaneously and, when persistent, can usually be controlled with endoscopic clipping or cauterization. Rarely, interventional angiography or colectomy is necessary. Bleeding risk should be minimized by stopping warfarin and aspirin 5 days before polypectomy and clopidogrel 7 days before and possibly holding these agents for several days after polypectomy, although stopping any of these agents must be tailored to the patient's risk profile (e.g., patient with a mechanical mitral valve with a high risk of stroke off anticoagulation therapy).

Colonic perforation after polypectomy occurs in 0.1% of patients, most of whom undergo successful treatment with conservative treatment that includes inpatient observation, bowel rest, and intravenous antibiotics. These patients need to be followed closely as inpatients for any sign of clinical deterioration warranting laparotomy. One alternative approach is early laparoscopic primary repair of the defect, with colonoscopic assistance if the perforation is not easily identified on laparoscopy. The patient should be in lithotomy position, and if colonoscopy is necessary, minimal insufflation with carbon dioxide should be used. Contraindications to this approach include peritonitis, malignancy, and presence of significant fecal soilage.

Postpolypectomy syndrome has been reported to occur in up to 0.3% of patients after polypectomy, most often when cauterization

has been used. The etiology is believed to be that the cautery causes a microperforation in the colonic wall and results in bacterial translocation. Patients typically present anywhere from 0 to 3 days after the polypectomy with abdominal pain and tenderness, fever, and leukocytosis. On computerized tomographic scan, fat stranding is typically seen in the mesentery and the colonic wall of the polypectomy site is thickened; however, unlike with colonic perforation, pneumoperitoneum is not present. Patients should be treated with bowel rest, intravenous antibiotics, and close observation until symptoms resolve. Recognition of postpolypectomy syndrome is important to avoid unnecessary laparotomy in these patients who may present with localized peritonitis.

Recommendations for surveillance after polypectomy are based on the risk of recurrent neoplasia after the index polypectomy. In 2008, the American Cancer Society, in collaboration with the U.S. Multisociety Task Force on Colorectal Cancer and the American College of Radiology, updated their guidelines for screening and surveillance for colorectal cancer and polyps (Table 1).

Increased risk of neoplasia is defined as: (1) three or more adenomas removed; (2) high-grade dysplasia present in polyp; (3) villous features in polyp; (4) adenoma of 1 cm or more; or (5) large adenoma removed piecemeal. These patients should have a repeat colonoscopy at 3 years. Lower risk is defined by one or two (<1 cm) tubular adenomas without high-grade dysplasia. These patients may safely defer colonoscopy to 5 to 10 years (if no family history). The presence of hyperplastic polyps does not change the recommendation of 10-year follow-up for those patients with average risk (Figure 2).

Colonoscopy is the best method for detection and removal of most polyps, but the miss rate of polyps greater than 1 cm may be as high as 14%. However, the miss rate of cancer is considered less than 5%. Evidence shows that slower withdrawal of the colonoscope to at least 6 minutes improves neoplasia detection rates. Because of the aforementioned miss rate, if patients have development of symptoms such as bleeding, abdominal pain, or change in bowel habits, repeat colonoscopy is typically warranted.

APPROACH TO THE MALIGNANT POLYP

Up to 5% of polyps that appear benign contain invasive cancer. This risk of cancer correlates with increasing polyp size such that polyps greater than 2 cm have an approximately 30% risk of cancer. For this reason, the colon should be tattooed at the site of any large polyp or any suspicious polyp in the event that further treatment and evaluation are necessary.

A malignant polyp is defined as adenocarcinoma that invades into, but no deeper than, the submucosal layer of the bowel wall,

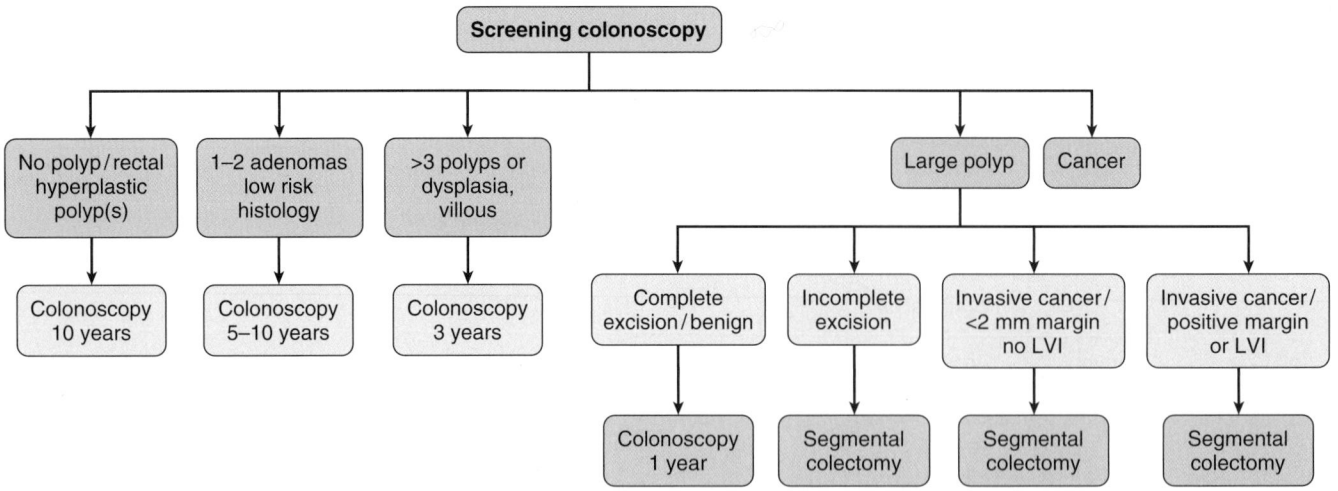

FIGURE 2 Algorithm for outcomes with screening colonoscopy. *LVI*, Lymphovascular invasion.

BOX 1: Summary of malignant colorectal polyps that should have an oncologic bowel resection

A. Lesions in Colon
  a. Pedunculated Haggitt level 4 with invasion into distal third of submucosa, or pedunculated lesions with lymphovascular invasion
  b. Lesions removed with margin <2 mm
  c. Sessile lesions removed piecemeal
  d. Sessile lesions with depth of invasion into distal third of submucosa (Sm3)
  e. Sessile lesions with lymphovascular invasion

B. Lesions in Middle Third and Upper Third Rectum
  Same as lesions in colon

C. Lesions in Distal Third Rectum
  a. Pedunculated Haggitt level 4 with invasion into distal third of submucosa, or pedunculated lesions with lymphovascular invasion
  b. All sessile lesions

An alternative may be a per anal full-thickness excision plus chemoradiation.
Reprinted with permission from Elsevier from Nivatvongs S: Surgical management of early colorectal cancer, Surg Clin North Am 82:950–966, 2000.

TABLE 2: Pathologic features of malignant polyps

Haggitt level	Submucosal invasion in polyp head (1), neck (2), stalk (3), and base (4) or submucosal invasion in a sessile polyp (4)
Submucosal invasion	Invasion in upper third of submucosa (Sm1), middle third (Sm2), or deep third (Sm3)
Tumor grade	Well, moderately, or poorly differentiated
Tumor budding	Absence or presence of clusters of malignant cells in the submucosa remote from the main site of submucosal invasion

Listed in order of escalating risk of lymph node metastasis.

making the lesion a T1 colon cancer. This is different than a polyp containing carcinoma in situ or high-grade dysplasia, in which changes are confined to the mucosa and lamina propria. These entities have no metastatic potential and are cured with complete polypectomy.

The main reason to proceed with formal segmental resection when a malignant polyp has been removed with negative margins is to harvest the associated mesenteric lymph nodes. The risk of lymph node metastasis in malignant polyps ranges from 8% to 15%. In some patients, this risk may approach the mortality rate associated with undergoing a formal resection.

Traditionally, the Haggitt level was used to classify malignant polyps and to predict lymph node metastasis (Box 1); however, the risk of lymph node metastasis in Haggitt level 4 lesions varies based on the depth of submucosal invasion. Because of this, the submucosal invasion classification is being increasingly used. The depth of submucosal invasion is stratified into three levels: Sm1 (upper third of submucosa), Sm 2 (middle third), and Sm3 (lower third). Haggitt levels 1 to 3 correspond with Sm1, but Haggitt level 4 can be Sm1, Sm2, or Sm3. A malignant polyp with a Sm3 classification is an

indication for formal resection. Other factors predictive of lymph node metastases or recurrence are high tumor grade, extensive tumor budding, and lymphovascular invasion (Table 2). In the absence of any of these features, the risk of adverse outcome is less than 1%; however, if a malignant polyp has one of these features, that risk increases to 20%. If two or more of these adverse features are present, the risk of adverse outcomes rises to 36%. Further evaluation of these features may better define patients who can be spared major surgery.

Criteria for close surveillance after endoscopic removal of a malignant polyp include: complete excision, a microscopic margin of greater than 2 mm, no lymphatic or vascular invasion, moderate to well differentiation, Haggitt level 1 to 3, or Sm level 1 to 2.

All other malignant polyps that do not meet the aforementioned criteria should be considered for surgical resection. However, even with some high-risk features, patients with serious medical comorbidities may be best managed with close surveillance and nonsurgical treatment. An alternative to patients at high risk with a malignant rectal polyp may be per anal full-thickness excision (either with transanal excision or TEM) with adjuvant chemoradiation.

SUGGESTED READINGS

Brooks D, Winawer D, Rex D, et al: Colonoscopy surveillance after polypectomy and colorectal cancer resection: consensus guidelines from the U.S.

Multi-Society Task Force on Colorectal Cancer and The American Cancer Society, *Am Fam Physician* 77(7):995–1002, 1003–104, 2008.

Huh KC, Rex DK: Advances in colonoscope technique and technology, *Rev Gastroenterol Disord* 8(4):223–232, 2008.

Nivatongs S: Surgical management of malignant colorectal polyps, *Surg Clin North Am* 82:959–966, 2002.

Noffsinger A, Hart J: Serrated adenoma: a distinct form of non-polypoid colorectal neoplasia? *Gastrointest Endosc Clin N Am* 20(3):543–563, 2008.

Soetikno RM, Kaltenbach T, Rouse RV, et al: Prevalence of nonpolypoid (flat and depressed) colorectal neoplasms in asymptomatic and symptomatic adults, *JAMA* 299(9):1027–1045, 2008.

MANAGEMENT OF PERITONEAL SURFACE MALIGNANCY

Marcello Deraco, MD, Dominique Elias, MD, PhD, C. William Helm MB.BChir, Olivier Glehen, MD, PhD, and Paul H. Sugarbaker, MD, FACS, FRCS

INTRODUCTION

Peritoneal metastases and peritoneal mesothelioma are included in a group of diseases collectively referred to as peritoneal surface malignancy. Over the past three decades, there has emerged an increasing optimism concerning improved management of cancer dissemination within the abdomen and pelvis. The results of treatment with systemic chemotherapy are poor, with an expected median survival time between 1 and 2 years. With a combination of cytoreductive surgery (CRS) and hyperthermic perioperative chemotherapy (HIPEC), long-term survival has been achieved in selected patients and the median survival of most diseases with peritoneal metastases (PM) has been doubled as a result of this multimodality treatment. In this chapter, five different diseases that frequently result in PM are discussed. The prognostic indicators useful in the selection of patients for treatment, the nature of these surgical interventions, and the results of treatment are presented.

PSEUDOMYXOMA PERITONEI AND PERITONEAL METASTASES FROM APPENDICEAL MALIGNANCY

The appendiceal malignant diseases constitute a wide spectrum of biologic aggressiveness. The tumors arising within this structure can be minimally aggressive or have invasive and metastatic capability. If a low-grade appendiceal malignancy is removed within an intact mucocele, recurrence does not occur. If rupture of the wall of the appendix occurs with either low-grade or high-grade disease, the tumor cells within are likely to disseminate to peritoneal surfaces. Sometimes, determination of whether intraperitoneal spread of mucus and neoplastic cells has occurred may be difficult or impossible. If the diagnosis of peritoneal dissemination of a high-grade or low-grade appendiceal malignancy disease has been established, a new treatment with curative intent is indicated in both groups of patients. Cytoreductive surgery is combined with HIPEC as a comprehensive management plan. In more than 1000 patients treated at the Washington Cancer Institute, the survival by quantitative prognostic indicators has been determined.

Management of Appendiceal Neoplasms With Peritoneal Dissemination

Current standard of care for patients with appendiceal mucinous neoplasms requires a comprehensive management plan. For patients with disseminated peritoneal adenomucinosis (DPAM), the first intervention is CRS and HIPEC. For patients with peritoneal mucinous carcinoma (PMCA), the first intervention is a short course of systemic chemotherapy with 5-fluorouracil and oxaliplatin. Cytoreductive surgery is a combination of visceral resections and peritonectomy procedures. After all visible evidence of abdominal and pelvic tumor has been surgically removed, an attempt to eradicate microscopic disease and small tumor nodules occurs with HIPEC. The CRS involves a series of visceral resections and peritonectomy procedures. The various combinations of surgical procedures are listed in Table 1. It should be emphasized that no organ or peritoneal surface is resected unless visible tumor is present. Oftentimes, with DPAM, the mucinous tumor is noninvasive and can be gauze débrided away from the involved visceral or parietal peritoneum; in this situation, the organ or peritoneal surface is not resected. These procedures have been diagrammed and described in several prior publications.

After CRS, several different local-regional chemotherapy regimens may be used to eradicate residual tumor nodules and free tumor cells within the peritoneal cavity. Over the past 23 years, an evolution of perioperative chemotherapy treatments has occurred at the Washington Cancer Institute. The regimen currently in use is hyperthermic intraperitoneal doxorubicin (15 mg/m^2) and mitomycin C (15 mg/m^2) plus systemic 5-fluorouracil (400 mg/m^2). As shown in Figure 1, *A*, an open method for chemotherapy administration that allows for manual distribution of the heat and chemotherapy solution is often used. In some clinical settings, a closed method may also be effective (Figure 1, *B*).

Outcome With Histopathology as a Quantitative Prognostic Indicator

The survival of patients with mucinous appendiceal neoplasm, when treated in a uniform fashion with CRS and HIPEC, is profoundly affected by the tumor's histologic type. With DPAM, noninvasive peritoneal surface tumor may become widely disseminate on peritoneal surfaces. In contrast, PMCA shows the same propensity for widespread intraperitoneal dissemination that is facilitated by large quantities of mucus, but this histopathology shows invasion into surrounding structures. Also, an intermediate (often called hybrid) type of disease exists in which 95% or more of the fields of view show DPAM but areas of PMCA exist. In the histologic assessment of prognosis presented in Figure 2, the intermediate type is included with the PMCA group. The figure includes all patients with a complete and an incomplete cytoreduction that are in the database.

Outcome With Peritoneal Cancer Index as a Quantitative Prognostic Indicator

The peritoneal cancer index (PCI) is a quantitative prognostic indicator that is determined at the time of surgical exploration of the abdomen and pelvis. The PCI is determined according to a diagram to be between 0 and 39 (Figure 3).

Appendiceal neoplasms that show the DPAM histology have an excellent prognosis, with 90% survival rate at 20 years follow-up if the PCI is less than 20. With DPAM histology with PCI greater than 20, the survival rate is 60% at 20 years. When the appendiceal neoplasm shows PMCA histology, the PCI continues to show a statistically significant effect on the survival rate $(P = 0.0004)$.

TABLE I. Visceral resections and peritonectomy procedures that may be required for complete cytoreduction

Cytoreductive surgery	
Visceral Resections	*Peritonectomy Procedures*
Resection of prior abdominal incisions	Anterior parietal peritonectomy
Greater omentectomy ± splenectomy	Left upper quadrant peritonectomy
Rectosigmoid colon resection	Pelvic peritonectomy
Hysterectomy and oophorectomy	Right upper quadrant peritonectomy
Cholecystectomy	Lesser omentectomy with stripping of the omental bursa

Outcome With Completeness of Cytoreduction as a Prognostic Indicator

The completeness of cytoreduction score (CC score) functions as a major quantitative prognostic indicator for patients with mucinous appendiceal neoplasms. The assessment is performed after the cytoreductive surgery is complete. For mucinous appendiceal neoplasms, a complete cytoreduction is defined as CC 0 or CC 1 with residual tumor nodules less than 2.5 mm. The survival of patients with appendiceal neoplasms by CC score has a profound effect on 10-year survival rates for both DPAM (complete vs incomplete, 75% vs 25%) and PMCA (complete vs incomplete, 27% vs 6%).

PERITONEAL METASTASES OF COLORECTAL ORIGIN

Outcome of Peritoneal Metastases Treated With Modern Systemic Chemotherapy

In patients with primary colorectal cancer (CRC), 5% to 10% present with synchronous peritoneal metastases (PM). Unfortunately, in 75% of these patients, PM are not diagnosed before the CRC resection. This fact shows the unsatisfactory preoperative radiologic detection of PM. With treatment with systemic chemotherapy, data from different registries show that the median survival time of these patients is currently only 8 months. The survival time is estimated at 4 months in the absence of surgery but at 14 months if the primary CRC is resectable.

In data from randomized trials in patients with many different anatomic sites of CRC metastases, the presence of PM is a poor prognostic factor. With folinic acid, 5-fluorouracil, and oxaliplatin (FOLFOX) or folinic acid, 5-fluorouracil, and irinotecan (FOLFIRI), median survival time was 12.7 months for patients with PM, whereas it was 17.6 months for patients without PM. All patients received the same mean number of treatment cycles in the two groups, indicating a relative resistance to treatment in the PM group. Addition of a targeted therapy (bevacizumab) prolonged median survival time by 3 months. In conclusion, systemic chemotherapy is a palliative treatment of PM of short duration, and patients with PM have an especially poor prognosis.

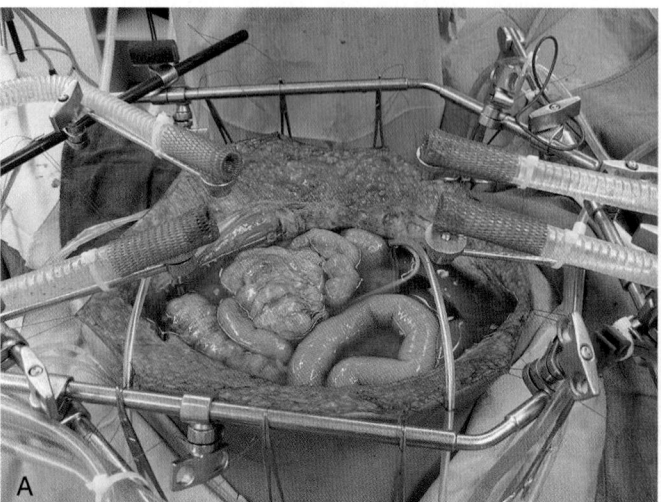 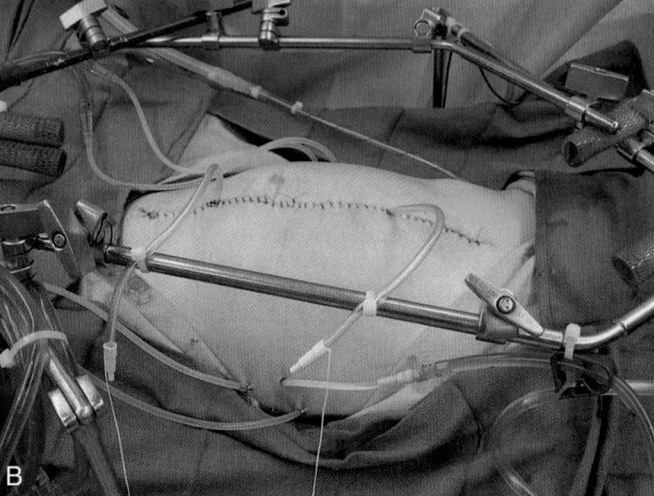

FIGURE I   A, Hyperthermic intraperitoneal chemotherapy administered with an open technique allows continued manipulation of the abdominal and pelvic contents to achieve uniform distribution of heat and chemotherapy. A vapor barrier above the chemotherapy solution is created by four smoke aspirators. **B,** The closed method for hyperthermic perioperative chemotherapy is preferred by some surgeons.

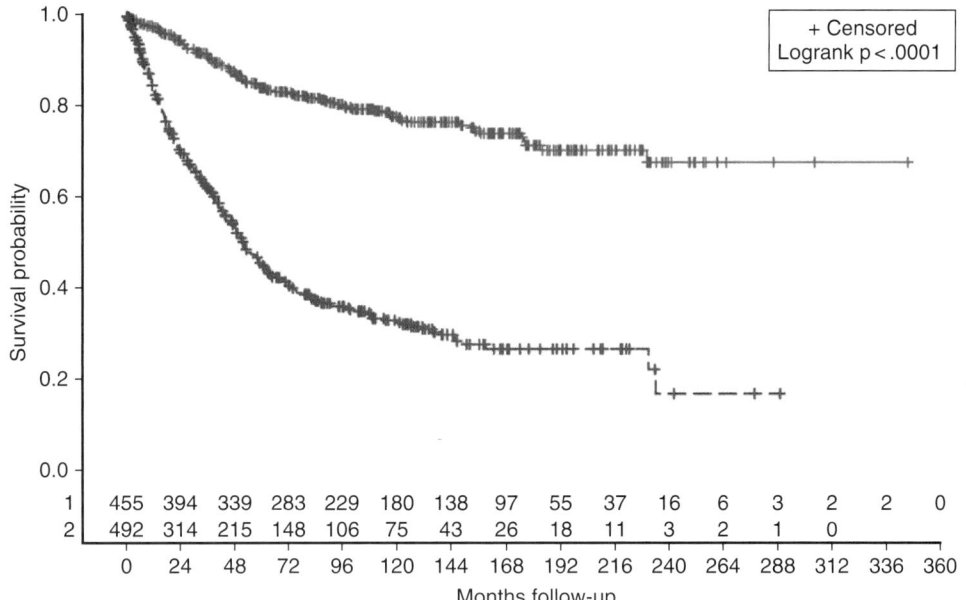

| 1 | 455 | 394 | 339 | 283 | 229 | 180 | 138 | 97 | 55 | 37 | 16 | 6 | 3 | 2 | 2 | 0 |
| 2 | 492 | 314 | 215 | 148 | 106 | 75 | 43 | 26 | 18 | 11 | 3 | 2 | 1 | 0 | | |

FIGURE 2 Peritoneal surface malignancy of appendiceal origin. Survival rate by histopathology of patients treated at Washington Cancer Institute. The graph includes all patients. The *blue line* (N = 455) indicates patients with disseminated peritoneal adenomucinosis (DPAM). The *red line* (N = 492) indicates patients with peritoneal mucinous adenocarcinoma (PMCA) and includes patients with intermediate type histology. *(From Sugarbaker PH: Epithelial appendiceal neoplasms,* Cancer J *15:225–235, 2009.)*

PERITONEAL CANCER INDEX

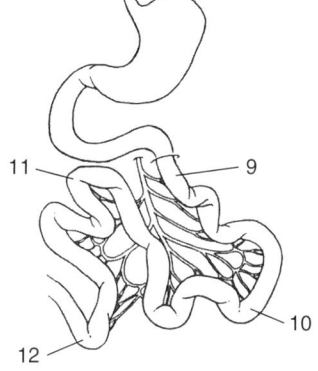

Regions   **Lesion size**

0	Central
1	Right upper
2	Epigastrium
3	Left upper
4	Left flank
5	Left lower
6	Pelvis
7	Right lower
8	Right flank
9	Upper jejunum
10	Lower jejunum
11	Upper ileum
12	Lower ileum

Lesion size score

LS 0   No tumor seen
LS 1   Tumor up to 0.5 cm
LS 2   Tumor up to 5.0 cm
LS 3   Tumor > 5.0 cm
       or confluence

PCI

FIGURE 3 Diagram for determining peritoneal cancer index *(PCI)* at the time of abdominal exploration. The distribution of tumor is recorded in 13 abdominal and pelvic regions, and the extent of disease is estimated in each region.

Complete Cytoreductive Surgery With Hyperthermic Perioperative Chemotherapy for Colorectal Cancer Peritoneal Metastases

This new approach, when complete cytoreductive surgery (CCRS) is possible, allows cure for approximately 25% of patients. The rationale requires resection of PM measuring more than 1 mm and then treatment of the remaining peritoneal disease with HIPEC. HIPEC penetrates into tumor nodules on peritoneal surfaces only 1 to 2 mm in depth; therefore, it can only be used after resection of the macroscopic disease. In animal models, many demonstrations suggest the efficacy of this approach. For example, in rats with PM of colon origin, median survival time was 43 days with CCRS alone, 75 days ($P = 0.003$) with CCRS + HIPEC (mitomycin, 15 mg/m^2), and 97 days with CCRS + HIPEC (mitomycin, 35 mg/m^2).

Concerning HIPEC technology for CRC PM, the two main strategies are: (1) use of intraperitoneal mitomycin C over a long duration (≥60 minutes) at 41°C; and (2) use of intraperitoneal oxaliplatin with a shorter duration (30 minutes) at a higher temperature (43°C) and with the addition of systemic 5-fluorouracil.

Outcome of Treatment for Peritoneal Metastases From Colorectal Cancer

The French Registry published in 2010 a report on the cumulative experience (523 patients) of 23 centers from 1990 to 2007. Of course, these early data showed less than optimal results. Median survival time was 33 months, and 5-year survival rate was 30%, with a postoperative mortality rate of 3% and a grade 3 to 4 morbidity rate of 30% during the first 30 days.

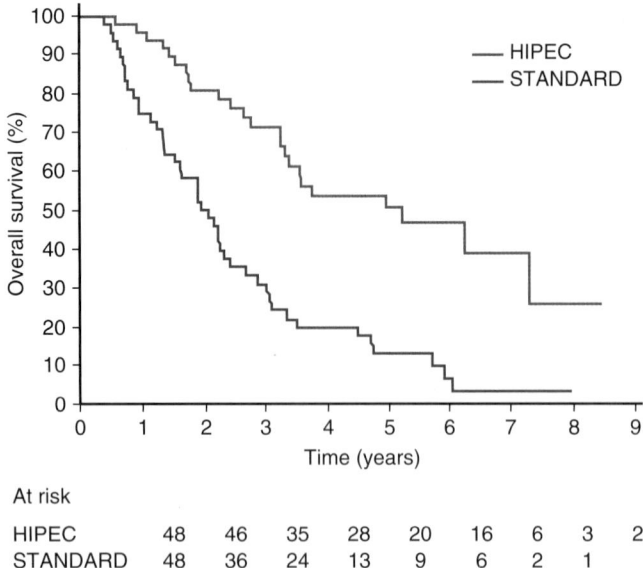

At risk

HIPEC	48	46	35	28	20	16	6	3	2
STANDARD	48	36	24	13	9	6	2	1	

FIGURE 4   Overall survival rates of 48 patients with peritoneal metastases treated with complete cytoreductive surgery plus hyperthermic perioperative chemotherapy *(HIPEC)*, compared with 48 patients with similar peritoneal metastases conventionally treated with systemic chemotherapy. *(From Elias D, Lefevre JH, Chevalier J, et al: Complete cytoreductive surgery plus intraperitoneal chemohyperthermia with oxaliplatin for peritoneal carcinomatosis of colorectal origin,* J Clin Oncol 27:681–685, 2008.)

Two major principles of management were demonstrated: (1) the need for CCRS; and (2) a low extent of disease measured by the PCI. After a CC-2 or CC-3 resection, the results were similar to those obtained with palliative chemotherapy alone. Also, when the PCI was more than 20, the results of treatment were similar to those obtained with palliative chemotherapy alone.

A retrospective study reported by Elias and coworkers compared patients with PM who had two different treatment strategies. All patients underwent a laparotomy that indicated that they had resectable PM. Forty-eight were conventionally treated with systemic chemotherapies, and 48 were treated with CCRS + HIPEC in an experienced center. After a mean follow-up period of 63 months, the 5-year overall survival rates were 13% in the systemic chemotherapy group and 51% in the CCRS + HIPEC group *(P* <0.05; Figure 4). A randomized trial (acronym: Prodige 7) is currently comparing CCRS alone versus CCRS plus HIPEC.

Currently, the indications for CRS plus HIPEC include: (1) patients with a good performance status; (2) patients presenting with minimal or moderate PM (PCI ≤20) and without other sites of metastases (except for a few liver metastases that are easily resectable); and (3) patients whose disease does not show rapid progression during treatment with systemic chemotherapy.

Improving Survival With Treatment of a Minimal Extent of Disease

Because the survival results yielded by CCRS + HIPEC are high for patients with a low PCI (indicating a small extent of disease), it is logical to propose this treatment early in the natural history of PM. Unfortunately, early PM does not produce symptoms, radiologic imaging is unreliable, and there are no reliable biomarkers. The only way to detect early PM is to perform second-look surgery. This strategy is currently proposed for patients at high risk for progression of PM. A review of the literature and a prospective study that the authors conducted on this topic allowed definition of the "high-risk" patients as: (1) patients with perforation at the time of resection of the primary tumor, (2) patients with ovarian metastasis, and (3) patients with minimally resected or residual PM.

Currently, sufficient evidence exists to consider patients for second-look surgery with the following features at the moment of the curative surgery of the primary: ovarian metastases, perforated tumor, and synchronous resected PM. For the three groups of patients at high risk defined previously, PM were documented at second-look surgery performed at 1 year in 60% of patients. The extent of PM was minimal, and CCRS + HIPEC was performed with a low complication rate. Experience suggested that HIPEC was indicated even if no macroscopic PM was detectable. The survival results of the 41 patients at high risk treated with this second-look strategy are promising, with a 5-year survival rate of 90%, a disease-free survival rate of 44%, and only 17% with relapse inside the peritoneum. Currently, an ongoing randomized trial (acronym: Prophylochip) is comparing, after 6 months of standard systemic chemotherapy in these patients at high risk, the traditional strategy (watchful waiting) with the new strategy (second-look surgery plus HIPEC).

DIFFUSE MALIGNANT PERITONEAL MESOTHELIOMA

Diffuse malignant peritoneal mesothelioma (DMPM) is an aggressive malignancy that arises from mesothelial cells within the serosal lining of the peritoneum. It is the most common primary peritoneal tumor. Throughout its natural history, it remains confined to the peritoneal cavity in most patients. It rarely metastasizes systemically; however, in advanced stages, direct extension to the pleural cavity may be noted. Most patients die of complications directly related to intra-abdominal disease progression, usually bowel obstruction. Incidence rates among men range from 0.5 to about 3 cases per million population. Incidence of DMPM has been rising worldwide since 1970, and a 5% to 10% increase in annual mortality rate is estimated worldwide at least until 2020. In contrast to pleural mesothelioma, only 58% and 20%, respectively, of men and women with DMPM have past asbestos exposure.

Patients are usually diagnosed with an advanced disease, and the most common symptoms are ascites and abdominal pain accompanied by weakness, weight loss, anorexia, abdominal mass, fever, diarrhea, and vomiting. Computed tomographic scan shows ascites, diffuse abdominal masses, and peritoneal thickening.

According to the World Health Organization (WHO) classification, peritoneal mesothelioma can be broadly categorized as benign-borderline mesothelioma including multicystic and well-differentiated papillary mesothelioma or DMPM. Within the DMPM category, the most frequent variants are epithelial, sarcomatoid, and biphasic. Differential diagnosis of DMPM is challenging and must be distinguished from benign reactive lesions, metastatic neoplasms, and particularly adenocarcinomas. Immunohistochemical studies represent an important diagnostic aid and depend on the use of panels of markers that may be positive (thrombomodulin [CD141], calretinin, keratin 5/6, D2-40, podoplanin, mesothelin, and Wilms' tumor 1 protein [WT1]).

Recently, a staging system form DMPM has been proposed. The PCI is used to define the T category: T1 (PCI 1-10), T2 (PCI 11-20), T3 (PCI 21-30), and T4 (PCI 31-39). T1 N0 M0 was designated as stage I. T2 and T3, in absence of N1 or M1 disease, were categorized as stage II. T4, N1, and M1 were categorized as stage III. The 5-year survival rates associated with stage I, II, and III diseases were 87%, 53%, and 29%, respectively. Currently, there are efforts to validate this proposal for a staging system through the accumulation of data within a prospective multiinstitutional registry.

Treatment of Diffuse Malignant Peritoneal Mesothelioma

This disease is generally considered nonchemoresponsive. Numerous single-drug and combination regimens have been tested over the past decades with modest results. Cisplatin alone and pemetrexed in association with cisplatin are the most effective regimens, with response rates of 12% to 28%. The multimodality treatment consisting of CRS and HIPEC evolved during the last two decades as the most effective approach for DMPM, with more than 50% long-term survival rates. Currently, the combined treatment of CRS and HIPEC is considered the gold standard for DMPM management.

Cytoreductive Surgery and Hyperthermic Perioperative Chemotherapy

Cytoreductive surgery with peritonectomy procedures and multivisceral resections allows the removal of all the visible tumor implants (macroscopic cytoreduction). Currently, patients with normal-appearing lymph nodes receive retroperitoneal and pelvic lymph node biopsies, whereas regional lymphadenectomy is suggested in patients with lymph node positive disease.

Local-regional drug administration with hyperthermia treats the free tumor cells and very small residual cancer nodules. At the authors' institution, the HIPEC is performed with the closed abdomen technique with cisplatin (45 mg/L of perfusate) and doxorubicin (15 mg/L of perfusate) for 90 minutes at a temperature of 42.5°C. Patients over 70 years of age or with relevant comorbidities and those who had undergone previous systemic chemotherapy or extensive cytoreductive surgery received a 30% dose reduction of both drugs. Perfusate volume is 4 to 6 L, and mean flow is 700 mL/min.

Results of Treatment of Diffuse Malignant Peritoneal Mesothelioma

Because DMPM involves a widespread tumor distribution on nearly all peritoneal surfaces and because most patients are diagnosed with advanced disease, a complete parietal peritonectomy is almost always required. Visceral resections are required when there is tumor encasement. The combined approach consisting of CRS and HIPEC has modified the natural history of DMPM with a dramatic improvement in outcomes. An international multiinstitutional study testing the combined treatment reported a median survival time of 53 months with 5-year overall survival of 47% (Figure 5). The most significant prognostic factors independently associated with improved survival were: epithelial subtype compared with the biphasic or sarcomatoid, the absence of lymph node metastasis, the completeness of cytoreduction scores, and HIPEC versus no HIPEC. Females consistently show a better prognosis.

Treatment of Benign/Borderline Peritoneal Mesothelioma

In the surgical management of benign/borderline peritoneal mesothelioma, a complete parietal peritonectomy is almost always required, whereas only rarely are visceral resections necessary. Fertility-sparing surgery should be considered in young patients. The 5-year overall and progression-free survival rates were 90% and 79%, respectively, at the National Cancer Institute of Milan. In the authors' experience, that has been corroborated at other centers, definitive tumor eradication by means of peritonectomy procedures and HIPEC is recommended as the optimal treatment to prevent disease progression or transition to DMPM.

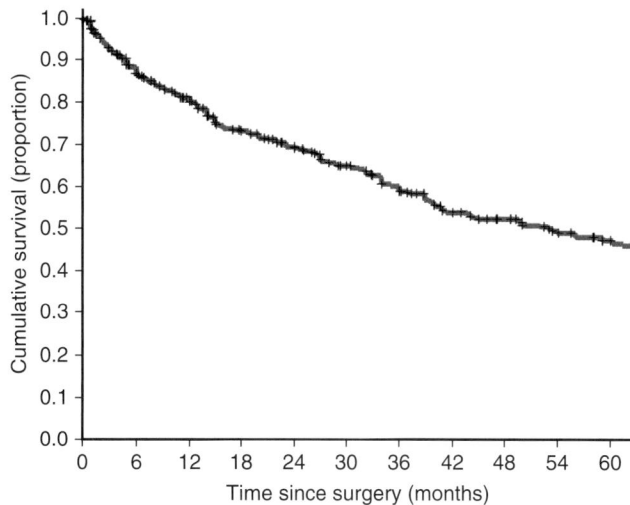

FIGURE 5 Survival with cytoreductive surgery and hyperthermic perioperative chemotherapy in patients with diffuse malignant peritoneal mesothelioma. Survival was determined from 401 patients in a multiinstitutional database. The 1-year, 3-year, and 5-year survival rates were 81%, 60%, and 47%, respectively. *(From Yan TD, Deraco M, Baratti D, et al: Cytoreductive surgery and hyperthermic intraperitoneal chemotherapy for malignant peritoneal mesothelioma: multi-institutional experience,* J Clin Oncol 20(27):6237–6242, 2009.)

PERITONEAL METASTASES FROM EPITHELIAL OVARIAN CANCER

Epithelial ovarian cancer (EOC) includes cancers of three origins: ovary, Fallopian tube, and peritoneum. Most commonly, these cancers show the serous histologic subtype and share similar behavior, treatment, and prognosis. These cancers disseminate to adjacent structures by direct extension and by exfoliation of cancer cells into peritoneal fluid, resulting in PM throughout the abdomen and pelvis. Retroperitoneal lymphatic involvement becomes more common with advanced disease, and hematologic spread may occur later. The prognosis of women with EOC remains poor, with less than 50% surviving 5 years. Survival rates have changed little over the last two decades.

Extent of Disease as a Prognostic Variable

It has been recognized for many years that patients with microscopic or small-volume peritoneal metastasis have better survival than those with large-volume disease. Multiple studies have shown that frontline treatment outcome is better for patients whose disease presents with, or is surgically reduced to, no visible disease or minimal visible disease (<5 mm if possible; <1 cm at worst). In the case of recurrent disease, surgery has traditionally been reserved for a select group of patients with isolated or limited sites of recurrence that occurs after a long interval from primary treatment and is resectable. A recent study from the German Arbeitsgemeinschaft Gynäkologische Onkologie Studiengruppe (AGO) suggests that for recurrent disease, surgical resection to no visible disease must be achieved for significant survival advantage.

Role for Intraperitoneal Chemotherapy

An important consideration for treatment planning for EOC is its confinement within the peritoneal cavity for much of its life history, not only at the time of diagnosis but also at the time of recurrence. Meta-analysis of seven randomized controlled trials in EOC investigating the use of intraperitoneal (IP) chemotherapy after frontline surgery has shown a survival advantage for IP chemotherapy. The Gynecologic Oncology Group 172 study recorded a median survival time of 66 months when IP treatments were used compared with 50 months in those receiving conventional intravenous (IV)–only chemotherapy after optimal surgery to less than 1 cm disease. Because adhesions form quickly after surgery, delay in delivery of the first dose of IP chemotherapy by even a few days after extensive surgery may prevent chemotherapy from reaching the entire peritoneal cavity and all cancer deposits. One way to overcome this deficiency is to use HIPEC at the time of surgery after all adhesions have been divided. HIPEC also treats free-floating cancer cells released by the surgery. In addition, the routine use of HIPEC eliminates the "lag time" after CRS before chemotherapy is usually given.

Series including well over 1000 patients with EOC treated with HIPEC have been reported. There are still no completed randomized controlled trials (RCTs), and the available studies are difficult to analyze and compare because of their heterogeneity, not only in populations treated but also in the variations in HIPEC technology. The HYPERO registry included 83 patients who had recurrent disease; 29% were platinum-resistant, and 85% had widespread peritoneal metastases. The median survival time of 23.5 months of patients treated with surgery and HIPEC was better than the 19.9-month median survival time for those with PM treated with surgery and further systemic chemotherapy in the AGO study. Not surprisingly, the amount of residual disease at the end of surgery before HIPEC is an important prognostic factor reported by many; this was supported in the initial report of the HYPERO registry (Figure 6).

Treatment of EOC, both frontline and at recurrence, requires combination treatment with surgery and chemotherapy. The principle aim of surgery is to prepare the patient for chemotherapy by leaving microscopic or small-volume disease. Because standard postoperative IV and IP chemotherapy has been shown to be less than curative in a large proportion of cases, HIPEC delivered at the time of optimal CRS alone or together with synchronous intraoperative intravenous chemotherapy and early postoperative chemotherapy should be further investigated. The results of several on going RCTs investigating HIPEC for EOC are awaited.

PERITONEAL METASTASES FROM GASTRIC CANCER

Peritoneal dissemination is the most frequent pattern of metastasis and recurrence with gastric cancers and occurs in 5% to 20% of patients being explored for potentially curative resection. Traditionally, there was a mutual agreement in the oncologic community that those patients with gastric peritoneal dissemination were incurable, with a median survival time of less than 1 year.

An Evolution of Curative Treatment Strategies for Gastric Cancer With Peritoneal Metastases

Since the 1980s, the development of CRS with peritonectomy procedures combined with HIPEC has given new hope for potential cure of PM. Recently, a collaborative effort of French institutions collected data from 159 patients and represents the largest experience of the treatment of PM from gastric origin. With a median follow-up period of 20.4 months, the overall median survival time was only 9.2 months, but the 5-year survival rate was 13% with some long-term survivors. These survival results are less encouraging than those obtained for other peritoneal surface malignancies, indicating a more aggressive disease process less responsive to this combined treatment modality and the need for improved patient selection. However, the combination of cytoreductive surgery with HIPEC is the only therapeutic strategy that can result in survivors at 5 years. Moreover, a recent phase III trial showed a significant benefit of HIPEC in addition to cytoreductive surgery for the treatment of gastric PM, especially when PM was synchronous.

Many prognostic factors have been identified for better patient selection for the combined procedure. The carcinomatosis extent assessed by the PCI demonstrated its significant influence on survival (Figure 7). Also, PCI was strongly correlated with the CC score. In the recent French study, a 5-year survival rate of 23% and a median survival time of 15 months were obtained in patients treated with complete macroscopic resection. Peritoneal metastases with localized or small tumor nodules seem to be the best indication for this combined procedure. In patients who had undergone complete cytoreductive surgery, the PCI represented the only strong prognostic factor. When the PCI was more than 12, despite a CCRS, no patient was alive at 3 years. These results suggest that this combined treatment for patients with extensive PM is not indicated even if complete cytoreductive surgery appears to be possible.

Laparoscopy may play an important role in the selection of patients by determining the extent of carcinomatosis. It may exclude patients with extensive small bowel involvement and avoid unnecessary laparotomy.

Another therapeutic method needs to be considered: neoadjuvant intraperitoneal and systemic chemotherapy (NIPS), developed by Yonemura, decreases the PCI and increases CCRS. These preliminary results from Japan are promising.

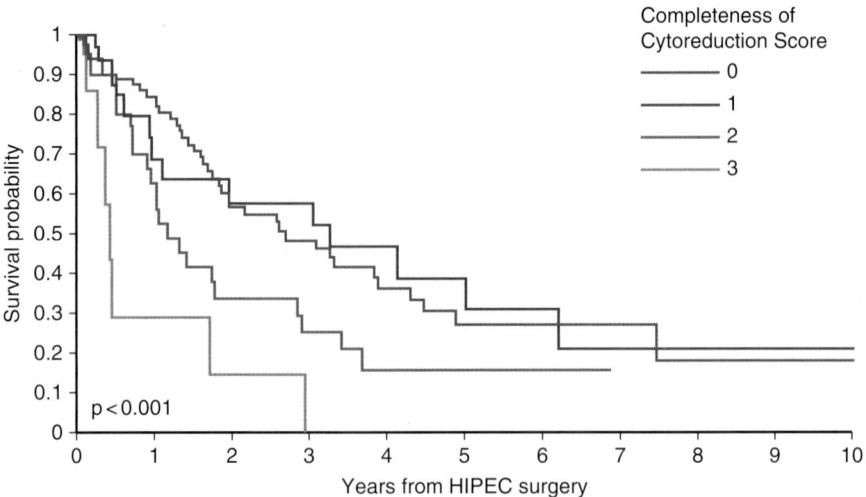

FIGURE 6 Overall survival by completeness of cytoreduction score in patients with peritoneal metastases from epithelial ovarian cancer. *0,* No visible disease; *1,* tumor nodules less than 2.5 mm in largest diameter; *2,* tumor nodules between 2.5 mm and 2.5 cm; *3,* tumor nodules greater than 2.5 cm. N=139 *HIPEC,* Hyperthermic perioperative chemotherapy *(From Helm CW, Richard SD, Pan J, et al: Hyperthermic intraperitoneal chemotherapy in ovarian cancer: first report of the HYPER-O registry,* Int J Gynecol Cancer *20:61–69, 2010.)*

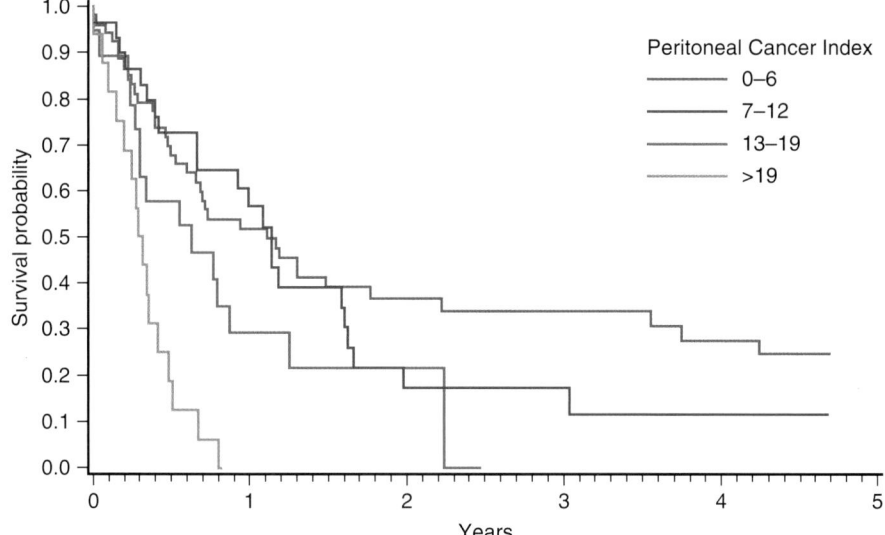

FIGURE 7 Survival of patients with peritoneal metastases from gastric cancer by the peritoneal cancer index. *Blue line,* peritoneal cancer index (PCI) 0-6; *red line,* PCI 7-12; *green line,* PCI 13-19; and *orange line,* PCI >19. *(From Glehen O, Gilly FN, Arvieux C, et al: Peritoneal carcinomatosis from gastric cancer: a multi-institutional study of 159 patients treated by cytoreductive surgery combined with perioperative intraperitoneal chemotherapy, Ann Surg Oncol 17:2370–2377, 2010.)*

Importance of the Surgical Learning Curve

The institution in which the procedure was performed plays an important role in determining the postoperative course and survival. The assumption is reasonable that experience provides better patient selection, improved surgical expertise with a higher rate of complete cytoreductive surgery, and more knowledgeable postoperative management. A learning curve has been reported by several authors and institutions performing the combination of CRS with HIPEC for the management of PM. All interventional complex procedures have an inherent risk that experience undoubtedly diminishes but can never be abolished. Morbidity and mortality reported may reach 60% and 6.5%, respectively.

In conclusion, long-term survival for patients with PM from gastric cancer is a realistic goal in selected patients, and PM should not be considered a terminal event. The principal prognostic factors are PM extent (PCI) and the CC score. The high mortality emphasizes the necessity of strict selection of patients younger than 60 years and with good performance status. Patients who may benefit from CRS and HIPEC are those with PCI less than 12 after response to neoadjuvant systemic chemotherapy or NIPS, with no diffuse small bowel involvement shown on computed tomographic scan and laparoscopy, and with a high probability of complete macroscopic cytoreduction.

Prevention of Gastric Carcinomatosis

For many Korean and Japanese researchers, HIPEC has been performed in an adjuvant setting. In the meta-analysis of Yan and associates, these phase III trials showed the benefit of HIPEC, especially for T3, T4, and lymph node positive gastric tumors as reported. Yonemura and colleagues conducted a randomized controlled study of 139 patients with T3 or T4 gastric tumor allocated to three groups: HIPEC plus surgery, intraperitoneal normothermic chemotherapy plus surgery, and surgery alone. After a follow-up period of more than 5 years, the 5-year survival rate of patients treated with the combination of HIPEC and surgery was significantly higher at 60% than those of the other two groups, with similar morbidity rates. In Western countries, some groups show the benefit of HIPEC as adjuvant treatment for the prevention of PM recurrence in advanced gastric cancer. Prospective randomized studies are needed in Western countries to demonstrate the benefit of HIPEC in advanced stage of gastric cancer to prevent PM development.

Suggested Readings

Elias D, Gilly F, Boutitie F, et al: Peritoneal colorectal carcinomatosis treated with surgery and perioperative intraperitoneal chemotherapy: retrospective analysis of 523 patients from a multicentric French study, *J Clin Oncol* 28:63–68, 2010.

Elias D, Lefevre JH, Chevalier J, et al: Complete cytoreductive surgery plus intraperitoneal chemohyperthermia with oxaliplatin for peritoneal carcinomatosis of colorectal origin, *J Clin Oncol* 27:681–685, 2008.

Glehen O, Gilly FN, Arvieux C, et al: Peritoneal carcinomatosis from gastric cancer: a multi-institutional study of 159 patients treated by cytoreductive surgery combined with perioperative intraperitoneal chemotherapy, *Ann Surg Oncol* 17:2370–2377, 2010.

Helm CW, Richard SD, Pan J, et al: Hyperthermic intraperitoneal chemotherapy in ovarian cancer: first report of the HYPER-O registry, *Int J Gynecol Cancer* 20:61–69, 2010.

Honoré C, Goéré D, Souadka A, et al: Definition of patients presenting a high risk of developing peritoneal carcinomatosis after curative surgery for colorectal cancer: a systematic review, *Ann Surg Oncol* 20(1):183–192, 2013.

Sugarbaker PH: Epithelial appendiceal neoplasms, *Cancer J* 15:225–235, 2009.

Yan TD, Black D, Sugarbaker PH, et al: A systematic review and meta-analysis of the randomized controlled trials on adjuvant intraperitoneal chemotherapy for resectable gastric cancer, *Ann Surg Oncol* 14:2702–2713, 2007.

Yan TD, Deraco M, Baratti D, et al: Cytoreductive surgery and hyperthermic intraperitoneal chemotherapy for malignant peritoneal mesothelioma: multi-institutional experience, *J Clin Oncol* 20(27):6237–6242, 2009.

The Management of Acute Appendicitis

Dylan Stewart, MD

OVERVIEW

Appendicitis is the most common cause of the acute abdomen. With more than 300,000 appendectomies performed in the United States annually, one expects surgeons to have great familiarity with the entity. However, no single abdominal condition presents in more different clinical scenarios than appendicitis, and it remains a source of diagnostic angst even in our modern surgical age. Appendectomy has long been the mainstay of treatment; however even this solid surgical dogma is now challenged by voices reporting successful nonoperative treatment. In addition, in the climate of increasing scrutiny of resource utilization, debates continue regarding the timing of surgery, the laparoscopic versus the open approach, and the duration of antibiotic therapy. Appendicitis continues to have significant morbidity and mortality, and debates aside, accurate diagnosis and timely intervention remain the goals of the evaluating surgeon.

HISTORICAL PERSPECTIVE

Appendicitis likely was as common at the dawn of surgery as it is today. However, its recognition as a clinical entity took a surprisingly long time, considering the relatively consistent pathologic features. One particular culprit may have been the highly influential French anatomist and surgeon Dupuytren, who attributed the disease to the cecum rather than the appendix. This French view of "perityphlitis" persisted despite decades of smaller, less authoritative voices championing a different pathologic explanation.

Hall of New York performed the first appendectomy in the United States in 1886, although his preoperative diagnosis was not appendicitis but an incarcerated hernia. The eventual recognition of appendicitis as the clinical entity was largely a result of the efforts of Harvard pathologist Reginald Fitz, who discarded the term typhlitis and presented 257 cases of appendicitis diagnosed pathologically. In his report, he also accurately predicted that appendectomy performed early in the disease process would likely provide ideal treatment.

ANATOMY AND PATHOPHYSIOLOGY

The appendix is considered a vestigial organ in humans, despite some evolutionary evidence to the contrary. It contains large amounts of lymphoid tissue but is thought to have no significant exocrine function. The appendix may be found in various anatomic positions, including under the ileocecal junction, in the pelvis or at the pelvic brim, and in the retrocecal space. The base is always located at the origin of the three taenia coli of the cecum. These anatomic positional differences make up part of the diagnostic challenge. Luminal obstruction is considered the pathologic hallmark of the process, either with lymphoid hyperplasia in children or with fecal concretions, adhesive bands, or tumors in adults. The obstruction leads to bacterial overgrowth, which causes an inflammatory response and may progress to venous congestion, arterial insufficiency, necrosis, and perforation.

PATIENT PRESENTATION AND DIAGNOSIS

History and Physical Examination

Much has been written about the presentation of acute appendicitis, and although "textbook" cases often are seen in emergency departments, in no way should deviation from the classic symptoms rule out the diagnosis. A feeling of malaise may be the first sign. Onset of pain is typically the first symptom, usually vague visceral pain that is described as epigastric. Nausea and anorexia then follow, and emesis, if it occurs at all, is usually noted after the onset of the pain. Emesis before onset of abdominal pain is considered much more typical of acute viral gastroenteritis. Anorexia is often thought of as a mainstay; however, many children are happily eating in the emergency department with right lower quadrant tenderness. As the inflammatory process progresses, somatic tenderness develops and localizes to the position of the appendix, be it in the right lower quadrant, the pelvis, or the retrocecal space. Either diarrhea or constipation may be reported, although a pelvic appendix is more likely to cause rectal irritation and loose stools. Urinary symptoms may also develop if the pelvic appendiceal inflammation irritates the bladder. Fever may not be present in the early stages (in fact, high fever is atypical) but may develop as the disease progresses to perforation or generalized peritonitis. Experienced clinicians know that the sequence of these symptoms (pain, nausea, followed by localized tenderness) is of paramount importance.

The differential diagnosis of appendicitis is vast and includes gastroenteritis, urinary pathology (infection or calculi), pelvic inflammatory disease, inflammatory bowel disease, diverticulitis, small bowel obstruction, cholecystitis, ovarian pathology including ectopic gestation, inflamed Meckel's diverticulum, and psoas abscess, to name but a few.

Patients in the earliest stages of appendicitis may not have tenderness on physical examination, but this becomes a near certainty as the disease progresses. Tenderness to moderate palpation in the right lower quadrant is the most convincing sign. A number of classical maneuvers to elicit pain in the evaluation of appendicitis are listed in Table 1.

Laboratory Examination

A single test value to confirm or rule out appendicitis does not exist. Typically, blood tests are ordered to search for other abnormalities and to learn of any fluid and electrolyte derangements in a potentially ill patient. The white blood cell count of the patient is normal or slightly elevated—significant elevation suggests perforation, abscess, or advanced disease. The differential may show predominance of neutrophils, even in relatively early cases. Urinalysis is usually obtained, but again results are nonspecific. Notation of pyuria may help to diagnosis pyelonephritis; however, this usually presents with higher fever and higher white blood cell count to begin with, and the pain is usually localized more to the costophrenic angle. Microscopic hematuria is quite common in appendicitis, although gross hematuria is more suggestive of nephrolithiasis. Urinary β-chorionic gonadotropin testing is mandatory in menstruating women and girls.

Imaging

In many patients, acute appendicitis is a clinical diagnosis, and no imaging is necessary. This is especially true for the young male patient, with a reliable and classic history of nausea, anorexia, and point tenderness in the right lower quadrant. No amount of imaging

TABLE 1: Physical examination maneuvers in the diagnosis of acute appendicitis

Test	Method
Iliopsoas test	Extension of right thigh with patient lying on left side elicits pain from retrocecal appendix on psoas muscle
Thigh rotation (obturator) test	Pain with internal rotation of thigh caused by inflammation of obturator internus by pelvic appendix
Rovsing's sign	Deep palpation in left lower quadrant elicits pain in right lower quadrant

should convince the surgeon to not operate on such a patient. Unfortunately, many of these children are irradiated to very minimal benefit and potentially significant risk. As the long-term dangers of ionizing radiation, especially in young children, are being discovered, the decision to image must be made thoughtfully and usually only after the emergency physician and surgeon have consulted.

Computed tomographic (CT) scan and ultrasound scan (US) have been extensively studied as diagnostic modalities for appendicitis. Both have clear advantages and disadvantages, and both examinations have a much better positive predictive value than their negative predictive value.

Ultrasound scan is fast, nonionizing, and relatively less expensive. It is also much more operator dependent and may be less useful in patients who are obese or in patients with overlying bowel gas. CT scan is more sensitive than US (94% vs 89% sensitivity), has less operator dependence, and may be more valuable in showing other intra-abdominal pathology. However, the dosage of radiation is significant, and early cases of appendicitis may not show significant findings. Significant interest exists in a limited abdominal CT scan with rectal contrast, but the accuracy of this method has not been proven superior to standard abdominal tomography and it fails to elucidate other potential pathologies.

In patients with a classic history, right lower quadrant pain, and no high suspicion for other pathology, exploration without further imaging remains perfectly appropriate. In patients with a less clear presentation, the author's practice is to proceed with US. If the US results are positive, the author proceeds to exploration. If the US results are normal and show no other pathology, it is the discretion of the surgeon to proceed with CT scan, observation, or exploration. Again, the key to the right imaging is to decide what tests to perform on the basis of early evaluation by the surgeon. A shotgun approach wastes time and resources and exposes the patient to excessive radiation. Often, even when the case is strongly suspicious for appendicitis, the patient has a CT scan to "get the attention" of the surgeon. Likewise, the fatigued surgeon may request scanning during early morning hours to "buy time." These practices should be condemned, and patients should undergo CT scan only when significant questions remain to be answered.

MANAGEMENT OF ACUTE APPENDICITIS

When appendicitis is suspected, patients should be appropriately resuscitated with fluids and electrolytes and prepared for the operating room. Antibiotics should be given; they have shown clear advantage in large systemic reviews. However, the decision to give antibiotics should be made only after the surgeon commits to operative exploration. Antibiotics may partially treat early appendicitis and therefore

are not appropriate for patients when the diagnosis is in doubt and observation is planned.

TIMING OF SURGERY

Historically, acute appendicitis has been considered a surgical emergency. However, in the new era of work hour restrictions and attention to issues such as physician fatigue, this commandment is changing. Multiple retrospective studies have suggested no increased morbidity in patients who have appendectomy delayed for up to 24 hours. A recent survey of pediatric surgeons showed that more than 90% believed postponement of an overnight appendectomy until the next morning was appropriate surgical care.

The author's practice, once the diagnosis has been made, is to schedule urgent appendectomy within the next 8 hours. Once the decision to operate has been made, antibiotics are given and the patient undergoes fluid resuscitation.

Laparoscopic Versus Open Appendectomy

Multiple meta-analyses have evaluated the question of laparoscopic versus open appendectomy. All show equivalent efficacy in terms of safety, with laparoscopy having a distinct advantage in terms of postoperative wound infection, pain, and cosmesis. The debate is likely to be moot: as more and more surgeons become facile with laparoscopy, it is likely to become the de facto standard, and open appendectomy will likely follow the fate of open cholecystectomy into surgical history.

MANAGEMENT OF NONPERFORATED APPENDICITIS

Laparoscopic Appendectomy

The patient is prepped from xiphoid to pubis, with gastric and bladder catheters placed for decompression. In larger patients, the left arm is extended for ease of laparoscopy from the left side. Usually, one monitor is sufficient at the patient's right side, as surgeon and assistant stand side by side during the laparoscopic dissection (Figure 1). Typically, a three-port technique is adequate. A 12-mL trocar is placed in the umbilicus via Hasson's technique or with the Veress needle, as per surgeon preference. Two 5-mL ports are then placed with direct vision: one in the left lower quadrant, and one in the suprapubic position. Even in small children, adequate triangulation can be achieved in this configuration. A 3-mL instrument without a trocar may be used in the suprapubic position for small children. An additional 3-mL or 5-mL instrument may be placed in the right upper or lower quadrant, if needed for additional retraction. A four-quadrant exploration is performed to quickly rule out other intra-abdominal pathology. This is particularly helpful in young women and girls. The appendix is reliably found by following the taenia coli proximally. The inflamed appendix is grasped, and a window is created in the mesoappendix at the cecal junction. The appendix is ligated here with a gastrointestinal endoscopic stapler. The base of the appendix is usually relatively uninflamed. However, if extensive cecal inflammation exists, safe ligation of the appendiceal base may not be possible, and the surgeon must decide between drainage or, rarely, performance of ileocecectomy. The mesoappendix is then ligated with a vascular stapler, and the appendix placed in a retractable bag and removed. Routine irrigation is not used.

Open appendectomy remains one of the classic exercises in general surgery. An incision lateral to the rectus muscle is mandatory, with layer-by-layer entrance into the abdomen via a muscle-sparing approach. The appendix is found by sweeping a finger from lateral

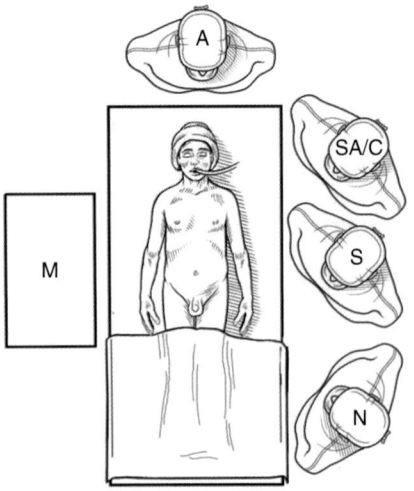
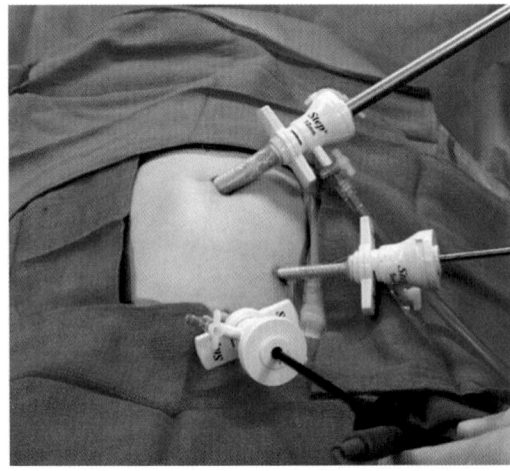

FIGURE 1   Arrangement for laparoscopic appendectomy. Surgeon *(S)* and surgical assistant/camera *(SA/C)* stand side by side once the diagnosis has been confirmed and the surgeon decides to proceed with appendectomy. The 3-port approach is shown in the photograph, with the largest (12-mm) port in the umbilicus and the 5-mm ports in the left lower quadrant and suprapubic positions. Positions of the anesthesiologist *(A)*, nurse *(N)*, and monitor *(M)* are also shown. *(Figure used with permission from Holcomb GW, Georgeson KE, Rothenberg SS: Atlas of pediatric laparoscopy and thoracoscopy, Philadelphia, 2008, Elsevier, Saunders p 77, Fig 14-2.)*

to medial in the right paracolic gutter, or by following the taenia as in a laparoscopic procedure. The appendix is externalized, ligated with absorbable suture, and resected, and a purse-string or Z-plasty–type suture is used to bury the appendiceal base into the cecum. The wound is closed in layers, and the skin is closed with absorbable suture. With perforation, the skin may be left partially open, or delayed primary closure may be used.

After surgery, most patients tolerate a diet immediately, and early ambulation and discharge should be the goal. Postoperative antibiotics in the setting of nonperforated appendicitis have no advantage and actually worsened clinical outcomes in a large, retrospective study.

MANAGEMENT OF PERFORATED APPENDICITIS

Typically, patients with ruptured or complicated appendicitis have either a delayed or unusual presentation. The diagnosis is confirmed with CT scan, which usually reveals right lower quadrant inflammation, phlegmon, or abscess (Figure 2). The surgeon must decide in these patients between early appendectomy and antibiotics and possibly percutaneous drainage, with interval appendectomy in 6 to 8 weeks time. A meta-analysis of 17 studies and more than 1500 patients published in 2010 suggested that patients treated with early appendectomy had more complications, including bowel obstruction, wound infection, and reoperation, than patients with delayed surgery and antibiotics. The vast majority of these studies were nonrandomized, however. Two recent randomized controlled trials (see Suggested Readings) in pediatric patients have addressed this issue. One trial found that the early appendectomy group had significantly reduced time away from normal activities as compared with the interval appendectomy group, and a reduced overall adverse event rate. Another study randomized children with a clear abscess on CT scan to immediate appendectomy versus percutaneous drainage and antibiotics. Here the authors concluded that early surgery was safe, with no differences in complications, length of stay, or hospital charges, and that in fact patients who went to the operating room immediately underwent fewer CT scans and had fewer healthcare visits.

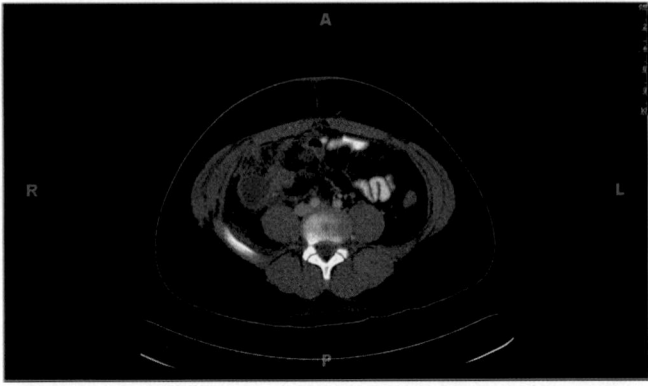

FIGURE 2   Computed tomographic scan of patient with an 8 day history of right lower quadrant pain. Fluid collection can be seen near the appendix.

Many studies have shown that laparoscopic appendectomy can be safely performed in the setting of abscess and right lower quadrant inflammation. As more surgeons develop experience with this technique, it seems likely to become the standard of care.

Antibiotics in Perforated Appendicitis

It is nearly universally accepted that patients with perforated appendicitis receive postoperative antibiotics. The well-known regimen of ampicillin, gentamicin, and clindamycin or metronidazole is the standard with which all others are compared. Length of treatment tends to vary by institution, and until recently, no prospective studies were available to guide the surgeon. Recently, a randomized, prospective trial in children looked at the efficacy of once-daily dosing of ceftriaxone and metronidazole, compared with the standard triple antibiotic regimen. The authors found no difference in the rate of abscess or wound infection and that the simpler regimen was more cost effective. In addition, the possible nephrotoxicity of the aminoglycoside is avoided.

In the future, postoperative antibiotic regimens will likely be based solely on the patient's condition, and not a predetermined time period. Many surgeons now believe that once the patient is afebrile, is tolerating a diet, and has a resolution of leukocytosis, the peritoneal inflammation is gone and antibiotics are no longer necessary or beneficial.

SPECIAL PATIENT SITUATIONS

Elderly

Appendicitis in the elderly is uncommon, with an estimated incidence rate in people more than 65 years old of 1 in 2000. As with children, diagnostic challenges may be found with patients unable to give a detailed history. The signs and symptoms of peritonitis at advanced ages may also be blunted, making the examination less reliable. CT scan is especially important in this group and may be instrumental in ruling out other pathologies in the elderly that can mimic appendicitis, such as diverticulitis and colonic neoplasms. Again, diagnostic laparoscopy can be extremely helpful in searching for alternate pathology if a healthy appendix is found.

Pregnancy

Acute appendicitis is the most common nonobstetric indication for surgery in the pregnant patient. As a disease primarily of young people of child-bearing age, it affects approximately 1 in 1500 pregnancies, with an equal distribution amongst all three trimesters. Diagnosis may be more difficult, however, later in gestation, as the appendix is moved cephalad by the expanding uterus and may reach the level of the gallbladder by the late third trimester. Patients tend to present with a more vague abdominal pain. Also, the physiologic leukocytosis of pregnancy makes laboratory evaluation less helpful. US is the first diagnostic test of choice. CT scan may be used, especially later in gestation, when the effects of ionizing radiation are less on the fetus, but should be reserved for very selected cases. Accurate and early diagnosis is especially important in these women because nonruptured appendectomy carries a low 5% fetal loss rate. Perforated appendicitis, however, may be associated with a fetal loss of more than 25%, which makes it best to err on the aggressive side when recommending surgical exploration.

Pregnancy is not a contraindication to laparoscopy, although a recent meta-analysis suggested it is associated with a higher risk of fetal loss. Access to the abdomen becomes more difficult when the uterus is in a more gravid state. Hasson's technique for entering the abdomen, minimized pneumoperitoneum pressures, dependent positioning, and mandatory obstetric consultation all help minimize the risks.

Negative Appendectomy

Historically, negative appendectomy rates of nearly 20% were expected and accepted, although this has changed in the era of CT scan and improved ultrasound imaging. If exploration is undertaken and a healthy appendix is discovered, a thorough search for alternate pathology must begin. Certainly, in open procedures, the appendix should be removed to avoid future confusion with a McBurney's incision.

Patients diagnosed with terminal ileitis and possibly Crohn's disease offer a special challenge because the rate of fistulization is high after appendectomy in patients with Crohn's disease. Generally, however, if the appendix appears uninvolved in the inflammatory process, it may be safely removed, again to help avoid future diagnostic confusion. If extensive involvement of the cecum or appendiceal base is found, the appendix should be left in situ with the rest of the inflammatory process. If uncomplicated inflammation of the ileum from Crohn's disease is suspected, ileocecectomy is not indicated. Only in cases of gross perforation of clear bowel obstruction should resection be performed.

SUGGESTED READINGS

Blakely ML, Williams R, Dassinger MS, et al: Early vs internal appendectomy for children with perforated appendicitis, *Arch Surg* 146(6):660–665, 2011.
Holcomb GW III, St Peter SD: Current management of complicated appendicitis in children, *Eur J Pediatr Surg* 22:207–212, 2012.
Similis C, Symeonides P, Shorthouse AJ, et al: A meta-analysis comparing conservative treatment versus acute appendectomy for complicated appendicitis (abscess or phlegmon), *Surgery* 147(6):818–829, 2010.
St Peter SD, Aguayo P, Fraser JD, et al: Initial laparoscopic appendectomy versus initial nonoperative management and internal appendectomy for perforated appendicitis with abscess: a prospective, randomized trial, *J Pediatr Surg* 45(1):236–240, 2010.
The SCOAP Collaborative, Drake FT, Florence MG, Johnson MG, et al: Progress in the diagnosis of appendicitis: a report from Washington State's surgical care and outcomes assessment program, *Ann Surg* 256:586–594, 2012.
Wilasrusmee C, Sukrat B, McEvoy M, et al: Systematic review and meta-analysis of safety of laparoscopic versus open appendicectomy for suspected appendicitis in pregnancy, *Br J Surg* 99(11):1470–1478, 2012.

HEMORRHOIDS

Vivek Chaudhry, MD, FACS, FASCRS, and Herand Abcarian, MD

ANATOMY

Hemorrhoids are a normal anatomy of the human anal canal. Fibrovascular cushions with subepithelial arteriovenous communications are present above the dentate line in all individuals. The three main cushions are located at the left lateral, right anterior, and right posterior positions. These cushions account for 15% to 20% of the resting anal pressure. During valsalva maneuvers, such as coughing and straining, they get engorged and aid in occlusion of the anal canal maintaining continence. Additionally, subepithelial sensory nerve endings in these cushions help individuals to discriminate among solid, liquid, and gas. Engorgement of the cushions during defecation allows safe dilation of the anoderm without tearing. *Internal hemorrhoids* arise from the superior hemorrhoidal plexus proximal to the dentate line and are covered by insensate columnar/transitional mucosa. Venous blood drains from the superior hemorrhoidal plexus to the superior rectal veins, through the inferior mesenteric vein draining into the portal system.

External hemorrhoids arise from inferior hemorrhoidal plexus below the dentate line and are covered by sensate skin. Venous blood drains into the middle or inferior rectal veins, through the pudendal veins, into the internal iliac veins draining into the systemic circulation.

ETIOLOGY AND PATHOPHYSIOLOGY

Hemorrhoids are considered to be pathologic when they produce symptoms. Prolonged constipation, diarrhea, and straining and faulty bowel habits lead to overengorgement and bleeding from the thin, friable mucosa and subsequent prolapse from disruption of the sensory Treitz's muscle. With aging, the collagen content of the connective tissue fixing the hemorrhoids to the anorectal muscular wall degenerates, allowing for caudal sliding of the hemorrhoids and distal rectal mucosa with the shearing force of defecation. The exposed mucosa secretes mucus, causing perianal skin wetness, irritation, pruritus, and difficulty with maintaining hygiene (Figure 1). External hemorrhoidal plexus can also get enlarged, causing combined internal and external hemorrhoidal disease. External hemorrhoids rarely produce symptoms. Occasionally they can develop painful acute thrombosis or large skin tags and can cause difficulty in hygiene. A tense clot under the sensitive anoderm is extremely painful. Acute prolapse may result in mucosal edema, engorgement, pain, sphincter spasm, thrombosis, and gangrene of the hemorrhoid (Figure 2). Rarely, pylephlebitis can develop. Hemorrhoids are graded by the degree of prolapse and reducibility (Table 1).

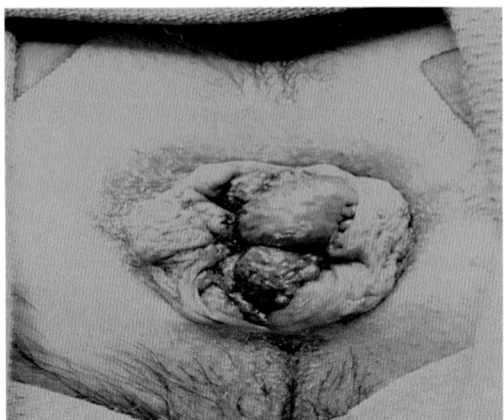

FIGURE 1   Grade II/III internal hemorrhoid.

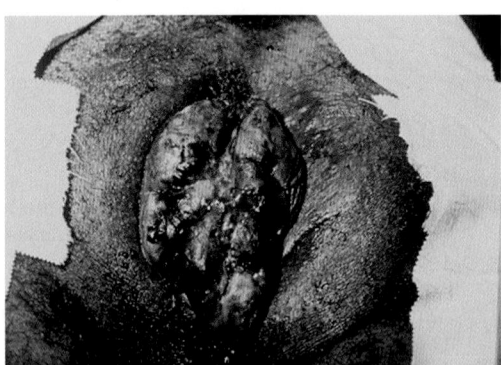

FIGURE 2   Grade IV strangulated hemorrhoids. These are treated with excisional hemorrhoidectomy (preferred). Alternatively, they can be treated with multiple thrombectomies and multiple rubber band ligations.

INCIDENCE

The exact prevalence of symptomatic hemorrhoids is unknown due to underreporting and self-medication. Symptomatic hemorrhoids have been reported to be present in 4.4% of the U.S. population. Males and females are equally affected, with the peak incidence in the fifth to seventh decades. Symptomatic hemorrhoids have a familial correlation, although the exact contribution of genetic inheritance is unknown. Pregnancy and the postpartum state increase the risk due to increased blood volume, decrease in vascular and muscle tone, and pressure from the gravid uterus impeding venous drainage.

EXTERNAL HEMORRHOIDS

Acute Thrombosis

Acute thrombosis is due to the rupture of a vein in the external hemorrhoidal plexus, with tense hematoma formation presenting as an exquisite painful perianal subcutaneous nodule, usually, but not always, after a vigorous valsalva maneuver, such as in straining at a bowel movement or a vigorous workout at the gym. The pain increases or remains constant for 2 to 3 days, after which the swelling and pain decrease either due to spontaneous reabsorption of the clot or, less commonly, due to pressure necrosis of overlying skin and gradual decompression of the clot (Figure 3).

If the patient is seen with a painful thrombosis within 24 to 48 hours, the treatment of choice is immediate excision of the hemorrhoid (not evacuation of the clot) under local anesthesia. The patient who presents later, when natural reabsorption of the clot has started, is treated with Sitz baths; stool softeners; and topical anesthetics, astringents, and steroids to aid in rapid resolution of symptoms.

Quiescent External Hemorrhoids

Perianal skin tags are often related to prior episodes of thrombosed external hemorrhoids or sentinel pile of a healed fissure. Small skin tags require no treatment unless they become large enough to interfere with proper anal hygiene. In the case of external hemorrhoidal tags, they can be excised under local anesthesia. Removal of minor skin tags in an occasional patient fixated on cosmesis is discouraged.

TABLE 1: Classification of hemorrhoids

External hemorrhoids	Origin below dentate line, covered by skin/anoderm, sensate
Internal hemorrhoids	Origin above dentate line, covered by columnar mucosa, insensate
Grade I	Bleed and prolapse into the lumen of anal canal
Grade II	Prolapse outside anal canal: reduce spontaneously
Grade III	Prolapse outside anal canal: requires manual reduction
Grade IV	Prolapse outside anal canal: irreducible

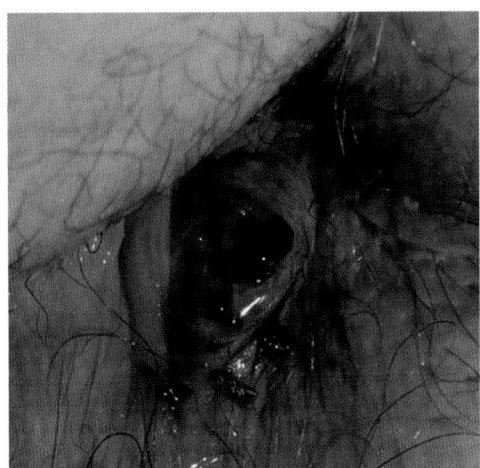

FIGURE 3 Thrombosed external hemorrhoid. Note that the clot is spontaneously extruding from pressure necrosis of the dome of the hemorrhoid.

INTERNAL HEMORRHOIDS

The management of internal hemorrhoids can be divided into non-operative (office) procedures and operative procedures.

Nonoperative Techniques

The principal of all nonoperative techniques is to produce fixation of the internal hemorrhoids to the muscular layer (Table 2). The most common nonoperative treatments of hemorrhoids include the following.

Rubber Band Ligation

Rubber band ligation (RBL) is suitable for Grades II and III hemorrhoids. This office procedure is performed in the Sims or prone jackknife position, using either a McGivney/Barron hemorrhoid ligator or a vacuum-assisted device (Figure 4). It is better to treat each hemorrhoidal complex individually to prevent postprocedural pain and undesirable protrusion. Placement of the band at least 5 mm cephalad to the dentate line reduces the incidence of postprocedural pain. Appropriately placed bans occasionally result in minor postprocedural discomfort for up to 24 hours, which is easily controlled by acetaminophen or nonsteroidal antiinflammatory drugs (NSAIDs). Severe pain immediately after the procedure usually indicates placement too close to the dentate line and is treated with cutting the band using a specifically designed cutting hook. Patients are instructed to rest for a few minutes after the procedure before assuming the upright posture to prevent vasovagal syncopal symptoms.

Minor complications of RBL include thrombosis of external hemorrhoids, which can be treated as described previously. Postband bleeding occurs in less than 1% of the patients and appears 3 to 7 days after banding. Rarely, if bleeding is more than a few drops and persists for a few hours, the patient must be examined and the source controlled with topical epinephrine followed by cauterization or suture.

Pelvic sepsis is a very rare (1 : 15,000) but life-threatening complication. Pain, fever, and urinary difficulty are the trifecta, which should serve as an early warning to this potentially lethal complication. Prompt examination under anesthesia, removal of the band with debridement of necrotic tissue, and hospitalization for intravenous (IV) antibiotics must be instituted. Failure to recognize this complication can result in death from overwhelming sepsis.

TABLE 2: Treatments of hemorrhoids by correcting bowel habits and patterns

Grades I and II	Grades II and III	Grades III and IV
• Dietary/lifestyle changes • High-fiber diet • Water • Stool softeners • Good stool habits • Office procedures	• Office treatments • Rubber band ligation • Sclerotherapy • Infrared coagulation • Transanal hemorrhoid ligation (THD)	• Surgical treatments • Ferguson hemorrhoidectomy utilizing scalpel, cautery, ligature • Stapled (PPH)

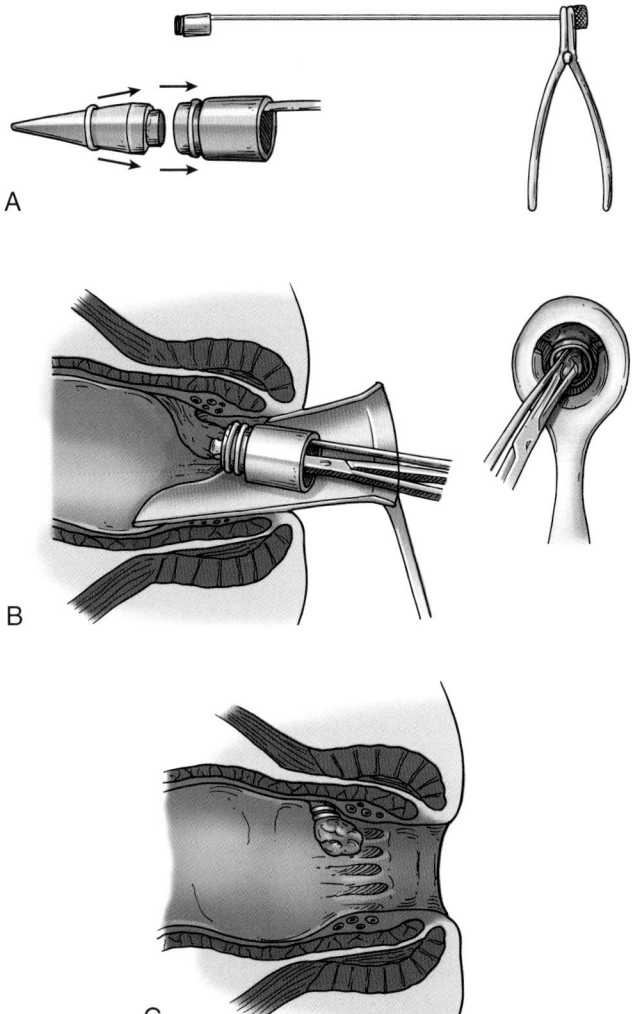

FIGURE 4 Rubber band ligation. **A,** Loading the rubber band on the applicator. **B,** Placement of the rubber band using a slotted anoscope. **C,** Appropriately placed band above the dentate line.

RBL enjoys universal acceptance. It is inexpensive, quick, well tolerated, and effective. A success rate of 80% to 100% has been widely reported, often with one session. It is superior to injection sclerotherapy in controlling prolapse, bleeding, and recurrent symptoms. Although multiple-band ligations at a single outpatient session have been reported to be safe and well tolerated, we continue to band a maximum two pedicles, especially during the first encounter. If more than three sessions are required to control symptoms, hemorrhoidopexy or hemorrhoidectomy should be offered.

Injection Sclerotherapy

The indications for its use include acutely bleeding Grades I and II hemorrhoids, especially in patients who are on anticoagulants and in patients who are immunocompromised or coagulopathic. Advantages of injection sclerotherapy include possibility of treating all hemorrhoids at one setting with no need to stop anticoagulant therapy. The disadvantage is the need for repeat injection at least two or three times to achieve the desired effect. Injection sclerotherapy is carried out by injecting 3 to 5 mL of phenol in vegetable (almond or arachis) oil in the submucosal space of each hemorrhoidal apex. An 18-gauge spinal needle (bent 30 degrees 2 cm from the tip) or an angled hemorrhoidal needle are used with the patient in the left lateral or prone jackknife position, using a strong light and a side or end viewing anoscope (Figure 5). Accurate submucosal injection at the hemorrhoidal apex causes swelling of the mucosa, with obvious vessels crossing it "striation sign." If the mucosa has no swelling, the injection is too deep and can result in prostatic abscess, erectile dysfunction, or pylephlebitis. Pale white mucosa is due to intramucosal injection with resultant sloughing and ulceration and must be avoided. The injection is painless and well tolerated other than a

sense of fullness. Though injection sclerotherapy can be repeated, it is more difficult to deliver therapeutic doses due to submucosal fibrosis and can result in stricture formation. It is encouraged to use an appropriate dose at the initial injection. An alternative is to use 1 to 2 mL of ethanolamine oleate directly into the hemorrhoid using a 25-gauge needle. Other sclerosants like 0.5 mL of 5% sodium morrhuate or 5% quinine urea have also been used. Efficacy is inferior to rubber band ligation.

Infrared Coagulation

Infrared coagulation (IRC) is most effective in Grades I and II hemorrhoids (Figure 6). Infrared light energy from a tungsten-halogen lamp is converted to heat, which causes coagulation of the vessels, tissue destruction, and scarring. Four mucosal applications of 1.5 seconds are placed at the apex of each hemorrhoid to produce scarring and fixation and to reduce distal sliding of the mucosa. IRC is quick, easy, and well tolerated, with less pain than RBL and minimal risk of delayed hemorrhage or ulceration. It is more expensive and less efficacious than RBL, especially in treating prolapse. Most surgeons prefer RBL over IRC.

Other treatments like laser, monopolar and bipolar coagulation, Ultroid, and cryotherapy have all been tried and eventually abandoned due to high cost and low success rates.

Operative Techniques

These procedures are based on excision of hemorrhoids, as well as fixation of mucosal prolapse. These operations are most suitable for Grades III and IV hemorrhoids and in cases of prolapsed gangrenous hemorrhoids requiring immediate excision.

Open Hemorrhoidectomy

Open hemorrhoidectomy (Milligan Morgan hemorrhoidectomy) has been used since the 1840s. The hemorrhoid is dissected off from the underlying sphincter complex with ligation of the hemorrhoidal vessel at its apex. Care is taken in leaving anoderm bridges intact to prevent anal stenosis. The wound is left open to heal by secondary intention. This procedure has not gained popularity in the United States.

Closed Hemorrhoidectomy

Closed hemorrhoidectomy (Ferguson hemorrhoidectomy) is the most popular excision technique in the United States (Figure 7). It is

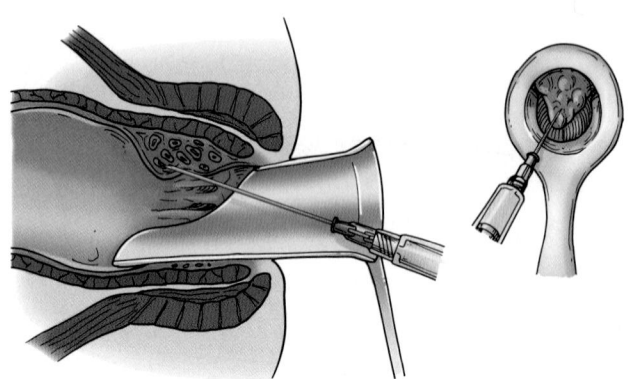

FIGURE 5 Injection sclerotherapy. Sclerotherapy needle (bent 2 cm from the tip) with bevel upward is inserted into the submucosa at the apex of the hemorrhoid bundle. "Striation sign" ensures correct plane of therapy. The mucosa swells without forming blebs or becoming "dead white."

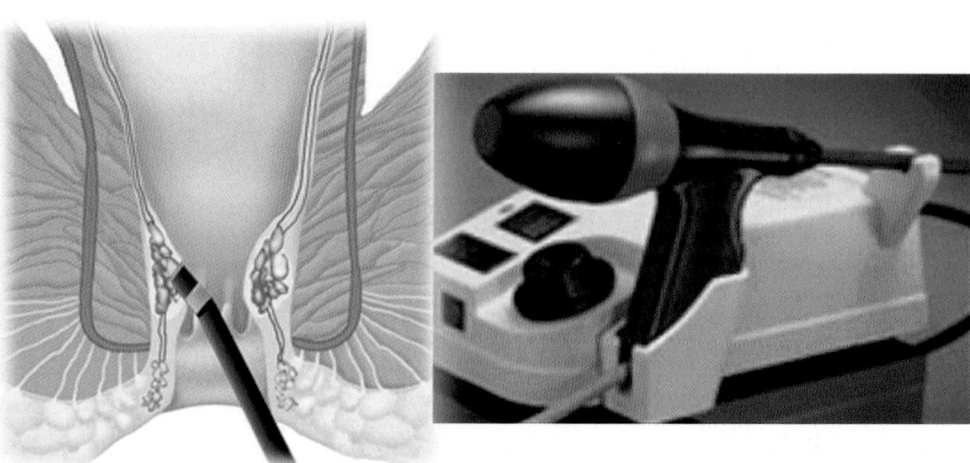

FIGURE 6 Infrared coagulation (IRC; Redfield Corporation). The sterile applicator is placed at the apex of the hemorrhoid bundle.

Excision technique for mixed hemorrhoids

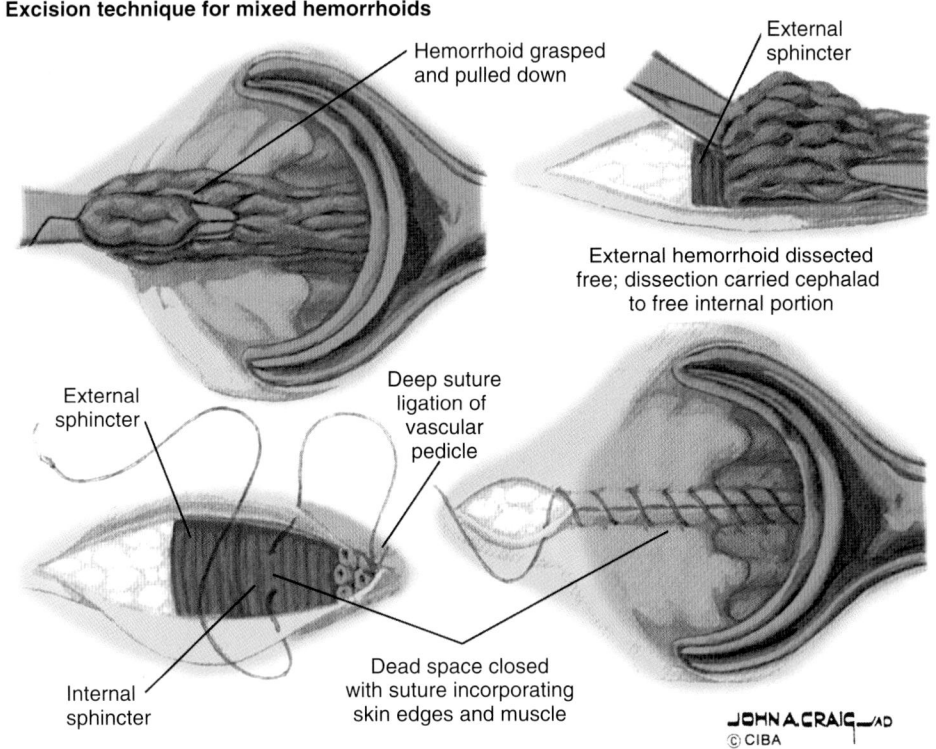

Hemorrhoid grasped and pulled down

External sphincter

External hemorrhoid dissected free; dissection carried cephalad to free internal portion

External sphincter

Deep suture ligation of vascular pedicle

Internal sphincter

Dead space closed with suture incorporating skin edges and muscle

JOHN A.CRAIG—AD
© CIBA

FIGURE 7 Ferguson hemorrhoidectomy (closed hemorrhoidectomy).

performed in the prone jackknife (preferred) or lithotomy position under local, regional, or general anesthesia, with the gluteal folds retracted with tape. Antibiotics are not administered routinely. A Hill-Ferguson retractor is placed in the anal canal and the hemorrhoid grasped at the perianal skin, the mucocutaneous junction, and the apex of the hemorrhoid. Dilute epinephrine solution is injected to reduce bleeding during dissection and to spare the superficial external sphincter. A diamond-shaped incision (scalpel/electrocautery) is made from the perianal skin into the anal canal and tapered toward the apex of the hemorrhoid. It is important to dissect superficial to the fibers of the internal sphincter, which is readily recognized due to its white muscle fibers. The apex of the hemorrhoid is clamped and suture ligated with 2-0 absorbable suture and the wound closed with accurate mucosa to mucosa approximation. The mucosa is fixed to the underlying sphincter muscle to recreate a new dentate line. The suture line continues into the perianal skin. The tail of the apical suture is left long for identification of the pedicle in case of postoperative hemorrhage. The same procedure is repeated at other major hemorrhoidal pedicles. Dibucaine-impregnated Gelfoam is placed in the anal canal. Patients are discharged the same day with narcotic and NSAID pain medications, Sitz baths, and stool softeners and are seen 10 days after surgery. They are instructed to keep dry gauze in between the buttocks and change it two or three times a day. The advantage of this technique is faster healing, but it also has the disadvantage of occasional wound infection and fistula formation. The success rate of this technique in the long-term follow-up period exceeds 90%.

The use of energy devices such as Harmonic Scalpel or Ligasure has been reported. There is no real advantage in using energy devices. It does increase the cost of the operation, and if the surgeon is not careful, excessive excision of the anoderm with subsequent fibrosis and scarring may lead to an anal stricture that is difficult to correct.

Park's Submucosal Excision

Park's submucosal excision is an attempt to remove the hemorrhoid and maintain the integrity of the overlying mucosa and anoderm.

However, the operation is tedious to perform and often associated with breakdown of the suture line and infection or fistulas. This procedure, despite its intended design, has not gained popularity.

The most common complication after excisional hemorrhoidectomy is urinary retention, followed by bleeding. Urinary retention occurs in 6% to 10% of patients and can be minimized by restricting fluid intake (IV or oral) for 4 to 6 hours postoperatively. Adequate pain control, relief of pelvic spasm with a warm bath, upright posture, privacy, and the sound of running water will often allow a patient to void without a Foley in the recovery room. Early bleeding is the result of a technical error, but bleeding occurring 5 to 7 days later is caused by slough of the suture line. If bleeding is severe and continues, the patient must be taken back to the operating room for resuturing of all hemorrhoidectomy suture lines.

Anal stenosis is a serious late complication from overaggressive excision of the anoderm. Treatment involves dilations or resection with flap anoplasty. Minor incontinence usually resolves over 3 months and can be minimized by preventing overzealous sphincter retraction. Major incontinence is very rare and indicates underlying sphincter damage.

Fixation Procedures

Stapled Hemorrhoidopexy

Stapled hemorrhoidectomy or procedures for prolapsed hemorrhoids (PPH) were popularized by Longo as a less painful alternative to excisional hemorrhoidectomy. It involves circular resection and anastomosis of a 1- to 2-cm ring of anorectal mucosa and submucosa at the top apex of the hemorrhoidal plexus. The operation (1) interrupts the superior hemorrhoidal vascular pedicles, (2) resuspends the prolapsing tissue at the anorectal ring, (3) preserves the vascular cushions (important for continence), and (4) avoids painful perianal wounds.

Patients are instructed to take an 8-oz. phosphosoda enema on the morning of the operation. Operations are performed under local, spinal, or general anesthesia in the prone jackknife (preferred) or lithotomy position. Preoperative antibiotics are not routinely administered.

The anal canal is dilated with a circular anal dilator. The circular anal dilator and obturator are inserted into the rectum. The obturator is removed, and the anal dilator is sutured to the perianal skin. The purse-string suture anoscope is inserted through the dilating anoscope to facilitate the placement of a circumferential purse-string suture.

Purse-string suture placement is the crucial part of this procedure. A 2 0 Prolene (polypropylene) purse-string suture is placed approximately 2 cm proximal to the apex of the hemorrhoids and 4 cm above the dentate line (Figure 8, *A*). This positions the purse-string suture approximately 4 cm proximal to the dentate line and the final staple line 2 cm above the dentate line. Care is taken to include only mucosa and submucosa at the same level circumferentially and to avoid gaps in the purse-string suture. In female patients the surgeon inserts a finger into the vagina, while placing the sutures in the anterior wall of the rectum to ensure that the suture is not accidentally placed too deep. Once completed, the purse-string suture is gently tightened to draw the redundant mucosa into the lumen of the rectum. The purse-string suture is deemed adequate if the rectum can be completely occluded with tension on the suture. The anvil of the stapler is inserted into the rectum and can be completely occluded with tension on the suture. The anvil of the stapler is inserted into the rectal lumen through the purse-string suture, which is then tied over the shaft of the stapler. The stapler is then closed slowly until it is fully tightened and the 4-cm mark on the head of the stapler is at the anal verge. In female patients the vagina is examined again to confirm that the posterior vaginal wall was not drawn into the head of the stapler. The stapler is held closed for 1 minute to assist in hemostasis, and then fired and removed.

The specimen retrieved from the stapler is inspected to verify that a complete "doughnut" of the tissue was excised. A digital examination confirms that the staple line is circumferential. The purse-string anoscope or a large Hill-Ferguson retractor is then inserted into the anus to examine the staple line and the sew areas for any bleeding.

A small role of Gelfoam (Pharmacia and Upjohn, Kalamazoo, MI) coated with anesthetic ointment is placed into the rectum. Patients are usually discharged home with oral analgesics and stool softeners.

PPH has been extensively studied. Several large randomized trials and systemic reviews have reached similar conclusions, and a representative systemic review is presented. In a review of 25 randomized controlled trials of 1918 patients with 1 to 62 months follow-up comparing conventional hemorrhoidectomy to stapled hemorrhoidopexy, PPH was associated with less operating rime (weighted mean difference: 11 minutes, $P = 0.006$); appeared to be less painful (37% reduction in analgesic requirement); required less time off work (weighted mean difference, j8.45 days; $P <0.00001$); enabled an earlier return to normal activities (weighted mean difference, j15.85 days; $P = 0.03$); and had better wound healing (odds ratio, 0.1; $P = 0.00006$). The patient satisfaction was significantly higher with stapled hemorrhoidopexy than conventional hemorrhoidectomy (odds radio, 2.33; $P = 0.003$). Although there was an increase in the recurrence of hemorrhoids at 1 year or more after the stapled procedure (5.7% vs 1%; odds ratio, 3.48; $P = 0.02$), the overall complication rate did not differ significantly from that of the conventional procedure (stapled vs conventional: 20.2% vs 25.2%; $P = 0.06$). Stapled hemorrhoidopexy had less postoperative bleeding (odds ratio, 0.52; $P = 0.001$), wound complications (odds radio, 0.05; $P = 0.005$), constipation (odds ratio, 0.45; $P = 0.02$), and pruritus (odds ratio, 0.19; $P = 0.02$). The overall need for surgical (odds ratio, 1.27; $P = 0.4$) and nonsurgical (odds ratio, 1.07; $P = 0.82$) reintervention after the two procedures was similar.

Unexplained persistent postoperative pain and major pelvic septic complications (pelvic sepsis, pneumoperitoneum, intra-abdominal sepsis, Fournier gangrene, rectovaginal fistula, and rectal perforation) have not been noted in any randomized trials. Most of these complications are probably related to technical errors, such as inappropriate placement of purse-string sutures that were too deep or too cephaled or distal in the rectum.

The ideal patient has circumferential Grade II/III internal hemorrhoids without significant external disease intra-abdominal (see Figure 8, *B* and *C*). Care should be taken in patients with narrow anal canals or previous sphincter injury. Additionally, Grade IV hemorrhoids treated with PPH have an increased risk of early recurrence. It is advisable that surgeons experienced in colon and rectal surgery perform this procedure.

Suture Hemorrhoidopexy

Pakravan and colleagues described open suture hemorrhoidopexy in 2009. This is a simple and inexpensive variation of stapled hemorrhoidopexy. An absorbable 3/0 suture (e.g., Vicryl) is placed above the dentate line horizontally and again in the same direction at the apex of hemorrhoid (Z stitch) 3 cm above the distal suture. A 1-cm window of rectal mucosa is excised in between the horizontal suture lines to allow adherence, scarring, and fixation. The suture is then tied. The same procedure is repeated in all quadrants when a prolapse is present. When all sutures are tied, the entire prolapsing complex of hemorrhoids and distal rectal mucosa is elevated and fixed at the anorectal ring. This is a cost-effective procedure most suitable for third-degree and very symptomatic second-degree hemorrhoids. The advantage of this operation is that it is simple and requires no special instrumentation and may be done again for additional hemorrhoids or future recurrences.

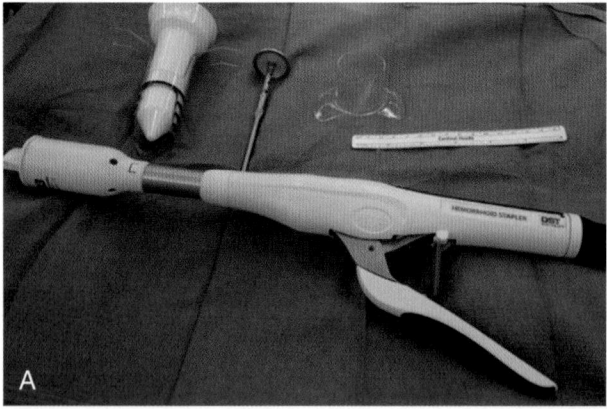
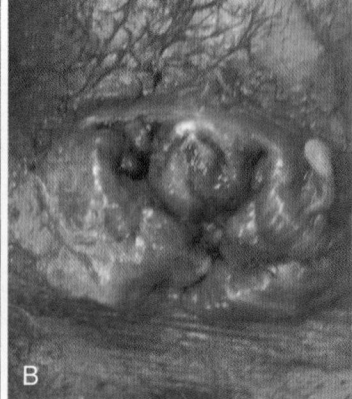
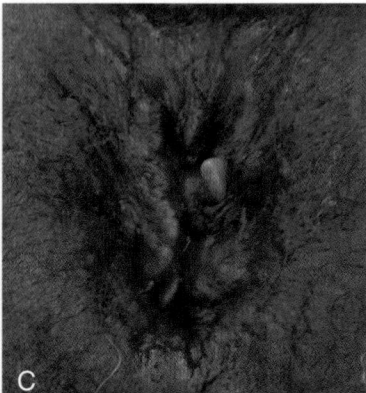

FIGURE 8   **A,** PPH—placement of purse-string 4 cm above the dentate line and resection and stapling of ring of rectal mucosa/submucosa. **B,** Preoperative view with prolapsed circumferential hemorrhoids. **C,** Postoperative result after application of the stapler.

Partial Stapled Hemorrhoidopexy

A recent variant of the stapled technique involves 1-3 quadrant resection and fixation using a special slotted stapler. Preliminary results promise decreased postoperative morbidity with equivalent efficacy.

Doppler Guided Transanal Hemorrhoidal Ligation

Hemorrhoidal artery ligation uses a special Doppler probe anoscope to identify and suture ligate the terminal branches of the superior hemorrhoidal artery, which feeds the major and minor hemorrhoidal plexus (Figure 9). Figure of eight absorbable suture ligation of an average of six pedicles is performed resulting in the reduction in the vascularity and size of the hemorrhoids.

In a systematic review of 150 patients in 3 randomized control trials (RCT) comparing PPH to transanal hemorrhoid ligation (THD), both procedures had similar efficacy with reduced postoperative pain in the THD group. The overall recurrence at 1 year is 11%, 10%, and 9% for prolapse, bleeding, and pain, respectively.

A recent modification of rectro-anal-repair (RAR) in conjunction with DGTHL is currently under investigation. RAR involves restoration of prolapsed tissue to their anatomic location with longitudinal absorbable sutures placed through a special slotted anoscope.

SPECIAL SITUATIONS

Strangulated Hemorrhoids

Incarceration of third- and fourth-degree hemorrhoids leads to edema, thrombosis, necrosis, and ulceration. Emergent hemorrhoidectomy in the operating room is safe provided all necrotic hemorrhoidal tissue is excised individually and care is taken to preserve viable anoderm. Injection of dilute epinephrine together with 150 to 200 IU of hyaluronidase aids in reducing the edema and facilitating the operation. Alternatively, massage/reduction of internal hemorrhoids with multiple rubber band ligations and external thrombectomies can provide immediate relief. Future hemorrhoidectomy is seldom needed. A randomized trial comparing excisional hemorrhoidectomy to incision and ligation showed both techniques to be safe with slightly improved early recovery after incision/ligation.

Hemorrhoids in Pregnancy

Constipation, lax sphincters, increased blood volume, and straining often result in exacerbation of hemorrhoids during the third trimester and postpartum and often resolve spontaneously after delivery. Generally the approach is conservative with Sitz baths, fiber, and stool softeners. The rare patient with acutely thrombosed prolapsed hemorrhoidal disease is operated on under local anesthesia in the left lateral position.

Hemorrhoids in Inflammatory Bowel Disease

Hemorrhoidectomy in patients with active anorectal Crohn's disease should not be performed because of an increased risk of nonhealing, local complications, major incontinence, and subsequent need for proctectomy. Patients with quiescent ileal or colonic disease undergoing conservative hemorrhoid surgery have a 90% healing rate at 2 months.

Hemorrhoids in the Immunocompromised

Anorectal complications are common in patients with HIV/AIDS. Infectious etiology and malignancy need to be ruled out using cultures, endoscopy, and biopsies. Many patients suffer from episodic or chronic diarrhea and incontinence. In selected patients with HIV infection under good control, excisional and nonexcisional therapies for proven symptomatic hemorrhoid disease can be safely accomplished with minimal complications. Surgery in patients with hematologic malignancies should only be offered as a last resort to relieve pain and sepsis.

Hemorrhoid Varices and Portal Hypertension

Contrary to popular belief, the incidence of hemorrhoidal disease is no greater in patients with portal hypertension than in the general population. Anorectal varices are seen in up to 80% of patients with portal hypertension but are implicated in less than 1% of massive gastrointestinal bleeding. Procedures used in the control of bleeding anorectal varices are direct suture ligation; stapled anopexy; transjugular portosystemic shunt; and mesocaval, mesorenal, and sigmoid to ovarian vein shunts.

SUGGESTED READINGS

Alonso-Coello P, Guyatt G, Heels-Ansdell D, et al: Laxatives for the treatment of hemorrhoids, *Cochrane Database Syst Rev* (4):CD004649, 2005.

Jayaraman S, Colquhoun PH, Malthaner RA: Stapled versus conventional surgery for hemorrhoids, *Cochrane Database Syst Rev* (4):CD005393, 2006.

Lin HC, He QL, Ren DL, et al: Partial stapled hemorrhoidopexy: a minimally invasive technique for hemorrhoids, *Surg Today* 42(9):868–875, 2012.

Pakravan F, Helmes C, Baeten C: Transanal open hemorrhoidopexy, *Dis Colon Rectum* 52(3):503–506, 2009.

Senagore AJ, Singer M, Abcarian H, et al: A prospective, randomized, controlled multicenter trial comparing stapled hemorrhoidopexy and Ferguson hemorrhoidectomy: perioperative and one-year results, *Dis Colon and Rectum* 45(11):1824–1836, 2004.

Walega P, Romaniszyn M, Kenig J, et al: Doppler-guided hemorrhoid artery ligation with recto-anal repair modification: functional evaluation and safety assessment of a new minimally invasive method of treatment of advanced hemorrhoidal disease, *Scientific World Journal* 324040, 2012.

Wolf BG, Fleshman JW, Beck DE, et al: The ASCRS textbook of colon and rectal surgery, ed 1, New York, 2007, Springer.

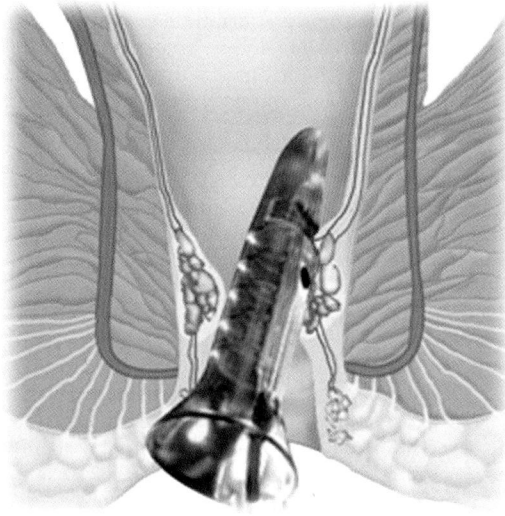

FIGURE 9 Doppler guided hemorrhoid artery ligation.

ANAL FISSURE

Susan L. Gearhart, MD, FACS, FASCAS

Anal fissure, or a longitudinal anal tear or ischemic ulcer, is a common cause of anal pain and bleeding in both infancy and adulthood. Symptoms associated with anal fissure usually occur following defecation. The pain can be short-lived or last several hours, and the bleeding is usually observed on the toilet tissue. Often patients will complain of hemorrhoids or anal tags because of the swelling around the anal fissure that occurs when the fissure is irritated. A history of constipation increases the likelihood for an anal fissure nearly threefold.

The cause of an anal fissure is believed to be related to trauma occurring to the anal canal with the passage of a hard stool. Fissures may also occur following a course of diarrhea. It has been demonstrated with anal manometric evaluation that trauma to the mucosa overlying the internal sphincter leads to a sustained increase in resting pressure within the anal canal. Furthermore, there is evidence to suggest an inverse relationship between anal resting tone and perfusion to the anoderm. A decrease in perfusion associated with increase in anal resting tone leads to poor tissue healing. Since the vascular supply to the anal canal enters laterally, posterior and anterior trauma to the anal canal will exhibit the slowest healing; this is due to increased relative ischemia. Currently, methods for treating anal fissures focus on decreasing anal resting pressure and therefore increasing perfusion of the anoderm.

Anal fissures occur up to 90% of the time in the posterior midline; however, fissures in women occur 25% of the time in the anterior midline. Acute fissures or fissures that have been present for less than 6 weeks have the appearance of a simple tear or ulcer in the anoderm, which starts at the dentate line. Chronic anal fissures, defined by symptoms present for more than 6 to 8 weeks, can be further characterized by the presence of an anal tag or "sentinel pile" at the distal end of the fissure and a hypertrophied anal papilla at the proximal end near the dentate line. Often the internal sphincter muscle is easily visualized in the fissure bed (Figure 1). Diagnosis of an acute or chronic fissure is made easily by the patient's history and physical exam findings. The physical exam is performed by gently spreading the buttocks with opposing thumbs while the patient is in the prone jackknife position. The typical anal fissure can be identified easily in the anterior or posterior position. Once a fissure has been identified, it would be prudent to avoid any further evaluation of the anal canal, which may worsen the patient's symptoms.

Anal fissures are frequently misdiagnosed. The most common diagnosis confused with anal fissures is hemorrhoids. Other diagnoses in the differential include a fistula in anorectal and perirectal abscess, inflammatory bowel disease, sexually transmitted diseases, and anal cancer. For this reason, all fissures that fail to heal with appropriate treatment should be biopsied. Atypical fissures are fissures not found in the midline and can be multiple, painless, and nonhealing (Figure 2). The associated diagnoses with lateral fissures include inflammatory bowel disease, syphilis, tuberculosis, leukemia, cancer, and human immunodeficiency virus (HIV). All atypical fissures should be biopsied or excised to rule out additional pathology.

TREATMENT

Acute Anal Fissure

The management of an acute posterior or anterior anal fissure that has been symptomatic less than 6 weeks is for the patient to improve bowel habits by increasing fiber supplements. The normal requirement for fiber consumption per day is 40 g. This amount may be obtained more easily by the addition of over-the-counter fiber supplements such as Metamucil or Fibercon. Patients can find dietary information about fiber from various websites. In addition, warm sitz baths after bowel movements and the addition of stool softeners if needed may aid in promoting healing.

Medical Therapy for Chronic Anal Fissure

For chronic anal fissure, there are several nonsurgical therapies. Most nonsurgical therapies are aimed at smooth muscle (internal sphincter) relaxation, antiinflammatory therapy, and pain control (Table 1). When evaluating the outcomes of different medical therapies, it is important to keep in mind that the natural history of anal fissures is a waxing and waning of symptoms. Furthermore, long-term follow-up of these patients is necessary to determine the success of these treatments. Therapies aimed at relaxation of the smooth muscle are designed to improve healing through improving blood flow to the anal canal. The role of antiinflammatory medication and topical anesthetics are to decrease pain that is due to inflammation and promote healing. The objective of these therapies is to provide quick relief through a short course of treatment. However, with diet modification and improvement in stool quality, in combination with antiinflammatory therapy, prolonged healing can occur.

Currently, several therapies are available that are effective at smooth muscle relaxation. Nitroglycerine, or glyceryl trinitrate (GTN), is a dimer of nitric oxide thought to locally release nitric oxide. Nitric oxide will then, in turn, bind to $3',5'$-cyclic guanosine monophosphate (cGMP), which results in a cascade of intracellular interactions ultimately leading to smooth muscle relaxation. In a similar fashion, L-arginine, an amino acid that is known to donate nitric oxide, leads to smooth muscle relaxation. The use of phosphodiesterase (PDE) inhibitors has been postulated to be an effective treatment for anal fissures. PDE is an enzyme important in the degradation of cGMP, which then, along a similar pathway as above, leads to smooth muscle relaxation (Figure 3).

Cytoplasmic calcium is important for smooth muscle contraction. By inhibition of calcium channel, smooth muscle relaxation occurs. The use of calcium channel antagonists first became popular in the treatment of esophageal spasm in conditions such as achalasia. Their use has also gained popularity in the treatment of anal fissures through this same mechanism. Botulinum toxin (Botox) prevents the release of acetylcholine from presynaptic nerve terminal and thus inhibits neuromuscular transmission in striated muscles such as the external anal sphincter. The exact mechanism that leads to induced relaxation of the internal anal sphincter from Botox is not known, but it is believed that relaxation of the external anal sphincter may bring about internal sphincter relaxation.

Nelson and colleagues (2012) evaluated 75 studies in which 5031 participants were randomized to a nonsurgical therapy for anal fissure. All atypical fissures, including inflammatory bowel disease, anal cancer, and infection, were excluded. The results of this review show that GTN was significantly better than placebo in healing anal fissure (49% vs 36%; $P < 0.0009$). However, the dose was listed as either 0.2% or 0.4%, 2 or 3 times a day, for 6 to 8 weeks; 30% of patients suffered from headaches; and recurrence occurred over time in 50% of patients. Botox and calcium channel antagonists were equivalent to GTN in efficacy but did not result in as many adverse events. However, Botox dosing was variable with anywhere from 10 to 100 units given intramuscularly in the external anal sphincter, internal anal sphincter, or the intersphincteric space (Figure 4). One author recommended Botox always be placed anteriorly even if the fissure is posterior. The studies evaluating calcium channel antagonists did not include long-term follow-up, and no study evaluated

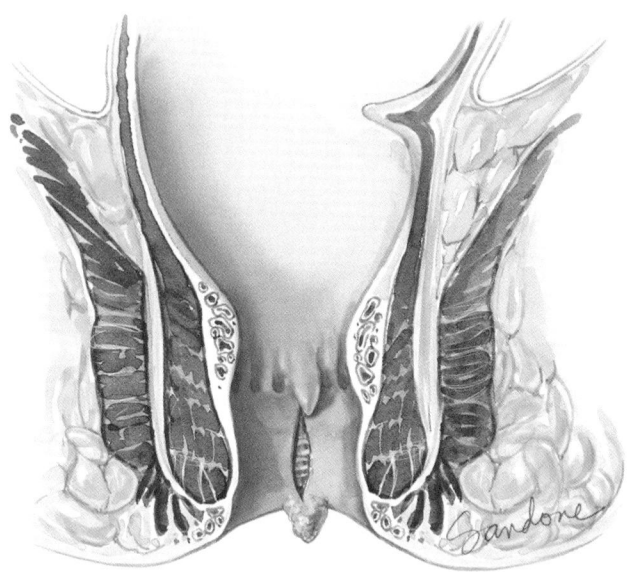

FIGURE 1 Chronic anal fissure exhibiting a sentinel pile and hypertrophied anal papilla. The internal sphincter muscle is seen within the bed of the fissure.

any patient past 1 year. Finally, no medical therapy came close to the efficacy of surgical sphincterotomy. However, none of the medical therapies in the randomized studies were associated with the risk of fecal incontinence.

Studies evaluating treatment for atypical anal fissures and anal fissures associated with inflammatory bowel disease are limited. It is important to emphasize the need for a biopsy, usually incisional or full thickness. If this is negative for infection, granuloma, or cancer, alternative therapies include fissurectomy or treatment with a local injection of steroid (Kenalog, Bristol-Myers Squibb, Princeton, NJ). Some authors have tried medical therapy aimed at reducing the anal resting tone. However, caution must be exercised in the use of medical therapy for the atypical fissure, since the pathophysiology of this fissure is unclear. Close follow-up is also recommended.

Surgical Therapy for Chronic Anal Fissure

The goal of the surgical approach to treatment of a chronic anal fissure is the relief of spasm of the internal anal sphincter. There are several operative techniques currently available to heal a chronic anal fissure by injuring the internal sphincter muscle. Historically, spasm of the internal anal sphincter muscle has been reduced with anal dilation. Because of the uncontrolled nature of this procedure, it has largely been replaced by the lateral internal sphincterotomy, which can be performed using an open or closed approach. In the open approach, a small incision is made in the intersphincteric groove (Figure 5). The internal sphincter muscle is identified and dissected

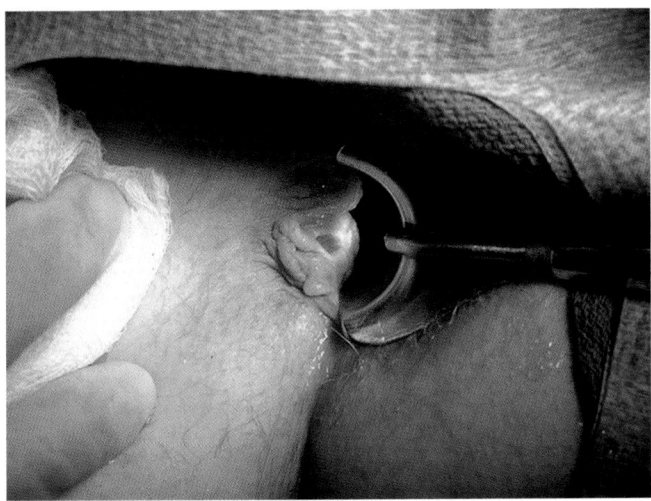

FIGURE 2 An exam under anesthesia reveals a prominent atypical lateral anal fissure or ulcer.

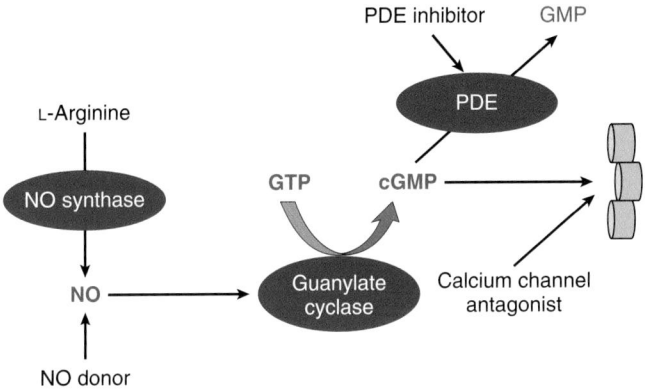

FIGURE 3 Biochemical mechanism for smooth muscle relaxation. *cGMP,* Cyclic guanosine monophosphate; *GMP,* guanosine monophosphate; *GTP,* guanosine triphosphate; *PDE,* phosphodiesterase.

TABLE 1: Nonsurgical therapy for anal fissure

Smooth muscle relaxation	Antiinflammatory	Pain control
Nitroglycerine ointment/patch	Topical hydrocortisone (Analpram-HC)	Topical anesthetic (Lidocaine)
Calcium channel antagonists (diltiazem, nifedipine)	Injectable steroid (Kenalog)	Clove oil
Phosphodiesterase inhibitors (sildenafil, minoxidil)		
α-Adrenoceptor antagonist (indoramin)		
Botulinum toxin injection		
Anal dilators		
L-Arginine		
Sitz baths		

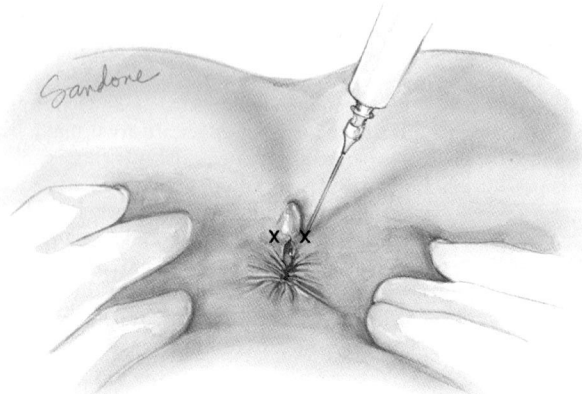

FIGURE 4   Botulinum toxin used in the treatment of a chronic anal fissure is injected here into the internal anal sphincter at both lateral edges of the fissure.

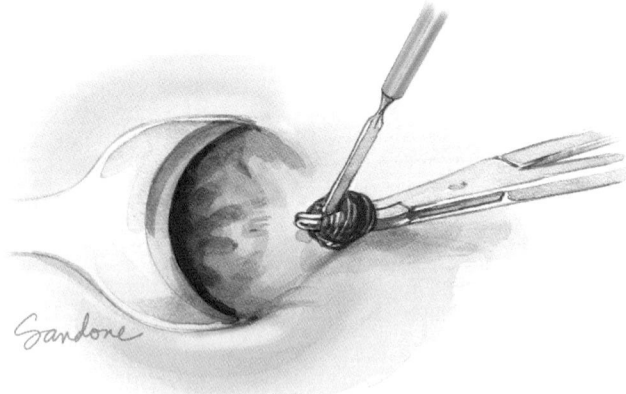

FIGURE 6   The hypertrophied internal sphincter is identified and elevated out of the wound. The sphincter is then divided using electrocautery.

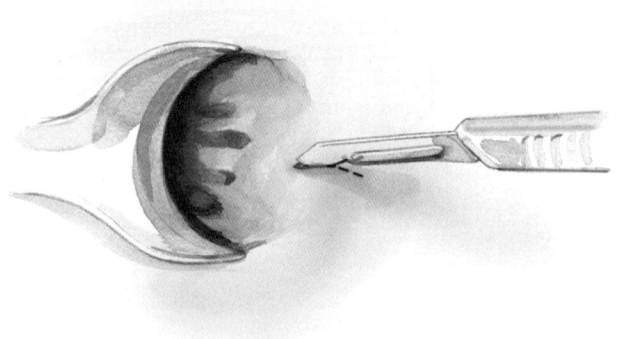

FIGURE 5   With the patient in the prone position, an incision is made in the intersphincteric grove on the right because less hemorrhoidal disease is found on the right side of the anus in the lateral position than on the left side.

free from the surrounding tissue and divided under direct vision with electrocautery (Figure 6). The wound is irrigated and closed with an absorbable suture. The closed technique has the same treatment goal; however, the procedure is performed with a scalpel blade, which is guided by palpation of the internal sphincter muscle (Figure 7). In both procedures, the sphincter muscle that is divided should at least include the muscle that is hypertrophied. It has been recommended by several investigators that the sphincter division should start at the dentate line. This procedure is associated with healing rates of greater than 90% and therefore remains the treatment of choice for those patients failing medical therapy.

The major drawback from surgical cutting or injury to the internal anal sphincter muscle is the risk of fecal incontinence. Recently, several reports have indicated that the rate of incontinence can be greater than 20%. However, it has recently been pointed out by a Cochrane review of surgery for anal fissure that although incontinence rates were reportedly higher, especially to flatus, that after fissure healing occurred, quality of life remained good despite the incontinence. Recently, a procedure introduced largely in Europe, the fissurectomy with or without advancement flap closure, has gained popularity because there is no direct injury that occurs to the anal sphincter muscles. In this procedure, the fissure is excised using a scalpel or scissors. If the wound edges are healthy, the anoderm is advanced downward or the skin is advanced upward to cover the sphincter complex. No internal sphincter muscle is cut; however, in

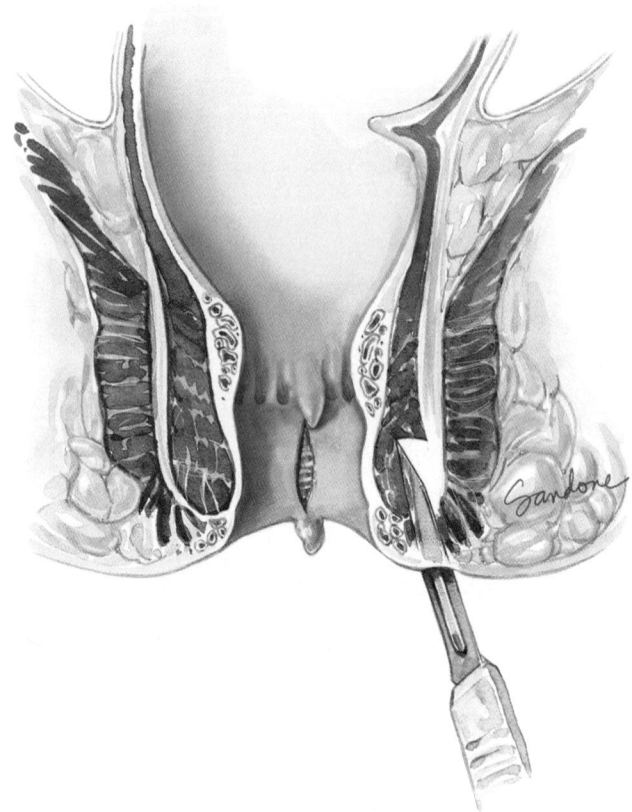

FIGURE 7   The closed lateral internal sphincterotomy is performed using an 11 blade scalpel along with gentle palpation of the anal sphincter complex.

some series, Botox was injected at the end of the procedure. The rate of incontinence associated with this procedure is less than 10%.

Treatment Algorithm

Once an anal fissure is diagnosed, it is important to determine the length of time it has been present. For any fissure that has been present for less than 6 weeks (acute), the treatment of choice is warm sitz baths, increased intake of dietary fiber, and stool softeners. Regardless of length of time, all patients with fissures should be educated on the benefits of a high fiber diet. If no healing of the anal fissure occurs, medical therapy with calcium channel antagonists for 6 weeks is the author's first choice. If a patient presents initially with a chronic anal fissure and has not tried medical therapy, medical therapy for a 6-week trial is initially attempted. If pain improves, then no further treatment is necessary. If pain recurs in less than 6 weeks, surgery should be considered. Otherwise, a repeat trial of medical therapy can be offered. The author favors medical approaches in female patients because of the increased risk of fecal incontinence. The surgical treatment of choice is lateral internal sphincterotomy. In this procedure, at a minimum, the hypertrophied portion of the internal anal sphincter should be divided. If the risk of incontinence is high, fissurectomy with advancement flap should be considered.

ACKNOWLEDGMENT

The author would like to acknowledge Corrine Sandone for her help in preparing the figures.

SUGGESTED READINGS

Garg P, Garg M, Menon G: Long term continence disturbance after lateral internal sphincterotomy for chronic anal fissure: a systematic review and meta-analysis, *Colorectal Dis* 2013 Epub.
Mousavi S, Sharifi M, Mehdikhah Z: A comparison between the results of fissurectomy and lateral internal sphincterotomy in the surgical management of chronic anal fissure, *J Gastrointest Surg* 13:1279–1282, 2009.
Nelson RL, Chattopadhyay A, Brooks W, Platt I, Paavana T, Earl S: Operative procedures for fissure in ano (review), *Cochrane Database Syst Rev* 11:1–39, 2011.
Nelson RL, Thomas K, Morgan J, Jones A: Non surgical therapy for anal fissure (review), *Cochrane Database Syst Rev* 2:1–91, 2012.
Poh A, Tan K, Seow-Choen F: Innovations in chronic anal fissure treatment: a systematic review, *World J Gastrointest Surg* 2(7):231–241, 2012.

ANORECTAL ABSCESS AND FISTULA

Jennifer Blumetti, MD, FACS, and
Jose R. Cintron, MD, FACS

INTRODUCTION

Anorectal abscesses and anal fistulas are very common, affecting thousands of patients annually, and were described in the literature as early as 400 BC by Hippocrates. The most common etiology is cryptoglandular, blockage of the anal crypts that leads to infection of the anal glands and results in suppuration. Abscesses result in anal fistula in 40% to 60% of cases, and the two entities may be considered a progression of the same disease, with abscess the acute state and fistula the chronic state. The treatment of abscesses has remained largely unchanged over time. Wide drainage remains the mainstay of treatment. The treatment of anal fistula has changed dramatically over the years. Fistulotomy with or without seton drainage has traditionally been the treatment for anal fistula. More recently, noncutting or sphincter-sparing techniques have been developed as a result of concerns for varying degrees of incontinence arising from division of the anal sphincter. Approaches to the patient with anorectal abscess and fistula are presented.

ABSCESS

Anorectal abscesses arise from cryptoglandular infection in up to 90% of patients, although other causes such as Crohn's disease or the downward progression of pelvic sepsis, such as diverticulitis or appendicitis, can also occur. Other uncommon causes of abscess are trauma and atypical infections such as tuberculosis. Abscesses are most commonly classified on the basis of location as perianal, ischiorectal, intermuscular, intersphincteric, submucosal, or supralevator

(Figure 1). Abscesses that originate in the deep postanal space may track to the ischiorectal fossa either unilaterally or bilaterally, resulting in a horseshoe abscess (Figure 2, *A*).

Diagnosis

Diagnosis of abscess is typically clinical, although imaging may be useful in selected cases. Patients typically report anal pain. Swelling and fever are also common symptoms. A thorough physical examination is necessary to rule out other causes of anal pain, such as fissure or thrombosed hemorrhoid. Erythema, palpable swelling, and tenderness are typically seen with perianal or ischiorectal abscesses. Fullness on digital rectal examination in the posterior anal canal is indicative of a deep postanal space abscess, and exquisite tenderness on digital examination without any external signs may be indicative of an intersphincteric abscess. If abscess is suspected but examination cannot be completed because of patient discomfort, then examination with anesthesia should be performed. Patients with systemic symptoms such as fever, tachycardia, and elevation of white blood cell count with few physical findings may have a supralevator abscess and could benefit from computed tomographic (CT) scan imaging to aid in diagnosis. Necrotizing soft tissue infection should be suspected if the patient has systemic signs combined with erythema, crepitus, induration, blistering, "dishwater" drainage, or overt gangrene of the tissue (Figure 3, *A*).

Treatment

The mainstay of treatment is adequate drainage of the abscess. Antibiotics alone do not play a role, although they may be indicated as an adjunct in patients with significant cellulitis, diabetes, or immunosuppression (patients with acquired immune deficiency syndrome (AIDS), chemotherapy, or transplant). Surgical drainage of simple perianal or superficial ischiorectal abscesses may be performed in the office or emergency room setting with a local anesthetic. Instillation of lidocaine with epinephrine is performed around the area to be drained. An elliptic incision is then made over the area of fluctuance to drain the abscess (Figure 4). Packing is typically not necessary for smaller abscesses. Some practitioners prefer to place a small mushroom catheter in the cavity to allow for drainage.

Larger ischiorectal abscesses and suspected intersphincteric abscesses should be drained in the operating room with regional or general anesthesia. Intersphincteric abscesses should be unroofed. Large ischiorectal abscesses should not be unroofed over the length of the abscess; rather, multiple counter incisions should be made and

Penrose drains placed between the incisions to allow for drainage. This prevents a large defect and allows for better wound healing. A horseshoe or hemihorseshoe abscess involving the deep postanal space should be managed with opening of the deep postanal space and counter incisions made over the lateral aspects of the abscess. This is done through a radial incision made in the posterior midline between the anus and the coccyx. The external sphincter and the anococcygeal ligament are spread in the midline, which allows for drainage of the deep postanal space. The responsible anal gland is drained by dividing the distal aspect of the internal sphincter in the posterior midline. Counter incisions are then made and connected to the deep postanal space with Penrose drains to fully drain the abscess. If a fistula is present, a seton should also be placed (see Figure 2, *B* to *D*).

Necrotizing infections are managed with broad-spectrum antibiotics to cover gram-positive, gram-negative, and anaerobic organisms. Prompt wide surgical débridement to healthy tissue should then be performed. Several reexaminations in the operating room may be necessary to adequately treat this aggressive disease (see Figure 3, *B*).

FISTULAS

Anal fistulas occur in almost half of the patients with anorectal abscess. They are most commonly cryptoglandular in origin with internal openings located at the level of the dentate line, but they can also occur with Crohn's disease, obstetric injuries, or trauma. Fistulas are typically classified by anatomic location as described by Parks in 1976 (Figure 5). Intersphincteric fistulas involve only partial amounts of the internal sphincter muscle, and transsphincteric fistulas involve varying amounts of both internal and external sphincter muscle. Transsphincteric fistulas can also be classified as low or high depending on the amount of sphincter muscle involved, with low transsphincteric fistulas involving the distal one third of the external sphincter and high transsphincteric fistulas involving more than half

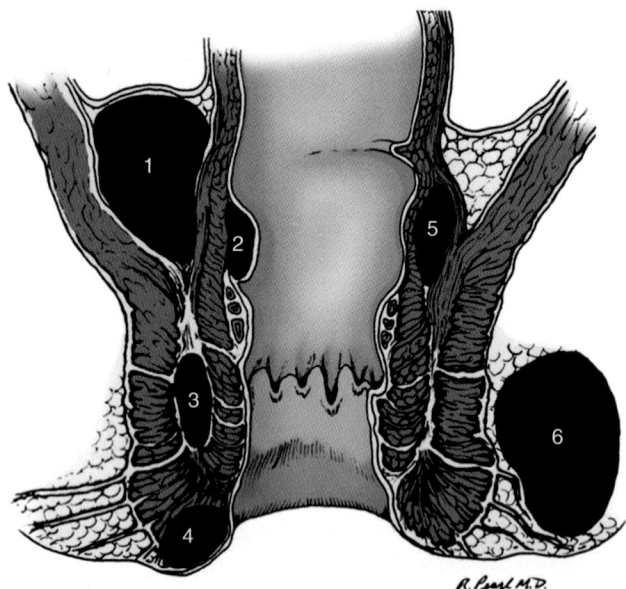

FIGURE 1 Abscess location: *1,* supralevator; *2,* submucosal; *3,* intersphincteric; *4,* perianal; *5,* intermuscular; *6,* ischiorectal. *(Original illustration provided by Dr. Russell Pearl.)*

FIGURE 2 Horseshoe abscess and fistula. **A,** Horseshoe abscess with arrows shows that the deep postanal space is a window to the bilateral ischiorectal fossa. **B,** Clamp in deep postanal space, with *arrow* pointing to the internal fistula opening. Seton is loosely encircling the fistula tract. **C,** Deep postanal space drained via a radial incision in the posterior midline, with seton in place. **D,** Teardrop-shaped counter incisions drain the ischiorectal fossa and are connected with Penrose drains. *(Original illustration provided by Dr. Russell Pearl.)*

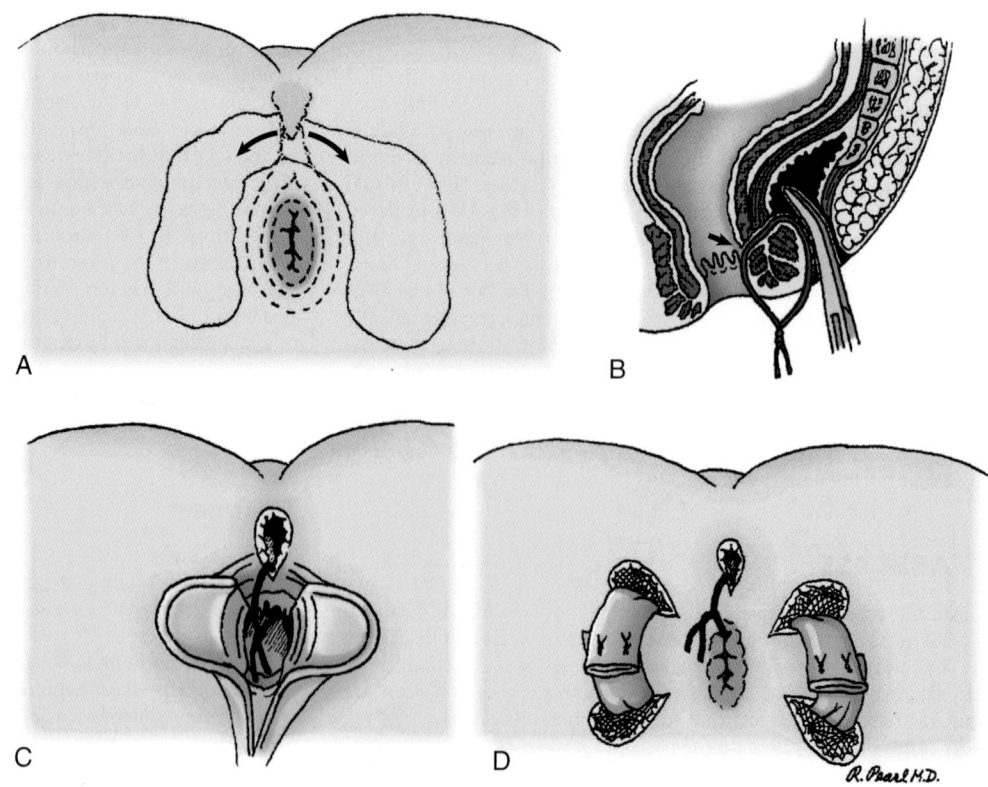

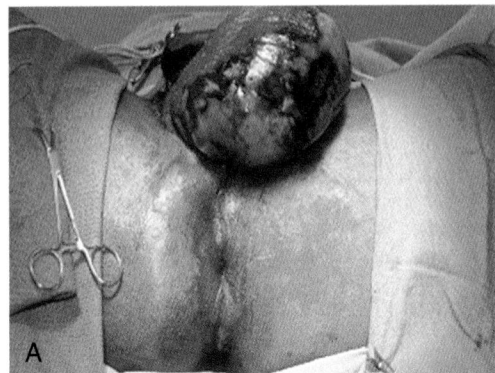
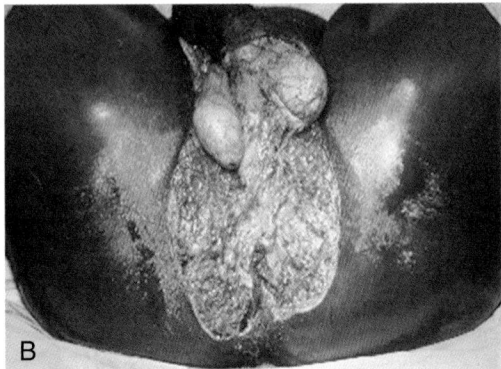

FIGURE 3 Necrotizing soft tissue infection. **A,** Necrotizing soft tissue infection involving the bilateral ischiorectal fossa and scrotum. **B,** Appearance after wide débridement. *(Photographs provided by Dr. Jose Cintron.)*

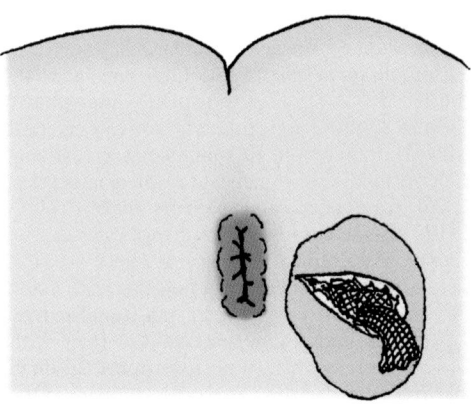

R. Pearl M.D.

FIGURE 4 Incision and drainage of abscess. An elliptic incision has been made to drain the abscess and packing placed. *(Original illustration provided by Dr. Russell Pearl.)*

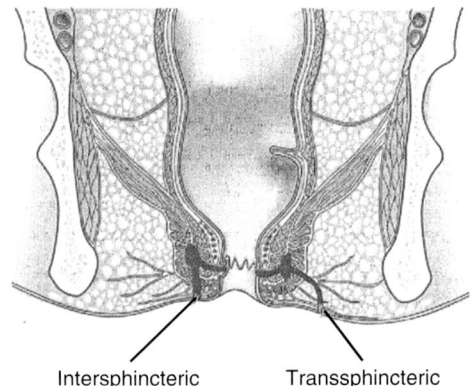
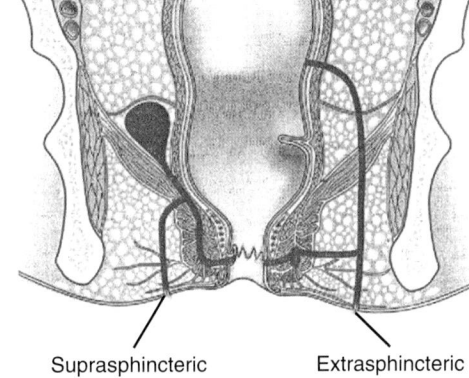

Intersphincteric   Transsphincteric   Suprasphincteric   Extrasphincteric

FIGURE 5 Park's classification of anal fistula.

of the external sphincter muscle. The less common suprasphincteric fistulas involve the entire external sphincter. Extrasphincteric fistulas are rare; they are typically not cryptoglandular in origin but may result from trauma, perforation of the rectum from foreign body, or Crohn's disease or can be iatrogenic.

Diagnosis

The diagnosis of anal fistula should be suspected in patients with a history of anorectal abscess that does not heal. A patient typically reports pain or purulent or bloody discharge and gives a history of a surgically or spontaneously drained abscess. Systemic signs are typically absent unless an undrained abscess is present. A history of prior anorectal surgery should be elicited, and the patient's continence should also be assessed before any intervention.

On examination, an external fistula opening is easily identified. A thorough examination should be made to evaluate for the number and location of the openings in relation to the sphincter complex. A palpable cord from the external opening toward the anal canal may be present. Internal examination with anoscopy should reveal the internal opening, although this may need to be performed with anesthesia because of patient discomfort. A history of a change in bowel habits, multiple external fistula openings, internal openings at a location other than the dentate line, or multiple internal openings should alert the examiner to the possibility of atypical causes of fistula such as Crohn's disease, human immunodeficiency virus (HIV), or malignancy.

Goodsall's rule (Figure 6) predicts the location of the internal opening based on the location of the external opening and is accurate in most cases. External fistula openings located posteriorly typically have internal openings in the posterior midline and a curved tract.

Anteriorly based fistulas typically have a radial course to the internal opening. Exceptions to Goodsall's rule may occur when the external fistula openings are located greater than 3 cm from the anal verge anteriorly. These likely have internal openings in the posterior midline.

Examination with anesthesia is an essential part of the diagnosis of suspected anal fistula. The accurate location and number of internal openings and their relationship to the sphincter muscles should be clearly delineated. Placement of a probe from the external opening to the internal opening should be performed, but with caution because aggressive probing may result in iatrogenic injury and creation of false tracts. The instillation of hydrogen peroxide into the external opening may help with identification of internal fistula openings. Endoanal ultrasound scan and fistulography may also aid in identification of internal openings in the operating room. Magnetic resonance imaging (MRI) can also be used if no internal opening can be identified in the operating room.

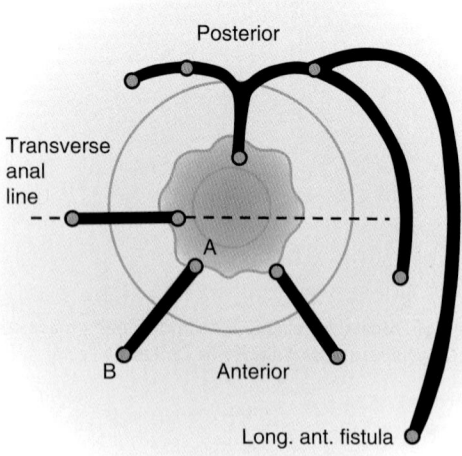

FIGURE 6 Goodsall's rule. A line is drawn transversely *(A)*. External openings anterior to this line track to the anus in a radial fashion *(B)*, and external openings posterior to this line track in a curvilinear fashion to the posterior midline. *(From Townsend CM, Beauchamp RD, Evers BM, et al, editors: Sabiston textbook of surgery, ed 19, Philadelphia, 2012, Elsevier Saunders, Fig 53-20.)*

Treatment

The treatment of anal fistula can be divided into cutting or noncutting (sphincter-sparing) procedures. Cutting procedures include simple fistulotomy or staged fistulotomy. Sphincter-sparing procedures include seton placement, endorectal or dermal advancement flap, fibrin sealant, anal fistula plug, and ligation of the intersphincteric fistula tract (LIFT). The choice of treatment is based on location of the fistula tract in relation to the sphincter muscles, the status of the patient's continence, and the number and type of prior anal procedures. These procedures are typically performed with regional or general anesthesia and with the patient in the prone jackknife position.

PRIMARY FISTULOTOMY

Fistulotomy has been considered the gold standard in the treatment of anal fistulas. Simple or primary fistulotomy can be safely performed in superficial fistulas (i.e., fissure fistulas), intersphincteric fistulas, and low transsphincteric fistulas (1/3 or less external sphincter muscle involved). Populations in which primary fistulotomy should not be performed are women with anterior fistulas, patients with disturbed continence, and patients with Crohn's disease or advanced HIV disease because incontinence rates can be high with this procedure. Fistulotomy is performed by placing a probe through the fistula tract and then unroofing the tract along its length (Figure 7). The wound can then be marsupialized by suturing the edges of the wound to the base of the tract with absorbable suture, which decreases the time for wound healing. Fistulotomy can be performed at the time of abscess drainage if the internal opening is readily visualized, such as in intersphincteric abscess or fistulas.

SETONS

A seton is commonly used in anal fistulas that cannot be treated with primary fistulotomy alone. High transphincteric fistulas, suprasphincteric fistulas, and anterior fistulas in women and in patients with HIV or Crohn's disease typically have a seton placed as part of the treatment. A seton can be used in one of three ways. First, setons can be used to drain sepsis and allow for identification of the tract at a subsequent operation. These setons are typically loosely tied, heavy-duty, nonabsorbable braided sutures that promote fibrosis and

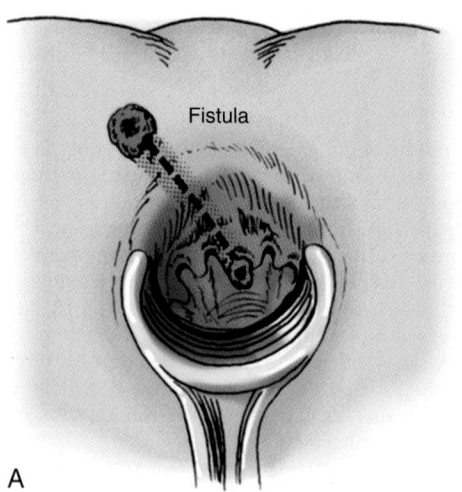
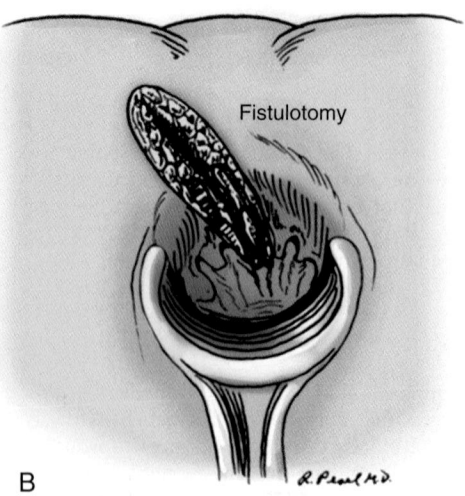

FIGURE 7 Primary fistulotomy. **A,** The fistula tract is identified. **B,** The tract is opened along its length. *(Original illustration provided by Dr. Russell Pearl.)*

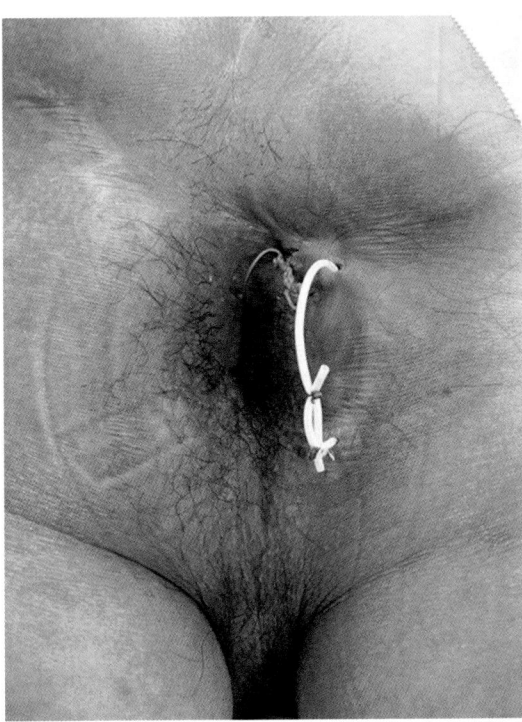

maturation of the tract before a definitive operation, either fistulotomy or a sphincter-sparing procedure (Figure 8). This may be performed in conjunction with a partial fistulotomy in which the distal part of the internal sphincter is divided and the seton placed in the remaining tract. The fistulotomy is then completed 8 to 12 weeks later once the first stage has healed. The second use of the seton is for patients in whom the seton may be the definitive procedure or in whom fibrosis is not desired (e.g., because of Crohn's disease or advanced HIV). In these patients, a vessel loop may be used as a seton to allow for drainage and prevent recurrent abscess formation (see Figure 8). The third technique is the use of a cutting seton. In this procedure, the skin overlying the fistula tract is opened, and a heavy braided suture, vessel loop, or rubber band is placed into the fistula tract and tied snugly. This is then tightened every 1 to 2 weeks with suture or rubber band placed via a hemorrhoid ligature, allowing for pressure necrosis to slowly cut through the sphincter muscles. This technique can result in significant incontinence rates and is used infrequently.

ADVANCEMENT FLAPS

Endorectal advancement flaps were originally described in 1912 by Elting and are used as an alternative to cutting procedures. Endorectal advancement flaps are commonly performed in high transsphincteric fistulas, in low transsphincteric fistulas in women, and in Crohn's fistulas if the patient has normal rectal mucosa. Endorectal flaps can be performed as a primary procedure or subsequent to seton drainage (Figure 9). The fistula tract should be curetted, and

FIGURE 8 Setons in place. The seton in the posterior midline is a nonabsorbable braided suture. The seton on the right is a vessel loop. *(Photograph provided by Dr. Jose Cintron.)*

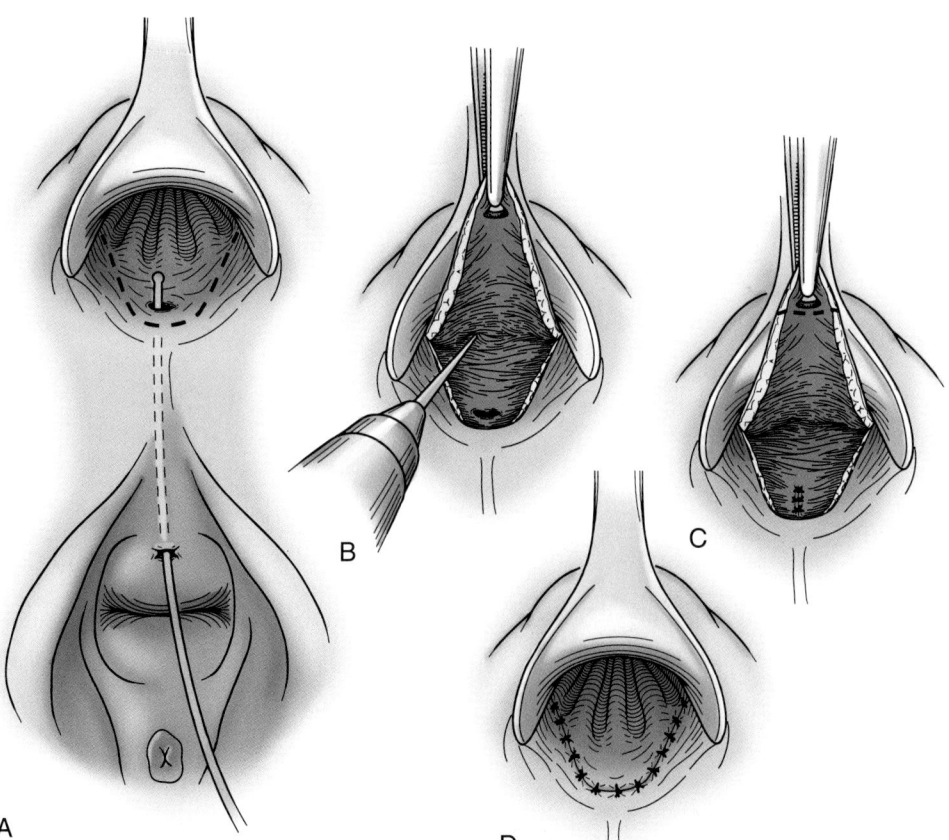

FIGURE 9 Endorectal advancement flap. **A,** A probe is placed through the tract. The flap extends distally to the internal opening. **B,** The flap is raised 4 to 6 cm. **C,** The distal aspect of the flap is excised, and the internal opening in the muscle is sutured. **D,** The flap is then sutured into place with interrupted suture. *(From Hyman N: Endoanal advancement flap repair for complex anorectal fistulas, Am J Surg 178:337–340, 1999.)*

the internal opening is then excised. A flap of mucosa, submucosa, and superficial circular muscle is created, extended 4 to 6 cm proximal to the internal opening to allow for a tension-free closure. The base of the flap provides the blood supply to the flap and should be twice the width of the apex of the flap. The internal opening is then closed with absorbable suture, and the flap then advanced and sutured to the dentate line. The external opening is widened to allow for drainage. This procedure is not appropriate for fistulas with internal openings that are distal to the dentate line. If the flap is sutured too distal, then the result is a mucosal ectropion. Success rates for this procedure range from 75% to 98%.

Dermal advancement flaps were originally used for mucosal ectropion and anal stenosis but were modified to treat anal fistulas. This technique involves creation of a pear-shaped incision that extends from just proximal to the internal opening and then to the external opening (Figure 10). The full-thickness flap is raised by deepening the incision lateral to the external sphincter muscle. Care is taken not to undermine the incision because the blood supply to the flap could become compromised. The internal opening is then excised and closed with absorbable suture. The flap is then advanced into the anal canal and sutured just proximal to the internal opening with interrupted absorbable suture. The donor site is left open to heal by secondary intention. This type of flap reduces the risk of mucosal ectropion and has a success rate of 77%.

FIBRIN SEALANT

The use of fibrin sealant is appealing because it has a low morbidity and no risk of incontinence and can be repeated if necessary. This technique is beneficial in longer rather than shorter fistula tracts. Typically, the patient has had a seton placed before the procedure to allow drainage of any infection. The fistula tract is then curetted. The commercially prepared product, such as Tisseel (Baxter Healthcare, Deerfield, Ill), is used. The two components of the sealant are injected through a dual-lumen catheter that has been inserted into the external opening and advanced to the internal opening. The catheter is slowly withdrawn during injection until a "pearly" coagulant is seen at the internal opening. Success rates with this procedure range from 14% to 40% (Figure 11).

FISTULA PLUG

The anal fistula plug is also a noncutting, sphincter-sparing technique and, similar to fibrin glue, has low morbidity and can be repeated if necessary. The ideal candidate for this procedure is one with a transsphincteric fistula who has had prior drainage with a

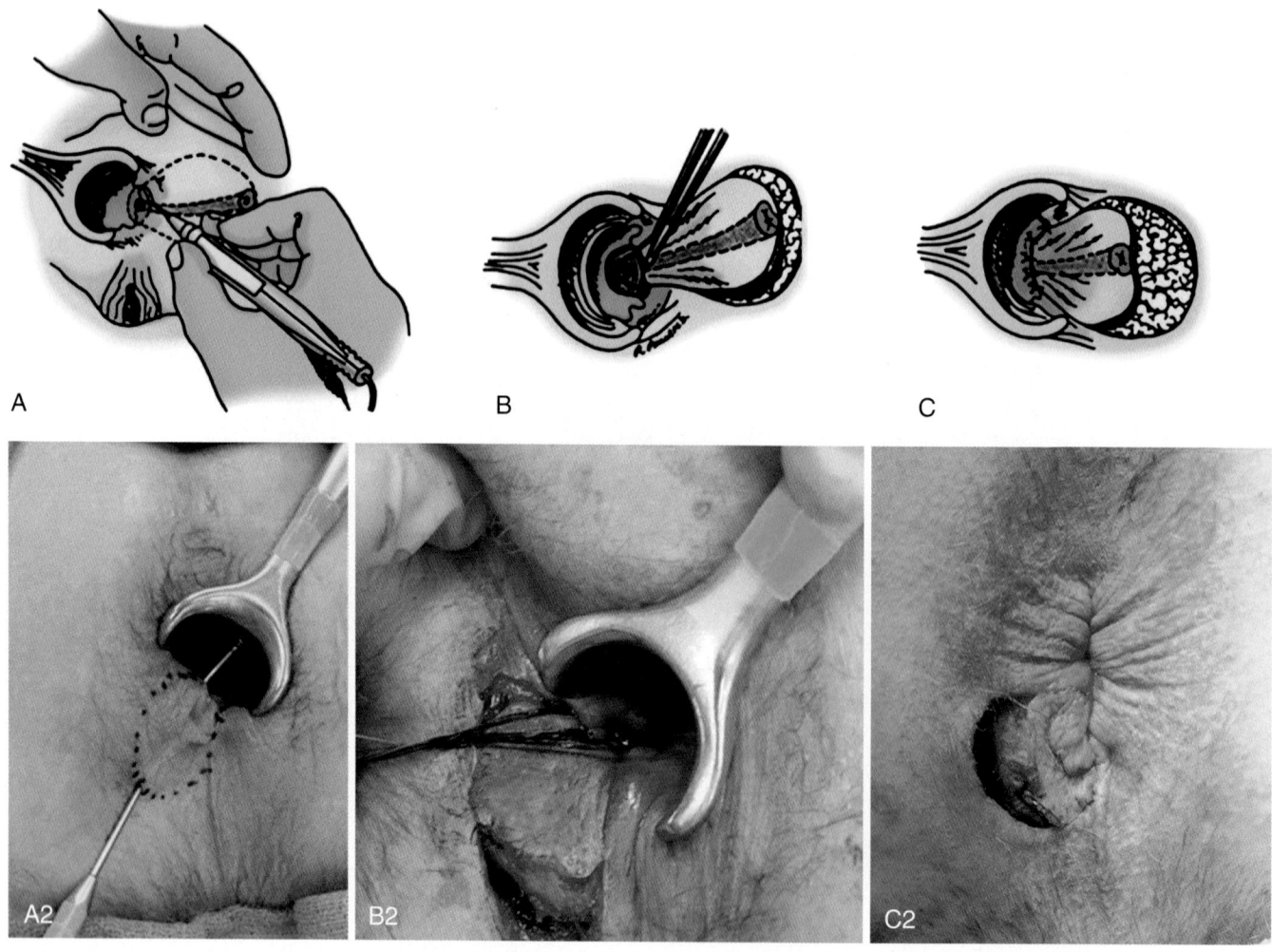

FIGURE 10   Dermal advancement flap. **A,** The U-shaped flap is created to encompass the external opening. **B,** The internal opening is excised, and the full-thickness flap is raised, advanced into the anal canal, and sutured into place. **C,** The final appearance of the flap. *(Illustrations from Nelson RL, Cintron J, Abcarian H: Dermal island-flap anoplasty for transsphincteric fistula-in-ano: assessment of treatment failures, Dis Colon Rectum 43:681–684, 2000. Photographs provided by Dr. Jose Cintron.)*

seton for 6 to 12 weeks before placement of the plug. Plugs may be made of treated porcine submucosa (Cook Biodesign; Cook Medical, Bloomington, Ind) or synthetic bioabsorbable polymer (Gore Bio-A; W. L. Gore and Associates, Flagstaff, Ariz; Figure 12) The fistula tract should be curetted, and the external opening débrided. The plug is then advanced from the internal opening to the external opening, until the base of the plug is seated at the internal opening. The plug is then sutured to the internal opening with absorbable suture to close the internal opening over the plug. The excess plug at the external opening is trimmed, and the external opening left open. Success rates have been reported primarily for the porcine submucosa plug and range from 43% to 87%.

LIGATION OF INTERSPHINCTERIC FISTULA TRACT

One of the more recently developed procedures for anal fistula, the ligation of the LIFT, was originally described by Rojanasakul in 2007. The procedure is ideal for transsphincteric fistulas with mature tracts, and most patients have had seton drainage before

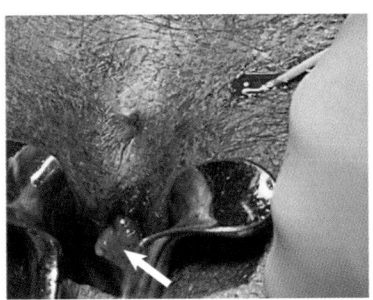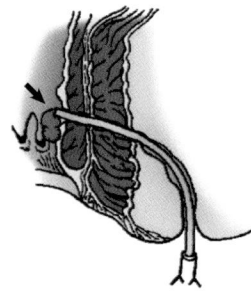

FIGURE 11 Fibrin sealant. The sealant is injected via a long catheter through the external opening and into the internal opening. The *arrow* shows the sealant at the internal opening. *(From Singer M, Cintron J: New techniques in the treatment of common perianal diseases: stapled hemorrhoidopexy, botulinum toxin and fibrin sealant, Surg Clin North Am 86(4):937–967, 2006, Fig. 2.)*

this procedure. A curvilinear incision is made just lateral to the intersphincteric groove. The internal and external sphincter muscles are separated in the intersphincteric space; no sphincter muscle is divided. A probe is placed within the fistula tract, and the tract is isolated circumferentially within the intersphincteric groove. It is then ligated proximally and distally with absorbable sutures after the probe is removed. The tract is then divided, or alternately a segment is excised. The incision is then closed with absorbable suture, and the external opening is widened to allow for drainage (Figure 13). Early success rates have ranged from 57% to 89%.

CHOICE OF PROCEDURE

A proposed treatment algorithm for anal fistula can be seen in Figure 14. Simple low-lying fistulas can almost always be treated with primary fistulotomy with high success rates and low incontinence rates, except in patients with Crohn's disease or HIV, in women with anterior fistulas, or in patients who have undergone sphincter division in the past. Fistulas with a significant amount of sphincter involvement and an associated abscess should first undergo drainage of the abscess and placement of a loosely tied seton, with a plan to return to the operating room for definitive surgery in 6 to 12 weeks. If there is a well-defined tract at reoperation, then a LIFT procedure is appropriate. Longer tracts may be amenable to fibrin sealant or fistula plug, which can be repeated if the fistula recurs. Endorectal flaps should be performed in fistulas with internal openings at the dentate line. Those with internal openings distal to the dentate line may be candidates for dermal flaps.

CONCLUSION

Anorectal abscesses and fistulas are very common diseases that result from infection of the anal crypts and glands. Wide drainage continues to be the mainstay of abscess treatment. Surgical procedures for anal fistula are trending toward more sphincter-sparing procedures and away from fistulotomy as the sole treatment. The surgeon should understand the various techniques used in the treatment of anal fistula so that treatment can be tailored to the individual patient.

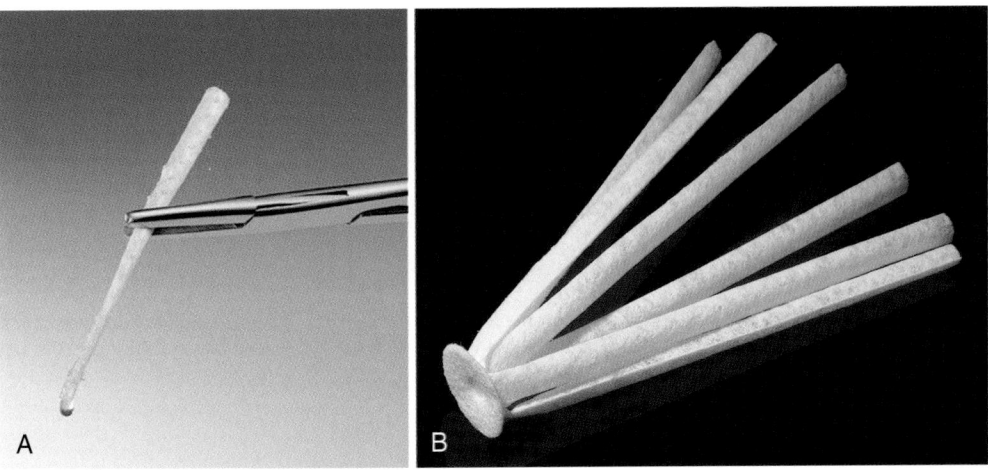

FIGURE 12 Fistula plugs. **A,** Porcine submucosa plug. **B,** Synthetic polymer.

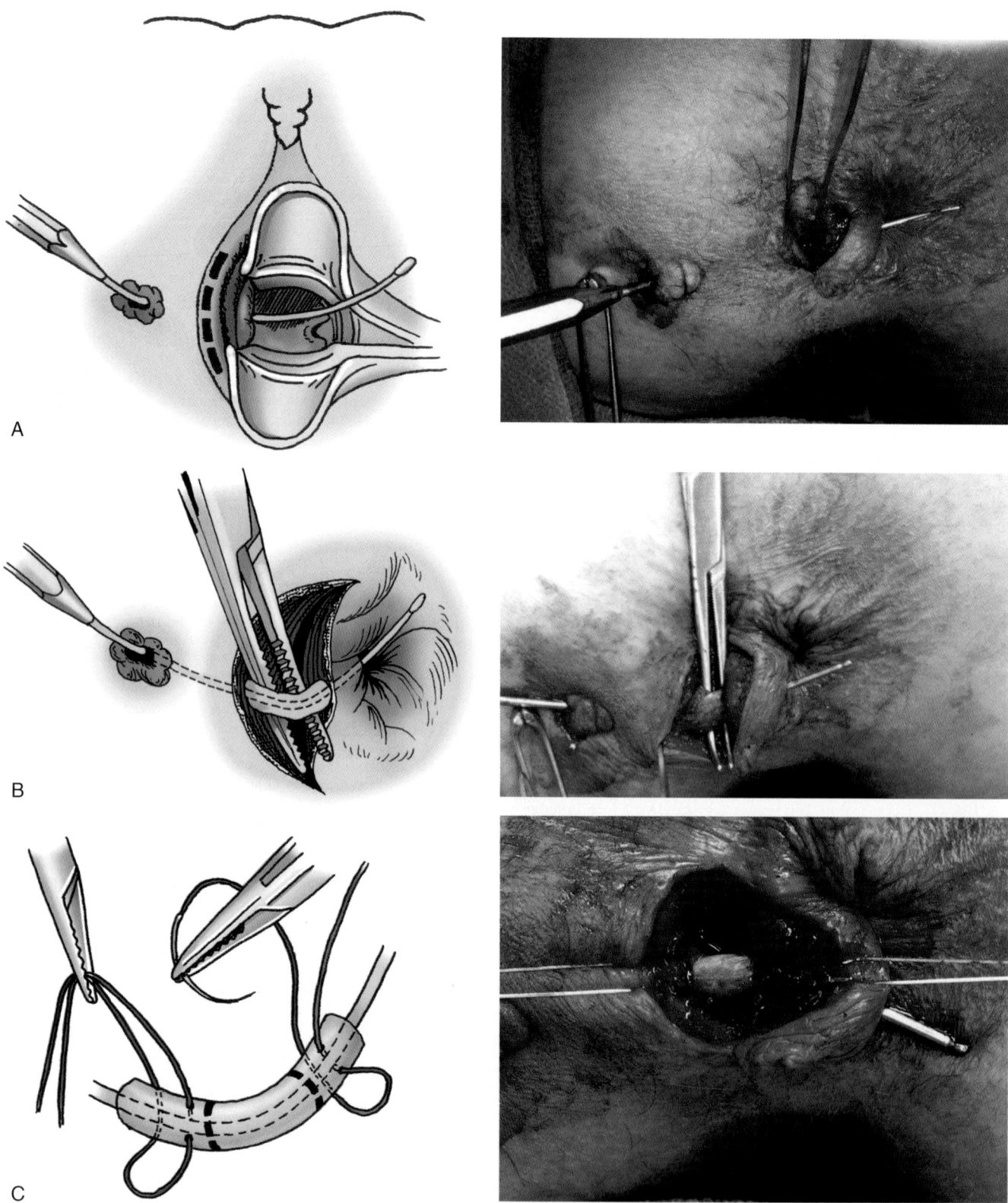

FIGURE 13 Ligation of intersphincteric fistula tract. **A,** A fistula probe is placed through the tract, a curvilinear incision is made, and the muscle is separated in the intersphincteric groove. **B,** The fistula tract is dissected free. **C,** Sutures are placed around the tract and tied once the probe is removed.

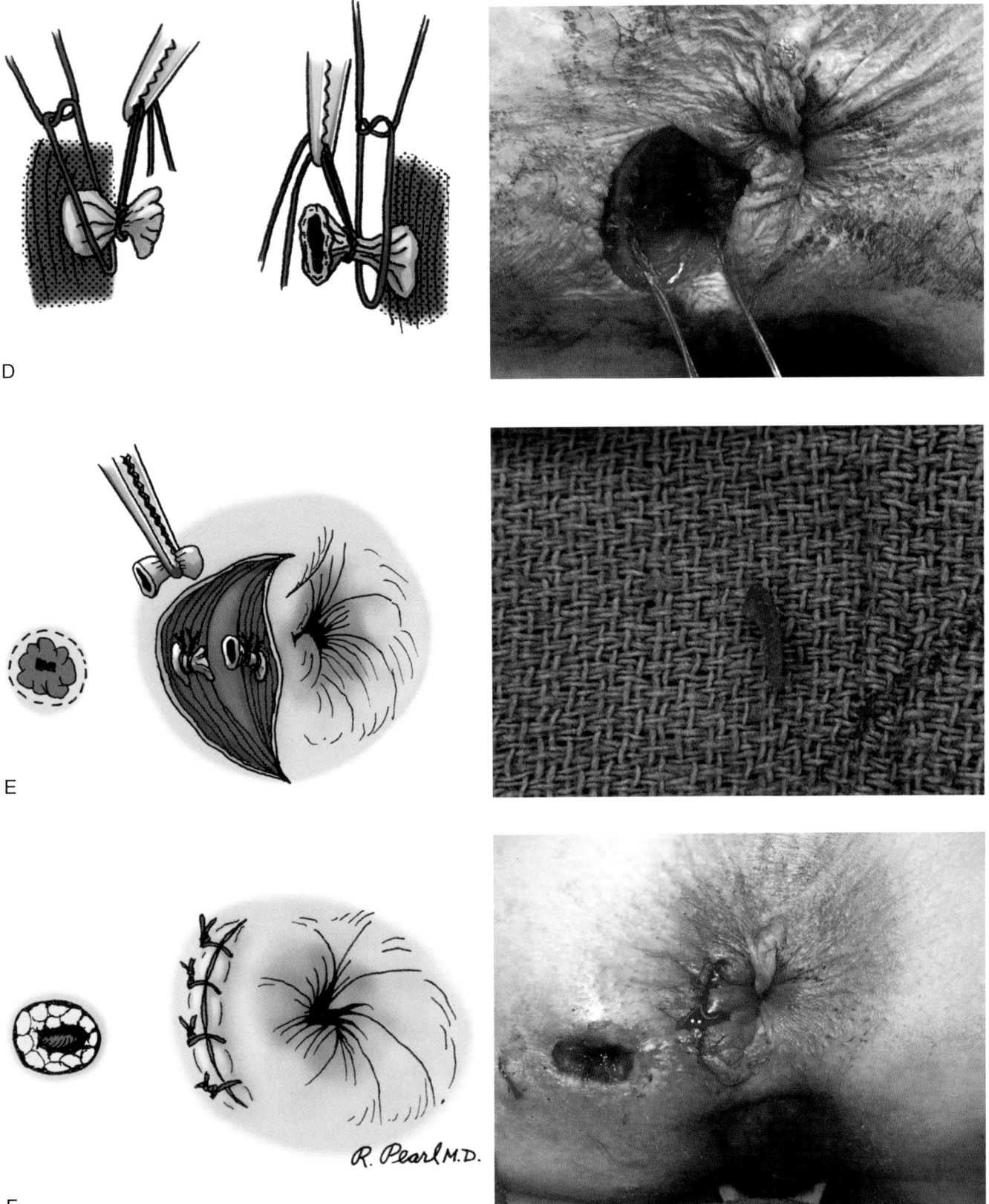

FIGURE 13 cont'd D, The tract is divided. **E,** A portion of the tract is excised if possible. **F,** The incision is closed, and the external opening is excised. *(Illustrations from Abcarian AM, Estrada JJ, Park J, et al: Ligation of intersphincteric fistula tract: early results of a pilot study, Dis Colon Rectum 55(7):778–782, 2012. Photographs provided by Dr. Jose Cintron.)*

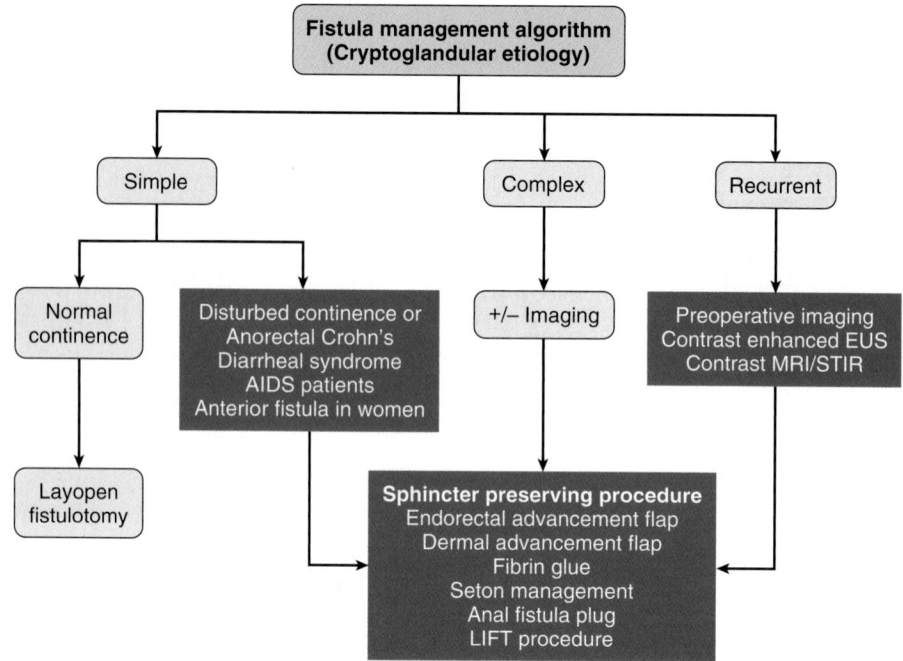

FIGURE 14 Algorithm for treatment of fistula. *EUS,* Endoscopic ultrasound scan; *LIFT,* intersphincteric fistula tract; *MRI,* magnetic resonance imaging; *STIR,* short T1 inversion recovery.

SUGGESTED READINGS

Abcarian AM, Estrada JJ, Park J, et al: Ligation of intersphincteric fistula tract: early results of a pilot study, *Dis Colon Rectum* 55(7):778–782, 2012.
Abcarian H: Anorectal infection: abscess-fistula, *Clin Colon Rectal Surg* 24:14–21, 2011.

Blumetti J, Abcarian A, Quinteros F, et al: The evolution of treatment of fistula in ano, *World J Surg* 36(5):1162–1167, 2012.
Vasilevsky C: Anorectal abscess and fistula. In Beck DE, Roberts PL, Saclarides, TJ, editors: *The ASCRS textbook of colon and rectal surgery,* New York, 2011, Springer, pp 219–244.

ANORECTAL STRICTURE

**Bard C. Cosman, MD, MPH, and
Yarah M. Haidar, MD**

DEFINITION

A *rectal stricture* is a nondistensible narrowing of the rectum that may interfere with free flow of the fecal stream. An *anal stricture* is a nondistensible narrowing of the anal canal that may interfere with defecation. The term *anorectal stricture* covers both conditions, although an individual patient typically has either one or the other and not both. Both conditions have been defined functionally as either the inability to pass a 12-mm diameter sigmoidoscope through the narrowed area or the inability to pass stool without pain because of partial obstruction of the lumen. Older sources describe benign and malignant stricture, but it is now customary to discuss only benign conditions under the heading of stricture; obstructing rectal and anal cancers are discussed under those headings. The term *stenosis,* synonymous with stricture, is most commonly applied to the muscle spasm that accompanies anal fissure—a functional rather than structural stenosis that is discussed under the heading of anal fissure. Congenital strictures are almost never seen in the adult patient, and they are covered in pediatric surgical texts as anorectal malformations or under the general heading "imperforate anus."

CAUSES

Benign, acquired anorectal strictures are caused by fibrosis, a nonspecific response to inflammation.

Rectal stricture may follow proctitis arising in inflammatory bowel disease (IBD), tuberculous or amebic proctitis, proctitis from venereal infections (syphilis, gonorrhea, *Chlamydia trachomatis, Herpes simplex),* radiation proctitis from prostate or cervical cancer treatment, and trauma from instrumentation. Suppositories, especially those that contain ergotamine or nonsteroidal antiinflammatory drugs, have been implicated. Probably the most common cause for rectal stricture in developed countries is iatrogenic, from a strictured surgical anastomosis.

Anal stricture may follow any inflammatory condition, including anal fistula, burns, and radiation injury from anal cancer treatment. Ulcerating anal infections such as chancroids and *H. simplex* may cause stricture, especially when they are chronic or recurrent. The most common cause for anal stricture is again iatrogenic, from excision of anoderm during anal operations for hemorrhoids, warts, and fistula.

CLINICAL PRESENTATION

Because of the extreme variability of fecal consistency and bowel habits, little correlation is found between the severity of anorectal stricture and the severity of symptoms. Symptoms may include pain, constipation, decreased stool caliber, difficulty in defecation, tenesmus, bleeding, diarrhea, urgency, and fecal incontinence. Pain is the most common symptom, followed by difficult defecation, followed by bleeding. Like stricture anywhere in the colon, rectal stricture may cause large bowel obstruction. Anal stricture almost never causes frank obstruction because patients seek treatment long before.

DIAGNOSIS

Rectal stricture may present insidiously because most processes that cause it are slow and chronic and the stricture may not be within reach of an examining finger. Anal stricture is always accessible to digital examination and is usually identified in the course of treatment for the causative condition. On the basis of digital anal and distal rectal examination, one can call a stricture mild, moderate, or severe. A *mild stricture* allows the passage of an index finger but feels abnormally tight to the examiner. A *moderate stricture* necessitates forceful and painful digital examination, prompting the examiner to refrain and consider examination with sedation or anesthesia. A *severe stricture* prohibits digital examination, mandating examination with anesthesia.

NONOPERATIVE MANAGEMENT

Medical Treatment

Many patients after anal operations such as hemorrhoidectomy have what amount to transient inflammatory strictures. Like a postoperative patient, anyone with an anorectal stricture may be helped with hydration, fiber, and stool softeners. Patients with IBD strictures should receive disease-specific medical treatment, which can help the inflammatory component but does not affect fibrosis. Infections should be identified and suppressed with antibiotics or antiviral medication.

Mechanical Dilation

Rectal strictures may be dilated in the endoscopy suite, the operating room, or even the office, depending on the location of the stricture and how painful it is to dilate. Tools for dilation include bougies, Hegar dilators, end-to-end anastomosis (EEA) sizers, and the rigid proctoscope. Today's version of the age-old "divulsion" treatment is balloon dilation, which can be done through a flexible sigmoidoscope.

Anal strictures can be dilated digitally, with the serial introduction of fingers. Severe anal strictures may respond to Hegar dilators of increasing diameter, followed by a finger. For many patients, defecation can be a form of autodilation, as long as the stool is solid; this argues for fiber rather than stool softeners for long-term use.

Stricture dilation is beneficial up to the point of injury that causes more fibrosis. In the words of the old-time "ambulant proctologist" Blanchard, "One cicatrix cannot be mended by the formation of another, any more than two wrongs make one right."

OPERATIVE MANAGEMENT

Stricturotomy and Stricturectomy for Rectal Stricture

These operations and their attendant controversies were the subject of whole books and monographs before the antibiotic era. As a measure of its prominence in the 19th century, the section on rectal (not anal) stricture comprises 15% of Allingham's anorectal surgical text. Today the rare stricture that does not respond to dilation is typically removed via anterior resection, a form of stricturectomy. Stricturotomy lives on in methods of fixing the rare membranous or short-segment stricture. These can be divided endoscopically with cautery or laser, and they can also be cored out with a circular stapler—something between stricturotomy and stricturectomy. The combination of effective treatment of underlying causes and endoscopic balloon dilation has made rectal stricture operations very rare today.

Anoplasty for Anal Stricture

Anoplasty is done for patients with moderate or severe stricture, or any symptomatic stricture refractory to dilation. The goal is to divide the stricture and correct the resulting defect. Anoplasty can be divided into three categories: transverse closure, simple random flaps, and full-thickness advancement flap.

1. *Transverse closure.* As in small bowel strictureplasty, the stricture is divided longitudinally, then sutured transversely. If there is substantial tension in bringing the edges together, as there often is, a flap repair is selected instead.
2. *Simple random flaps.* These receive their blood supply via a skin bridge. Examples include mucosal advancement, Y-V, and rotational S flaps.
   a. *Mucosal advancement flap.* A transverse incision is made at the dentate line, extending into the anal verge. The scar is excised, and the mucosa is sutured to the distal border of the internal sphincter at the anal verge. The external part of the wound is left open. This method is suitable for mid or high anal canal strictures.
   b. *Y-V advancement flap:* The initial incision is made radially at the level of the stricture, making the vertical limb of the Y. The bifurcation of the Y is located distally on the perianal skin. This flap is suitable for anal verge (low) strictures (Figure 1, *A*).
   c. *Rotational S flap:* In an S flap, the abnormal tissue is removed and replaced with skin, fixing the mucocutaneous junction at the normal position. The skin coverage is provided by a double-rotational flap, outlined by a large S, with the anal canal at the center. This more extensive flap is suitable for patients with recurrent strictures, high strictures, or strictures with mucosal ectropion (Figure 1, *B*).
3. *Full-thickness advancement flaps:* These receive their blood supply through the subcutaneous fat from the underlying muscle. Examples include the diamond, house, and V-Y flap. All three of these flaps are used in long strictures, high strictures above the dentate line, or strictures with mucosal ectropion.
   a. *Diamond flap:* Excision of scarred skin and anoderm leaves a roughly diamond-shaped defect. This is covered by a diamond-shaped flap that is advanced from distal to proximal, to the intraanal portion of the defect.
   b. *House flap:* A longitudinal incision extends from the dentate line to the distal end of the stricture. This incision corresponds to the walls of the house-shaped flap. It is

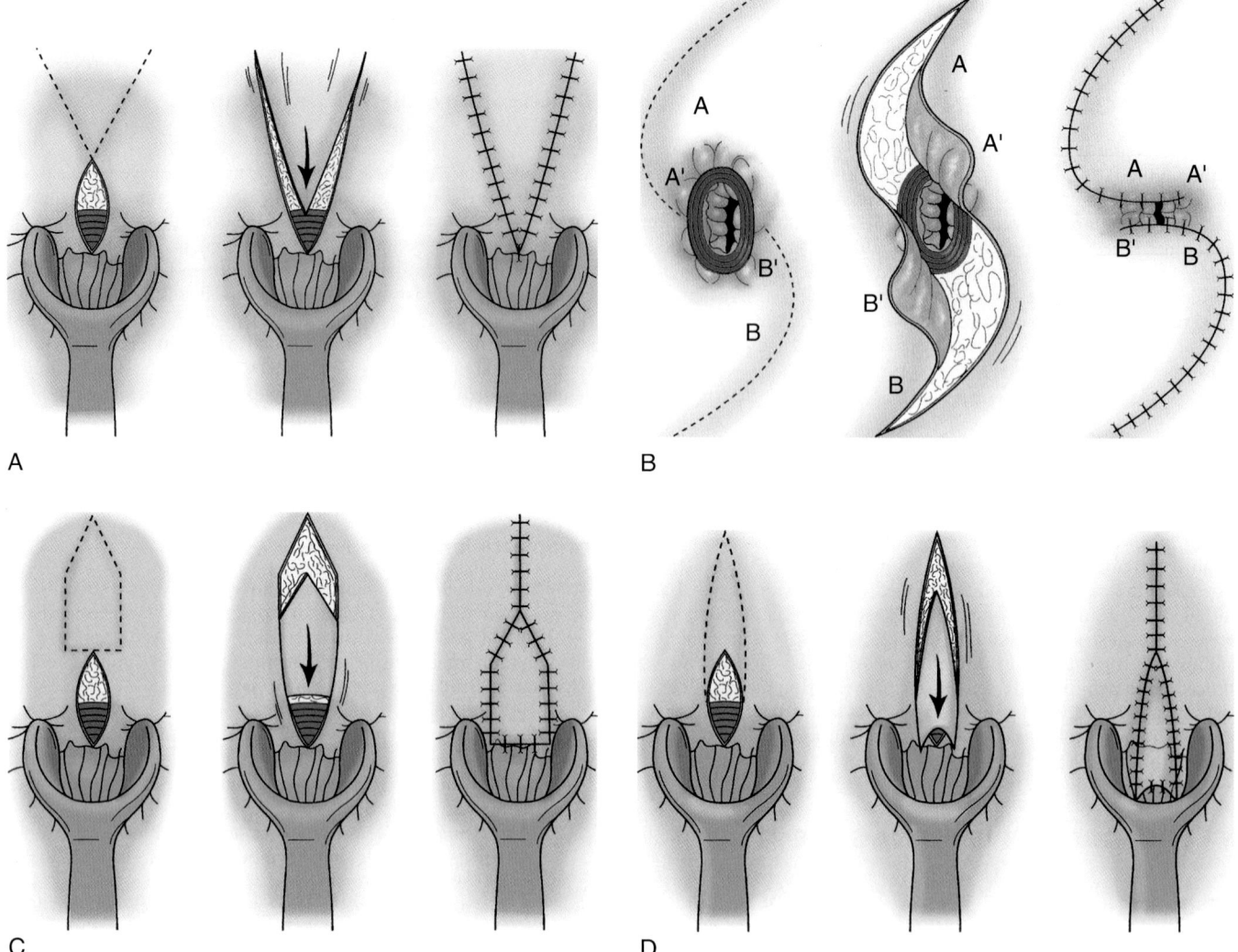

FIGURE I **A,** Y-V flap. **B,** S flap. **C,** House-shaped flap. **D,** V-Y flap. *(From Liberman H, Thorson AG: How I do it: anal stenosis, Am J Surg 179(4):325-329, 2000.)*

advanced proximally to line the entire length of the anal canal (Figure 1, *C*).

c. *V-Y advancement flap.* The strictured segment is excised radially, and then a V-shaped flap is advanced to the dentate line. Like the house flap, the V-Y's broad proximal edge can correct large deficiencies of anoderm (Figure 1, *D*).

SUMMARY

Anorectal strictures can develop from any cause of fibrosis, the most common of which is iatrogenic from previous anorectal surgery. Digital examination is used to categorize reachable strictures as mild, moderate, or severe. Symptoms do not correlate well with these categories. Treatment is based first on relieving symptoms, which commonly include pain, difficult defecation, and bleeding. Patients with mild symptoms can be treated with dietary modification, medication for the underlying condition (in the case of IBD or infection), and possibly dilation. Patients with severe symptoms and those with failed dilation may benefit from surgical treatment. For rectal stricture, this is primarily stricturectomy, although stricturotomy remains an option in rare cases. For anal stricture, various anoplasty options aim to incise the stricture and place distensible tissue in the resulting defect.

SUGGESTED READINGS

Allingham W: Ulceration and stricture of the rectum. In: *Fistula, hæmorrhoids, painful ulcer, stricture, prolapsus and other diseases of the rectum; their diagnosis and treatment,* ed 3, London, 1879, Churchill, pp 219–263.

Baatrup G, Svensen R, Ellensen VS: Benign rectal strictures managed with transanal resection: a novel application for transanal endoscopic microsurgery, *Colorectal Dis* 12(2):144–146, 2010.

Blanchard CE: Anal and rectal strictures. In: *An epitome of ambulant proctology,* Youngstown, Ohio, 1924, Medical Success Press, pp 129–131.

Brisinda G, Vanella S, Cadeddu F, et al: Surgical treatment of anal stenosis, *World J Gastroenterol* 15(16):1921–1928, 2009.

Duieb Z, Appu S, Hung K, et al: Anal stenosis: use of an algorithm to provide a tension-free anoplasty, *ANZ J Surg* 80(5):337–340, 2010.

Garcea G, Sutton CD, Lloyd TD, et al: Management of benign rectal strictures a review of present therapeutic procedures, *Dis Colon Rectum* 46(11):1451–1460, 2003.

Katdare MV, Ricciardi R: Anal stenosis, *Surg Clin North Am* 90(1):137–145, 2010.

Kelsey CB: *Stricture of the rectum: a study of ninety-six cases,* New York, 1890, [publisher unlisted].

Lawal TA, Frischer JS, Falcone RA, et al: The transanal approach with laparoscopy or laparotomy for the treatment of rectal strictures in Crohn's disease, *J Laparoendosc Adv Surg Tech A* 20(9):791–795, 2010.

The Management of Pruritus Ani

Mantaj S. Brar, MD, FRCSC, and
Anthony R. MacLean, MD, FRCSC, FACS

INTRODUCTION

Pruritus ani refers to the symptoms of itching and burning of the perianal skin. Patients often delay seeking medical attention, and their unsupervised attempts at treatment, including aggressive repetitive cleaning and the use of over-the-counter creams or ointments, typically only worsen symptoms. Although the estimated incidence rate of pruritus ani in the general population is 1% to 5%, it presents less often in clinical practice because many patients do not seek medical attention. This condition affects males more often than females, with a ratio of 4:1, and although also seen in children, most patients present in the fourth to seventh decades of life. Pruritus ani may be localized or diffuse in the perianal region. The onset of symptoms is typically gradual and is often worse at night or in warm, moist climates.

ETIOLOGY

Pruritus ani is classified as either idiopathic pruritus ani or secondary pruritus ani. The many secondary causes of pruritus ani include anorectal, infectious, and dermatologic and several systemic illnesses (Box 1). The diagnosis of idiopathic pruritus ani is only made after a thorough patient evaluation and exclusion of secondary causes. Although the authors' experience suggests that an overwhelming majority of pruritus ani is idiopathic, the proportion of patients with a secondary cause varies from 20% to 75% in the published literature.

Idiopathic Pruritus Ani

Several factors have been implicated in idiopathic pruritus ani, including local irritants, excess moisture, repeated trauma from wiping, and medications (Box 2). Fecal contamination is implicated as a local irritant in many cases, the presence of which may not be evident to the patient. Feces contain bacterial endopeptidases, allergens, and bacteria, which are capable of causing skin irritation. In addition, evidence from skin patch testing has shown that the perianal skin is particularly sensitive to irritation and pruritus from exposure to feces compared with skin at other areas of the body. Fecal contamination itself can be the result of poor hygiene, incontinence, chronic diarrhea, or loose stools and is also the mechanism by which several anorectal pathologies cause symptoms. Interestingly, physiologic studies in patients with idiopathic pruritus ani have shown a lower threshold for internal anal sphincter relaxation and lower retention capacity than in control subjects, suggesting that a functional abnormality may contribute to idiopathic pruritus ani. Several medications have been associated with idiopathic pruritus ani and cause symptoms either by causing diarrhea or loose stools, by inducing a histamine release, or by an idiopathic mechanism. The most commonly associated medications include colchicine, quinidine, tetracycline, erythromycin, and stool softeners (see Box 2). In addition, certain foods have also been associated with idiopathic pruritus ani, including coffee, cola, tea, chocolate, spicy foods, and citrus foods (see Box 2). Several proposed mechanisms include alteration of the pH of stool by citrus or spicy foods that cause local irritation, by histamine release, and by caffeinated foods that cause a transient inappropriate relaxation of the internal anal sphincter. Excess fluid intake may also cause pruritus ani by causing loose stools or diarrhea and subsequent fecal contamination and frequent wiping.

Secondary Pruritus Ani

Anorectal Conditions

A variety of anorectal conditions have been associated with pruritus ani, including prolapsing internal hemorrhoids, external hemorrhoids, anal fissures, fistula-in-ano, and neoplasms. Fistula-in-ano causes chronic irritation of the perianal skin from chronic drainage of fluid and a small amount of fecal debris. Prolapsing hemorrhoids and rectal prolapse lead to a chronic drainage of mucus at the level of the perianal skin and fecal contamination, which leads to irritation of the skin. In addition, prolapsed internal hemorrhoids, external hemorrhoids, and skin tags may impair good hygiene and result in feces left in the folds of the perianal skin after defecation, causing irritation. Other conditions that impair sphincter function, cause diarrhea, or decrease stool bulk may lead to fecal soiling and cause pruritus. Pruritus ani may be the presenting symptom of Paget's disease or Bowen's disease, and these neoplasms, although rare, should be considered in the differential diagnosis. Classically, the symptoms of pruritus are more severe and persistent in the setting of an underlying neoplasm.

Infectious Conditions

Infectious agents that cause pruritus ani include bacteria, viruses, fungi, and parasites. Bacterial infections most commonly associated with pruritus ani include *Corynebacterium minutissimum* (erythrasma), beta-hemolytic *Streptococcus* sp., and *Staphylococcus aureus*. Several sexually transmitted infections *(Gonococcus, Chlamydia,* and *Syphilis)* have also been implicated, although these pathogens are rarely responsible for chronic symptoms. Viral infections such as herpes simplex and human papillomavirus (HPV) can cause pruritus ani. With condylomata acuminata, functional changes of the anal sphincter may lead to fecal leakage and pruritus. Fungal infections with *Candida,* although usually a commensal organism in the perianal region, can lead to pruritus, particularly in patients with diabetes and immunosuppression and after treatment with antibiotics or steroids. However, the presence of dermatophytes in the perianal region is always considered pathologic in the setting of pruritus ani. The most common parasitic infection causing pruritus ani is *Enterobius vermicularis,* or pinworms; it usually affects children with nocturnal symptoms.

Dermatologic Conditions

The most common dermatologic causes of secondary pruritus ani are contact dermatitis, allergic dermatitis, lichen sclerosus, lichen planus, and psoriasis. Contact or allergic dermatitis may be the result of a number of possible irritants or allergens including soaps, deodorants, perfumes, topical medications, and foods. Patients with allergic dermatitis commonly have a history of asthma, hay fever, or eczema and may also have a family history. They present with dry scaly lesions that typically involve the face, neck, dorsum of the hands, and popliteal and antecubital fossa, and symptoms are usually worse with dry cold weather and stress. The etiology of lichen sclerosus and lichen planus are poorly understood but may be related to altered cell-mediated immunity. Lichen sclerosus commonly affects perimenopausal women, with involvement of the vulva and vagina in

BOX 1: Causes of secondary pruritus ani

Anorectal Conditions
Hemorrhoids (prolapsing internal or external)
Fistula-in-ano
Anal fissure
Hidradenitis suppurativa
Condylomata
Pilonidal sinus
Perianal Crohn's disease
Hypertrophied anal papilla
Anal canal cancer
Anal margin cancer
Paget's disease
Bowen's disease
Rectal adenoma
Rectal cancer
Rectal prolapse
Fecal incontinence
Chronic diarrhea
Skin tags

Infectious Conditions
Bacterial
Corynebacterium minutissimum (erythrasma)
Beta-hemolytic *Streptococci*
Staphylococcus aureus
Gonococcus
Chlamydia
Syphilis

Viral
Herpes virus
Human papillomavirus
Molluscum contagiosum

Parasitic
Pinworms *(Enterobius vermicularis)*
Scabies

Fungal
Candida
Dermatophytes

Dermatologic Conditions
Contact dermatitis
Allergic dermatitis
Lichen sclerosus
Lichen planus
Psoriasis
Radiation dermatitis

Systemic Conditions
Diabetes mellitus
Hepatic disease or jaundice
Leukemia
Lymphoma
Aplastic anemia
Renal failure
Hyperthyroidism

BOX 2: Factors associated with idiopathic pruritus ani

Local Irritants
Fecal contamination (poor hygiene, internal anal sphincter relaxation, incontinence, diarrhea)
Diet (coffee, tea, cola, chocolate, citrus fruits, spicy foods, tomatoes, beer, wine, dairy products)
Drugs (mineral oil, docusate, witch hazel, topical creams, "-caine" anesthetics)
Soaps, detergents, and perfumes

Moisture
Obesity
Heat
Athletic activity
Tight underwear

Trauma
Excessive wiping with toilet paper

Drugs
Colchicine
Quinidine
Tetracycline
Erythromycin

planus is associated with ulcerative colitis, lichen sclerosus, myasthenia gravis, and several hepatic diseases, namely hepatitis C, chronic active hepatitis, and primary biliary cirrhosis. Lesions usually begin on the volar aspects of the wrists and forearms, and involvement of the genitalia and mucous membranes is common. Lichen planus is characteristically a self-limiting disease that resolves over 8 to 12 months. Psoriasis commonly involves the scalp and the flexor surfaces of the elbows and knees and may also involve the perianal skin, but rarely exclusively.

Systemic Conditions

Several systemic diseases may be associated with pruritus ani, although it is uncommon as the sole presenting symptom. These diseases include diabetes mellitus, hepatic disease or jaundice, leukemia, lymphoma, aplastic anemia, renal failure, and hyperthyroidism (see Box 1).

PATIENT EVALUATION

A thorough history is imperative in the assessment of a patient with pruritus ani and should include details regarding location, frequency, and duration of symptoms; aggravating and alleviating factors; a dietary history, including fluid, coffee, and alcohol consumption; medication history; stool patterns, including frequency, stool consistency, and rectal bleeding; symptoms of incontinence; perianal hygiene patterns; history of skin lesions or dermatologic conditions; a medical history; and a review of any allergies.

Physical examination should include careful inspection of the perianal skin and genitalia, palpation of inguinal lymph nodes, a digital rectal examination, and a complete skin examination.

The appearance of the perianal skin can be classified with the Washington Hospital criteria: stage I consists of skin that is red and inflamed; stage II consists of white, lichenified skin; and stage III involves lichenified skin coincident with coarse ridges of skin and ulceration (Figure 1).

In addition, all patients should be evaluated with anoscopy and sigmoidoscopy. Colonoscopy should be considered in patients older than 40 years, with changes in bowel habits, with symptoms of gastrointestinal bleeding, or with a family history of colorectal cancer.

60% of patients. Although the symptoms are adequately treated with topical steroids, patients should be warned that the appearance of the skin may not change. In addition, the risk of squamous cell carcinoma in chronic nonresponders is reported to be 5%, and therefore, these patients should be followed closely and biopsies should be performed, particularly if symptoms of pruritus persist. Lichen

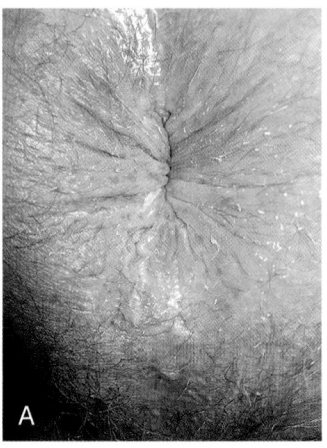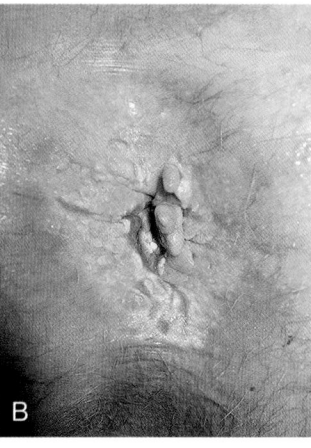

FIGURE I **A,** Washington stage II pruritus ani with white, lichenified skin. **B,** Washington stage III pruritus ani shows lichenified skin with ridges and ulcerations. *(From Markell KW, Billingham RP: Pruritus ani: etiology and management,* Surg Clin North Am *90(1):125–135, 2010. Courtesy of C. Os Finne, St. Paul, Minn.)*

Any suspicious lesions should be biopsied with a simple punch biopsy and should include both the lesion and the normal perianal skin if possible. If Bowen's disease is suspected, 3% acetic acid may be applied to the perianal region, causing whitening of the affected skin and mucosa, and may assist in demarcating the lesion and directing biopsies.

If infectious pathogens are suspected, aerobic, anaerobic, and fungal cultures should be taken, ideally before digital rectal examination because lubricants may have bactericidal activity. Infections caused by beta-hemolytic *Streptococcus* sp. present with a moist, bright, erythematous rash with distinct borders and can be confirmed with a rapid *Streptococcus* antigen test. Erythrasma appears as scaly patches of red to brown lesions, and if suspected, a Wood's lamp may be used to examine the groins, thighs, toe web spaces, and perianal region to confirm the diagnosis with the presence of coral-red fluorescence. False-negative results may result from recent washing, and if clinical suspicion is high, patients should return for reassessment and after refraining from washing for 48 hours. Herpes simplex is characterized by the presence of small, painful vesicles during an active eruption, and the diagnosis is confirmed with polymerase chain reaction (PCR) assay of vesicular fluid or serologic tests. The diagnosis of *Candida* infections may be difficult because they usually present with bright erythema commonly without the characteristic satellite lesions, and positive cultures may be misleading because *Candida* can be a commensal organism in the perineum. If pinworms are suspected, the diagnosis is confirmed with microscopic evaluation of cellophane tape applied to the perianal region in the early morning.

The diagnosis of dermatologic conditions may be difficult because of the atypical appearance of these conditions when involving the perianal skin and the absence of significant clinical exposure to these diagnoses. Contact dermatitis presents with extreme erythema with vesicles and scaly, macerated skin. If suspected, allergic dermatitis may be confirmed with skin patch testing. Psoriasis involving the perianal region has a so-called "inverse-psoriasis" appearance with a poorly demarcated, asymmetric, nonscaly lesion. Lichen sclerosus presents initially as a painful pruritic erythematous reaction and progresses into a thickened, indurated, raised, macular reaction and ultimately in sclerosis and atrophy of the affected skin. It classically appears in the figure-of-eight distribution around the vulva and anus. Lichen planus presents as shiny, pigmented, flat-topped papules and usually involves the volar aspects of the wrists and forearms.

For images of common dermatologic causes of pruritus ani, refer to the review by Zuccati and colleagues. If a dermatologic condition is suspected, consultation with a dermatologist should be obtained.

TREATMENT

Idiopathic Pruritus Ani

Idiopathic pruritus ani can be a difficult and frustrating condition for patient and physician alike. Patients commonly have chronic symptoms and social embarrassment and have had several unsuccessful attempts at self treatment. However, most patients respond to conservative measures, and patient reassurance about the benign nature and expected resolution of symptoms can be extremely helpful in alleviating the anxiety associated with the condition. In the authors' experience, patients with grade II or III skin changes generally need a longer course of conservative treatment for symptom resolution; these patients should be counseled accordingly.

Treatment begins with eliminating possible irritating factors, improving stool bulk, and educating the patient on perianal hygiene (Figure 2). Patients are instructed to discontinue all topical medications and any implicated oral medications if possible (see Box 2). Although no evidence exists for diet modification, all possible irritants from the diet should be eliminated (see Box 2), and a diary documenting dietary intake and symptoms should be instituted. Individual foods can then gradually be reintroduced after 2 weeks, one at a time, to identify foods that may aggravate symptoms. Patients should also be advised to wash undergarments with nonperfumed, hypoallergenic detergent. A high-fiber diet or fiber supplementation should be encouraged to increase stool bulk and help maintain regular bowel movements, which may minimize fecal soiling. In the setting of diarrhea or loose stools, antimotility agents, such as loperamide, may be considered and used judiciously to decrease stool frequency and reduce fecal contamination. In addition, if soiling is significant, tap-water enemas after bowel movements may be helpful in evacuating any residual feces in the distal rectum and anus and may further reduce contamination. Appropriate perianal hygiene and minimization of trauma and irritation to the perianal skin are paramount for effective conservative treatment. Whenever possible, patients should bathe after bowel movements. If bathing is not possible, patients should gently clean the perianal with premoistened wipes. The perianal skin should be dried after cleansing with a hair dryer at a low setting or, alternatively, gently patted dry with a soft towel. Vigorous rubbing or wiping should be strictly avoided. Patients should be instructed to keep the perianal skin as dry as possible, and strategies may include wearing loose-fitting cotton underwear, placing a cotton ball in the underwear, and using talcum powder on the perianal skin. Lastly, patients who have difficulty controlling nocturnal scratching should consider wearing a pair of soft cotton gloves at night.

Adjuncts to initial conservative management include use of topical steroids or antipruritic medications. The evidence of the efficacy of topical steroids is conflicting; a small cohort study showed no benefit when compared with a mild-cleansing agent, but a small randomized controlled trial (RCT) showed significant reduction in symptoms when compared with placebo. In the setting of local inflammation especially, 1% topical hydrocortisone cream applied twice daily may help relieve symptoms and promote healing. However, the use of topical steroids should be limited to 2 to 4 weeks because prolonged use may cause thinning and atrophy of the skin. Topical antipruritic medication may be applied at bedtime to prevent nocturnal itching and scratching, but topical "-caine" anesthetics should be avoided because they may worsen symptoms. In addition, oral antihistamines at bedtime may also be effective in reducing nocturnal symptoms.

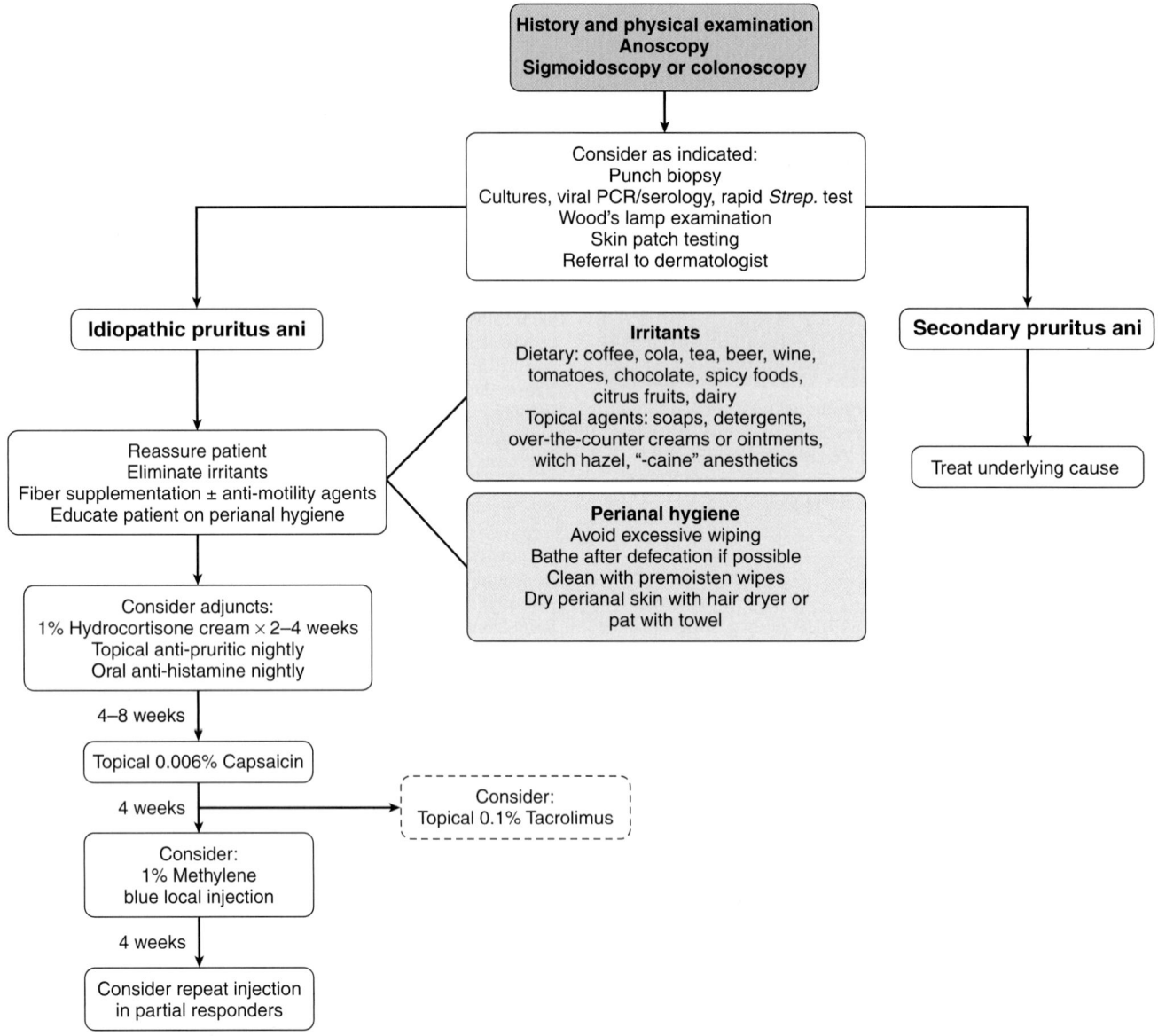

FIGURE 2 Management algorithm for pruritus ani. *PCR*, Polymerase chain reaction.

Patients with persistent symptoms despite conservative measures should be reevaluated at 4 to 8 weeks (see Figure 2). Secondary causes of pruritus ani should again be considered and excluded. This may include obtaining cultures if infectious etiologies are suspected, referral for patch testing to exclude an occult allergy, or punch biopsy of any persistent lesions, although the diagnostic yield of these investigations has been found to be extremely low.

Treatment options for refractory idiopathic pruritus ani include topical capsaicin, topical tacrolimus, and local injection of methylene blue. The use of topical agents before methylene blue injection is recommended for the ease of use and lower risk of adverse events. The use of 0.006% topical capsaicin has been shown in a recent small RCT to be effective at relieving symptoms when applied in a thin layer three times daily for 4 weeks. In patients with response to treatment, symptomatic relief occurred within 3 days, and after the treatment period, patients continued to use the preparation on an as-needed basis for long-term relief. The proposed mechanism of action of capsaicin is the inhibition of synthesis, release, and storage of the neuropeptide substance P, which mediates pain and itching impulses from peripheral sensory neurons. Patients should be warned that application of the cream causes a burning sensation and side

effects may include moderate to severe burning and urticaria. Alternatively, the use of 0.1% topical tacrolimus ointment applied daily for 4 weeks showed a significant reduction in symptom intensity and frequency in one small RCT, although long-term effectiveness was not reported. Side effects of topical tacrolimus include a minor burning sensation with application.

When topical therapies are ineffective for refractory cases, local injection of methylene blue may be considered. The exact mechanism of action in unknown, but it is postulated that methylene blue may be directly toxic to nerves supplying the perianal skin, a finding supported with electron microscopy. Several techniques have been described in the literature; the authors use a technique described by Mentes and associates. The symptomatic area is marked, patients are placed in prone jackknife position with the buttocks taped to retract them laterally, and then the perianal area is prepped. Fourteen to 20 mL of an equal parts solution of 2% methylene blue and 0.5% lidocaine is prepared and then injected with a 22-gauge needle intracutaneously targeting the dermoepidermal junction. Repeat injection may be performed at 4 weeks for partial response. Patients should be warned about the blue appearance of the perineum, which may last up to 6 weeks after injection, and numbness in the perianal skin, which may be persistent. Other possible side effects include a transient change in continence, cellulitis, and a small risk of skin necrosis requiring surgical débridement, which may be related to larger volume or superficial injections.

Secondary Pruritus Ani

The treatment of secondary pruritus ani is directed at the underlying anorectal, dermatologic, infectious, or systemic condition. For anorectal conditions (see Box 1), correction of the anorectal pathology, and the subsequent reduction of fecal contamination and moisture of the perianal skin, usually leads to resolution of symptoms. Local topical treatment or resection of Paget's and Bowen's disease alleviates symptoms, although the optimal treatment and follow-up of these lesions remains controversial (see Tumors of the Anal Canal chapter).

Bacterial infections are generally treated with appropriate oral antibiotics; however, longer courses may be necessary for successful eradication and symptom relief. For patients with erythrasma, the addition of topical betamethasone to the perianal skin and half-strength Whitfield's ointment to other involved areas may be helpful. Treatment of herpes simplex with oral acyclovir is usually effective, and condylomata are treated with topical podophyllin, topical 5-fluorocuracil, cryotherapy, fulguration, or surgical excision. Fungal infections with *Candida* or dermatophytes are successfully treated with topical imidazole, and in the setting of a moist rash, the addition of an antifungal powder may assist in keeping the perianal skin dry. In cases of suspected or confirmed pinworms, patients and all their household members are treated with 2 doses of oral mebendazole given 2 weeks apart to prevent reinfection.

If a dermatologic condition is suspected based on the appearance of perianal skin or the presence of other skin lesions, treatment should be initiated in consultation with a dermatologist. If contact or allergic dermatitis is suspected, the avoidance of the irritant or allergen is the most important intervention, in addition to reinforcing appropriate perianal hygiene (as in idiopathic pruritus ani). The addition of topical 1% hydrocortisone cream may also be helpful in contact dermatitis.

SUMMARY

Pruritus ani is a common condition that can often be successfully diagnosed and treated with a careful and thorough approach. Management of this condition consists of identifying and addressing the cause, minimizing further injury to the perianal skin, and maintaining close follow-up with the patient to ensure healing and relief of symptoms.

SUGGESTED READINGS

Daniel GL, Longo WE, Vernava AM: Pruritus ani: causes and concerns, *Dis Colon Rectum* 37:670–674, 1994.
Lysy J, Sistiery-Ittah M, Israelit Y, et al: Topical capsaicin: a novel and effective treatment for idiopathic intractable pruritus ani: a randomized, placebo controlled, crossover study, *Gut* 53:1323–1326, 2003.
Markell KW, Billingham RP: Pruritus ani: etiology and management, *Surg Clin North Am* 90:125–135, 2010.
Mentes BB, Akin M, Leventoglu S, et al: Intradermal methylene blue injection for the treatment of intractable idiopathic pruritus ani: result of 30 cases, *Tech Coloproctol* 8:11–14, 2004.
Zuccati G, Lotti T, Mastrolorenzo A, et al: Pruritus ani, *Dermat Ther* 18:355–362, 2005.

SURGICAL TREATMENT OF FECAL INCONTINENCE

Liliana Bordeianou, MD, MPH

Fecal incontinence is a sometimes devastating medical disorder that affects as many as 25% of elderly women; it may also be seen in younger women, particularly those who have experienced traumatic or obstetric injuries, and (more rarely) in males. Although it is not life threatening, fecal incontinence may have a profound effect on quality of life, leading to depression, anxiety, and agoraphobia. For the elderly, involuntary loss of feces is a common cause of entry into assisted living facilities and nursing homes.

The cause of fecal incontinence is frequently multifactorial and requires thoughtful etiologic evaluation. As part of this evaluation, after assessment of the severity of leakage, physicians commonly perform a physical examination, anorectal physiology testing, endoanal ultrasound scan, and, on occasion, defecography to exclude internal intussusception or rectal prolapse. Treatment for the condition, before any surgical intervention, may involve fiber supplementation to increase stool consistency, loperamide to decrease stool frequency, and amitriptyline to increase rectal sensory thresholds to fecal stimulation. These medical manipulations can also be combined with biofeedback, a series of specialized monitored exercises aimed at increasing anal sphincter strength and decreasing urgency through sensitivity retraining. Ultimately, most patients with mild fecal incontinence respond to these medical and biofeedback therapies. However, patients with severe leakage of solid and liquid stool frequently need further treatment, and fortunately, they can be offered several treatment options.

OVERLAPPING SPHINCTEROPLASTY

A leading cause of fecal incontinence is occult sphincter injury, which is experienced by nearly 10% of women who give birth vaginally. (Even higher rates are reported in women who experienced a difficult childbirth, requiring forceps or vacuum assistance, and in those who had episiotomies at delivery.) Some of these women have fecal incontinence develop immediately. In others, the clinical sequelae of injury only emerge with age. Therefore, the author recommends that all women with fecal incontinence and a history of vaginal delivery be evaluated for possible obstetric injury. The condition can sometimes be diagnosed by means of a regular physical examination but more often requires endoanal ultrasound scan, which provides a 360-degree image of the anal canal and permits one to clearly visualize both the internal and the external anal sphincter (Figure 1).

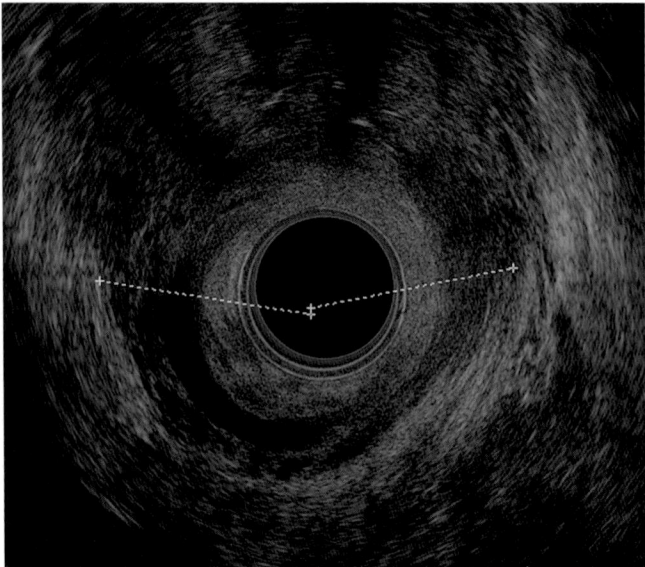

FIGURE I   Obstetric injury with internal and external sphincter disruption. The external sphincter injury is marked.

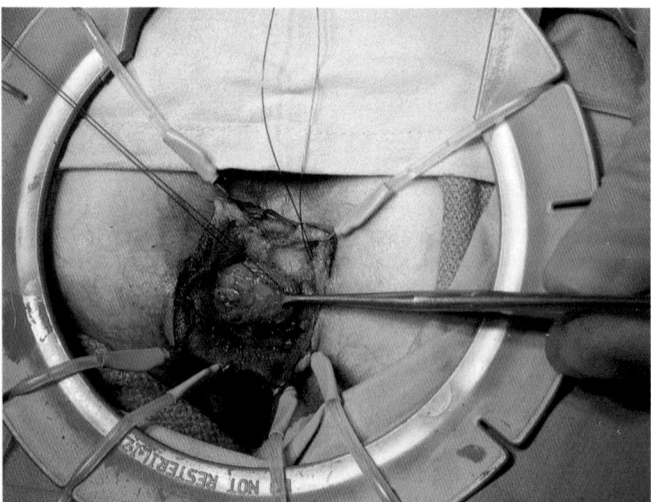

FIGURE 2   Overlapping external sphincteroplasty to correct obstetric injury.

In an appropriately selected patient, sphincter repairs (sphincteroplasty) can ameliorate or cure fecal incontinence. Nonetheless, sphincteroplasty is not appropriate for all patients who have been diagnosed with sphincter injury. The overall sphincter repair success rate is approximately 60%; it is lower in patients who have delayed pudendal nerve terminal motor latencies (which suggest a neurogenic cause of incontinence) and in patients with preserved anal sphincter pressures (which suggest an extrasphincteric cause). Careful evaluation is required to determine those patients for whom sphincteroplasty is a viable option and those for whom it may not be.

If sphincteroplasty is elected, the preparation includes bowel cleansing. The operation is best performed in the jackknife prone position. The surgeon makes an elliptic incision on the perineal body and separates the rectum from the vagina all the way to the levators. The surgeon then identifies and frees the snapped edges of the external anal sphincter to allow for an overlap of the edges. The scar tissue on the anterior aspect of the sphincter is not removed; instead, the scar is overlapped till the viable edges of the muscle are approximated. Interrupted mattress sutures of 2-0 polypropylene are then used to approximate the scar and the muscle in this overlapped position (Figure 2). Finally, the repair is covered with interrupted subcutaneous sutures, and the skin is loosely closed on top to allow drainage, which decreases the chance of a wound infection.

Patients are generally instructed to self administer a tap-water enema as part of the immediate postoperative course, to irrigate the rectum and stimulate a daily bowel movement. These patients are also placed on a bowel regimen aimed at decreasing the risk of postoperative constipation, which could lead to fecal impaction and eventually to wound dehiscence.

SACRAL NERVE STIMULATION

An alternative means of treatment for fecal incontinence, recently approved by the U.S. Food and Drug Administration (FDA), is sacral nerve stimulation (SNS). Its mechanism of action is unknown. The author generally offers SNS treatment to all patients who do not have a large sphincter injury that may be amenable to a simpler sphincter repair and who report full bowel movement loss more than twice a week.

The procedure is performed in two steps. At first, a small-tined lead is placed into the S3 foramen with fluoroscopic guidance. The wire is tunneled under the skin and connected to an external neurostimulator for a 2-week trial period. The patient is then asked to keep a bowel diary. Success is defined as a 50% reduction in the frequency of fecal incontinence episodes; if this rate is achieved, a permanent stimulator is connected to the previously tunneled lead and placed in the subcutaneous fat of the buttock.

The stimulator insertion procedure is simple, has low complication rates (aside from occasional infections of the wound and the device), and can be performed with light sedation. The device appears to ameliorate incontinence in at least 80% of the patients in whom it is implanted, with 40% reporting a return to full continence. At this time, the principal drawback of the procedure is the high price of the device, which is not covered by all insurance carriers, and the fact that its battery runs out in about 3 to 5 years, requiring further surgery to replace it.

INJECTABLES

Solesta (Salix Pharmaceuticals Inc., Raleigh, NC) is an FDA–approved, gel-like injectable dextranomer stabilized in hyaluronic acid. Studies comparing it with placebo treatment have found that Solesta, when injected into the anal submucosa, slightly reduces the number of fecal incontinence episodes and improves quality of life with minimal complications. However, the role and efficacy of this treatment remains open to debate. An argument can be made that the gel should be used before attempting a more expensive SNS implantation. However, the gel should not be used in those with severe incontinence who are being considered for an artificial bowel sphincter (see subsequent discussion) because the coexistent implants could potentially increase the rate of artificial bowel sphincter erosion and infection.

ARTIFICIAL BOWEL SPHINCTER

For patients with moderate to severe incontinence who do not respond to less intrusive approaches, an artificial bowel sphincter is sometimes considered. This device, which was approved by the FDA more than a decade ago, involves a fluid-filled cuff, which is placed around the anal sphincter and connected through tubing to a reservoir (usually placed in the space of Retzius). When filled with fluid, the cuff occludes the anus. When patients want to defecate, they squeeze a pump (generally hidden in the labia majora in the woman or the scrotum in the male) to temporarily transfer the fluid from the cuff to the reservoir. After the patient defecates, the cuff reinflates slowly to again pinch closed the anal canal.

Although the device is very effective, it presents risks as a result of its capacity to break or erode. This can lead to infection and even, on occasion, severe necrotizing infections. The author generally does not recommend the artificial bowel sphincter for any patients who have other added risk for perineal infections, such as prior radiation, obesity, or diabetes. Active research efforts are currently underway to modify and simplify the device and improve its durability.

OTHER

In some cases, fecal incontinence can be caused by full-thickness rectal prolapse or internal intussusception. The surgical approaches to these disorders are discussed in a separate chapter.

SUGGESTED READINGS

Graf W, Mellgren A, Matzel KE, et al: Efficacy of dextranomer in stabilized hyaluronic acid for treatment of faecal incontinence: a randomized, sham-controlled trial, *Lancet* 377:997, 2011.
Wexner SD, Coller JA, Devroede G, et al: Sacral nerve stimulation for fecal incontinence: results of a 120-patient prospective multicenter study, *Ann Surg* 251:441, 2010.
Wong MT, Meurette G, Wyart V, et al: The artificial bowel sphincter: a single institution experience over a decade, *Ann Surg* 254:951, 2011.

THE MANAGEMENT OF RECTOVAGINAL FISTULA

Ashwin L. deSouza, MS, MRCSEd, DNB, FCPS, MNAMS, and Herand Abcarian, MD

INTRODUCTION

Rectovaginal fistulae constitute one of the most frustrating conditions to treat. Although not life-threatening, they are associated with significant morbidity that greatly influences social well-being, sexual activity, and overall quality of life. With a limited number of surgeons conversant in its management, patients with rectovaginal fistulae often present to tertiary referral centers after multiple failed procedures.

Almost all reported literature on the management of rectovaginal fistula is made up of individual case series, each with a small number of patients. It is therefore difficult to objectively compare the results of the different treatment options available. The diverse etiology, numerous treatment options, and lack of randomized trials make it difficult to formulate evidence-based guidelines to optimally manage this condition.

This chapter emphasizes the surgical management of rectovaginal fistula and presents broad treatment guidelines based on current reported literature.

CAUSES

Obstetric injury is the most common cause of rectovaginal fistula. Approximately 2% of all vaginal deliveries are associated with third- and fourth-degree perineal tears, and 3% of these patients will subsequently develop a rectovaginal fistula. Fistulae arising from obstetric injury are often associated with anterior defects in the anal sphincter, leading to some degree of fecal incontinence.

Crohn's disease follows closely as the second most common cause, with 20% to 40% of patients developing either an anorectal or rectovaginal fistula. Rectovaginal fistulas are more likely to be associated with large bowel than with small bowel involvement and can occur in up to 10% of women with Crohn's disease. Rectovaginal fistulae associated with Crohn's disease have a high recurrence rate and often require multiple procedures before healing can be achieved.

Surgical trauma, anorectal infection, vaginal or anal neoplasm, and radiation therapy for malignancy constitute the other less common causes (Table 1).

CLINICAL MANIFESTATION

Patients usually present with symptoms of passage of gas or feces through the vagina, although this is often misinterpreted as anal incontinence. Sometimes the clinical presentation may be less obvious, with complaints of a persistent vaginal discharge, dyspareunia, or repeated urinary tract infections.

Because the majority of rectovaginal fistulae are below the level of the sphincter complex, digital examination can often locate the indurated fistulous tract. Meticulous examination with an anoscope or speculum usually reveals the granulation tissue around the opening of the fistula, which can be gently probed to delineate the tract. However, not all rectovaginal fistulas are evident on an initial clinical examination. If a high degree of clinical suspicion exists, a thorough examination with the patient under anesthesia is justified, especially in patients with Crohn's disease, in whom the activity of disease in the rectum can also be evaluated. On occasion, injection of dilute methylene blue in hydrogen peroxide into the primary opening of a fistula may aid in defining the secondary opening.

The goals of preoperative evaluation are to identify the fistula, determine the etiology, and evaluate the extent of the causative pathology and surrounding injuries. Endoanal ultrasonography (EAUS) is an important diagnostic tool to determine defects in the anal sphincter complex, and it can also serve to delineate additional occult collections in complex fistula tracts. Hydrogen peroxide–enhanced transanal ultrasonography has also been advocated to map complex fistulas. Pelvic magnetic resonance imaging (MRI) and endorectal MRI are useful diagnostic modalities that are especially popular in European countries.

Tests to determine the functional status of the pelvic floor and anal sphincter are indicated if there is a history of sphincter injury or any degree of incontinence. Anorectal manometry to determine

TABLE 1: Rectovaginal fistula etiology

Obstetric injury	Forceps delivery, episiotomy (posterior midline), prolonged labor, third- and fourth-degree perineal lacerations
Inflammatory bowel disease	Crohn's disease
Postsurgical	Anorectal surgery (fistulotomy) Vaginal surgery (hysterectomy, rectocele repair) Abdominal surgery (hysterectomy, low anterior resection, pouch procedure)
Infectious	Cryptoglandular abscess, diverticulitis, tuberculosis
Neoplastic	Anal canal, rectum, vagina, cervix
Radiation induced	External beam radiotherapy, brachytherapy

TABLE 2: Surgical options

Surgical approach	Procedures
Transanal	Fistulotomy Endorectal advancement flap Rectal sleeve advancement Fibrin glue Bioprosthetics
Transvaginal	Vaginal advancement flap
Transperineal	Episioproctotomy plus layered closure Overlapping sphincteroplasty Interposition flaps
Transabdominal	Primary repair plus omental flap Rectal resection plus coloanal anastomosis and omental flap

sphincter dysfunction and measurement of pudendal nerve terminal motor latency to detect nerve damage are two useful tests to evaluate the function of the pelvic floor. Undiagnosed sphincter injury or pudendal nerve damage could compromise an otherwise successful repair.

After complete workup of the perineum, an evaluation of the entire colon in cases of rectal malignancy, and of the small bowel in cases of Crohn's disease, is mandatory. Thus additional workup could include a small bowel series, colonoscopy, barium enema study, and a computed tomographic scan.

CLASSIFICATION OF RECTOVAGINAL FISTULAE

Rectovaginal fistulae may be classified according their relation to the sphincter complex as *high* (above the sphincter complex) or *low* (at or below the level of the sphincters, also known as *anovaginal*). The low fistula is almost always caused by obstetric trauma and is often associated with sphincter disruption.

Rectovaginal fistulae have also been classified as *simple* or *complex*. Simple fistulae are located in the middle or lower portion of the rectovaginal septum, are less than 2.5 cm in diameter, and are caused by local trauma or sepsis. A complex fistula, on the other hand, is usually greater that 2.5 cm, is located in the upper portion of the rectovaginal septum, and is secondary to causes other than trauma and infection, such as neoplasia, diverticulitis, or inflammatory bowel disease.

PREOPERATIVE PREPARATION

The type of preoperative preparation is largely subjective but usually varies with the type of procedure planned for the repair. For simple advancement flaps, a phosphate enema on the morning of the procedure is usually adequate. For more extensive repairs, such as an overlapping sphincteroplasty or an interposition flap, a full mechanical bowel preparation is preferred. Perioperative antibiotics and deep venous thrombosis prophylaxis can be administered as per institutional protocol.

SURGICAL MANAGEMENT

With fistulas due to obstetric injury, which occur in the immediate postpartum period, at least 3 months elapse before the acute inflammation subsides and fibrosis develops. In the interim, symptoms can be improved with stool-bulking agents or with induced mild constipation with loperamide or other antidiarrheals. Once inflammation subsides, a thorough evaluation of the sphincter mechanism should be undertaken to delineate the extent of sphincter disruption.

The presence of sepsis is an absolute contraindication to any attempt at surgical repair; thus drainage of abscesses and collections is the first step in management. A loose noncutting seton is usually placed through the fistula tract and kept in place until the infection subsides; this may take as long as 3 months and even longer in patients with Crohn's disease.

There are four surgical approaches to repair a rectovaginal fistula: *transanal, transabdominal, transvaginal,* and *transperineal.* Table 2 lists the various surgical options of each approach.

Transanal Approach

Fistulotomy

A fistulotomy involves laying open the fistula tract, which may or may not be excised. This is often performed as a two-stage procedure, in which a noncutting seton is first placed through the fistula to allow for drainage and fibrosis. In the second stage, the seton is removed by dividing the remaining tissue to lay open the tract.

Although a fistulotomy results in successful healing, it involves division of varying thicknesses of the external sphincter muscles. This causes a keyhole deformity, which almost always results in some degree of incontinence, often permanent. Hence a fistulotomy, although indicated only for superficial fistulas, is rarely used.

Endorectal Advancement Flap

Endorectal advancement flap forms the mainstay of treatment for low rectovaginal fistulas and is best suited for patients who do not have disruption of the sphincter muscles. The procedure is usually performed in the outpatient setting and with the patient in prone position, which offers excellent exposure of the anterior rectal wall. Both the anus and vagina are prepared, and a probe is inserted through the fistula from the vagina into the rectum. A trapezoid flap is then outlined with the base cephalad and twice the width of the apex. The flap consists of the rectal mucosa, submucosa, and a portion of the underlying internal sphincter, including the fistula opening at the apex; this is raised in cephalad manner with the use of needle-tip electrocautery. A sufficient length of flap should be mobilized 3 to 4 cm proximal to the fistula opening to ensure a tension-free closure after excision of the fistula. Injection of a dilute epinephrine solution facilitates dissection and minimizes blood loss.

After the flap is elevated, the fistula tract is curetted to remove all granulation tissue, and the defect in the remaining muscle layer (internal sphincter) is closed with a few interrupted absorbable sutures. The tip of the flap is then excised to remove the fistula opening, and the flap is advanced caudad and sutured in place with 3-0 interrupted absorbable sutures to close the wound. The vaginal opening is left open to facilitate drainage. Postoperative care includes a high-fiber diet, sitz baths, and stool softeners to avoid fecal impaction.

The endorectal advancement flap offers the advantages of performing the repair from the high-pressure side of the fistula and of preserving sphincter integrity. Short-term success rates for rectal advancement flaps alone vary from 42% to 68%, although higher success rates have been reported with the addition of a sphincteroplasty, if a sphincter defect exists.

Rectal Sleeve Advancement

In the presence of limited circumferential or stricturing disease in the distal rectum (e.g., Crohn's disease), a rectal sleeve advancement can be attempted. The procedure involves mobilization of the proximal rectum, resection of the involved distal portion, and restoration of continuity with an anorectal anastomosis.

Kraske Approach

The patient is placed in a semiprone jackknife position, and an incision is made just to the left of the midline, extending from the sacrococcygeal joint to the external anal sphincter. The incision is deepened, and the distal portion of the coccyx is excised. The pelvic floor muscles are then divided in the midline down to the rectum, which is circumferentially mobilized superiorly as far as possible and distally up to the anal canal. The rectum is then transected at the level of the pelvic floor. A circumferential mucosectomy is then performed from the level of the dentate line up to the level of rectal transection. The fistulous tract is completely excised, and the defect in the rectovaginal septum is closed with a few interrupted absorbable sutures. The vaginal defect may be left open for drainage. The mobilized rectum is then advanced to the dentate line and sutured in a single layer with interrupted sutures.

Fibrin Glue

Fibrin glue attempts to seal the fistula tract with a fibrin plug, which allows for ingrowth of fibrous tissue that permanently closes the fistula with minimal dissection and no sphincter disruption. However, experience with fibrin glue in rectovaginal fistulae has been very limited because of disappointing results. Extrusion of the fibrin plug as a result of the short length of the fistula tract is the predominant cause of failure.

Bioprosthetics

Two bioprosthetics have been used for rectovaginal fistulae: the bioprosthetic mesh (Surgisis ES; Cook Surgical, Bloomington, Ind) and the Rectovaginal Fistula Plug (RVP; Cook Surgical, Bloomington, Ind). Both products are made from lyophilized porcine intestinal submucosa, which provides a matrix for ingrowth of host connective tissue.

The bioprosthetic mesh is used as an interposition graft. The rectovaginal septum is dissected through a perineal incision, and the fistula is excised. After closure of the rectal and vaginal openings,

the rehydrated mesh is placed between the rectum and vagina with an adequate overlap over the rectal and vaginal closures; it is sutured in position with a few interrupted absorbable sutures, with the mesh kept as taut as possible.

The bioprosthetic rectovaginal fistula plug is tapered at one end to facilitate insertion. A fistula probe is introduced from the vaginal to the rectal opening, and the tapered end of the plug is tied to the probe with a suture. The probe is then withdrawn, the plug is pulled with it, and the button is lodged at the broader end at the rectal opening. The excess plug at the rectal end is then excised, and the plug is sutured in position with absorbable sutures, which closes the rectal mucosa over the plug. The vaginal opening is left open, and the excess plug is trimmed at this level. The short length of the fistula tract poses the same problem with the plug as with fibrin glue, which makes the plug suitable only for rectovaginal fistulas that are well over 1 cm in length.

The experience with bioprosthetics as a whole in rectovaginal fistulas is very small. Success rates of fistula closure by interposition techniques have been reported to be from 66% to 86%.

Transvaginal Approach

Vaginal Advancement Flap

In a technique similar to the rectal advancement flap, a flap of vaginal mucosa is raised, and the fistula tract is excised. The rectal mucosa is closed separately, over which the defect in the rectovaginal septum is approximated with interrupted absorbable sutures. The apex of the flap is then trimmed to excise the fistula opening and is sutured into position to close the wound.

The primary advantage of a vaginal flap is the use of healthy, pliable, and well-vascularized vaginal tissue, even though the repair is on the low-pressure side of the fistula. A vaginal flap is easier to mobilize than a rectal flap, especially in the presence of anorectal stenosis. In a comparative analysis of 11 studies, no difference was found in the closure rates between a rectal and vaginal advancement flap in rectovaginal fistulas due to Crohn's disease.

Transperineal Approach

Episioproctotomy and Layered Closure

This repair converts the fistula into a fourth-degree perineal tear by dividing all the tissue between the rectum and vagina through the perineal body. A layered closure is then performed to close the rectal mucosa, the rectal and vaginal muscular walls, and finally the vaginal mucosa. The greatest disadvantage of this procedure is the creation of a full-thickness defect in the anal sphincter. If the repair should fail, the patient will be fully incontinent. For this reason, this procedure should be attempted in only patients with documented existing sphincter disruption and incontinence.

Overlapping Sphincteroplasty

This technique is ideal for patients with concomitant sphincter injury. The detailed technique of an overlapping sphincteroplasty is described elsewhere in this text but essentially involves dissection and mobilization of the external sphincter through a transperineal approach. Very often the sphincter is so attenuated at the site of injury that the healthy ends of the sphincter can be overlapped and sutured into position without the need to divide or excise any tissue. This technique has the advantage of not worsening the degree of incontinence should the repair fail while still achieving the same end result. In the presence of sphincter injury, the addition of an overlapping sphincteroplasty to a rectal advancement flap has been reported to greatly increase the success rates.

Interposition Flaps

Patients with multiple failed attempts at repair usually have relative ischemia in the surrounding tissues. The interposition of healthy, vascularized tissue in the rectovaginal septum can theoretically increase the chance of successful closure but with a potential risk of de novo dyspareunia. The gracilis and bulbocavernosus flaps are the two most described pedicled flaps for rectovaginal fistula. Although not mandatory, fecal diversion is usually recommended, either before or at the time of the flap procedure.

The approach is usually via a perineal incision between the posterior fourchette of the vagina and the anal verge. The incision is deepened to expose the rectovaginal septum, which is then dissected proximal to the level of the fistula by about 2 cm. The fistula is then completely excised, and the rectal and vaginal defects are closed primarily.

The gracilis muscle has only vestigial function, and a reliable vascular pedicle enters the muscle laterally in its upper third. The muscle of either leg can be used and is harvested through an incision in the medial aspect of the thigh. The harvested muscle is then tunneled through the subcutaneous tissue at the groin and brought out at the perineal incision. This is then placed between the rectum and vagina and held in position with a few interrupted absorbable sutures. The success rate of the gracilis muscle flap has been reported to be as high as 75%.

A Martius flap, in which the bulbocavernosus muscle is used with the overlying fat in the labia majora, is based on the perineal branch of the pudendal artery and is placed in the rectovaginal septum in similar fashion. As with all interposition flaps, this repair has the potential risk for increased postoperative dyspareunia, but there are usually no complaints related to labial function or cosmesis. The success rate with this procedure has been reported to vary from 50% to 93.8%.

Transabdominal Approach

Rectal Sleeve Advancement

The patient is placed in the lithotomy position, and the rectum is mobilized anteriorly and posteriorly in standard fashion, right down to the pelvic floor, and the lateral vascular supply is kept intact. The rectum is then transected at the pelvic floor, which completes the abdominal part of the procedure. The transanal exposure and anastomosis is as described in the Kraske approach.

A rectal sleeve advancement can be offered only if the proximal rectum is normal and is most appropriate in patients with limited, circumferential disease in the distal rectum. Closure rates of 54% to 87% have been described for a rectal sleeve advancement flap in studies with a follow-up greater than 2 years.

Omental Interposition

This transabdominal approach is best suited to repair high rectovaginal fistulas, which are usually a complication of anterior resection, hysterectomy, or diverticulitis. The rectum is dissected down to the level of the fistula, which is then divided to expose the rectal and vaginal openings. If the rectal wall is healthy and pliable, the fistula opening can be débrided and closed primarily. However, if the surrounding rectum is unhealthy, a resection with primary coloanal anastomosis may be considered. The vaginal opening is then closed, and a pedicled omental flap is placed between the two closures and held in position with a few interrupted sutures.

Sometimes, a low rectovaginal fistula may require a transabdominal approach. After the failure of multiple local procedures, further attempts at repair with manipulation of local tissues have a very slim chance of success. A transabdominal approach in this setting has the advantages of resecting all ischemic tissue and bringing down well-vascularized tissues to the anal canal.

The procedure entails mobilization of the rectum and separation of the rectovaginal septum down to the pelvic floor. The fistula openings in the rectum and vagina are then débrided and closed perineally with interrupted absorbable sutures. An omental flap, based on either the left or right gastroepiploic artery, is prepared and placed in the pelvis. From the perineum, the lower rectovaginal septum is dissected free. The omental flap is then brought down into the rectovaginal septum and sutured to the subcutaneous tissue of the perineum. Additional sutures are placed to anchor the omentum to the levator ani along the lateral pelvic walls for tension-free interposition (Figure 1). Although this is a major surgical procedure, it brings vascularized omentum into the rectovaginal septum between the rectal and vaginal closures and may be the only option for successful closure in patients with multiple failed procedures.

TREATMENT GUIDELINES

Fecal Diversion

There is no consensus on the indications of proximal fecal diversion in rectovaginal fistulas, as it has been shown that a stoma does not necessarily ensure the success of a repair. However, after two failed attempts, surgeons are more inclined to place a diverting stoma prior to or at the time the third procedure is attempted. Repairs using interposition pedicle flaps are also more likely to be protected with a proximal stoma.

Choice of Repair

Considering the diverse etiology, the large number of surgical options, and the lack of randomized evidence, deciding on a line of treatment is often a daunting task. The choice of procedure is largely governed by the type of fistula (low or high, simple or complex), the etiology, the status of the sphincter mechanism, the number of prior failed attempts, and the functional status of the patient.

The results reported for each procedure vary greatly, and no procedure yields consistent results. It should be appreciated that almost any procedure for rectovaginal fistula is going to fail in a significant number of patients. This is why irreversible steps, such as full-thickness sphincter division, which might make the condition worse if the repair fails, are best avoided.

Probably the first point to consider in deciding on a line of treatment is the status of the sphincter mechanism. Documented defects in the anal sphincter with associated incontinence require an overlapping sphincteroplasty. This procedure is often combined with a rectal advancement flap and is the most commonly used first-line option in low fistulas resulting from obstetric trauma.

In the absence of sphincter injury, either a rectal or vaginal advancement flap can be considered as first-line options. Although the results for both procedures are more or less similar, a rectal advancement flap puts the repair on the high-pressure (rectal) side of the fistula and is often preferred over the vaginal flap. However, a rectal flap necessitates the presence of a healthy rectum and is best avoided in the presence of poorly controlled Crohn's proctitis or in the presence of rectal disease involving strictures.

If a rectal flap fails as the first procedure, it would probably be better to try the vaginal flap at the second attempt rather than to repeat the rectal flap. After failure of both a rectal and vaginal flap, the surgeon has the option of repeating a flap procedure or of considering an interposition pedicle flap. If the local tissues are still healthy and pliable, a repeat flap can be attempted. However, it should be appreciated that at every subsequent procedure, the success

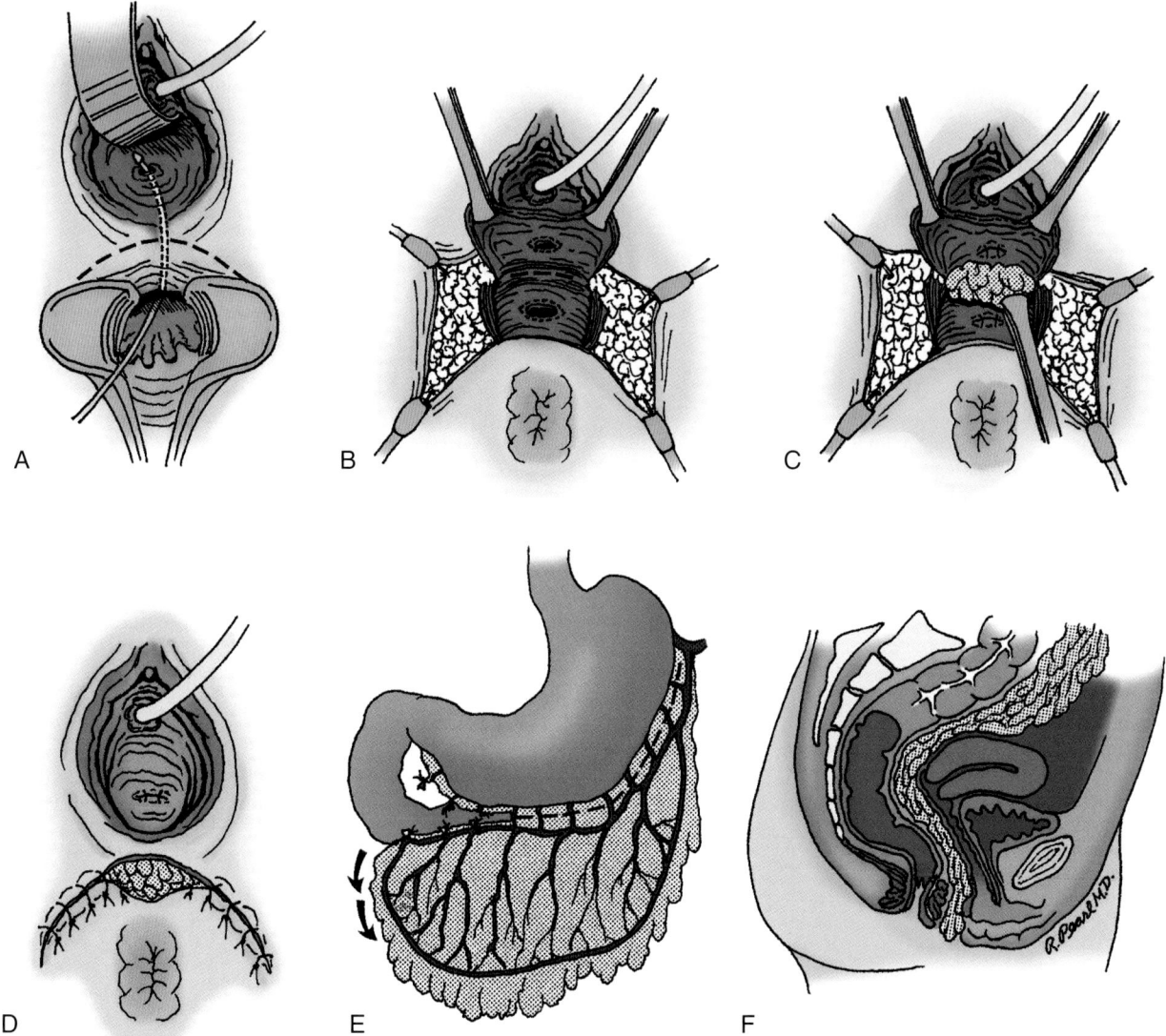

FIGURE 1 **A,** Probe delineating fistula. *Dashed line* indicates incision site. **B,** Posterior wall of vagina dissected from anterior rectal wall. Fistula sites débrided. Peritoneal cavity entered at apex of plane between vagina and rectum *(dashed line).* **C,** Fistula openings closed with interrupted polyglactin sutures. Mobilized omentum pulled down between vaginal and rectal repairs. **D,** Omentum sutured to subcutaneous tissue of perineum. Center of incision left open for drainage. **E,** Technique of omental mobilization based on left gastroepiploic artery as major blood supply. The dashed line represents the line of separation of greater omentum from the stomach. The arrows depict the downward rotation of the omentum for interposition. **F,** Lateral view showing completed interposition. *(Courtesy Russell Pearl, MD.)*

rate decreases further. Multiple failed attempts (more than three) render the rectovaginal septum and surrounding tissue ischemic, and further attempts at local repair are less likely to succeed. Interposition flaps should then be considered with appropriate counseling in view of the potential for de novo dyspareunia. Either a gracilis or Martius flap is an acceptable alternative.

Because experience with bioprosthetics is limited, definitive recommendation for their use is impossible. However, because bioprosthetics rely on tissue ingrowth from surrounding tissue, an ischemic rectovaginal septum would probably not be the best environment for a bioprosthetic mesh. If the proximal rectum is healthy, a distal proctectomy with a coloanal anastomosis will resect the diseased distal rectum, bring healthy proximal rectum to the anal canal, and also provide the opportunity to place a pedicled omental flap in the ischemic rectovaginal septum.

SPECIAL CONSIDERATIONS

Radiation-Induced Fistulae

With the increased use of both brachytherapy and external-beam radiation in the treatment of pelvic malignancies, radiation-induced complications are likely to increase. The first step in management of radiation-induced rectovaginal fistulas is to rule out the presence of residual or recurrent malignancy. This requires detailed imaging and an examination with the patient under anesthesia with multiple biopsies of areas of irregularity or random biopsies if no irregularity exists. Once the presence of malignancy has been ruled out, the condition of the rectum, vagina, and surrounding perineal tissues needs to be evaluated.

It is mandatory to wait at least 6 months after the completion of radiation treatment before any repair is attempted. This allows for the full effect of radiation to be realized and for the surrounding tissue to recover. If the local tissues are healthy, a rectal or vaginal advancement flap can be attempted. However, it should be appreciated that because the repair is being performed with radiated tissue, it is less likely to succeed. If one attempt at local repair fails, subsequent attempts will most likely be futile. Interposition flaps with nonradiated tissue (e.g., gracilis flap) or a resection of the involved rectum with a coloanal anastomosis and omental interposition then remains the best available option and is preferable to the classic Bricker procedure.

Crohn's Disease

Almost every patient with Crohn's proctitis and a rectovaginal fistula will require an examination under anesthesia and drainage with a noncutting seton until the infection and inflammation subsides. This is also essential to optimize medical therapy. After quiescence of the acute episode, definitive therapy for the rectovaginal fistula can be pursued.

Local repair is the initial choice in most cases of Crohn's disease–associated rectovaginal fistulae. If the rectum is relatively free from disease, and the rectal wall is pliable, a rectal advancement flap can be attempted. However, in the presence of rectal scarring, this procedure is best avoided. The alternatives include an anocutaneous flap, rectal sleeve advancement, or vaginal flap. An anocutaneous flap can be done only if the anal skin is soft and supple, which is often not the case in patients with Crohn's disease, although a success rate of 70% has been reported for this procedure. The vaginal advancement flap is another alternative for which good healing rates have been reported, especially when a portion of the levator ani muscle is interposed between the rectal and vaginal walls below the flap of vaginal mucosa. Closure rates with this technique have been reported to be as high as 92.3%; however, a 40% to 60% success rate is probably more realistic in Crohn's disease.

Crohn's disease–associated rectovaginal fistulae have an overall poor prognosis, with a recurrence rate that varies from 25% to 50%. It is therefore very important to elaborately counsel patients and set realistic treatment goals. In patients with poorly controlled proctitis, surgical options are very limited. Quite often patients are symptomatic from the abscesses associated with the repeated flare-ups of Crohn's proctitis. Prolonged seton drainage for 12 to 18 months epithelializes the fistula tract and limits further episodes of abscess. Very often, patients with multiple failed procedures prefer prolonged seton drainage to a total proctocolectomy and permanent ileostomy, which is the procedure of last resort.

Malignancy

The only definitive treatment of malignant rectovaginal fistulae is an en block surgical extirpation of the fistulous tract with the mass and any contiguous organs involved in the malignant process. This often requires a posterior or total pelvic exenteration. A diverting stoma is often placed to decrease symptoms, while the patient receives neoadjuvant therapy. The patient should then be reevaluated after adjuvant treatment to determine the extent of response and fitness for a major surgical procedure. In patients of good performance status with a satisfactory response to adjuvant therapy, a pelvic exenteration may be considered. However, very few patients fit this description, and treatment remains palliative in most cases.

ACKNOWLEDGMENTS

The authors wish to thank Russell Pearl, MD, for his contribution of the artwork for this chapter.

SELECTED READINGS

Ellis CN: Outcomes after repair of rectovaginal fistulas using bioprosthetics, *Dis Colon Rectum* 51(7):1084–1088, 2008.

Lefèvre JH, Bretagnol F, Maggiori L, et al: Operative results and quality of life after gracilis muscle transposition for recurrent rectovaginal fistula, *Dis Colon Rectum* 52(7):1290–1295, 2009.

Ruffolo C, Scarpa M, Bassi N, et al: A systemic review on advancement flaps for rectovaginal fistula in Crohn's disease: transrectal versus transvaginal approach, *Colorectal Dis* 12(12):1183–1191, 2010.

Schouten WR, Oom DM: Rectal sleeve advancement for the treatment of persistent rectovaginal fistulas, *Tech Coloproctol* 13:289–294, 2009.

Venkatesh KS, Ramanujam P: Surgical treatment of traumatic cloaca, *Dis Colon Rectum* 39(7):811–816, 1996.

THE MANAGEMENT OF CONDYLOMA ACUMINATA

Charles B. Whitlow, MD, and
David A. Margolin, MD

Human papilloma virus (HPV) is a DNA papovavirus that requires differentiating squamous epithelium for viral replication and is the most common sexually transmitted disease in the United States. The Centers for Disease Control (CDC) estimates that more than 20 million Americans are infected with HPV and that more than 6 million new cases will be reported each year as the prevalence approaches 50% in sexually active adults. Currently, more than 100 subtypes of HPV exist as determined by DNA typing.

Although HPV infections are most commonly located in the cervix, vagina, vulva, perineum, penis, and anus, the infection can affect any part of the body. Most HPV infections go unrecognized, but roughly one third of the HPV subtypes are associated with anogenital warts, accounting for about 10% of all HPV infections. Despite its indolent nature, HPV is responsible for a spectrum of perianal disease from asymptomatic infection, benign warts, and anal intraepithelial dysplasia to invasive anal squamous cell cancer.

Although one third of HPV subtypes are associated with anogenital warts, DNA subtypes 6 and 11 are the most common and are considered to be low-risk types with regards to malignant degeneration. Subtypes 16, 18, 31, and 35, although also seen in anogenital warts, are considered high risk because of their association with anal dysplasia and anal cancer. Because of the histologic similarities between the cervix and anus, a transition zone from columnar to squamous epithelium, the role of HPV in the development of anal dysplasia (AIN) and anal canal cancer is similar to the well-established role of HPV in the development cervical dysplasia and cervical cancer.

PRESENTATION AND EVALUATION

Morphologically, benign warty anogenital HPV infections or condyloma acuminata are the characteristic gray or pink, fleshy, cauliflower-like growths appearing on partially keratinized epithelium (Figure 1). However, HPV can also appear as small papules or as thick keratotic warts similar to common skin warts. They can be sessile or pedunculated and may range in size from several millimeters to giant Buschke-Löwenstein lesions. As condylomas enlarge and increase in number, they can encircle the anal margin and become confluent, sometimes making visualization of the anus difficult. Lesions may also be present in the anal canal and extend above the dentate line.

Most patients report a growth or growths in the perianal region. Like most types of anal pathology, a self diagnosis of hemorrhoids is common. Other frequent symptoms include pruritus, bleeding, chronic moisture or drainage, difficulty with hygiene, and pain. Physical examination must include inspection of the genitalia, groin folds, perineum, and perianal region. Anoscopy is needed to detect anal canal lesions and also allows for inspection of the distal rectal mucosa. Because of a higher incidence in patients with HPV, additional evaluation for other sexually transmitted diseases should be performed. Female patients should undergo vaginal speculum examination and Pap smear. Because condyloma acuminata, intraepithelial dysplasia, and anal squamous cell cancer are more common in patients with immunocompromise, a thorough history of high-risk behavior is mandatory and human immunodeficiency virus (HIV) testing should be considered. This chapter focuses on condyloma of the perianal skin and anal canal because these are the affected areas treated by general and colorectal surgeons.

THERAPY

Although spontaneous resolution of condyloma is reported, most patients need treatment. The goal of that treatment should be complete destruction of all condyloma; however, the underlying viral infection may persist. Patients should be counseled in advance that recurrence is common and generally occurs during the first 3 months. Many therapeutic options can be divided broadly into two categories: provider-administered ablative/cytodestructive therapies (including cryotherapy, laser ablation, and trichloroacetic acid [TCA]) and patient-administered topical therapies (such as podophyllotoxin, sinecatechins, and imiquimod). Other options such as interferon, topical 5-fluorouracil (5-FU), vaccines, and cidofovir are less well established.

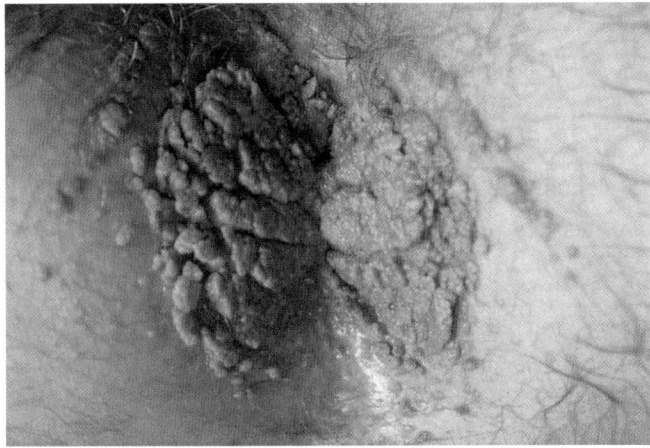

FIGURE I   Perinanal condyloma.

Topical Therapies

The mainstay of topical treatment for condyloma in the authors' practice is imiquimod (Zyclara, 3M Health Care, Loughborough, England). Imiquimod is an imidazoquinoline heterocyclic amine that functions as an immune response modifier. Imiquimod directly activates innate immune cells through Toll-like receptor 7, resulting in increased cytokine production, specifically increased interleukin-1 and tumor necrosis factor–alpha, and production of type I interferons (IFNs; IFN-alpha and IFN-beta). Indirectly, imiquimod enhances antigen-specific cell-mediated immunity. Imiquimod, an ointment, is applied at bedtime 3 times a week, left in place for 6 to 8 hours, and washed off in the morning. Treatment may take up to 16 weeks. A number of randomized controlled studies have shown that 5% imiquimod achieved a 50% complete response rate with a recurrence rate of 11%. The side effects of imiquimod are mostly local in nature and include burning, erythema, pain, and itching. However, these side effects are generally mild. Currently, imiquimod is not approved for use in the anal canal because of the possibility of significant ulceration and bleeding. The authors currently use imiquimod as their primary treatment modality. For patients with extensive warty disease, they use an 8-week to 10-week course before surgical treatment. Because of the high risk of recurrence in these patients, treatment for another 6 weeks is often continued after the surgical wounds are healed.

Podophyllin and Podophilox

Podophyllin is an amitotic agent obtained from the *Podophyllum* plant. It is an impure resin, generally suspended in tincture of benzoin in concentrations of 20% to 25%, and is applied to external warts by a provider on a weekly basis. The resin should be washed off 4 to 6 hours after application. Concerns about the use of podophyllin include local and systemic toxicity, teratogenicity, and mutagenicity. It is contraindicated in larger lesions and pregnancy. Clearance rates of most studies of podophyllin range from 40% to 60%, with recurrence rates as high as 60%.

Podofilox (podophyllotoxin) is the purified and standardized active component of podophyllin. It is available as a 0.5% topical gel or solution, which is applied by the patient twice a day for 3 days followed by 4 days with no treatment. This cycle is then repeated for 1 month, although at least one study shows safety for use up to 8 weeks. Local side effects include a burning sensation, pruritus, tenderness, and erythema but rarely are severe enough to require cessation of treatment. Total area of tissue treated should be less than 10 cm². Clearance rates in the 70% to 80% range are commonly reported, with recurrence rates of 10% to 20%. Podofilox has not been approved for anal canal or perianal condyloma; however, the gel has been studied in perianal warts with only 3% of patients discontinuing usage because of side effects.

Trichloroacetic acid

TCA is a corrosive chemical that denatures and precipitates protein. It is applied on a weekly basis directly to condyloma with an applicator. Because it destroys any tissue it contacts, normal adjacent skin should be protected with petrolatum. TCA is useful for small anal canal lesions; however, complete drying after application is important to protect unaffected anoderm. Few clinical trials exist that assess effectiveness, despite its fairly widespread use, but reported resolution rates range from 20% to 70%. It is ineffective for bulky disease, and the authors use it only for small lesions (<5 mm), few in number, in the anal canal.

Cryotherapy

Cryotherapy with liquid nitrogen is an appropriate technique for treatment of small perianal condyloma. This technique can be done in the office without anesthesia. Liquid nitrogen is applied with cotton-tipped applicator. The applicator is applied for 15 to 30 seconds. Care must be taken to limit the zone of injury because the application can cause significant pain. In an attempt to minimize local skin injury and pain, multiple smaller applications may be needed to achieve complete wart clearance. A specific advantage of cryotherapy compared with other modes of therapy is that it may be applied in the anal canal. A disadvantage to cryotherapy aside from local skin irritation is that intraanal applications may cause ulceration and significant rectal bleeding. The other drawback to office-based cryotherapy is maintenance of a ready supply of liquid nitrogen. The recurrence rate with cryotherapy is 20%.

5-Fluorouracil

5-Fluorouracil cream has been used as a topical treatment for anogenital condyloma. 5-FU is a pyrimidine antagonist that blocks the methylation of deoxyuridylic acid to thymidylic acid, interrupting DNA synthesis in the s-phase. Because of its mutagenic potential, 5-FU is contraindicated during pregnancy and should not be used by women of child-bearing age. No randomized controlled studies have evaluated its efficacy. Case studies have shown a 10% to 30% condyloma clearance rate. However, little data are available concerning recurrence.

Miscellaneous Treatments

The literature is filled with various other medical treatments for condyloma, including interferon, autologous vaccine, cidofovir, and many others. These have not proven to be effective in prospective trials, nor have they gained any widespread acceptance or usage.

Surgery

The goal of surgical treatment of condyloma is eradication of visible lesions with minimized destruction of normal adjacent tissue. This is accomplished through one of several techniques: tangential excision, electrocautery excision or fulguration, curettage, and laser excision. All of these techniques require some form of anesthesia and postoperative analgesics. These techniques are superior to the topical preparations listed previously for initial resolution of condyloma with cure rate of 60% to 90%. Recurrence rates of 20% to 30% are commonly reported.

Tangential excision with a scalpel or scissors can be performed as an office procedure and is especially useful for patients with smaller lesions that are few in number. The patient is placed in the lateral or prone jackknife position, and local anesthetic (lidocaine or bupivacaine with epinephrine) is injected subcutaneously or submucosally. Excision is performed at the level of the dermis, and hemostasis obtained with direct pressure or cauterization with silver nitrate. Cleansing with soap and water daily and after each bowel movement is all that is necessary for wound care.

Excision and fulguration with electrocautery is the optimal treatment for many anal condyloma. Smaller lesions can be treated with infiltration of local anesthesia; for larger lesions, outpatient general or spinal anesthesia is usually required. The patient is placed in lateral or prone jackknife position and then prepped and draped in the sterile manner. The superficial-most layer of the lesion is fulgurated with the electrocautery tip to a gray-white appearance that is then wiped with a dry gauze or a curette. This process of fulguration and tissue removal is repeated until the condyloma is completely removed without burning into the deep dermis or subcutaneous fat. Larger pedunculated warts are transected at the junction of the stalk with normal skin with a scalpel or electrocautery. In those patients with flat lesions, recurrent lesions, and those that do not have a benign appearance (ulcerated, friable, or hypervascular) and in patients who

are HIV positive, removed specimens should be sent for histopathologic evaluation. Postoperative care includes adequate oral analgesics and cleansing as described previously. An application of topical 5% lidocaine may be helpful for pain control. Because fulguration causes significant eschar formation, increasing pain and erythema may be a sign of bacterial infection. These infections are treated with either silver sulfadiazine or mupirocin. Full-thickness excision is discouraged for lesions than can be treated with the previous techniques. However, it may be necessary in larger flat lesions and especially in giant Buschke-Löwenstein tumors.

Surgical treatment of condyloma acuminata with the laser has been described. There is no benefit to the laser with regards to postoperative pain or clearance rates. Studies have shown higher recurrence in those patients treated with laser compared with electrocautery. Aside from the cost, the disadvantages of laser treatment include the need for special training and the exposure of operating room personnel to smaller viral particles in the laser plume compared with electrocautery smoke.

Treatment Recommendations

The goal of treatment for condyloma acuminata is eradication of visible disease with minimal morbidity and a low recurrence rate. Several factors should be considered in determining appropriate treatment. These include patient age, pain tolerance, compliance, and the size, number, and location of lesions to be treated.

For small lesions (<5 mm), regardless of the number, topical therapy should be the initial treatment. For a patient with a small number of lesions (<5), any topical preparation can be used. The authors currently use TCA in these cases. For patients with more extensive disease not involving the anal canal, imiquimod is the first-line therapy because intraanal application of imiquimod can cause severe mucosal ulceration. Small intraanal lesions can be treated with TCA or cryotherapy. Patients with intraanal lesions, those who are noncompliant with imiquimod, and those with failure of imiquimod therapy are offered excision and fulguration.

For more extensive disease, especially large multilobulated, cauliflower-like condyloma, surgery is the mainstay of treatment. The authors' preference for surgical treatment is excision and fulguration with the electrocautery as described previously. In these patients, after epithelial healing, imiquimod is used for treatment of any residual or recurrent disease. Although this is the authors' standard treatment, its efficacy in prevention of recurrence is still under investigation.

The treatment of anal condyloma and the prevention of anal canal cancer is an area of continued evolution. Currently, specific subtypes 16, 18, 31, and 35 are recognized to have an increased oncogenic potential; the histologic similarity between the anal transition zone and the cervical transition zone is also recognized. These are areas where immature metaplastic tissue susceptible to HPV infection can be found. It is important to recognize that oncogenic subtypes morphologically do not cause warty disease. Finally, some specific patient populations (individuals with immunocompromise [HIV, transplant] and men who have sex with men [MSM]) have been shown to have an increase in the rate of dysplastic lesions and anal canal cancer.

Currently, in conjunction with infectious disease colleagues, the authors screen and treat these patients aggressively. Individuals with HIV and immunocompromise undergo anal cytologic testing or Pap smear yearly. A key point to remember here is that this should be done with cotton-tipped swab, not polyethylene terephthalate swab, because of cellular adherence. Also, this should be done before a digital rectal examination because the lubricant used for the examination decreases cytologic results. Anal cytologic results can range from atypical cells of undetermined significance to low-grade squamous intraepithelial lesions (LSIL) to high-grade intraepithelial lesions (HSIL) to squamous cell cancer.

Once a cytologic diagnosis of HSIL is made, the patient then undergoes high-resolution anoscopy with biopsy and focal destruction of dysplastic lesions (Figures 2 to 4). Aside from treatment of normal warty tissue, this procedure allows for identification and treatment of potentially premalignant areas of AIN. This procedure involves high-resolution anoscopy with an operating microscope, acetowhitening with 3% acetic acid of the anal canal, and counter staining of the region with Lugol's solution. With direct vision, the anal canal is inspected for areas that do not stain brown with Lugol's

solution. The authors also look closely for cellular changes that would be seen on colposcopy, cellular mosaics and abnormal corkscrewing vessels. The areas are biopsied for confirmation and focal destruction. Biopsy allows for better quantification of the histologic diagnosis of anal intraepithelial neoplasia (AIN I, II, or III). These stained areas are then ablated with electrocautery. Although postoperative pain is a problem in roughly 50% of patients, there is a low chance of other significant morbidities. With use of high-resolution anoscopy and directed ablation, as opposed to radical excision, one can effectively eliminate AIN in individuals with HIV. The recurrence rate is high in patients with HIV (approximately 50%), but retreatment is safe and well tolerated (Figure 5).

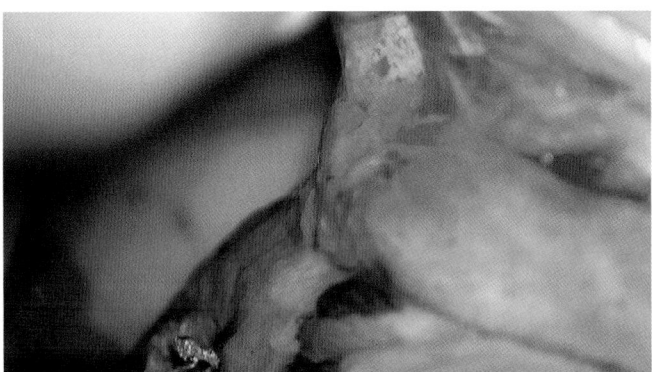

FIGURE 2 High-grade dysplastic lesion of anal transition zone seen on high-resolution anoscopy (HRA).

Human Papilloma Virus Vaccine

The quadrivalent HPV vaccine has been shown to be effective at preventing cervical infection and high-grade cervical neoplasia associated with HPV 6, 11, 16, and 18. CDC guidelines as of December 2011 recommend routine vaccination of males ages 11 and 12 years, vaccination of males ages 13 to 21 years not previously vaccinated, and vaccination for males ages 22 to 26 years based on increased risk factors such as HIV or anal-receptive intercourse. This vaccination showed reduced rates of anal intraepithelial neoplasia in homosexual males ages 16 to 26 years compared with placebo. The group studied did not have preexisting HSIL or warts, and the effect on vaccination in patients with existing disease is not known.

GIANT CONDYLOMA ACUMINATA

First described by Buschke and Löwenstein in 1925, giant condyloma acuminata (GCA) have been recognized as potentially malignant lesions. These large slow-growing painful cauliflower-like lesions located on the perineum and penis are sexually transmitted and associated with HPV types 6 and 11. These lesions were initially thought to be similar to ordinary condyloma because of their histologic similarity (benign histology, vacuolization of the cells of the superficial layer of the epidermis, parakeratosis, and infrequent mitotic figures). However, significant differences have been noted. GCA has marked papillomatosis, thickened rete ridges, increased acanthosis, and increased mitotic activity compared with ordinary condyloma. GCA also has shown infiltration of the surrounding tissues. This fact combined with GCA's histologic appearance can make it difficult to distinguish GCA from verrucous carcinoma. GCA has also been found to harbor areas of invasive squamous cell carcinoma, leading to the speculation that GCA represents part of the continuum from condyloma to invasive squamous cell cancer.

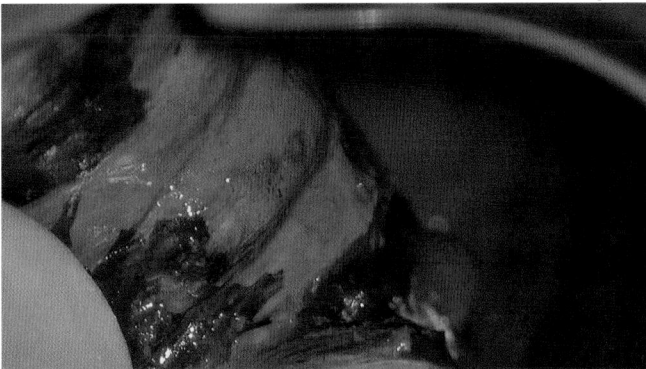

FIGURE 3 High-grade dysplastic lesion after aceto-whitening and Lugol's staining on high-resolution anoscopy (HRA).

The mainstay of treatment for GCA involves surgical excision. Ideally, wide local excision with a 1-cm margin is treatment of choice. This may require flap coverage or skin grafting to repair the defect. Rarely should this require fecal diversion for wound care and healing purposes (Figures 5 and 6). In lesions that involve the anal sphincters, abdominal-perineal resection is a viable option. In their review of the published literature, Trombetta and Place identified 45 patients in whom surgery was the primary therapy. This included simple excision, wide local excision, and abdominal-perineal resection. A 45% recurrence rate was seen with surgical treatment. This was a significant improvement from the 71% recurrence rate seen in those patients initially treated with nonsurgical therapy (podophyllin, intralesional interferon, and 5-FU).

The role of chemoradiation is an option in the treatment of extensive GCA in poor surgical candidates or where clear surgical margins are impossible. This is reasonable considering the relationship between HPV, GCA, and invasive non-GCA squamous cell-carcinoma. Similar to the treatment of anal canal cancer with 5-FU, mitomycin C and external beam radiation (XRT) has been shown to cause complete regression in cases of GCA (Figure 7).

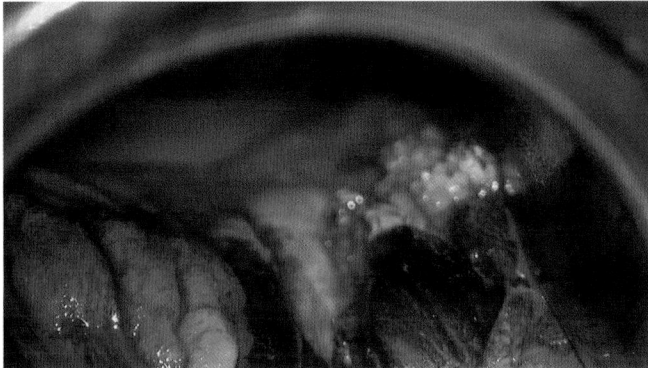

FIGURE 4 High-grade dysplastic lesion after focal destruction.

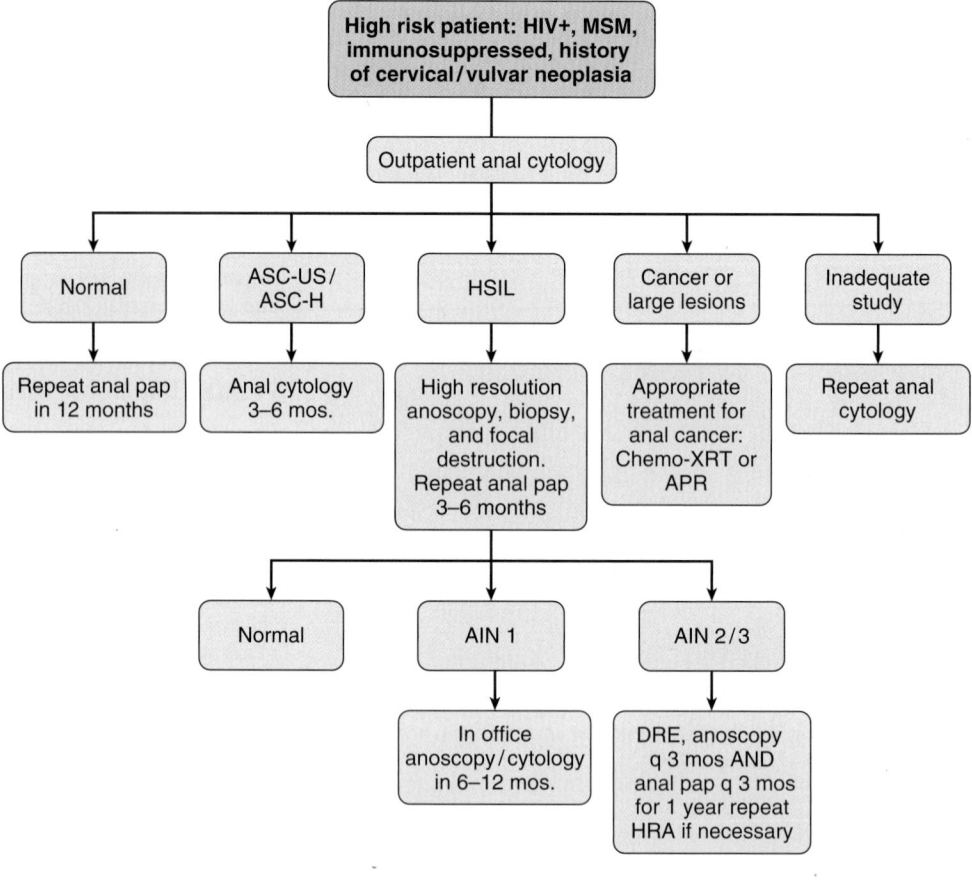

FIGURE 5 Treatment algorithm for anal Pap test and high-resolution anoscopy. *(Modified from Palefsky JM, Rubin M: The epidemiology of anal human papillomavirus and related neoplasia, Obstet Gynecol Clin North Am 36:187–200, 2009.)*

The algorithm shows:

High risk patient: HIV+, MSM, immunosuppressed, history of cervical/vulvar neoplasia → Outpatient anal cytology, branching to:

- Normal → Repeat anal pap in 12 months
- ASC-US/ASC-H → Anal cytology 3–6 mos.
- HSIL → High resolution anoscopy, biopsy, and focal destruction. Repeat anal pap 3–6 months
- Cancer or large lesions → Appropriate treatment for anal cancer: Chemo-XRT or APR
- Inadequate study → Repeat anal cytology

HSIL branch leads to:
- Normal
- AIN 1 → In office anoscopy/cytology in 6–12 mos.
- AIN 2/3 → DRE, anoscopy q 3 mos AND anal pap q 3 mos for 1 year repeat HRA if necessary

MSM – male having sex with male
HRA – high resolution anoscopy
ASC-US – atypical squamous cells of unknown significance
ASC-H – atypical squamous cells cannot rule out high-grade lesion
LSIL – low grade squamous intraepithelial lesion
HSIL – high grade squamous intraepithelial lesion
AIN 1 – low grade anal intraepithelial neoplasia
AIN 2/3 – high grade anal intraepithelial neoplasia
DRE – digital rectal exam
Chemo-XRT – combined modality chemo/radiation
APR – abdominoperineal resection

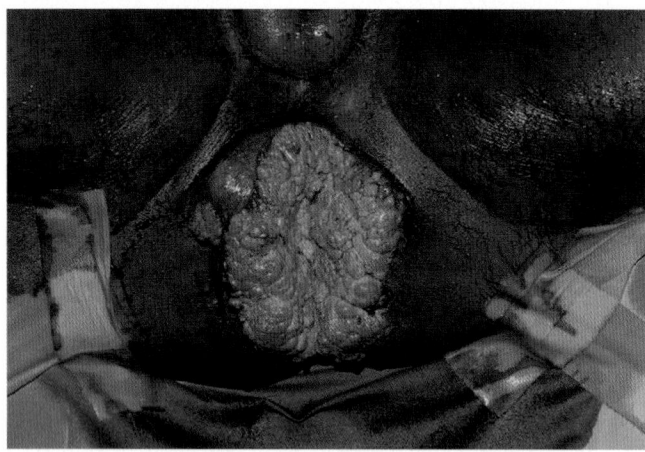

FIGURE 6   Giant perianal condyloma.

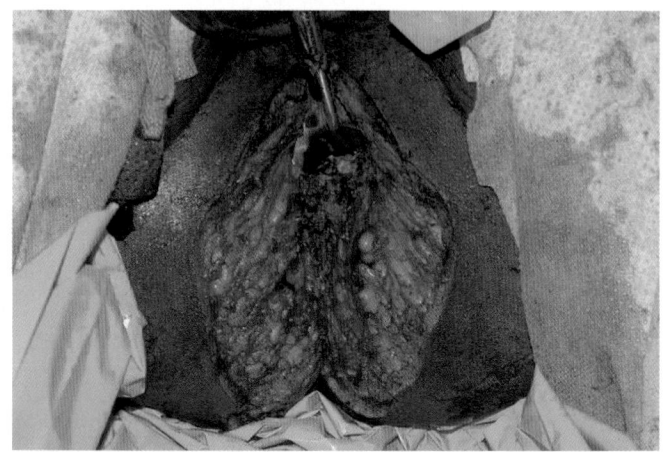

FIGURE 7   Resulting defect after wide local excision of giant perianal condyloma.

SUGGESTED READINGS

Centers for Disease Control: Recommendations on the use of quadrivalent human papillomavirus vaccine in males: advisory committee on immunization practices (ACIP), *MMWR* 60(50):1750–1758, 2011.

Echenique I, Phillips BR: Anal warts and anal intradermal neoplasia, *Clin Colon Rectal Surg* 24:31–38, 2011.

Palefsky J, Rubin M: The epidemiology of anal human papillomavirus and related neoplasia, *Obstet Gynecol Clin North Am* 36:187–200, 2009.

Paraskevas K, Kyriakos E, Poulios E, et al: Surgical management of giant condyloma acuminatum (Buschke-Lowenstein Tumor) of the perianal region, *Dermatol Surg* 33:638–644, 2007.

Trombetta LJ, Place RJ: Giant condyloma acuminatum of the anorectum: trends in epidemiology and management: report of a case and review of the literature, *Dis Colon Rectum* 44:1878-1886, 2001.

Whitlow CB, Gottesman L, Bernstein MA: Sexually transmitted diseases. In Beck DE, Roberts PL, Saclarides TJ, et al, editors: *The ASCRS textbook of colon and rectal surgery*, ed 2, New York, 2011, Springer, pp 295–307.

THE MANAGEMENT OF PILONIDAL DISEASE

Jeffrey A. Sternberg, MD, FACS, FASCRS

PILONIDAL DISEASE: COMMON AND CHALLENGING

Pilonidal disease is a common, acquired chronic infection of the skin and subcutaneous tissue overlying the sacrum and coccyx with an incidence of approximately 25 per 100,000. It typically affects people in their teens, 20s, and 30s. The disease rarely first becomes symptomatic after age 40. Men are affected at rates two to three times more frequent than those of women. The disease can manifest acutely, or individuals can live with intermittent symptoms for many years. In its most severe form, pilonidal disease can be severely debilitating, causing daily discomfort and limiting activity. Because pilonidal disease affects people in their most productive years, the socioeconomic effect of the disease is great because affected patients spend significant time away from school or work.

Pilonidal disease was originally described by Herbert Mayo in 1833 and initially thought to be of congenital origin. Unacceptably high recurrences despite seemingly adequate surgical interventions however, support the acquired as opposed to the congenital theory of etiology.

Pilonidal disease first gained public attention during World War II when more than 78,000 soldiers with this condition were admitted to U.S. Army hospitals for an average of 55 days. Surgical outcomes were so poor on these individuals that the U.S. military essentially banned further surgical procedures for this disease.

Pilonidal disease continues to be greatly misunderstood, and rates of recurrence and morbidity from traditional surgical approaches are unacceptably high. Because of this, the surgical treatment of pilonidal disease must change. Nonoperative treatment has gained popularity, but there is little evidence that nonsurgical treatments can cure significant pilonidal disease. More contemporary operations involving flaps and off-midline closure are gaining popularity among surgeons willing to move beyond surgical tradition. These more complex procedures may be performed in an outpatient setting, require minimal absence of patients from work or athletics, and have much lower recurrence rates than do conventional excisional procedures. Because many general and colon and rectal surgeons have limited experience with reconstructive procedures involving flaps, few have performed these rigorous but arguably superior operations. Asymmetric flap procedures should become the new norm for the treatment of advanced or recurrent pilonidal disease.

Because most recommendations regarding the treatment of this disease are derived from expert opinion or case report studies, the best treatment of pilonidal disease remains controversial.

ETIOLOGY AND CHARACTERISTICS

The Name

Pilonidal disease is an acquired condition of the natal cleft (Figure 1). There are two important ingredients in the development of pilonidal disease: a deep cleft and hair. The term *pilonidal* comes from the Latin *pilus*, meaning "hair," and *nidus*, meaning "nest." Most pilonidal abscesses contain hairs. Hairs that are shed from the scalp or back fall into and become lodged in an unusually deep cleft near the tailbone. The hairs in pilonidal abscesses are not ingrown. Hairs and debris are secondary invaders and not the cause of the condition. The shed hairs insert from their root end because barbs prevent them from inserting from their external apex. Local hair removal or eradication is therefore not preventive or curative.

Causes

Pilonidal disease most commonly occurs in hirsute individuals with deep natal clefts. The environment inherent in a deep natal cleft is the true cause of pilonidal disease. The cycle begins when an individual with a deep cleft sits. The stretch of the sitting motion ruptures hair follicles in the midline, and they become plugged with keratin. This follicular occlusive process is similar to what occurs in hidradenitis suppurativa. A subcutaneous abscess then develops. The moist, anaerobic nature of the cleft prevents healing, and a dilated pore or pit opens in the midline (Figure 2). Further sitting motions cause the skin of the cleft to tighten and lift off the sacrococcygeal fascia, which creates a suction force that pulls hair and debris through the holes, causing enlargement of the subcutaneous abscess. A foreign body reaction develops and contributes to the formation of pus and inflammation.

In the body's attempt to expel the infection, a secondary sinus may track to the cephalad aspect of the natal cleft (Figure 3). Such a secondary external opening is the result and not the cause of the disease, even though it may seem more impressive than the more anally located dilated pores. These pores, termed the *primary openings*, are the true source of pilonidal disease. The condition is less often observed in people with shallow natal clefts.

Not a Congenital Condition

Pilonidal disease is not caused by an infected congenital cyst. The abscess cavity in pilonidal disease does not have an epithelial lining

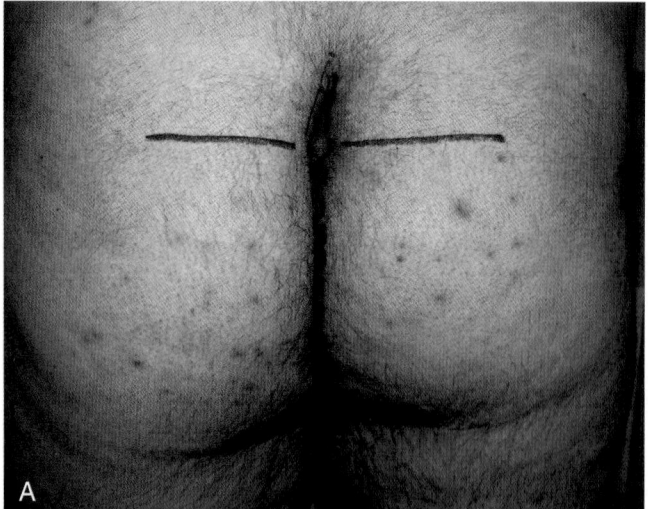

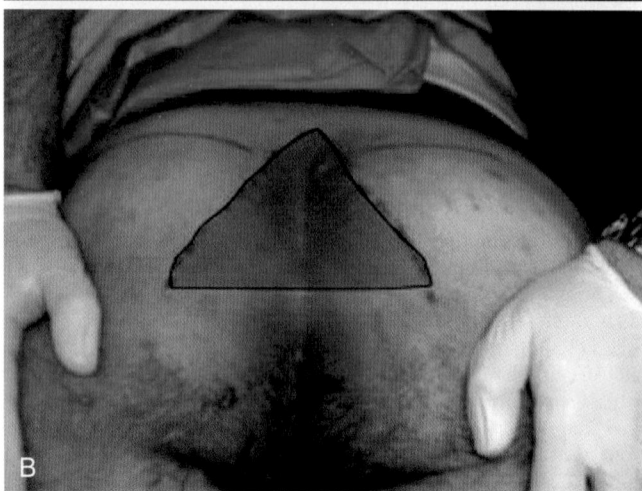

FIGURE 1 A, In a patient lying down, the edges of the buttock cheeks that touch when the person is standing are marked. The horizontal line is the contact point with the chair when the patient is seated. **B,** The buttock cheeks are spread to reveal the natal cleft, a 5- to 9-cm region bounded by the midsacrum and the perineum. The lateral borders are formed by the edges of the buttock cheeks that touch when the person is standing.

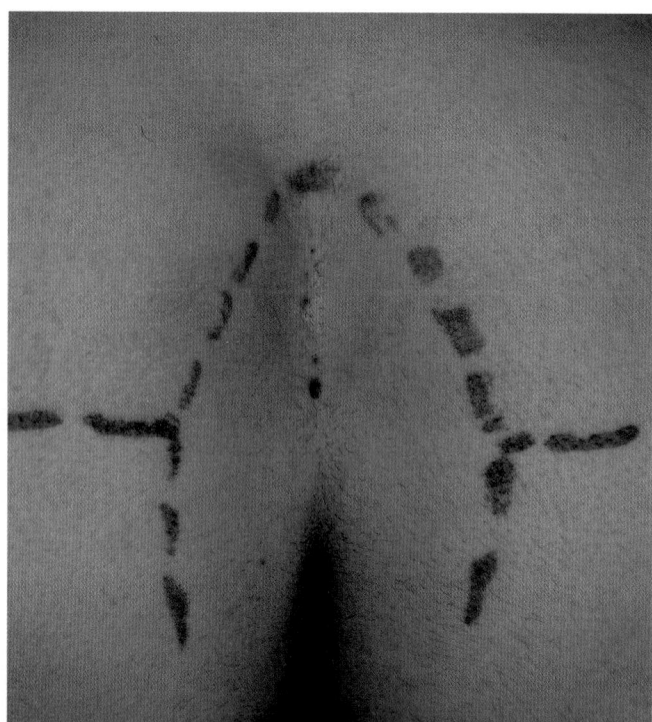

FIGURE 2 Five midline dilated pits in pilonidal disease.

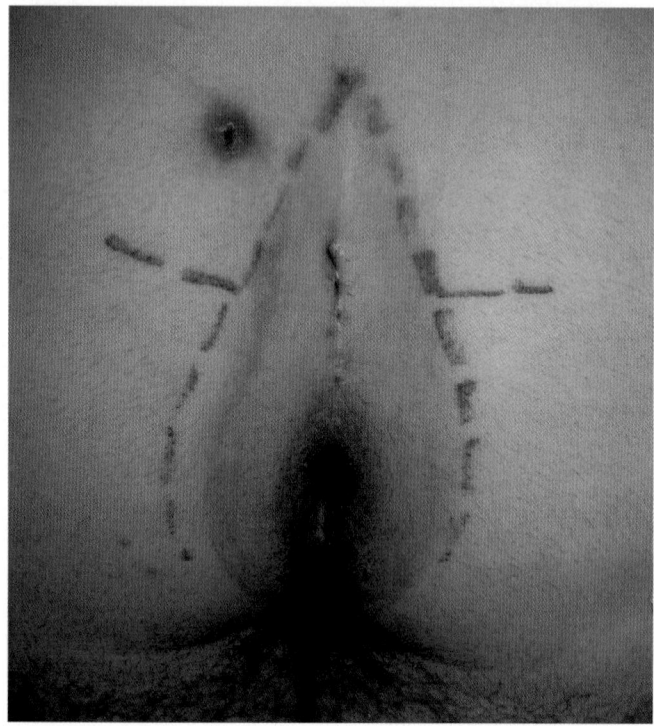

FIGURE 3 Chronic pilonidal sinus. Note four midline pits (the upper three contain protruding hairs) and left draining sinus tract cephalad to pits.

and is therefore not a cyst. Therefore, the term *pilonidal cyst* is a misnomer. The condition is simply a subcutaneous abscess filled with purulent material and debris, most often hair.

Implications of Anatomy on Surgical Approach

Failure to recognize that the depth of the cleft is the causative factor in this disease leads to misdirected surgical procedures. Wide excisions that attempt to remove a nonexistent cyst leave large midline wounds in persistently deep clefts that may not heal because of the anaerobic environment and repetitive shear forces (Figure 4). Such procedures often result in a larger wound that is even more difficult to treat than the original abscess. Even when such wounds heal, individuals remain at risk for recurrence of pilonidal abscess because the original cleft conditions remain hostile: the cleft remains deep.

Making the Diagnosis

Pilonidal disease can exist for months or years before it causes symptoms. The disease may manifest as an acute painful abscess or as a chronic draining sinus. To make the diagnosis, the clinician must recognize the dilated pits in the midline of the natal cleft with or

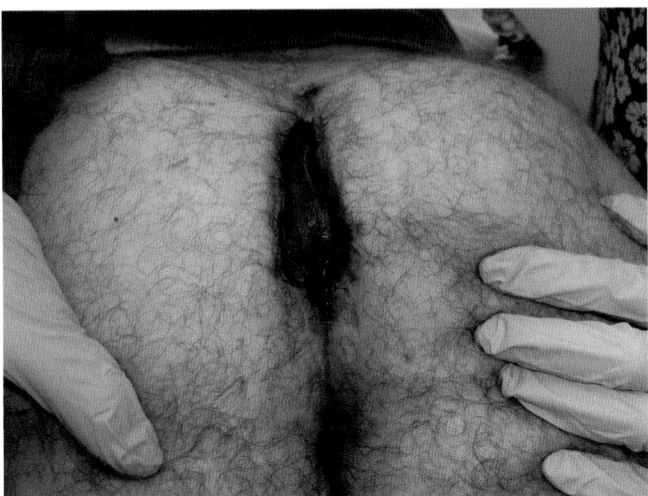

FIGURE 4 Large unhealed wound 6 months after wide excision and attempted midline closure in a 19-year-old male.

without an associated secondary sinus. Shed hairs are often seen protruding from these midline pits. Patients may report trauma to the coccygeal area before the development of symptoms. Trauma can cause an abscess to become inflamed or otherwise bring the patient's attention to the area. Pilonidal abscesses are not thought to be the direct result of acute trauma.

A CHANGING PARADIGM

Despite the currently accepted notion that pilonidal disease is a condition that is acquired rather than congenital, many surgeons continue to perform wide excisions in the midline deep cleft in an attempt to remove the nonexistent congenital cyst. Surgical procedures for pilonidal disease will continue to be unsuccessful until surgeons realize that the depth of the natal cleft in affected individuals is the cause of the disease. Therefore, for procedures to be routinely effective, the natal cleft must be made shallower. Traditional operations for pilonidal disease typically involve the unnecessary extensive excision of tissue down to the sacrum. Wounds are then left open to heal by secondary intention in the midline or closed in the midline in a residual deep cleft. Most midline incisions in a deep anaerobic environment will open because of trapped dead space and the hostile conditions in the cleft. Marsupialized wounds may heal but do so over a long period of time, and daily packing may be required. Many individuals with open sacral wounds are unable to sit, which results in significant morbidity that interferes with work, attending classes, or group living in school dormitories. A surgeon should not undertake an operation for pilonidal disease unless she or he is confident that the outcome is highly likely to be better than living with the disease itself. Often, overly aggressive surgical procedures make this condition worse and result in a more complex pilonidal condition or one or more large unhealed wounds that are more challenging to correct than the original problem (see Figure 4).

The Difficult Environment of the Cleft

Wounds in deep natal clefts are very resistant to healing. The reasons for this are not fully understood. Contributing factors include anaerobic conditions, a location and anatomy that challenge good hygiene, shear forces from movement, and mechanical forces from the natural contour and gluteal muscle tension. Aggressive débridement, cautery,

and dressing changes are rarely successful in healing chronic wounds in this region. Even negative-pressure wound therapy is typically unsuccessful. The best corrective therapy is asymmetric flap closure of these wounds that make the natal cleft shallow and leave operative incisions off the midline, where they are in the open air and can heal. Surgeons should be aware of the potential danger of creating midline wounds in the natal cleft, inasmuch as they often do not heal. Significant pilonidal disease or recurrent pilonidal disease necessitates a definitive surgical procedure to reduce the depth of the natal cleft to render it well aerated, dry, and shallow, so that hair and debris cannot be trapped.

DIAGNOSIS AND DIFFERENTIAL DIAGNOSIS

Recognition of midline pits with or without a chronic draining sinus clinches the diagnosis of pilonidal disease. On occasion, the sinus opening, if present, can be contained within the natal cleft, but typically it lies outside the boundaries of the natal cleft and above it on the right or left side. This location of the secondary opening probably results from the body's attempt to expel infection to the outside world (the "closed" nature of the cleft may be perceived as internal). With acute abscesses, edema can obscure the midline pits, and these pits may be visible only once the abscess has been adequately drained and the swelling subsides. If it is difficult to see the primary openings; placing upward traction on the natal cleft skin often reveals these pits because their deep apices are often tethered to the underlying abscess cavity.

Pilonidal disease must be distinguished from other processes such as perianal abscess, perianal fistula, hidradenitis suppurativa, or unusual skin infections. If the abscess extends down the natal cleft and approaches the anus, the condition can be difficult to differentiate from a perianal abscess. Draining openings in the lower part of the natal cleft without the dilated midline pits can be the result of a perianal fistula. Sometimes perianal fistulas do occur in individuals with quiescent pilonidal disease, in which case the focus of treatment should be on the symptomatic perianal fistula rather than the quiescent pilonidal disease. Pits off the midline sometimes indicate a different disease process such as hidradenitis suppurativa or unusual skin infections such as syphilis, tuberculosis, or actinomycosis.

Classification schemes exist for pilonidal disease, but they are not commonly referenced and are therefore not of significant clinical utility.

Imaging

Imaging is generally not required to evaluate or confirm the diagnosis of pilonidal disease. Only in rare circumstances during which chronically ill patients are suspected of harboring osteomyelitis of the sacrum should imaging such as magnetic resonance imaging (MRI) be employed. Findings on fistulograms and sinograms rarely change surgical therapy. In circumstances in which an anal fistula must be ruled out as a cause of a low-lying natal cleft pit, MRI or endoanal ultrasonography with hydrogen peroxide injected in the external opening of the suspected fistula may be helpful.

ACUTE PILONIDAL ABSCESS MANAGEMENT

Pilonidal disease may initially manifest as an acute abscess. The primary treatment of an acute pilonidal abscess is incision and drainage. Drainage should be performed 1 to 2 cm off the midline to avoid a large midline wound. A cruciate incision or an elliptical incision is needed to provide adequate drainage and prevent early closure of the draining incision. In such difficult-to-reach areas, packing is not recommended or required. Such procedures are usually safely performed in an office setting with local anesthesia and very rarely require an operating room setting. Antibiotics are usually not needed unless there is significant cellulitis or the individual is immunosuppressed or diabetic.

The flora of such wounds is usually represented by skin organisms, anaerobes, or both. These wounds do not typically contain resistant staphylococci unless they are recurrent.

After drainage, patients are instructed to soak in a warm tub several times a day for several days and to keep the area clean. Showering is permitted. They are asked to return in 3 weeks, at which time the primary openings are often seen.

Individuals who develop an acute abscess only once or who develop infrequent abscesses that necessitate only minor office-based drainage procedures are typically not advised to undergo surgical intervention. Over time, however, such conditions may progress to a chronic abscess with multiple dilated pits and chronic induration in the cleft without a drainable abscess. Patients with recurrent acute abscesses, those with a chronic abscess, and those who have a preference for definitive therapy should be evaluated or referred for surgical intervention.

CHRONIC PILONIDAL SINUS

A pilonidal sinus may develop after several acute abscess flares, or it may be initial presentation of the disease. Affected individuals have multiple dilated midline pits (some of which may be epithelialized as a result of their chronicity) and a chronic draining sinus that typically opens to the cephalad right or left aspect of the natal cleft.

Of importance is that the draining sinus at the top of the natal cleft is a secondary opening and that surgical treatment directed solely at this opening will fail to cure the condition because the more anally located primary pits are the source of the disease. Some individuals can live with a chronic pilonidal sinus with minimal symptoms and never require surgical intervention. However, in many cases, these sinuses are accompanied by annoying drainage and chronic pain, and therefore many patients desire definitive surgical therapy.

NONSURGICAL APPROACHES

Patients who have no symptoms despite the appearance of their pilonidal condition and those with minimal symptoms can be managed by observation. The best conservative approach involves doing nothing. There is little evidence that local shaving or hair removal is effective at preventing recurrent disease once primary openings have appeared. Some surgeons have advocated injecting phenol into sinus tracts to destroy them. This is quite painful and often has to be performed while the patient is under regional or general anesthesia, with a several-day hospitalization for postoperative pain control. The rationale for this treatment is that phenol destroys tissue and causes scarring. Because the scar tracts remain in the deep natal cleft, these individuals remain at risk for developing recurrent pilonidal disease. Few data support use of phenol in pilonidal disease.

SURGICAL APPROACHES

Indications for surgical intervention include recurrent acute abscesses, symptomatic chronic pilonidal sinuses, and patients' preference. Because of the demanding educational and employment activities of young individuals affected by the disease, many opt for surgery to try to eliminate the uncertainty of recurrent disease.

For early disease with several upper natal cleft pits and a short draining sinus, conservative surgical intervention consists of unroofing or pit-picking techniques.

Unroofing

In unroofing, a fistula probe is delivered through the lowest pit and out through either the highest pit or sinus if it is present (Figure 5). Electrocautery is used to perform a minimal elliptical incision over the probe and unroof the skin, connecting the midline pits and the sinus. The underlying abscess cavity is curetted to remove debris. The edges of the wound are best marsupialized. Packing can be performed but is cumbersome unless the patient has daily assistance. For short tracts, some patients can undergo these procedures under local anesthesia in an office setting, but procedures involving longer tracts necessitate regional or general anesthesia in an operating room. Wide excisions are unnecessary because the abscess cavities are rarely complex unless prior surgical procedures have been performed in this region. Injecting methylene blue is unnecessary because granulation tissue enables easy identification of the tract. Complete healing may take 6 weeks, but patients are permitted to be active during the healing period. Occasional silver nitrate treatments in the physician's office are useful in preventing the development of exuberant granulation tissue. The overall success rate of this procedure is unknown.

Pit Picking

Minimal excision of midline pits with débridement of the abscess cavity, often through a lateral wound as described by Bascom and Bascom, is a potentially curative procedure for early disease (Figure 6). Patients with several midline pits and perhaps a minor short tract sinus are candidates for this procedure. This procedure, performed with the patient under local anesthesia in the physician's office, involves small elliptical incisions (with a No. 11 blade or a 2-mm

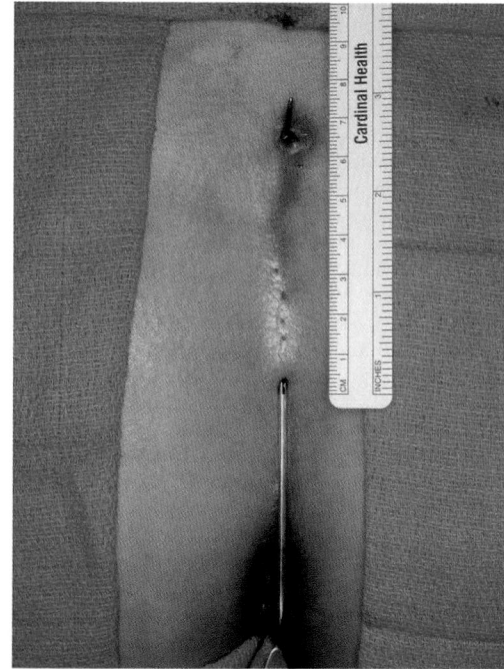

FIGURE 5 Probing the fistula tract: the first step before unroofing the pilonidal sinus.

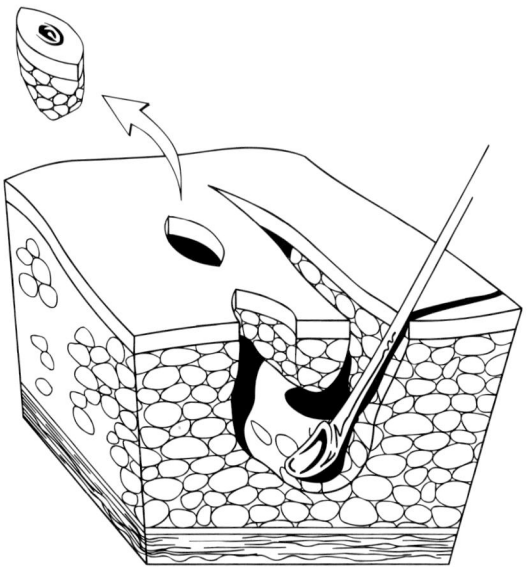

FIGURE 6 The incision is made lateral to the pilonidal sinus cavity, and the cavity is curetted. Pits are excised separately or en bloc. *(Adapted from Nivatvongs S: Pilonidal disease. In Gordon P, Nivatvongs S, editors: Principles and practice of surgery for the colon, rectum, and anus, St. Louis, 1992, Quality Medical.)*

punch biopsy blade) around the midline pits; these pits are closed with a fine monofilament suture. A lateral incision 1 to 2 cm off the midline enables access to the underlying abscess cavity. This abscess cavity is débrided with a curette and left open. Making the lateral wound elliptical enables adequate drainage and eliminates the need for packing. Patients return in 7 to 10 days for suture removal, and the wounds fully heal in approximately 2 weeks.

An alternative technique involves the use of trephines (small circular punch knives). In this technique, the midline pits are excised, as are their connections with the underlying abscess cavity, and the abscess cavity is débrided with the trephines. All wounds are left open.

The Goals of Surgery in Patients With Chronic Disease

The management of chronic pilonidal disease remains controversial. The first aim of surgery, however, is indisputably to eliminate the chronic infection and relieve pain and discharge in the least disfiguring manner possible with the shortest recovery possible. The second aim should be to decrease the possibility of future hair insertion into the vulnerable midline skin of the natal cleft by making it less deep. Unfortunately, many traditional surgical techniques have failed to adhere to these goals. Two commonly performed procedures are midline operations that involve a wide excision of the affected area in the natal cleft, often down to the sacrococcygeal fascia, with either a midline closure or marsupialization of the large resulting defect. Both these procedures introduce wounds in a persistently deep natal cleft. When wounds are closed in such environment, there is a high chance that the wound will open. Although open wounds may heal, they often do so at a high cost. Many of these wounds linger for months, necessitating daily meticulous care and packing. Data concerning the true recurrence rates after such procedures are limited. Evidence is increasingly in favor of a flap-based procedure with an off midline closure.

Asymmetric Flap Techniques

The Karydakis Flap

Dr. George Karydakis first developed the concept of eccentric excision for pilonidal disease and published his experience in 1973. In this technique, which is essentially an advancement flap procedure, an elliptical excision of skin encompasses the dilated midline pits and sinus tract and the underlying chronic subcutaneous abscess centered 2 cm off of the midline. After the excision, the skin and subcutaneous fat from the opposite side of the cleft is mobilized to produce a thick flap, which is advanced across the midline and sutured to the skin on the side of the excised tissue. The flap is further fixed to the underlying sacrococcygeal fascia. A Penrose or closed suction drain is placed at the upper end of the wound deep to the flap for several days to a week. This operation demonstrates some important concepts: wounds off the midline (where they are exposed to air) do heal, and shallower clefts help prevent recurrent disease because these clefts do not collect debris and do remain well aerated.

The results of a Karydakis flap operation are quite good, with a recurrence rate of only 1%, but complication rates are fairly high, at approximately 8% or 9%. Complications that occur include infections and fluid collections that necessitate drainage, but these rarely result in a failure of the operation. The operation, however, causes a significant degree of pain and can require a several-day hospitalization for pain control.

The Cleft Lift Procedure

The next evolution of the Karydakis operation, the cleft lift procedure, was originally developed by Dr. John Bascom. The goals of the cleft lift are to render the natal cleft shallow and to lateralize the incision. A cutaneous flap is both advanced and rotated across the midline of the natal cleft to make the cleft more shallow and therefore correct the anatomy that leads to recurrent pilonidal disease. In this procedure, the only tissue that is excised is an ellipse of skin rather than the skin, fat, and fascia of the Karydakis procedure. The abscess cavity wall is preserved and used in the closure to prevent dead space. Skin is necessarily removed so that the cleft has a smooth contour after the underlying tissue is brought together to eliminate the deep midline in the cleft. This operation is performed on an ambulatory basis and has become this author's preferred method of treating pilonidal disease that necessitates surgery.

The cleft lift operation requires meticulous planning and technique and is performed as follows. Preoperatively, the patient is asked to stand, and the line of skin contact of both buttocks is marked with an indelible marker. This defines the natal cleft lateral boundaries and serves as a guide for placing the wound so that it ends up in a well-aerated position. For orientation purposes, a second line perpendicular to the first is drawn where the patient's buttock cheek meets a chair in the seated position (see Figure 1, *A*).

General or regional anesthetic is used (a spinal anesthetic is preferred because patients can comfortably position themselves). Local anesthesia with sedation is not sufficient owing to the large size of the dissection. Patients are positioned prone (jackknifing is not necessary), and the buttocks are taped apart. The natal cleft, lower back, buttocks, and perianal tissues are shaven with clippers. The clinician must be careful not to injure fragile skin during this process because it can lead to wound complications. A field block with 0.5% bupivacaine with 1:200,000 epinephrine is administered.

An asymmetric ellipse of skin, which will eventually be excised, is marked on one side of the natal cleft, often the one that contains the sinus (Figure 7, *A* and *B*). The more scarred side is excised if the patient has undergone prior pilonidal surgery. The ellipse does not have to include the sinus, which will heal when the primary openings and underlying abscess have been removed. For a better cosmetic result, however, it is preferable to remove the sinus opening. The cephalad portion of the ellipse should be at least 2 cm above the top

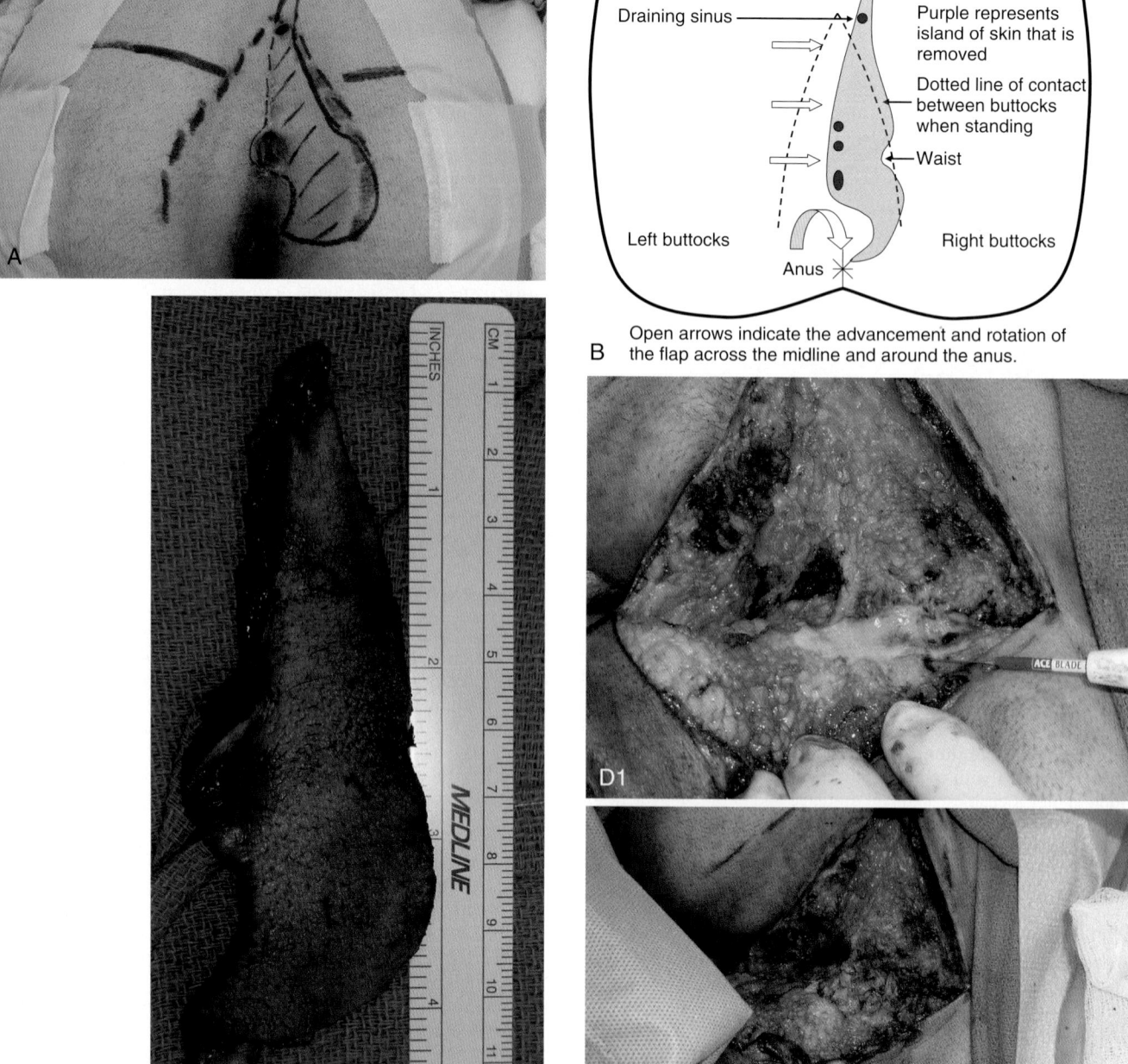

FIGURE 7 The cleft lift procedure. **A,** Operative planning photo showing markings of where buttocks meet (*dashed lines*), where the buttock meets the chair (*solid horizontal line*), and asymmetric ellipse of skin to be excised (*hatched area on right*). In this photograph, the right cephalad wound is the draining sinus, and the caudal wound is the large midline pilonidal opening. **B,** Operative planning diagram. **C,** Excised skin, including sinus opening at superior border and caudal wound in lower third (note that flap of skin shrinks in size after excision). **D,** Before and after cross-hatching: (1) intact fibrous abscess cavity wall, and (2) abscess wall after cross-hatching to disrupt fibrous fixation.

of the natal cleft to prevent the creation of a divot that can lead to recurrent disease. The anal aspect of the ellipse ends in a curve pointing toward the right or left posterolateral portion of the anus. It is important that the ellipse include all the primary midline openings. The lateral edge of the ellipse closely approximates the skin contact marking that was made preoperatively, but it comes in as a "waist" on a 45-degree angle to the lowest pit, inasmuch as this is the most challenging portion of the wound to close in a tension-free manner.

The medial line of the ellipse of skin to be removed is incised with electrocautery on the cutting mode or with a No. 15 blade. Cautery offers the advantage of being able to incise very precisely while remaining perpendicular to a contoured skin surface. It is very important that as much of the natal skin opposite from the excision is preserved for reconstructive purposes. The incision is made just to the opposite side of the dilated midline pits. The incision is carried around the lowest pit and ends in a comma-shaped or reverse

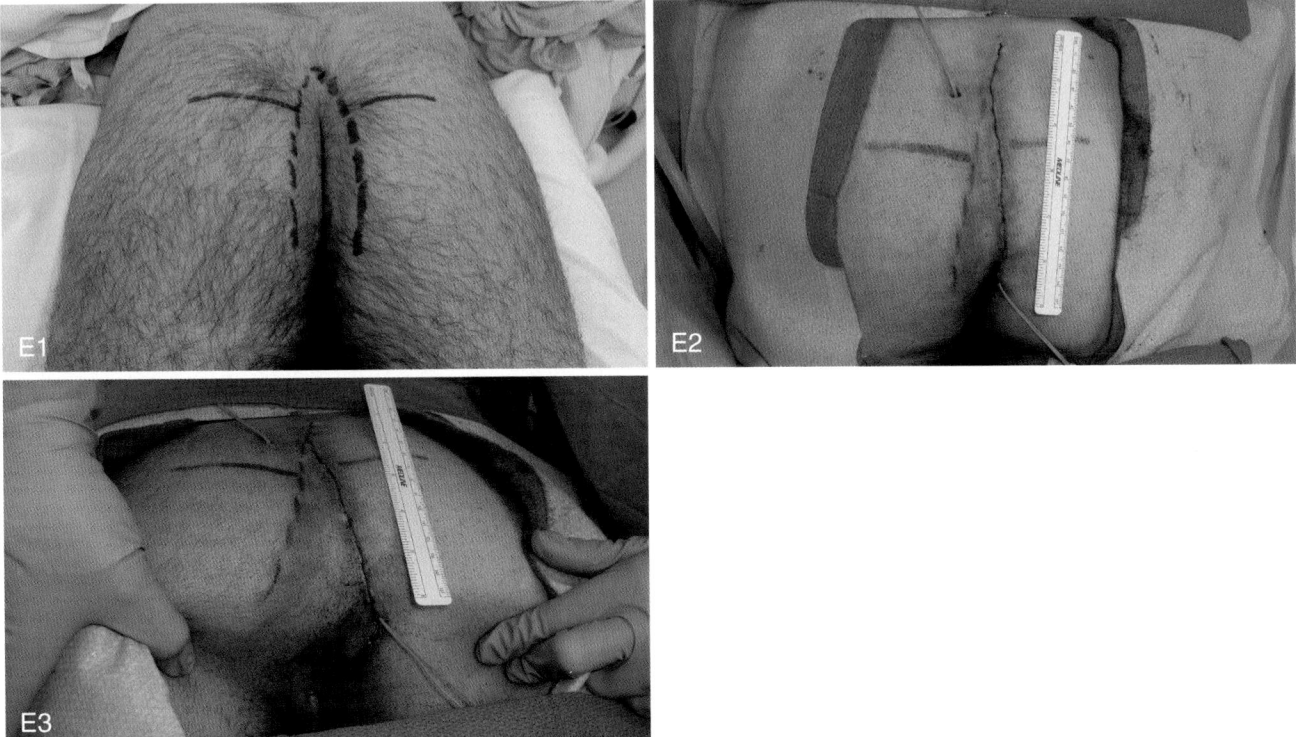

FIGURE 7, cont'd E, Comparison of the appearances of the natal cleft before and after surgery. (1) Preoperative deep and hirsute natal cleft; (2) immediate postoperative view of natal cleft that has been rendered significantly shallower with incision in open air, and (3) anus exposed to demonstrate lowest portion of incision.

comma-shaped curl pointing toward the corresponding posterolateral portion of the anus.

A skin flap is elevated off the opposite side of the natal cleft with electrocautery, extending out past the marked line of skin contact on that side. The flap is kept thin (3 to 5 mm in thickness, as in a mastectomy flap) at the cephalad aspect of the wound. The flap abruptly thickens toward the anal aspect. Dissection exposes the sacrococcygeal fascia overlying the coccyx. The anococcygeal ligament is exposed and divided to enable rotational mobility of the flap around the anus. This is the more challenging portion of the procedure (and an unfamiliar area for many surgeons), and care must be taken to avoid injuring the rectum, which lies immediately underneath the anococcygeal ligament. Once the flap is adequately mobilized, the ellipse of skin to be removed is elevated off that side of the natal cleft out to the lateral markings. This skin is dissected just beneath the dermis; all the underlying subcutaneous fat is preserved.

At this point, the tape is removed from the buttocks, and the coverage flap is draped across the midline while an assistant pushes the buttocks together and the lateral border of the ellipse of skin to be excised is marked again to ensure that the flap will adequately cover the resulting wound. The island of skin is then detached from its lateral attachment. The skin island typically measures 12 to 18 cm in length and 4 to 5 cm in width in the middle (depending on the body habitus of the patient and how close the lowest midline pit is to the anus; see Figure 7, *C*).

A large wound results from this excision. The abscess cavity and the long sinus tract can be seen (see Figure 7, *D1*). The abscess cavity and sinus tract are now unroofed and curetted free of debris. The abscess cavity wall is not removed, but occasionally the inner portion is excised if it contains a large amount of inspissated hair. Removal of the abscess cavity wall in its entirety would create dead space, in which infected fluid could accumulate and lead to an early recurrence of the abscess. The abscess cavity wall instead is cut into cubes of tissue left attached to the underlying tissue (see Figure 7, *D2*). This

is performed by making cross-hatch incisions to break up the scar to enable its rotational mobility during the next stage of the procedure. The wound is irrigated with antibiotic solution, and hemostasis is once again achieved with electrocautery.

The fibroadipose tissue of the buttock cheeks are next serially sewn together with numerous sutures of 2.0 absorbable monofilament suture as the assistant forcibly pushes the buttocks together. Numerous layers are required to take all tension off the flap. A passive drain (e.g., two Silastic vessel loops) is placed through a cruciate incision to the right upper aspect of the flap and is brought out through the wound itself at the inflection point where the wound dives down toward the anus (3 cm from the end of the anus). The superficial layers of the flap closure are created with 3.0 absorbable monofilament sutures, and the skin is closed with either interrupted or running 3.0 rapidly absorbing monofilament suture material (see Figure 7, *A* to *C*). Steri-Strips are applied to the wound, and the passive drain is tied to itself outside the patient to form a continuous loop. The incision often extends close to the anus to avoid a "dog ear" during the wound closure.

Patients are discharged the day of the procedure. They are instructed to have a caregiver roll gauze over the flap from the anal end to the upper margin to expel fluid from the upper drain hole three times a day. The drain is removed 9 days after the procedure, and patients are allowed to return to full activity at that time. The procedure does not cause significant pain because the flap is denervated during the procedure. Sensation is regained after a period of 6 to 9 weeks (see Figure 7, *E*).

Differences Between the Cleft Lift Procedure and Other Flap Procedures

The only tissue removed during the cleft lift procedure is skin. Hence, no dead space is created, and infected fluid does not have any place in which to accumulate. The procedure also seems to cause less pain than other procedures in which thick tissue flaps are moved. Patients are administered broad-spectrum antibiotics for 2 weeks after the procedure because these wounds are all chronically infected, many grossly so at the time of surgery.

Complications include stitch abscesses and, very rarely, wound breakdown. Even in the rare event that a wound fully opens, complete healing usually occurs within a month with dressing changes because these wounds are lateralized and now well aerated. The result of the cleft lift procedure appears to be durable. Recurrence rates are similar to those of the Karydakis flap procedure, but there seems to be fewer major complications that necessitate intervention. Healing of the closed wound is usually rapid, and patients recover quickly, often participating in sports within 2 weeks of surgery (Figure 8, *A* to *C*).

The Limberg Flap

Another flap procedure that is more invasive but successfully employed for treating pilonidal disease is the rhomboid, or Limberg, flap. The asymmetric variation of this flap is preferred because it keeps the incision away from the midline. In this procedure, the abscessed area is excised down to the presacral fascia by means of a diamond-shaped incision. Next, a rhomboid flap is mobilized full thickness down to the gluteal fascia and rotated to cover the defect. This flap procedure is complex, somewhat morbid, and leaves a disfiguring scar. It is rarely needed.

SURGICAL PITFALLS

The surgeon must keep the following pitfalls in mind:

1. Be sure the diagnosis is pilonidal disease. Pilonidal disease is common and can coexist with other infections of the natal cleft. Make certain that the pilonidal disease is active when a treatment is undertaken, to ensure that the episodes of abscess are indeed caused by the pilonidal pits rather than a concurrent perianal abscess. Be certain that the draining sinus tract does not represent hydradenitis suppurativa. In pilonidal disease, there are often multiple primary pit openings in the natal cleft midline, but if a draining sinus exists, it is usually singular. In hydradenitis suppurativa affecting the natal cleft area, there are often multiple draining sinuses or abscesses that can occur on both sides of the cleft. Also, ensure that openings draining close to the anus do not represent secondary openings of an anal fistula. Often, these openings can be gently probed in the physician's office with a lacrimal probe to determine whether they track toward the anus or upward to the midline pits, which would confirm their cause. Imaging studies, such as MRI, are almost never required unless underlying osteomyelitis is suspected.
2. Do not miss the lowest pit. Patients must be examined carefully in the physician's office to determine where the lowest midline pit is so that surgery can be well planned. This exercise can be difficult, particularly in very hirsute patients or those suffering pain from a chronic infection. The surgeon must spread the patient's buttocks widely (usually with the aide of an assistant), have good lighting, and be prepared to clean the area of debris in order to have an adequate view. The same holds true in the operating room. Failure to incorporate the lowest pit in the skin excision specimen will surely lead to a recurrence.
3. Surgical procedures (including flaps or soft tissue rearrangements) aimed at excising or flattening the cephalad aspect of the cleft but fail to address the causative primary pits will lead to treatment failure. In circumstances in which a pit lies within 1 to 2 cm of the anal verge and a cleft lift procedure is being performed, the pit can be excised and closed with fine absorbable sutures. These closed excisions will heal when the wound

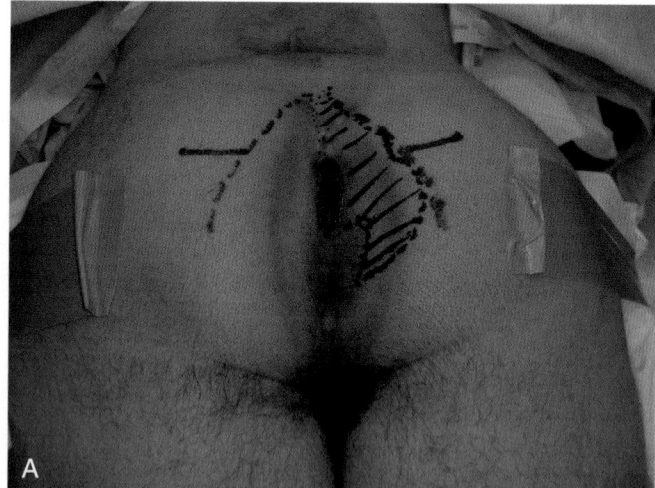
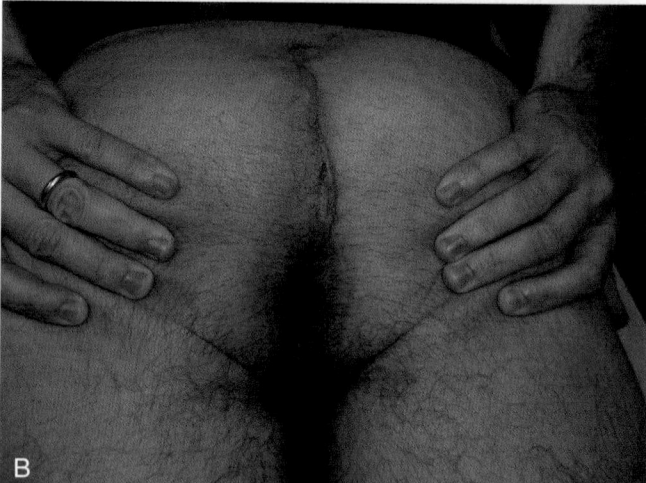
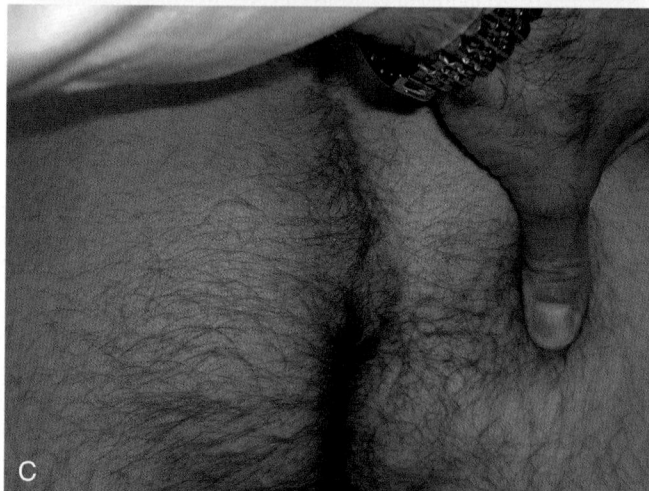

FIGURE 8 Before and after surgery. **A,** Before surgery: large pilonidal wound arising from confluent pits with preoperative planning markings. **B,** Seven weeks after surgery: postoperative shallowness of the natal cleft and near complete healing of wound. **C,** Four months after surgery: regrowth of hair, well-healed shallow natal cleft, and no recurrence of pilonidal disease.

has been rotated off the midline (around the anus) and detached from the sinus tract.

4. Failure to adequately rotate skin around the anus (often as a result of incomplete division of the anococcygeal ligament) during a flap procedure can result in a midline wound and lead to disease recurrence.

5. Avoid repeated wide excisions in the midline without rendering the cleft shallow.

6. Failure to excise an adequate length of skin during a flap procedure can lead to the creation of a midline divot in the residual cleft. Divots trap debris, and pits often develop in divots over time, leading to a recurrent pilonidal abscess. To avoid creating divots, the excision must start above the cephalad aspect of the natal cleft (generally 2 cm).

WHO SHOULD PERFORM SURGICAL PROCEDURES ON PILONIDAL DISEASE

Most general and colorectal surgeons have had little to no formal training in reconstructive flap procedures. Consequently, most are still performing outmoded procedures for pilonidal disease, including wide excisions with either midline closures or wide excisions with marsupialization. Earlier simple disease can be treated by any surgeon by unroofing of the sinus or by pit excision and lateral drainage.

If the disease recurs or if a patient has a complex primary pilonidal sinus, a flap procedure should be performed by an experienced surgeon. Unfortunately, few asymmetric flap procedures are currently being performed for more significant pilonidal disease. To offer patients optimal care for pilonidal disease, surgeons should feel comfortable in performing an asymmetric flap procedure. If a treating surgeon is not comfortable with one of these techniques, then the patient should be referred to a surgeon who is adept in performing flap procedures for complex pilonidal disease. Surgeons who do not perform surgery for pilonidal disease occasionally, have patient populations with high recurrence rates. Patients with advanced disease or recurrent disease from a failed procedure should be referred to a surgeon well versed in reconstructive flap procedures for this disease. There are many intricacies and tricks that can be learned only with experience. Furthermore, a surgeon performing a flap procedure should be very familiar with the cause and pathogenesis of pilonidal disease. Poorly performed flap procedures that leave a residual deep cleft or leave a low-lying pit are just as prone to failure as are misguided excisional procedures.

CANCER AND PILONIDAL DISEASE

Squamous cell carcinoma very rarely occurs in the setting of pilonidal disease. Those that arise are probably similar to scar carcinomas that result from chronic inflammation. The observation of a quickly expanding ulcer with heaped up edges or a fungating mass should prompt a biopsy of the edge of the lesion. If a cancer diagnosis is confirmed, treatment typically involves a wide local excision down to and including the sacrococcygeal fascia. A large flap is usually required to close the defect. Adjuvant chemotherapy or radiation therapy should be guided by the pathologic features and the general recommendations for squamous cell carcinoma.

SUMMARY

Pilonidal disease is a conceptually simple and common disease that affects young adults. It is thought to be an acquired disease, and the theory of congenital origin has fallen out of favor. The causes of pilonidal disease are a deep natal cleft and repetitive mechanical motion that lead to the trapping of hair or debris under the skin surface to form an abscess. Afflicted individuals may present with an acute abscess necessitating drainage or with the more chronic phase of the disease, a pilonidal sinus. Simple surgical procedures such as pit excision with lateral drainage or unroofing are reasonable first procedures to be performed. Major excisions in the midline should be avoided because they often do not heal, which makes the condition worse and more difficult to treat. More contemporary flap procedures that render the natal cleft shallow with off-midline closure are best used to treat advanced disease and have low recurrence rates. The cleft lift procedure is very effective, can be performed in an outpatient setting, has low morbidity and low recurrence rates, and may be considered the preferred flap procedure in treating pilonidal disease.

SUGGESTED READINGS

Al-Khamis A, McCallum I, King PM, et al: Healing by primary versus secondary intention after surgical treatment for pilonidal sinus, *Cochrane Database of Systematic Reviews* (1):CD006213, 2010.

Bascom J, Bascom T: Failed pilonidal surgery: new paradigm and new operation leading to cures, *Arch Surg* 137(10):1146–1150, 2002 (discussion, *Arch Surg* 137[10]:1151).

Bascom J, Bascom T: Utility of the cleft lift procedure in refractory pilonidal disease, *Am J Surg* 193(5):606–609, 2007 (discussion, *Am J Surg* 193[5]:609).

Karakayali F, Karagulle E, Karabulut Z, et al: Unroofing and marsupialization vs. rhomboid excision and Limberg flap in pilonidal disease: a prospective, randomized, clinical trial, *Dis Colon Rectum* 52(3):496–502, 2009.

Tezel E, Bostanci H, Anadol A, et al: Cleft lift procedure for sacrococcygeal pilonidal disease, *Dis Colon Rectum* 52(1):135–139, 2009.

LOWER GASTROINTESTINAL BLEEDING

Skandan Shanmugan, MD, and Sharon L. Stein, MD

DEFINITION

Lower gastrointestinal bleeding (LGIB) is bleeding that arises distal to the ligament of Treitz. LGIB accounts for approximately 20% of all major gastrointestinal bleeds. It is predominantly a disease of the elderly, with a mean age at presentation of 63 to 77 years. The incidence of hospital admission from LGIB is approximately 21 to 40 cases per 100,000 adults. Most patients have a self-limited course; in 80% to 90% of cases, bleeding stops spontaneously. However, as many as 25% of patients have rebleeding during or after hospital admission. The mortality rate from LGIB ranges from 2% to 4%. The successful management of LGIB depends on the accurate identification of the source of bleeding and definitive management, which may be medical, endoscopic, angiographic, or surgical.

The approach to LGIB can be challenging and requires a systematic algorithm for evaluation with concurrent stabilization of the patient and planning for definitive therapy (Figure 1). The management of LGIB necessitates a multidisciplinary approach with experienced endoscopists, radiologists, and surgeons. Although portions of the algorithm may be performed by nonsurgeons, the surgeon should follow the patient with significant LGIB and guide the diagnostic and therapeutic process. LGIB can range in severity from trivial to massive and from acute to chronic. Significant LGIB can be a serious and potentially life-threatening situation.

ETIOLOGY

The sources of LGIB are varied. Among the more common causes for bright blood per rectum or hematochezia (bloody stools) is upper gastrointestinal bleeding (UGIB), which occurs in approximately 10% to 15% of patients with LGIB. An additional 5% to 10% of bleeding may arise from small bowel sources such as Meckel's diverticulum, small bowel tumors, or angiodysplasia. Colonic sources of bleeding include diverticular bleeds, bleeding from neoplasia or polyps, and various types of colitis (Table 1). Approximately 10% to 20% of LGIB do not have a clear etiology and remain obscure despite thorough evaluation.

Diverticulosis

The prevalence of diverticulosis, or colonic outpouching, increases with age; in Western society, approximately two thirds of the population have diverticulosis by age 85 years. Twenty percent of patients with diverticulosis present with abrupt, painless bleeding or hematochezia during their lifetime, and 5% have severe hemorrhage. Although most diverticula are located in the sigmoid and descending colon, diverticular bleeding is fairly equally distributed between the right and left sides of the colon. Risk factors for bleeding diverticulosis include advanced age, the use of nonsteroidal antiinflammatory drugs (NSAIDs) or anticoagulation therapy, diabetes mellitus, and ischemic heart disease. The pathogenesis is believed to be the rupture

to the submucosal branch of the penetrating arteries or vasa recta into the colonic lumen as a result of stretching of the weakened diverticular wall. Observation alone is generally recommended after the first episode of diverticular hemorrhage. However, after a second episode, the risk of subsequent episodes is approximately 50%; thus, elective resection has been recommended after a second episode of diverticular bleeding. Surgical intervention consists of resection of the affected segment of colon.

Neoplasia

Occult bleeding, bright red blood per rectum, and hematochezia are all potential signs of benign adenomatous polyps and adenocarcinoma of the colon and rectum. Polyps account for 7% to 33% of cases of massive LGIB. Initial therapy is limited to biopsy of suspicious masses, local abatement of bleeding if possible, and the evaluation for a synchronous lesion via endoscopy before surgical resection. In cases of malignant disease, appropriate oncologic resection is warranted. If the patient's condition is hemodynamically stable, an appropriate staging workup should be done prior to resection.

Colitis

Colitis includes inflammatory bowel disease (IBD), ischemic colitis, and infectious colitis. Ulcerative colitis (UC) and occasionally Crohn's disease (CD) may manifest as bloody diarrhea, but less than 6% of patients have progression to massive LGIB that mandates an emergent operation. The recommended procedure is a total abdominal colectomy, with or without an end ileostomy; the rectum is generally not resected at this time because of the increased operative time and morbidity associated with the proctectomy. In addition, bleeding from the affected rectum dissipates greatly after diversion of fecal stream. Rectal preservation also allows for a formal proctectomy and ileal pouch–anal anastomosis (IPAA) for patients with UC or an ileoproctostomy for patients with rectal-sparing CD.

Ischemic colitis accounts for 3% to 12% of patients with LGIB, and these patients often present with an acute onset of cramping abdominal pain out of proportion to the physical examination results. Often ischemia follows surgical interventions such as abdominal aneurysm repair or cardiac procedures. Diagnosis can be confirmed via colonoscopy with visualization of edema, erythema, submucosal hemorrhage, necrosis, or ulceration at the watershed areas of the splenic flexure and sigmoid colon. Patients with signs of advanced ischemia should immediately proceed to surgical resection. In questionable cases, a gentle biopsy of the mucosa can be performed; if bleeding occurs, ischemia is generally still reversible. If no bleeding occurs, mucosa is nonviable and surgical resection is recommended. Nonoperative treatment is supportive with fluid resuscitation, antibiotics for bacterial translocation, and close observation. Surgical intervention is also warranted if the patient has signs of peritonitis or perforation develops or becomes hemodynamically unstable.

Infectious colitis may rarely cause hematochezia from pathogens such as *Escherichia coli*, *Salmonella*, *Shigella*, *Campylobacter jejuni*, *Entamoeba histolytica*, *Histoplasma*, and *Cytomegalovirus*. In infectious colitis, LGIB may be preceded by nonbloody diarrhea. Treatment is generally supportive with appropriate antimicrobial agents, bowel rest, and serial examinations.

Arteriovenous Malformation

Colonic arteriovenous malformation (AVM) includes vascular ectasia, angioma, and angiodysplasia and results from obstruction of

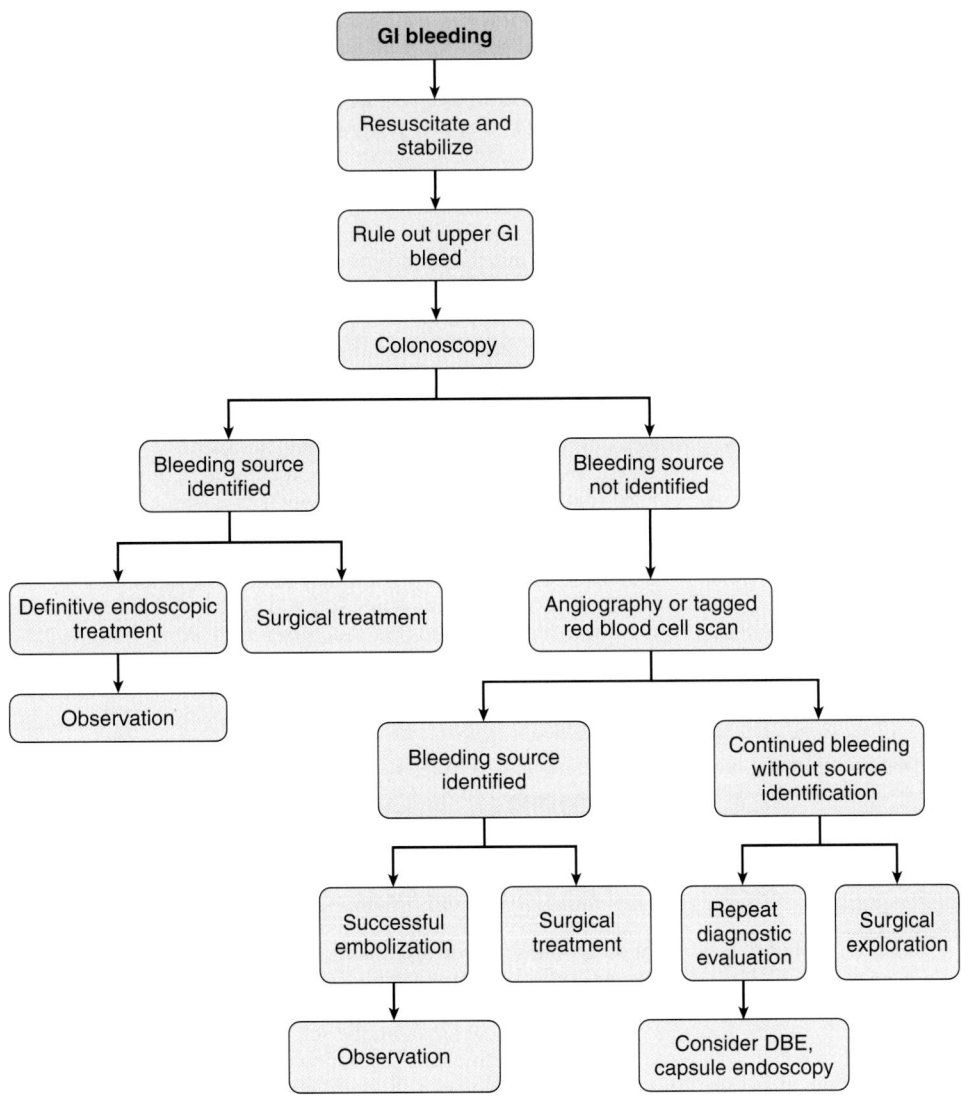

FIGURE 1 Approach to acute lower gastrointestinal *(GI)* bleeding. *DBE,* Double-balloon enteroscopy.

TABLE 1: Bleeding diagnoses in patients discharged with acute lower gastrointestinal bleeding in the National Inpatient Sample, 2002

Sources of acute lower gastrointestinal bleeding	
Diverticular	33.1%
Cancer/polyp	21.3%
Anorectal	21.0%
Colitis/ulcer	10.9%
Intestinal ischemia	6.6%
Angiodysplasia	6.0%

Adapted from Strate LL, Ayanian JZ, Kotler G, et al: Risk factors for mortality in lower intestinal bleeding, Clin Gastronenterol Hepatol 6(9):1004–1955, 2008.

the submucosal veins commonly found at the cecum. LGIB caused by AVMs can be slow, chronic, and intermittent. Bleeding from AVMs resolves spontaneously in 90% of the cases, although recurrence occurs in up to 70% of patients. Definitive surgical or colonoscopic treatment is required for identified sources.

Anorectal Disease

Hemorrhoids, fissures, anorectal fistula, and solitary rectal ulcers must not be overlooked as causes of a minor or major LGIB. A thorough anoscopy with good lighting can quickly eliminate anal sources of bleeding. Often treatment is supportive with appropriate bowel regimen, but occasionally surgical interventions are necessary, especially in patients with comorbidities and coagulopathies. Elimination of the possibility of a more proximal cause of hemorrhage is also important with a colonoscopic evaluation in patients who present with significant LGIB.

Small Bowel Bleeding

Small intestinal hemorrhage accounts for 5% to 10% of LGIB and should be considered as a potential source when the upper gastrointestinal tract, colon, and anorectum have been completely evaluated and excluded as a source for LGIB. The most common causes of small intestinal hemorrhage include angiodysplasia, jejuno-ileal diverticula, Meckel's diverticulum, neoplasia, enteritis, and aortoenteric fistulas.

Iatrogenic Cause of Bleeding

Other rare but sometimes life-threatening causes of LGIB include aortoenteric fistulas, postoperative hemorrhage, and post polypectomy bleeding. Aortoenteric fistula formation with severe hemorrhage has been reported from several weeks to years after aortic graft surgery. Fistulization to small bowel or duodenum at the junction of the aorta is the most frequent anatomic location and usually presents with a "herald bleed." These patients need immediate resuscitation and emergent operative management with resection and extraanatomic bypass.

Staple-line hemorrhage after colonic anastomoses is rare and usually self limited but occasionally may be severe enough to require endoscopic evaluation. Although endoscopy often reveals a spontaneously resolved bleeding site, treatment with epinephrine injection, coagulation, or clipping may obviate the need for operative revision in cases with ongoing bleeding. LGIB is a more common complication after colonoscopic polypectomy, with a reported incidence rate of 0.2% to 6%. Postpolypectomy hemorrhage is usually immediate but can occur up to 1 month after colonoscopy, especially in patients on anticoagulation therapy or antiplatelet agents. Postpolypectomy hemorrhage is generally managed with a repeat colonoscopy and endoscopic therapies such as snaring, thermal coagulation, epinephrine injection, or the application of a hemoclip.

DIAGNOSTIC ASSESSMENT AND THERAPY

Initial Evaluation and Resuscitation

Lower gastrointestinal bleeding may be acute or chronic in nature and can vary from minor, major, or massive in quantity and acuity. Patients with chronic LGIB may present with anemia, fecal occult positive stools, or intermittent hematochezia. If LGIB is acute, these patients may have hemodynamic instability or altered mental status. Patients with minor LGIB have hemodynamically stable conditions and can be evaluated and treated as an outpatient. These patients often present with anorectal disorders such as hemorrhoid disease and anal fissures, but more serious etiologies such as IBD, AVMs, and colon cancer should be considered as potential sources. Patients with major LGIB present with significant bleeding. By definition, a patient who needs 2 or more units of blood has a major LGIB. Patients with massive LGIB have an ongoing transfusion requirement, continued hemodynamic instability that necessitates intensive care monitoring, and possibly need vasoactive support.

Initial evaluation of the patient with an unstable condition must be accompanied by simultaneous resuscitation. The basics of cardiopulmonary resuscitation must be followed, including placement of two large-bore intravenous catheters and resuscitation to correct volume deficits. An immediate type and crossmatch should be sent to the blood bank along with pertinent laboratory tests, such as complete blood count, serum electrolyte values, creatinine values, CO_2 levels, prothrombin time, partial thromboplastin time, platelet count, and bleeding time. A thorough patient history and physical examination should include identification of any medications including typical anticoagulants (warfarin, antiplatelet agents, NSAIDs) and dietary supplements such as fish oil, ginseng, and gingko, which also affect the clotting cascade.

Description of the quality and color of blood may help identify upper or lower sources. Bright red blood per rectum is most typically from a lower gastrointestinal (GI) source; however, blood changes color as it is oxidized during its passage through the GI tract, and a brisk upper GI bleed may present as bright red blood per rectum. As many as 10% to 20% of patients initially believed to have a LGIB turn out to have an upper gastrointestinal source for the bleeding. For the patient with a hemodynamically unstable condition, a nasogastric tube and lavage should be included in the initial diagnostic evaluation. If clear bile is returned, indicating evaluation of the stomach and proximal duodenum, an upper GI source is significantly less likely. In addition, sources of anal bleeding should be promptly identified. A thorough anoscopy with adequate lighting can help identify bleeding hemorrhoids, fissures, and proctitis as part of the initial evaluation of LGIB.

The primary diagnostic tool for the evaluation of LGIB is colonoscopy. When colonoscopy fails to find the source of bleeding, mesenteric angiography can be used in a patient with significant bleeding, and radionuclide scanning if the patient's condition is stable. In cases where the bleeding source cannot be identified with these modalities, capsule endoscopy, small bowel enteroscopy, and computed tomographic (CT) angiography scans may have a role in establishing the etiology of the bleeding (see Figure 1). The specific diagnostic method selected depends on the presence of active bleeding, the severity of the bleed, the stability of the patient's condition, and the availability of these diagnostic modalities. Approximately 85% of all lower gastrointestinal bleeds resolve spontaneously.

Colonoscopy

Colonoscopy is an extremely valuable tool in the evaluation and management of LGIB and should be the first choice for most patients with LGIB. Colonoscopy has the advantage of being both diagnostic and therapeutic. Although patients typically undergo a bowel preparation before colonoscopy, blood acts as a strong cathartic. In the presence of major or massive LGIB, bowel preparation is often unnecessary and colonoscopy can be performed on an urgent basis. With a simple rectal washout, the source of left-sided bleed may be visualized. In addition, if the endoscopist is able to visualize the unprepped right colon with no signs of old or new blood, the left side of the bowel is strongly indicated to be the source of bleeding. If the endoscopist can pass into the terminal ileum and no blood is found, the discovery helps to eliminate the small bowel as the source of bleeding. For the patient with a hemodynamically stable condition, a bowel prep provides improved visualization of mucosal abnormalities such as vascular ectasia.

Definitive identification of the bleeding site requires visualization of active bleeding or fixed clot and is identified in 55% to 97% of cases. Visualization of blood or loose clot in the luminal surface without active bleeding can help localize the bleeding to one segment of the colon, but remember that blood may pass antegrade or retrograde in the intestines.

The endoscopist should be well prepared for the bleeding colonoscopy. Multiple flushes or power washer, endoclips, and various methods of cauterization should be available before the endoscopist starts the procedure. Treatment then depends on the etiology of bleeding. Benign etiology, such as diverticular bleeding or vascular ectasia, is treated locally when the bleeding source is identified. In these cases, injection of epinephrine, placement of a hemoclip, or thermal coagulation may be appropriate. Diseases such as ischemic colitis or UC may be amenable to medical therapy after identification. Bleeding polyps may be removed if they fail to show malignant characteristics; a malignancy can be treated with cauterization or endoclips to stop the bleeding but should be referred for more definitive surgical intervention. Internal hemorrhoids and rectal varices may also be treated with band ligation, and radiation proctitis can be treated with formalin fixation. Even if the endoscopist fails to treat the bleeding, a colonoscopy often provides information about the location of bleeding, which allows the surgeon to perform a limited resection if other treatment modalities are unsuccessful or inappropriate.

Disadvantages to colonoscopy include its relative contraindication in an unstable condition, the risk of perforation (especially in the setting of colonic inflammation, colitis, or therapeutic maneuvers), and the risks of sedation or anesthesia. In the case of massive LGIB, it may be impossible to identify or treat the source of bleeding endoscopically. In these cases, the next step is typically mesenteric angiography.

Selective Mesenteric Angiography

Selective or superselective mesenteric angiography has become widely used in the evaluation of LGIB because of its diagnostic and therapeutic benefits. The technique is performed via transfemoral placement of an arterial catheter. The superior mesenteric artery (SMA) is generally visualized first, followed by the inferior mesenteric artery (IMA) and the celiac axis. Radiologists often request a CT angiogram before angiography to limit the scope of invasive angiography and isolate the bleeding source.

Bleeding can be detected at rates as low as 0.5 to 1.0 mL per minute with angiography, with a sensitivity ranging from 40% to 95%. Although extravasation is unequivocal evidence of a bleeding source, angiography can also show more subtle findings such as tumor blush or angiodysplasia. When bleeding is identified, transcatheter therapy can be instituted to stop the bleeding, by means of either intraarterial vasopressin or transcatheter arterial embolization (TAE). Because vasopressin has a rebleeding rate that approaches 5%, most centers have adopted superselective TAE using microcoils or other agents. With superselective techniques, the rate of bowel ischemia and rebleeding after embolization is significantly low. Remember that even patients who have had bleeding controlled angiographically should have a colonoscopy because 5% to 30% have neoplastic lesions found.

At times, the angiographer may identify the source of bleeding but be unable to perform definitive therapy. Reasons include risk of ischemia to the bowel, inability to cannulate the vessel, and failure of embolic techniques. In these cases, the patient may require surgical intervention for treatment. The surgeon may request that the angiography catheter be left in place to allow the surgeon to identify the exact segment of bowel during surgery, which is particularly useful when a small bowel source may otherwise be difficult to identify.

Some investigators have used "provocative" measures such as the infusion of vasodilators, heparin, or thrombolytic agents to increase the accuracy and sensitivity of selective angiography, with acceptance of the risk of potential bleeding complications. This method is primarily used in patients with intermittent recurrent bleeding, for which other modalities have failed to show the source of bleeding. It has a sensitivity range of 29% to 40%, and typically, cases with positive test results go on to have embolization or surgery.

Technetium-Labelled Red Blood Scanning

Technetium-labelled red blood cell scanning (TcRBC) is a minimally invasive, high-sensitivity method to identify sources of bleeding. Blood is taken from the patient and labelled with technetium 99 m. The blood is then reinfused, and images are taken to evaluate the source of bleeding. Bleeding rates as low as 0.1 mL per minute can be detected. Images taken within the first 2 hours are most accurate for surgical intervention, but images can be taken over a 48-hour period and may be useful in intermittent or recurrent bleeding. Morbidity with TcRBC is minimal because this is a noninvasive study.

TcRBC has several significant disadvantages. TcRBC should not be used in a patient with a hemodynamically unstable condition because the process takes several hours to complete. In addition, TcRBC is unable to identify the source of bleeding in 25% to 60% of scans. Sources are identified by geographic location in the abdomen. Bleeding in the upper abdomen may be obscured by the uptake from the spleen and liver; identification of site in the small bowel is difficult as proximity to the ligament of Treitz or ileocecal valve is not provided. Surgical intervention based solely on TcRBC is frustrating; a false localization rate of approximately 25% has been reported. TcRBC has been suggested as a screening test to establish bleeding before angiography for confirmation. However, in practice, this is difficult to endorse; the time to obtain the TcRBC may significantly delay treatment, and a CT angiogram is now used preferentially to localize the site of bleeding. In the critically ill patient, radionuclide scanning should be bypassed in favor of selective mesenteric angiography.

Other Options

Newer modalities, including CT angiography and magnetic resonance imaging (MRI) angiography, have been studied more recently. They are promising, seem to provide good sensitivity and specificity, and may add additional anatomic information but are diagnostic and not therapeutic. Information gleaned from these examinations may help narrow the focus of angiography and speed treatment when used before superselective mesenteric angiography.

When no source of colonic bleeding has been identified, and blood is found proximal to the ileal cecal valve on endoscopy, the small bowel must be evaluated. Double-balloon enteroscopy (DBE) or "push-pull endoscopy" can be used to elucidate small bowel sources. With an over tube used to stabilize placement in the small bowel, the entire small bowel from ligament to Treitz to ileocecal valve can be visualized. DBE has a diagnostic yield of approximately 80%. DBE is not widely available, requires an experienced endoscopist with special equipment, and may take several hours to complete, but it allows for real-time analysis of the small bowel and therapeutic endoscopic treatment of sources. When DBE is not available, capsule endoscopy (CE) offers evaluation of the small bowel. Contraindications to a capsule study include small bowel obstruction, and a small bowel follow through is generally performed before ingestion to rule out an obstructing lesion. CE has a diagnostic yield of approximately 70% without any therapeutic benefits.

Surgery

Most patients with LGIB never need surgery; only approximately 10% to 25% of patients need operative intervention, either emergent or nonemergent. The surgical strategy depends on the intensity, cause, and localization of the bleeding. The indications for surgery include continued or recurrent hemorrhage despite nonoperative attempts at localization, ongoing hemodynamic instability, transfusion requirement of greater than 6 to 10 units, or pathologic finding requiring surgical intervention. There are no absolute predictors of who will need an operation, but 50% of patients who need 4 or more units of blood in the first 24 hours eventually need surgery. Morbidity and mortality increase significantly in patients who have received 10 or more units of blood.

Every effort should be made to localize the bleeding source before surgery. If the patient's condition remains stable, diagnostic tests should continue until the source of bleeding is identified. When the bleeding site has been localized to the colon, segmental resections may be performed based on appropriate treatment for the underlying pathology. In the case of diverticular disease, the affected segment should be removed; in the case of cancer, an appropriate oncologic resection should be performed. Smaller wedge resections may be performed for a single bleeding AVM or ectasia. In the case of segmental resection for preoperatively identified source of bleeding, the mortality rate is less than 10% in reported series. The rate of recurrent bleeding ranges from 0 to 15% after segmental colectomy for localized bleeding.

In cases where the bleeding cannot be localized before surgery, a thorough abdominal exploration may identify the source of bleeding. Running the small bowel during surgery may identify a small bowel lipoma or Meckel's diverticula. On-table colonoscopy and enteroscopy occasionally identify an intraluminal source of bleeding. To facilitate this, patients should be placed in the lithotomy position in the operating room. With the surgeon's assistance, an upper or lower endoscope may be advanced through the small bowel to evaluate for sources of bleeding. The surgeon gently manipulates the small bowel over the scope to advance the scope. If necessary, an enterotomy may be created for "on-field" insertion of the endoscope to complete evaluation of the small bowel. When found, the affected segment of small bowel can be resected, such as in the case of a Meckel's diverticula or small bowel AVM.

If localization techniques are not successful, but the bleeding appears to be originating from the colon, an emergency total abdominal colectomy (TAC) may be performed. TAC in this situation has a mortality rate of 10% to 30% but a rebleeding rate of less than 1%. If a more limited resection, such as segmental colectomy, is performed in this setting, the risk of rebleeding is approximately 35% to 75%, with a mortality rate of 20% to 50%.

Some surgeons advocate subtotal colectomy even if the bleeding source is identified because of the morbidity and mortality associated with reexploration from a repeat LGIB. Studies have shown comparable mortality rates for subtotal colectomy and segmental resection, and a frank discussion is warranted with the patient and family in regards to the risk and benefits of each approach and the postoperative effects on the quality of life. One of the often reported drawbacks to the TAC includes postoperative diarrhea and fluid losses. Preserving the distal terminal ileum may minimize this complication if a subtotal colectomy is necessary.

The choice of whether to perform a primary anastomosis should be based on three criteria: (1) definitive diagnosis of source of bleeding; (2) patient stability; and (3) patient comorbidities. In a patient with an unstable condition with a localized bleeding colonic segment, some have suggested a damage control approach; a temporizing surgical resection of the affected area is undertaken without an initial anastomosis or fecal diversion, accepting the necessity of a second-look operation. If the surgeon is not confident in the identification of the source of bleeding, an end ileostomy or colostomy is also suggested. Use of the end stoma helps elucidate the location of bleeding in the case of recurrence. In addition, use of temporary or permanent stoma should be based on the surgeon's clinical judgement of patient stability and ability to heal the anastomosis.

▍ SUMMARY

The approach to massive LGIB involves a thorough history and physical examination with concomitant resuscitation. A multidisciplinary effort including endoscopists, radiologists, and surgeons working together can most effectively diagnose and treat sources of LGIB. Although most bleeding resolves spontaneously or with nonoperative techniques, localization of bleeding helps limit morbidity and mortality for those who need surgery. Appropriate surgical intervention depends on underlying pathology and the overall clinical picture.

SUGGESTED READINGS

Czymek R, Kempf A, Roblick UJ, et al: Surgical treatment concepts for acute lower gastrointestinal bleeding, *J Gastrointest Surg* 12:2212–2220, 2008.

Green BT, Rockey DC: Lower gastrointestinal bleeding: management, *Gastroenterol Clin North Am* 34(4):665–678, 2005.

Hoedema RE, Luchtefeld MA: The management of lower gastrointestinal hemorrhage, *Dis Colon Rectum* 48:2010–2024, 2005.

Rios A, Montoya MJ, Rodriguez JM, et al: Severe acute lower gastrointestinal bleeding: risk factors for morbidity and mortality, *Langenbecks Arch Surg* 392(2):1665–1671, 2007.

Strate LL, Naumann CR: The role of colonoscopy and radiologic procedures in the management of acute lower intestinal bleeding, *Clin Gastroneterol Hepatol* 8(4):333–343, 2010.

THE LIVER

CYSTIC DISEASE OF THE LIVER

Cristina R. Ferrone, MD

OVERVIEW AND CLINICAL PRESENTATION

As a result of increased imaging, up to 5% of the population is diagnosed with one or more hepatic cysts. These cysts can be classified as benign or malignant, genetic or acquired, and infectious or parasitic. Most cysts are seen in women and are asymptomatic. When the cysts are symptomatic, patients often present with vague abdominal pain, fullness, or abnormalities in liver function tests. Depending on the location, large cysts may present with symptoms of early satiety, gastric outlet obstruction, intestinal obstruction, or liver function test abnormalities with or without jaundice from extrinsic compression of the bile ducts. If a patient has sudden intracystic hemorrhage develop, the patient may present with acute onset abdominal pain from sudden cyst enlargement and stretch of the Glisson's capsule. Rarely do cysts rupture or become torsive or infected. Luckily, most hepatic cysts are benign and asymptomatic and therefore do not require any intervention.

DIAGNOSTIC EVALUATION

The main reason to workup and treat hepatic cysts is to rule out malignancy or to treat symptoms. Routine laboratory tests are normal unless a very large cyst compresses the biliary system or synthetic compromise occurs from polycystic disease. If a parasitic etiology is suspected, *Echinococcus* serology should be performed. Patients with pyogenic abscesses often present with fevers, elevated white blood cell counts, and potentially positive blood cultures as a result of bacteremia.

Aspiration of cyst fluid is rarely helpful. Simple cysts contain a cellular thin straw-colored fluid, whereas the fluid is dark with intracystic hemorrhage. Bile-tinged fluid indicates a communication with the biliary tree, which needs to be addressed if an intervention is planned. Unfortunately, no markers have been identified to reliably diagnose a cyst with malignant potential or malignant disease.

Modern imaging modalities allow for assessment of the size, the location within the liver, and the relationship of the cyst to biliary and vascular pedicles. Imaging features that raise the suspicion of neoplasia include thickening or nodules of the cyst wall, multilocular lesions, septa, and papillary projections. Parasitic or hydatid cysts include "daughter" cysts or mural calcifications, and pyogenic cysts often present with edema and mural enhancement. Debris within the cyst requires a more extensive evaluation. Most frequently, it represents hemorrhage into the cyst, but it could be indicative of malignant disease or a parasitic infection.

IMAGING MODALITIES

The most inexpensive modality for evaluation of hepatic cysts is ultrasound scan (US). In the hands of an experienced operator, the sensitivity and specificity of US is greater than 90%. Simple cysts appear as homogeneous anechoic lesions with smooth borders. Nodules, septations, and echogenic areas should not be visualized. If a patient experiences hemorrhage into a simple cyst, blood can appear as echogenic material within a cyst, but unlike a neoplastic lesion, it should move with the patient.

Both computed tomographic (CT) scan and magnetic resonance imaging (MRI) are extremely useful in delineating the size and location of hepatic cysts. These modalities are not as operator dependent and can be compared with imaging done at different institutions and at different time points. CT scans should be performed with intravenous contrast so that the arterial/portal vein and delayed venous phase images can be used to fully assess the relationship of the cyst to the vasculature. Low-density fluid (<10 Hounsfield units) is seen in simple cysts (Figure 1). High-density fluid, nodules, septations, and an irregular thickened wall should raise the suspicion for malignancy. If cysts are very small, a CT scan may not be able to differentiate between a cyst and a mass.

Simple cysts may appear as hypointense lesions (T1-weighted image) or hyperintense lesions (T2-weighted image) on MRI (Figure 2). Hemorrhage into a cyst or the mucinous contents of a cyst adenoma increase the signal on T1-weighted images. If communication with the bile duct is suspected, a magnetic resonance cholangiopancreatography (MRCP) should be performed.

SIMPLE CYSTS

The most common type of hepatic cyst is a simple cyst. These congenital cysts are identified in up to 5% of the population. Most patients have a single cyst, but patients may also have multiple cysts (Figure 3). These cysts are lined with simple epithelium (single layer of cuboidal or columnar) that secretes fluid similar in composition and color to serum. They are thought to arise from aberrant intrahepatic bile ducts.

Simple cysts have no malignant potential; therefore, resection should only be considered for cysts in which there is diagnostic uncertainty or that are symptomatic. They usually do not communicate with the bile duct. Symptoms usually arise when the cyst is large (>5 to 8 cm) or pedunculated or when intracystic hemorrhage

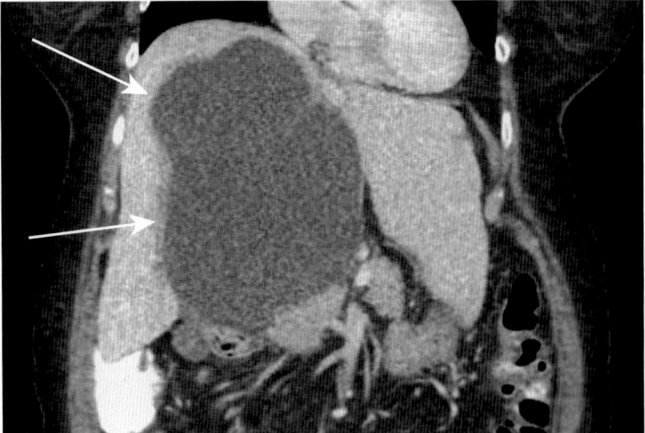

FIGURE 1   A single 16-cm simple hepatic cyst in a 73-year-old woman is shown on computed tomographic scan, with *arrows* indicating cyst.

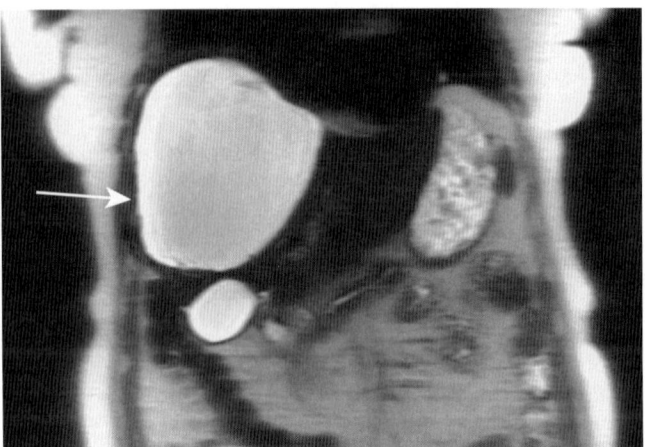

FIGURE 2   A 16-cm simple hepatic cyst is seen in a 63-year-old woman. The cyst is hyperintense on T2-weighted magnetic resonance images, with the *arrow* indicating the cyst.

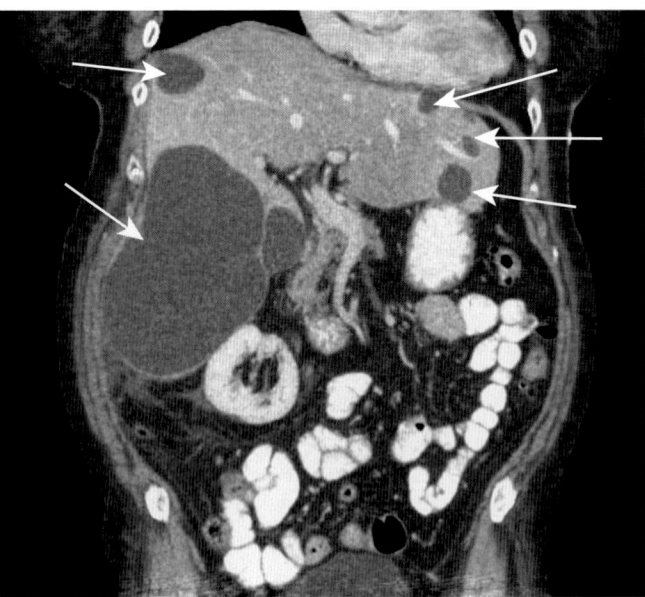

FIGURE 3   Multiple simple hepatic cysts in a 71-year-old woman are shown on computed tomographic scan, with *arrows* indicating cysts.

has occurred. Patients can present with abdominal fullness, pain, early satiety, or laboratory abnormalities. Percutaneous aspiration can be helpful in deciphering whether the abdominal pain is the result of the cyst. It is not a method for treatment of the cyst because recurrence occurs in 100% of patients and because there is a risk of infecting the cyst. Aspiration also allows for biochemical and cytologic analysis of the fluid. If mucin is seen in the fluid or cytology identifies atypical cells, a cystadenoma or cystadenocarcinoma is more likely. If bile is identified in the cyst fluid, the cystobiliary communication should be worked up with an MRCP or endoscopic retrograde cholangiopancreatography (ERCP).

Treatment of the hepatic cyst is warranted in patients with symptomatic cysts or with diagnostic uncertainty. Surgical deroofing (marsupialization, fenestration) is a very effective treatment and should be considered first-line treatment for medically fit patients in whom the cyst is not deep in the parenchyma. Either via laparoscopy or open technique, a large portion of the cyst wall is removed. Ideally as much cyst wall as possible should be removed without a liver resection. This allows for the fluid secreted by the epithelium to be reabsorbed by the peritoneum and for the cyst cavity to collapse over time. Surgical deroofing allows for pathologic evaluation of the cyst wall but also allows for visual inspection of the intrahepatic cyst wall, which is left in place. If any nodules are identified in the intrahepatic portion, they should be biopsied. If a bile leak is identified, it should

be oversewn. With a laparoscopic approach, the morbidity of the procedure is minimal. Usually 2 5-mm ports and a single 12-mm port are placed. A 5-mm laparoscope is used for visualization, and the other two ports are used as working ports to first aspirate the cyst contents (which are sent to cytology) and then resect the cyst wall. The cyst wall is then placed in a laparoscopic bag and taken out through the 12-mm port. Omentum can be sewn to the cyst cavity to prevent it from closing over and recurring. In very large cysts in which the amount of fluid secreted by the cyst wall is of concern, an electrocautery or argon beam can be used to fulgurate the cyst wall epithelium. A formal hepatic resection or enucleation can also be performed, but this increases the operative time, complexity, and morbidity of the procedure with an unclear benefit.

A potentially effective nonsurgical technique is aspiration and injection of a sclerosing agent. This can be performed percutaneously with radiologic guidance or laparoscopically with direct vision. The entire cyst contents need to be aspirated and sent for cytology to rule out malignancy and test for bile. If malignancy is not suspected and there is no communication with the biliary tree, a sclerosing agent, such as hypertonic saline, tetracycline, 95% ethanol, or other, can be injected into the cyst. The volume of sclerosing agent depends on the size of the cyst. Approximately 25% of the total cyst volume, but not more than 100 mL, is injected into the cyst. The sclerosing agent is left in the cyst for 10 minutes, with the patient changing position every few minutes to allow for contact of the agent with the entire cyst wall. After 10 minutes, the agent is aspirated. The sclerosing agent damages the epithelial lining, affecting its ability to secrete fluid and electrolytes into the cyst cavity. Symptomatic recurrence of the cysts occurs in approximately 5% to 10% of patients after sclerosis. However, in the patients with recurrence after sclerosis, a surgical intervention is more difficult and is associated with an increased morbidity.

POLYCYSTIC LIVER DISEASE

Differentiation of multiple simple cysts from polycystic liver disease (PCLD) can be difficult. Currently, no widely accepted definition of this rare condition exists; however, a familial pattern or involvement of other organs, such as the kidneys or the brain, is often found.

Isolated autosomal dominant polycystic liver disease (ADPCLD) is very rare, with a prevalence rate of 0.01%. It is associated with a mutation on chromosome 19 that affects hepatocystin. In patients who also have autosomal-dominant polycystic kidney disease (ADPKD), the mutation is in either chromosome 4 or 16 and results in alterations of the genes encoding the polycystin-1 and polycystin-2 proteins. These mutations result in bile duct overgrowth and failure of intralobular ducts to involute or connect with extralobular bile ducts. Cysts form from cell proliferation and fluid secretion into the biliary microhamartomas, which develop as a result of failure of duct development.

Most patients with PCLD are asymptomatic. Because of the great reserve of the liver, the remaining hepatic parenchyma is often sufficient. However, patients can rarely have liver failure develop. Often patients report abdominal fullness and distention, which can be associated with early satiety and shortness of breath. Rarely patients have development of obstruction of the portal vein, which results in portal hypertension and ascites, or obstruction of the inferior vena cava (IVC), resulting in lower extremity (LE) edema or Budd-Chiari syndrome. Cyst infection with gram-negative bacteria is very uncommon but potentially fatal. Patients should be treated with intravenous (IV) antibiotics and drainage of the infected cyst.

Cysts are staged via the Gigot classification, which is based on number, size, location, and remaining hepatic parenchyma via CT imaging (Table 1). Because most patients are asymptomatic, no treatment is recommended. For patients with symptoms, multiple options can be considered. If patients have large cysts, aspiration and sclerosis can be considered, but the recurrence rate is much higher (25% to 50%) than that for simple cysts. Laparoscopic or open fenestration can also be considered for large cysts, but because of the rigidity of the liver, they often do not collapse. In addition, the secretion of fluid and electrolytes can result in ascites. A more aggressive approach includes fenestration and resection. This is associated with higher morbidity but also a better chance at durable symptom relief. The most aggressive approach is liver transplantation. If transplantation is considered, it should occur before severe debilitation from pain, cachexia, and abdominal distention to limit the morbidity and mortality of the operation.

NEOPLASTIC CYSTS

Cystadenomas and Cystadenocarcinomas

Cystadenomas account for less than 5% of all hepatic cysts and are identified more frequently in women in their fourth or fifth decade. Originally, cystadenomas were described by Edmonson in 1958 as: (1) multilocular, (2) lined by columnar epithelium, and (3) accompanied by densely cellular ovarian-like stroma. Devaney and

colleagues broadened the definition by including unilocular cysts, a cuboidal epithelial lining, and those without an ovarian stroma.

Lesions with ovarian stroma, or true cystadenomas, occur frequently in segment IV of the liver and can become as large as 40 cm. The ovarian stroma contains estrogen and progesterone receptors. One hypothesis is that during embryonic development, ectopic ovarian cells shed into the liver as the gonads descend from the diaphragm into the pelvis. These cells then release hormones and growth factors, which promote epithelial proliferation and development of the cystadenoma. This is a theory similar to that of mucinous cystic neoplasms of the pancreas, which almost exclusively occur in the distal body and tail of the pancreas.

Cystadenomas without an ovarian stroma can occur in both genders. They tend to more commonly communicate with the biliary tree. In most patients, carbohydrate antigen (CA) 19-9 and carcinoembryonic antigen (CEA) levels in the cyst fluid are increased. The cysts have three distinct layers: epithelial layer, mesenchymal stroma, and an outer layer of collagen connective tissue. These cysts are surrounded by a dense pseudocapsule that allows them to be enucleated. Pathologically, cystadenomas are lined by mucin-secreting columnar or cuboidal epithelium. They have a dense layer of mesenchymal stroma composed of well-vascularized atypical spindle cells lying below the cuboidal cell layer. Early changes of malignant progression include intestinal metaplasia.

Most patients are asymptomatic, but patients are seen with abdominal distention, early satiety, and liver function test abnormalities. Radiologically, the findings are more likely to be complex cysts with mural nodularity, internal septation, or papillary projections. US and MRI are the best imaging modalities for these lesions because CT scan often does not show the septations (Figure 4). Aspiration of the cyst may aid in cyst characterization if mucin or elevated CEA/CA 19-9 is identified. However, CA 19-9 is also expressed by normal biliary epithelium and the epithelium of simple cysts, making it an unreliable marker. Cystadenomas are premalignant lesions; however, differentiation of cystadenoma from cystadenocarcinoma is difficult unless invasion of adjacent structures is identified.

In patients with benign cystadenomas, enucleation or resection should be considered. Fenestration and sclerosis are not good options because of the malignant potential of these lesions and the high recurrence rates. If malignancy is identified, a formal resection should be considered.

Cystadenocarcinomas are primary cystic cancers that do not communicate with the biliary tree and account for 0.4% of all hepatic malignancies. Cystadenocarcinomas with ovarian stroma occur exclusively in women, and those without ovarian stroma occur twice

TABLE 1: Gigot classification of polycystic liver disease

Category	Description
Type 1	Limited number (<10) of large cysts (>10 cm) with large areas of normal
Type 2	Diffuse involvement of the parenchyma by medium-sized cysts with large areas of uninvolved liver tissue
Type 3	Massive and diffuse involvement of the liver by small and medium-sized cysts with very little spared parenchyma

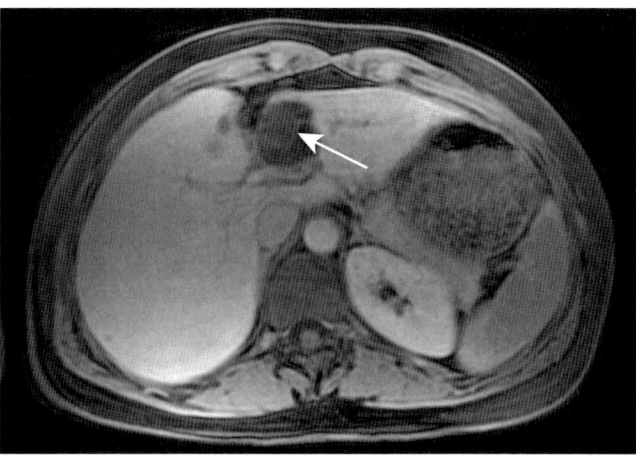

FIGURE 4 Hepatic cystadenoma lined by ovarian stroma in segment IV of the liver is seen in a 38-year-old woman. The *arrow* marks septation on the T1-weighted magnetic resonance image.

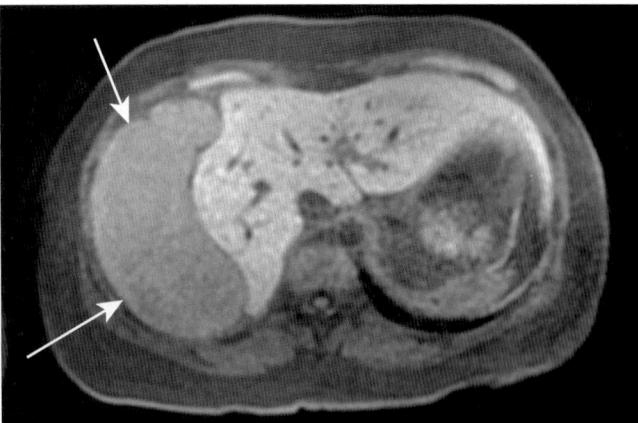

FIGURE 5 A 13-cm posttraumatic subcapsular hepatic cyst is seen in a 45-year-old man. The cyst is hyperintense on T1-weighted magnetic resonance images as a result of hemorrhage within the cyst (*arrows* indicating the cyst).

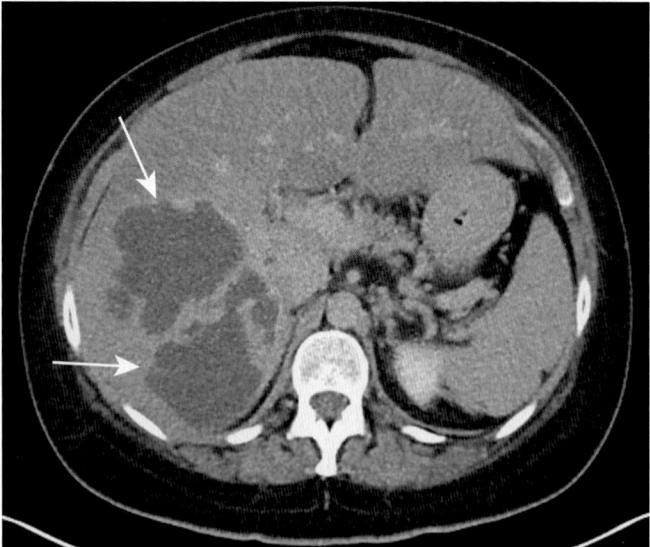

FIGURE 6 A large pyogenic abscess from *Escherichia coli* in a 57-year-old woman with diabetes is seen in delayed images on computed tomographic scan, with *arrows* indicating abscesses.

as often in men than in women. Most cases occur in patients in their 50s and 60s. Most patients present with nonspecific symptoms, such as abdominal pain or distention, and 20% present with biliary obstruction. On imaging, cystadenocarcinomas are more often large and have thicker septa, cystic debris, and bile duct dilation. Early changes of malignant progression include intestinal metaplasia in the epithelium that progresses to malignant tubopapillary epithelium. Patients should undergo a formal surgical resection because the tumor extension cannot reliably be assessed. Rupture of the cyst should be avoided as it may lead to carcinomatosis. Cystadenocarcinomas with ovarian stroma have a more favorable prognosis than those without ovarian stroma, as a result of less frequent parenchymal, vascular, and lymphatic invasion.

Intraductal Papillary Mucinous Neoplasm of the Bile Duct

Intraductal papillary mucinous neoplasm of the bile duct (IPMN-B) is a new pathologic classification for bile duct lesions with innumerable frond-like intraluminal papillary infoldings that produce mucin. Previously, these lesions were classified as biliary papilloma, mucin-producing peripheral cholangiocarcinoma, or intraductal variant of peripheral cholangiocarcinoma. These tumors are clinically, histologically, and phenotypically similar to intraductal papillary mucinous neoplasms (IPMNs) of the pancreas. Macroscopically, communication with the biliary system exists, and the tumors are divided into two types: the duct ectatic type with diffusely dilated bile ducts and the cystic type that presents as a large cystic mass. Invasive carcinoma is identified in 60% or more of the patients. An equal distribution is seen amongst gender, and the incidence peaks in patients in their sixth decade. Most patients present with nonspecific symptoms; however, mucobilia may result in obstruction of the biliary tree. Patients should undergo a formal hepatic resection and intraoperative cholangiogram to rule out biliary obstruction from mucus or tumor. In patients with a malignant component, the 5-year survival rate is between 60% and 80%.

TRAUMATIC CYSTS

Blunt trauma can result in intrahepatic hematomas or bilomas, which can develop into traumatic hepatic cysts (Figure 5). These are not true cysts because they lack an epithelial lining. They are usually managed conservatively. If patients have development of a persistent

bile leak or symptoms of pain or compression from progressive cyst enlargement, an intervention may be warranted. If biliary decompression via ERCP and sphincterotomy fails, surgical ligation of the leaking bile duct should be considered. Patients with compressive symptoms can be managed in a manner similar to that of simple cysts with unroofing or excision.

PYOGENIC LIVER ABSCESS

Pyogenic liver abscess is defined as a bacterial infection that results in single or multiple collections of pus within the liver (Figure 6). Hepatic infection can occur via five routes: (1) portal vein, (2) hepatic artery, (3) biliary tree, (4) adjacent organ infection, or (5) direct trauma to the liver. The most common causes of liver abscesses used to be appendicitis and diverticulitis. Currently, biliary malignancies and associated biliary interventions are the most common cause of liver abscesses. Patients usually present with fever, leukocytosis, and general malaise. Diabetes mellitus is associated with a tenfold risk for a liver abscess compared with the general population. CT scan is the most useful imaging modality because of its high sensitivity for detection of a liver abscess and for its ability with detection of other potentially contributing intraabdominal pathology. In Western series, *Escherichia coli* and *Streptococcus milleri* are the most common pathogen; in the East, the most common is *Klebsiella pneumoniae*. Treatment is centered on appropriate antibiotics and adequate drainage of pus. Percutaneous drainage is often sufficient for drainage. Surgical intervention should be considered if percutaneous drainage fails, if there is intraperitoneal rupture of the abscess, if the underlying cause needs to be addressed surgically, or if the abscess is large, multiloculated, and filled with debris.

SUGGESTED READING

Liu CH, Gervais DA, Hahn PF, et al: Percutaneous hepatic abscess drainage: do multiple abscesses or multiloculated abscesses preclude drainage or affect outcome? *J Vasc Interv Radiol* 20(8):1059–1065, 2009; Epub 2009.

The Management of Echinococcal Cyst Disease of the Liver

Susan C. Pitt, MD, and Henry A. Pitt, MD

Echinococcal cyst disease of the liver, also termed hepatic cystic echinococcosis or hydatid cyst disease, is a zoonosis caused by the canine tapeworm of the genus *Echinococcus*. The disease is endemic in the Mediterranean, Africa, the Middle East, South America, Asia, and parts of Europe in areas where sheep farming is predominant. Dogs (including wolves, foxes, and coyotes) are the primary host for this intestinal tapeworm, and sheep are the major intermediate host, although deer, elk, caribou, yaks, goats, camels, and other livestock also can carry the larval form. Infection in humans is generally incidental and is encountered most often in the United States either in immigrants or in Americans who have traveled to endemic areas. The combination of immigration and tourism has made hepatic echinococcosis a worldwide disease that may present many years after exposure. Antiparasitic chemotherapy with mebendazole or albendazole alone is not as effective as treatment combined with surgery. Percutaneous aspiration is another treatment option. This chapter reviews the available approaches to management of echinococcal cyst disease of the liver.

PATHOLOGY AND CLASSIFICATION

Hepatic hydatid disease results from fecal-oral transmission of the larval form of the dog tapeworm *Echinococcus granulosus*. Ova are shed in the feces of intermediate hosts (sheep, goats, or other herbivores) and inadvertently ingested in contaminated food and then penetrate the intestinal wall entering into the portal circulation. Once in the circulation, embryos can infect any tissue, such as the liver, where 55% to 80% of cases are reported, or the lungs (10% to 40% of human cases), the brain, or the bones. Another species found more commonly in elk or caribou, *Echinococcus multilocularis,* causes a hepatic infiltrative, potentially lethal form of the disease that is even less common in North America than *E. granulosus.* In the liver, *E. granulosus* has a two-layer cyst wall, an inner active cyst wall that consists of a single cell germinal layer where the echinococcal scolices and daughter cysts develop and an outer thicker acellular layer. This outer, reactive fibrous layer is called the pericyst and is calcified in approximately 50% of patients. Budding of the inner germinal layer within the cyst is termed daughter cysts or hydatid sand. The daughter cysts may float in the cystic fluid; and in approximately one third of patients, cyst expansion may result in rupture into the biliary tree, erosion through the diaphragm into the pleural cavity, or rarely, rupture into the peritoneum. On the other hand, mature cysts may become inactive, asymptomatic, and further calcified and have negative serology results.

Classification of echinococcal cyst disease of the liver has changed over the last 20 years. In the early 1980s, Gharbi published an ultrasound classification of hepatic echinococcal cysts that divides the cysts into five types (I to V) based on morphologic imaging appearance. However, in 2003, the World Health Organization Informal Working Groups on Echinococcosis (WHO-IWGE) put forth a standardized system to characterize the cysts that incorporates both the functional status of the parasite (active, transitional, or inactive) and the ultrasonographic (US) appearance of the cysts. Table 1 summarizes the WHO-IWGE classification system, which has aided the selection of optimal therapy and been applied to other imaging modalities, such as computed tomographic (CT) and magnetic resonance imaging (MRI) scans.

PRESENTATION AND DIAGNOSIS

Patients with echinococcal cyst disease of the liver can have a widely varied presentation that ranges from an extended asymptomatic period to rupture of the cyst into the peritoneal cavity with an acute abdomen and anaphylactic shock. Most patients, however, have uncomplicated disease that may be asymptomatic or present with right upper quadrant pain or fullness from cyst expansion, hepatomegaly, or fever. Obstructive jaundice, cholangitis, and productive cough from rupture into the pleural cavity and the lung are less common presenting symptoms. With the increase in abdominal imaging studies, incidental discovery of a cyst before symptom development is another common presentation. The diagnosis of this disease is centered on clinical findings, imaging, and serology and is confirmed with either demonstration of protoscoleces on direct microscopy or changes in US appearance that are pathognomonic for cystic echinococcosis.

Laboratory Tests

Evaluation may include various laboratory tests to help establish the diagnosis. A routine complete blood count (CBC) with differential may show eosinophilia in approximately 40% of patients, and assessment of liver function tests (LFTs) may reveal normal or mildly elevated transaminases. In addition, mild increases in the alkaline phosphatase or γ-glutamyltransferase (GGT) are seen in up to a third of patients. Classically, the Casoni's skin and Weinberg's complement fixation tests were used for diagnosis, but they have been replaced by a specific enzyme-linked immunosorbent assay (ELISA) that has sensitivity of 64% to100% depending on the antigen preparation. In patients with active cysts, complement fixation and indirect hemagglutination test results are positive 85% to 90% of the time. Immunoelectrophoresis also is diagnostic in approximately 90% of hepatic and 70% of pulmonary cysts, and hydatid antigen blotting can be used with 95% sensitivity and 100% specificity. Direct microscopic examination of protoscoleces from cyst fluid aspiration can help confirm the diagnosis and assess the viability of the cyst.

Imaging

US and CT scans are the most widely used imaging modalities for diagnosis of liver cysts, including echinococcal disease of the liver (Figure 1). These studies show position, size, number of cysts, proximity to vascular structures, and evidence of extrahepatic cysts. The WHO-IWGE's classification system which characterizes the cysts based on US appearance has standardized cyst description and attempted to facilitate the use of US as the primary diagnostic tool (see Table 1). Because of its low cost and its specificity of 90%, US is the preferred first-line imaging study worldwide. The classic findings for hydatid cysts are thick walls, unilocular or multilocular, often with calcifications, and daughter cysts.

When compared with US, CT scan may offer more detailed information about the location and depth of the cyst, which is useful for operative planning. MRI scans also can be used to demonstrate cyst characteristics and their relation to vascular and biliary structures. Magnetic resonance cholangiopancreatography (MRCP) offers further detail of the biliary tree and can delineate cystobiliary fistulae or associated abscesses in complicated cysts. MRI also can provide additional information about the liquid areas within the cyst matrix with T2-weighted imaging sequences when compared with CT scan. Hydatid cysts also need to be differentiated from simple congenital cysts, amebic abscesses, and cystadenomas (Table 2).

Endoscopic retrograde cholangiopancreatography (ERCP) also may be useful in the workup of hydatid cysts, especially in patients with cholangitis or jaundice, because communication with the biliary tract occurs in up to 25% of cases. ERCP delineates biliary anatomy, shows communication between the cysts and bile ducts, and can be used to drain the biliary tree before surgery (Figure 2). Routine use of ERCP is controversial but is advocated by the authors' group to completely define the bile duct anatomy and visualize any clinically silent connections between the bile ducts and the cysts. When operative treatment for hydatid disease is undertaken, intraoperative US (IOUS) also should be considered to confirm the relationship of bile ducts and vessels to the cyst with greater resolution than with a transabdominal probe.

TABLE 1: World Health Organization Informal Working Groups on Echinococcosis classification of hepatic echinococcal cysts

Cyst type (gharbi)	Status	Ultrasound features	Remarks	Treatment approach
CL (none)	Active	Unilocular, anechoic Usually round Cyst wall *not* visible	Early, not fertile Needs additional diagnostic tests	Needs diagnosis
CE 1 (type I)	Active	Unilocular, anechoic Round or oval Cyst wall *visible* Hydatid sand *(snowflake)*	Usually fertile *Pathognomonic*	<5 cm—ABZ >5 cm—PAIR + ABZ
CE 2 (type III)	Active	Multivesicular, septated Round or oval Cyst wall *visible* *Rosette, honeycomb-like*	Usually fertile *Pathognomonic*	PT or surgery + ABZ
CE 3 (type II)	Transitional	Detached floating membrane Less round, complex mass *Water lily sign*	Starting to degenerate *Pathognomonic*	PT, PAIR, or surgery + ABZ
CE 4 (type IV)	Inactive	Heterogenous, hypoechoic degenerating membrane No daughter cyst *Ball of wool*	Most not fertile Needs additional diagnostic tests	Surgery + ABZ, or watch and wait
CE 5 (type V)	Inactive	Thick, calcified wall Arch-shaped *Cone-shaped shadow*	Most not fertile *Highly suggestive* Needs diagnostic confirmation	Surgery + ABZ, or watch and wait

ABZ, Albendazole; *CE,* cystic echinococcosis; *CL,* cystic lesion; *PAIR,* puncture, aspiration, injection, and reaspiration; *PT,* percutaneous therapy.

FIGURE 1 A, Computed tomographic (CT) scan shows rupture of hepatic cyst through the diaphragm *(arrow)* into the pleural space. **B,** CT scan in the same patient shows a calcified cyst near the gallbladder fossa and a small superficial cyst on the left.

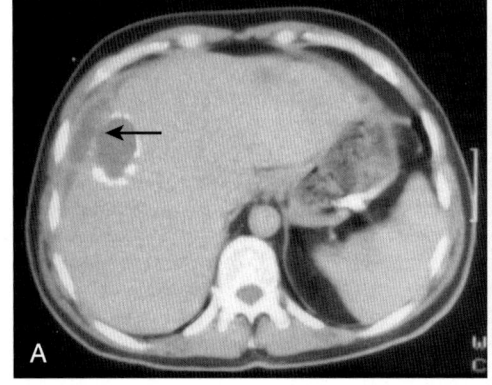
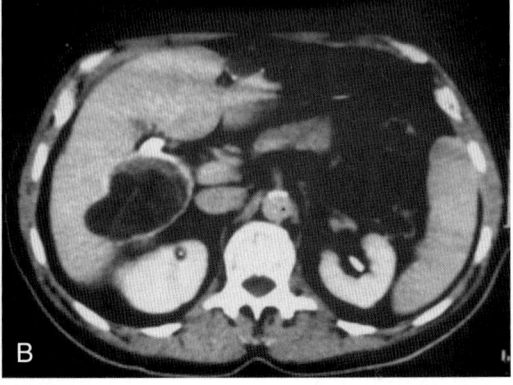

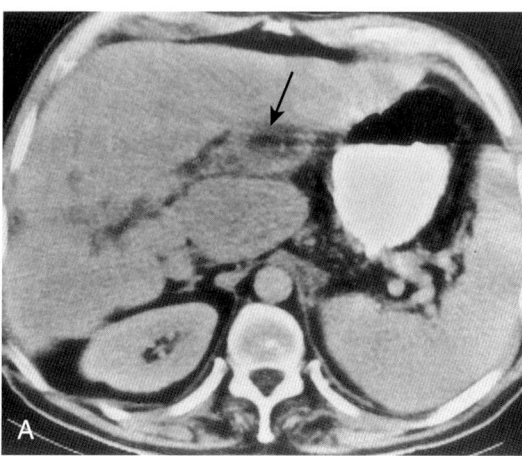
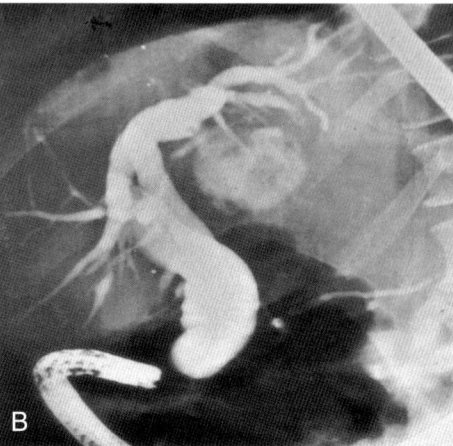

FIGURE 2 A, Computed tomographic scan shows a cyst in segment III of the liver. **B,** Endoscopic retrograde cholangiopancreaticography in the same patient shows biliary communication and an abnormally dilated biliary tree.

TABLE 2: Hepatic cyst differential diagnosis and imaging features

	Hydatid	Amebic	Congenital	Cystadenoma
Number	Single with daughter cysts	Single (or few)	Any	Single with loculations
Wall character	Thick, uniform, ± calcification	Thick, uniform	Thin, uniform	Variable, mural nodules, possible septations
Cyst contents	Clear or bilious, gelatinous; hydatid sand	Red-brown, "anchovy paste"	Clear, low-density	Green-brown, mucinous, low-density

TREATMENT

The principles of treatment of echinococcal cyst disease of the liver include early intervention to prevent secondary complications, eradication of the parasite, and prevention of disease recurrence with minimization of morbidity and mortality. Although most cysts are asymptomatic, complications such as cholangitis, anaphylaxis from cyst rupture, and pulmonary infection do occur and necessitate complete and thorough therapy. Protection of the patient against spillage of scolices and management of any complications that develop are imperative. Surgery remains the predominant therapeutic modality, but systemic chemotherapy; puncture, aspiration, injection, and reaspiration (PAIR); other percutaneous interventions; and watchful waiting also play a role in hydatid cyst management. Factors such as patient health, cyst characteristics, and the presence of complications all contribute to the decision over which treatment is most appropriate for each individual patient. The optimal or "best" treatment option for this disease has yet to be identified, and clinical trials comparing all of the available modalities do not exist. Therefore, available medical and surgical expertise and equipment, patient compliance, and the presence of recognized or national treatment centers should be weighed in the decision-making process.

Nonoperative Therapy

Benzimidazoles

Systemic chemotherapy with antihelminthic drugs, benzimidazoles, is the mainstay of medical treatment for echinococcal disease of the liver. Albendazole (10 to 15 mg/kg/d oral divided twice daily) is the drug of choice because it is readily absorbed from the gut, metabolized in the liver to its active form, and concentrated better in cystic fluid when compared with mebendazole. Formal assessment of the optimal treatment dose and regimen has not been performed, and recommendations vary from continuous treatment for 3 to 6 months with monotherapy to immediate discontinuation after surgery. These agents are not indicated for the treatment of inactive or calcified cysts except in complicated lesions. Monitoring of leukocyte counts and LFTs is essential because side effects include neutropenia, hepatotoxicity, nausea, and alopecia. More recent data suggest that albendazole combined with the antiparasitic drug praziquantel (a synthetic isoquinoline-pyrazine derivative, 40 mg/kg once a week) is more effective than albendazole alone. When used without other therapeutic modalities, the success rate of monotherapy with these drugs is approximately 30% and, thus, is only recommended in specific smaller (<5 cm) liver cysts (WHO cystic echinococcosis type 1 [CE1] and CE3). Therefore, additional percutaneous or surgical therapy should be used in conjunction with medical treatment (see Table 1). When combined with surgery, albendazole has been shown to both reduce the number of viable cysts at the time of surgery and decrease disease recurrence.

Percutaneous Therapy

Percutaneous treatment of hepatic cystic echinococcosis has become increasingly acceptable in recent years for carefully selected patients. Therapy can consist of either PAIR aimed at destroying the germinal cyst layer or needle decompression and catheter drainage with the goal of evacuating the entire endocyst. Catheter drainage is generally reserved for giant (>10 cm) unilocular cysts where the catheter is left in place until the daily output is less than 10 mL per day. Current consensus guidelines recommend PAIR for high risk patients, those who refuse surgery, those with failure of medical management alone, patients with infected cysts, and cyst recurrence after surgery. Cysts that are greater than 5 cm and classified as CE1 or CE3 are most amenable to primary treatment with PAIR plus a benzimidazole. PAIR is contraindicated in patients with biliary fistulae, complicated cysts, and inaccessible or high-risk locations (superficial), and those with CE2, CE4, CE5, inactive, or calcified cysts. Symptomatic pregnant women and children over 3 years of age should be evaluated with care and individual treatment decisions made with regard to the use of PAIR.

The PAIR procedure consists of percutaneous puncture and aspiration of the cyst with US guidance followed by injection or instillation of an indwelling scolicidal solution for 10 to 30 minutes, then reaspiration of the agent, and final irrigation with 0.9% saline solution. Protoscolicides typically used include either hypertonic 20% sodium chloride or 95% ethanol. The goal is to reduce the size and volume of the cyst, detach the inner germinal layer from the pericyst with the scolicidal agent, thicken the cyst wall, and eventually solidify the cyst. To prevent spillage of protoscoleces and improve efficacy of the therapy, albendazole should be administered at least 4 hours before PAIR (or up to 1 week before) and for 1 month after the procedure. Data have shown that combined treatment of PAIR plus albendazole is superior to either alone.

More than 4000 PAIR interventions have been performed over the last 20 years, proving the safety of the procedure. A 2003 meta-analysis compared PAIR plus albendazole or mebendazole with surgical therapy and found that PAIR and chemotherapy had a higher cure rate, less recurrence, fewer complications, and decreased length of stay. However, the surgical group was a historic control of mixed cases performed before 2001, and more than half of the patients did not receive any antihelminthic drug therapy, the standard of care, which makes interpretation of the results difficult. Thus, better data are needed comparing the various therapies before the optimal treatment of hepatic hydatid cysts can be fully determined.

Operative Therapy

Surgical management of echinococcal cyst disease of the liver was the only treatment option before the 1980s and has long been the primary therapeutic modality. The indications for surgery include large CE2 to CE3 cysts with multiple daughter cysts; superficial singular cysts at risk for spontaneous or traumatic rupture; infected cysts or those with biliary communication, particularly when percutaneous therapy is not available or possible; and cysts with a mass effect on adjacent vital organs. Evaluation of cyst type, size, location, presence or absence of complications, and patient factors (comorbidities, compliance) should be considered when choosing surgical intervention versus other therapies. Operative management is generally contraindicated in patients unfit for surgery and for inactive asymptomatic cysts, poorly located cysts, and very small cysts. The tenants of treatment with surgery remain to completely inactivate the scolices, eliminate the parasite and viable cyst contents, prevent recurrence or spillage of cyst contents, manage the cyst cavity, and prevent untoward morbidity and mortality.

A variety of surgical techniques exists, including open and laparoscopic cyst evacuation, pericystectomy, liver resection, and transplantation. Proper preoperative evaluation of the location of bile ducts and vascular structures with US, CT, or MRI should be obtained. If a bile duct connection is suspected, preprocedure ERCP should be performed. The use of IOUS also is helpful in identifying and avoiding key structures. These operative therapies should all be used in conjunction with a benzimidazole (administered for at least 1 day before surgery and for up to 1 month after surgery, if viable scolices are present) to decrease the risks of residual or recurrent disease.

Scolecoidal Agents

Inactivation of protoscolices and prevention of their spillage during surgery with scolecoidal agents is strongly recommended. In the past,

considerable controversy existed over the use and type of scolecoidal agents. Formalin, cetrimide, and chlorhexidine all have been used, but the safety and efficacy of these agents has not been established. The WHO recommends 20% hypertonic saline solution that should be in contact with the germinal layer of the cyst for at least 15 minutes before intervention. Hypertonic saline solution and other agents should be avoided in patients with cystobiliary fistulas because of the risk of chemically induced sclerosing cholangitis if it enters the biliary tract. Care should be taken to prevent the development of hypernatremia, another potential side effect of hypertonic saline solution that is seen with overuse. Peritoneal contents can be protected with protoscolicide-soaked surgical sponges. In addition, pre-evacuation injection of hypertonic saline solution into the cyst should be avoided because intracyst pressure is already high and may increase the likelihood of protoscolex spillage. A meticulous surgical technique is warranted rather than overreliance on scolecoidal agents.

Open Cyst Evacuation

As one of the safest surgical approaches, open evacuation of hydatid cysts is considered a conservative surgical therapy and is most suitable for peripherally located cysts on or near the surface of the liver. When anterior, an abdominal approach is best, whereas cysts in segments VI and VII are more amenable to a lateral flank approach. Figure 3, A, depicts evacuation of the cyst contents via aspiration; subsequent injection of a scolecoidal agent is optional at this time. Note, the field is lined with hypertonic saline solution–soaked gauze in the event of spillage. The cyst cavity is then opened, and the contents are aspirated with a large suction device with high negative pressure (Figure 3, B). Removal of daughter cysts, resection of the active cyst lining, and meticulous clearance of any remaining debris can be performed once the cyst is opened completely. The cyst may then be irrigated with a scolecoidal agent, as described previously. However, if the cyst fluid is bile stained or communication with the bile ducts was shown on preoperative ERCP, intracavity scolecoidal agents should be avoided. Simple closure of any biliary connection should be performed with absorbable sutures, and the cyst cavity filled with omentum. If the cystobiliary fistula cannot be easily closed, external drainage with a closed suction drain may be warranted.

Laparoscopic Cyst Evacuation

A laparoscopic approach to echinococcal liver disease uses the same principles as open surgery. Several reports have shown that carefully selected patients with peripherally located hepatic hydatid cysts may be safely managed with laparoscopic cyst evacuation. Anterior cysts without thick calcified walls and those in segments VI and VII (with a right lateral approach) are particularly amenable to this approach. One technique uses an 11-mm trocar placed just above the cyst, through which 10% povidone-iodine–soaked sponges are placed to act as a scolecoidal agent. The cyst is then punctured with a 14-gauge needle and aspirated, causing the endocyst to shrink away from the wall and rest at the bottom of the cyst. The 11-mm trocar is then upsized to 18-mm so that the germinal membrane can be aspirated. The laparoscope is then inserted directly into the cyst to identify any remaining daughter cysts or biliary fistulae, and the cyst cavity is irrigated with 20% hypertonic saline solution. Excision of the cyst wall followed by omentoplasty or closed suction drainage is then performed to complete the procedure.

Advantages to the laparoscopic approach include a reduced hospital stay, decreased hospital cost, and earlier return to productive activity. With laparoscopy, short operative times (less than 90 minutes) and low complication rates also have been reported. In properly selected patients with uncomplicated cysts, conversion to an open procedure should occur in less than 5% of cases. However, despite improved visualization, this approach has not gained widespread acceptance because of the relative inability to avoid or control peritoneal spillage in the setting of high intra-abdominal pressures from the pneumoperitoneum, a limited area for manipulation, and difficulty aspirating thick cyst contents. Techniques to minimize spillage of cyst contents include insertion of iodine-soaked sponges as described, fixing the cyst to the abdominal wall, lavage with scolicidal agents, and creation of a scolicidal pool around the liver by operating in the reverse Trendelenburg's position. Whatever approach is used, oral albendazole both before and after surgery is still indicated. In addition to simple drainage, laparoscopic partial cystectomy and even total pericystectomy also have been described.

Pericystectomy

The surgical literature divides the approaches to echinococcal cyst disease of the liver into conservative approaches, such as cyst evacuation, and more radical approaches, which include pericystectomy, liver resection, and transplantation. Pericystectomy involves complete resection of the cyst wall either closed, without entering the cyst cavity itself, or open, by sterilizing the contents with protoscolicidal agents, evacuating the cyst tissue, and then removing the pericyst tissue (see Figure 3, *A*). This procedure can be performed with electrocautery or a dissector either along a plane outside the pericyst or along the cyst wall itself. When dissecting around the cyst, some authors advocate use of a cleavage plane between the inner layer of the host's reaction towards the parasite and the outer layer, or adventitia, which limits damage to the liver parenchyma and allows safer removal (see Figure 3, *B*). Similar to cyst evacuation, pericystectomy is best performed on cysts along the periphery of the liver.

The advantage of this procedure over simple cyst drainage is a decreased risk of cyst content spillage into the peritoneal cavity when performed as a closed pericystectomy, which avoids potential anaphylaxis and decreases the risk of recurrence. Complete removal of the adventitia and elimination of the need for scolecoidal agents can be achieved with a closed procedure. The disadvantages of pericystectomy are an increased risk of bleeding or damage to bile ducts in proximity to the cyst wall because of the need for hepatic parenchymal transection. When encountered, vascular and biliary structures can be controlled with clips or sutures as illustrated in Figure 4, and the cavity may be closed over a drain. Pericystectomy is preferred to cyst evacuation because of a lower risk of secondary echinococcosis from protoscolex dissemination. However, the conservative approach of cyst evacuation is well suited for endemic areas where operations are performed by nonspecialty trained general surgeons and resources are limited.

Liver Resection/Transplantation

Another "radical" surgical approach to the management of hepatic echinococcal cyst disease is liver resection, which can range from nonanatomic wedge resection to formal hemihepatectomy. Although formal liver resection for benign disease may seem excessive, hepatic resection is now very safe, especially when performed by surgeons and centers with expertise in liver surgery. Multiple indications for liver resection exist, including complicated cysts with large biliary fistulae and small peripheral cysts where the cut surface of the liver is less with resection than with pericystectomy. Liver resection also should be considered for multiple cysts within proximity to one another or major structures, such as portal or hepatic veins or bile ducts, or when the resection would be relatively safe as seen with cysts confined to the left lateral segments II or III. Patients with recurrent disease who have failed more conservative management also are candidates for liver resection. Formal resection of the liver should be initiated only if complete excision of all cysts is possible. In one study, operative time, length of stay, postoperative morbidity, and cyst recurrence were shown to be increased in patients treated with liver resection compared with pericystectomy. However, resection avoids pedunculated ischemic hepatic tissue, which can be seen with pericystectomy.

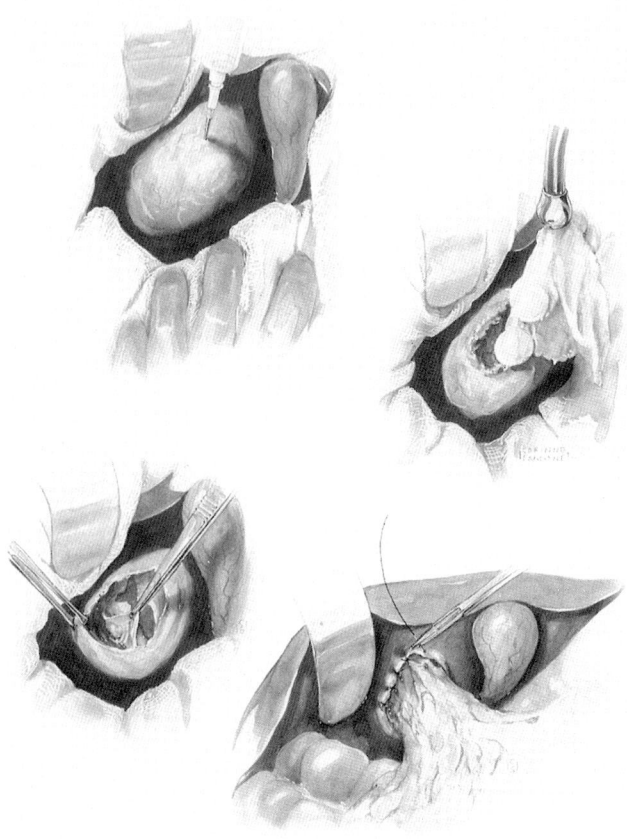

A

B

FIGURE 3   **A**, Open cyst evacuation shows cyst aspiration *(upper left)*, suction removal of daughter cysts *(upper right)*, resection of the active cyst lining *(lower left)*, and omental packing with suture tacking *(lower right)*. **B**, Operative picture shows the daughter cysts. *(From Cameron JL, Sandone C: Atlas of surgery: gallbladder and biliary tract, the liver portosystemic shunts, the pancreas, Philadelphia, 1990, BC Decker.)*

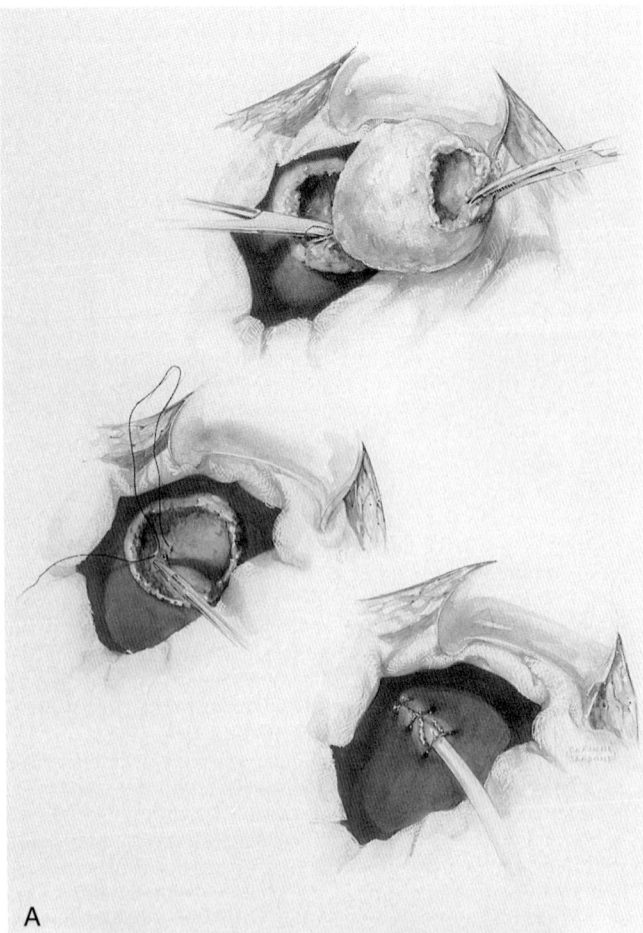

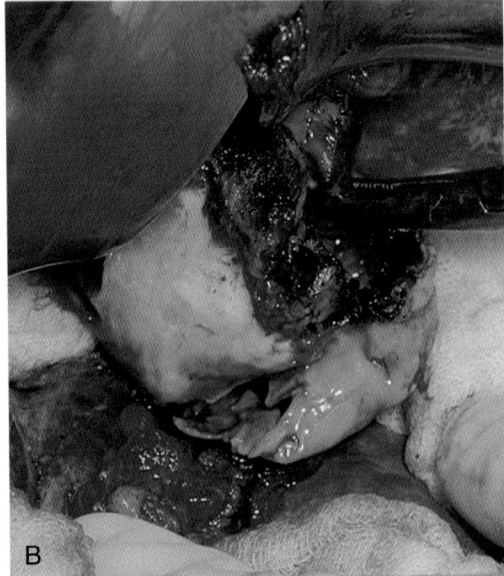

FIGURE 4 A, Pericystectomy is shown depicting removal of the calcified pericyst *(top right),* suture closure of a communicating bile duct *(middle left),* and (optional) closure of the cavity over a drain *(lower right).* **B,** Operative picture shows cyst removal. *(From Cameron JL, Sandone C: Atlas of surgery: gallbladder and biliary tract, the liver portasystemic shunts, the pancreas, Philadelphia, 1990, BC Decker.)*

Perhaps the most radical of surgical management options, liver transplantation, is rarely indicated in the treatment of hepatic hydatid disease not amenable to alternative therapies. As opposed to *E. granulosus,* which tends to form solitary cysts, *E. multilocularis* can produce a more complicated form of the disease with multiple cysts known as alveolar echinococcosis. These cysts can result in fulminant liver failure from sclerosing cholangitis, Budd-Chiari syndrome, or biliary sclerosis. In such unusual cases, orthotropic liver transplantation may be indicated.

Summary

Uncomplicated Disease

Patients with uncomplicated echinococcal cyst disease of the liver typically are asymptomatic with incidental cyst discovery on imaging or at abdominal surgery for other reasons. However, they may present with right upper quadrant pain without fever, chills, jaundice, or a cough. A complete history and physical examination should be performed, laboratory tests including LFTs and serology should be sent, and the WHO-IWGE type should be determined with US imaging or other available studies. For patients with CE1 or CE3 (Gharbi types I or II) cysts, particularly if they are anterior, peripheral, unilocular, less than 5 cm, and not heavily calcified, PAIR or laparoscopic cyst evacuation should be considered depending on local expertise (Table 3). Alternatively, uncomplicated cases with CE4 or CE5 (Gharbi types IV or V) cysts that are posterior, central, greater than three in number, large (>5 cm), or calcified should undergo open evacuation or resection when surgery is indicated. The WHO guidelines further suggest that in uncomplicated CE4 or CE5 cysts proven to be inactive, a watch and wait approach may be undertaken with long-term US imaging follow-up, especially if local surgical expertise is not available. WHO cystic lesions are frequently early hydatid or possibly other hepatic cysts and should not be treated until their parasitic origin has been confirmed. The decision to perform cyst evacuation, pericystectomy, or liver resection should be individualized on the basis of patient and cyst characteristics and surgeon experience.

TABLE 3: Treatment options summary

PAIR or laparoscopic evacuation	Open evacuation or liver resection
Uncomplicated Cases	
CE1 or CE3 cysts (Gharbi I or II)	CE 4 or CE 5 cysts (Gharbi IV or V)
Anterior location	Posterior or central location
Small size (<5 cm)	Large size (>5 cm)
Few number (1-3 cysts)	Multiple (>3 cysts)
Minimal or no calcification	Heavy calcification
Complicated Cases	
Infected cysts meeting previous criteria	Infected cysts meeting previous criteria
	Biliary or pulmonary communication
	Peritoneal rupture

Albendazole or mebendazole should be used in conjunction with all treatments.

CE, Cystic echinococcosis; *PAIR,* puncture, aspiration, injection, and reaspiration.

Complicated Disease

Patients with complicated hepatic hydatid cysts can be secondarily infected or have biliary obstruction, cystobiliary fistulae, or rupture into the biliary tree, peritoneal, or pleural cavities. Secondary bacterial infection usually occurs as a result of biliary communication and should be treated with appropriate systemic antibiotics and adequate cyst drainage. In carefully selected patients, percutaneous drainage may be needed before definitive surgical treatment. In the 5% to 15% of patients with hydatid cysts on imaging who present with jaundice or cholangitis, ERCP is indicated to both evaluate potential fistulae between the cyst and biliary tree and drain the biliary system with a stent. A sphincterotomy alone may not be adequate treatment. Once drainage is sufficient and cholangitis has resolved, open cyst evacuation should be performed and biliary fistulae closed as described previously. Cyst diameter greater than 7.5 cm is a risk factor for a biliary-cyst communication even in asymptomatic patients with an 80% likelihood of a fistula being present at surgery. Therefore, one should be prepared to deal with a biliary fistula in the operating room in patients with large cysts. A concomitant cholecystectomy and intraoperative cholangiogram to ensure complete cyst debris clearance from the bile ducts also may be required. In rare instances, a biliary-intestinal anastomosis or liver resection may be needed to fully treat cystobiliary fistulas.

Complicated disease also occurs occasionally when hydatid hepatic cysts rupture into the peritoneum or through the diaphragm into the pleura and lung (see Figure 1), which can result in widespread disseminated disease. Free rupture of a cyst into the peritoneal cavity presents with peritonitis, shock, and/or anaphylaxis. Treatment of the allergic reaction and surgical evacuation are necessary. In these situations, an open surgical approach is recommended to thoroughly control the spread of disease throughout the abdomen. Supportive and intensive therapy also is usually required for the care of these patients. On the other side of the diaphragm, the workup for patients with pulmonary complications includes imaging, serology, and bronchoscopy when bronchocystic fistulae are suspected. Benzimidazoles alone can be used for small, uncomplicated lung cysts. However, surgical management for these patients often includes evacuation of cysts from both the liver and the pleural spaces. Open cyst evacuation with closure of the diaphragm and drainage are indicated but should be as conservative as possible. For extended pulmonary involvement, severe suppuration, or other complications, pulmonary resection also may be required. In the chest, as in the abdomen, care must be taken to prevent spillage of cyst contents to avoid recurrent infection or anaphylaxis.

RESULTS

Morbidity and Mortality

Advances in the management of patients with echinococcal cyst disease of the liver have decreased the morbidity and mortality of the disease in recent years. In a 2003 meta-analysis of patients with all types of disease (uncomplicated and complicated) that compared 769 patients who underwent PAIR with 952 who had surgical intervention, minor and major morbidity rates for each modality were 8% and 13%, respectively, for PAIR as opposed to 25% and 33%, respectively, for surgery. The overall mortality rate reported in the same study was 0.1% for PAIR and 0.7% for surgery, demonstrating the relative safety of both approaches. Thus, in patients with uncomplicated hydatid cysts who undergo elective percutaneous or laparoscopic drainage procedures, open evacuation, pericystectomy, wedge resection, or left lateral sectionectomy, mortality should be very low, with morbidity rates ranging from 15% to 20%. A recent retrospective analysis of patients undergoing surgical treatment of hepatic echinococcal infection reported 0 mortality and 47% morbidity for resection procedures, but only a 17% morbidity rate for cyst evacuation. Not surprisingly, less invasive techniques were associated with reduced hospital stay and cost. In patients with complicated disease who undergo open evacuation, pericystectomy, or resection, morbidity is in the range of 40% to 50%, and mortality should be less than 5% (reports range from 0.5% to 4%). The presence of sepsis, peritoneal rupture, underlying comorbid disease, and malnutrition all are factors that increase mortality.

Long Term

Overall, the long-term cure rate for appropriately and adequately treated patients with echinococcal hepatic cysts is excellent and ranges from 90% to 95%. Medical treatment with benzimidazoles alone should only be used in patients who are otherwise not candidates for percutaneous or surgical therapy because recurrence rates are approximately 70% to 80%; therefore, when possible, medical therapy should be used in combination with a drainage or resection procedure. In uncomplicated cases, open surgical, laparoscopic, and percutaneous drainage techniques all have low recurrence rates around 10%. Because of the endemic nature of this disease and potential for reinfestation, long-term follow-up is necessary with serologic tests and imaging studies. WHO guidelines recommend follow-up visits including US imaging and laboratory tests (CBC and LFTs) every 3 to 6 months initially, then yearly once the situation is stable. Serologic tests also can be followed; but although a persistence of raised or a further increase in antibody levels may indicate residual or recurrent disease, these finding may occur even with full, adequate treatment. Currently, new antigens show promise in reliability for posttreatment monitoring. Patients with echinococcal cysts complicated by infection, cholangitis, pleura extension, or peritoneal rupture have unique problems. If the complication such as cholangitis can be treated before definitive cyst treatment, the long-term outcomes are similar to those of uncomplicated echinococcosis. However, patients with rupture into the pleural cavity or the peritoneum may have a recurrence rate as high as 25%.

SUGGESTED READINGS

Brunetti E, Kern P, Vuitton DA: Expert consensus for the diagnosis and treatment of cystic and alveolar echinococcosis in humans, *Acta Tropica* 114:1–16, 2010.

Motie MR, Ghaemi M, Aliakbarian M, Saremi E, et al: Study of radical vs. conservative surgical treatment of the hepatic hydatid cyst: a 10-year experience, *Ind J Surg* 72(6):448–452, 2010.

Nasseri-Moghaddam S, Abrishami A, Taefi A, Malekzadeh R, et al: Percutaneous needle aspiration, injection, and re-aspiration with or without benzimidazole coverage for uncomplicated hepatic hydatid cysts, *Cochrane Database of Systematic Reviews* 1, 2011.

Smego RA, Sebanego P: Treatment options for hepatic cystic echinococcosis, *Int J Inf Dis* 9:60–76, 2005.

WHO Informal Working Group: International classification of ultrasound images in cystic Echinococcus for application in clinical and field epidemiologic settings, *Acta Tropica* 85:253–261, 2003.

Cavernous Hepatic Hemangioma

Teviah E. Sachs, MD, MPH, and
Michael A. Choti, MD, MBA, FACS

Cavernous hemangiomas are the most common benign tumor of the liver. They are typically found incidentally during an evaluation for other reasons. With increasing use of cross-sectional imaging, surgeons are being asked to evaluate and manage these patients with increasing frequency. The reported incidence of hepatic hemangioma ranges from 0.4% to 20%, depending on autopsy studies, and they are more common in women with an approximate 3:1 ratio. Developing as congenital, non-neoplastic proliferation of vascular endothelial cells, the precise etiology of these tumors is unknown. Evidence to date shows that they have no malignant potential.

Hepatic hemangiomas can range from sub-centimeter in size to very large, sometimes encompassing the majority of the liver. Tumors of 5 cm or greater in diameter are typically referred to as giant hemangiomas (Figure 1). The term *cavernous* hemangioma is not related to size but rather is based on the histologic appearance, where a capacious vascular space is seen microscopically (Figure 2). Fibrous septa are seen between the vascular channels, as well as occasional calcifications and fibrosis in larger lesions. Hemangiomas can also display evidence of intraluminal microthrombus. On gross inspection, hemangiomas are well circumscribed, dark in color (often having a purplish hue), and soft and pliable, as one would expect from their vascular character (Figure 3). When found on the periphery of the liver, they often have a bulging appearance beneath the liver capsule.

PATHOPHYSIOLOGY AND CLINICAL PRESENTATION

Whereas there are no known specific causes of hepatic hemangiomas, their predisposition for females makes some suspect a hormonal association. Specifically, some evidence suggests that *growth* of hemangiomas can be related to steroid administration, pregnancy, or oral contraceptive use. In addition, exacerbation of symptoms can sometimes be seen with changes in estrogen milieu, such as pregnancy or hormone use.

The majority of hepatic hemangiomas are found incidentally during evaluation for other disease processes. They are asymptomatic in more than half of cases referred for surgical evaluation. Historically, the incidence of these tumors was based on autopsy series. However, the rise in number of imaging studies performed has made incidental identification the most common method of diagnosis. Whereas the age of onset is unknown, the majority of these tumors are diagnosed between the fourth and sixth decades of life. Hemangiomas are more commonly found in the right hemiliver and can be multiple in 10% to 40% of cases.

The natural history of cavernous hemangiomas within the liver is uneventful in most cases, and most remain asymptomatic. Although cavernous hemangiomas can grow and symptoms may develop (sometimes years or decades later), the majority remain stable. Regression can be seen in 10% to 15% of cases. For those patients who present symptomatically, symptoms are often variable. Any non-specific symptoms attributed to these lesions should be made with care, as other sources may be the cause. Right upper quadrant fullness and mild discomfort are the most common complaints. Patients will often describe symptoms that can be mistaken for symptoms of chronic cholecystitis or symptomatic cholelithiasis. The pathogenesis of this pain is unknown and likely multifactorial. Localized right upper quadrant pain can be due to infarction or thrombosis of the tumor itself. More commonly, patients may have more chronic or intermittent dull pain due to tumor engorgement and resultant stretching of Glisson's capsule. This stretching is transmitted via the autonomic C fibers and mediated by the celiac ganglion, resulting in nonspecific visceral pain that is difficult to differentiate from other intra-abdominal processes. In addition, diaphragmatic peritoneal irritation can cause referred pain to the right subscapular or shoulder region.

Less common presentations for symptomatic hepatic hemangiomas may include fever, nausea and vomiting, cardiac manifestations, jaundice, and, in rare cases, rupture. A patient with fever may undergo an intensive evaluation before a large hepatic hemangioma, often with thrombosis, is identified. Giant hemangiomas that cause compression of the duodenum or stomach may cause nausea, vomiting, early satiety, dyspepsia, or, in rare cases, gastric outlet obstruction. Pedunculated hemangiomas on the undersurface of the liver may be mistaken for tumors of the duodenum or kidney or as enlarged lymph nodes, compressing surrounding structures (see Figure 3). If large enough, giant hemangiomas can lead to development of arteriovenous shunting, which, in severe cases, can lead to cardiac hypertrophy and congestive heart failure. When these tumors compress the common bile duct extrinsically, the affected individual may have jaundice due to biliary obstruction.

Rupture is an exceedingly uncommon event, presenting variably with tachycardia, hypotension, anemia, and diffuse or focal abdominal pain. Such patients require immediate attention and, often, urgent intervention. Early reports estimated the mortality rate with rupture to be approximately 75%. However, with the advent of technology leading to earlier identification and therapy, more recent estimates of the mortality rate are as low as 30%. Often, giant asymptomatic hemangiomas are referred to a surgeon for resection because of a perceived risk of rupture by the physician or patient. Despite the large size and vascularity of these hemangiomas, the rate of spontaneous rupture is exceedingly rare with estimates of less than 1%. A recent review of the literature showed that only 46 cases of true spontaneous rupture have been reported. Similarly, even nonspontaneous rupture, such as that from trauma, anticoagulation, or comorbid disease, is rare, with only 38 cases reported in the literature during the same time period. Rupture has been associated with pregnancy and hormonal therapy, although this is not well described. Therefore, the risk of rupture should almost never be a reason for recommending surgical resection, regardless of size or risk factors.

There are no specific laboratory tests that are useful in diagnosing hepatic hemangiomas. However, abnormalities in liver function tests can be found, particularly when associated with proximity and compression of the biliary tree. In such cases, test findings may show bilirubin or alkaline phosphatase elevation. Thrombocytopenia can occur in rare cases due to platelet sequestration, as well as low fibrinogen levels due to fibrinolysis within the tumor itself (Kasabach-Merritt syndrome). Although this syndrome can occur at any age, it is more common in children. In addition, hepatic hemangiomas can be found in association with other vascular syndromes and disease states. Klippel-Trenaunay-Weber syndrome, in which patients display hepatic hemangiomas in conjunction with diffuse varicosities, most often affects the extremities. Although not a hallmark of diagnosis, hepatic hemangiomas are associated with von Hippel-Lindau disease, Osler-Rendu-Weber disease, Maffucci syndrome, and systemic lupus erythematosus.

The presence of hepatic hemangiomas can complicate the evaluation of patients with malignancy. Elevation in tumor markers alpha fetoprotein (AFP), CA-19-9, or carcinoembryonic antigen (CEA) in

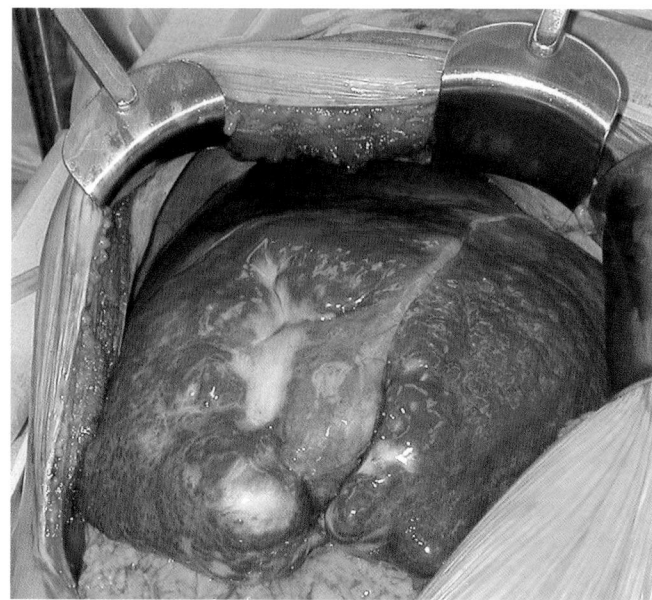

FIGURE 1 Giant hepatic hemangioma of the left hemiliver associated with abdominal pain.

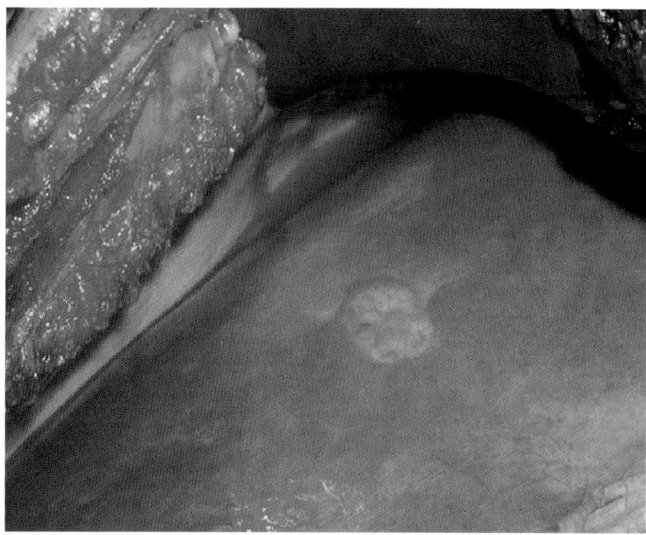

FIGURE 3 A small incidental hemangioma identified intraoperatively.

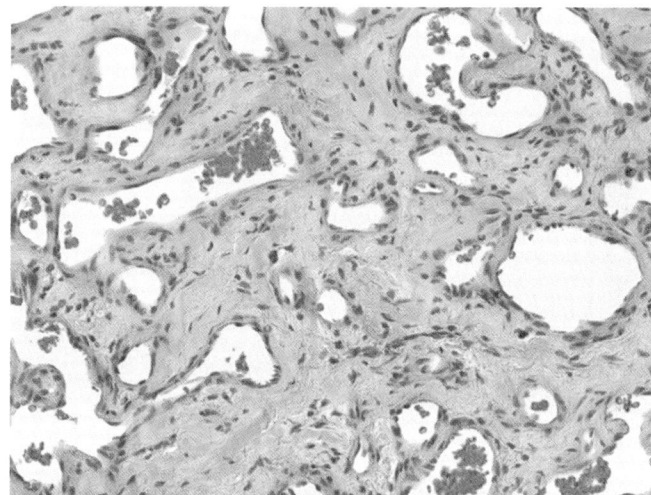

FIGURE 2 Photomicrograph of a section of a cavernous hepatic hemangioma, demonstrating the extensive vascularity and ill-defined network of capillaries and larger vessels.

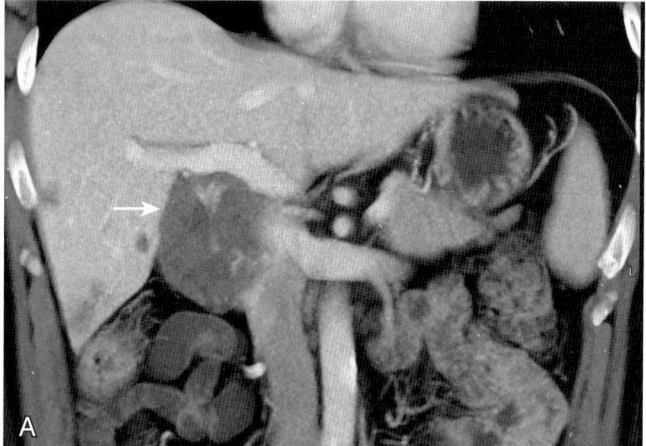

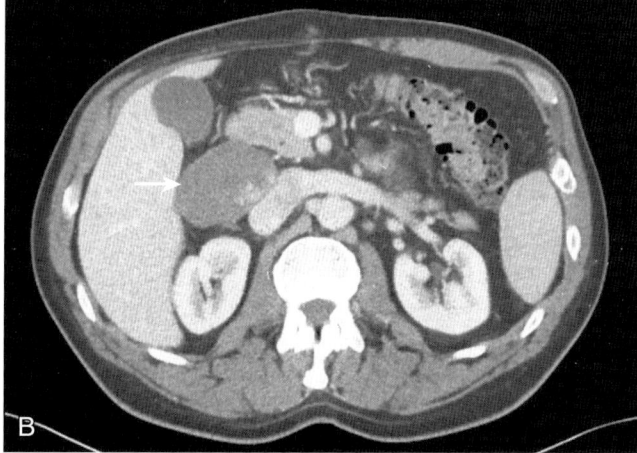

FIGURE 4 Contrast-enhanced, coronal (**A**) and axial (**B**) computed tomographic (CT) images showing an asymptomatic hemangioma (*arrow*) of the caudate lobe. Despite imaging, this mass was initially thought to be arising from the duodenum.

a patient with suspected hepatic hemangioma should question this diagnosis and raise the suspicion of a malignancy. In addition, in a patient being staged for extent of primary or metastatic disease within the liver, the presence of small hemangiomas can result in a false assumption of added malignancy, leading to overestimation of the extent of disease. These patients may be incorrectly excluded from resection of their malignancy.

DIAGNOSIS

Unlike some other benign tumors of the liver, hepatic hemangiomas are typically easy to diagnose on imaging evaluation. Contrast-enhanced computed tomographic (CT) scan is the most common way these lesions are identified and diagnosed. When getting a CT scan for evaluating for hemangioma, it is important to try to obtain a *delayed phase* as well as arterial and venous phases (Figure 4). This accentuates the late contrast puddling that is pathognomonic of these low-flow vascular tumors. The sensitivity of standard arterial and portal phase contrast CT scans is approximately 70%, while the addition of the delayed phase increases the sensitivity to over 90%. The classic CT findings are peripheral enhancement on arterial phase, with centripetal filling on portal venous phase and retention of contrast on washout or delayed phase.

Magnetic resonance imaging (MRI) is also a highly accurate method of diagnosing hepatic hemangiomas. These lesions display low signal intensity on T1 images and, importantly, a classic bright signal on T2-weighted noncontrast images due to their high water content. With use of contrast, much like CT scanning, hemangiomas display early peripheral enhancement and delayed centripetal filling (Figure 5). Studies report that MRI is superior to CT scan in sensitivity and specificity—both over 90%—for diagnosing hepatic hemangiomas. Availability, cost, and patient concerns may lessen the need for MRI as an additional required test, particularly if a multiple-phase CT scan confirmed the diagnosis. However, MRI should be considered in unclear cases. In addition, long-term surveillance with MRI may limit unnecessary radiation exposure.

Other imaging modalities have been described for diagnosing hepatic hemangioma, including planar scintigraphy (tagged red blood cell scans) and angiography. Although potentially helpful in selected cases, these studies are rarely necessary and currently uncommonly used. Ultrasound (US) imaging can also diagnose these tumors. The classic US appearance is that of a well-circumscribed, homogeneous, hyperechoic lesion (Figure 6). However, less than half of these lesions meet these criteria. Larger tumors often display fibrosis, thrombosis, and central necrosis, leading to heterogeneity on US. Larger lesions may have a hypoechoic center, and tumors can appear isoechoic on compression. Contrast-enhanced US can be useful in selected cases, increasing its sensitivity to 70% to 90%.

With use of quality contrast-enhanced cross-sectional imaging, the diagnosis of hemangioma is rarely in question, allowing for confidence in management strategy in most cases. However, in some situations, other tumors can be confused with this lesion. In particular, other vascular tumors such as angiosarcoma, epithelioid hemangioendothelioma, and hemangiopericytoma can mimic cavernous hemangioma. Unlike other solid lesions of the liver, biopsy of hemangiomas should be avoided because of risk of bleeding. In addition,

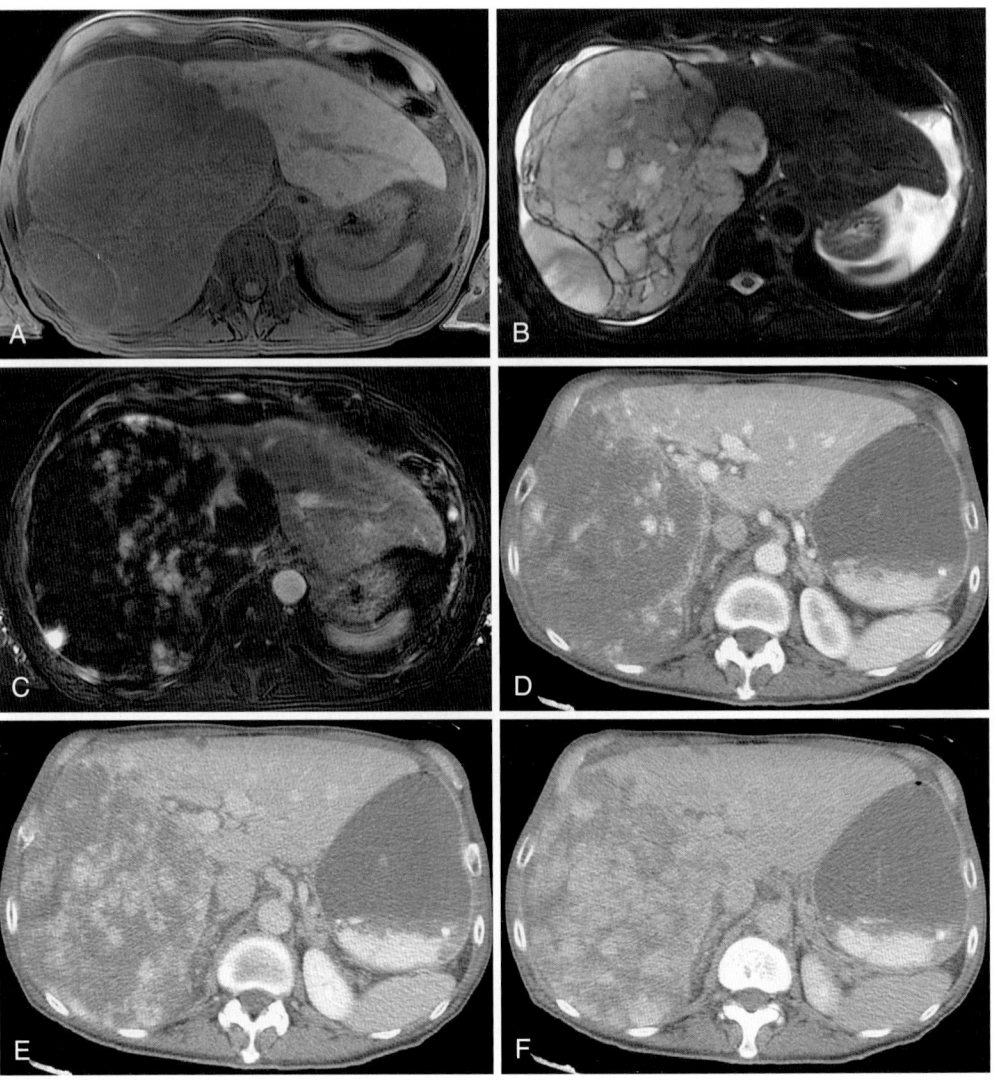

FIGURE 5 Giant cavernous hepatic hemangioma as seen on magnetic resonance imaging (MRI) (**A–C**) and CT scan (**D–F**). **A,** T1-weighted MRI without contrast. **B,** T2-weighted MRI without contrast. **C,** MRI with contrast, showing peripheral enhancement. **D,** Arterial phase computed tomographic (CT) scan showing classic peripheral enhancement. **E,** Portal venous phase CT scan showing centripetal enhancement. **F,** Delayed phase CT scan showing washout and equilibration.

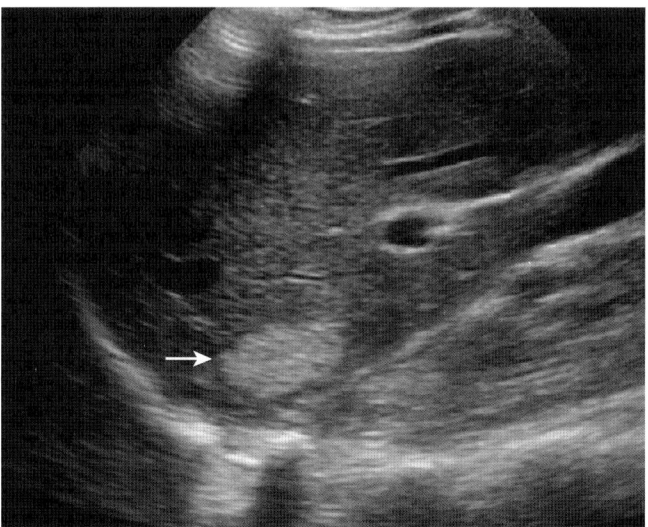

FIGURE 6 Ultrasound image demonstrating a small hepatic hemangioma *(arrow)* with classic findings of a well-circumscribed, homogeneous, and hyperechoic lesion.

percutaneous biopsy, either fine-needle or core, often will fail to provide evidence to support the diagnosis of hemangioma.

MANAGEMENT

As the preponderance of evidence suggests that cavernous hemangiomas rarely symptomatically progress or rupture, asymptomatic hepatic hemangiomas rarely require resection. Even large lesions can be reliably followed with serial imaging and patient follow-up, and rarely do they require subsequent intervention. Although CT scans can also be used for surveillance, the accumulated lifetime radiation risk makes this less appealing than US or MRI for monitoring. Importantly, image monitoring is less useful than symptom assessment in patient follow-up. Tumors that increase in size do not necessarily produce symptoms, and, in some cases, pain can develop even without a measurable growth in the lesion.

Intervention can be divided into acute and elective. Hemangiomas that are life threatening (e.g., in individuals with Kasabach-Merritt syndrome) or result in traumatic or spontaneous rupture or hemorrhage require acute intervention. In the case of acute hemorrhage, arterial embolization can be considered, but only as a temporizing measure, and should be followed by definitive resection when the patient is appropriately stable. If arterial embolization fails to control the hemorrhage, emergent operation is indicated. Surgical intervention, when performed, is done electively in most cases. It should be reserved for those who are clearly symptomatic or in rare cases where diagnosis is uncertain. When offering therapy to the symptomatic patient, the severity of the symptoms must be weighed against the morbidity of the procedure. Location, size, and approach are important factors when assessing surgical risk.

Surgical Resection

Various surgical techniques are available for use in the surgical resection of a hepatic hemangioma. In most cases, *enucleation* is the preferred approach to these tumors. Formal liver resection, whether anatomic or nonanatomic, is rarely necessary. Studies have

demonstrated a decrease in blood loss, operative time, and complications with enucleation over standard resection. The operation is carried out along the plane of the pseudocapsule, carefully and deliberately. Initially, it may be necessary to divide a centimeter or two of parenchyma before the pseudocapsule is defined. Staying near the tumor but avoiding entering the lesion will limit potential complications. Once the pseudocapsule has been identified, the surgeon can often use a gentle dissecting technique to separate the tumor from the parenchyma enough to identify vessels, which are then controlled using surgical clips, ties, or energy devices. As with standard liver resection, dissection can be achieved using blunt techniques, ultrasonic dissection devices, or an energy-based dissector. Staplers are useful for larger pedicles. Strict adherence to the plane of the pseudocapsule will minimize the risk of parenchymal injury and bile leak. In addition, care must be taken to avoid injury to pedicles within the liver that can often be splayed and immediately adjacent to the tumor. The use of a temporary inflow occlusion (Pringle maneuver) can be particularly helpful during enucleation of large hemangiomas to minimize blood loss and decompress the tumor engorgement, facilitating the dissection.

For lesions that are amenable to a laparoscopic approach, this technique may provide advantages over an open operation. Hemangiomas that are peripherally located are best suited to a laparoscopic resection. Lesions that are centrally located, are high on the dome, or are abutting major vascular and biliary pedicles may be more challenging when attempted by laparoscopy.

Intraarterial and Ablative Therapies

For patients who are unstable because of rupture, or for whom comorbid disease is prohibitive, bland transarterial embolization (TAE) is a therapeutic option. In more elective cases, some studies have reported transient pain relief with embolization of hemangiomas. However, TAE is rarely of durable benefit, in part likely due to the lack of dominant arterial pedicle. In selected cases, embolization can be used as a bridge to surgery in the unstable patient or in rare instances where a markedly symptomatic patient is not a candidate for surgery.

Percutaneous or intraoperative radiofrequency ablation and microwave ablation have also been reported as alternatives to surgery and have shown symptom improvement in some cases. Complete ablation is usually not possible in symptomatic patients because of the size and proximity to major vascular and biliary pedicles. Partial ablation might improve symptoms in some cases but should be reserved for highly selected situations.

INFANTILE HEPATIC HEMANGIOMA

Infantile hepatic hemangiomas are rare and the majority are detected incidentally. Although similar on imaging to adult hepatic hemangiomas, these tumors are pathologically distinct. They are composed primarily of endothelial cells, which has given rise to another name: hemangioendotheliomas. These are not to be confused with epithelioid hemangioendotheliomas, which are malignant; nor are they the same as adult hepatic hemangiomas, which are primarily vascular tumors. These hemangioendotherlial tumors are known to undergo interval periods of both rapid growth and involution. MRI is the most conclusive imaging modality for diagnosis of these lesions. Treatment has centered on steroids, immunomodulating agents, radiation therapy, and embolic therapy. When large enough, these tumors can cause significant symptoms in infants, including congestive heart failure, respiratory distress, gastric outlet obstruction, and coagulopathy. When coagulopathy and thrombocytopenia are encountered with these large hepatic lesions, known as the Kasabach-Merritt syndrome, treatment must be prompt.

SUMMARY

With the increased use of abdominal imaging, cavernous hepatic hemangiomas are being identified with increasing frequency. Fortunately, a definitive diagnosis can be made noninvasively in most cases, and asymptomatic patients can be managed conservatively with confidence. Biopsy is not necessary and should not be used for diagnosis. In cases where patients' symptoms affect their quality of life, or in the rare cases where malignancy cannot definitively be excluded, resection should be offered. When possible, enucleation is preferred to standard hepatic resection and can be done with minimal morbidity or mortality, even in large and centrally located tumors. Minimally invasive approaches can be considered in some cases.

SUGGESTED READINGS

Adam YG, Huvos AG, Fortner JG: Giant hemangiomas of the liver, *Ann Surg* 172(2):239, 1970.

Baer HU, Dennison AR, Mouton W, et al: Enucleation of giant hemangiomas of the liver; technical and pathologic aspects of a neglected procedure, *Ann Surg* 216:673–676, 1992.

Donati M, Stavron GA, Donati A, Oldhafer KJ: The risk of spontaneous rupture of liver hemangiomas: a critical review of the literature, *J Hepatobiliary Pancreat Sci* 18:797–805, 2011.

Kamaya A, Maturen KE, Tye GA, et al: Hypervascular liver lesions, *Semin Ultrasound CT MR* 30(5):387–407, 2009.

Yoon SS, Charny CK, Fong Y, et al: Diagnosis, management and outcomes of 115 patients with hepatic hemangioma, *JACS* 197(3):392–402, 2003.

THE MANAGEMENT OF BENIGN LIVER LESIONS

Kenzo Hirose, MD

Incidentally identified liver lesions are an increasingly prevalent issue in view of the growing frequency with which patients undergo imaging studies. Patients undergo computed tomographic (CT) scan of the abdomen and pelvis for a variety of indications, which leads to the identification of many liver lesions that otherwise would be clinically silent. The majority of these lesions are benign and require no further treatment or monitoring, but many will require specialized expertise for their diagnosis and management. A working knowledge of the diagnosis, natural history, and treatment of these lesions is important for any surgeon treating affected patients. A close working relationship with a radiologist, especially one with expertise in magnetic resonance imaging (MRI) of the liver, is particularly important because many of these lesions are diagnosed primarily on the basis of cross-sectional imaging.

DIAGNOSIS AND IMAGING OF BENIGN LIVER LESIONS

Although many benign liver lesions are identified incidentally, a full history and physical examination is mandatory in the initial evaluation of a patient with a liver lesion. Important points to document include symptoms of pain, weight loss, early satiety, anemia, a known history of liver disease or cirrhosis, use of oral contraceptive pills or anabolic steroid use, a history of malignancy, and prior attempts at biopsy or instrumentation. On physical examination, the physician should assess for signs of chronic liver disease, tenderness, palpable masses, and signs of other concomitant malignancy. Laboratory evaluation, including observation for tumor markers (alphafetoprotein, cancer antigen 19-9 [CA19-9], carcinoembryonic antigen, chromogranin) can be helpful if there is a suspicion of malignancy.

Ultimately, however, the mainstay of diagnosis of benign liver lesions is cross-sectional imaging, and a good working knowledge of imaging modalities and findings is important for assessing these patients. With contemporary imaging modalities, the need for biopsy of benign liver lesions has become relatively uncommon. The radiographic armamentarium that is available for characterization of liver lesions includes ultrasonography, multiphasic CT, MRI, sulfur colloid scintigraphy, fluorodeoxyglucose-labeled positron emission tomography (PET), and tagged red blood cell scanning. The major contemporary methods for evaluation of liver lesions are contrast–enhanced CT and MRI. Proper intravenous contrast phases must be used to characterize liver lesions. Rather than use of standard single-phase CT of the abdomen and pelvis, patients should undergo dynamic postcontrast imaging with precontrast, early arterial phase (30-second), portal venous phase (60-second), and equilibrium (90-second) phases. It is not uncommon for even a large liver lesion to be missed on single-phase CT but appear clearly on a dedicated liver protocol imaging study. Benign lesions of the liver are listed in Box 1; this chapter focuses on the most common diagnoses.

Characterization of the lesion as cystic or solid is the first step in radiographic assessment. Simple liver cysts have a very characteristic appearance on various imaging modalities, including anechogenicity and increased acoustic through-transmission on ultrasonography, water density on CT (−10 to 10 Hounsfield units), and homogeneous bright signal intensity on T2-weighted MRI. Cysts should be further assessed for signs of complexity, including internal septa, wall enhancement, and mural nodularity. Such findings should raise the suspicion of a biliary cystic neoplasm such as biliary cystadenoma or cystadenocarcinoma. Other findings, such as thickening of the wall, proteinaceous debris within the lesion, and loculation, in the correct clinical context, may be suggestive of liver abscess. Findings of a hydatid cyst would include the identification of endocyst/pericyst interface, calcification, and daughter cysts in the periphery of the main cyst.

Solid lesions can be further characterized by their enhancement pattern on postcontrast imaging. The most common benign neoplasm of the liver is hepatic hemangioma, characterized by high T2 signal intensity ("light bulb sign") on MRI and low attenuation on precontrast CT. On both MRI and CT, hepatic hemangiomas demonstrate peripheral nodular enhancement or "puddling" in early arterial phase contrast imaging with centripetal enhancement or filling in during portal venous and equilibrium phases. Figure 1 illustrates typical MRI findings of a hepatic hemangioma. Contrast agent–enhanced MRI has excellent diagnostic accuracy for hemangiomas larger than 2 cm, and, in general, no further diagnostic testing is necessary.

The two next most common benign lesions include focal nodular hyperplasia (FNH) and hepatic adenoma (HA). Differentiating these two entities is often a radiographic and diagnostic dilemma because they share many similar imaging characteristics. Furthermore, the natural history and management of these two lesions differ significantly, as discussed later in this chapter. FNH is a benign poly-clonal proliferation of all cellular elements of the liver, thought to be induced by an arterial malformation or a focal area of arterial hyperperfusion. HA on the other hand, is a monoclonal proliferation of hepatocytes that have the potential for spontaneous bleeding and malignant transformation. Figures 2 and 3 demonstrate the most typical findings seen in FNH and HA on contrast agent–enhanced

---

BOX 1: Benign lesions of the liver

Most Common
Hepatic cyst
Hepatic hemangioma
Hepatic adenoma
Focal nodular hyperplasia

Less Common
Biliary cystadenoma
Nodular regenerative hyperplasia
Angiomyolipoma
Endothelioid hemangioendothelioma
Bile duct hamartoma
Peliosis

MRI. FNH demonstrates hyperenhancement with arterial phase contrast agent and isointensity on venous phase imaging. These lesions can be relatively "stealthy" as they are composed largely of normal hepatocytes; they can be missed on standard, single-phase contrast CT because their attenuation is similar to that of background liver tissue during the venous phase. The classic finding is of a central scar, which is more often seen in larger lesions and may exhibit postcontrast enhancement as well.

The radiographic findings in HA can be varied, depending on whether they are the steatotic or inflammatory subtype. Adenomas tend to be hypointense on T1-weighted imaging, are also enhanced in the early arterial phase, and also tend to be isointense or hypointense on portal venous phases. Persistent enhancement through the portal venous and equilibrium phases is characteristic of an inflammatory adenoma. The presence of intralesional fat is characteristic of a steatotic HA and is useful for distinguishing adenoma from FNH. Fat-suppressed in-phase and out-of-phase imaging sequences can be helpful in assessing lipid content within the lesion. The presence of hemorrhage within the lesion also indicates HA rather than FNH.

Use of liver-specific contrast agents during MRI can also be especially useful in differentiating FNH from HA. Gadoxetic acid (Eovist) is an intravenous MRI contrast agent that is 50% cleared through hepatobiliary excretion. Hepatobiliary phase imaging with Eovist is typically performed 20 to 40 minutes after administration and

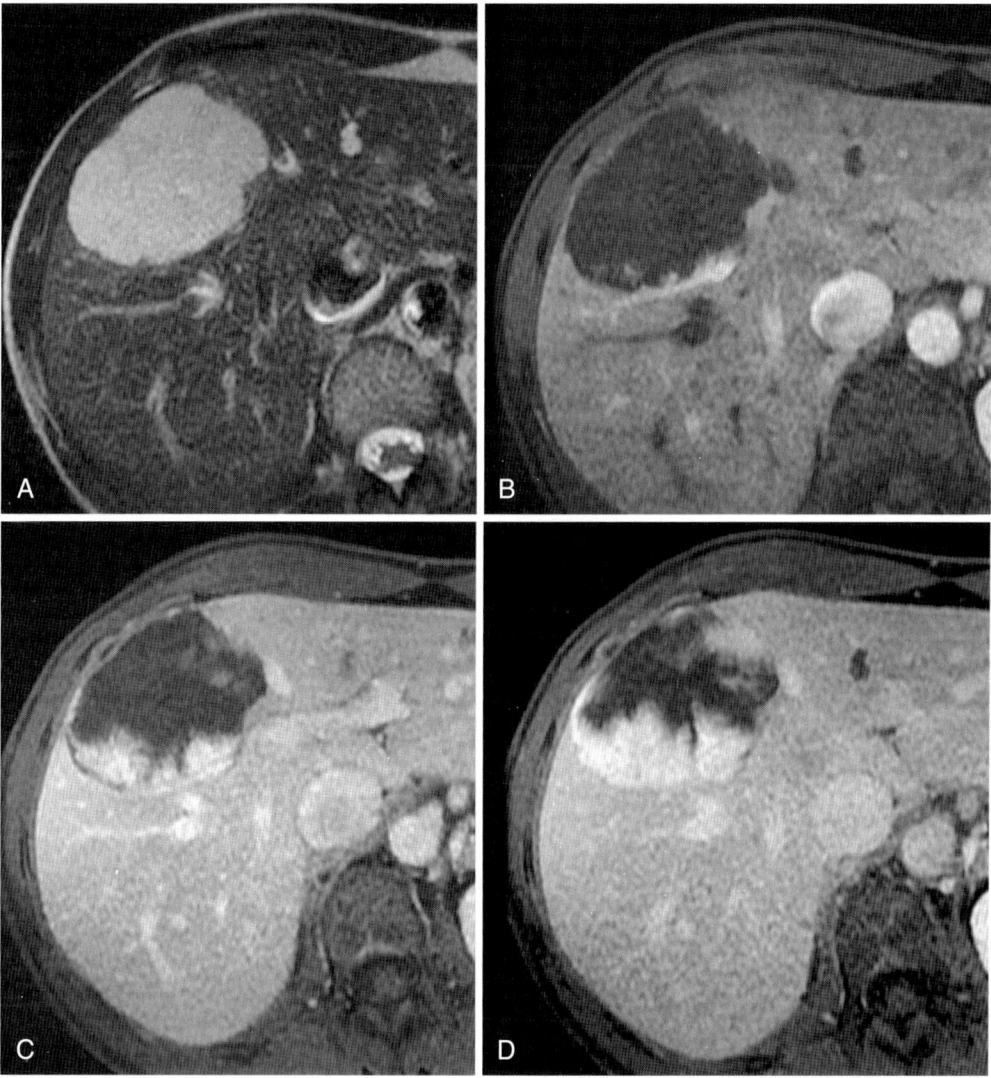

FIGURE 1 Typical magnetic resonance imaging (MRI) findings of hepatic hemangioma. **A,** T2-weighted sequence demonstrating homogeneous bright signal intensity. **B,** Early arterial phase postcontrast image demonstrating peripheral nodular enhancement **C,** Portal venous phase image demonstrating gradual filling in of the lesion. **D,** Equilibrium phase image demonstrating further centripetal enhancement.

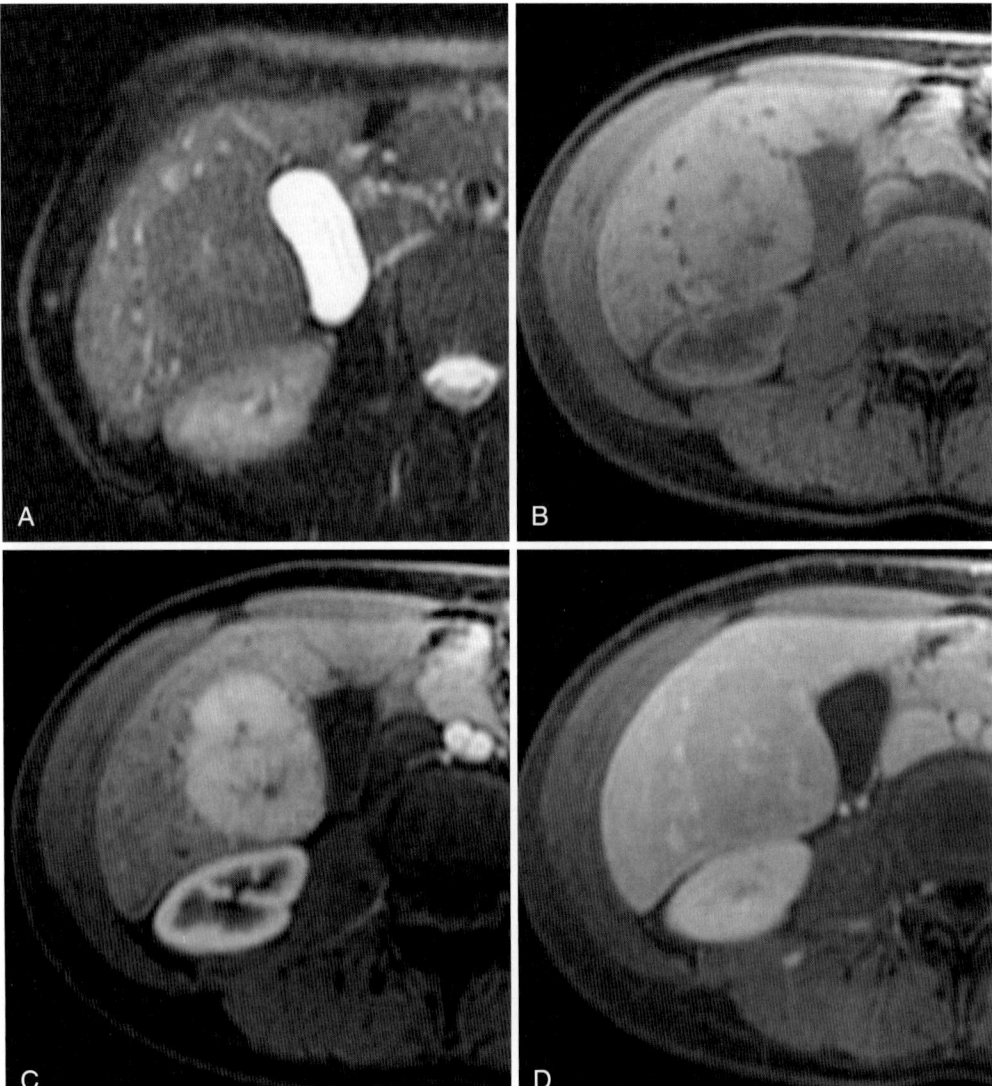

FIGURE 2 Typical magnetic resonance imaging (MRI) findings of focal nodular hyperplasia (FNH). **A,** T2 weighted sequence with slight hypoattenuation. **B,** Precontrast phase showing isointensity to background liver. **C,** Early arterial phase imaging sequence with clear hypervascularity and central scar. **D,** Portal venous phase with near isointensity to background. Note delayed enhancement of central scar.

demonstrates uptake by normal hepatocytes and excretion into the biliary tree. Uptake of the contrast agent on hepatobiliary phase imaging with Eovist is a finding highly specific for FNH. HA, on the other hand, consists of neoplastic hepatocytes whose function is abnormal and, consequently, do not take up Eovist in hepatobiliary phase imaging. These radiographic findings, coupled with the appropriate clinical context, can help reliably distinguish HA from FNH. Radiographic findings on cross-sectional imaging for the most common benign lesions of the liver are listed in Table 1.

The role of nuclear medicine in the diagnosis of benign liver lesions has gradually decreased as the specificity of cross-sectional imaging has increased. Technetium 99m–tagged red blood cell scans have traditionally been used to identify hepatic hemangiomas, but they are no longer commonly used, in view of the high specificity of dynamic postcontrast cross-sectional imaging. Radiolabeled sulfur colloid scintigraphy has also been used to distinguish FNH from HA because of specific uptake by Kupffer cells, which are present in the FNH but not in HA. In most patients, assessment with contrast agent–enhanced MRI is adequate, but when the findings are equivocal or when the patient has a contraindication to intravenous contrast agents, there may be a role for sulfur colloid scintigraphy.

When findings of imaging studies are equivocal, percutaneous biopsy may be warranted. However, the decision to perform biopsy

should be made carefully: the risks and benefits of biopsy should be weighed, and how the results will affect therapy should be considered. An absolute contraindication to biopsy is hepatic hemangioma because of the risk of massive hemorrhage. In most cases, high-quality, liver-specific cross-sectional imaging should enable the clinician to make this diagnosis. If the lesion is highly suspicious for malignancy on imaging and is amenable to surgical resection, then a percutaneous biopsy may not necessarily change management and, moreover, may lead to spreading of the tumor via the needle tract. In this case, the patient should undergo a diligent evaluation for a primary tumor, and if none is found, then the patient should undergo laparotomy and resection.

In the case of distinguishing FNH from HA, percutaneous biopsy may be helpful, but a few factors should be considered: these lesions may be difficult to identify on ultrasonography or noncontrast CT, which makes image-guided biopsy difficult; the histologic appearance of FNH can be difficult to distinguish from that of normal liver, which causes uncertainty about whether the actual lesion was sampled; HA are generally well vascularized, and biopsy significantly increases risk of bleeding; and both FNH and HA may have the appearance of a well-differentiated hepatocellular neoplasm and can be difficult to distinguish. In practice, percutaneous biopsy in the case of suspected FNH or HA often does not add information that aids

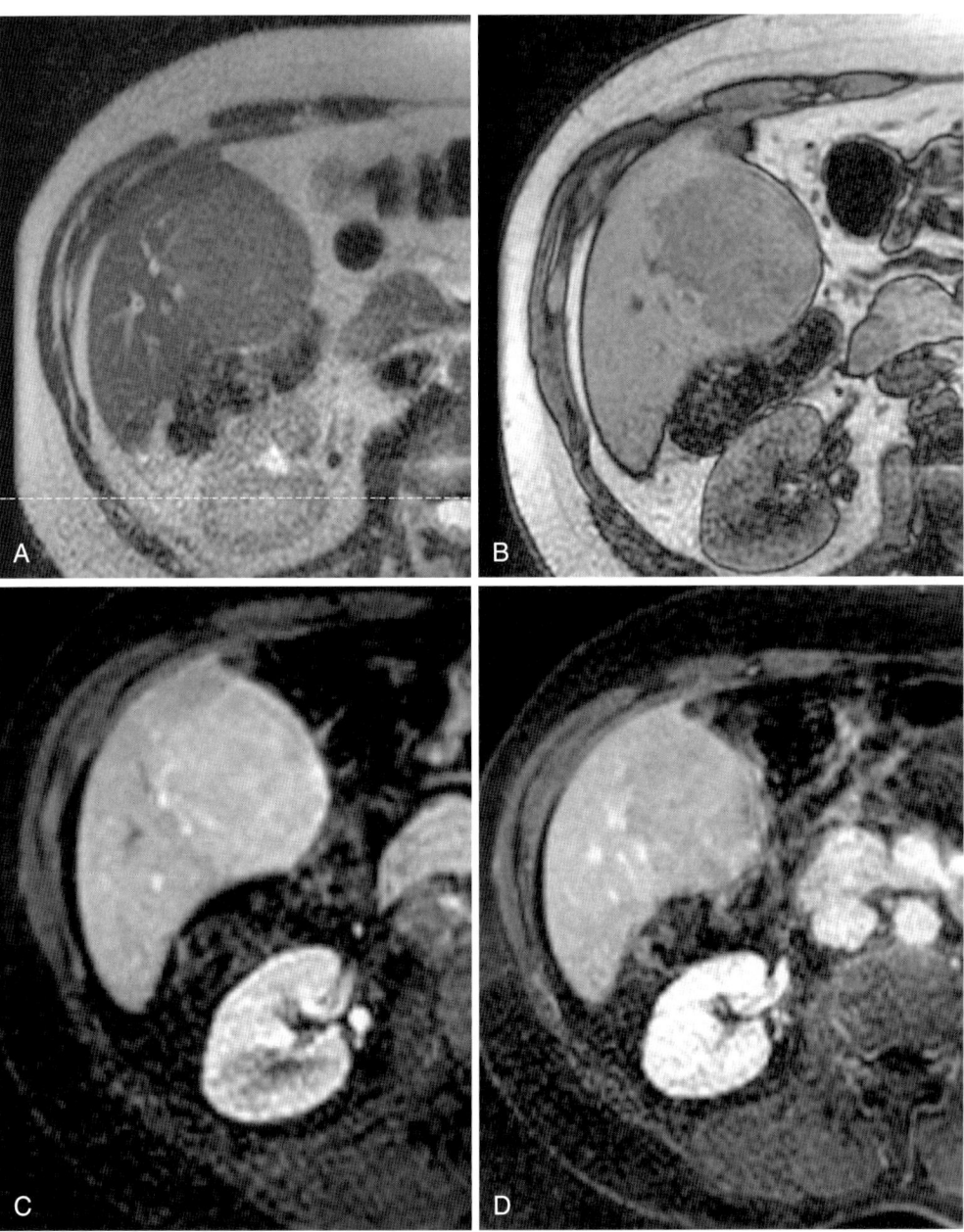

FIGURE 3 Typical magnetic resonance imaging (MRI) findings in hepatic adenoma. **A,** T2 weighted imaging with slight hypointensity. **B,** T1 weighted, out of phase, fat suppressed imaging sequence showing signal loss in lesion, suggestive of intralesional lipid content. **C** and **D,** Early arterial and portal venous phase post contrast sequences.

in clinical decision making. The field is in evolution, however, and more sophisticated molecular and genetic analysis of these biopsy specimens may lead to changes in clinical management, discussed in the following sections.

SURGERY FOR BENIGN LIVER LESIONS

In general, there are three indications for resection of benign liver lesions: (1) symptoms, (2) inability to rule out malignancy, and (3) prevention of malignancy or complications. Careful documentation of symptoms and review of imaging and or pathologic data are critical in deciding whether to proceed with resection.

Liver Cysts

Simple cysts of the liver are present in up to 5% of all adults, and most are benign. Asymptomatic cysts do not warrant intervention or serial examination. Potential symptoms may include pain, especially with cysts that are complicated by hemorrhage; shortness of breath, with lesions located in a subdiaphragmatic position; and early satiety or nausea, with lesions that cause mass effect on the stomach or duodenum. Symptoms are rare with cysts smaller than 5 cm. Liver cysts can manifest with acute symptoms when hemorrhage occurs within the cyst. These episodes of hemorrhage are rarely life-threatening and are generally self-limited. The cyst may take on a more complex appearance with an episode of bleeding, suggested by increased attenuation, heterogeneity, and layering of the fluid on cross-sectional imaging. It is important to distinguish these findings from those that may be suggestive of a biliary cystic neoplasm such as biliary cystadenoma or cystadenocarcinoma, as these lesions require a more formal resection.

When symptomatic, the ideal intervention for simple liver cysts is surgery. Needle aspiration of simple liver cysts should only be reserved to identify symptomatic response, as the cyst will inevitably recur and instrumentation of the cyst can lead to infection, bleeding, or inflammation that will make surgical intervention more difficult.

TABLE 1: Postcontrast cross-sectional imaging: typical findings of the most common liver lesions

Lesion	CT scan	MRI
Simple cyst	Density equivalent to water Does not communicate with biliary tree	Bright on T2-weighted imaging, water density May show proteinaceous density if prior hemorrhage has occurred
Hemangioma	Early peripheral nodular enhancement in arterial phase, centripetal filling in, follows blood pooling	Same contrast findings as for CT Bright on T2-weighted sequences ("light bulb" sign)
Hepatic adenoma	Hypervascular on early arterial imaging Isointense or hypointense on venous phase	Distinguished from FNH by presence of fat; may be appreciated on in-phase and out-of-phase imaging; lack of central scar
FNH	Hypervascular on early arterial phase imaging and isodense in comparison with surrounding liver on portal venous phase	Similar postcontrast findings as on CT; central scar may be enhanced on equilibrium phase images Will take up liver-specific contrast agents (e.g., gadoxetic acid [Eovist]) on hepatobiliary phase (20-30 min)

CT, Computed tomographic scan; *FNH*, focal nodular hyperplasia; *MRI*, magnetic resonance imaging.

Placement of a percutaneous drain into a simple liver cyst is almost never indicated.

The goal of surgery for simple liver cysts is elimination of symptoms. This is generally achieved by fenestration of the cyst, which entails excising a portion of the cyst wall, close to its margin with normal liver. This may be followed by ablation of the interior cyst wall with argon beam or electrocautery, although care must be taken not to damage any vascular or biliary structures that may be present along the inner wall of the cyst. Placement of a pedicled omental flap into the cyst cavity is a technique favored by some surgeons to prevent recurrence of the cyst. Complete resection of the cyst is generally not necessary except in cases in which an underlying cystadenoma or cystadenocarcinoma is suspected or in the setting of polycystic liver disease for which anatomic resection may be more effective. Simple cyst fenestration is often amenable to a laparoscopic approach with either ultrasonic shears or a bipolar vessel sealing device to excise the cyst wall. For cysts located in the right posterior sector, positioning of the patient in either the semilateral or full left lateral decubitus position can help optimize exposure laparoscopically.

Care should be taken in carrying the line of excision through adjacent liver parenchyma because large biliary and vascular structures can be compressed by the cyst and may not be clearly visualized on preoperative imaging. This is especially true in the setting of giant liver cysts (>20 cm) and may result in bile leakage or significant bleeding. Use of an Endo GIA vascular load stapler can help prevent this occurrence. If bleeding or bile leakage occurs, use of the stapler or clips or placement of a laparoscopic stitch can often remedy the situation. Bleeding from a rent in a major hepatic vein branch can be minimal in the presence of pneumoperitoneum, as the pressure of carbon dioxide often exceeds central venous pressure. If the patient becomes hemodynamically unstable or if laparoscopic maneuvers fail, then conversion to an open operation is necessary. If there was a prior episode of bleeding in the cyst, as evidenced by expression of thick chocolate-colored fluid from the cyst, there may be significant inflammatory adhesions of the cyst to the peritoneum or diaphragm. After completion of the fenestration, routine drainage of the resection bed is generally not performed. Short-term and long-term relief of symptoms in well-selected patients is excellent after surgery.

Hepatic Hemangioma

Hepatic hemangiomas are the most common benign neoplasm of the liver and can be definitively diagnosed with multiphasic (liver protocol) CT or MRI. Typical characteristics include peripheral "puddling" of early phase contrast agent in the lesion, followed by centripetal enhancement on later portal venous phase images, mirroring the blood pool. Hemangiomas are universally benign, with no risk of malignant degeneration and an exceedingly small risk of rupture or bleeding. Asymptomatic hemangioma may be managed safely with observation, without the need for serial imaging. Large hemangiomas can potentially cause symptoms from mass effect, including pain, shortness of breath, and early satiety. Lesions smaller than 5 cm rarely cause symptoms. Giant cavernous hemangiomas (>10 cm) of the liver are relatively rare but can be complicated by specific physiologic problems. Kasabach-Merritt syndrome can be observed with giant cavernous hemangiomas and is characterized by a consumptive coagulopathy, which leads to an appearance of disseminated intravascular coagulation. Typical findings include thrombocytopenia, hypofibrinogenemia, coagulopathy, and evidence of fibrinolysis. High-output cardiac failure resulting from arteriovenous shunting is usually observed only in the pediatric population.

In patients with symptoms or complications of hemangioma, intervention is warranted. Resection is the treatment of choice for patients who are healthy enough to undergo surgery. In many cases, enucleation is technically possible, as large hemangiomas tend to compress the adjacent liver parenchyma, creating a plane of dissection that is favorable to enucleation. Often a major arterial feeding branch can be identified that, when ligated, makes the hemangioma less tense and easier to manipulate. Extrahepatic clamping or ligation of the left or right hepatic artery can also facilitate dissection by decompressing the hemangioma. Formal anatomic resection is also an option and may be an appropriate choice with regard to the location and size of the hemangioma. For patients who are not candidates for surgery, bland embolization of giant hemangiomas has been performed in the past with some success. Pharmacologic therapies, including antiangiogenic medications, have been reported on an anecdotal basis and may represent another therapeutic modality for patients who cannot undergo surgery.

Focal Nodular Hyperplasia

FNH represents a nodular, polyclonal proliferation within the liver that contains all cellular elements of liver parenchyma. These lesions have no potential for malignancy or for spontaneous rupture or hemorrhage. The only two indications for resection of FNH are symptoms (e.g. pain, early satiety, weight loss) and inability to rule out malignancy. In general, the issue with this condition is establishing a definitive diagnosis, which can often be achieved with modern imaging technologies. Patients without symptoms who have typical imaging findings of FNH should not be offered resection and generally do not need long-term surveillance. Patients who do experience abdominal pain must have a careful evaluation to rule out other sources of pain, especially in patients with lesions smaller than 5 cm. A detailed history, physical examination, and correlation of the patient's complaints to the anatomic findings on imaging are necessary before surgical resection is offered for this condition. Resection must not be offered on the basis of anatomic or technical considerations alone.

Hepatic Adenoma

HAs are benign neoplastic growths of hepatocytes that typically occur in the setting of a normal background liver and tend to be hormonally sensitive. The classic clinical presentation is that of a young woman (aged 20s to 40s) with a history of oral contraceptive use. Anabolic steroid use in men can also lead to the development of HA. Other risk factors include glycogen storage disease and pregnancy. Patients may present with a hepatic mass incidentally identified on cross-sectional imaging, with abdominal pain, or more acutely with spontaneous rupture or hemorrhage. Contrast agent–enhanced MRI with in-phase and out-of-phase imaging is the optimum diagnostic imaging method for this entity. Typical findings include arterial hyperenhancement without washout and "dropout" in fat-suppressed imaging sequences, which suggest the presence of lipid within the mass. The radiographic diagnosis can be more difficult in the setting of a steatotic liver.

Patients with a diagnosis of HA who are taking oral contraceptives or anabolic steroids should discontinue those medications and undergo interval reassessment. The risk of malignancy in HA is correlated approximately with size; the risk of an occult hepatocellular carcinoma (HCC) within the lesion increases once the adenoma is larger than 5 cm. In most series of resected HA findings suggest that the risk of having a previously undiagnosed HCC is between 4% to 15% in affected patients. In men, the risk of HCC in HA can be as high as 47%, prompting some authorities to recommend that all HA in men who are not taking exogenous steroids should be considered for resection. Most of these series are retrospective case series of relatively small numbers of patients who have undergone resection, and thus they introduce an element of selection bias. Furthermore, very few studies, outside of anecdotal reports, have enabled the researchers to estimate the risk of malignant transformation of HA over time. Because of the relative rarity of this lesion, characterization of the long-term natural history is difficult. However, current indications for resection of HA include (1) size larger than 5 cm; (2) symptoms, including bleeding; (3) inability to rule out malignancy; and (4) male gender. Patients with HA who do not meet criteria for resection should be monitored with serial cross-sectional imaging and alpha-fetoprotein levels.

Data have helped categorize HA by molecular changes that are correlated with clinical behavior and may help stratify these lesions by risk. The most intriguing of these data involve the gene that encodes beta-catenin, *CTNNB1:* 15% to 19% of all HA harbor an activating mutation of *CTNNB1* and have a significantly higher incidence of HCC. In one series, 6 (46%) of 13 resected HA with activating mutations of *CTNNB1* were found on final pathologic study to have either HCC, HCC within a background of HA, or borderline HCC/HA. Of lesions that did not have a *CTNNB1* mutation, only 8% were thus characterized. Two other categories of HA have been proposed in addition to *CTNNB1* overexpression: (1) HA with *HNF1a* gene inactivation (30% to 50% of all HA), which show significant intralesional steatosis, and (2) those with *CRP/SAA* expression (30% to 35% of all HA) which demonstrate inflammatory HA histology, and are more common in the setting of obesity, hepatic steatosis, and alcohol use (previously categorized as telangiectatic

FNH). Of patients with either of these types, neither show as high a risk of HCC as those with *CTNNB1* overexpression. How these genotype-phenotype correlations will guide treatment is still in evolution, but risk stratification of HA with preoperative biopsy and genetic analysis may become a useful diagnostic test in the future.

In general, a wide margin of resection is not necessary for HA, as 90% of such lesions are benign. However, malignancy can be difficult to identify preoperatively, and frozen-section analysis is not reliable to distinguish well-differentiated HCC from HA. If possible, a negative margin resection should be performed in the case that HCC is identified on final histopathologic analysis. Aggressive vascular resection and reconstruction is not indicated in affected patients. HA characterized by high lipid content may be more difficult to palpate at operation; thus intraoperative ultrasonography and high-quality preoperative cross-sectional imaging are essential in guiding the resection plane. HA that manifest with acute bleeding are optimally treated with bland embolization to control the acute hemorrhage, followed by elective resection.

Formal resection at the time of acute hemorrhage is generally not recommended, although if the patient has life-threatening hemorrhage or if the lesion is refractory to transarterial interventions, then laparotomy may be necessary to achieve hemostasis. In these instances, the operation is analogous to a trauma laparotomy in which use of inflow occlusion (Pringle's maneuver), packing and pressure, topical hemostatic agents, and selective hepatic arterial ligation are potentially useful maneuvers. If formal resection is possible in an expeditious way, then it is also an option in the acute setting, although in patients with massive blood loss and hemodynamic instability, resection should not be attempted. Ethanol injection into the lesion, as well as radiofrequency energy (delivered either via ablation probe or a saline-linked radiofrequency device), can also be helpful to achieve hemostasis in this situation.

SUMMARY

Treatment of benign liver lesions requires a thoughtful assessment of clinical, radiographic, and pathologic data. The majority of these lesions do not require surgical intervention and can be managed safely by observation or monitored with serial imaging. Many affected patients require surgery, but clinicians must resist the temptation to recommend surgery simply on the basis of anatomic or technical considerations. The improvement in techniques of liver surgery, including the development of laparoscopic techniques, has reduced the rates of morbidity and mortality associated with these operations and in some ways has changed the risk/benefit balance of surgery. Although benign liver lesions represent a potentially ideal indication for laparoscopic liver resection, clinicians must be careful not to change the indications for surgery solely on the basis of ability to perform the operation.

SUGGESTED READINGS

Chun YS, House MG, Kaur H, et al: SSAT/AHPBA Joint Symposium on Evaluation and Treatment of Benign Liver Lesions, *J Gastrointest Surg* 17:636–644, 2013.
Farges O, Ferreira N, Dokmak S, et al: Changing trends in malignant transformation of hepatocellular adenoma, *Gut* 60(1):85–89, 2011.
Fergusson J: Investigation and management of hepatic incidentalomas, *J Gastroenterol Hepatol* 27(12):1772–1782, 2012.
Gore RM, Newmark GM, Thakrar KH, et al: Hepatic incidentalomas, *Radiol Clin North Am* 49(2):291–322, 2011.
Kneuertz PJ, Marsh JW, de Jong MC, et al: Improvements in quality of life after surgery for benign hepatic tumors: results from a dual center analysis, *Surgery* 152(2):193–201, 2012.
Zucman-Rossi J, Jeannot E, Nhieu JT, et al: Genotype-phenotype correlation in hepatocellular adenoma: new classification and relationship with HCC, *Hepatology* 43(3):515–524, 2006.

The Management of Malignant Liver Tumors

Laleh G. Melstrom, MD, MS, and Yuman Fong, MD

OVERVIEW

Hepatocellular carcinoma (HCC), fibrolamellar hepatocellular carcinoma, and intrahepatic cholangiocarcinoma (ICC) are the malignant tumors discussed in this chapter; the surgical management of metastatic liver tumors is discussed elsewhere in this book. Surgical therapy, in the form of resection or transplantation, results in the best outcomes and may result in cure. Many patients with HCC or ICC, however, have associated liver parenchymal disease such as cirrhosis from viral hepatitis. This and other comorbid conditions may increase the risk that surgical therapy.

Selection of patients with primary hepatic malignancies for resection is generally based on the localized nature of the tumor, whether it is technically resectable, and the adequacy of residual liver to support life. Patients with unresectable small tumors are offered liver transplantation or thermal ablation. Large or multiple unresectable disease and disseminated disease are treated with combinations of transcatheter embolization and systemic therapies.

HEPATOCELLULAR CARCINOMA

HCC represents the most common solid tumor worldwide, occurring in nearly 1 million patients yearly. In the United States, approximately 25,000 patients present with HCC annually. This cancer is associated with liver parenchymal injury, such as that from chronic hepatitis B or C viral infection. Overall, the long-term survival in HCC is poor, at less than 5%, because for most patients, the associated liver cirrhosis precludes resection.

Surgical Resection

Surgical resection is generally offered to patients with liver-localized disease and adequate hepatic reserve for recovery. In general, these patients have class Childs A cirrhosis. Outcome after resection for HCC depends on whether the resection margin is tumor-free, degree of cirrhosis, presence of vascular invasion, presence of satellite lesions, tumor size (>5 cm), bilobar involvement, and involvement of regional lymph nodes.

Among patients with resectable tumors, most Western (American and European) series have demonstrated 5-year survival rates ranging from 27% to 64%, and Eastern (Asian) series have documented 5-year survival rates ranging from 21% to 49%. The lower survival rates likely relate to the increased rate of cirrhosis and hepatitis B infection. In modern large series, morbidity rates range from 30% to 50% and mortality rates range from 1.6% to 5.3%.

Liver Transplantation

Liver transplantation is generally offered to patients with cirrhosis who do not have major cardiopulmonary comorbid conditions and whose local disease is limited. The Milan criteria (Lim et al., 2012) are the most commonly used tumor criteria for selection of patients for transplantation. The criteria include either one tumor less than 5 cm in size or three or fewer lesions, each less than 3 cm. Of patients with such limited disease, 60% to 80% are alive 5 years after transplantation.

Thermal Ablation

Small tumors can also be effectively killed by radiofrequency ablation or microwave ablation. Treatment effectiveness is directly related to the size of tumor and ease of access. Ablations can be performed during open surgery, through laparoscopy, or through percutaneous access. Proximity of the tumor to major blood vessels may attenuate effectiveness by a "heat sink" effect. There have been three randomized trials published to date demonstrating equal survival outcome among patients who underwent resection and those who underwent radiofrequency ablation for small HCC. The rate of morbidity from radiofrequency ablation is usually less than 10%, and the rate of mortality is less than 0.5%.

Embolization

If a lesion is found to be unresectable intraoperatively or preoperatively, other treatment options include transarterial chemoembolization (TACE), transarterial embolization (TAE), and radioembolization. Thrombosis of the portal vein is considered a contraindication to TACE or any transarterial modality because of the risk of severe hepatic insufficiency after the procedure. Risks associated with transarterial therapies include the postembolization syndrome, characterized by fevers and abdominal pain. Other serious complications can arise such as gallbladder infarction, pancreatitis, hepatic insufficiency, and sepsis. Response rates can be as high as 80%. In both TAE and TACE, patients require interval treatments approximately every 3 to 6 months.

FIBROLAMELLAR HEPATOCELLULAR CARCINOMA

Fibrolamellar HCC is very different from HCC. This cancer usually occurs in patient with no parenchymal liver injury or cirrhosis. It also occurs in young patients, with a median age of 27 years. These tumors secrete characteristic hormones and proteins, such as neurotensin and vitamin B_{12}–binding protein. Thus fibrolamellar tumors may be the primary neuroendocrine tumors of the liver.

These tumors also behave like neuroendocrine tumors in that they are well circumscribed and most often separate from adjacent blood vessels, even when they are large. Thus they are much more likely to be resectable than classic HCC. In addition, they are slow growing, and complete cytoreduction for multifocal disease can result in long-term survival. Surgical resection results in a 5-year survival rate of 30% to 50%.

Fibrolamellar HCC represents nodal metastases in 15% to 30% of cases. Thus the lymph nodes in the porta hepatis, celiac region, and peripancreatic areas should be examined and, if suspect, either sampled or dissected. In cases of nodal recurrence after previous liver resection, exploration and dissection of the recurrent lymph nodes represent rational therapy.

INTRAHEPATIC CHOLANGIOCARCINOMA

ICC is also known as *peripheral cholangiocarcinoma*. These tumors are also associated with viral hepatitis and cirrhosis and, consequently, are much more common in Southeast Asia. In the United States, the incidence of ICC is approximately 5000 cases yearly. The incidence is increasing, probably because, as a result of better pathologic diagnosis, many tumors that used to be called *metastases of unknown origin* have been determined to be ICC.

Surgical resection remains the best option and the only potentially curative option. Diagnostic laparoscopy should be considered for patients with ICC because of the high incidence of peritoneal metastases. Because up to one third of patients have nodal metastases, the regional nodes should be sampled and formally dissected if the samples are positive for cancer. Series published on outcomes after resection for ICC show that the 5-year survival rate for R0 resections ranges from 44% to 63%. The mortality rate has been documented at 2% to 7%.

Most patients at presentation are not candidates for resection because of peritoneal, lung, or bone metastases.

PREOPERATIVE ASSESSMENT

General Preoperative Assessment

Once a diagnosis is made, the patient's comorbid conditions, baseline liver function, tumor staging, and size of the future liver remnant (FLR) are all taken into consideration in the development of a treatment plan.

Assessment of medical condition and liver function is initiated with baseline blood work, including complete blood cell count, coagulation studies (prothrombin time/international normalized ratio [PT/INR]), complete metabolic panel, and hepatitis panel. Tumor markers (alpha-fetoprotein, carcinoembryonic antigen, cancer antigen 19-9) are studied to assist in diagnosis, as well as for determination of the usefulness of such markers for follow-up.

Defining tumor anatomy in relation to the healthy part of the liver is a key step in determining resectability. Imaging should include a triple-phase contrast computed tomographic (CT) scan of the abdomen and pelvis and a CT scan of the chest with intravenous contrast medium. Tumors that are hypervascular, such as HCC and metastatic neuroendocrine tumors, demonstrate increased uptake in the arterial phase, whereas tumors such as ICC and metastatic colorectal cancer demonstrate increased enhancement in the portal venous phase. CT scanning can be performed with concurrent magnetic resonance imaging of the liver in equivocal circumstances without a tissue diagnosis. A diagnosis of HCC can be made for lesions greater than 2 cm that appear hypervascular on two separate imaging modalities or for a focal hypervascular lesion greater than 2 cm and serum alpha-fetoprotein levels greater than 400 ng/mL. For larger high-risk tumors, a bone scan should also be considered for patients with HCC.

Comorbid conditions such as chronic renal failure, congestive heart failure, or severe chronic obstructive pulmonary disease may often preclude offering surgical management. In addition, comorbid conditions such as renal insufficiency, heart disease, and diabetes add a level of risk for postoperative morbidity and mortality.

Assessing liver function is important in determining whether a resection is feasible with acceptable morbidity and mortality risk. The Child-Turcotte-Pugh (CTP) score (Table 1)—which includes total bilirubin, serum albumin, PT/INR, the presence of ascites, and the presence of hepatic encephalopathy—subdivides liver disease into categories (A, B, and C) that translate into perioperative mortality risk for liver resection. CTP B and C scores imply risks for

TABLE 1: Child-Turcotte-Pugh score*

Measure	1 Point	2 Points	3 Points
Total bilirubin (mg/dL)	<2	2-3	>3
Serum albumin (g/L)	>35	28-35	<28
PT/INR	<1.7	1.71-2.30	>2.30
Ascites	None	Mild	Moderate to severe
Hepatic encephalopathy	None	Grades I-II (suppressed with medication)	Grades III-IV (refractory)

*The score employs five clinical measures: class A, 5-6 points; class B, 7-9 points; class C, 10-15 points.
PT/INR, Prothrombin time/international normalized ratio.

operative mortality of 30% and 80%, respectively. Traditionally, only patients with CTP A scores were considered candidates for surgical resection.

Other factors that ought to be taken into consideration include a platelet count of less than 100,000/mm³, radiologic indicators of cirrhosis or portal hypertension (such as the contour of the liver and splenomegaly), periportal and abdominal wall collateral vessels, and esophageal varices. The presence of these factors may make a large liver resection prohibitively risky.

The Future Liver Remnant

In order to minimize the risk of hepatic failure postoperatively, a minimum volume of liver is necessary for adequate hepatic function. In general, in a healthy, noncirrhotic liver, an FLR of 20% is adequate. In patients with chronic liver disease, a FLR of 40% is correlated with acceptable risk. This value is calculated most frequently on three-dimensional CT volumetry, whereby the FLR is the total liver volume (as calculated slice by slice) minus the planned resection volume. Another formula-based estimate is total liver volume (TLV) (cm³), which is calculated as $-794.41 + 1267.28 \times$ body surface area (m²). The ratio of the FLR volume measured on CT scan to calculated TLV is known as the "standardized FLR." Studies have demonstrated that a standardized FLR volume of less than 300 mL/m² is correlated with death and liver failure. Inadequate FLRs are correlated with increased hepatocellular injury and inadequate liver regeneration, which are correlated with subsequent morbidity and mortality secondary to hepatic failure.

In both healthy and diseased livers, a reasonable strategy to induce contralateral liver growth before resection has been to utilize portal vein embolization (PVE). PVE is performed through percutaneous access of the ipsilateral portal vein with particle embolization, with the use of microparticles and microcoils. By impeding portal venous blood flow to the side of the liver ipsilateral to the tumor, hypoxia-induced growth factors and shunted portal venous flow induce growth to the contralateral lobe and thus potentiate growth of the FLR before resection. In addition, PVE is used as an in vivo assessment of regenerative capacity. In patients with liver disease, PVE has been shown to decrease hepatic insufficiency, perioperative complications, and postoperative mortality. Furthermore, TACE for HCC followed by PVE several weeks later has been a useful strategy to optimize both perioperative and oncologic outcomes in these patients. Some centers are utilizing preoperative hepatic arterial embolization in primary HCC to induce necrosis and possibly to decrease tumor spillage and vascular spread of tumor cells intraoperatively. This may make resection more technically challenging secondary to the induced fibrosis.

OPERATIVE APPROACH TO RESECTION OF PRIMARY LIVER MALIGNANCIES

In general, the principles of liver resection revolve around controlling inflow and outflow vessels, parenchymal transection, and tumor clearance. These factors are all taken into account in the context of presumed adequate residual liver volume. Maintenance of a low central venous pressure is a key anesthetic principle to minimize backward bleeding from the hepatic veins during parenchymal transection. This entails accepting a urine output of 25 mL/hr and prompt reexpansion of intravascular volume after the resection is complete. The patient is kept in 15 degrees of the Trendelenburg position to maintain adequate cardiac preload and to decrease the risk of air embolism via openings in the hepatic veins during transection.

Incision and Access

Exposure is a key component of any hepatectomy. A right subcostal, hockey stick–type incision is the most commonly used for liver resection and gives excellent access and exposure for most right-sided tumors. For left-sided tumors, a midline incision extending superiorly to the xyphoid process should provide adequate exposure. Access to the suprahepatic portion of the inferior vena cava should be ascertained for particularly high-positioned tumors along the dome of the liver. The abdomen and chest should be prepared in such a way that a thoracoabdominal incision or sternotomy can be made intraoperatively if necessary.

Right Hepatectomy

After inspection of the peritoneal cavity, the falciform ligament is ligated and divided. The falciform ligament is tied with a long suture so that it can serve as a retraction handle. The liver is then mobilized by further dividing the falciform ligament to the dome of the liver. Intraoperative liver ultrasonography is performed to ascertain that all disease is identified. The triangular ligament is then divided. The liver is retracted to the patient's left side as the retroperitoneal attachments and the smaller branches from the right lobe to the inferior vena cava are ligated and divided. The gallbladder is then removed with suture ligation of the cystic duct stump.

Traditionally for major liver resections, the inflow and outflow vessels for the liver are dissected free outside the liver, controlled, and divided before liver parenchymal transection. The perforating veins to the retrohepatic portion of the inferior vena cava are usually dissected first. The right hepatic vein is then dissected and controlled by encircling it with a vessel loop. It is important not to divide the hepatic veins before the portal vein/hepatic artery (inflow). The right portal vein and right hepatic artery are then dissected free outside the liver and ligated with sutures or staples. Attention is then brought to the porta hepatis, where the hepatoduodenal ligament is controlled in preparation for a Pringle maneuver (intermittent occlusion of the inflow to the liver). The right hepatic vein is then divided before liver parenchymal transection.

More recently, the intrahepatic approach to vascular inflow control has been popularized. This technique is useful when the tumor is more than 2 cm from the hilus of the liver. When cancer is too close to the junction of the left and right inflow vessels, however,

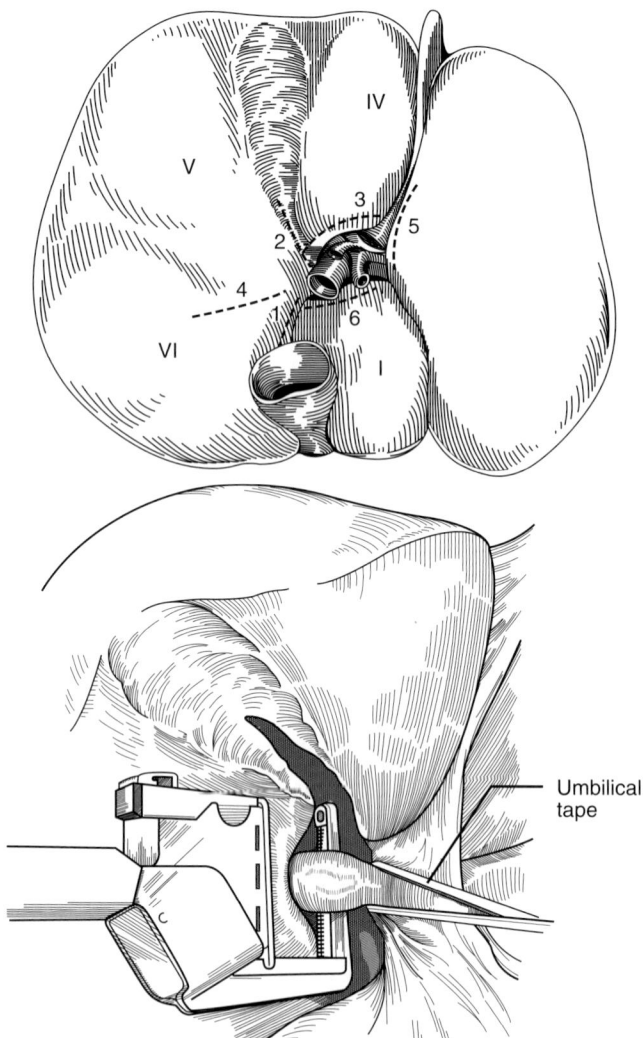

FIGURE 1 To access the right portal pedicle *(top),* hepatotomies are made in the gallbladder fossa (2) and in the caudate process (1). The pedicle is encircled with a renal pedicle clamp, and a vessel loop is passed around it. The vessel loop is used to retract the main portal vein/left portal vein to the left as a TA stapler is passed and fired to divide the right portal pedicle *(bottom). (From Fong Y, Blumgart LH: Useful stapling techniques in liver surgery,* J Am Coll Surg *185:93, 1997).*

the risk of causing a positive tumor margin is too great with the intrahepatic approach.

In the intrahepatic vascular approach, two incisions are made: one in the gallbladder bed and one in the caudate process. These are utilized to isolate the anterior and posterior sectoral inflow pedicles with umbilical tapes. The pedicles are then divided with a TA stapler (Figure 1, bottom). The advantages of this approach are that it is fast and it minimizes injury to the contralateral pedicle. Once the inflow is divided, the right hepatic vein can be ligated and divided. This is most frequently done with an endovascular stapler or by suture ligation.

For parenchymal transection, the authors place a 0 chromic suture on a large blunt needle through the gallbladder fossa and another just to the left of the transection line as handles for ease in liver mobility. The transection line is identified by the demarcation seen after the inflow is divided. This line appears primarily to the right of the course of the middle hepatic vein. The parenchyma can be divided with various coagulation devices. The authors utilize the

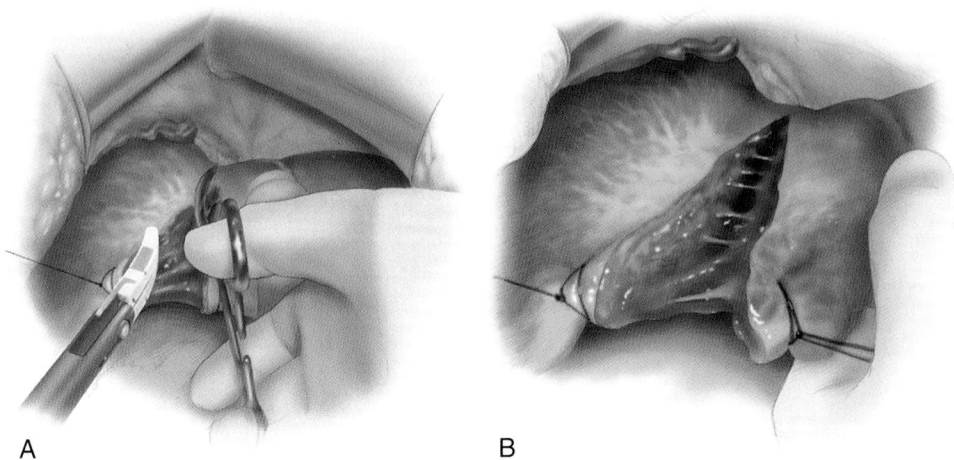

A   B

FIGURE 2 To divide the liver parenchyma, two stay sutures are placed for traction. The parenchyma is sequentially crush-clamped with a Kelly clamp; this demonstrates various size pedicles and veins. Those smaller than 5 mm are sealed and divided with the LigaSure device. If the structure is larger than 5 mm, the endovascular stapler, clips, and ties are used. *(From Patrlj L, Tuorto S, Fong Y: Combined blunt-clamp dissection and LigaSure ligation for hepatic parenchyma dissection: postcoagulation technique,* J Am Coll Surg *210:39, 2010.)*

traditional crush clamp technique with a Kelly clamp to sequentially crush liver parenchyma and reveal more prominent hepatic veins and pedicles (Figure 2). Vessels less than 5 mm in diameter can be divided with a LigaSure device (Covidien, Boulder, Colo) (see Figure 2). If they are larger, they should be tied or stapled. The parenchyma is methodically divided opening the line of transection like a book, layer by layer. As the authors approach the hepatic veins, the vein branches become more prominent, and the authors often utilize the vascular stapler.

After the specimen is delivered, the authors coagulate the surface with the argon beam, look for any profusely bleeding areas, and address those areas by coagulation or suture ligation. The authors then ask the anesthesiologist to initiate resuscitations to a central venous pressure of at least 8 cm H_2O in order to recognize any occult back bleeding from hepatic veins that are not adequately sealed.

Extended Right Hepatectomy

The principles of an extended right hepatectomy are the same as those for a right lobectomy except for the inclusion of segment IV of the left lobe and transecting the liver to the left of the middle hepatic vein. In this circumstance, the inflow is not completely controlled at the porta hepatis by dividing only the right portal vein and right hepatic artery. Recurrent inflow vessels arising in the umbilical fissure need to be ligated.

Left Lobectomy

The initial steps of a left lobectomy include mobilizing the falciform ligament and getting around the porta hepatis. The left triangular ligament is mobilized with care so as to not injure the left phrenic vein superiorly and the esophagus posteriorly. During mobilization of the left hepatic lobe, the ligamentum venosum is identified and divided after the liver is retracted to the patient's right. Branches from the left lobe and the caudate lobe to the inferior vena cava are identified and ligated to maximize mobility. The most challenging aspect of a left lobectomy is identifying and isolating the left and middle hepatic veins (particularly for large left-sided tumors).

The left lobe inflow has a much longer extrahepatic course than does the right. In extrahepatic control of inflow vessels, the left hepatic artery is identified, ligated, and divided first, followed by the left portal vein and then the bile duct. When intrahepatic pedicle ligation is used, hepatotomies are created in segments IV and II. The main left portal pedicle is then isolated and stapled.

Extended Left Hepatectomy

This will include a caudate resection and segments V and VIII. The challenging aspect of this procedure is defining the line of transection to the right of Cantlie's line that will remove segments V and VIII and not injure the right hepatic vein and the inflow to the posterior sector. In addition, often the segment VII inflow vessels arise from the anterior pedicle and not the posterior pedicle. Noting this anomaly and protecting the segment VII vessels are essential for saving enough functional liver.

Caudate Resection

The caudate can be approached from the right or left, depending on where the lesion is. The most tedious portion of resection of the caudate is meticulous isolation of perforating veins from the back of the caudate to the inferior vena cava. The most perilous aspect of this resection is losing control of the junction of the middle and left hepatic veins, where the highest caudate vein enters. In addition, the inflow from branches of the right and left portal vein need to be controlled.

Segmental and Wedge Resections

Lesions are often removed with wedge or segmental resections in order to preserve as much functional liver volume as possible. This is most relevant in the context of liver disease that precludes large anatomic resections. In segmental resections, vascular control is most often obtained in an intraparenchymal manner. (Figure 3 outlines the lines of segmental resection.)

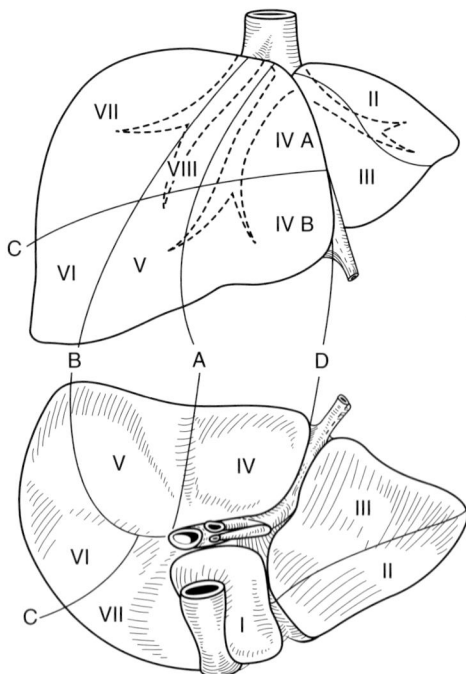

FIGURE 3 The lines of resection for the various segments. Segments VI and VII are resected in right posterior sectorectomy. Segments V and VIII are resected in right anterior sectorectomy. Segments IV, V, and VIII are resected in central hepatectomy. *(From Blumgart LH, editor: Video atlas: liver, biliary & pancreatic surgery, Philadelphia, 2011, Elsevier, p 73.)*

SUGGESTED READINGS

Blumgart LH, editor: *Video atlas: liver, biliary & pancreatic surgery*, Philadelphia, 2011, Elsevier.

Cauchy F, Fuks D, Belghiti J: HCC: Current surgical treatment concepts, *Langenbecks Arch Surg* 397(5):681–695, 2012.

Endo I, Gonen M, Yopp AC, et al: Intrahepatic cholangiocarcinoma: rising frequency, improved survival, and determinants of outcome after resection, *Ann Surg* 248(1):84–96, 2008.

Lim KC, Chow PK, Allen JC, et al: Systematic review of liver resection for early hepatocellular carcinoma within the Milan criteria, *Br J Surg* 99(12):1622–1629, 2012.

TREATMENT FOR HEPATOCELLULAR CARCINOMA: RESECTION VERSUS TRANSPLANTATION

**Jayme E. Locke, MD, MPH, and
Andrew M. Cameron, MD, PhD**

INTRODUCTION

Hepatocellular carcinoma (HCC) is the most common primary hepatic malignancy worldwide. It is three times more common in men and is most prominent in Asia and Africa. More than 80% of HCCs arise in the setting of cirrhosis, and patients with cirrhosis have an annual HCC incidence of 3% to 10%. It is thought that HCC arises from adenomatous hyperplasia, which progresses to atypical hyperplasia and ultimately deteriorates to overt malignancy. In addition to a cirrhotic liver, risk factors for the development of HCC include viral hepatitis (especially hepatitis B), aflatoxins, azo dyes, aromatic amines, N-nitrose compounds, chlorinated hydrocarbons, hydrosol compounds, pesticides, radiation, Thorotrast, smoking, porphyria, Budd-Chiari syndrome, oral contraceptives, anabolic androgenic steroids, and alpha-1 antitrypsin.

Over the past decade, the management of patients with chronic liver disease has improved, and in parallel, the prevalence of viral hepatitis, including hepatitis B and hepatitis C, has increased. As a result, there has been a dramatic increase in the number of patients diagnosed with compensated HCC. HCC is now well recognized as an important complication of cirrhosis and is a leading indication for liver transplantation. Currently, one third of patients with end-stage liver disease who are awaiting liver transplant carry the diagnosis of HCC. If left untreated, the 5-year survival is less than 10% and median survival is less than 6 months. As with most malignancies, HCC is amenable to cure when identified at an early disease stage, highlighting the importance of routine surveillance in patients who are at risk. Combining serum alpha-fetoprotein (AFP) levels with ultrasonography has proven to be the most sensitive and specific modality for HCC screening. AFP levels greater than 400 ng/mL are highly suggestive of HCC, and ultrasonography can detect 60% to 80% of lesions that are 1 cm or smaller and 90% of lesions 3 cm or larger. Early identification of HCC increases potential therapeutic options, which include liver resection and transplantation. Patient selection for a given modality is dependent on tumor pathology, including stage, size, number, and location, and the patient's associated medical comorbidities and degree of underlying liver dysfunction. Treatment requires a multidisciplinary approach, and multiple modalities may be employed.

EVALUATION

HCC can present with a palpable liver mass, abdominal pain, and deterioration in functional status, or the tumor may be found incidentally during routine surveillance. Although relatively uncommon, paraneoplastic syndromes can occur, including polycythemia, polymyositis, hypoglycemia, and diarrhea. A history and physical exam directed at identification of underlying liver disease should be performed in order to assess disease severity and stigmata of portal hypertension. History of prior hospitalizations for gastrointestinal bleeding and the presence of caput medusa, ascites, gynecomastia, and muscle wasting are important physical findings. In addition, basic laboratory testing directed at identification of viral hepatitis, coagulopathy, and hepatorenal syndrome should be performed.

The leading cause of death after hepatic resection for HCC is liver failure, and as such, determining the hepatic reserve is of high importance. The severity of liver disease can be estimated using the Child-Pugh classification (Table 1) and the Model for End-Stage Liver Disease (MELD). Patients with Child-Pugh A cirrhosis are predicted to have a perioperative mortality rate of less than 5% and can typically tolerate having up to 50% of their liver parenchyma resected. Patients who have Child-Pugh B cirrhosis have a predicted perioperative mortality rate of 10% to 15% and should have no more than 25% of their liver parenchyma resected. Patients with Child-Pugh C cirrhosis have a perioperative mortality that is in excess of 25%, and therefore, liver resection is contraindicated. The MELD score, introduced in 2002, is used to prioritize patients on the liver transplant waiting list. The score predicts 3-month mortality and the rate ranges from 6% to 40%. Serum creatinine, total bilirubin, and international normalized ratio are used to calculate the score. Patients with scores of 15 or higher typically benefit from liver transplantation. To shorten waiting times and to increase access to liver transplantation for patients with HCC, 22 MELD exception points are routinely awarded to these patients.

In addition to various classification systems, evaluation of the functional hepatic capacity may aid in the determination of hepatic reserve. Specifically, the indocyanine green (ICG) clearance test is a useful tool in predicting liver failure following resection. ICG is injected into the patient's bloodstream, and levels are then measured 15 minutes after injection. In patients with a normal functioning liver, less than 10% of ICG dye should be detected. Patients with 15% to 20% of the dye remaining are predicted to tolerate a two-segment resection, a single segment or wedge is indicated when 21% to 30% of the dye remains, and patients with more than 40% of the dye remaining are predicted to have postoperative liver failure independent of resection size.

IMAGING

HCC is diagnosed based on clinical and radiographic criteria, and a tissue diagnosis is not required. Percutaneous liver biopsy of the tumor is discouraged secondary to concern for seeding the biopsy track. Computed tomographic (CT) scan and magnetic resonance imaging (MRI) are the preferred imaging modalities for diagnosis of HCC. Triphasic hepatic CT imaging is ideal, as it allows for determination of tumor anatomy and proximity to major hepatic vasculature. Arterial enhancement followed by venous washout is the classic radiographic finding for HCC. In addition, CT imaging can be used to estimate the future liver remnant (FLR) and, as such, can help predict the likelihood of postoperative liver failure. FLR less than 40% is predictive of postoperative liver failure. MRI is equivalent to CT imaging in determining tumor anatomy and location, and it is an excellent alternative for patients with contrast allergies. In addition, both modalities have now replaced hepatic arteriography and can produce three-dimensional images that allow for estimation of liver volumes and perfusion territories and provide detailed intrahepatic anatomy. Ultrasonography is typically reserved for surveillance in patients at risk and, when needed, to assess intrahepatic and portal venous blood flow.

STAGING

The American Joint Committee on Cancer Tumor Node Metastasis (AJCC TNM) system uses tumor size, proximity to surrounding vasculature, local regional metastasis, and distant metastasis to determine prognosis for patients with HCC after liver resection (Table 2).

TABLE 2: AJCC/UICC TNM classification of hepatocellular carcinoma

T1	Single tumor without vascular invasion
T2	Single tumor with vascular invasion or multiple tumors, none >5 cm
T3	Multiple tumors, any >5 cm, or tumors involving major branch of portal or hepatic veins
T4	Tumors with direct invasion of adjacent organs other than the gallbladder, or perforation of visceral peritoneum
N1	Regional lymph node metastasis
M1	Distant metastasis

Stage	Tumor	Node	Metastasis
I	T1	N0	M0
II	T2	N0	M0
IIIa	T3	N0	M0
IIIb	T4	N0	M0
IIIc	Any T	N1	M0
IV	Any T	Any N	M1

AJCC, American Joint Committee on Cancer; *M,* distant metastasis; *N,* regional lymph node; *T,* primary tumor; *UICC,* International Union Against Cancer.
From American Joint Committee on Cancer: Cancer staging manual, *ed 6, New York, 2002, Springer-Verlag.*

TABLE 1: Child-Pugh classification of cirrhosis

Parameter	1 Point	2 Points	3 Points
Albumin (g/dL)	>3.5	2.8-3.5	<2.8
Bilirubin (mg/dL)	<2	2-3	>3
INR	<1.7	1.7-2.3	>2.3
Ascites	None	Slight	Moderate
Encephalopathy	None	1-2	3-4

Child-Pugh classification is calculated by summing the points per parameter to arrive at a total between 5 and 15.
INR, international normalized ratio.
Grade A = 5-6, Grade B = 7-9, Grade C = 10-15.

The AJCC TNM classification is an oncologic standard that provides useful prognostic information about survival and disease recurrence. However, it fails to account for the severity of underlying liver disease and patients' functional status, which are major considerations in choice of treatment modality for HCC. Most recently, the Barcelona Clinic Liver Cancer (BCLC) staging system has emerged as the standard staging system for HCC. The BCLC is the only classification system that accounts for tumor-related variables (size, number, vascular invasion, local regional and distant spread), liver function (Child-Pugh), and health status of the patient (Eastern Cooperative Oncology Group Performance Status) (Figure 1).

TREATMENT

Liver Resection

Liver resection is the treatment of choice for HCC in patients without cirrhosis and can be performed in patients with cirrhosis if they have preserved liver function and portal venous pressures of 10 mm Hg or less. The ability to resect a given tumor is determined, in part, by the absence of distant metastases and tumor location in relation to major hepatic vasculature. Intraoperative ultrasound is a useful adjunct to ensure that resection can be performed safely and adequate tumor-free margins can be obtained (~1 cm). Anatomic resection is preferable, as it is thought to prevent intrahepatic metastases

via the related portal vein tributary. Portal vein embolization can be used to increase the FLR and allow for resections that are more extensive. However, the effectiveness of portal vein embolization in patients with cirrhosis has not been established.

The main predictors of survival are tumor size, number, and presence of vascular invasion. In general, the survival rate is worse in patients with larger tumors, presence of micro- or macroscopic invasion, and in the setting of multiplicity, such that 5-year survival rates for patients with tumors up to 2 cm, 2 to 5 cm, and larger than 5 cm are 66%, 52%, and 37%, respectively (Table 3). Vascular invasion is the strongest predictor of tumor recurrence and correlates with tumor number and size. Approximately 70% of patients will experience disease recurrence within 5 years of resection. Neoadjuvant and adjuvant therapies have not been shown to afford any survival benefit in patients with HCC. Locoregional therapies, such as radiofrequency ablation (RFA), transarterial chemoembolization (TACE), and radiation, have been used to help downstage tumors initially regarded as unresectable.

Liver Transplantation

Over the past several decades, liver transplantation (LT) has evolved as the treatment of choice for patients with small HCC tumors, as it affords significant survival advantage over liver resection, particularly for patients with cirrhosis with limited hepatic reserve. LT simultaneously removes the tumor and corrects the underlying liver dysfunction.

FIGURE 1 The Barcelona Clinic Liver Cancer (BCLC) staging system for HCC. *CLT,* Cadaveric liver transplantation; *LDLT,* living donor liver transplantation; *M,* metastasis classification; *N,* node classification; *PEI,* percutaneous ethanol injection; *PS,* performance status; *RFA,* radiofrequency ablation; *TACE,* transarterial chemoembolization. *(From Khorsandi SE, Heaton N: Contemporary strategies in the management of hepatocellular carcinoma,* HPB Surg Epub 2012 Nov 4.)

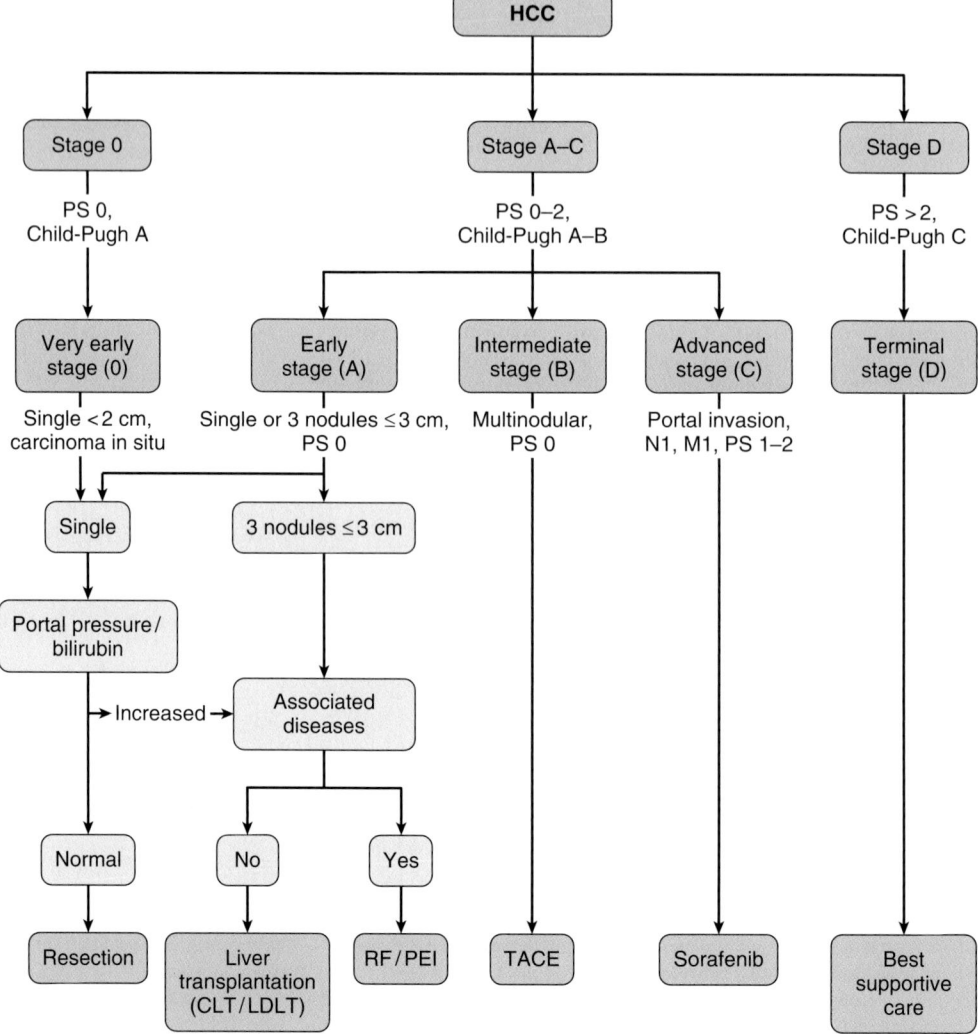

TABLE 3: Results of survival after hepatic resection for hepatocellular carcinoma in selected series

Author	Year	No.	1-Year survival (%)	3-Year survival (%)	5-Year survival (%)
Franco	1990	72	68	51	NR
Nagasue	1993	229	80	51	23
Llovet	1999	77	85	62	51
Zhou	2001	1000 (<5 cm)	91	77	65
		1366 (>5 cm)	76	48	37
Ercolani	2003	224	83	63	43
Shimozawa	2004	135	95	73	55

NR, Not reported.

TABLE 4: Survival following liver transplantation for hepatocellular carcinoma in selected series

Author	Year	No.	1-Year survival (%)	3-Year survival (%)	5-Year survival (%)
Mazzaferro	1996	48	90	84	NR
Hemming	2001	112	78	63	57
Roayaie	2002	43	90	58	44
Zavaglia	2005	155	84	75	72

NR, Not reported.

In addition, because HCC is often multifocal, total hepatectomy removes the source of potentially later-developing tumors.

During the late 1990s, the Milan criteria were introduced to help guide patient selection for LT. Adherence to the Milan criteria (solitary tumor up to 5 cm or three tumors up to 3 cm each) has improved the 5-year survival rate to over 70% and simultaneously decreased disease recurrence to less than 10% after LT (Table 4). The major limitation of LT as treatment for HCC is the scarcity of deceased donors, such that long waiting times increase the risk for disease progression. Currently, there is an approximate 20% dropout rate among patients waiting for LT that carry the diagnosis of HCC. As a result, bridging therapies, including RFA and TACE, have been introduced to maintain the tumor within listing criteria. Data from the International Liver Transplant Tumor Registry suggest that RFA combined with LT may improve overall survival. In addition, many have advocated for living donor LT to overcome the dropout rate experienced secondary to the shortage in donor organs. Although living donor LT reduces waiting time for the patient with HCC, reported outcomes have been inferior, with reduced survival and higher recurrence rates. Explanations for this phenomenon have included the loss of the observation period to assess tumor biology and less surgical oncologic clearance as the recipient inferior vena cava must be preserved.

The Milan criteria serve as a prognostic indicator of tumor biology. It has been suggested, however, that these criteria may exclude some patients with favorable biology. As a result, several efforts have been made to expand the Milan criteria. The University of California at San Francisco (UCSF) criteria include one tumor of 6.5 cm or less or multiple tumors of which the largest is 4.5 cm not to exceed 8 cm total. Alternatively, others have proposed downstaging tumors to within the Milan criteria using locoregional therapies such as RFA and TACE. Favorable results in terms of both survival and disease recurrence rates have been achieved using both the UCSF criteria and downstaging. However, these outcomes have been based on retrospective analysis of tumor burden at the time of explant, and no prospective validation has been performed.

LT has also been advocated as a salvage therapy for HCC recurrence after liver resection that is within the Milan criteria. Selected cases have shown similar 5-year survival rates among patients with salvage and primary LT. However, others have reported high operative mortality, higher recurrence rates, and a worse 5-year survival rate compared with primary LT. As a result, salvage LT remains controversial in the setting of a limited organ supply and unfavorable results.

SUGGESTED READINGS

Adam R, Zaoulay D, Castaing D, et al: Liver resection as a bridge to transplantation for hepatocellular carcinoma in cirrhosis: a reasonable strategy? *Ann Surg* 238:508–518, 2003.

Bismuth H, Chiche L, Adam R, et al: Liver resection versus transplantation for hepatocellular carcinoma in cirrhosis, *Ann Surg* 218:145–151, 1993.

Fuks D, Dokmak S, Paradis V, et al: Benefit of initial resection of hepatocellular carcinoma followed by transplantation in case of recurrence: an intention-to-treat analysis, *Hepatology* 55:132–140, 2012.

Graziadei IW, Sandmueller H, Waldenberger P, et al: Chemoembolization followed by liver transplantation for hepatocellular carcinoma impedes tumor progression while on the waiting list and leads to excellent outcome, *Liver Trans* 9:557–563, 2003.

Khorsandi SE, Heaton N: Contemporary strategies in the management of hepatocellular carcinoma, *HPB Surg* Epub 2012.

Llovet JM, Schwartz M, Mazzaferro V: Resection and liver transplantation for hepatocellular carcinoma, *Semin Liver Dis* 25:181–200, 2005.

Mazzaferro V, Regalia E, Doci R, et al: Liver transplantation for the treatment of hepatocellular carcinomas in patients with cirrhosis, *N Engl J Med* 334:693–699, 1996.

Olthoff KM, Forner A, Hubscher S, et al: What is the best staging system for hepatocellular carcinoma in the setting of liver transplantation, *Liver Trans* 17:S26, 2011.

Yao FY, Breitenstein S, Broelsch CE, et al: Does a patient qualify for liver transplantation after the down-staging of hepatocellular carcinoma? *Liver Trans* 17:S109–S116, 2011.

Yao FY, Ferrell L, Bass NM, et al: Liver transplantation for hepatocellular carcinoma: expansion of the tumor size limits does not adversely impact survival, *Hepatology* 33:1394–1403, 2001.

Radiofrequency Ablation of Hepatic Metastases from Colorectal Cancer

Anna M. Leung, MD, and Anton J. Bilchik, MD, PhD

OVERVIEW

Colorectal cancer is the third most common malignancy in the United States. Worldwide every year, 1 million people are diagnosed with colorectal cancer. Fifty percent of these patients eventually have hepatic metastases develop; half do not have other metastatic sites. Surgical resection is the only treatment with proven potential for cure. However, surgical resection is feasible in only 10% to 25% of patients with metastatic colorectal cancer. The need for alternative approaches has led to the development of local ablative techniques, such as radiofrequency ablation (RFA), ethanol injection, microwave ablation, photocoagulation, high-intensity focused ultrasound, and cryosurgical ablation. Of these, RFA has become one of the most frequently used modalities to clear liver metastases from colorectal and other cancers.

INDICATIONS AND PREOPERATIVE ASSESSMENT

Patients who are poor candidates for surgical resection of hepatic metastases from colorectal cancer include those with restrictive comorbid conditions or low performance status, surgically inaccessible tumors, large tumor burden, disease recurrence, and inadequate hepatic reserve. These conditions are not necessarily contraindications for RFA because ablation can be performed without general anesthesia and normal hepatic parenchyma can be preserved.

Candidates for surgical resection or ablative techniques should undergo laboratory assessment of hepatic function. They should also undergo computed tomographic (CT) scan, magnetic resonance imaging (MRI), or fluorodeoxyglucose (FDG) positron emission tomography (PET) to evaluate the size, location, distribution, and number of hepatic lesions; to identify any nonhepatic sites; and to estimate hepatic reserve after the tumor is removed or destroyed. Systemic therapy might be the most appropriate option for patients with more aggressive tumor biology or extrahepatic disease. RFA may be an alternative to resection for patients whose postoperative hepatic reserve would be compromised, especially those patients who have hepatotoxicity from prolonged exposure to systemic chemotherapy.

Proper preoperative assessment of hepatic functional reserve usually includes clinical assessment, liver biochemistry, coagulation profile, platelet count, and Child-Pugh classification. The indocyanine green clearance test can be used in patients with chronic liver disease. In addition, computed tomographic scan, volumetry, and laparoscopy are helpful in evaluation of whether the remnant liver is adequate. Adequate volume is usually described as a remnant of at least 25% to 50% depending on the health of the liver. Preoperative techniques to increase liver volume include portal vein embolization (PVE) to induce hypertrophy of the remnant liver. PVE can increase hepatic reserve by 10% to 15% within 6 weeks of treatment.

TECHNICAL CONSIDERATIONS

Unlike cryosurgery, which destroys tumors by freezing, RFA relies on thermal destruction. Heat is generated by radiofrequency energy delivered through a needle electrode (14 to 17.5 G) that is inserted into the tumor. Dispersive electrodes (adhesive grounding pads) are placed on the back or legs. Radiofrequency energy changes the direction of ions around an alternating electrode charge, resulting in high frictional energy, heat conduction, and thermal destruction. Tissue temperatures above 45°C cause apoptosis, and tissue temperatures above 90°C create an irreversible zone of coagulation necrosis.

Radiofrequency Ablation Devices

There are three major U.S. Food and Drug Administration (FDA)–approved devices for RFA (Figure 1). The RITA (AngioDynamics,

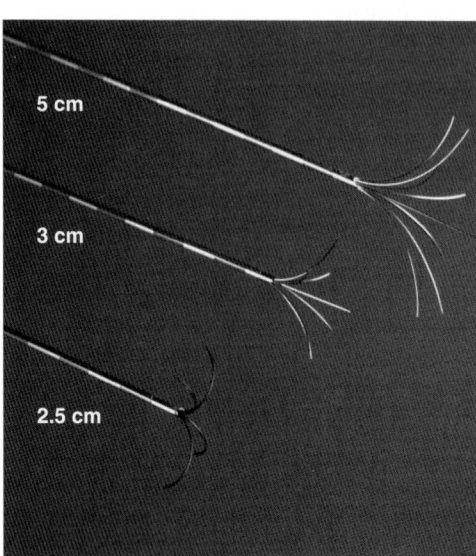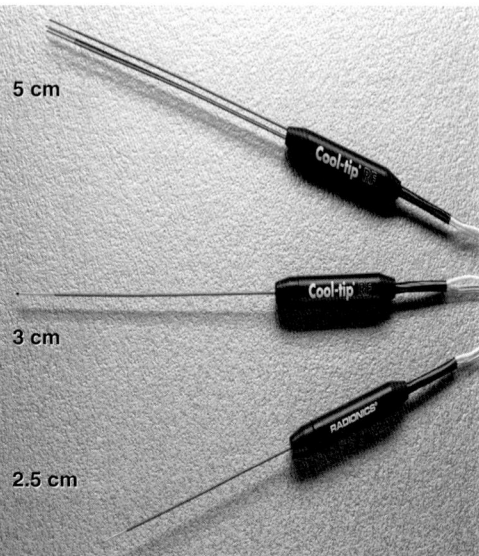

FIGURE I RITA *(left; AngioDynamics, Latham, NY)* and Cool-Tip *(right)*; Radionics, Burlington, MA probes used for radiofrequency ablation. *(Bilchik AJ, Krasny RM, Allegra D: Radiofrequency ablation for liver tumors. In Jarnagin WR, Belghiti J, Buchler MW, et al, editors: Blumgart's surgery of the liver, pancreas and biliary tract, vol 2, ed 5, Philadelphia, 2012, Saunders, p 1400, Fig. 85C.2.)*

Latham, NY) and Radiotherapeutics (Boston Scientific, Natick, Mass) use multiarray electrodes. The RITA has a single electrode through which multiple tines are deployed. The tines are deployed to varying depths, resulting in circumferential ablation. The tines have thermoprobes that measure temperatures in the ablation zone and maintain a steady temperature during ablation. The RITA system also uses saline solution to reduce impedance and can ablate tumors of up to 7 cm in diameter. The Radiotherapeutics system does not measure temperatures and instead adjusts ablation based on tissue impedance. This system has an ablation diameter of 4 cm. The third system, developed by Covidien (Mansfield, Mass), has a single-pronged or three-pronged electrode that is perfused with cold saline solution and has intermittent pulses that measure impedance and temperature. This system can produce ablation zones that reach 5 cm in diameter.

Radiofrequency Ablation Approaches

Radiofrequency ablation can be performed through percutaneous, laparoscopic, or open approaches. Each approach requires intraoperative imaging to monitor the ablation field during RFA.

Open or Laparoscopic Radiofrequency Ablation

The laparoscopic approach requires two ports in the right upper quadrant; the open approach requires a Chevron or midline incision, depending on previous scars (Figure 2). Both approaches allow visual inspection of the abdominal cavity, which is important because approximately 10% to 20% of patients have undiagnosed extrahepatic disease. If a laparoscopic approach is used, a 30-degree angled laparoscope is inserted to explore the abdomen; if an open approach is used, all parietal and visceral peritoneal surfaces, the lesser sac, omentum, and viscera should be manually palpated. Limited takedown of adhesions is indicated, and the liver should be mobilized with takedown of falciform and triangular ligaments. Adjacent viscera should be protected, and vital structures should be retracted to a distance of 2 cm from the ablation field. Finally, the porta hepatis should be evaluated; if necessary, portal nodes should be biopsied.

Open and laparoscopic approaches rely on ultrasound scan imaging to detect any undiagnosed hepatic disease because preoperative imaging can miss up to 30% of lesions. The liver should be examined with a flexible 7.5-MHz intraoperative ultrasound probe (Figure 3). Ultrasound scan also can identify the location of tumor with respect to major vascular pedicles and bile ducts. If a tumor is too close to large vessels, ablation is not complete because rapid blood flow produces a cooling or "heat sink" effect. Proximity to a central bile duct should be carefully evaluated because of the risk of ablation injury and the potential for fistula and stricture formation. If a tumor is too close to the gallbladder, cholecystectomy should be performed because of the risk of gallbladder perforation.

The RFA electrode is inserted with ultrasound guidance (Figure 4). The electrode should be placed parallel to and within the plane of the ultrasound probe, so that the electrode's tract can be visualized in its entirety. Many electrodes now are multiarray; additional electrodes deploy after placement of the main device into the tumor. During RFA, real-time ultrasonic monitoring shows hyperechogenicity within treated tissue, reflecting the formation of gas bubbles. However, ultrasound scan cannot reliably distinguish between ablated and normal tissue. For this reason, the ablation should start with the most posterior portion of the tumor and then the probe should be systematically withdrawn in 2-cm increments to create sequential overlapping zones of ablation that destroy the tumor and produce a surrounding 1-cm rim. If target temperatures are not reached, then tines can often be withdrawn slightly or rotated to increase the temperature in the region of ablation. Temporary vascular inflow occlusion (Pringle's maneuver) should be considered during laparoscopic or open RFA because it interrupts portal venous

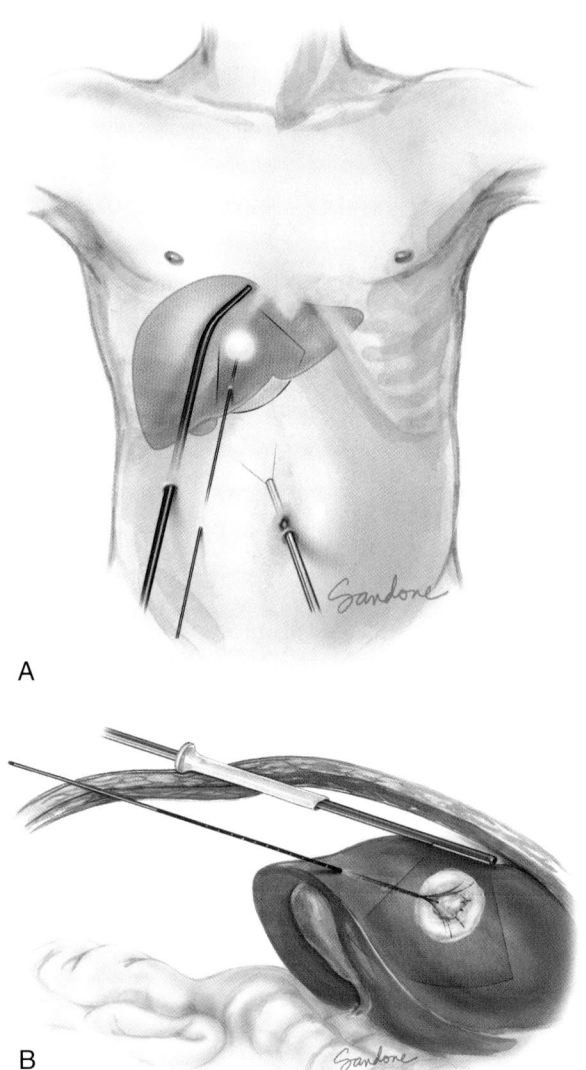

A

B

FIGURE 2 Laparoscopic approach in operative radiofrequency ablation (RFA) with intraoperative ultrasound scan guidance. **A,** Placement of ports. **B,** Intraoperative ultrasound scan and RFA probes. *(From Cameron JL, Sandone C: Atlas of gastrointestinal surgery, vol 1, ed 2, Hamilton, Ontario, 2008, BC Decker, p 182.)*

flow and decreases the heat sink during ablation, thereby increasing the ablation zone. After ablation, the probe track should be cauterized to minimize bleeding. The laparoscopic approach is associated with a shorter hospital stay, smaller incision, and less postoperative pain than the open approach. Both approaches require general anesthesia.

Percutaneous Radiofrequency Ablation

Percutaneous ablations are normally performed by interventional radiologists with ultrasound or CT scan guidance. Percutaneous ablation can be performed with a combination of minimal sedation and local anesthetic (Figure 5). CT scan guidance allows precise placement of the electrode and immediate assessment of the adequacy of ablation. On the other hand, the percutaneous approach does not allow visualization of the entire abdominal cavity or intraoperative ultrasound to identify additional lesions. Also, some hepatic lesions cannot be treated percutaneously. For example, ablation of tumors in the dome of the liver can damage the diaphragm, and ablation of peripheral liver lesions risks thermal injury to small bowel, stomach, or transverse colon. Finally, the percutaneous approach does not allow retraction to protect vital structures. Air, saline solution, or a balloon catheter can be introduced to separate vulnerable structures from the liver to avoid injury, but this can be technically difficult.

COMPLICATIONS

Radiofrequency ablation is relatively safe, with a low mortality rate (0 to 2%). Common complications are thermal, mechanical, septic, or anesthetic. Thermal complications include gastrointestinal perforation, biliary stenosis, and grounding pad burns. Mechanical complications encompass tumor seeding, pneumothorax, and bile duct or vessel injury resulting in hemorrhage or biliary leakage (Figure 6).

Septic complications are abscesses and wound infection. Finally, anesthetic complications include cardiac arrhythmias, myocardial infarction, and pneumonia. A common complication that occurs in 30% to 40% of patients is postablation syndrome, which likely reflects the release of cytokines from necrotic tissue. It is characterized by low-grade fever, malaise, chills, myalgia, delayed pain, nausea, and vomiting. This diagnosis is one of exclusion and should not be made until sinister complications have been ruled out.

MONITORING AND FOLLOW-UP

Laboratory Follow-up

Because elevated levels of carcinoembryonic antigen (CEA) are associated with local tumor recurrence, CEA levels should be monitored every 3 months after surgery. Although the absolute CEA value may be inconsequential, a rise in CEA level is concerning for recurrence.

Computed Tomographic Scan/Magnetic Resonance Imaging/Positron Emission Tomography

Ablation adequacy is assessed with CT scan or MRI. These scans are most informative with arterial and venous phases, with and without

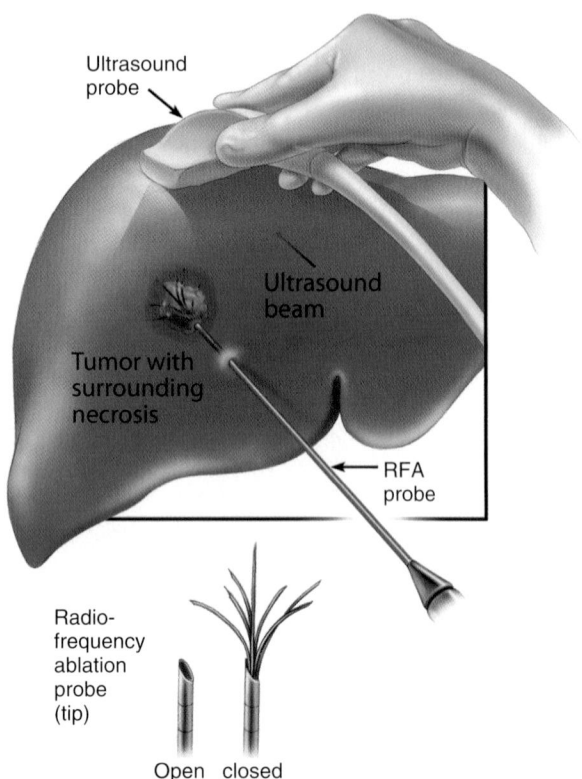

FIGURE 3 Radiofrequency ablation (RFA) during open laparotomy with intraoperative ultrasound scan guidance. (From Johns Hopkins Gastroenterology and Hepatology: Hepatocellular carcinoma (liver cancer): therapy. www.hopkins-gi.org. Accessed June 15, 2010.)

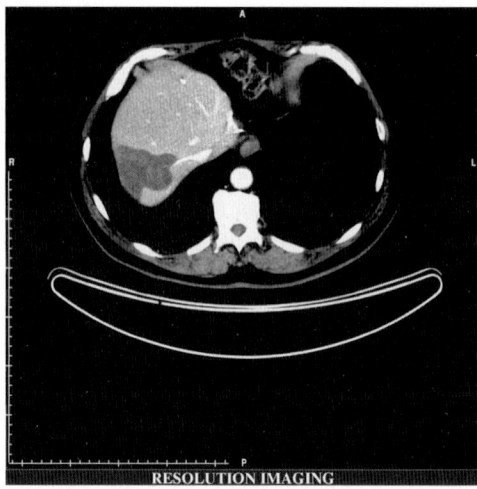

FIGURE 5 Percutaneous ablation performed adjacent to the diaphragm. (Bilchik AJ, Krasny RM, Allegra D: Radiofrequency ablation for liver tumors. In Jarnagin WR, Belghiti J, Buchler MW, et al, editors: Blumgart's surgery of the liver, pancreas and biliary tract, vol 2, ed 5, Philadelphia, 2012, Saunders, p 1401, Fig. 85C.5.)

FIGURE 4 Ultrasound scan–guided radiofrequency ablation. (Bilchik AJ, Krasny RM, Allegra D: Radiofrequency ablation for liver tumors. In Jarnagin WR, Belghiti J, Buchler MW, et al, editors: Blumgart's surgery of the liver, pancreas and biliary tract, vol 2, ed 5, Philadelphia, 2012, Saunders, p 1400, Fig. 85C.3.)

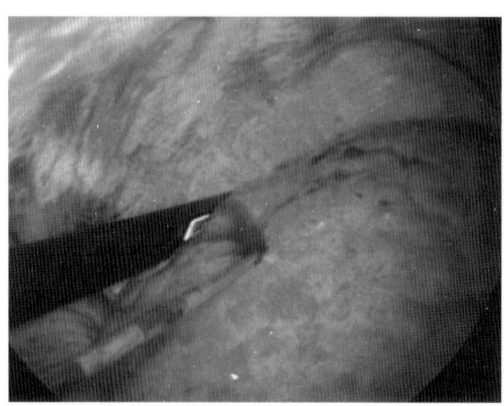

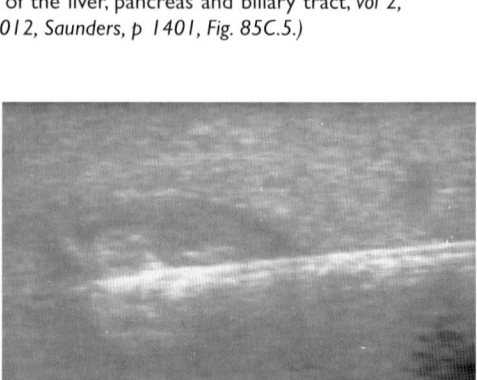

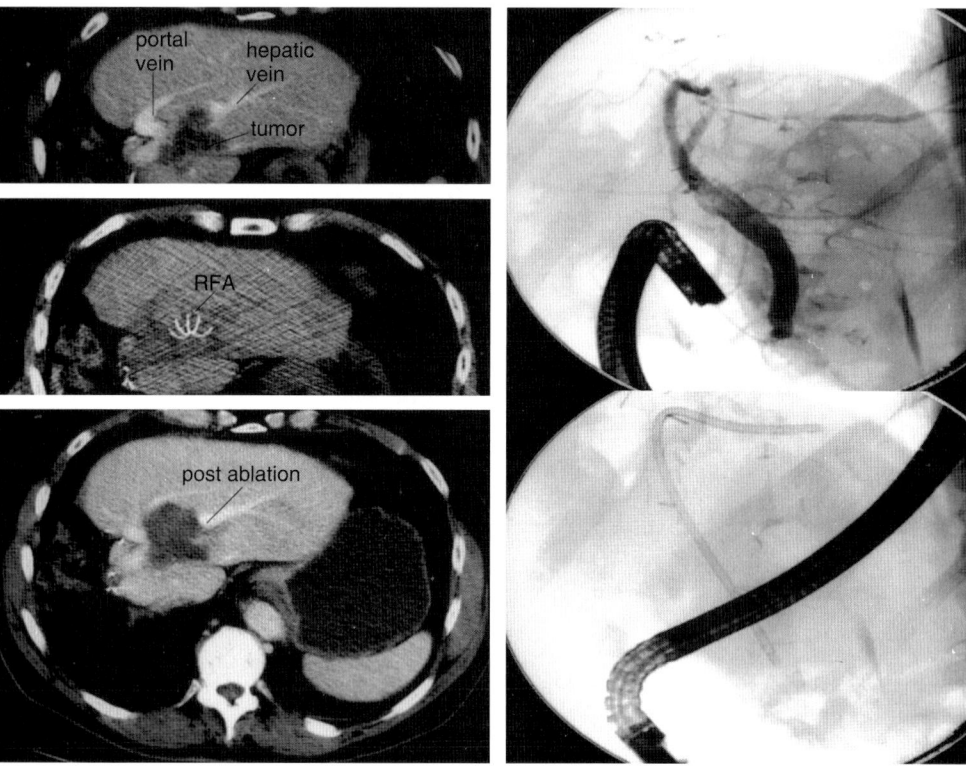

FIGURE 6 Biliary injury after radiofrequency ablation *(RFA)* treated with stent placement. *(Bilchik AJ, Krasny RM, Allegra D: Radiofrequency ablation for liver tumors. In Jarnagin WR, Belghiti J, Buchler MW, et al, editors: Blumgart's surgery of the liver, pancreas and biliary tract, vol 2, ed 5, Philadelphia, 2012, Saunders, p 1407, Fig. 85C.9.)*

intravenous contrast material. CT scans with intravenous (IV) contrast are obtained at 1 week (baseline), and then at 3-month intervals during the first year and 6-month intervals thereafter. The baseline image should reveal a hypovascular ablated field with a rim of hypervascular inflammatory tissue. Over the first several months, rim enhancement should disappear as inflammation resolves. Visible residual tumor within or immediately adjacent to the ablation zone within 6 months after ablation is considered a local recurrence or treatment failure. Recurrences usually appear as irregular nonenhancing areas on contrast CT scan. Serial imaging is essential for early detection of recurrence. Ideally, all imaging should be performed at the same institution where the ablation was performed. PET/CT scan is controversial for routine postablation follow-up imaging; however, PET appears to have good sensitivity for early detection of tumor recurrence.

RESULTS AND RESPONSE RATES

The response to RFA depends on the number and size of hepatic tumors. Response rates are higher when tumors are less than 5 cm in diameter and less than 3 in number. As might be expected, the best outcome is associated with RFA of a solitary lesion that is distant from vessels or biliary structures and is less than 3 cm in size. Response rates also are better with the newer generation probes and with increased physician experience. Although there are no randomized controlled trials of different RFA approaches, published results of nonrandomized comparisons suggest that open RFA results in the fewest local recurrences, followed by laparoscopic RFA and percutaneous RFA.

Radiofrequency Ablation Versus Surgical Resection or Systemic Therapy

Median postoperative survival time for patients with resectable colorectal liver metastases is 40 months, with a 10-year survival rate

of 20%. Median overall survival time after RFA ranges from 28 to 39 months, with a 5-year survival rate of 17% to 25%. However, published survival endpoints after RFA are difficult to assess because of variations in tumor size, missing data, and multiple treatment options before and after RFA. Comparison of RFA and surgical resection is difficult because candidates for surgical resection usually have a better health status, fewer comorbidities, less liver involvement, and more liver reserve. Even when comparisons of RFA and surgical resection are limited to patients with resectable disease, results are equivocal; some studies show comparable outcomes, whereas other studies show a survival advantage for surgical resection. Unfortunately, many of these studies preceded recent improvements in chemotherapy and catheter technology, and all of these studies were subject to the selection bias inherent in nonrandomized comparisons. Results from these studies are summarized in Table 1.

The first randomized trial to examine the efficacy of RFA was published in 2012. This phase II study randomly assigned patients with nonresectable colorectal liver metastases to systemic treatment alone or to systemic treatment plus RFA. Progression-free survival rate at 3 years was 27.6% for combined treatment versus 10.6% for systemic treatment only ($P = 0.025$). Median progression-free survival rate was 16.8 months (95% confidence interval [CI], 11.7 to 22.1) for combined treatment versus 9.9 months (95% CI, 9.3 to 13.7) for systemic treatment only. Although progression-free survival was significantly longer in the group treated with chemotherapy plus RFA, no difference was seen in overall survival for the two groups (median of 45.3 months for combined treatment vs 40.5 months for systemic treatment alone; $P = 0.22$).

NEWER TECHNOLOGIES

Microwave Ablation

During microwave ablation, electromagnetic waves at microwave frequencies are transmitted along a coaxial cable and through the tip

TABLE 1: Survival after radiofrequency ablation for colorectal liver metastasis

Article	Approach	No. of patients	Follow-up median (mo)	Median survival rate (%)			Overall median survival (mo)	Median disease-free survival (mo)
				1 y	3 y	5 y		
Solbiati L, *Radiology* (2001)	Percutaneous	117	6-52	93	69	46	36	12
Ianitti DA, *Arch Surg* (2002)	Percutaneous	52	20	87	50	–	–	–
Abdalla EK, *Ann Surg* (2004)	Open	57	21	–	37	22 (4 y)	–	–
Gillams AR, *Eur Radiol* (2004)	Percutaneous	167	17	91	40	17	32	
Jakobs TF, *Anticancer Res* (2006)	Percutaneous	68	21.4 (mean)	96	68	–	–	–
Siperstein AE, *Ann Surg* (2007)	Laparoscopic	234	24	–	20.2	18.4	24	–
Berber E, J *Gastrointest Surg* (2008)	Laparoscopic	68	23	–	–	30	24-34	9
Gleisner AL, *Surgery* (2008)	Open	55	–	–	72.7	–	–	3 y, 7.4%
Veltri A, *Cardiovasc Intervent Radiol* (2008)	Percutaneous open	122	24 (mean)	–	–	22		
Reuter NP, J *Gastrointest Surg* (2009)	Open	66	32 (mean)	–	–	21	27	12.2
Vyslouzil K, *Zentr Chir* (2009)	Open	31	–	87	26	–	–	–
Van Tilborg A, *Br J Radiol* (2011)	Open	100	29	93	77	36	56	–
Hamill CW, *Ann Surg Oncol* (2011)	Laparoscopic	64 (resectable) 37 (unresectable)	31.2	91.7 81.1	59 39.8	48.7 18.4	51 26	15 16.4

Bilchik AJ, Krasny RM, Allegra D: Radiofrequency ablation for liver tumors. In Jarnagin WR, Belghiti J, Buchler MW, et al, editors: Blumgart's surgery of the liver, pancreas and biliary tract, vol 2, ed 5, Philadelphia, 2012, Saunders.

of an electrode placed in the liver. Microwaves penetrate further into liver tissue than radiofrequency waves, and this ablative technique appears to overcome many of the problems that plague RFA. As compared with RFA, microwave ablation requires less time to achieve tumoricidal temperatures, decreases the heat-sink effect, and allows wider penetration and margins. It also does not require grounding pads or cooling systems, making it simpler to use. A recent study involving 14 Italian centers examined results of microwave ablation in 736 patients with 1037 lesions that included 187 colorectal metastases. The 2.9% major complication rate and 7.3% minor complication rate were equivalent to complication rates for RFA, which suggests that the two ablation techniques are equivalent with respect to safety. As more long-term data accumulate regarding the efficacy of microwave ablation, this modality may replace RFA as a faster and more effective means of destroying liver metastases.

High-Intensity Focused Ultrasound Scan

High-intensity focused ultrasound scan relies on the same principles as conventional ultrasound scan. It propagates harmlessly through living tissue, but if the ultrasound carries sufficient energy and is brought into a tight focus, the energy elevates local temperature and thereby causes necrosis of tumor without damage to the overlying tissue. Currently, little data are available on the safety or efficacy of this treatment.

Computer-Assisted Soft-Tissue Surgery

Computer-assisted soft-tissue surgery, which is performed with the CAS-One system (CAScination AG, Bern, Switzerland), is described by the manufacturer as the GPS for liver surgery. It involves a three-dimensional ultrasound technology planning model that allows interactive navigation of the liver and aligns image data with the patient. This new technology allows for greater precision, efficiency, and safety during placement of the RFA electrode in the tumor and can be used in conjunction with all ablation systems. The Cas-One is currently approved for use in Europe but not in the United States.

CONCLUSION

Ablation was initially used for local control of unresectable metastatic liver lesions, but advances in technology have given it curative

potential, particularly when combined with neoadjuvant or adjuvant administration of systemic agents. RFA has been used to destroy hepatic metastases during resection of primary colorectal cancer, and it also has been combined with liver resection to maximize residual liver volume and hepatic reserve and to treat recurrences.

Although hepatic resection is currently the gold standard for resectable liver tumors, some retrospective studies suggest that RFA can confer similar disease-free survival in carefully selected patients who have small tumors. Currently, the only randomized controlled trial assigned unresectable tumors to chemotherapy plus local ablation versus chemotherapy alone. It was sponsored by the European Organization for Research and Treatment of Cancer and was ultimately closed because of nonaccrual. Certainly, the time for a randomized study for resectable tumors is fast approaching.

Radiofrequency ablation can be a powerful tool, but certainly any treatment of colorectal metastasis to the liver should involve a multidisciplinary team to determine the best therapeutic options. This decision should be based on the institution's expertise, the tumor's location, and the patient's characteristics and comorbidities. In each case, the goal is individualized treatment that optimizes outcome.

SUGGESTED READINGS

Amersi F, McElrath-Garza A, Ahmad A, et al: Long-term survival after radiofrequency ablation of complex unresectable liver tumors, *Arch Surg* 141:581–587, 2006.
Bilchik AJ, Krasny RM, Allegra D: Radiofrequency ablation for liver tumors. In Jarnagin WR, Belghiti J, Buchler MW, et al, editors: *Blumgart's surgery of the liver, pancreas and biliary tract*, vol 2, ed 5, Philadelphia, 2012, Saunders.
Mulier S, Yicheng N, Jamart J, et al: Radiofrequency ablation versus resection for resectable colorectal liver metastases: time for a randomized trial? *Ann Oncol* 15(1):144–157, 2008.
Ruers T, Punt C, VanCoevorden F, et al: Radiofrequency ablation combined with systemic treatment versus systemic treatment alone in patients with non-resectable colorectal liver metastases: a randomized EORTC Intergroup phase II study (EORTC 40004), *Ann Oncol* 23(10):2619–2626, 2012.
Wong SL, Mangu PB, Choti MA, et al: American Society of Clinical Oncology 2009 clinical evidence review on radiofrequency ablation of hepatic metastases from colorectal cancer, *J Clin Oncol* 28(3):493–508, 2010.

THE MANAGEMENT OF HEPATIC ABSCESS

Fady Michael Kaldas, MD, and
Johnny C. Hong, MD, FACS

OVERVIEW

Hepatic abscesses are an uncommon disease with an annual incidence rate of approximately 3.6 per 100,000 in the United States. Although hepatic abscesses account for only 8 to 20 cases of every

100,000 hospital admissions, liver abscesses are uniformly fatal if untreated and require prompt recognition and treatment. Hepatic abscesses can be divided into three major categories: pyogenic, amebic, and fungal. Pyogenic abscesses represent the majority of liver abscesses in developed countries and tend to contain polymicrobial aerobic and anaerobic bacteria. Recently, liver abscesses secondary to hepatic tissue and tumor necrosis from ablative therapies for liver tumors have increasingly been seen because of the widespread utilization of these interventions. Amebic abscesses are the result of *Entamoeba histolytica,* which has a high endemic prevalence in Mexico, the Indian subcontinent, Indonesia, and tropical Africa. Most patients with amebic liver abscesses in the United States have a history of recent travel to an endemic area. Fungal abscesses are less common and are typically caused by *Candida* species. Fungal liver abscesses are being recognized with increasing frequency in patients with immunocompromise and those with malignant diseases.

The treatment of liver abscesses has evolved over the past decades from operative drainage as the only treatment modality to a multi-specialty approach with nonoperative or operative interventions that have significantly improved the care of patients. Although both interventional radiologists and biliary endoscopists may play a major role in the first-line management of these cases, surgeons need to be knowledgeable and must play an active role in the diagnosis and management of patients with liver abscesses because surgical intervention remains the salvage procedure in many of these cases.

PYOGENIC HEPATIC ABSCESS

Pyogenic abscesses are a rare but often lethal disease. The etiologies of the liver abscesses are multifactorial and associated with different disease processes. During the first three decades of the 20th century, pylephlebitis, from appendicitis, was the most common cause, with an overall mortality rate that approached 75% to 80%. During the 1950s to 1970s, biliary obstruction from both benign and malignant diseases accounted for most of the cases. Recently, the emergence of orthotropic liver transplantation (OLT) as the definitive therapy for end-stage liver disease and a more aggressive approach in the surgical therapy of hepatobiliary malignancies have resulted in yet another shift with regard to the etiology of hepatic abscesses.

Pathophysiology

Pyogenic abscesses can develop from multiple potential sources: (1) the biliary ductal system most commonly from ascending cholangitis, (2) the portal blood flow, from pylephlebitis originating from appendicitis or diverticulitis, (3) direct extension from adjacent disease, such as severe cholecystitis, (4) injury from trauma or liver-directed therapy, (5) the hepatic artery, from septicemia originating from a distant source, and (6) a cryptogenic process. In one of the largest Western series at Johns Hopkins Hospital, 40% of pyogenic liver abscesses were biliary in origin, and an underlying malignant disease was the cause in the majority of these patients in the non-OLT setting.

In liver transplant recipients, additional risk factors for pyogenic abscess include: (1) hepatic infarction from vascular thrombosis or anastomotic stenosis, (2) ischemic cholangiopathy (nonanastomotic biliary stricture) as a consequence of hepatic arterial compromise or the use of deceased-donor liver organs procured after circulatory death (donation after circulatory death [DCD]; Figures 1 and 2), and (3) biliary anastomotic stricture. The utilization of partial liver grafts (from live and deceased donors) carries an increased risk of biliary leak from the cut surface of the liver that may result in perihepatic

pyogenic abscess. Although the infectious organisms and initial diagnostic and treatment algorithms are similar to non–OLT-related causes, the definitive treatment is based on patency of the hepatic vessels, viability of the bile ducts, and function of the hepatic allograft. In severe cases, retransplantation of the liver is the only life-saving modality.

The types of bacteria isolated from the blood and the bile in patients with pyogenic hepatic abscesses vary with the underlying pathologic process (Table 1). *Escherichia coli, Klebsiella* spp., and *Enterococcus* are commonly isolated in cases related to choledocholithiasis, whereas *Pseudomonas* spp., other multiple resistant gram-negative aerobes, vancomycin-resistant *Enterococcus* (VRE), and yeast are the more likely pathogens in patients with biliary obstruction from unresectable biliary malignancy who received multiple courses of antibiotics. Although cases with liver abscesses from diverticulitis and appendicitis are attributed to gram-negative aerobes and *Bacteroides fragilis*, patients with severe forms of cholecystitis are likely to harbor anaerobes such as *Clostridium perfringens* and

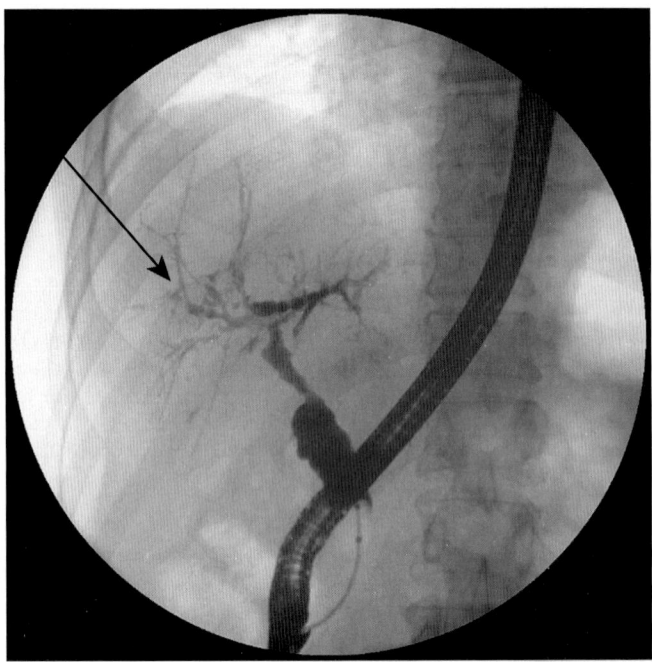

FIGURE I   An endoscopic retrograde cholangiopancreaticography showing intrahepatic ischemic cholangiopathy after orthotropic liver transplantation with a graft procured after circulatory death.

FIGURE 2   **A,** Endoscopic retrograde cholangiopancreaticography. **B,** Computed tomographic scan showing intrahepatic ischemic cholangiopathy progression to biloma and abscess formation.

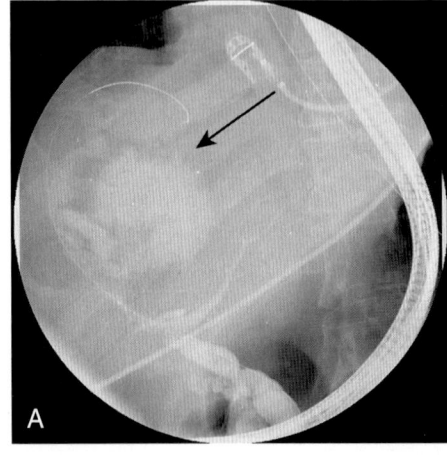

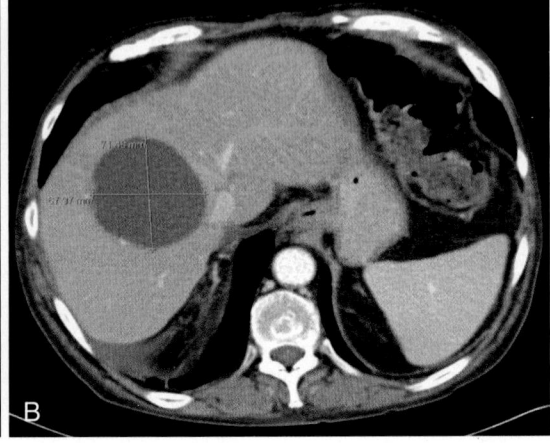

TABLE 1: Underlying etiology and bacteriology

Etiology	Bacteriology
Biliary, benign	*Escherichia coli* *Klebsiella* spp. *Enterococcus*
Biliary, malignant	*Pseudomonas* spp. Multiply resistant GN aerobes VRE Yeast
Diverticulitis/appendicitis	GN aerobes *Bacteroides fragilis*
Severe cholecystitis	See Biliary, benign *Clostridium perfringens* *Bacteroides* spp.
Subcutaneous abscess	*Staphylococcus* spp. MRSA
Endocarditis	*Enterococcus* spp. *Staphylococcus* spp.
Cryptogenic	Anaerobes

GN, Gram-negative; *MRSA,* methicillin-resistant *Staphylococcus aureus;*
VRE, vancomycin-resistant *Enterococcus.*

Bacteroides spp. Other pathogens frequently associated with specific conditions are *Staphylococcus* and methicillin-resistant *Staphylococcus aureus* (MRSA) from subcutaneous abscess, enterococcal and staphylococcal pathogens from endocarditis, and anaerobes in cryptogenic abscesses.

Diagnosis

The classic initial symptom of a pyogenic hepatic abscess is fever, which occurs in more than 90% of patients. Approximately one half of those with an abscess have abdominal or right upper quadrant pain. Other frequent symptoms include malaise, anorexia, and nausea. Occasionally, the diaphragm is involved, resulting in pleuritic chest pain, cough, or dyspnea. The mode of presentation may also include severe sepsis in patients with an underlying biliary malignancy and after liver-directed therapy or hepatic transplantation. On physical examination, the liver may be tender and enlarged, or the patient may appear jaundiced. Pyogenic liver abscesses rarely rupture, and frank peritonitis is unusual.

Over the past 40 years, advances in imaging have dramatically improved the diagnosis of pyogenic hepatic abscesses. Plain films may show an elevated right hemidiaphragm, right pleural effusion, right lower lobe atelectasis, abnormal extraluminal gas in the right upper quadrant, or portal venous gas if pylephlebitis is the source. Ultrasound scan (US) is a useful initial screening study for hepatic abscess because it has a sensitivity of 80% to 95% and is excellent in evaluation of the gallbladder and intrahepatic bile ducts. A computed tomographic (CT) scan is more sensitive (95% to 100%) in the detection of abscesses, and the presence of gas and rim enhancement with intravenous contrast is very suggestive of a hepatic abscess. CT scan also allows for a more thorough evaluation of the abdomen for detection of the underlying cause. Magnetic resonance imaging (MRI) of the liver is an equally sensitive technique in detection of liver abscesses and, in combination with magnetic resonance cholangiopancreatography (MRCP), provides detailed information with regard to the relationship of the hepatic abscess to the biliary system.

Treatment

Pyogenic hepatic abscesses are associated with a significant mortality rate, and prompt diagnosis and treatment of hepatic abscesses is crucial for good outcomes. Management must include treatment of both the liver abscess and the underlying source. Most pyogenic hepatic abscesses are managed with antibiotic administration and drainage.

Antibiotics

When a pyogenic hepatic abscess is suspected, blood cultures are drawn and empiric, broad-spectrum intravenous antimicrobial therapy is initiated. The antibiotic coverage is subsequently modified based on results of bacteriologic studies. A fluid sample obtained from the abscess is equally important in tailoring an antimicrobial regimen. If drainage is not undertaken, aspiration of the liver abscess may be performed to determine the bacteriology. As outlined previously, the bacteria found usually correspond to the source (see Table 1). As such, the choice of the initial antibiotic agents should be based on the presumed source of the hepatic abscess. For example, for a presumed biliary source, gram-negative aerobe and enterococcal coverage might include broad-spectrum single agents such as piperacillin-tazobactam, ticarcillin-clavulanate, or meropenem. However, if the patient has had multiple episodes of cholangitis and has indwelling stents, double coverage for pseudomonal species, and an agent such as linezolid for VRE, might be an appropriate start. For a presumed colonic source, the combination of fluoroquinolone or a third-generation cephalosporin with metronidazole provides appropriate coverage. For severe cholecystitis, a broad-spectrum penicillin should be included to cover *Clostridia,* and the addition of metronidazole for *Bacteroides* is a reasonable starting combination. If a subcutaneous abscess or endocarditis is the presumed source, inclusion of vancomycin for MRSA is appropriate.

Once the actual bacteria are isolated and sensitivities are determined, the antibiotic regimen should be adjusted to more specific, less broad, and less costly agents. Parenteral administration of antibiotics should be continued for 10 to 14 days. Classically, antibiotic treatment has been recommended for 4 to 6 weeks; however, shorter antibiotic duration may be appropriate if adequate drainage has been achieved. Even when prolonged antibiotics are indicated for multiple small abscesses with no abdominal source, oral antibiotics may be substituted for home intravenous antibiotics.

Drainage

Intravenous antibiotics have decreased the mortality rate of patients with pyogenic hepatic abscesses; however, most patients also need abscess drainage, either with percutaneous catheter placement, closed aspiration, or surgery. The surgical therapy of liver abscess has evolved to a multispecialty approach with rapid developments in minimally invasive surgery and ablative therapies, and advances in image-guided interventions.

Once the pyogenic abscess has been confirmed with CT scan and no intra-abdominal source necessitates operative intervention, the initial management should include systemic antibiotics and percutaneous drainage. At Johns Hopkins Hospital from 1973 to 1993, 45% of patients were treated with a percutaneous drain; many of these cases, especially later in the series, involved multiloculated abscesses. Rajak and colleagues (1998) compared catheter placement with percutaneous aspiration and found that the success rate was superior with catheter placement (60% vs 100%). Percutaneous catheter placement involves the insertion of an 8F to 14F pigtail catheter over a guidewire with imaging guidance. The abscess cavity is then studied with the injection of contrast through the catheter. Finally, the catheter is left to gravity or suction, until complete resolution of the drainage and collapse of the abscess cavity have occurred (Figure 3). Percutaneous drainage is not appropriate for patients with multiple large abscesses, a known intra-abdominal source that requires surgery, or ascites or in whom transpleural drainage is required.

Percutaneous needle aspiration involves imaging-guided drainage of the abscess without placement of the catheter. The benefits of needle aspiration are decreased cost, less invasiveness, and avoidance of drain discomfort. Yu and colleagues (2004) compared the outcomes after aspiration and drainage of liver abscesses and showed equivalent results between the two treatment modalities. Although aspiration resulted in less liver trauma, patient discomfort, and cost, this approach was associated with a higher recurrence rate requiring repeated aspiration procedures compared with catheter drainage.

Although patients with small hepatic abscesses and no biliary obstruction respond to prolonged intravenous antibiotics without drainage, a select group of patients requires surgical intervention.

When an intra-abdominal source for the infection requires an operation, the liver abscess can be drained surgically in concert with management of the primary problem (Figure 4). Surgical treatment is also required in cases of failed nonoperative therapies and remains the salvage procedure.

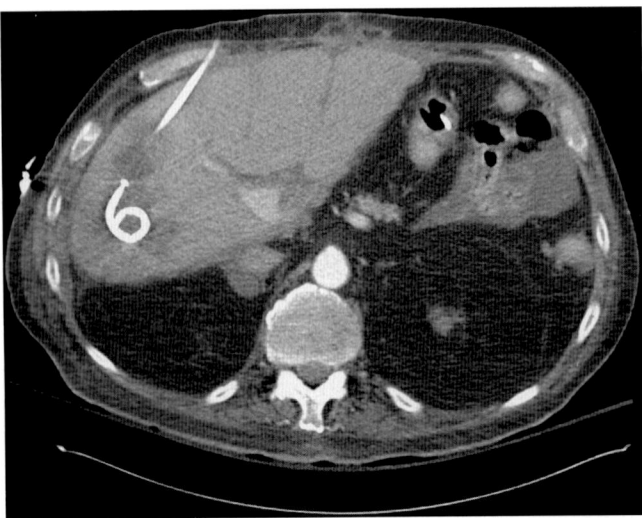

FIGURE 3 Radiograph showing percutaneous drainage of pyogenic abscess.

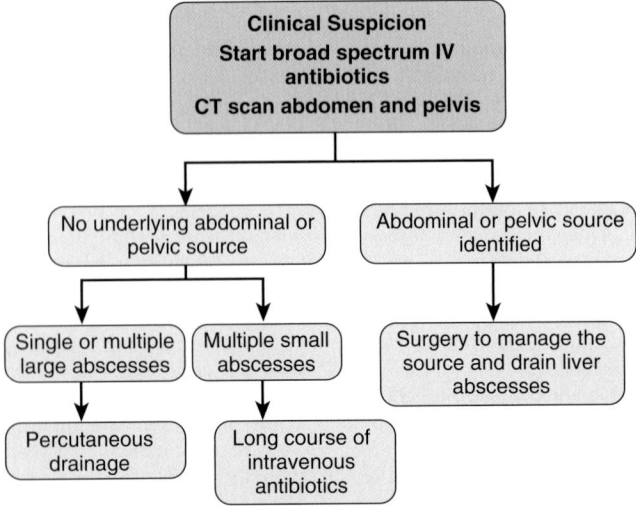

FIGURE 4 Algorithm for management of pyogenic hepatic abscesses. *CT*, Computed tomographic scan; *IV*, intravenous.

Before the availability of systemic antibiotics, an extraperitoneal approach for surgical drainage was performed to avoid contamination of the peritoneum. The availability of modern antibiotics and the current technique of a transperitoneal approach via a midline or right subcostal incision provides direct access to the liver abscess, abdomen, and pelvis. After the underlying pathology in the abdomen is addressed, the liver is evaluated and the hepatic abscess is located with palpation and intraoperative US. The area to be drained is then isolated from the rest of the abdomen with towels, and aspiration of the abscess is performed to obtain fluid for culture (Figure 5). A tract is then created through the hepatic parenchyma toward the cavity, ideally to drain the abscess in a dependent fashion. Next, the cavity is irrigated and suctioned to remove purulence and minimize contamination. The tract should then be enlarged and the abscess débrided to break up any loculated pockets of purulence. A large-caliber drain is placed in the abscess cavity, and the perihepatic area around the abscess may also be drained; however, these drains are brought out through separate incisions. All hepatic abscesses should be biopsied to rule out a tumor and to evaluate for trophozoites of *E. histolytica*.

Although drainage of a liver abscess in combination with systemic antibiotic is successful in most cases, hepatic resection is necessary in unusual circumstances. In patients in whom an inflammatory mass develops as a result of multiple percutaneous drainage procedures or chronic biliary obstruction from multiple biliary drainage procedures that involve one hemiliver, a hemihepatectomy is necessary to remove the diseased portion of the liver. However, these patients are prone to profound sepsis with liver manipulation; therefore, partial hepatectomy should be undertaken cautiously (Box 1).

AMEBIC HEPATIC ABSCESS

Amebiasis is a relatively common global parasitic infection caused by the protozoan *E. histolytica,* with the highest incidence in tropical and subtropical climates. Amebiasis typically affects men between the ages of 20 and 40 years. Although uncommon in the United States, amebic abscesses should be included in the differential diagnosis in patients with a history of travel to or immigration from endemic areas of the world and in the presence of human immunodeficiency virus (HIV).

The liver is the most common extraintestinal location of amebiasis, and amebic liver abscesses occur in 1% of patients with amebiasis. Human infestation occurs with the ingestion of a mature cyst in fecal contaminated food, water, or hands. Excystation occurs in the small intestine, and trophozoites are released and migrate to the large intestine. The trophozoites multiply by binary fission and produce cysts, which are passed in the feces. In many cases, the trophozoites remain confined to the intestinal lumen (noninvasive infection) of individuals who are asymptomatic carriers, passing cysts in their stool. In some patients, the trophozoites invade through the intestinal mucosa (intestinal disease), through the bloodstream, or via extraintestinal sites such as the liver, brain, and lungs (extraintestinal disease), where it forms into an abscess. The most common complication of amebic abscesses is rupture into the surrounding organs, such as direct extension into the pleuropulmonary space or rupture into the pericardium or peritoneum. The diagnosis and management of pyogenic and amebic abscesses differs, and these differences are reviewed.

Diagnosis

The presentation of amebic abscesses may be acute with fever and right upper quadrant pain or less specific with weight loss, fever, and abdominal pain. An amebic liver abscess usually does not present at the same time as colitis but within a year after the initial infection. Unlike a pyogenic abscess, the patient is not jaundiced and does not

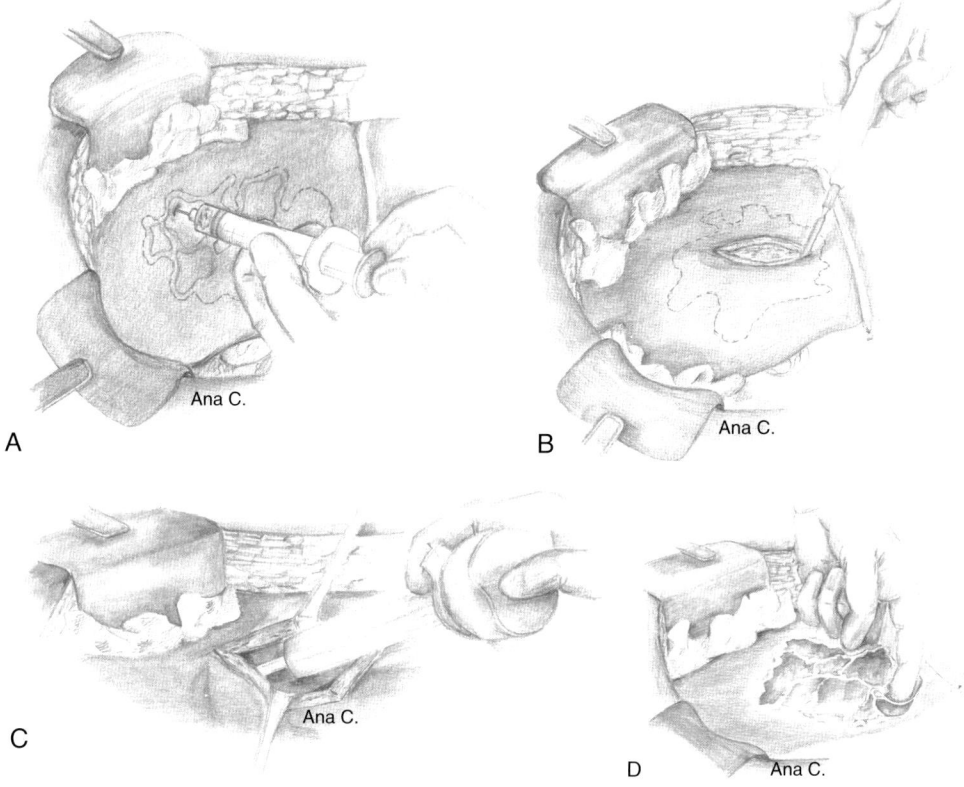

FIGURE 5 A, Abscess aspiration for aerobic and anaerobic culture. **B,** Incision of the liver capsule to drain the abscess. **C,** Irrigation of abscess cavity. **D,** Manual disruption of loculations. *(Illustrations by Ana Costache.)*

BOX 1: Pearls for pyogenic hepatic abscesses

- The most common organisms isolated from pyogenic liver abscess are gram negative; however, because of increased use of indwelling biliary stents, infection with other organisms, such as *Pseudomonas, Streptococcus,* and fungal species, has increased.
- Bacteriology and initial antibiotics should be tailored to the presumed underlying source.
- Aspiration of liver abscess should be undertaken in most patients, unless the abscess is small, because it provides rapid relief of symptoms and renders samples for culture.
- Percutaneous drainage is usually required, and open surgery should be reserved for selected patients.

---

have underlying biliary disease. Also, most patients are younger than 50 years and have a history of travel to an endemic location. The definitive diagnosis of an amebic liver abscess is by identification of *E. histolytica* trophozoites in the pus or serum antibodies to the ameba. The majority of amebic liver abscesses (75% to 80%) show up as a single focus in the right lobe.

Treatment

With the introduction of metronidazole decades ago, drainage procedures (surgical or percutaneous) are only necessary in circumstances in which a questionable diagnosis, bacterial coinfection, or complications from the amebic abscess exist.

Antibiotics

The mainstay for treatment of invasive amebiasis is metronidazole. Tinidazole and ornidazole are other nitroimidazole derivatives that are effective treatments; however, they are not currently available in the United States. Metronidazole is able to reach high concentrations in the liver. Current recommendations for metronidazole are 750 mg 3 times a day for 5 to 10 days. Caution should be taken in pregnant and breastfeeding mothers because metronidazole does cross the placenta and is secreted in breast milk. Ninety-five percent of patients respond after 10 days of therapy; however, 5% to 15% are resistant to metronidazole. Luminal antimicrobials, such as paromomycin and iodoquinol, should also be used to eradicate intestinal colonization because 10% of patients have relapse without luminal amebicidal agents.

A second-line luminal agent, diloxanide furoate, is available from the U.S. Centers for Disease Control for patients who clinically do not respond to paromomycin or iodoquinol. Follow-up stool examination is recommended after completion of therapy to ensure eradication of the infection.

Drainage

Blessmann and colleagues (2003) performed a prospective randomized trial to determine whether any significant benefit was obtained by adding aspiration to antibiotics for the treatment of amebic abscesses. In this study, aspiration did not improve the outcomes; therefore, image-guided percutaneous treatment is used only in the following circumstances: (1) if no clinical response is seen after 5 to 7 days of antibiotics, and (2) if an abscess, especially a large one, is at high risk for rupture. If the complication of rupture or extension does occur, percutaneous drainage is useful in treating pulmonary, peritoneal, and cardiac complications. Although surgical drainage is rarely required for this disease, surgical intervention is required in unusual situations such as hemorrhage, erosion into surrounding organs, or sepsis from a secondarily infected amebic abscess that has failed percutaneous treatment.

Outcomes

The vast majority of patients with amebic abscesses have defervescence and improvement after 3 days of therapy. However, if not treated in a timely fashion, this condition can be fatal, with mortality rates ranging as high as 15% to 20%. Several patient factors that are independent predictors of mortality include: (1) a bilirubin value greater than 3.5 mg/dL, (2) encephalopathy, (3) an abscess volume greater than 500 mL, (4) an albumin value less than 2 g/dL, and (5) multiple abscesses. In addition, patients with complications of the abscess, rupture, or direct extension as previously described have a worse outcome.

In conclusion, amebic abscesses have an excellent outcome with medical management, and drainage procedures are reserved for patients who do not respond to medical therapy. Patients have clinical improvement with amebicidal therapy more rapidly than radiologic resolution is observed. Complete radiologic resolution may take up to 9 months, and follow-up imaging is advised (Box 2).

FUNGAL HEPATIC ABSCESS

Bacteria and parasites constitute the majority of hepatic abscesses, but the incidence of fungal liver abscesses has been increasing. Most monomicrobial fungal abscesses are seen in patients with immune-compromise, such as with chemotherapy, with HIV infection, or after organ transplantation. Mixed bacterial and fungal abscesses typically occur in patients with biliary malignancies who have had long-term indwelling stents and have been frequently treated with antibiotics.

Treatment

Treatment of fungal abscesses follows the same principles as treatment for pyogenic hepatic abscesses, focusing on antimicrobial agents and drainage. Drainage is, again, with simple aspiration, percutaneous drainage, or surgical drainage. About 80% of fungal abscesses contain *Candida* spp.; the next most common fungal organisms are *Aspergillus* and *Cryptococcus*. Historically, amphotericin B was the first-line therapy, but micafungin and caspofungin are currently the agents of choice. An adequate course must be used; an earlier analysis suggested that inadequate treatment with amphotericin B was associated with a high mortality rate. Oral fluconazole may be used after initial intravenous therapy if *Candida albicans* is the cause. Patients with mixed fungal and bacterial abscesses also should receive appropriate antibiotics for the isolated bacteria.

BOX 2: Pearls for amebic liver abscesses

- Only 10% to 20% of patients with amebic liver abscess have a history of diarrhea.
- Treat the intestinal infection to prevent relapse of amebic liver abscess. Failure to use luminal amebicidal agents after metronidazole in cases of amebic abscess results in a 10% relapse rate.
- Failure to show response to antiamebic medication requires evaluation for polymicrobial infection with bacteria.
- Amebic abscess usually responds clinically to antimicrobial therapy in 3 to 7 days, although imaging takes several months to show resolution.
- Percutaneous drainage is rarely required.

Outcomes

Fungal abscesses of the liver are a significant source of mortality. The series from Johns Hopkins that analyzed fungal infections from 1973 to 1993 reported that all four patients with monomicrobial fungal abscesses with fungemia died. However, those patients who received a complete course of amphotericin B and did not have fungemia survived. In mixed fungal and bacterial abscesses, the overall mortality rate was 50%; however, adequate amphotericin B treatment resulted in a lower mortality rate (20% vs 62%). In conclusion, although fungal hepatic abscesses carry a high mortality rate, early administration of modern antifungal agents for the prevention of fungemia should improve survival.

SUGGESTED READINGS

Blessmann J, Binh HD, Hung DM, et al: Treatment of amebic liver abscess with metronidazole alone or in combination with ultrasound-guided needle aspiration: a comparative, prospective and randomized study, *Trop Med Int Health* 8:1030–1034, 2003.

Hong JC, Yersiz H, Petrowsky H, et al: Liver transplantation using organ donation after cardiac death: a clinical predictive index for graft failure-free survival, *Arch Surg* 146:1017–1023, 2011.

Huang CJ, Pitt HA, Lipsett PA, et al: Pyogenic liver abscess: changing trends over 42 years, *Ann Surg* 223:600–609, 1996.

Jay CL, Lyuksemburg V, Ladner DP, et al: Ischemic cholangiopathy after controlled donation after cardiac death liver transplantation: a meta-analysis, *Ann Surg* 253(2):259–264, 2011.

Lipsett PA, Huang CJ, Lillemoe KD, et al: Fungal hepatic abscess: characterization and management, *J Gastrointest Surg* 1:78–84, 1997.

Rajak C, Gupta S, Jain S, et al: Percutaneous treatment of liver abscess: needle aspiration versus catheter drainage, *Am J Roentgenol* 170:1035–1039, 1998.

Yu SC, Ho SS, Law WY, et al: Treatment of pyogenic liver abscess: prospective randomized comparison of catheter drainage and needle operation, *Hepatology* 39:932–938, 2004.

Transarterial Chemoembolization for Liver Metastases

Nikhil Bhagat, MD, and
Jean Francois H. Geschwind, MD

INTRODUCTION

According to the most recent epidemiologic data, the incidence of hepatocellular carcinoma (HCC) is rising worldwide. A number of therapeutic options exist for patients with liver cancer, whether primary or metastatic. The two definitive therapies are surgical resection and liver transplantation. However, surgical resection is often not possible because of multifocal tumors or poor hepatic reserve, and transplant recipients significantly outnumber donors. Transarterial chemoembolization (TACE) has been shown to improve survival in those patients with unresectable disease.

HISTORY

Yamada and associates first described the delivery of chemotherapy-soaked gel-foam pledgets within the hepatic arteries of those patients with HCC in the 1970s. The rationale for chemoembolization is as follows: normal liver tissue receives most of its blood supply (75% to 83%) from the portal vein, and liver tumors receive most of their blood supply (90% to 100%) from the hepatic artery.

Lipiodol, an iodine ester derived from poppy seed oil, began to be used in the 1980s as part of the chemoembolization cocktail. Lipiodol (or ethiodol) is taken up by the liver (normal hepatocytes and tumor cells), but it not metabolized by the tumors because of their lack of Kupffer's cells. As a result, lipiodol can be seen in tumors months after treatment and can be used to monitor treatment areas after TACE. In addition, lipiodol has been shown to have an embolic effect, which serves to decrease blood flow and retain chemotherapeutic agents in the tumor.

Although no data show increased efficacy of one chemotherapeutic agent over another, the most common cocktail used in the procedure is cisplatin, doxorubicin, and mitomycin. These agents have all been shown to have good liver extraction and low systemic drug concentrations when administered into the hepatic artery. In addition, the intratumoral concentration of chemotherapeutic drug is reported to be 10 times higher than if it was delivered through the hepatic artery as compared with the portal vein. The most common dosages of the medications are as follows: 50 mg doxorubicin (Adriamycin; Pharmacia-Upjohn, Kalamazoo, Mich), 100 mg cisplatin (Bristol Meyers Squibb, Princeton, NJ), and 10 mg of mitomycin C (Bedford Laboratories, Bedford, Ohio). This mixture is usually mixed in a 1:1 ratio with lipiodol.

Embolic agents are also usually used during the chemoembolization procedure, whether temporary agents (gel-foam slurry or pledgets) or more permanent agents (polyvinyl alcohol [PVA] or other particulates). The administration method for the embolic agent is not standard; some prefer to mix it with the chemotherapy, and others prefer to give the embolic agent at the end. Some data have suggested that postchemotherapy embolic agents help improve long-term arterial patency. Long-term arterial patency is necessary for repeated chemoembolization because its efficacy is related to the number of times it can be repeated.

As stated previously, the standard chemotherapy cocktail contains Adriamycin, cisplatin, and mitomycin. This cocktail is mixed with lipiodol (see previous mention for details) and administered through the microcatheter in a relatively superselective position. Although the lipiodol is embolic, further stasis is achieved after the administration of chemotherapy with another embolic agent; this agent is gel-foam slurry, PVA particles, or gelatin microspheres. The most commonly used agents include gel foam and PVA. The primary reason for the additional embolic agents is to help retain the chemotherapeutic agents within the tumor and to induce ischemic necrosis.

TECHNIQUE

A thorough preprocedure workup is necessary before chemoembolization. The diagnosis of HCC is made through either tissue diagnosis or imaging characteristics and elevated alpha-fetoprotein levels. A multiphasic cross-sectional imaging study, either magnetic resonance imaging (MRI) or computed tomographic (CT) scan, should be obtained to determine: (1) size of tumor; (2) extrahepatic tumor spread; (3) possible variant arterial anatomy supplying the tumor; (4) biliary ductal dilation; and (5) portal vein infiltration. Serum chemistry and hematology values also need to be ordered, including prothrombin time, international normalized ratio (INR), liver function tests, creatinine value, and alpha-fetoprotein level. Before the start of the procedure, intravenous fluids, prophylactic antibiotics (broad-spectrum to cover gram-negative and enteric), and antiemetics are administered.

Vascular access is typically obtained from one of the common femoral arteries in the groin. A vascular sheath is placed, and angiography of the superior mesenteric artery (SMA) is performed with delayed portal venous imaging. The purpose of visualization of this vessel is identification of any anomalous arterial supply to the liver parenchyma (originating from the SMA) and verification of the patency of the portal vein. Next, the celiac artery is catheterized and arteriography is performed to identify any anomalous vessels and primary supply to the tumor. Potentially dangerous locations for chemotherapy administration are identified on this angiogram (including left gastric artery, right gastric artery, cystic artery, and falciform artery). Many catheters can then be used for selective catheterization of the hepatic artery; usually, this is accomplished with a 5F reverse curve catheter, such as a Cobra, Simmons, or Sos. Superselection of the specific hepatic lobe (based on tumor burden) is performed with a microcatheter and microwire. On occasion, fluoroscopy is not sufficient to delineate the proper location of the microcather for embolization; in these cases, a CT scan can be obtained immediately after injection to verify optimal positioning (XperCT, Philips, Netherlands; DynaCT, Siemens Medical, Germany). Details are included in Figure 1.

PALLIATION FOR OTHER LIVER TUMORS

TACE is not only used in the setting of HCC; it has been used for palliation of cholangiocarcinoma. In addition, TACE has also been used for the palliation of numerous metastatic lesions to the liver, including ocular melanoma, neuroendocrine, colorectal carcinoma, renal cell carcinoma, some sarcomas, and breast cancer.

Cholangiocarcinoma

Cholangiocarcinoma is a rare hepatic malignancy with a typically poor prognosis. The only curative option for cholangiocarcinoma is

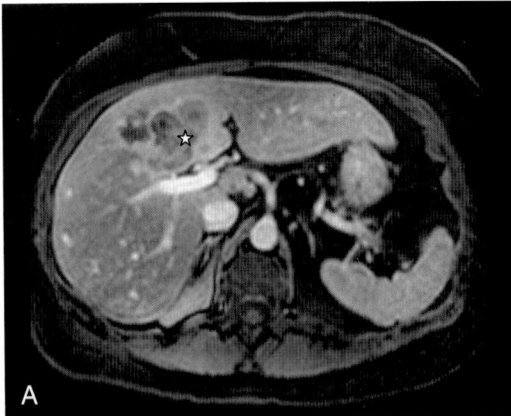

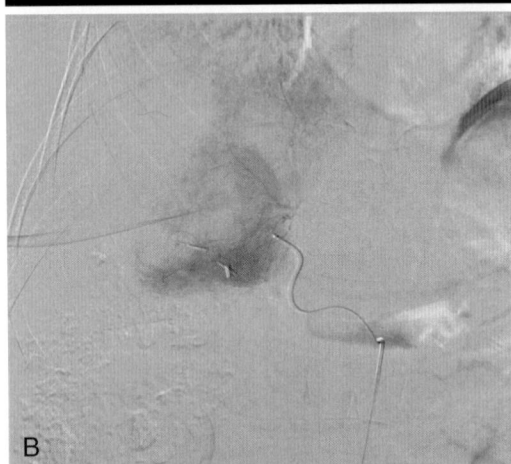

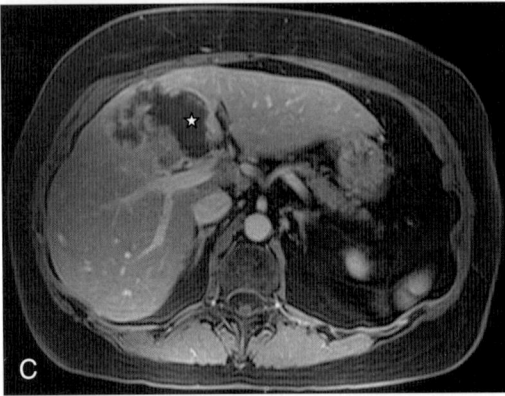

FIGURE 1 **A,** Magnetic resonance imaging (MRI) after contrast of 62-year-old woman showing segment IV cholangiocarcinoma with significant contrast enhancement *(star).* **B,** Angiogram before chemoembolization showing hypervascularity of lesion shown in **A.** **C,** MRI after contrast showing central necrosis in same lesion after chemoembolization *(star).*

surgical resection (see Figure 1). The prognosis is especially poor in those patients with unresectable disease (survival, 5 to 8 months), which usually comprises more than 70% of patients. Systemic chemotherapy has shown no impact on survival as compared with supportive care. Just like HCC, most of the blood supply to intrahepatic cholangiocarcinoma (ICC) is derived from the hepatic artery, making intraarterial therapy attractive. However, given the rarity of the disease, significant data have been difficult to accrue. In the study by Burger and colleagues, 17 consecutive patients were treated with conventional TACE (doxorubicin, cisplatin, mitomycin C, ethiodol,

and Embosphere particles [Biopshere Medical, Rockland, Mass]). These patients were relatively healthy (15 of 17 patients had Child-Pugh A; 14 of 17 had Eastern Cooperation Oncology Group (ECOG) 1-2). The median survival time in this group was 23 months. Two patients with unresectable disease went on to resection after TACE. In another retrospectively analyzed study of 15 patients treated for intrahepatic cholangiocarcinoma with TACE (single agent mitomycin C), Herber and associates found that the median survival time was 16.3 months and that 1-year, 2-year, and 3-year survival rates were 51%, 27%, and 27%, respectively. In this study, the patients were generally healthy with good liver function (14 of 15 had Child-Pugh A). Both of these studies have shown improved survival in those patients with intrahepatic cholangiocarcinoma after TACE therapy.

Ocular Melanoma

Ocular melanoma is the most common intraocular malignant tumor in adults. Up to 50% of those patients diagnosed with ocular melanoma have subsequent development of systemic metastases within 2 to 5 years. The metastatic disease tends to involve the liver; greater than 70% of cases of metastatic ocular melanoma involve the liver, and the liver is generally the first site of metastases. Once the melanoma metastasizes to the liver, the prognosis worsens, and survival is typically between 2 and 9 months. In a study by Sharma and colleagues in 2008, 20 patients with ocular melanoma were treated with cisplatin, doxorubicin, mitomycin C, and gel foam. After TACE, 13 of 20 patients had stable disease, with an overall survival time of 9 months. In another study by Vogl in 2007, 12 patients were treated with mitomycin C, ethiodol, and microspheres. Three of 12 had a partial response, and 5 of 12 had stable disease. The overall survival time in these patients was 21 months.

Colorectal Cancer

Colorectal cancer most commonly metastasizes to the liver and is the leading cause of death in these patients. At the time of initial diagnosis, 20% to 50% of patients already have liver metastases. Patients who only receive supportive therapy with colorectal metastases to the liver typically have a 7-month to 8-month survival time. The only curative option for these patients is surgical resection; surgical resection has a median survival time of 28 to 46 months, with 5-year survival rates from 24% to 40%. In a study by Vogl and associates in 2009, 463 patients with unresectable colorectal hepatic metastases that were refractory to systemic chemotherapy were treated with TACE. By imaging characteristics, 68 patients (14.7%) had partial response, 223 patients (48.2%) had stable disease, and 172 patients (37.1%) had progressive disease. The 1-year and 2-year survival rates after chemoembolization were 62% and 28%, respectively. Median survival times from date of diagnosis of liver metastases and date of first chemoembolization were 38 months and 14 months, respectively. In a study performed by Hong and associates, 36 patients were divided into two groups, those who received TACE therapy (n = 21) and those who received Y-90 therapy (n = 15). In these patients, the median survival times for the TACE and Y-90 groups were 7.7 months and 6.9 months, respectively (from the start of therapy). The 1-year, 2-year, and 5-year survival rates for the chemoembolization group were 43%, 10%, and 0, respectively. There were no significant survival benefits of TACE versus radioembolization.

Metastatic Neuroendocrine Tumors

Metastatic neuroendocrine tumors represent approximately 10% of metastatic disease of the liver. Carcinoid and pancreatic islet cell have a predilection to metastasize to the liver, and those patients with liver metastases have a poorer prognosis and quality of life. Surgical resection is curative but is only possible in less than 10% of patients. In a study performed by Gupta and colleagues in 2005, 69 patients with carcinoid metastases to the liver and 54 patients with pancreatic islet cell metastases to the liver underwent treatments with either hepatic arterial embolization (HAE) or chemoembolization (TACE). They found that carcinoid tumors had better outcomes than those with islet cell carcinomas in terms of response rate (66.7% vs 35.2%; $P = 0.001$), progression-free survival time (22.7 months vs 16.1 months; $P = 0.046$), and overall survival time (33.8 months vs 23.2 months; $P = 0.012$). Patients treated with TACE had a trend towards higher overall survival and improved response in islet cell tumors but not carcinoid tumors, but this difference was not statistically significant. Touzios and colleagues performed TACE with cisplatin, doxorubicin, and mitomycin C. The median survival time and 5-year survival rate were 50 months and 50%, respectively. Ruutiainen and associates performed TACE with cisplatin, doxorubicin, mitomycin, iodized oil, and PVA. The 1-year, 3-year, and 5-year survival rates were 86%, 67%, and 50%, respectively. Most recently, Vogl and associates (n = 15) compared two separate chemoembolization protocols, one with mitomycin C alone and the other with mitomycin C and gemcitabine. Their results showed that the combined mitomycin C and gemcitabine had significantly better 5-year and overall survival rates as compared with the mitomycin C alone (5-year survival rate, 46.67% vs 11.11%; overall survival time, 57.1 months vs 38.67 months).

Renal Cell Carcinoma

Renal cell carcinoma rarely is metastatic to the liver. However, its metastases are extremely vascular, making it an ideal candidate for intraarterial locoregional therapy. In a study performed by Nabil and colleagues in 2008, 22 patients were treated with TACE (either mitomycin C alone or mitomycin C with gemcitabine). Imaging showed a partial response in 13.7%, stable disease in 59%, and progression in 27.3%. Median survival times from diagnosis and from TACE were 68.6 months and 8.2 months, respectively. One-year and 2-year survival rates were 31% and 6%, respectively. Although these survival results are less than those achieved with surgery, those patients treated in this study had significantly more advanced disease as compared with those with surgical resection.

Breast Carcinoma

Distant metastases occur in approximately 6% to 7 % of all patients with breast carcinoma. The 5-year survival rate in these patients with stage IV disease is 10% to 18%. Of these patients (stage IV), 3% to 12% have metastases limited to the liver. In a study performed by Giroux and colleagues, eight patients with metastatic breast cancer were treated with TACE. On imaging, five patients had a partial response, one had stable disease, and two had disease progression. All patients died within 13 months after receiving the treatment, with a mean of 49 months from primary diagnosis.

Abdominal Sarcomas

Approximately 64% to 70% of abdominal sarcomas metastasize to the liver. Once the sarcoma metastasizes to the liver, there is a median survival time of 14 months in those patients who receive supportive care only. In a study published by Rajan and associates, 16 patients with a variety of gastrointestinal sarcomas were treated. Postprocedure imaging showed 2 patients had a partial response, 11 patients had stable disease, and 3 had progression. Survival rate from diagnosis was 81% at 1 year, 54% at 2 years, and 40% at 3 years. Median survival time was 20 months.

CONTRAINDICATIONS TO TRANSARTERIAL CHEMOEMBOLIZATION

Although there are no absolute contraindications to the TACE procedure, relative contraindications can be identified based on the exclusion criteria in most clinical trials: advanced liver disease (Child-Pugh classification C or above), active gastrointestinal bleeding, biliary obstruction, encephalopathy, refractory ascites, vascular invasion or portal vein invasion from tumor, extrahepatic metastases, portosystemic shunts, contraindication to arterial intervention (INR >1.8, platelets <50,000, creatinine >1.5), and poor performance status (ECOG >2).

In the case of biliary obstruction, care must be taken to avoid biliary necrosis of the obstructed segments, which could result in abscess formation. In a study by Kim and colleagues, the authors recommend a reduction in the amounts of oil/gelatin sponge particles to reduce the amounts of biliary complications after TACE (bilomas and focal biliary strictures). If a reversible cause is found for the biliary obstruction, a percutaneous biliary tube should be inserted before TACE. In addition, prior biliary reconstructive surgery has been identified as an independent risk factor for the formation of abscesses after TACE.

In regards to portal vein thrombosis, numerous studies have shown that TACE is safe in these patients. In a study by Pentecost and associates, nine patients with portal vein thrombosis underwent transarterial chemoembolization. In these patients, eight patients responded to treatment. No patient had development of hepatic infarction or insufficiency as a consequence of the procedure. A larger study was performed by Georgiades and colleagues in which 32 consecutive patients with portal vein thrombosis were treated with TACE. In these patients, the median overall survival time was 9.5 months. The 30-day mortality rate was 0, and there was no TACE-related hepatic infarction or acute liver failure. The 6-month, 9-month, 12-month, and 18-month survival rates were 60%, 47%, 25%, and 12.5%, respectively. The authors concluded that portal venous thrombosis should not be considered a contraindication to TACE.

Kothary and associates performed a study in which 52 patients underwent high-risk procedures. All patients had an elevated serum bilirubin values, 76.9% of patients had serum albumin levels less than 3.5 mg/dL, and 25% of the patients had portal vein invasion. Greater than 50% had a Child-Pugh score of 9 or greater. Although patients with multifocal disease and lobar invasion had significantly higher mortality rates, the 1-year and 2 year survival rates were 67.9% and 37.7%, respectively. The authors concluded that patients at high risk did not have a higher rate of mortality as a consequence of the procedure.

COMPLICATIONS

The most common complication after TACE is the postembolization syndrome (PES). It happens in approximately 2% to 7% of patients after the procedure. Symptoms of PES include abdominal pain, nausea, vomiting, and mild fevers. In a study performed by Leung and associates, the two factors associated with an increased risk of PES were gallbladder embolization and total chemoembolization dose administered. They also found that previous embolization was associated with a decreased risk of PES. Patel and colleagues performed a study where they showed that no patient factors (age, laboratory values) or bland versus chemoembolization were associated with a higher risk of PES. The treatment of PES is supportive care only.

The most important and serious consequence of TACE is hepatic insufficiency or failure. Chan and associates found that acute hepatic decompensation occurred in 20% of all patients treated with TACE, with 3% of cases irreversible. Patient factors associated with a higher rate of hepatic decompensation included: dose of cisplatin used, baseline bilirubin level, baseline prothrombin time, baseline aminotransferase (AST) level, and stage of cirrhosis.

Rarer (but equally as serious) complications of TACE include cerebral lipiodol embolism and pulmonary embolism or infarction. The former (cerebral lipiodol embolism) is caused by an arteriovenous shunt in the liver with either an intracardiac shunt or pulmonary shunt. Five total cases of cerebral lipiodol embolism have been reported in the literature. Pulmonary embolisms or infarctions can occur from an arteriovenous shunt occurring in the liver. A study by Chung and colleagues showed the incidence of pulmonary complications increase as the dose of lipiodol increases.

DRUG-ELUTING BEADS

The use of drug-eluting beads (DEBs) or microspheres signaled a new frontier in interventional oncology. This agent, which incorporates the chemotherapeutic agent on a microsphere, has a dual function: the capability to slowly release chemotherapy in a controlled fashion over time and embolization of the treated artery. The two types of drug-eluting microspheres are DC bead microspheres (Biocompatibles, Farnham, Surrey, United Kingdom) and Quadrasphere microspheres (Biosphere Medical Inc, Rockland, Mass). Much more data have been gathered regarding DC beads as compared with Quadrasphere; as a result, only DC beads are discussed here. The DC beads are derivatives of polyvinyl hydrogel and received European Conformity (CE) mark approval in 2003 for malignant hypervascular tumors. The DC beads are most commonly loaded with doxorubicin and are typically used for the treatment of HCC, cholangiocarcinoma, and neuroendocrine metastases. The beads can also be loaded with irinotecan; this agent is used for treatment of colorectal metastases to the liver.

CURRENT EVIDENCE

The pharmacokinetics of the profile of DEB-TACE is significantly different as compared with that of conventional TACE. The peak drug concentration occurs in both treatments within 5 minutes after injection, but it is significantly lower in the DEB-TACE group (78.97 ± 38.4 ng/mL vs 895.66 ± 653.1 ng/mL; $P = 0.001$). In addition, the variability of the maximal concentration of doxorubicin is considerably higher in the conventional TACE group as compared with the DEB-TACE group. In addition, the total systemic dose of doxorubicin of TACE is also significantly higher as compared with DEB-TACE. This improved pharmacokinetic profile of DEB-TACE allows more selective dose delivery to the tumor and a reduction of systemic toxicity.

One of the first studies to ascertain the effectiveness and safety of DC beads for unresectable HCC was performed by Malagari and associates. In this open-label study of 62 patients with unresectable HCC, mean tumor diameter was 5.6 cm and all patients were either at Okuda stage I or II. On the basis of imaging, after 9 months of treatment, a complete response was seen in 12.2% of patients, a partial response in 80.7%, progression of disease in 6.8%, and stable disease in 12.2%. Alpha-fetoprotein levels showed a mean decrease of 1123 ng/mL after the first session. Severe postprocedure complications were seen in two patients: one had cholecystitis, and one had a

liver abscess. Similar results were obtained in a study performed by Reyes and colleagues. In this study, 20 patients had doxorubicin-eluting beads TACE (DEB-TACE). On 1-month imaging, according to European Association for the Study of Liver Criteria (EASL), 12 patients had objective tumor response and 8 had stable disease. No patients had a progression of disease during treatment. Overall survival rates at 1 year and 2 years were 65% and 55%, respectively. Median overall survival time was 26 months.

In a prospective randomized trial comparing DEB-TACE with bland embolization, 41 patients were assigned to the DEB-TACE group, and 43 patients were assigned to the bland embolization group. Tumor response was evaluated with the EASL criteria and alpha-fetoprotein levels. The results showed that the recurrence rate was higher at 9 months with the bland embolization group as compared with the DEB-TACE group. There was also a longer time to progression (TTP) for the DEB-TACE group (42.4 ± 9.5 vs 36.2 ± 9.0 weeks; $P = 0.008$).

The Precision V trial is the only prospective randomized trial comparing the doxorubicin-eluting bead embolization (DEB-TACE) and conventional chemoembolization (administration of doxorubicin-oil emulsion followed by conventional TACE). In this study, there were 212 total patients, 102 in the DC-bead group and 110 in the conventional TACE (cTACE) group. All cases were Child-Pugh A/B and unresectable; the patients were randomized according to Child-Pugh status, performance status, extent of disease, and prior treatment. The primary endpoint was EASL (MRI criteria) 6 months after treatment. A trend towards improved EASL criteria was found in the DEB-TACE group, although this was not significant (DEB-TACE vs cTACE, respectively: complete response, 27% vs 22%; objective response, 52% vs 44%; disease control, 63% vs 52%; $P = 0.11$). A more sick subgroup analysis (Child-Pugh B, ECOG 1, bilobar disease) showed a significant increase in objective response in the DEB-TACE group versus cTACE ($P = 0.038$). Equally as important, the DEB-TACE group had reduced amounts of serious liver toxicity ($P < 0.001$) and significantly lower rate of doxorubicin-related side effects ($P = 0.0001$). The authors concluded that DEB-TACE is a safe procedure, with a better side-effect profile compared with conventional TACE, and is beneficial to patients with more advanced disease.

Many smaller trials have described the use of drug-eluting beads for metastatic liver disease, including primaries from colorectal cancer, neuroendocrine, and cholangiocarcinoma. A few promising trials have described the use of irinotecan-eluting beads for metastatic colorectal carcinoma.

In one study, 55 patients underwent 99 treatments with irinotecan drug-eluting beads. The median disease-free and overall survival time from the time of first treatment was 247 days and 343 days, respectively. A small trial with 11 patients performed by Aliberti and associates described preliminary results from treatment of intrahepatic cholangiocarcinoma with DEB-TACE. They reported a median survival of 13 months and 100% Response Evaluation Criteria in Solid Tumors (RECIST) response from DC-bead treatment.

Drug-eluting beads do carry the risk of complications, however. A recent study by Bhagat and colleagues showed that 7 of 13 patients had bilomas develop after DEB-TACE for neuroendocrine metastases (Figure 2). This rate of biloma formation was higher than previously reported. In the case of metastatic disease, there is a higher chance of biliary necrosis and biloma formation because of a less resilient biliary plexus as compared with those patients with cirrhosis (and HCC).

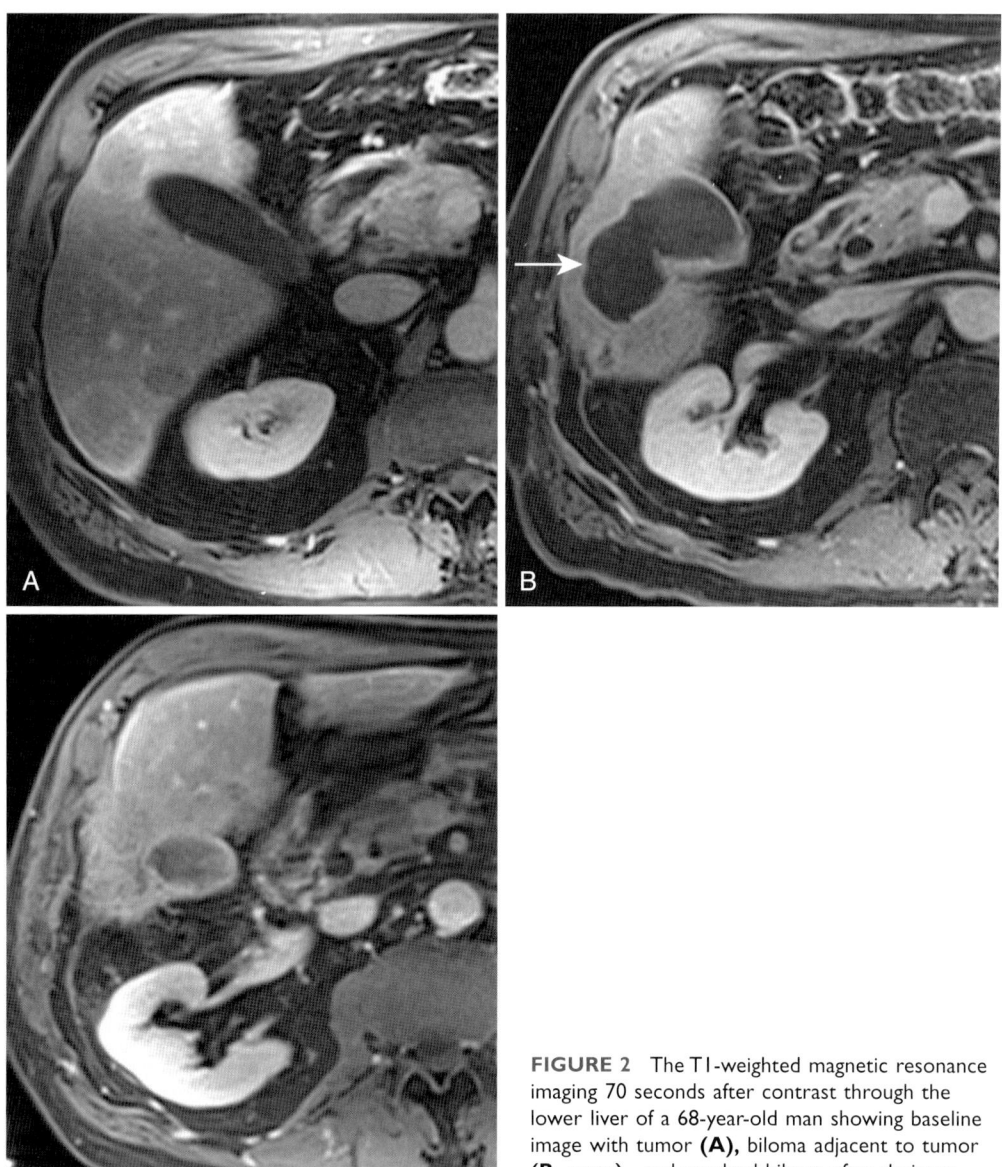

FIGURE 2 The T1-weighted magnetic resonance imaging 70 seconds after contrast through the lower liver of a 68-year-old man showing baseline image with tumor **(A)**, biloma adjacent to tumor **(B,** *arrow***),** and resolved biloma after drainage, now with mostly necrotic tumor **(C).**

SUGGESTED READINGS

Bhagat N, Reyes DK, Lin M, et al: Phase II study of chemoembolization with drug-eluting beads in patients with hepatic neuroendocrine metastases: high incidence of biliary injury, *Cardiovasc Intervent Radiol* 36(2):449–459, 2013, Epub 2012.

Geschwind JF, Ramsey DE, Cleffken B, et al: Transcatheter arterial chemoembolization of liver tumors: effects of embolization protocol on injectable volume of chemotherapy and subsequent arterial patency, *Cardiovasc Intervent Radiol* 26(2):111–117, 2003, Epub 2003.

Hong K, Geschwind JF: Locoregional intra-arterial therapies for unresectable intrahepatic cholangiocarcinoma, *Semin Oncol* 37(2):110–117, 2010, Epub 2010.

Llovet JM, Real MI, Montana X, et al: Arterial embolisation or chemoembolisation versus symptomatic treatment in patients with unresectable hepatocellular carcinoma: a randomised controlled trial, *Lancet* 359(9319):1734–1739, 2002, Epub 2002.

Sato T: Locoregional management of hepatic metastasis from primary uveal melanoma, *Semin Oncol* 37(2):127–138, 2010, Epub 2010.

PORTAL HYPERTENSION

PORTAL HYPERTENSION: THE ROLE OF SHUNTING PROCEDURES

Elaine Y. Cheng, MD, Jonathan R. Hiatt, MD, and
Ronald W. Busuttil, MD, PhD

Portal hypertension is a clinical syndrome defined by portal venous pressure that exceeds 5 to 10 mm Hg. The various etiologies of portal hypertension can be classified as prehepatic, intrahepatic, or posthepatic (Table 1). Of these, cirrhosis is the most common cause of portal hypertension in the United States, accounting for about 90% of cases.

Variceal hemorrhage is one of the most clinically significant manifestations of portal hypertension, with substantial morbidity and mortality. Varices are low-resistance venous collaterals formed from preexisting vascular channels dilated by portal hypertension. These collateral portosystemic channels arise at sites where portal and systemic veins normally meet (Table 2).

Gastroesophageal varices are present in approximately 50% of patients with cirrhosis; the incidence rate increases with the severity of liver disease. Variceal hemorrhage occurs at an annual rate of 5% to 15%, with size of the varices as the most important predictor of hemorrhage. The mortality rate for each episode of variceal bleeding approaches 20%, which underscores the importance of rapid and aggressive initial management and prevention of recurrent bleeding.

MANAGEMENT OF ACUTE VARICEAL HEMORRHAGE

An algorithm for management of patients with acute variceal bleeding is shown in Figure 1. These patients should be admitted to an intensive care unit for monitoring, resuscitation, and definitive treatment. Endotracheal intubation is often needed for airway protection, particularly during endoscopy and other procedures. Large-bore venous access should be secured, with rapid initiation of blood volume replacement. Packed red blood cells are transfused to a target hematocrit level of 25% to 30%; overtransfusion exacerbates portal hypertension and can increase the severity of bleeding. Coagulopathy is corrected with transfusion of fresh frozen plasma and platelets.

Patients with cirrhosis are at increased risk for infection as a result of impaired host defenses, particularly during or immediately after a major episode of gastrointestinal hemorrhage. Spontaneous bacterial peritonitis represents approximately half of these infections, with urinary tract infections and pneumonia comprising the remainder. Short-term antibiotic prophylaxis, usually with a third-generation cephalosporin, should be used routinely. The use of prophylactic antibiotics has been shown to reduce the risk both for rebleeding and for mortality in patients with acute variceal bleeding.

Various vasoactive medications can decrease blood flow to the gastroesophageal varices and help to control hemorrhage. Although vasopressin is the most potent available splanchnic vasoconstrictor, its clinical utility is limited by systemic vasoconstrictive properties that can produce hypertension, myocardial ischemia and subsequent cardiac failure, arrhythmias, ischemic abdominal pain, and limb gangrene. Consequently, vasopressin should always be used in conjunction with the venodilator nitroglycerin to reverse the systemic hemodynamic effects of the former medication without compromising the reduction in portal pressure.

Octreotide, a somatostatin analog with a longer half-life than its native counterpart, is a splanchnic vasoconstrictor and inhibitor of glucagon and other vasodilatory peptides. Octreotide is the only somatostatin analog available in the United States and often is used as an adjunct to endoscopic therapy in the control of acute variceal bleeding. The current regimen at the authors' center combines continuous infusions of octreotide with pantoprazole to suppress gastric acid secretion.

ENDOSCOPIC DIAGNOSIS AND THERAPY

Emergent esophagogastroduodenoscopy (EGD) plays a critical role in the diagnosis and therapy for suspected acute variceal hemorrhage. EGD is used to identify the presence of varices and to exclude other sources of bleeding, such as portal hypertensive gastropathy, gastritis, or ulcers. Endoscopic interventions in the form of sclerotherapy or variceal band ligation are effective in controlling hemorrhage in nearly 90% of patients.

In endoscopic sclerotherapy, a small amount of sclerosant is injected into the varix or adjacent tissues, causing thrombosis and obliteration of the varix. Complications associated with sclerotherapy occur in 10% to 40% of cases and include adverse pulmonary and renal effects, esophageal ulceration, stricture, and perforation.

Variceal band ligation is a newer therapeutic modality that involves suctioning the varix into a plastic sheath attached to the tip of the endoscope and then deploying a tight band around the varix to interrupt its blood supply. Endoscopic variceal band ligation is at least as effective as sclerotherapy in controlling bleeding, but it has a lower complication rate and therefore has largely replaced sclerotherapy as the preferred mode of endoscopic management.

TABLE 1: Causes of portal hypertension by location

Location	Etiologies
Prehepatic	Portal vein thrombosis Splenic vein thrombosis Congenital thrombosis of portal vein Arteriovenous fistula, resulting in excessive inflow
Intrahepatic	Presinusoidal Primary biliary cirrhosis Sinusoidal Cirrhosis Infiltrative liver diseases Idiopathic portal hypertension Congenital hepatic fibrosis Nodular regenerative hyperplasia Polycystic liver disease Postsinusoidal Venoocclusive disease
Posthepatic	Budd-Chiari syndrome Inferior vena cava webs or thrombosis Congestive heart failure Constrictive pericarditis Tricuspid valve diseases

TABLE 2: Common sites of varices

Portal inflow	Systemic outflow	Collaterals
Left gastric vein, short gastric veins	Intercostal, diaphragmatic, and esophageal veins	Gastroesophageal varices
Superior hemorrhoidal vein	Middle and inferior hemorrhoidal veins	Hemorrhoids
Left portal vein via falciform ligament	Umbilicus and abdominal wall veins	Caput medusa
Liver via lienorenal ligament	Left renal vein	Retroperitoneal collaterals

LUMINAL TAMPONADE

When medical and endoscopic measures fail to control variceal hemorrhage, the use of luminal tamponade with Sengstaken-Blakemore or Minnesota tubes can be a life-saving maneuver. Both of these devices have a large round gastric balloon, which compresses the gastroesophageal junction and reduces blood flow to the esophageal varices when the tube is placed on traction, and a distal port to evacuate luminal contents of the stomach. If the use of traction alone is insufficient to control the hemorrhage, the more proximal esophageal balloon is inflated to provide direct tamponade to the varices. Minnesota tubes are more modern devices that also contain an opening proximal to the esophageal balloon to remove swallowed saliva, obviating the need for the placement of a second tube for this purpose.

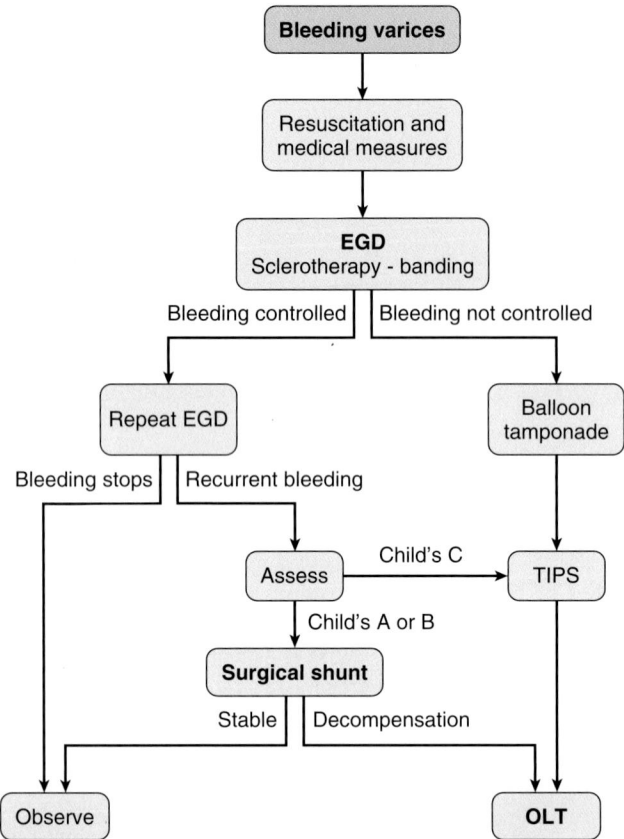

FIGURE 1   Management of acutely bleeding gastroesophageal varices. *EGD,* Esophagogastroduodenoscopy; *OLT,* orthotopic liver transplantation; *TIPS,* transjugular intrahepatic portosystemic shunt.

Aspiration pneumonia is the most common complication of luminal tamponade. Elective endotracheal intubation is often recommended to prevent aspiration, particularly in patients with encephalopathy. Other serious complications, such as airway obstruction or esophageal necrosis may occur, and therefore, the placement and maintenance of these tubes require experience and adherence to a strict protocol.

When properly applied, luminal tamponade can control bleeding in up to 90% of cases, but rebleeding occurs in 50% when the balloons are deflated. Moreover, the duration of balloon tamponade should not exceed 36 hours to avoid tissue necrosis. For these reasons, this treatment modality should only be considered a temporary bridge to more definitive measures of variceal hemorrhage control.

RADIOLOGIC INTERVENTIONS

Transjugular Intrahepatic Portacaval Shunt

Transjugular intrahepatic portacaval shunt (TIPS) is an interventional radiologic procedure by which a tract is created between the hepatic vein and portal vein and kept open with deployment of an expandable metallic stent covered with polytetrafluoroethylene (PTFE). This procedure creates a portacaval shunt within the liver, thereby reducing portal pressure. TIPS is an important modality for treatment of the complications of portal hypertension, such as variceal bleeding, portal gastropathy, ascites, or hepatic hydrothorax. The procedure has been shown to be highly successful in producing initial hemostasis in patients with acute variceal hemorrhage.

The most frequent complication after TIPS placement is worsening encephalopathy, which occurs in up to 30% of patients. A high rate of thrombosis also is seen and is attributed to intimal hyperplasia along the intrahepatic course of the metallic stent. Stenosis or occlusion occurs in the majority of cases by 1 year after TIPS placement, with recurrent variceal hemorrhage in 18% to 32% of patients. Repeated interventions such as dilation or restenting are often needed to maintain TIPS patency.

Balloon-Occluded Retrograde Transvenous Obliteration

The balloon-occluded retrograde transvenous obliteration (BRTO) procedure, used commonly in Asia since the 1980s, is now gaining popularity in the United States for the specific management of bleeding gastric varices in patients with spontaneous gastrorenal, splenorenal, or gastrocaval shunts shown on contrast-enhanced cross-sectional imaging. With a transjugular or transfemoral approach, a balloon-occlusion catheter is directed through the left renal vein into the spontaneous shunt; a sclerosing agent is then infused to obliterate the gastric varices. BRTO effectively controls gastric variceal hemorrhage and has the added advantage of preserving portal flow to the liver, thus reducing the risk of hepatic encephalopathy relative to TIPS. The occlusion of spontaneous gastrorenal shunts, however, can further exacerbate portal hypertension, precipitate hemorrhage from esophageal varices, and aggravate ascites. Nevertheless, BRTO can be a useful adjunct to TIPS in the management of gastric variceal bleeding, particularly for patients with poor hepatic reserve or a history of hepatic encephalopathy.

REBLEEDING PROPHYLAXIS

After the initial episode of variceal hemorrhage, untreated patients are at significant risk for rebleeding. The median rebleeding risk is approximately 70% within 2 years of the index hemorrhage, with an associated mortality rate of 33%. Secondary prophylaxis should therefore begin once the acute bleeding is controlled. Pharmacologic prophylaxis includes the use of nonselective beta blockers such as nadolol and propranolol, which reduce the risk of rebleeding by 40% and improve overall survival rate by 20%. The addition of endoscopic variceal band ligation to pharmacologic therapy further reduces the rebleeding risk. In patients with refractory variceal hemorrhage despite maximal pharmacologic and endoscopic prevention, TIPS or surgical shunting is warranted.

SURGICAL SHUNTS

Although surgical shunts are still considered in patients with recurrent variceal bleeding and preserved liver function, their use is much less common with the advent of endoscopic therapy, TIPS, and liver transplantation over the past several decades. Surgical shunts are categorized as total, partial, and selective. All provide decompression of gastroesophageal varices but differ in the maintenance of portal flow to the liver. The choice of surgical shunt should depend on the surgeon's familiarity with the procedure and the patient's native portal venous anatomy.

Total Portosystemic Shunts

These are large-caliber connections between the portal and systemic circulations with an end-to-side or side-to-side portacaval shunt, or alternatively with a mesocaval shunt with an interposition graft (Figure 2). Total portosystemic shunts effectively prevent variceal bleeding and control ascites, with additional advantages of ease of construction and durability. However, these shunts allow portal

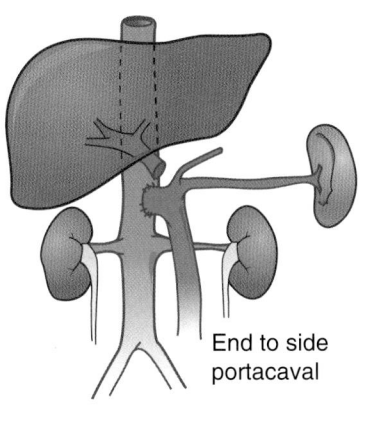

End to side portacaval

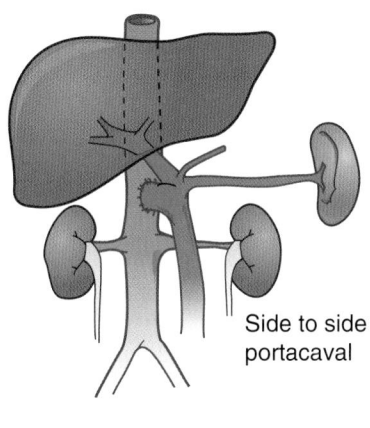

Side to side portacaval

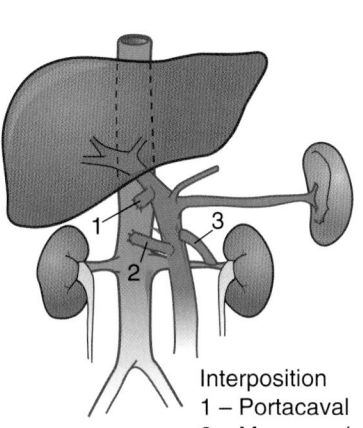

Interposition
1 – Portacaval
2 – Mesocaval
3 – Mesorenal

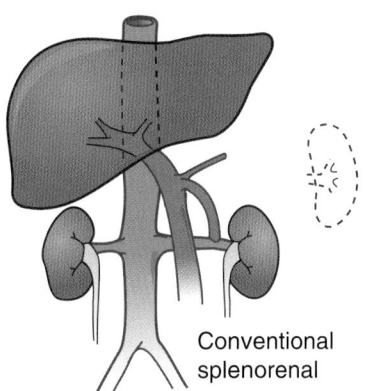

Conventional splenorenal

FIGURE 2 Total portosystemic shunts completely divert portal blood flow away from the liver. Various types of portosystemic shunts are illustrated, including the end-to-side or side-to-side portacaval shunts, interposition grafts, and the proximal splenorenal shunt. *(From Rikkers LF: Portal hypertension. In Moody FG, editor: Surgical treatment of digestive disease, Chicago, 1986, Year Book Medical, pp 409–424.)*

blood to bypass the metabolic actions of the liver, predisposing to development of hepatic encephalopathy and acute liver failure.

Portacaval shunting is discouraged in potential liver transplant candidates because scarring from previous dissection in the porta hepatis and the need for shunt dismantling significantly increases the technical complexity of the transplant operation. Portacaval shunts also have been associated with the development of a sclerotic portal vein, which is difficult to use for vascular anastomosis at the time of transplantation.

For these reasons, the mesocaval shunt has been advocated as a bridge to liver transplantation because it avoids dissection in the porta hepatis and is easily ligated during the transplant operation. The operative technique involves isolating the superior mesenteric vein at the root of the mesocolon; mobilizing the inferior vena cava below the third portion of the duodenum, which is reflected superiorly; and placing an interposition PTFE graft between these two vessels.

Partial Portosystemic Shunts

Partial, or small-diameter, portosystemic shunts have been advocated in place of total shunts to avoid the deleterious effects of portal blood flow deprivation on hepatic function. The operative strategy for a partial portosystemic shunt is similar to that for a complete shunt, with the exception that the shunt diameter is limited to 10 mm or less. In most instances, an 8-mm PTFE graft is placed between the inferior vena cava and the portal vein for portacaval shunts (Figure 3) or between the superior mesenteric vein and the inferior vena cava for mesocaval shunts. In comparison with complete portosystemic shunts, partial shunts have been reported to reduce the rate of encephalopathy, with maintenance of excellent long-term patency.

Selective Shunts

Selective shunts have excellent long-term patency and are effective at preventing recurrent variceal hemorrhage, while preserving portal blood flow, resulting in much reduced rates of encephalopathy and liver failure in comparison with total portosystemic shunts. First described by Warren in 1967, the distal splenorenal shunt (DSRS) is the most common type of selective shunt and serves to selectively decompress gastroesophageal varices while preserving blood flow to the liver.

The DSRS is constructed with mobilization of the splenic vein and the left renal vein, followed by ligation of the splenic vein near its junction with the superior mesenteric vein. The distal splenic vein is then anastomosed to the left renal vein, allowing gastroesophageal blood to decompress into the left renal vein and inferior vena cava. In addition, the coronary vein is ligated to complete the portal-azygous disconnection (Figure 4). Similar to the mesocaval shunt, the DSRS has the advantage of avoiding dissection of the porta hepatis in patients who may later become candidates for liver transplantation. The splenorenal shunt does not require inspection or ligation at the subsequent transplant operation.

One limitation of the DSRS is that new collateral venous channels may form with gradual reversal of flow, causing the shunt to lose its selectivity over time. Another potential drawback is the increase in splanchnic portal hypertension after complete portal-azygous disconnection, which may exacerbate existing ascites.

COMPARISON OF TRANSJUGULAR INTRAHEPATIC PORTACAVAL SHUNT WITH SHUNT SURGERY

A multicenter, prospective randomized controlled trial compared TIPS with the DSRS shunt in Child-Pugh class A and B cases with refractory variceal bleeding. The investigators found no significant differences in rebleeding, encephalopathy, or 2-year and 5-year survival rates between the two treatment modalities. The rates of thrombosis, stenosis, and reintervention were dramatically higher with TIPS (82%) than with DSRS (11%). Although this study illustrates that both procedures are effective in the control of refractory variceal

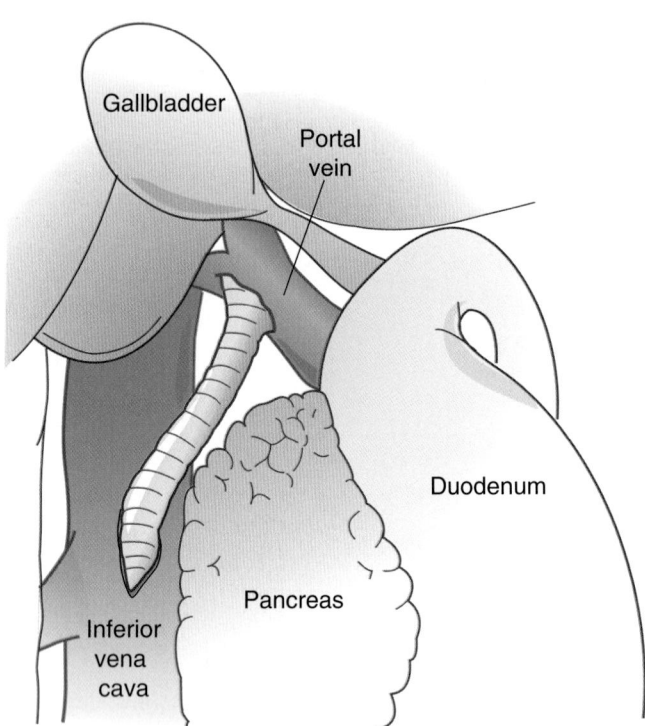

FIGURE 3 A small-diameter (8-mm or 10-mm) interposition portacaval shunt partially decompresses the portal venous system while preserving hepatic portal flow. *(From Sarfeh IJ, Rypins EB, Mason GR: A systematic appraisal of portacaval H-graft diameters: clinical and hemodynamic perspectives, Ann Surg 204(4):356–363, 1986.)*

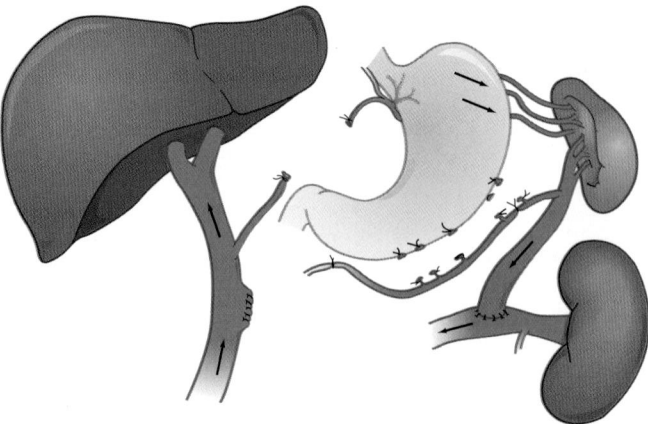

FIGURE 4 The distal splenorenal shunt allows selective variceal decompression into the left renal vein. Hepatic portal perfusion is maintained with complete portal-azygous disconnection, which is achieved by interruption of the coronary vein, gastroepiploic vein, and any other prominent venous collaterals. *(From Salam AA: Distal splenorenal shunts: hemodynamics of total versus selective shunting. In Baker RJ, Fischer JE, editors: Mastery of surgery, ed 4, Philadelphia, 2001, Lippincott Williams & Wilkins, pp 1357–1366.)*

bleeding in Child-Pugh class A or B cases, surgical therapy is preferred because of a less frequent need for reintervention, provided that the required expertise is available. Other patient factors, such as comorbidities, reliability to return for follow-up visits, and ongoing access to prompt medical care must also be considered when formulating a treatment plan for recurrent variceal bleeding.

SUMMARY

Bleeding from gastroesophageal varices causes significant morbidity and mortality in patients with portal hypertension. A multidisciplinary approach incorporating medical management, endoscopic interventions, and TIPS is the mainstay of therapy for control of variceal hemorrhage. Although now used rarely, surgical shunts can be safe and effective for recurrent, refractory bleeding in the carefully selected patient with preserved liver function.

SUGGESTED READINGS

Geevarghese SK, Hiatt JR, Busuttil RW: Management of portal hypertensive hemorrhage in the era of liver transplantation. In Busuttil RW, Klintmalm GB, editors: *Transplantation of the liver*, ed 2, Philadelphia, 2006, Elsevier Saunders.

Henderson JM, Boyer TD, Kutner MH, et al: DIVERT study group: distal splenorenal shunt versus transjugular intrahepatic portal systemic shunt for variceal bleeding: a randomized trial, *Gastroenterology* 130:1643–1651, 2006.

Warren WD, Salam AA, Hutson D, et al: Selective distal splenorenal shunt, *Arch Surg* 108:306–314, 1974.

THE ROLE OF LIVER TRANSPLANTATION IN PORTAL HYPERTENSION

Andrew Singer, MD, PhD, and
Susanna Nazarian, MD, PhD

The liver has a unique, dual circulation with roughly three quarters of flow supplied through the portal vein and the balance delivered via the hepatic artery. Portal inflow is itself derived from contributions from the splenic and superior mesenteric veins. Impedance to venous flow at any point along its path can result in increased portal venous pressures with morbid and potentially lethal consequences. Portal hypertension, a pathologic elevation of pressure within the portal venous system, is most commonly seen with cirrhotic, end-stage liver disease.

ETIOLOGIES OF PORTAL HYPERTENSION

Whereas in the United States chronic alcoholism and hepatitis C infection (HCV) are the most common causes of cirrhosis and portal hypertension, worldwide, hepatitis B infection (HBV) is the modal cause. Portal hypertension can, however, occur in the absence of cirrhosis. These noncirrhotic etiologies of portal hypertension can be divided into presinusoidal, sinusoidal, and postsinusoidal causes. That said, over time, all these processes may result in progression to cirrhosis. Prehepatic portal hypertension, seen with thrombosis of the portal vein, is often associated with hypercoagulable states or may occur in infants after umbilical vein cannulation. Schistosomiasis is an endemic parasite in some parts of the world, particularly in Asia, and can lead to both presinusoidal and sinusoidal portal hypertension. This fluke enters the skin and ultimately lodges in the superior or inferior mesenteric veins. Eggs from the adult worm flow into portal vein tributaries and elicit an immune response that leads to inflammation and eventual fibrosis. Portal hypertension in this setting is predominantly presinusoidal initially but eventually progresses to sinusoidal fibrosis. Noncirrhotic portal fibrosis, also known as idiopathic portal hypertension, is a sinusoidal variant of portal hypertension with dense portal fibrosis and dilated sinusoids in the absence of cirrhosis. Finally, postsinusoidal causes include hepatic vein thrombosis (Budd-Chiari syndrome), venous occlusive disease seen with allogeneic bone marrow transplant, and right heart failure.

PATHOPHYSIOLOGY OF PORTAL HYPERTENSION

Portal hypertension in the setting of cirrhosis is a result of both altered hepatic architecture and an imbalance of local vasodilators and vasoconstrictors. Hepatic fibrosis elevates intrahepatic resistance and increases portal pressures. Of the overexpressed vasoconstrictors, endothelin appears to play an especially critical role in the increased vascular tone seen with cirrhosis. Meanwhile, a relative deficiency in nitric oxide leads to contraction of septal fibroblasts and smooth muscle myocytes, further exacerbating the vascular tone imbalance. Portal hypertension is defined as a hepatovenous pressure gradient (pressure in the portal veins relative to the pressure in the vena cava) of at least 10 mm Hg. This pressure gradient can result in life-threatening morbidities, including the production of ascites, development of varices, and splenomegaly with associated thrombocytopenia from platelet sequestration and destruction.

With altered vascular tone, there is marked vasodilation of arterioles in the splanchnic organs and a decrease in the peripheral circulation resulting in relative hypotension and activation of the renin-angiotensin-aldosterone system. This causes salt and water retention, promulgating the production of ascites. Further, relative hypoperfusion of the kidneys and renal artery vasoconstriction may lead to hepatorenal syndrome and renal failure. Spontaneous bacterial peritonitis (SBP) complicating ascites, diagnosed with positive bacterial culture or an elevated polymorphonuclear white blood cell count in the peritoneal fluid, can be lethal, with a mortality rate that exceeds 30%. However, if SBP is recognized and treated early, best with a third-generation cephalosporin such as ceftriaxone, the mortality rate is less than 10%. Trials of antibiotic prophylaxis with either fluoroquinolones or co-trimoxazole in those with ascites have suggested a benefit in SBP reduction and overall patient survival.

The liver of a patient with portal hypertension is impaired in its ability to clear ammonia and other toxic metabolites, not only from its inherent parenchymal dysfunction but also from the shunting of blood around the liver. Hepatic encephalopathy ensues, which can range from mild fatigue, difficulty sleeping, and forgetfulness, to hepatic comas and even intracranial hypertension in acute liver failure. Treatment with lactulose or rifaximin can minimize hepatic encephalopathy and has been shown to reduce frequency and duration of encephalopathy-related hospitalizations. The most lethal consequences of portal hypertension, however, are bleeding complications. Twenty-five percent to 40% of patients with cirrhosis have gastroesophageal variceal hemorrhage develop. Acute bleeds from varices carry a mortality rate of 20% to 30% with the first bleed and up to 75% with recurrent bleeds.

MEDICAL MANAGEMENT OF PORTAL HYPERTENSION

Medical management can temporize and ameliorate the consequences of portal hypertension but does not treat the underlying causes. Diuretics, usually a combination of furosemide and spironolactone, help limit the production of ascites. The administration of albumin complements diuretic therapy by increasing oncotic pressure. Fluid restriction and compliance to a low-salt diet is also essential in controlling ascites. Nonselective beta-blockers, such as nadolol or propranolol, reduce the hepatoportal gradient and lower hepatic blood flow, curbing the progression of varices and reducing the bleeding risk. Other agents used to reduce portal pressure via splanchnic vasoconstriction or impedance of the renin-angiotensin-aldosterone system include octreotide, somatostatin, and midodrine. Repetitive large-volume paracenteses can improve patient mobility, respiratory status, and overall comfort.

Acute variceal bleeding can be torrential and rapidly fatal unless arrested with timely intervention. In the setting of such uncontrolled bleeding, a Sengstaken-Blakemore tube can be life saving. This nasogastric tube features a gastric balloon that can be pulled up against the gastroesophageal junction and an esophageal balloon that can be inflated to further tamponade bleeding. Care must be taken to deflate the balloon after 90 minutes to avoid pressure necrosis. With these tubes, it is possible to temporize vigorous bleeding and allow time for resuscitation, transfusion, correction of coagulopathy, and eventually definitive endoscopic banding and sclerotherapy. These endoscopic techniques are also crucial to the prevention of rebleeds, and surveillance esophagogastroduodenoscopy (EGD) should be undertaken at regular intervals to check for variceal recurrence and progression.

SURGICAL AND RADIOLOGIC MANAGEMENT OF PORTAL HYPERTENSION

Shunts to bypass portohepatic flow, and hence to limit the consequences of portal hypertension, were first introduced in 1903 by Vidal. Portosystemic shunts deliver splanchnic blood to the systemic system, circumventing the high-pressure portohepatic system. As a result, ascites production and variceal propagation are curbed. Shunts can be roughly divided into two categories: (1) nonselective shunts that completely divert blood from the portal venous circulation; and (2) selective shunts that divert the esophagogastrosplenic venous flow to the systemic circulation while maintaining portal flow from the upper intestinal circuit. The latter serve to minimize left-sided portal hypertension and esophagogastric varices with less exacerbation of encephalopathy as compared with nonselective shunts.

Until the early 1970s, shunts were exclusively a surgical undertaking. However, the introduction of the transjugular intrahepatic portosystemic shunt (TIPS) has revolutionized the management of portal hypertension, and the creation of surgical shunts is now rarely indicated. TIPS, a nonselective shunt, can be performed electively or created emergently in the setting of acute variceal bleeding. This interventional radiologic technique begins with access of the hepatic vein, most commonly the right, via the right internal jugular vein.

With fluoroscopy, needle access to the right portal system is attained, across hepatic parenchyma. The tract is then dilated, and a stent is introduced to connect the portal and systemic systems. The most feared complications related to TIPS are hepatic encephalopathy and frank liver failure. Although TIPS efficiently minimize ascites production and limit variceal bleeding, there is the risk of increased accumulation of toxic metabolites and in turn worsened encephalopathy as blood bypasses the hepatic parenchyma. In a similar fashion, the diversion of blood from the parenchyma may propel a compensated cirrhotic into acute liver failure.

Less catastrophically, TIPS are plagued with occlusion from endothelial proliferation, requiring repeated interventions. Stent patency, however, has markedly improved with the development of polytetrafluoroethylene (PTFE)–covered stents. When used judiciously, TIPS are highly effective at reducing the risk of bleeding from varices, with a rebleeding rate of 4% per year. Ascites is markedly decreased, with a reduced need for paracentesis and fewer episodes of spontaneous bacterial peritonitis. The incidence of hepatorenal syndrome is also lowered, and overall survival is increased. Absolute contraindications to TIPS include severely elevated right heart pressures, severe hepatic encephalopathy, and active infections. Relative contraindications include hepatic vein thrombosis, portal vein thrombosis, and poor hepatic reserve.

Although rare in the TIPS era, open surgical shunts are still performed when TIPS is not feasible or has failed. Examples of nonselective shunts include mesocaval shunts, which are fashioned by sewing a piece of prosthetic graft between the superior mesenteric vein and the vena cava, and the even more rarely performed total portosystemic shunt, which is created by side-to-side portocaval anastomosis. A splenorenal, or Warren shunt, is an example of a selective shunt. This shunt is created by disconnecting the splenic vein at its confluence with the superior mesenteric vein and anastomosing it to the left renal vein. In addition, the coronary vein and veins along the greater curvature of the stomach are ligated in an effort to minimize left-sided portal hypertension while maintaining some portal flow to the liver. Trials comparing surgical shunts and TIPS have shown roughly equivalent decrease in variceal bleeds and overall patient survival with similar impact on encephalopathy.

LIVER TRANSPLANTATION

Whereas medical treatments and shunting aim to temporize the sequelae of portal hypertension, with liver transplant, there is the promise of cure. This intervention, however, is limited by organ availability and the need for life-long immunosuppression after transplant. Accordingly, it is meted to those with advanced hepatic failure or to those who have primary hepatocellular carcinoma (HCC) in the setting of cirrhosis. The most common indications for adult liver transplantation in the United States are HCV and alcoholism. Others include nonalcoholic steatohepatitis (NASH), HBV, primary sclerosing cholangitis (PSC), autoimmune hepatitis, primary biliary cirrhosis (PBC), Wilson's disease, and hemochromatosis. In the pediatric population, biliary atresia is by far the leading indication for liver transplantation. Others include progressive fibrosing intrahepatic cholestasis (PFIC), acute hepatic failure from toxic exposures or viral infections, and rare inborn errors of metabolism.

The presence of portal hypertension complicates liver transplant and nontransplant surgeries. Disruption of varices within the esophagus, abdominal wall, peritoneal cavity, or retroperitoneum poses the threat of rapid and voluminous blood loss. The potential risk of esophageal and gastric variceal hemorrhage has limited the use of hemodynamic monitoring with transesophageal echocardiography (TEE) in patients with signs of portal hypertension undergoing liver transplantation. Splenic injury, given immense hypersplenism seen with portal hypertension, also brings the possibility of difficult-to-control bleeding. Likewise, the rapid removal of ascites during surgery may lead to hemodynamic instability. Despite correction of portal hypertension through liver transplant, ascites may persist in a subset of patients postoperatively. Although this phenomenon is incompletely understood, it is most often seen in those who had suffered from massive ascites before transplant. Hypersplenism, too, may take years to resolve.

With 16,000 people on the waiting list for liver transplantation and only 6000 transplants occurring annually, much thought has been given regarding the system for allocation of this precious resource. The United Network of Organ Sharing (UNOS) oversees the allocation of organs. The nation is divided into 10 regions and then subdivided into 58 organ procurement organizations (OPOs) within these regions. Within blood groups, livers are offered first within the OPO based on a scoring system for assessing the severity of liver disease, the Model for End-Stage Liver Disease (MELD), which predicts 90-day risk of death without transplantation. The MELD score ranges between 6 and 40 and is calculated from 3 measured laboratory values: bilirubin, international normalized ratio (INR), and creatinine. Nationally, the median MELD at transplant is approximately 26, yet it varies by blood group and transplant region. Because liver transplant has been shown to be a powerful tool in the treatment of early primary liver cancers, those with appropriately sized HCC are given 22 exception points, with additional points awarded quarterly while they remain on the wait list to facilitate timely transplantation. It is important to note that the degree of portal hypertension and associated morbidities are not components of the MELD score. That said, the organ allocation algorithm is continually under review to ensure fairness and achieve its goal of minimizing patient death on the waitlist.

Ninety percent of liver transplants in the United States use whole, cadaveric grafts. Pediatric transplantation requires either an appropriately sized graft, from a child or small adult, or a segmental graft from either a live or deceased donor. For adults unable to obtain timely deceased donor transplantation, often those underserved by the MELD allocation system, live donor liver transplantation of a hemiliver, most commonly the right lobe, from adult to adult may sometimes be an appropriate option. Significant recipient portal hypertension, however, may be a relative contraindication for use of these reduced sized grafts because it may result in portal hyperperfusion and allograft dysfunction.

Efforts to expand the organ pool have led to the use of expanded-criteria grafts with success. The donor pool now includes livers from elderly donors and those with elevated body mass index (BMI), allografts with prolonged cold ischemia time, those from donors with cancer history, and those procured from donation after cardiac death. Currently, nationwide 1-year graft and patient survival rates are approximately 84% and 88%, respectively. Liver transplantation remains the most efficacious and durable intervention for the treatment of portal hypertension in the setting of end-stage liver disease resulting from a heterogeneous collection of causes. As graft and recipient selection, operative techniques, perioperative and postoperative management, and immunosuppression continue to improve in the coming years so too will the safety and efficacy of liver transplantation.

SUGGESTED READINGS

Clavien PA, Lesurtel M, Bossuyt PM, et al: Recommendations for liver transplantation for hepatocellular carcinoma: an international consensus conference report, *Lancet Oncol* 13(1):e11–e22, 2012.

García-Pagán JC, Caca K, Bureau C, et al: Early use of TIPS in patients with cirrhosis and variceal bleeding, *N Engl J Med* 362(25):2370–2379, 2010.

Garcia-Tsao G, Bosch J: Management of varices and variceal hemorrhage in cirrhosis, *N Engl J Med* 362(9):823–832, 2010.

Ginès P, Cárdenas A, Arroyo V, et al: Management of cirrhosis and ascites, *N Engl J Med* 350(16):1646–1654, 2005.

Henderson JM, Boyer RD, Kutner MH, et al: Distal splenorenal shunt versus transjugular intrahepatic portal systematic shunt for variceal bleeding: a randomized trial, *Gastroenterology* 130(6):1643–1651, 2006.

Rosemurgy AS, Frohman HA, Teta AH, et al: Prosthetic H-graft portacaval shunts vs transjugular intrahepatic portasystemic stent shunts: 18 year follow-up of a randomized trial, *J Am Coll Surg* 214(4):445–453, 2012.

Wertheim JA, Petrowsky H, Saab S, et al: Major challenges limiting liver transplantation in the United States, *Am J Transplant* 11(9):1773–1784, 2011.

ENDOSCOPIC THERAPY FOR ESOPHAGEAL VARICEAL HEMORRHAGE

Justin A. Reynolds, MD, and
Francisco Antonio Durazo, MD, FACP

OVERVIEW

Gastroesophageal varices are the most important type of portosystemic collaterals that develop in the setting of portal hypertension. Variceal rupture is a well-known complication of portal hypertension and cirrhosis and is more common as the stage of liver disease progresses. Bleeding from esophageal varices can occur in up to 30% of patients with cirrhosis. Despite advances in medical and endoscopic therapy for variceal hemorrhage, the mortality rate associated with bleeding is as high as 20%.

All patients with suspicion of variceal bleeding should have adequate intravenous access established and undergo rapid resuscitation. Vasoactive medications such as octreotide are helpful in controlling bleeding and can be administered as a 50-µg bolus, followed by a 25-µg/h intravenous infusion. This should be continued for a minimum of 72 hours after definitive endoscopic therapy for a variceal bleed. Intravenous proton pump inhibitors (e.g., pantoprazole) are routinely given as well in case the source of bleeding is an ulcer rather than a varix. Blood products are often necessary for correction of thrombocytopenia and coagulopathy. Occasionally, the patient needs endotracheal intubation for airway protection or for lack of cooperation or encephalopathy.

Patients with cirrhosis who experience gastrointestinal (GI) bleeding are at greatly increased risk of infection-related complications such as bacteremia, pneumonia, and bacterial peritonitis from infected ascites fluid. These patients should receive empiric broad-spectrum antibiotics (e.g., ceftriaxone or norfloxacin) for at least 5 days.

Up to 25% of patients with known portal hypertension may present with upper GI hemorrhage that is not the result of esophageal varices. In these patients, common causes of bleeding include peptic ulcer disease, erosive esophagitis, Mallory-Weiss tears, portal hypertensive gastropathy, and gastric fundal varices. A careful diagnostic endoscopic evaluation should be performed in all such patients. In patients with documented esophageal varices but no other potential sources of bleeding identified at endoscopy, a variceal source of hemorrhage should be presumed.

ENDOSCOPIC THERAPY

Endoscopic Band Ligation

Endoscopic band ligation is a well-established, safe, and effective means of hemostasis for esophageal varices. Although preceded by sclerotherapy, band ligation has largely replaced it as a result of improved safety and equal efficacy. All band ligation devices are affixed on the tip of an endoscope that then uses suction against a mound of target tissue while a small, circular elastic band made of rubber or latex is deployed around the base of the target tissue. This compression results in hemostasis with subsequent sloughing of the necrotic tissue.

Several components are common to all band ligation devices, including a transparent cylindrical cap that carries up to 10 bands. A tripwire runs from the cap to a control knob assembly that is inserted into the accessory channel of the endoscope. When secured in place, the bands may be fired individually with the turn of a knob. Most endoscopists use a multiband device with at least six bands available to be deployed with one insertion of the endoscope. Single-fire devices are rarely used but are best with an overtube that allows for easy insertion and withdrawal of the endoscope for reloading and multiple-band applications.

After a diagnostic endoscopy has been done and varices amenable to band ligation have been identified, the endoscope is removed and the band ligation device is attached. After reinsertion, the endoscope is advanced until the banding cylinder is in 360-degree contact with the varix. Continuous suction is applied and maintained until the varix is drawn into the cap, fully causing a *red-out* appearance that obscures vision. The firing mechanism is then activated, and an elastic band is deployed around the base of the varix. Suction may then be withheld, and the banded varix disengages from the cylinder. Some transient bleeding may be encountered during band ligation as a result of variceal rupture. This process is then repeated until all varices have been banded, and the endoscope is then removed.

The optimal technique for ligation of esophageal varices begins with the largest column of varices at the most distal point, usually at or just below the gastroesophageal junction. Starting distally allows for better visualization and avoids the risk of band dislodgement during advancement of the endoscope. Subsequent ligations are applied to all columns at the same level and then repeatedly as the endoscope is withdrawn more cephalad. In the case of active hemorrhage, the bleeding varix is often targeted first, with band placement caudal and cephalad to the rent or directly on the rent itself. Large columns of varices frequently require multiple bands along the length for adequate ligation. With good technique, varices should decompress more proximally, signifying adequate compression and hemostasis.

After band ligation treatment, the patient may experience mild temporary chest pain that is generally alleviated with viscous lidocaine, or opiates in severe cases. The authors' practice is to allow the patient clear liquids that day, followed by soft-consistency foods for the ensuing 3 days before a normal diet resumes. Nasogastric or feeding tubes should be avoided so as not to dislodge any elastic bands. Repeat band ligation treatments are typically performed at 10-day to 14-day intervals until the varices are eradicated. This usually requires three to four treatment sessions for completion.

Endoscopic Sclerotherapy

Endoscopic sclerotherapy is still commonly used worldwide, although in the United States, it has largely been replaced by band ligation and now is used most often as salvage or an adjunct therapy during acute hemorrhage. Sclerosants are irritants that cause endothelial damage and thrombosis and lead to vascular obliteration. These can be injected directly into the lumen of the varix (intravariceal) or adjacent to the varix (paravariceal) or a combination of both.

After the diagnostic endoscopy is complete, an injector needle is advanced through the instrument channel of the endoscope. Most endoscopists then inject 1 to 5 mL of sclerosant directly into each varix. Treatment is confined to the distal esophagus unless a source of bleeding is identified elsewhere. The most commonly used sclerosants include ethanolamine, sodium morrhuate, and sodium tetradecyl sulfate. The maximum amount of sclerosant that may be used depends on the agent selected but should never be more than 5 mL per varix or 20 mL per session.

Patients with active bleeding from a discretely identified site should have that varix treated first with injection of sclerosant below the site of active bleeding. After hemostasis is achieved, the most distal varices near the gastroesophageal junction should then be treated and the injections should proceed proximally until all varices have been treated.

Complications of sclerotherapy may occur in up to 25% of patients. Common problems include chest pain, mucosal ulcerations and bleeding, esophageal strictures, and bacteremia. Patients with immunocompromise, those with a history of endocarditis, and those who have prosthetic valves, shunts, or ascites should all be considered for antibiotic prophylaxis before sclerotherapy.

Other Endoscopic Methods

Several other techniques for treatment of esophageal varices have been described. Most of these techniques, however, have been used either for salvage therapy of an acute bleed or in experimental studies.

For persistent variceal bleeding despite endoscopic therapy, an urgent transjugular intrahepatic portosystemic shunt (TIPS) or other type of portocaval shunt is often indicated. As a temporizing measure, the endoscopist may place a Sengstaken-Blakemore tube into the esophagus. This tube has a gastric balloon that compresses the gastroesophageal junction as traction is applied. An esophageal balloon is also inflated to provide temporary hemostasis as a bridge to more definitive therapy aimed at portal decompression. The use of covered esophageal stents has also been reported in several series as a salvage therapy to achieve hemostasis.

Tissue adhesives and fibrin glues have been studied for hemostasis and the prevention of variceal bleeding. Endoscopic injection of rapidly setting polymers such as cyanoacrylate is well described but not yet available in the United States. In such cases, the polymer is mixed with radiopaque contrast to slow hardening and allow for fluoroscopic monitoring for determination of proper injection location. Care must be taken to avoid gluing the injector needle into the varix or the endoscope.

Hemostatic sprays or powders have widely been used for the control of hemorrhage in battlefields, and one such compound is currently under evaluation for endoscopic use. With a through-the-scope delivery catheter, the powder is delivered with a pressurized CO_2 canister and applied to the site of hemorrhage until hemostasis is achieved. The coagulum later sloughs off and is naturally eliminated. Although this spray has been evaluated in other countries, it has not yet been evaluated or approved in the United States.

RESULTS

Endoscopic band ligation and sclerotherapy are successful in controlling variceal hemorrhage in upwards of 95% of patients. Band ligation is the preferred treatment for acute bleeding because of its lower risk of treatment-induced complications and also because of its excellent efficacy. Band ligation also requires fewer treatment sessions than sclerotherapy to eradicate varices and carries a lower incidence of recurrent bleeding.

Recurrent varices after initial eradication are common and occur more often in patients receiving band ligation than sclerotherapy. When encountered, one or two additional endoscopic treatment sessions are typically required. These patients frequently need routine endoscopic evaluations for surveillance. Nonselective beta-blockers such as propranolol or nadolol can also be used for prevention of variceal bleed if endoscopic therapy is not used. However, care should be exercised in beta-blockade for patients with advanced cirrhosis due to the potential risk of precipitating hepatorenal syndrome.

Complications

Endoscopic sclerotherapy is associated with a high risk of minor complications such as bacteremia, fever, pain, pulmonary infiltrates, and pleural effusions. These generally resolve spontaneously without intervention. Shallow mucosal ulcerations at the site of sclerosant injection are also common and occasionally result in recurrent bleeding or esophageal stricture formation (in up to 20% of patients). These strictures are typically responsive to balloon dilation or bougienage.

Endoscopic band ligation therapy has a lower overall risk of treatment-related complications. Shallow postbanding mucosal ulcers may form and result in recurrent bleeding in up to 5% of patients. However, most bleeding from ligation-induced ulceration is self limited. Temporary chest pain after banding is common and self limited. Esophageal strictures are very uncommon.

Prevention of First Variceal Hemorrhage

Endoscopic band ligation, nonselective beta-blockers, and a combination of both have all been shown to reduce the risk of hemorrhage from large esophageal varices in patients who have never bled before. However, prophylactic band ligation therapy is superior to beta-blockade medical therapy and also reduces the risk of a first variceal bleed by up to 70% compared with no treatment at all.

SUMMARY

Endoscopic treatment for variceal hemorrhage is safe and effective. Endoscopic band ligation is most commonly performed for acute variceal bleeding, although sclerotherapy may also be used as primary treatment or as salvage therapy. Other techniques for refractory hemorrhage are also available. Endoscopic band ligation compared with sclerotherapy is associated with more efficient eradication of esophageal varices and also fewer complications. However, recurrence of esophageal varices is more common after band ligation than after sclerotherapy. Prevention of a first variceal bleed is most effective with prophylactic band ligation, although nonselective beta-blockers may also be used.

SUGGESTED READINGS

American Association for the Study of Liver Diseases Practice Guideline: Prevention and management of gastroesophageal varices and variceal hemorrhage in cirrhosis, *Hepatology* 46(3):922–938, 2007.
American Society for Gastrointestinal Endoscopy Guideline: The role of endoscopy in the management of variceal hemorrhage, updated July 2005, *Gastrointest Endosc* 62(5):651–655, 2005.
American Society for Gastrointestinal Endoscopy Technology Committee: Sclerosing agents for use in GI endoscopy, *Gastrointest Endosc* 66(1):1–6, 2007.
American Society for Gastrointestinal Endoscopy Technology Committee: Endoscopic banding devices, *Gastrointest Endosc* 68(2):217–221, 2008.
American Society for Gastrointestinal Endoscopy Technology Committee: Emerging technologies for endoscopic hemostasis, *Gastrointest Endosc* 75(5):933–937, 2012.

TRANSJUGULAR INTRAHEPATIC PORTOSYSTEMIC SHUNT

Ezana M. Azene, MD, PhD, and Kelvin Hong, MD

OVERVIEW

The creation of a transjugular intrahepatic portosystemic shunt (TIPS) was put forth as a possible treatment for the symptoms of portal hypertension in the early 1970s. Over the ensuing 2 decades, the work of many pioneers—including Rosch, Uchida, Colapinto, Palmaz, and others, many of whom lent their names to relevant apparatus—culminated with the introduction of TIPS in mainstream clinical practice.

TIPS can be a life-saving procedure, as well as one that alleviates severe symptoms related to portal hypertension. TIPS is also a durable solution with a long-term efficacy of 90%. It is, however, a double-edged sword, demanding meticulous technique and stringent patient selection to keep what was once a high morbidity and mortality at a minimum.

INDICATIONS

The list of causes of portal hypertension is long and is summarized in Table 1. Whatever the causative pathophysiology, TIPS can reduce or normalize the portal pressure and ameliorate the associated symptoms. As the technique for placing a TIPS became more refined and safer, and the technology became more adapted to the specific physiology and anatomy of a portosystemic shunt, the indications for TIPS have gradually expanded. Table 2 shows the indications and contraindications for TIPS.

Variceal Bleeding

Portal hypertension can cause varices along the entire gastrointestinal tract, including the small bowel and colon (hemorrhoids). Varices are more apt to bleed through the mucosa of the gastroesophageal junction, where the coronary vein is particularly disposed to dilatation.

TABLE 1: Causes of portal hypertension

Presinusoidal	Perisinusoidal	Postsinusoidal
Portal, splenic, or superior mesenteric vein thrombosis	Cirrhosis	Budd-Chiari syndrome
Idiopathic portal hypertension	Congenital hepatic fibrosis	Venoocclusive disease (sinusoidal obstruction
Mass effect (i.e., tumor)	Cystic liver disease	syndrome)
Schistosomiasis	Sarcoidosis	Chronic passive congestion (nutmeg liver)
Precirrhotic stage, primary biliary cirrhosis		Mass effect (i.e., tumor)
Alcoholic central sclerosis		
Endotheliitis (liver rejection, radiation injury)		
Arterioportovenous fistula (traumatic or Osler-Weber-Rendu)		
Hyperdynamic splenomegaly (infectious or myelodysplastic)		
Nodular regenerative hyperplasia		
Congenital extrahepatic portal vein occlusion		

TABLE 2: Indications and contraindications for Transjugular Intrahepatic Portosystemic Shunt

	Indications		Contraindications	
	EMERGING INDICATIONS			
Standard of Care	*Supported by Controlled Studies*	*Supported by Noncontrolled Studies and Case Series*	*Absolute*	*Relative*
Portal variceal hemorrhage refractory to medical/endoscopic management	"Cirrhotic" portal vein thrombosis caused by slow blood flow in the portal vein	Hepatorenal syndrome (more so type II than type I)	Severely elevated right heart pressure	Hepatic vein thrombosis
Ascites refractory to medical management	Childs-Pugh B and C with acute esophageal variceal bleeding (simultaneously treated with medical and/or endoscopic interventions)	Hepatopulmonary syndrome	Severe tricuspid regurgitation	"Noncirrhotic" portal vein thrombosis caused by hypercoagulability or tumor thrombus
Budd-Chiari syndrome not responsive to anticoagulation		Portal gastropathy refractory to β-blockers	Severe pulmonary hypertension	Poor liver function reserve
Hepatic hydrothorax refractory to diuretics and salt restriction		Hepatic venoocclusive disease	Severe congestive heart failure	Polycystic liver disease
			Severe encephalopathy	Central liver mass
			Uncorrectable bleeding diathesis	Gastric antral variceal ectasia
			Active systemic or hepatic bacterial infection	
			Unrelieved biliary obstruction	

The primary treatment of bleeding gastroesophageal varices is medical management and/or endoscopic management. Even though endoscopic management is often successful, because of the progressive nature of chronic liver disease, recurrent bleeding should be expected in more than 50% of patients. Unlike medical or endoscopic management, shunting procedures like TIPS address the underlying cause of variceal bleeding (portal hypertension). Portosystemic shunting is therefore the only definitive treatment for portal variceal bleeding. Meta-analysis of the literature has shown that TIPS has a lower rate of both variceal rebleeding and death due to rebleeding, with a strong trend toward increased survival (at the expense of increased hepatic encephalopathy). Most of the studies included in these meta-analyses predate the era of polytetrafluoroethylene (PTFE)-covered TIPS stent-grafts, which have improved long-term patency over bare-metal stents with a trend toward better overall survival. Head-to-head comparisons of TIPS created with stent-grafts to endoscopic and medical management is lacking.

Currently, the primary indication for TIPS is to control portal variceal bleeding refractory to medical and endoscopic management.

However, there is evidence from one randomized controlled study supporting the early use of TIPS in selected patients with advanced cirrhosis (Childs-Pugh B and C) and acute esophageal variceal bleeding. Additional studies are needed to confirm this finding before TIPS can be accepted as a first-line therapy for bleeding esophageal varices in patients with advanced liver disease.

Ascites

Ascites is the most common complication of cirrhosis, and in addition to the severe limitations in lifestyle, it poses a risk for bacterial peritonitis and other infections, renal failure, and increased mortality. No single cause for cirrhosis-related ascites has been identified. However, it is likely that a combination of causes, including decreased plasma albumin levels, increased bowel permeability, and cirrhosis-related hemodynamic changes—such as increased cardiac output, vasodilatation, and increased plasma volume—factor together in the formation of ascites.

Initial management consists of sodium restriction and administration of loop diuretics and aldosterone antagonists. In advanced stages, ascites becomes refractory to medical management, and TIPS may be indicated. TIPS is very effective in eliminating ascites. Because the root causes are hemodynamic/hormone related, response to TIPS is not immediate. It may take 2 to 4 weeks after TIPS for ascites to resolve, during which time additional paracenteses may be necessary. Randomized controlled trials, meta-analyses, and systematic reviews of the literature have demonstrated that TIPS significantly improves transplant-free survival compared to repeated paracentesis.

Hepatic Hydrothorax

Hepatic hydrothorax is defined as the accumulation of at least 500 mL of pleural fluid in a patient with cirrhosis without cardiopulmonary disease. Even though this definition is not 100% specific to hepatic hydrothorax, additional signs, such as isolated right-sided hydrothorax and concurrent ascites, help confirm the diagnosis. It occurs in less than 10% of patients with cirrhosis, as peritoneal fluid permeates via small diaphragmatic communications. Again, initial management is sodium restriction and diuretics. In nonresponsive patients, TIPS will eliminate hydrothorax in most and decrease the frequency of thoracentesis in the rest.

Hepatorenal Syndrome

Hepatorenal syndrome portends a poor prognosis for the cirrhotic patient because it occurs during the late stages of the hemodynamic changes related to cirrhosis. Alterations in vasoactive hormones responding to these hemodynamic changes result in splanchnic vasodilation, renal arterial vasoconstriction, and the opening of small intrarenal arteriovenous communications. The end result is renal hypoperfusion and ensuing renal failure.

Two distinct forms of hepatorenal syndrome (HRS) have been identified: *type I HRS*, which is rapidly progressing, and *type II HRS*, which evolves slowly. Type I HRS is precipitated by an event that incites acute-on-chronic liver failure, an exaggerated systemic inflammatory response, and kidney dysfunction as part of a broader multiorgan failure. Targeting the precipitating event is the hallmark of treatment for Type I HRS. Type II HRS results in large part from a reduction in effective arterial blood volume created by a shift of fluid from the intravascular compartment to the extravascular compartment (i.e., ascites). Noncontrolled studies suggest that using TIPS to reduce the production of ascites may improve renal function in type II HRS. However, the use of TIPS in HRS should be undertaken after serious consideration because of the contrast load and acute hemodynamic changes it involves.

Hepatopulmonary Syndrome

Hepatopulmonary syndrome is the presence of intrapulmonary vasodilatation and multiple small, right-to-left shunts that result in impaired gas exchange. Because of the lack of data, TIPS cannot be recommended as a standard treatment for hepatopulmonary syndrome. In selected cases, however, especially in severely compromised patients on the liver transplant list, TIPS may prove to be a life-saving bridge to surgery.

Budd-Chiari Syndrome

Budd-Chiari syndrome is caused by mechanical obstruction of the hepatic venous outflow and gradually results in cirrhosis and portal hypertension. Excluding the hepatic venous web, which can successfully be treated with simple balloon angioplasty, treatment for the fulminant form of Budd-Chiari syndrome is liver transplantation, although anticoagulation may help stave off disease progression. TIPS has proven to be a valuable tool to bridge such patients to transplantation.

In the nonfulminant form of Budd-Chiari syndrome, anticoagulation is first-line therapy. When anticoagulation fails, TIPS is a reasonable and accepted next step. The use of TIPS in this patient population was studied in a large retrospective study that showed 1-year and 10-year transplant-free survival that was much greater than expected. The American Association for the Study of Liver Diseases (AASLD) now recommends creation of a TIPS in patients with Budd-Chiari syndrome who fail to improve with anticoagulation.

Portal Gastropathy

Portal hypertensive gastropathy (to be distinguished from vascular ectasia) is the diffuse dilatation of gastric veins that, along with the inflamed and fragile mucosa of the stomach, predispose the patient to bleeding. TIPS, which normalizes the portal pressure, and mucosal protection (avoiding nonsteroidal antiinflammatory drugs, alcohol) combine to minimize this risk.

TECHNIQUE

Patient Preparation

Many of the complications related to the placement of TIPS can be avoided by proper patient workup. Review of pertinent cross-sectional imaging will confirm a patent (nonthrombosed) portal vein and reveal the relative orientation of the hepatic and portal veins. This minimizes the number of attempts to engage the portal vein and therefore minimizes the associated bleeding risk. Good hydration will minimize the risk of acute renal failure, and initiation of metronidazole (Flagyl) and/or lactulose mitigates the risk of encephalopathy. Type and cross of blood may prove lifesaving if a bleeding complication is encountered. Finally, all involved should be cognizant of related risks, especially the 30-day mortality, which ranges from less than 5% for elective procedures in well-compensated patients to 50% for emergent procedures in unstable patients with advanced liver disease.

Access

Access through the right internal jugular vein is preferred, although the left internal jugular vein can also be used. Access is maintained with a long, large vascular sheath parked in the intrahepatic inferior vena cava to allow multiple catheter-wire exchanges without recrossing the right atrium (Figure 1).

Diagnostic Assessment

Optimizing the TIPS outcomes requires not only anatomic assessment but also functional assessment of the patient's hemodynamic status. One of the contraindications to TIPS is elevated right heart pressure. Ensuring that the right atrial pressure is not severely elevated is mandatory prior to shunting the portal venous blood to an already overburdened right heart. Right atrial pressures below 15 mm Hg are generally safe, whereas pressures above 20 mm Hg predispose the patient to acute right heart failure. There are no specific guidelines, and sound clinical judgment is important. For example, a right atrial pressure of 16 mm Hg should not preclude creation of a TIPS in an unstable patient with ongoing variceal bleeding.

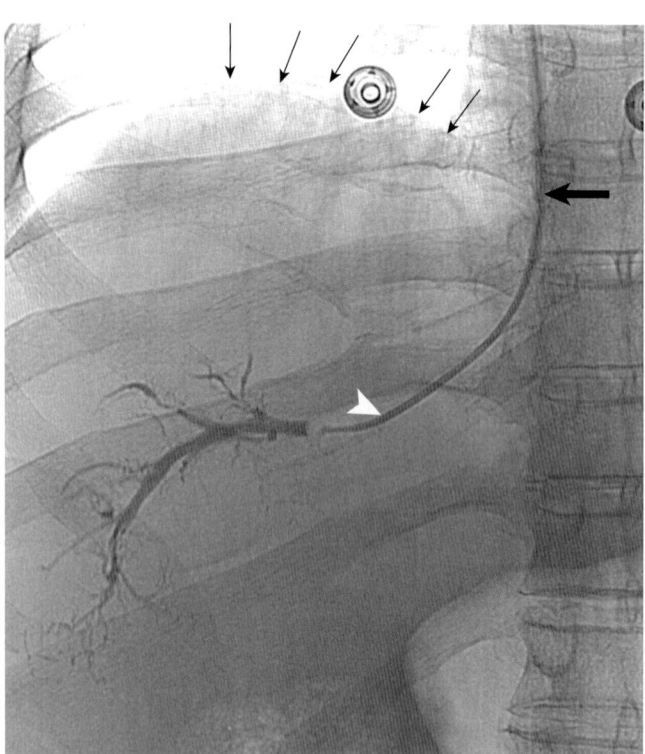

FIGURE 1 Right hepatic venogram performed via a selective catheter *(white arrowhead)*. The tip of the internal jugular sheath *(large black arrow)* is below the diaphragm *(black arrows)* to avoid catheter/wire manipulations in the right atrium. The steps of TIPS insertion outlined in Figures 1 to 9 are all from the same patient.

After selecting the right hepatic vein, free and wedged hepatic venous pressures are measured, which usually confirm portal hypertension. Normal corrected pressures should not necessarily terminate the procedure because these are not terribly accurate in general and are wholly inaccurate in cases of presinusoidal portal hypertension.

Delineation of the portal venous system is accomplished by injection of CO_2 via a catheter wedged into the hepatic vein. CO_2 is not nephrotoxic and can be given in virtually unlimited quantity. Frontal and lateral views show the anatomic relationships so the right portal vein can be targeted for access (Figure 2).

In the vast majority of patients, the TIPS is placed from the right hepatic vein into the right portal vein because this is the shortest and most direct path for shunt creation. However, a recent randomized controlled trial found that using the left portal vein resulted in a significant reduction in the incidence of encephalopathy and rehospitalization during two years of follow-up after TIPS creation. These data must be confirmed in additional studies before the standard approach of targeting the right portal vein is abandoned.

Shunt Placement

The next step is the cannulation of the right portal vein from the right hepatic vein. To accomplish this, a curved metallic sheath is advanced via the existing right internal jugular sheath in the right hepatic vein. The new catheter is rotated based on the anatomy revealed during CO_2 portography so it targets the right portal vein. When the operator judges the curved sheath to be directed toward the right portal vein, a long needle is advanced toward it. Aspiration of blood suggests intravascular location, and contrast injection confirms the tip to be in the portal vein (Figure 3).

Once it is confirmed that the tip of the needle is in the right portal vein, a wire is passed distally through the main portal vein into the superior mesenteric vein or splenic vein for security (Figure 4). The traversed liver parenchyma is fibrotic and difficult to cross unless predilated. A small-caliber (4 to 6 mm diameter) balloon is used to predilate the liver parenchyma between the right hepatic and right portal vein now crossed by the wire (Figure 5). A marking catheter is then passed over the wire into the portal venous system. This allows

FIGURE 2 Frontal **(A)** and lateral **(B)** digital subtraction views of a CO_2 hepatic venogram. CO_2 is injected via a balloon occlusion catheter to force the CO_2 retrogradely into the portal system. The right portal vein and its first-order branches, the left portal vein, and the main portal vein are easily visualized. In the lateral projection, the right portal vein is seen nearly en face. The operator usually targets the right portal vein from the right hepatic vein with a long needle introduced via the right internal jugular sheath. *BC,* Balloon occlusion catheter; *LPV,* left portal vein; *MPV,* main portal vein; *RAPV,* right anterior portal vein; *RPPV,* right posterior portal vein; *RPV,* right portal vein.

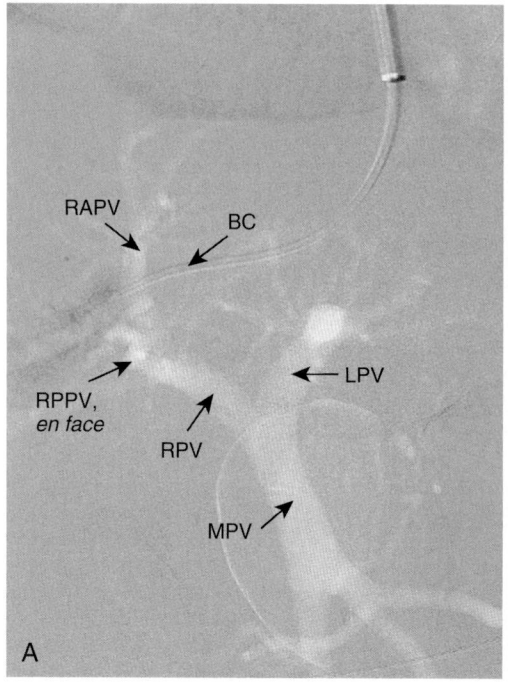

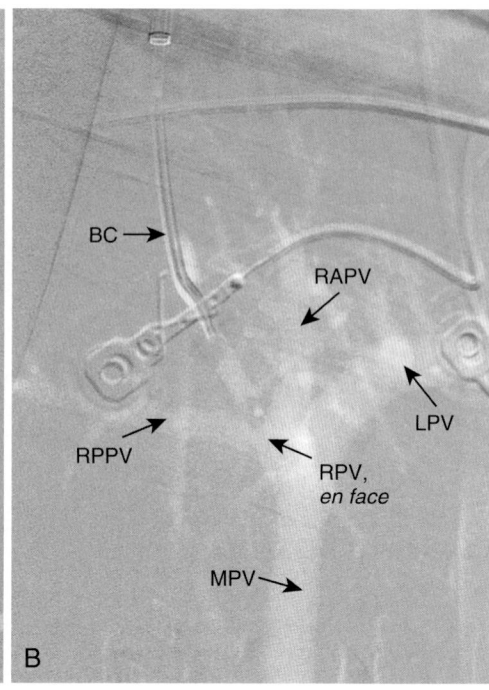

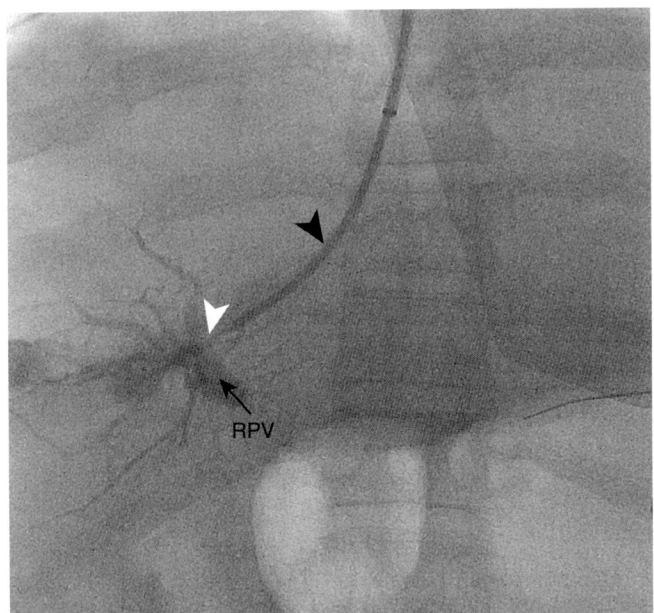

FIGURE 3 Frontal unsubtracted venogram via a needle *(white arrowhead)* after it was advanced from the right hepatic vein through a catheter *(black arrowhead)* toward the right portal vein (RPV). Contrast fills branches of the right portal vein with hepatopetal blood flow.

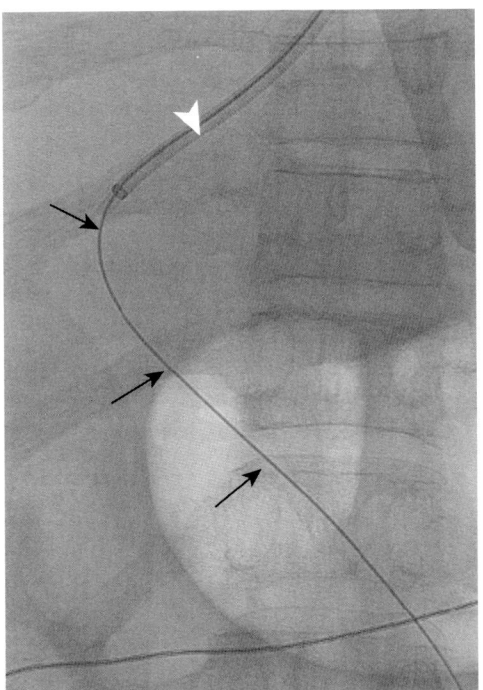

FIGURE 4 After the needle is confirmed to be in the targeted portal vein branch, a wire is advanced through it into the portal vein *(black arrows)*. Note the location of the right internal jugular sheath *(white arrowhead)*. The wire now crosses from the right hepatic vein, through a short segment of liver parenchyma, and into the right portal vein.

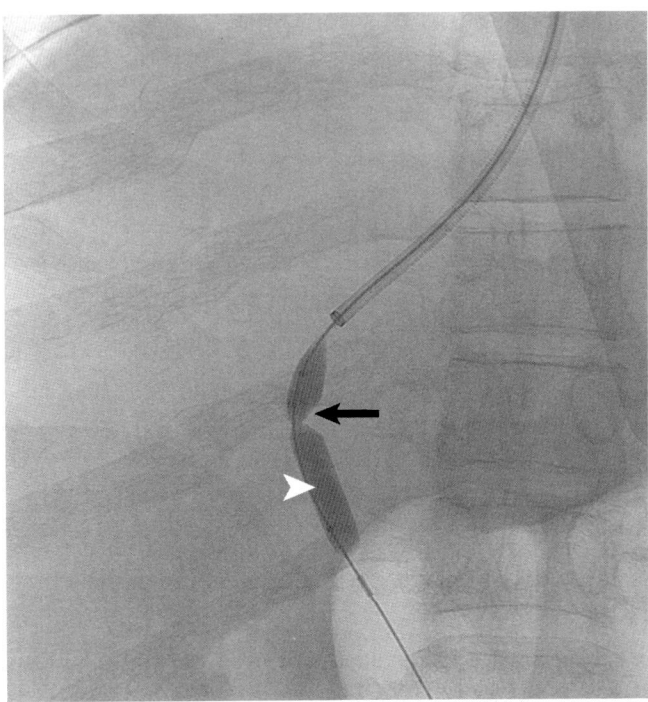

FIGURE 5 Because cirrhotic liver is difficult to cross, it is predilated with a small balloon *(white arrowhead)* to facilitate the necessary sheath exchanges. The "waist" *(black arrow)* in the middle of the balloon reveals just how hard the liver parenchyma can be.

for direct portal pressure measurement and a portal venogram. The venogram will be used to select the appropriate length stent to be placed (Figure 6).

If the direct portal pressure is within normal limits, TIPS creation is abandoned irrespective of the clinical picture. If a TIPS is not possible or is contraindicated, the gastroesophageal varices can be embolized via a catheter to stop the hemorrhage without placing a TIPS. Though this is very effective, it is nevertheless temporary; the ongoing portal hypertension will likely cause new varices to form.

The stent is advanced through the larger sheath, which keeps it constrained and in position. The sheath is pulled back into the right atrium, uncovering the stent. The distal 2 cm of the stent is uncovered and flares out upon withdrawal of the sheath. The rest of the stent is "rip-corded" open once it is in the appropriate position (Figure 7).

Shunt Evaluation

Usually, a 10-mm–diameter stent is used and initially balloon-dilated up to 8 mm in diameter. The direct portal pressure is measured again, and if it is not satisfactory, a 10-mm balloon is used to open the stent to capacity (Figure 8). The smaller the stent diameter, the less the chance for encephalopathy post procedure. A final portal venogram is performed to document flow and lack of variceal filling (Figure 9).

Special Cases

Budd-Chiari Syndrome

The creation of a TIPS in a patient with Budd-Chiari syndrome is especially challenging because the hepatic veins are thrombosed. This

FIGURE 6 Frontal unsubtracted **(A)** and subtracted **(B)** venograms. Simultaneous contrast injection **(A)** via the right internal jugular sheath *(white arrowhead)* and marker catheter *(black arrows)* in the portal vein allows for calculation of the required length of the stent. Note the esophageal varices *(white arrow)* arising from the left gastric vein. A wider field of view with digital subtraction **(B)** shows to greater effect the ominous esophageal *(black arrowhead)* and gastric *(asterisk)* varices. *IMV,* Inferior mesenteric vein; *LGV,* left gastric vein; *SMV,* superior mesenteric vein; *SpV,* splenic vein.

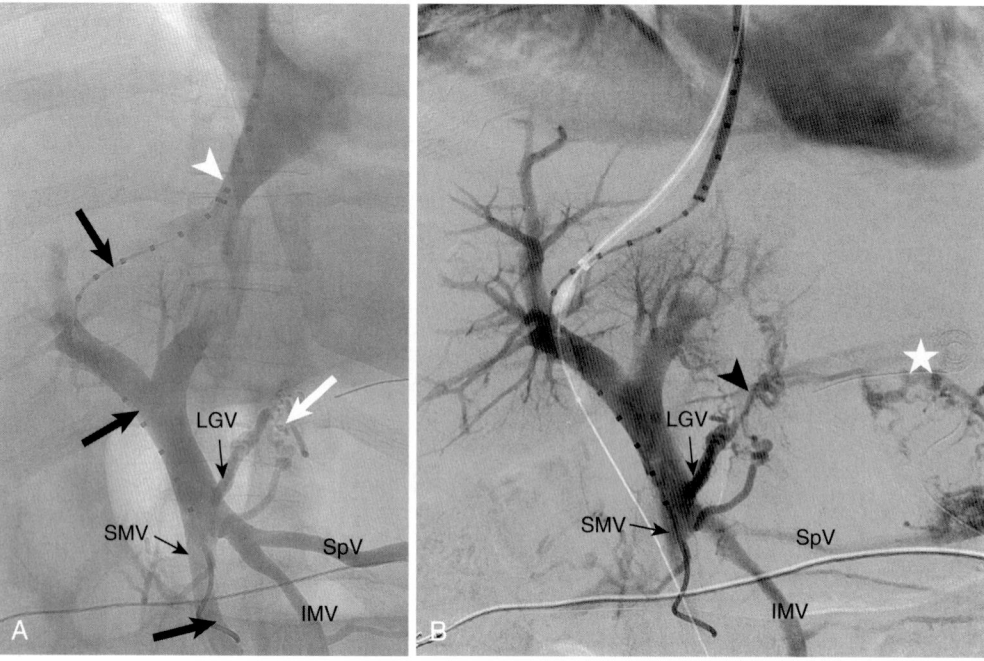

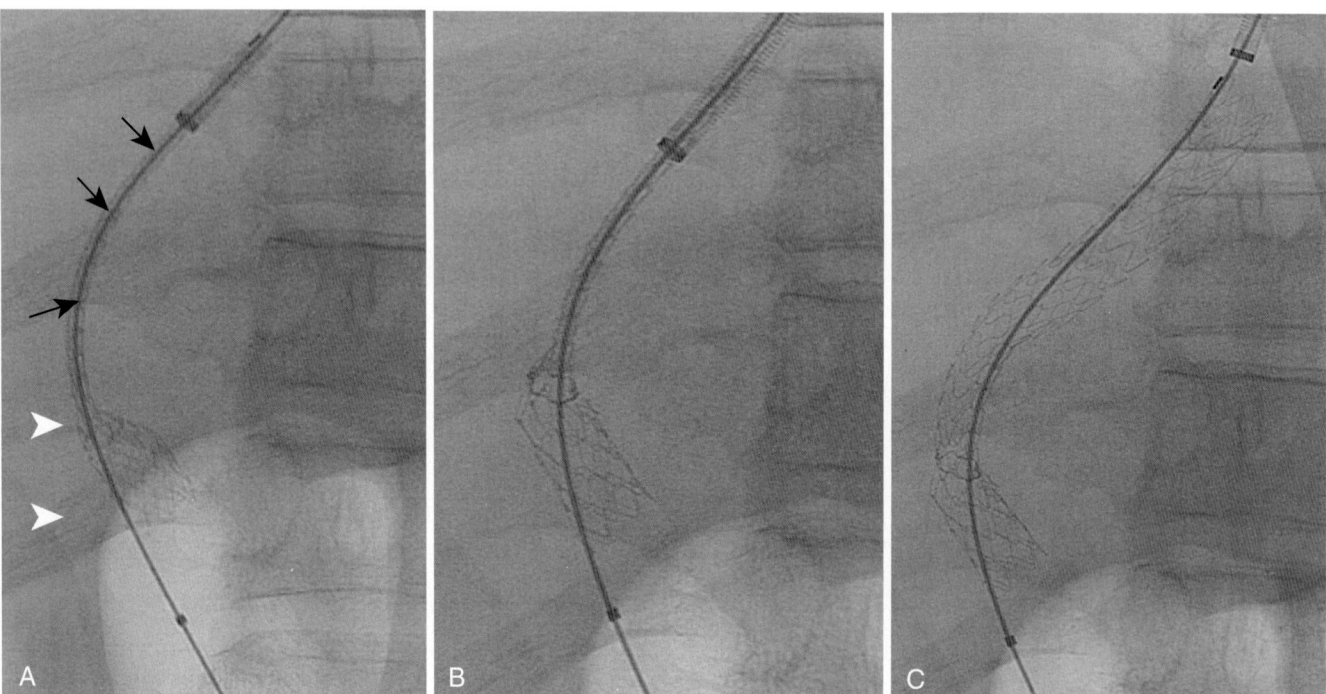

FIGURE 7 Frontal views of the deployment sequence of a TIPS stent. The stent is first advanced via a sheath through the right hepatic vein, across the liver parenchyma, and into the portal vein. **A,** The stent's distal 2 cm *(arrowheads)* are constrained only by the sheath, and once the sheath is pulled back, it springs open. The remainder of the stent *(black arrows)* remains undeployed. The entire system is then gently withdrawn until the proximal end of the distal 2 cm hits the parenchymal tract **(B)**. Once the operator judges the stent to be in proper position the remainder of the stent is opened by pulling on the rip cord **(C)**.

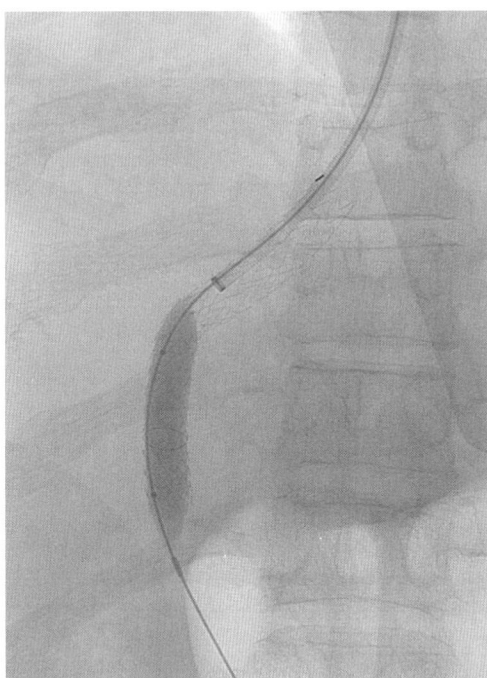

FIGURE 8   After TIPS placement, a balloon is used to open the stent to the desired diameter. The objective is to open the stent to the minimum diameter required to reduce the portal pressure to the desired level.

shows as the classic spider vein appearance on a hepatic venogram (Figure 10). Though it is best if the TIPS is placed from hepatic vein to portal vein, the lack of patent hepatic veins may necessitate an inferior vena cava (IVC) to portal vein TIPS through the caudate lobe, a so-called direct intrahepatic portocaval shunt (DIPS).

Parallel TIPS

Rarely, despite a previous TIPS, the patient's symptoms may not be completely alleviated. If portal hypertension and variceal bleeding are a persistent problem despite a TIPS, or if the first TIPS thromboses, a second TIPS may be placed utilizing the other hepatic and portal veins (Figure 11).

Transumbilical or Direct Portal Access

When access into the portal vein is challenging due to anatomy, the operator has two other options. First, access into the umbilical vein, which is usually dilated, provides a conduit into the left portal vein. A catheter there allows opacification of the portal venous system, which provides a better target for TIPS (Figure 12). Second, access through a naturally occurring portosystemic shunt, such as a splenorenal shunt, can sometimes be used to gain access to the portal circulation. When the umbilical vein is not accessible and a natural portosystemic shunt does not exist, direct percutaneous access into the right or left portal vein can allow for contrast opacification and targeting (Figure 13).

TIPS Reversal/Revision

Occasionally a TIPS reversal or revision is necessary. Limited liver reserve and/or overzealous shunting may result in liver failure or intractable encephalopathy. In such cases the interventionalist has the option to decrease the shunting or shut down the TIPS altogether. Several maneuvers exists to reduce shunting, including placing a stent

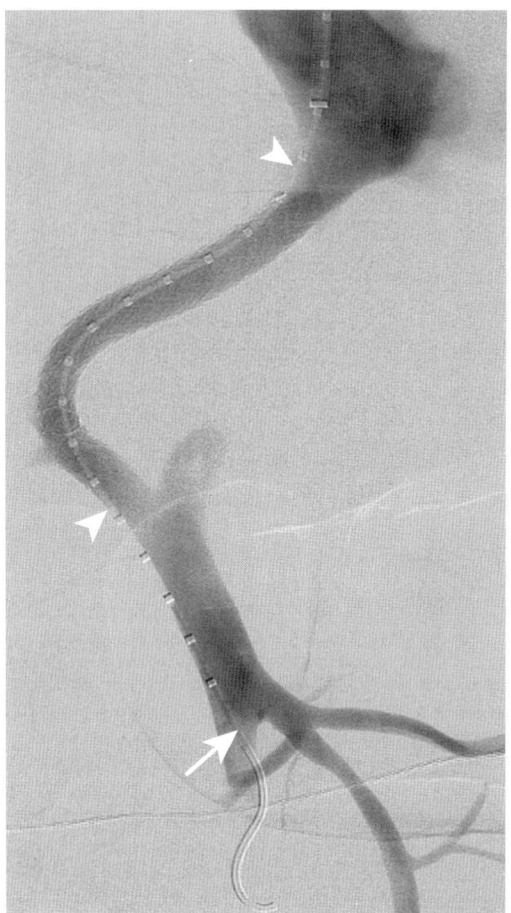

FIGURE 9   Frontal view of a portal venogram via a catheter *(arrow)* after TIPS placement *(arrowheads)*. Note the antegrade flow of contrast into the right atrium and no contrast filling the varices. Compare to Figure 6.

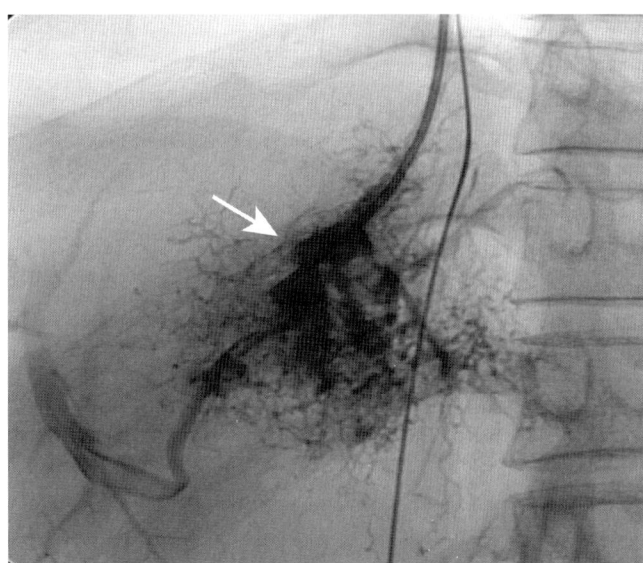

FIGURE 10   Frontal subtracted hepatic venogram in a patient with Budd-Chiari. Hepatic venogram shows the "spider-like" appearance *(arrow)* of multiple small collateral draining veins.

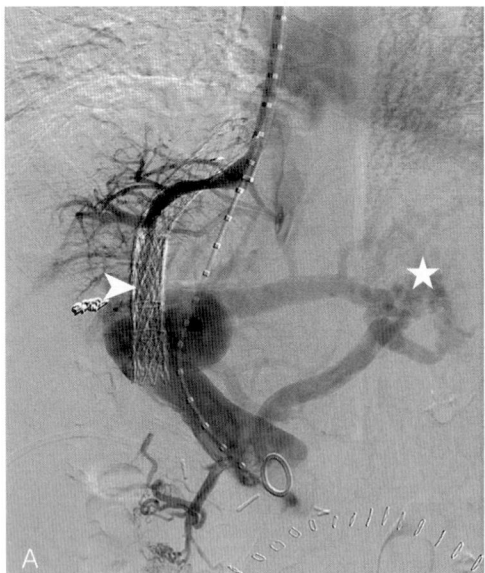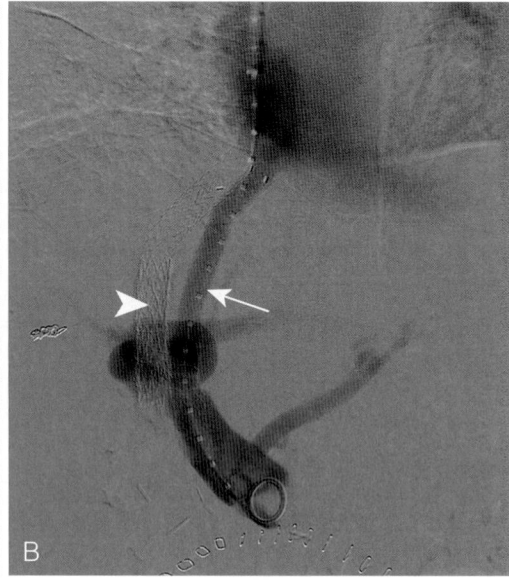

FIGURE 11 Frontal subtracted portal venogram **(A)** via a catheter placed through the middle hepatic vein shows the previously placed right hepatic to right portal vein TIPS (*arrowhead*) to be occluded. Because of this, the patient had recurrent bleeding from gastric varices (*asterisk*). Repeat portal venogram **(B)** after placement of a parallel TIPS (*arrow*) shows antegrade flow into the right atrium and decompression of the varices. The occluded right hepatic to right portal vein TIPS (*arrowhead*) is medial to the new parallel TIPS (*arrow*).

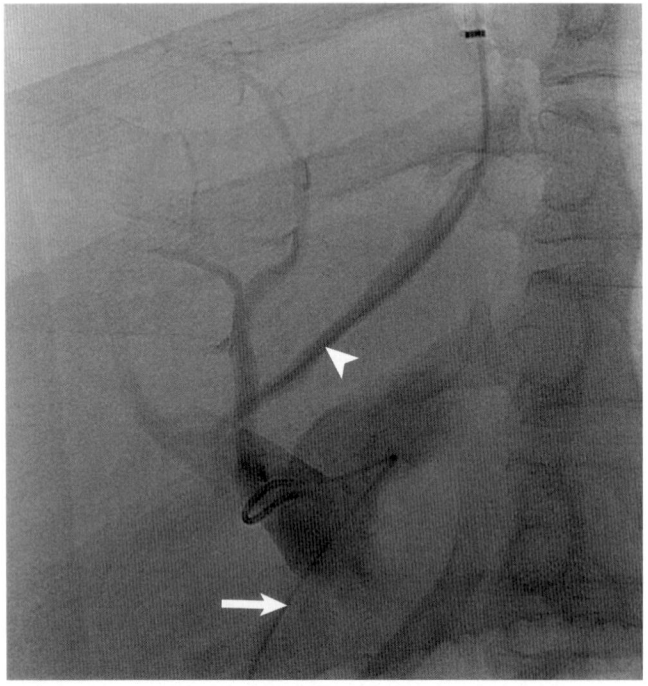

FIGURE 12 Superficially accessible portosystemic collateral vessels can be used to access and opacify the portal venous system for targeting prior to needle advancement. Here, a percutaneously placed transumbilical vein (*arrow*) opacifies the portal branches. A catheter (*arrowhead*) is seen traversing the parenchymal tract between the right hepatic vein and right portal vein.

within the TIPS, or two stents side by side, or even a "waisted" (hourglass-like) stent. If these interventions are not possible or are inadequate, then the entire TIPS can be shut down. TIPS shutdown is a rarely performed and is an advanced procedure beyond the scope of this text.

CLINICAL OUTCOMES

Clinical Response to TIPS

TIPS is the most effective option for treating gastroesophageal variceal bleeding. The rebleeding rate after TIPS placement is 4% per year—the lowest among all treatment options, including endoscopic management. TIPS is reserved after failure of endoscopic management only because of the greater risks associated with it, particularly encephalopathy. Cessation of bleeding is evident almost immediately after TIPS creation.

TIPS has also been shown to be very effective in treating ascites, and it reduces the risk of ascites by 50% to 80% over the life of the patient. Additionally, TIPS has been shown to improve survival and transplant-free survival compared to other treatment options. Resolution of ascites may take up to 4 weeks after TIPS placement.

In patients with hepatorenal syndrome, TIPS improves renal function in 62% of patients. However, it is occasionally difficult to distinguish non–cirrhotic-related chronic renal insufficiency from hepatorenal syndrome.

Complications and Management

The complications related to TIPS are shown in Table 3. The most feared complication is liver failure, which usually results from excessive portohepatic venous shunting in a liver with limited baseline reserve. If patients with no liver reserve are appropriately excluded, the risk of liver failure is 2% to 4%.

Encephalopathy can be seen in up to 12% of patients with compensated liver disease and in up to 50% of patients with noncompensated liver disease. Flagyl and/or lactulose provide significant relief for such patients, but a small percentage (~4%) will not respond and may require TIPS reversal.

Death from sepsis is rare (~4%) but very difficult to treat. Bacteremia results in TIPS stent seeding ("endotipsitis"), which can be very challenging or impossible to treat. Broad-spectrum antibiotics may

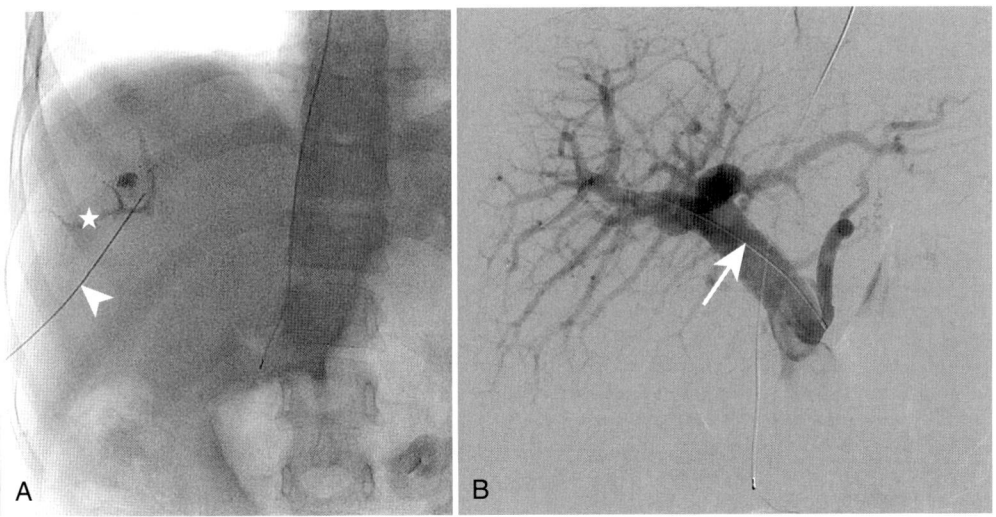

FIGURE 13   In cases where no other option is available, direct percutaneous portal vein access **(A)** can be useful. A needle *(arrowhead)* is placed under ultrasound guidance into the portal venous system, which is then opacified with contrast *(asterisk).* **B,** A catheter *(arrow)* is advanced into the main portal vein, where a portal venogram is performed and targeted for TIPS creation from the right hepatic vein.

TABLE 3: Complications related to TIPS

Complication	Frequency	Predisposing factors	Mitigating factors
TIPS dysfunction	Occlusion/stenosis: 18%-78% Thrombosis: 10%-15%	Uncovered stents Smaller-diameter stents Stent-migration/suboptimal placement	Choice of stent Precise deployment Venoplasty and/or restenting
Encephalopathy	In compensated liver disease: up to 12% In uncompensated liver disease: up to 50% Requiring TIPS reversal: 4%	History of encephalopathy High ammonia levels Limited reserve Increased age	Reduce or close the TIPS Metronidazole or lactulose
Bleeding	Hemobilia: <5% Intraperitoneal bleeding: 1%-2%	Difficult anatomy Abnormal coagulation profile	Correct coagulation profile
Sepsis	2%-10%	Active infection	Treat infection prior to TIPS
Renal failure	Highly variable	Elevated creatinine Dehydration Diabetes High contrast load	Hydrate Use carbon dioxide contrast
Liver failure/hepatic infarction	2%-4%	Limited reserve High bilirubin Overshunting	Reduce or close the TIPS

TIPS, Transjugular intrahepatic portosystemic shunt.

clear the bacteremia, but in some cases it recurs after cessation of treatment because the seeded stent elutes more bacteria. Active infection is an absolute contraindication to TIPS, and any infection must be cleared prior to intervention.

The overall post-TIPS 30-day mortality ranges from less than 10% to up to 40%. The higher mortality rate is seen in patients with poorly compensated liver disease who are having a TIPS created on an emergent basis, usually for life-threatening variceal bleeding. For patients with compensated liver disease who are having a TIPS

created on an elective basis, mortality is less than 5%. It is therefore important to carefully select patients and refer for TIPS placement before it manifests into an emergency.

The Model for End-Stage Liver Disease (MELD) score, routinely used to predict survival in patients with end-stage liver disease and to allocate liver transplants, was initially developed to predict poor survival in patients after creation of a TIPS. The cutoff score for high-risk short-term mortality (expected survival less than 3 months after TIPS creation) in the initial MELD study was 18. The MELDNa score, which incorporates serum sodium with the serum INR, bilirubin, and creatinine of MELD, has been shown to be a more accurate predictor of risk post-TIPS (MELDNa ≥15). Both versions of the MELD score are more accurate predictors of risk after TIPS than the Child-Pugh score.

Follow-up

TIPS follow-up is mostly based on clinical signs and symptoms. Ultrasound surveillance can be useful. However, false-positive reports (of occluded stent) can result if ultrasound is performed too soon after TIPS creation. The newly placed TIPS has air trapped within it, which limits ultrasound penetration and can simulate the sonographic appearance of an occluded TIPS. Waiting at least 2 weeks after TIPS for the air to be absorbed is generally adequate to avoid this problem. Recurrent variceal bleeding or ascites are a very specific indicator of TIPS restenosis or occlusion and should prompt a diagnostic venogram and/or intervention. There is a 10% rate of reintervention for stenosed or occluded TIPS. The 1-year primary unassisted patency rate for ePTFE covered stents is 80% to 85%. There is no role for the use of uncovered bare metal stents because their restenosis rate after TIPS creation is unjustifiably high.

SUMMARY

The most important determinant of clinical outcomes after TIPS placement is proper patient selection and preparation. Cirrhotic patients with portal hypertension should be under surveillance and should be referred for TIPS after conservative management fails but before the complications of portal hypertension manifest into an emergency. This, along with optimal patient preparation, can help reduce the morbidity and mortality related to TIPS to the lowest possible levels. Additionally, the introduction of expanded polytetrafluoroethylene stents has improved the efficacy and patency rate of TIPS, and many patients survive with a TIPS for many years. The benefits of a TIPS include reduced drop-off risk from the transplant list, improved lifestyle quality (i.e., resolution of ascites), as well as reduction in the many portal hypertension–related complications. But most importantly, TIPS often is a life-saving procedure for those with variceal hemorrhage.

Suggested Readings

Bai M, Qi X, Yang Z, et al: Predictors of hepatic encephalopathy after transjugular intrahepatic portosystemic shunt in cirrhotic patients: a systematic review, *J Gastroenterol Hepatol* 26(6):943–951, 2011.

Charon JP, Alaeddin FH, Pimpalwar SA, et al: Results of a retrospective multicenter trial of the Viatorr expanded polytetrafluoroethylene-covered stent-graft for transjugular intrahepatic portosystemic shunt creation, *J Vasc Interv Radio* 15(11):1219–1230, 2004.

Chen L, Xiao T, Chen W, et al: Outcomes of transjugular intrahepatic portosystemic shunt through the left branch vs. the right branch of the portal vein in advanced cirrhosis: a randomized trial, *Liver Int* 29(7):1101–1109, 2009.

Eesa M, Clark T: Transjugular intrahepatic portosystemic shunt: state of the art, *Semin Roentgenol* 46(2):125–132, 2011.

García-Pagán JC, Caca K, Bureau C, et al: Early TIPS (Transjugular Intrahepatic Portosystemic Shunt) Cooperative Study Group. Early use of TIPS in patients with cirrhosis and variceal bleeding, *N Engl J Med* 362(25):2370–2379, 2010.

Guy J, Somsouk M, Shiboski S, et al: New model for end stage liver disease improves prognostic capability after transjugular intrahepatic portosystemic shunt, *Clin Gastroenterol Hepatol* 7(11):1236–1240, 2009.

Hausegger KA, Karnel F, Georgieva B, et al: Transjugular intrahepatic portosystemic shunt creation with the Viatorr expanded polytetrafluoroethylene-covered stent-graft, *J Vasc Interv Radiol* 15(3):239–248, 2004.

Lo GH, Liang HL, Chen WC, et al: A prospective, randomized controlled trial of transjugular intrahepatic portosystemic shunt versus cyanoacrylate injection in the prevention of gastric variceal rebleeding, *Endoscopy* 39(8):679–685, 2007.

Malinchoc M, Kamath PS, Gordon FD, et al: A model to predict poor survival in patients undergoing transjugular intrahepatic portosystemic shunts, *Hepatology* 31(4):864–871, 2000.

Narahara Y, Kanazawa H, Fukuda T, et al: Transjugular intrahepatic portosystemic shunt versus paracentesis plus albumin in patients with refractory ascites who have good hepatic and renal function: a prospective randomized trial, *J Gastroenterol* 46(1):78–85, 2011.

Rössle M, Gerbes AL: TIPS for the treatment of refractory ascites, hepatorenal syndrome and hepatic hydrothorax: a critical update, *Gut* 59(7):988–1000, 2010.

Salerno F, Cammà C, Enea M, et al: Transjugular intrahepatic portosystemic shunt for refractory ascites: a meta-analysis of individual patient data, *Gastroenterology* 133(5):1746, 2007.

Senzolo M, M Sartori T, Rossetto V, et al: Prospective evaluation of anticoagulation and transjugular intrahepatic portosistemic shunt for the management of portal vein thrombosis in cirrhosis, *Liver Int* 32(6):919–927, 2012.

Silva RF, Arroyo PC Jr, Duca WJ, et al: Complications following transjugular intrahepatic portosystemic shunt: a retrospective analysis, *Transplant Proc* 36 (4):926–928, 2004.

Wong F: Recent advances in our understanding of hepatorenal syndrome, *Nat Rev Gastroenterol Hepatol* 9(7):382–391, 2012.

Yang Z, Han G, Wu Q, et al: Patency and clinical outcomes of transjugular intrahepatic portosystemic shunt with polytetrafluoroethylene-covered stents versus bare stents: a meta-analysis, *J Gastroenterol Hepatol* 25(11):1718–1725, 2010.

Zheng M, Chen Y, Bai J, et al: Transjugular intrahepatic portosystemic shunt versus endoscopic therapy in the secondary prophylaxis of variceal rebleeding in cirrhotic patients: meta-analysis update, *J Clin Gastroenterol* 42(5):507–516, 2008.

THE MANAGEMENT OF REFRACTORY ASCITES

Nyan L. Latt, MD, and Ahmet Gurakar, MD

INTRODUCTION

Ascites is defined as an abnormal accumulation of fluid in the peritoneal cavity due to portal hypertension, renal function, plasma hydrostatic-oncotic pressure imbalance, and endogenous vasoactive substances. Although cirrhosis of the liver is the primary etiology for more than 80% of patients with ascites, a small portion of ascites can be caused by other conditions such as malignancies (e.g., peritoneal carcinomatosis), infectious causes (e.g., abdominal tuberculosis), congestive heart failure, nephrotic syndrome, hepatic vein obstruction, pancreatic diseases, and miscellaneous disorders of the peritoneum. It is vital to diagnose the cause of ascites initially because the management can be very different, depending on the etiology. For a practicing surgeon, the presence of ascites is particularly important for preoperative risk assessment because most patients with ascites develop severe hepatic dysfunction, poor nutritional status, and electrolyte imbalances, which increase overall perioperative risks.

This chapter provides various pharmacologic and surgical treatment options and the rationale behind them in the management of refractory ascites. The pathophysiology of ascites and diagnostic modalities are briefly discussed to provide a better understanding of the different therapeutic approaches.

PATHOPHYSIOLOGY

The first hypothesis of ascites formation was the "backward theory" in early 1960s, in which portal hypertension and hypoalbuminemia lead to excessive splanchnic lymph formation, which causes the thoracic duct to flow backward to the heart and then extravasate into the peritoneal space. The backward flow theory was discredited later when it was found that systemic vasodilatation, caused by decreased systemic vascular resistance secondary to increased plasma volume and cardiac output. The "overflow theory," again, was dismissed later when studies showed that angiotensin-II blockade induced a significant reduction of the wedged hepatic venous pressure without any change in the hepatic blood flow. This finding suggests that arterial vasodilation is not systemic but rather confined to the regional splanchnic circulation.

The currently accepted hypothesis for the mechanism of ascites in cirrhosis is the "peripheral arterial vasodilation" theory. The primary causative effect is sinusoidal portal hypertension secondary to progressive hepatic fibrosis. Portal hypertension induces the release of nitric oxide and vasodilator peptides, which causes the splanchnic arterial vasodilation. The arterial vasodilation in the splanchnic circuit leads to reduced effective arterial blood volume, which activates vasoconstrictors and sodium-retaining systems, resulting in renal sodium retention. Therefore, high sodium concentration increases splanchnic capillary permeability and causes ascites formation.

Refractory Ascites

Ascites that are not responsive to sodium restriction and maximal diuretic therapy are called refractory ascites. The responsiveness to

therapy is determined by weight loss and the negative balance of sodium. Ascites of patients who develop complications such as hepatic encephalopathy, renal insufficiency, and hyponatremia after diuretics therapy are also considered refractory. Refractory ascites represent less than 10% of all ascites.

Diagnosis of Ascites

All patients with new-onset ascites or all patients with known ascites on admission should get diagnostic paracentesis because 10% to 25% of these patients can present with spontaneous bacterial peritonitis (SBP) without overt clinical signs and symptoms.

Analysis of ascitic fluid can help determine the etiology of the underlying conditions as well as detect causative microorganisms in infectious processes. Cell counts, gram stains, cultures, albumin, total protein, glucose, and LDH from ascitic fluid should be sent to the laboratory for analysis. Triglyceride levels should be added in suspected cases of chylous ascites. Cytology should be sent in suspected malignancies. Serum albumin, total protein, and LDH should be sent at the same time to compare serum-ascitic gradients. Testing serum for CA-125 is not necessary to make a diagnosis of ascites. Its use is not recommended in patients with ascites of any type.

To determine the etiology of ascites, the current recommendation is to calculate the serum-ascites albumin gradient (SAAG) rather than differentiate transudates from exudates. SAAG is based on the plasma oncotic-hydrostatic pressure balance and is directly related to portal pressure.

$$SAAG = Serum\ albumin - Ascitic\ albumin$$

The etiologies of ascites, according to SAAG, are shown in Table 1.

Paracentesis

Although most cirrhotic patients have prolonged prothrombin time and thrombocytopenia, there is no evidence supporting significant bleeding from paracentesis in this population. Routine transfusion of platelets or fresh frozen plasma is not recommended to perform paracentesis. The major contraindication for paracentesis is disseminated vascular coagulopathy (DIC).

The preferred site for needle entry is 3 cm medial and 3 cm superior to the anterior superior iliac spine on the left lower quadrant of the abdomen. The midline approach is not preferable because many patients are obese. The right lower quadrant also is not desirable because cecum can become distended in patients who take lactulose. The distended cecum has a higher risk of perforation. The needle should not be inserted in areas with cutaneous infection, abdominal wall hematoma, scars, or visibly engorged subcutaneous veins. Bedside ultrasound, if available, is useful, especially in ascites accumulated in compartments.

The paracentesis needle can be inserted by using either the angular technique or the Z-track technique. In the angular technique, the needle is inserted obliquely from the cutaneous site into the peritoneum. In Z-track, cutaneous tissues are pulled down, and the needle is inserted straight into the peritoneum. The purpose of these techniques is to ensure that cutaneous and peritoneal sites do not directly overlap each other, thereby minimizing ascetic fluid leakage (Figure 1).

Treatments of Ascites

The pathophysiology of ascites formation from cirrhosis is due to renal retention of sodium and water. Therefore, the goal of the treatment is to mobilize the ascitic fluid by creating a net negative balance

TABLE 1: Etiologies of ascites with or without portal hypertension

SAAG ≥1.1 g/dL: portal hypertension	SAAG <1.1 g/dL: no portal hypertension
• Cirrhosis • Alcoholic hepatitis • Vascular obstructions (Budd-Chiari syndrome or portal vein thrombosis) • Congestive heart failure • Metastasis to liver • Fatty liver disease of pregnancy • Myxedema	• Peritoneal carcinomatosis • Nephrotic syndrome • Pancreatitis • Peritoneal tuberculosis • Serositis

SAAG, Serum-ascites albumin gradient.

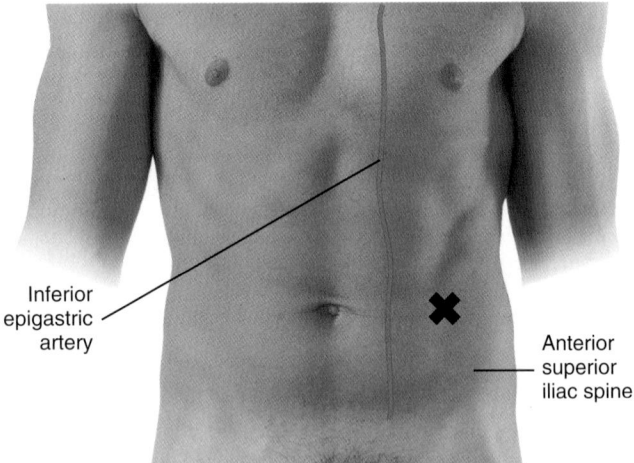

FIGURE 1 Preferred needle entry site for paracentesis. *(From Drake and Vogel: Gray's atlas of anatomy. Philadelphia: Churchill Livingstone, 2007.)*

of sodium. Net negative sodium balance can be achieved with decreasing sodium intake and increasing sodium secretion. Urinary sodium excretion in cirrhosis plays a role as a prognostic factor. While spot Ur Na++ less than 10 mg/dL represents only 20% in 2-year survival, Ur Na++ over 10 mg/dL represents 60% in 2-year survival among cirrhotic patients. The treatment of low-SAAG ascites should concentrate on underlying causes.

Nonpharmacologic Therapies

Dietary Sodium Restriction

Restriction of dietary sodium intake is one of the most important nonpharmacologic treatments of ascites because renal sodium retention is the key contributing factor of ascites formation. When sodium intake surpasses urinary and insensible losses of sodium, net positive sodium balance retains extra fluid, causing ascites and peripheral edema. The goal is to create a negative net balance of sodium, thereby contracting extracellular fluid volume. Fluid restriction is not necessary in patients with cirrhosis who are on diuretic therapy and sodium restriction.

A typical American diet usually contains 4 to 6 g of sodium per day. About one third of this sodium comes from salt, another one third comes from processed foods, and the rest is from water and other foods (meat, vegetables, etc.). Daily sodium restriction of 1.5

to 2 g is recommended. One teaspoon of table salt contains 2300 mg of sodium, which is more than the recommended daily sodium intake. It is very important for patients not to add any salt to their food at all. Staying away from all processed foods is also essential because processed foods contain a lot of sodium for preservation. Patients should be instructed to replace processed meats and vegetables with fresh or frozen and also to avoid eating at fast-food restaurants because processed food is their main ingredient.

Patients should keep a record of what they eat, including portion size and sodium content. Patients should weigh themselves and record their weight every day as well. Compliance is the most important part of this treatment because most patients fail to stick to a low-sodium diet. The progress of treatment can simply be monitored with daily weight, but there are objective measures to prove noncompliance in patients. Although the most accurate measurement is 24-hour urinary sodium, it is not practical to obtain, especially in outpatient settings. On the other hand, a spot urinary sample can easily be collected. It has been shown that a spot urinary Na+/K+ ratio of greater than 1 represents 24-hour sodium intake of greater than 2 g, indicating noncompliance. In such patients, nutrition counseling with a registered dietitian referral might be helpful.

In cirrhosis, only 15% to 20% of patients can achieve negative sodium balance by restricting dietary sodium intake, without diuretics. Therefore, diuretic therapy should be started on these patients, along with sodium restriction from the beginning of treatment.

Fluid Restriction

Restriction of daily fluid intake to 1 to 1.5 L per day is usually not necessary in patients with ascites because an adequate negative sodium balance can help eliminate excess free water. The only benefit of fluid restriction can be observed in patients with profound hyponatremia—that is, serum Na+ less than 125 mg/dL.

Pharmacologic Therapies

Diuretics

Most patients with cirrhosis need to take diuretic agents to control their ascites in addition to dietary sodium restriction. Diuretics increase renal sodium excretion, thereby achieving net negative sodium balance and eliminating excess fluid accumulated in extracellular spaces. The most commonly used diuretics are potassium-sparing aldosterone antagonists (e.g., spironolactone or amiloride) and loop diuretics (e.g., furosemide).

There are two strategies of treating ascites with diuretic agents. The first regimen begins with an aldosterone antagonist alone. The dose of spironolactone is increased every week to its maximal dose until the clinical response is achieved. If there is no response after maximal dose of spironolactone, furosemide should be added, and its dose should be increased every week. In the second approach, both spironolactone and furosemide are started as a combination from the beginning of treatment, and the doses are increased weekly with regard to clinical response and measurement of urinary sodium excretion. Studies have shown that there is no significant difference in terms of efficacy and incidence of complications between these two regimens.

The doses of diuretics are generally higher than doses started for hypertension or heart failure. The starting doses of spironolactone and furosemide are 100 mg and 40 mg per day, and the maximal doses are 400 mg and 160 mg per day, respectively. The therapeutic response can simply be monitored with daily weight. The goal of effective diuresis is losing 2 pounds per day in patients with peripheral edema and 1 pound per day without edema because the highest absorptive capacity of the peritoneal cavity is approximately 0.5 L per day. Overdiuresis can induce severe electrolyte imbalances and renal failure. A spot urinary Na+/K+ ratio of greater than 1 has a 90%

sensitivity in predicting a negative balance (>78 mmol/day sodium excretion).

The advantages of using aldosterone antagonists and loop diuretics together are counterregulatory effect on potassium reabsorption, greater natriuretic potency, and earlier onset of diuresis. Thiazide diuretics are not recommended, in general, despite their synergistic effect in blocking sodium reabsorption in distal tubules when used together with loop diuretics. Thiazides plus loop diuretics can cause significant hypokalemia and hyperammonemia via various mechanisms. In cirrhosis, hyperammonemia can result in hepatic encephalopathy. In individuals who develop gynecomastia due to spironolactone use, amiloride can be substituted. Other loop diuretic agents, such as torsemide and bumetanide, can also be used safely and effectively in cirrhotic patients with ascites. Diuretic agents should be discontinued when there are diuretic-induced complications, such as severe hyponatremia (serum Na^+ <120 mg/dL), renal failure, or hepatic encephalopathy.

Albumin

Hypoalbuminemia is a common complication of liver failure in cirrhosis because albumin is mainly synthesized in the liver. Albumin is a plasma volume expander, and it plays a crucial role in maintaining plasma oncotic pressure. On the other hand, as mentioned above, the pathogenesis of ascites is due to increased splanchnic arterial vasodilation, causing decreased effective plasma volume. In addition, intravenous albumin has a short half-life, and it is not cost-effective. Therefore, albumin should not be used routinely in the management of ascites. On the other hand, albumin infusions are very effective in preventing renal dysfunction associated with spontaneous bacterial peritonitis. Recently, concomitant use of albumin and vasoconstrictors has been shown to improve circulatory hemodynamics, renal function, and control of ascites.

Vasoconstrictors

Vasoconstrictors have been used in the management of hepatorenal syndrome and the prevention of hemodynamic instability after large volume paracentesis (LVP), along with albumin. Recent studies have shown that the use of vasoconstrictors in cirrhotic patients with preserved renal function improves sodium excretion, circulatory function, and ascites control. Various vasopressors have been studied for this purpose. Octreotide, a somatostatin analogue, can cause splanchnic vasoconstriction and improve renal perfusion. Midodrine, an α_1-receptor agonist, can also be used along with octreotide

and albumin. A randomized pilot study showed that midodrine plus standard medical therapy (sodium restriction, diuretics, and large volume paracentesis [LVP]) is superior to standard medical therapy alone for the control of ascites without any renal or hepatic dysfunction. Terlipressin, a vasopressin derivative, also induces splanchnic vasoconstriction and can be used to control ascites. Although terlipressin is not available in the United States, it has been widely used for hepatorenal syndrome in Europe and other parts of the world. A recent study showed that terlipressin plus diuretics and albumin might improve the outcomes of refractory ascites by increasing urinary sodium excretion and decreasing the need for LVP (Table 2).

Interventional Therapies

Patients with ascites, which are refractory to nonpharmacologic treatment options, often require additional interventional approaches to control their ascites. Interventional therapies include serial LVP, a transjugular intrahepatic portosystemic shunt (TIPS), a peritoneovenous shunt, and, ultimately, liver transplantation.

Large Volume Paracentesis

LVP, or therapeutic paracentesis, has been used in the management of cirrhosis patients with ascites for centuries, long before the discovery of diuretic agents. In LVP, 4 to 5 liters of ascitic fluid are removed. Randomized controlled trials have demonstrated that LVP can be performed safely and effectively every 2 weeks, even in patients with minimal urine sodium excretion. It can be performed either in an outpatient clinic or in a hospital setting. One controversy that has erupted over LVP is postparacentesis albumin infusion. Many studies have failed to reveal that albumin infusion after LVP has mortality or morbidity benefits, while significant improvements have been observed in electrolyte imbalances, plasma rennin, and creatinine levels. Since albumin is very expensive, it is not cost-effective to use routinely after LVP of 4 to 5 liters. In cases of larger amounts of ascitic fluid removal (i.e., 6 to 8 liters), however, albumin infusion should be considered to maintain homeostatic fluid balance.

Transjugular Intrahepatic Portosystemic Shunts

Although TIPS was pioneered by Dr. Josef Rosch in 1969, it was not in clinical practice until the late 1990s due to technical difficulties. Later, TIPS was used to decrease portal hypertension in the management of refractory variceal hemorrhage. However, it was found that

TABLE 2: Summary of medical therapy for refractory ascites

Category and action	Drugs	Dose	Remarks
Diuretics			
Aldosterone antagonist	Spironolactone	100 mg to 400 mg PO daily	Monotherapy or combination with furosemide
Epithelial sodium channel blocker	Amiloride	10 mg to 40 mg PO daily	Substitute for spironolactone in cases with gynecomastia
Loop diuretics (torsemide and bumetanide can be used)	Furosemide	40 mg to 160 mg PO daily	Combination with spironolactone
Vasoconstrictors			
Somatostatin analogue	Octreotide	300 mcg twice daily SQ	Can be used in combination with midodrine
α_1-receptor agonist	Midodrine	7.5 mg three times daily PO	Can be used in combination with octreotide and albumin infusion

PO, By mouth; *SQ,* subcutaneous.

TIPS might benefit in eliminating refractory ascites by means of increasing natriuretic effects. The TIPS procedure is essentially done by interventional radiologists in the United States, while some hepatologists perform TIPS in Europe. During the TIPS procedure, a shunt is created between the hepatic vein and the portal vein from a percutaneous jugular venous approach. A stent is then deployed across the shunt to maintain its patency. The major indications for TIPS placement are refractory ascites requiring LVP more frequently than every month, refractory variceal bleeding, and as a bridge to liver transplantation. The absolute contraindication for TIPS placement is worsening hepatic encephalopathy (Figure 2).

Recently, new synthetic fluoropolymer-covered stents have been used in TIPS procedures. A randomized trial showed that polytetrafluoroethylene-coated stents yielded more than twice the duration of patency of metal stents in 1 year. Meta-analyses have established that TIPS can provide better control of ascites and possible improvement in survival, although there are higher rates of hepatic encephalopathy. Reinitiating and titrating up the doses of diuretic agents in post-TIPS patients are reasonable because better natriuresis can be achieved after portal hypertension has been reduced.

Because favorable outcomes have been shown in recent studies, it is recommended that TIPS be performed earlier as a first-line treatment for acute and recurrent variceal bleeding in patients who have hepatic venous pressure gradients higher than 20 mm Hg. Additional benefits of TIPS are potential improvements in nutrition, body mass index, and quality of life in severely malnourished patients with end-stage liver disease.

Peritoneovenous Shunts

A peritoneovenous shunt (PVS) is a shunt that drains ascitic fluid from the peritoneal cavity to the systemic veins such as the internal jugular vein or the superior vena cava. It lies underneath the skin and runs from the abdomen to the upper part of the body. PVSs (also known as LeVeen shunts and Denver shunts) were introduced in the 1970s and were widely used until the late 1980s. Currently, PVSs are not used in clinical practice due to higher rates of complications and the development of newer and safer techniques such as TIPS. The complications associated with a PVS are obstructions (40% of shunt failure in first year) due to kinking/clogging of the shunts and thrombosis, serious infections such as peritonitis and bacteremia,

FIGURE 2 Transjugular intrahepatic portosystemic shunt placement. *(From Johns Hopkins Medical Institutions, used with permission.)*

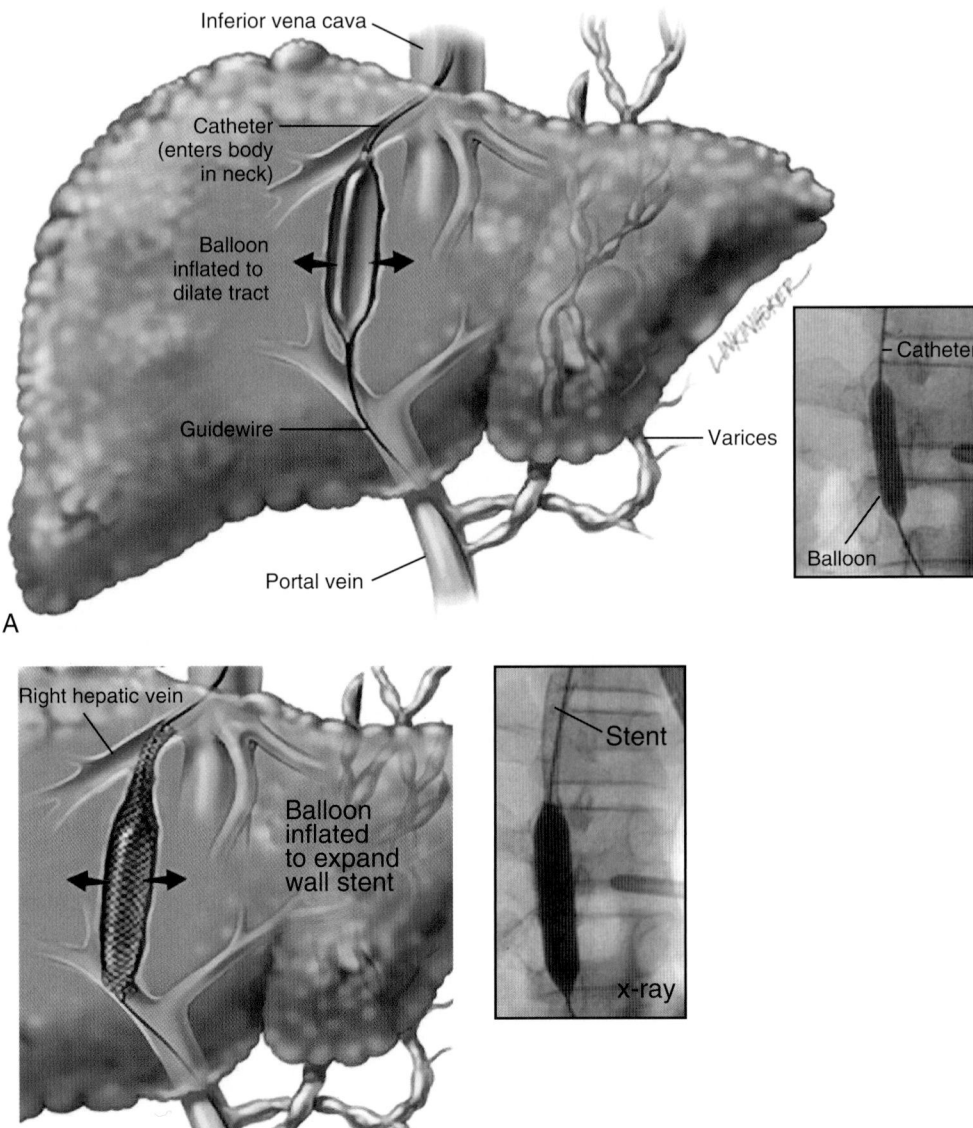

postshunt coagulopathy leading to DIC, pulmonary edema, and increased risk of variceal bleeding secondary to increased venous return and hepatic encephalopathy.

Spontaneous Bacterial Peritonitis

Spontaneous bacterial peritonitis (SBP) is an infection of the peritoneum that spontaneously occurs without any overt source that can be remedied surgically. It is a common complication in patients with portal hypertension and ascites. Approximately 30% of cirrhotic patients with ascites develop SBP, and it is associated with a 20% mortality rate. All hospitalized patients with ascites must have paracentesis for ascitic fluid analysis because clinical signs and symptoms are not sufficient to diagnose SBP. Patients with a previous normal ascitic fluid analysis who later develop abdominal pain, fever, encephalopathy, leukocytosis, or renal failure should have repeat paracentesis. Treating SBP only with empiric antibiotics, without a definitive bacterial culture, is not recommended because it can lead to inadequate therapeutic response and increased resistance of microorganisms.

Treatment of SBP

Ascitic fluid with absolute neutrophil counts more than 250 cells/mm³ is diagnostic for SBP. Empiric antibiotics need to be initiated as soon as possible before the result of bacterial culture is available. Most ascitic fluid culture will grow specific microorganisms, and the antibacterial therapy should be narrowed down. Patients who have negative culture results but have suspicious clinical symptoms of SBP should also be empirically treated with antibiotics. The recommended antibiotic therapies are summarized in Table 3.

Studies have shown that a decrease in mortality was observed in some patients with SBP who received intravenous albumin infusion along with empiric antibiotics. Current guidelines support giving 1.5 g/kg of albumin infusion within 6 hours of SBP diagnosis and 1.0 g/kg of albumin infusion on day 3 in patients with SBP who also have blood urea nitrogen less than 30 mg/dL, serum creatinine over 1 mg/dL, or total bilirubin less than 4 mg/dL.

Patients with ascites may also develop secondary peritonitis involving bowel perforation or intra-abdominal abscess. Clinical signs and symptoms are not helpful in distinguishing secondary peritonitis from SBP, although SBP infection can sometimes present with mild symptoms. It is recommended to perform ascitic fluid analysis for total protein, LDH, and glucose to assist in determination of secondary peritonitis. Elevated ascitic fluid absolute neutrophil counts (in thousands), multiple organisms on gram stains and cultures (including fungi and enterococcus), ascitic fluid total protein over 1 g/dL, ascitic fluid LDH more than half of the upper limit of the serum, and ascitic fluid glucose less than 50 mg/dL are suggestive of secondary peritonitis with 100% sensitivity and 43% specificity. These patients should be evaluated immediately with emergent abdominal x-rays and computed tomographic scanning to look for signs of intra-abdominal perforations or abscesses.

SBP Prophylaxis

Secondary prophylaxis with daily norfloxacin or trimethoprim-sulfamethoxazole is recommended in patients with ascites after the first episode of SBP. Primary prophylaxis for SBP in patients with cirrhosis and ascites is still controversial. Current guidelines support giving primary prophylaxis with oral norfloxacin to patients with ascitic fluid protein less than 1.5 g/dL and at least one of the following: serum creatinine over 1.2 mg/dL, blood urea nitrogen over 25 mg/dL, serum sodium below 130 mEq/L, or Child-Pugh over 9 with serum total bilirubin over 3 mg/dL. In patients with prior SBP who develop acute upper gastrointestinal bleeding, intravenous

TABLE 3: Summary of treatment and prophylaxis in spontaneous bacterial peritonitis

Antibiotics	Route and dosages
Empiric Antibiotics	
First-Line Therapies	
Cefotaxime	2 g IV every 8 hours (or)
Ofloxacin (patients with mild infection with no shock, vomiting)	400 mg PO every 12 hours
Second-Line Therapies	
Ceftriaxone	1 g IV every 12 hours (or)
Ciprofloxacin	400 mg IV every 12 hours (or)
Piperacillin-tazobactam	3.375 g IV every 6 hours (or)
Ertapenem	1 g IV every day for resistant pathogens (or)
Cefepime	1-2 g IV every 8 hours for resistant pathogens (or)
Prophylactic Antibiotics	
First-Line Therapy for Patients with GI Bleeding	
Ceftriaxone	1 g IV every day for 7 days
Secondary-Line Therapy for Patients with GI Bleeding	
Norfloxacin	400 mg PO every 12 hours for 7 days
Daily Primary Prophylaxis	
Norfloxacin	400 mg PO every 12 hours (or)
Trimethoprim-sulfamethoxazole	1 double-strength tablet PO every day

ceftriaxone therapy for 7 days is recommended. The antibiotic therapy for SBP prophylaxis is summarized in Table 3.

Hepatic Hydrothorax

Hepatic hydrothorax is a development of pleural effusion in a cirrhotic patient with portal hypertension, without any underlying cardiopulmonary diseases. It commonly presents on the right side, but left-sided and bilateral involvements can also be seen. The likely mechanisms for pathogenesis of hepatic hydrothorax are hypoalbuminemia, which reduces plasma osmotic pressure, azygos veins hypertension, transdiaphragmatic migration of ascitic fluid via lymphatic systems, and ascitic fluid leakage via diaphragmatic defects. Hepatic hydrothorax may occur in the absence of ascites. As in ascites, all patients who present with hepatic hydrothorax or pleural effusion with unclear etiology should have a diagnostic thoracentesis. Hepatic hydrothorax typically presents with transudative pleural effusions.

However, as in ascites and SBP, hepatic hydrothorax can become infected spontaneously, called spontaneous bacterial empyema (SBEM). In this case, the pleural fluid analysis becomes exudative. The diagnostic criteria for SBEM are serum-pleural albumin gradient over 1.1 g/dL, pleural fluid neutrophil counts over 500/mm³, with the absence of pneumonia or contiguous infectious process on chest radiography. SBEM occurs as a result of a direct microbial spread from the pleural cavity in the presence of portal hypertension. Rarely, SBEM can develop without clinically significant ascites. All patients with hepatic hydrothorax who develop fever, chest pain, dyspnea, and encephalopathy should have repeat thoracentesis to evaluate pleural fluid analysis.

The management of hepatic hydrothorax is basically the same as with refractory ascites. The conservative management includes sodium restriction and diuretic therapy. In refractory cases, therapeutic thoracentesis, TIPS, and peritoneovenous shunting can be performed. Tube thoracostomy with injection of a sclerosing agent can be a long-term management, but the evidence for its efficacy is not validated. In patients with documented SBEM, third-generation cephalosporins such as ceftriaxone (1 g intravenously daily for 10 days) can be given empirically. An antibacterial regimen should be narrowed down as soon as the results of bacterial cultures are obtained.

Hepatic hydrothorax is a late and serious complication of cirrhosis. Patients with hepatic hydrothorax generally have end-stage liver disease, and these individuals should be evaluated for liver transplantation.

SUGGESTED READINGS

Blumgart LH: *Surgery of the Liver, Biliary tract and Pancreas*, ed 4, Volume 2, Philadelphia, Elsevier, 2007.

Boyer TD, Haskal ZJ. American Association for the Study of Liver Diseases. The Role of Transjugular Intrahepatic Portosystemic Shunt (TIPS) in the Management of Portal Hypertension: update 2009, *Hepatology* 51(1):306, 2010.

Colombato L: The role of transjugular intrahepatic portosystemic shunt (TIPS) in the management of portal hypertension, *J Clin Gastroenterol* 41(Supp. 3):S322–S351, 2007.

Dhanasekaran R, West JK, Gonzales PC, et al: Transjugular intrahepatic portosystemic shunt for symptomatic refractory hepatic hydrothorax in patients with cirrhosis, *Am J Gastroenterol* 105(3):635–641, 2010.

Gordon FD: Ascites, *Clin Liver Dis* 16(2):285–299, 2012.

Khungar V, Saab S: Cirrhosis with refractory ascites: Serial large volume paracentesis, TIPS, or transplantation? *Clin Gastroenterol Hepatol* 9(11):931–935, 2011.

John McDonald, Andrew Burroughs, Brain Feagan, et al. *Evidence-based Gastroenterology and Hepatology*, ed 3, West-Sussex, UK, Wiley-Blackwell, 2010.

Bruce A. Runyon. AASLD Practice Guidelines: Management of Adult Patients with Ascites Due to Cirrhosis: An Update, *Hepatology* 2087–2107, 2009.

THE MANAGEMENT OF HEPATIC ENCEPHALOPATHY

David Victor, MD, and Ayman A. Koteish, MD

OVERVIEW

Hepatic encephalopathy (HE) is a complex, potentially reversible, neuropsychiatric syndrome observed in patients with cirrhosis or acute liver failure. Patients with HE may have symptoms ranging from subtle abnormalities, detectable only through specialized psychological testing, to frank coma. Generally accepted stages for the broad spectrum of clinical manifestations of encephalopathy are based on level of consciousness, cognitive function, behavioral disturbances, and neuromuscular features (Table 1). In milder cases, the encephalopathic patient may be unaware of any deficits, and symptoms such as sleep pattern reversal, mild confusion, irritability, or personality changes may be apparent only to close contacts. Consequently, it is often helpful to obtain a history from a cirrhotic patient in the presence of family members.

HE remains largely a clinical diagnosis; no specific signs, symptoms, or laboratory test results are diagnostic of this disorder. The symptoms commonly associated with HE also occur in other conditions, such as hypoglycemia, head trauma, and intoxication. Asterixis, a flapping tremor of the outstretched hands, is a common feature of HE but also occurs in other metabolic encephalopathies. Elevated plasma levels of ammonia are common but not universal in HE, and the level of blood ammonia concentration is not always correlated with the severity of encephalopathy. Electroencephalography testing results are always abnormal in overt HE, but observed changes, such as triphasic waves, are not specific. Focal neurologic deficits such as hemiplegia or hemiparesis are observed in fewer than 20% of patients with HE, and seizures are rarely observed. Consequently, other causes of altered mental status must be ruled out before the diagnosis of HE is confirmed, and any focal neurologic deficiency should prompt central nervous system (CNS) imaging to rule out structural lesions.

PATHOPHYSIOLOGY

The pathogenesis of HE is multifactorial, and despite extensive research in both humans and animals, it remains unclear. The basic tenet of most hypotheses is that the brain is exposed to toxic substances produced in the gut by the actions of bacteria on nitrogenous compounds, which are incompletely cleared from the blood by the compromised liver. Ammonia was the first such substance described and has been the most extensively studied. There is compelling evidence that ammonia is an important pathogenetic factor in HE. Most patients with overt HE exhibit elevated plasma levels of ammonia, and children with urea cycle enzyme deficits and otherwise normally functioning livers develop profound hyperammonemia and symptoms indistinguishable from those of HE.

Ammonia can affect CNS function through several mechanisms. After crossing the blood–brain barrier, ammonia enters CNS astrocytes and combines with the neurotransmitter glutamate to form glutamine through the action of glutamine synthetase. Astrocytic glutamine enters mitochondria, in which it is converted back to ammonia and glutamate. Mitochondrial ammonia contributes to the production of reactive oxygen species and upregulates aquaporin 4. This results in astrocytic swelling that causes histologic changes known as *Alzheimer type II astrocytosis*. Adverse effects of ammonia on cerebral perfusion and glucose metabolism additionally contribute to CNS impairment. There is evidence that γ-aminobutyric acid (GABA), the primary inhibitory neurotransmitter in the CNS, may also play an important role in the pathogenesis of HE. Increased GABA levels have been associated with liver injury and hyperammonemia. Increased production of endogenous benzodiazepine ligands by gut bacteria can result in increased GABAergic transmission and altered CNS function. This explains why some patients with HE respond to the benzodiazepine antagonist flumazenil even in the absence of exposure to exogenous benzodiazepines.

Other substances, such as mercaptans and neurosteroids, and manganese toxicity may also contribute to neuronal and astrocytic

TABLE 1: Clinical manifestations and severity of hepatic encephalopathy

Encephalopathy stage	Level of consciousness	Cognitive function	Behavioral disturbance	Neuromuscular feature
I (mild)	Abnormal sleep pattern	Shortened attention span, mildly impaired computations	Euphoria, depression, irritability	Tremor, muscular incoordination, impaired handwriting
II (moderate)	Lethargy, mild disorientation	Amnesia, grossly impaired computations	Overt change in personality, inappropriate behavior	Slurred speech, asterixis (flapping), hypoactive reflexes, ataxia
III (severe)	Somnolence, semistupor	Inability to compute	Paranoia, bizarre behavior	Hyperactive reflexes, nystagmus, Babinski sign, clonus, rigidity
IV (coma)	Stupor, unconsciousness	None	None	Dilated pupils, opisthotonus, coma

Modified from Conn H, Lieberthal M: The hepatic coma syndromes and lactulose, Baltimore, 1979, Williams & Wilkins.

injury in HE. In all likelihood, these factors have varying influences in individual patients, depending on the cause, acuity, and severity of the liver disease and hence the variable manifestations of HE.

CLASSIFICATION AND MANAGEMENT OF HEPATIC ENCEPHALOPATHY

HE can be classified according to the underlying disorder that leads to it. It is associated with cirrhosis and portal hypertension, the presence of shunts, and, more ominously, acute liver failure. In practice, HE is classified as overt encephalopathy, minimal HE, and encephalopathy associated with acute liver failure.

Overt Encephalopathy

HE is a common complication of cirrhosis and can be episodic, developing over a short period of time with fluctuations in severity, or it can be persistent, with continuous overt neurologic or behavioral abnormalities. In most patients with episodic encephalopathy, a precipitating factor other than liver disease can be identified (Box 1).

Gastrointestinal bleeding is a very common precipitant of HE. This occurs through a combination of decreasing hepatic and renal perfusion and a large protein load to the gut, which results in increased production of nitrogenous byproducts. Evaluation of gastrointestinal blood loss and control of active bleeding must be performed in all patients with episodic HE. Infection is also a common precipitating factor for HE. The clinician must search for a source of infection. Cirrhosis can make the signs of infection less apparent. The baseline neutropenia and impaired response to infection can obscure the source of infection. The authors recommend a basic workup for infectious disease and that patients with overt HE and ascites undergo a diagnostic paracentesis to rule out spontaneous bacterial peritonitis. If there is a high index of suspicion for infection, empiric antibiotic therapy should be started after culture samples have been obtained. Many cirrhotic patients take diuretics; intravascular volume depletion from vigorous diuresis can reduce renal perfusion and result in azotemia and increased ammonia production. A hypokalemic alkalosis can enhance renal ammonia production, thereby precipitating HE. Reestablishing intravascular volume and correcting electrolyte imbalances often reverses encephalopathy. Exposure to

BOX 1: Precipitating factors in hepatic encephalopathy

Gastrointestinal bleeding
Sedatives or analgesics
Dehydration
Renal failure
Hypokalemia
Metabolic alkalosis
Infection (spontaneous bacterial peritonitis, pneumonia, urinary tract infection)
Excessive dietary protein
Constipation

sedatives and analgesics, especially benzodiazepines, can potentiate the effects of putative neurotoxins in HE and should be avoided. In postoperative or critical care settings, HE is often blamed for the prolonged effects of sedation in patients with cirrhosis. In such patients, use of sedatives should be minimized as much as possible, and clinicians must be aware that these drugs may have prolonged effects.

Treatment for overt HE is designed to treat the inciting factors. If this is insufficient, then modulating the gut bacteria with medication is the mainstay of treatment. The medications used reduce the gut production of ammonia through a variety of mechanisms. Despite maximal medical therapy, HE is refractory in some patients. The medications used for treatment of overt HE are used for all types of HE but are best understood in the context of overt HE.

Oral Disaccharides

For many years, the nonabsorbable disaccharides lactulose and lactitol have been the mainstay of therapy for HE. Theoretically, lactulose increases ammonia clearance through its cathartic action and decreases ammonia absorption by increasing the stool pH. Many affected patients have an improvement in symptoms of HE within hours of lactulose administration. These agents improve symptoms of encephalopathy, but they do not reduce the mortality rate. Despite the limitations, these treatments are the "gold standard" of therapy for HE. Lactulose is typically administered orally and in multiple doses each day. The dosing schedule should be individualized for the patient to achieve three to five bowel movements per day. Excess bowel movements as a result of these agents can actually precipitate episodes of HE, probably through dehydration and electrolyte abnormalities. The side effects of these agents (bloating, nausea, flatus, diarrhea, abdominal pain) dramatically limit their use in many patients. In view of the transient changes in the gut from these medications, noncompliance with the therapy results in return of HE symptoms. When these drugs are used, patient education and monitoring are paramount in trying to ensure compliance.

In a patient with acute or worsened overt HE, administration of these agents should be carefully monitored because excessive administration can lead to significant bloating if the patient is not having bowel moments. This results from the consumption of the compound by the gut bacteria, which leads to bloating and further stasis of the gut. For patients unable to take lactulose orally, it can be administered per rectum as a retention enema (300 mL of lactulose with 700 mL of water).

Dietary Protein Restriction

The potential association between dietary protein intake and encephalopathy was first described decades ago. In theory, reducing dietary protein intake should reduce nitrogenous toxin production. Although improvement may occur in individual encephalopathic patients with dietary protein restriction, this benefit has been difficult to demonstrate in controlled trials. In fact, in several studies of severe acute alcoholic hepatitis, the administration of high-protein/high-calorie diets improved rather than exacerbated encephalopathy. In addition, protein restriction to less than 40 g/day can accelerate catabolism and contribute to malnutrition. In practice, monitoring for changes in HE is best in patients on a regular-protein diet.

Low-Absorbable Antibiotics

Suppression of toxin production by gut bacteria is the basis for the use of poorly absorbed antibiotics. In numerous clinical trials, researchers have assessed the efficacy of various antibiotics in patients with different classes of encephalopathy. Neomycin and metronidazole were classically used to treat HE; however, the side effects of these medications have limited their use. Limited effectiveness is noted with oral vancomycin.

Rifaximin, a derivate of rifamycin, was originally developed to treat traveler's diarrhea and has broad-spectrum activity against gram-negative rods and gram-positive cocci. Several studies show that rifaximin is equal to if not better than oral disaccharides in patients with both overt and minimal encephalopathy. Concerns about possible bacterial overgrowth or fungal colonization are unfounded. Rifaximin has been shown effective in long-term treatment of HE with minimal side effects. There is a theoretical risk of bacterial overgrowth and associated infections with long-term use of rifaximin, but this has not been confirmed in studies. In patients with intolerance to oral disaccharides, it is the medication of choice, and for some patients, its lower side effect profile makes it the primary medication for treatment of HE. The U.S. Food and Drug Administration approved the use of rifaximin for the reduction in the risk of the recurrence of overt HE in patients with advanced liver disease. The recommended dosage is 550 mg by mouth twice per day. The medication is effective in treating acute HE and maintaining a response to prevent overt HE. Rifaximin remains expensive, however, and patients are often unable to afford the medication in the long term. In practice, the combination of lactulose and rifaximin is known to be additive in its effect in some patients.

Other Therapies

Sodium benzoate combines with ammonia to produce hippurate, which is renally excreted. In limited trials, it compares favorably with lactulose. L-ornithine L-aspartate increases hepatic conversion of ammonia and is better than placebo at lowering plasma ammonia levels and improving encephalopathy grade. Flumazenil, a benzodiazepine antagonist, showed improvement in encephalopathy grade

but is not approved for this indication by the U.S. Food and Drug Administration. Zinc lowers plasma ammonia by increasing ornithine transcarbamylase activity, but its benefits in HE have been inconsistent. Branched-chain amino acids in several different formulations improve symptoms but not length of survival, and they are relatively expensive. Trials of probiotics, which are live organisms that confer a benefit on health, have yielded mixed results for benefit in treating encephalopathy. A meta-analysis suggested that probiotics might be beneficial in the treatment of HE. The evidence remains limited as to their effectiveness.

Hepatic Encephalopathy Associated With Acute Liver Failure

HE is a prominent and ominous component of acute liver failure, but it differs from that observed in cirrhosis and portal hypertension. Although marked hyperammonemia can occur in both disorders, cerebral edema with intracranial hypertension is common in acute liver failure but rarely occurs in chronic liver disease. The risk of cerebral edema is correlated with the encephalopathic grade in acute liver failure. It is very low in grades 1 and 2 HE but progresses to 35% in grade 3 HE and 75% in grade 4 HE. The reason for this association with acute liver failure is not entirely clear, because the consequences of hyperammonemia on cerebral function should be similar in acute and chronic liver disease. Some authorities have proposed that markers of systemic inflammation commonly observed in acute liver failure may be a contributing factor. Excess free water with hyponatremia may exacerbate ammonia-induced cerebral edema.

Accurately assessing intracranial pressure (ICP) on clinical grounds is difficult. Physical findings such as papillary changes, abnormalities in the oculovestibular reflex, and decerebrate posturing are indicators of intracranial hypertension but often are apparent only at an irreversible stage. Consequently, some medical centers advocate the use of invasive monitoring devices, which accurately measure ICP. However, there is significant risk in monitoring in patients with acute liver failure and related coagulopathy. Patients with acute liver failure who develop grade 2 HE should be admitted to an intensive care unit with integrated monitoring and multiorgan support. Patients with grade 3 encephalopathy should be ventilated for airway protection, and the head should be elevated to 30 degrees. Intravenous hypotonic solutions should be avoided because of the risk of hyponatremia-induced cerebral edema. Bolus infusions of mannitol (0.5 to 1 g/kg) or hypertonic saline should be given to patients with objective evidence of increased ICP. Temporary hyperventilation, with a goal $Paco_2$ of 25 mm Hg, may be helpful if the ICP cannot be adequately lowered with mannitol. Most patients require renal replacement therapy to lower ammonia levels because lactulose is ineffective in acute liver failure. Intracranial hypertension refractory to medical management should prompt consideration for liver transplantation. More detailed instructions for the management of patients with acute liver failure can be found in recommendations published by the U.S. Acute Liver Failure Study Group and by the American Association for the Study of Liver Diseases practice guidelines.

Minimal Hepatic Encephalopathy

Minimal HE is a milder form of HE in which impairment in cognitive function is detectable only through neuropsychological testing. It affects 20% to 70% of patients with cirrhosis. The number-connection test and block-design test have reasonable specificities for minimal HE and are easy to administer. The deficits in minimal HE are primarily related to visuospatial orientation, attention problems, and impaired short-term memory. Oral and written skills show little impairment. Neuroimaging studies have shown a correlation between minimal HE and changes in cerebral blood flow and abnormalities on neuropsychological testing. Although patients with minimal HE have no overt symptoms of encephalopathy, their capacity to work or drive may be diminished. When tested on a driving simulator, patients with minimal HE both overestimate their abilities to drive and show impaired performance. Other studies have shown that patients with minimal HE have more collisions and have difficulty with traffic rules and road signs. At present, there is no consensus as to whether driving restrictions should be mandated. Treatment with both lactulose and rifaximin improve neuropsychological testing and quality of life in patients with minimal HE. These therapies also show some benefit in driving performance as well.

SUGGESTED READINGS

Bass NM, Mullen KD, Sanyal A, et al: Rifaximin treatment in hepatic encephalopathy, *N Engl J Med* 362(12):1071–1081, 2010.

Holte K, Krag A, Gluud LL: Systematic review and meta-analysis of randomized trials on probiotics for hepatic encephalopathy, *Hepatol Res* 42(10):1008–1015, 2012.

Polson J, Lee WM: American Association for the Study of Liver Disease. AASLD position paper: the management of acute liver failure, *Hepatology* 41(5):1179–1197, 2005.

Sanyal AJ, Mullen KD, Bass NM: The treatment of hepatic encephalopathy in the cirrhotic patient, *Gastroenterol Hepatol (N Y)* 6(4 Suppl 8):1–12, 2010.

THE MANAGEMENT OF BUDD-CHIARI SYNDROME

Jennifer C. Price, MD, and James P. Hamilton, MD

OVERVIEW

Budd-Chiari syndrome (BCS) refers to any pathophysiologic process that results in hepatic venous outflow tract obstruction, but it most commonly refers to thrombosis of the hepatic veins or the intrahepatic or suprahepatic inferior vena cava (IVC). The vast majority of patients with BCS have an underlying risk factor for thrombosis, although usually this is unrecognized at the time of presentation. Myeloproliferative disorders are the most common underlying thrombotic risk factor for BCS; others include factor V Leiden mutation; G20210A prothrombin mutation; antiphospholipid syndrome; deficiencies of protein C, S, or antithrombin; paroxysmal nocturnal hemoglobinuria; Behçet's syndrome; hyperhomocystinemia; MTHFR mutation; ulcerative colitis; hypereosinophilic syndrome; granulomatous venulitis; recent pregnancy; and recent oral contraceptive use. For decades, the optimal treatment of BCS involved the creation of a surgical shunt or liver transplant to relieve the portal hypertension. However, improvements in outcomes with less invasive procedures (i.e., transjugular intrahepatic portosystemic shunt [TIPS]) have changed the management of this life-threatening condition.

PRESENTATION AND DIAGNOSIS

The presentation of BCS ranges from asymptomatic in 20% of cases to acute liver failure. Rapid recognition and diagnosis of BCS is critical for initiation of organ-saving and life-saving medical and interventional treatment strategies. Patients afflicted with this potentially devastating disorder are typically young (ages 20 to 40 years) and most often female. The female predominance (3:1) is thought to be related to the concomitant use of prothrombotic, estrogen-containing oral contraceptives in the setting of previously undiagnosed hypercoagulable state. The classic clinical presentation includes hepatomegaly, right upper quadrant pain, and ascites, followed by jaundice. These clinical findings are the direct consequence of the underlying pathophysiology: hepatic outflow obstruction. Lower extremity edema, portal hypertension-related gastrointestinal bleeding, and hepatic encephalopathy may occur. In acute and subacute presentations of BCS, ascitic fluid analysis typically reveals a serum-ascites albumin gradient of 1.1 g/dL or more with a total protein of more

than 3.0 g/dL. This pattern of laboratory values is indicative of hepatic congestion; thus, diagnostic transthoracic echocardiogram is required to help distinguish between BCS and right-sided heart failure. Ascitic fluid analysis in chronic BCS also reveals a serum-ascites albumin gradient of more than 1.1 g/dL, but the total protein value is usually lower than 2.5 g/dL. Serum laboratory abnormalities are often nonspecific. In acute presentations, serum transaminase values may be elevated up to 100 times the upper limit of normal. Alkaline phosphatase and bilirubin levels may also be elevated and gradually worsen with disease progression. Coagulation studies may be abnormal, with prolonged prothrombin time, indicating hepatic synthetic dysfunction, and elevated activated partial thromboplastin time (aPTT), signifying an underlying disorder of coagulation. Interpretation of the complete blood count often requires recognition of the overall disease process. In cases in which the hepatic vein thrombosis is caused by a myeloproliferative syndrome (i.e., essential thrombocytosis or polycythemia vera), the portal hypertension and associated splenomegaly/splenic sequestration may cause blood counts to fall into the normal range. Finally, a battery of laboratory tests is typically sent to diagnose a hypercoagulable state, with results specifying a diagnosis in approximately 50% of cases.

Doppler ultrasound scan is the initial study of choice in many centers to evaluate hepatic venous patency. Findings are highly correlated with venography, and it is relatively inexpensive and readily available. Other noninvasive imaging modalities for BCS include computed tomographic (CT) scan and magnetic resonance imaging (MRI), which in addition to characterizing hepatic outflow may also show parenchymal abnormalities, the degree of ascites, and the presence of caudate lobe hypertrophy. High-quality imaging can be diagnostic and used to help plan therapeutic intervention. For the best visualization of the hepatic vessels, it is critical that these cross-sectional imaging modalities are performed with intravenous contrast and with dedicated arterial, venous, and washout phases. A classic feature is caudate hypertrophy because the caudate lobe drains into the IVC and is spared from the outflow obstruction in BCS (Figure 1). Typical parenchymal perfusion patterns seen on CT scan or MRI in BCS are early central contrast enhancement with delayed patchy peripheral enhancement and prolonged peripheral retention of contrast. Ascites and splenomegaly may be seen; in addition, concomitant, extrahepatic portal vein thrombosis is present in approximately 15% of patients with BCS.

Hepatic venography remains the gold standard for diagnosis of BCS. In addition to diagnosis of difficult cases, venography can characterize the obstructive lesion and provides the opportunity to measure portal-caval pressures and perform a liver biopsy. Characteristic features of venography in BCS are occlusion of the hepatic veins and a "spider web" morphology of the small intrahepatic venules, which are thought to represent collateralization (Figure 2). Histologic findings of typical of BCS are centrilobular (zone 3) congestion, necrosis, fibrosis, and in some cases, cirrhosis. Intrahepatic

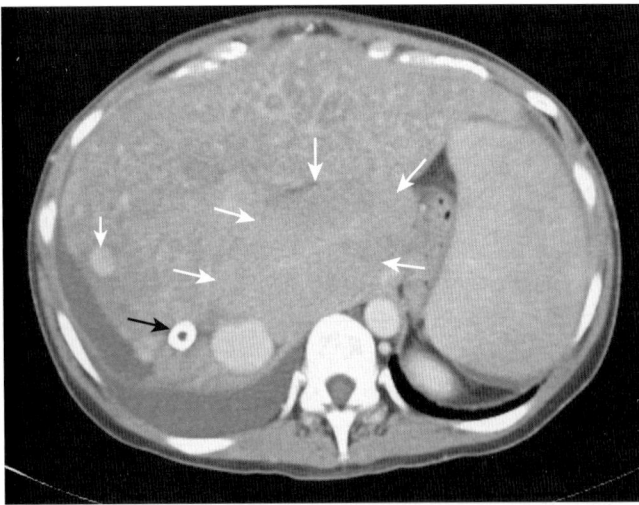

FIGURE 1 Typical computed tomographic scan of a patient with chronic Budd-Chiari syndrome. Note the heterogeneous appearance of the liver parenchyma, regenerative nodules *(small white arrow)*, and caudate lobe hypertrophy *(white arrows)*. The *black arrow* points to an occluded transjugular intrahepatic portacaval shunt.

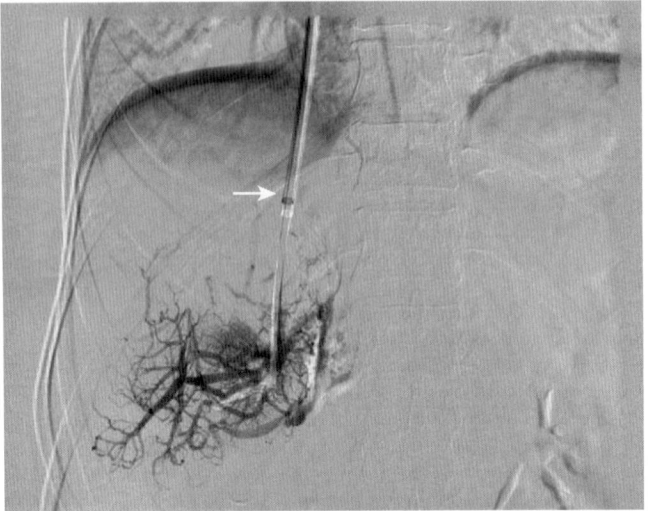

FIGURE 2 "Spider web" morphology of small portal venules in Budd-Chiari syndrome as seen on venography. A catheter is seen transcending the liver *(arrow)*.

portal vein thrombosis can occur and lead to portovenous and portoportal bridging fibrosis. Regenerative nodules are commonly seen in chronic BCS and may resemble focal nodular hyperplasia on histology and imaging. Hepatocellular carcinoma can develop in the setting of long-standing BCS and may be difficult to distinguish from regenerative nodules on imaging.

TREATMENT

The goals of treatment for BCS are to prevent clot propagation, restore vascular patency, decompress hepatic congestion, and treat complications of portal hypertension. The choice of therapy depends on a variety of factors, including the experience of the center, the availability of interventional radiology, and the patient's clinical presentation (Figure 3). The patency of the portal vein is often a critical factor because it may render TIPS or portal-caval shunt technically impossible.

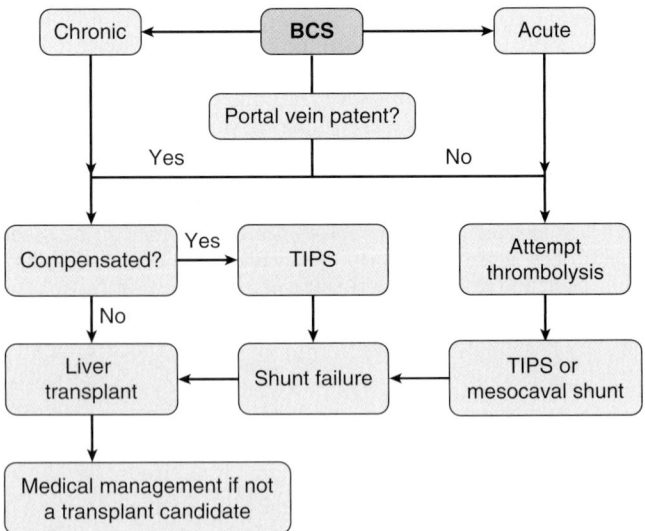

FIGURE 3 Treatment algorithm for patients with Budd-Chiari syndrome *(BCS)*. *TIPS*, Transjugular intrahepatic portacaval shunt.

MEDICAL THERAPY

Immediately after diagnostic imaging is performed, anticoagulation therapy with fractionated heparin should begin. The underlying cause of BCS should be thoroughly investigated and treated. The V617F point mutation in the tyrosine kinase Janus kinase 2 (JAK2) gene in myeloid cells is highly specific for myeloproliferative disorders and should be tested in all patients with BCS. Most patients with a predisposing thrombotic disorder require indefinite anticoagulation therapy, although hydroxyurea and aspirin may be as effective as anticoagulation at preventing thrombosis in some patients with myeloproliferative disorders. Medical treatment for portal hypertension, including sodium restriction and diuretic therapy, should also be initiated. Renal function should be monitored carefully because the acute portal hypertension caused by BCS may precipitate hepatorenal syndrome. A subset of patients may demonstrate steady clinical improvement and may avoid invasive treatment. However, anticoagulation therapy alone is unlikely to result in adequate venous recanalization, and patients receiving medical therapy only must be closely monitored for disease progression.

Systemic and in situ thrombolytic agents have been used to treat BCS, although this has been poorly studied in controlled trials. Some evidence shows that directed thrombolysis is effective, and it can be considered in acute forms of BCS for patients without contraindications. In acute presentation, tissue plasminogen antagonist (TPA) may be delivered directly into the hepatic vascular system through cannulation of the portal vein. This strategy is often used over a period of 12 to 24 hours, with careful monitoring for hemorrhagic complications in an intensive care unit. Thrombolytic agents should not be used in chronic BCS given the low chance of venous recanalization and increased risk of bleeding complications in the setting of portal hypertension.

Interventional Radiology

Most patients with BCS do not have improvement with medical treatment alone. The role of interventional radiology in managing these patients has become increasingly important. Balloon angioplasty can be used in cases of focal occlusions, such as IVC webs or short-length hepatic vein stenoses. Vascular reocclusion occurs commonly, and therefore, stent placement is recommended if feasible. However, careful consideration must be made before stent placement because it may interfere with vascular anastomosis if the patient eventually requires orthotropic liver transplantation (OLT). Successful stent placement leads to hepatic decompression, and clinical improvement can be sustained even despite reobstruction. Complications appear to be lower with the transluminal approach compared with the transhepatic approach.

Transjugular intrahepatic portosystemic shunt placement is now the standard of care for the treatment of BCS that has not responded to medical therapy. The rationale for TIPS is to create a intrahepatic shunt from the portal venous system to the proximal hepatic vein or IVC to bypass the obstructed hepatic veins (Figure 4). Historically, TIPS was not considered a durable therapy for BCS because of very high rates of stent occlusion (up to 75% at 1 year). At that time, TIPS was considered a bridge to definitive surgical therapies, such as liver transplant or creation of a surgical shunt. However, TIPS has been shown to be effective even in patients with severe BCS who have failed medical management. In 2008, Garcia-Pagan and colleagues showed an overall 84% 5-year survival rate after TIPS for BCS. This same series showed 88% and 78% 1-year and 5-year liver transplant-free survival rates. TIPS stents are now covered with polytetrafluoroethylene (PTFE). TIPS dysfunction from stent occlusion is less than 25% annually with these newer stents. TIPS can also be performed in the setting of BCS and portal vein thrombosis, although the success rate is lower in this setting, and the procedure may require an attempt of thrombolysis to the portal vein beforehand. TIPS remain a sophisticated procedure and is best performed by skilled interventional radiologists with much experience. Proper patient selection helps to increase the likelihood of success after TIPS. A right-sided echocardiogram should be performed, and TIPS should be avoided in patients with right heart failure. Patients with decompensated liver disease (e.g., Model for End-Stage Liver Disease [MELD] score of >17) often do very poorly after TIPS, and these patients should be considered for liver transplantation. The major complication after TIPS is the development of hepatic encephalopathy. This can be managed with nonabsorbable antibiotics and synthetic sugars to induce catharsis. Hepatic encephalopathy is typically not a problem in cases of acute BCS.

SURGICAL THERAPY

Portosystemic Shunting

Blakemore first described the portal-caval shunt in the late 1940s (Figure 5). Since then, multiple surgical variants have been developed, including splenorenal, mesocaval, and mesoatrial shunts. The choice of technique depends on individual patient factors such as patency of the IVC and extent of caudate lobe enlargement. Several studies show excellent short-term outcomes. However, among four multicenter retrospective analyses of patients with BCS who underwent portosystemic shunt, only one showed a survival advantage with portosystemic shunting after adjusting for Child-Pugh score. In 2012, Orloff and colleagues published results of their prospective cohort of 77 patients with BCS treated with surgical portosystemic shunt. Long-term survival rate was 95% among patients with isolated hepatic vein occlusion treated with side-to-side portacaval shunt after a mean follow-up period of 15 years. Mesoatrial shunt for IVC occlusion was associated with a high failure rate and thus discontinued in their series after 1990, but combined side-to-side portal-caval shunt with caval-atrial shunt in this population yielded a 100% survival rate at a mean follow-up period of 12 years.

Not surprisingly, shunt patency is essential to long-term success with portosystemic shunting. This was shown by Bachet and colleagues, who followed 39 patients a median of 100 months. Shunt dysfunction occurred in 20 patients and was associated with a significantly higher mortality (55% vs 16%). Shunt revision was successful for 7 of the 20 patients with shunt dysfunction, and none of these patients had refractory ascites develop or died during follow-up. Because of the increasing availability and success of TIPS for BCS, surgical portosystemic shunting has become less commonly performed at some centers. Nevertheless, surgical portosystemic

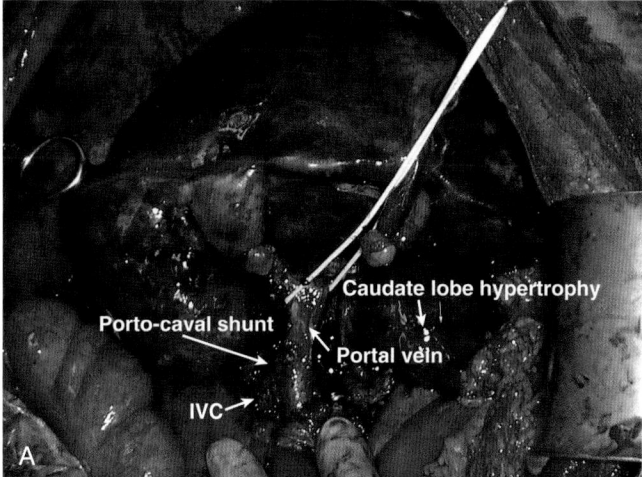

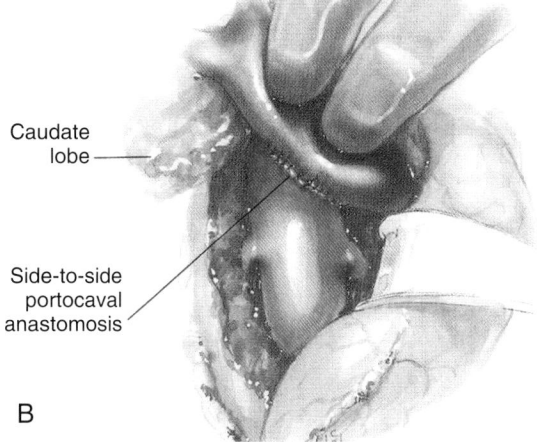

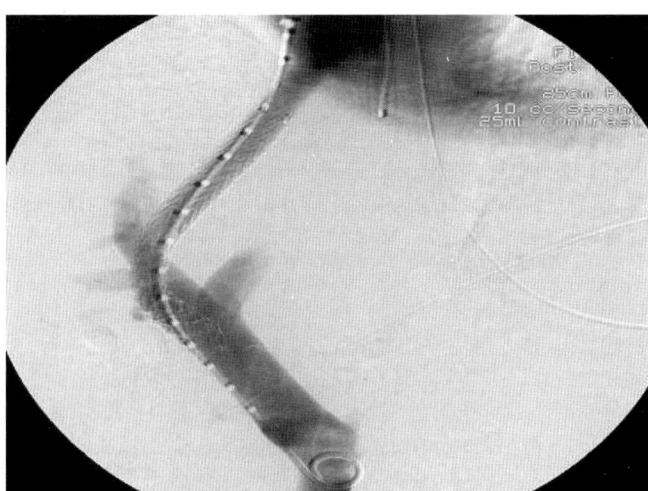

FIGURE 4 Transjugular intrahepatic portacaval shunt extending from right portal vein into the right atrium.

FIGURE 5 Budd-Chiari syndrome with previous portosystemic shunt procedure at the time of orthotropic liver transplantation. **A,** Caudate lobe hypertrophy. **B,** Side-to-side portal-caval shunt. *IVC,* Inferior vena cava.

shunting can be associated with excellent long-term outcomes if performed early in the course of the disease before the development of irreversible liver damage. Referral to an experienced surgeon is essential, and a liver transplant team should be consulted before a surgical shunt is performed.

Liver Transplantation

In patients with decompensated cirrhosis from BCS, OLT is the only curative option. In 1976, Putnam and Starzl reported the first case of OLT in a 22-year-old woman with acute hepatic venous occlusion, noting excellent results in 16-month follow-up. Since then, experience with OLT in the setting of BCS has undergone a dramatic evolution. Early experience with OLT for BCS yielded inferior outcomes, with 3-year survival rates as low as 45%. In general, two factors have modified the approach and positively influenced outcomes: (1) aggressive initiation of medical and interventional therapy; and (2) anticoagulation therapy. In the modern era of transplantation for BCS, survival has significantly improved. Mentha and colleagues evaluated 248 patients in the European Liver Transplantation Registry who underwent OLT for BCS and found 76%, 71%, and 68% 1-year, 5-year, and 10-year survival rates, respectively. Twenty-seven patients had venous thrombosis develop despite anticoagulation therapy, including six with recurrent venous outflow obstruction. Segev and colleagues examined 510 patients transplanted for BCS and found 81% graft and 85% patient survival rates at 3 years after OLT among those transplanted in the MELD era.

Liver transplantation in the setting of BCS poses several technical challenges. With acute or chronic disease, the liver may be markedly swollen and difficult to manipulate. Secondly, hyperplasia of the caudate lobe makes access to and dissection of the IVC a difficult endeavor. Concomitant stenosis of the IVC makes suprahepatic and infrahepatic control equally difficult. Although a prior TIPS procedure does not preclude OLT, distal migration of the stent may complicate the portal vein anastomosis. Substantial migration may require transection of the stent with the anastomosis performed directly to the portal vein remnant with the stent in situ. Noted by many institutional experiences, isolation of the hepatic veins for a piggyback anastomosis can be difficult with active outflow occlusion.

As mentioned in previous editions of this textbook, portal vein thrombosis can be a difficult problem, and it requires a strategic plan before transplant. At present, the authors find that the portal vein can routinely undergo thrombectomy and reasonable flow can be established, if the superior mesenteric vein (SMV) is patent. If this is not possible, a vein graft with donor iliac vein can be constructed between the donor portal vein and the SMV.

In the setting of complete mesenteric occlusion, two possibilities exist. First, many times, these recipients have an extremely large and patent coronary vein because of severe portal hypertension; this vein can be used for portal inflow. Second, anastomosis of the donor portal vein to the recipient's IVC (caval hemitransposition) with partial or total occlusion of the superior IVC superior is an option. Unfortunately, this approach can have extremely high morbidity and mortality.

Because of the aforementioned caudate lobe hyperplasia and caval stenosis, the recipient IVC may not be usable for live donor liver transplant (LDLT). In 2006, Yan and colleagues reported the first case of an adult-to-adult LDLT for BCS with a cryopreserved iliac vein graft. The authors highlight several important technical issues. In this case, it was necessary to incise the diaphragm and expose the pericardium to the level of the right atrium secondary to hepatic venous outflow occlusion. The iliac graft was then sewn to the suprahepatic and infrahepatic vena cavae. The right hepatic vein of the right hepatic lobe allograft was then sewn to the iliac graft in end-to-side fashion.

Alternatively, a large series from Japan reports the long-term outcome in eight patients with BCS who underwent LDLT. Of these, five patients underwent cavoplasty with a replacement vein graft after extensive resection of the thrombosed anterior IVC wall. Although the combined experience with LDLT for BCS is small, the current data suggest living donation as an emerging treatment option for this patient population.

Recurrence of hepatic venous outflow obstruction has been observed in up to 10% of patients, ranging from months to years after transplant. Consequently, lifelong anticoagulation therapy is currently recommended. Early experience with recurrent BCS after OLT carried an extremely high mortality rate. However, interventional techniques have provided some alternatives to retransplantation or death. In our experience, recurrent BCS can be approached in two ways. Primarily, retransplantation is an option in patients with mild to moderate thrombus burden in the hepatic veins and IVC refractory to an interventional approach. However, the anatomic features of the recurrent thrombus must be carefully delineated; recipients with a completed occluded IVC and portal vein are unlikely to be candidates for retransplant. In severe cases, TIPS can be used to reestablish flow in one or more hepatic vein in the setting of preserved liver function.

Finally, no evidence is found to suggest that OLT increases the risk of malignant transformation of underlying myeloproliferative disease in patients with BCS.

SUMMARY

The Budd-Chiari syndrome is a life-threatening condition that can be treated successfully when a timely diagnosis is made and the proper therapy applied. Initial treatment with anticoagulation therapy followed by placement of TIPS is the standard of care for patients with well-compensated liver function. Long-term follow-up studies of patients who undergo TIPS have shown excellent transplant-free survival rates, and stent failure is now uncommon. Although select centers have a robust experience with surgical portosystemic shunt procedures, the majority of institutions initially use interventional radiologic procedures for those with acute or subacute onset of disease.

Although long considered the most viable long-term treatment option for patients with all forms of BCS, liver transplant is typically reserved for patients with decompensated liver disease or recurrent stent/shunt failure.

SUGGESTED READINGS

Bachet JB, Condat B, Hagege H, et al: Long-term portosystemic shunt patency as a determinant of outcome in Budd-Chiari syndrome, *J Hepatol* 46(1):60–68, 2007.

Cameron JL, Maddrey WC: Mesoatrial shunt a new treatment for Budd-Chiari syndrome, *Ann Surg* 187:402–406, 1978.

Darwish MS, Plessier A, Hernandez-Guerra M, et al: EN-Vie (European Network for Vascular Disorders of the Liver) etiology, management, and outcome of the Budd-Chiari syndrome, *Ann Intern Med* 151:167–175, 2009.

Menon KV, Shah V, Kamath PS: The Budd-Chiari syndrome, *N Engl J Med* 350(6):578–585, 2004.

Mentha G, Giostra E, Majno PE, et al: Liver transplantation for Budd-Chiari syndrome: A European study of 248 patients from 51 centres, *J Hepatol* 44(3):520–528, 2006.

Molmenti EP, Segev DL, Arepally A, et al: The utility of TIPS in the management of Budd Chiari syndrome, *Ann Surg* 241(6):978–983, 2005.

Orloff MJ, Isenberg JI, Wheeler HO, et al: Budd-Chiari syndrome: 38 years' experience with surgical decompression, *J Gastrointest Surg* 16(2):286–300, 2012.

Srinivasan P, Rela M, Pracgalias A, et al: Liver transplantation for Budd-Chiari syndrome, *Transplantation* 73:973–977, 2002.

Zimmerman MA, Cameron AM, Ghobrial RM: Budd-Chiari syndrome, *Clin Liver Dis* 10(2):259–273, 2006.

GALLBLADDER AND BILIARY TREE

THE MANAGEMENT OF ASYMPTOMATIC (SILENT) GALLSTONES

Victor Zaydfudim, MD, MPH, Kengo Asai, MD, PhD, and Michael G. Sarr, MD

OVERVIEW

Gallstones and their sequelae are one of the most common problems managed and treated by the general surgeon. In the United States, between 30 and 45 million residents have gallstones, with an approximate prevalence rate of 1 in 10, depending on patient age. Approximately 80% remain asymptomatic throughout the patient's lifetime. Unfortunately, with modern and frequently overutilized cross-sectional imaging, these asymptomatic, previously unrecognized, and unsuspected gallstones are identified incidentally. Once discovered, the asymptomatic gallstones become a matter of discussion, more frequently from the patient's point of view than that of the surgeon. A recent Cochrane Hepato-Biliary Group review failed to identify any randomized clinical trials comparing cholecystectomy versus no cholecystectomy among patients (or any subset of patients) with asymptomatic cholelithiasis. Progression from asymptomatic cholelithiasis to symptomatic gallstone disease obviously occurs but seems rare, and prophylactic or incidental cholecystectomy in patients with asymptomatic gallstones is usually unnecessary and should not be performed in most patients. This chapter addresses existing evidence and exceptional cases in which cholecystectomy for asymptomatic cholelithiasis could be considered.

EPIDEMIOLOGY AND NATURAL HISTORY

Gallstone disease is the leading cause for hospital admissions and clinic visits for gastrointestinal symptoms in the United States, with more than 750,000 cholecystectomies performed annually. The burden of disease has increased by an estimated 20% since the 1980s, and currently, 10% to 15% of the adult population in the United States harbors gallstones. Most these gallstones are asymptomatic, and the majority of patients do not know that they have gallstones. Less than 20% of patients with gallstones have biliary colic or symptomatic cholelithiasis develop during their lifetime; even fewer patients develop the more severe cholecystitis or biliary pancreatitis. Only about 4% of patients with asymptomatic cholelithiasis have secondary sequelae of gallstone disease (e.g., cholecystitis, obstructive jaundice, or pancreatitis). Annual progression has been estimated at 0.3% for acute cholecystitis, 0.2% for obstructive jaundice, and 0.1% to 1.5% for biliary pancreatitis. In longitudinal cohort studies, biliary colic typically precedes other complications and, as such, is a harbinger of further symptoms of cholelithiasis. A series of landmark studies by Gracie and Ransohoff in the 1980s established the safety of expectant management among male patients with asymptomatic cholelithiasis, confronting historical medical and surgical beliefs that the presence of gallstones requires cholecystectomy.

Asymptomatic cholelithiasis, per se, can be a difficult diagnosis to suspect and establish, and the distinction between symptomatic and asymptomatic gallstones can on occasion be elusive. Abdominal imaging for diagnosis of abdominal pain, discomfort, or mass is, by definition, not performed in an asymptomatic patient. Incidentally discovered gallstones are those that are: (1) found during imaging for reports not related to gallstones (e.g., vague nonspecific complaints, staging for lymphoma or other neoplasms, screening for abdominal aortic aneurysm, etc.); or (2) discovered incidentally during abdominal exploration for an unrelated operation (e.g., colon resection for cancer or operation for morbid obesity). The truly asymptomatic patient should have no subjective symptoms related to gallstones. Although symptoms can be vague and varied, classic symptoms of gallstone disease that are relieved with cholecystectomy are biliary colic and epigastric crescendo/decrescendo abdominal pain in patients with cholelithiasis. When present, these symptoms improve in more than 90% and 70% of the patients, respectively. As both ultrasound and cross-sectional abdominal imaging become a more routine part of patient evaluation and as the dramatic and frightening incidence of overweight and obesity continues to surge, the recognized prevalence and the overall incidence of cholelithiasis will also increase.

Population-based risk factors for gallstone formation and gallstone disease have been studied widely. Native American populations in both North and South Americas have a significantly greater prevalence of cholelithiasis. Increasing age, female gender, obesity, and metabolic syndrome have all been associated with an increased risk of cholesterol gallstones. In addition, rapid weight loss, particularly after operations for morbid obesity, predisposes markedly to cholesterol stone formation. Pigment stones are common in patients with hemolysis, such as those with hemoglobinopathies (sickle cell disease, hereditary spherocytosis, thalassemia), and in patients with cirrhosis, cystic fibrosis, Crohn's disease, and recurrent infection or inflammation of the biliary tree. When gallstone disease is symptomatic, operative management is recommended in all patients. Management of asymptomatic cholelithiasis in specific populations is addressed further in this chapter.

PROPHYLACTIC CHOLECYSTECTOMY

A number of investigations have focused on size of gallstones and the association with progression from asymptomatic to symptomatic cholelithiasis. These studies attempted to establish a role for prophylactic cholecystectomy for patients with stones that are either "too small" (typically defined as less than 5 mm) or "too big" (typically defined as larger than 3 cm). Among patients with small stones, investigators tested the associations between small stones and biliary pancreatitis. For patients with large stones, investigators tested the associations between large stones and cholecystitis (from presumed impaction in the neck of the gallbladder or Hartmann's pouch) or as a possible contributing factor in development of adenocarcinoma of the gallbladder. Although both of these associations can be seen among patients with the diagnosis of disease (e.g., pancreatitis, cholecystitis, gallbladder cancer), causation has not been shown in cohort studies for any pathology among patients with either small or large stones.

The relationship between gallbladder cancer and the presence of large gallstones remains highly controversial. Published studies vary from a nearly tenfold increase in the relative risk of gallbladder cancer among patients with stones greater than 3 cm to no significant difference at all. The role of prophylactic cholecystectomy for patients with large gallstones remains undefined; however, cholecystectomy in an asymptomatic patient with either epidemiologic risk factors or patient anxiety and gallstones larger than 3 cm could at least be considered. Studies supporting expectant management of large gallstones recommend ultrasound surveillance with cholecystectomy in patients with development of symptoms or changing characteristics on imaging. Predictive models with simulation decision analysis provide inconclusive evidence to support prophylactic operations in an asymptomatic patient with either small or large stones. Size alone is not a criterion for cholecystectomy, and patients with incidentally discovered, asymptomatic gallstones do not require cholecystectomy. Patients with small or large stones who have symptoms develop, however, should be treated with cholecystectomy.

The prevalence of gallstones increases with age, but the risk of progression from asymptomatic to symptomatic gallstone disease, although low, seems to increase with the duration of gallstone presence. A 30-year-old patient with asymptomatic gallstones has a greater lifetime risk for development of symptomatic gallbladder disease than does an octogenarian with asymptomatic gallstones. Although routine prophylactic cholecystectomy in a patient with known asymptomatic gallstones and long life expectancy cannot be supported, an incidental cholecystectomy during an intraabdominal operation for unrelated pathology could be considered. Two caveats are: (1) the age cut-off is not well defined; and (2) the exact definition of a "younger" patient with "increased" life-time risk compared with the general population has not been identified. In addition, the risk-benefit analysis of a concomitant cholecystectomy in an asymptomatic patient varies with other patient-specific covariates. As such, the decision for a concomitant/incidental cholecystectomy should be individualized. Incidental cholecystectomy is addressed further in the chapter.

Minimally invasive techniques have markedly decreased postoperative pain, duration of hospital stay, and time to return to work among patients undergoing uncomplicated cholecystectomy. In addition, patient acceptance and physician willingness to offer cholecystectomy has also changed with the minimal access approach; after all, it is "just a lap chole." But, these operations are not risk-free. Access injuries (bowel or vascular) during trocar placement, albeit infrequent, are likely underreported and, when present, can be disastrous. Nonbiliary complications, such as risks of postoperative bleeding requiring reoperation or intraabdominal abscess requiring intervention, are low but nevertheless present. Biliary injury and postinjury complications have been studied extensively and are not trivial. Frequency of bile duct transection or obstruction requiring hepaticojejunostomy is approximately 1 in 500 cases; more patients are treated by interventional endoscopists and radiologists for less severe biliary injuries. Justification of such risk, albeit low, is more difficult to an asymptomatic patient.

INCIDENTAL CHOLECYSTECTOMY

Although prophylactic operation implies cholecystectomy to prevent future complications of gallstones in an asymptomatic patient, incidental cholecystectomy performed during an operation for an otherwise unrelated diagnosis is more common. The most accepted indication for incidental cholecystectomy among patients with asymptomatic cholelithiasis is the presence of other gallbladder pathology that mandates cholecystectomy. The most common gallbladder pathology not directly related to gallstones is a gallbladder polyp. The natural history and clinical diagnosis of gallbladder polyps have been scrutinized extensively. Patients with polyps greater than 10 mm, sessile rather than pedunculated polyps, adenomatous polyps with vascularity, and polyps that show rapid growth are considered at greater risk for development of gallbladder malignancy and should be referred for a cholecystectomy. Extensive literature and surgical dogma cover a rarer group of patients with porcelain gallbladder. A recent systematic review estimated a prevalence rate of gallbladder cancer of 0.2% in patients with a porcelain gallbladder. Indeed, with the exception of a single study from Argentina published in 1967, the incidence rate of gallbladder cancer among patients with calcified gallbladder is almost 0. Confusion between a true porcelain gallbladder (i.e., complete/diffuse intramural calcification seen immediately on abdominal imaging) and selective mucosal calcifications within the gallbladder wall (i.e., focal mucosal calcium deposition) should be addressed. The former (porcelain gallbladder) is likely not an independent risk factor for gallbladder cancer, and the latter (selective mucosal calcification) has been associated with an increased risk of gallbladder malignancy. Despite this lack of evidence, many surgeons continue to recommend cholecystectomy for patients with incidentally discovered porcelain gallbladder. In both groups of patients, those with gallbladder polyps and those with porcelain gallbladder, gallstones (if present) are removed during cholecystectomy. Unlike prophylactic cholecystectomy, incidental cholecystectomy for patients with stones that are large (>3 cm) or small (<5 mm) is more commonly accepted. In addition, incidental cholecystectomy during reoperative surgery, with the exception of revision abdominal hernia repairs with prosthetic mesh implantation, have also been accepted anecdotally but without significant evidence of benefit.

Incidental cholecystectomy during hepatic metastasectomy has also been advocated. Colorectal and neuroendocrine neoplasms constitute the most frequent metastases to the liver. Therapy depends largely on burden of disease; however, when feasible, hepatic resection can be the primary treatment modality. Incidental cholecystectomy, regardless of the presence of gallstones or extent of metastasectomy, is prudent for two reasons. First, recurrent, isolated metastases to hepatic segments IVB/V can be treated thereafter with ablation, without concern for the heat-sink effect or gallbladder wall injury. Second, systemic transcatheter therapy, such as transarterial chemoembolization or selective internal radiation therapy, poses a risk for cholecystitis, which can be avoided with a preemptive, incidental cholecystectomy during the initial metastasectomy.

Historically, clinical and physiologic studies suggested an increased rate of gallstone formation among patients undergoing an upper gastrointestinal operation involving vagotomy: esophagectomy, gastrectomy, or vagotomy for peptic ulcer disease. In addition, most studies that evaluated the utility of incidental cholecystectomy during major general alimentary tract, gynecologic, and vascular operations were performed among patients undergoing laparotomy. The results have been divergent. Some authors described a safe and potentially prophylactic operation, and others have shown a slight increase in risk without a clear benefit. A few considerations should be discussed. First, a number of these investigations were performed before routine use of therapeutic endoscopic retrograde cholangiography, and many patients in the control groups who needed postlaparotomy common bile duct explorations were treated currently with therapeutic endoscopy. Second, a number of patients in the control groups needed reexploration for an open cholecystectomy; currently, most of these patients would be candidates for minimally invasive cholecystectomy, alleviating much of the morbidity associated with relaparotomy. Third, abdominal access has evolved dramatically, and many operations are performed currently with laparoscopic or endovascular techniques.

The classic study by Ochsner, Cooley, and DeBakey published in 1960 pioneered the safety of concomitant incidental general surgery procedures for potential prophylaxis during abdominal aortic aneurysmectomy. Multiple subsequent studies showed the safety of cholecystectomy during open repair of abdominal aortic aneurysm, provided the retroperitoneum was closed over the prosthetic graft. Currently, however, more than 75% of aortic aneurysms are repaired endovascularly. No systematic studies have explored the need for, or the safety of, a concomitant cholecystectomy among patients with asymptomatic cholelithiasis undergoing endovascular aneurysm repair. Interestingly, one study evaluated development of gallbladder disease among 486 patients after endovascular abdominal aortic aneurysm repair (64 patients had known stones at the time of operation). Only three patients needed later intervention: one needed common bile duct exploration for an impacted stone 8 days after endovascular repair, another needed laparoscopic cholecystectomy for acalculous cholecystitis, and the third needed laparoscopic cholecystectomy for calculous cholecystitis 16 months after aneurysmorrhaphy. Data supporting any justification for a concomitant incidental cholecystectomy during endovascular operations are lacking, and currently the topic is moot.

Similarly, data to support concomitant incidental cholecystectomy among patients with asymptomatic cholelithiasis who are undergoing laparoscopic (or robotic) operations involving the gut, retroperitoneum, or pelvis are lacking. Has there been a shift in philosophy? One possibility is that trocar placement and triangulation, which are critical to a successful minimally invasive approach, limit the work area within the abdominal cavity. No studies have examined whether additional trocars and time during a laparoscopic colectomy or hysterectomy deter from "therapeutic" incidental cholecystectomy for asymptomatic gallstones. Second, the increasing subspecialization within general surgery creates the possibility that the surgeon performing colectomy or esophagectomy (not to mention hysterectomy) might be different than the one who usually performs a cholecystectomy. Third, the ability to perform a laparoscopic cholecystectomy later rather than the need for an open cholecystectomy has deflated the enthusiasm for a concomitant incidental cholecystectomy. As such, incidental cholecystectomy has lost favor largely by many surgeons among patients undergoing an intraabdominal operation. The morbid obesity population is an exception and is discussed separately.

SPECIAL POPULATIONS

The following section discusses populations in whom an incidental or prophylactic cholecystectomy for asymptomatic cholelithiasis has been considered. In most circumstances, the recommendation currently directs expectant management.

Diabetes

Historically, recommendations for prophylactic cholecystectomy in patients with diabetes with asymptomatic gallstones stemmed from clinical data that suggested two observations: (1) that these patients

were more likely to become symptomatic; and (2) that patients with diabetes have more complicated initial presentations of symptomatic cholelithiasis, in particular, acute cholecystitis. The clinical rationale argued for masked signs and symptoms of gallstone disease among patients with diabetic autonomic neuropathy, thereby leading to delayed diagnosis and worse outcomes. Historic reports described increased rates of severe cholecystitis (perforation, gangrene, and emphysematous cholecystitis) among patients with diabetes presenting with cholecystitis.

Subsequent studies from as early as 30 years ago failed to confirm that diabetes is an independent risk factor for adverse outcomes. Rather, the coexisting vascular, cardiac, and renal disease; obesity; and advanced age appear to play a greater role in outcomes than diabetes alone. Recent evidence including a 5-year prospective study of patients with non–insulin-dependent diabetics showed that only 15% of patients became symptomatic, congruent with the rate among the general population, and few presented with secondary sequelae of complicated gallstone disease. In addition, decision analysis models showed the superiority of expectant management over prophylactic cholecystectomy in most realistic modeling scenarios among patients with diabetes, with noninferiority and even possible improvements in life expectancy and quality of life. Thus, prophylactic cholecystectomy for asymptomatic cholelithiasis is not recommended in patients with diabetes. In the case of a patient with diabetes with asymptomatic gallstones discovered incidentally at the time of celiotomy for an unrelated condition (colon cancer, etc.), many surgeons would support a concomitant cholecystectomy.

Hemoglobinopathy

Hemoglobinopathies, including sickle cell disease, thalassemia, and hereditary spherocytosis, cause hemolysis and formation of pigment stones. Gallstones are most evident among patients with sickle cell disease. More than 55% of patients with sickle cell disease have gallstones by the age of 22 years, and up to 75% of these patients develop symptomatic cholelithiasis. In addition, more than 60% of patients with sickle cell disease have episodes of vasoocclusive, sickle cell crises. Symptom differentiation between biliary colic and cholecystitis and sickle cell crises can be difficult. As such, prophylactic cholecystectomy is recommended frequently in this population. Previous studies have suggested increased risks of vasoocclusive crises during the era of open cholecystectomy; however, laparoscopic approaches and improved perioperative management of patients at risk for crises (including hemoglobin optimization, hydration, pain control, and oxygenation) have improved markedly the safety of prophylactic cholecystectomy.

Patients with hereditary spherocytosis and thalassemia are also at increased risk of development of pigment gallstones. Fewer studies have examined the role of prophylactic cholecystectomy for asymptomatic cholelithiasis in these two patient populations. Current clinical evidence in patients with hereditary spherocytosis supports prophylactic cholecystectomy at the time of laparoscopic splenectomy. Asymptomatic patients should be screened for the presence of gallstones before splenectomy. Once the spleen is removed, no new stones should develop in this population. Patients with β-thalassemia pose a different challenge. Hepatomegaly is a frequent sequela of thalassemia major with hemosiderosis and secondary cirrhosis. Up to two thirds of patients with thalassemia major have pigment stones develop by the age of 15 years. Similar to patients with spherocytosis, concomitant prophylactic cholecystectomy can be performed safely during laparoscopic splenectomy. Laparoscopic cholecystectomy can also be performed safely in patients with thalassemia and symptomatic cholelithiasis. The role of prophylactic cholecystectomy for asymptomatic cholelithiasis as a stand-alone operation among patients with hereditary spherocytosis or thalassemia, however, has not been investigated adequately and is not recommended currently.

Transplant

Management of asymptomatic cholelithiasis among solid organ transplant recipients has been controversial. Chronic, posttransplant immunosuppression is associated with an increased risk of infection and a delay in the diagnosis of surgical pathology. In addition, the cholelithogenic effect of immunosuppressive calcineurin inhibitors (cyclosporine and tacrolimus) and early reports of substantial morbidity and mortality of cholecystectomy in symptomatic patients historically led to recommendations for prophylactic cholecystectomy in transplant candidates before transplant and for transplant recipients diagnosed with cholelithiasis after transplant. Subsequent studies, however, particularly in patients with kidney and pancreas transplant have shown the safety and efficacy of expectant management after introduction of laparoscopic cholecystectomy. Most patients with asymptomatic cholelithiasis after kidney or pancreas transplant remain asymptomatic; those few patients (~1%/y) in whom symptoms develop can and should be treated promptly with laparoscopic cholecystectomy. Treatment delays among symptomatic patients with immunosuppression can increase the risk of infectious complications. A decision analysis study by Kao, Flowers, and Flum provided convincing data to support the expectant management of asymptomatic cholelithiasis in patients with kidney or pancreas transplant. The mortality rate of expectant management was 2 deaths per 1000 patients compared with 5 deaths per 1000 prophylactic cholecystectomies. Expectant management was also favored in a wide range of adjustments considered during sensitivity analyses.

Risks and disease progression among patients with heart and lung transplants, however, appear different. Symptom progression among patients with known asymptomatic cholelithiasis before heart transplant has been documented in as many as 58% of heart recipients after transplant. Morbidity and mortality rates in this population can approach 40%, particularly in patients with secondary complications of gallstone disease. The decision analysis study by Kao and colleagues reported 5 deaths per 1000 patients who underwent prophylactic cholecystectomy after heart transplant compared with 44 deaths per 1000 patients modeled for expectant management. Thus, although expectant management is becoming the dominant strategy for patients with kidney and pancreas transplant, most patients with asymptomatic cholelithiasis after heart or lung transplant are managed currently with prophylactic cholecystectomy.

Gallbladder Cancer

Numerous risk factors for development of cholangiocarcinoma, including gallbladder adenocarcinoma, have been described. Some well-supported associations include ethnicity, including genetic and environmental predisposition (particularly American Indians, Native South Americans, and certain regions in North India), and the presence of concomitant pathology, such as choledochal cysts, gallbladder polyps (particularly larger vascular polyps), and selective mucosal calcifications in the wall of the gallbladder. As discussed, associations between large gallstones or porcelain gallbladder and development of malignant disease, although proposed in the past, are not supported by evidence. A number of studies evaluating "carcinogenesis" of gallstones have failed to control for other potential covariates such as ethnic predisposition. Presence of gallstones as the only potential risk factor for gallbladder adenocarcinoma in the non–Native American U.S. population does not merit cholecystectomy. There is no question that virtually all patients with gallbladder cancer have concomitant gallstones and the stones have some contribution to the pathogenesis of the gallbladder cancer, but the overall risk of development of gallbladder cancer when gallstones are present is negligible; therefore, other factors require consideration. Asymptomatic gallstones in conjunction with any other potential risk factor, such as ethnic or nongallstone pathologic predisposition, merit consideration for prophylactic cholecystectomy.

Spinal Cord Injury

Risk of gallstone formation is approximately two to three times greater among patients with spinal cord injury than in the general population. Multiple studies have evaluated the relationship between asymptomatic gallstones, symptomatic cholelithiasis, and secondary biliary complications in this patient population. Although the risk of cholelithiasis is greater, the risk of symptomatic progression is the same as in the general population. Regardless of level of injury, symptoms of biliary colic are not obscured typically among patients with spinal cord injury. Expectant management of asymptomatic gallstones should be advocated in this population, and cholecystectomy should be performed only in patients with symptomatic cholelithiasis.

Total Parenteral Nutrition

Two major factors predispose patients receiving prolonged total parenteral nutrition to an increased risk of gallstone formation. First is the decrease in overall gallbladder contractility. Although the gallbladder continues to undergo its cyclic pattern of contractions during fasting, the lack of postprandial contraction leads to biliary sludge and gallstone formation. Second is the altered composition of bile salts, particularly among patients with ileal pathology (either ileal Crohn's disease or resection) with a resultant disruption of the enterohepatic circulation.

Current evidence does not support prophylactic cholecystectomy among parenterally fed patients with asymptomatic gallstones. Reports from the early era of parenteral nutrition among chronically ill patients, almost half of whom needed an emergency open cholecystectomy, suggested routine ultrasound scan surveillance and consideration for early prophylactic cholecystectomy. In retrospect, the high rate of morbidity in that population was likely the result of a delay in diagnosis for a relatively new, pathophysiologic diagnosis. Modern understanding of hepatobiliary complications from parenteral nutrition precludes cholecystectomy in the asymptomatic patient. Patients with symptomatic cholelithiasis and those with acalculous cholecystitis (another well-known complication of parenteral nutrition) should undergo a prompt cholecystectomy.

Morbid Obesity

Obese patients have a greater incidence of gallstones than does the general population. In addition, rapid loss of excess body weight, common after operations for morbid obesity, has been linked to increased rates of gallstone formation. The reported prevalence rate of cholelithiasis after Roux-en-Y gastric bypass ranges from 28% to 71%, depending on how carefully patients were screened before surgery. In addition, altered anatomy after a Roux-en-Y gastric bypass or a duodenal switch/biliopancreatic diversion creates therapeutic challenges for the management of potential choledocholithiasis. Although preoperative prevalence and postoperative incidence of gallstones are clearly greater in this population, no consensus presently exists for management of patients with asymptomatic cholelithiasis. As such, current practice patterns vary, with a number of recommendations having been proposed, including: (1) routine prophylactic cholecystectomy in all patients at the time of bariatric surgery; (2) preoperative ultrasound screening followed by concomitant cholecystectomy at the time of bariatric operation if gallstones are identified; (3) postoperative use of oral ursodeoxycholic acid therapy for 6 months (the time of major weight loss and gallstone formation) among patients without gallstones; and (4) expectant management for all patients with asymptomatic gallstones.

Proponents of prophylactic cholecystectomy at the time of bariatric operation for all bariatric patients (whether gallstones are present or not) cite numerous advantages for routine cholecystectomy for all bariatric surgery patients: the high incidence of stone formation, the challenge of preoperative imaging in obese patients, the frequency of gallbladder pathology identified after cholecystectomy (e.g., chronic cholecystitis), and the difficulty of managing biliary complications, especially choledocholithiasis or cholangitis with the altered postoperative anatomy. Short additional operative time, less than 20 minutes in some reports, and the low incidence of morbidity and mortality associated with concurrent cholecystectomy favor prophylactic cholecystectomy. Most of these arguments were more prevalent and attractive in the era of open bariatric surgery, but they may remain pertinent currently in the rare patient who needs an open bariatric operation.

Others have adopted a more selective approach that includes preoperative ultrasound scan or intraoperative evaluation, with concurrent cholecystectomy if gallstones (or other biliary pathology) are identified. In a retrospective analysis of 1713 consecutive patients undergoing Roux-en-Y gastric bypass, the authors used selective cholecystectomy based on the presence of gallbladder pathology. In patients with normal preoperative ultrasound scan results, 8% needed subsequent postbypass cholecystectomy for symptomatic disease that developed during an average follow up of 31 months. Of the patients who had stones identified but did not undergo cholecystectomy because of surgeon or patient preference or because of technical factors, 18% subsequently needed cholecystectomy. These data are consistent with reports that describe rates up to 27% of symptomatic cholelithiasis after gastric bypass requiring cholecystectomy. Such data seem to support a more selective approach to concurrent cholecystectomy (limited to patients with known gallstones) at the time of gastric bypass.

Expectant management in bariatric surgery patients with or without asymptomatic gallstones is also safe. Another recent study reported 1050 "at-risk" patients after laparoscopic Roux-en-Y gastric bypass followed for a median of 32 months. Subsequent cholecystectomy was performed eventually in only 5% of patients for symptomatic cholelithiasis. There were no secondary biliary sequelae or complications. Post–gastric bypass choledocholithiasis is not a frequent complication and can be managed either with double balloon enteroscopy to reach the duodenum (provided the Roux limb is not too long) or with laparoscopic gastrotomy for insertion of the endoscope into the gastric remnant. Of 15 patients managed with this latter procedure at a quaternary interventional gastroenterology practice over a 7-year period, only 4 had choledocholithiasis (9 had unexplained biliary dilation with abdominal pain, 1 had type I sphincter of Oddi dysfunction, and 1 had recurrent acute pancreatitis).

The increased risk of stone formation related to rapid weight loss is thought to be greatest in the early postoperative period. Numerous studies have advocated the use of ursodeoxycholic acid (600 mg daily for 6 months after surgery). A recent meta-analysis of randomized control trials of 521 patients reported a decrease in the development of gallstones from 27% to 9% with the use of postoperative ursodeoxycholic acid. Cost and medication side effects, however, limit patient compliance with oral ursodeoxycholate, potentially inflating its true efficacy.

As such, the management of asymptomatic gallstones in the obese patient remains controversial. Multiple management approaches are safe. Prophylactic cholecystectomy can be performed safely for patients with asymptomatic gallstones at the time of initial bariatric operation but may require more trocars and can be challenging in patients with a large liver or marked visceral obesity. Expectant management with subsequent (laparoscopic) cholecystectomy in patients in whom symptoms develop is also safe.

SUGGESTED READINGS

Gracie WA, Ransohoff DF: The natural history of silent gallstones: the innocent gallstone is not a myth, *N Engl J Med* 307:798–800, 1982.

Gurusamy KS, Davidson BR: Surgical treatment of gallstones, *Gastroenterol Clin North Am* 39:229–244, 2010.

Kao LS, Flowers C, Flum DR: Prophylactic cholecystectomy in transplant patients: a decision analysis, *J Gastrointest Surg* 9:965–972, 2005.

Quesada BM, Kohan G, Roff HE, et al: Management of gallstones and gallbladder disease in patients undergoing gastric bypass, *World J Gastroenterol* 16:2075–2079, 2010.

Ransohoff DF, Gracie WA: Treatment of gallstones, *Ann Intern Med* 119:606–619, 1993.

Sakorafas GH, Milingos D, Peros G: Asymptomatic cholelithiasis: is cholecystectomy really needed? A critical appraisal 15 years after introduction of laparoscopic cholecystectomy, *Dig Dis Sci* 52:1313–1325, 2007.

Schmidt M, Hausken T, Glambek I, et al: A 24-year controlled follow-up of patients with silent gallstones showed no long-term risk of symptomatic or adverse events leading to cholecystectomy, *Scand J Gastroenterol* 46:949–954, 2011.

Stinton LM, Myers RP, Shaffer EA: Epidemiology of gallstones, *Gastroenterol Clin North Am* 39:157–169, 2010.

ACUTE CHOLECYSTITIS

James K. Elsey, MD, FACS, and
David R. Schmidt, MD, FACS

OVERVIEW

Acute cholecystitis is a complication of biliary tract disease, which can be differentiated from chronic cholecystitis in its presentation. Patients with acute cholecystitis commonly have a sudden onset of symptoms that persists greater than 4 hours and causes them to seek consultation in the emergency room, urgent care center, or their physician's office. Symptoms develop from the presence of acute inflammation in the mucosa and wall of the gallbladder, leading to distention of the wall and eventual ischemia. The inflammatory response begins as sterile but can lead to secondary bacterial infection. Rarely, untreated acute cholecystitis can lead to perforation with abscess formation and peritonitis.

Gallstones are most commonly associated with biliary tract disease and can lead to the development of acute cholecystitis when the gallstones become lodged in the cystic duct, causing obstruction of the gallbladder's release of its bile into the common bile duct. Symptoms can improve if the stones become dislodged back into the gallbladder, but more serious illness can occur if the stones pass into the common bile duct, which can result in jaundice and pancreatitis. Acute acalculous cholecystitis can occur where the cystic duct is obstructed in the absence of gallstones and is less common in the general population but more often associated with critically ill patients in the intensive care unit (ICU) and in patients receiving total parental nutrition. Cholelithiasis is estimated to be present in 10% of the population, and one third has development of symptoms. The risk of asymptomatic stones becoming symptomatic is reported to be 1% to 2% per year. Once symptoms of acute cholecystitis develop, these symptoms should be treated immediately to prevent the risk of development of a more serious medical illness.

CLINICAL PRESENTATION AND EVALUATION

Patients with acute cholecystitis should be differentiated from patients with symptomatic biliary colic because they need immediate evaluation, workup, and treatment to prevent the deleterious progression of the disease. The classic right upper quadrant pain is accompanied by signs of the inflammatory response, which include fever, nausea, and vomiting and signs of peritoneal inflammation, causing pain radiating to the back and right scapulae regions. In contrast, patients with biliary colic often have intermittent pain that lasts less than a few hours and do not classically have fevers. The distinction is important because acute cholecystitis requires immediate treatment and biliary colic can be treated with cholecystectomy on a nonemergent elective basis.

Patients with acute cholecystitis commonly present with fever, tachycardia, and right upper quadrant tenderness on the physical examination. A positive Murphy's sign occurs when the pain in the right upper quadrant causes a sudden inspiratory arrest during deep palpation. Local peritoneal signs may also occur in acute disease, but diffuse peritonitis suggests a more advanced stage of disease and possible perforation. A palpable tender mass is indicative of a possible phlegmon, which can be a sign of advanced local inflammation indicating a more difficult surgical approach to cholecystectomy. If jaundice is noted on examination, this suggests common bile duct obstruction by choledocholithiasis or possibly Mirizzi's syndrome caused by a large cystic duct stone with inflammation compressing the common bile duct.

After a thorough history and physical examination, the next step in a workup includes laboratory evaluation. A complete blood count typically reveals an elevated white blood cell count (WBC). Although a complete metabolic profile typically reveals normal liver function, mild elevation of transaminase may occur from local inflammation to the liver and mild hyperbilirubinemia can be seen in severe infections. Markedly elevated transaminase values may be the result of hepatitis, whereas hyperbilirubinemia may be indicative of common bile duct obstruction and choledocholithiasis. Amylase and lipase levels should be tested to rule out the development of acute pancreatitis in any patient with abdominal pain.

A right upper quadrant ultrasound scan is the radiographic study of choice for its specific findings, easy availability, and inexpensive costs. Gallstones are commonly seen along with other findings highly suggestive of acute cholecystitis, including a lodged stone in the neck of the gallbladder, gallbladder wall thickening of 4 mm or greater, and pericholecystic fluid. In the unusual case in which ultrasound scan is not helpful or is inconclusive, a hepatobiliary iminodiacetic acid (HIDA) scan can determine whether cystic duct obstruction is present. A HIDA scan that shows nonvisualization of the gallbladder is consistent with acute cholecystitis from cystic duct obstruction, although false-positive studies can occur in fasting patients. Abdominal computed tomographic (CT) scan can also illustrate changes in patients with acute cholecystitis but is less sensitive in milder disease of the gallbladder and should not be used as the initial study in uncomplicated acute cholecystitis. The CT scan may show gallstones, a thickened gallbladder wall, or pericholecystic fluid as seen on ultrasound scan, but it is most beneficial to rule out other intraabdominal pathology if the diagnosis of acute cholecystitis is unclear. A magnetic resonance cholangiopancreatogram (MRCP) can also show signs of acute cholecystitis but is used in the authors' institution in the evaluation of hyperbilirubinemia to rule out choledocholithiasis or malignancy.

DIFFERENTIAL DIAGNOSIS

Acute cholecystitis is most often associated with gallstones or cystic duct obstruction in calculus disease. The differential diagnosis in patients with acute right upper quadrant pain includes gastric, colonic, renal, pancreatic, liver, lung, cardiac, and appendiceal disease processes. These include peptic ulcer disease, gastritis, gastroenteritis, colitis, right or transverse colon diverticulitis, nephrolithiasis, renal infarction or infection, pancreatitis, hepatitis, liver abscess, pneumonia, myocardial ischemia, and appendicitis. A common consult occurs in patients who are admitted to rule out cardiac disease and who after a negative cardiac workup are found to have acute biliary tract disease.

MANAGEMENT

Once the diagnosis of acute cholecystitis is determined, the patient's condition is stabilized, comorbid risk factors are managed, and broad-spectrum antibiotics are given. More than 50% of patients with acute cholecystitis have positive bile cultures, with *Escherichia coli, Klebsiella, Enterobacter,* and Bacteroides species the predominant isolates, and antibiotic coverage should be broad enough to cover these organisms. Except in the instance of the patient with sepsis or immunocompromise, antibiotics are discontinued in the early perioperative period.

The debate over the timing of surgery in the patient with acute cholecystitis is one of mainly historic interest; it is now widely accepted that cholecystectomy should be performed within the first 72 hours of diagnosis. In the nonseptic, high operative risk case with reversible or improvable comorbid risk factors, it is often prudent to manage with supportive care, optimizing the clinical situation as best as possible and performing an elective cholecystectomy in 6 to 12 weeks.

Multiple studies have clearly shown the safety and the advantage of early cholecystotomy in the management of this process. No demonstrable difference is found in mortality rate, major bile duct injury, postoperative pain, or other significant complications in patients treated with early or delayed cholecystectomy. Early cholecystectomy halts the progressive inflammatory response and coincident tissue fibrosis that complicates tissue dissection and vital structure identification, allowing for the increased opportunity for a safe laparoscopic procedure and reducing the chances of open conversion. In addition, early cholecystectomy in patients with cholecystitis and systemic toxicity, emphysematous cholecystitis, and acute acalculous cholecystitis reduces the known tendency towards gangrene and perforation in this subset of patients.

LAPAROSCOPIC CHOLECYSTECTOMY

Laparoscopic cholecystectomy is now considered the procedure of choice in the operative management of acute cholecystitis. Multiple studies have confirmed that the overall morbidity rate, length of hospital stay, cost, and time to return to function are lower in the patient treated laparoscopically when compared with the standard open technique. That said, the variable and often severe inflammatory response seen in the patient with acute cholecystitis adds special technical challenges to the laparoscopic technique, potentially leading to devastating and lethal vascular and ductal injuries. Severe inflammation limiting the safe conduct of the laparoscopic procedure requires open conversion in up to 20% of these patients. Dramatic and ongoing improvements in optics, instrumentation, and laparoscopic skills have reduced the absolute contraindications of the technique to patients with adhesive hostile abdomens and those who cannot tolerate abdominal insufflation.

The primary guiding principle of laparoscopic cholecystectomy in the patient with acute cholecystitis is the safe removal of the gallbladder without vital biliary structure injury. Inherent challenges in this subset of patients include a lack of tactile sensation, a two-dimensional view of a three-dimensional field, lateral retraction techniques that distort the normal alignment of critical biliary tract structures, periodic difficulties in maintaining a dry field, and abnormal dissecting angles created by atypical and challenging body habitus. These limitations, combined with an often robust inflammatory response and the known frequent anatomic anomalies of the biliary structures, result in an inherently dangerous procedure of varying proportion. It is therefore essential to follow, without deviation, the time-honored proven techniques of laparoscopic cholecystectomy to avoid complications in these patients. Good visualization provided with a clear laparoscope with adequate illumination often aided by a 30-degree or directed device is essential. As in all operations, good exposure through adequate retraction is a fundamental requirement for success. The standard four-port approach is usually adequate; however, in more challenging cases, never hesitate to add more trocars and retractors to optimize exposure. Superolateral retraction on the dome of the gallbladder combined with inferolateral retraction of the infundibulum usually provides an adequate field to begin the dissecting process. In situations where the gallbladder is tensely distended, the retraction process can be greatly aided with needle drainage. Dissection is begun high on the gallbladder infundibulum with a goal of safely exposing and identifying the infundibular-cystic duct junction. The surgeon should avoid initial dissection efforts low on the gallbladder because it is very easy to become confused and lost in this area, creating a higher chance of vital structure injury. In cases of severe inflammation, it is often helpful to divide the inflamed or fibrotic gallbladder rind along the superior and inferior margins of the infundibulum before dissection, allowing for better mobilization and retraction of the infundibulum and, hence, safer dissection of the infundibular-cystic area. The top-down dissection should cautiously continue until the critical infundibular-cystic duct junction view is obtained. Dissection is only considered satisfactory when a complete and unobstructed 360-degree view of the infundibular-cystic junction is obtained, a clear space between the superior distal margin of the gallbladder and liver is seen, and the surgeon is absolutely certain that only two definite structures (cystic duct, cystic artery) are left entering the gallbladder. In no circumstance are any structures in this critical area to be clipped, cauterized, or divided until the surgeon has achieved this critical and certain level of dissection and exposure. In the circumstance when this cannot be achieved, an intraoperative cholangiogram through the distal infundibulum can sometimes clarify the anatomy. If this is not possible or not completely helpful, a dome-down dissection technique can be used. However, the surgeon must be very cautious in avoiding injury to the hepatic artery or the right hepatic duct while dissecting the distal superior edge of the gallbladder away from the liver. If the appropriate dissection techniques have not resulted in a certain and critical view of the anatomy, it is imperative to abort the laparoscopic procedure and convert to an open operation. Remember that the goal is the safe and uncomplicated removal of the gallbladder, and in this circumstance, conversion to an open procedure is not only the appropriate approach but is also the mark of a safe and mature surgeon. Finally, independent of the techniques used, the critically defined structures are individually ligated and the gallbladder is removed with the surgeon's energy source of choice.

One final note of caution involves the case of a short cystic duct. Injudicious dissection or cholangiography in the presence of a short cystic duct can lead to common duct injury or cystic duct postoperative bile leak. In this circumstance, it is better to perform cholangiography through the infundibulum and terminate the distal dissection by dividing the distal infundibulum by ligation or endostapling.

There has been an evolution in the use of intraoperative cholangiography from a routine standard to a more selective approach. Most surgeons today reserve cholangiography to situations of anatomic uncertainty or when choledocholithiasis is suspected. The overall incidence rate of common duct stones reported in conglomerate series of laparoscopic cholecystectomies is 4% to 11%; however, in patients with acute cholecystitis, the reported incidence rate has been as high as 18%. With use of cholangiography to help elucidate anatomic uncertainties, it is important to understand that the images can be misleading, especially when the right hepatic duct arises off of the cystic duct. Therefore, it cannot be overemphasized that intraoperative cholangiography, albeit often very helpful, should never be substituted for a definitive dissection creating the critical view of the vital biliary tract structures. In keeping with the noted increased incidence of ductal stones in patients with acute cholecystitis, some surgeons have advocated the routine preoperative use of MRCP or endoscopic retrograde cholangiopancreatography (ERCP). It is fair to say, however, that this practice is not mainstream, and most surgeons reserve this strategy for patients with hard signs of choledocholithiasis such as significant jaundice, cholangitis, ductal dilation, or radiologic findings of intraductal calculi.

When ductal stones are discovered during laparoscopic cholecystectomy, the growing consensus is that they should be definitively addressed at the time of the initial surgery. This is obviously more satisfactory to the patient and more cost effective and saves the patient from a potentially failed ERCP. Current options include laparoscopic common duct exploration and laparoscopic transcystic basket choledocholithotomy. Both procedures are difficult and require expertise that is not often available in every hospital. In such a situation, which is more common than not, it is well within the standard of care to plan for a postoperative ERCP choledocholithotomy.

OPEN CHOLECYSTECTOMY

Despite the mainstream acceptance of laparoscopic cholecystectomy as the procedure of choice in the management of acute cholecystitis, open cholecystectomy remains an important part of the surgical armamentarium in the treatment of this disease. The procedure is indicated when laparoscopy is contraindicated or when the laparoscopic procedure cannot be completed safely. The operation is performed through either a subcostal or a midline incision, both of which provide excellent exposure. Dissection is achieved through either a fundus-down or an infundibulum-down technique. In situations of severe inflammation, especially when the infundibular technique is too hazardous, the fundus-down technique is safer and advisable. As noted in the description of this technique done laparoscopically, it is important to proceed cautiously in the lower superior area of the gallbladder to avoid damaging the hepatic artery and duct, which can be retracted up in this dissection plane because of the inflammatory process often encountered in this situation. The principles of the rest of the operation are no different than those of the previously described laparoscopic procedure, with the exception of the situation where ductal stones are encountered. In this circumstance, the authors believe that definitive management of this problem should occur at the time of the initial open operation in the form of a common duct exploration and choledocholithotomy with T-tube drainage. If the technique of common duct exploration is not within the repertoire of the operating surgeon and not available in the hospital at the time of the surgery, it is then acceptable to close the patient and obtain a postoperative ERCP. The surgeon must be aware, however, that this exposes the patient to the possibility of a failed ERCP effort and the need of other difficult and dangerous ancillary procedures.

In the unusual, but periodic, case in which the inflammatory response is so severe as to preclude complete open safe dissection of the gallbladder, a partial cholecystectomy is the next best alternative. Key elements of this technique include leaving the back wall of the gallbladder intact, cauterizing the mucosa, and attempting, if possible, to close the distal infundibulum and place closed suction drains. Finally, for patients to whom partial cholecystectomy is deemed too hazardous or in patients with sepsis who are not operable candidates, tube cholecystotomy is the appropriate and often life-saving alternative.

NEW DEVELOPMENTS

In recent years and in keeping with the progressive minimally invasive theme in surgery, several reduced port or alternative port procedures for biliary surgery have been proposed. Single-port access surgery with one incision predominately at the umbilicus has gained some popularity. Although the procedure at the present time appears to be as safe in selected patients as a standard multiport laparoscopic cholecystectomy, the only proven advantage so far is possibly one of cosmesis. At the extreme end of this minimally invasive effort is incisionless, or natural orifice surgery (NOTES), which involves endoscopically created portals for surgery through the vagina or stomach. The NOTES procedures are currently investigational only but certainly highlight the ongoing miracles of surgical technologic development.

Finally, the application of the robot as an adjunct to the laparoscopic technique of cholecystectomy is gaining interest and popularity. Current robotic platforms allow for single-port access cholecystectomy with the advantage of three-dimensional optics, more achievable triangulation, markedly improved ergonomics, and a proposed reduction in the technical difficulty of the operation. The advantages and the appropriateness of this technology, and cost issues, are yet to be resolved and await further study.

COMPLICATIONS

A litany of recognized complications can occur after laparoscopic or open cholecystectomy. It is important to note and to be aware that the conduct of these common procedures in patients with acute cholecystitis with the coincident difficulties of dissection and anatomic recognition imposed by the inherent inflammatory process creates an environment of surgical difficulty and danger. Difficulties in structure recognition can lead to the delayed diagnosis of operative injuries, often with disastrous clinical results.

Subhepatic abscess most often occurs in patients with severely inflamed, gangrenous, or perforative gallbladders. The abscess results from the spillage of infected bile with often coincident hematoma and can be catalyzed by the presence of spilled stones that are left behind. The complication is best prevented by avoidance of bile spillage, obtaining of meticulous hemostasis in the liver bed, the retrieval of all spilled stones, copious irrigation of the subhepatic space, and the placement of closed suction drains if severe contamination has occurred. Most of these situations resolve after a short period of antibiotics, but definitive treatment with the placement of CT scan–directed drains is sometimes necessary.

Excessive bleeding, either from the bed of the dissected liver or from vascular injury, can be extremely problematic and challenging, particularly in the laparoscopic case. Liver bed bleeding, although often impressive, can almost always be controlled with the aggressive use of electrocautery and liberal use of topical chemical coagulant products. Vascular injuries often create a situation where control becomes difficult because of visual limitations from the ongoing hemorrhage and vessel retraction into areas of severe inflammation. Injudicious and poorly exposed dissection, blind clamping, or indiscriminate autoclipping often leads to ductal injury and should be avoided. In the circumstance of the laparoscopic case, if after a reasonable period of time, safe exposure and dissecting techniques have not achieved hemostasis, the patient should be rapidly converted to an open procedure. It is important to note that many bile tract injuries are complex and the surgeon should avoid missing a coincident ductal injury in this situation.

Bile duct leaks are unfortunately a common complication in this set of patients. They result from either persistent drainage of the interrupted ducts of Luschka or more commonly from a cystic duct leak from a dislodged clip. Clip dislodgement seems to occur when clips are placed across severely inflamed ducts or across ducts containing calculi. In efforts to prevent this complication, both of these maneuvers should therefore be avoided. If a good clip closure cannot be achieved, then closure of the biliary system can be accomplished by placing the endoGIA across the distal infundibulum. These patients present with low-grade fever, bloating, and hyperbilirubinemia, most commonly within the first postoperative week. The diagnosis is confirmed by the presence of a subhepatic fluid collection on ultrasound scan and a ductal leak on HIDA scan. Unless the patient presents with septic peritonitis and hemodynamic instability, the treatment is nonoperative and accomplished with CT scan drainage of the subhepatic space and endoscopic biliary stent placement.

Bile duct injury is an extremely serious and potentially catastrophic complication of cholecystectomy. The worldwide reported incidence rate of this complication is 0.1% to 0.2% in open procedures and 0.4% to 0.8% in those conducted laparoscopically. The classic injury occurs when the common bile duct is mistaken for the cystic duct, most commonly resulting from excessive cephalad retraction of the gallbladder, bringing the two ductal structures into parallel alignment. The incidence of this complication is markedly increased in situations of severe inflammation, anomalous anatomy, and excessive bleeding. As stated previously, it is important to note these injuries are often complex, with concomitant hepatic artery and portal vein branch injuries in up to 12% of patients. It is also interesting to note that the use of routine cholangiography has not been shown to prevent these injuries but certainly should be attempted after intraoperative bile duct injury has been discovered. Intraoperative recognition occurs in only about 25% of patients and is noted by evidence of a bile leak, abnormal cholangiogram, or obvious anatomic disruption at the time of surgery. In most patients, ductal injury recognition is delayed, presenting in the early postoperative period with jaundice and pain with or without sepsis, or 6 months to 1 year later, often with cirrhosis or liver failure from duct disruption or stricture. The management of this complication depends on the time of the diagnosis and the extent of the injury to the duct. The goal of treatment is the prevention of cholangitis, ductal stricture, and cirrhosis. When the common bile duct injury is discovered at the time of cholecystectomy, it is important to remain calm, not panic, and attempt to accurately define the nature, extent, and location of the injury. Minor nonelectrocautery lateral ductal injuries can be managed with simple T-tube drainage of the injury site. However, significant injuries from electrocautery and those involving damage to greater than 50% of the circumference of the bile duct wall require complex Roux-en-Y choledochojejunostomy reconstruction. Although immediate reconstruction of a major ductal injury is preferable at the time of the incident, this reconstruction requires the expertise of an experienced hepatobiliary tract surgeon who is facile in the management of this complication. If this level of expertise is not available in the hospital at the time of this injury, it is imperative not to attempt the repair but to define the injury, achieve drainage, and transfer the patient to a facility with these capabilities as soon as possible. In the patient in whom the diagnosis is delayed beyond the immediate operative period, the principles of drainage and ductal imaging also apply. Bile duct anatomy and drainage is often best accomplished in these patients with percutaneous transhepatic cholangiogram (PTC). Additional anatomic definition and drainage can be provided with ERCP and CT scan–directed catheters. In these circumstances, these patients are best treated with a delayed biliary tract reconstruction in 6 to 12 weeks, allowing for the resolution of sepsis and inflammation.

SUGGESTED READINGS

Clair DG, Brooks DC: Laparoscopic cholangiography: the case for a selective approach, *Surg Clin North Am* 74:961, 1994.

Elsey JK, Feliciano DV: Initial experience with single-incision laparoscopic cholecystectomy, *J Am Coll Surg* 210(5):L620–626, 2010.

Lo CM, Liu CL, Lai EL, et al: Early versus delayed laparoscopic cholecystectomy for treatment of acute cholecystitis, *Ann Surg* 223:37, 1996.

Rattner DW, Ferguson C, Warshaw AL: Factors associated with successful laparoscopic cholecystectomy for acute cholecystitis, *Ann Surg* 217:233, 1993.

Soper NJ, Flye MW, Brunt LM, et al: Diagnosis and management of biliary duct complications of laparoscopic cholecystectomy, *Am J Surg* 165:655, 1993.

Strasberg SM, Brunt LM: Rationale and use of the critical view in laparoscopic cholecystectomy, *J Am Coll Surg* 211(1):132–138, 2010.

THE MANAGEMENT OF COMMON BILE DUCT STONES

Rizwan Ahmed, MD, and Mark D. Duncan, MD

OVERVIEW

In the spectrum of biliary calculus disease, choledocholithiasis, or common bile duct (CBD) stones, provides diagnostic and therapeutic challenges to the surgeon. With advancements made in imaging and minimally invasive surgery, algorithms for optimal care have evolved. CBD stones are found in 8% to 10% of patients who have cholelithiasis. These are secondary CBD stones and are almost always cholesterol stones. Primary CBD stones are those found as a result of biliary stasis and infection; these stones are most often pigment stones composed of calcium bilirubinate. In only a small minority of these cases are CBD stones found in the absence of stones in the gallbladder.

The manifestation of choledocholithiasis is variable. Patients may have no symptoms, with either small stones passing through to the duodenum or with stones present. More commonly, stones obstruct the lumen of the CBD, causing clinical manifestations that may include obstructive jaundice, gallstone pancreatitis, or ascending cholangitis. Obstructive jaundice is evaluated to distinguish between calculus disease (CBD stone), stricture (which implies prior pancreatitis or prior surgery), and malignancy. In gallstone pancreatitis, levels of pancreatic enzymes typically rise and then rapidly fall. If the CBD is evaluated and cleared as described later, the authors perform laparoscopic cholecystectomy during the same admission.

The classic presentation of right upper quadrant pain, fever, and jaundice is described as *Charcot's triad,* after the French neurologist Jean-Martin Charcot's description of cholangitis. The presence of fever and jaundice may be indicators of locoregional infection confined to the CBD. When this condition progresses to include septic shock and mental status changes, termed *Reynold's pentad,* this indicates systemic infection, and decompression of the biliary tract is urgently needed. Fortunately, most patients with choledocholithiasis are spared this degree of illness.

Most often, cholelithiasis is detected as a result of clinical suspicion because of laboratory indicators, dilatation of the CBD on sonography or computed tomographic scan, or the history of jaundice or pancreatitis. The management of choledocholithiasis is dependent on when it is detected in relation to surgical treatment: (1) as a result of preoperative suspicion for or detection of CBD stones; (2) when CBD stones are found at the time of surgery, typically during intraoperative cholangiography (IOC); and (3) after cholecystectomy, when approximately 1% to 2% of patients who have undergone the procedure present later with symptomatic retained CBD stones. For the purpose of definition, previously undetected CBD stones found more than 2 years after cholecystectomy are defined as primary stones but are managed by the same postoperative algorithm.

CLINICAL LABORATORY FINDINGS

The classic laboratory findings with any biliary tract obstructions are elevation of the serum alkaline phosphatase level and direct hyperbilirubinemia. Elevations of the aspartate aminotransferase, alanine aminotransferase, and lactate dehydrogenase levels are often not present or are inconsistent and thus are of less diagnostic value. The finding of elevated pancreatic enzymes amylase and lipase levels in the presence of cholelithiasis raises the suspicion for gallstone pancreatitis, particularly in combination with a dilated CBD. Leukocytosis may be present with cholecystitis, cholangitis, or pancreatitis and is a nonspecific marker of biliary tract inflammation or infection. Any of the aforementioned laboratory abnormalities along with the physical signs and symptoms or with ductal dilatation observed on imaging warrant further investigation with imaging studies for treatment planning.

IMAGING WORKUP

Transabdominal Ultrasonography

The most common initial imaging modality for the evaluation of the gallbladder and biliary tract is transabdominal ultrasonography. The authors utilize the sonogram to answer the following questions. Are gallstones present? Is the gallbladder wall thickened, or is pericholecystic fluid present to suggest acute cholecystitis? Is there tenderness during the sonographic examination, the sonographic Murphy's sign? Is the CBD dilated? Is there sonographic evidence of acute pancreatitis? Ultrasonography has become the standard of care in diagnosing biliary tract dilation and biliary stones. The finding of dilation of the CBD to 1 cm or more in the presence of cholelithiasis raises the suspicion for choledocholithiasis. In at least half of patients presenting in the emergency department with suspicion of CBD stones, however, no stone is observed on subsequent definitive endoscopic retrograde cholangiopancreatography (ERCP). The sonogram itself may demonstrate actual calculi in the CBD, but this is less common. Endoscopic ultrasonography during upper endoscopy has been shown to be sensitive in 94% and specific in 95% of patients with choledocholithiasis, but this procedure requires special expertise and is rarely employed in the acute presentation.

Although hepatobiliary iminodiacetic acid (HIDA) may help clinicians detect obstructing CBD stones by virtue of nonvisualization of the duodenum and small bowel, it is seldom employed to evaluate the CBD directly.

Endoscopic Retrograde Cholangiopancreatography

The method routinely employed for diagnosis and therapeutic management of choledocholithiasis is ERCP. ERCP is standard practice for removing stones from the CBD; indeed, with the advent of ERCP, the frequency of surgical CBD exploration declined rapidly. When performed by a skilled endoscopist, ERCP and basket stone extraction, typically combined with sphincterotomy of the sphincter of Oddi, has satisfactorily cleared the CBD in 90% to 97% of cases. There are, however, consequences of ERCP, namely post-ERCP pancreatitis which is diagnosed on the basis of enzyme levels in up to 6% of patients and on the basis of clinical symptoms in 3%. As with any acute pancreatitis, the clinical course can be of short duration and inconsequential or develop into multisystem disease with life-threatening consequences. Other less common complications of ERCP—or with any biliary instrumentation, including percutaneous transhepatic cholangiography (PTC)—include sepsis from cholangitis, hemorrhage, or intestinal perforation. A rare, late complication is papillary stenosis. Furthermore, as already noted, approximately half of results of ERCP in the setting of suspected CBD stones are negative. Thus, to spare the risk of unnecessary diagnostic ERCP, the authors now routinely employ magnetic resonance imaging (MRI) or magnetic resonance cholangiopancreatography (MRCP).

Although some technically advanced laparoscopic surgeons may advocate for surgical clearance of the CBD by laparoscopic CBD exploration, the authors believe that preoperative ERCP is a better and safer approach when stones are documented in the CBD. In 2002, the National Institutes of Health published a consensus regarding the indications for ERCP and the contraindications to unnecessary procedures. For the purpose of this text, the key points addressed were as follows. Patients scheduled for elective cholecystectomy for cholelithiasis did not require ERCP if there was a low clinical suspicion for CBD stone. ERCP combined with sphincterotomy and stone removal was considered effective in the management of choledocholithiasis. Furthermore, in the consensus statement, postoperative ERCP was approved as an acceptable and effective means to clear CBD stones left behind after laparoscopic or open CBD exploration. This is in contrast to a previously stated surgical opinion that known choledocholithiasis identified in the operating room should be definitively addressed. An acceptable alternative to surgical CBD exploration is to complete the cholecystectomy procedure and to plan for postoperative ERCP. There is no demonstrable change in overall rates of morbidity or mortality between ERCP followed by laparoscopic cholecystectomy and laparoscopic cholecystectomy followed by ERCP. Some patients, particularly those with prior gastric bypass or with duodenal diverticula, are poor candidates for ERCP. Options for them are discussed as follows.

Magnetic Resonance Cholangiopancreatography

Advances in imaging have led clinicians to change the approach to suspected CBD stones. Although ERCP provides diagnosis and management in the same setting, it is not without complications, as outlined previously. MRCP has been found to be 93% specific and 94% sensitive in diagnosing choledocholithiasis and provides a noninvasive alternative to viewing stones missed in transabdominal ultrasonography. This attribute of MRCP provides the most utility in preoperative decision making for patients undergoing elective surgery for cholelithiasis in whom there is a question of a CBD stone, without subjecting the patient to ERCP. In particular, the half-Fourier acquisition single-shot turbo spin-echo (HASTE) MRI sequence provides excellent images that are more readily interpretable by surgeons than sonograms and is an ultrafast modality. Acquisition time is 13 seconds, which allows patients to hold their breath. The authors routinely employ MRCP for all patients in whom choledocholithiasis is suspected preoperatively (Figure 1). If the MRCP confirms a stone in the duct, the patient is then directed to therapeutic ERCP. If no stone is present, and the clinical course is consistent, the authors go ahead with the planned cholecystectomy, typically laparoscopically. In rare instances, rising bilirubin or alkaline phosphatase levels even after a negative MRCP prompt reconsideration of ERCP.

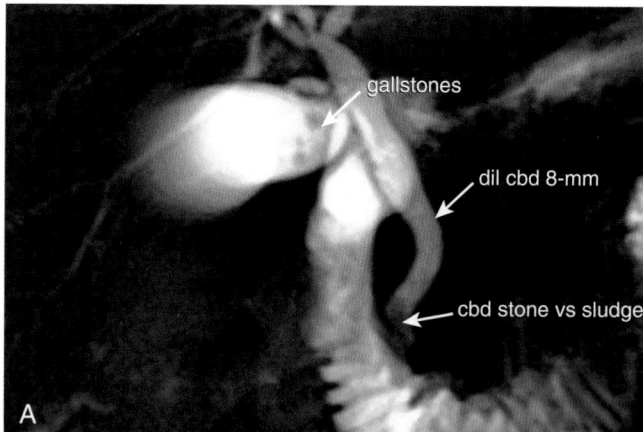

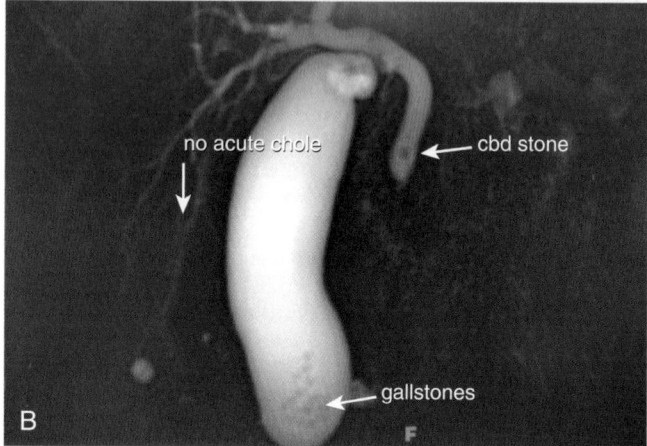

FIGURE 1   A, Magnetic resonance cholangiopancreatography demonstrating cholelithiasis and choledocholithiasis with mildly dilated common bile duct. **B,** Another patient with MRI demonstrating cholelithiasis and choledocholithiasis.

MANAGEMENT

Management of choledocholithiasis depends on when CBD stones were discovered in relation to surgery. The flowchart in Figure 2 demonstrates the algorithm for cholelithiasis suspected or discovered preoperatively, intraoperatively, or postoperatively.

Preoperative

Most patients will have already undergone ultrasonography before surgical evaluation for biliary tract disease. When choledocholithiasis is suspected on the basis of the findings of a dilated CBD or elevations in bilirubin, alkaline phosphatase, or pancreatic enzyme levels, the patient next undergoes MRCP. If CBD stones are confirmed by MRCP, or if they have already been demonstrated on ultrasonography, then ERCP is employed to clear the duct. If no stones are visualized on MRCP or during subsequent ERCP, then laparoscopic cholecystectomy is performed during the same admission. When choledocholithiasis is found and ERCP with endoscopic sphincterotomy is unable to clear the CBD of stones, several options are available to the surgeon. One is to proceed to surgery for laparoscopic cholecystectomy with laparoscopic CBD exploration. The technique for this is described in the Intraoperative section, but not all surgeons are capable of performing minimally invasive CBD exploration. Another consideration would be interventional radiologic studies for PTC. The initial PTC procedure is often diagnostic and not

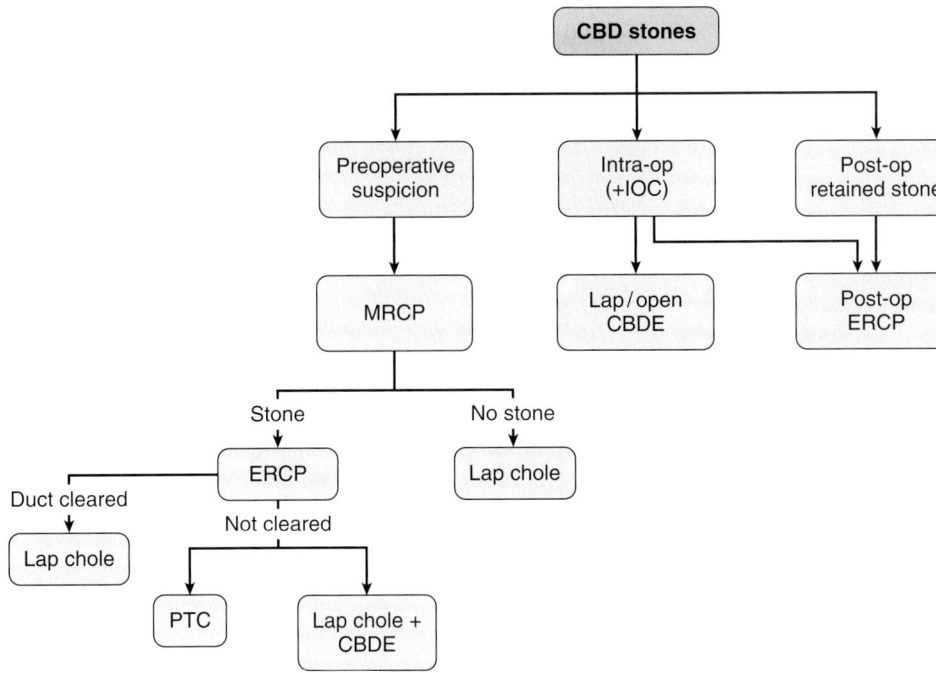

FIGURE 2 Algorithm for management of choledocholithiasis. *CBD*, common bile duct; *CBDE*, common bile duct exploration; *ERCP*, endoscopic retrograde cholangiopancreatography; *IOC*, intraoperative cholangiography; *Lap*, laparoscopy; Lap chole, laparoscopic cholecystectomy; *MRCP*, magnetic resonance cholangiopancreatography; *PTC*, percutaneous transhepatic cholangiography.

therapeutic, inasmuch as a catheter of adequate diameter to allow for instrumentation or manipulation is rarely available; thus repeated interventional radiographic studies with serial dilatation and upsizing is usually required. An effort at ERCP can also be repeated. The decision as to which option is best for a given patient is based on the clinical course of the condition and the availability of and local expertise with endoscopic, radiologic, and surgical techniques.

With the increasing number of patients undergoing bariatric procedures in which cholecystectomy is not always routinely performed, the ability to perform ERCP may be limited. In patients who have undergone Rou-en-Y gastric bypass, the duodenum and ampulla of Vater are no longer accessible to routine upper endoscopy. In this patient population, direct imaging, stent placement, or manipulation of the biliary tree may require a radiologic approach with PTC and catheter placement. Another option if PTC cannot be accomplished is to proceed to surgery: either laparoscopic cholecystectomy and CBD exploration or an open procedure. The history of previous foregut surgery does not preclude successful laparoscopic biliary tract surgery. The authors have employed, on rare occasion, placement of a polyethylene glycol (PEG) tube in the bypassed gastric remnant that can provide access for subsequent ERCP. This PEG tube can be placed either under computed tomographic guidance by an interventional radiologist or directly by a skilled endoscopist navigating up the Roux limb. In the latter case, the endoscopist may be able to reach the ampulla but, at extended endoscopy, is probably not able to cannulate and perform ERCP; instead, the endoscopist creates the more direct route via the PEG tube. These efforts to clear the CBD of stones in advance of surgery are warranted in a patient population who by virtue of either or both previous upper abdominal surgery and body habitus may be poorly suited for surgical CBD exploration. The same considerations apply to patients with prior gastric resection with gastrojejunostomy or in patients with known duodenal diverticulum.

Intraoperative

Choledocholithiasis may be suspected or found intraoperatively as a result of the presence of CBD dilation, which prompts IOC, or as a finding of IOC whether performed for specific indications or

routinely. Although the authors do not perform routine IOC with laparoscopic cholecystectomy, practices vary, and the frequency of IOC varies remarkably according to geography. Arguments in favor of routine IOC cite the detection of choledocholithiasis, the recognition of CBD anatomic variations, and, perhaps of most importance, the ability to identify CBD injury. Routine IOC, when reviewed in a meta-analysis of studies conducted nationwide, showed no reduction in rate of CBD injury compared to selective use of IOC. The authors conclude that routine IOC is not necessary.

Criteria for selective IOC are not uniformly accepted but typically include a history of jaundice, a history of pancreatitis, or elevation of hepatic enzyme levels. The essential components of IOC are visualization of right and left hepatic ducts, free flow of the contrast agent into the duodenum, visualization of any filling defect or obstruction, and identification of any CBD injuries. In the event that IOC does not reveal the intrahepatic ducts, the patient can be placed in the Trendelenburg position, and morphine sulfate can be administered intravenously to cause contraction of the sphincter of Oddi, thus preventing the flow of the contrast agent into the duodenum. If the concern is from the caudal flow of the contrast agent, the patient can be placed in the reverse Trendelenburg position and given glucagon. In practice, the authors have rarely found these maneuvers to be necessary. When IOC is successful, contrast material is visualized flowing into the duodenum and clearly into both hepatic ducts with no extravasation or filling defect.

Fluoroscopy is better than static images for intraoperative viewing. When choledocholithiasis is determined during surgery, the surgeon may elect to directly address this with laparoscopic CBD exploration. It is also considered acceptable practice to perform the laparoscopic cholecystectomy and plan postoperative ERCP for clearance of the CBD. Although this practice was previously controversial, it is now recognized that postoperative ERCP is usually successful, and as the National Institutes of Health consensus noted, the overall rate of morbidity is the same as when ERCP precedes surgery. The authors no longer recommend conversion to an open procedure solely to perform CBD exploration when cholecystectomy can be performed laparoscopically; the authors believe that the overall rate of morbidity of this approach exceeds that of morbidity after ERCP, in recognition of the small risk of unsuccessful ERCP and retained stones. For surgeons less familiar with minimally invasive techniques of CBD exploration, postoperative ERCP is the procedure of choice. Other potential barriers to a surgical approach to the CBD include the unavailability of a 3-mm endoscope/choledochoscope; the unavailability of appropriate sized Silastic tubes, biliary stents, or T-tubes; or simply the smallness of the CBD.

Technique of Laparoscopic Common Bile Duct Exploration

The simplest approach to laparoscopic CBD exploration is to avoid suture or incision in the CBD itself and instead go through the cystic duct to access the CBD (transcystic duct CBD exploration). During laparoscopic cholecystectomy, and before transsection of the cystic duct and removal of the gallbladder, a transverse opening is made sharply in the cystic duct, similar to what is done during IOC. The opening can then be dilated to directly engage the CBD, but the laparoscopic approach that the authors favor is to utilize a choledochoscope (2.5- or 3-mm endoscope) with a working channel for a basket stone extractor. This instrument may be more familiar to the operating room team as the *pediatric ureteroscope.* It allows direct visualization with constant saline flow in both the distal CBD and the proximal ducts. The choledochoscope may be directly inserted or placed over a guidewire with direct visualization in either setting. With saline flush alone, the surgeon may be able to flush a stone through the ampulla. It is more likely, however, that a Dormia basket will be passed through the 1.2-mm working channel of the choledochoscope. The disadvantage of using the basket is that once the stone is within the basket, the entire apparatus, including choledochoscope and basket, must be withdrawn together for extraction and then the choledochoscope reinserted after each effort.

A completion IOC helps confirm clearance of the duct. High success rates (up to 90%) have been reported for this approach. The great advantage of the transcystic duct approach is that after successful extraction of one or more stones, the cystic duct can then simply be doubly clipped proximal to the opening in the cystic duct, just as in typical laparoscopic cholecystectomy. Further options that may afford a more secure closure of the cystic duct stump include ligation and use of an Endo Stitch loop closure. If the CBD can be satisfactorily cleared in this scenario, a T-tube is not required.

Technique of Laparoscopic Direct Common Bile Duct Exploration

If limitations at the facility, of the surgeon's skill set, or of the patient's anatomy do not enable the transcystic duct approach, either a laparoscopic or open traditional CBD exploration can be performed. This may also be necessary in the case of large stones, small cystic duct, or stones in the proximal ducts. Laparoscopic direct CBD exploration requires more advanced laparoscopic training and skills than most surgeons performing general laparoscopic cholecystectomy possess. When either of these methods is employed, the laparoscopic surgeon must first expose the anterior surface of the CBD and, if need be, confirm the identity if the CBD with needle aspiration of bile. Next, fine (4-0) sutures laterally and medially (in the 3 and 9 o'clock positions) are placed on the CBD for traction and exposure. A 15- to 20-mm opening is made longitudinally on the anterior aspect of the distal CBD, and saline flush is instituted. This alone may dislodge stones. The surgeon may then place an endoscope directly, as described previously, or use a 4F biliary Fogarty catheter to try to remove one or more stones. After successful clearance of the duct, the choledochotomy is closed over a T-tube with interrupted 3-0 or 4-0 absorbable sutures; the tube exits the CBD at the inferior end of the choledochotomy opening away from the liver and caudal to the sutures. The authors bevel each end of the T-tube and also remove the back portion of the T-shaped end, or they cut a notch to facilitate extraction. T-tubes are customized from a 14F or smaller tube (Figure 3). If a commercial T-tube is unavailable, the surgeon can split one end of a straight Silastic catheter to create a "T" shape, but this type

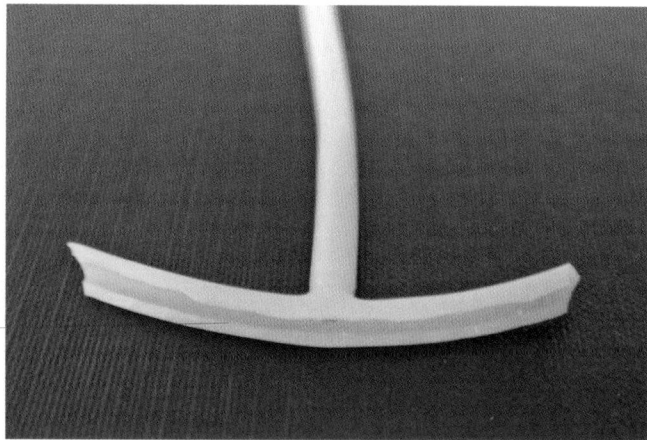

FIGURE 3 Customized 12F T-tube with beveled ends and portion of back wall removed.

of tube is more prone to be dislodged. The T-tube is brought out linearly through the abdominal wall to facilitate subsequent access for imaging or manipulation if needed.

The open CBD exploration follows the same steps with traction sutures on the duct, followed by a 15-mm to 20-mm anterior choledochotomy. The open approach affords more opportunities for stone extraction. These include direct saline flushing, digital palpation and manual massage of the duct, passage of Bakes dilators or Randall stone forceps, the use of a biliary Fogarty balloon catheter or a choledochoscope, and basket. Clearance of all stones from the duct can be demonstrated by removal of a known quantity of stones, by cholangiography, or by choledochoscopic visualization. The duct is closed with interrupted 3-0 or 4-0 absorbable suture over a T-tube in the inferior end of the choledochotomy caudal to the sutures.

The postoperative management of T-tubes depends on the clinical scenario and whether there is any suspicion of persistent stones in the duct. Clinical practice regarding removal of the T-tube varies widely, from 10 days to 6 weeks after placement. If multiple stones were found and extracted from the CBD at the time of surgery, there is a much higher incidence of residual stones, and the T-tube is left for a longer period and imaged with T-tube cholangiography before removal. It is the authors' practice to "internalize" the T-tube drain for most patients before discharge by clamping the tube externally and then monitoring the clinical and laboratory course. If the patient is recovering appropriately from the operation, and in the absence of fever, chills, increase in pain, or elevation of serum bilirubin or alkaline phosphatase levels, the tube remains clamped. This favorable and typical scenario indicates passage of bile from the CBD through the ampulla. The patient is then discharged with the T-tube clamped, and it is removed in 2 weeks in the outpatient clinic without T-tube cholangiography if the patient remains clinically stable. If, however, the patient has any of the aforementioned signs and symptoms after the T-tube is clamped, this implies pressure in the biliary tree from failure of the duct to empty through the ampulla, and the clamp is removed and the T-tube again drained externally to a bile bag until either the clinical scenario improves or T-tube cholangiography demonstrates patency without obstruction. In instances with known residual choledocholithiasis, the T-tube is the tract that allows interventional radiology to directly access the biliary tree for stone extraction, although dilation and upsizing of the drain may be required.

Postoperative

Patients may return to their physician after laparoscopic cholecystectomy with signs or symptoms suggesting a retained CBD stone. Such patients often present with recurrent or persistent pain, elevations of bilirubin and alkaline phosphatase levels, and ductal dilation on ultrasonography or computed tomographic scan. The workup in this scenario is very reminiscent of the preoperative workup, with liberal use of MRCP to help determine whether bile duct calculi are present. ERCP with endoscopic sphincterotomy is utilized to image and clear the duct of stones. In a single-institution retrospective analysis, 1085 patients who underwent cholecystectomies were studied; in 25 patients (2.3%), postoperative ERCP confirmed retained CBD stones, and these patients were subsequently treated with ERCP. The analysis also revealed that patients with small gallstones (<5 mm) were more likely to present later with retained CBD stones. In patients for whom a T-tube is present after CBD exploration, a radiographic approach to the extraction of retained stones is utilized. Once the T-tube tract is matured 4 to 8 weeks postoperatively, the duct is accessed in interventional radiology for attempted basket retrieval of stones. In the rare case in which neither endoscopic nor radiographic methods are capable of clearing stones nonsurgically, another operation, probably with open CBD exploration, may be needed.

SUMMARY

Choledocholithiasis manifests in a small population of patients undergoing cholecystectomy for cholelithiasis and persists in an even smaller number of patients after cholecystectomy. With the liberal application of MCRP imaging, the nearly ubiquitous utilization of laparoscopic cholecystectomy, and the advent of minimally invasive techniques for CBD exploration available to surgeons so trained,

there are now new algorithms to guide the management of CBD stones. Much of the decision making hinges either on the timing of presentation in relation to surgery or on the training and expertise of the surgeon in performing laparoscopic or open CBD exploration. The option of completing a cholecystectomy without performing CBD exploration with planned postoperative ERCP is also recognized as acceptable therapy. The availability of skilled endoscopists and interventional radiologists in the multidisciplinary approach to CBD stones further guides treatment choices. Optimal management of choledocholithiasis requires the surgeon to be cognizant of all treatment options so as to judiciously use the methods that take into account local expertise to best serve the patient's needs.

SUGGESTED READINGS

Andrew S: Gallstone size related to incidence of post cholecystectomy retained common bile duct stones, *Int J Surg* 11(4):319–321, 2013.

Bender JS, Duncan MD, Freeswick PD, et al: Increased laparoscopic experience does not lead to improved results with acute cholecystitis, *Am J Surg* 184:591–594, 2002.

Magnuson TM, Bender JS, Duncan MD, et al: Utility of magnetic resonance cholangiography in the evaluation of biliary obstruction, *J Am Coll Surg* 189:63–72, 1999.

Makary MA, Duncan MD, Harmon JW, et al: The role of magnetic resonance cholangiography in the management of gallstone pancreatitis, *Ann Surg* 241:119–124, 2005.

Martin DJ, Vernon DR, Toouli J: Surgical versus endoscopic treatment of bile duct stones, *Cochrane Database Syst Rev* (2):CD00327, 2006.

ACUTE CHOLANGITIS

Gaurav Sharma, MD, MS, Edward E. Whang, MD, and Jason S. Gold, MD

OVERVIEW

Acute cholangitis is a morbid condition characterized by infection and inflammation that affects the biliary tract. It usually occurs in the setting of biliary obstruction. The spectrum of clinical severity can range from mild to potentially life-threatening disease accompanied by septic shock and multiorgan dysfunction. Because of the propensity for rapid deterioration with untreated acute cholangitis, expeditious diagnosis and therapy are essential.

EPIDEMIOLOGY

The median age of patients diagnosed with acute cholangitis is reported to range from 50 to 60 years, and incidence increases with age. The most important risk factors are biliary stasis or obstruction, for which the most prevalent etiology is choledocholithiasis. In much of the world, secondary choledocholithiasis (caused by stones originating in the gallbladder) predominates. In Southeast Asia, however, where recurrent pyogenic cholangitis (Oriental cholangiohepatitis) is endemic, primary choledocholithiasis is an important cause of cholangitis. Interestingly, although malignant obstruction may cause acute cholangitis, the probability of its development in the absence of prior instrumentation of the biliary system is low. The etiologies of acute cholangitis are listed in Box 1.

PATHOGENESIS

Despite its communication with the small intestine, the biliary tree is usually sterile. Most cases of acute cholangitis are thought to arise from direct ascent of bacteria from the duodenum into the common bile duct; hematogenous seeding of the biliary tract is likely to play only a minor role. Bacterial proliferation within the biliary tract, together with its entry into the systemic circulation via lymphatic and venous channels, results in the infectious manifestations of acute cholangitis.

Obstruction to physiologic biliary outflow plays a critical role in the pathogenesis of acute cholangitis. Predominant causes of biliary obstruction resulting in cholangitis are secondary choledocholithiasis, gallbladder stones (2/3 to 3/4 of cases), and malignant disease. Benign strictures and primary sclerosing cholangitis also underlie a significant number of cases. An increasingly prevalent risk factor is iatrogenic biliary tract manipulation (see Box 1), which in some centers, particularly those with active liver transplantation programs, is associated with up to 50% of cases of acute cholangitis. Examples include endoscopic and percutaneous instrumentation of the biliary tract, indwelling biliary stents, anastomotic (bilibiliary or bilienteric) strictures, and ischemic strictures of the biliary tract. Endoscopic retrograde cholangiopancreatography (ERCP) has been implicated in 0.5% to 1.7% of cases of acute cholangitis, particularly when therapeutic interventions are undertaken.

Bile duct obstruction can be further categorized as "high" or proximal obstruction, versus "low" or distal. Outside of Southeastern Asia, the latter is most often the result of choledocholithiasis from gallstones, and the former is typically caused by cholangiocarcinoma. The site of obstruction is critical to determining the optimal treatment.

Polymicrobial infection is found in most patients with acute cholangitis. Bowel flora constitute the most common isolates. The most

BOX 1: Etiologies of acute cholangitis

Noniatrogenic

Benign Conditions

Choledocholithiasis
    Primary
    Secondary
Pancreatitis (chronic/acute), including pancreatic pseudocyst
Papillary stenosis
Mirizzi's syndrome
Choledochal cysts and Caroli's disease
Biliary strictures
    Ischemia
    Primary sclerosing cholangitis
    Recurrent choledocholithiasis
    Recurrent cholangitis
    Other inflammatory conditions

Malignancies

Pancreatic cancer
Cholangiocarcinoma
Duodenal/ampullary cancer
Primary tumor or metastasis to liver, gallbladder, or porta hepatis

Iatrogenic

Obstructed biliary endoprosthesis
Iatrogenic biliary stricture
    Direct surgical trauma
    Ischemia-induced stricture
    Anastomotic stricture (bilibiliary/bilienteric anastomosis)

BOX 2: Diagnostic criteria for acute cholangitis: Tokyo guidelines

A. Clinical Context and Clinical Manifestations
    1. History of biliary disease
    2. Fever or chills
    3. Jaundice
    4. Abdominal pain (right upper quadrant or upper abdominal)
B. Laboratory Data
    5. Evidence of inflammatory response*
    6. Abnormal liver function tests†
C. Imaging Findings
    7. Biliary dilation or evidence of an etiology (stricture, stone, stent, etc)
Suspected Diagnosis
    Two or more items in A
Definite Diagnosis
    a. Charcot's triad (2 + 3 + 4)
    b. Two or more items in A + both items in B + item C

*Abnormal white blood cell count, increased serum C-reactive protein level, and other changes indicating inflammation.
†Increased serum alkaline phosphatase, γ-glutamyl transpeptidase, aspartate aminotransferase, and alanine aminotransferase levels.
From Hirota M, Tadahiro T, Kawarada Y, et al: Tokyo guidelines for the management of acute cholangitis and cholecystitis, J Hepatobiliary Pancreat Surg 14:1–126, 2007.

frequently identified gram-negative bacteria are *Escherichia coli* (25% to 50% of cases), *Klebsiella* species (15% to 20% of cases), and *Enterobacter* species (5% to 10% of cases). The most commonly isolated gram-positive bacteria are *Enterococcus* species (10% to 20% of cases). The contribution of anaerobes, such as *Bacteroides* and *Clostridium* species, to the pathogenesis of acute cholangitis is controversial; however, anaerobes are not uncommonly cultured in specimens obtained from elderly patients and those who have undergone biliary instrumentation. Although bacteria are responsible for the great majority of cases of acute cholangitis, other pathogens, such as helminths, fungi, and viruses (e.g., cytomegalovirus and Epstein-Barr virus) can cause this syndrome. These organisms should be considered in the appropriate clinical setting (e.g., in areas where parasitic infections are endemic and among individuals with immunocompromise).

Repeated bouts of infection can lead to strictures and secondary biliary cirrhosis.

CLINICAL PRESENTATION

In 1877, Jean Charcot described the hallmarks of acute cholangitis: fever, jaundice, and right upper quadrant abdominal pain. Note that all three features of this eponymous triad are present in only 50% to 75% of patients with acute cholangitis. Fever and abdominal pain are the most common symptoms (present in more than 80% of cases), with jaundice being slightly less prevalent (60% to 70% of cases). Reynold's pentad (described by Reynold and Dargon in 1959) denotes the presence of mental status derangements and hypotension in addition to the features of Charcot's triad. This aggregate is present in less than 5% of cases of acute cholangitis and is suggestive of severe disease and systemic sepsis.

DIAGNOSIS

Acute cholangitis is a clinical diagnosis that is based on the presence of the clinical features discussed previously together with supportive data from laboratory tests and radiographic studies. Because acute cholangitis can present without abdominal pain, the absence of pain (or any of the individual symptoms and signs discussed previously) does not rule out this diagnosis. A high index of suspicion is warranted in elderly patients or patients with immunosuppression who may not exhibit the classic signs and symptoms of acute cholangitis until rapid decompensation and septicemia occur. Acute cholangitis should also be considered in patients who have attendant risk factors, such as choledocholithiasis or biliary strictures, with or without a history of instrumentation, and present with sepsis without abdominal pain or tenderness. The Tokyo guidelines provide criteria for diagnosis of acute cholangitis based on clinical, laboratory, and imaging findings (Box 2).

The differential diagnosis includes other conditions associated with right upper quadrant abdominal pain, jaundice, or fever such as cholecystitis, liver abscess, and hepatitis. Laboratory test findings typically associated with acute cholangitis include leukocytosis with neutrophilia and liver enzyme abnormalities suggestive of cholestasis (e.g., increased serum alkaline phosphatase, γ-glutamyl transpeptidase, and conjugated bilirubin concentrations).

Blood cultures should be performed in patients suspected of having cholangitis. In addition, cultures should be obtained from bile aspirated through percutaneous biliary catheters or obtained during biliary drainage and from any indwelling biliary prostheses that are removed. Although treatment should be initiated before culture results become available, these results can be used in directing specific antibiotic therapy.

Imaging studies have the following roles in patients with suspected acute cholangitis: (1) they can confirm the presence of dilated bile ducts (a finding present in most cases of acute cholangitis); (2) they may reveal the specific etiology responsible for biliary obstruction (e.g., gallstones); (3) they can exclude other conditions in the differential diagnosis (e.g., acute cholecystitis); and (4) they can be used to guide therapeutic interventions (e.g., biliary drainage or removal of an obstructed biliary stent).

Transabdominal ultrasound scan is the best initial imaging study in most patients with suspected acute cholangitis. It is noninvasive, rapid, and cost effective; it spares patients from exposure to ionizing radiation; and it is highly sensitive in the detection of biliary tract dilation. The absence of biliary tract dilation does not rule out acute cholangitis, especially if the ultrasound scan is obtained soon after acute onset of biliary obstruction before the bile ducts have had time to dilate. In cases of proximal bile duct obstruction, dilated intrahepatic ducts without dilated extrahepatic ducts may be noted. Transabdominal ultrasound scan is associated with relatively low sensitivity in the detection of choledocholithiasis but is very sensitive in finding stones in the gallbladder.

Cholangiography is often indicated for therapeutic and diagnostic purposes. When available, ERCP is the preferred method of cholangiography in cases of distal bile duct obstruction. If choledocholithiasis is suspected on the basis of ultrasound scan, further imaging is usually not necessary before ERCP. Unavailability or failure of ERCP should prompt percutaneous transhepatic cholangiography (PTC). PTC is often the preferred approach for cholangiography and drainage in proximal bile duct obstruction. Patients with

externally accessible indwelling biliary catheters (e.g., T-tubes or U-tubes) can undergo cholangiography with contrast instilled into these tubes.

Computed tomographic (CT) scanning can reveal biliary tract dilation and allows for global assessment of intraabdominal pathology, but it has poor sensitivity for the detection of intraductal stones. Magnetic resonance cholangiopancreatography (MRCP) has greater sensitivity for choledocholithiasis than CT scan (80% to 92% vs 33% to 40%, respectively) but is less widely available. MRCP can also be useful in assessing and characterizing biliary strictures. The prolonged duration of MRCP examination also limits the application in unstable conditions. CT scan or magnetic resonance imaging (MRI) may be useful when malignancy is in the differential diagnosis because these studies can identify masses and detect metastases. Endoscopic ultrasound scan (EUS) is another imaging option with excellent sensitivity for choledocholithiasis (93% to 95%).

THERAPY

Therapy for acute cholangitis consists of three main components: (1) resuscitation; (2) antibiotics; and (3) biliary drainage (Figure 1).

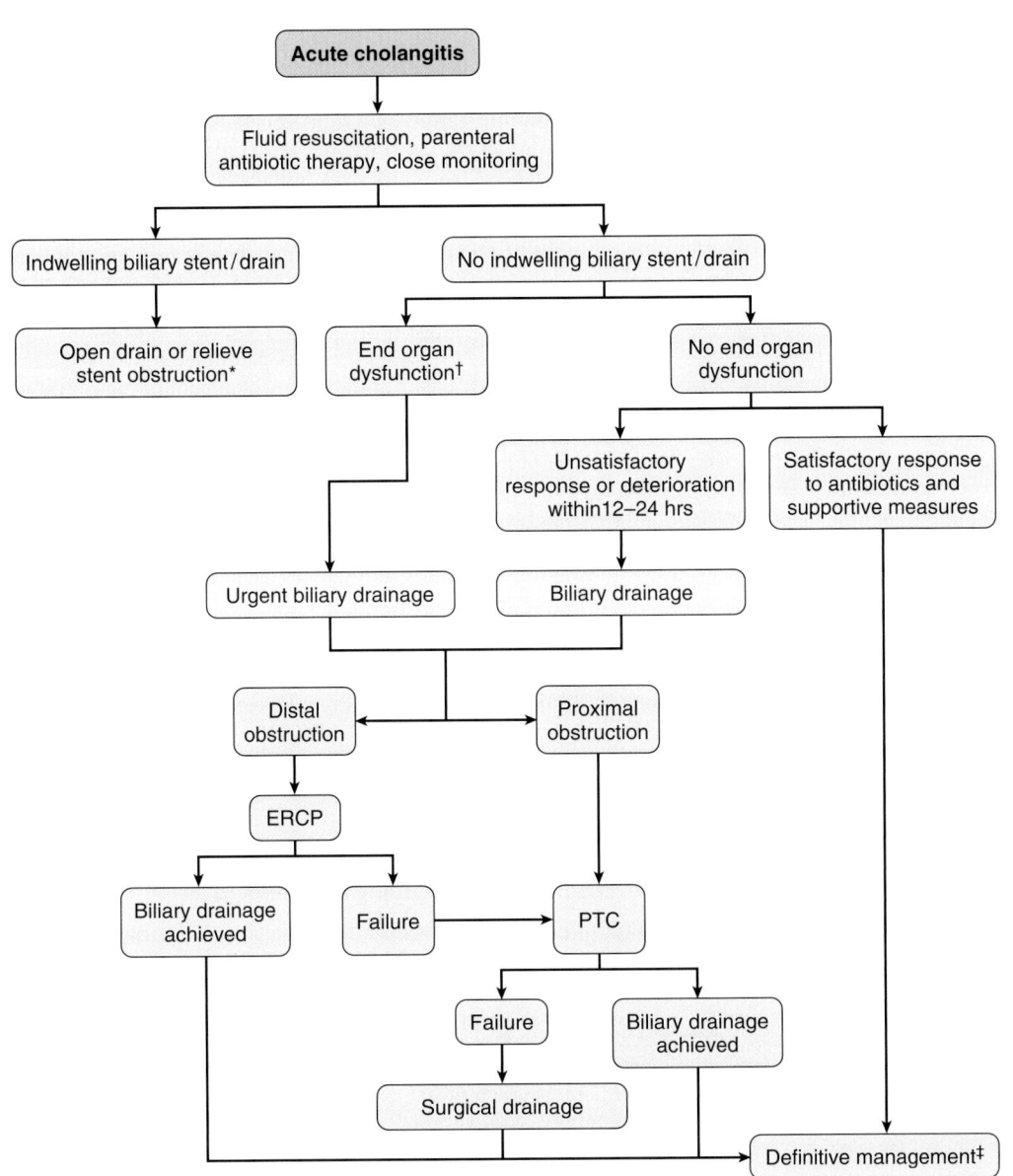

FIGURE I Clinical algorithm for management of acute cholangitis.
ERCP, Endoscopic retrograde cholangiopancreatography;
PTC, percutaneous transhepatic cholangiography.
*For changing internal stents, urgency is determined by presence or absence of end-organ dysfunction.
†For example, altered mental status or hemodynamic lability.
‡Timing of definitive management is determined by the severity of the episode of cholangitis and the comorbidities of the patient.

Resuscitation with administration of intravenous fluids and correction of electrolyte abnormalities should be initiated without delay. Patients with external biliary drains should have these drains placed to gravity drainage as soon as the diagnosis of acute cholangitis is considered. Given that urgent interventional or surgical procedures are often required, attention should be directed to identifying and correcting coagulopathies that may exist (e.g., those resulting from vitamin K deficiency or sepsis-induced thrombocytopenia). Vigilant monitoring to ensure adequacy of resuscitation and early recognition of clinical deterioration (e.g., end-organ dysfunction) is essential. Patients with significant comorbidities and those exhibiting signs of hemodynamic lability or end-organ dysfunction are best monitored in a dedicated intensive care unit (ICU), where invasive monitoring and inotropic support can be instituted.

When the diagnosis of acute cholangitis is considered, empiric broad-spectrum antibiotic administration should commence without delay once peripheral blood cultures have been drawn. The foremost concern in selection of empiric agents is effectiveness against both gram-negative and gram-positive bacteria (especially *Enterococcus*). A secondary concern is ability of the antibiotics to achieve high concentrations within bile even in the presence of biliary obstruction. Despite the low frequency with which anaerobes are isolated from bile cultures, coverage of anaerobes should be considered because standard culture techniques underestimate the true prevalence of anaerobic infections and anaerobes are prevalent in cultures of bile obtained from some patient groups (e.g., those with prior biliary instrumentation).

Several appropriate antibiotic choices exist for empiric therapy. Selection is often guided by institutional antibiotic stewardship policies. Options include the combination of ampicillin and gentamicin, fluoroquinolones (e.g., ciprofloxacin or levofloxacin) alone or with metronidazole, carbapenems (e.g., imipenem or meropenem), extended-spectrum penicillins (e.g., piperacillin), and penicillin/beta-lactamase inhibitor combinations (e.g., piperacillin-tazobactam, ampicillin-sulbactam, ticarcillin-clavulanate). Given the substantial risk of aminoglycoside-induced nephrotoxicity, the authors prefer to avoid gentamicin-based regimens unless specific reasons for their administration exist. Although they provide excellent activity against gram-negative bacteria, second-generation and third-generation cephalosporins provide poor coverage against *Enterococcus* species and are therefore not recommended. The authors often use piperacillin-tazobactam because of its broad gram-negative, gram-positive, and anaerobic coverage; penetration into bile; and ease of administration.

With resuscitation and empiric antibiotic therapy, up to 85% of patients with acute cholangitis have improvement, even in the absence of interventional therapy. When culture results become available, antibiotics should be tailored to sensitivity findings. The duration of antibiotic therapy should be based on clinical response; for patients documented to have bacteremia, antibiotic courses that last 1 to 2 weeks are recommended. Response to initial treatment with antibiotics and the presence or absence of infection-induced organ failure are critical in determining the need and timing of subsequent interventions.

Patients without end-organ dysfunction and with resolved signs of infection with initial antibiotic treatment usually require no further treatment beyond that for the underlying condition. Relapse after initial response requires biliary drainage. In patients with cholangitis caused by choledocholithiasis, drainage of the biliary tree is not indicated when the stone passes spontaneously.

Patients who do not have organ dysfunction but who do not have a satisfactory response to initial treatment with antibiotics of 12- to 24-hour duration require biliary drainage. Persistence or worsening of abdominal pain, fever, or leukocytosis despite antibiotic therapy indicates the need for biliary drainage. If required for choledocholithiasis, a cholecystectomy can often be performed on the same hospital admission in patients with cholangitis that does not result in end-organ dysfunction.

Patients with cardiopulmonary, neurologic, renal, hepatic, or hematologic dysfunction typically require organ support in an ICU setting and urgent biliary decompression without a prolonged trial of antibiotics. Interval treatment of the underlying condition typically occurs after recovery from the episode of cholangitis.

Techniques of Biliary Drainage

Considerations for selection of the optimal drainage technique in acute cholangitis are: (1) site of obstruction, (2) results of previous drainage attempts, and (3) availability of equipment and expertise for each drainage approach. ERCP is the first-line modality for establishing biliary drainage in most cases because the majority of cases of cholangitis are precipitated by distal obstruction as a result of choledocholithiasis. PTC is the preferred approach in cases in which ERCP fails or is unavailable and is often preferred for patients with proximal obstruction (e.g., as with hilar cholangiocarcinoma). Urgent surgical biliary drainage is associated with high mortality and is reserved for only those rare circumstances in which nonoperative techniques have been exhausted or are unavailable.

Endoscopic Drainage

ERCP is effective in establishing biliary drainage in 90% to 98% of cases, although this efficacy is lower in certain circumstances (e.g., cholangitis resulting from hilar cholangiocarcinoma). In procedures performed for acute cholangitis, bile should be aspirated from the common bile duct to decompress it *before* injection of contrast for cholangiography. Occlusive cholangiography performed before ductal decompression, particularly in cases of suppurative cholangitis, can induce bacteremia, sepsis, and rapid decompensation. Other complications of ERCP include pancreatitis, duodenal injury, and complications associated with upper endoscopy in general. For patients in whom endoscopic sphincterotomy is contraindicated, such as those with persistent coagulopathy, temporizing biliary drainage can be achieved by placement of a nasobiliary drain or an internal biliary stent without sphincterotomy. For instance, a 10F or smaller internal biliary stent can be safely placed across the major papilla without need for a biliary sphincterotomy. More definitive therapy (e.g., endoscopic sphincterotomy and removal of intraductal stones) can then be accomplished electively, after conditions have stabilized. If biliary access at ERCP is unsuccessful, an additional modality in some specialty centers is EUS-directed access of the biliary tree, followed by biliary drainage via this access. However, this is a consideration only in patients with stable conditions, and the same results are more commonly achieved with PTC. Other therapeutic applications facilitated by ERCP in patients with acute cholangitis include replacement of obstructed biliary stents and stenting or dilation of benign biliary strictures. ERCP with fluoroscopy-free methodologies (wire-guided cannulation or endoscopic ultrasound scan guidance) has been used to treat cholangitis during pregnancy, with varying results.

Percutaneous Transhepatic Drainage

Indications for PTC include: (1) proximal or intrahepatic biliary obstruction (e.g., hilar cholangiocarcinoma or hepatolithiasis), (2) unavailability of ERCP, (3) failed endoscopic drainage, and (4) challenging endoscopic access (e.g., complete obstruction or division of the bile duct; prior upper gastrointestinal surgery that altered intestinal anatomy, such as a Billroth 2 or Roux-en-Y reconstruction; or a large periampullary duodenal diverticulum). Furthermore, because PTC does not require oral passage of an endoscope, it can be performed in some patients with hemodynamically labile conditions without the requirement of sedation or airway protection. PTC involves fluoroscopically guided, percutaneous puncture of a peripheral bile duct; thus, this technique may be difficult in patients without dilation of the intrahepatic biliary system. PTC is reported to be successful in establishing biliary drainage in 90% of patients with biliary obstruction. Serious complications of PTC include intraperitoneal hemorrhage, hemobilia, and bile peritonitis. Percutaneous cholecystostomy is a technically easier alternative to PTC; however, it only provides drainage when the obstruction is distal to the junction of the cystic duct and the common hepatic duct, and it requires patency of the cystic duct.

Surgical Drainage

Because of the high efficacy of ERCP and PTC, surgical biliary decompression in the acute setting should be applied only if these nonoperative procedures fail to achieve biliary drainage or are unavailable. Historic series suggest that emergency surgery in unstable conditions with acute cholangitis is associated with perioperative mortality rates as high as 40%. If surgery is required in acutely ill patients, the initial approach should be limited to drainage of the bile duct. For distal bile duct obstruction, this can be most easily accomplished with choledochotomy and placement of a large-diameter (at least 16F) T-tube. Latex-free T-tubes are commercially available for allergic patients. Surgical drainage of proximal bile duct obstruction in patients with cholangitis is much more of a challenge. A hilar obstruction can be relieved with choledochotomy, dilation of the obstruction, and placement of a U-tube (in which the tube enters the biliary tree through a choledochotomy, traverses the obstruction, and the exits the intrahepatic biliary system through a rent in the liver, with both ends of the tube being brought out through the abdominal wall). More extensive procedures such as formal common bile duct exploration, transduodenal sphincteroplasty, and biliary enteric bypass are usually inappropriate in unstable conditions.

Principles of Management of Cholangitis Caused by Proximal Obstruction

Management of cholangitis is particularly challenging in the case of obstruction at or proximal to the biliary bifurcation and warrants special consideration. This should be suspected when initial imaging (e.g., ultrasound scan) shows dilation of the intrahepatic biliary tree without extrahepatic biliary dilation or in patients with previously known tumors, strictures, or surgery of the hepatic ducts or biliary confluence. In the setting where portions of the biliary system are obstructed and isolated from one another by the obstructions, multiple portions of the biliary tree that are infected and do not communicate with one another may require independent drainage to relieve cholangitis. In contrast, the overall approach to patients with isolation of different portions of the biliary tree is to minimize the extent of the biliary tree that is instrumented, particularly when the source of obstruction cannot be relieved (e.g., unresectable cholangiocarcinoma). In these cases, the risk of cholangitis incurred by instrumentation of an uninfected but obstructed division of the ductal system outweighs the loss of function of the parenchyma that occurs from unmitigated obstruction. Thus, before drainage is planned, a detailed anatomy of the biliary system should be constructed from records of prior procedures in combination with high-quality cross-sectional imaging such as CT scan or MRCP. Because cholangitis rarely develops from tumors or strictures without prior instrumentation, initial attention should focus on areas that have previously been instrumented. For instance, in a patient with cholangitis who has a hilar cholangiocarcinoma that originally isolated the right and left biliary systems and was drained with a stent draining the right anterior sectoral and main right hepatic ducts into the common hepatic duct, where the tumor has now progressed to isolate the right anterior and right posterior sectoral ducts, an initial attempt at drainage should address the right posterior sectoral duct because this was previously drained but is now isolated. Unlike ERCP, PTC facilitated by image guidance allows precise drainage of the area desired, minimizing unintended instrumentation of other divisions of the biliary tree. Considerations for drainage in the setting of proximal bile duct obstruction are best evaluated on an individualized basis with a multidisciplinary team approach.

Regardless of the etiology of acute cholangitis, patients should undergo definitive therapy, if indicated, on an elective basis. In this context, surgery plays an important role, most frequently as interval cholecystectomy for secondary choledocholithiasis and Mirizzi's syndrome, but also in the form of biliary reconstruction for benign biliary strictures and resection of periampullary tumors.

SUGGESTED READINGS

Hirota M, Tadahiro T, Kawarada Y, et al: Tokyo guidelines for the management of acute cholangitis and cholecystitis, *J Hepatobiliary Pancreat Surg* 14(1):1–126, 2007.

Van Delden OM, Lameris JS: Percutaneous drainage and stenting for palliation of malignant bile duct obstruction, *Eur Radiol* 18:448–456, 2008.

BENIGN BILIARY STRICTURES

**William G. Hawkins, MD, and
Steven M. Strasberg, MD**

Benign biliary strictures are usually the result of trauma or inflammation. Most traumatic biliary strictures result from iatrogenic operative injuries. These are the most common benign strictures requiring surgical treatment today. This chapter focuses on strategies for avoidance of iatrogenic injuries and management of the established injury. Inflammatory strictures are the result of pancreatitis and less commonly primary sclerosing cholangitis, septic cholangitis, and inflammatory pseudotumors. These noniatrogenic benign strictures are discussed at the end of the chapter.

IATROGENIC BILIARY INJURIES

Biliary injury during laparoscopic cholecystectomy and after conversion to open cholecystectomy continues to be an important clinical problem. Injury rates have decreased from levels in the early 1990s when laparoscopic cholecystectomy was introduced but have probably not fallen to levels recorded in the era of open cholecystectomy. Unfortunately, accurate current statistics for the incidence of biliary injuries are lacking, but a reasonable estimate is that there is 1 injury for every 300 cholecystectomies (0.3%). The anatomic injury classification used in this chapter was published in 1995 (Figure 1). It is a modification of the Bismuth classification adapted to better characterize injuries seen in the laparoscopic era.

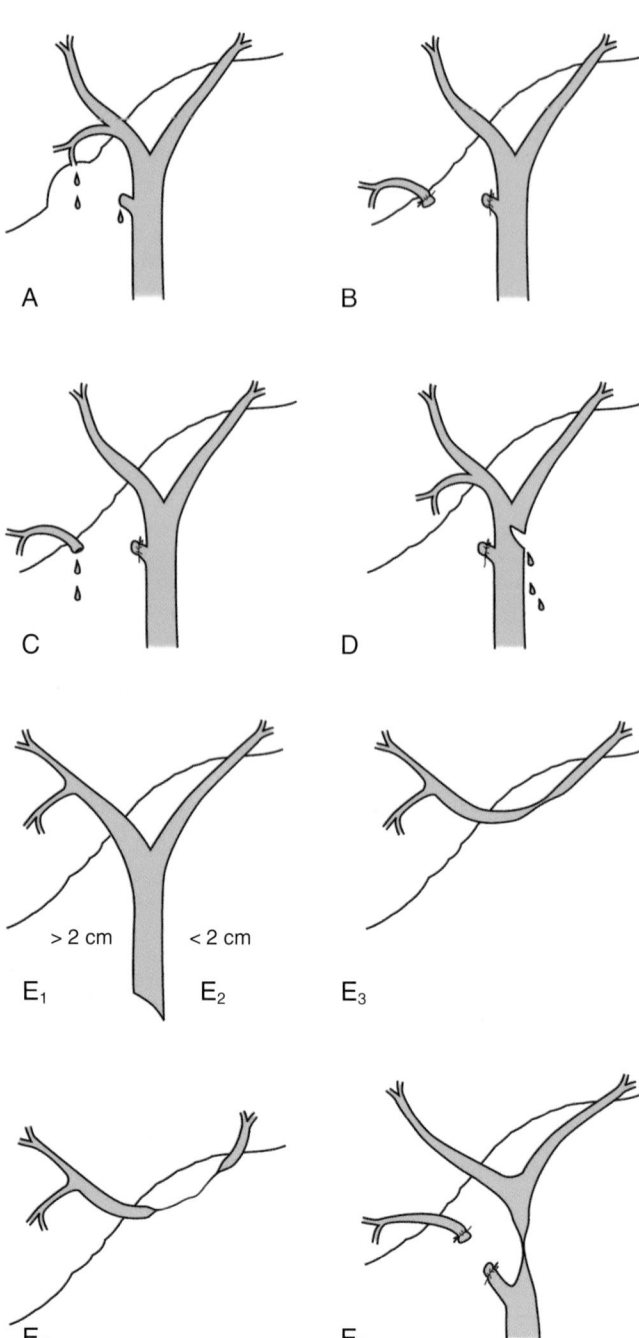

FIGURE 1   A classification of laparoscopic bile duct injuries. Type A injuries are leaks from the cystic duct or from ducts at the hepatic resection bed (e.g., ducts of Luschka). Types B and C involve injuries to aberrant right hepatic ducts. Type E injuries involve injuries to major bile ducts. *(From Strasberg SM, Hertl M, Soper NJ, et al: An analysis of the problem of biliary injury during laparoscopic cholecystectomy, J Am Coll Surg 180:101, 1995.)*

Risk Factors for Biliary Injuries

Patient-Related Factors

Inflammation

Acute Inflammation. In population studies, the incidence of biliary injury is higher when laparoscopic cholecystectomy is performed for acute cholecystitis than for elective indications. Acute inflammation causes thickening of tissues, increases friability and vascularity, and promotes adhesions. These factors obscure normal anatomic relationships and increase difficulty of exposure and dissection. Severe inflammation is more likely to be encountered when the time between onset of symptoms and surgery for acute cholecystitis is greater than 72 hours, when the white blood cell count is greater than 18,000 cells/mm^3, or when a definite tender palpable mass is present in the right upper quadrant.

Severe Chronic Inflammation. Repeated episodes of acute cholecystitis may result in marked scarring and contracture of the gallbladder and adjacent tissues with the result that the gallbladder may become shrunken and bound to surrounding viscera. Fibrosis and retraction may result in fusion of the gallbladder to the common hepatic duct and right hepatic artery, effectively obliterating the hepatocystic triangle and dissection planes between these structures, which then may appear to be part of the gallbladder. Such inflammation makes dissection very difficult and contributes to visual deception when certain techniques are used.

Congenital Abnormalities

Aberrant Right Hepatic Ducts. A low-lying aberrant right hepatic duct may cross through the hepatocystic triangle or even unite with the cystic duct 1 to 2 cm before terminating in a confluence with the common hepatic duct. The appearance of the confluence of the aberrant duct with the common hepatic duct is similar to the appearance of a normal confluence of the cystic duct with the common hepatic duct; consequently, great potential exists for misidentification of the aberrant duct as the cystic duct.

Other congenital abnormalities that may expose patients to a greater risk of biliary injury include parallel union cystic duct, in which the cystic duct runs parallel to the common hepatic duct and exposes the latter to injury during dissection of the cystic duct; aberrant high termination of the cystic duct into a normally positioned right hepatic duct, which exposes the latter to injury during dissection of the cystic duct; congenital adhesions between the gallbladder and common hepatic duct, which obscure the hepatocystic triangle and make the common duct appear as if it is emanating from the gallbladder like a cystic duct; and intrahepatic gallbladder, which is difficult to grasp and thus contributes indirectly to injury by making exposure of the cystic duct difficult. In extremely rare cases, a major duct such as the right hepatic duct or the common hepatic duct may enter the gallbladder directly. Injury to such a structure is virtually unavoidable.

Other Patient-Related Factors

Large Impacted Gallstones. Large impacted gallstones impair retraction and hide the cystic duct, which again gives the appearance that the common bile duct is coming out of the gallbladder. Large stones may also erode and efface the cystic duct, thus shortening or obliterating it ("absent cystic duct"), and in severe cases may cause common bile duct compression or erosion and with severe pericholecystic inflammation (Mirizzi's syndrome) and sometimes bile duct obstruction.

Obesity and Body Habitus. Morbid obesity and large body size make operative exposure more difficult, as do skeletal deformities.

Procedure-Related Factors

Misidentification: A Concept Problem

The two main types of bile duct misidentification are misidentification of the common bile duct as the cystic duct and misidentification of an aberrant right hepatic duct as the cystic duct, the latter discussed previously. The key to understanding why misidentification occurs rests with examining the rationale for identification of the cystic structures during cholecystectomy.

Infundibular Technique. In this fallible method, the putative cystic duct is traced to the gallbladder or the gallbladder is traced down to the cystic duct, at which point, after circumferential dissection of these structures, the infundibulum (funnel) is displayed. The bowl of the funnel is the gallbladder and the stem is the cystic duct. However, with severe inflammation in which the common hepatic duct is fused to the side of the gallbladder and the cystic duct is in the inflammatory mass (hidden cystic duct syndrome), a funnel shape may also be observed in which the bowl of the funnel is the fused gallbladder/common hepatic duct and the stem of the funnel is the common bile duct (Figure 2). This visual deception is most likely to occur when one or more inciting factors described previously are present. Once the common bile duct is divided, the surgeon naturally dissects up the left side of the common hepatic duct with the belief that the dissection is on the gallbladder. Then, to get to the cystic plate, the common hepatic duct must be divided. In this step, the right hepatic artery is frequently injured. This sequence is referred to as the classical injury (Figure 3).

Intraoperative Cholangiography. Intraoperative cholangiography (IOC) reduces the incidence of biliary injury. Operative cholangiography is best at detection of misidentification of the common bile duct as the cystic duct and prevention of excision injuries of bile ducts. Unfortunately, operative cholangiograms are sometimes misinterpreted. IOC is not usually effective at detection of aberrant right ducts, which unite with the cystic duct before joining the common duct.

Dissection of the Cystic Duct to the Confluence with the Common Hepatic Duct/Common Bile Duct. This is a common and usually safe technique in performance of open cholecystectomy. Its use during laparoscopic cholecystectomy has been associated with an increase in lateral injuries to the common hepatic duct (type D), especially in the presence of a parallel union cystic duct.

The Critical View of Safety Technique

In the critical view of safety (CVS) technique, the hepatocystic triangle is cleared of fat and fibrous tissue and the gallbladder is freed from the lower one third of its attachment to the cystic plate. Only two structures are connected to the lower end of the gallbladder once this is done. Raising the gallbladder off the lower one third of the cystic plate is an essential step, without which the critical view cannot be said to have been attained (Figure 4). It is equivalent in the open technique to taking the gallbladder off the gallbladder bed, before clipping the cystic duct and artery. No attempt is made to expose the common bile duct or common hepatic duct.

Top-Down Cholecystectomy. The cholecystectomy is started at the fundus, taking the gallbladder off the gallbladder bed before identification of structures in the hepatocystic triangle. Although this may be an effective technique of identification in most instances, the authors have shown that it may lead to serious vasculobiliary injuries when severe inflammation exists. The contracture associated with chronic inflammation results in loss of planes and an increased

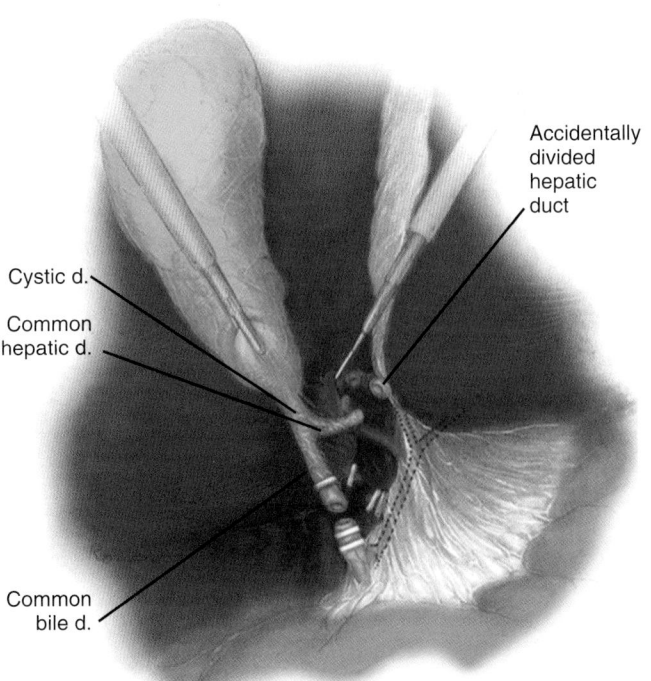

FIGURE 3 Classical bile duct injury. The steps in the classic injury are: 1, The common bile duct is mistaken to be the cystic duct and is divided; 2, the dissection proceeds along the left side of the common hepatic duct; and 3, to reach the cystic plate, the common hepatic duct is divided, often injuring the right hepatic artery at the same time. *(From Branum G, Schmitt C, Baille J, et al: Management of major biliary complications after laparoscopic cholecystectomy, Ann Surg 217:532, 1993.)*

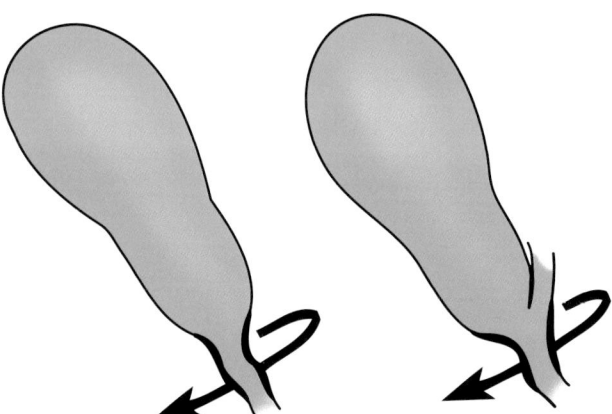

FIGURE 2 The deception of the hidden cystic duct and the infundibular technique of laparoscopic cholecystectomy. *Left:* Appearance to surgeon when a duct appearing to be the cystic duct is dissected first. Note that the duct appears to flare *(heavy black line)*, giving the appearance that the cystic duct has been followed on to the infundibulum. *Right:* True anatomic situation in the case of some classical injuries. The misleading flare or funnel *(heavy black line)* results from fusion of the common hepatic duct with the gallbladder and the hiding of the cystic duct in the inflammatory mass. *(From Strasberg SM, Eagon CJ, Drebin JA: The "hidden cystic duct" syndrome and the infundibular technique of laparoscopic cholecystectomy: the danger of the false infundibulum, J Am Coll Surg 191:661–667, 2000, Fig. 4.)*

chance of entering the right portal pedicle when the gallbladder is taken down from above under these conditions (Figure 5).

Technical Problems

Bile ducts may be injured in the course of dissection much in the same way that an enterotomy occurs in the course of dissecting

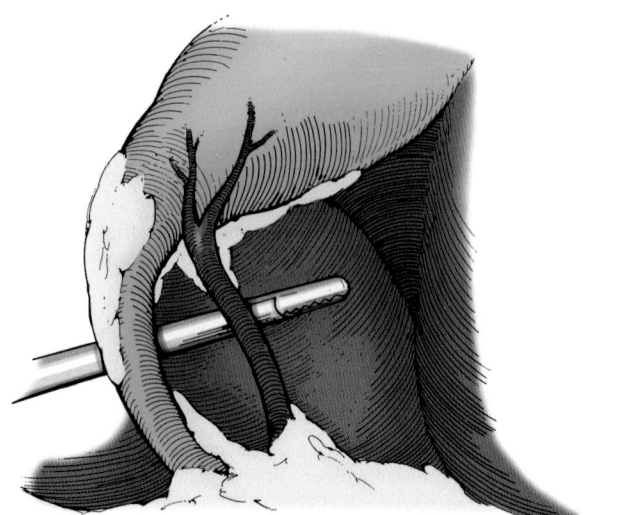

FIGURE 4 The three requirements of the Critical View of Safety are: 1, the hepatocystic triangle is dissected free of all tissue except for putative cystic duct and artery; 2, The lower one third of the gallbladder is dissected off the cystic plate; and 3, two and only two structures are seen to be attached to the gallbladder. It is not necessary to see the common bile duct. *(From Strasberg SM, Eagon CJ, Drebin JA: The "hidden cystic duct" syndrome and the infundibular technique of laparoscopic cholecystectomy: the danger of the false infundibulum, J Am Coll Surg 191:661–667, 2000, Fig. 1.)*

adhesions. Inflammation, aberrant anatomy, small duct size, and large body habitus contribute to the likelihood of this occurrence. About 10% of patients have a sizable hepatic duct that lies immediately deep to the cystic plate and is therefore prone to injury.

Failure to Obtain Secure Closure of the Cystic Duct. The cystic duct is normally occluded with metallic clips. When the duct is thick, rigid, or wide, clips may fail; their use should usually be avoided in these circumstances. Retained common duct stones may contribute to clip failure by raising bile duct pressure.

Thermal Injuries. Thermal injuries are more likely to occur in the presence of severe inflammation because hemorrhage is more common when dissecting in the face of acute inflammation and higher power settings may be used to control hemorrhage. These injuries are often not recognized at surgery and usually result in bile duct stenosis rather than loss of continuity. Avoidance requires use of low power settings and lifting of tissue off underlying structures and a culture of safety.

Tenting Injuries. The junction of the common bile duct and hepatic bile ducts may be occluded when clipping the cystic duct while pulling up forcefully on the gallbladder. This is an uncommon laparoscopic injury perhaps as a result of the magnification afforded by laparoscopy and is avoided by not pulling up strongly on the gallbladder during the act of clipping the cystic duct.

Surgeon-Related or Hospital-Related Factors

Learning Curve Effect

Inexperience with laparoscopic cholecystectomy was a well-documented cause of bile duct injuries in the 1990s. The likelihood of biliary injury was much greater during the early experience of a surgeon than subsequently. Inexperience with the procedure during acute cholecystitis possibly still contributes to injury.

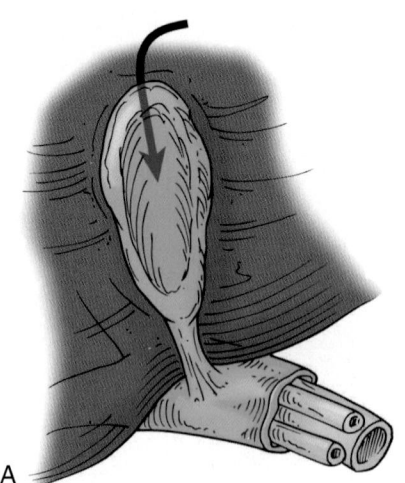
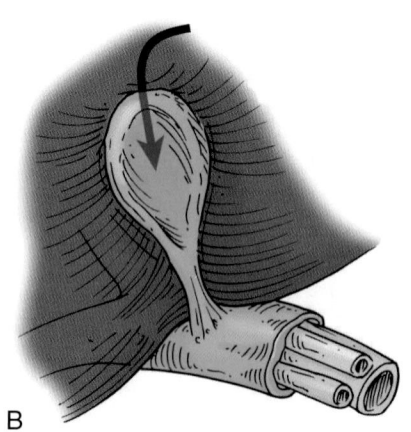

A   B

FIGURE 5 The relationship between the cystic plate and the right portal pedicle: **A,** under normal circumstances; and **B,** in the presence of severe contractive inflammation. The cystic plate attaches to the anterior surface of the right portal pedicle. Dissection downward in the plane deep to the plate *(arrow)* leads to the pedicle, with injury to the vessels and bile duct. When inflammation is mild, as in **A,** entry into the plane is usually readily detected with visualization of liver tissue. When there is severe contractive inflammation, the cystic plate is thickened, as in **B,** and determination of the position of the dissection in relation to the plate is difficult. In addition, the plate is foreshortened so that the distance from the top of the plate to the pedicle is very short. Both of these factors greatly increase the likelihood of injury to the pedicle. *(From Strasberg SM, Gouma DJ: "Extreme" vasculobiliary injuries: association with fundus-down cholecystectomy in severely inflamed gallbladders, HPB 14:1–8, 2012, Fig. 5.)*

The Psychology of Human Error

Certain traits of human behavior may contribute to biliary injury. Surgery is a complex task in which visual disorientation occurs occasionally, and persistence in error from a deadly mindset is a common human failing. The mindset error is the tendency to interpret information incorrectly after one has first made a decision. The point of departure of the authors with this view is that the visual disorientation is more likely to occur with certain methods of procedure and can be greatly diminished with the use of routine cholangiography or the critical view technique of identification.

Equipment

Laparoscopic equipment must be maintained in good operating condition. Focal loss of insulation on cautery instruments can result in arcing and thermal injuries to bile ducts or bowel.

Vasculobiliary Injuries

A vasculobiliary injury (VBI) is a combined injury to a bile duct and to a hepatic artery or portal vein. The bile duct injury is usually caused by direct operative trauma but also may be ischemic in origin or the result of both. Various degrees of hepatic ischemia may also be present. The most common VBI involves the right hepatic artery and a major bile duct such as the common hepatic duct. For instance, the right hepatic artery is probably injured in about 25% of type E biliary injuries. The right hepatic artery is injured more commonly than other arteries because it lies close to the common hepatic duct and the injury usually occurs as the common hepatic duct is divided in the classical injury described previously. Injury to the artery results in ischemia to the bile duct and may result in propagation of injury to a higher level than the mechanical injury. Consequently, repairs to the common bile duct when there has been an injury to the right hepatic artery tend to fail because of ischemia of that portion of the duct. As a result, assessment of the hepatic arteries should be part of the investigation of all major biliary injuries. In addition, in the face of a right hepatic artery occlusion, consideration should be given to delaying repair for about 3 months to give the ducts an opportunity to "die back" so that only adequately vascularized ducts remain. This avoids repair to an ischemic segment of duct. Right hepatic artery VBI may also result in hepatic ischemia. It is manifested as slow spotty infarction of the right liver, and the areas of infarct may become infected and develop abscesses. Another pattern is asymptomatic atrophy of the right liver.

Extreme Vasculobiliary Injuries

These injuries usually involve both a major hepatic artery and the main portal vein or one of its primary branches. Extreme VBIs account for only 5% of vasculobiliary injuries. However, they are important because their consequences are very serious. Hepatic infarction is frequent, often with rapid onset and frequently necessitating emergency hepatectomy or urgent liver transplantation. Death has occurred in about 50% of such cases. The pathogenesis involves two elements: severe inflammation necessitating conversion to an open procedure and the fundus-down technique. The gallbladder rests on the cystic plate, whose tapered lower end inserts into the front of the right portal pedicle (see Figure 5). If the plane of dissection in a cholecystectomy is behind rather than in front of the cystic plate and the dissection is continued downward in this plane, the sheath of the right portal pedicle containing the major vascular and biliary structures supplying the right liver is incised, exposing the structures to injury.

To prevent injury, surgeons should be aware that fundus-down cholecystectomy in the face of severe inflammation tends to bring the dissection onto the right portal pedicle with predicable

consequences. Contracture of the gallbladder, with puckering of the liver; dense adhesion of pericholecystic structures such as omentum, colon, and duodenum; and difficulty in finding the gallbladder are warning signs that can serve to steer the surgeon away from trying to take the gallbladder out from above. In the authors' opinion, fundus-down cholecystectomy in the face of severe inflammation should be avoided because it is an error trap.

The Culture of Safety in Cholecystectomy

Probably the most important part of prevention of biliary injury is the adoption of a culture in which the surgeon's mindset is tuned to safety first. This means adopting secure methods of ductal identification and meticulous dissection techniques, knowing when to get help from another surgeon, and knowing when to back away from completing a difficult cholecystectomy when local conditions are so adverse that the safety of the procedure is questionable. It includes readiness to switch strategies to perform lesser operations such as cholecystotomy or partial cholecystectomy. The warning signs of severe inflammation and indistinct anatomy should serve to direct the surgeon to perform a limited safe procedure such as cholecystotomy or subtotal cholecystectomy in which the gallbladder is not taken off the liver bed at all. This culture of cholecystectomy, which emphasizes safety, is much like that which is used throughout the aviation industry.

Presentation and Investigation

About one third of the more serious injuries are diagnosed during surgery. Most of the rest are identified within 30 days of surgery, but a few may appear years later. Intraoperative recognition may occur as a result of observation of bile in the field, by cholangiography, or rarely by actual visualization of the lacerated or divided duct. Sometimes the diagnosis is made after conversion for bleeding or inability to proceed in a difficult dissection.

Postoperative presentations of bile duct injury are influenced by the type of injury and whether a drain has been left. The most common presentations are pain with sepsis, with or without jaundice, and jaundice without other symptoms. Biliary fistula is also a common presentation. Some patients present only with abdominal distension and malaise. The latter is a particularly insidious presentation and is usually the result of bile ascites, which may not provoke much of an inflammatory reaction.

Pain and Sepsis

Computed tomographic (CT) scan is performed first to localize fluid collections, which may be aspirated to determine whether they contain bile. In most cases, a drain is placed in the biloma and an endoscopic retrograde cholangiopancreatography (ERCP) follows. Magnetic resonance imaging (MRI) with magnetic resonance cholangiography (MRC) has the potential to replace these investigations with a single one, but MRC does not show collapsed ducts well and is more likely to be useful with obstruction of the biliary tree than perforation with free drainage of bile into the peritoneal cavity. Many patients with pain or sepsis have type A or D injuries, and definitive treatment is possible at the time of endoscopy. Whether CT scan or MRI is used, an examination of the arteries and veins in the hepatoduodenal ligament should be part of the evaluation for all types of presentations.

Jaundice

The presence of jaundice suggests that the patient has sustained a type E injury. Duct occlusion is usually present if jaundice is the only symptom. Pain and sepsis from bile collections also tend to be present when a major duct is transected. ERCP is the first-line investigation, although some advocate starting with MRC. The duct may be found to be completely transected or occluded; often clips are seen at the point at which the dye column stops with loss of continuity to the upper biliary tract. Percutaneous transhepatic cholangiography (PTC) should then be performed to delineate the proximal ducts and to provide external drainage of bile. Often it is best to wait to perform the PTC until the biloma has contracted and the biloma drain can be injected in a retrograde manner to display the bile ducts for transhepatic puncture. If partially occluded (stenotic) rather than totally occluded ducts are found, the entire extent of injury may be diagnosed with ERCP.

Bile Fistula

The first-line investigation is a fistulogram. Subsequent management depends on anatomic findings.

Management of Biliary Injuries

Management of Injuries Recognized at the Initial Operation

Little has been written about the conduct of a laparoscopic cholecystectomy, subsequent to the discovery of a biliary injury. Highly suggestive evidence shows that repair of difficult biliary injuries frequently fails when performed by surgical teams engaged infrequently in surgery of the upper biliary tree.

When injury is suspected, it is helpful to ask for assistance from another surgeon. Intraoperative recognition of a biliary injury is an indication for conversion. The following two guidelines are suggested when laparotomy is undertaken for suspected injury: (1) repair should be attempted only if the techniques required for reconstruction are commonly used by the operating team, and (2) the injury should not be worsened by attempting a dissection for the purpose of an exact diagnosis. When appropriate expertise is not available, closed suction drains should be placed laparoscopically and the patient referred to a center of expertise in biliary surgery.

Type A injuries, recognized at the time of surgery, are repaired with suture of the cystic duct and drainage. Simple type D injuries are repaired by closure of the defect with fine absorbable sutures over a T-tube and placement of a closed suction drain, in the vicinity of the repair. The T-tube should be brought out through a separate incision in the duct, if possible. Avulsion of the cystic duct, a variant of type D injury, may be managed in the same manner. Type D injuries that are thermal in origin or that are complex (e.g., involving most of the circumference of the wall or with tissue loss) are best repaired with hepatojejunostomy. Complete transection should be repaired with a Roux-en-Y hepatojejunostomy, with application of the principles of anastomosis given subsequently.

Management of Biliary Injuries Diagnosed After Surgery

Management depends on type of injury, on type of initial management and its result, and on time elapsed since the initial operation or repair. This section focuses specifically on strictures or injuries that may lead to strictures.

Type A Injuries

These can almost always be managed with endoscopic sphincterotomy and stenting. A biloma drain may also be necessary for large collections of bile.

Type B Injuries

Type B injuries often remain asymptomatic or present only years later with right upper quadrant pain or cholangitis. Symptomatic patients need hepatojejunostomy or hepatic resection if biliary-enteric anastomosis is not possible. In asymptomatic patients, treatment is not recommended when the section of liver affected is small or the injury is remote and atrophy has occurred. When the injury is recent and the section of liver is large (e.g., the whole right liver), repair is empirically recommended.

Type C Injuries

Type C injuries require drainage of the bile collections and biliary-enteric anastomosis or ligation of the duct. If the duct is very small (e.g., 1 mm), then ligation is preferable. Occasionally, when reconstruction of the duct is not possible, resection of the part of the liver drained by the injured duct may be needed.

Type D Injuries

Treatment with ERCP and stenting is the treatment of choice in the postoperative period. When operation is necessary, the technique of repair is the same as when the problem is discovered at time of initial surgery.

Type E Injuries

The best chance for lasting repair is the first one. Strictures and sometimes clip occlusions may be treated with dilation and stents placed either with ERCP or percutaneously through the liver. In the authors' experience, nonsurgical therapy is most likely to be successful when the strictures are mild, appear months to years after surgery, or are of short length. Lillemoe and associates reported a 64% success rate with the use of stents.

Timing of Surgery

Factors that favor immediate repair are early referral, a stable patient, absence of bile collections, simpler injuries that can be rapidly diagnosed, and absence of a vasculobiliary injury. Often patients are referred several weeks after cholecystectomy when local inflammation may be expected to be great. In these patients, percutaneous tubes are placed to relieve obstruction of affected segments, drain subhepatic collections, and control sepsis. Repair is performed when inflammation has settled, usually about 3 months after the last operation. This delayed approach is sometimes used even when the patient is referred within the first week, especially in complex, hard-to-diagnose injuries an hose with a thermal or vasculobiliary injury. Immediate repair may also be undertaken when the injury is diagnosed months after surgery (e.g., after failure of stenting of a stenosis or late failure of a biliary-enteric anastomosis).

Preoperative Preparation

Complete diagnosis of the injury before operation is essential. Failure to do so may result in exclusion of bile ducts from the repair. The percutaneous transhepatic tubes placed to ensure biliary drainage from all liver segments also serve as guides to the position of the injured ducts at surgery. The authors' policy is to perform conciliation between CT scan and PTC studies to be sure that all ducts in the liver are accounted for.

Technical Aspects of Repair

Exposure

The incision must allow for good visualization of the porta hepatis. The authors prefer a right upper quadrant incision about 8 cm below the costal margin with extension up the midline to the xiphoid (hockey stick). If the dissection proves difficult or full mobilization of the liver is necessary, the incision may be extended further laterally or medially into a Mercedes type incision. If a previous Kocher incision has been made, this incision may be modified towards the midline and laterally to allow better visualization. A retractor fixed to the operative table is used to elevate the right costal margin and secure the abdominal exposure. Loupe magnification (2.5× to 3.5×) of the operative field is helpful.

Identification and Repair

The operative field is carefully examined, and the extent of the injury including vascular injury is documented. If the cholecystectomy is not completed, it is completed at this time. The principles of repair are that the anastomosis be tension free, have good blood supply, be mucosa-to-mucosa, and be of adequate caliber. Hepatojejunostomy is used in preference to either choledochocholedochostomy or choledochoduodenostomy because a tension-free anastomosis is always possible with hepatojejunostomy. Choledochocholedochostomy also fails frequently because blood supply to the upper end is inadequate in low transections and inadequate to the lower end in high transections. Whenever possible, an anterior longitudinal opening is created in the bile duct, and a long side-to-side anastomosis (sideways repair) is performed. Often this is done to the extrahepatic portion of the left hepatic duct after it is lowered by dividing the hilar plate (Hepp-Couinaud approach). This approach is particularly suitable for injuries at or just below the confluence of the right and left hepatic ducts (types E2 and E3).

When isolated right hepatic ducts exist, as in E4, E5, B, and C types of injury, the Hepp-Couinaud approach is not sufficient. For identification of the right ducts, the same initial steps to lower the hilar plate are followed, but then the dissection is extended to the right in the same coronal plane as the left duct (Figure 6). The liver capsule is divided, and then the cystic plate is encountered at its narrow lower end where it attaches to the right portal pedicle. The cystic plate is divided, exposing the sheath of the right main portal pedicle. Exposure of a larger area of the anterior surface of the sheath may be attained by coring out part of the overlying liver. Inside this sheath may be one or more ducts, depending on the level of injury and anatomic variances. Fine (5-0) holding sutures are placed in the duct, and then it is incised on the anterior surface to spatulate the orifice for anastomosis. The use of biliary probes helps ensure that all the segments are accounted for. Transhepatic drains that were placed to control leaks can be left in place during the dissection and facilitate identification.

Exposure is also facilitated during these procedures by dividing the bridge of tissue between segments 3 and 4 and fully opening the gallbladder fossa, which often collapses with adherence of its walls after cholecystectomy. If these maneuvers are not sufficient, resection of part of segment 4b or 5 opens the upper porta hepatis. The latter is an invaluable adjunct in the very difficult case.

The actual anastomosis is performed with fine absorbable sutures (usually 5-0). The order of suture placement is important. Usually, the anterior row of sutures is placed in the bile duct, and the ends of these sutures are laid upward over the patient's chest and kept in order on a spindle. If more than one duct is to undergo anastomosis, the anterior row sutures are placed in all the ducts, unless the ducts lie in a sagittal plane with one duct in front of the other, which is quite uncommon. Next, the posterior row is placed between the bile duct and the intestine, and the knots tied on the inside. The anastomosis is completed with use of the previously placed anterior row duct sutures to pick up the anterior lip of the opening in the bowel. When the ducts lay in the sagittal plane, the posterior duct is repaired first, followed by the anterior duct.

The use of postoperative stents is controversial. No evidence shows that they are helpful if a large mucosa-to-mucosa anastomosis has been achieved. The authors use them when very small ducts have undergone anastomosis.

Sometimes biliary reconstruction is not possible or advisable. When ductal reconstruction to a part of the liver is impossible,

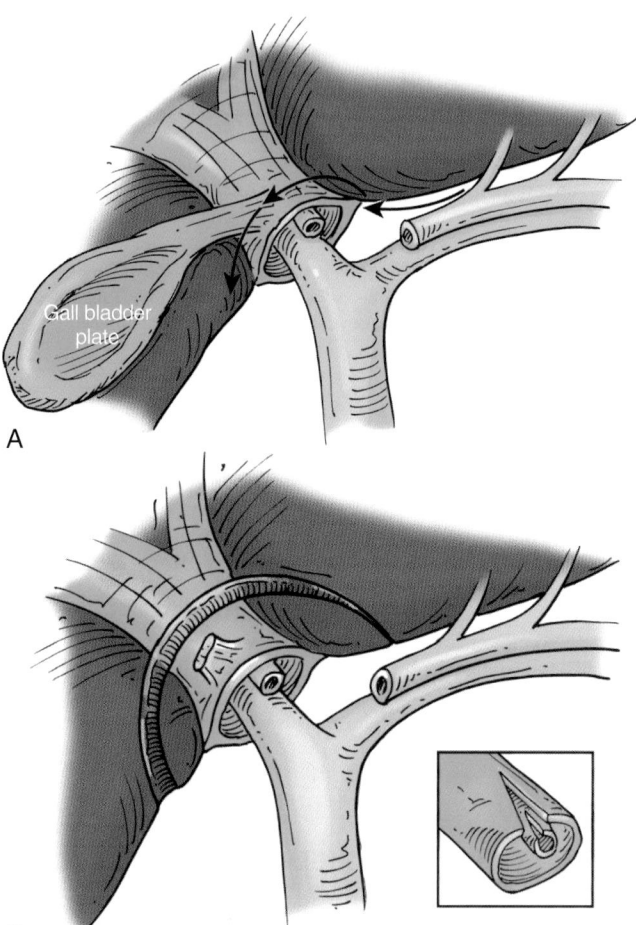

FIGURE 6 **A,** Operative technique for display of the isolated right ductal injuries. The amputated left and right ducts are shown, as are the portal vein and the sheath of the right portal pedicle. Note that the cystic (gallbladder) plate is a part of the Wallerian system of fibrous connective tissue that invests portal structures as they enter the liver. It attaches to the sheath of the right portal pedicle. The left and right hepatic ducts lie in the same coronal plane. The dissection is shown at a stage when the left hepatic duct has been isolated by the Hepp-Couinaud approach. The *arrows* indicate the direction of dissection from that point. **B,** A later stage in the dissection. The gallbladder plate has been cut and the liver pushed back off the right portal pedicle. The liver at the base of segment 5 has been cored away. The duct is isolated with the aid of the indwelling stent and opened on its anterior surface *(right and below on the diagram)*. *(Modified from Strasberg SM, Picus DD, Drebin JA: Results of a new strategy for reconstruction of biliary injuries having an isolated right sided component,* J Gastrointest Surg *5:266–274, 2001, Figs. 2 and 3.)*

resection should be performed. Occasionally, prior failure of reconstruction leads to secondary biliary cirrhosis and end-stage liver failure. Then, liver transplantation is required. In almost all examples of this unfortunate outcome, high reconstructions have been attempted by surgeons who lack experience in the procedures. Treatment of failed repairs with metallic stents gives very poor results in the long term, with 50% of treated patient having repeated cholangitis.

Treatment of Vasculobiliary Injuries

Immediate repair of the right hepatic artery has been performed either with end-to-end anastomosis or with a graft, usually taken from the inferior mesenteric vein. When a major arterial injury has been diagnosed, the size of the vessel, extent of injury, timing of the injury, and absence of pulsatile back bleeding all help determine the need for arterial reconstruction. If arterial repair is deemed necessary, this repair is performed first. The opportunity for repair is limited both because the procedure has to be done in close proximity to the injury, ideally within hours, and because the injury is frequently too severe to repair. Because only 10% of patients with a right hepatic artery/bile duct injury have clinically significant hepatic ischemia develop, the alternate strategy of allowing slow infarction to take place in a minority of patients and treating it with resection, if necessary, might result in better overall outcomes than routine early reconstruction.

Outcome of Treatment

Most surgical series cite very good short-term results. However, it is well known from older literature that there is a progressive restenosis rate. Two thirds of recurrences are diagnosed in the first 2 years after repair, but restenosis has been described after 10 years. Valid comparison among surgical series is difficult because of lack of standard reporting and effect of differences in the severity of injuries. Injuries above the confluence involving several bile ducts have a much worse prognosis than do injuries of the common hepatic duct, as do vasculobiliary injuries. Reporting of treatment failure is not uniform. Length of follow-up is another obvious variable that affects outcome and is not uniform among series.

OTHER BENIGN BILIARY STRICTURES

Biliary Strictures Secondary to Pancreatitis

Severe chronic pancreatitis such as alcoholic chronic pancreatitis and autoimmune pancreatitis may produce benign biliary strictures in the intrapancreatic segment of the common bile duct. Sometimes, the bile duct narrowing is the result of compression by a pseudocyst. In these cases, relief of compression or spontaneous resolution of the pseudocyst may relieve the stenosis.

Presenting symptoms are jaundice with or without pain. Diagnosis is made with CT scan or MRI combined with ERCP. ERCP permits brushings that may diagnose malignancy. Characteristically, the stricture is of the long smooth rat-tail type. One of the continuing conundrums in pancreatic surgery is the differentiation between benign and malignant causes of intrapancreatic bile duct stricture. Focal pancreatitis can produce a mass in the head of the pancreas, cause jaundice, and thereby mimic cancer. Cancer is more likely to arise in the chronically inflamed gland. The cancers are often scirrhous, making diagnosis with needle biopsy more difficult, especially in an already chronically inflamed gland. Endoscopic ultrasound scan (EUS)–guided fine needle aspiration (FNA) and core biopsies are very helpful in making the diagnosis, and the Ca19-9 level is also helpful.

Treatment depends on whether biliary stricture is an isolated problem or whether it is part of a more general problem such as unremitting pancreatic pain, whether a pseudocyst is present, or whether cancer is a serious consideration. For isolated strictures, endoscopic dilation and stenting with multiple stents has become the procedure of choice. When this fails, biliary enteric anastomosis with Roux-en-Y hepatojejunostomy or choledochoduodenostomy may be used. Treatment of the biliary stricture may simply require endoscopic drainage of a pseudocyst. Treatment may be part of a wider procedure such as the Frey's procedure that relieves the obstruction with removal of the surrounding compressive scar or with addition of biliary enteric anastomosis to the basic procedure.

Pylorus-preserving or standard Whipple's procedures, which relieve the biliary obstruction with resection, are sometimes used when cancer is suspected. Metallic stents should not be used in this or other benign strictures

Stricture From Noniatrogenic Bile Duct Injuries

Noniatrogenic bile duct injuries are usually caused by nonpenetrating trauma and are often a part of wider injuries. Isolated bile duct injury from penetrating trauma may occur, but more often, it is not isolated and is often fatal as the hepatic artery and portal vein are usually also injured. The injury is often missed, and diagnosis is delayed. The principles of complete diagnosis and repair enunciated previously apply to these injuries as well. Combined biliary and arterial injuries may occur, and the surgeon must be aware that the bile duct may be devascularized to a higher level than the laceration or transection.

Strictures From Calculous Disease

Oriental cholangiohepatitis is a disease associated with biliary parasite infestation leading to the development of intrahepatic and extrahepatic bile duct stones, usually of the brown pigment type. Recurrent pyogenic infections are common and lead to strictures. Treatment is with a combination of therapies, including eradication of the parasites, removal of the stones, dilation of the strictures, and occasionally local liver resection. Sometimes much of the therapy can be accomplished percutaneously. At other times, operative removal of stones and hepatojejunostomy is required; the Roux loop may be placed in proximity to the skin to permit later percutaneous access.

Choledocholithiasis occurring in Western countries may lead to biliary strictures through repeated bouts of cholangitis or local stone ulceration and resultant stricture formation often near the lower end of the bile duct. Such papillary stenosis is uncommon today. Endoscopic sphincterotomy (ES) is the treatment for low strictures, and biliary enteric anastomoses are used when unsuccessful or not applicable. Large stones within the gallbladder may cause biliary obstruction by external compression (Mirizzi's syndrome).

Primary Sclerosing Cholangitis

Primary sclerosing cholangitis (PSC) is an idiopathic autoimmune disease, frequently associated with inflammatory bowel disease. It causes biliary strictures, which are usually both intrahepatic and extrahepatic and multiple. Stones are not usually present. Degeneration to cancer may occur, and these cancers are difficult to diagnose early. Treatment of symptomatic localized strictures in the larger bile ducts is usually endoscopic. Resection of the confluence has been advocated when the major area of stricture is localized to that area. Many of these patients require liver transplantation as the definitive surgical procedure; this is done when end-stage liver disease appears or when cancer is suspected. Prior surgery on the bile ducts may make transplantation more difficult.

Benign Inflammatory Pseudotumors

Benign inflammatory tumors, also called hepatic inflammatory pseudotumors, mimic extrahepatic cholangiocarcinomas but consist of chronic inflammatory cells and fibrosis. They occur most frequently in extrahepatic upper ducts, and less commonly in lower ducts. About 10% of resected cholangiocarcinomas are actually pseudotumors.

SUGGESTED READINGS

Branum G, Schmitt C, Baille J, et al: Management of major biliary complications after laparoscopic cholecystectomy, *Ann Surg* 217:532, 1993.
Lillemoe KD, Martin SA, Cameron JL, et al: Major bile duct injuries during laparoscopic cholecystectomy: follow-up after combined surgical and radiologic management, *Ann Surg* 225(5):459–468, 1997.

Strasberg SM, Eagon CJ, Drebin JA: The "hidden cystic duct" syndrome and the infundibular technique of laparoscopic cholecystectomy: the danger of the false infundibulum, *J Am Coll Surg* 191:6617, 2000.
Strasberg SM, Helton WS: An analytical review of vasculobiliary injury in laparoscopic and open cholecystectomy, *HPB* 13:1–14, 2011.
Strasberg SM, Hertl M, Soper NJ: An analysis of the problem of biliary injury during laparoscopic cholecystectomy, *J Am Coll Surg* 180:101–125, 1995.

CYSTIC DISORDERS OF THE BILE DUCTS

Seth Goldstein, MD, Bulent Salman, MD, and Barish H. Edil, MD

OVERVIEW

Choledochal cyst disease is defined by dilation of the intrahepatic or extrahepatic biliary tree. Once thought to be exclusively a pediatric condition, it is now an increasingly recognized entity in adults. Regardless of age, choledochal cyst disease must be promptly recognized and treated to avoid biliary and hepatic complications. In addition, and most importantly, early intervention is necessary to prevent malignant degeneration.

CLASSIFICATION

Choledochal cyst is technically a misnomer because cystic dilations of the biliary tree often extend beyond the common bile duct (ductus choledochus). In this chapter, we refer to choledochal cysts with Todani's modification of the Alonso-Lej classification, which defines five types of cyst based on the pattern of biliary tree involvement as illustrated in Figure 1.

Type I (A, B, C) is the most common classification and consists of a dilation of the extrahepatic biliary tree: cystic, focal, and fusiform, respectively. Type II cyst is an extrahepatic supraduodenal saccular diverticulum of the common bile duct. Type III refers to dilation of the intraduodenal segment of the common bile duct, known as a choledochocele. Type IV cysts typically involve both intrahepatic and extrahepatic bile ducts (type IVA) or can be multiple extrahepatic dilations (type IVB). Type V, or Caroli's disease, is confined to intrahepatic ductal dilation alone and can be either unilobar or bilobar (see Figure 1).

ETIOLOGY

The exact pathogenesis of choledochal cyst is unknown; however, several theories exist to explain this unusual biliary disorder. The first hypothesis for the formation of choledochal cysts is a congenital defect in maturation and ductal plate malformation. The belief is that arrested or faulty bile duct plate remodeling takes place during embryogenesis and results in dilated bile ducts. This hypothesis relates primarily to the development of Caroli's disease and can be seen in either sporadic or inherited scenarios. The second hypothesis is an acquired condition as a result of biliary system obstruction from a stricture, web, or sphincter of Oddi's dysfunction. However, the most commonly accepted hypothesis is pancreaticobiliary

maljunction. Studies have indicated 57% to 96% of patients with choledochal cyst disease have this anatomic variant. The maljunction is defined by pancreatic and bile duct joining outside of the duodenal wall. A long common channel allows the milieu of pancreas and bile juice to mix and regurgitate up the biliary system, setting off a cascade of damage and inflammation and resulting in dilation of the ducts. Despite the association with pancreaticobiliary maljunction, no single theory can clearly explain the formation of different choledochal cyst types.

EPIDEMIOLOGY

Estimates of incidence range from 1 in 13,000 in East Asia to 1 in 2,000,000 in the United States. A female predominance of approximately 4:1 is found. The associated risk of malignancy at the time of diagnosis is 10%; the malignancy can be either gallbladder carcinoma or cholangiocarcinoma. The risk of malignancy also increases with age from 0.7% in the first decade, to 2.3% in the third decade, and up to 75% when diagnosed with a choledochal cyst disease in the ninth decade.

DIAGNOSIS AND PREOPERATIVE EVALUATION

The classic triad of abdominal pain, jaundice, and a palpable mass is actually observed in a minority of patients. In children, the usual symptoms are episodic abdominal pain, nausea with vomiting, and slowly progressive jaundice. Adults can present with signs of calculous biliary tract disease or pancreatitis and often have already undergone cholecystectomy before diagnosis.

Preoperative imaging is essential in determining the operative plan. Neonates and children are often evaluated first with abdominal ultrasound scan, which is safe and cost effective. Adults generally benefit from computed tomographic (CT) imaging, which defines the anatomy of the hepatobiliary and pancreatic regions. Magnetic resonance cholangiopancreatography (MRCP) can also be used to demonstrate biliary anatomy, including cyst pattern and pancreaticobiliary maljunction with a long common channel. In addition to biliary anatomy, cross-sectional imaging can evaluate for occult malignancy.

Cholangiography is the gold standard of choledochal cyst imaging and can be accomplished with endoscopic retrograde cholangiopancreatography (ERCP), with percutaneous transhepatic cholangiography (PTC), and now more commonly, with MRCP. This allows detail of the ductal dilation and shows whether a long common channel is present, which helps with the diagnosis of choledochal cyst.

Patients may have medical complications from choledochal cyst disease that necessitate attention before operative intervention. Cholangitis should be adequately treated with broad-spectrum intravenous antibiotics and, if necessary, with biliary decompression. Severe liver damage can be seen with long-standing choledochal cyst disease and can manifest as portal hypertension, uncorrected coagulopathy,

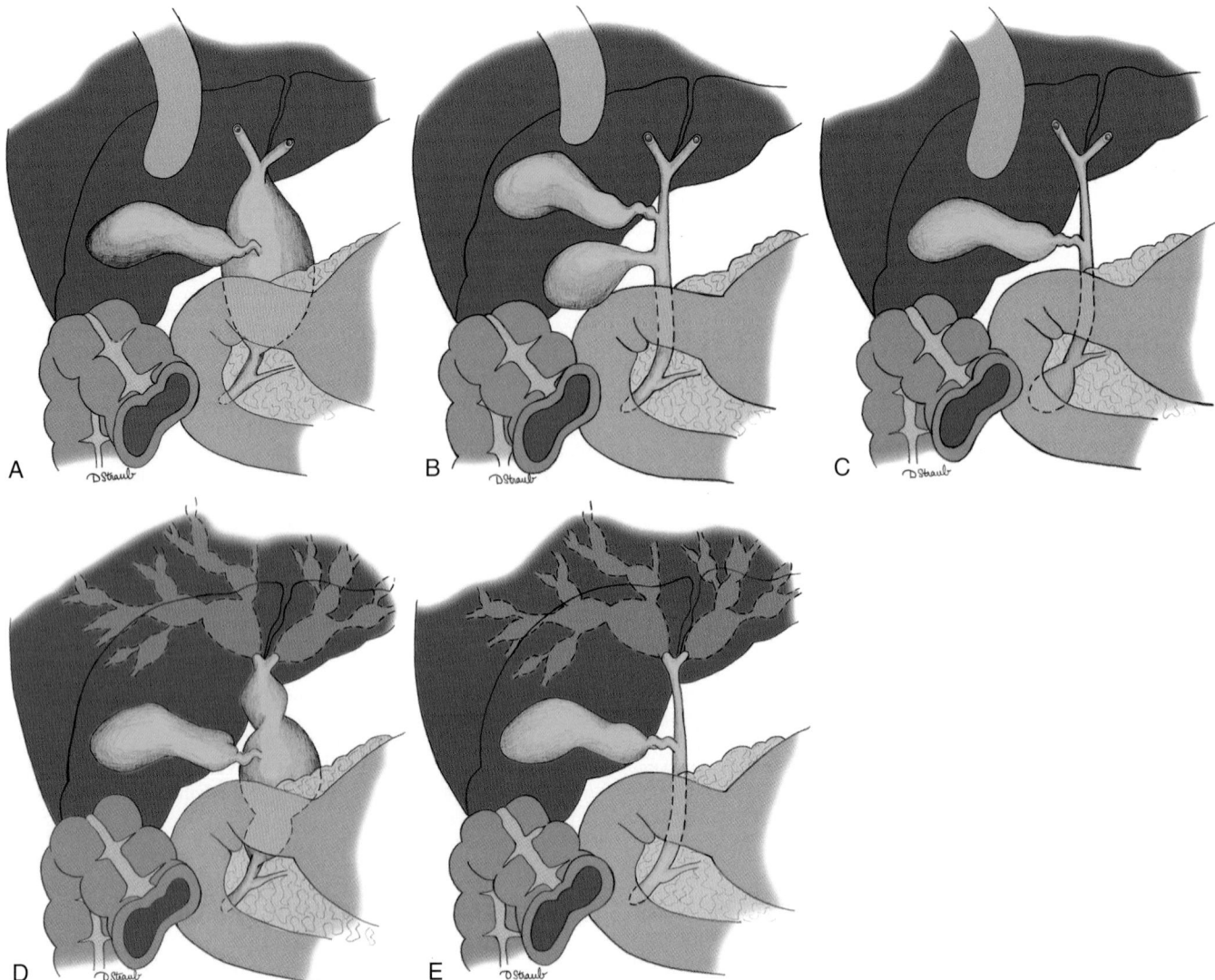

FIGURE 1   Classification of biliary cysts. **A,** Type I; **B,** type II; **C,** type III; **D,** type IVA; and **E,** type V. *(From Lipsett PA, Pitt HA, Colombani PM, et al: Choledochal disease: a changing pattern of presentation, Ann Surg 220:644, 1994.)*

and end-stage liver failure, which are contraindications for operative intervention.

MANAGEMENT

Treatment of choledochal cyst disease requires surgical excision of the abnormal biliary tree with biliary-enteric reconstruction. Surgical intervention most importantly removes the biliary tissue at risk for malignant transformation and excludes the liver from further pancreas and biliary juice exposure. In addition, it can relieve biliary obstruction, preventing future episodes of cholangitis, stone formation, or biliary cirrhosis that results in an interruption of the inflammatory injury cycle.

Type I: Extrahepatic Bile Duct Cyst

First, the peritoneal cavity is explored for signs of malignancy, either via laparoscopy or via midline or right subcostal incision. The gallbladder is removed in standard retrograde fashion from the liver bed with ligation of the cystic artery. The mobilization of the cystic duct to the common bile duct facilitates identification of the choledochal

cyst. The duodenum undergoes full kocherization to allow access to the posterior pancreas and distal bile duct/cyst. The dissection on the anterior cyst is continued down posterior of the duodenum and the head of the pancreas until the bile duct narrows at the inferior portion of the cyst, with care taken to not injure the pancreatic duct. This area is ligated and transected to allow for cephalad reflection and posterior dissection with identification of the portal vein. This dissection continues until the hepatic duct confluence is reached. Pathologic analysis of the resected specimen is obtained, along with frozen-section analysis of the proximal and distal margins, to exclude malignancy.

A standard 60-cm Roux-en-Y loop is used for an end-to-side hepaticojejunostomy. The anastomosis is constructed with a single layer of absorbable suture. Recent experiences of pancreaticobiliary surgeons have described cyst excision done laparoscopically. The experience and long-term outcomes of this approach have yet to be determined.

Type II: Extrahepatic Biliary Diverticulum

For type II cyst, complete excision of the cyst is again recommended. This can be performed with extrahepatic biliary resection and

Roux-en-Y reconstruction or complete excision with primary closure over a T tube. The defect in the wall of the common bile duct should be closed transversely to prevent narrowing of the lumen.

Type III: Choledochocele

Type III cysts are unusual; their malignant potential seems to be lower, but this is unclear. Typically, when a surgeon is faced with a type III cyst, it is because of obstructive symptoms. Complete excision can be done after kocherization through a lateral duodenostomy in the second portion of the duodenum. The common bile duct and pancreatic duct must be identified to prevent pancreatic duct injury. The cyst is excised, and a sphincteroplasty can be done with sewing of duct to duodenal mucosa with interrupted absorbable suture. ERCP with sphincterotomy is an alternative in patients who may not tolerate excision to facilitate drainage and potentially relieve symptoms. On a very rare occasion, the Whipple procedure may be necessary and may be considered if malignancy is suspected.

Type IV: Multiple Bile Duct Cysts

The surgical management of type IV choledochal cysts can be difficult because of the presence of intrahepatic cystic disease that makes complete excision of the disease impossible. In this situation, complete extrahepatic cyst excision with biliary enteric anastomosis is recommended. In addition, if one lobe of the liver is involved, then hepatectomy should be performed. However, in many situations, diffuse bilobar cyst disease remains, which is at risk for malignant transformation. Removal of the extrahepatic choledochal cyst and proper decompression of the intrahepatic disease may prevent or facilitate the management of long-term complications of biliary stasis, stones, cholangitis, cirrhosis, and malignant transformation in this condition.

Type V: Caroli's Disease

Type V choledochal cyst (Caroli's disease) is a difficult condition to manage and is unsettled. Initial management entails treatment of infectious complications with drainage, stone extraction, antibiotics, and ursodiol to help with the dissolution of stones to increase biliary flow. Occasionally, the ductal abnormalities are confined to one lobe of the liver, and in this situation, hepatic lobectomy can be considered. The main objective with diffuse disease is proper drainage of the liver to disrupt the inflammatory cycle and prevent further liver injury and malignancy. In the case of severe portal hypertension, or after failure of the biliary-enteric drainage procedure with or without partial hepatectomy, patients may be considered to be candidates for orthotopic liver transplantation.

PROGNOSIS

Surgical management has significantly changed over the last 30 years. Originally, surgical draining of the cyst with a cyst duodenostomy or Roux-en-Y cyst jejunostomy was advocated. This resulted in disease being left behind and continued risk of malignant degeneration. Complete cyst resection is necessary to mediate future cancer risks and should be done whenever possible. However, if this is not possible, as seen with type IV and V, then close surveillance and proper drainage is needed. Furthermore, patients with a history of enteric drained cysts without complete excision should be offered complete resection even if they are asymptomatic and technical challenges are anticipated to remove that cancer risk.

The perioperative complications are typical of hepatobiliary surgery and include bleeding, wound infection, and anastomotic leak. In the long term, the postoperative benign biliary stricture rate may be as high as 40%, commonly presenting as cholangitis. Patients should undergo lifelong surveillance, particularly if intrahepatic cystic disease remains because it is at risk for malignant degeneration.

SUGGESTED READINGS

Edil BH, Cameron JL, Reddy S, et al: Choledochal cyst disease in children and adults: a 30-year single-institution experience, *J Am Coll Surg* 206(5):1000–1008, 2008.

Lee SE, Jang JY, Lee YJ, et al: Korean Pancreas Surgery Club: choledochal cyst and associated malignant tumors in adults: a multicenter survey in South Korea, *Arch Surg* 146(10):1178–1184, 2011.

Tashiro S, Imaizumi T, Ohkawa H, et al: Committee for Registration of the Japanese Study Group on Pancreaticobiliary Maljunction: pancreaticobiliary maljunction: retrospective and nationwide survey in Japan, *J Hepatobiliary Pancreat Surg* 10(5):345–351, 2003.

PRIMARY SCLEROSING CHOLANGITIS

**Shirin Sabbaghian, MD, and
Steven A. Ahrendt, MD**

Primary sclerosing cholangitis (PSC) is a disease characterized by chronic inflammation and destruction of both intrahepatic and extrahepatic bile ducts resulting in multifocal strictures of the biliary tree, chronic cholestasis, and eventually biliary cirrhosis. Although etiology is uncertain, the disease is most likely an immune-mediated disorder influenced by genetic factors. Most patients (up to 80%) with PSC also have inflammatory bowel disease (IBD), more often ulcerative colitis (UC). Although many patients are asymptomatic at diagnosis and are only found to have the disease on investigation of persistently elevated liver function test results, typical initial symptoms on presentation include right upper quadrant pain, fatigue, pruritus, and weight loss. Symptomatic patients also commonly have jaundice on physical examination. The diagnosis of PSC is usually established with abnormal liver function test results and an abnormal cholangiogram (endoscopic or magnetic resonance) after secondary causes of sclerosing cholangitis are ruled out. The overall goals of treatment are to slow progression of disease and reduce the risks for cancer and end-stage liver disease. Liver transplant is the only effective therapeutic option for patients with this disease once cirrhosis develops.

DEMOGRAPHICS

A recent meta-analysis of studies from North America and Europe suggests that the incidence rate of PSC is 1 per 100,000 person-years at risk. The disease affects men predominantly, although patients with PSC who do not have IBD are more often women. PSC is most commonly diagnosed in the fourth decade of life.

ETIOLOGY

The cause of PSC remains unknown and is thought to be multifactorial; most investigators suspect the disease is an immune-mediated process, and some evidence suggests a genetic role. In support of an immune-mediated etiology, up to 80% of patients with PSC also have IBD, particularly UC. An increased frequency of other autoimmune diseases has also been observed in patients with PSC. In support of immune-mediated and non-Mendelian genetic causes, an increased frequency of certain genes in the human leukocyte antigen (HLA) complex and closely linked genes has been observed. These associated genes include HLA-B8 in the major histocompatibility complex (MHC) class I region; DR3, DR2, and DR6 in the MHC class II region; and certain MHC class I chain-related alleles (MICs). Other non–HLA-related genes have been suggested to play a role in this disease, although only conflicting evidence exists. Additional evidence of genetic influence for this disease is the finding of an approximately fourfold increased risk of PSC in first-degree relatives of patients with PSC.

ASSOCIATED DISEASES AND COMPLICATIONS

Primary sclerosing cholangitis has been associated with several diseases and potential complications (Table 1). The strongest association is with IBD, usually UC. Although as many as 80% of patients with PSC have IBD, only 3% to 8% of patients with IBD have PSC. Patients with both PSC and IBD are much more likely to have pancolitis than more limited colonic involvement. PSC has also been shown to be an independent risk factor for colon cancer in patients with UC. In addition, the risk of development of colorectal cancer in patients with PSC and UC appears to increase further after liver transplant. Colonoscopy is warranted in all patients with PSC either to exclude the diagnosis of IBD in patients without a history or for cancer surveillance in patients with UC or Crohn's disease.

An increased frequency of autoimmune disease has been found in PSC. This includes disorders unrelated to the liver and colon, such as type I diabetes mellitus and thyroid disease. Autoimmune hepatitis (AIH) has also been seen in up to 17% of patients with PSC and has been designated separately as PSC-AIH overlap syndrome.

TABLE 1: Diseases associated with primary sclerosing cholangitis

Disease	Frequency (%)
Ulcerative colitis	60-75
Gallstones	25
Autoimmune disease	20
Cholangiocarcinoma	7-14
Autoimmune hepatitis	1.4-17
Crohn's disease	5-10
Colon cancer	2

PSC is associated with an increased frequency of hepatobiliary malignancies, including cholangiocarcinoma (CCA), gallbladder cancer, and hepatocellular carcinoma (HCC). PSC is considered a risk factor for CCA, which is one of the most feared complications of this disease. In population-based studies, CCA has been shown to occur in 7% to 14% of patients with PSC. It is common (30% to 42% incidence rate) in autopsy series of patients with PSC, and it is has been diagnosed in up to 10% of patients undergoing liver transplant despite an extensive preoperative evaluation to exclude this diagnosis. CCA is often diagnosed early in the clinical course of PSC, with up to half of patients diagnosed within 1 year of a PSC diagnosis. The subsequent annual incidence rate is 0.5% to 1.5%. Unfortunately, CCA is usually not an operable lesion once discovered because it is diagnosed either at an advanced stage or because the background liver disease precludes resection as an option. Strong suspicion for malignancy should be maintained for patients with PSC and a dominant stricture (defined as a stenosis with a diameter of ≤1.5 mm in the common bile duct or of ≤1 mm in the hepatic duct) and for patients who have clinical signs of rapidly increasing jaundice, abdominal pain, and weight loss. Cytologic examination of biliary brushings and biopsies may be helpful, but they generally have low sensitivity for diagnosis of CCA. Periodic testing for carbohydrate antigen 19-9 (CA19-9) has been recommended by some investigators to evaluate for an elevated level, particularly a sustained elevation, although a high false-positive rate exists because of factors such as bacterial cholangitis.

Patients with PSC are predisposed to gallbladder disease, both benign and malignant. Gallstones have been found in 25% of patients with PSC. Gallbladder polyps are commonly seen on ultrasound scan in patients with PSC (4% to 6%), and more than half of these contain an invasive cancer. Cholecystectomy should be performed in patients with PSC with gallbladder polyps regardless of lesion size. Annual ultrasound scan screening of the gallbladder has been recommended for patients with PSC.

Hepatocellular carcinoma (HCC) is a risk among patients with PSC with end-stage liver disease. Two percent to 4% of explanted livers from patients with PSC were found to have concomitant HCC.

NATURAL HISTORY AND PROGNOSTIC MODELS

PSC affects both quality of life and life expectancy. Median survival time in symptomatic patients ranges from 10 to18 years after diagnosis, with patients dying of complications of PSC, such as liver failure or CCA, or of advanced associated disease, such as colorectal carcinoma in patients with IBD. Median survival in asymptomatic patients with PSC is longer than in patients presenting with symptoms, although survival is decreased when compared with matched, healthy individuals. The course of PSC is highly variable among individual patients; some patients have rapid progression to liver failure or development of a biliary malignancy early in their course, whereas others remain asymptomatic for years. Mathematic prognostic models have been developed to help determine when a patient should be considered for liver transplant and to help evaluate response to certain therapies. The revised Mayo Model, which considers age, total bilirubin level, serum aspartate transferase (AST) value, serum albumin value, and history of variceal bleeding, has been developed to estimate survival over 4 years.

PRESENTATION

PSC is more often diagnosed in men, typically during the fourth decade of life. Patients present with either abnormal liver function test results or manifestations of cholestatic liver disease. In earlier observational studies, 15% to 40% of patients were found to be asymptomatic at the time of diagnosis. Diagnosis is pursued in asymptomatic patients typically when persistently cholestatic biochemical tests are discovered. Symptomatic patients usually present with right upper quadrant pain, fatigue, pruritus, and weight loss. Cholangitis is uncommon on presentation in patients who have not undergone biliary surgery or biliary tract manipulation, such as endoscopic retrograde cholangiopancreatography (ERCP). Physical examination findings for symptomatic patients may include jaundice, hepatomegaly, and splenomegaly. Certain biochemical tests are commonly abnormal in patients with PSC. An elevated serum alkaline phosphatase is the "biochemical hallmark," although a normal value does not exclude the diagnosis. Serum aminotransferase levels are usually two to three times higher than normal, but again, normal values do not exclude the diagnosis. Total bilirubin level is normal in 60% of cases.

DIAGNOSIS

The diagnosis of PSC is normally supported with typical findings on cholangiogram. Magnetic resonance cholangiography (MRC) is the diagnostic procedure of choice when PSC is suspected. The diagnosis can usually be established noninvasively with MRC with a sensitivity and specificity exceeding 80%. The diagnosis may also be established with endoscopic retrograde cholangiography (ERC) or percutaneous transhepatic cholangiography (PTC). The typical cholangiographic findings in PSC include multifocal strictures with a resultant and characteristic beading pattern in both the intrahepatic and extrahepatic bile ducts. The hepatic duct bifurcation is often the most severely strictured segment of the biliary tree (Figure 1). Isolated involvement of the intrahepatic ducts and proximal extrahepatic

ducts occurs in approximately 20% of patients. Conversely, only 5% to 10% of patients have sclerosing cholangitis involving only the extrahepatic duct without intrahepatic duct involvement. Visualization of the entire biliary tree is critical to avoid missing a CCA.

The role of liver biopsy for the diagnosis of PSC has evolved. A liver biopsy often shows nonspecific findings in patients with PSC and rarely adds additional diagnostic information in patients with typical findings of the disease on cholangiography. However, a liver biopsy is warranted in patients with a cholestatic liver function panel and a normal cholangiogram to diagnose small duct PSC. Liver biopsy can also help diagnose patients suspected to have PSC-AIH overlap syndrome in whom immune suppressive therapy should be used for treatment.

PSC must be distinguished from secondary sclerosing cholangitis (SSC) that results from identifiable causes of biliary tree injury and stricture such as chronic obstruction, infection, chemical agents, drugs, and ischemia. Other diagnostic possibilities that are important to consider when pursuing a diagnosis of PSC are small duct primary sclerosing cholangitis, PSC overlap syndromes, and immunoglobulin G 4 (IgG4)–associated cholangitis. A cholestatic pattern to liver function studies supports the diagnosis of PSC and is useful for monitoring the course of the disease. Serum bilirubin is not commonly elevated early in the course of the disease but does increase as the disease progresses. The serum tumor marker CA19-9 may also be elevated in patients with PSC and CCA.

Occasionally, surgical resection may be necessary to make the diagnosis. For example, differentiation of localized sclerosing cholangitis from CCA can be difficult, especially when the stricture is in the perihilar region. Also, the combination of CCA and bacterial cholangitis may mimic sclerosing cholangitis. In cases like these, resection of the dominant stricture may be necessary to establish a diagnosis.

THERAPY

The overall goals of treatment of PSC are to slow progression of disease and reduce the risks for cancer and end-stage liver disease. A management algorithm is pictured in Figure 2. In general, asymptomatic patients should not be treated. No currently available medical therapy has shown any effect on disease progression. Symptomatic patients with persistently elevated liver function tests, pruritus, pain, or fatigue; evidence of significant extrahepatic or hilar strictures;

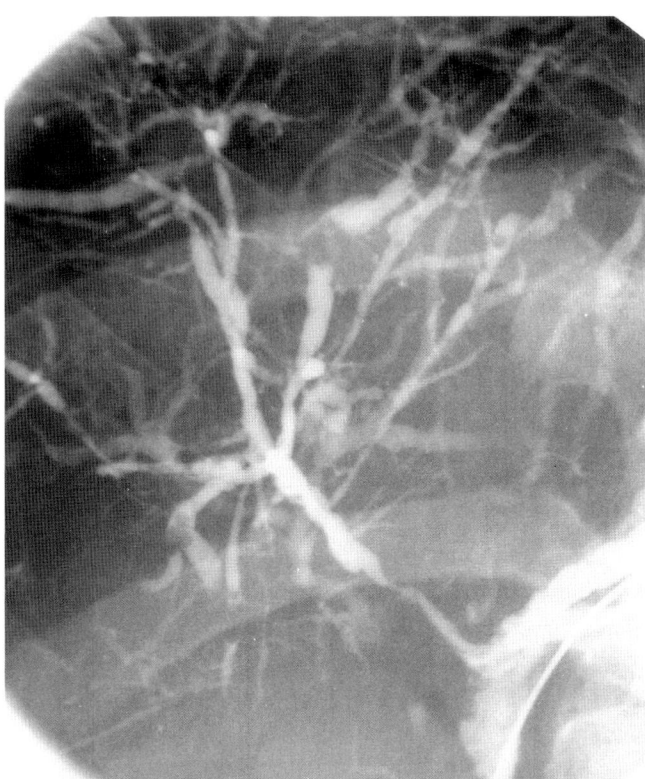

FIGURE 1 Percutaneous cholangiogram shows hepatic bifurcation *(lower right)* and right hepatic ducts in a patient with primary sclerosing cholangitis. Cholangiogram shows diffuse strictures of the intrahepatic bile ducts.

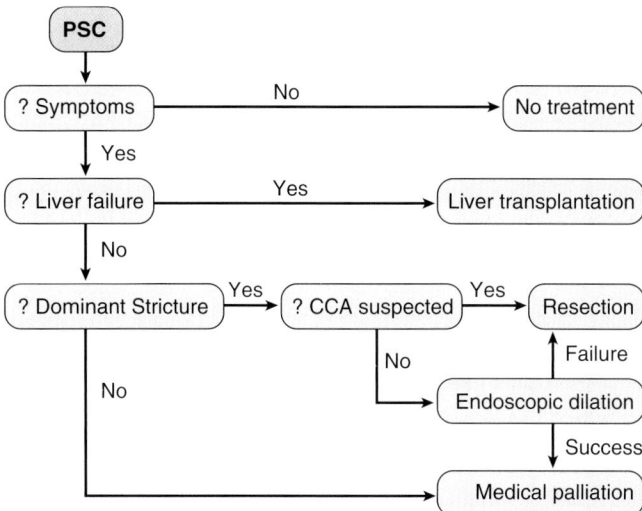

FIGURE 2 Management algorithm for primary sclerosing cholangitis *(PSC). CCA,* Cholangiocarcinoma.

and no clinical or imaging signs of cirrhosis are candidates for an endoscopic or surgical approach to improve biliary drainage. In addition, patients with dominant biliary strictures suspicious for CCA should undergo surgical exploration and resection of the extrahepatic bile ducts rather than prolonged efforts to establish a tissue diagnosis. When patients have cirrhosis develop, liver transplant is the only reasonable therapy.

Medical Therapy

Ursodeoxycholic acid (UDCA), which is used to treat primary biliary cirrhosis, initially showed promise as patients experienced improvement in liver function tests over time. However, in randomized studies that compared UDCA with placebo, the rates of treatment failure, including death, liver transplant, progression to cirrhosis, worsening of fatigue or pruritus, inability to tolerate the drug, or voluntary withdrawal from the study, were similar among the two treatment arms. Currently, the American Association for the Study of Liver Diseases (AASLD) recommends against use of UDCA as medical therapy for patients with PSC.

Antiinflammatory and immunosuppressive drugs, such as corticosteroids, penicillamine, azathioprine, colchicines, and anti–tumor necrosing factor (TNF) antibodies, have been tried in small studies. None of these drugs have proved to be beneficial in patients with classic PSC.

Symptoms of PSC are managed individually. Pruritus, for example, is managed with cholestyramine or UDCA and possibly antihistamines. Fatigue is managed symptomatically after hypothyroidism is ruled out. With advanced disease, fat malabsorption and steatorrhea may be present with subsequent deficiency of fat-soluble vitamins, vitamins A, D, E, and K. This can usually be treated with oral replacement of these vitamins.

Nonoperative Interventional Therapy

Dominant hilar and extrahepatic strictures occur in 15% to 20% of patients with PSC. They are defined as stenoses with a diameter of 1.5 mm or less in the common bile duct or of 1 mm or less in the hepatic duct. The initial approach to patients with a dominant stricture is endoscopic balloon dilation with or without stenting. The endoscopic approach avoids dissection of the porta hepatis before the need for hepatic transplant, allows treatment of both the right and left hepatic ducts simultaneously, and is associated with fewer complications than percutaneous or surgical procedures. Endoscopic therapies to treat dominant strictures include balloon dilation and stenting. Endoscopic stents are associated with a higher risk of complications, including cholangitis, and should be reserved for strictures that recur after balloon dilation. Endoscopic intervention can result in clinical improvement, and studies show that patients need fewer annual hospitalizations and have a short-term decrease in serum bilirubin and cholestatic symptoms after treatment. However, PSC is characterized by fluctuations in symptoms and degree of cholestasis, and to date, no controlled data show that endoscopic therapy alters the natural history of the disease.

The possibility of an existing CCA should be considered in all patients with a dominant stricture. Up to 9% of patients with dominant strictures managed endoscopically are ultimately diagnosed with CCA. Brush cytology or biopsy should be obtained at the time of dilation in all patients.

Dilation of biliary strictures also can be performed percutaneously in patients in whom an endoscopic approach has been unsuccessful. These strictures may be approached more easily via the percutaneous route than via the endoscopic route. In addition, the percutaneous approach may also be beneficial before surgery to aid in the intraoperative placement of large-bore transhepatic biliary

catheter. Morbidity for the percutaneous approach is higher when compared with endoscopic methods.

Operative Therapy

Surgical Resection

Surgical resection of the extrahepatic biliary tree is less commonly used now with the application of endoscopic therapy. In appropriately selected patients, resection of the extrahepatic biliary tract and hepatic duct bifurcation, which is frequently involved with a dominant stricture, may provide lasting relief from jaundice, may be used to exclude or make the diagnosis of CCA in a dominant biliary stricture, and may postpone the need for liver transplant. Operative management entails resection of the extrahepatic biliary tree, including the hepatic duct bifurcation, which is frequently involved with a dominant stricture. A cholecystectomy is performed if the gallbladder is still in place, and the distal common bile duct is divided at the level of the superior edge of the pancreas. Frozen sections are taken of each margin and of any suspicious areas to exclude the presence of CCA. If stents are planned for reconstruction, percutaneous stents can be placed before surgery to aid in the dissection of the hepatic duct bifurcation and to guide stent exchange with large-bore transhepatic biliary catheter at the time of surgery. Bilateral Roux-en-Y hepaticojejunostomies are created over these transhepatic stents, which are intended for removal approximately 1 year after placement if no obstruction exists at the anastomosis.

The overall morbidity rate after Roux-en-Y hepaticojejunostomy in PSC is 35%. Common complications include cholangitis, hemobilia, bile leak, and wound infection. Rarely, hepatic arterial bleeding related to the transhepatic stent has necessitated embolization for control. In a series of 40 patients without cirrhosis undergoing biliary reconstruction, the operative mortality rate was 2.5%.

Although used less frequently over the past decade, resection of the extrahepatic biliary tree in selected patients may delay the need for liver transplant. In a series of 77 patients followed for more than 5 years, the overall 3-year, 5-year, and 10-year survival rates after bile duct resection were 85%, 76%, and 53%, respectively. Patients without cirrhosis fared better with 1-year, 5-year, and 10-year survival rates of 95%, 83%, and 60%, respectively. Furthermore, in comparison of outcomes of surgical resection with endoscopic intervention, overall survival for patients without cirrhosis managed with bile duct resection was significantly longer than for a group of 35 concurrent patients without cirrhosis managed with endoscopic balloon dilation. Survival free of liver transplantation for the 40 patients who did not have cirrhosis at the time PSC was diagnosed was 95%, 92%, and 82% at 1, 3, and 5 years, respectively, after resection (Table 2). This was also significantly better than transplant-free survival in patients undergoing endoscopic intervention. None of the patients with surgical resection had CCA develop, with long-term follow-up exceeding 10 years, and only one patient (2%) needed a second operation for focal extrahepatic biliary obstruction and cholangitis.

Liver Transplant

Once cirrhosis develops, nonoperative biliary dilation or operative resection has little role in patient management because of the high morbidity. Complications of portal hypertension (e.g., variceal bleeding, ascites, hepatic encephalopathy, and recurrent cholangitis) are clear indications for liver transplant. Survival after hepatic transplant for PSC is similar to that for other end-stage liver disease. In three large series, 5-year patient and graft survival rates are approximately 70% to 80% and 60%, respectively. Patients with prior biliary tract or portal venous surgery do not appear to have increased hospital mortality after liver transplant.

TABLE 2: Survival in patients without cirrhosis with primary sclerosing cholangitis by treatment method

Overall Survival in Years (%)					
	No.	Risk score*	I Year	3 Year	5 Year
Resection	40	3.36 ± 0.12	95	92	85
ES/BD	26	3.13 ± 0.27	88	72[†]	58[†]
Percutaneous stenting	17	3.59 ± 0.28	87	79	63
Combined nonoperative	43	3.27 ± 0.21	87	74[‡]	59[‡]
Transplant-Free Survival in Years (%)					
	No.	Risk score*	I Year	3 Year	5 Year
Resection	40	3.36 ± 0.12	95	92	82
ES/BD	26	3.13 ± 0.27	83	56[†]	42[†]
Percutaneous stenting	17	3.59 ± 0.28	87	64[‡]	51[‡]
Combined nonoperative	43	3.27 ± 0.21	85	59[†]	46[†]

ES/BD, Endoscopic sphincterotomy plus balloon dilation.
*Multicenter risk score.
[†] $P < 0.01$ versus resection, overall survival includes patients undergoing liver transplant.
[‡] $P < 0.05$ versus resection, overall survival includes patients undergoing liver transplant.

The development of CCA before liver transplant significantly affects the long-term outcome. In the combined University of Pittsburgh and Mayo Clinic experience, 11 of 216 patients had an unsuspected CCA, and the survival rate was only 47% at 2 years. Preoperative diagnosis of CCA before transplant remains difficult. Long-term survival has been reported with a neoadjuvant regimen of external and bile duct luminal radiation therapy with concurrent chemotherapy before liver transplant for perihilar CCA.

Another potential problem after transplant is recurrent sclerosing cholangitis. Nonanastomotic biliary strictures are more common after liver transplant for PSC than for other diseases and have been diagnosed in up to 20% to 25% of patients within a median follow-up of 5 to 10 years after transplant. Male gender and the presence of intestinal inflammation after transplant in patients with IBD have been strongly associated with recurrent PSC in the transplanted liver.

SUMMARY

Medical therapy can improve liver function tests in patients with PSC but has not been proven to delay progression of disease to cirrhosis and the need for liver transplant, the development of CCA, or survival. Thus, patients managed medically should be included in clinical trials. Balloon dilation or stenting of dominant strictures has provided short-term symptomatic relief but has not been proven to improve survival and may, in fact, delay the diagnosis of CCA. Surgical resection of hilar and extrahepatic strictures in patients without cirrhosis may postpone or prevent the need for transplant in carefully selected patients. Surgical resection should be considered in patients particularly if CCA is suspected. Liver transplant is the treatment of choice for patients with PSC and cirrhosis. However, liver transplant has significant short-term and long-term morbidity and should not be used too early in the natural history of the disease.

SUGGESTED READINGS

Ahrendt SA, Pitt HA, Kalloo AN, et al: Primary sclerosing cholangitis: resect, dilate, or transplant? *Ann Surg* 227:412–423, 1998.
Ahrendt SA, Pitt HA, Nakeeb A, et al: Diagnosis and management of cholangiocarcinoma in primary sclerosing cholangitis, *J Gastrointest Surg* 3:357–368, 1999.
Chapman R, Fevery J, Kalloo A, et al: Diagnosis and management of primary sclerosing cholangitis, *Hepatology* 51:660–678, 2010.
Pawlik TM, Olbrecht VA, Pitt HA, et al: Primary sclerosing cholangitis: role of extrahepatic biliary resection, *J Am Coll Surg* 206:822–832, 2008.

Management of Cholangiocarcinoma

Sabino Zani, Jr., MD, and Theodore N. Pappas, MD

OVERVIEW

Cholangiocarcinomas consist of a rare group of malignancies that arise from the biliary epithelium. They consist of three distinct subclasses (intrahepatic cholangiocarcinoma, perihilar cholangiocarcinoma, and distal cholangiocarcinoma) determined by the location at which they arise in the bile duct. Historically, a nihilistic attitude has been seen toward treatment because of the relatively advanced stage of disease at initial presentation and the technically challenging aspects of diagnosis and surgical resection. Most patients with unresectable cholangiocarcinoma die within 6 months to 1 year of diagnosis. Surgical excision is the most effective form of therapy and the only potential for cure, without which patients die of hepatic failure or biliary obstruction.

Hepatobiliary malignancies account for 3% of the 560,000 annual cancer-related deaths within the United States, with cholangiocarcinoma accounting for only a small portion (10% to 20%). On average, presentation occurs in the seventh decade of life, with a slight male predominance (1.5:1). Autopsy series have reported an occurrence rate of 0.01% to 0.46%, with an actual incidence rate of 1 to 2 cases per 100,000. Cholangiocarcinoma is the second most common primary hepatic malignancy, with approximately 2500 cases of intrahepatic cholangiocarcinoma occurring yearly. An additional 2000 to 3000 cases/year consist of perihilar tumors (70%), periampullary tumors (20%), and multifocal or diffuse tumors (10%).

Although a number of identified risk factors have been linked to the development of cholangiocarcinoma, the overwhelming majority are likely sporadic. Patients with primary sclerosing cholangitis are at increased risk of cholangiocarcinoma with an associated prevalence rate of 30% to 42% and an annual incidence rate of 0.6% to 1.5%. Chronic inflammatory processes including hepatolithiasis, parasitic infestation *(Clonorchis sinensis),* bacterial infection *(Salmonella),* congenital biliary cystic disease (choledochal cyst, Caroli's disease), toxic compounds (thorium dioxide), and hepatitis C are associated with an increased risk of development of cholangiocarcinoma. Increasing evidence is linking a possible association between cholangiocarcinoma and alcohol use, obesity, and diabetes.

Cholangiocarcinomas represent a group of invasive, slow-growing tumors that have the potential to progress rapidly. This invasive nature allows for the subepithelial extension of tumor and characteristic spread via neural, perineural, and lymphatic routes. This makes nodal metastases a common occurrence. Most tumors are adenocarcinoma (>90%), with rare occurrences of additional malignant cell types arising within the biliary system leading to obstruction (i.e., carcinoid).

The three distinct morphologic subtypes of cholangiocarcinoma include sclerosing, nodular, and papillary. Sclerosing tumors account for 90% of tumors that occur mostly at the hilum. They consist of firm tumors associated with a dense desmoplastic reaction that contribute to the technical difficulties associated with surgical resection. Nodular tumors present as a firm, irregular nodule that project into the lumen of the bile duct. Many tumors present with a combination of these two subtypes, hence the classification of nodular-sclerosing. In contrast, papillary tumors are often soft and friable tumors that arise from a well-defined stalk. With occurrence commonly at the distal bile duct, these tumors account for less than 10% of all cholangiocarcinomas. This subtype is associated with a greater likelihood of resection and a more favorable prognosis.

CLINICAL PRESENTATION

Intrahepatic Cholangiocarcinoma

Patients with intrahepatic cholangiocarcinoma usually present with an asymptomatic liver mass, frequently characterized only by changes in liver function tests. Associated symptoms, when present, include pain, weight loss, early satiety, and anorexia. The presence of jaundice and cholangitis is rare in this patient population and is usually indicative of advanced disease from tumor compressing or invading the biliary confluence or portal vein, or extensive replacement of liver by tumor. Physical examination is usually unremarkable.

Perihilar and Distal Cholangiocarcinoma

More than 90% of patients with perihilar and distal cholangiocarcinoma present with obstructive jaundice. For the small subset of patients with early stage disease, obstruction may not be present and findings include vague abdominal pain and abnormal liver function test results. Patients with incomplete biliary obstruction of only the right or left hepatic duct or segmental duct do not present with jaundice. This delays tumor diagnosis and allows tumor growth, resulting in the potential for ipsilateral lobar atrophy. Often elevated alkaline phosphatase or γ-glutamyltransferase (GGT) levels may be the only signs to elicit further evaluation. The presence of a papillary tumor may cause intermittent jaundice via a ball valve mechanism of the tumor mass or as fragments of the tumor detach and pass to the distal common bile duct. Other symptoms may include weight loss, anorexia, acholic stool, pruritus, and fatigue. Cholangitis is rare in this population unless there is prior percutaneous or endoscopic biliary manipulation.

Physical examination often yields findings of jaundice with hepatomegaly associated with advanced disease. A distended gallbladder may be palpable in patients with distal cholangiocarcinoma. Abnormal live enzymes are often present, allowing the use of total bilirubin level to give insight into an underlying malignant or benign pathology. A malignant process often results in bilirubin levels of more than 10 mg/dL, with an average of 18 mg/dL. This is in contrast to benign processes such as choledocholithiasis associated with bilirubin levels of 2 to 4 mg/dL.

DIAGNOSIS

The diagnosis of cholangiocarcinoma can be technically difficult because pathologic confirmation can be daunting. Often surgical therapy is offered based on clinical suspicion and radiographic appearance. Patients with intrahepatic masses suspicious for cholangiocarcinoma are further evaluated with guidelines for the workup of a primary liver tumor. Patients with findings suspicious for perihilar and distal cholangiocarcinoma share many similarities as discussed subsequently.

Perihilar and Cholangiocarcinoma

Ultrasound Scan

Often initial investigation includes ultrasound scan as the evaluation of patients begins before consultation with hepatobiliary surgical specialists. It is a noninvasive cost-effective modality that can exclude benign pathology as the underlying cause of symptoms (i.e., cholelithiasis). Although findings are operator dependent, ultrasound scan is sensitive for confirming biliary duct dilation and localizing the site of obstruction. In cases of perihilar cholangiocarcinoma, typical findings include intrahepatic duct dilation with normal-caliber extrahepatic duct anatomy and a normal decompressed gallbladder. Findings of dilated intrahepatic and extrahepatic ducts are consistent with distal cholangiocarcinoma. The yield of this information may contribute to the ultimate diagnosis of disease but has minimal role in definitive diagnosis of cholangiocarcinoma.

Contrast-Enhanced, Triple-Phase, Helical Computed Tomographic Scan

The use of contrast-enhanced computed tomographic (CT) scan allows for greater understanding of the extent of disease process. Similarly sensitive for detection of the level of biliary obstruction, CT scan offers the added potential to assess vascular involvement, lymphadenopathy, and presence of lobar atrophy. The ability to evaluate metastatic disease is crucial because detection of bilobar metastases or extrahepatic disease precludes resection.

Magnetic Resonance Cholangiopancreatography

Similar to CT scan but with a greater sensitivity, magnetic resonance cholangiopancreatography (MRCP) offers a noninvasive modality that can assess the extent of bile duct invasion, vessel encasement, invasion of adjacent liver parenchyma with perihilar cholangiocarcinoma, lobar atrophy, lymphadenopathy, and distant metastases. Three-dimensional computerized reconstruction of the biliary tree provides superior imaging comparable with endoscopic retrograde cholangiopancreatography (ERCP) or percutaneous transhepatic cholangiography (PTC) with high positive and negative predictive values for detecting the level and features of biliary obstruction. This allows for defining the anatomy of tumors, assessing the potential for resection, and planning surgical treatment. Additional advantages over ERCP include the visualization of undrained bile ducts without injection of contrast, thus avoiding the risk of cholangitis.

Endoscopic Ultrasound Scan

Endoscopic ultrasound scan (EUS) offers the ability to evaluate the biliary system while avoiding contamination and potential for biliary sepsis. With an associated high sensitivity for detection of the level of obstruction and vascular involvement, this modality plays a crucial role in the staging of the disease process and predicting surgical resectability. The close proximity of the bile duct to the duodenum allows the added benefit of fine-needle aspiration (FNA) or core needle biopsy of tumor tissue or abnormal lymph nodes. This offers a greater sensitivity for detection of malignancy than brush cytology, increasing the diagnostic yield to 40% to 70%. This information is crucial to advise patients of surgical versus palliative options.

Tumor Staging

Optimal staging of cholangiocarcinoma allows the surgeon to formulate a treatment plan to accurately predict resectability, need for hepatic resection, and survival. Staging of cholangiocarcinoma requires careful patient selection and interpretation of imaging studies to accomplish this goal. Approximately 30% of cases are deemed not resectable based on this review. Laparoscopy is helpful for further assessment, as 25% to 30% of patients undergoing surgery are found to have unresectable disease, thereby minimizing surgical morbidity.

Radiologic review of surgical candidacy begins with evaluation of proximal and distal tumor margins to identify the potential for surgical resection. Identification of vascular encasement of the contralateral liver precludes surgical resection. Segmental or lobar atrophy may give insight to portal vein occlusion or obstruction in the assessment of vascular patency. Portal vein compression or narrowing, encasement, or occlusion as seen on ultrasound scan, CT scan, or magnetic resonance imaging (MRI) vascular studies are usually signs of tumor involvement. Patients with regional metastases are not candidates for surgical resection

Intrahepatic, perihilar, and distal cholangiocarcinoma are staged independently according to the 7th edition of the American Joint Committee on Cancer (AJCC) with the tumor node metastasis (TNM) staging system (Tables 1 to 3). Historically, perihilar cholangiocarcinoma have been classified based on the modified Bismuth-Corlette classification (Figure 1). Limitations to this system include critical information regarding vascular encasement or distant metastases. A more recent staging system based on this Bismuth-Corlette classification includes tumor size, extent of disease in the biliary system, vascular involvement, lymph node involvement, distant metastases, and functional liver remnant (Table 4).

PREOPERATIVE EVALUATION

Preoperative planning begins with a review of patient performance status. Surgical fitness of the patient is based on the extent of comorbidities, underlying liver disease, and nutritional status. Significant comorbidities including chronic liver disease or portal hypertension preclude resection, leaving palliation and biliary drainage options for therapy. Patients with unresectable conditions must have a tissue diagnosis before undergoing palliative treatments, including chemotherapy and radiation.

Patients determined to be adequate surgical candidates require meticulous review of radiologic studies to determine the potential success of tumor excision and need for concomitant liver resection, allowing an adequate future liver remnant. Selective ipsilateral portal vein embolization before resection can induce compensatory hypertrophy of the future liver remnant. Although controversial, this procedure is useful if the predicted liver remnant volume is less than 25%, reducing morbidity and mortality from liver dysfunction after resection.

Patients at high risk or those with sepsis are candidates for biliary stenting because it alleviates cholestasis. For the remainder of patients, biliary stenting remains controversial, predisposing to biliary infection and prolonging the postoperative hospitalization. Localized inflammatory effects of stenting may make the determination of tumor extent difficult at the time of operation. Patients requiring hepatic resection may benefit from stenting if the liver remnant is obstructed.

In the authors' practice, stenting is considered when the bilirubin value is more than 10 mg/dL or when the patient is malnourished and in need of nutritional support. The decision to use ERCP or PTC depends on local expertise and tumor location. ERCP is superior for distal cholangiocarcinoma. PTC is superior for perihilar cholangiocarcinoma as assessment of the biliary duct anatomy through proximally dilated ducts offers better visualization of the extent of perihilar stricture and perihilar anatomy. Each modality allows for biliary drainage, which is essential in the septic case. Additional advantages include the ability to obtain washings, brushings, and intraductal biopsies. Because of the desmoplastic nature of this disease, tissue-proven diagnosis remains low, yielding positive results in only one third of patients.

TABLE 1: Tumor node metastasis (TNM) staging for intrahepatic cholangiocarcinoma

Primary Tumor (T)		Distant Metastasis (M)			
TX	Primary tumor cannot be assessed	M0	No distant metastasis		
T0	No evidence of primary tumor	M1	Distant metastasis present		
Tis	Carcinoma in situ (intraductal tumor)	**Anatomic Stage/Prognostic Groups**			
T1	Solitary tumor without vascular invasion	Stage 0	Tis	N0	M0
T2a	Solitary tumor with vascular invasion	Stage I	T1	N0	M0
T2b	Multiple tumors, with or without vascular invasion	Stage II	T2	N0	M0
		Stage III	T3	N0	M0
T3	Tumor perforating the visceral peritoneum or involving the local extrahepatic structures by direct invasion	Stage IVA	T4	N0	M0
			Any T	N1	M0
T4	Tumor with periductal invasion*	Stage IVB	Any T	Any N	M1
Regional Lymph Nodes (N)					
NX	Regional lymph nodes cannot be assessed				
N0	No regional lymph node metastasis				
N1	Regional lymph node metastasis present				

Note: cTNM is the clinical classification; pTNM is the pathologic classification.
*The pathologic definition of periductal invasion is the finding of a longitudinal growth pattern along the intrahepatic bile ducts on both gross and microscopic examination.
Used with the permission of the American Joint Committee on Cancer (AJCC), Chicago. The original source for this material is Edge SB, et al: AJCC Cancer Staging Manual, ed 7, New York, 2010, Springer Inc, pp 252–253.

TABLE 2: Tumor node metastasis (TNM) staging system for perihilar cholangiocarcinoma

Primary Tumor (T)					
TX	Primary tumor cannot be assessed	N1	Regional lymph node metastasis (including nodes along the cystic duct, common bile duct, hepatic artery, and portal vein)		
T0	No evidence of primary tumor				
Tis	Carcinoma in situ	N2	Metastasis to periaortic, pericaval, superior mesenteric artery, or celiac artery lymph nodes		
T1	Tumor confined to the bile duct, with extension up to the muscle layer or fibrous tissue	**Distant Metastasis (M)**			
		M0	No distant metastasis		
T2a	Tumor invades beyond the wall of the bile duct to surrounding adipose tissue	M1	Distant metastasis		
T2b	Tumor invades adjacent hepatic parenchyma	**Anatomic Stage/Prognostic Groups**			
T3	Tumor invades unilateral branches of the portal vein or hepatic artery	Stage 0	Tis	N0	M0
		Stage I	T1	N0	M0
		Stage II	T2a-b	N0	M0
T4	Tumor invades main portal vein or its branches bilaterally; or the common hepatic artery; or the second-order biliary radicals bilaterally; or unilateral second-order biliary radicals with contralateral portal vein or hepatic artery involvement	Stage IIIA	T3	N0	M0
		Stage IIIB	T1-3	N1	M0
		Stage IVA	T4	N0-1	M0
Regional Lymph Nodes (N)		Stage IVB	Any T	N2	M0
NX	Regional lymph nodes cannot be assessed		Any T	Any N	M1
N0	No regional lymph node metastasis				

Note: cTNM is the clinical classification; pTNM is the pathologic classification.
Used with the permission of the American Joint Committee on Cancer (AJCC), Chicago. The original source for this material is Edge SB, et al: AJCC Cancer Staging Manual, ed 7, New York, 2010, Springer Inc, pp 270–271.

TABLE 3: Tumor node metastasis (TNM) staging system for distal cholangiocarcinoma

Primary Tumor (T)

TX	Primary tumor cannot be assessed
T0	No evidence of primary tumor
Tis	Carcinoma in situ
T1	Tumor confined to the bile duct histologically
T2	Tumor invades beyond the wall of the bile duct
T3	Tumor invades the gallbladder, pancreas, duodenum, or other adjacent organs without involvement of the celiac axis or the superior mesenteric artery
T4	Tumor involves the celiac axis or the superior mesenteric artery

Regional Lymph Nodes (N)

NX	Regional lymph nodes cannot be assessed
N0	No regional lymph node metastasis
N1	Regional lymph node metastasis

Distant Metastasis (M)

M0	No distant metastasis
M1	Distant metastasis

Anatomic Stage/Prognostic Groups

Stage 0	Tis	N0	M0
Stage IA	T1	N0	M0
Stage IB	T2	N0	M0
Stage IIA	T3	N0	M0
Stage IIB	T1	N1	M0
	T2	N1	M0
	T3	N1	M0
Stage III	T4	Any N	M0
Stage IV	Any T	Any N	M1

Note: cTNM is the clinical classification; pTNM is the pathologic classification.
Used with the permission of the American Joint Committee on Cancer (AJCC), Chicago. The original source for this material is the Edge SB, et al: AJCC Cancer Staging Manual, ed 7, New York, 2010, Springer Inc, pp 278–279.

SURGICAL TREATMENT AND OUTCOMES

Perihilar Cholangiocarcinoma

Appropriate candidates for resection based on radiologic criteria can undergo surgical exploration to determine whether the tumor is resectable. Laparoscopy allows the ability to evaluate for peritoneal metastases without the morbidity of a laparotomy. In the absence of

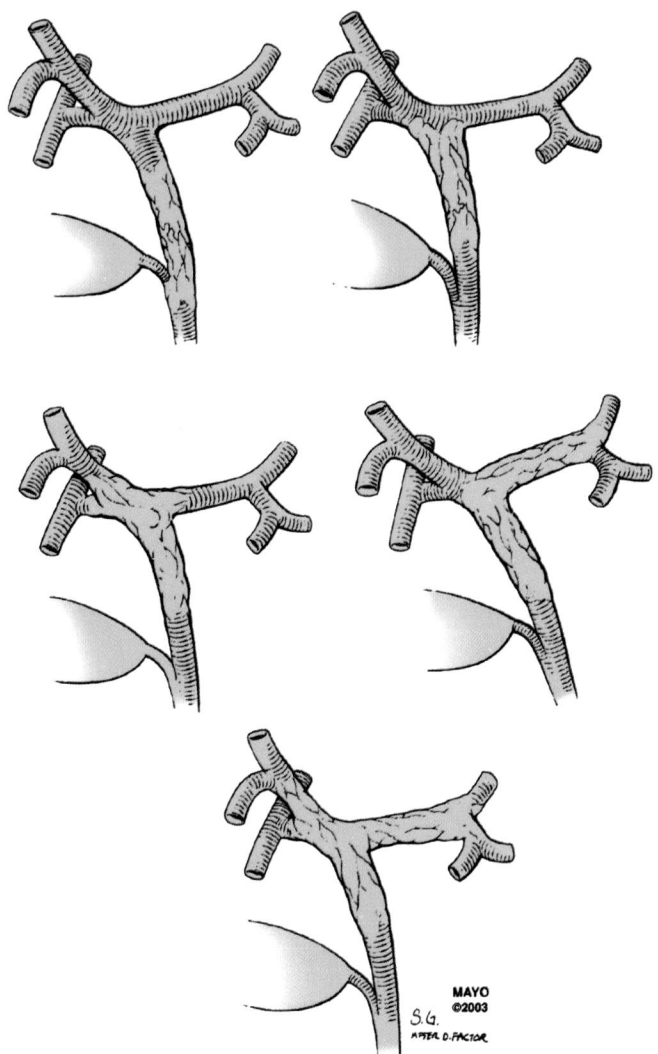

FIGURE 1 The Bismuth-Corlette classification of perihilar cholangiocarcinomas. Type I tumors are located distal to the hepatic ductal confluence. Type II cancers involve the junction of the right and left hepatic ducts. Type IIIA bile duct cancers involve the confluence and the right hepatic duct, whereas type IIIB tumors involve the confluence and the left hepatic duct. Type IV cancers involve both the proximal left and right hepatic ducts to the segmental bile ducts. *(Courtesy Mayo Clinic.)*

metastases, laparotomy is performed via a subcostal or J-type hockey stick incision.

Resection can be challenging because of the proximity to major vascular structures and the potential for extension into the right and left hepatic ducts. Initially, the distal bile duct is isolated at the level of the pancreas. A portion of the distal duct can be evaluated with frozen section to ensure negative margins. The bile duct is retracted cephalad and dissected off the portal vein posteriorly and the hepatic artery medial. Portal-caval lymphatic vessels are removed as part of this specimen. Cholecystectomy is then performed en bloc or separately. Bile duct bifurcation exposure is accomplished with individual dissection of the right and left duct to determine the extent of disease. The left hepatic duct is dissected proximal to the tumor, identified with stay sutures, and divided. Frozen section is obtained to ensure negative margins. If negative, the right hepatic duct is dissected, identified with stay sutures, and divided. Again, frozen section of the duct is obtained. If both ducts are found to be negative, resection is

TABLE 4: International cholangiocarcinoma group staging system for perihilar cholangiocarcinoma

Label	Side/location*	Description	Label	Side/location*	Description
Bile Duct (B)†			**Involvement (>180 degrees) of the Hepatic Artery (HA)**		
B1		Common bile duct	HA0		No arterial involvement
B2		Hepatic duct confluence	HA1		Proper hepatic artery
B3	R	Right hepatic duct	HA2		Hepatic artery bifurcation
B3	L	Left hepatic duct	HA3	R	Right hepatic artery
B4		Right and left hepatic duct	HA3	L	Left hepatic artery
Tumor Size (T)			HA4		Right and left hepatic artery
T1		<1 cm	**Liver Remnant Volume (V)**		
T2		1-3 cm	V0		No information on the volume needed (liver resection not foreseen)
T3		≥3 cm			
Tumor Form (F)			V%		Percentage of the total volume of a putative remnant liver after resection
Sclerosing		Sclerosing (or periductal)			
Mass		Mass-forming (or nodular)	**Underlying Liver Disease (D)**	**Fibrosis**	
Mixed		Sclerosing and mass-forming		Nonalcoholic steatohepatitis	
Polypoid		Polypoid (or intraductal)		Primary sclerosing cholangitis	
Involvement (>180 degrees) of the Portal Vein (PV)			**Lymph Nodes (N)‡**		
PV0		No portal involvement	N0		No lymph node involvement
PV1		Main portal vein	N1		Hilar or hepatic artery lymph node involvement
PV2		Portal vein bifurcation			
PV3	R	Right portal vein	N2		Periaortic lymph node involvement
PV3	L	Left portal vein	**Metastases (M)§**		
PV4		Right and left portal veins	M0		No distant metastases
			M1		Distant metastases (including liver and peritoneal metastases)

*R, Right; L, left.
†Based on the Bismuth classification.
‡Based on the Japanese Society of Biliary Surgery classification.
§Based on the tumor node metastasis classification.
From DeOliveira ML, Schulick RD, Nimura Y, et al: New staging system and a registry for perihilar cholangiocarcinoma, Hepatology 53(4):1363–1371, 2011.

completed and reconstruction via Roux-en-Y is performed with individual anastomoses to each duct.

Tumor extension from the left hepatic duct into the caudate requires a caudate lobectomy. Pancreatoduodenectomy may be performed in patients who are considered suitable candidates for positive tissue margin at the distal bile duct. Postoperative chemoradiotherapy is appropriate for the presence of positive tissue margins or positive lymph node status.

Patients with findings of metastases during laparoscopy can be appropriately palliated with biliary stenting, chemotherapy, or radiotherapy. Unresectable disease determined after laparotomy may undergo either segment III or IV bypass in conjunction with cholecystectomy.

Patients with locally advanced, unresectable cholangiocarcinoma without evidence of metastases pose a difficult problem. Reports of

liver transplantation in highly selected patients treated with neoadjuvant chemoradiation resulted in 5-year survival rates as high as 76%. The Mayo Clinic has pioneered this modality and developed a liver transplantation protocol that resulted in a 5-year disease-free survival rate of 82%. Currently, orthotropic liver transplantation (OLT) is not standard of care and is only performed for highly selected patients in specialized centers.

Although most patients are found to have unresectable disease at presentation, exploration should be offered to all patients with potentially resectable tumors. Associated perioperative morbidity (30% to 50%) and mortality (5%% to 10%) can be expected for patients undergoing surgery. Margin-negative 5-year survival rates range from 21% to 56% in various series. Tumor recurrence occurs in a majority of patients, commonly in the liver (37% to 70%), with additional sites involving lymph nodes, lungs, and bones (4% to

30%). Associated factors that influence the risk of recurrence include presence of multiple tumors, vascular invasion, and tumor size. Death usually results from liver failure or biliary sepsis.

Distal Cholangiocarcinoma

Appropriate candidates for resection based on radiologic criteria can undergo surgical exploration to determine whether the tumor is resectable. Laparoscopy allows the ability to evaluate for peritoneal metastases without the morbidity of a laparotomy. In the absence of peritoneal disease, laparotomy via a subcostal incision is performed to continue the evaluation for unresectability. Resection typically involves pancreatoduodenectomy with reconstruction as discussed elsewhere. Historically bile duct excision alone was performed but rarely successful as only 10% of patients obtained curative resection margins on final pathology.

Patients with findings of metastases during laparoscopy can be appropriately palliated with biliary stenting, chemotherapy, or radiotherapy. Unresectable disease determined after laparotomy can be treated with hepatojejunostomy or choledochojejunostomy as surgical bypass is associated with improved patency and fewer episodes of cholangitis than stenting.

Historically, distal cholangiocarcinoma was associated with a higher potential for resection and improved prognosis compared with perihilar cholangiocarcinoma. This was largely because of the delay in diagnosis associated with perihilar cholangiocarcinoma. Currently, adjusting for stage and completeness of resection, survival after resection for distal cholangiocarcinoma and perihilar cholangiocarcinoma is similar. After margin-negative resection, 5-year survival rates approach 30% to 50%. Tumor recurrence occurs commonly at the bile ducts, nodes, and liver. Associated factors that influence the risk of recurrence include margin positivity and positive nodal status.

PALLIATION

Patients with unresectable cholangiocarcinoma without evidence of metastatic disease who are not candidates for liver transplantation may benefit from photodynamic therapy (PDT). This process consists of intravenous administration of a photosensitizing agent (porphyrin) that accumulates within the tumor cells. Cholangioscopy then allows the introduction of a specific wavelength of light that activates the agent, resulting in cell destruction. PDT has been shown to improve cholestasis and quality of life. Patients require careful monitoring after therapy. The regional availability of this modality limits its utilization.

Although no chemotherapy is consistently effective, patients with unresectable cholangiocarcinoma are candidates for palliative chemotherapy. Historically, reports of 5-fluorouracil (5-FU)–based chemotherapy offered response rates of less than 10%. Additional studies that evaluated alternative regimens including mitomycin C, doxorubicin, gemcitabine, and capecitabine have shown minimal effect on response rates and increased associated toxicity. Similarly, patients without evidence for metastatic disease may be candidates for radiotherapy. Although few retrospective studies show a benefit to radiotherapy, further studies are needed to reach a consensus.

SUMMARY

The diagnostic and technical aspects of cholangiocarcinoma make this a challenging disease process to treat. Although surgical resection is the only effective therapy and potential for cure, most patients present with advanced disease that is often found to be unresectable. Patients who undergo resection face a high likelihood of recurrence, predicted by margin positivity and locoregional lymph node involvement. Liver transplantation is applicable to a highly selected patient population, which makes palliation a key component of care in most patients with unresectable disease. Key therapies include adequate biliary drainage, with the benefit of PDT offering reduced cholestasis and improved quality of life. Despite characteristic tumor resistance to chemotherapy and radiotherapy, these modalities may still serve a role in the treatment of unresectable cholangiocarcinoma.

SUGGESTED READINGS

Bismuth H, Nakache R, Diamond T: Management strategies in resection for hilar cholangiocarcinoma, *Ann Surg* 215:31–38, 1992.
Blechacz B, et al: Clinical diagnosis and staging of cholangiocarcinoma, *Nat Rev Gastroenterol Hepatol* 8:512–522, 2011.
DeOliveira ML, Schulick RD, Nimura Y, et al: New staging system and a registry for perihilar cholangiocarcinoma, *Hepatology* 53:1363–1371, 2011.
Edge SB, Byrd DR, Compton CC, et al: *American Joint Committee on Cancer Staging manual*, ed 7, New York, 2010, Springer.
Ito F, Cho CS, Rikkers LF, et al: Hilar cholangiocarcinoma: current management, *Ann Surg* 250:210–218, 2009.
Okabayashi T, Yamamoto J, Kosuge T, et al: A new staging system for mass-forming intrahepatic cholangiocarcinoma: analysis of preoperative and postoperative variables, *Cancer* 92:2374–2383, 2001.

GALLBLADDER CANCER

Reid B. Adams, MD, and Todd W. Bauer, MD

OVERVIEW

Gallbladder cancer (GBC) is a challenging disease, often due to its advanced stage at presentation and aggressive biology. An improved understanding of its natural history, however, has led to more appropriate patient selection for treatment; likewise, advances in surgical techniques have resulted in better long-term survival. Consequently, surgical therapy in appropriately selected patients is effective, and the past despair associated with GBC should be tempered. This discussion focuses on patient selection for treatment and an approach to therapy based on currently available data.

GBC incidence varies widely by geography and ethnicity throughout the world. In the United States, it is relatively uncommon, with fewer than 5000 cases per annum (1 to 2 per 100,000). However, it is the most common biliary tract malignancy and the fifth most common gastrointestinal malignancy. The incidence is higher for women (twofold to threefold) and whites (compared to African Americans); it increases with age and in those with obesity. Native Americans and Hispanic women have the highest incidence in the United States.

Chronic gallbladder inflammation is the most common unifying theme associated with potential risk factors for gallbladder cancer. In the United States, this association typically means cholelithiasis, which is present in 75% to 90% of GBCs. The presence of gallstones does not appear sufficient for malignancy, however, because only 0.5% to 3% of patients with cholelithiasis develop GBC.

NATURAL HISTORY, BIOLOGY, AND THE ROLE OF SURGICAL TREATMENT

The natural history of GBC has been defined by studies over the past 50 years leading to our solid understanding of the disease outcomes. Most of these reports have median survivals of 6 months or less, with overall 5-year survivals of 5%. Thus, the fatalistic mindset associated with GBC in the past is understandable. Only recently, based on reports beginning in the early 1990s, has a more optimistic attitude emerged based on evidence that radical surgical therapy can alter this dismal course. While randomized trials are lacking, cumulative evidence strongly supports the contention that liver resection and portal lymphadenectomy provide a survival advantage for selected groups of patients with GBC.

Poor survival in the past for GBC was likely due to the advanced stage of disease at presentation. Advanced disease results from its propensity to spread via the lymphatics, hematogenously, and by shedding into the peritoneal cavity. Tumor dissemination probably is facilitated by the structure of the gallbladder. Due to its thin wall, even minimal invasion permits penetration deep into the muscular layer, thereby allowing access to the lymphatic and vascular channels. This presents the possibility for dissemination early in the disease process. Similarly, minimal invasion can penetrate the connective tissue between the gallbladder and the liver (the cystic plate), ultimately allowing invasion of the adjacent liver. Therefore, dissection within this fibrous plane, as done during a standard cholecystectomy, typically leaves residual tumor at this site. Likewise, tumor penetration of the wall covered by peritoneum allows peritoneal seeding. The lymphatic drainage of the gallbladder is well described; it initially travels to the cystic and pericholedochal lymph nodes. From there, drainage leads to the retroportal and posterior-superior pancreaticoduodenal nodes. Finally, flow continues to nodes associated with the celiac and superior mesenteric arteries and the aortocaval region. However, direct drainage from the pericholedochal nodes to the aortocaval nodes does occur, possibly accounting for advanced disease early in the course.

STAGING

Understanding the patterns of spread and their relationship to outcomes is recognized by the recent changes for staging GBC published in the *American Joint Committee on Cancer Staging Manual* (Table 1). Changes to the current system correlate with resectability and patient survival. Based on this reorganization, the new staging correlates well with outcomes as validated with data from the National Cancer Data Base (Figure 1).

Thus, a detailed understanding of the patterns of spread and biology of the disease, combined with the outcomes associated with the new staging system, allow development of a rational approach for the evaluation and treatment of patients with GBC.

Clinical Scenarios

GBC presents as one of three common scenarios: suspicion prior to surgery based on symptoms and imaging or incidentally found on imaging done for an unrelated reason; discovered at the time of surgery; and discovered incidentally on the final pathology. Recent data show that approximately 50% of patients present with advanced or disseminated disease, and the other half are discovered incidentally following cholecystectomy.

TABLE 1: Gallbladder cancer stages

Primary tumor (T)

Tis	Carcinoma in situ
T1	Tumor invades lamina propria (T1a) or muscular layer (T1b)
T2	Tumor invades perimuscular connective tissue
T3	Tumor perforates serosa and/or invades the liver and/or one adjacent structure
T4*	Tumor invades main portal vein or hepatic artery or invades two or more extrahepatic structures

Regional lymph nodes (N)

N0	No regional lymph node metastasis
N1	Metastases to nodes along the cystic duct, common bile duct, hepatic artery, and/or portal vein
N2†	Metastases to periaortic, pericaval, superior mesenteric artery, and/or celiac artery lymph nodes

Distant metastasis (M)

M0	No distant metastasis
M1	Distant metastasis

Staging groups (TMN)

Stage 0	Tis	N0	M0
Stage I	T1	N0	M0
Stage II	T2	N0	M0
Stage IIIA	T3	N0	M0
Stage IIIB	T1-T3	N1	M0
Stage IVA	T4	N0-N1	M0
Stage IVB	Any T	N2	M0
	Any T	Any N	M1

*T4 denotes locally advanced, unresectable tumors.
†N2 nodes are considered distant metastatic disease.
Modified from AJCC cancer staging manual, *ed 7, New York, 2010, Springer.*

Suspicion Prior to Surgery

Abdominal imaging, whether done for right-upper-quadrant symptoms or unrelated reasons, may show gallbladder findings that raise concern for GBC. Typical findings range from diffuse wall thickening to an obvious infiltrative gallbladder mass. The nature of these findings influences the level of concern for GBC and affects the preoperative evaluation and treatment options.

In this situation, transabdominal ultrasonography (US) is commonly the initial study, although similar incidental abnormalities are increasingly being seen on computed tomographic (CT) and

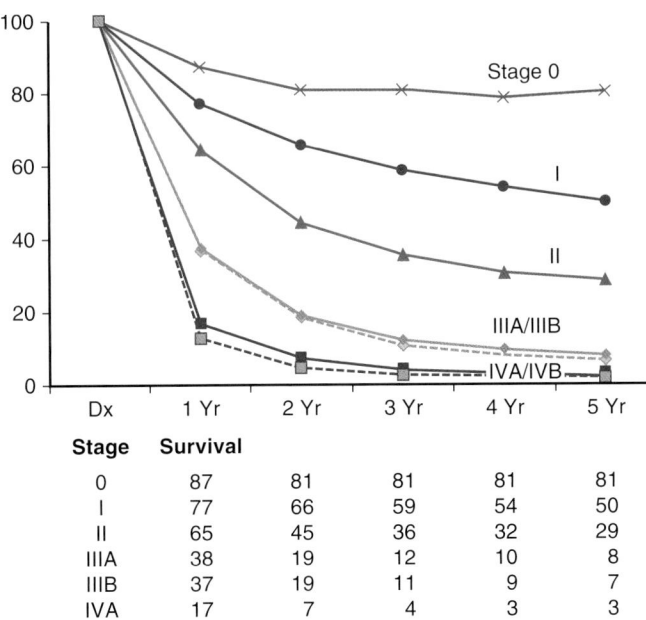

Stage	Survival				
0	87	81	81	81	81
I	77	66	59	54	50
II	65	45	36	32	29
IIIA	38	19	12	10	8
IIIB	37	19	11	9	7
IVA	17	7	4	3	3
IVB	13	5	3	2	2

FIGURE 1 Staging correlated to outcomes as validated with data from the National Cancer Data Base. *(From Fong Y, et al: Evidence-based gallbladder cancer staging: changing cancer staging by analysis of data from the national cancer database, Ann Surg 243(6):767–771, 2006.)*

magnetic resonance (MR) imaging. Findings of diffuse gallbladder wall thickening and cholelithiasis are common and rarely raise the specter of GBC. Consequently, the difficulty diagnosing GBC preoperatively stems from the similarity of symptoms to those of biliary colic, and/or chronic cholecystitis. The high rate of incidentally discovered disease likely results from this overlap.

Several studies reviewing GBC detection show that the rate of incidentally found GBC can be decreased; with modern imaging, a preoperative diagnosis can be made in approximately 80% of cases. However, to achieve this level of detection, a high index of suspicion is necessary because the overall preoperative detection rate in most series remains around 50%. Thus, preoperative review of the actual images by the operating surgeon can improve GBC detection.

On the other end of the spectrum are findings consistent with advanced disease. These include a heterogeneous mass replacing, or within, the gallbladder or infiltration of the surrounding liver. Between these extremes are findings that suggest, but are not diagnostic of, GBC. Concerning features include focal/asymmetric wall thickening, a disrupted mucosa, a fixed mucosal mass, or obliteration of the interface at the cystic plate.

Once a gallbladder abnormality is noted on US, the extent of additional evaluation is based on the findings and degree of suspicion for GBC. For instance, gallbladder polyps (GBPs) are common, seen in up to 4.5% of patients on US. The majority of GBPs are cholesterol followed by adenomyomas (adenomyomatosis), both nonneoplastic lesions. Less common are neoplastic polyps such as adenomas. Only adenomas are associated with a risk of malignancy, but the frequency with which they will progress to carcinoma remains unclear. The key feature related to malignancy is the size of the adenoma. Thus, the primary issue with polyps is distinguishing these from one another and from more ominous gallbladder abnormalities suggestive of GBC. The lack of firm guidelines for their evaluation hampers a standardized approach.

A general approach, then, is to examine the US features of polyps. These are very useful for distinguishing one from the other, and often, US is the only study required. Evaluation for mucosal vascularity by color Doppler ultrasound can differentiate indeterminate findings into benign or neoplastic lesions. Endoscopic ultrasonography also is reportedly helpful in delineating benign from neoplastic lesions, although its use in the United States appears limited. Cholesterol polyps characteristically are less than 5 mm, multiple, and frequently pedunculated. They are nearly always less than 1 cm in size and typically appear hyperechoic. Usually asymptomatic, they do not require treatment. Adenomyomatosis takes three forms: diffuse, segmental, and localized. All three can mimic GBC, so the diagnosis often is made at pathology. The localized type typically presents as a mass in the gallbladder fundus. These lesions often have characteristic features on US such as areas of cystic dilation, suggesting the diagnosis. If the diagnosis is likely but cannot be confirmed by US, MR imaging has typical features that can help confirm the diagnosis. If confirmed, adenomyomatosis does not require treatment. Adenomas are single, often sessile, polypoid lesions. Usually they are found in the absence of cholelithiasis. Although some debate persists, most studies report a low, to no, incidence of carcinoma in adenomas less than 1 cm. The incidence increases for adenomas between 10 and 18 mm; a high rate of carcinoma is reported in lesions 18 mm or larger, so all of these should be considered malignant.

Gallbladder imaging abnormalities suspicious for GBC should undergo high-resolution cross-sectional imaging, either CT or MRI, based on institutional expertise and experience. MRI is our choice for concerning lesions because it is more sensitive for detecting liver involvement or metastasis, and it allows cholangiography and angiography. This additional imaging can confirm GBC and assess its extent.

In general, laboratory studies are not useful. However, carcinoembryonic antigen (CEA) and carbohydrate antigen 19-9 (CA19-9) may be of value when lesions remain indeterminate by imaging. A CEA greater than 4 ng/mL is 93% specific and 50% sensitive for GBC. CA19-9 is 79% specific and sensitive for GBC. Together with the imaging features of an indeterminate lesion, these may modify the level of concern that a gallbladder abnormality is more likely to be benign versus malignant.

If the diagnosis of suspicious findings remains uncertain or GBC is suspected, there is no role for preoperative biopsy in patients with potentially resectable disease. GBC has a high propensity to seed biopsy tracts and the peritoneum, and an unnecessary biopsy increases this risk. When unresectable or metastatic disease is present, percutaneous biopsy is very accurate and appropriate if histologic confirmation will influence disease management.

Discovery at the Time of Surgery or Final Pathology

Due to the difficulty distinguishing GBC from benign disease, routine inspection of the gallbladder mucosa following cholecystectomy is recommended; suspicious areas should be examined by frozen section biopsy. If carcinoma is found, additional treatment may be required.

Incidentally discovered GBC on the final pathology is a common presentation. Treatment is based on the stage; staging prior to definitive therapy may be necessary.

RADIOLOGIC EVALUATION

When GBC is suspected or confirmed, CT or MR imaging is necessary for preoperative staging. The goals are to establish the diagnosis, evaluate its extent to plan definitive therapy, and limit patient exposure to nontherapeutic laparotomy. Based on the patterns of spread, imaging is directed primarily to the liver, adjacent organs, and regional/distant lymph nodes. While peritoneal disease is common in more advanced disease, it is difficult to identify preoperatively by imaging. Chest radiography should be done to complete the staging evaluation, although the risk of lung metastasis is rare unless locally advanced or abdominal metastatic disease is already present.

When patients have GBC discovered incidentally on pathologic review, staging as outlined for preoperatively suspected GBC may be indicated. The results of this imaging evaluation will dictate the treatment options.

While most GBCs are detectable by FDG-PET, its role in staging remains unclear. It appears most useful in detecting metastatic disease when evaluating primary GBC rather than recurrence. Several studies report PET altering surgical therapy 17% to 23% of the time. When GBC is incidentally discovered on pathology, PET has limited utility distinguishing residual tumor in the cholecystectomy bed from postoperative inflammation. If preoperative imaging suggests T1 disease, there is likely no benefit from PET. Because the likelihood of metastatic lymphadenopathy increases with T2 or greater GBC, PET may be more useful in this situation.

MANAGEMENT

Polyps

Cholecystectomy is the primary treatment for gallbladder polypoid lesions, and it should be considered in symptomatic patients. While polypoid lesions rarely cause symptoms, some patients have typical biliary symptoms such as colic or pancreatitis; cholecystectomy is indicated because the majority of them improve following surgery. The efficacy of cholecystectomy for polyps in patients with nonspecific upper-abdominal symptoms is less clear, and routine cholecystectomy should not be done unless another indication for polyp resection is present or no other cause for their pain is found. In the latter group, the expectation for symptom relief following cholecystectomy is low.

For patients with asymptomatic GBPs, the principal issue is determining which patients require treatment. As stated earlier, when asymptomatic cholesterol polyps or adenomyomatosis is confirmed, cholecystectomy is not indicated. Otherwise, for indeterminate polyps, cholecystectomy is recommended when specific criteria are met. When these criteria are absent, serial observation may be appropriate.

The main goal of cholecystectomy for polypoid lesions is to prevent malignant transformation or treat a GBC at its earliest stage. Features most consistently predicting malignancy include a single polypoid lesion larger than 10 mm in size in patients older than 50 years. These characteristics, coupled with other reported features, define several populations where routine cholecystectomy is recommended due to the increased risk of malignancy:

- Polyps larger than 10 mm
- Polyps in the presence of cholelithiasis, regardless of polyp size or symptoms
- Polyps in patients with primary sclerosis cholangitis

Several issues require attention when contemplating cholecystectomy for GBPs. The first consideration is the surgical approach, either laparoscopic or open cholecystectomy. We have favored open cholecystectomy in these patients to ensure no compromise in their oncologic outcome in the event GBC is present. There seems to be little justification for a smaller incision if it has the potential to contribute to a worse outcome. However, accumulated data support laparoscopic cholecystectomy alone as adequate treatment for Tis and T1a tumors. Additional evidence supports no difference in outcomes for patients treated with a laparoscopic cholecystectomy initially, followed by a delayed definitive operation for GBC if no perforation occurred. These findings support the contention that a properly done laparoscopic cholecystectomy is a reasonable approach for GBPs. Our primary concern remains, though, because approximately 20% to 30% of laparoscopic cholecystectomies are associated with an incidental cholecystotomy and bile spillage during the procedure. The aggressive biology and propensity for seeding of GBC makes

bile spillage an unacceptable risk, potentially converting a curative situation to an incurable one. Thus, if a laparoscopic approach is considered, a very low threshold for conversion to an open procedure should be adopted, and gallbladder perforation should be fastidiously avoided. If done laparoscopically, the specimen should be removed in an extraction bag.

A second issue to consider is readiness to perform definitive therapy. If a cholecystectomy is performed for a patient with a GBP, the specimen must be examined by frozen section biopsy at the time of surgery. If invasive (>T1a) GBC is present, the definitive procedure, an extended cholecystectomy, must be performed. Consequently, all patients undergoing cholecystectomy for GBP should be counseled about the risk of malignancy and consented for extended cholecystectomy at the same operation if GBC is found. If local expertise is not present to perform an extended cholecystectomy, the patient should be referred preoperatively to an experienced hepatobiliary unit.

The third issue is location of the polyp. Careful review of the preoperative imaging is important to identify the location of the polyp within the gallbladder. If it is adjacent to the cystic plate, we favor cholecystectomy with en bloc excision of the cystic plate to avoid dissection between the wall of the gallbladder and the cystic plate. If the polyp is not adjacent to the cystic plate, a standard cholecystectomy is performed.

When a polyp is 18 mm or larger, it should be considered malignant and treated as such. These patients should undergo preoperative staging as outlined previously. Appropriate treatment is an extended (radical) cholecystectomy.

The second important issue is surveillance for patients with polyps who do not undergo resection, a subject that remains unclear. This group primarily includes asymptomatic polyps less than 10 mm in size. The problematic issue for these patients is the lack of consensus regarding recommendations for the frequency and duration of follow-up. There is relatively uniform agreement that polyps in this group require serial ultrasound evaluation to ensure stability of the polyp. If a polyp increases in size during observation, cholecystectomy is indicated. There is general agreement that after initial discovery, repeat US should be done at 6 and 12 months. If no change is noted, then annual US is recommended. Emerging data suggest that ethnicity and geographic location modify the risks for GBC, likely explaining the wide variability in the risk of GBPs developing into GBC. For instance, Aldouri and colleagues reported a prevalence of GBC with GBP of 0.08% in a white population. Thus, some authors advocate no further surveillance after 2 years for a stable GBP. Another study observed neoplastic GBP growth over an 8-year surveillance period. Thus, some authors recommend annual US without a clear endpoint. Evidence exists that dysplasia to malignant transformation can take more than 10 years; this also suggests that a longer surveillance period may be appropriate. The tension in these discussions is balancing the substantial costs for surveillance with identification of a diminishingly small number of neoplastic GBPs.

Suspicious Findings Prior to Surgery

When the preoperative concern for GBC is greater than that described for GBPs, complete preoperative staging should be done and the patient prepared for a definitive oncologic operation. Findings precluding curative resection include a medically unfit patient or imaging showing metastatic disease (liver, peritoneum, extraabdominal), lymph node involvement outside the hepatoduodenal ligament, or encasement/occlusion of the main portal vein and hepatic artery. Jaundice in patients with GBC is a relative contraindication to curative therapy. While these patients may have technically resectable disease, a large study of this population reported 7% of patients with jaundice and GBC were resectable, and all those having resection died within 2 years of treatment. On the other hand, a more recent study reported a 45% resection rate and 5-year survival of 19%. Only patients with N0 disease had long-term survival; they recommended extensive lymph node sampling prior to resection. If any were positive, no resection should be done. These results were associated with a 16% operative mortality in patients undergoing curative resection for GBC presenting with jaundice. Thus, jaundice is an indicator of advanced disease in patients with GBC, and resection is feasible only in a highly selected population.

CT or MRI detects direct liver or adjacent organ involvement and guides treatment planning and counseling. If major hepatectomy may be necessary for complete resection, assessment of postoperative hepatic reserve is necessary to determine the need for portal vein embolization. If N2 nodal involvement is suspected preoperatively, PET scan or EUS and biopsy can determine disease presence, thereby avoiding unnecessary laparotomy.

Since the incidence of occult metastases is high, the procedure should start with staging laparoscopy for all patients. If negative, laparotomy and the definitive operation for GBC can proceed. In patients with a high degree of concern for GBC, a simple cholecystectomy to make the diagnosis is inappropriate. Thus, some patients may undergo partial hepatectomy for benign disease, a possibility they should be informed of preoperatively.

GBC Discovered at Time of Surgery

If a laparoscopic cholecystectomy is done and intraoperative frozen section shows GBC, several options are available. If this is truly incidental, the stage appears greater than T1a, and the operating surgeon has the necessary expertise, one option is to proceed to definitive resection. If the stage is uncertain or the expertise for definitive resection is not available, no further procedures should be done. The patient is recovered, the final pathology reviewed, appropriate staging completed, and then a definitive operation, if indicated, done. In this circumstance, our preference is to recover the patient and await the final pathology because accurate determination of the T stage on the frozen section can be difficult. In addition, this allows a full discussion with the patient and appropriate consenting. The patient is taken back to the operating room several days later for the definitive procedure.

During laparoscopic cholecystectomy, if GBC is suspected and this was unknown prior to the procedure, no dissection or biopsy should be done, a careful laparoscopic staging exam should be performed, and the patient should be closed and recovered. If a definitive resection cannot be done locally, the patient should be referred. Otherwise, completely stage the patient, appropriately consent him or her, and proceed to definitive resection. If GBC is suspected after the laparoscopic dissection has begun, we recommend stopping and converting to an open procedure. Usually, the issue in this case is difficulty dissecting the gallbladder from the fossa. We favor resecting a rim of liver around the gallbladder fossa in this case and doing a frozen section biopsy. If GBC is found, we proceed to a definitive resection at that procedure. If this circumstance is encountered and local expertise for a partial hepatectomy is not available, the dissection is stopped and the patient recovered, followed by transfer that day for definitive care.

GBC Incidentally Found on Final Pathology

When GBC is found incidentally on the final pathology, the need for additional treatment is based on the depth of tumor invasion. Hence, the slides should be carefully reviewed with the pathologist to verify this stage. Margin negative Tis and T1a tumors are adequately treated with simple cholecystectomy alone. Patients with tumors greater than T1a require more extensive resection. These patients should undergo complete staging, and if no contraindications are found, they should proceed to definitive surgery.

There is no role for port site resection of incidentally discovered GBC resected laparoscopically. While advocated by some in the past, port site disease is a marker for peritoneal disease and carcinomatosis. Excision is not curative or associated with improved overall or disease-free survival.

Definitive Surgical Therapy

Current data support partial hepatectomy and regional lymphadenectomy as essential elements of a definitive resection. This is referred to as an extended, or radical, cholecystectomy. It is appropriate treatment for T1b to T3 tumors. The principal components of the operation are resection of the liver around the gallbladder fossa and lymph node dissection of the hepatoduodenal ligament. While the goal of the liver resection is to obtain a margin of approximately 2 cm around the gallbladder fossa, a wedge resection of this site is often compromised as one approaches the hilum. Consequently, most major hepatobiliary programs, including ours, favor an anatomic resection of segments IVb/V.

Whether the extended cholecystectomy is the index operation or done for reresection of an incidentally found GBC, the approach is similar. We begin all these operations with staging laparoscopy, because the risk of disseminated disease is significant. If laparoscopy is negative, a right subcostal incision is made and used to explore the abdomen. Intraoperative ultrasonography is performed to define the extent of any liver involvement. A Kocher maneuver is done and a search for abnormal lymphadenopathy outside the hepatoduodenal ligament is made. Any suspicious nodes are excised and sent for frozen section. If nodes outside the N1 distribution are positive, the procedure is aborted because these represent distant metastatic disease. If the gallbladder is present, an en bloc cholecystectomy and segment IVb/V hepatectomy is completed. This is sent to pathology for frozen section biopsy of the cystic duct margin. If this is negative, there is no role for routine extrahepatic bile duct resection. Bile duct resection is only necessary to achieve a negative cystic duct margin. Likewise, routine hepatectomy larger than IVb/V is unnecessary, except when it is required to achieve a negative margin. This might be necessary for T3 tumors extending into the right lobe past segment V or for involvement of the right portal structures. The routine use of a larger hepatectomy or bile duct resection is associated with a higher morbidity and mortality without a concurrent improvement in survival. If a cholecystectomy was previously done, hepatectomy of segments IVb/V is done. While awaiting the frozen section results, the hepatoduodenal structures are skeletonized, removing all the soft tissue from the hepatic artery, portal vein, and extrahepatic bile ducts from the duodenum to the hepatic plate. If an adjacent organ has limited involvement by direct extension, en bloc resection is appropriate to achieve a negative margin. Extensive involvement may preclude a margin negative resection, and a debulking operation should not be performed. Involvement of more than one extrahepatic organ is T4 disease and considered locally unresectable.

Stage-Based Therapy

Tis and T1a: Simple cholecystectomy is sufficient because cure rates approach 100%. If the cystic duct margin is positive, additional cystic duct resection to a negative margin is required. If this is inadequate, then excision of the extrahepatic bile ducts and hepaticojejunostomy is appropriate.

T1b: The role of simple versus extended cholecystectomy for treatment has been controversial in the past. T1b tumors have a higher incidence of lymph node metastasis and locoregional recurrence. Current evidence shows improved survival compared to simple cholecystectomy in this group; thus, extended cholecystectomy is recommended for fit patients.

T2: Extended cholecystectomy is recommended for this group of patients. Patients with T2 tumors appear to derive the greatest benefit from radical resection. Long-term survival following extended cholecystectomy is 60% to 80% versus less than 50% with simple cholecystectomy.

T3: Extended cholecystectomy is recommended for these patients, with evidence supporting improved long-term survival around 15% to 20% in well-selected patients. A more extensive hepatectomy, such as an extended right hepatectomy, may be necessary to achieve negative margins when the right portal pedicle is involved. Likewise, resection of a single adjacent organ for direct extension may be necessary for margin clearance.

T4: These are considered locally unresectable tumors. Reports of resected T4 tumors are very limited and seem to be in the context of a finding at pathology when resection was done for what appeared to be a lower-stage tumor. Anecdotal cases of improved survival for these T4 tumors versus unresected T4 tumors have been published. Any improvement in survival is likely associated with a margin negative resection and N0 disease. In general, resection of T4 tumors is not feasible because these conditions are typically not present.

Adjuvant Therapy

Studies of recurrence following complete resection show that a majority of patients (85%) recur at a distant site, while only 15% have locoregional recurrence. This has implications for the choice of adjuvant therapy and suggests that systemic therapy should be part of any adjuvant strategy. However, no randomized phase III trials are available to establish a standard of care for patients with resected GBC. Several small studies and retrospective series suggest a survival benefit following radiotherapy for T2 or larger tumors or N1 disease. A recent phase III randomized trial showed a benefit for a gemcitabine-cisplatin combination versus gemcitabine alone when used for palliative therapy for metastatic biliary cancers. It is unknown whether this benefit would translate to the adjuvant setting.

PALLIATIVE CARE

Because a high proportion of patients with GBC are unresectable, providing palliation is an important role for the surgeon. Common symptoms include pain, jaundice, and bowel obstruction. Due to the poor prognosis and limited life expectancy, nonoperative approaches to palliation are optimal. We prefer endoscopic stenting for jaundice, when possible; a percutaneous approach is done when an endoprosthesis cannot be placed or provides inadequate palliation. A percutaneous gastrostomy with a jejunal feeding extension is preferable to operative bypass due to the short life expectancy in patients with duodenal or small bowel obstruction from direct extension or peritoneal disease.

SUGGESTED READINGS

D'Angelica M, Dalal KM, DeMatteo RP, et al: Analysis of the extent of resection for adenocarcinoma of the gallbladder, *Ann Surg Oncol* 16:806–816, 2009.

Duffy A, Capanu M, Abou-Alfa GK, et al: Gallbladder cancer (GBC): 10 year experience at Memorial Sloan-Kettering Cancer Centre (MSKCC), *J Surg Oncol* 98:485–489, 2008.

NCCN Guidelines: *Hepatobiliary Cancers. Version 2.* 2012. www.NCCN.org.

Pawlik TM, Gleisner AL, Vigano L, et al: Incidence of finding residual disease for incidental gallbladder carcinoma: implications for re-resection, *J Gastrointest Surg* 11:1478–1486, 2007.

GALLSTONE ILEUS

Ellen Hunter Bailey, MD, and
Kenneth W. Sharp, MD

Gallstone ileus is a rare cause of intestinal obstruction accounting for less than 3% of intestinal obstructions. It was originally described by Courvoisier in 1890 as an unusual cause of bowel obstruction. The most common cause is erosion of a large gallstone into the duodenum, where the stone passes until it lodges at the ileocecal valve. Other causes include erosion of a large gallstone into the stomach with obstruction of the stone at the pylorus or proximal duodenum causing gastric outlet syndrome, a condition also known as Bouveret's syndrome. Rare cases have been reported of the gallstone obstructing the colon (from cholecystocolic fistula) or lodging in small bowel strictures such as occurs with Crohn's disease.

Gallstone ileus is a disease of older adults, the average age at presentation exceeds 70. It is much more common in older women, and female-to-male ratios are between 3:1 and 5:1. The diagnosis should be suspected in the differential diagnosis of an older woman presenting with small bowel obstruction with no antecedent history of abdominal operations and without abdominal or inguinal hernias on physical examination.

PATHOGENESIS

Gallstone ileus requires a preceding biliary enteric fistula between the gallbladder and the intestine—most commonly the duodenum adjacent to the gallbladder—but may also exist between the gallbladder and the stomach, colon, or small bowel. It is theorized that a large stone impacts in the neck of the gallbladder and leads to inflammation, pressure necrosis, and then erosion into an adjacent hollow viscus. There are reports of coexisting fibrotic common hepatic or common bile duct obstructions (Mirizzi's syndrome) from the intense inflammatory reaction required for such fistulae to form. It is rare for stones smaller than 2 cm to cause obstruction, and the most common sites for impaction are the distal ileum, the sigmoid colon, and the second portion of the duodenum. The cholecystenteric fistula may close spontaneously after passage of the stone or may stay patent in some cases. Additional unusual cases have been described after endoscopic sphincterotomy for common bile duct stones has been performed, when large stones are extracted from the common duct and not endoscopically retrieved.

DIAGNOSIS

Patients will most often present with fairly classic symptoms of bowel obstruction such as abdominal pain, nausea, vomiting, and obstipation or constipation. The patients will rarely have fever, peritonitis, or signs of sepsis. A history of previous biliary colic is not commonly elicited, and a history of jaundice is rare. It may be possible to obtain a history suggestive of acute cholecystitis, but since the process is slow in progression, the episode may have happened years previously. Individuals present with crampy abdominal pain that may be sporadic in nature if the stone is not impacted; this pain has been attributed to the stone "tumbling" proximal to distal in the small bowel and causing intermittent obstruction. If the biliary enteric fistula is cholecystogastric, the gallstone may obstruct the gastric outlet. Individuals with this type of fistula complain predominantly of severe nausea and vomiting.

Laboratory evaluation of the patient is not diagnostic; there are no diagnostic findings in the electrolytes, liver tests (although elevated liver tests or bilirubin are not infrequent), amylase, lipase, or blood counts. Plain abdominal radiographs usually show dilated loops of small intestine with air fluid levels consistent with small bowel obstruction. Pneumobilia appears only half of the time on plain films and it is rarer still to see a radiopaque gallstone in the alimentary tract. The classic finding in gallstone ileus, Rigler's triad (distended loops of small bowel, air in the biliary tree, and a radiopaque stone in the right lower quadrant), is found in relatively few cases on plain radiographs. Computed tomographic (CT) scans are much more sensitive for visualizing pneumobilia and will show this finding more frequently than plain films. CT scans are used increasingly for the diagnosis of intestinal obstruction and can further delineate the cause of a bowel obstruction with air or even oral contrast in the biliary tract, a fistulous connection between the gallbladder and a surrounding hollow viscus, radiographic evidence of alimentary tract obstruction, and the obstructing stone (Figure 1).

Ultrasonography of the gallbladder shows cholelithiasis and choledocholithiasis in a variable number of patients. If there is air in the gallbladder, it will degrade the ultrasonographer's ability to visualize stones. Finally, a firm preoperative diagnosis of gallstone ileus is not essential. A proper diagnosis of bowel obstruction is sufficient to indicate the need for an operation. Many cases of gallstone ileus have not been diagnosed until the finding is made at laparotomy.

MANAGEMENT

Patients with gallstone ileus generally present dehydrated from poor oral intake and volume losses secondary to bowel distention and emesis. They frequently have significant electrolyte abnormalities. Initial therapeutic efforts should be focused on resuscitation: monitoring of vital signs and volume status, nasogastric decompression, judicious fluid resuscitation, and focused electrolyte correction. It is critical to focus on general physiologic optimization since this is an older patient population with significant preexisting medical comorbidities. Many of these patients fit into category 3 or 4 of the American Society of Anesthesiologists physical status classification system. Preoperative optimization of the dehydrated older patient with heart failure, coronary disease, renal failure, or respiratory failure may be best done in an intensive care unit for several hours prior to the stress of inducing a general anesthetic. Since these patients rarely present with sepsis or peritonitis, there is usually no need for truly emergent operation.

It is important to remember that there are always two separate disease processes present in the gallstone ileus patient: (1) a bowel obstruction and (2) an inflammatory biliary process that may be a chronic fistula or an active inflammatory phlegmon. The absolute priority is relief of the bowel obstruction by removing the obstructing gallstone. Biliary sepsis that demands drainage or cholecystectomy during the same operation is uncommon. Classically this is performed with a laparotomy during which the abdomen is thoroughly examined, the site of obstruction is identified, and the inflammatory process surrounding the gallbladder is assessed. The point of obstruction is found most commonly at the ileocecal valve, and the stone generally should not be forced distally through the obstructing point because of concern for splitting the bowel. The gallstone is milked backward and removed through a proximal longitudinal enterotomy in a healthy-appearing bowel, and the enterotomy is closed transversely. Some authors advocate for a transverse enterotomy and closure. If the stone is so tightly impacted it cannot be milked proximally, the bowel should be opened over the stone and the area resected (some advocate resection without opening the bowel in this circumstance). Although uncommon, any nonviable-appearing bowel is resected and anastomosed. It is unusual to perform bypass of an obstructed area rather than enterolithotomy. The remainder of the alimentary tract is examined for additional stones that are found in up to 5% of cases, and these should be removed. Repeat episodes of gallstone ileus are rare and occur in about 5% of postoperative patients (usually within 6 months of first presentation); more than 80% of recurrences resolve spontaneously.

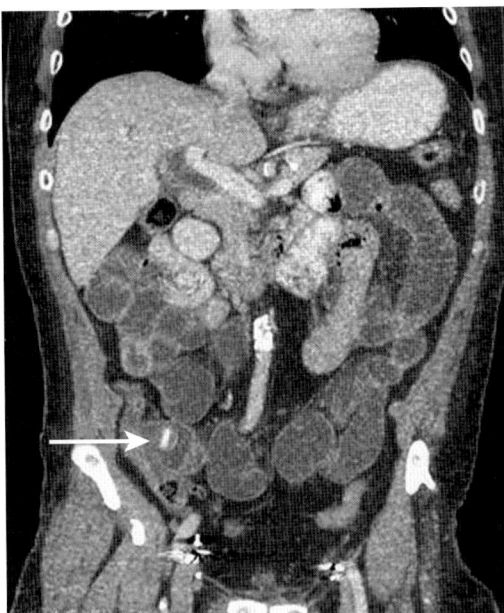
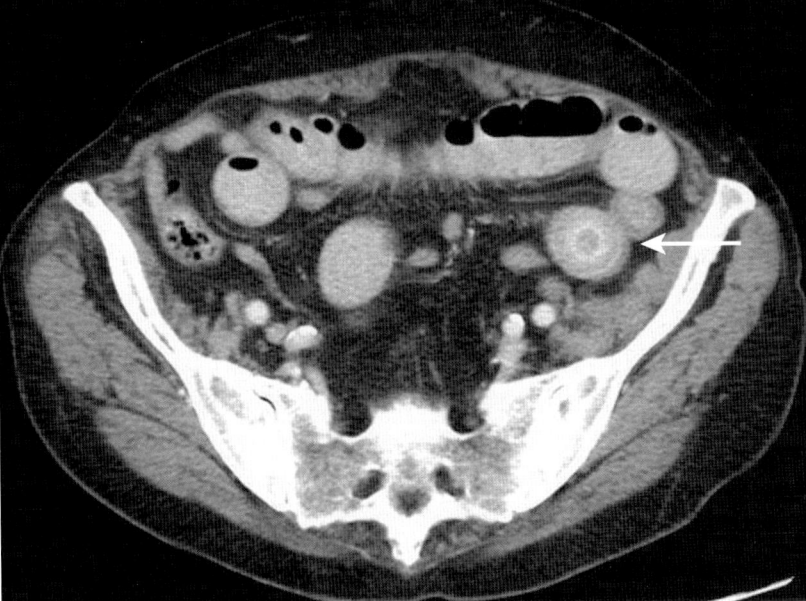

FIGURE 1   Coronal and axial images from a computed tomographic scan of the abdomen demonstrating gallstone ileus, with the gallstones (*arrows*) in the small bowel (photo shows two separate patients).

The management of duodenal or colonic obstruction is controversial. These cases are so unusual that there is little consensus as to proper management. Duodenal obstruction is problematic as the obstructing stone is often intimately associated with the inflammatory gallbladder process and may require taking down the fistula as well as making an extension of the duodenal fistula or a separate duodenotomy. If the area is extremely inflamed or there is an abscess, this is truly a formidable issue. Colonic obstruction is most common in the sigmoid, and several approaches have been described, including milking the stone back into the proximal colon with extraction and transverse colostomy formation as well as sigmoid resection and colostomy formation.

Performing a concomitant and definitive biliary procedure at the same time as management of the bowel obstruction (a "one-stage" operation) has been associated with significantly higher mortality rates in several review studies supporting enterolithotomy alone, and it remains controversial. Significant pericholecystic inflammation, fibrosis, and distortion of the normal biliary anatomic landmarks, duodenal fibrosis, and the presence of a fistula often complicate cholecystectomy in this process, and bile duct injuries have been sustained in this setting. Many of the fistulas (up to 80%) appear to close spontaneously, especially in the absence of residual cholecystolithiasis. It is rare that the management of the biliary process is emergent and must be done at the same operation as the enterolithotomy. It is unclear as to how many patients will have symptoms of biliary colic or symptoms from a persistent cholecystenteric fistula since many of these patients are older and have a limited life span. Many surgeons now opt to forgo a one-stage operation and instead offer interval cholecystectomy to patients who have persistent symptoms. The published experience with laparoscopic cholecystectomy as a staged second procedure after enterolithotomy for gallstone ileus is not large enough to determine how often a subsequent laparoscopic cholecystectomy may be performed instead of an open cholecystectomy (Figure 2).

Cholecystectomy at the time of enterolithotomy should be a careful and deliberated decision. Important considerations focus initially on the stability of the patient during the operation. Proceeding to cholecystectomy should not be done if the patient has any hemodynamic instability, poor urine output, hypothermia, significant uncorrected metabolic abnormalities, or unstable medical conditions. If the patient is stable and it is safe to add a significant amount of additional operative time, then a careful inspection of the right upper quadrant may be done. The amount of acute and chronic inflammation, edema, and anatomic distortion should be carefully assessed. Drainage should be the only procedure in the unusual situation when there is gross purulence. Cholecystostomy may be considered as part of the drainage procedure. Cholecystectomy and division of the enteric fistula is best done if the tissues have mature adhesions without significant edema and friability. The patient who has no pneumobilia on good preoperative imaging may indicate that the fistula has closed since the passage of the gallstone, and this may sway the surgeon to delay cholecystectomy. There is no consensus on the technical performance of the cholecystectomy as to a "dome down" versus an "infundibulum up" technique. Liberal use of intraoperative cholangiography should be pursued for two reasons: (1) there are a significant number of patients who will have common duct stone, and (2) it is useful in delineating the anatomy in a distorted field to avoid common duct injury. The experience of the operating surgeon in managing difficult open cholecystectomies should be an important judgment. If the surgeon has little experience in difficult open cholecystectomy, then the cholecystectomy should not be performed and the patient should be referred to a specialized hepatobiliary center for consideration of cholecystectomy at a later time.

The number of reports of laparoscopic approaches to managing gallstone ileus is increasing. Gaining safe laparoscopic entry to the abdominal cavity in the presence of distended loops of bowel can be fraught with difficulty, and open trocar placement is recommended to minimize the chance of injury to viscera. Just as in laparoscopic management of any small bowel obstruction, there may not be sufficient space to manipulate and run the bowel. The presence of hugely distended or edematous bowel loops may be a relative contraindication to use of laparoscopy. Two approaches are (1) laparoscopy with identification of the obstructing stone and exteriorization of the segment and extracorporeal management of the enterolithotomy and return of the repaired bowel segment to the abdomen, and (2) laparoscopy with intracorporeal enterotomy and stone extraction with intracorporeal repair of the enterotomy. The benefits of minimally invasive enterolithotomy to reduce morbidity or mortality have not yet been proven, but the technique seems attractive, especially in this patient population where mortality and morbidity have been reported to be between 10% and 30%.

Nonsurgical means of managing gallstone ileus have been described in highly selected cases. Lithotripsy of stones has been successful in a very small number of cases. This has been coupled with endoscopic fragment retrieval after electrohydraulic or extracorporeal lithotripsy. Upper endoscopy can be used for therapeutic maneuvers to remove proximal gallstones and to diagnose biliary proximal alimentary fistulas. Single-balloon enteroscopy, double-balloon enteroscopy, and colonoscopy are also described as successful endoscopic approaches to gallstone ileus.

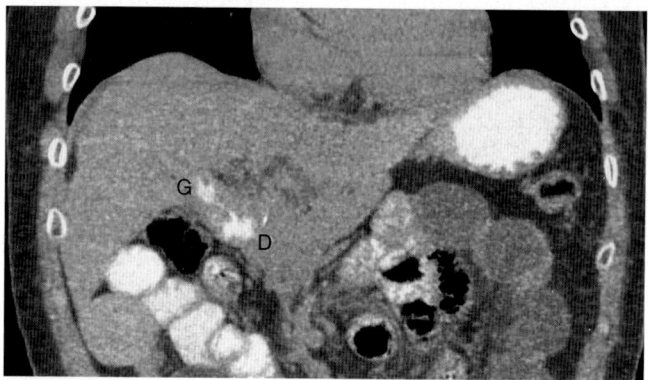

FIGURE 2 Coronal image of a computed tomographic scan of the abdomen showing cholecystoduodenal fistula. The oral contrast from the duodenum (*D*) has filled the gallbladder (*G*) through the fistula.

SUGGESTED READINGS

Muthukumarasamy G, Venkata SP, Shaikh IA, et al: Gallstone ileus: surgical strategies and clinical outcome, *J Dig Dis* 9:156–161, 2008.

Ravikumar R, Williams JG: The operative management of gallstone ileus, *Ann R Coll Surg Engl* 92:279–281, 2010.

Reisner RM, Cohen JR: Gallstone ileus: a review of 1001 reported cases, *Am Surg* 60:441–446, 1994.

Rodríguez-Sanjuán JC, Casado F, Fernández MJ, et al: Cholecystectomy and fistula closure versus enterolithotomy alone in gallstone ileus, *Br J Surg* 84:634–637, 1997.

Webb LH, Ott MM, Gunter OL: Once bitten, twice incised: recurrent gallstone ileus, *Am J Surg* 200:72–74, 2010.

Obstructive Jaundice: Endoscopic Therapy

Reem Zeyad Sharaiha, MD, MSc, and
Zhiping Li, MD

INTRODUCTION

Obstructive jaundice is caused by an interruption of bile flow through the biliary system. It can be the result of extrinsic compression or intrinsic obstruction and can be further divided into neoplastic and benign causes. Cholelithiasis and pancreatic cancer are the most common benign and neoplastic causes of jaundice, respectively, and comprise 40% of total cases. Other causes are listed in Table 1. Jaundice can be diagnosed on examination, based on the yellowness of the skin or the icterus of the cornea. (Total bilirubin levels of 4 mg/dL and above can be detected clinically). Biochemical liver function tests show an elevation in the direct bilirubin, alkaline phosphatase (ALP), and γ-glutamyltransferase (GGT) values and to a lesser degree, aspartate transferase (AST) and alanine transferase (ALT) values. Noninvasive imaging studies, such as transabdominal ultrasound scan (US), computed tomographic (CT) scan, and magnetic resonance cholangiopancreatography (MRCP) are common diagnostic modalities for the underlying cause of jaundice. Endoscopic studies, such as endoscopic ultrasound (EUS) and endoscopic retrograde cholangiopancreatography (ERCP), can be used for both diagnostic and therapeutic reasons.

Obstructive jaundice used to be mainly treated with surgical interventions or percutaneous transhepatic cholangiography (PTC) drainage. Endoscopic therapies have become a major component for management of obstructive jaundice. In many cases, it has become first-line therapy. This chapter focuses on the current standard of endoscopic therapy of obstructive jaundice.

ENDOSCOPIC THERAPIES FOR OBSTRUCTIVE JAUNDICE

Endoscopic Retrograde Cholangiopancreatography

ERCP was first introduced in 1968. It has quickly evolved from a purely diagnostic procedure to a mainly therapeutic one. Once the biliary system is accessed either directly through the papilla or, if the papilla is obscured, through EUS-guided needle puncture, both plastic and metal stents are used for endoscopic drainage. The advantage of a plastic biliary stent is the low cost and the large varieties of sizes available. However, plastic stents can be only used in the short term because they can occlude within 2 to 3 months from a small lumen (<3 mm). Recently, a plastic stent with a concept of drainage via enhanced surface area but without lumen (Wing stent) has provided a longer patency. Plastic stents can be removed endoscopically and reinserted as needed. Metal stents have the advantage of a large diameter (8-mm to 11-mm) lumen, longer patency, and an easier deployment option, but they are more expensive. Metal stents come in three different types: fully covered, uncovered, and partially covered. Uncovered and partially covered metal stents are permanent once they are deployed inside bile ducts. They are mostly used in malignant conditions when the life expectancy is greater than 6 months. The advent of fully covered metal stents has changed the paradigm for management of biliary strictures because they can be removed. The fully covered metal stents are now widely used in the setting of benign strictures.

The overall complication rate of ERCP ranges from 4% to 15%. The most common complication is pancreatitis, which occurs between 1.8% and 10%. Pancreatitis can be prevented with inserting a prophylactic pancreatic stent and giving 100 mg rectal indomethacin after the procedure, as shown in a recent randomized trial, especially for individuals at high risk. Risk factors for pancreatitis include female gender, young age, sphincter of Oddi dysfunction, difficult cannulation, pancreatic duct injection, precut sphincterotomy, and low endoscopic volume. Other complications include bleeding and perforation, especially after sphincterotomy, at rate of 1% to 2%. Most ERCP complications can be managed conservatively. Rarely do patients need surgical intervention.

Cholangioscopy

These miniature endoscopes and catheters permit direct visualization of bile ducts. They can access bile ducts directly (direct cholangioscopy) or are passed through the working channel of a duodenoscope during ERCP (mother and daughter scopes). The numerous indications for the use of cholangioscopy include evaluation of indeterminate biliary strictures, treatment of difficult bile duct stones, selective cannulation of obstructed bile ducts, and assessment of extent of cholangiocarcinoma. Multiple procedures can be performed during cholangioscopy, targeted biopsies of bile duct lesions can be obtained, and bile duct stones can be fragmented with electrohydraulic or laser lithotripsy probes that are applied directly to the stones. In patients with indeterminate strictures, cholangioscopy may lead to direct inspection of the epithelium to obtain biopsies. The sensitivity of conventional brush cytology and biopsy during ERCP for detection of malignancy in most series ranges from 30% to 50%. In prospective single-center case series, cholangioscopic visualization with or without biopsy was shown to have a sensitivity of 89% to 100% and a specificity of 79% to 96% for detection of biliary malignancy.

Endoscopic Ultrasound

The role of EUS in management of obstructive jaundice has evolved from staging and sampling tumors to accessing bile ducts. When an ERCP fails to cannulate bile ducts because of obstruction or variant anatomy, the biliary access can be achieved with EUS-guided bile duct puncture and cholangiogram. Then, it can be followed by either guidewire advancement for rendezvous ERCP in patients with duodenoscope-accessible papilla or direct drainage in patients with altered anatomy. Once access to the biliary tract is achieved via EUS techniques, the remainder of the procedure is very similar to ERCP. A plastic or a metal stent is left for drainage. In one study, EUS-guided cholangiography and EUS-guided rendezvous ERCP were successful in 97% and 75% of biliary procedures, respectively, that were failed previous standard ERCPs.

BENIGN BILIARY OBSTRUCTION

Choledocholithiasis

Gallstones are common and affect 5% of the population. Approximately 15% to 20% of cases eventually become symptomatic. Among those patients with symptomatic gallstone conditions, 15% have choledocholithiasis, which can result in obstructive jaundice and cholangitis. Choledocholithiasis can be diagnosed in several ways. MRCP has a sensitivity of 90%, similar to ERCP. MRCP has largely replaced

TABLE 1: Causes of obstructive jaundice

Benign	Choledocholithiasis
	Postsurgical stricture
	Pancreatitis
	Primary sclerosing cholangitis
	Primary biliary cirrhosis
	Parasites
Malignant	Pancreatic cancer
	Cholangiocarcinoma
	Ampullary cancer
	Gastric cancer
	Hepatoma
	Metastatic disease

ERCP as the method of choice for diagnosing choledocholithiasis. CT scan and abdominal ultrasound scan have similar sensitivities of 50% with nondilated ducts and 75% with dilated ducts. EUS is much more sensitive than any other modalities for stones that are less than 5 mm.

ERCP is indicated if choledocholithiasis is found on imaging, especially if cholangitis is present. During ERCP, biliary stones are removed with extractor balloon and basket after a biliary sphincterotomy. Baskets, especially lithotripsy baskets, are preferred for large stones (>1 cm). With extraction of the stones with a basket, stones should be removed one at a time, from the distal to proximal bile duct, to avoid impaction of the basket in the ampulla of Vater. With baskets that are compatible with an external lithotripsy system, basket impaction should also be avoided. Sphincteroplasty (balloon dilation of the sphincter) can be done to remove large stones, but only after a biliary sphincterotomy has been performed because it increases the rate of post-ERCP pancreatitis. Mechanical, electrohydraulic, or laser lithotripsies are used to breakdown large stones. The success rate of mechanical lithotripsy is 70% to 80%, and the factors associated with failure are the size of the stone (>30 mm), impaction of the stone at the bile duct, a ratio of stone to bile duct diameter greater than 1, and the type of lithotripter used. Electrohydraulic lithotripsy (EHL), laser-induced shockwave lithotripsy, and extracorporeal shockwave lithotripsy can be used for pulverizing stones. Cholangioscopy has increased the success of electrohydraulic and laser-induced shockwave lithotripsy. EHL can only be used with direct visualization with cholangioscopy to avoid ductal injury. In several retrospective series, clearance of difficult stones that have failed conventional ERCP treatments occurred in 90% to 100% of patients after one or two EHL sessions. The main risk of EHL is perforation, which has an overall risk of less than 1%. This occurs because of extreme elevation of the surface temperature of the stone and surrounding ductal tissues, which is usually caused by prolonged application of EHL. Bleeding can also occur. An alternative treatment is pulsed laser lithotripsy, which has success rates of 83% to 100% in removal of stones and clearing of bile ducts. A plastic stent is often left in situ if the duct is not clear of stones or until interval cholecystectomy is performed.

Postsurgical Complications

Biliary tract complications are an important cause of morbidity and mortality after liver transplants and laparoscopic cholecystectomy. The two main complications are biliary strictures and bile leaks. The incidence rate of these complications is very low (<2%) for postlaparoscopic cholecystectomy, but can reach between 10% and 25% after transplant. Risk factors include placement of T-tubes, acute hepatic artery thrombosis, hepatic artery stenosis, ischemia or reperfusion injury, technical factors during surgery (excessive dissection of periductal tissue during procurement, excessive use of electrocautery for biliary duct bleeding, and tension of the duct anastomosis), small caliber of the bile duct and mismatched size between donor and recipient bile ducts, prolonged cold and warm ischemia times, and primary sclerosing cholangitis. Initial evaluation should begin with Doppler ultrasound scan, followed by MRCP, which has a sensitivity of 96% and a specificity of 94% for diagnosing of postsurgical biliary complications.

Postsurgical Bile Leaks

Iatrogenic injury to the biliary tree after laparoscopic cholecystectomy occurs at a rate of 0.6%. Significant postoperative bile leaks occur in approximately 0.8% to 1.1% of patients. Patients with bile leaks usually present within the first postoperative week, with persistent bile discharge from an operatively placed drain or T-tube tract, symptoms of pain and fever, or abnormal liver function test results. Bile leaks may occur from the cystic stump or from transection of an anomalous duct that most commonly originate from the right hepatic lobe (ducts of Luschka, or subvesical ducts). Bile leak can be confirmed with measurement of bilirubin in the drainage.

Endoscopic cholangiography can delineate the site of the leak in more than 95% of patients. This is usually achieved with an occlusion cholangiogram. After a balloon catheter is inserted and inflated to the size of the duct, contrast is injected. The cholangiographic magnitude of contrast extravasation represents the size of the leak. Endoscopic therapy is successful in about 90% of patients with a postcholecystectomy biliary leak. The goal of endoscopic therapy is to decrease the transpapillary pressure gradient, leading to preferential transpapillary bile flow rather than extravasation at the site of the leak. The larger caliber plastic stent, or a fully covered metal stent used in about 10% of cases, is usually left in place for 4 to 8 weeks. If a percutaneous drain is in place, the drainage should be less than 10 mL per day before removal of the stent. A repeat ERCP at the time of stent removal should be performed to determine whether the leak is still present.

Bile leaks after liver transplant are thought to occur in 2% to 25% of patients. Leakage is thought to occur most commonly from the anastomotic site, from the cystic duct stump, from the surface of the liver (if living donor), or from the T-tube tract. Leaks can be diagnosed from the presence of bile from a drain or, if none are present, from MRCP or ERCP. Great caution should be taken with an occlusion cholangiogram in patients immediately after liver transplant (<7 days) to avoid overfilling and disrupting biliary anastomosis. The presence of a bile leak is an independent risk factor for the development of early or late strictures, and hepatic artery thrombosis, and requires prompt therapy. A biliary sphincterotomy or placement of a plastic stent in the common bile duct is successful in treating 90% to 95% of post–liver transplant bile leaks. Stents are preferred to be left in longer because of delayed healing from immunosuppression. Surgery or a percutaneous transhepatic approach is reserved for patients in whom the endoscopic approach is unsuccessful. Large bilomas that do not communicate with the bile ducts should be treated with percutaneous drainage and antibiotics.

Postsurgical Strictures

Postsurgical strictures are the most common cause of benign biliary strictures. Postlaparoscopic cholecystectomy is the culprit for more than 80% of these. Bile duct strictures also occur between 4% and 16% of cases after liver transplant. Early strictures are usually the result of technical problems with the operation, whereas late strictures are the result of ischemia and vascular insufficiency. Bile leak is an independent risk factor for the development of anastomotic strictures. Strictures are classified as anastomotic or nonanastomotic, depending on the stricture site. Most anastomotic strictures occur within the first year after liver transplant. The treatment of choice is serial endoscopic dilation and stenting. Response is usually seen by 3 months. However, an 18% rate of recurrence was shown in one study. Serial stenting with increasing diameter is usually done to prevent stent occlusion and cholangitis. Recently, a shift has been seen from the use of multiple plastic stents to fully covered metal stents that have a larger diameter, which reduces the number of reinterventions. Resolution of strictures occurs in 96% of cases; the rest require percutaneous treatment or surgical revision. Nonanastomotic strictures result mainly from ischemia. Less commonly, they can be from recurrence of the underlying disease, such as primary sclerosing cholangitis. Strictures occur anywhere from the hilum to the intrahepatic ducts and cause a beading appearance similar to primary sclerosing cholangitis. Sludge can develop proximal to the stricture and lead to recurrent episodes of cholangitis. Endoscopic treatment is the same, with a sphincterotomy, dilation, and large-caliber stent insertion. Time to response is longer, with a median time of 12 to 16 weeks versus 6 weeks for anastomotic strictures. Resolution of strictures is more problematic because only 50% have resolution and many patients may need retransplantation.

Primary Sclerosing Cholangitis

Primary sclerosing cholangitis (PSC) is a chronic disorder characterized by inflammation, fibrosis, and strictures of the intrahepatic and extrahepatic biliary tree. Ninety percent of those cases have underlying inflammatory bowel disease (mostly ulcerative colitis). Long-term complications of PSC include cholestasis, cholangitis, stricture formation, and eventually cirrhosis and hepatic failure. A high incidence of cholangiocarcinoma is found among patients with PSC. The diagnosis of PSC is established with the demonstration of characteristic multifocal stricture and dilation of intrahepatic or extrahepatic bile ducts on cholangiography. The biliary strictures may be focal, with normal intervening areas, or diffuse, with involvement of a long segment. Strictures can occur in any part of the biliary tree. MRCP has been proven to have the same sensitivity and specificity as ERCP for diagnosis of PSC.

Up to 60% of patients with PSC have development of a dominant stricture, defined as a stenosis with a diameter of 1.5 mm or less in the common bile duct or 1 mm or less in the hepatic ducts. Studies have shown reduced survival in patients with dominant strictures, and endoscopic therapies to relieve dominant strictures improve survival and slow disease progression. Endoscopic therapies include balloon dilation of the stricture with or without placement of plastic stents across strictures. Cholangioscopy can be used to selectively cannulate stricture bile ducts. Serial dilation is performed with fluoroscopy with high-pressure dilation balloons to match the downstream duct diameter. The patients should receive antibiotics before and after endoscopic therapies. The only definitive cure for PSC is liver transplantation. A small portion of patients have recurrence after the liver transplant.

MALIGNANT OBSTRUCTION

Endoscopic therapies are used in the setting of malignant biliary obstruction, either as a bridge to surgery or, in patients with unresectable disease, for palliation. They are mainly for patients with extrahepatic strictures and have limited impact in intrahepatic obstructions. The most common distal biliary malignant obstruction is from pancreatic cancer. In patients who are deemed potential surgical candidates, placement of distal pancreatic or short expandable fully covered metal stents do not interfere with subsequent surgery. The aim of biliary drainage is to relieve jaundice and prevent complications from cholestasis. Stents are also used in the setting of neoadjuvant therapy for locally advanced disease. Metal stents have been shown to be the treatment of choice.

In patients in whom access to the papilla is not possible, direct access to the bile duct via endoscopic ultrasound–guided puncture can be performed. A metallic or plastic stent is inserted to form either a hepatogastrostomy or a choledochoduodenostomy, depending on the site of puncture. These procedures have an overall success rate of 92% but are limited by complications that include biliary leak, pneumoperitoneum, and infection. Many studies have showed no difference in mortality between palliative surgery and endoscopic drainage groups.

Hilar obstruction may result from cholangiocarcinoma (Klatskin's tumor), gallbladder carcinoma, metastatic cancer, or compression from lymph nodes. Endoscopic biliary drainage is the preferred method for relief of biliary obstruction. When both hepatic ducts are occluded, the goal of endoscopic therapy is to place bilateral stents into the left and right common hepatic ducts. If bilateral stenting cannot be achieved, then unilateral stenting of the most dilated duct is performed. Cholangioscopy can be used to selectively cannulate the obstructive bile duct with a guidewire followed by balloon dilation and stent placement. Plastic biliary stents are commonly used as the initial endoscopic treatment because they are inexpensive and effective and can be easily removed or exchanged. Plastic stents, however, easily develop occlusion from sludge or tumor and require repeat ERCPs for stent exchange. Metal stents were introduced to help alleviate this problem by extending the duration of stent patency. Limitations of metal stents are the cost per procedure.

Endoscopic tumor ablations, such as photodynamic therapy or radiofrequency ablation, are also options for management of malignant biliary obstruction. Prospective randomized controlled trials have shown that photodynamic therapy in combination with stenting resulted in prolonged median survival and significantly improved performance status compared with stenting alone. Recently, endoscopic radiofrequency ablation of cholangiocarcinoma has also been tested as a palliative treatment modality.

SUGGESTED READINGS

Chapman R, Fevery J, Kalloo A, et al: Diagnosis and management of primary sclerosing cholangitis, *Hepatology* 51:660–678, 2010.

Gerges C, Schumacher B, Terheggen G, et al: Expandable metal stents for malignant hilar biliary obstruction, *Gastrointest Endosc Clin North Am* 21(3):481–497, 2011.

Itoi T, Sofuni A, Itokawa F, et al: Endoscopic ultrasonography-guided biliary drainage, *J Hepatobiliary Pancreat Sci* 17(5):611–616, 2010.

Terheggen G, Neuhaus H: New options of cholangioscopy, *Gastroenterol Clin North Am* 39(4):827–844, 2010.

Zepeda-Gómez S, Baron TH: Benign biliary strictures: current endoscopic management, *Nat Rev Gastroenterol Hepatol* 8(10):573–581, 2011.

THE PANCREAS

ACUTE PANCREATITIS

Nakul Valsangkar, MD, and
Sarah P. Thayer, MD, PhD

Acute pancreatitis accounts for 300,000 hospitalizations per year in the United States. The cause of 90% of cases can be attributed to alcohol and gallstones. Other causes include hyperlipidemia, hypercalcemia, trauma, heredity, drugs, and iatrogenic complications from procedures such as endoscopic retrograde cholangiopancreatography (ERCP). When a cause cannot be identified, the disease is termed *idiopathic* (Box 1).

The clinical manifestations of pancreatitis can be very broad, from mild to severe. The most common manifestation of acute pancreatitis is mild, with epigastric pain associated with nausea and vomiting, minimal organ dysfunction, and no parenchymal necrosis, and it usually has a self-limiting course. For approximately 15% of patients, however, pancreatitis can be severe and life-threatening. These cases of severe acute pancreatitis (SAP) are associated with organ failure involving the cardiovascular, renal, and/or respiratory systems. SAP is generally divided into two phases. The first phase is associated with the inflammatory response of the host as a result of tissue injury, which lasts approximately 1 week. During this time, the pancreatic edema and multiple-organ failure resolve or advance to peripancreatic ischemia and necrosis. The second phase, which can last weeks to months, is associated with this necrotizing process, and mortality in this case is usually associated with secondary infection.

The initial goal of assessment is to determine the cause, remove any ongoing stimulus that may continue to fuel pancreatitis (drugs, hyperlipidemia, or choledocholithiasis), and identify which patients will progress to SAP. The patient's history should focus on identifying the cause. Directed questions should concern history of alcohol consumption, cholelithiasis, hyperlipidemia, history of prior pancreatitis, and medications. It is important to obtain the ages and number of family members afflicted with AP. During physical examination, it is important to assess vital signs, oxygen saturation, and urine output. Depressed mentation, tachycardia, tachypnea, and low oxygen saturation are concerning signs of SAP. Abdominal examination usually reveals upper abdominal tenderness, particularly in the epigastrium. Affected patients may have peritonitis. Initial laboratory evaluation should include complete blood cell count and measurements of amylase, lipase, liver enzymes (alanine aminotransferase, aspartate aminotransferase, alkaline phosphatase, total and direct bilirubin), electrolytes (including ionized calcium), and the ratio of blood urea nitrogen (BUN) to creatinine. If oxygen saturations are found to be low, arterial blood gases should be measured. Ultrasonography should be considered when there is suspicion of choledocholithiasis, inasmuch as therapy is directed at early extraction. Early imaging by computed tomographic (CT) scanning is usually not needed if the diagnosis is clear; however, many physicians obtain a CT scan to exclude other diagnoses because many affected patients present with a toxic appearance, fever, peritonitis, and an elevated white blood cell (WBC) count. The initial management of patients with acute pancreatitis is to establish nothing by mouth (NPO) status and provide ample intravenous fluid hydration and pain control. Prophylactic antibiotics are no longer recommended and are used only in the setting of documented infection. It is important to identify patients who are likely to progress to more severe forms of pancreatitis. Several biochemical and imaging scoring systems have been developed to predict which patients are at greatest risk.

ASSESSMENT OF SEVERITY

Many scoring systems have been used to predict mortality in acute pancreatitis (Table 1). The first of these, Ranson's criteria, initially published in 1974, has been used worldwide as the standard in predicting outcome. This historical score is based on parameters (see Table 1) at hospital admission and at 48 hours to predict the likelihood of progression to SAP and overall mortality. The Ranson's score requires 48 hours of observation, which makes difficult the early identification of patients who are likely to have systemic complications and necrosis. The modified Glasgow or Imrie scoring system, like Ranson's, is based on biochemical factors such as age, WBC count, serum lactate dehydrogenase level, and blood glucose level, but the advantage is that it provides a complete assessment at the time of hospital admission (see Table 1). A significantly more detailed system, the Acute Physiology and Chronic Health Evaluation II (APACHE II) scoring system, has also been used. In spite of the complexity of APACHE II, numerous Web-based calculators make it possible to institute it routinely, such as the one at MDCalc. A published set of criteria is the bedside index for severity in acute pancreatitis (BISAP). Five simple clinical parameters (BUN, impaired mental status, systemic inflammatory response syndrome [SIRS], age, and pleural effusion) are used to obtain the BISAP score and thereby stratify patients within the first 24 hours of hospitalization into distinct groups by degree of risk for in-hospital mortality.

In addition to clinical scoring systems, there are systems based on imaging. Although contrast medium–enhanced computed tomography (CECT) is the diagnostic modality of choice in evaluating pancreatitis, it is best to wait at least 72 hours because early imaging is inaccurate in identifying necrotizing pancreatitis and grossly underestimates the extent of necrosis (Figure 1, *A* and *B*). Diagnostic yield is significantly better if CT scanning is performed at least 72 hours after the initial presentation. Examples of imaging-based systems are the Balthazaar score, the CT Severity Index (CTSI), and the Mortele score (modified CTSI). In the most recently published of these, the 10-point Mortele score, pancreatic inflammation and necrosis are evaluated with extrapancreatic complications. A score greater than

BOX 1: Causes of acute pancreatitis

Gallstone disease
Alcohol
Trauma
  Including intraoperative surgical trauma
Infections
Viruses (mumps, Coxsackie, hepatitis B, cytomegalovirus, varicella zoster, herpes simplex), bacteria (*Mycoplasma, Legionella, Leptospira, Salmonella* organisms), fungi (*Aspergillus* species), parasites (*Toxoplasma, Cryptosporidium, Ascaris* organisms)
Hyperlipidemia
At higher risk: patients with type I, type IV, and type V hyperlipidemia (Frederickson's classification)
Hypercalcemia
Hereditary pancreatitis
PRSS1: cationic trypsinogen with a gain of function mutation
Drugs
Didanosine, asparaginase, azathioprine, valproic acid, pentavalent antimonials, pentamidine, mercaptopurine, mesalamine, trimethoprim/sulfamethoxazole, sulfasalazine, furosemide, sulindac opiates, tetracycline, cytarabine, steroids
Post–endoscopic retrograde cholangiopancreatography (ERCP) status
Ischemic
Hypoperfusion, atheroembolic phenomena, vasculitides
Malignant tumors
Environmental toxins
Scorpion venom, insecticides, and organic solvents
Idiopathic

6 indicates SAP. These and other scoring systems are outlined in Table 1.

The revision of the Atlanta classification provides comprehensive definitions, in which both early clinical and later image-based scoring systems are used to assess acute pancreatitis. In this classification, clinical criteria are used to initially define pancreatitis into three grades of severity: mild pancreatitis, which is not associated with organ failure or with local or systemic complications; moderate pancreatitis, which includes organ failure that resolves in 48 hours or local or systemic complications without persistent organ failure; and SAP, which is characterized by single- or multiple-organ failure that lasts more than 48 hours.

It also uses an image-based classification system to morphologically classify the pancreas; this is usually used during the second phase of the inflammatory process. This classification specifies four types of pancreatic/peripancreatic collections: (1) interstitial edematous pancreatitis, (2) necrotizing pancreatitis, (3) acute peripancreatic fluid collection, and (4) pancreatic pseudocyst. Of all the assessments, no single system has yet been identified as the best overall predictor of disease severity. In general, clinical scoring systems are usually used initially, and radiologic (morphologic) criteria are used during the later phases of acute pancreatitis because these finding can be used to guide treatment.

COMPLICATIONS OF PANCREATITIS

Pancreatic and peripancreatic fluid collections are present in nearly 60% of the patients with acute pancreatitis; a third of these patients have three or more collections. They resolve spontaneously in half of patients, and intervention is usually not required. If a major duct has been disrupted, the fluid collection will probably give rise to a pseudocyst. These fluid collections contain high amylase levels. The management of pseudocysts is discussed elsewhere in this textbook. Of all patients with pancreatitis, 5% to 7% may progress to pancreatic necrosis, in which the mortality rate is 10%. In this necrotic tissue, secondary infection can develop in 40% to 70% of patients, and the mortality rate can be as high as 50% (Figure 2). Vascular complications among all patients with acute pancreatitis include thrombosis of the splenic vein (19%), superior mesenteric vein (14%), and portal vein (13%) and arterial hemorrhage (5%), which arises most commonly from the splenic artery, followed by the gastroduodenal artery.

MANAGEMENT OF PATIENTS WITH ACUTE PANCREATITIS

Supportive Care

Supportive care forms the cornerstone of the management of patients with acute pancreatitis. Patients are initially made NPO to limit pancreatic stimulation. Supportive measures also include volume replacement, maintaining electrolyte balance, and pain control. Patients can deteriorate rapidly, and it is crucial to closely monitor blood pressure, heart rate, BUN level, creatinine concentration, and urine output. Depending on the level of severity, the patient may be managed in a regular hospital room or in an intensive care setting. Several prospective studies have shown that SIRS, defined as alteration in heart rate, temperature, respiratory rate, and WBC, and if present for 48 hours or longer, is a predictor of pancreatic necrosis, multiple-organ failure, and death. On the basis of these clinical and laboratory markers, patients likely to suffer adverse outcomes must be identified early and transferred to an intensive care unit for specialized monitoring and care.

An admission to the intensive care unit should be considered if the patient has an APACHE II score of 8 or higher, a modified Glasgow score higher than 3 at 24 hours, a Ranson's score higher than 3, or C-reactive protein level higher than 150 mg/L 48 hours after admission, evidence of multiple-organ failure, or the presence of pancreatic necrosis.

Volume Resuscitation

Hemodynamic monitoring and fluid replacement are among the most important initial interventions in these patients because of a large volume ($\approx$10 L) of fluid sequestration, and increased vascular permeability in the pancreatic microcirculation. Worsening hemoconcentration 24 hours after hospital admission in these patients has been associated with a higher likelihood of developing pancreatic necrosis and multiple-organ failure. For replacement solutions, crystalloids such as normal saline or Ringer's lactate are preferred over colloids unless specifically indicated. Volume replacement can be titrated to a urine output of 0.5 mL/kg body weight/hour or higher after initial high-volume resuscitation.

Metabolic Imbalance in Acute Pancreatitis

Several electrolyte and metabolic abnormalities are common in acute pancreatitis. These include hyperglycemia, hypertriglyceridemia, hypoalbuminemia, hypocalcemia, and hypomagnesemia. Serum triglyceride levels higher than 1000 mg/dL may indicate underlying type I, IV, or V hyperlipoproteinemia as the cause of acute pancreatitis. Management of such patients entails establishing NPO status, restricting lipids if artificial nutrition is being provided, and administering lipid-lowering medications such as fibric acid derivatives. Plasmapheresis may be needed in some patients with very high levels

TABLE I: Scoring systems to predict disease severity and overall outcome in acute pancreatitis

Year	System	Notes
1974	Ranson's criteria	Historical score in which parameters at hospital admission and at 48 hours are used to define mortality Parameters at hospital admission: Age >55 WBC count >16,000/mm^3 Blood glucose level >200 mg/dL Serum LDH level >350 IU/L Serum AST >250 IU/L Ranson severity score: ≥3 is an indication of severe acute pancreatitis Parameters at 48 hours: Fall in hematocrit of >10% Fluid sequestration >6 L Hypocalcemia PaO$_2$ <60 mm Hg Increase in BUN by >5/dL after intravenous fluid hydration Base deficit >4 mmol/L Disadvantage: Can be read only at 48 h
1984	Modified Glasgow (Imrie scoring)	Parameters: Age >55 PaO$_2$ <60 mm Hg WBC count > 15,000/mm^3 Calcium level <8 mg/dL LDH level >600 IU/L Blood glucose level >10 mmol/L BUN >16 mmol/L Albumin level <3.2 g/L Modified Glasgow severity score: ≥3 is an indication of severe acute pancreatitis
1989	Acute Physiology and Chronic Health Evaluation II (APACHE II)	ICU-based scoring system to calculate morbidity and mortality Parameters/Chronic health points: Age >45 WBC count <3,000 or >14,900/mL Rectal temperature <36°C or >38.4°C MAP <70 or >109 mm Hg HR <70 or >109 mm Hg RR <12 or >24 bpm pH <7.33 or >7.49 Na$^+$ concentration <130 or >149 mM K$^+$ concentration <3.5 or >5.4 mM PO$_2$ <70 or >200 mm Hg Creatinine concentration <0.6/100 mL or >1.4 mg/100 mL Hct <30% or >45.9% GCS = 15-GCS APACHE severity score: ≥8 is an indication of severe acute pancreatitis Cumbersome to use and very complex; however, in comparison with the Ranson's and Glasgow systems, it can be calculated and recalculated daily
2004	Radiologic scoring: modified CT severity index (CTSI)	Based on contrast enhanced CT scan taken after at least 72 hours This score returns a total score based two grades: a *CT grade* (normal pancreas, 0; edematous pancreas, 1; mild extrapancreatic changes with pancreatic edema, 2; severe extrapancreatic changes and one fluid collection, 3; multiple collections, 4), and a *necrotic grade* (no involvement, 0; less than one third of pancreas involved, 2; one third to half involved, 4; more than half involved, 6) Severe pancreatitis indicated by a total score of >6 points

Continued

TABLE 1: Scoring systems to predict disease severity and overall outcome in acute pancreatitis—cont'd

Year	System	Notes
2006	Systemic inflammatory response syndrome (SIRS)	Criteria: Body temperature <36°C or >38°C Heart rate >90 Respiratory rate >20 or $PaCO_2$ <32 mm Hg WBC count < 4000/mm³ or >12,000/mm³ Generalized criteria for defining organ dysfunction: SIRS present at time of hospital admission (<48 hours) and persistent SIRS during hospitalization (present after 48 hours); when used in combination, they are correlated with likelihood of necrotizing pancreatitis, ICU admission, and in-hospital mortality in patients with pancreatitis
2008	Bedside Index for Severe Acute Pancreatitis (BISAP)	Parameters (each evaluated as 1 point on the 5-point BISAP score): BUN > 25 mg/dL Impaired mental status SIRS score >2 Age >60 Pleural effusion detected on imaging BISAP severity score: ≥3 is highly predictive of severe acute pancreatitis
2009	Japanese Scoring System (JSS)	Parameters: Base excess ≤3 mEq/L PaO_2 ≤60 BUN ≥40 mg/dL LDH ≥2 × upper limit of normal Platelet count ≤100,000/mm³ Serum calcium <7.5 mg/dL CRP ≥15 mg/dL SIRS criteria ≥3 Age ≥70 CT grade based on CT scan with contrast medium to measure pancreatic enhancement and extrapancreatic progression JSS severity score: ≥3, or CT grade ≥2, indicates that pancreatitis is severe
2012	Revised Atlanta Classification	Provides compressive definitions of morphologic features and of severity of pancreatitis; provides new information on cause, pathophysiologic features, and radiologic descriptions of pancreatic and peripancreatic collections Early clinical assessment of severity of pancreatitis: mild, moderate, or severe Mild: no evidence of organ failure and no local or systemic complications Moderate: organ failure resolving within 48 h or local or systemic complications Severe: organ failure that lasts >48 h Radiologic assessment of morphologic features of late phase of pancreatitis: CECT criteria identifying four types of pancreatic/peripancreatic collections: interstitial edematous pancreatitis, necrotizing pancreatitis, acute peripancreatic fluid collection (APFC), and pancreatic pseudocyst

AST, Aspartate aminotransferase; *BUN,* blood urea nitrogen; *CECT,* contrast medium–enhanced computed tomographic scan; *CRP,* C-reactive protein; *CT,* computed tomographic; *GCS,* Glasgow Coma Scale; *Hct,* hematocrit; *HR,* heart rate (beats per minute); *ICU,* intensive care unit; *LDH,* lactate dehydrogenase; *MAP,* mean arterial pressure; *PaO₂,* partial pressure of arterial oxygen; *PO₂,* partial pressure of oxygen; *RR,* respiratory rate (breaths per minute); *WBC,* white blood cell.

of serum triglycerides. Serum glucose levels should also be intensively monitored. The presence of hyperglycemia is a marker for poor prognosis and predisposes the patient to secondary infections by impeding neutrophil function. Hyperglycemia is treated with insulin as needed. Also present is hypoalbuminemia in association with hypocalcemia. Although the level of total calcium is low, ionized calcium levels are normal. Because total serum calcium measurements are inaccurate in these patients, ionized calcium levels should be monitored and treated if low.

Analgesia

Patients with acute pancreatitis experience debilitating pain. Patient-controlled analgesia pumps are frequently used. Parenteral narcotics are used, such as meperidine, hydromorphone, fentanyl, and morphine, along with the nonnarcotic buprenorphine. Morphine has been reported to cause a spasm of the sphincter of Oddi; although no definitive evidence for this has been found, some clinicians continue to avoid this narcotic. For pain control, patients can gradually

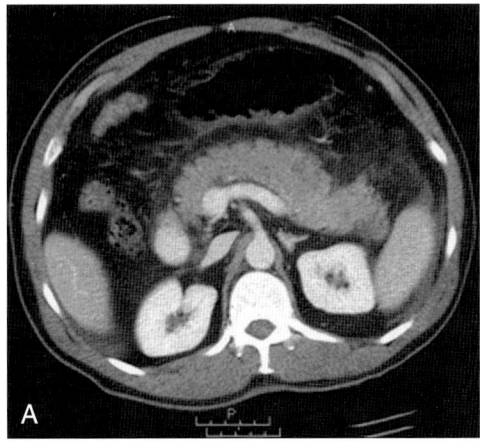
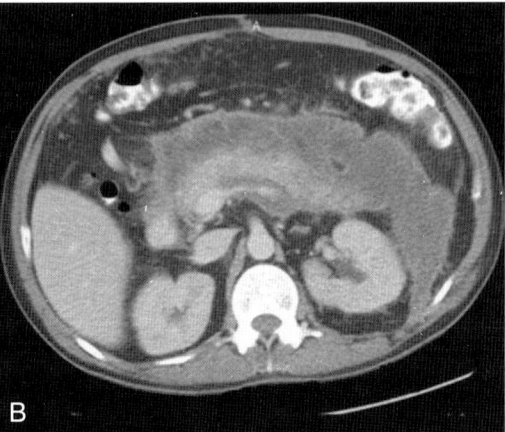

FIGURE 1 Contrast medium–enhanced computed tomographic (CECT) scan. **A,** CECT performed within the first week reveals enhancing pancreas with peripancreatic inflammation and edema with no evidence of necrosis. **B,** Delayed CECT from the same patient shows extensive pancreatic necrosis and perinecrotic fluid collection. These scans illustrate the fact that early imaging may grossly underestimate the extent of the pancreatic necrosis and injury.

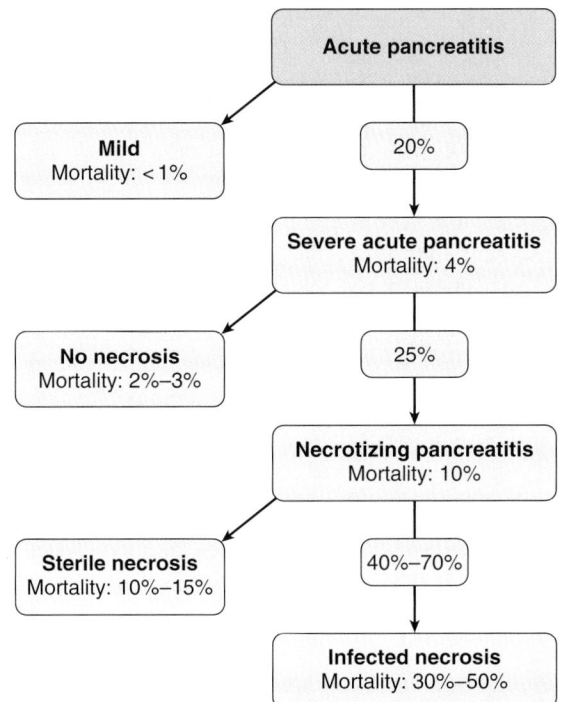

FIGURE 2 Progression of severity in acute pancreatitis. *(Adapted from Nicholson LJ: Acute pancreatitis: should we use antibiotics?* Curr Gastroenterol Rep *13(4):336–343, 2011.)*

be weaned off narcotics and shifted to nonsteroidal antiinflammatory drugs.

Nutrition

In contrast to patients with mild to moderate pancreatitis, in whom withholding enteral intake and bowel rest is one of the mainstays of treatment, patients with SAP require early initiation of nutrition. This has been demonstrated to affect outcome positively. In mild and moderate pancreatitis, patients usually advance to an oral diet within 1 week. In patients with severe pancreatitis, artificial nutrition should be considered early and initiated in the first 48 to 72 hours after hospital admission. For patients with SAP, early initiation of

nutrition (<48 hours) is associated with a decreased inflammatory response and has been shown to reduce length of hospital stay, infection (bacteremia, pneumonia, and infected necrosis), multiple-organ failure, need for surgical intervention, and mortality. A randomized controlled trial (International Standard Randomised Controlled Trial Number [ISRCTN] 18170985, "PYTHON"), currently underway, is designed to study whether initiation of very early enteral nutrition (<24 hours) reduces the incidence of infection and overall mortality in patients with SAP.

Enteral nutrition is preferred over total parenteral nutrition (TPN) because it is believed to preserve gut integrity, prevent bacterial translocation, and decrease the incidence of infectious complications of pancreatitis. An additional benefit is that it is more cost effective than TPN. Optimal enteral feeding regimens are rich in medium-chain fatty acids. Formulations enriched with these acids, such as Peptamen AF, are thought to be better tolerated by patients because of their minimal stimulation of the pancreas. In the past, there has been interest in the administration of probiotics in these patients; however, a prospective randomized controlled trial (ISRCTN38327949, "PROPATRIA") has shown patients treated with probiotic prophylaxis to have a higher risk of mortality.

Enteral nutrition can be administered via various routes. Between nasogastric and nasojejunal feeding, nasojejunal tubes are preferred because in theory they provide enteral nutrition but minimally stimulate pancreatic exocrine secretion, and they are tolerated better by patients. However, at least two randomized trials showed no difference between nasogastric and nasojejunal feeding with regard to outcome measures such as time to advancement to oral feedings, C-reactive protein levels, length of hospital stay, and analgesic requirements.

When enteral nutrition is not tolerated by the patient or does not fulfill the nutritional requirements, nutrition must be provided parenterally (TPN). Numerous studies have shown that with TPN, nutritional requirements are easily met with minimal technical and metabolic complications. In patients with severe pancreatitis, complication rates are reduced to one fourth and mortality rates to one third when TPN is initiated within 72 hours of the onset of symptoms. TPN is associated with complications such as hyperglycemia and catheter-related sepsis, however, and for these reasons, it is replaced by enteral feeding as early as tolerable. Finally, TPN may also be combined with low-volume enteral feeding, whereby trophic tube feeds are provided only for the purposes of gut epithelial integrity.

In summary, artificial nutrition is usually needed for patients with SAP. In these patients, the focus must be to provide nutrition by either route (enteral or parenteral) early (<3 days), and this improves overall outcome. As the pancreatitis resolves, attempts must be made to advance the diet back to enteral and then oral feeding.

Antibiotic Prophylaxis

The mortality rate among patients with infected pancreatic necrosis is up to 50%. The use of prophylactic antibiotics to reduce rates of infection and overall mortality has been controversial. However, results of meta-analyses and large multicenter, double-blind, randomized controlled trials suggest that prophylactic antibiotics have no role in the management of these patients. Thus, the use of antibiotics is reserved for patients in whom an infection has been documented.

Endoscopic Retrograde Cholangiopancreatography

ERCP should be considered when choledocholithiasis is suspected. Gallstone obstruction in pancreatitis is suspected when liver enzyme levels are elevated, bilirubin levels are elevated, and the common bile duct is dilated. ERCP is indicated in patients who have acute biliary pancreatitis with cholangitis and retained bile duct stones. Multiple randomized controlled trials have shown that in the subset of patients with severe pancreatitis of biliary origin and ongoing obstruction, there are significant benefits for morbidity and a trend for improved mortality rates when ERCP and biliary sphincterotomy are performed early.

MANAGEMENT OF COMPLICATIONS OF ACUTE PANCREATITIS

Pancreatic and Peripancreatic Fluid Collections

Pancreatitis may be associated with peripancreatic fluid collections in the abdomen in up to 60% of cases. If this is accompanied by signs and symptoms of infection, such as a fever and elevated WBC count that persists beyond 2 weeks, then the fluid may have to be drained and sent for microbiologic examination. If infection is documented, appropriate intravenous antibiotics must be administered. Care must be taken because occasional patients have a complex fluid collection and peripancreatic fluid collection can be diagnosed inappropriately, when in fact these cases represent pancreatic necrosis with perinecrotic fluid collection (see Figure 1, *B*), for which further technical considerations for treatment may be required.

Sterile and Infected Pancreatic Necrosis

Approximately 20% of all patients with pancreatitis develop SAP. Of these, 25% develop necrosis. The necrosis is initially sterile but can be secondarily infected in 40% to 70% of the cases. The mortality rates are 10% to 15% for sterile necrosis and can be as high as 30% to 50% for infected pancreatic necrosis. Pancreatic necrosis can be diagnosed by contrast-enhanced CT scan; the normal CT intensity of the pancreatic parenchyma is 100 to 150 Hounsfield units with intravenous contrast medium, and necrotic pancreas has a significantly lower (<40 Hounsfield units) CT intensity. Because patients with severe pancreatitis clinically appear extremely ill, with fever and an elevated WBC count, it can be challenging to determine whether sterile necrosis has become secondarily infected. CT imaging can be helpful especially when there are obvious signs of infection, such as gas in the necrotic cavity (Figure 3). If there is a question of infected necrosis, however, the patient should undergo CT imaging or ultrasonography-guided percutaneous fine-needle aspiration of the necrosis, followed by Gram stain and culture of the specimen. If the Gram stain is positive, appropriate broad-spectrum intravenous antibiotics should be started. Cultures and sensitivities can be used to narrow antibiotic coverage when available.

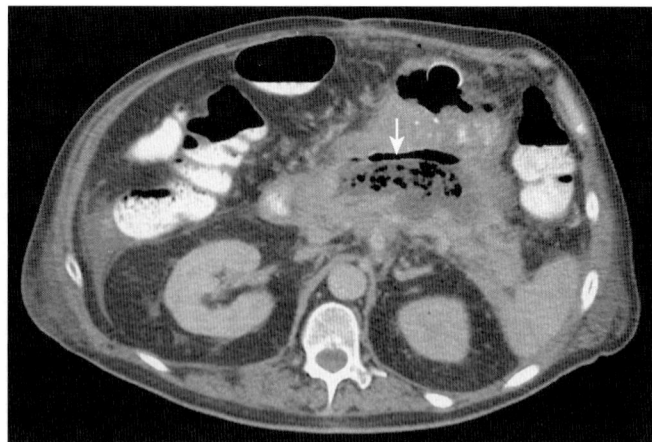

FIGURE 3 Contrast medium–enhanced computed tomographic (CECT) scan of the abdomen in a patient with infected necrotizing pancreatitis. The presence of extraluminal gas (*white arrow*) in an area of necrosis is suggestive of infection.

Infection of the pancreatic necrosis is one of the primary indications for intervention. This condition has traditionally been managed with an open necrosectomy along with an adequate drainage procedure. More recently, however, several advances in technique have expanded the potential therapeutic options for débridement. Techniques now include image-guided catheters, endoscopic and laparoscopic drainage, and standard open surgical débridement. Minimally invasive techniques are increasingly used first, with a conservative "step-up" approach, which is now more widely accepted in appropriately selected patients.

In patients with sterile necrosis, the indications for intervention include persistent pain, enteric or biliary obstruction, unresolving signs of SIRS, and persistent unwellness that last for more than 4 weeks. *Persistent unwellness* is a broad term that includes inability to tolerate oral feedings, persistent fever, nausea, vomiting, and hyperamylasemia. Nearly 50% of these patients are ultimately found to have infected necrosis. Infected pancreatic necrosis was traditionally thought to be fatal without mechanical removal of the infected tissue; however, surgeons have tried to avoid surgery and manage initially with percutaneous drainage. The rate of operative mortality for open necrosectomy is 15% for infected necrosis and 4.4% for sterile necrosis.

Regardless of the indications, pancreatic débridement should be delayed until there is a clear demarcation between the devitalized and normal tissues. This delay in intervening allows the necrosis to be organized and makes the intervention technically easier. The technical term currently used for this organized necrosis is *walled-off pancreatic necrosis* (Figure 4). Experience with numerous retrospective studies and at least one controlled trial has shown that waiting for at least 3 to 4 weeks after initial hospital admission is associated with lower rates of mortality than is an intervention carried out in the preceding period. In the only randomized controlled trial in which researchers analyzed the correlation between the timing of pancreatic débridement after onset of symptoms and the outcome, the mortality rates were 58% among patients who underwent early intervention (≤72 hours after onset of symptoms) and 27% among the patients who underwent late intervention (>12 days).

Percutaneous Drainage

Percutaneous drainage may be used to treat complications of pancreatitis. It has been shown to reduce the percentage of patients with necrotizing pancreatitis who need surgery, and it can be used to

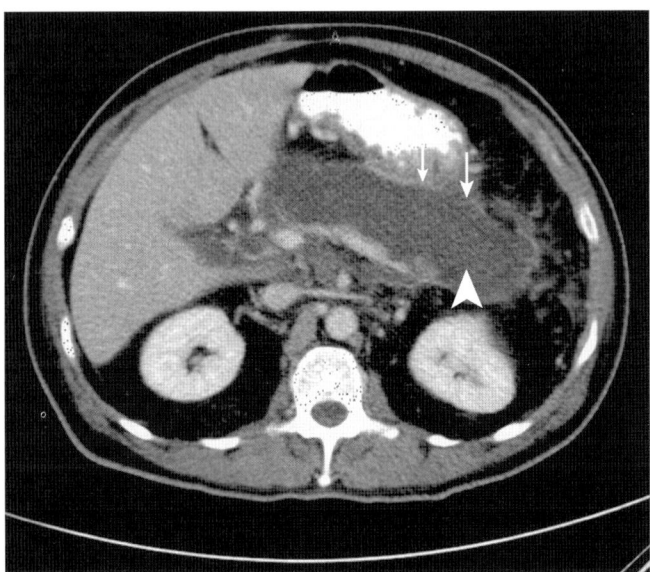

FIGURE 4 Contrast medium–enhanced computed tomographic (CECT) scan of the pancreas demonstrates walled-off pancreatic necrosis. This is a heterogeneous, well-encapsulated *(white arrows)* collection *(white arrowhead)* in the pancreatic and peripancreatic region.

stabilize critically ill patients in the 3-week to 4-week period before definitive surgery. It may be employed as an adjunct to other modalities such as endoscopic débridement. Percutaneous procedures are now part of a broader effort to minimize surgical trauma, and the aim is to reduce the source of infection rather than to evacuate all infected tissue. The "minimally invasive step-up" approach involves, as a first step, percutaneous or endoscopic drainage of infected collections. If there is no clinical response, the next step is minimally invasive retroperitoneal necrosectomy. In a large multiinstitutional randomized controlled trial by the Dutch Pancreatitis Study Group, this minimally invasive step-up approach was compared with open necrosectomy in patients with acute necrotizing pancreatitis (Minimally Invasive Step-Up Approach versus Maximal Necrosectomy in Patients with Acute Necrotising Pancreatitis [PANTER] trial). Preliminary data indicate that among patients with infected necrotizing pancreatitis who underwent the minimally invasive step-up approach, fewer major complications and deaths occurred.

A major drawback of percutaneous drainage is that it is resource intensive. After placement of the drains in the hospital, care includes frequent monitoring of the patient's status and evaluating the efficacy of the drainage. Drains may need to be repositioned or sized upward three or four times. This significantly increases the length of hospital stay. Additional catheters may also be needed. The biggest disadvantages of this technique are that it requires a dedicated and skilled interventional radiology team and that it is not appropriate for all patients. Percutaneous drainage is contraindicated in patients who have a pseudoaneurysm, are actively bleeding, have extensive solid necrosis, or are uncooperative.

Endoscopic Necrosectomy

Because of the high complication rate of open surgical necrosectomy, laparoscopic natural-orifice transluminal endoscopic surgery (NOTES) in the form of endoscopic transgastric or transduodenal necrosectomy offers a safer and minimally invasive technique for an appropriate subset of patients. In this technique, direct endoscopic drainage and necrosectomy are carried out under endoscopic ultrasound guidance.

The advantages of endoscopic transgastric/transduodenal necrosectomy are that it is less invasive, can be used in patients who are poor surgical candidates, and is associated with lower rates of morbidity and mortality. This procedure is most suitable for patients in whom the necrosis involves the lesser sac and in patients with walled-off pancreatic necrosis (WOPN). The disadvantages include a high risk of bleeding, which has been reported to be as high as 30%. Furthermore, some patients—those who have extrapancreatic necrosis, or multiple areas of necrosis that are not walled off, and those in whom the necrosis may extend into the paracolic gutters—are not candidates for this procedure. Patients undergoing endoscopic necrosectomy also have to undergo between two and six procedures for successful treatment, which increases costs significantly.

Endoscopic interventions have been compared directly with surgical interventions. Members of the Dutch pancreatitis study group compared endoscopic transgastric necrosectomy with video-assisted retroperitoneal débridement (VARD) or open necrosectomy for suspected or confirmed infected necrotizing pancreatitis in a randomized controlled trial (Pancreatitis, Endoscopic Transgastric vs. Primary Necrosectomy in Patients With Infected Necrosis [PENGUIN]). Patients were eligible for this trial if they could undergo either type of procedure, on the basis of CT imaging. The results of this study demonstrated that in comparable patients, endoscopic necrosectomy was associated with lower rates of multiple-organ failure, major complications, and mortality.

Videoscopic-Assisted Retroperitoneal Débridement

VARD was originally described as a hybrid between the endoscopic and the open translumbar approaches. In patients with pancreatic necrosis, if infection is suspected or confirmed, a 12F to 14F percutaneous drain is usually placed retroperitoneally. As described previously, a lack of clinical improvement after the placement of the drain leads to the decision of surgical intervention. The VARD surgical procedure involves a 5-cm incision in the left flank. This is followed by necrosectomy, performed with a suction device and grasping forceps under direct visualization, with the preoperative CT images and the previously placed percutaneous drain serving as a guide. After débridement can no longer be performed under direct vision, a long laparoscopic port is placed in the incision, followed by CO_2 inflation of the cavity, and a 0-degree videoscope is introduced. Additional débridement is then performed under videoscopic guidance. After the necrosectomy, irrigation is performed with saline. Two large-bore drains are introduced into the cavity, and continuous lavage is provided with normal saline (10 L/24 hours).

The proponents of this approach suggest that in comparison with pure retroperitoneal endoscopy, the small incision allows a part of the necrosectomy to be carried out under direct visualization with a shorter operative time and fewer numbers of procedures. In comparison with open necrosectomy, VARD is thought to decrease the physiologic stress of surgery to which patients with pancreatic necrosis are exposed.

Laparoscopic Surgical Necrosectomy

Laparoscopic surgical necrosectomy has been used for débridement in various approaches. In the transgastric approach, gastrotomies on the anterior and posterior gastric walls are used to enter the lesser sac. Visible pus is aspirated, and the retroperitoneum is irrigated and lavaged with normal saline. Suction and débridement with nontraumatic forceps are used to perform the necrosectomy. The lesser sac is irrigated after the débridement is complete, and the peritoneal cavity is lavaged before the abdomen is closed. In one series involving laparoscopic pancreatic necrosectomy, the mortality rate among noninfected patients was 10%. A hand-assisted laparoscopic surgical technique was also described. The surgical approach into the lesser sac was through the transverse mesocolon. The hand was used for enlarging the incision in the transverse mesocolon, while avoiding injury to the middle colic vessels, and the devitalized tissue was débrided by means of gentle finger dissection. After the completion of the débridement, postoperative drainage was provided by closed suction drain. The overall mortality rate was reported to be 11%.

Laparoscopic necrosectomy may be advantageous in carefully selected patients. It offers shorter lengths of stay, earlier postoperative recovery, and earlier return to work than does open surgery. However, laparoscopic necrosectomy has limitations, and patient selection is key to the success of the operation. Depending on the extent of necrosis, only a small subset of patients may be candidates for this approach.

Open Surgical Management of Acute Pancreatitis

Surgical Technique

There are numerous variations in the intraoperative technique and postoperative drainage of patients with acute pancreatitis. Each type of surgical procedure is best suited for a certain case; there are no guidelines or controlled data regarding which surgical procedure must be employed for a given patient. Nevertheless, the preoperative workup and the governing philosophy remain the same.

CECT is used as a guide to determine the location of the necrotic tissue and fluid collections. The incision used for the approach is either midline or subcostal. The lesser sac is approached through the gastrocolic ligament or by the transmesocolic route, depending on the surgeon's preference. In the transmesocolic approach, the preferred entry site into the lesser sac is the avascular region left of the ligament of Treitz (Figure 5, *A*). After the focus of necrosis is exposed, blunt dissection must be carefully performed to remove necrotic tissues that have separated, so as to avoid injury to large vessels in the area. If preoperative imaging suggests fluid collections in the perinephric and paracolic areas, these must also be entered and drained. After dissection, generous irrigation and gentle abrasion with sponge-covered fingertips must be performed. Significant bleeding may occur and must be dealt with via packing or suture ligature as appropriate. During the operation, samples of pancreatic and peripancreatic tissues must also be sent for microbiologic and bacteriologic testing. Methods to provide drainage after necrosectomy are (1) closed packing, (2) open packing, (3) planned staged repeat laparotomies, and (4) continuous lavage of the lesser sac.

Closed Packing

In the technique that is preferred at the Massachusetts General Hospital, the goal is for the initial débridement to be as complete as possible. Every effort is made to find, expose, and débride all foci of necrosis identified on preoperative CECT. The cavities resulting from

FIGURE 5 Open necrosectomy. **A,** Necrosectomy is performed through the transverse mesocolon. **B,** Multiple stuffed Penrose drains used for closed packing of the necrotic cavity after an open necrosectomy. **C,** The abdomen with stuffed Penrose and closed suction drains in place. **D,** Interval imaging with contrast medium–enhanced computed tomographic (CECT) scan of a patient after pancreatic necrosectomy, demonstrating the presence of the drains in the pancreatic bed and a collapsed necrotic cavity around the drains.

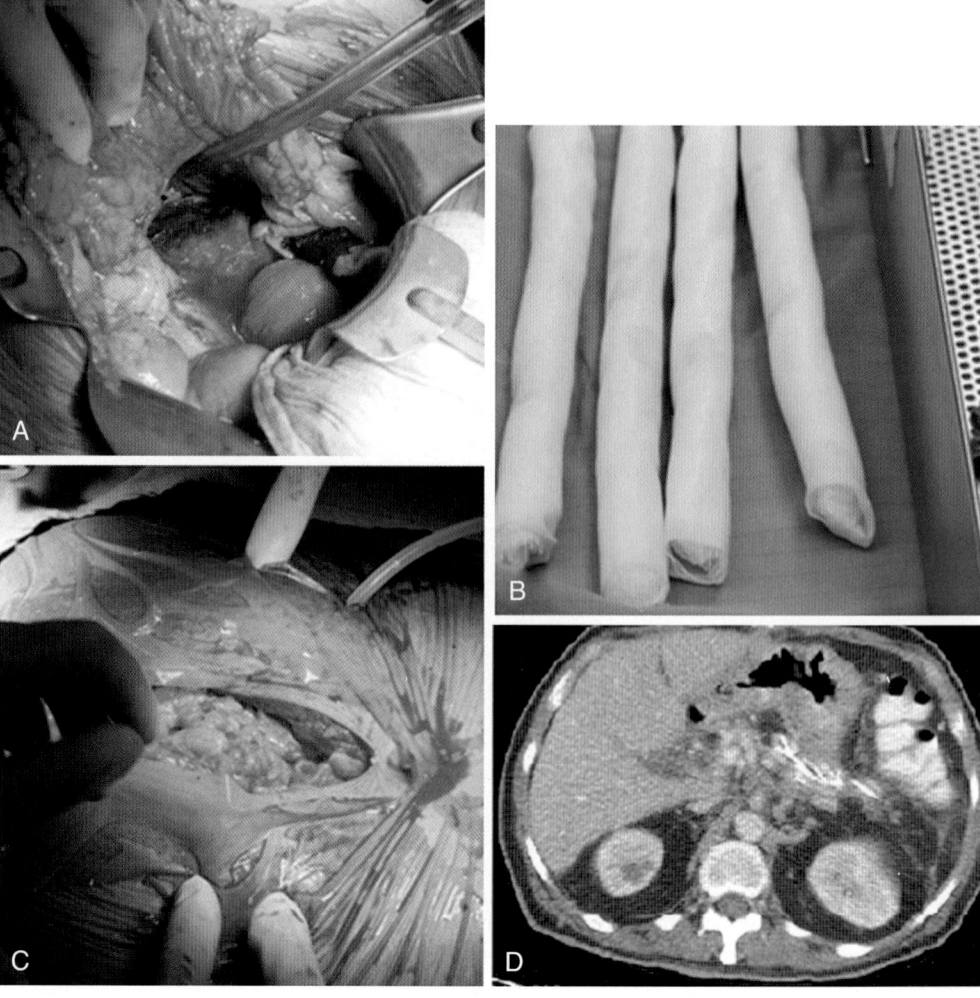

débridement are packed with gauze-stuffed ¾-inch Penrose drains and silicone rubber closed-suction drains (see Figure 5). The gauze-stuffed Penrose drains are removed first to allow the cavities to gradually collapse. The closed-suction drains are removed last, only after the drain output becomes minimal. In studies of this technique for patients with sterile and infected pancreatic necrosis, researchers have reported average postoperative lengths of stay between 27 and 34 days, reoperation rates as low as 15%, and mortality rates as low as 4% to 6%.

Open Packing, Planned Staged Relaparotomies With Repeated Lavage, and Continuous Lavage of Lesser Sac and Retroperitoneum

Certain techniques have been described historically, but these are no longer in widespread use. They are briefly described here. *Open packing* was reserved for patients in whom surgical intervention was necessary early. An overall mortality rate of 73% and procedural morbidity rate of 73% were described for this technique. *Planned staged repeat laparotomies* are associated with significant morbidity. This technique, like open packing, is used primarily when intervention has to be performed early and there is no clear demarcation between healthy and necrotic tissue. According to a published experience of this technique, the overall mortality rate was 17%, major complications included pancreatic fistula (78%) and hemorrhage (26%), and median length of stay in the hospital was 50 days. In addition to staged repeat laparotomies, the problem of leftover infection or necrotic tissue and subsequent intra-abdominal sepsis was previously addressed with continuous lavage of the lesser sac. This technique is not only cumbersome but also associated with increased rates of morbidity and mortality. It is generally accepted that closed packing is superior to open packing and staged repeat laparotomies; it causes less intra-abdominal and systemic trauma to the patient and results in better outcomes.

SUMMARY

Demographics

Pancreatitis causes 300,000 hospital admissions per year. Alcohol and gallstones account for 80% to 90% of all causes. Of all affected patients, 20% progress to SAP. One in four has necrosis, and 40% to 70% acquire infection. The mortality rate among patients with mild pancreatitis is less than 1%, and that among patients with infected necrosis can be as high as 50%.

Severity Assessment

Numerous scoring systems that are based on biochemical and clinical factors may help identify patients likely to develop severe pancreatitis. Imaging-based assessment of severity is usually more helpful during the second phase of pancreatitis.

Intensive Care Unit Admission

It is important to use objective metrics and determine early whether a patient needs to be admitted to the intensive care unit. This results in better outcomes for patients and better utilization of resources.

Supportive Care

Supportive care involves volume replacement, pain control, electrolyte balance, metabolic management, and achievement of euglycemia. No data suggest usefulness of prophylactic antibiotics.

Nutrition

NPO status and bowel rest are adequate for patients with mild pancreatitis. Early initiation of nutrition in patients with moderate and severe pancreatitis improves outcome. Although enteral nutrition is better with regard to gut integrity and has a lower incidence of infectious complications, TPN should be given when needed.

Minimally Invasive Step-Up Approach

In order to minimize the physiologic stress of surgery, the first step in management of infected pancreatic necrosis is percutaneous drainage. A gradual step-up approach is preferred, with minimally invasive and then open necrosectomy utilized successively in patients with no clinical response.

SUGGESTED READINGS

Banks PA, Bollen TL, Dervenis C, et al: Classification of acute pancreatitis—2012: revision of the Atlanta classification and definitions by international consensus, *Gut* 62(1):102–111, 2013.

Banks PA, Freeman ML: Practice guidelines in acute pancreatitis, *Am J Gastroenterol* 101(10):2379–2400, 2006.

Fernández-del Castillo C: Open pancreatic necrosectomy: indications in the minimally invasive era, *J Gastrointest Surg* 15(7):1089–1091, 2011.

MDCalc: *APACHE II score for ICU mortality* [online scoring calculator]. http://www.mdcalc.com/apache-ii-score-for-icu-mortality/. Accessed July 19, 2013.

Navaneethan U, Vege SS, Chari ST, et al: Minimally invasive techniques in pancreatic necrosis, *Pancreas* 38(8):867–875, 2009.

Nicholson LJ: Acute pancreatitis: should we use antibiotics? *Curr Gastroenterol Rep* 13(4):336–343, 2011.

van Santvoort HC, Bakker OJ, Bollen TL, et al: A conservative and minimally invasive approach to necrotizing pancreatitis improves outcome, *Gastroenterology* 141(4):1254–1263, 2011.

THE MANAGEMENT OF GALLSTONE PANCREATITIS

Alexandra Briggs, MD, and Stanley W. Ashley, MD

OVERVIEW

Gallstone disease remains one of the most common causes of acute pancreatitis in the United States, accounting for up to 40% to 60% of cases. Although the vast majority of patients have mild or moderate disease, up to 20% have a severe course marked by significant morbidity and mortality. Early determination of disease severity can help guide both medical and surgical management, and prediction systems based on both imaging and clinical data exist to help stratify patients into risk categories. Patients with mild disease should undergo cholecystectomy during the index admission because of a significant risk of recurrent symptoms associated with delayed intervention. In patients considered too high risk for surgical intervention, endoscopic interventions may help prevent recurrent episodes of gallstone pancreatitis. Severe disease requires admission to an ICU and aggressive medical management. In this cohort, some patients may benefit from endoscopic intervention, and cholecystectomy should usually be performed after resolution of the acute episode. The presence of pancreatic fluid collections, pseudocysts, or necrosis can alter the timing of both endoscopic and surgical intervention. This chapter discusses in detail the determination of the severity of disease and both endoscopic and surgical interventions for management.

PRESENTATION AND DIAGNOSIS

Diagnosis of acute pancreatitis according to the Atlanta Classification requires two of the following three criteria: (1) an elevation in the level of serum amylase or lipase to more than three times the upper limit of normal; (2) abdominal pain characteristic of pancreatitis; and (3) characteristic findings of pancreatitis on computed tomographic (CT) scan or other imaging. Typically, patients present with epigastric pain with radiation to the back, which can be accompanied by nausea and vomiting. The severity of the abdominal pain and tenderness on examination can vary widely depending on the extent of disease. Furthermore, in patients with severe disease, early signs of organ failure or systemic inflammatory response syndrome (SIRS) may be apparent even at the time of presentation. A full laboratory panel, including complete blood count (CBC), basic metabolic panel (BMP) with liver function tests (LFTs), and lipase tests, should be obtained. Measurement of serum lipase has been shown to be more sensitive and specific than serum amylase, given that the pancreas is the only source of serum lipase production. In patients with severe symptoms, an arterial blood gas value provides useful information regarding oxygenation and acid-base status. Although CT scan is not required for the workup of patients with acute pancreatitis, it can be helpful in diagnosis and can aid in the prediction of disease severity. Ultrasound scan can also provide useful information as to the etiology of acute pancreatitis with assessment for biliary disease.

Acute pancreatitis can have many potential causes, with alcohol abuse and gallstone disease accounting for most cases in the United States. The diagnosis of gallstone pancreatitis can be made with the confirmation of cholelithiasis, choledocholithiasis or gallbladder sludge with imaging and when other causes have been ruled out. Once a diagnosis has been made, patients should be promptly triaged based on severity of disease to either an inpatient ward or an ICU setting for further treatment.

Determination of Disease Severity

The treatment of gallstone pancreatitis should be guided by the severity of disease, given the disparate courses that the disease can take and the management strategies required. Severe disease occurs in 20% of patients, with significant acid-base disturbances, multiorgan failure, pancreatic necrosis and infection, and an increased mortality rate of up to 30%. Early identification of patients with severe disease allows for prompt intensive treatment and can help predict outcomes and the likelihood of complications. Both clinical and CT scan–based scoring systems exist for predicting severity in acute pancreatitis. A recent study of two clinical and seven CT scan–based scoring systems revealed no difference in the predictive accuracy between the two modalities. No consensus exists as to the best prediction system; however, the clinical scores that can be used in the first 24 hours may provide the most prompt and universally applicable assessment.

The most well-known clinical prediction system is the Ranson score, which is calculated with laboratory values both on admission and after 48 hours. A modified version of the Ranson criteria was developed specifically for biliary pancreatitis, with an initial score greater than 3 predicting severe disease. However, the full predictive value of this system requires the addition of data points 48 hours after admission, at which point the benefits of early identification and management of severe disease may already be lost.

One scoring system that can be used within the first 24 hours of presentation is the Acute Physiology and Chronic Health Evaluation II (APACHE-II) score. This is a complex system calculated with 12 data points that includes laboratory values, age, and mental status and also accounts for significant patient comorbidities. Although published cutoff values for severe pancreatitis vary, an APACHE-II score greater than 5 to 10 can be considered predictive of severe disease. This is a valuable tool, but it does require significant data collection and calculation to obtain.

The development of the Bedside Index for Severity in Acute Pancreatitis (BISAP) score has allowed for the simplified prediction of mortality within the first 24 hours of presentation (Table 1). A score between 0 and 5 is determined with criteria for age, blood urea nitrogen (BUN), presence of pleural effusions on imaging, presence of SIRS, and impaired mental status. BISAP scores of more than 3 correlate with higher rates of patient mortality and increased risk of organ failure, persistent organ failure, and pancreatic necrosis. Multiple validation studies have established the utility of this scoring system, and it may be more easily applied by clinicians given its relative simplicity in comparison with other systems.

Attempts have been made to use individual laboratory tests as predictors in pancreatitis. Although serial hematocrit values have been advocated as a useful marker of hemoconcentration and progression of disease, the sensitivity and specificity of this test has been highly variable in large scale reviews. One recent multicenter study showed that admission BUN value was an accurate marker for predicting mortality, with higher BUN values in nonsurvivors. In addition, it revealed that the odds ratio for mortality increased by 2.2 with each 5 mg/dL increase in BUN level during the first 24 hours. Although debate still exists on the utility of single laboratory studies in predicting disease severity and outcome, these easily measured values can provide additional information for clinicians during treatment.

Multiple scoring systems exist that use findings on CT scan as predictors of disease severity. The CT severity index combines the Balthazar CT scan score, based on the extent of pancreatic inflammation, with a separate point scale for the extent of pancreatic

TABLE 1: Bedside Index for Severity in Acute Pancreatitis (BISAP) score

Blood urea nitrogen (BUN)	>25 mg/dL
Age	>60 y
Impaired mental status	Glasgow Coma Scale (GCS) score <15
Systemic inflammatory response syndrome (SIRS)	Two or more of: Temperature, <36°C or >38°C Respiratory rate, >20 breaths/min; or P_aCO_2, <32 mm Hg Pulse, >90 beats/min White blood cell count, <4000 or >12,000 cells/mm^3 or >10% immature bands
Pleural effusion	Present on imaging

BISAP score ranges from 0 to 5, with 1 point for the presence of each variable within 24 hours of presentation.

TABLE 2: Computed tomographic scan severity index

Pancreatic inflammation		Points
Normal pancreas	Grade A	0
Pancreatic enlargement	Grade B	1
Pancreatic with inflammation of peripancreatic fat	Grade C	2
Single peripancreatic fluid collection	Grade D	3
Two or more fluid collections or retroperitoneal air	Grade E	4

Pancreatic necrosis	Additional points
None	0
≤30%	2
30%-50%	4
>50%	6

TABLE 3: Modified computed tomographic scan severity index

	Points
Pancreatic Inflammation	
Normal pancreas	0
Intrinsic pancreatic abnormalities with or without inflammatory changes in peripancreatic fat	2
Pancreatic or peripancreatic fluid collection or peripancreatic fat necrosis	4
Pancreatic Necrosis	
None	0
≤30%	2
>30%	4
Extrapancreatic Complications (One or More)	
Pleural effusion, ascites, vascular complications, parenchymal complications, or gastrointestinal tract involvement	2

undergo immediate CT scan on presentation; therefore, these systems may not always provide early guidance for patient care.

Timely determination of disease severity in acute pancreatitis can predict both mortality and complications and facilitate early triage of patients to the best treatment algorithms. Both clinical and CT scan–based scoring systems can be a useful adjunct in patient care, but they still have limitations in their predictive ability. However, careful clinical assessment of the patient on presentation combined with the use of these tools can aid in the appropriate initial course of treatment. Continued and dynamic assessment of patients over the first 24 to 48 hours of treatment can provide additional prognostic information and should guide subsequent therapy.

TREATMENT

Mild Disease

Initial management of mild gallstone pancreatitis involves resuscitation and electrolyte repletion in an inpatient monitored setting. Hydration with intravenous (IV) fluids should be adjusted as needed to maintain urine output (UOP) of 0.5 to 1 mg/kg/h, with boluses given as needed for oliguria or hypotension. Placement of a Foley catheter should be strongly considered for adequate monitoring of UOP and fluid status in patients in whom voids cannot be reliably measured. Electrolyte abnormalities should be corrected and followed with serial laboratory measurements at least daily. In addition, CBC, LFTs, and lipase values should be obtained daily. Additional laboratory tests may be obtained with changes in clinical status. Antibiotic therapy is not indicated in patients with mild disease. Patients should be kept on nothing by mouth (NPO), with serial abdominal examinations performed to follow the degree of abdominal tenderness. If a patient has worsening examination results, hemodynamic instability, or worsening laboratory values or fails to respond to treatment, transfer to the ICU is indicated for more aggressive management.

necrosis (Table 2). Severity is subsequently stratified with scores of 0 to 3 for mild disease, 4 to 6 for moderate disease, and 7 to 10 for severe disease. This method has since been modified (Table 3), and the cutoffs adjusted to 0 to 2, 4 to 6, and 8 to 10 for mild, moderate, and severe disease, respectively. The modified system accounts for extrapancreatic complications and also simplifies the stratification of inflammation and necrosis from the initial scoring system. These changes have resulted in improved correlation of severity with clinical parameters such as hospital stay, infection rate, and need for intervention and, unlike the original system, also correlated severity with the development of organ failure. However, not all patients

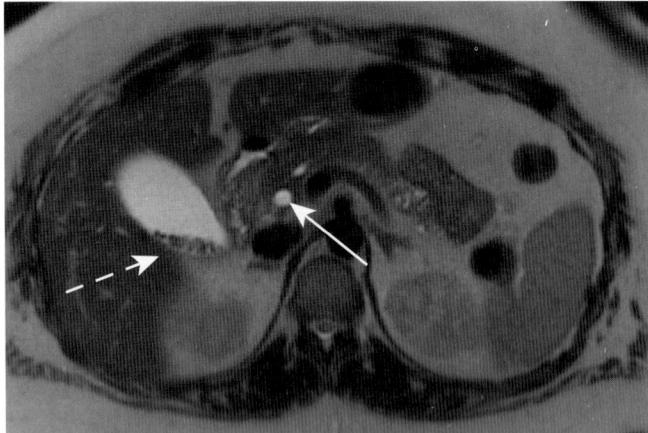

FIGURE 1 Magnetic resonance cholangiopancreatography image shows cholelithiasis *(dashed white arrow)* and a dilated common bile duct *(white arrow)*.

Definitive management for mild disease is either laparoscopic or open cholecystectomy during the index hospitalization once the acute symptoms have resolved. Given the well-established advantages of laparoscopy over laparotomy, a minimally invasive approach should be attempted in all suitable cases. Although initially there was much debate regarding the appropriate timing of cholecystectomy, multiple studies have shown an unacceptably high rate of recurrence of both gallstone pancreatitis (as high as 90% in some studies) and other biliary symptoms in patients awaiting interval cholecystectomy after discharge from the hospital. In one systematic review, up to 33% of patients awaiting interval cholecystectomy were readmitted with pancreatitis, biliary colic, or acute cholecystitis. Furthermore, the time to recurrence may be as short as within 2 weeks of discharge for more than one third of patients. Given this evidence, cholecystectomy should be performed during the index admission, once patients are adequately resuscitated and show clinical signs of improvement, including decreased abdominal pain. Both single-institution and nationwide studies in the United States and Europe have shown that compliance with this recommendation remains poor, with many patients discharged from the hospital without cholecystectomy. Steps should be taken to improve adherence to this guideline to prevent disease recurrences and complications.

Choledocholithiasis and Cholangitis

Choledocholithiasis may be suspected in patients with elevated alkaline phosphatase and total bilirubin values on presentation. Although ultrasound scan may reveal an enlarged common bile duct (CBD) or even the presence of CBD stones, its sensitivity is only 40% to 60% for the detection of choledocholithiasis. Magnetic resonance cholangiopancreatography (MRCP) is a more accurate method for the detection of CBD stones and has the advantages of being noninvasive and requiring no nephrotoxic contrast administration. A more invasive but highly sensitive and specific approach is endoscopic ultrasound (EUS). The most invasive approach is endoscopic retrograde cholangiopancreatography (ERCP), but it has the advantage of being both diagnostic and therapeutic (Figures 1 and 2). Stone retrieval can be completed at the time of ERCP, and when indicated, endoscopic sphincterotomy (ES) can also be performed. Approaches to the diagnosis of CBD stones vary among clinicians; there is no established standard for workup of these patients. In patients with mild symptoms, it is reasonable to trend liver function tests and only pursue additional imaging to diagnose CBD stones in those patients with persistently elevated results. If choledocholithiasis is diagnosed before cholecystectomy, ERCP and ES may be performed before surgery, avoiding the need to address the common duct during

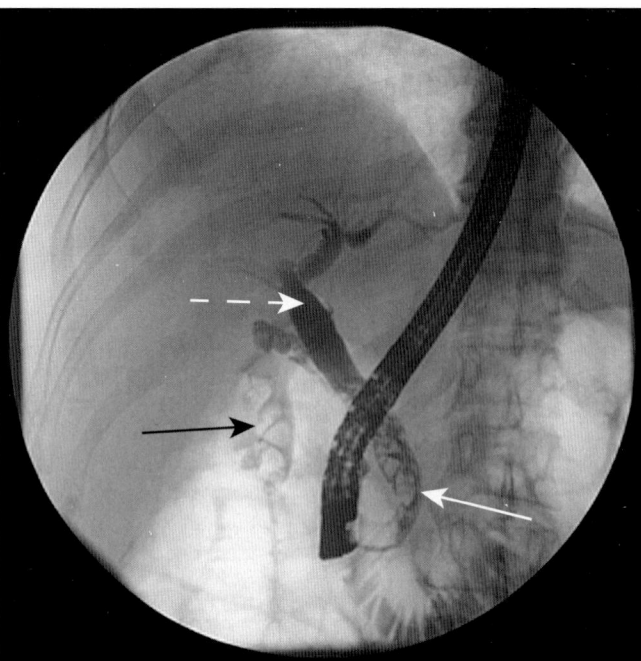

FIGURE 2 Endoscopic retrograde cholangiopancreatography image shows cholelithiasis *(solid black arrow)* and choledocholithiasis *(solid white arrow)* with associated common bile duct dilation *(dashed white arrow)* that requires decompression and stone removal.

surgery. If there is failure to retrieve the stones during ERCP, operative bile duct exploration with stone removal can be completed at the time of cholecystectomy. Several studies have suggested that if this can be accomplished laparoscopically, it may be the most cost-effective approach. Intraoperative cholangiography (IOC) can also be performed to confirm the patency of the CBD at the time of cholecystectomy. If filling defects are detected, laparoscopic transcystic duct bile duct exploration or even choledochotomy can be completed to remove visualized stones, but this depends on the skills of the surgeon, which can vary widely. Alternatively, in some cases, postoperative ERCP can be considered for stone retrieval after positive IOC; however, better outcomes have been shown in patients managed via laparoscopic bile duct exploration, and the unusual stone that cannot be removed endoscopically makes many surgeons uncomfortable with this approach.

Although the role of early ERCP in prevention of the evolution of gallstone pancreatitis remains controversial, all patients with evidence of cholangitis on presentation should undergo ERCP and ES. In addition to the characteristic abdominal pain seen on presentation, these patients have fever and jaundice, commonly known as Charcot's triad. More seriously ill patients can exhibit signs of shock and altered mental status in addition to the previous symptoms, a constellation of findings known as Reynold's pentad. Urgent or semi-urgent endoscopic decompression is indicated in most patients with evidence of biliary obstruction on imaging.

Patients at High Risk

In patients with mild disease who cannot safely undergo operative intervention, ERCP/ES can instead be used as a treatment modality. Age alone should not be used as a cutoff for laparoscopic or open cholecystectomy because outcomes in elderly patients without significant comorbidities are acceptable. However, if coexisting medical conditions suggest unacceptable risk to operative intervention in a patient of any age, alternatives should be considered. The use of ERCP and ES has been shown to significantly decrease the likelihood of recurrent biliary events, with published recurrence rates for gallstone pancreatitis between 0 and 6%, but because of healing of the sphincterotomy, the time interval may be limited; this has not been completely defined. However, although the risk of other biliary complications including colic or acute cholecystitis is lower in these patients than in those undergoing no intervention at all, the recurrence rate remains significant at up to 20%. Cholecystectomy provides the only definitive treatment for gallstone disease, but ERCP/ES can significantly decrease recurrence and is a useful alternative for those patients who cannot safely undergo operative intervention. As with cholecystectomy, this intervention should be completed during the index admission.

Pregnant Patients

Although physiologic changes during pregnancy can predispose women to the formation of gallstones, acute pancreatitis from all causes remains a rare event seen only in every 1 in 1000 to 5000 pregnancies. Initial management of gallstone pancreatitis should be similar to that of nonpregnant patients, with hydration, bowel rest, and careful monitoring. Obstetric consultation should be obtained when appropriate for fetal monitoring. Without definitive intervention during index hospitalization, pregnant patients are also at high risk of symptom recurrence. Laparoscopic cholecystectomy has been shown to be safe during all trimesters of pregnancy and should be pursued in accordance with current guidelines. Placing pregnant patients in the left lateral decubitus position and minimizing the use of reverse Trendelenburg's position can aid in the maintenance of adequate cardiac output, given the aortocaval compression that can occur with a gravid uterus and with insufflation. Additional precautions should be taken to limit the time and extent of insufflation, and entry into the abdomen should be carefully completed to minimize risk of injury to the uterus during the procedure. In patients in whom choledocholithiasis is suspected, MRCP can be safely used to assess the CBD without any radiation exposure to the fetus and to determine whether ERCP is indicated. There have not been large-scale studies of ERCP/ES in pregnancy; however it may be used safely in centers with sufficient experience, with precautions taken to minimize radiation exposure to the fetus. In pregnant patients deemed at high risk for cholecystectomy, ERCP/ES may be a feasible alternative to operative intervention until after delivery.

Severe Disease

Medical Management

Patients with evidence of severe gallstone pancreatitis should be immediately transferred to an ICU for aggressive medical management. Although insertion of a central venous catheter and arterial line are at the discretion of the clinician, they should be placed in critically ill patients for adequate monitoring and to facilitate care. Foley catheters should be inserted in all patients for careful monitoring of urine output. A constant IV fluid maintenance rate should be started, with additional boluses and adjustment as needed. Adequacy of resuscitation can be measured with the careful monitoring of acid-base status and through the maintenance of a mean arterial pressure (MAP) more than 60 mm Hg and urine output of at least 0.5 mg/kg/h. Electrolytes should be closely monitored and repleted because these may become significantly abnormal from both the fluid extravasation secondary to the disease process and the large volume resuscitation. In addition to serial electrolyte monitoring, CBC, LFTs and lipase values should again be followed. In these seriously ill patients, arterial blood gas (ABG) monitoring can provide valuable information regarding resuscitation status and oxygenation.

No role exists for antibiotics in patients with gallstone pancreatitis without proven necrosis. The use of prophylactic antibiotics in patients with necrosis remains controversial, with no clear consensus on whether any reduction results in either morbidity or mortality.

Concerns regarding possible fungal infection or antibiotic resistance with the use of prophylactic antibiotics have not been consistently proven, and there is no established role for the use of prophylactic antifungal therapy. A recent Cochrane review of antibiotic use in patients with acute pancreatitis and CT scan evidence of necrosis showed no statistically significant difference in mortality, pancreatic necrosis infection rates, or overall infection rates. However, an association was found between imipenem use specifically and a significant reduction in pancreatic infection rate, with a relative risk of 0.34 (confidence interval, 0.13 to 0.84.) Given these data, imipenem may be considered for use in patients with pancreatic necrosis; however, no adequately powered studies to date have provided definitive evidence of benefit. Antibiotics are indicated if cholangitis is a concern.

The role of nutrition in patients with severe pancreatitis has also been the subject of multiple studies. When possible, enteral administration is preferred to parenteral nutrition because it has been shown to decrease infection rates, organ failure, and operative interventions. Although the data are limited, mortality and length of hospital stay may also be lower in patients receiving enteral nutrition. No definitive evidence exists for whether gastric or jejunal feeding is the best route of enteral administration, although many have postulated that jejunal feeding is preferred to minimize pancreatic stimulation. At this time, there is also no current evidence to differentiate any specific type of diet or supplementation as preferable. If there is evidence of gastrointestinal complications such as severe ileus that preclude enteral feeding, parenteral nutrition should be initiated instead, given the overall benefits of providing nutrition in critically ill patients in a highly catabolic state.

Intervention in Severe Pancreatitis

Most patients in whom severe gallstone pancreatitis develops also require cholecystectomy for definitive management. However, in contrast to mild disease, intervention should be delayed until the acute episode has resolved and inflammation has decreased. Although little data exist, anecdotal experience suggests that the risk of recurrent pancreatitis in a patient with severe necrosis is low. In addition, patients with development of complications such as pseudocysts and fluid collections during the acute episode can be followed and reevaluated before interval cholecystectomy. In some cases, these may resolve spontaneously without additional intervention. However, if pseudocysts or collections are persistent, these can be addressed at the same time as the interval cholecystectomy.

The role of ERCP/ES in patients with severe pancreatitis remains a topic of significant debate. As previously mentioned, ERCP/ES should be performed urgently in patients with cholangitis. However, in patients without biliary obstruction and cholangitis, there may be no benefit to early endoscopic intervention. A recent Cochrane review showed no difference in complications or mortality between patients with gallstone pancreatitis managed medically versus those undergoing early ERCP. Although this review included patients with all levels of disease severity, no clear evidence shows that disease severity has any influence on ERCP outcomes.

Management of Pancreatic Necrosis

Patients with severe pancreatitis are at risk of development of infected pancreatic necrosis, which is associated with significant mortality as a result of sepsis and multiorgan failure (Figure 3). Differentiation between sterile and infected pancreatic necrosis is important because multiple studies have shown that a conservative approach to the management of sterile pancreatic necrosis can be successful. Repeat CT imaging in patients with systemic signs of infection such as fever and leukocytosis can be a useful tool in establishing the presence and extent of necrosis. If infected necrosis is suspected, fine-needle aspiration (FNA) can be used to establish this diagnosis. However, this could also introduce infection to a previously sterile collection.

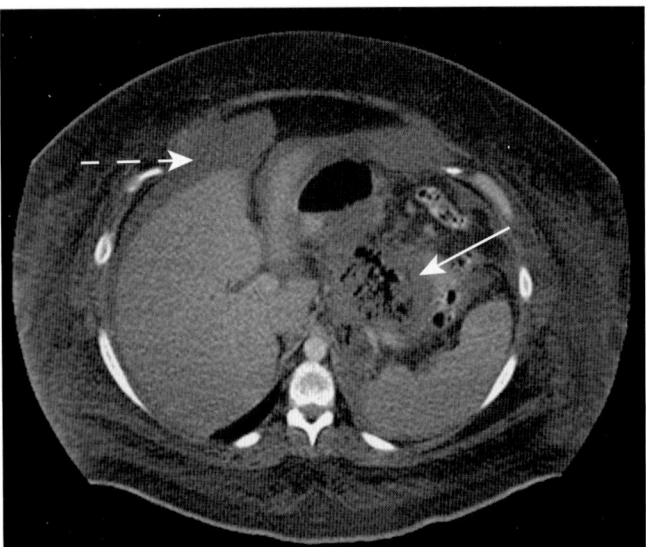

FIGURE 3 Computed tomographic scan image shows significant pancreatic necrosis *(white arrow)* and ascites *(dashed white arrow).*

The approach to patients with infected pancreatic necrosis has changed significantly with the use of percutaneous, endoscopic, and minimally invasive interventions. Prior studies have revealed that percutaneous drainage can be an effective first approach to infected necrosis, with 35% of patients in one randomized controlled trial

requiring only this intervention without the need for more invasive procedures. Less-invasive approaches are associated with decreased complication rates when compared with open necrosectomy. A recent randomized controlled trial of 22 patients compared endoscopic transgastric necrosectomy with surgical necronectomy and showed decreased serum levels of the inflammatory marker interleukin-6 (IL-6) and a decrease in a clinical composite endpoint composed of major complications and death. Multiple groups have now proposed a step-up approach to infected necrosis, starting with percutaneous drainage and then moving towards endoscopic or minimally invasive approaches as indicated. When feasible, these approaches should be considered in all patients with infected necrosis prior to open necrosectomy.

SUGGESTED READINGS

Bakker OJ, van Santvoort HC, van Brunschot S, et al: Endoscopic transgastric vs surgical necrosectomy for infected necrotizing pancreatitis a randomized trial, *JAMA* 307:1053–1061, 2012.

Bollen TL, Singh VK, Maurer R, et al: A comparative evaluation of radiologic and clinical scoring systems in the early prediction of severity in acute pancreatitis, *Am J Gastroenterol* 107:612–619, 2012.

Van Baal MC, Besselink MG, Bakker OJ, et al: Timing of cholecystectomy after mild biliary pancreatitis a systematic review, *Ann Surg* 255:860–866, 2012.

Van Santvoort HC, Besselink MG, Bakker OJ, et al: A step-up approach or open necrosectomy for necrotizing pancreatitis, *N Engl J Med* 362:1491–1502, 2010.

Villatoro E, Mulla M, Larvin M: Antibiotic therapy for prophylaxis against infection of pancreatic necrosis in acute pancreatitis, *Cochrane Database System Rev* 5, 2010.

PANCREAS DIVISUM AND OTHER VARIANTS OF DOMINANT DORSAL DUCT ANATOMY

**Robert Evans Heithaus Jr., MD, and
Steven B. Goldin, MD, PhD**

INTRODUCTION

Pancreas divisum refers to a variety of pancreatic ductal anatomic variations. Although commonly thought of in the context of pancreatitis, pancreas divisum is not a disease. "Normal" pancreatic ductal anatomy is present in approximately 80% of individuals. In people with normal anatomy, most pancreatic enzyme secretions (approximately 2 L/d) enter the duodenum via the ampulla of Vater or major papilla. People with pancreas divisum have a dominant dorsal duct that is responsible for draining most pancreatic enzyme secretions via the minor pancreatic duct or duct of Santorini. This condition occurs in up to 20% of the population, 95% of whom never have medical problems related to the ductal anatomy. Approximately 5% of those with pancreas divisum have pancreatitis develop as a result of the variant anatomy, which may be coupled to other predisposing

factors. Understanding how pancreas divisum predisposes to pancreatitis requires knowledge of the embryologic development of the pancreas. This knowledge allows the clinician to appropriately evaluate and treat individuals with pancreatitis as a result of variant anatomy.

PANCREATIC EMBRYOLOGIC DEVELOPMENT

At approximately 30 days' gestation, the endodermal lining of the duodenum forms separate ventral and dorsal pancreatic buds (Figure 1). As the duodenum changes in shape and size to form its C-shaped curve, the ventral pancreatic bud migrates clockwise into a location inferior to the dorsal pancreatic bud (see Figure 1). By the 6th week of gestation, the dorsal and ventral pancreatic buds are contiguous with each other; and by the 8th week, they fuse. The ventral pancreatic bud becomes the inferior portion of the head (also known as the uncinate process), and the dorsal bud forms the remaining portion of the head, body, and tail of the pancreas (Figure 2). The main pancreatic duct (duct of Wirsung) is formed by the fusion of the distal portion of the dorsal pancreatic duct with the entire ventral pancreatic duct. The main pancreatic duct then typically joins with the common bile duct to form a common channel that enters the duodenum at the major papilla (ampulla of Vater). The distal portion of the dorsal pancreatic duct (near the duodenum) may persist as the accessory pancreatic duct (duct of Santorini) or may be totally obliterated (Figure 3, *A* and *B*).

A number of variations in pancreatic ductal anatomy may occur during development. Pancreas divisum occurs when the ventral and dorsal ductal systems do not fuse completely. This condition happens

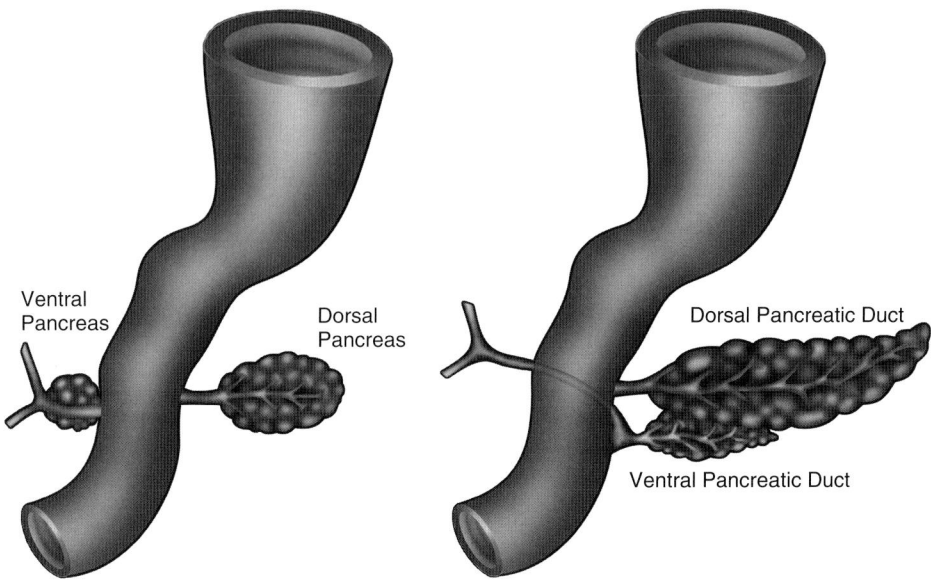

Ventral Pancreas

Dorsal Pancreas

Dorsal Pancreatic Duct

Ventral Pancreatic Duct

FIGURE 1 Dorsal and ventral pancreatic buds before migration *(left)* and after migration *(right)*. *(Lawrence PF: Essentials of general surgery, ed 5, Philadelphia, 2012, Lippincott Williams & Wilkins. Illustrations by Matthew Campbell.)*

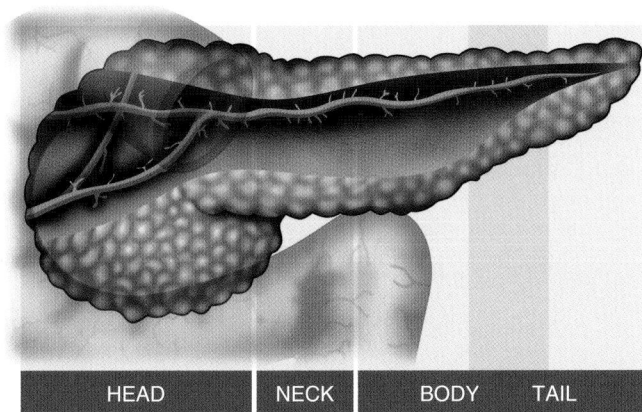

| HEAD | NECK | BODY | TAIL |

FIGURE 2 Divisions of the pancreas. *(Lawrence PF: Essentials of general surgery, ed 5, Philadelphia, 2012, Lippincott Williams & Wilkins. Illustrations by Matthew Campbell.)*

in up to 20% of the population. The classically described pancreas divisum has separate noncommunicating dorsal and ventral ducts. This classic variant occurs in up to 5% of the population (Figure 3, C). Other variations include an absent duct of Wirsung (Figure 3, D) and a filamentous communication between the ventral and dorsal ductal systems (Figure 3, E), which are seen in 4% and 10% of the population, respectively. All of these variants are typically lumped together under the heading of pancreas divisum because the dorsal duct that drains through the minor papilla is responsible for draining the majority of the pancreatic enzyme secretions into the duodenum.

CLINICAL SIGNIFICANCE

Pancreatitis is hypothesized to occur in those with ductal systems that are not able to adequately drain the pancreatic secretions from the gland into the duodenum. This occurs in only a small percentage of the 20% of individuals with some type of incomplete fusion, but the exact incidence rate of pancreatitis in this group is unknown. In most cases, the diameter of the major pancreatic duct ranges from 1.5 to 2 mm in the tail and 3 to 4 mm in the head of the gland. The

diameter of the minor duct is usually smaller, and when the minor duct is responsible for draining most of the gland (as in people with pancreas divisum), the potential for problems exists. Three primary pathologic conditions are associated with pancreas divisum: acute pancreatitis, chronic pancreatitis, and a pancreatic pain syndrome (midepigastric pain with radiation to the back). Although Goenei has shown pancreas divisum to be a predisposing factor in chronic and acute recurrent pancreatitis, most patients with pancreas divisum and pancreatitis have pancreatitis that is not the result of pancreas divisum. Remember that pancreas divisum may or may not be the cause of pancreatitis in any specific patient. Therefore, even if pancreas divisum is present, a careful investigation for other causes of pancreatitis is imperative. If no other cause for the patient's pancreatitis can be found, the diagnosis of pancreatitis from pancreas divisum should be entertained.

New research has shown an association between some genetic abnormalities and pancreas divisum. Bertin has recently shown that mutations in the cystic fibrosis transmembrane conductance regulator gene (CFTR), the serine protease inhibitor Kazal type 1 gene (SPINK1), and the cationic trypsinogen gene (PRSS1) are associated with both chronic pancreatitis and acute recurrent pancreatitis. In Bertin's study, pancreas divisum was found in 47% of patients with CFTR gene mutations. Another study by Choudari reported that 22% of patients with pancreatitis and pancreas divisum had CFTR mutations or polymorphisms. These genetic alterations likely result in increased viscosity of the pancreatic fluid, which may clog smaller ductal systems and predispose these individuals to pancreatitis. Although not completely understood, a multifactorial model is likely to evolve to explain how pancreatitis occurs in individuals with pancreas divisum that includes both anatomic changes and a variety of individual predisposing genetic factors.

DIAGNOSTIC STRATEGIES

Patients with acute bouts of recurrent pancreatitis, chronic pancreatitis, or pancreatic pain often undergo extensive evaluation to determine the etiology of their disease. The list of potential causes of pancreatitis is extensive, and every effort should be made to identify the cause. Biliary tract disease in patients without macroscopic cholelithiasis should also be considered. Ultrasound scan may not always detect sludge, small stones, and debris within the biliary system or gallbladder that can cause pancreatitis. Microscopic crystals in bile

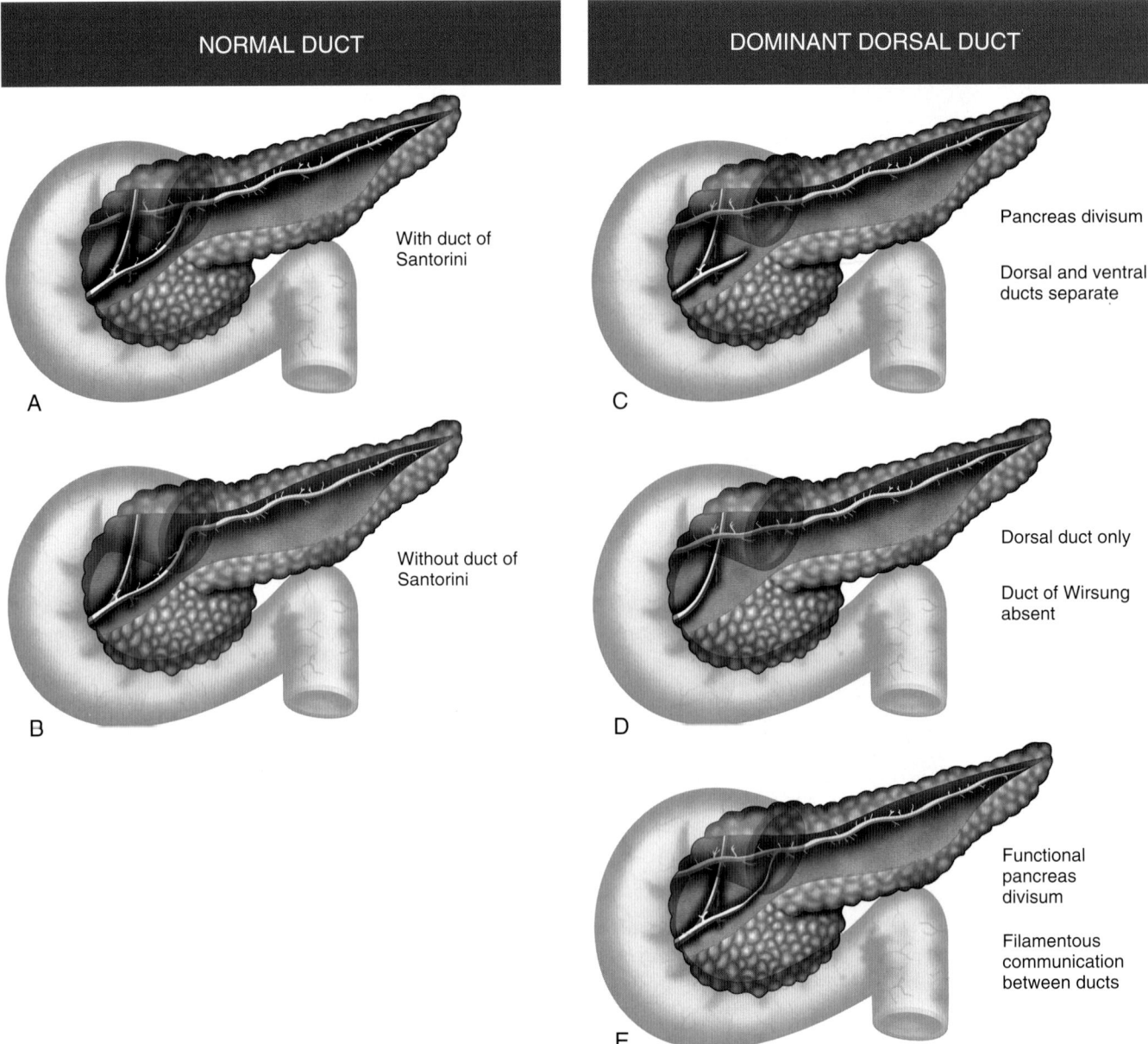

NORMAL DUCT

With duct of Santorini

A

Without duct of Santorini

B

DOMINANT DORSAL DUCT

Pancreas divisum

Dorsal and ventral ducts separate

C

Dorsal duct only

Duct of Wirsung absent

D

Functional pancreas divisum

Filamentous communication between ducts

E

FIGURE 3 **A** to **E,** Variations in pancreatic ductal anatomy. *(Lawrence PF: Essentials of general surgery, ed 5, Philadelphia, 2012, Lippincott Williams & Wilkins. Illustrations by Matthew Campbell.)*

have been identified in up to 85% of patients with idiopathic pancreatitis. Cholecystectomy is usually curative and can usually be completed during the same hospital admission if the episode of pancreatitis is not severe.

Numerous imaging modalities are available to aid the clinician. Ultrasound scan is probably the best diagnostic test for identification of gallstones. Endoscopic retrograde cholangiopancreatography (ERCP) is still considered the gold standard in diagnosing pancreas divisum. When an obvious cause for pancreatitis is missing, the ventral and dorsal ductile systems should be evaluated with imaging studies, and their respective papillae should be checked for stenosis. Pancreatic ductal manometry can be done but is difficult and beyond the expertise of many centers. Cannulation of the dorsal duct also causes complications in up to 8% of patients. The post-ERCP induced pancreatitis risk is less if only the major papilla is cannulated. Endoscopic ultrasound is another imaging technique that can also aid in the diagnosis of pancreas divisum through direct evaluation of the pancreatic parenchyma and the ductal response to increased

pancreatic enzyme secretion after intravenous (IV) secretin injection. Warshaw and colleagues have also shown the effectiveness of endoscopic ultrasound and secretin injection for evaluation of the papilla for a functional stenosis.

Multirow detector computed tomographic (CT) scan is also an effective means for evaluation of the pancreatic parenchyma and ductal anatomy. Asayama and associates showed that CT scan can reliably detect pancreas divisum in patients with Balthazar grade A acute pancreatitis (i.e., pancreatitis with no enlargement or inflammation involving the pancreas and peripancreatic fat seen on imaging). Magnetic resonance cholangiopancreatography (MRCP) may also be used in the evaluation of pancreatic ductile anatomy and does not subject the patient to ionizing radiation (Figure 4). Secretin stimulation can also be used with the MRCP and has been shown to increase the diagnostic yield of the test through enhanced visualization of the pancreatic ductal branches. One study by Ortega and colleagues compared endoscopic ultrasound scan (EUS) and MRCP and showed EUS to be superior in establishing a possible biliary

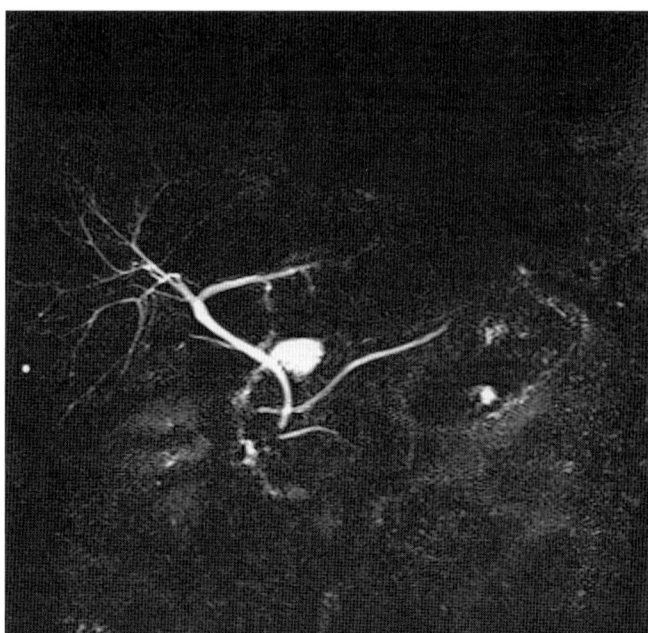

FIGURE 4   Magnetic resonance cholangiopancreatography shows pancreas divisum. *(Townsend, CM:* Sabiston textbook of surgery: the biologic basis of modern surgical practice, *ed 19, Philadelphia, 2012, Saunders.)*

etiology of pancreatitis in patients who had not undergone prior cholecystectomy; however, in patients whose gallbladder was surgically absent, MRCP seemed to be better.

TREATMENT

Treatment of patients with pancreatitis depends on identification of the etiology of the attack in the individual and then on focused intervention aimed at that etiologic agent. If pancreas divisum is a probable cause, both endoscopic and surgical treatment options exist. Unfortunately, only a handful of randomized controlled trials for endoscopic therapy have been performed, and none have been undertaken for surgical therapy. Also, no study has compared surgical with endoscopic treatment. Therefore, current treatment algorithms are based on a small number of retrospective studies.

Endoscopic Therapy

Endoscopic strategies include balloon dilation of the papilla, papillotomy, stent insertion, and endoscopic botulinum toxin injection into the papillae. These procedures can be extremely difficult to carry out because the minor papilla is often difficult to identify and hard to cannulate. These procedures have had limited success, are very operator dependent, and are dependent on various patient factors, including the type of pancreatitis and type of patient symptoms.

Balloon dilation by itself was associated with a high rate of postprocedure pancreatitis and has been largely abandoned. Pancreatic ductal stenting has also been used to treat a stenosis at the papilla, but the long-term success and the potential long-term problems that may accompany pancreatic ductal stenting are not fully known. Lans and associates, in a very small randomized controlled trial, showed that stenting might be superior to no intervention. Heyries and colleagues evaluated 24 patients who underwent sphincterotomy alone versus sphincterotomy plus stenting. The median duration of stenting was 8 months, and the median number of stent placements that

required an ERCP procedure was three. Patients were followed for a minimum of 2 years. Thirty-eight percent of participants experienced complications (44% of those with stenting vs 25% of those without). Complications included acute pancreatitis, acute cholecystitis, hemorrhage, stent migration, stent obstruction, and stenosis of the sphincterotomy. The authors concluded that both methods of treatment decreased the incidence rate of acute pancreatitis but the relief of chronic pain was less obvious. Another study for evaluation of the efficacy of minor pancreatic ductal stenting included 25 patients with pancreas divisum. Twenty-three of the 25 patients with stenting did not have further bouts of recurrent pancreatitis, but they did experience stent occlusion rates of 40.7%. After stent removal, 76% of the patients remained asymptomatic during a mean follow-up period of 24 months. Although these studies have shown promise, the long-term complications of pancreatic ductal stenting persist and include acquired chronic ductal changes, such as pruning and ectasia. Smith and colleagues have observed that more than 80% of patients have ductal changes consistent with chronic pancreatitis soon after insertion of a polyethylene stent. The significance of these changes is still unknown, as is their potential impact on later surgical intervention.

Besides endoscopic stenting, other endoscopic techniques have been used. Wehrmann and associates have reported a technique to inject botulinum toxin into the minor papilla. This treatment idea is based on techniques used to treat sphincter of Oddi dysfunction. Success with this technique has been reported in a nonrandomized group of five patients. Two of these patients relapsed within 1 year and subsequently underwent needle-knife sphincterotomy with relief of symptoms. One patient did not respond to therapy, and one patient required a second botulinum toxin injection Further studies need to be done to elucidate whether this procedure should be offered to patients with pancreatitis from pancreas divisum.

Patient or disease factors may also play a role in determining who obtains benefit from an endoscopic procedure. A small amount of data suggests that differences in response to endoscopic therapy might be based on the type of pancreatitis or pain a patient experiences. Borak and colleagues observed better responses to endoscopic therapy in older patients than in younger patients (median age, 58 years vs 46.5 years) and worse outcomes in patients with chronic pancreatitis treated endoscopically compared with those with acute recurrent pancreatitis or patients with pancreatic type pain. Similarly, a meta-analysis conducted by Liao and associates reviewed the response to surgery and to endoscopic therapy based on the type of pancreatitis or pain patients exhibited. The pooled overall response rate to endoscopic therapy and surgery were similar (69.4% vs 74.9%, respectively), suggesting that both treatment methods are effective in most patients. They also noted a better response in patients with acute recurrent pancreatitis compared with those with chronic pancreatitis or pancreatic pain.

Surgical Therapy

Transduodenal sphincteroplasty forms the cornerstone of surgical therapy for pancreas divisum. Other potential operative procedures include the Partington-Rochelle procedure (pancreaticojejunostomy), pancreaticoduodenectomy, and the Beger and Frey procedures. Most patients treated surgically have had failed previous endoscopic interventions because the majority of patients have been evaluated by a gastroenterologist before referral for surgery. In addition, the appeal of an endoscopic procedure is greater compared with one that requires a celiotomy.

Patient selection is essential when predicting operative success. A strong indication for surgical intervention includes endoscopic failure to cannulate the minor papilla via ERCP. When dorsal duct cannulation can be accomplished, patients that benefit from stenting of the pancreatic duct for a minimum of 3 months before surgery are more likely to have successful operative procedures.

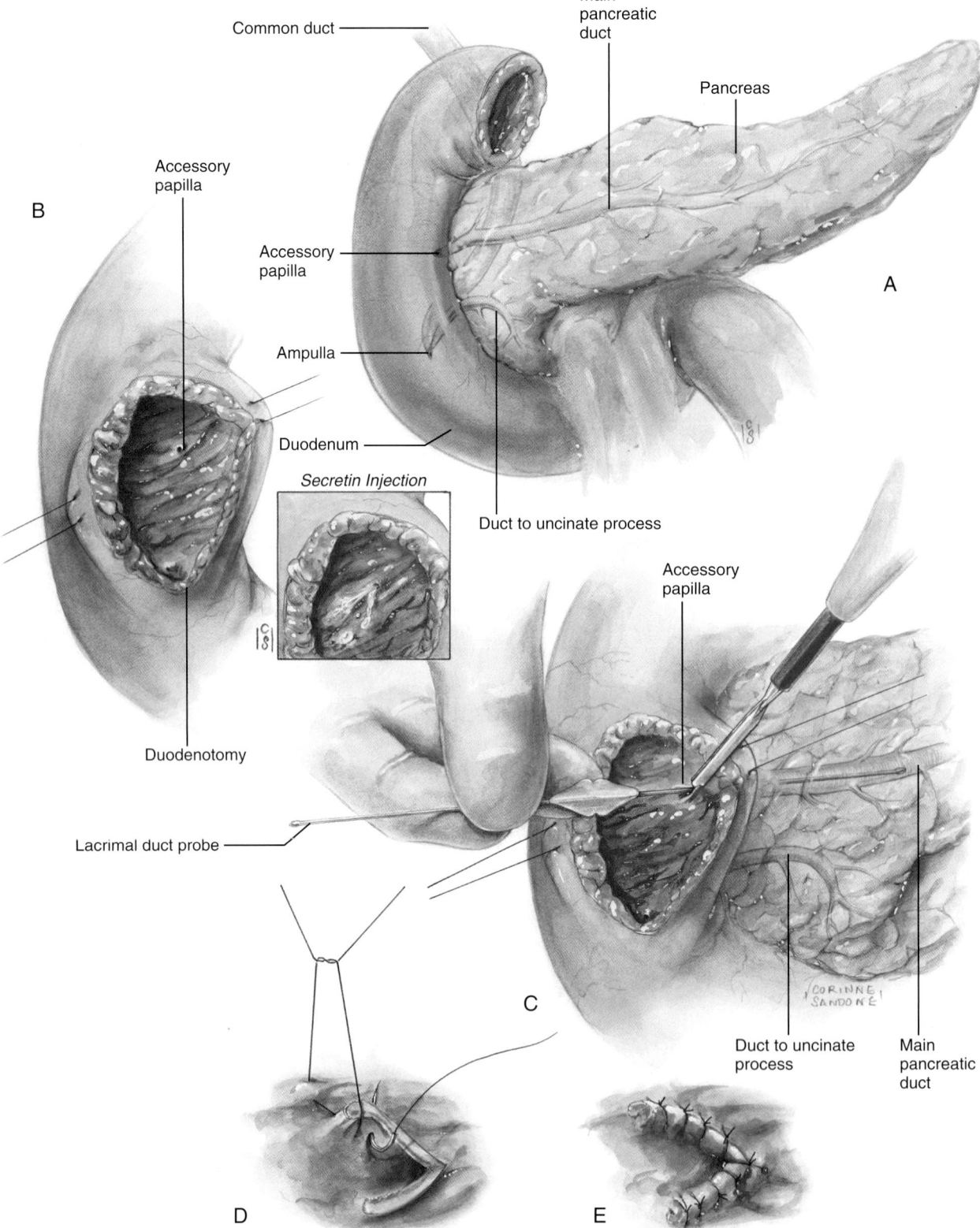

FIGURE 5 Dorsal duct sphincterotomy. **A,** Pictorial anatomy shows ampulla and accessory papilla in relation to duodenum and pancreas; **B,** longitudinal duodenotomy exposes accessory papilla; **C,** the dorsal duct is cannulated with a fine lacrimal probe, and the papilla is incised; and **D** and **E,** fine (5-0) absorbable sutures are placed in an interrupted fashion to approximate the mucosa from the duct to that of the duodenum. *(Used with permission from Cameron JL, Sandone C: Atlas of gastrointestinal surgery, ed 2, vol 2, Shelton, Conn, 2012, PMPH-USA.)*

Surgery can offer relief of symptoms with rates similar to those seen with endoscopic therapy. Morgan and associates retrospectively reviewed the outcome after transduodenal sphincteroplasty and showed that pain improved in 62% of patients. Patients who had a prior history of gastric surgery and had not undergone endoscopic sphincterotomy had better outcomes compared with those who had previous endoscopic interventions. Similar to endoscopic studies, younger patients with chronic pancreatitis had poorer outcomes.

Surgical Technique

Dorsal duct sphincterotomy is undertaken through a midline or right subcostal incision. A cholecystectomy should be done if the gallbladder is still present. A biliary Fogarty catheter may be inserted through the cystic duct to aid in the identification of the ampulla (Figure 5, A). This is often unnecessary because the papilla can usually be identified with careful palpation of the pancreaticoduodenal groove. Kocher's maneuver is done, and the pancreas is exposed to allow for visual inspection and palpation. A generous duodenotomy is made longitudinally opposite the ampulla of Vater (Figure 5, B). Exposure may be facilitated by placing stay sutures in the duodenum at either end of the incision. Palpation approximately 1 to 2 cm proximally and 0.5 cm anteriorly to the ampulla of Vater reveals the minor papilla. The papilla typically feels like a firm, tiny nodule. Intravenous secretin can be given at this time to help identify the minor duct by directly observing the outflow of pancreatic secretions. Secretin also helps ease cannulation through ductal dilation. Fine lacrimal probes are then carefully introduced into the dorsal pancreatic duct (Figure 5, C). Care should be taken to prevent traumatic cannulation because this can result in bleeding and hematoma formation. Minor trauma to this area can also make cannulation of the duct very difficult. Hence, atraumatic identification is very important because once this area has been traumatized, cannulation of the duct may be impossible. If indicated, a small catheter such as a 5F pediatric feeding tube can be inserted, and 2 to 3 mL of water-soluble contrast can be injected into the dorsal duct for further imaging.

After cannulation of the minor papillae, fine absorbable sutures (5-0 vicryl) should be placed in the duct 2 mm apart. The duct should be cut between the sutures until the diameter of the stoma is equal to the diameter of the minor duct. Absorbable 5-0 sutures are then placed in an interrupted fashion to approximate the mucosa from the duodenum and the duct (Figure 5, D and E). After sphincteroplasty, cannulation of the duct with a 3-mm or larger dilator usually indicates success.

The duodenotomy may be closed in a variety of manners with either one or two layers. The authors' preference is to use two layers with an inner layer of 3-0 vicryl placed in a Connell manner reinforced with a layer of 3-0 silk Lembert sutures. The duodenotomy may be closed longitudinally or transversely. Some surgeons advocate a sphincteroplasty of the sphincter of Oddi; however, if the patient's problems stem from stenosis of the dorsal duct, then this portion of the procedure is not indicated.

CONCLUSION

Pancreas divisum is seen in up to 20% of the population. To produce illness, other factors besides the anatomic variation seen with pancreas divisum are probably required. Treatment for patients symptomatic for pancreas divisum may be done either endoscopically or surgically. No randomized studies comparing endoscopic with surgical treatment exist. Success of any procedure is largely based on patient selection. Patients with pancreatic pain generally have worse outcomes than those with recurrent bouts of acute pancreatitis. Patients with chronic pancreatitis also seem to fair worse than those with pancreatic type pain. Patients with stenosis of the minor papilla and a soft pancreas without evidence of chronic pancreatitis usually have better outcomes with a good, fair, and poor response to therapy seen in 59%, 11% and 30%, respectively. In other studies, a good or fair outcome was seen in 85% of patients with documented stenosis at the papilla. Treatment depends on the ductal anatomy. Patients with chronic pancreatitis and a dilated pancreatic duct should undergo a pancreaticojejunostomy. Patients who have restenosis after surgical sphincteroplasty have success after revision only 50% of the time, and pancreatic head resection should be considered. Ultimately, the relief of outflow obstruction without restenosis generally results in successful symptom relief in most patients, which implies that surgical intervention is a definitive method of treatment in nearly all patients with pancreas divisum experiencing acute recurrent bouts of pancreatitis. Until a multicenter randomized control trial comparing surgery and endoscopic therapy is conducted, the treatment strategies surrounding this condition will continue to be debated.

SUGGESTED READINGS

Asayama Y, Fang W, Stolpen A, et al: Detectability of pancreas divisum in patients with acute pancreatitis on multi-detector row computed tomography, *Emerg Radiol* 19(2):121–125, 2012.

Bertin C, Pelletier AL, Vullierme MP, et al: Pancreas divisum is not a cause of pancreatitis by itself but acts as a partner of genetic mutations, *Am J Gastro* 107(2):311–317, 2012.

Bradley EL, Stephan RN: Accessory duct sphincteroplasty is preferred for long-term prevention of recurrent acute pancreatitis in patients with pancreas divisum, *J Am Coll Surg* 183:65, 1996.

Goldin S, Avgerinos D, Parikh A, et al: Pancreas. In Lawrence PF: editor: *Essentials of general surgery*, ed 5, Philadelphia, 2012, Lippincott Williams and Wilkins.

Gonoi W, Akai H, Hagiwara K, et al: Pancreas divisum as a predisposing factor for chronic and recurrent idiopathic pancreatitis: initial in vivo survey, *Gut* 60(8):1103–1108, 2011.

Heyries L, et al: Long-term results of endoscopic management of pancreas divisum with recurrent acute pancreatitis, *Gastrointest Endosc* 55:376–381, 2002.

Lia Z, Gao R, Wang W, et al: A systematic review on endoscopic detection rate, endotherapy, and surgery for pancreas divisum, *Endoscopy* 41:439–444, 2009.

Madura JA, Madura II JA, Sherman S, et al: Surgical sphincteroplasty in 446 patients, *Arch Surg* 140(5):504–513, 2005.

Morgan KA, Romagnuolo J, Adams DB, et al: Transduodenal sphincteroplasty in the management of shincter of Oddi dysfunction and pancreas divisum in the modern era, *J Am Coll Surg* 206:908–917, 2008.

Warshaw AL, Simeone JF, Schapiro RH, et al: Evaluation and treatment of the dominant dorsal duct syndrome (pancreas divisum redefined), *Am J Surg* 159:59–64, 1990.

Wehrmann T, Schmitt T, Seifert H: Endoscopic botulinum toxin injection into the minor papilla for treatment of idiopathic recurrent pancreatitis in patients with pancreas divisum, *Gastrointest Endosc* 50:545–548, 1999.

PANCREATIC NECROSIS

Jordan R. Stern, MD, and Jeffrey B. Matthews, MD, FACS

INTRODUCTION

Most patients who experience an attack of acute pancreatitis follow a benign course and recover without significant long-term sequelae. However, for the approximately 20% who do have complications, the outcome can be devastating. The most feared complication is the development of pancreatic necrosis, estimated to occur in 10% to 25% of all cases of acute pancreatitis and, in historic series, carrying a harrowing 10% to 20% mortality rate. Mortality in necrotizing pancreatitis is bimodal in temporal distribution. Early deaths, occurring within days of onset, are generally attributable to an exuberant systemic inflammatory response and the development of multisystem organ failure. Late deaths occur weeks later, typically in the setting of infection and sepsis. Infected pancreatic necrosis is associated with up to a threefold increase in mortality over sterile necrosis and has traditionally been considered an indication for urgent surgical intervention. However, operative débridement of necrotic pancreatic tissue carries a high mortality rate, and complications including abscess or pseudocyst formation, hemorrhage, bowel injury, pancreatic fistula, and late pancreatic exocrine and endocrine insufficiency are frequent. More recently, evidence has emerged that suggests that extended nonoperative management strategies are safe; this approach is now generally favored, even in the setting of infection. In those patients who cannot avoid surgical intervention, a multimodal approach including minimally invasive surgical techniques has become the preferred clinical strategy in many experienced centers. This chapter describes both the nonoperative and the operative management of pancreatic necrosis and outlines a strategy to optimize patient outcomes.

DEFINITIONS AND DIAGNOSIS

Considerable confusion has occurred over the nomenclature used to describe complications of severe acute pancreatitis. Terms such as necrosis, fluid collection, abscess, and pseudocyst are often used interchangeably. A more precise framework and definition of terms that distinguishes among these entities and facilitates communication between clinicians was developed at a multidisciplinary consensus conference in Atlanta in 1992. The Atlanta classification is outlined in Table 1.

Computed tomographic (CT) scan is particularly useful in establishing the presence of necrotizing pancreatitis and other peripancreatic complications (Figure 1). Administration of intravenous contrast is generally necessary to make the diagnosis. Criteria for the diagnosis of pancreatic necrosis are diffuse or focal areas of nonenhancement that involve greater than 30% of the pancreas or measure 3 cm in maximal dimension. Areas that contain gas should raise the suspicion of the presence of infected necrosis. Magnetic resonance imaging (MRI) may also be used, and the combination of T1-weighted and T2-weighted sequences in combination with magnetic resonance cholangiopancreatography (MRCP) can be of particular use in defining the extent of necrosis and assessing the bile ducts for anatomy and the presence of stones. MRI is particularly useful to distinguish fluid from solid collections of necrotic tissue, a distinct advantage over CT scan. Radiologically guided tissue sampling for bacterial culture is occasionally useful to distinguish between infected and sterile necrosis. This practice was originally based on prevailing surgical dogma of immediate operative intervention in infected necrosis.

Despite theoretic concerns for conversion of sterile necrosis to infected necrosis via instrumentation, rates of secondary infection are extremely low and image-guided needle aspiration should still be considered a safe and useful diagnostic tool. However, because initial nonoperative management is now generally favored regardless of infection status, this practice is no longer routine.

ROLE OF PROPHYLACTIC ANTIBIOTICS

Given the higher mortality rate for infected pancreatic necrosis, much attention has been paid to the potential benefit of prophylactic antibiotics to prevent secondary infection of initially sterile necrosis. Although the theoretic rationale is compelling, the supporting evidence is conflicting and concerns have been raised regarding the possible selection for resistant bacteria and the potential for the emergence of fungal infection. Given the potential concerns and lack of evidence to support their use, prophylactic antibiotic use should not be routine in clinical practice. Probiotic (rather than antibiotic) prophylaxis has been suggested as an alternative approach to the prevention of infection in pancreatic necrosis by maintaining normal gut flora, but recent evidence has unexpectedly shown an increased mortality in those patients undergoing probiotic therapy.

TIMING OF SURGICAL INTERVENTION

In the past, surgical intervention was generally undertaken early in the course of severe necrotizing acute pancreatitis, typically within a few days of onset. Early operation, particularly in cases of infected necrosis, was assumed to improve the otherwise dismal prognosis. However, a number of studies suggested that intervention within the first 48 to 72 hours was associated with particularly high mortality, and the International Association of Pancreatology (IAP) guidelines of 2002 recommended against surgical intervention within the first 14 days of onset of the illness unless there were specific overriding indications. Subsequent studies have provided evidence that mortality remains high even within the first 14 to 21 days of presentation but can be reduced to less than about 8% when operation is delayed beyond 28 to 30 days. One prospective, randomized trial that examined early versus late necronectomy was closed early because of high mortality in the early operative group. The benefit from delayed operation seems to come from the improved demarcation between normal and necrotic tissue over time, to the point where dissection can be less extensive, the risk of hemorrhage and injury to surrounding organs can be reduced, and unnecessary removal of otherwise viable pancreatic tissue can be limited. Given these findings, whenever possible, definitive surgical therapy should be delayed and patients managed nonoperatively for at least 28 days. As an added benefit, this practice obviates the need for surgery in a number of patients, especially those with sterile necrosis.

THERAPEUTIC INTERVENTION FOR PANCREATIC NECROSIS

Surgical intervention should be delayed whenever possible. However, the clinical scenario may dictate operation or other forms of intervention at earlier time points, particularly in patients who appear to have infected necrosis. In general, a clinical picture consistent with infection such as persistent fevers, tachycardia, adynamic ileus, and continued or progressive multisystem organ failure should be taken as sufficient evidence of infection even in the absence of confirmation with fine-needle aspirate and culture. A patient with failure to respond to supportive therapy, manifested by progressive multiorgan

TABLE 1: Atlanta classification for acute pancreatitis

Clinical entity	Definition	Clinical manifestation	Pathologic findings	Notes
Acute Pancreatitis	Acute inflammatory process, with variable involvement of other regional tissues or remote organ systems	Rapid onset with variable abdominal findings Often associated with emesis, fever, tachycardia, leukocytosis, and elevated pancreatic enzymes	Ranges from interstitial edema to macroscopic necrosis and hemorrhage See subsequent	Clinical diagnosis only
Severe Acute Pancreatitis	Associated with organ failure or local complications, such as necrosis, abscess, or pseudocyst	Increased abdominal tenderness and distention, hypoactive or absent bowel sounds, ≥ 3 Ranson criteria or ≥ 8 APACHE points with organ failure	Most often associated with necrosis, but also may occur with severe interstitial edema	Rapid onset, delayed progression from mild pancreatitis is rare
Mild Acute Pancreatitis	Minimal organ dysfunction and an uneventful recovery; lacking criteria for severe acute pancreatitis	Abdominal pain and tenderness but less severe Responsive to fluid resuscitation, usually within 48-72 h	Interstitial edema, with or without small areas of focal necrosis or peripancreatic fat necrosis	~75% of patients with acute pancreatitis have mild disease and an uncomplicated course
Acute Fluid Collection	Occur early in the course of acute pancreatitis, located in or near the pancreas, always lack a wall of granulation or fibrous tissue	Common in patients with severe disease (30%-50%), and usually discovered with imaging studies	No defined wall, precise fluid composition is unknown, and presence of bacteria is variable	Represents an early form of pseudocyst, but most regress and do not develop further
Pancreatic Necrosis	Diffuse or focal areas of nonviable pancreatic parenchyma, typically associated with peripancreatic fat necrosis	Severe pancreatitis with zones of nonenhanced (<50 Hounsfield units) parenchyma ≥ 3 cm or involving ≥ 30% of the pancreas on CT scan	Interstitial fat necrosis with vessel damage affecting acinar, islet, and ductal cells	Subclassified as infected and sterile pancreatic necrosis
Acute Pseudocyst	Collection of pancreatic juice enclosed by a wall of fibrous or granulation tissue, which arises as a consequence of acute pancreatitis, pancreatic trauma, or chronic pancreatitis	Occasionally palpable but most often develops several weeks after an episode of acute pancreatitis and discovered on repeat imaging	Well-defined wall of fibrous or granulation tissue present, may contain bacteria but does not contain pus	Develops at least 4 wk after attack and has defined wall, otherwise termed acute fluid collection (as described previously)
Pancreatic Abscess	Circumscribed intra-abdominal collection of pus, usually in proximity to the pancreas, containing little or no pancreatic necrosis, which arises as a consequence of acute pancreatitis or pancreatic trauma	Clinical picture usually that of systemic infection	Well-defined wall with presence of pus in the cavity and culture-positive aspiration for bacteria or fungi	Develops at least 4 wk after attack, and differentiated from infected pancreatic necrosis by lack of necrosis and presence of pus

This clinically based system of definitions was developed at the International Symposium on Acute Pancreatitis in Atlanta, in September 1992. It was created to standardize definitions among clinicians.
APACHE, Acute Physiology and Chronic Health Evaluation; *CT,* computed tomographic.
Adapted from Bradley E: A clinically based classification system for acute pancreatitis: summary of the International Symposium on Acute Pancreatitis, Atlanta GA, Sept 11-13, 1992, Arch Surg 128(5):586-590, 1993. Table reproduced from Stern JR, Matthews JB: Pancreatic necrosectomy, Adv Surg 45:155–176, 2011, Elsevier Science.

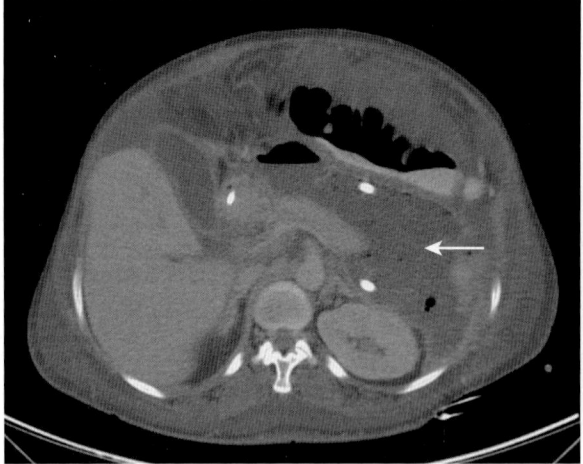
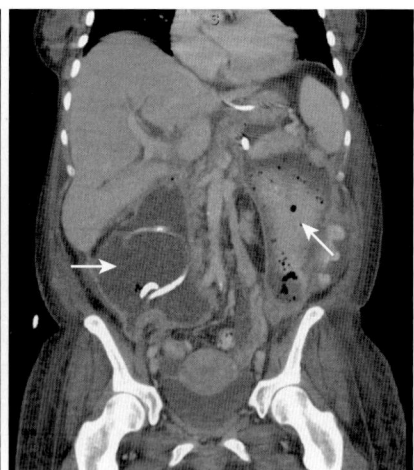

FIGURE 1 Computed tomographic (CT) scan of pancreatic necrosis. CT scan was performed with intravenous contrast on a 45-year-old woman with history of necrotizing pancreatitis. Axial and coronal images show extensive retroperitoneal collections containing air and fluid in addition to solid necrotic tissue (white arrows). A percutaneous drainage catheter is seen within the right-sided collection.

dysfunction and failure or other signs of clinical deterioration, should be considered a candidate for therapeutic intervention. The general principles of traditional "open" pancreatic necronectomy include complete débridement of necrotic tissue and wide drainage of infected compartments. However, in selected instances, temporization with percutaneous or endoscopic approaches may allow formal débridement to be deferred until a safer window of time.

Percutaneous Drainage

Primary intervention on patients with severe complications of acute pancreatitis may include image-guided drainage performed by interventional radiologists (see Figure 1). Large pseudocysts and abscesses containing little solid necrosis may be particularly amenable to percutaneous drainage, and this may circumvent the need for later surgical intervention in some patients altogether. Drains may be exchanged and upsized as needed. More commonly, though, percutaneous drainage is not definitive therapy but is instead used to gain source control to stabilize patients for delayed surgical intervention. In cases with a significant solid necrotic component, percutaneous drains may be inadequate to drain thick debris through even large-bore pigtail catheters. Nevertheless, occasionally, the combination of percutaneous drainage and prolonged antibiotic therapy may lead to complete resolution of such collections without the need for formal operative débridement, in apparent violation of long-held surgical dogma.

Endoluminal Drainage

Endoscopy has been used for some time in the management of pancreatic pseudocysts. Adequate definitive drainage may be accomplished through placement of transgastric, or occasionally transduodenal, drains into walled-off peripancreatic fluid collections abutting the stomach or duodenum. With advances in technology and endoscopic skill, drainage of more complex, heterogeneous collections extending into the retroperitoneal peripancreatic, pararenal, and paracolic spaces may be achieved. Pancreatic débridement with this approach is in essence a form of natural orifice transluminal endoscopic surgery (NOTES). An endoscope is passed through the mouth and into the stomach, where extrinsic compression from the necrotic cavity is indentified. Usually, endoscopic ultrasound scan is used to further characterize the space, the extent of solid versus fluid debris, and the presence of nearby vascular structures such as dilated or variceal short gastric veins. Entrance to the cavity is gained with electrocautery through the posterior stomach or medial duodenum

wall, and then the opening is enlarged to allow the endoscope to be passed directly into the cavity. Correct positioning is often confirmed with fluoroscopy (Figure 2, A). Endoscopic forceps can be used to remove solid material, followed by copious irrigation (Figure 2, B). Nasocystic catheters can be left in the cavity for irrigation, or double pigtail catheters (often multiple) can be left between the lumen of the stomach or duodenum and the cavity to allow for continued drainage through a controlled internal fistula.

Open Pancreatic Necronectomy

Open necronectomy with drain placement and continual postoperative lavage is effective to remove necrotic and infected tissues and has long been considered the standard against which newer approaches to infected necrosis should be judged. Mortality rates as high as 50% have been reported depending on the timing of intervention and patient selection, and the risks of bowel injury, postoperative fistula, recurrent abscess, and wound complications are considerable. Nonetheless, in modern series, the morbidity and mortality of open necronectomy are far lower when intervention is delayed and when it is performed in experienced centers. It remains an excellent, tried-and-true option in these patients.

A midline laparotomy or left-sided subcostal incision is used to gain peritoneal access, depending on radiologic findings of the extent of the necrosis and extension into retroperitoneal spaces. Blunt dissection is used to elevate the omentum, stomach, and transverse colon and mesocolon away from the inflammation and necrosis within the lesser sac, pancreatic body, and tail. On entering the involved peripancreatic spaces, significant amounts of fluid or necrotic tissue with extensive loculations are often encountered. Careful efforts to preserve the integrity of the transverse mesocolon are worthwhile, to avoid devascularization of the colon and to prevent internal adhesions, herniation, or fistulization of the small bowel. Access to the pancreatic head and uncinate process is gained via the lesser sac through Kocher's maneuver and extensive mobilization of the duodenum as possible. Necrotic tissue is often able to be finger-dissected away from the retroperitoneal vasculature and from viable pancreatic tissue, but clear definition of tissue planes is often impossible. The area posterior to the superior mesenteric vessels should be carefully and gently débrided and drained as well. Normal-appearing pancreas should be left undisturbed if possible, even at the expense of leaving a small amount of necrotic tissue behind. Depending on preoperative imaging, the pararenal spaces and paracolic gutters should be thoroughly explored for evidence of necrotic tracking. Once débridement is complete, attention should be turned to irrigation and establishment of adequate external drainage. Previously

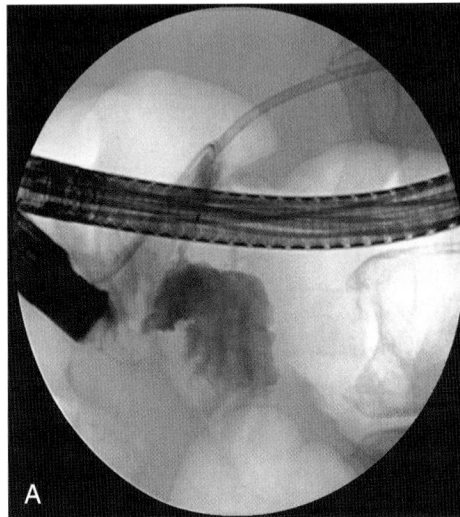
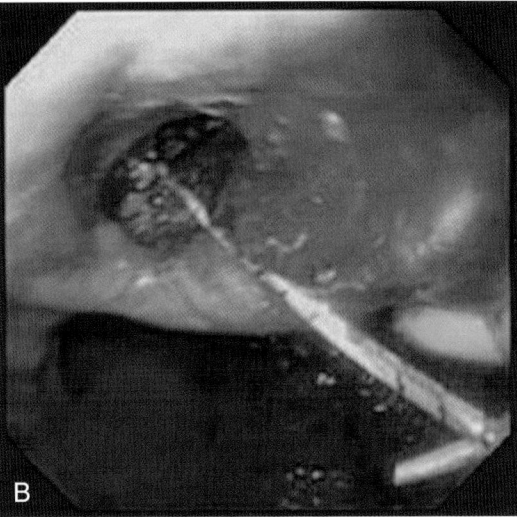

FIGURE 2 Endoscopic necronectomy. **A,** After the posterior gastrostomy is made with electrocautery, fluoroscopy is used to verify correct placement of the endoscope in the necrotic cavity. **B,** Endoscopic instruments are used to remove necrotic tissue through the opening in the stomach wall. *(Images courtesy of Irving Waxman, MD, Department of Gastroenterology, The University of Chicago Hospitals.)*

placed percutaneous catheters may be repositioned or exchanged. Additional catheters should be large bore (at least 28F) and should contain multiple large drainage holes to allow semisolid material to pass through. Ideally, the choice of surgical drainage catheter should allow for later exchange if necessary. Single-lumen closed-suction catheters can provide adequate drainage, and multiple-lumen catheters allow for continuous postoperative lavage with saline solution or peritoneal dialysis fluid if desired. The goal should be to achieve complete and thorough débridement at the time of initial operation. Planned reexploration every 48 to 72 hours is probably not necessary unless there has been significant hemorrhage or a question of viability of intestinal segments that may have been compromised by operative injury or mesenteric inflammation (particularly the transverse colon). Drains and packing should only be removed after a minimum of 7 days, allowing for the slow collapse of the necrotic cavity and resolution of pancreatic fistula.

Videoscopic Surgical Techniques

Several minimally invasive surgical alternatives to open necronectomy have evolved for the treatment of pancreatic necrosis, with both laparoscopic (transperitoneal) and intracavitary (retroperitoneal) approaches. Laparoscopic pancreatic necronectomy is analogous to the open technique, achieving the same goals of débridement and drainage. A larger incision can be used for a hand port to aid dissection, gain access to deeper loculations and compartments, and control bleeding if so desired by the operating surgeon. Drainage catheters are again left in the emptied cavities. Avoidance of full laparotomy while still achieving adequate débridement and drainage may be important in critically ill patients with compromised respiratory status, provided that they can tolerate pneumoperitoneum. Repeat laparoscopic intervention is simpler and safer than repeat laparotomy, and wound complications such as infection and hernia formation are less common. A retroperitoneal approach has variably been termed intracavitary or percutaneous necronectomy, or increasingly commonly, video-assisted retroperitoneal débridement (VARD) (Figure 3). VARD is touted to achieve lower operative mortality than open necronectomy and lower overall morbidity, postoperative organ failure, and need for intensive care unit (ICU) management. This approach is conceptually appealing, in that it avoids contamination of virgin spaces (most notably the peritoneal cavity), theoretically containing the infection with natural biologic compartment barriers and reducing the systemic inflammatory response, which can ultimately lead to multiple organ dysfunction and death.

Step-Up Approach

Because of the high morbidity and mortality of definitive surgical therapy for pancreatic necrosis, and the need to delay such interventions for a minimum of 4 weeks, a stepwise approach to these patients has been suggested. On presentation, patients with acute necrotizing pancreatitis often display signs of the systemic inflammatory response syndrome and sepsis, and timely implementation of supportive therapy in the ICU is paramount. After initial stabilization, attention should be turned to gaining source control and evacuating necrotic tissue and infected fluid collections. This can be achieved initially with percutaneous or endoscopic drain placement, which may improve patient stability and lead to clinical convalescence. Drainage procedures can achieve sufficient temporization such that definitive therapy can be delayed for the requisite time period as inflammation subsides and the necrosis becomes more organized. Perhaps even more importantly, drainage can obviate the need for necronectomy in approximately 35% of patients. For patients who do have organized necrosis that is not amenable to complete evacuation with percutaneous or endoscopic drains, definitive necronectomy should be undertaken first with minimally invasive approaches. On the basis of imaging and location of necrosis, and surgeon expertise with each technique, either VARD (retroperitoneal) or laparoscopic necronectomy can be performed at this time. This approach, with a progression of interventions with increasing invasiveness, led to decreased overall complications and death when compared with open necronectomy in a randomized trial.

SUMMARY

Pancreatic necrosis is a source of significant morbidity and mortality, and patients with this disease are often acutely and severely ill. Initial management should prioritize aggressive fluid resuscitation and supportive care in the intensive care unit. Prophylactic antibiotic therapy is no longer routinely used, but empiric therapy should be considered in patients who show signs of systemic infection (fever, leukocytosis) or with evidence of infection on imaging studies. Patients should be imaged with either infused CT scan or MRI to evaluate the location and extent of necrosis and associated fluid collections or abscesses, and temporizing percutaneous drainage procedures can be accordingly planned. Drains should be upsized if indicated with repeat imaging. With the "step-up" approach, in approximately one third of patients, percutaneous drainage alone suffices, and they recover without need for additional intervention. In patients with organized infected necrosis, either traditional open necronectomy, VARD, or

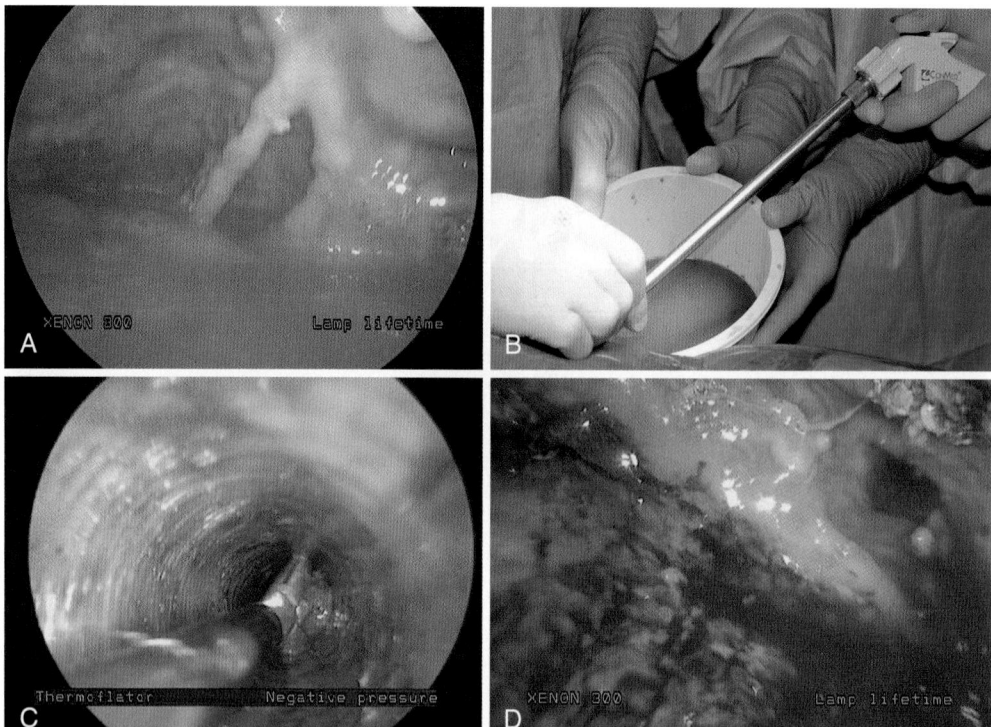

FIGURE 3 Video-assisted retroperitoneal débridement. The necrotic cavity is entered by following the tract of percutaneous drains, and a large amount of brown liquid and floating debris is encountered **(A)**, which is drained with a laparoscopic suction-irrigation device **(B)**. Solid material can be removed with graspers and other traditional laparoscopic instruments **(C)**. After débridement, healthy tissue is seen along the wall of the cavity **(D)**.

laparoscopic necronectomy should be performed after a minimum of 28 days to allow inflammation to subside and tissue planes to develop between necrosis and the remaining normal pancreas and underlying vasculature. The goals of débridement should be to completely evacuate all necrotic tissue and unroof any cavities throughout the retroperitoneal space and to leave large-bore drainage catheters to allow for continued drainage and irrigation. The step-up approach may represent a new standard of care in experienced centers, although open necronectomy continues to be a valid and acceptable approach.

Suggested Readings

Alverdy J, Vargish T, Desai T, et al: Laparoscopic intracavitary debridement of peripancreatic necrosis: preliminary report and description of the technique, *Surgery* 127(1):112–114, 2000.

Babu B, Sheen AJ, Lee SH, et al: Open pancreatic necrosectomy in the multidisciplinary management of postinflammatory necrosis, *Ann Surg* 251(5):783–786, 2010.

Seifert H, Biermer M, Schmitt W, et al: Transluminal endoscopic necrosectomy after acute pancreatitis: a multicentre study with long-term follow-up (the GEPARD Study), *Gut* 58(9):1260–1266, 2009.

Uhl W, Warshaw A, Imrie C, et al: IAP guidelines for the management of acute pancreatitis, *Pancreatology* 2(6):565–573, 2002.

van Santvoort H, Besselink MG, Bakker OJ, et al: A step-up approach or open necrosectomy for necrotizing pancreatitis, *N Engl J Med* 362(16):1491–1502, 2010.

The Management of Pancreatic Pseudocyst

Katherine A. Morgan, MD, and
David B. Adams, MD, FACS

"The fascination that pseudocysts hold for surgeons is beyond comprehension."

Robert Zollinger, MD

OVERVIEW

The pancreatic pseudocyst is a collection of pancreatic secretions contained within a fibrous sac comprised of chronic inflammatory cells and fibroblasts in and adjacent to the pancreas contained by surrounding structures. Why a fibrous sac filled with pancreatic fluid is the source of so much interest, speculation, and emotion amongst surgeons and gastroenterologists is indeed hard to understand. Do we debate so vigorously about bilomas, urinomas, or other abdominal collections of visceral secretions? Perhaps it is because the pancreatic pseudocyst represents a sleeping tiger, which though frequently harmless, still can rise up unexpectedly and attack with its enzymatic claws into adjacent visceral and vascular structures and cause life-threatening complications. Another part of the debate and puzzlement about pancreatic pseudocysts is related to confusion about pancreatic pseudocyst definition and nomenclature.

The Atlanta classification, developed in 1992, was a pioneering effort in describing and defining morphologic entities in acute pancreatitis. Since then, a working group has been revising this system to incorporate more modern experience into the terminology. In the latest version of this system, pancreatitis is divided into acute interstitial edematous pancreatitis (IEP) and necrotizing pancreatitis (NP), based on the presence of pancreatic tissue necrosis. The fluid collections associated with these two "types" of pancreatitis are also differentiated. Early (<4 weeks into the disease course) peripancreatic fluid collections in IEP are referred to as acute peripancreatic fluid collections (APFC), whereas in NP, they are referred to as postnecrotic peripancreatic fluid collections (PNPFC). Late (>4 weeks) fluid collections in IEP are called pancreatic pseudocysts, and in NP, they are called walled-off pancreatic necrosis (WOPN). These latter two entities are the subject of this chapter.

Acute pancreatitis represents a broad spectrum of disease. Although the disease course may smolder, typically an initial inciting event results in organ injury, which sets into play the evolving clinical course. The early phase of disease is marked by the inflammatory mediators from damaged pancreatic tissue, resulting in variable degrees of systemic inflammatory response. The later phase is determined by the morphology of organ injury, specifically with regard to tissue ischemia and necrosis. The outcome of this later phase is often impacted by local or systemic infection.

Peripancreatic fluid collections can occur in both the early and the late phases of disease. They presumably occur from injury to or ischemia of the main pancreatic duct or a side branch duct, although some, particularly early on, may be the result of third-space edema fluid. Peripancreatic fluid collections represent a heterogeneous entity. Definition of peripancreatic fluid collections is essential in determination of clinical decision making.

PATHOPHYSIOLOGY

Pancreatic pseudocysts develop as a consequence of pancreatic duct disruption and can occur in the setting of acute pancreatitis, chronic pancreatitis, or pancreatic trauma. In acute pancreatitis, ischemia, inflammation, and increased pressure may play a role in ductal injury. In chronic pancreatitis, ductal pathology from postinflammatory fibrosis can lead to ductal compromise. With duct disruption, pancreatic exocrine fluid leaks and pools. The pancreatic enzyme-rich fluid incites an inflammatory response with fibroblast-mediated extracellular matrix formation and the development of a fibrous capsule. Pseudocysts are defined microscopically by this inflammatory fibrous lining, which lacks an epithelial layer. The fluid content of walled-off pancreatic necrosis may develop from a similar pathophysiology, although in the presence of necrosis, or it may be the result of liquefaction necrosis of pancreatic or peripancreatic tissue after severe acute pancreatitis.

The natural history of the pseudocyst is determined by the resultant state of the underlying pancreatic duct. The duct injury may heal on its own, or a persistent fistula or ductal stricture may develop, which impedes resolution of the pseudocyst.

PRESENTATION

A pseudocyst may commonly present as persistent or worsening abdominal or back pain, bloating, early satiety, nausea, vomiting, or failure to thrive after a significant bout of pancreatitis or pancreatic trauma. A pseudocyst in the head of the pancreas can cause biliary obstruction with jaundice or duodenal obstruction with intolerance of oral diet. Mechanical compression from a pseudocyst or the associated inflammatory reaction can result in mesenteric venous thrombosis with variceal bleeding or ascites. The inflammatory pseudocyst

can erode into surrounding structures, including the small bowel or colon, to develop an enteric fistula. The pseudocyst can also erode into surrounding vessels (including the splenic artery, gastroduodenal artery, and superior mesenteric artery) to cause a pseudoaneurysm and potentially life-threatening hemorrhage. In addition, the cyst may rupture into the peritoneal cavity to result in pancreatic ascites or the thoracic cavity to result in a pleuropancreatic fistula. Finally, a pseudocyst may be asymptomatic and discovered incidentally on imaging.

DIAGNOSTIC EVALUATION

The goals of the diagnostic evaluation of the pancreatic pseudocyst include defining the disease process at hand, determining the need for intervention, and assessing the options for therapy. Distinguishing a pseudocyst or WOPN from a cystic neoplasm is an essential first step in this diagnostic process. Often history alone can make this determination, but radiography should be consistent with this distinction. Radiography is also effective in differentiating a pseudocyst from WOPN with the presence of necrosis. This important distinction has significant implications in the need for and approach to intervention. Finally, the evaluation of the anatomy of the underlying pancreatic duct and its relationship to the pancreatic pseudocyst is vital to clinical decision making.

Contrast-enhanced computed tomographic (CE-CT) scan is the modality of choice for the frontline evaluation of a pancreatic pseudocyst in the modern era. On CE-CT scan, a pseudocyst appears as a uniform, rounded, fluid-filled mass with a thickened, hyperdense capsule that may take on the morphology of the surrounding structures (Figure 1, A). WOPN is marked by associated necrosis, most often visualized as heterogeneity of the cyst fluid with solid matter and particulate debris (Figure 2, A). Pseudocysts most commonly occur in the lesser sac, although they may occur in the paracolic gutters, at the base of the mesentery, anterior to the stomach, or even more remotely from the pancreas deep in the retroperitoneum. CE-CT scan allows for the assessment of the pancreatic pseudocyst and its relationship to surrounding structures. It may show evidence of hyperdense material within the cyst, raising concern for hemorrhage from an associated pseudoaneurysm. It may show air within the pseudocyst, indicating infection or the presence of a fistula with the gastrointestinal tract. CE-CT scan can show evidence of pancreatic parenchymal atrophy or calcifications suggestive of underlying chronic pancreatitis. It can also show abnormalities of the underlying pancreatic duct or biliary system, although with less sensitivity and detail than magnetic resonance.

Magnetic resonance cholangiopancreatography with secretin stimulation (ssMRCP) is also a useful modality for the evaluation of a pancreatic pseudocyst (Figure 1, B). It can show more detailed morphology of cystic structures, improving the differentiation of the pseudocyst from neoplasm and detecting solid debris in WOPN, distinguishing it from the simple fluid of a pseudocyst (Figure 2, B). In addition, ssMRCP can help to delineate the anatomy of the pancreatic duct and its relationship to the pseudocyst.

Endoscopic retrograde cholangiopancreatography (ERCP) is used less commonly as a diagnostic tool in the modern era given the chance for inciting a bout of pancreatitis or for introducing enteric organisms into the pseudocyst or WOPN with the potential for infection. ERCP is well used therapeutically, however, in pseudocysts with a connection to the main pancreatic duct that may be amenable to endoscopic stenting or sphincterotomy for resolution.

Endoscopic ultrasound (EUS) may be useful in the evaluation of the pseudocyst, particularly in distinguishing it from a pancreatic cystic neoplasm. EUS examination can elucidate cyst morphology, including solid nodules or septations, and cyst relationship to the pancreatic duct and identify the presence of pancreatitis in the surrounding pancreatic parenchyma. EUS-guided fine-needle aspiration of fluid can also be helpful. High amylase fluid indicates the cyst is

FIGURE 1 A pancreatic pseudocyst is well visualized with contrast-enhanced computed tomographic scan **(A)** as a simple fluid-filled structure with a hyperdense fibrous capsule in the body of the pancreas and with magnetic resonance **(B)** on T2-weighted imaging as a round, homogeneously enhancing lesion.

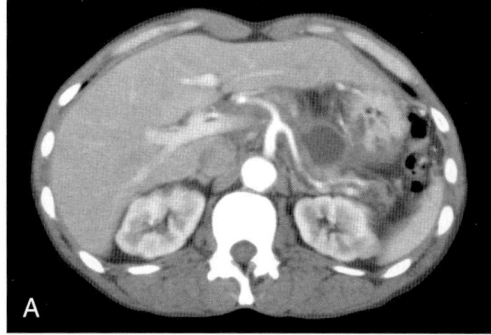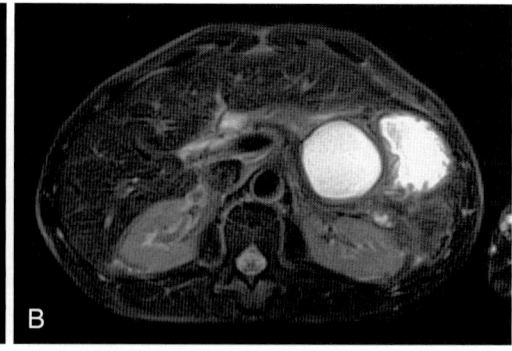

FIGURE 2 Walled-off pancreatic necrosis is shown on contrast-enhanced computed tomographic scan **(A)** as a peripancreatic fluid collection containing heterogeneous material representing solid necrotic debris and with magnetic resonance **(B)** on T2-weighted imaging as a rounded enhancing fluid-filled collection containing nonenhancing solid necrosis.

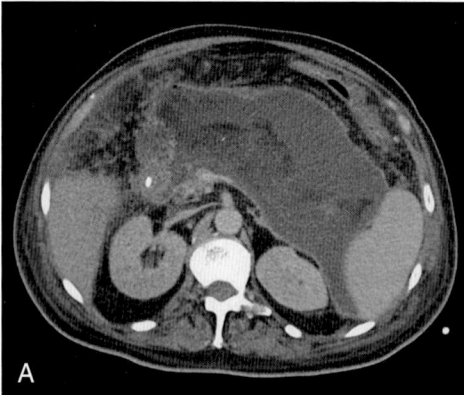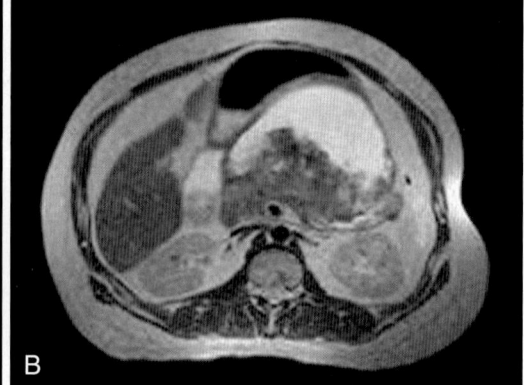

or has been in communication with the pancreatic duct. Cyst fluid high in carcinoembryonic antigen suggests the presence of a mucinous neoplasm. EUS can also be useful in the therapeutic management of pseudocysts in endoscopic cystoenterostomy.

MANAGEMENT

Pseudocysts (After Acute Interstitial Edematous Pancreatitis)

The natural history of pseudocysts in most cases involves spontaneous resolution over time. In persistent cases, however, intervention may be indicated. Historically, a pseudocyst greater than 6 cm or persistent over time (greater than 6 weeks) was considered to warrant intervention. Modern experience, however, has shown that watchful waiting is appropriate, particularly in small asymptomatic pseudocysts.

There are many reasons not to undertake operative internal drainage of a pseudocyst. The patient may be acutely and chronically unwell and a poor operative risk. The diagnosis may be incorrect despite evaluation with modern imaging studies. The collection may not be a pseudocyst as the acute fluid collection seen early in acute pancreatitis, the so-called pseudo-pseudocyst, does not need operative drainage. A sterile postnecrotic fluid collection or the pancreatic sequestrum may not need drainage. Beware of the cystic neoplasm. Many patients with mucinous cystic neoplasms have undergone cystogastrostomy with perilous outcomes. Most important is to remember that cyst internal drainage procedures do not correct an underlying pancreatic ductal disorder, and the cystoenteric or cystogastric anastomosis may not be effective long-term drainage of an obstructed pancreatic duct. A pancreatic pseudocyst that does not

communicate with the main pancreatic duct can be eradicated with a number of minimally invasive techniques.

Symptomatic pseudocysts that cause pain, obstruction (biliary, enteric, mesenteric venous), hemorrhage, or perforation (enteric fistula, pancreatic ascites, pleuropancreatic fistula) warrant intervention. Delineation of the anatomy with MRCP or ERCP is the first step in management. A pseudocyst in connection with the main pancreatic duct and with otherwise normal pancreatic duct anatomy can often be well treated with ERCP-guided sphincterotomy or transpapillary stent placement, altering the pressure differential across the ampulla and allowing for preferential drainage of the pseudocyst into the duodenum with resolution of the pancreatic duct disruption.

A pseudocyst without communication to the pancreatic duct or that has failed transpapillary endoscopic management can often be managed then with drainage. Endoscopic cystogastrostomy or duodenostomy involves placing a stent with endoscopic guidance through the back wall of the stomach or duodenum into a closely opposed retrogastric pseudocyst. Both open and laparoscopic surgical approaches to cystogastrostomy and duodenostomy are also well used, with the advantage of a larger anastomosis for a more durable drainage effect and better control of hemostasis. For all cystogastrostomies and cystoduodenostomies, the stomach or duodenum must be densely adherent to the pseudocyst, or the posterior enterotomy is at risk for postoperative leak and sepsis. In this procedure, an anterior gastrotomy is performed for access to the posterior gastric wall. The flat, firm, bulging surface on the back of the gastric wall represents the underlying pseudocyst. A posterior gastrotomy is then made with cautery (or another energy device for hemostasis). A cyst wall biopsy is included to rule out a cystic neoplasm and the cystoenteric anastomosis is oversewn to ensure hemostasis. The anterior gastrotomy is sewn or stapled securely closed. Open and laparoscopic Roux-en-Y cystoenterostomies are also used for drainage of the pseudocyst that is not well adherent to the stomach into a jejunal limb, with a similar technique.

In cases with the underlying pancreatic duct pathology visualized on preoperative MRCP or ERCP (stricture, obstruction), drainage alone may result in long-term failure of the operation with pseudocyst recurrence. If the pancreatic duct pathology is in the body or tail of the pancreas, distal pancreatectomy is a better, more durable operation than a cystoenterostomy.

Walled-Off Pancreatic Necrosis (After Acute Necrotizing Pancreatitis)

Walled-off pancreatic necrosis in many cases resolves spontaneously over time. In patients with evidence of infected necrosis, either by aspiration and culture or by visualized air within the collection on cross-sectional imaging, drainage or débridement is indicated. In the patient with sterile necrosis who is persistently unwell, marked by pain or nutritional failure with continued disease burden, intervention is also warranted.

The multiple approaches to the treatment of WOPN include the classic open necronectomy, the transgastric approach (either open, laparoscopic, or endoscopic), percutaneous drainage, and the retroperitoneal approach (open or videoscopic). The choice of approach is dependent on the anatomy and distribution of the necrosis, other patient-related factors (body mass index [BMI], surgical history, comorbidities), and importantly, surgeon experience and preference.

Similar to the pancreatic pseudocyst, the initial step in planning intervention in WOPN is to define the underlying pancreatic ductal anatomy with MRCP (or ERCP). Failure to address pancreatic ductal pathology may lead to primary operative failure and recurrent problems.

Open necrosectomy remains the mainstay of management of pancreatic necrosis. In this approach, the lesser sac is entered and gentle blunt débridement undertaken. The placement of large catheters for postoperative drainage and lavage is a classic component of this technique. Laparotomy allows for access to the entire peritoneal cavity for optimal débridement and safe accomplishment of hemostasis. In addition, concomitant cholecystectomy and enteral feeding access are easily obtained.

Open necrosectomy is always a good approach to pancreatic necrosis, even in this modern era. It is particularly suited for the patient with a large, diffuse disease burden, including both paracolic gutters and the root of the mesentery, which are not easily reached with less invasive techniques.

Transgastric necrosectomy emerges from the experience with transgastric drainage of pseudocysts. This technique can be accomplished in an open fashion or laparoscopically. An anterior gastrotomy is performed to gain access to the posterior gastric wall. The site of the WOPN is identified as a firm bulge in the wall of the stomach. The cavity is then entered with cautery or other energy sources (i.e., ultrasonic shears). This posterior gastrotomy is best made in a generous fashion to allow for thorough inspection and débridement of the necrosis cavity. The posterior gastrotomy and cavity wall opening are then secured together for hemostasis with a running absorbable suture. The anterior gastrotomy is closed either with a running suture or with a stapler. The endoscopic approach entails an endoscopically created posterior gastrotomy into the necrosum, often with the use of cautery and pneumatic dilation. Débridement is undertaken with endoscopic instrumentation and can be time and resource intensive.

The transgastric approach is well suited for the patient with disease burden primarily limited to the lesser sac and with a posterior mass effect on the gastric wall. An advantage of the transgastric approach includes the potential creation of a pancreatogastric fistula in cases of a disconnected left pancreatic remnant, potentially avoiding the need for distal pancreatectomy or fistula-enterostomy down the road.

In selected patients with pancreatic necrosis, image-guided percutaneous drainage can be an effective means of therapy. Percutaneous drains have the obvious advantage of avoiding the insult of surgical or even endoscopic intervention. Percutaneous drains serve to drain any liquid component of the necrosum but do not serve well to remove solid necrotic tissue. Several studies have shown significant percentages of patients with WOPN with response to percutaneous drainage alone without surgery (15% to 45%). At a minimum, percutaneous drainage can provide temporization for an ill patient early in the course of necrosis to allow for physiologic recovery and a delayed débridement. Drains are also an essential component of the retroperitoneal approach to pancreatic débridement.

The retroperitoneal approach to pancreatic débridement has been described with an open technique but is more commonly applied with laparoscopic guidance. It has been referred to as videoscopic-assisted retroperitoneal débridement (VARD) by the group in Seattle and as the step-up approach by the Dutch. This technique involves placing percutaneous catheters, typically in the left flank, as an initial attempt at drainage. In those patients with continued solid disease burden, the catheter track is then used as a guide into the necrosis cavity through the left flank into the lesser sac. The laparoscope is used for visualization, and laparoscopic instruments are used for the débridement. A large-bore catheter is left behind for postoperative irrigation and drainage. The retroperitoneal approach is best suited for patients with WOPN that extends into the left paracolic gutter. It can have limited effectiveness with disease burden at the base of the mesentery or into the right paracolic gutter.

Disconnected Left Pancreatic Remnant

In severe cases of acute pancreatitis, significant parenchymal inflammation and necrosis may result in obliteration of the main pancreatic duct, typically at the neck of the pancreas, resulting in a disconnected left pancreatic remnant. This viable body and tail tissue continues to have exocrine production, which does not have an avenue for drainage. The result is a midbody pseudocyst or persistent pancreatic fistula if a drain is in place (Figure 3). Patients with this problem may present several months after the resolution of severe pancreatitis with the signs and symptoms of a pseudocyst and are well treated with resection of the tail remnant. If there is a significantly large segment of disconnected pancreas, a cyst enterostomy can be undertaken to preserve pancreatic endocrine function. Alternatively, a distal pancreatectomy with islet autotransplantation is an option. If this anatomy is apparent at the time of initial débridement, the patient can undergo combined open distal pancreatectomy and débridement if they are physiologically fit for this potentially morbid operation. Alternatively, a transgastric débridement approach may be considered to allow for the creation of a pancreatogastric fistula and the internal drainage of this remnant.

Pseudocysts Associated With Chronic Pancreatitis

In the setting of chronic pancreatitis, delineation of the underlying pancreatic ductal anatomy is essential to the proper management of the pseudocyst. Unaddressed obstruction from stricture or stone is likely to result in long-term management failure. Endoscopic intervention with stenting or stricture dilation is a good initial approach, particularly in patients with small duct disease involving the pancreatic head. In small duct disease with a stricture in the body or tail, left-sided resection may be appropriate. In the setting of dilated duct pancreatitis, a drainage procedure consisting of a lateral pancreaticojejunostomy is a good option.

CONCLUSION

Peripancreatic fluid collections are heterogeneous. Most are benign and resolve spontaneously. Some, however, are complex, with significant potential for morbidity, and can be vexing in management. Proper categorization can aid in clinical decision making, as

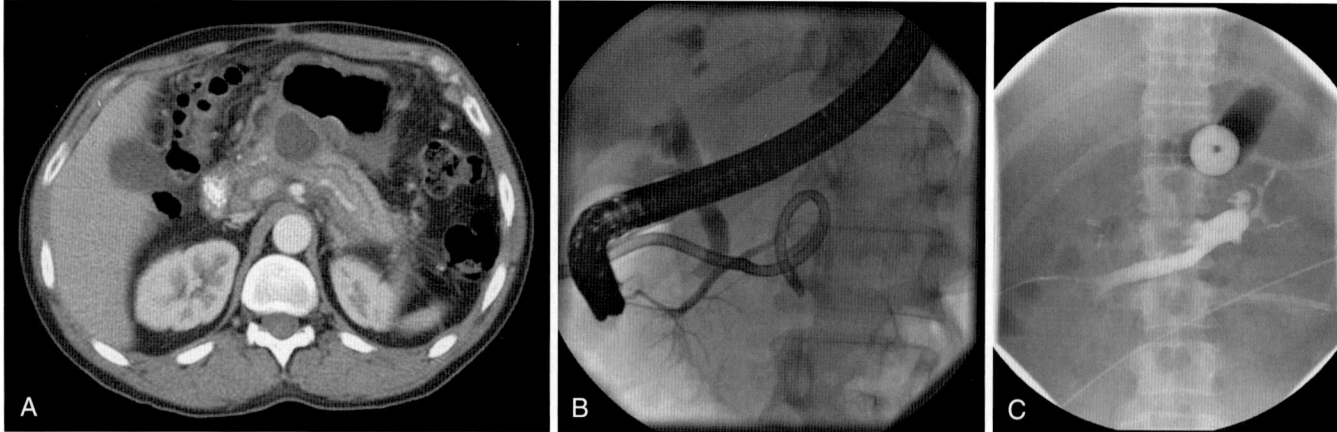

FIGURE 3 A disconnected left pancreatic remnant occurs after necrosis in the neck of the pancreas with resultant obliteration of the main pancreatic duct. The disrupted pancreatic duct from the viable left pancreas, now not in continuity, leaks and results in a midbody pseudocyst. This condition is visualized on contrast enhanced computed tomographic scan **(A)**. It is shown by an abrupt cut-off of the pancreatic duct at the neck on endoscopic retrograde pancreatography **(B)** and by a drain track fistulagram filling only a small tail remnant **(C)**.

can determination of the underlying pancreatic ductal anatomy. Symptomatic pseudocysts can be drained, but the underlying pancreatic duct pathology should be considered and may warrant a distal resection. Infected pancreatic necrosis and sterile necrosis with persistent illness require drainage or débridement. There are multiple effective approaches to pancreatic débridement in the modern era.

SUGGESTED READINGS

Bradley EL III, Allen K: A prospective longitudinal study of observation versus surgical intervention in the management of necrotizing pancreatitis, *Am J Surg* 161:19–25, 1991.

Freeny PC, Hauptmann E, Althaus SJ, et al: Percutaneous CT-guided catheter drainage of infected acute necrotizing pancreatitis: techniques and results, *Am J Roentgenol* 170:969–975, 1998.

Horvath K, Freeny P, Escallon J, et al: Safety and efficacy of video-assisted retroperitoneal debridement for infected pancreatic collections: a multicenter, prospective, single arm phase 2 study, *Arch Surg* 145:817–825, 2010.

Howard TJ, Moore SA, Saxena R, et al: Pancreatic duct strictures are a common cause of recurrent pancreatitis after successful management of pancreatic necrosis, *Surgery* 136:909–916, 2004.

Kozarek RA, Call TJ, Patterson DJ, et al: Endoscopic transpapillary therapy for disrupted pancreatic duct and peripancreatic fluid collections, *Gastroenterology* 100:1362–1370, 1991.

Nealon WH, Bhutani M, Riall TS, et al: A unifying concept: pancreatic ductal anatomy both predicts and determines the major complications resulting from pancreatitis, *J Am Coll Surg* 208:790–801, 2009.

Nealon WH, Walser E: Main pancreatic ductal anatomy can direct choice of modality for treating pancreatic pseudocysts (surgery versus percutaneous drainage), *Ann Surg* 235:751–758, 2002.

Uhl W, Warshaw A, Imrie C, et al: IAP guidelines for the surgical management of acute pancreatitis, *Pancreatology* 2:565–573, 2002.

van Santvoort HC, Besselink MG, Bakker OJ, et al: A step-up approach or open necrosectomy for necrotizing pancreatitis, *N Engl J Med* 362:1491–1502, 2010.

Warshaw AI, Rattner DW: Timing of surgical drainage of pancreatic pseudocyst, clinical and chemical criteria, *Ann Surg* 202:720–724, 1985.

PANCREATIC DUCTAL DISRUPTIONS LEADING TO PANCREATIC FISTULA, PANCREATIC ASCITES, OR PANCREATIC PLEURAL EFFUSION

Graham W. Donald, MD, and O. Joseph Hines, MD

INTRODUCTION

Pancreatic ductal disruptions represent a challenging clinical problem for the surgeon. The etiology, diagnoses, complications, treatments, and outcomes of ductal disruptions are highly variable. These are the result of or directed at the correction of one overarching problem—namely, leakage of caustic pancreatic enzymes outside of the ductal system into the pancreatic parenchyma or the peripancreatic space (pseudocysts, pancreatic necrosis, peripancreatic fluid collections) into other bodily cavities (pancreatic ascites, pancreatic pleural fistula) or externally through the skin (pancreaticocutaneous fistula).

Management of ductal disruption and the conditions that result require collaboration with multiple specialties, including gastroenterology, radiology, and surgery. Furthermore, current treatment strategies are evolving with special consideration for timing after the inciting event for intervention. Certainly when surgical intervention is being considered, the patient should be medically optimized and nutritionally replete, and the condition and ductal anatomy should be thoroughly defined.

ETIOLOGY AND COMPLICATIONS

Pancreatic ductal disruption can occur in the setting of pancreatic disease (acute and chronic pancreatitis), postoperatively after pancreatic surgery (e.g., pancreaticoduodenectomy, distal pancreatectomy, débridement for necrosis), or after trauma.

Ductal disruption occurring after an episode of acute pancreatitis or in the setting of chronic pancreatitis results in a variety of complications. *Peripancreatic fluid collections* refer to the presence of fluid around the pancreas with or without a semisolid debris component. The amount of fluid is likely a reflection of the caliber of the duct injured during the inflammatory process (minor peripheral ductule versus main pancreatic duct). *Pancreatic pseudocysts* are fluid collections that, unlike peripancreatic fluid collections, are classically described as having a thick wall that is lacking an epithelial lining and require several weeks to form.

Leakage of fluid beyond the confines of the pancreas or peripancreatic space—what can be called an internal pancreatic fistula—also occurs in cases of ductal disruption and usually in conjunction with the aforementioned problems (fluid collections, pseudocysts, necrosis). They also present unique problems, outlined below, requiring particular intervention related to anatomic considerations.

Pancreaticocutaneous Fistulae

Pancreaticocutaneous fistulae can occur, albeit rarely, in a spontaneous fashion after pancreatitis because there are no natural pathways from within the abdominal cavity to the skin. More commonly, these occur after drainage procedures for fluid collections or as a result of a drain placed at the time of surgery for operative débridement or resection.

Postoperative Fistulae

Pancreatic resection resulting in a pancreatic fistula or "leak" (i.e., iatrogenic ductal disruption) occurs in between 10% and 15% of pancreaticoduodenectomies and in around 20% to 30% of middle and distal pancreatectomies. After pancreaticoduodenectomy, pancreatic fistula is the result of a disruption of the anastomosis between the pancreatic remnant and the jejunum or stomach, and it can often be predicted based on the consistency of the pancreas and the diameter of the main pancreatic duct. It is well documented that the resection of a normal or soft pancreas has a much higher rate of fistula than resection of a firm or fibrotic pancreas and that a main duct of less than 3 mm increases the chance of postoperative fistula.

Pancreatic Ascites

Pancreatic ascites refers to enzyme-rich pancreatic fluid accumulated within the peritoneal cavity (Figure 1), and it often occurs with rupture of a pseudocyst in the face of a disrupted duct. The presence of pancreatic ascites may not be clear in a patient with ethanol-induced pancreatitis because these patients may have cirrhosis and some degree of ascites due to elevated portal vein pressures. Pancreatic ascites can also occur after splenectomy, distal pancreatectomy, or left nephrectomy wherein the tail of the pancreas has been damaged and the pancreatic fluid that leaks is not contained.

Pancreatic Pleural Fistulae

Pancreatic pleural fistulas can result in a pleural effusion or fluid within the mediastinum due to tracking of pancreatic juices from a fluid collection or pseudocyst in the abdominal cavity, usually through the foramina of the diaphragm and into the chest cavity. A rare clinical entity, it is infrequently associated with an acute episode of pancreatitis. More often, pancreatic pleural fistulae arise in the setting of chronic pancreatitis or in patients with recurrent attacks of acute pancreatitis with a history of alcohol abuse.

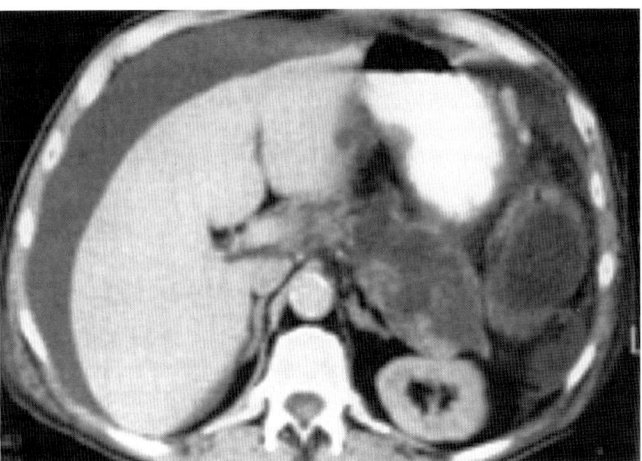

FIGURE I   Abdominal computed tomographic (CT) scan demonstrating pancreatic ascites with fluid around the liver and a fluid collection within the pancreas.

Trauma-Induced Ductal Disruption

A final etiology of ductal disruption is trauma. These injuries are associated with a high mortality rate and with blunt deceleration injury, oftentimes in patients who were wearing seatbelts when in a motor vehicle accident. Clinicians should therefore have a high index of suspicion for pancreatic injury in patients who are victims of this type of injury. These disruptions classically occur in the midbody of the pancreas where it traverses the spinal column, and it can lead to extravasation of the enzyme-rich fluid, resulting in a pseudocyst, a peripancreatic fluid collection, or any of the anomalous fistulous collections between the ductal system and bodily cavities heretofore mentioned.

CLINICAL PRESENTATION AND DIAGNOSIS

Pancreaticocutaneous/Postoperative Fistula

This clinical condition occurs when a drain placed percutaneously or surgically does not cease to drain enzyme-rich fluid. After pancreaticoduodenectomy, a leak is typically diagnosed if a surgical drain near the pancreaticoenteric anastomosis is draining greater than 30 mL/day of enzyme-rich fluid, with an amylase concentration of greater than three times the normal limit of serum amylase and after the fifth postoperative day. However, because of the wide variation in definitions of postoperative pancreatic fistula across the literature, an international study group (Bassi C, et al., 2005) recently established an all-inclusive definition of drain output of any measurable volume on or after postoperative day 3 with an amylase greater than three times the serum amylase level. The clinician should have a high index of suspicion for fistulae when a postoperative patient has any of the following: failure to convalesce in a normal fashion, nausea or vomiting, persistent fevers or unexplained sepsis, malnutrition or failure to thrive, or prolonged abdominal pain.

Pancreatic Ascites

Patients with pancreatic ascites typically complain of abdominal discomfort, and history and physical exam reveal weight loss, likely due to malnutrition in the setting of malabsorption. Examination reveals abdominal distention or fluid wave without tenderness.

Pancreatic Pleural Fistulae

Patients with a pancreatic pleural fistula may demonstrate dyspnea or cough, or show physical exam signs consistent with pleural effusion, such as decreased or absent breath sounds, decreased fremitus, and dullness to percussion. Radiograph may show fluid in the chest (Figure 2).

In all of these cases, failure to improve after the inciting event (pancreatitis, operation, or trauma) should prompt a computed tomographic (CT) scan to access for fluid collections (Figure 3). If the diagnosis is still unclear regarding the origin of fluid, the collection can be aspirated and tested for pancreatic amylase. Although there has been some discussion regarding the role of fluid analysis and the risk of introducing infection into a previously sterile collection, the likelihood of this is minimal. Aspiration of the pleural effusion may be both diagnostic and therapeutic, with the introduction of a tube thoracostomy.

Diagnostic Evaluation

CT is the most appropriate initial study when investigating suspected pancreatic ductal disruption. Optimal visualization of the pancreas is obtained with a pancreatic protocol CT, which involves images captured with a multidetector row helical scanner in three phases (arterial, late arterial, and venous) using thin slices. Sometimes oral contrast can be added to improve the quality of the image. Furthermore, CT guidance offers the ability to intervene percutaneously should any fluid collections or abscesses be apparent. In the case of pancreatic fistula, percutaneous drainage is essentially creating an iatrogenic, controlled pancreaticocutaneous fistula.

Endoscopic retrograde cholangiopancreatography (ERCP) is not recommended in the early period when ductal disruptions are suspected. The reasons are that first, ERCP carries with it a not insignificant risk of postprocedure pancreatitis that may exacerbate the inciting condition, and second, the risk of introducing infection via instrumentation may not outweigh the benefit of early characterization of ductal anatomy. Most importantly, however, is the fact that most of the conditions of pancreatic ductal disruption described above will resolve spontaneously over the course of a few weeks with conservative therapy alone. There is some literature advocating for ERCP because it has both diagnostic and therapeutic capabilities in the form of transpapillary stenting for persistent pancreatic fistula or for chronic pain associated with chronic pancreatitis. ERCP should instead be reserved for the chronic complication of a nonresolved ductal disruption with inadequate drainage into the gastrointestinal tract (see the "Management and Treatment" section). While classification systems for ductal disruption have been proposed, it is our opinion that the most important categorization of ductal anatomy is the distinction of whether or not the fluid collections that persist are in communication with the main duct and whether or not the duct is completely disrupted—that is, so-called *disconnected duct syndrome*—because definitive operative intervention is often necessary in these cases.

A safer and less invasive alternative to ERCP if CT scan images are equivocal is magnetic resonance cholangiopancreatography (MRCP). MRCP can delineate ductal anatomy (particularly of the main pancreatic duct), identify the majority of disruptions and fistulae without the need to instrument the duct, assess the need for ERCP or a step-up in therapy, be used in the setting of failed ERCP duct cannulation, or be used to monitor progression of a disruption over time without the need for repeat ERCP. Many institutions utilize MRCP to investigate persistent suspected ductal disruptions or ongoing fistulae prior to ERCP. Drawbacks of MRCP include possible lower spatial resolution of the ductal anatomy when compared to ERCP because MRCP depends on endogenous liquid within the duct for visualization, while ERCP takes advantage of the injection of dye as a contrast material. Secretin administration can stimulate pancreatic secretion and increase the sensitivity of MRCP.

MANAGEMENT AND TREATMENT

While the problem of pancreatic ductal disruption can lead to a variety of complications as previously mentioned, the management of this problem is largely dependent on the acuity or chronicity of the clinical problem. Early management in the acute phases in a majority of cases is conservative, because these disruptions and the anomalous fluid collections often resolve. Nasojejunal feeding or total parenteral nutrition to decrease pancreatic activity during the acute phase of pancreatitis that comes with oral or prepyloric alimentation, along with percutaneous management of fluid collections under CT or ultrasound guidance, are staples of early therapy. Repeat interval imaging at 4 to 6 weeks is obtained to assess the state of fluid collections as they respond to these interventions.

In cases where fluid collections and fistulas do not improve after being given adequate time to resolve or if patients' symptoms worsen, both of which indicate ongoing, large-caliber ductal disruption or superimposed infection, intervention is required and defined based on the inciting event and the condition to be addressed. Two of these—pseudocyst and postoperative leak—are unique clinical circumstances and will be addressed first.

Pseudocyst

As with necrosis, management of pseudocysts involves several specialties, each with varying degrees of invasiveness. Where traditionally operation was the gold standard intervention for mature pseudocysts with resolution in 90% to 95% of cases, percutaneous and endoscopic techniques to manage these problems are quickly gaining ground in terms of utilization. Percutaneous intervention is limited to simple drainage and carries the risk of an external fistula caused by an external drain and a higher recurrence rate. Endoscopic treatments involve transgastric and, rarely, transduodenal drainage. An additional modality that experienced endoscopists can employ is the placement of transpapillary stents during ERCP, which are small-caliber plastic catheters that traverse the sphincter of Oddi. Pancreatic fluid can then drain through the path of least resistance into the duodenum. This technique is most successful when there is radiographic evidence on ERCP or CT scan of connection between the main pancreatic duct and the pseudocyst.

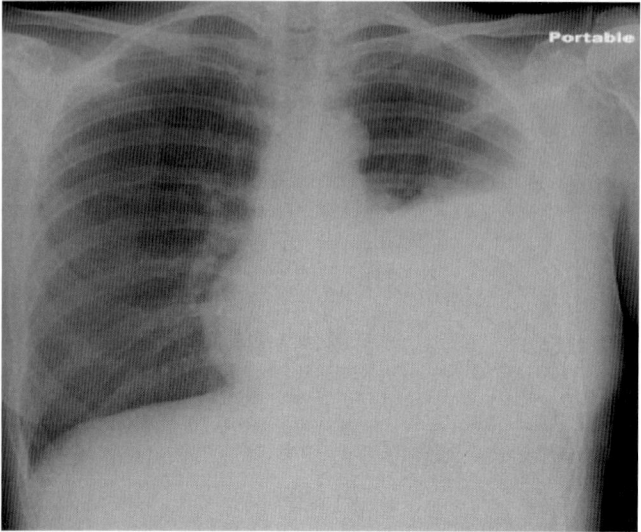

FIGURE 2 Chest x-ray demonstrating a left-sided pleural effusion secondary to a pancreaticopleural fistula.

Operative intervention includes cystogastrostomy or roux-en-Y cystojejunostomy, with postoperative hemorrhage and sepsis being more common after cystogastrostomy. Cystogastrostomy should be performed when the cyst is in close proximity or adherent to the posterior aspect of the stomach. After anterior gastrostomy, the pseudocyst is located with needle aspiration and drained into the stomach by excising a circle of the gastric wall into the cyst or by using a linear or circular stapler. If a portion of the gastric wall is excised, the cut edge of the stomach should be sewn with a running, locking absorbable suture to prevent postoperative hemorrhage. The anterior stomach is then closed in two layers. If the cyst is not near the stomach, a side-to-side cystojejunostomy should be performed and often positioned through the left transverse mesocolon.

Postoperative Pancreatic Fistulae/ Pancreaticocutaneous Fistulae

We previously discussed the association of pancreatic texture and main duct diameter in the development of postoperative pancreatic fistula after pancreaticoduodenectomy. Other risk factors include the underlying disease, with pancreatic fistula more likely in cases of

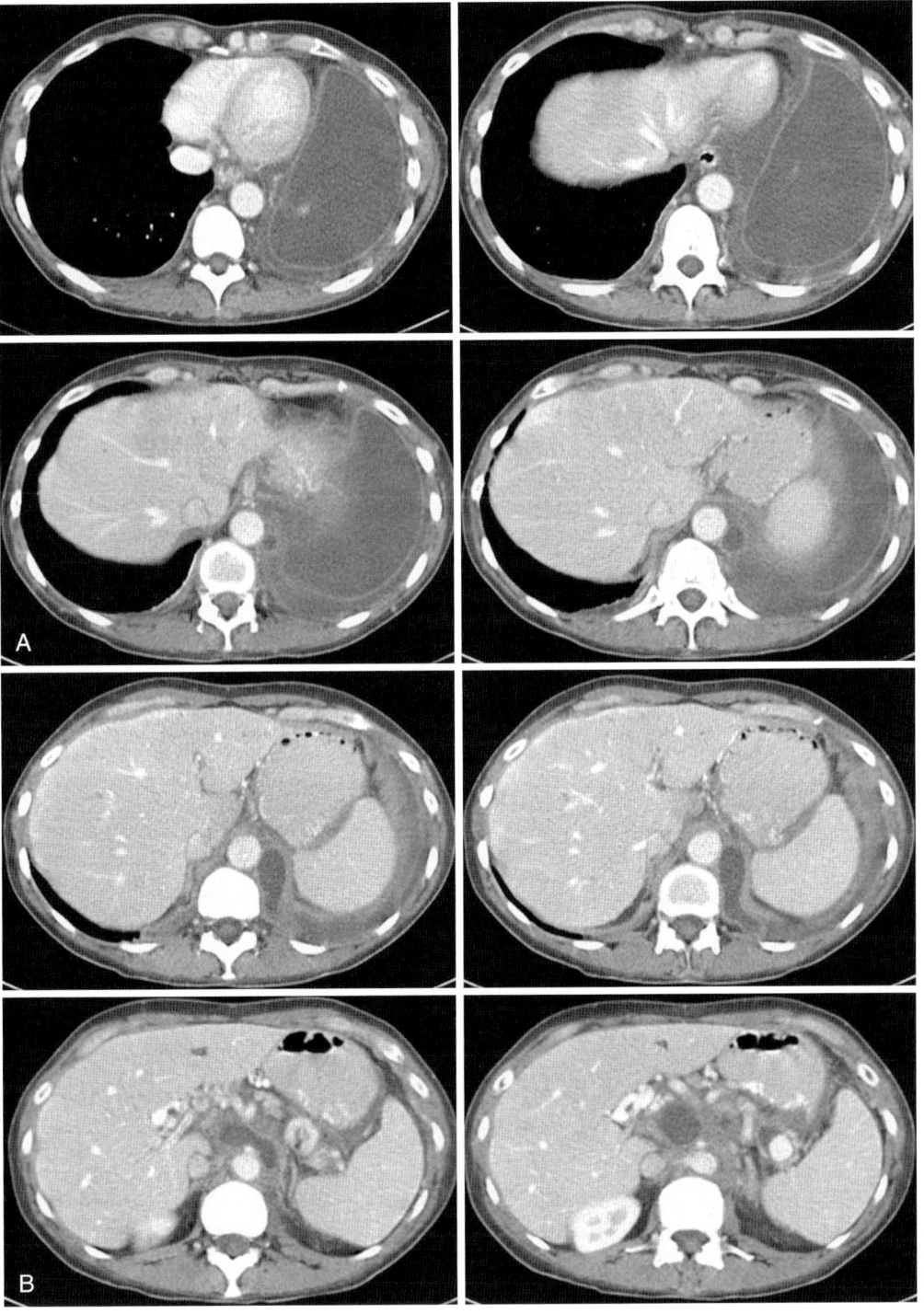

FIGURE 3 Computed tomographic (CT) scans showing a large pleural effusion **(A)**. There is a pancreatic pseudocyst communicating with this effusion **(B)**.

Continued

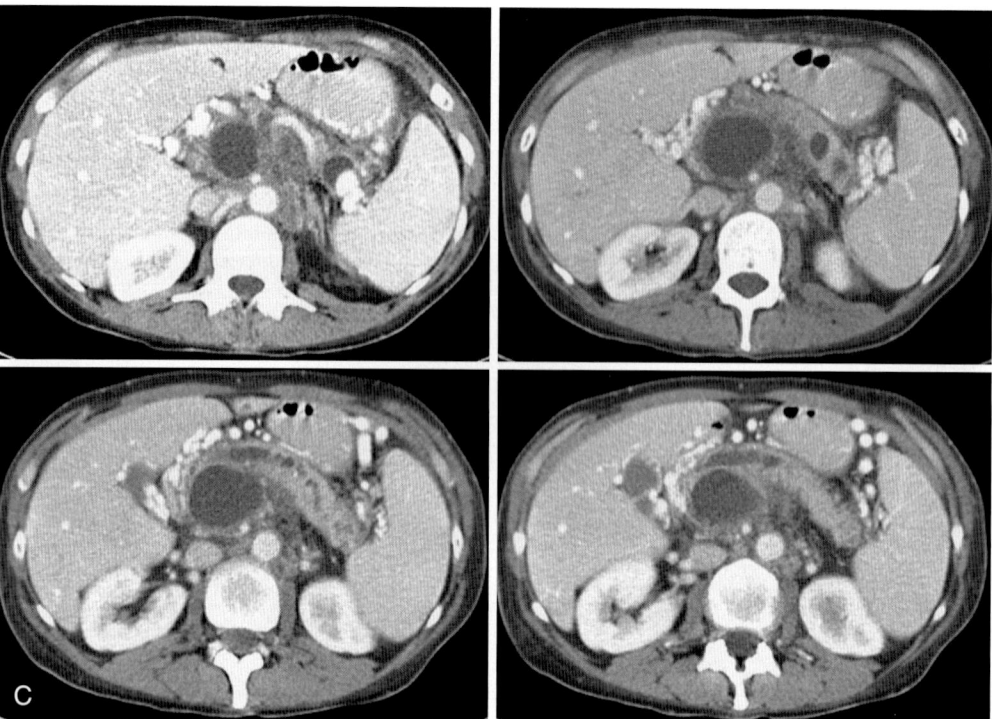

FIGURE 3, cont'd The final panel demonstrates chronic pancreatitis and a dilated pancreatic duct, as well as splenic vein thrombosis, a splenic artery aneurysm, and left-sided portal hypertension **(C)**.

benign cystic neoplasms and periampullary tumors and less likely in adenocarcinoma. Much research has been directed toward preventive measures to decrease the risk of these leaks developing.

Prophylactic somatostatin analogues have been widely studied. While individual studies show marginal benefit in reducing the rate of postoperative fistula after pancreaticoduodenectomy or distal pancreatectomy with administration of these analogues, subsequent meta-analyses of randomized controlled trials show no benefit. This is a testament to the heterogeneity of the studies, including differences in administration of the drug, the analogue used, and the definition of pancreatic fistula. A somatostatin analogue would, however, be useful in the case of high-output fistulae to control the volume and possibly lead to faster closure.

In regards to intraoperative measures, application of fibrin glue intraoperatively has garnered interest in the literature. Studies describing the use of fibrin glue on the pancreatic stump or circumferentially around the anastomosis after pancreaticoduodenectomy have varied results, overall showing no difference in fistula rates.

Methods of pancreatic reconstruction for pancreaticojejunostomy after pancreatic head resection include end-to-side duct-to-mucosa anastomosis or invagination of the pancreatic remnant. Results have shown, including one randomized controlled trial, that there is a significantly lower rate of fistula formation in the invagination group. In addition, some have advocated that a pancreaticogastrostomy may decrease postoperative leak. Validation studies are needed.

Prophylactic pancreatic duct stenting intraoperatively during pancreaticoduodenectomy theoretically decompresses the pancreatic duct and directs the flow of the enzyme-rich fluid into the enteric limb. As with the previous preventive strategies, this modality has mixed results in terms of decreasing fistula rate, and its role is not clear.

Once the diagnosis of a persistent pancreatic leak after resection is made, efforts should be directed at ensuring the patient is stable. Intravenous fluids should be administered liberally because these patients can suffer significant pancreatic fluid loss. Antibiotics should be empirically started for any patient with persistent fevers or an elevated white blood cell count. The management then depends on the nature of the initial operation (i.e., pancreatic head resection vs distal pancreatectomy vs enucleation, etc.). In the case of pancreatic fistula after pancreatic head resection, nearly 95% of fistula will resolve with conservative management alone—namely, prolonged tube drainage, which can be managed in the outpatient setting as long as the patient is eating and without fever.

In the case of an enucleation or distal pancreatectomy or in cases of débridement, MRCP or ERCP should be carried out to define the nature of the ductal disruption. It is at this point that transpapillary stents can be placed with the intent that stenting a downstream portion of the pancreatic duct will cause the enzyme-rich fluid to travel the path of least resistance into the intestine. Figure 4 demonstrates the successful stenting across a ductal disruption after enucleation of an insulinoma.

If a patient has a fever in the setting of a pancreatic fistula, a CT scan should be obtained to look for an intra-abdominal fluid collection, which could be drained during the same scan. If a patient has persistent fistula for several weeks after discharge, a fistulogram should be obtained and the original drain replaced with a red rubber catheter. At this point, nearly all fistulae close within 1 or 2 days because the rubber incites an inflammatory response, closing the fistula tract.

Late reoperation for persistent pancreatic fistula after a resection is thus rarely needed, but it would entail creating an anastomosis between a Roux limb to the fistula tract. At the time of laparotomy, the fistulojejunostomy is performed by first identifying the fistula tract. The tract is then traced toward and as close to the pancreas as safely possible and then sewn to a Roux limb of jejunum in an end-to-side fashion.

Early reoperation for pancreatic fistula is also rarely required but may be necessary in cases of hemorrhage caused by erosion of the fistula into an artery (a so-called "herald bleed") or for abscesses or fluid collections not amenable to percutaneous drainage. Reoperation consists of wide drainage of any fluid collections with drains left in place. In the case of hemorrhage, bleeding can be initially addressed by embolization through interventional radiology techniques.

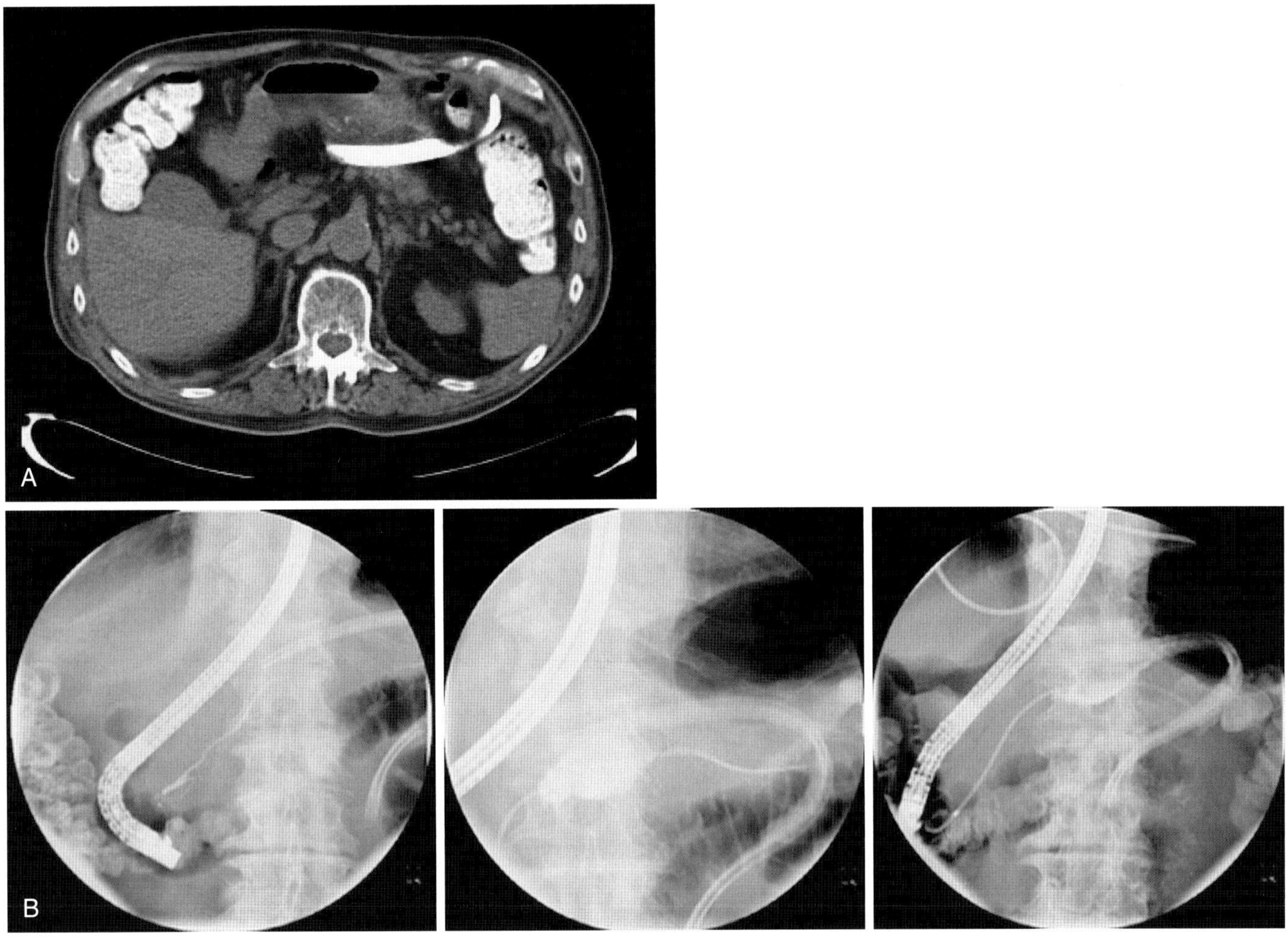

FIGURE 4 Pancreatic duct disruption at the pancreatic neck after an enucleation of an insulinoma followed by ERCP (demonstrating leak) **(A)** and placement of a long 5 French 15 cm pancreatic duct stent across the leak **(B)**.

Pancreatic Pleural Fistulae

Traditionally, pancreatic pleural fistulae are subjected to a nonoperative treatment trial for several weeks prior to any attempt at operative correction of the underlying ductal disruption. As with other pancreatic fistula, nonoperative treatment includes bowel rest and nutritional support. These patients may require repeated large-volume thoracentesis or tube thoracostomy. Medical management includes administration of antisecretagogues, including octreotide. If these fail to resolve the fistula, an interventional strategy may be attempted with ERCP and main duct stenting.

Conservative strategies, however, have low success rates in the case of pancreatic pleural fistula (with fistula resolution approximately only one third of the time), as well as high rates of recurrence and morbidity. We propose that appropriate patients be considered early on for surgical intervention with a Roux-en-Y limb pancreaticojejunostomy to the base of the fistula (Figure 5). In our experience, a majority of these patients will require no further therapy and will be subject to significantly shorter treatment duration.

Pancreatic Ascites

Initial management of pancreatic ascites entails nonsurgical, conservative strategies of nutritional support (nasojejunal feedings or total parenteral nutrition); antisecretagogues to diminish pancreatic secretions; and repeat, large-volume paracentesis. Salvage surgery is reserved for those cases that did not resolve in 6 weeks. Operative

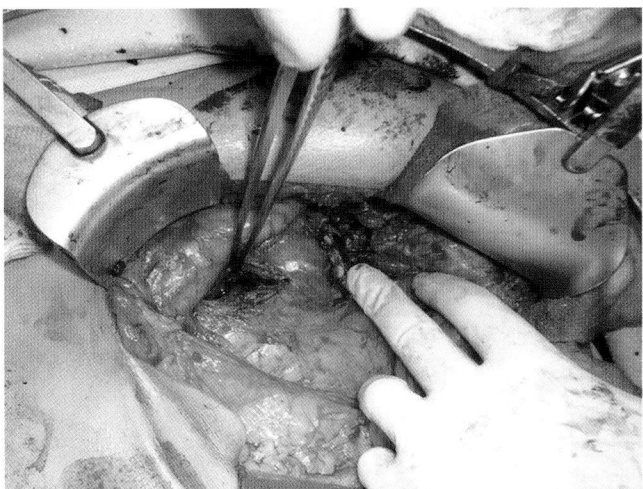

FIGURE 5 Exposed main pancreatic duct in the patient in Figure 3. A Roux-en-Y pancreaticojejunostomy was performed to control a pancreaticopleural fistula after a distal pancreatectomy, a splenectomy, and an excision of a splenic artery aneurysm.

management depends on the ductal anatomy. If the pancreatic ascites is due to a ductal disruption (defined by imaging or ERCP) without a pseudocyst, internal drainage into a Roux-en-Y limb is the operation of choice. If the ductal disruption is in the tail of the pancreas and the proximal duct is normal, distal pancreatectomy and oversewing of the remnant can be performed. If a ruptured pseudocyst is present, surgical therapy should be in the form of cystogastrostomy or Roux-en-Y cystojejunostomy.

It should be noted, however, that endoscopic therapy is becoming more advanced. Experienced endoscopists may be able to bridge a disruption with a stent via ERCP, with simultaneous endoscopic drainage of fluid collections or percutaneous drainage, thus precluding the need for surgery.

CONCLUSION

Overall, ductal disruption leading to pancreatic fistula, whether that be a thoracopancreatic, intra-abdominal (pancreatic ascites) or pancreaticocutaneous, the mainstay of therapy is ensuring first and foremost that the patient is receiving adequate nutritional support. Beyond that, the modalities of medical management, interventional procedures (radiologic and endoscopic), and surgery should all be considered. The optimal strategy or combination of strategies has changed considerably over recent years with advances in technique and is dependent on the etiology of the ductal disruption, the nature of the disruption, the overall condition of the patient, and access to resources.

SUGGESTED READINGS

Bassi C, Dervenis C, Butturini G, et al: Postoperative pancreatic fistula: an international study group (ISGPF) definition. *Surgery* 138(1):8–13, 2005.

Bhasin DK, Rana SS, Rao C, et al: Endoscopic management of pancreatic injury due to abdominal trauma. *JOP* 13(2):187–192, 2012.

Kazanjian KK, Hines OJ, Eibl G, et al: Management of pancreatic fistulas after pancreaticoduodenectomy: results in 437 consecutive patients. *Arch Surg* 140(9):849–854; discussion 854–856, 2005.

King JC, Reber HA, Shiraga S, et al: Pancreatic-pleural fistula is best managed by early operative intervention. *Surgery* 147(1):154–159. Epub 2009 Jun 9, 2010.

Nealon WH, Bhutani M, Riall TS, et al: A unifying concept: pancreatic ductal anatomy both predicts and determines the major complications resulting from pancreatitis. *J Am Coll Surg* 208:790–799, 2009.

THE MANAGEMENT OF CHRONIC PANCREATITIS

Timothy R. Donahue, MD, and
Howard A. Reber, MD

INTRODUCTION

Most patients with chronic pancreatitis seek medical care because of the pain that is commonly associated with the disease. This chapter reviews briefly the diagnosis, medical management, and endoscopic treatment of pain in these patients. A more detailed discussion of the surgical management and the operations for pain relief is provided, including the Peustow, Frey, and Beger procedures and pancreaticoduodenectomy.

DEFINITION AND TYPES OF CHRONIC PANCREATITIS

Chronic pancreatitis is characterized by progressive inflammatory changes in the pancreas that result in permanent structural damage. The inflammation is usually associated with epigastric abdominal pain, which is the most common presenting symptom. Nevertheless 5% to 10% of patients remain pain-free. The structural damage can result in impairment of endocrine and exocrine function. Patients may develop type I diabetes mellitus and fat malabsorption. Chronic pancreatitis contrasts with acute pancreatitis, which is an acute inflammatory response to pancreatic injury that often does not progress and is usually reversible. The two conditions may overlap, and patients with chronic pancreatitis can have intermittent episodes of acute inflammation. However the histopathologic features of the gland with chronic pancreatitis (acinar and islet atrophy, and chronic inflammation with fibrosis) do not return to normal when the episodes resolve. Less commonly, repeated episodes of acute pancreatitis can lead to chronic pancreatitis when they cause structural damage in the pancreas, such as ductal strictures or disruptions, or pseudocysts.

Due to the chronic inflammation, patients with chronic pancreatitis are at risk for pancreatic cancer. It has been shown that oncogenic KRAS mutations coupled with inflammation can lead to malignant transformation. Approximately 4% of patients with chronic pancreatitis develop pancreatic cancer in their lifetime.

Chronic pancreatitis has many causes. Alcohol abuse is the most common cause, particularly in the Western world, where it is the cause of 60% of cases. Caustic environmental insults also have been implicated. Certain anatomic changes that obstruct the pancreatic ducts also may lead to chronic pancreatitis. These include ductal strictures and disruptions, pseudocysts, stones, periampullary tumors, pancreas divisum, or mechanical and structural changes of the pancreatic duct sphincter. Chronic pancreatitis due to ductal obstruction is less likely to be associated with ductal calcification, which is more common in alcoholic chronic pancreatitis.

There are a number of genetic causes of chronic pancreatitis. These include mutations in the cystic fibrosis transmembrane receptor (CFTR), trypsin inhibitor (SPINK1), and trypsin-1 gene (PRSS-1).

Many less common causes complete the list. Autoimmune pancreatitis occurs in a small number of patients. It is usually associated with elevated serum levels of IgG4. Active flares can be relieved with systemic steroids. However, chronic and progressive inflammation can lead to the development of chronic pancreatitis. Tropical pancreatitis, another unusual cause, is rare in the Western world. Unfortunately, the exact cause of the disease often cannot be determined, and patients are diagnosed with "idiopathic" chronic pancreatitis in up to 30% of cases.

DIAGNOSIS AND SEVERITY CLASSIFICATION

The diagnosis of chronic pancreatitis can be difficult because other conditions may produce similar symptoms. If one is suspicious of the diagnosis, it is important to send these patients to a medical professional with experience in the management of pancreatic diseases. With disease progression, most patients experience abdominal pain; exocrine and endocrine dysfunction usually occur later. The pain is multifactorial; this may be due in part to increased intraductal and parenchymal pressure of the pancreas, which leads to ischemia of the gland. An increase in the number and sensitivity of intrapancreatic pain sensors also occurs. Exocrine function usually declines before endocrine function, but clinical evidence of insufficiency may not become evident for many years after the histopathologic changes begin. When exocrine function is impaired significantly, patients may no longer have elevations of pancreatic enzymes in the serum during episodes of acute inflammation.

Many imaging tests can be used to diagnose and "stage" chronic pancreatitis. On abdominal plain films, intraductal calcifications can be seen in 30% to 50% of patients. These are pathognomonic for the disease and are thought to be due to increased protein concentration in the pancreatic juice, which leads to concretions and proteinaceous plugs that eventually calcify (Figure 1).

Computed tomographic (CT) scan or magnetic resonance imaging (MRI)/magnetic resonance cholangiopancreatography (MRCP) are commonly used and are quite accurate for diagnosis. In most cases, there is characteristic beading of the main pancreatic duct with side branch ectasia (Figure 2) or ductal dilation. Endoscopic retrograde cholangiopancreatography (ERCP) is an invasive test that is now only occasionally used for diagnostic purposes. More often, it has a therapeutic role to manage ductal stones and strictures. The Cambridge Classification System (Table 1) was based on ERCP findings and used to divide patients into three categories according to the extent of the ductal changes. These correlate with pancreatic functional impairment. The categories include Cambridge I: equivocal; Cambridge II: mild to moderate; and Cambridge III: considerable changes (Figure 3). This classification can still be used today based on the ductal features evident from noninvasive imaging. Endoscopic ultrasound (EUS) is the highest-resolution test to visualize the pancreatic parenchyma and ducts, and it has been used to detect some of the earliest changes of chronic pancreatitis. EUS in the setting of more advanced chronic pancreatitis is used to obtain pancreatic tissue (fine needle aspiration) to differentiate chronic pancreatitis and pancreatic cancer. Cancer should always be excluded first in patients about to undergo endoscopic or surgical therapy.

MEDICAL MANAGEMENT

Patients with chronic pancreatitis are best managed at specialized centers because they often require experts from multiple disciplines such as radiology, gastroenterology, and surgery to coordinate their care.

In addition to pain control, a prime objective of patient management is to minimize the insults to the pancreas, which may slow the progressive inflammatory changes. Alcoholic patients with chronic pancreatitis should be strongly encouraged to stop all alcohol intake. While cigarette smoking has not been implicated as a cause of chronic pancreatitis, it can accelerate the disease. Smokers should be advised to stop smoking. Oral pancreatic enzymes that inhibit cholecystokinin (CCK) release have been used to decrease the frequency of acute attacks of inflammation, but their efficacy is doubted by most.

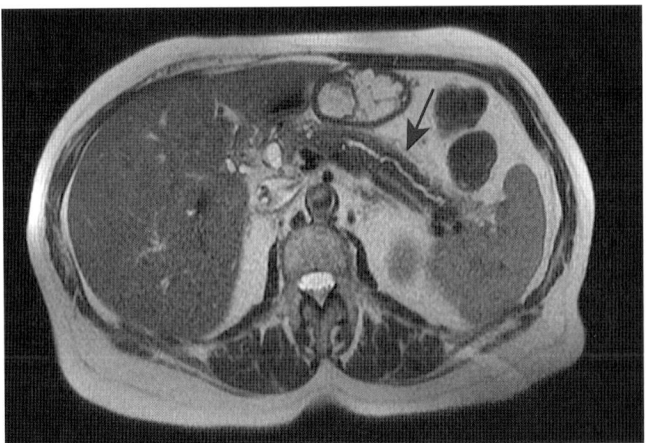

FIGURE 2 Abdominal MRI in a patient with chronic pancreatitis. T2 weighted images of an abdominal MRI with gadolinium contrast in a patient with chronic pancreatitis. The red arrow points to the pancreatic duct in the body/tail of the pancreas, which is moderately dilated and tortuous, both radiographic signs of chronic pancreatitis.

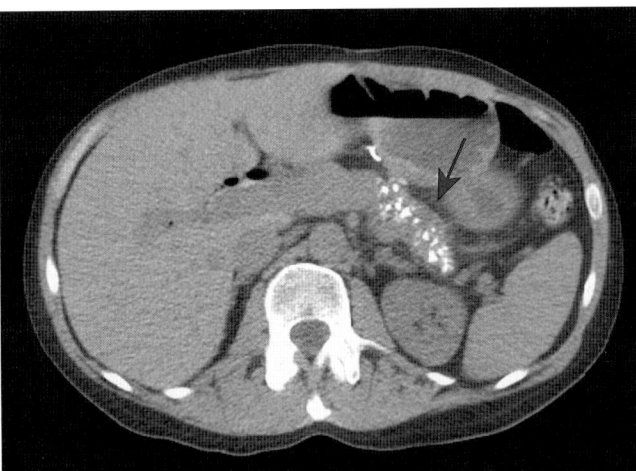

FIGURE 1 CT scan of a patient with chronic pancreatitis. Cross-sectional imaging without intravenous contrast of the body and tail of the pancreas reveals numerous calcifications within the pancreatic ductal system (*red arrow*).

TABLE 1: Cambridge classification of image severity for chronic pancreatitis

Cambridge class	Main pancreatic duct	Abnormal side branches
Normal	Normal	0
Equivocal	Normal	<3
Mild	Normal	>3
Moderate	Abnormal	>3
Marked	Abnormal*	>3

*Main pancreatic duct (MPD) terminates prematurely (abrupt, tapering, irregular), multiple MPD strictures, MPD dilated >10 mm, ductal filling defects (stones), intrapancreatic or extrapancreatic "cavities" are observed, or contiguous organ involvement (stenoses of common bile duct or duodenum, arterial venous fistula).

Modified from Axon ATR, Classen M, Cotton PB, et al: Pancreatography in chronic pancreatitis: international definitions, Gut 25:1107–1112, 1984.

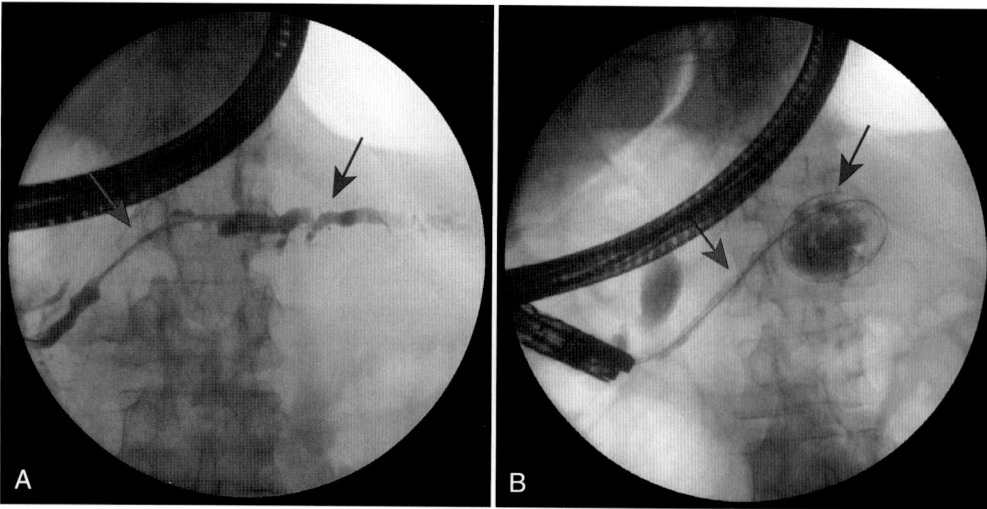

FIGURE 3 ERCP images in patients with Cambridge III chronic pancreatitis. **A,** Red arrow reveals a long pancreatic duct stricture with upstream ductal irregularity *(blue arrow)*. **B,** Long pancreatic duct stricture *(red arrow)* with an upstream ductal disruption. The patient in **(B)** presented with pancreatic ascites.

Proponents also believe that they will slow the progression of disease and improve chronic pain and acute exacerbations. We are skeptical. Of course, pancreatic enzyme supplements should be administered to patients with fat malabsorption manifested as diarrhea and steatorrhea. They should receive at least 30,000 IU of lipase with each meal and also be given medications to reduce gastric acid secretion, which can denature the non-enteric-coated enzymes and eliminate their activity. Most patients with chronic pancreatitis require analgesics for pain relief. Nonopioid medications should be used whenever possible. Referral to a pain specialist may be of value.

ENDOTHERAPY

By the time a patient has been referred for a surgical evaluation, most have been evaluated by a gastroenterologist, and many with strictures and dilated ducts have undergone some form of endoscopic intervention designed to relieve their pain. This usually takes the form of stricture dilation with or without stone removal, followed by the placement of a pancreatic duct stent. While strictures often can be dilated and stented effectively with endoscopic techniques, clearing the duct of stones is more challenging. Problems include difficulty with access to the stones because of stricture(s), adherence of the stone to the duct wall, and large size of the stone that precludes its removal. Fragmentation of the stone with endoscopic or extracorporal shock wave lithotripsy has been used with some success. The extracorporal approach is more frequently used in Europe compared to the United States. Multiple procedures may be required before a satisfactory result is obtained; often complete clearance is not possible.

Pain relief after endoscopic treatment is more likely in patients who have pancreatic duct strictures without stones. Stricture resolution may occur in one third of cases, and two thirds of patients experience improvement of pain. Most failures are due to recurrence of stricture after stents are removed, and there has been an unfortunate tendency for such patients to be managed with stents over long periods of time. Instead, such patients should be strongly considered for surgery. The results are worse for patients with pancreatic duct stones. In most series, at least one half of patients progress to surgery. Cahen and colleagues (Cahen D, et al., 2011) (Figure 4) recently reported in a randomized trial with 5-year follow-up that chronic pancreatitis patients with a dilated pancreatic duct who went straight to surgery had less hospitalizations and repeat procedures and better

long-term pain relief. Based on these results, those authors recommend that surgical therapy should be strongly considered at the outset and endotherapy reserved for those with multiple comorbidities who cannot tolerate the operation. We agree.

SURGICAL TREATMENT

Pain is the most common indication for surgery, but other reasons include biliary or duodenal obstruction or concern for cancer, usually in the head of the pancreas. Here we consider surgery for pain relief. Consideration of surgery requires an assessment of the significance of the pain for the individual patient, which is highly subjective; a determination of the type of surgical procedure that might be appropriate; and an evaluation of the ability of the patient to deal with any long-term morbidity that the operation itself might produce (e.g., diabetes or exocrine insufficiency).

In general, an operation may be indicated in patients whose pain interferes with the quality of their lives. For example, the attacks of pain may require frequent hospitalizations that interfere with school or employment. The patient may be unable to function productively because of the depression that often accompanies the chronic pain state. Nutrition may be impaired because oral intake is limited by the pain that eating produces. The patient may be addicted to narcotics.

The etiology of pain is not well understood, but it is probably multifactorial. Two pathogenic theories direct different surgical treatments. The first hypothesis relates the pain in chronic pancreatitis to the high pressure within the pancreatic ducts and the pancreatic parenchyma, which results in a compartment syndrome and gland ischemia. This is the rationale for *drainage* procedures in patients with dilated main pancreatic ducts. The second hypothesis relates the pain to the release of neurotransmitters in an "inflammatory mass" most often situated in the pancreatic head. This is the rationale for *resections* of the pancreatic head.

Most discussions about the choice of operation are centered on performing a resection versus a drainage procedure, or a combination of the two, and are influenced by the diameter of the main pancreatic duct and the size of the head of the pancreas. Normal duct diameters are 4 mm in the head, 3 mm in the body, and 2 mm in the tail of the pancreas. A pancreatic duct diameter greater than 7 mm in the body of the pancreas suggests that a pancreatic duct drainage procedure (lateral pancreaticojejunostomy or Puestow procedure)

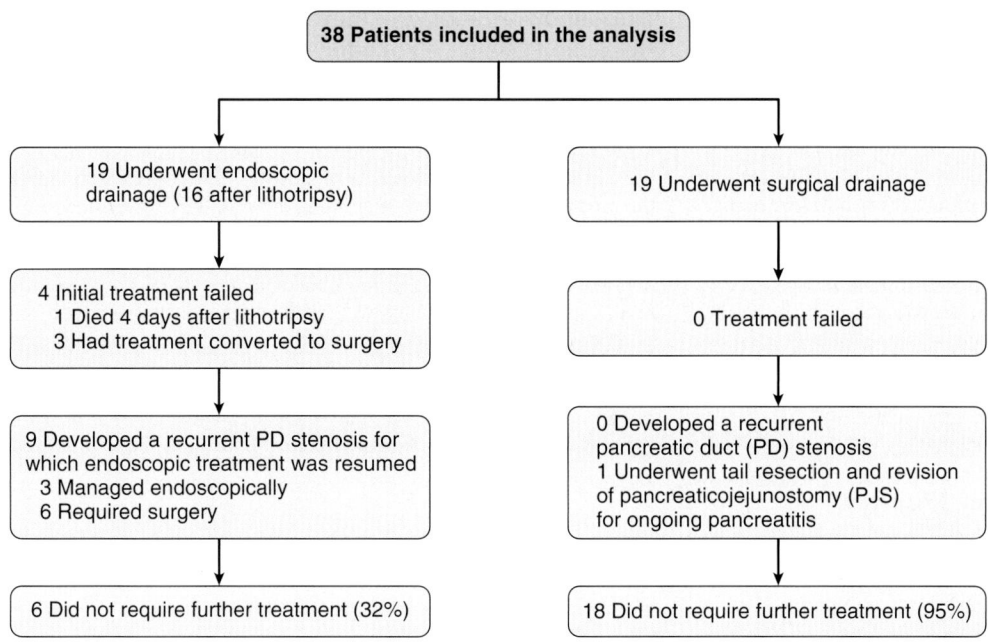

FIGURE 4 Randomized trial of endoscopic versus surgical therapy for patients with chronic pancreatitis and main pancreatic duct dilation. Ninety-five percent of patients who underwent surgical drainage did not require further treatment. In contrast, only 32% who had endoscopic therapy did not require further treatment. These results suggest that surgical therapy may be a more appropriate initial therapy. *(From Cahen DL, Gouma DJ, Laramee P: Long-term outcomes of endoscopic vs surgical drainage of the pancreatic duct in patients with chronic pancreatitis,* Gastroenterology *141:1690–1695, 2011.)*

would likely relieve pain. Indeed, prompt pain relief occurs in 80% to 85% of such patients, and endocrine and exocrine function are usually spared because no pancreatic parenchyma is removed. But because pain may recur in up to 50% of cases within 5 years, this operation is not ideal. If the pancreatic head exceeds 4 cm in its anterior-posterior diameter, some form of head resection should be considered. Most commonly, either a standard Whipple resection (pancreaticoduodenectomy) or its pylorus-preserving variant is done, which provides permanent pain relief in 85% to 90% of patients. However, because exocrine and endocrine insufficiencies occur in approximately 50% of cases, there may be reluctance to do the operation in certain patients who are judged to be incapable of managing these problems. A total pancreatectomy is sometimes considered, often in patients in whom multiple previous lesser operations have been done without pain relief. Of course, this guarantees endocrine and exocrine insufficiency, and the resulting diabetes may be brittle and difficult to manage. For this reason, this operation has been done only rarely. With improvements in the results of auto islet transplantation, this may be a more attractive alternative in the future.

If the duct and the head of the pancreas are both enlarged, often the best choice is an operation that combines drainage of the dilated duct along with a more limited resection of the pancreatic head and preservation of the duodenum, in an effort to minimize the risk of endocrine and exocrine insufficiency. Two procedures are available to achieve these goals: the so-called Beger procedure and the Frey operation. Randomized trials comparing the two procedures have shown equivalent permanent pain relief in 85% to 90% of patients and no endocrine or exocrine insufficiency precipitated by the surgery.

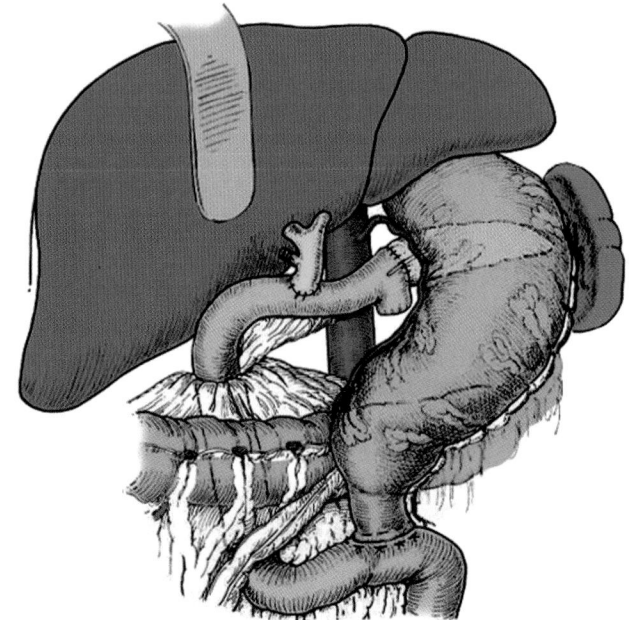

FIGURE 5 After pylorus-preserving pancreaticoduodenectomy (PPPD), reconstruction of the pancreatic duct and bile duct are in a retrocolic fashion. The pancreaticojejunostomy can be made in a side-to-side fashion if a chain-of-lakes ductal pattern exists in the pancreatic remnant. The end-to-side duodenojejunostomy is in an antecolic position to isolate the duodenal anastomosis from the pancreatic anastomosis and minimize delayed gastric emptying if the pancreatic anastomosis should leak. *(From Traverso LW: The surgical management of chronic pancreatitis: the Whipple procedure. In Cameron JL, editor:* Advances in surgery, *vol 32, St Louis, 1999, Mosby, p 33.)*

SURGICAL DRAINAGE AND RESECTION TECHNIQUES

Pancreaticoduodenectomy (Whipple Operation)

The Whipple operation (pancreaticoduodenectomy, pylorus-preserving pancreaticoduodenectomy) (Figure 5) is done most commonly for malignant or premalignant lesions in the head of the pancreas, but the technique for resection in patients with chronic pancreatitis is identical. However, in this latter group, repeated episodes of inflammation are common, so adherence of the peripancreatic tissues to various tributaries of the portal vein is frequent, and there may be some element of portal venous hypertension from venous compression in the head of the pancreas. Thus, operative blood loss is on average a bit higher than when the operation is being done for malignant disease. Pancreatic fistulae are uncommon because of the firm nature of the pancreas. In patients with chronic pancreatitis, a pancreaticoduodenectomy should *always* be done if there is also concern for the presence of cancer in the head of the pancreas, which may be difficult to diagnose with certainty in this setting. Otherwise, if the presence of cancer is not a concern, the choice for a Whipple resection is usually made on the basis of individual surgeon preference and consideration of the factors already discussed.

Lateral Pancreaticojejunostomy (Puestow Procedure)

The Puestow procedure is a lateral pancreaticojejunostomy between the main pancreatic duct and a Roux-en-Y limb of jejunum (Figure 6). The lesser sac is entered and the pancreas is exposed. The duodenum and head of the pancreas are mobilized (Kocher maneuver), and the gastroduodenal artery is ligated as it courses on the head of the pancreas at the point where it emerges from under the duodenum. The pancreatic duct is located by inserting a needle through the parenchyma on the anterior surface of the gland. The duct is then opened longitudinally by incising through the parenchyma. The duct must be opened over a long distance that begins in the head (even closer to the duodenum than shown in Figure 6) and through the entire length of the body and into the tail. Stones and concretions are removed from the duct lumen, and a retrocolic roux limb of jejunum is then anastomosed to the pancreatic duct in one or two layers. Although we routinely leave a closed suction drain along the anastomosis, fistulas are rare because the firm parenchyma holds sutures well.

Duodenum-Preserving Pancreatic Head Resection (Beger Procedure)

In Germany in 1972, Hans Beger performed a duodenum-preserving pancreatic head resection, or DPPHR, in patients with an inflammatory mass in the head of the pancreas. Many of these patients also had an enlarged pancreatic duct (Figure 7). The operation removes the inflammatory mass but maintains the viability of the duodenum and intrapancreatic common bile duct by preserving the posterior branch of the gastroduodenal artery. The neck of the pancreas is divided, and all but a small amount of pancreatic tissue along the medial aspect of the duodenum is removed. Reconstruction consists of an end-to-end pancreaticojejunostomy to the distal pancreas and pancreaticojejunostomy to the remnant of pancreatic tissue on the inner aspect of the duodenum. If the pancreatic duct is also dilated, it is longitudinally opened and a pancreaticojejunostomy is done to the body/tail portion of the pancreas.

Local Resection of the Head of the Pancreas With Lateral Pancreaticojejunostomy (Frey Procedure)

Charles Frey described a local resection of the head of the pancreas with lateral pancreaticojejunostomy in 1985. This is similar to the DPPHR, and it combines the pancreatic head resection with a duct drainage procedure, while preserving duodenal continuity (Figures 8 and 9). This operation is also indicated in patients with an enlarged inflammatory mass in the pancreatic head, and it preserves endocrine and exocrine function. The operation differs from the DPPHR in that the neck of the pancreas is not transected. Thus, inflammatory adherence to the superior mesenteric and portal veins, which may result in troublesome bleeding during the Beger operation, is not a problem. For that reason, many surgeons prefer it. The Frey procedure is more frequently performed in the United States, while the Beger procedure is more commonly done in Europe.

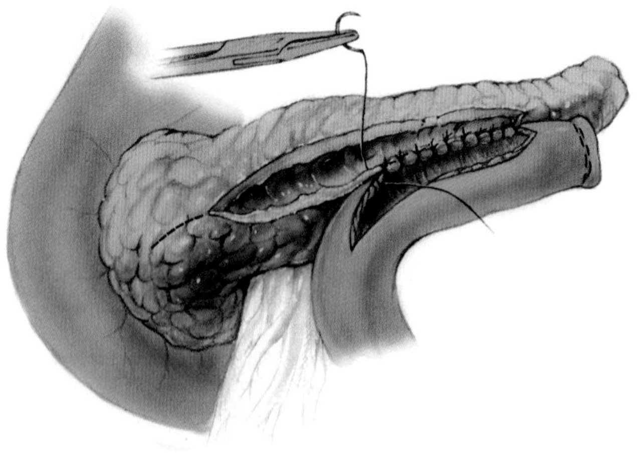

FIGURE 6 The Puestow procedure (lateral pancreaticojejunostomy) is depicted. Note the end of the limb is positioned toward the tail of the pancreas. If the Puestow procedure fails to relieve pain in long-term follow-up and a head resection is required, this position of the jejunal limb allows for the preservation of the pancreatic anastomosis and also allows addition of the biliary connection to the jejunal limb. *(Reprinted from Pancreaticojejunostomy [Puestow] for chronic pancreatitis. In Scott-Conner CEH, editor: Chassin's operative strategy in general surgery: an expositive atlas, ed 3, New York, 2002, Springer-Verlag. With kind permission of Springer Science+Business Media.)*

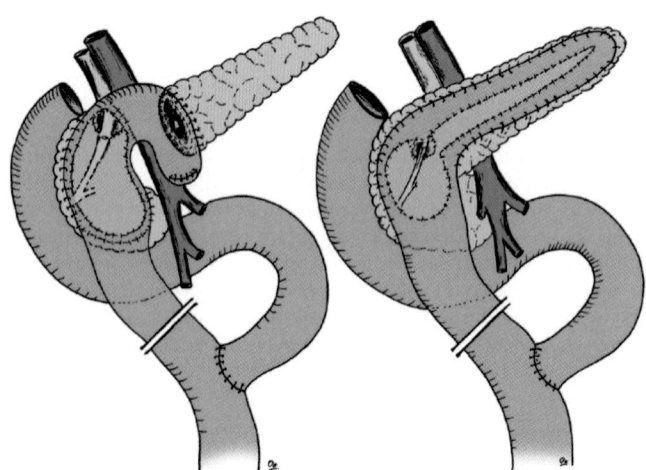

FIGURE 7 The Beger technique (duodenum-preserving pancreatic head resection) on the left is compared to the Frey procedure (LR-LPR, subtotal ventral head or local head resection combined with a lateral pancreaticojejunostomy). *(Reprinted from Köninger J, Seiler CM, Sauerland S, et al: Duodenum-preserving head resection: a randomized controlled trial comparing the original Beger procedure with the Berne modification, Surgery 143:490–498, 2008.)*

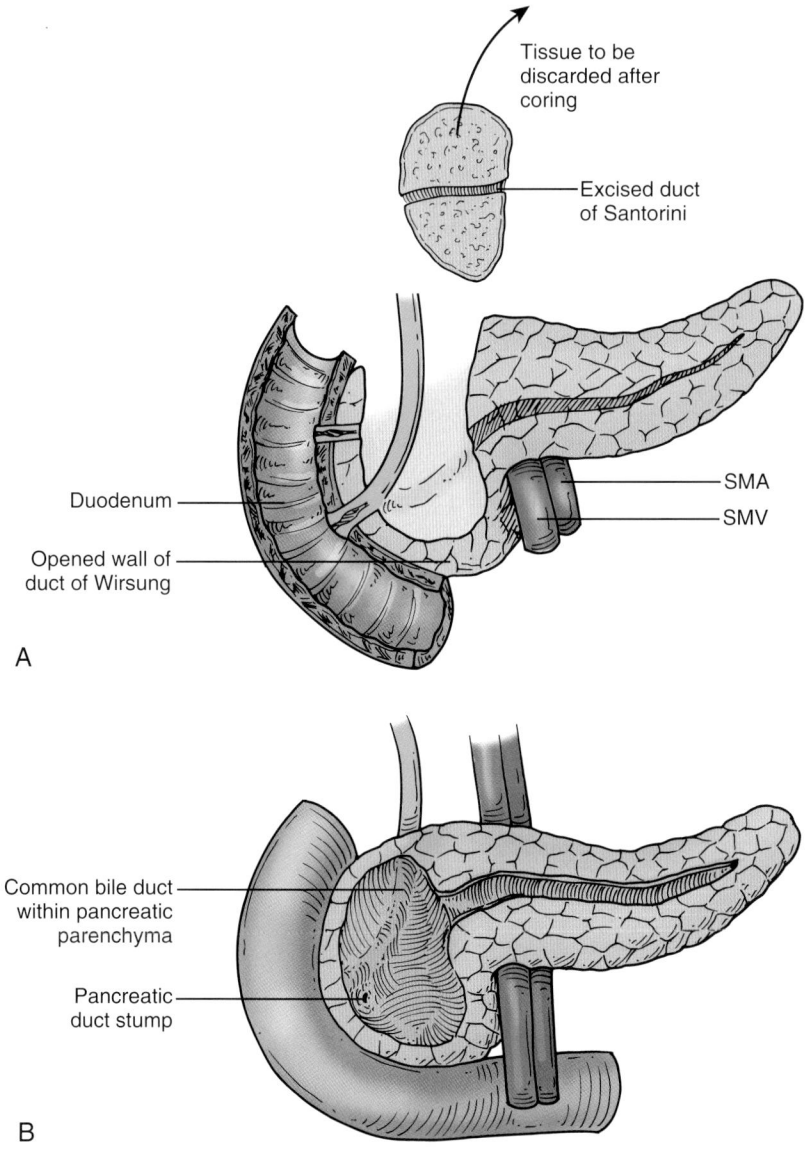

Tissue to be
discarded after
coring

Excised duct
of Santorini

SMA

SMV

Duodenum

Opened wall of
duct of Wirsung

A

Common bile duct
within pancreatic
parenchyma

Pancreatic
duct stump

B

FIGURE 8   A, Tissue removed from the head of the pancreas, including the duct of Santorini. Note that we do not try to remove this tissue as a single specimen as shown here, but rather in piecemeal fashion, taking slices outward from the opened duct of Wirsung and duct to the uncinate process. This technique allows us to assess the extent of resection by placing the thumb of the left hand within the head of the pancreas and with the fingers behind the Kocherized head. *SMA,* Superior mesenteric artery; *SMV,* superior mesenteric vein. **B,** Completed local resection of the head of the pancreas and decompressed main duct in the body and tail of the pancreas. It is unnecessary to ligate the pancreatic duct stump (Wirsung), shown at the bottom of the cavity created by the coring. The common duct is shown traversing the posterior head within the pancreatic parenchyma. The intrapancreatic location of the common duct is most frequently associated with clinical and biochemical evidence of biliary obstruction. When performing the local resection in such patients, it is best to place a metal Bakes dilator in the common duct so its position can be identified and injury prevented while freeing up the bile duct from obstructing scar tissue. *(From Frey CF, Reber HA: Local resection of the head of the pancreas with pancreaticojejunostomy,* J Gastrointest Surg *9(6):863–868, 2005.)*

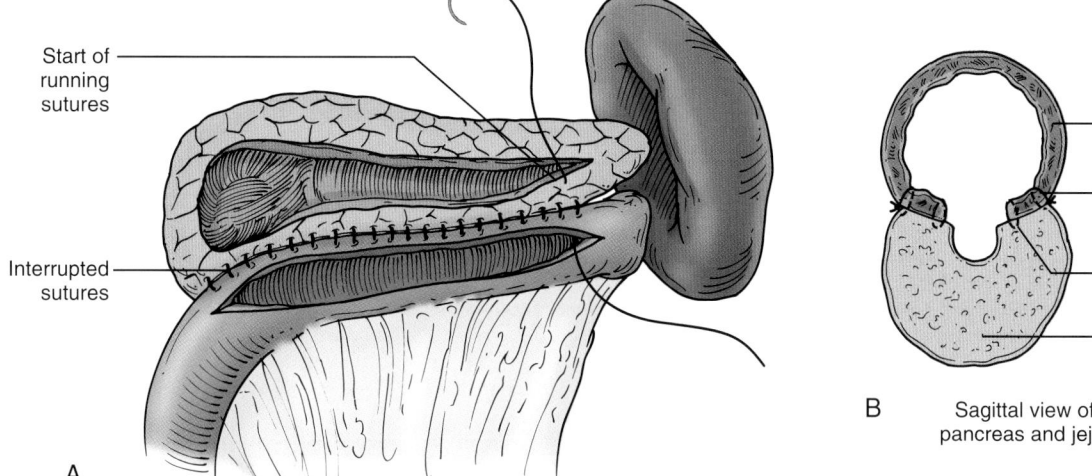

Start of
running
sutures

Interrupted
sutures

A

Boux jejunum

External
sutures
interrupted

Inter sutures
continuous

Body/tail of
pancreas

B   Sagittal view of the
pancreas and jejunum

FIGURE 9   A, The two-layer anastomosis approximates the opened jejunum to the circumference of the locally resected head and to the decompressed main duct in the body and tail of the pancreas. The inner layer is accomplished with running 3-0 or 4-0 absorbable sutures (e.g., PDS). Note: This layer approximates the capsule of the pancreas (not the wall of the duct) to the jejunum. The outer layer consists of 3-0 or 4-0 interrupted nonabsorbable sutures. **B,** Cross-sectional view of the completed two-layer anastomosis between the opened jejunum and the decompressed main duct in the body of the pancreas. *(From Frey CF, Reber HA: Local resection of the head of the pancreas with pancreaticojejunostomy,* J Gastrointest Surg *9(6):863–868, 2005.)*

Which Operation?

The majority of published studies on the outcomes of the surgical management of painful chronic pancreatitis are retrospective. Moreover, the patients who were analyzed were operated on at different stages of their disease, and often for more than a single indication. Thus, only limited guidance is available from those data. Only a few general guidelines that are derived from better studies are currently available. A meta-analysis of four randomized controlled trials comparing limited resections (Beger or Frey) to pancreaticoduodenectomy revealed that the drainage operations combined with duodenal-preserving limited head resections resulted in greater pain relief with lower perioperative morbidity (Figure 10) compared to the Whipple operation. Moreover, they were associated with lower rates of both early and late development of endocrine and exocrine dysfunction (Table 2). The choice between a Beger or Frey operation should depend on the individual preference and experience of the surgeon. However, if there is suspicion of the presence of a pancreatic cancer, any limited form of resection is contraindicated, and a pancreaticoduodenectomy should be done. Finally, the data from Cahen and colleagues (Cahen D, et al., 2011) (see Figure 4) suggest that early operations to surgically drain a dilated duct are probably better than prolonged efforts at endoscopic manipulations, stone extractions, and dilation of pancreatic duct strictures.

▌ SUMMARY

CP is a debilitating condition for many patients. They are best treated in high-volume centers with a multidisciplinary team of experts who are specialized in pancreatic diseases. At the time of diagnosis, all patients should be encouraged to stop the insulting substance in cases of acquired disease. The timing of intervention is not well established, but there is consensus that patients with a firm diagnosis of chronic pancreatitis and ductal obstruction with a dilated duct need to have ductal drainage. Early intervention *may* delay the progression of disease and development of endocrine and exocrine insufficiency. Endoscopic therapy with stone extraction and stent placement is an option for some prior to surgery, but many patients eventually need definitive surgical duct decompression. There are many factors that are considered when deciding the surgical treatment. The most prominent are the presence of an enlarged pancreatic head and dilated pancreatic duct. A limited resection with duodenal preservation and ductal drainage may be the best option for patients who have both findings.

TABLE 2: Meta-analyses comparing DPPHR versus PD, including sensitivity analyses

Outcome	Comparison	Effect size, RR/WMD (95% CI: P: I^2)
Pain relief	DPPHR vs PD	RR 1.08 (0.88-1.33; 0.46; 43%)
Morbidity	DPPHR vs PD	RR 0.54 (0.20-1.46; 0.22; 77.6%)
Blood replacement	DPPHR vs PD Frey vs ppPD[*,†]	WMD-1.28 (−2.32 to −0.25; 0.02; 88.7%) WMD-2.09 (−2.30 to −1.87; 0.01; 0%)
Operation time	DPPHR vs PD Frey vs ppPD[*,†]	WMD-53.03 (−134.96 to 28.89; 0.20; 99.2%) WMD-112.45 (−164.07 to −60.84; 0.01; 88.6%)
Pancreatic fistula	DPPHR vs PD	RR 0.39 (0.08-1.97; 0.26; 0%)
Delayed gastric emptying	DPPHR vs PD Frey vs ppPD[*,†]	RR 0.23 (0.05-1.11; 0.07; 32%) RR 0.06 (0.01-0.46; 0.01; 0%)
Hospital stay	DPPHR vs PD Exclusion of Buchler et al.[‡]	WMD-4.32 (−6.46 to −2.00; 0.01; 60.7%) WMD-5.26 (−6.67 to −3.86; 0.01; 0%)
Exocrine insufficiency	DPPHR vs PD	RR 0.20 (0.06-0.66; 0.01; 57.7%)
Endocrine insufficiency	DPPHR vs PD	RR 0.49 (0.22-1.09; 0.08; 0%)
Weight gain	DPPHR vs PD	RR 1.93 (1.33-2.81; 0.01; 46.1%)
Occupational rehabilitation	DPPHR vs PD	RR 1.36 (1.07-1.71; 0.01; 0%)
Quality of life	DPPHR vs PD	WMD-25.07 (18.83-31.31; 0.01; 57.1%)

P values of 0.01 include all data of <0.01.

CI, 95% confidence interval; *DPPHR*, duodenum-preserving pancreatic head resection; I^2, degree of statistical heterogeneity (0%-25% moderate, 26%-50% average, 51%-100% high statistical heterogeneity); *PD*, pancreaticoduodenectomy; *ppPD*, pylorus-preserving Whipple procedure; *RR*, relative risk; *WMD*, weighted mean difference.

[*]Farkas G, Leindler L, Daroczi M et al: Prospective randomized comparison of organ-preserving pancreatic head resection with pylorus-preserving pancreaticoduodenectomy. *Langenbecks Arch Surg* 391:338-342, 2006.

[†]Izbicki JR, Bloechle C, Broering DC, et al: Extended drainage versus resection in surgery for chronic pancreatitis: a prospective randomized trial comparing the longitudinal pancreaticojejunsotomy combined with local pancreatic head excision with the pylorus-preserving pancreatoduodenectomy. *Ann Surg* 228:771-779, 1998.

[‡]Buchler MW, Friess H, Muller MW, et al: Randomized trial of duodenum-preserving pancreatic head resection versus pylorus-preserving Whipple in chronic pancreatitis. *Am J Surg* 169:65-69, 1995.

From Diener MK, Rahbari NN, Fischer L, et al: Duodenum-preserving pancreatic head resection versus pancreatoduodenectomy for surgical treatment of chronic pancreatitis: a systematic review and meta-analysis, Ann Surg 247:950–961, 2008.

Review: Duodenum-preserving pancreatic head resection (DPPHR) vs pancreaticoduodenectomy (PD) for surgical treatment of chronic pancreatitis
Comparison: 01 DPPHR versus PD
Outcome: 01 Pain free patients

Study or sub-category	DPPHR n/N	PD n/N	RR (random) 95% CI	RR (random) 95% CI
Büchler 1995	12/16	06/15		1.88 [0.95, 3.71]
Klempa 1995	14/20	12/21		1.23 [0.77, 1.96]
Izbicki 1998	28/31	26/30		1.04 [0.87, 1.25]
Farkas 2006	17/20	18/20		0.94 [0.75, 1.19]
Total (95% CI)	87	86		1.08 [0.88, 1.33]

Total events: 71 (DPPHR), 62 (PD)
Test for heterogeneity: Chi^2 = 5.27, df = 3 (P = 0.15); I^2 = 43.0%
Test for overall effect: Z = 0.75 (P = 0.46)

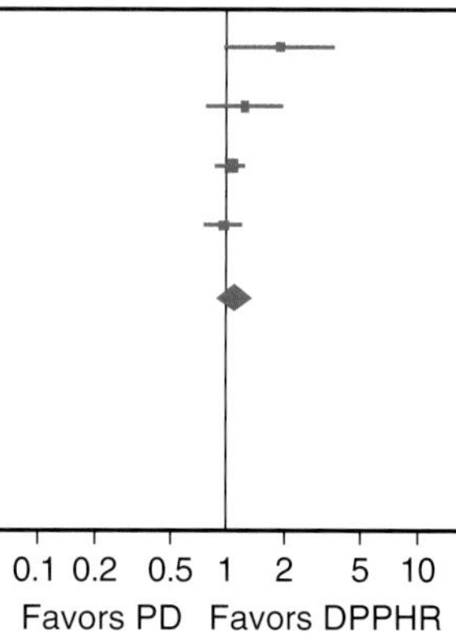

0.1 0.2 0.5 1 2 5 10
Favors PD   Favors DPPHR

FIGURE 10 Meta-analysis of complete pain relief. Combined analysis of four randomized clinical trials suggests there is no significant difference in pain relief between pancreaticoduodenectomy and limited resection (Frey or Beger). *(Extracted from Diener MK, Rahbari NN, Fischer L, et al: Duodenum-preserving pancreatic head resection versus pancreatoduodenectomy for surgical treatment of chronic pancreatitis: a systematic review and meta-analysis, Ann Surg 247:950–961, 2008.)*

SUGGESTED READINGS

Cahen DL, Gouma DJ, Laramee P, et al: Long-term outcomes of endoscopic vs surgical drainage of the pancreatic duct in patients with chronic pancreatitis, *Gastroenterology* 141:1690–1695, 2011.

Diener MK, Rahbari NN, Fischer L, et al: Duodenum-preserving pancreatic head resection versus pancreatoduodenectomy for surgical treatment of chronic pancreatitis: a systematic review and meta-analysis, *Ann Surg* 247:950–961, 2008.

Frulloni L, Falconi M, Gabbrielli A, et al: Italian consensus guidelines for chronic pancreatitis, *Dig Liver Dis* 42(Suppl 6):S381–S406, 2010.

Steer ML, Waxman I, Freedman S: Chronic pancreatitis, *N Engl J Med* 332:1482–1490, 1995.

PERIAMPULLARY CARCINOMA

Barish H. Edil, MD, Martin McCarter, MD, Csaba Gajdos, MD, and Richard D. Schulick, MD

OVERVIEW

Periampullary cancers are a set of neoplasms that arise in the pancreatic, biliary, ampullary, and duodenal tissues near the ampulla of Vater. Although these neoplasms arise from distinct tissues, they are often grouped together because of their anatomic proximity, common clinical presentation with signs and symptoms of obstructive jaundice, and surgical treatment requiring pancreaticoduodenectomy (when possible). Pancreatic ductal adenocarcinoma accounts for the majority of the cancers in the periampullary area, comprising nearly 85% of the cases. The other three periampullary cancers are cholangiocarcinoma of the distal bile duct, adenocarcinoma of the ampulla of Vater, and duodenal adenocarcinoma. In fact, it is common for the precise organ of tumor origin to be unknown prior to surgical resection. Taken together, these four cancers have an incidence of approximately 60,000 new cases per year in the United States. Long-term

survivals vary widely depending on the tissue of tumor origin, stage at diagnosis, degree of differentiation, and ability to perform a complete (R0) resection.

Besides the four cancers discussed earlier, other, less common tumors can arise in the periampullary region. These include neuroendocrine tumors, pancreatic cystadenocarcinoma, acinar cell and squamous cell carcinomas, gastrointestinal stromal tumors, sarcomas, lymphomas, and metastases from other primaries.

PERIAMPULLARY CANCER TYPES

Pancreatic Ductal Adenocarcinoma

Pancreatic ductal adenocarcinoma is the fourth leading cause of cancer death in the United States. In 2012 there were an estimated 44,000 new cases diagnosed, with 37,000 deaths from this disease. The median age at diagnosis is 71 years of age. African Americans have a higher risk of developing pancreatic ductal adenocarcinoma than do whites. There is a slightly higher incidence in men compared to women. The lifetime risk of developing pancreatic cancer is 1 in 68 men and women in the United States. Smoking and obesity are risk factors for the development of pancreatic ductal adenocarcinoma. Other factors have been suggested as risk factors, but these associations are not clear. These include diabetes, alcohol abuse, and radon exposure. It is estimated that between 5% and 10% of patients who develop pancreatic ductal adenocarcinoma have a familial form that is associated with mutations in BRCA-2 (familial breast cancer), PRSS1 (hereditary pancreatitis), p16 (familial atypical multiple mole and melanoma), or hereditary nonpolyposis colorectal cancer (HNPCC).

Surgical resection with pancreaticoduodenectomy is the only potentially curative therapy and typically yields 5-year survival rates from 15% to 25%. Only 20% to 30% of patients are able to undergo resection because of distant metastases at the time of diagnosis, locally advanced disease that typically involves the major hepatic and mesenteric blood vessels, or significant medical comorbidities.

Distal Bile Duct Adenocarcinoma (Cholangiocarcinoma)

Distal cholangiocarcinoma is the second most common periampullary cancer. These cancers arise in the most distal part of the bile duct from the junction of the cystic duct to the ampulla of Vater. It is distinguished from perihilar cholangiocarcinomas that arise near the union of the right and left hepatic ducts (also known as Klatskin tumors) or the more proximal intrahepatic cholangiocarcinomas. The incidence of cholangiocarcinoma is between one to two new cases per 100,000 persons per year in the United States. Approximately 30% of these cases are diagnosed as arising in the distal bile duct. It is a disease of the elderly with peak incidence in the seventh decade of life. Risk factors for the development of chlolangiocarcinoma include sclerosing cholangitis, choledochal cysts, hepatolithiasis, and liver flukes.

Surgical resection with pancreaticoduodenectomy is the most effective therapy for this disease, with 5-year survival rates ranging from 20% to 40%. About 1 out of every 10 pancreaticoduodenectomies are performed for distal bile duct cholangiocarcinoma.

Adenocarcinoma of the Ampulla of Vater

Ampullary adenocarcinoma is the third most common of the periampullary malignancies, occurring at a rate of slightly less than 1 per 100,000 per year in the United States. Peak incidence is in the seventh decade of life and is slightly more common in males. These lesions tend to be discovered at a smaller size compared to pancreatic adenocarcinomas because they cause obstructive jaundice early. Additionally they tend to have less biologic aggressiveness than pancreatic and distal bile duct adenocarcinomas. In studies that further subdivide these cancers into the intestinal versus pancreaticobiliary subtypes, it appears that those patients with the intestinal type have better long-term survival. Resection of ampullary adenocarcinomas with pancreaticoduodenectomy results in 5-year survival rates of 35% to 55%.

Duodenal Adenocarcinoma

Duodenal adenocarcinomas are relatively rare and only account for about 5% of all periampullary cancers. These cancers are equally prevalent in men and women and have a peak incidence in the seventh decade. These cancers are thought to arise from duodenal polyps as colorectal cancers tend to do. Duodenal adenocarcinomas tend to be larger at diagnosis than the other periampullary adenocarcinomas because of the ability for significant intraluminal growth prior to the development of symptoms. Duodenal adenocarcinomas have the most favorable biology compared to the other periampullary adenocarcinomas, with patients undergoing resection with pancreaticoduodenectomy with 5-year survival rates in the 40% to 60% range.

CLINICAL PRESENTATION AND PHYSICAL FINDINGS

Obstructive jaundice is the most common presenting sign of the periampullary adenocarcinomas. The earliest symptom is usually pruritus secondary to the deposition of bile salts in the skin. Patients then notice tea-colored urine; pale, chalk-colored stools; and scleral icterus. Patients also typically have anorexia and weight loss. Although the classic teaching is that these patients do not have pain, one third of patients will have some form of pain or discomfort. This pain is typically dull and constant midepigastric abdominal pain that radiates directly to the back. Severe pain may be caused by tumor infiltration of the celiac plexus, which portends a poor prognosis.

Patients may also present with signs and symptoms of pancreatic exocrine insufficiency, including abdominal discomfort, dyspepsia, and steatorrhea. They may also present with pancreatic endocrine insufficiency with the new onset of diabetes. Patients with ampullary or duodenal adenocarcinoma may also present with anemia or even frank gastrointestinal bleeding.

As in all patients, initial evaluation should include a complete history and physical examination to include past history of chronic pancreatitis and family history of cancers, including pancreatic, colon, and breast. In addition to the signs and symptoms of obstructive jaundice—pruritus, scleral icterus, jaundice, dark urine, pale stools, and self-inflicted excoriations due to scratching—patients may also have an enlarged palpable left supraclavicular (Virchow's) node or periumbilical (Sister Mary Joseph) node. They may also have a palpable nodule in the pelvis felt via a rectal examination. These three are signs of distant or metastatic disease. Hepatomegaly and a palpable gallbladder (Courvoisier sign) can be manifestations of distal bile duct obstruction. Ascites that manifests as shifting dullness or a fluid wave can be a sign of advanced liver disease or peritoneal dissemination.

LABORATORY STUDIES

The majority of patients diagnosed with a periampullary tumor present with signs or symptoms that may prompt additional investigations, including laboratory, imaging, endoscopy, and tissue biopsy. Basic laboratory testing includes a complete blood count, electrolytes, liver function tests, prothrombin time, albumin, and tumor markers (carbohydrate antigen, CA19-9, and carcinoembryonic antigen).

Distal biliary obstruction generally results in hyperbilirubinemia, with the direct (or conjugated) bilirubin being more elevated than the indirect (or unconjugated) bilirubin. Similarly, the alkaline phosphatase is generally more significantly elevated than the transaminases (alanine aminotransferase or aspartate aminotransferase). Other possible abnormalities include prolongation of the prothrombin time due to malabsorption of fat-soluble vitamins such as vitamin K. Malabsorption and weight loss may often manifest in the form of hypoalbuminemia. The tumor marker CA19-9 is frequently elevated, but its sensitivity and specificity are limited by several factors. First, the test for serum CA19-9 is dependent on the Lewis blood group antigen phenotype and therefore is not detectable in the 5% to 10% of the population with Lewis AB- phenotype. Second, biliary obstruction, inflammation, cholangitis, and other tumors such as stomach, ovarian, or colon are all associated with increased CA19-9 levels. Therefore, CA19-9 can be supportive of a diagnosis of periampullary carcinoma, but it should not be utilized to assume the diagnosis. If the CA19-9 happens to be elevated secondary to a periampullary tumor (estimated to be around 75%), it may be useful in monitoring for disease progression following treatment.

Imaging

The purpose of imaging periampullary tumors is to determine the extent of disease, obtain staging information, and assess the potential for resection. A three-phase pancreas protocol computed tomographic (CT) scan with fine cuts through the pancreas and liver provides valuable information regarding local and regional spread of disease (Figure 1). For patients with a contrast allergy or renal insufficiency, a magnetic resonance imaging study or magnetic resonance cholangiopancreatography (MRCP) study may be used to obtain similar information about the suitability for resection (Figure 2). If there are no obvious signs of metastatic disease (most commonly noted in the liver), then attention shifts to assessing the relationship of the tumor to the mesenteric vessels that course adjacent to the pancreas. Specific note is made of any abutment or invasion of the portal vein (PV), the superior mesenteric vein (SMV), the superior mesenteric artery (SMA), the celiac trunk, and the hepatic artery (HA). Involvement of these vessels does not prevent resection but is a biologic indicator of the extent of disease that may alter the preoperative treatment planning and the intraoperative approach. In general, unresectable locally advanced adenocarcinoma of the pancreas is defined as tumor abutting the celiac trunk, HA, or SMA by greater than 180 degrees or encasement/occlusion of the SMV/PV (Figure 3). These patients would be offered conversion therapy in the hope of downstaging the tumor and testing the biologic aggressiveness of any occult metastatic disease.

Endoscopic ultrasound (EUS) with fine needle aspiration (FNA) biopsy can sometimes add valuable information regarding the relationship of the tumor to the mesenteric vessels and has the advantage of being able to confirm a tissue diagnosis. The majority of pancreatic tumors are adenocarcinomas; however, the treatment approaches to neuroendocrine tumors, lymphomas, and other tumors that occur in the periampullary region vary significantly such that biopsy confirmation preoperatively may be helpful if there is a question about the diagnosis. For patients who present with unresectable or metastatic tumors, an EUS-guided celiac block may provide substantial pain relief.

The use of positron emission tomography combined with computed tomography (PET-CT) for periampullary tumors is still being debated. Assessment of the local vasculature involvement is superior with a pancreas protocol CT scan, but PET-CT may be useful in resolving potentially metastatic suspicious lesions noted on other imaging (Figure 4). Despite PET-CT and improvements in other imaging techniques, unsuspected distant metastatic disease is still

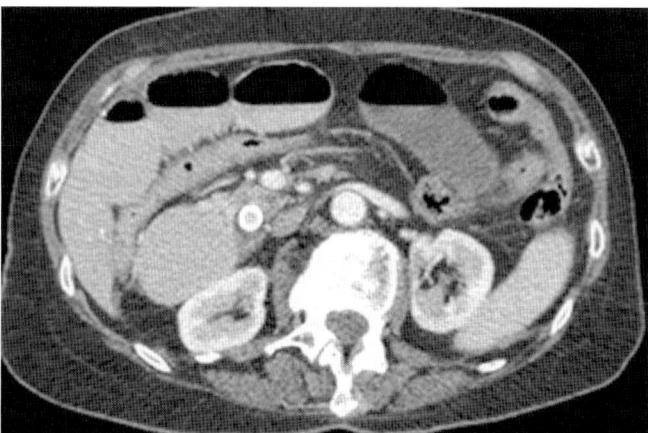

FIGURE 1 Computed tomographic scan demonstrating a resectable tumor in the head of the pancreas (note metallic biliary stent) with clear tissue planes around the superior mesenteric artery and portal vein.

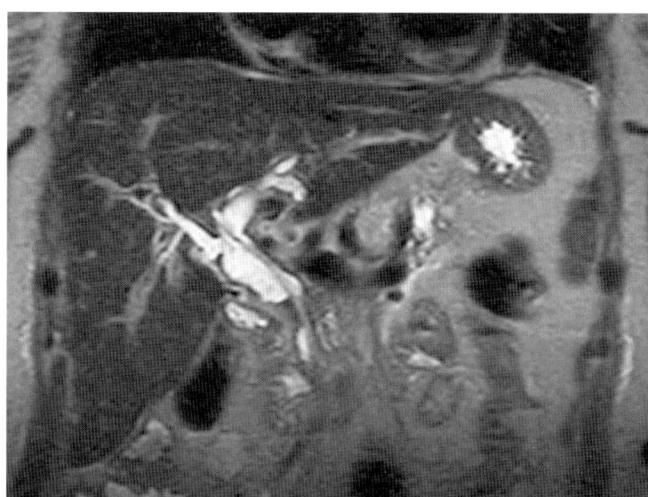

FIGURE 2 Magnetic resonance cholangiopancreatography (MRCP) demonstrating an abrupt cutoff in the common bile duct from a tumor in the head of the pancreas (note plastic biliary stent).

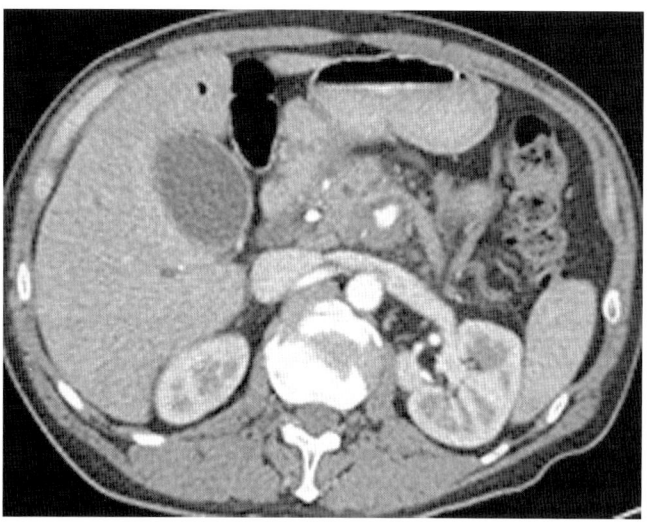

FIGURE 3 Cross-sectional computed tomography imaging demonstrating tumor encasement of the superior mesenteric artery and impingement of the splenic vein/portal vein confluence.

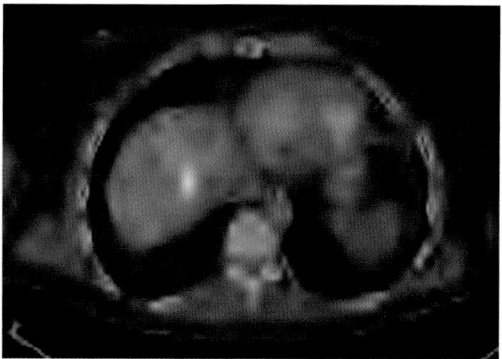

FIGURE 4 PET-CT scan demonstrating hypermetabolic activity in a small lesion at the dome of the liver consistent with metastatic adenocarcinoma of the pancreas.

encountered in roughly 10% to 20% of patients at the time of an operation. Most of these represent small (<5 mm) subcapsular liver nodules or peritoneal implants that are too small to detect with conventional imaging.

Biliary Stenting and Biopsy

Most patients presenting with periampullary tumors do so with evidence of jaundice that prompts further investigation. Endoscopic retrograde cholangiography (ERC) directly visualizes the ampullary region and provides an opportunity to relieve the obstruction while obtaining a provisional diagnosis. Ampullary adenomas or adenocarcinomas may present themselves for immediate biopsy. ERC may uncover benign causes of jaundice such as choledocholithiasis or inflammatory conditions such as primary sclerosing cholangitis. Tumors involving the distal common bile duct generally have features such as an abrupt cutoff that are consistent with malignancy (Figure 5). Obstruction of the common bile duct in conjunction with the pancreas duct (double duct sign) is frequently associated with malignancy (Figure 6). During ERC, attempts at biopsy or brushing of the duct may provide a tissue diagnosis, although the overall sensitivity and specificity of brushings are relatively low, and other approaches such as EUS with FNA or direct cholangioscopic biopsy may be needed.

For patients presenting with metastatic or locally advanced tumors, biliary stenting at the time of ERC provides immediate relief from the obstruction and allows for the patient's symptoms to improve while the remainder of the evaluation is undertaken. Complete resolution of jaundice-associated symptoms such as sclera icterus, pruritus, and changes in stool color may lag several days to weeks behind. The value of preoperative biliary stenting in patients with resectable disease remains controversial, although a prospective randomized trial in patients with pancreatic cancer presenting with a total bilirubin level of 2.3 to 14.6 mg/dL found that routine preoperative stenting was associated with an increase in serious complications with no change in mortality or length of stay. Preoperative stenting may be most valuable in patients with evidence of cholangitis, intractable pruritus, or significant nutritional deficiencies, or in whom surgery cannot be arranged in a timely (<7 days) fashion.

SURGICAL THERAPY

Pancreaticoduodenectomy is the preferred operation for potentially curable periampullary carcinomas. Access to the abdomen is carried out through an upper midline or bilateral subcostal incision. The initial assessment involves exploration of the entire abdomen, focusing on the liver, omentum, peritoneal surfaces, and base of the transverse mesocolon to rule out metastatic disease. The secondary assessment evaluates the relationship of the tumor to the mesenteric vessels. Although the exact sequence of investigation may vary, this phase generally involves a Kocher maneuver to assess the relationship of the tumor to the SMV and SMA and retroperitoneal structures such as the inferior vena cava, the right renal vein, and the aorta. Next, the SMV is identified, emanating from under the neck of the pancreas and followed proximally toward the portal vein. The gastroduodenal artery is dissected near its origin from the proper hepatic artery and test clamped to ensure adequate flow through the hepatic artery prior to being divided. Once divided, access to the PV above the neck of the pancreas allows for creation of a tunnel posterior to the neck of the pancreas to connect with the SMV. At this point a final assessment is made regarding the chances of achieving a margin negative resection (plus/minus vascular reconstruction), and the decision to proceed or abandon the procedure is confirmed.

A cholecystectomy is performed, and the common bile duct is dissected free and divided around the level of the cystic duct insertion. If the tumor is away from the pylorus, a pyloric-preserving approach may be taken by dividing the duodenum 1 to 2 cm beyond the pylorus with a stapling device. If tumor encroaches upon the pylorus, then a wider margin with division of the stomach to include the antrum with the specimen is undertaken. The right gastroepiploic vessels are divided to retract the stomach out of the field and expose the neck of the pancreas. The tunnel posterior to the neck of the pancreas overlying the SMV is developed, and stay sutures may be placed on the superior and inferior edges of the pancreas to control bleeding and provide additional retraction. The pancreas is divided sharply, with attention paid to identifying the location of the main pancreatic duct. If there is concern for potential tumor involvement, a frozen section is obtained from the cut surface of the gland, after which small bleeding vessels may be cauterized.

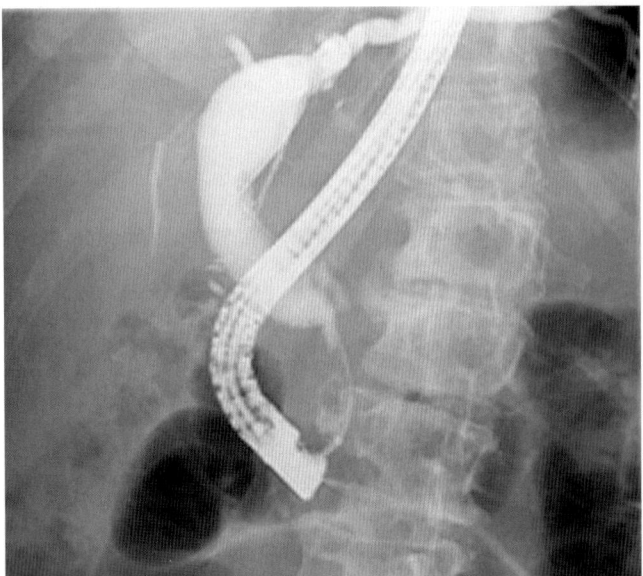

FIGURE 5 Endoscopic retrograde cholangiography demonstrating a narrow tapering of the common bile duct secondary to a tumor in the distal bile duct.

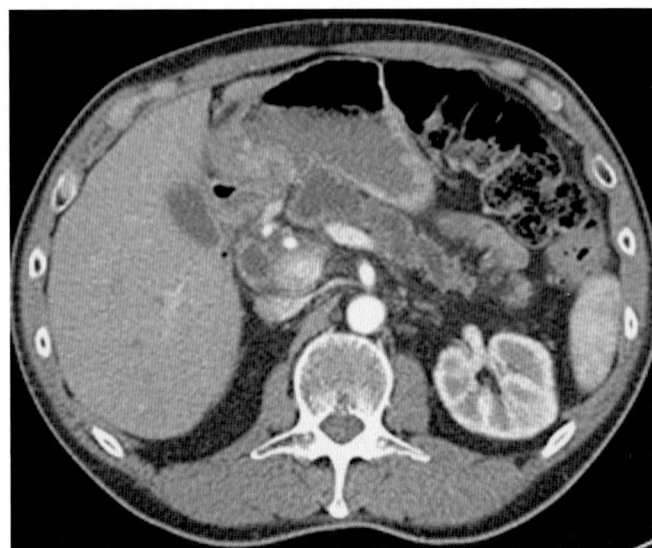

FIGURE 6 Computed tomographic scan with dilated common bile duct and main pancreas duct.

The proximal jejunum is identified and divided with a stapling device approximately 15 cm distal to the ligament of Treitz. The small vessels serving the proximal jejunum and fourth portion of the duodenum are controlled and divided prior to passing the intestine posterior to the mesenteric vessels to the patient's right side. Staying along the lateral border of the SMA and removing all pancreatic tissue from this area and the PV/SMV represent the retroperitoneal dissection, including the uncinate process. Local and regional lymph nodes are included with the specimen, although extended periaortic lymph node dissections have not been shown to improve survival. The specimen should be properly marked and oriented to facilitate pathologic analysis.

Reconstruction

The divided jejunum is passed through the transverse mesocolon to the right of the middle colic vessels to lay in the right upper quadrant as an upside-down "J." The pancreas body is mobilized off the splenic vein for 2 to 3 cm to facilitate the anastomosis. An end-to-side invaginated duct-to-mucosa pancreaticojejunostomy is fashioned in two layers, with a fine, absorbable monofilament used on the mucosa and a permanent suture used on the serosa and pancreatic capsule to buttress the pancreas against the jejunum. A pediatric feeding tube may be trimmed to serve as a pancreatic stent, especially in patients with a relatively small pancreatic duct.

An end-to-side hepaticojejunostomy is constructed 5 to 10 cm away from the pancreaticojejunostomy. In a common bile duct that is generally dilated and fibrotic, a running mucosa-to-mucosa layer is fashioned using an absorbable monofilament suture, with care being taken to avoid occluding the anastomosis. A stent is generally not needed for this anastomosis.

The duodenojejunostomy or gastrojejunostomy is performed in an antecolic fashion 15 to 20 cm downstream from the hepaticojejunostomy. A jejunal feeding tube is used only in select cases. Drains are placed posterior and anterior to the pancreatic and biliary anastomoses.

Recently, periampullary neoplasms at select centers are being approached by minimally invasive or laparoscopic techniques. At our institution, for the properly selected patients, laparoscopic pancreaticoduodenectomy is routinely done. Laparoscopic resection with periampullary and pancreatic tumors can decrease surgical risks, postoperative pain, and particularly wound complications compared to the open operation. This decrease in morbidity has facilitated the integration of surgery into the multimodality cancer care of these patients. There are no prospective randomized trials comparing minimally invasive techniques with open pancreaticoduodenectomy, but there have been studies comparing oncologic parameters that have shown that lymph node harvest and margin status are equivalent between the two approaches.

The laparoscopic approach does vary technically from the previously described open approach. Five ports are used to create a semicircle around the pancreas. After evaluating the abdomen for the absence of metastatic disease, the lesser sac is entered, allowing for the lifting of the stomach and the first portion of the duodenum. This permits evaluation and identification of the hepatic and gastroduodenal artery. Dissection and ligation of the gastroduodenal artery are done, allowing for orientation and evaluation of the portal vein below. At this point, attention is redirected to the superior mesenteric vein, which is found by cutting down on it along the lower edge of the pancreas in relation to the previously identified portal vein. This is followed by blunt dissection of the tunnel underneath the neck of the pancreas. The magnification and angle of visualization of the tunnel secondary to the laparoscope are excellent for assessing resectability. Once completed, the gallbladder is taken down from the gallbladder fossa and used for retraction to allow dissection and transection of the common bile duct. At this point, the colon is lifted, identifying the ligament of Treitz. The ligament of Treitz is dissected down under the root of the mesentery, staying on the duodenal wall. The proximal jejunum is then stapled and transected, but the two ends are sewn to each other loosely. This is an important step because as we remove the specimen, the jejunum will be pulled through the ligament of Treitz in proper orientation under the root of the mesentery, putting it in the perfect position for the pancreaticojejunostomy and hepaticojejunostomy.

Attention is brought back to the right upper quadrant, where the distal stomach is stapled and transected. The neck of the pancreas is also transected, paying attention to good hemostasis of the superior and inferior pancreaticoduodenal artery branches. The final steps include the Kocker maneuver and pulling the mobilized duodenum and sewn proximal jejunum through the ligament of Treitz. This leaves an excellent view of the superior mesenteric artery, allowing for transection of the uncinate process right along it.

Finally, the three anastomoses are completed, in similar fashion to the open technique, using intracorporeal knots in either a running or interrupted fashion to the jejunum, which is already in the proper position from the previous maneuvers. We have found that a pediatric feeding tube for both the pancreas and bile duct facilitates the anastomosis laparoscopically.

Laparoscopic pancreas surgery is a field that is in its infancy and continues to evolve. We currently offer it routinely for the properly selected patient at our institution, allowing for those patients to benefit from the minimally invasive approach.

Postoperative Care

A standardized approach to postoperative care has significantly improved surgical outcomes and reduced hospital stay in our experience. This includes close observation in a monitored unit for the first 24 hours postoperatively and transfer to a dedicated surgical nursing unit thereafter.

Nasogastric tubes are discontinued on postoperative day (POD) #1. Early ambulation, aggressive use of incentive spirometers, and tight blood sugar control are critical. Ice chips and sips of water are permitted early on. Formal introduction of clear liquids usually waits until POD #3 or #4. Diet is advanced to regular in the next 48 hours in the absence of nausea or vomiting. Patients may also receive prokinetic agents (erythromycin or reglan), but this is debated in the literature. Routine feeding tube placement at the time of the operation is unnecessary. While colonic ileus after Whipple procedure is infrequent, signs and symptoms could mimic delayed gastric emptying (DGE).

Systemic signs of infection (fever, elevated white count) on POD #4 to #5, or after, should prompt laboratory and radiographic workup, including cross-sectional imaging. Abdominal or retroperitoneal fluid collections should raise suspicion for an anastomotic leak. These fluid collections typically need to be drained and a sample sent for amylase levels and cultures for targeted antibiotic therapy under appropriate circumstances. With proper surgical techniques, the rate of bile leaks from hepaticojejunostomies should be minimal. Pancreatic leaks in the setting of dilated ducts and firm pancreas in pancreatic cancer patients should also be low. Patients with small pancreatic ducts and a soft pancreas with other types of periampullary cancers (bile duct, ampulla) are at higher risk for an anastomotic leak. Most of these patients can be treated conservatively or with percutaneous drains if necessary.

Surgically placed drains are tested for amylase levels and compared with serum levels after advancement to a regular diet. Low-volume pancreatic fistulas can be managed with little to no change in routine postoperative care as an outpatient. Drain output should be monitored daily, and drain amylase levels checked with postoperative visits. Drains are usually removed 1 to 3 weeks after discharge, depending on output. Management of high-output fistulas can be more challenging. Drains should be well secured to prevent accidental removal. The exact timing of drain removal depends on drain output and amylase levels. Decreasing drain output can be managed with slow, gradual removal of external drains, allowing enough time for the tissue around the drain to form a track. Alternatively, or in the setting of persistently high drain output, a drain injection study should be performed to rule out a large residual peripancreatic cavity, followed by fibrin glue injection into the drain track. The role of octreotide remains controversial.

A recent study from Europe found that early drain removal in a selected group of patients could be beneficial because it was associated with a decreased pancreatic fistula rate, fewer abdominal/pulmonary complications, a decreased hospital stay, and lower cost.

Postpancreatectomy hemorrhage several days after surgery is a rare but serious postoperative complication. It is frequently associated with pancreatic anastomotic leak and can present with blood loss via abdominal drains, hematemesis/melena, unexplained hypotension, or as a laboratory finding. Sentinel bleed (small amount of blood loss hours prior to massive hemorrhage) could be a warning sign. This is related to a pseudoaneurysm in the area of the gastroduodenal artery (GDA) stump, hepatic artery, or branch off the superior mesenteric artery. In this scenario the patient, if stable, should be evaluated by arteriography, which can be diagnostic as well as therapeutic.

SURGICAL OUTCOMES

Postoperative Complications

Perioperative morbidity and mortality for major pancreatic resections have declined significantly over the last 2 decades. While postsurgical mortality in high-volume centers is low (0% to 3%), postoperative morbidity continues to remain high (30% to 50%). The most frequent serious postoperative complications are DGE (15% to 40%), pancreatic anastomotic leak (10% to 20%), intra-abdominal abscess (8% to 10%), and postoperative hemorrhage (1% to 8%). The high variability in complication rates between studies can partially be attributed to lack of standardized reporting of postoperative adverse events.

The International Study Group of Pancreatic Surgery has greatly contributed to our understanding and better definition of postoperative complications. A series of recent publications by this group standardized definitions for postpancreatectomy hemorrhage (PPH), DGE, and pancreatic anastomotic leakage.

PPH has been categorized by three important parameters: onset (before or after 24 hours from the time of surgery), location (intra- or extraluminal), and severity (low or high). A combination of these variables categorized patients into A, B, and C categories, depending on the time of onset, the site of bleeding, and the clinical impact. DGE has been defined as the inability to return to a standard diet by the end of the first postoperative week. Categories A, B, and C have been established considering the inability to tolerate solid food by 7, 14, or 21 days, or nasogastric tube requirement by 3, 7, or 14 days postoperatively or reinsertion of the tube between the days mentioned above. DGE should also be differentiated from rare causes of mechanical obstruction with appropriate imaging. Postoperative pancreatic fistula has been defined as drain output of any measurable volume of fluid on or after postoperative day 3 with amylase content greater than three times the serum amylase activity. Further categories of leak with A (no clinical impact), B (deviation from normal postoperative course, percutaneous drain placement), and C (reoperation or death) have been established. Currently, existing leak definitions may still miss up to one third of pancreatic leaks. Also, achieving no measurable drain output by day 3 could be difficult, especially in the setting of intraoperative abdominal irrigation. Measurable drain output past 3 days with negative drain amylase signals no leak in the great majority of patients in our experience.

An increasing number of publications have addressed the surgical volume/outcome relationship worldwide. There is mounting evidence that complex pancreaticobiliary resections should be performed in high-volume centers to decrease postoperative complications, hospital cost, number of nontherapeutic laparotomies, and mortality, and to increase the number of patients receiving postoperative adjuvant therapy in a timely fashion. The exact definition of high-volume surgeon/center is debated: 10 to 12 cases per year usually qualify as high volume. While the overall postoperative complication rate between high-volume and low-volume centers could be comparable (likely secondary to the continued lack of standardization of reporting complications), the difference in postoperative mortality is substantial in most studies.

ADJUVANT AND NEOADJUVANT THERAPY AND SURVIVAL

The relative contribution of various treatment modalities to survival in periampullary cancers continues to be debated. Currently accepted treatment modalities include surgery, chemotherapy, and radiation in various combinations. A curative intent resection provides the only potential chance for cure or long-term survival. On the other hand, an up to 80% disease recurrence following pancreaticoduodenectomy argues against surgery alone being an adequate treatment modality. Preoperative or adjuvant chemotherapy likely increases the chances of survival, although the benefit is on the order of months rather than years. The role of radiation is even more debatable, especially in ampullary or biliary cancers. A controversial, prospectively randomized trial studying the effects of radiation in pancreatic cancer from Europe showed potentially detrimental effects of postoperative radiation. Other, retrospective reviews show potential benefit, but the effects of radiation are difficult to separate from the potential benefits of chemotherapy. Study outcomes have also been scrutinized by inclusion of patients with positive or unknown surgical resection margin status. Radiation may be best utilized in the setting of preoperative chemoradiation in pancreatic cancer for concerns of major vessel involvement or for close or involved resection margins in the postoperative setting for periampullary tumors, but the data, especially in ampullary-type or biliary-type cancers, are sparse.

While the safety of pancreaticoduodenectomies has come a long way, little progress has been made in terms of overall survival in periampullary tumors. Population-based studies show dismal results, with overall survival as low as 13 months in the setting of curative intent resection for pancreatic adenocarcinoma followed by adjuvant chemotherapy. Even today, selected centers of excellence continue to report a 24-month or shorter median survival for pancreatic cancer treated with curative intent surgery and adjuvant therapy. This translates into a 5-year survival of about 20%. Five-year survival of patients with resected invasive ampullary adenocarcinoma is significantly better at about 40% to 50%. Patients with resected distal bile duct tend to survive longer than pancreatic cancer patients but shorter than patients with invasive ampullary cancers (25%-35%). Surgical margin status and presence of lymph node metastasis continue to be strong predictors of long-term outcome.

The ideal adjuvant chemotherapy combination continues to be a search in progress. While gemcitabine showed promise in early clinical trials, the recent ESPAC-3 trial for surgically resected pancreatic adenocarcinoma showed no survival benefit over fluorouracil plus folinic acid in a prospective randomized trial, with both drugs resulting in a median overall survival of 23 months. Gemcitabine has been combined with various other drugs in multiple other studies without a significant improvement in overall survival. A recently published study from Europe compared single-agent gemcitabine (11% response rate) with a combination regimen (FOLFIRINOX, 31% response rate) in the setting of stage 4 pancreatic cancer. While results from this trial that involved patients with metastatic pancreatic cancer are not directly applicable to patients with resected pancreatic cancer, early clinical trials using neoadjuvant FOLFIRINOX in locally advanced pancreatic cancer are encouraging.

The benefits of adjuvant chemotherapy and radiation in resected, early-stage periampullary cancers are poorly studied. Most published trials lump various periampullary tumors together and frequently enroll metastatic and locally advanced patients together. The ABC-02 trial randomly assigned over 400 patients with locally advanced or metastatic cholangiocarcinoma, gallbladder cancer, or ampullary cancer to receive either cisplatin followed by gemcitabine or gemcitabine alone. Median overall survival was 11.7 months in the cisplatin-gemcitabine group compared with 8.1 months in the gemcitabine-only group. While combining cisplatin with gemcitabine appears to be beneficial in locally advanced or metastatic cholangiocarcinomas and ampullary cancers, the trial obviously provides no evidence for its use in resected, early-stage cancers.

A Phase-III EORTC trial studied adjuvant radiotherapy and 5-FU following curative intent resection of cancers of the pancreas and periampullary region. In the trial, 218 patients were randomized into adjuvant therapy versus observation. Over half of the patients had pancreatic cancer. When results were stratified for tumor location, the 2-year survival rate was 63% in the observation group and 67% in the treatment group, showing basically no advantage to adjuvant therapy in terms of overall survival. Progression-free survival was also similar between treatment groups.

Several studies examined the risks and benefits of neoadjuvant chemotherapy or chemoradiation in the setting of resectable and locally advanced pancreatic cancer. Arguments used for administration of neoadjuvant therapy include a high risk of undiagnosed stage 4 disease reflected by short postoperative disease-free survival, the conversion of locally unresectable disease to resectable, and whether preoperative radiation given in well-vascularized tissue may be more effective. Some investigators reported overall survival in the range of 3 years following administration of neoadjuvant chemoradiation to

patients with resectable pancreatic cancer, which is almost a year longer compared with survival curves reported from other major institutions in the United States in the setting of curative intent surgery followed by adjuvant therapy. However, these findings are not uniform, and recent meta-analyses of studies addressing the potential benefits of neoadjuvant treatment for pancreatic cancer found little to no evidence of survival benefit for resectable or borderline resectable tumors treated in a neoadjuvant fashion.

SUGGESTED READINGS

House MG, Yeo CJ, Cameron JL, et al: Predicting resectability of periampullary cancer with three-dimensional computed tomography, *J Gastrointest Surg* 8(3):280–288, 2004.

Katz MH, Wang H, Balachandran A, et al: Effect of neoadjuvant chemoradiation and surgical technique on recurrence of localized pancreatic cancer, *J Gastrointest Surg* 16(1):68–78, 2012.

Kennedy EP, Brumbaugh J, Yeo CJ: Reconstruction following the pylorus preserving Whipple resection: PJ, HJ, and DJ, *J Gastrointest Surg* 14(2):408–415, 2010.

Krishna N, Tummala P, Reddy AV, et al: Dilation of both pancreatic duct and the common bile duct on computed tomography and magnetic resonance imaging scans in patients with or without obstructive jaundice, *Pancreas* 41(5):767–772, 2012.

van der Gaag NA, Rauws EA, van Eijck CH, et al: Preoperative biliary drainage for cancer of the head of the pancreas, *N Engl J Med* 362(2):129–137, 2010.

Varadhachary GR, Tamm EP, Abbruzzese JL, et al: Borderline resectable pancreatic cancer: definitions, management, and role of preoperative therapy, *Ann Surg Oncol* 13(8):1035–1046, 2006.

Winter JM, Cameron JL, Campbell KA, et al: 1423 pancreaticoduodenectomies for pancreatic cancer: A single-institution experience, *J Gastrointest Surg* 10(9):1199–1210, 2006.

Winter JM, Cameron JL, Campbell KA, et al: Does pancreatic duct stenting decrease the rate of pancreatic fistula following pancreaticoduodenectomy? Results of a prospective randomized trial, *J Gastrointest Surg* 10(9):1280–1290, 2006.

VASCULAR RECONSTRUCTION DURING THE WHIPPLE OPERATION

Russell N. Wesson, MBChB, and
Andrew M. Cameron, MD, PhD

OVERVIEW

The importance of Whipple operation (pancreaticoduodenectomy) for pancreatic tumors with portal vein (PV) and superior mesenteric vein (SMV) resection and reconstruction lies in the ability to safely achieve outcomes that are equivalent to those of standard pancreaticoduodenectomy. Resection of these tumors, which, by nature of their location or size, involve the portal or mesenteric vein and classifies them as borderline resectable, allows the potential for complete clearance of disease and the avoidance of R2 resection. Thus, PV/SMV resection allows for R0 or R1 resection in tumors that would otherwise be unresectable.

With the increasing use of neoadjuvant therapy, previously unresectable tumors are now becoming resectable. Additionally, as the knowledge of indications for and outcomes after PV/SMV resection and reconstruction are being more widely disseminated and understood, the authors are seeing PV resection increasingly necessary and utilized. For both these reasons, PV resection and reconstruction is increasingly becoming an important element of pancreaticoduodenectomy and occasionally distal pancreatectomy.

RATIONALE FOR PV/SMV RESECTION

Proximity of the tumor to the SMV does not carry with it the implications that accompany arterial proximity. Tumors adjacent to or invading the superior mesenteric artery (SMA) are at risk of perineural invasion and extension along these autonomic nerves. Where tumors involve the artery, the periarterial neural plexus, together with the propensity of ductal adenocarcinoma for neural invasion, allows for the malignancy to extend locally through the nerve sheath into the retroperitoneum. This underlies the lack of added benefit from radical pancreatectomy in terms of survival and local recurrence rates, as findings from randomized trials show. Mesenteric or portal venous invasion does not in itself carry a worse prognosis as compared with similar tumors without PV/SMV involvement. As evidenced by the presence of circulating tumor DNA early in the course of the disease, tumors have access to the systemic circulation much earlier in the disease than when large enough to invade the PV or SMV. Additionally, resection of the vein does not carry the symptomatic implications of midgut denervation that accompany arterial resection.

Aside from the significant oncologic benefit in the borderline resectable tumors because of venous involvement, an approach to the vein is also an important technical aspect of pancreaticoduodenectomy. The ability to reconstruct the PV/SMV allows for the surgeon to deal effectively with venous injury, which may occur while attempting to mobilize the pancreatic neck off the PV and SMV where fibrosis or desmoplastic reaction makes this hazardous. Achieving a patent reconstruction avoids significant compromise to midgut venous outflow that results in bowel edema. Interruption of portal venous hepatic inflow can also result in extensive hepatic necrosis that can represent a serious morbidity or even mortality.

PREOPERATIVE IMAGING

The approach to PV resection at pancreaticoduodenectomy begins with interpretation of preoperative images and anticipation of surgical events and requirements.

High-quality computed tomographic (CT) and magnetic resonance (MR) imaging with three-dimensional vascular reconstruction, when performed according to established protocols, provides excellent images that allow for the preoperative determination of tumor resectability. Borderline resectable tumors describe those tumors where venous abutment or encasement by pancreatic tumors is present and, in rare cases, those tumors where a resectable short segment of occluded vein is present in the absence of arterial involvement. Abutment, compression or distortion, and encasement of the vein indicate increasing degrees of involvement. In these circumstances, the need for vascular resection and reconstruction should be anticipated and the venous anatomy and involvement appreciated.

Preoperative appreciation of venous involvement precludes the situation where vascular involvement is inadvertently discovered intraoperatively. Without this determination, attempting to mobilize the pancreatic head off the vein leads to two possible scenarios: either it becomes clear that there will be a grossly positive margin and R2 resection, or attempted mobilization of the pancreatic head results in a torn PV/SMV and potentially torrential hemorrhage. Anticipation of involvement precludes venous injury and is associated with lower blood loss and a technically easier reconstruction.

Preoperative imaging also allows for the defining of aberrant vascular anatomy, including the presence of a replaced right hepatic artery as well as a common hepatic artery originating from the SMA.

SURGICAL ANATOMY OF THE SUPERIOR MESENTERIC VEIN

The confluence of the superior mesenteric, splenic, and portal veins is posterior to the pancreatic neck. The main trunk of the SMV is constituted from a jejunal and an ileal branch that merge caudal to the pancreas. This main trunk receives the gastroepiploic and middle colic vein (which may or may not join as the gastrocolic trunk prior to entering the SMV).

The first jejunal branch of the SMV is usually found posterior to the SMA as it enters the posteromedial ileal branch where these merge to form the main trunk SMV. As the jejunal branch passes posterior to the SMA, it receives branches from the uncinate process. During mobilization of the pancreas from the vein, these branches are divided to release the main SMV and allow the SMA to be retracted laterally. Where the jejunal branch passes anterior over the SMA, the uncinate branches enter the ileal branch rather than the jejunal branch. In this situation, there are often variations of venous anatomy. This may include the inferior mesenteric vein draining

directly into the jejunal branch as opposed to the usual merging with the splenic vein.

SURGICAL TECHNIQUE

Mobilization of the portal and superior mesenteric veins above and below the pancreas, respectively, will allow for proximal and distal control of the mesenteric vasculature with vessel loops prior to reconstruction. The portal vein is mobilized by dividing the lymphoareolar attachment between the portal vein and the superior aspect of the pancreas as well as through division of small venous tributaries. Mobilization of the SMV is achieved by dividing the middle colic and right gastroepiploic venous tributaries, or their common trunk, the gastrocolic trunk, in addition to ligation of multiple tributaries from the inferior aspect of the uncinate process and pancreatic head. Perineural and lymphatic tissue between the SMA and the anterolaterally located superior MPV confluence is then divided.

Vein involvement is then addressed with one of several available techniques. Where tumor is adherent to a small area of vein, a Satinsky or DeBakey clamp can be applied to partially occlude the PV or SMV, and a small ellipse of vein can be longitudinally excised along the lateral aspect of the clamp (Figure 1). A running 5-0 nonabsorbable suture closes the defect in the vein (Figure 2). Should the repair result in a significantly narrowed vein with a risk of bowel edema, congestion, and PV thrombosis, the repair may be readdressed and converted from a longitudinal closure to a transverse closure. Other options include the placement of a venous patch, which may be fashioned using saphenous vein, or placement of an artificial (polytetrafluoroethylene [PTFE]) patch (Figure 3). Alternatively, the segment of vein may be resected after obtaining inflow and outflow control, usually with Blalock-Taussig–style clamps. Prior to venous occlusion, arterial inflow may be temporarily occluded with a Rummel tourniquet after the intravenous administration of 2500 to 3000 units of heparin with a circulation time of 2 to 3 minutes prior to occlusion. Some authors believe that arterial occlusion avoids bowel edema, which may complicate the biliary and pancreatic anastomoses; the

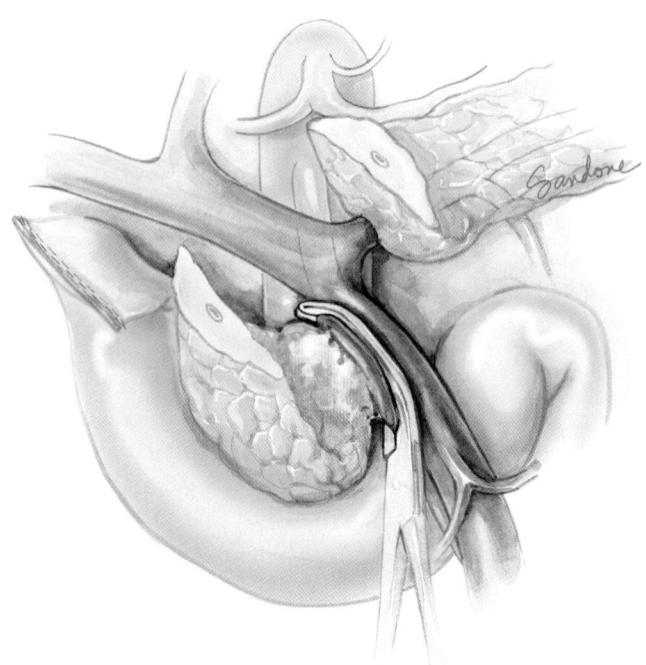

FIGURE 1   Side-biting vascular clamp to facilitate venous excision.

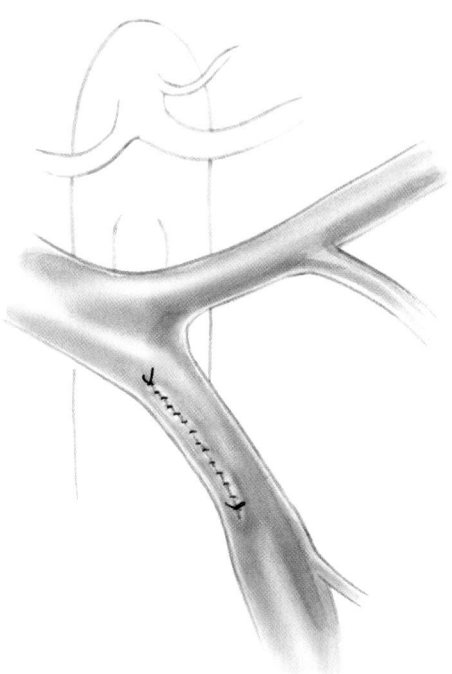

FIGURE 2   Primary repair of venotomy without compromise.

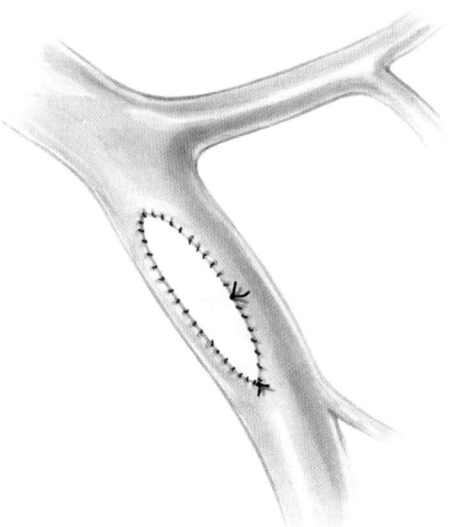

FIGURE 3   Repair with patch to avoid narrowing.

authors do not use heparin or arterial occlusion, as the venous resection and clamping is normally quite brief and well tolerated.

After excision of the affected area of vein, margins should appear grossly clear of disease, and frozen section should be sent for pathology review to ensure R0 resection where possible. Revision of the anastomosis and further resection of vein may be necessary should vein margins be microscopically positive. Mobilization of the proximal venous segment toward the liver and distal segment toward the bowel mesentery may enable primary anastomosis across a 2-cm to 3-cm gap directly. Division and ligation of the small venous tributaries to the SMV arising from the uncinate to the jejunal branch may

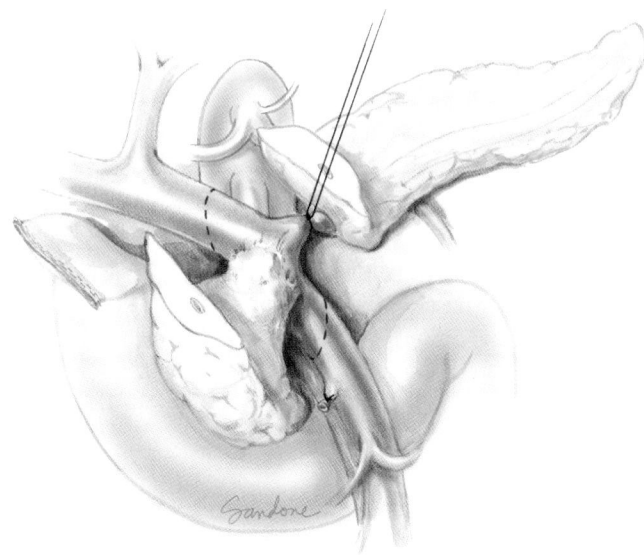

FIGURE 4   Division of splenic vein provides additional length for reconstruction.

be necessary for mobilization. The jejunal branch joining the medial SMV from the patient's left was exposed when the mesentery between the SMA and the SMV was dissected. The first jejunal branch may then be ligated if involvement by tumor necessitates resection, but the ileal branch must be of sufficient caliber to allow adequate venous flow. Involvement of these vessels with a need for reconstruction is a rare event. Where choices between reconstruction of either branch need to be made, the larger branch should be reconstructed with an interposition graft used as necessary.

Should primary reanastomosis initially not appear achievable because of the presence of a distance greater than 4 cm, various maneuvers may be used to facilitate this. The authors have found that interposition of a graft is rarely necessary. Splenic vein ligation and division will often facilitate primary anastomosis (Figure 4). The splenic vein tethers the SMV and prevents its mobilization to close the gap resulting from the resected vein. Division of the splenic vein frees the SMV and allows for closure of a gap 3 to 4 cm wide (Figure 5). Ligation of the splenic vein in the setting of a divided left gastric vein and inferior mesenteric vein that is a tributary to the splenic vein carries a risk of left-sided portal hypertension and the development of gastroesophageal varices. For this reason, some authors recommend construction of a splenorenal shunt at the time of surgery under these circumstances. However, the authors have found this to be a rare clinical consequence. In 42 instances of splenic vein ligation at PV resection, the authors have noted only 1 episode of variceal bleeding subsequent to this maneuver, occurring months after surgery with control via endoscopic injection.

Another technique facilitating primary anastomosis of the PV and SMV includes division of the hepatic coronary ligaments and the placement of a pack behind the liver that may facilitate caudal mobilization of the liver. Reconstruction is then carried out with a running suture leaving sufficient growth factor to allow for venous expansion and the avoidance of anastomotic constriction.

In rare cases, an interposition graft may be necessary. Many conduits have been used as interposition grafts, including internal jugular, left renal, splenic, and gonadal vein; the authors prefer the first two (Figure 6). Ringed PTFE grafts have been used but should be avoided because of a higher risk of venous thrombosis postoperatively. Although venous thrombosis acutely may cause hepatic ischemia and intestinal congestion necessitating thrombectomy and revision, thrombosis is rarely symptomatic if it occurs late postoperatively.

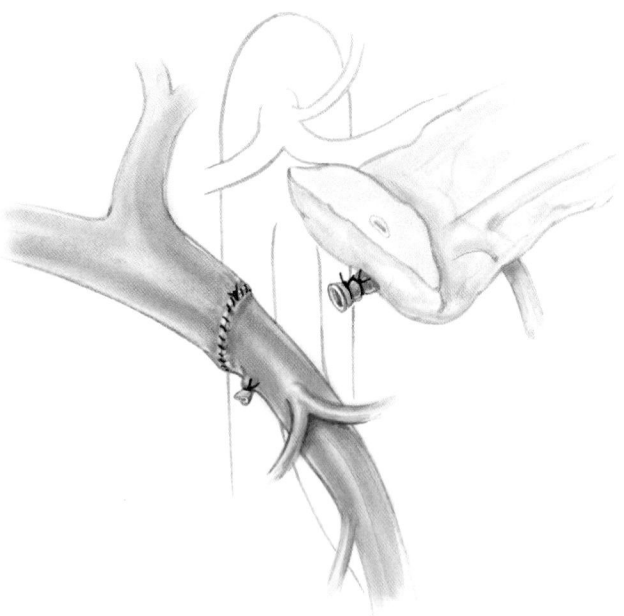

FIGURE 5 Primary anastomosis is usually possible when the splenic vein has been sacrificed.

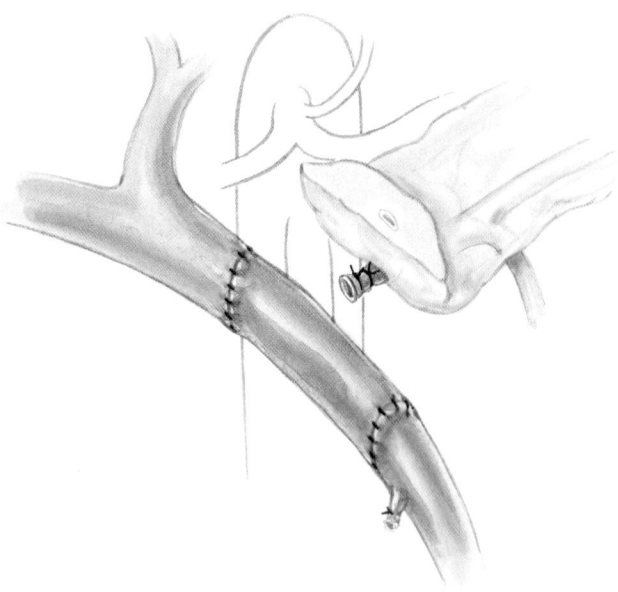

FIGURE 6 Interposition graft to avoid tension when necessary.

ARTERIAL RECONSTRUCTION

Preoperative imaging will show arterial involvement and define arterial anatomy, revealing the presence of replaced left or right hepatic arteries as they arise from the left gastric or SMA, respectively. Aberrant anatomy should be appreciated, and the chances of inadvertent injury of these vessels should be minimized. If a short segment of involved hepatic artery necessitates resection, mobilization of distal and proximal segments of redundant hepatic artery will often facilitate reconstruction with primarily anastomosis or use of conduit.

Where a replaced right artery is resected, reconstruction is performed to preserve common bile duct blood supply and avoid unnecessary compromise of hepatic arterial supply. If an aberrant common hepatic artery originates from the SMA and is involved by tumor, it should be recognized, preserved, or reconstructed. Finally, division of the gastroduodenal artery may compromise arterial supply to the liver if there is inadequate flow through the common hepatic artery via the celiac axis. Defining and dissecting the common hepatic artery down to the celiac axis will allow for division of the arcuate ligament and relief of extrinsic limitation of flow and an improved pulse and Doppler signal in the common hepatic artery.

SUMMARY

PV/SMV resection and reconstruction adds complexity to the already challenging operation of pancreaticoduodenectomy. However, it is increasingly being performed and can be performed safely, avoiding the catastrophic outcomes (through either residual disease or hemorrhage at injury) that may occur when vein involvement is not addressed appropriately or safely. Preoperative planning is an essential element of addressing venous involvement and allows for the anticipation of reconstruction with the performance of a safe and effective operation. In borderline resectable tumors due to venous involvement, outcomes can be achieved that are identical to those of patients without venous involvement who undergo standard pancreaticoduodenectomy. Resection of PV/SMV at pancreaticoduodenectomy gives rise to a median survival rate that equals that of patients undergoing standard pancreaticoduodenectomy. Vein resection therefore allows the possibility of curative treatment in an aggressive and otherwise fatal disease and should be undertaken in appropriately selected patients at high-volume centers and by surgeons experienced in venous resection and reconstruction techniques.

SUGGESTED READINGS

Lai EC: Vascular resection and reconstruction at pancreatico-duodenectomy: technical issues, *Hepatobiliary Pancreat Dis Int* 11(3):234–242, 2012.

Rehders A, Stoecklein NH, Güray A, et al: Vascular invasion in pancreatic cancer: tumor biology or tumor topography? *Surgery* 152(3 Suppl 1): S143–S151, 2012.

Wang F, Arianayagam R, Gill A, et al: Grafts for mesenterico-portal vein resections can be avoided during pancreatoduodenectomy, *J Am Coll Surg* 215(4):569–579, 2012.

PALLIATIVE THERAPY FOR PANCREATIC CANCER

Claudius Conrad, MD, PhD and
Keith D. Lillemoe, MD

INTRODUCTION

A surgeon's role in the treatment of pancreatic cancer in patients who are not candidates for resection with a curative intent remains very important, as a significant percentage of those patients will develop symptoms that need surgical or nonsurgical palliative procedures. The three most important symptoms that might require surgical palliation are (1) biliary obstruction, (2) gastric outlet obstruction, and (3) pain.

To put into perspective the role of surgery for palliation, we look to the following recent data from the National Cancer Institute: It was estimated that in 2012, 43,920 people in the United States would be diagnosed with pancreatic cancer and 37,390 would die of the disease. At diagnosis, 8% of the cancer would be localized, 27% would be locally advanced, and 53% would involve distant metastases. Even despite improvements in surgical outcomes and oncologic therapy, primarily with palliative chemotherapy, the corresponding 5-year survival rates for these stages will only be 23%, 10%, and 2%, respectively. Surgical resection with curative intent leads to significantly worse outcomes for patients with pancreatic cancer compared with patients with most other gastrointestinal cancers, with the median survival for resected patients being only 18.3 months and the 1- and 3-year survival rates being 58.4% and 34.8%. These data underscore the aggressive underlying biology of pancreatic cancer and illustrate that despite surgical, chemotherapeutic, and radiation-therapeutic advances, this deadly disease still carries a mortality rate that is dangerously close to the incidence.

Because the majority of pancreatic cancer patients do not undergo surgery with curative intent, addressing the potentially debilitating symptoms is of primary importance. A surgeon who cares for this population of patients needs to be versatile and competent in providing palliative care employing both operative and nonoperative techniques for palliation, including both improved endoscopic or percutaneous guided techniques and conventional open and newer, minimally invasive procedures. The improved outcomes (early success and durability of endoscopic palliation for malignant biliary obstruction) further improved with progress by the development of covered metallic stents, which have become the gold standard for management of this symptom. Further, minimal-access palliative surgical approaches have been developed over the past decade to offer surgical management of gastric outlet obstruction, biliary obstruction, and pain control via laparoscopic or robotic surgery, single-incision laparoscopic surgery (SILS), and even natural orifice transluminal endoscopic surgery (NOTES). Several studies have shown that laparoscopic surgery for pancreatic procedures results in less pain, decreased length of hospitalization, fewer wound infections, and other perioperative benefits that are of particular importance to patients whose survival is limited. Future technologic advances, such as articulating instruments, three-dimensional (3D) cameras, and a growing number of surgeons with advanced laparoscopic skills, likely will improve patient access to these minimally invasive options for palliation.

The management of pancreatic cancer today is an interdisciplinary team effort. Palliative therapy has been shown to improve quality of life, decrease symptom intensity, and elevate mood, as well as minimize unnecessary resource consumption by patients whose survival is limited. Considering the rising awareness and importance of financial responsibility in our healthcare system, a resource-conscious treatment approach to patients with advanced pancreatic cancer is expected to become increasingly significant. A greater integration of surgical input in the interdisciplinary care of these patients might help reduce rehospitalization and length of stay as well as facilitate cost containment.

In this chapter we list indications for palliative intervention and explain nonsurgical as well as surgical treatment options of the three most important symptoms: biliary obstruction, gastric outlet obstruction, and pain. We focus on the existing data with respect to palliative resection for "incurable pancreatic cancer." Finally, we touch on the medical treatment options (chemotherapy and chemoradiation) for patients with unresectable pancreatic cancer to comprehend the surgeon's role in providing care for patients receiving palliative chemotherapy and in managing potential complications.

INDICATIONS FOR PALLIATIVE INTERVENTIONS

It is our strong belief that an experienced pancreatic surgeon should be involved very early, at the first suggestion of the diagnosis of pancreatic cancer, well before invasive procedures such as biliary stenting or endoscopic ultrasound-guided fine-needle aspiration are performed, to ensure optimal timing, technique, or even the need for these procedures. Too often, the initial "knee-jerk" reaction to place a small plastic stent in jaundiced patients is either unnecessary or less optimal than a metal stent based on the overall plan for management. The surgeon should provide initial input as to the role of potentially curative resection and the need for palliative procedures. Comorbidities that render a patient unfit for major surgery, locally advanced disease with inability to achieve R0 resection, and disseminated disease are all contraindications for resection. Ideally this should be determined preoperatively on a high-quality computed tomographic (CT) scan with intravenous contrast with 1-mm thin sections administered as a "pancreas protocol" to depict both arterial and venous phases (Figure 1). The goal of the pancreatic protocol CT scan is to identify pancreatic tumor local extension and metastases, especially to the liver. An elevated CA 19-9 tumor marker value above 130 units/mL in the absence of jaundice has predictive value of radiographically occult systemic disease (26% of patients). In these patients, a staging laparoscopy might be considered before exploration.

The majority of patients (an estimated 80%) with pancreatic head adenocarcinoma seek medical attention for symptoms related to jaundice secondary to mechanical obstruction of the intrapancreatic portion of the distal common bile duct. As a consequence, jaundice is the most common and often the first symptom of pancreatic cancer. In addition to being a symptom for underlying pancreatic cancer, obstructive jaundice is a significant clinical problem in itself, leading to debilitating pruritus, anorexia and progressive malnutrition, liver malfunction and failure, and even premature death if not treated. Thus, relieving obstructive jaundice is of importance in all patients. The impact of successful biliary drainage on quality of life has been assessed prospectively in a cohort of patients with malignant biliary obstruction in the setting of unresectable disease. One month after relieving biliary obstruction via stenting, baseline bilirubin of greater than 14 mg/dL was associated with a lack of improvement in social function, while decreasing bilirubin levels were associated with improvements in social function and mental health.

Another common presenting symptom is gastroduodenal obstruction due to advanced tumor growth, a symptom that develops in 20% to 40% of patients during the course of their disease. Endoscopic or surgical intervention is required to relieve the obstruction.

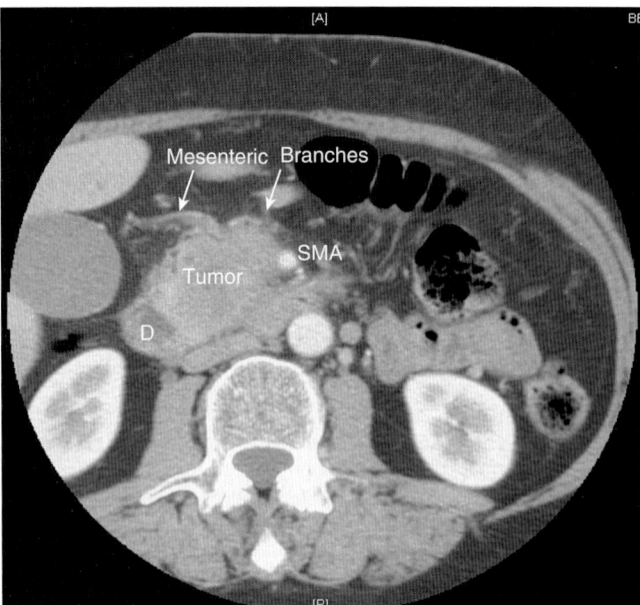

FIGURE 1 Pancreatic protocol CT scan of unresectable pancreatic cancer. This is an axial arterial phase CT image of a pancreatic head adenocarcinoma of a patient who, most surgeons would agree, is not eligible for resection. The superior mesenteric artery (*SMA*) is partially encased by the cancer that is also invading the colonic mesentery. The duodenum (*D*) is narrowed by the mass leading to gastric outlet obstruction, and the intrapancreatic portion of the common bile duct is completely obliterated by the mass, which is causing biliary obstruction and jaundice. *CT,* computed tomographic.

It is important to distinguish mechanical obstruction secondary to tumor growth from motility dysfunction of the stomach and duodenum due to infiltration of the celiac nerve plexus, which can lead to delayed gastric emptying. Motility dysfunction should be treated with pharmaceutical agents rather than surgery or stenting.

The question has been raised as to the role of biliary bypass and gastrojejunostomy in the presence of unresectable disease found at the time of operation. We and other groups have shown that if unresectable disease, with or without symptoms of gastric outlet obstruction, is found at exploration, a prophylactic gastrojejunostomy should be performed because as many as 20% of patients develop gastric outlet obstruction during the course of their disease. In contrast, due to the availability of endoscopic biliary stenting, if necessary, prophylactic biliary bypass is not indicated in nonjaundiced patients. The decision to add an open biliary bypass in a patient who has already been endoscopically stented is usually based on the operative findings for each patient. In a patient who is found to have unsuspected liver metastases, the authors likely would choose not to bypass the stented biliary tree. In contrast, in patients with locally advanced unresectable pancreatic cancer, the bile duct is often divided to assess for resectability. A biliary reconstruction must then be performed.

In contrast to other gastrointestinal cancers in general, where pain has been reported to occur at a relatively low frequency, pain in pancreatic cancer is a frequent symptom: about 20% to 40% experience pain at time of diagnosis and up to 80% experience pain during the course of their disease. The possible etiologies of the pain, which is usually dull and located in the back or upper abdomen, are infiltration of the mesenteric or celiac plexus, or pancreatic duct obstruction, although the precise pathophysiology has not been elucidated. Similar to pain treatment in general, palliating pancreatic cancer pain follows the World Health Organization's Pain Relief Ladder, which prescribes tiered increases in potency of administered analgesics starting with nonsteroidal antiinflammatory drugs (NSAIDs), followed by the addition of opioids and other adjuvant pain medication if needed. Pain medication should be administered on a schedule of every 3 to 6 hours rather than "on demand" and has been reported to have an efficacy of about 80%. Opioids, although more often underdosed than overdosed in the palliative setting, can lead to side effects such as altered mental status, constipation, nausea and vomiting, and loss of efficacy over time, especially if celiac or mesenteric plexus infiltration occurs.

Invasive treatment options should be considered when pharmacologic strategies to control cancer pain fail to provide adequate pain relief despite correct dosing or when treatment side effects become prohibitive. The principle behind these techniques is to interrupt transmission of nociceptive stimuli from the pancreas and infiltrated organs to the central nervous system. For pancreatic cancer, the celiac ganglion is the optimal site to interrupt the pain sensory process. Celiac plexus blocks or chemical splanchnicectomy can be performed percutaneously, endoscopically, or operatively while determining resectability via laparoscopy or laparotomy. Pain relief through these methods is effective, although diarrhea and orthostatic side effects have been reported in as many as 40% of the patients. With both percutaneous and endoscopic blockade of the celiac plexus available today, the surgeon's role in the palliation of pain due to pancreatic cancer is almost exclusively limited to the cases of patients undergoing operation for resection or for palliation of symptoms other than pain. Similar to biliary and gastric diversion, splanchnicectomy should be performed routinely during exploration if unresectability is discovered. We and others have shown that in patients who underwent prophylactic chemical splanchnicectomy with 50% ethanol, effective pain control can be achieved. Furthermore, the subgroup with severe pain showed improved survival following successful pain therapy.

The next three sections will discuss the specific surgical techniques in managing pancreatic cancer in patients with symptoms of (1) biliary obstruction, (2) gastric outlet obstruction, and (3) pain.

PALLIATIVE SURGICAL INTERVENTIONS

Palliation of Biliary Obstruction

Obstructive jaundice is amendable to endoscopic, percutaneous, laparoscopic, robotic, and open drainage procedures. There is good evidence that today the most efficacious initial strategy to relieve biliary obstruction is endoscopic stent placement. Although both surgery and endoscopy are equally effective palliative options, endoscopic drainage with the insertion of a stent into the bile duct has been shown to significantly reduce the length of initial hospitalization and is associated with lower procedural morbidity and mortality as well as improved quality of life. Plastic biliary stents, which have been used in the past, have a tendency to clog and therefore may require repeated endoscopic interventions. Today, self-expandable metal stents have a larger diameter and are associated with a lower occlusion rate than that of plastic stents. Therefore, the use of metal stents has been shown to be cost-effective in patients who are expected to survive longer than 6 months. Metal stents can be (1) uncovered, that is, simply a metal mesh; (2) covered, which were developed because tumor growth through the mesh decreased patency; or (3) partially covered, meaning that the ends consist of an uncovered metal mesh that holds the stent in place, and the middle segment is covered. Conflicting evidence from Europe and the United States exists as to which stent design is the most efficacious. A frequent concern of medical oncologists and gastroenterologists is that the placement of a self-expanding metal stent in a patient who requires drainage but whose resectability is unclear will make a possible pancreaticoduodenectomy challenging if not impossible. In our experience, metal stents are not a significant obstacle to either surgery for curative or palliative intent and should be deployed in patients whose life expectancy is estimated to be greater than 6 months or in those undergoing aggressive neoadjuvant therapy. Future research should explore the role of drug-eluding stents with, for example, Paclitaxel, with the idea that the chemotherapeutic drug will prevent obstruction secondary to tumor ingrowth.

Transhepatic percutaneous access should be reserved for patients in whom endoscopy fails or is not anatomically possible (e.g., prior gastric bypass). In most cases, after initial percutaneous access with external drainage, stents can be placed that can be totally internal or after initial transhepatic access, the so-called rendezvous-procedure can be performed where a transhepatic guidewire facilitates endoscopic stent placement.

Despite these clear advantages of endoscopic stent placement to relieve biliary obstruction, there are some advantages to having a patient undergo a surgical biliary bypass. Severe complications and readmissions, usually due to stent dysfunction, are more likely to occur in patients treated endoscopically. Furthermore, in patients with gastric outlet obstruction, consideration should be given to an operative approach to bypass both the obstructed biliary tree and duodenum, as the combination of both metallic biliary and duodenal stents is often problematic. Therefore, it is our practice to explain the advantages and disadvantages of both operative and endoscopic procedures, particularly to fit patients.

Our preference for surgical palliation of biliary obstruction is Roux-en-Y hepaticojejunostomy for open biliary diversion and a loop jejunostomy for a laparoscopic approach (Figure 2). The technical details are as follows. Cholecystectomy is performed, if it has not previously been performed, and the common bile duct is mobilized. An important technical point is that minimal mobilization of the bile duct should be performed with an understanding of the vascular supply to avoid ischemia, which can lead to stenosis or leak. The common bile duct or hepatic duct is then transected, and a frozen section of the margin is obtained. This is important to avoid leaving cancer at the anastomosis, which could lead to obstruction due to tumor regrowth. The distal end of the common bile duct is sutured closed. We routinely send aerobic and anaerobic cultures if the patient has had a prior biliary stent in order to have microbiology

data to initiate appropriate antibiotic therapy should biliary sepsis occur. The Roux-en-Y limb is created using a 40-cm jejunal limb that is usually anastomosed to a jejunal limb in end-to-side fashion approximately 20 cm distal to the ligament of Treitz. Alternatively, a loop hepaticojejunostomy with a proximal enteroenterostomy is a suitable option. The hepaticojejunostomy is completed with either interrupted 4.0 PDS or Vicryl sutures, or, if the duct diameter is large due to prior biliary obstruction, in running fashion. It is important to incorporate the jejunal mucosa into the anastomosis with great care to prevent transient biliary obstruction from an edematous mucosa. Other techniques for biliary drainage include choledochoduodenostomy or cholecystojejunostomy. These procedures performed via open surgical techniques have been almost entirely replaced by hepaticojejunostomy due to superior short- and long-term results. Patients undergoing gallbladder-enteric anastomosis are at substantially greater risk of requiring subsequent biliary drainage procedures compared to those undergoing a bile duct–enteric anastomosis. This discrepancy is secondary to frequent cystic duct involvement in tumor progression.

Laparoscopic biliary diversion requires advanced laparoscopic skills to safely mobilize the bile duct and to perform a stapled or handsewn hepaticojejunostomy. We construct a laparoscopic hepaticojejunostomy in a loop fashion. A loop of proximal jejunum is brought up to the hepatoduodenal ligament and anchored with a stitch. After transsection of the bile duct, a small enterotomy is made in the approximated jejunum. It is important to not make the enterotomy too large, as it tends to widen during fabrication of the anastomosis. This anastomosis can also be constructed in a side-to-side fashion, which might be technically easier in certain situations (Figure 3). Due to the magnification of a laparoscopic camera of about ×10, even a nondilated bile duct can routinely be anastomosed in a running fashion with double-armed 6.0 PDS sutures that have been shortened to a total length of 30 cm. Alternatively, as it is technically easier, a laparoscopic cholecystojejunostomy is an option for very select patients if the cystic duct is found to be well clear of tumor involvement.

Robotic surgery has recently been applied to the palliation of pancreatic and distal bile duct cancers. This resource intensive technology has the advantage of 3D vision and articulation of the

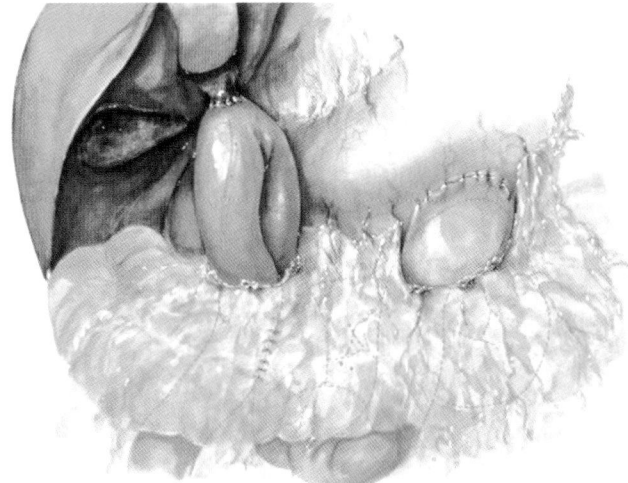

FIGURE 2 Anatomy after double bypass. The schema demonstrates a Roux-en-Y hepaticojejunostomy of 40 cm as well as a retrocolic loop gastrojejunostomy. We recommend this retrocolic position of the gastrojejunostomy, as it has been shown to have a lower rate of delayed gastric emptying. The gastrojejunal anastomosis should be delivered through the colonic mesentery to prevent obstruction, and care should be taken to avoid vagal branches, as severing them might lead to delayed gastric emptying.

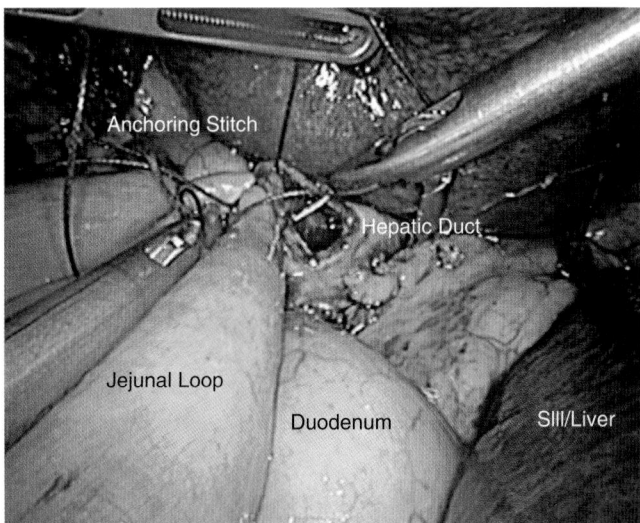

FIGURE 3 Laparoscopic view of a laparoscopic hepaticojejunostomy. A loop of jejunum is anchored at the hepatoduodenal ligament and a side-to-side hepaticojejunostomy constructed. Using a shortened double-arm suture facilitates running the suture for construction of the anastomosis. The magnification of the laparoscope might facilitate this anastomosis when a nonobstructed duct is small.

instruments. Because of these advantages, primarily open surgeons often find it easier to transition to offering patients a robotic approach over a laparoscopic one. However, the need for cost containment in health care today makes robotic palliation of pancreatic cancer an inefficient application of the technology at the present stage.

Palliation of Gastric Outlet Obstruction

We mentioned in the introduction that, based on level I evidence, a gastrojejunostomy should be performed regardless of symptoms if the patient is deemed ineligible for curative resection during operative exploration. Prophylactic surgical bypass at time of exploration does not increase postoperative morbidity or mortality and prevents late gastric outlet obstruction. A gastrojejunostomy can be performed either by laparoscopic or open technique as a simple loop side-to-side procedure or as a Roux-en-Y gastrojejunostomy (Figure 4). Complications of a Roux-en-Y gastrojejunostomy, such as Roux stasis syndrome, can occur; therefore, this technique is rarely indicated. The gastrojejunal anastomosis can be performed using a variety of techniques (handsewn vs stapled, running vs interrupted sutures, single layer vs double layer anastomosis); however, no technique has been shown to be superior over the others. Two different techniques of delivering the loop of jejunum are antecolic, which means ventral to the transverse colon, and retrocolic, where the loop of jejunum is delivered through the transverse colonic mesentery. It had been assumed that antecolic gastrojejunostomy avoids proximity to the tumor bed and therefore prevents late failure due to tumor ingrowth; however, delayed gastric emptying, despite a patent gastrojejunostomy, is a common postoperative problem following antecolic gastrojejunostomy. Retrocolic, isoperistaltic gastrojejunostomy, which has been shown to be associated with a lower incidence of postoperative delayed gastric emptying and even late-occurring gastric outlet obstruction, is therefore our recommendation (see Figure 2). The posterior gastrojejunostomy should be delivered below the transverse mesocolon and fixed in place at the level of the anastomosis to avoid obstruction at the mesenteric slit. Vagotomy of the gastric branches should be avoided during palliative gastrojejunostomy to prevent delayed gastric emptying. Long-term gastric acid suppression with a proton pump inhibitor is advised.

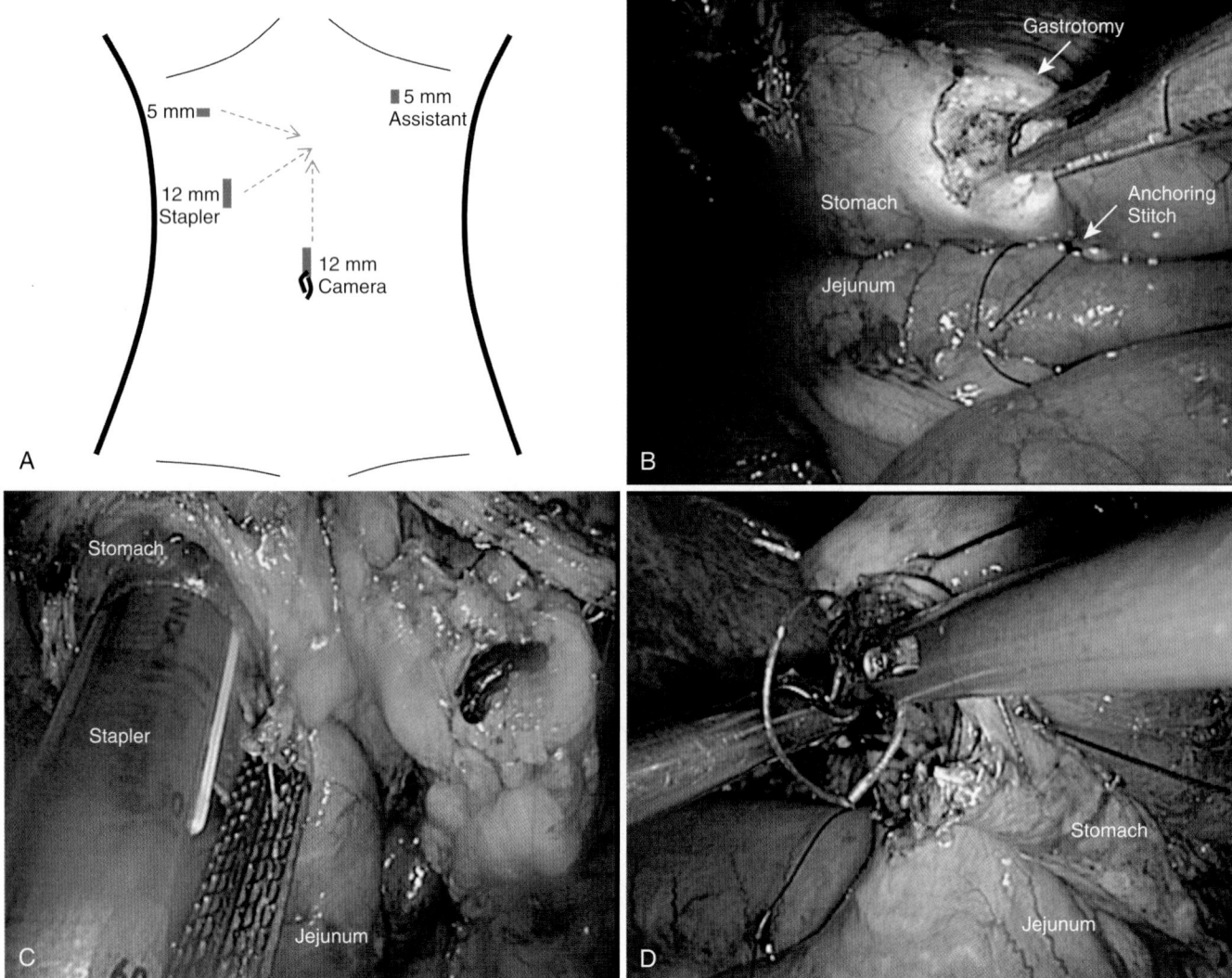

FIGURE 4   Laparoscopic gastrojejunostomy. **A,** Trocar positioning: two 12-mm trocars are used to accommodate camera and endoscopic stapler. The 5-mm port under the right costal margin is an operator working port, and the port under the left costal margin is used by the assistant for retraction. **B,** A loop of jejunum is anchored to the stomach, and a gastrotomy and an enterotomy are performed to accommodate the stapler. **C,** After the stapler is fired, an anastomosis between stomach and jejunum is created. **D,** The small whole that accommodated the stapler is sutured closed.

Duodenal stenting with self-expandable metallic stents is also an option in the treatment of gastroduodenal obstruction. The concept of the stent design is similar to that for the biliary tract, but duodenal stents are typically longer (6 to 12 cm) and of larger calibers (18 to 23 mm). To prevent spontaneous migration and avoid coverage of the ampullary opening, the stents are uncovered. Duodenal stents should be reserved for patients who are not surgical candidates for either an open or a laparoscopic approach because of either comorbidities or advanced disease. While endoscopic stenting for the palliation of malignant gastroduodenal obstruction is associated with early clinical success (i.e., shorter time to oral intake and shorter length of hospital stay), operative gastric bypass procedures are preferable in patients with an expected prognosis of several months, who are likely to benefit from the reliable durability of surgical palliation. Additionally, biliary obstruction leading to cholangitis occurs in 6% of patients if the major papilla is affected by the stent. Although the endoscopist will try to deploy the stent clear of the papilla, this is not always possible. Also, duodenal stenting across the ampulla will make the patient ineligible for endoscopic biliary drainage should biliary obstruction occur later in the disease. Duodenal perforation is yet another potential and catastrophic complication of duodenal stent placement, which occurs because of the need to dilate the stricture and then traverse it with a side-viewing endoscope. Mechanical irritation of the intestinal mucosa can also cause bleeding, erosion, and even perforation. If the ends of the duodenal stent rest at the intestinal curves, such as the duodenal bulb, junction between the second and third portions of the duodenum, or the ligament of Treitz, the fold can lead to stent obstruction. Finally, patients who undergo a surgical bypass can consume a more balanced diet afterward than can patients who undergo duodenal stenting. Therefore, although duodenal stents have their role in patients who are not surgical candidates, further studies and advancements in device technologies are necessary to assign this treatment option a definitive role in the treatment algorithm of palliation of gastrointestinal obstruction.

Palliation of Pain

Surgical procedures for pain management in patients with unresectable pancreatic cancer should be carried out only if an operation is indicated for possible resection or palliation of other symptoms. The surgeon should refrain from operating on patients with inoperable pancreatic cancer for the sole purpose of relieving pain. Our preferred method is chemical splanchnicectomy celiac plexus block with 50% ethanol, which we perform during open or laparoscopic exploration if unresectable disease is found. The procedure is indicated in both patients with and without significant pain, as level I evidence shows that celiac block both reduces pain and prevents the development of significant pain. In the open technique, we place our nondominant hand on the aorta, with index and middle finger on either side. We then move our finger downward along the aorta, and the first branch we encounter is the celiac trunk, where the celiac plexus is located. We then infiltrate 20 mL of 50% alcohol using a 22-gauge spinal needle into the retroperitoneum on both sides of the aorta. The small caliber of the needle will help to prevent leakage from the injection-side from the retroperitoneum into the abdominal cavity when the needle is removed. The laparoscopic approach to target the celiac plexus is performed under ultrasound guidance. A laparoscopic ultrasound probe that has a small channel to guide the needle directly facilitates safe celiac plexus blockade (Figure 5). The incidence of major complications following neurolytic celiac plexus block has been shown to be low at 1 out of about 700 cases, with the most severe complications being death, nonreversible and reversible paraplegia, and anterior spinal syndrome.

Celiac plexus neurolysis can be performed percutaneously via ultrasound, fluoroscopic, or CT guidance. The advantage of CT or ultrasound guidance, usually performed via an anterior approach, is that the target area can be directly visualized to avoid damage to the

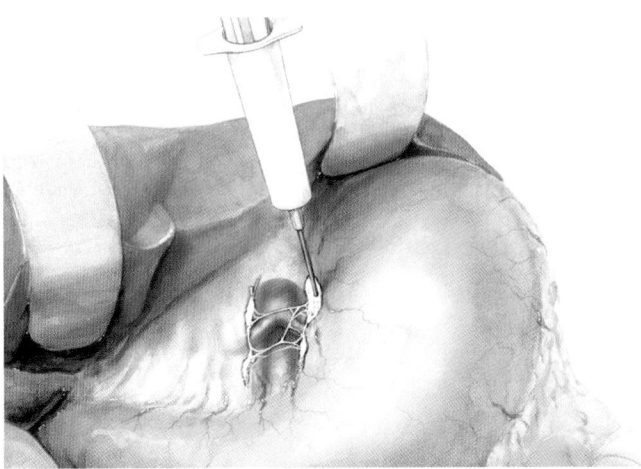

FIGURE 5 A chemical splanchnicectomy (celiac plexus block) can be accomplished by injecting 20 mL of 50% alcohol into the celiac ganglia on each side of the aorta at the level of the celiac axis. The use of a 22-gauge or smaller caliber spinal needle ensures containment of the injection wheal within the retroperitoneum. (Note: The celiac nerves are not frequently as nicely visualized as in this artist's rendition. More commonly the nerve fibers are not seen, and the alcohol is injected into the correct region, by palpating the aorta and celiac axis pulsation, and avoiding their puncture.)

surrounding structures, including the lung, pleura, liver, intestines, and blood vessels.

Celiac plexus blocks for abdominal pain management in pancreatic cancer patients can also be performed endoscopically. Endoscopic ultrasound–guided celiac and mesenteric plexus blocks are safe and effective. Real-time imaging and anterior access to the celiac plexus from the posterior gastric wall help to prevent complications related to the puncture of spinal nerves, the aorta and its branches, and the diaphragm.

OUTCOMES AFTER SURGICAL PALLIATION

Surgical palliation of a patient with unresectable pancreatic cancer has several advantages over an endoscopic approach to palliation. The key advantages are that (1) the three most important symptoms—biliary obstruction, gastric outlet obstruction, and pain—can all be addressed during one procedure; (2) the experienced pancreatic surgeon will be able to make a definitive assessment regarding resectability, which is often not possible based on cross-sectional imaging alone; and (3) surgical outcomes are generally more durable than nonsurgical options. The question then becomes what are the outcomes of surgical palliation. In a large series from the Johns Hopkins medical institutions, 1913 patients with pancreatic head adenocarcinoma were explored, and 30.5% underwent palliative procedures. The majority of the patients underwent a double bypass (64.5%), while a minority had either gastrojejunostomy (28.2%) or hepaticojejunostomy (7.2%) alone. The palliative failure rates were favorably low at 2.3% after hepaticojejunostomy and 3.1% after gastrojejunostomy. The overall complication rate was only 22%, and 95% remained free of recurrent duodenal or biliary obstruction. In contrast, in a recent 10-year retrospective analysis of 157 patients from the Memorial Sloan Kettering Cancer Center, the authors did not reach an equally positive conclusion regarding efficacy and morbidity of surgical palliation. In this series, only 38% underwent double bypass. Complications occurred in 28% of patients, 2% of whom died perioperatively, and 46% required interventions following exploration.

Surprisingly, the proportion of patients requiring interventions after surgical palliation was similar between double bypass or single bypass groups regardless of the procedure performed at the initial operation, as were the total number of inpatient days prior to death. Regardless, it is important that the surgical palliation for pancreatic cancer is performed with low morbidity, as complications have been shown to shorten survival after surgical palliation with an odds ratio of 3.

Data on outcomes for palliation using minimal access techniques such as laparoscopy or robotic surgery are limited. However, the limited data that are available indicate that the typical benefits of laparoscopic surgery, such as reduced length of stay and less pain, seem to be preserved for both laparoscopic and robotic surgery for palliation with a comparable or even lower morbidity.

Factors have been identified that help to predict survival after double bypass for palliation of pancreatic cancer. In a recent series of 397 patients with pancreatic adenocarcinoma from Johns Hopkins, four factors were found to predict early mortality: presence of distant metastatic disease (HR 2.59), poor tumor differentiation (HR 1.71), severe preoperative nausea and vomiting (HR 1.48), and lack of previous placement of a biliary stent (HR 1.36). These factors might be valuable in counseling patients regarding their survival, as patients who had all four of these risk factors lived less than 6 months.

In summary, surgical palliation performed with minimal complications is crucial in the treatment of pancreatic cancer to achieve the most efficient use of resources and, more important, to help patients maximize their quality of life for the limited time they have.

PALLIATIVE RESECTION VERSUS PALLIATIVE BYPASS

A question that has been the subject of debate in the past is whether palliative resection of pancreatic cancer is more beneficial for patients with advanced pancreatic cancer compared with the standard double bypass. Those favoring palliative resection contend that tumor debulking improves survival, minimizes or prevents pain from local tumor infiltration, and delays peritoneal and systemic spread. However, palliative resections are associated with significantly increased operative times, longer hospital stays, and higher overall morbidity and mortality rates compared with palliative bypass procedures as shown by cohort studies as well as pooled meta-analysis. Morbidity and mortality are 2 to 3 times higher in the R2 resection group. Although planned tumor debulking is beneficial for patients with other neoplasms such as ovarian carcinoma, the available data support the argument against palliative resection for pancreatic cancer because of the higher mortality and morbidity rates of resection compared with bypass. Therefore, we recommend performing a biliary and gastric bypass in the case of advanced disease during exploration and would strongly caution against planned palliative resection.

PALLIATIVE CHEMOTHERAPY AND CHEMORADIATION

A surgeon caring for patients with pancreatic cancer needs to be familiar with the treatment options of chemotherapy and chemoradiation in order to offer the best possible intervention to relieve symptoms in a context of limited survival and assist in the management of complications. In contrast to other gastrointestinal cancers where tumor size measurement is a good correlate to the efficacy of chemotherapy, the characteristic desmoplastic reaction and inflammatory response that develops around the pancreatic tumor makes this a less reliable predictor of objective response in pancreatic cancer. Metastases are an alternative for use to correlate to disease response and can be followed by serial imaging. We understand more and more that in addition to the objective tumor response and survival, the "clinical benefit" should be considered. For example, a comparison of gemcitabine with 5-fluorouracil (5-FU) showed that patients who did not exhibit a reduction in tumor size still showed threefold improvement in symptoms of a decreasing body mass index, pain, and/or performance status. Based on this information, gemcitabine became the standard chemotherapy for advanced pancreatic cancer. As every third patient treated with gemcitabine will develop symptoms such as diarrhea or fever, the surgeon should be cognizant of the side effect profile in case surgical consultation is requested.

Unfortunately, neither 5-FU in its intravenous or oral preparation nor gemcitabine nor any other single agent chemotherapeutic regimen has shown consistent response rates above 10%. This relative inefficacy led to the development of combination chemotherapeutic strategies, the most important one being a regimen with the acronym, FOLFIRINOX, consisting of the agents 5-FU, leucovorin, irinotecan, and oxaliplatin. In a French trial of 342 patients with metastatic pancreatic cancer, patients with a relatively good performance status were randomized to FOLFIRINOX versus a standard regimen with gemcitabine. In this trial, termed ACCORD-11, the median overall survival was 11.1 months in the FOLFIRINOX group as compared with 6.8 months in the gemcitabine group. Median progression-free survival was 6.4 months in the FOLFIRINOX group and 3.3 months in the gemcitabine group. However, more adverse events and a greater decline in patients' quality of life were noted in the FOLFIRINOX group. Although the median overall survival for patients with unresectable pancreatic cancer with best possible care remains low at less than 1 year, this combination chemotherapy increases the time of survival by almost 40% compared to standard chemotherapy. The trial was stopped after enrolling only 250 patients when a planned interim analysis showed that the primary trial endpoint (improved overall survival) had been met. Other combination chemotherapeutic regimens are not nearly as effective and researchers have difficulties showing any additional benefits of these regimens over single-agent therapy, among which the most efficacious might be gemcitabine plus oxaliplatin (GEMOX).

The prolonged survival of patients treated with FOLFIRINOX might translate into a greater need for durable palliation of symptoms. The surgeon needs to be familiar with this new regimen, as surgical consultation may be required in the presence of complications such as febrile neutropenia, thrombocytopenia, or diarrhea, which occur in 5% of patients undergoing FOLFIRINOX therapy. Prior to initiation of FOLFIRINOX therapy, patients must have normalized bilirubin levels, which usually require either endoscopic biliary stenting, with its associated risk of cholangitis, or surgical bypass. Thus, surgeons will have increasing involvement in the management of patients in the era of palliative FOLFIRINOX chemotherapy to ensure palliation of symptoms both prior to and after this more effective treatment.

Finally, it can be expected that as neoadjuvant regimens including FOFIRINOX have been increasingly employed, a higher percentage of patients with locally advanced pancreatic cancer may become candidates for resection. The data on the role of FOLFIRINOX as neoadjuvant therapy for patients with borderline resectable cancer are still limited, but one small retrospective series has shown that a R0 resection rate with the therapy can be achieved in as many as 44% of patients. If this experience is confirmed and use of FOLFIRINOX is expanded, more patients with locally advanced pancreatic cancer may undergo surgical exploration to attempt resection. As it is likely, some of these patients will still prove to be unresectable, at which point operative palliation will be appropriate.

Locally advanced pancreatic cancer is defined as locally unresectable cancer in the absence of distant metastasis; approximately one out of three patients presenting with pancreatic cancer have this type. Chemoradiation has been applied to this group to convert them to a status where resectability is possible. The precise role of applying chemoradiation to patients who have locally unresectable pancreatic cancer, however, still needs to be defined, as there is conflicting evidence regarding whether patients indeed benefit from chemoradiation. Treatment with high-dose radiotherapy can be difficult to tolerate, and the constraints of daily treatment with radiation for patients with only few months' range of survival can significantly compromise quality of life. In addition, radiation doses for palliation only of locally advanced pancreatic cancer beyond 30 Gy have been shown in retrospective trials to increase the rate of complications, including strictures, colitis, pancreatitis, and others, which might again require the expertise of a surgeon. Future direction might include the use of more focused energy such as proton beam radiation, which to date is available only at a few centers around the world.

CONCLUSIONS

A surgeon should be a central player in the multidisciplinary team caring for patients with advanced pancreatic cancer. This critical role is directed toward palliating the most common symptoms of advanced pancreatic cancer, which are biliary obstruction, gastric outlet obstruction, and pain, for which both surgical and nonsurgical options exist. Based on level I evidence, double biliary and gastric bypass and celiac axis chemical splanchnicectomy should be performed if unresectability is determined during an exploration, which may be the only way to definitively rule out unresectable disease. The first-line treatment of biliary obstruction is internal biliary drainage by endoscopic stent placement. If this is not possible, biliary bypass in the form of a hepaticojejunostomy should be performed by either an open or a laparoscopic approach. The stent technology for duodenal stenting is not yet at the level of biliary stenting, and therefore an open or laparoscopic surgical bypass for palliation of gastric outlet obstruction should be performed. Pain control via celiac plexus block, either percutaneously or via endoscopic techniques, provides excellent pain relief, and it is clear today that there is no benefit in planned palliative resection. Minimal-access techniques for palliation of advanced pancreatic cancer are excellent options with proven benefits in the perioperative period for patients undergoing pancreatic surgery. Furthermore, all patients with unresectable cancer and good performance status should be considered for FOLFIRINOX chemotherapy, and surgical input might be required to render a patient eligible for this regimen or to assist in the management of complications. Radiotherapy for locally advanced unresectable pancreatic cancer can be considered, but it should always be combined with chemotherapy, and higher dosages might lead to significant side effects in patients whose survival time is limited. In summary, it is expected that the already significant role of the surgeon in the team caring for patients with advanced pancreatic cancer will only expand with device development, improvements in imaging and staging, and new therapeutic agents.

SELECTED READINGS

Arcidiacono PG, Calori G, Carrara S, et al: Celiac plexus block for pancreatic cancer pain in adults, *Cochrane Database Syst Rev* (3):CD007519, 2011.

Conroy T, Desseigne F, Ychou M, et al: FOLFIRINOX versus gemcitabine for metastatic pancreatic cancer, *N Engl J Med* 364(19):1817–1825, 2011.

Gillen S, Schuster T, Friess H, Kleeff J: Palliative resections versus palliative bypass procedures in pancreatic cancer—a systematic review, *Am J Surg* 203(4):496–502, 2012.

Heinicke JM, Buchler MW, Laffer UT: Bilio-digestive double bypass for non-resectable pancreatic cancer, *Dig Surg* 19(3):165–167, 2002.

Hosein PJ, Macintyre J, Kawamura C, et al: A retrospective study of neoadjuvant FOLFIRINOX in unresectable or borderline-resectable locally advanced pancreatic adenocarcinoma, *BMC Cancer* 12:199, 2012.

Jeurnink SM, van Eijck CH, Steyerberg EW, Kuipers EJ, Stierma PD: Stent versus gastrojejunostomy for the palliation of gastric outlet obstruction: a systematic review, *BMC Gastroenterol* 8:18, 2007.

Kneuertz PJ, Cunningham SC, Cameron JL, et al: Palliative surgical management of patients with unresectable pancreatic adenocarcinoma: trends and lessons learned from a large, single institution experience, *J Gastrointest Surg* 15(11):1917–2716, 2011.

Koninger J, Wente MN, Muller MW, et al: Surgical palliation in patients with pancreatic cancer, *Langenbecks Arch Surg* 392(1):13–21, 2007.

Lillemoe KD, Cameron JL, Hardacre JM, et al: Is prophylactic gastrojejunostomy indicated for unresectable periampullary cancer? A prospective randomized trial, *Ann Surg* 230(3):322–328, 1999.

Lillemoe KD, Cameron JL, Kaufman HS, et al: Chemical splanchnicectomy in patients with unresectable pancreatic cancer. A prospective randomized trial, *Ann Surg* 217(5):447–455, 1993.

Lyons JM, Karkar A, Correa-Gallego CC, et al: Operative procedures for unresectable pancreatic cancer: does operative bypass decrease requirements for postoperative procedures and in-hospital days? *HPB (Oxford)* 14(7):469–475, 2012. doi:10.1111/j.1477-2574.2012.00477.x. Epub 2012 May 15.

Smith AC, Dowsett JF, Russell RC, Hatfield AR, Cotton PB: Randomised trial of endoscopic stenting versus surgical bypass in malignant low bileduct obstruction, *Lancet* 344(8938):1655–1660, 1994.

Sohn TA, Lillemoe KD, Cameron JL, et al: Surgical palliation of unresectable periampullary adenocarcinoma in the 1990s, *J Am Coll Surg* 188(6):658–666, 1999.

Neoadjuvant and Adjuvant Therapy of Pancreatic Cancer

Ana De Jesus-Acosta, MD, and Dan Laheru, MD

INTRODUCTION

Pancreatic ductal adenocarcinoma (PDA) is a lethal malignancy that remains the fourth leading cause of cancer-related mortality. Surgical resection of the primary tumor offers a potential cure when it is diagnosed at an early stage. Additional therapies are required in the preoperative (neoadjuvant) or postoperative (adjuvant) setting in an effort to achieve cure for this aggressive disease. This chapter focuses on the therapies given in the adjuvant and neoadjuvant setting with PDA.

Determination of resectability of the primary tumor is the most important objective at the initial staging evaluation. Ideally, these cases should be discussed in a multidisciplinary approach that includes surgical oncologists and medical and radiation oncologists. Pathologists and radiologists with experience in imaging of pancreas cancer should also be involved. These discussions are important for determining optimal selection and timing of surgical and nonsurgical interventions.

Imaging should include a specialized computed tomographic (CT) scan study or magnetic resonance imaging (MRI). CT scan should be performed according to a defined pancreas protocol, such as triphasic cross-sectional imaging and thin slices. Optimal multiphase imaging technique includes a noncontrast phase plus arterial, pancreatic parenchymal, and portal venous phases of contrast enhancement with thin cuts (3 mm) through the abdomen. This technique allows precise visualization of the relationship of the primary tumor to the mesenteric vasculature and detection of metastatic deposits as small as 3 to 5 mm. Pancreas protocol MRI is emerging as an alternative to CT scan.

On the basis of imaging, the pancreatic tumors should be classified as resectable (stage I or II), locally advanced (stage III), or metastatic (stage IV). In most institutions, patients with resectable disease with adequate performance status and comorbidities undergo surgery as the initial therapy followed by adjuvant chemotherapy or chemoradiotherapy after recovery. A subset of tumors have proven to be more challenging to definitively categorize as resectable or unresectable and have been classified as "borderline resectable" tumors. No uniform consensus exists as to the definition or management of borderline resectable and unresectable disease. Table 1 summarizes the anatomic staging described by several entities. Treatment sequences and selection of adjuvant versus neoadjuvant therapies focus on appropriate anatomic staging.

ADJUVANT THERAPY

Surgical resection is offered to patients diagnosed with resectable disease at the time of initial staging. This accounts for 10% to 20% of patients at the time of initial presentation. After resection, more than 80% of patients ultimately die of disease from either local or distant recurrence, which is the rationale for adjuvant treatment. Although the benefit of adjuvant therapy has been shown in the recent decades, the best choice of treatment modality remains highly controversial. For instance, within the North American hemisphere, chemoradiotherapy followed by chemotherapy, or vice versa, is considered a standard approach; chemotherapy alone is the current standard in Europe. Solid data support use of either 5-fluorouracil (5-FU) or gemcitabine as the standard chemotherapeutic option. In contrast, discussion continues regarding the role of adjuvant chemoradiation, specifically in the subgroup of patients with positive resection margins.

Adjuvant therapy should be given to patients who have not had neoadjuvant chemotherapy and who have adequately recovered from surgery and should be initiated within 4 to 8 weeks. Patients who have received neoadjuvant chemotherapy or chemoradiation are candidates for additional chemotherapy after surgery. If systemic chemotherapy precedes chemoradiation, systemic CT scan should be done after each treatment modality.

The Gastrointestinal Tumor Study Group (GISTSG) conducted a randomized clinical trial in the 1980s in which postsurgical patients were randomized to either observation or 5-FU–based chemoradiation followed by systemic 5-FU and leucovorin for 2 years or until evidence of recurrence. The results provided a statistically significant outcome that favored the patients treated with systemic chemotherapy. An additional randomized two-arm clinical trial was conducted by the Radiation Therapy Oncology Group (RTOG) 97-04 in which patients were assigned to receive postsurgical gemcitabine or infusion of 5-FU followed by the same 5-FU–based chemoradiation in both arms. The findings suggested a nonstatistical trend in favor of the gemcitabine arm. Subsequent studies comparing postsurgical treatments and observation supported the GISTSG findings and provided the basis for postoperative treatment.

The Europeans have contributed significantly to the field with several studies in the adjuvant setting. The European Study Group for Pancreas Cancer (ESPAC) and Charité Onkologie (CONKO) trials have further supported the role postoperative therapy over observation. Although the initial ESPAC-1 trial did favor postsurgical treatment over observation after resected pancreas cancer, it also suggested that radiation may not be a necessary component. The chemotherapy used in the initial ESPAC-1 trial was 5-FU and

leucovorin. Unfortunately, these results have not ended the controversy as to what should be the appropriate adjuvant treatment because this study was criticized for a complicated study design and the use of noncontemporary radiation therapy. However, it may have convinced the Europeans that chemotherapy alone should be the standard of care. Subsequently, the ESPAC-3 trial evaluated the value of gemcitabine versus 5-FU and concluded that either of these chemotherapy agents were equivalent with regards to overall and progression-free survival outcomes, although severe toxicities were less in the patients with gemcitabine treatment. The CONKO investigators conducted a randomized trial comparing gemcitabine for 6 months with observation in the CONKO-001 trial and showed a statistically significant improvement in disease-free survival in the patients treated with postoperative gemcitabine. Therefore, postoperative chemotherapy alone for a period of 6 months is widely accepted.

There are still unanswered questions in the adjuvant setting, such as the role of the addition of targeted therapy or more aggressive multiagent treatments. Although impressive 5-year survival rates of 55% were reported in regimens with immunochemotherapy (cisplatin, 5-FU, interferon alpha) combined with radiation, no survival difference as compared with 5-FU monotherapy was observed in a subsequent phase III trial. Regimens with substantial antitumor effect are still needed to improve long-term survival in patients with resected pancreas cancer.

Two positive phase III clinical trials for patients with advanced stage IV pancreatic cancer have been published and have again raised the question of use of multiagent chemotherapy or targeted therapy in the adjuvant setting. The first was a phase III clinical trial of gemcitabine versus gemcitabine plus erlotinib, which showed a small survival benefit for the combination therapy. A second phase III trial evaluated patients with stage IV disease treated with single-agent gemcitabine versus the combination of 5-FU, leucovorin, irinotecan, and oxaliplatin (FOLFIRINOX), which showed a significant survival benefit in the patients treated with the multiagent chemotherapy regimen. Given these results, several ongoing trials have been initiated to help to address these questions. The RTOG in collaboration with the European Organisation for Research and Treatment of Cancer (EORTC) has opened a phase III trial to evaluate the efficacy of the addition of erlotinib to gemcitabine and the addition of gemcitabine-based chemoradiation to this treatment in the postoperative adjuvant setting (RTOG 0848, EORTC 40084-22084). This trial will also help to establish the value of modern chemoradiotherapy. The CONKO investigators are evaluating the addition of erlotinib to gemcitabine in patients who have undergone a margin negative resection (CONKO-005). The FOLFIRINOX regimen has also been evaluated in a multicenter study in the adjuvant setting (NCT01526135) compared with single-agent gemcitabine.

As of now, the current standard of care in the United States includes 6 months of postoperative therapy with gemcitabine or 5-FU with leucovorin. Alternatively, chemotherapy with one of these two agents before or after chemoradiation (5-FU–based or gemcitabine-based) is also accepted. Although chemoradiation is still controversial, it is widely used in some academic centers in the United States. The data to support its use are based on large, single-institute series from Johns Hopkins University and the Mayo Clinic and the GISTSG trial designed in 1980s.

NEOADJUVANT THERAPY

The low rate of resectability, near absolute risk of recurrence, and poor long-term survival rate after pancreatectomy have led to the investigation of preoperative therapies. Only 10% to 20% of patients with PDA are candidates for resection at the time of diagnosis, and only 15% to 20% of these patients are alive after 5 years of an intended curative resection. Two group populations who potentially receive neoadjuvant therapy are discussed in this section: patients

TABLE 1: Classifications of resectability category

Category	AHPBA/SSO/SSAT Classification				M.D. Anderson Classification				NCCN			
	SMV/PV	SMA	CHA	Celiac Trunk	SMV/PV	SMA	CHA	Celiac Trunk	SMV/PV	SMA	CHA	Celiac Trunk
Resectable	No abutment* or encasement†	No abutment or encasement	No abutment or encasement	No abutment or encasement	Abutment or encasement without occlusion	No abutment or encasement	No abutment or encasement	No abutment or encasement	No abutment, encasement, or thrombus	Clear fat planes	Clear fat planes	Clear fat planes
Borderline	Abutment, encasement, or occlusion	Abutment	Abutment or short-segment encasement	No abutment or encasement	Short-segment occlusion	Abutment	Abutment or short-segment encasement	Abutment	Abutment, impingement, or encasement Short-segment occlusion with proximal/distal area suitable for reconstruction	Abutment	Short-segment encasement or abutment	No involvement
Locally advanced	Not reconstructible	Encasement	Long-segment encasement	Abutment	Not reconstructible	Encasement	Long-segment encasement	Encasement	Not reconstructible	Encasement		Abutment

AHPBA/SSO/SSAT, American Hepato-Pancreatico-Biliary Association/Society of Surgical Oncology/Society for Surgery of the Alimentary Tract; CHA, common hepatic artery; NCCN, National Comprehensive Cancer Network; PV, portal vein; SMA, superior mesenteric artery; SMV, superior mesenteric vein.

*Less than 180 degrees of vascular circumference.

†At least 180 degrees of vascular circumference.

TABLE 2: Neoadjuvant meta-analysis

	Group 1: resectable	Group 2: unresectable
Response Rates:		
Complete response/partial response	3.6%/30.6%	4.8%/30.2%
Resectability rate	73.6%	33.2%
Survival After Surgery	23.3 mo	20.5 mo
1-Year survival rate after surgery	77.9%	79.8%
2-Year survival rate after surgery	47.4%	50.1%

with resectable disease and patients with borderline resectable pancreatic cancer. Use of neoadjuvant therapy may also be reasonable in patients with indeterminate or questionable metastatic disease and in patients with suboptimal performance status or extensive medical comorbidities that necessitate prolonged evaluation and preclude immediate major abdominal surgery.

Neoadjuvant treatment offers hypothetic advantages over adjuvant therapy such as shorter duration of therapy, higher therapy completions rates, tumor downstaging with higher margin negative resections rates, decreased risk of lymph node positivity, and importantly, better patient selection. It may identify those patients (with both initially resectable and nonresectable disease) with rapid progressive or disseminated disease at restaging for whom surgery is unlikely to provide any benefit.

A recent consensus conference with representation from the Society of Surgical Oncology, the American Society of Clinical Oncology (ASCO), and the American Hepato-Pancreatico-Biliary Association attempted to define reproducible and clinically relevant criteria to better categorize resection classifications for nonmetastatic pancreatic cancers (see Table 1). Recommendations are that these patients be discussed in a multidisciplinary team before initiation of treatment and be encouraged to participate in clinical trials. In addition, the initial staging CT scan must be performed before biliary decompression procedures because postprocedure pancreatitis, if it occurs, may prevent detailed anatomic evaluation of tumor-vessel relationships and preclude accurate assessment of the extent of disease on CT scan.

No published phase III data exist for the use of neoadjuvant therapy in pancreatic cancer. However, a recent rigorous systemic meta-analysis reviewed a total of 111 studies (including 56 phase I and II clinical trials) involving 4394 patients with pancreatic cancer who received neoadjuvant therapy. It included patients with resectable disease (group 1) or nonresectable disease (group 2, borderline resectable and locally advanced disease). Chemotherapy was used in 96.4% of these studies as part of the neoadjuvant therapy, and radiation therapy was used in 93.7% of the studies. Patients with borderline resectable and unresectable disease were combined in one group because of the widely different definitions used on published studies for these two entities. Thirty-two percent of patients with nonresectable disease were able to undergo pancreatectomy after neoadjuvant treatment (Table 2). Their survival rates were comparable to patients who were staged as resectable before treatment. In the group of patients with resectable disease, the resection rates and survival rates after neoadjuvant therapy were similar to the ones observed in primarily resected tumors that are treated with adjuvant therapy. The meta-analysis highlights that further investigations are needed in this field and participation in prospective clinical trials should be encouraged.

Borderline Resectable Disease

For borderline resectable disease, although no high level evidence supports its use, an initial approach with neoadjuvant therapy is preferred as opposed to immediate surgery in many centers within the United States. In the largest report published, the M.D. Anderson Group retrospectively studied 160 patients with borderline resectable disease. With use of different types of neoadjuvant chemotherapy or chemoradiation, resection was achieved in 41% of the patients. The median survival time was significantly increased in the patients who were able to achieve resection: 40 months for the 66 patients with borderline disease who completed all therapy as compared with 13 months for the 94 patients who did not undergo pancreatectomy ($P = 0.001$).

Patients with borderline resectable disease may be at higher risk of perioperative complications because of the additional complexity of surgery, at higher risk for early systemic failure because of the advanced nature of the primary tumor, and at higher risk for margin-positive resection with surgery alone. This is important because studies have shown that in addition to nodal status, both completing resection and getting negative margins are factors that translate in increased survival. The survival rate remains poor for patients who undergo an incomplete (margin positive) resection, and the available data suggest that the survival duration of these patients is not different from that of patients with locally advanced, surgically unresectable disease treated with chemoradiation.

Limited evidence suggests any specific neoadjuvant treatment schema off study, although most investigators now agree on gemcitabine-based regimen followed by chemoradiation with either gemcitabine or 5-FU as chemosensitizer. Participation in clinical trials is encouraged. Guidelines from the National Comprehensive Cancer Network (NCCN) support the use of preoperative therapy in carefully selected patients falling into borderline resectable category. Newer regimens with 5-FU–based combinations used in the metastatic setting such as FOLFIRINOX are being explored now in the neoadjuvant setting (NCT01591733, NCT01595321).

Resectable Disease

Neoadjuvant therapy in this group remains experimental in the context of clinical trials. Even in this setting, a hypothetic rationale exists for its use with allowing patient selection. For example, the main limitation of multidetector CT scan is its low sensitivity for low-volume hepatic or peritoneal metastases. Studies suggest that up to 20% of patients who are thought to have resectable disease before surgery actually have CT occult metastatic disease found at laparoscopy or laparotomy. Once laparoscopic or laparotomy procedure is done, there is a delay on restarting systemic therapy until appropriate wound healing, which may further promote disease progression. Neoadjuvant therapy in this setting may allow appropriate patient selection for surgical therapies. Increasing literature is examining neoadjuvant strategies in resectable pancreas cancer, which have been reported in nonrandomized single-institution studies. Most large series have been published by the M.D. Anderson Cancer Center group and use a combination of gemcitabine-based chemoradiation with a short course of 30 Gy of radiation or gemcitabine combined with cisplatin followed by standard preoperative gemcitabine and rapid fractionation. Other groups are investigating neoadjuvant chemotherapy without preoperative chemoradiation. The strategy of neoadjuvant chemotherapy alone for resectable pancreas cancer is under investigation by the American College of Surgeons Oncology Group clinical trial.

Unanswered questions still exist and include the best definition for resectable and unresectable disease to justify its use and the best regimen and sequencing. In addition, a uniform approach for determining resectability on restaging imaging after the neoadjuvant therapy should be defined. Emerging data have recently advocated

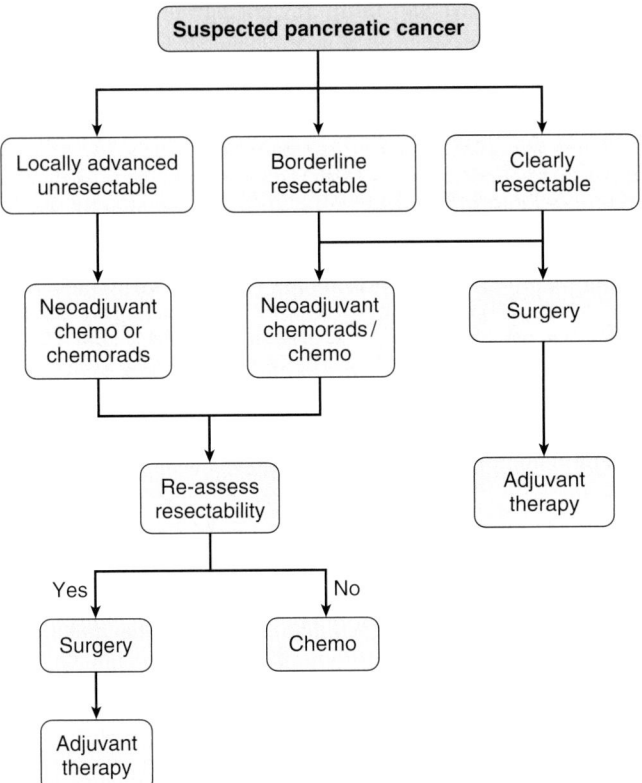

FIGURE 1 Algorithm for management of localized pancreatic cancer.

that response to neoadjuvant therapy is not reflected by traditional radiographic (RECIST) indicators. A recent retrospective study published by the M.D. Anderson group identified 122 patients who had borderline resectable pancreatic cancer and had their disease restaged after receiving neoadjuvant therapy. Of these, only one patient had downstaging to resectable disease based on reimaging studies; however, a total of 85 patients (66%) were able to undergo pancreatectomy, which resulted in increased survival as compared with patients who did not. These findings suggest that patients without evidence of metastases and with good performance status should undergo pancreatectomy after receiving initial neoadjuvant therapy. These findings may prompt more exploratory surgeries in the absence of disease progression.

Ongoing studies with more novel multiagent chemotherapy regimens with likelihood of significant response may further advance the field. Gemcitabine combined with nab-paclitaxel has been used as neoadjuvant therapy in patients with either resectable or borderline resectable PDA. Early reports at the ASCO 2012 annual meeting showed good resection rates for 6 of 16 patients (56%) as presented in national meetings. FOLFIRINOX was recently administered in the neoadjuvant approach in patients with borderline resectable pancreatic cancer and is being evaluated in prospective clinical trials.

At present, patients with borderline resectable disease are recommended to receive systemic chemotherapy for 2 to 4 months followed by chemoradiation; they should deviate from this course only in the event of radiographic evidence of disease progression or a decline in performance status. An algorithm for easy referral is provided in Figure 1.

FUTURE DIRECTIONS

The future for the development of new treatments is promising; significant progress has occurred in the understanding of the genetics and molecular biology of pancreatic cancer. It has been long appreciated that K-*ras* is often mutated in pancreatic cancer tumors. However, to date, there are no direct K-*ras* inhibitors, and targeting of K-*ras* either upstream or downstream has been largely unsuccessful. More recent strategies have included integrating downstream pathways such as *MEK, ERK,* and *AKT.* The development of a pancreatic cancer mouse model that reliably recapitulates human pancreatic cancer not only has allowed for opportunities to learn about how pancreatic cancer grows and develops and metastasizes but also has provided a unique platform with which to test new treatments in a methodic and systematic manner. In addition, much has been learned about the supportive tumor-stromal cell environment that is thought to not only influence the development of pancreatic cancer progression but also support mechanisms for resistance to effective treatment given its inherent protective properties. There is also significant new understanding in the complex relationship and role between inflammation and the immune suppressive tumor microenvironment in pancreatic cancer. Already new treatment opportunities are targeting small molecules that can reverse immune suppression or whole cell immunotherapy approaches that lead to immune activation. Advances in these areas may provide opportunities to test these approaches in the adjuvant and neoadjuvant setting.

SUGGESTED READINGS

Callery MP, Chang KJ, Fishman EK, et al: Pretreatment assessment of resectable and borderline resectable pancreatic cancer: expert consensus statement, *Ann Surg Oncol* 16:1727–1733, 2009.

Conroy T, Desseigne F, Ychou M, et al: FOLFIRINOX versus gemcitabine for metastatic pancreatic cancer, *N Engl J Med* 364:1817–1825, 2011.

Evans DB, Varadhachary GR, Crane CH, et al: Preoperative gemcitabine-based chemoradiation for patients with resectable adenocarcinoma of the pancreatic head, *J Clin Oncol* 26:3496–3502, 2008.

Gillen S, Schuster T, Meyer Zum Buschenfelde C, et al: Preoperative/neoadjuvant therapy in pancreatic cancer: a systematic review and meta-analysis of response and resection percentages, *PLoS Med* 7:e1000267, 2010.

Katz MH, Pisters PW, Evans DB, et al: Borderline resectable pancreatic cancer: the importance of this emerging stage of disease, *J Am Coll Surg* 206:833–848, 2008.

Marten JS, Debus J, Harig S, et al: Final results of the open-label, multicenter, randomized phase III trial of adjuvant chemoradiation plus interferon-α2b (CRI) versus 5-FU alone for patients with resected pancreatic adenocarcinoma (PAC), *J Clin Oncol* 28(Suppl):18s, 2010.

Picozzi VJ, Abrams RA, Decker PA, et al: Multicenter phase II trial of adjuvant therapy for resected pancreatic cancer using cisplatin, 5-fluorouracil, and interferon-alfa-2b-based chemoradiation: ACOSOG Trial Z05031, *Ann Oncol* 22:348–354, 2011.

Picozzi VJ, Kozarek RA, Traverso LW: Interferon-based adjuvant chemoradiation therapy after pancreaticoduodenectomy for pancreatic adenocarcinoma, *Am J Surg* 185:476–480, 2003.

Varadhachary GR, Tamm EP, Abbruzzese JL, et al: Borderline resectable pancreatic cancer: definitions, management, and role of preoperative therapy, *Ann Surg Oncol* 13:1035–1046, 2006.

Varadhachary GR, Wolff RA, Crane CH, et al: Preoperative gemcitabine and cisplatin followed by gemcitabine-based chemoradiation for resectable adenocarcinoma of the pancreatic head, *J Clin Oncol* 26:3487–3495, 2008.

Unusual Pancreatic Tumors

Casey Boyd Duncan, MD, MS, and
Taylor S. Riall, MD, PhD

OVERVIEW

Ductal adenocarcinoma is the most common pancreatic tumor, but a variety of less common pancreatic tumors may be encountered by the surgeon. This chapter covers unusual pancreatic tumors, both nonneoplastic and neoplastic, that may present the surgeon with a diagnostic dilemma.

Because of increasing use of radiographic imaging, the incidental diagnosis of pancreatic lesions, especially cystic lesions, has become more common. Cystic lesions of the pancreas, such as serous cystadenoma, mucinous cystic neoplasms, intraductal papillary mucinous neoplasms, and pancreatic pseudocysts, can have similar radiographic appearances and presenting symptoms. Signs and symptoms such as abdominal pain, nausea, vomiting, fatigue, weight loss, bloating or abdominal fullness, jaundice, and early satiety may be present with any of the tumors or disease processes discussed in this chapter and are therefore not always helpful in making a diagnosis. Differentiating between these lesions can be difficult, and the diagnosis must be accurate because the management often varies.

Rare solid tumors of the pancreas, including solid pseudopapillary tumors, acinar cell carcinoma, and adenosquamous carcinoma, also have similar symptoms to those of ductal adenocarcinoma and may not be suspected preoperatively. Similarly, autoimmune pancreatitis and pancreatic lymphoma can present with a mass or focal pancreatic enlargement. The management of these entities is not surgical, and accurate diagnosis is critical. Finally, masses that are not of pancreatic origin, such as intrapancreatic accessory spleen and metastatic tumors to the pancreas, are discussed.

The goal of this chapter is to help the surgeon differentiate between unusual tumors of the pancreas, with particular emphasis on differential diagnosis and management. Table 1 details the laboratory, radiographic, and pathologic findings and recommended management of each of the unusual pancreatic tumors mentioned in this chapter.

NONNEOPLASTIC PANCREATIC CYSTS

Lymphoepithelial Cysts

Lymphoepithelial cysts of the pancreas are a rare entity, making up approximately 0.5% of pancreatic cysts. These cysts are benign lesions composed of mature keratinizing squamous epithelium surrounded by an external rim of lymphoid tissue. They are thought to arise from the inclusion of ectopic pancreatic tissue in a peripancreatic lymph node that has subsequently undergone squamous metaplasia.

Lymphoepithelial cysts of the pancreas are more common in men and occur primarily in the sixth decade of life. Serum laboratory values are typically normal in these patients, although cyst fluid may have high levels of carcinoembryonic antigen (CEA) and carbohydrate antigen 19-9 (CA 19-9).

Sonographically, lymphoepithelial cysts appear hypoechoic with internal debris. Lymphoepithelial cysts have low attenuation and are typically well circumscribed and sharply demarcated from the surrounding pancreatic tissue on computed tomographic (CT) scan. Magnetic resonance imaging (MRI) can be helpful in visualizing the internal keratin component of the cyst (high T1 and low T2 signal). Multiple loculi within a single cyst are common, but the presence of more than one cyst at a time is rare. Pancreatic ductal dilation is uniformly absent. Endoscopic biopsy reveals stratified squamous epithelium, lymphocytes, and the absence of neoplastic cells. The peripheral lymphoid tissue often contains organized follicles and germinal centers, characteristic of a lymph node. The cysts almost uniformly contain dense keratinous debris, often described as "caseous" or "curd-like." The surrounding pancreatic parenchyma and lymph nodes are typically normal, except in cases of cyst rupture, where inflammatory changes and fibrous tissue may be present.

Accurate diagnosis of this entity is crucial and can usually be achieved by means of radiologic imaging and endoscopic biopsy. Lymphoepithelial cysts are truly benign and need only be resected in cases of severe symptoms. In cases where the diagnosis of lymphoepithelial cyst is certain, asymptomatic patients can be observed. In symptomatic patients of acceptable surgical risk, laparotomy should be performed with intraoperative frozen section biopsy of the mass. Enucleation, resection, and biliary drainage (in cases of pancreatic head lesions) are options for symptomatic cysts, depending on the location. Survival is excellent, and recurrence is rare.

Pancreatic Pseudocysts

Pancreatic pseudocysts (Figure 1) are not uncommon and can be confused with other cystic neoplasms of the pancreas. Pancreatic pseudocysts do not have an epithelial lining and are not true cysts. Pseudocysts are surrounded by a wall of collagen and fibrous and granulation tissue. Symptoms of pancreatic pseudocysts are similar to those of other pancreatic cysts. Complications of a pseudocyst may result in upper gastrointestinal bleeding, fever, jaundice, sepsis, or pleural effusion.

CT scan is the imaging modality of choice for visualizing pancreatic pseudocysts, with sensitivity and specificity approaching 100%. CT scan findings consistent with a pseudocyst include a round, fluid-filled cavity, typically surrounded by a thick wall. Pseudocysts are frequently unilocular (see Figure 1).

When the diagnosis is unclear, upper gastrointestinal endoscopy may be used to aspirate cyst fluid for analysis. Cyst fluid levels consistent with pancreatic pseudocyst include a high amylase (>250 U/L), low CEA (<5 ng/mL), and low CA 19-9 (<37 U/mL). Endoscopic retrograde cholangiopancreatography (ERCP) can be helpful in evaluating communication with the pancreatic duct, which influences treatment decisions.

Intervention (endoscopic, percutaneous, or surgical) is indicated in the case of symptomatic pseudocysts, complicated pseudocysts (vascular, gastrointestinal, or biliary compression, fistula, infection, or hemorrhage), and pseudocysts that are large (>5 cm) and have been unchanged for 6 weeks. Importantly, pseudocysts that communicate with the main pancreatic duct are unlikely to resolve spontaneously and require a definitive internal drainage procedure. Endoscopic drainage can be performed with a transpapillary or a transmural approach (cystogastrostomy, cystoduodenostomy) in suitable candidates. Surgical drainage in the form of a cystogastrostomy or cystojejunostomy can be performed with an open or laparoscopic technique. Surgical resection of the cyst may be necessary in cases of a disconnected duct. External (percutaneous) drainage is not routinely performed but can be successful if no ductal connection is present.

TABLE 1: Laboratory, radiographic features, and management of unusual pancreatic tumors

	Serum laboratory values	Cyst fluid laboratory values	Ultrasound scan	ERCP	CT scan/MRI	Pathology/histology	Management
Lymphoepithelial cyst	Normal	High CEA, CA 19-9	Hypoechoic, internal debris	Ductal dilation absent	Low attenuation; internal keratin (high T1-weighted, low T2-weighted)	Squamous epithelium, germinal centers	Surgical resection when symptomatic
Pancreatic pseudocyst	Normal	High amylase; low CEA, CA 19-9	Anechoic, smooth, round	Ductal communication variable	Round, fluid-filled, smooth, unilocular	Wall composed of collage and granulation tissue, no epithelial lining	Endoscopic or surgical drainage for pseudocysts with ductal communication, older than 6 weeks, symptomatic
Serous cystadenoma	Normal	Low CEA, CA 19-9, amylase	Septations, calcifications	Duct disruption or obstruction	Septations, honeycomb pattern, central scar, hypervascular	Mitoses absent	Resection when symptomatic or enlarging
Serous cystadenocarcinoma	Elevated CA 19-9	Low CEA, CA 19-9, amylase	Septations, calcifications	Ductal disruption or obstruction	Septations	Mitoses may be present, although local invasion and distant metastases not uncommon	Resection when diagnosed before surgery or when malignancy cannot be ruled out
Mucinous cystadenoma	Normal	High CEA, CA 19-9	Round, smooth, loculi	Ductal communication absent	Round, well-encapsulated, septation, macrocystic	Columnar epithelium, ovarian stroma, ER/PR +	Surgical resection
Mucinous cystadenocarcinoma	Normal	High CEA, CA 19-9 (higher than benign MCN)	Calcifications and mural nodules more common with malignancy	Ductal communication absent	Septation, macrocystic, calcifications, mural nodules	Columnar epithelium, ovarian stroma, ER/PR +, mitotic figures	Surgical resection
Intraductal papillary mucinous neoplasm	Normal	High CEA	Mural nodules, ductal dilation	Ductal communication and dilation	Mural nodules, ductal dilation	Various levels of dysplasia, ductal invasion	Surgical resection for all invasive, main duct, and symptomatic IPMN; small, asymptomatic branch duct IPMN may be observed
Cystic neuroendocrine tumor	Normal, unless functioning	Low or normal CEA, CA 19-9	Smooth, round, unilocular or multilocular	Normal ductal anatomy	Round, smooth, internal fluid, hypervascular, hyperintense on T2-weighted	Stain positive for chromogranin and synaptophysin	Surgical resection

Continued

TABLE I: Laboratory, radiographic features, and management of unusual pancreatic tumors—cont'd

	Serum laboratory values	Cyst fluid laboratory values	Ultrasound scan	ERCP	CT scan/MRI	Pathology/histology	Management
Solid pseudopapillary tumor	Normal	NA	Well-defined, hypoechoic, posterior enhancement	Ductal disruption rare	Cystic degeneration, calcifications, hemorrhage, solid and cystic	Vimentin, NSE, CD10/56, synaptophysin, α-1 antitrypsin, β-catenin	Surgical resection
Acinar cell carcinoma	High pancreatic enzymes, LFTs; low or normal CEA, CA 19-9	NA	Cystic or solid	Ductal invasion rare	Exophytic, hypodense, cystic or solid	Zymogen granules; stains positive for trypsin, chymotrypsin, amylase, lipase, synaptophysin, chromogranin	Surgical resection
Adenosquamous carcinoma	Elevated LFTs, CEA, CA 19-9	NA	Solid, internal necrosis	Ductal disruption rare	Solid, internal necrosis	At least 30% squamous epithelium	Surgical resection
Autoimmune pancreatitis	Elevated IgG, IgG4, CA 19-9	NA	Diffusely enlarged pancreas	Long segment strictures, strictures from side branches, no ductal dilatation or abrupt cutoff	Diffusely enlarged pancreas with delayed enhancement	Lymphoplasmacytic infiltrate, storiform fibrosis, obliterative phlebitis, IgG4 positive	Steroids, azathioprine or rituximab for relapse
Pancreatic lymphoma	Elevated LFTs, LDH, β2-microglobulin, CA 19-9	NA	Solid, hypodense pancreatic mass	Ductal dilation rare	Solid mass, peripancreatic lymphadenopathy	Large lymphocytes, CD20, CD30, EBV positive	Chemotherapy, radiation, surgical resection debatable
Intrapancreatic accessory spleen	Normal	NA	Solid, posterior acoustic enhancement, similar echogenicity to spleen, vascular pedicle on Doppler scan	NA	Well-circumscribed, zebra-striped pattern of enhancement, low T1-weighted, high T2-weighted	Lymphoid follicles, red and white pulp, CD8 positive	Resection only if diagnosis unclear, symptomatic, or with treatment of hematologic disorders
Metastatic tumors to the pancreas	Elevated CA 19-9	NA	Solid mass in head of pancreas	With or without dilation of pancreatic ducts and biliary tree	Hypervascular, displacement of surrounding structures	Similar to primary	Resection if isolated pancreatic metastases or from renal cell carcinoma primary

CA 19-9, carbohydrate antigen 19-9; CEA, Carcinoembryonic antigen; CT, computed tomographic; EBV, Epstein-Barr virus; ERCP, endoscopic retrograde cholangiopancreatography; ER/PR, estrogen receptor/progesterone receptor; IgG, immunoglobulin G; IPMN, intraductal papillary mucinous neoplasm; LDH, lactate dehydrogenase; LFTs, liver function tests; MCN, mucinous cystic neoplasm; MRI, magnetic resonance imaging; NA, not applicable; NSE, neuron-specific enolase.

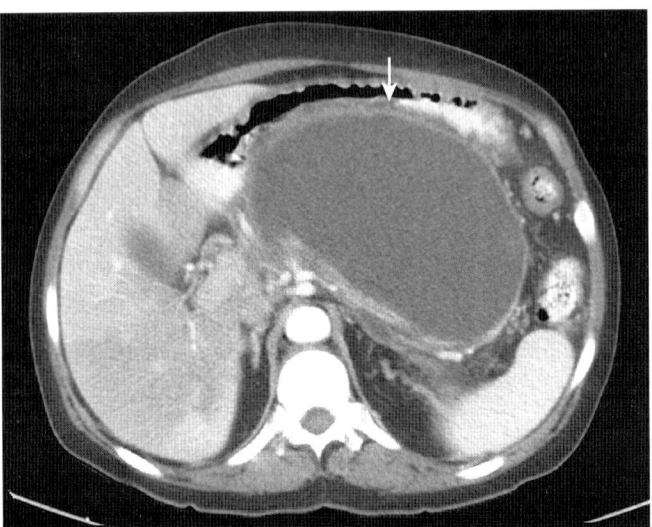

FIGURE I   Computed tomographic scan shows a large, unilocular pancreatic pseudocyst *(arrow)* in a patient with a history of severe necrotizing pancreatitis 3 months previously. Compression of the stomach is noted.

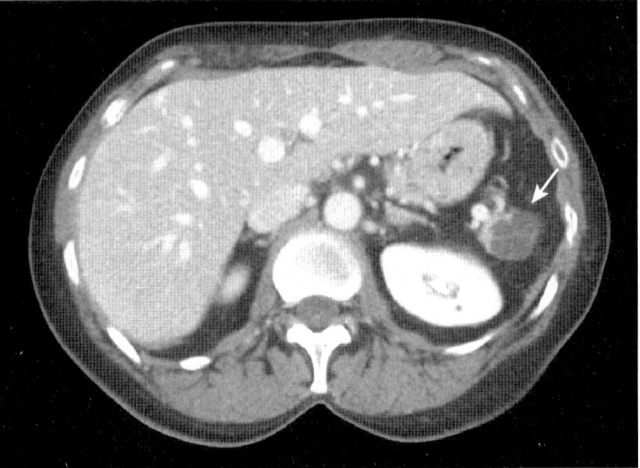

FIGURE 2   Computed tomographic scan shows a large serous cystadenoma of the pancreas *(arrow)*. The mass has multiple septations and a honeycomb appearance.

PANCREATIC CYSTIC NEOPLASMS

Serous Cystadenoma

Serous cystadenomas (Figure 2) of the pancreas are typically benign tumors composed of a single layer of glycogen-containing cuboidal or flattened epithelial cells. Serous cystadenomas have been reported to constitute 14% of incidentally discovered asymptomatic pancreatic lesions.

Serous cystadenomas are more common in women and present at a mean age of 56 to 65 years. Up to 56% of serous cystadenomas are asymptomatic, with many found incidentally on imaging done for other purposes. Approximately 41% to 56% of serous cystadenomas occur in the body or tail of the pancreas.

The classic CT scan findings in serous cystadenoma include septations, central calcifications, clusters of small cysts, a "honeycomb" or "sponge" pattern, and a central scar or sunburst calcification (see Figure 2). A serous cystadenoma may be visualized as a hypervascular mass on arteriography. Pancreatic duct distortion or obstruction may be seen on ERCP.

Serous cystadenomas are benign. The key component in management of serous cystadenomas of the pancreas is differentiating these from mucin-producing cystic tumors of the pancreas, which have malignant potential. This can often be achieved with CT imaging alone. In cases of diagnostic uncertainty, endoscopic ultrasound scan (EUS) can be used to biopsy the cyst wall or aspirate cyst fluid for cytologic examination, although sufficient specimen volume to make a diagnosis is obtained in less than 50% of procedures. Cyst fluid from a serous cystadenoma tends to be acellular with glycogen-rich epithelial cells. Mucinous, inflammatory, or malignant cells should be absent. Serous cystadenoma fluid typically has low levels of CEA (<5 ng/mL), CA 19-9 (<37 U/mL), and amylase (<250 U/L; see Table 1).

In asymptomatic patients, observation with serial imaging can safely be performed. Surgical resection of a serous cystadenoma is indicated in patients who are symptomatic, in those with enlarging tumors, and when malignancy or malignant potential cannot be ruled out. After surgical resection, survival is excellent and reoperation or recurrence is rare.

Serous Cystadenocarcinoma

Serous cystadenomas are almost uniformly benign, although a few cases (<20) of their malignant counterpart, serous cystadenocarcinoma, have been reported in the literature. Serous cystadenocarcinomas compose only 1% of all cystic pancreatic neoplasms. Patients with serous cystadenocarcinoma present with symptoms similar to patients with serous cystadenoma. Serum CA 19-9 levels may be elevated but are not helpful in differentiating between pancreatic lesions. Because of its nonspecific signs and symptoms, serous cystadenocarcinoma is frequently misdiagnosed before surgery as serous cystadenoma, ductal adenocarcinoma, or gastrointestinal stromal tumor. The recurrence rate after surgical resection for serous cystadenocarcinoma is low, and long-term survival is achievable. Because of the rarity of serous cystadenocarcinoma, surgical resection for serous cystadenomas is currently indicated only in those with symptoms or enlarging tumors and in cases where malignancy cannot be definitively ruled out.

Mucinous Cystic Neoplasms

Mucinous cystic neoplasms (MCNs; Figure 3) occur almost exclusively in women, with a mean age at diagnosis that ranges from 44 to 66 years in various studies. MCNs of the pancreas can be benign (mucinous cystadenoma), borderline, or malignant (mucinous cystadenocarcinoma), based on the degree of epithelial dysplasia within the cyst. Up to 40% of patients with MCNs have invasive malignancy at the time of diagnosis. Most patients with MCNs are symptomatic. Patients with malignant MCNs are more likely to exhibit symptoms, although an absence of symptoms does not necessarily eliminate the possibility of malignancy. Most MCNs are located in the body or tail of the pancreas.

Microscopically, MCNs have an inner columnar epithelial layer and an outer, dense layer composed of ovarian-type stroma, which differentiates them from other cystic neoplasms. Immunohistochemistry of MCNs is frequently positive for estrogen and progesterone receptors. Macroscopically, MCNs appear as round cystic lesions with a smooth surface and fibrous pseudocapsule. Multiple loculi may be present (see Figure 3, A).

On CT scan or MRI (see Figure 3, B), MCNs appear as round, well-encapsulated, septated, macrocystic tumors. Calcifications may be visualized within the wall of the tumor and occur more frequently in malignant MCNs. Similarly, mural nodules, biliary obstruction,

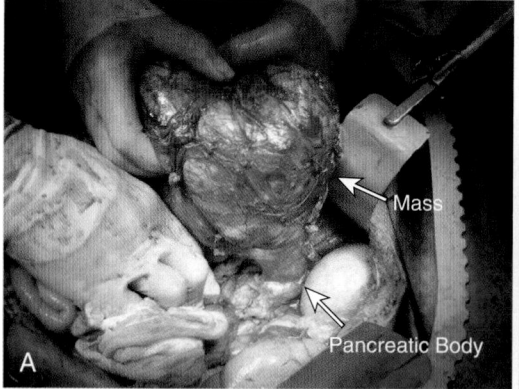
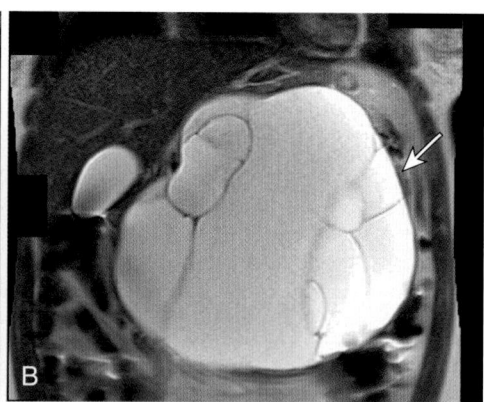

FIGURE 3   A, Intraoperative photograph shows a large mucinous cystic neoplasm originating from the body of the pancreas. **B,** Coronal T2-weighted magnetic resonance image shows a large, multilocular mucinous cystic neoplasm of the pancreas *(arrow),* displacing the liver, stomach, and spleen.

invasion of vascular structures, extrapancreatic lesions, ascites, and obliteration of fat planes around the pancreas increase the likelihood of invasive malignancy within the MCN. ERCP shows an absence of pancreatic ductal communication in MCNs. An elevated cyst fluid CEA level strongly suggests a mucinous neoplasm (MCN or intraductal papillary mucinous neoplasm [IPMN]) rather than a nonmucinous cyst, and MCNs with malignancy have even higher CEA levels compared with benign MCNs. A cyst fluid CA 19-9 level greater than 37 U/mL suggests a mucinous lesion (either cystadenoma or cystadenocarcinoma) rather than a serous cystadenoma or pseudocyst.

Because of the risk of occult malignancy within the lesion and future malignant transformation, the treatment of choice for all MCNs is complete surgical resection. Laparoscopy can be used in patients with small MCNs (<4 cm) without mural nodules on imaging. Nonoperative management is only indicated in patients who cannot tolerate surgery. Enucleation or partial resection of MCNs should be avoided, particularly in those with large tumors, because the intraoperative or preoperative recognition of underlying malignancy is limited.

Prognosis is largely determined by the presence or absence of an invasive component. Recurrence after resection of benign MCN has been reported to be less than 5%, but this increases to as high as 37% in those with invasive carcinoma. The 5-year disease-specific survival rates are 100% and 57% for noninvasive and invasive MCN, respectively, and long-term survival even with tumor recurrence has been reported. Patients with resected malignant MCN should undergo surveillance CT scan or MRI every 6 months.

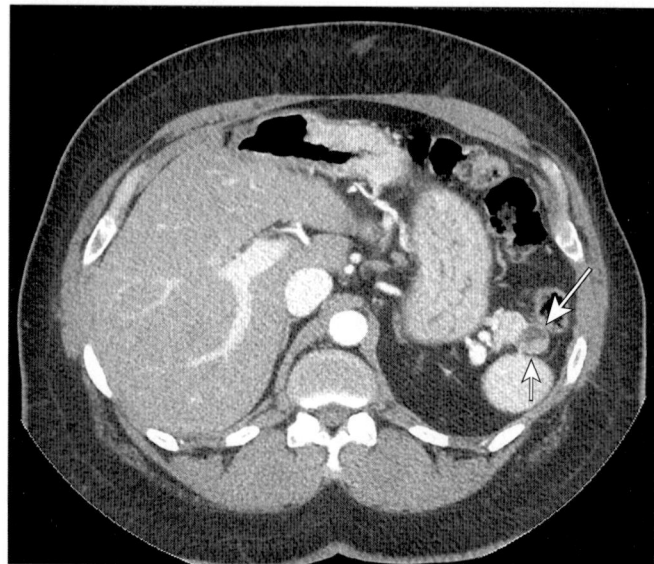

FIGURE 4   Computed tomographic scan shows a cystic intraductal papillary mucinous neoplasm *(large arrow)* with internal solid component *(small arrow)* in the tail of the pancreas.

Intraductal Papillary Mucinous Neoplasms

Intraductal papillary mucinous neoplasms (IPMNs; Figure 4) are defined as intraductal mucin-producing neoplasms that extensively involve the main pancreatic ducts or side branch ducts. IPMNs lack the ovarian stroma characteristic of MCNs of the pancreas. Although both are mucinous neoplasms of the pancreas, MCNs and IPMNs must be differentiated, as the recurrence patterns and surveillance recommendations vary between the two. Compared with MCN, IPMNs occur more commonly in men, present later in life, and are less often located in the body or tail of the pancreas.

IPMNs have been shown to follow a progression from adenoma to borderline IPMN with dysplasia, to IPMN with carcinoma in situ, to invasive carcinoma. IPMNs are classified as main duct IPMN and branch duct IPMN, with the former more likely to harbor invasive carcinoma. Recent guidelines have lowered the threshold for the definition of main duct IPMN. Main pancreatic duct size greater than 5 mm in diameter, segmental or diffuse, without ductal obstruction is highly suggestive of main duct disease. Communication with the pancreatic duct can be seen on ERCP, CT scan, or magnetic resonance cholangiopancreatography (MRCP). The absence of main duct dilation in the presence of IPMN or a cyst greater than 5 mm in

diameter that communicates with the main pancreatic duct indicates branch duct disease. Endoscopically, mucin can be visualized extruding from the ampulla. EUS or CT scan may show mural nodules (see Figure 4) within the cyst, which are more likely to be associated with IPMN (versus pseudocyst or serous cystadenoma) and with the presence of invasive carcinoma. Elevated cyst fluid CEA values are indicative of a mucin-producing neoplasm of the pancreas (MCN or IPMN). Preoperative fine-needle aspiration has been shown to have an accuracy of 84%, a sensitivity of 78%, and a specificity of 88% in diagnosing of IPMN.

The management of patients with IPMN has recently changed according to 2012 International Consensus Guidelines. Surgical resection is recommended for all patients with main duct IPMN, preoperatively diagnosed invasive IPMN (main duct or branch duct), and symptomatic patients with IPMN (main duct or branch duct). For patients with branch duct IPMN, those with "high-risk stigmata" (obstructive jaundice, an enhancing solid component within the cyst, pancreatic duct size ≥10 mm) should undergo surgical resection. Those patients without high-risk stigmata but with "worrisome features" (cyst size ≥3 cm, thickened cyst walls, main pancreatic duct size of 5 to 9 mm, mural nodules, distal pancreatic atrophy, lymphadenopathy) should undergo EUS to further characterize the cyst. If EUS shows a mural nodule, main duct features consistent with main duct involvement (thickened walls, intraductal mucin, or mural nodules), or cytology suspicious or consistent with malignancy, surgical resection should be performed. Patients without worrisome features or suspicious EUS findings should undergo surveillance imaging (CT scan, MRI, or EUS) depending on the size of the largest cyst. In summary, observation is indicated in patients with branch duct disease who meet international consensus guidelines: (1) asymptomatic condition, (2) tumors of less than 3 cm, (3) main duct diameter of less than 10 mm, (4) no mural nodules, and (5) benign cytology.

Patients who do not undergo surgical resection for IPMN require regular surveillance because these tumors have malignant potential. In addition, IPMN is thought to be a field defect in the pancreatic ductal epithelium. Patients with both resected noninvasive and resected invasive IPMN are at increased risk for recurrence in the pancreatic remnant independent of surgical margin status and should undergo routine surveillance. Survival in patients with IPMN is based on the presence of invasive cancer.

Cystic Neuroendocrine Tumors

Cystic neuroendocrine tumors of the pancreas compose approximately 10% of pancreatic neuroendocrine tumors and between 2% and 14% of cystic pancreatic tumors in the literature. These tumors are rare and are frequently confused with other cystic tumors of the pancreas. Cystic neuroendocrine tumors may secrete insulin, glucagon, or gastrin, but most tumors are nonfunctional and nonmalignant. The cystic nature of these tumors may be related to intratumoral hemorrhage.

CT scan findings consistent with cystic neuroendocrine tumors of the pancreas include a round, smooth-walled, cystic lesion, most commonly in the body or tail of the pancreas, with internal fluid of variable density. MRI may show a hyperintense lesion on T2-weighted imaging. Mesenteric angiography may reveal a hypervascular lesion in the pancreas. ERCP shows normal biliary and pancreatic ducts. Cystic neuroendocrine tumors may be unilocular or multilocular. EUS may be used to further visualize the tumor and obtain cyst fluid for analysis. Cyst fluid CEA and CA 19-9 levels may be low or normal. This is similar to pancreatic pseudocysts and serous cystadenomas but is in contrast to mucinous cystic neoplasms, which have elevated CEA and CA 19-9 levels. Tumor cells stain positive for chromogranin and synaptophysin in all cases. Lymph node involvement and distant metastases are rare. Like all pancreatic neuroendocrine tumors, cystic neuroendocrine tumors should be resected.

RARE SOLID PANCREATIC TUMORS

Solid Pseudopapillary Tumor

Solid pseudopapillary tumors (SPTs) are infrequent, typically benign tumors of the pancreas. SPTs represent 1% to 3% of all pancreatic neoplasms, although the incidence rate has been increasing over the last decade. First described by Frantz in 1959, SPTs of the pancreas were first defined by the World Health Organization in 1996. SPTs are distinct in having both solid and cystic components, which may be accompanied by cystic degeneration, necrosis, and hemorrhage. Malignant SPTs are rare and are associated with invasion of surrounding blood vessels, neural tissue, or pancreatic parenchyma. Although distant spread is rare, the most common locations for metastases are the liver, mesentery, peritoneum, portal vein, and spleen.

SPTs occur most commonly in young women, with a mean age at diagnosis ranging from 22 to 38 years. Most commonly, SPTs are located within the tail of the pancreas. More than 80% of patients with SPTs present with symptoms. Serum laboratory values, including alpha-fetoprotein (AFP), CEA, CA 19-9, and CA 125, are typically normal in patients with SPTs.

Abdominal ultrasound scan, CT scan, and MRI are the most commonly used imaging modalities for the diagnosis of SPTs. An SPT appears as a well-defined hypoechoic mass with solid and cystic components. Calcifications, intratumoral hemorrhage, cystic degeneration, and posterior enhancement may be identified.

Preoperative tissue biopsy may be performed with endoscopic guidance, although the correct diagnosis is made in only 50% of patients who undergo biopsy. Most SPTs stain positive for vimentin, neuron-specific enolase, CD10, CD56, synaptophysin, alpha-1 antitrypsin, and β-catenin.

Surgical resection remains the mainstay of treatment for SPTs. SPTs are frequently completely resectable, with most patients undergoing a margin negative (R0) resection and up to 95% cured after surgery. Enucleation is not indicated. Recurrence of disease in patients with SPTs is rare, and the median disease-free survival time has been shown to be 40 months. Patients with locally unresectable or metastatic SPTs can still benefit from surgical resection. Surgical debulking of metastatic disease, including hepatic lobectomy or enucleation of metastatic deposits, can result in long-term survival. Chemotherapy and radiation therapy are not routinely used because of the rarity of this disease and the success of surgical resection in the treatment of SPTs.

Acinar Cell Carcinoma

Acinar cell carcinoma (ACC) of the pancreas is a rare malignant tumor of the exocrine pancreas. ACC is predominantly diagnosed in men, with a mean age at diagnosis ranging from 56 to 64 years. Patients with ACC are almost always symptomatic. Lipase hypersecretion syndrome, a paraneoplastic syndrome characterized by elevated lipase levels, subcutaneous fat necrosis, polyarthralgia, and eosinophilia, has been reported. Laboratory values are nonspecific in patients with ACC and may include elevated liver enzymes and anemia. CEA and CA 19-9 levels can be low or normal and thus are not helpful in diagnosis. ACC has been associated with elevated levels of pancreatic enzymes, including trypsin, chymotrypsin, lipase, and amylase.

The diagnosis of ACC based on radiologic imaging alone is rare. Internally, ACC may be cystic or solid. Larger tumors are more likely to be cystic because of central necrosis, which develops as they outgrow their blood supply. Ductal dilation is uncommon. There is no predilection for location within the pancreas for ACC.

Microscopically, ACC appears hypercellular with granular, eosinophilic cytoplasm. Periodic acid-Schiff (PAS) staining is positive for zymogen granules within the tumor cells. Specifically, ACC tumor cells frequently stain positive for trypsin, chymotrypsin, amylase, lipase, synaptophysin, or chromogranin.

In the Surveillance, Epidemiology, and End Results (SEER) population, 57% of patients with ACC presented with metastatic disease and were not candidates for surgical resection. When compared with patients with pancreatic adenocarcinoma, patients with ACC were more likely to present with localized disease and less likely to have unstaged disease compared with patients with pancreatic adenocarcinoma. In a small case series, one third of patients with ACC had positive lymph node involvement and more than half had metastatic disease at presentation. Portal vein invasion has been shown in 35.1% of patients with ACC, arterial invasion in 21.2%, and extrapancreatic nerve plexus invasion in 15.6%.

Patients with locoregional ACC should undergo evaluation by a surgeon, as surgical resection is the only curative option. Adjuvant and neoadjuvant chemotherapy and radiation have been used in the treatment of ACC, but benefit is unclear.

Patients with ACC have a median survival time that ranges from 19 to 47 months. Overall 5-year survival rates for ACC are approximately 40%. Patients with ACC who undergo surgical resection have significantly improved survival. In population-based data, patients without resection with locoregional ACC have a 5-year survival rate of 22% compared with 75% in patients with resection. As expected, patients with distant disease have worse survival compared with patients with local or regional ACC.

Adenosquamous Carcinoma

Adenosquamous carcinoma of the pancreas accounts for 1% to 4% of exocrine pancreatic malignancies. According to the Armed Forces Institute of Pathology, pancreatic adenosquamous carcinoma is defined as a neoplasm of the pancreas that is comprised of at least 30% malignant squamous cell carcinoma mixed with ductal adenocarcinoma.

The mean age at diagnosis of adenosquamous carcinoma ranges from 55 to 71 years, similar to that of pancreatic adenocarcinoma. Patients with adenosquamous carcinoma also present with symptoms similar to adenocarcinoma of the pancreas, making a preoperative diagnosis difficult. Bilirubin, alkaline phosphatase, CEA, and CA 19-9 levels may be elevated in patients with adenosquamous carcinoma of the pancreas; however, these values are not helpful in differentiating this lesion from the more common adenocarcinoma.

CT and MRI findings of adenosquamous carcinoma include a large, solid lesion with variable amounts of internal necrosis. Invasion of surrounding organs or distant metastases are not uncommon. Typically, one cannot differentiate adenosquamous carcinoma from adenocarcinoma radiographically. EUS-guided fine-needle aspiration biopsy can be performed, but an adequate sample of tissue must be obtained to make an accurate diagnosis before surgery, as the amount of squamous differentiation in the tumor can range from 10% to 90%.

Compared with adenocarcinoma, adenosquamous carcinoma is more likely to occur in the body or tail of the pancreas and is more likely to be poorly differentiated. Lymph node involvement, perineural invasion, and vascular involvement are common. No significant difference in the stage at presentation is found between patients with adenosquamous carcinoma and patients with adenocarcinoma of the pancreas, with more than half of all patients presenting with distant stage disease.

Although the adenosquamous variant may be difficult to differentiate from adenocarcinoma before surgery, differentiation is not really necessary because surgical resection offers the only chance for cure for both entities. The median overall survival time for patients with adenosquamous carcinoma of the pancreas is 4 to 7 months, similar to that of patients with adenocarcinoma. Median survival is improved to 12 months after surgical resection of locoregional

adenosquamous carcinoma, which is worse than that of patients with resected adenocarcinoma. Adjuvant chemotherapy or radiation has been used in the treatment of adenosquamous carcinoma, although the survival benefit is unclear. Palliative chemotherapy may provide some survival benefit for patients with metastatic adenosquamous carcinoma.

AUTOIMMUNE PANCREATITIS

Autoimmune pancreatitis (AIP; Figure 5), also known as lymphoplasmacytic sclerosing pancreatitis (LPSP), is the pancreatic manifestation of a systemic immunoglobulin G 4 (IgG4)–mediated fibroinflammatory disease. Most patients with AIP are male and over the age of 50 years. AIP is uncommon and occurs with a prevalence rate of 2.2 cases per 100,000 people. Patients can present with a pancreatic mass, obstructive jaundice, and abdominal pain; AIP can easily be confused with pancreatic adenocarcinoma. Patients may have a biliary stent placed for obstructive jaundice associated with AIP before a definitive diagnosis is made (see Figure 5, A). AIP must be differentiated from pancreatic cancer for two reasons: first, AIP, when definitively diagnosed, should be treated with steroids and not surgical resection; and, second, pancreatectomy can be extremely difficult because of the severe inflammation in the pancreas of patients with AIP.

In the late stages, patients can have both exocrine and endocrine insufficiency develop. Other organ systems can be similarly affected by the systemic inflammatory state, which may result in sclerosing cholangitis, sialadenitis, retroperitoneal fibrosis, interstitial nephritis, thyroiditis, or lymphadenopathy.

The current diagnostic criteria for AIP include a combination of radiographic, serologic, histologic, and clinical findings. Level 1 criteria for the diagnosis of type 1 AIP include: diffuse enlargement of the pancreatic parenchyma, or sausage-like pancreas (see Figure 5, B), on radiographic imaging; long strictures or multiple strictures on ERCP; serology (IgG4 more than twice the upper limit of normal); and specific histologic findings (lymphoplasmacytic infiltrate with fibrosis, storiform (swirling) fibrosis, obliterative phlebitis, and IgG4-positive cells [>10 cell/high power field (HPF)]). Type 2 AIP is definitively diagnosed with histologic confirmation of idiopathic duct-centric pancreatitis (IDCP). Serologic findings are absent in type 2 AIP. In addition, extrapancreatic involvement is exhibited in type 1 AIP only and is absent in type 2 AIP.

Radiographic (CT scan, MRI, and ultrasound scan) findings consistent with AIP include a diffusely enlarged (sausage-shaped) pancreas (see Figure 5, B) with delayed enhancement, pancreatic calcifications, irregular ductal narrowing, and the absence of

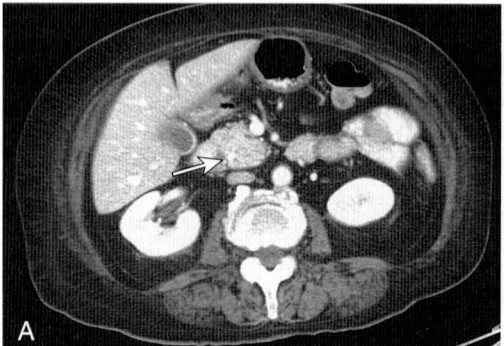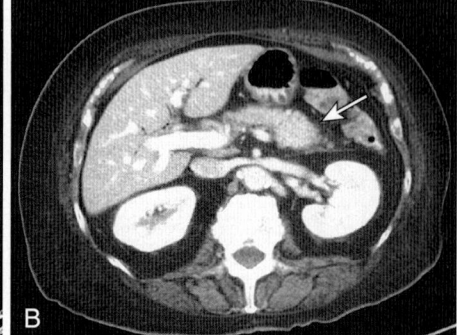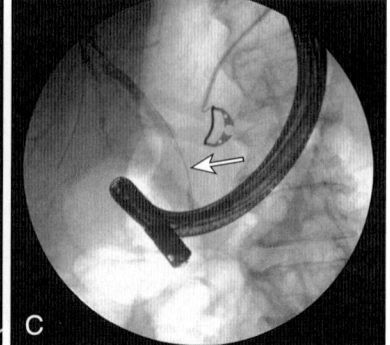

FIGURE 5   **A,** Preoperative computed tomographic scan shows diffuse enlargement of the head of the pancreas without a focal lesion in a patient with elevated serum immunoglobulin G 4. Note the biliary stent *(arrow)* placed for obstructive jaundice. **B,** The body and tail of the pancreas are shown in the same patient. Note the diffuse enlargement or sausage-like shape of the body and tail of the pancreas *(arrow).* **C,** Endoscopic retrograde cholangiopancreatography is shown in a patient with autoimmune pancreatitis and jaundice. Note the long segment stricture *(arrow)* in the common bile duct that is difficult to differentiate from pancreatic adenocarcinoma.

pancreatic ductal dilatation or abrupt cutoff of the pancreatic duct. A mass or focal enlargement of the pancreas may be seen and may lead the practitioner to suspect pancreatic cancer. ERCP features consistent with AIP include long-segment strictures (see Figure 5, *C*) or multiple noncontiguous strictures with side branches arising from the strictures and without upstream dilation.

Serum total IgG levels may be elevated in patients with AIP, although an elevated IgG4 level is more frequently observed and is more sensitive and specific for the diagnosis of AIP. Specifically, an IgG4 level greater than twice the normal value (>134 mg/dL) is strongly suggestive of AIP, although a normal value should not exclude the diagnosis. Elevations in antinuclear antibodies and γ-globulin may occur but are much less common. Serology alone is not sufficient to make a diagnosis of AIP. Especially in the setting of biliary obstruction, CA 19-9 values may also be elevated in AIP, further confusing the clinical picture with that of pancreatic adenocarcinoma.

Histology is required for diagnosis of AIP and is helpful in excluding the presence of malignancy, although a definitive diagnosis is often not made until the time of surgical resection. EUS can be used to obtain a fine-needle aspirate (FNA) or core biopsy of the pancreas. Similar findings may be seen on pathologic examination of extrapancreatic lesions of AIP, such as salivary glands and lymph nodes.

AIP is notoriously steroid responsive. However, steroids should not be given if malignancy has not been definitively ruled out. A steroid trial (40 mg or 0.6 to 1.0 mg/kg daily) can be given with reassessment of imaging and laboratory work after 2 weeks. Symptomatic improvement alone after steroid administration does not confirm the diagnosis of AIP. Response to steroids is defined as improvement in radiographic abnormalities, including biliary strictures and pancreatic enlargement, and resolution of obstructive jaundice and extrapancreatic manifestations. Rising CA 19-9 levels should prompt investigation for malignancy. IgG4 levels may be falsely elevated in other pancreatic diseases, and a decrease in IgG4 level does not necessarily indicate treatment success. In patients who have a definitive diagnosis of AIP, a total of 12 weeks of oral prednisone should be completed, including an 8-week taper. Restoration of normal pancreatic function and anatomy may not occur in all patients with AIP, even with steroid treatment.

Up to 40% of patients experience disease relapse after an initial course of steroids. Relapse can occur in the pancreas or extrapancreatic sites. Patients with clinical or radiographic relapse require an additional 12-week course of oral steroids, in addition to azathioprine (2 to 2.5 mg/kg) for up to 2 years. Rituximab is currently being studied and may be of benefit in patients with refractory AIP.

PANCREATIC TUMORS/MASSES NOT OF PANCREATIC ORIGIN

Pancreatic Lymphoma

Primary pancreatic lymphoma is defined as extranodal lymphoma originating in the pancreas, and secondary pancreatic lymphoma occurs from direct extension from adjacent peripancreatic lymphadenopathy. Criteria for primary pancreatic lymphoma include: no palpable superficial lymphadenopathy, no enlargement of mediastinal lymph nodes, normal leukocyte count, a pancreatic mass with grossly involved peripancreatic lymph nodes, and the absence of splenic or hepatic involvement.

The mean age at diagnosis of pancreatic lymphoma is 57 years. Nonradiating abdominal pain is the most common symptom, and B symptoms (fever and chills) are uncommon. A palpable abdominal mass or hepatosplenomegaly may be noted on physical examination. Symptoms have been reported for up to 18 months before definitive diagnosis as a result of the difficulty in differentiating this disease from the more common pancreatic adenocarcinoma.

Liver enzyme levels (bilirubin, aspartate transaminase, alanine transaminase, alkaline phosphatase) are typically elevated in patients with jaundice from pancreatic lymphoma. CA 19-9 values may be increased but are not helpful in making the diagnosis or differentiating from adenocarcinoma. Serum lactate dehydrogenase (LDH) and β2-microglobulin levels are useful but are not routinely ordered in the workup of a pancreatic mass.

The CT scan findings of pancreatic lymphoma can be indistinguishable from adenocarcinoma, with a solid hypodense mass with peripancreatic lymphadenopathy, with or without extrahepatic biliary dilation. A large, infiltrating lesion with ill-defined borders may also be seen. Invasion or encasement of the superior mesenteric artery is not uncommon.

Accurate diagnosis of primary pancreatic lymphoma is crucial to ensure appropriate treatment but requires a high index of suspicion based on an atypical history for pancreatic adenocarcinoma. Tissue biopsy is necessary and endoscopic FNA biopsy can be performed. Unfortunately, the sensitivity of FNA biopsy in diagnosing pancreatic lymphoma is 71%, and in many cases, the diagnosis is not made before surgery. CT scan–guided percutaneous or endoscopic core biopsy or laparoscopic surgical biopsy provide actual histology (versus cytology) and may serve as alternative methods to obtain a tissue diagnosis and avoid the high morbidity and mortality of an open operation or pancreatic resection. Tissue samples of primary pancreatic lymphoma typically stain positive for CD20 and may also be positive for CD30 and Epstein-Barr virus (EBV). Large lymphocytes with irregular nuclei and prominent nucleoli are characteristic.

Diffuse large B-cell lymphoma (DLBCL) is the most common histologic subtype of pancreatic lymphoma. Most patients present with stage I or II disease, confined to the abdomen. Historically, treatment for lymphoma has included radiation and chemotherapy without surgery. Chemotherapy regimens include a combination of cyclophosphamide, doxorubicin, vincristine, prednisone, bleomycin, and rituximab. The use of surgical resection for pancreatic lymphoma has been debated by several authors. A study by the Mayo Clinic reports a median survival of 13 months, 22 months, and 26 months for patients with pancreatic lymphoma treated with chemotherapy alone, radiation therapy alone, and combination chemotherapy and radiation therapy, respectively. However, all patients in this study experienced recurrence of disease; the authors recommend surgical resection in an effort to improve local control of disease. A large review by Koniaris and colleagues showed that patients treated with chemoradiation alone have a cure rate of 46%, compared with 94% for patients treated with surgical resection (distal pancreatectomy or pancreatoduodenectomy) and adjuvant therapy. Improvements in pancreatic surgery techniques have led these authors to propose a treatment algorithm, whereby patients with resectable disease (pancreatic lymphoma confined to the pancreas or duodenum and without vascular invasion) should undergo initial surgical resection with or without adjuvant chemoradiation. However, this analysis may be limited by selection bias, in which patients with resectable disease have a better prognosis compared with patients with adenopathy or distant disease who do not undergo surgical resection and have worse survival. Behrns and associates suggest that, because of the low success rate with chemotherapy and radiation alone, patients with localized, bulky lymphoma confined to the pancreas may benefit from surgical debulking with possible neoadjuvant or adjuvant chemoradiation. Surgical biliary and enteric bypass may be necessary to alleviate symptoms associated with pancreatic lymphoma.

Intrapancreatic Accessory Spleen

Accessory splenic tissue has been reported in up to 10% of the general population, with the majority of accessory spleens located at the splenic hilum. Intrapancreatic accessory spleen (IPAS; Figure 6)

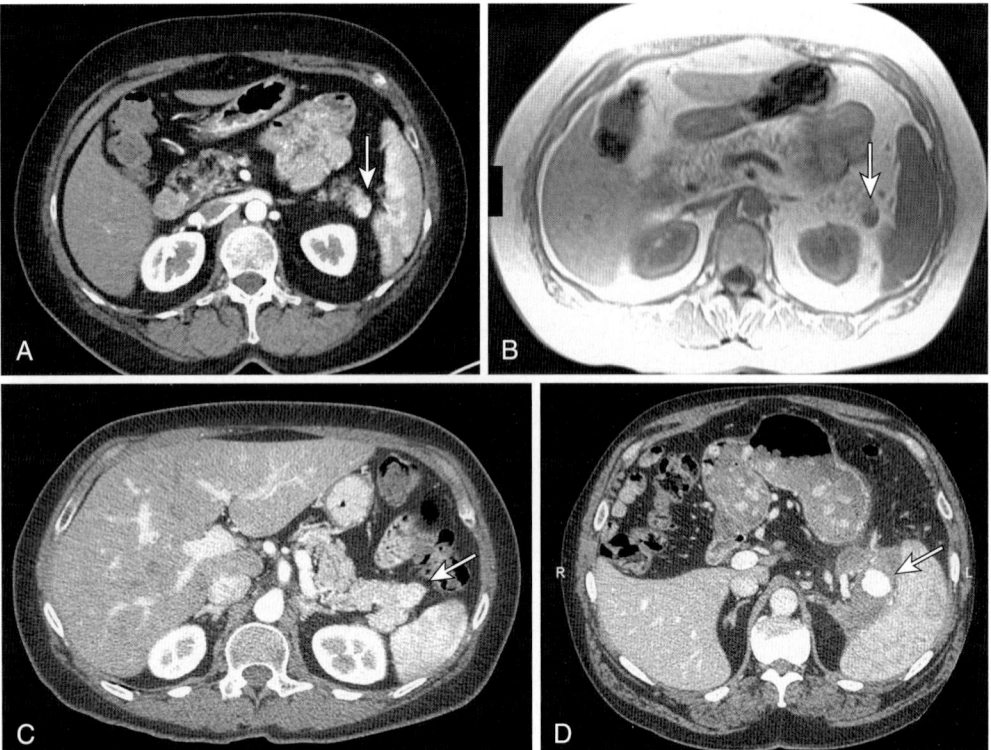

FIGURE 6   A, Computed tomographic (CT) scan of a patient with intrapancreatic accessory spleen (IPAS; *arrow*), originally interpreted as neuroendocrine tumor of the pancreas. Note the zebra-striped pattern and similar enhancement to the neighboring spleen on the arterial phase CT scan. **B,** Magnetic resonance imaging on the same patient as in **A** shows IPAS *(arrow)* with similar signal intensity as the spleen. **C,** CT scan shows pancreatic neuroendocrine tumor located in the tail of the pancreas *(arrow)*. The tumor enhances greater than the spleen and lacks the zebra-striped pattern of enhancement of the spleen, which may help to differentiate these tumors from IPAS. **D,** Splenic artery aneurysm *(arrow)* is shown. This can be differentiated from neuroendocrine tumors and IPAS because of the enhancement greater than that of the spleen and similar to the abdominal aorta. A pool of blood is noted around the aneurysm.

accounts for almost 20% of accessory splenic tissue and occurs most frequently in the tail of the pancreas. IPAS is frequently identified incidentally during imaging for another etiology. Patients with IPAS are frequently asymptomatic.

Accurate diagnosis of IPAS is vital to avoid unnecessary surgery. Characteristic findings on radiographic imaging can help elucidate the diagnosis. Sonographically, IPAS appears as a round, solid, homogeneous, hypoechoic mass within the pancreas. A fibrous capsule with posterior acoustic enhancement may be seen. Doppler ultrasound scan may show a vascular pedicle entering the mass, as most of the blood supply to IPAS originates from the splenic artery and vein. In all cases, the echogenicity of IPAS should be higher than that of the pancreas and similar to that of the anatomic spleen.

IPAS appears as a well-circumscribed mass on CT scan. An arciform or "zebra-striped" pattern of enhancement is typically present in the normal spleen as a result of varying flow rates of contrast through the red and white pulp, and this pattern, when seen in the pancreas, should point toward the diagnosis of IPAS (see Figure 6, *A).* MRI findings consistent with IPAS include a low-signal intensity mass on T1-weighted images and a high-signal intensity mass on T2-weighted images (see Figure 6, *B).* Superparamagnetic iron oxide-enhanced MRI and Tc-99m heat-damaged red blood cell are additional modalities used to accurately localize IPAS.

IPAS is most frequently misdiagnosed as a pancreatic neuroendocrine or other pancreatic vascular lesions because of the hypervascular, hyperattenuating features on CT scan (see Figure 6, *A).* Of note, pancreatic neuroendocrine tumors enhance greater than the spleen and have a characteristic ring-like enhancement during the arterial

phase of CT scan. The zebra-striped pattern of enhancement is notably absent in neuroendocrine tumors (see Figure 6, *C).* A splenic artery aneurysm can be seen on CT scan as a vascular lesion with enhancement similar to the abdominal aorta (see Figure 6, *D).* Metastases to the pancreas are typically hypervascular and rapidly enhance, and splenic vein involvement may be present. A history of previous cancer, especially renal cell carcinoma, can help differentiate metastatic lesions from other hypervascular lesions.

IPAS should only be resected in three circumstances. First, resection should be performed when the diagnosis is unclear and IPAS is misdiagnosed as malignancy. Second, resection is indicated if IPAS causes symptoms, including torsion, infarct, rupture, or cyst formation. Finally, IPAS should be resected during the treatment of hematologic disorders, in which all splenic tissue should be removed. Because of the location of IPAS in the tail of the pancreas, distal pancreatectomy is the most commonly performed procedure.

CANCER METASTASTIC TO THE PANCREAS FROM OTHER SITES

Metastatic tumors to the pancreas are rare, accounting for approximately 2% of all pancreatic tumors. More than 60% of metastatic tumors to the pancreas originate from renal cell carcinoma (Figure 7), although colon cancer, lung cancer, breast cancer, and melanoma are also frequently identified. Typically, widespread metastatic disease is seen at the time of diagnosis, with less than 5% of cases having

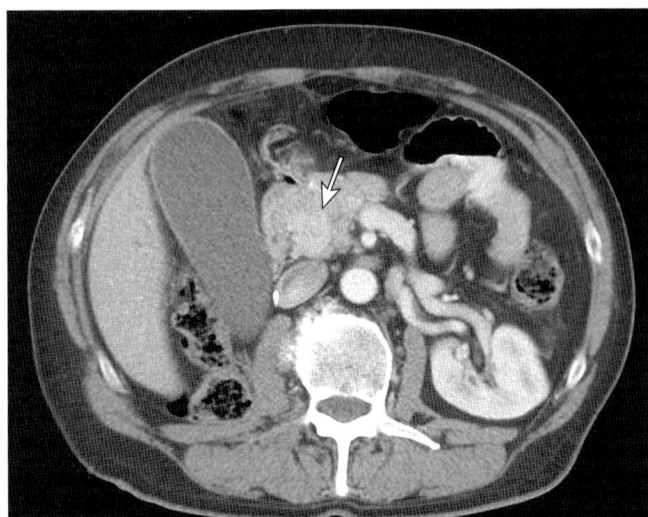

FIGURE 7 Computed tomographic scan shows a patient with a history of renal cell carcinoma status after right nephrectomy who presented with 2 weeks of painless jaundice. Hydropic gallbladder is noted with a hypervascular lesion in the head of the pancreas (arrow). Pancreatoduodenectomy was performed, with final pathology showing renal cell carcinoma metastatic to the pancreas.

isolated pancreatic metastases. The time interval from resection of the primary tumor to the diagnosis of pancreatic metastasis is typically long, ranging from 36 months to 19 years.

Nearly 50% of patients with metastatic tumors to the pancreas are asymptomatic, and thus, a good portion of these tumors are identified on imaging performed for routine surveillance or an alternate reason. When symptoms are present, they depend on the location of the tumor and are similar to those of pancreatic cancer.

Most patients with metastatic lesions undergo CT scan, although MRI and angiography may also be performed. Hypervascular lesions of the pancreas are more likely to be metastatic rather than primary pancreatic carcinoma, which typically presents as a hypovascular lesion. Metastatic tumors may also demonstrate rim enhancement. Displacement of surrounding vascular structures may be more likely than invasion in the case of metastatic lesions.

The most common location for metastatic lesions is the head of the pancreas, and tumors may be solitary or multiple. Tissue diagnosis via percutaneous or endoscopic biopsy may be performed, although a correct diagnosis is not always obtained before surgery. Preoperative tissue diagnosis to distinguish between primary and metastatic pancreatic lesions is not necessary in the case of isolated, resectable disease because the surgical intervention is not altered based on the diagnosis.

Surgical resection can provide survival benefit in patients with metastatic lesions of the pancreas. In one large single-institution study, a margin negative (R0) resection was possible in all 49 patients with metastatic lesions to the pancreas. Survival after pancreatic resection for metastatic lesions depends largely on the site of the primary tumor. Median overall survival for patients with metastatic lesions to the pancreas has been estimated between 19 months and 3.7 years. Patients with renal cell carcinoma metastatic to the pancreas have markedly improved survival compared with patients with primary tumors from other sites; survival may be longer than 10 years in some cases. Pancreatic resection for metastatic renal cell carcinoma is associated with a median survival of 70 to 105 months, with 2-year and 5-year survival rates of 78% and 65%, respectively. Patients with resected colorectal carcinoma metastatic to the pancreas have a median survival of 54 months, and patients with resected metastatic melanoma and lung cancer have the worst prognosis, with a median survival of 14 months and 6 months, respectively. Selection bias and small sample sizes likely play a role in these survival data, with those patients who present to surgeons having resectable disease and improved survival.

Surgical resection for metastatic lesions to the pancreas should be considered in patients who are fit for surgery and who have no additional extrapancreatic disease. No single cancer type is a contraindication for surgical resection. However, patients with more biologically favorable tumors, and those patients who have a long interval between diagnosis of the primary disease and pancreatic metastasis, are more likely to benefit from pancreatic resection.

SUGGESTED READINGS

Ahrendt SA, Komorowski RA, Demeure MJ, et al: Cystic pancreatic neuroendocrine tumors: is preoperative diagnosis possible? *J Gastrointest Surg* 6(1):66–74, 2002.

Bassi C, Salvia R, Molinari E, et al: Management of 100 consecutive cases of pancreatic serous cystadenoma: wait for symptoms and see at imaging or vice versa? *World J Surg* 27(3):319–323, 2003.

Behrns KE, Sarr MG, Strickler JG: Pancreatic lymphoma: is it a surgical disease? *Pancreas* 9(5):662–667, 1994.

Boyd CA, Benarroch-Gampel J, Sheffield KM, et al: 415 Patients with adenosquamous carcinoma of the pancreas: a population-based analysis of prognosis and survival, *J Surg Res* 174(1):12–19, 2012.

Holen KD, Klimstra DS, Hummer A, et al: Clinical characteristics and outcomes from an institutional series of acinar cell carcinoma of the pancreas and related tumors, *J Clin Oncol* 20(24):4673–4678, 2002.

Koniaris LG, Lillemoe KD, Yeo CJ, et al: Is there a role for surgical resection in the treatment of early-stage pancreatic lymphoma? *J Am Coll Surg* 190(3):319–330, 2000.

Papavramidis T, Papavramidis S: Solid pseudopapillary tumors of the pancreas: review of 718 patients reported in English literature, *J Am Coll Surg* 200(6):965–972, 2005.

Reddy S, Edil BH, Cameron JL, et al: Pancreatic resection of isolated metastases from nonpancreatic primary cancers, *Ann Surg Oncol* 15(11):3199–3206, 2008.

Sachs T, Pratt WB, Callery MP, Vollmer CM Jr: The incidental asymptomatic pancreatic lesion: nuisance or threat? *J Gastrointest Surg* 13(3):405–415, 2009.

Shimosegawa T, Chari ST, Frulloni L, et al: International consensus diagnostic criteria for autoimmune pancreatitis: guidelines of the International Association of Pancreatology, *Pancreas* 40(3):352–358, 2011.

Tanaka M, Fernandez-Del Castillo C, Adsay V, et al: International consensus guidelines 2012 for the management of IPMN and MCN of the pancreas, *Pancreatology* 12(3):183–197, 2012.

van der Waaij LA, van Dullemen HM, Porte RJ: Cyst fluid analysis in the differential diagnosis of pancreatic cystic lesions: a pooled analysis, *Gastrointest Endosc* 62(3):383–389, 2005.

Intraductal Papillary Mucinous Neoplasms of the Pancreas

Klaus Sahora, MD and
Carlos Fernandez-del Castillo, MD

Intraductal papillary mucinous neoplasms (IPMNs) were first described in 1982 by Ohashi and colleagues, and in the last 30 years, the disease has become one of the most common diagnoses in the field of pancreatology. Although many new insights have been gained recently, its epidemiology, natural history, and proper management remain in a state of flux, and therefore treatment is not standardized.

In its classic form, IPMN presents as a dilated main pancreatic duct (MD-IPMN), full of mucus that extrudes through a bulging ampulla (this was previously referred to as mucinous ductal ectasia; Figure 1). Patients have recurrent episodes of pancreatitis-like pain, with or without hyperamylasemia, and commonly have steatorrhea, diabetes, and weight loss. Not surprisingly, this clinical picture has led to the diagnosis of chronic pancreatitis in many of these patients. Other patients present with jaundice, and still others have no symptoms at all and the disease is detected incidentally. In this form of IPMN, the neoplasm originates in the main pancreatic duct (Figure 2), more commonly in the cephalic portion, and from there spreads to the rest of duct, up to the secondary branches. IPMNs affecting the main pancreatic duct have a high malignant potential, and more than 60% of those resected, regardless of the presence of symptoms, harbor carcinoma in situ or invasive cancer.

It is now well recognized that IPMNs can also originate in the side branches (BD-IPMN) of the pancreatic ductal system (Figure 3). These occur frequently in the uncinate process and neck, but they can be found anywhere in the pancreas. Depending on the imaging method, 40% to 60% of BD-IPMNs are multifocal, involving all pancreatic regions, probably representing a pancreatic "field defect" (Figure 4). A large proportion of patients with BD-IPMN are asymptomatic, and most BD-IPMNs are detected by computed tomographic (CT) scan or ultrasound that was done for other reasons, but other patients can present with abdominal pain, pancreatitis, or jaundice. This variant of IPMN is much more frequent (perhaps 10:1), and, more importantly, the risk of cancer is far less. Currently, most branch duct IPMNs are managed expectantly (see guidelines below), and of those that are resected, the risk of cancer is about 25%. There are also IPMNs that affect both the main duct and its branches. This subvariant, called combined or mixed-type IPMN, shares epidemiologic features with main duct IPMN and has a similar rate of malignancy.

Both main/combined and branch duct IPMN occur typically in the seventh and eighth decades of life. Initial reports suggested a strong male predominance, but more recent series indicate an equal distribution in the United States. The main differential diagnosis of main duct IPMN is with chronic pancreatitis and that of branch duct IPMN with mucinous cystic neoplasms (MCN). The latter occur almost exclusively (>90%) in women, with a mean age of 50 years, and are located predominantly in the tail of the pancreas. Although both entities can form multilocular cysts lined by mucinous epithelium, MCNs have no obvious communication with the ductal system of the pancreas and typically show an ovarian-like stromal layer around the cysts.

Histopathologically, IPMNs encompass a spectrum of epithelial changes ranging from low-grade lesions (adenoma) to invasive adenocarcinoma, with borderline tumors harboring high-grade dysplasia in between. Oftentimes, the entire spectrum can be found in the same specimen, and therefore thorough sampling is required for these tumors. The pathologic classification of IPMN has evolved over the last decade, revealing complex cellular diversity in the mucinous epithelium. Nonmalignant IPMNs can be subclassified into the gastric (most BD-IPMN), intestinal (most MD-IPMN), pancreatobiliary, and oncocytic types, whereas invasive IPMNs are divided into the colloid and tubular types. It has been shown that the histopathologic subtype in invasive IPMN is an important prognostic factor, with a much more favorable outcome in colloid carcinoma. Tubular carcinomas, which primarily originate in the gastric epithelial neoplasia found in BD-IPMN, have a behavior and prognosis that are similar to conventional ductal adenocarcinoma.

Overall, the average age of patients with malignant main duct IPMNs is 6 years older than those with low-grade or high-grade dysplasia. This supports the current view that most, if not all, main duct IPMNs eventually become malignant. By contrast, this age differential is not seen in branch duct IPMNs.

PREOPERATIVE WORKUP

The extent and type of preoperative workup in patients with IPMN depends on the nature of the presenting symptoms, the certainty of the diagnosis, the likelihood that malignancy is present, and the age and surgical risk of the patient.

CT or MRI

Pancreatic protocol CT or gadolinium-enhanced magnetic resonance imaging (MRI) are indispensable, and they can give very precise information on the type, location, and extent of the tumor (see Figure 1). Both modalities are comparable in detecting associated masses, adjacent organ infiltration, and lymph node or organ metastases. MRI is the procedure of choice of many radiologists, being superior in the recognition of septae and nodules. In addition, magnetic resonance cholangiopancreatography (MRCP) provides a noninvasive way to assess the biliary and pancreatic ducts, and it can detect the small communication between the cyst in side branch IPMNs and the main pancreatic duct.

All surgically fit patients with "high-risk stigmata" (obstructive jaundice, enhanced solid component, main pancreatic duct [MPD] size of >10 mm) on CT or MRI should proceed with surgery without further radiologic or cytopathologic workup.

Indications for EUS

IPMNs with "worrisome features" (cysts ≥3 cm; thickened, enhanced cyst walls; MPD size of 5-9 mm; nonenhanced mural nodules; abrupt change in the MPD caliber with distal pancreatic atrophy; and lymphadenopathy) should undergo endoscopic ultrasound (EUS) for further evaluation.

EUS with fine-needle aspiration allows for sampling of both fluid and solid components of the tumor and can also assess the extent of involvement and detect small nodules (see Figure 4). For side-branch IPMN, which often presents as an asymptomatic isolated cyst or cluster of cysts in the pancreas, this is the optimal method to confirm diagnosis and distinguish them from small oligocystic serous cystadenomas (SCN). Sampling of the fluid will typically show mucus, a high amylase level, an elevated carcinoembryonic antigen (CEA) (a marker that is always low in SCN), and cytology with mucinous

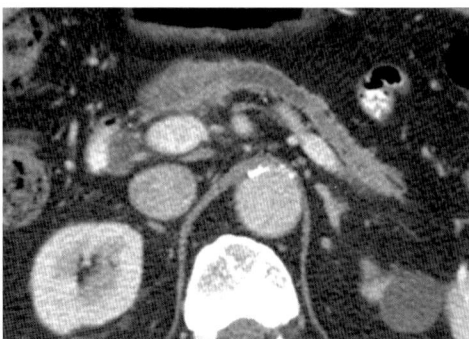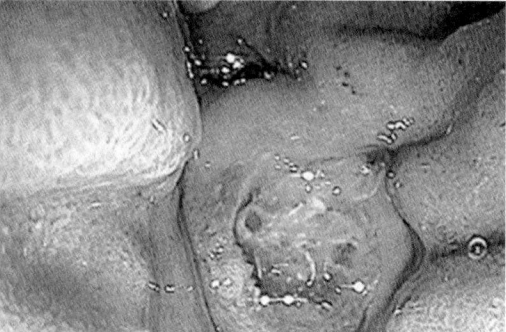

FIGURE 1 Computed tomographic scan (*left*) and endoscopic image (*right*) of a main duct intraductal papillary mucinous neoplasms (IPMN) demonstrating main duct dilation and mucus protruding out of the papilla vateri. The patient presented with three episodes of moderately severe upper abdominal pain. The pancreatic duct is dilated throughout the neck and proximal body, and tapers throughout the distal body and tail. The patient underwent a Whipple procedure, and final pathology revealed mixed-type IPMN with invasive tubular carcinoma.

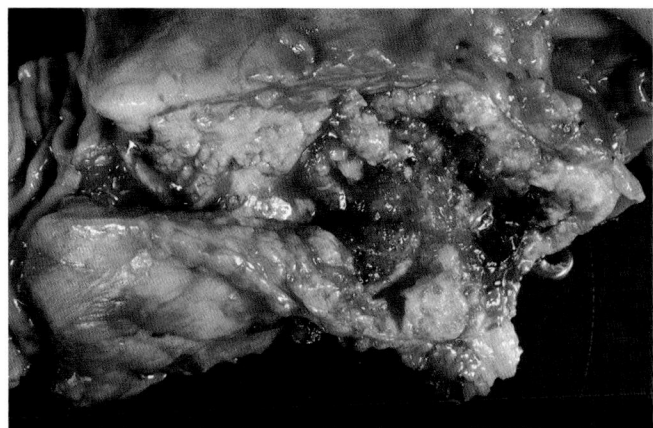

FIGURE 2 Resected main duct-intraductal papillary mucinous neoplasms (MD-IPMN) revealing typical intraductal papillary growth after opening of the main pancreatic duct.

epithelium and papillae. In recent years, the use of molecular markers has evolved. It has been demonstrated that K-RAS mutations are found in approximately 50% of mucinous lesions compared to non-mucinous, but they do not correlate with the grade of atypia. Recent studies showed that GNAS mutations can be found in 66% (KRAS or GNAS in 96%) of IPMNs but not in MCN or SCN, and therefore this may offer a promising tool to distinguish these cystic neoplasms from one another.

ERCP

The role of endoscopic retrograde cholangiopancreatography (ERCP) has widely been displaced by MRCP. ERCP may disclose a bulging papilla with a patulous orifice extruding mucus. While this image is pathognomonic of IPMN, it is seen in only about 25% of cases. According to the 2012 International Association of Pancreatology (IAP) guidelines, routine ERCP for sampling of fluid or brushings in IPMN is no longer recommended. In patients who present with jaundice, ERCP will allow temporary stenting if surgery will be delayed for any reason or Wallstent placement if the tumor is unresectable or if the patient is not an operative candidate.

Because the majority of these tumors are now being identified as an incidental finding during a CT or ultrasound done for other reasons, in many cases it will be important to document the diagnosis

before proceeding with surgery, and this may require EUS and/or ERCP.

INDICATIONS FOR RESECTION

Because of the well-documented frequency of malignancy (mean 62%) in MD-IPMN, surgical resection is recommended in all fit patients. In patients with BD-IPMN, the indication for surgical resection has changed over the last decade, and it is still the subject of controversy. Nevertheless, there is a consensus that all young and surgically fit elderly patients with BD-IPMNs should be resected if they present with obstructive jaundice, an enhanced solid component, an MPD size of greater than 6 mm, or cytology that is suspicious or positive for malignancy (Figure 5).

Approach to Multifocal BD-IPMN

Indications for resection in multifocal BD-IPMNs are the same as for unifocal. In cases where all cysts are located in a pancreatic region, segmental anatomic resection should be performed. In patients presenting with multifocal BD-IPMN in different locations (i.e., the head and the tail of the pancreas), a segmental resection should be performed to remove the lesion with the highest oncologic risk.

OPERATIVE STRATEGY

The surgical management of IPMNs is different from other pancreatic tumors. In the latter, the surgeon can accurately locate the tumor from preoperative studies and accordingly plan a segmental pancreatic resection (Whipple, distal, or middle pancreatectomy), but that is not always the case in IPMNs. In IPMNs, the preoperative studies will show a dilated pancreatic duct in the main duct variety but not necessarily the intraductal mass, which is often small. Due to the overproduction of mucus, dilation can occur both proximally and distal to the tumor, making location problematic. This difficulty is compounded by the propensity of the tumor to spread microscopically along the duct.

With the available preoperative studies, the surgeon can determine which portion of the pancreas is primarily affected and plan the surgical intervention, but he or she should be prepared to change this plan depending on the intraoperative findings. At Massachusetts General Hospital, we have not found that intraoperative ultrasound adds much more to the preoperative imaging, but we rely heavily on the frozen section diagnosis of the transection margin of the

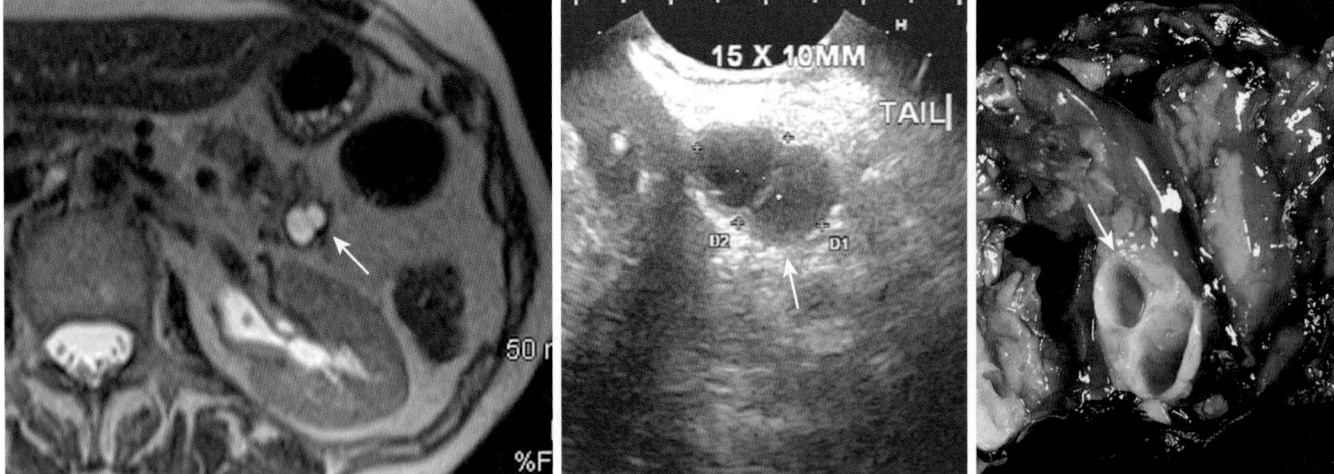

FIGURE 3 T2 magnetic resonance imaging (MRI) (*left*), endoscopic ultrasound (EUS) (*middle*), and pathologic specimen (*right*) of a bilobed branch duct intraductal papillary mucinous neoplasms (BD-IPMN). The patient was incidentally diagnosed with a cystic lesion (15 to 10 mm) in the tail of the pancreas during workup for diverticulitis. Fine-needle aspiration (FNA) revealed high-grade, atypical epithelial cells. The patient underwent distal pancreatectomy, and the final diagnosis was BD-IPMN with moderate dysplasia.

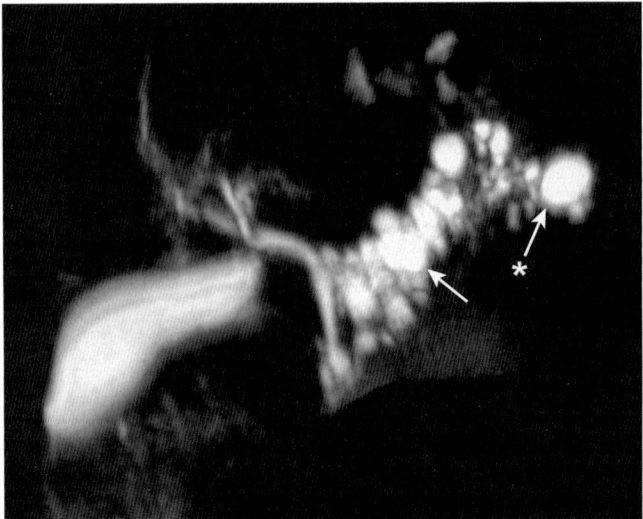

FIGURE 4 Magnetic resonance cholangiopancreatography (MRCP) of a patient with multifocal intraductal papillary mucinous neoplasm (IPMN) involving the whole pancreas. The largest lesion is located in the junction of the head and body of the pancreas and measures 30 mm in diameter. A smaller lesion can be seen* in the junction of the body and tail. Cytology of the smaller cyst suggested that it had at least high-grade dysplasia. The patient underwent distal pancreatectomy, and the final diagnosis after histologic workup was BD-IPMN with low-grade dysplasia. This patient is now being followed for the remaining lesions, which are still stable 2 years after surgery.

pancreas. Because IPMN extends along the pancreatic duct and can do so without obvious macroscopic tumor, it is important to rule out the presence of tumor at the margin so no tumor is left behind. A denuded epithelium in the duct is not uncommon in this pathology, and deepithelialization should not erroneously be interpreted as a "negative" margin because recurrence has occurred in this setting. To reduce operative time, we have found it useful to excise a segment of pancreas from the end to be examined intraoperatively before we remove the entire specimen, thus giving the pathologist ample time to perform this exam. A 3- to 4-mm slice is enough, and it should be

done with a scalpel rather than cautery to facilitate the interpretation, which can often be challenging for the pathologist. If the margin shows tumor is present, we extend the resection a few centimeters and obtain a new margin. The process is usually continued until a negative margin is obtained, and it can potentially lead to total pancreatectomy (see later discussion).

We also use intraoperative pancreatoscopy whenever there is a dilation of the pancreatic duct. This allows for inspection of the ductal system of the remaining pancreas and can potentially identify "skip" lesions if they are macroscopic. The presence of these skip lesions has been proposed based on recurrence of IPMN in the remaining pancreas in the setting of a truly negative transection margin. Pancreatoscopy can be done using the laparoscopic choledochoscope, which is small enough to fit in a 4-mm pancreatic duct.

Because of the potential to modify or extend the surgical resection plans at the time of surgery, it is important that the surgeon discuss and evaluate preoperatively the risks and consequences of a total pancreatectomy with the patient. This obviously needs to be individualized carefully. Whereas a total pancreatectomy may be appropriate in a young, fit patient who has an IPMN with carcinoma in the head of the pancreas that is extending into the body and tail, it may not be the right operation for an elderly or frail patient with an IPMN that is only an adenoma or borderline tumor, even if present at the transection margin. In our experience with 404 patients, 59% required a Whipple resection, 3% an extended pancreaticoduodenectomy, 5% a total pancreatectomy, 25% a distal pancreatectomy, and 8% resection of the middle segment of the pancreas.

Although preoperative determination of malignancy is sometimes available from ERCP brushings or the EUS-aspirate of the fluid or solid component, most often this is not the case. Patients with malignant IPMN tend to have larger tumors, a larger portion of solid component, and a higher incidence of jaundice, recent-onset diabetes, or steatorrhea. If malignancy is not anticipated based on the preoperative imaging and clinical presentation, the surgeon can consider more conservative resection, such as middle pancreatectomy or a distal pancreatectomy without splenectomy.

PROGNOSIS AND FOLLOW-UP

The prognosis of patients with resected IPMN is quite good. In our series, the median survival for all patients is over 10 years. The survival in patients who had high-grade dysplasia is very similar to

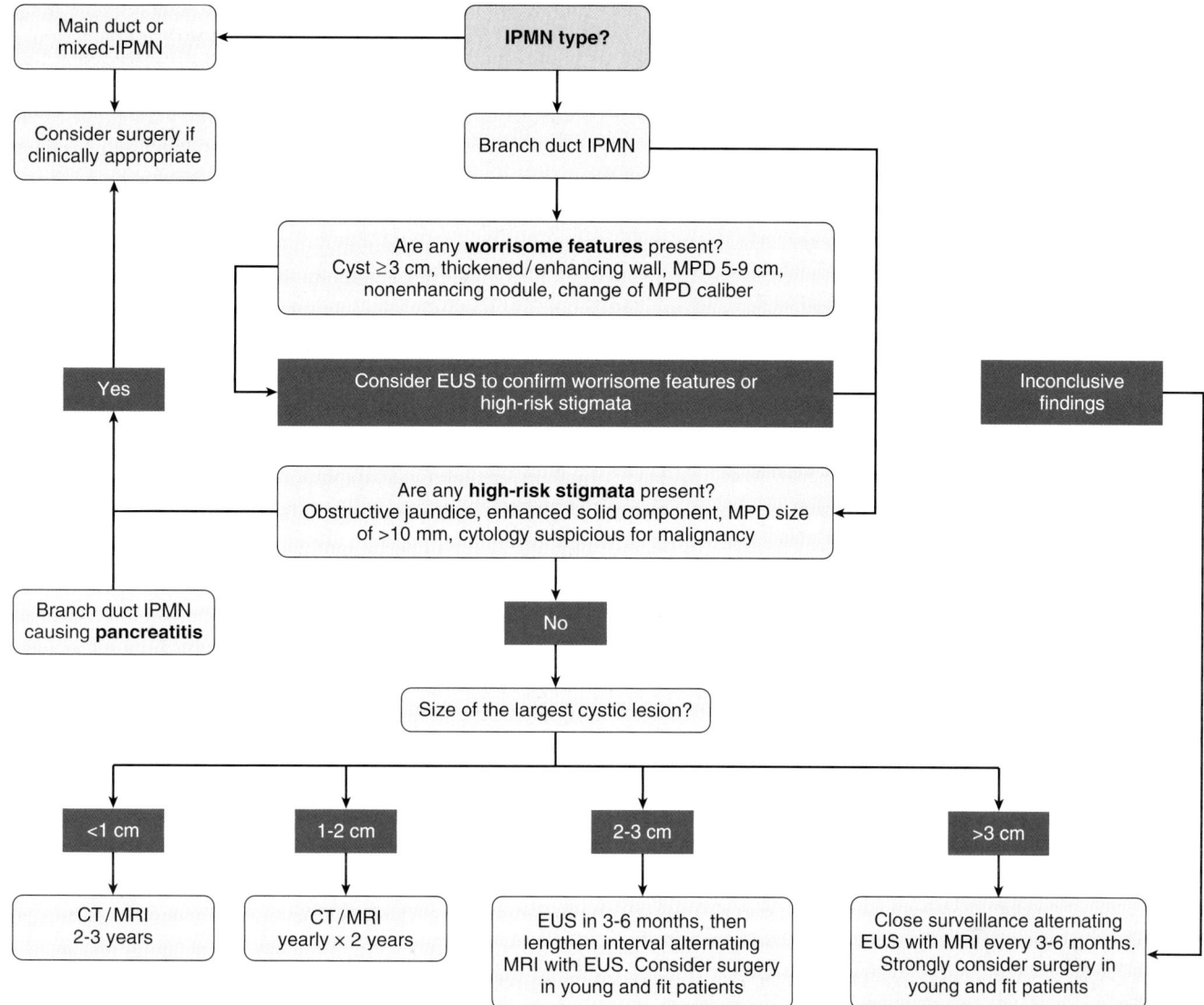

FIGURE 5 Algorithm for the management of intraductal papillary mucinous neoplasms (IPMN) according to International Association of Pancreatology (IAP) 2012 guidelines. *CT*, computed tomographic; *EUS*, endoscopic ultrasound; *IPMN*, intraductal papillary mucinous neoplasms; *MPD*, main pancreatic duct; *MRI*, magnetic resonance imaging.

that of patients with low-grade dysplasia. Depending on the histopathologic subtype of invasive IPMN, median survival in patients with colloid cancer is much more favorable (median 132 months) than in patients with tubular carcinoma (median 35 months), which is only marginally better than in pancreatic ductal adenocarcinoma.

The recurrence rate of IPMN in the remaining pancreas (when no known lesions are left behind and the margin is negative) ranges in the literature from 0 to 20%. Often it is not clear if ductal dilation in the pancreatic remnant is IPMN recurrence or is caused by postresectional anastomotic stenosis. Several studies, mostly from Japan, have shown an increased incidence of conventional ductal adenocarcinoma of the pancreas both in patients being followed with branch duct IPMN and in those that have been resected. The actual frequency of this phenomenon is unclear, but it has been described as 3% to 10%.

Follow-up of patients who underwent resection for IPMN depends on multiple factors. Patients with clear resection margins and without a known remaining IPMN in the pancreatic remnant should be followed at 2 years and 5 years to rule out recurrence.

Those with low-grade or high-grade dysplasia at the resection margin should be closely followed twice a year by MRCP, CT, or EUS. Patients with multifocal IPMN and a known lesion left behind should be followed according to the guidelines for nonresected IPMNs. In the case of invasive IPMN carcinoma (stage II/III), the follow-up schedule is the same as that of ductal adenocarcinoma.

Suggested Readings

Falconi M, Salvia R, Bassi C, et al: Clinicopathological features and treatment of intraductal papillary mucinous tumour of the pancreas, *Br J Surg* 88(3):376–381, 2001.

Fernandez-del Castillo C, Adsay NV: Intraductal papillary mucinous neoplasms of the pancreas, *Gastroenterology* 139(3):708–713, e702, 2011.

Fernandez-del Castillo C: Surgical treatment of intraductal papillary mucinous neoplasms of the pancreas: the conservative approach, *J Gastrointest Surg* 6(5):660–661, 2002.

Matthaei H, Norris AL, Tsiatis AC, et al: Clinicopathological characteristics and molecular analyses of multifocal intraductal papillary mucinous neoplasms of the pancreas, *Ann Surg* 255(2):326–333, 2012.

Mino-Kenudson M, Fernandez-Del Castillo C, Baba Y, et al: Prognosis of invasive intraductal papillary mucinous neoplasm depends on histological and precursor epithelial subtypes, *Gut* 60(12):1712–1720, 2011.

Partelli S, Fernandez-Del Castillo C, Bassi C, et al: Invasive intraductal papillary mucinous carcinomas of the pancreas, *Ann Surg* 251(3):477–482, 2010.

Sohn TA, Yeo CJ, Cameron JL, et al: Intraductal papillary mucinous neoplasms of the pancreas: an increasingly recognized clinicopathologic entity, *Ann Surg* 234(3):313–321; discussion 321–312, 2001.

Tanaka M, Fernandez-Del Castillo C, Adsay V, et al: International consensus guidelines 2012 for the management of IPMN and MCN of the pancreas, *Pancreatology* 12(3):183–197, 2012.

THE MANAGEMENT OF PANCREATIC ISLET CELL TUMORS EXCLUDING GASTRINOMAS

Scott P. Albert, MD, Mark Bloomston, MD, and E. Christopher Ellison, MD

OVERVIEW

Pancreatic neuroendocrine tumors (PNETs), also termed islet cell tumors, are rare and represent about 3% of all pancreatic tumors. Modern analyses have suggested that the incidence has been increasing over the last three decades, in part because of the growing use of endoscopic and radiographic examinations. The peak incidence for PNET is between the ages of 40 and 69 years, which is earlier than with pancreatic adenocarcinoma. Most tumors are sporadic, but they can be associated with syndromes such as multiple endocrine neoplasia (MEN), neurofibromatosis type I, tuberous sclerosis, von Recklinghausen's disease, and von Hippel-Lindau syndrome. In patients with MEN 1, pancreatic tumors occur between 20% and 40% of the time and are often multiple in nature.

Recent evidence suggests that PNETs arise from pluripotent stem cells and have a distinct tumor development pathway as compared with pancreatic adenocarcinomas. PNETs commonly contain mutations in MEN and mammalian target of rapamycin (mTOR) signaling pathways, and K-*ras* mutations are associated with pancreatic adenocarcinomas. These mutational differences allow for more systemic therapeutic options in patients with neuroendocrine cancers.

PNETs are a diverse group with a wide spectrum of biologic behavior that ranges from low-grade indolent tumors to high-grade aggressive tumors with propensity to metastasize. These tumors can also be broadly classified into nonfunctional or functional types based on symptoms, although most are capable of producing any type of hormone. Functional tumors are commonly named after the dominant hormone-related syndrome, such as insulinomas, gastrinomas, vasoactive intestinal polypeptide-secreting tumors (VIPomas), glucagonomas, somatostatinomas, and other rare functional tumors (Table 1). Nonfunctional tumors compose 40% to 90% of all pancreatic neuroendocrine tumors and are more common than their functional counterparts. Serum levels of pancreatic polypeptide are not infrequently elevated in nonfunctional PNET, but there is no associated clinical syndrome. Current neuroendocrine tumor staging uses American Joint Committee on Cancer (AJCC) tumor node metastasis (TNM) classification guidelines that are based on the previously developed staging system used for exocrine pancreas cancers.

TABLE 1: Summary of functional tumor types

Tumor	Annual incidence	Presentation	Location	Malignant	MEN associated
Insulinoma	0.1 per million	Whipple's triad: neuroglycopenia, hypoglycemia, symptom improvement with glucose administration	Entire pancreas	10%	5%
Glucagonoma	Rare	Necrolytic migratory erythema	Tail	>70%	Occasional
VIPoma	Rare	Watery diarrhea, hypokalemia, achlorhydria	Tail	50%	Occasional
Somatostatinoma	Extremely rare	Diabetes, diarrhea, cholelithiasis	Pancreas, duodenum, small bowel	70%	Rare
Nonfunctional	2.2 per million	Variable	Entire pancreas	>50%	Rare

MEN, Multiple endocrine neoplasia; *VIPoma*, vasoactive intestinal polypeptide-secreting tumor.

Consideration for other classification systems has been evaluated, including a European staging classification that may be more prognostic of overall survival. In addition, PNETs can be further characterized by tumor grade (i.e., NET1, NET2, NET3) which is determined by the mitotic index or Ki-67 activity during pathologic assessment. Tumor grade can be helpful information in making further treatment decisions. High-grade neuroendocrine cancers behave very aggressively and are treated more like small cell lung cancers.

DIAGNOSIS

Patients with functional tumors frequently present with symptoms related to the type of hormone produced in excess, whereas nonfunctional tumors are often asymptomatic until later in the disease course. Nonfunctional tumors are often an incidental finding on imaging or result from mass effect symptoms, such as abdominal pain, weight loss, anorexia, nausea, or jaundice. About 50% of patients with nonfunctional tumors have liver metastases as part of the initial presentation. Although this implies a greater metastatic potential for nonfunctional tumors, recent data suggest a lead-time bias with patients harboring functional tumors that present earlier in their course rather than a true difference in tumor biology.

High-quality cross-sectional imaging is necessary for diagnosis and allows for assessment of the primary tumor and evaluation of the liver for metastatic disease. PNETs appear as hypervascular lesions on computed tomographic (CT) scan; on magnetic resonance imaging (MRI), these tumors are best visualized on fat-suppressed T1-weighted images with contrast enhancement. Somatostatin receptor scintigraphy (octreotide scan) can be used selectively for tumor detection in challenging cases, monitoring of tumor response, or definition of metastatic disease (Figure 1). This test uses a radiolabeled somatostatin analog and can image the entire body, which makes it especially useful for identification of distant metastatic disease. Endoscopic ultrasound scan (EUS) is another effective diagnostic tool for localization of small hormonally active tumors and obtainment of tissue samples (Figure 2). Other tests to include in the workup are serum electrolyte levels, liver function tests, measurement of 24-hour urine 5-hydroxyindoleacetic acid (5-HIAA) and serum chromogranin-A (CGA) levels. CGA is frequently elevated in both functional and nonfunctional types. Plasma levels of CGA and pancreastatin, a functional split product of CGA, have been shown to be useful markers for monitoring tumor response to various treatments. Awareness that CGA levels can be falsely elevated in patients

with renal insufficiency or liver disease or in patients taking proton pump inhibitors is important.

FUNCTIONAL TUMORS

Insulinoma

Presentation

Insulinomas are the most common functional tumor and are more common in women. Approximately 90% of insulinomas present with limited local disease, which makes them amenable to curative surgery. The most frequent presentation corresponds to symptoms related to hypoglycemia, such as headaches, blurred vision, and incoherent thinking. The release of catecholamines from the associated hypoglycemia may result in excessive sweating, tachycardia, and nervousness. The classic presentation, Whipple's triad, consists of neurologic symptoms of hypoglycemia (neuroglycopenia), plasma glucose of less than 50 mg/dL at the time of symptoms, and relief of symptoms with administration of glucose. Patients may present with sudden or rapid weight gain as a result of compensatory eating to offset fasting hypoglycemia. The differential diagnosis in these patients includes hepatic insufficiency, factitious hypoglycemia, chronic adrenal insufficiency, and hypopituitarism.

Diagnosis

The first step in diagnosis is demonstration of elevated insulin to glucose ratio during fasting and associated elevated C peptide levels. Measurement of levels of sulfonylurea is often necessary if factitious hypoglycemia is suspected. An insulin to glucose ratio greater than 0.4 is consistent with an insulinoma. The preferred diagnostic test is a 72-hour fast with the measurement of glucose, insulin, and C peptide levels every 6 hours, until symptoms of hypoglycemia appear. This requires in-hospital monitoring. Symptoms develop in 75% of afflicted patients after 24 hours, and 95% of patients have symptoms after 48 hours of fasting if an insulinoma is present.

The next challenge is often localization because most are less than 1.5 cm in diameter and occur equally throughout the pancreas. CT scan or MRI is often adequate for localization, although EUS can be valuable if localization of the lesion becomes difficult. Occasionally, indium 111 diethylenetriaminepentaacetic acid (DTPA)-octreotide

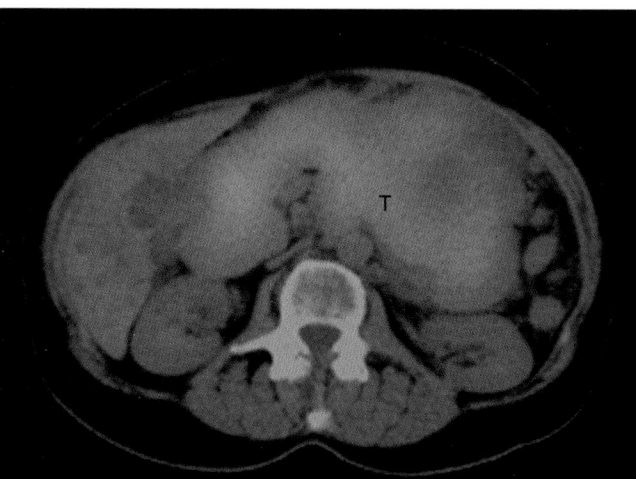

FIGURE 1 Octreotide scan shows increased activity in the pancreatic tumor *(T)*. The patient is administered octreotide radiolabeled with indium 111. Note the tumor enhancement caused by the uptake of octreotide by tumor-bearing somatostatin receptors.

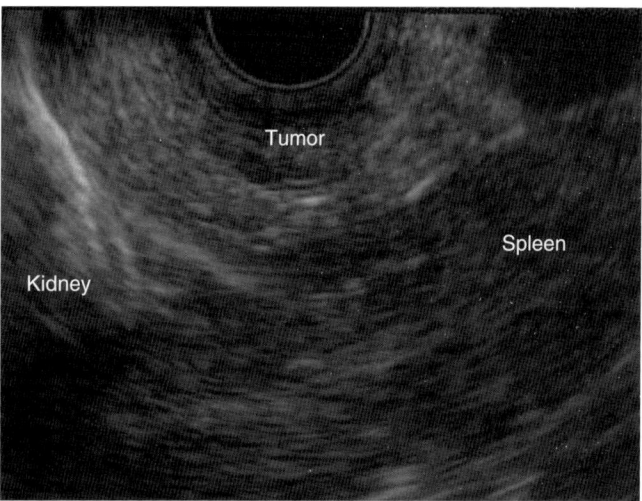

FIGURE 2 Endoscopic ultrasound scan image shows a neuroendocrine tumor in the tail of the pancreas. The spleen and left kidney are in view.

(octreotide scan) can be helpful for localization, although insulinomas are less likely to have a positive scan as compared with other PNETs. An invasive procedure that requires selective cannulation of pancreatic arteries followed by the injection of calcium and measurement of insulin levels in the portal circulation can be performed in difficult cases or for recurrent disease. However, most can be localized with modern cross-sectional imaging.

Treatment

Preoperative hypoglycemia can be managed with frequent small meals. Octreotide should be used with caution because it can worsen hypoglycemia by suppressing glucagon secretion. Diazoxide can be used to suppress insulin secretion. Surgical resection is the mainstay of treatment, with enucleation or pancreatectomy appropriate depending on the size and location of the tumor. Figure 3 shows a robotic enucleation of a small insulinoma in the body of the pancreas. Blind pancreatic resection is not indicated, and rarely surgical exploration with intraoperative ultrasound scan is required to make the diagnosis.

Glucagonoma

Presentation

Patients often present with diabetes, anemia, stomatitis, weight loss, and diarrhea. Two thirds of patients present with necrolytic migratory erythema, a severe rash with raised, scaly, erythematous patches that sometimes begins on the perineum and progresses to the trunk and extremities (Figure 4). The differential diagnosis for this type of rash includes psoriasis, pemphigus, eczema, zinc deficiency, pellagra, end-stage liver disease, and epidermal necrolysis. Deep venous thrombosis occurs in 30% of patients. Patients frequently have deficient amino acid levels as a result of stimulation of gluconeogenesis and associated amino acid oxidation.

Diagnosis and Treatment

The diagnosis can be made with measurement of glucagon to blood glucose ratios. A fasting glucagon level greater than 1000 pg/mL (normal, 0 to 150 pg/mL) is consistent with the diagnosis of glucagonoma. Cross-sectional imaging is used to identify the mass and assess resectability. These tumors most often arise from the tail of the pancreas (Figure 5). Glucagonomas have a high incidence of metastatic disease (60%), with the liver the most common site for metastases. Other conditions that can cause elevated glucagon levels include fasting, sepsis, pancreatitis, Cushing's syndrome, renal failure, and hepatic failure. Nutritional supplementation and replacement of

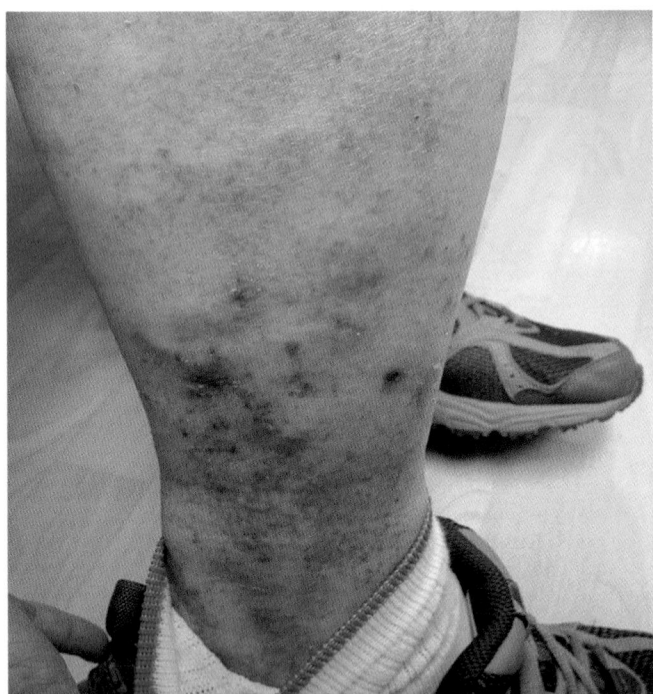

FIGURE 4   Patient with characteristic rash from a glucagonoma. The rash is erythematous and scaly and located on the pretibial region but can also affect the perioral and intertriginous areas.

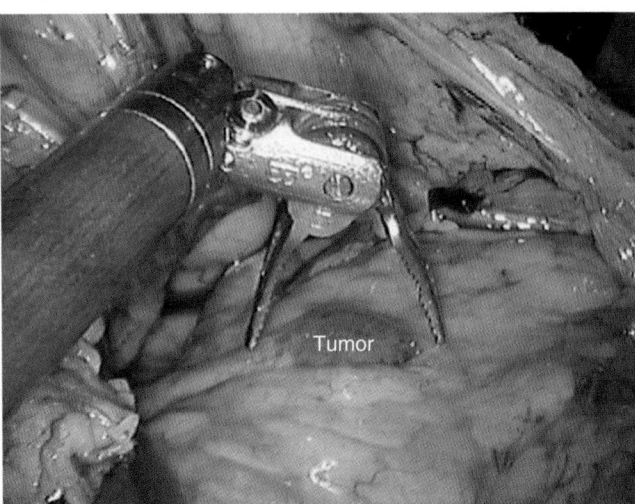

FIGURE 3   Minimally invasive robotic enucleation of an insulinoma in the tail of the pancreas. On preoperative cross-sectional imaging and intraoperative ultrasound, the mass was noted to be away from the main pancreatic duct.

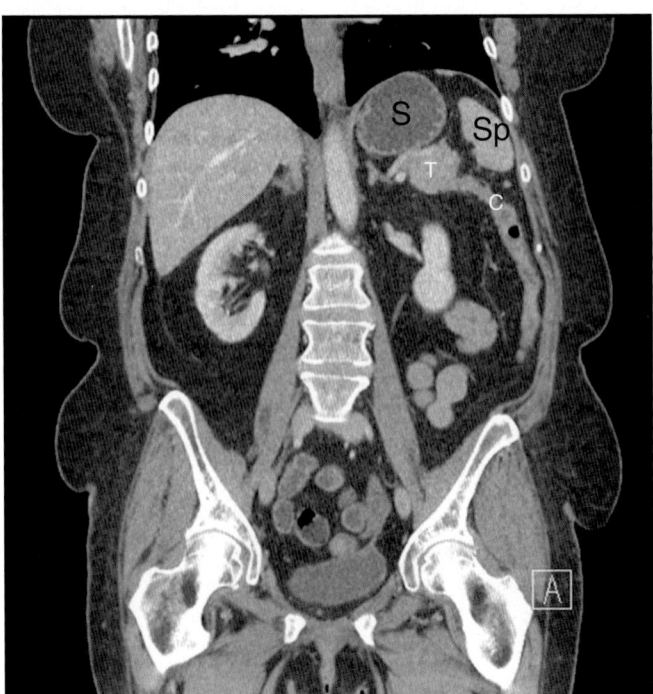

FIGURE 5   Coronal computed tomographic scan image shows a tumor (T) in the tail of the pancreas consistent with the patient's diagnosis of a glucagonoma. The stomach (S), spleen (Sp), and colon (C) can be seen adjacent to the mass.

amino acid losses may be necessary before any surgical intervention. Patients should also receive supplemental zinc. Octreotide can be used in the management of symptoms. Formal pancreatectomy is usually required for the management of glucagonomas.

Vasoactive Intestinal Peptide-Secreting Tumor

Presentation

First described in 1958 by Verner and Morrison, the classic presentation of a VIPoma is known as WDHA (watery diarrhea, hypokalemia, and achlorhydria) syndrome. Patients present with profuse diarrhea with volumes of 10 L/d that persists despite fasting. Not surprisingly, because of the severe diarrhea, patients are frequently hypokalemic and acidotic. Rarely, patients may also present with neurocognitive symptoms.

Diagnosis and Treatment

Plasma vasoactive intestinal peptide levels greater than 200 pg/mL are suggestive of a VIPoma, but typically levels are closer to 1000 pg/mL in most cases. These tumors are often located in the tail of the pancreas and are commonly metastatic (~50%). Cross-sectional imaging is needed to localize the tumor and determine resectability. The initial step in treatment is correction of severe electrolyte abnormalities. Octreotide can be used to help with symptoms before surgery.

Somatostatinoma

Presentation, Diagnosis, and Treatment

Patients most often present with diabetes, cholelithiasis, steatorrhea, and diarrhea. The inhibition of insulin, cholecystokinin, and pancreatic enzyme secretion by somatostatin leads to the associated disorders commonly seen in this syndrome. Somatostatin levels are greater than 100 pg/mL. Most somatostatinomas (70%) are metastatic at presentation. Seventy percent of these tumors are located in the pancreas, but they can also be found in duodenum and proximal small bowel.

Other Rare Functional Tumors

Other rare pancreatic functional tumors include adrenocorticotrophin-producing tumors (ACTHoma) parathyroid hormone-related peptide (PTH-RP) secreting tumors, and pancreatic polypeptide-producing tumor (PPoma). The treatment of these tumors is similar to the management of nonfunctional tumors.

Surgical Considerations

Localized

Surgery is central to the treatment of PNETs, and formal pancreatic resection is usually required, although small tumors (<2 cm) can be treated with enucleation in select cases. Minimally invasive approaches can be used for resection at institutions with experience (see Figure 3). For patients with small tumors and multiple comorbidities, close observation may be appropriate, although progressive disease should be resected, if feasible. Studies have shown that small tumors (<2 cm) are less likely to behave in a malignant fashion, but short-term follow-up is required to confirm tumor stability. The goal of surgical intervention is to achieve a complete resection with negative margins (i.e., R0). Often, removal of contiguous organs (e.g., stomach, colon,

kidney) is necessary to achieve complete resection (Figure 6). If incidental liver metastases are found at the time of primary tumor resection, resection and cholecystectomy (in anticipation of future octreotide or liver-directed embolic therapy) is recommended if it can be completed safely and with minimal added morbidity.

Metastatic

Patients with neuroendocrine tumors can present late in the disease course and often with synchronous liver metastases. As such, quality and quantity of life is often determined by the hepatic disease burden. In cases of synchronous liver disease, the goals of surgical treatment should be palliation of symptoms in hormonally active tumors or complete surgical resection of both the primary and the liver metastases. Complete surgical resection of all disease should be the goal. Debulking surgery is more controversial, especially in the asymptomatic patient with bulky liver metastases. In the symptomatic patient, complex approaches combining surgical resection with ablation or embolic therapy might be used to achieve symptom control. In cases where the primary pancreatic tumor is readily resectable, it may be appropriate to proceed with resection if complete primary tumor removal is expected, thus allowing treatment, namely regional embolic therapies, to focus entirely on the liver disease. A recent multicenter analysis showed that patients with low-volume disease or symptomatic high-volume liver disease benefited most from palliative cytoreductive hepatectomy. Asymptomatic patients with a larger (>25%) liver tumor burden benefited equally with surgery or transarterial chemoembolization (TACE). The role of neoadjuvant systemic treatments is still evolving, but with the development of more effective systemic therapies, more patients might be converted to surgical candidates (Figure 7).

Metastatic liver tumors derive most of their blood supply from the arterial circulation, whereas portal circulation supplies the healthy liver. These differences in blood supply allow for effective regional liver therapies that include TACE, bland arterial embolization (transcatheter arterial embolization [TAE]) and radioembolization with radionuclide-laden spheres (e.g., Yttrium-90). Objective responses to regional therapy are variable (usually >50%), with stabilization of progressing disease commonplace (80% to 90%). Perhaps more importantly, most patients experience improvement in their symptoms from functional tumors. Peptide receptor radiation therapy (PRRT) with a radiolabeled somatostatin analog potentially treats somatostatin receptor-positive tumors. This novel therapy specifically delivers a cytotoxic dose of radiation directly to active tumor

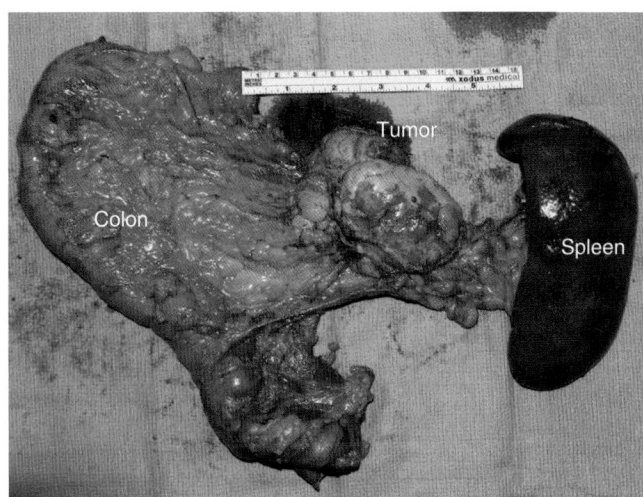

FIGURE 6 En bloc resection specimen after treatment with capecitabine and temozolomide. The colon and spleen along with the distal portion of pancreas were removed.

FIGURE 7 **A,** Axial contrast-enhanced computed tomographic scan images shows a large pancreatic neuroendocrine tumor (T). **B,** A dramatic response to preoperative treatment with capecitabine and temozolomide is shown. Multiple liver metastases (M) are seen in **A.** The stomach (S) is less compressed after treatment, and there was resolution of early satiety symptoms. The resection specimen is seen in Figure 6.

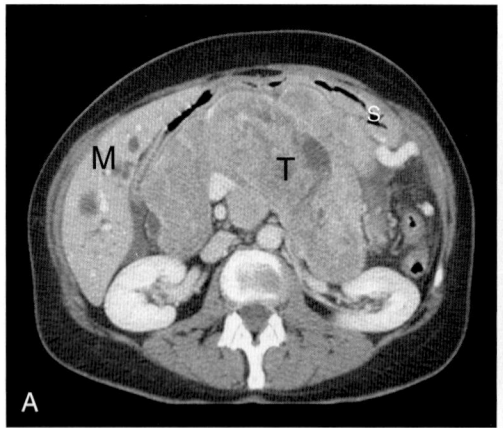
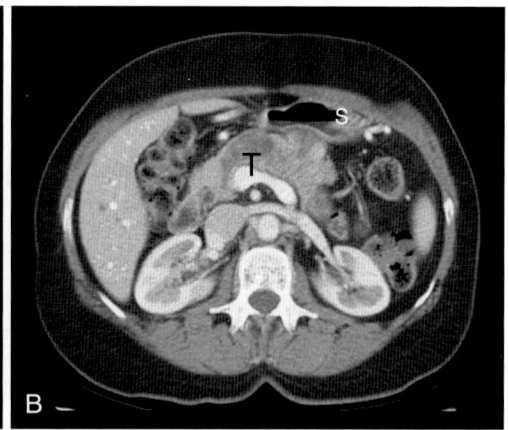

and is gaining popularity in Europe, although it is currently only available in the United States in clinical trials.

Systemic Treatments

An improved understanding of neuroendocrine tumor biology has led to new systemic therapies and a more targeted approach to treatment. Several encouraging clinical trials that include patients with metastatic pancreatic neuroendocrine tumors have recently been completed. These newer treatment options include somatostatin analogs, tyrosine kinase inhibitors, mTOR inhibitors, and novel combinations of chemotherapeutic agents.

Somatostatin Analogs

Somatostatin analogs inhibit the growth of tumor cells that express somatostatin receptors; thus, these drugs have been shown to have a stabilization effect on tumor growth. A randomized clinical trial evaluated the use of long-acting octreotide in patients with metastatic midgut carcinoid tumors. This study included a significant proportion of patients with pancreatic neuroendocrine tumors. The group that received long-acting octreotide had a significantly longer time to disease progression as compared with the placebo group. Although the use of somatostatin analogs for tumor stasis is still an open debate, its use in reducing symptoms, especially in patients with metastatic disease, is the standard of care.

Targeted Treatments

Multiple recent randomized trials have shown promising results with the use of targeted drug therapies for PNETs. Sunitinib, a multikinase inhibitor that blocks the VEGF receptor, has shown activity against PNETs. In a phase II study, patients with PNETs achieved a 17% partial response rate with minimal significant side effects. A follow-up phase III trial in which patients were randomized to sunitinib or placebo was stopped early because of clear benefit in the study group. The median progression-free survival time was 11.4 months in the sunitinib group compared with 5.5 months with placebo. Overall survival was also significantly better with sunitinib. Another targeted agent, everolimus, blocks a separate kinase along the *Akt* pathway known as mTOR. This pathway has been shown to be involved in

PNET cell growth. A phase III trial randomized patients to everolimus or placebo, and again, the targeted treatment group showed encouraging results. The median time to progression was significantly better in the treatment group (11.0 months vs 4.6 months). Patients included in both the everolimus and sunitinib trials had low-grade or intermediate-grade PNETs and were deemed to have unresectable or metastatic disease.

Chemotherapy

The only chemotherapy drug currently approved in the United States for metastatic PNETs is streptozocin. Additional older regimens have included doxorubicin or 5-fluorouracil (5-FU). Early promising phase II data combine capecitabine with temozolomide. Capecitabine is an oral prodrug for 5-FU, and temozolomide is an oral alkylating agent. In patients with metastatic pancreatic neuroendocrine tumors treated with this drug combination, the objective response rate was a surprising 70% (21 of 30 patients), and progression-free survival was improved over historic controls. In some cases, patients may show a dramatic response to newer combinations of systemic therapy as seen in Figure 7. The continued understanding of the various biologic pathways in neuroendocrine cancers allows for more options in targeted and chemotherapeutic treatments. More studies are looking at various combinations of regional therapies, targeted treatments, and chemotherapy agents.

SUGGESTED READINGS

Mayo SC, de Jong MC, Bloomston M, et al: Surgery versus intra-arterial therapy for neuroendocrine liver metastasis: a multicenter international analysis, *Ann Surg Oncol* 18(13):3657–3665, 2011.

Raymond E, Dahan L, Raoul J-L, et al: Sunitinib malate for the treatment of pancreatic neuroendocrine tumors, *N Engl J Med* 364(6):501–513, 2011.

Rinke A, Muller HH, Schade-Brittinger C, et al: Placebo-controlled, double-blind, prospective, randomized study on the effect of octreotide LAR in the control of tumor growth in patients with metastatic neuroendocrine midgut tumors: a report from the PROMID study group, *J Clin Oncol* 27(28):4656–4663, 2009.

Strosberg JR, Fine RL, Choi J, et al: First-line chemotherapy with capecitabine and temozolomide in patients with metastatic pancreatic endocrine carcinomas, *Cancer* 117(2):268–275, 2011.

Yao JC, Shah MH, Tetsuhide I, et al: Everolimus for advanced pancreatic neuroendocrine tumors, *N Engl J Med* 364(6):514–523, 2011.

TRANSPLANTATION OF THE PANCREAS

Niraj M. Desai, MD and
James F. Markmann, MD, PhD

INTRODUCTION

Type 1 diabetes mellitus, formerly known as *juvenile diabetes,* is characterized by hyperglycemia resulting from destruction of the insulin-producing beta cells of the pancreatic islets of Langerhans. This loss of beta cells is caused by T lymphocyte–mediated autoimmune destruction that typically occurs during childhood or early adolescence. Insulin replacement can lead to acceptable control of blood glucose levels; however, affected individuals are subject to the development of various secondary complications, including cardiac disease, stroke, retinopathy and blindness, nephropathy and renal failure, peripheral and autonomic neuropathy, and amputation. Although careful blood glucose control has been demonstrated to decrease the number of diabetes-related secondary complications, it has also been shown to lead to an increased number of dangerous hypoglycemic episodes. Technological advances (insulin pumps and continuous glucose sensors) may help reduce the incidence of secondary complications and the number of hypoglycemic episodes.

Transplantation therapy for type 1 diabetes was developed as an alternative to insulin administration with the goal of reducing or eliminating the development of secondary complications of the disease by perfecting glycemic control. The pancreas—both the whole organ and isolated pancreatic islets—is being transplanted into individuals with type 1 diabetes. Clinical islet transplantation remains experimental and is available at only select centers, but it is expected to become an approved therapy in the United States during 2015. It has proven efficacy in diabetic individuals with severe hypoglycemia unawareness. In contrast, whole-organ pancreas transplantation is an established and widely available therapy for the treatment of type 1 diabetes. Whole-organ pancreas transplantation is the focus of this chapter.

WHOLE-ORGAN PANCREAS TRANSPLANTATION

History and Early Results

On December 20, 1893, Dr. P. Watson Williams grafted pieces of a sheep pancreas into the subcutaneous tissues of a diabetic child who died 3 days later of unrelenting diabetic ketoacidosis. This first attempt to treat diabetes with transplantation, although unsuccessful, preceded decades of animal experimentation in which investigators developed the methods necessary to perform a vascularized pancreas transplantation.

The first vascularized pancreas transplant in a patient was performed on December 17, 1966, by Drs. William Kelly and Richard Lillehei at the University of Minnesota. The patient achieved temporary insulin independence but eventually required graft removal and ultimately died of postoperative complications. The subsequent early experience with pancreas transplantation was characterized by some technical success, but no graft functioned beyond 1 year. Most pancreas grafts that were successful from a technical perspective were lost as a result of rejection. The initial enthusiasm for this procedure dwindled so much that it was nearly abandoned by the mid-1970s. However, further technical refinements and the introduction of more potent immunosuppressive medications (first cyclosporine and then tacrolimus) allowed for better outcomes after pancreas transplantation. Throughout the 1980s and early 1990s, the number of pancreas transplants performed in the United States increased dramatically, peaking at nearly 1500 transplantations during 2004. However, this number has declined since, with fewer than 1100 transplants performed in the United States during 2012.

Indications and Patient Selection

The majority of patients undergoing pancreas transplantation have type 1 diabetes mellitus and end-stage renal disease. In these individuals, pancreas transplantation is performed with simultaneous kidney transplantation (SPK) or after successful kidney transplantation (pancreas after kidney [PAK] transplantation). The normal blood glucose control achieved by the transplanted pancreas should protect the transplanted kidney from recurrent diabetic nephropathy and is beneficial from an overall quality-of-life perspective. In a small proportion of patients with difficult-to-control diabetes but with preserved renal function, pancreas transplantation alone (PTA) is performed. In the United States for the 3-year period ending in 2011, 75% of pancreas transplantations were SPK, 12% PAK, and 13% PTA. SPK and PAK recipients require immunosuppressive therapy to protect both the kidney and pancreas from rejection, whereas in the case of PTA recipients, the need for immunosuppression is solely for the pancreas itself. For this reason, careful individual risk to benefit consideration is essential in selecting PTA recipients.

Potential pancreas recipients are carefully screened for contraindications to transplantation, such as an ongoing infectious process or malignancy. These candidates almost always have medical comorbid conditions resulting from secondary complications from diabetes; therefore, a thorough assessment of a candidate's cardiovascular status is essential. Cardiac contraindications to pancreas transplantation include the presence of noncorrectable coronary artery disease, ejection fraction of less than 40%, or myocardial infarction within the previous 6 months. Recipient age is also important, although there is no consensus as to what an upper age limit should be for undergoing pancreas transplantation. National data indicate that almost all pancreas transplantations in the United States are performed in recipients younger than 65 years.

The Donor Operation

Selection of an appropriate deceased donor for pancreas procurement includes standard donor selection criteria. In addition, there is a bias toward using organs from younger, leaner, and hemodynamically stable deceased donors. Donor organs that require high doses of vasopressor are considered higher risk for complications in the recipient. In addition, pancreata with significant infiltration of fat in the parenchyma are usually avoided because they are associated with a greater likelihood of postoperative complications such as pancreatitis, peripancreatic fat necrosis, and infection. On the basis of these relatively stringent selection criteria, only a fraction of deceased donors are deemed suitable for whole-organ pancreas donation. In the United States, there were 8143 deceased donors during 2012; however, only 1079 pancreata were transplanted (from 13% of all deceased donors, in comparison with 5941 livers (73%) and 11,991 kidneys (75% of all deceased donors).

Pancreas procurement from a deceased donor is performed in careful conjunction with liver procurement. The blood supply to the liver is identified to ensure that both organs can be removed and transplanted. In most cases, aberrant blood supply should not preclude the transplantation of both organs. Initial dissection involves division of the gastrocolic ligament, so as to expose the anterior surface of the pancreas. Visual inspection is considered an important element in pancreas procurement because this is an opportunity to assess the organ for the presence of infiltrating fat, fibrosis, or hematoma that might preclude transplantation. The portal triad is carefully dissected, with division of the common bile duct and the gastroduodenal artery. In addition, the common hepatic, the proximal left gastric, and the proximal splenic arteries are all dissected free from surrounding lymphatic tissues. Further dissection of the pancreas includes performing Kocher's maneuver to mobilize the pancreatic head and dividing the lienophrenic and lienocolic ligaments to mobilize the pancreatic body and tail. Of note, the spleen is left in continuity with the pancreas to minimize manipulation of the gland, and it is removed later during backbench preparation. The duodenum is decontaminated by flushing of a solution containing povidone-iodine, an antibiotic, and an antifungal through a nasoduodenal tube.

After the donor has been prepared with heparin, the abdominal aorta is ligated at the iliac bifurcation, and a cannula is placed in a retrograde direction for perfusion. The liver surgery team may also place a cannula into a portal vein tributary, such as the inferior mesenteric vein, for portal perfusion. The supraceliac aorta is crossclamped, the vena cava is vented, and the abdominal organs are flushed in situ with preservation solution (Belzer UW Cold Storage Solution) at 4° C. In addition, topical cooling of the organs is performed. Once the organs have been adequately flushed, the liver and pancreas are removed either en bloc and divided on the back table or removed separately from the donor. In the latter situation, the liver is removed first, by division of the portal vein 1 cm cephalad to the superior margin of the pancreatic head (approximately at the level of the coronary vein), and division of the splenic artery 5 mm beyond its origin, which thus preserves the entire celiac axis with the liver. Next, removal of the pancreas proceeds. The proximal duodenum (just beyond the pylorus) and the distal duodenum (near the ligament of Treitz) are divided with GIA staplers. The small bowel mesentery and transverse colon mesentery that lie inferior to the pancreas are divided. The superior mesenteric artery is divided at its origin from the aorta. Long segments of iliac arteries and veins are removed for vascular reconstruction on the back table.

Backbench Preparation of the Pancreas

In relation to other solid organs, the pancreas requires more preparation before transplantation into the recipient. This back table preparation is performed in ice-cold preservation solution to minimize further ischemic injury to the organ. The duodenum is often shortened with a GIA stapler, with care to exclude any gastric tissue and also not to compromise the opening of the ampulla of Vater. The surgeon divides the small bowel mesentery by firing a stapler across this mesentery and then reinforcing it with Prolene suture. The transverse colon mesentery is divided in a similar manner. The surgeon removes the spleen by dividing the vessels in the splenic hilum, being careful not to injure the tail of the pancreas. Finally, the arterial inflow to the graft is reconstructed because the organ has two major sources of blood supply that are not in continuity: the splenic artery, which supplies the pancreatic body and tail, and the superior mesenteric artery, which supplies the pancreatic head. In most instances, arterial reconstruction can be performed with a donor iliac artery as a Y-graft. The internal iliac artery is joined to the splenic artery, and the external iliac artery to the superior mesenteric artery. Both anastomoses are performed in an end-to-end manner with fine Prolene (6-0) sutures. The common iliac artery of the Y-graft can then be anastomosed to the recipient artery to provide the arterial inflow to the pancreas. In rare instances, it is necessary to create a portal vein extension graft on the backbench with donor iliac vein; however, this

technique is avoided when possible because it may increase the risk of venous thrombosis of the pancreas graft.

The Recipient Operation

Unlike the techniques for most solid-organ transplantations, those for transplanting the pancreas have evolved significantly. Partial segmental grafts containing only the pancreatic body and tail were once common; however, this technique is rarely used now. Exocrine secretions were previously managed by pancreatic duct ligation or by injection of a polymer that would cause duct obliteration; today the exocrine secretions are handled by internal drainage.

The two significant areas in pancreas transplantation in which current techniques differ are the drainage of exocrine secretions and the venous drainage of the graft. Exocrine drainage is performed either via the intestinal tract or via the bladder. Throughout most of the 1980s and 1990s, drainage of the pancreatic secretions into the recipient bladder was the most common form of exocrine drainage. This technique is convenient for monitoring organ function by measurement of amylase levels in the urine. However, problems with hematuria, cystitis, bicarbonate loss, and dehydration are all associated with bladder drainage. These complications necessitate surgical revision to enteric drainage in 20% of bladder-drained pancreas recipients. Because of these issues and the lower rejection rates observed with newer immunosuppressive medications, the majority of transplant centers now perform enteric drainage of exocrine secretions. This enteric drainage is either directly into a loop of jejunum in a side-to-side manner or into a Roux limb of jejunum.

The venous drainage of the graft is either to the systemic circulation (via an iliac vein or the inferior vena cava) or to the portal circulation. Portal venous drainage has the advantage of delivering insulin in a more physiologic manner inasmuch as insulin undergoes a "first pass" through the liver and the hyperinsulinemia that results from systemic drainage is avoided. An immunologic advantage of portal drainage has also been observed in several experimental studies in which the delivery of foreign antigen via the portal system results in diminished immune responses. Despite these theoretical advantages, there has been no demonstrable difference in outcomes between portal and systemic venous drained pancreatic transplants in humans, and systemic venous drainage is how the majority of pancreas transplants are performed.

There are two common locations in the abdomen where a pancreas transplant is placed, on the basis of the type of venous drainage planned: either in the pelvis (most commonly the right side) for systemic venous drainage or in the midabdomen for portal venous drainage. When the graft is placed in the pelvis, the donor portal vein is anastomosed to the external iliac vein, the common iliac vein, or the inferior vena cava. In this pelvic position, the graft is oriented with the duodenum inferiorly if bladder drainage is planned (Figure 1, *A*) or with the duodenum in either the superior (see Figure 1, *B*) or inferior direction if enteric drainage is planned. Alternatively, for portal venous drainage, the pancreas is placed in the midabdomen below the transverse colon with the duodenum oriented superiorly. The portal vein of the pancreas is anastomosed to the major branch of the superior mesenteric vein found in the small intestine mesentery in an end-to-side manner (Figure 2). Enteric drainage for exocrine secretions must be used with portal venous drainage. With either technique, the arterial Y-graft of the pancreas is anastomosed in an end-to-side manner with either the iliac artery (common or external) or the aorta.

COMPLICATIONS

The major complications after pancreas transplantation are often technical in nature. Thrombosis (arterial or venous) is more frequent in pancreatic grafts than in other solid-organ transplants, and the

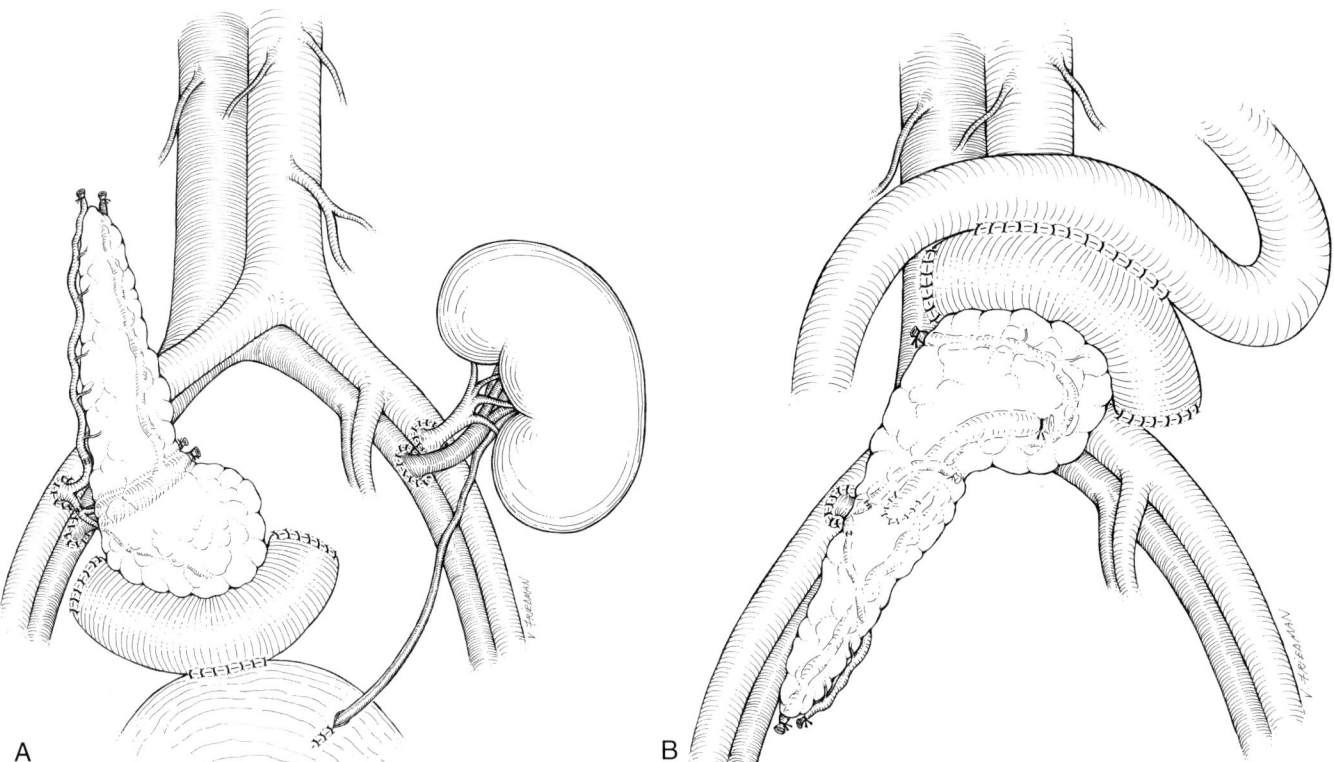

FIGURE 1 Whole-organ pancreas transplantation with systemic venous drainage. The pancreas is placed in the right side of the pelvis with anastomosis of the donor portal vein to the recipient iliac vein for venous drainage. The donor iliac artery Y-graft is sewn to the recipient iliac artery for arterial inflow to the graft. Kidney transplantation can be performed simultaneously with the left-sided iliac vessels. **A,** The donor duodenum is oriented inferiorly to allow anastomosis to the recipient bladder *(shown)* or to the recipient small intestine *(not shown)* for pancreatic exocrine drainage. **B,** Alternatively, the donor duodenum is oriented superiorly to allow anastomosis to the recipient small intestine for pancreatic exocrine drainage.

reported incidence is approximately 5% to 10%. Thrombosis often occurs within the first week after transplantation and is characterized by a sudden increase in serum glucose level. In most instances of thrombosis, graft removal is necessary. Early pancreatitis occurs in 10% to 20% of cases and is largely a reflection of ischemic damage to the gland during preservation and subsequent reperfusion injury. Elevated serum amylase levels and graft edema are characteristic, and graft pancreatitis is usually treated with octreotide. Leakage at the site of pancreatic exocrine drainage is another early complication, with management often dictated by the method of drainage. Bladder-drained transplants with a small leak at the duodenocystostomy can often be managed by Foley catheter drainage of the bladder, which allows the site of leakage to heal over time. Leaks at the duodenojejunostomy in transplants with enteric drainage usually result in peritonitis, and operative intervention is necessary to control the leak.

Rejection after pancreas transplantation was once very common. The diagnosis of pancreas rejection is often difficult, and a variety of indicators are used to help establish the diagnosis. These include increased serum amylase levels, decreased urinary amylase excretion (if bladder drainage is used), biopsy of the pancreas, and the presence of hyperglycemia. Hyperglycemia is a late indicator of rejection, however, and the pancreas is often difficult to salvage once hyperglycemia has occurred. If SPK transplantation is performed, then renal allograft dysfunction can often assist with the diagnosis of pancreatic rejection, since the rejection process is usually occurring in both organs. As a result of the high incidence of rejection and the difficulty in establishing the diagnosis, pancreas transplant recipients usually receive potent induction immunosuppression with a T cell–depleting agent and maintenance therapy with tacrolimus, mycophenolate mofetil, and corticosteroids.

The total amount of immunosuppression that pancreas transplant recipients receive is among the highest for any solid-organ transplant. As a result, they are more susceptible to the complications of immunosuppressive therapy. These complications include infection with opportunistic bacteria, viruses, and fungi; malignancy; and gastrointestinal complications. The high incidence of these complications highlights the importance of effective prophylaxis strategies.

RESULTS

Patient and graft survival after pancreas transplantation have improved significantly since the 1990s. The rates of patient survival are approximately 97% at 1 year and 92% at 3 years after SPK transplantation. Similar patient survival rates are reported for PAK and PTA recipients. Graft survival is variable, depending on the type of pancreas transplant performed (Figure 3). For SPK recipients, 1- and 3-year pancreas graft survival rates are 89% and 80%, respectively. For PAK and PTA recipients, 1- and 3-year pancreas graft survival rates are 84% and 66%, respectively.

The effect of a successful pancreas transplant on the complications associated with diabetes mellitus is debated. Because the successful transplant restores euglycemia and normal hemoglobin A_{1C} levels, most proponents argue that diabetic complications should cease and the damage perhaps be reversed. Neuropathy appears to stabilize and often improve after pancreas transplantation, whereas retinopathy progression is slowed after several years of graft function. The development of diabetic nephropathy in the transplanted kidneys of SPK and early PAK recipients appears to be prevented by successful pancreas transplantation. In PTA recipients, diabetic

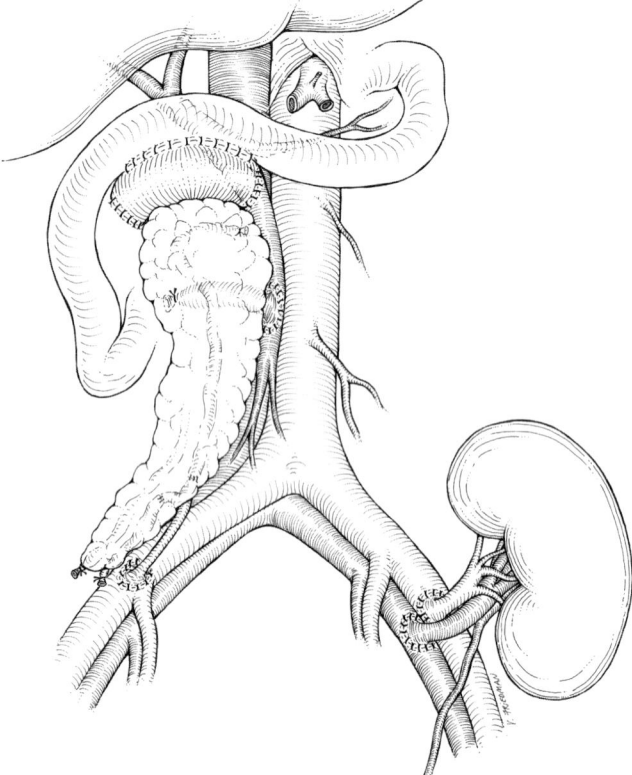

FIGURE 2 Whole-organ pancreas transplantation with portal venous drainage. The pancreas is placed in the midabdomen with anastomosis of the donor portal vein to the major branch of the recipient superior mesenteric vein for venous drainage. The donor iliac artery Y-graft is sewn to the recipient iliac artery for arterial inflow to the graft. The donor duodenum is oriented in the superior direction for anastomosis to the recipient small intestine. Kidney transplantation can be performed simultaneously with either the left *(shown)* or right iliac vessels.

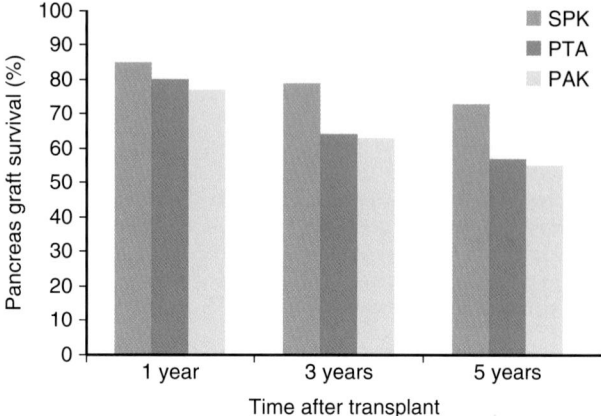

FIGURE 3 Pancreas graft survival rates at 1, 3, and 5 years after whole organ transplantation by transplantation category. *PAK*, pancreas-after-kidney (transplantation); *PTA*, pancreas transplantation alone; *SPK*, simultaneous kidney (and pancreas) transplantation.

nephropathy appears to stabilize after the transplantation; however, the renal benefit is probably outweighed by the detriment to renal function caused by the maintenance immunosuppressive agents, specifically tacrolimus or cyclosporine.

RISK/BENEFIT CONSIDERATIONS

Considerable evidence suggests that a pancreas transplant can stabilize the secondary complications of diabetes and, in some cases, reverse the damage. Despite this evidence, the procedure is considered appropriate for only a subset of patients with type 1 diabetes because of its highly invasive nature in comparison to insulin therapy and because of the potential for significant surgical complications. Therefore, risk/benefit considerations are of utmost importance in pancreas transplantation and play an essential role in the recipient selection processes.

In several important studies, researchers have evaluated the survival benefit of pancreas transplantation by examining large data sets to compare the survival of pancreas recipients with that of patients who were on a waiting list for transplantation but did not receive a pancreas. In this study design, the two patient groups were as similar as possible. Because the indications, risks, and benefits differ depending on whether a patient has underlying renal failure, these analyses were stratified according to whether a patient remained waitlisted or underwent an SPK, PAK, or PTA procedure. All studies revealed a marked survival benefit for patients who received simultaneous pancreas and kidney transplants, with more than a 50% reduction in mortality at 4 years, in comparison with similar patients who remained on the waiting list.

In contrast to the clear survival benefit of SPK transplantation, the data for PAK and PTA recipients are less clear. In one study, the rate of mortality among both PAK and PTA recipients was increased 4 years after transplantation; PAK recipients exhibited a 42% increase in mortality and PTA recipients exhibited a 57% increase in mortality, in comparison with the patients who remained on the waiting list. However, another study demonstrated no difference in mortality rates among PAK and PTA recipients, with a trend toward improved survival in the PAK and PTA recipients in comparison with patients who remained on the waiting list.

There are two important caveats to these risk/benefit studies. The first is that the effect of pancreas transplantation on quality of life was not evaluated in these nonrandomized retrospective analyses and would probably heavily favor the PAK and PTA recipients. Whether this factor would outweigh any survival disadvantage in the short term and the significant cost of these complex procedures has not been evaluated. A second critical outcome measure that is lacking from these studies is the long-term effect of successful pancreas transplantation on the secondary complications of diabetes. There is considerable evidence that diabetic nephropathy, neuropathy, and retinopathy may be positively affected by the long-term normoglycemia conferred by transplantation.

These results substantiate the marked clinical benefit observed in the care of patients who receive simultaneous pancreas and kidney transplants. The relative contributions of the transplanted kidney and of the transplanted pancreas to the overall survival benefit have not been differentiated. This issue is significant because of the marked survival benefit that has been documented in the setting of kidney transplantation alone in diabetic recipients.

Although the survival benefit for SPK recipients is clear, the data demonstrating a lack of survival benefit for PAK and PTA recipients remain controversial. At a minimum, the studies available to date suggest a narrow therapeutic margin for PAK and PTA recipients. Perhaps the most meaningful conclusions that can be drawn at present are that recipients should be selected with the utmost care, donor organs should be optimal, and the surgery should be performed at transplantation centers with good outcomes. The field is dynamic as a result of both improvements in surgical techniques and in perioperative care, and the frequent introduction of new immunosuppressive agents with more favorable safety profiles. It is expected that a clear survival benefit for pancreas transplantation will be established with further advances in the field.

SUGGESTED READINGS

Gruessner RWG, Sutherland DER, editors: *Transplantation of the pancreas*, New York, 2004, Springer.

Gruessner RWG, Sutherland DER, Gruessner AC: Mortality assessment for pancreas transplants, *Am J Transplant* 4:2018–2026, 2004.

Kandaswamy R, Stock PG, Skeans MA, et al: OPTN/SRTR 2011 Annual data report: pancreas, *Am J Transplant* 13(Suppl 1):47–72, 2013.

Venstrom JM, McBride MA, Rother KI, et al: Survival after pancreas transplantation in patients with diabetes and preserved kidney function, *JAMA* 290:2817–2823, 2003.

HEMATOLOGIC INDICATIONS FOR SPLENECTOMY

Tiffany Stoddard, MD, and
Adrian Park, MD, FRCSC, FACS, FCS (ECSA)

OVERVIEW OF SPLENIC STRUCTURE AND FUNCTION

Although the spleen is not an essential organ, it does perform a variety of significant functions. These functions include filtration of blood, destruction of senescent or malformed erythrocytes and the removal of inclusion bodies, antigen processing and clearance, antibody production, hematopoiesis, and storage of erythrocytes, lymphocytes, and platelets. The splenic architecture is designed to maximize its ability to perform these functions. The white pulp is the portion that contains lymphoid nodules, which expand in response to infection or inflammation. The red pulp contains venous sinuses that ultimately drain into the splenic vein. The sinusoids are lined by a fibrocellular network that contains macrophages. The absence of tight junctions between the endothelial cells facilitates diapedesis and further enhances the filtering abilities of this portion of the spleen. The red and white pulps are divided by a marginal zone that contains white blood cells.

Given the functions of the spleen, that this organ has a central role in many hematologic disorders is no surprise. The hematologic indications for splenectomy have evolved throughout history, but there are still many diseases for which this surgery remains an integral part of their management. These disorders cover a broad spectrum of pathologies involving erythrocytes, white blood cells, platelets, and bone marrow.

ERYTHROCYTE DISORDERS

Red blood cell (RBC) disorders can be divided into membrane defects, hemoglobinopathies, enzyme deficiencies, and autoimmune phenomena.

Membrane Defects

This category includes a spectrum of disorders characterized by a deficiency or dysfunction of cytoskeletal elements that results in altered RBC morphology, which increases the susceptibility to destruction. The end result is varying degrees of hemolysis and anemia. The best known disorder in this group is hereditary spherocytosis (HS). It is the most common inherited chronic hemolytic disease in northern Europe and North America. It can be associated with abnormalities in spectrin, ankyrin, band 3 protein, and protein 4.2 that result in a more spherical RBC morphology and render it more susceptible to destruction within the spleen. HS is associated with varying degrees of hemolysis and anemia, but most commonly the anemia is compensated (i.e., normal hemoglobin, reticulocytosis). The severity of HS is measured with hemoglobin and bilirubin levels, the spectrin content, and reticulocyte count. Splenectomy is generally indicated in children with severe cases (hemoglobin, 6 to 8 gm/dL), should be considered in cases of moderate disease, and probably should not be performed in mild cases. Although splenectomy does not correct the membrane deformity, it is curative in that it eliminates the problem of hemolysis and resultant anemia.

Other membrane disorders are elliptocytosis, ovalocytosis, and stomatocytosis. Splenectomy is not necessarily indicated for these conditions, and in the case of stomatocytosis, splenectomy may actually be contraindicated as a result of some reports of an increased incidence of thromboembolic events after splenectomy in this patient population.

Hemoglobinopathies

Various disorders of hemoglobin organization also result in hemolysis. Sickle cell disease and the thalassemias are representative of this category.

Sickle Cell Anemia

Initially described in 1904 by James B. Herrick after his intern found "peculiar elongated and sickle shaped" erythrocytes in a patient's blood smear, sickle cell disease is a defect in hemoglobin that results from a single amino acid substitution on the beta chain that leads to the incorporation of valine instead of glutamic acid. This results in an unstable molecule that is more susceptible to oxidative stresses and makes the red cell less deformable and more susceptible to splenic sequestration and destruction. The spleen is enlarged in the first decade of life but usually atrophies from repeated episodes of vascular occlusion and infarction. Splenectomy may be indicated in a variety of circumstances, such as persistent splenomegaly, acute severe or recurrent sequestration crises, hypersplenism, massive infarction, and splenic abscess. Splenectomy does not reverse sickling.

Thalassemia

The thalassemias comprise a group of disorders that arise from defective synthesis of the alpha and beta globin subunits such that they may simply be reduced or absent. Hemoglobin production and erythrocyte survival are reduced as a result of unstable homotetramers that precipitate as inclusion bodies. These disorders are characterized by varying degrees of hemolysis, ineffective erythropoiesis, lymphadenopathy, and hepatosplenomegaly. The mainstay of treatment is chronic transfusion, but significant risks are associated with iron overload. Splenectomy may be indicated in the setting of painful splenomegaly and in cases of hypersplenism that are associated with transfusion volumes exceeding 225 to 250 mL/kg/y. Splenectomy can be beneficial in protecting against extramedullary hematopoiesis and in decreasing the transfusion requirement. Unfortunately, these patients have very high rates of overwhelming postsplenectomy sepsis. Splenectomy should be individually considered in this population.

Autoimmune Hemolytic Anemias

Autoimmune hemolytic anemias (AIHA) are very rare; when they do occur, they are mostly seen in association with other autoimmune phenomena, such as lupus. AIHA is characterized by the presence of autoantibodies to RBC antigens. Whether the antibodies are associated with a secondary cause must first be determined. In addition, the antibody isotype and the optimal binding temperature for the antibody must be determined. Warm AIHA is defined by an optimal antibody binding temperature of 37°C, and cold AIHA is characterized by an optimal binding temperature of 30°C. Splenectomy has no role in the management of cold AIHA.

Steroids are the primary treatment of choice in warm AIHA. They decrease autoantibody formation and decrease the density of Fc receptors on splenic macrophages. They result in remission in 70% to 85% of patients, but most cases that respond need maintenance steroids to maintain a normal hematocrit value. Splenectomy is considered to be second-line therapy and may be necessary in patients who require high doses of steroids (>15 mg/d) for maintenance of hemoglobin levels. Splenectomy is associated with decreased anti-RBC antibody production and decreased RBC destruction. After splenectomy, as many as 20% of patients experience long-term remission or cure and 50% have a significant decrease in the steroid requirement, but the remainder of patients experience little significant remission.

Enzyme Deficiencies

Erythrocyte enzyme deficiencies are rare, and splenectomy generally has a limited role in their management. Pyruvate kinase deficiency is the only disorder in this group for which splenectomy has shown consistent benefit. It is usually reserved for patients who have severe anemia or who do not tolerate anemia. Although it does not eliminate hemolysis, splenectomy usually results in a 1 to 3 g/dL increase in hemoglobin and may reduce or eliminate the transfusion requirement.

PLATELET DISORDERS

Idiopathic Thrombocytopenic Purpura

Idiopathic thrombocytopenic purpura (ITP) is the most common indication for elective splenectomy. It is characterized by the formation of platelet autoantibodies and the subsequent removal of the platelet-antibody complexes by the reticuloendothelial system. The spleen manufactures the anti-platelet immunoglobulin G (IgG) and plays a major role in the removal of those complexes. Splenomegaly is rarely part of the clinical presentation. The childhood and adult forms differ. The childhood form tends to follow an acute infectious process and commonly spontaneously resolves; adults tend to have a

more chronic course that rarely resolves without medical intervention. Usually no therapy is necessary if the patient does not have any bleeding complications and the platelet count is above 30,000/mm³. Corticosteroids are the first line in management in adult patients who need therapy, but the long-term response rate is about 20% to 30%. Many other medical therapies including intravenous immunoglobulin, various immunosuppressive therapies, and thrombopoietin receptor agonists, have been used as second-line therapies. However, many of these agents require continuous administration to achieve a response and therefore can be associated with toxicities.

Before the introduction of glucocorticoids in 1950, splenectomy was the only treatment modality available. Although it is no longer first-line therapy, it is still indicated in cases of medically refractory disease and in cases that require prolonged steroid therapy. The initial response to splenectomy has been reported to be as high as 80% to 90%, but the sustained response rates to splenectomy are consistently reported lower at around 60%, and some patients may need additional therapy such as thrombopoietin receptor agonists or rituximab to increase platelet counts. Many studies have sought to determine whether there are factors predictive of the response to splenectomy, but the findings have been inconsistent.

Thrombotic Thrombocytopenic Purpura

Thrombotic thrombocytopenic purpura (TTP) is a disease that has been characterized by a deficiency of the metalloproteinase that cleaves the large multimers of von Willebrand's factor and results in platelet clumping in the vasculature and subsequent deleterious effects. The classic features include fever, thrombocytopenia, anemia, renal dysfunction, and neurologic sequelae all secondary to the pathology in the microvasculature. Although the condition is rare, with approximately 11 cases per million per year, early recognition and intervention is critical; the outcome is dramatically improved when timely therapy is implemented.

Historically, splenectomy and steroids in combination was the treatment of choice and resulted in a response rate of only 50% and a mortality rate of 40%. The exact mechanism of the benefits of splenectomy is not completely understood, but it has been postulated that removal of the spleen eliminates a potential source of antimetalloproteinase antibody production and a site of platelet sequestration. Plasma exchange was introduced in 1977 and yielded remission rates of 70% to 80%. Splenectomy continues to play a role in the management of TTP as 20% to 30% of patients have disease resistant to or recurrent after plasma exchange. However, of those patients who undergo splenectomy, as many as 8% to 17% experience relapsing disease.

Myeloproliferative Neoplasia

This category includes essential thrombocythemia, polycythemia vera, primary myelofibrosis, and chronic myelogenous leukemia. These diseases involve proliferation of one or more of the myeloid, erythroid, or megakaryocytic cell lines. Splenomegaly is a common feature of these proliferative disorders because the spleen is a site of extramedullary hematopoiesis. However, splenectomy does not cure any of these disorders and is usually only indicated in cases of symptomatic portal hypertension, drug-refractory splenomegaly associated with severe symptoms (e.g., pain and early satiety), transfusion-dependent anemia, severe thrombocytopenia, and uncontrollable hemolysis.

White Blood Cell Disorders

Similar to the myeloproliferative neoplasias, splenectomy does not correct the disease process but may be indicated in cases of symptomatic splenomegaly or hypersplenism. Some diseases in this category include chronic lymphocytic leukemia (CLL), hairy cell leukemia (HCL), Hodgkin's disease (HD), and non-Hodgkin's lymphoma (NHL).

HCL and HD deserve special mention because splenectomy was historically central to the management of these diseases. HCL is a chronic B cell lymphoproliferative disorder associated with characteristic cells displaying cytoplasmic projections. Splenomegaly and pancytopenia are frequent features of the disease. Before advances in medical therapy, splenectomy was the treatment of choice and resulted in improvement in or normalization of the peripheral smear in 40% to 75%. However, purine analogues are associated with significantly higher hematologic response rates and are the mainstay of therapy currently.

HD is a disorder characterized by the presence of Reed-Sternberg cells and is often associated with bulky lymphadenopathy but less so with massive splenomegaly. Historically, splenectomy was a part of the staging process for HD but, with the introduction of more advanced imaging techniques and the more liberal use of chemotherapy splenectomy, is no longer considered routine in the management of the disease.

PREOPERATIVE CONSIDERATIONS

There are special considerations in preparation for splenectomy. Laparoscopic splenectomy is considered the gold standard technique for most indications for splenectomy, but this technique increases in difficulty with increasing size of the spleen and may be impossible in cases of massive splenomegaly. Therefore, preoperative imaging is helpful to provide information regarding splenic anatomy. The guidelines of the European Association for Endoscopic Surgery suggest that all patients should undergo preoperative imaging, which may be an ultrasound scan to evaluate splenic size and volume. However, computed tomographic (CT) scan may be preferable when more information is needed about splenic anatomy and vasculature. CT scanning may also facilitate the search for accessory splenic tissue, but obtaining this study should not preclude a thorough intraoperative search. Although preferred by some surgeons, the routine use of preoperative splenic artery embolization is not recommended and may in fact lead to severe pain and ischemic complications if performed too far in advance of splenectomy.

Perhaps the most important preoperative consideration is that of vaccination. Patients who have undergone splenectomy have an extremely high risk of septic events compared with the general population, and every precaution should be taken to minimize the risk of these events. In the setting of elective splenectomy, preoperative vaccination against the most common encapsulated pathogens that may cause overwhelming postsplenectomy sepsis is paramount. In addition, antibiotic prophylaxis should also be administered at the time of splenectomy. Another point of consideration is the risk of thrombosis in this population, especially of the portal and splenic venous systems. Therefore, all patients should receive appropriate perioperative prophylaxis.

LAPAROSCOPIC SPLENECTOMY

Since it was initially described in 1991, laparoscopic splenectomy has been adopted as the standard of care for most indications for splenectomy. Although more technically challenging than open splenectomy, the laparoscopic technique has been shown repeatedly to be safe when performed by experienced surgeons, and no difference is found in hematologic outcomes when compared with open splenectomy. There have been concerns that this approach is not amenable to patients with splenomegaly, but again, when performed by experienced surgeons, laparoscopic splenectomy remains the preferred method even in this setting.

POSTOPERATIVE CONSIDERATIONS

Infection is the most common complication after splenectomy. Although rare, the most feared infectious complication is overwhelming postsplenectomy sepsis (OPSS). Although all patients have a significant risk for this commonly fatal complication after splenectomy, patients undergoing splenectomy for hematologic or malignant indications have the greatest risk, and patients who undergo splenectomy for trauma or iatrogenic injury have the lowest risk. The risk is also highest within the first 2 years after surgery; it declines over time but never reaches zero.

Because of the special adaptations of splenic macrophages, they have an increased avidity for antigens that other macrophages lack. Therefore, patients after splenectomy are more susceptible to infections caused by encapsulated organisms, the most common being *Streptococcus pneumoniae*, *Haemophilus influenzae*, and *Neisseria meningitidis*. OPSS rapidly progresses from a febrile illness to circulatory collapse and death within a matter of hours. Because of the rapid progression of disease and often fatal course despite antibiotic therapy, the best management of OPSS includes educating patients and families about the features of the disease and the necessity of prompt evaluation of febrile illness and prevention.

Although difficult to quantify in the literature, vaccination of asplenic patients against the most commonly encountered pathogens is accepted as the mainstay of preventive therapy. The benefits of vaccination against pneumococcus have been reported, and one study observed a decrease in the risk of postsplenectomy sepsis from 7.8% in unvaccinated patients to 2.4% of vaccinated patients during a 17-year follow-up study.

In the setting of elective splenectomy, patients should be vaccinated 2 weeks before surgery to optimize antigen recognition and processing. If splenectomy is performed emergently, vaccinations can be administered after surgery; some advocate delaying administration for 2 weeks to avoid the transient immunosuppression associated with general anesthesia and surgery.

Thromboembolic events are also cited as fairly common and potentially devastating complications after splenectomy. These events include arteriothrombosis (myocardial infarction, stroke), venous thrombosis, and pulmonary hypertension. Some studies have reported an increased risk of arteriosclerotic events in patients who have undergone splenectomy for trauma, HS, and thalassemia. Venous thrombotic events have been more commonly reported. Interestingly, the risk of portal venous thrombosis has been reported to range from 5% to 37% after splenectomy. This phenomenon appears to occur most commonly within the first 2 weeks after surgery, may be related to the technical aspects of surgery, and has not been clearly shown to be influenced by the degree of postoperative thrombocytosis. The rates of deep venous thrombosis and pulmonary embolism have also been noted to occur with increasing frequency after splenectomy, with the greatest risk appearing to be associated with a history of thalassemia. Finally, the incidence of pulmonary hypertension has been reported to be increased after splenectomy. Again, patients with thalassemia appear to have the greatest risk compared with the general population. Various pathologic mechanisms have been proposed to explain these thromboembolic events, including alterations in the lipid profile, a relative hypercoagulable state, and potential alterations in platelet and endothelial activation. No evidence suggests that specific antithrombotic therapy beyond routine perioperative prophylaxis is necessary after splenectomy.

CONCLUSION

Despite medical advances, splenectomy continues to play a significant role in the management of many hematologic disorders. With the appropriate prophylactic measures and careful evaluation of each patient, splenectomy will continue to be a safe procedure.

SUGGESTED READINGS

Crary SE, Buchanan GR: Vascular complications after splenectomy for hematologic disorders, *Blood* 114(14):2861–2868, 2009.

Habermalz B, Sauerland S, Decker G, et al: Laparoscopic splenectomy: the clinical practice guidelines of the European Association for Endoscopic Surgery (EAES), *Surg Endosc* 22(4):821–848, 2008.

Romano F, Garancini M, Ciravegna AL, et al: The implications for patients undergoing splenectomy: postsurgery risk management, *Open Access Surg* 4:21–34, 2011.

Silecchia G, Boru CE, Fantini A, et al: Laparoscopic splenectomy in the management of benign and malignant hematologic diseases, *JSLS* 10:199–205, 2006.

Spelman D, Buttery J, Daley A, et al: Guidelines for the prevention of sepsis in asplenic and hyposplenic patients, *Intern Med J* 38:349–356, 2008.

CYSTS, TUMORS, AND ABSCESSES OF THE SPLEEN

**Thomas McIntyre, MD, and
Michael E. Zenilman, MD**

Cysts, tumors, and abscesses of the spleen are entities that occur rarely but often require surgical treatment (Box 1). Splenectomy in cancer surgery for tumors or processes in other organs, such as pancreatic and gastric, is much more common, as is a splenectomy for trauma and its complications.

CYSTS

Splenic cysts are classified as either primary (true) or secondary (false) based on the presence of an epithelial lining of the lumen. False cysts are also referred to as pseudocysts. The diagnosis of cyst is now made more frequently as a result of the increased use of abdominal imaging. Both true and false cysts can become quite large and symptomatic and can even rupture.

Primary (True) Cysts

Primary cysts with an epithelial lining are either parasitic or nonparasitic. In the United States, approximately 5% of splenic cysts are parasitic. However, in geographic regions where hydatid disease is endemic, such as South America and parts of the Mediterranean region, most splenic cysts are parasitic.

Parasitic

Parasitic cysts occur after infection with the *Taenia echinococcus*. The most common organism is *Echinococcus granulosus,* which forms a unilocular cyst. Rare infections from *E. multilocularis* and *E. vogelii* form multiloculated cysts. These cysts are typically asymptomatic and are associated with manifestations of echinococcal (hydatid) disease elsewhere. The most commonly affected organ is the liver, followed by the spleen and lungs. A parasitic cyst should be suspected if the splenic cyst has wall calcifications and internal daughter cysts. Serologic testing for parasite antibodies should be sent to confirm the diagnosis. In all cases, splenectomy is indicated to avoid the potential complications of rupture and bacterial superinfection.

Splenectomy should be combined with medical management of echinococcal disease. Appropriate intraoperative precautions and surgical techniques should be used to minimize cyst rupture and intraperitoneal contamination.

Nonparasitic

Nonparasitic epithelial-lined cysts account for 20% of all splenic cysts and can be congenital or neoplastic. Neoplastic splenic cysts are exceedingly rare. Congenital cysts are either epidermoid or dermoid

---

BOX 1: Classification of splenic cysts, tumors, and abscesses

Cysts
Primary (true)
  Parasitic
  Nonparasitic
    Congenital
      Epidermoid
      Dermoid
    Neoplastic
Secondary (false), or pseudocysts

Tumors
Malignant
  Lymphoproliferative disease
    Non-Hodgkin's lymphoma
    Hodgkin's disease
    Hairy cell leukemia
    Chronic lymphocytic leukemia
  Myeloproliferative disease
    Chronic myelogenous leukemia
    Myelofibrosis
  Primary tumors
    Angiosarcoma
  Metastatic tumors
Benign
  Hemangioma
  Hamartoma
  Lymphangioma
  Littoral splenic angioma

Abscesses
Bacterial
Fungal
Lymphangioma

Reprinted from McIntyre T, Zenilman ME: Cysts, tumors and abscesses of the spleen. In Cameron J, editor: Current surgical therapy, *ed 9, Philadelphia, 2008, Elsevier Saunders.*

and are usually detected in children or young adults. Epidermoid cysts account for 90% of all nonparasitic true cysts.

Symptomatic splenic cysts can cause left upper quadrant pain, early satiety, and postprandial nausea and vomiting. Of the asymptomatic patients, half have a palpable mass on physical examination. Computed tomographic (CT) scan typically shows a solitary cyst with occasional wall calcifications.

Secondary (False) Cysts or Pseudocysts

Secondary cysts or pseudocysts account for the vast majority of splenic cysts seen in the United States. The spleen is the most commonly injured organ after abdominal trauma, and most secondary cysts are posttraumatic in origin. They may also occur in association with a pancreatic pseudocyst after acute pancreatitis and splenic infarcts or infections. The diagnosis of splenic pseudocysts is increasingly common because of the widespread nonoperative management of splenic trauma and increased use of diagnostic abdominal imaging for trauma.

Treatment

Indications for treatment of splenic cysts are based on the patient's symptoms and cyst diameter. Possible complications of an untreated cyst include: spontaneous rupture with peritonitis or bleeding, abscess formation, hypersplenism, and portal hypertension. For asymptomatic cysts less than 5 cm, conservative treatment is advocated because these cysts often resolve. If the cyst is greater than 5 cm or symptomatic, surgical intervention is recommended. Percutaneous drainage should be avoided because of the high incidence of recurrence and subsequent inflammatory reaction that ensues and renders subsequent operations difficult.

Surgical options include complete or partial splenectomy, unroofing of the cyst, and fenestration. All of these can be accomplished with open or minimally invasive techniques. A spleen-preserving minimally invasive procedure is recommended if possible. Splenic preservation is advocated because the spleen plays an important role in regulation of the circulating blood volume, hematopoiesis, and protection against infection and malignant disease.

Splenectomy

Complete splenectomy is recommended in polycystic cases and when cysts are inaccessible for fenestration or partial splenectomy. Splenectomy should be performed laparoscopically when possible. The laparoscopic procedure is typically performed with the patient in the lateral position and uses four subcostal ports. The spleen is first mobilized from its attachments to the colon and retroperitoneum. The short gastric vessels can be clipped and divided or transected with a Harmonic scalpel (Ethicon Endo-Surgery, Cincinnati, Ohio) or Ligasure device (Covidien, Covidien, Mansfield, Mass). The vascular pedicle can then be isolated and divided. The specimen is placed in a bag, morcellation is performed, and the specimen is removed from one of the subcostal port sites.

Partial Splenectomy

It is believed that at least 25% of the splenic parenchyma should be preserved to ensure adequate postoperative splenic function. Partial splenectomy is recommended if the cyst cavity is deep within the splenic parenchyma. In general, splenic cysts respect the segmental blood supply of the spleen, which makes partial splenectomy possible without major blood loss. Control of splenic arterial inflow and complete splenic mobilization are first performed. Segmental vessels are ligated until a desired line of ischemic demarcation is achieved. Transection and hemostasis of the splenic parenchyma is undertaken

within the cyanotic area with a variety of techniques that include: parenchymal fracture, electrocautery, clips, endoscopic gastrointestinal anastomotic staplers, argon beam coagulation, sutures, and topical hemostatic agents. The use of high-energy tools such as the Harmonic scalpel (Ethicon Endo-Surgery, Cincinnati, Ohio) or Ligasure device (Covidien, Covidien, Mansfield, Mass) make this operation more feasible. Polar lesions are more amenable to a laparoscopic approach.

Unroofing or Fenestration

These techniques are recommended for superficial and peripherally located cysts and can almost always be done laparoscopically. The major problem with unroofing and fenestration is a slightly higher risk of recurrence. In most cases, however, the residual cysts are small and asymptomatic. To reduce the risk of reappearance, the surgeon should remove as much cyst wall as possible and fill the resulting parenchymal defect with omentum.

In traumatic pseudocysts, however, most conservation treatment, such as fenestration or unroofing, ultimately fails, and splenectomy is required.

TUMORS

Malignant

Malignant tumors of the spleen can be grouped into these categories: lymphoproliferative disease, myeloproliferative disease, primary splenic (nonlymphoid) neoplasm, and metastatic lesion. In lymphoproliferative and myeloproliferative diseases, the spleen is rarely the primary site of malignancy and is usually secondarily involved (Figure 1).

Lymphoproliferative Disease

Non-Hodgkin's lymphoma (NHL) is the most common malignant disease that involves the spleen. It is rarely the primary site of

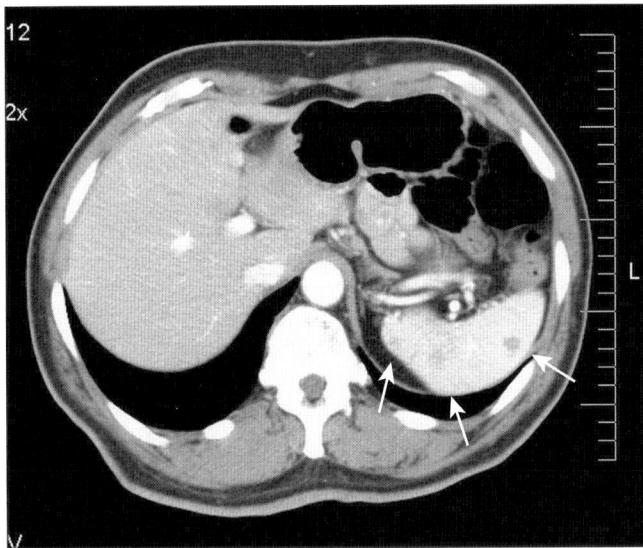

FIGURE 1 This abdominal computed tomographic scan of a 72-year-old man with weight loss and weakness shows multiple hypodense lesions in the spleen *(arrows)*. Splenectomy was performed and revealed non-Hodgkin's lymphoma. Typically in this disease, the diagnosis is made before splenectomy, and surgery is for symptoms, not diagnosis.

malignancy (as seen in Figure 1) but is secondarily involved in up to 40% of all patients with NHL. Once a diagnosis is made, multiagent chemotherapy with or without radiation is the primary mode of treatment. Splenectomy is reserved for patients with development of cytopenia or symptomatic splenomegaly. Splenectomy in these patients does improve peripheral blood counts but has no effect on long-term survival.

Hodgkin's disease is a highly curable disease that progresses in a predictable fashion from one nodal group to another. Critical to effective treatment is accurate staging based on extent of disease. Determination of the presence of infradiaphragmatic disease is difficult in patients with clinical stage I or II supradiaphragmatic disease. Up to 35% of all patients with stage I and II disease have occult splenic disease or upper abdominal nodal involvement. This was the rational for staging laparotomy in the past. Because of the dramatic improvements in radiographic imaging and chemotherapeutic regimens, currently less than 5% of patients require staging laparotomy. An abdominal CT scan is currently the principal investigational tool for infradiaphragmatic disease, although staging laparotomy is still considered the most accurate technique to determine abdominal disease. Staging laparotomy should be performed only if results would change the final treatment regimen. The staging procedure can be safely done laparoscopically and should include inspection of the peritoneum, splenectomy, and wedge; core biopsies of the liver; and biopsies of the para-aortic, iliac, portal, and mesenteric lymphatic node basins.

Hairy cell leukemia is a lymphocytic leukemia that manifests as splenomegaly and pancytopenia. In patients with symptomatic hypersplenism, splenectomy is beneficial. It is associated with improved overall survival, likely because of the reduced risk of complications associated with pancytopenia.

Chronic lymphocytic leukemia (CLL) is treated with splenectomy only in patients with symptomatic splenomegaly or cytopenia resulting from hypersplenism. No increase in survival is seen; however, there is a substantial reduction in peripheral lymphocyte count and transfusion requirements.

Myeloproliferative Disease

Chronic myelogenous leukemia (CML) accounts for 30% of all adult leukemia. Splenectomy during the blastic or accelerated phase of the disease has been shown to improve quality of life and decrease transfusion requirements. Myelofibrosis is a rare disorder that is universally fatal, with mean survival time of 5 years. Splenectomy has a palliative role in reducing transfusion requirements and improving quality of life.

Primary (Nonlymphoid) Neoplasms

Angiosarcoma is the most common nonlymphoid malignant tumor of the spleen. These tumors grow rapidly and metastasize early and thus carry a poor prognosis. Splenectomy is indicated but rarely curative. Other exceedingly rare malignancies include fibrosarcoma, leiomyosarcoma, plasmacytoma, malignant fibrous histiocytoma, and vascular tumors, such as hemangiosarcoma and lymphangiosarcoma.

Metastatic Tumors

Metastatic involvement of the spleen from nonlymphoid malignant disease is rare and usually a manifestation of disseminated disease. Splenic metastases are usually seen in association with widespread visceral metastases. The infrequent involvement of the spleen may be a function of the immunologic role of the spleen and its ability to eliminate microscopic metastatic disease. Cancers known to metastasize to the spleen include breast, lung, melanoma, ovarian, endometrial, gastric, colonic, and prostate. Splenectomy is acceptable when thorough workup reveals solitary splenic metastases and the primary tumor is controlled. Splenectomy can also be justified in conjunction with an abdominal debulking procedure for ovarian carcinoma.

Benign

The discovery of benign splenic tumors has become more common as a result of improvements in CT technology and its widespread use. They are usually found incidentally and are seldom symptomatic. Hemangiomas are the most common benign tumors of the spleen. They are typically associated with hemangiomas of other intra-abdominal organs, particularly the liver. The associated risks include rupture and hemorrhage. These tumors do not require treatment unless they become symptomatic as a result of splenomegaly or they produce a consumptive coagulopathy, thrombocytopenia, microangiopathic anemia, or disseminated intravascular coagulation. There have been recent reports of treated hemangiomas with radiofrequency ablation, but this should only be considered in small tumors and only if symptomatic.

A tumor called littoral splenic angioma, described in 1991, is comprised of the sinus-lining cells of the spleen, also called littoral cells. These solid tumors are almost always asymptomatic and are diagnosed at pathology. They are vascular in origin and may be related to the integrity of the immune system. Interestingly, splenic littoral angiomas have been described in patients undergoing anti–tumor necrosing factor (TNF) alpha antibody therapy; a therapy commonly used for patients with inflammatory bowel disease and sarcoidosis.

Hamartomas of the spleen can be either cystic or solid. These lesions very rarely become symptomatic because of their size, and splenectomy is reserved only as a necessary diagnostic maneuver.

Lymphangiomas are benign cystic tumors that are rare and occasionally lead to hypersplenism. They are commonly associated with lymphangioma of the liver and lesions in other parts of the body, including the lung, skin, and bone. Splenectomy is only indicated to alleviate symptoms or confirm a diagnosis. Other benign tumors of the spleen include lipoma, angiomyolipoma, leiomyoma, hemangioendothelioma, and hemangiopericytoma.

Treatment

Splenectomy is accepted as the surgical procedure for nearly all tumors of the spleen that require treatment. Some small benign lesions might be amenable to partial splenectomy, but for malignant disease, splenectomy is the rule. Several series comparing splenectomy for benign and malignant tumors have shown that splenectomy can be safely performed laparoscopically for malignant disease with similar outcomes.

ABSCESSES

Splenic abscesses are rare, with reported incidence rates after intra-abdominal abscesses of less than 0.5%. In untreated patients, mortality rates can approach 100%; but with appropriate treatment, mortality rates are reduced to only 10% to 15%. Interestingly, recent reports document splenic rupture after intra-abdominal abscess, pelvic abscess, and splenic abscess (see subsequent discussion), which increases mortality.

Most abscesses arise from hematogenous spread from a distant primary septic focus, such as bacterial endocarditis, infected splenic arterial aneurysms, intra-abdominal infections including fecal peritonitis, diverticulitis, appendicitis, pyelonephritis, and direct introduction of bacteria into the bloodstream from intravenous drug use. They may also arise as a secondary infection in a splenic hematoma after a noninfectious embolic event or trauma. Recent reports have documented splenic abscess after sleeve gastrectomy for bariatric surgery; so, with the increase in upper abdominal gastric surgery, more reports may be seen.

Finally, there can also be direct penetration of the splenic parenchyma from an adjacent intra-abdominal process, such as a perforated ulcer, pancreatitis, or colon cancer. Because of the increased incidence of human immunodeficiency virus (HIV) and more aggressive chemotherapy and immunosuppression for organ transplantation, immunodeficiency has become a more frequent risk factor.

Most patients present with fever, fatigue, abdominal pain, and leukocytosis. Only about half of patients have positive blood cultures. CT scan is the diagnostic procedure of choice; it shows a low-density lesion that does not enhance with intravenous (IV) contrast. The gram-positive aerobic organisms *Staphylococcus* and *Streptococcus* are the most common bacteria cultured. Gram-negative organisms like *Salmonella* are also seen, as is polymicrobial flora. Fungal organisms such as *Candida* and *Aspergillosis* represent approximately 8% of all cases and are more commonly found in patients with immunosuppression.

Splenic Rupture

Recent reports of splenic rupture have followed not only abscesses or infarcts but also colonoscopy. So, the presentation of a patient with severe abdominal pain, hypotension, and decreased hematocrit should suggest this diagnosis. These patients also present with nausea, emesis, and dizziness (Figure 2).

Splenic rupture after chemotherapy for hematologic disease has also been observed (Figure 3).

Splenic Infarct

Splenic infarction can occur after upper abdominal surgery such as pancreatectomy, bariatric surgery, splenic torsion (e.g. the wandering spleen), and sepsis. Spontaneous infarction has been associated with collagen vascular diseases, sarcoidosis, and, of course, chronic autoinfarction in sickle cell disease. Recently, a number of patients have been reported with acute splenic infarction after high-altitude travel (e.g., airplane); they are typically carriers of the sickle cell trait (Figure 4). Hypoxemia of altitude is believed to induce sickling and infarction. Although typically limited to only portions of the spleen and with a benign course, acute infarction as depicted can require surgery.

Treatment

Splenectomy is the definitive treatment for splenic abscesses. Treatment with IV antibiotics remains a cornerstone of treatment as well. Broad-spectrum antibiotics should be used once the diagnosis is made until the regimen can be tailored to specific culture data. Percutaneous aspiration can be used to direct antimicrobial therapy. Percutaneous drainage is increasing in popularity as a treatment option and is safe in carefully selected patients. Failure rates for percutaneous drainage range from 50% to 60%, and patients require lengthier hospital stays. It should be reserved for patients unable to tolerate surgery or as a temporizing measure for patients needing stabilization. Despite the rarity of these lesions, several series have shown that splenectomy can be done laparoscopically in this cohort of patients. The authors typically begin laparoscopically to perform an "intact" splenectomy, but many times the abscess is entered during surgery and easily drained with the laparoscopic suction. One can expect the patients to need intensive monitoring after surgery, both for infection and bleeding. Use of energy sources such as described earlier and argon beam electrocoagulation make surgery more straightforward.

Treatment of splenic rupture can also be performed laparoscopically; the authors' preference is with hand-port assistance. However, the open technique still gives the best exposure, control of vessels, lavage, and drainage.

When no tumor is present or a benign process is suspected, the spleen can be removed from a laparoscopic port with morcellation.

OVERWHELMING POSTSPLENECTOMY SEPSIS

Splenectomy increases a patient's risk for routine bacterial infection and, more importantly, overwhelming systemic sepsis usually associated with gram-positive encapsulated organisms. The incidence rate of overwhelming postsplenectomy sepsis (OPSS) is highest in children, as high as 4%, but adults are also considered to be at risk. The mortality rate of OPSS is approximately 50%. Vaccinations against *Streptococcus pneumoniae, Haemophilus influenzae*, and *Neisseria* meningitis should be given 2 weeks before surgery. If this is not possible, vaccination should be delayed until 2 week after surgery. Given that the highest incidence of overwhelming postsplenectomy sepsis has been shown to be in the first year after splenectomy, some advocate providing low-dose prophylactic penicillin to patients at high risk in the first year after operation.

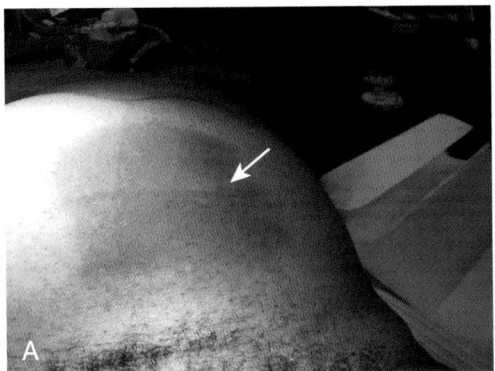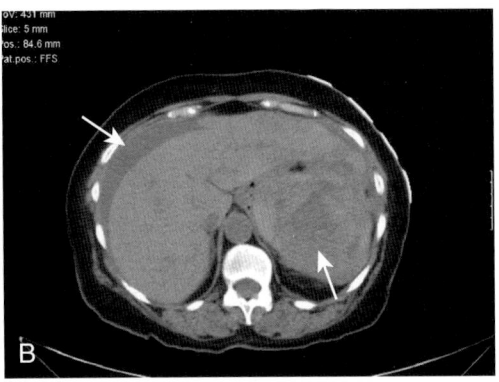

FIGURE 2 Splenic rupture after colonoscopy. This 55-year-old patient was seen 24 hours after colonoscopy with abdominal pain, hypotension, and decreased hematocrit values. **A,** She presented with a Cullen's sign; and **B,** computed tomographic scan showed ruptured spleen *(bottom arrow)* and hemoperitoneum *(top arrow)*. Open splenectomy was performed, and the patient was discharged from the hospital within 1 week. *(Photographs courtesy of Lisa Dresner, MD.)*

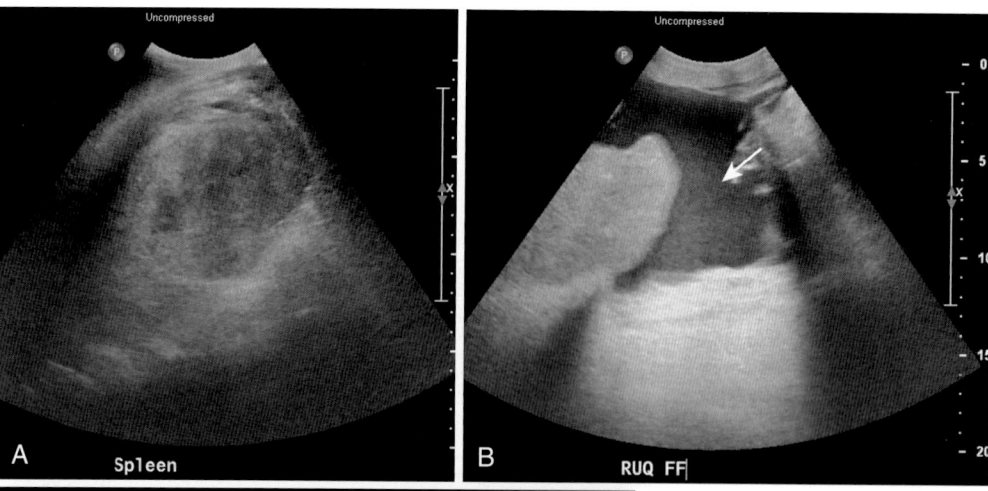

FIGURE 3 A 73-year-old patient presented with syncope, hypotension, and acute anemia 2 weeks after completing chemotherapy for appendiceal B-cell lymphoma. A computed tomographic (CT) scan 2 days before presentation was normal. After presentation to the emergency room, Focused Abdominal Sonography for Trauma (FAST) showed: **A,** splenic parenchymal disruption; and **B,** free fluid in the abdomen around the liver. **C,** CT scan showed the same. Emergency surgery confirmed ruptured spleen *(Photographs courtesy of Enrique Daza, MD.)*

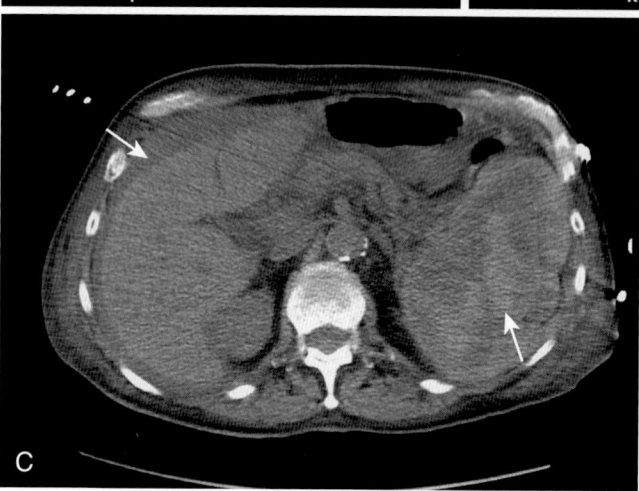

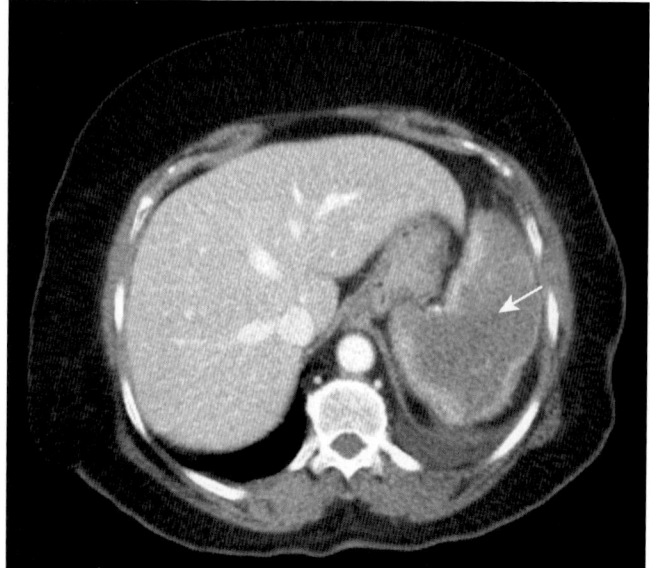

FIGURE 4 Computed tomographic scan of a patient with sickle cell trait who presented with left upper quadrant pain, nausea and vomiting, leukocytosis, and splenic infarct *(arrow)* 7 days after a 4-hour airplane trip. Open splenectomy confirmed the diagnosis.

SUGGESTED READINGS

Carbonell A, Kercher K, Matthews B, et al: Laparoscopic splenectomy for splenic abscess, *Surg Laparosc Enodosc Percutan Tech* 14(5):289–291, 2004.

Cordesmeyer S, Pützler M, Titze U, et al: Littoral cell angioma of the spleen in a patient with previous pulmonary sarcoidosis: a TNF-α related pathogenesis? *World J Surg Oncol* 19(9):106, 2011; PubMed PMID: 21929754; PubMed Central PMCID: PMC3187736.

Feldman LS: Laparoscopic splenectomy: standardized approach, *World J Surg* 35(7):1487–1495, 2011; PubMed PMID: 21424869.

Koshenkov VP, Németh ZH, Carter MS: Laparoscopic splenectomy: outcome and efficacy for massive and supramassive spleens, *Am J Surg* 203(4):517–522, 2012; Epub 2011; PubMed PMID: 21924403.

Singla S, Keller D, Thirunavukarasu P, et al: Splenic injury during colonoscopy: a complication that warrants urgent attention, *J Gastrointest Surg* 16(6):1225–1234, 2012; Epub 2012; PubMed PMID: 22450952.

Splenic Salvage Procedures: Therapeutic Options

Hadley K. H. Wesson, MD, MPH, and
Kent A. Stevens, MD, MPH

The management of splenic injury in the setting of trauma has changed over the past five decades and continues to evolve as our understanding of therapeutic options improves. Since the 1960s, we have shifted from an era in which blunt splenic injuries in both adults and children were treated with splenectomy to an era in which nonoperative management (NOM) has become the dominant modality for splenic salvage.

The advantage of splenic salvage arises from concerns regarding risks associated with the asplenic state, including overwhelming post-splenectomy infection, a well-known but rare complication. While the focus of this chapter is on splenic salvage methods, including NOM, splenorrhaphy, and partial splenectomy, the role of definitive operative management with splenectomy in the hemodynamically unstable patient with splenic injury cannot be overemphasized.

NONOPERATIVE MANAGEMENT

Selective NOM of blunt splenic injuries in children has been practiced for more than four decades, first described in 1968 by Toronto's Hospital for Sick Children as an alternative to splenectomy in hemodynamically stable children. Despite the acceptance of this approach within the pediatric population, there was initial reluctance to adapt this to the adult population. Considerable advancements have since occurred. The American Association for the Surgery of Trauma developed the Organ Injury Scale for the spleen to aid in therapeutic and research decisions (Table 1), and computed tomographic (CT) sacn for blunt injury has become the standard of care. By the mid-1990s, NOM in the adult population had increased fivefold.

As NOM continued to develop as a mainstay option, surgeons sought to determine appropriate candidates for NOM. NOM was attempted for clinical conditions in which it was previously contraindicated, including hypotension responsive to fluid, high-grade splenic injury; neurologic impairment; a requirement for more than 2 units of blood; immunologic disease; and advanced age. While some conditions were associated with poor outcomes, others appeared acceptable. The need for a clear and standardized approach to NOM prompted the Eastern Association for the Surgery of Trauma (EAST) to generate evidence-based guidelines regarding NOM in 2003 and subsequently updated in 2011 (Table 2). As a result, today between 53% and 77% of patients with blunt splenic injury are managed nonoperatively.

Guidelines for Nonoperative Management

Patients with blunt splenic injuries must meet five criteria to be considered for NOM: (1) hemodynamic stability; (2) CT documentation and classification of the injury; (3) absence of intra-abdominal or retroperitoneal injuries mandating operative intervention; and (4) transfusion of fewer than 2 units of packed red blood cells (pRBC); and (5) be managed in a hospital facility that can provide continuous monitoring and serial exams. Exclusion criteria include patients in whom coagulopathy cannot be reversed and patients who must receive urgent anticoagulation therapy, such as in the setting of a vascular injury requiring anticoagulation.

The 2011 EAST guidelines use level II evidence to recommend that in a hemodynamically stable patient, the severity of the splenic injury (according to the grade of the injury or degree of hemoperitoneum), and age are not contraindications for NOM. The guidelines also state abdominal CT scan is the most reliable method to identify and assess the severity of the injury to the spleen in hemodynamically stable patients.

Approach to Nonoperative Management

An approach to management of splenic injuries is illustrated in Figure 1. The first step in deciding to pursue NOM is determined by the patient's hemodynamic stability. Thus it is important to establish standardized definitions and degrees of hemodynamic instability. In an effort to address this, the Western Trauma Association proposed a scoring system in 2006 to improve management and consistency of definitions of hemodynamic stability:

Grade 0: No significant hypotension (systolic blood pressure < 90 mm Hg) or serious tachycardia (heart rate > 130 beats/minute)

Grade 1: Hypotension or tachycardia by report but not reported in the emergency department

Grade 2: Hypotension or tachycardia responsive to initial volume loading with no ongoing fluid or pRBC requirement

Grade 3: Hypotension or tachycardia responsive to initial volume loads with modest ongoing fluid (<250 mL/hr) or pRBC transfusion

Grade 4: Hypotension or tachycardia only responsive to more than 2 liters of volume loading and the need for vigorous ongoing fluid infusion (>250 mL/hr) and pRBC transfusion

Grade 5: Hypotension unresponsive to fluid and pRBC transfusion

This scoring system can guide further management. For patients who are hemodynamically unstable on initial presentation, remain unstable despite fluid administration (e.g., grade IV or V), and have a positive result from a focused assessment with sonography for trauma (FAST) examination, emergent operative management and splenectomy are necessary. For patients whose FAST exam result was negative but who are hemodynamically unstable, intra-abdominal hemorrhage and operative intervention should be promptly initiated.

For hemodynamically stable adult patients with an isolated blunt splenic injury, NOM is currently the standard of care. NOM in adults is attempted in approximately 85% of all patients with blunt splenic injury. Failure rates are dependent on the grade of the injury and range from 8% to 38%. The optimal success rate of NOM is achieved when CT scanning is combined with serial clinical examinations. Patients should be actively observed with serial physical examinations, continuous monitored vital signs, and serial hemoglobin levels. During this period of active observation, if patients become hemodynamically unstable, need 2 or more units of blood, or develop peritonitis, emergent splenectomy is indicated. If the patient is stable, a repeat CT scan should be obtained. If the CT scan shows a larger hemoperitoneum or active bleeding, the patient should be taken to the operating room.

Role of Angioembolization

If the initial abdominal CT scan shows evidence of ongoing bleeding, splenic angiographic embolization (SAE) should be considered. SAE

525

TABLE I: Organ injury scale for the spleen by the American Association for the Surgery of Trauma

Grade	Injury type	Description of injury
I	Hematoma	Subcapsular, nonexpanding, <10% surface area
	Laceration	Capsular tear, nonbleeding, <1 cm parenchymal depth
II	Hematoma	Subcapsular, nonexpanding, 10%–50% surface area; intraparenchymal, <5 cm in depth
	Laceration	Capsular tear, active bleeding, 1–3 cm parenchymal depth that does not involve a trabecular vessel
III	Hematoma	Subcapsular, >50% surface area or expanding; ruptured subcapsular or parenchymal hematoma with active bleeding; intraparenchymal hematoma ≥ 5 cm or expanding
	Laceration	>3 cm parenchymal depth or involving trabecular vessels
IV	Laceration	Laceration involving segmental or hilar vessels producing major devascularization (>25% of spleen)
V	Laceration	Completely shattered spleen
	Vascular	Hilar vascular injury with devascularized spleen

TABLE 2: Criteria for nonoperative management of blunt splenic injury

1. Hemodynamic stability
2. Documented computed tomographic classification of injury
3. Absence of additional injuries requiring operative intervention
4. Transfusion of fewer than 2 units of packed red blood cells

Source: East Associated for the Surgery of Trauma (EAST) AdHoc Committee on Practice Management Guideline Development. Non-operative management of blunt injury to the liver and spleen 2003. Available at: http://east.org.tpg.

is an adjunct in NOM. Based on level II evidence, EAST guidelines suggest SAE is appropriate in hemodynamically stable patients with CT scan findings of contrast extravasation, pseudoaneurysm or arteriovenous fistula, moderate hemoperitoneum, high-grade injury (grades IV–V), or persistent splenic bleeding..

A 2004 multicenter study by the Western Trauma Association showed the grade of splenic injury was the strongest predictor of successful SAE. More than 90% of patients with grade III splenic injuries and 80% of patients with grades IV and V splenic injuries were successfully managed with SAE. This is significantly higher than NOM success rates that did not use SAE: the 2000 EAST multi-institutional trial found observation alone (i.e. without SAE) had successful splenic salvage rates of only 80%, 66.7%, and 25% for grades III, IV, and V injuries, respectively.

While SAE can extend the application of NOM, the impact of SAE in the algorithmic approach to splenic trauma has not been well studied. Consensus has not been reached on either the indications for embolization or the optimal site (proximal vs segmental) of embolization. In theory, proximal (main) splenic artery embolization enables clot formation by decreasing distal flow into the parenchyma. Through selective distal coil embolization, a catheter is placed over a wire adjacent to the intraparenchymal vascular injuries, which are then embolized with Gelfoam (Pfizer, New York, NY) or a small coil. In practice, proximal embolization appears to be more common than distal embolization.

Complications associated with proximal and distal embolization are under investigation. Current studies show rebleeding following embolization ranges between 4.7% and 9.0%. Perfusion pressure to the spleen can also decrease, and this results in splenic ischemia. While hemostasis can be achieved this way, concerns about splenic function remain, and avoidance of surgical splenectomy may not result in the preservation of a functional spleen. Following proximal embolization, patients may face the same impaired immune response risks and infectious complications as those faced by patients who underwent splenectomy.

Progression of Care

The 2011 EAST Guidelines Update recommend that the need for follow up imaging be based on the patient's clinical status. Patients managed nonoperatively can be discharged in as early as 3 to 4 days. However, guidelines recommending the duration of hospitalization, duration the patient should remain NPO (nothing by mouth), duration of bed rest, initiation of deep venous thromboembolism prophylaxis, and resumption of normal activity have not been established. Surgeons' attitudes and practices regarding these issues have been surveyed. In 2005, 50% of polled EAST members recommended patients with grade I or II splenic injuries return to light normal activity in 2 weeks, while patients with higher-grade injuries wait at least 4 to 6 weeks.

Results of Nonoperative Management

NOM has been highly successful in hemodynamically stable patients. An EAST 2000 multicenter trial showed an 89% success rate of NOM without the use of SAE. More recent studies incorporating SAE as a standard of care show higher rates of success: a recent retrospective review of 398 patients found a 97% success rate of NOM that included SAE in those that qualified. Common causes of failure are bleeding in the first 96 hours, abscess formation, and splenic artery pseudoaneurysm.

OPERATIVE SPLENIC SALVAGE

When the patient's condition necessitates operative intervention, the surgeon should be aware of options to pursue splenectomy versus splenic salvage techniques. Operative splenic salvage should be approached cautiously. It should not be attempted in unstable patients undergoing damage control surgery or patients whose injuries warrant expeditious splenectomy, such as patients with severe head injury. In the author's experience, splenorrhaphy and partial splenectomy is relatively infrequent: in the past 5 years at the Virginia Commonwealth University Medical Center's level I trauma center of the 683 splenic injuries, 158 were managed operatively, of which 146 were managed with splenectomy, 12 were managed with splenorrhaphy, and none were managed with partial splenectomy.

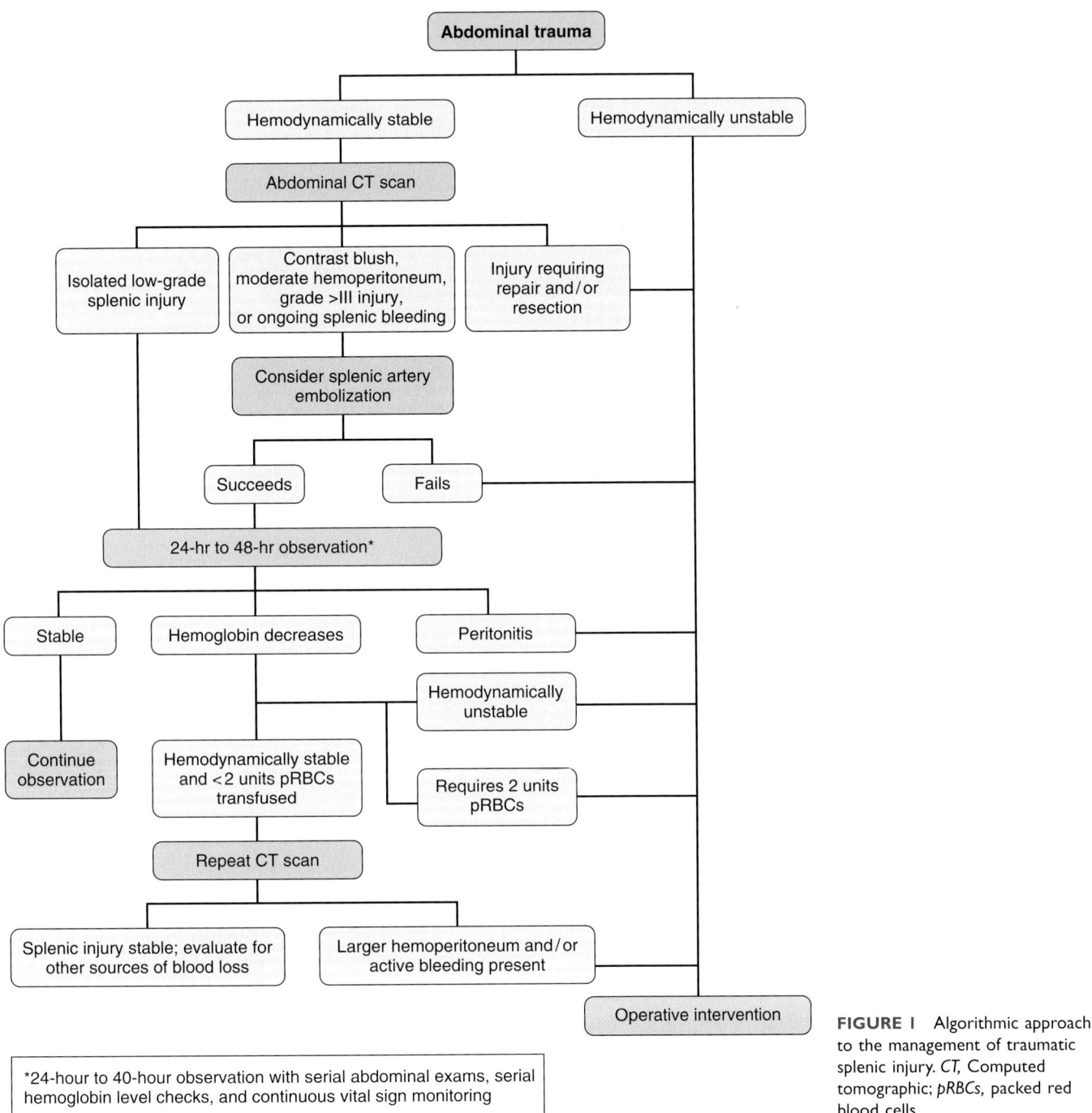

FIGURE I Algorithmic approach to the management of traumatic splenic injury. *CT,* Computed tomographic; *pRBCs,* packed red blood cells.

*24-hour to 40-hour observation with serial abdominal exams, serial hemoglobin level checks, and continuous vital sign monitoring

Operative management should be performed through a midline incision. The abdomen should be thoroughly examined to evaluate for other intra-abdominal injuries. To visualize the extent of splenic injury, adequate exposure and mobilization are mandatory. Dividing the avascular lienophrenic, lienorenal, and lienocolic ligaments allows the spleen to be mobilized from the retroperitoneum. The lesser sac is entered by removing the omentum from the left transverse colon. If the only injury is to the spleen and the patient is hemodynamically stable, splenic splenorrhaphy or partial splenectomy can be considered.

Splenic Splenorrhaphy

Small capsular tears may be managed with argon beam coagulation, an electrocoagulation system that achieves hemostasis using inert gas as a medium to conduct radiofrequency energy. Hemostasis can also be achieved using hemostatic agents such as microfibrillar collagen (Avitene; Davol, Cranston, RI), absorbable gelatin sponge (Gelfoam, Pfizer, New York, NY), or methylcellulose (Surgicel; Johnson & Johnson, New Brunswick, NJ). Deep lacerations can be repaired by placing horizontal mattress sutures using a 2-0 synthetic monofilament such as Prolene (Ethicon, Piscataway, NJ). Sutures can be placed either directly or over Dacron strips or pledgets (Invista Inc, Wichita, Kans) (Figure 2). Omentum can also be placed into the laceration to act as a hemostatic agent before approximating the defect with mattress sutures.

A technique that is occasionally applicable to patients with macerated splenic injuries not amenable to hemostatic agents or suture splenorrhaphy is to use a mesh wrap. Once the spleen is mobilized, a sheet of synthetic absorbable polyglycolic mesh is wrapped around

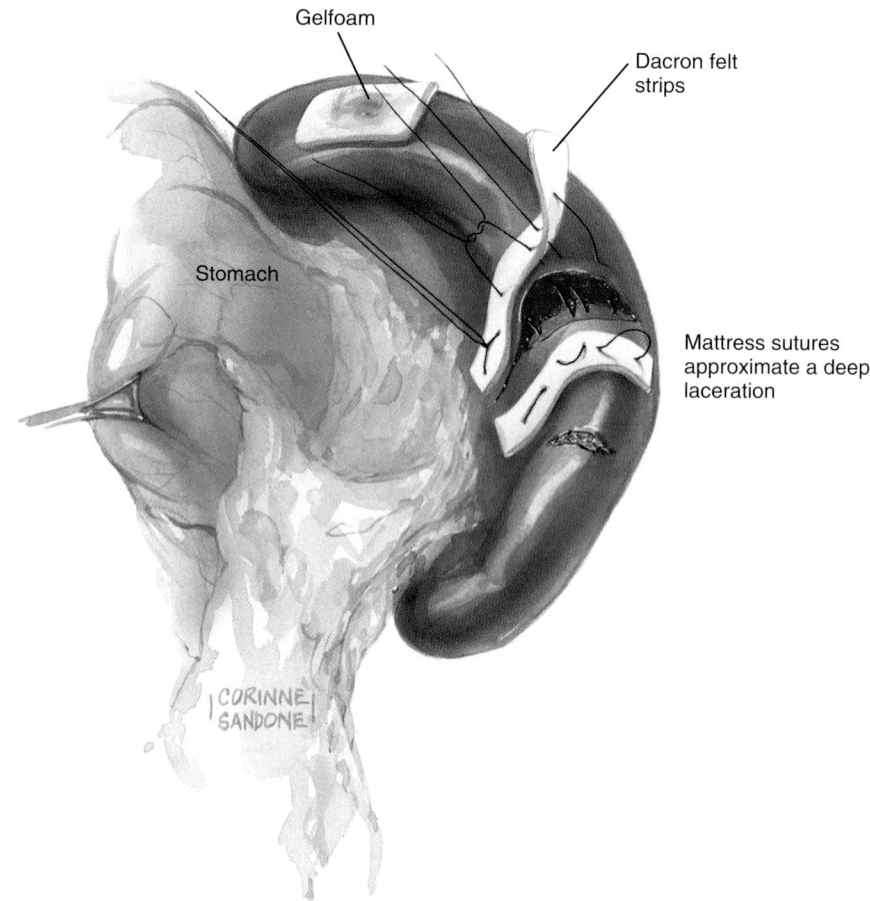

FIGURE 2 Horizontal mattress sutures with Dacron strips approximate the laceration. *(From Cameron JL, Sandone C: Atlas of gastrointestinal surgery, 2nd ed, vol 2, 2013; used with permission from PMPH-USA, Shelton, Conn.)*

the spleen and gathered at the hilum, where a purse string suture is placed, thereby compressing the spleen to achieve hemostasis. Care should be taken to ensure the vasculature at the hilum is not compressed.

Partial Splenectomy

If the splenic laceration is more substantial and extends into the splenic hilum, maneuvers to control hemorrhage and preserve the spleen in its entirety may not be adequate. In such cases, a partial splenic resection can be performed by removing the nonsalvageable portion of the spleen. A partial splenectomy may be performed if ligating of a branch of the splenic artery results in significant hemostasis and at least half of the splenic parenchyma attached to an identifiable vessel is viable.

Manual compression of the spleen with a Mikulicz pad and/or temporarily cross-clamping the splenic hilum with a DeBakey bulldog clamp may be required to control the bleeding laceration. After the bleeding from the laceration has been controlled, the omentum can be divided anterior to the splenic hilum and the short gastrics ligated. By exposing the spleen, the extent of the splenic laceration and involvement of the splenic hilum can be assessed (Figure 3). The branch of the splenic artery feeding the lacerated pole is ligated and divided. The corresponding splenic vein branch is likewise ligated and divided (Figure 4). The residual splenic parenchyma is then divided with electrocautery, and the resected margin of the spleen can be oversewn using mattress sutures with Dacron stripes or omentum.

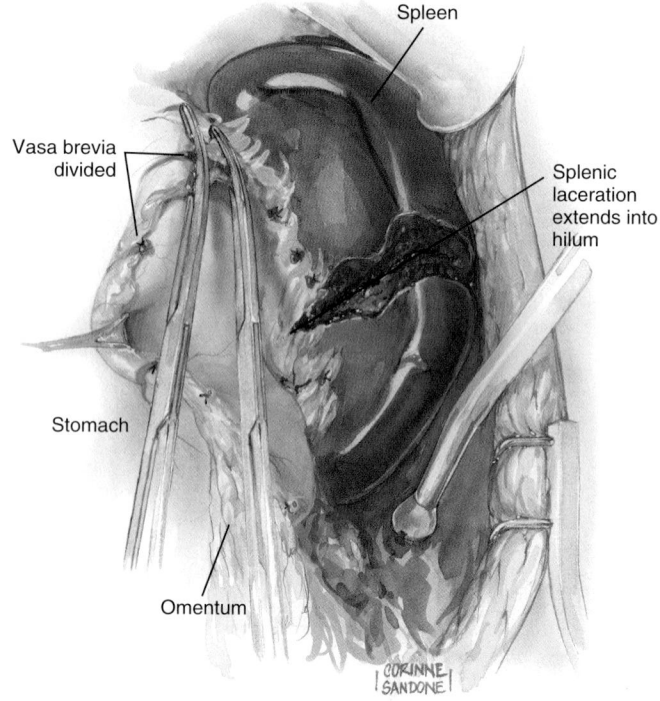

FIGURE 3 Deep laceration extending into the splenic hilum. *(From Cameron JL, Sandone C: Atlas of gastrointestinal surgery, 2nd ed, vol 2, 2013; used with permission from PMPH-USA, Shelton, Conn.)*

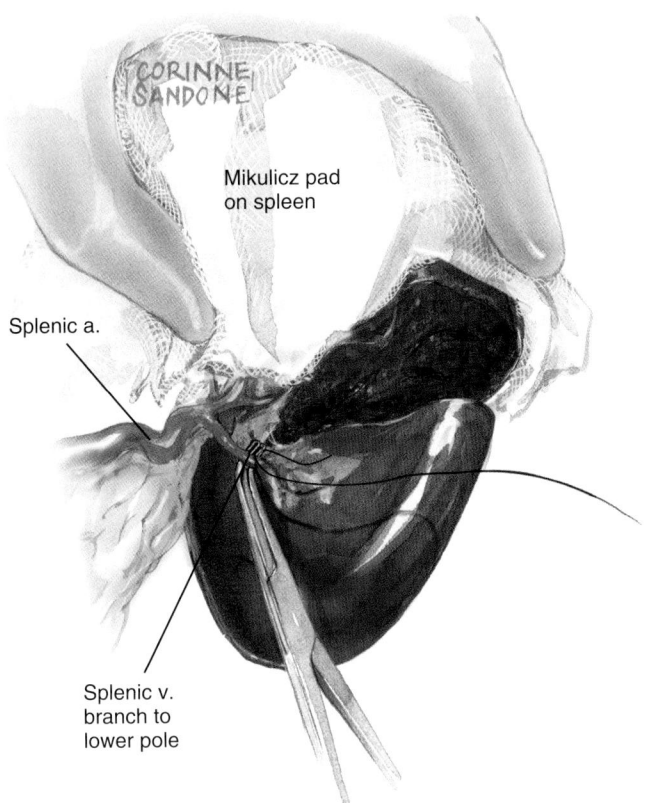

Mikulicz pad
on spleen

Splenic a.

Splenic v.
branch to
lower pole

FIGURE 4   Partial splenectomy involves ligating and dividing the branches of the splenic artery and vein while applying manual compression as necessary. *(From Cameron JL, Sandone C:* Atlas of gastrointestinal surgery, *2nd ed, vol 2, 2013; used with permission from PMPH-USA, Shelton, Conn.)*

RECOMMENDATIONS

Careful selection, CT scan imaging, and serial clinical examinations are crucial to the successful NOM of patients with blunt splenic injuries. The use of angioembolization has furthered our ability to salvage a patient's spleen without operative intervention, and angio-embolization should be used liberally when indicated and available.

SUGGESTED READINGS

Haan HM, for the Western Trauma Association Multi-Institutional Trials Committee: Splenic embolization revisited: a multicenter review, *J Trauma* 56:542, 2004.

Peitzman AB, Heil B, Rivera L, et al: Blunt splenic injury in adults: multi-institutional study of the Eastern Association for the Surgery of Trauma, *J Trauma* 70:1026–1031, 2011.

Schnuriger, B, Inaba K, Konstantinidis A, et al: Outcomes of proximal versus distal splenic artery embolization after trauma: a systematic review and meta-analysis, *J Trauma* 70:252–260, 2011.

Stassen NA, Bhullar I, Cheng JD, et al: Selective nonoperative management of blunt splenic injury: An eastern associated for the surgery of trauma practice management guideline, *J Trauma* 73:S294–S300, 2012.

HERNIA

INGUINAL HERNIA

Shirin Towfigh, MD, and Leigh Neumayer, MD, MS

OVERVIEW

Inguinal hernia repair remains the most common general surgical procedure in the United States, with over 800,000 performed annually. It has a long history, and thus a wide variety of techniques have been described. The goals of inguinal hernia repair, however, remain the same for all techniques: to provide long-lasting, secure closure of the pelvic floor defect, reduce pain, and improve quality of life. In modern-day repair, recurrence after hernia repair has remained fairly low. A concerning trend is the increase in chronic pain seen after inguinal hernia repair. Though mesh implantation has been associated with this trend, most believe that chronic pain is a result of surgical technique, difficulty with identification of hernia anatomy, and other unknown patient factors. In this chapter, we review diagnosis of inguinal hernias among adults, common procedures for inguinal hernia repair and their expected outcomes, and the issue of chronic postinguinal herniorrhaphy pain.

DIAGNOSIS

Patients with inguinal hernias may present with complaints of a painless bulge, pain in the groin without a bulge, or some variation in between. It is very important to accurately document the preoperative symptoms and confirm that they are consistent with an inguinal hernia. Some patients may have other causes for their symptoms, such as epididymitis, testicular pain, or endometriosis. Symptoms from an inguinal hernia may include a burning or pinching sensation in the groin. The pain may radiate into the scrotum, labia, or vagina, down the leg, or around the back. They may have worsening pain with prolonged sitting, prolonged standing, bending, coughing, straining, getting out of a car, or toward the end of the day. Lying flat almost always results in improvement of their symptoms. Women may also report worse pain during their menses. Obstructive symptoms may include bloatedness, nausea, and vomiting.

Inguinal hernias are most commonly seen in men and are of the indirect type—that is, the result of a patent processus vaginalis. These hernias typically present with a bulge in the groin that may extend into the scrotum or labia. A less common variant, an interstitial hernia, dissects within the oblique muscle layers and presents with an oblong bulge extending superolaterally. Direct hernias are a result of weakness in the transversalis fascia and are more commonly seen in older males. Femoral hernias are rare and typically seen in women, as their pelvis is broad and the femoral space is wider. This compares to the narrow pelvis of males where the myoaponeurosis attaches at a different angle, resulting in downward forces merging onto a larger myopectineal orifice of Fruchaud (Figure 1).

Hernia development is considered to be due to genetic factors as well as acquired factors. Patients with inguinal hernias have been shown to have a higher proportion of immature type III collagen as compared to type I collagen. Patients with a family history of hernia are four times more likely to have an inguinal hernia. Medical diseases that have been associated with a higher risk of inguinal hernia include aneurysmal disease, other collagen disorders, hiatal hernia, and sleep apnea. In addition, it is commonly believed, though never scientifically proven, that increases in abdominal pressure contribute to the development of hernia. Such activities include straining due to constipation or prostatic hypertrophy, chronic cough or clearing of the throat, and heavy lifting as part of a daily job. Exercise has been shown to have a protective effect on hernia development. It is important to control for these risk factors preoperatively in order to improve outcomes after hernia repair.

Diagnosis of a hernia is based primarily on physical exam. The patient is examined in the standing position to allow for gravity to accentuate any findings. Standing alone may demonstrate a bulge, and attempts should be made to reduce it. In men, the examiner's digit is used to follow the spermatic cord cephalad into the inguinal canal by using the redundancy of the scrotal skin. There, the internal ring may be entered, and also the direct space can be examined for weakness. A cough or valsalva by the patient may be necessary if the initial exam is not diagnostic. The femoral space is examined by pressing medially in the groin just cephalad to the pubic bone. In women, the inguinal exam is often not as obvious, because many do not have a palpable bulge, defect, or reducible mass. If that is the case, the examiner may be able to elicit pain while pressing at the internal ring. This is suggestive of a hernia as the cause of the patient's pain, and further workup may be necessary. Femoral hernias, when palpable on examination, present as bulges below (caudad) the inguinal ligament. The bulge can be found just medial to the femoral pulse and frequently feels like a lipoma or lymph node. The differential diagnosis for a mass in this location must include femoral hernia.

If the exam is suggestive of a hernia, such as pain or mild fullness at the internal ring, without palpable mass or defect, and the history is also suggestive of a hernia, then radiologic studies may be considered before proceeding to surgery. These include ultrasound, herniogram, computed tomographic (CT) scan, or magentic resonance imaging (MRI). All of these studies can be performed in dynamic mode, with valsalva, to accentuate small hernias.

INGUINAL HERNIA REPAIR

Repair of the inguinal hernia should be timed to provide the most benefit to the patient and the least risk from the procedure. It was considered at one time that all inguinal hernias should be repaired

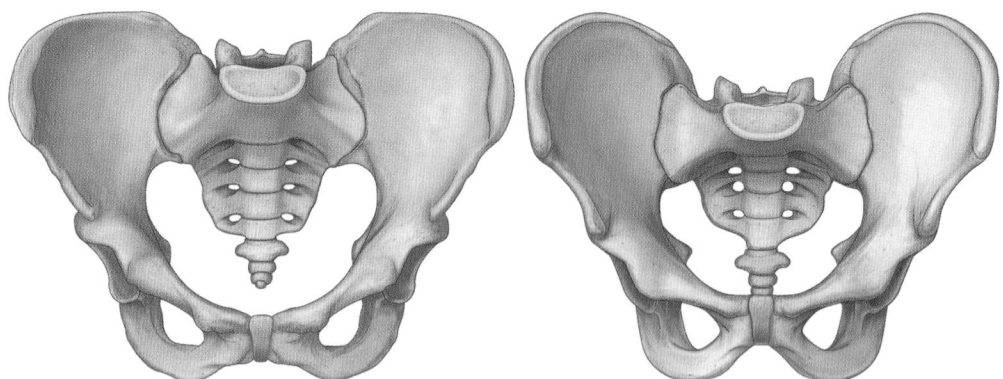

FIGURE 1   Female pelvis (left) and male pelvis (right). *(From Drake RL, Vogl AW, Mitchell AWM, et al: Gray's atlas of anatomy, Philadelphia, 2007, Churchill Livingstone.)*

to reduce the morbidity and mortality associated with potential incarceration or strangulation. Based on two prospective clinical trials in men with asymptomatic or minimally symptomatic inguinal hernias, the option of watchful waiting has been shown to be of low risk. In one trial, the risk of incarceration among patients randomized to the watchful waiting arm was calculated as 0.18% per year. No patient had a strangulated hernia during the trial period (2-4.5 years). In the second trial, only males age 55 and over were enrolled. Among this population, patients in the watchful waiting trial were more likely to suffer from a debilitating medical complication such as stroke or heart attack, thus rendering them poor candidates for elective inguinal hernia repair in the future. However, there were no hernia-related complications during the watchful waiting period. A commonly accepted practice now is to offer elective inguinal hernia repair to patients physically fit for surgery and to patients with symptomatic inguinal hernias. The timing of the repair is rarely urgent unless there is a known incarceration episode. In those at higher risk for perioperative complications or for minimally symptomatic patients not wishing to undergo repair at this time, watchful waiting is considered a safe option.

Femoral hernias, unlike other inguinal hernias, are associated with a much higher risk of incarceration or strangulation. One third of all femoral hernias are repaired emergently, compared to 6% of all inguinal hernias. Thus, repair is recommended for all patients with femoral hernias.

Tissue Repair

The technique of nonmesh or tissue repair dates back to ancient Egypt. Hundreds of techniques have been described since. Though mesh repair has become the standard in the United States, tissue repair remains the primary technique across the world and is growing in its application in the United States due to the increased concern with chronic pain. Tissue repair is considered to be superior to mesh repair in terms of chronic pain, though most studies show that acute postoperative pain and hernia recurrence are significantly worse when mesh is not used. Tissue repair is indicated for patients at risk for mesh infection, such as with a strangulated hernia requiring bowel resection. Also, it should be considered for patients at higher risk for chronic pain, such as women and those who present with a history of chronic pain.

The type of tissue repair and its outcome is dependent on technique and surgeon experience. No single technique is considered to be superior. The surgeon should be familiar with at least one or two techniques and perfect them in order to have the best outcome. All tissue repairs share a similar concept: closure of the defect and reinforcing the pelvic floor. A relaxing incision is often incorporated to reduce the tension on the repair. Repairs are performed with permanent suture.

The Marcy repair is a primary closure of the internal ring defect alone, without any further reinforcement of the pelvic floor. It is most often used for children because the recurrence rate is considered too high among adults.

The Bassini and McVay repairs involve opening the pelvic floor transversely and reducing all preperitoneal contents and the hernia sac back into the abdominal cavity. It is not necessary to resect the hernia sac if it can be successfully reduced. For the Bassini repair, one reapproximates the tissues by sewing the conjoint tendon to the inguinal ligament. For the McVay repair, the conjoint tendon is sutured to Cooper's ligament, thus patching the femoral space as well. Then, at the level of the femoral vein, a transition suture is used to continue the approximation from the conjoint tendon to the inguinal ligament. The suture line for both repairs starts medially at the anterior rectus fascia overlying the pubic tubercle and ends laterally at the internal ring. Suturing is in interrupted fashion using permanent suture. Care must be taken not to entrap the ilioinguinal, iliohypogastric, and genitofemoral nerve branches. The external oblique is then closed over this repair.

The Shouldice repair involves step-by-step layered closure of the pelvic floor. Pelvic floor dissection is similar to the Bassini and McVay (Figure 2, *A*). Classically, the cremasteric muscle is resected, including the genital branch of the genitofemoral nerve. For the hernia repair, starting medially at the pubic tubercle, the lower edge of transversalis fascia is sutured in running fashion to the underside of the upper edge, with partial thickness bites of the transversus abdominis and internal oblique (Figure 2, *B*). This continues laterally. At the internal ring, the proximal stump of cremasteric muscle enveloping the spermatic cord is included, and the suture line is reversed (Figure 2, *C*). In this second suture line, full-thickness bites of the upper edge of the transversalis fascia is sutured to the inguinal ligament below (Figure 2, *D*). Once completed medially, this suture end is tied to the tail of the first suture line. The third suture line begins laterally at the internal ring. The external oblique just above the inguinal ligament is sutured to partial-thickness bites of the internal oblique from the superior flap (Figure 2, *E*). This is continued medially toward the anterior rectus fascia overlying the pubic tubercle and reversed for the fourth and final suture line, which involves another layer of external oblique from the lower edge sewn to the internal oblique of the superior flap (Figure 2, *F*). To prevent ptosis of the testicle, the distal end of the cremasteric muscle stump is sutured to the anterior rectus fascia at the pubic tubercle or included in the external ring closure.

Mesh Repair

The gold standard in the United States involves implantation of mesh. It has been shown to provide a secure repair with little or no tension, as compared with tissue repair. Also, since most patients have

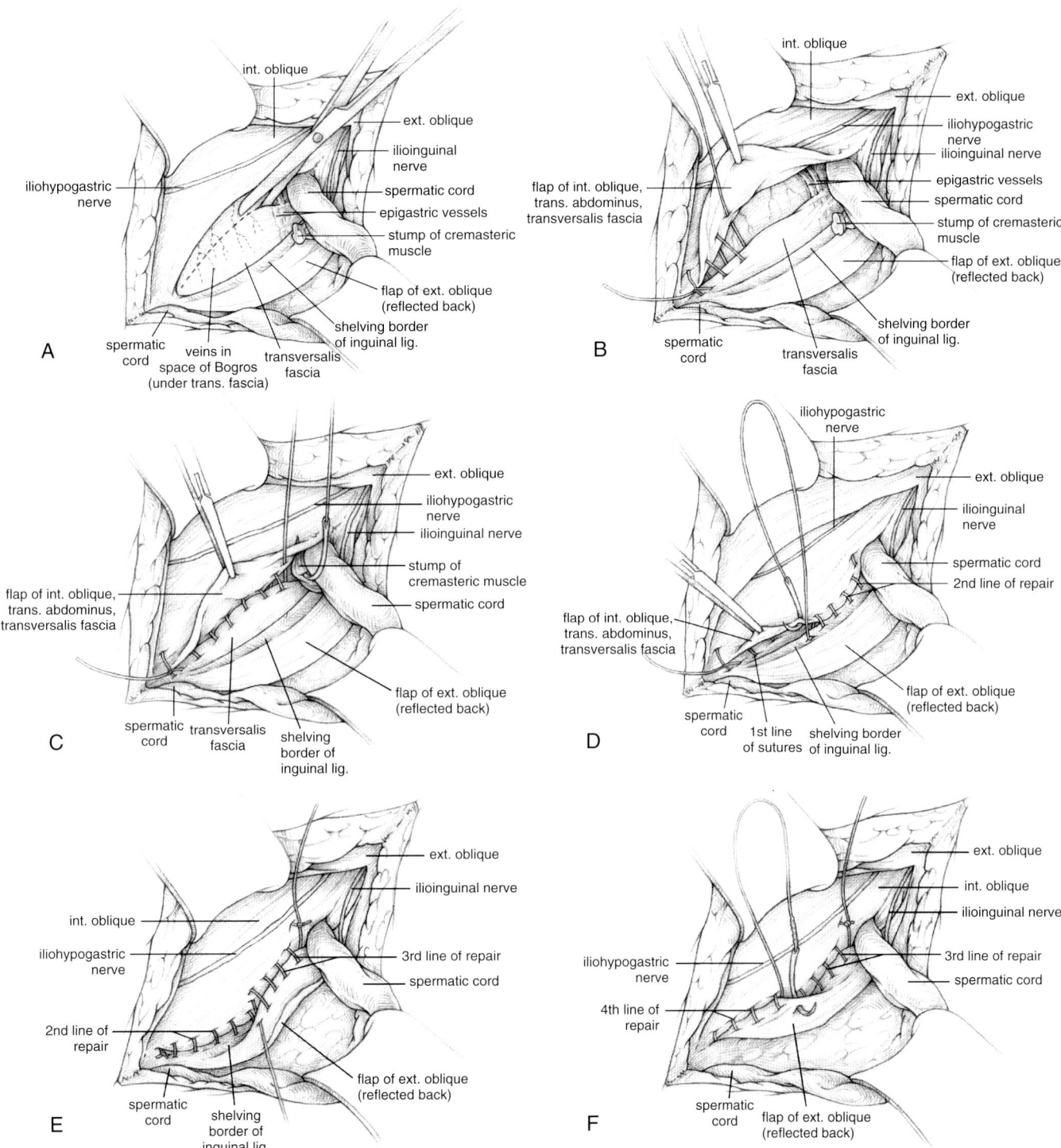

FIGURE 2 Shouldice hernia repair. **A,** Splitting of the transversalis fascia from the internal ring to the pubic crest as far as desired. **B,** First suture line continues to tack the lateral flap of transversalis fascia to the transversalis fascia lying medially beneath the rectus, transversus abdominis, and internal oblique muscles. **C,** Reconstruction of the internal ring incorporating transversalis fascia and the proximal stump of cremasteric muscle. **D,** Second suture line "carrying" the previously established medial flap of tissue to the curved or shelving edge of the inguinal ligament. **E,** The undersurface of the external oblique close to inguinal ligament is now in this third line of sutures being tacked over the internal oblique. **F,** The fourth line of sutures tacks more of the lower flap of the external oblique over the internal oblique. *(From Shouldice EB: The Shouldice repair for groin hernias, Surgical Clinics of North America 83:1163–1187, 2003.)*

intrinsically weak pelvic floor tissue or may have a wide defect with absent tissue, the implant can augment the security of repair by bolstering the muscles or bridging the defect. Hernia recurrence rates using mesh implantation are typically under 5% nationally and are reported by experts to be less than 1%. This compares to recurrence after elective tissue repair, which may reach as high as 15% to 20%, depending on the patient characteristics and surgical technique performed. There are a multitude of hernia mesh biomaterials and techniques that have been developed. Outcomes are variable and dependent on surgeon technique and expertise. No single repair is considered to be superior. For the best outcome, it is important that the surgeon be informed about the risks and benefits of each implant and to know the correct surgical technique recommended for the chosen mesh biomaterial.

The onlay patch repair, reported by Lichtenstein and modified by Amid, is one of the most commonly performed inguinal hernia repairs with mesh. After the hernia sac and fat are reduced, flat mesh, 8×15 cm or 3×6 inches, is sutured in running fashion starting inferomedially at the anterior rectus fascia over the pubic tubercle and continuing along the ilioinguinal ligament, stopping at the internal ring. A few interrupted sutures are placed at the superior edge of the mesh. Care is taken to place sutures only in conjoint tendon and anterior rectus fascia, as the iliohypogastric nerve runs through the internal oblique muscle layer and can be entrapped if sutures are placed through this muscle. A lateral slit in the mesh accommodates the spermatic cord or round ligament. The round ligament can be sacrificed in most women, so a slit may not be necessary. In the Amid modification of this repair, the tails of the mesh are sutured to each other laterally at the level of the inguinal ligament, thus forming a three-dimensional tunnel for the recreated internal ring (Figure 3). This conforms to the contour of the pelvis and has lower risk of ring tightness as compared to the keyhole technique. The lateral tails of the mesh are tucked under the external oblique. For large indirect hernias, some advocate narrowing the internal ring with absorbable suture. For direct hernias, it is recommended to imbricate the

redundant transversalis fascia, using absorbable sutures prior to placing the onlay patch.

The multi-institutional European TIMELI trial compared the traditional Lichtenstein repair with sutures to a similar repair spraying fibrin glue to anchor the mesh. Patients had body mass index (BMI) under 35 kg/m² and nonscrotal, nonincarcerated inguinal hernias. Results showed no significant difference in recurrence between the two groups (0.94% overall). The patients with fibrin glue had significantly lower moderate to severe pain or groin discomfort at 12 months (8.1% vs 14.8%). More experience is being gained with nonsuture techniques of mesh repair using tissue glue or implanting self-adhering mesh.

The mesh plug technique was introduced to reduce the amount of dissection necessary and thus reduce postoperative pain. Plugs are variable in their construction. They are typically placed through the defect after highly dissecting out the hernia sac and confirming wide retromuscular dissection free of retroperitoneal fat. Some plugs have an outer leaflet that can be positioned in this retromuscular space, essentially resulting in a small sublay repair. Other plugs are developed as a space occupying implant, thus requiring an onlay mesh repair with a second flat patch of mesh.

The sandwich repair, such as that pioneered by Gilbert, involves a two-layer mesh repair. The anterior leaflet of this mesh is placed as an onlay, similar to the Lichtenstein repair. It may or may not require suturing. Gilbert recommends only an anchoring stitch placed medially. The posterior leaflet of the mesh is placed in the retromuscular, preperitoneal space, providing a sublay repair. With this repair, it is important that the hernia sac is dissected highly and that the retromuscular preperitoneal space is widely dissected free of all fat and adhesions in order to accommodate this mesh.

Since mesh implantation induces an inflammatory process in the groin, chronic pain and postoperative swelling can be greater with this procedure than with tissue repair. Recent studies are suggesting a lower inflammatory response and less postoperative chronic pain and swelling with lightweight mesh biomaterials, defined as weighing less than 40 g/m². The recurrence rate of these products may be slightly higher than that of normal-weight mesh, also referred to as heavyweight mesh, defined as weighing 90 g/m² or greater. One study reports a 3% absolute increase in hernia recurrence rate when using lightweight mesh.

Laparoscopic repair is growing in popularity as more surgeons are gaining experience with the preperitoneal anatomy and the surgical technique. It has been associated with shorter recovery time and less postoperative pain. The learning curve is high and directly related to outcome. Expert surgeons with experience performing 250 or more laparoscopic cases can provide this repair to their patients with lower complication rates and lower recurrence rates as compared to the open repair. Laparoscopic repair involves dissection of the peritoneal sac and preperitoneal fat from the posterior abdominal wall and pelvic floor. The dissection can be performed totally extraperitoneally (TEP) or transabdominally with a preperitoneal dissection (TAPP). No single technique is considered superior, and the outcome is dependent on surgical technique and surgeon experience. It is important, however, that the surgeon performing the TEP technique also be facile with the TAPP technique, because conversion from TEP to TAPP may be necessary due to adhesions, scarring, large hernia, or other confounding factors.

The principles of laparoscopic technique include safely reducing the peritoneal hernia sac without injuring the external iliac vessels, bladder, or intraperitoneal organs. For this reason, most large scrotal hernias and some incarcerated hernias are not performed laparoscopically. The mesh is placed retromuscularly and extraperitoneally. It is important that the dissection be complete and wide, examining all three potential areas of hernia development in the myopectineal orifice: indirect, direct, and femoral spaces. Also, spermatic cord lipomas should be carefully dissected off prior to mesh placement. This may not be as evident during laparoscopic dissection as with an open dissection. The mesh size used is 10×15 cm or 4×6 inches.

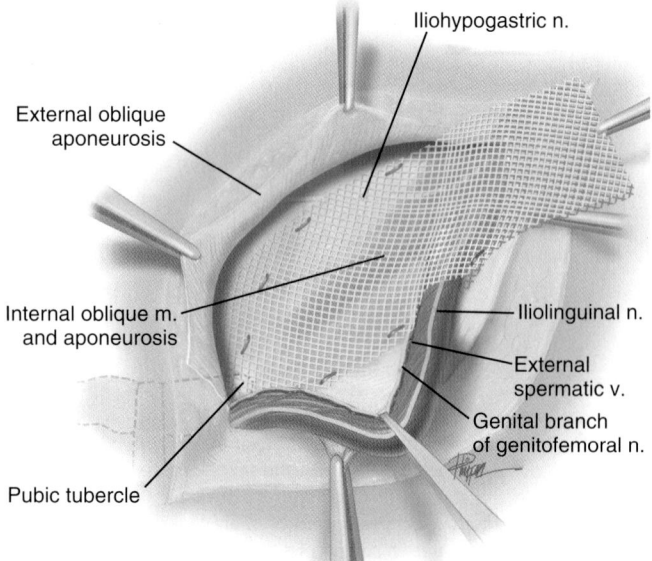

Iliohypogastric n.

External oblique aponeurosis

Internal oblique m. and aponeurosis

Iliolinguinal n.

External spermatic v.

Genital branch of genitofemoral n.

Pubic tubercle

FIGURE 3 Amid modification of Lichtenstein open inguinal hernia repair with mesh. Mesh is sized to overlap with pubic tubercle, inguinal ligament, and conjoint tendon, typically 3×6 inches. Note the interrupted sutures or staples placed in conjoint tendon, with care not to entrap iliohypogastric nerve. Laterally, the tails of the mesh are secured to each other and the inguinal ligament with a single suture or staple. *(Image courtesy of PK Amid, MD.)*

For most indirect hernias, the mesh can be placed without fixation or with the use of tissue glue alone. For direct hernias, the mesh should provide wide overlap medially and be fixed with permanent fixation. When using a fixation device, care should be taken not to injure the bladder inferomedially; external iliac vessels, genitofemoral nerves, and lateral femoral cutaneous nerves inferolaterally; and the ilioinguinal and iliohypogastric nerves superolaterally.

For patients with large scrotal hernias, with loss of pelvic floor domain, or with bilateral inguinal hernias that are not amenable to laparoscopic repair, the Stoppa repair is a tension-free technique that can offer long-lasting repair. It is also known as a giant prosthetic reinforcement of the visceral sac. Essentially, it is a wide preperitoneal repair that involves implantation of a flat piece of mesh from left to right anterior superior iliac spine in the transverse dimension and from mid-anterior rectus muscle to sacrum in the longitudinal dimension. It can also be modified for unilateral hernias.

CHRONIC POSTINGUINAL HERNIORRHAPHY PAIN

Surgical techniques for inguinal hernia repair have advanced rapidly in the past few decades. With the introduction of mesh implantation in the 1980s, average hernia recurrence rates have dramatically reduced. Recurrence rates are now less than 5% overall and less than 1% as reported by most experts. Thus, most of the efforts toward advancement of hernia repair have been concentrated on developing techniques and biomaterials that reduce operating time, reduce surgical incision length and dissection, and reduce postoperative pain and recovery time.

We are now dealing with the phenomenon of chronic postinguinal herniorrhaphy groin pain, or inguinodynia. Chronic pain, defined as persistent pain lasting longer than 3 months postoperatively, is reported to be 15% to 33%. Three percent of patients suffer from severe debilitating pain. With over 800,000 inguinal hernia repairs performed annually in the United States, a large number of patients are suffering from pain due to their operation. A recent hernia database using the Caroline Comfort Scale for preoperative and postoperative evaluation of patients followed patients for up to 2 years postoperatively. Results showed that young patients and women are at highest risk for chronic pain. It is important to carefully evaluate the symptoms of all patients preoperatively, counsel patients about the risk of chronic pain as part of the informed consent process, and tailor the surgical plan and technique to meet the patient's specific needs.

The four main causes of chronic postoperative pain include hernia recurrence, mesh-related pain, nerve-related pain, and infection. Patients with chronic pain after hernia repair may suffer from one or a combination of these causes.

Hernia recurrence, if not obvious from exam and history, can be confirmed by radiologic studies if necessary. These patients typically complain of recurrence of their preoperative pain. Their pain may be activity-related. The pain is relieved when lying flat. Some may have new pain due to a missed femoral hernia or a new direct inguinal hernia. Repair of the recurrent hernia will treat this problem.

Patients with mesh-related pain may have pain due to a persistent inflammatory reaction to the mesh. In most patients, the inflammation associated with mesh resolves with time. In a small subset, the inflammatory reaction persists, resulting in swelling and chronic pain in the affected area. CT scan or MRI may show an abnormal inflammatory reaction in the groin that is not typical of postoperative changes after mesh repair. In most patients, antiinflammatory treatments such as ice packs, nonsteroidal antiinflammatory medications, or steroid injections may relieve their discomfort. In rare cases, the mesh must be removed.

A more common mesh-related complication is termed *meshoma*, and it is due to the folding or balling of mesh (Figure 4). This is perceived by the patient as a mass in the groin and can sometimes

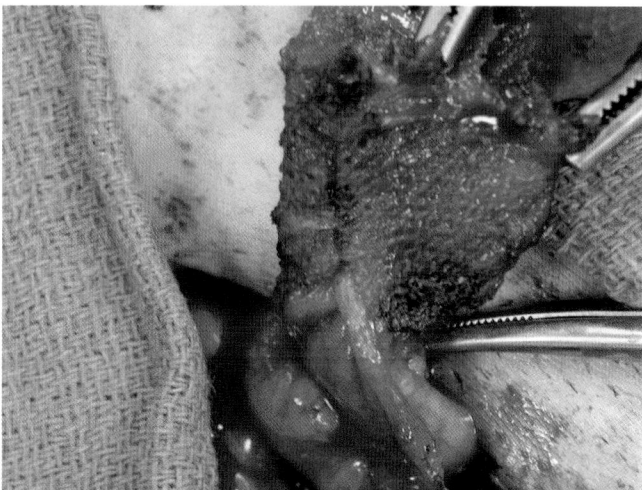

FIGURE 4 Meshoma (ball of mesh) folded, with ilioinguinal nerve entrapped within its fold (at 5:00 position).

be felt on exam. The patient typically has pain with hip flexion. Activities such as sitting, driving, and bending are uncomfortable. It is not unusual for the patient to prefer to stand or to slouch back when sitting, with ipsilateral leg extended. Radiologic studies may confirm this diagnosis by showing a thickened pelvic floor or a foreign body mass with adjacent mass effect, such as distortion of the bladder. Removal of the mesh is the only treatment for this problem.

Neuropathic pain may be due to direct nerve injury at the time of hernia surgery, ingrowth of the mesh into a nerve, entrapment of the nerve by suture, fixation material, scar tissue or a fold in the mesh (see Figure 4), or impingement on the nerve from the mass effect of a meshoma. These patients typically have a burning pain or electrical shooting sensation in the dermatome of the affected nerve. Any external pressure from belts, jeans, or underpants causes discomfort. Diagnostic testing includes a local nerve block. Treatment may include serial nerve blocks, topical lidocaine patch, nerve ablation, or neurectomy. The mesh may or may not need to be removed.

An active infection of the mesh will present with purulent drainage from the wound or a fluid collection around mesh implant. In some patients, their mesh can be seeded from bacteremia, such as tooth infection. They may present with a chronic infection, resulting in pain and intermittent swelling in the groin. They may also have associated constitutional symptoms such as fever, night sweats, fatigue, or joint pain. Radiologic study may show an inflammatory reaction, thickening of the soft tissue, or a fluid collection with or without gas. Antibiotics alone will improve their symptoms. In most cases, mesh removal is necessary.

Regardless of the cause of the chronic pain, it is important that the surgeon address this issue in a timely manner. Urologists and pain management specialists may also be consulted to help address the patient's needs. Early treatment of the cause of chronic pain provides the best outcome.

SUGGESTED READINGS

Alfieri S, Amid PK, Campanelli G, et al: International guidelines for prevention and management of post-operative chronic pain following inguinal hernia surgery, *Hernia* 15:39–49, 2011.

Amid PK: Lichtenstein tension-free hernioplasty: its inception, evolution, and principles, *Hernia* 8:1–7, 2004.

Campanelli G, Pascual MH, Hoeferlin A, et al: Randomized, controlled, blinded trial of Tisseel/Tissucol for mesh fixation in patients undergoing Lichtenstein technique for primary inguinal hernia repair. Results of the TIMELI trial, *Ann Surg* 255(4):650–657, 2012.

Fitzgibbons RJ Jr, Giobbie-Harder A, Gibbs JO, et al: Watchful waiting vs repair of inguinal hernia in minimally symptomatic men: a randomized prospective clinical trial, *JAMA* 295(3):285–292, 2006.

Neumayer L, Giobbie-Harder A, Jonasson O, et al: Open mesh versus laparoscopic mesh repair of inguinal hernia, *N Engl J Med* 350:1819–1827, 2004.

O'Dwyer PJ, Norrie J, Alani A, et al: Observation or operation for patients with asymptomatic inguinal hernia: A randomized clinical trial, *Ann Surg* 244(2):167–173, 2006.

Shouldice EB: The Shouldice repair for groin hernias, *Surg Clin North Am* 83:1163–1187, 2003.

Simons MP, Aufenacker T, Bay-Nielsen M, et al: European Hernia Society guidelines on the treatment of inguinal hernia in adult patients, *Hernia* 13:343–403, 2009.

RECURRENT INGUINAL HERNIA

Robert Moesinger, MD

INTRODUCTION

Inguinal hernia repair is the most frequently performed operation by general surgeons. An inguinal hernia is present in 4 to 5 million Americans (prevalence rate, 1.5%). The lifetime risk of inguinal hernia is approximately 27% for men and 3% for women. At least 770,000 inguinal hernia repairs are performed in the United States annually. The recurrence rate is relatively low but difficult to pin down because it is nearly impossible to truly follow these patients long term. Many large series of inguinal herniorrhaphy cases show recurrence rates of 1% to 3%. The true lifetime recurrence rate is probably around 5%, but it may be higher. On the basis of that rate, it should be safe to assume that 30,000 to 40,000 inguinal hernia repairs for recurrence are performed annually in the United States. The rate of recurrence after a second inguinal repair is definitely higher and may approach 10%.

Recurrent inguinal hernia, particularly an early recurrence, is frustrating for both surgeon and patient. The inevitable thought that "something went wrong" is present and can be difficult to explain. At the time of repair of the initial hernia, it is important to explain to patients that hernia recurrence is a possibility at any point in their lives.

PREVENTION

Obviously, prevention of recurrence wherever possible is ideal. Classic surgical teaching emphasizes careful handling of tissue and avoiding tension as key aspects of a durable repair. The advent of tension-free repairs, initially via open techniques and now also with laparoscopic techniques, with synthetic mesh to buttress the inguinal floor has clearly improved recurrence rates compared with classic sutured repairs (Bassini's, McVay's, etc). Whether an open anterior repair is superior to a laparoscopic posterior repair remains controversial, and in terms of recurrence rates, the repairs are probably equivalent.

Multiple risk factors for poor healing can lead to hernia recurrence. Diabetes mellitus, wound infection, vascular disease, connective tissue disorders, ascites, and immunosuppression are all implicated in poor wound healing and hernia recurrence. Some evidence shows that family history of recurrent hernia can predispose a patient to recurrence, suggesting genetic wound-healing problems. Obesity is an important risk factor for hernia recurrence because it puts increased tension on the repair. Glucocorticoids clearly interfere with wound healing by suppressing the inflammatory response. Wherever possible, risk factors should be identified and minimized before elective hernia repair. For example, patients with chronic renal failure who are treated with peritoneal dialysis can be converted to temporary hemodialysis for hernia repair and the early postoperative period. Tapering of glucocorticoids, better diabetes control, and other methods may help obtain a more durable repair.

Smoking is a particularly important risk factor in hernia recurrence. Smoking clearly interferes with collagen synthesis and alters extracellular matrix proteins. Smoking also causes tissue ischemia. Perhaps the worst effect of smoking is the smoker's cough. The Valsalva maneuver associated with coughing creates a large amount of tension on the abdominal wall, and with a smoker's cough, this tension is applied constantly to the fascia every day that the patient continues to smoke.

Technical problems that can result in hernia recurrence include: (1) failure to notice an indirect hernia when a direct hernia is repaired or inadequate dissection and reduction of an indirect sac, (2) failure to notice a direct hernia when an indirect hernia is repaired, (3) excessive tension on the suture line of a sutured primary repair, (4) failure to adequately reinforce the inguinal canal at its most inferomedial portion, leading to the classic medial recurrence, near the pubic tubercle, and (5) failure to seat the mesh correctly during a laparoscopic repair, allowing recurrence through the unprotected portion of the inguinal floor.

ANATOMY

Recurrent hernias are most common direct hernias through the transversalis fascia, which is the floor of the inguinal canal. The classic recurrence seen in the era of open suture repair is in the inferomedial portion of the inguinal floor near the pubic tubercle. This can still happen with mesh repair, if the mesh is not seated and secured into the pubic tubercle. However, recurrences at many places in the inguinal floor have been seen, including quite laterally, near the internal ring, lateral to the edge of a previous mesh repair, and even lateral to the iliofemoral vessels.

In a recurrent hernia, particularly after multiple recurrences, exact anatomic structures can become nonexistent, and even the spermatic cord may be unrecognizable. In these cases, intraoperative palpation usually reveals the defect in the inguinal floor that requires repair. If the patient is awake, having the patient bear down or cough can help pinpoint a defect. In particularly perplexing cases, laparoscopy can be used to directly visualize the inguinal region and find elusive defects.

DIAGNOSIS

Like primary hernias, the hallmark of recurrent inguinal hernia is a bulge in the groin, usually over the pubic tubercle and often extending down into the scrotum. The degree of symptoms varies from none to severe. Distinguishing recurrent hernia from chronic inguinodynia is important. As more patients undergo groin surgery for hernias, it has become very clear that a certain number will develop chronic groin pain. This is often described as a "twinge" or "an electric shock" that begins in or near the scar and goes onto the lateral scrotum or medial thigh. It is often triggered by certain movements or activities. The frequency can vary from occasional to multiple times a day. It is often very aggravating, but it is not associated with a bulge on the affected side. Its cause is sometimes difficult to determine. Some patients clearly develop pain from an ilioinguinal neuroma or entrapment, and in others, the pain is secondary to chronic groin strain.

Physical examination in these patients reveals no evidence of a hernia, but often a trigger point can be identified that reproduces the pain when it is palpated. These patients should have a hernia excluded with imaging, and then a variety of medical therapies can be helpful. Fortunately, this chronic inguinodynia often resolves over time; reassuring the patient that there is no recurrence and that nothing is seriously wrong is often adequate therapy. The first therapy of choice after exclusion of hernia is injection of the trigger point with a mixture of 9 mL of 0.25% bupivacaine and 1 mL (40 mg) of depo-methylprednisolone. This injection provides long-term relief surprisingly often and can be repeated as needed, or referral for a more permanent nerve block can be made. Neuromodulators like gabapentin (Neurontin, Pfizer, New York, NY) or amitriptyline can be helpful. Some patients, particularly those with complicated worker's compensation issues, benefit from referral to a chronic pain specialist. In some cases, groin exploration with section of the ilioinguinal nerve can provide good pain relief, but this is generally a last resort.

Imaging of the groin in cases where the diagnosis of recurrence is unclear can be helpful. Computed tomographic scan can show a defect in the fascia or a knuckle of bowel or fat in the inguinal canal. Ultrasound scan is useful, but sensitivity varies with experience and skill of the ultrasonographer. Ultrasound scan of the groin with the patient supine, then standing, and then during a Valsalva maneuver can show evidence of very small defects in patients with groin pain but no obvious bulge.

The most accurate (and most invasive) imaging is diagnostic laparoscopy, which has been used in particularly perplexing cases and frustrated patients to definitively rule in or out an abdominal wall defect. This has the advantage of allowing one to look at the entire abdominal wall; if found, the hernia can be fixed at the time of laparoscopy. This is a great tool in patients who are difficult to examine, like the obese patient.

PATIENT PREPARATION

As with all surgery, adequate patient preparation helps to obtain a superior result. The surgeon needs to look for causes of the recurrence and try to eliminate risk factors where possible. Smokers should be strongly encouraged to quit before repair of recurrent hernia. Male patients need to be told that there is a higher risk of damage to cord structures during recurrent repair than during primary repair with resultant testicular atrophy. The likelihood of damage to the ilioinguinal nerve is also much higher during recurrent repair. Perhaps the most important point of discussion is informing patients that the risk of another recurrence after the second repair is not trivial, even if an excellent technical result is achieved. For these reasons, the author does not try to convince the hesitant patient with an asymptomatic recurrence to have another repair. Waiting until the patient is symptomatic, or the hernia exhibits a substantial growth rate, is acceptable and safe, particularly in elderly patients. Good studies show that the rate of strangulation of inguinal hernia is less than 1% per year.

ANESTHESIA

General, regional, and local anesthesia with sedation are all acceptable for recurrent hernia repair. The patient, when awake, is able to cough to help locate a defect and to ensure it is adequately closed. Laparoscopic repair inevitably requires general anesthesia. Large recurrences should probably not be attempted with local anesthesia because it usually proves inadequate.

REPAIR OPTIONS

Emergent

Fortunately, recurrent groin hernias rarely present as an emergency. Even when the hernia is incarcerated, the neck of the hernia is usually generous and strangulation is extremely unusual. Acutely incarcerated hernias often spontaneously reduce at the induction of anesthesia. They can then be repaired normally. These patients need to be closely watched after surgery to ensure that there is no resultant damage to the bowel. Alternatively, transinguinal laparoscopy has been performed to look at the bowel and ensure its viability after it has spontaneously reduced from incarceration.

True strangulated hernias require resection of the affected bowel, and this is usually done via a laparotomy incision, often in addition to the groin incision. There is no role for synthetic mesh in this situation. The hernia defect can be loosely "closed" from the inside to prevent reincarceration with definitive repair at some future time if necessary.

Laparoscopic

Laparoscopic inguinal hernia repair is almost as common as open hernia repair (40% vs 55% in population-based studies) for primary and recurrent inguinal hernias, although advantages and disadvantages compared with open repair remain a subject of ongoing study. Many laparoscopic approaches are now used, the most common of which is probably the laparoscopic total extraperitoneal (TEP) hernia repair. Other approaches include a single port variant of the TEP repair and laparoscopic transabdominal preperitoneal repair (TAPP). Advantages include the ability to repair both sides or to examine the contralateral side during a primary repair. A laparoscopic approach allows the surgeon to avoid going through the scar tissue and altered anatomy of a previous anterior approach. A physical advantage is suggested for preperitoneal mesh, which is pushed *into* the defect when the patient strains as opposed to being pushed *away* from the defect as is the case with an anteriorly placed mesh. Laparoscopic repair may be of particular benefit in recurrent inguinal hernias for these reasons. Many studies have compared open and laparoscopic approaches, but none have shown such clear benefits as to lead to the abandonment of the other approach; for now, and probably the foreseeable future, surgeons should use the technique with which they feel most comfortable.

Stoppa Procedure

The Stoppa procedure, or giant prosthetic reinforcement of the visceral sac, has been described by a number of authors. Essentially, a large mesh is placed in the preperitoneal space, replacing the transversalis fascia in containing the abdominal viscera. It may be the ideal approach for large, multiply recurrent groin hernias or groin hernias with multiple defects in which the transversalis fascia has become so shredded that traditional repair is hopeless. This procedure is well

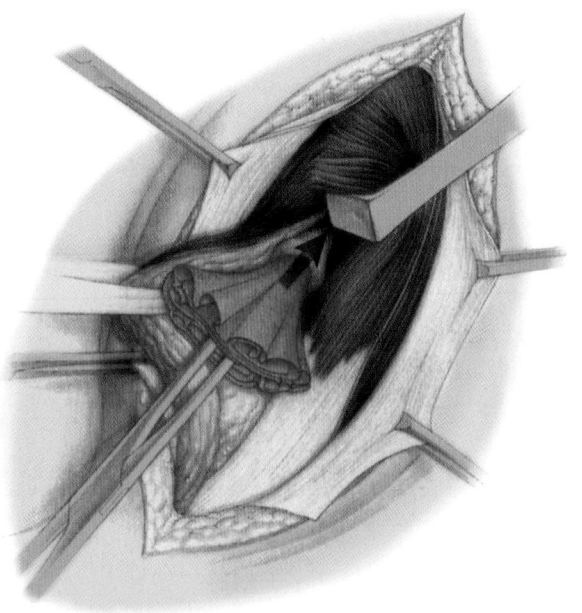

FIGURE 1   Placement of a prefolded mesh plug into a patulent internal ring.

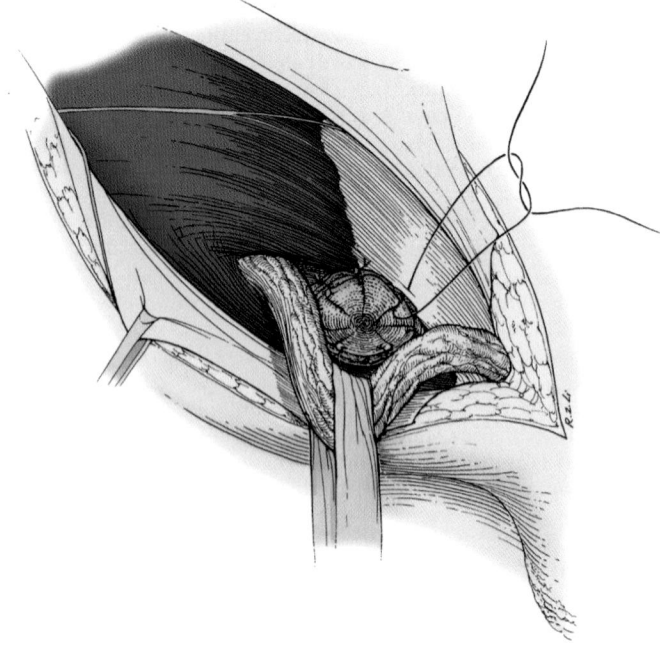

FIGURE 2   Mesh plug in position in a direct defect. Although the spermatic cord is shown retracted away from the defect, often the spermatic cord is scarred down or unidentifiable and a meticulous dissection of the spermatic cord is not necessary.

described and illustrated by Drs. Wantz and Fischer in the seventh edition of *Current Surgical Therapy* and is not replicated here.

Plug and Patch

The vast majority of recurrent groin hernias are relatively small discrete defects, either in the inguinal floor itself or as part of a loose internal ring. The edges are usually readily palpable from an anterior approach, and except for the defect, the remaining inguinal tissue is competent. Plugging and patching these defects is an easily learned technique with near universal application that requires minimal dissection and results in a tension-free repair.

Local, regional, or general anesthesia is effective. An incision is made through the previous scar. The subcutaneous tissue is divided until the aponeurosis of the external oblique is found. Although the anatomy is always distorted from previous repair, usually the external oblique is recognizable and is opened parallel to its fibers along the length of the incision. Sometimes the spermatic cord is identifiable. If it can be done easily, it should be mobilized as in primary repair. However, if it is scarred in, then no attempt to mobilize it should be made. If the patient is awake, the patient can cough to identify the hernia defect. These defects are also palpable. An indirect sac, if found, can be dissected away from the cord if it is not difficult. If it is tightly adherent, then it should be divided, allowing the distal sac to stay open in the wound. The proximal sac is then ligated at the internal ring as in primary repair. Extensive dissection of a tightly adherent sac injures the venous plexus of the testicle and can lead to testicular swelling and then atrophy. Blunt finger dissection of the preperitoneal tissue away from the sides of the defect is usually adequate to prepare the defect for repair, and little formal dissection is required. If previously placed mesh is encountered, it should generally be left undisturbed because removing it is usually difficult and traumatic. An appropriately sized synthetic plug is inserted into the defect and sutured in place. This can be through a direct defect or through a loose internal ring for an indirect recurrence (Figures 1 and 2). Then, a mesh patch is used as an overlay over the defect, securing the plug in place and reinforcing the inguinal floor (Figure 3). It is secured to the inguinal ligament and conjoint tendon where

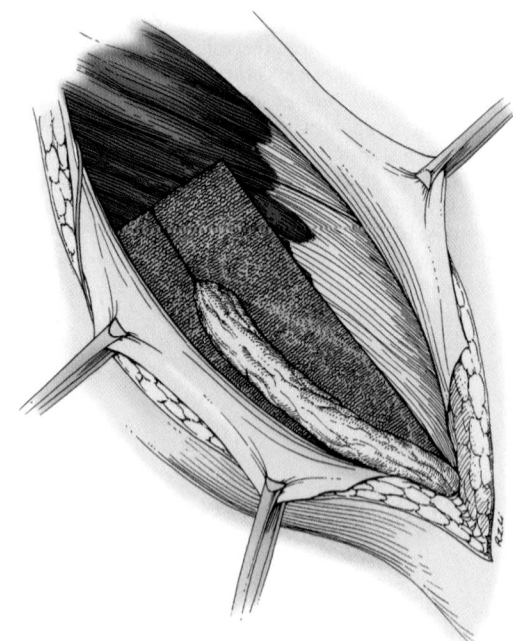

FIGURE 3   Onlay patch in position in the inguinal canal.

identifiable. Otherwise, it is secured to any good solid tissue. In an inguinal floor with no identifiable anatomy, the laparoscopic tacker has been used to secure the mesh to the pubic tubercle and to any solid shelves of tissue found. Some meshes are designed with tiny barbs to hold themselves in place, requiring little if any further fixing in place. The awake patient can be instructed to cough before the wound is closed.

After surgery, patients are instructed that they cannot drive until they no longer take narcotics. They should not lift anything heavier than 10 to 15 lbs for 2 to 3 weeks, after which, if they are doing well, they are instructed to begin normal activity as they are able.

COMPLICATIONS

Complications of recurrent hernia repair are essentially the same as for primary repair. Recurrence is the most troublesome complication, but large series of patients suggest that the recurrence rate is not more than 10%. Chronic groin pain can also be a problem as discussed previously. Hematomas and seromas are more common after recurrent hernia repair. Testicular swelling and atrophy are also more common after recurrent hernia repair, particularly after aggressive dissection of a hernia sac from the cord structures, which is to be avoided. Infectious complications are fortunately rare. Superficial wound infection, stitch abscess, and cellulitis can occur. They are treated with opening of the wound or antibiotics as indicated. Removal of the mesh is virtually never necessary.

SUMMARY

Recurrent groin hernia is a common problem. A number of strategies exist for fixing these hernias; the best strategy is usually the one with which the surgeon is most comfortable. Anterior open placement of mesh and laparoscopic techniques are both safe and effective for recurrent inguinal hernia repair. Gentle handling of the tissues, the avoidance of tension, and appropriate reinforcement of hernia defects and patient preparation are the key principles in repairing recurrent hernias.

SUGGESTED READINGS

Deysine M, Deysine GR, Reed WP Jr: Groin pain in the absence of hernia: a new syndrome, *Hernia* 6:64–67, 2002.
Eker HH, Langeveld HR, Klitsie PJ, et al: Randomized clinical trial of total extraperitoneal inguinal hernioplasty vs Lichtenstein repair: a long-term follow-up study, *Arch Surg* 147:256–260, 2012.
Junge K, Rosch R, Klinge U, et al: Risk factors related to recurrence in inguinal hernia repair: a retrospective analysis, *Hernia* 10:309–315, 2006.
Robbins AW, Rutkow IM: The mesh-plug hernioplasty, *Surg Clin North Am* 73:501–512, 1993.
Wantz GE, Fischer E: Recurrent inguinal hernia. In Cameron JL, editor: *Current surgical therapy*, ed 7, St Louis, 2001, Mosby, pp 605–611.

INCISIONAL, EPIGASTRIC, AND UMBILICAL HERNIAS

Paul G. Curcillo II, MD, FACS

INCISIONAL HERNIAS (VENTRAL HERNIAS)

The term *ventral hernia* is often used to describe incisional hernias. In fact, a ventral hernia is any defect within the anterior abdominal wall. Incisional hernias make up only a portion of all the hernias that can occur from the xyphoid process to the pubic bone and between the most lateral aspects of the oblique muscles.

Unlike all other hernias that surgeons evaluate and repair, incisional hernias are unique in that surgeons contribute to the source and cause of the disease. In this regard, attention should always be given to appropriate closure because prevention is always better than treatment. Of all surgical incisions, 10% to 15% will develop a hernia in time. In patients developing a wound infection, this rate can double. In view of that, attention to detail with adequate fascial stitches, appropriate suture to tissue length, and complete aseptic technique is the best way to reduce this disease. Internal or external retention sutures in patients with risk factors for hernia development (obesity, diabetes, immunosuppression, advanced age) often prevent hernias as well.

The discussion of incisional hernias also requires attention to other ventral hernias: namely, umbilical and epigastric hernias. Repair techniques are similar, but often, if such hernias are present before a patient's first surgery, they can predispose the patient to development of an incisional hernia after surgery.

Because nearly 150,000 patients a year undergo repair of ventral hernias, this number would be expected to decrease as repair techniques improve and more laparoscopic procedures are developed. However, this decrease has not yet materialized. When one considers that two of the most common surgical procedures performed are cholecystectomy and hysterectomy/oophorectomy, hernia occurrence rate would have been expected to decreased since 1990 with the advent of laparoscopy. The fact that it has not actually proves that it is still the midline incision that has the highest rate of hernia occurrence. Cholecystectomy routinely involves a right upper quadrant incision, and gynecologic procedures generally were performed through Pfannenstiel incisions. Incisions in both these regions rarely result in hernia formation. In fact, midline incisions account for almost 90% of all incisional hernias. With regard to the anatomy, a discussion of the other two topics of this chapter shows why incisional hernias can also be caused by underlying patient anatomy if not identified and included in primary closure of the initial wound.

UMBILICAL HERNIAS

Umbilical hernias are most often detected and repaired in children. However, in some patients, umbilical hernias, both known and undetected, continue to occur into adulthood. An important aspect of diagnosing and treating an umbilical hernia in adults is to determine how it has developed. In an adult who has had one in his or her entire life, assessment and repair are relatively straightforward. However, in the adult with a new-onset umbilical hernia, then anything that can increase intra-abdominal pressure needs to be considered as a potential causative agent. New-onset increasing constipation, difficulty with urination, and chronic cough can not only lead to the development of a new hernia but also stress the repair postoperatively and need to be addressed. After ruling out cancer of the colon or urinary tract, physicians need to consider the stress postoperatively that will continue and thus be placed on the repair. The age-old primary closure or "tensioned" repair becomes a much less viable option.

Any patient undergoing a midline or even a laparoscopic incision needs to be assessed for umbilical hernia. Such hernias should always be noted preoperatively or, at the very least, before the incision, so that closure can incorporate the repair of the native hernia. A common hernia is an umbilical hernia after laparoscopy. When it is repaired laparoscopically, closure is often made from the umbilical port, and a hernia is noted just above it that was clearly stretched from the tension of the wound closure. A small, unappreciated defect can develop postoperatively into a larger defect that could have been prevented. Equally as common is the umbilical hernia that develops at the top of a low midline incision from pelvic surgery that is not included in the closure.

EPIGASTRIC HERNIA

One of the most confusing areas for both diagnosis and repair of ventral hernias is the epigastrium. This area from the xyphoid process down to the umbilicus is often an area of weakness from the separation of the right and left rectus muscles (diastasis recti). The separation of the muscle with the fascial envelope left intact produces the classic appearance of a hernial bulge, but no true defect hole is present. It manifests during isolated contraction of the rectus muscles rather than increased intra-abdominal pressure such as during cough or a Valsalva maneuver as with a hernia. This is best demonstrated by having the patient lie back and then sit up on the examination table. During *inclining* and *reclining* (Figure 1), the bulge appears and promptly resolves once the recti are relaxed. This separation is often a cosmetic concern but does not need to be repaired. However, once a true defect, or a break in the fascial integrity, occurs, an epigastric hernia has developed. This usually manifests as a bulge or protrusion in the midepigastrium surrounded by the diastasis recti and is most often properitoneal fat or a portion of the falciform ligament. This repair now needs to be more extensive than simple closure of the defect because the lateral tissue will be too weak to hold the sutures and may result in a recurrence.

Like an umbilical hernia, an epigastric hernia should be noted preoperatively in a patient about to undergo a midline incision. Closure from the planned surgery must account for the weakened tissue that will be grasped with every placement of the suture, as well as the perforating effect of needle punctures too closely placed. Failure to account for this weakness will certainly result in an incisional hernia with time.

The most important aspect of treating incisional hernias is often to prevent them and plan wound closure appropriately.

APPROACH TO THE REPAIR OF VENTRAL HERNIAS

To Repair or Not to Repair

The first question in evaluating a patient with a ventral hernia is whether it should be repaired. The traditional teaching was to "repair every hernia." Certainly an incarcerated hernia needs to be addressed in a timely manner, and few authorities would argue against repair. The decision is more involved with regard to elective evaluation and consideration for repair.

Box 1 lists the indications for repair of hernias. In patients with small hernias, or those simply referred because they were found on routine examination or computed tomographic scan, observation with follow-up is an option. Particularly in patients with other comorbid conditions, repairing a hernia is not without complications. If a hernia does not grow with time, then routine office follow-up can be a safe option in a compliant patient. An important aspect of this is the size of the hernial defect and the size of the hernial sac. A large-mouthed hernia that spontaneously reduces can be monitored, whereas a small defect with a larger sac raises the concern of eventual incarceration. Naturally, any report that a hernia has become firm or is not reducing should raise concern and prompt repair.

The patients' concerns also need to be a consideration in the evaluative and planning process. Many patients are concerned about the appearance. Not only is repairing hernias from a cosmetic standpoint acceptable but also the final appearance and outcome must be considered as surgeons plan the approach and technique.

Techniques of Hernia Repair

All hernia repairs can be classified into two categories: *tensioned* and *tension-free*. It is important to remember that simply placing a piece of mesh does not necessarily make a repair tension-free, nor is a laparoscopic repair necessarily a tension-free repair (Table 1).

BOX 1: Indications for hernia repair

Expanding hernia
Loss of abdominal domain
Cosmesis
Thinning of soft tissue and skin on anterior abdominal wall
Nonhealing wound on scar

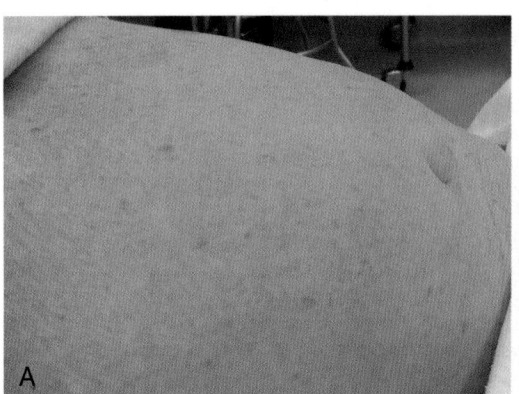
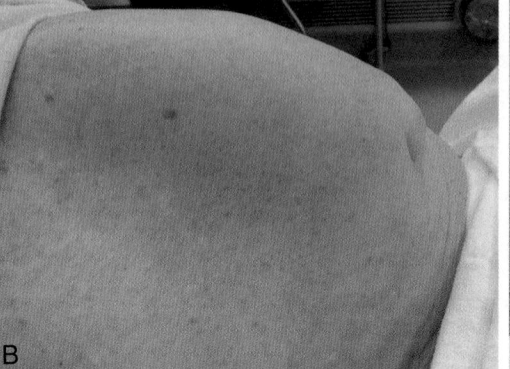
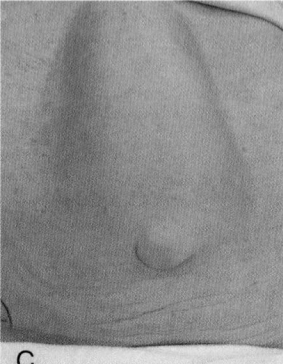

FIGURE 1 Diastasis recti versus hernia. **A,** Patient supine. **B,** Patient actively inclining or reclining. **C,** Umbilical hernia within diastasis recti.

TABLE 1: Tensioned and tension-free repairs

Tensioned repairs	Tension-free repairs
Primary tissue-to-tissue closure	Sublay mesh placement Open Laparoscopic
Inlay mesh placement	Onlay mesh placement
Advancement flap closure	Plug and patch repair
Onlay mesh placement over flap closure	

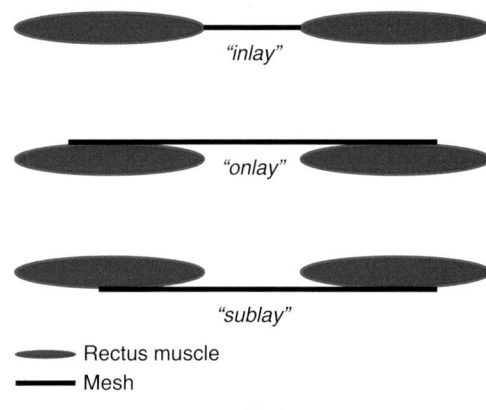

FIGURE 2   Mesh positions.

Tensioned Repair

The primary repair is rarely ever performed except for small hernias because defects greater than 2.5 or 3 cm repaired primarily have a high recurrence rate. A surgeon should keep in mind that although a primary repair is perhaps slightly more painful and somewhat more restrictive postoperatively than a mesh repair, it eliminates the need to place a foreign body. For a young patient with a small umbilical hernia or perhaps a small trocar hernia, primary repair should still be offered as a first choice. Should the hernia recur, then mesh can be offered. However, the presence of the diastasis recti should always be determined before repair because the recurrence rate can dramatically increase if the muscle is close to the actual defect. This scenario is often best approached with a mesh repair. The same holds true for epigastric hernias.

Tension-Free Repairs

Perhaps one of the most important steps in understanding the best way to repair a hernia was the development of laparoscopic inguinal hernia repair. As laparoscopists turned the camera to the pelvis and inguinal region and saw an opportunity to repair inguinal hernias from within, one of the early stumbling blocks was attempting to form, cut, and shape the mesh for the defect. Before this, most meshes were placed in an inlay manner (Figure 2). However, difficulties in planning the mesh shape and size extracorporeally and in trimming the mesh intracorporeally led to the concept of simply placing a piece of mesh larger than the defect with a wide overlap. In addition, and probably of most importance, the mesh was being placed in a sublay position (see Figure 2). This allowed for wide coverage of the area with decreased tension. In the likely event of continued intra-abdominal pressure from constipation, urinary difficulties, or chronic cough, the hydrostatic pressure would be directed towards the mesh against the abdominal wall and fascia; thus the mesh would be secured to the wall around the defect rather than protruding into the wound. For virtually all hernias repaired in a tension-free technique, both laparoscopically and with open surgery (i.e., with mesh plugs), a piece of mesh is cut larger than the defect and placed posterior to the defect. Recurrence of hernias has clearly decreased with this concept applied.

Mesh

For hernia repairs with mesh, a wide variety of mesh types and combinations are available (Box 2). Synthetics (both reactive and nonreactive), coated meshes, and biologic materials are all used in hernia surgery. A surgeon needs to be knowledgeable of all the types and be able to apply them where and when appropriate. The ideal mesh placed within the abdomen would be completely inert on the bowel side to prevent adhesions and completely reactive on the abdominal wall side to promote tissue ingrowth. An ideal biologic mesh would

BOX 2: Mesh types and coatings

Type
Nonreactive
Expanded polytetrafluoroethylene (ePTFE)

Reactive
Polypropylene
Polyester

Biologic
Porcine dermis
Bovine dermis
Human cadavaric
Porcine intestine

Coatings
Hyaluronic acid
Omega fatty acids
Modified polysaccharides
Collagen
Cellulose
Titanium

promote formation of new fascia; the current development simply of new scar tissue can lead to the "pseudo"-hernia observed when the defect is still present, but is now simply spanned by scar tissue and sac, rather that sac and fatty tissue. Although a defect may not be present to allow bowel to incarcerate, patients may not understand that the development of laxity is not a recurrence, and they may wish to have it revised.

In simple cases with minimal adhesions, coated mesh or polytetrafluoroethylene (PTFE)–based meshes may help prevent adherence to the bowel and omentum. However, regardless of the mesh type used, if extensive adhesiolysis is necessary to expose the defect, then the inflammatory response that ensues will lead to adhesion with virtually any mesh placed. In these cases, combined PTFE/polypropylene or coated meshes offer some relief. Although adhesions will still develop, lysing them on reoperation if necessary is often easier than with polypropylene-only or biologic meshes placed intra-abdominally.

Combined Approach

A hernia surgeon needs to be facile in all aspects of surgery. Not every hernia can be repaired with the same method. Although it seemed as though the 1990s were giving rise to repairing all hernias laparoscopically, it soon become evident that laparoscopic repair was sometimes not appropriate. The decision can often be made preoperatively; however, the plan can change once the defect is visualized. Most hernias should be approached laparoscopically, albeit if only as an initial step. First, the laparoscopic approach allows better visualization not only of the defect but also of the entire area to assess whether there are any other defects along the incision, whether the defect is isolated or within a large lax area, and whether the diastasis recti will ultimately affect the repair. Furthermore, adhesiolysis is often best performed laparoscopically. In patients with extensive adhesions, even if the repair is open with muscle flaps and mesh, a laparoscopic adhesiolysis allows most of the surgery to be performed without opening of the wound. Thus less exposure of the primary wound minimizes the chance of wound and, ultimately, mesh infection. In some cases, once the adhesiolysis is complete, it may become evident that a laparoscopic mesh placement would be the *wrong* repair (Box 3).

BOX 3: Contraindications to laparoscopic ventral hernia repair

Large defect
- Mesh not large enough
- No lateral space to allow 3-cm to 5-cm overlap beyond defect

Skin thinning
- Loss of tissue below skin = loss of protection for mesh

Infection
Fistula
Concurrent contamination

Laparoscopic Repair

Hernia repair has been altered by the current changes and evolution of laparoscopic surgery. Although fewer than 50% of ventral hernias are repaired laparoscopically, surgeons are showing a trend to using even less invasive techniques. Reduced port techniques introduced in 2002 limit the approach to only two trocars. Along with the single-port access repairs, with only one port site, these advanced procedures have offered the benefit of limiting not only postoperative pain and scarring but also the number of potential hernia sites in the future. Repairs have also been completed using natural orifice transluminal endoscopic surgery (NOTES) approaches; with instruments and mesh place Transvaginally completely avoiding cutaneous incisions in an attempt to limit scarring. Regardless of the approach, the concept and techniques are identical for all minimally invasive approaches.

A safe entry laparoscopically is always the first step (Figure 3). In a patient with an umbilical hernia, a separate access site is necessary. A subxyphoid position or lateral abdominal wall entry in the open technique is often the safest approach. Trocars need to be placed widely enough in the abdominal wall and with enough distance so that the surgeon can see the entire defect, as well as position the tacking devices along the outer rim of the mesh at least 3 to 5 cm from the defect edge. Once entry is obtained, additional trocars are placed to proceed with the adhesiolysis. Sharp and blunt dissection and energy dissection are acceptable methods if the same techniques and care are taken laparoscopically that would be taken with open surgery. Instruments that are sharp or hot should never be out of view and should avoid touching other instruments during activation. Failure to be vigilant in this regard can result in missed bowel injuries. An injury to the bowel during laparoscopic dissection can be

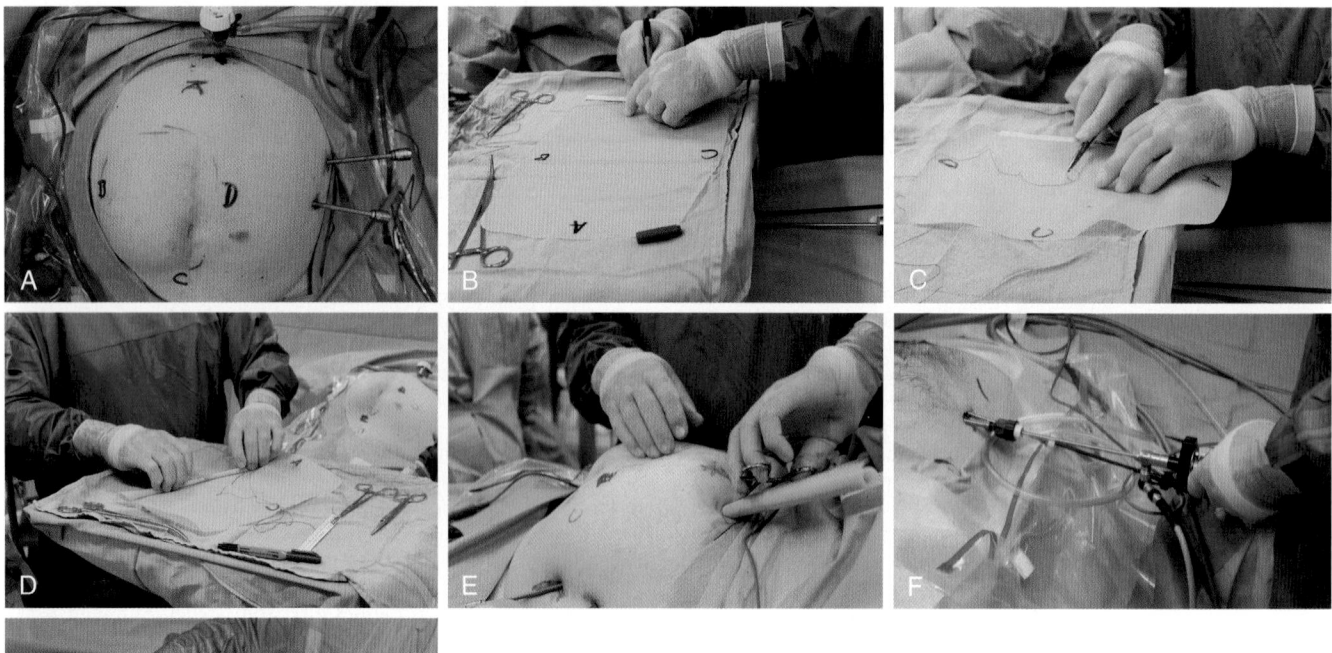

FIGURE 3 Laparoscopic repair of hernia. **A,** Perimeter of defect marked externally. **B,** Mesh marked with corresponding points to skin. **C,** Central suture placed. **D,** Mesh rolled tightly on hard surface. **E,** Mesh inserted through port site with large Kelly clamp to guide. **F,** Trocars inserted in single-port access technique. **G,** Counterpressure held (with hand) perpendicular to tacker.

repaired just as with open surgery. As with open surgery, a bowel injury may manifest itself postoperatively; therefore, with extensive adhesiolysis, the patient should be monitored closely after surgery.

Once the adhesiolysis is complete, the entire defect or incision, or both, should be visualized. If a laparoscopic placement of mesh is appropriate, then the defect should be measured. A thin ruler can be inserted, with counter pressure placed on the abdominal wall, and marked while the edge of the defect is observed from within. Once the defect size is measured, the mesh size can be determined. A 3-cm to 5-cm overlap in all directions is recommended in order to ensure wide coverage and allow for migration that may occur. The use of polypropylene meshes can minimize migration, but some still occurs with time. In general, simply adding 6 to 10 cm to the defect size helps guide the decision as to which size of the precut meshes to be applied. It is good practice to choose a size larger than estimated, to ensure wide overlap. Not only does the defect need to be widely covered with overlap, but also any laxity of the abdominal wall and musculature, such as diastasis recti, needs to be covered. This is one of the clear benefits of the laparoscopic approach for exposure of the defect from within.

The mesh can then be inserted directly through the trocar site or through a large trocar. The mesh should be centered on the defect with either a centrally placed suture or with the use of instrumentation to a position correlating with the marks on the abdominal wall.

The mesh can be secured with either tacks or transfascial sutures. If a reactive mesh with tissue ingrowth is utilized, tacks generally suffice. Both absorbable and nonabsorbable tacks are acceptable. Tacks should be placed every 2 to 3 cm around the perimeter and then a "double crown" technique utilized with the tacks placed around the outer edge of the fascial defect. If the mesh used does not have tissue ingrowth, then transfascial suture are advised at least at four points and nonabsorable tacks are recommended.

The author and colleagues always attempt to pull the mesh off the abdominal wall at the end of the procedure. Our philosophy is that if we can pull the mesh off, it is not secure. Tugging on the mesh to move the abdominal wall externally demonstrates enough force to determine whether the tacks and mesh are secure.

On exsufflation, the mesh is observed to ensure it does not crimp or fold. Once the abdomen is reexplored and proven to have no injuries, the trocars are removed and wounds closed. The patient is placed in an abdominal binder to decompress the hernia sac, which is not removed. Virtually all patients develop seromas in the sac as the mesh adheres. On examination at 1 week, seromas are usually not yet present. At approximately 2 weeks, the seroma is palpable, indicating that the reactive mesh has adhered to the underlying wall, and the fluid created by the sac can no longer extravasate into the abdomen. The abdominal binder is worn 24 hours a day, except during showers, and can help prevent and minimize the seroma. If one does develop, it can generally be monitored and will be resorbed with time. Occasional aspiration may be necessary if a seroma clinically becomes symptomatic. It is best to wait 2 to 3 months to ensure that the mesh has scarred to minimize the possibility of infection.

Open Repair/Abdominal Wall Reconstruction

In some patients, although the laparoscopic approach to perform the adhesiolysis is the first step, an open repair (Figure 4) may be necessary. A large sac may have to be excised, the patient may have extensive scarring or old mesh that needs to be excised, or the hernia size may be too large for adequate placement of a piece of mesh. In many cases, reapproximation of fascia may be necessary. With the exception of small primary hernias, tissue-to-tissue primary closure is rarely adequate to prevent a high rate of recurrence. As a result, a number of methods have been developed to bring fascial edges together, with focus on decreasing the tension. Component separation or advancement flaps of the overlying muscle can be used.

A benefit to this type of repair is tissue-to-tissue reapproximation in which the bowel and abdominal contents come into contact only with peritoneum and the mesh can be placed on the outer side of the defect. Although not in a sublay position, the mesh in this repair serves to reinforce the primary repair. The laterally placed sutures create a "suspension bridge" across the primary closure, absorbing some of the tension. In addition, should the tissue-to-tissue closure

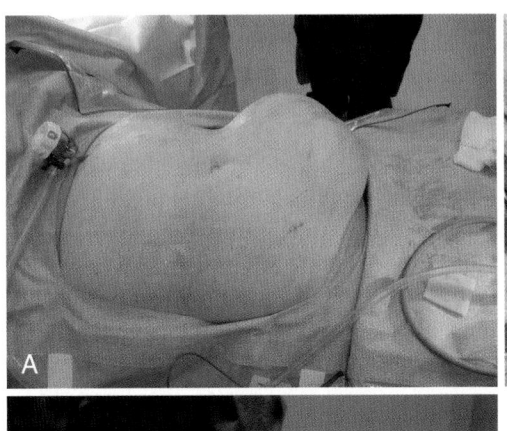
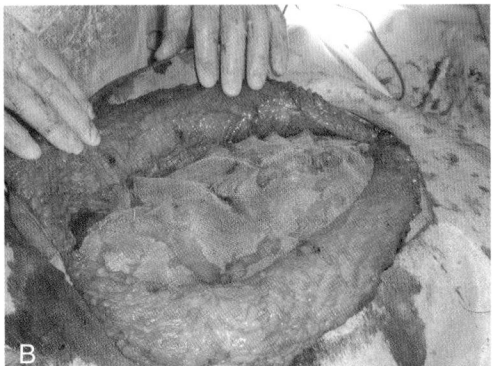
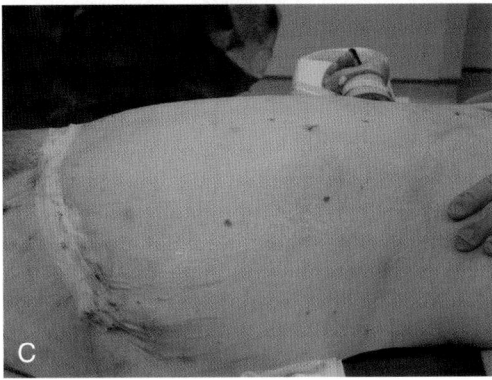

FIGURE 4 Open hernia repair with abdominal wall reconstruction. **A,** Multiple defects demonstrated on insufflation. **B,** Component separation complete with polypropylene mesh overlay (3 to 5 cm). C, Final closure.

develop a defect with time, the reinforcing mesh atop acts as a barrier to hernia formation and does not expand as does a hernia sac. Of more importance is that plain polypropylene can be used to promote tissue ingrowth on both sides because it is not in contact with the abdominal contents.

In this technique, once the defect is cleaned and identified, the fascial edges need to be grasped with Kocher clamps and pulled toward the contralateral side. The fatty tissue overlying the rectus sheath and external oblique muscle is then raised in the avascular plane. This maneuver alone allows the fascial edge to advance across midline. Depending on the size of the defect and the amount of fascia present from prior surgeries, the distance to the lateral side of the abdominal wall may be a few centimeters, or it may track back to the level of the pelvic brim. A similar release on the contralateral side brings the other side across midline as well.

On occasion, a releasing incision needs to be made along the lateral edge of the rectus muscle fascia for very large hernias, although this often times leads to replacing the midline hernia with lateral laxities. In general, the relaxing incisions are not necessary. If the fascia from each side can be brought approximately 3 to 4 cm across midline with good overlap, the relaxing incision is not necessary.

Reapproximation is performed with a running long-term absorbable suture, with several interrupted absorbable sutures placed along the incision. Care should be taken during the closure to monitor the peak inspiratory pressures the PIP and to ensure that they do not increase by more than 25%. Although an abdominal compartment syndrome is rare, an increase in the PIP would be an early indicator.

A piece of polypropylene mesh is placed over the incision with 5-cm overlap in all directions, including top and bottom portions of the incision. Absorbable sutures are placed in a mattress fashion laterally around the perimeter and across the midline incision. Closed-suction drains are placed in the dead space, and the wound is closed. Excess skin and soft tissue can often be excised to eliminate the old scar and offer clean fat planes to close. As in the laparoscopic procedure, an abdominal binder is placed.

In the rare patient in whom the defect is too large to close primarily, the defect may have to be spanned by a piece of mesh. A coated or dual-layer mesh is preferred for the same reasons mentioned previously. The sublay position is the best position, and this is one of the few situations where a sublay mesh should be placed in the open technique. A wide defect allows good exposure and visualization of the mesh before closure. In smaller hernias that can be repaired laparoscopically, sublay mesh is harder to place, and there is generally one corner portion that is not visualized at the end and often causes a problem with bowel entrapment or recurrent hernia (Figure 5).

FOLLOW-UP

In general, patients are seen by the surgeon the first 2 weeks to evaluate seromas and drains. Binders are maintained for 4 to 6 weeks, and then their use is tapered off with time. Longer applications of the binder are common with open repairs. Activity is unrestricted for laparoscopic repairs and restricted to no heavy lifting or strenuous activity for open repairs.

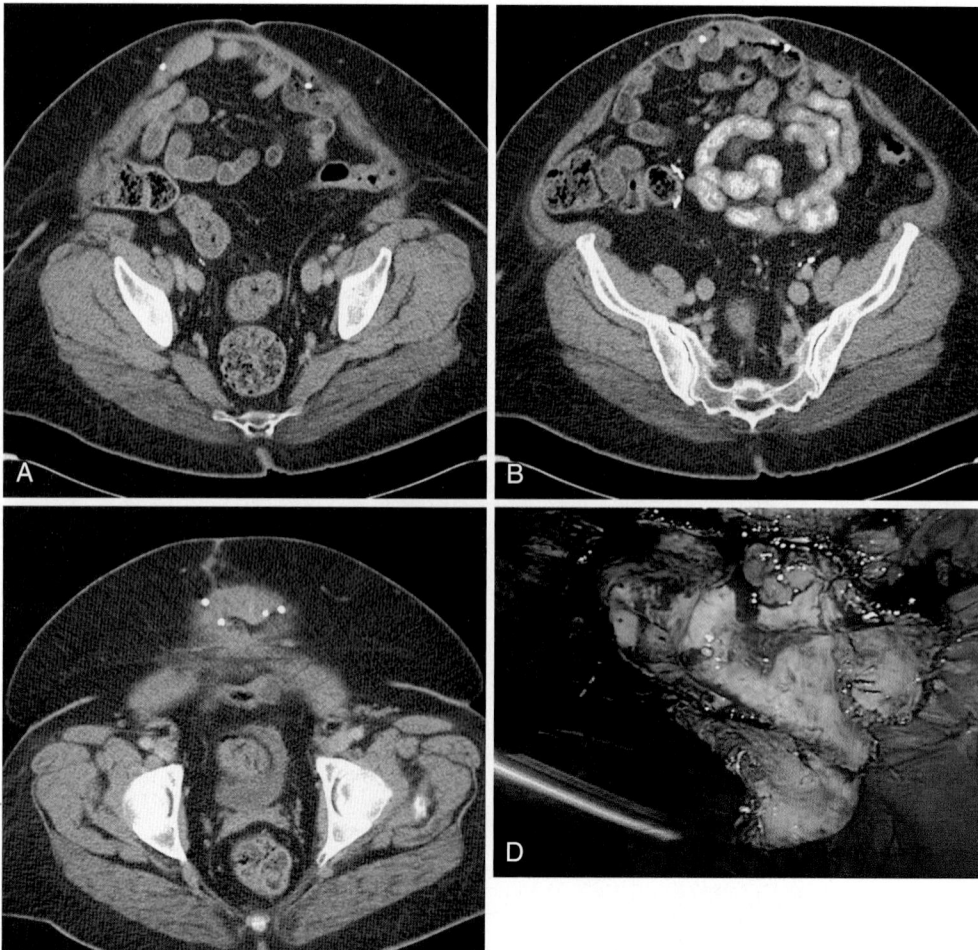

FIGURE 5 Open sublay mesh repair. **A** to **C,** Computed tomographic scans. **D,** Intraoperative photo.

CONCLUSION

Hernia repair has always been a common surgical procedure. Since 2000, it has developed into its own field for complex and difficult hernias. However, hernia repairs still make up a fair portion of most general surgeons' practice. With the trend toward laparoscopy and abdominal wall reconstructions, surgeons need to be facile in both so that they can adapt the surgery to the patient and be versatile in their ability to change plans in the operating room if necessary. With small, simple hernias, a laparoscopic procedure should be attempted first. Unlike most other laparoscopic surgeries, however, ventral hernias are approached differently surgeons are working "up" toward the abdominal wall, and around the entire abdominal area and often times in opposition to the camera. Easier cases will pave the way for repair of more difficult cases, and mesh applications will expand. Adhesiolysis may also become easier than open surgery as skill develops. In the current environment, a hernia surgeon needs to be versed in both laparoscopy and open procedures.

SUGGESTED READINGS

Curcillo PG: Laparoscopic ventral hernia repair—a simplified technique for laparoscopic ventral hernia repair—one stitch, two port technique. In Fitzgibbons R, editor: *Operative Techniques in General Surgery*, 6(3):200–208, Philadelphia, 2004, Elsevier.

Curcillo PG: Ventral hernias. Limited advancement flaps and onlay polypropylene mesh for primary and recurrent. *American Hernia Society*, New Orleans, May 2001.

LeBlanc KA: Current considerations in laparoscopic incisional and ventral herniorrhaphy, *SLS* 4(2):131–139, 2000.

Podolsky ER, Curcillo PGC: Single port access (SPA) surgery—a 24 month experience, *Jour Gastrointestinal Surgery* 14(5): 2009.

Podolsky ER, Moulas A, Wu AS, et al: Single port access (SPA) laparoscopic ventral hernia repair: initial report of 30 cases, *Surg Endosc* 24(7):1557–1561, 2010.

THE MANAGEMENT OF SEMILUNAR LINE, LUMBAR, AND OBTURATOR HERNIATION

John Paige, MD

INTRODUCTION

Semilunar line, lumbar, and obturator hernias all share common features that make their diagnosis and management challenging. First, they comprise a small percentage of all forms of herniation, and, as such, they are encountered rarely during a surgeon's career. Second, they are often difficult to diagnose on physical examination because most of these defects do not extend through all layers of the overlying musculature. As a consequence, these hernias are often encountered by the surgeon in the emergency setting after incarceration or strangulation of their contents, limiting therapeutic options and increasing both morbidity and mortality. Additionally, all three types of hernias can result in a so-called Richter's herniation (i.e., partial entrapment of a portion of an involved organ or tissue through the defect), altering presentation and making diagnosis even more challenging. Finally, eponyms for particular types of these hernias abound, requiring surgeons to have an intimate knowledge of the anatomic borders and location associated with each one (Table 1).

Computed tomographic (CT) scanning has become the preferred modality for the preoperative diagnosis of these uncommon hernias because it is useful in characterizing both the defect itself as well as the contents within the hernia sac (Figure 1). Ultrasonography (US) can also be useful as a rapid means of evaluation in the emergent setting; it should not, however, delay operative exploration in patients with peritonitis. Both open and minimally invasive surgical (MIS) repairs have been described for each type of hernia, and primary as well as tension-free options exist. In general, synthetic prostheses should be avoided in the presence of strangulation or contamination, and the approach undertaken should be based on the clinical situation and the surgeon's experience and expertise with the technique chosen. As with many aspects of general surgery, successful diagnosis and management of these challenging hernias require a high index of suspicious, a clear understanding of the surgical anatomy, and familiarity with several options for repair.

SEMILUNAR LINE (SPIGELIAN) HERNIATION

The linea semilunaris, or linea Spigeli, extends from the tip of the ninth cartilage to the pubic spine and serves as the lateral border of the aponeurotic zone in which Spigelian hernias form (Figure 2). This zone is bordered medially by the lateral edge of the rectus abdominis muscles, and it is widest in the so-called Spigelian hernia belt, a zone extending 6 cm above the anterior superior iliac interspinal plane. In this region, the arcuate line, or line of Douglas, marks the caudal end of the posterior aponeurotic sheath of the rectus muscles; its intersection with the semilunar line creates a weak point. Ninety percent of semilunar line hernias form within this belt, protruding through various layers of the abdominal wall musculature, depending on their relation to the arcuate line (Figure 3). In addition

TABLE 1: Anatomic borders, incidence, and demographic characteristics of some uncommon abdominal wall and pelvic floor hernias

Anatomic location of herniation	Eponym	Anatomic borders of defect	Incidence, demographics
Semilunar line	Spigelian hernia	Within the aponeurosis of transverse abdominal muscle between the lateral edge of the rectus abdominis and the linea semilunaris	1%-2% of all hernias Female predominance Left > right
Lumbar			<2% of all hernias Left > right
Superior triangle	Grynfelt hernia	Base: twelfth rib Medial border: erector spinae muscle Lateral border: internal oblique muscle	Most common location for herniation Short, obese individuals
Inferior triangle	Petit hernia	Base: iliac crest Medial border: latissimus dorsi muscle Lateral border: external oblique muscle	Less common location for herniation Women with wide hips
Obturator	N/A	Superolateral: obturator groove of pubic bone Inferior: free edge of obturator membrane; internal and external obturator muscles	<1% of all hernias Thin, old women (female predominance) Right > left

to spontaneous creation, iatrogenic herniation is possible when surgical drains or laparoscopic ports are placed within this vulnerable aponeurotic zone between the semilunar line and the lateral edge of the rectus muscles, especially in the area of weakness along the hernia belt. Care, therefore, should be taken when choosing the location for these devices.

Abdominal pain is a common presenting symptom of semilunar line hernias. Such pain is exacerbated by increases in intra-abdominal pressure and relieved with rest. On physical exam, a lump may be palpable in the appropriate aponeurotic zone; it can increase in size with patient Valsalva and disappear spontaneously when the patient lies supine. Such spontaneous reduction of the hernia can lead to diagnostic difficulties because CT of the patient in the supine position might not reveal a hernia sac. Hence, diagnostic laparoscopy may be required to confirm the presence of a hernia if CT or US studies are equivocal. Defects tend to be small in size and oval in shape, and, consequently, incarceration of contents commonly occurs. Often, diagnosis is made upon operative exploration for obstructive symptoms.

Given the high rate of incarceration, repair is indicated for all diagnosed semilunar line hernias. Contraindications to operative intervention are limited to those situations in which patient comorbidities preclude general anesthesia. Examples include recent myocardial infarction, severe pulmonary disease, and severe coagulopathy. An open approach should be undertaken in emergent cases or when laparoscopy is contraindicated (e.g., portal hypertension with coagulopathy). In cases involving complete obstruction or frank peritonitis, open exploration should be undertaken expeditiously after the initiation of appropriate resuscitative measures.

Open repair typically consists of anterior hernioplasty with or without prosthesis (Figure 4). If a mass is present, a skin incision is made over it and carried down through the aponeurosis of the external oblique in cases when it is not penetrated. When a mass is not present or in cases of diagnostic uncertainty, a midline incision should be made. For incarcerated hernias, a medial incision of a small, constricting ring extending to the rectus abdominis will aid in the reduction of sac contents. The sac should be opened to inspect its contents after its complete dissection from surrounding tissues. It

is reduced in toto or excised. Following reduction, the peritoneal surface of the adjacent semilunar line should be palpated for additional defects because multiple hernias can exist. Small defects can be repaired primarily with reapproximation of the transversis abdominis and internal oblique aponeuroses using nonabsorbable suture. In cases of larger orifices, multiple defects, thin or weak aponeuroses, or recurrence, tension-free repair should be undertaken using a synthetic mesh (e.g., polypropylene or expanded polytetrafluoroethylene [ePTFE]); it should be placed in an extraperitoneal underlay position and secured with interrupted nonabsorbable sutures. The repair is then reinforced anteriorly by primary closure of the external oblique aponeurosis; skin closure completes the procedure.

MIS options for repair of semilunar line herniation do exist. In general, they are variations of MIS incisional and inguinal hernia repair techniques applied to the setting of a Spigelian hernia and, as such, follow the same principles for exposure, dissection, and mesh placement and fixation. The intraperitoneal onlay mesh (IPOM) repair follows the same steps as a laparoscopic ventral hernia repair. Access is obtained via direct exposure and opening of the fascia with port placement and insufflation (i.e., the Hasson technique) or with Veress needle insufflation with port placement via direct visualization. A combination of 5 and 10 mm ports is placed intraperitoneally according to the principle of triangulation of instruments with the laparoscope (Figure 5). The abdomen is then explored, the hernia defect identified, contents are reduced via gentle traction, and an approximately 3-cm to 5-cm circumferential area cleared around the edges of the defect(s). Mesh is then placed into the abdomen after placing four interrupted sutures in the cardinal locations and rolling the mesh. Typically, a composite synthetic mesh with an antiadhesive layer is chosen to promote scarring to the abdominal wall and decrease adhesion formation to intra-abdominal organs; ePTFE can also be employed. Authors have advocated rolling the mesh in the form of a scroll to assist with securing it to the anterior abdominal wall by unrolling each side sequentially. The mesh is initially secured to the abdominal wall via the four interrupted transabdominal sutures. Following this maneuver, fixation tacks are placed circumferentially around the mesh in one or two rows. Further

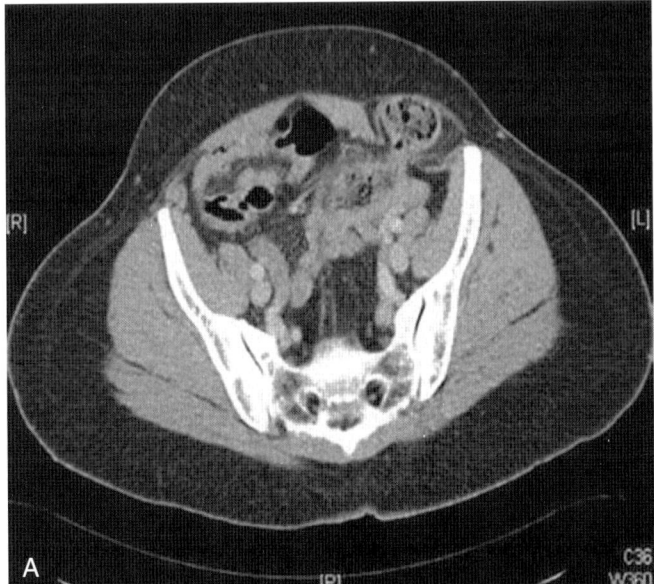

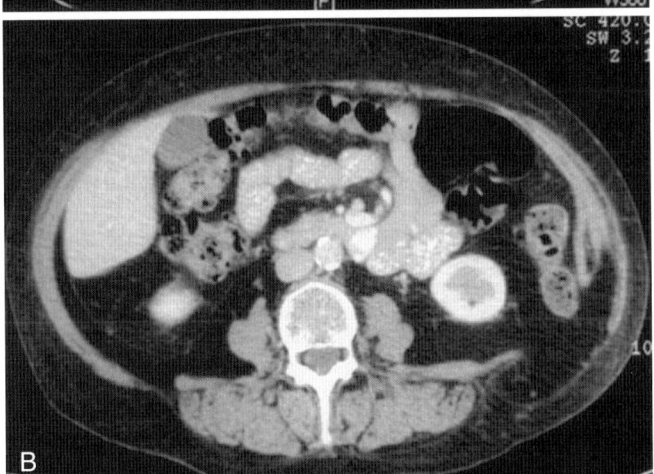

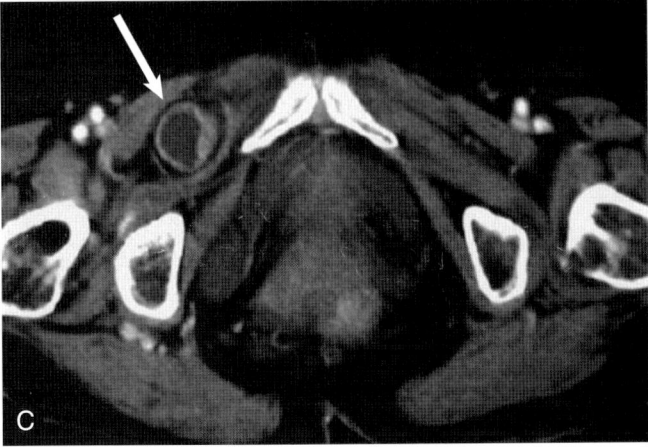

FIGURE 1   A, Computed tomographic (CT) scan of the abdomen demonstrats a left-sided Spigelian hernia containing sigmoid colon. **B,** CT scan reveals the presence of a left Petit hernia involving extraperitoneal fat and partially descending colon. **C,** CT scan demonstrates a right-sided obturator hernia revealing a fluid-filled mass located between the pectineus and the right external obturator muscles. (**A** *From Sheu EG, Smink DS, Brooks DC: Spigelian hernia. In Jones DB, editor:* Mastery techniques in surgery: hernia, *Philadelphia, 2013, Wolters Kluwer/Lippincott, Williams & Wilkins, pp 385–392;* **B** *from Cavallaro G, Sadighi A, Mecili M, et al: Primary lumbar hernia: the open approach,* Eur Surg Res *39:88–92, 2007;* **C** *from Chang SS, Shan YS, Lin YJ, et al: A review of obturator hernia and a proposed algorithm for its diagnosis and treatment,* World J Surg *29:450–454, 2005.)*

creation of a preperitoneal workspace using a balloon pump. Its advantage is the placement of mesh preperitoneally, preventing intra-abdominal adhesion formation. It requires midline placement of ports; mesh is secured with tacks. The TAPP repair creates a preperitoneal flap intra-abdominally. Mesh is placed and secured using tacks and sutures (i.e., transabdominal or intra-abdominal). The flap is sutured close, covering the mesh and protecting the intra-abdominal contents from contact with it. Both of these repairs can be technically more challenging, given the preperitoneal placement of the mesh. They require a 3-cm to 5-cm overlay over the defect and can employ synthetic mesh alone (i.e., without an antiadhesive layer composite).

As already mentioned, the decision regarding the approach for repair depends on multiple factors. A randomized controlled trial comparing open versus MIS repair of elective Spigelian hernias demonstrated an advantage for the MIS approach in terms of hospital length of stay and morbidity. It did not show an advantage, however, regarding recurrence rates or mortality. Current recommendations advocate MIS repair, preferably via TEP, in elective cases when such expertise is available. Laparoscopy is also advocated in cases where the diagnosis is in doubt or if another intraperitoneal procedure is being contemplated. Anterior hernioplasty is reserved for more complicated cases (i.e., strangulation) or in the setting of recurrence.

Complications related to repair are similar to those encountered for other types of ventral hernia repair, including bowel injury, bleeding, mesh migration/shrinkage, infection, and recurrence. Thankfully, recurrence rates are rather low, owing to the layered closure of open repairs. One recent review found only a 0.7% rate among over 800 repairs.

LUMBAR HERNIATION

Lumbar hernias can be congenital or acquired. Acquired hernias are by far the most common, approaching 80% of all lumbar hernias. Primary acquired hernias occur spontaneously and are commonly found in the superior lumbar triangle (i.e., Grynfelt hernias). Secondary acquired hernias arise following surgical incision (e.g., from denervation after retroperitoneal aortic aneurysm repair), infection (i.e., after lumbar abscess), or trauma (e.g., deceleration and sheering after a motor vehicle crash); they are not typically confined to an anatomically defined region in the lumbar area. Age over 60 years, hard labor (i.e., heavy lifting), conditions causing increased intra-abdominal pressure, and morbid obesity are all recognized risk factors for lumbar herniation.

Lumbar hernias typically present as a painless mass or protrusion in the lumbar region that may increase in size with straining. Associated back pain and/or vague abdominal symptoms may be present.

transabdominal sutures are then placed at 4- to 6-cm intervals. Mesh should overlap the defect by 3 to 5 cm from all edges. Fascial closure of all 10-mm port defects is then undertaken, and the procedure is completed.

In addition to the IPOM technique, both total extraperitoneal (TEP) and transabdominal preperitoneal (TAPP) repairs have been described for semilunar line hernias. The TEP repair requires the

Contents can contain either extraperitoneal fat or intraperitoneal structures. In severe cases, whole organs such as the kidney and/or spleen may be involved. Additionally, sliding hernias can occur. Incarceration is present in approximately a quarter of cases, and strangulation can approach 20%. Given such rates, many authors recommend repair when the diagnosis of lumbar hernia is made. In the case of superior lumbar triangle hernias, the latissimus dorsi muscle covers the defect anteriorly, making clinical diagnosis more difficult. For inferior lumbar triangle hernias, no overlying muscular layer is present. CT and US are the preferred modalities for delineation and diagnosis of lumbar hernias.

Open repair is conducted with the patient in a prone position. An incision is made over the hernia defect with exposure of the sac and defect. The sac is then dissected free from surrounding structures. Small defects (i.e., those less than 2.5 cm in diameter) may be repaired primarily with nonabsorbable sutures. Musculoaponeurotic flaps can also be used to cover larger defects. In general, however, tension-free repair using synthetic mesh is preferred for most defects (Figure 6). Mesh should overlap the edge of the defect by 3 to 5 cm. It is secured to surrounding structures using interrupted nonabsorbable sutures and then covered by reapproximating overlying muscle. If mesh remains exposed after such reapproximation, a rotational fascial or musculoaponeurotic flap can be fashioned for coverage, especially for inferior lumbar triangle defects. Otherwise, a second layer of mesh can be placed. Recently, a sutureless meshplasty repair has been described in which mesh is placed over the defect without fixation and loosely covered by overlying tissue.

MIS repairs consist of transabdominal or retroextraperitoneal approaches. The patient is typically positioned in a semilateral position in order to allow repositioning in the supine or true lateral position as needed (Figure 7). For the transabdominal approach, a periumbilical port is placed and pneumoperitoneum established. Additional ports are then placed based on the size and location of the hernia. Typically a supraumbilical and infraumbilical port in the midline is sufficient. The hernia is exposed after mobilization of the ipsilateral colon and kidney as needed. The contents are then gently reduced, and the defect is dissected free from surrounding tissue. Synthetic or composite mesh is then placed and secured with tacks and transabdominal sutures. Some authors have advocated the placement of bone anchors to the iliac crest and/or an encircling suture around the twelfth rib to secure the mesh. The extraperitoneal approach involves the creation of a workspace within the

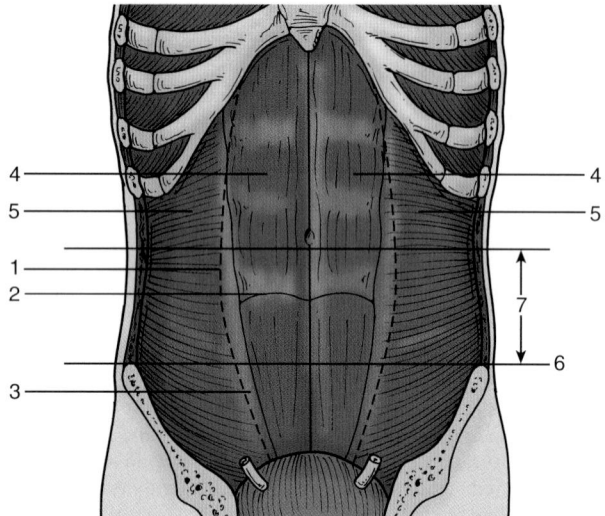

FIGURE 2   Posterior view of the abdominal wall. (1) Semilunar line of Spiegel. (2) Semicircular line of Douglas. (3) Spigelian aponeurosis. (4) Posterior rectus sheath. (5) Transversus abdominis muscle. (6) Interspinal line connecting the anterior superior iliac spines, forming the caudal border of the (7) Spigelian belt, where the majority of Spigelian hernias occur within the Spigelian aponeurosis. *(From Sheu EG, Smink DS, Brooks DC: Spigelian hernia. In Jones DB, editor: Mastery techniques in surgery: hernia, Philadelphia, 2013, Wolters Kluwer/Lippincott, Williams & Wilkins, pp 385–392.)*

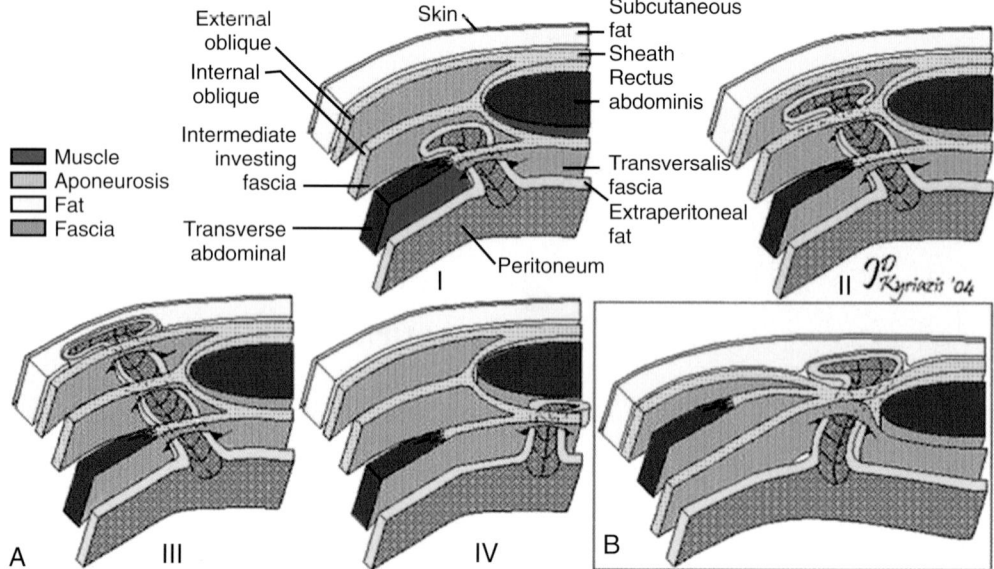

FIGURE 3   Three-dimensional schematic presentation of cross section of the abdominal wall in vicinity of the left border of the sheath of the rectus abdominis muscle, posterior view. Spigelian hernia sac is shown at various surgical levels. **A,** Above the semicircular line (of Douglas). *I,* Superficial to the aponeurosis of the transverse abdominal muscle. *II,* Superficial to the aponeurosis of the internal oblique muscle. *III,* Superficial to the aponeurosis of the external oblique muscle. *IV,* Penetrating the posterior lamina of the rectus sheath. **B,** Below the semicircular line (of Douglas). *(From Skandalakis PN, Zoras O, Skandalakis JE, et al: Lumbar hernia: surgical anatomy, embryology, and technique of repair, Am Surg 27:42, 2006.)*

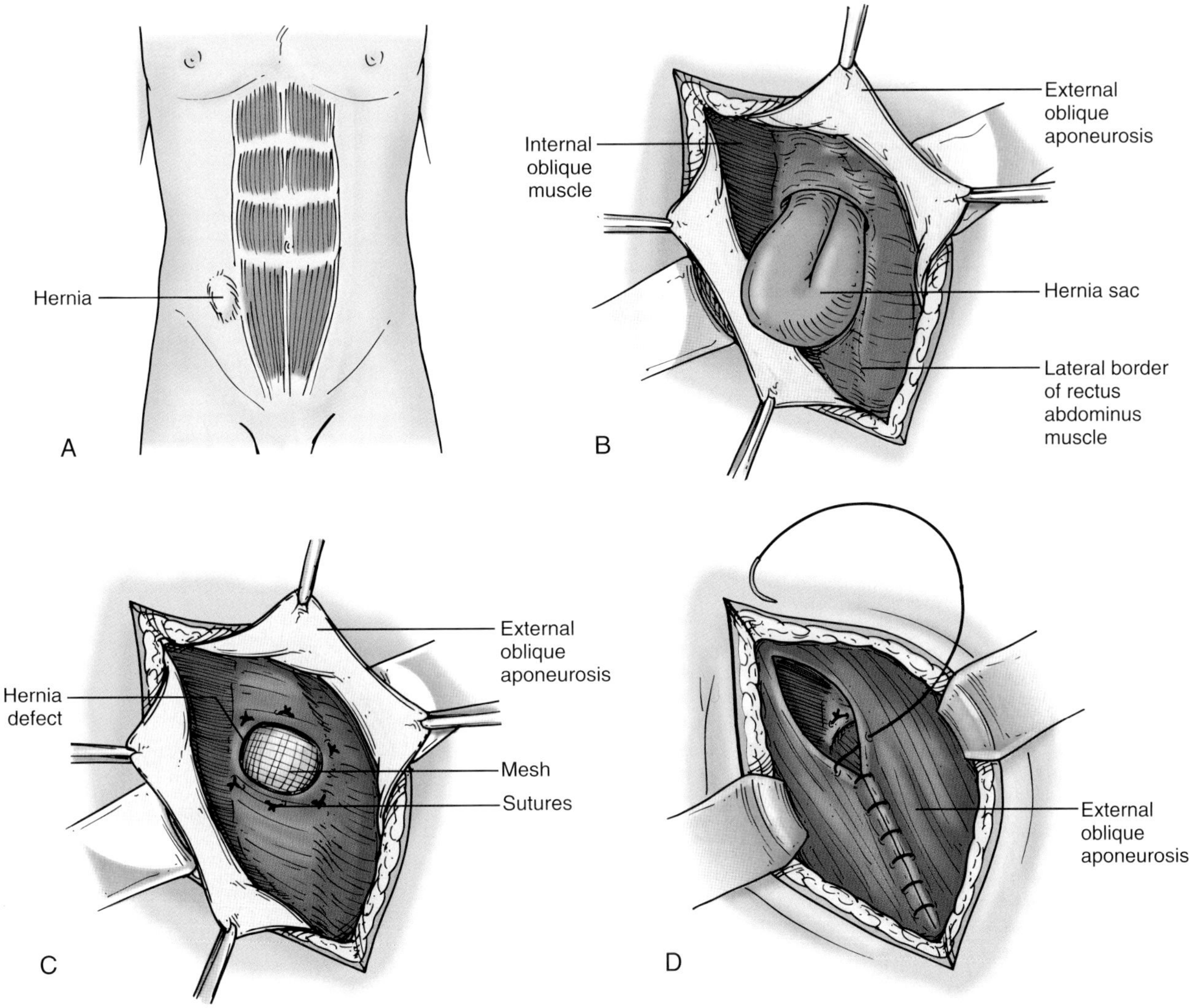

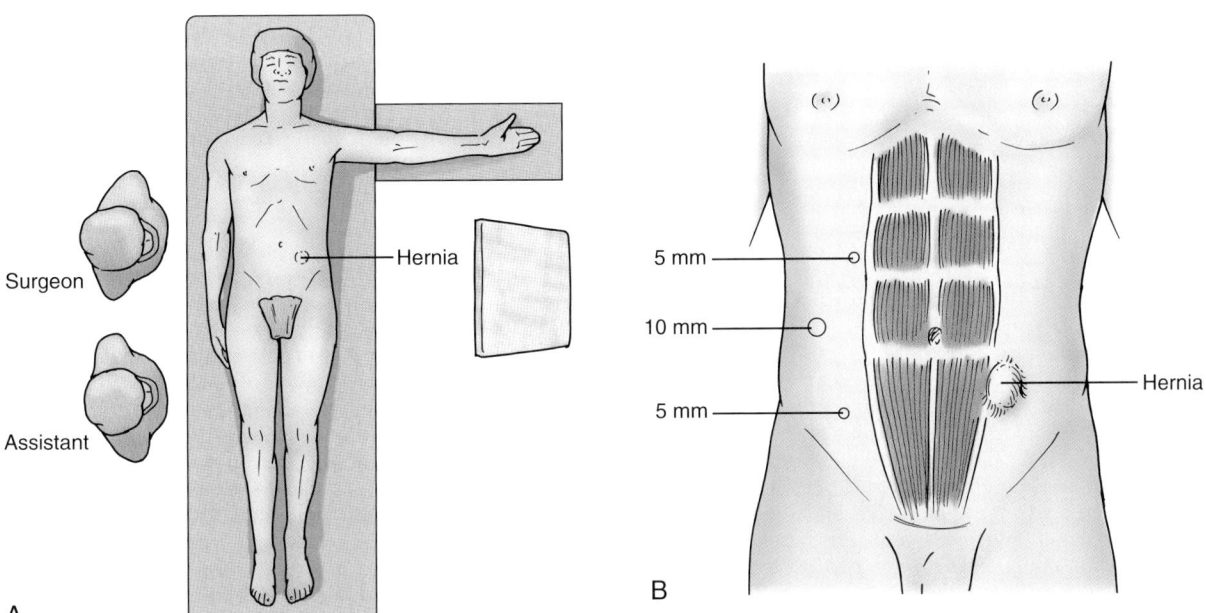

FIGURE 4 Schematic representation of open Spigelian hernia repair. **A,** Typical location of Spigelian hernia at the lateral border of the rectus, inferior to the umbilicus. **B,** Exposure of the hernia sac and fascial defect. The external oblique aponeurosis has been divided. **C,** After the hernia sac has been reduced and/or excised, an underlay mesh is placed to cover the hernia defect and is secured in place with interrupted sutures. **D,** The external aponeurosis is reapproximated to cover the hernia defect and mesh. *(From Sheu EG, Smink DS, Brooks DC: Spigelian hernia. In Jones DB, editor:* Mastery techniques in surgery: hernia, *Philadelphia, 2013, Wolters Kluwer/Lippincott, Williams & Wilkins, pp 385-392.)*

FIGURE 5 Laparoscopic repair of Spigelian hernia: equipment and trocar placement. **A,** The patient is placed in a supine position. The contralateral arm is tucked to enable free movement of the surgeon and the assistant, who stand opposite the hernia. **B,** Example of trocar placement. At least one 10-mm port is required to introduce the mesh. Placement of the working ports as far lateral facilitates securing the proximal side of the mesh. *(From Sheu EG, Smink DS, Brooks DC: Spigelian hernia. In Jones DB, editor:* Mastery techniques in surgery: hernia, *Philadelphia, 2013, Wolters Kluwer/Lippincott, Williams & Wilkins, pp 385–392.)*

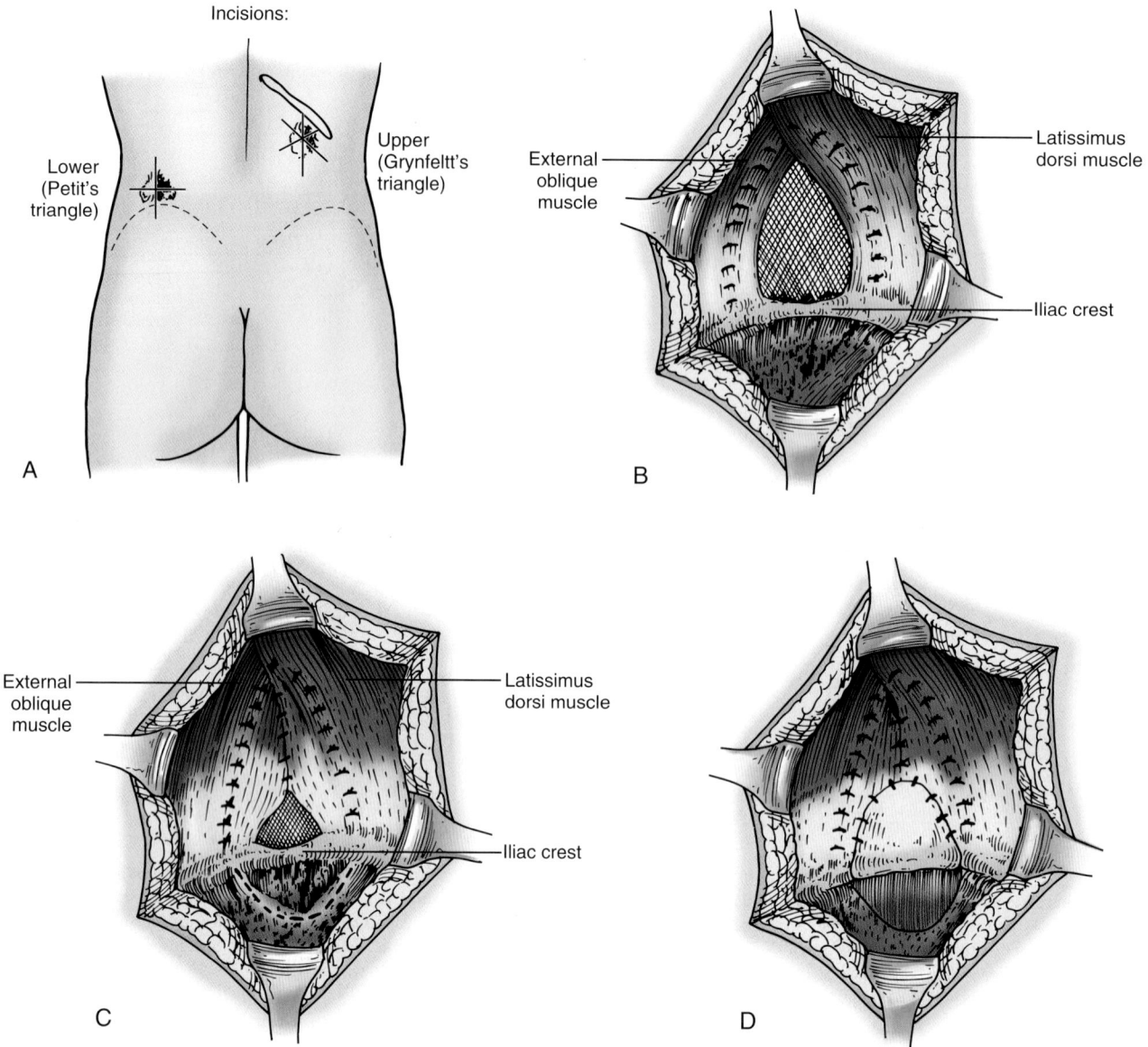

FIGURE 6 A, Oblique or vertical incision over the lumbar hernia site. **B,** Patch over the defect, anchored to muscles and periosteum. **C,** External oblique latissimus dorsi muscles approximated over the mesh. A flap of gluteal fascia is cut (dotted line). **D,** Rotation of the flap of gluteal fascia to complete coverage of the mesh. *(Originally from Skandalakis JE, Gray SW, Mansberger AR Jr, et al: Hernia: surgical anatomy and technique, ed 2, New York, 1989, Springer, with permission. From Stamatiou D, Skandalakis JE, Skandalakis LJ, Mirilas P: Lumbar hernia: surgical anatomy, embryology, and technique of repair, Am Surg 75:202–207, 2009.)*

retroperitoneum with reduction of the hernia sac and mesh repair of the defect.

Although randomized trials are lacking, longitudinal prospective studies have demonstrated an advantage in MIS repair of lumbar hernias in terms of overall cost, pain control, and return to normal activity. Recurrence rates for repair can approach 15%. Diffuse hernias, large defects, local morbidity, and muscle atrophy increase the risk of recurrence. Moreno-Egea and colleagues have recently suggested an algorithm for repair of acquired lumbar hernias based on type. Primary hernias should be repaired either via an open or laparoscopic approach based on surgeon expertise. Secondary hernias arising from trauma should undergo laparoscopic repair if chronic, open repair via laparotomy if acute. Finally, postincisional hernias should undergo laparoscopic repair if less than 10 cm in size and open double mesh repair if greater than 15 cm. Those hernias ranging from 10 to 15 cm in size should undergo laparoscopic versus open repair based on the degree of muscular atrophy present.

OBTURATOR HERNIATION

Although obturator herniation accounts for only 0.2% to 1.6% of all small bowel obstructions, 90% of patients presenting with an obturator hernia have signs and symptoms of small bowel obstruction (i.e., nausea, vomiting, crampy abdominal pain). Oftentimes, patients report previous attacks with spontaneous resolution. Known as the "little old lady" hernia, it occurs predominantly in older, thin women with concomitant illness. Risk factors include multiparity, malnutrition, chronic illness, and conditions associated with increased abdominal pressure. Gangrenous bowel can be present on exploration in up to 50% of cases, resulting in high perioperative morbidity and mortality. Hence, all obturator hernias should be repaired once diagnosed. Additionally, because bilaterality can occur, exploration of the obturator region opposite the hernia should be undertaken at the time of repair.

Herniation can follow the path of the anterior or posterior branch of the obturator nerve (Figure 8). Its compression by the sac contents leads to its irritation and associated medial thigh pain radiating to behind the knee and into the hip. The pain is relieved with hip flexion and exacerbated with extension, abduction, or medial rotation of the thigh, the so-called Howship-Romberg sign. Some authors consider its presence as pathognomonic for obturator herniation. In some cases, a tender mass is present in the upper inner thigh or felt antero-laterally on rectal examination. Ecchymosis in the femoral triangle below the inguinal ligament can also be present. In cases of bowel necrosis and perforation, patients will have frank peritonitis.

CT remains the diagnostic modality of choice in patients who do not require immediate operative intervention. It has high sensitivity and accuracy. US of the inguinal region and inner thigh is a fast,

inexpensive way to diagnose an incarcerated obturator hernia in the emergency department, but it should not delay surgery. In certain situations, plain radiograph can reveal intraluminal air overlying the obturator canal or at the level of the superior pubic ramus, suggesting the presence of an obturator hernia. Herniography (i.e., placement of iodinated contrast within the peritoneal cavity) is effective in diagnosing obturator herniation without incarceration. Finally, laparoscopy has been advocated in cases of obstruction to assist with diagnosis. Repair can then be undertaken via open or laparoscopic means based on findings and/or the presence of contamination.

Depending on the patient presentation, open repair can be via a transabdominal or extraabdominal approach. Laparotomy via lower midline incision should be undertaken in cases of peritonitis, diagnostic uncertainty, complete intestinal obstruction, suspected gangrenous bowel, or deteriorating clinical condition. The patient should be placed in the Trendelenburg position to assist with exposure. Gentle dorsal and medial traction is used to reduce incarcerated bowel. In cases in which such a maneuver is unsuccessful, the deep ring of the obturator canal can be incised in a downward and medial direction at its lower margin because 50% of the time the nerve and vessels will be lateral to the sac. Care must be taken, however, because they can lie anterior, medial, or posterior in the remaining cases. Hip flexion and adduction after finger stretching of the obturator canal can assist with reduction as well. In extreme cases, a counter incision medial to the femoral vein is required with disinsertion of the pectineus muscle in order to reduce the hernia. After reduction, any necrotic bowel should be resected. The hernia sac itself should be inverted and excised. This maneuver decreases the rate of recurrence. Small defects can be repaired with interrupted or purse-string closure. Larger defects require tissue flaps in the setting of strangulation or contamination. Periosteum, muscle aponeurosis, costal cartilage, round ligament, uterus, ovary, and bladder have all been used; bioprostheses are an alternative.

Extraabdominal open repair is indicated when the preoperative diagnosis of an obturator hernia has been made and contamination is not anticipated. The obturator approach is useful when a palpable mass can be felt. It involves an incision over the mass with division of the fascia lata, retraction of the pectineus and adductor longus muscles, reduction of the hernia sac, and closure of the defect. Preperitoneal exposure of an obturator hernia can also be undertaken via an inguinal, suprapubic, or lower midline incision (Figure 9). The midline approach has the advantage of allowing exploration of the obturator region opposite to the hernia. When strangulation or contamination is not present, synthetic mesh repair can be employed for large defects.

MIS repair is generally recommended in the setting of elective repair, although some authors have advocated its use in the presence

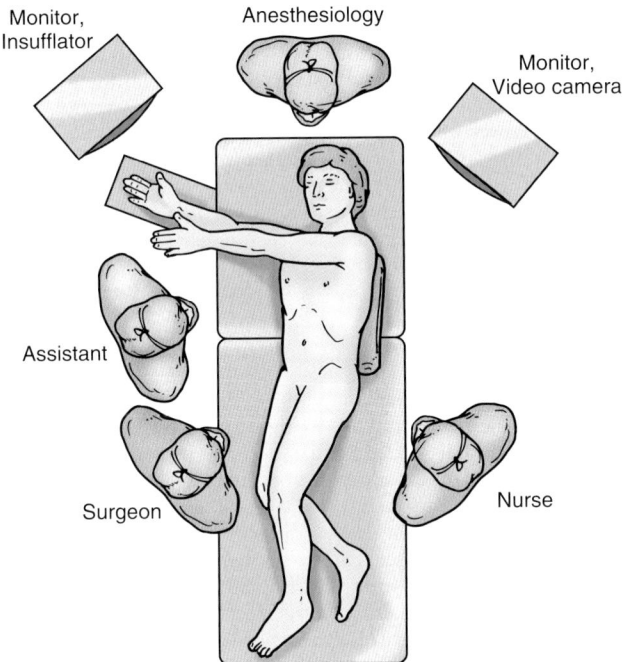

FIGURE 7 Patient position for laparoscopic left lumbar hernia repair. The patient is placed at a 45-degree angle from the horizontal. A rolled blanket is used as a posterior wedge. *(From Arca MJ, Heniford BT, Pokorny R, et al: Laparoscopic repair of lumbar hernias, J Am Coll Surg 187:147–152, 1998.)*

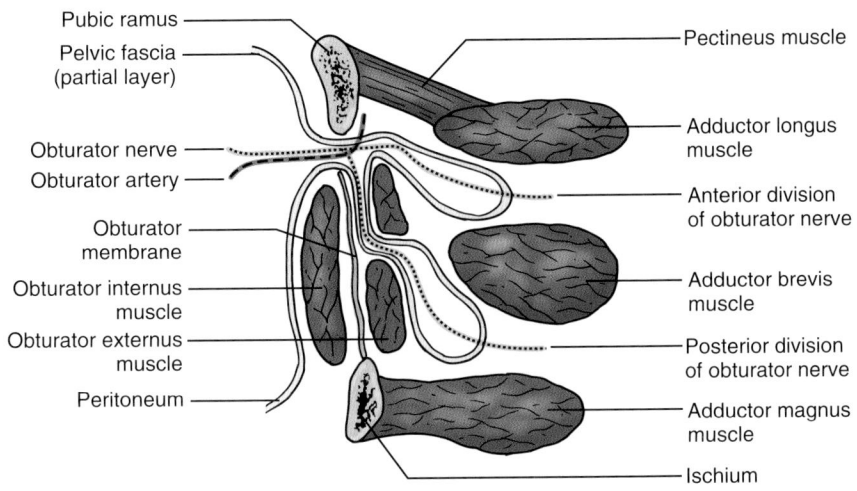

FIGURE 8 Herniation can follow the path of the anterior or posterior branch of the obturator nerve. *(From Stamatiou D, Skandalakis LJ, Zoras O, Mirilas P: Obturator hernia revisited: surgical anatomy, embryology, diagnosis, and technique of repair, Am Surg 77:1147–1156, 2011.)*

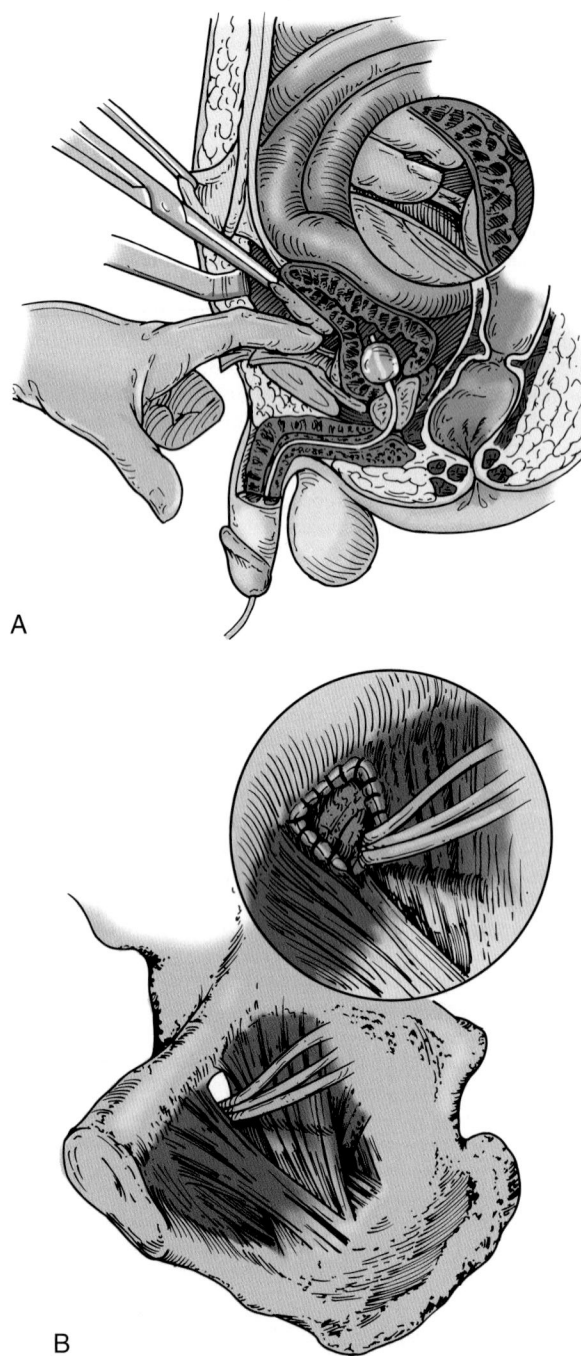

of obstruction without evidence of bowel necrosis, ischemia, or contamination. TAPP and TEP approaches have been described and are similar in technique as for inguinal hernia repair. For the TAPP approach, the obturator space is exposed via a parietal peritoneal incision and flap creation. In the TEP approach, the preperitoneal fat overlying Cooper's ligament must be swept away with medial retraction of the bladder. Both approaches allow for easy exploration of the opposite obturator space, concomitant repair of inguinal or femoral hernias, and better visualization. The TAPP approach also allows for close inspection of the bowel to rule out necrosis, but care must be taken to completely close the peritoneal flap to prevent contact of mesh with intra-abdominal contents. Additionally, mesh must adequately cover the obturator opening. As with Spigelian and lumbar hernias, MIS repair of obturator hernias results in shorter lengths of stay, less pain, and less morbidity (i.e., fewer pulmonary complications and lower postoperative ileus rates in the case of obturator hernias).

Postoperative morbidity rates for obturator hernia repair can approach 40% given the high rates of gangrenous bowel and peritonitis on presentation. Complications described in the literature include sepsis, pneumonia, wound infection, mesh migration, fistulae, small bowel obstruction, urinary tract infection, pulmonary embolism, myocardial infarction, and congestive heart failure. Mortality can range from 12% to 70%. As a result, intensive care is often required in the postoperative period, especially following emergent presentations. Recurrence rates are fortunately low, occurring less than 10% of the time following repairs.

SUMMARY

Management of semilunar line, lumbar, and obturator herniation remains a challenge for the practicing surgeon given their uncommon nature, unusual anatomy, and high risk of incarceration. CT and US are useful modalities for diagnosing and delineating these hernias that can be difficult to identify on physical exam. Repair of these hernias is indicated when they are discovered because incarceration and strangulation of contents are not infrequent events. Fortunately, surgical options include multiple open and MIS approaches with or without the use of prosthesis. Management is guided by the clinical situation, surgeon experience, and anatomic considerations.

SUGGESTED READINGS

Sheu EG, Smink DS, Brooks DC: Spigelian hernia. In Jones DB, editor: *Mastery techniques in surgery: hernia*, Philadelphia, 2013, Wolters Kluwer/Lippincott, Williams & Wilkins, pp 385–392.

Stamatiou D, Skandalakis JE, Skandalakis LJ, Mirilas P: Lumbar hernia: surgical anatomy, embryology, and technique of repair, *Am Surg* 75:202–207, 2009.

Stamatiou D, Skandalakis LJ, Zoras O, Mirilas P: Obturator hernia revisited: surgical anatomy, embryology, diagnosis, and technique of repair, *Am Surg* 77:1147–1156, 2011.

FIGURE 9   A, Exploration of the retropubic space. *Inset:* Identification of the structures that pass through the obturator canal. **B,** A relatively large defect of the obturator canal. *Inset:* Closure with the use of mesh. *(Originally from Skandalakis LJ, Gadacz TB, Mansberger AR, et al: Modern hernia repair: the embryological and anatomical basis of surgery, New York, 1996, Parthenon Publishing Group, pp 286–296, with permission. From Stamatiou D, Skandalakis LJ, Zoras O, Mirilas P: Obturator hernia revisited: surgical anatomy, embryology, diagnosis, and technique of repair, Am Surg 77:1147–1156, 2011.)*

ATHLETIC PUBALGIA: THE "SPORTS HERNIA"

**Bruce Ramshaw, MD, FACS, and
Issa Mirmehdi, MD**

INTRODUCTION

The diagnosis and management of a sports hernia, or athletic pubalgia, is a complex undertaking. Even the terminology to describe the condition has been controversial, primarily because the most commonly used term, *sports hernia*, is not an accurate description of the underlying disease for most cases. For most patients who are diagnosed with a sports hernia, no true hernia defect is present. The management can be a long and frustrating process, and the decision to proceed with more aggressive treatment, including surgery, can be complex. The basic strategies and techniques for surgical management also vary, and although most patients do well with surgical management from those surgeons who are experienced treating this condition, regardless of the technique, there are also failures with all approaches. This chapter discusses the background, diagnosis, and management of a sports hernia, and it presents a concept for learning and improving care for treating complex conditions such as sports hernias.

BACKGROUND

Sports hernia or athletic pubalgia is defined as chronic groin pain (lasting more than 6 to 8 weeks without improvement or the patient not able to return to normal activities) in an individual who frequently engages in athletic and/or strenuous activity. It is diagnosed in the absence of a palpable hernia and when other causes of inguinal pain are excluded. Due to the lack of a visible or palpable hernia defect, this syndrome has not been well understood by many general surgeons. Only recently, perhaps due to the increasing media coverage about professional athletes whose careers have been interrupted or ended as a result of this condition, attempts to better understand the complex nature of sports hernia have been made. Although this condition has been popularized by the experience of professional athletes with this condition, it also affects athletes in college and high school, as well as recreational athletes and people who perform other strenuous activities.

In 1980, Gilmore (Gilmore OJ, 1991) recognized chronic groin pain in professional athletes, mostly soccer players, and undertook to surgically repair the disruption. This condition was subsequently referred to as Gilmore's groin. A similar condition was also reported in Europe and Australia. Many investigators have described the chronic lower abdominal and groin pain in professional athletes as a syndrome secondary to muscular injury or incipient inguinal hernias. In 1991, Taylor and colleagues (Taylor D, et al., 1991) concluded that while the majority of groin pain in athletes was caused by muscle strains, inguinal hernias, or subclinical abdominal wall defects without herniation, in a smaller subset of cases there was no palpable hernia or any other cause of groin pain. Following the terminology used in the European literature, they referred to this condition as *pubalgia*.

ANATOMY, PATHOPHYSIOLOGY, AND DIFFERENTIAL DIAGNOSIS

Etiology

Gilmore identified torn external oblique aponeurosis, torn conjoint tendon, and dehiscence between the torn conjoint tendon and inguinal ligament as the underlying causes of chronic groin pain. Meyers and colleagues (Meyers W, 2007) suggested that hyperextension injury with the pivot point being the anterior pelvis or pubis symphysis is the most likely etiology of sports hernia. Tendons of the rectus abdominis and adductor longus insert on the pubis symphysis so they pull against each other. This anatomic apparatus, when combined with sport activities that involve rapid pelvic movements such as hyperextension, can potentially injure weaker abdominal wall muscles. This group has documented over 20 distinct anatomic defects from magnetic resonance imaging (MRI) results with surgical recommendations based on each abnormality.

A different perspective on the mechanism of sports hernia focuses on the notion that the syndrome is an incipient hernia, with the defect being in the transversalis fascia comprising the posterior wall of the inguinal canal. Polglase and colleagues found substantial derangement in the posterior wall of the inguinal canal in 61 out of 72 professional athletes, mostly Australian Rules football players who presented with chronic groin pain and underwent surgical exploration of the inguinal canal.

While a general consensus on the complex nature of sports hernia is yet to be established, a third viewpoint combines both mechanisms of muscle tear and incipient hernia and categorizes this condition as one component of a broader pattern of "groin disruption injury." According to this school of thought, sports hernia is an occult or incipient direct hernia, which is derived from pelvic instability. This underlying mechanism also gives rise to other groin syndromes such as osteitis pubis, conjoint tendinopathy and/or tear, adductor tendinopathy and/or tear, and nerve entrapment and/or irritation of the variety of nerves in the groin and pelvic area.

People at Risk

A sports hernia is more likely to occur in athletes who engage in sports that require sudden turns and pelvic movements and/or those that require the athlete to push hard against resistance. It is thought that the highest prevalence occurs in athletes who are professional soccer players, ice hockey players, and football players, respectively. Men are more frequently affected than women. However, there seems to be an increase in the number of female athletes experiencing chronic groin pain as more women engage in competitive sports. It has also been postulated that gender-specific anatomic variation may play a role in predisposing male athletes, more than female athletes, to developing chronic groin pain. Brophy and colleagues demonstrated that male soccer players tend to generate a greater activation of the iliacus muscle in the kicking limb, and this difference may contribute to a higher susceptibility to developing sports hernia. Other risk factors include limb length discrepancy, poor pelvic muscle balance, reduced hip range of motion, and pelvic instability.

Presentation and Differential Diagnosis

Patients with sports hernia present with lower abdominal pain on exertion. Most can recall a distinct injury during exertion prior to the onset of the pain. The pain is usually located in the inguinal region around the insertion point of rectus abdominis muscle on the pubis or along the course of the ilioinguinal nerve. Most patients experience unilateral pain, although in some athletes, their symptoms begin with unilateral pain and subsequently progress to bilateral pain. The pain may also radiate to the lower abdomen, perineum, scrotum, or thigh. At rest, there is usually minimal or no pain. Valsalva maneuvers such as coughing or bearing down may sometimes reproduce the pain. Also, adduction against resistance can exacerbate the pain in some patients. The majority of these patients report that their groin pain preceded their adduction pain. Patients will experience these symptoms for many months, and some present having suffered from their pain for more than 1 year. At the time of presentation, the majority of athletes have stopped competitive physical activity, or they are limited in their ability to compete.

On physical examination, a localized tenderness can be elicited near the rectus abdominis insertion above the pubic tubercle on the affected side or on both sides, depending on the course of the pain progression. This finding is more pronounced during resisted sit-up. Additional findings may include inguinal canal tenderness or tenderness at the hip adductor origin. A pain along the adductor longus tendon on the affected side may also be elicited on forceful adduction. Occasionally, a cough impulse can be palpated at the rectus abdominis origin when the patient is standing. It is uncommon to palpate a cough impulse at the external inguinal ring. A thorough physical exam should generally rule out inguinal hernia.

The different diagnosis for groin pain without a hernia bulge can be extensive (Figure 1). The patient can have more than one condition, including inguinal (direct and/or indirect), femoral, obturator, or other more rare hernias in the groin and pelvic region. A lipoma of the spermatic cord may also be present. For most sports hernias, however, the patient is otherwise healthy, and the duration of the pain, the location of the pain, and the activities that bring on the pain will differentiate a sports hernia from other conditions.

Diagnostic Approach

Sports hernia is primarily diagnosed by history and physical examination. Most data in the literature indicate that imaging studies have relatively poor diagnostic value. However, they can be helpful to rule out other causes of groin pain and may identify specific musculoskeletal injuries causing pain in some cases.

MRI is an imaging modality that can occasionally provide helpful data in diagnosing sports hernia, particularly when the underlying mechanism is muscle or tendon tear. Yet, its reported sensitivity can vary greatly, likely due to the experience of the radiologist reading the film and to the many false positives that may occur when injuries are identified but are not actually causing the symptoms. MRI may also be helpful to rule out osteitis pubis, occult stress or avulsion fracture, and other etiologies of groin pain.

Another imaging technique that may be helpful in diagnosing sports hernia in the setting of inguinal canal posterior wall defect is dynamic ultrasonography. In this technique, the probe is placed on the medial aspect of the inguinal region, first along the plane of the inguinal canal and then perpendicular to the initial position. At each position, the patient is asked to cough or bear down, and if a defect is present, ballooning of the posterior wall of the inguinal canal will be present.

Computed tomographic (CT) scan or plain radiograph are usually normal in patients with sports hernia. They may, however, provide information to rule out bony fractures or other causes of pain.

MANAGEMENT

Nonsurgical

Most cases of groin pain in athletes will resolve with conservative management strategies. When pain does not resolve after 6- to 16-week period of rest and conservative management strategies, surgery is often the most definitive management for patients with a sports hernia. Conservative management includes rest, core strengthening exercises, stretching, and antiinflammatory medications. The initial rest period is usually 1 to 4 weeks, and during this period, the athlete may receive steroids or platelet-rich plasma injections to the rectus abdominis, adductor longus origin, or both. If injections are not desired, the patient may receive a short course of oral steroids, which is quickly tapered. At the end of the 4-week period, a functional trial of an athletic regimen appropriate for the athlete's sport is performed to evaluate the patient's response to the conservative management. Core strengthening exercises may emphasize the development of a strong single-limb stance and pelvic rotation exercises against resistance. Some of the works listed in Suggested Readings describe in more detail the prophylactic and conservative physical training exercises and strategies to prevent and manage sports hernias nonoperatively.

Surgical

There are a variety of surgical approaches based on the philosophies about the causes and the documented pathologies found for patients with a sports hernia. We present the laparoscopic approach first, and then the various open methods are described.

Laparoscopic Approach

The concept behind a laparoscopic approach for sports hernia is to reinforce the groin from the inside or behind the groin to block intra-abdominal pressure and allow healing of any musculoskeletal injury. This approach may be most helpful for patients with groin weakness and occult hernias, which might contribute to the patient's symptoms. Although a total extraperitoneal approach is used typically, a transabdominal approach may be used in patients with atypical pain or two different types of pain for which a diagnostic laparoscopy may be indicated.

The technique involves exposure of the entire myopectineal orifice, including reduction of any preperitoneal fat from the indirect space (lipoma of the cord), the femoral space, or obturator foramen. Other rare hernias of the groin may also be visualized and reduced. The most common finding during a laparoscopic approach is a weak transversalis over the direct space. Occasionally actual tears can be visualized. A mesh is used to cover the entire myopectineal orifice and provides a barrier to intra-abdominal pressure that may contribute to the lack of healing of the groin. This would also cover any true hernia defect. The type of mesh used may be extremely important. Chronic groin pain after mesh hernia repair can be a devastating complication. Our hernia program has evaluated hundreds of mesh explants, and for the patient with a sports hernia, we now offer a variety of alternatives to the standard heavyweight polypropylene mesh. The wider-pore, lightweight polypropylene mesh has become a popular option. There are also other polymers, such as polyester, which is relatively hydrophilic, and nonwoven polypropylene and coated polypropylene, both of which may result in less inflammation and better biocompatibility. Today, long-term resorbable meshes (synthetic and biologic) are available that can provide the necessary support for the groin during healing and recovery and will resorb over many months or years to leave no permanent material in the groin. We provide patients with these options with the most current information available so they can make their own decision. A polyester mesh and a long-term resorbable synthetic mesh used for sports hernia repair are shown in Figures 2 and 3. Fixation of mesh may include no fixation, absorbable tack fixation, or glue fixation. Although permanent tack or staple fixation might be used, this may increase postoperative pain.

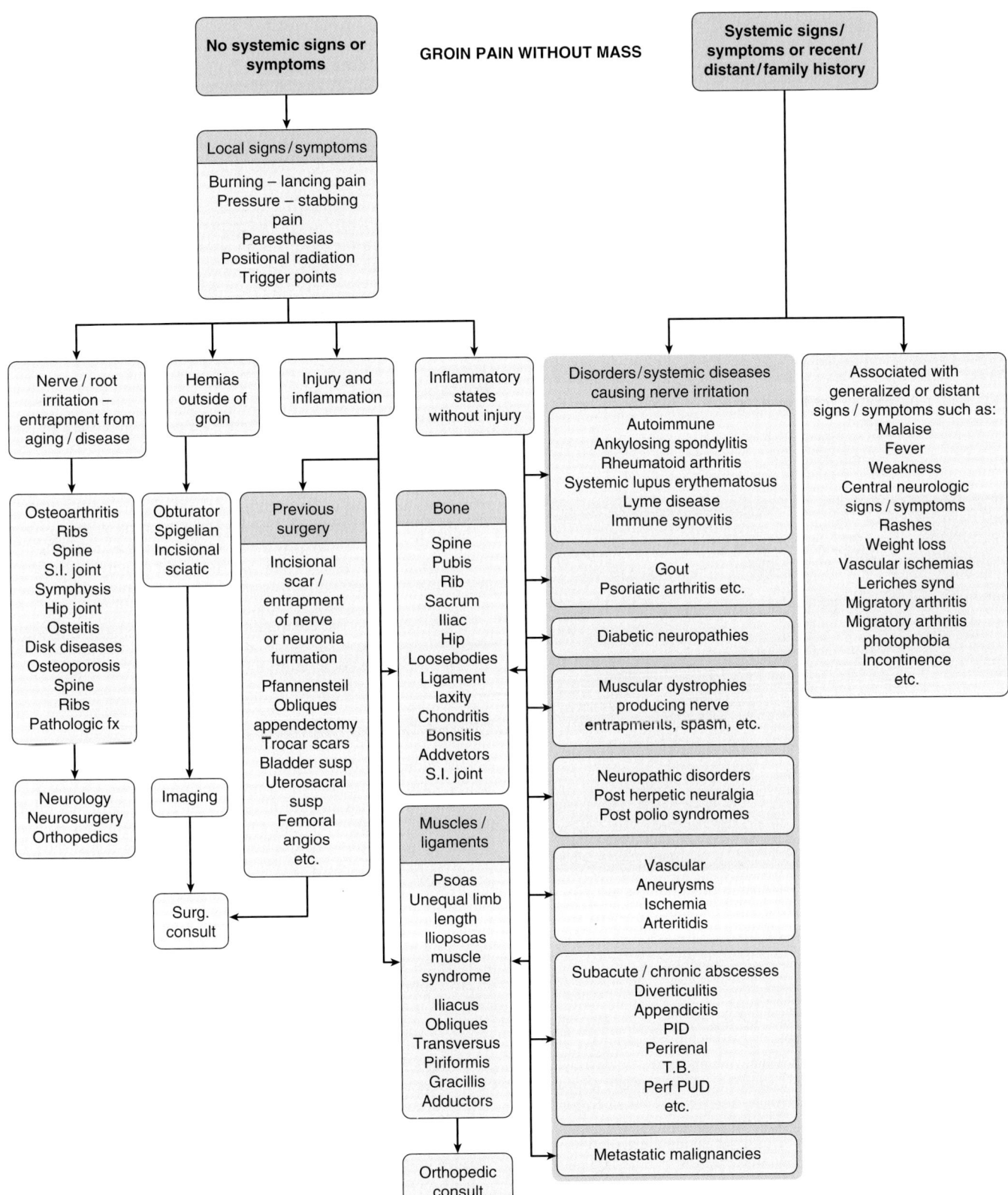

FIGURE 1   A partial list of possible differential diagnoses and potential related systemic symptoms for a patient with groin pain and no groin mass. *Fx,* Fracture; *Perf PUD,* perforated peptic ulcer disease; *PID,* pelvic inflammatory disease; *S.I.,* sacroiliac joint; *T.B.,* tuberculosis.

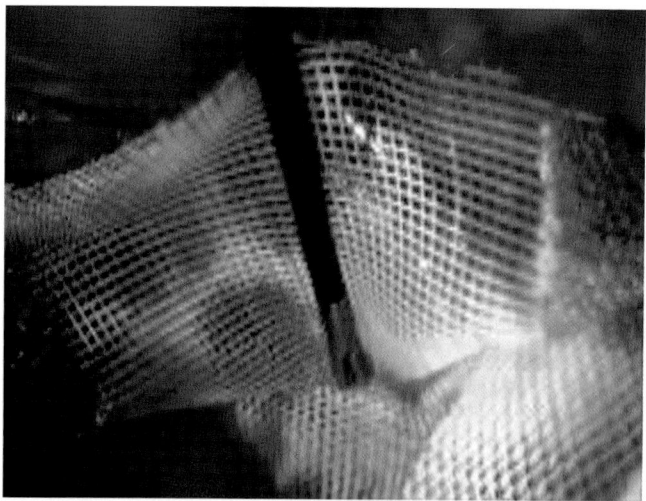

FIGURE 2 A polyester mesh used for laparoscopic sports hernia repair of the right groin.

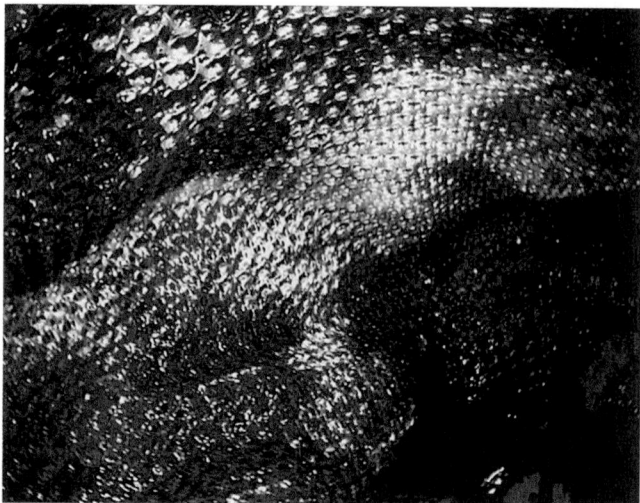

FIGURE 3 A long-term resorbable mesh used for laparoscopic sports hernia repair of the left groin.

Open Mesh Approach

Similar to the laparoscopic approach, the focus of an open mesh placement is to reinforce the floor of the groin to allow for groin stability and musculoskeletal healing. A lightweight polypropylene mesh is typically used and placed similar to a Lichtenstein approach for inguinal hernia repair. Other mesh alternatives described for the laparoscopic approach could also be utilized. One advantage of the open mesh approach is the opportunity to divide the genital branch of the genitofemoral, the ilioinguinal, and/or the iliohypogastric nerves if they are observed to be entrapped in scar tissue or in the tissue disruption caused by musculoskeletal injury. Alternatively, a neurolysis may be performed if a scar tissue release appears appropriate.

Open Nonmesh Approaches

A variety of open nonmesh approaches have been described. One approach popularized by Muschaweck (Muschaweck U, 2010) is presented as an open "minimal repair" technique. The procedure involves a repair of the posterior inguinal floor with two running sutures, including lateralization of the rectus muscle with the second suture. Selectively, the genital branch may be divided if it is impinged by the scar or damaged tissue. The internal ring is reinforced with a buttress of internal oblique muscle to protect the pampiniform plexus.

Myers has presented a more targeted approach to repair of the groin with a variety of techniques utilized, depending on the finding on the MRI and at surgery. General descriptions of these approaches include a variety of repair, release, and excision procedures that may include the reconstruction of the rectus abdominis to the pubis and a selective adductor tenotomy as indicated by the radiographic, clinical, and surgical findings. An adductor tenotomy may include a partial release of the fibers approximately 1 to 2 cm from its attachment to the pubis. Transection with or without reattachment of the adductor longus has also been described.

Postoperative Course

In general, the postoperative recovery is quicker with the less invasive approaches. The laparoscopic approach is the least invasive and has the quickest recovery, with the open reconstructive approaches often requiring the longest recovery. Many factors, however, can impact recovery. The degree of preoperative pain; the nature of the athletic activity; and the decisions of the athletic trainer, athlete, team owner, coach, and so on all may play a role in the timing of return to full activity. In general, athletes may return to light activity in the first 1 to 2 weeks and may try their regular training regimen within 1 to 4 weeks. After appropriate strength, endurance, and flexibility are obtained, return to full competition is appropriate. For very high-level athletes, appropriate game conditions may be simulated to test the appropriateness of a return to full competition.

Clinical Quality Improvement

As mentioned, when performed by surgeons with experience treating sports hernias, all of the procedures described achieve a relatively high rate of success in returning an athlete to his or her sport. However, all of these techniques have failures as well. This demonstrates the reality that a sports hernia, like most problems in health care, is a complex medical problem. For complex problems, a one-size-fits-all solution will not work for every patient. In addition, the most aggressive, costly treatment cannot be used for every patient due to wasteful use of limited resources. The ideal situation would be to learn which patient subpopulations would be best treated with nonsurgical approaches, which would be best treated with minimally invasive approaches, and which would require the most aggressive or costly approaches requiring the longest recovery.

A relatively new science is now being applied to health care that can begin to determine the appropriate indications for the various presentations of complex medical problems such as the sports hernia. Complex adaptive systems science concepts have produced the principles of continuous learning and clinical quality improvement (CQI) in health care. The first step in applying CQI is to define the dynamic processes of care for the entire cycle of care for a specific complex medical problem. In this case, the processes of care would be defined for an athlete from the time of the initial symptom of groin pain until the ability to return to full competitive activity with no future incidence of groin pain. All appropriate treatment options would be included in the dynamic care processes, and the outcomes measures that determine the value of care would be determined and documented. These outcomes measures would include the costs for the entire cycle of care; the quality of the outcomes measure, such as the relief of pain symptoms after treatment; and the patient's and family's experiences with their care. By defining and documenting the care processes and measuring the outcomes that determine the value of care, we can then use these results to provide feedback to improve the processes of care iteratively over time. With more and more data and experience, this will allow for a better understanding of what the best value of care will be for what type of patient.

Another element of complex adaptive systems science applied to health care is the emergence of care communities on the Internet for guidance in caring for complex medical problems such as sports hernias. Through websites, blogs, chat rooms, and other communication methods, more and more people experiencing the symptoms of sports hernias are sharing their stories and experiences with symptoms and treatments. For complex medical problems, these groups and this body of information have been a relatively untapped resource as we strive to improve the value of care for sports hernias and other complex medical problems.

SUMMARY

Sports hernias are complex problems that can be very frustrating for athletes suffering from pain and the inability to return to an activity they enjoy. This is usually a quality of life issue, but for high-level athletes, this can also be a serious economic problem as well. More information about this problem is coming forth, both in the traditional medical literature as well as through emerging care communities on the Internet. As with any complex medical problem, we must apply new scientific thinking to better understand which patients will receive the most value from the variety of surgical and nonsurgical treatment options available and to develop innovative strategies to attempt to prevent this condition and to continuously improve the value of care for this group of patients.

Suggested Readings

Brophy RH, Chiaia TA, Maschi R, et al: The core and hip in soccer athletes compared by gender, *Int J Sports Med* 30(9):663–667, 2009.

Caudill P, Nyland J, Smith C, et al: Sports hernias: a systematic literature review, *Br J Sports Med* 42:954–964, 2008.

Ekstrand J, Ringborg S: Surgery versus conservative treatment in soccer players with chronic groin pain: a prospective randomised study in soccer players, *Eur J Sports Traumatol Rel Res* 23:141–145, 2001.

Garvey JFW, Read JW, Turner A: Sportsman hernia: what can we do? *Hernia* 14:17–25, 2010.

Genitsaris M, Goulimaris I, Sikas N: Laparoscopic repair of groin pain in athletes, *Am J Sports Med* 32:1238–1242, 2004.

Gilmore OJ: Gilmore's groin: ten years experience of groin disruption–a previously unsolved problem in sportsmen, *Sports Med Soft Tissue Trauma* 1(3):12–14, 1991.

Kachingwe AF, Grech S: Proposed algorithm for the management of athletes with athletic pubalgia (sports hernia): a case series, *J Orthop Sports Phys Ther* 38(12):768–781, 2008.

Litwin DE, Sneider EB, McEnaney PM, Busconi BD: Athletic pubalgia (sports hernia), *Clin Sports Med* 30(2):417–434, 2011.

Meyers WC, McKechnie A, Philippon MJ, et al: Experience with "sports hernia" spanning two decades, *Ann Surg* 248(4):656–665, 2008.

Meyers WC, Yoo E, Devon ON, et al: Understanding "sports hernia" (athletic pubablgia): The anatomic and physiologic basis for abdominal and groin pain in athletes, *Oper Tech Sports Med* 15:165–177, 2007.

Minnich JM, Hanks JB, Mushcaweck U, Brunt LM, Diduch DR: Sports hernia: Diagnosis and treatment highlighting a minimal repair technique, *Amer J Sports Med* 39:1341–1349, 2011.

Muschaweck U, Berger LM: Sportsman's groin- diagnostic approach and treatment with the minimal repair technique, *Sorts Health* 2:216–221, 2010.

Nam A, Brody F: Management and therapy for sports hernia, *J Am Coll Surg* 206(1):154–164, 2008.

Polglase AL, Frydman GM, Farmer KC: Inguinal surgery for debilitating chronic groin pain in athletes, *Med J Aust* 155:674–677, 1991.

Swan KG, Wolcott M: The athletic hernia: a systemic review, *Clin Orthop Relat Res* 455:78–87, 2007.

Taylor DC, Meyers WC, Moylan JA, et al: Abdominal musculature abnormalities as a cause of groin pain in athletes. Inguinal hernias and pubalgia, *Am J Sports Med* 19:239–242, 1991.

Werner J, Hagglund M, Walden M, et al: UEFA injury study: a prospective study of hip and groin injuries in professional football over seven consecutive seasons, *Br J Sports Med* 43:1036–1040, 2009.

ABDOMINAL WALL RECONSTRUCTION

Anthony P. Tufaro, DDS, MD, FACS, and
Kurtis A. Campbell, MD, FACS

The need for complicated reconstruction of the abdominal wall is a growing problem in many hospitals large and small. Improvement in trauma care, oncologic surgery, and critical care of surgical patients has led to a host of new problems. Survival of these patients has demanded a comprehensive approach to reconstruction and rehabilitation of the devastated abdominal wall. The problem list that needs to be reviewed includes enterocutaneous fistulas, loss of domain, loss of soft tissue coverage, chronic infection and colonization, deconditioning of the patient, and long-term disability. The trunk is surrounded by a very well designed multilayered wall that first and foremost protects the solid and hollow viscera from injury. The wall, made up of skin, fat, fascia, muscle, and peritoneum must be impervious to water, flexible, resistant to trauma of all kinds, and capable of expanding, contracting, and helping resist infection from the inside environment as well as the outside world. Any attempt at reconstruction of the abdominal wall must take all of these things into consideration and try to incorporate as many of them as possible into the new construct.

ANATOMY

The composite nature of the abdominal wall demands that a number of specialized tissues must work in concert to maintain normal function.

Skin and Adipose Tissue

The skin is the first line of defense for the deeper structures. The skin is the primary barrier to infection, and is vital for fluid control and temperature regulation (Figure 1). The loss of abdominal wall skin may be the result of thermal injury, avulsive trauma, oncologic resection, and necrotizing soft tissue infections and chronic wounds associated with unstable soft tissue coverage. Perhaps the most common cause of skin "loss" seen in patients requiring reconstruction is a relative loss. If we take the patient who suffers an abdominal

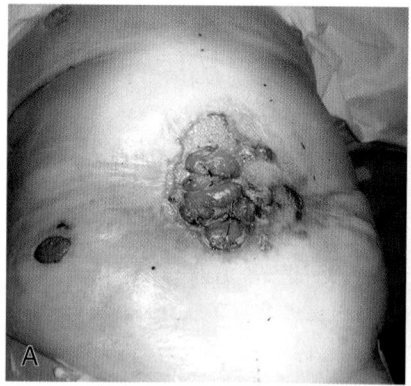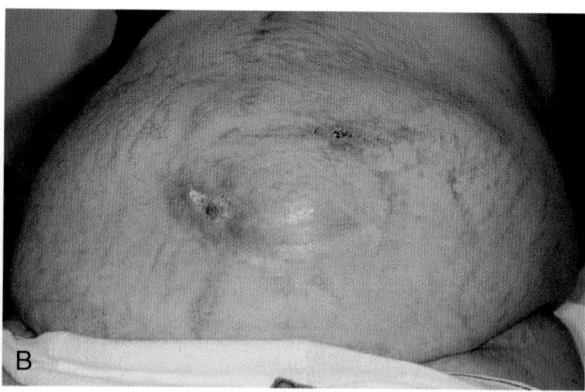

FIGURE I **A,** A devastated abdominal wall with small bowel fistulae. The problem is complicated by the loss of stable skin and soft tissue coverage. **B,** Unstable skin coverage associated with skin graft on bowel and chronic draining wound.

catastrophe of any etiology, subject them to 6, 8, or even 10 hours of surgery or more, administer many liters of colloid and crystalloid fluids, and then attempt to close this multilayered structure over the viscera, we quickly see that it becomes an impossibility. The management of the open abdomen is now a relatively common problem. The longer-term problem of skin retraction and fibrosis is a challenge that can be quite vexing. If the deeper structures can be advanced over the viscera, and fascia and muscle are intact, then the problem can be solved with a split-thickness skin graft on a healthy bed. Fluid loss, infection, the need for complex dressing changes, and disability will be cured in short order. The subcutaneous fat has a protective function in that it offers padding and thermal protection. The loss of the fat layer will not be of great consequence in the short term. However, the skin graft will be tighter and can restrict the movement of the underlying muscles. The skin graft without the fat layer will not be able to move freely and will be fixed to the muscles, fascia, or both. There will be a cosmetic depression at the site of fat loss. If the fascia and muscle are closed over abdominal cavity contents, hernias should not be an acute problem.

The cosmetic and some of the functional problems of skin grafts, which some patients find unacceptable once their major medical issues have been solved, can be addressed with secondary procedures such as excision of all or part of the graft and closure of the defect created with advancement of adjacent skin and subcutaneous fat. Tissue expanders can be placed in an effort to increase the available lipocutaneous coverage to attain a primary closure after excision of the skin graft.

Fascia

Fascia is an important component of the multilayered nature of the abdominal wall. The abdominal wall musculature functions within the tough fibrous envelope of the fascia. The fascia of the rectus sheath is formed mainly by the aponeuroses of the external oblique, internal oblique, and transversus abdominis muscles. The aponeuroses join to form the linea semilunaris at the lateral edge of the rectus and pass anterior and posterior to the rectus abdominis muscles. The posterior rectus sheath ends at the arcuate line, which is often described as being found 2 cm cranial to a horizontal line drawn between the anterior superior iliac spines. The fascial sheaths meet and intersect in the midline at the linea alba, which runs from the xiphoid process to the pubic symphysis. This concept of paired lateral muscle groups exerting forces on and across paired vertical muscles and fixed together in the midline is important in understanding the concepts of loss of domain, functional shortening of muscles, and reconstruction failures.

Fascia is a difficult material to replace. Fascial grafts from the legs (fascia lata) were used extensively in the past. With the advent of freely available, large sheets of acellular dermis, both allograft and xenograft, the need for the morbidity of harvesting fascia from the legs has almost been eliminated. These acellular dermal matrices act as a biologic substitute. A true loss of fascia is fairly unusual. This is primarily seen when fascia is directly excised, as seen in tumor resection such as desmoids and sarcomas, or necrotizing soft tissue infections. The majority of cases of fascial loss are actually relative losses due to retraction of the fascial edge secondary to the unopposed action of the lateral muscles. The layered lateral muscular wall inserts at the linea semilunaris and will exert a lateral vector on the rectus muscle when the linea alba closure fails in the midline. This midline hernia will assume a "C" shape with the rectus muscles fixed at the xiphoid and pubic symphysis. The muscles will not function as efficiently at their new shorter working length. There will be fibrosis of the muscle, scarring of the soft tissue, and a relative lack of fascia in the midline. As more and more viscera exits through the hernia, a loss of domain will develop with a resultant inability to return the viscera back into the abdominal cavity and close muscle and fascia over the top (Figure 2). The release of the lateral fascia and musculature, via a component separation will allow the rectus fascia and muscles to be brought together in the midline.

Muscles

The paired muscle groups of the abdominal wall are designed to work together for the most efficient functioning. As discussed in the previous section, when a group of muscles is allowed to function independent of the stabilizing action of its mirrored group, dysfunction and lack of coordinated movement ensue. A true loss of muscle tissue is most commonly seen in the case of tumor resection or soft tissue infection requiring débridement (Figure 3). The dynamic action of the muscle is not easily replaced. The gap left by the loss of muscle tissue can be closed using any prosthetic material of choice; however, this will be a static patch replacing a dynamic structure. Replacement of muscle tissue with dynamic muscle tissue would require a free tissue transfer with motor nerve repair. This is not practical and is not done.

Peritoneum

The peritoneum represents a unique serous membrane that lines the abdominal cavity and is reflected over the contained viscera. In its undamaged state, it allows the viscera to glide freely against the wall of the abdominal cavity and the adjacent viscera with the least possible friction. Violation of the peritoneum can and does lead to adhesions of the viscera to adjacent structures. This is exacerbated by acute and chronic inflammation, as is often seen in patients requiring abdominal wall reconstruction. There is no practical way to reconstruct the peritoneum when there is a relative loss of this tissue, as in the case of the open abdomen or the large ventral hernia with a loss of domain. The important point is that this specialized tissue

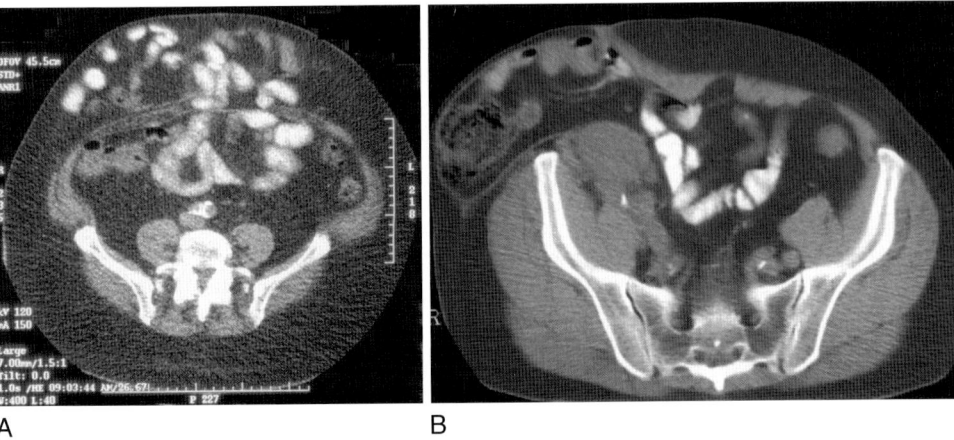

A   B

FIGURE 2   Large ventral hernia with loss of domain.

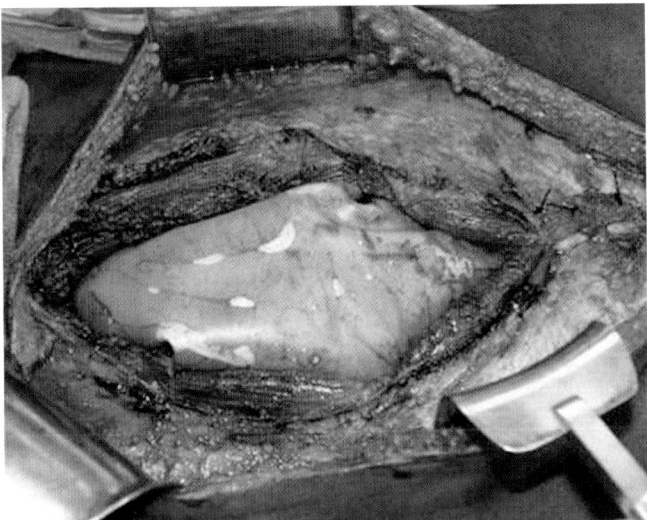

FIGURE 3   Defect of abdominal wall following tumor resection. Resection of rectus abdominis muscle and associated fascia.

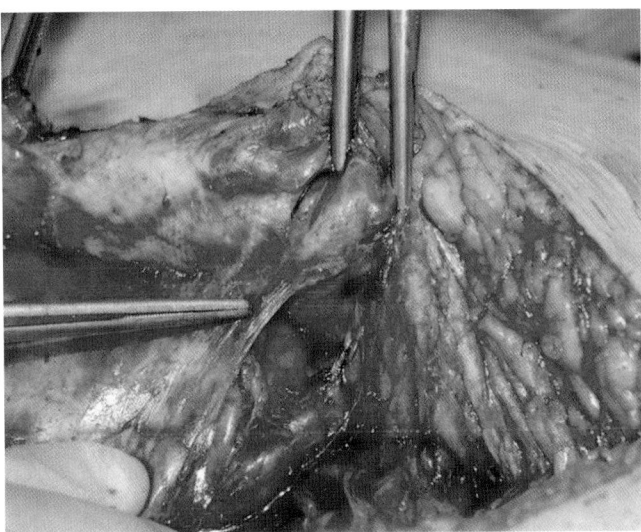

FIGURE 4   Adhesions secondary to prosthetic mesh placed in contact with viscera.

protects the delicate abdominal viscera. Any reconstruction must address this, and care must be taken so that materials that may be in contact with the viscera cause a minimum of inflammation. Prosthetic materials such as polypropylene cause inflammation, adhesions, and fistulae if placed in direct contact with the bowel (Figure 4). It is our policy always to obtain biologic tissue coverage over the viscera prior to placing any prosthetic mesh. This can be autologous or allogeneic.

PATIENT EVALUATION

The patient who presents for abdominal wall reconstruction often presents with multiple problems that must be addressed if there is any hope of reasonable long-term outcome that includes durable anatomic reconstruction, restoration of thoracoabdominal dynamics to allow high levels of activity, and satisfactory quality of life. The etiology of the defect is important. Is the patient an otherwise healthy young individual who sustained a gunshot wound or a morbidly obese patient who underwent an oncologic surgical procedure and went on to have an open abdomen with skin graft on the bowel? The initial evaluation should include a computed tomographic scan with oral and possibly intravenous contrast. Problems such as fistulae, abscesses, stoma issues, and history of obstruction will need to be addressed either before or at the time of the definitive reconstruction.

Something as ubiquitous as cholelithiasis must be considered prior to final reconstruction. A thorough understanding of the problem list is an absolute requirement for success. Begin with evaluating what is missing and why, starting in a layered fashion. Is there a skin defect, actual or relative? Can the myofascial layer be advanced to close the hernia? Is the bowel in continuity? These things should be understood prior to entering the operating room.

APPROACH TO REPAIR

The term *abdominal wall reconstruction* usually implies multiple problems that need to be addressed. Often there is a large defect of the myofascial component with unstable skin coverage. The myofascial deficits may be secondary to resection or retraction and scarring. The major question to be asked is can the native tissue be closed over the viscera? Attempting to obtain a primary fascial closure in the face of a large composite defect can almost ensure recurrence of the hernia. The closure of the tissues under excessive tension leads to necrosis at the suture line, increased intra-abdominal pressures, and recurrence with a larger defect. In many cases of relatively smaller defects, the skin and subcutaneous tissue can be elevated off of the fascia for the full length of the midline incision. Care must be taken in the face of stomas and multiple parallel and/or crossing incisions. By separating the lipocutaneous layer from the myofascial layer, the components can now move independently of each other. Often, previously placed prosthetic materials are the source of ongoing problems of infection and unstable skin coverage (Figure 5). This prosthetic material will need to be removed.

Fascial Closure

If undermining and separation of the skin and subcutaneous fat from the myofascial layer does not allow for fascial closure without tension, a thorough understanding of all the available options will need to be reviewed.

Freeing of the skin and fat from the fascia will allow for evaluation of the abdominal wall areas at risk. Care must be taken when undermining the lipocutaneous layer. The aggressive elevation of the tissue can compromise the vascular supply to large areas of the abdominal wall. Approach perforating vessels carefully and preserve as many as possible. Areas of attenuated fascia or previously unidentified hernias can be addressed at the time of reconstruction. Lysis of intra-abdominal adhesions is also an important factor in getting the fascia closed. The deep surface of the abdominal wall musculature must be evaluated for defects, foreign material, and adhesions. The fascial edges are then approximated without tension. As much of the cranial and caudal fascia as possible is closed. The retraction of the fascia is

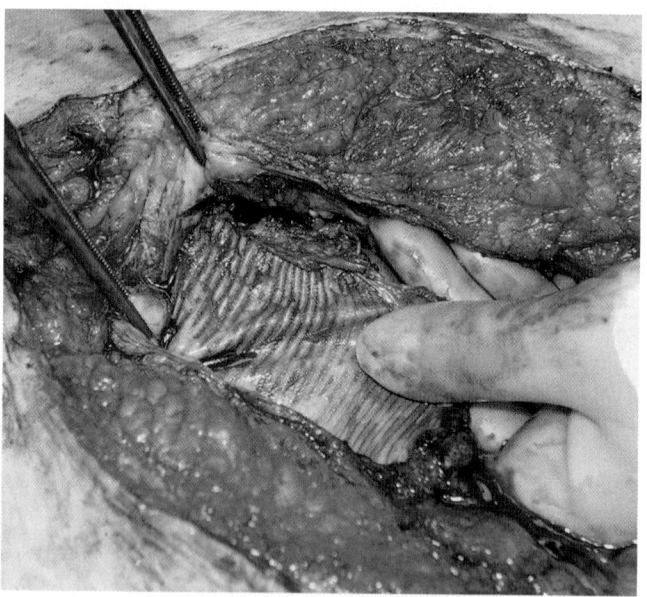

FIGURE 5 Multiple layers of prosthetic material with chronic draining wound.

maximal in the center of the C-shaped defect. This area is best addressed with a biologic "inset" (Figure 6). This will replace the viscera back into the peritoneal cavity with a "no tension" fascial closure.

The list of choices of implant material for the fascial patch grows longer every day. An understanding of some basic principles is important. We can consider the choices to be broken into two main divisions: biologic and synthetic. The biologic implants can be autologous, but, as mentioned earlier, the widely available allografts render autologous choices somewhat unimportant. The use of a biologic implant is advisable in contaminated fields. Many patients who present for reconstruction have open infected wounds and chronic bacterial colonization. Patients who will require bowel resection, stoma revision, or have large enterotomies at the time of reconstruction should be managed with a biologic of choice. We place our biologic inset at the time of the initial reconstruction and obtain stable soft tissue coverage (skin and subcutaneous fat) over the abdominal wall. The implant is fixed to the native fascia with interrupted mattress sutures set back about 2 cm from the edge of the defect. This ensures that if one suture fails, there is not a total loss of integrity of the construct. We do not consider the biologic implant to render long-term stability; failure is often seen at the interface of the inset with the native tissue. Furthermore, the concept of a static implant material fixed to dynamic abdominal wall musculature is a problem that is not solved by using a biologic implant alone. The patient is advised to have a planned return to the operating room in 3 to 4 months. At that time, the now stable soft tissue is opened, and a sheet of polypropylene mesh is used to cover the biologic implant and fixed to the fascia of the anterior abdominal wall across the entire area at risk. In cases when there is no significant contamination, the biologic implant will be placed and then a sheet of polypropylene mesh is placed over the abdominal wall. The mesh is quilted in place with multiple sutures (Figure 7). The mesh is also quilted to the biologic implant. The quilting ensures rapid soft tissue ingrowth to stabilize the two materials and decreases the chance of fluid accumulation between the mesh, the native tissues, and the biologic implant. The idea of wide coverage with mesh and fixation to stable structures outside the area at risk allows for a transfer of lateral forces from the midline to the mesh and thus the entire abdominal wall. Often the lipocutaneous flaps will be sutured to the mesh, again in an effort to encourage rapid tissue ingrowth and eliminate the possibility of large fluid accumulations. Multiple large closed suction drains are used.

Fascial Defects

The inability to close the fascia is not an uncommon situation. The retraction of the fascia can be addressed with an inset of acellular dermis as described previously. The other widely used option is the use of component separation. A lateral release of the external oblique should not be mistaken for a component separation. Ramirez and

FIGURE 6 **A,** Placing sutures for acellular dermal inset. **B,** Acellular dermal inset in position.

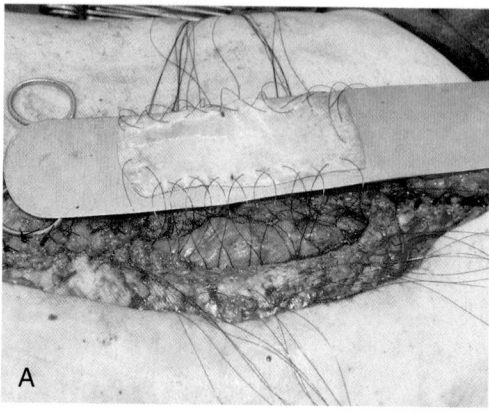

A

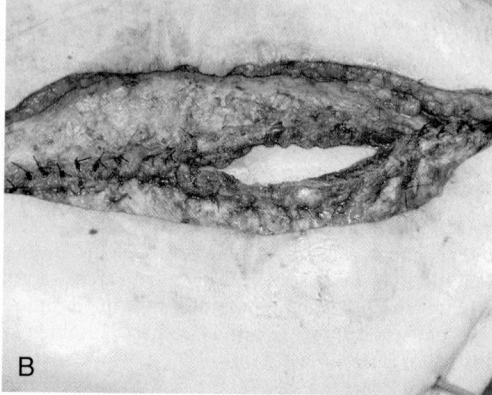

B

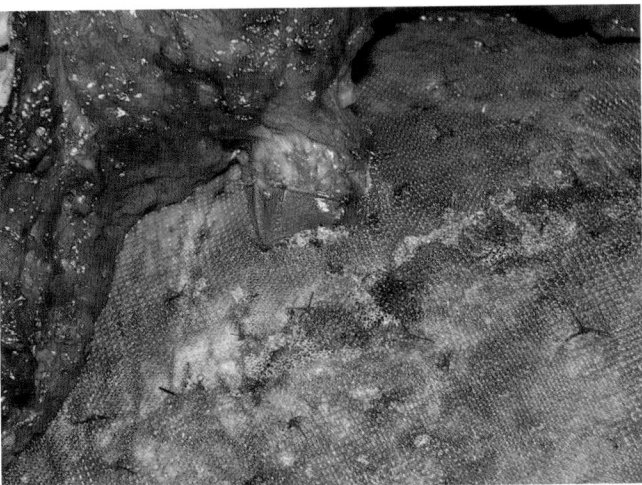

FIGURE 7   Quilted mesh onlay.

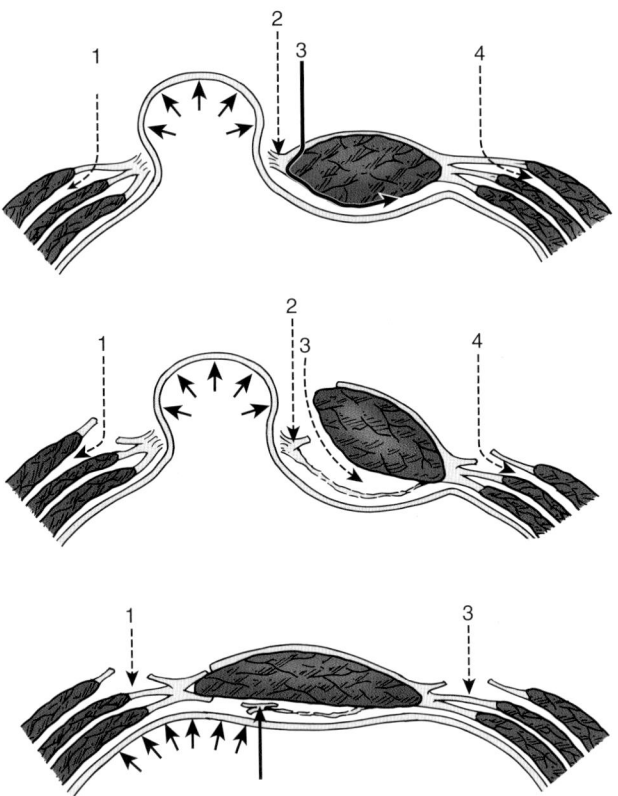

FIGURE 8   Component separation. *1,* Separation of the external oblique muscle from the underlying internal oblique. *2,* The internal oblique muscle is adherent to the transversus abdominis muscle. *3,* The rectus can be easily separated from the posterior rectus sheath. *4,* The anterior rectus sheath is adherent to the rectus muscle at the tendinous inscriptions above the umbilicus. The segmental neurovascular bundle of the rectus muscle travels in the deep surface of the internal oblique muscle, between this and the transversus muscle not at its lateral margin but at a variable distance (10-25 mm) from the margin close to the axis formed by the deep superior and inferior epigastric arteries. The external oblique muscle alone can be advanced toward the midline 2 cm in the upper and lower third, and 4 cm in the middle third in the midline around the waistline. Each rectus muscle with the overlying rectus sheath can be advanced 3, 5, and 3 cm, respectively, in the upper, middle, and lower thirds. For this advancement to occur, the muscle has to be removed from its encasement in the posterior rectus sheath. The rectus muscle with the overlying rectus sheath and its attached internal oblique and transversus muscles can be advanced 5 cm in the epigastrium, 10 cm at the waistline, and 3 cm in the suprapubic region. *(From Ramirez OM, Ruas E, Dellon AL: "Components separation" method for closure of abdominal-wall defects: an anatomic and clinical study,* Plast Reconstr Surg *86:519, 1990.)*

colleagues first described the technique of component separation with their landmark publication in 1990. Multiple variations on the original technique have been tried, but the original description still appears to be the most widely used and effective (Figure 8). The basic technique is predicated by the fact that the external oblique muscle can be separated from the internal oblique muscle in a relatively avascular plane. Once the external oblique is released, the rectus abdominis muscle can be separated from the posterior rectus sheath. The muscle will be held in place to the anterior sheath by the muscular inscriptions. The external oblique fascia is carefully separated from the linea semilunaris just lateral to its insertion into that structure. Careful dissection will release the external oblique muscle and its restricting fascia from the internal oblique and transversus abdominis muscles. They will remain attached to the linea semilunaris. The entire composite construct of muscle and fascia can be moved to the midline. With the release of the external oblique muscle and fascia, the rectus muscle and fascia can be moved medially 10 cm at the waistline. Because the muscle and fascia are fixed to the ribs cranially and the pubic symphysis caudally, one can expect to achieve 5 cm of medial movement in the epigastrium and 3 cm in the suprapubic area. In our experience, the component separation can get significant midline defects closed; however, there is a price to be paid. The procedure can lead to significant lateral "bulges," particularly in larger patients. We will onlay polypropylene mesh out past the medial edge of the now released external oblique. The mesh is then fixed across the abdominal wall from xiphoid to pubic symphysis with a quilting technique. In cases of gross contamination, we would obtain biologic closure over the patient's viscera using the component separation and close the skin/fat flaps over large closed suction drains. The plan would be for the patient to come back in 3 to 4 months when we would place a large mesh onlay to ensure the stability of the reconstruction.

In cases of a lateral fascial defect such as in tumor resection, necrotizing infection, or avulsive wound, the feasibility of using component separation alone is reduced. In these cases, the peritoneal defect is reconstructed with acellular dermis sutured with interrupted mattress sutures placed 1 to 2 cm back from the edge of the defect. This material will maintain the viscera in the abdominal cavity and separate it from the polypropylene mesh onlay. The mesh will be applied widely and fixed to stable structures such as the anterior superior iliac spine, pubic symphysis, inguinal ligament, and/or ribs. The mesh will be quilted in place for the previously mentioned reasons. By fixing the mesh to stable structures and quilting it in place, we are able to transfer the forces across the entire construct and decrease stress at the interface of the construct with native tissue (Figure 9).

PROSTHETIC MATERIALS

The choices of prosthetic materials that can be used in abdominal wall reconstruction essentially fall into two categories: synthetic and biologic. The history associated with synthetic materials extends back over 100 years to 1903 with the first reported use of a silver wire mesh. This material fell from favor quickly due to erosion, fragmentation of material, and secondary infection. Thereafter, both polyvinyl and nylon products were used. However, these were found to have unacceptable high levels of tissue reactivity and increased infection rates as well. Polypropylene was first used in this medical application

FIGURE 9 **A,** Large abdominal wall soft tissue tumor. **B,** Acellular dermal inset being trimmed to size. **C,** "Patch" sutured in place. **D,** Quilted mesh onlay for reinforcement.

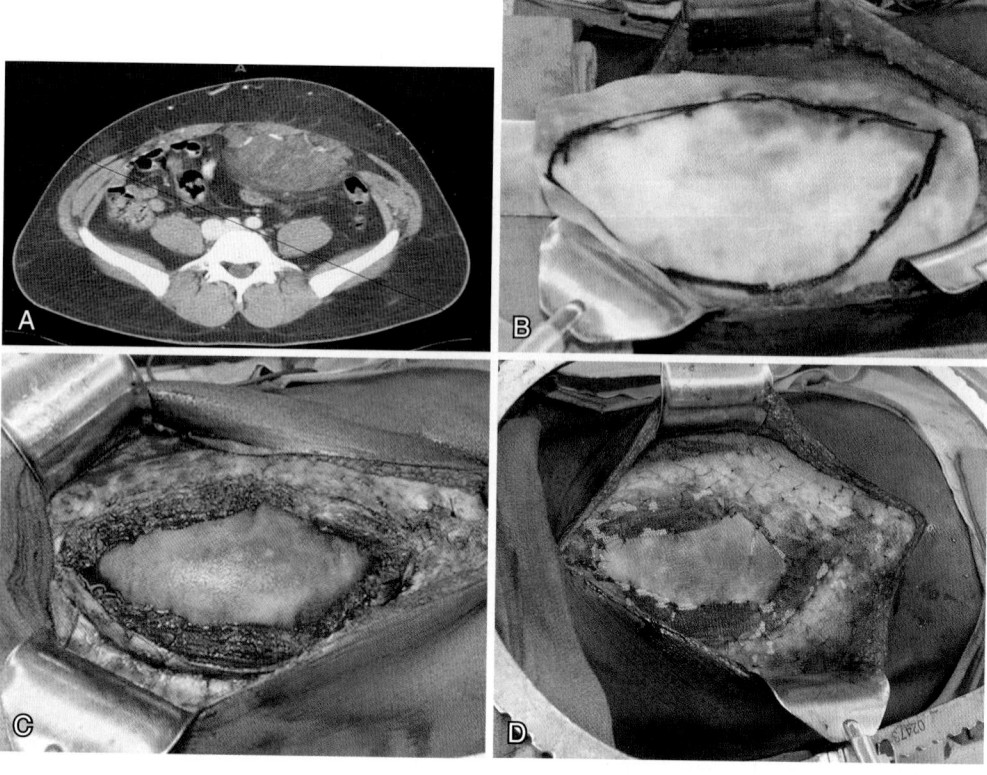

in 1959. Subsequent to that, other materials such as polytetrafluoroethylene (PTFE) have been produced and used. In addition, absorbable synthetic materials, including polyglactin 910 and polyglycolic acid, have been developed and used.

Synthetic Materials

Polypropylene mesh products have been used extensively in abdominal wall reconstruction. This material results in significant tissue ingrowth and fibroblast proliferation. The typical remodeling that occurs due to the reduction of cellular content and corresponding increased production of extracellular matrix is in fact inhibited to a great extent by implantation of artificial meshes. The balance between neosynthesis and protease-mediated degradation of extracellular matrix surrounding these implanted materials remains shifted toward neosynthesis. These are important concepts in that cellular migration and cell proliferation are the basic growth factor–dependent mechanisms of wound healing. Transforming growth factor beta 1 (TGF-β 1) appears to play a prominent role in wound healing and is known as a powerful growth factor for mesenchymal cells and a growth inhibitor of epithelial cells. Low levels of TGF-β 1 terminate growth inhibition and correspondingly result in an increase in the proliferation of fibroblasts. Fibroblasts play a significant role in the formation of defective tissue in wound healing. The synthetic hernia meshes have now evolved to include lighter weight meshes, which likely offer several advantages, including increased abdominal wall compliance, reduced inflammatory reactivity, and subsequent improvement in tissue incorporation.

Sheet-like synthetic products such as PTFE have been used as well. These have been shown to reduce intra-abdominal adhesions. These laminar products are associated with decreased tissue incorporation and increased risk of seroma. This may be due to the micropore nature of these sheet-like products, which results in resistance to the passive movement of fluid through the material. The incidence of

seroma may be linked to increased risk of infection as well as increased likelihood of chronic pain, in that the host inflammatory response to the implanted material may contribute to the formation of the seroma. In keeping with this, PTFE products have been shown to have a tendency to encapsulate with little tendency to integrate into the host abdominal wall. With this lack of integration into the native tissue, there is a tendency toward insufficient anchorage of the material to the underlying or adjacent fascia, leading to failure of the repair. We therefore do not recommend the use of these materials to achieve a durable long-term outcome.

Absorbable Materials

The use of absorbable products has little application in the durable reconstruction of large abdominal wall defects. They may play a role when there is no identifiable method of achieving a biologic reconstruction of a large myofascial defect over which a macroporous mesh product can then be applied to achieve a durable reconstruction. It is our preference, however, to use bioprosthetic products in that particular application.

Bioprosthetics

Many bioprosthetic products are available. In broad categories these fall into either autologous tissue versus acellular dermal products, which are available as both allograft and xenograft products. The use of autologous materials such as tensor fascia lata has been essentially replaced by the widespread availability and ease of use and handling of the off-the-shelf acellular products. Varying products have specific material processing characteristics and reported advantages. The choice, however, should be based on the surgeon's experience and familiarity with a specific product. We have used these products many times to achieve restoration of the myofascial component of the abdominal wall when the patient's native tissue cannot be reapproximated in an acceptable fashion. Their use as a reinforcing material to address the reconstruction of the entirety of the abdominal wall may be cost prohibitive, at the present time, given the relatively low-cost, favorable material handling characteristics and known excellent tissue incorporation of other synthetic macroporous products.

CONCLUSIONS

Large abdominal wall defects may represent seemingly simple surgical problems, which are, in fact, quite complex. The techniques are simple, but the approach requires careful forethought and attention to detail to afford the patient the best possible outcome, which will be durable and lead to normal function and a high quality of life. The fact that the recurrence rates for recurrent hernias approaches 50% in patients who are at high risk should be proof enough that the management is not simple at all. The surgeon must make a comprehensive problem list at the outset. These are not challenges that are amenable to the quick fix. The execution of the operative plan must be carried out with an understanding of the causes of failure.

The procedures and details presented in this chapter are the culmination of our experience in the management of almost 500 complex abdominal wall reconstructions. We have analyzed our successes and, more important, our failures. Following the steps outlined here will help to ensure predictable outcomes and long-term success.

SUGGESTED READINGS

Choi JJ, Palaniappa NC, Dallas KB, et al: Use of mesh during ventral hernia repair in clean-contaminated and contaminated cases: outcomes of 33,832 cases, *Ann Surg* 255:176, 2012.

Matthews BD, Pratt BL, Pollinger HS, et al: Assessment of adhesion formation to intra-abdominal polypropylene mesh and polytetrafluoroethylene mesh, *J Surg Res* 114:126, 2003.

Morris LM, LeBlanc KA: Components separation technique utilizing an intraperitoneal biologic and an onlay lightweight polypropylene mesh: "a sandwich technique", *Hernia* 17:45, 2013.

Ramirez, OM, Ruas, E, Dellon AL: "Components separation" method for closure of abdominal-wall defects: an anatomic and clinical study, *Plast Reconstr Surg* 86:519, 1990.

Reynolds D, Davenport DL, Korosec RL, et al: Financial implications of ventral hernia repair: a hospital cost analysis, *J Gastrointest Surg* 17:159, 2013.

Weyhe D, Hoffmann P, Belyaev O, et al: The role of TGF-β1 as a determinant of foreign body reaction to alloplastic materials in rat fibroblast cultures: comparison of different commercially available polypropylene meshes for hernia repair, *Regul Pept* 138:10, 2007.

THE MANAGEMENT OF BENIGN BREAST DISEASE

Lisa Jacobs, MD, and Rosemarie Hardin, MD

Benign breast disease accounts for a significant number of referrals to a breast surgeon and a source of substantial anxiety for patients. These conditions include mastalgia, nipple discharge, palpable solid masses and cysts, fibrocystic disease, and infections. These conditions must be appropriately managed to provide patients with the necessary care to either cure the disease or provide symptomatic relief to make them manageable. It is important to be able to discern when a coexisting suspicious pathology develops and when further imaging and biopsy are indicated.

EVALUATION OF BENIGN BREAST COMPLAINTS

The evaluation of benign breast complaints begins with a focused history and clinical breast examination. The history should include a detailed assessment of the symptoms, aggravating and alleviating factors, duration of symptoms, and presence of associated symptoms. The goal of documenting this history is not only to ascertain pertinent information to appropriately diagnose the patient's condition but also to help guide the selection of diagnostic testing that will have the most yield, especially with regard to the age of the patient. Furthermore, this information helps identify patients who are at high risk for development of breast cancer in the future and are candidates for screening. Clinicians must maintain clinical suspicion of atypical findings because patients with seemingly benign presentations could harbor findings suggestive of malignancy, and, of course, some patients with benign disease may be at risk for later development of breast cancer.

Detailed documentation of the history is followed by a thorough bilateral breast examination, including examination of regional lymph node basins. The physical examination should begin with visual inspection for asymmetries, skin or nipple changes, nipple inversion, breast edema, and breast erythema. This is followed by superficial and deep palpation in an orderly manner to carefully examine all quadrants of the breast, including the axillary tail. It is useful to ascertain whether any nipple discharge is present and to characterize it in terms of color and location, especially if it involves a single duct or multiple ducts and if a trigger point can be identified.

Diagnostic imaging is selected on the basis of clinical suspicion of the underlying cause of a patient's symptoms and includes the same studies available for evaluation of a patient with suspected breast cancer, including mammography, ultrasonography, and magnetic resonance imaging (MRI), all of which can be used with biopsy to help establish the diagnosis. It is important to consider the age of the patient as well. In a young patient with dense parenchyma who presents with typical benign symptoms suggestive of a cyst or fibroadenoma, an ultrasound study may prove more useful than mammography, which would be less sensitive with dense parenchyma. As with patients suspected of having breast cancer, negative results of imaging should not deter the recommendation of aspiration or biopsy of suspect palpable abnormalities detected on physical examination.

On occasion, imaging findings are abnormal but no changes are found on physical examination. In these cases, biopsy may be required if there are features suspect or indeterminate for malignancy. Abnormalities that can be visualized with ultrasonography should be subjected to ultrasonography-guided biopsy because this is the most comfortable positioning for the patient. If abnormalities are visible only by mammography, a stereotactic biopsy must be considered. For abnormalities identified only on MRI, MRI-guided biopsy is the only option. If the target lesion is deep in the breast along the chest wall or in a superficial location close to the nipple, or if the patient cannot tolerate the positioning for an image-guided biopsy, then a needle-localized surgical excisional biopsy may be warranted.

BREAST MASSES

Palpable breast masses are one of the most common complaints. In premenopausal women, most breast masses are benign, especially when they have been present over several months to years. However, any suspect palpable breast mass necessitates additional imaging and diagnostic biopsy. Palpable abnormalities could represent dense breast parenchyma with fibrocystic changes, cysts, lipomas, or fibroadenomas. On the basis of the initial history and physical examination findings, the differential diagnosis is usually evident. If a lesion is suspected to be cystic in nature, this can be confirmed on ultrasonography, and a cyst aspiration can be attempted. If the cyst expresses serous fluid and is completely collapsed at the end of the aspiration, no further biopsy is warranted. However, if the cyst fails to resolve completely, or if it appears to be complex in nature with a solid component, additional biopsy is warranted. If a lesion appears to be solid, benign versus malignant characteristics can be determined on the basis of imaging criteria. Benign fibroadenomas are well circumscribed and do not have spiculated, irregular margins typical of malignant lesions. These are generally identified with the aid of ultrasonography, and a biopsy sample can be obtained under ultrasound guidance. If a patient presents with a benign history with imaging findings supportive of a fibroadenoma and the mass is asymptomatic, then close observation with short-term interval imaging remains an option.

FIBROADENOMAS

The majority of palpable breast masses are benign, especially in younger women, and the most frequently encountered solid benign mass is a fibroadenoma. These lesions are well circumscribed with smooth edges and are mobile with rubbery consistency. Many patients have multiple fibroadenomas, either synchronous or metachronous. They can be mildly symptomatic, with patients complaining of tenderness or pain at the site, often worse at the time of menstruation. Fibroadenomas are believed to be hormonally sensitive and can increase in size or become more symptomatic at the time of menstruation or with hormonal changes associated with pregnancy or the use of oral contraception. They usually become less symptomatic with age and often calcify in postmenopausal women.

Ultrasonography is a useful diagnostic test for these lesions because they are more commonly diagnosed in younger women, and ultrasonography-guided biopsy can confirm the diagnosis. Small asymptomatic lesions can be observed and monitored, but larger symptomatic lesions usually warrant excision, especially when more than 2 cm in diameter. Furthermore, if a lesion enlarges rapidly or if any suspect pathologic process is associated with the fibroadenoma, such as increased cellularity of the lesion, excision is warranted in order to rule out a more aggressive variant of a fibroepithelial lesion known as a *phyllodes tumor*. Phyllodes tumors can be locally aggressive and recurrent, and wide local excision is required. Of course, as with any growing palpable mass, excision is also warranted to ensure that a breast cancer was not misdiagnosed. In summary, indications for resection include size greater than 2 cm, increasing size, pain associated with the lesion, increased cellularity on biopsy, or anxiety caused by the presence of the mass.

BREAST CYSTS

Breast cysts can also manifest as a palpable abnormality or a cause of breast pain. The physical examination usually reveals benign findings of a lesion with well-circumscribed borders, similar to a benign solid breast mass. Ultrasonography is a useful tool for diagnosis of a breast cyst. Cysts that are well circumscribed without septations or debris and have thin walls are referred to as *simple cysts*. An asymptomatic simple cyst with typical benign imaging features does not require intervention other than reassurance. If symptomatic, such cysts can be observed or aspirated in the physician's office under ultrasound or palpation guidance. Aspiration of serous fluid confirms the diagnosis of a simple cyst, and ultrasonography is used to document complete resolution of the cyst. If the cyst aspirate is bloody in nature, it should be sent for cytopathologic evaluation for possible malignancy. If the cyst has septations and is thought to be more complex with potentially a solid component or a thick wall, then tissue biopsy is warranted. This can be performed with ultrasonography-guided core biopsy, with a clip left in place to mark the location in case an excisional biopsy is warranted in the future.

BREAST PAIN

Breast pain, or *mastalgia*, remains a challenge to breast surgeons because the cause is not always clear and the symptom spectrum ranges from vague pain to debilitating pain. It may also be difficult to ascertain whether an associated pathologic process is contributing to the mastalgia, such as underlying bone disease, costochondritis, or fibromyalgia, all of which can contribute greatly to the sensation of mastalgia.

It is important to document a timeline of the patient's symptoms, alleviating and aggravating factors, associated symptoms, and whether it is cyclical in nature. The history should reveal whether the pain affects both breasts or whether the symptoms are unilateral. Breast pain can be hormonally driven, with escalation of symptoms during reproductive years or at the time of menses. Hormonally driven mastalgia may also be associated with fibrocystic breast disease. If cyclical in nature, mastalgia tends to be bilateral and diffuse in nature, and it often improves after the onset of menses. Noncyclical pain has no relation to the menstrual cycle, and affected patients therefore do not experience the relief from breast pain at the start of menses. The most common causes of noncyclical breast pain include cysts, fibroadenomas, and chest wall syndromes such as costochondritis.

Breast pain may resolve on its own with little intervention. Conservative measures are often helpful; they include well-fitted, appropriately-sized, supportive bras; warm compresses; and dietary modifications to reduce high fat intake and lower caffeine intake. Nonsteroidal antiinflammatory agents are very useful for persistent pain. Vitamin E, fish oil, and evening primrose oil may be helpful to women who suffer from mastalgia. Topical nonsteroidal antiinflammatory drugs (NSAIDs) are also a consideration for persistent, severe breast pain. It is important to realize that at times no further treatment is necessary other than reassurance and helping to reduce a patient's anxiety by explaining that breast pain is not a typical sign of breast cancer.

NIPPLE DISCHARGE

Nipple discharge is another common presenting complaint that can be quite worrisome to patients. Benign physiologic nipple discharge is present in many women; in many cases, it can be induced from several ducts by nipple manipulation, and it typically does not warrant any further evaluation. Nipple discharge that is spontaneous, recurrent, unilateral, and involving a single duct necessitates further diagnostic evaluation and, on occasion, surgical intervention. If pathologic discharge is present, evaluation should begin with diagnostic mammography and ultrasonography. Cytologic study and occult blood testing of nipple discharge is often insufficient for accurate diagnosis, and low diagnostic yield can produce misleading information. If a specific lesion is identified on imaging, then tissue biopsy is warranted for diagnosis. In some cases, ductography is a useful diagnostic study. The fluid-producing duct is cannulated and contrast material is injected. This is followed by mammography in an attempt to identify filling defects within the duct. The advantage of ductography is identification of lesions that are a greater distance from the nipple than would normally be excised by a resection of retroareolar tissue. If mammography and ultrasonography fail to identify suspect abnormalities, then an excisional biopsy of the duct is warranted. Cannulation of the duct with a lacrimal probe is often helpful. Another option is subareolar ductal exploration with duct ligation and excision. It is important to inform the patient that she may be unable to breastfeed after this procedure.

Nipple discharge is most commonly a result of benign intraductal lesions, specifically papillomas, duct ectasia, and fibrocystic breast disease, and it does not necessarily imply the presence of a malignancy. Of course, although it is rare, physiologic nipple discharge can develop from hyperprolactinemia, as can occur with a primary pituitary tumor, hypothyroidism, or medication. The discharge may be copious, bilateral, and milky, and it is typically expressed from multiple ducts. No breast surgical intervention is required, and affected patients should be referred to an endocrinologist for further evaluation.

In summary, a suspect nipple discharge is unilateral and spontaneous, comes from a single duct, and is bloody or clear. These discharges necessitate further evaluation because they may be the result of malignancy. However, even with these manifestations, the majority are benign.

BREAST INFECTION

Breast infections are more common in women who are premenopausal and those who are lactating. These infections are often very painful and manifest with systemic symptoms such as fever, malaise, and leukocytosis. Mastitis in a lactating woman is often caused by skin flora such as *Staphylococcus* infection. Such flora respond to oral antibiotics and conservative measures such as application of warm compresses if diagnosed promptly. Lactating women should be encouraged to continue breastfeeding and ensure that the breast is emptied with each feeding. However, many women present late with fluctuant abscesses that necessitate surgical incision and drainage. This procedure can be very painful, and drainage procedures should be performed in the operating room with the patient under sedation if possible, especially for larger abscesses. In view of the acidic environment of the abscess cavity, it is often difficult to attain adequate local anesthesia, which would significantly affect the ability to drain the cavity thoroughly.

Ultrasonography is useful for detecting the true extent of the abscess cavity and for evaluation of recurrent abscesses, inasmuch as these may be caused by undrained pockets or retained debris and may necessitate more formal débridement to prevent recurrence. It is important to submit the exudate to Gram stain and culture to help direct antibiotic therapy. Ultrasonography can also be a useful therapeutic modality if the breast infection is caught in early stages of development with a free-flowing collection of aspirate. Ultrasonography can be used to aspirate abscess cavities that have not organized into multiloculated collections, which are harder to drain completely. This conservative strategy, in combination with antibiotic therapy, may help prevent the need for operative intervention. It is important, however, to document resolution of the cavity after the aspiration and to ensure that there is no residual cavity or undrained loculations, which would predispose to recurrent infection.

Breast infections in nonlactating women are generally caused by bacteria introduced through the nipple. These infections are typically retroareolar and are managed with antibiotics and drainage if necessary, as described previously. It is of utmost importance to consider inflammatory breast cancer in the differential diagnosis. Patients with mastitis should quickly show some improvement in symptoms with the initiation of treatment. If the symptoms are not improving with antibiotics, then any underlying abnormality should be subjected to biopsy. Inflammatory breast cancer should always be suspected when the affected patient is nonlactating and postmenopausal and has no precipitating factors or systemic signs of infection.

ABNORMAL SCREENING MAMMOGRAMS

As technology continues to improve with better mammographic imaging, many suspect findings may be identified on mammography. These may include new microcalcifications, densities, architectural distortions, or developing masses. These mammographic abnormalities are typically not appreciated on clinical breast examination, and the patient has no symptoms. In these cases, an image-guided biopsy is necessary to establish the diagnosis and rule out a malignancy. The findings, such as typical ductal hyperplasia, are often benign and warrant no additional intervention. On occasion, biopsy may demonstrate a benign but indeterminate result. In these cases, additional tissue is needed to assess for a coexisting malignancy, which can occur in 10% to 15% of cases. Women with these indeterminate lesions should undergo an excisional biopsy with needle localization. An excisional biopsy is typically recommended for patients found to have atypical ductal hyperplasia, atypical lobular hyperplasia, papillomas, or sclerosing adenosis with radial scarring.

Similarly, lobular carcinoma in situ—which is considered a marker for increased risk of developing breast cancer but not an early noninvasive breast cancer, like its counterpart, ductal carcinoma in situ—should be subjected to excisional biopsy. The purpose of the excisional biopsy in all of these cases is to decrease the risk of sampling error. Affected women, although the biopsy finding is considered benign, should be offered high-risk screening with the goal of early detection of any subsequent malignancies. These women should also be offered antiestrogen therapies for risk reduction. Some women, however, refuse to undergo excisional biopsy after image-guided biopsy with the findings just described. Several studies have demonstrated that if mammotomy biopsy is performed instead of a core biopsy, then observation can be considered if more tissue is available for pathologic assessment and if patients did not experience adverse outcomes. However, the standard of care is recommendation of excisional biopsy.

SUMMARY

Patients with benign breast problems commonly present to surgeons for evaluation. The main goal is to establish the presence of a benign condition with appropriate history and physical examination, imaging, and, when necessary, biopsy. This protocol also helps ensure that the problems are not being misdiagnosed, which could result in missed early breast cancers, including inflammatory breast cancer, which masquerades as mastitis. Once the diagnosis is confirmed to be benign, then the decision regarding surgery is individualized to the patient according to the presence of symptoms amendable to surgical intervention. Patients require scheduled follow-up to ensue that no interval problems develop. Those with benign biopsy results that pose an increased risk for the development of breast cancer in the future should be appropriately screened for breast cancer. Patient education and reassurance are vital.

Suggested Readings

Amin AL, Purdy AC, Mattingly JD, et al: Benign breast diseases, *Surg Clin North Am* 93(2):299–308, 2013.

Flynn GB, Tipton C: An algorithm for managing breast pain, *Clin Advisor* September 15, 2011. Available at www.clinicaladvisor.com.

Guray M, Shahin A: Benign breast diseases: classification, diagnosis and management, *The Oncologist* 11(5):435–449, 2006.

Pearlman M, Griffin J: Benign breast disease, *Obstet Gynecol* 116(3):747–758, 2010.

SCREENING FOR BREAST CANCER

Michele A. Gadd, MD

OVERVIEW

Breast cancer is the most common noncutaneous cancer diagnosed in women, accounting for more than 1 in 10 new cancer diagnoses each year. Breast cancer is the second most common cause of death from cancer among women in the world. In 1989, the American Cancer Society (ACS), the National Cancer Institute (NCI), and nine other organizations joined to issue a uniform set of guidelines for breast cancer screening. The guidelines have remained largely intact over the years, with the addition of magnetic resonance imaging (MRI) to improve screening in subgroups of women at high to moderate risk. As a result of breast cancer screening, death rates in the United States have decreased by 30% since the 1990s.

Mammography remains the gold standard for breast imaging. The cost-benefit relationship associated with screening has become increasingly scrutinized as imaging technologies evolve and breast cancer treatment improves. Growing concern exists that increased utilization of alternative breast imaging technologies has resulted in an increased number of false-positive findings. These false-positive findings in turn lead to more imaging, more biopsies, and more costs, without a proven benefit towards decreasing breast cancer mortality. In 2009, the United States Preventive Task Force (USPTF) issued a modification of their 2002 screening guidelines. Their current recommendations have not been widely adapted, but this reanalysis of the benefits versus harm of screening is an important part of maintaining up-to-date recommendations as medical technology evolves. This chapter outlines standard screening practices and a brief description of cutting-edge technology used in diagnostic imaging.

SCREENING RECOMMENDATIONS

The American Cancer Society recommendations for breast cancer screening are maintained on the ACS web site (http://www.cancer.org/docroot/CRI/content/CRI_2_4_3X_Can_breast_cancer_be_found_early_5.asp; Table 1). For women at average risk, screening includes annual clinical breast examination beginning at age 40 years, counseling to raise awareness of breast symptoms, and regular annual mammography beginning at age 40 years. Breast self examination is an option starting at age 20 years and between the ages 20 and 40 years. A clinical breast examination should be done as part of a regular health examination at least once every 3 years.

Guidelines from the U.S. Preventive Services Task Force (USPSTF; http://www.ahrq.gov/clinic/uspstf/uspsbrca.htm) were revised in November 2009 to recommend screening mammograms every 2 years for women between the ages of 50 and 74 years and decisions to start regular mammograms before age 50 years on an individual basis, taking into account the benefits and harms (see Table 1). These recommendations have led to significant controversy, and most centers in the United States continue to follow the ACS guidelines. At this time, no finite age at which mammography should be discontinued exists. Mammograms for older women should be based on the individual and her overall health. As long as the individual is a candidate for treatment and her life expectancy is greater than 5 years, she should continue to be screened.

The recommendations for women whose risk is estimated to be higher than average include an increased intensity of screening depending on estimated risk level. High risk is defined as a more than 20% lifetime risk, and moderately increased risk is a 15% to 20% lifetime risk. Risk estimates can be obtained with one or more risk-prediction models. Women at high risk should have an annual mammogram, annual MRI, and breast examination every 6 months. Individuals with a strong family history should initiate screening 5 to 10 years before the youngest age at diagnosis in a relative. Individuals who are known *BRCA* mutation carriers should begin screening at age 25 years with MRI and add mammography at 30 years. Individuals with a moderate risk should discuss with their doctor the benefits of adding MRI screening to annual mammography.

SCREENING MODALITIES

Breast Self Examination

Breast self examination (BSE) was advocated in the past; however, recent updates have listed it as optional or have removed it from the screening guidelines. Clearly, some breast cancers are mammographically occult or develop between imaging sequences. In these cases, there is added value to a self examination, or at least recognition of a change, and medical attention soon after the abnormality is identified. Large randomized trials have failed to show a reduction in the breast cancer–specific or all-cause mortality from regular BSE in large populations of average risk. The current opinion is that evidence is insufficient to recommend for or against teaching or performing routine BSE. If patients are performing a routine self breast examination, a review of the examination and a discussion of findings during the clinical examination is worthwhile to improve an individual's technique and address anxiety.

Clinical Breast Examination

Clinical breast examination is a key component of breast cancer screening because approximately 10% to 20% of all breast cancers are not visible on screening mammography. Beginning at age 20 years, women should have a clinical breast examination every 2 to 3 years and then annually after age 40 years. If a suspicious or questionable finding is identified based on a clinical breast examination, often a diagnostic mammogram or ultrasound scan can assist in the evaluation. If the finding is believed to represent something other than normal breast tissue or a simple cyst, a biopsy should be performed, even if imaging is normal. Patients at high risk (*BRCA* mutation, family history, history of radiation to the chest wall, past breast cancer, lobular carcinoma in situ and atypia) should have a breast examination twice a year.

At the time of clinical examination, family history of breast cancer, the benefits of early detection, and the importance of regular mammography can be discussed. Although breast self examination has become an option in the ACS recommendations, it is useful to provide instruction on how to perform a self examination. This is also a time to inform individuals about the potential benefits, risks, and limitations of the breast examination. Individuals should be made aware that most questionable findings on a self breast examination are benign and that in some cases additional imaging or perhaps even a biopsy may be recommended to exclude an underlying breast cancer.

Screening Mammography

Mammography is the foundation of breast imaging and is used to screen asymptomatic women for breast cancer. Two-view

TABLE 1: Comparison of American Cancer Society (ACS) and U.S. Preventive Services Task Force (USPSTF) breast cancer screening recommendations

Variable	ACS guidelines	2009 USPSTF guidelines
Age to begin mammograms	40 y	50 y
Frequency of mammograms	Annually	Every 2 y
CBE	Annually	Insufficient evidence to assess additional benefits and harms of CBE beyond screening mammography in woman aged ≥40 y
SBE	Optional	Recommends against SBE

CBE, Clinical breast examination; *SBE*, self breast examination.

TABLE 2: Breast Imaging, Reporting, and Data System (BIRADS) classification of breast imaging

Category	Assessment	Recommendation
0	Incomplete	Need additional imaging or prior studies for comparison
1	Negative	Resume routine screening mammography
2	Benign	Resume routine screening mammography
3	Probably benign	Risk of malignancy, <2%; short-term interval follow-up at 6 months recommended
4	Suspicious abnormality	Intermediate risk of malignancy; biopsy recommended
5	Highly suggestive of malignancy	Chance of malignancy, >95%; appropriate action should be taken
6	Known biopsy-proven malignancy	Treatment of known malignancy

mammography has been shown in numerous studies to decrease the mortality of breast cancer as a result of earlier diagnosis. Screening mammograms provide two views of each breast: the mediolateral oblique (MLO) projection images the breast from a medial to lateral approach, and the craniocaudal (CC) projection images the breast from a superior to inferior view. Individuals generally stand for the test, and each breast is imaged separately. The breast is compressed between two firm plates, and the corresponding arm is raised or wrapped around the device. The technician requests that the individual withhold breathing for a few seconds while the image is taken. The use of two views allows physicians to localize an abnormality to a particular quadrant within the breast and increases the sensitivity of mammography. To help standardize reporting and recommendations, the American College of Radiology added a Breast Imaging, Reporting, and Data System (BIRADS) classification (Table 2). The BIRADS categories classify mammographic findings by level of suspicion. Each category is associated with guidelines for patient management to aid clinicians in their decision making about the need for a subsequent biopsy and follow-up recommendations.

Digital Mammography

A rapid influx of full-field digital mammography into screening centers has been seen over the past few years in the United States. Full-field digital mammography compared with screen film mammography offers the ability to maximize the performance of detection and display and the ability to manipulate contrast and brightness. These features have been shown to improve detection of low-contrast findings in dense breast tissue. Studies that compared digital with film-screen mammography in Europe and in the United States have produced conflicting results. The Digital Mammographic Imaging Screening Trial (DMIST) performed film-screen and digital mammography in asymptomatic women at the same screening encounter. The overall accuracy was similar, but the digital method was more accurate in premenopausal and perimenopausal women younger than 50 years with mammographically dense breasts and was less accurate in women aged 65 years or older with nondense breasts.

Another study was done by the Breast Cancer Surveillance Consortium (BCSC) among women aged 40 to 79 years in a large population-based cohort of community-based imaging facilities in the United States. Cancer detection rates were similar in women aged 50 to 79 years. Women 40 to 49 years with extremely dense breasts benefited the most from digital mammography.

Biopsies

The preferred method of biopsy is a percutaneous core needle biopsy or, in some cases, a fine-needle aspiration biopsy. The choice between these two techniques depends on the indications, location, and institutional cytologic and pathologic support within the clinic. In either case, a diagnosis of benign versus malignant disease and even markers for estrogen receptor, progesterone receptor, and *Her-2 neu* can be established on both types of samples with an adequate cell yield. In the case of a nonpalpable finding seen on imaging, a stereotactic core biopsy is preferred. Stereotactic biopsies are performed with a stereotactic device that allows for two-dimensional orientation and targets the lesion, which is then biopsied with a 3-mm core needle. The patient generally lies on her abdomen, and the breast is placed through a hole within the stereo table. If the abnormality is considered relatively vague mammographically, is not seen with ultrasound scan (or MRI), or is deemed too posterior or too close to the nipple or the individual breast is too small to adjust safely within the stereotactic unit, then a needle localized breast biopsy is recommended. In this case, a guidewire is placed into the breast while the patient is sitting in a chair with the breast in compression. A surgical biopsy is then performed with the guidewire for accurate targeting of the questionable lesion. When a breast biopsy is performed, pathologic and radiologic findings should be correlated. Discordance requires additional evaluation. For a BIRADS 5 lesion on imaging, if benign with needle biopsy, a surgical excision should be performed to exclude the possibility of breast cancer. Similarly, a clinically suspicious palpable finding that is mammographically and ultrasonographically occult and benign on needle biopsy should also be removed surgically to exclude breast cancer.

HIGH-RISK SCREENING

Several national medical organizations have developed guidelines and recommendations for screening women at high risk. The ACS published guidelines for screening with MRI as an adjunct to mammography in 2007 (Table 3). The National Comprehensive Cancer Network (NCCN) issued parallel guidelines followed by recommendations for mammography, MRI, and ultrasound scan jointly by the Society of Breast Imaging (SBI) and the American College of Radiology (ACR). In general, annual screening mammography is recommended for women of appropriately high risk beginning at 30 years, supplemental screening with breast MRI is recommended for a subset with very high risk, and screening ultrasound scan is recommended for women in whom MRI is unavailable. The results of a recent study with computer-simulated modeling concluded that annual MRI at age 25 years, alternating every 6 months with digital mammography beginning at age 30 years, may be the most effective screening strategy for mutation carriers.

Women at a substantially greater than average risk for development of breast cancer can be defined by a number of factors. Genetic abnormalities account for 5% to 10% of all cases of breast cancer. *BRCA 1* or *2* mutation carriers have a 37% to 87% risk of development of breast cancer by the age of 70 years. A variety of models are available to predict risk. The most widely used is the Gail model, which is based on age, number of first-degree relatives with breast cancer, age of menarche, age of first live birth, number of previous biopsies (including presence of atypia), and race or ethnicity. The Claus model includes a more comprehensive family history. The BRCAPRO model is based on personal history and family history data, including breast and ovarian cancer and Jewish ancestry. The BOA-DICEA model incorporates family history of breast, ovarian, prostate, and pancreatic cancer, and finally the Tyrer-Cuzick model uses family history plus gynecologic history.

TABLE 3: American Cancer Society (ACS) recommendations for breast magnetic resonance imaging (MRI) screening as an adjunct to mammography

Recommend Annual MRI Screening (Based on Evidence*)

BRCA mutation

First-degree relative of *BRCA* carrier but untested

Lifetime risk ~20% to 25% or greater, as defined by BRCAPRO or other models that largely depend on family history

Recommend Annual MRI Screening (Based on Expert Consensus Opinion†)

Radiation to chest between age 10 and 30 years

Li–Fraumeni syndrome and first-degree relatives

Cowden and Bannayan-Riley-Ruvalcaba syndromes and first-degree relatives

Insufficient Evidence to Recommend for or Against MRI Screening‡

Lifetime risk 15% to 20% as defined by BRCAPRO or other models that largely depend on family history

Lobular carcinoma in situ (LCIS) or atypical lobular hyperplasia (ALH)

Atypical ductal hyperplasia (ADH)

Heterogeneously or extremely dense breast on mammography

Women with a personal history of breast cancer, including ductal carcinoma in situ (DCIS)

Recommend Against MRI Screening (Based on Expert Consensus Opinion)

Women at <15% lifetime risk

*Evidence from nonrandomized screening trials and observational studies.
†Based on evidence of lifetime risk for breast cancer.
‡Payments should not be a barrier. Screening decisions should be made on a case-by-case basis, as there may be particular factors to support MRI. More data on these groups is expected to be published soon.
From Saslow D, Boetes C, Burke W, et al: American Cancer Society guidelines for breast screening with MRI as an adjunct to mammography, CA Cancer J Clin *57:75–89, 2007. © 2007 American Cancer Society. This material is reproduced with permission of Wiley-Liss, Inc., a subsidiary of John Wiley & Sons, Inc.*

OTHER IMAGING MODALITIES

Ultrasound Scan

Ultrasound scan is primarily used in diagnostic evaluation of findings on mammography, clinical examination, or MRI. Focused breast ultrasound scan characterizes palpable or screening-detected lesions and can be used to perform an image-guided needle biopsy of sonographically visible lesions. The role of whole-breast screening ultrasound scan was evaluated by the American College of Radiology Imaging Network National Breast Ultrasound Trial (ACRIN 6666). After screening of 2809 women at very high risk, an additional 4 cancers per 1000 women were detected with ultrasound scan alone. The downside of ultrasound scan is the increased numbers of false-positive findings that lead to an increased biopsy rate, the length of time that it takes to perform an ultrasound scan, and its user-dependant variability. There has been recent emphasis on screening with ultrasound scan after mammography in women at high-risk or with dense breast, or both, who may not meet the recommendations for screening MRI.

Magnetic Resonance Imaging

Breast MRI adds an additional element to the detection of cancer: tumor physiology. Most breast cancers display enhancement after administration of intravenous paramagnetic contrast, which makes them highly detectable. This feature largely results from tumor neovascularity and tumor-specific characteristics of these new blood vessels. Unfortunately, some hormonally active fibrocystic tissue and benign tumors may also enhance. Low specificity is a major limitation to screening MRI. False-positive callbacks are associated with additional mammographic imaging or ultrasound scan, biopsies, and interval repeat imaging, which adds to screening costs. Evolving technologies undoubtedly will improve this aspect of MRI.

The efficacy of MRI as a screening tool in patients at high risk has been validated in multiple studies. In 2007, the ACS recommended annual screening MRI as a supplement to screening mammography for women with high risk for breast cancer based on a known *BRCA* mutation or a lifetime risk of 20% to 25% or greater with breast cancer risk models. On the basis of expert consensus opinion, the ACS also recommended annual MRI screening for those individuals who received radiation to the chest between the ages of 10 and 30 years; those with Li-Fraumeni, Cowden, or Bannayan-Riley-Ruvalcaba syndromes and their first-degree relatives. Data are still insufficient for recommendation for or against MRI screening for individuals with a lifetime risk of 15% to 20%, those with lobular carcinoma in situ (LCIS), atypical ductal or lobular hyperplasia

(ADH or ALH), and dense breast on mammography and those with a personal diagnosis of breast cancer, including ductal carcinoma in situ (DCIS).

Tomosynthesis

The key challenge to cost-effective screening is increasing sensitivity and specificity of imaging. The controversy between various screening guidelines largely arises from the additional costs incurred by follow-up diagnostic imaging and biopsies to evaluate the large number of false-positive results noted primarily in individuals with dense breasts. Tomosynthesis addresses the issue of dense breasts and overlying superimposed densities, which often hide breast cancers. Tomosynthesis involves the acquisition of multiple images of the breast recorded at difference angles while the detector is held stationary. As a result, the reader is presented with a series of images (0.05-mm slices) through the breast. Research has shown that masses are more visible in these reconstructed slices than in standard film-screen mammography. The potential benefits of tomosynthesis include improved screening sensitivity, improved lesion size detection, better characterization of vague findings, and decreased recall rates.

FUTURE

Companion digital technologies continue to be developed due to the advent of digital mammography and computer reconstruction. Stereo-digital mammography offers the potential to produce a three-dimensional image of the breast, and early studies look promising for reducing the number of false-positive results. MRI specificity may be improved with diffusion-weighted imaging or spectroscopy and also eliminate the need for intravenous contrast injection. Similarly, ultrasound scan specificity may be improved with sheer wave technology and elastography to measure the stiffness of lesions.

SUGGESTED READINGS

Berg WA, Blume JD, Cormack JB, et al: Combined screening with ultrasound and mammography versus mammography alone in women at elevated risk of breast cancer, *JAMA* 299(18):2151–2163, 2008.

D'Orsi CJ, Newell MS: On the frontier of screening for breast cancer, *Semin Oncol* 38(1):119–127, 2011.

Kerlikowske K, Hubbard RA, Miglioretti DL, et al: Comparative effectiveness of digital versus film-screen mammography in community practice in the United States: a cohort study, *Ann Intern Med* 155:493–502, 2011.

Lee CH, Dershaw DD, Kopans D, et al: Breast cancer screening with imaging: recommendations from the Society of Breast Imaging and the ACR on the use of mammography, breast MRI, breast ultrasound, and other technologies for the detection of clinically occult breast cancer, *J Am Coll Radiol* 7(1):18–27, 2010.

US Preventive Task Force: Screening for breast cancer: US Preventive Services Task Force recommendation statement, *Ann Intern Med* 151(10):716–726, 2009.

THE ROLE OF STEREOTACTIC BREAST BIOPSY IN THE MANAGEMENT OF BREAST DISEASE

Alexandra June Gordon and Nora Hansen, MD

INTRODUCTION

With the increase in mammography in the United States, stereotactic breast biopsies have become more common. Formerly, image-detected abnormalities required mammographic localization and excision, resulting in many surgical excisions for benign pathology. In contrast to an open biopsy, stereotactic biopsy can be done with a local anesthetic through a small incision with less significant parenchymal and skin scarring, and it is more cost effective. It leaves little or no deformity as long as the incision is made in an appropriate location and orientation.

In 2005, the National Accreditation Program for Breast Centers (NAPBC) was formed as a way to accredit breast programs, with the ultimate goal of improving breast cancer management and outcomes. The NAPBC set 27 standards required for accreditation of a breast center. One of them is that 90% of cancers must be diagnosed using a minimally invasive biopsy technique. Many other organizations support this concept as well.

HISTORY

In 1908, a neurosurgeon and a physiologist at University College London Hospital developed the stereotactic method and tried it on animals. They called it the Horsley-Clarke apparatus. However, the poor quality of the images limited its use. Between 1947 and 1949, using known anatomic landmarks, Ernest A. Spiegel, Henry T. Wycisand, and Lars Leksell developed the first stereotactic devices for brain surgery in humans. For neurosurgery, however, further improvements were necessary. Russell A. Brown, a computer scientist, invented a way to target stereotactic surgery using computed tomographic (CT) scan. Because CT could capture anatomic details in the brain, this greatly improved the accuracy and usefulness of stereotactic procedures. For breast biopsies, however, imaging was not the problem. Mammograms were able to produce a clear image of breast tissue, but the biopsy tools used needed refinement. With the advent of a spring-loaded core biopsy device, and later a vacuum-assisted, rotating blade biopsy probe, stereotactic biopsy became very accurate and useful. Stereotactic breast biopsy technology was introduced in the United States in the late 1980s by Dr. Kambiz Dowlat. As a result of the accuracy of stereotactic biopsy, it has become the predominant method for biopsy of nonpalpable breast lesions (Table 1).

Although many studies have reported the accuracy of stereotactic biopsies, the core needle biopsy sample may not provide complete characterization of the histologic findings, and this can lead to an underestimation of the presence of cancer (Table 2). This occurs most commonly in high-risk lesions such as atypical ductal hyperplasia (ADH), flat epithelial atypia (FEA), radial scars, and papillary and lobular lesions. These findings on a core biopsy require further investigation with an excisional biopsy to rule out the possibility of an associated cancer.

TABLE 1: Accuracy of stereotactic percutaneous core needle biopsy

Investigator	Year	Number of cases	Concordance with surgical biopsy
Parker	1991	102	96%
Dronkers	1992	5?	91%
Elvecrog	1993	100	94%
Gisvold	1994	104	90%
Pfari	2002	214	97%
Zuiani	2007	171	98%

TABLE 2: False negative rate of stereotactic percutaneous core needle biopsy

Investigator	Year	Method	Number of cases	Underestimation rate
Burak	2000	Stereo 11G-VAB	201	11.8%
Zuiani	2007	Stereo 11G-VAB	171	17.2%
Lourenco	2007	Stereo 11G-VAB	168	28.6%
Lourenco	2007	Stereo 9G-VAB	71	25.4%

CERTIFICATION

There is some controversy as to who should perform stereotactic biopsies—surgeons or radiologists. Regardless of who performs the biopsy, certification should be mandatory to ensure that the physician performing the biopsy is capable and meets certain standards. Certification not only ensures that the physician is capable, but it confirms that the equipment meets certain standards as well. Certification can be achieved through several avenues, but the most common certification process is through the American Society of Breast Surgeons (ASBS). ASBS certification requirements are outlined in Table 3. Upon completion of the prerequisites and a clinical application, each applicant for certification must successfully pass a written and practical examination.

PATIENT SELECTION, INDICATIONS, AND CONTRAINDICATIONS

A complete history and physical exam are important in any patient being considered for a stereotactic breast biopsy. Patients are usually advised to stop taking aspirin or nonsteroidal antiinflammatory agents prior to the procedure, although patients who must continue anticoagulation drugs can still have a stereotactic biopsy.

TABLE 3: American Society of Breast Surgeons certification requirements

Stereotactic Breast Procedure Certification

Requirements
1. A clinical application
2. A written exam
3. A practical exam

Prerequisites
1. Must have attained board certification via American Board of Surgery (ABS) or American Osteopathic Board of Surgery (AOBS) or evidence of international equivalent, upon completion of training.
2. Must document an appropriate level of training and a minimum of 1 year of experience in the performance of stereotactic breast procedures.
3. Must document performance of no fewer than 12 stereotactic breast procedures per year and evaluation of a minimum of 480 mammography exams in the last 2 years.
4. All applicants must have a minimum of 4 hours of AMA PRA Category 1 CME in medical radiation physics or can attest to the review of Radiation Physics and Safety by Howard Snider, MD, which is included in application. Applicants with less than 5 years of experience must have a minimum of 15 hours of AMA PRA Category 1 CME in breast imaging, including a minimum of 7 hours in stereotactic breast procedures during the last 5 years.

OR

Applicants with 5 or more years of experience must have a minimum of 5 hours of AMA PRA Category 1 CME in breast imaging or breast intervention during the last 5 years.

TABLE 4: Breast Imaging Reporting and Data System (BI-RADS) mammography categorizing system

BI-RADS 1	Normal mammogram
BI-RADS 2	Benign finding
BI-RADS 3	Probably benign, short interval follow-up suggested
BI-RADS 4	Suspicious for malignancy
BI-RADS 5	Strongly suggestive of malignancy
BI-RADS 6	Imaging in a patient with known malignancy
BI-RADS 0	Additional imaging evaluation or comparison with previous films suggested

TABLE 5: Indications for stereotactic biopsy

1	Lesions that are highly suggestive of malignancy, BI-RADS 5
2	Lesions that are suspicious, BI-RADS 4
3	Lesions that are BI-RADS 3 when there are other clinical reasons to perform a biopsy or in cases where a short-term follow-up would not be practical
4	Multiple suspicious lesions
5	Mammographic lesions that correspond to suspicious areas on MRI
6	A nonpalpable suspicious solid mass on mammography that is not seen on ultrasound
7	Suspicious microcalcifications that are new or at site of prior lumpectomy
8	Suspicious architectural distortion

Before the biopsy, a complete diagnostic workup must be performed. It is important to rule out pseudolesions that could lead to discordant biopsy results and require further surgical intervention for benign lesions. Additional mammographic views and ultrasound can help eliminate abnormalities caused by overlapping densities or clusters of calcifications that may appear to be suspicious. Mammograms are classified according to the American College of Radiology (ACR) Breast Imaging Reporting and Data System (BI-RADS) (Table 4).

Mammogram reports are required to categorize a mammogram according to the BI-RADS system by the Mammography Quality Standards Act and Program (MQSA). A BI-RADS 4 or 5 will likely require a stereotactic biopsy if the lesion is nonpalpable and cannot be seen on ultrasound. A BI-RADS 4 lesion is one with an intermediate risk. The majority of these lesions are benign, so a stereotactic biopsy can alleviate the need for a surgical excision and can be done under a local anesthetic. For those patients with BI-RADS 5 lesions, a stereotactic biopsy can decrease the number of trips to the operating room, and the surgeon can perform a definitive operation in a single surgery. If the lesion cannot be seen on the mammogram, a stereotactic biopsy cannot be performed.

Other contraindications to a stereotactic biopsy are limited to the patient's body habitus and the patient's ability to remain in the required position during the biopsy. Obese patient may be too heavy for a stereotactic table. Upright units that are attached to the mammography unit may make biopsy possible in this group of patients. Other relative contraindications include patients with severe kyphosis, making it impossible to position the breast deep enough through the hole in the biopsy table to localize the lesion, or patients who are unable to lie prone and still for the length of the biopsy, which may be the case with patients with a chronic cough or very anxious patients. If there is not enough breast tissue to compress and the breast compresses to less than 2.2 cm, the patient is not a good candidate for this approach and a needle localization procedure may be necessary. There are also circumstances when the breast is very large and the lesion very deep so the stereotactic needle cannot reach it. If the lesion is too close to the chest wall or the skin, it may be impossible to adequately or safely perform a stereotactic biopsy. However, the vast majority of mammographic lesions are amenable to stereotactic biopsy, and this should be the biopsy mode of choice for these patients. Table 5 lists current indications for a stereotactic breast biopsy recommended by the American College of Radiologists, the American Society of Breast Surgeons, and the Radiological Society of North America.

THE FUNDAMENTALS

Four terms a surgeon must be familiar with in order to perform a stereotactic biopsy are *targeting, pullback, stroke,* and *stroke margin.* Targeting is how the surgeon interprets the stereotactic images in order to sample the appropriate area of the breast. The surgeon must interpret a pair of images that are obtained at a 15-degree angle (Figures 1 and 2).

Stroke and stroke margin are related but are not identical. The stroke of a needle is the amount that it advances when fired. This can be calculated as the postfire position minus the prefire position of the tip of the needle. The stroke margin is the distance between the image receptor (i.e., the support behind the breast) and the tip of the needle after the needle has been fired. You want to have a *positive* stroke margin—that is, the stroke margin must be larger than the stroke. A negative stroke margin occurs when lesions are close to the image receptor and the stroke is larger than the stroke margin. This should be avoided because the needle can pass completely through the breast and damage the image receptor. While most machines calculate the stroke margin for you, easy-to-use stroke margin calculators are available online (Figures 3 and 4).

Pullback is related to the initial position of the needle relative to the area of interest. To understand this, it is important to be familiar with the features of a hollow biopsy needle. The portion of the needle that does the cutting is termed the *biopsy aperture,* and it is set back slightly from the tip of the needle. Because of this design, it is the biopsy aperture that needs to pass through the lesion and not the tip of the needle. It is imperative that the center of the biopsy aperture be in the middle of the target. In this instance the biopsy needle passes through the center of the lesion by half the length of the biopsy aperture plus the length of the tip of the needle. If the needle is placed too close to the target, when it is fired, the needle can advance past the lesion, pushing it forward and resulting in an inaccurate sample (Figures 5 and 6).

THE PROCEDURE

There are many types of stereotactic tables; the most common ones are manufactured by Hologic, Fischer, and Siemens. Stereotactic units consist mostly of tables with a circular aperture through which

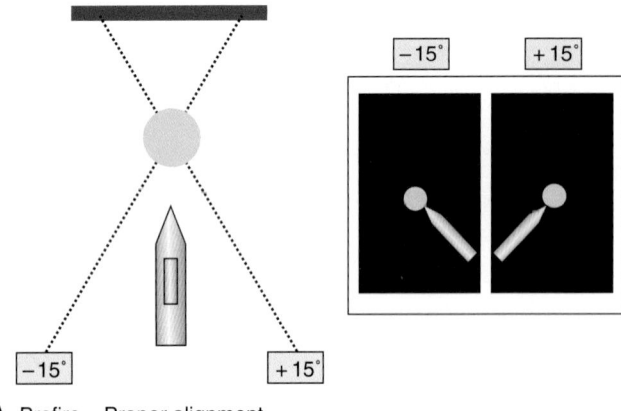

A Prefire – Proper alignment

B Postfire – Proper alignment

FIGURE 1 A, Prefire views of the biopsy needle properly aligned relative to the target. **B,** Postfire views. *(Based on drawings courtesy of Beth A. Boyd, RN.)*

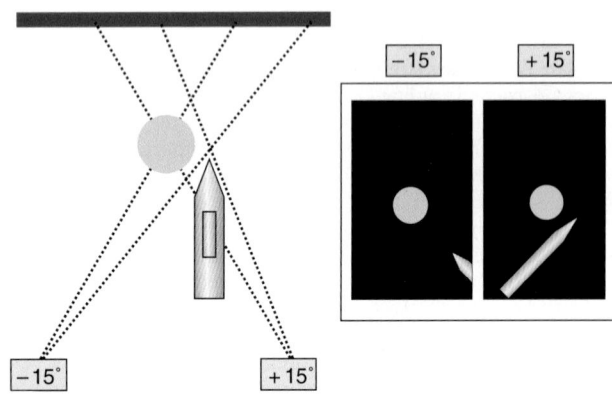

Prefire – Needle to the right

FIGURE 2 Prefire view of the needle to the right of the target. Understanding the 15-degree offset projection will help interpret the location of a misaligned biopsy needle. *(Based on drawings courtesy of Beth A. Boyd, RN.)*

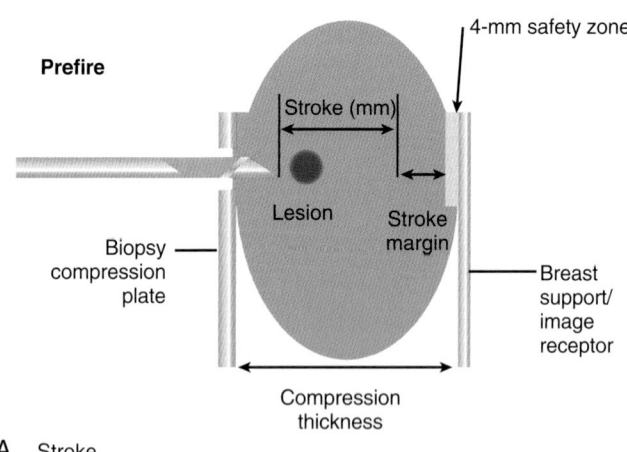

A Stroke

B Positive stroke margin

FIGURE 3 A, When fired, the needle will advance a preset distance, called the *stroke.* **B,** The distance of the tip of the needle from the back plate once the needle has been fired is the *stroke margin.* It should always be a positive number to avoid damage to the image receptor. *(Based on drawings courtesy of Beth A. Boyd, RN.)*

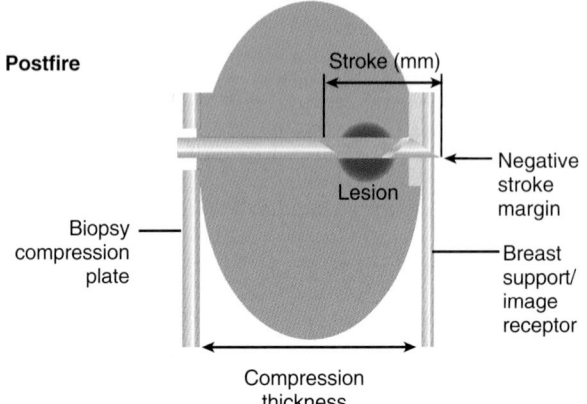

FIGURE 4 Negative stroke margin. The fully deployed needle is accurately placed but damages the image receptor. *(Based on drawings courtesy of Beth A. Boyd, RN.)*

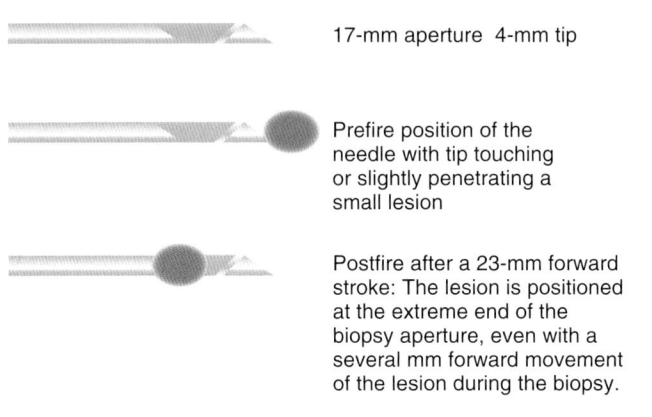

17-mm aperture 4-mm tip

Prefire position of the needle with tip touching or slightly penetrating a small lesion

Postfire after a 23-mm forward stroke: The lesion is positioned at the extreme end of the biopsy aperture, even with a several mm forward movement of the lesion during the biopsy.

FIGURE 5 Needle without pullback. The core biopsy needle is positioned too far into the lesion; when fired, it may pass too far to adequately sample the target. *(Based on drawings courtesy of Beth A. Boyd, RN.)*

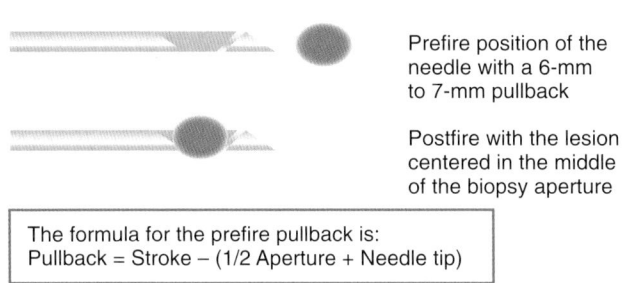

Prefire position of the needle with a 6-mm to 7-mm pullback

Postfire with the lesion centered in the middle of the biopsy aperture

The formula for the prefire pullback is:
Pullback = Stroke – (1/2 Aperture + Needle tip)

FIGURE 6 Needle with pullback. Proper position of the core biopsy needle to center the biopsy aperture within the lesion. (Note that the stereotactic machine will calculate the proper position of the biopsy device, including the required pullback.) *(Based on drawings courtesy of Beth A. Boyd, RN.)*

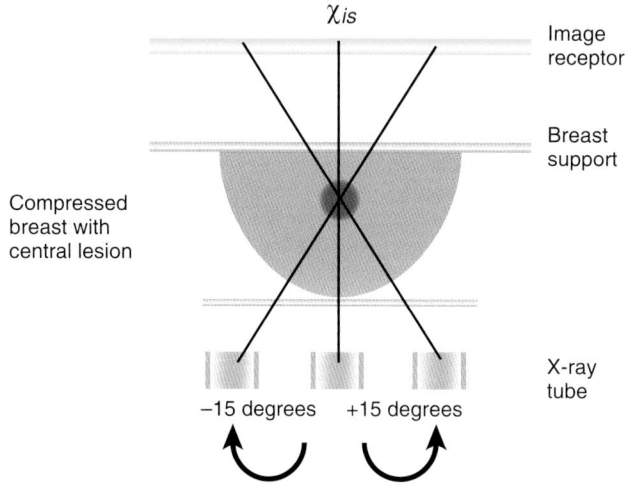

$\chi$is

Image receptor

Breast support

Compressed breast with central lesion

X-ray tube

–15 degrees   +15 degrees

FIGURE 7 The computer calculates the position of the lesion in the breast based on the difference in the 15-degree offset views. *(Based on drawings courtesy of Beth A. Boyd, RN.)*

the breast is suspended. It is occasionally desirable to use an upright table when the patient's body habitus or other concerns prevent the patient from lying prone. Despite the type of table used, the technique is similar. The first step in a stereotactic procedure is to select the best approach for the needle insertion. This is usually based on the shortest approach to the lesion so as little breast tissue as possible is penetrated. The approach could be from the lateral, medial, cranial, or caudal direction. If more than one lesion is to be biopsied, it would be important to determine if all the lesions could be approached from the same direction so repositioning could be limited during the procedure. To keep it immobilized during the biopsy, the breast is lightly compressed between a compression plate and a support behind the breast (the image receptor). It is imperative that the lesion be identified, and based on the location of the lesion, an approach for the biopsy is chosen. At times it can be difficult to position the lesion within the field of view, and it may take several attempts to reposition the compression plate so the lesion can be seen. Landmarks on the mammogram, such as vessels or macrocalcifications, can sometimes help guide the surgeon in identifying the lesion to be biopsied. If a blood vessel is in the path of the biopsy needle, a different approach may be necessary because there is a possibility of injuring the vessels with the biopsy needle, resulting in a hematoma. The lesion is initially imaged in the center of a 5 × 5 cm cutout in a compression plate. A scout image, taken perpendicularly to the compression plate, is obtained and then used to center the target in the field of view.

After the perpendicular scout image, two more x-rays are obtained 30 degrees apart—one at +15 degrees and the other at –15 degrees. The two images are viewed on a monitor, and the physician uses a cursor to select the target lesion on both images. Stereotactic imaging uses the principle of parallax to locate the three-dimensional location of a target within the breast from a pair of two-dimensional images. Derived from the Greek word *parallaxis*, which means "alteration," parallax is a difference in the apparent position of an object when viewed from two locations—in our case, a right (+15 degrees) and left (–15 degrees) eye location. We can use this parallax to determine distances (Figure 7).

Two targeting systems are currently used in stereotactic equipment, and the type of system used depends on the manufacturer. The polar coordinate system is used by Siemens and defines a target by distances from a fixed point and angular distances from a reference line. The depth of the targeted lesion is determined from the back compression plate and is expressed in millimeters, while the horizontal and vertical axes are expressed in degrees. Hologic uses a Cartesian system that defines the exact position of the target in three-dimensional space in millimeters in three axes that intersect at right angles (z-depth, x-horizontal, and y-vertical), and the depth is determined by a reference point in front of the breast on the front compression plate. A z-value of zero indicates the level of a reference point on the compression plate in front of the breast or at the opening through which the biopsy is performed. The z-value corresponding to the level of the image receptor behind the breast will equal the thickness of the compressed breast, so it is important to understand that you should not attempt a biopsy of a lesion if the calculated z-value is greater than the compression of the breast. This would result in the biopsy needle traversing the breast and into the image receptor. When the center of rotation is behind the breast, a larger parallax will correspond to a *shallower* target, one closer to the compression plate. When the center of rotation is in front of the target, a larger parallax will instead be a deeper target, closer to the back support of the breast. After the computer has calculated the location in three dimensions from the initial images, an appropriate biopsy device is selected and the skin is sterilely prepared.

Several types of biopsy needles are now available for stereotactic biopsies. Guidelines from the American College of Surgeons state that stereotactic biopsy should be performed with a vacuum-assisted biopsy device to reduce sampling error and minimize the false negatives. Despite the advent of the rotating, vacuum-assisted cutting device, approximately 10% to 20% of patients thought to have atypia at the time of biopsy demonstrate ductal carcinoma in situ (DCIS) or invasive carcinoma at the time of excision. Stereotactic biopsy is typically performed with a Mammotome-type needle, an 8-gauge to 11-gauge vacuum-assisted rotating cutting device. As the probe spins, the sample passes through the device into a hollow collection chamber. Because the device samples directionally, multiple specimens can be collected without having to remove and reinsert the device. While an 8-gauge to 11-gauge needle is typical, devices range from 18 gauge to 1.5 cm. The patient and reason for the procedure dictate the aperture of the needle used. Smaller needles would be used for a patient who required ongoing anticoagulation therapy to minimize the bleeding risk. Multiple studies suggest that false negatives are least common among biopsies with an 11-gauge needle. Larger needles would be used to remove intact tissue samples of calcifications or other mammographic densities. Prior to the biopsy, the surgeon should be familiar with the type of needle being used.

It is very important to be familiar with the biopsy device used because different devices require different amounts of breast tissue in front of and behind the lesion. Local anesthesia is administered—typically a 30-gauge needle injecting lidocaine without epinephrine into the skin, followed by a 25-gauge to 22-gauge needle for lidocaine with epinephrine deeper into the breast tissue. The addition of epinephrine helps reduce bleeding.

The biopsy device is placed in a small incision made with a scalpel, and the appropriate location of the device is verified in both the prefire and postfire views. Some biopsy devices do not require a skin nick and can be advanced directly into the breast. Specimens are obtained to sufficiently sample the target. Typically there are 10 to 15 samples taken from an 11-gauge device or 6 to 8 samples for an 8-gauge needle. Confirmation that the sample is sufficient and accurate is made by both the radiographic review of the biopsy specimens and the stereotactic views. If the biopsy was targeting calcifications and there are no calcifications in the stereo specimens, then additional biopsy samples should be obtained. It is always advisable to place a biopsy marker—a small, radiographically detectable clip—into the biopsy site if the patient requires further procedures or treatment. This marking is vital if the lesion is determined to be malignant. The most commonly used clip is stainless steel, but there are many options, including those that are deployed within the biopsy cavity rather than into the surrounding breast tissue, which may be less likely to move. Approximately 2% to 28% of traditional, stainless-steel clips are more than 1 cm away from the desired location, and the thinner the breast, the more likely there will be clip movement. Furthermore, if the clip is deployed when the breast tissue is compressed, upon release of the tissue, the clip may move a considerable amount. It is also possible that the clip may not deploy. Accurate placement is then verified with additional stereotactic views or with a two-view follow-up mammogram. If more than one lesion is biopsied, it is important to use different-shaped markers to identify each site, which is then correlated with the final pathology. If one is benign and one is malignant, the clip that marked the malignant lesion could be localized accurately for the definitive surgical procedure. The puncture site is generally closed with a Steri-strip, and dry gauze is placed either inside the patient's bra or held in place with an Ace wrap (Figures 8 to 12).

CHALLENGING CLINICAL SCENARIOS

A thin breast can be problematic for two reasons: there can be a negative stroke margin, and it may be impossible to center the lesion in the biopsy aperture, causing the sample of interest to be a small portion at the proximal end of the removed tissue. Generally a modification of the approach will resolve this issue, and the shortest approach will provide enough tissue to sample. It is also helpful to compress or bolster the breast in order to give a thin breast more volume. This can be done with anything that won't interfere with the radio waves: saline or gel bags, gauze, or Ace bandages.

A lesion that is close to the chest wall can be difficult to visualize and often necessitates a change in the patient's position. First, a chest wall lesion is most easily visualized with an medial lateral oblique (MLO) and lateral (LAT) view. It can be helpful to pull the breast downward with some force. If neither this nor repositioning helps, it is possible to put the patient's arm through the opening in the table along with the breast. In this scenario, it is important to avoid injuring axillary structures.

Lesions that are subareolar are difficult to biopsy because of the vascularity and often insufficient image quality. However, it is still possible to biopsy lesions in this location, but it may require a different approach.

Most complicated procedures occur because of the location of the lesion in the breast. It is helpful to remember that the image (especially of a faint lesion) will be better if the lesion is closer to the image receptor (breast back support) and farther from the source of the

FIGURE 8 Digital mammography.

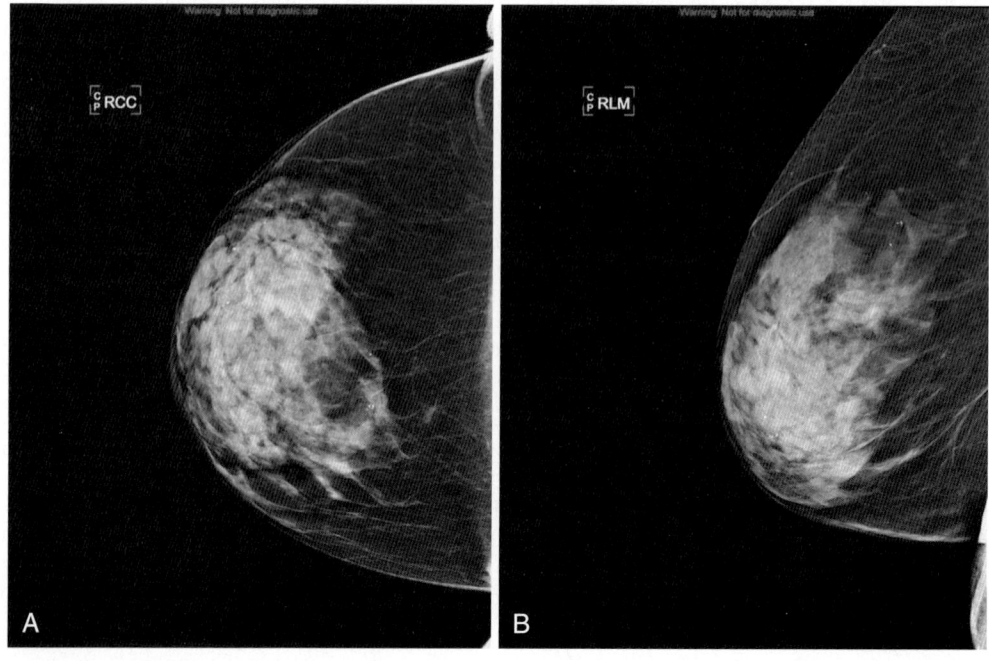

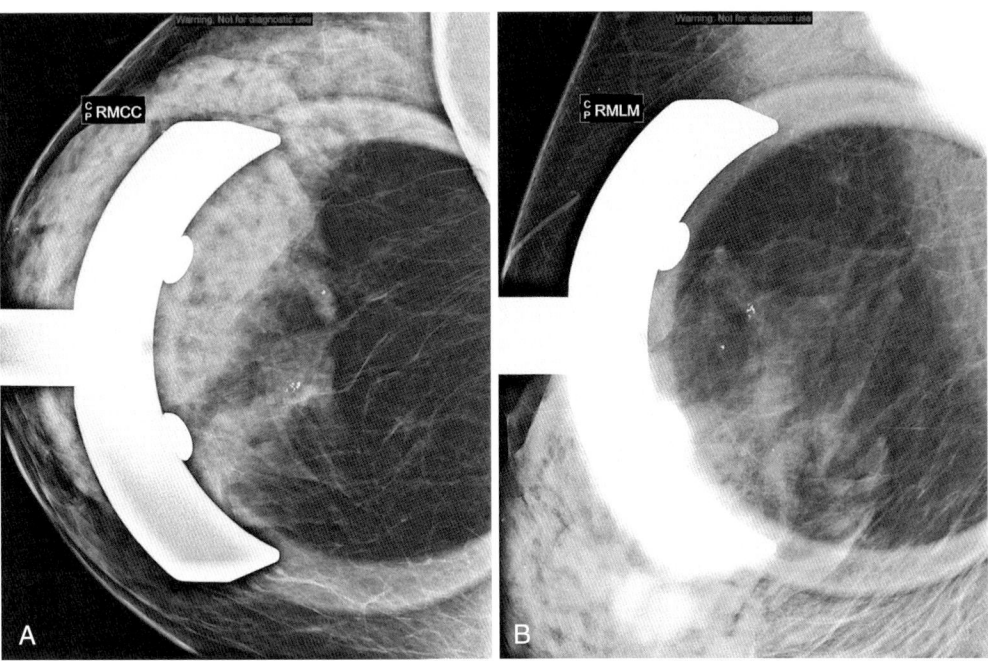

FIGURE 9 Digital mammography magnification view.

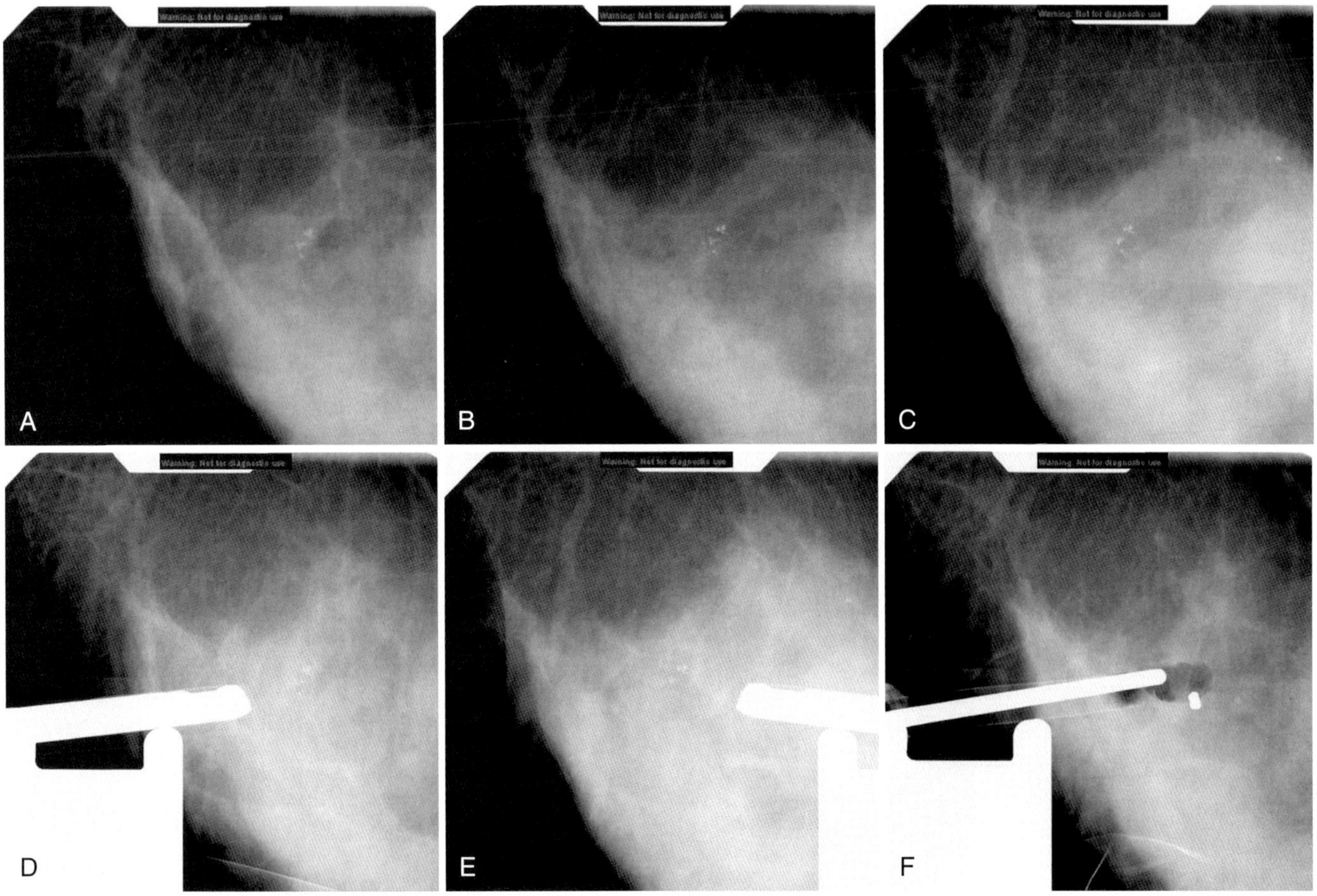

FIGURE 10 Stereotactic biopsy images.

x-ray beam. For example lesions at 6 o'clock are best approached craniocaudally.

PATHOLOGIC CORRELATION

The most important step in the biopsy procedure is to correlate the images from the procedure with the anticipated pathologic findings. If the images are not concordant with the pathology, the surgeon cannot trust the quality of the biopsy. The success of the procedure depends on accurate targeting and adequate tissue sampling. In addition to imaging before and during the procedure, the surgeon x-rays

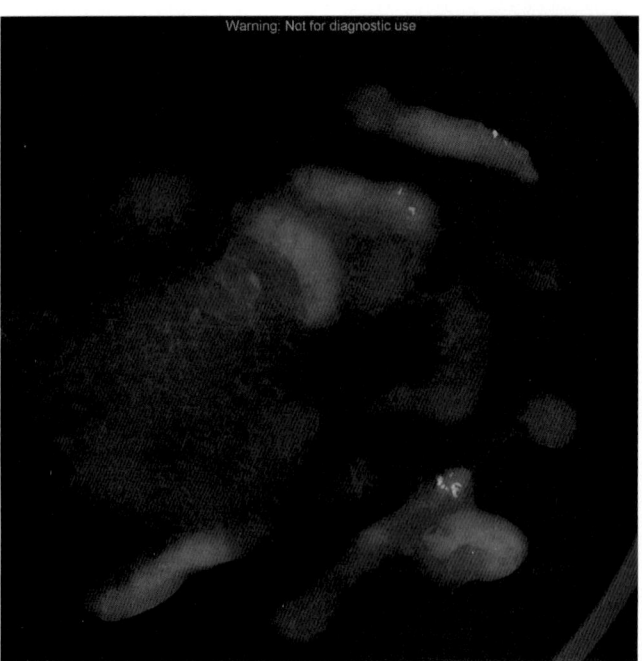

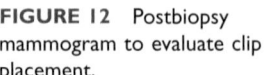

FIGURE 11   Specimen radiograph.

the core samples to make sure they include the area of interest. Indications that the procedure was unsuccessful would be an entirely benign tissue sample in a malignant-looking lesion. In this instance, surgical follow-up would be recommended because the targeting may have been insufficient.

Certain findings place women at a higher risk of developing breast cancer or suggest there is an adjacent malignant lesion and more surgery is required. Because the risk of coexisting malignancy is more important, the surgical excision is primarily for the purpose of ruling this out as opposed to complete excision of the atypical focus. In most instances, except those with a large radiographic area, both are accomplished. The following lesions identified on core biopsy should undergo an excisional breast biopsy to rule out the possibility of an associated malignancy. Pathologic findings that do not correspond to breast imaging findings (discordance) are outlined in Table 6.

CONCLUSIONS AND FUTURE DIRECTIONS

Stereotactic biopsies have essentially replaced excisional breast biopsies for nonpalpable mammographic abnormalities. These biopsies can be performed by both radiologists and surgeons, but it is imperative that any physician performing these biopsies be properly trained and certified. Pathologic correlation is essential to minimize false-negative results, and if the pathologic findings are discordant with the imaging findings, further investigation of the abnormality is required. This can be achieved either through a repeat stereotactic biopsy or with an excisional breast biopsy. As technology continues to improve in the area of both imaging and device development, the stereotactic approach may become not only a diagnostic tool but also a therapeutic one. Several types of tumor ablation are being explored, including cryoablation, radiofrequency ablation, and laser ablation, which may be able to utilize the stereotactic approach and increase the indications for the stereotactic apparatus. Further investigation is needed in these areas before they can be incorporated into the management of the breast cancer patient. However, the stereotactic approach offers a direct route of access to tumors in the breast and may in the future change the way we manage the breast cancer patient.

FIGURE 12 Postbiopsy mammogram to evaluate clip placement.

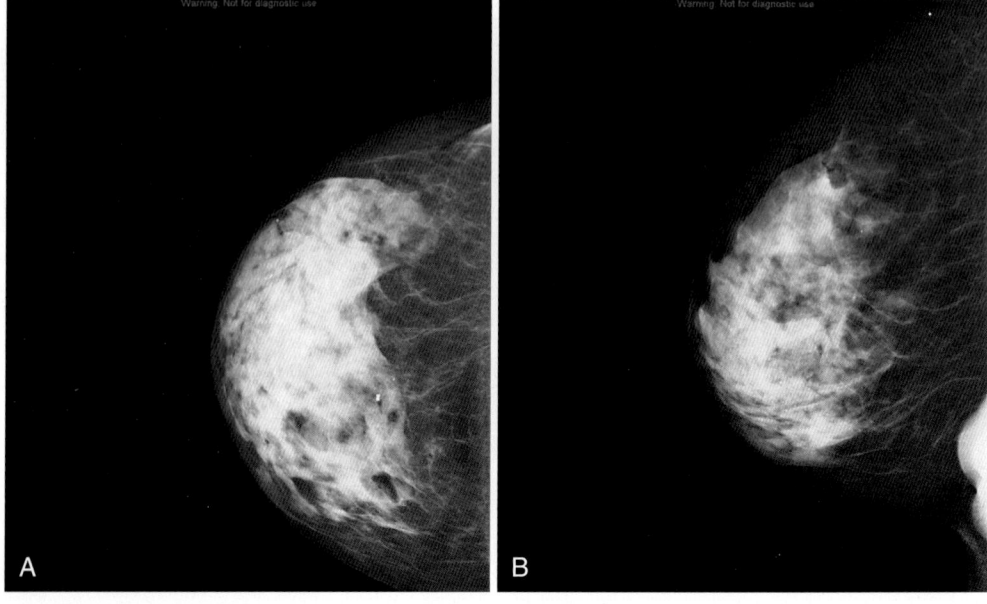

TABLE 6: Discordance

Atypical ductal hyperplasia (ADH)	Those with ADH have an upgrade rate of 15% to 20%, requiring most to be excised. Furthermore, a diagnosis of ADH carries a fourfold risk of developing cancer and thus requires close observation.
Lobular neoplasia	Note that this includes lobular carcinoma in situ (LCIS), pleomorphic LCIS, and atypical lobular hyperplasia (ALH). The distinction between these two types of lobular carcinoma is quantitative and not qualitative and thus hard to distinguish adequately on biopsy. Not all institutions excise LCIS or ALH, the decision to excise is made on an individual basis.
Radial scar	Excision is recommended unless the lesion is small and was completely removed on biopsy. If atypia is present, however, excision is always recommended.
Papillary lesions	Papillary lesions when asymptomatic are associated with DCIS about 10% to 20% of the time. When atypia is present, the upgrade rate increases and thus all lesions should be excised.
Phylloides tumor	Often impossible to diagnose a phylloides tumor on a needle biopsy. Often the core biopsy will be reported as a fibroepithelial lesion, and this should be excised to determine if this represents a phylloides tumor.

SELECTED READINGS

Allison KH, Eby PR, DeMartini WB, Lehman CD: Atypical ductal hyperplasia on vacuum-assisted breast biopsy: suspicion for ductal carcinoma in situ can stratify patients at high risk for upgrade, *Hum Pathol* 42(1):41–50, 2011. PMID 20970167.

American Society of Breast Surgeons: Website (http://www.breastsurgeons.org) for the statement on performance and practice guidelines for stereotactic biopsy for information on stereotactic certification and accreditation programs, and for a Web-based program to track stereotactic procedures, "The Mastery of Breast Surgery Program."

Head JF, Elliott RL: Stereotactic radiofrequency ablation: a minimally invasive technique for nonpalpable breast cancer in postmenopausal patients, *Cancer Epidemiol* 33(3-4), 2009. PMID 19699164.

Reynolds A: Stereotactic breast biopsy: a review, *Radiol Technol* 80(5), 2009. PMID 19457848.

MOLECULAR TARGETS IN BREAST CANCER

Helen Krontiras, MD, Oluwafunmi O. Awonuga, MD, and Kirby Bland, MD

The current knowledge for the complex molecular and genetic pathways involved in breast carcinogenesis has increased exponentially over the last few decades. We now know that breast cancer is a diverse and heterogeneous disease composed of an ever-enlarging number of biologic subtypes, each with differing clinical behaviors and outcomes. This chapter focuses on the clinically relevant cellular and molecular targets important for the practicing surgeon involved in the care of breast cancer.

MOLECULAR PROFILING

Contemporary advancements in molecular biology and genetics show that breast cancer has complex and diverse biologic behavior that influences its natural history and response to therapy. The introduction and widespread use of sophisticated high through-put technologies, such as gene expression arrays, coupled with effective analytic tools, has allowed for breast cancer characterization, or profiling, on a molecular level, beyond the traditional methods of anatomic stage and histologic grade.

With the use of microarrays and hierarchal cluster analysis, Perou and colleagues first described in 2000 the molecular classifications of breast cancer known as the intrinsic subtypes. These include three main subtypes of estrogen receptor (ER)–negative tumors: (1) basal-like; (2) human epidermal growth factor receptor–2 (HER2) enriched; and (3) normal-like. The two subtypes of ER-positive tumors, luminal A and luminal B, are evident, and a sixth breast cancer subtype, termed claudin-low, has also been defined. These subtypes differ significantly in prognosis and in the therapeutic targets they express. The subtypes important in the clinical setting are described subsequently (Table 1).

TABLE 1: Intrinsic subtypes of breast cancer

Type	Characteristics	Markers
Luminal A	Low grade High ER 50% of all breast cancer	ER+, PR+, HER2–, CK8+, CK18+
Luminal B	Higher grade Lower ER 10% of breast cancer	ER+, PR+/–, HER2+/–
HER2	High grade P53 mutations 5% to 10% of breast cancer	ER–, PR–, HER2+
Basal	High proliferation 30% of breast cancer	ER–, PR–, HER2–

*CK,*Cytokeratin ; *ER,* estrogen receptor; *HER2,* human epidermal growth factor receptor–2; *PR,* progesterone receptor.

Luminal Subtypes

The term *luminal* derives from the similarity in expression between these tumors and the luminal epithelium of the breast. Luminal subtypes comprise the majority of ER-positive breast cancer and are characterized by expression of ER, progesterone receptor (PR), and other genes associated with ER activation. The luminal subtypes are further divided into luminal A and luminal B subtypes.

Luminal A tumors usually have high expression of ER-related genes, low expression of the HER2 cluster of genes, and low expression of proliferation-related genes. They are typically low to moderate tumor grade. Luminal A tumors are the most common of all the subtypes (50%) and carry the best prognosis of all breast cancer subtypes. Luminal B tumors are less common (10%) and have a worse prognosis than luminal A tumors; luminal B have superior prognosis to the nonluminal subtypes basal-like and HER2-enriched. Luminal B tumors have a relatively lower (although still present) expression of ER-related genes, variable expression of the HER2 cluster, and higher expression of the proliferation cluster, including Ki67.

HER2-Enriched

The HER2-enriched subtype is characterized by high expression of the HER2 and proliferation gene clusters and low expression of the luminal cluster. This subtype is uncommon and represents only about 10% of all breast cancers. These tumors are typically negative for ER and PR and positive for HER2. Most tumors that are positive for ER and HER2 fall into the luminal B subtype. Before HER2-targeted therapy, this subtype carried a poor prognosis. However, this unfavorable outcome has been significantly improved with HER2-directed therapy.

Basal-Like

The basal-like subtype derives its name from similarity in expression to that of the basal epithelial cells. It is characterized by low expression of the luminal and HER2 gene clusters. These tumors are typically ER, PR, and HER2 negative on clinical assays that are termed triple-negative. Most triple-negative tumors (TNBC) are basal-like; however, not all TNBC are basal-like, and not all basal-like breast cancer possess triple-negative receptors. Approximately 20% of breast cancers are basal-like. The basal-like tumors have high expression of the proliferation cluster of genes and high expression of the epidermal growth factor receptor (EGFR) and the basal cluster, which includes basal epithelial cytokeratins 5, 14, and 17.

Basal-like breast cancer and triple-negative breast cancer are similar in clinical characteristics, but practically, clinical assays currently only identify TNBC; thus, triple-negative is a surrogate of the basal-like subtype in the clinical setting. Both are associated with aggressive phenotypes. In comparison with all the other subtypes of breast cancer, TNBCs present at an earlier age of onset and are seen more often in premenopausal women of African ancestry. They tend to be large, high-grade tumors with frequent lymph node positivity. They often present as interval cancers, between mammograms or on clinical examination. As a result, TNBC is characterized by poorer survival outcomes and higher relapse rates than non–triple-negative breast cancers. Distant metastases most often occur in visceral sites. Recurrences rates typically peak in the first 3 years after diagnosis and rapidly diminish thereafter, confirming the aggressive natural history of the disease. Although TNBCs often carry a poor prognosis, they tend to have an improved rate of complete pathologic response compared with luminal subtypes in studies of neoadjuvant therapy, the so-called triple-negative paradox that indicates significant heterogeneity even with the basal-like/TNBC subtype. Lehman and associates in 2011 subclassified this group into seven subtypes, each

with potential specific therapeutic implications. Interestingly, most breast cancers that occur in women with the BRCA1 mutation are basal-like and triple-negative. This is being exploited in clinical trials of targeted therapy discussed later in this chapter.

Clinical Gene Expression Assays

Multiple limited-set gene expression profiling assays have been validated and are in clinical use today. First described in 2002, these gene expression profiles identify tumors with high and low risk for recurrence and provide independent prognostic information beyond the anatomic and immunohistochemical classification of breast cancer. Genetic expression profiles are commercially available and covered by most insurance carriers. These assays are typically considered in ER-positive and HER2-negative breast cancer as an *adjunct* to traditional prognostic parameters.

The 21-gene reverse-transcriptase polymerase chain reaction assay (Oncotype DX; Genomic Health, Redwood City, Calif) is performed on formalin-fixed paraffin-embedded tissue and evaluates 16 cancer-related genes (Ki67, STK15, survivin or BIRC5, CCNB1 and MYLB2, ER, PGR, BCL2, SCUBE2, HER2, GRB7, MMP11, CTSL2, GSTM1, CD68, and BAG1) and 5 reference genes. An individualized risk estimate or recurrence score (0 to 100) is provided for each tumor sample submitted: low risk, <18; intermediate risk, 18 to 30; and high risk, ≥31 (Figure 1).

Should the recurrence score indicate a low risk score, hormone therapy alone may be considered, sparing chemotherapy; if the recurrence score indicates a high-risk category, chemotherapy followed by hormonal therapy may provide a better outcome. Studies show that associations of recurrence score with survival were independent from standard clinicopathologic factors. Current National Comprehensive Cancer Network (NCCN) breast cancer clinical practice guidelines recommend considering Oncotype DX for patients with ER-positive, node-negative breast cancer to aid decision making regarding adjuvant systemic therapy. Recent studies indicate that Oncotype DX may be useful in node-positive ER-positive HER2-negative breast cancer as well.

MammaPrint (Agendia; Amsterdam, Netherlands) or the Amsterdam 70-gene profile is also validated and commercially available. This microarray assay is performed on freshly collected tissue and provides similar information regarding the potential benefit of chemotherapy in selected patients with ER-positive or ER-negative disease.

ESTROGEN RECEPTOR SIGNALING PATHWAYS

Beatson in 1896 reported regression of advanced breast cancer with removing ovaries in patients with premenopausal breast cancer after observing that rabbits that had ovaries removed stopped producing milk, indicating a relationship between the breast and the ovary. However, not all breast cancers responded to oophorectomy. It was not until the 1970s, when the estrogen receptor was discovered, that the reason became known. Jenson developed the hypothesis that some breast cancers contain the estrogen receptor and others do not. Those that did not have the receptor would not respond to endocrine manipulation. Since that time, the ER has been extensively studied, and endocrine therapy remains one of the most important modalities in breast cancer treatment for ER-positive cancers.

The ER is a ligand-dependent transcription factor and is actually composed of two receptors. The estrogen alpha receptor (ER-α) is a class I nuclear receptor located on chromosome 6q, and the estrogen receptor beta (ER-β) is located on chromosome 14q. Both ER-α and ER-β are members of the steroid receptor family of proteins, and both share common structural and functional domains, except that ER-β lacks a portion of the C-terminal domain. They bind with high

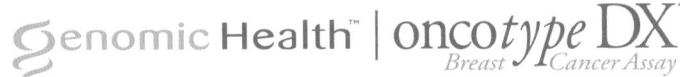

Genomic Health, Inc.
301 Penobscot Drive
Redwood City, CA 94063 USA
Toll Free Tel 866-ONCOTYPE (866-662-6897)
Worldwide Tel +1 650-569-2080
www.oncotypeDX.com

PATIENT REPORT

Patient/ID: Doe, Jane
Sex: Female
Date of Birth: 01-Jan-1950
Medical Record/Patient #: 556677771
Date of Surgery: 25-Sep-2008
Specimen Type/ID: Breast/SURG-0001

Requisition: R00003G
Specimen Received: 05-May-2009
Date Reported: 15-May-2009
Client: Community Medical Center
Ordering Physician: Dr. Harry D Smith
Submitting Pathologist: Dr. John P Williams
Additional Recipient: Dr. Sally M Jones

BREAST CANCER ASSAY DESCRIPTION

Onco*type* DX Breast Cancer Assay uses RT-PCR to determine the expression of a panel of 21 genes in tumor tissue. The Recurrence Score® is calculated from the gene expression results. The Recurrence Score range is from 0-100.

RESULTS

Breast Cancer Recurrence Score = **12**

The findings summarized in the Clinical Experience sections of this report are applicable to the patient populations defined in each section. It is unknown whether the findings apply to patients outside these criteria.

CLINICAL EXPERIENCE: PROGNOSIS FOR NODE NEGATIVE, ER-POSITIVE PATIENTS

The Clinical Validation study included female patients with Stage I or II, Node Negative, ER-Positive breast cancer treated with 5 years of tamoxifen. Those patients who had a Recurrence Score of 12 had an Average Rate of Distant Recurrence of **8% (95% CI: 5%-10%)**

The following results are from a clinical validation study of 668 patients from the NSABP B-14 study. *N Engl J Med* 2004; 351: 2817-26.

Recurrence Score vs Distant Recurrence in Node Negative, ER-Positive Breast Cancer Prognosis

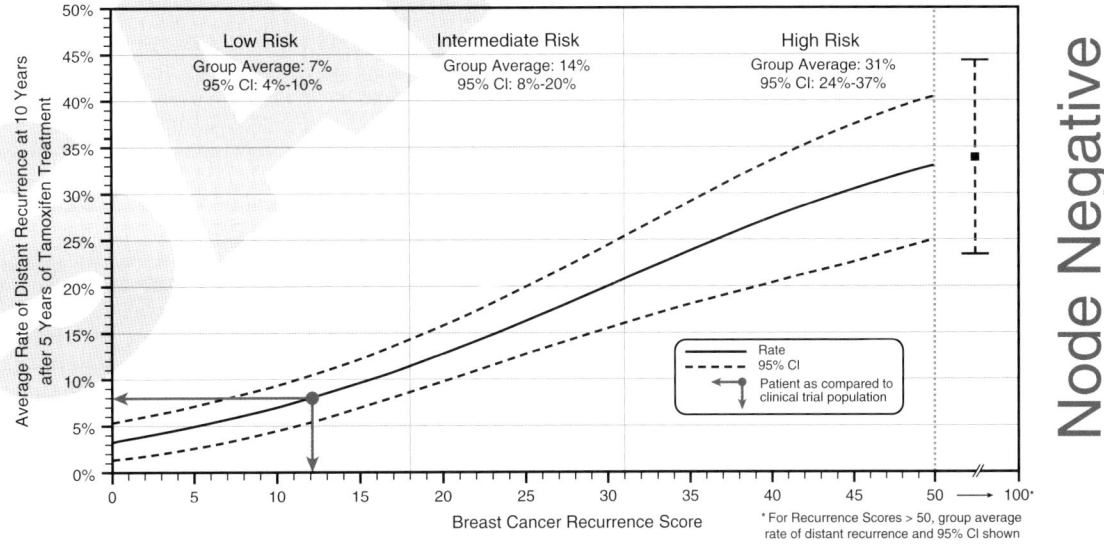

FIGURE 1 Oncotype DX Recurrence Score (RS) Report. The report provides a RS on a scale of 1 to 100. The RS result is correlated with a specific likelihood of distant recurrence at 10 years based on the average 10-year distant recurrence rate for that RS in the clinical trial population. Of note, the clinical trial population was treated with 5 years of tamoxifen. In addition, the report does provide a quantitative single gene report for estrogen receptor, progesterone receptor, and human epidermal growth factor receptor–2 scores. *(Oncotype DX and Recurrence Score are registered trademarks of Genomic Health Inc, Redwood City, Calif.)*

affinity to the ligand estrogen. Estrogen binds the receptor, causes dimerization, and facilitates interaction of the receptor with promoter regions in the DNA. These regions are termed *estrogen response elements*, which function by regulating the activation or repression of gene transcription. Currently, little is known about the role of ER-β in breast cancer. Approximately 60% of tumors coexpress ER-α and ER- β. Some evidence suggests that a high ratio of ER-α to ER-β at a target site is important, and high ratios are associated with high levels of cellular proliferation and tamoxifen resistance.

The assays used for ER determination in clinical practice measure ER-α levels, the "classic ER." Approximately 70% to 80% of all invasive breast cancers and nearly all intraductal breast cancers express the ER-α protein (ER positive). Traditionally, ER positivity has been measured quantitatively with immunohistochemistry (IHC). Approximately 60% of ER-positive tumors are also progesterone receptor (PR) positive. Although patients with ER-positive tumors have a better prognosis than patients with ER-negative tumors, expression of the estrogen receptor is more useful as a predictor for response to endocrine therapy. In ER-positive/PR-positive tumors, 70% respond to endocrine therapy. In addition, 50% of ER-negative tumors express PR, perhaps indicating downstream activation of the endocrine pathways; of these, 30% respond to tamoxifen therapy.

Selective estrogen receptor modulators (SERMs) are competitive ER antagonists with partial agonist activity. Tamoxifen is the most widely used SERM for breast cancer treatment. Tamoxifen competitively inhibits the binding of estradiol to estrogen receptors in some sites and maintains agonist activity in some tissues.

Given in an adjuvant setting, tamoxifen reduces the risk of breast cancer recurrence and death in premenopausal and postmenopausal women with ER-positive disease. Specifically, the Early Breast Cancer Trialists Collaborative Group (EBCTCG) overview and meta-analysis of randomized trials of adjuvant tamoxifen found that this SERM reduced the 15-year probability of breast cancer recurrence (from 46% to 33%, a 39% reduction in the annual recurrence rate) and breast cancer mortality (from 33% to 24%, a 30% reduction in the annual mortality rate). It is given daily (20 mg). The side-effects profile is notable in some women for symptomatic hot flashes and vaginal dryness or discharge related to the antiestrogenic effect of the medication. More worrisome but rare side effects include an increased risk for the development of uterine cancer and thromboembolic events in postmenopausal women. Tamoxifen treatment may also offer beneficial side effects in postmenopausal women, including an improvement in bone density and lipid profile.

Although they do not directly interfere with the ER, aromatase inhibitors (AIs) are the mainstay of endocrine therapy in postmenopausal ER-positive breast cancer. Landmark trials have shown that AIs are superior to tamoxifen in reducing breast cancer recurrence in postmenopausal women. Specifically, 12 prospective randomized studies show that the use of an AI in this patient population reduces the risk of local recurrence and improves disease-free survival when compared with tamoxifen alone. AIs block conversion of adrenally synthesized androgens to estrogen with the aromatase enzyme, thus suppressing estrogen levels. This is the last step in steroid conversion to active hormones and does not interfere with production of corticosteroids or mineralocorticoids. Production of estrogen in the ovary is not suppressed, however, and AIs are currently indicated only for postmenopausal women with ER-positive breast cancer. Currently, three AIs are used in clinical practice: exemestane (Aromasin; Pfizer, New York, NY) anastrozole (Arimidex; Astra-Zenaca, London, England), and letrozole (Femara; Novartis, Basel, Switzerland).

AIs have been studied as initial and sequential therapy after tamoxifen and also as extended therapy. Initial use of an AI, in comparison with tamoxifen, was studied in the anastrozole, tamoxifen, alone or in combination (ATAC), trial of postmenopausal women with ER-positive breast cancer. With a median follow-up period of 120 months, there was significantly longer disease-free survival with anastrozole than with tamoxifen (hazard ratio [HR], 0.91; 95% confidence interval [CI], 0.83 to 0.99). Anastrozole was also associated

with a prolonged time to recurrence (HR, 0.84; 95% CI, 0.75 to 0.93), fewer recurrences (absolute reduction of 2.7% at 5 years and 4.3% at 10 years), and fewer contralateral breast cancers (HR, 0.68; 95% CI, 0.50 to 0.91). In addition, in comparison with tamoxifen, treatment with anastrozole causes significantly fewer episodes of hot flashes, vaginal discharge, vaginal bleeding, endometrial cancer, strokes, and thromboembolic events. However, women on anastrozole in this study reported more musculoskeletal problems than those on tamoxifen, and a significantly increased number of fractures were seen in the women in the anastrozole group.

GROWTH FACTOR RECPTOR PATHWAYS AND DOWN STREAM PATHWAYS

The epidermal growth factor receptor family is made up of four receptors: HER1 (erbB1/EGFR), HER2 (erbB-2), HER3 (erbB-3) and HER4 (erbB-4). These receptors are transmembrane proteins with three cellular domains and function primarily as tyrosine kinases that activate the phosphatidylinositol 3-kinase (PI3K)/AKT and RAS/RAF/MAPK pathways.

Perhaps the best characterized of the EGFR family receptors is HER2. The HER2 gene, also known as *Her 2 neu* or c-erbB2, is located on chromosome 17q and is normally involved in regulation of cell proliferation. The HER2 gene is a protooncogene a normal gene with the potential to become an oncogene with molecular alterations, such as mutation, amplification, or overexpression of its protein product. HER2 overexpression is an early event in breast cancer development. HER2 is overexpressed or gene amplified (or both) in approximately 20% of invasive breast cancers. Patients with overexpression of HER2 often have high-grade tumors, axillary lymph node involvement, and decreased expression of estrogen and progesterone receptors. These characteristics are associated with an increased risk of recurrence and decreased survival; however, HER2 overexpression is also independently associated with poor prognosis.

Trastuzumab (Herceptin; Genentech, South San Francisco, Calif) is a recombinant humanized monoclonal antibody that targets the extracellular domain of the HER2 protein. Multiple randomized controlled trials of trastuzumab in the adjuvant setting have shown that trastuzumab given in combination with chemotherapy to patients with tumors that overexpress HER2 significantly improves disease-free and overall survival compared with chemotherapy regimens that do not contain trastuzumab. Used in the neoadjuvant setting, trastuzumab plus chemotherapy improves pathologic complete response (approximately 65% with trastuzumab and 25% without trastuzumab). Significant cardiac events occur in approximately 2% of patients who have received trastuzumab plus chemotherapy compared with 0.3% with standard chemotherapy according to a meta-analysis of almost 11,000 patients in the adjuvant setting. Data suggest that the cardiac toxicity observed with trastuzumab therapy is reversible in most cases. Those cases with tumors that possess low or negative levels of expression or amplification are not likely to have significant benefit from treatment with trastuzumab, but studies are underway examining the role of Herceptin in HER2-negative cases. Current guidelines recommend that trastuzumab be given in the adjuvant setting in conjunction with chemotherapy for invasive HER2 overexpressing tumors more than 1 cm and for HER2-positive node-positive disease. Consideration for systemic adjuvant therapy with trastuzumab is recommended for invasive HER2 overexpressing tumors between 5 and 10 mm and for HER2-positive micrometastatic nodal disease. Evaluation is ongoing to determine the optimal duration, combination, and sequencing.

Lapatinib is an oral, reversible, small-molecule dual inhibitor of both EGFR (HER1) and HER2 kinases. In 2007, lapatinib was approved for use in combination with capecitabine in trastuzumab-refractory HER2-positive metastatic breast cancer. Pertuzumab, another monoclonal antibody, targets the extracellular domain of HER2 at a different site. This drug was approved for use in metastatic HER2-positive breast cancer in combination with docetaxel and trastuzumab in 2012.

Data from clinical trials suggest that dual blockade of the HER pathways may be superior to single therapy targeting. Trials testing different combinations of both new and approved targeted HER pathway blockers without cytotoxic chemotherapy are underway to determine whether chemotherapy and its associated additional toxicity may be avoided in this patient population. Ongoing studies of new agents and combinations will likely result in a number of new agents being approved for the metastatic, adjuvant, and neoadjuvant settings in the near future.

PI3K/AKT PATHWAY

Phosphatidylinositol 3-kinase (PI3K) is a major signaling hub downstream of HER2 and other tyrosine kinases and activates AKT, serum/glucocorticoid regulated kinase, mammalian target of rapamycin (mTOR), and several additional molecules involved in cell cycle regulation, progression, and survival. Uncontrolled activation of the PI3K/AKT/mTOR pathway occurs in more than 70% of breast cancers and appears to be involved with both endocrine and HER2-targeted therapy resistance. Combination therapy with PI3K pathway inhibitor is a promising new avenue in breast cancer treatment. In 2012, everolimus, an mTOR inhibitor, was approved for advanced hormone receptor-positive, HER-negative breast cancer in combination with exemestane after failure of treatment with letrozole or anastrozole.

ANGIOGENESIS

Angiogenesis or the growth of new blood vessels is fundamental for tumor growth and metastasis. Tumors with volumes less than a few cubic millimeters exist in a prevascular state with continued cycle of proliferation and cell death, receiving oxygen and nutrients through diffusion. Tumor angiogenesis is the proliferation of a network of blood vessels that penetrate into cancerous growths, supplying nutrients and oxygen and removing waste products.

The primary promoter of tumor angiogenesis is vascular endothelial growth factor A (VEGF-A or VEGF). VEGF is synthesized in tumor cells and is expressed in most types of human cancer. Increased expression of VEGF in tumors is usually associated with diminished prognosis. Although the VEGF family of growth factors and receptors have three known receptors, VEGF signals principally through VEGF receptor 2 (VEGFR-2) and activates a series of proteins that transmit a signal into the nucleus to initiate new endothelial cell growth, differentiation, and apoptosis. In addition, VEGF mediates vascular permeability and allows deposition of angiogenic proteins into the surrounding tissue, perpetuating angiogenesis and sustaining tumor growth. Studies by Folkman and others more than 40 years ago showed in preclinical models that inhibition of angiogenesis could inhibit cancer growth. This led to the development of agents to inhibit angiogenesis for therapeutic intention.

Bevacizumab (Avastin; Genentech/Roche) is a humanized monoclonal antibody that inhibits VEGF. It was the first angiogenesis inhibitor approved by the U.S. Food and Drug Administration (FDA). It is approved for advanced solid organ malignancies, including lung, colon, and kidney. Approval for breast cancer was withdrawn in November 2011 because of increased toxicity and a lack of survival benefit in overall survival across all breast cancer subtypes in the initial clinical trials.

Small molecule multityrosine kinase inhibitors that target, among others, the VEGF-2 receptor are currently being investigated. Studies are ongoing as to the appropriate patient subset, schedule, and partner chemotherapies; however, because of lack of specificity, successful outcomes with these targeted therapies may hinge on the work exploring response prediction.

DNA REPAIR PATHWAYS

Poly(ADP-ribose) Polymerase Inhibitors

Multiple distinct DNA repair pathways exist to maintain stability of the genome. Single-stranded DNA damage is repaired with base excision repair (BER), nucleic acid excision repair (NER), mismatch repair, or direct repair. Double-stranded breaks are repaired with homologous recombination and nonhomologous end joining.

Poly(ADP-ribose) polymerases (PARPs) are a family of enzymes involved in chromosome stability, regulation of apoptosis, cell division, and transcriptional regulation and differentiation. There are 17 enzymes in the PARP family. The best known are PARP1 and PARP2, which are important in the function of BER. PARP inhibitors interfere with DNA damage repair by inhibiting BER. DNA repair is optimal for healthy cells, but the opposite effect is desired in cancer cells that experience DNA damage from therapy such as chemotherapy and radiation.

BRCA1 and 2 genes are tumor suppressor genes that play a crucial role for maintenance of genomic stability by promoting repair of double-stranded breaks by homologous repair. Most people with the BRCA deleterious gene mutation are heterozygous for the mutation, meaning they have one normal and one mutated allele. Tumors with DNA repair defects including BRCA mutations appear to have particular sensitivity to PARP inhibition. Loss of PARP1 protein function in a BRCA1-defective or BRCA2-defective background cripples the cell's ability to repair double-strand DNA damage, leading to cell cycle arrest or cell death. Therefore, PARP inhibitors could be selectively lethal to cells deficient in BRCA1 and BRCA2. In addition to BRCA mutations, some sporadic breast cancers, including some TNBC, also exhibit similarity to BRCA1 mutant tumors, a concept referred to as BRCAness. These tumors also appear to be sensitive to PARP inhibition, and exploiting this similarity could have significant therapeutic promise for TNBC, which as of yet has no specific target. A number of PARP inhibitors are in clinical development and multiple ongoing trials to test the efficacy of this approach.

SUGGESTED READINGS

Arteaga C, Sliwkowski M, Osbirne C, et al: Treatment of HER2-positive breast cancer: current status and future perspectives, *Nat Rev Clin Oncol* 29(9):16–32, 2011.

Foulkes W, Smith I, Reis-Filho J: Triple-negative breast cancer, *N Engl J Med* 363:1938–1948, 2010.

Perou C, Sorlie T, Eisen M, et al: Molecular portraits of human breast tumours, *Nature* 406:747–752, 2000.

Breast Cancer: Surgical Management

Megan K. Baker, MD

INTRODUCTION

Breast cancer surgical management continues to evolve in response to evidence-based clinical research and burgeoning basic science investigations. The surgeon's role, however, remains constant. It is our role to ensure a proper diagnosis, timely treatment planning, and patient care follow through. With reliance on a multidisciplinary model, surgeons are best able to provide patients with state-of-the-art care and thereby improve the patient's chance for successful outcome.

DIAGNOSIS AND WORKUP

In addition to the technical aspects of diagnosis and imaging, the importance of a thorough history and physical examination cannot be overstated. Elements of the history and examination should strongly influence decisions on genetics referral, staging evaluation, and care planning. The gold standard for the diagnosis of breast cancer is image-guided or palpation-guided core biopsy. The routine use of fine needle aspiration (FNA) and excisional biopsy as diagnostic tools is no longer recommended. In an era in which the histology and biologic features of a breast cancer so strictly dictate treatment, FNA of a breast mass is an unnecessary and typically incomplete evaluation. At the same time, excisional biopsy subjects the patient to a needless level of intervention that may compromise aesthetic outcome or result in a delay or abdication of neoadjuvant chemotherapy options. Similarly, routine or indiscriminate use of radiologic staging studies is discouraged because this has not been shown to change outcome. Thorough bilateral breast imaging remains essential and commonly consists of diagnostic digital mammography. It is often augmented with ultrasound scan (US) or magnetic resonance imaging (MRI) where appropriate. The routine use of preoperative MRI has not been shown to improve outcome in terms of overall survival, disease-free survival, or margin reexcision rates in randomized studies. At the author's center, MRI has been useful in situations with discordance between physical examination and routine imaging, in cancers with lobular histology, in patients with predisposing genetic conditions, and in cases with unexpected involved margins or planned neoadjuvant chemotherapy.

TREATMENT

Noninvasive and Invasive Breast Cancer

As established by the National Surgery Breast and Bowel Project (NSABP) B06 and NSABP B17, breast-conserving therapy (BCT) may be used in the surgical management of the breast for most non-invasive and invasive breast cancers. Partial mastectomy, most commonly complemented with radiation therapy, may be conducted via excisional, wire-guided, hematoma, or ultrasound scan–guided techniques. The principles are the same: localization of the lesion, surgical excision of the cancer with adequate margins, and maintenance of the breast aesthetic. Contraindications to breast-conserving surgery include multicentric disease, locally advanced breast cancer, inflammatory breast cancer, unfavorable breast-to-tumor ratio, and any contraindication to radiation therapy.

Breast Incision and Procedure Selection

Incision style and placement depends both on the location of the tumor and on the strategy for radiation therapy. Historically, incisions have been placed directly overtop the tumor, and only the most superficial skin layers have been closed, leaving a wound seroma to resolve spontaneously. In the setting of partial breast irradiation therapy, this seroma cavity is instrumental. When present in the context of whole breast irradiation, this seroma can lead to an unfavorable cosmetic result. For some patients who plan to undergo partial breast irradiation therapy with an after-loading catheter technique, the shape of the partial mastectomy cavity and the distance from cavity-to-skin or cavity-to-rib surface are relevant. These considerations may be mitigated by the type of after-loading balloon catheter chosen or avoided with three-dimensional (3D) conformal radiation. Careful coordination with radiation oncology is essential to ensure the safest treatment plan and to optimize patient eligibility, safety, and cosmesis. In the author's practice, after-loading balloon catheters are used. These catheters are placed with US guidance at the time of the patient's postoperative visit after final pathology results and adequacy of resection are reviewed. For minimization of discomfort at the time of catheter removal, a short track, 2 to 3 cm, between the catheter skin entry and the cavity is favored.

Depending on the amount of tissue excised, location of the tumor, and degree of ptosis, oncoplastic surgical techniques may be useful and favorable. These techniques often reduce, if not eliminate, the seroma cavity. Parallelogram technique is well suited to upper outer quadrant wounds, and crescent or batwing mastopexy excision planning can offer an improved aesthetic outcome for more centrally located lesions (Figure 1). The principles of ensuring glandular coverage of the pectoralis muscle and removal of any redundant skin envelope can mitigate many potential concave results that often become exaggerated after radiation therapy.

Localization

Localization of the lesion can be completed with standard palpation when the lesion is easily noted on examination. In the nonpalpable setting, US guidance, hematoma guidance, wire localization, or more recently, radioactive nucleotide seed implant may be used. At the author's institution, US guidance for nonpalpable solid mass localization and stereotactic wire-guided localization of calcifications are often used. More recently, the availability of biopsy clip markers with coating visible on ultrasound scan has reduced the need for stereotactic wire placement in many centers.

Surgical Margins

The definition of an *adequate margin* remains controversial. The most historical clinical trial data commonly required no tumor on ink, but many institutions, like the author's, rely on a more conservative 2-mm margin. Recent studies have looked at margin-to-tumor ratio as a method to predict adequacy of resection. Ultimately, the heterogeneity of much of the level I data renders any conclusion difficult. Nonetheless, most agree that clear margins are necessary and surgeons should strive to minimize need for reexcision. Multiple strategies exist to reduce the need for reexcision of margins and

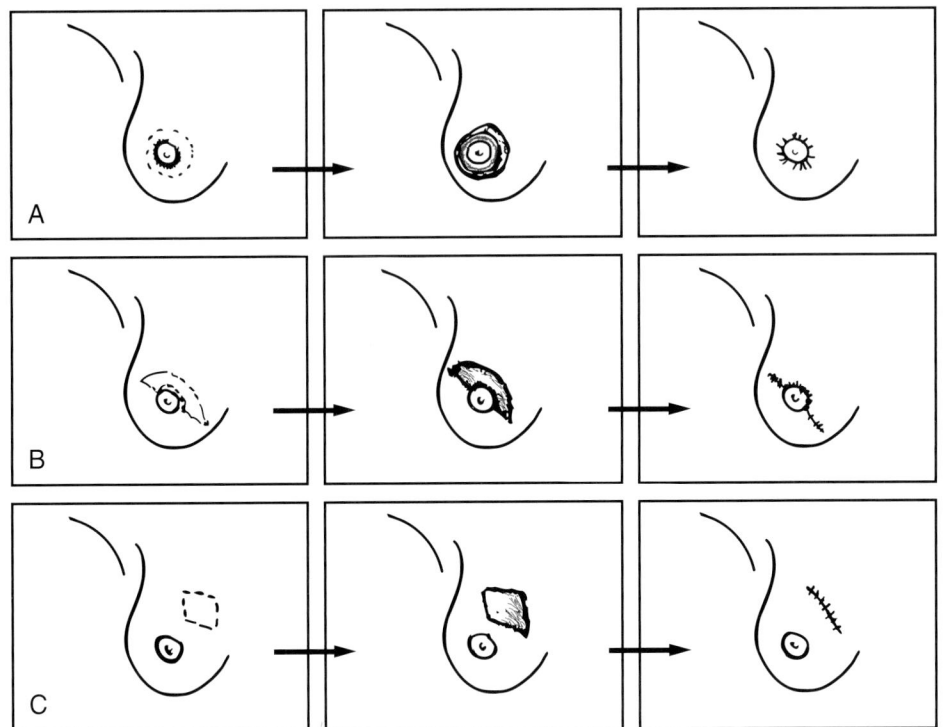

FIGURE 1   A, Parallelogram technique. **B,** Batwing mastopexy technique. **C,** Oncoplastic incision planning. *(A and B from Anderson BO, Masetti R, Silverstein MJ: Oncoplastic approaches to partial mastectomy: an overview of volume-displacement techniques, Lancet Oncol 6(3):145–157, 2005. C Hussein O, El-Khodary T: "Diamond" mammoplasty as a part of conservative management of breast cancer: description of a new technique, Int J Surg Case Rep 3(6):203–206, 2012.)*

include routine cavity reexcision or, as in the author's practice, selective reexcision based on intraoperative specimen radiograph imaging. Alternatively, intraoperative US assessment of the excised specimen may be instrumental. Attention to margins can significantly reduce reexcision rates without compromising breast contour.

All surgical lumpectomy specimens should be carefully oriented in a two-point orientation system and handled carefully so as not to distort margin integrity. The wounds are generally closed in two layers with absorbable suture. In the setting of oncoplastic closures, deeper pexing sutures may be necessary and, on occasion, a drain if a large tissue rearrangement was undertaken.

Staging the Axilla

The surgical management of the axilla has undergone recent and dramatic change. In the late 20th and early part of the 21st century, stage I and II breast cancers typically underwent axillary staging via sentinel lymph node (SLN) biopsy. In the event that any SLN was then found to have tumor, completion lymph node dissection was then undertaken, classically involving level I and II axillary lymph nodes. With the publication of American College of Surgeons Oncology Group (ACOSOG) Z0011 trial results, the further management of the axilla in the setting of a positive SLN has changed considerably. For those patients who meet inclusion criteria and for whom whole breast irradiation and standard of care adjuvant therapy are planned, further axillary lymph node dissection can be avoided. This strategy has been shown to have equivalent overall and disease-free survival rates but 30% less morbidity when compared with the dictum of complete node dissection (Table 1).

The use of SLN biopsy for in situ disease is less well defined. SLN biopsy is commonly used in the setting of an in situ diagnosis for any patient with suspicion for microinvasive disease and for those undergoing mastectomy. SLN biopsy is selectively offered to patients with high-grade ductal carcinoma in situ. The latter is a reflection of the 15% to 20% increased risk for upstaging to invasive carcinoma after complete excision of an area diagnosed as ductal carcinoma in situ (DCIS) on core biopsy.

TABLE 1: Patient selection criteria for avoidance of axillary lymph node dissection

Avoidance of axillary lymph node dissection patient selection guidelines (ACOSOG Z0011)
Tumor size <5 cm (T1 or T2)
Fewer than three positive SLN
No evidence of extracapsular tumor extension in SLN
Planned whole breast radiation therapy
Planned standard of care adjuvant therapy

ACOSOG, American College of Surgeons Oncology Group; *SLN,* sentinel lymph node.

In an era of ever increasing use of preoperative axillary ultrasound scan staging, patients who are found to have abnormal pathologic lymph node characteristics may undergo FNA or core biopsy. In the event that that regional axillary metastasis is identified, the SLN biopsy may be avoided. The use of preoperative axillary US has become more challenging given the results of the ACOSOG Z0011 trial and has not yet been reconciled in the literature.

Lastly, the timing of SLN biopsy in the setting of neoadjuvant chemotherapy is debated. Proponents of staging the axilla before neoadjuvant therapy stress the advantage of most accurately predicting benefit from postmastectomy radiation therapy. Many centers commonly perform the SLN biopsy after neoadjuvant chemotherapy, embracing the decreased need for complete node dissection in the commonly downstaged axilla. To date, no definitive consensus exists, so planning in concert with the multidisciplinary team is imperative.

Sentinel Lymph Node Technique

In the absence of clinically positive or US biopsy positive axillary lymph nodes, the SLN is identified and removed to stage the axilla.

It may be effectively identified with vital blue dye, with radionucleotide tracer, or, as at the author's center, with the combination of both. When dye technique is used, 5 mL are typically injected in the subareolar parenchyma of the ipsilateral breast, followed by 5 minutes of massage. A small incision is made at the base of the axillary hair line and dissection is taken deep to the clavipectoral fascia, and careful attention is paid to the identification of a blue lymphatic or focus of tracer uptake. Once the SLN is identified and removed, the bed to ex vivo tracer counts ratio are 10% or less, and no other blue nodes or clinically worrisome nodes are palpated, the SLN may be sent to pathology. The author's practice is to send SLN for frozen hematoxylin and eosin (H&E) staining should patients desire partial breast irradiation therapy or concomitant mastectomy. With respect to the former, accelerated partial breast radiation is not offered in the setting of a positive SLN; and as such, surgeons may choose to close the partial mastectomy cavity in such a way to obliterate the seroma cavity. If the SLN is negative, the skin is simply closed, with the seroma cavity left intact to facilitate future placement of an afterloading balloon.

Axillary Lymph Node Dissection Technique

In situations in which axillary lymph node dissection is required, level I and II dissections are classically performed. The boundaries of level I are as follows: anterior, clavipectoral fascia; posterior, subscapularis muscle; inferior, axillary tail; superior, axillary vein; medial, lateral edge of pectoral major muscle; and lateral, anterior border of the latissimus dorsi muscle. Level II lymph nodes are located just deep to pectoralis minor muscle. During the dissection, care should be taken to avoid skeletonizing the axillary vein, which can increase lymphedema risk. At the same time, careful identification of the long thoracic and thoracodorsal nerves is paramount to avoid future muscle weakness. When feasible, attention to the preservation of the intercostal nerves minimizes postoperative paresthesias. The wound is closed primarily, and a drain, typically a 15F closed suction drain, is placed and maintained on closed suction until daily output drops below 20 mL.

Mastectomy Technique

For those patients who are not candidates for BST or who prefer mastectomy, several options are available depending on the decision for or against reconstruction and what type. In any of these scenarios, the necessary extent of glandular excision is similar for traditional total mastectomy, skin-sparing mastectomy, and nipple-sparing mastectomy (NSM; barring removal of the nipple areolar complex [NAC]). Unlike the historic subcutaneous mastectomy, the axillary tail is removed and the gland is excised to its superior extent at the clavicle, medially to the lateral edge of the sternum, laterally to the latissimus muscle, inferiorly at the inframammary fold, and posteriorly deep to the pectoralis fascia. Preservation of the inframammary fold depends on whether or not the patient is undergoing reconstruction. The author's practice is to remove the inframammary fold if a patient is not undergoing reconstruction to better facilitate ease of prosthesis fitting in the future.

The thickness of the skin flap varies between patients. The skin flap should represent not only the skin but its supporting subcutaneous adipose tissue, which varies depending on body habitus. The tenet of dissection in the relatively avascular plane between the superficial breast fascia and the subcutaneous dermal fat remains true today. At the author's center, adequate exposure is achieved with Adair clamps and blunt rake retractors. This method of retraction is efficient but also minimally harmful to the skin flap. The mastectomy wounds are closed primarily, and two 15F round JP drains are placed. The drains are maintained on closed bulb suction until their daily output is less than 20 mL.

Reconstruction

In the author's practice, barring comorbid conditions that represent contraindications to reconstruction, all patients undergoing mastectomy are offered consultation with plastic and reconstruction surgery. In the event that patients choose reconstruction, their options typically include implant reconstruction or autologous tissue options. In most cases, utilization of donor muscle and its resultant muscle weakness can be avoided in favor of perforator flap techniques, such as deep inferior epigastric perforator (DIEP) or gluteal arterial perforator (GAP) flaps. If necessary, either approach can be preceded with tissue expander placement. Further, for optimal cosmesis for those women undergoing reconstruction, they may be safely offered skin-sparing mastectomy or at times nipple-sparing mastectomy where the inframammary fold and the majority or entirety of the skin envelope are preserved.

Nipple-Sparing or Total Skin-Sparing Mastectomy Technique

Emerging data support the use of NSM or total skin-sparing mastectomy (TSSM) techniques. The author's practice most commonly uses an inframammary incision, oriented and centered laterally at 7:30 and 4:30 on the patient's right or left side, respectively, just above the inframammary fold (Figure 2). Unlike a radial incision, these are slightly longer, averaging 8 to 9 cm, but rarely visible with the patient in the upright position. Either strategy allows for excellent exposure and access to internal mammary vessels for autologous reconstruction. Attention should be paid to avoid incisions that involve the nipple areolar complex, as this has been associated with an increased risk of nipple necrosis.

Exclusion criteria for NSM include extensive DCIS, large tumor of more than 4 cm, less than 2 cm proximity to NAC, inflammatory breast cancer, or locally advanced disease. Several operative techniques are quite helpful during this procedure: use of a lighted retractor, early dissection at the pectoralis fascia, and countertraction of the skin envelope by an operative assistant. The author typically instills local anesthetic liberally behind the NAC to facilitate easier dissection, which is sharply undertaken in this location. The tissue immediately behind the nipple is sent for intraoperative frozen section. In the event that atypia or malignancy is identified, the NAC is resected. Given the rare rate of nipple recurrence and the natural history of breast cancer most commonly developing in the terminal duct units, the author does not find it necessary to core out the

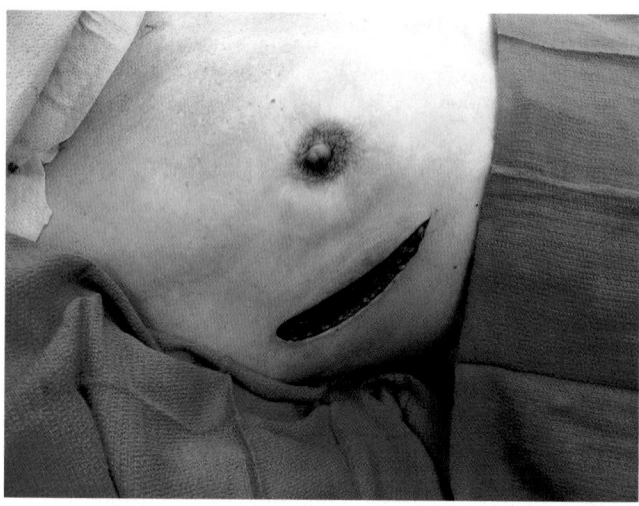

FIGURE 2 Nipple-sparing mastectomy incision.

nipple. A SLN biopsy is commonly performed through a separate small axillary incision. For those patients who desire immediate autologous reconstruction, the SLN is often performed in advance of the mastectomy to elucidate those patients who will need postmastectomy radiotherapy and therefore identify those patients who should have a temporizing tissue expander placed.

ADJUVANT THERAPY

Both local and systemic adjuvant therapy should be considered at the same time as surgical planning in the context of a multidisciplinary care model. Biologic factors such as hormone receptor status, *Her 2 neu* status, and gene signature assay results often dictate need for systemic therapies and impact surgical decision making. Likewise, the incorporation of partial breast irradiation therapy into the treatment paradigm mandates cooperative surgical treatment planning with the radiation oncology colleagues. The standard duration of radiation therapy varies depending on type of radiation technique: 5 days for accelerated partial breast and 6 weeks of whole breast external beam. Additional consideration may be given to the use of a boost, accelerated whole breast technique, or avoidance of radiation therapy all together. The author's center's practice is to avoid radiation therapy for those women over 70 years of age who have undergone breast-conserving surgery for small tumors (<2 cm), who have node-negative hormone-receptor positive disease, and who are able to undergo endocrine therapy.

PROPHYLACTIC SURGERY

A significant increase in the utilization of prophylactic mastectomy has occurred in parallel with an improved understanding of high-risk breast cancer genetic syndromes (i.e., BRCA, p53, PTEN) and improved reconstruction techniques. Immediate breast reconstruction is often performed in this setting. The author strongly encourages a complete diagnostic workup and examination and detailed consultations before surgery with a genetics counselor to delineate a patient's risk for cancer, a medical oncologist to explore chemoprophylaxis options, a plastic surgeon, and at times a psychologist to review issues of body image, risk, and family planning. Prophylactic

mastectomy has been shown to be effective in reducing the risk of subsequent breast cancer in this high-risk setting by more than 95%.

Even more recently, the use of contralateral prophylactic mastectomy (CPM) has dramatically increased. No large study has shown an overall survival benefit with this approach, and several have noted improved disease-free survival and improved patient satisfaction. The author strives to prioritize the therapeutic principles of the ipsilateral breast at all times and attempts to reduce risk that prophylactic intervention might compromise therapeutic intent. For example, the author's preference is for a patient who desires both mastectomy and CPM and who will be receiving systemic chemotherapy to do so in the neoadjuvant setting. This decreases the risk that an unintended complication on the prophylactic side might delay systemic therapy.

SUMMARY

The surgeon is central to the multidisciplinary treatment of breast cancer. A surgeon must work collaboratively with the breast cancer team to optimize the patient's options and outcome.

SUGGESTED READINGS

Anderson BO, Masetti R, Silverstein MJ: Oncoplastic approaches to partial mastectomy: an overview of volume-displacement techniques, *Lancet Oncol* 6(3):145–157, 2005.

Bevers T, Anderson BO, Bonaccio E, et al: NCCN clinical practice guidelines in oncology; breast cancer screening and diagnosis, *J Natl Compr Canc Netw* 7(10):1060–1096, 2009.

Giuliano AE, McCall L, Beitsch P, et al: Localregional recurrence after sentinel lymph node dissection with or without axillary dissection in patients with sentinel lymph node metastases: the American College of Surgeons Oncology Group Z0011 randomized trial, *Ann Surg* 252(3):426–433, 2010.

Hughes KS, Schnaper LA, Berry D, et al: Lumpectomy plus tamoxifen with or without irradiation in women 70 years of age or older with early breast cancer, *N Engl J Med* 351(10):971–977, 2004.

Turnbull L, Brown S, Harvey I, et al: Comparative effectiveness of MRI in breast cancer (COMICE) trial: a randomized controlled trial, *Lancet* 375(9714):563–571, 2010.

Warren PA, Foster RD, Stover AC, et al: Outcomes after total skin-sparing mastectomy and immediate reconstruction in 657 breasts, *Ann Surg Oncol* 19(11):3402–3409, 2012.

ABLATIVE THERAPIES IN BENIGN AND MALIGNANT BREAST DISEASE

John Cox, MD, Paul Toomey, MD, Evan Tummel, MD, Robert Gabordi, MD, and Charles Cox, MD

OVERVIEW

As the management of breast cancer evolves toward improved cosmetic results and minimally invasive surgery, the possibility of removing the primary tumor through ablative techniques is being

investigated. Ablative techniques have been based on two methods: heat through radiofrequency ablation (RFA) or cold cryoablation through the use of liquid nitrogen. Material science improvements and software modeling have led to commercial development of these two technologies, which allow discrete control of the size and shape of the tissue destruction. One aspect that remains unpredictable is the adequacy of margins in the pathologic destruction of cancer. This uncertainty has led to the investigation of the efficacy of the cryoablation technique for the cancers that are discrete lesions with clearly defined margins. Most ductal breast cancers are a mixture of ductal carcinoma in situ (DCIS) and invasive ductal carcinoma (IDC). Early-stage, low-grade discrete tumors exhibiting minimal DCIS show promise for ablative techniques.

The current cryoablation study of the American College of Surgeons Oncology Group (ACOSOG), the Z1072 trial, is being conducted to evaluate the feasibility of applying this technology to the treatment of primary breast tumors. Before the application of an ablative technique, it is critical to identify the tumor's histologic features, percentage of DCIS, genomic tumor markers, and hormone receptor status for estrogen, progesterone, and *HER-2/neu*.

Radiographic concordance with ultrasonography and magnetic resonance imaging (MRI) are essential in defining the tumor size, margins, and adequacy of tumor destruction both before and after ablative procedures. An understanding of the imaging modalities typically applied to breast cancer will also help in the evolution of ablative techniques. Precise imaging techniques to visualize the extent of the breast cancer also remain elusive. Combined pathologic and radiologic understanding of breast cancer may allow ablative techniques to safely and effectively destroy the primary breast tumor while also eliminating the need for surgical resection of the breast tumor.

CRYOABLATION

Controlled tissue destruction by freezing was first described by James Arnott in 1845 when he used a mixture of salt and ice to alleviate pain and bleeding, as well as to decrease tumor size. At the Great Exhibition of 1851 in London, Arnott displayed his cryotherapy apparatus for its use on readily accessible cancers such as breast, cervical, and skin tumors. There has been resurgence in the utilization of cryotherapy since 2000 in the treatment of benign fibroadenomas, and investigation of its use for cancer therapy continues.

Cryoablation for patients with a biopsy-proven fibroadenoma was approved by the U.S. Food and Drug Administration in 2001. The Fibroadenoma Cryoablation Treatment (FACT) registry reported on 444 patients with fibroadenomas who were treated with cryoablation. Overall patient satisfaction was 88% to 91%. One year after cryoablation, 35% of patients reported palpable masses, and 29% had residual masses visualized by ultrasonography. Palpability after cryoablation correlated with the size of the initial fibroadenomas. Only 25% of patients exhibited a palpable mass for fibroadenomas measuring less than 2 cm in diameter, whereas 59% of patients with masses greater than 2 cm demonstrated a residual palpable mass at 1 year.

The use of cryoablation for the treatment of breast cancer remains investigational. In the current studies, prerequisites for cryoablation treatment of IDC include a discretely imaged mass less than 2 cm at largest dimension and a minimal component of DCIS on core biopsy. The insidious nature of the margins for DCIS necessitates careful pathologic review to qualify the patient for ablative techniques alone. The technical limit of the freezing mechanism achieves a maximum "ice ball" diameter of 4 cm, which allows up to a 1-cm margin for a 2-cm tumor.

Complete ablation has been achieved for early-stage IDC. In the largest series, needle localization excision was compared with ultrasonography-guided cryoablation for patients with biopsy-proven IDC. The maximum tumor size was 1.7 cm and the goal ice ball created an 8-mm margin around the mass. The degree of DCIS on preoperative core biopsy was not limited in this study. After cryoablation with a single freeze cycle, the negative margin rates were significantly lower than those for needle localization for IDC (11% vs 20%, respectively). However, margins positive for DCIS were found more frequently in patients who underwent cryoablation (30% vs 18%). Achieving a minimum 6-mm freeze margin beyond the tumor has been shown to reduce positive margins to 6%.

More recently, a cohort of 29 patients with a maximum tumor diameter of 1.5 cm underwent cryoablation with two freeze cycles and an interposing thaw cycle to create a 6-mm margin. Two freezing cycles were performed during the same procedure, with an interposing thaw cycle to increase cellular destruction within the ice ball. All patients had microscopically negative margins for invasive cancer on pathology review. Five patients (17%) displayed margins positive for DCIS.

Ongoing Cryoablation Trials

The ACOSOG's Z1072 study is a phase II trial for treatment of IDC with cryoablation technology and was scheduled for completion in March 2013. In this study, the utility of MRI was also evaluated to detect residual IDC or DCIS after cryoablation. Another phase II trial involving cryoablation after neoadjuvant therapy for IDC is scheduled for completion in 2014.

Cryoablation Technique and Mechanism

The current U.S. Food and Drug Administration–approved Visica system for cryoablation of breast fibroadenomas allows technical limits of tissue destruction in a 4-cm diameter (Figure 1). Another system is the IceCure in its third generation. It is a liquid nitrogen system that offers fast procedure times (3 to 12 minutes) and two probe sizes (freeze zone 2.5 cm or 4.0 cm) for tailored tissue treatment. Other systems are also under development. Ultrasound guidance is utilized to place the cryoprobe tip in the center of the desired target. A continuous stream of liquid nitrogen flows throughout the probe and creates a spherical freezing zone measuring 4 cm in diameter (Figure 2). The initial freeze cycle is followed by a period of passive thawing before the final freeze cycle. Cytotoxic temperatures are achieved during the freezing process. The freezing target temperatures are −160°C to −190°C[15]. The passive thaw between the first and second freeze is continued until the probe is warmed to approximately −1°C. Peritumoral injection with saline may be utilized to increase the distance away from adjacent epidermis or the chest wall so as to protect them from cold injury (Figure 3).

Cells closest to the cryoablation probe die immediately as a result of intracellular ice formation. Farther away from the probe, the extracellular ice formation results in direct mechanical destruction and osmotic damage from dehydration. Ischemia is also induced as a result of blood vessel damage, platelet activation, and thrombosis. Moreover, mitochondrial damage ensues in cells not completely destroyed and subsequently compels cells to undergo programmed cell death. Repeated freeze-thaw cycles increase the efficacy of these mechanisms, inasmuch as the thawing allows for an influx of

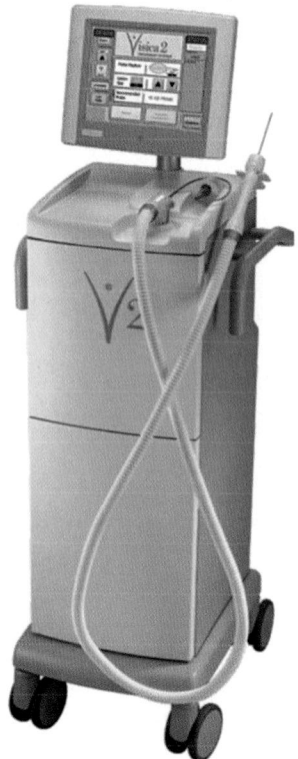

FIGURE 1 Visica II machine is liquid nitrogen based. *(Courtesy Sanarus Technologies LLC, Pleasanton, Calif.)*

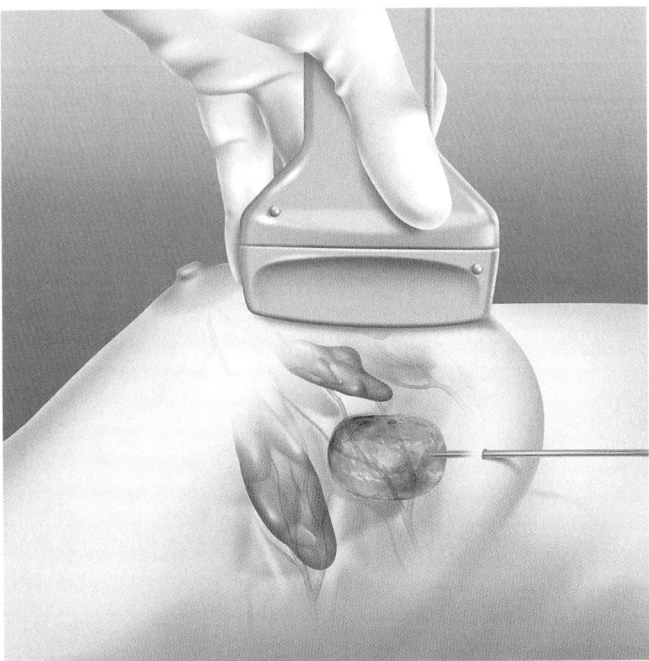

FIGURE 2 Ultrasonography is used to monitor the developing cryogenic zone created by the cryoprobe. *(From Kaufman C, Littrup P, Freman-Gibb L, et al: Office-based cryoablation of breast fibroadenomas: 12 month follow-up,* J Am Coll Surg *198[6]:914–923, 2004.)*

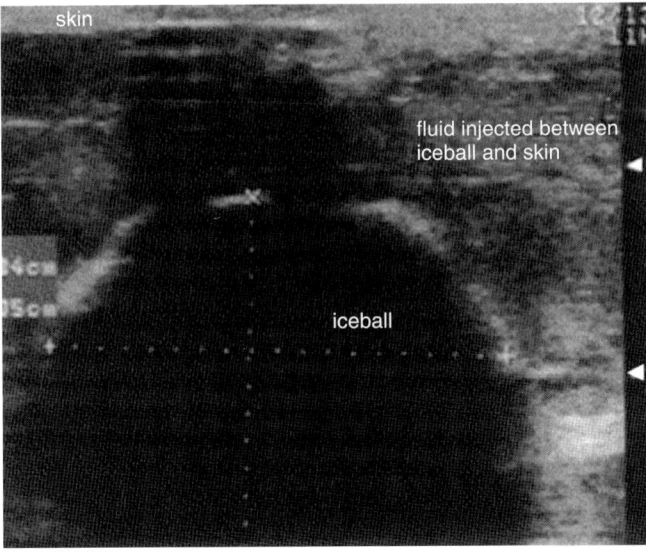

FIGURE 3 Ultrasound image of hypoechoic ice ball and protective saline injection. *(From Kaufman C, Bachman B, Littrup P, et al: Office-based ultrasound-guided cryoablation of breast fibroadenomas,* Am J Surg *184[5]:394–400, 2002.)*

extracellular fluid into the cells; as a consequence, the cells swell, which causes them to burst (Figure 4).

The technique itself requires insertion of the probe precisely into the lesion and automatically freezing the lesion to attain the correct ice ball size to engulf the lesion with adequate freezing of margins. The freezing process takes 10 to 30 minutes, depending on the size. Technologic advancements have increased the ease and speed of cryoablation especially on smaller lesions. Commercial offerings from Sanarus Technologies and IceCure Medical have enabled this procedure to reach production levels.

Cryoablation Benefits

One of the major benefits of cryoablation is its convenience of use in the clinical setting under ultrasound guidance. Local anesthesia is usually sufficient because the cryogenic process further anesthetizes the breast tissue. Furthermore, the financial burden associated with operating room costs and risks of general anesthesia can be avoided. Cosmesis is maximized and the rate of infection is minimized with ablative technology, in contrast to surgical excision.

Oncologically, perhaps the most exciting potential benefit occurs with the subsequent biologic immune response and tumor necrosis after cryoablation. Tumor proteins and tumor-associated antigens are preserved, which potentially initiates an antitumor immune response to develop through T-cell stimulation. This immune response is directed against tumor cells and has even been shown to attack distant disease, which leads to regression after cryoablation. As cellular destruction occurs, inflammatory cytokines, heat shock proteins, DNA, and RNA are released from the tumor cells. These substances, partially destroyed proteins, along with other proteins, attract granulocytes, macrophages, and natural killer cells, which in turn provide additional immune responses that stimulate release of cytokines and chemokines. This proinflammatory environment attracts dendritic cells, a type of antigen-presenting cell (APC), which capture, process, and present tumor antigens to tumor-specific T cells. Once these APCs reach the tumor bed and are activated, they undergo a change in phenotype with upregulation of cell surface markers and eventually travel to nearby lymphatic vessels to present tumor antigens to tumor-specific T cells. The activated T cells are then able to destroy major histocompatibility complex class II+ tumors and provide help to a variety of antitumor effector cells, including CD8+ cytotoxic T cells, B cells, and macrophages.

There is anecdotal evidence of the regression of metastatic disease in patients after cryoablation of the primary tumor. Unfortunately, these antimetastatic effects have not been consistently replicated. The immune system also has several mechanisms in place that seem to inhibit the mentioned antitumor immunity. Some of these mechanisms include regulatory T cells, suppressive or tolerogenic APCs, and an unfavorable tumor environment. It has been suggested that in order to capitalize on the tumor-fighting immune response after cryotherapy, clinicians must first find a way to counteract the inhibitory influence of metastatic cancer on antitumor immunity. This is a topic of intense laboratory research. One method involves injecting activated dendritic cells loading with specific tumor antigens simultaneously with cryoablation in order to enhance antigen presentation for the generation or augmentation of antitumor immunity. In addition, clinical trials for renal and prostate cancer have shown some success with vaccines consisting of irradiated tumor cells transduced with granulocyte-macrophage colony–stimulating factor (GM-CSF). Other immune modulators act to disrupt the inhibitory influences on antitumor immunity (e.g., decreasing the number or function of regulatory T cells, which act to block the function of antitumor T cells).

Cryoablation clearly has the potential to stimulate the immune system through a variety of pathways by either enhancing antitumor immunity or suppressing the inhibitory influences on the antitumor immune system. A better understanding of innate immunity after cryoablation may lead to antitumor vaccines. Further research on adjuvant cellular immunotherapy and improved comprehension as to why such a complex immune response exists after cryoablation may lead to promising therapies in the fight against cancer. In addition, current investigation of cryoablative therapy for antitumor immune modulation involves preoperative injection of intratumoral immunomodulatory ipilimumab (human monoclonal anti–CTLA-24 antibody) for early-stage, resectable IDC, with results expected in 2013.

Two other techniques being investigated for breast cancer treatment include laser and microwave ablation. In laser ablation, heat is generated for tissue destruction. The laser device is also placed under

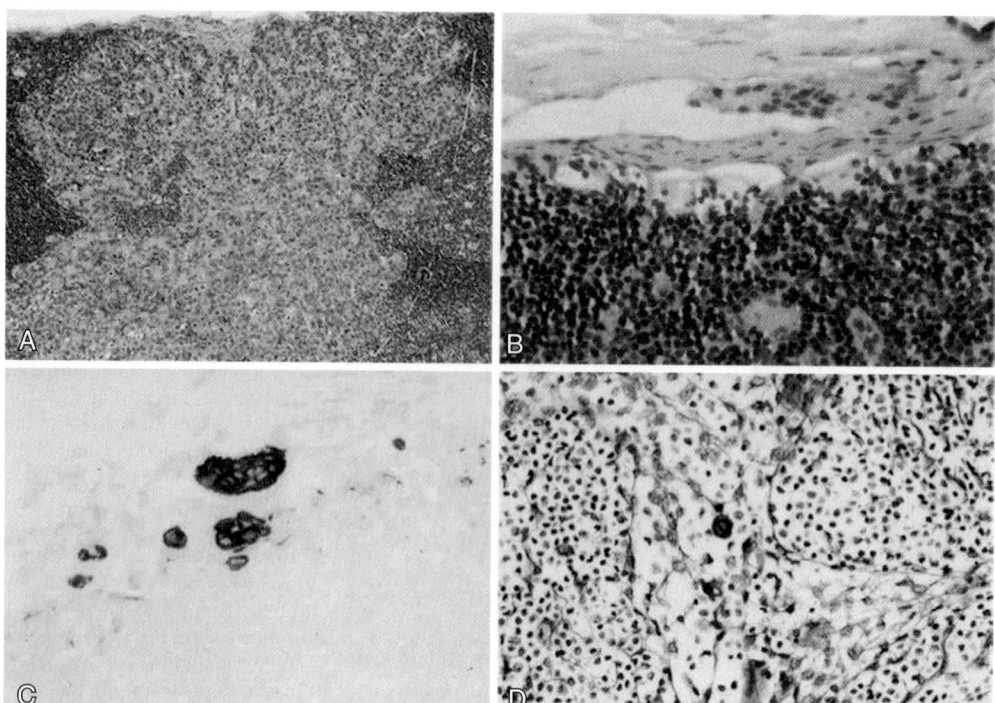

FIGURE 4 Photographs of mucinous invasive carcinoma after cryoablation, demonstrating histologic tumor destruction. *(Courtesy of Dr. Fred Odere, Raleigh Community Hospital, Raleigh, North Carolina. From Bland KI, Copeland EM, editors: The breast: comprehensive management of benign and malignant disorders, ed 3, Amsterdam, 2003, Elsevier, Figure 55-7, p 1133.)*

image guidance with stereotactic mammography or MRI. The high water content of breast cancer tissue enables focused microwaves to achieve specific tissue ablation.

RADIOFREQUENCY ABLATION

RFA is a technique in which thermal energy is applied to a specific location in order to cause focal tissue destruction. The tissue damage is achieved through the generation of intense heat by an alternating electric current running through one or more uninsulated electrode tips in the frequency range of radio waves (460 to 500 kHz). This current creates penetrating electromagnetic waves that agitate charged ions in adjacent tissue, creating an intense frictional heat, which in turn induces the desired effect: cellular protein denaturation and coagulation necrosis. As the temperature within the tissues become elevated beyond 45°C to 50°C, the tumor cells begin to die, and a localized region of necrosis around the electrode is created.

The technical means by which RFA is delivered to breast lesions is relatively straightforward. Local anesthesia and occasionally light sedation are used for patient comfort in preparation for the procedure. Some authorities have proposed either sterile saline or 5% dextrose solution to be locally infused peritumorally when there is less than 1 cm of margin from tumor edge to skin or from tumor edge to chest wall/pectoralis muscle. This infusion, whether superficial or deep to the tumor, is resistant to heating by RFA because of its high impedance; thus skin burns and chronic chest pain from inadvertent radial damage are minimized. A grounding pad is placed on the patient's skin as a reference electrode, which completes the electrical circuit and prevents electrical shock. The RFA probe with the uninsulated electrode is introduced into the tumor under ultrasound guidance. There are limits to the size of the ablation field that can be generated by a single electrode, and thus the use of secondary electrodes that deploy out of the distal end of the primary electrode has been the treatment standard (Figure 5). Initially the temperature of the tissue rises as the power through the electrode is gradually increased. The thermal zone of injury is monitored by ultrasonography and is delineated by a hyperechoic region, and at times the

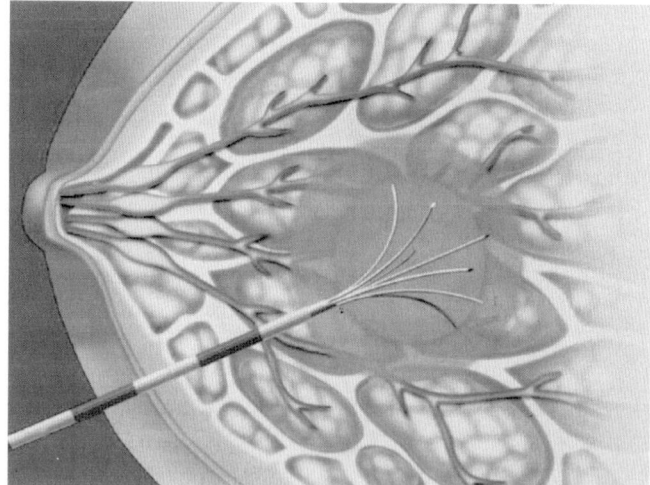

FIGURE 5 Representation of radiofrequency ablation, showing star array probe with breast and surrounding frozen ablation zone. *(Courtesy of RITA Medical Systems. From Simmons R: Ablative techniques in the treatment of benign and malignant breast disease, J Am Coll Surg 197[2]:334–338, 2003. Copyright by the American College of Surgeons.)*

Doppler function is used as adjunct for hypervascular tumors. The RFA device continuously monitors impedance and power throughput during the treatment cycle, and once the involved region of tissue nears complete ablation, the impedance begins to rise, and the power delivered drops accordingly (Figure 6).

Breast cancer treatment by means of RFA has been studied only since 2000; researchers have attempted to duplicate its success in treating other tumors. The initial results of Jeffrey and colleagues (Jeffery SS, et al., 1999) in their pilot study were inspiring and paved the way for additional studies. Izzo and associates (Izzo F, et al., 2001) used ultrasonography-guided RFA for stages T1 and T2 breast cancers, followed by immediate resection, on 26 patients. They

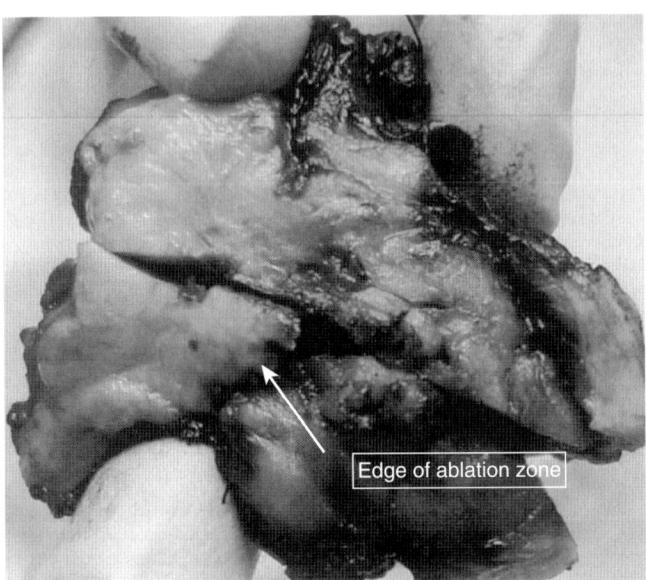

Edge of ablation zone

FIGURE 6 Excised breast cancer after radiofrequency ablation. *Arrow marks outer red rim of ablation. (From Simmons RM: Image-guided ablation of breast tumors. In Bland KI, Copeland EM, editors: The breast: comprehensive management of benign and malignant disorders, ed 3, Amsterdam, 2003, Elsevier.)*

efficacy in treating liver, lung, and renal cancers, and results in pancreas, bone, brain, and prostate carcinomas have been encouraging as well. RFA is currently approved for the treatment of several cancers, including unresectable liver cancer and metastatic bone cancer, and has been under investigation for its utility in malignant breast disease.

In the majority of the initial studies of RFA in patients with breast cancer, investigators used intraoperative ablation immediately before surgical excision. RFA in these patients was delivered in the operating room with patients under a general anesthetic. Because of the risks of general anesthesia alone, some authorities question the benefits of RFA over lumpectomy. Moreover, with immediate resection, the true zone of necrosis could be underestimated. In the testing of pathologic margins for tumor viability, investigators utilized differing markers for immunohistochemical staining, and such testing has been inconsistent across studies. Of most importance, rates of short-term and long-term survival with RFA as a substitute for surgical resection cannot be accurately extrapolated from studies in which immediate or subsequent resection was undertaken.

Clearly RFA is a promising noninvasive technique for management of primary breast cancer; however, its use is still in its infancy at this point. Although the results are encouraging, some limitations in study design constrict clinical applicability. It appears as though stringent patient selection and a standardized method of delivery will be necessary to maximize patient safety and to obtain a consistent therapeutic effect. Additional studies are necessary before this treatment modality becomes mainstream.

demonstrated complete coagulation necrosis in 25 (96%) of 26 patients. One patient had remaining tumor cells adjacent to the needle penetration site, and one patient was found to have full-thickness burn of the skin overlying the tumor. Burak and colleagues (Burak WE, et al., 2003) demonstrated that RFA can be safely performed in the outpatient setting under ultrasound guidance and with local anesthesia, with accurate tumor ablation and good patient tolerance. Their series of 10 patients, all with stage T1 tumors, underwent RFA with delayed excision (1 to 3 weeks later). One patient had residual tumor, which was seen on post-RFA MRI and confirmed histologically.

Some of the later studies had difficulties in reproducing the results of their predecessors. Up through 2007, most of the large published series have shown that more than 85% of patients had complete ablation of the index lesion. However, in 2008, Medina-Franco and associates reported a mere 76% rate of complete target lesion ablation as reviewed by histopathology in their 25-patient study. This may have resulted in part because the tumors treated were larger, with a mean size of 20.8 mm (range, 9 to 38 mm). Garbay and colleagues (Garbay JK, et al., 2008) aborted their phase II clinical trial of RFA in recurrent breast cancer because of poor efficacy. They were able to show only 60% complete ablation rate in their first 10 patients, with a mean tumor size of 14 mm (range, 10 to 22 mm). Significant complications in almost 30% of study patients was reported by Imoto and associates (Imoto S, et al., 2009). Thirty patients were enrolled for the RFA study involving clinical stage I breast cancers. Of the 30, 9 had complications: 2 with skin burns and 7 with pectoralis major burns.

In 2012, Wilson and colleagues were able to reduce margin reexcision rates to less than 5% with a combination of local excision (lumpectomy) with immediate intraoperative RFA to the cavity site. The margins that were ablated were 1 cm circumferentially under ultrasound guidance. Only 3 of 73 patients in the study needed reexcision of margins after initial resection with immediate RFA treatment.

Currently it is believed that RFA is one of the most promising noninvasive techniques that have been proposed for treatment of breast cancer. It has already been demonstrated to have significant

SUGGESTED READINGS

Bland K, Gass J, Klimberg S: Radiofrequency, cryoablation, and other modalities for breast cancer ablation, *Surg Clin North Am* 87:539–550, 2007.

Burak WE, Agnese DM, Povoski SP, et al: Radiofrequency ablation of invasive breast carcinoma followed by delayed surgical excision, *Cancer* 98:1369–1376, 2003.

Cooper SM, Dawber RP: The history of cryosurgery, *J R Soc Med* 94(4):196–201, 2001.

Gage AA: History of cryosurgery, *Semin Surg Oncol* 14(2):99–109, 1998.

Garbay JR, Mathieu MC, Lamuraglia M, et al: Radiofrequency thermal ablation of breast cancer local recurrence: a phase II clinical trial, *Ann Surg Oncol* 15(11):3222–3226, 2008.

Gazelle GS, Goldberg SN, Solbiati L, et al: Tumor ablation with radiofrequency energy, *Radiology* 217:633, 2000.

Hamazoe R, Maeta M, Merakami A, et al: Heating efficiency of radiofrequency capacitative hyperthermia for treatment of deep-seated tumors in the peritoneal cavity, *J Surg Oncol* 48:176–179, 1991.

Imoto S, Wada N, Sakemura N, et al: Feasibility study on radiofrequency ablation followed by partial mastectomy for stage I breast cancer patients, *Breast* 18(2):130–134, 2009.

Izzo F, Thomas R, Delrio P, et al: Radiofrequency ablation in patients with primary breast carcinoma: a pilot study in 26 patients, *Cancer* 92:2036–2044, 2001.

Jeffrey SS, Birdwell RL, Ikeda DM, et al: Radiofrequency ablation of breast cancer: first report of an emerging technology, *Arch Surg* 134:1064–1068, 1999.

Kachala, S, Simmons, R: Ablative therapies in benign and malignant breast disease. In Cameron JL, Cameron AL, editors: *Current surgical therapy*, ed 10, Philadelphia, 2011, Elsevier.

Klimberg S, Kepple J, Shafirstein G, et al: eRFA: excision followed by FRA—a new technique to improve local control in breast cancer, *Ann Surg Oncol* 13(1):1422–1433, 2006.

Littrup PJ, Freeman-Gibb L, Andea A, et al: Cryotherapy for breast fibroadenomas, *Radiology* 234(1):63–72, 2005.

Maccini M, Sehrt D, Pompeo A, et al: Biophysiologic considerations in cryoablation: a practical mechanistic molecular review, *Int Braz J Urol* 37(6):693–696, 2011.

Medina-Franco H, Soto-Germes S, Ulloa-Gómez JL, et al: Radiofrequency ablation of invasive breast carcinomas: a phase II trial, *Ann Surg Oncol* 15(6):1689–1695, 2008.

Nath S, Haines D: Biophysics and pathology of catheter energy delivery systems, *Prog Cardiovasc Dis* 37:185–204, 1995.

Nurko J, Mabry CD, Whitworth P, et al: Interim results from the FibroAdenoma Cryoablation Treatment Registry, *Am J Surg* 190(4):647–651, 2005;
discussion, *Am J Surg* 190(4):651–652, 2005.

Pfleiderer SO, Freesmeyer MG, Marx C, et al: Cryotherapy of breast cancer
under ultrasound guidance: initial results and limitations, *Eur Radiol*
12(12):3009–3014, 2002.

Pfleiderer SO, Marx C, Camara O, et al: Ultrasound-guided, percutaneous
cryotherapy of small (< or = 15 mm) breast cancers, *Invest Radiol*
40(7):472–477, 2005.

Sabel MS, Kaufman CS, Whitworth P, et al: Cryoablation of early-stage breast
cancer: work-in-progress report of a multi-institutional trial, *Ann Surg
Oncol* 11(5):542–549, 2004.

Sidana A, Chowdhury W, Fuchs E, et al: Cryoimmunotherapy in urologic
oncology, *Urology* 75(5):1009-1014, 2010.

Simmons R: Ablative techniques in the treatment of benign and malignant
breast disease. *J Am Coll Surg* 197(2):334-338, 2003.

Singletary SE, Dowlatshahi K, Dooley W, et al: Minimally invasive operation
for breast cancer, *Curr Probl Surg* 41(4):394–447, 2004.

Tafra L, Fine R, Whitworth P, et al: Prospective randomized study comparing
cryo-assisted and needle-wire localization of ultrasound-visible breast
tumors, *Am J Surg* 192(4):462–470, 2006.

Tafra L, Smith SJ, Woodward JE, et al: Pilot trial of cryoprobe-assisted breast-
conserving surgery for small ultrasound-visible cancers, *Ann Surg Oncol*
10(9):1018–1024, 2003.

Wilson M, Korourian S, Boneti C, et al: Long-term results of excision followed
by radiofrequency ablation as the sole means of local therapy for breast
cancer, *Ann Surg Oncol* 19(10):3192–3198, 2012.

LYMPHATIC MAPPING AND SENTINEL LYMPHADENECTOMY

**Melissa S. Camp, MD, MPH, and
Barbara L. Smith, MD, PhD**

INTRODUCTION

Patients diagnosed with invasive breast cancer typically require evaluation of the axillary lymph nodes. This information is important
for staging purposes and has prognostic and treatment implications.
Before the advent of sentinel lymph node biopsy (SLNB), axillary
staging consisted of a level I and II axillary lymph node dissection
(ALND). Although complete axillary node information is obtained
from a full ALND, it comes at the risk of complications, including
lymphedema, paresthesias, and arm dysfunction.

In the 1990s, SLNB was shown to reliably predict axillary nodal
status in breast cancer. In the breast, the lymphatic anatomy consists
of lymphatic channels that converge as they leave the breast, delivering fluid and cells to a specific node or small group of nodes referred
to as the sentinel nodes. These are the first lymph nodes to receive
drainage from the breast. Sentinel lymph node (SLN) mapping takes
advantage of this anatomic arrangement, as radioactive or blue dye
particles injected into the breast travel through the lymphatic channels and accumulate in the sentinel nodes first. Identification of the
sentinel nodes is important because they are the most likely nodes to
contain metastatic tumor if metastasis to the lymph nodes has
occurred. If the sentinel nodes do not contain evidence of metastatic
tumor, there is a very low risk of clinically significant axillary lymph
node involvement.

Multiple studies have shown that SLN mapping for SLNB is successful approximately 95% of the time and is accurate in prediction
of the presence of positive axillary nodes, with a false-negative rate
of approximately 10%. No difference has been shown in axillary
recurrence or survival for patients with a negative SLNB as compared
with a negative ALND. Moreover, SLNB has been shown to have a
significantly lower risk of lymphedema and the other complications
associated with ALND. Therefore, if the SLNB results are negative, a
full ALND can be omitted. If the SLNB results are positive, a full
ALND may or may not be indicated.

INDICATIONS AND CONTRAINDICATIONS FOR SENTINEL LYMPH NODE BIOPSY

Patients eligible for SLNB include patients with clinically node-
negative diagnosis of T1 to T3 invasive breast cancer who are undergoing lumpectomy or mastectomy. Certain patients with ductal
carcinoma in situ (DCIS) may have an indication for SLNB, including those with suspicion of microinvasion and those with extensive
DCIS requiring mastectomy. Patients with palpable DCIS or large
areas of high-grade DCIS may also be considered for SLNB.

Patients with inflammatory breast cancer, T4 breast cancer, and
biopsy-proven positive nodes are generally not eligible for SLNB. If
patients are found to have clinically positive axillary nodes on physical examination, they should undergo an axillary ultrasound and
biopsy (either fine-needle aspiration [FNA] or core biopsy) of any
suspicious-appearing nodes to confirm axillary metastases. A level I
and II ALND is indicated if clinically positive lymph nodes are found
to contain metastatic disease on biopsy.

As imaging modalities improve, more patients with clinically
negative nodes will have evidence of suspicious-appearing nodes on
ultrasound or magnetic resonance imaging (MRI). For patients with
suspicious nodes based on imaging criteria and a FNA result positive for malignancy, many recommend proceeding with a full ALND.
Some, however, consider these patients with clinically negative but
imaging and FNA positive nodes eligible for SLNB and tangent radiation if they meet the eligibility criteria for the American College of
Surgeons Oncology Group (ACOSOG) Z0011 trial.

TECHNICAL ASPECTS

Mapping of the SLN can be achieved with either blue dye (isosulfan
blue or methylene blue) or radioisotope (technetium-99 m sulfur
colloid). The blue dye or radioisotope can be injected in a subareolar,
subdermal, or peritumoral location. The blue dye is typically injected
in the operating room after the induction of anesthesia and is followed by 5 minutes of breast massage, whereas the radioisotope can
be injected up to 24 hours before surgery. Although each technique
can be used individually with good success, use of blue dye and

radioisotope in combination increases the success of mapping and identifying the SLN.

If radioisotope is used for SLN mapping, a lymphoscintigram can be obtained to show whether mapping has been successful and to show the location of the sentinel lymph nodes. Lymphoscintigrams do not need to be ordered routinely, however, because a handheld gamma probe can be used in the operating room before the start of the procedure to determine whether mapping was successful. If a strong signal is not detected with the gamma probe, blue dye can be injected at the start of the procedure to aid with localization of the sentinel lymph node.

If a lymphoscintigram is obtained, nonaxillary sentinel lymph nodes (such as internal mammary nodes) can be identified up to 10% of the time. In general, the probability that a nonaxillary sentinel node would be the only positive node or that the status of a nonaxillary sentinel node would alter decisions about adjuvant therapy is small (~6%). Resection of nonaxillary sentinel nodes is typically not recommended, given the increased morbidity associated with internal mammary SLNB and the fact that clinical management algorithms are based on the status of the axillary sentinel nodes.

Isosulfan blue has been associated with a 1% to 3% incidence rate of allergic and anaphylactic reactions. No anaphylactic reactions have been reported with methylene blue, but skin necrosis has been reported with injection of methylene blue in an intradermal location. Methylene blue dye is contraindicated for use in pregnant women (U.S. Food and Drug Administration [FDA] pregnancy category X: studies have shown evidence of fetal abnormalities or fetal risk, contraindicated for use in pregnant women), and isosulfan blue is a FDA pregnancy category C agent (no adequate studies in pregnant women, but can be used if potential benefit to mother justifies potential risk to fetus). Technetium-99 m sulfur colloid can be used for mapping in pregnancy because the total radiation exposure to the fetus is low, particularly with adequate hydration to facilitate excretion via the urine.

The operative technique for performing a SLNB involves a 2-cm to 3-cm incision in the axillary skin over the point of maximal gamma probe signal. If blue dye but not radioactive dye is used, the incision is made at or just above the lower aspect of the hairline in the axilla. Dissection is carried down through the subcutaneous fat and clavipectoral fascia to enter the axillary fat pad. If radioisotope is used, a gamma probe is used to identify "hot" nodes. Any nodes with counts of more than 10% of the hottest node are considered to be hot. If blue dye is used, blue lymphatic channels can be followed and blue nodes identified with visual inspection. All hot or blue nodes should be removed, as should any other nodes that appear suspicious via palpation. Palpable suspicious nodes, for example, may be nodes that are completely replaced with tumor and that no longer have the ability to take up blue dye or radioisotope. If the SLN fails to map with either radioisotope or blue dye, a level I and II ALND is recommended. Failure to map most commonly occurs in the setting of previous breast or axillary surgery that may have altered the lymphatic drainage.

The sentinel nodes that are removed are sent to pathology for evaluation and can be evaluated with an intraoperative frozen section or permanent section. Sentinel lymph nodes removed during mastectomy should be sent for evaluation with intraoperative frozen section. If SLN are positive on frozen section, a level I and II ALND can then be performed at the time of mastectomy. On the basis of the recently published results of the ACOSOG Z0011 trial (discussed in greater detail subsequently), it is now recommended that sentinel lymph nodes removed during breast-conserving surgery be sent for permanent section only. Exceptions to this recommendation include patients in whom intraoperative palpation of the axillary lymph nodes is suggestive of gross extranodal extension or three or more positive nodes and patients who have received neoadjuvant therapy. These patients do not meet Z0011 eligibility criteria, and a second procedure can be avoided if a positive frozen section is followed by an immediate completion ALND. An intraoperative frozen section is

also appropriate if patients undergoing breast conserving surgery do not receive systemic therapy and radiation therapy as per Z0011 guidelines.

SPECIAL CONSIDERATIONS

Neoadjuvant Chemotherapy

For patients undergoing neoadjuvant chemotherapy, discussion continues as to whether SLNB should be performed before or after completion of neoadjuvant treatment. If SLNB is performed before neoadjuvant chemotherapy and evidence is found of nodal disease, then ALND is generally performed regardless of the response to treatment. SLNB performed after neoadjuvant chemotherapy, on the other hand, allows for a single operative procedure, and ALND can be avoided if neoadjuvant chemotherapy has eradicated whatever nodal disease may have been present.

One concern with SLNB performed after neoadjuvant chemotherapy is whether it is as accurate as SLNB performed before therapy. Neoadjuvant chemotherapy has been suggested to potentially alter the lymphatic drainage pathway, interfering with the ability of the radioisotope or blue dye to accurately map the location of the sentinel nodes. Moreover, the effects of chemotherapy may not be uniformly distributed across all nodes, raising the question of whether there may still be residual disease in nonsentinel lymph nodes even if the sentinel node has had a complete response and is negative.

Several studies have addressed the issue of whether SLNB is accurate after neoadjuvant chemotherapy. Within the National Surgical Adjuvant Breast and Bowel Project (NSABP) B-27 trial, the success rate for SLN mapping after neoadjuvant chemotherapy was 95.6% and the false-negative rate was 10.7%, very similar to the rates obtained with SLNB performed before chemotherapy. Another study by Hunt and colleagues showed that after neoadjuvant therapy the SLN was identified 97.4% of the time, compared with 98.7% in the group who had SLNB before chemotherapy. The false-negative rate was 5.9% in the neoadjuvant group, compared with 4.1% in the group who had SLNB before chemotherapy. Moreover, they showed that SLNB after neoadjuvant chemotherapy resulted in fewer positive SLNB and therefore decreased the rates of ALND. Other studies have had similar findings, confirming that SLNB is feasible and accurate after neoadjuvant chemotherapy.

More recently, studies have addressed the question of whether SLNB is accurate after neoadjuvant chemotherapy in patients who initially present with clinically positive axillary nodes. Small studies to date have concluded that SLNB is accurate in predicting the status of the axilla in these patients and can correctly identify patients who have been downstaged to node negative status and therefore can avoid an ALND. The ACOSOG Z1071 trial is currently accruing patients to determine the reliability of SLNB after neoadjuvant chemotherapy in patients with biopsy proven axillary nodal disease at presentation.

Another important consideration with SLNB and neoadjuvant chemotherapy is the impact on decisions about postmastectomy radiation therapy (PMRT). Historically, decisions about the need for PMRT and inclusion of additional radiation fields (such as axillary or supraclavicular fields) have been made based on axillary staging performed before systemic therapy. With neoadjuvant therapy and the potential for downstaging or complete pathologic response, debate exists about how to interpret posttreatment axillary nodal status when making decisions regarding the need for PMRT or additional radiation fields. Some radiation oncologists prefer SLNB before neoadjuvant therapy to help guide radiation decisions. The need for PMRT can also impact reconstruction options, so advance knowledge of a positive SLN can allow for appropriate planning in terms of delayed rather than immediate reconstruction or choices regarding use of autologous tissue versus tissue expanders or implants.

Implications of Micrometastatic Disease and Isolated Tumor Cells Detected with Sentinel Lymph Node Biopsy

Positive SLN detected with SLNB is classified into one of three categories: isolated tumor cells (ITC; N0[i+]), which are 0.2 mm or less in size; micrometastases (N1mic), which are more than 0.2 mm but not more than 2.0 mm in size; and macrometastases, which are more than 2.0 mm in size. Micrometastases and macrometastases are typically seen on routine hematoxylin and eosin (H&E) staining, but ITC often cannot be identified without the use of immunohistochemistry (IHC). The Z0010 trial found that 10.5% of SLN that were negative with H&E had evidence of occult metastasis with IHC, but no difference was found in overall survival between patients with IHC-positive and IHC-negative SLN. The NSABP B-32 trial found that 15.9% of SLN that were negative with H&E were positive with IHC for occult metastasis. Patients with IHC-positive nodes were found to have a small but statistically significant 1.2% decrease in overall survival at 5 years compared with those with IHC-negative nodes. This difference was deemed clinically insignificant, however, and the trial concluded that IHC analysis of negative SLN is not warranted. On the basis of subgroup analysis, the NSABP B-32 trial also showed that the risk associated with ITC was lower than the risk associated with micrometastases for all outcomes evaluated.

Although the presence of macrometastases in SLNB has traditionally led to a completion ALND, the need for ALND when micrometastases are found on SLNB is debated. One study with patients in the Surveillance Epidemiology and End Results (SEER) database diagnosed from 1998 to 2004 found that the proportion of patients with micrometastases who underwent SLNB alone increased from 21% to 37.8%. There was no statistically significant difference in overall survival for patients with micrometastases who underwent SLNB alone compared with SLNB followed by completion ALND. This study concluded that there was a trend towards foregoing completion ALND in patients with micrometastases on SLNB even before the publication of the ACOSOG Z0011 trial.

ALTERNATIVES TO AXILLARY LYMPH NODE DISSECTION FOR POSITIVE SENTINEL LYMPH NODES

ACOSOG Z0011 Trial

The ACOSOG Z0011 trial, published in 2010, has resulted in a paradigm shift in the management of the axilla for patients undergoing breast-conserving therapy. The trial was designed to evaluate the need for completion ALND in patients with low-volume metastatic disease on SLNB and randomized 446 patients to SLNB alone and 445 patients to SLNB plus ALND. The primary outcome was overall survival, and secondary outcomes included disease-free survival and locoregional recurrence.

Eligibility criteria included patients with T1 or T2 clinically node-negative breast cancer who were treated with lumpectomy and SLNB, had one or two positive SLN detected with H&E staining (on frozen section, touch prep or permanent section), received whole breast radiation but no specific axillary radiation, and received systemic therapy as determined by the treating physician. Although the trial closed in 2004 because of slow accrual (planned accrual of 1900 patients) and a low event rate, at a median follow-up of 6.3 years, there were no statistically significant differences in overall survival, disease-free survival, or locoregional recurrence between the SLNB alone and SLNB plus ALND groups.

The ACOSOG Z0011 study concluded that completion ALND provided no benefit in locoregional control or survival, despite the removal of additional positive lymph nodes. Of the patients in the SLNB plus ALND group, 27.4% were found to have additional positive nodes beyond the SLN, so it can be assumed that a similar proportion of patients in the SLNB alone group had additional positive nodes that were not removed. The rate of axillary recurrence in the two groups, however, was similar (0.9% in the SLNB alone group vs 0.5% in the SLNB plus ALND group). This suggests that adjuvant radiation and systemic therapy have a significant impact on any remaining positive nodes and contribute to effective local control without ALND.

One clinical implication of the Z0011 trial is that the use of intraoperative frozen section for SLNB is no longer indicated for patients undergoing lumpectomy and SLNB who meet Z0011 eligibility criteria. Patients who are found on permanent section to have one or two positive SLN are able to forego ALND, and those found to have three or more positive SLN are recommended to undergo delayed completion ALND. The Z0011 trial is not applicable, however, to patients receiving neoadjuvant chemotherapy, patients suspected to have extranodal extension or three or more positive nodes based on intraoperative assessment, or patients undergoing mastectomy. For these situations, the use of intraoperative frozen section for SLN is still warranted, and completion ALND is indicated if SLN are found to be positive.

IBCSG-23-01 Trial

The International Breast Cancer Study Group, IBCSG-23-01 trial was designed to address whether differences in survival exist between patients with micrometastases who undergo SLNB only versus those who undergo completion ALND. Preliminary results suggest that there is no difference in 5-year disease-free survival between the two groups. In addition, the rate of axillary relapse at 5 years was about 1% in patients with micrometastases who underwent SLNB only.

AMAROS Trial

The After Mapping of the Axilla: Radiotherapy or Surgery? (AMAROS) trial enrolled 4767 patients undergoing lumpectomy and SLNB and randomized those with positive SLN to either ALND or axillary radiotherapy. This trial is ongoing and the results are not yet available.

COMPLICATIONS

Complications associated with SLNB include paresthesias from disruption of sensory nerves, seroma, lymphedema, hematoma, and wound infections. All of these complications occur much less frequently after SLNB than after ALND. In the Z0011 trial, for example, adverse effects were reported in 25% of patients who underwent SLNB alone compared with 70% of patients who underwent SLNB plus ALND. With respect to specific complications, patients in the SLNB plus ALND group had more wound infections (8% vs 3%), seroma (14% vs 6%), paresthesias (39% vs 9% at 1 year), and subjective lymphedema (19% vs 6% at 1 year) compared with patients in the SLNB alone group. Other studies have also shown that the risk of complications with SLNB is about half that of ALND.

FUTURE DIRECTIONS

With publication of the data from Z0011 and the anticipation of results from trials such as AMAROS and IBCSG-23-01, debate about management of the axilla in the setting of a positive SLN continues. Can the results of Z0011, for example, be extrapolated to other clinical scenarios? If a patient is clinically node negative but has a node suspicious on ultrasound and positive on FNA, can they be considered for SLNB and not automatically undergo a full ALND if all other Z0011 eligibility criteria are met? Other clinical situations that are being debated include whether patients undergoing mastectomy with positive SLN need a completion ALND if they will be receiving PMRT, whether all patients with positive SLN after neoadjuvant chemotherapy need a completion ALND, and whether patients with more than two positive SLN can forego a completion ALND. Future studies in these areas will hopefully provide answers to these questions.

CONCLUSION

Currently, SLNB is the standard of care for axillary staging in patients with T1 to T3 invasive breast cancer and for patients with DCIS undergoing mastectomy. SLNB has been shown to reliably and accurately predict nodal status with significantly decreased morbidity compared with ALND. Completion ALND for positive SLN is still indicated in certain clinical situations, but radiation and systemic therapy contribute to local control, allowing omission of axillary dissection in selected patients with a positive SLN.

SUGGESTED READINGS

De Boer M, van Dijck J, Bult P, et al: Breast cancer prognosis and occult lymph node metastases, isolated tumor cells, and micrometastases, *J Natl Cancer Inst* 102:410–425, 2010.

Giuliano A, McCall L, Beitsch P, et al: Locoregional recurrence after sentinel lymph node dissection with or without axillary dissection in patients with sentinel lymph node metastases: The American College of Surgeons Oncology Group Z0011 Randomized Trial, *Ann Surg* 252(3):426–433, 2010.

Hunt KK, Yi M, Mittendorf EA, et al: Sentinel lymph node surgery after neoadjuvant chemotherapy is accurate and reduces the need for axillary dissection in breast cancer patients, *Ann Surg* 250(4):558–566, 2009.

Krag DN, Anderson SJ, Julian TB, et al: Sentinel lymph node resection compared with conventional axillary lymph node dissection in clinically node negative patients with breast cancer: overall survival findings from the NSABP B-32 randomized phase 3 trial, *Lancet Oncol* 11(10):927–933, 2010.

Lucci A, Mackie McCall L, Beitsch PD, et al: Surgical complications associated with sentinel lymph node dissection (SLND) plus axillary lymph node dissection compared with SLND alone in the American College of Surgeons Oncology Group Trial Z0011, *J Clin Oncol* 25(24):3657–3663, 2007.

Mamounas EP, Brown A, Anderson S, et al: Sentinel node biopsy after neoadjuvant chemotherapy in breast cancer: results from National Surgical Adjuvant Breast and Bowel Project Protocol B-27, *J Clin Oncol* 23(12):2694–2702, 2005.

Veronesi U, Viale G, Paganelli G, et al: Sentinel lymph node biopsy in breast cancer: ten year results of a randomized controlled study, *Ann Surg* 251(4):595–600, 2010.

THE MANAGEMENT OF THE AXILLA IN BREAST CANCER

Jennifer H. Lin, MD, and
Armando E. Giuliano, MD, FACS, FRCSEd

OVERVIEW

Axillary nodal status remains one of the most important factors predictive of long-term survival in patients with breast cancer. Axillary nodal metastases are associated with a poorer prognosis and often prompt more aggressive systemic and local treatment. Although the standard for staging and treatment has been levels I and II axillary dissection for invasive breast cancer, the surgical management of the axilla has evolved. Aggressive dissection of the axilla is no longer necessary for most patients with early breast cancer.

Nineteenth century theories of breast cancer championed by William Halsted maintained that breast cancer metastasized sequentially from the primary tumor to regional lymphatics, then to distant metastatic sites. He proposed that the radical mastectomy, with removal of the pectoralis major and minor muscles, complete axillary node dissection, and supraclavicular node dissection, would lead to higher cure rates. Bernard Fisher disputed this theory in the 1970s, proposing instead that breast cancer was a systemic disease at the time of diagnosis. Fisher's National Surgical Adjuvant Breast and Bowel Project (NSABP) B-04 prospective randomized clinical trial proved that extensive local treatment aimed at the removal of axillary node metastases did not, in fact, lead to improved survival. This pivotal study, with 25 years of follow-up, compared radical mastectomy with simple mastectomy with nodal and chest wall radiation, and with simple mastectomy alone, and showed no difference in overall survival between the three treatment arms.

Axillary lymph node dissection (ALND), once consistently used for staging and treatment of breast cancer, is no longer routinely indicated. This procedure has significant morbidities, including lymphedema, pain, neuropathy, cosmetic deformity, and decreased range of motion. Sentinel lymph node biopsy (SLNB), with its decreased morbidity, has replaced axillary dissection as a highly accurate axillary staging procedure in patients with clinically node-negative early-stage breast cancer.

CLINICALLY NODE-NEGATIVE INVASIVE BREAST CANCER

Sentinel node biopsy has been validated in numerous clinical studies and has replaced axillary dissection for clinically node-negative breast cancer. This technique is based on the hypothesis that the first node draining the primary tumor reflects the status of the remaining lymph nodes in that basin. This procedure is highly predictive (96%) of the tumor status of the remaining axillary nodes in which a sentinel node is identified, with an acceptably low false-negative rate (0 to 11%). This was determined from a comparison of results of patients randomized to SLNB or ALND and from studies that compared sentinel node status with completion ALND status in the same patient.

Management of Patients With Pathologically Negative Sentinel Nodes

Patients with tumor-free sentinel nodes are adequately treated with SLNB only, and no further axillary treatment is needed. Axillary recurrence rates are less than 1%, with greatly decreased morbidity compared with ALND.

This has been validated in a number of prospective randomized trials. The NSABP trial B-32 was the largest multicenter randomized control trial designed to examine whether SLNB was equivalent to ALND in breast cancer with tumor-free sentinel lymph nodes. This trial showed that overall survival, disease-free survival, and regional control were all equivalent in patients who had SLNB plus ALND or SLNB alone. Other trials from Europe have shown the same results.

Management of Patients With Sentinel Node Micrometastases

Sentinel node biopsy has allowed for more intensive examination of the draining lymph nodes. Complete histologic analysis of these nodes has involved serial sectioning with three to five sections per node examined. Tumor deposits in lymph nodes may be detected with routine hematoxylin and eosin (H&E); immunohistochemical (IHC) methods, which stain breast epithelial cytokeratins and facilitate identification of small tumor deposits; or even polymerase chain reaction (PCR). These staging procedures have led to the detection of micrometastases (>0.2 mm to 2.0 mm, or more than 200 cells; N1mi) and isolated tumor cells (ITCs; defined as small clusters of cells ≤0.2 mm, single tumor cells, or nonconfluent or nearly confluent clusters of cells not exceeding 200 cells in a single histologic cross section; N0[i+]; American Joint Committee on Cancer [AJCC] Breast Cancer Staging, ed 7). Although the most recent guidelines from the American Society of Clinical Oncology (ASCO) Consensus Statement in 2005 recommend completion axillary dissection when either micrometastatic disease or isolated tumor cells in lymph nodes is found regardless of the method of detection, recent studies show this to be unnecessary, especially for patients treated with breast-conserving surgery and whole-breast irradiation.

A cohort analysis of the NSABP B-32 randomized trial examined whether patients with occult sentinel lymph node micrometastases and ITCs had worse survival compared with patients without micrometastases or ITCs, assessed with both H&E and IHC analysis. Although this study showed a small statistically significant but clinically insignificant decrease in 5-year overall survival rate of 1.2% in patients with occult sentinel lymph node metastases, this difference was concluded to be insufficient to cause alterations in adjuvant systemic treatment or justify the use of routine IHC.

Similarly, the American College of Surgeons Oncology Group (ACOSOG) Z0010 trial, one of the largest multicenter prospective trials to examine the significance of occult sentinel node metastases, showed that IHC-detected occult sentinel node metastases were not associated with survival differences in women undergoing breast-conserving surgery, sentinel node biopsy, and whole-breast irradiation for treatment of T1 or T2 clinically node-negative breast cancer. Long-term follow-up study may eventually reveal small differences in outcome, but these too are likely to be of no clinical significance. Most patients in the ACOSOG Z0010 trial and NSABP B-32 trial received adjuvant systemic therapy, which demonstrates practice patterns independent of IHC findings because IHC results were blinded to clinicians in both studies.

The findings of these two trials are confirmed by the 2011 preliminary results of the randomized International Breast Cancer Study Group (IBCSG) Trial 23-01 that compared axillary dissection versus no axillary dissection in patients with sentinel node micrometastases and have important implications for current clinical practice in the management of micrometastases and ITCs. Patients with micrometastases or ITCs should not have additional axillary node dissection or systemic therapy solely on the basis of the findings of sentinel lymph node (SLN) micrometastases or ITCs.

Management of Patients With Sentinel Node Macrometastases

The management of patients with lymph node macrometastases, defined as tumor deposits of more than 2.0 mm, has also undergone recent radical changes. Although the 2005 ASCO guidelines recommend routine axillary dissection for patients with a positive SLN, recent data from the ACOSOG Z0011 trial show this to be unnecessary for many patients.

In the ACOSOG Z0011 trial, patients with early breast cancer and H&E-detected sentinel node metastases were randomized to SLNB alone versus ALND. The patients who were enrolled had clinical T1 or T2 invasive breast cancer, no palpable lymphadenopathy, and one or two sentinel nodes with macrometastases and underwent breast-conservation surgery (BCS) and received whole-breast irradiation. This multicenter randomized trial showed no difference in local control, disease-free survival, or overall survival for patients with H&E-detected sentinel node macrometastases who were randomized to SLNB alone versus SLNB plus ALND. The results of this trial indicate that axillary node dissection is not necessary after SLNB in women undergoing BCS and whole-breast irradiation, with one or two tumor-involved SLNs, a T1 or T2 tumor, and no significant extranodal extension. No axillary specific radiation was given, and 96% of the patients received adjuvant systemic therapy (chemotherapy or hormonal therapy or both). These findings have resulted in a change of the 2012 National Comprehensive Cancer Network (NCCN) guidelines, which no longer recommend mandatory completion ALND for macrometastases, micrometastases, or ITCs in patients who meet *all* of the following criteria: T1 or T2 tumor, one or two positive sentinel lymph nodes, breast-conserving surgery, whole-breast irradiation planned, and no neoadjuvant chemotherapy. These results are not applicable for patients treated with mastectomy, partial breast irradiation, prone radiation, neoadjuvant chemotherapy, or T3 cancers. These women undergoing mastectomy who are found to have sentinel node macrometastases still should undergo completion axillary node dissection.

CLINICALLY NODE-POSITIVE INVASIVE BREAST CANCER

In patients with grossly palpable nodes, the standard remains axillary node dissection with the removal of level I and II axillary nodes. In patients with suspicious palpable axillary nodes, however, clinical examination is often unreliable and can be falsely positive in up to 40% of patients. In these circumstances, axillary ultrasound scan with needle biopsy is a reliable technique. Alternatively, patients with clinically suspicious axillary nodes can undergo sentinel node biopsy with removal and evaluation of the palpable nodes.

Traditional level I and II axillary dissection requires that at least 10 lymph nodes be evaluated for accurate staging of the axilla. Axillary dissection should not include level III nodes unless gross disease is apparent.

Other Indications for Axillary Node Dissection

Axillary node dissection should be performed in patients when many clinically suspicious nodes are present in the axilla after all sentinel nodes have been removed. In addition, a complete axillary node dissection should be done if no sentinel node is identified or if the SLNB is technically unsatisfactory. Although the indications for completion axillary dissection in patients with tumor-involved sentinel nodes have been altered by recent data from the ACOSOG Z0010 and Z0011 trials, those undergoing mastectomy with tumor-involved sentinel nodes still need completion axillary dissection. Axillary dissection remains indicated in women undergoing BCS and whole-breast irradiation found to have more than two tumor-involved sentinel nodes or gross extranodal extension.

In patients with inflammatory breast cancer, sentinel node biopsy should not be performed because the subdermal lymphatics can be partially obstructed with tumor emboli, leading to an unacceptably high false-negative rate. Thus, in patients with inflammatory breast cancer, an axillary node dissection should be performed.

Axillary dissection, and even SLNB, may be omitted in patients who have particularly favorable tumors, patients for whom the selection of adjuvant systemic therapy is unlikely to be affected, the elderly, and those with serious comorbid conditions, with the understanding that they may be at increased risk for ipsilateral lymph node recurrence.

AXILLARY MANAGEMENT FOR DUCTAL CARCINOMA IN SITU

Sentinel node biopsy in patients with ductal carcinoma in situ (DCIS) is generally not indicated because of the low risk of axillary node metastases; however, it can be performed in selected clinical situations. Although up to 15% of patients with DCIS are found to have involved sentinel nodes, usually ITCs or occasionally micrometastases, this finding is of no clinical significance. In retrospective and prospective studies, these sentinel node ITCs and micrometastases are not associated with increased local or distant recurrence in patients with pure DCIS or even microinvasion. Because these rates of sentinel node involvement in DCIS are not consistent with the pathogenesis of DCIS, these small deposits are thought to represent tumor debris, perhaps from biopsies, rather than viable metastatic tumor cells in the nodes.

SLNB in patients with DCIS may be performed selectively in certain clinical circumstances. Because DCIS is now frequently diagnosed with core needle biopsy, invasive carcinoma is subsequently found on definitive excision in up to 15% to 20% of patients. Mastectomy precludes sentinel node biopsy if an invasive tumor is subsequently found, so SLNB is recommended for patients with DCIS undergoing mastectomy. This avoids the need for axillary dissection if an invasive cancer is identified and no sentinel node biopsy was performed. Selective use of SLNB is recommended in patients with large (>4 cm), palpable, or high-grade DCIS diagnosed with core-needle biopsy who are having BCS to avoid a second operation if invasive cancer is subsequently found.

AXILLARY MANAGEMENT IN PREGNANT PATIENTS

Radiolabeled colloids for sentinel node biopsy for pregnant patients are safe based on the rapid clearance and uptake of the colloid. The dose of radiation received by the fetus with standard technetium 99m (Tc-99m) sulfur colloid has been shown to be minimal and falls well below National Council on Radiation Protection and Measurements threshold guidelines for pregnant patients. Limited studies document the safety of SLNB during pregnancy with low-dose lymphoscintigraphy (10 MBq) with Tc-99m and recommend the use of injection on the same day as the operation to reduce the dose of radiation. Some centers advocate the use of Tc-99m sulfur colloid with hydration and placement of a bladder catheter to avoid accumulation of excreted isotope in the pelvis.

Blue dye should not be used for sentinel node biopsy in pregnant patients because it is currently classified as a category C drug and limited data exist on its teratogenic effects and its low risk of anaphylactic maternal reaction.

AXILLARY MANAGEMENT IN THE ELDERLY

For elderly patients with clinically negative nodes, careful consideration must be given before surgical staging of the axilla. SLNB should be considered only if the nodal status will alter treatment decisions. SLNB can be omitted in elderly or frail patients with estrogen receptor-positive, clinically node-negative tumors in which chemotherapy is not an option and endocrine therapy will be used regardless of nodal status. In elderly patients, axillary recurrences after BCS and endocrine therapy are low (1% at 5 years), even with the omission of radiation and axillary surgery.

Age greater than 70 years was found to be associated with increased SLNB difficulty and failure rates. SLNB should be performed in elderly patients based on their health and need for information of axillary nodal status. SLNB should be performed in healthy elderly patients with clinically node-negative breast cancer in whom chemotherapy is under consideration. Axillary dissection should be performed in elderly patients with clinically positive nodes.

AXILLARY MANAGEMENT IN MALE BREAST CANCER

Because the delayed diagnosis of breast cancer in men often leads to the presentation with more advanced tumors, the most common surgical procedure in these patients is a modified radical mastectomy, followed by radiation therapy for large tumors, nodal metastases, or skin involvement. The feasibility and accuracy of SLNB in male patients with breast cancer, however, has been supported by numerous small institutional studies. The SLNB procedure has been shown to be reliable in male patients with breast cancer, sparing many patients unnecessary axillary node dissections.

POSITIVE AXILLARY NODES WITH AN OCCULT PRIMARY TUMOR

Up to 1.0% of breast cancer patients may present with only enlarged axillary nodes and an occult primary tumor not present on physical examination, breast ultrasound scan, or mammography. A core or fine-needle biopsy of the suspicious axillary node should be obtained and appropriate immunohistochemistry performed (i.e., estrogen receptor [ER]/progesterone receptor [PR] and human epidermal growth factor receptor–2 [HER2]) to help identify a breast origin. Other tumor types, such as lymphoma, ovarian cancer, melanoma, and occasionally lung, thyroid, or neuroendocrine tumors, should be ruled out with an expanded panel of immunohistochemical markers. If axillary node histology is consistent with a breast origin, breast magnetic resonance imaging (MRI) is indicated for identification of the primary tumor in 50% of such patients. A staging workup should be performed to rule out distant metastases.

In patients with histopathologic evidence of breast cancer in axillary nodes, but no primary breast lesion identified after additional imaging, complete axillary node dissection should be performed. Subsequent treatment of the breast with whole-breast irradiation without mastectomy has shown low rates of local failure. Alternatively, mastectomy may be performed. In patients with bulky or fixed axillary nodes, neoadjuvant systemic therapy followed by axillary dissection may be considered.

AXILLARY MANAGEMENT AFTER NEOADJUVANT CHEMOTHERAPY

Neoadjuvant chemotherapy is often considered in women with large clinical stage IIA, IIB, and T3N1M0 tumors who wish to undergo

BCS. The appropriate timing of SLNB in women treated with neoadjuvant chemotherapy remains under debate; initial early data showed mixed results of feasibility and accuracy of SLNB in this setting.

Proponents of SLNB after neoadjuvant chemotherapy cite the benefits of a single operative staging procedure. Furthermore, because neoadjuvant chemotherapy may eradicate nodal disease in up to 40% of patients, many patients can theoretically be spared from a complete ALND.

However, concerns exist that SLNB after neoadjuvant chemotherapy may decrease the accuracy of identification of SLN and increase the false-negative rate. Chemotherapy may cause fibrosis and obstruction of tumor-involved lymphatic channels, which may lead to inaccurate mapping. Furthermore, the response to chemotherapy may not occur uniformly in lymph nodes, leaving residual disease in nonsentinel lymph nodes and limiting the accuracy of SLNB in this setting. The false-negative rate of sentinel node biopsy in the preneoadjuvant or postneoadjuvant chemotherapy setting is low; however, a pathologic complete response after chemotherapy may occur in lymph node metastases previously undetected with clinical examination. The information gained from prechemotherapy axillary staging may have implications on further clinical treatment decisions, such as the need for completion axillary dissection, postmastectomy radiation, and axillary nodal irradiation.

Patients with a negative sentinel node after neoadjuvant chemotherapy are often recommended to undergo axillary irradiation because the true axillary status was unknown. A negative sentinel node found before neoadjuvant chemotherapy spares the patient axillary irradiation.

The largest series to examine the feasibility of SLNB after neoadjuvant chemotherapy was completed as part of the NSABP B-27 trial. These patients underwent SLNB with radioactive colloid, blue dye, or both and had an identification rate of 84.8%. The study suggested that the use of SLNB after neoadjuvant chemotherapy could be most applicable to patients who had a complete clinical response after therapy. Nevertheless, no convincing evidence shows that patients with previously tumor-involved axillary nodes, which subsequently become negative after neoadjuvant chemotherapy, can be spared axillary dissection.

A recent prospective study, ACOSOG Z1071, showed higher than expected false-negative rates with SLNB after neoadjuvant chemotherapy. This study, however, does not answer the important question of the outcome of the untreated axilla after conversion from positive to negative with neoadjuvant therapy and the impact on survival.

In patients with clinically negative axillary nodes anticipated to undergo neoadjuvant chemotherapy, sentinel node biopsy may be performed for accurate staging of the axilla before initiation of systemic treatment. For those with clinically suspicious axillary nodes, needle biopsy of the nodes before treatment is recommended, along with SLNB before neoadjuvant chemotherapy if the needle biopsy results are negative.

If the prechemotherapy SLNB is histologically negative, axillary dissection may be omitted. If the prechemotherapy needle biopsy or SLNB is histologically positive, then a completion axillary dissection should be performed at the time of definitive surgical therapy. A clip may be placed at the time of needle biopsy to ensure the removal of the affected node at the time of axillary dissection. Alternatively, if prechemotherapy nodes are initially positive and then convert to negative on SLNB after chemotherapy, axillary-specific irradiation can be considered as an alternative to completion axillary nodal dissection.

MANAGEMENT AFTER PRIOR AXILLARY SURGERY

SLNB after prior axillary surgery is less successful because of the disruption of the lymphatic drainage pattern. Multiple studies,

however, have shown that reoperative SLNB is feasible after previous axillary surgery. In patients who have had previous complete axillary dissection, the success of reoperative SLNB is between 29% and 38%. Because nonaxillary lymphatic drainage can occur in up to 30% of patients being considered for reoperation after a prior complete axillary dissection, preoperative lymphoscintigraphy is necessary to identify aberrant nonaxillary drainage patterns.

MANAGEMENT OF AXILLARY TUMOR RECURRENCE

Patients with isolated axillary recurrence have 5-year survival rates of approximately 60% to 80%. In patients with involved supraclavicular nodes, internal mammary nodes, or multiple sites of nodal disease, the prognosis is worse. Nodal recurrences may present up to 10 years after initial treatment but are usually seen in the first 2 to 3 years.

Axillary node recurrences often present as an asymptomatic mass in the axilla. This can indicate regional recurrence of the prior cancer, in-breast tumor recurrence occurring in the axillary tail, or a new breast primary. A tissue diagnosis with needle biopsy confirms the presence of recurrence. Should a regional recurrence be found, a search for a new breast primary, and a full metastatic workup, is indicated. A completion axillary node dissection is indicated, usually with regional radiation and additional systemic therapy.

AXILLARY RADIATION AFTER AXILLARY DISSECTION

After ALND, axillary and supraclavicular nodal irradiation is used in select patients who are at high risk for local recurrence. Patients with multiple tumor-involved axillary nodes (usually four or more) or significant extranodal tumor deposits usually require axillary-specific radiation with an additional radiation field that includes the supraclavicular nodes. Occasionally, a fourth field is added posteriorly to bring up the dose in the posterior axilla (known as the posterior axillary boost [PAB] field). A total dose of 45 to 50 Gy is given, over 1.8 to 2.0 Gy fractions daily. This dose is typically what is necessary to eradicate microscopic disease. Higher doses are sometimes needed with gross disease remaining or with extensive extranodal spread.

The morbidity after ALND increases significantly with the additional axillary radiation therapy, with reported lymphedema rates up to 30%. Brachial plexus injury may be seen after axillary irradiation. These morbidities are significantly reduced with modern techniques, such as intensity-modulated radiotherapy (IMRT) and image-guided radiotherapy (IGRT).

ALTERNATIVES TO AXILLARY SURGERY

Alternative nonsurgical methods of axillary treatment are being investigated in patients with clinically negative lymph nodes to avoid the morbidities of ALND. These alternatives include radiation, systemic therapy, and observation only.

Axillary irradiation has been shown to be effective in several studies. In standard tangential whole-breast irradiation, approximately 80% of level I and of level II axillary lymph nodes are treated to 95% of the prescribed dose. Similarly, systemic therapy contributes to local control. This has been shown in the ACOSOG Z0011 trial, which effectively compared the efficacy of tangential whole-breast irradiation and adjuvant systemic therapy with ALND with whole-breast irradiation and adjuvant systemic therapy for patients with positive sentinel nodes. Randomized control trials have shown the efficacy of axillary radiation therapy. Studies of ALND versus axillary radiation therapy show axillary failure rates of 1% to 3%, with no impact on survival rates. Axillary observation, with no treatment specific to the axilla for patients at low risk, show low failure rates and no difference in 5-year survival rate (96%) compared with ALND.

Several trials investigating axillary irradiation are still in progress. The European Organization for Research and Treatment of Cancer (EORTC) 10981 AMAROS (After Mapping of the Axilla: Radiotherapy or Surgery) trial is a phase III study to compare completion ALND with axillary irradiation in patients with positive sentinel nodes. This study aims to prove equivalence of axillary surgery and axillary radiation therapy for locoregional control in the setting of a tumor-involved sentinel node. A new EORTC trial, the POWER trial (Positive Sentinel Node: Wait & See, Excision, or Radiotherapy), aims to identify axillary recurrence rates in patients with sentinel node micrometastases if no further axillary therapy is offered.

In frail patients with node-negative breast cancer and estrogen receptor-positive tumors, endocrine therapy only without axillary surgery or axillary radiation may be applicable. Axillary radiation therapy without surgical staging may also be considered in patients with clinically node-negative disease whose nodal status will not alter adjuvant treatment plans.

TECHNICAL ASPECTS OF AXILLARY LYMPH NODE DISSECTION

The ALND is best performed when the patient is positioned supine, with the ipsilateral upper extremity prepped and wrapped free to allow for elevation and adduction. This maneuver provides better exposure to the upper levels of the axilla by decreasing tension on the pectoral muscles. The incision is placed transversely in the mid axilla, posterior to the pectoralis major margin. The dissection begins with the exposure of the lateral border of the

pectoralis minor with dividing the interpectoral tissues. Division of the clavipectoral fascia medially along this border and transversely in line with the coracobrachialis muscle releases the specimen and exposes the axillary vein. Effort should be made to preserve median pectoral nerve whenever possible. The inferior branches of the axillary vein are divided, releasing the specimen cranially. Care should be taken to remove only axillary tissue inferior to the axillary vein to avoid brachial plexus injury. Blunt dissection of the remaining attachments of the specimen along the serratus and subscapularis muscles releases it inferior and posteriorly. Preservation of the upper intercostal nerves is often possible, but sensation may be altered after mobilization and retraction of these branches. The long thoracic and thoracodorsal nerves are carefully identified and preserved. A marking stitch for orientation is often placed at the apex of the specimen. A drain is often left in place and removed after surgery.

SUGGESTED READINGS

Giuliano AE, Hawes D, Ballman KV, et al: Association of occult metastases in sentinel lymph nodes and bone marrow with survival among women with early-stage invasive breast cancer, *JAMA* 306:385–393, 2011.

Giuliano AE, Hunt KK, Ballman KV, et al: Axillary dissection vs no axillary dissection in women with invasive breast cancer and sentinel node metastasis: a randomized clinical trial, *JAMA* 305:569–575, 2011.

Hunt KK, Ballman KV, McCall LM, et al: Factors associated with local-regional recurrence after a negative sentinel node dissection: results of the ACOSOG Z0010 trial, *Ann Surg* 256:428–436, 2012.

Krag DN, Anderson SJ, Julian TB, et al: Sentinel-lymph-node resection compared with conventional axillary-lymph-node dissection in clinically node-negative patients with breast cancer: overall survival findings from the NSABP B-32 randomised phase 3 trial, *Lancet Oncol* 11:927–933, 2010.

Veronesi U, Viale G, Paganelli G, et al: Sentinel lymph node biopsy in breast cancer: ten-year results of a randomized controlled study, *Ann Surg* 251:595–600, 2010.

INFLAMMATORY BREAST CARCINOMA

Rosemarie Hardin, MD, and
Julie R. Lange, MD, ScM

INTRODUCTION

Inflammatory breast cancer (IBC) is a rare and aggressive form of breast cancer that warrants special consideration. It accounts for less than 5% of invasive breast cancers in the United States, but accounts for a disproportionate number of breast cancer deaths. It has unique diagnostic criteria, and the history and physical exam are central in determining whether a patient has inflammatory breast cancer. This subtype of breast cancer is mainly diagnosed on clinical suspicion and physical exam and then confirmed with diagnostic biopsy and breast imaging. The rapid progression of symptoms differentiates IBC from neglected, locally advanced invasive breast cancer with skin involvement. IBC demonstrates aggressive behavior from the outset and requires multimodality treatment, including systemic

chemotherapy, surgery, radiation therapy, and hormonal therapy and trastuzumab when appropriate. Long-term survival rates remain well under 50%.

CLINICAL PRESENTATION

Compared to other types of breast cancer, IBC tends to be diagnosed at younger ages, with a median age of 57 years, compared to a median age of 62 years for other types of breast cancer, according to the National Cancer Institute statistics. It is also more common among African American women and tends to occur at somewhat younger ages in this population, with a median age of 54 years.

The clinical presentation of IBC is unique and is the key to its proper diagnosis. IBC has rapid onset, typically from several weeks up to 6 months. The usual clinical presentation of IBC is with erythema, swelling, and warmth involving at least one third of the breast, giving an "inflamed" look to the breast. The swelling and edema of the breast can in some cases be quite noticeable, with an increase in the size of the breast over a short time; patients may report a growing sense of heaviness in the breast. The skin of the breast often displays the classic thickening referred to as *peau d'orange*. These skin changes result from blockage of the cutaneous lymphatics. A skin biopsy often demonstrates adenocarcinoma invading the dermal lymphatics. However, there is no direct correlation between the presence, number, or size of the emboli and the degree of erythema present. Although nipple involvement is not a defining clinical feature of IBC, there may be nipple changes evident, such as retraction or swelling, and certainly the skin changes affecting the breast can also affect the nipple-areolar complex. The skin changes are often the most notable feature of IBC and can rapidly progress in some cases from a vague pinkish discoloration to deep or bright red in a matter of days and can involve the breast diffusely. There may or may not be a distinct tumor mass on exam. The striking erythema of IBC can be mistaken for breast infection. While mastitis or cellulitis can occur in women of any age, it is more common around the time of lactation. Clinical concern should be raised regarding the possibility of IBC among nonlactating women presenting with erythema and swelling of the breast.

Most women diagnosed with IBC have regional nodal involvement at the time of diagnosis; therefore, it is common to find palpable or matted axillary lymph nodes. It is estimated that the frequency of involvement of axillary and supraclavicular lymph nodes in IBC ranges from 60% to 85%.

IBC is a distinctly separate clinicopathologic entity from locally advanced breast cancer (LABC). While the presentation of LABC can include skin thickening, erythema, peau d'orange, and axillary adenopathy, these changes in LABC are generally found after a long clinical history of a slowly enlarging (and neglected) breast mass. IBC, however, is characterized by a very short clinical history, with rapid development of skin changes usually prior to (or without) the development of a distinct mass. The clinical history is the key to distinguishing these two entities.

DIAGNOSIS AND STAGING

Evaluation of the woman with suspected inflammatory breast cancer includes history and physical exam, diagnostic breast imaging, biopsy, liver function tests, and systemic staging studies. The main goals of diagnostic breast imaging are to identify a possible primary breast tumor, evaluate the regional nodes, and enable image-guided biopsy for pathologic confirmation of IBC. Image-guided needle biopsy also allows for evaluation of estrogen receptor, progesterone receptor, and *Her 2 neu* status. The goals of systemic staging are to properly evaluate regional disease and determine whether distant metastatic disease is present.

Initial breast imaging includes diagnostic mammogram and breast ultrasound as needed. The most common mammographic findings in a patient with IBC include skin thickening, diffusely increased density unilaterally, discrete mass, axillary adenopathy, architectural distortion, and suspicious calcifications. If a lesion is identified in the breast parenchyma or a suspicious regional lymph node is identified, then an image-guided core biopsy can be performed to confirm the diagnosis and provide information regarding histologic grade, estrogen and progesterone receptor status, and *Her 2 neu* status. Breast ultrasound can also be useful in detecting signs of the disease and in particular can be helpful for evaluation of tumor burden in the regional lymph nodes. Ultrasound guidance is frequently used for needle biopsy to establish the status of abnormal-looking axillary nodes. Magnetic resonance imaging (MRI) has found increasing use in the diagnosis and evaluation of breast cancer in general. MRI is not necessary for all cases of IBC, but it can be used selectively when helpful, such as for women with dense breast parenchyma that might limit the sensitivity of mammograms.

Skin punch biopsy is sometimes done as part of the initial evaluation. Punch biopsy of the skin may reveal dermal lymphatic invasion of the papillary and reticular dermis, resulting from lymphovascular tumor emboli. If a skin punch biopsy is chosen, it is recommended that at least two biopsies between 2 and 8 mm in diameter be performed in a representative area of the breast with skin changes. While dermal lymphatic invasion is considered to be strongly supportive of a diagnosis of IBC, it is neither necessary nor sufficient. A negative skin biopsy does not rule out IBC if clinical suspicion is strong.

Essential findings to establish a diagnosis of IBC include a history of rapid development of breast erythema with skin edema with duration of symptoms less than 6 months (and usually less than 3 months); diffuse changes, usually including at least a third of the skin of the breast; and pathologic confirmation of invasive mammary carcinoma.

At diagnosis approximately one fourth of patients with IBC will have distant metastases. Systemic radiologic staging is an essential part of the initial evaluation of patients diagnosed with IBC. Minimally, this can include liver enzymes; computed tomographic (CT) scan of chest, abdomen, and pelvis; and bone scan. The proper role of positron emission tomography-computed tomographic (PET-CT) scan for staging of breast cancer is evolving. It is most helpful in situations where conventional staging studies are equivocal and when the result of PET-CT would alter treatment decisions. There is some suggestion that PET-CT may have a role in the early assessment of response to systemic therapy. At present the use of PET-CT must be decided on an individual basis.

In the seventh edition AJCC TNM staging system, IBC is the only primary tumor classified as T4d. Patients with N0, N1, or N2 disease without evidence of distant disease are designated as stage IIIB. Those with evidence of metastases to supraclavicular, infraclavicular, or internal mammary nodes but without distant disease are stage IIIC. Patients with distant disease have stage IV disease. About 20% to 35% of patients with IBC have identified distant disease at the time of presentation.

TREATMENT

IBC requires a multimodality approach involving systemic therapy as the first treatment, given the aggressive nature of this disease, followed by locoregional therapies with surgery and radiotherapy, as well as the addition of systemic hormonal therapy when indicated.

Neoadjuvant Chemotherapy

Given the presentation of IBC and its propensity for rapid progression and distant metastasis, the cornerstone of therapy remains the prompt institution of systemic therapy with anthracycline-based neoadjuvant chemotherapy. The benefit of taxanes is also recognized for this population, as it is for other breast cancer patients. Trastuzumab should be included for patients whose tumor is positive for *Her 2 neu* overexpression. Neoadjuvant chemotherapy allows systemic treatment as expeditiously as possible and often results in decreased disease burden in the breast, improving operability and completeness of resection. Furthermore, the clinical response to neoadjuvant chemotherapy can be a good indicator of prognosis. Response to neoadjuvant chemotherapy should be carefully monitored with a combination of physical examination and radiologic imaging. Patients responding to chemotherapy (with a decrease in locoregional tumor burden) will proceed on to surgery as the next step. Patients who do not respond to neoadjuvant chemotherapy should be considered for alternate additional chemotherapies and/or preoperative radiation therapy. Those responding to these secondary treatments can then proceed on to surgery. Patients with stage IV disease can be restaged after initial chemotherapy; surgery is considered on an individual basis, depending on the estimation of systemic disease control versus the need for expectant palliation of the primary site.

Surgery

Surgery plays an important role in the multimodal approach to the treatment of IBC and is done for the purpose of locoregional control following response to neoadjuvant chemotherapy. Patients who fail to respond to neoadjuvant chemotherapy should be considered for radiotherapy to improve local control; if improvement is seen, they can then be considered for surgical intervention. Appropriate surgery for patients with IBC is a modified radical mastectomy—that is, total mastectomy along with levels I and II axillary dissection. Sentinel node biopsy has been shown to be an unreliable method of assessing the regional lymph nodes in patients with IBC, and it is recommended that patients have an axillary dissection of levels I and II even if the initial clinical evaluation of the axillary nodes was negative. Lumpectomy is not used for patients with IBC, even in the case of complete response to neoadjuvant therapy, given the diffuse nature of this disease within the breast. Similarly, skin-sparing mastectomy is not used in patients with IBC, given the likelihood of diffuse skin involvement at diagnosis. If reconstruction is desired, it is considered in a delayed fashion, once the patient has completed all chemotherapy and radiation therapy, and demonstrated lack of systemic progression on follow-up staging studies.

Decision making regarding surgery for patients who fail to respond to neoadjuvant therapies and for those with stage IV IBC remains difficult. These patients require careful restaging after initial systemic therapy, multidisciplinary discussion, and sound judgment about the potential benefit of surgery for expectant palliation. Even in the face of chemotherapy-resistant local disease or established distant disease, there may be a role for surgery as a palliative measure for select patients.

Radiation Therapy

Following modified radical mastectomy, patients with IBC are recommended to receive radiation to the chest wall, axilla, and supraclavicular fossa, with consideration of radiation to the internal mammary nodes if there is concern about involvement of that basin. The primary purpose of such radiation is for locoregional control because its effect on survival in this population is unclear. Radiation is also used as a local control treatment in patients who do not respond well to neoadjuvant therapy and may make subsequent surgery more complete.

Targeted Therapy With Trastuzumab

A higher incidence of *Her 2 neu* overexpression has been documented in IBC. *Her 2 neu* is overexpressed or amplified in approximately 36% to 60% of patients with IBC. Trastuzumab should be given in combination with systemic chemotherapy regimens for *Her 2 neu* positive IBC and continuing beyond the end of chemotherapy to extend to a year of trastuzumab. The largest series of patients with *Her 2 neu* positive IBC treated with neoadjuvant trastuzumab were part of the NOAH (neoadjuvant trastuzumab) trial. A significantly higher pathologic complete response was noted in women who received

neoadjuvant chemotherapy in combination with trastuzumab (54%) than in women who did not receive trastuzumab (19.3%).

Hormonal Therapy

The result of hormone receptor status on the original core biopsy can drive decision making for adjuvant hormonal therapies, which are generally started once the locoregional therapies have been completed. Most IBC are estrogen- and progesterone-receptor negative. This may contribute to the difficulty in obtaining durable control of this aggressive disease. In the subset of patients with receptor positive tumors, hormonal therapy with either an aromatase inhibitor or tamoxifen for 5 years is an important part of the overall therapeutic plan.

PROGNOSIS AND FOLLOW-UP

As with other types of breast cancer, prognosis is dependent on lymph node status and stage; the presence of distant metastatic disease is strongly associated with poorer outcome. Women with stage III IBC have a better prognosis than those with stage IV IBC. Women with stage III disease have a 40% 5-year survival compared to 11% in women with stage IV; both of these are significantly worse than survival in other types of breast cancer.

The response to neoadjuvant chemotherapy is an important indicator of prognosis. In a study conducted at MD Anderson Cancer Center, patients who achieved a pathologic complete response had a far better 5-year survival than those with residual disease. Similarly, patients with a pathologic complete response in the axillary lymph nodes had a better overall survival and disease-free survival than those with residual nodal disease.

Given the infrequency of this disease and the advanced stage at presentation of most patients, IBC remains a challenging clinical problem. Many patients with IBC may benefit from evaluation and treatment at an established breast program with clinical trials available. More research to better define the molecular and genetic characteristics of IBC is needed, with the hope that a more complete understanding of the disease will lead to improved treatments.

S U G G E S T E D   R E A D I N G S

Dawood S, Merajver SD, Veins P, et al: International expert panel on inflammatory breast cancer: consensus statement for standardized diagnosis and treatment, *Ann Oncol* 22:515–523, 2011.

Robertson FM, Bondy M, Yang W, et al: Inflammatory breast cancer: the disease, the biology and the treatment, *Ca Cancer J Clin* 60:351–375, 2010.

Yamuchi H, Woodward WA, Valero V, et al: Inflammatory Breast Cancer: What we know and what we need to learn, *Oncologist* 891–899, 2012.

Ductal and Lobular Carcinoma in Situ of the Breast

Thomas N. Wang, MD, PhD, and
Marshall M. Urist, MD

Ductal carcinoma in situ (DCIS) and lobular carcinoma in situ (LCIS) of the breast are noninvasive cancers with dissimilar implications. Whereas DCIS is a precursor lesion to invasive ductal carcinoma, LCIS is considered a marker of increased risk for breast cancer development. Malignant cell proliferation in both entities is confined to the basement membrane. Because the risk of systemic metastases is virtually nonexistent, the prognosis for DCIS and LCIS is excellent. The goal of treatment of in situ breast carcinoma is to prevent the development of invasive disease. The challenge in management is determining which patients are at risk for subsequent invasive breast cancer (IBC) and providing the appropriate therapy that minimizes recurrence without causing unnecessary morbidity. Personalization of treatment necessitates careful patient evaluation and multidisciplinary planning.

DUCTAL CARCINOMA IN SITU

DCIS is a clonal proliferation of malignant epithelial cells confined within the basement membrane of the mammary ducts. It represents a spectrum of pathologic lesions with variable malignant potential predetermined by histologic architecture, presence of necrosis, and nuclear grade. Two major histologic subtypes of DCIS exist: comedo (presence of central necrosis, many mitotic figures, and large pleomorphic nuclei) and noncomedo (absence of central necrosis and mitotic figures, presence of specific papillary, micropapillary, or cribriform architecture) carcinoma. Nuclear grade is classified as low, intermediate, or high grade as determined by nuclear morphology and mitotic index. High-grade DCIS is commonly associated with necrosis and has the most aggressive biologic characteristics with the highest local recurrence rates. Regardless of nuclear grade or histologic subtype, the long-term prognosis of DCIS is excellent, with survival rates at 10 years exceeding 95%. Therefore, the challenge in the treatment of DCIS is to balance the risk for local recurrence with unnecessary surgical morbidity.

DCIS incidence rates have increased 7.2-fold from 1980 to 2007. In 2008, the incidence of DCIS was approximately 67,000 new cases in the United States, making it the fastest growing subtype of breast cancer. The growing incidence is a result of the increasing use of screening mammography. DCIS currently accounts for over 20% of all mammographically detected breast cancers. DCIS usually presents as microcalcifications detected by screening mammography with confirmation of the diagnosis by histologic examination of biopsy specimens. IBC develops at or near the same site in the ipsilateral breast as the index DCIS lesion in the majority of women in whom DCIS goes untreated. Therefore, management of DCIS aims to rule out concurrent IBC (present in 10% to 25% of cases of DCIS) and prevent the future development of IBC. The optimal treatment of DCIS is complete surgical excision by either breast-conserving surgery (BCS) and adjuvant radiation therapy or mastectomy. Areas of controversy include adequate margin size of excision, the role of sentinel lymph node biopsy to assess for regional metastasis, the need for adjuvant radiation therapy after lumpectomy, and the need for systemic therapy with hormonal agents.

Diagnosis

The majority (90%-95%) of cases of DCIS present as suspiciously grouped, pleomorphic, or fine linear microcalcifications on mammograms. In rare cases, patients with DCIS have a palpable mass, a mammographically detected mass, Paget's disease of the nipple, or suspicious nipple discharge. Indeterminate calcifications are further evaluated with magnification views of the breast. Breast cancer that is diagnosed by detecting incidental calcifications on mammography is pure DCIS in 65% of cases, DCIS with a focus of invasion in 32% of cases, and IBC in 4% of cases. The presence of invasive foci is more often associated with large areas of calcifications (>10 mm) and linear versus granular calcifications. All mammographically detected lesions are confirmed by pathologic evaluation of breast tissue obtained through biopsy. Stereotactic core needle biopsy has replaced needle-localized excisional biopsy as the optimal diagnostic tool as it permits the acquisition of tissue for accurate strategic planning without an additional operation that may be potentially deforming. However, breast biopsy with needle localization is still necessary in cases where lesions are not amenable to stereotactic core needle biopsy (too superficial, adjacent to the chest wall, too close to breast implants, or not enough breast tissue necessary for compression).

The role of breast magnetic resonance imaging (MRI) in the diagnosis of DCIS is evolving. Currently, mammography remains the standard of care for the detection and diagnosis of noninvasive breast cancer. Because MRI often misses small, mammographically visible foci, it is not an adequate replacement for mammography as a tool for diagnosing DCIS.

Treatment

Similar to IBC, management of noninvasive breast cancer has evolved with the application of multimodality therapy and less aggressive surgery. In the past, DCIS was often treated with simple mastectomy or even modified radical mastectomy. However, when overwhelming evidence demonstrated that BCS and adjuvant radiation therapy for IBC achieved survival rates similar to those of total mastectomy, investigators questioned whether mastectomy for DCIS was overtreatment and unnecessary. Unlike IBC, no randomized trial is currently being conducted that compares total mastectomy with BCS as treatment for DCIS. Retrospective studies have shown that total mastectomy for DCIS is superior to BCS in terms of disease-free survival. Silverstein and colleagues compared local recurrence among 227 patients with DCIS. They reported a disease-free survival rate of 98% in patients undergoing mastectomy versus 81% in those receiving BCS ($P = 0.0004$). Recently, Tunon-de-Lara and colleagues reported similar results in a review of 676 patients with DCIS. They reported a local recurrence rate of 2.6% for the mastectomy group, 7.5% for the lumpectomy plus radiation therapy group, and 14.5% for the lumpectomy only group. Involved surgical margins and young patient age were predictive of local recurrence after BCS. Nevertheless, there was no significant difference in survival in any subgroup comparison, regardless of treatment. Thus, the standard therapy for DCIS is BCS followed by radiation therapy or mastectomy alone.

Surgical Therapy

In choosing the optimal management of DCIS, physicians and patients need to take into consideration the patient's risk of local recurrence associated with BCS. Although the long-term prognosis of DCIS is excellent with low mortality rates regardless of treatment, the psychologic impact of a local recurrence, especially an invasive recurrence, is devastating for any patient. Therefore, the aim of BCS for DCIS is complete excision with clear margins and a cosmetically acceptable result. Mastectomy should be considered for multicentric DCIS, large lesions, centrally located disease, inadequate margins after repeated attempts at breast conservation, in patients who prefer to have a mastectomy, or if adjuvant radiation therapy is contraindicated. Certainly, deciding between BCS and mastectomy involves extensive discussion among the patient, surgeon, radiologist, medical oncologist, and radiation oncologist. A multidisciplinary approach allows for the personalization of care. Finally, all patients requiring total mastectomy for DCIS should be offered the option of immediate breast reconstruction, which is associated with a psychologic benefit and a similar oncologic outcome. In the United States, approximately one third of patients with DCIS undergo mastectomy.

The size of the negative margin remains controversial because there are no prospectively acquired definitive data defining an adequate margin. Silverstein and colleagues retrospectively evaluated margin status in 469 patients with DCIS, 256 of whom were treated with BCS alone and 213 treated with BCS and adjuvant radiation therapy. They acquired precise data on margin size by analyzing samples with three-dimensional reconstruction. The authors observed that with a margin width of 10 mm or more, the incidence of local recurrence was only 2.3%, and there was no added benefit from adjuvant radiation therapy. Patients with margin widths between 1 and 10 mm benefited from adjuvant radiation therapy to an acceptable risk of recurrence. However, patients treated with a margin width of less than 1 mm had a suboptimal outcome with or without adjuvant radiation therapy. Although adjuvant radiation therapy significantly decreased the incidence of local recurrence from 58% to 30% in this group, such a recurrence rate is unacceptably high, suggesting that adjuvant radiation therapy is not adequate treatment. More recently, Neuschartz and colleagues also showed that a margin width of less than 1 mm was associated with an increased rate of local recurrence despite adjuvant radiation therapy. Margin widths greater than 1 mm were associated with a 5-year recurrence rate of 10.9% for BCS alone and 4.6% for BCS plus adjuvant radiation therapy. Therefore, we recommend at least a 2- to 3-mm margin of excision for DCIS if adjuvant radiation will be administered. Further excision, or possibly mastectomy, may be indicated in patients with an excision margin of less than 2 mm.

Traditionally, axillary dissection and sentinel lymph node biopsy have had no role in the management of DCIS. The risk for nodal metastases in patients with DCIS is less than 3%. The low rate of nodal metastases, the high survival rate of patients with DCIS, and the significant morbidity rate of patients with an axillary lymph node dissection makes axillary nodal dissection unnecessary. However, the evaluation of axillary nodes by sentinel lymph node biopsy may be considered in certain situations, such as the presence of large DCIS lesions (>4 cm), palpable breast lesions, high-grade disease, microinvasive disease, or suspicious-appearing axillary lymph nodes on physical examination or by ultrasound examination. These particular features may increase the chances of finding an invasive cancer in the lumpectomy specimen to as much as 20%. Sentinel node biopsy performed at the same time as the lumpectomy may save the patient an additional operation. In addition, all patients undergoing a mastectomy for DCIS should undergo a concomitant sentinel node biopsy because a sentinel node biopsy would not be possible after a mastectomy.

Radiation Therapy

Three prospective randomized controlled trials have investigated the role of adjuvant radiation therapy in patients with DCIS after lumpectomy (Table 1). The National Surgical Adjuvant Breast and Bowel Project (NSABP) study B-17 enrolled 818 patients with DCIS between 1985 and 1990. The patients were randomized to undergo

TABLE 1: Clinical trials evaluating radiation therapy in patients with DCIS after breast-conserving surgery

Trial	Follow-up (years)	Breast recurrence rate	
		No radiation	Radiation
NSABP B-17	12	17%	8%
EORTC	4	16%	9%
UK/ANZ	5	14%	6%

DCIS, Ductal carcinoma in situ; *EORTC,* European Organization for Research and Treatment of Cancer (*P* < 0.005); *NSABP B-17,* National Surgical Adjuvant Breast and Bowel Project B-17 (*P* < 0.001); *UK/ANZ,* United Kingdom and Australia and New Zealand (*P* < 0.0001).

either lumpectomy alone or lumpectomy followed by breast irradiation to a total dose of 50 Gy. Through 12 years of follow-up, the investigators observed a 58% lower incidence of ipsilateral breast tumor recurrences associated with the use of adjuvant radiation therapy. Local recurrence rates were 17% in patients who did not receive radiation and 8% in patients who did. All subsets benefited from radiation therapy, regardless of the clinical or mammographic tumor characteristics. These data led to the recommendation that all patients with DCIS treated with BCS receive adjuvant radiation therapy. There was no difference in the distant disease-free or overall survival. Two other randomized controlled trials, the European Organization for Research and Treatment of Cancer (EORTC) study and the United Kingdom and Australia and New Zealand (UK/ANZ) study, demonstrated similar findings, as summarized in Table 1. Together, these three prospective trials show that adding radiation to lumpectomy of DCIS statistically decreases a patient's risk for developing recurrent breast cancer.

Although adjuvant radiation therapy significantly decreases local recurrence in BCS, it does not provide a clear survival advantage for patients with DCIS. In addition, radiation therapy is time consuming and condemns the patient to potential morbidities. Therefore, many clinicians are interested in identifying a subset of patients that can be treated with BCS alone. Silverstein and colleagues evaluated the effect of pathologic features (tumor size, margin width, nuclear grade, and the presence or absence of necrosis) on local recurrence. Patient age was later included to improve the accuracy of predicting local failure. By assigning a numeric score to each parameter, this group devised the University of Southern California/Van Nuys Prognostic Index (USC/VNPI; Table 2). In a retrospective review of a prospective database, which included 12-year surveillance of 706 women who had BCS for pure DCIS, they found that USC/VNPI scores of 4, 5, and 6 had an average recurrence rate of 2%, of which 0% was invasive. USC/VNPI scores of 7, 8, and 9 had an average recurrence rate of 22%, of which 46% were invasive. USC/VNPI scores of 10, 11, and 12 had an average recurrence rate of 52%, of which 43% were invasive. Based on these findings, Silverstein and colleagues recommended lumpectomy alone for scores of 4, 5, and 6; lumpectomy and radiation for 7, 8, and 9; and mastectomy for 10, 11, and 12.

Wong and colleagues from the Dana-Farber Cancer Institute conducted a single-arm prospective study of the use of wide excision alone for patients with favorable DCIS, defined as non–high-grade DCIS without necrosis, diameter less than or equal to 2.5 cm, and excision margins greater than or equal to 1 cm. They accrued patients from May 1995 to July 2002. These patients were treated with surgery alone and no radiation. The trial was terminated early when the number of local recurrences met the predetermined stopping boundary. Only 158 patients had been enrolled (the initial target had been

TABLE 2: The USC/Van nuys prognostic index scoring system for DCIS

	SCORE		
	1	2	3
Size	< 15 mm	16-40 mm	> 40 mm
Margin	> 10 mm	1-9 mm	< 1 mm
Pathology	Non–high nuclear grade without necrosis	Non–high nuclear grade with necrosis	High nuclear grade with or without necrosis
Age	> 60	40-60	< 40

DCIS, Ductal carcinoma in situ; *USC*, University of Southern California.

200 patients). The rate of ipsilateral local recurrence was 2.4% per patient-year, corresponding to a 5-year recurrence rate of 12%. Thirty-one percent of these recurrences were IBC. Despite the use of margins greater than or equal to 1 cm, the local recurrence rate was substantial in patients with small, low- to intermediate-grade DCIS lesions treated with excision alone. These findings contradict Silverstein's evaluation and question the validity of the USC/VNPI.

Criticisms of the Dana-Farber study include the fact that this was a single-arm study that was not compared with studies of treatment with adjuvant radiation therapy. In addition, the number of patients enrolled in the study was small, and the follow-up time was relatively short due to its required early termination. Undoubtedly, the USC/VNPI is a simple and reliable scoring system that has been confirmed by other groups to accurately identify a subset of patients who are at risk of local recurrence and benefit from radiation therapy or mastectomy. However, only prospective randomized trials can precisely predict the risk of local recurrence of conservatively treated DCIS. Except in a controlled trial adopting uniform criteria for margin evaluation, USC/VNPI should not be used to determine which patients can be treated with local excision alone. To date, no subset of patients from prospective randomized clinical trials has been identified that does not benefit from radiation therapy when undergoing BCS for DCIS.

Hormonal Therapy

Similar to the success of tamoxifen in the treatment of early IBC, the NSABP B-24 trial demonstrated a benefit from tamoxifen for women with DCIS after treatment with BCS and adjuvant radiation therapy. Conducted from 1991 to 1995, investigators randomized 1804 patients with DCIS treated with excision and radiation to receive either tamoxifen or placebo for 5 years. Tamoxifen and radiation were administered concurrently. In that trial, surgical margins were allowed to have tumor involvement. At 7 years of follow-up, the women treated with tamoxifen had a 27% reduction in the annual incidence rate of all breast cancer–related events and a 48% reduction in IBC. The cumulative incidence of all IBC events in the tamoxifen group was 4.1% (2.1% ipsilateral, 1.8% contralateral) versus 7.2% (4.2% ipsilateral, 2.3% contralateral) in the placebo-treated group. Additionally, a retrospective analysis of estrogen receptor (ER) expression in the NSABP B-24 trial demonstrated that increased levels of ER expression predict for a better tamoxifen benefit with respect to improved risk reduction for the development of breast cancer following BCS. Therefore, tamoxifen treatment should be considered as a strategy to reduce the risk of breast cancer recurrence in women with DCIS treated with BCS, especially in those women with ER-positive DCIS.

Recently, retrospective evaluation of the NSABP B-24 database corroborates the belief that adjuvant tamoxifen reduced subsequent ipsilateral breast cancer only in patients with ER-positive DCIS. Allred and colleagues from the Washington University School of Medicine retrospectively reviewed the hormone receptor status of patients enrolled in the NSABP B-24 clinical trial. The investigators evaluated the receptor status in 732 patients with DCIS and known receptor status by immunohistochemistry. They found a significant discrepancy between the ER results from an experienced central laboratory, which used a comprehensively validated assay for ER, and other institutional laboratories. Assuming that the central laboratory results were correct, the authors demonstrated that the false negative rate from institutional laboratories was 30% to 40%, which may be responsible for the benefit observed in ER-negative patient cases observed in the NSABP B-24 database. We advocate adjuvant tamoxifen therapy for the treatment of patients with ER-positive DCIS unless medically contraindicated.

Surveillance

Surveillance of patients previously treated with DCIS includes physical examination every 6 months for 5 years and then annually. A diagnostic mammogram should be performed yearly. Evaluation of both breasts is paramount, and special attention should be paid to the ipsilateral breast following BCS. Most recurrences occur in close proximity to the site of prior disease. Often, mastectomy is necessary in patients who have a DCIS recurrence initially treated with BCS and adjuvant radiation therapy. Local recurrences following a mastectomy for DCIS should be treated with a negative margin resection followed by chest wall radiation, if possible. Finally, patients with local recurrences that present as IBC should receive the appropriate systemic therapy after the indicated surgical treatment. Figure 1 outlines our management algorithm of patients with DCIS.

LOBULAR CARCINOMA IN SITU

Foote and Stewart first coined the term *lobular carcinoma in situ* in 1941 to emphasize the similarity between cells of LCIS and cells of invasive lobular carcinoma. In addition, they noted that the foci of neoplastic cells in LCIS were contained within the basement membrane similar to those in DCIS. They believed that LCIS was a premalignant lesion to invasive lobular carcinoma and recommended mastectomy as the primary treatment. Later, the term *atypical lobular hyperplasia* (ALH) was introduced to describe morphologically similar but less well developed lesions. Over the past 60 years, it has become clear that LCIS and ALH are not precursor lesions for invasive carcinoma in the same way that DCIS is a precursor lesion to invasive cancer. The diagnosis of LCIS represents a marker for increased risk for subsequent carcinoma. Radical surgery has fallen out of favor, but recommendations for treatment are not uniform and vary from close surveillance with mammography to surveillance alone to bilateral mastectomy in some cases. Recently, new data suggesting that LCIS may be an obligate precursor lesion for IBC may have significant implications for the future management of patients with LCIS.

Pathophysiology

The histologic features of LCIS and ALH are well established. LCIS is divided into two specific subtypes: classic and pleomorphic. Classic LCIS consists of a monomorphic population of small, round, polygonal or cuboidal cells with a thin rim of clear cytoplasm and a high nuclear-to-cytoplasmic ratio. The cells are loosely cohesive and regularly spaced, and they fill and distend the acini. The nucleus is characterized by small nucleoli and few mitotic figures. Pagetoid spread, in which the neoplastic cells extend along adjacent ducts, is

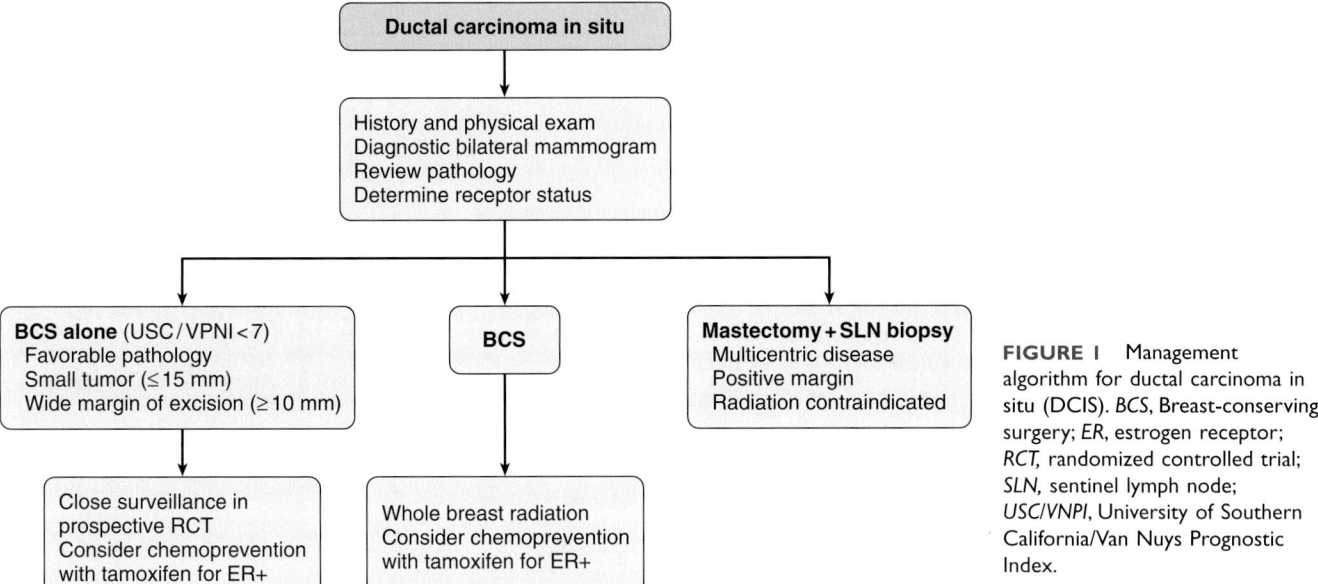

FIGURE I   Management algorithm for ductal carcinoma in situ (DCIS). *BCS,* Breast-conserving surgery; *ER,* estrogen receptor; *RCT,* randomized controlled trial; *SLN,* sentinel lymph node; *USC/VNPI,* University of Southern California/Van Nuys Prognostic Index.

frequently seen. Pleomorphic LCIS exhibits cells with distinctly larger nuclei and prominent nucleoli with frequent mitotic figures. Central necrosis and calcification within lobules are common. For a diagnosis of LCIS, more than half of the acini in an involved lobular unit must be filled and distended by the LCIS cells, leaving no central lumina. A lesion is regarded as ALH when the characteristic cells fill less than half of the acini with no or only mild distension of the lobule and the lumina are visible.

Natural History

Women with LCIS are usually in their fifth decade of life with a mean age of diagnosis between 44 and 46 years of age, 10 years younger than women with DCIS. Only 10% of women with LCIS are postmenopausal. The risk of developing IBC in patients with LCIS is 7 to 18 times higher than that of the general population. The SEER data between 1973 and 1998 revealed that the minimum cumulative risk of developing IBC after LCIS was 7.1% at 10 years, with a lifetime risk of 30% to 40%. It was a common belief that this increased risk was equal for both breasts. However, studies that are more recent demonstrate that carcinoma is 3 times more likely to develop in the ipsilateral breast compared to the contralateral breast. Furthermore, the SEER data between 1988 and 2002 revealed that women with LCIS are also 5.3-fold more likely to develop invasive lobular carcinoma and 0.8-fold less likely to develop invasive ductal carcinoma. These new data suggest that LCIS may behave as both a precursor lesion to invasive lobular cancer and a risk indicator for IBC.

Diagnosis

The diagnosis of LCIS is often an incidental finding after a breast biopsy is performed for another reason. There are no specific clinical abnormalities that would alert a physician to LCIS on breast examination or patient symptomatology, and rarely is LCIS visible on mammography or other imaging modalities. Therefore, the true incidence of LCIS in the general population is unknown. The incidence of LCIS in otherwise benign breast biopsies is between 0.5% and 3.8%. Similar to DCIS rates, LCIS rates have also increased since the 1980s as a result of the increasing numbers of screening mammograms and biopsies being performed, in some series as much as a threefold increase. Characteristically, LCIS is multifocal and bilateral

in many cases. Over 50% of patients contain multiple foci in the same breast, and 30% will have LCIS in the contralateral breast. It is this multifocality in a clinically undetectable lesion that makes management of this disease a significant challenge.

Treatment

As previously mentioned, new epidemiologic data support the premise that LCIS may be a precursor lesion to invasive lobular carcinoma as well as a risk indicator for IBC. In addition, recent studies comparing the molecular signatures of LCIS and coexisting invasive lobular carcinoma also support the hypothesis that LCIS may act as a precursor. Therefore, advocates for the precursor role of LCIS suggest that a more definitive treatment strategy with BCS and adjuvant radiation may be necessary for patients with LCIS. Recently, Ciocca and colleagues challenged this premise and hypothesized that if LCIS were a precursor, its presence in the lumpectomy specimen, particularly at the margin, would increase local recurrence after BCS. They evaluated 2894 patients treated with BCS at the Fox Chase Cancer Center for DCIS, stage I or stage II breast cancer, of which 290 patients also exhibited findings of LCIS, with 84 LCIS present at the margin of excision. Five- and 10-year local recurrence rates were not statistically different among patients with LCIS at the margin, LCIS within the lumpectomy specimen but not at the margin, or no LCIS. The presence of LCIS at the lumpectomy margin did not have an impact on local recurrence, unlike the increase in local recurrence rates found in patients with positive or close lumpectomy margins for DCIS. These findings do not support LCIS as a precursor to the development of IBC. In addition, their results also confirm that reexcision of a positive margin for LCIS is not necessary. Until further studies can definitively clarify the precursor function of LCIS, we maintain that LCIS should still be managed as a risk indicator for the development of IBC.

Specimen Evaluation

Stereotactic core needle biopsy has become the most common method for breast tissue sampling after a suspicious mammogram. Controversy exists as to the need for surgical excision after the finding of LCIS or ALH on a core needle biopsy specimen. Elsheikh and colleagues prospectively studied 33 cases of core biopsies that underwent follow-up surgical excision. Surgical excision of the tissue surrounding a core biopsy of LCIS revealed IBC in 4 of 13 cases (31%). Five of the 20 cases (25%) of ALH revealed carcinoma, including 4 DCIS and 1 invasive lobular carcinoma. Underestimation of cancer when a core biopsy showed LCIS or ALH was found in 28% of prospectively examined patients, including 20% of those with ALH and 38% of those with LCIS. The authors recommended surgical excision in all patients with core needle biopsy specimens exhibiting findings of LCIS or ALH to rule out malignancy. We believe that the best strategy for the management of LCIS or ALH found on core needle biopsy is a multidisciplinary team approach to determine whether there is discordance between the radiologically identified abnormality and the pathologic findings. If LCIS is identified in a core specimen with other high-grade lesions or the imaged abnormality has not been adequately explained by the pathology found (radiologic-pathologic discordance), then further surgical excision is necessary. If LCIS is a true incidental finding with no suspicious findings or discordance, further excision is not necessary.

Management of surgical excision specimens exhibiting LCIS is also an area of some controversy. If LCIS only is seen in an excisional biopsy, no further excision is required. Finally, a finding of LCIS at the margin of an excisional biopsy in association with an IBC also does not warrant further excision if the IBC has been completely excised.

Treatment Options

Counseling regarding LCIS necessitates informing patients of their increased risk for IBC and the need for close follow-up. The risk of IBC is 0.5% to 1.0% per year. Because the risk is low, observation is the preferred treatment option for patients diagnosed with LCIS. In addition, patients should understand that the biology of the potential IBC tends to be favorable and deaths from an early detected IBC unlikely. Prophylactic bilateral mastectomy should be considered in special circumstances, such as in women with a BRCA1 or BRCA2 mutation or a strong family history. Nevertheless, the decision to pursue prophylactic mastectomy for risk reduction should be made only after careful evaluation and multidisciplinary counseling. Women treated with bilateral mastectomy are appropriate candidates for breast reconstruction.

Two studies, the NSABP P-1 Breast Cancer Prevention Trial and the NSPBP P-2 Study of Tamoxifen and Raloxifene (STAR), examined chemoprevention of invasive and noninvasive breast cancer for patients with LCIS. The NSABP P-1 trial evaluated the use of tamoxifen for the prevention of breast cancer in 13,388 women at high risk. High risk was determined by the Gail model risk assessment based on the patient's age, age at menarche, age at first live birth, family history of breast cancer, and number of breast biopsies, including diagnosis of atypical hyperplasia and/or diagnosis of LCIS. Of the participants, 8.4% had a diagnosis of LCIS. The study found that tamoxifen decreased the risk for developing IBC by 49% in all enrolled women at high risk. Subset analysis of patients with LCIS had an even greater risk reduction of 56%. The STAR trial enrolled 19,747 high-risk women also determined by the Gail model. All of the women studied were postmenopausal, of which 9% had a diagnosis of LCIS. They were randomized to receive daily doses of tamoxifen or raloxifene. The two drugs were equally effective for the prevention of IBC in the postmenopausal women with a history of LCIS. Women taking raloxifene had a lower risk of thromboembolic events and fewer uterine cancers as compared with women taking tamoxifen. However, unlike tamoxifen, which reduced the incidence of DCIS and LCIS by half, raloxifene had no effect in the prevention of noninvasive breast cancer occurrences.

The present National Comprehensive Cancer Network guidelines (2009) recommend observation as the primary treatment for women

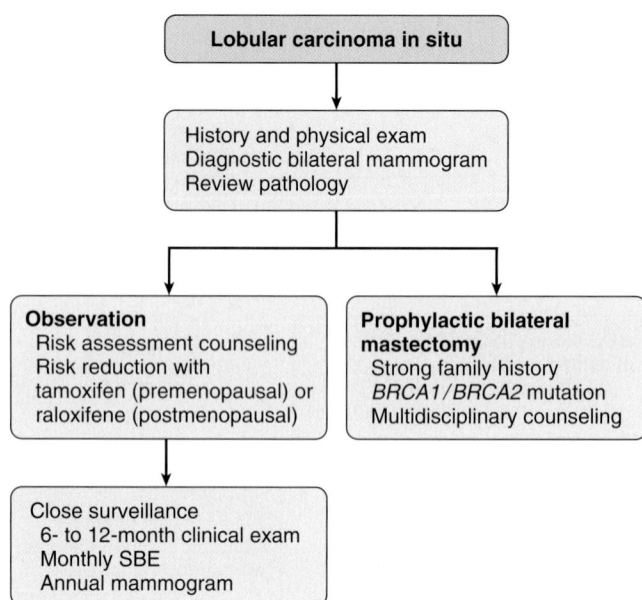

FIGURE 2   Management algorithm for lobular carcinoma in situ. *SBE*, Self-breast examination.

with LCIS. The use of tamoxifen in premenopausal women or tamoxifen or raloxifene in postmenopausal women should be considered as a risk-reduction strategy in women with LCIS. Risk-reduction or prophylactic bilateral mastectomy may be considered as an option for women with a history of LCIS, especially in women with a BRCA1 or BRCA2 mutation or a strong family history of breast cancer, only after careful evaluation and counseling. Surveillance of patients with LCIS should include interval breast examinations by a physician every 6 to 12 months and periodic self-breast examinations. All patients being followed by close observation should undergo annual diagnostic mammography (Figure 2). Finally, all patients with LCIS should be offered the option of participation in clinical research protocols evaluating screening or risk assessment.

SUGGESTED READINGS

Allred DC, Anderson SJ, Paik S, et al: Adjuvant tamoxifen reduces subsequent breast cancer in women with estrogen receptor-positive ductal carcinoma in situ: a study based on NSABP protocol B-24, *J Clin Oncol* 30:1268–1273, 2012.

Ciocca RM, Li T, Freedman GM, Morrow M: Presence of lobular carcinoma in situ does not increase local recurrence in patients treated with breast-conserving therapy, *Ann Surg Oncol* 15:2263–2271, 2008.

Daly MB: Tamoxifen in ductal carcinoma in situ, *Semin Oncol* 33:647–649, 2006.

Schwartz GF, Allen KG, Palazzo JP: Biology and management of lobular carcinoma in situ of the breast. In Bland KI, Copeland EM, editors: *The breast*, ed 4, Philadelphia, 2009, Elsevier Science.

Silverstein MJ: Ductal carcinoma in situ: treatment, controversies and oncoplastic surgeries. In Bland KI, Copeland EM, editors: *The breast*, ed 4, Philadelphia, 2009, Elsevier Science.

Vogel VG, Costantino JP, Wickerham DL, et al: Effects of tamoxifen versus raloxifene on the risk of developing invasive breast cancer and other disease outcomes: the NSABP Study of Tamoxifen and Raloxifene (STAR) P-2 trial, *JAMA* 295:2727–2741, 2006.

Wong JS, Kaelin CM, Troyan SL, et al: Prospective study of wide excision alone for ductal carcinoma in situ of the breast, *J Clin Oncol* 24:1031–1036, 2006.

ADVANCES IN NEOADJUVANT AND ADJUVANT THERAPY FOR BREAST CANCER

Nicole Kounalakis, MD, and
Christina Finlayson, MD

OVERVIEW

Systemic therapy for breast cancer is evolving rapidly. The medical treatment of cancer includes chemotherapy, endocrine therapy, and therapy with targeted biologic agents. In the past, a patient's stage, based on tumor size and nodal involvement, would determine the recommendations for medical therapy, whereas now the biologic features of the tumor direct the treatment plan. As a result of advances in the understanding of these biologic features, individualized systemic therapy is effective, less toxic, and directed at the tumor profile. Systemic treatment may influence the surgical and radiation options; thus surgeons should be involved with these medical decisions in both the neoadjuvant and adjuvant settings. In view of the many treatment options available, a multidisciplinary approach, starting at the time of diagnosis, can provide a tailored plan that results in the best outcome for patients. The adjuvant and neoadjuvant therapy for operable stages I, II, and III breast cancer are described in this chapter.

NEOADJUVANT SYSTEMIC THERAPY

Neoadjuvant systemic therapy has many proven benefits. Its effectiveness offers valuable prognostic information, and the rates of disease-free and overall survival are equivalent to those for adjuvant therapy. Clinicians can alter therapy if the tumor does not respond and can also distinguish a subset of patients who have an improved outcome: pathologic complete response (pCR). In addition, neoadjuvant therapy has the potential to improve surgical outcomes. For women in whom at presentation mastectomy appears to be the best option, it increases the possibility for breast-conserving surgery by approximately 16%. For women who are potential candidates for breast conservation at presentation, it limits the area of resection, and cosmesis is better. Neoadjuvant systemic therapy can be delivered either as chemotherapy, with or without biologic therapy, or as hormonal therapy.

Neoadjuvant Chemotherapy

The safety and efficacy of neoadjuvant chemotherapy have been demonstrated in several randomized controlled trials. Patients who are candidates for adjuvant therapy can also be considered for neoadjuvant therapy. Neoadjuvant chemotherapy does not increase the surgical complication rate, worsen survival by delaying surgical treatment, or decrease the accuracy of findings in the sentinel lymph node biopsy (Table 1).

There is no difference in overall survival or disease-free survival benefit between neoadjuvant and adjuvant therapy. Benefits for the patient include improved prognostic information and increased opportunities for breast conservation. Patients with a pCR after neoadjuvant therapy have an improved prognosis, and patients with no response have a considerably worse prognosis. The most immediate benefit from the neoadjuvant approach occurs in patients who are candidates for mastectomy at presentation but whose treatment can potentially be converted to breast conservation if the tumor has a favorable response to treatment; the best results occur with tumors more likely to achieve a pCR. Patients more likely to have a pCR tend to be younger (<40 years of age), have a high-grade tumor with a Ki67 protein level greater than 20%, and have tumor receptors that do not have estrogen receptor (ER), progesterone receptor (PR), or *Her 2 neu* (triple negative) or are ER-negative and PR-negative and *Her 2 neu*-positive (Table 2).

For breast cancers that are either ER+ or ER– but also *Her 2 neu*–negative, standard neoadjuvant chemotherapy is a doxorubicin (Adriamycin)–based regimen for 3 to 4 months before surgery. If the patient is *Her 2 neu*–positive, trastuzumab (Herceptin) is administered with a taxane (e.g., docetaxel) and carboplatin; doxorubicin is usually omitted because of the potential for increased cardiac toxicity. The patient should be monitored during therapy with a clinical examination after each cycle. If the tumor is not clinically responding after two to three cycles, chemotherapy should be stopped, and the patient should proceed to surgery.

Neoadjuvant Endocrine Therapy

Historically, the use of neoadjuvant endocrine therapy was limited to patients whose conditions were not suitable for chemotherapy. However, several trials demonstrated similar overall response rates in postmenopausal ER/PR-positive patients treated with neoadjuvant endocrine therapy or chemotherapy. Certain tumor characteristics are predictive of a poor response to neoadjuvant chemotherapy but could be considered for neoadjuvant endocrine therapy: low-grade tumors with high ER/PR positivity, low Ki67 protein proliferative index, and certain histologic features such as lobular, tubular, and low-grade mucinous tumors (see Table 2).

For postmenopausal patients who are candidates for neoadjuvant endocrine therapy, aromatase inhibitors are recommended over tamoxifen. Several trials have shown increased rates of response, which lead to a higher rate of breast-conserving therapy with aromatase inhibitors. The P024 trial was the first to compare neoadjuvant use of letrozole with tamoxifen in postmenopausal women with locally advanced ER/PR-positive disease. The overall response rates were 55% for letrozole and 36% for tamoxifen ($P < 0.001$). Significantly more letrozole-treated patients underwent breast-conserving surgery (45% vs 35%, respectively; $P = 0.022$). Based on the American College of Surgeons Oncology Group's (ACOSOG's) Z1031 trial, no particular aromatase inhibitor is preferred in the neoadjuvant setting; exemestane, letrozole and anastrozole all had equivalent outcomes.

The duration of neoadjuvant endocrine therapy must be at least 4 months to produce an optimal response; this time period varies among patients. In those who desire a lumpectomy and are showing a good clinical response, neoadjuvant endocrine therapy can safely be extended to a maximum duration of 8 months with carefully monitoring.

At this time, premenopausal women are not considered candidates for neoadjuvant endocrine therapy outside of a clinical trial. Future research will reveal whether such patients could also benefit from this treatment approach.

Surgery After Neoadjuvant Therapy

Before the initiation of systemic therapy, the tumor must be adequately marked with clips, and biopsy samples must be taken from any lesions of concern. Tumor response should be assessed with

TABLE 1: Considerations in the timing of sentinel lymph node biopsy

Timing of sentinel lymph node biopsy	Advantages	Disadvantages
Before neoadjuvant chemotherapy	More data on false-negative rate More data to support choice of chemotherapy on basis of nodal staging Assists in preoperative decisions: need for postmastectomy radiation	ALND may be unnecessary Additional surgical procedure
After neoadjuvant chemotherapy	False-negative rate: 10% in clinically node-negative patients Reduces the need for ALND by 30% in clinically node-negative patients at presentation For clinically node-positive patients at presentation, according to findings of ACOSOG Z1071 study, the axilla can be restaged with a sentinel lymph node biopsy after chemotherapy; in 40% of patients, disease converts to node negative, and ALND may be avoided	Not as much data on false-negative rates No long-term data on rates of axillary recurrence, disease-free survival, or overall survival

ACOSOG, American College of Surgeons Oncology Group; *ALND,* axillary lymph node dissection.

TABLE 2: Tumor characteristics and responsiveness to neoadjuvant chemotherapy

Patient and clinical characteristics	Increased likelihood of pCR	Decreased likelihood of pCR
Age	<40 years	>60 years
Tumor size	<2 cm	>4 cm
Histologic features	Ductal	Lobular
Grade	High	Low
Ki67 protein level	High score >20	Low score <20
Estrogen receptor	Negative	Positive
Her2/neu	Positive	Negative

pCR, Pathologic complete response.

bimonthly clinical exams. If the clinical response is ambiguous, the breast can be imaged with ultrasonography or mammography. Evaluation of treatment response during or after neoadjuvant chemotherapy is also an accepted indication for breast magnetic resonance imaging (MRI). If the patient is receiving chemotherapy, the authors normally wait 2 to 3 weeks after the last dose of therapy or until the white blood cell count is within normal range before surgery is performed. For neoadjuvant endocrine therapy, no waiting period is necessary before surgical resection.

After the completion of systemic therapy, the surgeon and patient must decide whether a lumpectomy is feasible. Imaging with ultrasonography, mammography, or MRI, or a combination of these, can help guide this decision, but the ultimate surgical goal is to achieve negative margins, remove all malignant calcifications, and produce a cosmetically acceptable result. To achieve negative margins, a second margin excision may be necessary. In women with larger breasts, an oncoplastic approach can be used to achieve acceptable cosmesis after a larger resection. If negative margins cannot be achieved, a mastectomy with or without reconstruction should be performed.

If metastatic disease to the axilla is diagnosed before the initiation of chemotherapy, either through sentinel lymph node biopsy or through image-guided biopsy, the standard of care is to perform a lymph node dissection at the time of the tumor resection after the completion of neoadjuvant systemic therapy. The results of ACOSOG's Z1071 study, presented in abstract form at San Antonio

Breast Cancer Symposium 2012, demonstrated that with at least two nodes recovered in a sentinel lymph node biopsy after neoadjuvant chemotherapy, clinicians can accurately assess tumor response in the axilla and can reasonably assess nodal status in node-positive cases. Because neoadjuvant chemotherapy eradicated nodal disease in 40% of patients in this study, further research will dictate whether an axillary lymph node dissection can be omitted if the sentinel lymph node is negative in these patients after systemic therapy. Until that information is available, the authors recommend an axillary node dissection for most patients who had node-positive disease before neoadjuvant chemotherapy and absolutely when nodal disease persists after neoadjuvant chemotherapy.

ADJUVANT THERAPY

Endocrine Therapy

Estrogen and progesterone receptor–positive tumors constitute 75% of all breast cancers. Stimulation of these receptors by estrogen is a critical step in the development of breast cancer. Three treatment options exist to target ER/PR receptors: tamoxifen, aromatase inhibitors, and ovarian suppression or ablation.

Defining ER/PR-positive breast cancers has been a controversial topic because of the heterogeneity of expression. It is now understood that any degree of positivity qualifies patients for estrogen-targeted treatment, although the greater the degree of expression of estrogen and progesterone receptors, the greater the response to treatment.

Premenopausal Patients

Approximately one fifth of all new cases of breast cancer occur in women younger than 50 years of age, and 60% of these cases are ER-positive. Options for these patients include tamoxifen, ovarian suppression or ablation, or a combination of ovarian suppression with tamoxifen. Tamoxifen is a selective estrogen receptor modulator, and it inhibits the growth of breast cancer cells by competitively binding to the estrogen receptor. It should be offered for at least 5 years. If it is tolerated well and the tumor is aggressive, tamoxifen can be given for up to 10 years.

The benefits of tamoxifen in the adjuvant setting were clearly demonstrated from the 2011 Early Breast Cancer Trialists Collaborative Group's (EBCTCG's) meta-analysis of randomized trials. In ER-positive patients, breast cancer mortality was reduced by 30% in the first 15 years of follow-up when tamoxifen was used in the adjuvant setting for 5 years. Breast cancer recurrence was reduced by 39%. This benefit was seen in both premenopausal and in postmenopausal patients. Side effects of tamoxifen are a nonsignificant increase in stroke-related deaths and an increase risk of uterine cancer (3.8% vs 1.1% in the control group). There was a trend toward a lower incidence of cardiac deaths.

Ovarian suppression in addition to tamoxifen has shown benefit in reducing rates of breast cancer recurrence and mortality. Ovarian suppression can be accomplished with the use of luteinizing hormone–releasing hormone (LHRH) agonists. For premenopausal women, the 2007 EBCTCG meta-analysis showed that LHRH agonists alone showed a trend toward reducing recurrence (28% relative reduction, $P = 0.08$) in comparison with no further systemic treatment. When LHRH agonists were administered with tamoxifen, the risk of both recurrence and death was significantly decreased.

In a more recent trial, the North American Intergroup trial INT 0101, premenopausal patients with node-positive disease were randomly assigned to receive one of three protocols: (1) chemotherapy alone: cyclophosphamide, doxorubicin, 5-fluorouracil (CAF); (2) CAF followed by 5 years of an LHRH agonist, goserelin; or (3) CAF with both goserelin and tamoxifen. With a median follow-up period of 9.6 years, addition of tamoxifen and goserelin to CAF improved disease-free survival but not overall survival. There was no benefit to the addition of LHRH agonists to chemotherapy without tamoxifen in premenopausal women. Thus the role of LHRH agonists alone or with chemotherapy but without tamoxifen requires further investigation. There is proven benefit to administering LHRH agonists over tamoxifen and chemotherapy or tamoxifen alone. In the ongoing Suppression of Ovarian Function Trial (SOFT), treatment with tamoxifen alone is being compared with ovarian suppression plus either tamoxifen or exemestane.

For adjuvant endocrine treatment in premenopausal women with ER-positive breast cancer, current guidelines recommend the use of tamoxifen alone or in combination with ovarian suppression or ablation for at least 5 years. Aromatase inhibitors are contraindicated in premenopausal women.

Postmenopausal Patients

Standard of care for postmenopausal women with ER/PR-positive breast cancer is at least 5 years of adjuvant therapy with an aromatase inhibitor. Aromatase inhibitors decrease plasma levels of estrogen by inhibiting the synthesis of estrogens from androgenic substrates. The benefit of aromatase inhibitors over tamoxifen in postmenopausal women was demonstrated in the 2010 EBCTCG meta-analysis, which showed a reduction in both breast cancer recurrence and mortality when aromatase inhibitors were used instead of tamoxifen. There are several aromatase inhibitors and they all have similar efficacy in the adjuvant setting; no particular agent is preferred. The optimal duration of adjuvant aromatase inhibitor therapy is at least 5 years, but this duration is still being evaluated in ongoing trials. For women who do not tolerate, have a contraindication to, or decline aromatase inhibitor therapy, tamoxifen for 5 years is recommended. Women taking an aromatase inhibitor may have difficulty with joint pain, which is the most common reason for discontinuation. They should have a dual energy x-ray absorptiometry (DEXA) scan at initiation of therapy and every 1 years to evaluate bone density because progression of osteoporosis is a known side effect. Addition of a bisphosphonate to the adjuvant regimen can decrease the osteoporosis risk, as well as decrease risk of bone metastasis.

Adjuvant Chemotherapy

Molecular and Genomic Profiling

Molecular profiling has one of the longest track records as therapy for breast cancer. With the advent of measureing the presence or absence of estrogen and progesterone receptors, medicine could be personalized with antiendocrine therapy for patients who had the appropriate tumor-based targets for response. The addition of *Her 2 neu*–targeting agents and the biologic agent trastuzumab (Herceptin) further refined this patient- and tumor-specific approach to adjuvant therapy.

Genomic profiling is now used for risk stratification and therapeutic decision making. For women with ER-positive breast cancer, genomic profiling may be helpful in selecting which patients should receive adjuvant chemotherapy. Genomic profiling should not be used in patients already determined to benefit from chemotherapy or in patients with multiple comorbid conditions who would be unable to tolerate chemotherapy. Patients must be cautioned that for a favorable recurrence score, chemotherapy can be omitted only if the patient commits to 5 years of antiendocrine therapy.

The best validated prognostic molecular test is the Oncotype DX (Genomic Health, Redwood City, Calif), which is used to analyze 21 genes and has been on the commercial market since 2003. One of its benefits is that paraffin-embedded fixed tissue is used, and the test can be ordered at any time in the diagnostic process. It provides a recurrence score that is predictive of responsiveness to chemotherapy and relapse rate. The activity of 16 genes and 5 control genes on breast cancer tissue is measured, and a proprietary mathematical formula is used to develop a single recurrence score to predict the risk of distant relapse despite 5 years of tamoxifen therapy. The recurrence score was validated with the use of tissue samples and the clinical database from the National Surgical Adjuvant Breast and Bowel Project (NSABP) B-14 study, which was a prospective randomized controlled trial in which the adjuvant treatment of tamoxifen alone was compared with tamoxifen plus chemotherapy in patients with ER-positive, node-negative early-stage breast cancer. The individual recurrence scores are further stratified into low-risk (score, <18), intermediate-risk (score, 18 to 30), or high-risk (score, >30) groups. The rates of distant recurrence at 10 years were 7%, 14%, and 31%, respectively, in these groups. Not only does the Oncotype DX test provide prognostic information, but it also demonstrated that there was no additional benefit to adding chemotherapy to the treatment regimen of a woman in the low-risk group. Other studies have shown similar scores and results when aromatase inhibitors are used instead of tamoxifen for postmenopausal women.

The true cutoff for the recurrence score number that defines who would benefit from chemotherapy is in the process of further refinement. The Trial Assigning IndividuaLized Options for Treatment

(Rx) (TAILORx) is an evaluation of differences in response for women with recurrence scores from 11 to 25. In this study, patients with ER-positive, node-negative, *Her 2 neu*–positive cancer and recurrence scores in the range of 11 to 25 are randomly assigned to receive either endocrine therapy alone or chemotherapy followed by endocrine therapy.

Oncotype DX has also expanded testing to patients who are ER positive with one to three positive lymph nodes. The study set which validated this application was much smaller, with 367 participants. A retrospective analysis of the NSABP B-28 trial presented at the 2012 Breast Cancer Symposium calculated the Oncotype recurrence score in 1065 node positive, ER/PR+ patients who had received chemotherapy plus adjuvant TAM. The recurrence score was a significant independent predictor of disease free and overall survival. Since all of these patients had received chemotherapy, the data suggests that Oncotype DX may be useful in assessing the risk of locoregional recurrence and therefore may guide the decision of adjuvant radiation therapy. The final published results from this NSABP study will have to be reviewed prior to using the Oncotype in node positive ER+ patients.

Another molecular profiling product is the Amsterdam 70-gene profile, Mammaprint (Agendia, Amsterdam, Netherlands), in which a microarray analysis of gene expression is used on breast cancer tissue. It is used to determine the prognosis of patients with breast cancer and can be used for all tumors, including node-positive, *Her 2 neu*–positive, and ER/PR-negative disease. A low score is correlated with an increased risk of distant metastasis at 10 years, although it does not provide information on the responsiveness to chemotherapy. Although this test previously required fresh tissue, paraffin-embedded tissue can now be used, which has extended the clinical situations in which the test can be performed. The clinical utility of this test is still unclear. A large international study, Microarray In Node Negative Disease May Avoid Chemotherapy (MINDACT), is underway to test node-negative tumors with the Mammaprint. Patients with discordant clinical and genomic characteristics are randomly assigned to either receive or not receive chemotherapy. The results of this trial are still pending.

Several other molecular tests are in use. All breast cancer molecular tests should be used to augment, not replace, known prognostic clinical factors. Despite the ability of these tests to assign prognosis or responsiveness to chemotherapy, they do not assist in determining the optimal chemotherapeutic agent for individuals. Current guidelines indicate that adjuvant therapy should be considered on the basis of clinical and tumor characteristics, life expectancy, and comorbid conditions.

Chemotherapy

Several regimens of adjuvant chemotherapy are accepted for the *Her 2 neu*–negative tumor. These agents are usually represented by their first letter, and the medical record often looks like alphabet soup. An early standard—cyclophosphamide, methotrexate, and 5-fluorouracil—gave way to regimens based on anthracycline (doxorubin or epirubicin) and a taxane (Taxol and Taxotere). More recently, the regimen of docetaxel plus cyclophosphamide has been added to the menu of options because it confers excellent survival and fewer long-term sequelae. There also is no single standard dosing regimen for these drugs. The recent Eastern Cooperative Oncology Group (ECOG) 1199 trial showed that out of four possible dosing strategies, doxorubicin plus cyclophosphamide followed by 12 weekly doses of paclitaxel proved to be the superior regimen in terms of both disease-free and overall survival rates, at the cost of an increase in peripheral neuropathy. The duration of this regimen is approximately 4 months. Dose-dense chemotherapy is another schedule commonly utilized for early-stage breast cancer. This decreases the time interval between cycles of doxorubicin plus cyclophosphamide from the traditional 3 weeks to 2 weeks. This schedule has been associated with an improvement in disease-free survival rates but more on-treatment

side effects. Patients with triple-negative tumors derive the greatest benefit.

The role of anthracyclines in treating early-stage breast cancer has become controversial. It is unclear whether adding a taxane to the standard regimen decreases the need for an anthracycline in certain patients. Anthracyclines have been associated with increased cardiac toxicity, especially in patients with a history of either cardiac disease or radiation therapy. Patients are now living longer as breast cancer survivors, and the seriousness of cardiac toxicity should not be minimized. In US Oncology Adjuvant Trial 9735, patients with stages I to III *Her 2 neu*–negative cancers were randomly assigned to receive either a regimen of docetaxel plus cyclophosphamide or a regimen of doxorubicin plus cyclophosphamide. This trial has had a median follow-up period of 7 years, and docetaxel plus cyclophosphamide improved disease-free survival (81% vs 75%) and overall survival (87% vs 82%).

Her 2 neu–Targeted Therapy

Approximately 20% of all breast cancers demonstrate amplification of the *Her 2 neu* oncogene. Women with stages I to III breast cancer and *Her 2 neu* overexpression should be considered for adjuvant treatment with chemotherapy and trastuzumab.

Before the use of trastuzumab, several studies had shown that patients with *Her 2 neu*–positive tumors smaller than 1 cm have a higher risk of recurrence than women with *Her 2 neu*–negative tumors of the same size. The current National Comprehensive Cancer Network guidelines recommend that trastuzumab and chemotherapy be administered for node-negative, *Her 2 neu*–positive tumors larger than 6 mm (stage T1b) and for all node-positive tumors.

Trastuzumab is the only *Her 2 neu*–directed agent to result in a survival benefit when administered with chemotherapy in the adjuvant setting. In a joint analysis of data from the North Central Cancer Treatment Group's (NCCTG's) N9831 trial and the NSABP's B-31 trial, treatment of *Her 2 neu*–positive disease with chemotherapy alone (doxorubicin plus cyclophosphamide followed by paclitaxel) was compared with chemotherapy with trastuzumab; the latter produced an improvement in disease-free survival and a 39% significant reduction in death.

Trastuzumab does increase the risk of congestive heart failure and decreases left ventricular ejection fraction. The choice of which chemotherapy regimen to administer with trastuzumab depends on the patient's preexisting cardiac condition. Some regimens include anthracyclines (anthracycline, carboplatin, and taxotere [ACT]) and others do not (taxotere carboplatin: docetaxel plus cyclophosphamide). In comparison with ACT and trastuzumab, docetaxel plus cyclophosphamide with trastuzumab was found to produce a higher incidence of congestive heart failure (0.4% vs 2%) and a lower incidence of sustained loss of mean left ventricular ejection fraction (18.6% versus 9.%; Table 3). Because cardiac toxicity is known to be associated with trastuzumab alone and when combined with anthracyclines, there is a shift toward regimens that do not include anthracyclines, inasmuch as they appear to be equivalent in efficacy.

Trastuzumab is administered intravenously concomitantly with chemotherapy and then after the completion of the chemotherapy, for a total of 52 weeks. No data support the use of trastuzumab with endocrine therapy instead of chemotherapy for patients with triple-positive disease. Endocrine therapy should be administered with trastuzumab after the completion of chemotherapy.

Lapatinib is an oral *Her 2 neu*–directed agent. The current data show that there is no role for lapatinib in the adjuvant setting after chemotherapy for stages I to III breast cancer. Whether the combination of lapatinib plus trastuzumab with chemotherapy will improve survival in the adjuvant setting is currently being investigated in the Adjuvant Lapatinib and/or Trastuzumab Treatment Optimization (ALTTO) study.

TABLE 3: Timing and major side effects of systemic therapy

Systemic agent class: specific agent	Time of treatment	Side effect
Taxanes: docetaxel, paclitaxel	Neoadjuvant, adjuvant	Cutaneous reaction Motor and sensory neuropathy Embryo-fetus toxicity Myelosuppression
Anthracyclines: doxorubicin (Adriamycin), epirubicin	Neoadjuvant, adjuvant	Cardiomyopathy, congestive heart failure Myelosuppression
Carboplatin	Neoadjuvant, adjuvant	Neuropathy Myelosuppression
Trastuzumab	Neoadjuvant, adjuvant	With doxorubicin: cumulative risk of congestive heart failure; decreased left ventricular ejection fraction Cardiomyopathy, embryo-fetus toxicity, pulmonary toxicity
Aromatase inhibitors: anastrozole, exemestane, letrozole	Neoadjuvant, adjuvant	Arthralgias, myalgias, osteoporosis, embryo-fetus toxicity
Tamoxifen	Adjuvant	Blood clots, endometrial cancer, ovarian cysts, embryo-fetus toxicity

SUMMARY

The array of systemic options and treatment regimens available to patients with breast cancer is progressing rapidly. These options include endocrine, cytotoxic, and targeted agents that can now be administered with improved efficacy and less toxicity. Molecular profiling has become a valuable asset in creating a treatment plan. Patients who will benefit most from chemotherapy or targeted biologic agents can be identified and treated accordingly. In contrast, patients who derive minimal benefit from chemotherapy can now avoid this toxicity and be treated instead with antiendocrine therapy. Determining the appropriateness of neoadjuvant therapy for a particular patient can improve surgical outcomes and provide prognostic information.

For surgeons, an understanding of how these therapies will affect patients' local control options is important. The authors recommend that each patient with cancer be seen by a multidisciplinary team to allow discussion of these various options. Sometimes these teams practice in one location, but often the multidisciplinary approach requires close collaboration among colleagues who do not practice in physically adjacent spaces. Close coordination and integration of breast cancer specialists through a multidisciplinary team leads to improved outcomes for patients. A dialogue between diagnostic specialists (imagers, pathologists) and therapeutic specialists (breast and plastic surgeons, radiation and medical oncologists) can lead to the optimal treatment strategy. The most significant advances in breast cancer have resulted from physicians' ability to provide an individualized treatment plan, and this can be realized only through a multidisciplinary approach.

SUGGESTED READINGS

Alba E, Calvo L, Albanell J, et al: Chemotherapy (CT) and hormonotherapy (HT) as neoadjuvant treatment in luminal breast cancer patients: results from the GEICAM/2006-03, a multicenter, randomized, phase-II study, *Ann Oncol* 23:3069–3074, 2012.

Dowsett M, Cuzick J, Ingle J, et al: Meta-analysis of breast cancer outcomes in adjuvant trials of aromatase inhibitors versus tamoxifen, *J Clin Oncol* 28:509–518, 2010.

Moja L, Tagliabue L, Balduzzi S, et al: Trastuzumab containing regimens for early breast cancer, *Cochrane Database Syst Rev* (4):CD006243, 2012.

Montagna E, Bagnardi V, Rotmensz N, et al: Pathological complete response after preoperative systemic therapy and outcome: relevance of clinical and biologic baseline features, *Breast Cancer Res Treat* 124:689–699, 2010.

Paik S, Shak S, Tang G, et al: A multigene assay to predict recurrence of tamoxifen-treated, node-negative breast cancer, *N Engl J Med* 351:2817–2826, 2004.

Peto R, Davies C, Godwin J, et al: Comparisons between different polychemotherapy regimens for early breast cancer: meta-analyses of long-term outcome among 100,000 women in 123 randomised trials, *Lancet* 379:432–444, 2012.

Rastogi P, Anderson SJ, Bear HD, et al: Preoperative chemotherapy: updates of National Surgical Adjuvant Breast and Bowel Project Protocols B-18 and B-27, *J Clin Oncol* 26:778–785, 2008.

Slamon D, Eiermann W, Robert N, et al: Adjuvant trastuzumab in HER2-positive breast cancer, *N Engl J Med* 365:1273–1283, 2011.

The Management of Recurrent and Disseminated Breast Cancer

Edwin O. Onkendi, MB, ChB, and
Judy C. Boughey, MD

INTRODUCTION

Invasive breast cancer remains the most common malignancy among females in the United States, constituting 30% of all new cancer cases and 15% of all cancer deaths among women. With the current advances in breast cancer screening, many breast cancers are diagnosed at an early stage, which, together with advances in neoadjuvant and adjuvant systemic and regional therapies, has resulted in most patients with breast cancer having longer survival than before. About 10% to 20% of stage I to III breast cancers recur locoregionally, with the risk of relapse higher with lymph node–positive and larger tumors. Despite this fact, no significant differences in disease-free survival, distant disease-free survival, or overall survival have been shown by multiple randomized controlled trials with long-term follow-up between mastectomy and breast conservation therapy (BCT; breast-conserving therapy, lumpectomy with adjuvant radiation therapy). The Early Breast Cancer Trialists' Collaborative Group (EBCTCG), however, performed an overview of randomized trials and showed that local recurrence and survival are linked. The EBCTCG estimates that for every 4 local recurrences prevented at 5 years, 1 death is prevented at 15 years.

BCT is known to be associated with higher rates of ipsilateral in-breast tumor recurrence (IBTR) compared with mastectomy. Isolated IBTR rates range from 8.8% at 20 years in the Milan study to 14.3% at 20 years in the National Surgical Adjuvant Breast and Bowel Project (NSABP-06) trial to 22% at 18 years in the National Cancer Institute study. The difference in IBTR rates across the studies is explained by the differing inclusion criteria and methods, specifically tumor sizes, and margin status. IBTR has been shown to be associated with poorer survival and distant metastasis. Advances in our understanding of tumor biology and improvements in early detection, operative techniques, systemic therapies, and radiation delivery have resulted in improvement in the locoregional control rates over historical studies.

RELAPSE PATTERNS AND DEFINITIONS

Breast cancer relapse can occur in various forms. The most common forms of relapse are:

1. Local recurrence (in-breast tumor recurrence [IBTR] or chest wall).
2. Regional recurrence (axillary, internal mammary, or infraclavicular lymph nodes).
3. Distant recurrence (metastasis to bone, lung, liver, brain, and other sites).

IBTR refers to breast cancer recurrence within the ipsilateral preserved breast after breast-conserving surgery. IBTRs are classified by location into:

1. True recurrence (a recurrence at the original lumpectomy site or within the boost volume of the preserved breast).
2. Marginal miss (a recurrence close to but not within the boost volume).
3. Elsewhere recurrence, or recurrence in other quadrants, other than the quadrant previously involved by the original breast cancer.

True recurrences and marginal misses constitute about 80% of IBTRs. True breast cancer recurrences and new ipsilateral primary breast cancer have been shown to have different natural histories and prognoses. These two entities can be distinguished based on histologic subtype, hormone receptor status, human epidermal growth factor receptor–2 (HER2) overexpression, tumor location, and discordant DNA flow cytometry. New ipsilateral primary breast cancer is associated with significantly better survival and lower rates of distant metastases than true recurrences. New ipsilateral primary breast cancer has been defined as tumor located more than 3 cm from the original primary tumor site (with breast imaging or clinical examination) that is of a different histology from the primary tumor or whose estrogen receptor (ER)/progesterone receptor (PR) or Her 2 neu status is different from the original primary tumor. On the other hand, a true recurrence has been defined as tumor located within 3 cm of the primary tumor bed or whose histologic subtype or ER/PR and Her 2 neu status is consistent with the primary tumor. Some authors have suggested that molecular classification is a reliable method of distinguishing these two entities.

Chest wall recurrence denotes recurrence that occurs in the preserved skin, nipple-areolar complex, subcutaneous tissue, remaining breast tissue, pectoral muscle, fascia, ribs, or intercostal muscles after any of the different types of mastectomy with or without reconstruction.

Regional recurrence refers to recurrence in the draining lymph nodes, usually axillary or supraclavicular and occasionally in the infraclavicular or internal mammary lymph nodes. Distant metastases most commonly involve bone or visceral organs (lung, liver, brain, and abdominopelvic organs).

THERAPEUTIC PRINCIPLES AND STRATEGIES

Ipsilateral Breast Tumor Recurrence After Breast-Conserving Therapy

Preoperative Considerations

IBTR after BCT is resectable in up to 85% of cases. When patients present with localized IBTR that is amenable to operative resection, mastectomy is the standard approach and can be performed once the patient has undergone staging with positron emission tomography (PET) scan or computed tomographic (CT) scan and bone scan to rule out distant metastases. Repeat breast-conserving surgery may be technically feasible. However, it is associated with a higher rate of re-recurrence, especially if the first recurrence occurred within 5 years of resection of the primary tumor, with 90% of these invasive. Many of the recurrences after 5 years following treatment of primary tumor are second primary cancers. Repeat breast-conserving surgery is also not recommended for these patients because repeat adjuvant breast radiation therapy to prevent future recurrence cannot be administered to the previously irradiated tissues. Patients who did not receive radiation after the initial breast-conserving surgery may be candidates for BCT with full-dose radiation of the whole breast, although data are limited. About 10% to 20% of patients are classified as inoperable because of advanced local or regional recurrences or synchronous distant metastases. Patients with locally advanced recurrences (large or fixed tumors, skin or chest wall involvement, or inflammatory carcinomas) or regionally advanced disease should undergo neoadjuvant systemic therapy before consideration of surgical intervention. Skin recurrences are associated with higher incidence of distant metastases and uncontrolled local disease and a poor overall outcome.

Choice of Operation

Mastectomy is the standard treatment recommended for operable IBTR after BCT.

A standard simple/total mastectomy is often recommended because these patients have had previous breast radiation, which complicates options for immediate reconstruction. For patients who wish to pursue immediate reconstruction, discussion with a plastic and reconstructive surgeon and counseling of the patient regarding potential risks and complications associated with reconstruction in a radiated field is needed. Use of autologous tissue flap is recommended in these situations. The choice depends on patient preferences, extent of tumor, skin involvement, and timing of breast reconstruction. Skin-sparing mastectomy can be performed as long as there is no skin involvement. Use of nipple-sparing mastectomy in patients with IBTR and previous radiation has not been studied and lacks oncologic safety data.

The choice of incision depends on the type of mastectomy, location of the tumor, previous surgical scars, and skin involvement by tumor. For most cases, a standard simple mastectomy incision can be used. Care should be taken when designing the incision so the old surgical incision and any involved skin is resected along with the skin incorporated in the mastectomy incision where possible to avoid multiple scars on the chest wall.

Occasionally, patients treated with lumpectomy decline adjuvant radiation therapy and present with recurrent disease in the breast. In these cases, the lack of previous radiation simplifies the management. Mastectomy remains the standard recommendation. Although repeat breast conservation can be performed, the oncologic safety of this approach is not established. In addition, depending on breast size, tumor size, and extent of previous lumpectomy, cosmesis may be challenging with a second lumpectomy in the same breast. If lumpectomy is performed for recurrence, clips should be placed in the lumpectomy bed to mark the cavity for the delivery of the radiation boost. Adjuvant whole-breast radiation is strongly recommended, and patients who remain unprepared to consider adjuvant radiation are better served with mastectomy.

Technical Factors During Mastectomy for In-Breast Tumor Recurrence

In patients who have previously undergone breast-conserving surgery and adjuvant breast radiation, care should be taken during the development of the skin flaps because of radiation-associated microvascular changes that result in a tenuous blood supply to the skin and predispose the flaps to a higher risk of flap ischemia and necrosis. Because of the fibrosis from the previous radiation, the plane between the breast tissue and subcutaneous tissue may be harder to visualize. Care is necessary in the area of the previous lumpectomy scar to avoid skin flap necrosis. Attention is also required in the area of the recurrent tumor to ensure adequate margins are achieved, with resection of the skin overlying the tumor or the underlying muscle if needed. With dissection of the breast from the underlying pectoralis muscle, this plane is often fibrosed from the previous radiation and requires additional attention to avoid leaving breast tissue behind or damaging the muscle.

Complications and Their Prevention

An increased risk of seroma and wound healing complications is found in patients who have had prior breast radiation. The surgeon should attempt to minimize the risk of these complications. The risk of seroma formation may be reduced with use of quilting sutures, which involves mastectomy flap fixation with absorbable sutures.

Because of the microvascular changes that occur after breast radiation, there is an increased risk of skin flap necrosis. Meticulous surgical technique during mastectomy should be maintained to minimize this risk. SPY angiography (Novadaq Spy angiography system; Novadaq Technologies, Inc, Concord, Ontario, Canada) may be performed to evaluate breast cutaneous blood flow before surgery to assist in operative planning or during surgery to evaluate mastectomy flap viability and perfusion after mastectomy before reconstruction (Figure 1). This technique has been described in the literature for evaluation of reconstructive flaps and coronary artery bypass grafts. It is performed with intravenous injection of 5 mL of indocyanine green and then use of the SPY angiography camera to evaluate the perfusion of the mastectomy flaps. Preoperative SPY images usually show the decreased blood flow to the mastectomy flaps on the radiated side compared with the contralateral nonradiated side (see Figure 1). SPY angiography can be used to guide plastic surgeons regarding the appropriate volume of fluid to place in an expander and minimize risk of skin flap necrosis.

Recurrence After Mastectomy

Preoperative Considerations

Breast cancer recurrence after mastectomy is less common than recurrence after breast-conserving surgery. However, local recurrences after mastectomy can be more difficult to manage and are associated with a higher rate of distant metastasis and grave prognosis. Feasibility of resection should be assessed with physical examination, ultrasound scan, and magnetic resonance imaging (MRI). Local

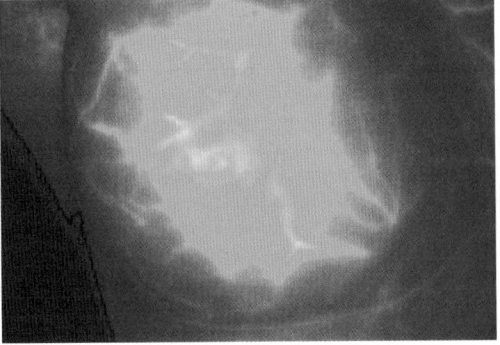
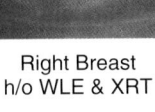

Right Breast
h/o WLE & XRT

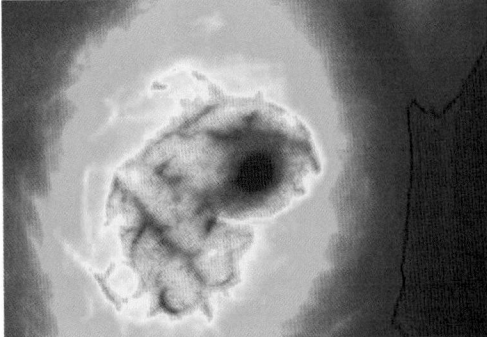

Left Breast

FIGURE 1 SPY angiography shows perfusion of breast skin. This patient had a history of lumpectomy and radiation on the right. In comparison of the perfusion on the right with the left before any surgical intervention, the SPY angiography clearly documents decreased perfusion on the side with the previous radiation.

recurrence may involve the skin, chest wall, muscle, or ribs and requires wide local excision of the involved structures. Preoperative evaluation should include a multidisciplinary team discussion including medical and radiation oncology, breast surgeon, and plastic surgeon. The patient should be evaluated for distant disease with use of PET scan and additional imaging as indicated. Systemic neoadjuvant chemotherapy or hormonal therapy or both should be considered for large recurrences to decrease the extent of surgery necessary. After systemic therapy, if no evidence of distant disease is found, curative resection should be considered if complete resection is feasible. These patients often end up with large wound defects after excision of the recurrence and may require input from a plastic surgeon to close the resulting wounds. Therefore, before surgery, the surgeon should carefully estimate the extent of resection that will be required. A thoracic surgeon should be involved if the tumor involves the bony chest wall and resection of involved rib cage is anticipated.

Technical Tips

Patients with skin or chest wall recurrence require wide resections to obtain negative margins; closure of the resulting wound may be difficult primarily depending on the size of the lesion and laxity of the skin at the mastectomy site and any prior radiation to the area. Often the recurrent disease, especially recurrence in the skin, may extend further histologically than can be seen with visual and imaging evaluation of the chest wall. In planning the incision either before or during surgery, multiple punch biopsies of skin areas beyond those areas that are hyperemic or contain petechiae or other suspicious skin changes may be performed with pathologic analysis for disease. After resection to grossly normal margins, intraoperative frozen analysis is

helpful to guide the intraoperative decision making regarding further resection of the adjacent tissue and skin and evaluation of the deep margins.

In patients in whom resection resulted in large skin defects, different options exist for achieving wound closure (Figure 2, A). The goal is to achieve closure of the wound with skin to allow for subsequent adjuvant radiation in many cases. These options include local skin primary closure, local advancement flaps, DermaClose device-assisted delayed primary closure (DermaClose RC, Wound Care Technologies, Inc., Chanhassen, Minn), skin grafts, local vascularized pedicle flaps, and free flaps.

Local advancement skin flaps can be created by undermining the skin and subcutaneous tissues to the clavicle superiorly, the sternal border medially, the posterior axillary line posteriorly, and onto the abdomen inferiorly. After this mobilization, the wound edges may be temporarily approximated with clamps. If too much tension arises during this process, the skin flap perfusion may be assessed with the SPY angiography described previously and tense areas of skin with poor perfusion should be identified and tension decreased in these areas. Well-perfused areas may then be approximated with interrupted vertical mattress sutures starting in the peripheries. Often, a defect remains in the center of the wound that cannot safely be approximated. In this case, a DermaClose device may be applied to this defect and appropriate tension applied (Figure 2, B). SPY angiography may again be used to reassess the perfusion of the skin flaps and the wound edges. The tension of the DermaClose may be progressively increased over several days to approximate the wound edges to facilitate subsequent delayed primary closure (Figure 2, C).

When a positive deep margin is found at the level of the ribs, rib resection may be necessary (Figure 3, A). This is associated with a high rate of pneumothorax, usually from parietal pleural disruption.

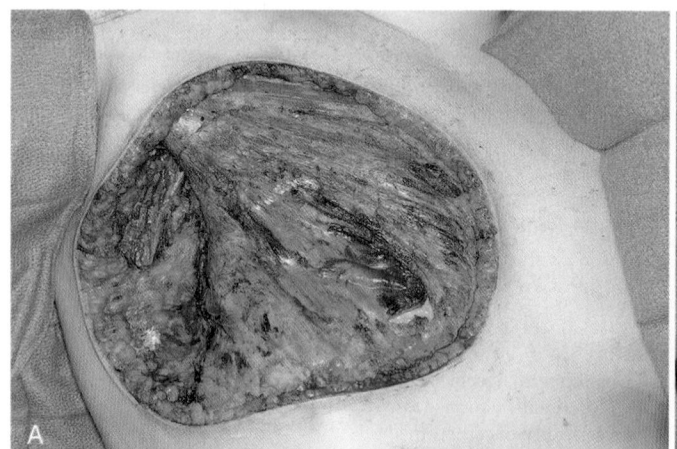

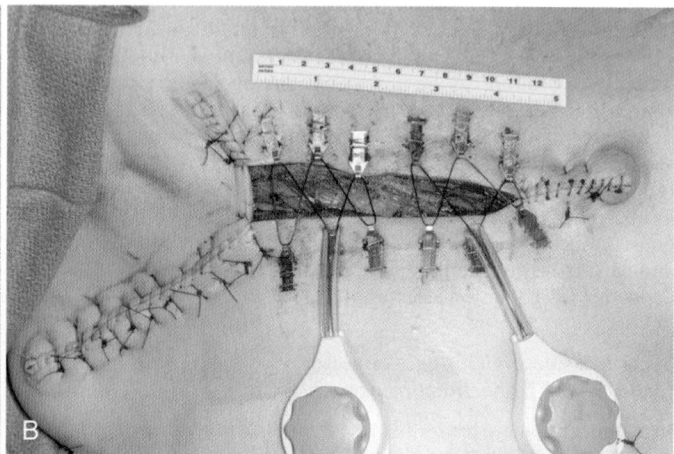

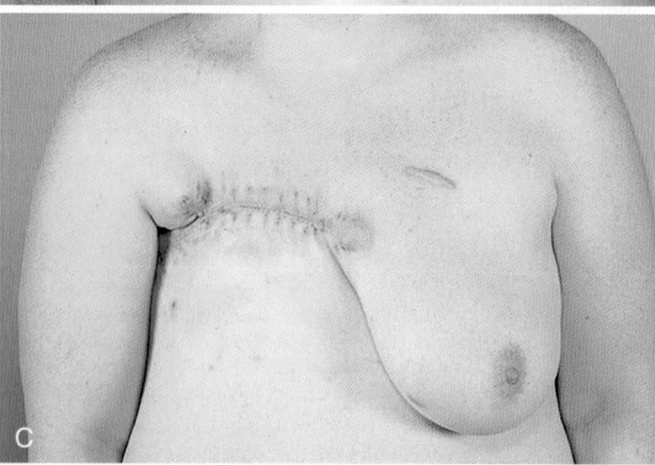

FIGURE 2 **A,** Surgical bed after mastectomy in a patient who underwent mastectomy for a local recurrence that involved a large area of the breast and overlying skin and the ipsilateral axilla without any evidence of distant metastatic disease. The figure shows the exposed pectoralis major muscle and lack of any overlying or adjacent skin for closure. **B,** Skin flaps were undermined inferiorly onto the abdomen and laterally to create advancement flaps and allow the skin edges to come together. A DermaClose device (DermaClose RC, Wound Care Technologies, Inc., Chanhassen, Minn) was then placed to apply continuous tension across the skin flaps to bring them together. **C,** Final results. The entire defect is covered with full-thickness skin without requiring a split-thickness skin graft or autologous tissue flap for closure.

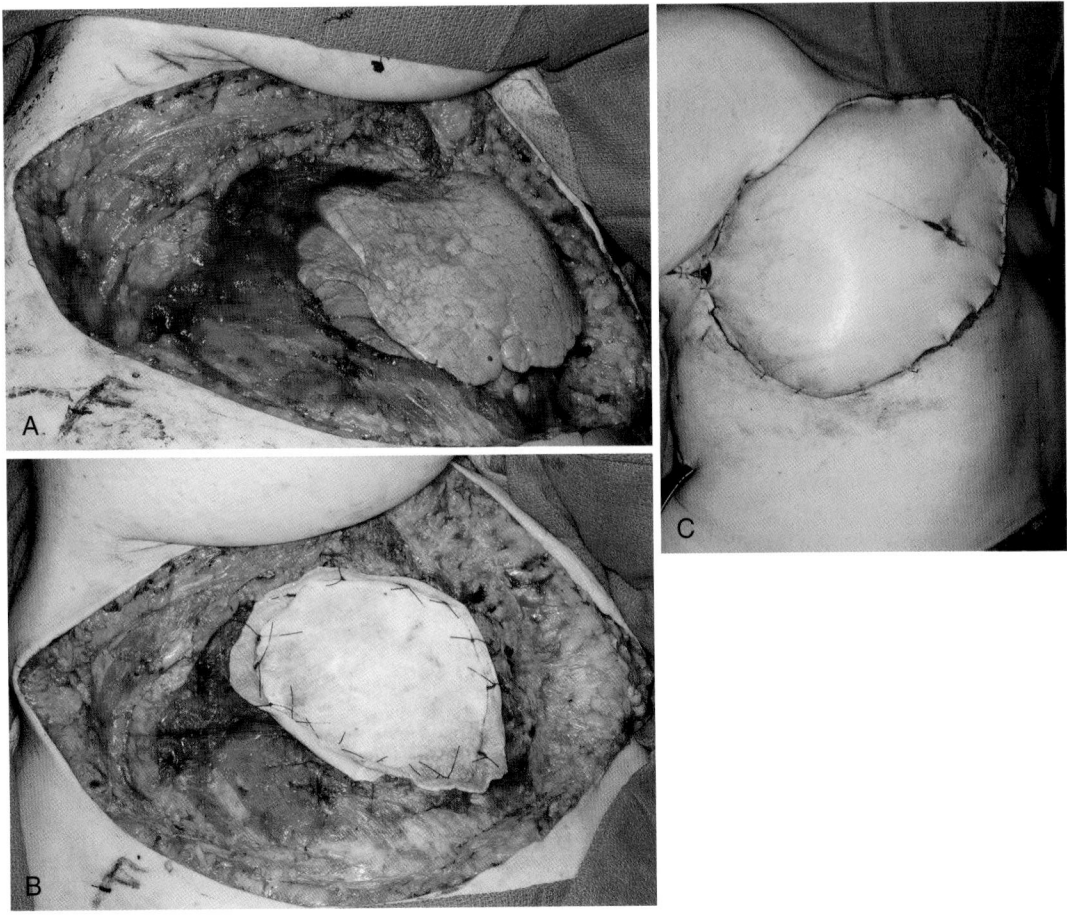

FIGURE 3   A, Resection of local recurrence includes skin, muscle, and en bloc resection of underlying ribs, resulting in exposed lung. **B,** Coverage of chest wall defect with mesh. **C,** Closure of soft tissue defect with use of a transverse abdominis musculocutaneous (TRAM) flap.

It may also be associated with hemothorax. A chest tube should be placed if there is disruption or en bloc resection of the parietal pleura. In this case, however, the cause of a pneumothorax is external atmospheric air gaining entry into the pleural space and not a visceral pleural leak, unless a visceral pleural disruption is known to have occurred. Therefore, airtight closure and dressing help prevent persistence of the pneumothorax. The resulting chest wall defects after en bloc resection of ribs with exposed lung may be closed with mesh, typically a biologic mesh (Figure 3, *B),* and covered with a local advancement flap, pedicled flap, or free flap (Figure 3, *C).*

Nodal Staging of Recurrent Breast Cancer after Breast Conservation or Mastectomy

Ability to perform repeat nodal staging at the time of recurrence depends on the extent of the previous nodal surgery performed for the index breast cancer and prior breast surgery and radiation therapy received. Physical examination and ultrasound scan examination of the regional nodal basins to include ipsilateral axilla, supraclavicular nodal basin, and internal mammary nodes is recommended with fine-needle aspiration or core needle biopsy of any suspicious lymph nodes. Patients with positive axillary lymph nodes should undergo axillary lymph node dissection.

In patients with clinically negative lymph nodes (i.e., no palpable lymph nodes and sonographically negative nodes), sentinel lymph node (SLN) mapping should be considered and has been shown to be feasible, although limited data are found on the false-negative rate in this situation.

SLN can provide valuable information to assist in planning adjuvant therapy and potentially avoiding the morbidity of axillary lymph node dissection (ALND). However, previous breast surgery and radiation with SLN surgery or ALND may have interfered with the native lymphatic drainage patterns and resulted in contralateral axillary drainage or extra-axillary drainage to the internal mammary or other nodal basins (Figure 4).

Therefore, a preoperative lymphoscintigraphy with imaging should be performed to map out the lymphatic drainage of the current tumor, even in patients who have previously undergone an ipsilateral ALND. Blue dye injection in addition to radiolabeled colloid should be used during surgery to assist in lymph node mapping.

Studies have shown that SLNs could be identified in 65% of patients with IBTR after BCT. SLNs were identified in 70% of patients in whom less than 10 lymph nodes (LNs) had been removed during the initial surgery, and the SLN success rate was 67% if more than 10 LNs had been removed at the initial surgery. The incidence of alternative lymphatic drainage (extra-axillary or internal mammary) increased as the number of axillary lymph nodes removed during the initial surgery increased or if mastectomy or radiation was part of the initial treatment. A similar study from Memorial Sloan-Kettering Cancer Center reported success in identification of a SLN in 75% of patients who had less than 10 LNs removed at the initial surgery and 44% in those who had had more than 10 LNs removed. SLN identification rates in the literature in patients with local recurrence after initial mastectomy range from 40% to 50%. In patients with a previously undissected axilla with large tumors and high-risk disease,

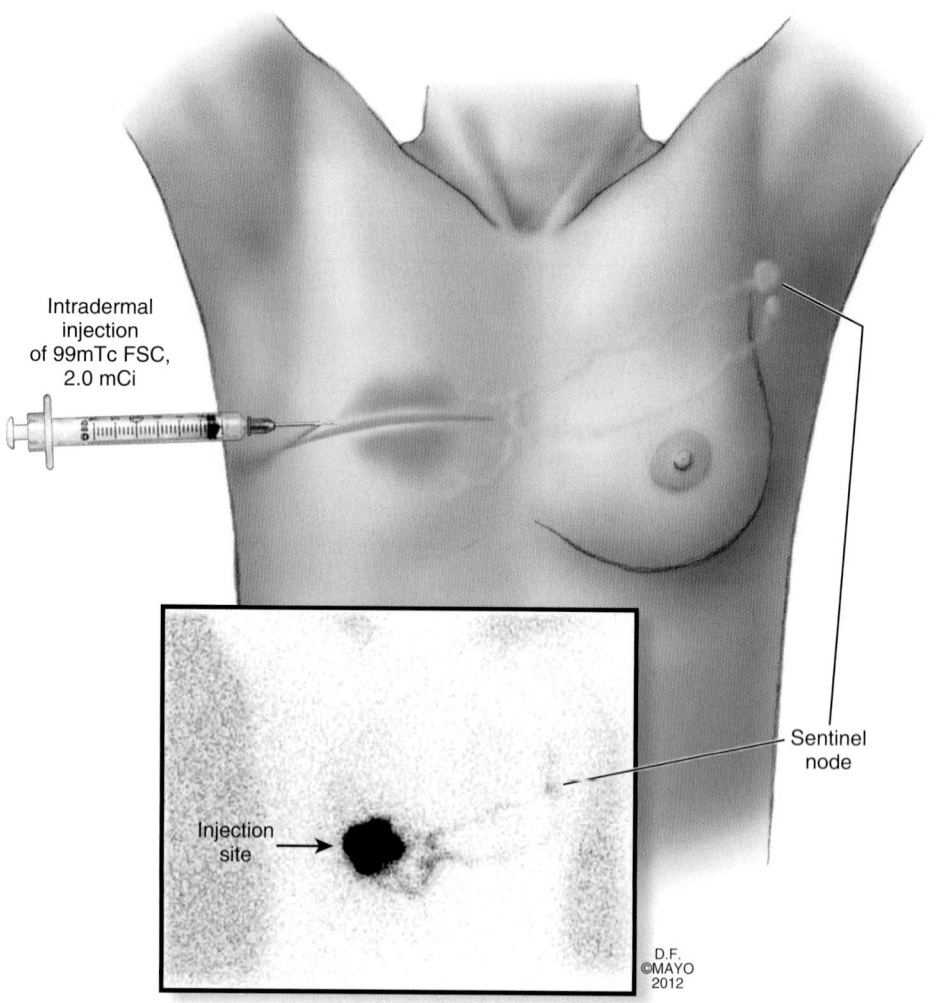

Intradermal injection of 99mTc FSC, 2.0 mCi

Injection site

Sentinel node

D.F.
©MAYO
2012

FIGURE 4 Injection at the site of recurrent breast cancer after previous right mastectomy with lymphoscintigraphic mapping showing drainage to the contralateral (left) axilla. *(Courtesy of Mayo Clinic.)*

ALND can be considered given the lack of false-negative data on SLN in this situation.

Adjuvant chemotherapy or hormonal therapy should be strongly considered. If the patient has not had prior radiation therapy, adjuvant radiotherapy should also be considered in addition to systemic therapy. In patients with unresectable tumors, palliative chemotherapy may be the only option.

Lymph Node Recurrence

The incidence of axillary and supraclavicular lymph node recurrences in patients who have undergone previous axillary lymph node dissection is 0.7% and 1.3%, respectively, at 7 years. In the presentinel lymph node era, the incidence rate of axillary nodal recurrences in patients who did not undergo ALND was about 20%. In the current sentinel lymph node sampling era, patients with SLN-negative disease had nodal recurrences develop less than 1% of the time.

On the basis of the results of the American College of Surgeons Oncology Group (ACOSOG) Z0011 randomized controlled trial, the use of ALND in patients with a positive SLN is decreasing. ACOSOG Z0011 enrolled patients with clinical T1 or T2 breast cancer treated with breast-conserving surgery with one or two positive SLNs and receiving whole-breast radiation and randomized them to either completion ALND or no further axillary surgery (SLN alone without any specific axillary treatment). This study showed no significant difference in the rate of ipsilateral axillary nodal recurrences in

patients with positive SLNs who underwent ALND (0.5% at 6.3 years) compared with those with positive SLNs who did not undergo ALND (0.9% at 6.3 years). There was also no difference in survival between the two groups.

Patients who present with axillary recurrence and who were previously SLN-negative or those who did not undergo ALND should undergo axillary lymph node dissection. For patients with axillary recurrence treated with a prior ALND, a redo axillary dissection can be performed if residual tissue is present, or a localized excision of the recurrent disease is possible in cases with minimal residual axillary tissue. Patients with nodal recurrence benefit from subsequent adjuvant systemic therapy and radiation therapy if not contraindicated based on previous radiation fields.

Technical Tips

Axillary Lymph Node Dissection

The incision from the previous sentinel node surgery or previous axillary dissection should be used if present and extended as needed for adequate exposure in the axilla. If no prior scar is found, a curvilinear or a lazy S incision 1 cm below the hair-bearing portion of the axilla is used. The extent of the previous axillary surgery and the amount of scar tissue present affect the complexity of dissection. Paralytics should be avoided so the nerves can be easily identified, and dissection should be performed slowly and meticulously to avoid damage to the nerves. The nerves can be difficult to identify and may not be in their usual anatomic location depending on scarring from prior surgery and any prior radiation. Use of clips and scissors rather than electrocautery is recommended.

Superior and inferior subcutaneous flaps are created, and the axilla is entered by incising the clavipectoral fascia. Adequate exposure is obtained with medial and cephalad retraction of the pectoralis major muscle. Two other retractors are used to triangulate the wound. The next step should be to define the axillary dissection borders and identify the important structures. The borders of axillary dissection are the axillary vein superiorly, the pectoralis muscles superomedially, the latissimus dorsi posterolaterally, and the serratus anterior and fascia medially. The initial dissection of the axilla should begin with the identification of the axillary vein superiorly. The medial pectoral nerve is then identified and preserved. The surgeon should avoid dissection cephalad to the inferior border of the axillary vein. Dissection is begun along the inferior border of the axillary vein with ligation or clipping of small venous or lymphatic vessels. The thoracoepigastric vein should then be identified because it is a very important landmark to identify and protect the thoracodorsal neurovascular bundle, which usually lies deep to this vein. The thoracoepigastric vein may invariably be ligated. The thoracodorsal neurovascular bundle is isolated and preserved. Dissection continues along the pectoralis minor muscle to the chest wall, with identification and protection of the medial pectoral nerve. Dissection along the pectoralis minor muscle to the chest wall with retraction of this muscle medially allows the level II lymph nodes to be dissected away and the intercostobrachial nerves to be identified coursing from the chest wall laterally. The long thoracic nerve of Bell enters the axilla deep to the axillary vein and courses posterior to the intercostobrachial and along the lateral border of the serratus anterior deep to the superficial fascia. It is identified deep to the serratus anterior fascia on the medial chest wall and should be preserved. Sometimes, in the lower axilla, a small vein that is a tributary of the thoracodorsal vein may course from the long thoracic nerve and help in identification. Once these major structures have been identified, one is then ready to proceed to removal of the axillary nodal tissue. With the thoracodorsal neurovascular bundle and the long thoracic nerve kept visible at all times, the fibrofatty tissue between them that contains the axillary nodes is bluntly dissected from the axilla, starting from the inferior border of the axillary vein and proceeding caudally and off the subscapularis muscle with skeletonization of the thoracodorsal neurovascular bundle and ligation of the multiple arterial and venous branches from and into the fibrofatty tissue, respectively. All visible and palpable lymph nodes, normal and abnormal, should be removed, with care taken to clip the small lymphatic channels to minimize lymphocele formation. The specimen is amputated and submitted for pathologic analysis.

In cases with significant scarring, an alternative approach is to dissect laterally to identify the latissimus dorsi muscle first. From here, enter the axilla and identify the thoracodorsal nerve, vein, and artery. Access from this direction can be helpful if there is scarring around the axillary vein and less scarring laterally in the axilla. From here, the thoracodorsal bundle can be followed cephalad to where the thoracodorsal vein enters the axillary vein, with care to preserve the adjacent thoracodorsal nerve. Inferiorly in the axilla, a tributary of the thoracodorsal vein, which crosses over to the serratus muscle, enters the muscle at the level of the long thoracic nerve of Bell, and aids identification of the long thoracic nerve.

Internal Mammary and Supraclavicular Lymph Node Metastasis

An isolated breast cancer recurrence that involves an internal mammary lymph node occurs rarely (<1%). Although no consensus exists regarding the management of internal mammary node recurrences, randomized controlled trials have shown that radiation or resection of internal mammary lymph node recurrences is not associated with improved survival. Internal mammary and supraclavicular nodal disease can often be treated with systemic therapy and radiation, although sometimes surgical resection of these nodes may be recommended and multidisciplinary discussion is important.

Metastatic Breast Cancer

Patients with metastatic breast cancer should be managed by a multidisciplinary team that includes a medical oncologist, radiation oncologist, breast surgical oncologist, plastic surgeon, palliative care specialist, psychosocial support, pathologist, and radiologist.

Intact Primary Tumor in Patients with Metastatic Breast Cancer

Approximately 5% of women in the United States with breast cancer have stage IV disease at diagnosis. Considerable interest is now found in changing the traditional approach to these patients, which has been primarily systemic chemotherapy, with operative resection used only as a palliative procedure in cases with locally advanced disease (toilette mastectomy). Current data show that one third to one half of patients with stage IV breast cancer undergo surgical resection of the primary tumor, and retrospective studies have shown an improved survival in these patients compared with patients in whom the primary tumor is not resected. All of these studies have intrinsic selection bias, which makes interpretation of these data complex. The hypothesis is that uncontrolled local disease may act as a source of continued systemic seeding for distant metastasis.

The treatment options for patients with stage IV disease with an intact breast primary include the traditional approach of systemic chemotherapy only, with local therapy of the breast primary limited to those patients that develop uncontrolled local disease. Alternatively, in recent years, interest has been seen in early local operative resection of the intact primary to free margins supported by data from retrospective studies and experiences from other cancers like colon cancer and renal cell cancer. As a result, prospective clinical trials are underway to gather data regarding benefit of resection of the primary tumor in patients with stage IV breast cancer.

Given that the data so far have only been from retrospective studies, randomized trials are needed to provide better unbiased data. One such randomized trial by the Eastern Cooperative Oncology Group (ECOG; NCT01242800) is ongoing and will look at whether patients with intact primary breast cancer with stage IV disease who receive optimal systemic therapy with no evidence of progression receive a survival benefit from early local therapy of the primary disease (surgery and radiotherapy of the primary tumor after induction systemic chemotherapy) compared with those who receive only palliative local therapy and systemic therapy. Other ongoing randomized controlled trials include one sponsored by Turkish Federation of the National Societies for Breast Diseases (NCT00557986) and another by Tata Memorial Hospital, India (NCT00193778). The results of these randomized controlled trials will better define the criteria for early local therapy and the survival benefit achieved.

Isolated Distant Metastatic Disease

The mainstay of treatment of stage IV breast cancer is systemic chemotherapy. Metastasectomy may be feasible and may render patients disease free in a highly select group of patients. Ability to resect metastatic disease is dependent on extent of metastatic disease (number of foci of metastasis and number of sites of metastatic disease).

Hepatic Breast Cancer Metastases

The liver is the third most common site for breast cancer metastasis, after bone and lung. About 10% to 15% of patients with newly diagnosed metastatic breast cancers have hepatic metastases, with about 5% of these having isolated hepatic metastases as the only site of distant metastasis. Systemic chemotherapy is the standard treatment often with a palliative intent. However, recent studies have shown that resection of hepatic breast cancer metastasis does improve survival. Only a highly select group of patients are candidates for hepatic metastasectomy; these are patients with hormone-receptor positive tumors, with a disease-free interval of more than 1 year, who have a good response to chemotherapy and undergo subsequent surgical resection with negative margins. Five-year survival rates after R0 resection of hepatic metastases range from 34% to 37%, with recurrence-free rates from 12% to 22%. The morbidity and mortality of hepatic resection is 1% to 5% and less than 1%, respectively. Given that these patients are usually on systemic chemotherapy, and hormonal therapy in some cases, the exact survival benefit of metastasectomy may be difficult to filter from that achieved from systemic therapy without a randomized controlled trial.

Pulmonary Metastases

Lung is one of the most common sites of breast cancer metastasis, along with bone. About 15% to 25% of patients present with isolated lung metastases. A select number of patients may benefit from combined operative resection of metastases along with systemic chemotherapy and hormonal therapy. From existing literature, factors that have been shown to be associated with better survival after lung metastasectomy of breast cancer are a long disease-free interval between the primary tumor and the appearance of metastases

(>3 years), R0 resection, estrogen receptor–positive disease, and solitary metastases. Of these, a long disease-free interval was the most consistent, likely indicating an indolent type of breast cancer. Overall survival rates at 5 and 10 years have been reported to be 38% and 22%, respectively, by Friedel's study of 467 patients in the International Registry of Lung Metastases, and 54% and 40% from Yoshimoto's study of 90 patients. For the same reasons as stated previously, it is difficult to single out the survival benefit obtained by addition of metastasectomy to the traditional chemotherapy in these patients and further studies are needed to better define this.

SUGGESTED READINGS

Babiera GV, Rao R, Feng L, et al: Effect of primary tumor extirpation in breast cancer patients who present with stage IV disease and an intact primary tumor, *Ann Surg Oncol* 13(6):776–782, 2006.
Boughey JC, Mittendorf EA, Solin LJ, et al: Controversies in breast surgery, *Ann Surg Oncol* 17(3):230–232, 2010.
Brooks JP, Danforth DN, Albert P, et al: Early ipsilateral breast tumor recurrences after breast conservation affect survival: an analysis of the National Cancer Institute randomized trial, *Int J Radiat Oncol Biol Phys* 62(3):785–789, 2005.
Khan SA, Stewart AK, Morrow M: Does aggressive local therapy improve survival in metastatic breast cancer? *Surgery* 132(4):620–626, 2002.
Pockaj BA, Wasif N, Dueck AC, et al: Metastasectomy and surgical resection of the primary tumor in patients with stage IV breast cancer: time for a second look? *Ann Surg Oncol* 17(9):2419–2426, 2010.

MALE BREAST CANCER

Rosemarie Hardin, MD, and
Theodore Tsangaris, MD

OVERVIEW

Carcinoma of the male breast is an exceptionally rare entity and accounts for less than 1% of all breast cancers and 0.1% of cancer mortality in men. The American Cancer Society estimates that in 2012, 2190 new cases of invasive breast cancer will be diagnosed in men and 410 men will die of breast cancer. Male breast cancer (MBC) warrants special consideration to foster prompt diagnosis and institution of appropriate therapies. Because of low clinical acuity and suspicion in men with breast symptoms, breast cancer tends to be diagnosed at later stages, with at least half of the cases presenting with stage 2 or higher breast cancer. It is not surprising then that approximately half of patients have regional spread of disease to the axillary lymph nodes at the time of diagnosis. Fortunately, the 5-year survival rates are similar across stages, comparable with women, although the overall survival rate in men tends to be lower than in women. This is thought to be largely because of the older age at diagnosis and resulting increased comorbidities.

Given the rarity of this disease, whether male breast cancer has its own distinct biology is difficult to ascertain. Treatment strategy for male breast cancer and determination of prognosis is extrapolated from our understanding of female breast cancer, with adjustments made for differences in anatomy and hormonal variations in men.

RISK FACTORS

Because of the rarity of this disease, establishment of causative links to development of MBC has been challenging. Similar to female breast cancer, the risk of MBC is increased twofold to threefold in patients with a positive family history of breast cancer and can be significantly higher in those with a known genetic predisposition. The most familiar gene mutation responsible for MBC is the *BRCA 2* gene. However, many other genetic mutations and syndromes can predispose to MBC, including mutations in the *AR* gene, cytochrome p45017 *(CYP17)*, *PTEN* tumor suppressor gene associated with Cowden syndrome, *CHEK2* gene, and Klinefelter's syndrome (XXY karyotype).

Inherited MBC is most commonly associated with the *BRCA 2* mutations, which account for approximately 40% of MBC. The lifetime risk of development of male breast cancer in a *BRCA 2* carrier is approximately 7%, which is 80 to 100 times that of the normal population. *BRCA 1* can also predispose to MBC, but at a much lower risk of approximately 1%, and can account for approximately 4% of MBC cases. Other risk factors for the development of MBC include alterations in the estrogen-testosterone ratio, history of radiation exposure, and some occupational hazards. It is speculated that men who are exposed to high-temperature environments may be predisposed to early testicular failure and that the resulting estrogen-testosterone imbalance may predispose to breast cancer.

Increased estrogen exposure or androgen insufficiency can predispose men to breast cancer. The most well-known associated syndrome with such a hormonal imbalance is Klinefelter's syndrome (XXY), which accounts for 3% of MBC cases. Males with this syndrome have testicular dysgenesis, gynecomastia, low testosterone levels, normal to low estrogen levels, and increased gonadotropin levels. This condition results in a high estrogen to androgen ratio, leading to a fiftyfold increased risk of development of breast cancer. Interestingly, this can be the outcome of abnormal hormonal stimulation resulting in proliferation of mammary duct epithelium or it may result from increased estrogen from the conversion of exogenous therapeutic testosterone in adipose tissue.

Men with undescended testes, congenital inguinal hernia, or orchitis or who have undergone orchiectomy are also at increased risk. Interestingly, obesity increases the estrogen-testosterone ratio and is considered a risk factor for MBC. Other considerations are increased estrogen levels in patients with cirrhosis with liver failure, in men treated for prostate cancer, and in transsexuals taking exogenous estrogens.

PRESENTATION

Male breast tissue is predominately made up of ductal elements, stroma, adipose tissue, and subcutaneous fat. Lobular tissue, which in women is responsible for lactation, is usually absent in males unless they have increased estrogen exposure. Normal male breast anatomy lacks terminal lobules found in females; therefore, lobular carcinomas are rarely if ever encountered. Most male breast cancers are low-grade and intermediate-grade invasive ductal cancer; the remaining cases present with ductal carcinoma in situ (DCIS). Paget's disease and inflammatory breast cancer, rare entities in female patients, have been reported to occur in male patients as well. Most MBCs are hormone receptor positive and *Her 2 neu* negative, which translates into better prognosis if detected early.

Most men with breast cancer present at older ages compared with women with breast cancer, with the peak incidence occurring between ages 68 and 71 years, with a painless breast mass, localized to the subareolar area. It is sometimes difficult to discern this from changes associated with gynecomastia. However, gynecomastia tends to be bilateral and can be associated with tenderness. The tissue tends to remain soft and mobile as opposed to the firm lesions associated with malignancy. Of note, no definitive link between gynecomastia and MBC has been proven, and at present, gynecomastia is not considered a risk factor for the development of carcinoma. Other findings suggestive of breast cancer in females may be evident on examination, including regional lymphadenopathy, nipple retraction, or nipple discharge. Nipple discharge, if present in men, should alert the physician to a more ominous finding. Given the smaller amount of breast tissue in men, cancers can involve the local adjacent tissues, specifically the overlying skin and chest wall musculature.

DIAGNOSIS

The evaluation of a palpable breast abnormality in a male should proceed in a similar manner as with female patients (Figure 1). A careful history and physical examination is conducted. Physical examination should include both breasts, the chest wall, and the regional nodal basins. This is followed by diagnostic imaging with mammography and ultrasound scan. Mammography has been shown to be 92% sensitive and 90% specific for detection of male breast cancer. Mammography remains the diagnostic tool of choice in men presenting with breast symptoms. Given the rarity of MBC, it is not justified as a screening modality except for those at particularly high risk, such as those with the *BRCA 2* mutation. Ultrasound scan can help to better delineate palpable abnormalities, assess involvement of underlying musculature, and accurately assess regional nodal basins for nodal disease. It follows that any palpable lesion identified should be biopsied with image-guided core biopsy for confirmation of pathologic diagnosis and receptor status of malignant tumors. Patients with palpable lymphadenopathy or suspicious nodes identified on ultrasound scan should undergo fine-needle aspiration to determine management strategy. Evaluation of distant metastases follows the same strategy as for women and should

be based on clinical assessment of symptoms suggestive of metastatic spread or in cases of locally advanced disease.

Of note, given the rarity of male breast cancer, a careful family history should be obtained and patients should be strongly considered for genetic counseling and testing. This test is performed to determine risk of development of additional cancers in the male patient, with heightened awareness of other cancer screenings that may be warranted, and also provides useful information to family members regarding their associated risk and possible preventative strategies. Male relatives discovered to have the *BRCA* mutation should be followed as high-risk cases and should closely adhere to strict surveillance programs with consideration of screening mammography for early detection. Given the rarity of MBC, little data exist regarding prophylactic surgery. However, it can be discussed with men who are *BRCA 2* carriers for risk reduction in the same manner as female BRCA mutation carriers. Interestingly, males who have a family history of breast cancer and whose female relatives are proven to be *BRCA+* are sometime not informed of these genetic test results. This is an important consideration in counseling female patients who undergo genetic testing.

TREATMENT

Although many surgical options are available for women diagnosed with breast cancer, the options available to men are more limited. If women are deemed candidates for breast conservation, they are often offered lumpectomy with sentinel lymph node biopsy (SLNBX) followed by radiation; and those that require mastectomy can be offered skin-sparing mastectomy to facilitate reconstruction and nipple-sparing mastectomies that offer a pleasing cosmetic outcome. The anatomy of the male breast does not necessarily lend itself to breast conservation, with lesions that are typically located deep in the subareolar tissue, and the cosmetic outcome is improved with mastectomy. However, there is no specific contraindication to breast conservation in men if so desired and if it can be accomplished without disfigurement. Men do not undergo reconstructive procedures; therefore, skin-sparing and nipple-sparing mastectomies are not considered. Men diagnosed with breast cancer typically undergo total mastectomy. Axillary staging is an important component of surgical management, as studies have shown that men who underwent mastectomy without axillary dissection developed nodal recurrence and had poorer prognosis. Therefore, sentinel lymph node biopsy is appropriate in men and follows the same algorithm as used in female patients.

The decision for local radiation therapy follows the same guidelines as for women. This includes patients who present with large tumors, have microscopically positive margins that cannot be surgically improved, and who have four or more positive lymph nodes. Decision for systemic therapy is considered for the patients with advanced disease who are at risk of recurrence and death from breast cancer.

Given that most male breast cancers are hormonally sensitive, adjuvant hormonal manipulation is a crucial adjuvant therapy, with tamoxifen reducing the risk of recurrence. Similar to women, tamoxifen can lead to hormonal changes in men and is poorly tolerated by some. These changes include hot flashes, mood changes, and decreased libido and are present in approximately 20% of men. They are likewise at risk of venous thromboembolism. These side effects are in part responsible for the low compliance with hormonal therapy reported in male patients with breast cancer.

Patients with metastatic disease are managed in the same fashion as female patients. Given that most MBCs are estrogen receptor positive, hormonal therapy is often considered first-line therapy in the metastatic setting. Tamoxifen has established efficacy with a 50% response rate in metastatic male breast cancer. For males who are estrogen receptor negative who present with rapid progression of disease, chemotherapy can be considered for palliation. Trastuzumab

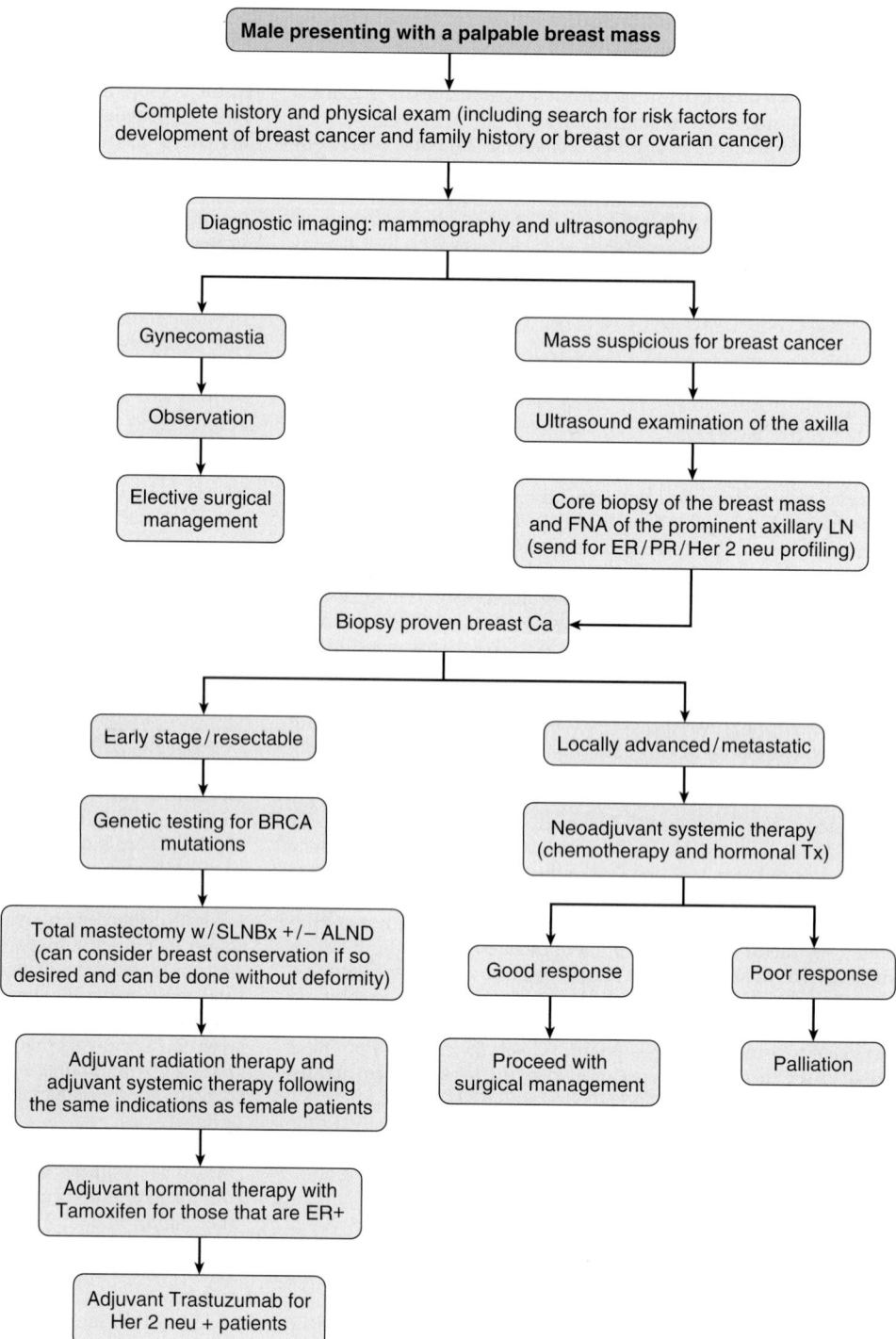

FIGURE 1   Treatment algorithm for a male with a palpable breast mass. *ALND*, axillary lymph node dissection; *ER*, estrogen receptor; *FNA*, fine needle aspiration; *LN*, lymph node; *PR*, progesterone receptor; *SLNBX*, sentinel lymph node biopsy.

should be considered in those that are *Her 2 neu* positive, extrapolating from evidence in female patients.

PROGNOSIS

As with female breast cancer, staging follows the American Joint Committee on Cancer tumor node metastasis (TNM) staging system. Tumor size, grade of tumor, presence of lymph node metastases, and distant disease determine outcome. As in women, predictors of locoregional failure include positive margins, increased tumor size, and involvement of the axillary lymph nodes. Estrogen, progesterone status, and overexpression of *Her 2 neu* also help to predict prognosis and guide adjuvant therapies.

Even in those patients who do not have a genetic predisposition, those diagnosed with male breast cancer are at risk for subsequent cancers, which can include contralateral breast cancer, melanoma, and prostate cancer among others. Close follow-up for health maintenance is especially crucial for these patients.

The diagnosis, surgical treatment, and use of adjuvant therapies for patients diagnosed with male breast cancer remain largely extrapolated from our experience with female breast cancer patients; fortunately, this has been met with success. However, as MBC is increasingly recognized with treatment modifications accounting for differences in anatomy and hormonal balance, our knowledge regarding this disease will be broadened. This will advance our understanding of the disease and help to better determine optimal male specific treatment algorithms.

SUGGESTED READINGS

Johansen Taber K, Morisy L, Osbahr A, et al: Male breast cancer: risk factors, diagnosis and management (review), *Oncol Rep* 24:1115–1120, 2010.

Weiss JR, Moysich KB, Swede H: Epidemiology of male breast cancer, *Cancer Epidemiol Biomarkers Prev* 14:20–26, 2005.
White, J, Kearins O, Dodwell D, et al: Male breast carcinoma: increased awareness needed, *Breast Cancer Res* 13:219–225, 2011.
Yamauchi H, Woodward W, Valero V, et al: Inflammatory breast cancer: what we know and what we need to learn, *Oncologist* 17:891–899, 2012.

BREAST RECONSTRUCTION FOLLOWING MASTECTOMY: INDICATIONS, TECHNIQUES, AND RESULTS

Hakim K. Said, MD, FACS, Sara H. Javid, MD, Shannon Colohan, MD, Otway Louie, MD, David W. Mathes, MD, Benjamin O. Anderson, MD, and Peter C. Neligan, MD

Early treatment of breast cancer centered on removal of disease, prevention of recurrence, and life expectancy. Since then, early detection and multimodal treatment have proven very effective, and breast cancer is currently one of the most curable forms of cancer. Survival without breast restoration, however, has a dramatic negative impact on self-image and lifestyle. Advances in the quality of care have focused on quality of life after treatment, particularly on returning women to their former lives before they were diagnosed with cancer. Today, the options for restoring a breast are better than ever, with natural tissues, organic matrices, or synthetic implants, especially when used in novel combinations.

INDICATIONS

The surgical treatment options for both noninvasive (ductal carcinoma in situ) and invasive breast cancer include breast-conserving surgery (lumpectomy) and mastectomy. Approximately 70% of patients with early-stage invasive breast cancer are candidates for and elect breast-conserving surgery, but many will require or choose mastectomy due to the extent of malignant disease in the breast, prior radiotherapy exposure, contraindication to or desire to avoid radiotherapy, and/or risk reduction for subsequent breast cancers. Various technical approaches to mastectomy differ primarily with respect to the amount of the skin envelope that is preserved.

A non–skin-sparing ("standard") mastectomy is performed when a patient does not desire or cannot undergo immediate reconstruction. A wide elliptical incision is made, excising the nipple areolar complex (NAC) and the skin overlying the tumor, ultimately leading to a long transverse or oblique scar. The goal should be to minimize postoperative skin redundancy that might interfere with the wearing of a prosthesis. In contrast, in a skin-sparing mastectomy, the breast is removed through a much smaller circumareolar incision narrowly encompassing the NAC in order to preserve the skin envelope for the reconstructed breast mound. A newer variation of this skin-sparing approach is the "nipple-sparing," or "total skin-sparing," mastectomy. The nipple-sparing mastectomy, previously termed the *subcutaneous mastectomy* in the 1970s and 1980s, was an operation that fell into disrepute out of concern that excessive fibroglandular tissue would be left behind the NAC, but it is now being reevaluated for the purpose of cancer prophylaxis and in carefully selected breast cancer cases.

Because the perfusion to the skin and the nipple comes primarily from the breast that must be removed, the remaining skin may be relatively ischemic and prone to healing challenges. As the mastectomy plane grows closer to the skin, the chance increases of causing damage to the subdermal plexus that is the only remaining source of perfusion. Whereas in a standard mastectomy, this ischemic central breast skin would be removed, in skin-sparing mastectomy, most of these skin flaps are preserved. Nipple-sparing mastectomy leaves essentially all the breast skin intact, regardless of how far away the nearest intact blood vessels lie. This further increases the amount of ischemic skin, the chance of healing problems, and the risk of complications after either of these kinds of mastectomy. Reliably preserving an intact and undamaged subdermal plexus is a challenge in skin-sparing mastectomy, and critically important in nipple-sparing mastectomy, in order to avoid complications after mastectomy. Moreover, while leaving fibroglandular tissue behind poses an oncologic risk, excessively thinning the dermal subcutaneous tissue negatively impacts the appearance and quality of the reconstructive outcome.

In general, both skin-sparing and nipple-sparing mastectomies are only performed in the setting of breast reconstruction, whether that reconstruction is performed during the same operation or shortly thereafter as a separate procedure once the skin has recovered and the surgical pathology results are known.

Several studies have demonstrated that post-mastectomy breast reconstruction affords several benefits, including improved body image, psychological health, and reduced concern for cancer recurrence. Although most patients are eligible to undergo reconstruction in a "delayed" fashion following completion of their breast cancer treatment, many patients are eligible to begin reconstruction at the time of their mastectomy ("immediate" reconstruction). The decision to proceed with immediate reconstruction depends on patient and disease factors, as well as treatment-related factors. In some cases, the mastectomy is performed as a separate procedure, with reconstruction to be performed a few weeks later ("delayed-immediate"), in order to allow pathologic examination of the specimen before proceeding with the reconstructive procedure.

Immediate reconstruction, with either a prosthetic device or autologous tissue, requires a preserved skin envelope with a skin-sparing mastectomy. The majority of patients with early-stage (0, I, II) breast cancer can undergo this approach. Immediate reconstruction is contraindicated in a patient with skin involvement, such as skin ulceration (T4b) or inflammatory (T4d) breast cancer. In addition, if a patient is expected to require post-mastectomy radiation therapy (PMRT), such as those with locally advanced (stage III) cancers, immediate reconstruction with autologous tissue is to be avoided to prevent the deleterious effects of radiation on the reconstruction. However, in such cases, skin-sparing mastectomy with immediate reconstruction using a temporary prosthesis (tissue expander) is often possible, with the understanding that this expander may need to be deflated prior to radiation. Other relative contraindications for immediate reconstruction include active smoking history and medical comorbidities such as morbid obesity or cardiopulmonary disease.

RECONSTRUCTIVE TECHNIQUES

Women who elect to undergo reconstruction have two main reconstructive options: prosthetic devices (tissue expanders, implants) or autologous tissue reconstruction using tissue transferred from a distant donor site to the chest wall. The choice can sometimes be driven by the breast cancer treatment plan, such as patients who will require PMRT, which largely eliminates the option of immediate autologous reconstruction. More commonly, reconstruction reflects the patient's choice and the reconstructive surgeon's recommendation. For instance, very slender women may not have ample donor tissue available for autologous reconstruction, and women with a history of prior radiation (e.g., mantle radiation for lymphoma) may not be candidates for implant-based reconstruction because of the significantly higher risk of implant complications in a radiated setting.

Implants

Implants are selected by many women because of the desire to avoid a second surgical scar and recovery associated with the donor site or because it entails less extensive surgery. Downsides of implant-based reconstruction include higher risk of infection due to presence of a foreign body, risk of capsular contracture, and risk of leak or rupture, which would require removal or replacement.

Two Stages

Historically, the two-stage implant approach is the earliest form of breast reconstruction, although implants have gone through many iterations. Today the great majority of implants are placed in two stages. First, an adjustable implant called an *expander* is placed subpectorally, either deflated or partially filled. Typically, over the next 3 months, the expander is inflated with saline on a weekly basis to reach an appropriate goal size. At that point, the expander is replaced by a softer and more aesthetic implant, saline or silicone. Although in the United States, between 1994 and 2007, a moratorium prohibited use of silicone gel implants, elsewhere in the world their use has continued. In 2007, the safety data were convincing enough to warrant rerelease of silicone gel implants on the U.S. market. Subsequent studies have documented significantly improved patient satisfaction and better aesthetic outcomes in the setting of breast reconstruction using silicone gel implants versus saline implants. Most patients currently choose the silicone implants, and the outcomes are closer to the results obtained with autologous reconstruction (Figure 1).

One Stage

An alternative to this approach is one-stage reconstruction using a permanent silicone implant placed subpectorally at the time of the mastectomy. This reduces the number of surgeries required but poses several risks. First, there must be sufficient skin redundancy after

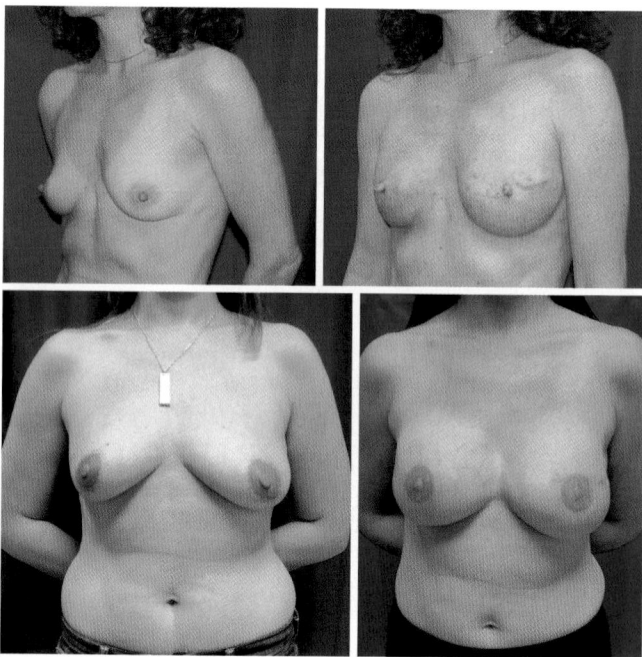

FIGURE I   Implant reconstruction.

mastectomy to permit construction of a full breast of the desired size. Second, the mastectomy skin must be of sufficient viability to tolerate the weight and expansion produced by a full-size implant. Third, the patient's desired goals in terms of the final implant must be explicitly known and achievable at this point. Many patients lose enough skin through mastectomy to reduce the volume that can be reached, or they have delicate skin flaps that would be compromised by or even necrose as a result of excessive tension from a full-size implant. Patients generally are better served by placement of an adjustable expander with a lower fill volume and a two-stage reconstruction. In addition, the second stage implant exchange allows the patient to choose her desired implant size and type and allows for another chance to adjust the pocket for a more optimal breast shape.

Tissue Matrices

Offered by a number of manufacturers, tissue matrices are organic substrates derived from human, porcine, or bovine origins, processed to produce an implantable organic scaffold. They are commonly placed in conjunction with an expander at the time of mastectomy as a "sling," which offloads the skin by bearing the weight of the implant. In addition, these matrices allow a significant degree of control over the size and shape of the implant pocket, including definitive positioning of the inframammary fold. Evidence suggests they may have a beneficial effect on capsular contracture rates, which are especially high among patients who have undergone radiation (Figure 2).

Autologous Methods of Breast Reconstruction

Some women do not like the idea of having implants, while others, for any number of reasons, may not be candidates for that type of reconstruction. The most common reason that a patient may not be eligible for implant reconstruction is because of a history of radiation. Using the patient's own tissues to reconstruct the entire breast is an attractive option for these patients. Natural tissue has the potential to provide durable reconstruction of the full breast volume, often without the vulnerability of implants, which can fail or require replacement eventually.

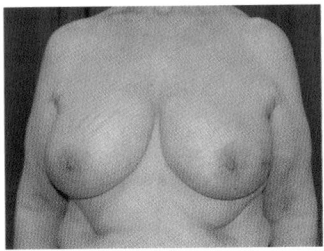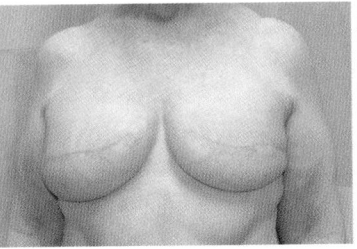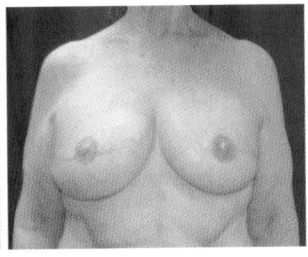

FIGURE 2 One-stage implant reconstruction with tissue matrix.

There are many ways to reconstruct a breast using autologous tissue. All involve incisions for harvesting tissues from various donor sites elsewhere on the body. These methods can be divided into three broad categories: (1) fat grafting, (2) pedicled flap reconstruction, and (3) free flap reconstruction. The last of these requires microsurgical skills.

Fat Grafting

The use of fat grafting in breast reconstruction is a relatively new technique. Fat grafting has been used in aesthetic surgery for a number of years. Structural fat grafting involves harvesting adipose tissue from other areas on the body through a series of tiny nick incisions. Small amounts of fat are carefully prepared and then injected in multiple planes into areas to be treated. Depending on the site, 30% to 70% of the fat injected with this technique can be retained and engrafted long-term. Overcorrection, subsidence, and retreatment are the keys to reaching the goal size with this method. It is an extremely useful technique for reconstruction of lumpectomy defects, where one treatment may be all that is necessary (Petit et al., 2011).

It has also gained favor for contour correction and volume adjustment in conjunction with implant reconstruction. Some of the issues associated with implants, such as implant rippling or edge step-off deformities, can be addressed easily with lipofilling using fat harvested from other sites of redundancy, without significant scars or deformity at the donor sites.

More recently, Khouri has introduced the concept of external expansion using a suction cup device worn by women called the Brava bra (BRAVA LLC, Miami, Fla). This expands the recipient site, creating an edematous mound that can accommodate larger volumes of fat injection. Typically, patients will undergo 3 to 4 sessions of fat grafting over a number of months, in conjunction with a regimen of external expansion before and after each surgery. With persistence, the entire breast mound can be reconstructed to a reasonable volume with repeated rounds of this method.

Pedicled Flap Reconstruction

A pedicled flap is one in which the vascular supply remains intact and is transferred into the breast from an adjacent region. The two most common pedicled flaps in use for breast reconstruction are the latissimus dorsi myocutaneous flap and the transverse rectus abdominis myocutaneous (TRAM) flap. Other flaps exist based on perforators from the thoracodorsal vessels and the intercostal vessels. These will be discussed later. Many of these flaps are also extremely useful for reconstructing partial mastectomy defects or defects resulting from lumpectomy.

The Latissimus Flap

The blood supply of the latissimus dorsi is from the thoracodorsal artery. Because of the favorable position of this pedicle, the latissimus muscle and its overlying skin can be pivoted on the pedicle and rotated from the back to the chest. The skin paddle of the latissimus can be oriented obliquely or transversely to hide the donor site scar under the bra line. In most cases, the latissimus flap is combined with placement of a breast implant, as there usually is insufficient bulk to create a breast mound. This is particularly useful in patients who have been through radiation treatments. The addition of nonradiated tissue from the back can make implant reconstruction possible in patients who otherwise might not be candidates for implants.

The TRAM Flap

Introduced by Hartrampf, the TRAM flap takes advantage of the blood supply of the abdominal skin. Based on the superior epigastric artery, an ellipse of lower abdominal skin and fat, along with underlying rectus abdominis muscle, is mobilized. This flap is tunneled from the abdomen into the chest, where it is folded and inset to reproduce the breast shape. The abdominal donor site is treated similarly to a tummy tuck, by undermining the upper abdominal skin and advancing it to facilitate closure. Critics of the pedicled TRAM flap point out that, with sacrifice of one or both rectus muscles, there is significant potential weakening of the abdominal wall and careful reconstruction of the abdomen to prevent future development of a ventral hernia is critical.

Free Flap Breast Reconstruction

Free flap breast reconstruction has undergone an evolution over the past 20 years. Because of concerns with abdominal wall integrity following pedicled TRAM flap reconstruction, the free TRAM was developed, based on the deep inferior epigastric vessels. The rationale was that less muscle could be harvested, and the expectation was that donor morbidity would be less. As our knowledge of vascular anatomy improved, the free TRAM became the muscle-sparing free TRAM, harvesting less and less muscle. Ultimately, with the introduction of perforator flaps, we learned how to dissect the vascular pedicle out of the rectus muscle with minimal disruption of the muscle and preservation of the segmental nerves. This evolved to become the deep inferior epigastric perforator (DIEP) flap (Figure 3). In each of these flaps, the major pedicle, the deep inferior epigastric artery, is divided and reanastomosed in the chest to the internal mammary vessels.

In patients who are not candidates for abdominal-flap breast reconstruction, either because of insufficient tissue availability or because of previous surgery, there are several other options. These include the transverse upper gracilis (TUG) flap (Figure 4), which includes skin and subcutaneous fat from the upper inner thigh, or the superior and inferior gluteal artery perforator (SGAP and IGAP) flaps. Each relies on a donor site and removal of excess tissue at a respective site on the patient. All of these flaps require advanced microsurgical expertise as well as an intimate knowledge of the vascular anatomy of the flap involved based on preoperative computed tomographic scan imaging evaluation. Each donor site also represents a particular set of benefits or drawbacks depending on the site and the patient.

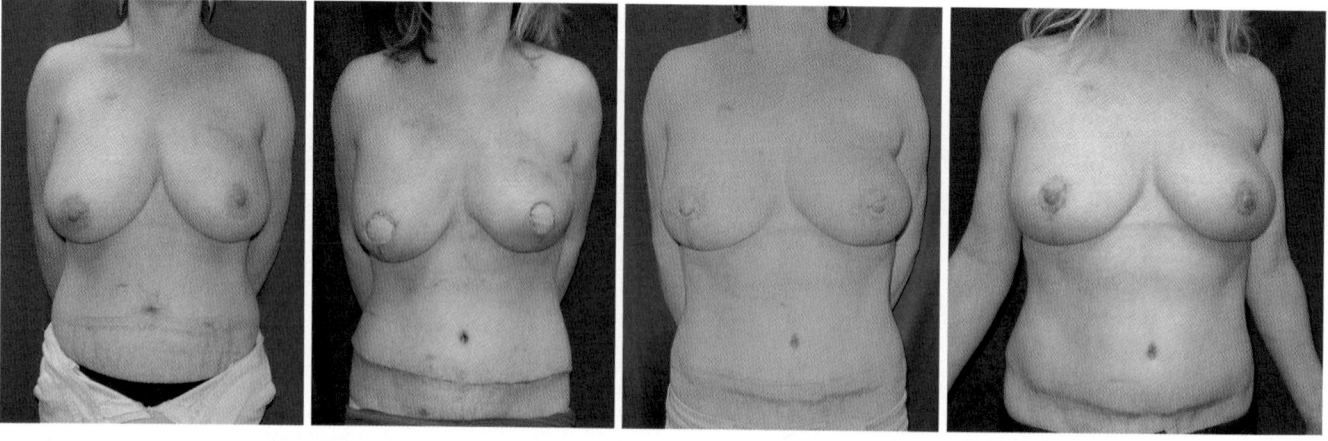

FIGURE 3   Immediate deep inferior epigastric perforator (DIEP) flap reconstruction.

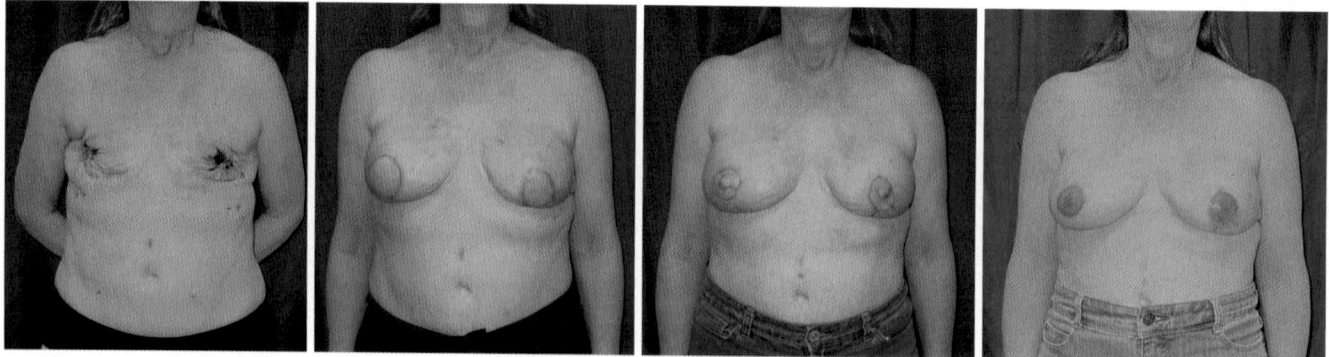

FIGURE 4   Delayed transverse upper gracilis (TAG) flap reconstruction.

SUGGESTED READINGS

Boneti C, Yuen J, Santiago C, et al: Oncologic safety of nipple skin-sparing or total skin-sparing mastectomies with immediate reconstruction, *J Am Coll Surg* 212(4):686–693; discussion 693–685, 2011.

Khouri RK, Eisenmann-Klein M, et al: Brava and autologous fat transfer is a safe and effective breast augmentation alternative: results of a 6-year, 81-patient, prospective multicenter study, *Plast Reconstr Surg* 129(5):1173–1187, 2012.

Lambert K, Mokbel K: Does post-mastectomy radiotherapy represent a contraindication to skin-sparing mastectomy and immediate reconstruction: an update, *Surg Oncol* 21(2):e67–e74, 2012.

Laronga C, Lewis JD, Smith PD: The changing face of mastectomy: an oncologic and cosmetic perspective, *Cancer Control* 19(4):286–294, 2012.

Petit JY, Lohsiriwat V, Clough KB, et al: The oncologic outcome and immediate surgical complications of lipofilling in breast cancer patients: a multicenter study—Milan-Paris-Lyon experience of 646 lipofilling procedures, *Plast Reconstr Surg* 128(2):341–346, 2011.

Salzberg CA: Focus on technique: one-stage implant-based breast reconstruction, *Plast Reconstr Surg* 130(5 Suppl 2):95S–103S, 2012.

Wagner JL, Fearmonti R, Hunt KK, et al: Prospective evaluation of the nipple-areola complex sparing mastectomy for risk reduction and for early-stage breast cancer, *Ann Surg Oncol* 19(4):1137–1144, 2012.

Warren Peled A, Foster RD, Stover AC, et al: Outcomes after total skin-sparing mastectomy and immediate reconstruction in 657 breasts, *Ann Surg Oncol* 19(11):3402–3409, 2012.

ENDOCRINE GLANDS

ADRENAL INCIDENTALOMA

Alan P. B. Dackiw, MD, PhD

OVERVIEW/CLINICAL PROBLEM

An adrenal "incidentaloma" is an adrenal mass, usually measuring 1 cm or more in size, that is discovered incidentally during a radiologic examination performed for indications other than a suspected adrenal problem. The widespread use of abdominal ultrasonography, computed tomographic (CT) scanning, and magnetic resonance imaging (MRI) has resulted in the findings of adrenal incidentaloma, which necessitates the subsequent workup. Numerous autopsy studies have revealed that the overall frequency of adrenal adenomas is approximately 6%; abdominal CT identification has demonstrated similar numbers. The prevalence of adrenal adenomas increases with age. The probability of finding an unsuspected adrenal adenoma on abdominal CT scans in a patient between 20 and 29 years of age is approximately 0.2%, in comparison with approximately 7% in a patient older than 70 years.

The majority of adrenal incidentalomas are clinically nonfunctioning, benign adrenal cortical adenomas. Other frequently reported diagnoses include cortisol-secreting adrenal cortical adenoma, aldosteronoma, pheochromocytoma, adrenal cortical carcinoma, and metastatic carcinoma. In the evaluation of the adrenal incidentaloma, three important questions must be asked: (1) Is the mass functioning or nonfunctioning? (2) Is the mass benign or malignant? (3) If malignant, is it primary or secondary? If the clinician directs the history, physical examination, and laboratory evaluation to answering these three questions for each zone of the adrenal cortex and the adrenal medulla, all incidentally discovered massed will be thoroughly and correctly evaluated (Figure 1). Because these masses are discovered initially on abdominal imaging, the imaging characteristics and size in evaluation of these masses are discussed first.

IMAGING

Density/Hounsfield Unit Assessment

The primary goal of imaging is to distinguish among adrenal adenoma, adrenal carcinoma, and pheochromocytoma (Figure 2), as well as metastatic lesions. Imaging cannot, however, reliably distinguish between nonfunctioning and functioning adrenal adenomas. The diagnosis of an adenoma relies on the presence of lipid content in the adrenal lesion, which can be identified by density measurement

on noncontrast CT scans or on in-phase and out-of-phase MRI. Alternatively, an adenoma can be identified by measuring contrast washout on CT scans. Lesions that have attenuation values below 10 Hounsfield units (HUs) on noncontrast CT scans and loss of signal on out-of-phase MRI are adenomas. The differential diagnosis can be further delineated by CT scans obtained immediately after intravenous administration of a contrast agent and then again after a 10-minute to 15-minute delay. Benign adrenal lesions are commonly enhanced up to 80 to 90 HUs and are washed out more than 50% on the delayed scan, whereas lesions such as metastatic tumors, carcinomas, or pheochromocytomas do not washout. Pheochromocytomas usually show enhancement to more than 100 HUs, which diagnostically distinguishes them from adenomas. On noncontrast CT scans, some benign adrenal lesions do not have attenuation values of less than 10 HUs and may have values of 20 to 40 HUs. This result is found in lipid-poor adenomas, often of smaller size. In these cases, a washout of more than 50% may enable the diagnosis of an adenoma. These masses may also be further evaluated by MRI; however, they may remain indeterminate.

Size

The size of the adrenal mass, as measured on CT scans or MRI, remains the single best indicator of malignancy. In a clinical review of six reported series, Copeland reported that 105 (92%) of 114 adrenal cortical carcinomas were more than 6 cm in diameter. In contrast, large adrenal adenomas (>6 cm) are relatively uncommon, although the exact frequency is unknown. In an important study, Ross and Aron assumed that 1% of adenomas were more than 6 cm in diameter and, on the basis of this assumption, calculated that fewer than 1 per 10,000 adrenal neoplasms smaller than 6 cm in diameter would be an adrenal cortical carcinoma (in the absence of CT characteristics suggesting malignancy, such as irregular borders and lack of homogeneity). They further estimated that the likelihood of adrenal cortical carcinoma increases to 35% to 98% in patients with an adrenal mass larger than 6 cm.

Ross and Aron's widely read 1990 article established the routine practice of operating on patients with nonfunctioning unilateral adrenal neoplasms greater than 6 cm in size and considering observation in patients with smaller lesions. However, there are reasonable concerns about this recommendation: (1) Their calculations were based on an estimate of the frequency of large (>6 cm) adrenal adenomas, a number that, although probably low, is unknown; (2) adrenal cortical cancer is an aggressive malignancy, and no data support the safety of observing an enlarging adrenal cancer (until it reaches 6 cm); and (3) small (<5 cm) adrenal cortical cancers have been documented in a number of reported series. Therefore, clinical reality suggests that few endocrine surgeons would merely observe a 4- or 5-cm unilateral adrenal mass (regardless of CT characteristics) in an otherwise healthy 40- to 50-year old patient.

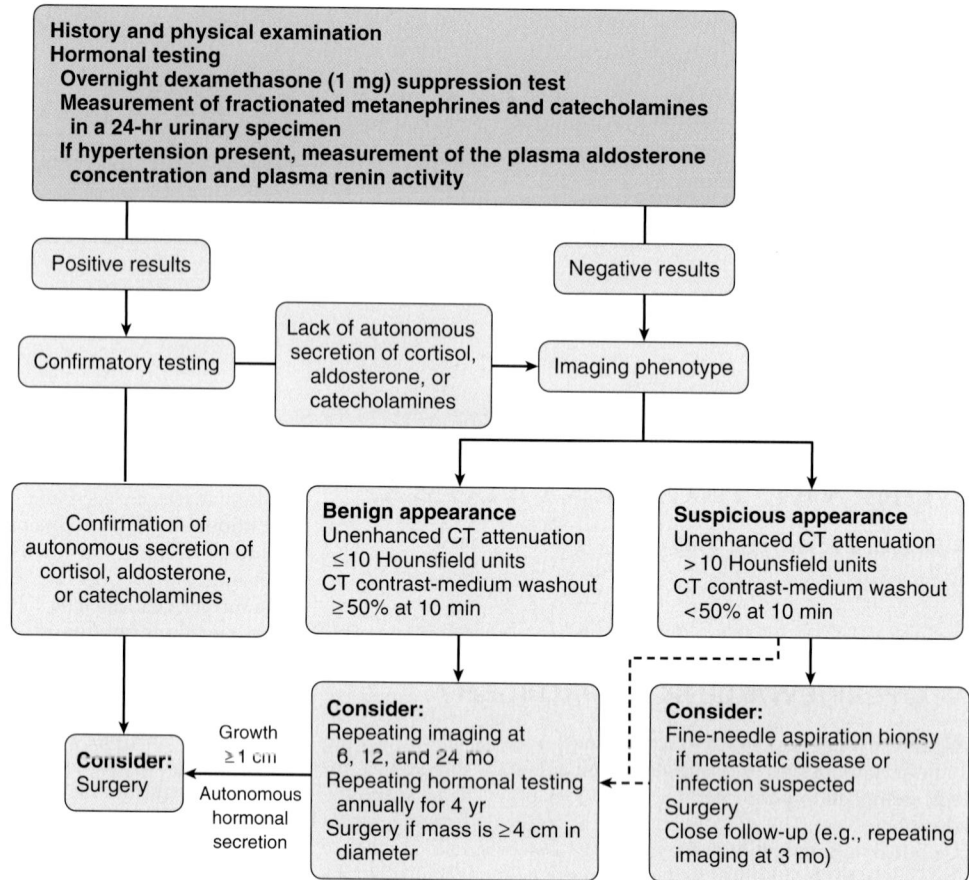

FIGURE 1 Algorithm for the evaluation of patients with an adrenal incidentaloma. *(From Young WF Jr: Clinical practice: the incidentally discovered adrenal mass, N Engl J Med 356:601–610, 2007.)*

Indeed, updated clinical guidelines since have recommended operating on adrenal masses that are 4 cm in size or greater. This point was emphasized by the results of a multiinstitutional retrospective study of incidentally found (and nonfunctional) adrenal neoplasms reported by Terzolo and colleagues. Of the 210 patients in the study, 115 (55%) underwent adrenalectomy and adrenal cortical carcinoma was found in 15 patients (13% of patients who underwent surgery and 7% of patients with incidental adrenal neoplasms). Of the 15 cancers, 3 were smaller than 6 cm in diameter (2.6% of surgical patients and 1.4% of patients with incidental adrenal neoplasms). In all three of these patients, the radiographic characteristics suggested malignancy (i.e., inhomogeneous density, irregular shape and margins). Thus tumor diameter was highly correlated with the risk of cancer; for a diameter of 5 cm, the sensitivity was 93% and the specificity was 64% for identifying adrenal cortical carcinoma. Furthermore, if the 5-cm size criterion had been used as an indication for adrenalectomy, one carcinoma less than 5 cm (diameter, 3.7 cm) would have been observed among the 15 patients with cancer. The CT characteristics of this tumor, as noted previously, did provide an adequate indication for adrenalectomy.

Most guidelines now recommend surgical excision of adrenal neoplasms larger than 4 cm in diameter and those of any size with suspect imaging characteristics. The CT and MRI criteria assume greater importance in the evaluation of nonfunctioning tumors 3 to 5 cm in diameter. CT characteristics of malignancy include tumor inhomogeneity/heterogeneity, irregular shape, irregular margins, and hemorrhage with underlying mass, lack of fat suppression on MRI on T2 out-of-phase gradient imaging or heterogeneous signal intensity on T2-weighted MRI. As noted previously, MRI characteristics of malignancy include the signal intensity on T2-weighted images. Adenomas have low signal intensity in comparison to the liver (adrenal mass/liver ratio ≤1.4), cortical carcinomas and metastases are moderately bright (adrenal mass/liver ratio, 1.2 to 2.8), and

pheochromocytomas usually are extremely bright (adrenal mass/liver ratio >3.0). However these ratios overlap in some cases, and thus size of the mass, other imaging characteristics, and the overall clinical picture must be considered.

Current practice is to recommend adrenalectomy for all biochemically confirmed functioning cortical neoplasms and those with suspect radiographic findings, regardless of tumor size. Nonfunctioning tumors 4 cm in size or larger with benign radiographic characteristics are considered for surgical resection if patient age and general health are acceptable. The radiographic assessment of tumor size cannot be the only consideration; nonfunctioning, radiographically benign adrenal cortical neoplasms approximately 4 cm in diameter necessitate individualized treatment that is based on patient age and comorbid conditions. For example, adrenalectomy is a reasonable recommendation in a healthy 50-year-old woman (adrenal cortical cancers cluster in the 40-year to 50-year age range and are more common in women) with a 3.8-cm to 4.0-cm unilateral nonfunctioning adrenal neoplasm. For such a patient, no data suggest that careful follow-up, no matter how frequent, can detect malignancy, if it were to exist, at a curable stage. Such a patient has a relatively long life expectancy, multiple serial CT scans or other abdominal imaging are needed, and the risk of death from disease is high if the adrenal cortical cancer is not cured at the first surgical procedure; therefore, adrenal resection is reasonable in this patient. In contrast, in a 75-year-old man with multiple comorbid conditions with a similar 4-cm unilateral nonfunctioning adrenal neoplasm, observation would probably be recommended unless radiographic criteria were strongly suggestive of malignancy.

Fine-needle aspiration (FNA) biopsy of an isolated adrenal mass should be performed only in patients with a history of cancer or if there is clinical, laboratory, or radiographic evidence of a primary extraadrenal malignancy and if biopsy findings would result in a change in the clinical management. There is no indication for adrenal

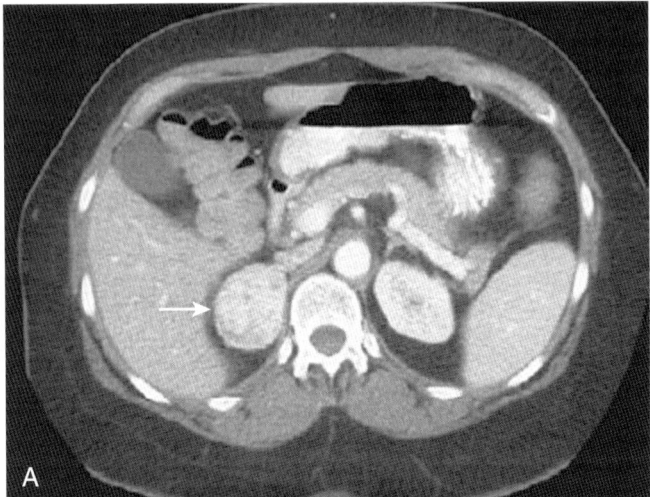

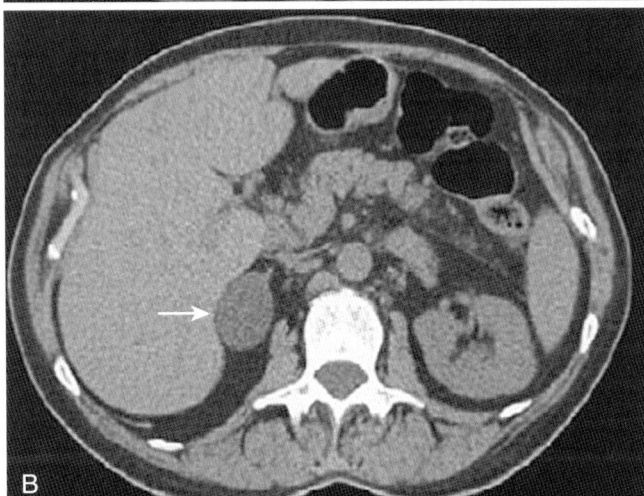

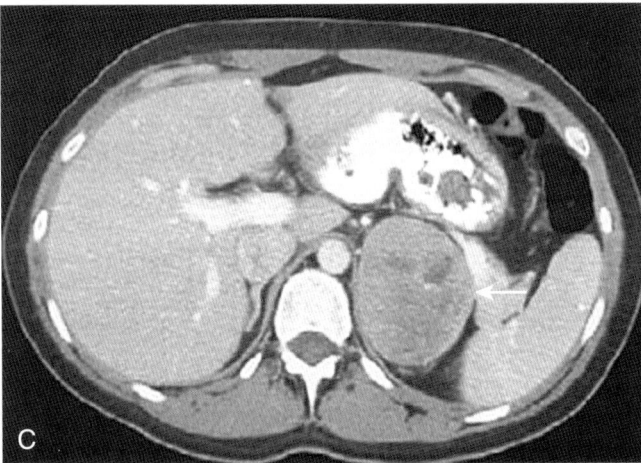

FIGURE 2 Imaging characteristics of adrenal masses: pheochromocytoma (**A**), benign cortical adenoma (**B**), and adrenocortical carcinoma (**C**). Imaging phenotypes and characteristics are as discussed in text. *(From Young WF Jr: Clinical practice: the incidentally discovered adrenal mass,* N Engl J Med *356:601–610, 2007.)*

biopsy in the absence of presumed metastasis to the adrenal glands. It is critically important to rule out pheochromocytoma before a biopsy is performed because of the risk that percutaneous biopsy may trigger severe hypertension in a patient with a catecholamine-secreting tumor. Furthermore, the manifestation of an occult metastatic cancer as a small, unilateral, asymptomatic adrenal mass is rare; thus, investigating all hormonally inactive adrenal masses to detect occult metastatic cancer would result in a large number of unnecessary fine-needle aspiration biopsies.

▮ RAPID OFFICE BIOCHEMICAL EVALUATION (SUMMARY)

The diagnostic evaluation of a patient with a unilateral adrenal mass includes measurement of serum electrolyte levels to rule out hypokalemia secondary to aldosterone excess, an overnight 1-mg dexamethasone suppression test, a 24-hour urine collection for 17-ketosteroids if a masculinizing or feminizing adrenal tumor is suspected, and a 24-hour urine collection to measure catecholamine (and metanephrine) concentrations if pheochromocytoma has not been ruled out. In the author's institution, rapid office evaluation begins with obtaining an afternoon blood sample for cortisol and electrolyte measurements and for plasma metanephrine, normetanephrine, and catecholamine measurements, and a 24-hour urine collection to measure vanillylmandelic acid, metanephrine, and catecholamine concentrations. Dexamethasone (1 mg) is then taken at 10:00 PM that evening, and the following morning at 8:00 AM, blood is obtained for plasma cortisol analysis. During the afternoon of the second day, patients return their timed urine collection specimen. If the patient's plasma cortisol level is not suppressed below 5.0 mcg/dL, the patient undergoes a second timed 24-hour urine collection, this time to measure the cortisol, 17-hydroxysteroid, and 17-ketosteroid concentrations.

▮ CLINICAL EVALUATION

Cortisol Production (Zona Glomerulosa)

History/Symptoms

In documenting the history, the clinician should note weight gain, fatigue, depression, other emotional and cognitive changes, sleep disturbances, menstrual irregularities, high blood pressure, glucose intolerance, and easy bruising.

Physical Examination

On physical examination, the patient should be evaluated for hypertension, evidence of central obesity, supraclavicular fat accumulation, a dorsocervical fat pad ("buffalo hump"), facial plethora, thinned skin, purple striae, acne, ecchymoses, hirsutism, and proximal muscle weakness or wasting. Patients may offer photographs demonstrating changes in appearance over several years.

Biochemical Evaluation

Adrenal autonomy is best assessed by an overnight dexamethasone (1 mg) suppression test. Although the optimal cutoff value is controversial, a cortisol level greater than 5 mcg/dL or 138 nmol/L is an acceptable criterion for defining an abnormal result. If the result is abnormal, confirmatory testing should be performed, including midnight salivary cortisol measurements, adrenocorticotropic hormone (ACTH) measurement, 24-hour urine cortisol measurement, and possibly a 2-day dexamethasone suppression test.

Aldosterone Producing Adenoma (Zona Fasciculata)

History/Symptoms

Affected patients may have symptoms of nocturia, polyuria, muscle cramps, and palpitations, in addition to a history of hypertension often difficult to control with multiple medications.

Physical Examination

Physical examination will reveal hypertension (mild, moderate, or severe).

Biochemical Evaluation

Measurement of the plasma aldosterone concentration and plasma renin activity is the critical screening and diagnostic test. Patients may be hypokalemic or normokalemic. A ratio of plasma aldosterone concentration to plasma renin activity ratio that is 20 or higher and a plasma aldosterone concentration of 15 ng/dL are positive results. These levels and ratios can be determined while the patient is receiving antihypertensive drugs, with the exception of aldosterone antagonists such as spironolactone end eplerenone. If this screening test result is positive, the diagnosis can be confirmed by aldosterone suppression testing with either a saline infusion test or 24-hour urinary aldosterone excretion test while the patient maintains a high-sodium diet. To confirm that the adrenal mass (and not bilateral adrenal hyperplasia) is the source of aldosterone excess in patients with documented primary aldosteronism, adrenal venous sampling should be considered in patients with bilateral adrenal abnormalities on CT scans and in patients older than 40 years.

Sex Steroid Production (Zona Reticularis)

Measurement of 17-hydroxysteroid and ketosteroid levels are performed only in patients with suspected masculinizing or feminizing tumors.

Pheochromocytoma (Adrenal Medulla)

History/Symptoms

Patient may have no symptoms or may have episodic spells or paroxysms with classic symptoms that include headache, palpitations, and diaphoresis. Other symptoms reported are tremor and anxiety.

Physical Examination

Signs on physical examinations include hypertension (paroxysmal or sustained), evidence of orthostatic hypotension, pallor, and possibly retinopathy.

Biochemical Evaluation

Most pheochromocytomas secrete the catecholamines norepinephrine or epinephrine and, more rarely, dopamine. Routine testing for pheochromocytoma has included a 24-hour urine collection for catecholamines, total and fractionated metanephrines, and vanillylmandelic acid, as noted previously. In a 24-hour urine collection, a total metanephrine level above 1800 mcg in the appropriate clinical setting is highly suggestive of a pheochromocytoma, and a plasma metanephrine level exceeding three or four times normal is also highly suspect for a pheochromocytoma. The measurement of plasma free metanephrine and normetanephrine levels has the highest sensitivity (97% to 100%) and specificity (85% to 89%) and is often the best initial test in screening for pheochromocytoma. Because of the very high sensitivity of this test, if the result is negative, it is highly unlikely that the detected adrenal incidentaloma is a pheochromocytoma. If the result is positive, the diagnosis is corroborated by assessment of the patient history, a confirmatory 24-hour urine collection, the previously noted imaging phenotype, and possibly a nuclear medicine (metaiodobenzylguanidine [MIBG]) scan in select cases.

Adrenalectomy

Adrenalectomy is indicated in any patient with a hormonally active adrenal tumor, enlarging mass, or suspected malignancy. Adrenal tumors can be generally categorized as *functional* or *nonfunctional*. Most functional adrenal tumors are less than 6 cm in diameter, and patients with functional tumors are excellent candidates for laparoscopic adrenalectomy (Figure 3). Functional tumors include aldosterone- and cortisol-producing adenomas and pheochromocytomas. The main indication for performing an adrenalectomy with an open approach is the size of the tumor or mass in the adrenal gland. It may be technically feasible to remove larger tumors up to 14 cm with a laparoscopic approach; as a general rule, however, if a large adrenal tumor is suspected to be an adrenal cortical carcinoma preoperatively because of size and imaging characteristics, an open approach is recommended. These tumors are often soft, friable, and easily penetrable, with indistinct tissue planes. An open approach to these tumors is often safer, to avoid possible tumor disruption or violation of tissue planes that may occur with a laparoscopic approach.

▌ PREOPERATIVE PREPARATION

The importance of documenting and diagnosing function of an adrenal neoplasm preoperatively cannot be overemphasized, inasmuch as the preoperative, intraoperative, and postoperative medical management of patients with hormonally active tumors is extremely important.

Pheochromocytoma

Patients with pheochromocytoma are treated preoperatively for 2 to 4 weeks with α-adrenergic blockade. Phenoxybenzamine, usually at 10 mg by mouth twice daily, has been the drug of choice at the author's institution, inasmuch as intraoperative blood pressure control has been good with this regimen. The addition of β-adrenergic blockade may prove necessary after institution of α-adrenergic blockade if hypertension is persistent or tachycardia ensues. Close intraoperative communication with anesthesiology colleagues cannot be overemphasized, with availability of nitroprusside, phentolamine, and adrenergic agents after tumor removal to control blood pressure intraoperatively.

Aldosteronoma

Patients with aldosterone-producing adenomas require electrolyte monitoring and correction before surgery, which may necessitate aggressive potassium replacement. This must be done with caution and closely monitored in patients who also may be receiving spironolactone or eplerenone. In some patients, it may be difficult to completely normalize potassium levels preoperatively.

Cortisol-Producing Adenoma (Cushing)

Affected patients may be treated preoperatively for a brief period (5 to 7 days) with ketoconazole in an attempt to decrease and eliminate

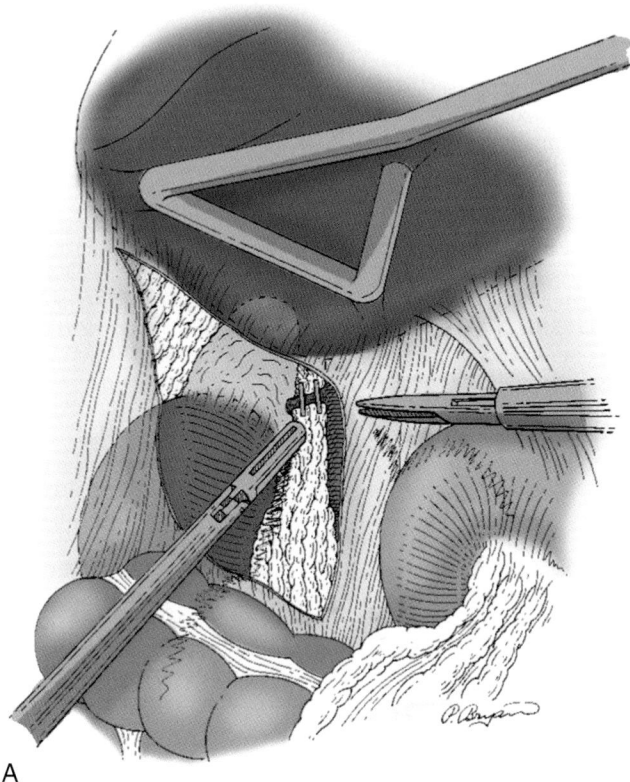

A

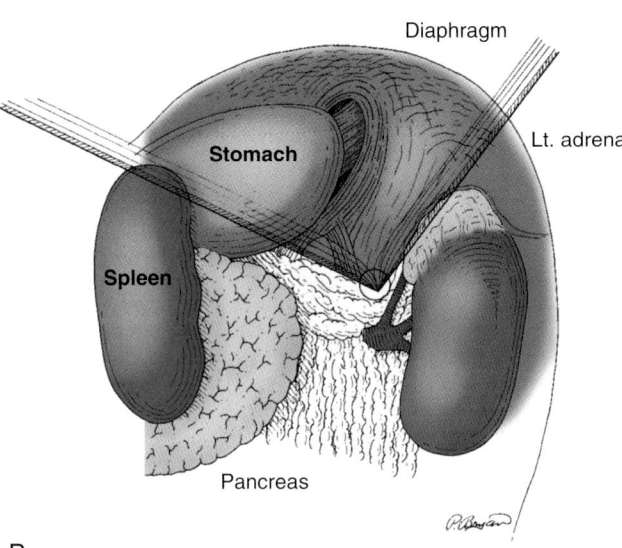

Diaphragm

Stomach

Lt. adrenal

Spleen

Pancreas

B

FIGURE 3 Laparoscopic adrenalectomy. *(From Dackiw APB: Laparoscopic adrenalectomy. In Cameron JL, editor:* Current surgical therapy, *10th ed, Philadelphia, 2011, Elsevier.)*

the significant hypercortisolemia perioperatively, which theoretically may affect blood vessel fragility and bleeding, as well as wound healing. Patients are treated with 100 mg of intravenous hydrocortisone at induction of anesthesia and after tumor removal, followed by a dose every 8 hours until oral replacement and taper begin.

OPERATIVE TECHNIQUE AND POSTOPERATIVE CARE

As noted previously, if a large adrenal tumor is suspected to be an adrenal cortical carcinoma preoperatively because of size and imaging characteristics, an open approach is recommended. The two main techniques used today for laparoscopic adrenalectomy are the lateral transabdominal approach popularized by Gagner and the posterior retroperitoneal approach popularized by Walz. Interestingly, laparoscopic left adrenalectomy and laparoscopic right adrenalectomy are two anatomically and technically distinct procedures (see Figure 3). The lateral transabdominal approach is the author's preferred approach (used in approximately 300 cases) for several reasons, except in certain clinical circumstances, such as in patients who have undergone multiple prior abdominal operations. These reasons include familiarity with laparoscopic intra-abdominal anatomy, the potential to remove larger tumors, and the ability to perform laparoscopy. Most patients who undergo laparoscopic adrenalectomy may be discharged 24 to 48 hours postoperatively. An ileus may persist for 24 to 48 hours. Patients with pheochromocytoma require postoperative hemodynamic monitoring in an intensive care unit, and those with Cushing's syndrome require postoperative stress-dose steroids, followed by an oral tapering dose often over several months for up to 2 years. Patients with aldosterone-producing adenomas often experience significant diuresis postoperatively and require close monitoring of their fluid balance and electrolytes because some may develop significant hyperkalemia.

SUGGESTED READINGS

Dackiw APB: Laparoscopic adrenalectomy. In Cameron JL, editor: *Current surgical therapy*, ed 10, Philadelphia, 2011, Elsevier.

Dackiw APB, Lee JE, Gagel RF, et al: Adrenal cortical carcinoma, *World J Surg* 25:914–926, 2001.

NIH state-of-the-science statement on management of the clinically inapparent adrenal mass ("incidentaloma"), *NIH Consens State Sci Statements* 19(2):1–25, 2002.

Young WF Jr: Clinical practice: the incidentally discovered adrenal mass, *N Engl J Med* 356:601–610, 2007.

Zeiger MA, Thompson GB, Duh QY, et al: The American Association of Clinical Endocrinologists and American Association of Endocrine Surgeons medical guidelines for the management of adrenal incidentalomas, *Endocr Pract* 15(Suppl 1):1–20, 2009.

THE MANAGEMENT OF ADRENAL CORTICAL TUMORS

Peter D. Peng, MD, Danielle A. Bischof, MD, Douglas Ball, MD, and Nita Ahuja, MD

OVERVIEW

The adrenal glands are paired retroperitoneal endocrine organs located superior to the kidneys. The left adrenal gland lies superomedial to the left kidney with venous drainage into the left renal vein, and the right adrenal gland lies superomedial to the right kidney and drains into the inferior vena cava. The adrenal cortex comprises 80% to 90% of the adrenal gland, and the zona glomerulosa, zona fasciculata, and zona reticularis are responsible for production of aldosterone, cortisol, and sex hormones, respectively.

Adrenal cortical tumors in patients referred for surgery generally fall into one of four categories: (1) incidentalomas; (2) functional hormone-secreting tumors that cause a clinical syndrome such as Cushing's syndrome, Conn's syndrome, or virilizing/feminizing syndromes; (3) adrenocortical carcinoma; or (4) adrenal metastasis. Evaluation of these patients should consist of a thorough history, physical examination, cross-sectional imaging, and functional evaluation that includes:

- Plasma renin activity (PRA), plasma aldosterone concentration (PAC), and PAC/PRA
- Serum adrenocorticotropic hormone (ACTH) *and* 24-hour urine cortisol *or* 1-mg dexamethasone suppression test *or* midnight salivary cortisol
- 24-hour urine catecholamines and metanephrines *or* plasma metanephrines

An adrenal protocol computed tomographic (CT) scan is the imaging modality of choice in the diagnostic assessment of adrenal masses. Lesion size, appearance of margins, heterogeneity, precontrast attenuation levels, percent washout on delayed images, and local extent of the lesion can distinguish lesions that are likely benign from malignant lesions and metastases. Magnetic resonance imaging (MRI) may also help differentiate an adenoma from an adrenocortical carcinoma or a metastasis and may be superior to CT scan in determination of local extent of the lesion and invasion of adjacent structures.

The role of image-guided percutaneous biopsies of the adrenal gland is limited because biopsy is unable to distinguish an adenoma from adrenocortical carcinoma. However, in patients with a history of malignancy, after a pheochromocytoma is ruled out, percutaneous biopsy may be useful to distinguish between a primary adrenal tumor and a metastatic lesion.

INCIDENTALOMA

The increasing use of cross-sectional imaging in medicine has resulted in the frequent incidental finding of adrenal masses in up to 5% of imaging studies. The evaluation and management of an incidentaloma focuses on (1) functional status and (2) likelihood of malignancy. As mentioned previously, the workup should begin with evaluation to determine whether the lesion secretes active endocrine hormones. Although history and clinical examination may provide some insight, biochemical evaluation is essential. *All functional lesions should be resected.*

Nonfunctional lesions should be evaluated for the likelihood of malignancy. Cross-sectional imaging with an adrenal protocol CT scan is useful to stratify the risk of malignancy. Empiric data have shown size to be an important criteria, with lesions less than 4 cm likely to be benign and those more than 6 cm with a significant probability of malignancy. The imaging phenotype of the lesion can also be helpful in determination of malignancy risk. Adrenal lesions have been shown to appear approximately 25% smaller on cross-sectional imaging when compared with pathologic analysis. Lesions with a precontrast density of less than 10 Hounsfield units are virtually all benign adenomas. Benign adenomas also typically display rapid washout, with more than 50% washout 10 minutes after contrast administration. Adrenocortical carcinomas, pheochromocytomas, and metastases typically have delayed washout, with less than 50% washout on delayed images. Some investigators have advocated for resection of all nonfunctional incidentalomas of more than 3 cm, and others believe that nonfunctional incidentalomas of more than 5 cm in size and those between 3 and 5 cm with imaging features not consistent with a benign adenoma should be resected. The authors recommend taking the imaging phenotype and patient factors, including age and comorbidity, into consideration when deciding on management for nonfunctional incidentalomas between 3 and 5 cm.

FUNCTIONAL HORMONE-SECRETING TUMORS

Functional hormone-secreting tumors are identified either through history and clinical examination or through the biochemical workup of an incidentally identified adrenal mass.

Aldosteronoma

Primary hyperaldosteronism accounts for 1% of all cases of hypertension and results in Conn's syndrome, which is characterized by hypertension, hypokalemia, and polyuria. Hypokalemia may result in muscle weakness, cramping, and periodic paralysis. The diagnosis is initially suggested through measurements of elevated PAC, depressed PRA, and PAC:PRA ratio greater than 30. A persistently elevated aldosterone value after salt loading (either a 2-L saline solution infusion over 4 hours or 2 days of oral sodium loading) confirms the diagnosis.

Cases of primary hyperaldosteronism are commonly caused by either an aldosteronoma (65%) or bilateral idiopathic hyperaldosteronism (25%); it is crucial to distinguish between the two because unilateral adrenalectomy in the setting of idiopathic hyperaldosteronism is not curative. High-resolution CT scanning and selective adrenal venous catheterization are used to distinguish the two diagnoses. Most clinically significant aldosteronomas are hypodense on CT scan, measuring 0.5 to 2 cm. In older patients, the risk of nonfunctional adrenal adenomas is increased, and many advocate for selective adrenal venous catheterization in patients over the age of 40 years with hyperaldosteronism to rule out bilateral hyperaldosteronism before surgery. If bilateral nodules, adrenal hypertrophy, or no lesions are found on CT scan, then selective adrenal venous catheterization with aldosterone sampling is essential to localize the lesion. Adrenal vein sampling is accomplished through measurement of aldosterone and cortisol levels in both adrenal veins and the inferior vena cava. Sensitivity of adrenal vein sampling is improved with ACTH infusion. The ratio of cortisol in the adrenal vein samples compared with inferior vena cava sample is used to confirm successful cannulation of the adrenal veins. The aldosterone/cortisol ratios from both adrenal veins are then compared. Generally, an elevation of aldosterone/cortisol ratio of greater than fourfold on one side confirms lateralization and indicates a unilateral process amenable to cure through adrenalectomy. If the ratios are similar, bilateral hyperplasia should be suspected. Bilateral adrenal hyperplasia resulting in Conn's syndrome is treated with aldosterone antagonists and surgery is not indicated. Spironolactone is the most commonly used aldosterone antagonist; eplerenone is an alternative aldosterone antagonist that can be used in males who have development of gynecomastia on spironolactone.

Laparoscopic adrenalectomy is preferred for localized aldosteronomas. Blood pressure should be optimized before surgery through administration of spironolactone, and additional antihypertensive medications can be given as needed. Potassium levels should also be normalized before surgery with potassium replacement. After resection, hypokalemia is corrected in more than 95% of patients, and 75% have improvement in hypertension. Spironolactone should be discontinued after the operation.

Cushing's Syndrome

As described by Harvey Cushing in 1932, Cushing's syndrome is caused by glucocorticoid excess and is characterized by central obesity, moon facies, hypertension, polyphagia, polydipsia, easy bruising, and skin changes. The most common causes of Cushing's syndrome are exogenous steroid use, pituitary adenomas or hyperplasia (known as Cushing's disease), ectopic ACTH-secreting tumors (small cell lung cancer, bronchial carcinoid tumors, thymomas), and ACTH-independent adrenal tumors. ACTH-independent adrenal tumors directly hypersecrete glucocorticoids and include adrenal adenomas, adrenocortical carcinomas, and more rarely, primary pigmented nodular adrenal dysplasia and macronodular adrenal hyperplasia.

The initial biochemical workup for Cushing's syndrome shows elevated 24-hour urinary-free cortisol or elevated 1-mg dexamethasone suppression test results. The 24-hour urine-free cortisol test is the most sensitive and specific test for Cushing's syndrome. Further workup aims to characterize the disease as either pituitary, ectopic, or adrenal. Low plasma ACTH levels (<5 pg/mL) through feedback inhibition can distinguish ACTH-independent adrenal tumors, whereas high levels suggest pituitary or ectopic disease. The dexamethasone suppression test can help distinguish between Cushing's disease, ectopic ACTH-secreting tumors, and ACTH-independent adrenal tumors.

CT scan and MRI complement biochemical tests by localizing pituitary and adrenal lesions. Pituitary tumors can be resected transsphenoidally or irradiated. Occasionally, patients with ACTH-dependent Cushing's disease with failed transsphenoidal resection or radiation require bilateral adrenalectomy. For cases of adrenal Cushing's syndrome, high-resolution CT scan can differentiate a unilateral adenoma from bilateral hyperplasia. Adrenal Cushing's syndrome is most commonly caused by a unilateral adrenal adenoma, which is small and amenable to laparoscopic adrenalectomy. Ketoconazole can be used to control cortisol excess before surgery. For prevention of adrenal crisis, perioperative stress dose steroids should be initiated with hydrocortisone 100 mg intravenously (IV) every 8 hours and can be tapered to an oral dose after surgery. The contralateral adrenal gland may remain suppressed for several weeks after an operation, and gradual oral steroid tapers are recommended, with close monitoring for signs of adrenal insufficiency. Perioperative antibiotics are recommended because patients are more susceptible to infectious complications. Cases of bilateral nodular hyperplasia are very rare and should be initially treated with medical management, with bilateral adrenalectomy reserved for patients with severe Cushing's syndrome who have failed medical management. After bilateral adrenalectomy, patients must be maintained on lifelong glucocorticoid and mineral-corticoid replacement.

Virilizing/Feminizing Tumors

Virilizing or feminizing tumors are rare and secrete androgen or estrogens. Approximately 50% of androgen-secreting tumors are malignant, and all feminizing tumors are malignant. Women with virilizing tumors most commonly present with hirsutism, irregular menses, or other virilizing signs. The diagnosis of an androgen-secreting tumor is established with documented elevated serum testosterone and dehydroepiandrostenedione (DHEA-S) values, with an adrenal protocol CT scan that shows an adrenal mass. Estrogen-secreting adrenal tumors can result in feminization in men, characterized by gynecomastia, gonadal atrophy, and loss of libido. In women, feminizing tumors can result in precocious puberty or postmenopausal bleeding. Feminizing adrenal tumors are characterized by elevated serum estradiol levels with suppressed gonadotropins (follicular-stimulating hormone and luteinizing hormone) and an adrenal mass on CT scan. If the appearance of a virilizing tumor on CT scan is benign, it can often be safely removed laparoscopically with a low threshold for conversion to open if evidence of local invasion or other evidence of malignancy exists. Feminizing tumors and virilizing tumors with a CT scan appearance suspicious for adrenocortical carcinoma should be removed with an open approach (see Adrenocortical Carcinoma).

ADRENOCORTICAL CARCINOMA

With an incidence rate of less than two cases per million per year, adrenocortical carcinomas (ACCs) are rare and are associated with a poor prognosis. Sixty percent of patients with ACC present with symptoms of hormone excess. Most commonly, adults with hormone-secreting ACC present with glucocorticoid excess alone (45%) or with both glucocorticoid excess and androgen excess (25%). A minority of patients with hormone-secreting ACC presents with sex-steroid excess alone; aldosterone-secreting ACC is exceedingly rare. More than 40% of patients with ACC present with metastatic disease at the time of diagnosis and are not candidates for curative-intent surgical resection. On CT scans, ACCs tend to be heterogenous with irregular borders and areas of necrosis or hemorrhage (Figure 1). CT imaging of adrenal lesions with precontrast density of more than 20 Hounsfield units and delayed washout are more likely to be malignant. More than 90% of ACCs are greater than 6 cm in size on presentation.

Preoperative staging imaging, including CT scan, of the chest and abdomen should be obtained for all patients with adrenal lesions suspicious for ACC to identify distant metastases. The most common sites for metastatic adrenocortical carcinoma are lung, liver, peritoneum, and bone. Complete surgical resection of adrenocortical carcinoma is the cornerstone of curative intent therapy for patients with stage I-III disease (Table 1); this involves en bloc resection of any involved adjacent organs for patients with locally advanced disease. Invasion into the inferior vena cava should be considered regional disease, and consideration should be given to resection and thrombectomy, which may require cardiopulmonary or veno-venous bypass. Although the experience has been mixed, in some series, laparoscopic resection of adrenocortical cancer has been associated with increased rates of tumor rupture and positive margins and decreased time to recurrence. The authors, therefore, advocate for open resection of lesions that are highly suspicious for adrenocortical carcinoma.

The overall survival rate for adrenocortical carcinoma is poor, and mean survival times are 22 to 47 months. Survival is, however, stage specific and improved with R0 resection. The 5-year survival rate with complete resection of stage I and II tumors is 40% to 60%, but only 10% of patients with stage IV disease survive beyond 1 year. Even with complete resection, recurrence of ACC is common, with up to 85% of patient having local recurrence or metastatic disease develop. Complete resection of recurrent or metastatic disease may mineralocorticoid replacement is recommended. The role of adjuvant radiation in the management of adrenocortical carcinoma is controversial. On the basis of data from retrospective case series, adjuvant radiation has been suggested for patients with positive resection margins and those with stage III disease.

ADRENAL METASTASES

Adrenal masses in patients with a history of cancer are metastatic lesions in 30% to 75% of cases. The most common cancers that metastasize to the adrenal gland are lung cancer, renal cell carcinoma, melanoma, gastrointestinal cancers, breast cancer, lymphomas, and hepatocellular carcinoma. Features of adrenal metastases on CT scan include bilateral disease, irregular shape, heterogeneity, unenhanced attenuation of more than 20 Hounsfield units, and delayed washout after contrast administration. For confirmation of the diagnosis of a metastatic lesion, fine-needle aspiration can be undertaken once pheochromocytoma has been ruled out. Imaging should be undertaken to rule out extraadrenal disease, which precludes resection.

Adrenalectomy in selected patients with isolated adrenal metastases has been associated with improved survival in retrospective series. Metachronous presentation with a long disease-free interval has been associated with improved outcomes. Most adrenal metastases are small and well encapsulated; laparoscopic adrenalectomy is believed to be as effective as open resection for these lesions. En bloc resection is recommended for lesions with local invasion of adjacent structures. Survival and recurrence rates after resection of adrenal metastases vary according to disease histology.

LAPAROSCOPIC ADRENALECTOMY

Laparoscopic adrenalectomy has become the standard technique at many institutions for small, localized adrenal tumors with benign appearance on imaging and for adrenal metastases. Many surgeons advocate the open approach for lesions suspicious for adrenocortical carcinoma and those associated with extracapsular invasion or lymphadenopathy. Laparoscopic adrenalectomy can be performed through a lateral transabdominal or a posterior retroperitoneal approach. Patient outcomes with both approaches are comparable, with improved postoperative pain requirements, resumption of regular diet, and length of stay when compared with the open approach.

The lateral transabdominal approach is the most commonly used approach for adrenalectomy. After induction of general anesthesia, a Foley catheter is placed. In addition, an orogastric tube is placed to decompress the stomach and duodenum. The patient is then positioned in the lateral decubitus position, with the affected side up, on a beanbag (Figure 2). An axillary roll is placed, and the table is flexed to increase the space between the costal margin and the iliac crest. The patient's chest and legs are taped to the operating room table. A 10-mm port is first inserted just inferior to the costal margin at the level of the midclavicular line. A 10-mm 30-degree laparoscope is used. Two additional 5-mm working ports are introduced, flanking the camera port. All trocars should be at least 5 cm apart. A right adrenalectomy often requires placement of a fourth port for liver retraction. On insertion of trocars, a diagnostic laparoscopy is performed.

The right and left adrenalectomy differs in the exposure of the adrenal gland and the adrenal vein. The authors favor early identification and ligation of the adrenal vein when possible. For large adrenal lesions, this sometimes is not possible and the gland must be mobilized before identification and division of the vein. For a left adrenalectomy, mobilization of the colon inferiorly and the spleen medially allows access to the superior pole of the kidney and the adrenal gland (Figure 3). The lateral attachments of the spleen should be mobilized superiorly until the stomach is visible for adequate

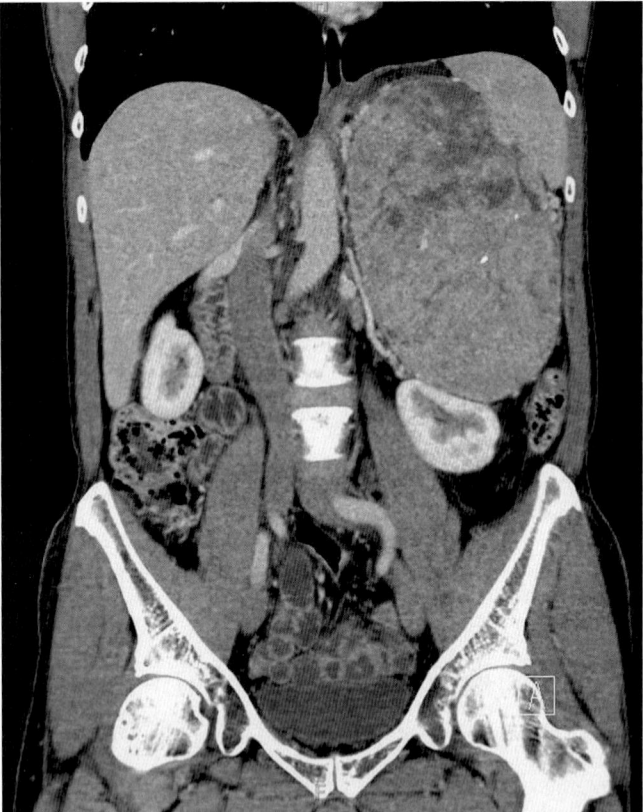

FIGURE 1 Left retroperitoneal mass replacing the left adrenal gland measures 18 × 15 × 11 cm with heterogeneous attenuation, central calcifications, and necrotic changes suspicious for adrenocortical carcinoma. On final pathology, the mass was described as an adrenocortical oncocytic neoplasm of indeterminate malignant potential, but it was treated as malignant given its size.

TABLE 1: Tumor node metastasis (TNM) staging for adrenocortical carcinoma

TNM

T1: <5 cm, no invasion
T2: >5 cm, no invasion
T3: Any size, locally invading (but not adjacent organs)
T4: Any size, locally invading adjacent organs
N0: No regional positive nodes
N1: Positive regional nodes
M0: No distant metastatic disease
M1: Distant metastasis present

Stage

I: T1N0M0
II: T2N0M0
III: T1N1M0, T2N1M0, T3N0M0
IV: T3N1M0, T4N1M0, TXNXM1

improve survival in selected patients and provides palliation from symptoms of hormone excess.

In retrospective studies, adjuvant mitotane has been shown to improve recurrence-free and overall survival in patients with resected adrenocortical carcinoma. Patients may have adrenal insufficiency develop during treatment with mitotane, and glucocorticoid and

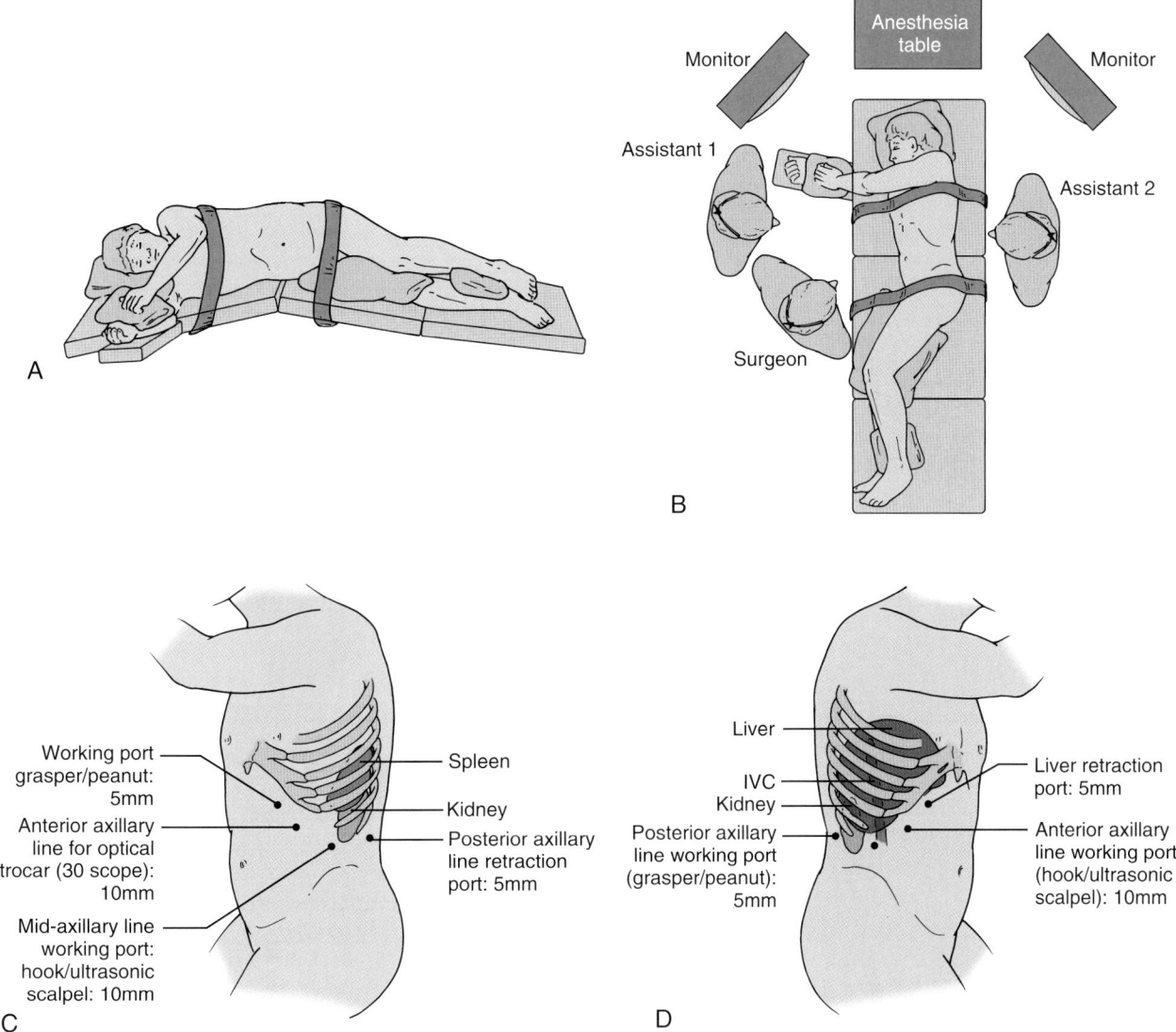

FIGURE 2   Positioning and trocar placement for laparoscopic adrenalectomy. The patient is in full lateral decubitus position, and the table is flexed to open up the flank. **A,** Patient positioning for a laparoscopic left adrenalectomy. **B,** Positioning of patient, surgical team and monitors for a laparoscopic left adrenalectomy. **C,** Trochar placement for a laparoscopic left adrenalectomy. **D,** Trochar placement for a laparoscopic right adrenalectomy. *IVC,* Inferior vena cava. *(Current Surgical Therapy, ed 10, Fig 129-3.)*

exposure of the retroperitoneum. The peritoneum is incised at the inferior aspect of the tail of the pancreas, and the plane between the tail of the pancreas and the adrenal gland and kidney is opened. The left adrenal vein is identified as it joins the left renal vein along the superior aspect of the left renal vein. The left adrenal vein is then isolated, clipped, and divided.

In a right adrenalectomy, a liver retractor is inserted to lift the right hepatic lobe anteromedially (Figure 4). The right triangular ligament and lateral hepatic attachments are divided so the right hepatic lobe can be retracted medially to allow visualization of the right adrenal gland. Dissection then begins in the plane between the lateral inferior vena cava and the right adrenal gland. This dissection is continued until the right adrenal vein is identified as it enters posterolateral aspect of the inferior vena cava. The right adrenal vein is short and broad. Dissection along the superior and inferior aspects of the right adrenal vein towards the adrenal gland can often lengthen the vein to facilitate clipping and division of the vein. The vein is then isolated, clipped, and divided (or stapled with an endoscopic vascular stapler). The plane between the lateral inferior vena cava and the

medial aspect of the right adrenal is then further developed, with care taken to identify and ligate an accessory adrenal vein (generally superior to the main adrenal vein) when present.

For both approaches, after the adrenal vein is divided, the adrenal is then dissected out from surrounding retroperitoneal structures with a Harmonic scalpel (Ethicon Endosurgery, Cincinnati, Ohio). Adrenal arteries, which can be highly variable, are divided with the Harmonic scalpel or are clipped, depending on the size of the vessel. Minimized grasping of the adrenal is essential to avoid tumor rupture and nuisance bleeding. Once the adrenal gland is freed, it is placed in a specimen bag and extracted from the camera trocar site.

SUMMARY

The indications for operative resection of adrenocortical tumors are evidence of functional hormone secretion and risk of malignancy. Biochemical tests and cross-sectional imaging are thus essential for diagnosis and operative planning. Localized adrenocortical

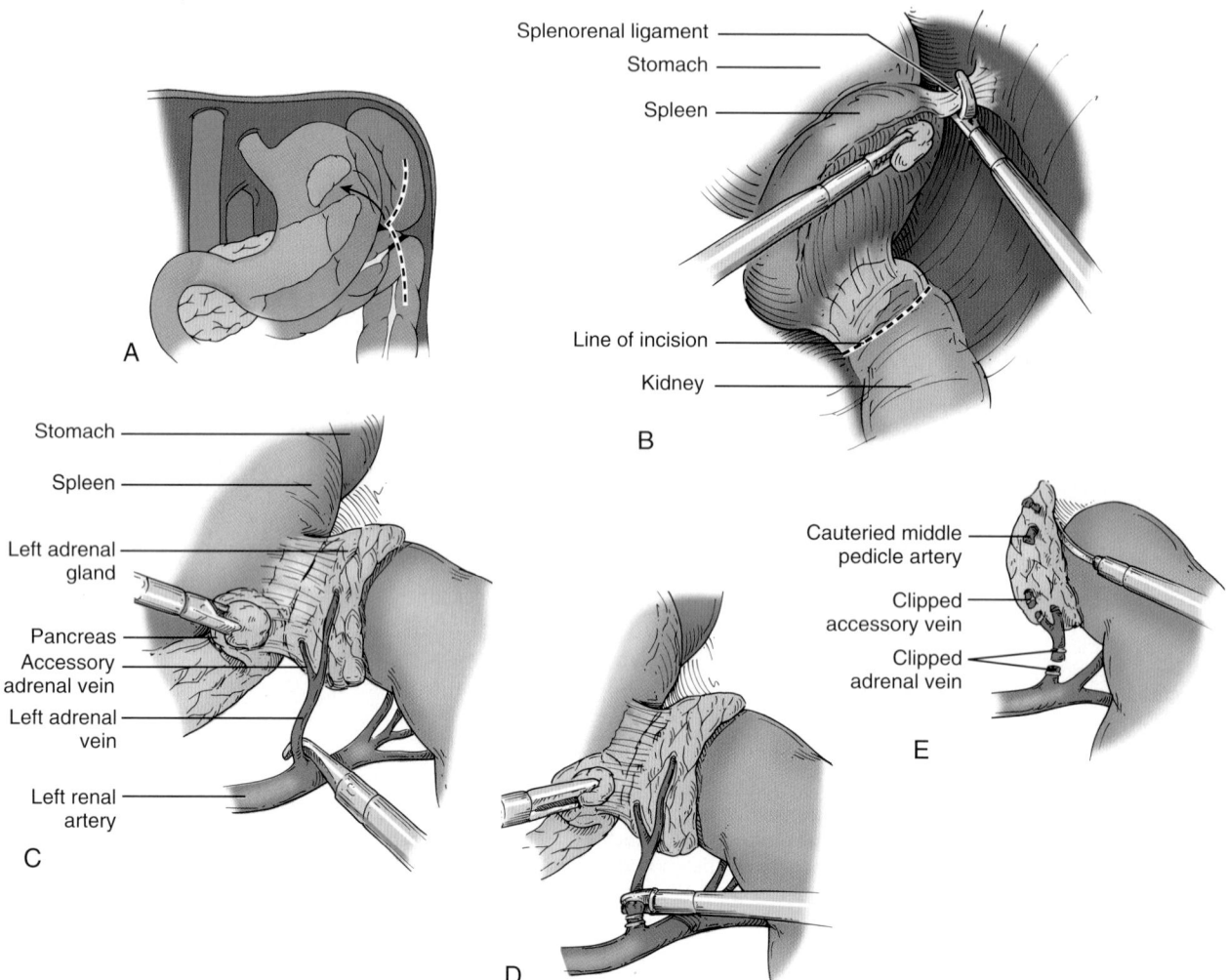

FIGURE 3 Technique of laparoscopic left adrenalectomy. **A,** The splenic flexure is mobilized; the splenorenal ligament must be completely mobilized to the left crus of the diaphragm. **B,** Incise the peritoneum along the inferior border of the pancreas to expose the adrenal gland. **C,** Dissect along the superior border of the renal vein to identify the main adrenal vein. **D,** Divide the main adrenal vein between 10-mm clips. **E,** Mobilize the remainder of the adrenal gland with the ultrasonic scalpel. (Current Surgical Therapy, ed 10, Fig 129-4.)

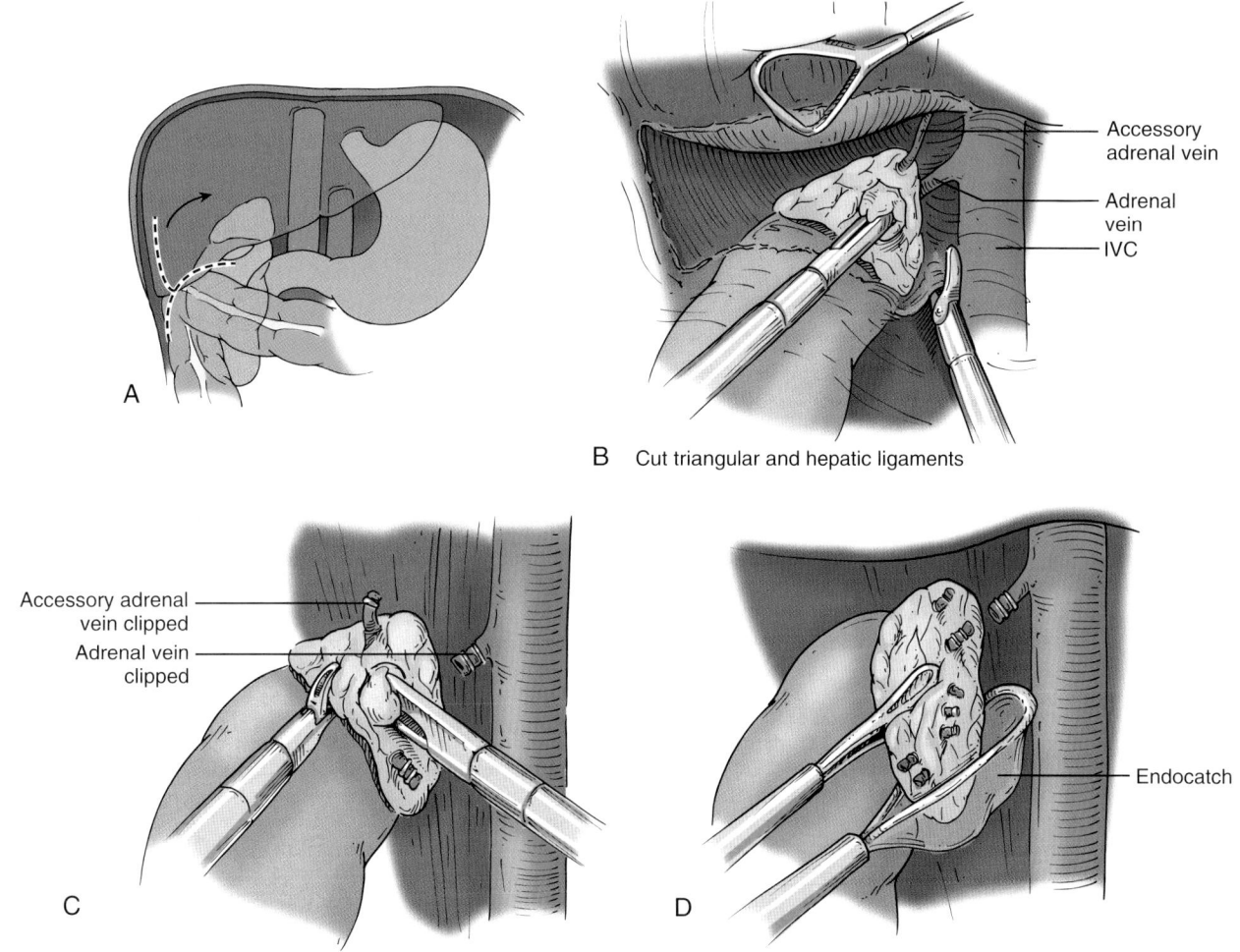

Accessory
adrenal vein

Adrenal
vein

IVC

B   Cut triangular and hepatic ligaments

Accessory adrenal
vein clipped

Adrenal vein
clipped

Endocatch

FIGURE 4   Technique of laparoscopic right adrenalectomy. **A,** The right hepatic lobe is mobilized to completely expose the right adrenal gland and vein. **B,** Dissect along the lateral wall of the vena cava until the right adrenal vein is identified. **C,** Mobilize the remainder of the gland with the ultrasonic scalpel. **D,** Remove gland with sterile impermeable bag. *IVC,* Inferior vena cava. *(Current Surgical Therapy, ed 10, Fig 129-5.)*

carcinomas should be resected en bloc through an open approach. Laparoscopic adrenalectomy is appropriate for smaller noninvasive lesions and for metastatic adrenal tumors.

SELECTED READINGS

Johnson PT, Horton KM, Fishman EK: Adrenal mass imaging with multidetector CT: pathologic conditions, pearls, and pitfalls, *Radiographics* 29(5):1333–1351, 2009.

McKenzie TJ, Lillegard JB, Young WF Jr, et al: Aldosteronomas: state of the art, *Surg Clin North Am* 89(5):1241–1253, 2009.

Miller BS, Ammori JB, Gauger PG, et al: Laparoscopic resection is inappropriate in patients with known or suspected adrenocortical carcinoma, *World J Surg* 34(6):1380–1385, 2010.

Shen WT, Sturgeon C, Duh Q: From incidentaloma to adrenocortical carcinoma: the surgical management of adrenal tumors, *J Surg Oncol* 89:186–192, 2005.

Zeh HJ 3rd, Udelsman R: One hundred laparoscopic adrenalectomies: a single surgeon's experience, *Ann Surg Oncol* 10(9):1012–1017, 2003.

Zeiger MA, Thompson GB, Duh QY, et al: American Association of Clinical Endocrinologists and American Association of Endocrine Surgeons medical guidelines for the management of adrenal incidentalomas: executive summary of recommendations, *Endocrine Pract* 15(5):450–453, 2009.

The Management of Pheochromocytoma

James C. Cusack, Jr., MD, and
Roy Phitayakorn, MD, MHPE (MEd)

OVERVIEW

Until recently, rare tumors arising from chromaffin cells of neural crest origin and located in sympathetic and parasympathetic paraganglia were called pheochromocytomas. In 2004, the World Health Organization more specifically classified these tumors based on their origin and designated the more common tumor that arises approximately 90% of the time in the adrenal medulla as pheochromocytoma. In contrast, the term paraganglioma is now used to describe the less common extraadrenal tumor that arises from the para-aortic sympathetic chain, the sympathetic and parasympathetic chain of the neck (including the carotid body) and posterior mediastinum, the organ of Zuckerkandl, or the urinary bladder. Most commonly, patients with pheochromocytoma/paraganglioma present with non-specific symptoms of catecholamine excess, such as hypertension, headaches, palpitations, and sweating, although 10% of tumors are asymptomatic. Serious complications associated with catecholamine storm, including myocardial infarction, cardiac failure, aortic dissection, and takotsubo cardiomyopathy, may first occur during induction of general anesthesia or surgery. The incidence rate of pheochromocytoma and paraganglioma is two to eight per million persons per year and is equally distributed between males and females, most commonly in their third to fifth decade. Although rare, these tumors are present in up to 1% of patients with hypertension and up to 5% of patients with incidentally discovered adrenal masses. The historical "10% rule" no longer pertains to pheochromocytoma and paraganglioma. Although 10% of these tumors are extra-adrenal in location, 15% to 20% are now estimated to be malignant, defined by the presence of metastases not local invasion, and as many as 25% of these tumors occur in the setting of a hereditary syndrome such as multiple endocrine neoplasia types 2A and 2B, von Hippel-Lindau disease, neurofibromatosis type 1, and hereditary paraganglioma syndrome. These changes have implications in the workup, management, and surveillance of the patient newly diagnosed with pheochromocytoma or paraganglioma. For example, genetic testing should be considered for patients diagnosed with pheochromocytoma or paraganglioma, particularly those with bilateral or multifocal disease, sympathetic and malignant extra-adrenal disease, family history suggestive of a hereditary pheochromocytoma-paraganglioma syndrome, and age less than 50 years. Effective leadership by the well-informed surgeon, who coordinates the efforts of the multidisciplinary team that includes the endocrinologist, radiologist, anesthesiologist, surgeon, and genetics counselor, is requisite to the successful management of the patient with pheochromocytoma and paraganglioma.

CLINICAL PRESENTATION

With the current frequency of radiographic imaging, one of the most common presentations of a patient with pheochromocytoma is an incidentally found adrenal mass. Clinical signs or symptoms of functional pheochromocytomas include hypertension, blurred vision, headaches, sweating, dyspnea, chest pain, constipation, tachycardia/palpitations, nausea/vomiting, and psychiatric symptoms including anxiety, aggression, and a feeling of impending doom. However, approximately 20% of patients may have a pheochromocytoma that is biochemically inactive. Some patients may also present after hypertensive complications upon receiving general anesthesia for an unrelated operation.

DIAGNOSIS

All patients with a suspected pheochromocytoma or paraganglioma should undergo biochemical screening that typically includes 24-hour urinary catecholamines and metabolites (vanillylmandelic acid, total and fractionated metanephrines, epinephrine, norepinephrine, and dopamine). These results can be confirmed with measurements of plasma catecholamine and metabolite levels and chromogranin A. Figure 1 illustrates an example of a biochemical workup algorithm. Alternatively, some centers use plasma metanephrines to *exclude* a biochemically functional pheochromocytoma and then proceed with urinary catecholamine and metabolite measurements only for patients with plasma catecholamines that are three to four times the upper limits of normal. Table 1 lists various foods and medications that may lead to falsely elevated urinary or plasma catecholamine or metabolite levels.

Once the biochemical diagnosis of pheochromocytoma or paraganglioma is confirmed, localization studies include either adrenal-protocol computed tomographic (CT) imaging or magnetic resonance imaging (MRI). An adrenal-protocol CT scan includes 2-mm to 5-mm scanning slices with 3 phases of imaging (noncontrast, with contrast, and delayed washout). Pheochromocytomas and paragangliomas are typically dense on CT scan (Hounsfield units, >10) and retain contrast on delayed washout images. An MRI may be more useful in patients who cannot receive radiation (pregnancy, children) or have contrast allergies. Pheochromocytomas and paragangliomas are typically hyperintense on T2-weighted images and isointense to hypointense relative to liver on T1-weighted images. Radiographic signs associated with malignancy include large size, gross invasion of surrounding structures, and metastases.

If neither CT scan nor MRI is able to locate a pheochromocytoma or paraganglioma or metastatic disease is suspected in a patient with positive biochemical testing, an ^{123}I-metaiodobenzylguanidine (MIBG) image is often obtained next because of its excellent specificity for pheochromocytoma. Importantly, patients who undergo ^{123}I-MIBG imaging should receive a short course of either supersaturated potassium chloride (SSKI) or potassium perchlorate to prevent postprocedure thyroid complications. Similarly, [^{18}F] fluorodeoxyglucose (FDG) positron emission tomography (PET) may be useful to localize possible metastases in cases of malignant pheochromocytoma, but false-positive results from retroperitoneal brown fat are common.

PREOPERATIVE MANAGEMENT

Before adrenalectomy, patients with a pheochromocytoma should have a complete blood count, basic metabolic panel, and an electrocardiogram (EKG). The EKG frequently shows repolarization abnormalities, which are the result of the toxic effects of excessive catecholamines on the myocardium. A preoperative echocardiogram may be of value in patients with a significant cardiac history or a new cardiac murmur to aid in risk stratification.

General recommendations are that all patients with pheochromocytoma undergo alpha-adrenergic blockade, which should be started 1 to 2 weeks before surgery. An exception to alpha-adrenergic blockade may be patients with a pheochromocytoma that only secretes dopamine. The clinical goal of alpha-blockade is postural hypotension, but patients may experience other side effects, including fatigue, reflex tachycardia, loose stools, dizziness, somnolence, or

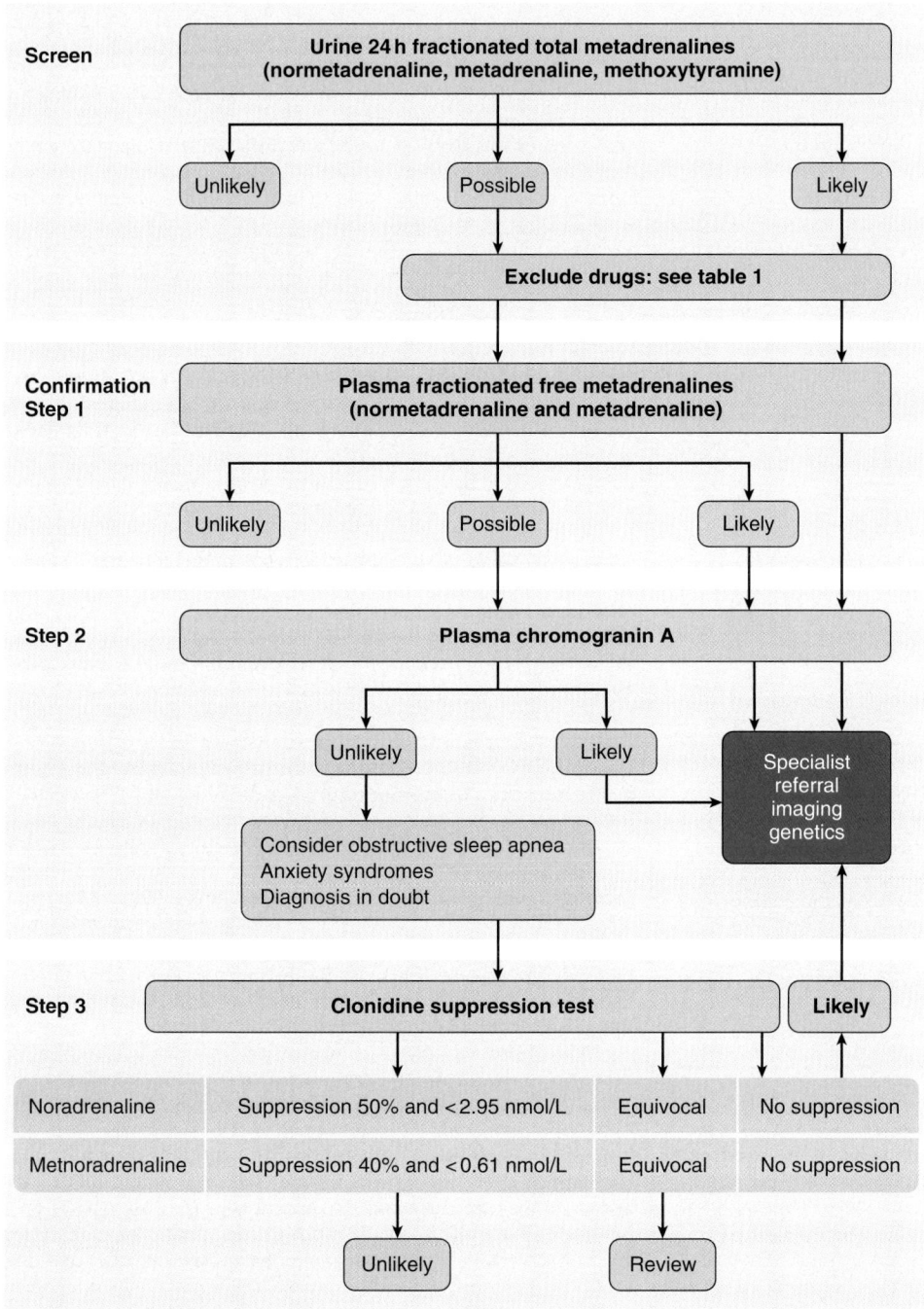

Screen — Urine 24 h fractionated total metadrenalines (normetadrenaline, metadrenaline, methoxytyramine)

Unlikely — Possible — Likely

Exclude drugs: see table 1

Confirmation Step 1 — Plasma fractionated free metadrenalines (normetadrenaline and metadrenaline)

Unlikely — Possible — Likely

Step 2 — Plasma chromogranin A

Unlikely — Likely

Specialist referral imaging genetics

Consider obstructive sleep apnea
Anxiety syndromes
Diagnosis in doubt

Step 3 — Clonidine suppression test — **Likely**

Noradrenaline	Suppression 50% and <2.95 nmol/L	Equivocal	No suppression
Metnoradrenaline	Suppression 40% and <0.61 nmol/L	Equivocal	No suppression

Unlikely — Review

FIGURE 1 A sample biochemical workup algorithm for patients with a suspected functional pheochromocytoma or paraganglioma. *(Used with permission from Barron J: Phaeochromocytoma: diagnostic challenges for biochemical screening and diagnosis, J Clin Pathol 63:669-674, 2010.)*

nasal congestion. Several alpha-blockers are commonly used in patients with pheochromocytoma. The authors most commonly use phenoxybenzamine (Dibenzyline), which is a long-acting, noncompetitive alpha-antagonist. Patients are started on a 10-mg dose twice a day, and the dose is gradually increased by 10 mg every other day until the patient becomes orthostatic. Most patients become orthostatic with a total dosage of 40 to 120 mg/d (1 mg/kg), but dosages up to 240 mg/d may be necessary. The authors typically titrate alpha-blockade on an outpatient basis, but some patients need inpatient admission to achieve successful blockade. Phenoxybenzamine can lead to tachycardia from increased norepinephrine release by cardiac sympathetic nerve endings. This side effect can be ameliorated with the concomitant usage of beta-blockers. Beta-blockers are typically started several days before surgery after alpha-adrenergic blockade and subsequently titrated to a goal heart rate of around 60 beats per minute. Beta-blockers should not be given before alpha-adrenergic blockade to avoid unopposed alpha-adrenergic receptor stimulation, which can cause hypertensive crisis.

Selective short-acting alpha-adrenergic blockers (doxazosin, prazosin, and terazosin) are competitive α_1-receptor antagonists and have a shorter duration of action, less associated reflex tachycardia, and a lower incidence of postoperative hypotension compared with phenoxybenzamine. However, incomplete alpha-adrenergic blockade may occur with prazosin or terazosin because they require more frequent dosing than doxazosin.

Dihydropyridine calcium-channel blockers, amlodipine, nifedipine, or nicardipine, may also be used as part of the preoperative preparation for patients with pheochromocytoma as an adjunct to alpha-adrenergic blockade or in patients who are intolerant to alpha-blockers. Preferential use of calcium channel blockers before surgery

TABLE 1: Foods and medications associated with false-positive elevations in catecholamine levels

Chocolate
Beers and wine
Cured or smoked meats
Aged cheeses (including yogurt and sour cream)
Fermented soy bean or fish products (tofu, soy sauce, fish sauce, shrimp paste)
Nuts (peanuts, coconuts, Brazil nuts)
Certain fruits (raspberries, red plums, pineapples, bananas, and figs)
Certain vegetables (avocados, eggplants, fava beans, snow peas, green beans, and sauerkraut)
Opioid analgesics (oxycodone, morphine, tramadol, heroin) and naloxone
Corticosteroids
Antidepressants such as tricyclic antidepressants (amitriptyline, nortriptyline, imipramine, clomipramine), norepinephrine reuptake inhibitors, type-A monoamine oxidase inhibitors (phenelzine and deprenyl), and selective serotonin reuptake inhibitors (fluoxetine, duloxetine, paroxetine)
Antibiotics such as linezolid
Antipsychotics such as droperidol, sulpiride, chlorpromazine
Antiemetics such metoclopramide and prochlorperazine
Nasal decongestants that contain pseudoephedrine or phenylpropanolamine
Weight-loss supplements that contain fenfluramine, amfepramone, phendimetrazine, phenylethylamine, or phentermine
Antinarcolepsy medications that contain dextroamphetamine
Attention-deficit hyperactivity disorder medications that contain amphetamine or methylphenidate
Anti-impotence supplements that contain yohimbe bark extract
Illegal recreational drugs such as ketamine and cocaine
Chewing tobacco

may be of more value in patients with normotensive conditions who have intermittent paroxysmal hypertensive episodes to avoid the side effects of orthostatic hypotension associated with the alpha-adrenergic blockers.

Metyrosine (alpha-methyl-para-tyrosine) is also used for preoperative preparation of patients with pheochromocytoma. Metyrosine depletes adrenal catecholamine stores by inhibiting tyrosine hydroxylase, the rate-limiting enzyme in catecholamine synthesis. However, metyrosine may also cause extrapyramidal side effects, sedation, depression, and galactorrhea. Because of its greater toxicity, including potential negative effect on cardiac function, the authors reserve metyrosine for patients who cannot tolerate alpha and beta blockade or who have hypertension that is refractory to alpha-adrenergic blockade.

Patients with pheochromocytoma require preoperative intravascular volume resuscitation with a balanced oral electrolyte solution after starting alpha-blockade. Some clinicians also advocate a high sodium diet (>5 g/d), and others admit patients with pheochromocytoma the day before surgery to supplement intravascular volume with isotonic intravenous fluids. Ideally, a patient should receive enough preoperative volume resuscitation to have a hematocrit value that has been reduced into the normal range before surgery. These measures likely help to minimize severe postoperative hypotension after resection of the pheochromocytoma, but no randomized controlled studies exist to confirm their efficacy.

INTRAOPERATIVE MANAGEMENT

Careful preparation for the potentially dramatic hemodynamic swings that may accompany resection of pheochromocytoma and paraganglioma is requisite to the safe intraoperative management of these patients. Before induction of general anesthesia, large-bore intravenous access is established to facilitate rapid volume resuscitation and an intraarterial catheter is placed for continuous blood pressure monitoring. Although a pulmonary artery catheter is reserved for patients with underlying systolic or diastolic cardiac dysfunction, a central venous catheter may be helpful in select patients. A urinary catheter is placed routinely. The management plan for intraoperative acute catecholamine excess before ligation of draining veins of the pheochromocytoma or paraganglioma, and intraoperative acute catecholamine deficiency after control or ligation of the draining veins, should be discussed by the anesthesiologist and surgeon as a component of the Universal Protocol. The pharmacologic agents to be used during the procedure are mixed in advance, and the lines are fed through pumps.

Short-acting antihypertensive agents are used for rapid control of hypertension. Sodium nitroprusside, a potent direct-acting vasodilator favored for this purpose because of its rapid onset of action (within seconds) and short duration of effect (3 to 4 minutes), may be titrated at doses of 0.5 to 8 µg/kg/min. Transient dose increases up to 8 µg/kg/min to control acute hypertension should never exceed 10 minutes because of potentially toxic accumulation of cyanide ion. Other agents such as esmolol, nicardipine, and nitroglycerine have less desirable properties of a somewhat slower onset of action or a longer duration of effect but may be used to supplement the antihypertensive effects of sodium nitroprusside. Fenoldopam mesylate, a benzazepine derivative and selective dopamine-1–receptor agonist is a more recently developed agent used to manage hypertensive crisis that has both an intermediate time to onset and duration of effect. Intravenous magnesium has recently been advocated as a safe and effective adjunct in the intraoperative management of pheochromocytomas and paragangliomas because it provides a catecholamine blockade and protection against life-threatening cardiac arrhythmias. Lidocaine bolus followed by continuous infusion may also be used to manage ventricular arrhythmias.

Hypotension that may accompany ligation of the adrenal vein or draining vessels of a paraganglioma results from a rapid drop in serum levels of vasoactive catecholamines. The likelihood of significant hypotension after ligation of the venous drainage from the tumor is associated with large tumor size and the presence of high circulating levels of catecholamines. Hemodynamic instability appears to be less dependent on surgical approach, the type of preoperative adrenergic blockade used, or the specific type of tumor syndrome. Resultant hypotension after ligation of the draining vessels typically responds to immediate cessation of all vasodilatory agents, titration of exogenous catecholamines (epinephrine, norepinephrine, or dopamine) or phenylephrine, and rapid volume resuscitation with crystalloids or blood as indicated.

Refractory hypotension as may occur in the setting of intraoperative hemorrhage or massive serum catecholamine levels may be rescued with transfusion or vasopressin therapy, respectively. Most importantly, minimization of manipulation of the adrenal gland or paraganglioma before ligation of the draining veins and close communication between surgeon and anesthesiologist at the critical step of ligation of the venous drainage minimize hemodynamic lability during surgery.

OPERATIVE TECHNIQUE

Selection of the surgical approach (transabdominal or retroperitoneal) and technique (open, minimally invasive laparoscopic, or single-port access) used to manage pheochromocytoma depends to a large degree on whether the tumor is unilateral, bilateral, or multifocal and whether the patient has hereditary or sporadic pheochromocytoma. Factors that influence the choice of an open surgical approach include a suspicion of local invasion as determined by size greater than 6 cm or radiographic evidence of vascular invasion and the location of a paraganglioma in a region not easily accessed with minimally invasive techniques. Minimally invasive adrenalectomy is the preferred technique because it is associated with less postoperative pain, shorter hospital stays, and quicker return to work compared with open adrenalectomy.

Recent technical advances have led to changes in the specific approach used to treat pheochromocytoma, and posterior retroperitoneoscopic adrenalectomy is preferentially used in certain centers for the resection of sporadic pheochromocytoma less than 5 cm and unilateral hereditary pheochromocytoma in the presence of a normal contralateral adrenal. Although both approaches have proven to be safe and have comparable blood loss, the posterior retroperitoneoscopic approach offers early control of the adrenal vein and requires less manipulation of the adrenal and adjacent soft tissue structures and therefore requires less operative time. Patients with hereditary disease and evidence of bilateral adrenal involvement are generally treated with an open technique, comprised of a total adrenalectomy and a contralateral cortical-sparing adrenalectomy. Cortical-sparing adrenalectomy is also used in the setting of contralateral metachronous pheochromocytoma in patients who have undergone prior adrenalectomy.

Transabdominal Laparoscopic Adrenalectomy

The patient is administered intravenous antibiotics and sequential compression devices are placed for deep venous thrombosis (DVT) prophylaxis. The patient is administered general endotracheal anesthesia in the supine position and then placed in the lateral decubitus position with the bed flexed to increase the distance between the ribs and iliac crest. After a pneumoperitoneum is established, 3 10-mm trocars are placed with direct visualization 2 cm below and parallel to the costal margin and spaced equidistant from the midclavicular line medially to the midaxillary line laterally. A 30-degree laparoscope is placed through the middle trocar, and the peritoneal reflection of the kidney is dissected to facilitate placement of a fourth trocar at the costovertebral angle.

In the case of a left adrenalectomy, the splenic flexure is taken down medially to facilitate displacement of the colon away from the inferior aspect of the adrenal. The lienorenal ligament is incised 1 cm from the spleen, and the dissection continues up to the diaphragm, stopping at the short gastric vessels posterior to the stomach. The tail of the pancreas and spleen fall medially to expose the adrenal gland. The lateral and anterior portions are dissected free with careful grasping and retracting of the perirenal fat, with care to leave the adrenal capsule intact. The adrenal vein, which drains into the left renal vein, is clipped, as is the adrenal artery, and divided. The smaller branch vessels are divided with a Harmonic scalpel (Ethicon Endosurgery, Cincinnati, Ohio), EnSeal device (SurgRx, Inc, Redwood City, Calif), or LigaSure (Covidien, Boulder, Colo) vessel-sealing device. Once separated from the remainder of the retroperitoneal attachments, the adrenal is placed into an EndoCatch bag (Ethicon Endosurgery) and removed. All trocar sites are closed with absorbable suture.

For a right adrenalectomy, the lateral peritoneal attachments to the liver and the triangular ligament are taken down, and the liver is retracted with a fan retractor placed through the medial port. The adrenal gland, identified at the medial aspect of the superior pole of the kidney, is dissected circumferentially after incising Gerota's fascia. The right adrenal vein, which drains into the vena cava, is identified, clipped, and divided. The adrenal artery is similarly divided, and the smaller vessels are controlled with a vessel-sealing device. The right adrenal gland may then be removed as described for the resection of the left adrenal gland.

Posterior Retroperitoneoscopic Adrenalectomy

The principle advantage of posterior retroperitoneoscopic adrenalectomy (PRA) over anterior laparoscopic approaches is direct access to the adrenal glands without the need to enter the peritoneal cavity or displace adjacent organs. Another noteworthy advantage to this approach includes access for potential bilateral adrenalectomy. Furthermore, insufflation of the retroperitoneal space may be better tolerated from a cardiac and pulmonary perspective than insufflation of the peritoneal cavity used in the laparoscopic transabdominal approach. This approach is rapidly becoming the preferred approach for benign pheochromocytomas up to 6 cm in diameter. Disadvantages of this approach are difficulty controlling significant hemorrhage because of the small working space and a paucity of anatomic landmarks during the initial phases of the dissection. Contraindications to this approach include malignant pheochromocytoma and any evidence of invasion of the tumor into surrounding structures on preoperative imaging studies. Morbid obesity with a body mass index (BMI) of more than 45 is a relative contraindication. Single-access techniques with this approach are also in development.

The patient receives preoperative antibiotics and DVT prophylaxis as in the case of the laparoscopic approach. The patient is first positioned in the supine position for the administration of general endotracheal anesthesia. The patient is then repositioned in the prone jackknife position on a Cloward table (Cloward Surgical Saddle, Surgical Equipment International, Honolulu, Hawaii), which supports the anterior iliac crests laterally and allows the abdomen to hang anteriorly between the saddle to reduce pressure on the retroperitoneal space (Figure 2). Knees and hips are bent at a 90-degree angle, and the knee rest is lowered to minimize pressure on the knees. The face is padded, and the arms are flexed on arm boards with the elbows bent at a 90-degree angle.

Relative to careful patient positioning, port placement is equally important. A 1.5-cm incision is made immediately adjacent to the tip of the 12th rib, and the subcutaneous tissues are dissected to facilitate entry into the retroperitoneal space (see Figure 2). This site subsequently is used as the middle port site. A small space 5 cm medial and 5 cm lateral is developed in the retroperitoneal space with blunt dissection. The medial (10-mm) trocar is placed just lateral to the paraspinous muscles and 5 cm medial to the middle port site. The trocar is aimed at the adrenal gland and angled at 45 degrees cephalad. The lateral (5-mm) trocar is placed inferior to the 11th rib and 5 cm lateral to the middle trocar and aimed medially toward the adrenal. A 12-mm trocar with an inflatable balloon and adjustable sleeve is then placed into the middle trocar site. A pneumoperitoneum is created with CO_2 to a pressure of 20 to 24 mm Hg to minimize venous bleeding in the operative field. A 10-mm, 30-degree videoscope is placed into the middle trocar, and the retroperitoneal space below the diaphragm is dissected with sharp and blunt technique. The videoscope is placed through the medial trocar, and the surgeon works through the middle and later trocars to reveal Gerota's fascia. The fascia is then dissected to reveal the superior pole of the kidney. With further dissection, the paraspinous muscles are retracted to reveal the adrenal gland. On the right side, the inferior vena cava (IVC) is identified, and the liver may be visible through the peritoneum. On the left side, the posterior wall of the stomach and spleen may be appreciated through the peritoneum. A tear in the peritoneum during the course of dissection does not compromise the pneumoperitoneum and need not be repaired.

With the Harmonic scalpel or the EnSeal device, the adrenal gland is dissected first along its inferior aspect overlying the superior aspect of the kidney by gently retracting the adrenal gland in the cephalad direction and the kidney in the caudal direction. Dissection of the medial attachments then reveals the adrenal vein, which on the right side drains medially into the IVC (Figure 3) and on the left side drains inferiorly into the renal vein (Figure 4). The adrenal vein is clipped and divided. The dissection of the superior and medial aspects of the adrenal gland is then completed. The gland is placed

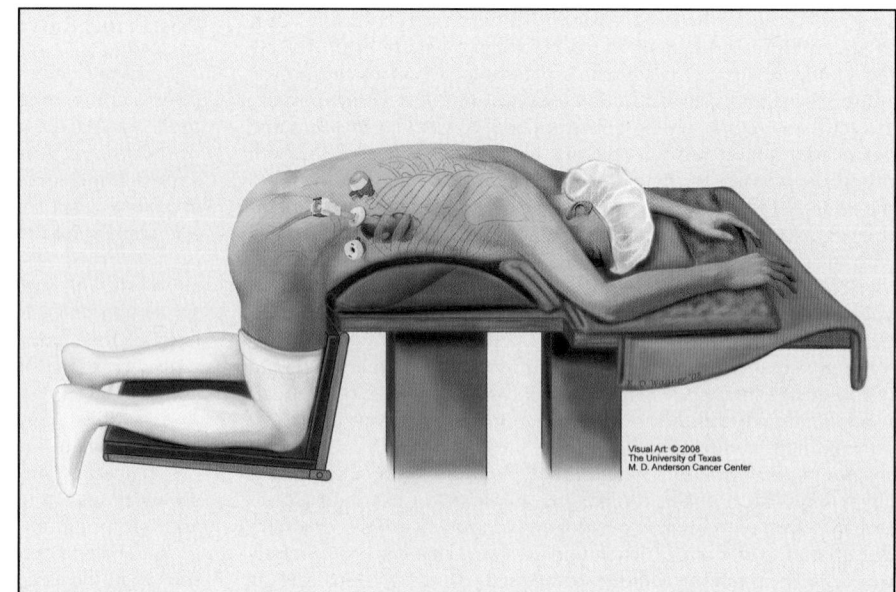

FIGURE 2 The Cloward table (Cloward Surgical Saddle, Surgical Equipment International, Honolulu, Hawaii) allows the patient's abdomen to hang anteriorly to decrease pressure on the retroperitoneal space. *(Used with permission from Callender GG, Kennamer DL, Grubbs EG, et al: Posterior retroperitoneoscopic adrenalectomy, Adv Surg 43(1):147-157, 2009.)*

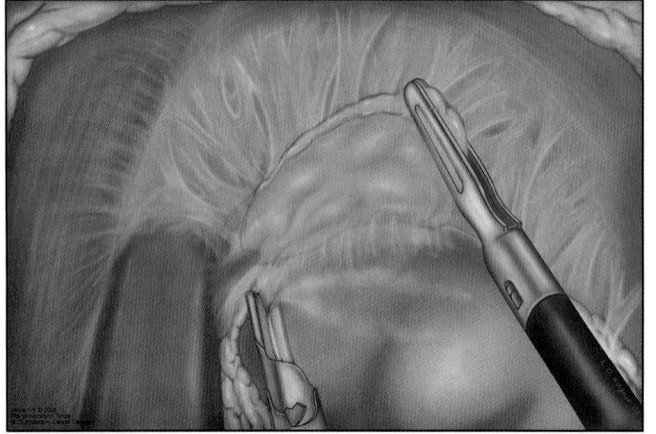

FIGURE 3 Right posterior retroperitoneoscopic adrenalectomy. After identification of the paraspinous muscles *(left)*, the inferior vena cava, and the superior pole of the right kidney, the adrenal is dissected inferiorly off the kidney, leaving the superior and medial attachments intact. The adrenal vein is identified medially, then clipped and divided. The medial and superior dissection can then proceed. *(Used with permission from Callender GG, Kennamer DL, Grubbs EG, et al: Posterior retroperitoneoscopic adrenalectomy, Adv Surg 43(1):147-157, 2009.)*

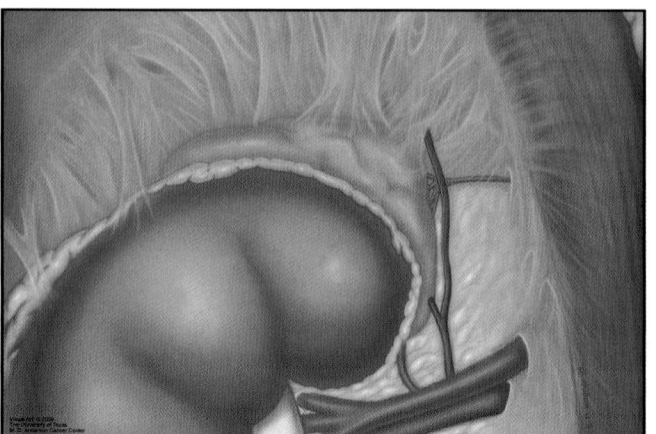

FIGURE 4 Left posterior retroperitoneoscopic adrenalectomy. After dissection of the inferior aspect of the adrenal gland from the left kidney, the adrenal gland can be gently retracted laterally by grasping the periadrenal fat to reveal the adrenal vein, which drains inferiorly into the renal vein. The adrenal vein is clipped and divided before dissecting the gland superiorly and medially. *(Used with permission from Callender GG, Kennamer DL, Grubbs EG, et al: Posterior retroperitoneoscopic adrenalectomy, Adv Surg 43(1):147-157, 2009.)*

into an EndoCatch device passed through the middle trocar and removed. The retroperitoneal space is inspected for bleeding as the insufflation pressure is reduced to 10 mm Hg. Once hemostasis is obtained, the ports are removed and the sites are closed with absorbable sutures.

Open Adrenalectomy and Cortical-Sparing Adrenalectomy

When an open adrenalectomy is considered, a standard operative approach through either a long subcostal, bilateral subcostal, or upper midline incision is used. Although the classic

thoracoabdominal incision, which extends from the abdomen up through the seventh or eighth intercostal space and through the diaphragm, provides excellent exposure to the retroperitoneum, it is associated with increased morbidity and is rarely used. Critical steps involved in a right adrenalectomy include superior and medial mobilization of the liver to expose the inferior vena cava and right hepatic vein. This facilitates complete visualization of the adrenal gland. Dissection is performed along the superior and inferior aspect to expose the adrenal vein at the superomedial aspect of the gland. Dissection of the retroperitoneal soft tissues along the IVC above the duodenum toward the tumor is performed, and small veins draining the caudate lobe into the IVC are ligated and divided. Gentle traction on the adrenal gland laterally and inferiorly combined with medial and anterior traction of the IVC with a vein retractor expose the short, broad adrenal vein as it enters the posterior aspect of the IVC. The adrenal vein may be suture ligated or clipped and divided. The adrenal artery branch from the inferior phrenic artery may be identified at the superomedial aspect of the gland. This vessel should be ligated and divided, followed by division of the small arterial and venous branches located inferomedially, connected to the renal artery, aorta, and renal vein.

The open left adrenalectomy is approached through a long left subcostal or upper midline incision. The omentum is mobilized from the left transverse colon and splenic flexure. Adhesions from the posterior wall of the stomach to the pancreas are lysed, and the inferior border of the pancreas is dissected free from retroperitoneal soft tissues with careful blunt technique. The lateral peritoneal attachments to the spleen are divided, and the spleen and the body and tail of pancreas are reflected toward the right upper quadrant. The adrenal vein, located inferomedially, may be visualized early in the course of dissection, in which case it should be ligated and divided. Often a large tumor may obscure visualization of the adrenal vein, in which case the gland needs to be mobilized along the superior border. Similar to the right, the arterial branch from the left phrenic artery may be controlled. The left renal vein is dissected with care to protect a branch of the renal artery, which courses adjacent to the posterolateral aspect of the gland. The adrenal vein is then identified, ligated, or clipped and divided. The remaining branch vessels along the inferomedial aspect of the gland are then divided.

Planning for a cortex-sparing adrenalectomy requires accurate preoperative imaging of the vascular supply of the adrenal gland, particularly that portion to be preserved. Although the adrenal gland typically receives its blood supply from the renal artery, inferior phrenic artery, and aorta, it is the blood supply from the phrenic artery that must be preserved when in situ preservation of the adrenal cortex is considered. The open technique has been used traditionally for cortex-sparing adrenalectomy, but experience with minimally invasive approaches has recently been reported. Whether performed with an open approach or a minimally invasive approach, cortex-sparing adrenalectomy should result in the preservation of approximately one third of the cortex that is well perfused. With resection of the medullary portion of the adrenal gland, the retroperitoneal attachments to the superior portion of the gland must be left intact to avoid devascularization of the preserved cortex.

POSTOPERATIVE MANAGEMENT

The mortality rate for adrenalectomy in all patients with a pheochromocytoma should be less than 1% for an elective operation in a properly prepared patient. Potential postoperative complications after pheochromocytoma resection include life-threatening arrhythmias, splenic injury, prolonged intubation, renal dysfunction, hypoglycemia, and persistent hypotension. Interestingly, the rate of postoperative myocardial infarction or stroke is very low. Severe hypoglycemia after resection of pheochromocytoma is related to catecholamine-induced depletion of glycogen stores, overstimulation of insulin production by preoperative alpha-blockade, and hyperinsulinemia after loss of catecholamine inhibitory effect on the beta$_2$-receptors of the pancreatic islet cells. Cardiac beta-blockade and the residual effects of anesthesia may mask any clinical signs or symptoms of hypoglycemia, so patients may initially present with seizures. As a result, blood glucose levels should be monitored for at least 24 hours after surgery and intravenous fluids should include dextrose.

The average length of stay for laparoscopic adrenalectomy for pheochromocytoma is 1 to 2 days; the authors typically discharge patients on beta-blocker therapy and reduced levels of antihypertensive medications. These medications are carefully weaned on an outpatient basis. Repeat catecholamine levels are typically checked on the first postoperative visit to confirm curative resection.

PALLIATIVE THERAPY

The current World Health Organization classification defines malignancy of pheochromocytomas and paragangliomas as the presence of metastases to a site where paraganglionic tissue is not normally present, most commonly the liver, lung, bone, and retroperitoneal or mediastinal lymph nodes. Importantly, local invasion into surrounding soft tissues, despite its potential lethality, is a poor predictor of metastases, and conversely, the absence of invasion does not preclude development of metastases. The development of recurrence at the site of origin in 6.5% to 16.5% of patients with sporadic pheochromocytoma and paraganglioma up to 15 years after initial resection further defies a clear distinction between benign and malignant disease. Locally advanced pheochromocytoma that involves the kidney, liver, spleen, pancreas, diaphragm, or inferior vena cava should be managed with margin negative resection of surrounding soft tissues. Preservation of adjacent organ function should be considered when feasible with early control of tumor venous drainage.

Despite the lack of consensus on how to determine malignant potential based on the histologic and immunohistochemical characteristics of the primary tumor, 15% to 20% of these tumors are estimated to be malignant. In addition, 50% of patients with development of recurrent disease experience distant metastasis. The 5-year survival rate in the setting of metastatic disease identified at the time of initial diagnosis or diagnosed after surgery as recurrent disease is approximately 45%.

As in the case for primary tumors, surgical resection is the treatment of choice for recurrent, multifocal, and metastatic tumors if all identifiable disease can be resected. Palliative resection of large tumors in the setting of multifocal metastatic disease may be considered for symptom relief but does not improve survival. Alternative interventions such as arterial embolization, cryoablation, external-beam radiation therapy, and radiofrequency ablation may offer effective symptom relief with less potential morbidity in this scenario. For the 60% of patients with metastatic pheochromocytoma or paraganglioma sites that are MIBG-avid, treatment with ^{131}I-MIBG has improved 5-year survival rates to as high as 65%. Patients with unresectable or multifocal metastatic disease may also be considered for systemic therapies. Although systemic therapy has not been shown to improve survival in patients with metastatic disease, it may provide effective symptom relief. The most frequently used cytotoxic chemotherapy regimen with cyclophosphamide, vincristine, and dacarbazine offers a biochemical response rate of 72% and a median survival of 3.3 years. The more recently used targeted therapy with the tyrosine kinase inhibitor sunitinib also offers promising response rates.

Suggested Readings

Amar L, Servais A, Gimenez-Roqueplo AP, et al: Year of diagnosis, features at presentation, and risk of recurrence in patients with pheochromocytoma or secreting paraganglioma, *J Clin Endocrinol Metab* 90(4):2110–2116, 2005.

Callender GG, Kennamer DL, Grubbs EG, et al: Posterior retroperitoneoscopic adrenalectomy, *Adv Surg* 43(1):147–157, 2009.

Dickson PV, Alex GC, Grubbs EG, et al: Posterior retroperitoneoscopic adrenalectomy is a safe and effective alternative to transabdominal laparoscopic adrenalectomy for pheochromocytoma, *Surgery* 150(3):452–458, 2011.

Graham GW, Unger BP, Coursin DB: Perioperative management of selected endocrine disorders, *Int Anesthesiol Clin* 38(4):31–67, 2000.

Huang H, Abraham J, Hung E, et al: Treatment of malignant pheochromocytoma/paraganglioma with cyclophosphamide, vincristine, and dacarbazine: recommendation from a 22-year follow-up of 18 patients, *Cancer* 113(8): 2020–2028, 2008.

Joshua AM, Ezzat S, Asa SL, et al: Rationale and evidence for sunitinib in the treatment of malignant paraganglioma/pheochromocytoma, *J Clin Endocrinol Metab* 94(1):5–9, 2009.

Kinney MA, Warner ME, vanHeerden JA, et al: Perianesthetic risks and outcomes of pheochromocytoma and paraganglioma resection, *Anesth Analg* 91(5):1118–1123, 2000.

Lord MS, Augoustides JG: Perioperative management of pheochromocytoma: focus on magnesium, clevidipine, and vasopressin, *J Cardiothorac Vasc Anesth* 26(3):526–531, 2012.

Organization PaPRS: Pheochromocytoma: recommendations for clinical practice from the First International Symposium on Pheochromocytoma, *ISP2005* 2011: 2005.

Pacak K: Preoperative management of the pheochromocytoma patient, *J Clin Endocrinol Metab* 92(11):4069–4079, 2007.

Tischler AS: Pheochromocytoma and extra-adrenal paraganglioma: updates, *Arch Pathol Lab Med* 132(8):1272–1284, 2008.

Walz MK, Alesina PF, Wenger FA, et al: Posterior retroperitoneoscopic adrenalectomy: results of 560 procedures in 520 patients, *Surgery* 140:943–948, 2006.

THE MANAGEMENT OF THYROID NODULES

Daniel W. Karakla, MD, and Matthew J. Bak, MD

The incidence of well-differentiated thyroid carcinoma (WDTC) is increasing, and estimates are that more than half of those of us over age 50 years have a thyroid nodule. The dilemma and challenge lie in determination of who truly has a malignancy. At times, malignant disease is obvious. For instance, a 70-year-old man with a rapidly enlarging right thyroid mass, progressive hoarseness, and dyspnea has anaplastic (undifferentiated) thyroid cancer until proven otherwise. At other times, disease is much less obvious. Take for instance a 36-year-old woman with an asymptomatic 2-cm left thyroid nodule and no family history of thyroid disease.

A thyroid nodule is a discrete lesion that with physical examination or radiography (ultrasound scan [US], computed tomographic [CT] scan, magnetic resonance imaging [MRI]) is distinct from its surrounding thyroid parenchyma. Palpable nodules are more common in women (5%) than in men (1%). More thyroid nodules are detected radiographically, and the incidence of WDTC is increasing, likely because of this. Fortunately, the mortality from WDTC has not really increased.

HISTORY

A pertinent history of thyroid nodules should always include duration, mode of discovery, associated pain, and voice changes. Many patients may describe intermittent hoarseness, which may be related to reflux or vocal abuse (prolonged voice strain or speaking). The voice change that persists and is progressive is more concerning for laryngeal or recurrent laryngeal nerve pathology.

Does the patient have symptoms of hyperthyroidism, such as anxiety, tremor, weight loss, muscle weakness, diarrhea, palpitations, or heat intolerance? Hypothyroid symptoms include fatigue, weight gain, cold intolerance, constipation, and dry or brittle skin and hair.

Compressive symptoms may be obvious, such as dyspnea or dysphagia. Patients can sometimes localize these symptoms to the location of the thyroid but, unfortunately, may not be able to accurately explain the symptom. The patient may describe a pressure sensation, choking feeling, difficulty finding a comfortable position to sleep, or a nagging cough, unrelated to reflux or respiratory infection. Another sometimes subtle but potentially worrisome report is aspiration.

Personal history of neck radiation should always be sought. Children exposed to radiation at lower doses are counterintuitively at increased risk for development of thyroid malignancy. Radiation for lymphoma treatment, occupational exposure, fallout from Chernobyl or other nuclear accidents, and even remote childhood radiation for acne or thymus enlargement done in years past are risk factors for thyroid malignancy.

Family history of thyroid disease especially should be elicited. Medullary thyroid carcinoma (MTC) may be familial or sporadic, associated with multiple endocrine neoplasia (MEN) 2a and MEN 2b. Papillary thyroid carcinoma (PTC) is usually isolated, but one should consider Cowden disease, familial adenomatous polyposis, and familial nonmedullary thyroid cancer.

PHYSICAL EXAMINATION

A thorough head and neck examination should be performed. Unfortunately, this is not always done. Without ever thinking about it, surgeons immediately assess for visual asymmetry or visible goiter or neck mass and listen for dysphonia or stridor. Although rare in the general thyroid nodule patient population, oral mucosal neuromas should prompt consideration of MEN 2b. Every patient evaluated for a thyroid nodule, especially before surgery, should have a laryngeal examination. This may be with mirror (indirect laryngoscopy) or fiberoptic nasopharyngolaryngoscopy to assess vocal cord mobility. Not every patient with vocal cord paresis or paralysis has a perceptible voice change, so a laryngeal examination only in patients with hoarseness may miss this important finding. Is there stridor, and is it inspiratory, expiratory, or biphasic? Inspiratory stridor tends to be associated with glottic or supraglottic obstruction. Expiratory stridor tends to be related to obstruction below the level of the glottis.

Obviously, palpation of the neck is the key element of the examination. A methodic examination sometimes elicits pathologic metastatic lymphadenopathy, but this is may be extremely difficult in the thick, obese, or muscular neck. Assessment should be made of the airway anatomy for deviation from the thyroid. The thyroid nodules should be assessed for mobility, firmness, tenderness, size, and location. If one cannot palpate the inferior extent of the mass, then significant substernal extension may exist, and imaging to investigate that is warranted.

LABORATORY ASSESSMENT

The single most useful test is a thyroid-stimulating hormone (TSH) level. If the TSH value is low or high, then a free T4 and free T3 should be assessed. Elevated TSH level may represent subclinical or clinical hypothyroidism, and further testing of thyroid antibodies and thyroid hormone replacement may be indicated. Suppressed TSH values may represent subclinical or clinical hyperthyroidism. Patients with hyperthyroidism may need medical treatment. Patients with toxic nodules, toxic multinodular goiter (MNG), and Graves' disease have an extremely low incidence of malignancy. Measurement of vitamin D and calcium levels is probably also reasonable in patients before surgery. Measurement of serum calcitonin in patients with suspected or known MTC is certainly indicated, but not in every patient with a thyroid nodule.

RADIOLOGY ASSESSMENT

Ultrasound Scan

Thyroid or neck US is being done more commonly than ever before. US is done by surgeons and should be considered as an extension of your fingers or physical examination. US is done by endocrinologists and, of course, by radiologists as well.

Thyroid nodules can be examined with US to determine size, cystic versus solid nature, location, and concerning characteristics. Characteristics concerning for malignancy include ill-defined or irregular borders, microcalcifications, internal vascularity, absence of colloid halo sign, hypoechogenicity, and suspicious lymph nodes. The presence of two or more of these characteristics likely increases the risk for malignancy, but US characteristics alone are rarely pathognomonic. US-guided fine-needle aspiration (FNA) has been shown to yield more diagnostic specimens than free-hand nodule palpation FNA.

Nuclear Medicine

Thyroid scintigraphy used to be included in most algorithms describing the workup of thyroid nodules. It should really only be used for patients with hyperthyroidism and is an unnecessary expense for euthyroidism or hypothyroidism.

Computed Tomographic Scan

In the authors' opinion, CT scan of the neck with contrast is an extremely valuable imaging modality in the workup of patients with a larger thyroid mass, question of substernal extension, or malignancy, lymphadenopathy, or a difficult thyroid or neck examination. The authors have regretted *not* obtaining a neck CT scan at surgery but cannot ever recall regretting that a CT scan was obtained. One should consider that obtaining a CT scan with iodinated contrast may delay the administration of I_{131} after surgery. However, in practical use, I_{131} treatment has not been meaningfully delayed. Urinary iodine can be assessed usually within 2 to 3 months, and I_{131} administered after that. CT scan is rapid and cheaper than MRI, gives multiple reformatted views, and defines relevant relationships of the thyroid and nodes to the airway, alimentary tract, vessels, and mediastinum. It, in essence, provides an excellent road map in the more surgically challenging cases.

Magnetic Resonance Imaging

MRI is more costly than CT scan. It usually requires more time in the scanner for the patient, who may not be comfortable supine or may have claustrophobia, and some motion artifact may occur (Table 1).

MRI gives excellent anatomic and soft tissue information and multidimensional views without the concern for iodine treatment that may be considered with CT scan contrast.

Fine-Needle Aspiration

Fine-needle aspiration biopsy has become a mainstay in the workup of a patient with a thyroid nodule. Typically, a 25-gauge (or 23-gauge) needle is placed into the thyroid nodule without negative pressure to

TABLE 1: Charges for imaging procedures (including professional fee)

US	$585
CT scan neck with contrast	$1906
MRI with contrast	$4358

CT, Computed tomographic; *MRI,* magnetic resonance imaging; *US,* ultrasound scan.

obtain a less bloody specimen. Several aspirations are taken, and the slides are air dried or immediately fixed for further cytopathologic staining and interpretation. As mentioned previously, US guidance has been shown to give a higher yield of diagnostic FNA specimens. The cytopathologist typically wishes to see at least six groups of cells in an adequate sampling.

A core needle biopsy may be indicated in the occasional patient with a thyroid mass. Patients suspected of having anaplastic thyroid carcinoma, thyroid lymphoma, metastatic disease to the thyroid, or unresectable primary thyroid carcinoma may be candidates for core needle biopsy and the further treatment planning, without the need for open incisional biopsy.

Thyroid FNA has been assigned a sensitivity ranging from 65% to 98% and a specificity from 72% to 100%. Its utility really lies in "ruling in" cancer, so that appropriate surgery can be planned and expedited, and in "ruling out" cancer, so that patients and surgeons can avoid unnecessary and potentially morbid surgery.

Unfortunately, although FNA has certainly helped with more appropriate decisions with and for patients, it is still imperfect. The various terminologies assigned to FNA cytopathologic interpretation have been inconsistent and difficult to interpret. The Bethesda System for Reporting Cytopathology has been promulgated in an attempt to facilitate uniformity, communication, and research (Box 1 and Table 2).

The atypia of undetermined significance (AUS) and follicular lesion of undetermined significance (FLUS) categories have been studied. These indeterminate specimens comprise a significant proportion of patients with thyroid nodule. A panel of molecular tests can be examined, such as BRAF, RET/PTC, PAX8/PPARG1, and Ras. The cytologic evaluation can be evaluated in conjunction with these molecular results, and it may increase the predictive power regarding cancer versus benign diagnosis. The hope is that this testing may allow some patients to avoid potentially unnecessary diagnostic surgery.

SURGICAL CONSIDERATIONS

Patients with a thyroid nodule considered for surgery include those with compressive symptoms, radiographic airway or esophageal compression, substernal extension, and malignant, suspicious, or indeterminate cytopathology. When the decision for surgery and appropriate preoperative counseling, consent, and clearance are obtained, one must give strong consideration to airway management (Figure 1).

Discussion with the anesthesia team is paramount before induction of anesthesia. Most patients can be induced, masked, and intubated in the standard way. However, a simple and somewhat predictive evaluation can be done in the preoperative area. Ask patients whether they can sleep supine at night. Do they have to wake up and sleep semi upright? Do they have choking episodes? Can they lie supine without difficulty in the preoperative area? Patients with large, compressive thyroid nodules, who cannot lie flat, with Mallampati III/IV airways, trismus, poor cervical extension, prior C-spine fixation, or

BOX 1: Recommended diagnostic categories for reporting thyroid cytopathology

I. Nondiagnostic or Unsatisfactory
Cyst fluid only
Virtually acellular specimen
Other (obscuring blood, clotting artifact, etc.)

II. Benign
Consistent with a benign follicular nodule (includes adenomatoid nodule, colloid nodule, etc.)
Consistent with lymphocytic (Hashimoto's) thyroiditis in the proper clinical context
Consistent with granulomatous (subacute) thyroiditis
Other

III. Atypia of Undetermined Significance or Follicular Lesion of Undetermined Significance

IV. Follicular Neoplasm or Suspicious for a Follicular Neoplasm
Specify whether Hürthle cell (oncocytic) type

V. Suspicious for Malignancy
Suspicious for papillary carcinoma
Suspicious for medullary carcinoma
Suspicious for metastatic carcinoma
Suspicious for lymphoma
Other

VI. Malignant
Papillary thyroid carcinoma
Poorly differentiated carcinoma
Medullary thyroid carcinoma
Undifferentiated (anaplastic) carcinoma
Squamous cell carcinoma
Carcinoma with mixed features (specify)
Metastatic carcinoma
Non-Hodgkin's lymphoma
Other

From Ali SZ, Cibas ES: The Bethesda System for Reporting Thyroid Cytopathology, *New York, 2009, Springer.*

TABLE 2: The Bethesda System for Reporting Thyroid Cytopathology: implied risk of malignancy and recommended clinical management

Diagnostic category	Risk of malignancy (%)	Usual management*
Nondiagnostic or unsatisfactory	1-4	Repeat FNA with ultrasound scan guidance
Benign	0-3	Clinical follow-up
Atypia of undetermined significance or follicular lesion of undetermined significance	~5-15[†]	Repeat FNA
Follicular neoplasm or suspicious for a follicular neoplasm	15-30	Surgical lobectomy
Suspicious for malignancy	60-75	Near-total thyroidectomy or surgical lobectomy[‡]
Malignant	97-99	Near-total thyroidectomy[‡]

FNA, Fine-needle aspiration.
*Actual management may depend on other factors (e.g., clinical and sonographic) besides the FNA interpretation.
[†]Estimate extrapolated from histopathologic data from patients with "repeated atypicals."
[‡]In the case of "suspicious for metastatic tumor" or a "malignant" interpretation indicating metastatic tumor rather than a primary thyroid malignancy, surgery may not be indicated.
From Ali SZ, Cibas ES: The Bethesda System for Reporting Thyroid Cytopathology, *New York, 2009, Springer.*

challenging full or obstructive dentition, may require special airway management, such as fiberoptic intubation.

The choice of endotracheal tube should also be a joint decision, made by the surgeon and the anesthesia team. An oversized endotracheal tube can lead to laryngotracheal injury, even with a relatively short intubation duration. Electrophysiologic recurrent laryngeal nerve (RLN) monitoring tubes may help decrease the incidence of RLN injury during thyroid surgery. Guidelines for its use have been developed. However, RLN monitoring tubes at this time can be viewed as an adjunct to RLN visualization during thyroid (parathyroid) surgery and are not uniformly standard of care across various geographic institutions (Figure 2).

When should the surgeon consider an incisional biopsy? Incisional biopsy should be considered in situations where a core needle biopsy might be considered: that is, in patients suspected of having anaplastic thyroid carcinoma, thyroid lymphoma, metastatic disease to the thyroid, or unresectable primary thyroid carcinoma not diagnosed with FNA or core needle biopsy.

When should the surgeon consider a level 6 (central compartment) neck dissection? Ideally, the thyroid surgeon will foresee the need for a level 6 node dissection before starting the surgery. Warning or predictive indicators before surgery include medullary thyroid carcinoma diagnosis, US/CT scan/MRI findings of likely pathologic lymphadenopathy, physical examination finding of firm or fixed

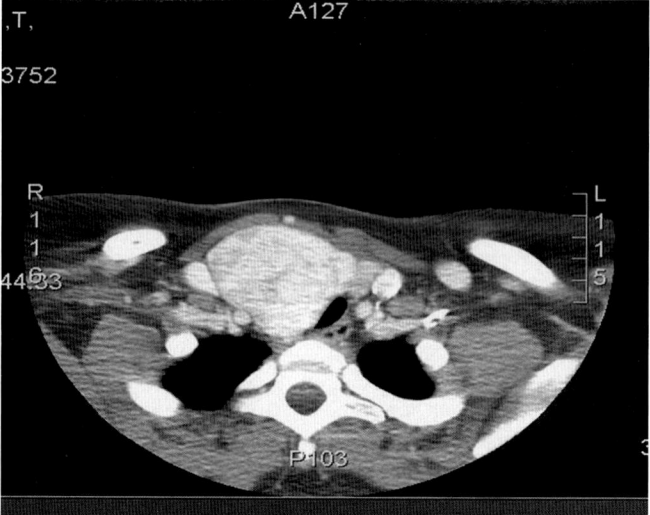

FIGURE 1   Computed tomographic scan of compressive nodule. *(From Randolph GW, Dralle H, et al: Electrophysiologic recurrent laryngeal nerve monitoring during thyroid and parathyroid surgery: international standards guideline statement, Laryngoscope 121(Suppl 1):S5, 2011, Fig 1.)*

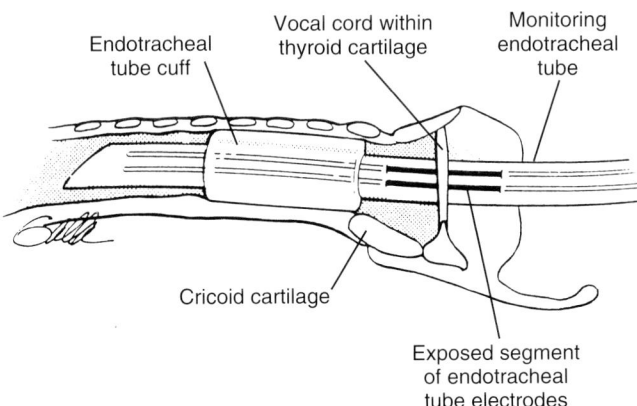

FIGURE 2 Monitoring endotracheal tube in place. The tube's cuff is in the subglottis; *black lines* on the side of the tube represent the exposed segment of electrodes that come into contact with the luminal surface of the vocal cord. *(From Randolph GW: Surgery of the thyroid and parathyroid glands, ed 2, Philadelphia, 2013, Saunders, p 327, Fig 33-15B.)*

thyroid mass, palpable pathologic lymphadenopathy, and RLN paresis or paralysis.

During surgery, the finding of pathologically enlarged level 6 lymphadenopathy, lateral neck (levels 2, 3, 4) lymphadenopathy, T3 or higher primary papillary carcinoma, or MTC should prompt the surgeon to perform a level 6 dissection. By definition, this dissection should include the soft tissues from hyoid bone to manubrium and carotid to carotid. Realistically, most of the concerning node-bearing tissue lies at an axial plane inferior to the typical superior parathyroid location, so that the superior parathyroids may be maintained in situ with their blood supply. The inferior parathyroid glands typically lie within the node-bearing soft tissues and should be identified, dissected, and reimplanted. A thorough level 6 dissection should also entail the superior mediastinum (level 7). The old adage "do it right the first time" here pays dividends, as reoperative surgery in the central neck puts the recurrent laryngeal nerves and parathyroid glands at significant risk.

There is rarely a role for subtotal thyroid lobectomy. Near total or total thyroid lobectomy is the appropriate surgery for a patient with a solitary thyroid nodule that meets indications for surgery. Meticulous dissection and preservation of the parathyroid glands and recurrent laryngeal nerves should be routine. Generally, the external branch of the superior laryngeal nerve is avoided by careful dissection directly on the thyroid superior pole.

The definition of minimally invasive thyroid surgery in unclear. The techniques of minimally invasive video assisted thyroidectomy (MIVAT), minimally invasive thyroid surgery, and robotic transaxillary and periauricular/retroauricular thyroidectomy are being promoted and marketed. Whatever technique is used, it should result in complete thyroid surgery, with an extremely low incidence of recurrent laryngeal nerve and parathyroid injury, acceptable scar, competitive cost, and rapid patient recovery.

INTRAOPERATIVE FROZEN SECTION

Frozen section should not be used when a diagnosis of malignancy papillary thyroid carcinoma (PTC) has already been made with FNA. It is not useful in diagnosis of follicular carcinoma and infrequently useful in diagnosing the follicular variant of PTC. It is useful in diagnosing PTC, medullary, anaplastic, lymphoma, and malignancies metastatic to the thyroid. The cost of intraoperative frozen section at the authors' institution is $200 for the initial block and $100 for each subsequent block, so cost should be factored into the decision-making algorithm.

An intraoperative diagnosis of PTC on frozen section may enable the surgeon, if indicated, to perform a total or near-total thyroidectomy at the initial surgery, instead of a lobectomy alone. The advantages here are a single anesthetic, less cost than two surgeries, not having to deal with healing changes or fibrosis from the first surgery, and, importantly, less emotional and psychologic distress for the patient. Surgeon-pathologist discussions, intraoperative touch prep for cytology, comparison with previous FNA slides, and an experienced thyroid pathologist help to maximize frozen section utility in intraoperative decision making.

Intraoperative parathyroid hormone (PTH) assessment may prove useful in predicting which patients may have clinically significant hypoparathyroidism or hypocalcemia. A baseline PTH is drawn before incision, and another rapid PTH is drawn approximately 15 minutes after either a total thyroidectomy or a completion thyroidectomy. If a greater than 70% drop in the PTH is seen, then these patients may be at increased risk and can be started on prophylactic supplemental oral calcium and vitamin D. Patients with a stable PTH can be released home sooner and safely. Other surgeons have found that placing all patients with completion or total thyroidectomy on a supplemental calcium and vitamin D regimen and releasing them home on the day of surgery, with detailed reinforced instructions has proven safe and cost effective.

SUMMARY

The management of thyroid nodules is truly a team effort, incorporating the knowledge and skills of the surgeon, endocrinologist, pathologist, and radiologist. Thoughtful treatment plans can be developed individually for each patient, incorporating newer technologies before and during surgery, as warranted.

SUGGESTED READINGS

Cibas ES, Ali SZ: The Bethesda System for Reporting Thyroid Cytopathology, *Thyroid* 19(11):1159–1165, 2009.

Hassel LA, Gillies EM, Dunn ST: Cytologic and molecular diagnosis of thyroid cancers: is it time for routine reflex testing? *Cancer Cytopathol* 1120(1):7–17, 2012. doi:10.1002/cncy.20186. Epub 2011.

Higgins TS, Gupta R, Ketcham AS, et al: Recurrent laryngeal nerve monitoring versus identification alone on post-thyroidectomy true vocal fold palsy: a meta-analysis, *Laryngoscope* 121(5):1009–1017, 2011. doi:10.1002/lary.21578.

Randolph GW, Dralle H, Abdullah H, et al, International Intraoperative Monitoring Study Group: Electrophysiologic recurrent laryngeal nerve monitoring during thyroid and parathyroid surgery: international standards guideline statement, *Laryngoscopy* 121(Suppl 1):S1016, 2011.

Singer MC, Bhakta D, Seybt MW, et al: Calcium management after thyroidectomy: a simple and cost-effective method, *Otol Head Neck* 146(30):362–365, 2011.

NONTOXIC GOITER

Gerard M. Doherty, MD, FACS

OVERVIEW

Goiter is a nonspecific term referring to any enlargement of the thyroid gland. However, in common use, it mainly denotes benign causes of thyroid enlargement, such as toxic multinodular goiter, diffuse toxic goiter (Graves' disease), or nontoxic multinodular goiter. Though malignant enlargement of the thyroid gland can technically be considered a goiter, it is usually referred to as a mass or nodule.

Nontoxic goiter is a benign condition. Though some thyroid glands resected because of nontoxic goiter may contain small cancers within them (up to 20% contain microcarcinomas), the predominant process and the decision making are based upon the benign enlargement. In some areas of the world, nontoxic goiters are endemic due to iodine deficiency, though public health efforts have reduced this somewhat.

PATHOGENESIS

A nontoxic multinodular goiter is defined as an enlargement of the thyroid gland containing follicles that are morphologically and functionally altered. The pathogenesis is multifactorial and can include iodine deficiency, goitrogens such as bamboo shoots, maize and sweet potatoes, genetic factors, and dyshormonogenesis. A family history of nontoxic goiter could indicate environmental, dietary, or dyshormonogenesis as causes. Aside from severe iodine deficiency, the cause in an individual is typically not evident, nor does it often influence management.

CLINICAL FEATURES

Nontoxic goiters may remain asymptomatic, or they may give rise to compressive features such as dyspnea, dysphagia, or venous congestion/discomfort with certain movements. A change in the voice can occur from direct pressure on the larynx or from stretching of the laryngeal nerve. Direct effects on the nerve causing paresis of the ipsilateral vocal fold are uncommon from benign goiter because nerve paresis is much more commonly associated with malignant infiltration of the nerve. Sudden changes in the goiter, as from hemorrhage into a nodule, can cause transient, intermittent, or permanent hoarseness. Thyroidectomy can often assuage voice changes due to direct pressure on the larynx, but the benefits for more uncommon changes due to effects on the nerve are less consistent.

On physical examination, the size of the gland, the features of diffuse enlargement or nodularity, tracheal deviation, extension of the gland below the sternum or clavicular heads, or high up into the neck near the angle of the mandible are all important for treatment planning. Associated lymphadenopathy should raise suspicion of malignancy (Figure 1).

EVALUATION

Thyroid stimulating hormone (TSH), free T4, and T3 levels should be checked to identify subclinical or overt thyrotoxicosis, hypothyroidism, or a euthyroid state. Fine-needle aspiration should be performed with ultrasound guidance for any suspicious thyroid nodule. Ultrasound features that raise the risk of malignancy include hypoechogenicity, microcalcifications, hypervascularity, and solid components of complex (cystic and solid) nodules.

Plain chest films can demonstrate tracheal deviation, retrotracheal and retrosternal extension, airway compression, and gross calcifications. However, cross-sectional imaging, such as computed tomographic (CT) scan or magnetic resonance imaging (MRI), is more informative for these findings. In particular, evaluating the extent of airway compression, the precise geometry of goiter position in the chest, and any associated lymphadenopathy that might indicate a clinically significant malignant component is much more effective with CT or MRI.

Radioiodine scans, pulmonary function tests, flow volume loops, and barium swallow studies may each be useful in specific situations, but they are not typically necessary in the era of accurate cross-sectional imaging.

Preoperative assessment of vocal cord movement should be considered for each patient. Deliberate voice assessment is mandatory, and fiberoptic laryngoscopy should be considered for patients with any voice alteration or any prior neck operation.

INDICATIONS FOR TREATMENT

Nontoxic goiter that causes local discomfort, such as tightness or a choking sensation, especially with certain movements, or that has caused mechanical partial obstruction of the upper aerodigestive tree should be considered for treatment. Substantial extension of the goiter into the chest, even in the absence of symptoms, should be considered a relative indication for treatment, because further enlargement of the thoracic component can lead to the need for a more disruptive operation to resect it in the future. Cosmesis alone is rarely an isolated concern or indication for therapy, as most patients with goiter of sufficient size to be bothersome also have other symptoms.

TREATMENT MODALITIES

TSH-suppression therapy with thyroxine has little role in the management of an established goiter. Prospective trials have failed to demonstrate a benefit for management of multinodular goiter. The side effects of TSH-suppression, including bone density loss and atrial arrhythmias, negate the theoretical value, particularly in the elderly patients for whom nonoperative therapy might be most attractive.

Radioiodine administration can cause goiter size reduction of 40% to 60% within 2 years, decreasing compressive symptoms. Complications include radiation thyroiditis and hypothyroidism, as well as a temporary enlargement of the gland that may be important in some clinical situations. Recent experience with the use of exogenous TSH administration to increase the efficiency of radioiodine administration in goiters with limited iodine uptake is promising, but follow-up to date is limited. These approaches may be useful for patients who have comorbidities that affect the safety of operative management, but those same comorbidities must be considered if the patient may become temporarily hyperthyroid from treatment or as the time course of correction of the local pressure symptoms of the goiter is extended.

Surgical management remains the mainstay of treatment for symptomatic, nontoxic goiter, and it is generally well tolerated, even in patients with limited physiologic reserve. The operation should typically be a bilateral procedure, removing all, or nearly all, of both thyroid lobes, in addition to any substernal extension. The operation is nearly always limited to a cervical incision, with median

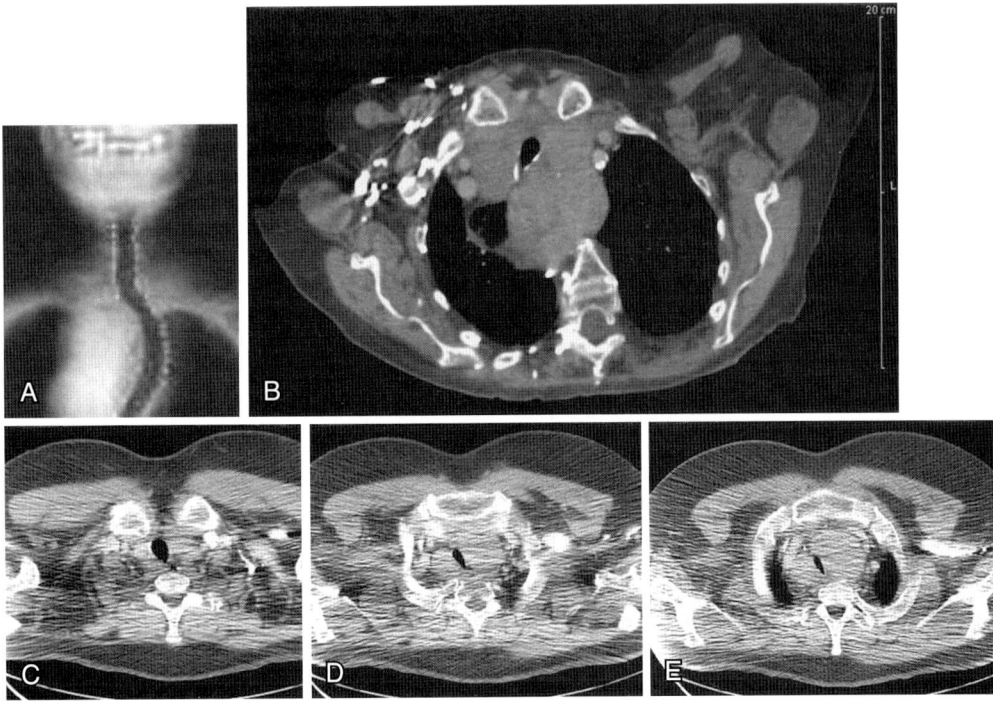

FIGURE 1 Images of goiters. **A,** Standard chest radiograph can demonstrate a goiter mainly by the displacement of the path of the trachea. In this image, a large substernal goiter displaces the trachea to the left. **B,** Posterior extension of the mediastinal goiter can make the resection more complicated. This patient has a large posterior extent from the left thyroid lobe, which must be managed carefully to avoid stretch injury to the left recurrent laryngeal nerve. The esophagus is also compressed distally and at the level of this image is displaced to the right, and contains both air and debris. **C, D,** and **E,** These images demonstrate that though the thyroid may be relatively normal in the neck on examination, ultrasound, and CT scan (**C**), the retrosternal portion (**D** and **E**) can be quite bulky. This patient presented with respiratory compromise of unclear etiology until the CT scan was obtained.

sternotomy or posterolateral thoracotomy being necessary only very rarely in previously unoperated patients. In experienced centers, complication rates are low (<2%) with techniques that include careful hemostasis and liberal parathyroid autotransplantation. For patients with significant airway compression or deviation, securing the airway can be the most critical part of the operation and may require conscious fiberoptic intubation under topical anesthesia to begin the procedure.

The thyroid gland should be exposed by a sufficient incision; though many thyroid operations can be done through very limited incisions, the geometry of the large multinodular goiter often requires long incisions in order to safely expose and remove the gland. Subplatysmal flaps improve the exposure of the limits of the gland, especially superiorly for glands with upper poles that extend high in the neck. The strap muscles can be separated in the midline or divided near the upper pole, as necessary, in order to expose the thyroid gland. The larger the cervical portion of the gland, especially the upper poles, the more likely it is that transverse division of the sternohyoid and sternothyroid muscles will be helpful.

The author typically starts the operation on the side of the larger lobe if the goiter is asymmetric. The upper pole of the gland is isolated by first separating the lateral aspect of the upper portion of the thyroid gland from the carotid sheath. If recurrent nerve monitoring is used, then the sheath is opened and the vagus nerve stimulated to establish baseline electromyography (EMG) function. The plane between the larynx and the upper pole of the thyroid gland is then opened, exposing the superior thyroid artery. The external branch of the superior laryngeal nerve (EBSLN) can be identified during some operations by direct inspection or by nerve monitor stimulation. However, in any case, the delicate fascia over the cricothyroid muscle

should be kept intact because the nerve is deep to this. As the plane is followed superiorly, the nerve should stay medial and superior to the upper pole of the thyroid and its vessels. The upper pole vessels can then be divided safely using any number of hemostatic strategies, including ligatures, clips, and powered dissection tools. The branches of the superior thyroid artery should be individually controlled immediately adjacent to the thyroid parenchyma to minimize the risk to the EBSLN.

Once the upper pole is fully mobilized, the thyroid is partially rotated anteriorly to continue dissecting the lateral portion of the thyroid gland. The middle thyroid vein, if present, is divided and the thyroid separated from the carotid sheath along its entire extent. The dissection can then be carried posteriorly to the deep muscles of the neck. The ability to rotate the thyroid gland may be limited by a large substernal component. The decision of whether to proceed with the dissection of the tracheoesophageal groove, recurrent laryngeal nerve, and parathyroid glands next (the author's preference) or dissect the substernal portion of the goiter in order to create the necessary mobility is dictated by the geometry of the particular patient and goiter. Occasionally, dividing the isthmus of the thyroid gland immediately anterior to the trachea can provide a needed degree of freedom to rotate the gland sufficiently.

The tracheoesophageal groove is dissected to identify the recurrent laryngeal nerve (RLN). The author tries to identify the RLN as low in the neck as possible, because this is the area where the nerve is least tethered to surrounding structures and least likely to be stretched during dissection and identification. The nerve is identified by its appearance, by it location and course, and by stimulation if nerve monitoring is used; however, stimulation alone is not sufficient to identify the RLN. In particular, the absence of an EMG signal does not demonstrate that a stimulated structure is not the RLN. Although intraoperative nerve monitoring is used by many experienced thyroid surgeons as an intraoperative adjunct, large trials have failed to show a benefit to patients as measured by RLN injury rates. The use of intraoperative nerve monitoring is a reasonable adjunct at the discretion of the surgeon, but it is not a standard of care.

Once the nerve is identified, it can be separated from the posterior aspect of the thyroid gland, and the intrathoracic portion can be safely delivered into the wound. The arterial supply to the thyroid goiter comes entirely from branches in the neck; there is no intrathoracic arterial supply to be concerned with. The only risk, then, is traction on the RLN as the substernal or paraesophageal intrathoracic portion of the goiter is delivered into the cervical wound by blunt dissection and gentle traction.

An important note of caution: in posteriorly displaced goiters with a component that extends inferiorly along the esophagus, especially on the right, the RLN may pass anterior to some portion of the goiter and may appear to be buried within the thyroid parenchyma because it has been trapped between nodules. This configuration makes the RLN especially vulnerable to stretch injury if this possibility is not recognized and anticipated early in the dissection.

Once the nerve is identified and the inferior portion of the thyroid gland mobilized, the RLN is traced up to its insertion into the larynx under the inferior border of the cricothyroid muscle. The small branches of the inferior thyroid artery are divided along the parenchymal surface of the gland, with the RLN always in view and protected. The parathyroid glands typically become evident during this portion of the dissection. Their blood supply from the inferior thyroid artery should be preserved if possible. If not, then the glands should be removed and grafted into the sternocleidomastoid muscle. As the dissection approaches the insertion of the RLN into the larynx, the RLN becomes progressively more fixed by surrounding tissues, including branches of the inferior thyroid artery, the fascial attachments of the thyroid gland to the trachea, and the insertion itself. Great care is necessary to safely dissect the thyroid gland away from the RLN without directly injuring or stretching the RLN. Once the RLN is fully separated from the thyroid gland, then the final attachments of the thyroid gland to the trachea can be divided. If intraoperative nerve monitoring was used, then the EMG signal with vagus nerve stimulation should be assessed at the completion of the dissection.

The process is then repeated on the opposite side. If there has been difficulty with the dissection on the initial side, then the contralateral procedure may be modified to reduce the risk of complications. For example, if the RLN lost function as documented by intraoperative nerve monitoring, then the contralateral RLN dissection may be modified to leave the RLN segment near the laryngeal insertion undisturbed by leaving a portion of the thyroid lobe in place at that position.

Devitalized parathyroid tissue should be cut into small (1- to 2-mm) pieces and grafted into small pockets in the sternocleidomastoid muscle. It is best to close each pocket with a suture to hold the graft in place while it develops a blood supply over the ensuing 6 to 12 weeks. It is not necessary to attempt to mark the site with permanent sutures or clips because subsequent reoperation to remove these remnants is extremely rare and best guided by ultrasound if necessary.

Meticulous hemostasis is important because bleeding in the confined space of the neck can compress the airway. The strap muscles are reapproximated in some fashion, depending on how they were opened or divided, but the closure should not be occlusive. The platysma muscle is reapproximated to align the skin edges and remove tension from the wound. The skin is closed according to the preference of the surgeon; the author's current preference is to approximate the skin edges with a running 3-0 polypropylene pull-out subcuticular suture, followed by skin glue. The suture is removed after the glue is dry (about 2 minutes). This provides a cosmetic closure that requires no further attention until after the glue peels away at about postoperative day 14.

POSTOPERATIVE CARE

In the author's practice, patients remain hospitalized overnight after removal of a nontoxic goiter in order to manage their limited pain and to monitor them for neck hematoma or hypocalcemia. All patients are managed with oral calcium supplements (calcium carbonate 1250 mg orally TID) beginning on the morning after surgery. If they are symptomatic with numbness or tingling, or if their calcium on the morning after surgery is below 8 mg/dL, then the dose is doubled (2500 mg TID). If their symptoms persist, either before or after discharge, or if there is special concern about the immediate parathyroid function—for example, if two or more parathyroid glands were grafted—then activated vitamin D is added to increase the gastrointestinal absorption of calcium (calcitriol 0.5 to 1.0 mcg daily in two divided doses).

Postoperative voice assessment is mandatory in all patients. Most patients have some immediate voice changes, but these nearly all resolve within 2 weeks of operation. Laryngoscopy to document vocal cord motion should be performed for all patients with significant voice changes that persist beyond 2 weeks and for all patients who have a change in their intraoperative nerve monitoring findings during the procedure if that adjunct has been used. While some have advocated for more broad use of laryngoscopy preoperatively and postoperatively, there is no evidence that this changes patient outcomes, so most experienced surgeons focus this effort in a more selective way.

SUGGESTED READINGS

Alesina PF, Rolfs T, Hommeltenberg S, et al: Intraoperative neuromonitoring does not reduce the incidence of recurrent laryngeal nerve palsy in thyroid reoperations: results of a retrospective comparative analysis, *World J Surg* 36(6):1348–1353, 2012.

Melin M, Schwarz K, Lammers BJ, et al: IONM-guided goiter surgery leading to two-stage thyroidectomy-indication and results, *Langenbecks Arch Surg* 398(3):411–418, 2013. Epub 2012 Nov 23.

Pieracci FM, Fahey TJ 3rd: Substernal thyroidectomy is associated with increased morbidity and mortality as compared with conventional cervical thyroidectomy, *J Am Coll Surg* 205:1–7, 2007.

Rayes N, Steinmüller T, Schröder S, et al: Bilateral subtotal thyroidectomy versus hemithyroidectomy plus subtotal resection (dunhill procedure) for benign goiter: long-term results of a prospective, randomized study, *World J Surg* 37(1):84–90, 2013.

White ML, Doherty GM, Gauger PG. Evidence-based surgical management of substernal goiter, *World J Surg* 32(7):1285–1300, 2008.

THE MANAGEMENT OF THYROIDITIS

Charles Parker, MD, and David Steward, MD

OVERVIEW

Thyroiditis refers to a diverse group of inflammatory disorders that affect the thyroid gland. Categorization of these conditions can be based on the presence or absence of pain, suspected etiology, or duration of disease (Table 1). Diagnosis can often be suspected on the basis of a thorough history and physical examination, although laboratory or radiologic workup may be necessary for confirmation. Management requires an understanding of the evolution of the ensuing disease process and thyroid pharmacology.

CHRONIC LYMPHOCYTIC THYROIDITIS

Overview

Chronic lymphocytic thyroiditis (Hashimoto's thyroiditis) is the most common inflammatory condition of the thyroid gland and the most common cause of hypothyroidism in the United States. The disease results from an autoimmune process characterized by lymphocytic infiltration and follicular destruction of the gland. Progression of thyroid destruction can lead to chronic thyroid failure and an atrophic gland in approximately 10% of patients. Up to 95% of chronic lymphocytic thyroiditis occurs in women, usually between the ages of 30 and 50 years. Presentation is typically asymptomatic, but symptoms of hypothyroidism can be present in approximately 20% of patients at the time of diagnosis. Even fewer (~5%) have thyrotoxicosis develop during the early phase of the disease. Patients with euthyroidism with Hashimoto's disease have development of hypothyroidism at a rate of approximately 5% per year. Physical examination generally reveals a firm, irregular, and nontender goiter. Some patients may report a feeling of tightness or fullness in the neck.

Diagnosis is suspected on the basis of clinical examination finding of a goiter and is confirmed with laboratory findings of hypothyroidism (elevated thyroid-stimulating hormone [TSH] and low free thyroxine [FT4] values) and elevated thyroid peroxidase antibody, which is present in 90% of patients with Hashimoto's thyroiditis. Thyroid ultrasound scan is obtained for suspicion of a dominant nodule on examination or family history of thyroid malignancy. Ultrasound scan shows an enlarged gland with a heterogenous or diffusely hypoechogenic pattern in most patients depending in part on the extent of lymphocytic infiltrate. The heterogenous hypoechogenicity may result in pseudonodularity, which may be difficult to distinguish from nodular disease. Infrathyroidal lymph nodes are frequently present, especially in younger patients, and may be mistaken for nodular disease.

Management

Management of Hashimoto's thyroiditis is primarily medical. Indications for thyroid hormone therapy include symptomatic or biochemical hypothyroidism. Levothyroxine therapy is initiated, with the dose determined by the patient's TSH level, age, and body mass; the dose can be up to approximately 1.6 μg/kg/d, with a goal for the TSH in the lower half of the reference range (1 to 3 mIU/L). TSH level should be rechecked 6 weeks after initiation of therapy and then every 6 to 12 months. If dose changes are needed, they should be made in increments of 12.5 μg to 25 μg or higher depending on the TSH level. A TSH test should be repeated in 6 weeks to ensure adequate replacement. Patients may not experience complete relief of hypothyroid symptoms until after 3 to 6 months of therapy. For patients with persistent hypothyroid symptoms despite TSH levels in the range of 1 to 3 mIU/L, FT3 levels may be checked; if levels are low, liothyronine (LT3) therapy should be considered. In patients with progressively enlarging goiter and compressive symptoms despite adequate replacement therapy or with suspected malignancy, surgical management is indicated. Total thyroidectomy is often performed for the compressive goiter, with more than 90% of patients experiencing symptomatic relief after surgery. Two-stage surgery with hemithyroidectomy and completion thyroidectomy may reduce the risk of bilateral recurrent laryngeal nerve injury or hypoparathyroidism and is a reasonable alternative. If thyroid malignancy is suspected because of suspicious findings on ultrasound scan, diagnostic evaluation should include an ultrasound scan–guided fine-needle biopsy. Coexistence of Hashimoto's thyroiditis does not significantly alter the management of thyroid nodules, which is determined by the results of fine-needle biopsy. Rarely, a rapidly enlarging goiter may represent primary lymphoma, which requires core or incisional biopsy for diagnosis.

SUBACUTE LYMPHOCYTIC THYROIDITIS

Overview

Subacute lymphocytic thyroiditis (subdivided into silent or postpartum thyroiditis) may represent a variant of Hashimoto's thyroiditis with a similar autoimmune etiology. Subacute lymphocytic thyroiditis should be suspected in the patient with goiter and self-limiting thyrotoxicosis. As a result of follicular destruction, patients may experience a transient period of thyrotoxicosis as a result of the release of stored hormone. This phase may last from 2 to 4 months. A period of hypothyroidism may follow from depletion of stored hormone and typically lasts up to 6 months before the patient returns to a euthyroid state. However, up to 20% of patients may experience chronic hypothyroidism and need life-long hormone therapy. Diagnosis is suspected based on a history of transient thyrotoxicosis and the laboratory findings of evolving thyroid function studies. Unlike subacute granulomatous thyroiditis, systemic symptoms such as fever, thyroid tenderness, and an elevated erythrocyte sedimentation rate are unusual in subacute lymphocytic thyroiditis. If Graves' disease is suspected, a radioiodine uptake study can differentiate between the two hyperthyroid states. Graves' disease is associated with elevated uptake from increased hormone synthesis, and subacute lymphocytic thyroiditis shows decreased uptake. Anti-TSH receptor antibodies in Graves' disease are not present in subacute lymphocytic thyroiditis. Anti-thyroid peroxidase (anti-TPO) and anti-Tg antibody testing is often positive in subacute lymphocytic thyroiditis (silent and postpartum), but on average, lower levels are seen then in Hashimoto's thyroiditis.

Postpartum thyroiditis is similar to silent thyroiditis but is defined as the development of thyroid dysfunction within 12 months after pregnancy in a previously euthyroid female. Postpartum thyroiditis can also develop after spontaneous or induced abortion. Approximately 20% to 40% of patients exhibit the characteristic triphasic course of an initial hyperthyroid phase, followed by subsequent

TABLE 1: Features of thyroiditis*

Form of thyroiditis	Duration of disease	Etiology	Presence of pain	Thyroid function	Management
Chronic lymphocytic thyroiditis (Hashimoto's)	Chronic, progressive	Autoimmune	Painless	Hypothyroid	Levothyroxine
Subacute lymphocytic thyroiditis (silent and postpartum)	Subacute, transient, or progressive	Autoimmune	Painless	Triphasic	Beta-blockers, levothyroxine
Subacute granulomatous thyroiditis (de Quervain's)	Subacute, transient	Viral	Painful	Triphasic	NSAIDs, beta-blockers, levothyroxine
Acute suppurative thyroiditis	Acute	Bacterial	Painful	Euthyroid	Antibiotics, surgical drainage
Invasive fibrosis thyroiditis (Reidel's)	Chronic, progressive	Idiopathic	Rarely painful	Euthyroid or hypothyroid	Steroids
Drug-induced	Acute/subacute, transient, or progressive	Pharmacologic	Painless	Hyperthyroid or hypothyroid	Thionamides, steroids, beta-blockers, levothyroxine, surgery

*Diseases listed in descending order of frequency.
NSAIDs, Nonsteroidal antiinflammatory drugs.

hypothyroidism and then a return to the euthyroid state. Another 20% to 30% experience only hyperthyroidism, and 40% to 50% only hypothyroidism. Management is similar to that of silent thyroiditis.

Management

Management is towards alleviation of symptoms. Symptoms of thyrotoxicosis, such as palpitations, tachycardia, tremors, anxiety, and heat intolerance, are best controlled with beta-blocker therapy. Antithyroid medications are not helpful because the thyrotoxicosis is not the result of excess hormone production but of release of prestored hormone. Common therapeutic agents include propranolol 10 mg to 40 mg 3 to 4 times daily or atenolol 25 mg to 100 mg daily or twice daily. Symptomatic hypothyroidism can be managed with levothyroxine therapy. Thyroid function laboratory results should be monitored every 4 to 6 weeks to confirm resolution of thyrotoxicosis and detect onset and resolution of hypothyroidism.

SUBACUTE GRANULOMATOUS THYROIDITIS

Overview

Subacute granulomatous thyroiditis (de Quervain's thyroiditis) is the most common cause of a painful thyroid gland. It is most likely caused by a viral infection and is generally preceded by an upper respiratory tract infection. Numerous etiologic agents have been implicated, including mumps virus, echovirus, coxsackievirus, Epstein-Barr virus, influenza, and adenovirus. Women between the ages of 30 and 50 years are most likely to be affected. Typical presentation is that of acute thyroid pain and low-grade fevers. Pain may be exacerbated with turning of the head or swallowing and may radiate to the jaw, ear, or occiput. Similar to subacute lymphocytic thyroiditis, patients may experience a triphasic course in relation to

thyroid function. About 50% of patients present with symptoms of thyroidotoxicosis from follicular disruption and release of stored thyroid hormone. This phase may last 4 to 6 weeks before thyroid stores are depleted and the patient experiences hypothyroidism. Symptoms of hypothyroidism may last up to 6 months. As follicles repair, normalization of thyroid studies and euthyroidism develops. About 5% to 15% have persistent hypothyroidism after 12 months. Laboratory evaluation reveals a mildly elevated erythrocyte sedimentation rate (ESR) early in the disease course, normal white blood cell count (WBC), and evolving thyroid function tests. Antithyroid antibodies are normal.

Management

Management is directed against symptom control similar to subacute lymphocytic thyroiditis. Pain is often managed with nonsteroidal antiinflammatory drugs (NSAIDs). Rarely, severe pain refractory to NSAIDs may be managed with steroids. Median time for resolution of pain is 5 weeks. Beta-blockers are used to control symptoms of thyrotoxicosis, and levothyroxine is used during the hypothyroid phase.

ACUTE SUPPURATIVE THYROIDITIS

Overview

Acute suppurative thyroiditis is a rare disorder most commonly caused by bacterial infection from *Staphylococcal* and *Streptococcal* species. In the patient with immunocompromise, fungal, mycobacterial, or parasitic sources should also be suspected. The disorder is rare because of the intrinsic resistance the thyroid has to infection as a result of its rich lymphovascular supply, fascial encapsulation, and high iodine content. Mechanisms for infection include lymphovascular spread, direct trauma, or more commonly, a persistent piriform sinus fistula. In children with acute suppurative thyroiditis, a left piriform sinus fistula is the most common cause. In adults, the condition is more likely to occur in patients with preexisting thyroid disease, such as Hashimoto's thyroiditis, nodular goiter, or thyroid cancer. Presentation is that of acute neck swelling, pain, and high fevers. Some may present in acute airway distress from a compressive abscess requiring intubation and emergent drainage. Laboratory workup reveals an elevated WBC, elevated ESR, and normal thyroid function studies. Human immunodeficiency virus screening should be performed in patients because of its association with an immunocompromised state. Computed tomographic (CT) scan of the neck with contrast is often the first diagnostic test performed. CT imaging allows for identification of any fluid collection, its accessibility to needle aspiration, extrathyroidal extension, and the possibility of a piriform sinus fistula. Ultrasound scan with needle aspiration is performed next to obtain fluid for culture and antibiotic sensitivity testing.

Management

Management begins with broad-spectrum empiric antibiotics. Common agents include penicillinase-resistant penicillins and beta-lactamase inhibitors (piperacillin/tazobactam or ampicillin/sulbactam) or clindamycin for a penicillin allergy, plus vancomycin if methicillin resistant *Staphylococcus aureus* is suspected. Antibiotics are narrowed once sensitivity data are obtained. Duration of antibiotics is determined by clinical response; however, 14 days of therapy is reasonable in most patients. In the unstable airway, emergent transcutaneous incision or open-surgical drainage is needed. If the patient's condition is stable and CT imaging has identified the thyroid as the site of infection, then ultrasound scan with needle aspiration may be more appropriate. If fluid accumulation recurs or clinically the patient's condition fails to improve, the decision needs to be made to determine the success of repeat needle aspiration versus surgical drainage and possible partial or total thyroidectomy. Thyroid resection may be necessary in patients with persistent disease or when multiple poorly defined abscesses are present. Management of a piriform sinus fistula often requires direct endoscopy for identification and complete fistula tract excision with hemithyroidectomy after resolution of the acute illness.

INVASIVE FIBROUS THYROIDITIS

Overview

Invasive fibrous thyroiditis (Reidel's thyroiditis) is a rare idiopathic disorder characterized by progressive fibrosis and inflammation of the thyroid gland and adjacent cervical structures. The mean age at presentation is 50 years, and 80% of all cases occur in females. A hard fixed mass involving the thyroid with compressive symptoms or neck pain is common. Extension into adjacent structures may cause dyspnea, hoarseness, dysphagia, and restricted neck movement. Association with systemic fibrosis is seen in up to one third of patients, with common sites being the retroperitoneum and mediastinum. Evaluation requires thyroid function studies and ultrasound scan. Ultrasound scan shows a diffuse, hypoechoic, hypovascular appearance from the extensive fibrosis. Unique to the patient with Reidel's thyroiditis is the finding of carotid artery encasement, which is not typically seen in other benign goiter diseases. Hypothyroidism is present in 80% of patients during the course of disease. Ultrasound scan–guided fine-needle aspiration is often nondiagnostic but may reveal inflammation and fragments of fibrous tissues. Definitive diagnosis with open biopsy to rule out possible thyroid malignancies is often needed.

Management

Management is often with both surgical and medical therapy. Surgery to relieve compressive symptoms may initially be performed at the time of open biopsy. Total thyroidectomy is difficult because of the extrathyroidal extension of disease and loss of fascial planes. Debulking surgery, limited to an isthmectomy, is often performed to prevent surgical complications from a more aggressive dissection and to reduce airway constriction. Prednisone is the first step in medical therapy and has been shown to have a more dramatic effect in reducing the size of the mass and compressive symptoms when initiated early in the disease course. Doses may range from 15 mg to 100 mg daily and may be required for years, with tapering and withdrawal based on clinical response. In cases refractory to prednisone, the addition of tamoxifen has been reported to be successful. A recent report describes the use of mycophenolate mofetil in combination with prednisone to successfully reduce the size of a mass.

DRUG-INDUCED THYROIDITIS

Overview

Several drugs are known to cause thyroid inflammation, including amiodarone, interferon-alfa, interleukin-2, and lithium. A thorough history often reveals the suspected agent. Patients may present with either symptoms of hypothyroidism or hyperthyroidism depending on the pharmacologic agent and length of use. Baseline thyroid function tests are needed before the start of any of the previous medications and should be monitored every 6 months with continued therapy. Amiodarone is associated with both hypothyroidism and hyperthyroidism. In iodine-deficient areas, amiodarone-associated hyperthyroidism is more common; however, in iodine-sufficient areas, amiodarone-associated hypothyroidism is more common. Thyroid dysfunction may occur acutely after initiation of amiodarone therapy or may develop after several years of therapy. There are two types of amiodarone-induced thyrotoxicosis. Type 1 is from the increased thyroid hormone production, often from the iodine load exacerbating underlying thyroid disease, and type 2 is from follicular destruction and release of stored hormone. Differentiating between the two types can be difficult because of the similarity in presentation. Characteristics of type 1 amiodarone-induced thyrotoxicosis are a detectable radioactive iodine uptake level, hypervascularity on color flow Doppler scan, and a multinodular or diffuse goiter seen on ultrasound scan. Characteristics of type 2 amiodarone thyrotoxicosis are a nondetectable radioactive iodine uptake level, absent vascularity on color flow Doppler scan, and no goiter or small goiter on ultrasound scan. Lithium is more commonly associated with hypothyroidism from chronic use; however, several reports have described thyrotoxicosis from chronic lithium use. Both interferon-alfa and interleukin-2 can be associated with hypothyroidism and thyrotoxicosis.

Management

Often these medications can be continued, and the patient is treated for thyroid symptoms with either levothyroxine or beta-blockers. In type 1 amiodarone-induced thyrotoxicosis, hyperthyroidism is the result of increased thyroid synthesis. Effective management requires thionamides, methimazole 30 mg to 40 mg daily, along with potassium percholorate at 1 g daily, to prevent further hormone production. Type 2 amiodarone-induced thyrotoxicosis is best treated with several months of glucocorticoids. In both types, if thyrotoxicosis persists despite medical therapy and amiodarone cannot be discontinued, then total thyroidectomy may be necessary.

SUGGESTED READINGS

Aslam R, Steward D: Surgical management of thyroid disease, *Otolaryngol Clin North Am* 43:273–283, 2010.

Fatourechi MM, Hay ID, McIver B, et al: Invasive fibrous thyroiditis (Riedel thyroiditis): the Mayo Clinic experience, 1976-2008, *Thyroid* 21:765–772, 2011.

McManus C, Lou J, Sipple R, et al: Should patients with symptomatic Hashimoto's thyroiditis pursue surgery, *J Surg Res* 170:52–55, 2011.

Paes JP, Burman KD, Cohen J, et al: Acute bacterial suppurative thyroiditis: a clinical review and expert opinion, *Thyroid* 20:247–255, 2010.

Pearce EN, Farwell AP, Braverman LE, et al: Thyroiditis, *N Engl J Med* 348:2646–2655, 2003.

HYPERTHYROIDISM

William S. Duke, MD, and David J. Terris, MD

INTRODUCTION

Hyperthyroidism refers to thyrotoxicosis specifically caused by hyperactivity of the thyroid gland. This state of metabolic excess is the result of elevated levels of the thyroid hormones, tetraiodothyronine (thyroxine, T4) and the metabolically active triiodothyronine (T3). Signs and symptoms of this condition reflect the underlying hypermetabolic state, which if left untreated may progress to heart failure and arrhythmia, significant neurologic derangements, thyroid storm, and even death (Table 1). The incidence rate of hyperthyroidism in the United States is approximately 0.5 to 1 per 1000, with women affected 10 times more often than men.

Graves' disease is the most common cause of hyperthyroidism, accounting for more than 50% of all cases. This autoimmune condition is caused by antibodies directed against the thyroid-stimulating hormone (TSH) receptor, resulting in thyroid enlargement, an increase in thyroid vascularity, and increased production and secretion of thyroid hormone.

Hyperthyroidism may also be caused by a toxic multinodular goiter, which usually arises within the background of a longstanding nontoxic multinodular goiter, or by a solitary toxic nodule, which is the result of a hyperfunctioning adenoma. Less commonly, hyperthyroidism may be associated with excess iodine intake, as in the case of amiodarone-induced hyperthyroidism and the Jod-Basedow effect,

or may be the result of high levels of human chorionic gonadotropin (gestational thyrotoxicosis), which is structurally similar to TSH. Hyperthyroidism may also be present during the early phase of Hashimoto's thyroiditis, another type of autoimmune thyroiditis.

Regardless of etiology, the goal of management of hyperthyroidism is to decrease the hyperfunctioning state of the thyroid gland, mitigate the immediate and long-term sequelae of exposure to excess thyroid hormone, and return the patient to a euthyroid state. This can be achieved through the use of medications, radiation therapy, or surgery.

ASSESSMENT AND DIAGNOSIS

The thyroid gland secretes T4 and T3 in response to TSH stimulation in a feedback cycle. As T4 and T3 levels increase, the anterior pituitary gland decreases the amount of TSH produced. Primary hyperthyroidism occurs when the thyroid gland no longer responds appropriately to falling levels of TSH by decreasing the synthesis and release of T4 and T3.

Patients with symptoms concerning for hyperthyroidism should have serum TSH and free thyroxine (T4) tests obtained, and if indicated, free T3. Primary hyperthyroidism is associated with a TSH level generally below 0.1 mU/L with an elevated T4. Subclinical hyperthyroidism is present when the TSH is suppressed but the thyroid hormone levels are normal. Measurement of serum TSH receptor antibodies may be useful in the management of patients with Graves' disease.

Imaging studies are often beneficial in evaluation of patients with thyroid disease. Radioactive iodine uptake scans, performed with either ^{123}I or ^{131}I, may help elucidate the etiology of thyrotoxicosis. In Graves' disease, diffuse homogeneous uptake is seen throughout the gland, whereas toxic nodular disease shows intense uptake in the pathologic nodules. Hashimoto's thyroiditis and conditions of exogenous excess thyroid hormone intake result in decreased uptake on radioactive thyroid scans. Most patients should undergo a thyroid ultrasound scan to evaluate for the presence of nodules, which may suggest toxic nodular disease or lesions concerning for concurrent malignancy.

NONSURGICAL TREATMENT

The treatment of hyperthyroidism is separated into three principal modalities: medications to suppress thyroid function, radioactive iodine (RAI) ablation of the thyroid gland, and surgery. The choice of therapy depends on many factors, including the natural history of the disease and the wishes of the patient. Antithyroid medications and RAI are more common in the United States, with surgery generally reserved for failures or complications of other modalities, concern for a coexisting thyroid malignancy, an obstructive or cosmetically significant goiter, or patient preference.

The thionamides, methimazole and propylthiouracil (PTU), are the primary agents for the medical control and preoperative management of hyperthyroidism. They impair thyroid hormone production.

TABLE 1: Clinical manifestations

Symptoms	Signs
Palpitations	Tachycardia
Heat intolerance	Arrhythmia
Diaphoresis	Valve disease
Anxiety/nervousness	Congestive heart failure
Restlessness	Dyspnea
Emotional lability	Hyperreflexia
Psychosis	Hyperkinesis
Increased appetite	Weight loss
Diarrhea	Stare, lid lag
Hair loss	Proptosis
Fatigue	Dermopathy
Muscle weakness	Bone demineralization
Insomnia	
Pathologic fracture	
Reproductive impairments	

PTU also functions to inhibit the peripheral conversion of T4 to T3, which makes it particularly useful in patients with life-threatening thyrotoxicosis. The effects of thionamide therapy may become apparent after several weeks, although maximal efficacy may take 2 months or more to achieve. Both agents cross the placenta, and methimazole has been associated with certain birth defects. Severe reactions such as agranulocytosis may occur with either agent. PTU carries an additional risk of severe hepatotoxicity, and in 2009, the U.S. Food and Drug Administration (FDA) recommended reserving PTU for patients in the first trimester of pregnancy or who are allergic to or intolerant of methimazole.

Beta-blockers are frequently used to control the catecholamine-mediated symptoms of hyperthyroidism. Propranolol is especially useful because it assists in blocking the peripheral conversion of T4 to T3. Beta-blockers should not be administered in isolation without other medications to suppress thyroid function and should not be used in patients who have concurrent congestive heart failure, unless tachycardia caused by the hyperthyroidism is the cause of the heart failure.

Radioactive iodine treatment with ^{131}I achieves a hypothyroid state in approximately 80% of patients. This effect may take several months to achieve, during which time patients should be continued on the pretreatment medical regimen to control the hyperthyroidism. RAI is contraindicated during pregnancy and lactation and may exacerbate the ophthalmologic manifestations of Graves' disease.

SURGICAL INDICATIONS AND CONTRAINDICATIONS

Surgical management of hyperthyroidism may be appropriate in several circumstances. The decision to proceed with surgery over other forms of therapy should be based on several factors, including response to and tolerance of medical therapy, the patient's candidacy for RAI, comorbid disease, and patient preference.

Medical treatment of hyperthyroidism with thionamides may be complicated by allergy or severe side effects that preclude their continued use. Some patients do not have the disease adequately controlled with medical therapy, and approximately 50% of patients treated with thionamides have relapse once therapy is discontinued.

Surgery may be favored in those patients who continue to manifest symptoms of hyperthyroidism despite prior treatment with thionamides and RAI. Although no studies have shown a consistent significant risk of secondary malignancy with RAI, some patients are reluctant to have any form of radiation therapy and favor surgery over long-term medical treatment. RAI is used with caution in young children with hyperthyroidism.

Several other factors may favor surgery over medical therapy. Patients with thyroid nodules that are concerning for or proven to be malignant should undergo surgical treatment. Surgery may be the preferred treatment option for patients desiring to become pregnant soon after treatment or in patients who are already pregnant but who are either resistant to thionamide treatment or whose symptoms are so severe that they cannot wait several weeks for the medications to reach efficacy. Surgery may also be appropriate for young children, patients with compressive goiters, and patients who are deemed poor candidates for long-term follow-up.

SURGICAL PREPARATION

Thyroid storm is a severe, life-threatening exacerbation of thyrotoxicosis that may be triggered by surgery. This hypermetabolic state may be manifested by fever, tachycardia and other arrhythmias, cardiovascular collapse, gastrointestinal disturbances, mental status changes including coma, and death. Every effort should be made to control hyperthyroidism and convert the patient to a euthyroid state before surgery. Coordination of preoperative medical management of the patient's hyperthyroidism with an endocrinologist who can assist in medication selection and dosing is essential (Table 2).

Thionamide treatment should begin several weeks before surgery, although achieving a euthyroid state may require several months in some patients. Elective surgery should be postponed until a euthyroid state is reached to avoid precipitating thyroid storm.

Methimazole may be started at 20 to 40 mg once daily or twice daily in divided doses. No parenteral form is available. PTU may be started at 300 to 600 mg/d, divided every 8 hours. PTU may be given rectally in patients with severe thyrotoxicosis who are unable to take medications orally. Higher doses may be needed for acute thyroid storm, and both agents may be decreased to lower maintenance doses as the hyperthyroidism resolves.

Iodine-containing agents are useful adjuncts in achieving a euthyroid state before surgery and for controlling acute thyrotoxicosis. Lugol's solution (8 mg of iodide per drop) and saturated solution of potassium iodide (SSKI; 50 mg iodide per drop) work by transiently inhibiting thyroid hormone production and release. An initial response may be present within 24 hours, with peak efficacy reached

TABLE 2: Medications for treatment of hyperthyroidism

Class	Mechanism of action	Medication	Starting dose
Thionamide	Impair thyroid hormone production	Methimazole	20-40 mg PO daily or divided twice daily
		Propythiouracil	300-600 mg PO divided every 8 h
Beta-blocker	Block catecholamine-mediated hyperthyroid symptoms	Propranolol	20-40 mg PO every 6 to 8 h
Iodine preparation	Inhibit thyroid hormone synthesis and release	Lugol's solution	2-5 drops PO 1 to 3 times daily
		Saturated solution of potassium iodide (SSKI)	1-2 drops PO 1 to 3 times daily
Steroid	Support metabolic function in critical illness	Hydrocortisone	50-100 mg IV every 8 h
		Dexamethasone	2 mg IV every 8 h

IV, Intravenously; *PO,* orally.

within 2 weeks. These medications should be administered concurrently with a thionamide to decrease the risk of accelerated release of stored thyroid hormone and rebound hyperthyroidism once the iodine solution has been withdrawn. SSKI is started at 1 to 2 drops by mouth (PO) 1 to 3 times daily, and Lugol's solution is started at 2 to 5 drops PO 1 to 3 times daily. These agents cross the placenta, and their use in pregnancy may result in fetal harm.

Beta-blockers are used perioperatively to control the catecholamine-mediated cardiovascular symptoms of hyperthyroidism. As mentioned previously, propranolol (20 to 40 mg PO every 6 to 8 hours) is especially useful because it also assists in blocking the peripheral conversion of T4 to T3.

Treatment with steroids may also be necessary, as patients in thyroid storm have both increased cortisol metabolism and inadequate cortisol secretion to meet metabolic demands. When given with iodine-containing agents and thionamides, steroids may also help decrease thyroid hormone synthesis and peripheral conversion of T4. Hydrocortisone (50 to 100 mg intravenously [IV] every 8 hours) or dexamethasone (2 mg IV every 8 hours) may be given to meet the steroid requirement in these critically ill patients.

SURGICAL OPTIONS

The appropriate surgical intervention for patients with hyperthyroidism depends on the underlying cause of the disease. Patients with Graves' disease, toxic multinodular goiter, and other processes that affect the entire gland should undergo total thyroidectomy. Total thyroidectomy removes all identifiable thyroid tissue, resulting in a hypothyroid state and the need for thyroid hormone replacement.

Subtotal thyroidectomy is mentioned only so that it may be condemned. It is a procedure done historically for logical reasons but has little role in a modern thyroid practice. It purports to preserve 3 to 6 g of thyroid tissue superiorly near the insertion of the recurrent laryngeal nerve (RLN), with the thought of protecting the RLN and endeavoring to avoid permanent hypothyroidism. After several decades of this surgery, a high risk of recurrent hyperthyroidism has been recognized; now, wide consensus exists that the RLN should be identified in all cases to avoid inadvertent injury.

Patients with a toxic nodule may be eligible for a unilateral thyroid lobectomy to remove the pathologic adenoma (if the contralateral lobe is normal), which is nearly always permanently curative. Attempts to extirpate just the nodule from the surrounding normal tissue are discouraged.

SURGICAL ANATOMY

The thyroid is a bilobed gland that resides in the anterior neck. The lobes are connected by a central isthmus, which crosses the trachea approximately at the level of the third tracheal ring. Occasionally, a pyramidal lobe, a remnant of the thyroglossal duct, may extend superiorly from the isthmus. The gland is posterior to the sternothyroid and sternohyoid muscles and medial to the carotid sheath. Each lobe is about 4 cm in height, 2 cm wide, and 2 cm deep; the total gland typically weighs approximately 20 g. Glands affected by Graves' disease, large nodules, or diffuse goiter can be significantly larger and extend into the chest or posterior to the esophagus. The gland is held tightly adherent to the trachea by a suspensory ligament, Berry's ligament.

Blood supply to the gland is provided by the superior thyroid artery, which arises from the external carotid artery, and the inferior thyroid artery, which branches off the thyrocervical trunk. These vessels contribute to the superior and inferior vascular pedicles, respectively.

The superior laryngeal nerve (SLN) exits the vagus nerve and gives off an external branch that supplies the cricothyroid muscle. Although significant variation can be found in the course of this nerve, it typically crosses posterior to the external carotid artery and travels to the cricothyroid muscle in close proximity to the superior thyroid artery and along the inferior constrictor muscle. This nerve is not routinely exposed during thyroidectomy, and transecting the superior vascular pedicle near its insertion into the thyroid gland decreases the risk of nerve injury.

The RLN, also a branch of the vagus, provides some laryngeal sensation and supplies motor innervation to all of the intrinsic laryngeal muscles except the cricothyroid. This nerve must be protected during dissection to avoid postoperative hoarseness or, in the case of bilateral injury, acute respiratory distress. The left RLN recurs around the aortic arch and ascends the neck in the tracheoesophageal groove (Figure 1). The right RLN recurs around the subclavian artery and approaches the larynx from a more lateral location, making its location more variable. The nerve is usually deep to the inferior thyroid artery. Identification of the nerve in the soft tissue near the inferior pole of the gland can be difficult. The nerve may be more consistently identified near its insertion under the inferior constrictor muscle near the cricothyroid joint.

Preservation of parathyroid integrity is of paramount importance in thyroid surgery. There are usually two superior and two inferior parathyroid glands, although some patients may have supernumerary glands. The exact location of the parathyroid glands varies,

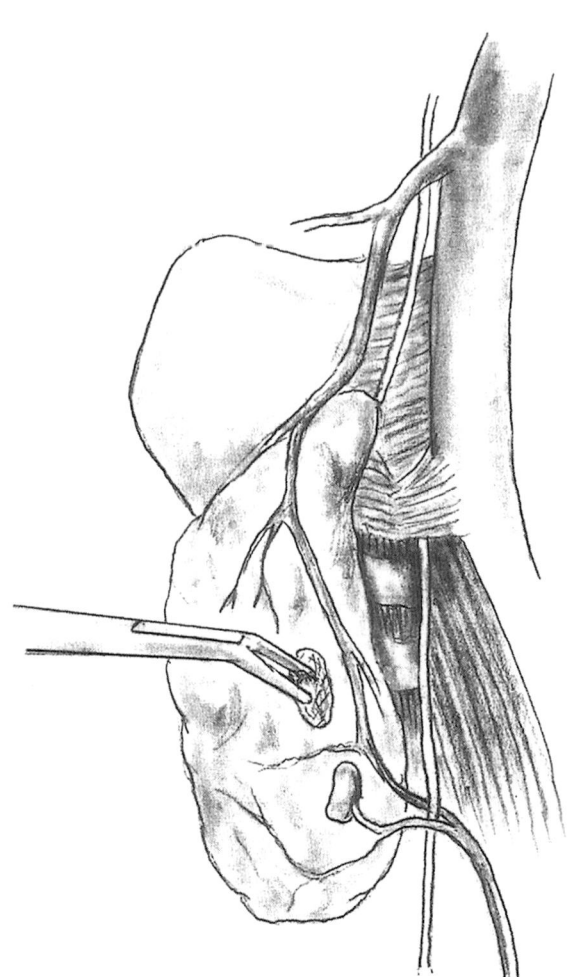

FIGURE 1 The left superior laryngeal nerve is identified posterior to the superior thyroid artery along the inferior constrictor. The left recurrent laryngeal nerve is located in the tracheoesophageal groove deep to the inferior thyroid artery. *(Reprinted with permission from Terris DJ, Gourin CG: Thyroid and parathyroid diseases: medical and surgical management, New York, 2009, Thieme Medical Publishers, Inc.)*

but they are closely associated with the superior and inferior poles of the thyroid gland. The superior parathyroid gland is found approximately 1 cm superior to the junction of the RLN and the inferior thyroid artery, tightly adherent to the posterior aspect of the gland. The location of the inferior parathyroid glands is more variable, usually adjacent to the inferior pole of the thyroid gland. The parathyroid glands tend to be oval, flat, or bean-shaped and have a reddish brown or rust-colored appearance. Both the superior and inferior glands receive their vascular supply from the inferior thyroid artery, which should be preserved during dissection.

SURGICAL TECHNIQUE

Conventional Thyroidectomy

The traditional approach to thyroidectomy has evolved considerably over the past 10 years. It involves placing the intubated patient supine on the operating room table without extension. A horizontal incision, rarely longer than 6 cm long, is centered on the midline and marked previously with the patient upright in the holding area. Once the skin and subcutaneous tissues have been divided, the platysma is identified and divided horizontally. Subplatysmal flaps are no longer raised (as was classically taught). Instead, the midline raphe between the strap muscles is simply divided vertically, with exposure of the underlying thyroid gland. The strap muscles are elevated off the anterior face of the thyroid lobes and retracted laterally. The superior extent of each thyroid lobe is identified, and the vessels of the superior vascular pedicle are ligated and transected as a single bundle with an advanced energy device such as Harmonic shears (Ethicon Endosurgery, Cincinnati, Ohio) or the LigaSure (Covidien, Boulder, Colo;

Figure 2). Care should be taken during this portion of the dissection to avoid injuring the external branch of the SLN or the superior parathyroid gland.

Once the superior vascular pedicle has been divided, the lobe is retracted medially and the posterior and lateral surface aspect of the gland is dissected. The superior parathyroid gland should be identified along the mid to upper third of the gland, dorsal to the RLN, and reflected posterolaterally.

The middle thyroid vein is ligated and transected, and the inferior parathyroid is dissected away from the thyroid. Once the inferior pole is fully mobilized, the RLN can be readily identified distal along its course, just deep to the tubercle of Zuckerkandl. The easiest method is to find the nerve dissecting perpendicular to its course with blunt elevators (Terris Blunt Elevators, Medtronic, Minneapolis, Minn).

Once the RLN has been identified, the ligament of Berry can be divided and all remaining attachment to the trachea released.

The isthmus is ligated and divided if only a lobectomy is necessary. If a total thyroidectomy is necessary, the ipsilateral lobe may be removed or the isthmus left intact, and the procedure is repeated on the opposite side. The pyramidal lobe, if present, is removed in continuity. Once the gland is resected, hemostasis is ensured and the integrity of the RLNs and parathyroid glands are verified. Parathyroid glands that have become devascularized are reimplanted by mincing the affected gland into 1-mm pieces, then placing the pieces into a small pocket created in the anterior aspect of the sternohyoid muscle. The pocket is closed and its location marked with either a surgical staple or a nonabsorbable suture.

The strap muscles are reapproximated in the midline with a single 3-0 vicryl figure-8 suture (Ethicon, Inc, Somerville, NJ; Figure 3). The subcutaneous tissues are closed with buried interrupted 4-0 vicryl sutures, and the skin edges are sealed with tissue adhesive and horizontal ¼-inch Steri-Strips (3M Corporation, St Paul, Minn).

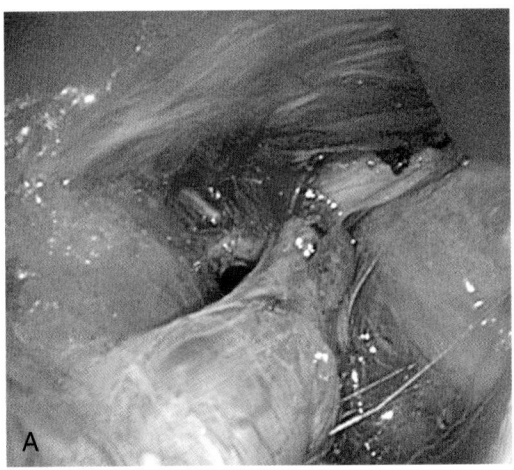
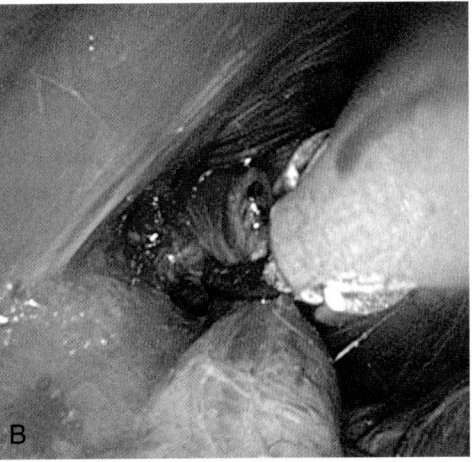

FIGURE 2 **A,** The superior vascular pedicle is isolated. **B,** The vessels are simultaneously ligated and divided immediately adjacent to the superior border of the gland with a Harmonic-ACE 23E (Ethicon Endosurgery, Cincinnati, Ohio). *(Reprinted with permission from Terris DJ: Novel surgical maneuvers in modern thyroid surgery, Operative Techniques Otolaryngol 20(1):23-28, 2009.)*

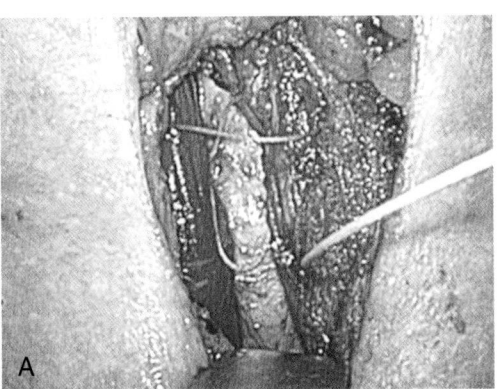
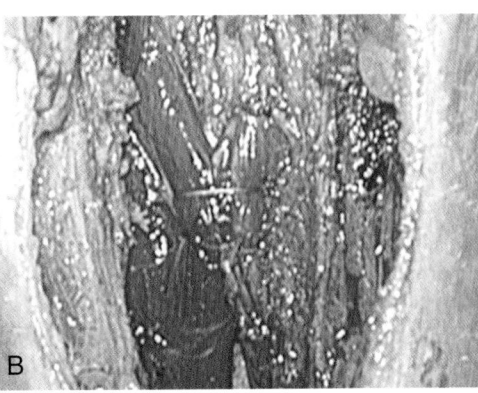

FIGURE 3 **A,** The midpoint of the strap muscles is identified. **B,** The muscles are closed with a single figure-8 3-0 vicryl suture (Ethicon, Inc, Somerville, NJ). *(Reprinted with permission from Terris DJ: Novel surgical maneuvers in modern thyroid surgery, Operative Techniques Otolaryngol 20(1):23-28, 2009.)*

The conventional approach to thyroidectomy offers the surgeon wide exposure of the operative field. However, this procedure results in a long scar and the extent of dissection frequently necessitates drain placement and overnight hospitalization. Most patients heal well, and with proper placement, the scar fades over time and may be nearly imperceptible. Despite the acceptable long-term healing outcomes, many patients are reluctant to consent to a longer incision and are uncomfortable and inconvenienced with a drain after surgery. As technology has evolved, new techniques and approaches have emerged to mitigate the cosmetic impact and extent of dissection frequently associated with the conventional thyroidectomy technique.

Minimally Invasive Nonendoscopic Technique

The minimally invasive nonendoscopic procedure uses a smaller incision than the conventional technique and eliminates elevation of the subplatysmal flaps. A 3-cm to 5-cm incision is marked in a low cervical skin crease while the patient is awake and upright (usually in the holding area). Anesthesia is established, and the neck is maintained in a neutral position without use of a shoulder roll. An incision is made in the previously marked skin crease and carried down through the platysma, with exposure of the sternohyoid and sternothyroid muscles. The muscles are separated in the midline and retracted laterally, with liberal lateral and posterior mobilization of the thyroid gland.

The superior pole is isolated and the upper pedicle ligated as a single bundle. Care is taken to avoid injury to the superior laryngeal nerve. The superior lobe is mobilized and the superior parathyroid gland identified. The middle thyroid vein is ligated. The inferior lobe is mobilized sufficiently to identify the inferior parathyroid gland and the recurrent laryngeal nerve. The inferior pole vessels are then ligated where they enter into the capsule of the thyroid gland. The remainder of the gland is dissected off of the trachea, with the recurrent laryngeal nerve kept under direct vision. Vessel ligation and hemostasis are accomplished with the ultrasonic shears (Harmonic ACE-23P or Focus; Ethicon Endosurgery).

For unilateral lobectomy, the isthmus is divided adjacent to the contralateral lobe. When total thyroidectomy is performed, the contralateral lobe is dissected as mentioned previously. The strap muscles are approximated with a single figure-8 suture of 3-0 vicryl (Ethicon, Inc). The subcutaneous tissues and platysma muscle are closed with interrupted 4-0 vicryl sutures. The skin is closed with skin adhesive. No drain is used.

Minimally Invasive Video-Assisted Thyroidectomy

The minimally invasive video-assisted thyroidectomy (MIVAT) is similar to the nonendoscopic minimally invasive approach except that an endoscope is necessary to achieve the magnification needed to reduce the incision to below 3 cm.

A 15-mm to 20-mm low horizontal cervical incision is used. The procedure begins much like the nonendoscopic approach until the superior pole is addressed. The room lights are darkened, and a 5-mm 30-degree laparoscope is introduced into the wound to visualize the superior pole of the thyroid gland with the scope angled upward. Harmonic-ACE shears (ACE23P; Ethicon Endosurgery) are used to coagulate and divide the superior pole vessels close to the thyroid capsule.

After the middle thyroid vein is ligated and the inferior pole mobilized, the endoscope is angled downward to facilitate identification of the recurrent laryngeal nerve, which is traced for a length of approximately 20 or 30 mm. The inferior parathyroid gland is identified and dissected away from the thyroid.

The lobe is then exteriorized with liberal use of hemostat clamps placed directly on the gland itself. The recurrent laryngeal nerve is then traced to its entrance under the inferior constrictor muscle as with open surgery. The Harmonic-ACE shears are used to ligate vessels and divide tissue during this dissection. The isthmus is then divided with electrocautery or the harmonic shears.

The contralateral lobe is removed in similar fashion if indicated by clinical circumstances. Closure is the same as for minimally invasive nonendoscopic surgery, and the procedure is accomplished on an outpatient basis.

Remote Access/Robotic Thyroidectomy

Advances in robotic surgical technology now allow access to the thyroid gland through incisions placed remotely, with cosmetically conspicuous anterior cervical scars avoided. This remote access, robotically assisted surgery was originally described in South Korea with an axillary point of entry. This concept has been further refined, and now the procedure can be accomplished via a postauricular incision, similar to the facelift incisions with which most head and neck surgeons are familiar. This robotic facelift thyroidectomy (RFT) is most appropriate for patients with nodules smaller than 4 cm who have unilateral disease and are not morbidly obese.

The patient is marked sitting upright in the holding area. A proposed cervical incision is outlined in the unlikely event that conversion to open surgery is necessary. The postauricular hair is trimmed. A facelift incision is then outlined, hidden by the postauricular crease. The incision crosses over to the occipital hairline at a level that will be obscured by the ear. The incision is continued inferiorly approximately 1 cm within the occipital hairline so that it will be completely concealed once the hair grows back. The patient is placed supine on the operating table. After induction and intubation with an electromyographic endotracheal tube (for laryngeal nerve monitoring), the head is turned 30 degrees away from the anticipated side of lobectomy and supported with a soft cushion to prevent excessive neck rotation. The operating table is placed in reverse Trendelenburg's position and tilted away from the surgeon to facilitate the open dissection.

Development of an ample surgical pocket during the open dissection facilitates the robotic portion of the procedure. The open dissection involves the sequential identification of a series of structures, starting with the sternocleidomastoid muscle (SCM) and including the great auricular nerve, then the external jugular vein, then the omohyoid muscle. The omohyoid and strap muscles are retracted ventrally while all other structures remain dorsal (Figure 4). The triangle bounded by the anterior surface of the SCM, the posterior sternohyoid muscle, and the superior border of the omohyoid muscle is widely opened, providing superb access to the superior pole of the thyroid gland. A series of progressively deeper retractors is used to achieve this dissection. Once the anteromedial surface of the SCM is dissected to the clavicle, a customized retractor blade, which is compatible with the modified Chung fixed retractor system (Marina Medical, Sunrise, Fla), is introduced and placed underneath the omohyoid and the other strap muscles to maintain the operative pocket.

With the retractor fixed in position, the daVinci surgical robotic system (Intuitive Surgical Inc., Sunnyvale, Calif) is deployed. The robotic pedestal is angled approximately 30 degrees to the operating table, with its long axis parallel to the retractor system. Fine positioning adjustments are more easily made by moving the operating table rather than the robot. Three arms are used. The camera arm is positioned first, holding a 30-degree down endoscope parallel to the retractor system, or angled slightly upward. A Maryland grasper is placed in the nondominant arm, and a Harmonic device (Ethicon Endosurgery) is placed in the dominant arm. These instruments are positioned on either side of the endoscope.

The robotic phase of dissection is characterized by a step-by-step series of landmark identification. This begins with ligation of the superior vascular pedicle with the Harmonic device. The superior

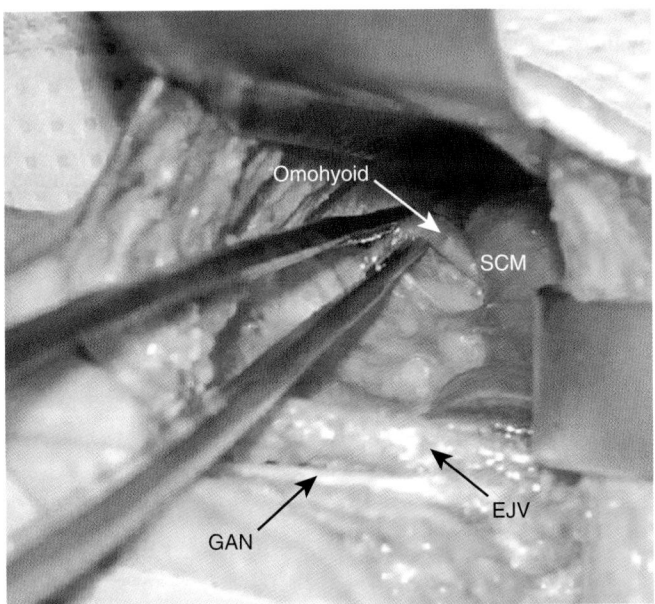

FIGURE 4 Surgical approach for robotic facelift thyroidectomy procedure. The vector of approach is superficial to the great auricular nerve *(GAN)* and external jugular vein *(EJV)*. The superior pole of the right lobe is medial to the sternocleidomastoid muscle *(SCM)* and deep to the omohyoid. *(Reprinted with permission from Terris DJ, Singer MC, Seybt MW: Robotic facelift thyroidectomy: II: clinical feasibility and safety,* Laryngoscope *121(8):1636-1641, 2011.)*

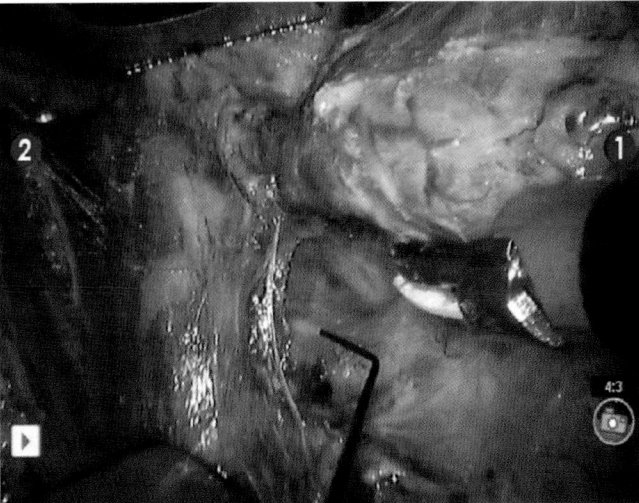

FIGURE 5 The recurrent laryngeal nerve, seen by the tip of the lower forceps, is identified under the inferior constrictor near its insertion into the larynx as the superior pole of the gland is retracted inferiorly. *(Reprinted with permission from Terris DJ, Singer MC, Seybt MW: Robotic facelift thyroidectomy: patient selection and technical considerations,* Surg Laparosc Endosc Percutaneous Techniques *21(4):237-242, 2011.)*

pole is reflected inferiorly and ventrally, and the inferior constrictor muscle is traced until the lower border is encountered. The external branch of the superior laryngeal nerve can usually be seen running along the inferior constrictor muscle. The superior parathyroid gland is visualized on the posterior surface of the thyroid and is dissected posterior-superiorly. The recurrent laryngeal nerve is seen laterally passing underneath the inferior constrictor muscle (Figure 5). After the nerve is dissected for a small distance inferiorly, the ligament of Berry may be safely divided with the Harmonic device, and the isthmus is transected at the midline. The middle thyroid vein is ligated with the Harmonic device, and then the inferior pole is fully mobilized. The inferior parathyroid gland is dissected inferiorly, and the inferior pole vessels are divided. The remaining attachments to the trachea are divided, and the thyroid lobe is retrieved.

After thorough irrigation and inspection of the thyroid bed and pocket, Surgicel (Ethicon, Inc) is placed in the thyroid compartment. The subcutaneous tissues are closed with interrupted sutures of 4-0 vicryl (Ethicon, Inc). Dermaflex skin adhesive (Chemence Medical Products, Inc, Alpharetta, Ga) is placed to seal the wound. The Quarter-inch Steri-Strips (3M Corporation) are placed horizontally along the incision.

POSTOPERATIVE MANAGEMENT

A great diversity exists in the postoperative management of patients for thyroidectomy, particularly in regards to drain utilization, calcium supplementation, the timing of postoperative discharge, and thyroid hormone replacement. Emerging evidence-based trends may help guide care during the postoperative period.

The use of drains after thyroidectomy is a long-held practice of conventional thyroid surgery. Meticulous attention to hemostasis and vessel ligation is more important for the prevention of hemorrhage, and the presence of a drain has no impact on hematoma

formation. Nevertheless, some surgeons still advocate the use of drains (especially in patients with large goiters or substernal extension). Motivated patients may be instructed in outpatient drain care, eliminating their need for a protracted hospital stay. Patients may undergo follow-up in the office for drain removal.

Hypocalcemia is one of the most common complications of thyroid surgery. Transient hypocalcemia lasting less than 6 months may be seen in up to 36% of patients. Hypocalcemia may be related to excessive manipulation, devascularization or removal of the parathyroid glands, renal disease, or inadequate calcium or vitamin D intake. Patients undergoing surgery for hyperthyroidism are at increased risk for postoperative hypocalcemia. This may result from increased renal excretion of calcium and phosphorous and direct stimulation of osteoclasts by T3.

The two principal options for addressing this potential complication include: routine supplementation with calcium and vitamin D (typical dosing is a 3-week taper of calcium carbonate starting at 1 g three times a day [tid]) and serial calcium level acquisition to inform intervention.

Parathyroid hormone (PTH) levels may also be used to guide management. Patients with a postoperative PTH level greater than 30 pg/mL are at a low risk for requiring supplementation and may be observed. Patients should be counseled about the early symptoms of hypocalcemia, including perioral and distal extremity numbness and tingling. Patients experiencing these symptoms should be counseled to self medicate with calcium and to seek medical attention if they fail to resolve. In rare cases, addition of calcitrol (0.25 to 0.5 mg twice daily [bid]) may be necessary.

Although thyroid surgery has traditionally been performed on an inpatient basis, it is now clear that the vast majority of patients can be managed as outpatients. The Surgical Affairs Committee of the American Thyroid Association recently drafted a position paper providing guidance on this issue.

Finally, patients who undergo total thyroidectomy require thyroid hormone replacement. A number of considerations for arriving at an optimal starting dose exist, but the authors have found it easier to simply prescribe 100 mcg per day for most patients and allow the endocrinologist or primary care provider to titrate the level.

COMPLICATIONS

Modern thyroid surgery is generally regarded as a safe procedure; however, even experienced surgeons encounter a range of potential postoperative complications from poor wound healing and keloid formation to postoperative infections and mortality. Fortunately, most of these complications are rare. Some risks that are inherent to thyroid surgery warrant specific discussion.

Hematoma is one of the most feared complications of thyroidectomy. Although the risk is low (less than 2%), the consequences can be disastrous. Because of the relationship of the thyroid bed to the larynx, blood that is trapped beneath the strap muscles causes venous and lymphatic outflow obstruction, then supraglottic edema, then airway obstruction, then death. The best way to avoid airway compression is to close the strap muscles loosely (single point of fixation) so the blood can escape the thyroid compartment.

The most critical aspect of postthyroidectomy hematoma is early recognition. Patients may report increasing pain or dysphagia, and dyspnea and frank respiratory distress with visible neck swelling often occur later. Hematomas typically present within 24 hours of surgery, but the presentation may be delayed for even several days in some cases. The first step in management of compressive/expanding hematomas is expeditious opening of the wound to achieve decompression. The airway should be evaluated; if it is compromised, it should be secured by either intubation or temporary tracheostomy. The patient can then be returned to the operating room for exploration of the surgical field and definitive control of bleeding.

Hypocalcemia is the most common complication of thyroid surgery, with transient hypocalcemia occurring in up to 40% of patients and permanent hypocalcemia reported in as many as 15% of patients in some series. Early signs include numbness and paresthesias of the fingers and perioral region. Patients may demonstrate Chvostek's sign (facial nerve spasm when lightly tapping the cheek) or Trousseau's sign (carpal spasm when the upper arm is compressed with a blood pressure cuff). Later findings include worsening tetany, respiratory distress, mental status changes and neurologic impairments, and cardiac arrhythmias. Treatment involves rapid replacement of calcium (either orally or intravenously) and vitamin D and magnesium as indicated.

Nerve injury is an important potential complication of thyroid surgery. Injury to the SLN impairs contraction of the cricothyroid muscle, reducing the patient's dynamic pitch range. This injury rarely affects the conversational voice, and patients may be unaware of any changes until they attempt to sing. Patients with symptomatic SLN injury may benefit from speech therapy.

Recurrent laryngeal nerve injury is a more noticeable condition than SLN injury. Transient RLN injury may occur in up to 15% to 20% of patients, and permanent injury occurs in 1% to 3% of cases in expert case series. The risk of nerve transection is higher in patients with thyroid malignancy, large substernal goiters, and thyroiditis. The clinical manifestations of unilateral nerve injury depend on the extent of the damage and the ability of the patient to compensate for the injury. Injury patterns vary from asymptomatic mild paresis to complete paralysis with severe dysphonia, impaired speech fluency, and dyspnea from excess air escape. Because some patients with unilateral vocal cord paresis may be asymptomatic, consideration should be given to preoperative laryngoscopy to evaluate vocal cord mobility, especially in cases of revision or completion surgery.

Patients with unilateral paresis may be observed, treated with voice therapy, or referred for a temporary medialization procedure to improve glottic closure. An observation period of 6 to 12 months is recommended before definitive treatment. When the nerve is observed to be transected, repair should be performed. Although neurorrhaphy results in synkinesis and fails to produce meaningful movement of the vocal cord, it helps to maintain the bulk and tone of the cord, which helps to maintain the voice.

Bilateral RLN injury is a much more serious condition. The RLN provides innervation to the posterior cricoarytenoid muscles, which are the sole abductors of the vocal cords. Injury to both RLNs may result in acute airway obstruction. The patient may need immediate reintubation or urgent tracheostomy until a more definitive procedure to open the airway can be performed by an otolaryngologist.

Recurrent hyperthyroidism may occur in patients who undergo less than total thyroidectomy for surgical treatment of disease. Although very rare in the case of a solitary toxic adenoma, up to 2% of patients undergoing subtotal thyroidectomy for Graves' disease or toxic multinodular goiter may have recurrence of hyperthyroidism. The incidence rate of this complication should be close to zero for patients who undergo total thyroidectomy.

CONCLUSION

Medical treatment with antithyroid drugs and RAI therapy are the primary treatment modalities for treatment of hyperthyroidism in the United States. Surgery may be an appropriate option and provides a more durable cure in selected patients. Care should be taken to achieve a euthyroid state before surgery whenever possible. Complications are low when the surgery is performed by experienced surgeons with meticulous adherence to surgical principles. Surgical techniques continue to evolve, particularly with the advent of new technologies, and may make surgery easier, faster, or safer. Nevertheless, careful vigilance for complications and early intervention is mandatory. Recent advances continue to advance this surgical discipline, making it safer and more cosmetically acceptable to a growing number of patients.

SUGGESTED READINGS

Hopkins B, Steward D: Outpatient thyroid surgery and the advances making it possible, *Curr Opin Otolaryngol Head Neck Surg* 17(2):95–99, 2009.

Melmed S, Polonsky KS, Larsen PR, et al: *Williams textbook of endocrinology*, ed 12, Philadelphia, 2011, Elsevier.

Terris DJ: Novel surgical maneuvers in modern thyroid surgery, *Operative Techniques Otolaryngol* 20(1):23–28, 2009.

Terris DJ, Gourin CG: *Thyroid and parathyroid diseases: medical and surgical management*, New York, 2009, Thieme Medical Publishers, Inc.

Terris DJ, Gourin CG, Chin E: Minimally invasive thyroidectomy: basic and advanced techniques, *Laryngoscope* 116(3):350–356, 2006.

Terris DJ, Singer MC, Seybt MW: Robotic facelift thyroidectomy: patient selection and technical considerations, *Surg Laparosc Endosc Percutaneous Techniques* 21(4):237–242, 2011.

Wang TS, Roman SA, Sosa JA: Postoperative calcium supplementation in patients undergoing thyroidectomy, *Curr Opin Oncol* 24(1):22–28, 2012.

SURGICAL APPROACH TO THYROID CANCER

Tammy M. Holm, MD, PhD, Diana Caragacianu, MD, and Gregory W. Randolph, MD

BACKGROUND

Goiter has been described since ancient times, with the first surgical resection recounted by Paulus in 500 AD. Initially a bloody, disordered procedure with significant morbidity and mortality, the surgery has since evolved in large part through the seminal work of Theodor Kocher, the father of modern thyroid surgery. Today, thyroidectomy is a precise, elegant operation with low operative morbidity and virtually nonexistent mortality.

Although nodular thyroid disease is relatively common, existing in approximately 4% to 7% of the general population with palpation criteria and up to 50% of elderly adults with ultrasound scan criteria, only 5% of these nodules are ultimately found to be malignant. Thyroid malignancies are thus relatively rare and constitute only 2% of all cancers. The incidence of thyroid cancer has been increasing at a higher rate than any other cancer in the United States. Study of the Surveillance, Epidemiology and End Results (SEER) database has revealed a 2.4-fold increase in thyroid cancer between 1973 and 2002. The National Cancer Institute (NCI) estimates 56,460 new cases of thyroid cancer in 2012 alone.

Thyroid cancers are generally classified into follicular cell–derived and nonfollicular cell–derived variants based on their cell type of origin (Table 1). Papillary thyroid cancer (PTC), follicular cancer (FC), Hürthle cell cancer (HCC), and anaplastic cancer (AC) are considered to be follicular cell–derived, whereas medullary thyroid cancer (MTC) and lymphoma are nonfollicular cell-derived. A detailed discussion of the characteristics of these different thyroid cancers is beyond the scope of this surgically oriented text, and the reader is referred to the Suggested Readings section for further details. However, the authors stress the importance of a basic understanding of the epidemiology, histopathology, clinical behavior, and prognosis of these thyroid cancers in evaluating, managing, and counseling affected patients (see Table 1).

PTC is far and away the most common thyroid cancer, comprising approximately 80% of all thyroid cancers. PTC may be associated with several hereditary diseases or syndromes, such as familial adenomatous polyposis (FAP), Gardner's syndrome, Cowden disease, Werner's syndrome, and Carney's complex, all of which should raise the index of suspicion for PTC in any patient presenting with a thyroid mass. PTC, FC, and HCC are also classified as well-differentiated thyroid cancers (WDTCs), which like other histologically well-differentiated cancers, generally have a relatively indolent course, with rather high 10-year survival rates. WDTC arises from the follicular cells of the thyroid gland and shares ionizing radiation as a common risk factor, an important piece of history to ascertain during the initial workup. As a whole, these slow-growing nonaggressive WDTCs account for approximately 95% of all thyroid malignancies. Staging for WDTC as described by the American Joint Committee on Cancer Staging (AJCCS) is unique in that age is a factor in determination of stage. Stage II is the highest possible stage in patients under the age of 45 years old. Tumor size, extrathyroidal spread, lymph node involvement, and metastatic disease allow for further classification in older patients. Notably, tumor node metastasis (TNM) staging is intended to provide information regarding survival and does not reliably predict disease recurrence, which, given the relatively indolent nature of WDTC, is the more clinically relevant endpoint as compared with mortality.

MTC, AC, and lymphoma are, in contrast, more aggressive malignancies with poorer prognoses. MTC is notable for its association with the multiple endocrine neoplasia (MEN), types 2A and 2B. Familial medullary thyroid carcinoma (FMTC) is now considered a variant form of MEN 2A. A diagnosis of medullary thyroid cancer should therefore be entertained in patients with a thyroid mass and family history of MTC. Moreover, MTC or the potential for MTC should be considered in any patient with stigmata of MEN 2A and 2B, such as pheochromocytoma, hyperparathyroidism, or mucosal neuromas.

The treatment of all thyroid cancers with the intention of cure is based on the foundation of complete surgical excision vis-à-vis total thyroidectomy. The plan and extent of surgery, however, depends on the type of thyroid cancer, locoregional spread, and the presence of distant metastatic disease.

DIAGNOSIS AND SURGICAL MANAGEMENT

Patients with thyroid cancer typically present with a palpable thyroid nodule. Surgical management of thyroid cancer is determined in large part by histologic data obtained from fine-needle aspiration biopsy (FNAB) of the thyroid nodule. The six distinct categories of thyroid fine-needle aspiration (FNA) cytology on which surgical management may be based are: (1) benign; (2) nondiagnostic; (3) suspicious for follicular/Hürthle neoplasm; (4) atypia of undetermined significance/follicular lesion of undetermined significance; (5) suspicious for malignancy; and (6) malignant.

With clearly benign cytology, surgery is usually deferred and serial ultrasound scan surveillance is appropriate. In some cases (i.e., when the nodule is particularly large [>4 cm] or the patient desires removal), lobectomy may be considered. For nondiagnostic results, repeat aspiration with ultrasound scan–guidance is warranted because half of all repeated aspirates are diagnostic. If multiple attempts at biopsy are nondiagnostic, core needle biopsy or diagnostic lobectomy should be considered. Patients should be counseled that approximately 10% of such nodules are malignant.

FNAB results that are suspicious for follicular or Hürthle cell cancer require resection of the nodule with hemithyroidectomy. Intraoperative frozen section is generally unreliable for confirmation of FC or HCC and is not recommended for a real-time confirmation of the cancer diagnosis because the issue of vascular invasion cannot be definitively settled with limited section and analysis available during frozen section. Approximately 20% of patients need second stage completion thyroidectomy for final histopathologic diagnosis of FC or HCC. In cases of significant contralateral lobe nodularity, history of head and neck radiation, or substantial perceived risk with a second anesthesia, total thyroidectomy can be recommended at the first operation.

Atypical or follicular lesions of undetermined significance have a 5% to 10% risk of malignancy. If repeat biopsy fails to clarify the diagnosis, lobectomy with or without intraoperative frozen section is warranted. In follicular lesions that are described as microfollicular with reduced colloid but no nuclear abnormalities, diagnostic lobectomy without frozen section is justified. In such lesions, if substantial nuclear abnormalities are noted, the potential for PTC exists. In these cases, frozen section analysis during lobectomy may be warranted because papillary cancers can be diagnosed in some of these cases on touch prep during frozen section analysis.

In addition to preoperative FNA, thyroid function blood testing studies are mandatory. The authors believe that all patients undergoing thyroid surgery must undergo preoperative laryngeal

TABLE 1: Thyroid cancer overview

	Cell of origin	FNA or histologic characteristics	Mean age at presentation (y)	Female:Male ratio	10-Y survival rate	Metastases	Response to RAI	Risk factors
Papillary (80%)	Follicular cell	Orphan Annie Eye nuclear changes, psammoma bodies*	40-50	3:1	>90%	Bone, lung (only 5% at time of presentation)	Yes	Ionizing radiation
Follicular (11%)	Follicular cell	Microfollicular pattern with reduced colloid cytologically with capsular invasion†	50-60	3:1	85%-92%	Lung, bone, brain (approximately 15% at time of presentation)	Yes	Iodine deficiency, ionizing radiation
Hürthle (3%-4%)	Follicular cell	>75% Hürthle cells‡ with capsular invasion†	50-60	2:1	75%	Lung, bone, CNS	Variable	Ionizing radiation
Medullary (5%-10%)	Parafollicular C cells	Uniform polygonal cells with fine, granular eosinophilic cytoplasm staining for calcitonin	30-40, 10 for MEN2B	1:1	70%-90%	Lung, liver, bone, brain	No	Family history, RET mutation
Anaplastic (1%-2%)	Follicular; dedifferentiated thyroid cancer	Spindle, giant, and squamoid cells	70-80	2-3:1	5%-10%§ at 5 y	Lungs, bone, brain	No	May arise from preexisting goiter or cancer
Lymphoma (1%-5%)	B/T cells	Multiple subtypes	60-80	3-4:1	50%-70%	—	No	Hashimoto's thyroiditis

B/T, Bone (B) cell/Thymus (T) Cells; *CNS,* central nervous system; *FNA,* fine-needle aspiration; *MEN2B,* multiple endocrine neoplasia type 2B; *RET,* RET protooncogene.
*Multiple histologic variants of papillary thyroid cancer exist.
†Minimal invasive versus invasive variants are differentiated by degree of vascular and capsular invasion.
‡Large polygonal cells with prominent nucleoli.
§Survival at 5 years.

examination to determine vocal cord functional status. This is especially true in cases of past thyroid, parathyroid, or other surgery that may have jeopardized the recurrent or vagus nerves. It is also important in all cases of thyroid malignancy given the potential for invasive disease. One must note that not all vocal cord paralysis is symptomatic, and so only routine laryngeal examination identifies all cases of preoperative vocal cord dysfunction. This information is of dramatic importance in the conduct of the subsequent surgery and in an operative plan that avoids bilateral vocal cord paralysis as an outcome. Preoperative workup must also include evaluation of cervical spine pathology (arthritis, degenerative joint disease, atlantoaxial subluxation, etc.) to allow for appropriate positioning for resection. Preoperative radiographic evaluation with ultrasound scan of the neck for assessment of not only the thyroid gland but also pathologically enlarged lymph nodes suspicious for metastasis should be performed. In the case of WDTC, only evidence of lymph node macrometastases serves as an indication for compartmental neck dissection (i.e., central neck dissection or ipsilateral lateral neck dissection).

Approximately 60% to 80% of aspirates read as suspicious for PTC are positive. Lobectomy for removal of the thyroid nodule followed by total thyroidectomy as a single-stage procedure when frozen section findings are consistent with malignancy is recommended. Total or near total thyroidectomy is currently recommended by the American Thyroid Association (ATA) for management of PTC of more than 1 cm in the absence of surgical contraindications. The National Comprehensive Cancer Network (NCCN) recommends total thyroidectomy for all patients with biopsy-proven PTC and any one of the following criteria: (1) age less than 15 years or greater than 45 years; (2) radiation history; (3) known distant metastases; (4) bilateral nodularity; (5) extrathyroidal extension; (6) tumor with greater than 4 cm diameter; (7) cervical lymph node metastases; or (8) aggressive histologic variant.

Total thyroidectomy coupled with remnant radioactive iodine ablation allows for easier detection of nodal or metastatic recurrent disease. The rationale for and primary goal of total thyroidectomy in the setting of malignancy is to remove the gross primary tumor in its entirety along with any associated locoregional macroscopic nodal disease. Approximately 35% of patients presenting with PTC have macroscopic nodal disease at presentation. Ultrasound scan and, in some centers, axial computed tomographic (CT) scanning are tools to preoperatively map out nodal disease in both central and lateral compartments so that a rational surgical nodal plan can be developed. Microscopic nodal disease may be present in up to 80% of patients with PTC. Most believe such microscopic disease is of little significance and does not require prophylactic compartmental surgery.

Biopsy results read as suspicious for or diagnostic of MTC, AC, or lymphoma require further workup for appropriate management. All patients with suspected or confirmed MTC should undergo preoperative evaluation to exclude associated genetic disease (i.e., MEN 2A/B). Approximately one quarter of all MTC cases are hereditary; the remainders are sporadic. Sporadic disease tends to be more unilateral (68%), and familial disease tends to be bilateral or multifocal (94%) and usually presents at an earlier age.

Workup of MTC includes screening for pheochromocytoma and hyperparathyroidism and serum calcitonin, carcinoembryonic antigen (CEA), RET protooncogene analysis, and neck ultrasound scan with lymph node mapping. Patients with palpable lymph nodes or serum calcitonin greater than 150 to 400 pg/mL should undergo further imaging (CT scan of neck, chest, abdomen) to evaluate for distant metastatic disease.

Total thyroidectomy with compartment-oriented nodal dissection is the mainstay of therapy for MTC. Prophylactic thyroidectomy is recommended within the first year of life for children with MEN 2B and between 3 and 5 years of age in children with MEN 2A and familial MTC. The exact timing of prophylactic thyroidectomy relates to the risk of malignant transformation within C cell clones and the likelihood of the development of nodal disease. The ATA has made

recommendations as to the timing of prophylactic thyroidectomy based on the risk for these events as it relates to the specific codon mutation. Pheochromocytoma must be evaluated for and, if present, must be addressed before thyroid resection.

In the case of FNAB suspicious for anaplastic thyroid cancer, early recognition and intervention is vital. Because of extensive necrosis, isthmectomy may be required to provide a tissue diagnosis and should not be delayed. Isthmectomy may need to be combined with tracheostomy depending on airway status, which can quickly deteriorate. Although palliative tracheostomy was once standard of care for all patients with unresectable disease, more recent data suggest that tracheostomy does not improve survival or quality of life in all patients. Today, the authors recommend palliative tracheostomy selectively in patients whose respiratory compromise is imminent and unresponsive to steroids.

The role for surgery is limited in anaplastic thyroid cancer (ATC) because of advanced disease at presentation. A large burden of distant metastases is a contraindication to surgery, although neoadjuvant radiation may transition inoperable disease to resectable disease. In the best case scenario, a full resection may be performed, followed by a full course of radiation therapy (XRT) 2 to 4 weeks after surgery. Positron emission tomography (PET)/CT scan should be performed on completion of XRT, with subsequent initiation of chemotherapy with paclitaxel or another taxane. Monthly restaging should be continued during chemotherapy and then every other month if the patient remains disease free for 6 months. After 2 years without recurrence, attention may be returned to underlying remnant PTC/FC and remnant radioactive iodine ablation (RRA) may begin.

Given the rapidly fatal progression of unrecognized ATC and the similarities in presentation between ATC and lymphoma, distinguishing the two processes is paramount for appropriate management. Definitive diagnosis is made with flow cytometry and occasional core needle biopsy. Open biopsy with isthmectomy is usually necessary for determination of the specific cell type of lymphoma. Surgery is otherwise not indicated for management of lymphoma, which is a medically managed entity. Thyroid lymphoma is generally sensitive to chemoradiation (rituximab, cyclophosphamide, doxorubicin, vincristine, and prednisolone [R-CHOP], 40 to 60 Gy). Typically, patients undergo one cycle of R-CHOP followed by radiation and five additional cycles of R-CHOP.

Although results of FNAB largely drive the surgical management of thyroid cancers, these results must also be considered in the context of the patient's clinical picture as a whole for appropriate surgical decision making. Additional clinical parameters regarding the extent of thyroidectomy include: (1) age of the patient, given increased risk of malignancy in patients over 60 years and under 20 years; (2) gender of the patient, with males generally having increased risk of malignancy; (3) family history of thyroid malignancy; (4) personal history of exposure to ionizing radiation; and (5) rapidly growing thyroid mass. Qualities such as size, firmness, and fixation of the thyroid mass, nodal disease, and vocal cord paralysis are also important indicators of malignant potential.

SURGICAL APROACH

The goals of effective operative therapy are constant between all types of thyroid cancer: (1) effective treatment of the disease; (2) minimized long-term side effects and complications; and (3) minimization of postoperative discomfort. The overriding principle is to encompass all gross disease and neck nodes at first resection, understanding that microscopic disease in the contralateral lobe and nodes likely has little significance towards overall survival. The extent of thyroidectomy is tailored to the patient's risk group (as detailed previously), intraoperative findings, and the progress of the surgery itself, particularly in cases where the contralateral lobe is not involved by cancer. Resection should always begin on the side of the nodule or the side with the most disease burden. Because injury to the recurrent laryngeal nerve (RLN) on one side may be an indication for aborting a total thyroidectomy, initiation of the thyroidectomy on the affected side ensures that most, if not all, gross disease can be resected regardless of RLN injury.

For appropriate identification and preservation of the recurrent laryngeal nerves, nerve monitoring is recommended. Good communication between the anesthesiologist and surgeon is vital to ensuring a smooth case and postoperative recovery. The patient should be positioned supine with arms tucked and padded. The neck should be extended with the assistance of inflatable balloon or shoulder roll (Figure 1). The patient should then be placed in reverse Trendelenburg's position to reduce venous pressure. After positioning, the surgeon should assess the monitor for appropriate impedance value (<5 kΩ) and event threshold (100 μV) with the stimulator probe set

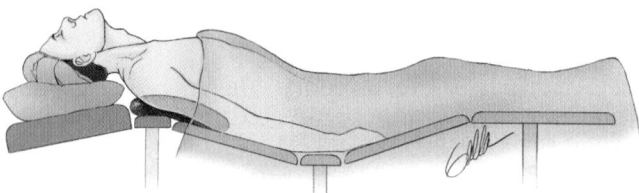

FIGURE 1 The neck is extended with a shoulder roll but adequately supported with a sponge donut. Twenty degrees of reverse Trendelenburg's position is maintained to avoid venous engorgement in the neck. *(From Randolph GW: Surgery of the thyroid and parathyroid glands, Philadelphia, 2002, WB Saunders.)*

at 1 to 2 mA. No paralytics should be used after induction to allow for appropriate nerve monitoring during surgery. This last point should be specifically vocalized and stressed to the anesthesia team. Once the team is satisfied that the patient is appropriately positioned and the nerve monitor is suitably situated and functional, the skin should be prepared from chin to sternum and bilateral neck to lateral clavicles in standard sterile fashion. The field should be draped to include the chin, bilateral neck, and suprasternal notch.

The authors find it helpful to consider thyroidectomy as a logical sequence of steps progressing through the neck from anterior/ventral to posterior/dorsal. A small, 4-cm to 5-cm horizontal incision should be placed within a natural skin fold of the neck approximately 1 fingerbreadth below the cricoid cartilage's anterior arch. The platysma is then incised, reflecting a flap superiorly, with care taken to preserve the anterior jugular veins. The strap muscles are then encountered and divided along the midline raphe. Special attention is paid to the ease with which the strap muscles are dissected from the ventral aspect of the gland, with consideration of malignant infiltration in cases of difficulty. In cases where better exposure is required, the authors recommend dividing the strap muscles superiorly to prevent denervation. Continuing laterally, the middle thyroid vein is divided, which, together with lateral retraction of the strap muscles and sternocleidomastoid muscle (SCM), exposes the lateral thyroid region (Figure 2).

With use of a dry sponge to prevent slippage, the thyroid and larynx are retracted medially, with the thyroid rotated slightly up and over the trachea, to expose the parathyroid and RLN (Figure 3). The dissection is then continued inferiorly, with the inferior thyroid veins ligated to allow for visualization of the inferior parathyroid gland,

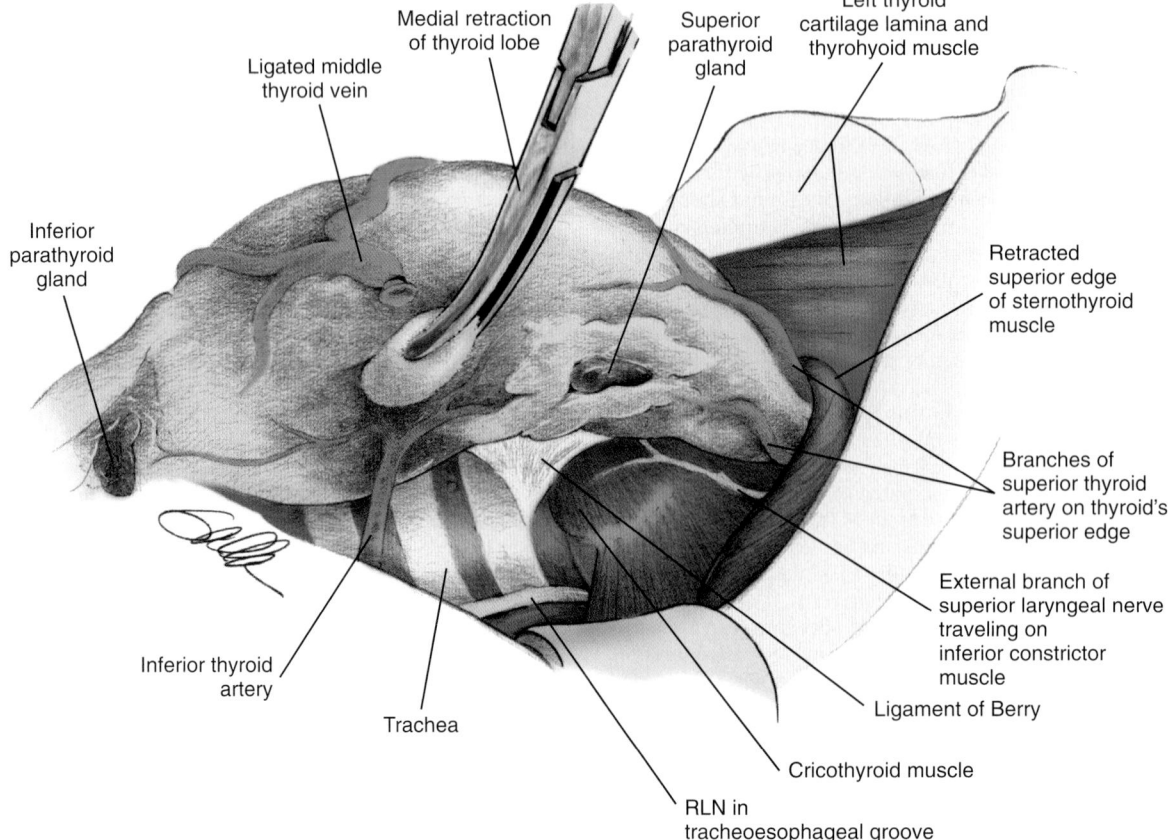

FIGURE 2 Left lateral view of lateral thyroid region shows exposure. Exposure of the region is facilitated by ligation of the middle thyroid vein and lateral retraction of strap musculature. Once this is performed, the thyroid lobe is retracted medially. As this is done, deeper anatomy, including the inferior thyroid artery, parathyroid glands, and recurrent laryngeal nerve *(RLN)*, becomes apparent. *SLN*, superior laryngeal nerve. *(From Randolph GW: Surgery of the thyroid and parathyroid glands, Philadelphia, 2002, WB Saunders.)*

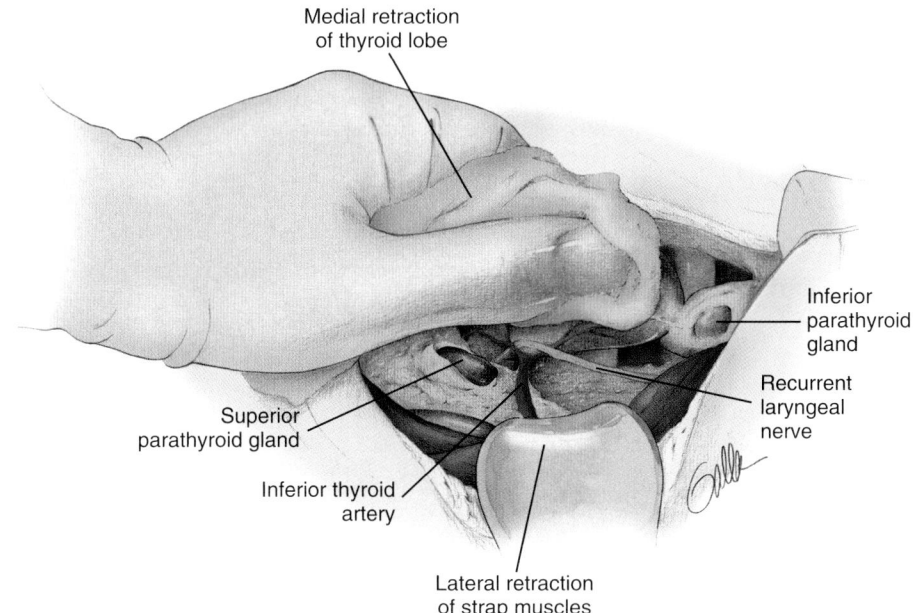

Medial retraction
of thyroid lobe

Inferior
parathyroid
gland

Recurrent
laryngeal
nerve

Superior
parathyroid gland

Inferior thyroid
artery

Lateral retraction
of strap muscles

FIGURE 3 Appropriate traction on the thyroid gland in an anteromedial direction places the inferior thyroid artery under tension and facilitates exposure of the recurrent laryngeal nerve. The inferior parathyroid is usually located anterior to the nerve and approximately 1 cm inferior to the point at which the inferior thyroid artery crosses the nerve. The superior parathyroid gland is usually located superior to the inferior thyroid artery and posterior to the nerve, where it passes deep to the inferior constrictor muscle. *(From Randolph GW: Surgery of the thyroid and parathyroid glands, Philadelphia, 2002, WB Saunders.)*

which is usually situated anterior/ventral to the RLN just below the point at which the inferior thyroid artery crosses over the RLN. Visual identification of the RLN is confirmed with the nerve stimulator, and then the inferior thyroid artery is divided, with care taken to preserve the blood supply to the inferior parathyroid. With the inferior lobe freed before dissection of the superior pole, better lobe mobilization is facilitated and greater visualization is allowed of the superior pole region and the external branch of the superior laryngeal nerve (EBSLN), which supplies motor function to the cricothyroid muscle.

With dissection of the RLN superiorly, the ligament of Berry is encountered; this anchors the thyroid to the inferior aspect of the cricoid cartilage. Great care must be taken to avoid RLN injury at this point in the dissection because varying degrees of thyroid tissue may infiltrate the ligament, bringing thyroid tissue directly adjacent to the nerve, which lies deep to the ligament. Remember the less than 1% risk of a nonrecurrent right-sided nerve that is at risk for injury in this location. The superior pole vessels are divided individually, low on the thyroid to avoid damage to the EBSLN (Figure 4). After ligation of the superior pole vessels, the superior parathyroid should be seen at the ligament of Berry and tubercle of Zuckerkandl. Meticulous hemostasis is achieved with gentle pressure; clamping should be avoided until the RLN has been identified and confirmed. Pledgets soaked in diluted epinephrine or fine-tipped bipolar cautery may also be used.

Once the superior and inferior aspect of the thyroid lobe is freed, the thyroid lobe can be sharply dissected from trachea. The thyroid may be removed with or without isthmus division. In hemithyroidectomy, the isthmus and pyramidal lobe are taken as part of the final specimen. Special care must be taken with dissection of the ligament of Berry, pyramidal lobe, and the superior pole because these are the sites where thyroid remnants most frequently occur.

Once the specimen has been removed, the authors examine the neck for nodal disease visually and with palpation and reassess parathyroid viability. If the parathyroids appear marginal, they should be biopsied for confirmation and then reimplanted in the SCM. By invoking the mantra, "Every parathyroid is the only parathyroid," we continually remind ourselves of the importance of meticulous dissection and preservation, thereby reducing our risk for injury.

Once the thyroid has been removed, hemostasis is assessed for through irrigation and intermittent sustained Valsalva's maneuver to at least 30 mm Hg. Any sites of bleeding may be controlled with bipolar cautery, once again with care taken to avoid RLN injury. The

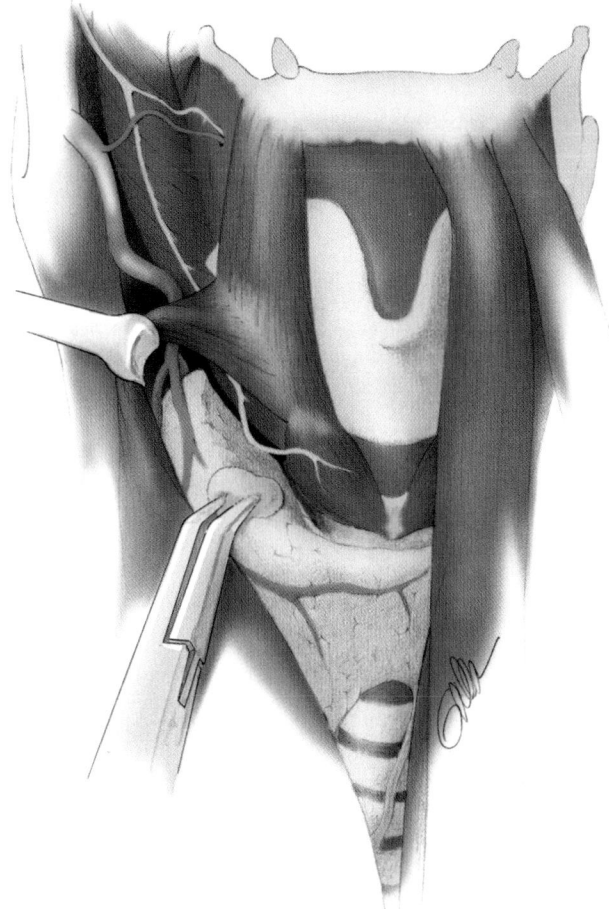

FIGURE 4 The external branch of the superior laryngeal nerve must be protected during dissection of the superior pole and ligation and division of superior pole vessels. The superior pole vessels are ligated and divided directly on the thyroid capsule of the superior pole to avoid inadvertent injury to the external laryngeal nerve. *(From Randolph GW: Surgery of the thyroid and parathyroid glands, Philadelphia, 2002, WB Saunders.)*

strap muscles are then reapproximated, with an open space kept inferiorly to allow for drainage in the rare case of hematoma. The platysma is then closed, followed by the skin. Drains are generally not indicated.

RECURRENT LARYNGEAL NERVE MONITORING

Recurrent laryngeal nerve trauma is one of the most serious complications of thyroid and parathyroid surgery. Unilateral vocal cord paralysis can result in vocal changes severe enough to necessitate change in vocation, significant dysphagia, and pulmonary complications. Bilateral vocal cord paralysis is a surgical emergency because of loss of airway. Rates of injury to the RLN are generally reported at 2% to 5%, although a systematic review of more than 25,000 patients showed an average of immediate postoperative vocal cord paralysis of 10%. Surgical exposure and visualization of the RLN is the gold standard of injury prevention and has been shown to lower the incidence rate of nerve injury to less than 1% in benign thyroid disease. Intraoperative nerve monitoring (IONM) is a valuable adjunct to visual nerve identification, serving as an aid to dissection and mapping of the RLN and as a tool to prognosticate the function of the nerve at the end of surgery.

The potential for unrecognized RLN injury, even in the setting of visual identification, is particularly high in cases of malignancy, substernal goiter, and revision surgery. Neural stimulation is superior to visual inspection in determination of intraoperative injury. Hence, intraoperative monitoring to establish functional status of the nerve remains an important tool for timely identification of injuries, especially in the context of bilateral surgery. Although the positive predictive value (PPV) varies in the literature from 10% to 90%, with an average of 45%, the PPV increases as a result of routine application of neural monitoring. In addition, aggressive endotracheal tube placement and troubleshooting algorithms can increase the PPV to 75% or higher.

Various intraoperative methods of monitoring the RLN exist, including continuous electromyography (EMG) monitoring, stimulation-evoked EMG monitoring, surface endotracheal tube–based EMG monitoring, and hook wire electrodes. The authors found the noninvasive surface electrode system with intermittent stimulation-evoked EMG monitoring ideal, accurate, and simple to use. On the basis of normative parameters of EMG amplitude and threshold, intraoperative EMG criteria can be formulated, which, when present, imply normal vocal cord function after surgery. These criteria are divided into: (1) initial/setup criteria, which inform the surgeon that the nerve has been appropriately identified and that the monitoring system is working; and (2) final/prognostic EMG parameters, which if satisfied, correlate with normal vocal cord function after surgery (Box 1).

IONM is a safe and reliable technique that can be predictive of and may lessen the risk of RLN morbidity by guiding intraoperative surgical decision making. Recognition of intraoperative EMG signal change can allow reexploration of the nerve to identify any site of potential injury and staging of the second side to avoid potential bilateral cord paralysis and airway compromise.

LYMPH NODE DISSECTION

The lymph nodes of the neck are divided into six levels (Figure 5). In thyroid cancer, the pertinent levels are the central (level VI) and lateral (levels II to IV) neck. Nodal malignancy is most frequently found within the central compartment. The central neck includes the prelaryngeal, pretracheal, and paratracheal nodes extending from the hyoid bone superiorly to the suprasternal notch inferiorly and the carotid arteries laterally. The anterior border of the lateral neck is comprised of the lateral edge of the carotid sheath, and the

---

BOX 1: Recurrent laryngeal nerve (RLN) monitoring: prognostic function

Electrophysiologic Findings That Predict Normal Postoperative Vocal Cord Function
A. Initial Setup Criteria
   Average initial stimulation at 1 mA, 900 μV (range, 144 to 2050 μV)

B. Final Prognostic Criteria
   Final average stimulation at 1 mA, 1200 μV (range, 247 to 3607 μV)
   Final average threshold at 0.37 mA (range, 0.15 to 0.80 mA)

If A and B are met, expect normal postoperative vocal cord function; contralateral surgery can be considered.
If A and B are not met, consider neural injury, especially if there is a gradient of evoked waveform around possible injured segment with less than 100 μV for evoked EMG proximal to injury.
If RLN injury is considered via stretch in upper mediastinum with substernal goiter, then test ipsilateral vagus to ensure that entire ipsilateral circuit is intact.

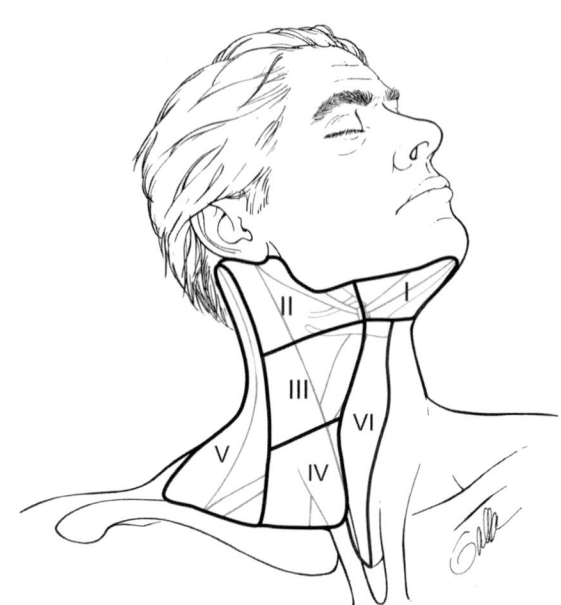

FIGURE 5 The level system for describing location of lymph nodes in the neck. *Level I*, Submental and submandibular group; *level II*, upper jugular group; *level III*, middle jugular group; *level IV*; lower jugular group; *level V*, posterior triangle group; *level VI*, anterior compartment group. *(With permission from Janfaza P, Nadol JB, Galla RJ, et al, editors: Surgical anatomy of the head and neck, Philadelphia, 2001, Lippincott Williams & Wilkins.)*

posterior border is the posterior border of the SCM. The superior border is the skull base, and the inferior border is the clavicle. The level V nodes make up the posterior triangle between the posterior border of the SCM and the anterior border of the trapezius muscle. The apex of these muscles forms the superior border; the clavicle lies inferiorly.

Central neck dissection involves removal of all nodes and fibrous fatty tissue within level VI. Modified lateral neck dissection involves removal of all nodes and fibrous fatty tissue within levels II to V, with preservation of the spinal accessory nerve, the internal jugular vein, and the sternocleidomastoid muscle in the absence of malignant invasion. Nodal thyroid metastases in the lateral compartment do not frequently invade these structures; therefore, avoidance of their removal remains oncologically sound.

Therapeutic resection of clinically positive nodal metastases, identified either with ultrasound scan, CT scan, or palpation, by compartment-oriented resection has been shown to decrease subsequent nodal recurrence. "Berry picking" selected lymph nodes is associated with higher rates of regional node recurrence and is no longer recommended.

Although clear evidence exists for therapeutic lymph node dissection, prophylactic dissection for WDTCs, which commonly metastasize to the central and lateral neck (i.e., PTC and HCC), remains controversial. Both the ATA and NCCN recommend consideration of prophylactic resection in patients at high risk as defined by age older than 45 years old, male gender, increased invasiveness or extent of disease, and size larger than 4 cm. Proponents for prophylactic resection argue that preoperative ultrasound scan fails to identify up to 50% of malignant lymph nodes and that their identification may alter postoperative management, including the implementation of RRA. Opponents for prophylactic resection argue that the risk for recurrent nerve injury and hypoparathyroidism outweigh an unclear benefit given the low rate of development of clinical disease in the neck despite high rates of micrometastatic disease. Moreover, should clinically significant disease develop subsequent to thyroidectomy without lymph node dissection, the risk of injury to the recurrent nerve or parathyroid glands is no different between primary and reoperative central neck dissection in skilled hands.

OPERATIVE OUTCOMES

Complications of thyroid surgery include nerve injury (RLN, EBSLN), hypoparathyroidism, and bleeding or hematoma. In general, morbidity from thyroidectomy remains low with even further reduction of complications when performed by experienced thyroid surgeons. Hypoparathyroidism, as defined by calcium levels less than 8 mg/dL within 6 months of thyroidectomy, occurs in 1% to 6.5% of patients. Experienced centers report hematoma rates at less than 1%.

POSTOPERATIVE MANAGEMENT

Postoperative RRA destroys residual microscopic disease and removes remnant thyroid tissue to facilitate thyroglobulin monitoring as a proxy for recurrent disease. Although the recurrence and mortality benefit in patients at low risk is unclear, consistent benefit has been shown in patients with high-risk WDTC. As such, RRA is recommended in select patients with incomplete resection, aggressive histology, and extrathyroidal, nodal, or distant metastases.

Thyroid-stimulating hormone (TSH) stimulates follicular cell growth, invasion, and angiogenesis. Thyroid hormone replacement both suppresses TSH production and prevents the development of hypothyroidism. Standard dosing begins at 2 μg/kg/d and is titrated according to TSH level. The recommended level of TSH suppression is determined by primary tumor stage.

Well-differentiated thyroid cancer recurs in approximately 10% to 30% of patients after initial treatment, with the majority recurring within the first 2 years. Surveillance includes physical examination, ultrasound scan, and measurement of thyroglobulin and TSH levels every 6 months for 2 years and then annually if the patient remains disease free. Most patients have recurrent disease develop in the neck alone, and 20% have recurrence develop with distant metastases, typically the lung or bone. Approximately half of patients who undergo a second operation are rendered disease free.

In contrast to WDTC, postoperative RRA, external beam radiation, hormone suppression therapy, and chemotherapy are not effective in MTC. More than half of the patients with MTC and palpable tumor have nodal metastases at presentation, most frequently to the central neck. Serum calcitonin is a sensitive and specific tumor marker for disease and is also useful for follow-up surveillance. A direct correlation is found with calcitonin level and tumor mass.

Surveillance of MTC includes monitoring of calcitonin and CEA levels after surgery and then semiannually. If calcitonin is high, a metastatic workup should be initiated and can include CT scan of the neck, chest, abdomen, and pelvis.

In patients with advanced local disease and extensive distant metastases, palliation is the goal with preservation of the airway and speech and swallowing capabilities. Current clinical trials are exploring the benefit of external beam radiation (EBRT) for bone metastases and hepatic embolization in the case of liver metastases. Targeted molecular therapies are also being explored for systemic management of disease. Tyrosine kinase inhibitors (TKIs) make up the majority of current immunotherapy-based treatments and include sorafenib, which selectively targets RET, and vandetanib, which targets vascular endothelial growth factor receptor and epidermal growth factor receptor and RET.

Unfortunately, ATC remains a rapidly fatal disease, with median survival ranging between 3 and 5 months. The 5-year survival rate is approximately 5% to 10%, with "cure" being defined as survival longer than 2 years. Emerging therapies for ATC include small-molecule tyrosine kinase inhibitors and vascular disrupting agents. All patients should be referred to the physician data query (PDQ) database for appropriate clinical trials: http://cancernet.nci.nih.gov/search/searchclinical trialsadvanced.aspc.

SUGGESTED READINGS

American Thyroid Association Surgery Working Group: Consensus statement on the terminology and classification of central neck dissection for thyroid cancer, *Thyroid* 19(11):1153–1158, 2009.

Guerrero MA, Clark OH: Controversies in the management of papillary thyroid cancer revisited, *ISRN Oncol* 303128, 2011.

Layfield LJ, Cibas ES, Baloch Z: Thyroid fine needle aspiration cytology: a review of the National Cancer Institute state of the science symposium, *Cytopathology* 21(2):75–85, 2010.

Pitt SC, Moley JF: Medullary, anaplastic and metastatic cancers of the thyroid [review], *Semin Oncol* 37(6):567–579, 2010.

Randolph GW, editor: *Surgery of the thyroid and parathyroid glands*, ed 2, Philadelphia, 2012, Elsevier Saunders.

Randolph GW, Dralle H, International Intraoperative Monitoring Study Group, et al: Electrophysiologic recurrent laryngeal nerve monitoring during thyroid and parathyroid surgery: international standards guideline statement, *Laryngoscope* 121(Suppl 1):S1–16, 2011.

Primary Hyperparathyroidism

Nishant D. Patel, MD, and Martha A. Zeiger, MD

BACKGROUND AND EPIDEMIOLOGY

Primary hyperparathyroidism is the most common cause of hypercalcemia. Parathyroid surgery has evolved from the identification of the first parathyroid gland in 1849 by Sir Richard Owen in an Indian rhinoceros to a variety of safe and effective surgical procedures for the management of primary hyperparathyroidism. The first parathyroidectomy was performed by Felix Mandel in 1925, and to this day, surgery remains the definitive treatment for primary hyperparathyroidism. Primary hyperparathyroidism is present in approximately 1% of adults in the United States, and the incidence increases to 2% after the age of 55. Women are two to three times more likely to have primary hyperparathyroidism than men.

PATHOPHYSIOLOGY, PRESENTATION, AND DIAGNOSIS

Primary hyperparathyroidism is characterized by hypercalcemia resulting from excessive parathyroid hormone production by one or more parathyroid glands. It is caused by a single adenoma in approximately 80% to 85% of patients, multigland hyperplasia in 10%, double adenoma in 4%, and parathyroid carcinoma in 1%. It is present in nearly all patients with multiple endocrine neoplasia type I and in 25% of patients with multiple endocrine neoplasia type 2A.

The clinical presentation of primary hyperparathyroidism results from the effects of excess parathyroid hormone, which in turn causes bone resorption of calcium and phosphorous, increased intestinal absorption of calcium, renal reabsorption of calcium, and hypercalciuria. Although most patients are asymptomatic, common signs and symptoms can include bone pain, osteopenia/osteoporosis, bone fractures, joint pain, kidney stones, urinary frequency/incontinence, fatigue, proximal muscle weakness, poor concentration, depression, nausea, and vomiting. Severe complications include renal dysfunction, hypertension, and severe neurologic dysfunction such as delirium or coma. The risk of developing symptoms or complications from primary hyperparathyroidism in patients who are asymptomatic at the time of initial diagnosis ranges from 23% to 62% by 10 years. Untreated disease may also lead to premature death from cardiovascular disease. The underlying physiologic basis is still under investigation but may involve decreased glucose tolerance, changes in vasomotor tone, hypertension, abnormal lipid metabolism, and obesity. The risk of premature death also increases with worsening hypercalcemia.

The diagnosis is most often made in the outpatient setting on routine laboratory evaluation. It is then confirmed by documenting the presence of high or high-normal calcium and concomitant elevated or high normal (nonsuppressed) parathyroid hormone levels. Associated laboratory abnormalities include decreased serum phosphate and increased or high-normal serum chloride levels. In addition, a 24-hour urinary calcium and creatinine should be collected to rule out familial hypercalcemic hypocalciuria (FHH), a disorder resulting from an autosomal dominant loss of function of the calcium-sensing receptor gene. A 24-hour urinary calcium to creatinine ratio of less than 0.01 distinguishes FHH from primary hyperparathyroidism. A family history of members younger than 10 years of age with hypercalcemia is also suggestive of FHH. Urinary calcium level is elevated in primary hyperparathyroidism (unlike FHH, which is <100 mg/24 hours); excretion that exceeds 400 mg in 24 hours is predictive of complications from primary hyperparathyroidism.

INDICATIONS FOR SURGERY

Currently, surgical management is the only curative therapy for patients with primary hyperparathyroidism, and patients who are symptomatic should undergo parathyroidectomy. With regard to asymptomatic patients, the most recent guidelines published in 2009 recommend parathyroidectomy for asymptomatic patients younger than 50 years of age, with serum calcium levels over 1 mg/dL above the upper limit of normal, creatinine clearance less than 60 mL/min, bone mineral density T score of 2.5 or lower at any site, or previous bone fracture fragility (Table 1). It is important to recognize that the symptoms of hyperparathyroidism are often subjective and subtle. Therefore, some patients who are considered "asymptomatic" and do not meet the criteria for surgical intervention may still benefit from parathyroidectomy.

LOCALIZATION

Most cases of primary hyperparathyroidism are due to a single parathyroid adenoma. Once the biochemical diagnosis of primary hyperparathyroidism is made, all patients should undergo localization studies to identify the abnormally functioning parathyroid gland(s) in preparation for minimally invasive parathyroidectomy. The two best preoperative localizations studies include the technetium-99m sestamibi scan (Figure 1) with single photon emission computed tomography (SPECT) and a neck ultrasound. A neck ultrasound will also identify any suspicious thyroid nodules.

Sestamibi with SPECT has a reported sensitivity of 80% to 90% in identifying a single adenoma (Figure 2). The sensitivity decreases with double adenomas and multigland hyperplasia. We routinely perform ultrasonography to localize parathyroid glands preoperatively. When findings are concordant with sestamibi scintigraphy, the sensitivity of preoperative localization improves to 94% to 99%. Although tumor biology influences the false-negative rate of sestamibi scans, the experience of the institution is also a critical factor. Successful visualization of a parathyroid adenoma can be as low as 50% to 60% in some centers. We recently reported on the subtleties or "shadows" discovered on sestamibi scans that had been initially read as negative or indeterminate. These subtleties include asymmetry of the thyroid gland, subtle posterior extension on a lateral view, or prominence of a thyroid lobe on early or delayed imaging. In our study "shadows" were found in 41% of cases with negative sestamibi and 76% of cases with indeterminate sestamibi scans. We showed that identification of these subtleties on sestamibi scan resulted in a successful minimally invasive approach in 91% of patients and a cure rate of 98%.

MINIMALLY INVASIVE PARATHYROIDECTOMY WITH INTRAOPERATIVE PARATHYROID HORMONE MONITORING

With a positive preoperative localization study (either sestamibi, ultrasound, or both), a unilateral or minimally invasive parathyroidectomy can be performed. A large-bore intravenous catheter is placed

TABLE I: Indications for parathyroidectomy

Age	<50 years
Serum calcium	1.0 mg/dL above upper limit of normal
24-hour urinary calcium	Not indicated
Creatinine clearance	<60 mL/min
Bone mineral density	T score <−2.5 at any site, or previous bone fracture fragility

Adapted from 2009 NIH Consensus Development Conference recommendations.

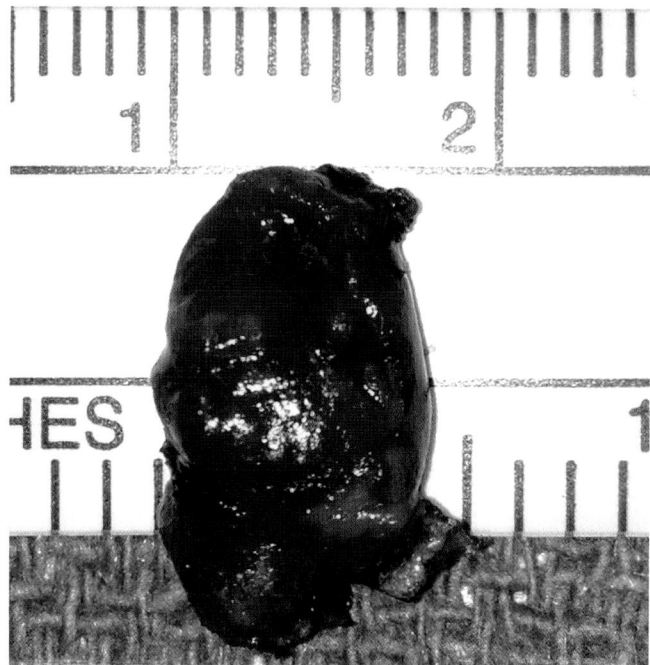

FIGURE 2   Excised parathyroid adenoma weighing 256 mg.

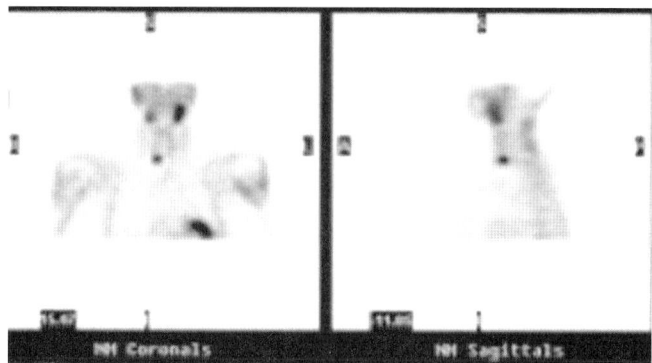

FIGURE I   Anterior-posterior and lateral view of technetium-99m sestamibi scan with single photon emission computed tomograph (SPECT) showing parathyroid adenoma in the right inferior position.

preoperatively to allow for blood sampling, and a baseline parathyroid hormone level is measured. Under general anesthesia, a lateral or midline 2-cm to 4-cm transverse incision within a skin crease is made on the same side as the localized hyperfunctioning parathyroid adenoma. The platysma is divided and subplatysmal flaps are raised. The strap muscles are separated vertically and dissected off the thyroid gland. The thyroid gland is gently rotated medially. The parathyroid adenoma is identified, and its vascular pedicle is divided. Upon excision of the parathyroid gland, intact parathyroid hormone levels are measured at baseline and 5- and 10-minute intervals thereafter. Based on the Miami criteria, a drop of 50% or more in the intact parathyroid hormone level from the baseline or time 0 is considered successful. The strap muscle is closed with 2-0 running suture, the platysma reapproximated with 3-0 interrupted suture, and the skin closed with running 4-0 monofilament suture.

BILATERAL NECK EXPLORATION

Failure to achieve the 50% drop in the intact parathyroid hormone level suggests multigland disease and necessitates further operative exploration. If unilateral exploration fails or preoperative imaging does not localize, one should proceed with conventional bilateral neck exploration. Bilateral neck exploration is also the procedure of choice for multiple endocrine neoplasia. A slightly longer 3- to 5-cm transverse incision is made within a skin crease. All four parathyroid glands are identified, and a 3.5-gland parathyroidectomy (subtotal parathyroidectomy) or 4-gland excision with autotransplantation in the nondominant brachioradialis muscle is performed. Ectopic

parathyroid adenomas can be located in the trachea-esophageal groove, the thymus, within the thyroid, or, finally, in the carotid sheath. Failure to achieve biochemical cure once these areas have been explored should lead to termination of the operation. Reexploration is then planned for a later date following further imaging studies (sestamibi-SPECT, computed tomographic scan, magnetic resonance imaging).

OUTCOMES AND FOLLOW-UP

The benefits of surgical management of primary hyperparathyroidism are well documented and include improvement in renal function, bone density, quality of life, survival, and a reduction in cardiovascular events. For bilateral neck exploration, the complication rate, including the risk of recurrent laryngeal nerve injury, remains low (4%), with success rates of 95% or better. Minimally invasive parathyroidectomy has comparable results with success rates of 98% and complication rates between 1% and 3%. The minimally invasive approach provides the additional advantages of smaller incision, improved cosmetic outcome, decreased pain, shorter operating time, same-day discharge, lower risk of nerve injury, and lower risk of postoperative hypocalcemia. Documentation of biochemical cure consists of eucalcemia 6 months postoperatively.

CONCLUSION

Parathyroidectomy remains the gold standard treatment for primary hyperparathyroidism. Minimally invasive parathyroidectomy has supplanted the traditional bilateral approach. Bilateral exploration is used, however, in patients with multigland disease, multiple endocrine neoplasia, and in the event that intraoperative parathyroid hormone levels do not drop appropriately or preoperative imaging fails to localize an adenoma. The majority of patients will be cured with minimal operative morbidity and will experience resolution of symptoms and excellent long-term health benefits.

SUGGESTED READINGS

AACE/AAES Task Force on Primary Hyperparathyroidism: The American Association of Clinical Endocrinologists and the American Association of Endocrine Surgeons position statement on the diagnosis and management of primary hyperparathyroidism, *Endocr Pract* 11:49–54, 2005.

Augustine, MM, Bravo PE, Zeiger MA: Surgical treatment of primary hyperparathyroidism, *Endocr Pract* 17:75–82, 2011.

Irvin GL III, Sfakianakis G, Yeung L, et al: Ambulatory parathyroidectomy for primary hyperparathyroidism, *Arch Surg* 131:1074–1078, 1996.

PERSISTENT AND RECURRENT HYPERPARATHYROIDISM

Michael J. Campbell, MD, and Quan-Yang Duh, MD

INTRODUCTION

Most patients with primary hyperparathyroidism (HPT) are cured with parathyroidectomy. About 5% of patients, however, have persistent or recurrent disease. The risk of a failed parathyroidectomy is higher when performed by low-volume surgeons and at low-volume centers. Reoperations for persistent or recurrent hyperparathyroidism present a challenge to the endocrine surgeon; the diseased glands are harder to find, and the complication rates are higher because of scarring from the prior operation. A systematic approach to evaluation and treatment of these patients is therefore crucial. The approach, sequentially, should include confirmation of the diagnosis, reassessment of the indication for parathyroidectomy, localization of the diseased glands, and planning for a safe and successful reoperation.

DIAGNOSIS OF PERSISTENT OR RECURRENT HYPERPARATHYROIDISM

Persistent hyperparathyroidism is defined as hyperparathyroidism that did not resolve after the initial parathyroidectomy or that recurred within 6 months of the initial operation. Recurrent hyperparathyroidism is defined as the return of disease after an apparent cure more than 6 months subsequent to the initial parathyroidectomy. Although some overlap exists, the designation of persistent and recurrent hyperparathyroidism separates two relatively distinct groups of patients. Persistent disease accounts for 80% of reoperations and is the result of inadequate resection. This can be caused by failure to find a parathyroid adenoma, failure to identify a second adenoma or inadequate resection of an adenoma (partial resection of a "dumbbell" adenoma), or hyperplastic parathyroid tissue (insufficient subtotal parathyroidectomy). Recurrent disease accounts for 20% of reoperations and is usually the result of an abnormality that is intrinsic to all the parathyroid tissue. Recurrent hyperparathyroidism commonly occurs in patients with familial HPT (with or without multiple endocrine neoplasia [MEN] type 1) and in those with multigland disease (MGD) at the initial operation (double adenomas or hyperplasia). Development of a second adenoma (in a gland observed as healthy during the initial operation) is rare but has been reported in patients with a history of neck irradiation. Other rare causes of recurrent disease are parathyroid carcinoma or parathyromatosis from a ruptured capsule and regrowth of parathyroid tissue in the operative field.

In evaluation of patients for persistent or recurrent HPT, reconfirmation of the diagnosis of hyperparathyroidism, with documentation of concurrent hypercalcemia with an inappropriately elevated serum parathyroid hormone (PTH) value, is important. Five percent to 10% of patients who are cured with a parathyroidectomy have persistently elevated serum levels of PTH with normocalcemia. This results from secondary hyperparathyroidism that may be caused by bone hunger, vitamin D deficiency, inadequate calcium intake or absorption, reduced peripheral sensitivity to PTH, underlying chronic kidney disease, or a renal leak of calcium. Isolated high serum PTH value alone without concurrent hypercalcemia is not diagnostic of persistent or recurrent hyperparathyroidism.

Because 2% to 10% of failed parathyroidectomies result from an incorrect diagnosis, it is imperative to revisit the initial diagnostic workup and reconfirm the diagnosis of primary hyperparathyroidism by documenting concurrently elevated serum calcium and PTH levels. Patients with a diagnosis of normocalcemic hyperparathyroidism deserve closer scrutiny. Ionized calcium and 25-hydroxyvitamin D (25OHD) levels also need to be measured. Ionized calcium is not affected by hypoalbuminemia and is a more accurate measurement of physiologically active free serum calcium. Most patients with normocalcemic hyperparathyroidism have a normal plasma level of total calcium but an elevated ionized calcium value. Because 1,25-dihydroxyvitamin D is the most potent suppressor of PTH secretion, patients with vitamin D deficiency commonly present with a normal serum calcium value but an elevated PTH level. Vitamin D replacement resolves the secondary hyperparathyroidism in such patients and may obviate the need for parathyroidectomy.

Because of the high prevalence of vitamin D deficiency in patients with HPT, the Third International Workshop on Asymptomatic Primary Hyperparathyroidism recommended measurement of 25OHD in all patients with HPT and repletion of levels less than 20 ng/mL before any surgical decision is made. These patients may have a varying degree of primary and secondary hyperparathyroidism that may become more obvious after vitamin D replacement. Vitamin D replacement in patients with hypercalcemia hyperparathyroidism may worsen hypercalcemia or hypercalciuria, so it needs to be carefully monitored. Finally, patients should have a 24-hour urinary calcium and creatinine measurement to rule out benign familial hypocalciuria hypercalcemia (FHH), which is caused by a heterozygous germline mutation of the calcium sensor gene. Parathyroidectomy is not indicated in patients with FHH. FHH is suspected in patients with a family history of failed parathyroidectomy, if the 24-hour urine calcium excretion is less than 100 mg/24 hours or if the urinary calcium:creatinine clearance ratio is less than 1%.

INDICATIONS FOR REOPERATIVE PARATHYROIDECTOMY

In general, the indications for reoperation in patients with persistent or recurrent HPT are the same as those for initial parathyroidectomy. However, one needs to rebalance the potential benefits of a successful reoperation with the potential increased risks associated with a reoperation. Reoperative parathyroidectomy is associated with a higher risk for a failed operation (10% vs 5%), permanent recurrent nerve injury (5% vs 1%), and hypoparathyroidism (5% to 10% vs 1%) when compared with initial parathyroidectomy.

Nephrolithiasis, fractures from osteoporosis/osteopenia, severe hypercalcemia or hypercalcemia-related pancreatitis, and peptic ulcer disease are strong indications for parathyroidectomy. Indications for parathyroidectomy in asymptomatic patients with milder disease are more controversial. The recommendations from the Third International Workshop on the Management of Asymptomatic Primary Hyperparathyroidism in 2009 for parathyroidectomy are summarized in Box 1. More subtle indications for parathyroidectomy include the nonspecific symptoms of muscle aches, weakness, nocturia, and neurocognitive derangements such as depression, emotional lability, and impaired cognition.

In patients with borderline indications, although the initial operation may have been indicated, a reoperation may not be. The surgeon and the patient should weigh the increased risks of a reoperative parathyroidectomy against the potential benefits when deciding on a reoperation.

PREOPERATIVE CONSIDERATIONS

Persistent HPT is most commonly caused by an inadequate initial operation. Most missed parathyroid adenomas are in the neck, and many are in their normal anatomic positions. The usual causes of persistent HPT are, therefore, inadequate exploration or failure to recognize the adenoma during the initial operation. Ectopic glands account for half of reoperative parathyroidectomies, and 80% of patients need resection of a single parathyroid adenoma. The most common ectopic locations are listed in Table 1 and shown in Figure 1. Some common ectopic locations, such as the cervical thymus for the lower glands and tracheoesophageal groove for the upper glands, are more likely to have already been explored by an experienced surgeon during the initial exploration. Incomplete resection of multiple abnormal glands accounts for about one third of patients with persistent HPT.

Recurrent HPT is most commonly associated with parathyroid hyperplasia in which all glands are abnormal or potentially abnormal. Many are caused by familial diseases such as MEN type 1 or familial HPT. In these patients, a "cure" for hyperparathyroidism depends on how much parathyroid tissue remains after the initial operation and how fast the remnants grow. During the initial operation and subsequent reoperation, the surgeon needs to balance the risk of recurrence from remnant parathyroid tissues versus the risk of hypoparathyroidism. When hyperplasia was recognized at the initial parathyroidectomy, the patients may have undergone a subtotal parathyroidectomy or a total parathyroidectomy and autotransplantation of parathyroid tissue to the forearm, thus determining where the recurrent disease is located.

Less than 1% of patients with primary HPT have parathyroid cancer, but more than half have recurrence. Persistent or recurrent disease from parathyroid carcinoma tends to occur at or near the primary tumor site, including the regional lymph nodes. Parathyromatosis is usually caused by capsular rupture and spillage of parathyroid cells during initial parathyroidectomy. Both parathyroid cancer and parathyromatosis have a high risk of re-recurrence and may require multiple reoperations.

PREOPERATIVE EVALUATION

After confirmation of the diagnosis of persistent or recurrent HPT and the indications for reoperation, attention is turned toward localization of the parathyroid tumor. Previous operative and pathology reports provide insights as to which glands have already been identified, biopsied, or removed. Review of the pathology slides shows whether the parathyroid tissue previously removed is hypercellular (adenoma or hyperplasia), normal, or parathyroid cancer. It is useful to correlate previous localization studies with the finding during the initial operation and pathology report. Discrepancies among them may provide clues as to the location of a missed gland or the likelihood of MGD. The history and physical examination should focus on the indications for parathyroidectomy and personal or family history of endocrinopathy that may suggest MGD.

Because reoperative parathyroidectomy is associated with a fivefold increased risk of injury to the recurrent laryngeal nerve, laryngoscopic evaluation of vocal cord function is mandatory. Approximately 7% of patients undergoing reoperative parathyroidectomy already have vocal cord palsy before the reoperation; some of these patients may not be hoarse or otherwise symptomatic. Because of the increased risk of bilateral vocal cord paralysis, bilateral reexploration should be avoided if possible.

PREOPERATIVE LOCALIZATION STUDIES

Bilateral four-gland exploration is a time-tested approach for initial parathyroidectomy, with a high success rate and a low complication rate. Reoperative parathyroidectomy, on the other hand, is best performed with a precise, targeted approach with minimal blind exploration. Scarring from the prior operation not only makes the parathyroid tumors harder to find but also increases the risk of injury to the recurrent laryngeal nerve and the healthy parathyroid glands. Thus, reoperative parathyroidectomy requires as precise as possible preoperative localization of the diseased gland.

BOX 1: Indications for surgical treatment in asymptomatic hyperparathyroidism

1. Total serum calcium greater than 1.0 mg/dL above the upper limit of normal
2. Creatinine clearance less than 60 mL/min
3. Bone mineral density T score ≤ 2.5 at any site
4. Age <50 years
5. Inability or unwillingness to undergo biannual biochemical surveillance

Modified from Bilezikian JP, Khan AA, Potts JT, et al: Guidelines for the management of asymptomatic primary hyperparathyroidism, J Clin Endocrinol Metab 94(2):333-334, 2009.

TABLE 1: Location of ectopic glands identified during reoperation

Location	%
Paraesophageal	28
Mediastinal	26
Intrathymic	24
Intrathyroidal	11
Carotid sheath	9
High cervical/undescended	2

Data from Shen W, Duren M, Morita E, et al: Reoperation for persistent or recurrent primary hyperparathyroidism, Arch Surg 1996;131:861-869.

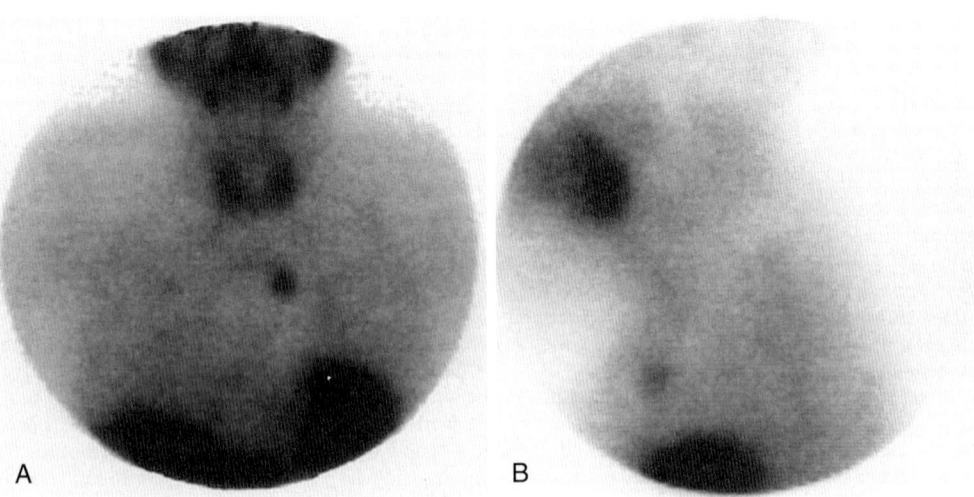

FIGURE 1 Technitium 99m sestamibi scan shows a mediastinal parathyroid adenoma. **A,** Frontal view. **B,** Lateral view of the same patient shows a parathyroid adenoma in the anterior mediastinum. *(From Arici, C, Cheah, WK, Ituarte, PHG et al: Can localization studies by used to direct focused parathyroid operations? Surgery 129(6):720-729, 2001.)*

With good preoperative localization, the success rate of reoperation can be similar to that of initial parathyroidectomy. Because of potential false-positive and false-negative results, the authors recommend obtaining two concordant localization studies before proceeding with reoperative parathyroidectomy. The two most commonly used localization studies are ultrasound scan and sestamibi scan (MIBI). Computed tomographic (CT) scan and magnetic resonance imaging (MRI) may also be used. Selective venous sampling (SVS) for PTH is more invasive and is only used on rare occasions.

Ultrasound scan is widely available, well tolerated, inexpensive, and excellent for identification of parathyroid tumors in the neck. Ultrasound scan, however, is operator dependent and cannot penetrate air and bones to detect ectopic glands located deep in the neck or in the mediastinum. The reported sensitivity for detection of parathyroid tumors in patients with persistent or recurrent HPT is 57% to 74%, with a positive predictive value (PPV) of 52% to 92%. Ultrasound scan has an added advantage: to guide fine-needle aspiration (FNA) of suspected lesions. Because of occasional difficulty in distinguishing follicular thyroid tumors from parathyroid tissue with cytology, the needle aspirate should to be sent for both cytology and PTH tests. An elevated PTH level in the aspirate (in the range of hundreds or thousands) is nearly 100% specific for parathyroid tissue. In addition, ultrasound scan can be used during surgery to confirm preoperative findings and to guide exploration.

MIBI is more successful than ultrasound scan for localization of ectopic parathyroid glands (Figure 2) but is more expensive and requires use of radionucleotide. Sensitivity for MIBI in recurrent or persistent HPT is 79% to 85%, with a PPV of 89% to 96%. The addition of single photon emission computed tomography (SPECT-MIBI) increases the sensitivity and specificity of sestamibi scanning.

When ultrasound scan and MIBI suggest the same site (concordant), the accuracy of localization of a parathyroid tumor approaches 95%. When ultrasound scan and MIBI results are negative, inconclusive, or discordant, then additional localization studies, such as MRI and CT, are necessary.

MRI identifies parathyroid adenomas with its intermediate to low signal intensity on T1-weighted imaging and high intensity on T2-weighted imaging. Unfortunately, cervical lymph nodes have similar imaging characteristics and may cause false-positive findings. MRI has the advantage of not requiring contrast or exposing the patient to ionizing radiation, but it is expensive. Use of gadolinium (Gd) increases the accuracy of localization. MRI has a sensitivity of 47% to 82% and a PPV of 80% to 89% in patients with persistent or recurrent HPT.

CT scan detects parathyroid adenomas based on their relative enhancement over surrounding structures. Standard CT scan has a

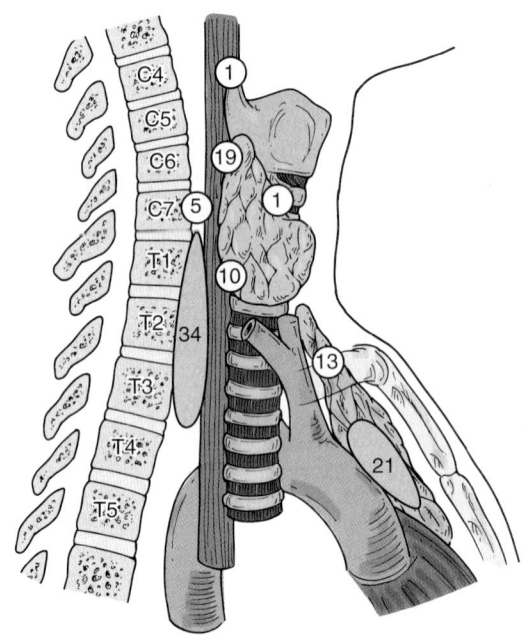

FIGURE 2 Anatomic locations of ectopic parathyroid glands with the number in each location given (n = 104). *(From Wang CA: Surgical management of primary hyperparathyroidism, Curr Prob Surg 22(11):37, 1985.)*

sensitivity of 40% to 86% for detection of parathyroid adenomas. Recently, four-dimensional computed tomographic (4D-CT) scan has been shown to accurately localize hyperfunctioning parathyroid glands that have otherwise been difficult to localize. The fourth dimension of the 4D-CT scan is a timed study of contrast perfusion. Parathyroid tumors have a more rapid uptake and washout of contrast compared with healthy parathyroid glands. 4D-CT scan has 88% sensitivity for localizing hyperfunctioning glands in patients undergoing reoperative parathyroidectomy. 4D-CT scan is quick and produces excellent anatomic details of the adenoma and surrounding structures, but it exposes the patient to ionizing radiation and is limited by metal clips, which cause scattering artifacts. The choice of MRI versus CT scan for patients with persistent or recurrent HPT is usually institution dependent.

If the noninvasive localization studies are inconclusive or conflicting, then SVS for PTH may be helpful. SVS does not precisely localize the parathyroid tumor but instead uses the gradient of PTH drainage to predict the side (lateralize) of the adenoma. Venous drainage with a twofold gradient in PTH levels is considered positive. SVS is 77% sensitive for lateralizing a hyperfunctioning parathyroid gland. Previous dissection can disturb normal venous drainage pathways and cause inaccuracy. Table 2 summarizes the sensitivities, benefits, and disadvantages of various localization studies.

OPERATIVE TECHNIQUE

After a review of the patient's history, previous operative and pathology reports, and localization studies, the surgeon can usually determine whether the patient has a solitary adenoma or multigland disease and the most likely location of the tumor(s). A missing upper gland must be distinguished from a lower gland because it may dictate the surgical approach (see subsequent discussion). More than two thirds of patients undergoing reoperation for hyperparathyroidism have a single adenoma. In these patients, with two concordant localization studies, a focused approach with intraoperative parathyroid hormone monitoring (ioPTH) can produce cure rates comparable with those of the primary (not reoperative) parathyroidectomy. A focused approach to reoperative parathyroidectomy, which minimizes unnecessary exploration, is less likely to injure the recurrent laryngeal nerve and the healthy parathyroid glands.

Most reoperative parathyroidectomies (85%) can be performed through the same cervical incision as the initial operation. Parathyroid glands in the neck can be explored via a central approach, between the strap muscles, or a lateral approach, between the strap muscles and the ipsilateral sternocleidomastoid muscle. Depending on the approach of the initial parathyroid exploration, the alternate approach can be used to minimize the need to dissect through scar tissue.

Most of the time, the neck has been previously explored through a central approach. In such cases, a lateral approach, with the previous cervical skin incision, usually works well and avoids previously violated surgical planes (Figure 3). In the lateral approach between the sternocleidomastoid muscle and the strap muscles, the carotid is retracted laterally, exposing the posterior border of the thyroid where most upper glands are found. The lateral approach also allows for a more direct approach to the tracheoesophageal groove and paraesophageal or retroesophageal area where many ectopic upper

parathyroid glands are found. Because the upper glands are usually located behind the recurrent laryngeal nerve, the lateral approach is ideal, allowing for direct access and avoiding the nerve anteriorly. The inferior glands are located anterior to the recurrent laryngeal nerve and are usually easier to reach through a central approach with the same incision.

Normal-appearing parathyroid glands should be protected. They can be marked with a clip and biopsied. Because uncertainty always exists about the number and location of remaining healthy parathyroid glands, reoperative excision of even a single adenoma may risk permanent hypoparathyroidism. If available, a sufficient amount of the excised parathyroid tissue should be cryopreserved for potential

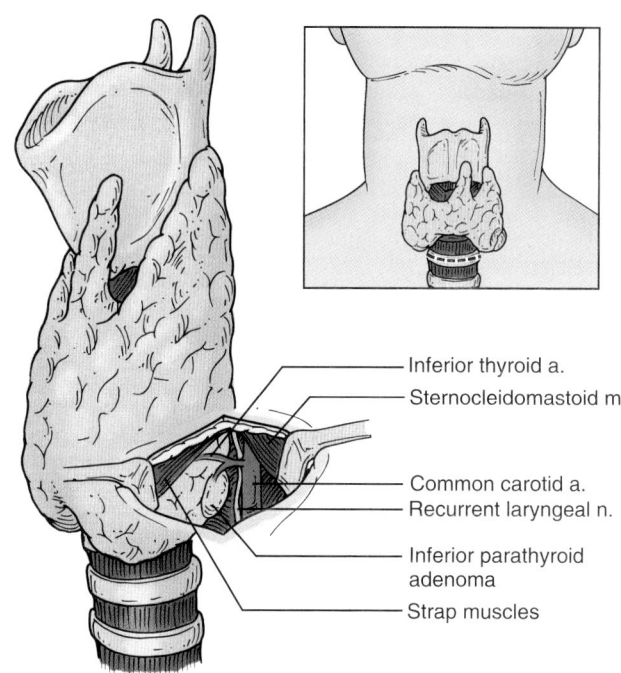

FIGURE 3 A lateral approach to identification of a posteriorly located parathyroid adenoma. *(From Wang TS, Udelsman R: Remedial surgery for primary hyperparathyroidism,* Adv Surg *41:1-15, 2007, Fig 5.)*

Labels in figure:
- Inferior thyroid a.
- Sternocleidomastoid m.
- Common carotid a.
- Recurrent laryngeal n.
- Inferior parathyroid adenoma
- Strap muscles

TABLE 2: Summary of the sensitivities, benefits, and drawbacks to localization tests in patients with persistent or recurrent hyperparathyroidism

Test	Sensitivity (%)	Benefit	Drawbacks
Ultrasound scan	57-74	No radiation, inexpensive	Unable to locate mediastinal glands, user dependent
^{99mTc}Sestamibi scan with or without SPECT	79-85	Able to locate ectopic glands	Radiation exposure, time-consuming
MRI	47-82	No radiation exposure	Expensive
CT scan	40-86	Readily available, inexpensive	Radiation exposure, artifact from previous clips
4D-CT scan	88	More specific than standard CT scan	Less available, radiation exposure
Selected venous sampling for PTH	77-93	Good sensitivity in the face of otherwise negative localization	Invasive, expensive

CT, Computed tomographic; *4D-CT,* four-dimensional computed tomographic; *MRI,* magnetic resonance imaging; *PTH,* parathyroid hormone; *SPECT,* single photon emission computed tomography.

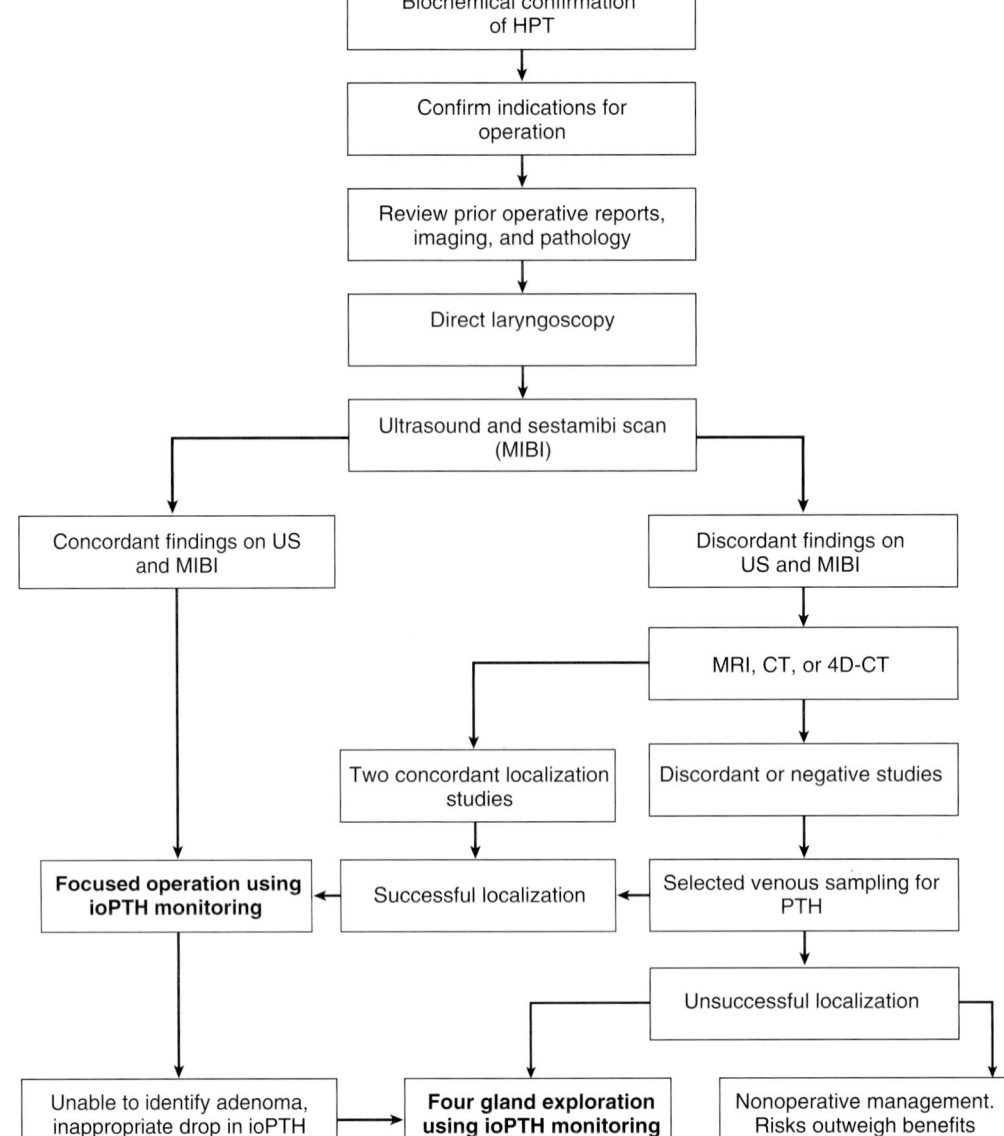

FIGURE 4 Algorithm for the diagnosis and management of recurrent and persistent hyperparathyroidism.
CT, Computed tomographic scan; *4D-CT,* four-dimensional computed tomographic scan; *HPT,* hyperparathyroidism; *ioPTH,* intraoperative parathyroid hormone monitoring; *MIBI,* sestamibi scan; *PTH,* parathyroid hormone; *US,* ultrasound scan.

future autotransplantation. If cryopreservation is not available and the anticipated risk for hypoparathyroidism is high, then immediate autotransplantation can be considered. Abnormal parathyroid tissue should be autotransplanted to an area that is easily accessible, in case of need for reexcision if disease recurs, usually in the nondominant brachioradialis muscle. Immediate autotransplantation has a 90% success rate, whereas autotransplantation of cryopreserved parathyroid tissue is 60% successful.

Occasionally, because of MGD or inconclusive localizing studies, a more extensive exploration is necessary. In such situations, a systematic approach to searching for missing parathyroid glands is pursued based on which glands have been identified, biopsied, or removed during previous operations. The normal anatomic locations should be considered first. The upper glands are often found cephalad to the inferior thyroid artery, posterolateral to the recurrent laryngeal nerve at the level of the cricoid cartilage. The lower parathyroid glands have a more variable location, but they are most often found caudal to the inferior thyroid artery and anteromedial to the recurrent laryngeal nerve. If a missing upper parathyroid gland is not found in its usual location, then one can search for an ectopic gland along its path of descent from its forth pharyngeal pouch origin. The most common locations for ectopic upper glands are in the

tracheoesophageal groove, paraesophageal or retroesophageal space, carotid sheath, or high cervical position. The most common locations for ectopic inferior glands are in the thymus, anterior mediastinum, or intrathyroidal. Figure 4 shows the authors' algorithm for workup and management of these patients.

For patients with parathyroid hyperplasia found at the initial operation, subtotal parathyroidectomy is usually preferred, with approximately 50 mg of tissue left from the most normal-appearing gland. For reoperations, however, where the number and location of remaining glands are likely to be uncertain, complete resection of the abnormal glands with cryopreservation is preferred. If intraoperative PTH shows that the patient is likely to have hypoparathyroidism (<10 pg/mL), then immediate autotransplantation to the forearm is considered.

POSTOPERATIVE MANAGEMENT

The results of reoperative parathyroidectomy are usually worse than for initial operation, both because of patient selection (more likely to have ectopic glands and MGD) and scarring that necessitates more limited exploration. Large series from tertiary referral centers have success rates of approximately 90%. Historically, the risk of permanent recurrent laryngeal nerve injury was estimated to be 3% to 10%, and the risk of permanent hypoparathyroidism 10% to 20%. With the newer localization studies, intraoperative PTH monitoring, and intraoperative recurrent laryngeal nerve monitoring, more modern series have 1% risk of recurrent laryngeal nerve injury and 2% risk of permanent hypoparathyroidism. Transient hypoparathyroidism is common after reoperative parathyroidectomy, and many patients need at least temporary oral calcium and vitamin D replacement. Even after an apparently successful reoperation, these patients need close follow-up for HPT because they are at higher risk of having, again, persistent or recurrent disease.

CONCLUSION

Reoperation for persistent or recurrent hyperparathyroidism is challenging. Before the operation, the diagnosis and indication for operation need to be confirmed. Review of prior operative and pathology reports and results of localization studies usually allows for a focused exploration. Preoperative laryngoscopy, intraoperative monitoring of the recurrent nerves and PTH levels, and cryopreservation of parathyroid tissue all need be considered to mitigate the expected higher risks of operative complications.

SUGGESTED READINGS

Caron, NR, Sturgeon C, Clark OH: Persistent and recurrent hyperparathyroidism, *Curr Treatment Options Oncol* 5:335–345, 2004.

Jaskowiak N, Norton, JA, Alexander JR, et al: A prospective trial evaluating a standard approach to reoperation for missed parathyroid adenoma, *Ann Surg* 224(3):308–321, 1996.

Richards ML, Thompson GB, Farley DR, et al: Reoperative parathyroidectomy in 228 patients during the era of minimal-access surgery and intraoperative parathyroid hormone monitoring, *Am J Surg* 196:937–943, 2008.

Shen W, Duren M, Morita E, et al: Reoperation for persistent and recurrent primary hyperparathyroidism, *Arch Surg* 131:861–869, 1996.

Udelsman R, Donovan PI: Remedial parathyroid surgery: changing trends in 130 cases, *Ann Surg* 244:471–479, 2006.

SECONDARY AND TERTIARY HYPERPARATHYROIDISM

**Jason D. Prescott, MD, PhD, and
Antonia Stephen, MD**

OVERVIEW

Primary hyperparathyroidism is the overproduction of parathyroid hormone (PTH) by abnormal parathyroid glands, and secondary hyperparathyroidism (2°HPT) refers to the excess secretion of serum PTH by normal parathyroid glands in response to perturbations in calcium homeostasis. The most common pathologic process that affects normal calcium metabolism, and thus stimulates increased parathyroid gland function, is chronic renal failure. Other causes of 2°HPT include vitamin D deficiency, inadequate calcium ingestion, calcium malabsorption, and idiopathic hypercalciuria. 2°HPT is common; population studies suggest a prevalence rate as high as 6.6% in some cases. Reversibility is an implicit feature of this disorder, and correction of the underlying abnormality should result in disease resolution. Cases in which this does not occur either represent misdiagnosis (e.g., primary hyperparathyroidism) or indicate development of tertiary hyperparathyroidism (3°HPT). 3°HPT occurs when chronically stimulated parathyroid tissue in a patient with 2°HPT becomes autonomous, producing elevated and unsuppressed levels of PTH even after correction of abnormal calcium metabolism. The development of 3°HPT therefore represents an additional pathologic event, superimposed on a background of 2°HPT, that produces autonomous parathyroid gland function. The most common clinical scenario in which this develops is in a patient with 2°HPT and chronic renal failure who undergoes renal transplantation. Despite a functional kidney in such cases, and therefore normalization of calcium metabolism, the parathyroid glands continue to overproduce PTH, which results in a condition similar to primary hyperparathyroidism.

Chronic renal failure (CRF) is the most important cause of 2°HPT, and 2°HPT develops in the majority of patients with CRF. Most 2°HPT cases are successfully managed medically; surgical treatment for 2°HPT (parathyroidectomy) is almost always reserved for those cases in which medical management fails. Medical treatment in these cases is complex, however, and unlike most other causes of 2°HPT, parathyroidectomy can play a therapeutic role. In this chapter, we review the pathophysiology and current treatment strategies for CRF-associated 2°HPT and 3°HPT, including medical and surgical approaches.

PATHOPHYSIOLOGY

The pathologic mechanisms resulting from renal failure that lead to hyperparathyroidism are complex and incompletely understood. The primary known stimulus for PTH secretion is low serum ionized calcium, and persistently low serum calcium measurements may well be expected in patients with 2°HPT. Interestingly, patients with CRF and 2°HPT often have serum calcium levels in the normal (or low normal) range, which indicates that more complex biochemical interactions are at play. At least four interdependent factors that affect calcium homeostasis contribute to the development and progression of 2°HPT: hypocalcemia, impaired vitamin D activation, hyperphosphatemia, and parathyroid resistance to fibroblast growth factor 23 (FGF23; Box 1). In the absence of renal disease, absorption of urinary calcium is extremely efficient, reaching 98% in individuals with eucalcemia. As renal failure progresses, however, absorption of urinary calcium is correspondingly impaired and hypocalcemia develops. Renal failure progression also results in impaired vitamin D activation. In normal circumstances, the kidneys convert 25-hydroxyvitamin D to its most active form, 1,25-dihydroxyvitamin D. This compound then acts directly on the small intestine, stimulating calcium absorption, and on the parathyroid glands, where it inhibits PTH gene expression. As loss of functional renal parenchyma progresses in CRF, vitamin D activation capacity is proportionally compromised, which results in both hypocalcemia and direct activation of PTH synthesis.

Hyperphosphatemia, which is common in patients with renal failure, also contributes to hypocalcemia by titrating ionized calcium from the serum as calcium phosphate and by directly inhibiting renal activation (hydroxylation) of 25-hydroxyvitamin D.

A recent discovery was the elucidation of FGF23 function in phosphate metabolism. FGF23 acts on the kidney, stimulating phosphate excretion, and on the parathyroid gland, inhibiting PTH synthesis and secretion. As progressive hyperphosphatemia develops during chronic renal failure, serum FGF23 levels correspondingly increase. Despite this increase, however, FGF23 receptor concentrations in the parathyroid gland decline as renal failure progresses. Thus, the abnormal parathyroid tissue characteristic of 2°HPT becomes progressively resistant to FGF23, and hyperparathyroidism results.

3°HPT is diagnosed when the inciting cause for 2°HPT is corrected, and, nonetheless, the parathyroid glands continue to overproduce PTH. This typically manifests biochemically as elevated serum calcium and PTH levels. The inability of the parathyroid glands to revert to their normal inhibitory feedback response, as mediated by elevated serum calcium levels, may relate to the hyperplasia that originally developed during the preceding 2°HPT and CRF.

CLINICAL MANIFESTATIONS OF SECONDARY AND TERTIARY HYPERPARATHYROIDISM

The clinical sequelae of 2°HPT and 3°HPT can be both debilitating and life threatening. All cause and, in particular, cardiovascular-related mortality rates are increased in 2°HPT. Periarticular calcium deposition can produce arthritis, joint space effusion, and impaired joint function. 2°HPT-associated bone disease in the context of CRF, termed renal osteodystrophy, is an additional source of significant morbidity in this patient population. The development of nephrocalcinosis can exacerbate kidney failure and produce a vicious cycle that accelerates the progression of both renal dysfunction and 2°HPT. Finally, calcification of cutaneous arterioles, with associated subcutaneous tissue inflammation, is the hallmark of calciphylaxis, a rare but highly morbid condition associated with CRF-mediated 2°HPT. This condition is characterized by progressive cutaneous ischemia that presents as painful erythematous skin lesions, usually on the distal extremities or trunk, which progress to frank gangrene and subsequent sepsis. Mortality rates in affected patients can reach 80%.

MEDICAL MANAGEMENT

Curative management in patients with CRF-related 2°HPT requires renal transplantation, which, when successful, results in normalization or near normalization of serum calcium, phosphorous, and PTH levels in up to 95% of patients. Demand for donor renal grafts, however, far exceeds supply, and the vast majority of patients with 2°HPT are therefore managed medically. Curative medical therapy remains to be developed, so current medical treatment strategies thus focus on control of serum PTH, calcium, and phosphorous levels.

Consensus treatment guidelines for the management of CRF, including associated 2°HPT, have been published by the National Kidney Foundation (Kidney Disease Outcomes Quality Initiative [KDOQI]) and by the Kidney Disease: Improving Global Outcomes (KDIGO) foundation. These treatment algorithms are designed to minimize cardiovascular (KDOQI) and bone/extraskeletal calcification (KDIGO)–related mortality in CRF-associated 2°HPT. Most experts use one or both algorithms in the management of these patients.

Management of Hyperphosphatemia

Treatment of hyperphosphatemia should be initiated when serum phosphate levels exceed 5.5 mg/dL in stage 3, stage 4, or stage 5 CRF (glomerular filtration rate [GFR], 30-59, 15-29, and <15 mL/min/1.73 mol/L^2, respectively). The treatment goal in these cases is stabilization of serum phosphate levels between 3.5 and 5.5 mg/dL. Management should begin with restriction of daily dietary phosphate intake to less than 900 mg and, when end-stage renal disease is present, dialysis. Phosphate-binding medications should be added when dietary restriction and, if applicable, dialysis fail to consistently produce serum phosphate levels below 5.5 mg/dL.

Management of Serum Parathyroid Hormone Levels and Hypocalcemia

Optimal overall outcomes among patients with CRF requiring dialysis have been associated with serum PTH maintenance between 150 and 300 pg/mL. Treatment in these patients therefore focuses on stabilization of serum PTH levels within this range. Activated vitamin D analogs can lower serum PTH levels, and use of these agents is indicated when serum PTH levels rise above 300 pg/mL in end-stage renal disease or exceed the upper limit of normal in nondialysis CRF cases. Because vitamin D may exacerbate hyperphosphatemia, however, and may produce hypercalcemia, activated vitamin D treatment is contraindicated when serum phosphate levels exceed 5.5 mg/dL or the corrected serum calcium concentration is greater than 9.5 mg/dL. In addition, vitamin D therapy should be discontinued if corrected serum calcium levels exceed 10.2 mg/dL or if serum phosphate levels rise above 5.5 mg/dL. Finally, vitamin D supplementation should be stopped if serum PTH levels fall below 150 pg/mL in patients with dialysis-dependent 2°HPT.

The calcimimetics are a relatively new medication class and function to increase the sensitivity of the calcium-sensing receptor (CaSR) protein to calcium, thus acting to inhibit secretion of parathyroid hormone. Use of cinacalcet, the prototype agent, in the management of patients on dialysis with 2°HPT is associated with improved serum phosphate, calcium, and PTH control. Moreover, cinacalcet appears to attenuate fracture risk, rates of parathyroidectomy, and hospitalization rates in these patients. Cinacalcet therapy should be considered for patients on dialysis in whom phosphate binders provide inadequate serum PTH suppression. Hypocalcemia contraindicates calcimimetic therapy, and treatment should be discontinued if corrected serum calcium levels fall below 8.4 mg/dL. In addition, cinacalcet has not been approved for use in patients with CRF before dialysis; and although cinacalcet is associated with improvements in serum PTH in such patients, its efficacy and safety in this population remain to be established.

The medical management of 2°HPT in patients with CRF is challenging, and the combination and dosage of phosphate binders, vitamin D analogs, calcium supplements, and calcimimetics chosen is patient specific. Treatment assessment and medication dosage titration therefore require careful monitoring of serum calcium, phosphate, and PTH levels. Serum total calcium, phosphate, and PTH should be measured weekly until stable levels are achieved with a given medication regimen, and then every 1 to 3 months. Serum 25-hydroxyvitamin D levels tend to change slowly and should be evaluated every 3 to 6 months in this patient group.

SURGICAL MANAGEMENT

Surgical resection of hyperplastic parathyroid tissue can provide durable resolution of 2°HPT in patients with CRF, with consequent symptomatic improvement, reversal of bone demineralization, and decreases in long-term mortality rates. Because 2°HPT develops when otherwise healthy parathyroid tissue responds inappropriately to pathologic external stimuli, all parathyroid tissue is affected and four-gland hyperplasia results. Thus, the aim of parathyroid surgery in 2°HPT is to remove enough hyperplastic parathyroid tissue to improve calcium homeostasis and treat otherwise unremitting symptoms, without producing hypoparathyroidism.

Indications

Parathyroid surgery for CRF-associated 2°HPT is indicated when: (1) medical therapy fails to control serum PTH levels, hypercalcemia, or hyperphosphatemia; (2) 2°HPT-related symptoms become refractory to medical therapy; (3) intractable rapid turnover bone disease develops; or (4) calciphylaxis is present (Box 2). Patients in whom serum PTH levels exceed 800 pg/mL and in whom serum calcium levels are greater than 10 mg/dL or in whom serum phosphate levels are above 5.5 mg/dL, despite maximal medical therapy, should be offered surgery. Similarly, intractable symptoms in a background of medically refractory 2°HPT merit surgical intervention. These include refractory pruritus, bone pain, muscle pain, anemia, abdominal pain, and weakness. Rapid turnover bone disease that does not respond to medical management should also prompt surgical intervention, especially when associated with pathologic fracture. Finally, biopsy-confirmed calciphylaxis is an absolute indication for emergent parathyroidectomy, which may arrest disease progression and improve wound healing.

Tertiary Hyperparathyroidism

Instances in which PTH levels remain elevated after renal transplantation represent 3°HPT; posttransplantation parathyroid surgery remains the primary management strategy in these cases. Recent studies, however, question this approach. Multiple contemporary series show a significant risk of transplant dysfunction and rejection when parathyroid surgery is performed after renal transplantation. The underlying mechanisms to explain these findings remain unknown, and graft dysfunction does not occur in all postparathyroidectomy transplant cases. Nonetheless, some experts now advocate parathyroid surgery before renal transplantation to potentially avoid postparathyroidectomy renal graft dysfunction. This strategy remains controversial because those patients with CRF in whom 3°HPT does not develop and who therefore do not need parathyroidectomy cannot be identified before transplantation and thus are subjected to unnecessary parathyroid surgery. In addition, renal graft function among patients undergoing pretransplant parathyroid surgery, relative patients receiving parathyroid surgery after renal transplantation, remains to be objectively defined.

BOX 2: Indications for parathyroidectomy in patients with chronic renal failure

1. Persistent hyperphosphatemia, hypercalcemia, or elevated parathyroid hormone, despite maximal medical therapy
2. Refractory hypercalcemic symptoms
3. Intractable renal osteodystrophy
4. Calciphylaxis

Medical therapy for 3°HPT continues to improve. Cinacalcet, for example, has shown efficacy in lowering both serum calcium and PTH levels in 3°HPT cases. Nonetheless, small studies that compare medical therapy with parathyroid surgery for 3°HPT suggest that parathyroidectomy affords superior serum PTH, calcium, and phosphate control. Until long-term outcome data comparing these interventions become available, parathyroid surgery remains the preferred intervention for 3°HPT. Medial therapy should be reserved for patients who are not surgical candidates or for stabilization in anticipation of parathyroidectomy.

Preoperative Assessment

In addition to verification of both the diagnosis of 2°HPT and the presence of associated surgical indications before surgery, the operative candidacy of all patients with CRF-associated 2°HPT should be formally assessed with preoperative risk stratification. Patients in whom severe preexisting comorbidities contraindicate surgery should be managed medically. In addition, imminent renal transplantation is a relative contraindication to parathyroidectomy, at least among those experts who do not ascribe to routine pretransplantation parathyroidectomy (see Tertiary Hyperparathyroidism).

Formal preoperative imaging for purposes of localizing abnormal parathyroid glands is unnecessary in both 2°HPT and 3°HPT, as pathologic involvement of all four glands is expected and four-gland exploration is therefore indicated. Localization imaging should be limited to rare cases in which supernumerary or ectopic parathyroid glands are suspected. All patients with 2°HPT and 3°HPT should, however, receive a formal preoperative thyroid ultrasound scan, both for identification of any potentially malignant coincident thyroid nodules that may be present and for assessment of parathyroid anatomy. Discovery of suspicious thyroid nodules should prompt an appropriate preoperative malignancy workup, and failure to identify all four parathyroid glands is a reasonable indication for additional localization imaging. Preoperative sestamibi or four-dimensional computed tomographic (CT) scanning can be used to localize ectopic parathyroid glands that are not visualized with ultrasound scan.

Operative Technique

Adequate surgical management of 2°HPT and 3°HPT requires either subtotal parathyroidectomy, in which 3.5 parathyroid glands are resected, or total parathyroidectomy with autotransplantation. Despite ongoing debate, the balance of reported data does not demonstrate relative superiority for either procedure, and surgeon preference thus dictates technique selection.

The procedure begins with semi-Fowler patient positioning. The cervical spine is placed in extension, and after application of sterilizing skin preparation, a 4-cm to 6-cm symmetric Kocher's incision is made approximately 2 fingerbreadths above the sternal notch. The relatively prominent anatomic location of this incision should always prompt careful consideration of cosmesis, and whenever possible, postoperative scarring should be minimized by placing the incision within a preexisting skin crease. Dissection is carried through the platysma muscle and subplatysmal flaps are elevated, exposing the underlying strap musculature. The median raphe defining the plane of symmetry between the strap musculature on either side of the neck is then incised, and the sternohyoid muscle is dissected free from the underlying thyroid gland. The thyroid is then carefully mobilized to avoid injury to associated branches of the inferior thyroid artery, which supply both the thyroid and the parathyroid glands. Systematic examination of all four parathyroid glands is then performed. If subtotal parathyroidectomy is planned, all four parathyroid glands should be visualized before resection. This allows selection of the least abnormal-appearing parathyroid tissue for remnant creation. An approximately 40-mg parathyroid remnant, marked with a nonabsorbable suture or a titanium clip, is left attached to its associated vascular pedicle. The identity of this tissue should be verified with frozen section analysis of its resected component, and the remnant should be carefully observed for signs of inviability. Cases in which the remnant appears inviable should prompt either autotransplantation of remaining parathyroid tissue or creation of a new remnant from a separate parathyroid gland.

The most fragile structure associated with the ipsilateral parathyroid glands, and thus at risk for iatrogenic injury during parathyroid exploration, is the recurrent laryngeal nerve (RLN). Identification and preservation of both RLNs, which supply motor function to the vocal cords, is thus a critical component parathyroid surgery. Although parathyroid gland anatomy can be highly variable, the inferior parathyroid gland is generally situated just anterior to the course of the ipsilateral RLN, and the superior parathyroid gland tends to localize posteriorly relative to this nerve. Cases in which total parathyroidectomy is performed should generally prompt intraoperative parathyroid reimplantation. Although omission of autotransplantation decreases the probability of disease recurrence, most experts prefer to accept an increased recurrence risk in exchange for minimization of permanent postoperative hypocalcemia risk. For autotransplantation, the most normal-appearing parathyroid gland is selected; this tissue is sharply minced into 1-mm fragments. The identity of this tissue should be verified with frozen section analysis before autotransplantation. Appropriate autotransplant acceptor sites include the sternocleidomastoid muscle, the brachioradialis muscle of the nondominant forearm, and the subcutaneous soft tissue of the chest wall. Site selection depends on surgeon preference, although autotransplantation distant from the neck allows either biochemical or imaging-based differentiation between cervical and implant-associated disease in cases of recurrence. Three or 4 pockets adequately sized to accept 5 to 10 parathyroid tissue fragments are then created with blunt dissection at the donor site, and approximately 10 mg of minced parathyroid tissue is placed into each pocket. The aperture of each implantation site is closed with nonabsorbable suture or with titanium clips. Cases in which recurrent disease develops from progressive hyperplasia of autotransplanted tissue may be managed with resection of one or more of the implantation pockets with local anesthesia.

Special Considerations and Intraoperative Adjuncts

Gland ectopy is a relatively common finding in parathyroid surgery. Ectopic inferior glands are most frequently found within the ipsilateral thymus, and ectopic superior parathyroids are often paraesophageal. Other ectopic localization sites include the carotid sheath, the anterior mediastinum, adjacent to the cervical vertebral bodies, and within the ipsilateral thyroid lobe parenchyma. Failure to localize any of the four parathyroid glands in their typical anatomic positions should prompt careful exploration of potential ectopic sites. Cases in which an ectopic parathyroid gland localizes to the anterior mediastinum may require partial sternotomy.

A number of adjunctive intraoperative strategies have been proposed for improving the success of parathyroid surgery. These include ultrasound scan and gamma probe-assisted intraoperative gland localization and titration of parathyroid tissue resection on the basis of serial intact PTH measurements. Although data that support the value of these techniques have been reported, the adoption of these data remains controversial, and the use of intraoperative adjuncts during surgery for 2°HPT remains surgeon specific. The presence of supernumerary glands, although rare, may confound the adequacy of subtotal parathyroidectomy or total thyroidectomy with

autotransplantation for 2°HPT and 3°HPT. This potential pitfall may be avoided through intraoperative PTH monitoring, as associated persistent serum PTH elevation prompts further surgical exploration and gland resection. In addition, some experts include routine intraoperative cervical thymectomy in the operative management of 2°HPT and 3°HPT because supernumerary parathyroid gland localization is often thymic.

POSTOPERATIVE MANAGEMENT

2°HPT exists in the context of severe hypocalcemia; thus, rapid decreases in serum PTH levels that occur after successful parathyroid surgery can result in the rapid and profound bony absorption of serum calcium. The sequelae of this process, termed hungry bone syndrome, can produce significant symptoms, including tetany, seizures, and heart failure. Patients after 2°HPT surgery must therefore be carefully monitored for signs and symptoms of hypocalcemia. Although the hypocalcemia may have been corrected in 3°HPT, the bone loss is often present and these patients are also at risk for hungry bone syndrome. Routine postoperative oral supplementation with 4 to 6 g of calcium, divided into 3 or 4 daily doses, should be initiated immediately after surgery, and serum calcium levels should be serially monitored. Patients with persistent hypocalcemia, despite these interventions, need intravenous (IV) calcium gluconate administration. Postoperative hypocalcemia in patients who previously needed dialysis may also be controlled by increasing dialysate bath calcium concentration. Postoperative supplementation with activated vitamin D (e.g., calcitriol) should be started if preoperative vitamin D deficiency is present, if hypocalcemia persists despite aggressive oral calcium supplementation, or if intravenous calcium infusion is necessary. Finally, hypomagnesia can accompany hypocalcemia and interfere with normalization of low serum calcium concentrations. Serum magnesium levels should thus be monitored after surgery, and hypomagnesia should be corrected with oral or intravenous magnesium sulfate. The hypocalcemic nadir after parathyroidectomy for 2°HPT generally occurs 2 to 4 days after surgery, with most patients showing improving serum calcium levels thereafter. A small number of these patients have persistent hypocalcemia, however, presumably as a result of parathyroid remnant or autotransplant failure. These patients need ongoing calcium and vitamin D supplementation. Finally, all patients after 2°HPT and 3°HPT surgery must be followed for the development of recurrent or persistent disease. Serum calcium and PTH concentrations should be measured 1 week after surgery, 6 months later, and then annually. Rising serum calcium and PTH concentrations are suggestive of recurrent or persistent disease and should prompt evaluation for additional medical or surgical therapy.

SUGGESTED READINGS

Goldfarb M, Gondek SS, Lim SM, et al: Postoperative hungry bone syndrome in patients with secondary hyperparathyroidism of renal origin, *World J Surg* 36(6):1314–1319, 2012.

Kidney Disease: Improving Global Outcomes (KDIGO) CKD-MBD Work Group: KDIGO clinical practice guideline for the diagnosis, evaluation, prevention, and treatment of Chronic Kidney Disease-Mineral and Bone Disorder (CKD-MBD), *Kidney Int Suppl* (113):S1–S130, 2009.

Pitt SC, Panneerselvan R, Chen H, et al: Secondary and tertiary hyperparathyroidism: the utility of ioPTH monitoring, *World J Surg* 34(6):1343–1349, 2010.

Shen WT, Kebebew E, Suh I, et al: Two hundred and two consecutive operations for secondary hyperparathyroidism: has medical management changed the profiles of patients requiring parathyroidectomy? *Surgery* 146(2):296–299, 2009; Epub 2009.

Metabolic Changes Following Bariatric Surgery

Ali Tavakkoli, MD, and Robert N. Cooney, MD

METABOLIC CONSEQUENCES OF OBESITY

Obesity is an excess accumulation of body fat, and is commonly defined as a body mass index (BMI) of more than 30. Although BMI is easy to calculate, assessing obesity based on BMI has several limitations. For example, athletic individuals may have an elevated BMI because of increased muscle mass instead of excess fat. Although one can calculate body fat and define obesity as percentage body fat more than 32% in women and more than 25% in men, these calculations are difficult. More importantly, neither BMI nor percentage of body fat definitions of obesity provides any information on the regional distribution of excess body fat. This is important because the metabolic consequences of obesity are influenced by both the amount and the distribution of body fat. Abdominal or visceral obesity leads to a chronic inflammatory state caused in part by the release of free fatty acids and cytokines from adipose tissue. Visceral obesity is associated with increased risk of insulin resistance, hyperlipidemia, hypertension, cardiovascular disease (CVD), and stroke. This pattern is also referred to as android obesity and is more commonly seen in men. The gynecoid pattern of obesity is characterized by an excess accumulation of subcutaneous fat in the gluteal and buttock areas, more commonly seen in women, and is less frequently associated with adverse metabolic effects. The importance of central obesity is highlighted in populations who, despite relatively low BMI, have high levels of visceral obesity (e.g., Asians) and are prone to adverse effects of obesity at a lower BMI.

Although the obesity epidemic in the United States is well documented, affecting 36% of the adult population and nearly 20% of children, the problem is an international one, with many Western countries reporting similar rates. The highest rate of obesity is observed in Samoa, where it affects 75% of adults. The global epidemic of obesity is multifactorial and has genetic, environmental, and epigenetic roots. The recent exposure of humans to an environment with excess cheap food is thought to have led to an imbalance between caloric intake and energy expenditure, resulting in pathologic excess fat deposition. The risk of reaching this detrimental state of fat accumulation in our current environment is modulated by genetic risk factors, diet, exercise, and lifestyle.

Although adipose tissue was originally thought to be a relatively quiescent accumulation of stored calories, more recent studies indicate adipose tissue to be metabolically and hormonally active. In severe obesity, excess lipid accumulates in these metabolically active adipocytes, and in hepatocytes and muscle cells. Excess accumulation of nutrients and fat within these cells leads to increased secretion of adipocyte-derived peptides (e.g., leptin, adiponectin, resistin) and cytokines (e.g., tumor necrosing factor–α [TNF-α], interleukin-6 [IL-6]) collectively referred to as adipokines. The paracrine and endocrine actions of these adipokines contribute to a state of chronic low-grade inflammation, which in turn interferes with many physiologic cellular processes (such as insulin signaling) and leads to the metabolic derangements seen in obesity (such as insulin resistance and type 2 diabetes).

The obesity-induced inflammatory state adversely affects most organ systems in the body and contributes to a shortened life expectancy. Each 5-unit increase in BMI is associated with a 30% increase in all cause mortality, with BMIs of more than 40 associated with a reduced life expectancy of 8 years. Obese individuals have a poor quality of life with increased risk of many life-threatening conditions, including: cancers, heart disease, type 2 diabetes, hypertension, stroke, hyperlipidemia, and sleep apnea. The prevalence of these comorbidities often increases with the severity of obesity (Table 1). This is most evident with type 2 diabetes. At age 18 years, women with a BMI of 30 to 35 have a 54.6% lifetime risk of development of diabetes, which is increased to 74.4% for those with BMI of more than 35.

Although modest weight loss (5% to 10% excess weight) can lead to reductions in the risk of these chronic diseases, nonsurgical weight loss is often unsuccessful or short lived in 90% to 95% of patients. As a result, bariatric surgery has become the standard of care in the treatment of medically complicated or morbid obesity. A variety of weight loss operations are in common practice.

METABOLIC IMPROVEMENTS AFTER WEIGHT LOSS SURGERY

Weight Loss

The term excess body weight loss (EBWL), calculated with the actual and ideal body weight, is commonly used to describe weight loss. Not surprisingly, the degree of EBWL varies between procedures. The mean EBWL is 70% to 80% for biliopancreatic diversion (BPD) with or without duodenal switch, 60% to 70% for Roux-en-Y gastric bypass (RYGB), 50% to 60% for sleeve gastrectomy (SG), and 40% to 45% for laparoscopic adjustable gastric banding (LAGB) at 2 years. In general, procedures with higher weight loss are also associated with increased short-term and long-term complications. The balance between the desired weight loss and surgical risk influences the patient when choosing an operation and the surgeon when offering the procedure.

The mechanisms underlying the weight loss are multifactorial and vary by procedure. The proposed mechanisms for postsurgical weight loss are summarized in Table 2. Of critical importance are long-term changes in appetite and hunger after surgery. In contrast, nonsurgical weight loss leads to increased hunger and reduced energy expenditure, which presumably contribute to the ultimate failure of dieting in achieving long-term weight reduction. Weight loss surgery prevents such physiologic responses and maintains hunger control despite limited calorie intake.

Long-term follow-up studies such as the Swedish Obesity Study show significant long-term weight loss in surgical patients compared with control subjects, with up to 20 years of follow-up. The durability of postsurgical weight loss is a concern for patients and clinicians. Definition of successful weight loss for bariatric surgery varies depending on the procedure but for RYGB is described as losing and maintaining 50% or more EBWL. Most patients regain some weight after reaching their nadir weight, with pathologic weight regain (>20% of the maximal weight loss) reported in 15% to 20% of patients. This observation highlights the fact that bariatric surgery is not a replacement for long-term lifestyle changes that are needed to help maintain weight loss. A commitment to changes in diet and exercise are critical for long-term success. The importance of such changes and the need for regular postoperative follow-up examination with the bariatric team should be discussed with patients before surgery.

TABLE 1: Risks of cardiovascular and metabolic disorders with obesity

Life expectancy	30% increase in mortality rate for each 5-unit increase in BMI. In patients with BMI > 40, life expectancy is reduced by 8 years.
Hypertension	5-fold risk of hypertension in obese individuals. 85% of patients with hypertension have a BMI > 25.
Cardiovascular disease	A 9% increase in cardiovascular mortality rate with each unit increase in BMI.
Type 2 diabetes	Men with BMI ≥ 35 have 42-fold increase in risk of diabetes compared with men with BMI < 23. 74% lifetime risk of type 2 diabetes if BMI > 35.

BMI, Body mass index.

TABLE 2: Proposed mechanisms for weight loss after bariatric procedures

Physical restriction of food intake	Although a common belief, especially in case of LAGB, little data support this. Food transit through the stomach is only minimally altered after LAGB, and the supraband compartment is empty of food within 1-2 min after ingestion. BPD has a large gastric reservoir and yet leads to best weight loss results.
Malabsorption	Although a degree of this occurs after BPD, little malabsorption is seen after LAGB, SG, or RYGB as measured with stool calorimetry and nitrogen balance.
Decreased hunger signals and reduced food intake	This is true for all bariatric procedures and the result of hormonal changes along the gut-brain axis after surgery.
Increased energy expenditure and diet induced thermogenesis	Although this has been documented in rodents, little data support this in humans.
Changes in food preference	Changes in food preference have been documented and are related in part to alterations in reward and taste and concerns about physiologic implications of ingestion of certain foods that may lead to dysphagia or dumping syndrome.
Changes in gut microbiota	Animal studies show a role for intestinal microbacteria in obesity and diabetes. Definitive human data are currently lacking, but this is an area of significant scientific interest.

BPD, Biliopancreatic diversion; *LAGB*, laparoscopic adjustable gastric band; *RYGB*, Roux-en-Y gastric bypass; *SG*, sleeve gastrectomy.

Nonalcoholic Fatty Liver Disease

Nonalcoholic fatty liver disease (NAFLD) is present in more than 70% of individuals with a BMI of more than 35 and represents a spectrum of disease characterized initially by the accumulation of liver fat (steatosis), which if severe, causes inflammation and nonalcoholic steatohepatitis (NASH) and later fibrosis or cirrhosis. Hepatic steatosis and NASH, markers of central adiposity, are thought to be important in the pathogenesis of obesity-related metabolic disorders, often referred to as the metabolic syndrome (visceral adiposity, insulin resistance, hyperinsulinemia, hypertension, hyperlipidemia). NASH is a leading cause of cirrhosis in the United States and one of the main indications for liver transplantation. Therefore, resolution of NASH-related hepatic injury is an important endpoint in bariatric and metabolic surgery. Studies have shown weight loss operations lead to a near universal improvement in the severity of hepatic steatosis, inflammation, and fibrosis. A few cases of worsening fibrosis and inflammation have been reported, although in most cases, this is transient and is thought to be related to the rate of postoperative weight loss. Although all bariatric procedures lead to improvements in the severity of liver injury, a recent study showed patients who underwent RYGB had significantly greater improvement in grade of liver disease compared with those who underwent restrictive-only procedures (SG and LAGB; 95% vs 66%) as a direct result of better weight loss seen after RYGB.

Lipid Profiles

Dyslipidemia is seen in up to 50% of patients who undergo bariatric surgery, with more than 70% experiencing an improvement or resolution of this comorbidity within 2 years of surgery. Surgery leads to reductions in total cholesterol and low-density lipoprotein (LDL) and also increases high-density lipoprotein (HDL) levels. Variation is found in the remission rate of dyslipidemia between the common bariatric procedures, and better results are achieved with the more malabsorptive operations, with BPD leading the way with a 90% remission/improvement rate. In a recent study that compared SG and RYGB, gastric bypass led to a reduction in cholesterol and LDL and an increase in HDL, and the SG only increased HDL without altering LDL levels. Both operations result in a significant reduction in triglyceride levels.

Hypertension

Hypertension is common in obesity and rises in prevalence with increasing weight. The odds ratio for hypertension is 1.7 for individuals who are overweight compared with those of normal weight and is 2.6 for BMI 30 to 34.9, 3.7 for BMI 35 to 39.9, and 4.8 for BMI 40 or more. Elevated blood pressure is seen in up to 50% of patients who undergo bariatric surgery, with 60% to 70% documenting an improvement or remission after weight loss surgery. Improvements in blood pressure are also linked to weight loss, and the remission rates vary between the bariatric procedures.

A meta-analysis of several studies showed improvement in hypertension in 58% of patients undergoing LAGB. These improvements were less evident when gastric banding was studied in randomized fashion with control arms. In a small Australian study of obese adolescents randomized to LAGB, systolic blood pressure (BP) was reduced by 12.5 mm Hg compared with baseline values; however, this was not significant when compared with the control group. The Swedish Obesity Study, a study cohort that consisted mainly of adjustable or vertical banding, also showed no significant improvement in hypertension at 10 years after surgery compared with control subjects, although a modest improvement was seen at the 2-year time point.

For patients who undergo RYGB, hypertension has been shown to improve or resolve in 60% to 70% of cases compared with baseline, an observation that has been further confirmed in a nonrandomized study. A European study of patients undergoing RYGB or intensive medical therapy showed the rate of hypertension remission was 49% for the surgical group versus 23% for the medical therapy group. BPD has also been shown to resolve hypertension in 60% to 80% of patients.

Cardiovascular Risk and Mortality

CVD remains the leading cause of mortality in the United States. Several risk scores have been developed to calculate an individual's risk of having a cardiovascular event and are widely used to help guide strategies for primary prevention. Of these risk scores, the Framingham risk score (FRS) is most commonly used. This risk score is calculated on the basis of age, gender, and smoking status and cholesterol, HDL, and systolic blood pressure. These parameters are all improved after bariatric surgery; therefore, it is not surprising that weight loss procedures have been shown to reduce FRS and the 10-year risk of a cardiac event by 40%. Serum and laboratory risk predictors, such as creactive protein (CRP), have also been shown to decline after surgery by about 60%.

Two large cohort studies have shown the reductions in risk factors also translate to reductions in mortality rate. In a large cohort study from Utah, at a mean follow-up of 7.1 years, cardiovascular mortality rate was decreased by 56% compared with control groups. Similar improvements in cardiovascular mortality have also been reported in the Swedish Obesity Study.

Type 2 Diabetes

Of all metabolic changes after bariatric surgery, none have been as impressive as the improvements in glucose homeostasis. Type 2 diabetes has reached epidemic proportions in the United States, and despite significant investments in preventive measures, the rate is set

to continue to climb. New pharmacologic therapies (glucagon-like peptide-1 [GLP-1] analogues and dipeptidyl peptidase-IV [DDP-IV] inhibitors) have been disappointing, and most patients with diabetes do not reach the therapeutic goals set by the American Diabetic Association and other endocrine societies (glycosylated hemoglobin [HbA$_{1c}$], <7%). These trends and the remarkably rapid improvement in diabetes seen after bariatric interventions have pushed surgery to the forefront of the diabetes treatment and created the field of *metabolic surgery*, defined as the operative manipulation of a *normal* organ or organ system to achieve a biologic result for a potential health gain.

The observation that alterations in gastrointestinal anatomy can lead to diabetes resolution was noted more than 50 years ago, and improvements in glycemic control after weight loss operations have been well documented for the past 20 years. Several large studies and meta-analyses have confirmed that all bariatric procedures lead to significant improvements in glucose control and diabetes remission, although success rates vary between the different operations with RYGB and BPD offering the best chance of disease remission (Table 3). Although improvements in glycemic control are expected after any form of weight loss (surgical or diet-induced), studies have confirmed weight-independent effects on diabetes after RYGB and BPD.

Three randomized studies have now confirmed that LAGB, RYGB, SG, and BPD lead to better diabetes control than intensive medial therapy. In the study that compared LAGB with medical therapy, surgery led to a diabetes remission rate of 73% versus 13% for the medical arm at 2 years. The improved outcomes in the surgical arm were linked to improved weight loss. Mingrone and colleagues compared medial therapy with RYGB or BPD and showed that at 2 years diabetes remission (defined by fasting glucose <100 mg/dL and HbA$_{1c}$ <6.5% in the absence of pharmacologic therapy) was seen in 0 in the medical arm compared with 75% in RYGB and 95% for BPD. Interestingly, weight loss did not predict glycemic improvement after these procedures. Schauer and associates compared medical therapy with RYGB or SG and showed that after 12 months of follow-up, diabetes remission (defined as HbA$_{1c}$ <6% with or without medications) was 12% in the medical group versus 42% in the RYGB and 37% in the SG arms.

These data have prompted many of the diabetes societies to alter their treatment guidelines for management of type 2 diabetes and recommend surgery in patients with poorly controlled diabetes and BMI of more than 35. The International Diabetes Federation, an umbrella organization that represents many national societies, in their 2011 position statement went one step further, recommending that patients with BMI of more than 30 and diabetes that is poorly controlled with medication should also be considered for surgery.

Although the antidiabetic effects of LAGB are directly linked to weight loss, the studies point to a weight-independent effect for RYGB and BPD. This topic has received significant scientific attention over the last few years with many proposed mechanisms (Table 4). Although many hormones have been investigated to help elucidate the mechanisms of weight-independent effect of RYGB on glucose homeostasis, GLP-1 has emerged as a likely explanation, with several

TABLE 3: Weight changes and metabolic improvements 2 years after bariatric procedures

	Weight loss	Lipid improvement	Hypertension	T2D improvement
BPD	70%-80%	90%	80%	90%
RYGB	60%-70%	60%-70%	60%	80%
SG	50%-60%	50%-60%	60%	70%-80%
LAGB	40%-45%	60%	58%	50%-60%

BPD, Biliopancreatic diversion; *LAGB*, laparoscopic adjustable gastric band; *RYGB*, Roux-en-Y gastric bypass; *SG*, sleeve gastrectomy; *T2D*, type 2 diabetes.

TABLE 4: Proposed mechanisms for anti-diabetic effects of RYGB and other similar procedures

Restriction and acute decrease in food intake after surgery	Unlikely. Food intake is reduced after many GI surgeries where patients are kept nothing by mouth. Most of these surgeries, however, lead to a state of insulin resistance rather than sensitivity.
Malabsorption	Unlikely. No evidence that RYGB leads to enough nutrient malabsorption to account for the rapid improvement in diabetes.
Changes in postprandial incretin response	Postprandial GLP-1 levels are increased after these surgeries, leading to enhanced insulin release. This is likely from earlier delivery of food to the distal small bowel where GLP-1 is primarily secreted.
Isolation of proximal bowel from nutrient flow	Evidence points to a role for proximal bowel in sensing nutrient availability and quality. Isolation of this region of the intestine from nutrient exposure can lead to alterations in nutrient absorption and glucose homeostasis. This idea is behind some of the metabolic devices currently in development.
Intestinal gluconeogenesis	Rodent studies have suggested that ability of proximal bowel to generate glucose and release it to the portal circulation leads to changes in hepatic insulin sensitivity and glucose homeostasis. Human studies are lacking.
Changes in circulating bile acids	Human and animal studies have shown increased circulating bile acid levels in patients after RYGB and linked this to improved glucose homeostasis.

GI, Gastrointestinal; *GLP*, glucagon-like peptide; *RYGB*, Roux-en-Y gastric bypass.

studies showing increased postprandial levels after RYGB and BPD. GLP-1, an incretin hormone, leads to enhanced insulin secretion and satiety. However, it likely is not the only contributing factor; isolation of the proximal bowel from nutrient exposure also appears to play a critical role by altering nutrient sensing. Alterations in vagal signaling have been identified as a potential mechanism that leads to the metabolic benefit of surgery.

Although more work is needed to help understand the mechanism of diabetes improvement after RYGB and other weight loss operations, we have entered an era of metabolic surgery where surgical outcomes are assessed by improvements in diabetes and cardiovascular risk factors.

METABOLIC SURGERY AND FUTURE DIRECTIONS

The slow progress in finding effective new medical therapy for type 2 diabetes, the increasing prevalence of the disease, and increasing data that confirm effectiveness of bariatric surgery in diabetes remission have been the impetus behind recommendations to lower the BMI threshold for surgical intervention in patients with diabetes to 30, and possibly below. An intense interest also exists in understanding the scientific mechanisms that underlie the antidiabetic effects of these procedures to help develop less invasive alternatives that can replicate the metabolic benefits of these procedures. Alternative surgical procedures have been tested, and significant investment has been seen in developing endoluminal devices for treatment of diabetes, heralding with it the emerging field of "interventional diabetology."

Surgery in Patients With Diabetes and Low Body Mass Index

The 1991 National Institutes of Health (NIH) consensus statement recommends bariatric surgery in patients with BMI of more than 35 and type 2 diabetes. Although most patients with type 2 diabetes are overweight or obese, around 70% have a BMI of less than 35 and fail to qualify for surgical intervention on the basis of BMI. They struggle with their chronic disease, which is often poorly controlled with medications alone. Considering the impressive results of bariatric

surgery, the immense interest to lower the BMI threshold for patients with diabetes who are interested in surgical intervention is not surprising. The proposal has been to lower the BMI to 30, with this number lowered to 27 for those of Asian ethnic origin, where adverse metabolic effects are seen at a lower BMI.

Several small studies have confirmed the safety of bariatric procedures in this patient population, although long-term data are lacking. There is also no consensus as to the best surgical procedure for this patient population. In a randomized study from Taiwan that involved patients with diabetes with a BMI of 25 to 34, RYGB was shown to be more effective than SG in achieving diabetes remission (93% vs 47%). The mean postoperative BMI was 22.8 for RYGB and 24.4 for SG, both within normal weight range.

Data, however, have suggested that our current surgical interventions are less effective in achieving glycemic control in patients with diabetes and low BMI. Other studies have documented cases of diabetes recurrence in patients after bariatric procedures, including RYGB. A few cases of pancreatic β-cell hypertrophy (nesidioblastosis) that lead to hypoglycemic episodes and necessitated pancreatic resection have also been documented. These observations have been cited as reasons for caution in declaring surgery the treatment of choice for the low-BMI and diabetes group and highlight the need for more studies to confirm success, safety, and durability of surgical procedures in patients with low BMI.

Alternative Surgical Procedures

Surgical steps in the rearrangements of gastrointestinal anatomy are thought to be critical to the metabolic success of most bariatric surgical procedures. These include (1) isolation of duodenum and proximal bowel from nutrient exposure and (2) earlier exposure of distal bowel and ileum to undigested food (see Table 4). Some surgical groups have worked on developing alternative novel procedures that achieve one or both of the previous goals and could have therapeutic value in patients with diabetes and low BMI. Of these procedures, duodenal-jejunal bypass and ileal interposition with or without sleeve gastrectomy have received the most attention and have been tested in human subjects with good early results. These procedures are, however, complex, and whether they offer any advantages in terms of effectiveness, durability, or safety over the more standard procedures, such as RYGB, is not clear.

TABLE 5: Broad categories of endoluminal devices in development for weight and diabetes

Device category	Mechanism of action	Examples
Restrictive devices	This category includes devices that change gastric volume or shape or modulate transit to induce earlier and prolonged satiety. Most of these devices are placed for a short period of time and lead to modest weight loss.	Intragastric balloons (e.g., BIB, Allergan, Irvine, Calif)
Barrier devices	These devices prevent nutrient contact with the proximal gut, in effect reproducing elements of RYGB. The devices are marketed as metabolic devices. They are designed for temporary placement and, although they have shown promising results, do not have the long-term effect of surgery.	Duodenal-jejunal bypass liner (e.g., EndoBarrier, GI Dynamics, Lexington, Mass)
Neuromodulators	These devices involve a generator that sends signals via laparoscopically placed electrodes to targeted organs, which can be stomach, intestine, or nerves. Signals can be stimulatory or inhibitory. Although device placement involves a surgical procedure, it is less risky than traditional bariatric procedures.	Gastric stimulators (e.g., Tantalus system, Metacure, Raleigh, NC) Vagal blockers (e.g., VBLOC, Enteromedics, St. Paul, Minn)

RYGB, Roux-en-Y gastric bypass.

Endoluminal Devices and the Interventional Diabetologist

With the recognition that gastrointestinal manipulation can lead to improvements in glycemic control, several endoluminal devices are in development to replicate the metabolic success of bariatric surgery without the need for an invasive procedure. Many such devices are in various stages of development, and a few have received regulatory approval in Europe or Australia; none have as of yet received approval in the United States. This is, however, likely to change in the near future. Their induction will herald an era when diabetes management will not be only handled by the endocrinologists but also by surgeons who will help manage obese diabetes with surgery and by advanced interventional endoscopists (interventional diabetologists) who will deploy endoluminal devices to manage patients with poorly controlled diabetes who do not qualify for surgery or wish to avoid it.

The devices in development can be broadly divided in to three groups, as summarized in Table 5. Of these, many achieve modest weight loss and with it an improvement in diabetes; a few however, are marketed as metabolic devices with a primary indication for diabetes management and not weight loss.

SUGGESTED READINGS

Dixon JB, le Roux CW, Rubino F, et al: Bariatric surgery for type 2 diabetes, *Lancet* 379(9833):2300–2311, 2012.

Dixon JB, Zimmet P, Alberti KG, et al: International Diabetes Federation Taskforce on Epidemiology and Prevention: Bariatric surgery: an IDF statement for obese type 2 diabetes, *Surg Obes Relat Dis* 7(4):433–447, 2011.

Mingrone G, Panunzi S, De Gaetano A, et al: Bariatric surgery versus conventional medical therapy for type 2 diabetes, *N Engl J Med* 366(17):1577–1585, 2012.

Schauer PR, Kashyap SR, Wolski K, et al: Bariatric surgery versus intensive medical therapy in obese patients with diabetes, *N Engl J Med* 366(17):1567–1576, 2012.

Sjöström L, Peltonen M, Jacobson P, et al: Bariatric surgery and long-term cardiovascular events, *JAMA* 307(1):56–65, 2012.

GLYCEMIC CONTROL AND CARDIOVASCULAR DISEASE RISK REDUCTION AFTER BARIATRIC SURGERY

Fady Moustarah, MD, MPH, FRCS(C) General Surgery, Stacy A. Brethauer, MD, and Philip R. Schauer, MD

INTRODUCTION

Obesity and cardiovascular disease (CVD) are two chronic conditions that remain leading causes of morbidity and mortality; therefore, there is a need for effective therapeutic strategies to reduce their public health burden on individuals and societies. Bariatric surgery is emerging as an efficient, cost-effective solution to address these two associated chronic diseases. The objective of this chapter is not to present an exhaustive overview of bariatric surgical procedures and their therapeutic effectiveness, as this has been the subject of many comprehensive systematic reviews since 2000. The commonly performed bariatric procedures in North America are reviewed briefly, and the focus is on their effect in reducing CVD risk, especially in terms of improving glucose metabolism and diabetes control. Evidence from controlled trials published in 2012 are highlighted. In addition, results demonstrating reduced CVD incidence and mortality in large population studies, such as the Swedish Obese Subjects (SOS) project, are discussed.

The Obesity Epidemic

Obesity, or excess body fat, is now recognized as a global public health problem. According to the World Health Organization, rates have doubled since 1980; more than 1.4 billion adults, 20 years of age and older, are estimated to have been overweight and obese in 2008. The United States has the highest rates of obesity in the developed world. The World Health Organization and the U.S. National Institutes of Health use body mass index (BMI) to define overweight and obesity along a clinical continuum of increasing severity: overweight is defined as a BMI of 25 kg/m^2 or more and obesity as a BMI of 30 kg/m^2 or more, whereby BMI is a measure of body weight in kilograms divided by the square of body height in meters. On the basis of these definitions, the most recent data on obesity prevalence in the United States, from the National Health and Nutrition Survey, show that more than one third of adults and almost 17% of children and adolescents in the United States were obese in the period 2009 to 2010.

Obesity and Risk for Cardiovascular Disease

These rates not only are alarming but carry additional implications, in view of the adverse clinical effect of excess body fat, especially in relation to CVD risk and death. Many large population studies have now shown that obesity is associated with increased rates of mortality; CVD and cancer are responsible for much of this excess mortality over time. Evidence now implicates obesity as an *independent risk factor* for coronary heart disease (CHD) and show BMI to predict

CHD beyond what is expected with measurement of traditional risk factors included in the risk score derived from the Framingham Heart Study (Box 1). Cardiovascular conditions associated with obesity are numerous and include hypertension, early and accelerated coronary atherosclerosis, myocardial infarction, congestive heart failure, and atrial fibrillation (Box 2). The clinical burden of these conditions is more pronounced and difficult to treat in severely obese patients.

Obesity and the Metabolic Syndrome

Beyond being recognized by the American Heart Association as an independent predictor of CVD risk, obesity, particularly the visceral type, is a key component of the metabolic syndrome. This syndrome represents a cluster of metabolic disorders that together increase CVD risk. As defined by the National Cholesterol Education Project Adult Treatment Panel III (ATP III), the concurrence of any three of the five features listed in Box 3 defines the metabolic syndrome. Visceral obesity is often associated with a proinflammatory metabolic state characterized by insulin resistance and hyperinsulinemia, which leads to impaired glucose tolerance, dyslipidemia, atherosclerosis, and progression to type 2 diabetes mellitus (T2DM).

Obesity and Diabetes

Among the modifiable risk factors for CVD (see Box 1), T2DM is a powerful independent predictor of risk. Obesity is strongly associated with T2DM: about 90% of affected patients are overweight or obese, and about 65% die of a cardiovascular event. Although initially part of the Framingham risk score, diabetes was excluded from the updated version in 2002 because it was deemed to be a CHD risk equivalent. In fact, in patients with diabetes mellitus, but no prior cardiovascular events, the risk for future myocardial infarction is equivalent to that in nondiabetic patients with established ischemic heart disease. This fact highlights the importance of effective prevention and treatment strategies in diabetic patients, especially in those who also suffer from clinically severe obesity or have features of the metabolic syndrome, which together increase CVD risk and pose a significant threat to life.

The Therapeutic Role of Weight Loss

Weight loss has been shown to be one of the most effective nonpharmacologic means of reducing risk in obese patients with diabetes. It contributes to lowering blood pressure; raising high-density lipoprotein (HDL) cholesterol levels; decreasing blood glucose, triglyceride, and insulin levels; and preventing the development of T2DM. In fact, the weight loss does not have to be substantial. Even a small (5% to 10%) weight loss, secondary to dietary and behavioral interventions, has been shown to improve blood pressure and decrease the risk of developing diabetes in people in whom glucose tolerance is already subclinically impaired. Evidence regarding the efficacy of lifestyle and behavioral modification in achieving weight loss and improving CVD risk profile is starting to emerge from large-scale randomized controlled prospective studies. The Action for Health in Diabetes ("Look AHEAD") trial is such a study (the largest of its kind, with more than 5000 enrolled patients), which published its interim 4-year results. It showed the promise of intensive lifestyle interventions in keeping overweight and obese patients with T2DM at lower CVD risk and for longer periods of time in comparison with the control group when results were averaged over the 4-year timeline of the study (Table 1). Whether this will translate into lower incidence of CVD and mortality is yet to be established on follow-up. Of

BOX 1: Cardiovascular disease risk factors

Traditional Nonmodifiable

Age (men ≥45 years; women ≥55 years)*
Family history of premature CHD (CHD in male first-degree
    relative aged <55 years; CHD in female first-degree relative
    aged <65 years)*
Gender*
Race

Traditional Modifiable

Smoking*
High blood pressure (≥140/90 mm Hg or patient taking
    antihypertensive medication)*
High cholesterol levels (low HDL cholesterol level: <40 mg/dL)*
Diabetes
Prediabetes condition

**Emerging Nontraditional CVD Risk Factors (Associated
With Visceral Obesity)**

Insulin resistance/hyperinsulinemia
Dyslipidemia with elevated triglyceride levels, low HDL level, and
    increased apolipoprotein-B serum concentrations
Procoagulation and abnormal fibrinolysis with increased serum
    fibrinogen concentrations and increased production of
    plasminogen activator inhibitor
Inflammation with increased serum levels of C-reactive protein,
    tumor necrosis factor, interleukin-6
Endothelial dysfunction
Premature atherosclerosis
Microalbuminuria

*These risk factors include major independent factors accounted for in the Framingham
risk score. The current version of the Framingham risk score was published in 2002. The
score is used to estimate the 10-year cardiovascular risk of an individual on the basis of
data obtained from the Framingham Heart Study. The score is *gender*-specific. Individuals with *low risk* have <10% risk for CHD at 10 years; those with *intermediate risk* have
a 10% to 20% risk for CHD; and those with *high risk* have more than a 20% risk for
CHD. In the current version of the FRS, diabetes was removed from the score. If the
person has type 2 diabetes, this person is classified as having a CHD risk equivalent.
CHD, Coronary heart disease; *CVD,* cardiovascular disease; *HDL,* high-density
lipoprotein.

BOX 2: Cardiovascular conditions associated with obesity

Early and accelerated atherosclerosis
Hypertension
Myocardial infarction or acute coronary syndrome
Structural heart changes and congestive heart failure
Atrial fibrillation
Sudden cardiac death
Stroke

importance, however, is that the Look AHEAD trial was stopped
because no reduction in cardiovascular events were observed over the
course of the study.

Despite the importance and effectiveness of weight loss in reducing CVD risk, the problem remaining is that sustaining weight loss
over time is more of an elusive goal than the weight loss itself. This
has been a consistent result of previous weight loss studies, and the
data from the Look AHEAD trial constitutes level 1 evidence to
support this finding. The trial showed that the maximum mean
weight loss of 8.6% achieved at 1 year with intensive lifestyle intervention was reduced to 4.7% at 4 years. Pharmacotherapy for obesity
has also been disappointing, inasmuch as it failed to meet weight loss
expectations and has been plagued with multiple medication with-
drawals from the market because of undesirable side effects. At
present, bariatric surgery is the only established treatment that allows

BOX 3: Diagnostic criteria for the metabolic syndrome*

Three or more of the following five cardiovascular risk factors:

1. Central obesity (waist circumference): ≥102 cm in men;
   ≥88 cm in women
2. Hypertriglyceridemia: triglyceride levels ≥1.7 mmol/L
   (≥150 mg/dL)
3. Low levels of high-density lipoprotein (HDL): <1.03 mmol/L
   (<40 mg/dL) in men; <1,29 mmol/L (<50 mg/dL) in women
4. Systemic hypertension: blood pressure ≥130/85 mm Hg or
   necessity for medication
5. Elevated fasting plasma glucose level: ≥5.5 mmol/L
   (≥100 mg/dL)

*As defined by the National Cholesterol Education Program Adult Treatment Panel III
(ATP III).

for significant and durable long-term weight loss, along with associated "cures" or sustained long-term improvements in weight-related
comorbid conditions. Systematic reviews have previously summarized the weight loss effect of different procedures, and the durability
of this weight loss has been reported in multiple-case series and
large-scale population studies.

BARIATRIC PROCEDURES

Bariatric surgery has evolved considerably since the 1960s. Commonly performed bariatric procedures today can be classified according to their anatomic and physiologic features. Traditionally,
procedures have taken one of two forms, or both: reduction in the
size of the stomach, so as to mechanically restrict food ingestion, and
bypass of varying lengths of intestine, so as to cause malabsorption
of ingested nutrients. Increased recognition of the hormonal contribution to the observed biochemical effects of the practiced procedures has led to the adoption of the term *metabolic gastrointestinal
surgery*. Common restrictive procedures include adjustable gastric
banding (AGB) and sleeve gastrectomy; combination restrictive/
malabsorptive procedures include Roux-en-Y gastric bypass (RYGB)
and biliopancreatic diversion (BPD), with or without duodenal
switch (BPD±DS) (Table 2 and Figure 1). Procedures vary in terms
of their surgical techniques (laparotomy or laparoscopy), magnitude
of weight loss and extent of its durability, resolution rate of associated
comorbid conditions (Table 3), and risk profile (Table 4). Detailed
descriptions of these procedures with technical drawings can be
found in the chapter titled "Laparoscopic Surgery for Severe Obesity."

Effect of Bariatric Surgery on Risk Factors for Cardiovascular Disease and Components of the Metabolic Syndrome

Improving glucose and lipid metabolism and alleviating systemic
inflammation are among the principal biochemical mechanisms by
which bariatric surgery reduces CVD risk. The surgically induced
weight loss and associated improvement in blood pressure also contribute independently to decreasing CVD risk. The rest of this chapter
highlights the biochemical improvements observed after bariatric
surgery, and some of the clinical evidence for such favorably altered
metabolism is reviewed.

Glycemic Control

Insulin resistance and T2DM are remarkably improved after bariatric
surgery. The American Diabetes Association defines diabetes in

TABLE 1: Mean 4-year changes in weight and cardiovascular disease risk factors: Look AHEAD trial

Measure	Study group		Between-group mean difference	P value
	Diabetes Support and Education	Intensive Lifestyle Intervention		
Weight, % initial weight	−0.88	−6.15	−5.70	<0.001
HbA$_{1c}$ level	−0.09	−0.36	−0.27	<0.001
Systolic blood pressure	−2.97	−5.33	−2.36	<0.001
Diastolic blood pressure	−2.48	−2.92	−0.43	0.01
High-density lipoprotein cholesterol level	1.97	3.67	1.70	<0.001
Triglyderide levels	−19.75	−25.56	−5.81	<0.001
Low-density lipoprotein cholesterol level (adjusted for medication use)	−9.22	−8.75	0.47	0.42

HbA$_{1C}$, Hemoglobin A$_{1C}$.

TABLE 2: Classification of common bariatric procedures

Procedure	Examples
Restrictive	Adjustable gastric band Sleeve gastrectomy
Gastric restriction combined with diversion	Roux-en-Y gastric bypass
Diversionary malabsorptive procedures with gastric volume reduction	Biliopancreatic diversion with or without duodenal switch

non-pregnant adults based on the following glycemic criteria: (1) symptomatic hyperglycemia with a random plasma glucose ≥11.1 mmol/L (200 mg/dL), (2) a plasma glucose >11.1 mmol/L (>200 mg/dL) 2 hours after a 75-gram oral glucose tolerance test, (3) a fasting plasma glucose ≥7 mmol/L (126 mg/dL), or (4) HbA1c ≥6.5%. Even though improvements in glycemic control after gastrointestinal surgery were reported as long ago as the 1960s, it was in 1995 that in a landmark paper, Pories and colleagues described the durable effect of bariatric surgery in controlling T2DM more than a decade after the operation. Since then, many reports have confirmed the therapeutic effect of the various bariatric procedures in obese prediabetic patients (with impaired fasting glucose) and in patients with frank T2DM.

In fact, bariatric surgery has been shown to improve insulin sensitivity and play a role in prevention by halting the development of diabetes in patients at high risk for T2DM. Today, the mechanisms for such postoperative improvement in glucose metabolism as a function of time remain an active area of research. Clinically, however, glycemic control improves within days after surgery, even when the amount of weight loss is insufficient to explain the observed improvement. In one series, Schauer reported immediate postoperative independence from oral hypoglycemic agents on post-RYGB discharge from the hospital in 30% of patients who were on such medication preoperatively. What is more remarkable than the ability of bariatric surgery to completely reverse established diabetes is the ability to put the condition into remission for prolonged periods of time. In a study published by Pories, 83% of 165 diabetic patients experienced remission of diabetes at a mean follow-up of 9.4 years after RYGB.

The best evidence for the durability of remission over time came from a large-scale controlled observational study, the SOS project. This study showed reversal of diabetes in 72% of the patients who underwent surgery, in comparison with only 21% of the control group, at 2 years of follow-up. The durability of this remission was related to maintenance of weight loss. At 10 years, as weight regain was observed, diabetes remission rates remained impressive but were decreased to 36% in the surgery recipients and 13% in the control subjects. The odds ratios for surgical recovery from diabetes at 2 and 10 years were 8.42 (95% confidence interval [CI]: 5.68 to 12.5) and 3.45 (95% CI: 1.64 to 7.28), both significant at $P < 0.001$ respectively.

Meta-analyses of smaller scale studies also demonstrate the durability of diabetes remission after bariatric surgery. In a meta-analysis, Buchwald and colleagues (2009) reviewed the results of 621 studies and observed an overall 78.1% resolution of clinical manifestations of diabetes after surgery, noting that the proportions of patients with diabetes resolution or improvements were similar before and after 2 years of follow-up. Diabetes resolution was reported to be the most extensive for patients undergoing BPD with or without duodenal switch (95.1%), followed by RYGB (80.3%), and AGB (56.7%). A limitation of this study rests in its use of clinical reports of diabetes remission rather than hard biochemical markers of glucose control.

The superiority of bariatric surgery to conventional medical therapy in achieving improved glycemic control in diabetic patients is still being documented. Evidence is available from three well-designed randomized control trials that addressed this question through the use of hard biochemical markers of glucose metabolism, such as fasting plasma glucose and hemoglobin A$_{1C}$ (HbA$_{1C}$) levels as endpoints (Table 5). In Dixon and associates' (2008) study, 30 diabetic patients who underwent surgery were compared with a matched control group of 30 patients over a period of 2 years. They found that remission of diabetes occurred in significantly higher numbers of patients who underwent laparoscopic AGB than in those who received standard treatment (73% vs 13%), on the basis of achieving a HbA$_{1C}$ level lower than 6.2%, attaining a fasting plasma glucose level lower than 7 mmol/L, and taking no antidiabetic medications. In 2012, Schauer and associates released the first report from the STAMPEDE (Surgical Therapy And Medications Potentially Eradicate Diabetes Efficiently) randomized clinical trial. This study randomly assigned 150 patients with T2DM (mean age, 49; 68% female; mean preoperative HbA$_{1C}$ level, 9.2%), with equal duration of diabetes before surgery, to receive either intensive medical therapy alone or medical therapy plus RYGB or sleeve gastrectomy; 50 patients were assigned to each of the three groups. After 1 year, weight loss was

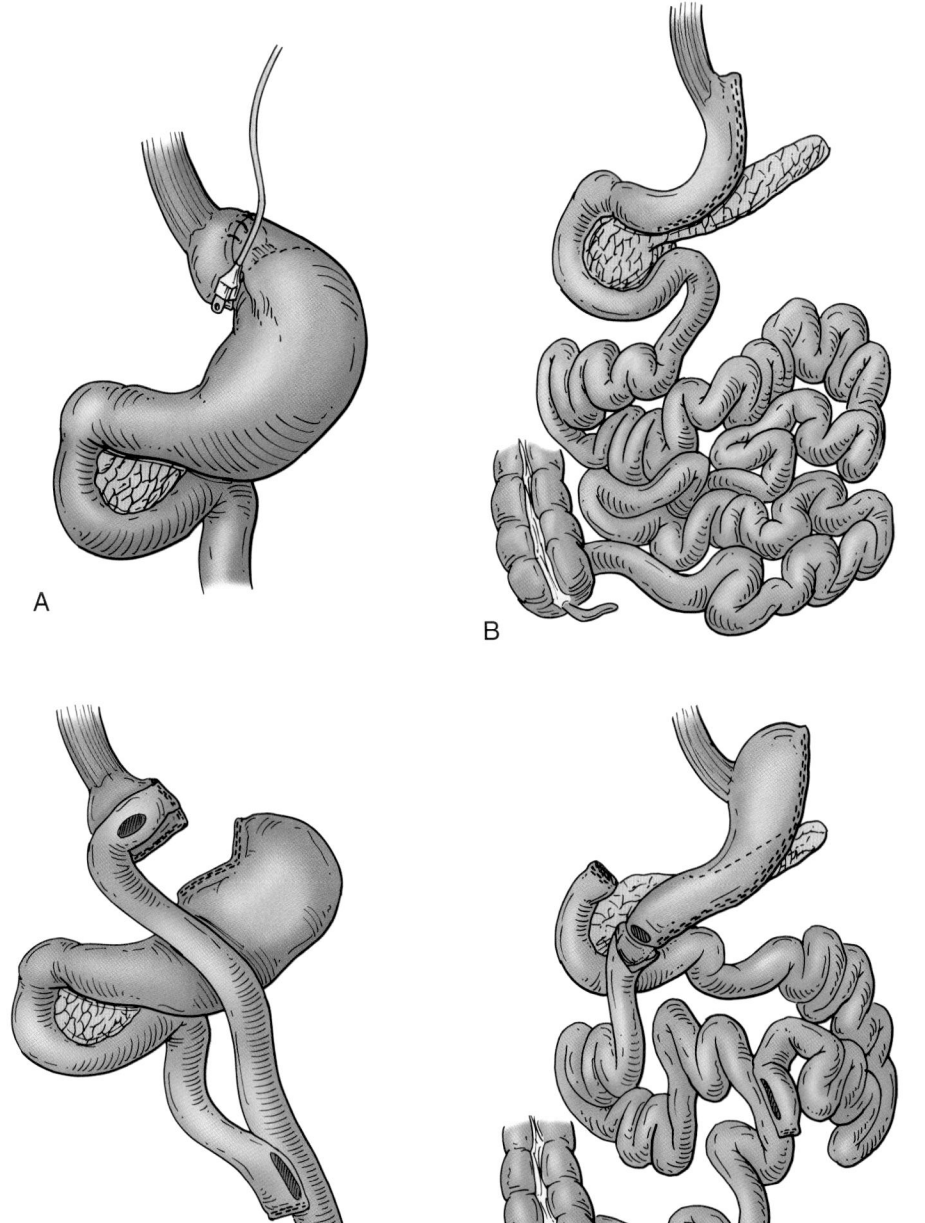

FIGURE 1   Illustrations of commonly performed bariatric procedures. **A,** Adjustable gastric banding. **B,** Sleeve gastrectomy. **C,** Roux-en-Y gastric bypass. **D,** Biliopancreatic diversion (shown with duodenal switch). *(Reprinted with permission from Cleveland Clinic Center for Medical Art & Photography, copyright 2005-2010. All rights reserved.)*

TABLE 3: Weight loss and resolution rates of obesity-associated comorbid conditions after weight loss surgery[*]

Outcome	Gastric banding	Gastric bypass	BPD or DS	Total
Excess weight loss	47%	62%	70%	61%
Resolution of type 2 diabetes mellitus	48%	84%	99%	77%
Resolution of hyperlipidemia	59%	97%	99%	79%
Resolution of hypertension	43%	68%	83%	62%
Resolution of sleep apnea	95%	80%	92%	86%

[*]According to procedure performed as summarized by a 2004 systematic review of 22,094 patients.

BPD, Biliopancreatic diversion; *DS,* duodenal switch type biliopancreatic diversion.

From Buchwald H, Avidor Y, Braunwald E, et al: Bariatric surgery: a systematic review and meta-analysis, JAMA *292(14):1724–1737, 2004.*

TABLE 4: Bariatric procedure related postoperative complications

Procedure	Complications	
	Early Postoperative Period (<30 Days)	*Late*
Laparoscopic RYGB	Anastomotic leak with peritonitis Abdominal abscess Pulmonary embolism Bleeding Pulmonary complications Acute distal gastric dilation Roux limb obstruction Wound infection	Stomal stenosis Marginal ulcer Dumping syndrome Intestinal obstruction Internal hernia Incisional hernia Cholecystitis Vitamin and mineral deficiencies Weight regain Hypoglycemia
Laparoscopic BPD ± DS	Same as those of laparoscopic RYGB	Same as those of laparoscopic RYGB; the following are more common in the BPD procedure than in RYGB if aggressive prophylactic measures are not followed postoperatively: Anemia Protein-calorie malnutrition Vitamin B_{12} deficiency Hypocalcemia Osteoporosis Fat-soluble vitamin deficiency Night blindness
Laparoscopic sleeve gastrectomy	Staple line leak Abscess Hemorrhage Sleeve stricture Wound infection	Intractable nausea with or without vomiting Reflux symptoms Gastric dilation Weight loss failure Weight regain
Laparoscopic AGB	Hemorrhage Wound infection Food intolerance Reflux Nausea with or without vomiting Slippage Wound infection	Reflux symptoms Erosive esophagitis Esophageal dilation Pouch enlargement Band slippage Gastric prolapse Vomiting Tubing-related problems Leakage of the reservoir Band erosion Weight loss failure Lower average weight loss

AGB, Adjustable gastric banding; *BPD±DS*, biliopancreatic diversion with or without duodenal switch; *RYGB*, Roux-en-Y gastric bypass.

greatest in the RYGB recipients, and a HbA_{1C} level lower than 6% (primary endpoint) was achieved in 42% of patients who underwent RYGB, in 37% of patients who underwent sleeve gastrectomy, and in only 12% of those who received only medical therapy.

Also in 2012, Mingrone and colleagues published results of their study on bariatric surgery versus conventional medical therapy for T2DM. Their primary endpoint was diabetes remission at 2 years, as measured by a fasting plasma glucose level lower than 5.6 mmol/L and a HbA_{1C} level lower than 6.5% in the absence of diabetic drug therapy. Patients (mean age, 43.4 years; 47% female; mean preoperative HbA_{1C} level, 8.65%) were randomly assigned to undergo RYGB, BPD, or medical therapy. Better glycemic control was observed in the surgery recipients after 2 years, and although diabetes remission rates were 95% and 75% after BPD and RYGB, respectively, no remission occurred in patients who received only medical therapy. An important post hoc analysis also showed that, in contrast to the previous

results with the laparoscopic AGB in Dixon and associates' trial, initial BMI and postoperative weight loss were not predictive of the improvement in hyperglycemia observed after surgery.

For patients with poorly controlled T2DM and BMIs of 35 kg/m^2 or more, bariatric surgery is currently considered as acceptable therapy; however, such treatment remains controversial for patients with class 1 obesity or BMIs between 30 and 35 kg/m^2 (Table 6). In 2011, the International Diabetes Federation (IDF) released its position statement recognizing a role for bariatric surgery as a treatment option alternative for patients with class 1 obesity in whom diabetes cannot be adequately controlled by optimal medical regimens, especially in the presence of other major CVD risk factors. The American Diabetes Association remained conservative on this issue and indicated that surgery for class 1 obesity and diabetes should be restricted to approved research protocols. In 2012, the American Society for Metabolic and Bariatric Surgery (ASMBS) also reviewed the

TABLE 5: Comparison of three randomized trials of surgery versus medical therapy for obese diabetic patients*

Characteristics	Dixon et al. (2008)	Schauer et al. (2012)	Mingrone et al. (2012)
Country	Australia	United States	Italy
Protocol	Laparoscopic AGB vs MTx	RYGB vs SG vs MTx	BPD vs RYGB vs MTx
Study			
Sample sizes	AGB: 30 MTx: 30	RYGB: 50 SG: 50 MTx: 50	BPD: 20 RYGB: 20 MTx: 20
Mean age (years)	47.0	49.8	43.5
Mean BMI_i (kg/m^2)	37.0	37.0	45.0
Diabetes duration (years)	<2	8	6
Study duration (years)	2	1	2
Primary outcome	FBG <7 mmol/L HbA_{1C} <6.2%	HBA_{1C} <6.0%	FBG <5.6 mmol/L HbA_{1C} < 6.5%
Outcomes			
Weight loss	AGB: 25.0 MTx: 1.5%	RYGB: 29% SG: 25% MTx: 5.4%	BPD: 33% RYGB: 33% MTx: 5%
Diabetes remission	ABG: 73% MTx: 13%	RYGB: 42% SG: 37% MTx: 12%	BPD: 95% RYGB: 75% MTx: 0%

*Based on biochemical marker of glucose metabolism.
AGB, Adjustable gastric banding; *BMI$_i$*, initial body mass index; *BPD*, biliopancreatic diversion; *FBG*, fasting blood glucose; *HbA$_{1C}$*, hemoglobin A$_{1C}$; *MTx*, medical therapy; *RYGB*, Roux-en-Y gastric bypass; *SG*, sleeve gastrectomy.

currently available clinical evidence and released a position statement highlighting the emerging role of bariatric surgery in treating class 1 obesity and T2DM. In summary, the ASMBS stated that AGB, sleeve gastrectomy, and RYGB have all been shown to be safe in randomized trials and are effective in patients with BMIs of 30 to 35 kg/m^2 in the short and medium term. It also stated that patients with class 1 obesity who are unable to achieve substantial and durable weight and comorbidity control with nonsurgical therapeutic methods should be considered eligible for surgery.

Lipid Metabolism

As visceral adiposity diminishes and insulin resistance improves after bariatric surgery, so does the metabolic syndrome with its associated components, including dyslipidemia, thereby decreasing CVD risk. Batsis and colleagues (2008) performed a population-based

retrospective study and showed that over a mean follow up period of 3.4 years, the prevalence of metabolic syndrome decreased from 87% to 29% of 180 surgically treated patients, whereas the risk reduction was only 10% in patients who had been treated nonsurgically. Postoperative improvements in serum lipid profiles have been documented in numerous reports and include reductions in total cholesterol, low-density lipoprotein cholesterol, and triglyceride levels and increases in HDL cholesterol. These changes are observed in the majority of patients and are more frequent after procedures with a malabsorptive component. In one study, for example, Nguyen and associates (2006) found that 82% of patients on lipid-lowering therapy were able to discontinue such drugs 1 year after RYBG. A much larger retrospective study performed in 949 patients showed that plasma concentrations of triglycerides, HDL cholesterol, and low-density lipoprotein cholesterol all significantly improved over a similar 1-year time frame after RYGB. At the Cleveland Clinic, a smaller study demonstrated improvement in apolipoprotein B levels as early as 3 months postoperatively. After BPD, long-term 5-year to 10-year improvement in dyslipidemia is particularly impressive; resolution rates of 95% to 100% have been reported.

Inflammatory State

Many investigators have described the favorable modulation of a number of obesity-associated inflammatory markers after bariatric surgery. Adipose tissue is no longer viewed as inert energy storage tissue; it is now appreciated as an endocrine organ that produces a spectrum of adipokines that have important inflammatory and immune functions. Obesity, particularly the central or abdominal type, is seen as a state of chronic systemic inflammation contributing to various aspects of CVD risk, including accelerated atherosclerosis and endothelial dysfunction. Surgically induced weight loss; the resultant improvement in visceral adiposity, insulin resistance, and dyslipidemia; and the reduction in inflammatory molecules all contribute to improving the inflammatory state. High sensitivity C-reactive protein levels, for example, show consistent decreases after bariatric procedures by up to 89%. In one study in which more than 430 patients were monitored for approximately 1 year, C-reactive protein levels were above the 3-mg/dL cutoff level in only 10% of patients after RYGB, in comparison with 35% of patients before RYGB.

Although interleukin-6 levels have been shown to decrease by up to 41% after bariatric surgery, the authors observed no such decreases in interleukin-6 or interleukin-10 levels after RYGB in a prospective study of inflammatory markers in patients evaluated at the Cleveland Clinic; leptin, plasminogen activator inhibitor 1, and C-reactive protein levels decreased significantly, however, at 3 and 6 months of follow-up. Fibrinogen and interleuken-1 receptor antagonist levels also decreased, and adiponectin levels significantly increased at 6 months in the authors' study. Adiponectin is an important adipose tissue–derived cytokine, levels of which are decreased in obesity and increased from 30% to 140% after weight loss surgery, according to some reports. The function of adiponectin is not fully understood at this time, but its presence is correlated positively with improved insulin sensitivity. It can also cause vasodilation by stimulating nitric oxide in endothelial cells and can contribute to decreased atherogenesis and lower CVD risk.

Reduced Cardiovascular Disease and Mortality After Bariatric Surgery

It is now recognized through multiple observational studies that surgically induced weight loss is associated with a reduction in overall mortality. The strength of available evidence varies and is limited by study design, surgical procedure, and patient selection. In 2004, the McGill Bariatric Cohort Study—a retrospective case–control analysis

TABLE 6: American and international guidelines for bariatric surgery eligibility in adults

Guideline	ASMBS (2012)*	American Diabetes Association (2012)	International Diabetes Federation (2011)†
Prioritization for surgery *recommended*	BMI >40 kg/m² or BMI >35 kg/m² with one serious weight loss–responsive comorbid condition	Surgery *not* prioritized for any group	BMI >40 kg/m² or BMI >35 kg/m² when diabetes and other comorbid conditions not controlled by optimum medical treatment
Eligibility for surgery can be *considered*	BMI >30 kg/m² when substantial and durable weight loss and comorbidity improvement are unachievable with nonsurgical methods	BMI >35 kg/m², especially if diabetes or other comorbid condition is not controlled by lifestyle and pharmacologic treatment	BMI >35 kg/m², or BMI >30 kg/m² when diabetes and other comorbid conditions are not controlled by optimum medical treatment
Comment	AGB, SG, and RYGB have been shown in randomized controlled trials to be safe and effective in patients with BMIs of 30-35 kg/m² in short and medium term	Little evidence for patients with BMIs between 30 and 35 kg/m²; use should be restricted to research protocols	Adjustment of BMI for patients of Asian ethnic origin is advised

*Based on biochemical marker of glucose metabolism from American Society for Metabolic and Bariatric Surgery (2012).
AGB, Adjustable gastric banding; *ASMBS*, American Society for Metabolic and Bariatric Surgery; *BMI*, body mass index; *RYGB*, Roux-en-Y gastric bypass; *SG*, sleeve gastrectomy.
†*Dixon JB, Zimmet P, Alberti KG, et al: Bariatric surgery: an IDF statement for obese type 2 diabetes,* Diabet Med *28(6):628-642, 2011.*

in which more than 1000 surgically treated obese patients were compared with more than 5700 obese control subjects—was the first to report that a 67% excess weight loss at 5 years was associated with an 89% reduction in relative risk for mortality. A retrospective case-control matched study from the University of Utah also showed a survival advantage in their surgical group after RYGB with a mean follow-up of 7.1 years: The adjusted rate of long-term mortality in the surgical cohort of 7925 patients decreased by 40% in comparison with the same-size matched control group (hazard ratio, 0.6; P <0.001). The rate of coronary artery disease–related mortality decreased by 56% among the patients who underwent surgery. Other researchers also demonstrated survival benefits over a 2-year follow-up even in the higher risk Medicare patient population. Specifically, a survival advantage was observed as early as 6 months postoperatively among patients older than 65 years and as early as 11 months in patients aged 65 years or younger. Studies from Europe and Australia have also confirmed survival advantages with AGB.

Despite the evidence for improved CVD risk profile and survival in general after bariatric surgery, what remains to be established is whether this risk reduction translates into decreased incidences of CVD and of related mortality. The best evidence to address this question at present came from the SOS project, an ongoing, nonrandomized, matched, prospective observational study in which more than 4000 patients were enrolled and monitored over time in Sweden. Reports on the primary endpoint (overall mortality rate) of the SOS project were published in 2007 by Sjöström and associates (Figure 2). At 10 years, a 23.7% overall unadjusted (30.7% adjusted) decrease in mortality was observed among patients who had undergone bariatric surgery in comparison with a well-matched control population of patients who did not undergo surgery. This improvement in overall mortality after bariatric surgery, along with the repeated observations of the beneficial effect of such surgery on diabetes, dyslipidemia, and hypertension, suggest that bariatric surgery directly influences CVD.

In fact, in the most recent report from the SOS project, Sjöström and associates (2012) described the effect of obesity surgery on the predefined endpoints of myocardial infarction and stroke, reported as incidence rates of fatal and total (fatal and nonfatal) cardiovascular events (Figure 3). The study groups included 2010 patients who

underwent one of three forms of bariatric surgery (BMI ≥ 34 kg/m² in men; BMI ≥ 38 kg/m² in women): gastric bypass (13.2%), gastric banding (18.7%), or vertical banded gastroplasty (68.1%); and 2037 contemporaneously matched obese control subjects who received usual medical care. Over a median follow-up period of 14.7 years (range: 0 to 20 years), bariatric surgery was associated with a reduction in the number of cardiovascular deaths and first-time cardiovascular events (fatal or nonfatal), after the cardiometabolic risk profile at baseline was controlled. In comparison with control subjects, the adjusted hazard ratio of bariatric surgery for total cardiovascular events was 0.67 (95% CI: 0.54 to 0.83, P <0.001); for fatal cardiovascular events, the adjusted hazard ratio was 0.47 (95% CI: 0.29 to 0.76; P = 0.02). It is noteworthy that weight loss was only about 16% at 15 years in the patients who had undergone surgery, whereas over time the control group showed weight changes around a maximum of 1%. Of interest, secondary subgroup analyses of the SOS data failed to demonstrate an association between initial BMI and postoperative health benefits of bariatric surgery. Even the magnitude of surgery-induced weight loss was not predictive of cardiovascular events in this cohort. This puts into question the current clinical practice of using BMI as a main indication and eligibility criteria for bariatric surgery, when cardiovascular benefits are realized independent of differences and changes in body weight. Further post hoc analysis of the SOS data revealed that, unlike baseline BMI or the magnitude of postoperative weight loss, a high baseline insulin level was in fact a predictor of cardiovascular events in the study. This suggests that weight-independent mechanisms rather than the magnitude of weight loss alone may explain part of the cardiometabolic benefits of surgery.

In an attempt to obtain further insight into the role of bariatric surgery in reducing CVD risk and improving cardiac structure and function, investigators at the Cleveland Clinic performed and published a systematic review of more than 19,500 bariatric surgery patients in 73 clinical studies. Although diagnostic criteria, cardiovascular risk factor reporting, and cardiac imaging parameters varied across published reports evaluated by the review, results were useful. Baseline preoperative prevalence of hypertension, diabetes, and hyperlipidemia were 44%, 24%, and 44%, respectively. On mean

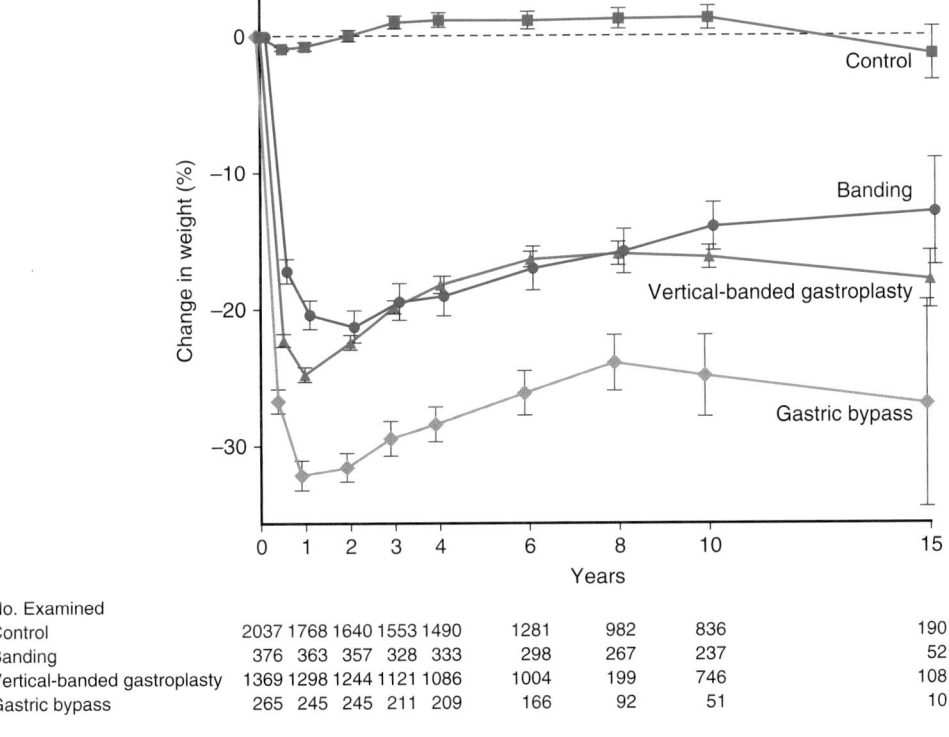

No. Examined

Control	2037	1768	1640	1553	1490	1281	982	836		190
Banding	376	363	357	328	333	298	267	237		52
Vertical-banded gastroplasty	1369	1298	1244	1121	1086	1004	199	746		108
Gastric bypass	265	245	245	211	209	166	92	51		10

A

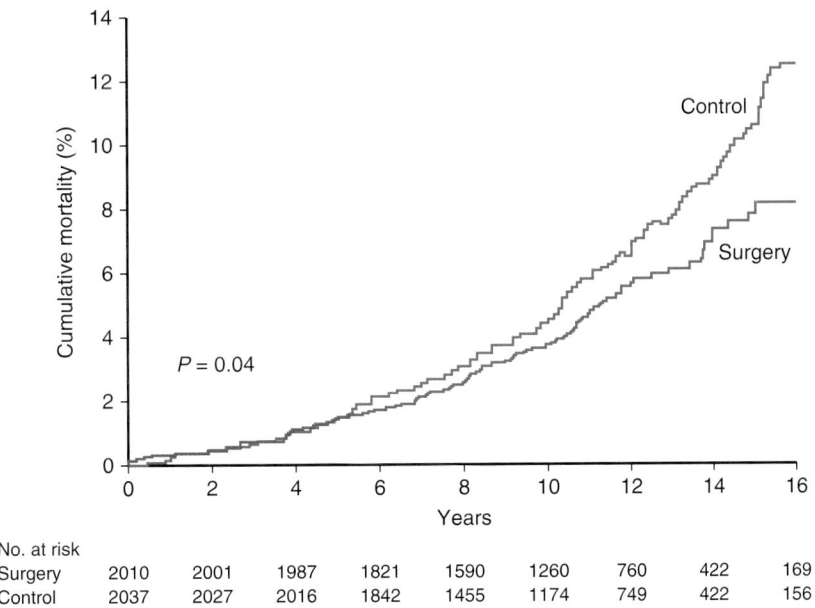

No. at risk

Surgery	2010	2001	1987	1821	1590	1260	760	422	169
Control	2037	2027	2016	1842	1455	1174	749	422	156

B

FIGURE 2 The 2007 report of the Swedish Obese Subjects study, describing the effects of bariatric surgery on mortality: **A,** Weight change over time according to bariatric procedure used in the study. **B,** Cumulative mortality rate over course of study. *(From Sjöstrom L, Narbro K, Sjöstrom CD, et al: Effects of bariatric surgery on mortality in Swedish obese subjects, N Engl J Med 357:741–752, 2007.)*

follow-up of 58 months (range, 3 to 176 months), an average of 54% excess weight loss was reported, and this was associated with a post-operative resolution of or improvement in hypertension, diabetes, and hyperlipidemia in 63%, 73%, and 65% of patients, respectively. What is more remarkable about the review is that echocardiographic data from 713 patients revealed significant improvements in left ventricular function, with regression in hypertrophy after surgery and improved diastolic function. This finding adds to current evidence that bariatric surgery enhances future cardiovascular health and may in fact be doing so by having direct physiologic end-organ effects on the heart.

CONCLUSIONS

Severe clinical obesity and chronic medical illnesses associated with it are no longer the sole preoccupation of patients and their internists. The pandemics of obesity, diabetes, and cardiovascular heart disease have multidimensional effects on individuals and societies, and the surgeon's current role cannot be understated as research into improving therapeutic interventions, understanding mechanisms of bariatric procedures, and developing preventive strategies continue. Beyond achieving weight loss, bariatric surgery is proving to have remarkable metabolic and cardiovascular effects in the short and

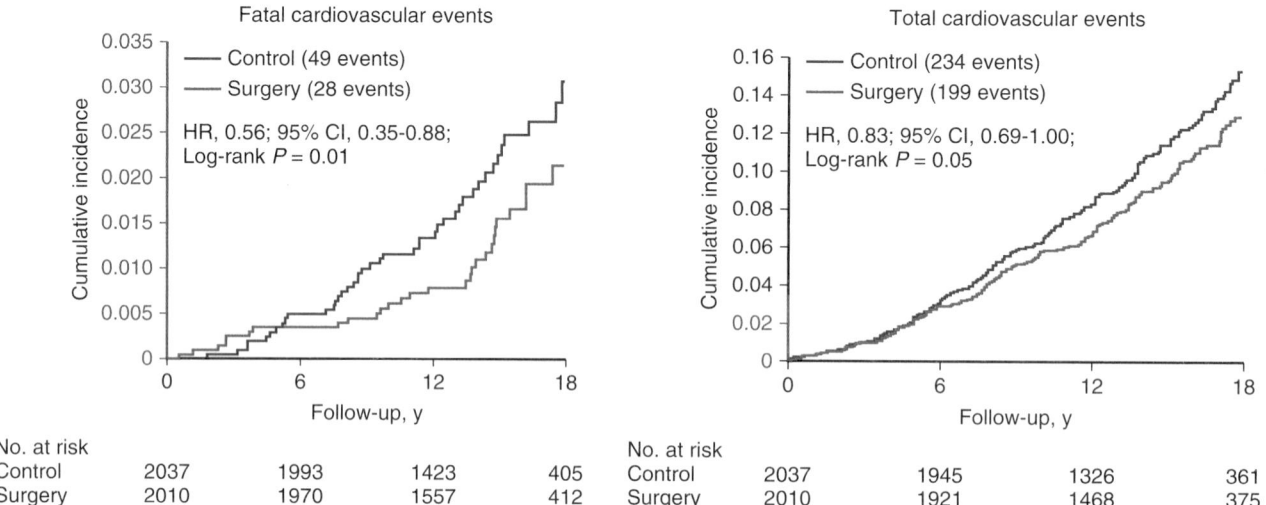

FIGURE 3 Incidence rates of cardiovascular events. The combined endpoint was myocardial infarction and stroke, whichever came first; fatal cardiovascular events and total (fatal and nonfatal) cardiovascular events are shown. The incidence data are based on observations until December 31, 2009. Follow-up time was truncated at 18 years because the number of persons at risk beyond this point was low. All persons are included in the calculation of hazard ratios (HRs). The incidence rates per 1000 person-years for fatal cardiovascular events were 0.9 (95% confidence interval [CI]: 0.6 to 1.3) among patients who underwent surgery and 1.7 (95% CI: 1.3 to 2.2) in the control group; for total cardiovascular events, the rates were 6.9 (95% CI: 6.0 to 8.0) and 8.3 (95% CI: 7.3 to 9.4), respectively. X-axis regions shown in *blue* indicate range from 0 to 0.035. *(Data from Sjöström L, Peltonen M, Jacobson P, et al: Bariatric surgery and long-term cardiovascular events, JAMA 307(1):56–65, 2012.)*

long term, and its safety profile continues to improve. National and international societies have started to advocate a role for bariatric surgery even in patients with class 1 obesity and poorly controlled T2DM, especially in the presence of other CVD risk factors. Results of large-scale systematic reviews and important long-term prospective studies, such as the SOS project, all point to the important role of bariatric surgery in improving cardiovascular risk profile and decreasing the overall incidence of cardiovascular events in severely obese patients over long follow-up periods. Although the majority of patients in the SOS surgical cohort underwent procedures infrequently offered today, similar positive results are expected, and perhaps with greater magnitude, when the more frequently performed malabsorptive procedures, such as RYGB and BPD with duodenal switch, are offered today, while surgeons and scientists continue to find innovative ways to study and serve patients with severe obesity and CVD.

SUGGESTED READINGS

Adams TD, Gress RE, Smith SC, et al: Long-term mortality after gastric bypass surgery, *N Engl J Med* 357(8):753–761, 2007.

American Diabetes Association: Standards of medical care in diabetes—2012, *Diabet Care* 35(Suppl 1):S11–S63, 2012.

American Society for Metabolic and Bariatric Surgery: Position statement: bariatric surgery in class 1 obesity (BMI 30-35 kg/m2), Gainesville, FL, September 2012.

Batsis JA, Romero-Corral A, Collazo-Clavell ML, et al: Effect of bariatric surgery on the metabolic syndrome: a population-based, long-term controlled study, *Mayo Clin Proc* 83(8):897–907, 2008.

Buchwald H, Avidor Y, Braunwald E, et al: Bariatric surgery: a systematic review and meta-analysis, *JAMA* 292(14):1724–1737, 2004.

Buchwald H, Estok R, Fahrbach K, et al: Weight and type 2 diabetes after bariatric surgery: systematic review and meta-analysis, *Am J Med* 122(3):248–256, 2009.

Cristou N, Sampalis J, Liberman M, et al: Surgery decreases long-term mortality, morbidity, and health care use in morbidly obese patients, *Ann Surg* 240:416–423, 2004.

Dallal RM, Hatalski A, Trang A, et al: Longitudinal analysis of cardiovascular parameters after gastric bypass surgery, *Surg Obes Relat Dis* 8(6):703–709, 2012. doi:10.1016/j.soard.2011.09.020

Dixon JB, O'Brien PE, Playfair J, et al: Adjustable gastric banding and conventional therapy for type 2 diabetes: a randomized controlled trial, *JAMA* 299(3):316–323, 2008.

Dixon JB, Zimmet P, Alberti KG, et al: Bariatric surgery: an IDF statement for obese type 2 diabetes, *Diabet Med* 28(6):628–642, 2011.

Expert Panel on Detection, Evaluation, and Treatment of High Blood Cholesterol in Adults: Executive Summary of the Third Report of the National Cholesterol Education Program (NCEP) Expert Panel on Detection, Evaluation, and Treatment of High Blood Cholesterol in Adults (Adult Treatment Panel III), *JAMA* 285(19):2486–2497, 2001.

Favretti F, Segato G, Ashton D, et al: Laparoscopic adjustable gastric banding in 1,791 consecutive obese patients: 12-year results, *Obes Surg* 17(2):168–175, 2007.

Grundy SM, Brewer HB Jr, Cleeman JI, et al: Definition of metabolic syndrome: report of the National Heart, Lung, and Blood Institute/American Heart Association conference on scientific issues related to definition, *Circulation* 109(3):433–438, 2004.

Hu FB: *Obesity epidemiology*, New York, 2008, Oxford University Press.

Longitudinal Assessment of Bariatric Surgery (LABS) Consortium, Flum DR, Belle SH, et al: Perioperative safety in the longitudinal assessment of bariatric surgery, *N Engl J Med* 361(5):445–454, 2009.

Marceau P, Hould FS, Simard S, et al: Biliopancreatic diversion with duodenal switch, *World J Surg* 22(9):947–954, 1998.

Mingrone G, Panunzi S, De Gaetano A, et al: Bariatric surgery versus conventional medical therapy for type 2 diabetes, *N Engl J Med* 366(17):1577–1585, 2012.

Moustarah F, Brethauer S, Schauer P: Laparoscopic surgery for severe obesity. In Cameron JL, Cameron AM, editors: *Current surgical therapy*, ed 10, Philadelphia, 2011, Elsevier Saunders, pp 1304–1316.

Moustarah F, Gilbert A, Despres JP, et al: Impact of gastrointestinal surgery on cardiometabolic risk, *Curr Atheroscler Rep* 14(6):588–596, 2012.

Pontiroli AE, Folli F, Paganelli M, et al: Laparoscopic gastric banding prevents type 2 diabetes and arterial hypertension and induces their remission in morbid obesity: a 4-year case-controlled study, *Diabet Care* 28(11):2703–2709, 2005.

Pories WJ, Swanson MS, MacDonald KG, et al: Who would have thought it? An operation proves to be the most effective therapy for adult-onset diabetes mellitus, *Ann Surg* 222(3):339–350, 1995 (discussion, *Ann Surg* 222(3):350–332, 1995).

Schauer PR, Burguera B, Ikramuddin S, et al: Effect of laparoscopic Roux-en-Y gastric bypass on type 2 diabetes mellitus, *Ann Surg* 238(4):467–484, 2003 (discussion, *Ann Surg* 238(4):484–465, 2003).

Schauer PR, Kashyap SR, Wolski K, et al: Bariatric surgery versus intensive medical therapy in obese patients with diabetes, *N Engl J Med* 366(17):1567–1576, 2012.

Schauer P, Shirmer B, Brethauer S: *Minimally invasive bariatric surgery*, New York, 2008, Springer.

Sjöström L, Narbro K, Sjöström CD, et al: Effects of bariatric surgery on mortality in Swedish obese subjects, *N Engl J Med* 357(8):741–752, 2007.

Sjöström L, Peltonen M, Jacobson P, et al: Bariatric surgery and long-term cardiovascular events, *JAMA* 307(1):56–65, 2012.

Vest AR, Heneghan HM, Agarwal S, et al: Bariatric surgery and cardiovascular outcomes: a systematic review, *Heart* 98(24):1763–1777, 2012.

Wing RR: Long-term effects of a lifestyle intervention on weight and cardiovascular risk factors in individuals with type 2 diabetes mellitus: four-year results of the Look AHEAD trial, *Arch Intern Med* 170(17):1566–1575, 2010.

Skin and Soft Tissue

Nonmelanoma Skin Cancers

Paul N. Manson, MD

Common nonmelanoma skin cancers include basal and squamous cell carcinoma. The common forms of skin cancer arise from the upper layers (epidermis) of the skin:

1. Basal cell: the basal layer of the epidermis
2. Squamous cell: the superficial layer of the epidermis
3. Melanoma: the basal pigmented cells of the skin

In the United States, basal cell and squamous cell skin cancers are especially common in individuals of Northern European heritage, and it is estimated that more than 3 million cases of nonmelanoma skin cancers occur in every year. The frequency of these cancers is such that almost everyone in the United States living to age 80 will have one, and their incidence exceeds those of the other common visceral cancers combined. As the life span increases, these malignancies become more common because of the effects of sun exposure and other causative factors. The incidence of basal cell cancers (BBC) is four times higher than that of squamous cell cancers (SCC). Although most of these skin lesions behave rather benignly in comparison with other cancers, certain subtypes need to be identified; these subtypes (more aggressive lesions) must be treated differently, with wider excisions, sentinel lymph node biopsy, and continued periodic observation for regional and metastatic spread. Specifically, with these subtypes, complete negative peripheral and deep margins must be confirmed at the time of resection before reconstruction and recurrence excluded during frequent postoperative observation of the patient. Less commonly, some of these patients need, in addition to surgery, postoperative radiation treatment.

Many patients ignore their initial lesions (Figure 1), which enables development of large tumors. In these cases, and especially on the face, disfigurement may result because they can involve not only soft tissue structures but also muscle, nerves, cartilage, and bone. Statistics indicate that the annual cost of treating basal and squamous cell cutaneous cancer reaches $1 billion.

RISK FACTORS AND PRECURSER LESIONS

Risk factors for basal and squamous cell cancer include a number of carcinogens. The most agreed upon is sunlight. Cumulative exposure to sun, especially tropical sun, without protection, in fair-skinned individuals who "burn" rather than tan, is the risk most generally agreed upon. Although there is a clear relationship between sun exposure and the incidence of nonmelanoma skin cancers, clinicians debate the exact relationship; most agree that sun exposure is linked more closely to the development of squamous cell carcinoma than to that of basal cell carcinoma. Patients who have had sunlamp treatment for psoriasis are especially prone to squamous cell cancers. Some clinicians believe that microtrauma to the skin contributes to the origin of basal cell cancers. Tumors are more common on sun-exposed surfaces such as the face, scalp, and neck. Radiation exposure, such as that delivered commonly at one time for acne, is also known to predispose to the development of skin cancer and thyroid cancer.

Certain lesions are assumed to be precancerous. Actinic keratoses (Figure 2) are red, crusty lesions that weep and sometimes develop cutaneous horn proliferation. At least 15% develop into in situ and/or invasive squamous cell cancer. Therefore, treatment of these lesions with desiccating treatment such as liquid nitrogen, curettage, or excision seems reasonable in appropriate patients. Other authorities believe that topical chemotherapy such as fluorouracil (Efudex) can eliminate superficial lesions.

Because sun exposure has been implicated in the predisposition to these lesions, there has been considerable attention to programs aimed toward preventing excess exposure, especially sunburns. Two guides to this prevention are "Safe Sun Guidelines" and "Skin Protection from Ultra Violet Light Exposure" (avaialble form the Skin Cancer Foundation at www.skincancer.org). The exact effectiveness of this prophylaxis is not known, but it is under study.

Genetics may also contribute to the development of these lesions. Hereditary conditions such as basal cell nevus (Gorlins) syndrome predispose to the development of hundreds of cutaneous basal cell cancers. People of Northern European descent, such as those of Irish and English heritage, also seem more prone to the development of skin cancer. Certain oncogenes (*RIS* and *DOS*) have been implicated, as have the sonic hedgehog signaling pathway for basal cell cancer. The *PTCH* (patched) gene on chromosome 9q has been suggested in the genesis of these lesions as well.

The literature has emphasized that certain infiltrative subtypes of BCC and SCC tend to be incompletely resected, and therefore the lesions carry a high risk of persistence, recurrence, and metastasis. Such lesions are described later in this chapter, so that they may be managed with greater attention to margins.

Immune suppression, such as that utilized for organ transplantation, leads to a greatly increased frequency of cutaneous skin cancer after a period of 10 to 15 years. It is not unusual for individuals who have undergone immunosuppression to eventually suffer hundreds of aggressive skin cancers as a result, which may be lethal. Those who are immunosuppressed also tend to experience more aggressive lesions, which are less differentiated, have a higher recurrence and a lower cure rate.

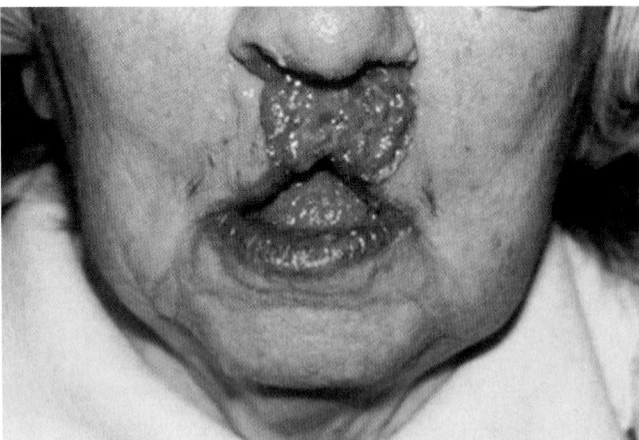

FIGURE 1   Neglected basal cell cancer originating in the lip, invading the anterior maxilla and the floor of the nose.

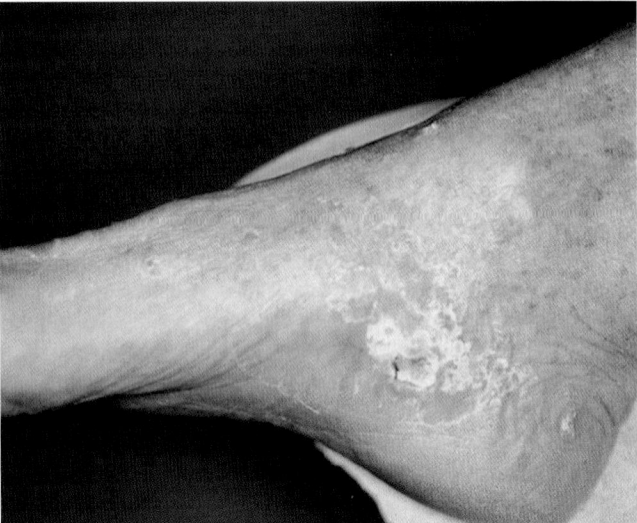

FIGURE 2   Actinic keratoses are premalignant in 15% of cases and represent precancerous squamous cell lesions. They are characterized by slight thickening in the skin, redness, and crusting or flaking. They may be capable of cutaneous horn formation.

Ultraviolet light exposure, such as that used in psoriasis treatment, frequently causes sunburns that impair local skin immunity. Certain medications can also predispose to skin cancers.

Although occurrence at a young age has been implicated by some authorities to have an adverse effect on prognosis, there is no general agreement that this is a significant risk factor for a poorer outcome.

CLINICAL EVALUATION OF BASAL CELL AND SQUAMOUS CELL CANCERS

The physical examination and evaluation of basal cell (Figure 3, *A* and *B*) and squamous cell (Figure 4, *A* and *B*) cancers first includes an analysis of tumor location and size. The tumor should be characterized by its appearance as a probable skin cancer type. The borders of the tumor, the entire local and regional area, and local lymph nodes should be evaluated. A generalized skin examination and a complete history and physical examination would indicate whether the lesion is primary, is recurrent, or has less common features. The general health of the patient dictates other treatment considerations. Certain anatomic areas are predisposed to incomplete resection and recurrence, for example, fusion planes (areas where the primitive parts of the face come together) in the head and neck, such as the areas of the nasal labial fold and the groove between the nose and the cheeks. Certain areas such as the ear, mucosal surfaces, genitalia, and lip tend to be affected by squamous cell cancers, which possess a greater capacity for metastasis. The "mask area" of the face is known have deeper skin cancers, which are more likely to be resected incompletely, and therefore they have a higher risk of recurrence or persistence. Lesions that are larger than 2 cm in diameter carry more risk of persistence and recurrence than do smaller lesions. In general, for all lesions that carry higher risk, complete disease-free margins should be determined surgically or postsurgically, as described previously.

Although curettage and desiccation were formally appropriate for small (6-mm to 10-mm or less) low-risk lesions, a higher recurrence rate has been noted, and the practice is becoming distinctly less common in academic medical centers as an acceptable treatment. Tumors that have occurred in areas of prior radiation treatment, those that occur in areas of prior scarring or persistent ulcers, and basal cell or squamous cell cancers that have perineural involvement have a lower cure rate, lower overall survival rates, and higher recurrence rates. Lesions in which large nerve perineural involvement is

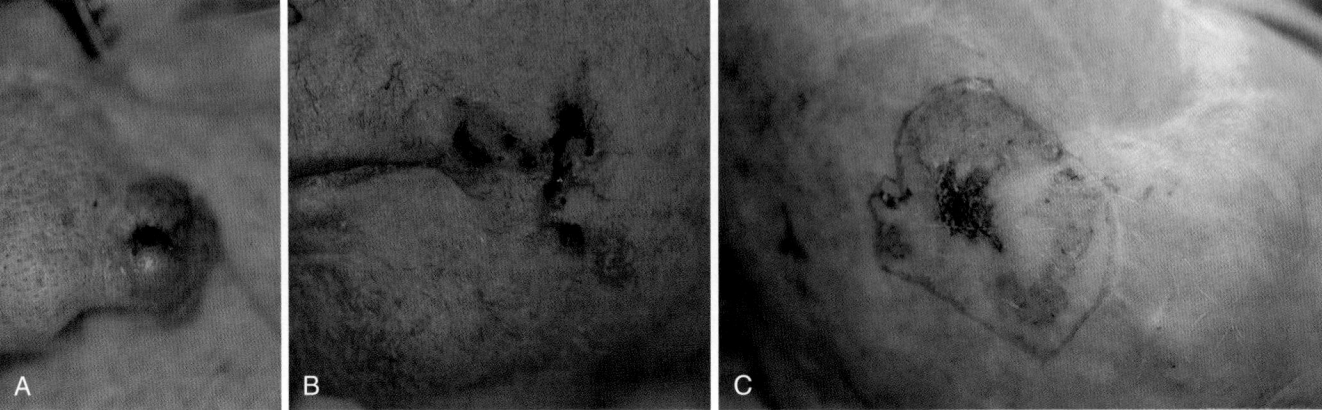

FIGURE 3   Basal cell carcinoma. **A,** Nodular basal cell carcinoma manifests as a nodule of pink, firm, opalescent, generally well-circumscribed tissue in the skin. It may be accompanied by telangiectasia and some redness of surrounding skin. **B,** Micronodular and **C,** Infiltrative and morpheaform basal cell cancer have a flat, red, crusty appearance with poorly defined borders.

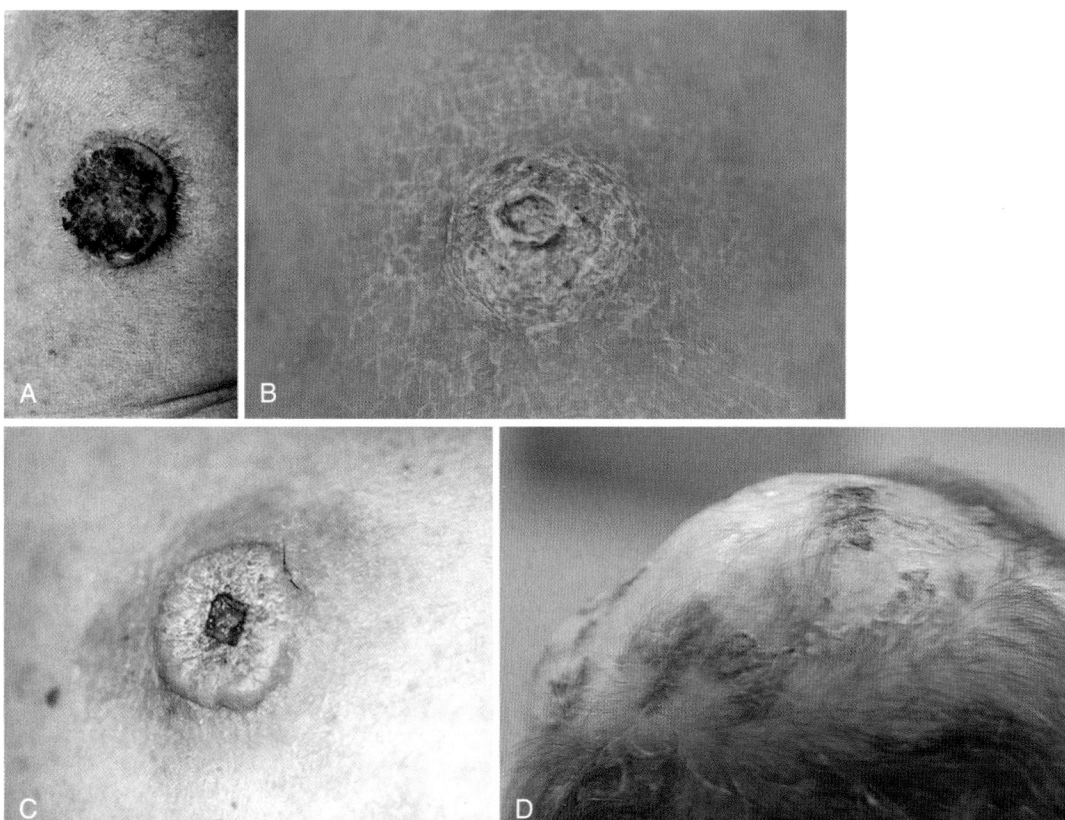

FIGURE 4   Squamous cell cancer. **A** to **C,** Squamous cell cancer, keratoacanthoma variant, has a nodular appearance with scaly superficial margin and some surrounding erythema. It grows rapidly, often from week to week, and is frequently ulcerated in the center. **D,** Squamous cell cancer has a red, scaly appearance with occasional cutaneous horn formation. Frequently, there is bleeding. Some thickening of the skin in the area of tumor is seen.

confirmed should be evaluated with magnetic resonance imaging (MRI) with gadolinium to rule out significant more distant perineural spread. The author has yearly had patients with facial poorly differentiated squamous cell carcinomas who present with sensory symptoms (numbness) and in whom MRI reveals perineural spread along the cranial nerves up to the skull base. In these lesions, and for those with higher risk of infiltrative spread, the peripheral and deep margins may be increased to accommodate these unfavorable histologic characteristics.

With regard to squamous cell cancer, moderate and poorly differentiated lesions have a higher recurrence rate and a greater potential for infiltrative local spread and local or regional lymphatic or systemic (or both) metastasis. Originally, squamous cell cancer was categorized in several grades; however, most pathologists currently believe that two general groups of behavior can be identified for squamous cell cancers:

1. Well differentiated
2. Moderately differentiated, poorly differentiated, and undifferentiated.

Although the prognosis within the latter group is dramatically worse, especially for the poor and undifferentiated lesions, the tendency is to treat these as high-risk lesions with wider and deeper resection margins, perhaps sentinel lymph node biopsy, and histologic confirmation of negative peripheral and deep margins before defect closure or flap reconstruction.

Just as squamous cell carcinoma has higher risk types characterized by less differentiated lesions, basal cell cancer has been characterized into various histologic subtypes, some of which carry a higher risk of more infiltrative spread and, in particular, frequent spread beyond the apparent clinical margins. Basal cell cancers can be divided into two broad groups on the basis of their activity and tendency for subtle infiltrative spread. It is very unusual for basal cell cancers to exhibit lymph node or systemic metastasis, and these lesions are frequently neglected, previously irradiated, multiply recurrent lesions. Nonaggressive subtypes of basal cell cancers include the following:

1. Keratotic
2. Infundibulocystic
3. Nodular
4. Superficial

The primary lesions in this group may generally be managed with 5-mm resection margins.

The subtypes that carry more risk include those with more aggressive growth patterns:

1. Micronodular
2. Infiltrative
3. Sclerosing
4. Morpheaform
5. Desmoplastic
6. Basosquamous carcinoma

Basosquamous tumors have the histologic appearance of both basal cell and squamous cell cancer in some parts of the lesion, and this process probably represents a "collision-type" lesion, which should be treated according to the differentiation of the squamous cell type.

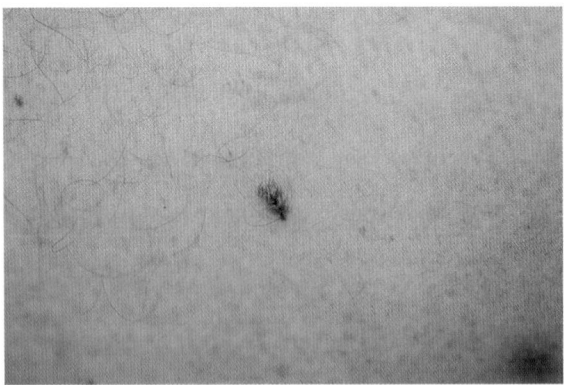

FIGURE 5 Pigmented basal cell cancers resemble melanomas in appearance; the difference is defined only histologically. They frequently demonstrate redness, bleeding, and brown-black pigmentation.

Some basal cells are pigmented (Figure 5) and are easily confused with melanoma by appearance.

Basal cell or squamous cell cancers that develop in an area of chronic ulceration or chronic scarring (Marjolin's ulcers), such as burn scars and pressure sores, have a worse prognosis, perhaps partly because of the difficulty in establishing the diagnosis and therefore late detection and the larger size of these lesions.

The clinician should note the rapidity of growth according to the history provided by the patient because some lesions, such as the keratoacanthoma variant of squamous cell carcinoma, double in size quite rapidly. The more rapidly growing lesions should be removed for diagnosis as soon as feasible because most of these lesions are malignant, and it is impossible to differentiate the benign lesions clinically.

Nerve symptoms are especially concerning; they include numbness, pain, burning sensation, paresthesias, and, in the case of motor nerves, paralysis or muscular symptoms, such as weakness or double vision. These symptoms immediately connote high risk in the treatment of the tumor.

Subtypes of squamous cell cancers, such as adenoid or adenosquamous carcinoma, and those producing squamous cell variants are tumors whose characteristics increase the risk of incomplete resection, recurrence, and metastasis. Desmoplastic cutaneous squamous cell carcinoma similarly is often incompletely resected and thus has a higher risk of recurrence because of deeper extensions along fascial planes with failure to achieve clear margins. Some authorities have suggested that invasion of a tumor into the fat, or invasion deep enough to penetrate lymphatic vessels, constitutes (as is known with melanoma) more potential for recurrence and metastasis through invasion of blood and lymph vessels; confirmation of this opinion is as yet incomplete. These characteristics certainly should be noted by the treating physician, and more extensive treatment and evaluation locally, regionally, and systemically should be contemplated.

Squamous cell carcinoma in situ represents full-thickness atypia of the upper skin layer (epidermis), but the lesions are still noninvasive and may be treated by simple complete excision. Because dermal invasion is not characteristic of this lesion, metastasis is not possible, and so complete excision is all that is necessary. Some authorities believe that topical chemotherapy agents such as fluorouracil (Efudex) can be utilized for squamous carcinoma in situ; however, complete excision is always the treatment of choice and especially for those demonstrating any evidence of recurrence, persistence, or failure of treatment.

Clinical Appearance and Patient Examination

The clinical appearances of lesions such as squamous cell and basal cell are characteristic. Their features include color change, nodularity,

and ulceration (see Figures 3, 4, and 5). Scaling and telangiectasis are frequent. In general, the skin is reddened and thickened. Flaking or keratoses may be present, and both types of lesions frequently demonstrate surrounding premalignant lesions, such as keratosis. Frequently, squamous cells arise in area of actinic keratoses, which are known to be precursor lesions.

Once the diagnosis is suspected, a complete regional examination of the skin and lymph nodes should be completed. A complete, careful skin examination is always recommended because of the frequency of additional lesions. Attention should be directed particularly to sun-exposed skin sites. Patients with basal and squamous cell carcinoma are at increased risk for developing melanoma, as well as additional nonmelanoma skin cancers.

In order to determine the best treatment for a particular skin cancer, a full-thickness skin biopsy is often necessary or desirable. This information can usually help establish lesion type, differentiation, and histologic features. Although shave biopsy is commonly employed, it may not reveal the full extent of penetration of the tumor and may miss areas that enable accurate classification of the tumor. Biopsy samples that include the deep reticular dermis help more accurately identify deeper processes and characterize the lesion. Infiltrative histologic features or deeper penetration will be missed by more superficial biopsy, and, in particular, higher risk lesions may be incompletely diagnosed on shave biopsy. For instance, the specimen from a shave biopsy of a squamous cell cancer is frequently interpreted as squamous cell carcinoma in situ, and the invasive component of the lesion is not confirmed. Squamous cell carcinomas with poorly differentiated or undifferentiated histologic characteristics and those larger than 2 cm carry more risk for infiltrative spread and lymph node involvement. Some practitioners, on the basis of histologic confirmation of aggressive characteristics, perform a sentinel lymph node examination for these lesions. Clinically enlarged nodes can be subjected to needle aspiration biopsy; however, a negative result does not preclude the need for excisional biopsy of an enlarged lymph node.

Research since 1990 has resulted in improved treatment of both basal and squamous cell cancers. This improvement is related to accurate pathologic characterization of the tumor. Although either surgery or radiation can be utilized for early lesions, surgery is generally preferred because diagnosis can be confirmed, the completeness of disease-free margin can be evaluated, and it is (usually) a one-step definitive, efficient treatment. In some cases, age, cosmetic, or functional considerations of the part affected may cause the patient to choose radiation. In general, treatment by surgery should include a complete excision of the lesion with an additional margin, whereby margin size is related to the differentiation or subtype and thus the behavior of the tumor. The margins and accuracy of pathologic confirmation of complete resection are much more important in more serious lesions.

In the past, curettage or desiccation was used for many skin cancers, whereas today this treatment is becoming less common because of the desire to achieve a complete histologic examination. Most skin lesions should be excised with confirmation of the diagnosis and the excision margins, especially for more aggressive cancers. For cancers carrying higher risk, complete excision must be confirmed with standard pathologic peripheral- and deep-margin evaluation (either Mohs' microsurgery or standard pathologic study in which frozen section and permanent sections confirm negative deep and peripheral margins).

With curettage or electrodesiccation, if the lesion extends to subcutaneous (fat) tissue, surgical excision should be performed. The effectiveness of treatment of superficial lesions by curettage depends on the clinicians' perception of reaching appropriate normal dermis tissue. Fat, being less dense than dermis, cannot be utilized to determine the characteristics of normal skin tissue. In addition, if some of the curetted tumor is sent for biopsy, the identification of a higher risk lesion should prompt a secondary surgical excision. Curettage does not provide pathologic confirmation of negative margins or a complete evaluation of the lesion.

Complete Excision and Peripheral Margin Evaluation

For low-risk basal cell carcinomas (less than 2 cm in diameter) with well-differentiated and nonaggressive characteristics, the general cure rate is greater than 90% to 95% with 4-mm to 5-mm clinical margins. The perception of a negative margin depends on identification of the edge of clinically normal skin without erythema, telangiectasis, or any characteristics of the tumor. A nodular lesion with a surrounding rim of erythema must be treated beyond the erythema, which could represent invasion of skin by cancer. With regard to squamous cell carcinoma, margins of 5 to 7 mm are considered more appropriate. Recurrent lesions generally necessitate more margin, such as 1 cm. Careful tracing of the exact margin of the tumor with marking ink under good illumination is required. The proper peripheral margin for cure is then added to the exact lesion border of the tumor, with a second line of marking ink indicating the resection margin. Excision of larger lesions or of those originating in fusion planes may necessitate 10-mm margins, with confirmation of clear deep and peripheral margins.

Reconstruction of the Defect

In most cases, elliptical excision, with the long axis oriented in the relaxed lines of skin tension, and layered primary closure, with careful side-to-side approximation, are appropriate. In some areas, healing can be by secondary intention. The scar from such healing may be more depressed, shiny, and obvious than that occurring from primary layered wound closure. Skin grafting, either partial or full thickness, is a simple method of closing larger defects for which side-to-side approximation cannot be obtained. In the face, considerations of appearance may lead to closure of defects with local flaps, and for more extensive lesions, distant flap reconstruction is required, with secondary procedures for cosmetic improvement. In all cases, the author believes that absolute confirmation of negative surgical margins is always necessary before any complex closure, such as a flap, is accomplished.

Confirmation of Negative Margins

Techniques for rapid or intraoperative evaluation of margins include intraoperative frozen-section assessment and Mohs' surgery. In Mohs' technique, the full length of each margin is determined immediately. In either of these techniques, the immediate margin evaluation may be supplemented by a further determination of permanent margins when more confirmation is desired. Finally, with higher risk lesions, especially those for which a more complex reconstruction is required, margins can be confirmed by immediate permanent analysis techniques before reconstruction is undertaken. The wound may be left open or dressed with an allograft while the final pathologic opinion is awaited. Another technique that has been suggested, in which the size of the lesion would produce a large open, difficult-to-manage wound, is to resect a small strip of tissue at each of the four peripheral margins anticipated for the lesion and immediately close the defect edge to the remaining central specimen; the major portion of the lesion is left intact as the four samples are evaluated. The margins can then be altered appropriately and the remainder of the lesion removed at the definitive resection and reconstruction.

In a complete assessment of the deep and all peripheral margins, the surgeon must be careful to label these clearly so that they can be analyzed by the pathologist in proper sequence and in proper orientation. For all high-risk lesions, all peripheral and deep margins must be confirmed, and this should be completed before any reconstruction is accomplished. If the margins are equivocal in such lesions, a repeat assessment is performed, and the results are awaited before any reconstruction is initiated. An allograft can be placed into the defect until the permanent complete margin evaluation is available. The author prefers sentinel node evaluation for poorly differentiated high-risk squamous cell cancers, although the benefit of this technique routinely and certainly in less differentiated squamous cell cancers has yet to be proven.

Enlarged Regional Nodes

Positive results of needle or excisional biopsy of an enlarged regional lymph node or of sentinel node biopsy confirm the need to remove regional lymph nodes. The sentinel node biopsy technique, in high-risk lesions, has minimized the use of elective regional node dissection, thereby limiting morbidity to cases of proven lymph node metastasis.

Radiation Therapy as Primary or Adjunctive Treatment

Radiation therapy is not generally utilized alone for lymph node treatment or for treatment of high-risk lesions that frequently recur in the absence of initial surgical clearance, but it may be added as adjunctive treatment (for instance, in the management of poorly differentiated squamous cell lesions with the possibility of in transit spread). Sometimes, radiation therapy with or without concurrent chemotherapy is used after lymph node dissection in high-risk cases. Radiation therapy has also been utilized as adjunctive treatment in cases in which the margins are histologically but not clinically positive, for perineural involvement, and when the risk of intralymphatic spread into adjacent skin is high. Patients who have extranodal penetration of tumor—for instance, in extracapsular spread of tumor beyond lymph nodes—are also candidates for postoperative radiation therapy.

Radiation therapy in many cases of primary straightforward, non-melanoma skin cancer can produce good cure rates and excellent cosmetic results. Many treatments are required, and there is no confirmation of negative margins, nor is there complete assessment of the entire tumor for its histologic characteristics. Of course, as in surgery, proper treatment techniques must be applied. Radiation therapy is often reserved for older patients or for cosmetically sensitive areas that are difficult to reconstruct. Some physicians prefer it for thin, wider intraepithelial lesions, such as Bowen's disease, and for patients who have multiple extensive lesions or who refuse surgery.

Patients with disease remaining after radiation therapy and chemotherapy may be candidates for vismodegib, a hedgehog pathway inhibitor, when further surgery and radiation therapy are contraindicated.

Long-Term Follow-up of Basal and Squamous Cell Cancers

All patients with basal and squamous cell carcinoma, especially those with high-risk lesions, should have a complete skin examination periodically with special attention to the area where recurrence, either locally or regionally, is likely. Although most recurrences of lesions develop within a 2-year period, a tumor can recur, in rare cases, after 5 to 10 years. Of patients who have a basal or squamous cell cancer, one third to half develop another lesion within the next 5 to 10 years. Follow-up schedules should be tailored to the particular severity and extent of disease in the patient, to the risk of recurrence, and to the severity of the original lesion.

With lesions that are capable of in-transit metastases, such as poorly differentiated and undifferentiated squamous cell cancer, an additional margin of tissue, perhaps 1 cm, must be excised to account for the possibility of in-transit and invasive spread beyond clinically obvious boundaries. These lesions behave like melanoma in that they are capable of intralymphatic spread, which can appear adjacent to the lesion or in regional lymphatic vessels or lymph node drainage areas.

Superficial therapies for actinic keratosis, very superficial basal cells, or in situ squamous cell carcinoma include 5-fluorouracil or imiquimod. It is difficult to predict the cure rate of these treatments because they are not predicated on complete excision, follow-up is generally incomplete, and biopsy proof of eradication is lacking.

DERMATFIBROSARCOMA PROTUBERANS

Dermatofibrosarcoma protuberans is an uncommon fibrotic skin lesion. The most frequent age range of affected individuals is between 20 and 50 years. Most lesions are located on the trunk or proximal extremities; the head and neck area are affected less commonly (Figure 6). Some patients provide a causal history of trauma; however, the relationship to trauma has not been proved. The lesion grows slowly as a rule and does not metastasize; however it has a strong tendency for local fascial extension along tissue planes in small, thin finger-like projections that evade clinical perception. After conservative surgical excisions, the recurrence rate is up to 60%; therefore, it is recommended that 3-cm to 4-cm clinical margins or Mohs' surgery be utilized.

Dermatofibrosarcoma protuberans manifests clinically as a painless, firm, red to brown or purple plaque (see Figure 6). It can have soft areas or protrusions. This indolent manifestation is often enough to prevent early diagnosis because of its benign nature. The diagnosis can prove difficult, and differentiating it from other fibrotic skin processes can require special stains. Negative results of biopsy in one area should not be reassuring but should prompt more biopsy or complete excision of a suspect lesion. Immunostaining with CD34 factor, factor XIIIA (anti-metallothionein), tenascin, and stromelysin-3 is helpful in making the diagnosis. The lesion is frequently misdiagnosed both clinically and pathologically, and resection is frequently incomplete.

Treatment

Treatment of dermatofibrosarcoma protuberans is surgical excision with wide margins. Up to 4 cm has been recommended. Currently, Mohs' micrographic surgery is the surgical method of choice, which has reduced recurrence rates to about 2%. Regional lymph node biopsy is not indicated because the incidence of metastatic spread is so low (probably 1%). Although adjuvant radiation has been recommended after standard surgical treatment, achieving widely negative margins surgically is highly recommended. The value of radiation therapy in patients who have widely negative surgical margins has yet to be established.

CUTANEOUS T-CELL LYMPHOMA

Lymphomas may manifest as cutaneous lesions and include mycosis fungoides and Sézary disease, which are cancers originating from T4 helper cells. These rare tumors appear as reddish patches, plaques, or reddish lumps. They are sometimes oozing or have a psoriatic appearance. Itching is a prominent clinical symptom. Diagnosis is commonly delayed because its appearance overlaps with those of many other benign cutaneous lesions. In some patients, the lesions progress to frank systemic lymphoma over time, and 5-year survival rates thereafter vary from 50% to 100%.

Therapy includes excision; chemotherapy agents; topical irradiation, such as skin electron beam therapy; and combined chemotherapy and radiation treatment. In some cases, surgery provides control of local symptoms and apparent cure for limited lesions.

BASAL CELL NEVUS SYNDROME

Basal cell nevus syndrome (also known as *Gorlin's syndrome* or *nevoid basal cell carcinoma*) is an inherited autosomal dominant disorder that manifests with multiple cutaneous basal cells, jaw cysts, musculoskeletal and neurologic abnormalities, odontogenic keratocysts, calcification of the falx cerebri, and palmar and plantar pits. The lesions behave as basal cell cancers and are usually managed with surgical excision. It is not infrequent that palmar and plantar pits contain basal cell cancer. The pits are usually small, being 3 mm or less in depth. Usually, affected patients have hundreds of basal cell cancers over the course of their lives. Topical chemotherapy agents such as fluorouracil (Efudex) have been used in an attempt to eradicate early superficial nonfacial basal cells, but surgical excisions are the treatment of choice.

BOWEN'S DISEASE

Bowen's disease is an erythematous, plaquelike lesion that represents a low-grade, slow-growing intraepithelial variant of squamous cell

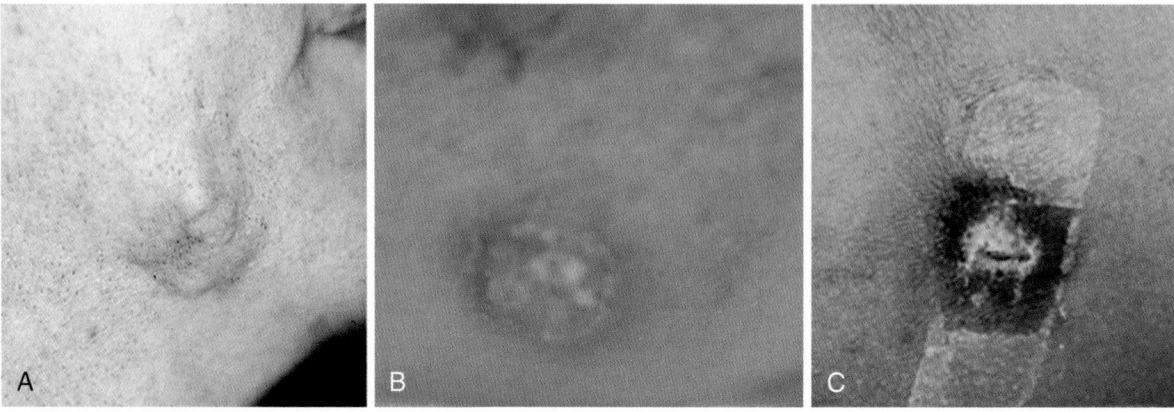

FIGURE 6   A–C, Dermatofibrosarcoma protuberans looks like lumps of fibrous scar tissue. Its indolent appearance belies its invasive character, and the diagnosis must be confirmed by biopsy. Wide margins are necessary because of the tumor's tendency for local invasion.

carcinoma. In essence, the growth of this tumor is intraepidermal, and its history and progression are similar to those of other intradermal carcinomas such as erythroplasia of Queyrat. It is a less common malignancy that appears as a circumscribed, red or pink patch that can weep and look scaly. Many such lesions occur on the trunk or lower extremities and genitalia, but they can involve the head and neck area. The progression of these lesions is limited and normally extends over years. Invasive squamous cell carcinoma can arise in these lesions, and if so, metastasis is eventually possible. Excision with an initial 5-mm margin is recommended. Lesions that occur in cosmetically sensitive areas may necessitate flap coverage; lesions that are large may necessitate skin grafting. In the head and neck, cosmetically sensitive flap reconstructive techniques are preferred when primary closure is not possible.

MERKLE CELL CARCINOMA

This rare neuroendocrine skin cancer is characterized by rapid growth and is a firm, intradermal, red nodule that rapidly progresses to ulceration (Figure 7). Lesions can be traced to a polyomavirus infection, and the disease is definitely more frequent among patients who undergo immunosuppression. The disease progresses rapidly by intravascular and lymphatic spread. Therefore, initial positron emission tomographic (PET) imaging should be performed to evaluate the possibility of regional and distant spread. Positive regional nodes,

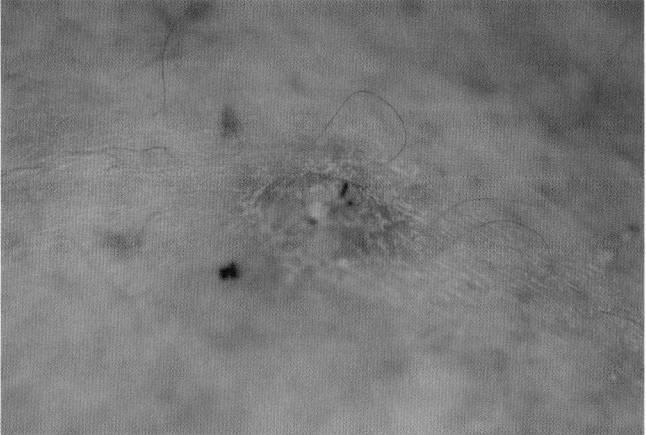

FIGURE 7 Merkle cell skin cancer looks like a tumor lump that frequently grows rapidly. It must be differentiated by biopsy and confirmed by immunohistochemical staining.

which occur in 50%, are predictive of poor survival rates; the disease tends to be undertreated by limited surgical resections, and thus local failure is common (in up to one third of patients). Local control may be improved by larger resection margins of 3 to 5 cm, which often generate the need for skin grafting. Sentinel node biopsy is routinely recommended.

Periodic follow-up with local, regional, and systemic monitoring is recommended. Although most recurrences are detected in the first 2 to 3 years, survival is best predicted by nodal and distant disease. The behavior of Merkle cell cancer is usually more aggressive than invasive melanomas, and in fact, the mortality rate exceeds that of melanoma. The histologic diagnosis is confirmed with immunohistochemical staining. Because of the frequency of local failure in treatment when surgical margins are compromised, some authorities have recommended postoperative radiation therapy for the primary tumor, draining lymphatic vessels, and regional lymph node basins. The added value of this treatment when surgical margins are generous, sentinel lymph node biopsy is obtained, and PET scans are negative has not been established. Adjuvant chemotherapy for regional disease has also been recommended (for positive regional node disease) in addition to surgery.

ANGIOSARCOMA

This rare vascular tumor of the skin generally occurs as a rapidly enlarging nodule or plaque, sometimes simulating a bruise (Figure 8). In-transit metastasis occurs quickly, and initial manifestation with satellite nodules is common. There is a predilection for occurrence in the head and neck area and in elderly persons. In one series, the mean age was 70 years, and affected patients were predominantly male. Aggressive treatment is indicated with 3-cm to 5-cm margins; flap or skin graft reconstructions are frequently required. Sentinel lymph biopsy is recommended. Local recurrence is frequent because of the tendency for in-transit metastasis, and the prognosis is quite limited with 20% survival being routine. These statistics and the proven aggressive behavior of this tumor have generated the recommendation that radiation and chemotherapy accompany the planned surgery. Despite these additions, the prognosis remains largely unaffected by additions to the surgical treatment proposed.

ADENEXAL TUMORS OF THE SKIN

Adnexal tumors arise from skin appendages such as eccrine, apocrine, and sebaceous glands and hair follicles. Some arise from fibrous or neural tissues. Sebaceous carcinomas usually manifest as slightly reddened nodules whose diagnosis is dependent on biopsy. The prognosis varies with the aggressiveness of the lesion, and wide

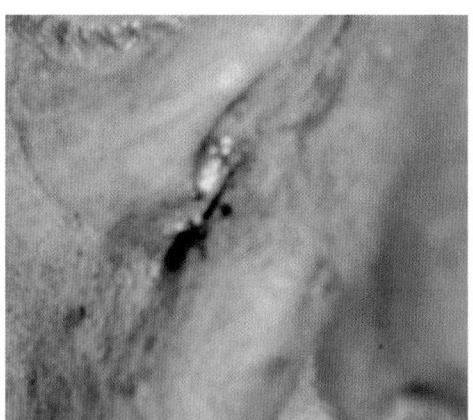
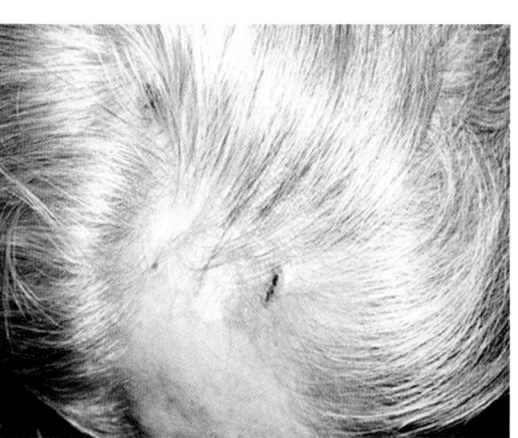

FIGURE 8 Angiosarcoma is a rapidly growing aggressive cancer that often initially appears as a reddish streak or lump, a bruise or hemangioma. It is capable of early intralymphatic and systemic metastasis.

excision with 2-cm margins to fascia is recommended. Some practitioners perform sentinel lymph node evaluations in these more aggressive lesions, but the value of these interventions remains to be proven.

CONCLUSION

Nonmelanoma skin cancers vary in severity from the relatively common and benign varieties to very aggressive and frequently lethal lesions. Treatment favors surgical resection predicated on accurate diagnosis and classification, and the aggressiveness of treatment should be based on good pathologic definition of the lesion type.

ACKNOWLEDGMENTS

The author thanks and acknowledges the panels who created the National Comprehensive Cancer Network (NCCN) Guidelines, (www.nccn.org) which form an excellent and carefully considered basis of the recommendations for diagnosis and

treatment in these lesions. The author recommends these guidelines in the strongest terms for readers wishing further information and clarification because they serve as a yearly updated summary of current recommendations for evaluation and treatment. The author has extensively relied on NCCN Summaries, Clinical Practice Guidelines, Classifications and Recommendations in preparing this chapter.

SUGGESTED READINGS

Barton R: Malignant tumors of the skin. In Mathes SJ, editor: *Plastic surgery*, vol 5, Philadelphia, 2006, Saunders/Elsevier, pp 273–304.
Calonje JE, Brenn T, Lazar AJ, et al: *McKee's pathology of the skin*, Philadelphia, 2012, Elsevier Saunders.
Farmer E, Hood A: *Pathology of the skin*, Englewood Cliffs, NJ, 1990, Appleton & Lange.
Miller, SJ, Maloney ME: *Cutaneous oncology—pathophysiology, diagnosis and management*, Malden, MA, 1998, Blackwell Science.
National Comprehensive Cancer Network: *NCCN Guidelines*. Available at http://www.nccn.org.
Thorne CH: General plastic surgery techniques. In Thorne CH, Bartlett SP, Beasley RW, et al, editors: *Grabb and Smith's plastic Surgery*, ed 7, Philadelphia, in press, Walters Kluwer/Lippincott Williams & Wilkins.

THE MANAGEMENT OF CUTANEOUS MELANOMA

Anna M. Leung, MD, Mark B. Faries, MD, and Donald L. Morton, MD

OVERVIEW

Melanoma is not the most common skin cancer, but it is the deadliest, causing more than 75% of skin cancer deaths. This year melanoma will strike more than 76,000 Americans and kill more than 8790 patients. Despite these bleak statistics, prognosis is excellent with early diagnosis and treatment. Surgery provides the best option for cure of stage I to III melanoma. Surgery is also indicated for certain patients with stage IV disease; in these cases, metastasectomy can prolong survival.

Melanoma risk factors include sun exposure, family history, prior melanoma, blistering sunburn, fair complexion, and dysplastic nevi. Suspicious lesions can be recognized with the ABCD characteristics (Asymmetry, irregular Borders, variegated Color, and large Diameter). Rapidly changing lesions or lesions that differ significantly from the patient's other nevi also may be suspicious for melanoma.

BIOPSY TECHNIQUES

Any lesion suspicious for melanoma should be biopsied to provide pathologic information (depth and diagnosis) for management. Excisional biopsies should be done for small lesions, and punch biopsies (4-mm to 6-mm punch) should be performed for larger lesions or lesions in cosmetically sensitive areas. These techniques are preferable to shave biopsies because the base of the lesion should be included for histologic evaluation and final margin determination. If

a punch is performed, it should be taken at the thickest, most palpable area of darkest pigmentation. Because reexcision is necessary for a lesion that has been confirmed as melanoma with pathologic evaluation, the original excisional biopsy should be oriented in the direction of any subsequent wide local excision. Longitudinal incisions should be made on the extremities, and incisions on the trunk and back should be oriented to minimize distracting tension on the wound.

TREATMENT OF PRIMARY LESION

Margins

Wide local excision is the treatment of choice for the primary melanoma. Excision should include all affected skin and subcutaneous tissue plus a margin of normal skin around the edge of the previous biopsy site or the widest area of pigmentation. Margin width is based on lesion depth (Table 1). The excision should reach down to the midsubcutaneous region for confirmed in situ lesions and down to the fascia for deeper lesions, with removal of the fascia and underlying muscle if the lesion is more than 4 mm thick or if concern exists for invasion of the muscle.

Elderly patients with chronically sun-exposed skin frequently have abnormal melanocytic proliferation, often clinically unapparent, which makes determination of boundaries of excision difficult. Several punch biopsies should be performed at the proposed margin. If no evidence of abnormality is found, then these punch biopsy sites are used as the margins of resection.

Incision and Reconstruction

The wide local excision is often done through an elliptic incision with a length-to-width ratio of 3:1. If orientation of the excision can be determined initially, then the incision is an ellipse. If orientation cannot be determined, then a circular incision is made preliminarily and final flaps are oriented subsequently. Most wide local excisions can be closed with straightforward local advancement flaps with a two-layered dermal and subcuticular closure. If the wound cannot be closed primarily with local advancement flaps, then a rotational rhomboid flap, complex V-Y or Z-plasty flap, or skin grafting can be considered (Figure 1).

Although skin grafts provide excellent coverage, healing can take many weeks and the risk of graft loss is always present. Skin grafts can either be full or split thickness. Split-thickness skin grafts (STSGs) can cover larger areas; they have better neovascularization and thus a higher chance of graft acceptance. The most common donor site for STSG is the upper lateral thigh. If the recipient site is also the leg, the donor site should be the contralateral thigh because wide local incision is usually accompanied by a lymphatic procedure. Bolster dressings and negative wound vacuum systems can be used to promote postoperative graft healing. In general, split-thickness skin grafts should not be used in cosmetically sensitive areas such as the face, head, and neck because of mismatch of skin color and type.

Full-thickness skin grafts provide the best cosmetic outcome for the scalp and face. The graft is taken from a matching area of skin, usually the upper chest or postauricular neck. The donor skin must be trimmed of all subcutaneous tissue to the level of the dermis. Reconstruction options should always be discussed thoroughly with the patient. Plastic and reconstructive surgeons may be consulted, but the oncologic portion of the operation should never be compromised for cosmetic reasons.

Special Sites

Nail Bed

Wide local excision for subungual melanoma is based on the same principles as wide local excision for any other cutaneous melanoma. The margins are again based on depth (see Table 1). Removal generally requires a partial amputation at the midproximal phalanx. If the primary lesion is on the foot, preservation of the metatarsophalangeal joint of the great toe is usually sufficient to prevent functional compromise. Subungual melanoma of the distal finger typically requires amputation of one phalanx proximal to the melanoma; melanoma of the proximal finger can be managed with soft tissue excision, skin grafting, and attempted preservation of bone and tendon. If a tendon must be resected, it can be reimplanted by securing the cut ends of the tendon to the distal remaining phalanx with nonabsorbable suture. This helps prevent paradoxical motion of the digit after surgery. Resection for melanoma of the hand must balance the two goals of functional preservation and optimal oncologic outcome.

Sole of Foot

Melanoma of the sole of the foot requires wide local excision down to plantar fascia, with either full-thickness skin grafting or flap coverage. If the melanoma is on an area such as the instep that is not weight bearing then a thinner, split-thickness skin graft can be used. In weight-bearing areas, acral skin may be rotated into the excision site, with skin grafting of the secondary defects.

TABLE 1: Wide excision margins for primary melanoma

Thickness of primary	Excision margin
Melanoma in situ	5 mm
≤1 mm	1 cm
1.01-2 mm	1-2 cm
2.01-4 mm	2 cm
>4 mm	≥2 cm (dependent on location and ease of larger margin)

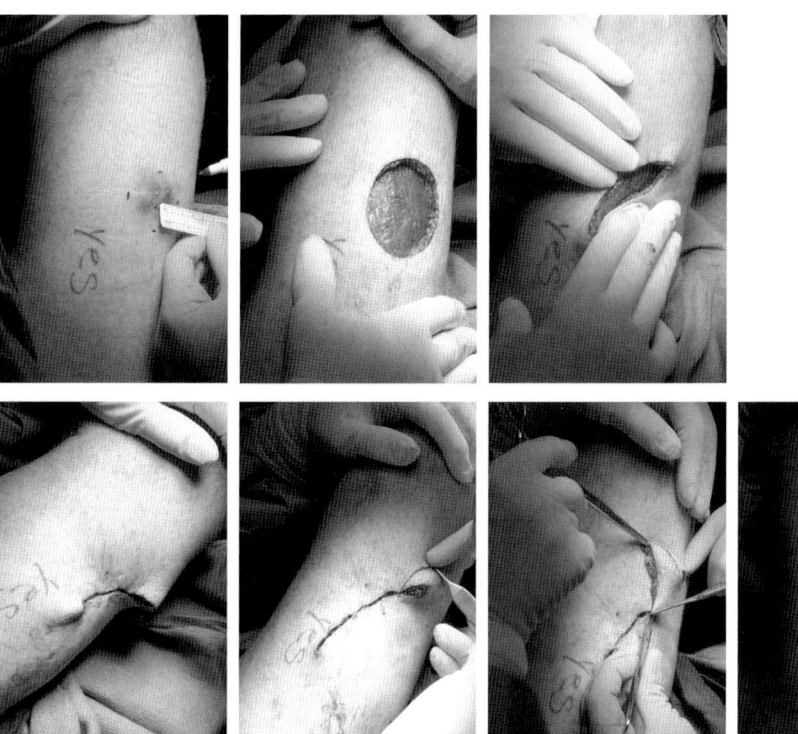

FIGURE 1 Wide local excision of an extremity melanoma. *Top row (left to right):* Measurement of circumferential margin; after excision; assessment of lines of tension. *Bottom row (left to right):* Wound closure after flap mobilization; marking of redundant skin; extension of redundant skin across wound; final closure.

Ear

Wide local excision of ear melanoma is dependent on the location of the lesion. Lesions at the top of the ear can usually be removed with a simple wedge excision. Cartilage is closed with interrupted nonabsorbable sutures, and the skin can easily be reapproximated. By contrast, resection of melanomas on the lower ear usually leaves a defect that requires skin grafting or flaps.

TREATMENT OF REGIONAL NODES

Regional lymph nodes are the most likely first site of melanoma spread. In the past, all patients with intermediate-thickness melanoma and clinically normal nodes underwent elective regional lymph node dissection, but most basins were pathologically clear. Thus, elective nodal dissection subjected patients to a potentially morbid major operation that in many cases had no benefit. In the late 1980s, Donald L. Morton developed the technique of intraoperative lymphatic mapping and sentinel lymph node biopsy (SNB) as a minimally invasive, low-morbidity alternative for identification of patients with occult nodal metastasis. Since then, this technique has been established as a new standard for the management of melanoma.

The Multicenter Sentinel Lymphadenectomy Trial I (MSLT-I) confirmed the accuracy and clinical impact of SNB. Patients with primary melanoma and clinically normal nodes were randomized to treatment with wide local excision (WLE) plus nodal observation, with regional lymphadenectomy for clinical evidence of nodal metastasis during follow-up, or to WLE plus SNB, followed immediately by regional lymphadenectomy for a positive sentinel node. The trial confirmed that the sentinel node's tumor status was the most important prognostic factor for these patients. Among those patients who had nodal disease, disease-free and overall survival rates were significantly improved by early removal, which was made possible with SNB.

Sentinel Node Biopsy

SNB is indicated for patients whose primary lesions are more than 1 mm in depth. Rates of sentinel node positivity are 12% to 20% for 1-mm to 2-mm melanomas, 28% to 33% for 2-mm to 4-mm melanomas, and 28% to 44% for melanomas more than 4 mm. For patients with thin melanomas (<1 mm), other considerations for SNB include young age, male gender, Clark level IV lesion, ulceration, regression, incomplete biopsy (e.g., shave biopsy), or mitotic rate 1 or more.

SNB is conceptually simple but can be technically challenging and requires experience for optimal accuracy. The rate of false-negative lymphatic mapping/SNB in MSLT-I, determined by nodal recurrence in tumor-negative dissected sentinel node basins, was 10.3% for the first 25 cases versus 5.2% in the subsequent 25 cases. The surgeon, nuclear medicine physician, and pathologist must work as a team to ensure a low false-negative rate. Because of the steep learning curve for SNB in melanoma, if facilities are not proficient in all aspects of this procedure, then these cases should be referred to a specialized center. The accuracy and morbidity of SNB are optimized if WLE and SNB are performed at the same operation.

Because the sentinel node is the first lymph node to receive lymphatic drainage from the primary tumor site, if this node is free of disease, then remaining (downstream) lymph nodes also should be free of disease (Figure 2). As a result of the variability of lymphatic drainage from a primary cutaneous melanoma, two tracers are used:

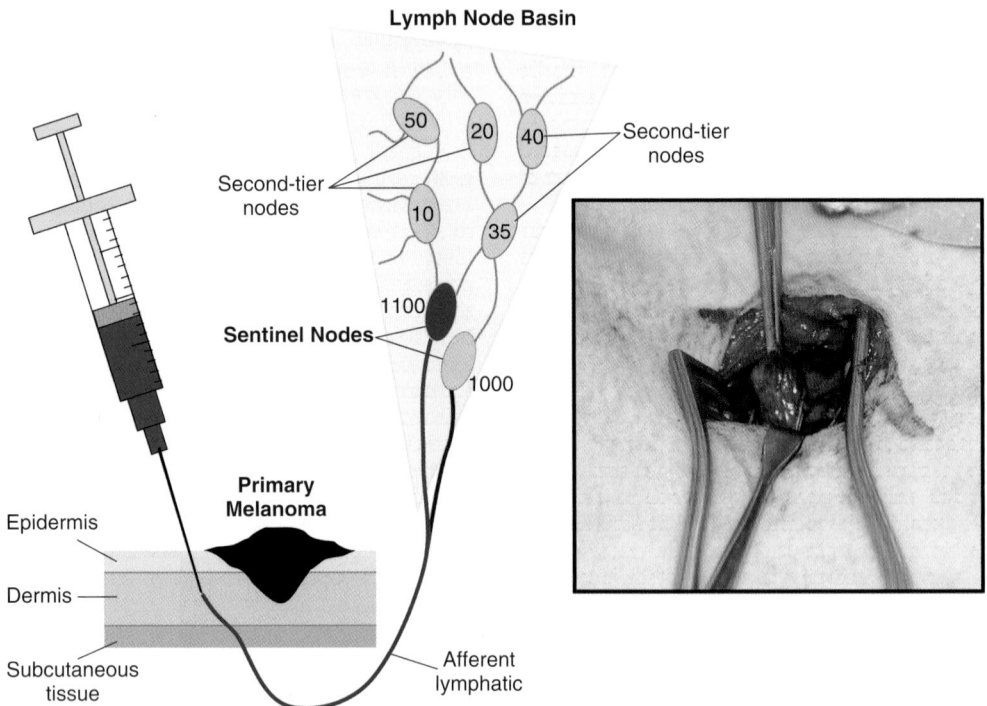

FIGURE 2   At different times, blue dye and radiotracer are injected intradermally at the site of the primary tumor (radiotracer is injected immediately before preoperative lymphoscintigraphy, and blue dye is injected immediately before the surgical procedure). During intraoperative lymphatic mapping, blue-stained afferent lymphatics are visualized and followed to the first blue-stained node (i.e., the sentinel node *[inset]*). A hand-held gamma probe confirms higher radioactive counts within this sentinel node and can identify additional sentinel nodes that are not stained blue. *(Reprinted with permission from Bagaria SP, Faries MB, Morton DL: Sentinel node biopsy in melanoma: technical considerations of the procedure as performed at the John Wayne Cancer Institute,* J Surg Oncol *101(8):669-676, 2010.)*

a radiocolloid and a vital blue dye. Lymphoscintigraphy is performed before surgery on the day of surgery, or the day before surgery, with injection of technetium sulfur colloid intradermally in the skin of the primary site. Because approximately 10% of mapping procedures identify a sentinel node in an ectopic location, imaging of potential drainage basins should include popliteal, epitrochlear, supraclavicular, and internal mammary sites, plus the intramuscular triangle of the upper back. The skin is marked over the sentinel node, and a film identifying this node's location is sent with the patient to the operating room. In some instances, the primary melanoma drains to more than one basin.

In the operating room, before prepping and draping, 1 to 2 mL of isosulfan blue is injected into the intradermal tissue of the operative site. Allergic reactions to isosulfan blue are rare (<1%) but can be as serious as an anaphylactic reaction. Blue dye should not be injected outside the boundaries of the wide local excision because blue-stained skin can remain blue for several months. Injection should always be intradermal rather than subcutaneous because relatively few lymphatic channels are found within the subcutaneous tissue. The density of lymphatic channels within the intradermal tissue allows rapid transit (minutes) of the tracer to lymph nodes; no massage is necessary. A gamma probe confirms the location of the sentinel node, and an incision is made in a location convenient for SNB and compatible with a subsequent completion dissection if that were to prove necessary. Intermittent use of the gamma probe guides the surgeon to the location of the sentinel node, which is identified with color and radioactivity (see Figure 2). The node is removed from the surrounding fatty tissue, with ligation of vessels and lymphatic channels to prevent lymphocele and seroma formation. For radioactive nodes after resection, the point of greatest radioactivity should be marked with a suture to aid the pathologist in the identification of the most likely area of metastasis.

Once the node is removed, the basin should be examined to rule out significant radioactivity, blue-stained nodes, or palpably abnormal nodes. Multiple sentinel nodes can be present, and all nodes that are hot (radioactivity >10% of the hottest node) and blue should be removed. Once the sentinel node dissection is complete, the nodal basin should be irrigated and inspected for hemostasis and the wound should be closed in two layers. Gloves and instruments should be changed before wide local excision of the primary melanoma.

Technically difficult areas include the head and neck, where lymphatic drainage is variable and unpredictable. Also, because the primary lesion is close to the draining basin, there is often a very high background radioactivity. Discussion with the nuclear medicine physician is important to ensure evaluation of all potential nodal locations. During surgery, the gamma probe should be used to confirm identification of all pertinent sites, and nodal basins should also be reexamined with the probe after wide local excision because this removes the high background that the primary lesion produces (Figure 3).

Frozen section examination is not routine because its accuracy for melanoma is low and it uses a large portion of the specimen. Final staining uses hematoxylin-eosin and immunohistochemistry with antibodies to several melanoma marker epitopes (S-100, HMB-45, and MART-1).

SNB is a relatively benign procedure. Complications occur approximately 10% of the time but are generally transient and mild in nature. The most common complications include seroma, hematoma, and infection. Depending on the location of the node, nerves in close proximity can be inadvertently injured. Morbidity can be decreased by avoiding disruption of lymphatic channels and nonsentinel lymph nodes during SNB. The rate of lymphedema associated with SNB is only 1%.

Completion Lymphadenectomy

Because most patients with sentinel node metastasis have no additional positive nodes, the second Multicenter Selective

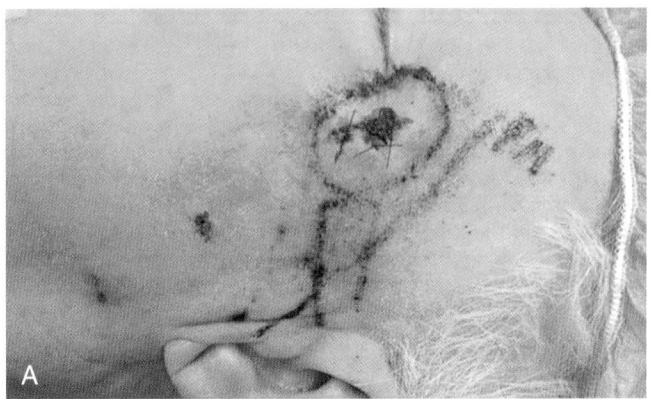

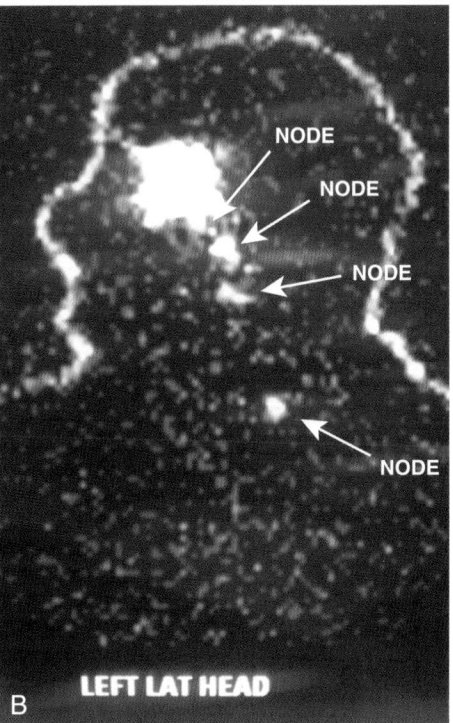

FIGURE 3 **A,** primary lesion *(circled);* and **B,** lymphoscintigraphy of a head and neck melanoma. Note the multiple draining nodes and the high background radioactivity of the primary lesion.

Lymphadenectomy Trial (MSLT-II) is randomizing patients with sentinel node metastasis to either nodal observation (ultrasound scan imaging and clinical examination) or completion dissection. Results will determine whether completion lymphadenectomy is necessary for patients with limited nodal involvement. Until then, completion lymphadenectomy remains the standard of care for all patients with a positive sentinel node or other evidence of regional nodal metastases.

Before completion lymphadenectomy, patients with proven nodal disease should be evaluated for systemic disease. Laboratory values including serum lactate dehydrogenase (LDH), complete blood cell count (CBC), and liver enzymes should be drawn; elevations are suggestive but not diagnostic of systemic involvement. In cases of high concern for systemic involvement (e.g., a patient with clinical evidence of nodal disease), imaging with magnetic resonance imaging (MRI) of the brain; computed tomography (CT) of the chest, abdomen, and pelvis; and full-body positron emission tomography (PET) should be performed to rule out systemic disease. If evidence of systemic disease is found on imaging, then the patient may be a candidate for clinical trials or systemic therapy.

The first step in completion lymphadenectomy is excision of the previous sentinel node scar and the creation of skin flaps. Sharp dissection rather than electrocautery is preferred because it decreases the chances of thermal injury to subdermal vessels that supply the skin flaps. Because melanoma is a cutaneous disease, the skin flaps should be as thin as possible without compromising perfusion. Visible lymphatic channels should be secured with ties or clips to prevent seroma or lymphocele. Lymphadenectomy should be performed as much as possible in an en bloc manner with preservation of motor nerves and muscle. Two closed-suction drains are placed in the basin after dissection through two separate stab incisions. These drains are left in place until the output is below 25 mL/d for 2 consecutive days. Patients can perform gentle range of motion exercises after completion dissection, but strenuous activity should be avoided until after the closed-suction drains are removed and healing is complete. An adequate number of lymph nodes should be evaluated (Table 2).

Neck Dissection

The extent of lymph node dissection in the neck is dependent on location and indications for the procedure. Clinically gross disease requires more aggressive resection, which occasionally may include removal of the internal jugular vein, spinal accessory nerve, and sternocleidomastoid if affected by extracapsular invasion. If nodal involvement is microscopic or limited to the sentinel node, usually all functionally important structures can be preserved. Removal of parotid lymph nodes with superficial parotidectomy should be performed in patients with primary lesions of the face or scalp anterior to the coronal suture or if lymphoscintigraphy reveals drainage to a preauricular node. Bipolar electrocautery should be considered in neck dissection because it allows for better control of current and heat transmission, thus preventing nerve injury.

Axillary Dissection

Axillary dissection is more extensive for melanoma than for breast carcinoma. Dissection should include all three levels of the axilla and skeletonization of the axillary vein. The superior border of dissection is the axillary vein from the thoracic inlet (Halsted's ligament) to the latissimus dorsi tendon. Medially the dissection extends to the serratus anterior and intercostal muscles and should include

interpectoral (Rotter's) nodes if the primary lesion is on the anterior chest. The lateral border of dissection is the edge of the latissimus dorsi muscle, and the inferior border is the fourth intercostal space. The subscapularis forms the posterior border of the dissection. The pectoralis minor muscle may be transected or removed if necessary to ensure complete dissection of level III. The lateral thoracic and thoracodorsal neurovascular bundle should be preserved unless directly involved with tumor. Often branches of the intercostobrachial sensory nerves need to be sacrificed, resulting in sensory loss of the posterior upper arm.

Inguinal Dissection

Superficial inguinal dissection involves the inguinofemoral basin. Superficial inguinal dissection extends 5 to 6 cm superior to the inguinal ligament and clears the tissue superficial to the abdominal fascia. The medial border is the adductor magnus, and the lateral border is the sartorius. All lymphatic tissue overlying or surrounding the femoral vessels is removed. Motor branches of the femoral nerve should be spared, but some sensory branches may be included. Sacrifice of the sensory branches may result in numbness on the anterior thigh. Cloquet's node, which is the highest superficial lymph node and lowest node in the iliac chain, is taken from the femoral canal and identified as such. If Cloquet's node contains tumor, then dissection of the deep inguinal basin is indicated.

Closure of the superficial inguinal dissection includes closure of the femoral canal with interrupted nonabsorbable sutures to prevent a femoral hernia. In addition, transposition of the sartorius muscle over the femoral vessels is indicated if the femoral vessels are exposed and at risk for injury. The sartorius is mobilized and transected at its insertion from the anterior iliac spine, and the muscle is then secured to the inguinal ligament. The wound is then closed in several layers, and closed suction drains are placed.

Deep inguinal dissection involves the iliac and obturator inguinal basins. Indications for deep dissection include positive Cloquet's node, palpable nodes, positive nodes on imaging, extracapsular extension of tumor, and more than four positive nodes on superficial dissection. Deep dissection can be performed by extending the incision for superficial dissection in a superolateral direction onto the lower abdomen, with transection of the inguinal ligament. An alternative method is to use a separate muscle-splitting incision obliquely on the lower abdomen, 5 cm above the inguinal ligament. The musculature of the abdomen is split, and the retroperitoneal space is entered anteriorly. The peritoneum and ureter are preserved and swept superiorly. All lymphatic tissue along the iliac, hypogastric, and obturator vessels is removed. Complications from inguinal dissection include wound infection in 10% to 15% of cases and lower extremity lymphedema in 20% of cases. Techniques to prevent postsurgical edema include leg elevation and graduated compression stockings.

Popliteal Dissection

The popliteal basin is bordered laterally and superiorly by the biceps femoris, medially and superiorly by the semimembranosus and semitendinosus muscles, and inferiorly by the medial and lateral heads of the gastrocnemius. The popliteus muscle creates the deep floor. This basin is considered part of the inguinal basin, and positive lymph nodes in the popliteal basin mandate superficial inguinal lymphadenectomy.

Ectopic Sentinel Nodes

Not uncommonly, lymphatic mapping identifies sentinel nodes in the epitrochlea, flank, or intramuscular triangle of the back or outside the axilla. If these nodes contain tumor, the surgeon should perform complete lymphadenectomy (CLND) of the ectopic basin and CLND of adjacent basins.

TABLE 2: Recommended number of evaluated nodes by basin

Basin	Number of nodes
Axillary	15
Inguinal, superficial	8
Inguinal, deep	6
Cervical, anterior	15
Cervical, posterior	15
Supraclavicular	6
Suprahyoid	4
Parotid	3
Popliteal	2-3

Adjuvant Radiotherapy and Adjuvant Interferon-alpha After Completion Dissection

Although melanoma is classically considered radioresistant, radiotherapy may be helpful for patients who have a high risk of regional nodal relapse because of large palpable metastases (>3 cm), extracapsular extension, or more than five involved lymph nodes. Complications from radiotherapy vary by basin. Systemic recurrence is common after lymphadenectomy if the patient has a large number of positive nodes. Interferon alpha slightly improves disease-free survival but not overall survival. Clinical trials are evaluating systemic adjuvant treatment after lymphadenectomy.

IN-TRANSIT DISEASE

In-transit melanoma metastases are unique lesions that represent foci of tumor cells that have spread via the dermal and subdermal route. The risk for in-transit disease is based on the characteristics of the primary melanoma rather than margin of the wide local excision or nodal management. Unfortunately, in-transit disease can be quite extensive, which makes management challenging (Figure 4). In-transit metastasis requires staging to rule out distant disease. Treatment decisions are based on the extent of the lesions (size and number), anatomic location, quality of surrounding skin, depth of in-transit (dermal or subcutaneous) disease, and presence of additional disease. Methods of treatment include local, regional, and systemic therapies.

Local Therapies

Local therapies include topical therapies, intralesional injection, electrochemotherapy (ECT), radiotherapy, and surgery. Topical therapy, intralesional injection, and ECT should be considered in the setting of extensive lesions, lymphedema, or induration of surrounding skin. Topical therapy is noninvasive but tends to be effective only in patients with very superficial in-transit disease. The most common topical agent is imiquimod.

Intralesional injection has been used since the 1960s. At the authors' institution, bacille Calmette-Guérin (BCG) has been injected intralesionally to induce regression of in-transit metastases. Other investigators have reported significant side effects such as systemic toxicity and death; however, the authors' experience indicates that when BCG regimens are based on skin responsiveness to purified protein derivative, side effects are usually mild and limited to local inflammation, erythema, edema, and ulceration. Other intralesional injection agents include cytokines (interferon-alpha 2b and interleukin-2), and rose bengal disodium.

ECT involves electroporation with high-intensity electric pulses to facilitate intracellular delivery of cytotoxic drugs (bleomycin and

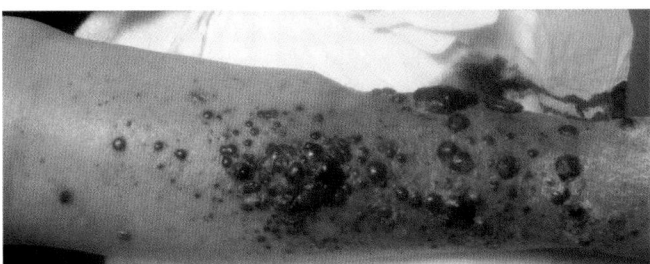

FIGURE 4 In-transit melanoma of the leg. The extensive nature of these lesions makes this patient ineligible for surgical resection for cure. However, this is an ideal candidate for regional hyperthermic perfusion chemotherapy.

cisplatin). ECT is not an option in patients with kidney failure, and bleomycin is contraindicated in patients with pulmonary fibrosis.

Simple excision with negative margins should be performed if just a few small in-transits are surrounded by normal skin. A combination of resection and laser ablation can be considered for wider areas. Radiation is generally not effective for gross disease but can be used after resection for prevention of recurrence.

Regional Therapies

Regional therapies can be considered if extensive lesions are isolated to a limb. Methods include isolated limb perfusion (ILP) and isolated limb infusions (ILI), which both use the chemotherapeutic agent melphalan. Both perfusion and infusion can deliver a concentration of chemotherapy that is 25 times higher than that delivered with systemic administration, with limited systemic toxicity. ILP requires open cannulation of the vessels and use of an oxygenated extracorporeal circuit. ILP can result in fairly high locoregional toxicity such as erythema, edema, lymphedema, and even extensive damage to the deep tissues resulting in functional loss or need for amputation. ILI is a percutaneous method that does not require open cannulation. In addition to locoregional toxicity being much lower, ILI also uses a hypoxic and acidotic environment that may contribute to the effectiveness of melphalan.

Systemic Therapies

Systemic chemotherapy including dacarbazine has also been used in the treatment of patients with in-transit melanoma. Unfortunately, response rates with the use of chemotherapy have been low and are often coupled with systemic toxicity.

METASTATIC DISEASE

Resection in the setting of metastatic disease is generally contraindicated, but metastasectomy can improve outcomes of carefully selected patients with melanoma. Optimal candidates have slow-growing tumors (tumor doubling times, >40 days), one to three metastases, and good performance status. Although conventional systemic therapy for melanoma yields dismal results, resection with adjuvant vaccine therapy has produced 5-year survival rates of 40%; many patients have survived longer than 10 years. In 2011, the U.S. Food and Drug Administration (FDA) approved two new therapies for stage IV disease: ipilimumab, which blocks CTLA4, and vemurafenib, which is a B-raf inhibitor. In addition, PD-1 inhibitors (programmed death 1 ligand blockade) have shown promise in early-phase studies.

FOLLOW-UP

Recurrence after surgical resection for melanoma is common, especially in patients with thick melanomas or nodal disease. Thus, follow-up with clinical examination and routine laboratory work (LDH, CBC, and liver enzymes) is important. All patients should have routine lifelong dermatologic screening because patients with one melanoma have a 5% to 10% risk of development of a second primary melanoma and an increased risk of basal cell and squamous cell carcinoma. After removal of a thin primary with no nodal involvement, follow-up with the surgeon should be scheduled every 6 months for the first 3 years and then yearly for the following 2 years. For patients with intermediate or thick melanoma and positive or negative regional nodes, the follow-up should be every 3 months for the first 3 years then every 6 months for the next 2 years. After a disease-free interval of 5 years, follow-up can be conducted yearly.

Recurrence usually occurs near the wide local excision site or the regional nodal basin, so these areas should be examined with special care. Distant recurrence can also occur. Because melanoma has an unpredictable metastatic pattern that can target any area of the body, symptoms or abnormality on routine laboratory workup should warrant further imaging.

MANAGEMENT OF RECURRENT DISEASE

Local recurrence is based on either: (1) radial extension of abnormal melanocytes, which results in recurrence at the area of original excision; or (2) local dissemination (metastasis) of tumor cells through lymphatic channels, resulting in satellite or in-transit metastasis. These two types of local recurrence are prognostically distinct. The risk of local recurrence depends not only on the width of surgical excision but also on the pathologic characteristics of the primary lesion. Factors such as depth, ulceration, and neurotropism are associated with higher local recurrence rates. Although local recurrence is dependent on resection margins in radial extension, pathologic characteristics of the primary lesion (thickness, >4 mm), ulceration, and desmoplastic melanoma with neurotropism and spread along nerves are the reasons for satellite or in-transit metastasis.

CONCLUSION

Surgery is curative for early-stage melanoma, but the approach to advanced melanoma is less straightforward. Recent breakthroughs in immunotherapy and improved surgical techniques have introduced the possibility of multimodal regimens tailored to the patient's melanoma and timed to produce synergistic effects. In addition to vemurafenib and ipilimumab, PD-1 and MEK inhibitors have shown promise in early trials and are being tested in combination with existing regimens to provide maximal therapeutic benefit. Ipilimumab, which is approved for stage IV disease, is being considered as a postoperative adjuvant to improve disease-free and overall survival in patients with resected high-risk melanoma (IIIb, IIIc, M1a, M1b). For decades, little progress has been made in the treatment of melanoma, but now aggressive and innovative clinical trials have been designed to create new strategies of treatment and we have the potential for significant improvements in outcome.

SUGGESTED READINGS

Bagaria SP, Faries MB, Morton DL: Sentinel node biopsy in melanoma: technical considerations of the procedure as performed at the John Wayne Cancer Institute, *J Surg Oncol* 101(8):669–676, 2010.
Howard JH, Thompson JF, Mozzillo N, et al: Metasectomy for distant metastatic melanoma: analysis of data from the first Multicenter Selective Lymphadenectomy Trial (MSLT-I), *Ann Surg Oncol* 19(8):2547–2555, 2012.
Leung AM, Hari DM, Morton DL: Surgery for distant melanoma metastasis, *Cancer J* 18:176, 2012.
Morton DL, Thompson JF, Cochran AJ, et al: Multicenter Selective Lymphadenectomy Trial Group: sentinel node biopsy versus nodal observation for primary melanoma, *N Engl J Med* 355:1307, 2006.

THE MANAGEMENT OF SOFT TISSUE SARCOMA

Chandrajit P. Raut, MD, MSc, and Alessandro Gronchi, MD

OVERVIEW

Soft tissue sarcomas (STS) are malignant tumors that arise from mesoderm-derived tissue, including fat, smooth and skeletal muscle, blood vessel, and connective tissue. Additional tumors classified as STS include malignant tumors of nerve sheath origin, derived from ectoderm. Approximately 11,000 new cases of STS, representing 1% of all malignancies, with a slight male predominance, lead to approximately 3900 deaths per year in the United States. Although considered rare at all ages, STS is the third most common solid malignancy in children and accounts for 15% of all pediatric cancers.

STS are a heterogeneous group of neoplasms that may be subclassified into more than 70 specific histologies and may be distributed throughout the body. Approximately one half arise in the extremities, and one third arise in the abdomen, pelvis, and retroperitoneum. The most common histologic subtype in adults is now recognized to be gastrointestinal stromal tumor (discussed elsewhere), followed by liposarcoma and leiomyosarcoma. In contrast, these subtypes are relatively less common in children, in whom pediatric (embryonal/alveolar) rhabdomyosarcoma accounts for nearly half of all STS diagnoses.

Tumor-related factors predictive of recurrence or survival include size, grade (low, intermediate, or high), and depth (superficial or deep according to the involvement of the investing fascia), although the impact of these and other risk factors may vary depending on histology and site of origin. The most important treatment-related factor predictive of recurrence is quality of surgical margins (negative/positive). This factor has shown to be the strongest prognosticator of local failure, but it also plays a role in distant failure and final outcome. Pattern of failure depends on tumor grade and histology and site of origin because it influences the possibility of achieving clear surgical margins. In general, low-grade tumors tend to recur locally or locoregionally, with only a low risk of distant spread; high-grade tumors may also recur locally but have a much higher propensity for distant failure. Extremity STS most commonly spread to the lung when they metastasize, whereas retroperitoneal sarcomas generally recur in a locoregional pattern. Some histologic subtypes have peculiar natural histories. For example, myxofibrosarcomas tend to recur locally repeatedly before spreading to distant sites, myxoid/round cell liposarcomas may spread to other organs (lungs, abdominal cavity, soft tissue, and bone) early in the course of the disease, and angiosarcomas are generally multifocal and difficult to control surgically and can give rise to lymph node metastases and distant spread very early in the course of the disease.

Traditionally, surgical textbooks and peer-reviewed literature have discussed the surgical management of STS based on site of origin. Although site of origin remains an important consideration, it has become increasingly clear that surgery must also be tailored to specific sarcoma histology to more accurately reflect tumor biology and pattern of recurrence.

This chapter covers the management of nongastrointestinal stromal tumor (non-GIST) STS. Surgical management is discussed both by specific histology and by site of origin. Although the focus of this chapter is surgery, additional treatments, such as radiation therapy or chemotherapy, and imaging are considered as appropriate.

ETIOLOGY

Most sarcomas arise sporadically, without recognizable etiologic factors. Various chemical agents and herbicides have been associated with specific STS. For instance, vinyl chloride and thorium dioxide (Thorotrast) have been linked to hepatic angiosarcomas. Another well-recognized risk factor is chronic lymphedema in the development of angiosarcoma, a phenomenon known as Stewart-Treves syndrome. Therapeutic and environmental exposure to radiation is associated with development of sarcomas within the treatment field at a median interval of approximately 10 years, with the most common histologies being angiosarcoma and unclassified pleomorphic sarcoma (formerly called malignant fibrous histiocytoma [MFH]; see subsequent discussion).

Germline genetic mutations and molecular alterations have been associated with the development of sarcomas. Li-Fraumeni syndrome, the result of mutations of *p53*, is associated with both STS and osteosarcoma. Neurofibromatosis type I (von Recklinghausen's disease), the result of mutations of *NF1*, is associated with an approximately 15% risk of development of malignant peripheral nerve sheath tumors and an increased risk of development of gastrointestinal stromal tumors. Familial adenomatous polyposis, the result of mutations in *APC*, is associated with desmoid tumors.

Chromosomal rearrangements may lead to gene fusions associated with sarcomas, such as the *SSX-SYT* rearrangement seen in synovial sarcoma. Similarly, chromosomal amplification may be associated with specific sarcoma histologies, such as increased levels of MDM2 and CDK4 proteins in association with chromosomal 12 amplification in well-differentiated and dedifferentiated sarcoma.

GRADING

The American Joint Committee on Cancer (AJCC) has developed a staging system for sarcomas. The AJCC staging system not only incorporates the traditional variables of tumor size, nodal disease, and metastatic disease but also tumor grade. Unlike the more common grading based on differentiation (well, moderate, or poor), STS grading is based on histology specific features, including differentiation, necrosis, and mitotic count, and is most commonly classified as low (grade I), intermediate (grade II), or high (grade III). Tumor stage incorporates both size (T1, ≤5 cm; T2, >5 cm) and depth with respect to fascia (superficial, T1a or 2a; deep, T1b or 2b). True nodal spread is rare.

However, considerable variability is found in outcome amongst patients within each stage, in part because a critical factor, histology, is not incorporated into the AJCC staging system. Other prognostic factors, such as site of origin and patient age, are also not weighted. To address this, several institutions have created nomograms based on STS histology or site that consider specific prognostic factors as continuous rather than categoric variables; in the long run, these may be more useful at identifying prognostically similar cohorts for future studies.

TREATMENT

Surgery remains the standard and only potentially curative therapy in the management of STS. In general, wide or radical resections are necessary to achieve negative margins. In other words, the tumor must be resected en bloc, with a cuff of healthy tissue all around, to avoid contamination from tumor surface and removal of tumor microsatellites that may be present in the healthy tissues surrounding the pseudocapsule. The extent of resection and adequacy of margins depends on a variety of factors, including histology and presence of an intact biologic barrier, such as muscular fascia, vascular adventitia, periosteum, or epineurium.

Patients with STS should undergo evaluation at a sarcoma center because the administration of neoadjuvant or adjuvant therapy may be indicated. Generally, this involves multidisciplinary evaluation by a surgical oncologist and, depending on histology, a medical oncologist and a radiation oncologist. Reevaluation of pathology slides by a pathologist specializing in sarcomas is critical to confirm the exact histology and determine the most appropriate treatment. In fact, approximately 25% of all sarcomas are initially designated with the incorrect histology, and approximately 15% are assigned the wrong histology in a clinically significant manner that impacts the treatment plan. Given the complexity of many operations needed, support from other specialists, including plastic and reconstructive surgery, vascular surgery, urology, thoracic surgery, and anesthesia, is commonly required.

IMAGING

Histology-specific and site-specific imaging recommendations are discussed in further detail in the subsequent individual sections. For better definition of the extent of extremity and truncal STS, including depth of invasion and relationship with neurovascular structures, magnetic resonance imaging (MRI) of the affected site is the preferred imaging study. Further staging studies for patients with extremity STS should include chest imaging: chest x-ray for low-grade lesions and chest computed tomographic (CT) scan for intermediate-grade or high-grade lesions. Patients with abdominal visceral, pelvic, and retroperitoneal sarcomas should undergo CT imaging of the abdomen and pelvis and, in most cases, chest. Those with primary STS of the rectum or metastases to the liver may need further evaluation with MRI of those sites. STS involving vascular structures, such as leiomyosarcoma arising in the wall of inferior vena cava, are usually sufficiently characterized with the standard MRI or CT imaging of the site and (CT) angiography is not necessary. Patients with breast STS should undergo MRI to define depth of extension; mammography is not routinely useful. Those with scalp STS may undergo either a CT scan or MRI. Routine head CT scans are not needed as a staging study. Although much has been written about the use of positron emission tomography (PET) in some sarcomas and many other malignancies, it is rarely indicated in routine sarcoma care. PET scans should only be ordered selectively, when attempting to resolve an ambiguous finding on other imaging or gauging treatment responses under specific circumstances.

HISTOLOGY-SPECIFIC TREATMENT

Atypical Lipomatous Tumor/ Well-Differentiated Liposarcoma

Atypical lipomatous tumor (ALT)/well-differentiated liposarcoma is a low-grade tumor that, when arising in the extremity, has a relatively low rate of recurrence, may not recur for quite some time, and has no risk of distant metastatic spread and death, unless dedifferentiation occurs over its natural history. Dedifferentiation, if it occurs, in fact entails a risk of metastatic spread as high as 20%. In contrast, low-grade locally recurrent ALT may grow slowly for years. Therefore, such tumors that arise in the extremity can be resected with a limited negative or even a positive margin, especially when preservation of limb function is an issue (Figure 1). Radiographically, ALT may be difficult to distinguish from an intramuscular lipoma, a benign entity that can also arise in deep muscle tissue. ALT/well-differentiated liposarcoma is a more threatening neoplasm when located in the retroperitoneum, even in absence of areas of dedifferentiation. In fact, as discussed subsequently, local control is an issue at this site, and patients often die of locoregional failure, without development of distant metastases (Figure 2).

Dermatofibrosarcoma Protuberans

Dermatofibrosarcoma protuberans (DFSP) is a superficial tumor that infiltrates soft tissue for centimeters beyond the obvious margins of the lesion and can recur locally after an inadequate resection. However, the more common variety of DFSP does not display metastatic behavior. Therefore, the goal of surgery should be negative margins, often necessitating reconstruction with plastic surgery. When cosmesis is an issue, limited positive margins may be accepted and a wider resection postponed until DFSP locally recurs. Because of the relatively indolent nature of the growth of DFSP, a tissue expander may be placed and resection may be delayed to allow a single-stage resection and reconstruction (Figure 3). DFSP is usually a relatively superficial tumor, so resection of muscle deep to the tumor is not often necessary. Intraoperative frozen-section margin analysis is not generally helpful because the surrounding fat rarely freezes well for analysis. Mohs' micrographic surgery has been reported as a treatment for this neoplasm, but long-term results are lacking. Radiation therapy is not usually recommended. Follow-up should consist of a physical examination, and imaging may be reserved for patients with a suspicious mass in the tumor bed. Approximately 5% to 10% of patients with DFSP have a more aggressive fibrosarcoma variant that may recur locally and potentially spread. Those individuals should be treated as with a "conventional" sarcoma with more aggressive local therapy (including radiation) and followed with systematic imaging.

Malignant Fibrous Histiocytoma

MFH is an archaic term that covered a variety of sarcoma histologies with very different clinical behavior and treatment approaches. The term MFH has been largely replaced by specific sarcoma histologies, including myxofibrosarcoma, fibromyxosarcoma, etc. Those that do not fall into known histologies and would have otherwise been termed MFH are now typically called unclassified pleomorphic sarcoma.

Myxofibrosarcoma

This tumor when located superficially infiltrates through soft tissue (subcutaneous fat and investing fascia) centimeters beyond the ostensible margins of the visible or palpable mass (Figure 4). When located intramuscularly, the extension of the infiltration is usually limited by anatomic barriers, although it has a higher propensity to invade into those anatomic boundaries compared with other histologic subtypes. Myxofibrosarcoma most commonly arises in the extremities of elderly individuals. It has a 30% rate of local recurrence and a 16% rate of distant recurrence. Multiple local recurrences have been associated with eventual amputation. Therefore, aggressive local therapy is critical. Wide surgical margins (2-cm to 4-cm radial margins beyond the clinical boundaries of the palpable mass, especially in more superficial tumors) should be the goal of surgery, which often requires complex wound closure or flap reconstruction by a plastic and reconstructive surgeon and resection and reconstruction of vessels or nerves. Radiation therapy, either before or after surgery (described subsequently), may be considered, although the direct impact on this specific histology remain unknown. Follow-up imaging should include the primary site (usually with an MRI) and the lungs (with chest CT scan).

Low Grade Fibromyxoid Sarcoma

The similar nomenclature of this lesion to those listed previously belies its behavior. Local recurrence is again a problem, but interval to relapse may vary. These malignant neoplasms follow a more indolent course, and the risk of relapse persists well beyond 5 years. Therefore, patients may be followed at longer intervals early in the postoperative course, but follow-up should continue for a decade or more.

Angiosarcoma

Management of primary and radiation-associated (secondary) angiosarcoma of the breast is discussed in the subsequent section on breast sarcomas. Scalp angiosarcoma (Figure 5) is a particularly

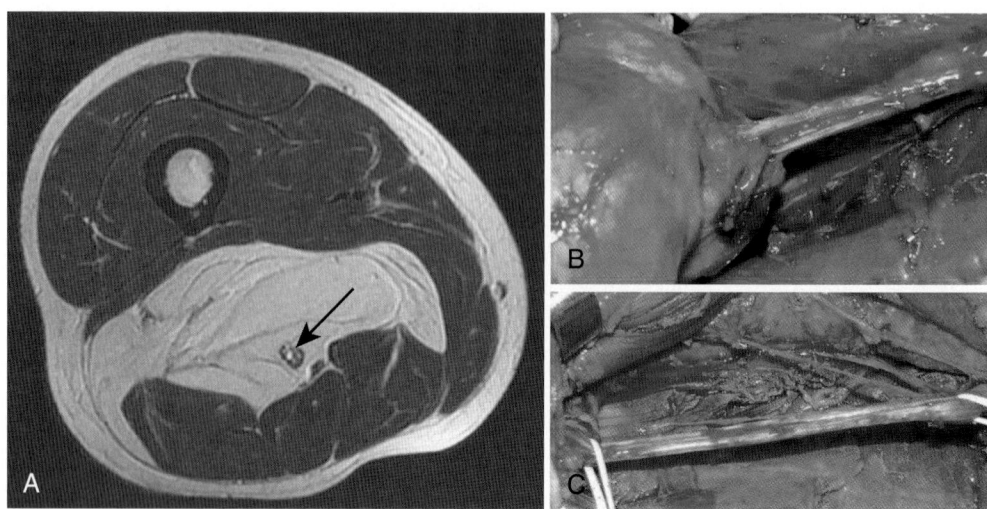

FIGURE 1 **A,** Axial magnetic resonance imaging of the thigh shows a well-differentiated liposarcoma encasing the sciatic nerve *(arrow)*. **B,** Tumor peeled off of sciatic nerve. **C,** Surgical field after resection of the tumor, with skeletonized nerve.

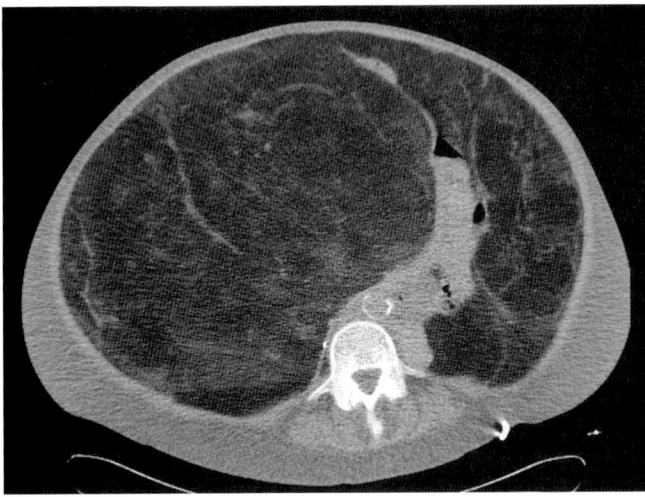

FIGURE 2   Locally advanced well-differentiated liposarcoma.

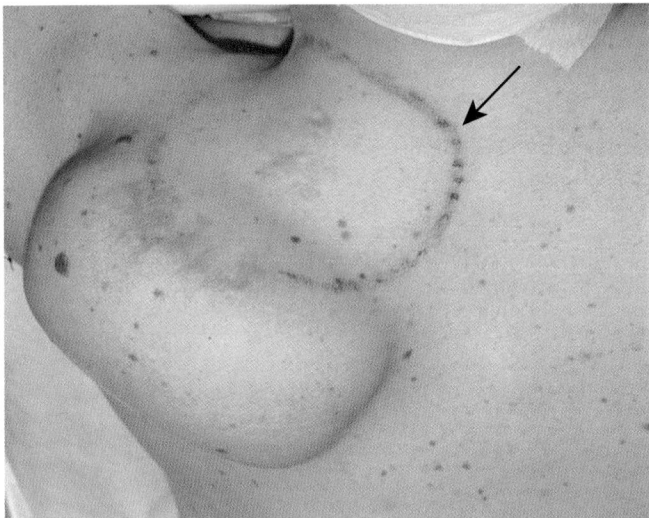

FIGURE 3   Dermatofibrosarcoma protuberans repaired with a rotational flap after prior tissue expander placement. Intended line of incision line marked in black *(arrow)*.

insidious malignancy. Scalp angiosarcomas are commonly multifocal, with both clinical examination and CT scan or MRI. Although radical surgery is possible (requiring complex flap reconstructions), it is not uncommon for patients to have local recurrences develop immediately outside the margins of resection even if the margins of the initial resection were widely negative and with or without radiation therapy. Angiosarcoma is sensitive to systemic chemotherapy and to radiation therapy. Because surgery is rarely curative, it should not be considered first-line therapy for scalp angiosarcoma. Surgery may be reserved for patients who are experiencing problems with local control (bleeding from a fungating tumor) or who only appear to have a solitary site of disease with both clinical examination and imaging while undergoing systemic therapy.

Radiation-Induced Sarcomas

Radiation-induced sarcomas are rare and include a variety of histologic subtypes, the most common of which are unclassified pleomorphic sarcoma, angiosarcoma, malignant peripheral nerve sheath tumors, and leiomyosarcoma. Beside the intrinsic characteristics of each histologic subtype, they are all characterized by a high propensity to locally recur, given the difficulty of obtaining clear margins. This is the result in part of the difficulty in distinguishing tumor infiltration of healthy tissues from radiation-induced soft tissue changes around the tumor site and in part of the discontiguous and multifocal involvement of tissue within the radiation field (Figure 6). The tumor should be excised with as much tissue around it as possible. This often if not always requires reconstruction and coverage by a plastic surgeon and potentially a more liberal policy of neurovascular resection and reconstruction. Systemic chemotherapy and reirradiation are often considered, given the overall dismal prognosis, although the use of the latter must be weighed with caution.

Malignant Peripheral Nerve Sheath Tumors

Malignant peripheral nerve sheath tumors (MPNST) often arise from a major peripheral nerve, which can be identified macroscopically. They can occur sporadically or in the context of neurofibromatosis type 1 (von Recklinghausen's disease). The high-grade variant is marked by an early propensity for distant metastases. When originating from a peripheral nerve, MPNST also may spread along the nerve fibers proximally or distally. Wider margins at this level should

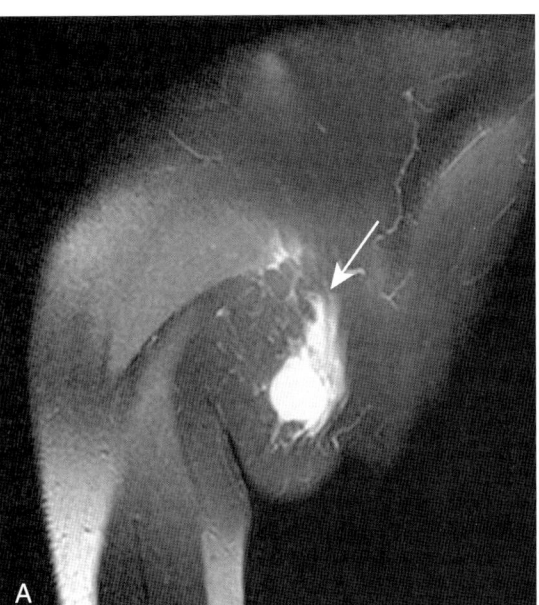

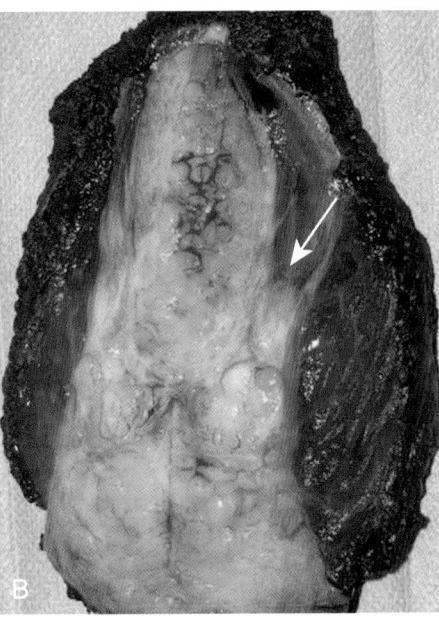

FIGURE 4   Periscapular superficial myxofibrosarcoma on sagittal view on: **A,** magnetic resonance imaging; and **B,** surgical specimen, showing infiltration of the surrounding tissues extending 2 to 3 cm from the mass *(arrow)*.

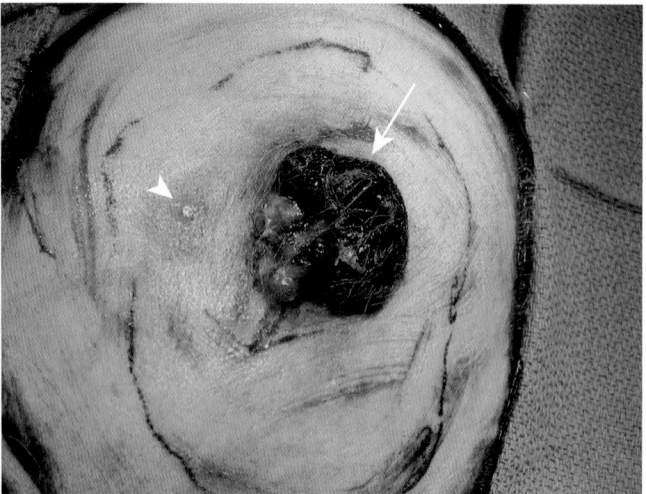

FIGURE 5 Multilobulated angiosarcoma *(arrow)* on the vertex of a shaved scalp with satellite lesion nearby *(arrowhead)*.

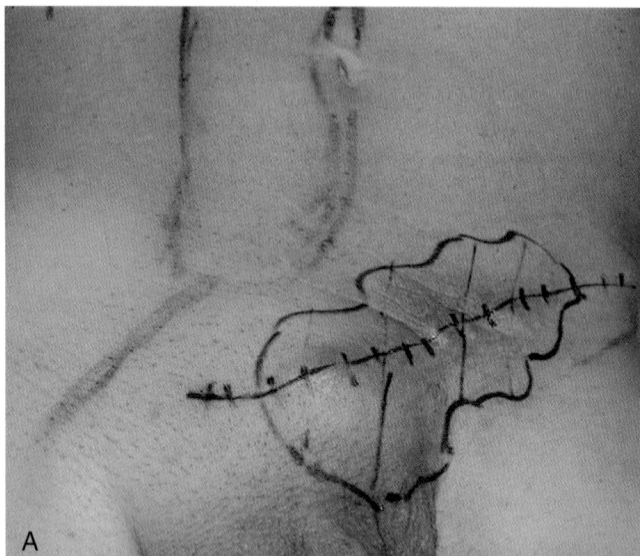

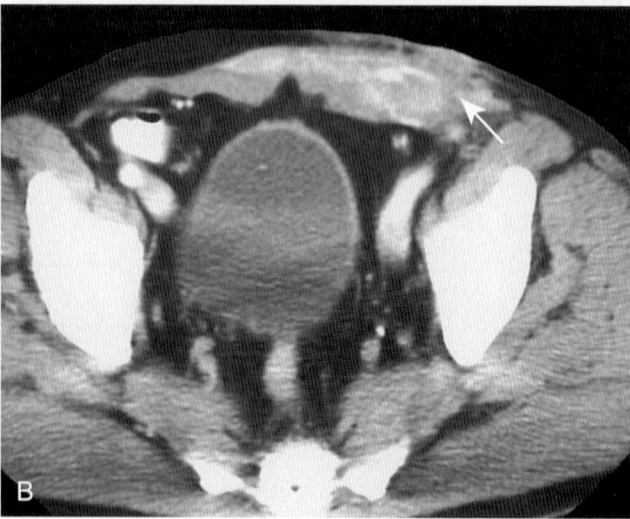

FIGURE 6 **A,** Clinical and **B,** radiographic appearance *(arrow)* of a radiation-induced sarcoma of the left groin.

be obtained (if possible, at least 4 cm of macroscopic healthy nerve; Figure 7) to limit locoregional failure, which eventually may reach the spinal cord. Intraoperative frozen-section analysis may help ensure clear margins. Systemic chemotherapy is used on an individualized basis.

EXTREMITY SOFT TISSUE SARCOMA

Clinical and Diagnostic Evaluation

Patients with extremity STS commonly present with a palpable mass. Initial clinical evaluation should include a thorough history and physical examination, with attention directed to size, precise location, and evidence of neurovascular compromise. No tumor markers are known for STS histologies at present. After a thorough examination, an MRI (or CT scan) of the affected site is indicated for most lesions; small superficial lesions may be directly excised at the discretion of the surgeon. MRI generally provides more detailed soft tissue definition but is less readily accessible, may be problematic for patients with claustrophobia, and cannot be performed in patients with embedded shrapnel and certain types of aneurysm clips, cardiac devices, or other implants. Staging evaluation is completed with a chest x-ray (for low-grade malignancies) or a chest CT scan (for intermediate-grade or high-grade malignancies). Routine head CT scan (other than for alveolar soft part sarcoma) and PET scan are not needed.

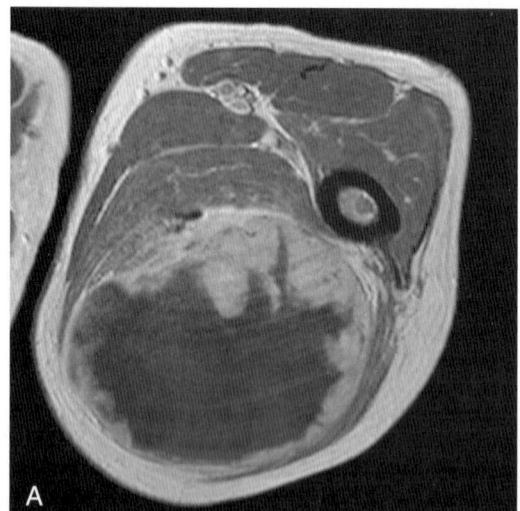

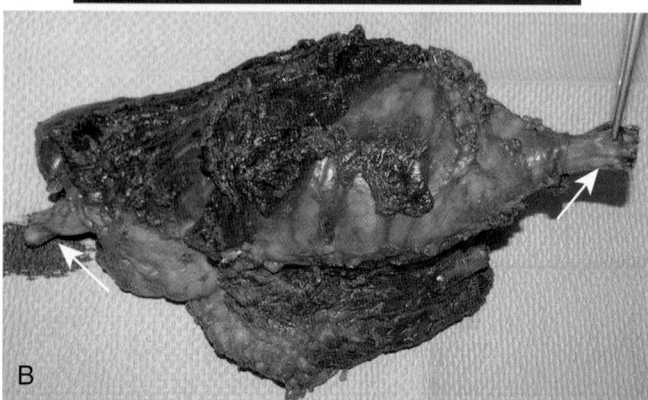

FIGURE 7 **A,** Preoperative magnetic resonance imaging and **B,** surgical specimen showing malignant peripheral nerve sheath tumor arising from the sciatic nerve *(arrows* indicate nerve stumps).

Imaging alone is rarely diagnostic of the specific sarcoma histology, with the exception of well-differentiated liposarcoma (also known as atypical lipomatous tumors). Well-differentiated liposarcomas have a radiographic density similar to normal surrounding fat but tend to be well encapsulated with thick internal septations. Such tumors may be treated with resection (complete excision with a margin of normal surrounding muscle, fat, or fascia to minimize risk of local recurrence) and do not require a biopsy.

Other neoplasms suspicious for sarcoma should be biopsied. The authors prefer to obtain core needle biopsies with radiographic guidance, although they may be performed without imaging depending on location. Although biopsy tract recurrences are exceedingly rare, the site selected for the core needle biopsy should be planned such that it can be included in the incision used during the subsequent definitive resection or at least in the radiation field. Thus, coordination between the surgeon and the interventional radiologist is necessary. It is important to specify core needle biopsy rather than fine-needle aspiration because the latter rarely yields enough tissue and architecture information to distinguish between different sarcoma histologies. A key advantage of core needle biopsy over an open biopsy is that the former can be directed towards a specific portion of the tumor. If a core needle biopsy fails to yield a diagnosis, an open incisional or excisional biopsy should be obtained. Although incisional biopsies have been used for diagnosis commonly, they are often performed improperly in inexperienced hands. Incisional biopsies should be performed through longitudinally oriented incisions placed such that the incision can be included in the final resection when a definitive resection is planned. If a transverse incision is used, then when subsequent reexcision is required, challenges for reconstruction and risk of lymphatic disruption (depending on location) are magnified. Excisional biopsies should be confined to lesions less than 2 cm in size and superficial in location.

Surgical Treatment

Until the early 1980s, the standard of care for patients with extremity sarcomas was amputation. That changed after a seminal randomized controlled trial conducted by Rosenberg and colleagues at the National Cancer Institute. In that trial, patients with high-grade extremity STS were randomized to undergo amputation or limb-sparing surgery with adjuvant radiation therapy. Those undergoing limb-sparing surgery trended towards a higher rate of local recurrence. Importantly, however, no difference was found in overall survival. This altered the standard treatment for extremity STS.

Currently, the goal of surgery is not only limb sparing but also function sparing, with appropriate biologic margins achieved. Surgical resection should be carefully planned based on preoperative imaging. Resections should include not only the entire tumor (without rupture or violation of the surrounding pseudocapsule) but also an adequately wide margin (1 to 2 cm) of normal, nonneoplastic tissue. Resections performed with positive margins do result in higher risk of local recurrences and, to a lesser extent, of distant metastases and death. If the STS is close to the superficial skin, then an adequate skin paddle overlying the tumor should be resected en bloc with the tumor (Figure 8). The surgeon should not compromise the margin by minimizing the skin resection just to avoid a skin graft or flap. Tumors that extend towards but do not involve the fascia should include the fascia as a margin. Superficial tumors that involve the fascia should include the fascia and generally an additional margin of underlying muscle. By definition, when the investing fascia is infiltrated, the tumor is considered deep, even if it is mainly located in the superficial tissues. Similarly, deep tumors that extend superficially to the fascia should include a margin of overlying subcutaneous and cutaneous tissues as a margin. It is uncommon for primary STS to violate a fascial plane, but not recurrent STS. Deep tumors that do not extend in superficial tissues do not need large resection of superficial tissues (Figure 9). The tumor specimen should be oriented with marking sutures. When possible, additional margins may be sent separate from the main specimen, representing the superior, inferior, medial, lateral, superficial, and deep margins of dissection, with the true margins appropriately marked for orientation. Tumors that abut bone may include the periosteum as a margin if the bone is not directly invaded (Figure 10). If necessary, vascular resection and reconstruction should be considered for involved vessels (Figure 11). If a critical nerve is encased, reconstruction with an interposition nerve graft should be considered (Figure 12). Such reconstructions may be compromised if radiation is administered after surgery; therefore, preoperative radiation may be warranted. The specimen should be reviewed with the pathologist for optimal orientation.

Furthermore, it is critical to take into account the specific histology, as described previously. For instance, resection for myxofibrosarcoma requires wider margins than resection for ALT. Thus, the surgeon must understand the different sarcoma histologies, confirm the accuracy of the diagnosis, and review the treatment plan in a multidisciplinary consultation.

Wound closure should be meticulous to minimize risk of wound complications, which can be considerable as described in the next section. Drains may be necessary, particularly after preoperative

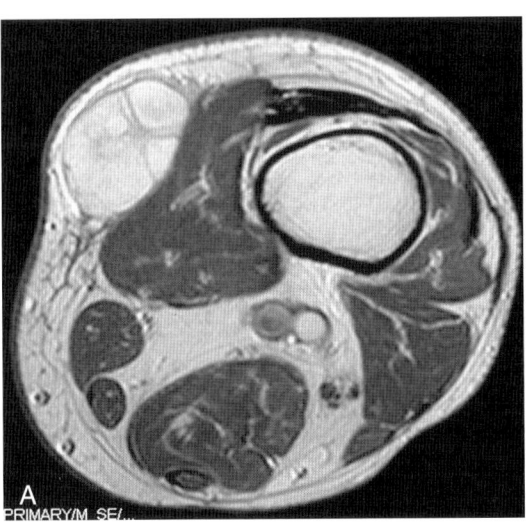
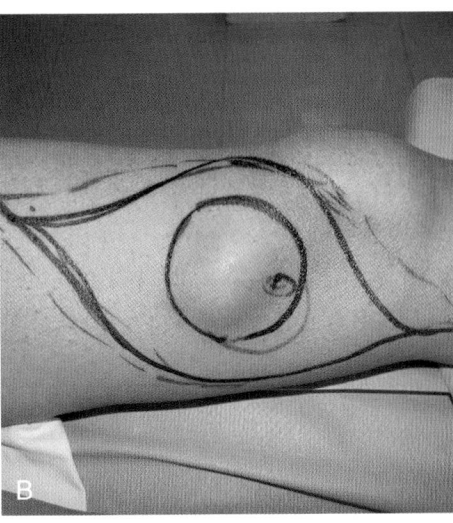

FIGURE 8 A, Axial magnetic resonance imaging of a superficial unclassified pleomorphic sarcoma. **B,** Planned wide skin incision around the visible mass to achieve adequate skin margin.

FIGURE 9 A, Axial magnetic resonance imaging of malignant solitary fibrous tumor of the thigh shows deep location. **B,** Because of its deep location, only a minimal skin paddle around biopsy tract is needed at resection.

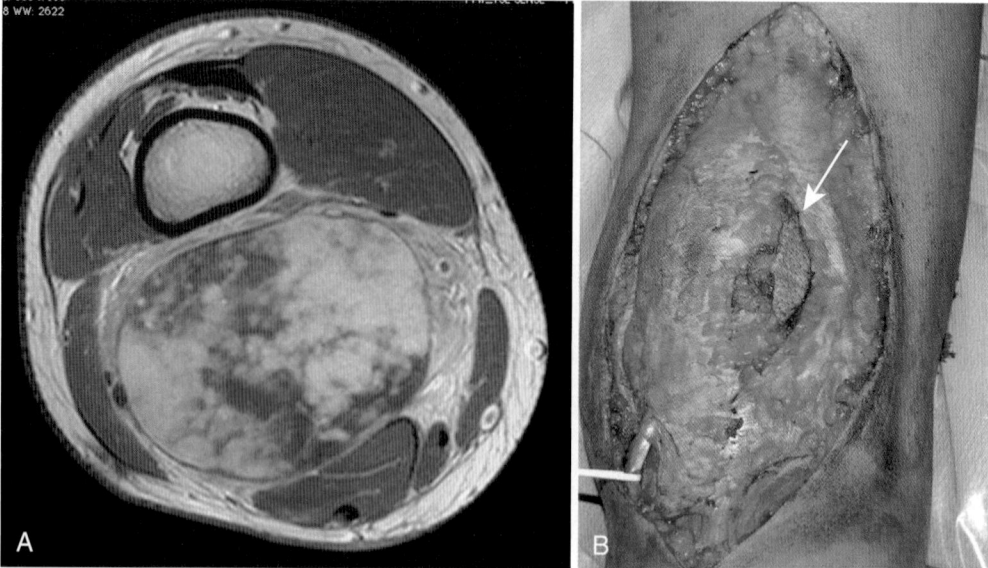

FIGURE 10 A, Axial magnetic resonance imaging of an unclassified pleomorphic sarcoma of the anterior compartment of the thigh partially encasing the femoral shaft. **B,** Intraoperative image shows periosteum stripped off en bloc with the tumor. **C,** Surgical specimen shows the deep margin over the bone *(arrow).*

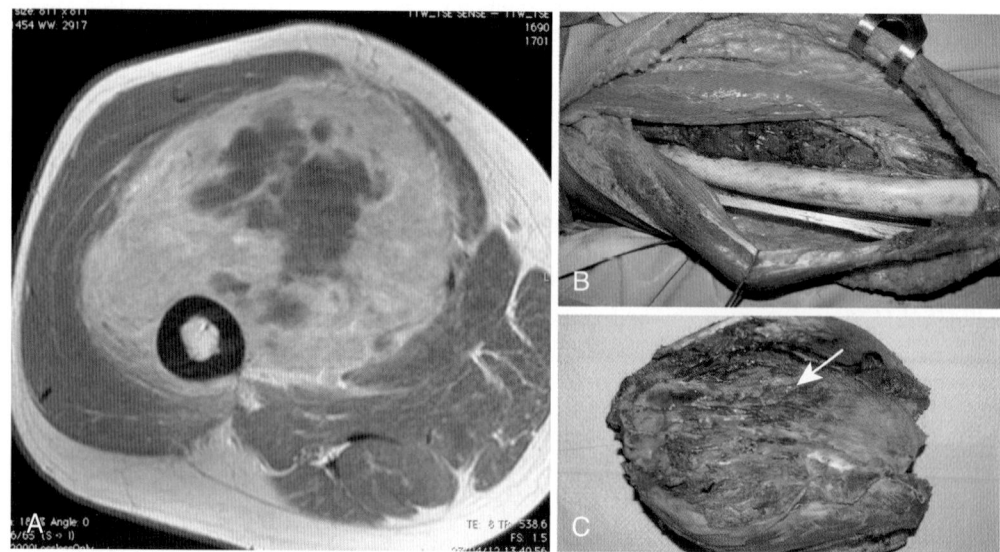

FIGURE 11 A, Axial magnetic resonance imaging of a monophasic synovial sarcoma of the thigh involving the femoral vessels *(arrow).* **B,** Intraoperative image of the surgical field with vascular replacement of both artery and vein.

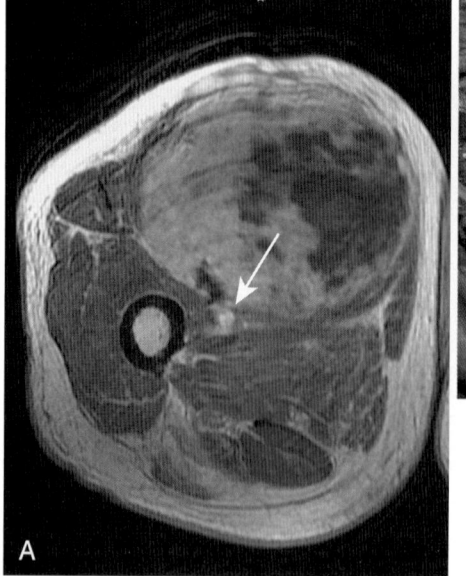
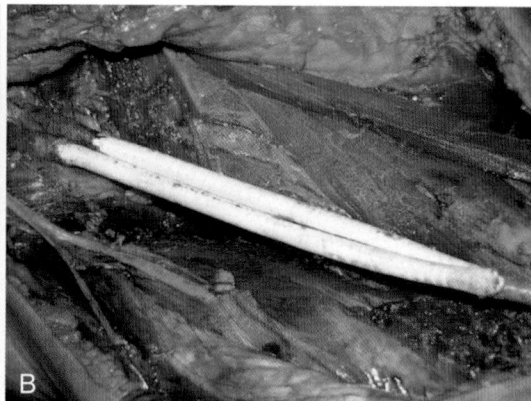

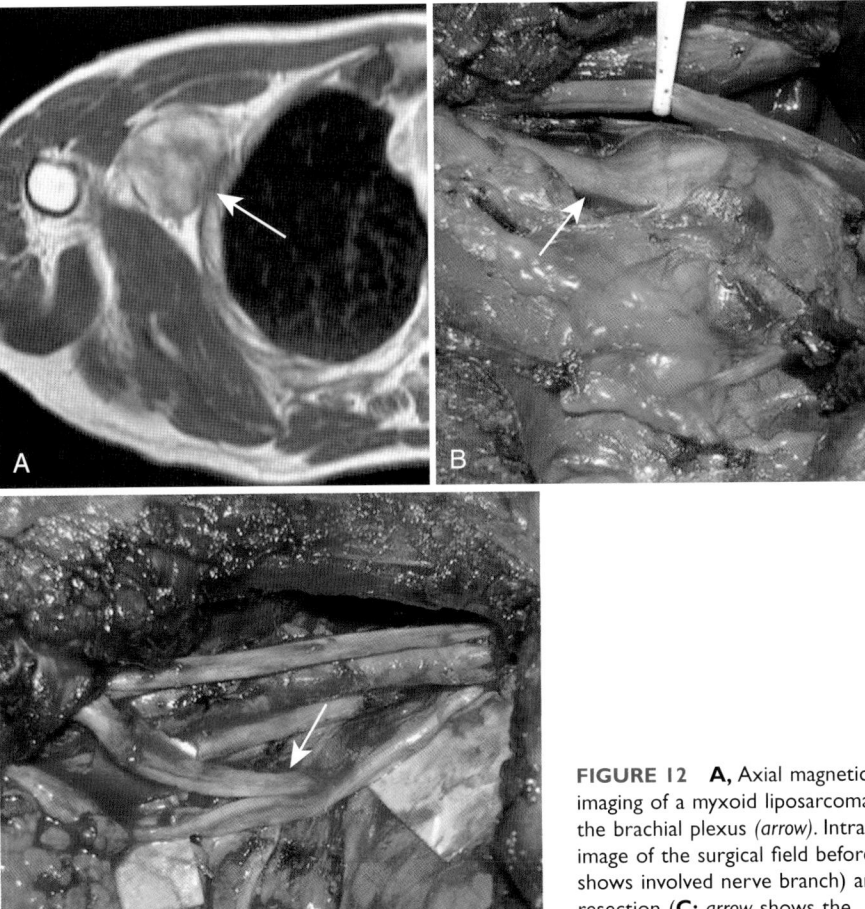

FIGURE 12   **A,** Axial magnetic resonance imaging of a myxoid liposarcoma involving the brachial plexus *(arrow)*. Intraoperative image of the surgical field before (**B**; *arrow* shows involved nerve branch) and after resection (**C**; *arrow* shows the reconstruction with autografts).

radiation therapy or in the setting of recurrent tumors, because ongoing serous drainage may continue for weeks after surgery. Flap reconstruction may be necessary for proper wound closure or if a large, potential dead space is left behind (especially if preoperative radiation therapy had been administered).

Adjuvant/Neoadjuvant Radiation Therapy and Chemotherapy

Limb-sparing surgery generally relies on adjuvant/neoadjuvant radiation therapy to minimize risk of local recurrence, as seen in the National Cancer Institute (NCI) trial. The goal of radiation is to treat the margin to minimize the risk of recurrence, not necessarily to reduce the size of the tumor per se. Radiation therapy reduces the risk of local recurrence from greater than 30% to less than 10% in most series but does not impact distant failure or overall survival.

Radiation therapy may be delivered as external beam radiation therapy (EBRT) or brachytherapy. EBRT may be delivered before or after surgery. One randomized trial, by O'Sullivan and colleagues and sponsored by the Canadian NCI, compared preoperative EBRT with postoperative EBRT. No difference was found in local recurrence rates. Preoperative EBRT was associated with a doubling in the rate of wound complications (35% vs 17%) but importantly with a lower rate of late complications and tissue fibrosis and better functional outcomes. Postoperative EBRT generally covers a larger field (including drain sites) and is higher dose than preoperative EBRT. This is particularly important in young adults of child-bearing age with proximal thigh STS; preoperative EBRT may spare the gonads, whereas postoperative radiation may not.

Brachytherapy may be delivered through afterloading catheters placed across the tumor bed at the end of surgery. The goal of brachytherapy is to deliver additional radiation to a close margin (including neurovascular structures) with minimal treatment to surrounding tissue, particularly when further EBRT is no longer feasible. When the final pathologic margins are confirmed, the appropriate catheters may be loaded with radioactive seeds once or twice a day for a defined treatment period concentrated over the close margins. To minimize wound complications, catheters should not be loaded until at least postoperative day 5. To minimize the risk of dislodging the catheters, any drains placed at the time of surgery should remain in place until the catheters have been removed.

Patients with small (<5 cm), superficial, well-circumscribed STS resected with an appropriately wide margin (>1 cm) of nonneoplastic tissue or biologic barrier (fascia) may not need radiation therapy, provided that they can be reliably followed.

Approximately 25% to 50% of patients with extremity STS have distant metastatic disease develop. Those with large (>10 cm), deep, high-grade STS may be considered for preoperative or postoperative chemotherapy, usually with active agents such as doxorubicin and ifosfamide (response rates of 20% to 40% in patients with metastatic disease). However, no consistently convincing data are found that such an approach improves overall survival for most STS histologies. Some data have suggested limited benefit for specific histologies, such as myxoid liposarcoma and synovial sarcoma, but no consensus exists amongst sarcoma experts about the routine use of chemotherapy in the adjuvant setting for extremity sarcomas.

Hyperthermic isolate limb perfusion (ILP) and infusion (ILI) have been investigated in several institutions as treatment for patients with locally advanced STS in whom limb-sparing, function-sparing surgery may not be possible. These procedures involve placement of vascular access catheters into the main artery and vein of the affected extremity and perfusion with high-dose chemotherapy (usually melphalan) and tumor necrosis factor-alpha under hyperthermic conditions. ILP is generally performed as an open procedure with cut down directly onto the vessels. ILI uses percutaneously placed catheters and is conducted in hypoxic conditions. Although both have proven efficacy in melanoma, the data for STS are more limited. No randomized trials have compared either technique with aggressive limb-sparing resection with EBRT for STS. Arguably, patients under consideration for ILP and ILI usually have locally advanced or multifocal STS and are not necessarily candidates for surgery with EBRT at first evaluation. ILP and ILI should be considered as potential therapies in appropriately selected patients, and eligible patients should be referred to centers where this therapy is available.

RETROPERITONEAL SOFT TISSUE SARCOMA

Clinical and Diagnostic Evaluation

Patients with retroperitoneal STS are often asymptomatic until the mass reaches a large size (often 15 cm or greater). Symptoms include a palpable mass, early satiety, abdominal discomfort, or occasionally a new varicocele in men. Others may be incidental findings during abdominal imaging for other reasons. Initial clinical evaluation should include a thorough history and physical examination, with attention directed to ruling out other diagnoses in the differential, including lymphoma, primary germ cell tumor, and testicular cancer metastatic to retroperitoneal lymph nodes (if male). Although no tumor markers are known for STS histologies at present, screening studies for other diagnoses include lactate dehydrogenase, human chorionic gonadotropin, and alpha fetoprotein. After a thorough examination, a CT scan of the abdomen and pelvis is indicated. Staging evaluation is completed with a chest CT scan. Routine head CT and PET scans are not needed.

Imaging alone is rarely diagnostic of the specific sarcoma histology, with the exception of well-differentiated liposarcoma. As described in the previous extremity STS section, well-differentiated liposarcomas have a radiographic density similar to normal surrounding fat but tend to be well-encapsulated with thick internal septations. Giant lipomas are only identified anecdotally in the retroperitoneum; therefore, any mass consisting of very well-differentiated fatty tissue should be considered as well-differentiated liposarcoma and treated as such (Figure 13). These tumors do not require a biopsy. Other lesions suspicious for retroperitoneal STS should be biopsied. The authors prefer to obtain core needle biopsies with radiographic guidance. Biopsy tract recurrences are exceedingly rare and biopsy tracts do not need to be reexcised during definitive surgery. Furthermore, if preoperative EBRT is planned, the biopsy site is usually included within the radiation field. Again, it is important to specify core needle biopsy rather than fine-needle aspiration because the latter rarely yields enough tissue and architecture information to distinguish between different sarcoma histologies.

Anatomic Features of Retroperitoneal Sarcomas

In patients with extremity STS, distant failure is a common pattern of recurrence. In contrast, retroperitoneal sarcomas (RPS) more commonly recur in a locoregional manner, and mortality in RPS is more often associated with locoregional recurrence. Proper resection of RPS requires appreciation of the anatomic boundaries of the

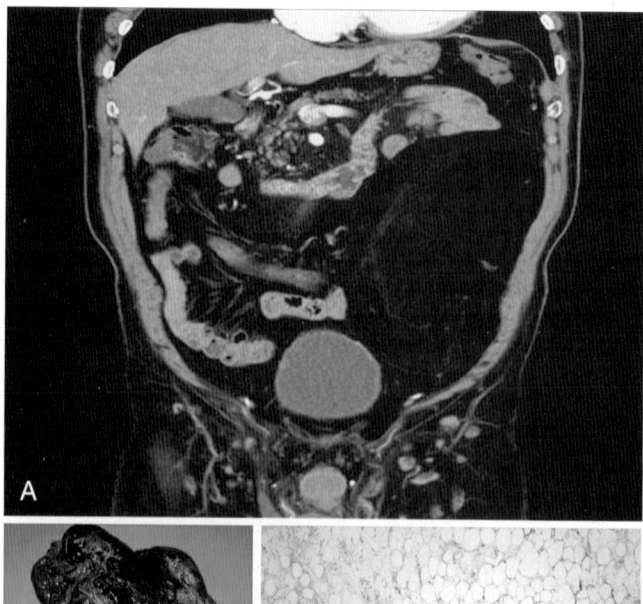

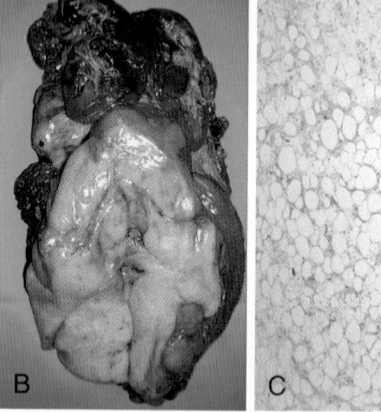
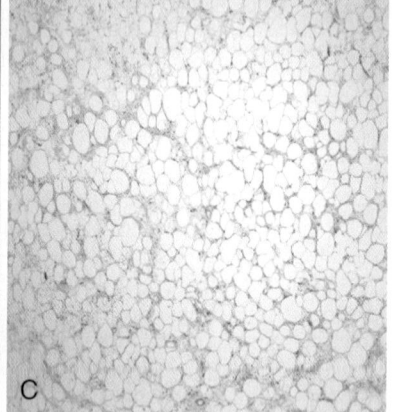

FIGURE 13   **A,** Coronal computed tomographic scan view of a left-sided retroperitoneal well-differentiated liposarcoma, together with **B,** macroscopic and **C,** microscopic appearance.

tumor. CT imaging should be reviewed to identify landmarks defining the extent of the mass to determine which structures may be safely resected and which ones cannot. The *anterior* margin of a RPS is generally the ipsilateral colon and mesocolon, pancreas, liver, or stomach. The *posterior* margin is generally the psoas and iliacus muscles inferiorly, the ipsilateral kidney and diaphragm superiorly, and the ipsilateral ureter and gonadal vessels medially. However, this may vary from tumor to tumor, and some or all of these structures could be anterior to the mass, in which case they constitute a portion of the anterior margin. The *medial* margin usually includes the spine and paraspinous muscles, the inferior vena cava (for right-sided tumors), and the aorta (for left-sided tumors). The *lateral* margin is constituted by the lateral or flank musculoskeletal sidewall, although depending on the size and location of the tumor, the kidney or colon could also border the lateral portion of the mass. The *superior* margin is similarly dependent on the size and location of the mass and may include the diaphragm on either side, the right lobe of the liver, the duodenum, and the head/uncinate process of the pancreas for right-sided tumors and pancreatic tail, spleen, and splenic vessels for left-sided tumors. The *inferior* margin may include the iliopsoas muscle; the femoral nerve; the common, internal, and external iliac vessels; and the pelvic sidewall. Clearly, the size and specific location of the mass determine which of the many structures mentioned constitute which specific margin.

In general, the ipsilateral kidney, colon, and mesocolon and at least a portion of the psoas can be safely and relatively easily resected without much difficulty. Resection of the pancreatic tail and spleen can usually be performed with relatively low short-term morbidity. Resection of other structures, including but not limited to the aorta, inferior vena cava, iliac vessels, femoral nerve, diaphragm, duodenum, pancreatic head or uncinate process, and liver, entail more significant resections, with ensuing greater morbidity.

Technical Aspects of Retroperitoneal Sarcoma Resection

Before surgery, contralateral renal function should be assessed with a nuclear scan if an ipsilateral nephrectomy is planned. Patients should undergo bowel preparation. Patients may be placed in either a supine or modified lateral decubitus position. The abdomen may be entered through a midline, oblique, flank, or thoracoabdominal incision, depending on the precise anatomic location. It is important to adjust the incision to the extent of tumor to provide optimal exposure.

The goal of surgery should be an aggressive multiorgan resection, with removal of involved or attached surrounding organs and retroperitoneal fat en bloc with the tumor in an effort to maximally clear the margins and avoid spilling tumor (Figures 14 and 15). Because of the size of the tumors, exposure and retraction may need to be

shifted periodically. Ideally, the operation is conducted with carefully circumferential dissection around the expected specimen, enabling systematic exposure on a broad front. It is important to approach surgery with curative intent. A macroscopically incomplete resection is no more beneficial than nonoperative management.

The resection specimen should be reviewed with the pathologist immediately after removal for orientation and identification of margins of concern.

Radiation Therapy

The role of radiation therapy is controversial, in the absence of phase III randomized controlled trial data. Radiation therapy unequivocally reduces the risk of local recurrence in patients with extremity STS, but this has not been proven in RPS. Furthermore, the proximity of radiosensitive tissues and organs, such as liver and small intestine, together with the large size of the radiation field limits its utility in some patients. Those who use radiation therapy generally favor delivering it before surgery, when the bulk of the tumor itself displaces uninvolved organs out of the radiation field. One ongoing randomized trial is evaluating the utility of preoperative radiation therapy in patients with RPS, based in Europe and open in selected North American centers.

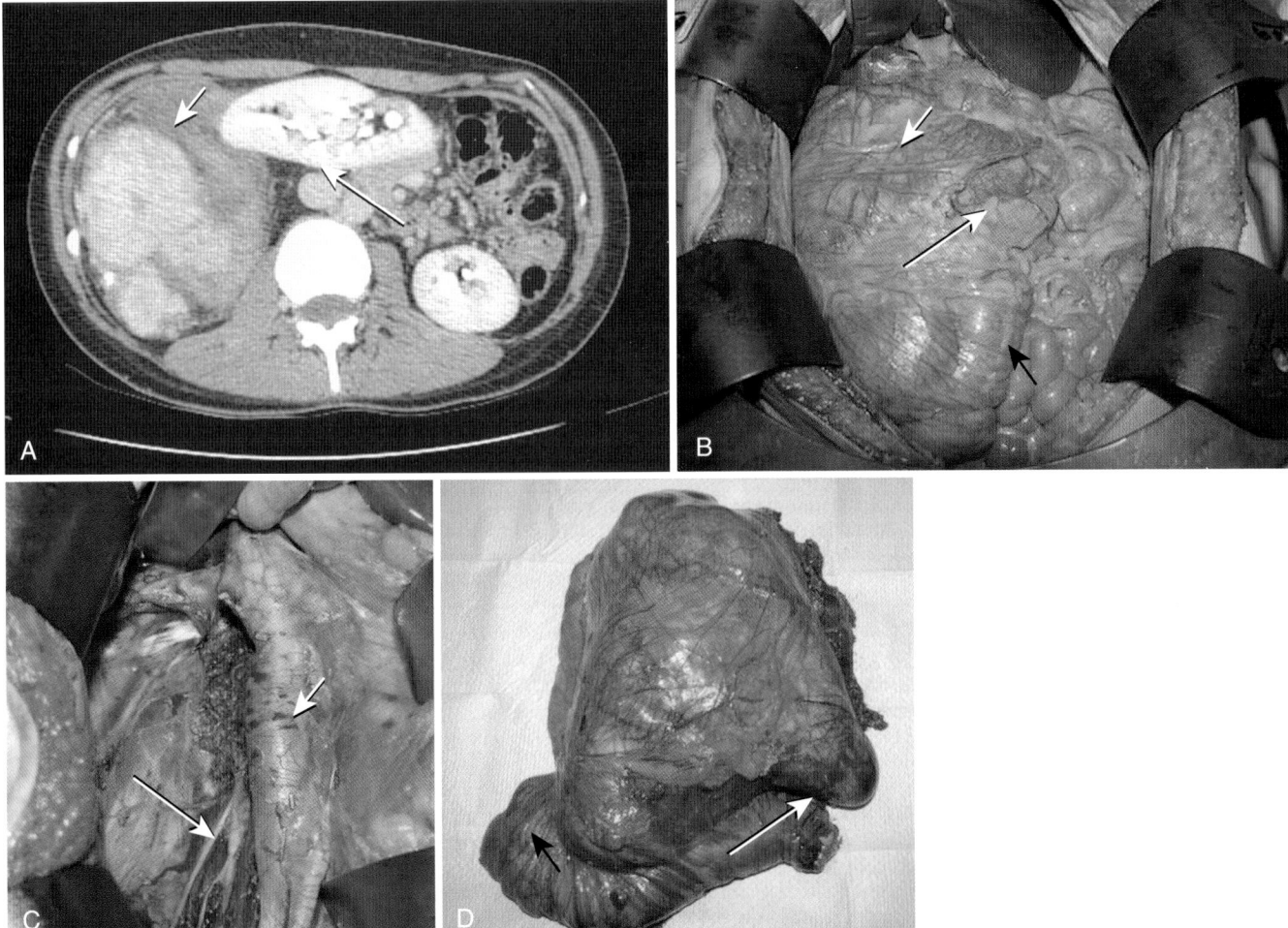

FIGURE 14   A, Axial computed tomographic scan image of a conventional right retroperitoneal liposarcoma *(short white arrow)* displacing the right kidney anteriomedially *(long white arrow)*. **B,** Intraoperative image of the same right retroperitoneal sarcoma *(short white arrow)* with the kidney displaced anteromedially *(long white arrow)* and the right colon displaced medially *(short black arrow)*. **C,** Surgical field after tumor removal shows a clean right retroperitoneal space with visible femoral nerve roots *(long white arrow)* after psoas resection and exposed inferior vena cava. **D,** Surgical specimen including right colon *(short black arrow)* and right kidney *(long white arrow)*; psoas not shown, but present.

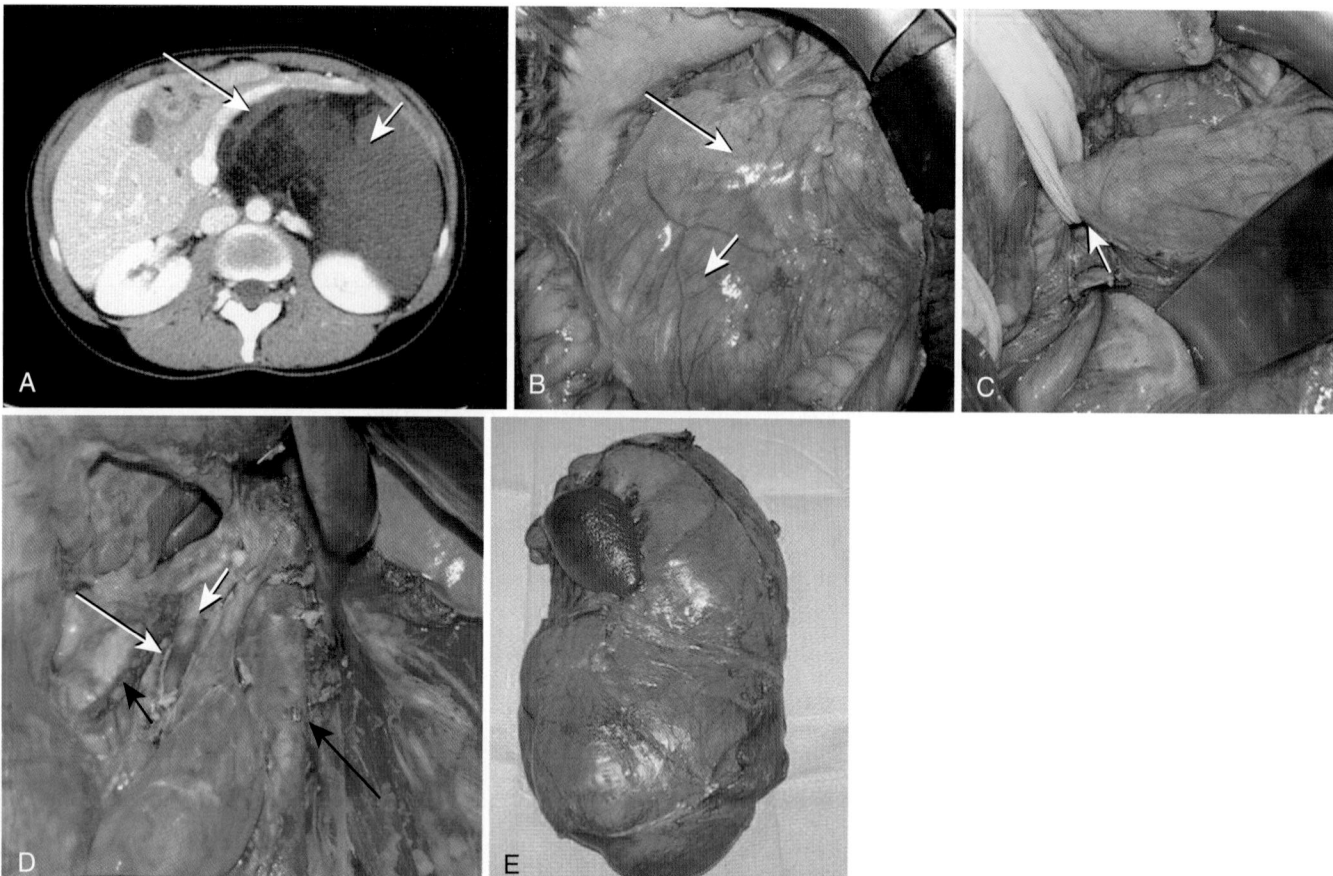

FIGURE 15 **A,** Axial computed tomographic scan and **B,** intraoperative image of a conventional left retroperitoneal liposarcoma *(short white arrow)* displacing the pancreas anteriorly *(long white arrow)*. **C,** Preparation of pancreatic body for transaction *(white arrow)*. **D,** Surgical field after tumor removal shows a clean right retroperitoneal space with visible portal vein *(long white arrow)*, superior mesenteric artery *(short white arrow)*, pancreatic stump *(short black arrow)*, and aorta *(long black arrow)*. **E,** Surgical specimen including left colon, left kidney, left psoas, distal pancreas, and spleen.

BREAST SARCOMA

The most common sarcoma histologies arising in the breast are angiosarcoma and phyllodes. Angiosarcoma may arise either primarily within the breast parenchyma or secondarily within the breast skin as a consequence of lymphedema or more commonly radiation therapy delivered as a part of breast conservation therapy for breast cancer. Each of these malignancies is considered individually.

Primary Angiosarcoma

Primary angiosarcoma is a disease of the breast parenchyma that arises in young women. Angiosarcoma, irrespective of site, is in general responsive to systemic chemotherapy. However, once chemotherapy is stopped, the disease tends to regrow. Furthermore, despite its sensitivity to chemotherapy, there is no proven survival benefit from systemic therapy. The only potentially curative therapy is surgery. Although breast cancer may be treated with breast conservation limited surgery because of the proven benefit of radiation therapy and hormonal therapy, no such proven beneficial adjuvant therapies are found for primary breast angiosarcoma. Therefore, patients should be offered a simple mastectomy instead of lumpectomy. Partial resection of pectoralis major may be necessary to achieve negative margins. The skin may be closed primarily. Before surgery, the patient should undergo staging with a chest, abdomen, and pelvic CT scan and MRI of the breast. Initial physical examination should include a contralateral breast examination. The

contralateral breast may be a site for metastatic disease, but to date, a contralateral prophylactic mastectomy has no proven benefit.

Secondary Breast Angiosarcoma

Secondary breast angiosarcoma is a disease that affects older women. Historically, secondary angiosarcoma arose in the setting of lymphedema. Now, it is more commonly seen as a consequence of radiation therapy. Radiation therapy-associated angiosarcoma is a cutaneous malignancy that may extend into breast parenchyma, whereas primary angiosarcoma is a disease of the breast parenchyma. Thus, the operation for secondary angiosarcoma is different than that for primary angiosarcoma. Patients with secondary radiation therapy-associated angiosarcoma should undergo not only a total mastectomy but, more importantly, resection of the affected organ—all of the breast skin. This disease is often multifocal, and therefore, as much of the irradiated skin should be removed en bloc with the breast as possible. This is critical; a simple mastectomy alone does not remove the organ (skin) involved, and recurrences may be noted within weeks to months. If tumor extends to pectoralis major, then the muscle should be removed as well. All patients need extensive reconstruction, including skin grafting, just to restore a flat, closed chest wall. Preoperative staging should include MRI of the breast and a CT scan of the chest, abdomen, and pelvis. Follow-up imaging should include CT scan of the chest, abdomen, and pelvis. MRI of the chest wall is not usually necessary because local recurrences are often apparent on clinical examination alone.

Phyllodes Tumor

Phyllodes tumors of the breast can grow to be quite large. Surgery alone is the primary therapy. Tumors should be resected with a negative margin; for smaller tumors, a lumpectomy may be possible, but for larger tumors, a simple mastectomy may be necessary. Lymph node biopsy is not necessary. Recurrences may be observed in approximately 15% of patients, including local recurrences in the ipsilateral breast and distant recurrences in locations such as lung and liver. Contralateral breast recurrences are exceedingly rare; thus, contralateral prophylactic mastectomy is not indicated.

DESMOID FIBROMATOSIS

Desmoid fibromatosis is a nonmetastatic neoplasm that displays malignant local behavior. Desmoids may arise in the context of familial adenomatous polyposis (FAP), concurrent with a pregnancy or sporadically. Those that arise in the context of FAP may be quite aggressive, often involving the bowel mesentery and occasionally encasing the mesenteric vessels. In fact, local complications secondary to desmoids are the most common cause of death after colon cancer in individuals with FAP. Those that arise during pregnancy may grow during pregnancy, but often this growth stabilizes postpartum.

Recently, there has been a trend towards less radical surgery and more nonoperative management. The natural history of desmoids may vary, and some tumors may stop growing or even shrink without intervention. Therefore, nonoperative management is justifiable, particularly for tumors situated in difficult locations. Systemic therapy, including cytotoxic intravenous chemotherapy with different agents and schedules, oral tyrosine kinase inhibitors, nonsteroidal antiinflammatory drugs, and hormonal agents such as tamoxifen, has varying degrees of efficacy (Figure 16).

When surgery is undertaken, it is important to avoid compromising function when possible. Mesenteric desmoids may be particularly problematic to resect, especially those associated with FAP, and surgery should be approached with caution. Systemic therapy with cytotoxic intravenous chemotherapy may be effective in shrinking the tumor sufficiently to avoid extensive bowel resection. Wide margins are usually not possible. Extraabdominal desmoids may be more easily resected, but again, achieving wide margins may be challenging, given the infiltrative nature of these tumors. Reconstruction is often necessary.

METASTATIC DISEASE

Unlike adenocarcinomas, STS rarely spread to lymph nodes (<5%). Consequently, sentinel lymph node biopsy (SLNB) and lymphadenectomy are rarely indicated. However, SLNB may be considered in patients with sarcomas known to have a higher propensity for lymph node spread (epithelioid sarcoma, clear cell sarcoma). Importantly, SNLB has no proven therapeutic or long-term survival benefit.

Patients with distant metastatic disease should undergo systemic therapy. Doxorubicin and ifosfamide are two of the most effective agents in STS and may be used in combination. Doxorubicin dosing is limited lifetime by risk of cardiotoxicity. A liposomal formulation of doxorubicin does not seem to have a similar risk. Paclitaxel, gemcitabine, vinorelbine, and dacarbazine, and in Europe, trabectedin (also known as ET743), are additional agents with activity in sarcoma. In general, although response rates are approximately 20% at best, some histologies do have higher response rates to certain agents. For instance, vascular tumors such as angiosarcoma respond to taxanes and gemcitabine, leiomyosarcoma to dacarbazine and trabectedin, and liposarcoma to trabectedin.

Targeted therapies, similar to imatinib mesylate in gastrointestinal stromal tumors, are under investigation. The only established targeted therapy at present is imatinib in DFSP (in this circumstance, it

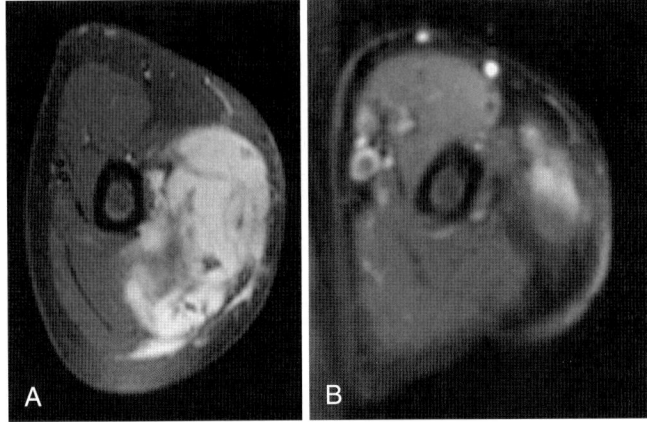

FIGURE 16 Axial magnetic resonance imaging of proximal thigh desmoid-type fibromatosis treated with chemotherapy (specifically, methotraxate plus vinorelbine for 45 cycles over 21 months): **A,** before and **B,** after chemotherapy.

is only rarely needed because DFSP is a surgical disease with a very high cure rate).

SUMMARY

Soft tissue sarcomas may arise in a variety of body sites and within a variety of tissues. The management of STS requires a thorough understanding of the biology of the different histologies. Limb-sparing and function-sparing approaches should be used when feasible, but extent of surgery should not be compromised for ease of closure. Margins of resection and use of adjuvant radiation therapy and chemotherapy are contingent on accurate histologic diagnosis. However, adjuvant therapy after a marginal resection is not an appropriate substitute for a margin negative operation. Treatment planning should include multidisciplinary consultation to determine optimal therapy, taking into consideration the site and extent of the disease, its natural history and sensitivity to available treatments, surgical challenges, and of course, the wishes of the patient.

SUGGESTED READINGS

Ardoino I, Miceli R, Berselli M, et al: Histology-specific nomogram for primary retroperitoneal soft tissue sarcoma, *Cancer* 116(10):2429–2436, 2010.

Bonvalot S, Raut CP, Pollock RE, et al: Technical considerations in surgery for retroperitoneal sarcomas: position paper from E-Surge, a master class in sarcoma surgery, and EORTC-STBSG, *Ann Surg Oncol* 19(9):2981–2991, 2012.

Enneking WF, Spanier SS, Goodman MA: A system for the surgical staging of musculoskeletal sarcoma, *Clin Orthop Relat Res* (153):106–120, 1980.

Haglund KE, Raut CP, Nascimento AF, et al: Recurrence patterns and survival for patients with intermediate- and high-grade myxofibrosarcoma, *Int J Radiat Oncol Biol Phys* 82(1):361–367, 2012.

Kattan MW, Leung DH, Brennan MF: Postoperative nomogram for 12-year sarcoma-specific death, *J Clin Oncol* 20(3):791–796, 2002.

Nascimento AF, Raut CP: Diagnosis and management of pleomorphic sarcomas (so-called "MFH") in adults, *J Surg Oncol* 97(4):330–339, 2008.

Raut CP, George S, Hornick JL, et al: High rates of histopathologic discordance in sarcoma with implications for clinical care, *Proc Am Soc Clin Oncol* 29(suppl), 2011, abstract 10065.

Rosenberg SA, Tepper J, Glatstein E, et al: The treatment of soft-tissue sarcomas of the extremities: prospective randomized evaluations of (1) limb-sparing surgery plus radiation therapy compared with amputation and (2) the role of adjuvant chemotherapy, *Ann Surg* 196(3):305–315, 1982.

Sanfilippo R, Miceli R, Grosso F, et al: Myxofibrosarcoma: prognostic factors and survival in a series of patients treated at a single institution, *Ann Surg Oncol* 18(3):720–725, 2011.

Evaluation of the Isolated Neck Mass

Philip W. Smith, MD, and John B. Hanks, MD

OVERVIEW

An isolated neck mass is a common clinical scenario in patients of all ages. Management varies widely with the many etiologies. Success in this scenario requires familiarity with cervical anatomy, an organized approach to differential diagnosis, and a stepwise evaluation as summarized in Figure 1. Tissue acquisition for diagnosis often is required, and surgical treatment is indicated for many etiologies of neck mass. Therefore, the prepared surgeon is well positioned to play a central role in the clinical evaluation, diagnostic workup, and management of neck masses.

Although benign thyroid nodules are common and thyroid malignancy is an important consideration for neck masses, thyroid lesions are addressed elsewhere in this text.

DIFFERENTIAL DIAGNOSIS

The differential diagnosis of the isolated neck mass is broad and includes congenital, inflammatory, and neoplastic processes (Box 1.) Between 2% and 9% of head and neck cancers present as cervical masses without a known primary. Although malignancy must be considered in all cases of neck mass, the likelihood varies significantly with age. In the pediatric population, less than 10% of neck masses are neoplastic, whereas as many as 80% of neck masses that occur outside of the thyroid are neoplastic in adults over the age of 40 years.

WORKUP

History

The clinical history gives indications as to the likelihood that a given neck mass is benign or malignant. The importance of patient age was highlighted previously. Other history items that raise the probability of malignancy include a known personal history of malignancy, strong family history of malignancy, smoking or other tobacco use, heavy alcohol use, sun exposure, and radiation exposure. Neck-specific history items that are concerning for malignancy include persistent mass, dysphagia, hoarseness or other neurologic deficit, epistaxis, and radiating pain, including otalgia. Constitutional symptoms such as sweats, fevers, fatigue, and weight loss are concerning for lymphoma or other malignancy but also may be present with infectious etiologies. Rapidly developing tender masses are often infectious or inflammatory.

One also should ask about prior treatments, biopsies, and surgical interventions. More often in children, but also in adults, lymphadenopathy may already have been treated with antibiotics. Persistence of lymphadenopathy after antibiotics should be considered concerning for malignancy. Retrieval of relevant prior imaging, operative reports, pathology reports, and pathology specimens is imperative whenever possible.

A history of severe or episodic hypertension rarely may be associated with a head and neck paraganglioma, although only a small minority of head and neck paragangliomas are functional. A history of cough with pressure on the mass has been associated with schwannoma of the vagus nerve. This can be confirmed with palpation on physical examination.

Physical Examination

A thorough physical examination is warranted in all cases of neck mass. On general examination, one should note presence of cachexia and stigmata of alcoholism or tobacco abuse. Examination of skin, lungs, and abdomen may provide clues as to a primary source of metastatic disease to the neck. Axillary and femoral lymph node basins should be examined and may be revealing in a systemic disease process. General examination also helps the surgeon understand a patient's general fitness to tolerate medical and surgical interventions. The clinician also should seek any prior incisions that indicate diagnostic or therapeutic interventions that the patient may have neglected to describe.

Patients and even referring physicians may commonly mistake normal structures for pathology. Such structures may include ptotic salivary glands, the horn of the thyroid cartilage, the hyoid bone, or spinal transverse processes (particularly C2). Therefore, examination of the neck should first confirm the presence of a pathologic finding. If an abnormality is present, a detailed examination ensues. The mass should be measured in at least two dimensions with a tape measure and documentation of the findings. Photographs for the medical record may also be valuable. The location of the mass should be precisely defined. The location should be defined not only in a descriptive fashion relative to normal anatomy (e.g., "at the anterior border of the sternocleidomastoid muscle [SCM] at the level of the cricothyroid") but also by the nodal level based on the system outlined in Figure 2 and Table 1. This system of nodal levels is of value for several reasons: (1) it allows reproducible communication between caregivers and relevant boundaries with physical examination, imaging, and operative anatomy; (2) nodal levels are diagnostically important because malignancies of different origins spread characteristically to different nodal levels (see Table 1); and (3) lymph node levels are important therapeutically because lymph node dissection typically proceeds based on nodal level compartment based dissection.

Other important examination findings include firmness, tenderness, symmetry to the contralateral neck, and fixation to surrounding structures. Neurologic function also should be evaluated, including cranial nerve (CN) function. This evaluation should include facial symmetry (marginal mandibular branch of the facial nerve/CN VII), voice (superior and recurrent laryngeal branches of the vagus nerve/CN X), atrophy and function of the SCM and trapezius (spinal accessory/CN XI), tongue deviation (hypoglossal nerve/CN XII), symmetric air movement (phrenic nerve), and neural and sensory upper extremity function (brachial plexus). Physical examination findings that are concerning for malignancy include firmness, fixation to surrounding tissue, unilateralism, and neurologic deficit.

All other aspects of the neck also should be examined, including the thyroid, salivary glands, and all nodal basins. Visualization of the mucosal surfaces of the upper aerodigestive tract is important, as is evaluation of the skin of the head and neck, including the scalp and auditory canal. Palpation with the gloved hand, including bimanual palpation of the floor of the mouth, may help with identification of abnormalities that exist deep to normal-appearing mucosa. Examination of dentition also is important because dental infection can lead to cervical lymphadenopathy.

With appropriate training, mirror examination or flexible fiberoptic laryngoscopy allows significantly improved visualization and can be performed in the office setting. Evaluation of all mucosal surfaces is possible, from the nasal cavity to the vocal cords. The location of the neck lesion that is concerning for metastatic

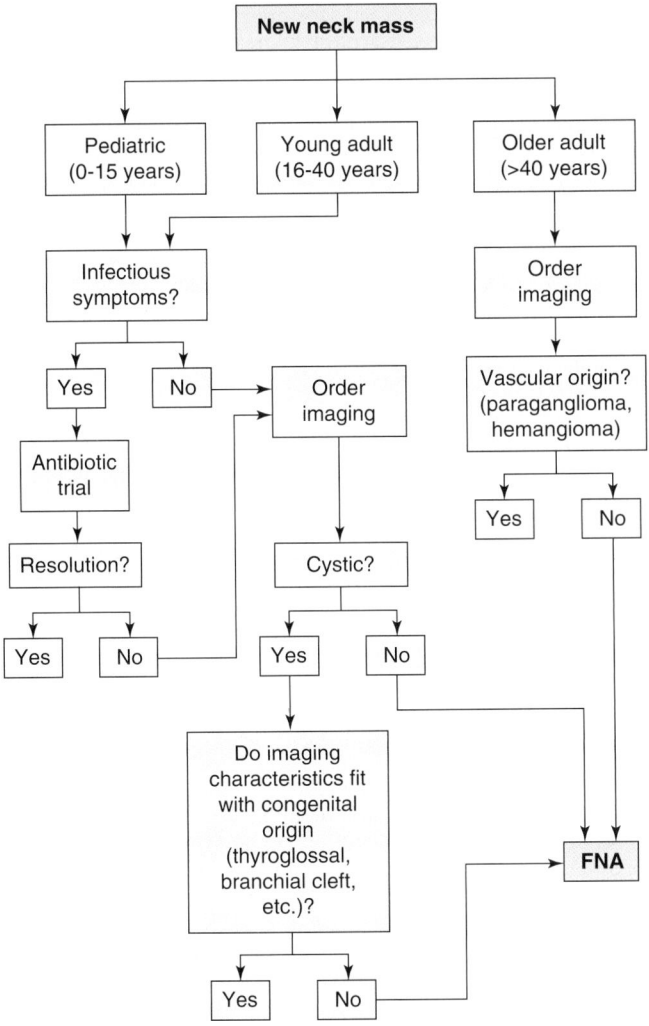

FIGURE 1 Diagnostic algorithm for a new neck mass. The distinction made based on age of 40 years should be taken as a general guideline to be adjusted based on clinical evaluation and not as an absolute rule. *FNA*, Fine-needle aspiration. *(Adapted from Flint PW, Haughey BH, Lund VJ, et al:, editors:* Cummings otolaryngology: head & neck surgery, *ed 5, Philadelphia, 2010, Elsevier, Fig. 166-2.)*

BOX 1: Differential diagnosis of neck masses

Developmental
Inclusion cyst
Thyroglossal duct cyst
Congenital vascular malformations
Branchial cleft cyst
Cystic hygroma
Laryngocele
Teratoma
Bronchogenic cyst

Infectious
Bacterial lymphadenitis (*Staphylococcus aureus, Streptococcus pyogenes, Bartonella, Brucella*)
Viral (Ebstein-Barr, HIV, other common viruses)
Protozoal (toxoplasmosis, leishmaniasis)
Fungal (histoplasmosis, blastomycosis, coccidioidomycosis)

Other Miscellaneous
Sialadenitis, sialolithiasis
Sjögren's syndrome
Sarcoidosis
Aneurysm

Benign Neoplasia
Lipoma
Thyroid nodule/diffuse goiter
Parathyroid adenoma (rarely palpable)
Fibroma
Neurofibroma
Sebaceous cyst
Benign salivary tumors (pleomorphic adenoma, Warthin's tumor)

Malignancies
Lymphoma
Carotid body tumor
Thyroid cancer
Malignant salivary tumors (mucoepidermoid, adenoid cystic)
Parathyroid cancer
Plasmacytoma
Carcinoid
Metastasis to cervical lymph nodes (thyroid, squamous cell carcinoma, adenocarcinoma, melanoma)

lymphadenopathy helps to determine the most likely primary sites and so can guide this evaluation. Attention should be paid to all visible surfaces, especially the lymphoid region of the nasopharynx, base of the tongue, and oropharynx (Waldeyer's ring). This evaluation also allows assessment of potential airway difficulties for future surgical interventions.

Two congenital lesions are worth highlighting for their specific physical examination findings. The first is a thyroglossal duct cyst. These cysts occur along the thyroglossal tract between the thyroid and the base of the tongue. They may become infected, which leads to presentation with typical inflammatory symptoms and frequently follows an upper respiratory infection, or they may present as an asymptomatic mass. Most are diagnosed before adulthood, but initial presentation in adults is not uncommon. Thyroglossal duct cysts are found in or near the midline of the neck and typically just below the hyoid bone. Protrusion of the tongue typically results in cephalad movement of the mass. This feature may be more easily appreciable by first applying slight inferior digital pressure on the mass before tongue protrusion. Thyroglossal duct cysts may create a mass effect or develop recurrent infection, and about 1% harbor malignancy. Therefore, when these cysts are found, excision of the cyst, pyramidal

lobe if present, and the tract up to the base of the tongue including the central portion of the hyoid bone is indicated (the Sistrunk procedure). Confirmation of the presence of normal thyroid tissue in the thyroid bed with examination or imaging before excision is important.

The other group of congenital lesions is branchial cleft cysts. Similar to thyroglossal duct cysts, these may present in an inflamed fashion after an upper respiratory infection. These cysts are almost always diagnosed before age 20 years and account for 20% of pediatric neck masses. First branchial cleft cysts present inferior to the auricle or just below the angle of the mandible. These may communicate with the auditory canal and may be closely associated with the facial nerve. Second branchial cleft cysts are the most common (95%). They are found inferior to the angle of the mandible on the anterior border of the SCM and communicate with the tonsillar fossae. Third branchial cleft cysts also present on the anterior border of the SCM, lower than a second cleft cyst, and communicate with the pharynx at the thyrohyoid membrane or piriform sinus. Branchial cleft cysts and their tracts are typically excised with care given to the relationship of these tracts to cranial nerves and other deep structures.

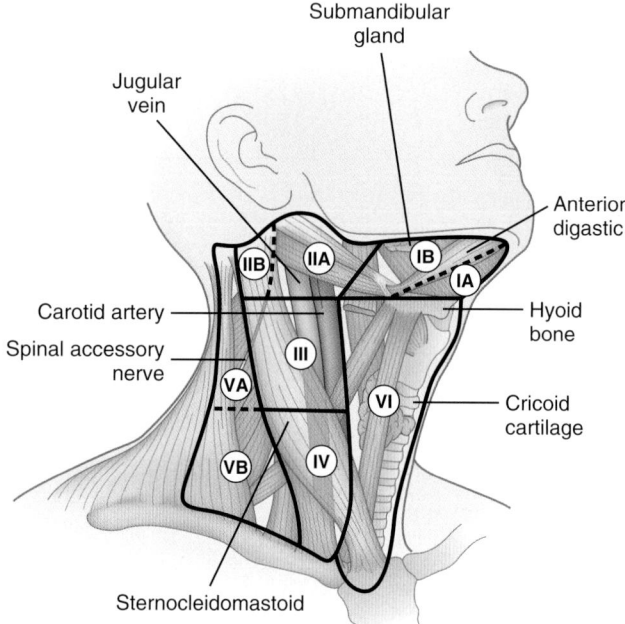

FIGURE 2 Numbered lymph node levels of the neck. Boundaries are given in Box 1. Criteria exist to define these levels clinically, radiographically, and surgically. *(From Townsend CM Jr, Beauchamp RD, Evers BM, et al: Sabiston: Textbook of surgery, ed 19, Philadelphia, 2012, Fig. 38-3.)*

Imaging

Imaging may be valuable at several steps in the evaluation and management of a neck mass. It can be valuable in characterizing the primary lesion, in searching for a primary source of a metastasis, and in follow-up after an intervention. Communication with radiologists before a study helps ensure that the optimal study and protocol are performed and maximizes information garnered from each study.

Anteroposterior (A/P) and lateral chest radiographs should be obtained if concern exists that the neck mass is related to an atypical infectious or inflammatory source and in those with history of cough or travel. Chest imaging also is indicated for those masses whose location and biopsy findings are concerning for a thoracic primary malignancy, such as lung cancer, and for patients with a new diagnosis of cancer to evaluate for pulmonary metastasis. Abnormalities identified on chest film often require a computed tomographic (CT) scan of the chest for further delineation.

Ultrasound scan can serve as an extension of the physical examination during the initial office evaluation of the mass. Alternately, formal radiology-performed ultrasound scan may be used. Ultrasound scan allows precise measurements of size and definition of the relationship to normal anatomy, distinguishes cystic from solid lesions, allows assessment of vascularity, and may help distinguish whether the mass is invasive into surrounding structures. Ultrasound scan also allows characterization of lymph nodes based on features other than just size, which can help distinguish benign from pathologic adenopathy; this ability exceeds that possible with CT scan. Ultrasonographic features that suggest malignancy include loss of the normal hyperechoic fatty hilum, hyperechogenicity or hypoechogenicity, cystic degeneration, punctuate calcifications, unclear borders with surrounding structures, and perinodal edema (Figure 3). Ultrasound scan also is ideal for evaluation of thyroid nodules and has the advantage of not exposing the patient to ionizing radiation or intravenous contrast.

CT scan of the neck requires ionizing radiation to the thyroid and is most valuable if performed with intravenous contrast. Contrast may be contraindicated because of renal disease or allergy and may

impair delivery of radioactive iodine therapy in the case of thyroid pathologies. Despite this, contrast CT scan is an excellent and widely available imaging modality and is superior to ultrasound scan in providing three-dimensional resolution of the anatomy of the lesion and evidence of invasion or distortion of normal anatomy. Also, if the presenting lesion is thought to be nodal metastasis from a head and neck primary malignancy, high-quality CT scan of the head and neck can identify a primary source in 20% of cases. Therefore, contrast CT scan of the head and neck is valuable and is indicated in many neck masses in which the diagnosis or primary source is not already defined. This scan should encompass at least the region from the skull base to the aortic arch.

Magnetic resonance imaging (MRI) is helpful in some situations and often is better than CT scan in defining the presence or absence of invasion by the mass into surrounding structures, particularly vascular and neural structures. It may also be helpful in patients with significant dental artifact, in pregnant patients, in those with iodinated contrast reactions, and in those in whom iodinated contrast is undesirable because of expected future need for therapeutic radioiodine therapy. MRI is helpful in the diagnosis and evaluation of carotid body tumors, glomus tumors, and schwannomas. Outside of these scenarios, MRI is not routinely indicated for initial evaluation of neck mass.

The role of positron emission tomography (PET) or fusion imaging of PET with CT scan (PET/CT) continues to be elucidated. PET and PET/CT are not appropriate first-line studies for the initial evaluation of a neck mass. However, PET is an appropriate secondary imaging technique for patients who are being evaluated for a metastatic squamous cell carcinoma of unknown primary when CT scan or MRI have been unrevealing. On the basis of specific pathologies, PET and PET/CT also may be appropriate for further workup once a diagnosis has been made or for the monitoring of a patient being followed for malignancy. However, a PET may commonly be obtained for other reasons, and a PET avid lesion may be discovered that is distinct from the primary process. The clinician must then evaluate whether this lesion represents a neoplasm or whether this is a false-positive finding resulting from other hypermetabolic conditions (infection, inflammatory process). This process should proceed similarly to a neck mass discovered on clinical grounds. Remember that PET is not specific for malignancy; inflammation, infection, and muscle activity can lead to false-positive results.

With improvements in the capabilities of CT scan and MRI, diagnostic arteriography is rarely necessary for neck masses. Arteriography may be indicated therapeutically, particularly for embolization of some highly vascular lesions before resection.

Tissue Diagnosis

The presence of an isolated neck mass in an adult over age 40 years should be considered malignant until proven otherwise. These masses frequently are metastatic squamous cell carcinomas from the upper aerodigestive tract. Fine-needle aspiration (FNA) biopsy plays a central role in the diagnostic evaluation of neck masses and should be considered the standard of care in undiagnosed adult neck masses. FNA can be performed with simple equipment, is widely available, is generally safe, and is diagnostic in 90% or more of cases. Samples can be evaluated both for pathology and for microbiology depending on the clinical scenario. Risks associated with this procedure including bleeding and sampling error.

Readily palpable lesions may be amenable to simple manual biopsy, but ultrasound scan is now readily available and real-time ultrasound guidance should most often be used to decrease risk and increase diagnostic yield. In cases of a cystic lymph node, ultrasound scan should be used to ensure that the wall is sampled. Ultrasound guidance also helps to avoid needle biopsy of vascular lesions that are mistaken as a solid mass with examination if imaging is not already completed.

TABLE 1: Boundaries of cervical lymph node levels and considerations for primary site for metastatic disease

	Boundaries and contents	Metastatic primary sites
Level I	Submandibular and submental nodes. Bounded by the mandible superiorly, the midline anteriorly, the hyoid inferiorly, and the stylohyoid muscle posteriorly. Subdivided into IA and IB by the anterior belly of the digastric muscle. IA crosses the midline to the contralateral anterior belly of the digastric.	IA: Floor of mouth, lower lip, anterior tongue, lower gum. IB: Oral cavity, anterior nasal cavity, submandibular gland, midface soft tissues.
Level II	Upper jugular nodes. Bounded by the skull base superiorly, the stylohyoid muscle anteriorly, the inferior border of the hyoid bone inferiorly, and the posterior border of the SCM posteriorly. Subdivided into IIA and IIB by the spinal accessory nerve.	Oral cavity, nasal cavity, nasopharynx, oropharynx, hypopharynx, larynx, parotid gland.
Level III	Middle jugular nodes. Bounded by the inferior border of the hyoid bone superiorly, the sternohyoid muscle anteriorly, the inferior border of the cricoid cartilage inferiorly, and the posterior border of the SCM posteriorly.	Oral cavity, nasopharynx, oropharynx, hypopharynx, larynx, cervical esophagus, thyroid.
Level IV	Lower jugular nodes. Bounded by the inferior border of the cricoid cartilage superiorly, the sternohyoid muscle anteriorly, the clavicle inferiorly, and the posterior border of the SCM posteriorly.	Hypopharynx, thyroid, cervical esophagus, larynx, Virchow's node (lung or abdominal malignancy).
Level V	Posterior triangle nodes. Bounded by the junction of the trapezius and SCM superiorly, the posterior border of the SCM anteriorly, the clavicle inferiorly, and the anterior border of the trapezius laterally. Subdivided into VA and VB by the plane of the inferior border of the cricoid cartilage.	Nasopharynx, oropharynx, thyroid, cutaneous structures of scalp and neck, breast.
Level VI	Also known as the central compartment. Pretracheal, precricoid (Delphian), paratracheal nodes, and parathyroidal nodes. Bounded by the hyoid bone superiorly, the carotid sheath laterally, and the sternum inferiorly.	Thyroid, glottic and subglottic larynx, piriform sinus, cervical esophagus.
Level VII (variably defined)	This level is variably defined and is the substernal extension of level VI to the level of the innominate artery.	Similar to level VI.

SCM, Sternocleidomastoid muscle.

FNA typically can be performed on an outpatient basis. Because multiple passes should be taken, the use of local anesthetic is suggested. If manual palpation guidance is used, the mass should be transfixed between the thumb and forefinger of the nondominant hand. If ultrasound scan is used, a 12.5-MHz probe is appropriate in most cases (Figure 4). The needle should be passed along the long axis of the probe at an oblique angle so that the entire needle course can be imaged in real time. Needle guides are available with some ultrasound equipment and may be used if desired. A 22-gauge to 25-gauge needle is affixed to a 10-mL syringe with several milliliters of air already in the syringe. The syringe may be placed in a special control handle, but this is not required. The mass should be entered with negative pressure on the syringe. Three to four aspirates should be made per pass, and multiple angled passes should be made to ensure adequate sampling. Suction on the syringe plunger should be relieved before exiting the mass to avoid aspiration of the sample into the body of the syringe. The syringe is then removed from the needle, filled with air, and placed back on the needle. The specimen is then expelled from the needle onto a glass slide. The slide containing the specimen is immediately smeared with another slide. The specimen is then promptly placed in formalin or ethanol to prevent desiccation. The presence of a cytologist for immediate review of the slides helps ensure that adequate specimen is achieved and increases diagnostic yield.

If initial FNA biopsy results are nondiagnostic, the surgeon should communicate with the pathologist to determine whether the specimen is inadequate or whether a different type of biopsy is needed. If inadequate biopsy is the problem, then repeat FNA with ultrasound guidance and immediate cytopathology review is indicated.

FNA biopsy provides the cytopathologist with the opportunity to comment on abnormalities at the cellular level but with minimal ability to comment on architectural characteristics. This may render specific diagnosis impossible, which is particularly a challenge for lymphoma and follicular thyroid cancer. In situations in which FNA biopsy is inadequate, core needle biopsy provides a small "plug" of tissue with some preservation of architectural features. A conversation with the pathologist familiar with the case is the best approach to ascertain if a core needle biopsy is expected to be helpful beyond an FNA and therefore worth the slightly increased risk of hematoma or other injury. Core biopsy also typically should be performed with real-time ultrasound guidance. If lymphoma is suspected, this should be communicated to the pathologist to ensure appropriate specimen handling, including sending the specimen unfixed.

Excisional biopsy may be necessary in a minority of cases, roughly 10% of those with malignant neck mass. Advantages include excellent tissue acquisition for pathologic analysis and the potential of therapeutic benefit in some cases. Disadvantages include cosmesis;

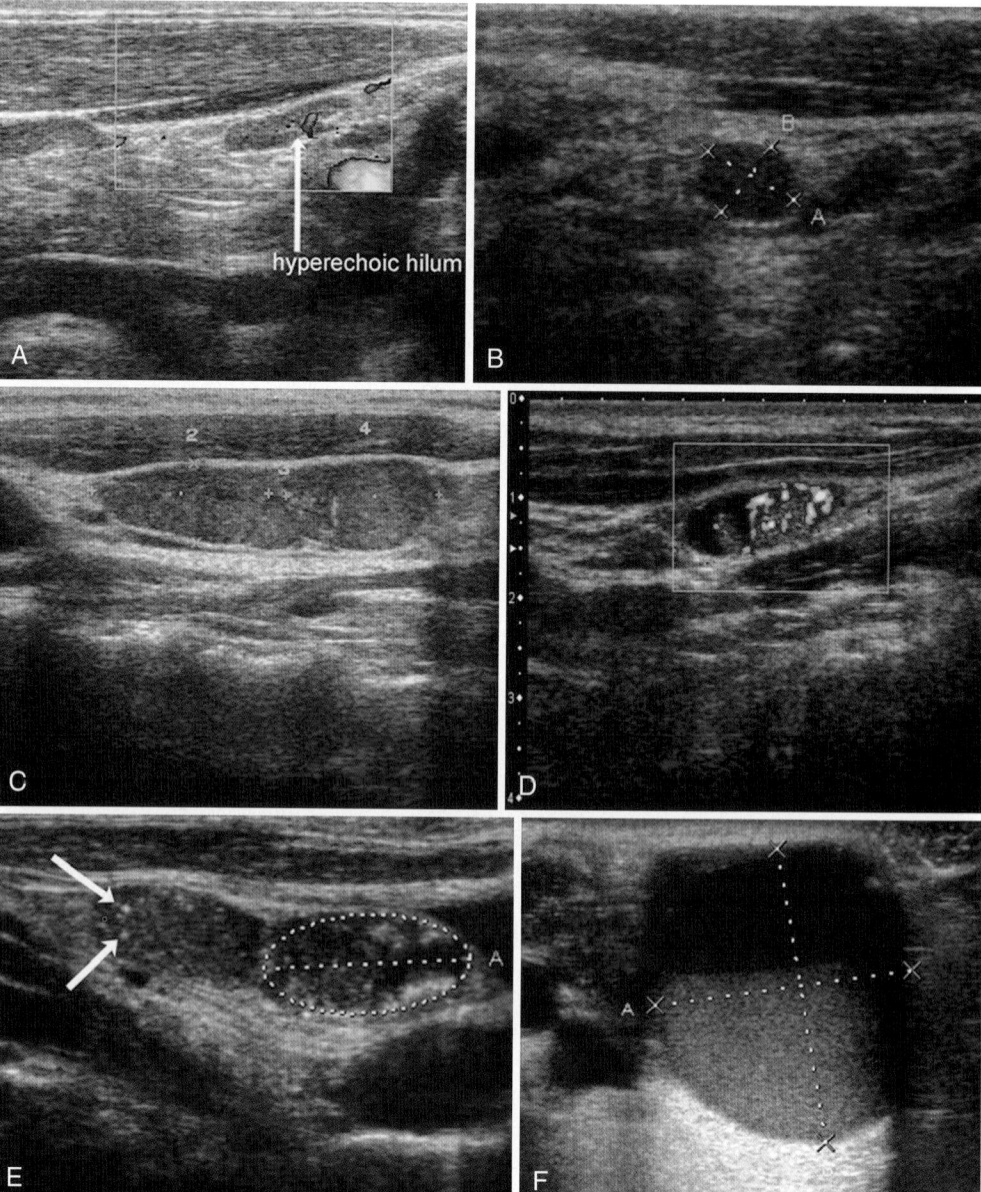

FIGURE 3 A, Benign lymph node shows hyperechoic hilum. **B,** Malignancy rounded and hyperechoic lymph node. **C,** Malignant lymph node with loss of hyperechoic fatty hilum. **D,** Malignant lymph node with peripheral and central vascularization. **E,** Malignant lymph node with hyperechoic punctuate calcifications. **F,** Malignant lymph node with cystic degeneration. *(From Leboulleux S, Girard E, Rose M, et al: Ultrasound criteria of malignancy for cervical lymph nodes in patients followed up for differentiated thyroid cancer, J Clin Endocrinol Metab 92(9):3590-3594, 2007.)*

potential poor wound healing, particularly if therapeutic radiation may ensue; potential spread of disease; need for anesthetic; risk of surgical complication, such as nerve injury; and creation of a reoperative field if subsequent compartment-based dissection proves necessary. With the excellent success of FNA in diagnosis of squamous cell cancer, open biopsy should very rarely be necessary. Not only does it expose the patient to anesthetic and procedural risks, but it may worsen the prognosis and increase the local failure rate. If squamous cell cancers remain a possibility and an excisional biopsy is planned, the surgeon should discuss proceeding directly to formal compartment-oriented neck dissection with the same anesthetic if squamous cell carcinoma ultimately is identified. Obviously, a thorough examination for a primary malignancy should be completed before this approach; this should be a rare event given the utility of FNA.

Although most thyroid masses are benign, a thorough and thoughtful evaluation of thyroid nodules should be pursued. This workup is detailed elsewhere in this text, but FNA also plays a prominent role for thyroid lesions and is particularly effective in diagnosis of papillary thyroid cancer. On occasion, a biopsy of a lateral neck mass shows thyroid follicular cells in a patient without known thyroid

disease. This finding should be considered an indication for a primary thyroid malignancy within the thyroid, most often a papillary thyroid cancer. The concept of benign embryologic rests of thyroid cells in the lateral neck, or lateral aberrant thyroid, has largely been disproved.

Carotid body paragangliomas typically can be diagnosed on the basis of classic imaging features on CT/CTA, MRI, or angiogram, including splaying of the internal and external carotid arteries. These lesions are highly vascular. Biopsy of carotid body tumors is not needed and should be discouraged.

Endoscopy and Biopsy

When FNA of a neck mass reveals squamous cell cancer, the surgeon must seek the primary lesion. As previously reviewed, the nodal level may direct the initial evaluation. A thorough history and physical examination, including mirror examination or flexible fiberoptic laryngoscopy, should be completed. Initial imaging consists of CT scan of the neck, which results in identification of a primary malignancy in 20% of cases. Chest imaging (plain x-ray or CT scan) aids

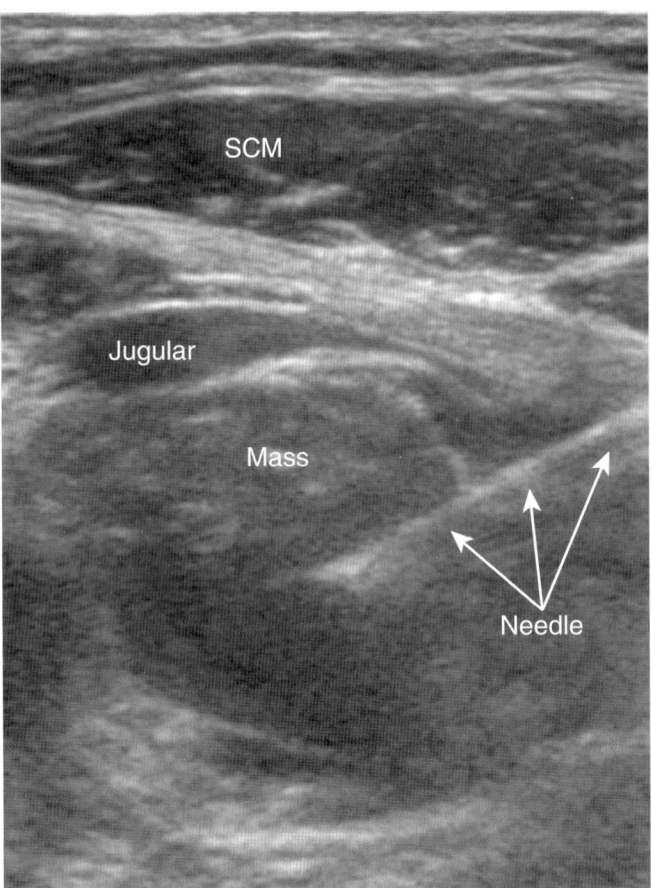

FIGURE 4   Ultrasound-guided fine-needle aspiration biopsy of a neck mass lying posterior to the jugular vein. This biopsy was performed with a 22-gauge needle and confirmed metastatic papillary thyroid cancer. *SCM,* Sternocleidomastoid muscle.

in the search and is particularly useful for lower neck nodal disease. PET may be a useful secondary imaging study. If PET is used as part of the diagnostic approach, it should be completed before endoscopy and biopsy both to aid in targeting the evaluation and to prevent false-positive PET findings from recently manipulated tissue.

When the primary tumor site remains occult after these studies, panendoscopy and biopsy should follow. Panendoscopy includes laryngoscopy, bronchoscopy, and esophagoscopy. If a primary tumor still is not identified, then at the same setting, biopsies should be performed. If the tonsils are still present, ipsilateral tonsillectomy should be performed; tonsils are found to be the primary source in 20% to 40% of these patients. Bilateral tonsillectomy also is a reasonable, but if this is not performed, then the contralateral tonsil should at least be biopsied. Directed biopsies also should be performed of the nasopharynx, hypopharynx, tongue base, and piriform sinus. Special attention should be paid to any area that was at all suspicious on the imaging evaluation.

■ SURGICAL CONSIDERATIONS

Anesthesia and Airway Considerations

Many neck masses feel superficial on examination but can be misleading. Neck masses usually lie deep to the platysma, and major neurovascular structures are in the operative field. Local anesthetic can impair motor response of nerves at risk. Therefore, most neck mass surgical biopsies or excisions are performed with general anesthetic, typically via orotracheal intubation. Although neck masses may commonly displace structures, including the airway, a standard intubation usually can be achieved; however, skilled anesthesiologists and the availability of adjuncts such as the difficult airway cart are important. In cases in which clinical or radiographic evaluation suggests significant airway compromise or distortion, communication with the anesthesiologist is imperative. Awake fiberoptic intubation or other strategies may be used. If the airway is markedly compromised, a planned tracheotomy may be appropriate and should be performed before extremis develops. Communication again is important regarding avoidance of long-acting paralytics to permit monitoring of motor nerve response.

Incisions

Transverse skin incisions that are preferentially placed in a preexisting skin crease are preferred for optimal cosmetic results. When possible, the incision should be placed along the same line as would be used if a subsequent more radical procedure, such as neck dissection, followed the initial procedure. If a small incision is initially used and a need for more exposure occurs, neck incisions can be widened with either transverse or oblique extensions (e.g., along the anterior border of SCM) for better visibility. Although cosmesis is important, it is more important to have adequate exposure to identify anatomic landmarks and protect vessels and nerves.

Potential Nerve Injuries

Neurologic injury may occur with both diagnostic and therapeutic interventions. An understanding of the anatomy is essential to minimize the rate of injury, as is discussion of all potential temporary dysfunction or permanent injury with the patient before intervention. Low-energy nerve-stimulating devices may aid in identification of motor nerves in the course of dissection but cannot substitute for knowledge of anatomy and meticulous technique. Among the most frequently at risk and commonly injured nerves in the neck are the spinal accessory nerve (CN XI) and the marginal mandibular branch of the facial nerve (CN VII). Both injuries cause significant morbidity.

The marginal branch of CN VII is at risk below the body of the mandible. It courses from the main trunk of the nerve in the parotid gland over the body of the mandible (at the area of the facial artery) onto the fascia of the submandibular gland, deep to the platysma. The nerve then courses superiorly to cross over the mandible and ultimately becomes more superficial to the level of the platysma and innervates the depressors of the lower lip. The nerve thus lies below the inferior aspect of the mandible for several centimeters. Avoiding the region of the body of the mandible can minimize chances of injury to this nerve. To avoid injury to this nerve, which may be diminutive in size, incisions should be made at least two fingerbreadths below the inferior edge of the body of the mandible. In dissection of the submandibular region, the fascia of the gland should be elevated with the skin flap and the facial vein should be isolated and divided low. Dissection should proceed bluntly, spreading in the expected direction of the nerve.

The vagus nerve (CN X) descends within the carotid sheath, typically posterior to the vascular structures. Unlike division of the vagus in the chest or abdomen, a vagal injury or sacrifice in the neck carries the added morbidity of creating an ipsilateral vocal fold paralysis and atrophy of the vocal fold. This occurs because the recurrent laryngeal nerve has not branched from the vagus nerve until after the latter has descended from the neck. If a vagus nerve injury occurs, neurorrhaphy is not expected to restore normal function but may help to prevent atrophy of the vocal cord, which improves the functional result of subsequent vocal cord medialization procedures. In the right neck, the potential exists for a nonrecurrent laryngeal nerve that courses directly medially from the vagus. This aberrant nerve may course with the superior thyroid artery or more inferiorly. Nonrecurrent right laryngeal nerves occur in the setting of an aberrant right subclavian artery, arteria lusoria, and could be injured in the carotid sheath or central compartment if not recognized.

The spinal accessory nerve (CN XI) is at risk for surgical injury in cervical levels II and V. It exits the jugular foramen together with the vagus and glossopharyngeal nerves and courses inferior laterally deep to the posterior belly of the digastric. It passes either superficial or deep to the internal jugular vein. It gives off branches to the SCM and passes either through or deep to the SCM into the posterior triangle. It exits the posterior border of the SCM at approximately the junction of the upper and middle third of the posterior border of the SCM, typically 5 to 8 cm from the mastoid tip. This is approximately 1 cm cephalad to Erb's point, where cutaneous nerves including the greater auricular nerve can be found at the posterior border of the SCM. CN XI then runs superficially, overlying the levator scapula muscle in the posterior triangle to the trapezius and crosses, and may connect with branches of the cervical plexus in its course. It frequently has a meandering course in level V, and the absence of a defined platysma in the posterior triangle renders it even more susceptible to injury.

The hypoglossal nerve (CN XII) provides motor innervation to the tongue. It traverses levels I and II. It descends between the internal jugular vein and the carotid artery and then courses medially. It runs deep to the posterior belly of the digastric muscle, where is it surrounded by the ranine veins. Injuries to this nerve may occur during attempts to control bleeding from these veins.

Other Potential Complications

Although these procedures are usually clean, wound infection sometimes occurs and may be related to the smoking and nutritional status of the patient or irradiated tissue. Chyle leak also may occur and is most likely with procedures in the left level IV. The thoracic duct runs deep to the carotid artery low in the left neck and empties into the internal jugular vein deep to its junction with the subclavian vein. All tissue divided in this area lying between the phrenic and vagus nerves should be carefully ligated. When they occur, chyle leaks are initially managed conservatively with a low-fat diet and medium chain triglyceride diet. High-volume or persistent leaks occasionally require reoperation for definitive repair, which usually is accomplished with the placement of Weck clips once the leak is identified and isolated from other structures.

Suggested Readings

Chen A, Otto KJ: Differential diagnosis of neck masses. In Flint PW, Haughey BH, Lund VJ, et al: editors: *Cummings otolaryngology: head & neck surgery*, ed 5, Philadelphia, 2010, Elsevier.

Gleeson M, Herbert A, Richards A: Management of lateral neck masses in adults, *BMJ* 320(7248):1521–1524, 2000.

Shah JP, Strong E, Spiro RH, et al: Surgical grand rounds: neck dissection: current status and future possibilities, *Clin Bull* 11:25–33, 1981.

HAND INFECTIONS

Derek L. Masden, MD, and
Christopher L. Forthman, MD

INTRODUCTION

Hand infections are common and are often managed by a wide range of medical professionals. These infections can range from isolated and simple to complex with great potential for extensive damage, particularly in select patient populations such as diabetics and the immunocompromised. Early recognition of these infections with implementation of treatment is imperative to avoid more complex sequelae and tissue destruction. As with most infections, antibiotic therapy has a central role, but if there is more than just superficial cellulitis, these infections often require surgical therapy for complete eradication (Table 1).

Any patient presenting with a possible hand infection should undergo a thorough history and complete hand examination, including neurovascular status and evaluation of motion. In addition, specific attention should be paid to hand and finger posture, swelling, skin changes, and focal pain and tenderness, and an examination should be made both proximal and distal to the area of concern. Comparison should be made between both the adjacent nonaffected tissue (for example, the other fingers) and the contralateral hand.

Hand x-rays should be performed to evaluate for skeletal abnormalities such as bony destruction, to determine the presence of any gas formed by bacteria, and to rule out a foreign body. Routine lab studies including a complete blood count, erythrocyte sedimentation rate, and C-reactive protein may be performed. The physician should be reminded that often lab studies may be indeterminate, and clinical judgment will ultimately decide which patients require surgical intervention regardless of specific lab results. When possible, cultures should be taken to help tailor antibiotic coverage.

MICROBIOLOGY

By far the most common pathogen cultured in hand infections is *Staphylococcus aureus*, accounting for up to 80% of hand infections in some series. Anaerobes or mixed flora typically make up the remainder of the cultures and are more common in select patient groups such as diabetics and the immunocompromised (such as those with human immunodeficiency virus). Human bites often contain oral flora such as *Eikenella corrodens*, whereas dog and cat bites may contain *Pasturella multocida*. Cat scratches may be associated with *Bartonella henselae* and be associated with regional lymphadenopathy. Infections resulting from interactions with marine animals may contain *Vibrio* species or *Mycobacterium marinum*.

Methicillin-Resistant *Staphylococcus Aureus*

The rate of methicillin resistance in *Staphylococcus aureus* hand infections ranges from 34% to 78%. Community acquired methicillin-resistant *Staphylococcus aureus* (MRSA) infections are becoming more common, and these patients often experience a delay in appropriate antibiotic treatment. In many communities, empiric coverage for MRSA may be warranted in the patient presenting with a hand infection (Figure 1).

TABLE I: General recommendations for hand infections

Infection	Likely organism(s)	Initial antibiotic therapy*	Surgical therapy
Cellulitis	*Staphylococcus* or *Streptococcus*	Cephalexin. Use clindamycin or trimethoprim/sulfamethoxazole (Bactrim) for suspected MRSA.	Only indicated for associated abscess
Abscess	*Staphylococcus*	Vancomycin. Add piperacillin/tazobactam (Zosyn) for diabetic/immunocompromised patients.	Immediate drainage (no closure), soaks and motion the day after surgery
Flexor tenosynovitis	*Staphylococcus*, anaerobes, polymicrobial	Ampicillin/sulbactam (Unasyn). Replace Unasyn with Zosyn for diabetic/immunocompromised patient and add vancomycin if possible MRSA.	Consider 12-24 hours observation for early signs; otherwise, drainage of flexor sheath (no closure), soaks, and motion the day after surgery
Septic arthritis	*Staphylococcus*	Vancomycin. Add ceftriaxone if *Neisseria gonorrhoeae* is suspected.	Immediate drainage (no closure), soaks, and motion the day after surgery
Animal bite	*Pasteurella multocida* is classic, but staph, strep, and anaerobes are common	Unasyn or PO equivalent. If penicillin allergic, then consider fluoroquinolone and clindamycin.	Clean thoroughly in ER and observe closely for signs of a deep infection. Cat teeth inoculate the deep tissues, so consider incising the puncture site to facilitate drainage. Dog teeth tear local tissues and will usually drain spontaneously.
Human bite	*Eikenella corrodens* is classic, but staph, strep, and anaerobes are common	Unasyn or PO equivalent. If penicillin allergic, then consider fluoroquinolone and clindamycin.	Clean thoroughly in ER and observe closely for signs of a deep infection (e.g., abscess, FTS, etc.). "Fight bites" require immediate drainage, even in the absence of overt infection.
Necrotizing fasciitis	*Streptococcus* or *polymicrobial*	Vancomycin *and* clindamycin *and* piperacillin/tazobactam (Zosyn)	Emergent radical débridement(s), hemodynamic monitoring, possible amputation
Gas gangrene	*Clostridium perfringines, Strep pyogenes, Staph aureus, Vibrio vulnificus*, polymicrobial	Vancomycin *and* clindamycin *and* piperacillin/tazobactam (Zosyn). Consider high-dose penicillin.	Emergent radical débridement(s), hemodynamic monitoring, possible amputation

*Antibiotic coverage should be adjusted once cultures are back to decrease the creation of antibiotic-resistant organisms and to minimize drug side effects to the patient.

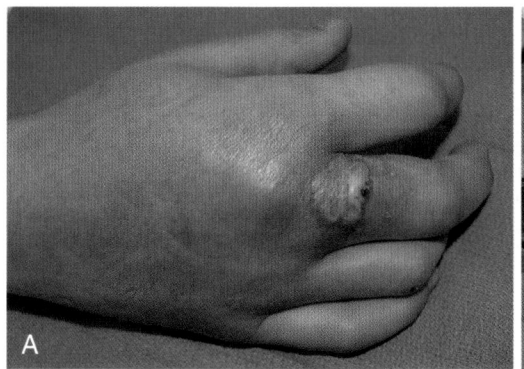
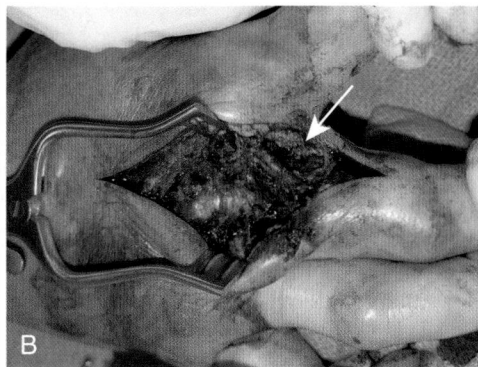

FIGURE I A, MRSA abscess. The red, swollen region with central necrosis or "spider-bite appearance" is typical. **B,** Infection has entered the webspace *(arrow),* a "collar-button" abscess, and will require a palmar incision for adequate drainage.

The Diabetic and Immunocompromised Hand

The rising population of diabetic and immunocompromised patients mandates that physicians be aware of the rapid downward course they may encounter once these patients are infected. These patients may develop polymicrobial abscesses or abscesses with especially virulent bacteria such as pseudomonas or other Gram negatives. This fact should be considered when choosing antibiotic coverage. Additionally, infection spread can be rapid in this patient population, leading to challenges in treatment and greater morbidity and mortality. Even the simplest infections can lead to devastating complications and impairment in these individuals. These factors necessitate swift evaluation and require a low threshold for surgical exploration to prevent progressive tissue damage.

Bite Wounds

Bite wounds, most commonly from domesticated pets or other humans, are a significant contributor to hand infections. With the vast amount of bacteria found in the animal or human mouth, these wounds have the propensity to produce serious infections that, if left untreated, may have serious consequences. There are approximately 2 million cases of animal bite wounds every year, accounting for 1% of emergency room visits each year in the United States. Although the vast majority of these bites are from dogs, only a small amount of dog bites result in infection, in part due to the destructive nature of canine teeth, which usually leave open wounds. In contrast, cat bites more frequently become infected because feline teeth cause small puncture wounds that can inoculate the deeper structures of the upper extremity. These small puncture-type wounds can be the source of a flexor tenosynovitis, dorsal abscesses, or other deep hand infections.

Human "bites" are more often associated with an altercation that involves a direct blow to a person's mouth with a hand. The so-called "fight bite" can result in septic arthritis if the injury inoculates bacteria into an underlying joint. Septic arthritis presents as a swollen joint that is painful with limited motion. Similar to other hand infections, *Staph* is the most common organism, although other flora may be present, particularly if related to a bite wound. If the diagnosis is in doubt, the joint may be aspirated and the fluid sent for white count and Gram stain. Suspected septic arthritis, particularly after a "fight bite," requires immediate surgical drainage aimed at preventing damage to the articular cartilage (Figure 2).

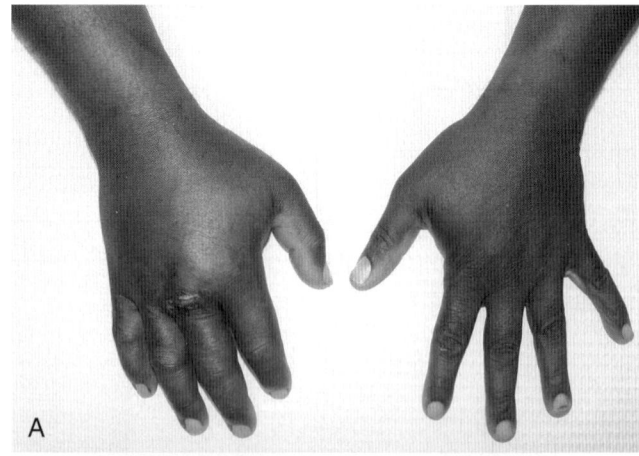

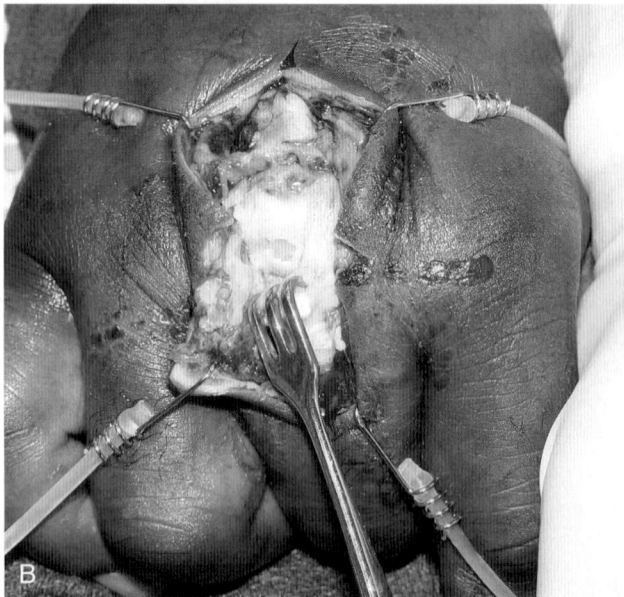

FIGURE 2 A, Human bite to the metacarpophalangeal joint of the right long finger following a fight. **B,** Surgery revealed a complete laceration of the extensor digitorum communis, violation of the joint space, and damage to the articular cartilage.

FINGER INFECTIONS

Many finger infections that require surgical drainage can be treated under local anesthesia using a digital block. Care should be taken to critically evaluate the patient to be certain that the infection is localized to only the finger and that a more proximal infection (such as a flexor tenosynovitis) is not present. If there is an indication of a more proximal infection, a wrist block or general anesthesia should be considered to allow formal operative débridement.

A digital block is performed by inserting the needle through the flexor tendon at the level of the palmar digital crease of the affected digit, contacting the underlying bone and then slowly injecting 2 mL of lidocaine without epinephrine into the space between the periosteum and the flexor tendon as the needle is withdrawn. Alternatively, the digit can be approached dorsally with the needle entering the dorsal skin of the finger over the metacarpal head of the affected digit and then introducing 2 mL of lidocaine without epinephrine volarly into each webspace flanking the digit. A digital tourniquet can then be made by clamping a penrose drain around the base of the digit. Care must be taken to remove the tourniquet at the completion of the drainage procedure.

Paronychia

Diagnosis

A paronychia is an infection involving the tissue surrounding the lateral fingernail (paronychial fold), proximal nail fold (eponychial fold), or extending into the nail matrix (Figure 3). Risk factors include nail biting, hangnails, and manicures. The most common inciting organism is *Staphyloccocus aureus*, but it can also include oral flora. Typically a painful swollen area with erythema along the lateral border of the fingernail or beneath the proximal nail fold is the hallmark of an acute paronychia. Purulent drainage or failed conservative therapy with warm soaks necessitates surgical drainage.

Treatment

Early paronychia can be treated with warm soaks several times a day. Simple paronychia that have developed an abscess are treated with incision and drainage. This can be done at the bedside or in the office with a digital block. Superficial paronychia can be treated by simple elevation of the paronychial/eponychial fold off of the nail plate with an elevator or scalpel to drain the abscess. Infections that have spread

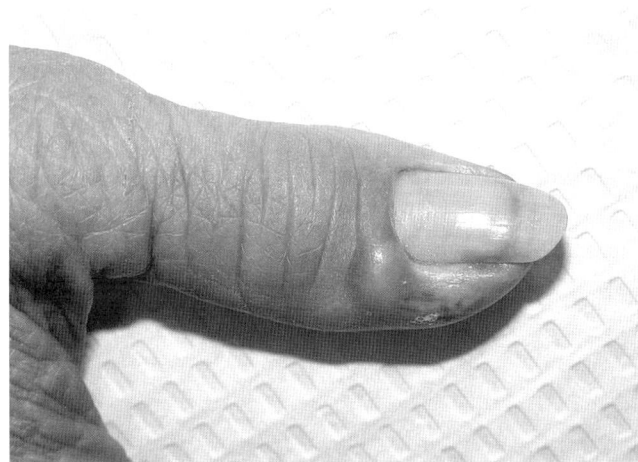

FIGURE 3 Acute paronychia of the thumb involving the inferior aspect of the thumb nail fold.

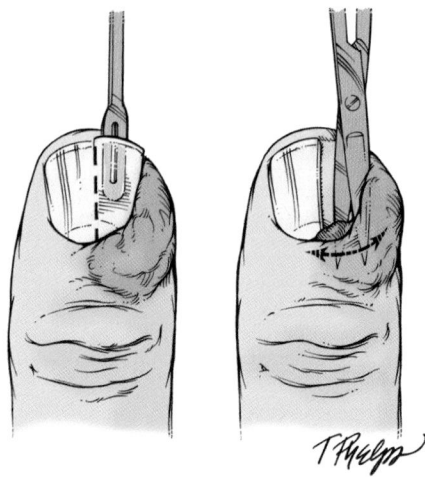

FIGURE 4 Surgical drainage of acute paronychia. The lateral nail on the affected side is gently elevated from the nail bed, and a longitudinal strip of nail is removed. If this does not decompress the infection adequately, the margins of the nail fold are opened gently to drain the adjacent soft tissues.

below the nail plate require removal of at least part of the nail plate. The nail fold is elevated, and a longitudinal strip of nail is cut away on the affected side (Figure 4). If needed, the entire nail is removed. The wound should be irrigated and dressed with daily soaks in warm, soapy water or diluted hydrogen peroxide beginning soon thereafter. Empiric antibiotics treatment should be initiated with either cephalexin or amoxicillin/clavulanate (Augmentin) to cover the most common pathogens. In areas with frequent community-acquired MRSA, trimethoprim/sulfamethoxazole (Bactrim) or clindamycin should be used.

Felon

Diagnosis

A felon represents a compartmentalized abscess in the fat pad of the distal phalanx. There are numerous vertical septae that extend from the distal phalanx to the dermis, and once inoculated with bacteria, small abscesses can develop. The patient usually presents with a swollen fingertip, throbbing pain, and erythema (Figure 5). The swelling is mostly distal to the distal interphalangeal (DIP) joint, and any extension proximally should raise the suspicion of a flexor tendon sheath infection.

Care should be taken to distinguish a felon from herpetic whitlow, which can have a similar appearance when present at the fingertip. Herpetic whitlow is a viral lesion caused by the herpes simplex virus. Whitlow is common in children, dental workers, and other populations frequently exposed to saliva. The disease appears as clear vesicles and mild finger swelling that may resemble a felon. Although the fluid may be turbid or hemorrhagic, it is not purulent, and unlike a felon, the pulp space does not have increased tension. The diagnosis can be made by sending scrapings from an open vesicle for a Tzanck smear.

Treatment

In the earliest stages of a felon, a trial of warm soaks, elevation, and antibiotics may be initiated; however, surgical decompression is often necessary. Surgical drainage requires a thoughtful skin incision and then blunt dissection with disruption of the pulp septae. Multiple incisions have been described, and care and planning should be performed in order to adequately treat each patient. A distal-based fish mouth incision at the tip of the finger should be avoided because it may result in painful scarring and deformation of the fingertip. If the felon is located along the volar midline, then a volar longitudinal

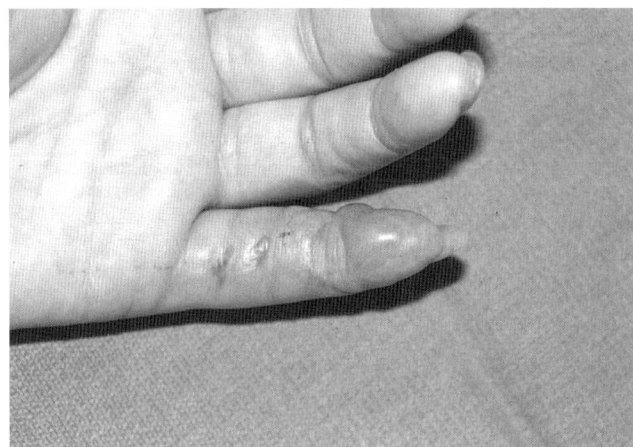

FIGURE 5 Acute felon. Blistering is evident distally, where tissue pressure is significantly elevated.

incision can be made. Otherwise, a high lateral incision just below the nail can be performed, avoiding the digital artery or nerve (Figure 6). This incision should be placed on the noncontact side of the affected digit (radial for the thumb and ulnar for the remaining digits) to avoid painful scarring that interferes with pinch. Once careful disruption of the septae has been performed and the fingertip is adequately decompressed, it should be packed and dressed. Empiric antibiotics are started, followed by soaks and dressing changes the next day.

Pyogenic Flexor Tenosynovitis

Diagnosis

Bacteria that inoculate the flexor tendon sheath, often from penetrating trauma, may lead to a pyogenic flexor tenosynovitis. The flexor sheath runs from the distal interphalangeal joint to the A1 pulley over the metacarpal head, and bacteria may enter the sheath anywhere along this course. Failure to institute treatment in a timely manner can have devastating consequences, ranging from tendon adhesions to finger necrosis. Kanavel described four cardinal signs of flexor tenosynovitis: tenderness along the course of the sheath, fixed flexed position of the finger, extreme pain with passive extension of the finger, and fusiform swelling of the affected digit (Figure 7). All of these signs may not be present, but the clinician should evaluate for each and have a low threshold to begin treatment. Early infections (<24 hours) in healthy individuals may be managed with a trial of antibiotics; however, failure to respond or delayed presentation is an indication for surgical débridement.

Treatment

Surgical treatment of flexor tenosynovitis includes operative exploration, débridement of necrotic tissue, and flushing of the tendon sheath. Surgery should be performed in the operating room and may consist of either open or closed sheath irrigation. In open sheath irrigation, the flexor sheath is exposed using either a Brunner-type or midlateral incision, taking care not to injure the digital neurovascular bundles that reside laterally. The tendon sheath is opened in order to remove all infectious material. Care should be taken to preserve the critical annular pulleys of the digit, with the A2 pulley being located over the proximal part of the proximal phalanx and the A4 pulley located over the midportion of the middle phalanx. The sheath is copiously irrigated with sterile saline until all purulent material is removed. Any large incisions should be loosely closed.

The alternative method is the closed sheath technique, which involves limited incisions located proximally and distally to allow access to the sheath. The proximal incision is located at the level of the A1 pulley volarly, and the distal incision is placed either midlaterally or volarly at the distal interphalangeal crease. The sheath is then accessed at both sites, and a pediatric feeding tube or other small intravenous catheter is introduced to allow copious antegrade irrigation. Catheters can be left in place for postoperative irrigation, but this technique is messy and cumbersome and has not proved to be more useful than routine wound care.

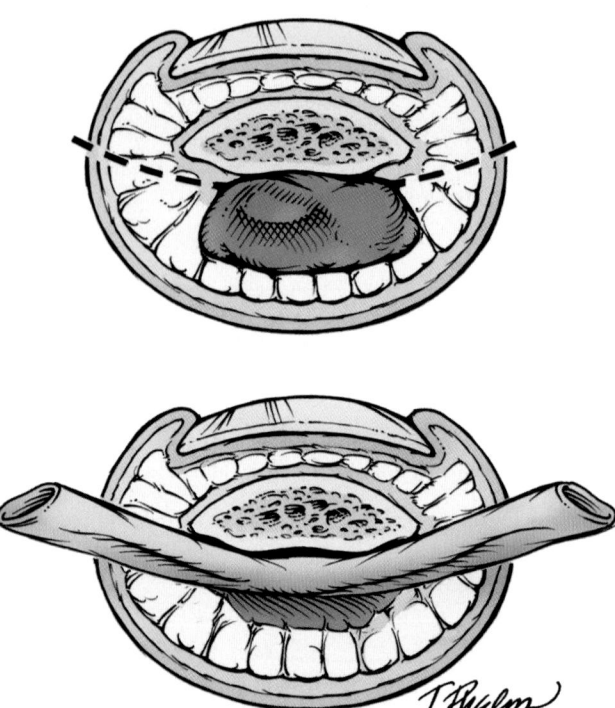

FIGURE 6   Through-and-through drainage of a felon ensures complete decompression and minimizes the risk of incomplete treatment. A drain is placed and maintained for 48 hours.

After open or closed tendon sheath irrigation, the hand should be splinted and elevated, and a course of antibiotics should be prescribed. Wound soaks are then performed several times a day. The wounds can be dressed with gauze and allowed to heal secondarily.

HAND INFECTIONS

Some hand infections, such as a dorsal abscess, may be treated in the emergency room with just a local field block. The patient requires débridement in the operating room when the infection involves closed volar spaces or joints.

Bursal Infections

Diagnosis

The flexor tendon sheath of the thumb is continuous with the radial bursa, a thin envelope extending from the flexor pollicis sheath at the level of the metacarpophalangeal joint through the carpal canal into the forearm. The small finger flexor sheath is continuous with the ulnar bursa, another fine envelope tracking ulnar to the flexor tendons and into the carpal canal and forearm. Infections of the thumb and small finger flexor tendons may propagate along these bursa and into the distal forearm. The "Parona space," a potential space that lies between the pronator quadratus and flexor tendons, may communicate infections between the radial and ulnar sides of the hand. This space may also communicate with the thenar and midpalmar spaces deep in the palm. Bacterial extension through this communication is generally associated with a severe generalized deep volar infection. Sometimes the result is a more limited but nonetheless serious radial and ulnar bursal space infection referred to as a "horseshoe" abscess. It is important for the surgeon to be aware of the potential spaces and communications when treating the infected hand. Failure to recognize bacterial extension into these spaces can lead to an incomplete débridement and increased morbidity (Figure 8).

Treatment

Infections that spread along bursa require aggressive débridement in the operating room under general anesthesia. The infected digits should be thoroughly debrided as previously described in flexor tenosynovitis. Often the extent of the disease is not recognized until the time of surgery. Because the infection is followed proximally, care should be taken to avoid making large, continuous incisions across the hand. Separate thenar or hypothenar incisions can be made in the palm, in line with skin creases, while another incision can be placed on the distal volar forearm to inspect for infection in the Parona space. The most severe infections will require an extended carpal tunnel release in order to adequately debride necrotic tissue and infected tenosynovium. After copious irrigation, the wounds can be closed loosely over a drain and the hand splinted. Postoperative care includes appropriate antibiotics, daily dressing changes and soaks, and hand therapy.

Deep Space Infections: Thenar, Hypothenar, and Midpalmar Space Abscesses

Diagnosis

Three potential spaces exist in the palm that can become infected with resultant abscess formation. The interosseous muscles are deep to these spaces, and the flexor tendons are superficial (Figure 9). The thenar space is bordered by the adductor pollicis dorsally, the index finger flexor volarly, the adductor pollicis insertion on the proximal

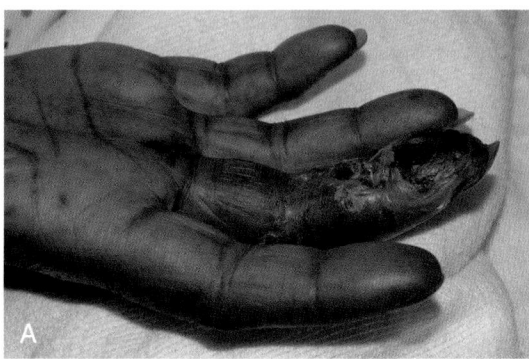
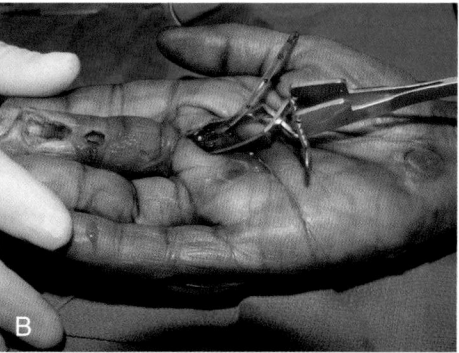

FIGURE 7 **A,** Late pyogenic flexor tenosynovitis in a diabetic immunocompromised patient. Swelling and a slightly flexed posture are evident. **B,** Necrotic tissue has been debrided, and the sheath is irrigated in a closed fashion.

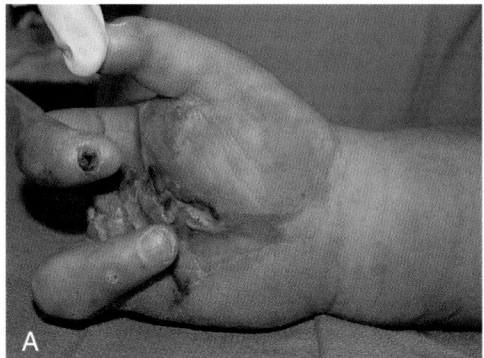
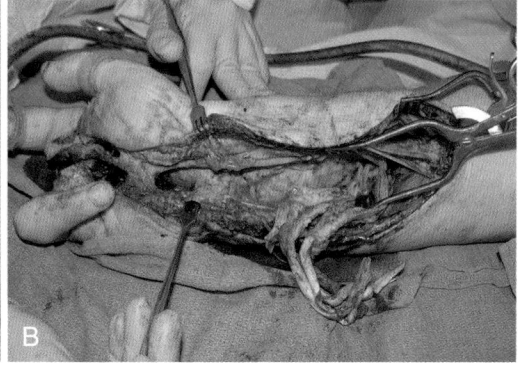

FIGURE 8 **A,** Inadequate treatment of "finger infections" is manifest as generalized hand and forearm swelling. **B,** Bacterial extension through the carpal tunnel and the Parona space results in a severe generalized deep volar forearm infection.

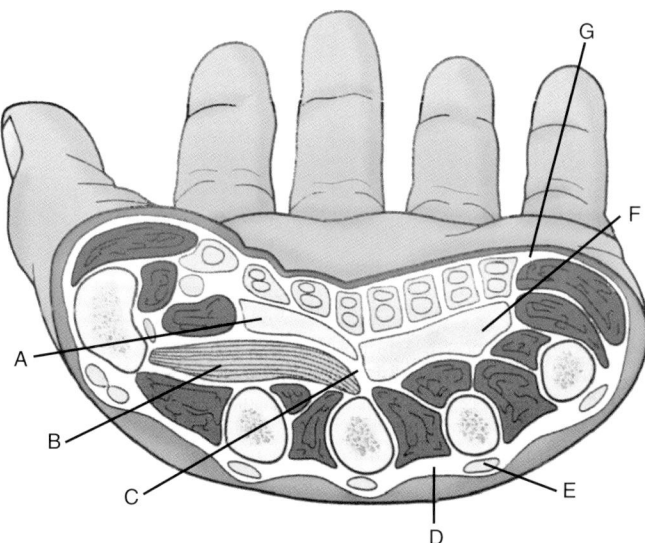

FIGURE 9 Cross-section anatomy of the hand. **A,** Thenar space. **B,** Adductor pollicis. **C,** Midpalmar septum. **D,** Dorsal subaponeurotic space. **E,** Extensor tendon. **F,** Midpalmar space. **G,** Hypothenar space.

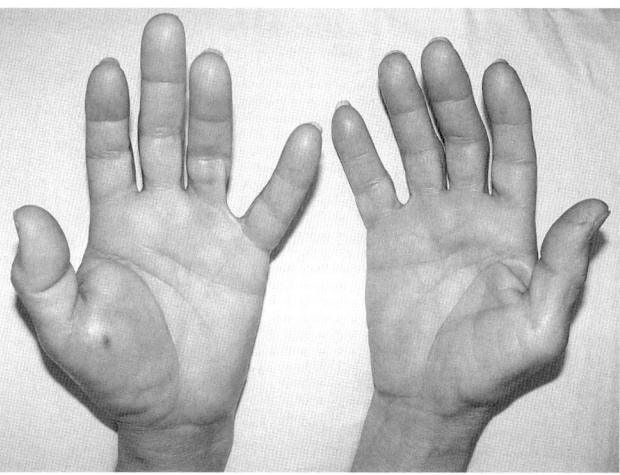

FIGURE 10 Thenar space infection resulting from a cat bite, showing thenar edema and abduction of the thumb.

phalanx radially, and the midpalmar septum ulnarly. Infections are often the result of penetrating trauma. The first webspace area becomes swollen and exquisitely tender to palpation as the potential space becomes filled with purulent fluid. The thumb may be abducted with extreme pain on passive adduction or opposition (Figure 10).

The midpalmar space lies between the thenar and hypothenar eminences. The floor is the fascia of the second and third volar interosseous, and the superficial border is the flexor sheaths of the long, ring, and small fingers. The radial and ulnar borders are defined by septae running from the third and fifth metacarpals to the dermis.

These septae are termed the oblique septum and the hypothenar septum, respectively. Infections are most often a result of penetrating trauma or extension from an adjacent infection.

The hypothenar space lies between the hypothenar septum and the hypothenar muscles, with the periosteum of the fifth metacarpal as the floor. Infection of this space is rare, as is spread of infection to adjacent areas. The patient may present with localized pain and swelling along the hypothenar eminence, with absence of swelling elsewhere in the palm or fingers.

Treatment

The thenar space can be approached either dorsally or volarly (Figure 11). The volar approach typically involves an incision along the

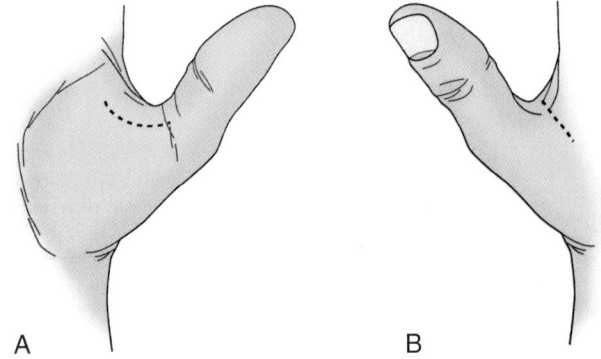

FIGURE 11 Surgical approach for incision and drainage of a thenar space infection. **A,** Transverse incision. **B,** Dorsal longitudinal incision.

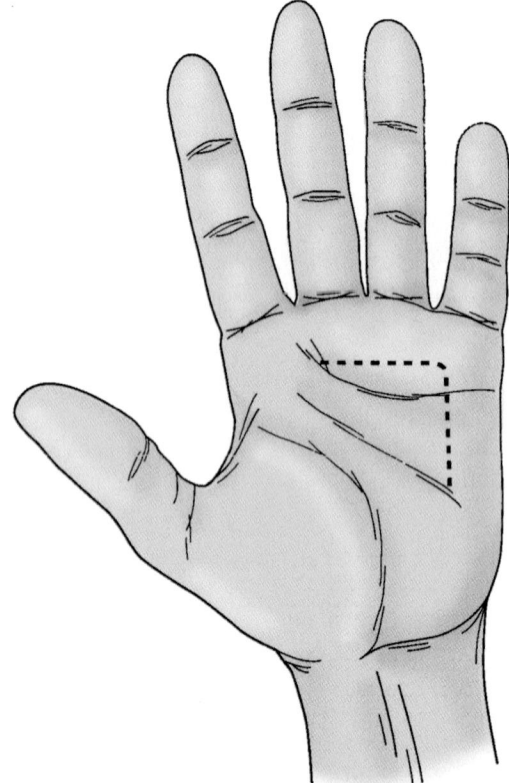

FIGURE 12 Combined longitudinal and transverse incision for drainage of midpalmar space abscess.

thenar crease approximately 1 cm proximal to the webspace and proceeding proximally. Blunt dissection is then carried out to the adductor pollicis, and the abscess is drained. Care should be taken proximally where the motor branch from the median nerve may be encountered. Dorsal incisions may be transverse or longitudinal, and blunt dissection is then performed to the interval between the first dorsal interosseous and the adductor pollicis, where the abscess should be encountered. The radial artery may be encountered in this region.

The midpalmar space is approached volarly, with a transverse incision at or about the distal palmar crease, a longitudinal incision, or a combination of the two (Figure 12). Blunt dissection is again used to avoid damage to the palmar neurovascular bundles and then carried out longitudinally on either side of the flexor tendons until the abscess is expressed.

Similar to the thenar space, the hypothenar space can be accessed with an incision along the hypothenar eminence, parallel to the fifth

metacarpal. The dissection is carried to the level of the hypothenar fascia, where the abscess should be encountered and drained.

After drainage and irrigation, all wounds should be closed loosely over drains or packing, and the hand should be splinted. Dressing changes, soaks, or irrigation should be begun the next day, along with therapy attempts to restore hand function.

Web Space Abscesses

Diagnosis

Often referred to as "collar-button abscesses" because of their hour-glass shape, these infections may result from a fissure in the skin between adjacent fingers, from a distal palmar callus, or track from dorsal to volar. There is localized pain and swelling in the affected webspace, and classically the adjacent fingers are abducted away from the abscess.

Treatment

Drainage of a webspace abscess can be performed with a single dorsal incision or a combined dorsal and volar approach. Care should be taken not to place the incision across the webspace or to connect the dorsal and volar incisions because this will decrease the ability of the fingers to abduct due to the contracting scar. After skin incision, dissection is performed bluntly to allow full egress of purulent material. After irrigation, a drain should be placed in each incision, but a through and through drain for both incisions should be avoided. The hand should be splinted, and daily dressing changes and soaks should begin the following day.

Dorsal Hand Abscesses

Diagnosis

Dorsal hand abscesses can be either deep—occupying the so-called "subaponeurotic" potential space below the extensors—or subcutaneous. The depth of the abscess may be difficult to distinguish clinically. The patient typically presents with focal pain, swelling, and erythema. Dorsal abscesses may also develop in the fingers (Figure 13).

Treatment

While simple cellulitis responds favorably to antibiotics, fluctuant infections must be drained. Most dorsal hand abscesses may be drained in the emergency department under a local field or regional block. If the clinician is certain that the abscess is in the subcutaneous tissue, a simple longitudinal incision can be made over the most prominent part of the abscess in order to fully express the infectious material. If the abscess seems deep, a longitudinal incision should be biased toward the region over the second metacarpal or the space between the fourth and fifth metacarpal to avoid the extensor tendons. Blunt dissection is then performed to expose the abscess below the extensor tendons and fully express the pus. Irrigation is performed, followed by loose closure and a splint. Early hand motion is initiated when possible.

NECROTIZING FASCIITIS OF THE UPPER EXTREMITY

Diagnosis

Necrotizing fasciitis is a rapidly progressive, potentially fatal bacterial infection that most commonly spreads along the fascial planes of the

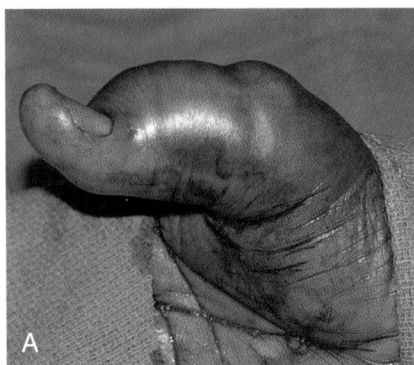

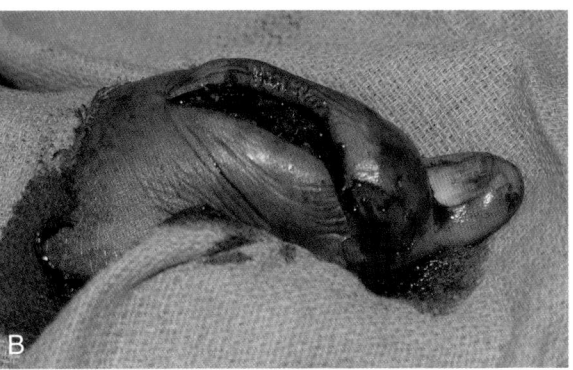

FIGURE 13 **A,** A large dorsal abscess is anatomically separated from the palmar tissues by finger ligaments (Cleland and Grayson). **B,** The abscess is drained by a linear incision made over the path of greatest fluctuance.

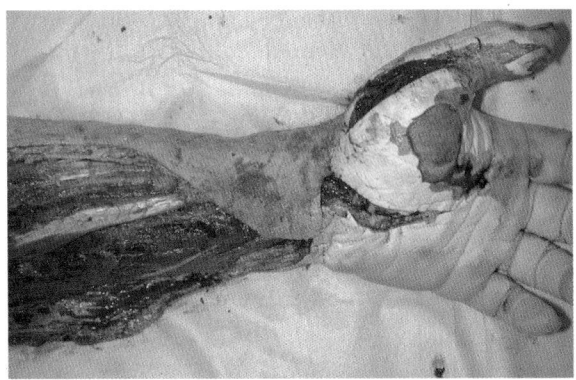

FIGURE 14 A 78-year-old man presented with systemic illness and a rapidly progressing dominant arm soft tissue infection. Early and aggressive management with serial wide surgical débridement, negative pressure therapy, and subsequent delayed closure allowed for preservation of the limb. Tissue sample confirmed the diagnosis of necrotizing fasciitis. *(From McDonald LS, Bavaro MF, Hofmeister EP, et al.: Hand infections,* Journal of Hand Surgery *36(8):1403-1412, 2011.)*

muscles (Figure 14). In the upper extremity it is most common in diabetics, alcoholics, and intravenous (IV) drug users, with some reports showing more than half of these infections being precipitated by self-injection. The presentation may be delayed several days after initial symptoms. It is essential that the clinician maintain a high suspicion for this disease in patients presenting with severe upper-extremity infections. Symptoms may include extreme pain, blistering and bullae, skin hemorrhage or loss, rapid progression, and crepitus. If there is any suspicion for necrotizing fasciitis, immediate resuscitation and empiric intravenous antibiotics should be initiated, followed immediately by surgical débridement. The most common pathogen is *Streptococcus pyogenes* (Group A strep), although some cases may be polymicrobial or contain other bacteria such as anaerobes. With the rising incidence of MRSA, more MRSA-related necrotizing fasciitis cases are being encountered.

Treatment

After resuscitation, the patient should be urgently taken to the operating room. Patient outcomes for necrotizing fasciitis are directly linked to adequacy and timing of débridement. Exsanguination of the extremity should be avoided so as not to milk the bacteria proximally. Débridement requires longitudinal incisions along the affected extremity, with liberal removal of infected and devitalized tissue. Amputation may be necessary. Tissue samples should be taken for culture. The classic finding is "dishwater pus," a thin, foul-smelling fluid along the fascial planes, along with thrombosis of the microvasculature in the affected area. The fascia may appear gray or grayish-green and swollen. The surgeon should have a low threshold for extending incisions and further débridement because the possibility of missing large pockets of purulent material can have devastating consequences. After removal of all infected tissue, the wounds should be copiously irrigated out and left open. Dressing changes should be started within the next 24 hours and be done two to three times a day. The patient will likely require multiple débridements occurring every couple of days until it is certain that all infectious and devitalized tissue has been removed. These patients may require soft tissue reconstruction once the infection is eradicated.

OSTEOMYELITIS

Diagnosis

Osteomyelitis in the hand can result from penetrating trauma, septic arthritis, other deep infections, or seeding of the bone from bacteremia. Injured bones, either from trauma or surgery, are particularly susceptible due to the damaged cortex, which allows pathogen penetration. Plain x-rays may show signs of bony destruction, although this typically appears several weeks after the infection has begun (Figure 15). MRI or bone scan will help with early detection. The gold standard for diagnosis is tissue culture and bone biopsy with pathologic confirmation.

Treatment

Although it is possible for early cases of osteomyelitis to be treated with IV antibiotics alone, treatment often requires surgery. Draining wounds, abscesses, and areas of necrotic bone should be washed out and debrided to a margin of healthy bone and soft tissues. Necrotic soft bone is easily debrided with a rongeur or osteotome until hard bone is encountered. The presence of hardware may make eradication of the infection difficult. Any implantable hardware should be considered for removal, especially if it is loose or no longer needed for stability. External fixators can provide provisional fixation during the interim. Antibiotics should be culture driven when possible and should be administered intravenously for 4 to 6 weeks. The surgeon should have a low threshold for an infectious disease consultation to aid with antibiotic tailoring and duration.

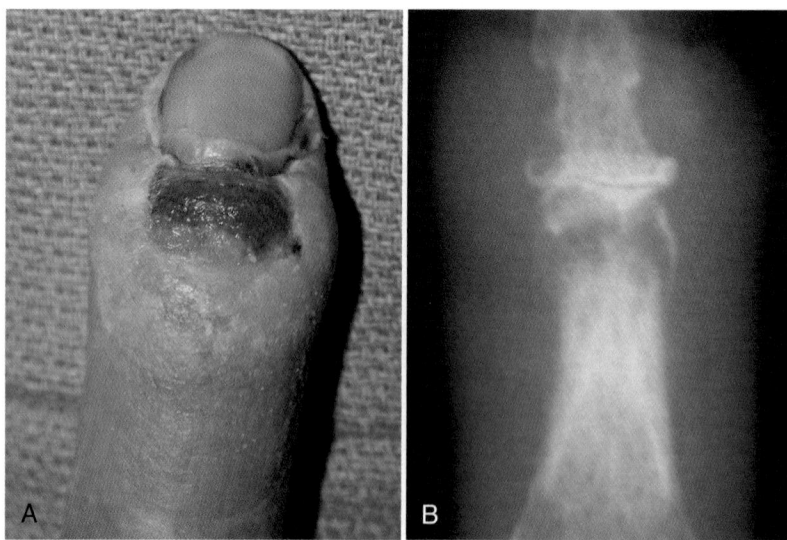

FIGURE 15 Osteomyelitis. *(From Wolfe SW, Hotchkiss, RN, Pederson WC, et al:* Green's operative hand surgery, *ed 6, Philadelphia, 2010, Churchill Livingstone.)*

SUGGESTED READINGS

Cornwall R, Waitayawinyu T: Infections. In Trumble TE, editor: *Hand Surgery Update IV*, Rosemont, IL, 2007, American Society for Surgery of the Hand, pp 543–562.

Honda H, McDonald JR: Current recommendations in the management of osteomyelitis of the hand and wrist, *J Hand Surg Am* 34:1135–1136, 2009.

Kwo S, Agarwal JP, Meletiou S: Current treatment of cat bites to the hand and wrist, *J Hand Surg Am* 36:152–153, 2011.

McDonald LS, Bavaro MF, Hofmeister EP, et al: Hand infections, *J Hand Surg Am* 36:1403–1412, 2011.

O'Malley M, Fowler J, Ilyas AM: Community-acquired methicillin-resistant Staphylococcus aureus infections of the hand: prevalence and timeliness of treatment, *J Hand Surg Am* 34:504–508, 2009.

Sunderland IR, Friedrich JB: Predictors of mortality and limb loss in necrotizing soft tissue infections of the upper extremity, *J Hand Surg Am* 34:1900–1901, 2009.

NERVE INJURY AND REPAIR

Pablo A. Baltodano, MD, and Gedge D. Rosson, MD

INTRODUCTION

During the past 40 years, and mainly due to the availability of surgical operating microscopes, surgeons have been routinely repairing nerves. This has paralleled the advance of microvascular free flap reconstruction and digital replantations. Performing optimal nerve repairs requires meticulous microsurgical operative techniques and the use of both the science and the art of peripheral nerve surgery.

Nerve repair is an exercise in patience and delayed gratification. The surgeon must exercise patience and care to appropriately direct sensory fibers into sensory end organs and motor fibers into appropriate muscles. In many cases, it can take months or even years for the final results.

GENERAL PRINCIPLES

Basic Anatomy

Prior to embarking on peripheral nerve surgery, it is critical to understand the basics of peripheral nerve anatomy (Figure 1) and physiology. Knowing the anatomy and physiology for potentially injured nerves enables the clinician to adequately assess the magnitude of peripheral nerve injuries. Additionally, an adequate understanding of the histology of peripheral nerves sets the basis for performing optimal nerve repairs.

The most basic subunit of the peripheral nerve is the axon. Each axon is surrounded by the endoneurium. Axons are grouped into fascicles, and these fascicles are surrounded by a thin perineurium. The grouped fascicles are also surrounded by interfascicular epineurium. The main nerve itself is surrounded by an external epineurial

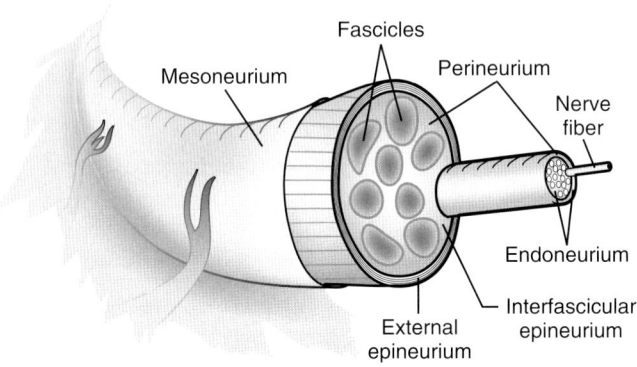

FIGURE 1   The normal anatomy of the peripheral nerve.

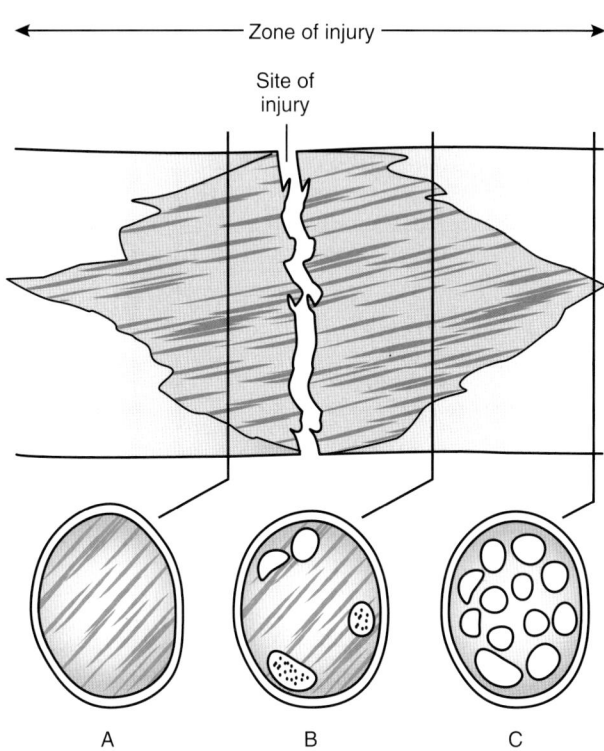

FIGURE 2   Following nerve injury, the zone of injury may extend well beyond the site of injury. **A,** The nerve consists entirely of scar tissue. **B,** Scar tissue and a fascicular pattern are seen in the more remote zones of injury. A fascicular pattern may be seen, but it may be scarred (stippled). **C,** Normal fascicle (clear) will protrude from the plane of the cut nerve because of increased endoneurial pressure.

sheath. The external segmental blood supply to the nerve travels through a final layer of connective tissue referred to as the mesoneurium, which also allows nerve gliding during normal range of motion.

Fascicular Topography

When performing nerve repairs, it is important to understand the difference between the fascicular topography in the proximal nerve trunk and the fascicular topography in the distal nerve. Most nerves have a significant intermingling of sensory and motor fibers with plexus formation in the nerve trunks proximally. The more distal nerve fascicles have usually become groups of sensory fibers and groups of motor fibers. This partially explains why more distal nerve repairs have better long-term functional outcomes. For example, repairing facial nerve injuries within the temporal bone often leads to a significant amount of disabling synkinesis and dyskinesis due to the lack of distinctive fascicular architecture in the proximal facial nerve trunk. This is in contradistinction to repair of the facial nerve in the parotid gland branches or distally because these fascicles are now in their final configuration.

Pathophysiology of Nerve Injury

The surgeon willing to perform a successful nerve repair should have a clear concept of the mechanism of injury, zone of injury (Figure 2), degree of injury, and the nerve components involved. Based on the mechanism of injury, lesions may be classified as open (sharp or raggedy laceration) or closed (overstretching, blunt, or compressive trauma). Gunshot wounds, although technically open, behave more like closed injuries because the nerve damage is more likely due to the blast effect than to transection. Second, the zone of injury should be determined. A very clean injury to the nerve such as that with a scalpel will have a small zone of injury, whereas avulsion nerve injury with a table saw can have a very wide zone of injury. It is nearly impossible to accurately detect the zone of injury during the initial exploration if there is any crush or avulsion component.

Subsequently, the degree of injury may be classified as neurapraxia, axonotmesis, and/or neurotmesis using the Seddon's classification or as degrees I to V by the Sunderland's classification. Mackinnon and Dellon added a degree VI (combined nerve injury) to the Sunderland's classification. Determining the degree of nerve injury provides guidance as to when nerve injury requires surgical intervention (Table 1).

Regarding the nerve components injured, three scenarios are possible. The first is when there is focal or segmental demyelination with preservation of the axons (clinically manifested as neurapraxia). In this scenario, functional recovery will occur spontaneously (as the

myelin heals, within minutes or days but up to 6 weeks). Thus, no surgical intervention is required. Hitting your "funny bone" is an example of an ulnar nerve neurapraxia that lasts minutes. The so-called "Saturday night palsy" (radial nerve injury with wrist drop) is another common example of neurapraxia.

The second scenario is characterized by axonal injury (axonotmesis). In this context, the axon itself will die back to the nearest node of Ranvier. Once the injury has stabilized over the next several hours, the injured axon will begin to grow. These axons form multiple "growth cones" (nerve sprouting) and attempt to grow at a rate of approximately 1 mm per day or 1 inch per month into the distal endoneurial tubes, if available. The segment of the nerve distal to the injury will undergo Wallerian degeneration. In this case, the myelin sheath and cellular debris are phagocytosed, and the axon is completely replaced over a period of 3 to 6 weeks.

Axonotmesis can result in a range from complete recovery to no recovery; the ultimate recovery is based on the degree of damage to the axonal surrounding tissues (endoneurium, perineurium, and epineurium) and the scar tissue that may result from it. Axonotmetic injuries may have intact or partially severed surrounding tissues. If the surrounding tissues remain intact (Sunderland's degree II), the axon sprouts will likely reach the distal endoneurial tubes and spontaneous recovery will occur. In contrast, if the surrounding tissues are partially severed (Sunderland's degree IV), the axonal sprouts will not reach the distal endoneurial tubes and a neuroma in continuity will develop.

The third scenario is when the axons and their surrounding tissues are completely injured (neurotmesis). After a transection injury, the regenerating axonal sprouts will not reach the distal endoneurial tubes and a neuroma will develop. Whenever substantial

TABLE 1: Classification and expected recovery of nerve injuries

Classification		Nerve component injured					Expected recovery		Surgery indicated
Seddon's	Sunderland's Degree (Modified)	Myelin	Axon	Endoneurium	Perineurium	Epineurium	Extent	Rate	
Neurapraxia	First	Yes	No	No	No	No	Complete	Fast	None
Axonotmesis	Second	Yes	Yes	No	No	No	Good	Slow	None
Axonotmesis	Third	Yes	Yes	Yes	No	No	Variable	Slow	None or neurolysis
Axonotmesis	Fourth	Yes	Yes	Yes	Yes	No	None	None	Nerve repair
Neurotmesis	Fifth	Yes	Yes	Yes	Yes	Yes	None	None	Nerve repair
	Sixth	Combination of injury					Variable	Variable	Variable

damage to the surrounding tissues precludes the axonal sprouts from reaching the distal endoneurial tubes (as is the case with Sunderland's degrees III to VI), a neuroma will develop and surgery will be required.

It is critical to highlight that the distal nerve segment will still have viable axons, which can transmit electrical stimulation for up to 72 to 96 hours. This is most important when repairing small motor nerves such as distal branches of the facial nerve. Thus, when confronted with a sharp facial laceration with nerve injury, it is critical to bring the patient to the operating room within 72 hours, if at all possible, because the distal nerve endings can be located with electrical stimulation.

It has also been found that the changes in the denervated muscles are different from the changes in the sensory end organs. When muscles are denervated, the muscles suffer from both disuse atrophy and denervation atrophy. Also, most of the motor endplates themselves will die within 12 months, and by 18 to 24 months they will all be gone. After that time, even if a functional axon could reach the muscle, the muscle cannot be reinnervated. At this point, reconstructive repairs addressing muscles, tendons, bones, and joints remain the only options. The sensory end organs, on the other hand, do not undergo degeneration, and reports have been made of reinnervating sensory targets and improving sensibility even many years after the original injury.

Timing

Optimal surgical timing is an essential factor for successful nerve repair. Closed injuries must be approached differently from open injuries. Additionally, with a limited time window for repair, "the earlier the better" remains a fundamental concept. Surgical timing for nerve repair can be summarized by the "3 plus 1" rule (Table 2), with early repair occurring within 3 days, subacute repair around 3 weeks, delayed repair around 3 to 6 months, and late repair after 1 year.

Whenever a *subacute repair* (around 3 weeks) is being considered, but another team (e.g., an orthopedic surgical team) is performing an acute surgery, it makes sense to explore the nerve at the same time. Nerve action potential (NAP) testing helps to determine recovery across a nerve injury by evaluating the capacity of a nerve segment to conduct an action potential (i.e., proximal and distal to an injury). Lesions-in-continuity with (+) NAP should be observed for several months. If a blunt or ragged transection is found, or after injuries with a significant crush or avulsion component, performing the repair at a second stage allows time for better definition of the zone

of injury. The scarred, damaged nerve endings are not readily apparent until 2 or 3 weeks after the injury, and scarred nerve endings should not be sutured together because the axons cannot regenerate through scar tissue. Nerve endings should be fixed under tension using radiopaque clips, staples, or a small Prolene. This will prevent retraction and allow easy identification of the nerve stumps during the second-stage surgery (subacute repair).

Delayed repair (around 3 to 6 months) is indicated when it is difficult to determine whether the injury will recover spontaneously. A closed injury may be a simple stretch traction injury with neurapraxia and regenerate well on its own. Therefore, these patients must be followed clinically every month, and sensation should be monitored by noninvasive neurosensory testing of the skin distal to the nerve injury. A formal nerve conduction study and electromyography should be performed at 6 weeks and 12 weeks following significant closed injury of a motor nerve. Observation can be continued in patients with signs of spontaneous recovery. An important concept is that 90% of the spontaneous nerve recoveries occur within 4 to 6 months, so it is reasonable to wait for that period (especially with distal injuries) before proceeding with nerve reconstructive surgery. Surgery is indicated when there is no evidence of clinical or electrophysiologic recovery after this period of observation. Motor nerves should be repaired within 4 to 6 months to give the regenerating axons time to grow into the target muscles.

As said before, gunshot wounds, although technically open, behave more like closed injuries because the nerve damage is more likely due to the blast effect than to transection. This often results in neurapraxia or axonotmesis, and it may not require surgical repair. Similarly, close observation should be implemented, and surgery should be performed if there are no signs of improvement.

Lesions-in-continuity can be evaluated with intraoperative NAP testing. As mentioned above, lesions-in-continuity with (−) NAP should undergo early repair. On the other hand, lesions with (+) NAP should be observed for a period of 4 months, after which surgery is performed if no signs of recovery are evident.

Late repair (after 1 year) may be considered a salvage procedure for patients presenting late or patients with incomplete recovery or failure to recover. Some surgeons consider repairs performed 9 months after the injury as late repairs. Especially in the case of motor nerves, the results of late repair are typically suboptimal because of permanent changes at the muscular level.

Treatment Options

Several treatment options for nerve injuries are available (Table 3).

TABLE 2: "3 plus 1" rule for timing of nerve repair

Timing	Time	Indications	Injury classification
Early	3 days	• Nerve transection with sharp injuries • Lacerations of the face (repairing in <72 hours adds the benefit of intraoperative nerve stimulation) • Acute nerve compression due to vascular (e.g., hematoma, pseudoaneurysm) and/or bony injuries • Acute neurologic worsening under close observation • Lesions-in-continuity with (−) NAP	Neurotmesis
Subacute	3 weeks	• Blunt or ragged transections (e.g., propeller blades, chain saws) • Injuries with significant crush or avulsion component	Neurotmesis
Delayed	3 months	• Nonpenetrating injuries (stretching injuries, contusive injuries, gunshot wounds) • Lesions-in-continuity with (+) NAP without adequate recovery	Axonotmesis
Late	>1 year	• Salvage procedures	Neurotmesis or axonotmesis

TABLE 3: Treatment options and indications for the repair of nerve injuries

Options	Indications
Observation	• Recovering nerve injury • Partial nerve injury
Neurolysis	• Lesion-in-continuity with positive NAP
Direct coaptation	• Laceration • Tension-free direct coaptation possible
Nerve graft or conduit	• Laceration with retracted stumps (delayed repair) • Direct repair without tension not possible
Nerve transfer	• Avulsions (e.g., brachial plexus avulsion) • Specific cases of nerve injury for which nerve transfer may lead to a more rapid or reliable recovery (i.e., because of proximity to the end-organ) than proximal nerve grafting • Innervation of free-functioning muscle transfers
Direct neurotization	• Under investigation/used for direct muscle reinnervation after severe trauma
Tendon and/or muscle transfers	• Delayed (>1 year) for improvement of function
Bony and/or joint procedures	• Delayed (>1 year) for improvement of function
Amputation	• Rarely indicated; sometimes desired by patients

NAP, Nerve action potential.

PREOPERATIVE MANAGEMENT

Patient Education

Patients must be adequately informed and well educated as to realistic expectations. Microsurgical techniques can yield good functional outcomes; unfortunately, patients rarely obtain excellent results in terms of motor and sensory regeneration. Several limitations to nerve repair exist. The speed of regeneration (up to 1 mm/day or 1 inch/month), a large distance from repair site to end organ, muscle atrophy or neuromuscular junction degeneration, limited availability of functional donors or graft materials, and unrealistic expectations may all result in unsatisfactory outcomes.

These limitations become evident depending on the clinical scenario. When treating an individual distal sensory nerve injury, these limitations are reduced. When treating a single, simple distal sensory nerve injury, success is more likely and these limitations are not as critical. Conversely, these limitations severely impact the outcome of multiple proximal motor nerve injuries, such as proximal brachial plexus lesions. Making patients aware of the limitations of nerve reconstruction surgery can produce more realistic expectations and more satisfied patients.

Preoperative Assessment

The optimal approach to nerve injury assessment includes a detailed history of the mechanism of injury and the onset of the deficit; a physical exam (neurologic, vascular, and musculoskeletal examination); and electrodiagnostic studies, such as electromyelogram and nerve conduction studies. These three pillars (history, physical exam, and electrodiagnostic studies) help the clinician to determine the extent and severity of the nerve injury. Additionally, imaging studies (radiographs, ultrasound, computed tomographic scan, magnetic resonance imaging and neurography, and/or myelogram) can further enlighten the clinical scenario and the operative

planning. Specifically, high-resolution (3 Tesla) magnetic resonance neurography (MRN) has been increasingly used to better define the anatomy of injured nerves. MRN provides a substantial benefit for the evaluation of large proximal nerve elements such as the brachial plexus, the lumbosacral plexus, the sciatic nerve in the pelvis, and other nerves that follow deep or complex courses, where electrodiagnostic studies are difficult to use. The clinician must also remember to use sensory and motor function grading scales, which will facilitate follow-up and assessment of the results of interventions (including observation).

Equipment

Prior to any nerve exploration or repair, proper equipment must be readily available. Nerve repairs should be performed only on medically stable patients. The surgical team should be well rested and well trained in microsurgical techniques. The equipment and room setup is similar to microvascular surgery as needed for free flap reconstruction. A well-maintained operative microscope or a minimum of 4× loupe magnification should be available. Microsurgical instruments such as microforceps, microscissors, microbipolar, and microsurgical needle drivers are required, as well as 9-0 or 10-0 nylon sutures. Heparinized saline solution is needed if a nerve conduit will be utilized.

Positioning and Planning

Patients must be positioned on the operating room table to allow ease of access to both the site of injury and any potential donor sites if nerve grafting will be required. These areas should be simultaneously prepped and draped for ease of access. For nerve repairs in the upper extremities, the patient's arm is placed on an arm board, and comfortable seating should be available. Nerve repairs of the lower extremities can also be performed with the surgeons seated if the patient is placed on the operating table so there is room under the table for the surgeon and the assistant to sit comfortably across from each other. If the operating room table is not positioned appropriately, the base of the table will be at the same level as the surgeon's knees. Common potential donor sites for nerve grafting include the sural nerve in the leg, the medial or lateral antebrachial cutaneous nerves, the superficial sensory radial nerve, the superficial peroneal nerve, the distal posterior interosseous nerve, the great auricular nerve, and the cervical plexus nerves.

The initial exploration should be under loupe magnification and tourniquet control if possible. If repair of a motor nerve is planned (and it is within 72 hours of the original injury), it is critical to remember that a tourniquet applied longer than 30 minutes can cause ischemia of the distal nerve, and intraoperative nerve stimulation will no longer be possible. Thus, the initial dissection must be well planned, focused, and directed to make sure there is enough time to dissect the putative distal nerve and apply stimulation for 30 minutes afterward.

OPERATIVE TECHNIQUE

Both an organized approach to exposing the injured nerve (Table 4) and a thorough knowledge of the anatomy are essential, especially when significant scarring is expected. To expose the injured segment of the nerve, dissection should be performed between two muscle groups parallel to the long axis of the nerve to identify a normal segment of the nerve, both proximally and distally, before dissecting to expose the injured segment. If it is near a compression site, such as the ulnar nerve near Osborne's band, then the site of compression should be released at this time. The regenerating nerve will become swollen during the regenerative phase, and potential future compression should be prophylactically removed.

After exposing the injured segment, there are two possibilities: the identification of a lesion-in-continuity versus nerve stumps. Intraoperative inspection of a lesion-in-continuity does not necessarily predict outcomes. A very firm lesion, particularly if a preoperative MRN showed a severe injury, most likely should be resected and reconstructed. However, if a lesion-in-continuity is identified, intraoperative NAP testing can be performed. If NAP (+), conservative management is indicated (observation will render better outcomes than resection, so only neurolysis should be performed). If NAP (−),

resection of the lesion followed by nerve reconstruction will improve outcomes.

If nerve stumps are identified, reconstruction is indicated. NAP, somatosensory-evoked potentials (SSEP), and motor-evoked potentials (MEP) may be used to help determine if the proximal nerve stump can be used for reinnervation.

Preparation of Nerve Endings

The most critical step is the preparation of the nerve endings. In fact, nerve resection is nerve repair's most neglected technique. Care must be made to adequately resect damaged nerve endings; this will be based on the mechanism of injury and the zone of injury. As previously mentioned, if there is any crush or avulsion, then it may be wise to tag the nerve endings using radiopaque clips, staples, or a small Prolene suture and come back in 3 weeks to adequately assess the scar formation. If the nerve repair was done 3 weeks or more after the original injury, it should be possible to adequately assess the scarred nerve endings. Any neuroma and scar are excised sharply using a scalpel, with the nerve placed on a flat, sterile wooden tongue depressor. The nerve stumps should be sliced proximally and distally (like slicing a loaf of bread) until a healthy fascicular pattern is visualized. This is called *les yeux d'escargot* (snail's eyes) (Figure 3). This pattern of healthy fascicles protruding from the cut nerve endings is due to the pressure within the endoneurium. The fascicles that protrude past the cut nerve ending should be further divided until all the fascicles lie flush with the epineurial sheath. This is critical so that the fascicles do not overlap once the epineurium is sutured. Any overlap of fascicles could lead to failure of the axonal sprouts to find the distal endoneurial tubes.

Tension-Free Nerve Coaptation

Direct coaptation is the traditional gold standard for nerve reconstruction. This technique delivers the axonal sprouts into their distal targets via a single suture line, which increases the feasibility of fascicular alignment. Thus, by decreasing fascicular mismatch, it theoretically improves outcomes (Figure 4).

Following meticulous preparation of the nerve endings, the tourniquet is usually deflated. Nerve coaptation by direct end-to-end suture of nerve stumps is then performed using several interrupted 9-0 or 10-0 nylon sutures. As a rule of thumb, the smaller the number of sutures used to approximate the nerve accurately, the better the outcome. Good results with fibrin glue have been reported, and it

TABLE 4: Key operative principles of nerve repair

Preparation for repair	Know the anatomy Plan adequate exposure, and plan for the possible need for additional exposure Plan for nerve graft harvest
Repair	Expose the normal segment of nerve first, then find the pathologic segment Dissect down to the nerve, then dissect along the nerve Dissect between the muscle groups Preserve vascular structures Use NAP to evaluate neuroma-in-continuity Prepare nerve endings Employ microsurgical technique Perform a tension-free nerve repair Simpler is better

NAP, Nerve action potential.

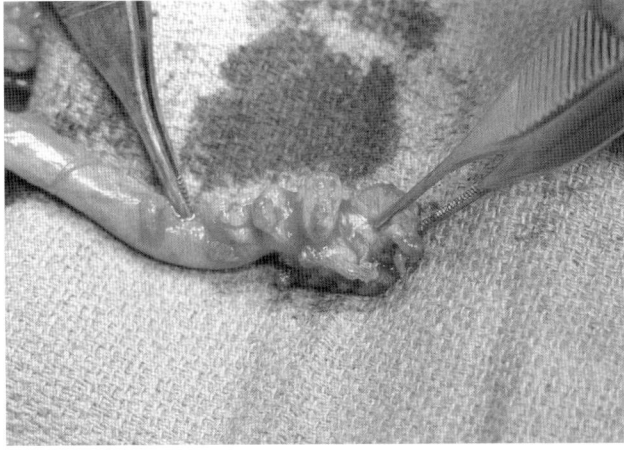

FIGURE 3 The damaged nerve ending, which in this case is a neuroma, is cut back until healthy fascicles are visualized, called *les yeux d'escargot*.

can be combined with minimal interrupted nylon sutures. Nerves are generally repaired with an end-to-end coaptation.

It is extremely critical that there be no tension whatsoever on the repair. One recent significant finding in nerve repair studies is that nerve repair success decreases significantly if there is any tension on the repair. It is more important to have a tension-free repair than to perform a primary nerve coaptation. Some studies have reported that leaving a submillimeter gap between the nerve stumps can improve axonal migration, reduce fascicular mismatch and improve outcomes. If needed, a nerve graft or interpositional bioabsorbable nerve conduit can be used. Some additional length on the nerve can be achieved for certain nerves such as the ulnar nerve at the elbow, which can be transposed anteriorly to the medial humeral epicondyle to give several centimeters of extra length. Most nerves do not have the ability to be transposed to add length. It is critical to never use positioning of joints, such as flexion of the elbow, to give added length to the nerve. This will result in stretching of the nerve and poor outcome when the limb is straightened later.

Epineurial Versus Grouped Fascicular Repair

For primary nerve repair, an epineurial repair is usually the most predictable (see Figure 4). The external epineurial vessels can be arranged to ensure that the fascicles are appropriately aligned. Additionally, to facilitate restoration of fascicular orientation, it is important to be familiar with the serial cross-sectional fascicular topography, fascicular stimulation, histochemical stains, and gross fascicular matching. Often, only two or three interrupted sutures are necessary to align and coapt the nerve endings. It is critical at this stage to ensure there is no overlapping of the fascicles (Figure 5). The fascicles should just be gently coapted within the epineurium. It is also important to make sure the needle passes only through the epineurium and does not catch a portion of one of the fascicles because this can lead to a small intraneural neuroma, and the fascicle will not heal properly.

Occasionally, it is appropriate to perform fascicular or grouped fascicular repairs. In a large nerve where the fascicles are easily identifiable, it may be possible to suture the internal epineurium between the fascicles with a few small, interrupted nylon sutures and then perform the epineurial repair. Some researchers have reported that grouped fascicular repair results in more intraneural scarring, so most peripheral nerve surgeons continue to use the epineurial repair.

Management of the Nerve Gap

Most often the resection of the scarred nerve endings will result in some amount of nerve gap. Nerve gaps require alternative methods of nerve repair such as interpositional nerve grafting or use of an off-the-shelf bioabsorbable nerve conduit, which is excellent for gaps less than 3 cm (Figure 6). Prospective double-blind trials have shown that using a bioabsorbable nerve conduit results in better two-point

discrimination than primary repair with nerve grafts in digital injuries with gaps less than 3 cm. Nerve transplants and decellularized nerve allografts have been reported, and the specific indications and outcomes are still evolving.

Using a nerve conduit requires an entubulation technique. The nerve conduit must be the correct diameter to accommodate the nerve. The nerve conduit should be approximately 10 mm longer than the nerve gap (e.g., a nerve gap of 3 cm would require up to a 4-cm nerve tube). The entubulation technique involves placing the proximal nerve ending 5 mm within one end of the nerve tube and the distal nerve ending 5 mm within the distal end of the nerve tube. Using a horizontal mattress suture, enter the nerve conduit 5 mm from the ending, suture the epineurium of the nerve ending itself and pull it 5 mm into the nerve tube, and tie the suture on the outside of the nerve conduit. A couple of extra epineurial interrupted sutures can be placed from the epineurium to the end of the nerve tube. This, of course, should be performed without the tourniquet so perfect hemostasis can be determined. Blood from the nerve ending must not be allowed to enter the nerve tube and coagulate. The final step is to flush any blood or debris out of the nerve conduit with heparinized saline. If a synthetic, biodegradable nerve conduit is not available, an acceptable alternative is autogenous vein grafting. These do tend to collapse, however, and the final results are not as predictable.

For nerve gaps greater than 3 cm, an interpositional nerve graft should be used. There are many potential donor sites for nerve grafts, and the patient must give consent preoperatively if a nerve graft is a possibility.

To calculate the length of the graft, measure the gap and add 10%. Calculating the graft length by this method will prevent tension on the reconstruction. To maximize the surface area at the repair sites, one or several "cable" grafts may be used (Figure 7). Either individual suturing or grouped suturing of the cable grafts is acceptable.

The nerve graft should be sutured into place in a reversed fashion from its usual anatomic course (i.e., the more distal end of the nerve graft should be sutured to the proximal end of the nerve gap being repaired, and the proximal end of the nerve graft should be sutured to the distal end of the nerve gap). This ensures that axons will not be lost through small side branches in the nerve graft as the axons grow through the graft. When the diameter of the nerve at the site of repair is much larger than the diameter of the nerve graft, grouped fascicular repair may be utilized. As mentioned before, it is critical to know the appropriate anatomic topography of the fascicles in the nerve to guarantee that motor fascicles are grafted to motor fascicles

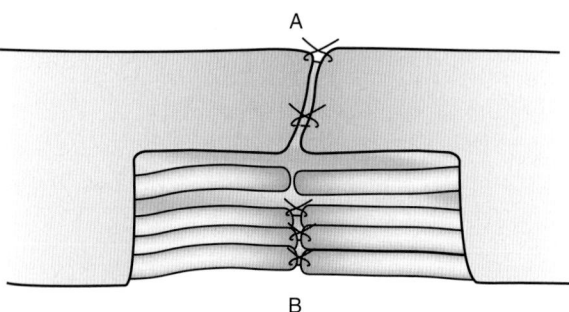

FIGURE 4 Nerve repairs. **A,** Epineurial repair. Note that the visible fascicles under the epineurium are opposed without overlap, and epineurial vessels are used to align nerve ends. **B,** Grouped fascicular repair.

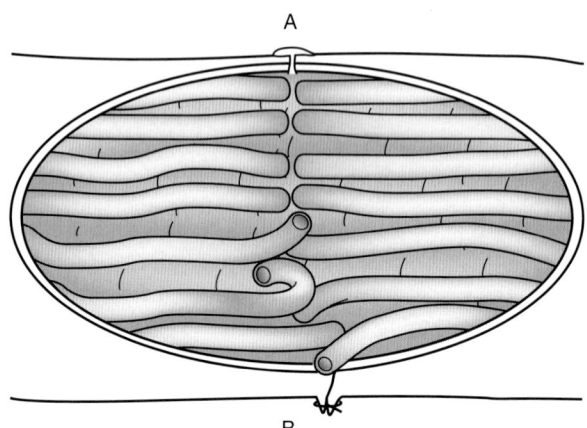

FIGURE 5 A, Appropriately trimmed fascicles will lightly oppose when the epineurium is gently approximated. **B,** Fascicular overlap and disorder may arise when fascicles have not been trimmed and protrude from the epineurium or when the epineurial repair is too tight.

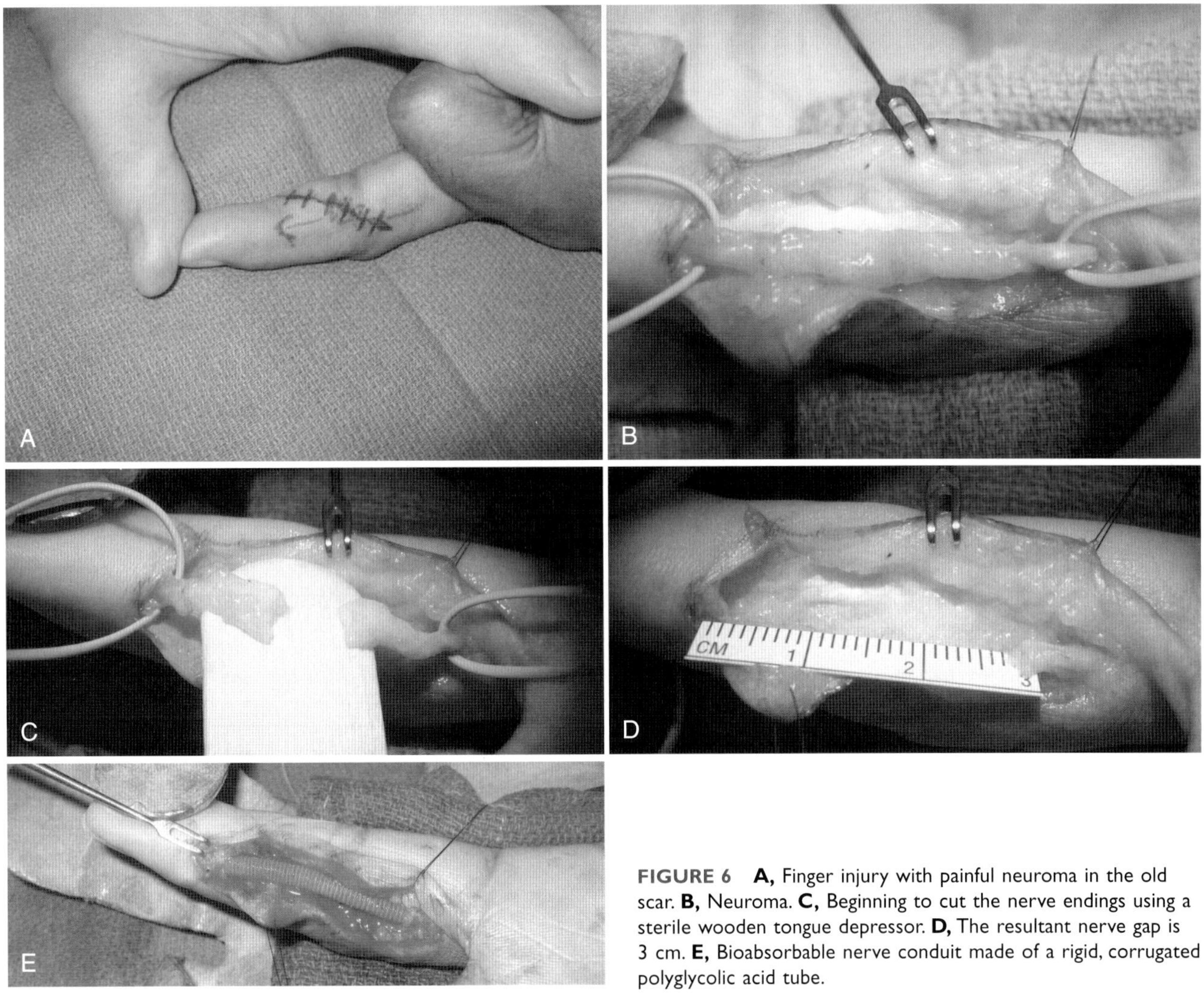

FIGURE 6 **A,** Finger injury with painful neuroma in the old scar. **B,** Neuroma. **C,** Beginning to cut the nerve endings using a sterile wooden tongue depressor. **D,** The resultant nerve gap is 3 cm. **E,** Bioabsorbable nerve conduit made of a rigid, corrugated polyglycolic acid tube.

and sensory fascicles are grafted to sensory fascicles. An inevitable disadvantage of nerve grafting is donor site morbidity. Permanent sensory loss is expected, and a small chance of neuropathic pain exists. The practice of using vascularized nerve grafts to improve the speed and quality of regeneration remains controversial.

Nerve Transfers

Nerve transfer *(neurotization)* refers to the procedure of transecting an expendable working nerve, branch, or fascicle in the vicinity of an injured nerve to coapt it to the nonfunctioning nerve. The main advantages of nerve transfers are better proximity to the end organ (which in turn decreases the time to reinnervation) and the fact that distal nerves contain a larger number of relatively "pure" (motor or sensory) axons (i.e., since nerve transfers involve the distal components of the nerve, at this level the axons are either motor or sensory). Indications for nerve transfers are summarized in Table 3.

When nerve transfer is indicated, outcomes are improved because this can be performed more distally and closer to the muscles in question than other repair techniques (i.e., proximal reconstruction with coaptation, conduits, and grafts). For example, an upper trunk brachial plexus injury would result in a loss of flexion of the elbow. If the lower trunk is intact, redundant fascicles of the ulnar nerve to the flexor carpi ulnaris muscle or from the median nerve going to

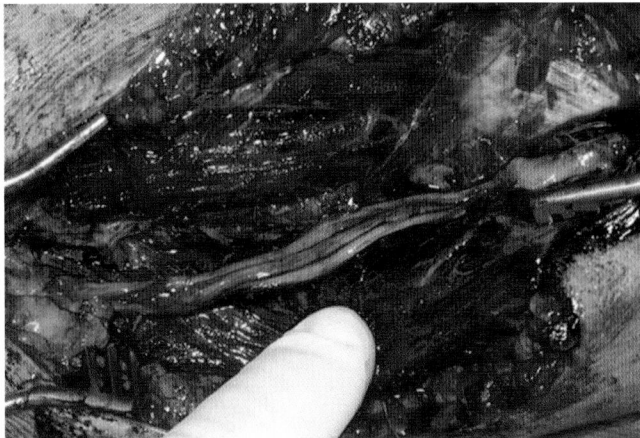

FIGURE 7 Intraoperative photograph of three sural nerve segments bridging a radial nerve gap in the distal arm following a humeral fracture.

superficial flexor muscles can be transferred to either the brachialis or the biceps motor nerve. This will result in faster reinnervation of the muscles than if a repair of the upper trunk of the brachial plexus was performed because it would take many months for the axons to grow all the way down into the arm.

Based on the expected time to reinnervation, the benefits of nerve transfers versus nerve grafts should be carefully evaluated for each clinical scenario. Most surgeons advocate distal nerve transfers closer to the end organ as opposed to proximal nerve grafting farther from the end organ.

Nerve Compression

Some nerve injuries do not result in interruption of the nerve but rather in a lesion-in-continuity with a (+) NAP. These nerve injuries do not need resection of the nerve with grafting, but rather they can improve dramatically with appropriate decompression of the nerves with neurolysis (i.e., releasing scar tissue and compressive bands or fascia surrounding the injured nerve). Generally, external neurolysis completed during the nerve exposure will suffice.

POSTOPERATIVE MANAGEMENT

Postoperative management begins in the operating room, even before closing the skin. Once the nerve has been repaired, the joints should go through the full range of motion to look for any signs of nerve tension. It is critical to detect tension on the nerve repair at this stage because tension can greatly diminish the functional outcome. Once the skin closure is complete, the extremity should be immobilized in a very well-padded, protective splint for 7 to 10 days. At this point, gradual protective range of motion to promote neural gliding can begin under the careful direction of a physical therapist or occupational therapist experienced in nerve injuries. Range of motion

should be gradually increased over the next 6 to 8 weeks. Physical therapists are integral to keeping the limb supple and free from contractures. Occasionally, patients have paraesthesia/dysesthesias of the neurosensory territories. These can be treated with Neurontin or Lyrica, and the occupational therapist or physical therapist can begin desensitization programs. Follow-up of nerve repairs is required for at least 2 years in children and up to 5 years in adults. The regeneration period is longer, and sensory/motor reeducation is more challenging in adults.

Sensory and Motor Reeducation

Any sensory nerve repair can have an improved outcome if sensory reeducation regimens are implemented. When motor nerves are repaired, it is critical for a physical therapist and occupational therapist to assist the patient with motor retraining as the muscles become reinnervated.

SUMMARY

A thorough knowledge of anatomy, the nerve injury process, and available repair and reconstructive options along with specific microsurgical skills in the context of a multidisciplinary team are required for optimal nerve injury management. The basic tenets of nerve repair are summarized in Table 5, and the expected outcomes are provided in Table 6. Figure 8 summarizes the proposed nerve injury management algorithm.

TABLE 5: Principles of nerve repair

1. Medical stability of patient
2. Preoperative and postoperative quantitative assessment of sensory and motor function
3. Early surgical exploration if open injury for microsurgical repair with appropriate magnification, sutures, and instrumentation
4. Bloodless field under tourniquet control, when possible
5. Extent of zone of injury assessed appropriately. All scarred nerve must be resected.
6. Primary nerve repair when clinical and surgical judgment permits
7. Secondary repair if zone of injury indeterminate at initial exploration
8. Tension-free nerve repair
9. Interpositional nerve graft or bioabsorbable nerve conduit, if direct repair would result in tension
10. Avoidance of positional or postural maneuvers to facilitate tension-free repair
11. Epineurial repair unless intraneural topography dictates group fascicular repair
12. Postoperative immobilization for 7 to 10 days, followed by early-protected motion
13. Postoperative sensory and motor reeducation
14. Routine postoperative monitoring with noninvasive neurosensory testing

TABLE 6: Expected outcomes from repair and reconstruction

Relevant factors	Functional outcomes
The "best surgery is no surgery"	Spontaneous recovery > nerve repair
Patient age	Younger patient > older patient
Level of injury	Distal > proximal
Type of nerve injured	Pure nerves > mixed nerves
Specific nerve involved	Radial nerve > median nerve > ulnar nerve Nerves C5 and C6 and those of the upper trunk > nerves C8 to T1 and those of the lower trunk Tibial nerve > peroneal nerve

TABLE 6: Expected outcomes from repair and reconstruction—cont'd

Relevant factors	Functional outcomes
Mechanism of injury	Lacerations > low-velocity gunshot injuries > high-velocity gunshot injuries Transections > crush or avulsion injuries Stretch injuries > ruptures > avulsions
Timing of repair and reconstruction	The "earlier the better." Waiting 2 to 3 weeks might be reasonable in some instances (blunt or ragged transections or injuries with significant crush or avulsion component) to allow time for better definition of the zone of injury.
Type of repair or reconstruction	Neurolysis alone because of a (+) NAP has good results 90% of the time. Direct end-to-end nerve repair > interpositional nerve grafting Distal nerve transfer > proximal nerve grafts Direct nerve transfers > nerve transfers with interpositional grafts

NAP, Nerve action potential.

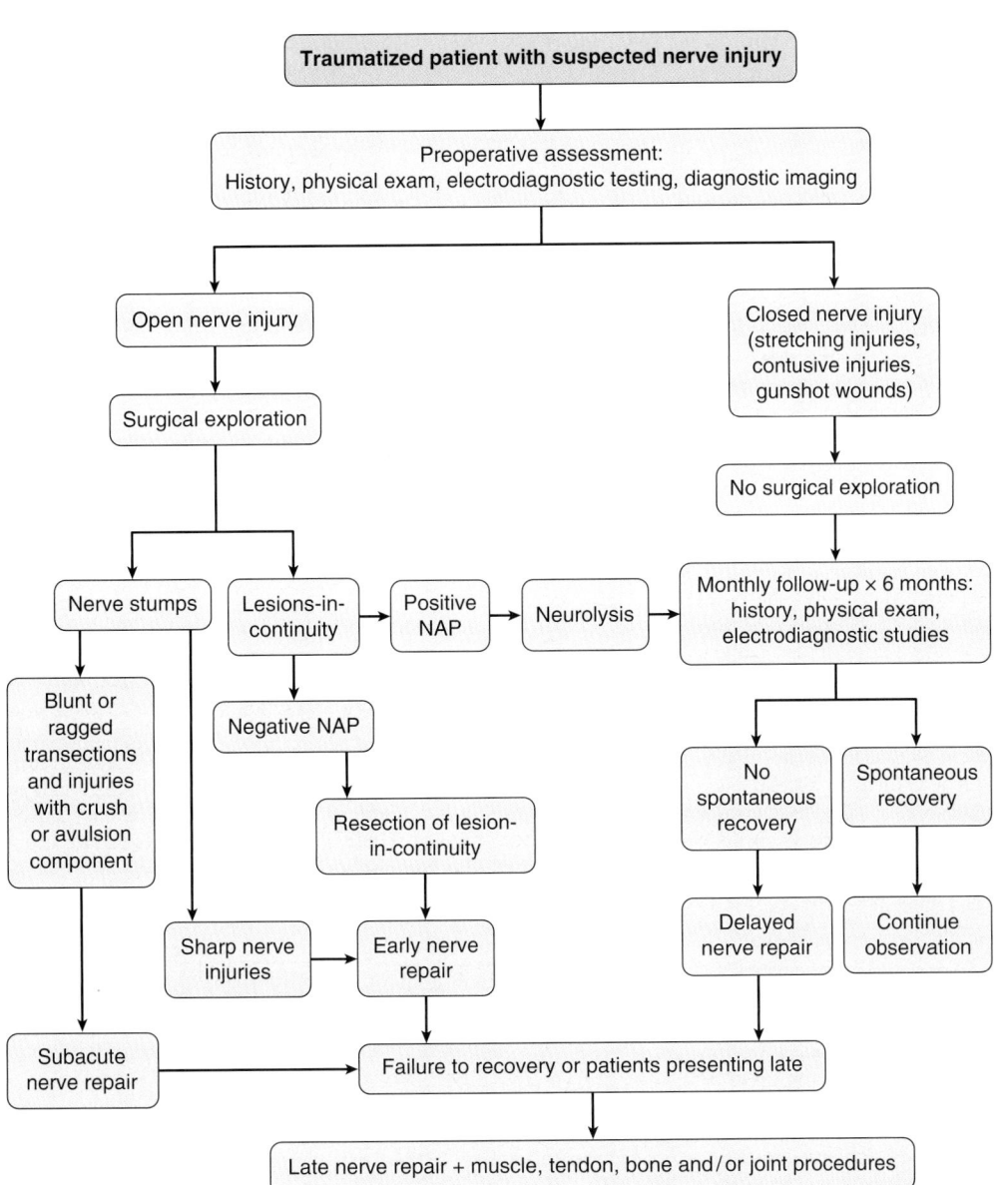

FIGURE 8 Nerve injury management algorithm. *NAP*, Nerve action potential.

SUGGESTED READINGS

Cohen MD, Dellon AL: Computer-assisted sensorimotor testing documents neural regeneration after ulnar nerve repair at the wrist, *Plast Reconstr Surg* 107(2):501–505, 2001.

Dellon AL: Resection: nerve repair's most neglected technique, *Plast Surg Tech* 1(3):191–199, 1995.

Dellon AL: *Somatosensory testing and rehabilitation*, Baltimore, 2000, Kirby Lithographic.

Kline DG, Happel LT: Penfield lecture: A quarter century's experience with intraoperative nerve action potential recording, *Can J Neurol Sci* 20(1):3–10, 1993.

Mackinnon SE, Dellon AL: *Surgery of the peripheral nerve*. New York, 1988, Thieme.

Midha R, Lee P, Mackay M: *Surgical techniques for peripheral nerve repair. Neurosurgical operative atlas: spine and peripheral nerves*, ed 2, New York, 2007, pp 402–408.

Millesi H: The nerve gap. Theory and clinical practice, *Hand Clin* 2(4):651–663, 1986.

Sunderland S: A classification of peripheral nerve injuries producing a loss of function, *Brain* 74(4):491–516, 1951.

Oberlin C, Durand S, Belheyar Z, et al: Nerve transfers in brachial plexus palsies, *Chirurgie de la Main* 28(1):1–9, 2009.

Spinner RJ, Kline DG: Surgery for peripheral nerve and brachial plexus injuries or other nerve lesions, *Muscle & Nerve* 23(5):680–695, 2000.

Weber RA, Breidenbach WC, Brown RE, et al: A randomized prospective study of polyglycolic acid conduits for digital nerve reconstruction in humans, *Plast Reconstr Surg* 106(5):1036–1045, 2000.

EXTREMITY GAS GANGRENE

Sharon Henry, MD

INTRODUCTION

Hippocrates in 5 BC provided the earliest description of the generic disease process of a severe necrotizing soft tissue infection (NSTI). Many additional descriptions appeared later in the medical literature, especially around the time of the Civil War. The term gas gangrene is used specifically to describe clostridial myonecrosis. These infections are rare and may only be seen a few times in the career of a community surgeon. An estimated 1000 to 3000 cases occur annually in the United States. Furthermore, these infections are life and limb threatening. Prompt identification and quick and efficient treatment are imperative.

The presentation of patients with infection from clostridium is frequently dramatic. The infection can begin innocuously but progresses rapidly. The initial signs are nonspecific and include erythema, swelling, and pain. The erythema transforms into necrosis, often first becoming violaceous or purpuric. The swelling becomes indurated, and the pain abates as the tissue necrosis progresses. Systemically, the patient often describes flulike symptoms of nausea, vomiting, fever, and muscle aches. The patient may describe lightheadedness and present to the hospital with full-blown sepsis.

The infection occurs most commonly in traumatic or postoperative wounds. Cases have also been described after illicit and therapeutic drug injection, and in some studies, as many as 50% of cases are idiopathic. Some patients with development of gas gangrene have no underlying medical conditions. Others have a variety of medical conditions (Table 1).

BACTERIOLOGY

Clostridia bacilli are toxin-producing bacteria that invade tissue and cause tissue necrosis, gas formation, and tissue destruction. They are anaerobic, spore-forming, gram-positive bacteria that are found in the soil. The spores are heat resistant and can persist in the environment for extensive time periods. Areas of tissue hypoxia are fertile sites for growth that can be rapid. More than 150 species of clostridia have been identified, but perfringens, novyi, histolyticum, septicum, bifermentans, and fallax are most commonly involved with infection.

Infections caused by *C. septicum* are frequently associated with malignancy, either overt or occult. These are frequently gastrointestinal malignancies. All species produce a variety of exotoxins (Table 2), but the alpha toxin is most associated with the tissue destruction that allows the organism to invade the muscle. The toxins produce capillary and small vessel thrombosis, which results in necrosis of tissue augmenting the hypoxic environment and facilitating the spread and growth of the organisms. The toxin also has a direct negative effect on movement of neutrophils to the site of injury or infection.

DIAGNOSIS

Clinical Examination

The challenge of treatment of gas gangrene begins with the challenge of the diagnosis. Tissue crepitus is pathognomonic but not always present. The skin findings of multiple bullae with violaceous or purpuric skin discoloration occur late. Systemic sepsis is also a late finding. The objective is identification of the process early, before the patient has suffered significant tissue damage and is in profound shock.

Laboratory Tests

Laboratory tests may reveal profound derangements as a result of damage from toxin elaboration. Severe leukocytosis or leukopenia, hyponatremia, lactic acidosis, thrombocytopenia, coagulopathy, elevation of C-reactive protein, creatine kinase, and liver function tests can be seen but are nonspecific. Some attempts have been made to use routine diagnostic laboratory tests to discriminate necrotizing soft tissue infection from cellulitis. Wall and associates found serum sodium (Na) <135 mEq/L, white blood cell count (WBC) ≥15 × 10^9/L, and blood urea nitrogen (BUN) >15 mg/dL to be found more commonly in patients who are diagnosed with NSTI than those with cellulitis. Wong and his colleagues created a scoring system based on C-reactive protein, leukocyte count, hemoglobin, sodium, creatinine, and glucose measured at admission. Patients with scores of more than six had an increased likelihood of NSTI.

Diagnostic Radiography

Diagnostic radiology can be helpful. Plane x-rays may show air in the soft tissues not appreciated on physical examination. Ultrasound

TABLE 1: Possible etiologies for gas gangrene

Posttraumatic	Postprocedural	Spontaneous
Penetrating wounds	Surgical procedures: gastrointestinal tract or biliary tract, open or laparoscopic Gynecologic	Gastrointestinal cancer
Crush injuries	Subcutaneous injection	Diabetes mellitus
Battlefield injuries	Intramuscular injections	Hepatic dysfunction
Farm injuries	Gastrointestinal perforations	Leukemia
Open fractures	Bone marrow transplant	Lymphoproliferative disorders

TABLE 2: Selected clostridial toxins

Gas gangrene–causing organisms and their toxins

Species	Toxins	Activity
Clostridium perfringens (welchii)	Alpha	Phospholipase C/ myonecrosis
	Beta	Lethal, necrotic/ enterotoxemia
	Epsilon	Lethal, permease/ enterotoxemia
	Kappa	Collagenase
	Lambda	Protease
	Mu	Hyaluronidase
Clostridium sordelii (bifermentans)	Alpha	Phospholipase C
	Beta	Lethal
	Hemolysin	Oxygen-labile hemolysin
Clostridium novyi (hemolyticum)	Alpha	Lethal
	Beta and gamma	Phospholipase C
	Delta	Oxygen-labile hemolysin
Clostridium septicum	Alpha	Lethal, necrotizing
	Beta	DNase
	Gamma	Hyaluronidase
	Delta	Oxygen-labile hemolysin
Clostridium histolyticum	Alpha	Necrotizing
	Beta	Collagenases
	Gamma	Proteinase
	Epsilon	Oxygen-labile hemolysin

Modified from Hathaway CL: Toxigenic Clostridia, Clin Microbiol Rev 3(1):66-98, 1990.

TABLE 3: Antimicrobial therapy for necrotizing fasciitis

	First-line	Alternative
Polymicrobial		
Gram-negative	Beta-lactam/ beta-lactamase inhibitor or fluoroquinolone	Third or fourth generation cephalosporin, carbapenem, aminoglycoside
Gram-positive	Clindamycin or beta-lactam/ beta-lactamase inhibitor	Third or fourth generation cephalosporin
MRSA	Vancomycin	Linezolid, daptomycin
Clostridia		
	Penicillin G high dose	Clindamycin
	Clindamycin	Metronidazole

MRSA, Methicillin-resistant Staphylococcus aureus.

intramuscular fluid collections. When performed with intravenous contrast, it can also identify unperfused muscle. Magnetic resonance tomography can also show gas, fluid collections, and edema and perfusion abnormalities of the muscle, which may aid in the diagnosis of NSTI. These studies are frequently most useful for demonstrating the extent of disease, which helps to guide operative intervention. Unfortunately, nonspecific findings on radiologic studies are not necessarily helpful in excluding the infection. Thus, a CT scan that shows only tissue edema in a patient with severe cellulitis and blistering with a high WBC and hypotension does not rule out the possibility of an NSTI.

TREATMENT

The approach to the treatment of patients with NSTI in general or gas gangrene specifically begins with resuscitation. These patients often experience significant delays in reaching medical therapy because the diagnosis was missed early, either because they were thought to have simple cellulitis or they did not present for medical evaluation until physiologic decompensation had already occurred. In either case, a rapid and aggressive attempt to correct the abnormal physiology should be undertaken. Volume resuscitation begins, with the administration of isotonic crystalloid. Blood, fresh frozen plasma, platelets, or other component therapy is given to begin correction of abnormalities identified. Adequate quantities of blood and components should be available for the operating room (OR) because extensive blood loss is possible. Even after adequate volume resuscitation, shock can commonly persist. This can result from the inflammatory response to the sepsis or toxemia. In these cases, addition of pressors and inotropes may be necessary to allow for safe administration of anesthesia. Broad-spectrum antibiotics should be given to cover the suspected pathogens. Clostridia are generally responsive to penicillin G, but resistance is increasing. Many other antimicrobials are also effective against clostridia (Table 3). The combination of penicillin and clindamycin is considered the most effective. Gram-negative and methicillin-resistant staphylococcus coverage should be added until definitive diagnosis has been made. Placement of large-bore intravenous access for resuscitation and monitoring is necessary.

scan with duplex of the extremity can show venous and arterial occlusions. Sonography can also show air and fluid collections that may not be appreciated on physical examination. Computed tomographic (CT) scan is even more sensitive for the identification of air in the tissues. In addition, it is capable of identifying subfascial or

An arterial line is frequently necessary, especially if pressors or inotropes have been required.

Tetanus immunization status should be assessed and the patient appropriately treated (Table 4).

Operative Treatment

Although these patients present with severe physiologic derangements and some attempt at correction must occur before surgery, it is important to recognize that the physiology will not be restored with medical therapy alone and proceeding to the OR, even with persistent abnormalities, is a risk that must be taken. The resuscitation can continue into the operative phase of treatment. The extremity must be circumferentially prepped and draped, extending to the joint above and below the involvement. When the diagnosis is in question, exploration of the extremity can be diagnostic. Vertical skin incisions are made usually over the area of maximal skin abnormality because the skin has to be removed with evidence of necrosis or purpura. The dissection must continue through the deep fascia and muscle thoroughly inspected. Tissue cultures should be obtained; if any diagnostic uncertainty exists, pathology should also be sent. Stat gram stains can give an indication of the types of bacteria present and influence antibiotic choice. Frequently the subcutaneous fat and superficial fascia are involved. Extensive débridement of this layer often produces skin compromise that results in large surface area wounds that require skin grafting for closure. Toxin production and bacterial spread along the fascial plane make blunt dissection easy, with the superficial layers separate from the deep, offering minimal resistance. With operation on patients with intravenous drug use, needles may be found in the subcutaneous tissues, and tissues should be handled preferentially with instruments rather than finger dissection. Compromised muscle either has a congested appearance or is very pale, depending on the time course of the process. Nonviable muscle is friable and peels away easily, offering little resistance to removal. The cut edges often do not bleed or produce only venous blood. The muscle does not contract when stimulated with the cautery; this is independent of muscle relaxation. Knowledge of the distribution of the neurovascular bundles in the compartments is important when performing these débridements because functional outcome can be impaired through inadvertent or unnecessary transection of blood vessels or nerves. Historically, amputation has been the only procedure recommended to treat gas gangrene. The goal is to get ahead of the infection. The limb is removed above the level of gross involvement of the infection. If amputation is planned, through joint amputation should be considered because it is frequently less time consuming and results in lower blood loss. It also spares tissue that can be used for reconstruction or closure. Blood loss can also be diminished through the use of a tourniquet during surgery. Tourniquet use is generally discouraged in the patient with vascular disease or diabetes undergoing an amputation; however, in a patient with an unstable condition with coagulopathy or thrombocytopenia, use of this device may prevent further destabilization from blood loss. Unfortunately, if hip or forequarter amputation is necessary, tourniquets are not an option. There is a balance between aggressive débridement to remove compromised tissue and arrest growth of bacteria and extension of the infection with tissue preservation for future reconstruction. Reexploration is the rule rather than the exception. Caring for these patients is resource intense. Hospital and intensive care unit stays are long. The patients are initially returned to the operating room within 24 to 72 hours, and sooner if they have progression of the infection. Repeated operating room washouts and inspections are necessary in these large wounds. Reconstruction or stump closure is only performed when the infection is well controlled and the patient has been assessed for adequacy of blood flow, arterial and venous. Sepsis and the large surface area of the wound combine to increase the basal metabolic rate and increase nutritional requirements. Supplemental tube feeding is frequently necessary. Reconstruction should be delayed until markers of nutrition are improving.

Hyperbaric Oxygen

When available, hyperbaric oxygen (HBO) is used to aid the treatment of this infection. Very high levels of dissolved oxygen are produced and may result in bacterial killing of anaerobic organisms. Some animal data suggest that HBO is synergistic with antibiotics and deactivates exotoxin. Resuscitation, antibiotic administration, and surgical débridement should never be delayed to allow for the use of HBO.

OUTCOME

Elliot and colleagues found that mortality correlated with the presence of organ failure at admission and delay in first débridement. Anaya and associates found death to occur more commonly in patients who had a WBC >30 × 10⁹/L, serum creatinine >2 mg/dL, or preexisting heart disease. Others have found that mortality increased with the presence of premorbid conditions. Mortality was more than 50% in patients who had three or more of the following risk factors: age more than 50 years, malnutrition or obesity, diabetes, injection drug use, and hypertension.

SUGGESTED READINGS

Anaya DA, McMahon K, Nathens AB, et al: Predictors of mortality and limb loss in necrotizing soft tissue infections, *Arch Surg* 140:151–157, 2005.

Carter PS, Banwell PE: Necrotising fasciitis: a new management algorithm based on clinical classification, *Int Wound J* 1:189–198, 2004.

Elliott D, Kufera JA, Myers RAM: Necrotizing soft tissue infections: risk factors for mortality and strategies for management, *Ann Surg* 224:672–683, 1996.

Graves C, Saffle J, Morris S, et al: Caloric requirements in patients with necrotizing fasciitis, *Burns* 31:55–59, 2005.

Hatheway CL: Toxigenic Clostridia, *Clin Microbio/Rev* 3(1):66–98, 1990.

Jallali N, Withey S, Butler PE: Hyperbaric oxygen as adjuvant therapy in the management of necrotizing fasciitis, *Am J Surg* 189:462–466, 2005.

McGillicuddy E, Lischuk A, Schuster K, et al: Development of a computed tomography-based scoring system for necrotizing soft-tissue infections, *J Trauma* 70:894–899, 2011.

Mills MK, Faraklas I, Davis C, et al: Outcomes from treatment of necrotizing soft-tissue infections: results from the National Surgical Quality Improvement Program database, *Am J Surg* 200:790–797, 2010.

Morgan MS: Diagnosis and management of necrotising fasciitis: a multiparametric approach, *J Hosp Inf* 75:249–257, 2010.

Schneider J: Rapid infectious killers, *Emerg Med Clin North Am* 22:1099–1115, 2004.

Stevens DL, Bisno AL, Chambers HF, et al: Practice guidelines for the diagnosis and management of skin and soft-tissue infections, *Clin Infect Dis* 41(10):1373–1406, 2005.

TABLE 4: Tetanus toxoid recommendations for high-risk wounds

	Yes	No	Never immunized or immunocompromised
Immunized within 5 years	No booster	Booster	Vaccine and tetanus immunoglobulin 250 IU

Wall DB, De Virgilio C, Black S, et al: Objective criteria may assist in distinguishing necrotizing fasciitis from non-necrotizing soft tissue infection, *Am J Surg* 179:17–21, 2000.

Wilkinson D, Doolette D: Hyperbaric oxygen treatment and survival from necrotizing soft tissue infection, *Arch Surg* 139:1339–1345, 2004.

Wong CH, Khin LW, Heng KS, et al: The LRINEC (Laboratory Risk Indicator for Necrotizing Fasciitis) score: a tool for distinguishing necrotizing fasciitis from other soft tissue infections, *Crit Care Med* 32:1535–1541, 2004.

Necrotizing Skin and Soft Tissue Infections

Patrick B. O'Neal, MD, and
Kamal M.F. Itani, MD, FACS

OVERVIEW

Necrotizing skin and soft tissue infections (NSTIs) represent a range of infectious conditions that cause deep tissue necrosis. NSTI is described by terms based on location of infection, pathogen, and depth of necrosis. The most frequently used terms are necrotizing fasciitis, Fournier's gangrene, clostridial myonecrosis, synergistic necrotizing cellulitis, and gas gangrene. Necrotizing fasciitis represents infection that extends through the deep fascia below the subcutaneous layers. Fournier's gangrene is a similar condition that originates in the perineum, whereas clostridial myonecrosis and synergistic necrotizing cellulitis extend into the deep muscle compartments and cause muscular necrosis. These diseases have received extensive media attention and have been lumped under the catchy rubric of "flesh-eating" bacterial disease. Hippocrates (500 BC) acknowledged necrotizing fasciitis as "diffuse erysipelas caused by trivial accidents, where flesh, sinews, and bones fell away in large quantities, leading to death in many cases." The elaborate categorization of these conditions has caused confusion regarding this disease. Put simply, the pathophysiology of these infections in all categories is the same and is the result of bacterial penetration of skin defenses causing widespread necrosis and leading to rapid systemic deterioration and death. Any patient with signs or symptoms concerning for NSTI should raise a sense of urgency in the clinician for rapid diagnosis and early treatment. Unfortunately, the diagnosis of NSTI can be difficult and tempt the clinician to postpone lifesaving treatment while obtaining time-consuming diagnostic studies. This should be absolutely avoided in favor of urgent operative management.

PATHOPHYSIOLOGY

NSTI occurs when bacteria gain entry into the subcutaneous layers of the body where areas of relatively poor blood flow and relative hypoxia exist. Such conditions allow for poor immune response to infection and rapid overgrowth and spread of bacteria. Often, these microorganisms elaborate toxins that lead to both direct necrosis and indirect necrosis through thrombosis of perforating vessels and vasoconstriction increasing tissue hypoxia. Furthermore, these bacteria elaborate exotoxins that can lead to shock and multiorgan dysfunction.

DIAGNOSIS

Necrotizing fasciitis is a rare disease with an incidence rate estimated at 0.4 cases per 100,000 individuals by the U.S. Centers for Disease Control. Because delay in adequate treatment can have tremendous deleterious effects on outcome with increased morbidity and mortality, early diagnosis is paramount with necrotizing soft tissue infections. A thorough history and physical examination should be performed because this diagnosis relies more on clinical judgment rather than diagnostic testing. Certain comorbidities may predispose patients to this disease. Such conditions include advanced age, obesity, diabetes mellitus, alcoholism, cirrhosis, chronic debilitation, vasculopathy, intravenous drug use, immunosuppression, malignancy, chemotherapy, hypertension, chronic obstructive pulmonary disease (COPD), congestive heart failure (conditions that impair oxygen delivery), end-stage renal disease, perirectal abscess, perforated viscus, and recent surgery. A thorough history for assessment of patient comorbidities and risk factors may help raise suspicion of this problem. Despite this extensive list of predisposing conditions, as many as 20% of NSTIs occur in patients with no apparent predisposing factor. Although NSTI may seem to occur spontaneously without any clear injury or portal of entry, NSTI often originates in the perineum, diabetic foot ulcers, decubitus ulcers, incision sites, and puncture and traumatic wounds and as a result of perforated viscus with subsequent seeding of soft tissues.

Initial physical examination findings may range from minimal to quite dramatic (Table 1). One may appreciate swelling, induration, mild to exquisite tenderness, mild to violaceous erythema, tenderness beyond areas of erythema, cutaneous anesthesia, necrotic tissue or skin with a blue or purplish hue, and wounds with exuding purulent, gray, or foul-smelling drainage (Figure 1). The skin may blister or slough, and crepitus may be present, indicating gas formation in the tissues. Crepitus, however, is present in only a fraction of patients and should not be relied on for diagnosis. One must keep in mind that obvious stigmata of NSTI may be subtle. Any patient with soft tissue pain out of proportion to examination findings should be considered to be potentially harboring an elusive deep NSTI that has yet to make itself obvious because early skin changes may be minimal despite extensive subcutaneous fat, fascia, or muscle destruction. Tenderness beyond areas of erythema may be particularly ominous because it is indicative of rapidly progressive infection in the deep layers beneath the skin.

The hallmark of NSTI is its rapidly virulent and destructive behavior. Tracking within the fascial planes beneath the skin, a place with poor vascularity and thus host defenses, allows for the rapid spread of bacteria and overwhelming infection. Most patients have quick development of signs of systemic toxicity, which include high fever, nausea, vomiting, malaise, tachycardia, hypotension, shock, mental status changes, and oliguric renal failure.

Laboratory values are nonspecific. White blood cell counts may reveal extreme leukocytosis, leukopenia, and high bandemia. Other common laboratory abnormalities include those that indicate

TABLE 1: Necrotizing fasciitis signs and symptoms

Early	Late
Local	
Skin puncture or injury	Hematic/gas bullae
Erythema	Necrosis
Warmness	Purple/blue skin color
Tenderness	Crepitus
Myalgia	Hypoesthesia
Hypersensitive skin	Sensory/motor deficit
Systemic	
Pain out of proportion	Fever (sometimes hypothermia)
Swelling	Hypotension
Fever	Mental confusion Multiorgan failure

Wang YS, Wong CH, Tay YK: Staging of necrotizing fasciitis based on evolving cutaneous features, Int J Dermatol 46:1036-1041, 2007.

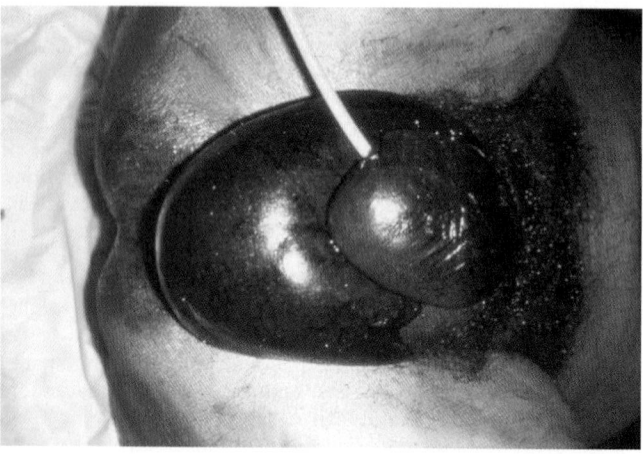

FIGURE 1 Black discoloration of penile, scrotal, and perineal skin in a patient with necrotizing infection of the perineum. Erythema, edema, and severe tenderness are also seen over the lower abdomen. *(From Dolghi O, Itani KMF: Necrotizing infection of the perineum,* Hosp Physician 44(1):39-45, 2008.)

TABLE 2: Laboratory Risk Indicator for Necrotizing Fasciitis (LRINEC) score system

LRINEC Score

LRINEC variable	Value	Score points
C-reactive protein (mg/L)	<150	0
	>150	4
White blood cell count (cells/mm³)	<15	0
	15-25	1
	>25	2
Hemoglobin (g/dL)	>13.5	0
	11-13.5	1
	<11	2
Sodium (mmol/L)	≥135	0
	<135	2
Creatinine (mg/dL)	≤1.6	0
	>1.6	2
Glucose (mg/dL)	≤180	0
	>180	1

LRINEC Score

Points, sum	Risk category	Nectrotizing fasciitis probability
≤5	Low	<50%
6-7	Intermediate	50%-75%
≥8	High	>75%

For patients at intermediate and high risk, the model has positive predictive value of 92% and negative predictive value of 96%.
Wang YS, Wong CH, Tay YK: The LRINEC [Laboratory Risk Indicator for Necrotizing Fasciitis] score: a tool for distinguishing necrotizing fasciitis from other soft tissue infections, Crit Care Med 32:1535-1541, 2004.

dehydration/fluid sequestration, such as low bicarbonate levels, elevated blood urea nitrogen, creatinine, and lactate levels. In addition, patients may present with hypoalbuminemia, elevated creatine phosphokinase, hyponatremia, and coagulopathy. The Laboratory Risk Indicator for Necrotizing Fasciitis (LRINEC) score system (Table 2) can be used as an adjunct for assessment of probability of necrotizing fasciitis. This should not, however, discourage operative débridement when clinical suspicion is high.

Because of the rapid lethality of necrotizing soft tissue infection, one should be cautious about obtaining advanced radiographic evidence of disease as this can delay lifesaving operative treatment. If obtained quickly in patients with relatively stable conditions, plain films may reveal air tracking in the soft tissues. Computed tomographic scan and magnetic resonance imaging may show air tracking in soft tissues, fascial separation, and abscess formation, but often these studies do not add much because they may only reveal nonspecific fat stranding. In patients with unstable conditions, these studies should be avoided in favor of rapid transfer to the operating room.

Biopsy of involved tissue typically reveals liquefaction necrosis of subcutaneous tissues and fascial layers with polymorphonuclear infiltrates and thrombosis of the perforating vessels to the skin. The fascial plains may weep a dishwater-appearing or hemorrhagic fluid.

MICROBIOLOGY

Necrotizing fasciitis has recently earned a classification system based on the pathogen of origin. Type I represents polymicrobial infections, type II represents monomicrobial infections, type III represents marine organisms, and type IV represents fungal organisms. In all classifications, the organisms gain entry to the subcutaneous spaces, multiplying in areas of relative hypoxia and low blood flow and allowing for rapid proliferation.

As many as 75% of necrotizing soft tissue infections are polymicrobial, with an average of four organisms in a single infection (Table 3). For this reason, initial antibiotic treatment should be broad

TABLE 3: Organisms recovered from 198 consecutive patients with necrotizing soft tissue infections

Organism	No. of cultures	No. of isolates (% of cultures)
Aerobic		
Streptococci	182	83 (45.6)
Enterococci	182	61 (33.5)
Staphylococci	182	64 (35.2)
Escherichia coli	182	57 (31.3)
Proteus spp.	182	38 (20.9)
Other gram-negative bacilli*	182	76 (41.8)
Anaerobic		
Peptostreptococci	131	45 (34.4)
Bacteroides spp.	128	70 (54.7)
Clostridium perfringens	129	12 (9.3)
Other clostridia	128	17 (13.3)
Other anaerobic species	128	27 (21.1)
Fungal species	171	9 (5.3)

*In order of prevalence: *Klebsiella* spp., *Enterobacter* spp., *Pseudomonas*, *Acinetobacter* spp., *Eikenella corrodens*, *Citrobacter feundii*.
Elliott DC, Kufera JA, Myers RA: Necrotizing soft tissue infections: risk factors for mortality and strategies for management, Ann Surg 224:672-683, 1996.

in spectrum. Polymicrobial infections often cause extensive local damage but on the whole are less lethal than other highly virulent monomicrobial infections. The most commonly isolated gram-positive organisms in polymicrobial infections include *Staphylococcus aureus*, *Streptococcus pyogenes*, and *Enterococcus*. *Escherichia coli* is the most common gram-negative organism isolated, whereas *Bacteroides* and *Peptostreptococcus streptococcus* are the most common anaerobes isolated from polymicrobial infections.

The patient's history and physical examination may provide clues as to which organisms may be the culprit of the soft tissue infection. Soft tissue infections located in the perineum, those secondary to perforated viscus, and those secondary to decubitus ulcers or diabetic foot ulcerations tend to be polymicrobial in nature. These infections may contain all three, gram-positive, gram-negative, and anaerobic, organisms.

Bite wounds and water-borne infections are unique subdivisions of polymicrobial infections that, in addition to the more common bacteria species, tend to harbor unusual organisms, including *Pasteurella multocida* in cat and dog bites and *Capnocytophaga carnimorsus* from dog bites. In human bite wounds, *Eikenella corrodens* is common. Water-borne infections often contain *Vibrio* and *Aeromonas* species.

Monocrobial infections tend to be more aggressive, commonly presenting with acute onset and rapid progression to fulminant infection. Highly virulent pathogens include *Streptococcus pyogenes* (group A β-hemolytic *Streptococcus*), *Clostridium* species, community-acquired methicillin-resistant *Staphylococcus aureus* (MRSA), *Vibrio vulnificus*, and *Pseudomonas aeruginosa*.

Group A β-hemolytic *Streptococcus*, by far the most common monomicrobial isolate, can result in a rapidly progressive NSTI with systemic toxicity and high mortality rates. These bacteria produce exotoxins that independently cause systemic toxicity and result in multisystem organ failure. In addition, exotoxins released include powerful proteolytic enzymes such as hemolysins, fibrinolysins, hyaluronidases, antiphagocytic M proteins, leukocidins, and streptolysins O and S. These allow for rapid tracking through otherwise healthy tissue.

Clostridium species such as *Clostridium perfringens* are of particular concern in puncture and traumatic wounds and in intravenous drug users. *Clostridium* also produces exotoxins that are responsible for its rapid destructive spread, systemic toxicity, and high mortality. Clostridium reproduces every 8 minutes and produces α-toxin (phospholipase C) and θ-toxin (perfringolysin). These toxins cause direct tissue injury, kill neutrophils and impede migration, lead to hemolysis and microvascular thrombosis, and increase vascular permeability, which leads to rapid destruction of soft tissues including muscle tissue. In addition, α-toxin directly inhibits myocardial contractility, resulting in shock.

With the rise in MRSA in the community, the practitioner now sees NSTI as a result of MRSA infection. Community-acquired MRSA is able to produce coagulases that lead to direct tissue invasion and necrosis. In addition, these bacteria have the ability to produce Panton-Valentine leukocidin, which is a potent white blood cell and dermonecrotic toxin. Common populations affected with this disease include contact sports teams, prisoners, military recruits, injection drug users, institutionalized residents, and those who attend child and adult day care centers.

TREATMENT

Support

On identification of patients with necrotizing soft tissue infection, rapid operative management should be made the priority treatment and not be delayed for other therapeutic or monitoring measures. Nonetheless, supportive measures should be initiated as soon as possible, and these cases can be labor intensive from a supportive standpoint. Appropriate antibiotic therapy should be immediately delivered. Invasive monitoring should be implemented, including arterial lines for blood pressure monitoring and central venous lines for the delivery of medications and central venous pressure monitoring. Patients should receive aggressive fluid resuscitation and vasopressor and inotropic support when needed. Aggressive glycemic control can improve outcomes; thus, an insulin drip may be appropriate. Serial laboratory values should be obtained because these patients can have rapid fluid and electrolyte shifts. Foley catheter placement and lactic acid measurements can be used to direct fluid resuscitation. Urine myoglobin and creatine kinase levels should be obtained when myonecrosis is suspected. Blood products should be made available because development of coagulopathies or excessive operative blood loss is not unusual. Early parenteral or enteral support should be initiated on a patient-dependent basis. These patients exhibit high protein and caloric requirements because of their highly catabolic state.

Antibiotic Therapy

Antibiotic therapy should be initiated immediately on presentation and continued until no further evidence of infection in the involved tissues or sign of systemic toxicity is found. Antibiotic choice should initially be broad spectrum and then tailored to microbiology obtained from samples retrieved at the time of surgery (Table 4). One should acknowledge the likely origin of infection in choosing antibiotics. For example, infections from perineal and intraabdominal sources or from diabetic foot ulcers and pressure sores are more likely

TABLE 4: Suggested empiric antimicrobial therapy for necrotizing infections based on suspected causative organism

Agent	Dose	Comments
Infections from Mixed Organisms (e.g., intraabdominal source, diabetic foot infections)		
Piperacillin/tazobactam (Zosyn)	3.375 g IV q6h	Use aminoglycoside with anaerobic coverage in patients with severe penicillin allergy
Ertapenem (Invanz)	1 g IV q24h	Also provides MRSA coverage; may require added anaerobic coverage
Meropenem (Merrem IV)	1 g IV q8h	
Imipenem/cilastatin (Primaxin)	1 g IV q6-8h	Requires added anaerobic coverage
Tigecycline (Tygacil)	100 mg IV, then 50 mg IV q12h	Requires added anaerobic coverage
Ciprofloxacin (Cipro)	400 mg IV q12h	
Cefotaxime (Claforan)	1 g IV q8h	Provides anaerobic coverage and inhibits bacterial exotoxin production by ribosomes
Consider adding to any of these regimens:		
Clindamycin	600-900 mg IV q8h	
Infections from Streptococci (e.g., upper extremity/torso infections not associated with intraabdominal source)		
Penicillin	2-4 MU IV q4-6h	Use vancomycin, linezolid (Zyvox), or daptomycin (Cubicin) in patients with severe penicillin allergy
Plus:		
Clindamycin	600-900 mg IV q8h	Inhibits bacterial exotoxin production by ribosomes
Infections from Methicillin-Resistant *Staphylococcus aureus* (MRSA; e.g., institutionalized patients, athletes, IV drug users)		
Vancomycin	1 g IV q12h	Does not inhibit toxin production
Linezolid	600 mg IV q12h	Bacteriostatic; inhibits toxin production
Daptomycin	4 mg/kg IV q24hr	Bactericidal, myopathy, excellent tissue penetration
Ceftaroline	600 mg IV q12h	Bactericidal
Infections from *Clostridium* spp. (e.g., puncture wounds, traumatic wounds, severe early postoperative wound infection)		
Penicillin	2-4 MU IV q4-6h	
Plus:		
Clindamycin	600-900 mg IV q8h	
Infections from Animal and Human Bites		
Ampicillin/sulbactam	1.5-3 g IV q6-8h	
Cefuroxime (Ceftin, Zinacef)	1 g IV q24h	Good activity against *Pasteurella multocida* and *Eikenella corrodens*
Cefoxitin	1 g IV q6-8h	
Ciprofloxacin	400 mg IV q12h	
Infections from *Vibrio* spp. (water-borne infections; e.g., shellfish workers)		
Cefotaxime	2 g q8h	
Plus:		
Minocycline	200 mg IV load then 100 mg q12h	

h, Hour; *IV,* intravenous; *q,* every.

to be polymicrobial, whereas extremity infections are more likely to be monomicrobial. Extremity infections, infections related to intravenous drug use, and infections in patients from certain backgrounds, including prison inmates, Alaskan natives, institutionalized individual, and athletes, are more likely to harbor community-acquired MRSA.

Infections that are likely polymicrobial should be treated with broad-spectrum agents, such as imipenem-cilastin, meropenem, piperacillin-tazobactam, ticarcillin-clavulanate, and tigecycline. In patients with rapid spread or severe systemic toxicity, multiagent therapy should be considered. *Streptococcal* and *Clostridial* infections should generally be treated with high-dose penicillin and high-dose clindamycin. In addition to toxicity to said pathogens, evidence suggests clindamycin's ribosomal inhibitory properties may reduce toxin production responsible for widespread organ dysfunction, thus reducing toxicity. Infections at high risk for MRSA should be treated with antibiotic combinations including vancomycin or other anti-MRSA agent. Like clindamycin, linezolid also has ribosomal-blocking properties that may reduce toxin production.

A combination of penicillin and clindamycin with a gram-negative agent as empiric therapy provides several advantages, such as covering of a polymicrobial infection, the high prevalence of streptococcus in polymicrobial and monomicrobial infections, a better antibiotic tissue penetration, and the reduction in bacterial toxin production.

Surgery

Surgery should focus on rapid identification of affected tissue with complete excision of all devitalized skin and soft tissue (Figure 2). Reports show a sevenfold to ninefold increased risk of death with inadequate or delayed initial débridement. Incision should be made with dissection through all soft tissue layers until the deep muscle layers are encountered. A thorough probing of all tissue and fascial planes to assess for tracking should be made to direct further dissection. Typical findings that indicate devitalized tissue include murky dishwater-appearing fluid in the subcutaneous fat and fascial layers, tissue that dissects from deeper tissue with minimal resistance, nonbleeding tissue, and vascular thrombosis. Noncontractile muscle indicates devitalized muscle tissue. All tissue overlying involved fascial planes should be immediately débrided along with the affected fascia. Easy separation of fascia from underlying tissue with use of

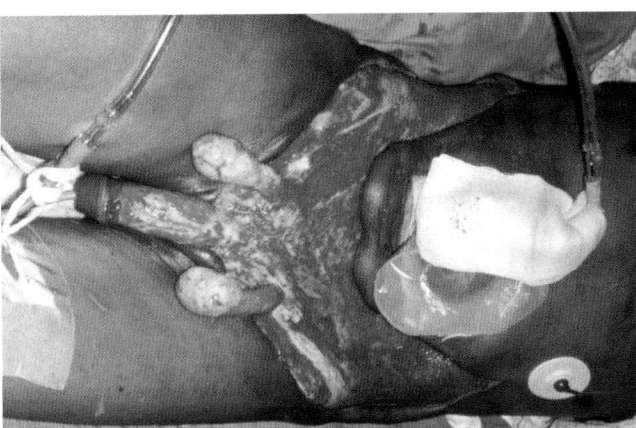

FIGURE 2 Extensive débridement of the scrotum, penis, perineum, and lower abdomen was performed. A sigmoid loop colostomy was also created. *(From Dolghi O, Itani KMF: Necrotizing infection of the perineum,* Hosp Physician *44(1):39-45, 2008.)*

the "finger test" indicates active infection and indicates tissue that should be débrided. All fluid collections should be drained. Débridement should extend back to viable soft tissue and muscle that exhibit brisk bleeding. Tissue (including fascia) should be sent to microbiology for Gram stain and culture for aerobic, anaerobic, and fungal organisms to help tailor antibiotic usage.

In certain patient populations and NSTI presentations, operative management should be further tailored. Amputation may be necessary for infections that rapidly progress toward the trunk, involving major joints, or for extensive myonecrosis. Guillotine amputations of lower extremities should be considered, especially in patients with peripheral vascular disease for rapid containment of infection. In patients with Fournier's gangrene, all affected perineal soft tissue, including the scrotum and penile skin, should be débrided and colonic diversion considered. Colonic diversion may need to be delayed until a second operation depending on patient stability. Testicles can usually be preserved because they have an independent blood supply, although removal should not be delayed if they are involved. Patients with perforated viscus need the intraperitoneal injury to be addressed, likely with diversion if secondary to perforated colon.

Return to the operating room within 24 hours or earlier for a second look should strongly be considered, and débridement of any missed devitalized tissues performed. Patients may need multiple trips to the operating room before the infection is eradicated completely, with a median number of returns around four.

Wounds should be treated with serial wet-to-dry dressing changes until all infection has been cleared. Some authors prefer Dakin's solution–soaked or iodine-soaked gauze dressings, and some authors recommend the use of topical antibiotics, such as silver sulfadiazine. No tissue grafting should be attempted until the infection is fully treated and the patient's condition has stabilized.

Adjunct Treatments

Although urgent surgical débridement is the most important therapeutic maneuver for NSTI and should never be postponed in favor of other treatment modalities, it is worth mentioning a number of mostly theoretic adjunct treatments. These include hyperbaric oxygen therapy, intravenous immunoglobulin, and plasmapheresis. Hyperbaric oxygen therapy works on the premise that increased oxygen supply to infected tissues inhibits bacterial growth and improves host response to infection. Evidence supporting hyperbaric oxygen therapy is limited. Furthermore, because urgent surgical débridement is the most lifesaving therapy, no patient should be transferred to a facility housing a hyperbaric oxygen chamber without first undergoing adequate surgical débridement. Intravenous immunoglobulin works on the premise that the immunoglobulin binds exotoxins that cause systemic toxicity. Plasmapheresis works on the premise that it filters bacterial exotoxins that result in shock and multiorgan dysfunction. By reducing circulating toxin, intravenous immunoglobulin and plasmapheresis may hasten recovery from systemic shock. Again, evidence for these treatment modalities is controversial.

RECONSTRUCTION

Reconstruction should be initiated as soon as possible once all infection has been eradicated and systemic toxicity has subsided. This aids in restoring hemostasis, speeds healing, decreases fluid losses, and improves final cosmetic outcome. Split thickness skin grafts are favored. Staging reconstructions are used for complex reconstructions. The assistance of a plastic surgeon or urologist may be beneficial for difficult areas such as the hands, face, and perineum, particularly if flaps are needed or pockets need to be made for uncovered testicles.

COMPLICATIONS

Multiple complications can occur with NSTI. Despite attempts at improving recognition and speed to surgical management of necrotizing fasciitis, improvement in mortality has been plagued with death rates remaining around one in four. Obviously, with the extent of débridement necessary, disfigurement and disability are considerable. Contractures can occur in involved limbs. Secondary infections in the critically ill are common and include line infections, pneumonias, urinary tract infections, and secondary soft tissue infections. For those with Fournier's gangrene, impotence and decreased sperm count or motility are common. In addition, débridement of the perirectal muscles may result in fecal incontinence and the need for a permanent colostomy.

CONCLUSION

Necrotizing soft tissue infections should be promptly recognized to expedite surgical treatment and minimize morbidity, long-term disability, and death. Diagnosis can be difficult, and no firm diagnostic criteria exist. The clinician must recognize the clues and have a low threshold for surgically exploring areas of concern.

SUGGESTED READINGS

Dolghi O, Itani KMF: Necrotizing infection of the perineum, *Hosp Physician* 44(1):39–45, 2008.

Elliott DC, Kufera JA, Myers RA: Necrotizing soft tissue infections: risk factors for mortality and strategies for management, *Ann Surg* 224:672–683, 1996.

Lancerotto L, Tocco I, Salmaso R, et al: Necrotizing fasciitis: classification, diagnosis, and management, *J Trauma* 72(3):560–566, 2012.

May A, Stafford R, Bulger E, et al: Treatment of complicated skin and soft tissue infections, *Surg Infect* 10(5):467–499, 2009.

Roje Z, Roje Z, Matic D, et al: Necrotizing fasciitis: literature review of contemporary strategies for diagnosing and management with three case reports: torso, abdominal wall, upper and lower limbs, *World J Emerg Surg* 6(46):1–17, 2011.

Stevens DL, Bisno AL, Chambers HF, et al: Practice guideline for the diagnosis and management of skin and soft-tissue infections, *Clin Infect Dis* 41:1373–1406, 2005.

Wang YS, Wong CH, Tay YK: Staging of necrotizing fasciitis based on the evolving cutaneous features, *Int J Dermatol* 46:1036–1041, 2007.

Wong CH, Khin LW, Heng KS, et al: The LRINEC (laboratory risk indicator for necrotizing fasciitis) score: a tool for distinguishing necrotizing fasciitis from other soft tissue infections, *Crit Care Med* 32:1535–1541, 2004.

THE MANAGEMENT OF PRIMARY CHEST WALL TUMORS

George J. Arnaoutakis, MD, and
Avedis Meneshian, MD

OVERVIEW

A chest wall mass may represent any one of a broad spectrum of entities, ranging from benign or malignant primary chest wall tumors; locally invasive tumors originating from the lungs, pleura, mediastinum, or breast; metastatic lesions; and nonneoplastic (infectious or inflammatory) lesions. Of these, primary chest wall tumors, whether benign or malignant, are the least common; they comprise only 5% of all thoracic neoplasms. They are best classified according to their tissue of origin and are further subdivided as either benign or bearing malignant potential (Box 1). In this chapter, we review the most common primary chest wall tumors and focus on surgical management options, including chest wall resection and reconstruction.

DIAGNOSIS

The vast majority of patients with primary chest wall tumors present with a painless, enlarging mass. Other patients who are entirely asymptomatic may have a primary chest wall tumor detected with thoracic imaging studies performed for unrelated indications. Pain in a patient with a primary chest wall tumor likely represents bony erosion or involvement of adjacent nerves and is often a harbinger of malignant tumor behavior. Workup includes a history and physical examination, with attention directed to a history of other malignancies, radiation exposure (therapeutic or environmental), and overt signs of infection or inflammation on physical examination.

A plain film chest radiograph may reveal a soft tissue or bony abnormality. Contrast-enhanced thoracic computed tomographic (CT) scan can help delineate the extent of bony, soft tissue, pleural, lung, or mediastinal involvement and can also exclude nodal or pulmonary metastatic disease. Contrast-enhanced magnetic resonance imaging (MRI) can help delineate vascular or nerve involvement. A freely mobile mass less than 2 cm in size can generally be excised with clear margins, with achievement of both diagnostic and therapeutic purposes. In contrast, larger lesions or those that are fixed to the underlying bone or soft tissue should undergo core needle biopsy or open incisional biopsy before definitive resection. Care must be taken to plan these biopsies with a subsequent curative resection in mind, with incisions placed appropriately so as not to preclude subsequent complete resection as indicated. Tissue diagnosis before surgical resection can help exclude infectious or inflammatory lesions in which resection may not be necessary for treatment and may allow for neoadjuvant radiation or chemotherapy in the induction setting if the lesion is malignant.

BENIGN BONY AND CARTILAGINOUS TUMORS

Fibrous Dysplasia

The most common benign bony tumor of the chest wall, fibrous dysplasia represents a lesion in which normal marrow and cancellous bone is replaced with a fibrous stroma. It typically presents as a painless mass of the rib, commonly located posteriorly or laterally on the chest wall. Radiographic findings are variable but often include a central ground-glass appearance with punctate calcifications and peripheral cortical thinning. The tumors most commonly present as a solitary lesion in otherwise healthy individuals 20 to 30 years of age. However, these lesions can rarely be multiple and associated with the McCune-Albright syndrome, which includes cutaneous manifestations and endocrine abnormalities in the context of short stature and precocious puberty. No surgical therapy is indicated, unless the diagnosis remains questionable or the lesion is symptomatic. If so, limited partial rib resection is the definitive treatment.

Osteochondroma

A benign bony lesion that typically presents in the third decade of life, an osteochondroma classically involves the costochondral junction. These lesions can present either as a palpable painless mass or can grow unnoticed within the chest cavity to a larger size. Punctate central calcifications with a mineralized hyaline cartilage cap are characteristic radiologic findings. When these lesions are asymptomatic or small, observation with serial imaging is appropriate. Symptomatic or enlarging lesions can be resected with local excision. Although malignant degeneration is rare (<1% of patients), if the cartilage cap becomes greater than 2 cm in thickness, resection should be considered because malignant transformation to chondrosarcoma or osteosarcoma has been reported.

Chondroma

Chondromas are benign cartilaginous tumors that originate from the medullary cavity. They are more commonly found anteriorly in the rib and have no gender predilection. They too present either as a painless mass or an incidentally documented lesion on imaging. On chest radiograph, characteristic findings include an osteolytic lesion with well-defined sclerotic margins. On CT scan or MRI, punctate calcifications and cortical scalloping may be seen. These benign lesions are difficult to differentiate from low-grade chondrosarcomas, radiographically and often histologically, and therefore should be resected with wide local excision.

MALIGNANT BONY AND CARTILAGINOUS TUMORS

Chondrosarcoma

The most common malignant chest wall tumor, chondrosarcomas most commonly occur in the fourth to seventh decades of life. Most

involve the costochondral junction or the sternum. On imaging, irregular margins and bony destruction are typical (Figure 1). Early stage lesions can retain a thickened cortical cap, whereas more advanced tumors progress to complete cortical destruction and an associated soft tissue mass. Suspected benign chondromas in which the cortical cap thickens over time may be in the process of malignant degeneration into chondrosarcoma. All suspected chondrosarcomas should undergo wide local excision; they often require chest wall reconstruction. Poor prognostic factors include hypercellularity, cytologic atypia, high mitotic index, and tumor size. High grade tumors have a 75% chance of distant spread at the time of diagnosis. Because these tumors respond poorly to chemotherapy or radiation, complete surgical (wide-local) excision is the primary modality of therapy.

Osteosarcoma

Osteosarcomas of the chest wall generally present at puberty as a rapidly expanding mass and arise from the rib, scapula, or clavicle. Environmental factors (fluoride exposure, farm workers) and genetic predispositions (young age at puberty, familial history, retinoblastoma gene defect, Li-Fraumeni syndrome) increase the lifetime risk of development of osteosarcoma. Radiographic findings include bony destruction with an associated large heterogeneous mass comprised of necrotic tumor and hemorrhage. There is often central punctate calcification. Because distant metastasis (typically to the lung) is common and good systemic options for therapy exist, biopsy for tissue confirmation is indicated for suspected osteosarcomas. Induction chemotherapy followed by surgical resection (wide local excision with reconstruction as needed) is the treatment of choice; however, overall 5-year survival rates remain poor, at less than 20%.

Ewing's Sarcoma

These malignant, small, round cell tumors have in common the genetic translocation between chromosomes 11 and 22 and include both Ewing's sarcomas and primitive neuroectodermal tumors (PNETs; also known as Askin's tumors). With a typical occurrence in children and young adults, 15% of Ewing's sarcomas and up to 50% of PNETs arise in the chest wall and can involve a single rib, the clavicle, or the scapula, in descending frequency. They often present as a painful enlarging chest mass with constitutional symptoms that include fever, weight loss, and generalized malaise. Associated pleural effusions are also common. On imaging, radiographic findings include a large noncalcified mass with bony destruction. As with osteosarcomas, systemic disease at diagnosis is frequent, and therapy should include neoadjuvant chemotherapy followed by complete surgical resection and chest wall reconstruction. Postoperative radiation should be reserved for a margin-positive resection. Bilateral whole lung irradiation may be used in the adjuvant setting to improve

---

BOX 1: Primary chest wall tumors

Soft Tissue

Benign
Lipoma
Hemangioma
Lymphangioma
Fibroma
Rhabdomyoma
Neurofibroma
Desmoid tumor

Malignant
Malignant fibrous histiocytoma
Rhabdosarcoma
Liposarcoma
Neurofibrosarcoma
Leiomyosarcoma
Synovial sarcoma

Bony and Cartilaginous

Benign
Fibrous dysplasia
Osteochondroma
Chondroma

Malignant
Chondrosarcoma
Osteogenic sarcoma
Ewing's sarcoma
Askin's tumor (primitive neuroectodermal tumor)
Plasmacytoma

FIGURE 1 Computed tomographic scans of a patient with malignant tumor of the chest wall. Both *white arrows* denote the chest wall tumor. The image on the left shows soft tissue involvement with soft tissue settings. The image on the right shows extent of bony involvement and destruction with bone windows.

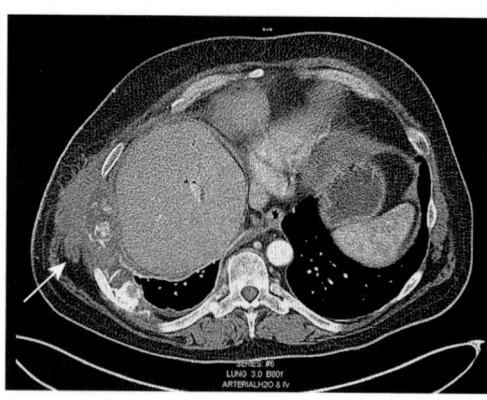
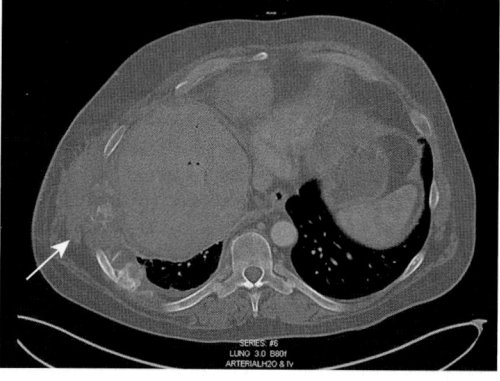

event-free survival in patients with documented pulmonary metastases. Overall 5-year survival rates for Ewing's sarcoma can approach 65%, whereas for PNETs, long term survival remains approximately 15%.

Solitary Plasmacytoma

Plasmacytomas tend to occur in men in their 60s and 70s and present with pain, typically without a palpable mass. Imaging documents an expansile multicystic mass. Plasmacytoma is associated with multiple myeloma but is not necessarily a systemic disease. After tissue diagnosis is confirmed, local therapy with radiation is indicated. Up to two thirds of patients may have development of systemic involvement with multiple myeloma; the 5-year survival rate is 25% to 35%. However, solitary plasmacytomas that are successfully irradiated and do not progress to systemic multiple myeloma have an excellent long-term prognosis. Indications for surgical resection as local therapy include those patients in whom radiation therapy is not an option.

BENIGN SOFT TISSUE TUMORS

Lipomas

Chest wall lipomas are typically larger and deeper than those soft tissue lipomas found in other anatomic locations. They are rarely symptomatic. Imaging reveals homogenous masses consistent with mature fatty tissue. Resection is only indicated for symptomatic or enlarging lesions or for suspicion of low-grade liposarcoma.

Fibromas (Desmoid Tumors) and Fibromatosis

Desmoid tumors arise from fibroblasts deep within the chest wall musculature and often occur in patients in their teenage years to early 30s. They present as a slowly growing, sometimes painful mass, often in the context of prior trauma or prior thoracotomy or in the context of systemic fibromatosis (Gardner's syndrome). Complete surgical resection with wide margins (up to 4 cm if possible) with chest wall reconstruction is the optimal therapy because local recurrence rates are quite high. Adjuvant radiation therapy can be used both prophylactically and in the context of microscopically positive margins. Recurrence rates for margin-positive disease, despite radiation therapy, remain as high as 90%.

Hemangiomas

Hemangiomas of the chest wall are benign proliferations of blood vessels that form in the context of muscle, rib, or subcutaneous tissues. They typically occur in children. MRI or ultrasound scan can be used to confirm the diagnosis. Resection is only indicated if symptoms develop, such as bleeding, ulceration, or rarely heart failure from arteriovenous malformation and shunting (cavernous hemangiomas). When indicated, local excision is curative, with chest wall reconstruction reserved for larger lesions.

Benign Peripheral Nerve Sheath Tumors

Chest wall schwannomas are encapsulated tumors that develop from intercostal nerves or thoracic spinal nerve roots. They are typically asymptomatic and identified incidentally during thoracic imaging. CT scan and MRI are usually sufficient for diagnosis, and in asymptomatic cases, serial imaging and observation suffice. If the diagnosis is in doubt, needle biopsy can be confirmatory. Resection is reserved

for symptomatic or enlarging lesions. This may require contiguous chest wall or vertebral body resection and reconstruction.

MALIGNANT SOFT TISSUE TUMORS

Malignant Fibrous Histiocytoma

Malignant fibrous histiocytoma (MFH) has two age peaks at diagnosis: 20 to 30 years and 50 to 60 years, with the latter the more common period of diagnosis. They rarely arise from the chest wall; when they do, they are generally associated with prior radiation exposure. Imaging reveals a heterogeneous mass with irregular borders; bony involvement is rare. Tissue confirmation with a well-planned needle biopsy is indicated because induction chemotherapy followed by surgical resection and reconstruction is the therapy of choice. Postoperative radiation can be reserved for margin-positive disease. Even with complete resection and systemic therapy, metastases can be documented in 30% to 50% of patients and 5-year survival rates remain less than 40%.

Synovial Sarcomas

These malignant tumors rarely present as a primary chest wall malignancy, and the thoracic surgeon is more typically involved with the management of oligometastatic lung involvement from systemic disease. Nevertheless, primary synovial cell sarcomas of the chest wall can occur, typically in early adulthood. Imaging generally reveals heterogeneous centers as a result of necrosis or hemorrhage within cystic components. Nearly 50% may have calcification. Treatment involves complete surgical resection with adjuvant chemotherapy or radiation. Induction paradigms with chemotherapy or chemoradiation followed by surgical resection have also been used. Five-year survival rates approach 50%.

Rhabdomyosarcomas

Rare in adults, rhabdomyosarcomas are the second most common malignant primary chest wall tumor in children. The vast majority of cases present with distant metastases, and complete staging should be undertaken to determine which patients are candidates for primary site resection. Staging in children can include CT scan of the thorax, abdominal ultrasound scan, and bone scan, although positron emission tomography (PET)/CT scans are being increasingly used. Tissue confirmation is important because when these aggressive tumors are resectable, they are treated with induction chemoradiation, followed by wide local excision with chest wall reconstruction, and adjuvant chemotherapy or radiation as indicated. Five-year survival rates remain poor with surgical resection alone; trimodality therapy has resulted in significant improvement in 5-year survival rates, with rates as high as 75% in selected series in patients without documented metastases at the time of diagnosis.

SURGICAL TREATMENT OF CHEST WALL TUMORS

Chest Wall Resection

Surgical resection remains the mainstay of therapy for primary chest wall malignancies, whether benign or malignant. Benign lesions should be resected to microscopically clear margins. Many malignant chest wall lesions have high recurrence rates; therefore, aggressive wide local excision with chest wall reconstruction as indicated has been advocated. The general guidelines for planning surgical resection of primary chest wall tumors are as follows. Primary malignant tumors of the chest wall should be resected with a 4-cm margin. This margin width has been shown to afford better long-term survival. Tumors arising from adjacent structures (most commonly lung cancers) should be resected to include the involved rib and a rib above and below the area of invasion. Metastatic lesions can generally be resected to microscopically clear margins but only in carefully selected patients in whom the solitary chest wall metastasis is thought to be the only site of systemic disease.

Given the large defects often left with wide local excision of these lesions, careful planning to ensure an adequate oncologic operation and excellent functional and cosmetic results from reconstruction is critical. Planning for resection must begin at the time of original tissue diagnosis, with care taken to place biopsy incisions in areas that can subsequently be incorporated into wide local excisions. Therefore, the involvement of the surgeon in planning therapy for these patients, and collaboration with plastic and reconstructive surgeons as needed, must occur early in the treatment course.

Chest Wall Reconstruction

The thorax is a rigid structure that protects the underlying viscera, supports the upper extremities and shoulder girdle, and allows for ventilation. Anatomic defects in the bony framework of the chest may result in exposure of vital structures to the external environment or alteration of chest wall mechanics that leads to subsequent ventilatory impairment. Large defects may result in lung herniation, contraction of the resected hemithorax, scapular entrapment, and suboptimal cosmesis. The goals of reconstruction are to mitigate these alterations of the chest wall and their potential complications.

No formal guidelines exist for mandating skeletal reconstruction after chest wall resection, thus rendering surgical judgment essential. General preference as discussed in textbooks and the authors' own practice takes into account defect location, size, local tissue condition, and patient comorbidities. Posterior defects, which are supported by the overlying scapula and back musculature, may be left without skeletal reconstruction if less than 10 cm in diameter. If the posterior rib defect encompasses the fourth or fifth ribs, special attention must be paid to the location of the scapular tip because it may become entrapped within the chest if no reconstructive support is provided. Anterior and lateral defects of two consecutive ribs with a resultant defect less than 5 cm in size are generally well tolerated with no functional consequence. Anterior resections of the first through third ribs may be especially well tolerated without reconstruction because of the support provided by the overlying pectoralis muscles. When more than three adjacent ribs in the anterolateral location are resected, or the resulting defect is 5 cm or greater, the possibility of paradoxical chest wall motion and its inherent complications arises, suggesting reconstruction should be undertaken. The authors' practice is to reconstruct defects 4 cm in size if pulmonary function is borderline, thus minimizing the chance of postoperative pulmonary insufficiency in these patients with marginal reserve. In patients who have dense underlying adhesions or pulmonary scarring from prior radiation or surgery, the authors may leave defects larger than 5 cm unreconstructed as ventilation may not be affected. Tolerance for defect size also increases in the setting of infection, as graft infection may develop.

OPTIONS FOR CHEST WALL RECONSTRUCTION

After the decision has been made to perform skeletal stabilization, a suitable graft option must be selected for the bony defect and the overlying soft tissue coverage needed. Options for chest wall reconstruction include autogenous fascia and bone, metals, plastics, and prosthetic meshes and patches, with or without muscle flap reconstruction. The authors' preference is to use acellular dermal matrices (ADM) for skeletal reconstruction in conjunction with muscle flaps for soft tissue coverage of defects as needed (Table 1).

The authors' greatest clinical experience with ADMs for chest wall reconstruction has been with AlloDerm (Lifecell Corporation, Bridgewater, NJ) (Figure 2). At times, the resection is small, and soft tissue coverage is the major issue facing the team of surgeons. At other times, the defect is massive, and chest wall stabilization is critical. Based on the estimated size of the defect during surgery before resection, the authors request the AlloDerm be brought to the operating room (OR) for rehydration, which can take on average 30 to 40 minutes. The authors recently moved to the use of the extra-thick (2.30-mm to 3.30-mm) noncrosslinked graft because this seems to provide better skeletal support, although this observation is based on anecdotal evidence and objective data do not currently exist. Size selection is based on the defect, and multiple grafts may be sutured together for additional coverage.

After skeletal resection is complete, rib margins are blunted to avoid sharp ends, which may injure the graft or underlying viscera. Thorough inspection for hemostasis is performed, and the wound is irrigated with copious saline solution. The authors generally do not prestretch the graft more than 10% to 15% before implantation but undersize the graft relative to the defect to allow for ideal tension when placed. A tense, drum-like feel of the graft is ideal to prevent redundancy and leaking. During sizing, it is essential to account for patient positioning. Most surgical approaches are with the patient in a lateral decubitus position on the OR table, with maximal table flexion to increase interspace distance for chest entry. Restoration of the OR table to a neutral position during determination of allograft size reduces the chance of inadequate graft tension. The AlloDerm matrix has two distinct surfaces, and proper orientation of the allograft before insertion is important. The authors use a number 1

TABLE 1: Flaps used to cover thoracic soft tissue defects after chest wall resection

Type of flap	Arterial supply	Indications
Latissimus	Primary: thoracodorsal Secondary: perforating vessels from posterior intercostal vessels	Anterolateral and posterior defects
Pectoralis major	Primary: Thoracoacromial artery Turnover flap: internal mammary perforators	Anterior chest wall defects
Serratus	Subscapular artery	Intrathoracic coverage
Rectus abdominis	Deep superior or inferior epigastric artery	Lower sternal defects
External oblique	Segmental blood supply from posterior intercostal arteries	Inframammary fold defects

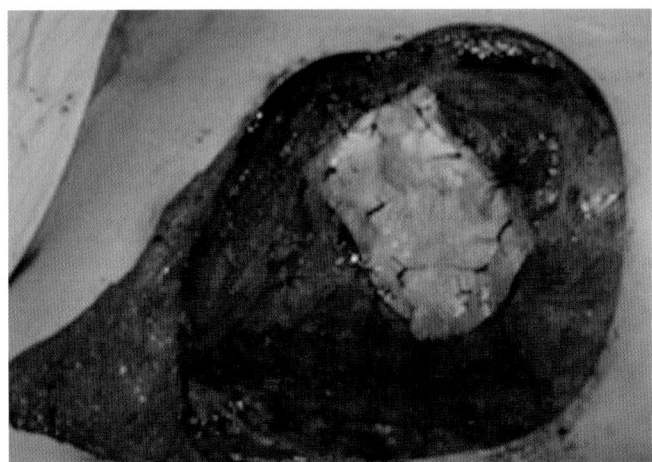

FIGURE 2 Intraoperative photograph of a chest wall reconstruction with AlloDerm (Lifecell Corporation, Bridgewater, NJ) acellular dermal matrix. The periphery of the AlloDerm is sutured to the chest wall with interrupted, nonabsorbable Prolene sutures.

polypropylene (nonabsorbable) suture with a cutting $\frac{1}{2}$-circle 40-mm needle for graft implantation. This suture allows for ease of passage through the dense dermal graft and facilitates bone penetration when necessary. Single interrupted sutures for secondary support are placed in four quadrants or at any area where there is pleating and a tighter seal is desired. A combination of running or interrupted sutures is then placed circumferentially depending on the surgeon's preference. Suture is passed through fascia when available or directly through the adjacent rib when fascia is not in proximity, and the superficial portion of the tissue flap is sutured to the ADM to obliterate the dead space.

After implantation, the graft is thoroughly irrigated and tested for leakage by insufflating the underlying lung after submersion of the graft in saline solution. Once the acellular dermal matrix has been placed to provide the structural support, soft-tissue coverage generally with a muscle flap with healthy well vascularized tissue is critical.

It is the overlying soft tissue flap that allows for cellular infiltration and revascularization and therefore preserves viability of the ADM. The type of tissue flap and the method for reconstruction is based on the surgeon's preference (see Table 1). The authors then place a 28F chest tube in a posteroapical position through the interspace ideally two ribs below where the ADM is secured. The pleural tube is managed as for any standard lung resection. To prevent seroma formation, 19F subcutaneous closed-suction drains are placed to close the dead space below the tissue flap and ADM. The drains remain in place until the patient has been ambulating for 24 to 48 hours and once the drain output is less than 30 cm³ over 24 hours. If the postoperative course is complicated by a wound infection or infected seroma, the ADM, unlike synthetic mesh, can be treated conservatively and salvaged. This is accomplished oftentimes with percutaneous drainage of the fluid collection, débridement of infected tissue, antibiotics, negative pressure wound vacuum placement, and local wound care without implant removal.

SUMMARY

Primary chest wall tumors are rare. When therapy is indicated, surgical resection remains the primary modality of treatment, alone or in combination with chemotherapy or radiation, in the neoadjuvant or adjuvant setting. Margin-negative resection affords the best chance of cure. Careful planning and collaboration to ensure outstanding oncologic outcomes with optimal functional and cosmetic results after reconstruction are critical for the surgical therapy of primary chest wall tumors.

SUGGESTED READINGS

Mansour KA, Thourani VH, Losken A, et al: Chest wall resections and reconstruction: a 25-year experience, *Ann Thorac Surg* 73(6):1720–1725, 2002.
Rocco G: Chest wall resection and reconstruction according to the principles of biomimesis, *Semin Thorac Cardiovasc Surg* 23(4):307–313, 2011.
Shah AA, D'Amico TA: Primary chest wall tumors, *J Am Coll Surg* 210(3):360–366, 2010.
Skoracki RJ, Chang DW: Reconstruction of the chest wall and thorax, *J Surg Oncol* 94(6):455–465, 2006.

MEDIASTINAL MASSES

Ashok Muniappan, MD, and Douglas Mathisen, MD

INTRODUCTION

The mediastinum extends from the thoracic inlet to the diaphragm and is surrounded by the pleural cavities, spine, and sternum. The mediastinum is commonly and arbitrarily divided into anterior, middle, and posterior compartments. According to Shields's system, introduced in 1972, the anterior compartment contains all of the structures anterior to the heart and great vessels, including the thymus, fat, lymph nodes, and connective tissue (Figure 1). The middle compartment, also called the visceral compartment, contains the heart, trachea, main-stem bronchi, great vessels, esophagus, vagus nerves, thoracic duct, and lymph nodes. The posterior compartment

refers to the paravertebral sulci, which contain the proximal intercostal nerves, intercostal vessels, thoracic spinal ganglion, sympathetic trunk, and lymph nodes. There are slightly different definitions of the mediastinal compartments in the anatomic, radiologic, and surgical literature. In anatomy texts, the mediastinum also includes a superior compartment, which is arbitrarily defined as occupying the space above a line connecting the sternomanubrial joint and the caudal border of the fourth vertebra. Other descriptions place certain structures in different compartments. For instance, classification systems that predate Shields's often place the proximal esophagus in the middle compartment and the distal esophagus in the posterior compartment.

A wide variety of masses, of both benign and malignant origin, arise in the mediastinum. A systematic approach to diagnosis is necessary to select appropriate therapy. Careful documentation of the patient's age, symptoms, and physical signs, as well as critical review of pertinent imaging, can greatly simplify the differential diagnosis. Although a biopsy often refines the differential, occasionally the diagnosis is uncertain until definitive resection.

CLINICAL PRESENTATION AND DIAGNOSIS

Signs and Symptoms

Only about one third of mediastinal masses present with symptoms, while most are found incidentally on imaging performed for other reasons. The most common symptoms are chest pain, cough, or shortness of breath, and are related to compression of normal structures by the mass. Invasion of the stellate ganglion can lead to Horner's syndrome, compression of the superior vena cava (SVC) can result in SVC syndrome, and involvement of the phrenic nerve can present as diaphragmatic paralysis. Malignant masses are more likely to be symptomatic, given their potential for invasion and rapid growth. Some mediastinal masses are also associated with characteristic paraneoplastic syndromes.

Imaging

Chest computed tomographic (CT) scan is the ideal imaging modality to evaluate mediastinal masses. The resolution of CT imaging precisely localizes the mass and establishes its relationship to normal structures. Moreover, CT imaging can distinguish whether the mass is cystic, solid, fatty, or vascular. Magnetic resonance imaging (MRI) is an adjunctive imaging modality that improves soft tissue assessment, but it is not routinely necessary. MRI can reliably identify the presence of bronchogenic and enteric cysts, evaluate involvement of the neural foramen by posterior mediastinal masses, and assess involvement of the heart and great vessels. Specialized studies such as sestamibi scanning (mediastinal parathyroid), octreotide scanning (thymic carcinoid), and metaiodobenzylguanidine scanning (mediastinal paraganglioma) are useful when these diagnoses are suspected.

Tumor Markers

Circulating tumor markers are elevated in patients with certain mediastinal masses. Malignant germ cell tumors (GCTs) of the anterior mediastinum produce elevations of alpha fetoprotein (AFP),

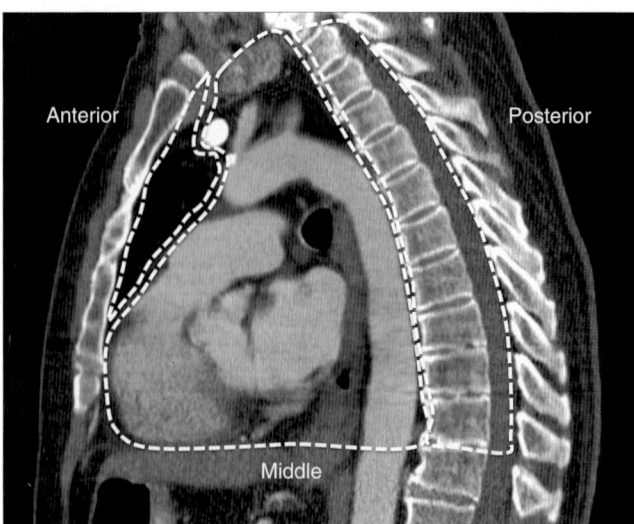

FIGURE 1 A sagittal view of the mediastinum and its anterior, middle, and posterior compartments. The posterior compartment includes the paravertebral sulci, while excluding the spine itself.

beta human chorionic gonadotropin (β-HCG), and lactate dehydrogenase (LDH). The pretreatment marker levels in patients with GCTs correlates with prognosis, while the posttreatment level measures response to therapy. Thymic carcinoids produce ectopic adrenocorticotropic hormone in about 50% of patients, which may be associated with Cushing's syndrome. Malignant ganglionic tumors and pheochromocytomas of the posterior mediastinum can produce excess catecholamines, leading to abnormal elevations of catecholamine metabolites such as dopamine, vanillylmandelic acid, and homovanillic acid. Ectopic mediastinal parathyroid glands produce increased parathyroid hormone.

Biopsy Techniques

Pretreatment biopsy of mediastinal masses is not always necessary. A well-encapsulated mass in the anterior mediastinum, with imaging features consistent with a thymoma, is resectable without preoperative biopsy. Biopsy of an early thymoma may seed the pleura or mediastinum, increasing the chance of recurrence. Other masses of the anterior mediastinum that appear resectable and show no signs of invasion should undergo resection, which is both diagnostic and therapeutic.

Similarly, posterior mediastinal masses, with benign features on imaging, are resectable without a biopsy. Biopsy of a mediastinal cyst is also unnecessary and can complicate resection if the biopsy causes hemorrhage or infection of the cyst.

In contrast, advanced thymoma, lymphoma, malignant germ cell tumors, and other malignant-appearing lesions of the mediastinum require a pretreatment histopathologic diagnosis to guide therapy. CT-guided needle biopsy is especially suitable for masses in the anterior or posterior mediastinum. Core needle biopsy is superior to fine-needle aspiration (FNA), as some preserved architecture is necessary to reliably distinguish between thymoma and lymphoma. Needle biopsy is often inadequate for establishing a diagnosis of lymphoma, and additional tissue obtained with an open incisional biopsy is necessary to perform flow cytometric and cytogenetic tests to allow lymphoma subclassification. In this situation, a Chamberlain procedure (anterior mediastinotomy) is the optimal procedure to perform an incisional biopsy of a mass in the anterior mediastinum.

The middle mediastinum can be accessed with cervical mediastinoscopy, as is frequently done in staging lung cancer or evaluating mediastinal lymphadenopathy. Increasingly, endoscopic ultrasound, either with endobronchial ultrasound (EBUS) or endoesophageal ultrasound (EUS), complements cervical mediastinoscopy and provides a noninvasive technique for biopsy of a mass in the middle mediastinum. Recent reports suggest that EBUS is useful for biopsy of indeterminate mediastinal masses that are adjacent to the central airway and may make open biopsy unnecessary (Yasufuku K, et al., 2011).

Diagnosis

The identity of the mass is surmised by evaluating its location and radiographic features and accounting for the patient's age, signs, and symptoms. The most common mediastinal masses and location are presented in Table 1. In adults, thymomas and thymic cysts are the most commonly encountered primary mediastinal mass (approximately 25% of all mediastinal masses, and almost 50% of anterior mediastinal masses), while in children neurogenic tumors are the most common (approximately 40%). In both adult and pediatric series, mediastinal masses are malignant in approximately 35% to 50% of patients. The mediastinal location of masses in adults is approximately 55% in the anterior mediastinum, 20% in the middle mediastinum, and 25% in the posterior mediastinum. The increased proportion of neurogenic tumors in pediatric patients explains why

TABLE 1: Common mediastinal masses and their usual locations

Anterior	Middle	Posterior
Thymoma	Bronchogenic cyst	Schwannoma
Lymphoma	Lymphoma	Neurofibroma
Substernal thyroid goiter	Pericardial cyst	Ganglioneuroma
Parathyroid adenoma	Neuroenteric cyst	Ganglioneuroblastoma
Germ cell tumor		Neuroblastoma Pheochromocytoma

the majority of pediatric masses are seen in the posterior mediastinum (35% in the anterior mediastinum, 15% in the middle mediastinum, and 50% in the posterior mediastinum). Evaluation of tumor markers and biopsy results refines the differential diagnosis. In some patients, final diagnosis is not established until the lesion is resected.

Anterior Mediastinum

Thymic Tumors

Although thymomas are relatively rare tumors, they are the most common anterior mediastinal tumor. The mean age at presentation is approximately 55 years, and there is no gender predilection. Approximately 50% of patients present with chest pain, dyspnea, cough, or one of the paraneoplastic syndromes, while the remainder are incidentally discovered masses. Thymoma is associated with myasthenia gravis (~30% to 50%), aplastic anemia (~5%), and agammaglobulinemia (~1%). While a thymoma is present in only about 15% of patients with myasthenia gravis, up to 50% of patients with thymomas have myasthenia gravis.

CT imaging usually reveals a well-circumscribed soft tissue mass in the anterior mediastinum, often adjacent to the ascending aorta. The mass may ascend into the neck, approach either pulmonary hilum, or descend to the diaphragm. Lymphadenopathy is atypical for thymoma and if present suggests a diagnosis of lymphoma or an advanced thymic malignancy. Both pleural spaces should be carefully examined on CT imaging, looking for evidence of pleural metastases. Advanced thymic tumors are bulky, encase vascular structures, and have irregular borders on CT imaging.

The World Health Organization (WHO) classification system for thymic epithelial neoplasms correlates with tumor biology and prognosis. In order of worsening prognosis, there are Type A (medullary thymoma), Type AB (mixed thymoma), Type B1 (predominantly cortical thymoma), Type B2 (cortical thymoma), Type B3 (well-differentiated thymic carcinoma), and Type C (thymic carcinoma) thymic tumors. Not surprisingly, surgical resection of the tumor is more accurate for WHO classification than core needle biopsy. Types A and AB thymomas are quite benign, and complete resections are associated with freedom from recurrence and significant chance of cure.

The Masaoka system stages resected thymomas (Masaoka A, 2010). As CT imaging does not reliably assess capsular invasion, surgical resection and histopathologic assessment are necessary to distinguish between stage I and II thymomas (Table 2). The Masaoka stage also predicts survival.

A median sternotomy and total thymectomy is the most appropriate operation for the majority of early-stage thymomas. As mentioned earlier, preoperative biopsy is not necessary for anterior mediastinal masses that appear resectable; biopsy is relatively contraindicated, given the risk of tumor seeding. Transcervical thymectomy, video-assisted thoracic surgery (VATS), and robotic thoracoscopic techniques are also utilized for thymoma resection. Although a recent

TABLE 2: Masaoka staging system of thymoma

Stage	Criteria
I	No evidence of capsular invasion
II	Microscopic capsular invasion or gross involvement of surrounding fat or pleura
III	Gross involvement of adjacent organs including pericardium, great vessels, and lung
IVa	Pleural or pericardial metastases
IVb	Hematogenous or lymphogenous metastases

multicenter report suggested that robotic thymectomy can safely resect early-stage thymomas and is associated with low morbidity, long-term oncologic outcome is unclear because the median follow-up was relatively short (Marulli G, et al., 2012). For now, minimally invasive thymectomy for thymoma is most suitable for centers with a clinical research protocol.

Thymic tumors that appear unresectable at presentation (Masaoka stages III and IV) should undergo CT-guided core needle biopsy or a Chamberlain procedure to establish the diagnosis (Figure 2). Resection follows induction chemotherapy, with adjuvant radiation for concerning margins. SVC or innominate vein reconstruction may be necessary for resection of tumors that extensively involve the innominate vein or SVC (Lanuti M, et al., 2003).

Recurrent disease is usually local, either in the anterior mediastinum or in the pleural spaces. Consideration of resection is usually appropriate, and control of the disease can be possible given the slow growth of most thymomas. In small single-center series, pleuropneumonectomy has been undertaken in highly selected patients in an attempt to eradicate extensive unilateral pleural recurrences (Wright C, 2011).

Germ Cell Tumors

The anterior mediastinum is the most common extragonadal site of a GCT. Tumors are histologically either seminomas or nonseminomatous GCTs, which differ markedly in terms of prognosis and treatment. Mature teratomas of the mediastinum behave in a benign manner and are not associated with any elevation of tumor markers. Nonseminomatous masses, including yolk-sac tumors, choriocarcinomas, embryonal carcinomas, and mixed tumors, are malignant. AFP and β-HCG are often significantly elevated in patients with malignant GCTs, while patients with seminomas have normal or minimally elevated levels. A clinical picture with elevations of AFP and β-HCG, as well as characteristic CT imaging, is pathognomonic,

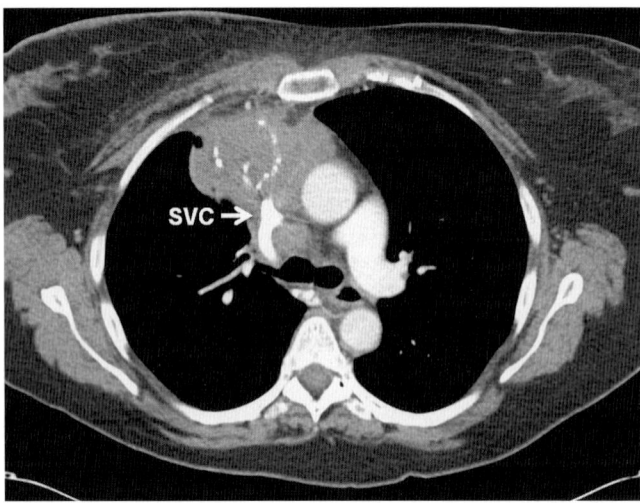

FIGURE 2 Axial computed tomography image of 66-year-old patient with a WHO B3 thymoma encasing the superior vena cava *(SVC)*. After neoadjuvant chemotherapy, the patient underwent sternotomy and resection of the mass, which required SVC reconstruction. Adjuvant radiotherapy was administered to close margins in the right pulmonary hilum.

although CT-guided core biopsy is usually performed to confirm the diagnosis.

Mature Teratomas

Mature or benign teratomas occur equally in men and women, and the mean age at presentation is approximately 30. Mature teratomas are the most common germ cell neoplasm of the mediastinum and account for approximately two thirds of such tumors. CT imaging is typically very suggestive, revealing characteristics such as bone, teeth, and fat within a well-defined cystic structure. A median sternotomy enables complete resection and cure. Although these lesions are benign, resection is indicated, as the mass may continue to grow and cause respiratory or cardiovascular compromise from compression or rupture.

Seminomas

Primary mediastinal seminomas occur predominantly in men, and the mean age at presentation is approximately 30. They account for approximately one third of mediastinal GCTs. Testicular seminomas also metastasize to the mediastinum, although this is typically associated with significant retroperitoneal disease. While small mediastinal seminomas may be diagnosed after complete resection, most seminomas are bulky and appear to be infiltrative or "pushing" surrounding structures on CT imaging. A core needle biopsy, or in some cases a Chamberlain procedure, establishes the diagnosis. At presentation, seminomas are often metastatic. Metastases are common in local lymph nodes and slightly less often in lungs or liver. Seminomas are very sensitive to platinum-based chemotherapy and radiotherapy. Chemotherapy is preferable to avoid cardiac toxicity of mediastinal radiation. Residual masses are often observed, while surgery is occasionally considered in selected patients. Treated patients who present without visceral metastases are expected to have greater than 90% 5-year survival.

Nonseminomatous Germ Cell Tumors

Primary mediastinal nonseminomatous germ cell tumors (PMNS-GCTs) are rare tumors (1% to 5% of mediastinal masses) that occur predominantly in young men aged 20 to 40. Patients present with symptoms such as chest pain, cough, and dyspnea, caused by a large mass in the anterior mediastinum. CT imaging reveals a large, bulky tumor that appears infiltrative and pushes adjacent structures, including the aorta, brachiocephalic vein, SVC, heart, and lung. The central airways may be narrowed, and it is important to recognize this before delivering an anesthetic; access to rigid bronchoscopy and appropriate anesthetic techniques are vital in these patients, as severe respiratory or cardiac compromise may occur with anesthetic induction. Although elevations in AFP or β-HCG are virtually diagnostic combined with the imaging findings, needle biopsy is usually performed to confirm the diagnosis. When biopsy findings return with benign features consistent with a mature teratoma, the elevation of tumor markers is due to malignant elements within the mass that were not sampled, and a mixed tumor with benign and malignant elements is diagnosed. Primary surgical therapy is rarely undertaken, as these masses are often metastatic at presentation and the bulky and infiltrative presentation precludes a complete resection. Cisplatin-based combination chemotherapy regimens such as VIP (ifosfamide, etoposide, and cisplatin) and BEP (bleomycin, etoposide, and cisplatin) produce responses in most patients, with normalization of tumor markers and regression of the mass on CT imaging. Bleomycin is associated with pulmonary toxicity and should be avoided when pulmonary resection is anticipated. In patients with normalized markers, surgical resection of the remaining mass is recommended if technically feasible. While the anterior mediastinal mass is typically approached via median sternotomy, alternative incisions such as a posterolateral thoracotomy or a sternothoracotomy (clamshell incision) are useful when the mass involves the pulmonary hilum or lung. In a patient with continued marker elevation, second-line chemotherapy is appropriate, and surgical resection is rarely undertaken. Five-year survival is approximately 50% for all patients with PMNSGCTs, with an improved prognosis for patients who undergo resection and no viable malignant tissue remains.

Lymphoma

Lymphomas represent about 20% of anterior mediastinal masses. They can also occur in the middle mediastinum and rarely in the posterior mediastinum. Lymphomas are often not confined to the mediastinum, and disease may be seen elsewhere. Patients may present with symptoms related to compression as well as harbor "B" symptoms (fevers, night sweats, and weight loss).

Hodgkin's lymphoma is the most common primary mediastinal lymphoma, with nearly half of all Hodgkin's disease occurring in the mediastinum. It has a tendency to occur in thymic tissue, but it can also involve lymph nodes in the middle mediastinum. Patients are typically younger than patients with thymomas (20s to 30s) and are slightly more often female. While needle biopsy may identify lymphoma, it usually fails to provide enough tissue for lymphoma subclassification. Differentiating from thymoma may also be difficult on a needle biopsy. Additional tissue obtained by a Chamberlain procedure, VATS, or cervical mediastinoscopy is necessary to distinguish between Hodgkin's lymphoma and non-Hodgkin's lymphoma. Obtaining tissue is the primary role for the surgeon, as these tumors are typically treated with a combination of chemotherapy and radiation, and resection is usually not indicated. Greater than 90% of patients are cured if they present with low-volume disease.

Primary mediastinal B-cell lymphoma (PMBL) and lymphoblastic lymphomas are the other lymphomas frequently encountered in the anterior mediastinum (Figure 3). These non-Hodgkin's lymphomas are more likely to present with SVC syndrome, compared with Hodgkin's lymphoma. Chemotherapy regimens are chosen based on lymphoma subclassification. While prognosis is typically inferior to that of Hodgkin's lymphoma, cure is still possible.

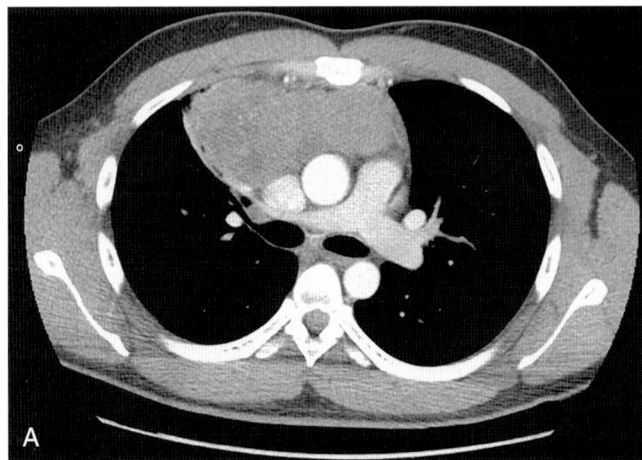

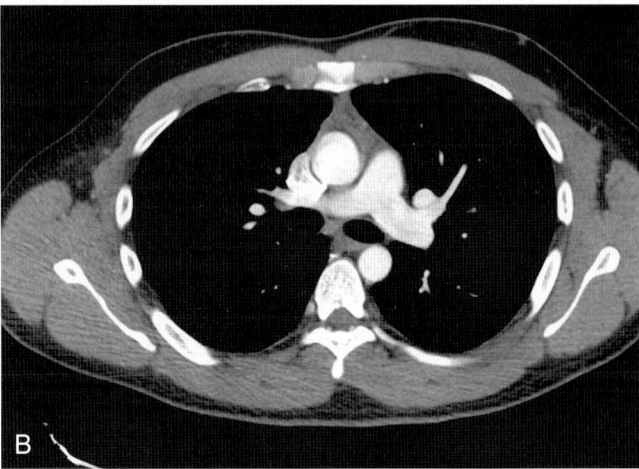

FIGURE 3 A, Axial computed tomography image of a 28-year-old man with a primary mediastinal B-cell lymphoma. The diagnosis was established with a biopsy performed through a right Chamberlain procedure. **B,** The patient received six cycles of multiagent chemotherapy (R-CHOP) with a complete response.

Thyroid and Parathyroid

Substernal goiters are typically extensions of cervical thyroid tissue that descend into the anterior mediastinum. Occasionally, large substernal goiters can also wrap around the trachea and approach the esophagus. Rarely, substernal goiters arise in ectopic thyroid tissue, and the diagnosis may not be suspected preoperatively. While substernal goiters are not universally symptomatic, many patients report dyspnea or dysphagia, secondary to compression. Substernal goiters do not have a higher incidence of occult carcinoma compared with cervical goiters. When a substernal goiter is identified, subtotal thyroidectomy is typically indicated and is easily performed through a low cervical collar incision. Medical therapy for symptomatic goiters only delays definitive therapy and may complicate resection. Extremely large goiters occasionally require a partial upper sternotomy to facilitate resection. A total sternotomy would be excessive in most patients. The vasculature of a substernal goiter originates in the neck, except in the case of an ectopic thyroid, which derives perfusion from the internal mammary or innominate arteries, or even the aorta in some cases. While postoperative morbidity is minimal, recurrent laryngeal nerve injury and hypoparathyroidism may occur.

Ectopic mediastinal parathyroid adenomas are responsible for 5% of primary hyperparathyroidism. By far, the most common location for a mediastinal parathyroid adenoma is in the thymus or anterior mediastinum. Rarely, parathyroid adenomas are found in the middle mediastinum in a paratracheal position or in the posterior

mediastinum, adjacent to the esophagus. A common clinical scenario is one in which a patient has persistent hyperparathyroidism after cervical exploration. Localization studies such as Sestamibi scanning, CT imaging, and selective venous sampling help to detect the mediastinal parathyroid adenoma. While median sternotomy has historically been the procedure of choice, increasingly, minimally invasive techniques such as VATS and mediastinoscopy reliably remove mediastinal parathyroid adenomas. Intraoperative documentation of at least 50% reduction in parathyroid hormone and histologic confirmation of resection ensure correction of hyperparathyroidism (Wei B, et al., 2011).

Middle Mediastinum

Castleman's Disease

Castleman's disease is a rare lymphoproliferative disorder that produces benign lymph node masses. While Castleman's disease may occur virtually anywhere in the body, in 70% of patients the nodal masses develop in the chest. They predominantly occur adjacent to the central airways or in the pulmonary hilum, and occasionally in the anterior or posterior mediastinum. They commonly appear as enhancing masses on CT imaging, and patients are often asymptomatic. There are characteristic histopathologic findings, with the hyaline vascular follicular form being the most prevalent type. Castleman's disease is often discovered at the time of incisional biopsy and frozen section analysis. If the patient has unicentric disease and resection is technically feasible, the mass should be resected, and cure is achieved in the vast majority of patients. Systemic therapy with an agent such as rituximab that targets proliferating B-cells in the mass is more appropriate for multicentric disease (Talat N, et al., 2012). Long-term prognosis is inferior in patients with multicentric disease, as recurrences and progression are likely.

Mediastinal Lymphadenopathy

The most common benign conditions that produce mediastinal lymphadenopathy are sarcoidosis and granulomatous disease. Sarcoidosis is a systemic inflammatory disorder that occurs usually in patients aged 30 to 40. CT imaging reveals significant paratracheal, subcarinal, and hilar lymphadenopathy. While patients are often asymptomatic, they may have symptoms related to involvement of organ systems such as the lungs, liver, skin, and nervous system. The diagnosis is supported by an elevation in circulating angiotensin-converting enzyme. Biopsy of the involved lymph nodes reveals non-caseating granulomas. Ultimately, sarcoidosis is a diagnosis of exclusion, once other disorders are ruled out.

Granulomatous disease causing mediastinal lymphadenopathy is especially prevalent in regions where fungal infections such as coccidiomycosis (e.g., southwestern United States) and histoplasmosis (e.g., Ohio and Mississippi River Valleys) are prevalent. While patients are often asymptomatic, airway obstruction or hemorrhage may occur due to erosion by broncholiths, which are heavily calcified mediastinal lymph nodes. Biopsy of these nodes is often necessary to establish the diagnosis, and the characteristic histopathologic finding is the presence of necrotizing granulomas. Resection is typically unnecessary, and systemic therapy, with antibiotics, is occasionally indicated.

The most common malignant cause of mediastinal lymphadenopathy is metastatic lung cancer. While CT and PET imaging are often suggestive of mediastinal lymph node metastases, tissue diagnosis is often required to avoid false positive diagnosis. Mediastinal lymph node involvement represents a higher stage of disease and influences various treatment decisions. Cervical mediastinoscopy readily samples the lymph nodes adjacent to the trachea and proximal main-stem bronchi in the middle mediastinum. The Chamberlain procedure or VATS are necessary to sample nodes in the aortopulmonary window.

Increasingly, EBUS is used to complement, and in some cases replace, cervical mediastinoscopy in mediastinal staging. Although EBUS can reliably assess a number of benign and malignant abnormalities in middle mediastinal lymph nodes, FNA needle biopsy is usually inadequate for subclassification of lymphoma, and mediastinoscopy is indicated.

Mediastinal Cysts

Mediastinal cysts typically occur in the middle mediastinum and represent approximately 20% of mediastinal masses. Bronchogenic cysts are the most common type of mediastinal cyst (approximately 60%), while esophageal duplication cysts and pericardial cysts make up the remainder. Mediastinal cysts are lined with epithelium responsible for secretion of fluid. Communication with the adjacent airway, foregut, or pericardium is possible but rare. CT imaging reveals a smooth and homogenous mass of soft tissue density adjacent to the airway or esophagus. MRI is occasionally useful to confirm that the cyst is fluid filled.

Bronchogenic and esophageal cysts are typically resected, even in asymptomatic patients. The precise natural history of bronchogenic and esophageal cysts is unknown, but there are anecdotal reports of malignant degeneration. The primary indications for resection are that these lesions often become symptomatic during the patient's lifetime, and infection or hemorrhage makes resection more complicated. While minimally invasive VATS and robotic techniques are increasingly employed to resect mediastinal cysts, the safe and complete resection of the cyst remains the primary goal. When cysts cannot be completely resected without injuring the adjacent airway or esophagus, the residual epithelium is fulgurated to reduce the likelihood of recurrence.

Pericardial cysts typically occur in the right cardiophrenic border and are often asymptomatic. Pericardial cyst resection is appropriate when a patient is symptomatic or the cyst is rapidly growing; the majority of patients can be observed. VATS techniques are particularly suited for resection of pericardial cysts.

Posterior Mediastinum

Neurogenic tumors in the posterior mediastinum account for approximately 15% of mediastinal masses in adults and nearly 50% in children. They are typically asymptomatic and benign in adults and are discovered incidentally on chest imaging. Neurogenic tumors most often occur in the paravertebral sulcus and originate from cells in the peripheral nerves, the ganglion, or the paraganglionic cells. Malignancy is more common in pediatric patients.

Schwannomas and neurofibromas are benign tumors that account for the majority of posterior mediastinal neurogenic tumors. They arise from the nerve sheaths of the peripheral nerves. Ganglioneuromas are also benign tumors, but they arise from the ganglia. Ganglioneuroblastomas and neuroblastomas are malignant tumors arising from the ganglia and are encountered in children far more often than in adults. Symptomatic masses are more likely to be malignant. CT imaging best characterizes these masses, which usually appear as solid, round, and well-demarcated lesions. Extension into the neural foramen is carefully assessed, and findings such as neural foramen widening should be further evaluated with an MRI. Dumbbell tumors are those that originate in the paravertebral sulcus but have significant neuroforaminal extension (Figure 4). While most posterior mediastinal masses are easily removed by a standard posterolateral thoracotomy or VATS, dumbbell tumors require a coordinated approach with a spine surgeon to achieve a safe resection (Shadmehr M, et al., 2003). Paraplegia is a known, but very preventable, complication of dumbbell tumor resection; unrecognized hemorrhage and hematoma formation in the foramen or foreign bodies such as bone wax and antithrombotic agents may result in spinal cord compression and injury. Malignant tumors may require adjuvant

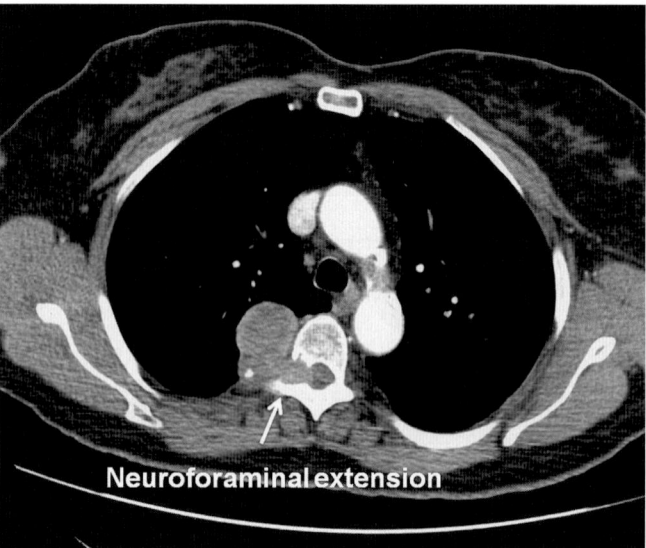

FIGURE 4   Axial CT image of 66-year-old woman with right posterior mediastinal schwannoma with neuroforaminal extension (dumbbell tumor). Resection was accomplished by a combined approach (staged laminectomy followed by thoracotomy).

radiation for positive or close surgical margins and adjuvant chemotherapy for metastatic disease.

Pheochromocytomas and chemodectomas arising in the posterior mediastinum are less common and are derived from paraganglionic cells. Mediastinal pheochromocytomas require preoperative preparation to avoid hemodynamic complications, as with those that are located in the abdomen. Chemodectomas are typically very vascular tumors, and consideration of preoperative embolization is warranted to reduce operative blood loss.

CONCLUSION

Expert diagnosis and management of mediastinal masses require familiarity with a diverse set of diagnostic tools and therapeutics. Imaging is the cornerstone for forming the differential diagnosis, and CT imaging, in particular, is the most versatile test. Diagnosis is facilitated by familiarity with various biopsy techniques, including needle biopsy by CT guidance or EBUS, mediastinoscopy, the Chamberlain procedure, and VATS. Minimally invasive techniques are perfectly suited for resecting many mediastinal masses, reducing morbidity and recovery time. Invasive or bulky masses still require conventional approaches, such as median sternotomy, to safely resect the lesion and occasionally reconstruct adjacent structures. Surgery alone is inadequate for mediastinal masses such as germ cell tumors, and close collaboration with medical and radiation oncology is necessary.

SELECTED READINGS

Lanuti M, De Delva PE, Gaissert HA, et al: Review of superior vena cava resection in the management of benign disease and pulmonary or mediastinal malignancies, *Ann Thorac Surg* 88:392–398, 2009.

Marulli G, Rea F, Melfi F, et al: Robot-aided thoracoscopic thymectomy for early-stage thymoma: a multicenter European study, *J Thorac Cardiovasc Surg* 144:1125–1130, 2012.

Masaoka A: Staging system of thymoma, *J Thorac Oncol* 5:S304–S312, 2010.

Shadmehr MB, Gaissert HA, Wain JC, et al: The surgical approach to "dumbbell tumors" of the mediastinum, *Ann Thorac Surg* 76:1650–1654, 2003.

Talat N, Belgaumkar AP, Schulte KM: Surgery in Castleman's disease: a systematic review of 404 published cases, *Ann Surg* 255:677–684, 2012.

Wei B, Inabnet W, Lee JA, Sonett JR: Optimizing the minimally invasive approach to mediastinal parathyroid adenomas, *Ann Thorac Surg* 92:1012–1017, 2011.

Wright CD: Stage IVA thymoma: patterns of spread and surgical management, *Thorac Surg Clin* 21:93–97, 2011.

Yasufuku K, Nakajima T, Fujiwara T, Yoshino I, Keshavjee S: Utility of endobronchial ultrasound-guided transbronchial needle aspiration in the diagnosis of mediastinal masses of unknown etiology, *Ann Thorac Surg* 91:831–836, 2011.

PRIMARY TUMORS OF THE THYMUS

Michal Hubka, MD, and Douglas E. Wood, MD

ANATOMY

The thymus is located in the anterior mediastinum. It lies just posterior to the sternum and anterior to the pericardium; the upper horns of the H-shaped gland extend into the neck. The arterial blood supply comes from small branches of the inferior thyroid arteries, and venous drainage is via a single or multiple branches into the left innominate vein. Bilateral phrenic nerves are intimately associated with the upper aspect of the thymus, inasmuch as they course distally on the pericardial surface. Understanding the location of the phrenic nerves is of critical importance during surgical resection.

PATHOLOGY

Thymic tumors are the most common anterior mediastinal neoplasms and include both thymomas and thymic carcinomas. No risk factors are known to predispose a person to thymic disease, although there is an association of thymomas and myasthenia gravis. In addition to thymic neoplasms, the differential diagnosis of an anterior mediastinal mass includes intrathoracic thyroid tumors, parathyroid tumors, lymphomas, and germ cell tumors.

Thymomas can be associated with a wide variety of systemic syndromes. The neuromuscular disease myasthenia gravis is caused by autoantibodies' blocking acetylcholine receptors in the neuromuscular junction. The disease manifests as weakness that tends to worsen with activity, and its effects can be observed in the muscles that control speech, respiration, the eyes, and limbs. It is estimated that 30% to 50% of patients with a thymoma have myasthenia, whereas only 15% of patients with myasthenia have a thymoma. Thymectomy improves the symptoms in up to 60% of patients with myasthenia, but this improvement occurs slowly over time and is variable in degree. Thymectomy results in a decreased incidence of exacerbations and a decrease in the need for medications, as well as a higher incidence of long-term remission. Because the improvement in symptoms is not immediate, thymectomy is not undertaken in the midst of a myasthenic crisis. Patients with severe neurologic symptoms should be treated with plasmapheresis or intravenous gamma globulin before surgery. Serum levels of antiacetycholine receptor antibodies can be measured if the diagnosis of myasthenia is unclear. Management of patients with severe symptoms should be in conjunction with a neurologist.

Thymomas are also associated with hematologic abnormalities, especially red blood cell aplasia, immunodeficiencies, and collagen vascular diseases. Resection of the thymoma does not reliably improve the symptoms in such patients.

Thymic carcinoid is a rare tumor. It can be associated with multiple endocrine neoplasia type 1 (MEN 1) and Cushing's syndrome. Many patients have nodal metastases or distant metastases, or both, at the time of presentation. Other rare thymic neoplasms include small-cell tumors and sarcomas.

Unlike thymoma, thymic carcinoma is an aggressive tumor with a poor prognosis. There are two histologic types: squamous and lymphoepithelioma. Median length of survival of all patients with thymic carcinoma is only 2 years, but this can be improved when complete surgical resection is accomplished. Aggressive resection is warranted, but overall results remain poor. Partial responses to chemotherapy and radiation therapy have been reported.

EVALUATION

About half of thymic tumors are initially asymptomatic and found on radiographs obtained for other reasons. Patients with symptomatic tumors typically report chest pain, but less commonly compression of the airway or venous return is observed, or compromise of the phrenic or recurrent laryngeal nerves is evident. Patients with a thymoma may also show symptoms and signs of paraneoplastic syndromes. Beta-human chorionic gonadotropin and alpha-fetoprotein levels should be evaluated to rule out germ-cell tumors. Serum levels of antiacetylcholine antibodies should be examined in patients with even mild symptoms suggestive of myasthenia gravis.

Computed tomographic scan of the chest with intravenous contrast agent is the most valuable diagnostic procedure (Figure 1), although magnetic resonance imaging is occasionally helpful in evaluating invasion into the chest wall and vascular structures. CT and positron emission tomography can be helpful in evaluating for distant metastasis in advanced-stage thymic carcinoma. It is most important to distinguish lesions that can be treated primarily by resection from those that can be treated primarily with chemotherapy. Frequently, these lesions can be differentiated by their radiographic appearance. Thymic tumors tend to originate in the area of the thymus itself, rarely extend into the neck, and usually do not produce associated adenopathy. Thymomas tend to have smooth contours, whereas thymic carcinomas often contain necrotic centers or calcifications. In contrast, mediastinal lymphoma is generally a more bulky and infiltrative tumor and is usually associated with additional adenopathy. Thyroid goiter or tumors usually have characteristic radiologic features and continuity with the cervical thyroid. Radiologic suspicion of thymoma can be established with a high degree of reliability in a majority of affected patients. Pleural or pericardial effusions are the most common manifestation of locally advanced disease and may also cause thoracic symptoms. The pleural surfaces should be carefully examined for evidence of possible pleural "drop" metastases.

For resectable lesions, it is appropriate to forgo biopsy and proceed directly to complete resection to make the diagnosis. Tissue sampling should be reserved only for locally advanced or unresectable cases or in patients in whom an alternative diagnosis, such as lymphoma, is the primary diagnosis. This can be done with a CT-guided core needle biopsy or an incision via an anterior mediastinotomy. For an anterior mediastinotomy, or Chamberlain's

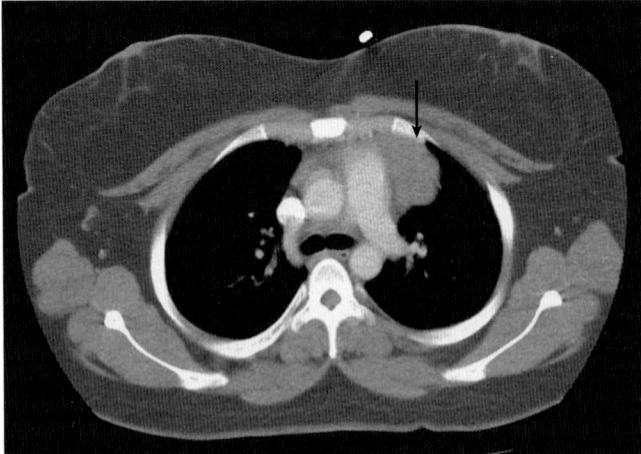

FIGURE 1   Computed tomographic scan of a thymoma (arrow) in the left anterior mediastinum.

TABLE 1: World Health Organization staging: histologic categories	
A	Spindle cell or medullary thymoma
AB	Mixed thymoma
B1	Lymphocyte-rich or predominately cortical thymoma
B2	Cortical thymoma
B3	Epithelial thymoma
C	Thymic carcinoma

procedure, an incision is made over the second rib, and the second costal cartilage is optionally excised for additional exposure. Biopsy samples can usually be obtained directly, and a video mediastinoscope can be inserted into the wound to allow for further visualization if necessary. Videoscopic transpleural tissue sampling short of complete (R0) resection should be avoided because of the major concern of pleural space seeding and the possible tragic consequences of iatrogenic spread of tumor. If the mass compresses the airway, great care must be used in administering a general anesthetic.

STAGING

A number of different staging systems have been proposed for thymomas. At this time, two systems are used in conjunction: the World Health Organization (WHO) histologic classification and the Masaoka system, which describes invasion and metastasis. The WHO classification is outlined in Table 1. Tumors with A, AB, and B1 histologic features carry a better prognosis. The Masaoka classification is shown in Table 2. Most affected patients initially present with early-stage disease, and these patients have an excellent overall prognosis when treated. The incidence of distant metastasis is very low.

PRINCIPLES OF THERAPY

Treatment of thymomas and thymic carcinomas should be carried out in tertiary and quaternary medical centers by a multidisciplinary team consisting of thoracic surgeons, medical oncologists, and radiation oncologists.

The primary treatment for early-stage thymoma is surgical resection. Patients who have Masaoka stage I disease should undergo resection; R0 resection is correlated with excellent rates of 5-year survival. Stage II disease—microscopic (IIA) or macroscopic (IIB) invasion through the tumor capsule—found on final pathologic studies after an R0 resection also carries a very good prognosis with regard to 5-year survival. However, adjuvant radiation therapy can be considered in cases with increased risk of recurrence: close surgical margins, WHO grade B tumor, or both. Adjuvant chemotherapy for stages I and II thymomas is reserved for patients with microscopically and macroscopically positive margins of the resected specimen.

Stage III disease includes tumor invasion into the pericardium or lung, with or without great vessel invasion; stage IVa involves metastatic disease localized to pleura or pericardium. Patients with stage III or IVa disease should be treated with multimodality therapy. Resectable tumors with solitary pleural or pulmonary metastasis

(IVa) can be treated with upfront surgery followed by chemotherapy or with neoadjuvant chemotherapy followed by a resection. Neoadjuvant chemotherapy is preferred for stage III disease. Most chemotherapy regimens that have been used for neoadjuvant therapy are cisplatin-based. Response to neoadjuvant chemotherapy is seen in over two thirds of patients with most patients proceeding to resection. Complete pathologic response at the time of resection was seen in 14% of patients treated with neoadjuvant cisplatin, doxorubicin, and cyclophosphamide plus prednisone. A complete resection should be then attempted after restaging imaging. Patients who are found not to be candidates for an R0 resection intraoperatively should undergo maximum debulking followed by postoperative radiation therapy. Unilateral phrenic nerve resection is usually appropriate if needed to accomplish a complete resection. However, bilateral phrenic nerve resection should be avoided because of the high likelihood of respiratory compromise. Postoperative radiation therapy regimens vary from 45 to 50 Gy for microscopic residual disease or close surgical margins and up to 60 Gy for gross residual disease.

Adjuvant radiation therapy with completely resected stages II and III disease is controversial because there is no evidence for improved survival or decreased recurrence rates.

Stage IVb thymomas, unresectable tumors, and biopsy-proven thymic carcinoma are treated with definitive platinum-based chemotherapy. Thymic carcinoma metastasizes to the liver, bone, and brain as well as the thorax. No randomized trials have been conducted to guide the choice of treatment because of the rarity of the disease. Regimens studied include cisplatin, doxorubicin, and cyclophosphamide; partial and complete response rates of 50% and 10% were observed, and the median length of survival was 37.7 months. Etoposide with cisplatin appears to produce slightly better results, with partial and complete response rates of 56% and 31%, respectively. Median length of survival was also better, at 52 months.

OPERATIVE MANAGEMENT

Before surgical resection, pulmonary function testing should be performed both to stratify the risk for perioperative pulmonary complications and to obtain baseline values.

Classically, the surgical approach to early-stage thymomas is usually through a partial or complete median sternotomy. With solitary pulmonary or pleural metastasis, a separate thoracotomy or videoscopic approach can facilitate access to the pleural space. However, invasive or locally disseminated thymomas, Masaoka stage III or IV, should be approached through a sufficiently large incision. A clamshell incision affords improved exposure to bulky tumors that obscure important mediastinal structures and renders access to bilateral pleural spaces. Thoracoscopic and robotic approaches have been developed and can facilitate complete resection of early-stage thymomas. However, it is very important to not violate the primary

TABLE 2: Masaoka staging system and survival

Stage	Definition	Frequency at presentation	5-year survival rate	10-year survival rate
I	Macroscopically encapsulated, no microscopic invasion of the capsule	40%	92%	88%
II	IIa: Macroscopic invasion into mediastinal fat or pleura IIb: Microscopic invasion of the capsule	25%	82%	70%
III	Invasion into neighboring organs	25%	68%	57%
IVa	Pleural or pericardial metastasis	10%	61%	38%
IVb	Lymphatic or hematogenous metastasis	1%-2%	0%	0%

Data summarizing the results from multiple large studies from Detterbeck FC, Parsons AM: Thymic tumors, Ann Thorac Surg *77:1860–1869, 2004.*

principles of surgical resection in the enthusiasm to perform a minimally invasive procedure. Excessive tumor manipulation or disruption of the tumor capsule may result in spread of tumor into the mediastinum or pleural space. Minimally invasive approaches are not appropriate for larger thymomas (>4 cm) or outside of centers without substantial experience in robotic or thoracoscopic thymectomy. Transcervical thymectomy in the presence or suspicion of a thymoma should be avoided because of concern for incomplete mediastinal resection.

Transsternal Thymectomy

The chief goal of every surgical approach is to achieve a complete resection of all thymic tissue and the tumor, which is crucial for a good outcome. After sternotomy, the mediastinum and bilateral pleural spaces are evaluated for unanticipated metastatic disease. The tumor is evaluated to ensure that it can be completely resected and to see what, if any, structures need to be removed en bloc. In cases of myasthenia gravis, all anterior pericardial fat should be resected because it can contain ectopic thymic tissue.

Dissection can begin at the inferior poles of the thymus to clear it of the pericardium cranially until the left innominate vein is encountered. Invasion of the pericardium necessitates anterior pericardiectomy. This procedure can be performed without any consequences. The thymic venous branches draining into the innominate vein are then divided after ligation. The dissection should extend laterally to the phrenic nerves on both sides. The arterial blood supply from the internal mammary arteries can usually be divided with electrocautery. The superior horns of the thymus are then dissected, and division of the thyrothymic ligament liberates the gland.

Transsternal thymectomy remains the "gold standard" in surgical treatment of both myasthenia gravis and thymoma. The ability to achieve direct tumor visualization, palpation, and delicate direct handling suggests that transsternal thymectomy remains the sole approach for advanced-stage thymomas and thymic carcinomas. The limitation of this approach is increased hospital stay and outpatient postoperative recovery in comparison with approaches that do not require sternal division.

Video-Assisted Thoracic Surgery: Thymectomy

The use of minimally invasive thoracoscopic and robotic approaches for resecting small thymomas has increased. Thoracoscopic thymectomy can be approached via either the right or left side, depending on surgeon's preference and lateral dominance of the thymus. After intubation with a double-lumen tube, the patient is then placed in the lateral decubitus position, as for a conventional thoracotomy. A port is introduced along the midaxillary line between the sixth and eighth intercostal spaces according to the site of the tumor. In addition, two or, in rare cases, three other operative ports are positioned along the anterior and posterior axillary line to triangulate the working space around the lesion.

The dissection starts inferiorly, on the ipsilateral side, at the pericardiophrenic angle until the inferior horn is dissected, and then it proceeds to the contralateral side until the contralateral inferior horn is reached. Subsequent dissection continues upward similarly to the transsternal approach until the left innominate vein is encountered.

The thymic veins are identified, clipped, and divided, and then the upper horns are dissected. This technique results in removal of all thymus and perithymic fat. The specimen is then liberated from the patient via a port incision and a protective pouch.

Robotic Thymectomy

Robotic thymectomy offers improved visualization and depth perception via a binocular thoracoscope and carbon dioxide insufflation, as well as improved dexterity from wristed instrumentation (EndoWrist; Intuitive Surgical, Sunnyvale, Calif). This method, however, lacks haptic feedback; thus insinuation of tissue tension must be performed visually.

Robotic thymectomy can also be performed via either the right or left side, depending on surgeon's preference and lateral dominance of the thymus. The advantage of a left-sided approach is improved visualization of the left brachiocephalic vein. The right-sided approach affords better protection of the right phrenic nerve, which courses more anteriorly than the left and hence tends to be more intimately involved with the thymus.

The patient is positioned at a 30-degree angle. The camera is then introduced in the fifth intercostal space at the midaxillary line, with two working ports introduced in the third intercostal space at the midaxillary region and the fifth intercostal space at the midclavicular line, so that all instruments are triangulated to be 8 to 10 cm apart. The right arm of the EndoWrist has a spatula with electric cautery function in order to perform dissection, and the left arm dominant instrument is a Cadière forceps, an instrument for grasping the thymus atraumatically.

The dissection follows the same principles as basic videoscopic thymectomy. Starting inferiorly, the inferior horns and perithymic epicardial fat are freed, and dissection proceeds upward until the left innominate vein is encountered. The dissection is completed by dividing the thymic veins and dissecting the upper horns. The specimen is then placed in a protective pouch and removed via a port incision.

Minimally invasive surgical approaches to thymic disease are becoming more common. Video-assisted thoracic surgery (VATS) thymectomy was reported to produce results equivalent to those of transsternal thymectomy in early-stage thymomas, with a 5-year overall survival rate of 100%. The advantage of decreased hospital stay and fewer analgesia requirements in comparison with transsternal thymectomy is especially important in patients with myasthenia gravis and impaired respiratory mechanics.

Robotic thymectomy can be considered a natural progression of VATS, offering high-definition binocular vision, and improved maneuverability of robotic instruments enabled by wrist articulation of the instruments inside the chest cavity. These features enable precise isolation of the anatomic structures and safe manipulation of the tissues. Since the early 2000s, the robotic system has facilitated extension of a minimally invasive approach to cases of malignant tumors. In cases of myasthenia gravis, improvement in symptoms is observed in more than 90% of cases, on par with a transsternal approach. Complete remission is achieved in up to 30% of patients after robotic thymectomy and has surpassed the results of VATS. This probably results because resection is more complete, involving all prepericardial fat that contains ectopic thymic tissues.

The main limitations of robotic thymectomy are lack of long-term data, pressure for inappropriate use, and cost. Initial investment in the robot itself, as well maintenance of the robotic instrumentarium, is high. Some hospitals attempt to overcome the high cost by multidisciplinary use of the robotic system.

The surgeon's experience and technical aptitude with both VATS and robotic thymectomies is correlated directly with decreased operative times and comfort with resection of larger tumors. Some authorities argue that adequate level of competence is not reached until after 70 minimally invasive thymectomies.

SUMMARY

Thymic pathologic processes range from benign gland disease associated with symptoms of myasthenia gravis to thymoma to thymic carcinoma. Surgical management of thymic disorders should be included in every case in which cure is the goal because chemotherapy alone is almost never curative.

The thymus gland lies in a precarious anatomic location; thus it is amenable to a variety of surgical approaches. Transsternal thymectomy remains the most oncologically sound approach in locally advanced thymomas and thymic carcinomas. Minimally invasive approaches are becoming options for early-stage thymomas in centers with substantial experience. A thoracic surgeon should possess technical equipoise with all approaches and tailor them as appropriate to individual clinical cases.

SUGGESTED READINGS

Detterbeck FC, Parsons AM: Thymic tumors, *Ann Thorac Surg* 77:1860–1869, 2004.
Goldstein SD, Yang SC: Assessment of robotic thymectomy using the Myasthenia Gravis Foundation of America Guidelines, *Ann Thorac Surg* 89(4):1080–1085, 2010.
National Comprehensive Cancer Network Guidelines: http://www.nccn.org/professionals/physician_gls/f_guidelines.asp#thymic

THE MANAGEMENT OF TRACHEAL STENOSIS

Cameron D. Wright, MD

Tracheal stenosis is usually the result of endotracheal tube cuff ischemic necrosis of the underlying trachea. The ischemic area of trachea involves varying depths of injury that cause a spectrum of injury from mucosal to full thickness, including the cartilage. Cuff lesions are circumferential and usually become progressively stenosed until reepithelialization occurs. The site of a tracheostomy stoma may become stenosed, usually as a result of a combination of factors: excessive removal of anterior tracheal wall at the time of tracheostomy, peristomal infection, or excessive lateral pressure from the ventilator tubing. Stomal stenosis is usually triangular in shape with a collapse of the two lateral tracheal walls to the center, often with a relatively normal posterior membranous wall. The narrowest portion of the airway is the cricoid in the lower larynx. Selection of an endotracheal tube that is too large relative to the size of the cricoid can lead to circumferential injury to the cricoid mucosa, which may lead to subglottic (laryngeal) stenosis. Stenosis that involves the larynx is more complex to repair, and the results are less certain than with simple tracheal resection. Stenosis also may involve the glottis from endotracheal tube damage to the vocal cords and arytenoids. An abnormal glottis must be corrected before correction of any tracheal problem because the glottis must provide an adequate airway at the conclusion of a tracheal resection. Malacia may be present in the trachea around the stenotic area and if severe must be resected as well.

TIMING OF THERAPY

Resection should be deferred until the patient fully recovers from the original illness that precipitated mechanical ventilation. All necessary operations that require general anesthesia (e.g., burn cases that need multiple excisions and scar releases) should be completed before tracheal resection. Often steroids are mistakenly administered to treat new-onset "asthma" after prolonged intubation. Steroids should be rapidly weaned because they play no role in amelioration of postintubation stenosis and they interfere with healing of the tracheal anastomosis. Glottic pathology should be corrected before treatment of tracheal pathology. Mucosal inflammation identified with bronchoscopy should be allowed to resolve before resection to reduce the chance of an anastomotic problem. A simple stomal stenosis rarely progresses to life-threatening airway obstruction, so these patients usually can be safely observed while they recover from their critical illness. Tracheal cuff stenosis often gradually scars to the point of airway obstruction, leading to the need for urgent treatment. If the patient is in otherwise good shape, definitive treatment with resection may be performed. The airway can be temporarily improved with bronchoscopic dilation if only a short period of time (i.e., weeks) is needed before definitive treatment. Laser bronchoscopy often further injures the airway and should be avoided when one wishes to temporize before proceeding to definitive resection. If months are needed before resection can be contemplated, tracheostomy should be strongly considered. Tracheostomy must be carefully planned and performed so as not to needlessly injure normal trachea, which could jeopardize the proposed tracheal resection. The stoma should be constructed through the most severely damaged trachea, which eventually is resected so as not to waste good trachea. Self-expanding metallic stents should not be used for postintubation stenosis because they effectively lengthen the airway injury and often convert a simple short resection to a very long resection, which has a much greater failure rate. Silicone tracheal T tubes are useful in patients who need tracheostomy to maintain an airway because they allow for normal airflow through the mouth and nose. These tubes are relatively nonreactive with the tracheal mucosa and do not usually lead to extension of the injury to the airway.

INDICATIONS FOR RESECTION

In general, any patient with obstructive airway symptoms and tracheal stenosis after intubation should have definitive tracheal resection and reconstruction. Absolute contraindications are few and include a nonreconstructible airway (usually because of excessive length of the damaged airway), severe comorbidities, and a continued need for ventilation. Relative contraindications include a history of radiation to the trachea, continued mucosal inflammation beyond the area of resection, and active steroid use.

FACTORS TO CONSIDER FOR TRACHEAL RESECTION

Anatomic and demographic factors influence how much trachea can be safely resected and reconstructed. Probably the most important factor is body habitus; young, tall, thin patients with long necks have an abundance of trachea and are the most straightforward candidates for surgery. Alternatively, elderly kyphotic, short, obese patients with short necks and a cricoid that is at the sternal notch are the most challenging cases. Recent high-dose steroid use and insulin-dependent diabetes are risk factors for anastomotic problems, so special attention needs to be paid to the amount of tension on the anastomosis in these patients at higher risk. Pediatric patients tolerate anastomotic tension less well than adults; ideally resections only under 30% should be done in children, whereas some adults can tolerate resections up to 50% of the length of the trachea. Previous tracheal surgery causes relative fixation of the remaining trachea and thus limits any possible reresection to less than normal. Previous radiation therapy to the trachea also limits tracheal mobility and impairs microvascular blood supply, both of which place constraints on how much trachea can be safely removed.

AIRWAY MANAGEMENT

Patients who present with critical airway obstruction almost always can be managed with bronchoscopic dilation. A tracheostomy very rarely is needed to establish an airway acutely in postintubation tracheal stenosis. Patients should be promptly taken to the operating room for urgent bronchoscopic dilation. If the airway is judged to be critical, muscle relaxants are avoided and induction of anesthesia is done with an inhalational technique, which allows the patient to breathe spontaneously until the airway is secured with bronchoscopy. The surgeon must be present during induction of anesthesia with all equipment immediately available and absolute competence to establish an airway. When the patient's condition is deep enough to allow airway manipulation, rigid bronchoscopy is commenced with an adult #7 or #8 rigid bronchoscope to visualize the airway and stenosis. Dilation is begun with plastic small-diameter Jackson dilators through the bronchoscope until the maximal size is reached (about 6 mm). At this point, the airway is open enough to allow suctioning of retained distal secretions and to allow the anesthesiologist to ventilate the patient enough to return the end-tidal CO_2 to normal. The

airway can be further dilated with passage of serial-sized rigid bronchoscopes from a pediatric #3 up to an adult #9. The surgeon can appreciate the degree of resistance with the passage of each size scope to decide exactly how far to dilate so as to avoid tearing the airway. The surgeon should select the proper sized bronchoscope that is just a little too big to fit through the stenosis to begin dilation with. This allows for a graded stretching of the stenosis. If too large a size is selected, the lip of the bronchoscope can instead tear the mucosa, leading to development of a flap that can occlude the end of the bronchoscope and lead to loss of the airway. Alternatively, the trachea can be dilated with balloon dilation. If dilation is planned as a temporizing measure, in general the dilation should be to the largest size possible so it lasts for as long as possible. If dilation is being done just before a resection, usually one dilates just enough to accept a #6 or #7 endotracheal tube.

TRACHEAL RESECTION AND RECONSTRUCTION

The patient is placed supine with an inflatable bag under the shoulders and the head placed in a soft gel ring that provides stability. At the beginning of the operation, the inflatable bag is inflated to extend the neck almost to the point of causing the head to float. An inflatable bag is used as when the trachea is to be reapproximated the bag is deflated and the head is flexed forward to cause the larynx and trachea to devolve toward the carina, which reduces tension on the anastomosis. The neck and anterior chest are prepped and sterilely draped. Usually a low collar incision is made just above the clavicles (Figure 1). If a stoma is present and is close to the incision, it is incorporated into the incision and excised. If it is inconveniently far away, it is ignored in terms of incision placement and later excised and closed separately. Some elderly kyphotic cases require access to the upper mediastinum for adequate exposure to the trachea; in such cases, all that is needed is a partial upper sternotomy through the manubrium only for access. Access is achieved below the pretracheal plane; the innominate vein and artery are simply retracted away from the trachea for excellent exposure all the way to the carina. Full sternotomy or lateral thoracotomy is never needed to deal with postintubation stenoses. Once the collar incision is made, subplatysmal flaps are elevated from the top of the thyroid cartilage to the clavicles. The strap muscles are separated in the midline and retracted laterally. The thyroid isthmus is divided if it has not already been done. The fatty tissue below the thyroid covering the airway is divided in the midline to complete the exposure of the entire anterior aspect of the airway present in the neck. The pretracheal fascia is elevated off the trachea at the sternal notch, and dissection is carried down to the carina, staying directly on the trachea as if for mediastinoscopy. This pretracheal mobilization facilitates reapproximation of the trachea and reduces tension on the anastomosis.

The anterior surface of the trachea is exposed from about 3 o'clock to 9 o'clock, which still preserves the blood supply that comes directly to the tracheal rings in a low lateral fashion. The area of the stenosis is now dissected in a circumferential fashion, staying exactly on the wall of the trachea so as to avoid injury to the recurrent nerves. The recurrent nerve is never dissected out and exposed. Injury to the nerve is rare if dissection is kept close to the trachea. Sometimes subtle cuff stenoses are difficult to see externally to know where to dissect. In such cases, intraoperative flexible bronchoscopy with pulling the endotracheal tube back to the cricoid allows precise identification of the limits of the stenosis. The surgeon on the field can pierce the trachea with a fine 25-gauge needle, which can be seen by the bronchoscopist to precisely localize the lesion. The trachea should be dissected no more than 1 cm beyond the stenosis to limit ischemia to the two cut ends of the divided trachea, which survive by collateral submucosal vascular supply. With high lesions, transection is carried out below the lesion. The endotracheal tube cuff is deflated before

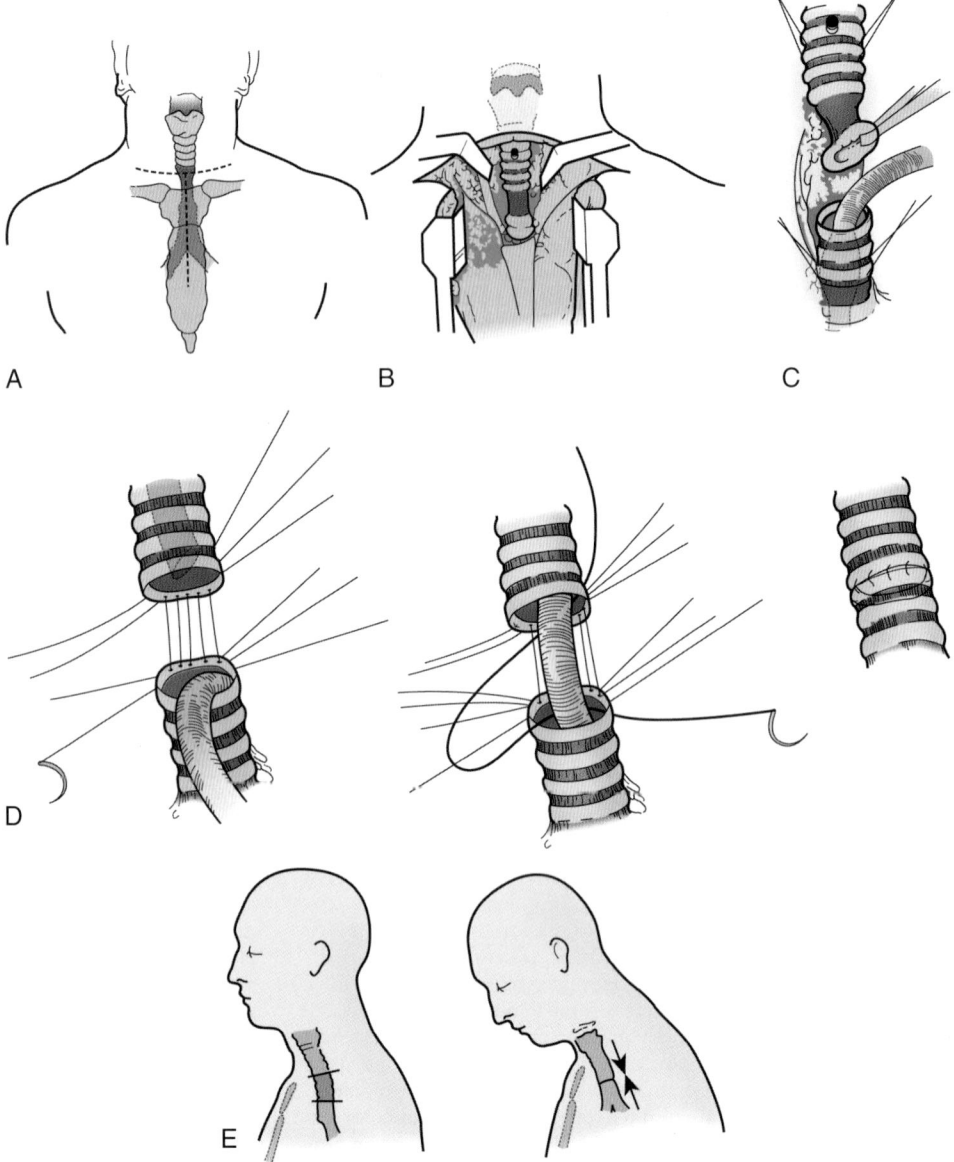

FIGURE 1 Tracheal resection and reconstruction for postintubation stenosis. **A,** A collar incision is used for most cases of postintubation stenosis. For very low lesions or for older patients with kyphosis, the upper sternum is split to provide better access. **B,** Access to the distal trachea is achieved by retracting the vessels forward and inferiorly. The innominate vein is never divided, and the innominate artery is left in its investing sheath to separate it from the eventual anastomosis. **C,** Once the trachea has been divided, ventilation is carried out with a sterile armored endotracheal tube on the field and is controlled by the assistant. **D,** The technique of anastomosis with fine 4-0 interrupted absorbable sutures. The native endotracheal tube can be faintly seen in the proximal trachea in the first drawing. After the posterior sutures are placed, the native endotracheal tube can be advanced into the distal trachea to allow placement of the anterior sutures. **E,** Cervical flexion reduces tension on the anastomosis by devolving the trachea toward the carina. *(From Grillo HC: Surgery of the trachea,* Curr Probl Surg *1970;7:2-59).*

the trachea is incised so the cuff inflates at the end. The tip of the endotracheal tube is pulled into the proximal airway out of the operative field. The stenotic trachea is elevated off the esophagus and dissected toward the larynx until relatively normal trachea is reached for the proximal tracheal transection. The distal airway is intubated with a separate sterile long armored endotracheal tube and is typically held in place and manipulated by the assistant. The distal airway must be kept clear of blood by the assistant to maintain good pulmonary hygiene. With a low lesion, the trachea is usually transected just above the stenosis and the stenotic trachea is dissected downward off the esophagus to the more normal distal trachea. In general, for all but the shortest lesions, it is better to remove less rather than more trachea and then rejudge both the quality of the remaining trachea against the degree of tension that will be required to perform the anastomosis. A balancing act is almost always necessary between the desire to achieve a normal trachea for anastomosis and the desire for an increased level of tension for the anastomosis. Sometimes mildly abnormal tracheal mucosa must be left behind to allow the anastomotic tension to be at an acceptable level. This judgment of how

much to resect in all but the shortest stenoses is critical and takes experience to develop.

Lateral stay sutures of 2-0 Vicryl (Ethicon, Inc, Somerville, NJ) are placed at 3 o'clock and 9 o'clock about 2 tracheal rings from the cut edge, which will be tied outside the airway to loosely approximate the trachea and help reduce tension on the anastomotic sutures. If the resection is very short and thus the anastomotic tension minimal, the anastomotic sutures are placed next. If a fair amount of tension is expected, a trial approximation is usually done to decide whether additional release measures are needed. This judgment takes experience to develop and is critical to a successful result. If the tension is judged to be excessive, the distal trachea is mobilized to the maximal extent as a first step. If this is not enough, then usually a suprahyoid laryngeal release as described by Montgomery needs to be performed. A suprahyoid release usually translates to an additional 1 to 1.5 cm of tracheal length. Once the surgeon is assured the trachea can be safely reapproximated, the anastomosis is begun. Circumferential fine 4-0 Vicryl sutures are placed starting in the posterior midline and working out to the lateral stay sutures at 3 o'clock and 9 o'clock on both sides. The sutures are placed so that the knots are on the outside and are about 3 to 4 mm deep from the cut edge and 3 mm apart from each other. Each suture is placed in a snap after the needle is cut off and then tagged to the drapes in successive order so that the more superficial sutures can be tied first followed by the deeper ones. Once the posterior sutures are placed, the remaining anterior sutures are placed again from one stay to another. Ventilation during the anastomosis is intermittent, with the assistant removing the endotracheal tube while the surgeon places a suture and then replacing the tube to allow ventilation while another suture is being readied. Once all the sutures are placed, the inflatable bag under the shoulders is deflated and the head elevated to reduce tension on the anastomosis. Ventilation is then switched back to the native endotracheal tube by carefully advancing the tube past the anastomosis into the distal trachea. Care must be taken to avoid entrapping or tangling the anastomotic sutures. The assistant then takes tension off the suture line by maintaining tension on the lateral stay suture and all the anterior sutures while the surgeon ties the lateral stay suture on the surgeon's side of the table. The opposite stay is then tied, followed by the anterior sutures and then finally the posterior sutures.

The endotracheal tube cuff is then deflated, and a large tidal volume breathe is given to an airway pressure of about 30 cm of water to test the anastomosis to ensure it is airtight. The author also pulls back the endotracheal tube and rebronchoscopes the patient to inspect the anastomosis from the inside as well. The anastomosis is covered with available vascularized tissue: the thyroid, a pedicled thymus flap, or a pedicled strap muscle. The wound is then irrigated, a suction drain placed, and the wound closed. A heavy guardian suture is placed between the chin and chest to prevent inadvertent neck extension by the patient. The suture is placed so that the neck is in a neutral position, not in a severe flexion position. The patient is awakened and extubated in the operating room and observed long enough to ensure a good airway. Patients are usually kept in the hospital 5 to 7 days for observation. A bronchoscopy is usually done on the anticipated day of discharge to carefully inspect the anastomosis and ensure there are no impending anastomotic complications. Recovery is usually quick and uneventful.

RESULTS

Results of tracheal resection have been quite satisfactory. From 1965 to 1992, 503 patients underwent tracheal resection and reconstruction for postintubation stenosis. This included the author's early experience before standardization of the operation was accomplished. Fifty-three of these patients had previous attempts at tracheal resection. A total of 521 resections were done, 13 for restenosis after initial repair. Lengths of resection averaged 3.5 cm and extended up to 7.5 cm. Results were good in 87.5% and satisfactory in 6%; failure occurred in 4%, and deaths in 2.4%. Failures were treated with tracheostomy in 11 patients, with T tubes in 7 patients, and with dilations in 2 patients. Prior resection increased the failure rate from 2.1% to 9.7% and the mortality rate from 2.1% to 3.8%. The level of the airway anastomosis is also a predictor. Trachea to trachea anastomoses faired best with a failure rate of 2.2%, trachea to cricoid anastomoses led to a 6% failure rate, and trachea to thyroid cartilage had a failure rate of 8.1%. Laryngeal releases were only performed in 46 patients. Dehiscence or restenosis occurred in 29 patients with 7 deaths. A subsequent publication from the author's group identified the risk factors for anastomotic failure: length, >4 cm; diabetes; age, <17 years; preoperative tracheostomy; reoperation; and laryngeal anastomosis.

SUGGESTED READINGS

Grillo HC, Donahue DM, Mathisen DJ, et al: Postintubation tracheal stenosis: treatment and results, *J Thorac Cardiovasc Surg* 109:486–493, 1995.
Montgomery WW: Suprahyoid release for tracheal stenosis, *Arch Otolaryngol* 99:255–260, 1974.
Wright CD, Grillo HC, Wain JC, et al: Anastomotic complications after tracheal resection: prognostic factors and management, *J Thorac Cardiovasc Surg* 128:731–739, 2004.

THE MANAGEMENT OF ACQUIRED ESOPHAGEAL RESPIRATORY TRACT FISTULA

Jahan Mohebali, MD, and
Christopher R. Morse, MD

OVERVIEW

Acquired esophageal respiratory tract fistulas present clinicians with significant diagnostic and management challenges. These fistulas result from myriad causes, both benign and malignant, and can involve the trachea or lower airways. Benign fistulas can be further separated into iatrogenic and noniatrogenic etiologies. In even the mildest circumstances, patients have chronic symptoms that include cough, aspiration, and recurrent bronchopulmonary infections. In severe cases, they may be in a clinical state of rapid and precipitous decline. Multiple approaches to treatment have been described in the literature and range from endoscopic stenting to surgical resection and reconstruction. Regardless of the underlying etiology, or chosen surgical approach, optimal management depends on early diagnosis and definitive repair. In cases in which definitive repair must be delayed, initial intervention should focus on fistula control and patient stabilization.

BENIGN ESOPHAGEAL RESPIRATORY FISTULAS

Benign acquired esophageal respiratory fistulas arise from both iatrogenic and noniatrogenic causes. The most common iatrogenic cause is tracheoesophageal fistula (TEF) formation in the setting of prolonged mechanical ventilation. This well-described clinical entity results from tissue pressure necrosis from the endotracheal tube cuff. The risk of fistula formation is increased when a concomitant nasogastric tube is present, presumably from opposing pressure exerted on the esophageal wall. Patients prone to poor tissue healing (e.g., with diabetes or on high-dose steroid therapy) are particularly susceptible to this complication. High-volume, low-pressure endotracheal tube cuffs have mitigated, although not eliminated, these fistulas. Other patients at risk for iatrogenic fistulas are those who sustain injury to the airway or esophagus, including those undergoing esophageal dilation; surgery of the esophagus, airway, or cervical spine; and chronic stent placement.

Noniatrogenic causes are many and may affect any part of the esophagus and airway. Common etiologies include perforation of esophageal diverticula and mediastinal inflammatory processes, such as infectious and granulomatous disease. Fistula formation may also occur as a complication of caustic ingestion, foreign bodies, and trauma. Rare cases of fistula formation in patients with underlying immunodeficiency and esophageal Crohn's disease are also reported in the literature.

Timely diagnosis of benign esophageal respiratory tract fistulas requires a high index of suspicion. The cardinal symptoms of chronic cough, aspiration, and recurrent respiratory infection are nonspecific, and although fistulas are considered in the differential diagnosis in the setting of known esophageal or respiratory malignancy, benign fistulas are rarely considered as the underlying etiology in patients without neoplasm. As a result, many of these patients present after years of persistent symptoms that have been misdiagnosed as adult onset asthma or recurrent community-acquired pneumonia.

In patients on mechanical ventilation, signs of TEF include inability to achieve adequate tidal volumes, a persistently dilated stomach, or an unusually high level of air escaping from either a nasogastric or gastrostomy tube. In severe cases, patients may experience respiratory failure and sepsis that is refractory to standard therapy.

When suspicion for an underlying fistula is high, diagnosis is best achieved with barium swallow. Although this study requires patient cooperation, and thus precludes use in patients on ventilation, it remains the most highly sensitive diagnostic test. Bronchoscopy and esophagoscopy should always accompany a contrast study for direct visualization and characterization of the fistula in preparation for operative intervention.

TREATMENT OF BENIGN FISTULAS

Successful repair depends on appropriate timing and preoperative planning. Historically, a multistep procedure was used for surgical repair; however, Grillo pioneered a one-step procedure that showed no difference in recurrence rates with simultaneous elimination of the morbidity of esophageal diversion. Patients on mechanical ventilation represent a significant challenge in that their rate of fistula recurrence is often higher after surgical repair. This is primarily the result of positive pressure on the airway suture line. Although it is not an absolute contraindication, repair in these patients should ideally be delayed until successful weaning from the ventilator has been accomplished.

Repair of Benign Tracheoesophageal Fistula

A variety of techniques have been described to surgically repair TEF. These include direct closure of the tracheal and esophageal defects (Figure 1), segmental tracheal resection and primary anastomosis with direct esophageal closure, tracheal closure with an esophageal patch, and as previously mentioned, a two-stage approach with esophageal diversion and primary closure of the tracheal defect. Regardless of the approach used, repair must take into account any underlying tracheal stenosis or tracheomalacia. If a stoma is present, the decision to include it in the repair depends on the distance between the stoma and the fistula. In the case of TEF resulting from prolonged endotracheal intubation, the surgeon must understand

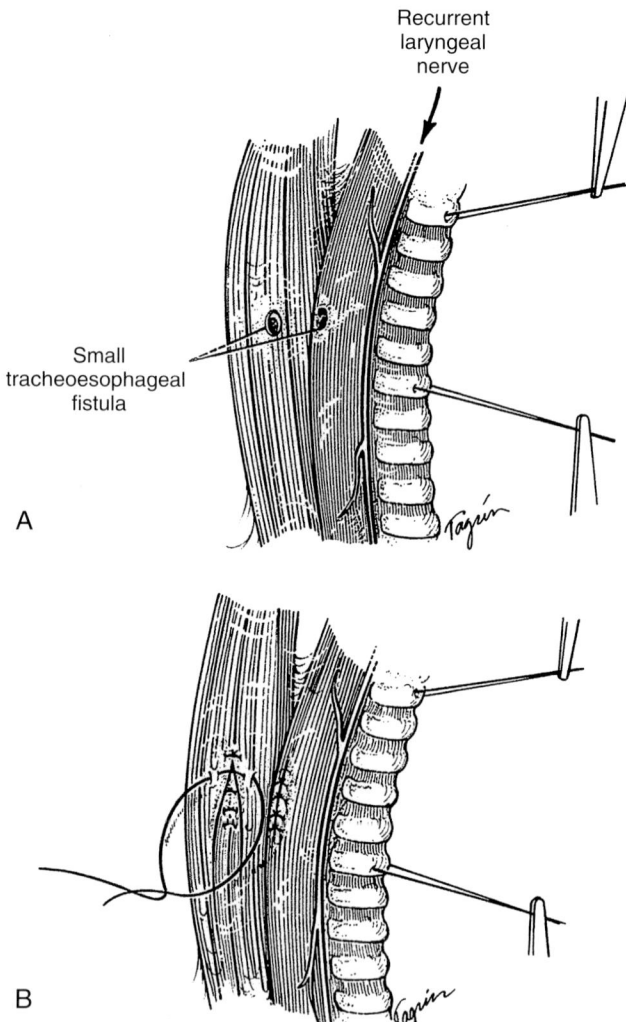

FIGURE 1   Small tracheoesophageal fistulas can be managed with division of the fistula and direct repair of the trachea and esophagus. **A,** The fistula is approached laterally, and the recurrent nerve is elevated with the trachea. **B,** The esophagus is closed in two layers. *(With permission from Mathisen DJ, Grillo HC, Wain JC, et al: Management of acquired nonmalignant tracheoesophageal fistula, Ann Thorac Surg 52:759, 1991.)*

that there is often circumferential tracheal necrosis from the cuff that is best addressed with concomitant tracheal resection and reconstruction. Toward this end, Grillo's anterior cervical approach allows for adequate survey of the tracheal defect and is ideal if resection and reconstruction become necessary. Furthermore, transection of the trachea regardless of whether resection is planned facilitates assessment and repair of the esophageal defect. If no tracheal tissue is resected, the ends of the trachea can simply be primarily reanastomosed after esophageal repair.

The operation begins with the patient placed supine with the neck extended. A low cervical collar incision should incorporate any stoma and provides excellent exposure for proximal fistulas (Figure 2). If the fistula lies lower, a partial sternotomy improves exposures. Subplatysmal flaps are then raised, strap muscles are separated, and the thyroid isthmus is ligated and divided. The boundaries of the involved tracheal segment are confirmed with introduction of a 25-gauge needle through the anterior trachea with direct bronchoscopic vision. Circumferential tracheal dissection is then carried out in the area of anticipated transection, typically at the distal boundary of the fistula orifice. Direct dissection on the trachea minimizes nerve palsy.

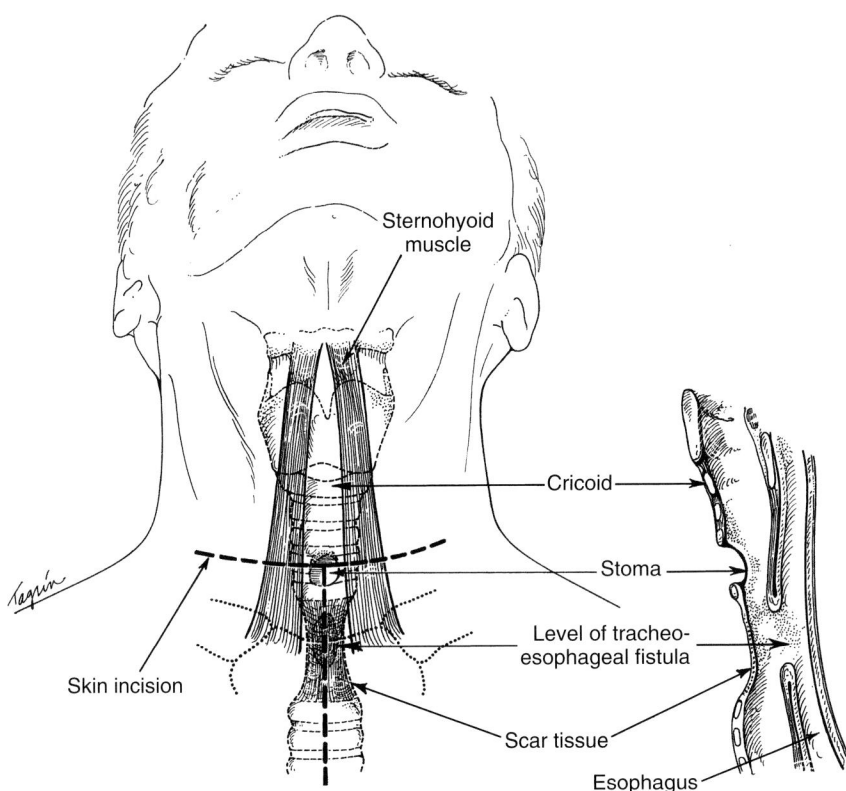

FIGURE 2 Exposure for most tracheoesophageal fistulas is through a low cervical collar incision. Splitting the manubrium might facilitate distal tracheal exposure. *(With permission from Mathisen DJ, Grillo HC, Wain JC, et al: Management of acquired nonmalignant tracheoesophageal fistula, Ann Thorac Surg 52:759, 1991.)*

When dissection is complete, the trachea is divided (Figure 3). Cross-field ventilation is then achieved with intubation of the distal trachea. The orotracheal tube is pulled back, and a plane is developed between the esophagus and the membranous trachea. Once the esophageal defect is visualized, the mucosal edges are freshened and a two-layer longitudinal repair is carried out over a nasogastric tube. The inner layer is closed with inverting, interrupted 4-0 silk sutures through the full thickness of the mucosa. The knots should lie within the esophageal lumen. The outer layer consists of interrupted 4-0 silk sutures to reapproximate the esophageal muscle over the mucosal closure. A muscle flap, most often the sternohyoid, is used to cover the esophageal suture line to reduce the rate of fistula recurrence (Figure 4).

Next, attention is turned to the trachea. If circumferential tissue necrosis or concomitant tracheal stenosis or tracheomalacia is found, resection with reconstruction should be performed. If this is unnecessary, simple primary reanastomosis is performed. First, stay sutures are placed laterally to secure the proximal and distal trachea. Interrupted 4-0 vicryl sutures are then used to reanastomose the trachea, beginning with the membranous wall posteriorly and moving circumferentially forward (Figure 5). At this point, the endotracheal tube is advanced so that the cuff lies distal to the suture line and the neck is maintained in a flexed position to reduce tension. The stay sutures are tied first followed by the anastomotic sutures. An additional strap muscle flap is used to cover the anterior tracheal suture line. A drain is placed, and the cervical incision is closed in layers over it.

Occasionally, the length of the tracheal defect prohibits resection and reconstruction. In this case, the trachea is still divided to facilitate esophageal repair. No tracheal resection, however, is performed; the tracheal defect is instead closed over a T tube. A pediatric endotracheal tube can be passed through the side arm of the T tube to provide mechanical ventilation.

As mentioned, repair should ideally be delayed until the patient is weaned from mechanical ventilation. However, in some cases, the fistula itself may be responsible for ongoing respiratory failure and ventilator dependence. In these challenging circumstances, control of the fistula is critical to achieve extubation before definitive surgical repair. The patient's current endotracheal tube should be replaced with an extra long cuffed tube that allows the cuff to sit distal to the tracheal defect. This maneuver simultaneously minimizes additional tissue necrosis and excludes the fistula from both positive airway pressure and the lower respiratory tract. A nasogastric tube should be pulled back so that the tip sits just proximal to the esophageal orifice of the fistula to control oropharyngeal secretions. A gastrostomy tube and jejunostomy tube should be placed for drainage of gastric secretions and nutritional support, respectively. In cases in which these measures are insufficient to control the fistula, tracheal or esophageal stents have been described as temporizing methods. Although stents typically deliver unacceptably high rates of recurrence and complications when used as definitive therapy for benign fistulas, recent studies support their use as adjuncts in the particularly challenging scenario of patients on mechanical ventilation. These stents can often be removed later at the time of definitive surgical repair. It should be emphasized, however, that in the case of benign TEF, the esophagus and trachea should typically not be stented simultaneously because the two opposing stents are likely to contact one another, thereby introducing a foreign body into the fistula tract and subsequently impeding healing and closure.

Repair of Benign Bronchoesophageal Fistulas

In the case of lower esophageal airway fistulas, successful operative repair begins with the accurate definition of fistula anatomy. This requires examination with barium swallow, coupled with direct visualization with bronchoscopy and esophagoscopy in the operating room. Bronchoscopy often shows an area of inflammatory change with heaped up granulation tissue at the fistula orifice. Esophagoscopy, in turn, typically reveals a papilla or dimple at the esophageal defect. Literature reviews have shown that the vast majority of noniatrogenic, benign bronchoesophageal fistulas, which usually arise

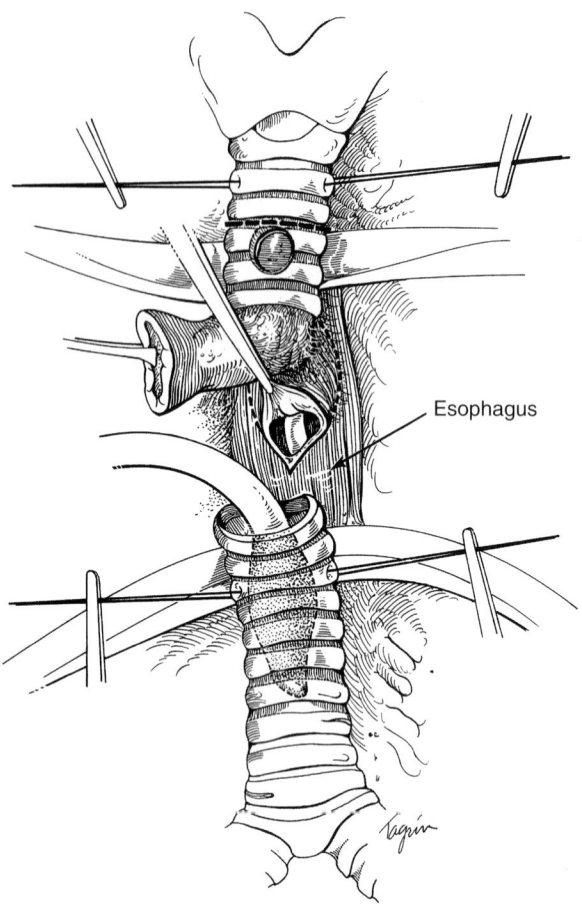

FIGURE 3 Circumferential dissection of the trachea allows the recurrent laryngeal nerves to fall laterally away from the trachea. Transection of the trachea exposes the esophagus. Ventilation is achieved across the operative field with placement of a sterile Tovell tube into the distal trachea. *(With permission from Mathisen DJ, Grillo HC, Wain JC, et al: Management of acquired nonmalignant tracheoesophageal fistula, Ann Thorac Surg 52:759, 1991.)*

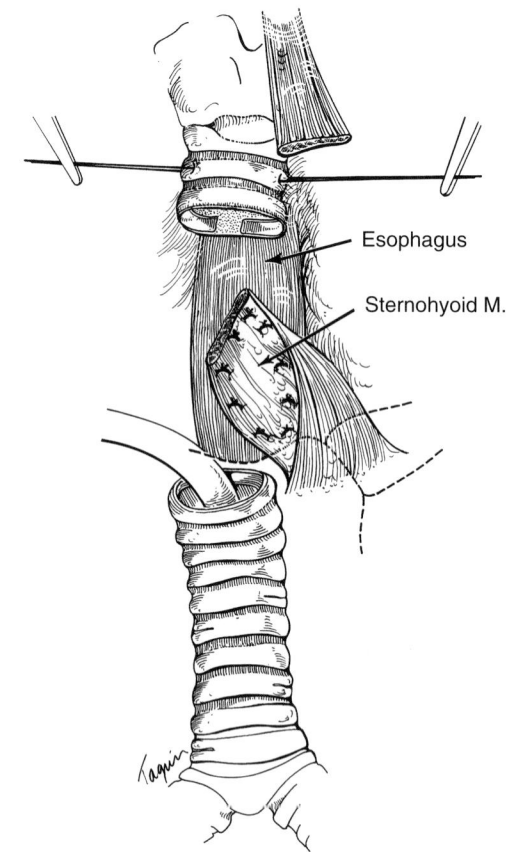

FIGURE 4 A pedicled strap muscle is used to buttress the esophageal repair and separate the esophageal suture line from the tracheal anastomosis. *(With permission from Mathisen DJ, Grillo HC, Wain JC, et al: Management of acquired nonmalignant tracheoesophageal fistula, Ann Thorac Surg 52:759, 1991.)*

from mediastinal granulomatous or infectious processes, involve the right bronchial tree and distal esophagus. The more obtuse angle of the right mainstem bronchus, with its subsequent proximity to inflamed mediastinal nodes and the esophagus, may explain this pattern. Conversely, fistulas that result from intrinsic esophageal disease, or iatrogenic esophageal injury, are more likely to involve the left bronchial tree. These rules are not concrete, however, and fistulas can adopt unusual or tortuous paths.

After fistula characterization, repair begins with a right posterolateral thoracotomy. The fistula is then exposed and divided. Primary repair of the esophagus and bronchus can typically be achieved; however, it is of utmost importance to address any underlying esophageal or airway disease with resection if indicated. A pedicled tissue flap consisting of intercostal muscle, omentum, pericardial fat, or thickened pleura should be interposed between the esophageal and airway suture lines to prevent dehiscence and recurrence.

MALIGNANT ESOPHAGEAL RESPIRATORY TRACT FISTULA

The most common cause of malignant esophageal airway fistulas is esophageal malignancy, closely followed by lung cancer, although other intrathoracic neoplasia may result in the development of fistulas. By definition, fistula formation implies metastatic disease, and

therefore, prognosis is exceedingly poor. As opposed to the case of benign disease, malignant fistula treatment focuses on palliation rather than cure. Historically, esophageal diversion or exclusion was the mainstay of treatment; however, the modern cornerstone of management is endoscopic stent placement. Use of stents to definitively manage benign fistulas is typically discouraged because of high rates of recurrence and complications related to stent migration. As previously mentioned, the exception is in the case of patients on mechanical ventilation with failed traditional techniques of fistula control. Stent use in the setting of malignant fistulas, however, relieves obstruction and becomes fixed in the malignant stricture that is often present to seal the fistula and prevent stent migration.

Esophageal Stents

Esophageal stents have evolved significantly from early models that consisted of rigid plastic to self-expanding metal stents (SEMS), to covered SEMS, and most recently, to hybrid self-expanding plastic stents. Each model has distinct advantages and shortcomings. Rigid plastic stents required significant dilation and often led to subsequent complications. SEMS have largely replaced plastic precursors; however, they are associated with significant tumor ingrowth and a subsequent decreased rate of retrievability. A newer generation of covered SEMS has higher retrieval rates but is also associated with an increased incidence of stent migration. Other complications reported in the literature include hemorrhage, obstruction, and perforation, with the complication rate rising with increasing stent dwell

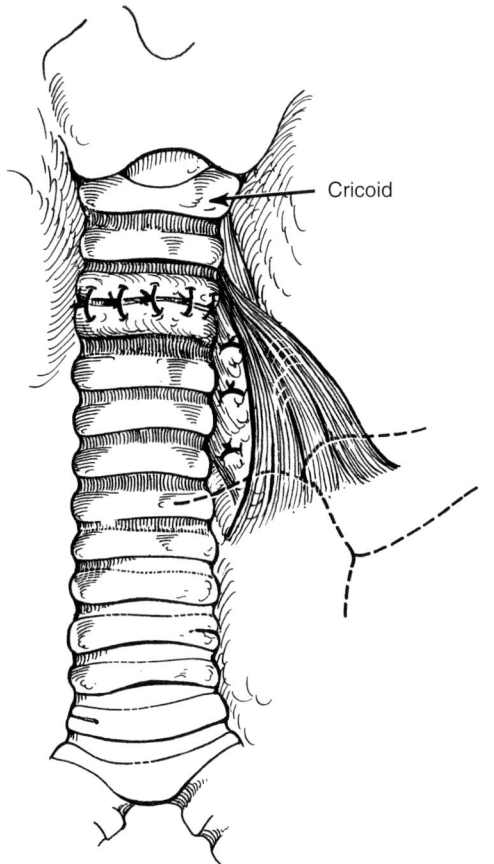

FIGURE 5 Tracheal anastomosis is performed with interrupted fine absorbable sutures (4-0 polyglactin). Four later traction sutures (2-0 polyglactin) are not shown. *(With permission from Mathisen DJ, Grillo HC, Wain JC, et al: Management of acquired nonmalignant tracheoesophageal fistula,* Ann Thorac Surg *52:759, 1991.)*

time. Each manufacturer provides a variety of stents with different lengths, diameters, and expansile forces that can be tailored to the clinical situation.

Although esophageal stent deployment can be performed with monitored anesthesia care, general anesthesia with endotracheal intubation ensures patient comfort and optimizes safety. The first step is to perform esophagoscopy to define the extent of esophageal involvement, locate the fistula orifice, and mark the boundaries of the associated malignant stricture. This is typically done in combination with fluoroscopy, whereby external clips are placed on the thorax to coincide with the proximal and distal ends of the stricture. Because many patients have underlying dysphagia, some degree of concurrent stricture dilation is also performed. In doing this, the surgeon should be cautious against overdilation of the stricture, which can decrease the possibility of achieving an adequate seal and increase the stent

migration rate. After dilation, a guidewire is passed across the stricture and a stent expected to overlap the ends of the stricture by 1 to 2 cm is selected. The stent is then deployed into position with fluoroscopy using the external thoracic clips as markers. After recovery from anesthesia, barium swallow confirms sealing of the fistula tract before initiation of oral intake.

Airway Stents

Comparable to their esophageal counterparts, fistulas that arise from primary lung or respiratory tract neoplasms often require stenting for fistula occlusion. These fistulas, however, are optimally addressed by stenting of the airway rather than the esophagus because an obstructing airway stricture is likely. Concomitant esophageal stenting is occasionally required to ensure complete fistula occlusion.

A variety of airway stents that are similar to esophageal stents can be tailored to each clinical situation, and methods of deployment are analogous. Stent placement begins with evaluation of the airway and fistula orifice with bronchoscopy. Any necessary dilation is performed, and the stent is slowly deployed with direct bronchoscopic visualization. A baseline postoperative chest x-ray is useful to document stent position and to assess lung volumes. Barium swallow should confirm successful exclusion of the airway from the fistula tract.

SUMMARY

Acquired esophageal respiratory tract fistulas represent an uncommon and challenging clinical scenario. The presentation and pathophysiology of this disease entity is variable; however, treatment is based on fundamental principles: defining fistula anatomy, early intervention when feasible, and concomitantly addressing any underlying esophageal or airway pathology at the time of surgery. In patients who are ventilator dependent, initial interventions should focus on controlling the fistula and its consequent morbidity to facilitate extubation before definitive surgery. Although benign fistulas are primarily treated with operative repair, endoscopic stenting has become the palliative treatment of choice for fistulas that arise in the setting of neoplastic processes.

SUGGESTED READINGS

Eleftheriadis E, Kotzampassi K: Temporary stenting of acquired benign tracheoesophageal fistulas in critically ill ventilated patients, *Surg Endosc* 19:811–815, 2005.

Mangi A, Gaissert H, Wright C, et al: Benign-broncho-esophageal fistula in the adult, *Ann Thorac Surg* 73:911–915, 2002.

Mathisen D, Grillo H, Wain J, et al: Management of acquired nonmalignant tracheoesophageal fistula, *Ann Thorac Surg* 52:759–765, 1991.

Pennathur A, Chang A, McGrath K, et al: Polyflex expandable stents in the treatment of esophageal disease: initial experience, *Ann Thorac Surg* 85:1968–1973, 2008.

Shen K, Allen M, Cassivi S, et al: Surgical management of acquired nonmalignant tracheoesophageal and bronchoesophageal fistulae, *Ann Thorac Surg* 90:914–919, 2010.

REPAIR OF PECTUS EXCAVATUM

Kimberly M. Lumpkins, MD,
Paul Colombani, MD, MBA, FACS, FAAP, and
Fizan Abdullah, MD, PhD

Pectus excavatum (PE), historically known as funnel chest, is the most common chest wall deformity. It occurs in approximately 1 in 500 live births, with a male predominance of 2:1 to 9:1 in various series. The sternum is depressed towards the vertebral column with the greatest depression typically at the level of the xiphoid process. The implications of PE may range from cosmetic deformity with psychologic distress to significant cardiopulmonary impairment from decreased thoracic cavity capacity and compression of the heart. Although the exact etiology of PE is unclear, the condition is believed to result from abnormal development of the costal cartilages. Overgrowth of the costal cartilages, especially cartilages 4 through 7, leads to progressive dorsal displacement of the sternum. PE is associated with connective tissue disorders such as Marfan disease. PE often runs in families, but no specific genetic etiology has been identified.

EVALUATION OF THE PATIENT WITH PECTUS EXCAVATUM

Initial evaluation of the patient with PE requires a careful history and physical examination. One third of patients with PE have a defect evident from early childhood, and the remainder first appreciates the problem during the adolescent growth spurt. A history of worsening deformity around this time is often elicited. Symptoms at rest are rare, but the patient may report impaired exercise tolerance with shortness of breath. On physical examination, the chest should be examined for symmetry and location of the deepest point of the pectus. Asymmetry is not uncommon, and the defect is often slightly skewed to the right side. Patients with PE have a typical kyphotic posture with a protuberant abdomen. Calipers can be used to measure the chest diameter at both the deepest point of the deformity and the lateral chest wall to get an approximate indication of the severity of the pectus. Stigmata of collagen vascular disease, such as long fingers and toes, myopia, and easy bruising, may be observed. Patients who have clinical stigmata of Marfan disease but do not carry this diagnosis may benefit from referral for diagnostic evaluation.

Further diagnostic examination including chest computed tomographic (CT) scan, pulmonary function tests, and transthoracic echocardiogram is indicated to assess the degree of cardiopulmonary impairment caused by the PE. A chest CT scan without intravenous contrast allows the calculation of the Haller index, a quantification of the severity of the PE defect. For determination of the Haller index, the anteroposterior (AP) diameter of the chest is measured from the inner ribcage to the spine at the greatest point of the defect. The transverse diameter of the chest is measured from the inside of the ribs at the same location. The index is the ratio of the transverse to the AP diameters of the chest. PE repair is generally recommended at a Haller index of 3.5 or greater. An exercise pulmonary function test (PFT) is performed for assessment of lung volumes at rest and exercise. Typically, a mild to moderate restrictive defect is seen in these patients. Finally, an echocardiogram may show right ventricular

compression or mitral valve prolapse. A subset of patients with PE with narrow chests exists for whom the Haller index fails; an improved corrective index has been developed to help grade the severity of their disease.

The extent of cardiopulmonary involvement in PE remains a subject of debate. Increasing Haller index has been associated with worse impairments in pulmonary function, but many patients with PE have spirometry values within the normal range. Many patients report subjective improvement in exercise tolerance after repair despite having normal PFT values both before and after surgery. In many cases, insurance requires documentation of objective measures of cardiopulmonary impairment or significant PE-related symptoms before authorization of repair. The operation is otherwise considered cosmetic in nature and is not covered.

OPEN REPAIR

The first widely adopted technique for repair of PE was the Ravitch operation. In this procedure, a midline sternal (in males) or fourth interspace transverse incision (in females) is performed and skin flaps are elevated to expose the sternum and the costal cartilages. The abnormal costal cartilages are resected in the subperichondrial plane. An anterior sternal osteotomy is performed to flatten the sternum. A metal strut is often placed retrosternally to provide more secure fixation. Historically, the Ravitch procedure was performed as early as age 4 years. However, a very small but significant subset of patients who underwent repair at such an early age subsequently had acquired Jeune's syndrome (asphyxiating thoracic dystrophy) develop as they progressed through puberty. These patients' thoracic cavities failed to expand with growth, presumably as a result of abnormal fixation of the growth plates in the costochondral joints. Correction of acquired Jeune's syndrome is complex and often unsatisfying. Most authors recommend delay of open PE repair until puberty to avoid this complication (Figure 1).

MINIMALLY INVASIVE PECTUS EXCAVATUM REPAIR (NUSS PROCEDURE)

In 1997, Nuss introduced a minimally invasive approach to PE repair. This approach relies on the natural flexibility of the costal cartilages to enable repair from the inside of the chest. Advantages include a shorter operative time and less disfiguring scar. The patient is placed supine with arms extended. The site of deepest depression of the sternum is identified and traced laterally. Incisions of 4 cm in length are made bilaterally along this line at its intersection with the anterior axillary line and are deepened until the pleura are entered with direct vision. In the original description, an introducer is then passed with thoracoscopic guidance from the left chest just retrosternally into the right chest. The thoracoscope is transferred to the right chest to observe passage of the introducer. Remaining strictly in the immediate retrosternal plane and using thoracoscopic guidance minimizes the chance of cardiac perforation or other mediastinal injury. However, in the authors' practice, thoracoscopy is no longer used during passage of the introducer. With use of slightly medial incisions, the pericardium is seen and bar passed without difficulty. In difficult cases, sternal elevation can be used to facilitate transmediastinal passage of the introducer. An umbilical tape is tied to the introducer as the tip exits the right-sided skin incision. The introducer is then withdrawn back through the left chest so that the umbilical tape traces its transthoracic passage. A pectus bar is selected based on the patient's body habitus. Ideally the bar should extend just beyond the edge of the rib cage on each side without protruding

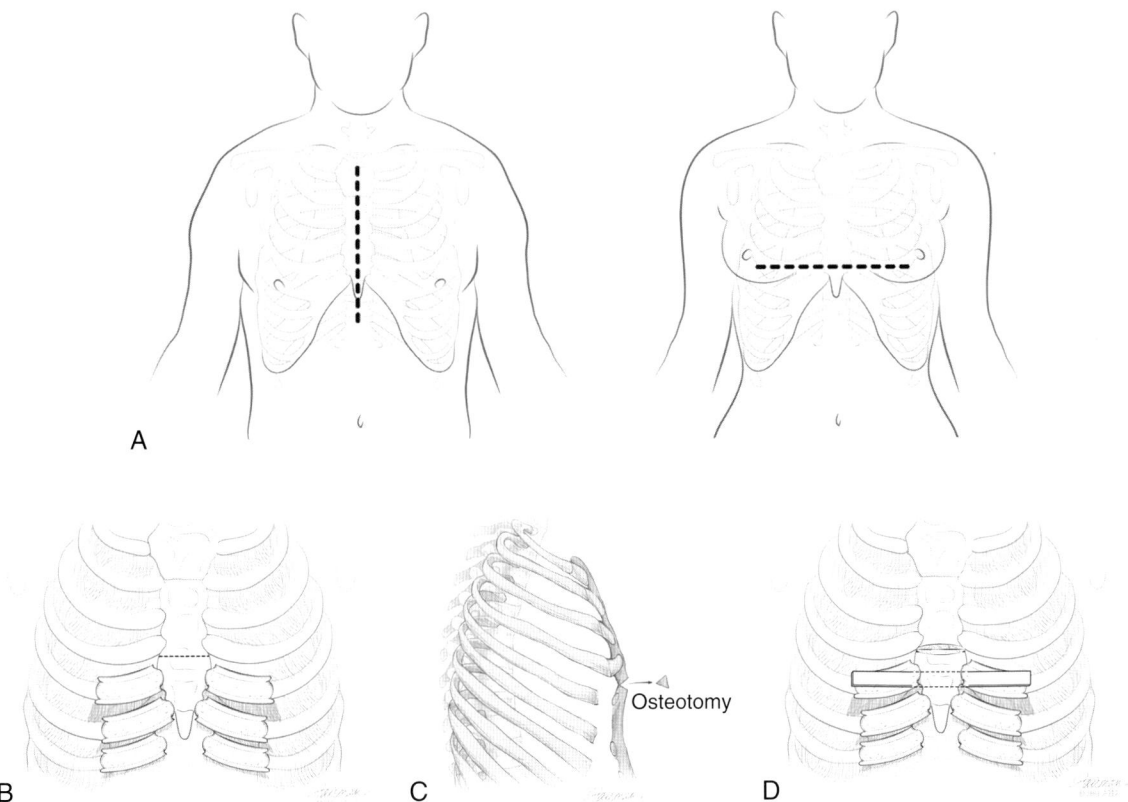

FIGURE 1   Open repair of pectus excavatum. **A,** *Left,* midline incision; *right,* submammary incision for cosmetic use in females. **B,** The costal cartilages are freed circumferentially from the perichondrium and divided at the junctions with the sternum and with the ribs. **C,** The sternal osteotomy allows the sternum to rise to a level position. **D,** Rehbein strut in place behind sternum. *(John Hopkins University Illustrations courtesy of Jennifer E. Fairman, CMI, FAMI.)*

too far beyond the ribcage, typically 2.5 cm shorter than the distance between the midaxillary lines. The exact degree of bend that must be applied to each side of the bar is a matter of judgment, but the goal is to slightly overcorrect the sternum rather than undercorrect it. The umbilical tape is tied to one end of the bar and is then withdrawn through the chest with the bar upside down (concave side up). After the bar is grasped exiting the right chest, it is flipped 180 degrees so that the convex side is elevating the sternum. Bar stabilizers are placed over the ribs on both sides to secure the bar above the ribcage. Wire or heavy polydioxanone (PDS) suture fixation of the stabilizers around the ribs is used bilaterally to avoid bar displacement. Patients with complex asymmetric defects, patients with Marfan's disease, and patients with suboptimal elevation of the sternum after placement of a single bar may benefit from placement of a second bar to improve sternal elevation. Placement of a second bar follows the principles of placement of the initial bar. A chest x-ray is obtained routinely in the recovery room. Small bilateral pneumothoraces are commonly observed as a result of air introduced during bar placement and in general may be managed expectantly without further imaging as long as the patient is clinically well (Figure 2).

Preoperative counseling is essential before repair. Postoperative pain can be considerable during the first few postoperative weeks, and some patients continue to experience pain for the entire period while the bar is in place. In severe cases, this can require removal of the bar with likely recurrence of the PE defect. Postoperative use of ketorolac and gabapentin can limit the use of narcotic analgesics. In general, the authors limit physical activity for the first 6 weeks after bar placement. After this point, there are no specific activity restrictions.

The ideal age for minimally invasive PE repair continues to be debated. A shift has been seen over the years towards repair at an older age, especially late adolescence into early adulthood. The authors typically perform the repair at 14 years of age. Recent reports suggest that patients over 30 years of age are more likely to require placement of two bars.

The correct length of time for the bar to remain in place remains debated. At least 2 years is recommended to allow adequate time for the costal cartilages to remodel in their new position. The authors have had rare immediate recurrences with bar removal at 2 years that have led them to favor leaving the bar in position for 3 years. At this point, the bar may be removed as an outpatient procedure. With general anesthetic, the previous incisions are reopened and the wires and stabilizers are exposed. The wires are cut and removed, followed by the stabilizers. The bends at either end of the bar are removed, and the bar can then be pulled out one side of the chest. The deep layers of the incision are closed with 2-0 vicryl suture and tied while a Valsalva's maneuver is performed to evacuate any introduced air. After routine subcuticular skin closure, the patient is returned to the recovery room. A postoperative chest x-ray is obtained. Small bilateral pneumothoraces may be seen and do not require intervention in the absence of clinical symptoms. The patient is discharged home with narcotic analgesia after a suitable observation period in recovery.

COMPLICATIONS OF MINIMALLY INVASIVE REPAIR

Although asymptomatic pneumothorax is commonly observed after PE repair, symptomatic pneumothorax may rarely result from inadvertent injury to lung parenchyma during bar placement. Enlarging

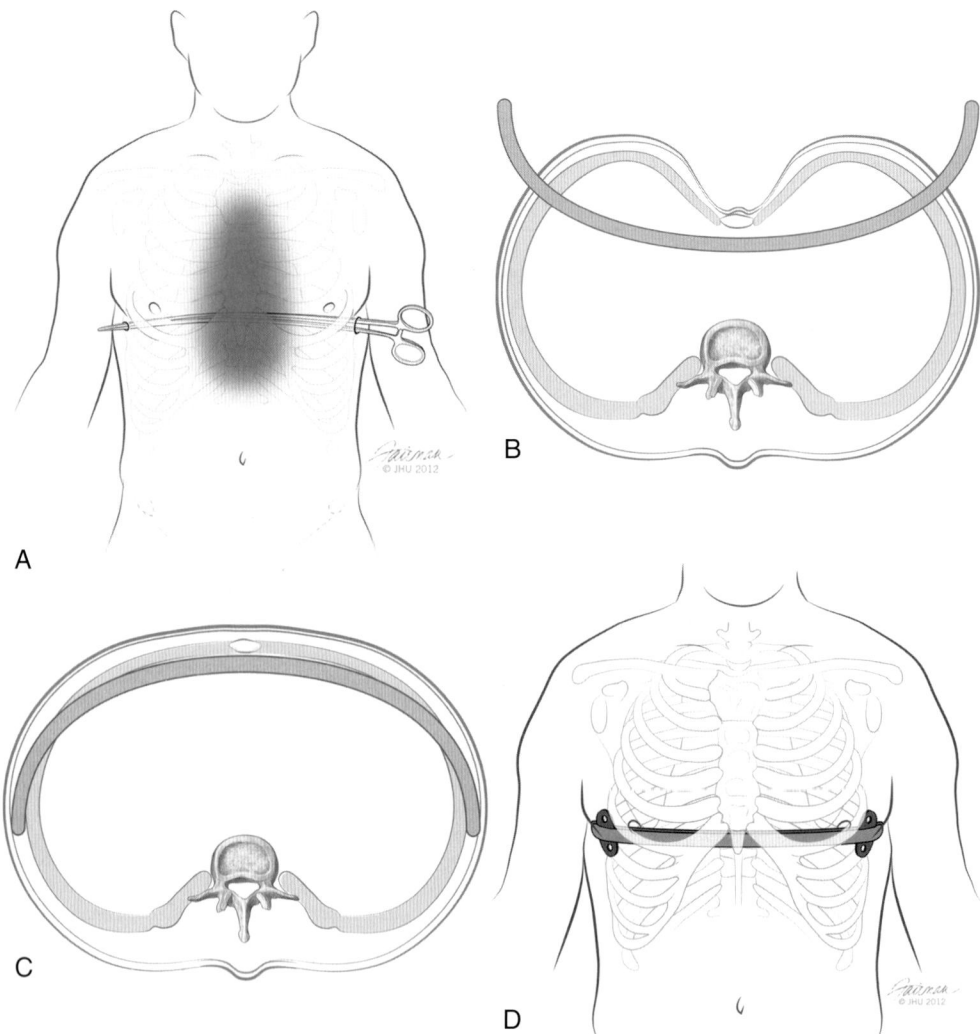

FIGURE 2 Minimally invasive pectus excavatum repair. **A,** Schematic of long clamp passing posterior to the sternum through bilateral intercostal incisions. **B,** Initial orientation of bar after passage through chest. **C,** Position of bar after flipping. **D,** Bar stabilizers in position. (John Hopkins University, Illustrations courtesy of Jennifer E. Fairman, CMI, FAMI.)

pneumothorax in the setting of clinical deterioration requires placement of chest tubes, often bilaterally. Urinary retention is frequently noted after surgery at a rate that exceeds that seen with other operations. The cause of this finding is uncertain, but this generally resolves within several days.

Intraoperative cardiac perforation is the most dreaded complication of minimally invasive repair. Although this is exceptionally rare, it is highly lethal. Immediate median sternotomy and cardiac repair are indicated in this setting.

Displacement of the bar can occur in as many as 5% of patients, often leading to immediate recurrence. Reoperation is required to flip the bar back into the appropriate position and resecure the bar to the rib cage. Additional wires may be necessary to adequately secure the bar in position. Wound infection is rare, occurring in less than 2% of patients, and can often be treated with antibiotics. Surgical drainage is sometimes necessary for more extensive infections.

Most pectus bars are composed of stainless steel, although titanium bars are available by special order. Unsuspected allergy to nickel may lead to localized skin reaction at the incisions or pericarditis. Symptoms may not occur for many months after placement, and these patients can often be treated medically with corticosteroids until it is time to remove the bar. Metal salt patch testing can be used before surgery to identify patients with allergies. A titanium bar is used in these individuals; however, it cannot be bent to shape as with a stainless steel bar. It must be molded to the correct shape by the manufacturer with guidance from the preoperative CT scan.

OUTCOME OF PECTUS EXCAVATUM REPAIR

Neither open nor minimally invasive repair of PE has been shown to be clearly superior in the repair of PE. Both have a higher than 94% success rate in improving psychologic perceptions and subjective assessment of exercise tolerance. No difference is seen in length of stay, although the rate of pneumothorax and reoperation is higher in the minimally invasive repair. Since its introduction, the minimally invasive repair has far surpassed the open repair in popularity and is used for the majority of PE repairs. However, the open repair may still be preferable in patients with severely asymmetric defects and in patients with mixed carinatum/excavatum phenotype. Failures of open repair have been successfully corrected with the minimally invasive approach, as have previous failures of minimally invasive repairs.

Suggested Readings

Croitoru DP, Kelly RE, Goretsky MJ, et al: The minimally invasive Nuss technique for recurrent or failed pectus excavatum repair in 50 patients, *J Pediatr Surg* 40:181–187, 2005.

Frantz F: Indications and guidelines for pectus excavatum repair, *Curr Opin Pediatr* 23:486–491, 2011.

Kelly RE, Goretsky MJ, Obermeyer R, et al: Twenty-one years of experience with minimally invasive pectus excavatum by the Nuss procedure in 1215 patients, *Ann Surg* 252:1072–1082, 2010.

Lawson ML, Mellins RB, Paulson JF, et al: Increasing severity of pectus excavatum is associated with reduced pulmonary function, *J Pediatr* 159:256–261, 2011.

Papandria DJ, Arlikar J, Sacco Casamassima MG, et al: Increasing age at time of pectus excavatum repair of children: emerging consensus? *J Pediatr Surg.* 48:191–196, 2013.

St Peter SD, Juang D, Garey CL, et al: A novel measure for pectus excavatum: the correction index, *J Pediatr Surg* 46:2270–2273, 2011.

VASCULAR SURGERY

OPEN REPAIR OF ABDOMINAL AORTIC ANEURYSMS

**Babak J. Orandi, MD, MSc, and
James H. Black III, MD**

OVERVIEW

Abdominal aortic aneurysm (AAA) affects as many as 8% of people over 60 years of age, and AAA rupture accounts for 15,000 deaths annually in the United States. Given that the natural history of AAA is progressive growth and eventual rupture and that the survival of rupture is rather dismal, the clinical aim is to detect AAAs and repair them when the risk of rupture begins to outweigh the risk of repair. The advent of the endovascular era has drastically changed AAA management. Many patients are willing to accept the increased risk of secondary interventions associated with endovascular aneurysm repair (EVAR) because of the minimally invasive nature of EVAR; however, a number of situations exist in which open surgical repair (OSR) is preferred. Unsuitable anatomy, lack of available endovascular capabilities, and uncertainty about long-term endograft durability in young patients are situations in which OSR may be the preferred approach (Box 1).

A number of large studies have characterized the phenotype of the typical patient with AAA. Risk factors include increased age, male gender, family history of AAA, increased height, hypertension, hyperlipidemia, coronary artery disease, peripheral arterial disease, cerebrovascular disease, and smoking history. The factors associated with an increased likelihood of rupture are female gender, increased mean arterial blood pressure, current smoking, diminished forced expiratory volume in 1 second, and aneurysm size.

The vast majority of patients with AAA are asymptomatic, and disease is detected incidentally or with screening. However, patients may present with thromboembolic symptoms, particularly lower extremity digital ischemia. Occasionally, patients report a pulsatile sensation in the chest, abdomen, or back. Large aneurysms can lead to compressive symptoms. Compression of the ureter results in hydronephrosis, and compression of the bowel or stomach leads to obstructive symptoms or early satiety. Although a rare presentation, aortic dissection in the setting of AAA can cause severe abdominal or back pain and mandates expedient repair because of the exceptionally high risk of rupture. AAA rupture presents with severe abdominal or back pain and, if uncontained, hemodynamic instability.

INDICATIONS FOR REPAIR

AAA symptoms typically mandate repair; however, the clinical decision making can be more nuanced in the asymptomatic patient. Because of the inherent risks of aortic interventions, the risk of rupture must exceed the risk of the proposed treatment to be justified. Several large randomized controlled trials have helped to define the aneurysm size at which repair is beneficial for the asymptomatic patient.

The United Kingdom Small Aneurysm Trial (UKSAT) randomized 1090 patients 60 to 76 years old with AAAs between 4.0 and 5.5 cm to either early OSR or surveillance and repair if the AAA grew to exceed 5.5 cm. The early OSR group had a 5.8% 30-day mortality rate with no long-term overall survival benefit. Of note, 76% of the patients in the surveillance group ultimately needed aneurysm repair.

The results of the UKSAT were mirrored in the Aneurysm Detection and Management (ADAM) trial. Five hundred sixty-nine patients within the U.S. Veterans Affairs healthcare system ages 50 to 79 years with aneurysms 4.0 to 5.4 cm in size were randomized to early OSR or surveillance. The investigators had a lower 30-day mortality rate (2.7%) for patients with OSR than that seen in the UKSAT, but patients for early OSR did not obtain benefit compared with the surveillance group. In the surveillance group, nearly 62% of patients eventually underwent AAA repair.

The advent of EVAR, with its associated lower operative mortality rate, has not changed the 5.5-cm threshold. Cao and colleagues recently showed that this size cut point holds true for patients with small aneurysms (4.1 to 5.5 cm) randomized to surveillance versus early EVAR in the Comparison of Surveillance Versus Aortic Endografting for Small Aneurysm Repair (CAESAR) trial. Only 50% of the planned 740 patients were randomized, and the trial was terminated prematurely for low enrollment, although follow-up is ongoing. At 3 years after randomization, no difference was found in mortality between the two groups, although the study may be insufficiently powered because of poor enrollment. Recently, the Positive Impact of Endovascular Options for Treating Aneurysms Early (PIVOTAL) trial randomized 728 patients with 4.0-cm to 5.0-cm AAAs to surveillance or early EVAR. At interim analysis, no difference was found between the two groups in terms of survival at a mean follow-up time of 20 months. A recent Cochrane review of treatment for small AAAs confirmed the findings of these larger studies. Namely, patients with small asymptomatic AAAs who undergo treatment, whether OSR or EVAR, have a higher 30-day mortality rate than those who undergo surveillance, and no difference is seen in overall long-term survival. Of note, nearly all the patients in these trials have been male. Given the lack of study of AAAs in women and that female gender is a risk factor for rupture, a slightly lower threshold for intervention of 5.0 cm is generally accepted.

Briefly, it is appropriate to consider the preferred imaging modalities for surveillance. In general, ultrasound scan (US) is the preferred method for AAA screening and surveillance because it is noninvasive, is relatively inexpensive, and obviates the need for intravenous contrast administration. It is nearly 100% sensitive and specific, although AAA visualization can be limited by bowel gas or truncal obesity. Despite these benefits, computed tomographic (CT) imaging is the mainstay for operative planning (Figure 1). It allows for better delineation of the vascular anatomy, including evaluation of a potential landing zone to determine suitability for EVAR, and the presence of aberrant vessels and renovascular and aortoiliac disease.

PREOPERATIVE PLANNING

Because of the high-risk nature of aortic surgery and the frequent existence of comorbid conditions in this patient population, a thorough preoperative workup with medical optimization is warranted, particularly in terms of cardiovascular risk. For patients with significant coronary artery disease, the definitive trial on the timing of coronary revascularization, if needed, is the Coronary Artery Revascularization Prophylaxis (CARP) trial. In this study, patients at high risk for perioperative cardiac complications who were undergoing major elective vascular surgery were randomized to undergo revascularization or no revascularization before their vascular surgery. Revascularization before vascular surgery did not alter long-term mortality, with close to 20% of patients in either group having development of a myocardial infarction or related cardiac morbidity. Of note, this study's results do not apply to patients with unstable

---

BOX 1: Factors to consider for the patient with an abdominal aortic aneurysm

Indications for Abdominal Aortic Aneurysm Repair
- Greater than 5.5 cm in males, 5.0 cm in females
- Growth more than 0.5 cm/6 months
- Symptomatic

Indications for Open Surgical Repair of Abdominal Aortic Aneurysm
- Hostile neck
- Neck less than 1.5 cm
- Significant angulation of the neck, typically more than 60 degrees
- Suprarenal aneurysm
- Young patient (relative)
- Endovascular capabilities unavailable

---

angina, aortic stenosis, or severe dysfunction of the left ventricle; these patients may benefit from cardiac intervention before AAA repair.

For current smokers, smoking cessation at least 2 weeks before surgery is ideal to prevent respiratory complications such as pneumonia. Patients with chronic obstructive pulmonary disease or other baseline pulmonary disease may benefit from the institution of bronchodilator therapy.

For patients with AAA with baseline renal insufficiency, care must be taken during and after surgery to avoid hypotension. Accordingly, some patients may need preoperative admission for intravenous fluid hydration. In addition, the administration of intravenous contrast in obtaining imaging studies must proceed judiciously to avoid contrast-induced nephropathy.

Preoperative communication with the anesthesia team is critical to ensure that any concerns can be addressed in a timely fashion. Epidural anesthesia in conjunction with general anesthesia ought to be considered for better postoperative pain control and fewer respiratory complications. The possibility of intraoperative and postoperative bleeding mandates the availability of a robust supply of blood products and appropriate vascular access to administer them and arterial blood pressure monitoring. Cell saver is helpful to prevent hemodilution if significant blood loss is to be expected. Maintenance of normothermia throughout the case with the use of warmed fluids and external warming devices reduces coagulopathy.

For patients undergoing AAA surveillance rather than immediate repair, studies have examined the role of beta-blockers, statin therapy, and angiotensin converting enzyme inhibitors in slowing aneurysm growth with mixed results. Because many of these patients are at significant risk of cardiovascular disease, these measures are frequently appropriate regardless of their possible beneficial effects on AAA growth. Studies of antimicrobial therapy with doxycycline or roxithromycin to eradicate *Chlamydophila pneumoniae*, which has been implicated in AAA pathogenesis, have yielded disappointing results to reduce AAA growth rate. The most effective measure to decrease aneurysm growth is smoking cessation for current smokers, as tobacco has been shown to accelerate AAA growth and is an independent risk factor for AAA rupture.

SURGICAL REPAIR

Surgical Approaches

Open surgical repair can be accomplished with a transperitoneal (TP) or left retroperitoneal (RP) incision. The TP approach is generally performed via a generous midline incision (Figure 2), although a transverse incision near the level of the umbilicus is infrequently

---

FIGURE 1 **A,** Extensive mural atheroma at the origin of the right renal artery can be fractured with aortic cross clamping, making an infrarenal cross-clamp location prone to produce renal interaction. **B,** The same patient shows a healthy aortic wall at the level of the celiac artery.

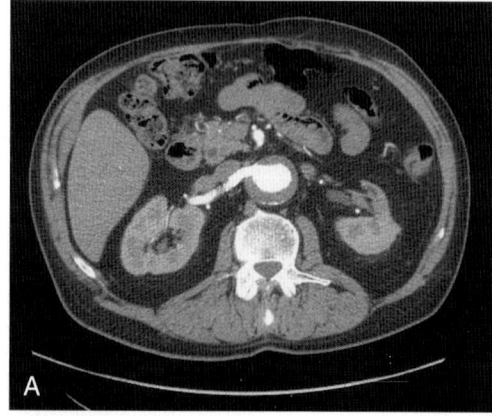
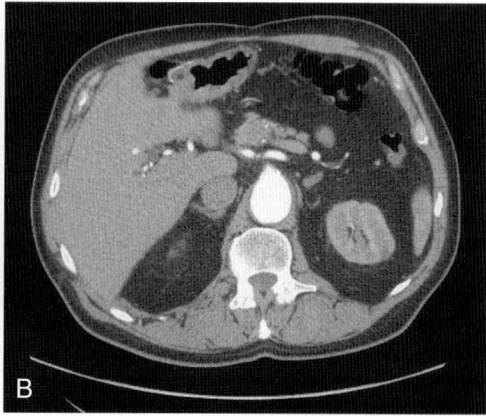

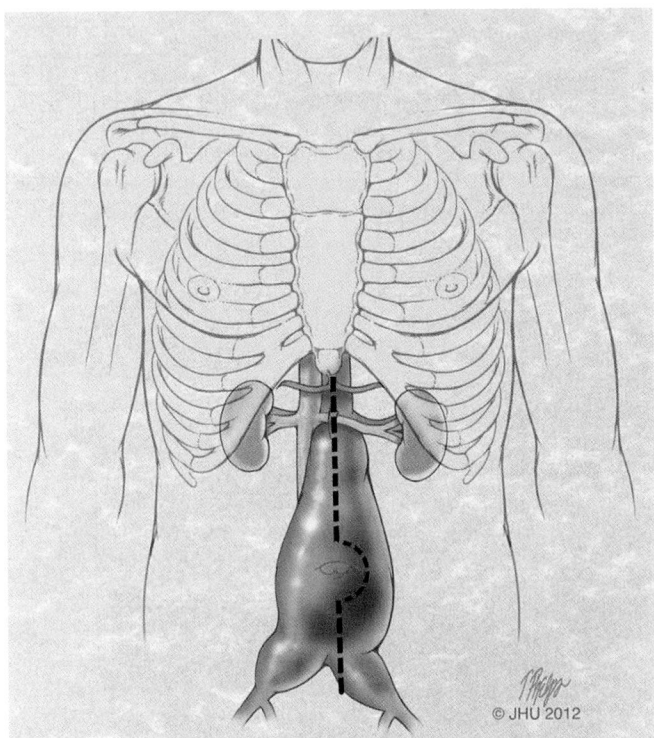

FIGURE 2 The transperitoneal approach provides wide access to the infrarenal aorta and allows inspection of the peritoneal contents.

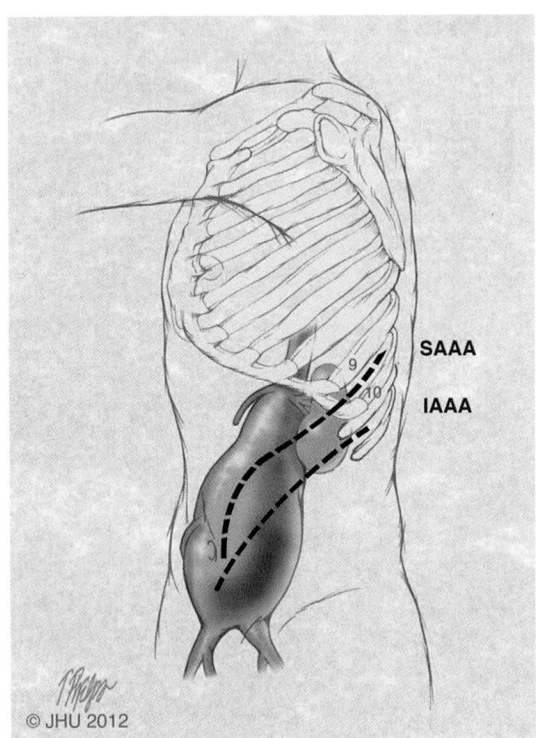

FIGURE 3 Incisions for exposure of infrarenal abdominal aortic aneurysm *(IAAA)* and suprarenal abdominal aortic aneurysm *(SAAA)* via left flank approach.

performed. Advocates of the latter approach claim that there is less postoperative pain and respiratory compromise, although the popularity of this approach has not caught on. The RP incision can be extended through the intercostal space between the ninth and tenth ribs to allow for a thoracoabdominal exposure (Figure 3). Extension of the incision between the 11th and 12th ribs allows for a purely retroperitoneal approach.

The TP approach has the advantages of wide access, the ability to offer full evaluation of the abdomen, and usually fairly rapid performance. In addition, it allows for easier access to the iliac arteries to treat occlusive or aneurysmal disease involving these vessels (Figure 4). These advantages must be tempered with the disadvantages of longer ileus, more insensible fluid losses, and more difficult access to proximal control for juxtarenal and suprarenal AAAs. On the other hand, the RP approach offers the advantages of avoiding a difficult dissection and lysis of adhesions for patients with multiple prior abdominal surgeries or other reasons to have a hostile abdomen, decreased insensible fluid losses, possibly shorter ileus duration than the TP approach, and enhanced access to proximal control of juxtarenal and suprarenal AAAs (Figure 5). Indeed, the latter is perhaps the most compelling reason to perform a RP approach; however, this approach makes access to the iliac and right renal arteries difficult, does not allow for exploration of the abdomen, takes longer to position the patient and gain access to the aorta, and may be associated with more chronic pain, wound problems, and incisional hernias.

Transperitoneal Approach

A longitudinal incision that uses the full length of the abdomen is performed. The colon is retracted in a cephalad direction, and the small bowel is retracted to the right and superiorly. Division of the ligament of Treitz enhances the rightward retraction of the small bowel. Blunt and sharp dissection along the anterior aspect of the aneurysm aids in identifying the left renal vein, which is gently

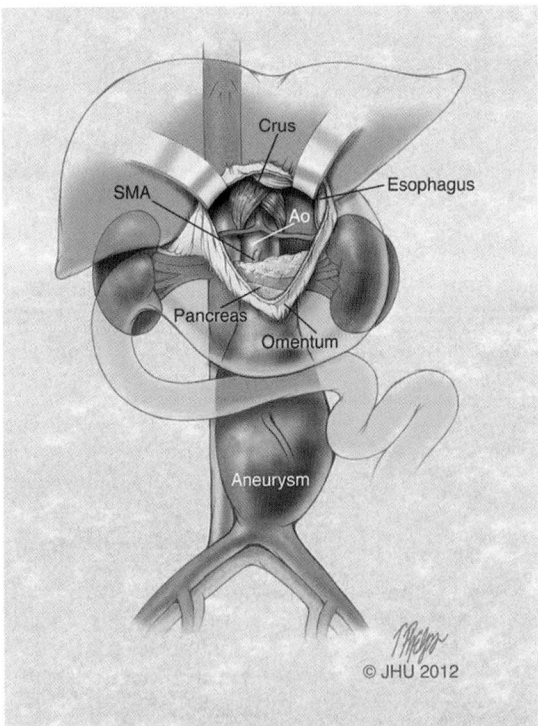

FIGURE 4 In a transperitoneal approach, the suprarenal aorta can be controlled through the gastrohepatic ligament and with division of the crus. This may be helpful in proximal aortic control during contained infrarenal aortic rupture when blood staining and hematoma obliterates the retroperitoneal anatomy. *SMA,* Superior mesenteric artery.

retracted cephalad. If necessary, ligation of the adrenal, gonadal, and lumbar arteries further mobilize the left renal vein. Avoid sacrificing the left renal vein because of the subsequent venous hypertension and increased bleeding and because of the risk of postoperative renal failure. Dissection of the aneurysm neck in anticipation of cross clamping is performed, with extension of the dissection in a caudad direction. Several variations and their indications of the transperitoneal approach are described in Table 1.

Retroperitoneal Approach

With the patient in the right lateral decubitus position, an incision is made at the level of the 11th rib from the posterior axillary line to the lateral rectus abdominis muscle. The retroperitoneum is entered laterally, and the peritoneal sac and posterior Gerota's fascia are retracted anteromedially to further open the retroperitoneal space and expose the aorta (Figure 6). If greater cephalad exposure is

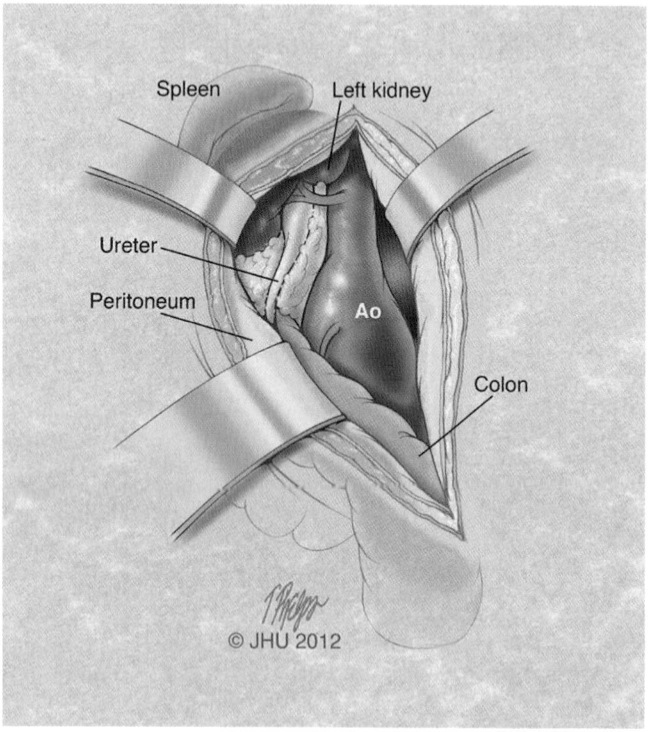

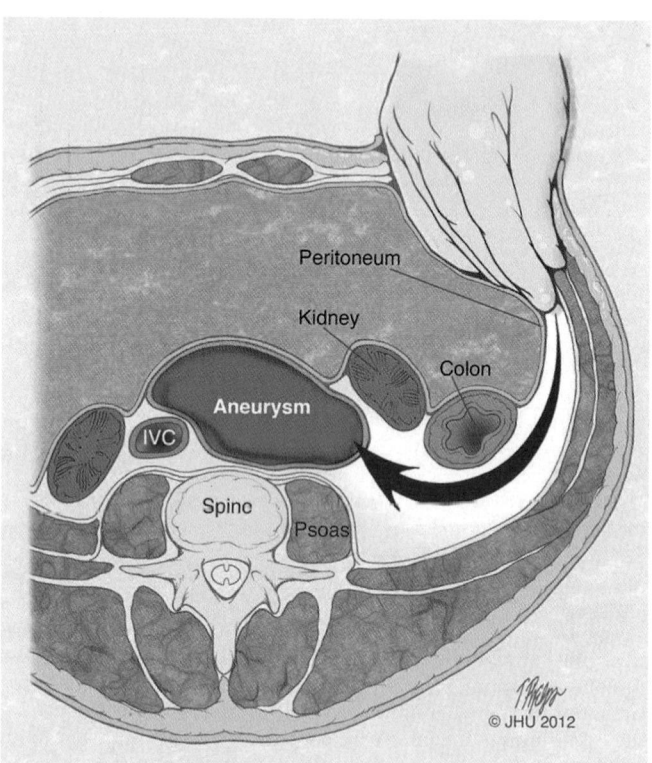

FIGURE 5 The abdominal aorta (Ao) is easily controlled in the retroperitoneal approach. The left kidney can be reflected anterior and the left lateral crus opened to expose the suprarenal region.

FIGURE 6 The plane of entry into the retroperitonal space is easily developed with manual blunt dissection behind the left kidney. *IVC,* Inferior vena cava.

TABLE I: Transperitoneal approach variations

	Indications	Steps
Transperitoneal approach with supraceliac clamping	Rupture Juxtarenal AAA Heavy atherosclerotic disease in neck of the aorta precluding infrarenal/suprarenal clamping	Extend incision superiorly, with lower sternal split if needed Retract left hemiliver Divide gastrohepatic ligament Mobilize esophagus to the left Divide the right crus of the diaphragm
Transperitoneal approach with right medial visceral rotation	Juxtarenal AAA Concomitant right renal artery bypass or transaortic renal endarterectomy	Divide the hepatic flexure Mobilize the right colon by dividing the peritoneal reflection Retract right-sided viscera medially and superiorly Superior mesenteric artery is perpendicular to the aorta Divide the posterior crus of the diaphragm
Transperitoneal approach with left medial visceral rotation	Need for continuous exposure of the abdominal aorta and retroperitoneal approach is contraindicated	Divide the splenorenal and phrenocolic ligaments Mobilize the left colon by dividing the peritoneal reflection Left-sided viscera, with or without the kidney, are mobilized toward the right

AAA, Abdominal aortic aneurysm.

needed for suprarenal pathology, division of the median arcuate ligament and the crural fibers of the left hemidiaphragm can be performed.

Operative Conduct

Once the continuously diseased segment of the aorta is exposed and just before cross clamping, the patient undergoes systemic anticoagulation with intravenous heparin, except in the case of AAA rupture. Minimally diseased segments of the aorta are identified proximal and distal to the aneurysm as clamp sites using the knowledge of the preoperative CT scan, and the visceral and iliac vessels are clamped before clamping of the nonaneurysmal proximal aorta to prevent atheromatous embolization. After the clamps have been placed, the aneurysm sac is opened via a longitudinal arteriotomy. Mural thrombus is carefully removed, and lumbar vessel back bleeding is controlled with suture ligatures. At this point, the interior of the AAA should be inspected for delineation of healthier aortic wall for suture placement. Oftentimes the less diseased pararenal and suprarenal intimal surface is apparent as uninvolved by the mural thrombus burden (Figure 7).

The aortic reconstruction proceeds with a graft, typically composed of Dacron or polytetrafluoroethylene, which may be bifurcated in the event that aneurysmal disease extends to the iliac or femoral vessels. The graft is sized to fit the defect, and in the case of a bifurcated graft, care is taken to keep the main body of the graft short to prevent limb kinking and subsequent outflow obstruction. The proximal anastomosis is then performed with a double-armed 3-0 nonabsorbable continuous suture. In the situation of a suprarenal AAA, the aortotomy should be taken posterior to the left renal artery. Thereafter, a bevel is taken across the Dacron graft to allow the lateral wall of the graft more length to reconstruct the suprarenal region (Figure 8).

The distal anastomoses are performed in a similar fashion. Just before finishing the distal anastomosis, release the proximal clamp temporarily to flush out any clots that might otherwise embolize distally. The proximal clamp is closed, and the anastomosis is completed. This step is performed near the completion of the first distal anastomosis in the case of a bifurcated graft. Flow can now be reestablished to the just-completed limb, and with the other outflow limb occluded by a clamp, the final anastomosis can be performed and the final clamp removed. After hemostasis is ensured, the aneurysm sac is reapproximated over the graft if a TP exposure was used. This measure, in addition to flap coverage with omentum, helps minimize the risk of graft erosion and fistulization with surrounding structures, particularly small bowel.

Several points are worth noting regarding visceral vessel reimplantation. When reimplantation is anticipated, grafts with side arms for vessel reimplantation can be used to minimize clamp time and expedite visceral reperfusion. Usually the inferior mesenteric artery (IMA) can be sacrificed without consequence because it is often occluded; occasionally, however, it is the major source of flow to the left colon, particularly in the setting of significant occlusive disease of the iliac and mesenteric vessels and in patients with history of colon surgery. Poor back bleeding of the IMA should prompt reimplantation to prevent life-threatening ischemia of the colon.

At this point in the operation, a thorough evaluation for hemostasis to prevent postoperative hemorrhage is mandatory. The usual culprits are lumbar and intercostal vessels and undetected intraoperative iatrogenic splenic injury. The reconstructed vessels are palpated for a pulse, the viscera are inspected for perfusion, the wound is closed, and the patient is transferred to the intensive care unit for postoperative care.

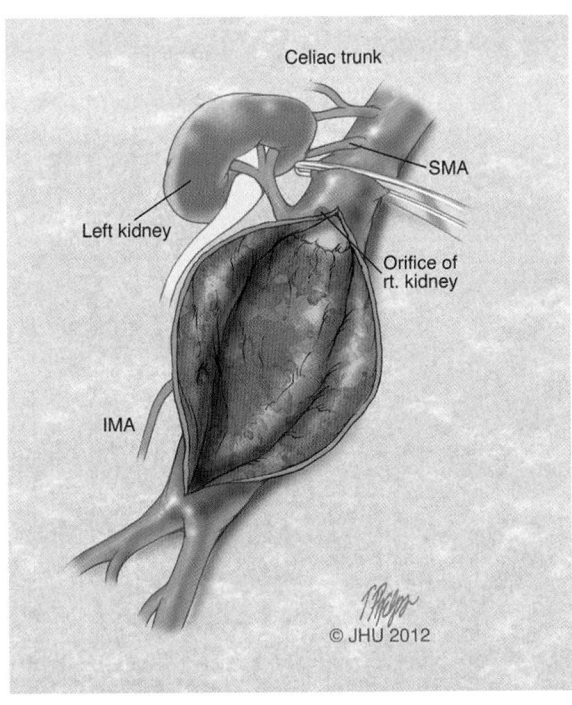

FIGURE 7 Juxtarenal abdominal aortic aneurysm after aortotomy. The aortic cross clamp is placed suprarenal to avoid embolizing material off the thrombus-laden infrarenal segment. *IMA,* Inferior mesenteric artery; *SMA,* superior mesenteric artery.

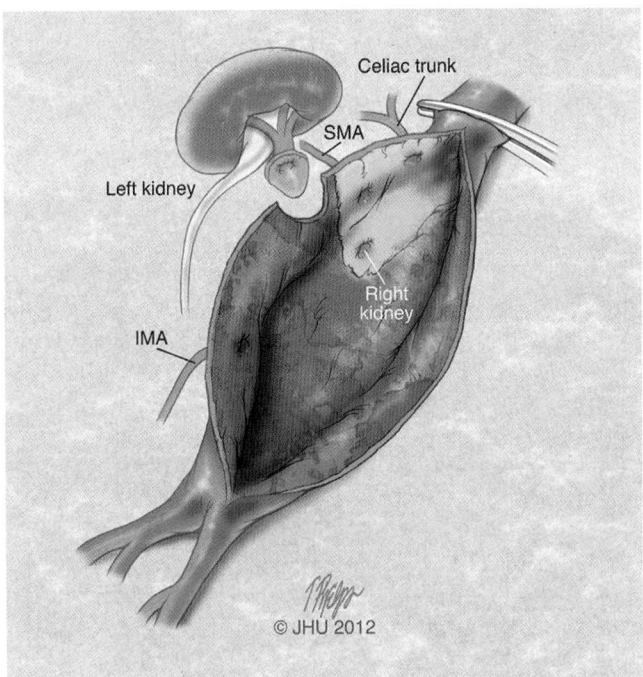

FIGURE 8 The aortotomy after suprarenal abdominal aortic aneurysm opening is taken posterior to the left renal artery. If the left renal origin cannot be directly reimplanted onto the surgical graft, an interposition 6-mm to 8-mm diameter graft can be used. *IMA,* Inferior mesenteric artery; *SMA,* superior mesenteric artery.

COMPLICATIONS

On the basis of the large randomized controlled studies mentioned previously, the 30-day operative mortality rate associated with OSR of 2.0% to 5.8% is generally favorable. In a study with a large administrative database, surgeon volume, hospital volume, and vascular surgery specialty were all found to be independently associated with a lower in-hospital mortality rate. Approximately one third of patients undergoing elective OSR have some sort of complication develop. Because of the magnitude of the operation and the baseline comorbidities of this patient population, there are a number of major complications specific to AAA repair to be aware of when caring for these patients in the perioperative period.

Ischemic colitis is a relatively rare but highly lethal complication after AAA repair; it most commonly involves the sigmoid colon and may be seen in 20% to 40% of patients after surgery for ruptured AAA. As mentioned previously, ligation of the IMA is usually safe but can be problematic for patients with insufficient collateral flow. For this reason, some surgeons advocate routine IMA reimplantation. Occasionally, patients with IMA borderline blood flow become symptomatic after surgery (Figure 9, *A,B*) after diuresis or an episode of hypotension. Patients can present in the postoperative period with hemoccult-positive or grossly bloody diarrhea. Other signs may be nonspecific, and symptoms include abdominal pain and distension, leukocytosis, metabolic acidosis, and fever. The diagnosis is made with flexible sigmoidoscopy. Treatment includes supportive care with intravenous fluid resuscitation, broad-spectrum antibiotics, bowel rest, total parenteral nutrition, and in the case of transmural ischemia or lack of improvement in patients with only mucosal involvement, colon resection with end colostomy. Primary anastomosis is not recommended because a leak may lead to fecal contamination of the aortic graft. Patients with spontaneously resolving ischemic colitis are at risk for colonic strictures.

Lower extremity complications can be either paralytic or ischemic in nature. Paraplegia, although dreaded and often irreversible, is thankfully a very rare occurrence. In elective cases, it occurs approximately in 1 of 100 to 2500 patients. The incidence rate is much higher in the case of AAA rupture—1.4%. It is thought that the underlying mechanism is spinal artery thrombosis, embolization, loss of forward flow through the iliac arteries, or disruption of an aberrantly low spinal artery. Ischemia of the lower extremities is a much more common complication than paraplegia. Debris inside the aneurysm sac may embolize distally during the course of the operation, necessitating cautious handling of the aorta during dissection, careful clamping of the distal vessels, flushing of the vessels, and sequential clamp removal. Large debris may need to be mechanically extracted; however, smaller emboli lodge distally, and little can be done to ameliorate this problem after the fact, underscoring the importance of prevention with careful operative technique. Thrombosis occasionally is the etiology of lower extremity ischemia and may be secondary to inadequate intraoperative anticoagulation, a preexisting hypercoagulable state, or technical error. Thrombectomy, anticoagulation, or revision of the distal anastomosis may be necessary.

Sexual dysfunction is a relatively common complication after AAA repair and occurs in 10% to 20% of patients. During surgery, care must be taken to avoid injury to the autonomic nerves that course along the lateral side of the distal aorta and cross into the pelvis near the left common iliac artery to minimize disruption of pelvic parasympathetic control of the bladder neck during orgasm. Loss of such nerve innervations produces retrograde ejaculation. The possibility of retrograde ejaculation, reduced male fertility, and difficulty achieving orgasm should be discussed with patients as part of the informed consent process.

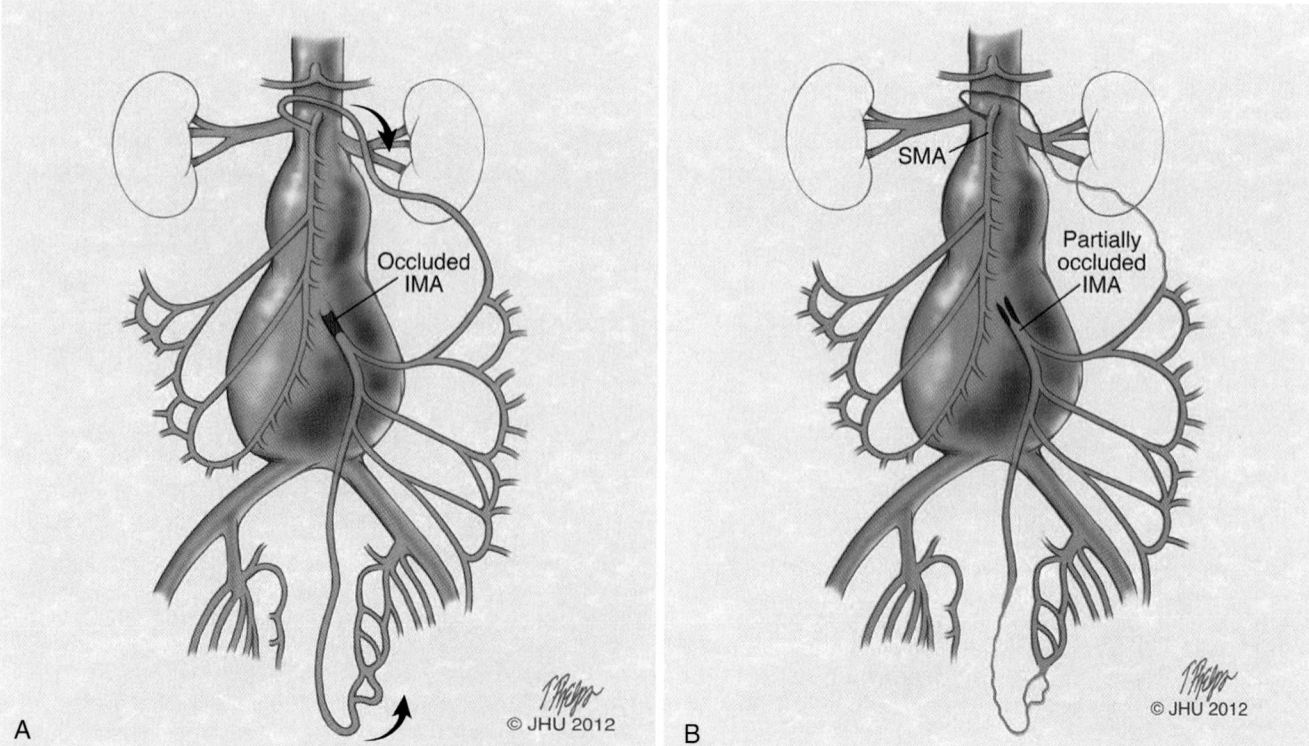

FIGURE 9 **A,** When the inferior mesenteric artery *(IMA)* is chronically occluded, collateral flow from the superior mesenteric artery *(SMA)* via the marginal artery or from internal iliac artery via the rectal and sigmoid arcade preserves colon viability during open surgical repair. **B,** In cases of preserved IMAs, the collateral network may be insufficient to maintain viability of the colon after surgery.

CONCLUSION

The advent of EVAR and the increasing expansion of its indications have forever altered the treatment of AAA. Even so, OSR is frequently necessary, particularly for patients with anatomy not amenable to endovascular repair. In addition, a number of questions remain as to the long-term durability and cost effectiveness of EVAR, rendering OSR perhaps a less commonly used operation yet still an important modality in the treatment of AAA.

SUGGESTED READINGS

Cao P, DeRango P, Verzini F, et al: Comparison of surveillance vs aortic endografting for small aneurysm repair, *Eur J Vasc Endovasc Surg* 41:13–25, 2011.

Chaikof EL, Brewster DC, Dalman RL, et al: The care of patients with an abdominal aortic aneurysm: the Society for Vascular Surgery practice guidelines, *J Vasc Surg* 50:1S–49S, 2009.

Dimick JB, Cowan JA Jr, Stanley JC, et al: Surgeon specialty and provider volumes are related to outcome of intact abdominal aortic aneurysm repair in the United States, *J Vasc Surg* 38(4):739–744, 2003.

Filardo G, Powell JT, Martinez MA, et al: Surgery for small asymptomatic abdominal aortic aneurysms, *Cochrane Database Syst* 2012, Issue 3. Art. No.: CD001835. DOI: 10.1002/14651858.CD001835.pub3.

Gloviczki P, Cross SA, Stanson AW, et al: Ischemic injury to the spinal cord or lumbosacral plexus after aorto-iliac reconstruction, *Am J Surg* 162(2):131–136, 1991.

Huber TS, Wang JG, Derrow AE, et al: Experience in the United States with intact abdominal aortic aneurysm repair, *J Vasc Surg* 33:304–310, 2001.

Lederle FA, Wilson SE, Johnson GR, et al: Immediate repair compared with surveillance of small abdominal aortic aneurysms, *N Engl J Med* 346:1437–1444, 2002.

Ouriel K, Clair DF, Kent KC, et al: Endovascular repair compared with surveillance for patients with small abdominal aortic aneurysms. *J Vasc Surg* 51:1081–1087, 2010.

United Kingdom Small Aneurysm Trial Participants: Long-term outcomes of immediate repair compared with surveillance of small abdominal aortic aneurysms, *Lancet* 352:1649–1655, 1998.

ENDOVASCULAR TREATMENT OF ABDOMINAL AORTIC ANEURYSM

Fahad Shuja, MD, and Christopher J. Kwolek, MD

INTRODUCTION

An abdominal aortic aneurysm (AAA) is defined as a focal dilatation of 50% or greater than the adjacent nonaneurysmal aorta. This disease affects primarily patients in the sixth to eighth decades of life. Other risk factors include smoking, male gender, Caucasian race, chronic obstructive pulmonary disease, and a positive family history. Increased use of modern imaging modalities may contribute to the increase in the diagnosis of AAAs since the diagnosis is often made incidentally when the patient is being evaluated for other problems. In a Veterans Affairs screening study of more than 73,000 patients 50 to 79 years old, the prevalence of AAAs greater than 3 cm was 4.6% and the incidence of those 4 cm or greater in size was 1.4%.

The primary determinant of rupture risk is maximum aneurysm diameter. Despite minor differences in estimated risks, there is general consensus that the rupture risk increases substantially with a AAA diameter between 5 and 6 cm. Surgical repair is indicated when the risk of aneurysm rupture outweighs operative risks, and therefore a size of 5.5 cm is considered appropriate for repair in most circumstances. Other indications for repair include symptomatic aneurysms and aneurysms that grow more than 0.5 cm within a 6-month interval. Two recent prospective randomized trials have shown no difference in outcomes between early endovascular treatment and delayed treatment of asymptomatic aneurysms between 4 and 4.9 cm (Pivotal Trial, Medtronic, Minneapolis, Minn) and between 4 and 5.4 cm (Caesar Trial, Cook, Bloomington, Ind).

PREOPERATIVE CONSIDERATIONS

The long-term success of aortic endografts depends heavily on appropriate patient selection. Different devices vary in their specific anatomic requirements, but the basic principles remain the same. These include an appropriate aortic neck, a distal sealing zone, and a suitable path for the endograft to be placed through. Computed tomographic angiography with reformatted three-dimensional reconstructions is the most widely used preoperative imaging assessment tool for this purpose.

Aortic Neck Anatomy

The aortic neck is defined as the area of the aorta cephalad to the aneurysm, below the level of the renal arteries, in which the endograft will be placed. This area serves as the site of proximal fixation that will prevent the device from distal migration. It is important to obtain a circumferential seal in this region to prevent blood leakage into the aneurysm sac. For this reason, the graft is typically oversized by 10% to 20% relative to the diameter of the aneurysm neck. The minimal length needed varies among devices, but it is typically 15 mm. The largest neck diameter that can be treated with a Food and Drug Administration (FDA)–approved device is 32 mm. The presence of circumferential thrombus or severe aortic wall calcification can negatively affect the ability to obtain seal and fixation. Other factors that are important in determining whether a patient is a candidate for endovascular aneurysm repair (EVAR) include the angulation and shape of the aortic neck. Angulation is the angle formed between the vertical plane and a line that transects the long axis of the aneurysm. Angulation of greater than 60 degrees may lead to endoleaks, kinking, and stent migration and is therefore considered a contraindication for EVAR. A conical-shaped neck, defined as an increase in diameter of the neck by more than 10%, is also considered a contraindication to routine endografting.

Iliofemoral Access

The iliofemoral arterial system provides access for endograft placement. The presence of thrombus, calcifications, and tortuosity can significantly hinder a distal seal. Most available endografts require at least a 15-mm segment of iliac artery to be of adequate caliber and free of significant disease. The largest iliac diameter currently treated by an FDA-approved device is 25 mm. A minimum common femoral artery diameter of 6 mm is required to accommodate the smallest delivery system available. The configurations of the most recently approved endografts in the United States are listed in Table 1.

TECHNICAL DETAILS OF THE PROCEDURE

1. Prep the patient's abdomen from xiphoid to mid thighs to allow for both femoral and retroperitoneal access for placement of an iliac conduit if necessary.
2. For open exposure of the femoral arteries, use bilateral oblique groin incisions halfway between the inguinal ligament and the groin crease just over the femoral pulse, to optimize wound healing in heavy patients. These can be extended inferiorly, if necessary, using a hockey stick incision. Only use a vertical incision if you are planning to perform an iliofemoral endarterectomy. Use a 19G entry needle and a 0.035-inch 3J guidewire to enter the common femoral artery.
3. For percutaneous access to the femoral arteries, use ultrasound to identify a noncalcified entry site for the micropuncture needle and guidewire. Upsize to a 5F sheath over a 0.035-inch guidewire. Then use two ProGlide closure devices (Abbott, Abbott Park, Ill) over a 0.035-inch 3J guidewire prior to inserting your working sheath.
4. Systemically heparinize the patient with 75 to 100 mg/kg of heparin.
5. Using a Kumpe catheter (Cook Medical, Bloomington, Ind) or a Berenstein catheter (Boston Scientific, Natick, Mass), direct the guidewire into the descending thoracic aorta and exchange for a 0.035-inch Lunderquist guidewire (Cook Medical, Bloomington, Ind) on the side for placement of the main body of the stent graft.

6. After gaining access on the contralateral side, advance an 8F sheath into the bottom of the aneurysm sac and place a marking pigtail catheter at the L1 vertebral level, checking the position of the renal arteries with a gentle hand injection of contrast.
7. If uncertain about your stent graft measurements and lengths, you can proceed to perform a power injection run with the marking pigtail catheter in place to obtain total length measurements. Otherwise, you can proceed to insert the main body of the graft over the Lunderquist wire on the ipsilateral side and perform the first power injection run at the level of the renal vessels. You can then proceed to adjust the image intensifier cranially to correct for parallax and repeat a power injection run at a rate of 20 mL/sec for a total of 10 mL of volume. This will allow you to position the fabric of the stent graft just at the level of the renal arteries. You must know the relationship of the graft to the proximal markers for the stent graft that you are using.
8. For Gore, Cook, and Medtronic grafts, you then proceed to deploy the proximal portion of the graft just above the renal arteries and pull down into the final position. Both Cook and Medtronic grafts also have a proximal bare spring that is deployed for fixation.
9. Do not forget to pull down the marking catheter into the aneurysm sac. This can also be performed over a 3J wire after the proximal graft has been deployed. You then proceed to cannulate the contralateral gate with a Kumpe catheter, Cobra-2 catheter (Cook Medical, Bloomington Ind), or a reversed curve catheter such as a visceral selective, depending on the position of the contralateral gate. Do not forget to rotate the image intensifier if necessary to get different orientations of the contralateral gate.
10. Once the wire and catheter are in the contralateral gate, advance both into the descending thoracic aorta and exchange for a 0.035-inch Lunderquist guidewire. Confirm that you are actually in the contralateral gate by advancing a sheath and performing an injection of contrast into the graft. Inflate a 12-mm balloon within the contralateral gate and rotate the

TABLE 1: FDA-approved devices for endovascular repair of abdominal aortic aneurysms

Device/type (Avg # pieces)	Manufacturer	Main body diameter (mm)	Aortic treatment diameter (mm)	Main body delivery size (F)	IFU neck length/angle (degrees)	Iliac treatment diameter (mm)	Material	Suprarenal stent
Zenith Flex/ modular (2-3)	Cook Inc. (Bloomington, Ind)	22-36	18-32 Outer to outer	18-22 ID 20-24 OD	15 mm ≦60	7.5-20	Stainless steel– polyester	Yes
AFX/Unibody (1-2)	Endologix (Irvine, Calif)	25-34	18-32 Inner to inner	19 OD	15 mm ≦60	10-23	Cobalt-chromium-PTFE	Optional
Excluder/ modular (2-3)	WL Gore (Flagstaff, Ariz)	23-35	19-32 Inner to inner	18 ID 20 OD	15 mm ≦60	8-25	Nitinol-PTFE	No
Endurant II/ modular (2-3)	Medtronic (Minneapolis, Minn)	23-36	19-32 Inner to inner	18-20 OD	10 mm ≦60	8-25	Nitinol-polyester	Yes
Ovation Prime/ modular (3)	Trivascular (Santa Rosa, Calif)	20-34	16-30 Inner to inner	14-15 OD	10 mm ≦60	8-20	Nitinol-PTFE-polyethylene glycol	Yes

FDA, Food and Drug Administration; *ID*, inner diameter; *IFU*, instructions for use; *OD*, inner diameter; *PTFE*, polytetrafluoroethylene.

image intensifier laterally in both directions to make sure that the balloon remains within the iliac limb. Then, rotate a pigtail catheter in the main body of the graft and advance cranially to prove that the catheter is not trapped between the stent graft and the aortic wall.

11. Reinsert the marking catheter to measure the distance from the contralateral gate limb to the hypogastric artery. Perform a hand injection of contrast via the ipsilateral sheath, which has been pulled back into the external iliac artery. For the left internal iliac artery, rotate the image intensifier to the right and caudally. For the right internal iliac artery, rotate the image intensifier to the left and caudally.

12. Choose the appropriate length and diameter iliac graft limb, making sure that the proximal portion lands between the minimal and maximal overlap zones.

13. Deploy the ipsilateral iliac graft limb for Gore, Cook, and Medtronic grafts.

14. If extending to the external iliac artery is necessary, an additional iliac extension limb will often be used. If the common iliac aneurysm extends down to the iliac bifurcation, then embolization of the internal iliac artery will also be necessary to prevent an endoleak from occurring.

15. Using a compliant CODA (Cook Medical, Bloomington, Ind) or Reliant (Medtronic, Santa Rosa, Calif) balloon, you should perform balloon angioplasty of the proximal attachment zone, the graft overlap sites, and the distal attachment zones.

16. Completion angiogram should be performed using the marking pigtail catheter and a power injection with a rate of 20 to 25 mL/sec for a total volume of 25 or 30 mL. Delayed views will also be necessary to evaluate for late endoleaks. Other things to evaluate include the following:
    a. Filling of the renal and visceral vessels
    b. The position of the proximal endograft with the distance to the renal arteries and the presence of a type I endoleak
    c. Blood flow through the main body and the iliac limbs
    d. Distal flow into the iliac vessels and runoff vessels, including the presence of a type IB endoleak and status of the internal iliac artery.
    e. Delayed flow into the aneurysm sac via lumbar collaterals and the inferior mesenteric artery, leading to a type II endoleak

17. Hints for improved angiography. (A) Remove all stiff guidewires and replace them with softer catheters or wires that will not straighten the vessels. (B) Pull back the sheaths into the external iliac arteries and draw back on them with a 30-mL syringe while performing a power injection to simulate flow in the native external iliac arteries.

18. Remove the sheaths over a stiff wire if the access was difficult. Watch for a drop in pressure, potentially signifying a tear in the iliac artery. If this occurs, place an occlusion balloon across the iliac artery on the affected side. If this is unsuccessful, you can also place an aortic occlusion balloon via the contralateral side.

19. Perform repair of the femoral artery using primary closure with either two running 5-0 Prolene sutures (Ethicon, Somerville, NJ) or multiple interrupted Prolene sutures, or using femoral endarterectomy with bovine pericardium angioplasty closure.

A selection of endograft bodies, iliac limbs, proximal aortic cuffs, and distal extensions will be critical to safely performing these procedures. In addition, a selection of large compliant aortic angioplasty balloons (e.g., CODA, Reliant) and noncompliant aortic balloons (Z-MED, B. Braun, Bethlehem, Pa) and bare metal 3010 or 4010 Palmaz stents (Cordis, Bridgewater, NJ) will be helpful to address proximal or distal endoleaks.

Of the currently available endografts on the market, all perform well when used within the parameters of the instructions for use (IFU) of the device. We performed a device-specific analysis within and outside the IFU on three endografts in commercial use at the time: Cook Zenith, Gore Excluder, and Medtronic AneuRx. There was no difference between the devices in intraoperative technical factors, perioperative mortality, graft failure, and aneurysm-related mortality within the IFU. However, EVAR procedures performed outside of IFU had higher rates of aneurysm-related mortality, reintervention, and graft thrombosis.

POSTOPERATIVE CARE AND FOLLOW-UP

Intraoperative anesthesia management involves a regional anesthetic in over 90% of cases in our institution with general anesthetic reserved for those patients with airway problems who cannot lie flat for several hours. In some instances, the procedure can be performed under local anesthesia, particularly in patients with good access vessels, which may be amenable to percutaneous closure. This trend will increase as the diameter of delivery systems continues to decrease to less than 14F.

Patients no longer require a stay in the intensive care unit or even a prolonged stay in the recovery room. After patients are transferred to the floor, the epidural catheter is removed and the patients are encouraged to ambulate. Ice bags can be used for control of local swelling over the groin incisions, and oral pain medications are used. Patients are provided with preoperative teaching information with plans for discharge on postoperative day (POD) 1. Visiting nurses check on their status at home. No routine postoperative imaging is obtained.

Patients are seen in follow-up evaluation at 30 days with an abdominal/pelvis computed tomographic angiogram with intravenous contrast. This will be used as the new baseline exam for assessing aneurysm sac size and volume as well as the presence of an endoleak. Patients are routinely seen at 6 and 12 months with similar studies done to evaluate sac size and the presence or absence of an endoleak. If the sac is stable or shrinking with stable anatomy, we will often switch to surveillance using a graft duplex to assess for flow in the stent graft, measure aneurysm sac size, and determine the presence of flow outside the graft signifying an endoleak. Plain films of the stent graft can also be obtained to assess for stent graft position and the presence of stent fractures. Follow-up will continue on an annual basis. If the aneurysm sac is obliterated after 5 years, then we will often switch to a follow-up regimen of every 2 years.

COMPLICATIONS

A number of complications can be seen following EVAR. These are often related to issues with access at the time of the procedure or longer term issues with the exclusion of the aneurysm sac.

The primary route of insertion for most endografts is the iliofemoral arterial system. In cases of iliac artery atherosclerosis, the lumen may not permit the passage of the delivery system. Advancement of the device despite resistance can cause dissection, thrombosis, or even vessel rupture in 1% to 2% of cases. The iliac artery can be treated with balloon angioplasty or dilatation prior to advancement of an endograft. An alternative is to place an endovascular or open iliac conduit. The final solution is to use a hybrid of these two techniques by using the SoloPath balloon-expandable sheath (Terumo, Ann Arbor, Mich) to simultaneously dilate the vessel and provide a pathway to the aorta.

An endoleak is the persistence of blood flow outside of the endograft within the aneurysm sac. Endoleaks result when there is incomplete isolation of the aneurysm sac from systemic circulation resulting in aneurysm sac expansion and potential rupture. Endoleaks are the most common cause of secondary interventions and aneurysm-related morbidity following EVAR. They are classified according to their etiology. Five different types of endoleaks have been described (Table 2).

Type I

Type I endoleaks result from inadequate seal at either the proximal aortic or distal iliac attachment sites. This can result from a size mismatch between the graft and the vessel, severe aortic neck angulation, or applying the graft to a vessel wall with heavy calcification or thrombus. Type I endoleaks are usually visualized on angiography immediately after deployment. Delayed type I endoleaks are thought to be secondary to aneurysm sac reconfiguration, as the sac diameter decreases over time. Type I endoleaks rarely close spontaneously and are therefore repaired as soon as they are discovered. Treatment may involve reballooning the attachment site, using proximal or distal extension grafts, or placing a balloon-expandable Palmaz stent to obtain better graft expansion and wall apposition.

Type II

These are the most common type of endoleaks, occurring in up to 25% of EVAR patients. They occur from retrograde filling of the aneurysm sac from a patent aortic branch vessel, such as the inferior mesenteric artery or a lumbar artery. Patients are often asymptomatic and diagnosed on postoperative surveillance imaging. The endoleaks may not be visible during the arterial phase since the sac fills retrograde through a collateral network; therefore, delayed images are often necessary. These will show pooling of contrast outside of the endograft wall and within the aneurysm sac. Management of a type II endoleak may consist of close observation, and spontaneous resolution is reported in 30% to 90% of cases. However, in patients where the aneurysm sac increases in size, we have had success treating these patients with embolization using Onyx Glue (EV3, Covidien, Mansfield, Mass) via a direct translumbar approach.

Type III and Type IV

Type III endoleaks are caused by defects in the fabric of the graft or at the junction of modular components. Treatment consists of placing covered stents to exclude the aneurysm sac from systemic pressure. Type IV endoleaks are due to leaking of blood between the interstices of the fabric or where the graft is sutured to the stent.

TABLE 2: Types of endoleaks

Type of endoleak	Definition
I	Inadequate sealing at either proximal or distal attachment sites
II	Flow into the aneurysm sac from patent branch vessels (e.g., inferior mesenteric artery or lumbar artery)
III	Defect in the fabric of the graft or failure of seal between graft components
IV	Leaking of blood between the interstices of the graft fabric
V	The aneurysm sac remains pressurized in the absence of a visible endoleak, also termed *endotension*

When seen at the time of initial implantation, these usually resolve with reversal of anticoagulation. However, relining of the endograft may also be necessary if this persists.

Endotension

Endotension, or type V endoleak, is defined as elevated aneurysm sac pressure resulting in sac expansion in the absence of a radiographically demonstrable endoleak. The exact etiology is unknown, and treatment is largely undefined. Secondary conversion to open repair is sometimes necessary but carries a significant mortality rate in some series.

Limb Thrombosis

Thrombosis of an iliac limb occurs in up to 11% of cases. The lack of stent support within an iliac limb increases the risk of thrombosis by eightfold, compared with intrinsically supported limbs. Most patients experience ipsilateral buttock and/or limb claudication within the first 6 months following their EVAR. Management is dictated by patient symptoms. Asymptomatic patients can be observed while symptomatic patients might require attempts at thrombolysis or a femoral-femoral bypass.

Migration

Migration of stent grafts is a known risk factor for development of a delayed type I endoleak and subsequent aneurysm rupture. Conrad published our 10-year results with EVAR in 2009. The overall incidence of graft migration in more than 800 EVAR patients was 1.7%. Neck angulation and neck diameter have been cited as important risk factors for device migration. Treatment usually involves placement of a proximal extension graft or conversion to open repair.

SUMMARY

Parodi and colleagues reported the first repair of an aortic aneurysm with a stent graft in 1991. Since then, EVAR has emerged as the procedure of choice for 70% to 80% of patients with AAA treated in the United States. While the elective mortality rate for open repair has remained consistent at 4% to 5% when based on data from large administrative databases, the perioperative morbidity and mortality rates of EVAR have continued to decrease. These differences are even more pronounced in patients over the age of 80.

There are three widely quoted randomized trials comparing endovascular repair to open repair of AAA. The EVAR 1 trial compared 543 EVAR patients with 539 open repair patients. There was a significant increase in the 30-day mortality rate for open repair versus EVAR (4.7% compared with 1.7%). The EVAR group had a significantly higher rate of secondary intervention (9.8% compared to 5.8%); however, procedures related to the original open operation, such as bowel obstruction and hernia repair, were not included in the analysis. After 8 years of follow-up, the aneurysm-related survival rate was 93% in both groups. The DREAM trial comprised 351 patients with aneurysms larger than 5 cm randomized to EVAR versus open repair. The rates of aneurysm-related deaths were 5.7% and 2.1% for open and endovascular repair, respectively. However, there was no survival advantage after the first postoperative year. The largest of the three trials, OVER, followed 881 patients for a mean of 5.2 years within the Veterans Affairs hospital system. The trial had similar conclusions: an upfront survival advantage with EVAR with "mortality catch-up" later. Another important similarity among all three trials is the remarkably low aneurysm-related mortality rate (<5%) up to 6 years of follow-up.

A trial comparing EVAR to medical management in 338 patients unfit for open surgical repair (EVAR 2 trial) showed a similar 30-day mortality rate (9%) as well as a 4-year AAA-related mortality rate (14%) between the two groups. The study was criticized for a 25% crossover rate from nonoperative to EVAR arm. Furthermore, 52% of the perioperative deaths in the EVAR group occurred preoperatively. The Society for Vascular Surgery published their own data on patients at high risk in 2006. A total of 565 EVARs and 61 open repairs were compared in patients at high risk. The definition of "high risk" was the same as that in EVAR 2 (age > 60, aneurysm > 5.5, and one of the following: symptomatic congestive heart failure, valvular heart disease, cardiac arrhythmia, chronic obstructive pulmonary disease, chronic renal failure, or serum creatinine value > 2.6 mg/dL). The 30-day mortality rate for EVAR was 2.1% compared with 5.1% for open repair. This difference was not statistically significant. There was no difference in rates of AAA-related death at 4 years (4% vs 5%). This study helped alleviate the initial concerns that had emerged after EVAR 2 about the safety of EVAR in patients at high risk.

NEW DEVICES ON THE HORIZON

Key limitations to successful EVAR relate to patient's anatomy and device design. Short/angulated necks, occlusive/tortuous iliofemoral arterial system, preservation of hypogastric inflow, endograft migration, and endoleaks pose major challenges for future progress in the area of EVAR.

Several companies have developed lower profile devices to allow treatment of patients with smaller and more tortuous iliac access vessels. The Trivascular Ovation (Trivascular, Santa Rosa, Calif) device has a 14F outer diameter (OD) delivery system and was recently approved for use in the United States. The Cook low-profile device (LP) (Cook, Bloomington, Ind) has an 18F OD introducer system while the Cordis Incraft device (Cordis, Bridgewater, NJ) also has a 14F OD delivery profile. Both are currently in clinical trial within the United States.

The Terumo Anaconda stent graft (Terumo, Ann Arbor, Mich) has a retrievable proximal delivery system that allows for repositioning of the stent graft in the proximal seal zone. Both the Anaconda graft and the Lombard Aorfix graft (Lombard Medical, Oxfordshire, UK) are designed to accommodate more severe angulation in the proximal aortic neck. Both have completed clinical trials in the United States.

Fenestrated stent graft technology is now available to address juxtarenal aneurysms with neck lengths of less than 10 mm. The Cook Zenith fenestrated stent graft (Cook Inc, Australia) is now approved for use in the United States, and the Endologix Ventana endograft is currently being evaluated as part of an FDA-approved Investigational Device Exemption trial (Endologix, Irvine, Calif).

Two new stent grafts currently being evaluated outside of the United States have the potential to revolutionize the management of AAAs. The Cardiatis multilayer stent (Cardiatis, Isnes, Belgium) is designed to divert flow away from the aneurysm sac while allowing for persistent patency of critical side branches without the need for any branched grafts or fenestrations. This stent has been approved for use in Europe where further data are being accumulated on the treatment of AAA. The Nellix stent graft system (Endologix, Irvine, Calif) relies on the use of two balloon-expandable stents to maintain a flow channel through the aneurysm sac to the iliac arteries. Two attached endobags are then filled with a polymer, which completely obliterates the aneurysm sac, theoretically eliminating the risk of endoleaks since the aneurysm cavity is filled. This device is commercially available in Europe and will soon enter clinical trial in the United States.

Current endograft technology has allowed between 70% and 80% of current AAAs in the United States to be treated with stent graft technology. Although initial results are excellent, long-term follow-up remains critical since up to 25% of patients may require a secondary intervention. The majority of these interventions can be performed with a catheter-based procedure, and the need for open conversion with graft explantation remains low. Next-generation endografts are now being designed to address these shortcomings and may prove more durable than current devices.

SUGGESTED READINGS

Abbruzzese TA, Kwolek CJ, Brewster DC, et al: Outcomes following endovascular abdominal aortic aneurysm repair (EVAR): an anatomic and device-specific analysis, *J Vasc Surg* 48:19–28, 2008.

Abularrage CJ, Patel V, Conrad MF, et al. Improved results for the management of type II endoleaks with Onyx Glue, *J Vasc Surg* 56:630–636, 2012.

Brewster DC, Cronenwett JL, Hallett JW Jr, et al: Guidelines for the treatment of abdominal aortic aneurysms: report of a subcommittee of the Joint Council of the American Association for Vascular Surgery and Society for Vascular Surgery, *J Vasc Surg* 37:1106–1117, 2003.

Conrad MF, Adams AB, Guest J, et al: Secondary intervention after endovascular abdominal aortic aneurysm repair, *Ann Surg* 250:383–389, 2009.

Giles KA, Pomposelli F, Hamden A, et al: Decrease in total aneurysm-related deaths in the era of endovascular aneurysm repair, *J Vasc Surg* 49:543–551, 2009.

Greenhalgh RM, Brown LC, Kwong GP, et al: Comparison of endovascular aneurysm repair with open repair in patients with abdominal aortic aneurysm (EVAR 1 trial), 30-day operative mortality results: randomised controlled trial, *Lancet* 364:843–848, 2004.

Lederle FA, Wilson SE, Johnson GR, et al: Immediate repair compared with surveillance of small abdominal aortic aneurysms, *N Engl J Med* 346:1437–1444, 2002.

Ouriel K, Clair DG, Kent KC, et al: Endovascular repair compared with surveillance for patients with small abdominal aortic aneurysms, *J Vasc Surg* 51:1081–1087, 2010.

Prinssen M, Verhoeven EL, Buth J, et al: A randomized trial comparing conventional and endovascular repair of abdominal aortic aneurysms, *N Engl J Med* 351:1607–1618, 2004.

Schermerhorn ML, O'Malley AJ, Jhaveri A, et al: Endovascular versus open repair of abdominal aortic aneurysms in the Medicare population, *N Engl J Med* 358:464–474, 2008.

Sicard GA, Zwolak RM, Sidawy AN, et al: Endovascular abdominal aortic aneurysm repair: Long-term outcome measures in patients at high-risk for open surgery, *J Vasc Surg* 44:229–236, 2006.

The Management of Ruptured Abdominal Aortic Aneurysm

Natalia O. Glebova, MD, PhD, and
Mahmoud B. Malas, MD, MHS, FACS

INTRODUCTION

Ruptured abdominal aortic aneurysm (rAAA) is a lethal condition, with mortality rates estimated at 90% for all patients and at 40% to 70% for those patients who reach the hospital. rAAA is the 13th leading cause of death in the United States. The incidence of rupture has decreased over time, likely because of the implementation of screening and aggressive repair of asymptomatic enlarging abdominal aortic aneurysms (AAAs). The mortality rate of rAAA, on the other hand, has remained high, albeit with recent trends toward decline thought to result from the increase in endovascular repair of rAAA.

The risk factors for AAA rupture are aneurysm diameter, female gender, chronic obstructive pulmonary disease (COPD), cigarette smoking, and hypertension. Peak wall stress is a better predictor of rupture than aneurysm diameter but is more difficult to determine in clinical practice. Rupture of an AAA, defined as bleeding outside the adventitia of the dilated aortic wall, may be free into the peritoneal cavity or contained in the retroperitoneal space. Retroperitoneal rupture is in general thought to result in better outcome than free intraabdominal ruptures because the retroperitoneum may tamponade the hemorrhage and thus allow patient survival to definitive care.

DIAGNOSIS AND EVALUATION

The classic symptoms of a patient presenting with a rAAA are severe back pain, hypotension, and a pulsatile abdominal mass. This combination is infrequent, and other symptoms, such as abdominal or chest pain or a syncopal episode, may constitute the presentation. Differential diagnoses of patients with rAAA often include perforated viscus or ulcer, renal stones, or myocardial infarction. The nonspecific nature of the symptoms, coupled with the dire prognosis should diagnosis of a rAAA be delayed or missed, underscore the need for high suspicion of rAAA as the etiology for any patient presenting with severe abdominal or back pain.

Patient evaluation is concomitant with resuscitation, further diagnostic studies, and treatment planning. Physical examination should include not only the usual cardiac, respiratory, and abdominal examinations but also assessment of popliteal pulses to ascertain the presence of other aneurysms and of femoral and pedal pulses to evaluate distal perfusion and establish the patient's baseline values. Carotid arteries should be auscultated for bruits. An electrocardiogram (ECG) should be performed if the patient's condition is stable and time allows, and blood should be drawn for chemistries, blood counts, and crossmatch.

If the patient's condition is stable, imaging helps confirm the diagnosis and determine the treatment approach. If a plain abdominal or chest x-ray is obtained (likely in consideration of a perforated viscus), a calcified AAA may be visible. Ultrasound scan is useful for identification of an AAA but is not sensitive for detection of rupture. Computed tomographic (CT) scan is the best imaging modality for

evaluation of rAAA. On the basis of several studies, patients with conditions that are stable enough on presentation to the emergency department with a rAAA are likely to survive 2 to 11 hours before intervention. Thus, if the patient's condition is stable, enough time is generally available to obtain a CT scan. This scan confirms the diagnosis and delineates anatomy (e.g., identification of a retroaortic left renal vein anomaly helps to avoid injury during cross clamping). If endovascular repair is a consideration, a CT scan with intravenous contrast should be performed (Figure 1). Alternatively, an angiogram may be performed once the patient is in the operating room.

When the patient is diagnosed with rAAA, preoperative resuscitation should be centered on permissive hypotension, with a systolic blood pressure goal of 50 to 70 mm Hg concomitant with an appropriate level of consciousness. Aggressive resuscitation may raise the blood pressure enough to overcome the existing tamponade and result in profuse bleeding, with the ensuing instability and increased use of blood products contributing to the cycle of coagulopathy.

TREATMENT

In the operating room, if the patient's condition is unstable, further bleeding from the rAAA should be halted with the selective percutaneous placement of an occlusive balloon in the suprarenal aorta proximal to the rupture. This is done with local analgesia to avoid the hemodynamic instability that is likely to take place on induction of general anesthesia in a patient with a hypovolemic, and likely already hypotensive, condition. Access is obtained via the common femoral artery, and a sheath is introduced through which a compliant balloon is advanced and inflated with fluoroscopy (see subsequent discussion). This effectively establishes proximal control. An angiogram may be performed with temporary balloon deflation to delineate anatomy and evaluate for endovascular repair or rAAA.

Endovascular Repair

Although results are not uniform, some studies have found the endovascular repair of rAAA is associated with less morbidity and mortality (long-term follow-up of endovascular aneurysm repair [EVAR] for rAAA is lacking). A fine-cut CT scan with and without intravenous contrast is necessary to determine whether the patient is a candidate for endovascular repair on the basis of iliac artery diameter, calcification, and tortuosity, as well as aneurysm neck diameter, thrombus load, and angulation. Alternatively, angiography may be performed to evaluate for EVAR versus open repair. General contraindications for EVAR are infrarenal neck length of less than 10 mm, neck diameter greater than 32 mm, angulation greater than 60 degrees, external iliac artery diameter less than 6 mm, and extensive calcification or thrombus present at the landing zones.

If the patient's condition is stable, a standard EVAR may be performed. This procedure can be done entirely with local anesthesia with intravenous sedation as needed. Access is gained via puncture of the common femoral artery anterior to the femoral head. Ultrasound scan–guided puncture may be helpful in patients with weakly palpable femoral pulses. After sheath placement, a 180-cm Benston wire (Cook Medical, Bloomington, Ind) is advanced into the thoracic aorta with fluoroscopic guidance. Next, a glide catheter (Terumo Medical Corporation, Somerset, NJ) is advanced over the Benston wire with fluoroscopic guidance. Then, a 260-cm Amplatz super stiff wire (Cook Medical) is introduced through the glide catheter. Next, a 14F or 16F 35-cm sheath is placed in the femoral artery over the stiff wire, with the tip of the sheath kept in the suprarenal aorta. A compliant occlusion balloon is then placed through the sheath and inflated proximal to the rupture up to the contour of the aortic wall

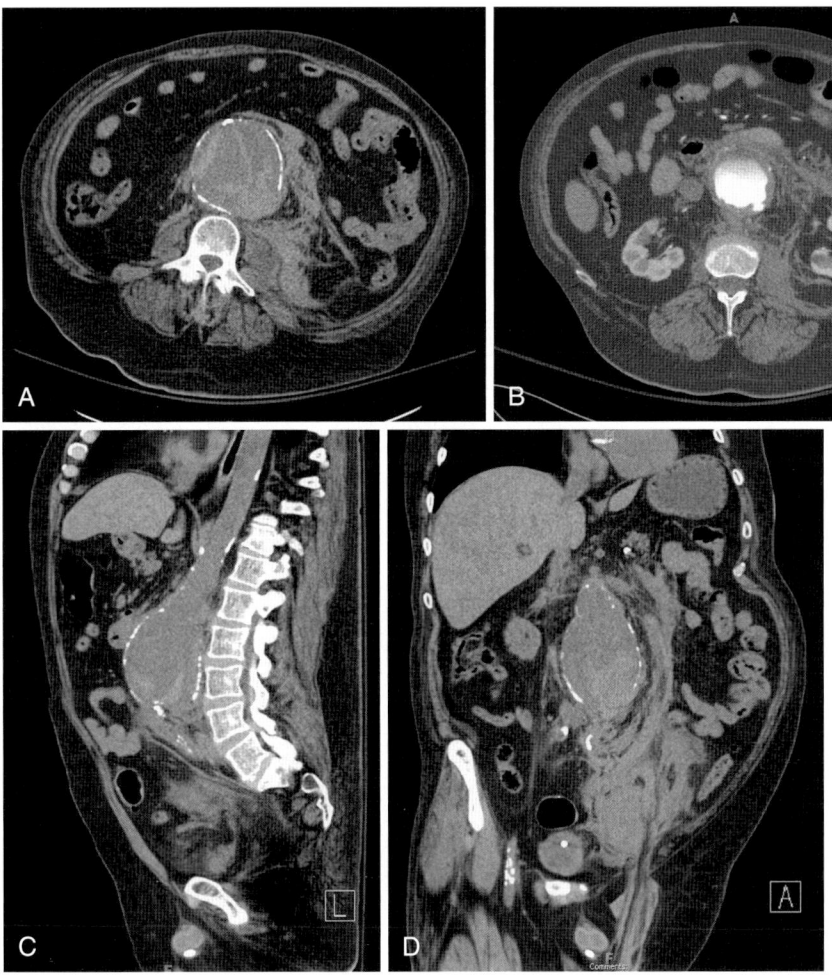

FIGURE 1 Computed tomographic (CT) scan of abdomen and pelvis shows ruptured infrarenal abdominal aortic aneurysm (AAA) with contained left retroperitoneal hematoma. **A,** CT scan without intravenous contrast shows rupture of the aneurysm. **B,** CT scan with intravenous contrast shows the area of rupture. **C,** Saggital views of same aneurysm. **D,** Coronal view of the ruptured AAA. *(Images courtesy of Dr. T. Reifsnyder; used with permission).*

to achieve complete occlusion and immediate hemodynamic improvement (Figure 2). The sheath tip should be placed under the balloon's shoulders and the sheath secured outside the patient to prevent distal migration of the balloon under the mounting proximal pressure.

A multihole catheter is inserted over a hydrophilic guidewire through the same sheath to perform an aortogram with bilateral iliac artery runoff to delineate the anatomy. This process may be difficult given the absence of aortic flow with a proximal occlusion balloon. Identification of the orifice of each renal artery is imperative to prevent coverage during endograft deployment. Either CO_2 angiography or temporary deflation of the occlusion balloon may be necessary to achieve this goal. Alternatively, aspiration off the sheath site port during contrast injection can simulate blood flow.

The stent graft is inserted via the contralateral common femoral artery after percutaneous access is obtained as described previously or via cut down approach. A stiff wire is then used to introduce the stent graft via an appropriate sheath. Of note, the tip of the ipsilateral sheath that supports the balloon should be above the stent graft to allow eventual withdrawal of the balloon into the sheath after stent deployment (see Figure 2). The stent graft is positioned based on angiography data. Once the endograft has been deployed, a second occlusion balloon may be inflated inside the graft main body and the proximal balloon deflated and withdrawn through its sheath, thus minimizing visceral ischemia time.

Usually, a bifurcated stent graft is used for EVAR of rAAA. At least one internal iliac artery needs to be preserved to minimize the risk of colon ischemia. In patients with unstable conditions, one may choose to rapidly place an aortouniiliac endograft with a contralateral iliac occluder followed by a femorofemoral crossover bypass graft. Once the aneurysm is excluded, the occlusion balloon is retrieved through its sheath. If the patient's condition becomes hemodynamically unstable with balloon deflation, one can inflate a smaller balloon in one of the endograft limbs to allow enough time for resuscitation with perfusion of at least one of the lower extremities.

Endoleaks are evaluated with angiography and treated expeditiously because their presence may result in ongoing hemorrhage. If hemodynamic instability is encountered despite aneurysm exclusion confirmed with angiography and the patient exhibits hypotension with difficulty in ventilation, peaked airway pressures, and decreased urine output, the cause of instability may be abdominal compartment syndrome from a large hematoma. The authors' experience is to create a small retroperitoneal incision to evacuate the hematoma, which successfully stabilizes the patient's condition during endovascular repair of rAAA after exclusion of the aneurysm.

Open Repair

If an open repair approach is chosen, the patient should be prepped and draped before the induction of general anesthesia. Large-bore peripheral intravenous catheters, an arterial line, a nasogastric tube, and a Foley catheter should all be placed. Every attempt should be made to keep the patient warm to minimize coagulopathy. One may choose between the transabdominal and the retroperitoneal approach, usually determined by the surgeon's typical approach to elective AAA repair.

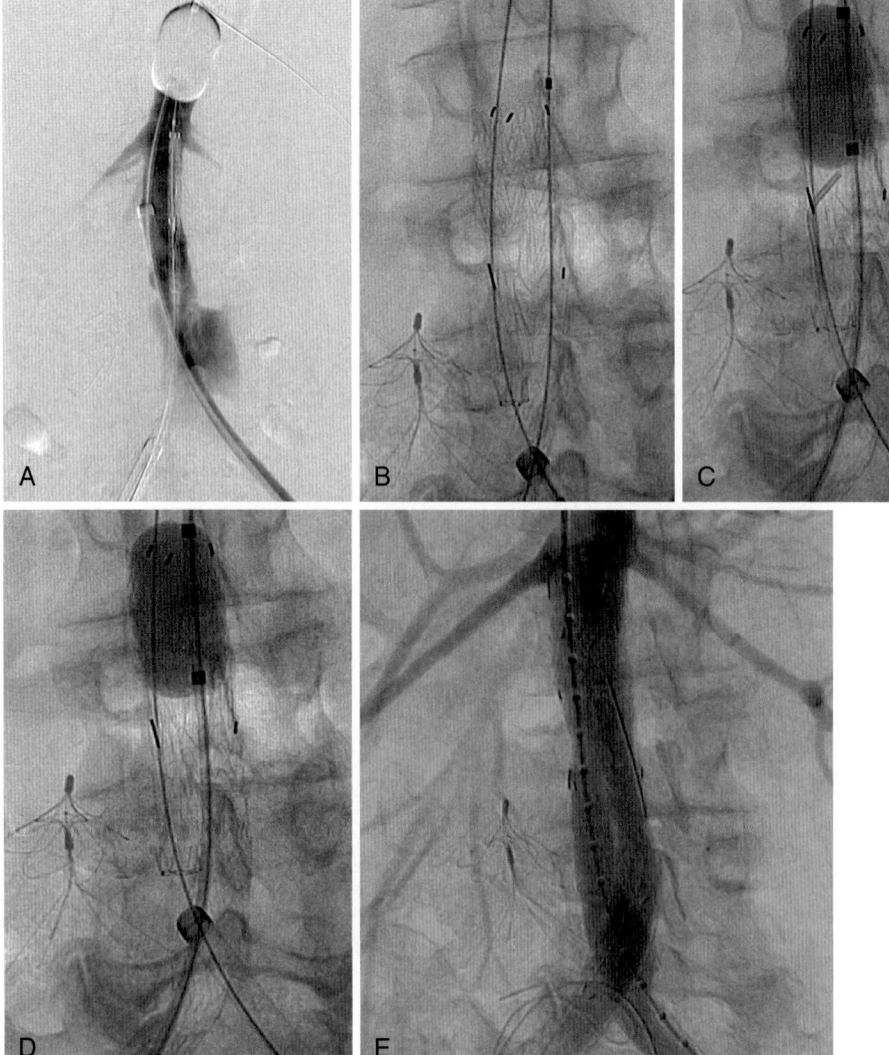

FIGURE 2 Endovascular repair of ruptured abdominal aortic aneurysm. **A,** Inflated suprarenal aortic occlusion balloon and stent graft shown before deployment, with angiogram revealing the area of rupture. **B,** Aortic occlusion balloon has been deflated and retracted, and the stent graft subsequently deployed. **C,** Reinflation of aortic occlusion balloon below the renal arteries in the endograft main body before contralateral gate cannulation. **D,** Contralateral gate cannulation with inflated aortic occlusion balloon. **E,** Completion angiogram with no evidence of endoleak and compete exclusion of the rupture. *(From Mehta M, Kreienberg PB, Roddy SP, et al Ruptured abdominal aortic aneurysm: endovascular program development and results, Semin Vasc Surg 23(4):206-214, 2010, Fig. 4.)*

A transabdominal approach allows evaluation of intestinal ischemia. With a midline incision, the abdomen is entered, and the supraceliac aorta is exposed by dividing the left triangular ligament of the liver, retracting the left lobe of the liver to the right, and incising the gastrohepatic ligament. The stomach and esophagus (identified with the nasogastric tube) are reflected to the left. If the balloon occlusion technique described previously has not been used, the supraceliac aorta is identified at the diaphragmatic crus and clamped, or alternatively compressed against the spine with a sponge stick. The clamp should be moved to an infrarenal location as soon as possible to minimize visceral ischemia time. Care is taken to identify the left renal vein. After clamping, further resuscitation is allowed before the aneurysm sac is entered.

On opening of the aneurysm, retrograde bleeding from the lumbar arteries is controlled with suture ligation. Distal control is achieved by clamping the iliac arteries or distal aorta. Alternatively, 5F Fogarty occlusion balloons may be placed into each iliac artery through the aneurysm sac. The proximal anastomosis is then completed with a tube graft and 3-0 doubled armed polypropylene sutures. Pledget reinforcement may be necessary if the wall of the aorta is severely diseased. Once the proximal anastomosis is completed, the clamp should be moved distally to the graft. Good communication with the anesthesia team is imperative because hypotension may result from visceral reperfusion. A bifurcated graft

should be used only if the iliac arteries are severely diseased. An aortobifemoral graft increases the risk of graft infection; thus, the authors prefer to perform the anastomosis to distal external iliac arteries and stay in the pelvis. For minimized risk of pelvic and colonic ischemia, at least one internal iliac artery should be reperfused. This may be achieved with retrograde perfusion from the distal external iliac artery or antegrade flow from the common iliac artery, depending on the aortic reconstruction configuration. If systemic heparinization is not used to minimize bleeding, the iliac arteries should be flushed copiously with heparinized saline solution to avoid distal thrombosis before completion of the distal anastomosis.

Care must be taken at the conclusion of open rAAA repair to examine the colon and evaluate the blood supply with Doppler scan at the antimesenteric border if intestinal viability is in doubt. Abdominal closure is then performed in the routine manner, although one may have to leave the abdomen open with a negative-pressure dressing if organ edema is concerning for development of abdominal compartment syndrome.

A retroperitoneal approach may be chosen for open repair of rAAA. This approach is thought to be associated with less morbidity and is helpful in patients with prior abdominal surgery and in those with a suprarenal AAA. A curvilinear incision is made from the umbilicus to the 12th rib. The anterior rectus sheath and muscle is divided, followed by the external oblique, and the retroperitoneum is best entered at the 12th rib level. The peritoneum is then mobilized bluntly to the right, and the left ureter is identified and retracted medially. The operation proceeds similarly to the repair described previously.

Postoperative management after either open or endovascular repair of rAAA requires attention to possible complications. Bleeding, abdominal compartment syndrome, myocardial infarction, arrhythmias, congestive heart failure, respiratory failure, renal failure, liver dysfunction, and ischemia of multiple organs including colon, spinal cord, and extremities are some of the more severe complications encountered after these operations.

DISCUSSION

Ruptured AAA remains a highly morbid and lethal condition. Those patients who survive to reach the hospital and undergo repair of rAAA have exceedingly high rates of morbidity and mortality. Several patient characteristics are known to be associated with death after rAAA: hypotension, advanced age, cardiac arrest, elevated serum creatinine, anemia, and ischemic heart disease.

The multiorgan failure (MOF) that not infrequently occurs in these patients is thought to result from the ischemia-reperfusion injury that occurs during rAAA repair. The "two-hit" hypothesis stipulates that two ischemic events, rupture that results in total body ischemia from hemorrhagic shock and aortic cross clamping that leads to lower torso ischemia, are followed by reperfusion, which leads to the release of inflammatory mediators and further tissue injury.

Several prospective randomized trials have shown dramatic decreases in operative mortality and morbidity rates after elective AAA repair with the endovascular approach but with higher long-term reintervention rates compared with open repair. However, the most recent randomized trial in the United States, the Open Surgery versus Endovascular Repair of Abdominal Aortic Aneurysm (OVER) trial, has shown similar reintervention rates between open elective AAA repair and EVAR. Because rAAA is less common, no level I evidence is found regarding the role of EVAR in the repair of ruptured AAA. Nevertheless, endovascular repair of rAAA is associated with less blood loss, ischemia, and shock. Centers with high volumes of elective EVAR have published encouraging results that show a decrease in operative deaths from rAAA to 20% to 30% with the endovascular approach described previously. An important note is that those patients who undergo EVAR may have a higher rate of reintervention, which requires close follow-up.

SUMMARY

Ruptured AAA is a morbid and lethal condition characterized by patient presentation with back or abdominal pain, hypotension, and sometimes a palpable pulsatile abdominal mass. Evaluation should be concomitant with treatment. A key feature of resuscitation is permissive hypotension, with a systolic blood pressure goal of 50 to 70 mm Hg concomitant with an appropriate level of consciousness. Repair may be approached in the open fashion or with endovascular means. CT scan with intravenous contrast or an angiogram is necessary if endovascular repair is planned. With either approach, if the patient's condition is unstable, a suprarenal occlusive balloon percutaneously placed in the aorta before the induction of anesthesia helps decrease bleeding and stabilizes the patient. Whether endovascular or open repair is the best approach in rAAA is not entirely clear at this point. Further research will help determine which approach is preferable in which patients.

SUGGESTED READINGS

Giles KA, Pomposelli F, Hamdan A, et al: Decrease in total aneurysm related deaths in the era of endovascular aneurysm repair, *J Vasc Surg* 49:543–550, 2009.

Hinchliffe RJ, Bruijstens L, MacSweeney ST, et al: A randomized trial of endovascular and open surgery for ruptured abdominal aortic aneurysm: results of a pilot study and lessons learned for future studies, *Eur J Vasc Endovasc Surg* 32:506–513, 2006.

Hoornweg LL, Storm-Versloot MN, Ubbink DT, et al: Meta analysis on mortality of ruptured abdominal aortic aneurysms, *Eur J Vasc Endovasc Surg* 35:558–570, 2008.

Malas MB, Freischlag JA: Interpretation of the results of OVER in the context of EVAR, DREAM and the EUROSTAR registry, *Seminars Vasc Surg* 23:165–169, 2010.

Malina MM, Veith F, Ivancev K, et al: Balloon occlusion of the aorta during endovascular repair of ruptured abdominal aortic aneurysm, *J Endovasc Ther* 12(5):556–559, 2005.

Mayer D, Pfammatter T, Rancic Z, et al: 10 Years of emergency endovascular aneurysm repair for ruptured abdominal aortic aneurysms: lessons learned, *Ann Surg* 249(3):510–515, 2009.

Mehta M, Kreienberg PB, Roddy SP, et al: Ruptured abdominal aortic aneurysm: endovascular program development and results, *Seminars Vasc Surg* 23(4):206–214, 2010.

Saqib N, Park SC, Park T, et al: Endovascular repair of ruptured abdominal aneurysm does not confer survival benefits over open repair, *J Vasc Surg* 56(3):614–619, 2012.

ABDOMINAL AORTIC ANEURYSM AND UNEXPECTED ABDOMINAL PATHOLOGY

Junaid Malek, MD, and Michael T. Watkins, MD

OVERVIEW

Abdominal aortic aneurysm (AAA) is a common, typically asymptomatic, potentially life-threatening condition. In the elective operative setting, management revolves around excluding the dilated segment of aorta from pressurized blood flow to prevent further growth and eliminate the risk of rupture. Currently, two major approaches exist for treating AAA: open surgical repair via either anterior or retroperitoneal approaches and minimally invasive endovascular aneurysm repair (EVAR).

Prior to the advent of endografting, open repair remained the long-standing gold standard for treating AAA, with proven long-term efficacy. However, EVAR has quickly replaced open AAA as a first-line treatment in suitable candidates because of the significantly decreased risk of perioperative morbidity and mortality. Continued evolution of stent grafts and delivery systems has made endovascular repair feasible in progressively more unfavorable aneurysm anatomy. As EVAR grows in popularity, fewer patients are undergoing laparotomy for repair of their aneurysms; thus, the discovery of unexpected, coincident intraabdominal pathology at the time of operation has become less common. Furthermore, the frequent preoperative use of noninvasive imaging modalities—including computed tomographic (CT) scan, Doppler ultrasound, and magnetic resonance imaging (MRI)—has increased the likelihood of discovering coexisting conditions well before the patient ever sees the operating room. Nevertheless, indications for open AAA repair still exist, and surgeons who encounter unexpected conditions at the time of repair must prioritize their findings and develop an operative strategy that minimizes the overall risk to the patient.

Clinical scenarios involving aortic aneurysms and coincident intraabdominal pathology may be generally separated into four distinct categories: elective operation for aortic pathology with incidental finding of asymptomatic nonvascular pathology; emergent operation for presumed symptomatic aortic pathology with incidental findings of nonvascular pathology; emergent operation for abdominal pathology with incidental finding of an aortic aneurysm; and elective operation for abdominal pathology with incidental finding of an aortic aneurysm. This chapter describes each of these scenarios, focusing on those clinical entities most commonly encountered.

ELECTIVE ABDOMINAL AORTIC ANEURYSM REPAIR AND ASYMPTOMATIC ABDOMINAL DISEASE

Virtually every patient undergoing an elective aneurysm repair, either EVAR or open, has undergone a preoperative CT scan. When asymptomatic intraabdominal disease is discovered on CT scan prior to EVAR, the surgeon is generally able to choose whether to proceed with EVAR or to treat the concomitant pathology first. Because EVAR is so well tolerated and causes minimal physiologic derangement, the aneurysm can typically be repaired without significantly delaying the subsequent treatment of other time-sensitive pathology, such as cancer. Furthermore, the peritoneal cavity is left untouched by EVAR, permitting a clean laparotomy for other intraabdominal interventions. Even in an era of extensive preoperative imaging prior to elective open AAA repairs, unrecognized pathology is occasionally discovered. Frequently this identified pathology will have either been too small to appear on CT scan or will have been of a nature making it unlikely to appear. At this point the surgeon has three options: continue the open AAA without any other concomitant surgical procedure, abandon the AAA and treat the concomitant condition first, or attempt simultaneous treatment of both AAA and the unexpected pathology. The decision depends on the type and severity of abnormality found. If the surgeon elects to continue the AAA repair without synchronous treatment of concomitant disease, it must be recognized that the patient may not have another opportunity for the secondary disease process to be safely addressed for quite some time because of the need for the patient to recover from the physiologic insult of a major open vascular procedure in the immediate postoperative period and the well-recognized risk of reoperative laparotomy because of adhesion formation in the intermediate term. If the surgeon elects to treat only the concomitant pathology without treating the AAA, the increased risk of aneurysm rupture caused by delay in repair must be considered. Because open AAA repair is almost always reserved only for those aneurysms large enough to exhibit an elevated risk of rupture, this risk should not be considered insignificant. If the surgeon chooses to address both problems simultaneously, he or she must be willing to accept the potentially increased morbidity of putting a patient through two procedures instead of one, lengthening anesthetic time and increasing blood loss. Furthermore, resection of the concomitant pathology may require opening the gastrointestinal or biliary tracts, thereby potentially increasing the risk of an aortic prosthetic graft infection, a devastating complication. The most commonly encountered abnormalities include cholelithiasis, appendix and Meckel's diverticulum, gastrointestinal malignancies, genitourinary malignancies, and solid organ tumors.

Cholelithiasis

Cholelithiasis is found in up to 20% of AAA laparotomies. When noted, the surgeon must choose whether to leave the gallstones alone because simultaneous treatment may increase the chances of graft infection or perform a cholecystectomy to avoid the risk of postoperative cholecystitis or choledocholithiasis. Because cholecystectomy can generally be performed quickly with a minimum of blood loss, the greatest factor at play is the elevated risk of graft infection associated with opening the biliary tract.

This topic was once a subject of much debate in the literature, with some citing an elevated risk of cholecystitis in the postoperative period. However, as advances in minimally invasive and interventional radiologic techniques have improved our ability to treat gallbladder disease, the weight of opinion has shifted away from synchronous cholecystectomy. Laparoscopic cholecystectomy, transhepatic biliary stenting, and endoscopic retrograde cholangiopancreatography (ERCP) have permitted symptomatic cholelithiasis and choledocholithiasis to be safely treated almost always without the need for second laparotomy.

Because any AAA repair, open or endovascular, requires close postoperative follow-up, the patient may be screened in the postoperative period for any signs or symptoms suggestive of symptomatic cholelithiasis and referred for elective laparoscopic cholecystectomy when indicated. Patients with recognized gallstone disease should be educated in dietary modification and should be considered for treatment with ursodiol.

Appendix and Meckel's Diverticulum

Because of the significant risk of aortic prosthetic infection associated with opening the gastrointestinal tract, asymptomatic appendices and Meckel's diverticula should unequivocally be left alone during an open AAA repair. Incidental discovery of acute appendicitis during an open AAA repair would be a rare occurrence indeed, but if discovered, it would certainly need to be resected. A more challenging dilemma arises if evidence of a chronically inflamed appendix or Meckel's diverticulum is discovered. The risk-benefit ratio would still argue against synchronous resection, *unless the inflammation indeed appears to be acute*. Advances in laparoscopic management of appendix and Meckel's diverticula have made resection following AAA repair, even in the immediate postoperative period, quite feasible, with a low likelihood of need for repeat laparotomy. In the setting of acute appendicitis with gross purulence, appendectomy followed by interval aneurysms repair is the preferred approach.

GASTROINTESTINAL MALIGNANCIES

Gastrointestinal (GI) malignancies are notoriously difficult to identify on CT scans. Furthermore, aortic aneurysms and GI malignancies tend to occur in the same patient populations: in smokers and in those older than age 50 years. Thus, the discovery of previously unrecognized colorectal or small bowel malignancies at the time of laparotomy for AAA repair is a relatively common occurrence. Colorectal cancers (CRCs) are most common, with an estimated frequency of concurrence with AAA of between 0.49% and 2.1%. Therefore, the occasional discovery of synchronous GI malignancies would most certainly be encountered in high-volume vascular centers.

Concomitant surgical correction of both CRC and AAA is considered controversial because of the magnitude of a combined operation. Generally, a staged procedure is recommended, with the order of treatment depending on the judged severity of each condition; a 4- to 6-week period of convalescence between open operations is usually required to maximize the patient's physiologic reserve. However, intervention for CRC can often be accelerated by employing less invasive laparoscopic and endovascular methods. Unfortunately, during this period, the untreated pathology may worsen or become symptomatic. Repairing the AAA first postpones colectomy and risks metastasis of colorectal cancer, whereas starting with colectomy leaves the patient at risk of death from rupture of the aneurysm. Synchronous treatment, on the other hand, avoids the need for a second operation, which may not be well tolerated in the frail vascular surgical population; postoperative recovery may be faster from a psychological point of view as well.

Lin and colleagues (Lin P, et al., 2008) published a multicenter retrospective review of 108 patients with concomitant CRC and AAA. Among the 35 cases in which CRC was treated first followed by staged open aneurysm repair, Lin observed that two patients (6%) died after their initial CRC resection with autopsy results of both patients confirming aortic aneurysm rupture as the cause of death. Among the 11 patients who underwent CRC resection first followed by staged EVAR, two (18%) developed sigmoid ischemia after EVAR, requiring immediate laparotomy and sigmoidectomy. Among the 26 patients who underwent AAA repair first, the time to subsequent colectomy was significantly delayed when compared to other cohorts and averaged 115 days. Finally, those patients who underwent EVAR as either the primary or staged operation required a significantly shorter cumulative hospital length of stay. While no graft infections were identified during the study period in the eight patients undergoing combined open AAA repair and CRC resection, the authors argued that the possibility of such infections is a substantial enough concern to prompt avoidance of a combined approach. Lastly, because of the increased risk of aortic rupture after abdominal operations, Lin recommended that patients with asymptomatic synchronous CRC and AAA of greater than 5 cm undergo aneurysm repair first to reduce the risk of perioperative aneurysm rupture.

Shalhoub and colleagues (Shalhoub J, et al., 2009) published a review of 24 cases from prospectively maintained databases of patients with concurrent colorectal malignancy and abdominal aortic aneurysms. In patients undergoing staged management with colectomy first, they documented no interval aneurysm ruptures. However, in their series, patients with large aneurysms underwent EVAR prior to colectomy. The authors concluded that staged management is a reasonable approach with a low risk of aneurysm rupture, though simultaneous repair may be performed in patients with obstructing CRC with an aneurysm that is less than 6 cm, where the risk of interval AAA rupture is significant. They also stressed the usefulness of EVAR in preventing delay of CRC management. It may be preferable to perform EVAR first for a large aneurysm; the patient is discharged home within 24 hours and is able to undergo colectomy, usually via laparoscopic approach, in the next 2 to 4 weeks. In one case, an 8-cm AAA was discovered incidentally on preoperative CT scan for colon adenocarcinoma in a 72-year-old man. He underwent EVAR followed by laparoscopic hemicolectomy 3 weeks later and was cancer free with a stable aneurysm at his 2-year follow-up.

Should the surgeon opt to proceed with synchronous resection, excellent surgical technique with control of peritoneal contamination is a must if graft infection is to be avoided. Preoperative administration of antibiotics and aggressive bowel preparation should also be performed if the cancer was recognized preoperatively. If EVAR is not an option in the setting of a nearly obstructing left-sided colorectal lesion, a temporary transverse colostomy can be performed at the conclusion of open AAA repair.

Discoveries of small bowel and gastric tumors have also been reported, with patients undergoing simultaneous enterectomies or gastrectomies. In such cases, a management algorithm similar to that described above for colorectal malignancies is best followed. Patients should be staged when possible, unless the acuity of each condition individually is felt to be so high as to mandate synchronous intervention.

Genitourinary Malignancies

Renal carcinoma, unless large or invasive, may go unrecognized if aneurysms are approached via midline laparotomy. The chance of discovering a synchronous renal mass is increased with the retroperitoneal approach.

Synchronous repair of AAA and nephrectomy have been described, with a low risk of bacterial graft contamination. Although synchronous treatment avoids necessitating a second retroperitoneal exploration, a staged approach should be used if the AAA repair is particularly difficult or if intraoperative blood loss is significant. Additionally, patients with known reduced preoperative kidney function may benefit from a staged approach with more meticulous operative planning. In Figure 1, a frail vasculopath presented with a tender abdominal aneurysm, right flank pain, and a right renal mass on CT scan. He underwent endovascular AAA repair, followed by catheter-directed radiofrequency ablation of the renal tumor.

In cases of bladder or prostate cancer, the risk of urinary bacterial contamination is higher. Although there are reports of simultaneous resection of aggressive bladder cancer and aneurysm repair, a staged approach would be considered most prudent to minimize the risk of bacterial graft contamination.

A prospective study by Grego (Grego F, 2003) compared simultaneous aneurysmectomy and radical cystoprostatectomy with a staged procedure and found no statistically significant difference in the outcome and morbidity. Preoperative renal function must be assessed before a concomitant operation, as an early trend toward increased mortality was found by Grego in those patients with preoperative moderate renal insufficiency. Again, aneurysm size matters here: an AAA greater than 5 cm may undergo a simultaneous operation, and smaller AAAs may be staged, also considering EVAR if possible.

Solid Organ Tumors

Solid tumors of the spleen, liver, and adrenal gland have also been documented and successfully resected at the time of AAA repair.

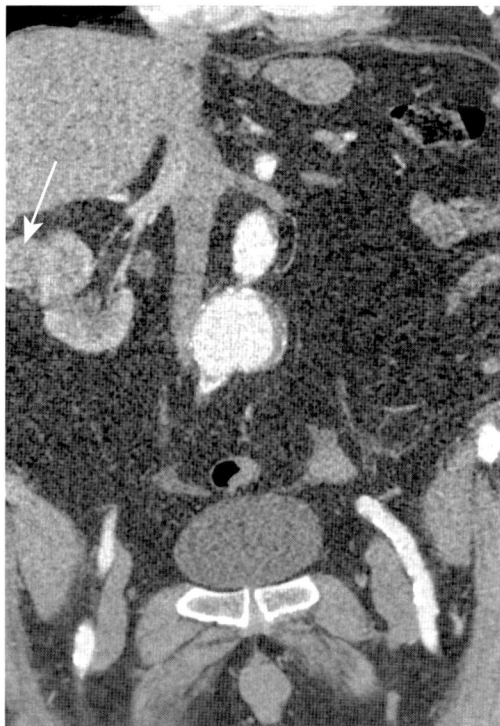

FIGURE 1   Abdominal aortic aneurysm (computed tomographic scan).

Given the typically sterile nature of these organs, simultaneous resection appears reasonable as long as the patient can physiologically tolerate the blood loss and additional anesthetic time associated with the second procedure.

EMERGENT ABDOMINAL AORTIC ANEURYSM REPAIR AND CONCOMITANT DISEASE

Emergent AAA repair is indicated in two situations: with symptomatic AAA and ruptured AAA (rAAA). Imaging studies are usually available in the first case but not necessarily in the latter because of the extreme urgency of the condition and need for prompt transport to the operating room. In either case, the first priority is aneurysm repair, after which the major goal should be for prompt and aggressive resuscitation in the intensive care unit. Pursuing other intraabdominal findings at this time would be ill advised unless they were deemed to be life threatening in nature.

Among patients with a symptomatic but unruptured AAA and a synchronous intraabdominal lesion, the prioritization of conditions should depend on the severity and related mortality risk of each. Symptomatic AAAs are believed to represent aneurysms in the initial stages of rupture, suggesting that the risk of leaving them untreated would be significant. However, if a concomitant intraabdominal condition is considered life threatening or extremely urgent, aneurysm repair could conceivably be temporarily delayed. If the AAA is massive or is demonstrating early signs of rupture on visual inspection, synchronous open repair would be necessary. Thankfully, the concurrence of two such unrelated yet life-threatening conditions is a rare event.

The treatment of ruptured AAAs is shifting away from open repair toward EVAR when technically possible, with studies indicating a 30% mortality rate reduction in EVAR cohorts. Unexpected concomitant disease may be evident on preoperative imaging conducted for EVAR planning but is otherwise unlikely to be discovered. Even if other pathology is noted preoperatively, treatment of the aneurysm always takes first priority. However, if suspicion develops during EVAR of a synchronous intraabdominal catastrophe, aneurysm repair may need to be followed by diagnostic laparoscopy or exploratory laparotomy prior to transport to the ICU.

Unfortunately, patients in whom control of aneurysmal bleeding has been achieved and aortic continuity restored may nevertheless have suffered enough visceral ischemia during the procedure to develop bowel necrosis. In such cases, clearly nonviable bowel should be resected prior to returning the patient to the ICU for resuscitation, and the abdomen should be left open for marginal bowel to be inspected 24 to 48 hours later.

EMERGENT LAPAROTOMY FOR SYMPTOMATIC ABDOMINAL PATHOLOGY WITH INCIDENTAL ASYMPTOMATIC ABDOMINAL AORTIC ANEURYSM

A broad spectrum of emergent intraabdominal pathologies may bring a patient to the operating room without prior CT imaging. Possible scenarios include blunt or penetrating abdominal trauma, severe lactic acidosis of suspected intraabdominal origin, obvious bowel obstruction in a virgin abdomen, or clear perforation with peritonitis, to name only a few.

Clearly, acute intraabdominal pathology must be prioritized and treated first, and any life-threatening conditions should be addressed promptly. If the aneurysm is found to be exceedingly large or at imminent risk for rupture, either an intraoperative or prompt postoperative vascular surgical consult should be sought.

Operations for intraabdominal infectious conditions, such as perforated viscus or infected necrotizing pancreatitis, make open aneurysm repair in the near-term time frame prohibitively dangerous given the high likelihood of graft infection. If at all possible, the patient should be considered for endovascular repair, as this prevents infected peritoneal contents from ever coming into contact with prosthetic material.

If the patient did not undergo preoperative imaging or was taken for laparotomy based solely upon clinical impression, it is important to ascertain whether the patient's acute presentation (e.g., abdominal pain) was actually a result of the anticipated nonvascular pathology or was rather stemming from the aneurysm. If laparotomy is otherwise negative for findings explaining severe abdominal pain, a symptomatic aneurysm in the early stages of rupture should be added to the differential diagnosis, and a vascular surgeon should be consulted intraoperatively for prompt assessment. Consideration for abdominal closure and prompt CT imaging for possible EVAR should be made in the absence of a ruptured AAA.

Necrotic small bowel with superior mesenteric artery (SMA) compromise in the setting of AAA should also prompt an urgent vascular surgical consultation. Aneurysmal thrombus or dissection could account for a sudden SMA ostial thrombosis. This life-threatening condition would require emergent revascularization, with or without concomitant aneurysm repair.

ELECTIVE LAPAROTOMY FOR ABDOMINAL PATHOLOGY WITH INCIDENTAL ASYMPTOMATIC ABDOMINAL AORTIC ANEURYSM

With the frequent use of preoperative imaging studies in preparation for elective intraabdominal surgeries, the unexpected discovery of AAA at laparotomy is rare. The discovery of an unexpected aneurysm may be alarming, especially to an operating surgeon who in all likelihood is not a vascular specialist. Unless the aneurysm is exceedingly large or appears to be at imminent risk for rupture, it is probably reasonable for the surgeon to proceed with the planned abdominal operation. A vascular surgeon should be consulted either intraoperatively or promptly following the conclusion of the operation to assess the aneurysm and the patient's suitability for repair. Given the need for high-quality preoperative CT angiography, as well as specialized equipment including fluoroscopy, synchronous EVAR in such a situation is generally not feasible. However, patients with aneurysms larger than 5 cm may be considered for prompt endovascular repair in the perioperative period. Patients with unfavorable anatomy for EVAR may do better with a more extended convalescent interval provided they are followed closely and warned about the signs and symptoms associated with AAA expansion or rupture.

SUMMARY

Although several case series and theoretical models do exist in the literature addressing the topic of AAA repair and synchronous disease management, much of the decision making depends on basic surgical principles of infection control, relative risk of the underlying pathologies encountered, and minimization of patient morbidity. Several general recommendations may be followed:

1. Emergent AAA repair takes priority over any concomitant disease.
2. Any nonlethal, nonvascular pathology discovered during elective AAA repair may be left alone at that time.
3. Incidental AAA found during emergent or elective laparotomy should be promptly evaluated by a vascular surgeon in the

immediate perioperative period; if large enough to represent a rupture risk, it should be addressed soon thereafter, preferably via EVAR.

4. Meticulous surgical technique must be followed if the gastrointestinal or biliary tracts are to be violated during a synchronous aneurysmectomy, as aortic graft infection is a highly lethal complication.

SUGGESTED READINGS

Baxter NN, Noel AA, Cherry K, et al: Management of patients with colorectal cancer and concomitant abdominal aortic aneurysm, *Dis Colon Rectum* 45:165, 2002.

Grego F, Lepidi S, Bassi P, et al: Simultaneous surgical treatment of abdominal aortic aneurysm and carcinoma of the bladder, *Vasc Surg* 37(3):607–614, 2003.

Lin PH, Barshes NR, Albo D, et al: Concomitant colorectal cancer and abdominal aortic aneurysm: Evolution of treatment paradigm in the endovascular era, *J Am Coll Surg* 206:1065–1075, 2008.

Matsumoto K, Nakamaru M, Obara H, et al: Surgical strategy for abdominal aortic aneurysm with concurrent symptomatic malignancy, *World J Surg* 23(3):248–251, 1999.

Ouriel K, Ricotta JJ, Adams JT, et al: Management of cholelithiasis in patients with abdominal aortic aneurysm, *Ann Surg* 198:717, 1983.

Prusa AM, Wolff KS, Sahal M, et al: Abdominal aortic aneurysms and concomitant disease requiring surgical intervention: simultaneous operation versus staged treatment using endoluminal stent grafting, *Arch Surg* 140:686, 2005.

Shalhoub J, Naughton P, Lau N, et al: Concurrent colorectal malignancy and abdominal aortic aneurysm: a multicentre experience and review of the literature, *EurJ Vasc Endovasc Surg* 37:544–556, 2009.

Sung HH, Park BK, Kim CK, et al: Comparison of percutaneous radiofrequency ablation and open partial nephrectomy for the treatment of size- and location-matched renal masses, *Int J Hyperthermia* 28(3):227–234, 2012.

Valanovich A, Andersen CA: Concomitant abdominal aortic aneurysm and colorectal cancer: a decision analysis approach to the therapeutic dilemma, *Ann Vasc Surg* 5:449, 1991.

THE MANAGEMENT OF THORACIC AND THORACOABDOMINAL AORTIC ANEURYSMS

R. Todd Lancaster, MD, MPH, and Richard P. Cambria, MD

INTRODUCTION

Descending thoracic aortic aneurysms (DTAAs) involve the segment of the aorta bounded by the origin of the left subclavian artery and the diaphragm. Thoracoabdominal aortic aneurysms (TAAAs) involve the visceral aortic segment and varying degrees of the thoracic and abdominal aortas in accordance with the anatomic classification devised by Crawford (Figure 1). These aneurysms are uncommon when compared with isolated infrarenal aneurysms, comprising no more than 2% to 5% of the spectrum of aortic aneurysms.

In contrast to degenerative aneurysms associated with the abdominal aorta, the thoracic aorta is involved in a broader spectrum of pathologies, which are potentially etiologic in the formation of aneurysms. Examples of these include dissection, connective tissue disorders, aortitis, and trauma. Open surgical management of diseases of the thoracic aorta is accompanied by significant morbidity and mortality rates compared with repair of abdominal aortic aneurysms (AAAs). The emergence of stent-graft repair of the thoracic aorta, however, has substantially diminished the morbidity of surgical repair for many patients; although its role in certain pathologies such as degenerative aneurysm of the descending thoracic aorta and acute traumatic tear is well established, its ultimate utility in acute and chronic dissection remains the subject of ongoing study.

Patients with aneurysms in these locations are often diagnosed incidentally on radiographic imaging; however, up to 40% of patients will present with symptoms. These symptoms are related to compression or erosion of nearby structures or to inflammation of the mediastinal pleura. When symptomatic, patients with aneurysmal dilation of the thoracic aorta may manifest back pain, hoarseness, dysphagia, cough, and, of course, rupture. The final point to be made in this regard is that such back pain mediated by large thoracic aneurysms can be chronic in nature, somewhat different from the paradigm typically associated with symptomatic AAA. In particular, large aneurysms involving the visceral aortic segment can lead to a syndrome of both epigastric and back pain; the latter can be severe when vertebral body erosion occurs. As would be intuitively expected, such symptoms have been correlated in natural history studies with increased rupture risk.

INDICATIONS FOR SURGERY

Longitudinal studies have found that the mean rate of growth for all thoracic aneurysms is 0.1 cm per year. Not surprisingly, increasing aneurysm size is associated with higher rupture risk. Rupture, which carries a 90% mortality rate, accounts for 30% of all deaths in patients with thoracic aneurysms, occurring with an incidence rate of 3.5 per 100,000 patient-years. Risk factors for rupture include increasing patient age, pain (including atypical pain), other symptoms attributable to the aneurysm, a history of chronic obstructive pulmonary disease (COPD), and dissection developing within a degenerative aneurysm. Population-based studies have indicated an overall 5-year rupture risk of 20%, with 80% of ruptures occurring in women. In fact, female gender has been identified as an independent variable predicting aneurysm rupture (relative risk [RR] 6.8; 95% confidence interval [CI], 2.3-19.9; $P = 0.01$).

DTAAs appear to expand at more rapid rates as they become larger, and several investigators have correlated increased expansion rates with rupture. Furthermore, studies have indicated that rupture risk is negligible in aneurysms less than 5 cm, equivalent to the risk of surgical morbidity in the 5-cm to 6-cm range, and increases substantially at aneurysm diameters larger than 6 cm and/or growth rates of 10 mm or more per year. These natural history observations have led to the acceptance of 6 cm as a generally appropriate size threshold for recommendation of surgical intervention in patients with degenerative DTAAs and TAAAs. Increasing expansion rate is used as an indicator of heightened rupture risk, as is the presence of symptoms, and in such cases, consideration is given to earlier operation. In the cases of chronic dissection and Marfan's syndrome, a 5-cm size threshold is maintained because of rupture proclivity at

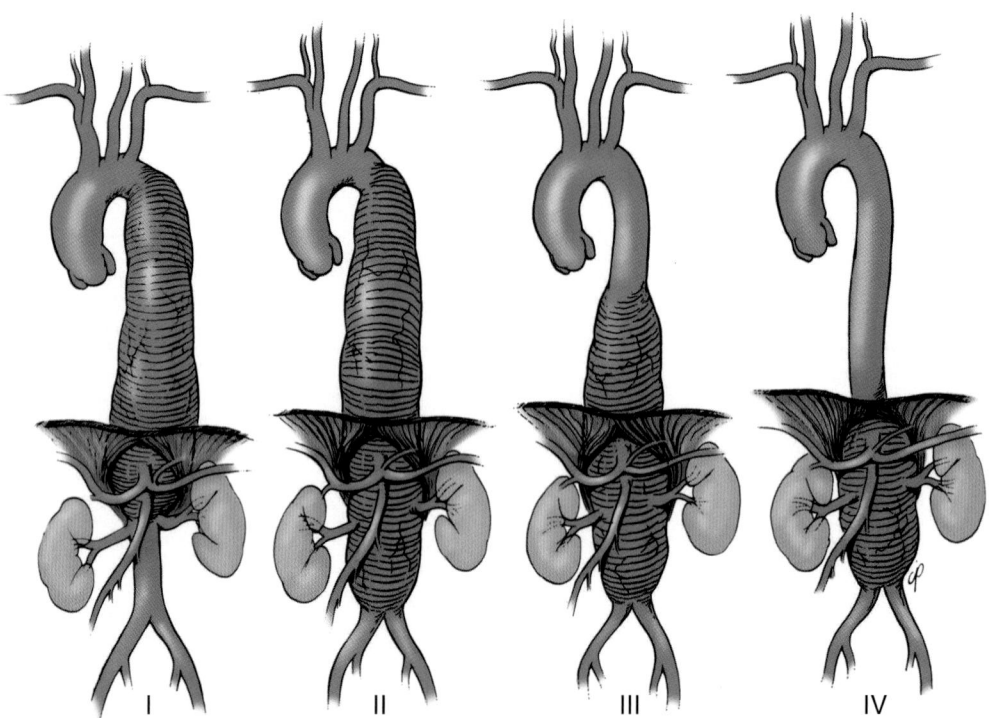

FIGURE 1 Crawford classification scheme for thoracoabdominal aortic aneurysm.

I   II   III   IV

smaller sizes; in addition, many such patients are considerably younger than the typical patient with a degenerative lesion.

PREOPERATIVE RISK ASSESSMENT

The Crawford classification describes TAAA based on the extent of aortic resection and, in many cases, can be considered caudal extension of a descending thoracic aortic (DTA) lesion (e.g., extent I TAAA) or cephalad extension of a total abdominal aneurysm (e.g., extent IV TAAA). This classification is useful clinically since it has direct implications for both the technical conduct of operation and the incidence of operative complications, especially ischemic spinal cord injury (SCI).

An accurate assessment of associated comorbid conditions (especially cardiac, pulmonary, and renal comorbidities) is mandatory to guide appropriate decision making with respect to recommending open surgical repair. All patients should be evaluated with dipyridamole thallium scanning, or the equivalent thereof, to assess perioperative myocardial ischemic potential. In addition, patients with a history of symptoms suggestive of heart failure should have an assessment of left ventricular function. Cardiac catheterization may be appropriate for patients with evidence of coronary ischemic potential on physiologic testing, or with an ejection fraction of less than 30%. However, ischemic cardiomyopathy in this range generally precludes open operation. Patients who have severe coronary disease and asymptomatic aneurysms may undergo myocardial revascularization prior to aneurysm repair, as the clinical scenario dictates.

While patients with significant impairments of pulmonary reserve can usually be detected on the basis of history alone, we have a low threshold for obtaining preoperative pulmonary function studies in patients with extent I-III TAAA. Limited pulmonary reserve is a common consideration in deciding to forego formal open repair. Yet COPD itself is a well-documented risk factor for aneurysm expansion and rupture. Advanced age is an important component only inasmuch as it is accompanied by overall fragility and impaired functional status.

The coexistence of renovascular disease and some degree of renal insufficiency is especially commonplace in patients with TAAA and has important implications for accurate assessment of perioperative risk and long-term preservation of renal function. In our experience, 15% of patients had significant renal insufficiency as manifested by a preoperative serum creatinine of 1.8 mg/dL or higher. In many series, the presence of an abnormal preoperative serum creatinine is at least a univariate correlate of perioperative mortality, largely related to an increased risk of perioperative renal failure. Although the potential for restoration of renal function by correction of renovascular lesions exists in some patients, advanced renal dysfunction constitutes a relative contraindication to elective operations.

Associated vascular diseases and comorbid conditions are commonplace in patients presenting for treatment of thoracic aneurysms. Synchronous aneurysms typically involving the ascending aorta or arch have been observed in some 10% of patients being evaluated for DTAA or TAAA repair. Prior operation for aortic aneurysm disease is seen in one third of patients, and the most common of these is a previous infrarenal aneurysm repair. Additionally, up to one quarter of patients with thoracic aortic disease have concomitant AAA; therefore, all patients should undergo baseline imaging of the entire aorta at the time of initial diagnosis.

OPEN SURGICAL MANAGEMENT

The choice of surgical technique varies as a function of aneurysm extent and complexity. The two general approaches involve a clamp-and-sew technique (often supplemented by adjuncts to minimize complications related to spinal cord, renal and visceral ischemia) versus the use of distal aortic perfusion through an atriofemoral bypass (AFB) circuit. Although distal perfusion has been favored as a technique for repairing isolated thoracic aneurysms, some centers report comparable results using both clamp-and-sew and distal perfusion techniques. Variations in operative technique largely have been driven by the effort to minimize the major complications of SCI and renal failure. Sufficient experience and review of end results support the selective application of adjuncts such as cerebrospinal fluid (CSF) drainage, distal aortic perfusion, intercostal reconstruction, and renal hypothermic perfusion.

Adjuncts for Organ Protection

Our institutional experience over the past quarter-century has evolved from a clamp-and-sew technique (with adjuncts such as epidural cooling) to one that favors distal aortic perfusion with motor evoked potential (MEP) monitoring for extent I-III TAAA. The clamp-and-sew technique, with emphasis on surgical simplicity and expediency, continues to be applied for extent IV TAAA with favorable results. Among spinal cord protective adjuncts, only CSF drainage is supported by a robust evidence base. The benefits of routine intercostal reconstruction have been questioned in the context of the "collateral network concept," which de-emphasizes the importance of individual intercostals arteries, since these vessels are generally interconnected in the paraspinous musculature and well collateralized via the hypogastric arteries, as demonstrated in magnetic resonance imaging studies. Based on these data, our approach to TAAA repair has evolved to emphasize intraoperative support of the collateral network through distal aortic perfusion and selective intercostal reconstruction based on MEP monitoring. The latter provides real-time assessment of spinal cord nutritive circulation during the conduct of operation.

Renal protection is achieved through the direct installation of renal preservation fluid (4° C lactated Ringer's with 25 g of mannitol per liter and 1 g methyl prednisolone per liter) into the renal artery ostia after the aorta is opened, thus causing a rapid decline of renal core temperature. This is important because of the significant impact of postoperative renal failure (defined as a doubling of baseline creatinine or absolute level >3.0 mg/dL) on operative mortality. Indeed, in our experience, patients who sustained significant postoperative renal failure had an eightfold increase in their mortality risk (OR 7.8; 95% CI, 3.4-17.9; P <0.0001). Equally important to renal protection is renal artery reconstruction, either secondary to their location with respect to the aneurysm or because of orificial stenosis. Whereas the left renal artery is generally managed with a side-arm bypass graft, treatment of right renal artery stenosis is more challenging through a left flank incision. Our practice is to use balloon-expandable stents placed directly into the ostia for right renal artery reconstruction during TAAA repair for either orificial stenosis or, if technical issues arise with inclusion, button reconstruction of the right renal artery (Figure 2). Review of our own experience shows that after a mean follow-up of 405 days, 98% of renal stents were patent, suggesting that placement of balloon-expandable stents is a durable form of renal artery reconstruction during TAAA repair.

The final adjunct in our overall approach involves in-line mesenteric shunting, again also selectively applied in accordance with aneurysm complexity, anticipated duration of mesenteric ischemia, or both. As displayed in Figure 3, immediately after performance of the proximal anastomosis, pro-grade pulsatile perfusion can be established into either the celiac axis or superior mesenteric artery (preferred) to minimize visceral ischemic time and its potential contribution to coagulopathic bleeding. When combined with distal aortic perfusion during performance of the proximal anastomosis, such in-line mesenteric shunting often results in 10 minutes or less of visceral ischemia. Obviously, the same concept can be achieved by creating a Y-circuit on the AFB cannulae setup, but this can be clumsy to position intraprocedurally.

Operative Technique

Irrespective of individual preferences concerning protective adjuncts, the key to operative success remains the provision of broad, continuous exposure of the entire left posterolateral aspect of the

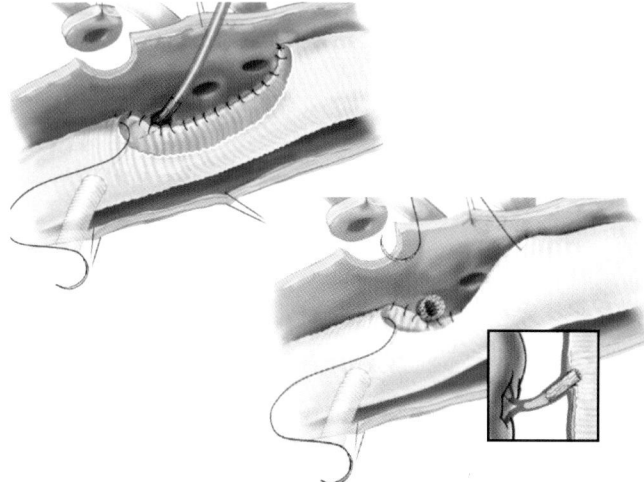

FIGURE 2 Treatment of right renal artery stenosis via a left flank incision. Placement of a balloon-expandable stent is favored over orificial endarterectomy.

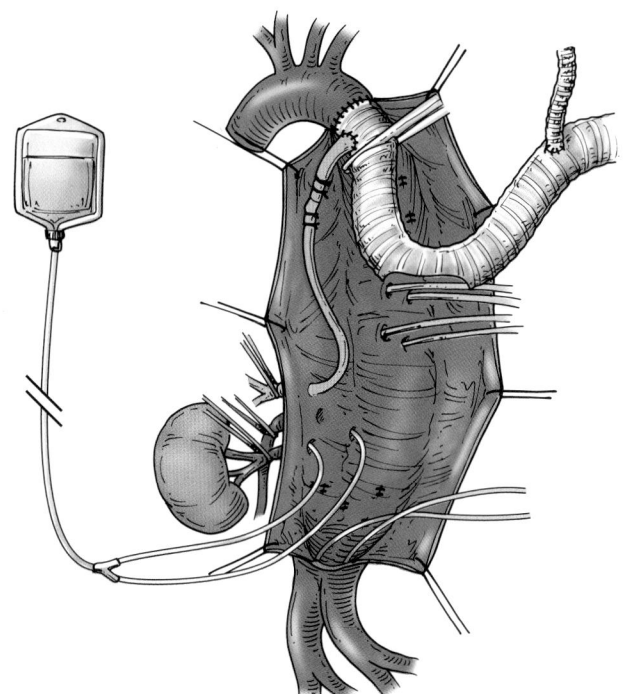

FIGURE 3 After completion of the proximal anastomosis, in select cases, a side-arm graft is used for in-line mesenteric shunting to the celiac or superior mesenteric artery.

thoracoabdominal aorta (Figure 4). The patient is positioned on the table in the right lateral decubitus position. The location and extent of the thoracic portion of the incision is determined by the proximal extent of the aneurysm as the posterior portion of a standard posterolateral thoracotomy incision is only necessary for type I and type II aneurysms. We keep the thoracic portion of the incision low and have found that the fifth or sixth interspace with posterior division of the sixth or seventh ribs provides adequate exposure for even the more proximal aneurysms. The costal margin is divided at the level of the sixth interspace, and a self-retaining retractor system is placed to ensure continuous exposure of the entire operative field (Figure 5). A thoracoabdominal incision at the eighth interspace will usually provide adequate exposure for a type IV aneurysm, and a double

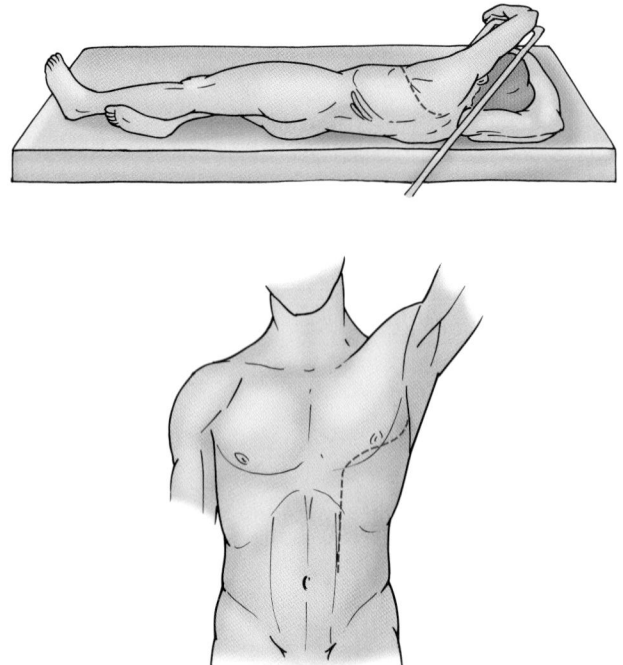

FIGURE 4   Thoracoabdominal incision. The patient is positioned in the right lateral decubitus condition. The interspace through which the incision is carried is determined by the proximal and distal extent of the aneurysm.

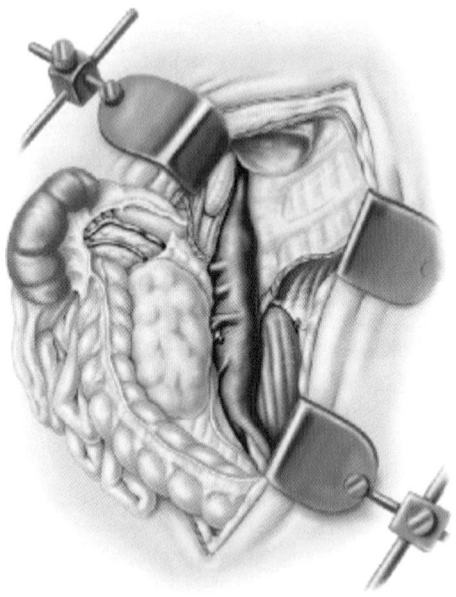

FIGURE 5   A self-retaining retractor is used to provide broad, continuous exposure of the left posterolateral aspect of the thoracoabdominal aorta.

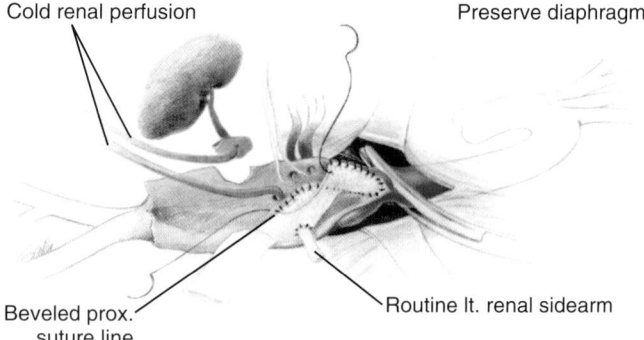

Cold renal perfusion   Preserve diaphragm

Beveled prox. suture line   Routine lt. renal sidearm

FIGURE 6   In the majority of extent IV TAAA repairs, the anatomy is suitable for a simplified reconstruction with a beveled proximal anastomosis with a left renal side-arm graft.

lumen tube for deflation of the left lung is generally not necessary in these cases. The abdominal portion of the incision is not extended to the midline; rather, it is kept well lateral on the abdominal wall. The advantage of this approach is that it allows the visceral contents to lie within the abdominal cavity, thus decreasing evaporative fluid and heat losses. The abdominal portion of the incision is transperitoneal, thus allowing direct inspection and assessment of the visceral circulation when the case is completed. We have found no advantage,

and indeed increased bleeding, when attempting to keep the abdominal portion of the incision extraperitoneal.

In the repair of extent IV TAAA, we use limited lateral division of the diaphragm, preserving its phrenic innervation. Subsequently, for the majority of these lesions, the operative field is set up in a totally infradiaphragmatic orientation. The repair is undertaken using a clamp-and-sew technique with routine renal hypothermic perfusion. We do not employ the use of a double-lumen endotracheal tube or that of CSF drainage. In the majority of our experience (93%), the patient's anatomy is suitable for a simplified reconstruction with a single-beveled proximal anastomosis (Figure 6).

For repair of extent I-IV TAAA, exposure of the left posterolateral aspect of the abdominal aorta is obtained by entering the plane posterior to the spleen, left kidney, and left colon (Figure 7). The abdominal contents are then reflected to the patient's right, and the left ureter is identified and preserved under laparotomy pads. The retroperitoneal fatty and lymphatic tissues overlying the aorta are transected with electrocautery, and the large posterior branch of the left renal vein that courses across the aorta is identified and divided. Located topographically close to this vein is the left renal artery (Figure 8). Once identified, the left renal artery is dissected back toward its origin on the aorta, which serves as a suitable point to initiate the cephalad and caudad division of the retroperitoneal tissues over the aorta inferiorly and division of the median arcuate ligament and diaphragmatic crura superiorly.

There are several methods by which the incision in the diaphragm may be managed (Figure 9). The quickest and simplest method that affords excellent exposure is direct radial division of the central tendon of the diaphragm from underneath the costal margin to the aortic hiatus. This approach, however, will irrevocably paralyze the left hemidiaphragm and ultimately contribute to postoperative respiratory embarrassment. A second approach involves the circumferential division of the diaphragm through its muscular portion, leaving a few centimeters attached laterally to the chest wall; this method is both time consuming and bloody. When the surgeon elects to preserve diaphragmatic innervation in an extent I-III lesion, a large Penrose drain can be passed around the diaphragm pedicle and used to retract superiorly and inferiorly as needed during the reconstruction. We have applied this method liberally, particularly in patients with evidence of preoperative pulmonary compromise.

After deflation of the left lung, the thoracic component of the dissection is typically straightforward. Electrocautery is used to divide the mediastinal pleura over the aneurysm and proximal aorta. For type I and type II aneurysms, proximal control of the aorta in the region of the left subclavian artery origin is necessary. Mobility of the vagus nerve is gained by dividing it distal to the origin of the left recurrent nerve, which should be identified and preserved. Should more proximal control be necessary, the ligamentum

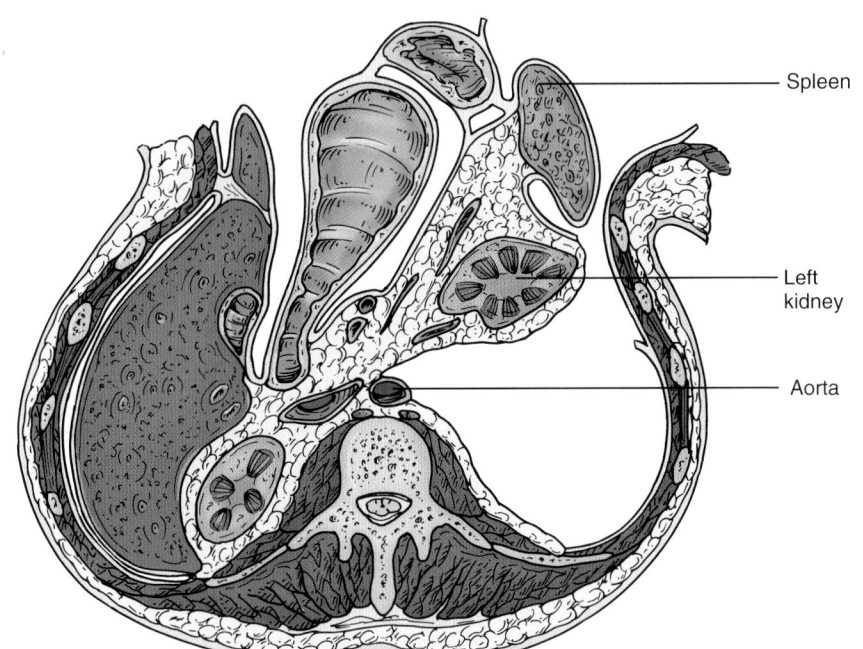

Spleen

Left
kidney

Aorta

FIGURE 7 Exposure of the left posterolateral aspect of the thoracoabdominal aorta is obtained by entering the plane posterior to the spleen, left kidney, and left colon.

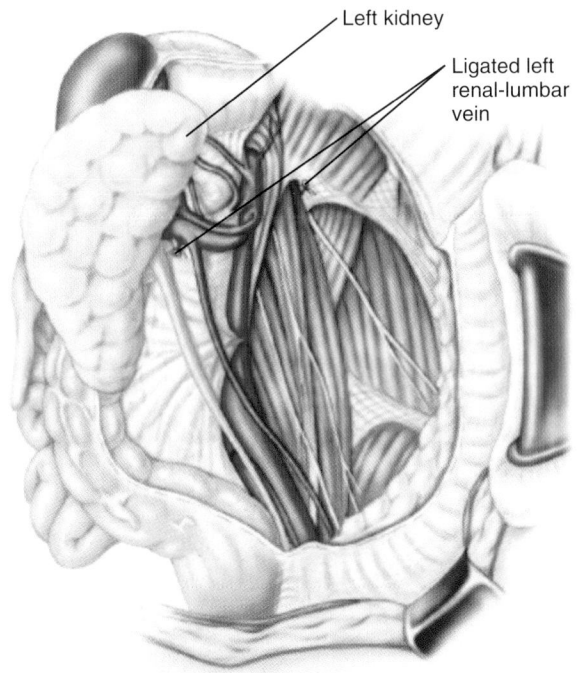

Left kidney

Ligated left
renal-lumbar
vein

FIGURE 8 The posteriorly coursing left renal-lumbar vein is divided as it lies across the aorta. This vein is located topographically close to the left renal artery.

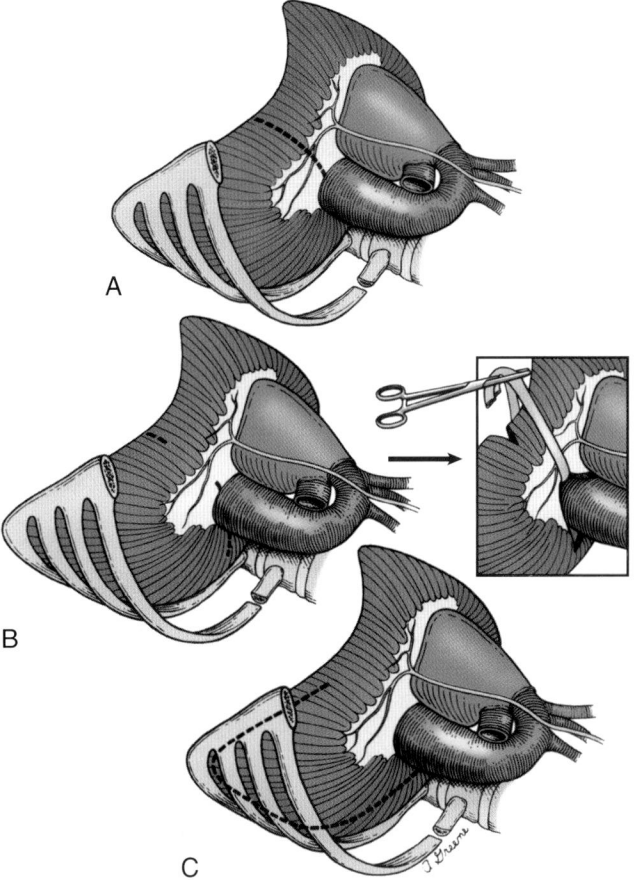

A

B

C

FIGURE 9 Various methods for management of the diaphragm. **A,** Direct radial division, including division of the phrenic nerve. **B,** Radial division of the diaphragm with preservation of the phrenic nerve. **C,** Circumferential division of the diaphragm through the muscular portion.

arteriosum is divided on the underside of the aortic arch. Care must be taken to keep the dissection directly on the aortic arch to avoid injuring the left main pulmonary artery. When degenerative aneurysm is the underlying pathology, exposure in this area is usually straightforward. However, in patients with chronic dissection, the prior inflammation from the dissecting process makes exposure more difficult. The aorta is surrounded with a vessel tape on either side of the left subclavian artery depending on the proximal extent of the aneurysm. Blunt dissection on the posterior aspect of the aorta is used to clear sufficient normal aorta to allow placement of the cross clamp while maintaining adequate length of aorta for an accurate proximal aortic anastomosis. There are circumstances wherein proximal aortic cross clamp application is either not technically possible or is hazardous (e.g., in the case of a shaggy or highly calcified aorta). In such cases, deep hypothermic circulatory arrest (DHCA) can be used for the proximal reconstruction with resumption of brain perfusion after the anastomosis has been performed. Indeed a few champion this technique as "preferred" in TAAA surgery. However, the "majority" opinion, which we share, is that the consequences of DHCA (specifically, bleeding and lung dysfunction) are such that this method should be used only when no other technical option exists to repair the aneurysm. In fact, this has been rare in our experience. External control of the left subclavian artery is desirable but not mandatory, as intraluminal balloon control can be obtained if the aortic clamp is placed proximal to the left subclavian artery. The celiac artery and superior mesenteric artery (SMA) are controlled externally as this is required for in-line mesenteric shunting and facilitates subsequent visceral Doppler interrogation.

Next, the aortic prosthesis is prepared by attaching a 6-mm polytetrafluoroethylene (PTFE) side-arm graft that will serve as the conduit for left renal artery reconstruction. An additional side-arm graft of 10-mm Dacron (Atrium; Hudson, NH) is placed proximally to provide inflow for the in-line mesenteric shunt (Figure 10). For most aneurysms, a Dacron prosthesis is the preferred conduit. However, a PTFE conduit is used to repair mycotic aneurysms because of its decreased susceptibility to infection. At this point, the surgeon begins the clamping sequence in close cooperation with the anesthesiologist. It is important to avoid abrupt, severe increases in afterload coincident with proximal thoracic aortic cross-clamping,

which can be accomplished with the judicious use of pharmacologic afterload reducing agents in anticipation of placement of the aortic clamp. Abrupt and severe increases in afterload that occur with proximal aortic cross-clamping can lead to left ventricular strain, myocardial ischemia, and an increase in CSF pressure.

If indicated, AFB is initiated by cannulation of the left atrium through a purse string suture in the left inferior pulmonary vein, and the arterial return is established via the left common femoral artery (Figure 11). Typically a single small dose of heparin is used. It is unnecessary to monitor activated clotting times, and heparin is redosed only if flow in the bypass circuit needs to be turned off for a period of time (e.g., to dissect out a prior aortic graft). Flow through the bypass circuit is such that distal mean perfusion pressures of at least 60 to 70 mm Hg are maintained; a gauge to the adequacy of the distal perfusion pressure is persistent urine output and the status of MEPs. MEPs are monitored by a dedicated neurologist who is able to address technical issues such as patient response to anesthetic agents and electrode failure. Any true deterioration in MEPs prompts either an increase in the stimulus intensity or an increase in distal perfusion pressures. If MEPs do not respond to the initial hemodynamic maneuvers, reconstruction of lumbar or intercostal vessels via an inclusion button is performed (Figure 12). Depending on TAAA extent and topography, multiple sequential clamp sites are often utilized; with "isolation" of the DTA between clamps, deterioration of MEP is rather rare. In cases using AFB, sequential clamping allows continuous renal and visceral perfusion during the creation of the proximal anastomosis.

After the establishment of AFB, the aneurysm is opened initially in the chest. When the entire descending thoracic aorta is resected,

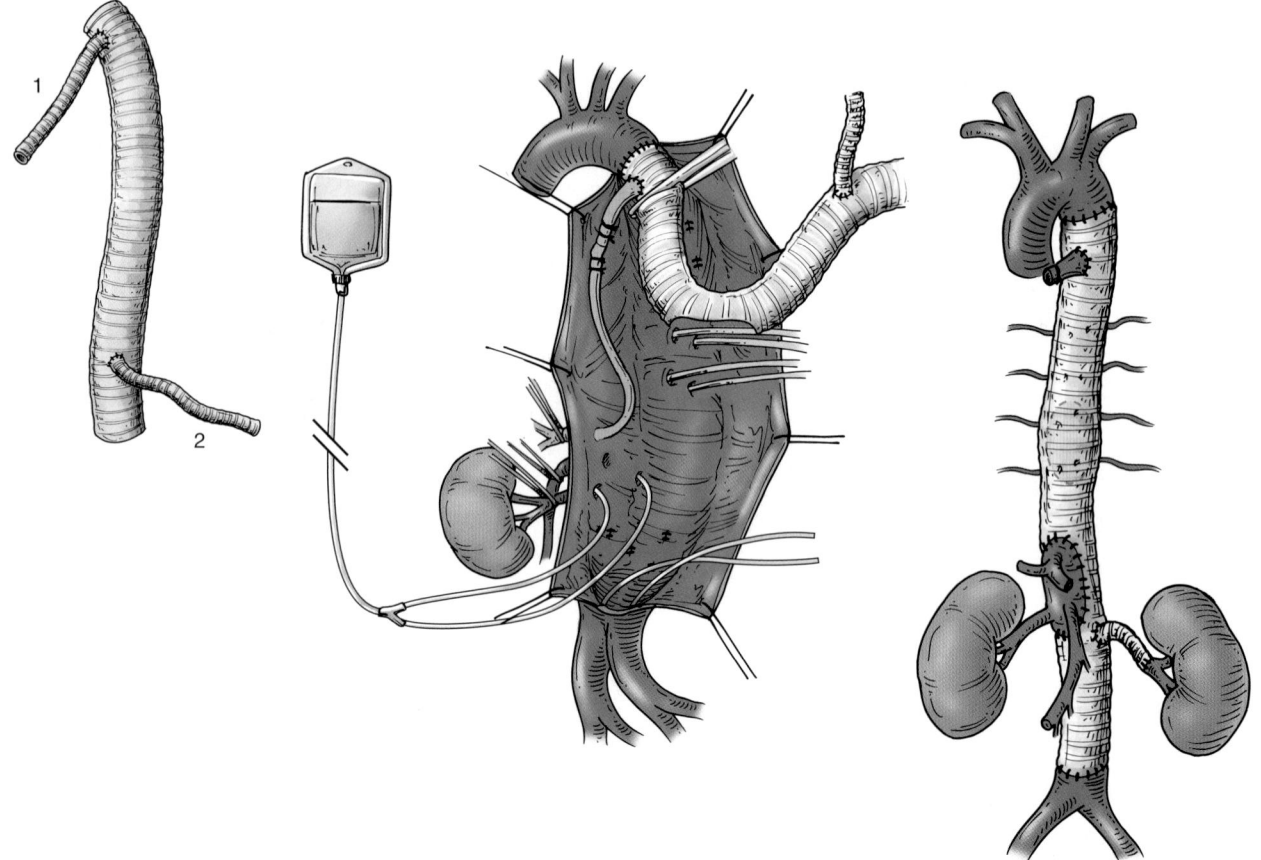

FIGURE 10   Preparation of the aortic prosthesis. A 10-mm Dacron graft *(1)* is attached proximally for in-line mesenteric shunting, and a 6-mm polytetrafluoroethylene (PTFE); *(2)* side-arm is attached for the left renal artery reconstruction. Sequential clamping allows for mesenteric perfusion during visceral reconstruction.

proximal intercostal vessel orifices between T_4 and T_8 are usually backbleeding profusely and are quickly oversewn. Intercostal arteries in the T_9 to L_1 aortic segment are evaluated for potential reimplantation into the main body of the graft. These vessels are controlled with intraluminal balloons to prevent backbleeding and the negative "sump" effect on net spinal cord perfusion caused by exposure of these orifices to atmospheric pressure (Figure 13). Even without deterioration in MEP, the decision to reconstruct or eventually oversew these vessels is deferred to later stages in the operation. The proximal aortic neck is prepared for reconstruction, and circumferential division of the aorta is generally preferred, and is mandatory in chronic dissection, to avoid the late complication of suture line esophageal erosion. Reinforcement of the suture line with an external Teflon felt (Bard; Murray Hill, N.J.) collar is a frequently applied adjunct.

A clamp is placed on the main aortic graft distal to the mesenteric shunt side-arm, flow is then established in the shunt, and mesenteric perfusion (typically into the SMA origin with a 20F arterial perfusion catheter) is confirmed by assessing arterial backbleeding from the other mesenteric vessel origin. The next step of the operation may be reconstruction of the intercostal vessels in the T_9 to L_1, if so indicated by deterioration of MEP, but in fact, this is uncommon. These can be reconstructed through an inclusion button anastomosis, or intercostal arteries in the region of a proximal or distal aortic anastomosis can be reconstructed using a long beveled suture line. Other methods of intercostal vessel reanastomosis include the attachment of additional short side-arm grafts to the main aortic graft, or, in cases where vessel origin is rotated superiorly and to the patient's left side, implantation to the main aortic graft using Carrel patches of aorta that contain the intercostal vessels may be feasible but can be technically clumsy (see Figure 12).

Visceral and renal artery reconstruction is carried out next. Orificial endarterectomy can be performed when significant occlusive lesions of the right renal and superior mesenteric arteries exist (Figure 14). This involves incising the diseased intima and media and developing a proper endarterectomy plane that can be verified by noting the pinkish color of the inner adventitia. While such orificial endarterectomy has been the standard method for clearing visceral vessel ostial stenoses, we have largely abandoned this in favor of direct orificial balloon-expandable stenting. This is particularly true with

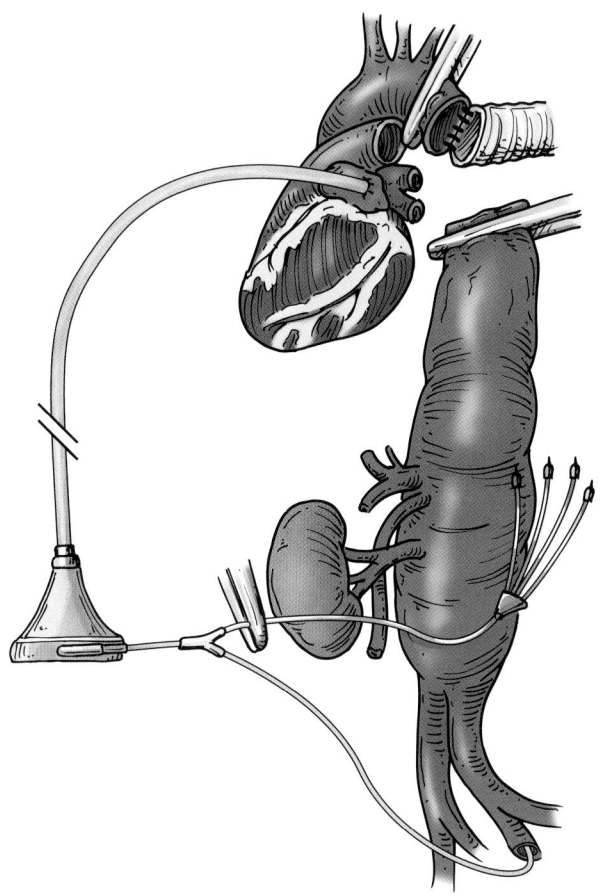

FIGURE 11 Atriofemoral bypass is initiated by cannulation of the left atrium (via the left inferior pulmonary vein), and arterial return is established vial the left common femoral artery. A Y-connector may be applied to the arterial return tubing for perfusion of visceral or intercostal arteries.

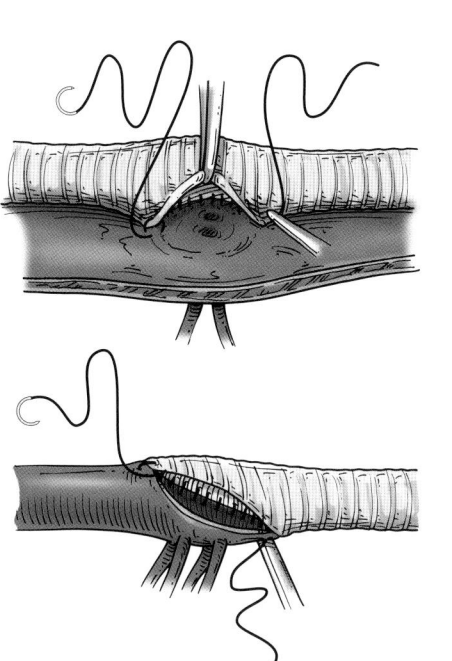

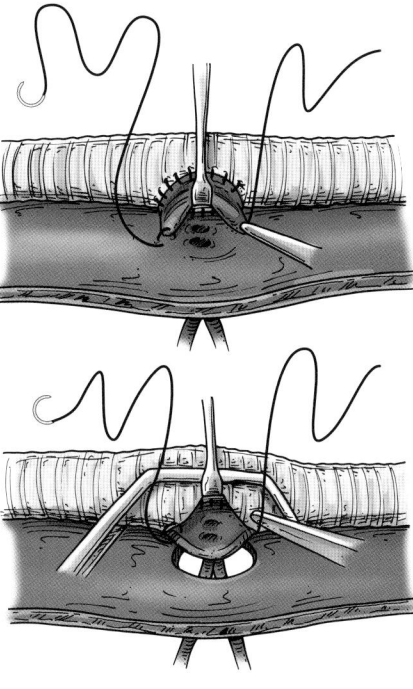

FIGURE 12 If indicated, reconstruction of lumbar or intercostal vessels may be performed via inclusion button, short side-arm graft, beveled anastomosis, or Carrel patch.

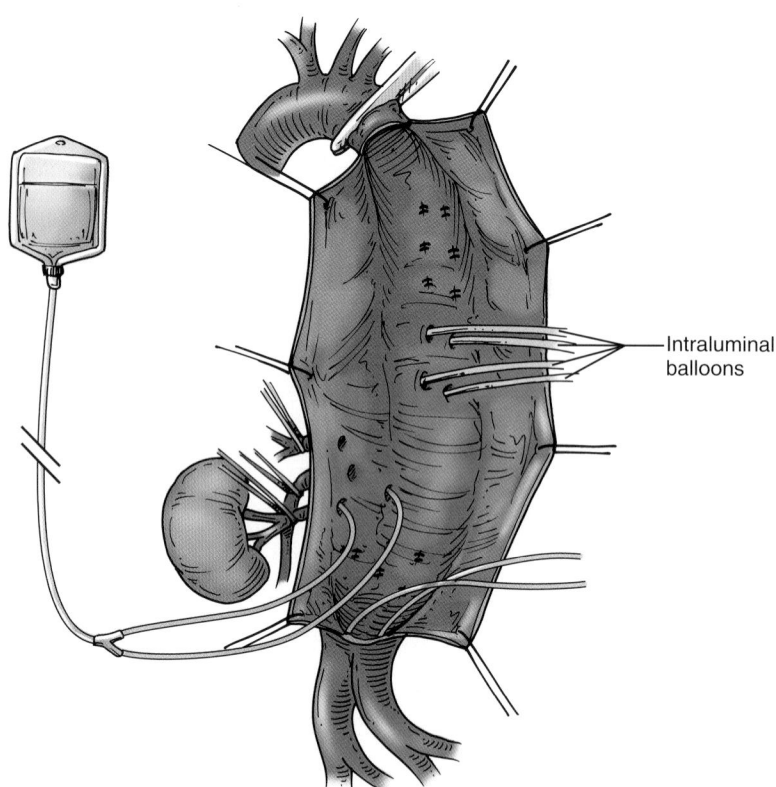

Intraluminal balloons

FIGURE 13 After the aneurysm is opened, back-bleeding intercostal arteries are controlled with Pruitt intraluminal balloons. *(LeMaitre Vascular, Burlington, Mass.)*

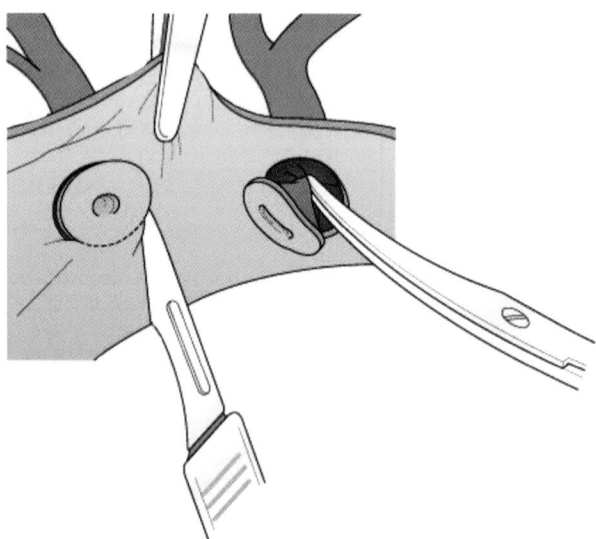

FIGURE 14 During visceral artery reconstruction, orificial endarterectomy may be performed in the setting of significant occlusive lesions.

respect to the right renal artery (see Figure 2). This method is simple, and certainly expeditious when compared with the endarterectomy; our follow-up studies have also verified its durability.

The most common method of visceral and renal artery reconstruction, especially in extent II and III TAAA, is a single inclusion button that encompasses the origins of the celiac, superior mesenteric, and right renal arteries (Figure 15). In extent I TAAA, a beveled distal anastomosis incorporating all renal/visceral vessels and the distal aorta is often possible (Figure 16); alternatively, either the celiac superiorly or the left renal artery inferiorly can be reconstructed with

separate side-arm grafts. If the aneurysm is excessively large in the visceral aortic segment, the wide separation of the visceral/renal ostia may necessitate individual inclusion button anastomoses for each vessel. Alternatively, the superior mesenteric artery and right renal artery can be reimplanted as a single inclusion while reconstruction of the celiac trunk with a side-arm graft is deferred until later. The aortic graft is placed under tension, and an elliptical side island is excised from the main aortic graft. This ellipse usually begins on the lateral aspect of the graft and spirals posteriorly in the region of the right renal artery reconstruction. With the graft under tension, it is possible to complete the posterior portion of the anastomosis using single bites of the suture passing through both the aorta and the Dacron graft. Suture bites are taken close to the origin of the visceral vessels to avoid leaving excess aneurysmal aortic wall. As the posterior aspect of this suture line continues around the inferior border of the right renal artery, we exchange the 6F renal cold perfusion catheter for a 12F perfusion catheter to temporarily stent the origin of the right renal artery. The catheter is gently agitated up and down as the suture line moves around the renal artery orifice to ensure that it is not compromised by generous suture bites as they pass outside of the aorta. It is important to identify the course of the right renal artery with this indwelling catheter in order to avoid renal artery occlusion in circumstances where the right renal artery drapes over a large infrarenal component of the aneurysm (Figure 17). Just prior to completion of this suture line, backbleeding and patency of the celiac, superior mesenteric, and right renal arteries are verified, and the in-line mesenteric shunt is clamped and removed. A single flush of the proximal aortic cross-clamp is performed to ensure that no clot or debris has built up in the graft.

Reconstruction of the left renal artery is now accomplished with a separate side-arm graft of 6-mm PTFE. This provides a direct deliberate anastomosis in end-to-end fashion while allowing flexibility to deal with the spectrum of occlusive lesions, multiple renal arteries, and other wrinkles that may be encountered. It is important to orient this side-arm graft so that it will not kink when the left renal artery is returned to its anatomic position (see Figure 17). Some

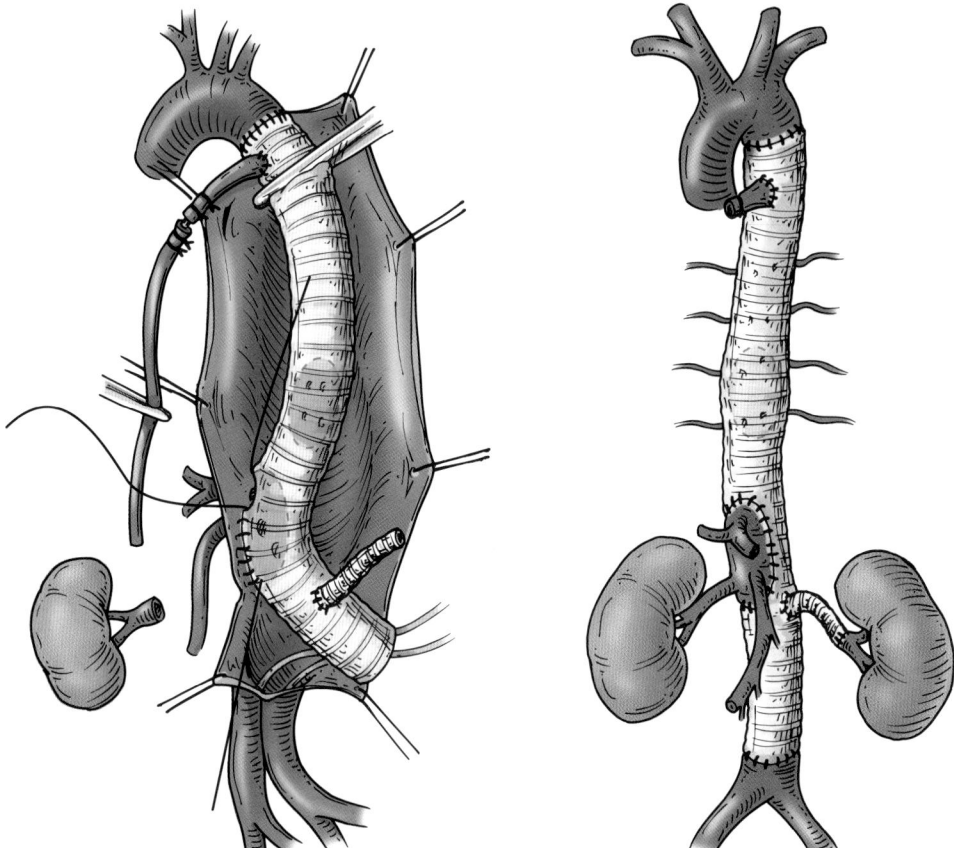

FIGURE 15 A single inclusion button is often used for efficient reconstruction of the celiac, superior mesenteric, and right renal arteries.

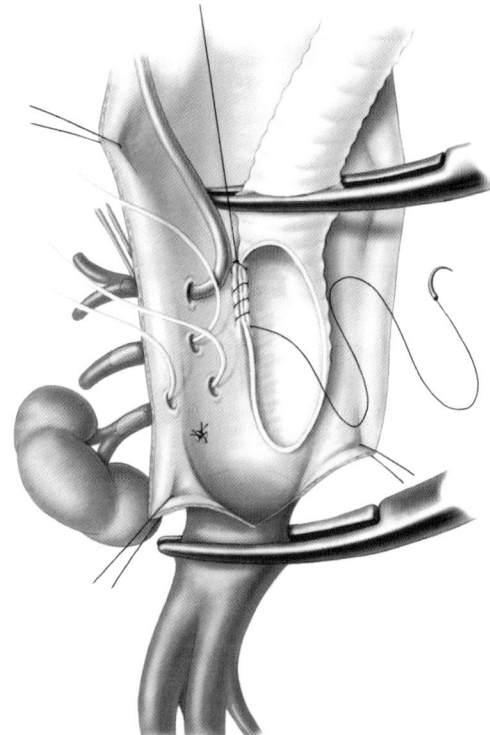

FIGURE 16 For extent I TAAA, a beveled distal anastomosis incorporating all renal and visceral vessels is often possible. As shown, the most caudal extent of the graft can often be tucked just posterior to the left renal artery origin when the aorta is not frankly aneurysmal at the renal artery level. Alternatively, the left renal caudally and/or the celiac axis superiorly can be reconstructed with separate side-arm grafts. Note in-line mesenteric shunt in celiac axis origin.

surgeons advocate the use of a single inclusion button that contains ALL renal and visceral vessels. This often requires the inclusion of too great an area of the native, aneurysmal aorta and has contributed to a so-called patch aneurysm, which has been rare in our experience.

We make every effort to perform tube type of reconstructions to the aortic bifurcation unless there is gross aneurysmal disease of the proximal common iliac arteries. After reestablishment of flow to the lower extremities and verification of adequate lower extremity perfusion by intraoperative pulse volume recordings, Doppler signals in the left renal, celiac, and superior mesenteric vessels are checked in addition to palpation of the superior mesenteric artery pulse in the root of the mesentery. A final verification of MEP is made; in rare cases, a deferred intercostal reconstruction is performed at that time. Hemostasis will usually be adequate at this point but protamine and infusions of platelets and fresh frozen plasma are typically increased at this point in the operation when a final check for hemostasis is made. Careful inspection of the inferior aspect of the aneurysm sac in both the chest and abdomen is necessary to detect backbleeding lumbar and/or intercostal vessels, which can be a source of significant postoperative hemorrhage. The redundant aneurysm sac is then sutured securely over the aortic prosthesis in the abdomen and the chest. The left kidney is returned to its anatomic position, and perinephric fat suffices to provide adequate coverage of the aortic graft in the region of the visceral aortic segment. Prior to closure, renal artery reconstructions are interrogated one final time. Closure of extensive incisions typically takes close to an hour, and two teams are utilized.

Outcomes

Treatment results as reported in the literature can be misleading; grouping patients at wide variance for complication risk leads to

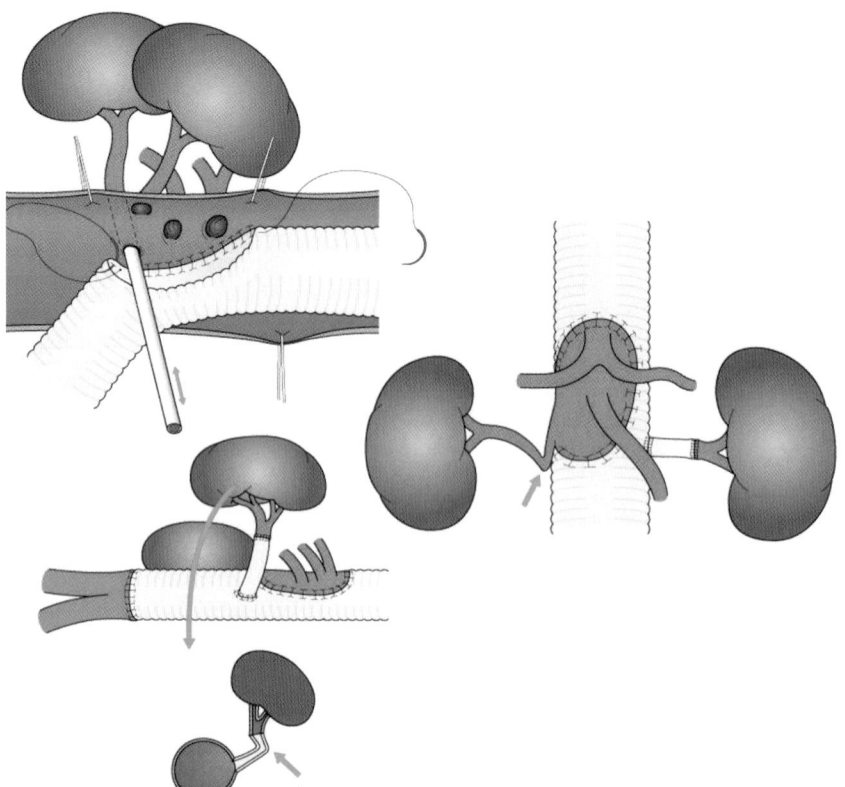

FIGURE 17 During reconstruction of the right renal artery (*top left*), a 12F perfusion catheter is used to temporarily stent the origin of the vessel. As the suture line courses around the inferior and caudal end of the right renal artery ostium, the 12F perfusion catheter is agitated to direct the operator to the course of the artery outside the aneurysm (see *Operative Technique*). This prevents the suture line from impinging or occluding the right renal artery outside the aneurysm. *Bottom left:* The orientation of the left renal artery side-arm graft is critical; it must not kink as the left kidney is returned to its anatomic position.

imprecision. For example, it is axiomatic that SCI risk is highest in extent II TAAA, whereas we and others have reported considerably reduced morbidity and mortality for type IV TAAA repair.

A review of our experience with open repair of extent IV TAAA included 179 patients, 87% of whose surgeries were completed in an elective setting. Thirty-day mortality was 2.8%, and any degree of spinal cord injury occurred in 2.2%. Five-year survival was 62% plus or minus 4%. Results of multivariate analysis showed only preoperative renal insufficiency was associated with mortality or major complications.

The initial review of our experience with the use of AFB/MEP in the repair of extent I-III TAAA demonstrated improved results, when compared with our own institutional historical controls, most of whom were treated with a clamp-and-sew technique and epidural cooling for spinal cord protection. After propensity-score matching, the 30-day mortality in the AFB/MEP group was not significantly different (2% vs 5%; $P = 0.38$), but none of those patients treated in the AFB/MEP group suffered postoperative paraplegia (vs 5% in the clamp-and-sew [CS] group). The composite death/paraplegia rate was decreased from 9% (CS) to 2% (AFB/MEP) ($P = 0.01$).

In the recent update of our experience, the impact of atriofemoral bypass with MEP, over a standard CS technique was evaluated in a retrospective, risk-adjusted series of patients undergoing extent I-III TAAA repair. One hundred patients undergoing TAAA repair with AFB/MEP were compared with 385 patients undergoing repair with the CS technique. There was no difference in the rate of intraoperative death (MEP = 1.0% vs CS = 0.5%; $P = 0.50$), length of intensive care unit stay (MEP = 9.6 ± 8.6 days vs CS = 9.5 ± 12.3 days; $P = 0.95$), or length of hospital stay (AFB/MEP = 19.9 ± 12.6 days vs CS = 21.6 ± 23.5 days; $P = 0.49$). However, the composite outcome of perioperative death and paraplegia rate was lower in the AFB/MEP cohort (7% vs 19%; $P = 0.004$). The multivariate model for predictors of this composite outcome showed that AFB/MEP was protective (OR = 0.39 [0.17, 0.9]; $P = 0.028$). Long-term (4-year) survival was

improved in the AFB/MEP group as well (73 ± 6% vs 60 ± 3%; $P = 0.004$).

It has become almost fashionable to emphasize, perhaps unduly, the morbidity of and recovery from open surgical repair. Indeed, one California administrative database study reported an overall mortality of 19% one year after operation and suggested that reporting perioperative outcomes considerably understated the negative potential of surgical repair. Alternatively, we have consistently reported late outcomes in terms of both survival and functional status. These studies indicate late survival in our cohort either equates or is superior to that seen after AAA repair, indicating that the resource commitment to bring these patients through operation is indeed justified. Furthermore, permanent loss of functional status has been a rare outcome after operation.

ENDOVASCULAR SURGICAL MANAGEMENT

Stent graft repair in the thoracic aorta (thoracic endovascular aorta repair [TEVAR]) bears many comparisons with the parallel experience of such repair in the abdominal aorta, but there are important technical, anatomic, and pathologic distinctions between the two technologies. First, the significantly increased morbidity of open surgical repair in the thoracic aorta, as compared with open AAA repair, solidified the important clinical need for TEVAR. With respect to design and engineering considerations, thoracic devices are proportionately larger and thus require larger bore delivery devices when compared with those of endovascular aorta repair (EVAR). Furthermore, unless the surgeon is treating pathology in the relatively straight portion of the descending aorta, considerations of engineering, accuracy of deployment, and the like are a constant when TEVAR needs to involve the aortic arch. Indeed, overall results of TEVAR, including the potential for complications such as stroke, are highly dependent on the proximal extent or proximal seal zone applicable in any individual case. As shown in Figure 18, a widely promulgated classification scheme stratifying the proximal seal zone is readily correlated with procedural complexity, the need for debranching, or even trans-sternal approaches, and the risk of neurologic complications, in particular, stroke. The other important distinction when compared with EVAR is that TEVAR, to date, has been applied to the spectrum of thoracic aortic pathologies beyond degenerative aneurysm and including entities such as traumatic aortic tear and acute/chronic aortic dissection.

After a series of industry-sponsored studies focusing on degenerative aneurysm, commercial applicability of a TEVAR device dates only since mid-2005. Thereafter, rapid adoption of TEVAR across the spectrum of thoracic aortic pathologies occurred. We previously reported this phenomenon in an examination of thoracic aortic repair in Medicare beneficiaries during the interval 2004 to 2007 (Table 1). Not only was there a rapid shift from open repair to TEVAR, but across the spectrum of pathologies, this transition was accompanied by significantly reduced perioperative mortality.

TEVAR (Figure 19) offers the benefit of aortic repair without the physiologic insult associated with thoracotomy and clamping of the proximal aorta. The success of TEVAR is predicated on obtaining quality aortic imaging, careful patient selection, and appropriate preprocedural planning.

Similar to endovascular AAA repair, there are several anatomic barriers to thoracic stent grafting. First and foremost, the proximal and distal seal zones should be at least 15 mm in length to ensure an adequate fixation and seal. Conventional thoracic stent graft landing zones are depicted in Figure 18; ideally the seal zone is achieved in the area from zone 2 to zone 4. Additionally, the delivery systems for thoracic endografts are larger than their abdominal counterparts. In the presence of extensively calcified or narrow iliac arteries, a prosthetic conduit sewn to the common iliac artery or aorta may be required for successful device delivery and should be planned in advance.

Outcomes

Clinical results after TEVAR for degenerative aneurysm were initially available in the form of European registry studies. Data from 249 patients undergoing endovascular repair for degenerative thoracic aneurysms in the European EUROSTAR and the United Kingdom Thoracic Endograft registries (prospectively gathered databases of aortic pathology) showed a 30-day mortality of 5.3% and paraplegia rate of 4% with an 80% one-year survival.

In North America, three industry-sponsored multicenter trials were conducted to assess the efficacy of TEVAR as compared with open surgical repair for degenerative aneurysm of the descending thoracic aorta, where anatomy was potentially amenable to repair with either open repair or TEVAR. None of these studies were randomized, and in fact, their value was somewhat diluted by the irreconcilable limitations of retrospective control groups. Nonetheless, as displayed in Table 2, the summary results from these three industry-sponsored trials allow comparison of some 500 patients treated with TEVAR, as opposed to 350 who underwent open surgical repair for isolated aneurysm of the descending thoracic aorta. The overall results strongly favor TEVAR with respect to significantly reduced perioperative mortality and SCI complications. It is worth emphasizing the fact that these trials were conducted at either

TABLE 1: Use of TEVAR versus open repair for degenerative TAAA in medicare beneficiaries

Year	TOTAL COHORT (n = 11,166)		
	TEVAR	Open	Total
2004	467 (21%)	1798 (79%)	2265
2005	1012 (38%)	1627 (62%)	2639
2006	1630 (52%)	1503 (48%)	3133
2007	1729 (55%)	1400 (45%)	3129
Total	4838 (43%)	6328 (57%)	11,166

TAAA, Thoracoabdominal aortic aneurysm; *TEVAR,* thoracic endovascular aorta repair.

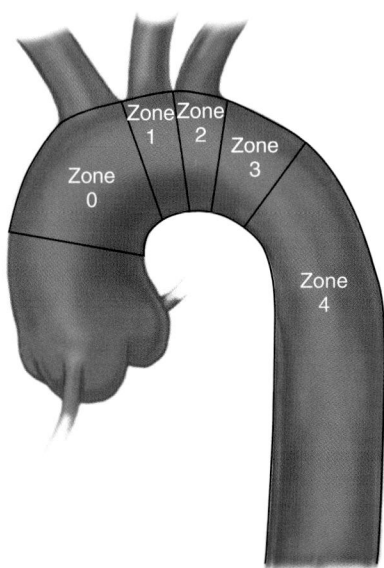

FIGURE 18 Proximal landing zone classification for thoracic endovascular stent grafts. The site of the proximal landing zone is correlated with procedural complexity and the risk of neurologic event.

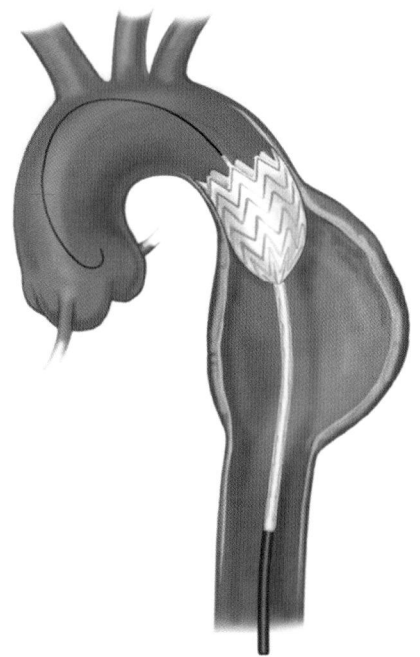

FIGURE 19 Endovascular repair of thoracic aortic anuerysms (TEVAR) allows for repair of thoracic aortic aneurysms without the physiologic insult associated with clamping the proximal aorta.

TABLE 2: Summary of composite clinical trial results for TEVAR versus open repair for degenerative TAAA

	TEVAR (n = 495)	Open (n = 353)	P value
Mortality	10 (2%)	30 (8.5%)	<0.001
Paraplegia/ paraparesis	31 (6.2%)	46 (13%)	0.007
Total paraplegia	8 (1.6%)	18 (5.1%)	0.0037

TAAA, Thoracoabdominal aortic aneurysm; *TEVAR*, thoracic endovascular aorta repair.

major academic medical centers or high-volume thoracic aortic centers. Stated differently, both the open and endovascular operations were, in general, performed by very experienced, expert surgeons. Accordingly, the favorable comparative results with TEVAR versus open operation have created the milieu where, in the eyes of most surgeons, a descending thoracic degenerative aneurysm whose anatomy is amenable to TEVAR is generally treated with this endovascular approach. Certainly, our posture is consistent with this general trend.

Recently, we compiled our own experience with 105 patients undergoing thoracic aortic stent-grafting and compared the results with those of 93 patients treated with open surgery during the same time period. Despite borderline statistical significance, the operative mortality was halved in the stent graft group when compared with the open surgery group (7.6% vs 15.1%; P = 0.09). While a 7.6% mortality lies in the lower end of reported rates for thoracic endografts, which have been as high as 20%, it is substantially higher than that of our updated experience with 873 infrarenal AAA endovascular repairs (1.8%) and may be related to the fact that 30% of the endograft patients were not considered candidates for open surgery. The spinal cord ischemia rate was 6.7% in our stent graft population with two patients experiencing transient paraparesis that resolved after discharge. These results are similar to those of other multicenter trials that reported spinal cord ischemia rates of 3%. In addition, available reviews suggest that 8% to 43% of landing sites in DTAAs will not allow an appropriate 15-mm length for secure proximal fixation. Indeed, in 20% of our patients, the left subclavian artery was intentionally covered (11.5% underwent preprocedural subclavian artery bypass). The 4-year survival for this group was 54% and freedom from reintervention rate was 81%. Similarly, the celiac axis may be covered, in some cases, in order to achieve an adequate distal seal zone. It is generally agreed that coverage of the celiac axis is acceptable as long as there is a large SMA and patent gastroduodenal artery that can collaterize the celiac branches.

As endovascular repair has become more widely used for ruptured AAA, thoracic stent grafting may have an analogous role in ruptured DTAAs. A recent prospective series of 59 patients undergoing endovascular thoracic stent grafting using the Gore TAG device for descending thoracic aortic catastrophes included 20 patients with ruptured thoracic aortic aneurysms. The 30-day mortality was 15%, which is nearly one half the mortality rate for open repair of ruptured aneurysms cited in the literature from centers of excellence and nearly one third the mortality rate based on data from the National Inpatient Sample. Twenty-five percent of patients had a device-related event, which included one graft infection and three endoleaks. The 1-year actuarial survival was 37%, which largely reflects the advanced age and multiple comorbidities in this group of patients.

ALTERNATIVE APPROACHES

Prior to commercial availability of TEVAR in 2005, open operation was the only technical option for most TAAAs. Thereafter, arch and/or visceral debranching with subsequent TEVAR enabled a hybrid surgical approach to many patients. Indeed, early proponents of this technique often cited unsatisfactory results with open repairs as the rationale. As intuitively expected, the reported results vary widely as a function of the patient cohorts. We applied this method to a group of some 25 patients deemed unsuitable for conventional repair and showed that hybrid repair is not without significant morbidity and mortality. In addition to a mortality rate of 21.7% (trending toward two times that for open repair at our institution), hybrid repairs presented new concerns, including a 10% rate of visceral bypass graft thrombosis. Looking specifically at renal artery bypass, grafts performed during hybrid procedures had a significantly higher rate of thrombosis (19%) as compared with those done for open repairs (1.6%). In a series of 252 patients undergoing thoracic stent graft procedures, one group reported that a debranching procedure was an independent risk factor for late mortality overall and specifically in the subgroup of asymptomatic patients. Hybrid procedures may be appropriate for certain high-risk groups, but the morbidity and mortality associated with visceral debranching is not insignificant. Corroborative data are available from the North American Registry; Oderich and colleagues reviewed results with hybrid operation in 208 patients with extent I-IV TAAA and noted a 14% mortality and a 10% rate of paraplegia.

For DTAAs extending into the visceral aorta, branched and fenestrated stent grafts may provide novel options for previously excluded anatomy. Many of the initial fenestrated trials have focused on juxtarenal AAA and type IV TAAAs. It is logical to assume that total endovascular repair will be an important advance in the treatment of TAAA, just as has occurred with DTAA. However, the technology has been slow in advancing. Fenestrated grafts are custom designed stent grafts with three types of fenestrations (small, large, and scalloped) through which visceral artery stents are placed, thus preserving the patency of the artery (Figure 20). The French multicenter trial of the Cook fenestrated stent graft involved 80 patients in whom 237 visceral arteries were perfused through fenestrations. During follow-up (which ranged from 1 to 38 months with a mean of 10 months), there were no ruptures and no open conversions. Ten percent of patients required secondary procedures to correct endoleaks or to treat threatened visceral vessels. Most of these patients however did not have true TAAA.

In the United States, although slow to evolve from an engineering and regulatory perspective, total endovascular repair of extensive TAAA is on the horizon. Yet the scant available information from the true experts advancing this technology indicates overall outcomes have still not equaled those of open repair with spinal cord protection strategies. Greenberg and colleagues reported a series of 633 patients undergoing endovascular repair of TAAA or juxtarenal abdominal aortic aneurysms. In that cohort, 188 patients underwent repair of extent I-III TAAA. Of that subset of patients, the 30-day mortality was 5.9%, and the 4-year survival was estimated to be 59%.

A direct comparison by Greenberg and colleagues of open and endovascular outcomes for TAAA was reported in 2008. That series reported a borderline improvement in spinal cord ischemia rates for those undergoing endovascular repair. It is noteworthy, however, that there was a significant difference in the extent of aneurysms between the groups, with more extent IV aneurysms found in the endovascular group. Nonetheless, the incidence of spinal cord ischemia for those with extent I-III TAAA in the endovascular group was 10%.

A parallel series outlining the experience of Chuter's group, reported early and intermediate results of endovascular TAAA repair in 81 patients. There were zero extent I aneurysms in this series, and 40 patients with extent II and III disease. The overall mortality in that study was 6.2%. Permanent paraplegia occurred in three patients

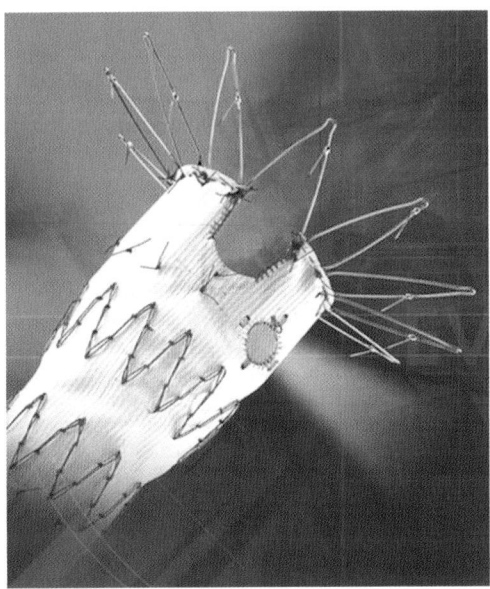

FIGURE 20   Fenestrated stent grafts employ fenestrations and scallops to preserve patency of branch vessels.

(3.7%), and transient paraplegia/paraparesis occurred in 16 patients (19.8%). Sixteen branches occluded (nine renal, two celiac) or developed stenoses (four renal, one superior mesenteric artery), requiring stenting. Multicenter trials evaluating the role of branched totally endovascular repair for TAAA will soon be underway.

SUGGESTED READINGS

Conrad MF, Ergul EA, Patel VI, et al: Evolution of operative strategies in open thoracoabdominal aneurysm repair, *J Vasc Surg* 53(5):1195–1201, 2011. e1. Epub 2011 Feb 11.

Conrad MF, Ergul EA, Patel VI, et al: Management of diseases of the descending thoracic aorta in the endovascular era: a Medicare population study, *Ann Surg* 252(4):603–610, 2010.

Lancaster RT, Conrad MF, Patel VI, et al: Further experience with distal aortic perfusion and motor-evoked potential monitoring in the management of extent I-III thoracoabdominal aortic aneurysms, *J Vasc Surg* 58(2):283–290, 2013.

Patel VI, Ergul E, Conrad MF, et al: Continued favorable results with open surgical repair of type IV thoracoabdominal aortic aneurysms, *J Vasc Surg* 53(6):1492–1498, 2011. Epub 2011 Apr 22.

Patel VI, Lancaster RT, Conrad MF, et al: Open surgical repair of thoracoabdominal aneurysms – the Massachusetts General Hospital experience, *Ann Cardiovasc Surg* 1(3):320–324, 2012.

THE MANAGEMENT OF ACUTE AORTIC DISSECTIONS

Karen M. Kim, MD, and
Thomas E. MacGillivray, MD

OVERVIEW

Acute aortic dissection is the most common catastrophe of the human aorta. With a reported incidence of 3 out of 100,000 patients each year, aortic dissections are a deadly disease with an early mortality of 1% to 2% per hour. Without appropriate treatment, the 2-week mortality of aortic dissections involving the ascending aorta is approximately 90%. While the presentation may be classic, symptoms can be nonspecific and can occur in patients with no evident risk factors. Misdiagnosis leading to even a slight delay in treatment is associated with increased mortality. Therefore, proper diagnosis and expeditious therapy are essential for improved survival.

CLASSIFICATION

Acute aortic dissection can manifest in several different patterns, which have different therapeutic and prognostic implications. There are two classification schemes in use worldwide to describe aortic dissection: the DeBakey and Stanford systems (Figure 1). The DeBakey system categorizes the dissection based on the origin of the intimal tear and the extent of the dissection. Aortic dissections involving the ascending and descending aortas and the aortic arch are DeBakey type I. Dissections confined only to the ascending aorta are DeBakey type II. Aortic dissections that originate and propagate distal to the left subclavian artery are DeBakey type III (IIIa is limited to the descending thoracic aorta, whereas IIIb extends below the diaphragm).

The Stanford classification system divides dissections into two categories: those that involve the ascending aorta (proximal to the innominate artery) and those that do not. Stanford A dissections include all dissections involving the ascending aorta (DeBakey types I and II) regardless of the site of origin. Stanford B dissections describe dissections not involving the ascending aorta, including those involving the aortic arch.

"Acute" dissections are those present for 14 days or less, whereas "chronic" dissections describe those present for more than 2 weeks. Acute Stanford A dissections account for more than 60% of all dissections and are considered to be surgical emergencies requiring immediate operation. Acute Stanford B dissections are further classified as "complicated" or "uncomplicated." Complicated Stanford B dissections include approximately 20% of patients with rupture or impending rupture, malperfusion, and/or refractory pain or hypertension for whom open surgical or endovascular therapy is recommended. Uncomplicated Stanford B dissections are managed effectively with aggressive medical therapy.

Intramural hematoma (IMH) represents approximately 10% to 20% of patients who present with the clinical picture of acute aortic dissection but, on imaging, have no blood flow in the false lumen or any identifiable intimal lesions. It is sometimes inappropriately referred to as a dissection with a thrombosed false lumen. IMH may result from a microscopic intimal tear, hemorrhage of the vasa vasorum, or a penetrating aortic ulcer. Although it is a matter of discussion and debate, the authors manage IMH the same way as acute aortic dissection.

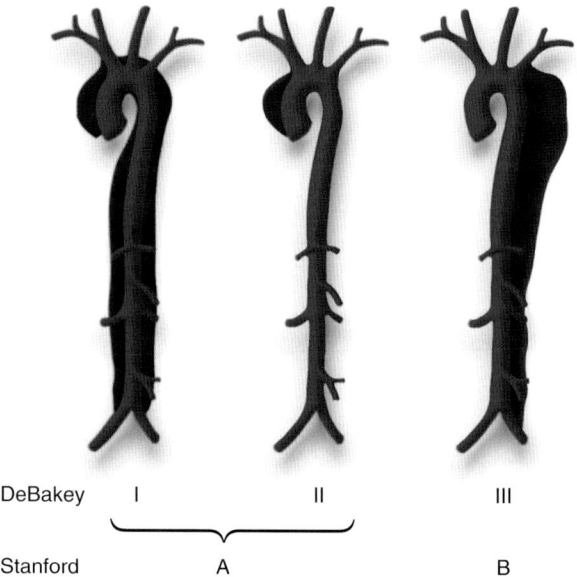

FIGURE 1   Anatomy and classification of aortic dissection: DeBakey and Stanford systems. *(Modified from Cambria RP, Brewster DC, Gertler J, et al: Vascular complications associated with spontaneous aortic dissection, J Vasc Surg 7(2):199-209, 1988.)*

PRESENTATION AND DIAGNOSIS

An acute aortic dissection results from a sudden aortic intimal disruption, which leads to the pressurized propagation of blood flow plowing through the false lumen within the media of the aorta. Circulatory collapse and death can occur within seconds as a result of aortic rupture frequently misdiagnosed as a massive myocardial infarction. The classic presentation is acute, severe, "10/10," "tearing," or "ripping" chest pain radiating to the back between the scapulae. Occasionally, patients will present with little or no pain. Afflicted patients often appear listless and possess a sense of impending doom.

Because blood flow in the false lumen can disrupt and occlude branching vessels of the aorta, patients can present with symptoms and signs of malperfusion. A new neurologic deficit or a pulseless extremity can distract the unsuspecting clinician, who may be focusing on just the tip of the iceberg. Electrocardiographic changes or a new diastolic murmur can occur from retrograde dissection into the coronary arteries or the aortic valve which may result in myocardial ischemia or congestive heart failure. Acute paralysis, abdominal pain, renal insufficiency, and syncope are all well-recognized atypical presentations of acute dissection. Difficult-to-control hypertension can be a risk factor and a presenting sign in patients with aortic dissection. Hypotension and shock are concerning signs of tamponade, cardiac dysfunction, or ongoing hemorrhage. A high index of suspicion for aortic dissection is imperative for any patient with asymmetric pulses or differential blood pressures in the extremities.

High-resolution contrast-enhanced computed tomographic angiography (CTA) has replaced conventional aortography as the gold standard diagnostic study to confirm or exclude the diagnosis of acute aortic dissection. CTA has a diagnostic sensitivity and specificity of 90% to 100% and is readily available in most hospitals. False positive diagnoses can occur because of artifactual lines resulting from mistiming of contrast boluses or inappropriate gating with the cardiac cycle. Although scans limited to the thoracic aorta can confirm the diagnosis, it is helpful to scan the entire aorta and iliofemoral vessels to assess for subclinical malperfusion and to assist in planning the surgical strategy.

Transesophageal echocardiography (TEE) is a valuable tool used to diagnose and manage patients with acute aortic dissection.

Although TEE requires special expertise, it can rapidly assess for tamponade, valvular dysfunction, and cardiac wall motion abnormalities, particularly in the hemodynamically unstable patient transported directly to the operating room. Magnetic resonance imaging, conventional aortography, and coronary angiography have a very limited role in the acute management of patients with aortic dissection.

MANAGEMENT

Once the diagnosis of acute aortic dissection is suspected, invasive hemodynamic monitoring and aggressive antiimpulse therapy should be instituted without delay. A radial or femoral arterial monitoring cannula should be placed in the extremity with the best pulse and blood pressure. Intravenous beta-blockade should be the medication of first choice to decrease the aortic dP/dT by titrating the infusion to a goal heart rate of 60 to 70 beats per minute and a systolic blood pressure of 100 to 110 mm Hg. Once adequate beta-blockade has been achieved, vasodilators can be added to further control hypertension. Initial blood pressure control with vasodilators like nitroprusside or hydralazine should be avoided. Although vasodilators will lower the blood pressure, they can increase the dP/dT and shear forces in the aorta, thereby increasing the risk of rupture. Acute Stanford A dissection patients with a diastolic murmur or TEE evidence of significant aortic valve regurgitation should not be managed with beta-blockers because of the high risk of exacerbating congestive heart failure.

Acute aortic dissection can be a very dynamic disease with a rapidly evolving clinical course. Patients diagnosed with acute type A aortic dissection should be emergently transferred to a cardiac surgical center for immediate surgical repair. Time is critical. Unnecessary testing or optimizing medical therapy should not be allowed to delay definitive treatment, which is surgery. Even patients with cerebral, renal, visceral, and/or extremity malperfusion should be managed with central aortic reconstruction as a first step, which will frequently correct the malperfusion syndrome. Although nonoperative management carries a very high risk of death, good clinical judgment always has an important role in the management of patients at very high risk.

SURGICAL MANAGEMENT OF STANFORD A DISSECTIONS

The goal of surgical therapy for patients with acute type A aortic dissection is to prevent imminent death from exsanguination or tamponade due to aortic rupture, acute aortic insufficiency, or malperfusion to the coronary, cerebral, and systemic circulations. The primary technique to accomplish these goals is to replace the ascending aorta with a tube interposition graft, thereby reestablishing flow in the true lumen of the aorta.

Invasive arterial and central venous pressure monitoring are helpful in the induction and conduct of general anesthesia. Temperature monitoring of the nasopharynx, central venous or pulmonary arterial blood, and bladder can ensure uniform perfusion and cooling. TEE, electroencephalogram, and cerebral oximetry are useful adjuncts for monitoring.

Cardiopulmonary bypass is required, so the surgeon must determine the site of arterial perfusion. Traditionally, the common femoral artery has been the most common approach for arterial cannulation given its size, easy accessibility, and surgeons' familiarity. In recent years, experienced aortic surgeons have been using the right axillary/subclavian artery as the preferred site for arterial perfusion. The arterial cannula can be connected to an 8-mm to 10-mm Dacron graft that is anastomosed in end-to-side fashion to the axillary artery. This approach allows for antegrade systemic perfusion and the option of selective antegrade cerebral perfusion during circulatory arrest should extensive arch reconstruction be required. Some experienced surgeons advocate the use of direct central ascending aortic cannulation with the use of TEE guidance. This approach can be challenging, but central aortic cannulation can be lifesaving in the management of an unstable patient.

Through a median sternotomy, the heart and ascending aorta are readily exposed. The right atrium is cannulated easily for venous drainage to initiate cardiopulmonary bypass. Most aortic surgeons recommend deep hypothermia in preparation for an open distal aortic anastomosis. During cooling, it is imperative that the surgical, anesthesia, and perfusion teams monitor the patient to ensure uniform perfusion and cooling. Occasionally, cannulation strategies must be altered to manage malperfusion during cardiopulmonary bypass. Given the increased frequency of aortic insufficiency and coronary malperfusion, the surgeon should be prepared to vent the left ventricle on bypass and meticulously protect the myocardium with direct antegrade coronary ostial and retrograde coronary sinus cardioplegia strategies.

Although there is considerable debate about the optimal temperature for profound hypothermia and circulatory arrest, the author achieves 18°C in the nasopharynx before turning off the circulation. With the patient in reverse Trendelenburg position, the entire ascending aorta from the sinotubular junction up to the innominate artery is resected. The aortic tissues are extremely fragile, and they should be delicately handled. Without an aortic cross clamp, the aortic arch can be inspected for complex intimal disruptions and to confirm that the brachiocephalic branches are intact and arising from the true lumen. All of the layers of the proximal aortic arch are then reconstructed, obliterating the false lumen to allow flow through the true lumen once central perfusion has been reestablished. Some surgeons reconstitute the aortic wall between two felt strips and anastomose a Dacron graft to the aortic-felt sandwich (Figure 2, A). The author prefers to sew the Dacron graft to the aortic wall buttressed with a strip of Dacron around the adventitia. The use of glues during these operations. Although glues allow for easier tissue handling, they can be destructive to the aorta and promote late pseudoaneurysm formation.

With the distal anastomosis completed, the aortic arch is de-aired, the proximal end of the graft is clamped, and cardiopulmonary bypass is resumed through the Dacron graft to promote true lumen flow (see Figures 2,B and 2,C). Generally, aortic arch replacement is not routinely necessary for managing most patients with acute type A aortic dissection. Arch replacement increases the complexity and length of the procedure, which can add to the already high-risk operation. Situations when the aortic arch should be considered for

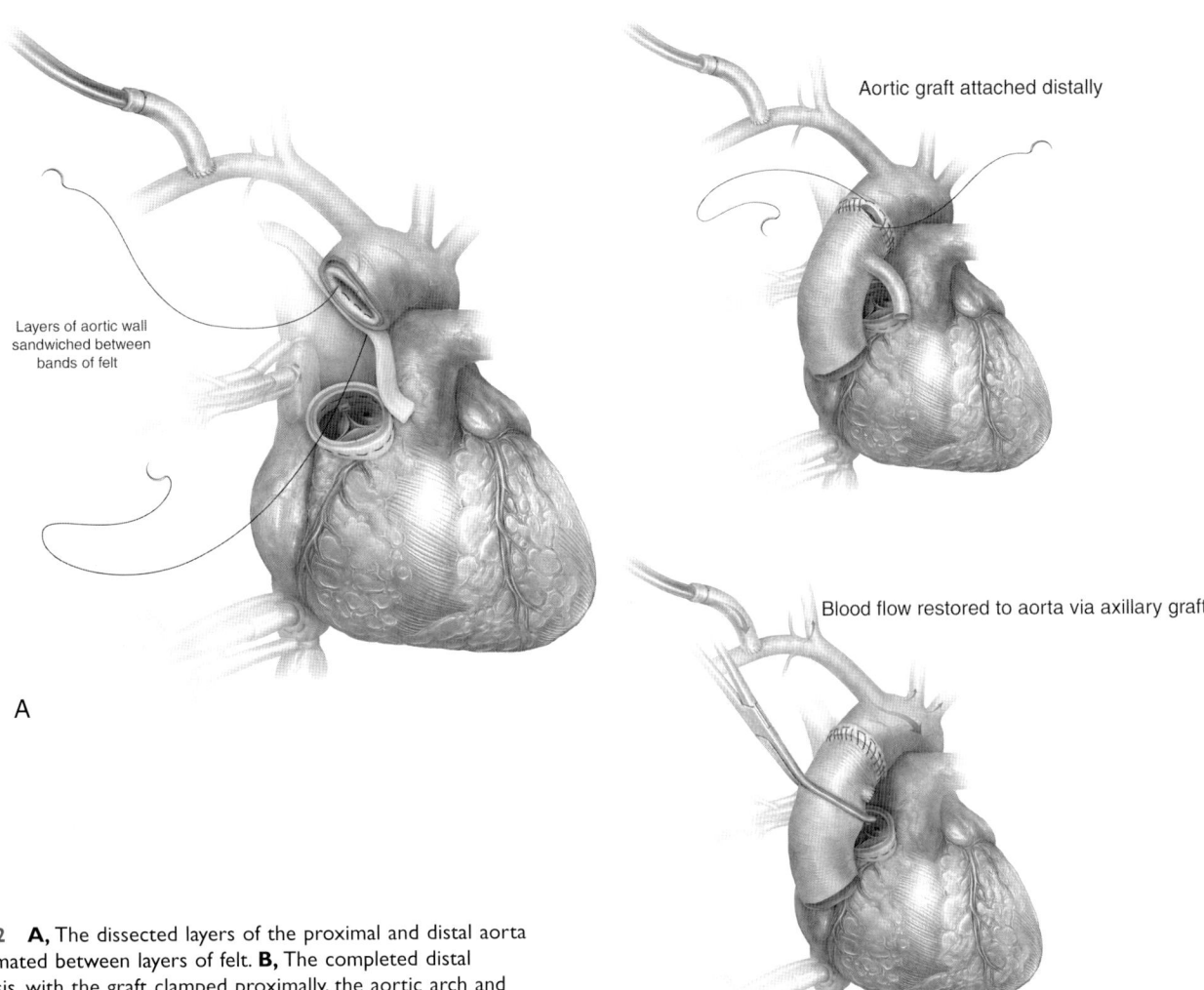

FIGURE 2 **A,** The dissected layers of the proximal and distal aorta reapproximated between layers of felt. **B,** The completed distal anastomosis, with the graft clamped proximally, the aortic arch and branches de-aired, and flow restored to the patient's head and body via axillary artery inflow.

Continued

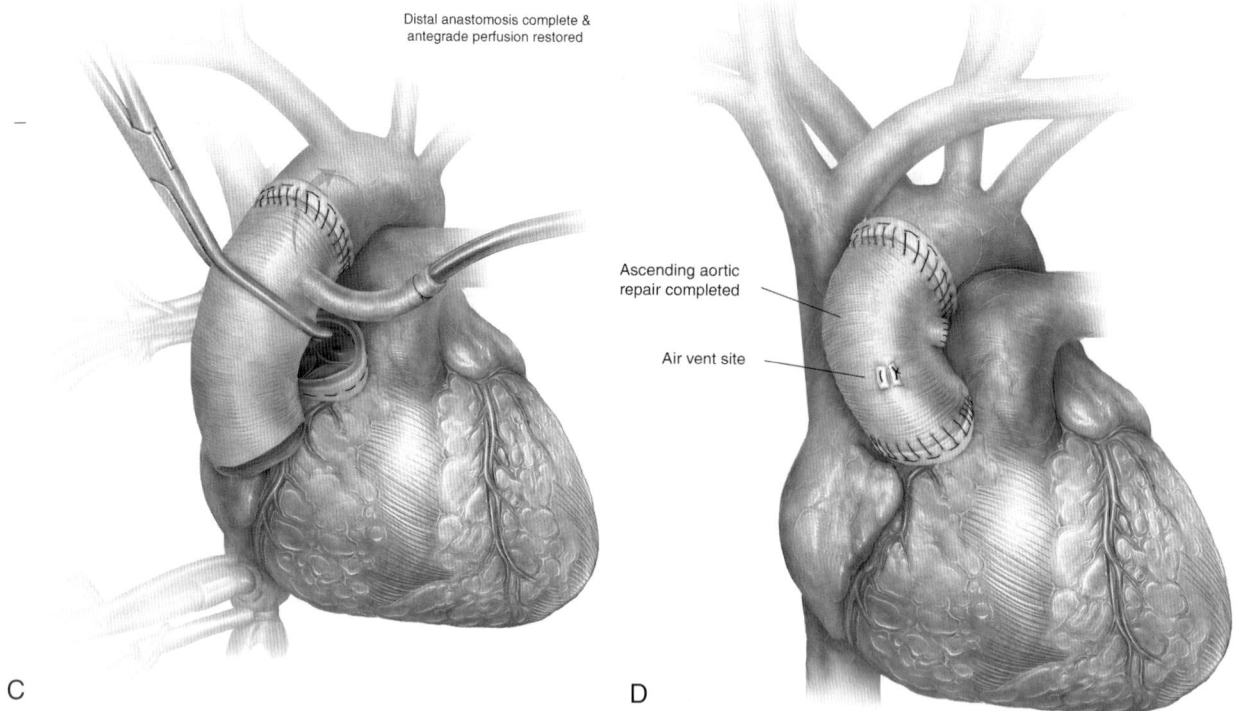

FIGURE 2, cont'd C, Distal reperfusion reinitiated through a side-arm of the ascending graft. **D,** The completed procedure, with the dissected ascending aorta removed, the valve resuspended, all air evacuated from the left circulation, and the patient decannulated. *(From Bolman RM 3rd: Acute type A aortic dissection,* Oper Tech Thorac Cardiovasc Surg 14(2):124 135, 2009.)

replacement in patients with acute dissection include when there are complex intimal disruptions in the arch, arch aneurysms larger than 5 cm, or connective tissue syndromes (e.g., Marfan, Loeys-Dietz, Ehlers-Danlos). Arch replacements should be performed with the use of selective antegrade cerebral perfusion, which has been demonstrated to improve outcomes.

During rewarming, the aortic root and proximal ascending aorta are assessed and reconstructed (see Figure 2,D). Often, the aortic root is minimally involved with the dissection, and the sinotubular junction can be reconstructed in a similar sandwich-type fashion as the distal anastomosis. Attention is required when operating on patients who present with aortic regurgitation and in those who have complex aortic root dissections approaching the coronary ostia. Aortic regurgitation is the most common cardiac complication associated with acute type A dissection. There are three possible dissection-related mechanisms that can contribute to aortic regurgitation. Acute dilation of the sinotubular junction and root caused by the expanding false lumen can result in incomplete coaptation of the valve cusps. The dissection can also extend into the aortic root, disrupting the commissural posts and resulting in prolapse of the valve cusps. Additionally, an aortic flap can itself prolapse through the valve in diastole, thereby preventing appropriate valve function. In most patients, the sinotubular junction can be reconstructed, the aortic valve commissures resuspended, and the aortic root left alone. Situations when composite aortic root replacement with coronary button reimplantation should be considered include when patients have aneurysms of the aortic root exceeding 5 cm, complex aortic valve pathology, dissection approaching the coronary ostia, or connective tissue syndromes (e.g., Marfan, Loeys-Dietz, Ehlers-Danlos). Valve-sparing aortic root replacement should be reserved for highly experienced aortic surgeons in this setting.

SURGICAL RESULTS WITH ACUTE TYPE A DISSECTIONS

According to the International Registry of Acute Aortic Dissection (IRAD) database, the overall surgical mortality of acute type A aortic dissection is 25%. In unstable patients (preoperative presence of tamponade, shock, congestive heart failure, stroke, coma, myocardial ischemia/infarction, acute renal failure, or mesenteric ischemia), the surgical mortality is 31%. Postoperatively, patients with aortic dissection are at risk for coagulopathic bleeding requiring transfusions and reexploration. Transient neurologic dysfunction, stroke, renal insufficiency, acute lung injury, new malperfusion syndromes, multiorgan system failure, and refractory hypertension are some of the possible early postoperative complications requiring intensive care and prolonged hospital care of these complicated patients. There is variability of outcomes reported from different centers, but the fact remains that acute type A aortic dissection is a highly lethal condition which, even when appropriately managed, has a high risk of morbidity and mortality.

MANAGEMENT OF ACUTE TYPE B DISSECTIONS

Medical management of patients who have uncomplicated type B dissections with antiimpulse therapy remains the preferred treatment, resulting in reported in-hospital mortality rates of less than 10%. Historically, the results of open surgical therapy for patients with acute type B dissection have been associated with a higher mortality rate than medical therapy, perhaps due to patient selection or complications requiring surgery. For patients with complicated type B dissections, thoracic endovascular aortic repair (TEVAR) has largely replaced open surgery and has improved results. Whether TEVAR proves to be superior to medical management in high-risk patients with uncomplicated type B dissection remains to be proven.

SUGGESTED READINGS

Hiratzka LF, Bakris GL, Beckman JA, et al: 2010 ACCF/AHA/AATS/ACR/ASA/SCA/SCAI/SIR/STS/SVM Guidelines for the diagnosis and management of patients with thoracic aortic disease: executive summary, *JACC* 55(14):1509–1544, 2010.

Loeys BL, Chen J, Neptune ER, et al: A syndrome of altered cardiovascular, craniofacial, neurocognitive and skeletal development caused by mutations in TGFBR1 or TGFBR2, *Nat Genet* 37(3):275–281, 2005.

Nienaber CA, Rousseau H, Eggebrecht H, et al: Randomized comparison of strategies for type B aortic dissection: the Investigation of STEnt grafts in Aortic Dissection (INSTEAD) trial, *Circulation* 120(25):2519–2528, 2009.

Stevens LM, Madsen JC, Isselbacher EM, et al: Surgical management and long-term outcomes for acute ascending aortic dissection, *J Thorac Cardiovasc Surg* 138(6):1349–1357, 2009.

Trimarchi S, Nienaber CA, Rampoldi V, et al: Contemporary results of surgery in acute type A aortic dissection: the International Registry of Acute Aortic Dissection experience, *J Thorac Cardiovasc Surg* 129(1):112–122, 2005.

Tsai TT, Nienaber CA, Eagle KA: Acute aortic syndromes, *Circulation* 112(24):3802–3813, 2005.

CAROTID ENDARTERECTOMY

Robert J. Beaulieu, MD, and
Christopher J. Abularrage, MD, FACS

OVERVIEW

Stroke was the third most common cause of death in the United States in 2010, with an estimated annual cost of $73.7 billion. Approximately 800,000 strokes occur every year, with up to 35% of strokes causing death or severe disability. Extracranial carotid disease represents the most common preventable cause of ischemic stroke. Thus, carotid endarterectomy (CEA), since it was first performed by DeBakey in 1954, occupies a prominent position in stroke prevention.

CLINICAL PRESENTATION

Clinical Status

Clinical status and degree of stenosis are the two most important factors in determination of the appropriate treatment for patients with known carotid disease. Clinical status, determined by the presence or lack of symptoms, confers differing degrees of future stroke risk. Indeed, most patients with carotid disease are completely asymptomatic. This group of patients is frequently identified with an asymptomatic carotid bruit or with screening duplex ultrasound scan. The finding of a carotid bruit, however, is insensitive as only 30% to 50% of patients have high-grade carotid stenosis. Moreover, only 20% to 50% of patients with carotid stenosis have a bruit. Thus, anatomic imaging is imperative to confirm the diagnosis of carotid stenosis in patients with a carotid bruit.

Symptomatic clinical status is defined by temporary or permanent neurologic deficit as a result of an ischemic, embolic event. Although only a small minority of patients has symptoms, the events can often have devastating consequences. Temporary ischemic events include amaurosis fugax, transient ischemic attack (TIA), and reversible ischemic neurologic deficit (RIND). Amaurosis fugax involves monocular blindness from temporary occlusion of the ophthalmic artery. Patients frequently report a shade coming down over the eye. TIA is a temporary interruption in normal neurologic function that resolves within 24 hours (80% resolve within 2 hours). TIA is characterized by temporary numbness, paresthesia, paralysis, or difficulty with speech. RINDs are similar to TIA except they last between 24 and 48 hours. Finally, symptoms of a stroke last beyond 24 hours and are most often permanent.

In determination of a patient's symptomatic status, other causes of stroke, such as cardiac thrombus, endocarditis, and intracranial cerebrovascular disease, are important to rule out. Also imperative is confirmation that a patient's symptoms are referable to the anatomic finding of carotid stenosis because the threshold for performing a CEA would be different. Symptoms of amaurosis must be ipsilateral to a carotid stenosis, and symptoms from TIA, RIND, or stroke are typically contralateral.

Imaging Studies

Carotid duplex ultrasound scan is currently the imaging modality of choice in evaluation of carotid artery disease. It allows for the evaluation of both anatomy (B-mode analysis) and flow-velocity patterns (duplex mode or spectral analysis) for determination of the degree of stenosis (Figure 1). When compared with catheter angiography, duplex ultrasound scan is more than 90% accurate. Duplex ultrasound scan is operator dependent, and frequent comparisons with measurements on the basis of catheter angiography are necessary for quality assurance.

Other noninvasive means of providing anatomic data beyond duplex scan include computed tomographic angiography (CTA) and magnetic resonance angiography (MRA). CTA can be performed in an expeditious manner and provides data on the aortic arch, common carotid artery, tortuosity, and unusual lesion anatomy. MRA, similarly, defines lesion anatomy and has the added benefit of helping with determination of cerebral infarction in the early hours after a stroke. As many as 10% of asymptomatic patients and 30% of symptomatic patients have evidence of cerebral infarct on magnetic resonance imaging (MRI) or computed tomographic scan. MRA can be limited by the fact that it may overestimate degree of stenosis, especially in the absence of intravenous contrast.

Catheter angiography is the gold standard for determination of degree of stenosis and is defined as: % stenosis = [1 − minimal residual lumen/normal distal cervical internal carotid artery diameter] × 100 (Figure 2). Angiography, however, is associated with a 1% to 2% risk of stroke and is now most often used in cases of concerns about vascular anatomy or when noninvasive tests are discordant.

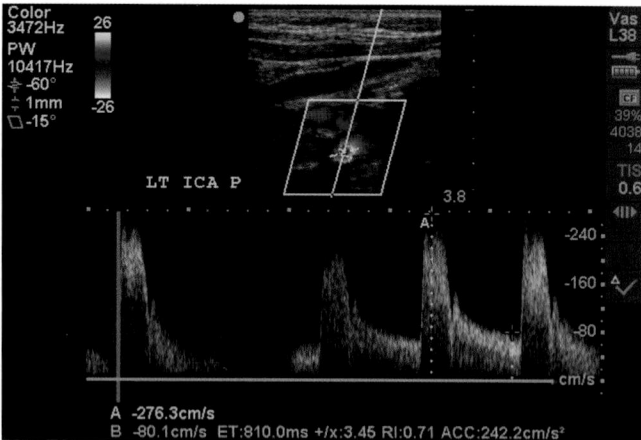

FIGURE 1 Preoperative duplex ultrasound scan shows increased velocities at the area of a high-grade carotid stenosis.

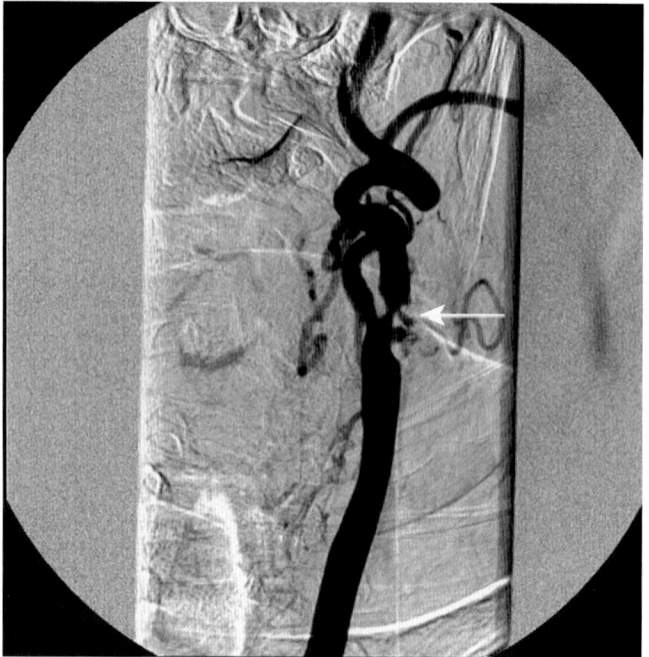

FIGURE 2 Preoperative angiogram shows a high-grade carotid stenosis with normal distal internal carotid artery.

INDICATIONS

Carotid endarterectomy is one of the best studied peripheral vascular surgical operations, with indications based on multiple randomized trials (Table 1). The Asymptomatic Carotid Atherosclerosis Study (ACAS) trial randomized asymptomatic patients with more than 60% stenosis to CEA and medical management versus medical management alone. The 5-year stroke rate among patients managed with surgery was 5.1% compared with 11% for those undergoing medical management alone, which accounted for an absolute ipsilateral stroke risk reduction of 5.9% and a relative risk reduction of more than 50%. The Asymptomatic Carotid Surgery Trial (ACST) confirmed these findings with an absolute any stroke risk reduction of 5.4% and a relative risk reduction of 46%. One should note that best medical management in these studies was antiplatelet therapy alone as the studies were performed before the statin era. Comparisons of antiplatelet therapy and statins with surgery have not been performed.

The estimated 5-year incidence rate of stroke among patients who have had a TIA is 35% to 45%. Several large center trials have explored the benefit of surgically treating this patient population. The North American Symptomatic Carotid Endarterectomy Trial (NASCET) compared surgery and medical management with best medical management alone in symptomatic patients with carotid stenosis. Patients treated with best medical management were shown to a have 2-year cumulative risk of ipsilateral stroke of 26%, whereas patients treated with surgery had a 9% risk, a 17% absolute risk reduction. In those with moderate stenosis (50% to 69%), a decrease was seen in the 5-year ipsilateral risk of stroke from 22.2% to 15.7%. The European Carotid Surgery Trial (ECST) further confirmed these results with an absolute ipsilateral stroke risk reduction of 13.8%.

Current recommendations from the Society for Vascular Surgery (SVS) recommend CEA and best medical management for the treatment of asymptomatic disease with carotid stenosis greater than 60% and symptomatic disease with greater than 50% stenosis. A joint statement from the SVS and the American Heart Association released updated recommendations for 2011 to further clarify these standards. Currently, high-level evidence recommends CEA for the symptomatic patients (TIA or nondisabling ischemic stroke) with more than 50% stenosis within 6 months of symptoms provided the anticipated rate of perioperative stroke or mortality is less than 6%. According to the American Association of Neurological Surgeons and the American Stroke Association, treatment with CEA within 2 weeks of presentation for acute stroke is reasonable and appropriate. For asymptomatic patients, CEA for stenosis greater than 60% is recommended as long as the perioperative risk of stroke and death is less than 3%.

TABLE 1: Randomized trials comparing carotid endarterectomy with medical management of carotid stenosis

Trial	Stenosis indication	Medical stroke risk	Surgical stroke risk	Risk reduction	Time period
Asymptomatic					
ACAS	≥60%	11.0%	5.1%	5.9%	5 y
ACST	≥60%	11.8%	6.4%	5.4%	5 y
Symptomatic					
NASCET	≥70%	26%	9%	17%	2 y
	50%-69%	22.2%	15.7%	6.5%	5 y
ECST	70%-99%	20.6%	6.8%	13.8%	3 y

ACAS, Asymptomatic Carotid Atherosclerosis Trial; *ACST*, Asymptomatic Carotid Surgery Trial; *ECST*, European Carotid Surgery Trialists; *NASCET*, North American Symptomatic Carotid Endarterectomy Trial.

Carotid Endarterectomy Versus Carotid Stenting

As the technique of carotid artery stenting (CAS) becomes more widespread, comparison of the outcomes with the gold standard of endarterectomy is important. CAS was initially used for patients with high-risk medical or anatomic criteria; however, it is now being applied to those with both symptomatic and asymptomatic disease.

Although multiple trials have examined the outcomes of CAS, perhaps the most accepted study is the Carotid Revascularization Endarterectomy Versus Stenting Trial (CREST) trial. This trial encompassed a group of 2502 symptomatic and asymptomatic patients. The periprocedural stroke rate was higher in the CAS group (4.1% vs 2.3%; $P = 0.01$); however, the periprocedural myocardial infarction rate was higher in the CEA group (2.3% vs 1.1%; $P = 0.03$). After this period, the ipsilateral stroke rate was similar between the CAS and CEA groups (2.0% and 2.4%, respectively; $P = 0.85$). In comparison of symptomatic and asymptomatic patients, the difference in the periprocedural stroke rate was accounted for by the symptomatic group. With examination of the 4-year study period outcomes, however, a trend was found towards an increased risk of stroke in the asymptomatic patients ($P = 0.07$) but not in the symptomatic patients ($P = 0.25$). Although decisions must be made on an individual basis and newer stent technologies could bring differing results, these data are a reminder that CEA remains the gold standard for treatment of carotid occlusive disease.

CAROTID ENDARTERECTOMY: OPERATIVE TECHNIQUE

Preoperative Medical Regimen

Optimization of the medical management of patients with carotid disease is essential to reduce risk of perioperative stroke. Before surgery, all patients should be placed on antiplatelet therapy with aspirin or clopidogrel. The dosing of aspirin therapy has been extensively examined, and clear evidence exists that 81 mg or 325 mg daily is an appropriate dose, with no additional benefit (and possible increased risk) with an increase to 650 or 1300 mg daily. Perioperative clopidogrel use results in decreased number of observed embolic events with transcranial Doppler scan in patients undergoing CEA, a surrogate measure that correlates with the risk of stroke. Clopidogrel is not associated with an increased risk of perioperative bleeding, and dual perioperative antiplatelet therapy may be associated with a decreased risk of stroke compared with single antiplatelet therapy.

Statin therapy has also been shown to benefit patients with carotid disease both before and after surgery. The author's institution has shown a lower rate of cerebrovascular symptoms among patients with known carotid disease presenting for CEA. Further, among 1600 patients undergoing CEA in a large series, statin use decreased the 30-day risk of stroke and TIA, and mortality. The protective effects

of statin therapy appear largely related to its pleiotropic arterial effects rather than the lipid-lowering effects; therefore, all patients should be started and subsequently continued on statin therapy regardless of serum lipid profile. On hospital discharge, antiplatelet and statin therapies are continued long term in the patient for CEA.

Dextran has been used for its antiplatelet effects during carotid endarterectomy. A dextran-40 drip can be started just before clamping of the internal carotid artery at a rate of 5 to 10 mL per hour and continued in the immediate postoperative period. Although dextran therapy was common years ago, more recent evidence suggests that it may be associated with an increased risk of congestive heart failure and other perioperative complications without decreasing the risk of stroke.

Anesthesia

CEA may be performed with a variety of anesthetic methods, including general, regional, and local anesthesia. Selection of anesthetic method requires consideration of several factors. General anesthesia provides a secure airway in a patient asleep, which allows the surgeon to operate without the patient having undue anxiety. Despite suggestion from early reports that patients undergoing CEA with general anesthesia need longer hospital lengths of stay, current evidence does not show a significant difference compared with patients undergoing CEA with regional anesthesia. Many reports have shown improved cardiac stability in patients undergoing CEA with regional anesthesia, but evidence does not support a subsequent reduction in the incidence of myocardial infarction compared with general anesthesia. Regional anesthesia may be inappropriate in the anxious patient who is unlikely to tolerate the necessary surgical positioning and technique. Among regional anesthesia techniques (deep versus superficial or intermediate blocks), equal efficacy appears to exist in analgesia; however, regional anesthesia with deep block is associated with a significantly higher rate of conversion to general anesthesia, with approximately 2% of patients needing conversion. One proposed benefit among regional or local methods versus general anesthesia may be in regards to selective shunting (see subsequent discussion). The author's current practice is to perform CEA with general anesthesia unless the patient has excessive cardiac risk and is not a candidate for carotid stenting.

Patient Positioning

Appropriate patient positioning is fundamental to achieve adequate exposure and reduce risks of complications, including loss of orientation, hyperextension injury, and unnecessary extension of skin incision. The patient is placed in the supine position at the edge of the bed on the operative side, and a roll is placed behind the scapula to achieve some hyperextension of the neck (Figure 3). A padded ring is placed under the head to prevent neck injury from extreme

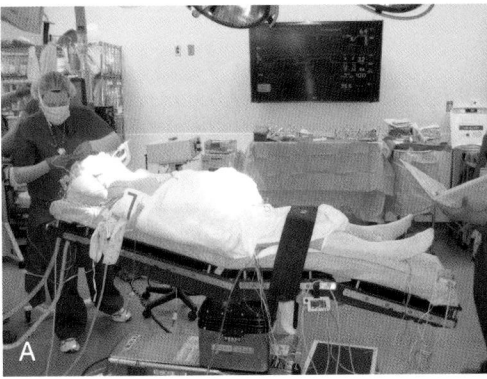
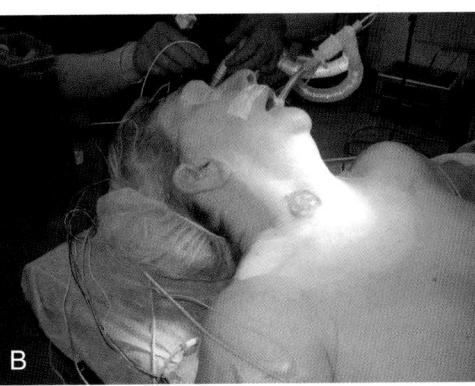

FIGURE 3 **A,** The patient is positioned supine on the operating room table in the "beach-chair" position. **B,** The patient's neck is then extended and turned to the contralateral side to assist with exposure. Note the electroencephalogram electrodes and wires placed for selective shunting and draped away from the operative field.

hyperextension. If local or regional anesthesia is used, a Mayo stand is placed over the patient's head so that the surgical drapes may be suspended away from the patient's face in an effort to prevent sensations of claustrophobia. With general anesthesia, the endotracheal tube is secured to the corner of the mouth opposite the side of the operative field. Nasotracheal intubation may be necessary for a high lesion or a high bifurcation. The operating table is then adjusted to the "beach chair" position, with a moderate amount of reverse Trendelenburg's position to decompress the venous system. The prepped area should be from the base of the earlobe and the mastoid process down to the sternal notch.

Skin Incision

The standard incision for CEA is a longitudinal incision parallel to the medial border of the sternocleidomastoid muscle. If the preoperative evaluation indicates the need for more cephalad exposure above the angle of the jaw, the upper portion of the incision is angled posterior to the earlobe in an effort to avoid the parotid gland. Improved cosmesis may be obtained from a transverse incision placed within a skin crease 1 to 2 cm inferior to the angle of the jaw. However, difficulty with exposure may be encountered if this incision is made in an improper location. Proper location can often be determined with identification of the location of the carotid bifurcation on preoperative imaging and the transverse incision made over this point.

Operative Technique

Fundamental principles of good surgical technique are paramount to a successful CEA. Obscuration of vital structures of the neck with unintentional bleeding can result in injury and disastrous consequences. The dissection begins with division of the platysma and mobilization of the medial border of the sternocleidomastoid muscle with electrocautery. Care should be taken to avoid severing the external jugular vein, which runs immediately deep to the platysma, in the event that it is needed for patching. Dissection through a transverse skin incision is more likely to encounter the external jugular than it is through a longitudinal incision. The greater auricular nerve exits at the lateral border of the sternocleidomastoid muscle and heads towards the ear. Transection of this nerve in the superoposterior aspect of the wound results in a cutaneous sensory deficit of the earlobe.

Once the sternocleidomastoid muscle is retracted laterally, the carotid sheath is then entered. The internal jugular vein is identified and dissected along its entire medial length. The facial vein commonly serves as a landmark for the carotid bifurcation and is identified medially crossing the base of the wound. Division of the facial vein allows lateral retraction of the internal jugular vein. At this point, the vagus nerve should be identified in its typical course running between the carotid artery and internal jugular vein. An important consideration is that the vagus nerve may be located anterior to the common carotid artery (CCA) in approximately 5% of patients. The patient is then given 80 U/kg of heparin. An activated clotting time (ACT) is maintained at 200 to 250 seconds.

Circumferential control is obtained around the CCA with an umbilical tape and Rummel tourniquet (Figure 4). The ansa cervicalis can then be identified running medial to the distal CCA. Preservation of the ansa is not necessary, but it may be useful to track it superiorly to its junction with the hypoglossal nerve in an effort to identify the hypoglossal, which crosses medially from a superior to inferior location.

Sharp dissection is continued along the anterior aspect of the CCA to its bifurcation. Manipulation of the carotid artery should be minimized in this region to reduce the risk of intraoperative embolization. The carotid bulb may be injected with 1% lidocaine to

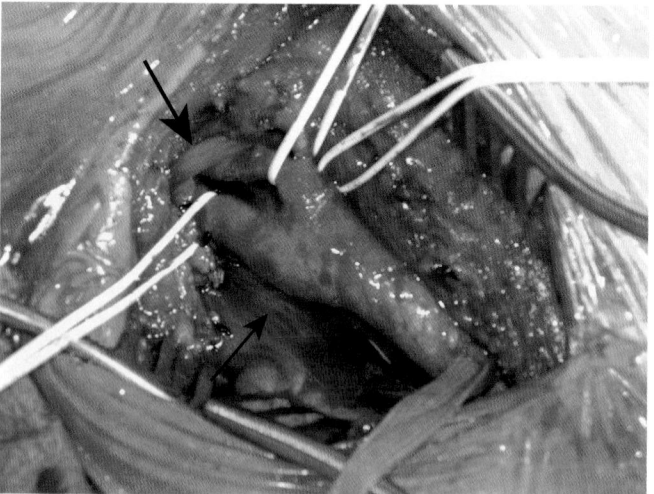

FIGURE 4 Intraoperative exposure of the carotid bifurcation. The common carotid artery is encircled with an umbilical tape, and the internal carotid, external carotid, and superior thyroid arteries are encircled with vessel loops. Care is taken to identify and avoid the vagus nerve (*small arrow*) and the hypoglossal nerve (*large arrow*).

anesthetize the carotid body and reduce hemodynamic instability. The superior thyroid artery is typically the first branch of the external carotid artery (ECA). It is identified coming off the medial border of the carotid bifurcation or proximal ECA and is controlled with a vessel loop in Potts fashion. The ECA is dissected and encircled with a vessel loop.

As sharp dissection is continued along the internal carotid artery (ICA), it is imperative to ensure the ICA is controlled beyond the distal extent of disease process. This may require ligation of small crossing veins, ligation of the occipital artery, or working superior to the hypoglossal nerve. Once superior to the plaque, the ICA is encircled with a vessel loop.

The superior thyroid is controlled with the vessel loop, and the ICA is clamped first to prevent distal embolization during clamping of subsequent vessels. As with vessel loop placement, the clamp must be placed beyond the distal aspect of carotid plaque to reduce the risk of embolization or incomplete endarterectomy. The CCA and ECA are subsequently clamped. A longitudinal arteriotomy is made with an 11 or 15 blade and extended with Potts scissors from normal CCA to normal ICA.

At that point, a determination must be made whether to shunt. The type of shunt used is based on surgeon preference, but it should be opened and available if necessary. The author prefers to use the Argyle shunts (Covidien, Mansfield, Mass) because they can be sized to the ICA (Figure 5). The shunt, when needed, is first placed in the distal ICA and allowed to back bleed. The proximal end is then placed into the CCA. Certain surgeons choose to shunt all patients; however, the author prefers selective shunting to reduce the small risk of stroke or ICA dissection associated with shunt insertion. If local or regional anesthesia is used on a patient, a decrease in hemispheric or global neurologic function signifies poor cerebral perfusion that necessitates shunting. With general anesthesia, electroencephalogram (EEG) monitoring can be used to identify cerebral ischemia. A 50% decrease in fast background activity, an increase in delta wave activity, and a complete loss of EEG signals constitute the criteria for shunting. Patients with a recent stroke, TIA, or amaurosis are routinely shunted to avoid cerebral hypoperfusion of at risk regions.

Less common methods for cerebral monitoring include carotid stump pressure measurement and cerebral oxygen saturation. Carotid stump pressure measurement is performed after clamps are placed on both the ECA and the CCA, with the ICA remaining patent. A needle is connected to a pressure line and inserted into the distal CCA

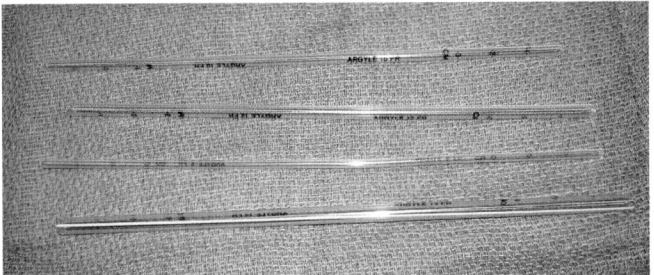

FIGURE 5 Argyle shunts (Covidien, Mansfield, Mass) come in different sizes that can be matched to the internal carotid artery.

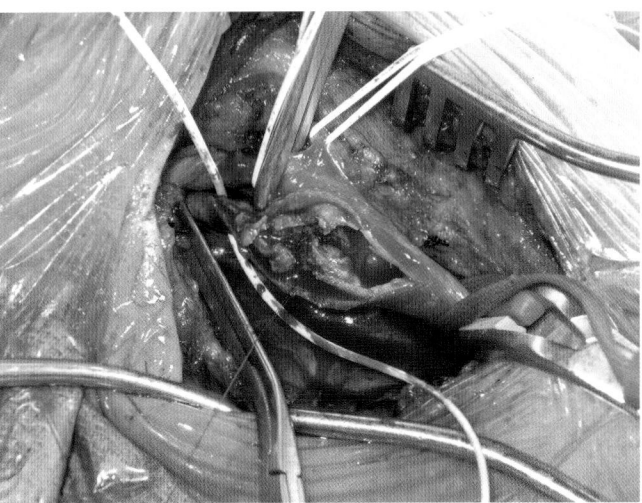

FIGURE 6 Intraoperative photograph shows the plaque within the carotid artery.

below the carotid bifurcation. A stump pressure of 50 mm Hg is used as a threshold for shunting. Stump pressure measurements are limited by the risk for embolization with clamping of the CCA or insertion of the needle, and watershed cerebral hypoperfusion despite adequate pressures. Cerebral oxygen saturation is measured with near-infrared spectroscopy probes placed before surgery on the patient's right and left forehead. An ipsilateral baseline cerebral oxygen saturation less than 55% or a decrease of greater than 15% with clamping is predictive of ischemia requiring shunting. Although this technique is associated with a 94% specificity, sensitivity is only 68%, resulting in unnecessary shunt placement in certain patients.

The endarterectomy is begun with a Freer or Penfield elevator in the plane between the media and adventitia, starting within the mid plaque (Figure 6). Once an endpoint in the distal CCA is established, the plaque is transected. The endarterectomy is then continued up into the ICA. At the endpoint of the plaque, it can either be flared across the ICA by pulling the plaque off transversely or transected with Iris scissors. Either way, a smooth transition from endarterectomized surface to normal intima is mandatory to prevent embolization or dissection with reperfusion. Gentle injection of saline solution onto the surface may reveal an intimal flap that must be remedied with further endarterectomy or 7-0 polypropylene tacking sutures. Tacking sutures should be avoided unless absolutely necessary because these are potentially thrombogenic and may increase the risk of perioperative stroke. The endarterectomy is continued back towards the ECA. The ECA clamp is removed, and the remainder of the plaque is endarterectomized in eversion fashion. Once the endarterectomy is complete, a Schmidt or pediatric intestinal clamp is passed up into the external carotid artery to remove any remaining debris. The endarterectomized surface is then carefully inspected, and all residual fragments of intima and media are removed with DeBakey forceps.

The current body of literature supports closure of the arteriotomy with a patch because it is associated with a decreased rate of restenosis compared with primary closure. A variety of patch materials are available, including autologous vein, polytetrafluoroethylene (PTFE), woven polyester (Dacron; Atrium Medical Corporation, Hudson, N.H.), and bovine pericardium (Figure 7). Recent comparisons of closure methods report no difference in perioperative bleeding, infection, or pseudoaneurysm formation between patch materials, and surgeons may therefore use the material with which he or she is most proficient. Autogenous vein or bovine pericardium should be used in infected fields.

At that point, antegrade and retrograde flushing maneuvers should be performed. If a shunt was used, it is removed before final closure of the artery and back bleeding from the ICA can occur to clear debris created with shunt manipulation. The arteriotomy is then closed, and the clamp on the ICA is briefly released to fill the vessel with blood. It is then replaced while the clamps on the CCA and ECA are released. This directs any remaining debris or air up the ECA before reperfusion of the ICA. Finally, the ICA clamp is removed.

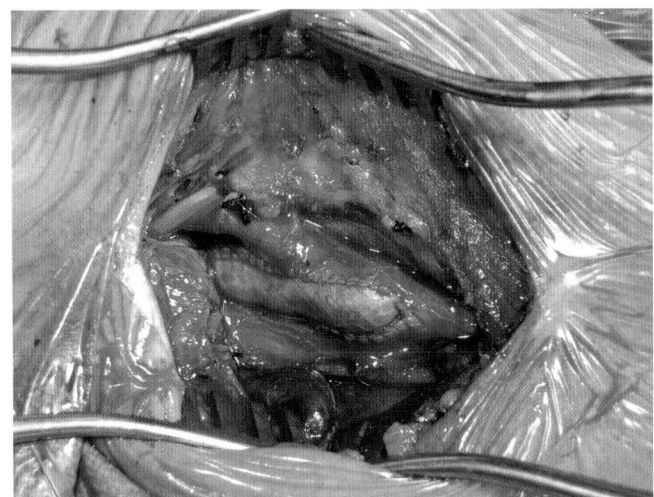

FIGURE 7 Completion intraoperative photograph shows the bovine pericardial patch sewn with 6-0 polypropylene sutures in running fashion.

Eversion Endarterectomy

Eversion endarterectomy is an alternative technique for carotid revascularization. Exposure of the carotid artery is performed in a similar manner to the previous description. It is technically difficult to shunt, and the authors therefore advocate performing a test clamp of the ICA before committing to this technique. If there is no indication of cerebral ischemia and no need for shunting, one may proceed with the eversion technique. If the patient does need shunting, the author falls back on the conventional endarterectomy with patch technique.

For performance of eversion, the ICA is obliquely transected at its origin and everted. The plaque is pulled away from the rolled back adventitia until the distal limit is exposed and is then transected. The ECA/CCA is then endarterectomized. The ICA is then reanastomosed to the carotid bifurcation with running 6-0 polypropylene suture. Advantages of eversion endarterectomy include a shorter clamp time, no lengthening of the ICA, and no need for patching. Disadvantages include the difficulty in shunting. Eversion endarterectomy has also been purported to have lower restenosis rates; however, a recent systematic review of the literature showed no difference in stroke or clinically significant restenosis rates. Surgeons should use the technique most familiar to them to decrease the risk of perioperative stroke.

Completion Studies

Among the several potential etiologies of stroke in patients undergoing CEA, thromboembolism and carotid artery thrombosis from inadvertent technical error remain preventable. The most common intraoperative completion studies, including handheld continuous Doppler scan, duplex ultrasound scan, and intraoperative angiography, have all been used to mitigate this risk.

Handheld continuous Doppler scan evaluation can be rapidly used to assess for areas of high turbulence and velocity changes in the repair. However, it is highly operator dependent and less sensitive than duplex ultrasound scan, especially to small intimal flaps and subtle stenoses. Duplex ultrasound scan is a sensitive tool that provides both anatomic imaging and real-time physiologic information regarding blood flow through the endarterectomy repair. Both duplex ultrasound scan and intraoperative angiography are equally sensitive in detecting "major" technical defects. However, duplex ultrasound scan has been shown to be more sensitive in detecting "minor" flaws (87% vs 59%).

Although the author regularly performs completion duplex ultrasound scan, an interesting note is that certain studies have not found completion imaging to decrease the risk of perioperative stroke but rather to only decrease the rate of restenosis. Moreover, no consensus exists as to criteria for reexploration. Most studies agree that "minor" technical abnormalities should be left alone because of a significant association between intraoperative revision and perioperative stroke. "Major" abnormalities may need to be addressed. These may include a peak systolic velocity in the ICA greater than 125 cm/s, an ICA/CCA velocity ratio greater than 2.0, spectral broadening throughout systole, a B-mode flap in the ICA 2 mm, or any other obvious major anatomic problem, such as a severe kink or intravascular thrombus.

Unexpected Intraoperative Findings of the Internal Carotid Artery

High Carotid Bifurcation

Occasionally one encounters a high carotid bifurcation or a superiorly ending plaque that necessitates further cephalad exposure of the internal carotid artery. When it is anticipated before surgery, nasotracheal intubation is the simplest maneuver to gain better exposure. This leaves the mouth closed and obtains a few extra centimeters. Preoperative anterior subluxation of the mandible by an otolaryngologist also provides superior exposure. For more exposure once the operation has started, the hypoglossal nerve can be dissected out, which allows the surgeon to work on both sides of it. One must be careful not to cause traction injury when doing so. Ligation and division of the occipital artery may also afford the surgeon a bit more working room. Division of the digastric muscle is the next step to gain exposure; however, care must be taken to avoid the hypoglossal nerve, which frequently lies directly posterior to the muscle belly. If the aforementioned maneuvers are insufficient, assistance should be obtained from an otolaryngologist in performing resection of the styloid process.

Hypoplastic Internal Carotid Artery

Severe stenosis of the internal carotid artery may lead to the findings of a small ICA distal to the lesion. This can result from one of two things: either the artery is normal but underfilled because of poor perfusion pressure, or the artery itself is hypoplastic (Figure 8). A normal artery should look normal on the outside. If one suspects a

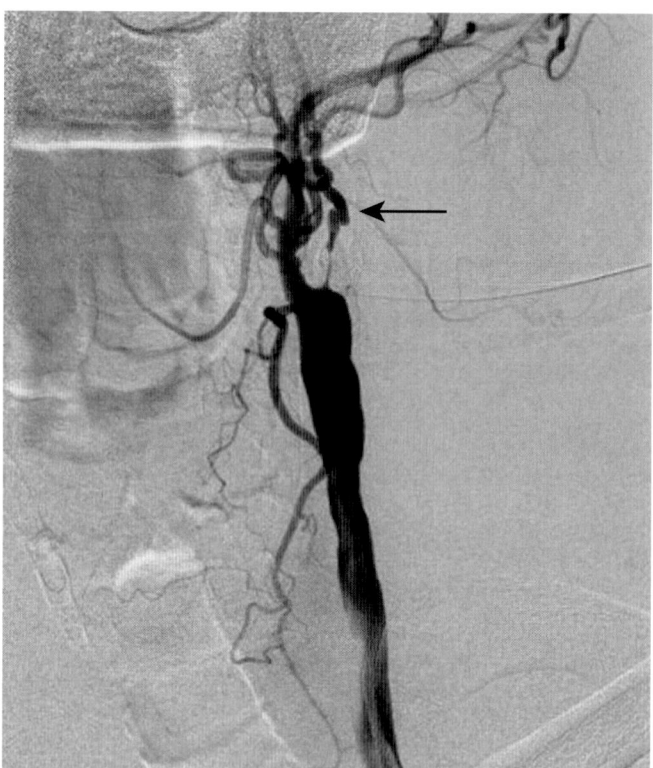

FIGURE 8 Angiogram shows a string sign with a hypoplastic distal internal carotid artery *(arrow)*.

hypoplastic artery, however, an on-table angiogram can be performed. If the hypoplasia extends to the skull base, then anticoagulation therapy is indicated. If the artery has already been opened, then one should proceed with ligation with postoperative anticoagulation therapy.

Thrombosed Internal Carotid Artery

Occlusion of the internal carotid artery is never treated surgically because this is associated with an increased risk of stroke. However, lesions may progress during the preoperative period. The author tries to ensure that the patient has a duplex ultrasound scan within 6 weeks of surgery to avoid this scenario. An acutely thrombosed artery found at the time of surgery should lead to abandonment of the case. Manipulation of the ICA in this case increases the risk of stroke.

COMPLICATIONS

Stroke

The risk of perioperative stroke is directly related to the indication for the operation. A recent large, multicenter trial showed perioperative stroke rates of 3.2% among symptomatic patients and 1.4% in asymptomatic patients. Commonly, these strokes are ipsilateral to the side of operation; however, significant risk of contralateral stroke remains, and symptoms in this distribution should be investigated thoroughly in the postoperative period. The observation of contralateral stroke after endarterectomy has supported the belief that many of these neurologic events result from emboli or microemboli that enter cerebral circulation during the manipulation of the carotid artery. Through observation with transcranial Doppler monitoring during endarterectomy, the periods of highest risk for embolic events are immediately before institution of cerebral protection through applying vascular clamps and immediately on removal of the clamps. Therefore, the principals of delicate tissue manipulation and minimal plaque disruption before protection are of extreme importance in reducing the risk of stroke during endarterectomy.

Changes in the patient's neurologic status recognized in the immediate postoperative period should be considered the result of thrombosis until proven otherwise. In the author's center, the protocol for stroke recognized in the recovery room is to urgently obtain a carotid duplex scan. The surgeon can then make the decision regarding to proceed directly to the operating room or, in the case of negative duplex scan results, to obtain an MRI to look for acute ischemic changes that necessitate the involvement of the neurology team.

Nerve Injury

Cranial nerve injuries are the most frequent complications after CEA, with rates in large prospective trials between 4% and 9%. Because of their anatomic relationship to the carotid arteries, the hypoglossal, recurrent laryngeal, superior laryngeal, and marginal mandibular nerves are subject to traction and minor trauma during the operation. Injuries to these nerves are usually transitory, typically resolving in a few days or weeks.

Myocardial Infarction

The presence of carotid disease serves as a marker for widespread arterial disease in most patients. In fact, the most common cause of death after CEA is cardiac disease. In the CREST trial, the rate of postoperative myocardial infarction was shown to be 2.3% among a combined group of symptomatic and asymptomatic patients. Maximization of the preoperative risks of patients undergoing CEA is essential with correct modification of cardiac risk factors, including the introduction of aspirin and statin therapy to the patient's current regimen, when appropriate. In patients with multiple cardiac risk factors, including diabetes, hypertension, recent history of coronary intervention, and creatinine greater than 2.0 mg/dL, cardiology workup before carotid surgery may be indicated.

Hyperperfusion Syndrome

A small percentage of patients have an entity known as hyperperfusion syndrome after CEA. This clinical syndrome involves loss of autoregulation of the cerebral vessels as a result of chronic dilation under the ischemic conditions produced by long-standing stenosis. After restoration of normal blood flow, the increased pressure in the cerebral vasculature causes cerebral edema and hemorrhage. Clinical sequelae typically occur within 2 weeks of CEA and consist of headache ipsilateral to the side of repair, focal seizures, and radiographic evidence of intracerebral hemorrhage. Prevention of hyperperfusion syndrome consists of strict blood pressure control in the immediate postoperative period, especially in patients who were treated for high-grade stenosis. If clinical signs develop, patients should be immediately admitted to an intensive care unit for antihypertensive and antiseizure therapy.

RECURRENT CAROTID STENOSIS

After endarterectomy, patients are followed in the clinic with carotid duplex scan within 6 weeks. In the author's practice, if initial imaging shows an intact repair, the next follow-up appointment is scheduled for 6 months. Recurrent stenosis occurs in approximately 5% to 22% of patients. Analysis suggests that the rate of recurrence may be dependent on the time from CEA, with a 10% restenosis rate in the first year, 3% rate in the second, and 2% rate in the third year after surgery. Neointimal hyperplasia is the most common cause of restenosis, although early restenosis may result from an inadequate endarterectomy. Serial carotid duplex scan examinations in patients with neointimal hyperplasia show that up to one third spontaneously regress, and therefore, restenosis within the first 6 months should not be operated on and should be followed up with a repeat duplex scan at 1 year confirming persistence of the restenosis. Lesions that develop after 36 months most likely represent recurrent atherosclerotic disease.

Populations with increased risk of restenosis include women, patients who continue to smoke, and those with cardiovascular risk factors such as hypertension, hypercholesterolemia, or diabetes mellitus. Technical factors during the operation may also influence the rate of restenosis. In particular, injury from intraluminal shunt placement, arterial clamping, or placement of tacking sutures in the vessel may predispose to early intimal hyperplasia. Restenosis is more common with primary closure of the arteriotomy; however, no difference in restenosis was found in a recent comparison of eversion endarterectomy with conventional endarterectomy with patch closure.

In the setting of recurrent stenosis, repeat carotid endarterectomy has the potential to be performed successfully with excellent results. Several large studies have shown low stroke and death rates (combined measure of 3.7%) after repeat CEA. However, additional challenges with technique and dissection increase the risks of injury to surrounding structures. Intimal hyperplasia is a firm, rubbery plaque rich in fibroblasts and smooth muscle cells surrounded by dense accumulation of collagen and acid mucopolysaccharide. It is less prone to ulceration or thromboses than primary lesions or late restenotic, atherosclerotic lesions. No prospective randomized trials exist to support repeat CEA, but most available evidence encourages treatment of symptomatic and very high-grade asymptomatic recurrent stenoses.

Carotid angioplasty and stenting (CAS) has been proposed as an alternative to mitigate these risks, but recent trials have not confirmed a therapeutic benefit of CAS compared with CEA. Ultimately, careful planning and technique are of paramount importance in obtaining excellent results in repeat CEA.

COMBINED CAROTID ENDARTERECTOMY–CORONARY ARTERY BYPASS

Still another class of patients has asymptomatic carotid disease that is found in the course of preoperative workup for coronary artery bypass grafting (CABG). Although no consensus exists regarding the best timing for both surgeries, meta-analyses suggest that the risk of stroke, myocardial infarction, or death varies depending on which procedure is performed first. Staged CEA-CABG or CABG-CEA is associated with a lower cumulative risk of stroke/myocardial infarction/death than synchronous CEA-CABG, but these subgroups had a lower incidence of acute preoperative cardiac or neurologic symptoms. At the author's institution, synchronous CEA-CABG is typically performed because the operative stroke risk is less than 5%. Because patients are heparinized for the CABG, a drain is left in the surgical bed and the skin is not closed until the CABG is completed.

SUGGESTED READINGS

Asymptomatic Carotid Atherosclerosis Study Collaborators: Endarterectomy for asymptomatic carotid stenosis: Executive Committee for the Asymptomatic Carotid Atherosclerosis Study, *JAMA* 273(18):1421–1428, 1995.

Brott TG, Hobson RW 2nd, Howard G,et al: Stenting versus endarterectomy for treatment of carotid-artery stenosis, *N Engl J Med* 353(1):11–23, 2010.

Giangola G, Migaly J, Riles TS, et al: Perioperative morbidity and mortality in combined vs. staged approaches to carotid and coronary revascularization, *Ann Vasc Surg* 10(2):138–142, 1996.

NASCET Collaborators: Beneficial effect of carotid endarterectomy in symptomatic patients with high-grade stenosis, *N Engl J Med* 325(7):445–453, 1991.

Yadav JS, Wholey MH, Kuntz RE, et al: Protected carotid-artery stenting versus endarterectomy in high-risk patients, *N Engl J Med* 351:1493–1501, 2004.

THE MANAGEMENT OF RECURRENT CAROTID ARTERY STENOSIS

Timothy K. Williams, MD, and
Bruce A. Perler, MD, MBA

INCIDENCE OF RESTENOSIS

Estimates are that approximately 140,000 carotid endarterectomy (CEA) procedures are performed annually in the United States alone. Despite a low risk of periprocedural complications and well-documented durability after CEA, a small minority of patients have recurrent stenosis develop in the treated artery over time. For example, in the Asymptomatic Carotid Atherosclerosis Study, the recurrent stenosis rate after CEA was approximately 7% at 60 months of follow-up. In a meta-analysis that included 55 studies, the rate of recurrent carotid stenosis after CEA ranged from 6% to 14% and documented an annual incidence rate of 1.5% to 4.5%. In another analysis, the rate of restenosis was 10% within the first year, 3% within the second year, and 2% in the third year after CEA, which indicates that the rate of restenosis is not linear.

Carotid angioplasty and stenting (CAS) is increasingly performed as an option for patients deemed to be unacceptable candidates for CEA. Although the incidence of restenosis after CAS is not as well defined in the literature, the rate of restenosis appears to be higher than after CEA. For example, a recent study documented an in-stent restenosis rate of 15% at 4 years (defined as >60% luminal narrowing). In the study with the longest follow-up period reported to date, the rate of 70% or more restenosis was 19% after CAS, including 16% who underwent reintervention, and 0 after CEA at a mean follow-up period of 5 years. However, symptomatic recurrence is rare, occurring in only 1% to 5% of patients after either CEA or CAS.

TIMING OF RESTENOSIS AND PATHOGENESIS

The pathophysiology of recurrent carotid stenosis, and the necessity for reintervention, is related to the timing of presentation. It is important to differentiate early recurrent stenosis from residual stenosis or stenosis from technical imprecision in the performance of the CEA. Technical issues include performance of an incomplete endarterectomy, residual dissection flaps, clamp-related intimal injury, and stenosis related to the suture line. Although considerable debate and conflicting data are found with respect to its efficacy, the authors believe performance of a completion study before the neck incision is closed markedly reduces the likelihood of leaving the patient with residual defects from technical error; the authors' preference is the performance of a completion duplex scan (Figure 1). Technical issues after CAS are largely related to residual stenosis after stent placement. Identification and correction of these immediate technical imperfections are crucial to reduce acute thrombotic complications in addition to later restenosis.

Early recurrent stenosis generally develops within the first 2 years after CEA and results from the development of myointimal hyperplasia. Although the pathophysiology of this process is not completely understood, it is believed to represent a variable response of the vessel wall to injury. The process involves the proliferation of vascular smooth muscle, collagen, and a variety of other extracellular matrix proteins. The luminal surface of this lesion is typically lined

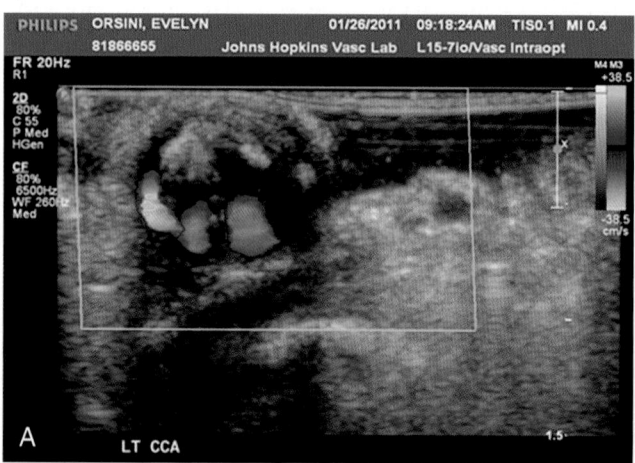
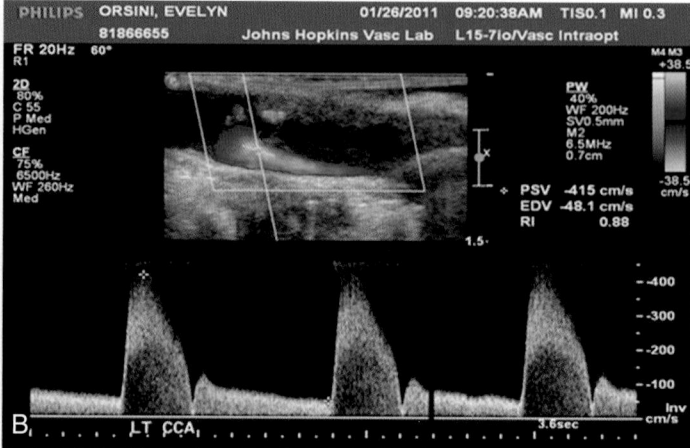

FIGURE 1 **A,** Completion carotid duplex scan. Note the intimal dissection in the common carotid artery from clamp injury on this transverse image. **B,** Note the elevated velocities at the site of intimal dissection from the clamp injury during carotid endarterectomy.

with endothelium. As such, it tends to be nonthrombogenic with a low thromboembolic potential. Myointimal hyperplasia accounts for most cases of recurrent carotid stenosis and usually peaks around 1 year after surgery. This lesion often has a smooth tapered appearance on duplex ultrasound scan or angiography. In a small percentage of patients after both CEA and CAS, myointimal hyperplasia can result in a hemodynamically significant lesion. The molecular basis for this process may be linked to the inflammatory process of the initial atherosclerotic lesion. Some studies have shown that lipid-rich and heavily macrophage-infiltrated plaques result in a more robust myointimal proliferation in the postoperative setting, likely related to an abundance of various inflammatory molecules including specific matrix metalloproteases.

Late recurrent stenoses, defined as developing more than 2 years after CEA, and usually much later, typically result from progressive or new atherosclerotic disease, although these lesions may have a component of underlying intimal hyperplasia. Although myointimal hyperplastic lesions are characteristically smooth, recurrent atherosclerotic plaques have a varied appearance similar to that of primary plaques. They typically are irregular and heterogeneous in both gross and radiographic appearance.

RISK REDUCTION

Multiple factors, modifiable and nonmodifiable, have been associated with the development of recurrent carotid stenoses. Most studies have examined risk factors specific for patients undergoing CEA; less long-term follow-up data are found on CAS.

The most important nonmodifiable risk factor is female gender, very likely related to the relatively smaller diameter of the carotid vessels in women. In addition, chronic renal insufficiency has been associated with an increased risk of early recurrent stenosis. The most robust risk factor associated with late restenosis is hyperlipidemia. Statin therapy has been associated with a significantly reduced rate of both early and late restenosis after CEA. In addition to the benefit of lowering lipid levels, the so-called pleiotropic effects of statins may also be operative in ameliorating the pathophysiologic process of restenosis. A reduction in the rate of recurrent stenosis associated with statin use has not been identified in patients undergoing CAS, however.

On the other hand, typical risk factors for atherosclerosis, such as ongoing smoking, hyperhomocysteinemia, hypertension, and diabetes, have not been shown to have strong links to the development of myointimal hyperplasia. Furthermore, although platelet inhibition with agents such as aspirin and clopidogrel has clearly been associated with a reduced risk of cardiovascular and cerebrovascular events in patients with carotid stenoses, these medications do not have a clear impact on the natural history of recurrent carotid stenosis. Conversely, some recent evidence suggests that cilostazol, a phosphodiesterase inhibitor commonly used to treat intermittent claudication, may modify the progression of myointimal hyperplasia and has shown some benefit in patients undergoing CAS. More study is warranted to validate this finding.

Without question, the most important modifiable factor in reducing the incidence of restenosis after CEA is technical. In addition to avoiding technical imperfection at the time of the endarterectomy as noted previously, closure of the arteriotomy with a patch has consistently been shown to be associated with a significantly lower incidence of restenosis compared with primary closure. In a Cochrane review, the use of a Dacron or vein patch reduced the rate of restenosis by 76% compared with primary closure. In the only large randomized trial to compare standard endarterectomy with eversion endarterectomy, the Eversion carotid endarterectomy versus standard (EVEREST) trial, the 4-year cumulative risk of restenosis was 3.5%, 1.7%, and 12.6%, for eversion, conventional endarterectomy with patch, and conventional endarterectomy with primary closure, respectively. On the basis of the reported experience to date, no consensus exists on the superiority of a particular patch material (i.e., Dacron, polytetrafluoroethylene [PTFE], bovine pericardium, greater saphenous vein, or cervical vein).

DIAGNOSIS OF RESTENOSIS

Duplex ultrasound scan, the gold standard diagnostic modality for the detection and monitoring of carotid artery disease, is likewise the noninvasive method of choice for the diagnosis of recurrent carotid stenosis after both CEA and CAS. Although no consensus exists with respect to the most appropriate timing of baseline and interval evaluations after surgery, most clinicians obtain an initial postoperative study within the first 6 to 12 months. Retrospective studies have shown that evaluations earlier than 6 months rarely diagnose a clinically significant abnormality. The authors' preference is to obtain a completion duplex scan in the operating room and then a postoperative duplex scan at 6 and 12 months and then yearly thereafter. The scanning interval may be dictated by other factors such as the status of the contralateral carotid artery (e.g., a high-grade contralateral stenosis). When a greater than 50% stenosis is present, the authors' practice is to perform duplex scan examinations at 6-month intervals.

Duplex criteria for the quantification of the degree of stenosis in the native carotid artery do not correlate directly with the velocity criteria for establishing the degree of carotid restenosis after CEA or CAS. After CEA with patch angioplasty, a funneling or bottleneck effect is believed to be created, whereby blood flowing through the relatively large diameter carotid bulb is funneled down into the narrow lumen of the internal carotid artery (ICA), creating turbulent high-velocity flow. This is believed to result in an artifactually higher peak systolic velocity (PSV) than would be expected in a native ICA of a similar diameter. With respect to CAS, the relatively noncompliant, nondistensible stent appears to create an architecture that more closely resembles the hemodynamic pattern seen within a rigid tube. Therefore, this serves to artificially elevate the PSV above what would be expected for a given degree of stenosis in a native ICA.

The effects of these hemodynamic changes have been rigorously examined, and correlation of duplex scan findings with computed tomographic angiography (CTA) and traditional angiography has been used to validate these findings. A recent study examined duplex ultrasound scan in patients after CEA with patch closure and showed that a PSV of 213 cm/s or more and an end-diastolic velocity (EDV) of 60 cm/s or more were optimal for detection of a greater than 50% restenosis, with a sensitivity of 99% and a specificity of 100%, respectively. In addition, an ICA to common carotid artery (CCA) PSV ratio of 2.25 or higher was found to be most accurate for detection of a 50% or greater restenosis. For detection of a stenosis of greater than 70%, a PSV of greater than 274 cm/s and an EDV of 80 cm/s had a sensitivity of 99% and a specificity of 91%, respectively. The optimal ICA:CCA PSV ratio for detection of a 70% or greater stenosis was 3.34.

Revised duplex scan criteria after CAS have also been reported and include a PSV of greater than 220 cm/s for detection of a greater than 50% stenosis, with a sensitivity of 100% and a specificity of 96%, respectively. A PSV of greater than 340 cm/s or an ICA:CCA PSV ratio of greater than 4.15 was ideal for determination of an 80% or greater restenosis after CAS, with a sensitivity of 100% and a specificity of 98%, respectively.

Other diagnostic modalities may be performed when doubt exists regarding the degree of restenosis with duplex scan. CTA provides excellent visualization of the neck and cerebral vasculature and has largely obviated the need to perform conventional angiography. However, CTA may yield equivocal results when a very severe preocclusive stenosis exists so that conventional angiography may be indicated to definitively assess the vessel. Magnetic resonance angiography (MRA) is also a useful option but requires longer acquisition time and may overestimate the degree of stenosis. It is also not a desirable option after CAS because the metal stent produces significant artifact. MRA may be beneficial in assessment of plaque morphology, a factor that is increasingly recognized as a predictor of embolic risk.

INDICATIONS FOR REINTERVENTION

Only a minority of patients in whom a recurrent carotid stenosis develops after endarterectomy needs reintervention. For example, in an institutional series of 950 CEAs, reintervention was necessary in only 3.8%, with a mean follow-up period of 4.5 years. The decision to reintervene in a patient with recurrent carotid stenosis depends on several factors, including the patient's symptomatic status, the degree of stenosis, progression in the degree of stenosis, associated comorbidity, and the anticipated risk of the procedure. No level I evidence exists, and therefore, no definitive guidelines exist to establish absolute indications for reintervention. Thus, this clinical judgment must be individualized.

The most compelling indication for reintervention is the symptomatic patient with a greater than 50% restenosis on the ipsilateral side, regardless of the type of previous procedure or the time of presentation of the restenosis. Among asymptomatic patients, the decision to reintervene is most dependent on the timing of the development of restenosis, which implies the underlying pathologic lesion and also the severity of the stenosis.

Within the first 24 to 36 months after CEA, restenosis is most likely the result of myointimal hyperplasia. These lesions are typically very smooth and rarely ulcerated and have low thromboembolic potential. In addition, the development of myointimal hyperplastic lesions is a dynamic process, and many of these lesions regress over time as documented with serial duplex scan examinations. In fact, some studies have indicated that as many of one third of these lesions significantly regress over time. Therefore, the threshold for reintervention within the first 2 to 3 years in the asymptomatic patient is very high. The authors follow patients with serial duplex scan examinations, unless there is a greater than 80% to 90% stenosis, and are even more conservative in the patient with considerable associated comorbidity. Other considerations include the rate of progression of the stenosis during follow-up and the status of the remainder of the cerebral circulation.

On the other hand, recurrent stenoses that develop more than 3 years after the CEA are likely the result of progressive atherosclerosis. Similar to early recurrent stenoses from myointimal hyperplasia, most symptomatic patients warrant reintervention. On the other hand, the threshold for reintervention for the asymptomatic patient with a late recurrent stenosis should be lower than for early asymptomatic recurrent stenoses. Although the natural history of late recurrent stenosis after endarterectomy is not as well documented as for primary carotid atherosclerotic disease, one can assume that the thromboembolic potential is similar.

INTERVENTION FOR RECURRENT CAROTID STENOSIS

Once a decision to reintervene has been reached, the next decision is whether to perform a reoperative CEA or a CAS procedure. This decision should be based on a number of factors, including the anatomic location of the carotid bifurcation and the extent of the recurrent lesion, the timing of the restenosis (early versus late), and associated comorbidity. Although duplex ultrasound scan is the diagnostic modality of choice to identify recurrent carotid stenoses and follow patients long term, the authors believe that further imaging is usually required before undertaking a reoperative procedure. In most cases, the necessary anatomic information may be obtained with a CTA, although angiography remains the gold standard to provide the most definitive information. These contrast studies define the

bifurcation location and the extent of the recurrent lesion and, in conjunction with the duplex scan, characterize the underlying pathology (myointimal hyperplasia versus atherosclerosis).

To date, most patients treated for recurrent carotid stenoses have undergone reoperative endarterectomy. CAS has been reserved for patients with high bifurcations or very distal recurrent lesions, previous radiation therapy, or radical neck surgery, and the authors have had a lower threshold for electing CAS for early, myointimal hyperplastic lesions where the risks of CAS appear lower than in the treatment of atherosclerotic lesions. Furthermore, for patients who have undergone bilateral CEA procedures, knowledge of the status of the contralateral recurrent laryngeal nerve is important before considering reoperative CEA. CAS is the preferred option in the setting of contralateral recurrent laryngeal nerve paresis. Finally, this decision should also weigh the patient's overall severity of comorbidity, electing CAS for patients with prohibitive operative risk, although this is rarely encountered in the authors' practice.

REOPERATIVE CAROTID ENDARTERECTOMY

Reoperative CEA is associated with increased risk when compared with primary CEA. These challenges include the difficulty of dissection and identification and protection of crucial structures in a scarred field and technical challenges with respect to the method of arterial repair. However, with proper preoperative evaluation and careful attention to operative technique, excellent results have been achieved in this clinical setting.

Before undertaking a reoperative CEA, one must know as much as possible about the original procedure (e.g., whether the patient underwent a primary closure, patch closure, or eversion endarterectomy). One also should identify whether any cranial nerve injury or other complications occurred. Before surgery, a regimen of aspirin 81 mg per day and a statin should be started, and a beta blocker may also be indicated depending on the patient's cardiovascular risk profile.

Technical Details

The operative approach to reoperative CEA is very similar to that of the initial operative intervention with certain caveats. In the case of an unusually cephalad exposure during the initial operation or concern for very distal disease at the time of reoperation, nasotracheal intubation should strongly be considered. With the jaw closed in the absence of an endotracheal tube in the mouth, several millimeters of additional distal arterial exposure are afforded. The authors prefer a longitudinal incision through the original incision, but with extension proximally and distally. Dense scar tissue is likely to be encountered, so one should try to expose the common carotid artery proximal and the internal carotid artery distal to the previous operative field through unscarred tissues. Division of the posterior belly of the digastric muscle may be necessary to gain further distal exposure, with care exercised to identify the crossing glossopharyngeal nerve. Resection of the styloid process or mandibular subluxation represents further options to gain additional distal exposure. The sternocleidomastoid muscle should be sharply dissected off its medial attachment from the adjacent vascular structures. The internal jugular vein should be carefully dissected free from the previously endarterectomized carotid artery to which it is typically quite adherent. The operator should be constantly vigilant to identify the vagus nerve that not infrequently is encased more anteriorly or superficially than usual in the perivascular scar tissue and the hypoglossal nerve at the apex of the incision. It is not necessary to dissect free the entire length of the carotid artery; this increases the risk of injury to surrounding structures, particularly for the external carotid artery, which can typically be controlled with a clamp after anterior exposure or intraluminally after the arteriotomy is made. One should avoid subadvential dissection of the arterial structures. Once proximal and distal control is achieved, one can then proceed with the dissection of the carotid bifurcation and external carotid artery.

After administration of systemic heparin anticoagulation and clamping, a longitudinal arteriotomy is performed, through the patch if previously patched, or the native artery if not, or if there was a previous eversion endarterectomy. Once the artery is opened, the incision is carried proximally and distally with Potts scissors until healthy artery is reached beyond the disease process in the common and internal carotid arteries. The placement of an intraluminal shunt is dependent on surgical preference, following the same guidelines as used for a primary CEA.

If the recurrent stenosis results from atherosclerosis, a clean dissection plane is usually achievable and endarterectomy is performed in similar fashion to the initial operation; it then is repaired as a patch angioplasty. Others have performed eversion endarterectomy in this setting with comparable results. When dealing with myointimal hyperplasia, the fibrous tissue is generally very adherent to the underlying vessel wall so that a clean dissection plane is not easily established and therefore a conventional endarterectomy may not be possible. In this situation, a generous patch angioplasty is usually sufficient to restore a widely patent lumen (Figure 2).

On the other hand, when a long-segment stenosis is encountered, especially when it is dense and fibrotic, another useful option is to simply resect the segment and replace it with an interposition common-internal carotid graft with a prosthetic graft or greater saphenous vein (Figure 3). The shunt can be temporarily removed and replaced through the graft while the anastomoses are performed. The external carotid artery may then be reimplanted into the graft, or simply ligated. Finally, in some cases in which the intensity of scar

tissue around the carotid artery makes the dissection excessively risky, one can preferentially perform a bypass from the common carotid to the internal carotid artery in relatively unscarred tissues. The authors have preferentially used a 6-mm ringed PTFE graft for carotid interposition bypass procedures with excellent long-term results (see Figure 3).

In the patient with a significant restenosis after CAS, CEA can often be performed. In many cases, the carotid stent is not well incorporated and can easily be removed with a conventional endarterectomy with patch angioplasty. In some cases, however, a dense neointimal hyperplastic response is encountered with a smooth vessel lumen. In this case, the anterior wall of the artery and stent can be opened or partially excised, and a patch closure can be performed. For atherosclerotic lesions with dense incorporation of the stent, extraction of the stent from the vessel is sometimes not possible, requiring excision and performance of an interposition bypass as described previously. In the rare case in which a common-internal carotid bypass is not feasible because of extensive common carotid disease after either CEA or CAS, an ipsilateral subclavian-internal carotid artery bypass is an option.

Results

Reoperative CEA is more risky than a primary operation. Whereas the American Heart Association guidelines include a stroke and death rate of less than 3% for asymptomatic and less than 6% for symptomatic patients undergoing primary CEA, the acceptable stroke and death rate for reoperative CEA is less than 10%. Numerous series have documented acceptable results in properly selected patients in the hands of experienced vascular surgeons. For example, a recently published review of 28 series that included nearly 2000

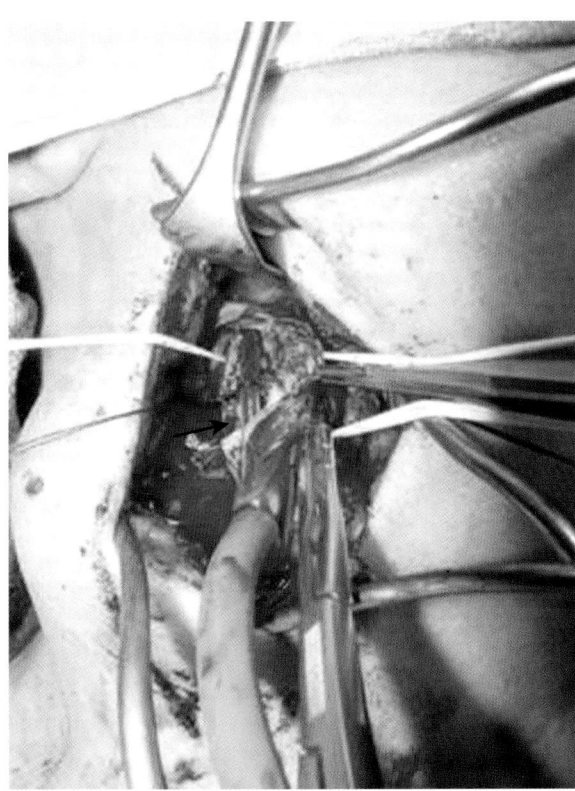

FIGURE 2 Completed reconstructions with Dacron patch angioplasty (Maquet Getinge Group, Atrium, Hudson, NH). *(From Cronenwett J, Johnston W, editors: Rutherford's vascular surgery, ed 7, Philadelphia, 2010, Saunders.)*

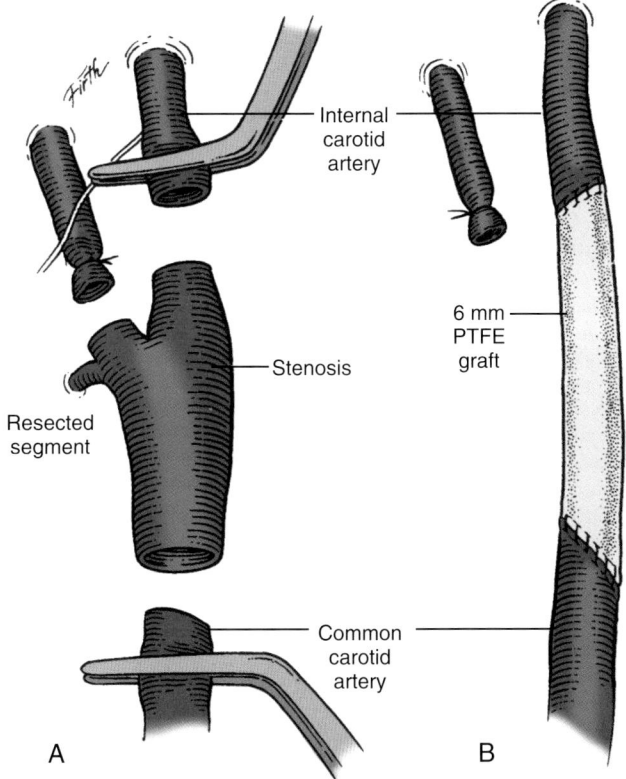

FIGURE 3 A, Resection of diseased segment of carotid artery with ligation of external carotid artery. **B,** Continuity restored with placement of interposition polytetrafluoroethylene (PTFE) common-internal carotid artery bypass graft.

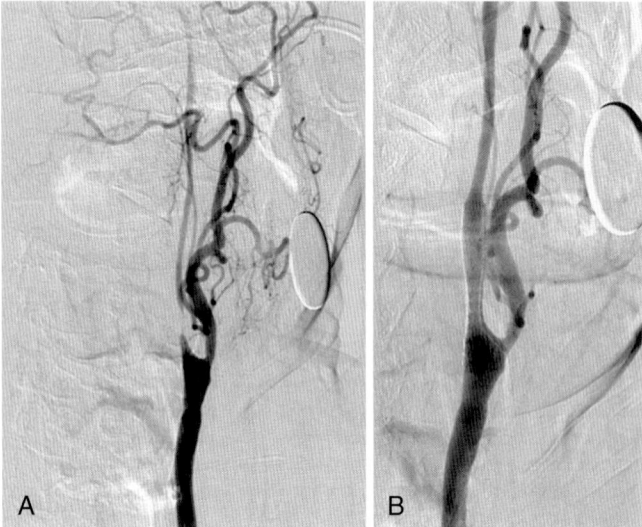

FIGURE 4 **A,** Diagnostic arteriogram shows high-grade recurrent internal carotid stenosis. **B,** Completion arteriogram after successful angioplasty and stent placement.

cases documented a combined perioperative stroke and death rate that ranged from 0 to 10.5%, with a rate of 0 to 5.6% in 26 of the 28 series. In a series of 59 patients who underwent eversion CEA for recurrent stenoses, the 30-day stroke rate was 4.5%.

The greatest risk of reoperative CEA is cranial nerve injury. Although the incidence rate of cranial or cervical nerve injury has been reported to be as high as 21% after CEA for restenosis in one prospective cohort study, most recent studies have documented a cranial nerve injury rate of 0 to 7%. In the review of 28 series that included nearly 2000 patients noted previously, the rate of cranial nerve injury ranged from 0 to 19% in the 25 reports in which this complication was reported. The rate of cranial nerve injury was 7% or less in 17 of the 25 reports. In a series of 59 patients undergoing eversion CEA, the cranial nerve injury rate was 4.5%.

Furthermore, reoperative CEA has been shown to yield extremely durable long-term results. In a review of 13 series, the 5-year stroke-free rate ranged from 82% to 96%. The restenosis-free survival rate ranged from 83% to 95% at a 5-year follow-up and from 68% to 86% at a 10-year follow-up.

CAROTID ANGIOPLASTY AND STENTING

The techniques and devices for CAS have continued to evolve over the past decade. To date, this endovascular therapy has been used primarily in patients at high risk, and recurrent carotid stenosis has been a relatively common indication. CAS represents an attractive option, especially when the recurrent stenosis has resulted from myointimal hyperplasia (Figure 4). This includes fibrous lesions that develop after CEA and in-stent restenosis after CAS. In general, these types of lesions are thought to be less prone to distal embolization during CAS than restenotic plaques formed later by the progression of atherosclerosis.

Relative contraindications to CAS for recurrent disease are similar to those for treatment of primary atherosclerotic disease. These include anatomic factors related to the aortic arch, such as a type III arch and bovine arch anatomy, severe vessel tortuosity, circumferentially calcified plaque, suspected plaque rupture with thrombus formation, and inability to achieve safe vascular access. Other relative contraindications include a recent major stroke, a contraindication to systemic anticoagulation therapy or appropriate antiplatelet therapy, a severe contrast allergy, and stage IV chronic renal failure.

Technical Details

The patient should begin a regimen of clopidogrel 75 mg daily 7 days before the procedure or receive a loading dose of 300 mg the morning of the procedure in addition to aspirin 81 mg daily. These medications are continued in the postoperative period; however, the duration of dual-antiplatelet therapy for CAS is not well established. The authors routinely continue dual antiplatelet therapy for a minimum of 3 months.

The techniques used to perform CAS for recurrent disease after CEA are essentially the same as those used for treatment of primary disease and are outlined in greater detail elsewhere in the text. For the patient with a recurrent stenosis after CAS, repeat carotid angioplasty or stenting is a viable option. Evidence suggests that balloon angioplasty alone has an unacceptably high repeat recurrence rate of approximately 25%, so additional stent placement is usually necessary. However, use of a cutting balloon may provide a significant benefit over traditional angioplasty in this clinical scenario.

Results

Although reported clinical experience is limited, the available evidence suggests that CAS is a safe and effective treatment option for patients with recurrent carotid stenoses. In a multicenter study that included 358 CAS procedures for recurrent stenosis, the 30-day stroke and death rate was 3.7% and the 3-year freedom-from-stroke rate was 96%. In a recent institutional series that included 83 CAS procedures performed for recurrent stenoses in 75 patients, the periprocedural stroke rate was 3.6%. With a mean follow-up period of 22 months, recurrent stenoses occurred in 4 cases (5%).

SUMMARY

Recurrent stenosis is a relatively uncommon complication after carotid interventions and appears to occur more commonly after CAS as compared with CEA. The decision to reintervene in the patient with a recurrent carotid stenosis must be individualized on the basis of the patient's symptomatic status, the severity of the stenosis, the timing of presentation of the restenosis and underlying responsible pathology, the status of the cerebral circulation in general, and the patient's overall comorbidity. Likewise, although reoperative CEA has been the standard of care, CAS has emerged as an important endovascular option with acceptable clinical outcomes.

SUGGESTED READINGS

AbuRahma AF, Abu-Halimah S, Hass SM, et al: Carotid artery stenting outcomes are equivalent to carotid endarterectomy outcomes for patients with post-carotid endarterectomy stenosis, *J Vasc Surg* 52:1180–1187, 2010.

de Borst GJ, Ackerstaff RG, de Vries JP, et al: Carotid angioplasty and stenting for postendarterectomy stenosis: long-term follow-up, *J Vasc Surg* 45:118–123, 2007.

de Borst GJ, Moll F: Biology and treatment of recurrent carotid stenosis, *J Cardiovasc Surg* 53(Suppl 1):27–34, 2012.

de Borst GJ, Zanen P, de Vries J-P, et al: Durability of surgery for restenosis after carotid endarterectomy, *J Vasc Surg* 47:363–371, 2008.

New G, Roubin GS, Iyer SS, et al: Safety, efficacy, and durability of carotid artery stenting for restenosis following carotid endarterectomy: a multicenter study, *J Endovasc Therap* 7:345–352, 2000.

Perler BA: Carotid endarterectomy: still the "gold standard" in the endovascular era, *Adv Studies Med* 4:433–435, 2004.

van Lammeren GW, Peeters W, de Vries J-P PM, et al: Restenosis after carotid surgery: the importance of clinical presentation and preoperative timing, *Circulation* 42:965–971, 2011.

Balloon Angioplasty and Stents in Carotid Artery Occlusive Disease

Charles S. O'Mara, MD, MBA

BACKGROUND

The approximately 800,000 strokes each year in the United States make stroke the nation's third leading cause of death. On average, a stroke occurs every 20 seconds in this country. Nearly three quarters of patients with stroke are over the age of 65 years, and this condition is a leading cause of permanent disability. The estimated direct and indirect costs of stroke of $70 billion per year are indeed staggering. Atherosclerosis of the internal carotid artery (ICA) is the cause of stroke in 20% to 40% of cases. These facts indicate that prevention of stroke from carotid occlusive disease is a major national health issue.

Carotid endarterectomy (CEA) for treatment of carotid artery atherosclerosis was first performed about 60 years ago. The efficacy of this operation later came under scrutiny but in the early 1990s was confirmed by two large multicenter randomized trials, the North American Symptomatic Carotid Endarterectomy Trial (NASCET) and the Asymptomatic Carotid Atherosclerosis Study (ACAS), both of which compared CEA with medical therapy alone and showed significant benefit from the surgery.

After the development of endovascular interventions for other arterial occlusive lesions, carotid artery balloon angioplasty and stenting (CAS) was proposed as an alternative to CEA for treatment of carotid atherosclerosis. Although both CAS and CEA can be performed with local anesthesia with similar operative and hospitalization times, CAS offers the advantage of percutaneous groin arterial access rather than a neck incision for direct carotid artery exposure, which carries risk of incisional pain, cranial nerve injury, wound infection, and neck hematoma.

This potential advantage of CAS led to its initial limited clinical use and then to the performance of several randomized trials that compared CAS with CEA (Table 1). These trials produced varied results and often showed poor performance for CAS. However, the studies were criticized because of inconsistent operator skill and experience with CAS, nonuniformity of embolic protection device (EPD) use, and incomplete use of periprocedural antiplatelet therapy.

In 2010, results were reported for the Carotid Revascularization Endarterectomy versus Stenting Trial (CREST), which is the largest prospective randomized trial to date comparing CAS with CEA. This National Institutes of Health (NIH)-funded study enrolled 2502 symptomatic and asymptomatic patients from 117 U.S. and Canadian centers. The rate of achieving the primary composite endpoint of any stroke, myocardial infarction (MI), or death during the periprocedural period or ipsilateral stroke in follow-up was 7.2% for CAS versus 6.8% for surgery, a difference that was not significant (Table 2). However, periprocedural stroke rate was significantly higher with stenting at 4.1% versus 2.3% with surgery, and MI was significantly higher with CEA at 2.3% versus 1.1% with CAS. Quality of life after recovery for those patients who had a stroke was worse than for those patients who had an MI. Rate of ipsilateral stroke during a mean follow-up period of 2.5 years was not significantly different between groups with 2.0% for CAS and 2.4% with CEA. Counterintuitively, younger patients tended to have better results with stenting, and older patients did better with surgery. The study showed a higher risk for periprocedural stroke with stenting in patients of advanced age (more than 70 years) and with recent (within 2 weeks) neurologic ischemic symptoms.

CREST results are encouraging in showing that both procedures are effective in long-term stroke prevention. However, certain components of CREST have been intensely debated and interpreted differently according to one's bias for or against CAS or CEA. Stenting enthusiasts argue that statistical similarity in the primary composite endpoint establishes equipoise for the procedures. In contrast, others question the inclusion of MI as a component of the primary endpoint for procedures that have stroke prevention as their principal objective. They argue for the use of only stroke and death as a more appropriate composite endpoint, which significantly favors endarterectomy in CREST.

Suffice it to say, CREST has produced valuable level I data comparing CAS with CEA but has not fulfilled the expectation by some of proving undeniably that CAS is better than or even equal to CEA. Hopefully, additional data analysis from CREST and results of future clinical trials will facilitate the decision process of applying each procedure to its most appropriate clinical situation. In addition, recent information about treatment of carotid occlusive disease with a combination of antiplatelet agents and statins, along with healthy lifestyle habits such as regular exercise, dietary discretion, and tobacco abstinence, suggests that medical management alone may assume an increasingly important role in the future for this patient population.

TECHNICAL CONSIDERATIONS IN PERFORMANCE OF CAROTID ARTERY STENTING

Preprocedural assessment includes a complete history focused on cardiovascular elements and on symptoms of neurologic or ocular ischemic events. Thorough physical examination is essential, with an emphasis on palpation of pulses, auscultation for bruits, and complete neurologic assessment. Preprocedural imaging often includes carotid ultrasound scan, computed tomographic angiography, and magnetic resonance imaging and angiography (MRI/MRA). These imaging modalities give important information about the presence and hemodynamic significance of carotid occlusive disease, the condition of the brain parenchyma, the presence of additional intracranial or extracranial vascular anomalies (e.g., saccular aneurysms, vascular malformations), and the anatomy of the aortic arch.

Before CAS, patients should begin dual antiplatelet therapy. The author's regimen typically consists of clopidogrel 75 mg daily and aspirin 81 mg daily beginning 3 to 5 days before the procedure. In emergency circumstances, when antiplatelet therapy has not been started before the procedure, the author uses a loading regimen of clopidogrel 600 mg and aspirin 325 mg given at the time of the procedure. In addition, for patients who have been taking antiplatelet therapy on a chronic basis, the author typically gives a smaller loading dose of clopidogrel 150 to 300 mg immediately after the procedure. If oral administration is not possible, clopidogrel can be given via nasogastric tube; aspirin can be given similarly or per rectum (300 or 600 mg suppository).

Femoral arterial access is accomplished with care to avoid distracting and potentially dangerous access site complications, especially in patients with severe peripheral artery disease. The author routinely uses fluoroscopic assistance and has a low threshold for ultrasound scan guidance and initial micropuncture to facilitate safe femoral artery access. A limited femoral arteriogram in ipsilateral

TABLE 1: Randomized multicenter trials comparing carotid artery stenting (CAS) and carotid endarterectomy (CEA)

Trial	Year	No. of patients	MAE rate for CAS	MAE rate for CEA	Length of follow-up
CAVATAS	2001	504	10.0%	9.9%	3 y
SAPPHIRE	2008	334	24.6%	26.9%	3 y
SPACE	2008	1214	9.5%	8.8%	2 y
EVA-3S	2008	527	11.1%	6.2%	4 y
ICSS	2010	1713	8.5%	4.7%	120 d

CAVATAS, Carotid and Vertebral Artery Transluminal Angioplasty Study; *EVA-3S*, Endarterectomy Versus Angioplasty in Patients with Symptomatic Severe Carotid Stenosis; *ICSS*, International Carotid Stenting Study; *MAE*, major adverse event (stroke, death, or myocardial infarction, varied by trial); *SAPPHIRE*, Stenting and Angioplasty with Protection in Patients at High Risk for Endarterectomy; *SPACE*, Stent-Protected Angioplasty versus Carotid Endarterectomy.

TABLE 2: Results of Carotid Revascularization Endarterectomy versus Stenting Trial (CREST; 2502 patients)

Endpoint	CAS	CEA	P value
Primary composite endpoint of periprocedural stroke, death, or MI or ipsilateral stroke in 4 y	7.2%	6.8%	0.51
Periprocedural death	0.7%	0.3%	0.18
Any periprocedural stroke	4.1%	2.3%	0.01*
Periprocedural MI	1.1%	2.3%	0.03*
4-y rate of stroke or death	6.4%	4.7%	0.03*
Ipsilateral stroke after periprocedural period	2.0%	2.4%	0.85

CAS, Carotid artery stenting; *CEA*, carotid endarterectomy; *MI*, myocardial infarction.
*Statistically significant difference.

oblique orientation is routinely done through the sheath immediately after its placement to document a satisfactory entry site into the common femoral artery.

After arterial access is achieved, systemic anticoagulation therapy is initiated either with intravenous heparin bolus administration (100 units per kg body weight) or with bivalirudin (Angiomax; Medicines Company, Persippany, NJ) via continuous infusion (0.75 mg/kg intravenous [IV] bolus, followed by 1.75 mg/kg/h IV infusion) to maintain during the procedure activated clotting times in the range of 250 to 300 seconds. Introduction of a J wire always includes fluoroscopically following the tip during its passage from the femoral sheath to the aortic arch to avoid an errant course with resultant arterial injury. A 6F pigtail catheter passed over the J wire and into the aortic arch is used to perform arch aortography in 35-degree to 40-degree left anterior oblique orientation of the fluoroscopy unit. The author usually hand injects 10 mL of contrast with a closed manifold system to provide sufficient anatomic mapping for subsequent selective catheter placement, while limiting the amount of contrast media used. However, if preprocedure imaging leaves questions about arch anatomy or pathology, power injection of 15 to 20 mL of contrast gives additional angiographic detail to resolve such issues.

On the basis of aortic arch anatomy, an appropriately shaped angiography catheter is chosen for selective cannulation of the aortic arch branches. Typical aortic arch anatomy allows for use of a selective catheter with a simple curve (Berenstein, vertebral; Merit Medical, South Jordan, Utah), and increasingly complex and tortuous aortic arch anatomy requires the use of selective catheters that have either an intermediate curve (H1; Cook Medical, Bloomington, Ind, JR4;

Cordis, Hialeah, Fla) or a complex curve (Simmons; Cook Medical, Bloomington, Ind, Vitek; Cook Medical, Bloomington, Ind). All catheter exchanges are done over a guidewire. Extreme care is given to avoid the introduction of microthrombi and tiny air bubbles with frequent guidewire wiping with heparinized saline sponges and with meticulous heparinized saline solution flushing of catheters and sheaths.

In general, complete four-vessel cerebral arteriography with digital subtraction technique is performed before proceeding with stenting to document baseline vascular anatomy and recruited collateral pathways. However, the approach to each patient's arteriographic requirements is individualized based on preprocedure imaging information and on individual clinical circumstances, such as need to expeditiously complete the procedure (patient discomfort or anxiety) or need to minimize total contrast media administered (renal insufficiency). These considerations are tempered by the understanding that incidental lesions discovered with angiography (intracranial carotid stenosis or aneurysm) may alter the therapeutic plan.

After completion of selective arteriography for the target carotid artery, the external carotid artery (ECA) is selectively cannulated with an angle-tipped angiography catheter over a soft, angled hydrophilic guidewire that is then exchanged for an exchange-length, floppy-tipped 0.035-inch stiff wire (Supracore; Abbott Vascular, Abbot Park, Ill). Extreme caution is taken to avoid passing the wire too far and causing vessel perforation with resultant neck hematoma. A posterior ECA branch is selected so that if perforation were to occur, it could be manually compressed easily in the back of the neck (Figure 1). In contrast, anterior ECA branch perforation is difficult to manually

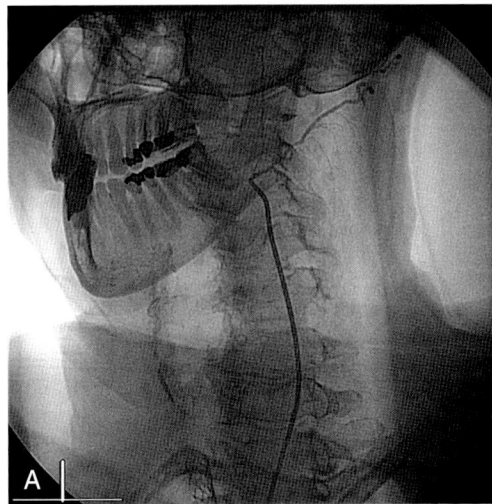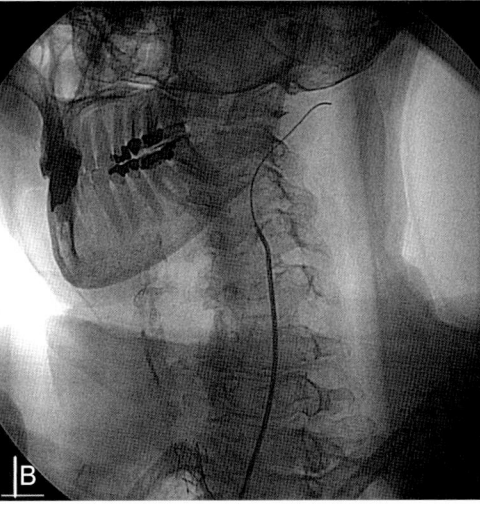

FIGURE I   A, Selective injection to document catheter location in a posterior branch of the external carotid artery before placement of the exchange-length wire used for positioning of the long sheath into the distal common carotid artery. **B,** Wire placement into the external carotid artery branch through the selective catheter. Inadvertent vessel perforation by the wire could be readily managed with manual compression against the posterior neck muscles.

compress and has been reported to produce an expanding hematoma with resultant airway compression and respiratory compromise. If concern arises about wire crossing of a worrisome carotid bifurcation lesion or if the ECA is occluded, curling the floppy tip of the wire before its introduction usually allows adequate purchase of the stiff portion of the wire for subsequent passage of the sheath into the common carotid artery (CCA) without the wire extending beyond the distal CCA.

Once the long stiff wire is in place, the angiography catheter is removed and the femoral sheath is exchanged for a 6F hydrophilic-coated, 90-cm sheath (Shuttle; Cook Medical, Bloomington, Ind) with its tip in the distal CCA. The sheath dilator and the stiff wire are removed. Currently, a distal filter typically is used for embolic protection. The distal filter, attached to a 0.014-inch wire, is passed through the sheath, carefully maneuvered through the carotid stenosis, and placed in the distal cervical ICA, where it is deployed with removal of its covering sheath. Very tight carotid stenoses that cannot be safely negotiated with the tip of the embolic protection device may require use of a low-profile microcatheter (Prowler; Johnson & Johnson, New Brunswick, NJ) and steerable microwire (Transcend; Boston Scientific Corp., Miami, Fla). Occasionally, predilation of a tight stenosis with a low-profile coronary angioplasty balloon may be necessary to allow subsequent crossing of the lesion with the distal filter. Also, problems imposed by vessel angulation and tortuosity can be resolved with use of a "buddy wire" to slightly straighten the anatomy and facilitate crossing of a lesion by the distal filter, angioplasty catheter, or stent. Furthermore, in situations in which passage of the distal filter is difficult, maneuvers such as having the patient take deep breaths, having the patient turn the head far to one side or the other, or careful manual pressure on the side of the patient's neck by an assistant can be helpful. Obviously, to avoid embolization of plaque material, manual pressure should not be applied directly to the carotid bifurcation.

The carotid lesion is predilated if stenosis is severe enough to impair stent positioning or to constrain it after deployment. Predilation is done with an angioplasty balloon that is 3 or 4 mm in diameter and 15 or 20 mm in length, depending on the anatomy of the lesion. For reduction of risk of associated bradycardia and hypotension, intravenous atropine 1.0 mg is routinely administered several minutes before this balloon predilation, which is done with a rapid inflation-then-deflation sequence. Patients with severe aortic stenosis may be intolerant of even mild bradycardia and hypotension with balloon inflation. Therefore, consideration should be given in such patients to anesthesia monitoring and a temporary pacemaker in place for the procedure.

The self-expanding stent is positioned precisely to cover the carotid lesion and is deployed with withdrawal of its constraining cover. Carotid bifurcation lesions typically are best treated with a tapered stent that has a larger diameter proximally to match the CCA and a smaller diameter distally to match the ICA. The stent often crosses the ECA origin, but flow into that artery continues through the interstices of the stent (Figure 2). Occasionally, more than one stent is necessary to treat a long carotid stenosis, but preference is given to use of only one stent if possible.

Postdeployment balloon angioplasty is typically done with a balloon that is 5, 5.5, or 6 mm in diameter and 20 mm in length. Diameter selection is made according to size of the ICA. Care is taken to inflate the balloon only within the confines of the stented segment of the artery. Postdeployment balloon angioplasty is used to achieve an angiographically acceptable but not necessarily perfect result. If a residual stenosis of less than 30% is present after stent placement alone, poststenting balloon angioplasty is forgone based on knowledge that nitinol stents tend to expand slowly after deployment and that embolic events may occur during balloon angioplasty even after stent deployment (Figure 3).

The balloon angioplasty catheters and the carotid stent are passed into position over the wire attached to the distal filter. The same wire is used for passage of a retrieval sheath that captures the filter along with any microemboli that have been trapped during the procedure. After retrieval and removal of the filter and its wire, completion arteriograms are obtained of the treated carotid artery and of the cerebral territory that it supplies with injection of contrast through the long sheath. The long sheath is then removed over its dilator and a guidewire to avoid vessel trauma during exit. Systemic anticoagulation therapy is discontinued. After sheath removal, the femoral artery puncture site is sealed with either manual compression or use of a closure device.

Current practice is to observe patients for several hours after CAS in a cardiovascular recovery suite where personnel are trained and experienced in perioperative cardiovascular and neurologic assessment. The patient is then transferred to a step-down cardiovascular unit for observation over night and discharged the following morning.

DESIGN OF CAROTID STENT SYSTEMS

Carotid Stents

Endovascular stents are constructed in two basic configurations: balloon-expandable and self-expanding. Balloon-expandable stents are appropriate for lesions located at the origin of the CCA and the innominate artery (Figure 4), where precise placement of the proximal end of the stent relative to the artery orifice is critical and where the possibility of compression is not an important consideration. In

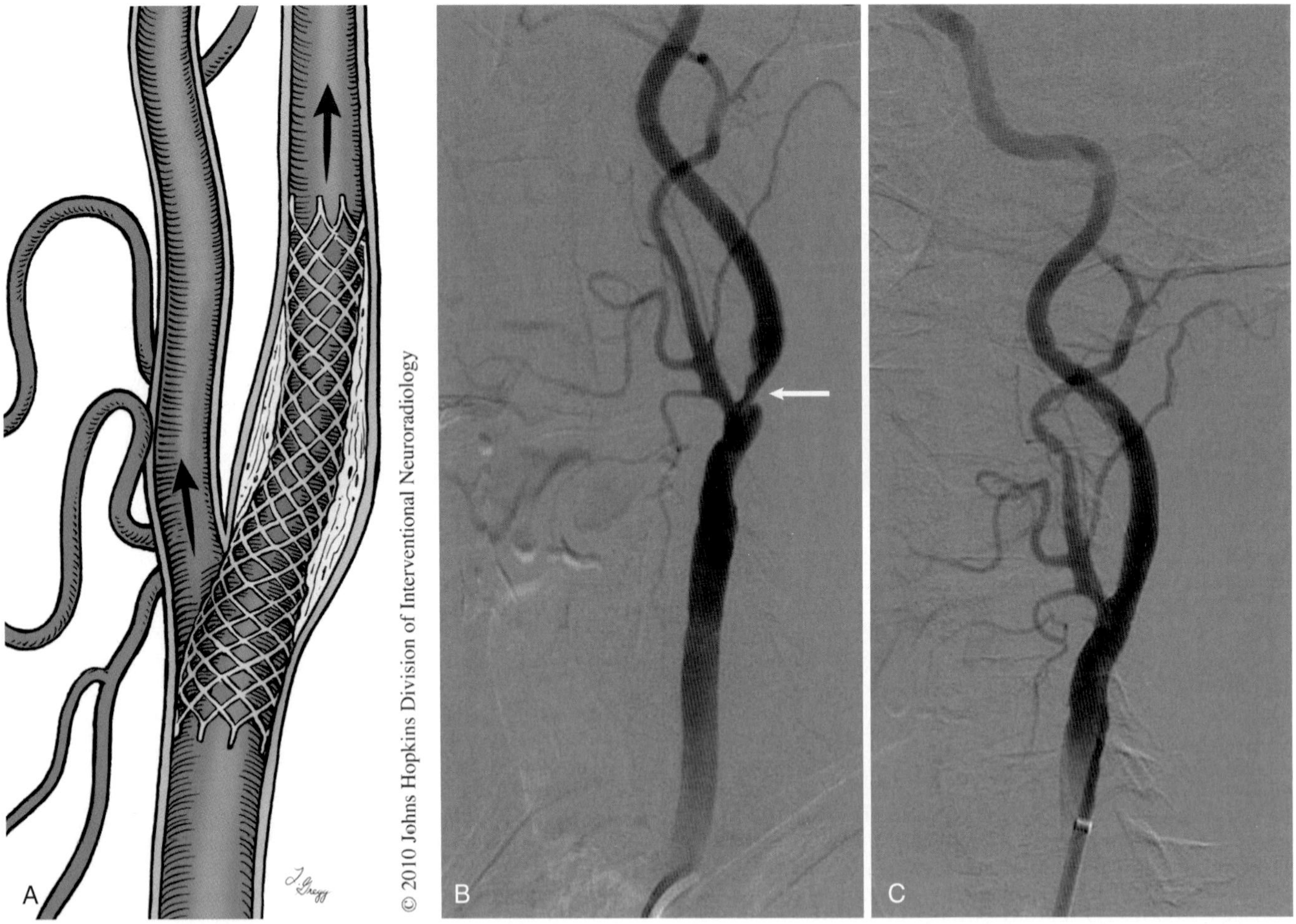

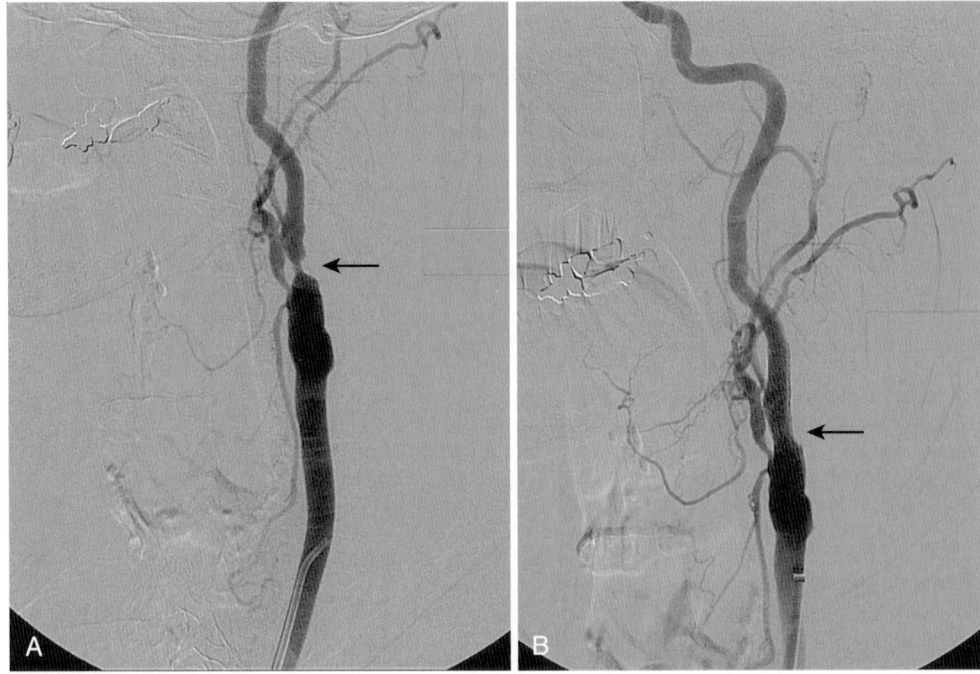

FIGURE 2   **A,** Schematic representation of a stent deployed across the carotid bifurcation to treat a proximal internal carotid artery lesion. Blood flow continues into the external carotid artery through the interstices of the stent. **B,** Digital subtraction arteriogram (DSA; left common carotid injection, lateral neck projection) showing a severe stenosis in the proximal internal carotid artery *(arrow)*. **C,** Completion DSA after placement of a stent across the carotid bifurcation. Note correction of the internal carotid artery stenosis with continued perfusion of the external carotid artery and its branches. (**A,** *Illustration courtesy of Lydia Gregg, 2010 Johns Hopkins Interventional Neuroradiology.*)

FIGURE 3   **A,** Digital subtraction arteriogram (DSA; left common carotid injection, lateral neck projection) showing severe stenosis in proximal internal carotid artery *(arrow)*. **B,** Completion DSA after carotid artery stenting. Notice the residual mild stenosis *(arrow)* at the site of the lesion, which was judged acceptable even though not angiographically perfect.

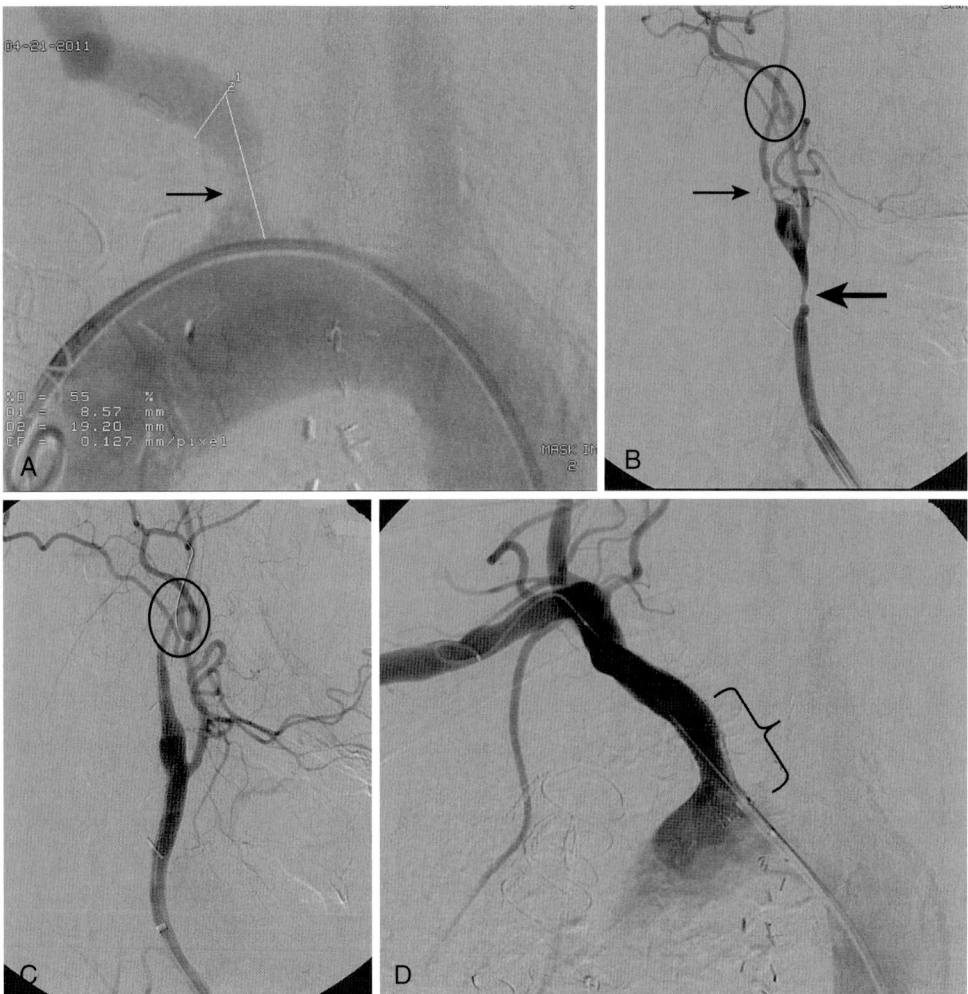

FIGURE 4 **A,** Arch aortogram (40-degree left anterior oblique orientation) showing severe stenosis of the proximal innominate artery *(arrow)*. Note white linear markings of electronic calibrations for length and diameter measurements for planning of subsequent innominate stent placement. **B,** Digital subtraction arteriogram (DSA; right common carotid injection, lateral neck projection) showing high-grade recurrent stenosis after carotid endarterectomy in the distal common carotid artery *(larger arrow)* and the proximal internal carotid artery *(smaller arrow)*. Note the 360-degree loop *(circled)* in the internal carotid artery distal to the stenosis; the external carotid artery is superimposed in this projection. **C,** DSA after the lesions were successfully treated with two overlapping carotid stents. Distal internal carotid artery tortuosity precluded use of a distal filter. Note the wire still in this segment of the artery *(circled)*. **D,** Completion DSA after treatment of the innominate stenosis with a balloon-expandable stent based on electronically calibrated measurements done previously (see **A**). Innominate stenting was done immediately after the carotid stenting was accomplished. The bracket depicts the extent of the stent.

contrast, cervical carotid lesions are better treated with self-expanding stents that are tolerant of neck mobility and that spontaneously reexpand if externally compressed.

Self-expanding stents are made in two basic designs: open-cell and closed-cell. The advantage of an open-cell design is a greater flexibility that permits better vessel wall apposition and easier navigability through tortuous vascular anatomy. However, open-cell stents have the disadvantage of lower radial force that may limit stent expansion as a result of recoil, especially in heavily calcified lesions. Open-cell design may be more prone to in-stent restenosis. Closed-cell stents offer the advantage of greater radial force, but they are less flexible and more prone to result in kinking when used in tortuous arteries. The Space-Protected Angioplasty versus Carotid Endarterectomy (SPACE) trial suggested a higher rate of embolic complications with open-cell carotid stents. However, recent data show no

differences in specific carotid stent cell designs with respect to risk of stroke or mortality.

Embolic Protection Devices

From the inception of CAS, the greatest concern has been the potential for atheroembolic stroke associated with the procedure. EPDs were incorporated into the CAS procedure to minimize this risk. Despite the absence of robust clinical or trial data establishing efficacy, use of an EPD during CAS has become generally accepted. EPDs provide temporary cerebral protection by one of the following methods (Figure 5): (1) balloon occlusion of the distal cervical ICA; (2) placement of a filter in the distal cervical ICA; and (3) balloon occlusion of the CCA combined with balloon occlusion of the ECA

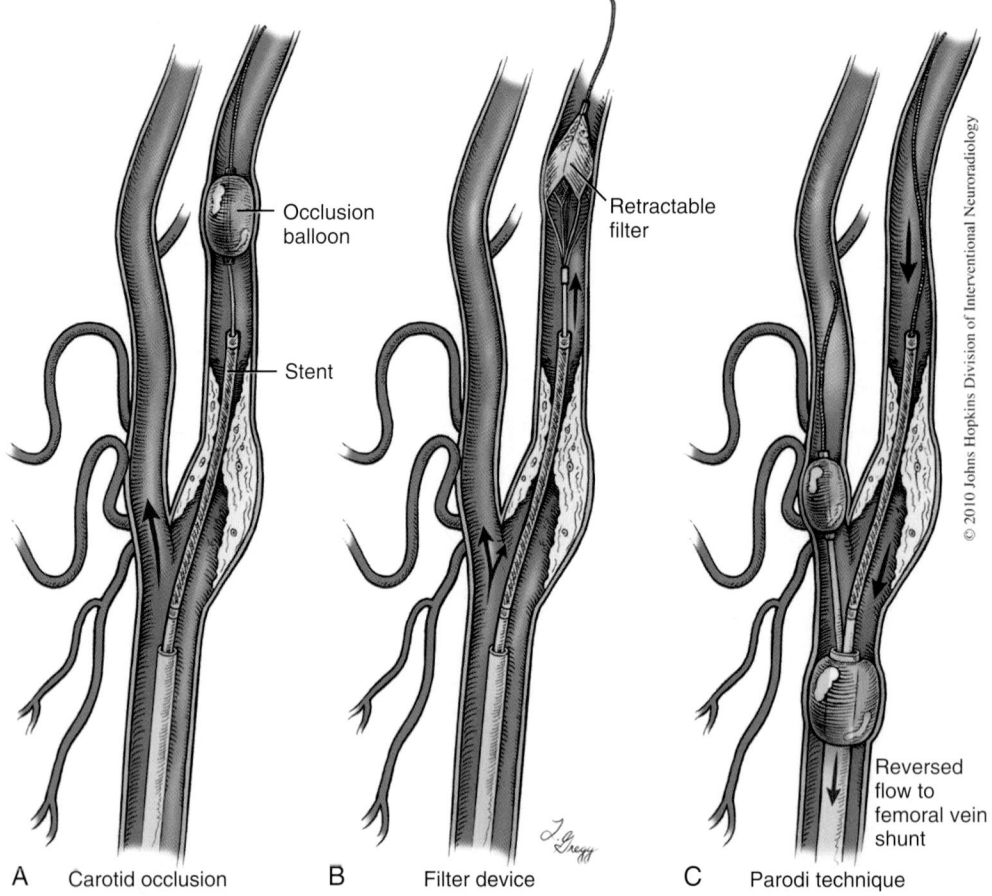

FIGURE 5 Schematic representation of the different methods of embolic protection devices. *Arrows* indicate the direction of blood flow. **A,** Distal occlusion. Stenting is performed with internal carotid artery flow temporarily interrupted by inflating a balloon within the distal internal carotid artery. After stent deployment and after dilation, stagnant blood proximal to the balloon, which may contain plaque debris, is aspirated through the delivery catheter. After aspiration, the dead space below the balloon is flushed with saline solution to chase any remaining material into the external carotid artery. The balloon is then deflated and removed. **B,** Distal filtration. A filter is delivered through the stenosis and deployed in the distal internal carotid artery by withdrawing its constraining sheath. After stenting, a recovery catheter is used to retrieve the filter and its contents. **C,** Proximal protection. During stenting, two occluding balloons are inflated, one in the common carotid artery and the other in the external carotid artery. Flow reversal is created either with active aspiration from the delivery catheter in the common carotid artery distal to the common carotid artery balloon or with directing flow from this catheter to a catheter in the femoral vein. With use of a system that returns blood to the femoral vein, a filter is used within the connection to trap debris from the carotid plaque. *(Illustration courtesy of Lydia Gregg, 2010 Johns Hopkins Interventional Neuroradiology.)*

and either aspiration or flow reversal in the ICA (proximal protection). Various EPDs are currently commercially available (Table 3).

Distal protection with either balloon or filter has the disadvantage that the carotid lesion must be crossed before initiation of cerebral protection. Nevertheless, because of simplicity and ease of use, and the avoidance of carotid flow interruption, distal protection with a filter has evolved as the most common method currently used for cerebral protection. However, transcranial Doppler scan studies have shown that particles smaller than the pore size of the filters (60 to 140 μm) can evade capture because of flow through the filter. Such microemboli may be associated with new white lesions on the diffusion-weighted MRI of the brain, but the clinical consequences of this "controlled embolization" are unclear. In addition, incomplete apposition of the filter rim to the vessel wall may allow emboli of various sizes to pass around the filter. Finally, filters occasionally can

be difficult to retrieve and they may become occluded from obstructing debris captured during CAS.

With the distal balloon occlusion method, after the stent is deployed, a catheter is advanced across the treatment site and is used to aspirate debris before deflating and recovering the balloon. With the distal filter method, after stent placement, the filter attached to the working wire is recovered, bringing with it any plaque debris trapped in its mesh. In contrast, proximal protection methods involve the inflation of a balloon in the ECA and another on the guiding catheter in the CCA. With the Gore Flow Reversal System (W.L. Gore & Assoc., Newark, Del), a closed circuit is then established between the guiding catheter and the venous system by way of the femoral vein to create retrograde flow in the ICA being treated. A filter in the tubing that connects the guiding catheter to the femoral vein traps any embolic debris dislodged from the site of carotid stenting. With

TABLE 3: Commercially available embolic protection devices

Method	Device	Manufacturer
Distal occlusion	GuardWire	Medtronic (Minneapolis, Minn)
Distal filtration	RX Accunet	Abbott Vascular (Abbott Park, Ill)
	Angioguard RX	Cordis (Cordis, Hialeah, Fla)
	Emboshield NAV6	Abbott Vascular
	FilterWire EZ	Boston Scientific (Miami, Fla)
	FiberNet	Medtronic
	Gore Embolic Filter	W.L. Gore & Associates (W.L. Gore & Assoc., Newark, Del)
	SpiderFX	Covidien (Mannsfield, Mass)
Proximal protection	Gore Flow Reversal System	W.L. Gore & Associates
	Mo.Ma Ultra	Medtronic

the Mo.Ma Ultra device, (Medtronic, Minneapolis, Minn), after stenting, blood in the ICA is aspirated until clear of debris.

The concept of proximal protection is appealing because crossing the lesion with the protection device is not required. Recent reports suggest that proximal protection, in experienced hands, is associated with low risk of microembolic events during CAS, acceptable 30-day stroke and death rates, low incidence of femoral access complications, and low (less than 1%) rate of patient intolerance to temporary proximal occlusion. In addition, proximal embolic protection provides an option when marked arterial tortuosity or a limited landing zone precludes use of distal protection. Nevertheless, clinicians have been slow to adopt proximal protection devices because they require larger sheath access (9F or 9.5F), are more complicated to use than distal filter devices, and may be poorly tolerated by patients with poor intracranial collateral circulation. Also, this method of embolic protection has the disadvantage of limiting the ability of the operator to visualize angiographically the precise location of the lesion during stent deployment.

Special attention is appropriate for the small but important incidence of cerebral atheroembolization remote from the target lesion being stented, a situation for which an EPD is not helpful. These events probably result from catheter manipulation in a diseased aortic arch or branch vessel, sometimes involving the cerebral hemisphere contralateral to the site of treatment. This potential occurrence warrants extreme care and meticulous attention to catheter manipulations in these patients, who often have diffuse atherosclerotic disease. In patients who have a markedly diseased aortic arch or hostile arch anatomy for branch vessel access, transcervical access to the proximal CCA through a small incision low in the neck may provide safer access for CAS than a transfemoral approach.

PERIPROCEDURAL MANAGEMENT

Antiplatelet Therapy

As mentioned previously, antiplatelet therapy is essential for success of CAS. Dual antiplatelet therapy with clopidogrel (75 mg daily) and aspirin (81 or 325 mg daily) is the current standard. The considerable individual variation in the degree of platelet inhibition provided by antiplatelet therapy is now well known. Information is accumulating about the impact of clopidogrel or aspirin resistance on long-term stent patency and restenosis rates. Testing for such resistance may become a more common practice in the future to foster individualization of antiplatelet therapy. Ticlopidine (250 mg twice daily) can be used in patients who cannot tolerate clopidogrel. If a patient cannot take antiplatelet therapy, carotid stenting should be reconsidered, as the postprocedural stroke risk is unacceptably high. Dual antiplatelet therapy should be continued for at least 3 months after the stent procedure, and daily aspirin should be continued indefinitely thereafter.

Glycoprotein IIb-IIIa inhibitors are associated with increased risk of intracranial hemorrhage after carotid stenting, and their role should be confined to the treatment of acute thrombus formation during or immediately after the procedure. For management of acute in-stent thrombosis, abciximab is administered by giving one half of the 0.25-mg/kg bolus dose intraarterially near the clot and administering the second half of the bolus dose intravenously over 5 minutes, followed by an intravenous infusion of 0.125 µg/kg/min for 12 to 24 hours.

Hemodynamic Instability

Periprocedural bradycardia caused by carotid sinus stimulation has been associated with inflation of the angioplasty balloon in the proximal ICA. It is rarely seen in patients who have previously undergone CEA, probably because of the denervating effect of surgical dissection near the carotid bulb. Periprocedural bradycardia has been infrequent in the author's practice, possibly related to routine use of atropine intravenously just before angioplasty balloon inflation. However, bradycardia, profound hypotension, and asystolic cardiac arrest can occur. Refractory periprocedural bradycardia is managed with cardiac pacing in addition to atropine administration.

Arterial hypotension may accompany periprocedural bradycardia and is usually managed with volume expansion. Moderate bradycardia and mild hypotension, similar to that seen occasionally after CEA related to carotid baroreceptor stimulation, are best treated with fluid supplementation, close observation for any neurologic dysfunction, and occasional use of low-dose vasopressor support.

Control of postprocedural hypertension is important to minimize risk of cerebral hyperperfusion syndrome (CHS). Severe headache associated with hypertension after CAS should heighten suspicion of CHS, which can also present with seizures and focal neurologic deficits. Proper management of CHS entails early diagnosis, rapid control of hypertension, anticonvulsant therapy, osmotic diuresis, and neurologic consultation.

Distal cervical ICA vasospasm is sometimes induced with catheter or wire manipulation or with distal filter or balloon placement. Avoidance of movement of the distal filter once deployed helps to minimize vasospasm at the site. Resolution of the vasospasm often occurs spontaneously but can be hastened with transcatheter administration of nitroglycerin (200-µg bolus) into the involved artery.

Periprocedural Neurologic Assessment

Distal embolization is one of the main complications of CAS, but the consequences of cerebral embolic events vary widely. Microemboli may produce white lesions on diffusion-weighted MRI scan without apparent neurologic sequelae. Larger emboli may produce a small stroke with MRI yet remain clinically silent or they may cause devastating neurologic deficit, depending on the function of the cerebral tissue that has been damaged. Therefore, operators who perform CAS must be familiar with the anatomy of the brain and its vasculature so that intracranial cerebral branch vessel occlusion can be readily identified. It is equally important that operators be thoroughly familiar with normal neurologic function and the clinical manifestations of stroke. In addition, dedicated expert neurologic support is essential for a successful carotid stenting program.

Follow-up

Patients are usually discharged from the hospital on the day after undergoing CAS. Follow-up office visit occurs 4 to 6 weeks after surgery, again 6 months later, and annually thereafter. Follow-up includes a complete neurologic assessment and carotid ultrasound scan examination. Each visit also includes a global cardiovascular evaluation with emphasis on possible coronary, renal, and peripheral arterial occlusive problems. Hypertension and hypercholesterolemia are managed aggressively. Because of antiinflammatory and plaque stabilization effects, statin therapy is advised for almost all patients, even in the absence of laboratory evidence of cholesterol abnormalities. Healthy lifestyle habits are encouraged, with emphasis on regular aerobic exercise, dietary discretion, and complete abstinence from tobacco use.

SUMMARY AND PERSPECTIVE

Results of clinical trials have shown that both CAS and CEA are effective procedures for stroke prevention; each has an important place in carotid disease management. Defining the clinical situations treated best with one procedure or the other, or with medical management alone, continues to be an evolving process.

Currently, concerns about higher stroke risk with CAS, coupled with reimbursement restrictions and cost-effectiveness issues for CAS, make CEA the standard, and much more commonly performed, method of treating carotid occlusive disease when intervention is warranted. In the author's practice, CAS is reserved for patients with recurrent stenosis after CEA, a history of neck irradiation or radical neck dissection, lesions located high in the neck (above the level of the C2 cervical vertebra), and contralateral vocal cord paralysis. Most of the author's patients undergoing CEA are at "high risk" with traditional trial criteria, and only rarely is the author compelled to use CAS because of extreme cardiopulmonary risk factors that make surgical treatment prohibitive.

CAS should be used with reservation in situations where the risk of periprocedural stroke is higher than usual. These circumstances involve both clinical and anatomic factors. Clinical factors include age older than 80 years and recent (within 2 weeks) neurologic ischemic symptoms. Anatomic factors include vessel angulation greater than 60 degrees, heavily concentrically calcified lesions, heterogeneous plaque composition as assessed with grayscale ultrasound scan, and a severely diseased aortic arch, especially when combined with branch vessel configuration that is hostile for sheath access.

In the future, technologic advances will probably make CAS safer and more attractive as a replacement for CEA in many cases. Also, more frequent use of proximal embolic protection, replacement of bare metal stents with covered stents, and selective use of transcervical access may lower the stroke risk of CAS. In the meantime, skilled vascular surgeons who are trained and experienced in performing both CAS and CEA bring a unique perspective and ability to judge the multiple variables that must be weighed carefully in deciding which of these two good procedures is the better choice for an individual patient.

SUGGESTED READINGS

Bonati LH, Jongen LM, Haller S, et al: New ischaemic brain lesions on MRI after stenting or endarterectomy for symptomatic carotid stenosis: a substudy of the International Carotid Stenting Study (ICSS), *Lancet Neurol* 9:353–356, 2010.

Brott TG, Hobson RW, Howard G, et al: Stenting versus endarterectomy for treatment of carotid artery stenosis, *N Engl J Med* 363:11–23, 2010.

Matsumura JS, Gray W, Chaturvedi S, et al: Results of carotid artery stenting with distal embolic protection with improved systems: Protected Carotid Artery Stenting in Patients at High Risk for Carotid Endarterectomy (PROTECT) trial, *J Vasc Surg* 55:968–977, 2012.

Murad MH, Shahrour A, Shah ND, et al: A systematic review and meta analysis of randomized trials of carotid endarterectomy vs stenting, *J Vasc Surg* 53:792–797, 2011.

Stabile E, Salemme L, Sorropago G, et al: Proximal endovascular occlusion for carotid artery stenting: results from a prospective registry of 1,300 patients, *J Am Coll Cardiol* 55:1661–1667, 2010.

Sternbergh WC, Crenshaw GD, Bazan HA, et al: Carotid endarterectomy is more cost-effective than carotid artery stenting, *J Vasc Surg* 55:1623–1628, 2012.

THE MANAGEMENT OF ANEURYSMS OF THE EXTRACRANIAL CAROTID AND VERTEBRAL ARTERIES

Jerry Goldstone, MD, FACS, FRCSEd (hon), and
Virginia L. Wong, MD, FACS

INTRODUCTION

Atherosclerotic occlusive and ulcerated lesions of the cervical carotid arteries are extremely common, but aneurysms of these vessels are rare, particularly when compared to the frequency of aneurysms involving the intracranial carotid arteries and their branches. Contemporary reports indicate that only 0.2% to 2% of all carotid procedures are performed for aneurysms. In the most recent review, there were 19 operations for aneurysms during an interval in which over 3000 procedures were performed for occlusive disease. Vertebral artery aneurysms are even rarer. Thus, there are no randomized or even large studies available, leaving relatively small, single-institution case series as all that are available to guide management and predict outcomes.

CAROTID ARTERY ANEURYSMS

Etiology

In early reports there was a predominance of infectious causes of extracranial carotid aneurysms, many associated with pharyngeal and other head and neck septic lesions. These occurred mostly in younger patients who had tonsillar and pharyngeal infections, such as peritonsillar abscess. With the availability of antibiotics, infected carotid aneurysms have largely disappeared except for those caused by infected prosthetic patches after carotid endarterectomy. The majority of carotid aneurysms now are either atherosclerotic or degenerative in nature. These are true aneurysms, commonly saccular rather than fusiform in shape and involve the carotid bifurcation and first portion of the internal carotid artery. About 15% of carotid aneurysms are pseudoaneurysms caused by patch infection following carotid endarterectomy or trauma (blunt, penetrating, and iatrogenic). Patch angioplasty–related aneurysms occur at the carotid bifurcation. There have been a few reports of infected carotid stents causing carotid aneurysms. Blunt traumatic injuries tend to involve the distal extracranial internal carotid artery, whereas most penetrating injuries, which can cause A-V fistulas as well as pseudoaneurysms, tend to involve the common carotid. The increased use of computed tomographic (CT) scans and magnetic resonance (MR) scans in trauma centers has identified carotid aneurysms that were previously not detected, so the proportion caused by trauma may be underestimated. Less frequent causes include dissection, fibromuscular dysplasia, Becet's disease, and other collagen vascular diseases. A recent report from South Africa described the emergence of human immunodeficiency virus (HIV)-related vasculopathy as an increasing cause of carotid aneurysms. In addition, extensive head and neck surgery and radiation have been cited as etiologic factors in carotid aneurysms.

Presentation and Diagnosis

Due to the changing etiology, most carotid aneurysms now occur in adults. For atherosclerotic aneurysms, the average age is over 60 years, with a 2:1 male preponderance. Patients are frequently asymptomatic at presentation, with a pulsatile neck mass being the most frequently encountered sign, present in more than 90% in some series. Symptoms, when present, vary depending on the size, location, and etiology of the aneurysm. They often consist of ischemic neurologic events such as transient monocular or hemispheric ischemic attacks or frank stroke caused by thromboembolic phenomena. Compressive symptoms from the aneurysm itself can cause neck pain and facial pain, headache, cranial nerve palsy, Horner's syndrome, hoarseness, and dysphagia. Patients with an infectious etiology may have leukocytosis and other signs of local sepsis such as peritonsillar abscess or overlying cervical cellulitis. Rupture, which was common in the preantibiotic era, is now rare, but may occur into the pharynx or externally through a draining sinus (as might occur with an infected pseudoaneurysm following carotid endarterectomy). Victims of penetrating trauma are mostly young adults with obvious cutaneous wounds but who rarely have isolated carotid injuries and who may not be actively bleeding when initially evaluated. This makes probing cervical wounds potentially dangerous and is why it should be avoided until adequate imaging has been performed.

The differential diagnosis of a pulsatile neck mass includes carotid artery redundancy (kink, coil, loop), carotid body tumor, paraganglioma, malignant neoplasm, lymphadenopathy, brachial cleft cyst, and peritonsillar abscess. A pulsatile mass at the base of the neck is one condition frequently misdiagnosed as a common carotid aneurysm. It is almost always a dilated tortuous subclavian artery, and almost always on the right side in middle-aged hypertensive women.

Duplex ultrasound should be the initial diagnostic modality (Figure 1). It is useful for vessels from the clavicle to just above the mandible and can determine aneurysm size, extent, flow characteristics, presence of mural thrombus, and dissection. Due to the presence of the mandible, lesions located high in the neck or near the skull base cannot be interrogated by ultrasound and may be missed altogether with this modality. The same is true for proximal common carotid aneurysms due to the clavicle. CT and MR are invaluable for visualizing these lesions and surrounding structures. In most centers, CT or MR angiography (CTA, MRA) can be quickly performed,

allowing three-dimensional image reconstruction that provides a high-quality, detailed definition of arterial anatomy that is essential for proper treatment planning. These studies can be obtained more quickly than and can avoid the risks of catheter-based angiography, but angiography is still required when endovascular therapy is being considered. One major advantage of catheter angiography is that it allows for the measurement of carotid back pressure and balloon occlusion testing, which is helpful if carotid ligation is a possible treatment alternative.

Indications for Intervention

Intervention for carotid artery aneurysms is appropriate for the relief of symptoms caused by local compression as well as for the treatment of hemorrhage that, although rare, is associated with high rates of morbidity and mortality. The natural history of asymptomatic extracranial carotid aneurysms is not known, but the primary indication for treatment is the prevention of new or recurrent neurologic events caused by embolism of aneurysm contents into the cerebral circulation. In Winslow's classic 1926 article, nonoperative management resulted in a 70% mortality rate due to thrombosis, embolism, and rupture. Contemporary reports have not refuted these data, although some suggest that anticoagulation and antiplatelet therapy may be sufficient for selected asymptomatic patients with small, distal aneurysms caused by blunt trauma or dissection. These reports present follow-up imaging that demonstrated stabilization or resolution of the arterial pathology without clinical consequences in at least some of the patients. This approach requires close monitoring of the patients with prompt intervention for lesions that enlarge or become symptomatic. This type of observational approach is quite controversial, with most authors favoring treatment of all of these aneurysms, regardless of size, because of their potential to cause neurologic symptoms.

Treatment

A careful baseline neurologic evaluation should be performed before undertaking repair by any method. For patients with atherosclerotic aneurysms, cardiac risk assessment is appropriate. For open surgical repair, the need for intraoperative cerebral perfusion monitoring and protection should be taken into account because carotid clamp times are generally longer than required for carotid endarterectomy. Electroencephalography, transcranial Doppler, carotid back (stump) pressure measurement, and routine shunting have all been used successfully for this purpose. If an interposition vein graft is going to be used, a small, short shunt should be selected so that it can be placed through the vein. Although carotid endarterectomy using local-regional anesthesia can be successfully performed, general anesthesia is recommended for the treatment of carotid aneurysms because of the time required for a more difficult and extensive dissection and the need for more extensive cervical exposure and complex arterial reconstruction.

The objectives of treatment for most patients are to exclude the aneurysm from the circulation and restore cerebral blood flow to prevent neurologic events. The treatment selected will depend on the location and etiology of the aneurysm. As discussed earlier, the location varies with etiology. Atherosclerotic aneurysms most commonly occur at or near the bifurcation of the common carotid artery, as do pseudoaneurysms following endarterectomy (Figures 2 and 3). Injuries due to blunt trauma and arterial dysplasia occur much higher in the internal carotid artery toward the base of the skull (Figure 4). Proximal exposure of the common carotid artery and its bifurcation can be achieved through a standard longitudinal incision along the anterior border of the sternocleidomastoid muscle. This incision can be extended behind the ear if necessary to gain more distal exposure. Care must be taken to avoid manipulation of the aneurysm itself to

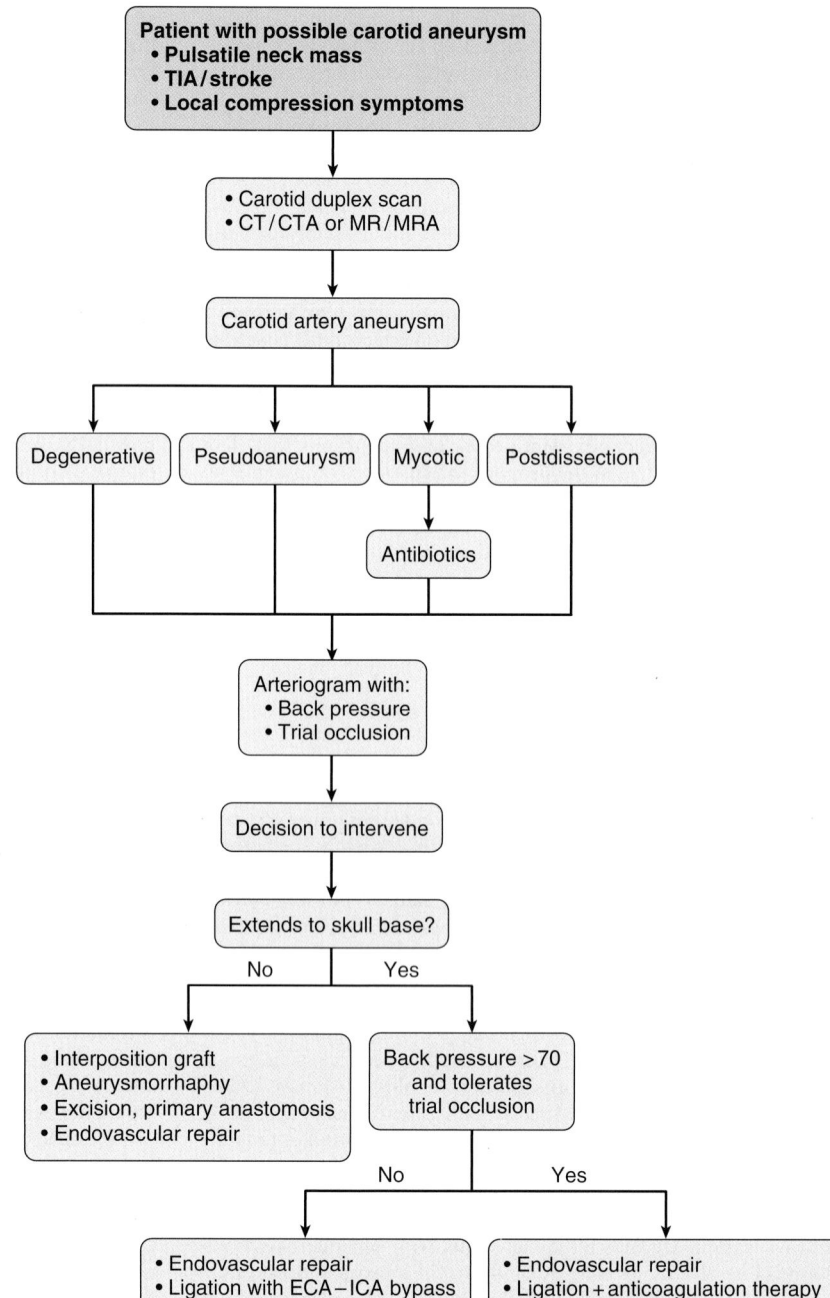

FIGURE 1   Algorithm for diagnosis and treatment of carotid aneurysms. *CT/CTA,* Computed tomographic/CT angiography; *ECA,* external carotid artery; *ICA,* internal carotid artery; *MR/MRA,* magnetic resonance/MR angiography; *TIA,* transient ischemic attack.

prevent dislodgement of thrombotic material before application of a distal occluding clamp (or vessel loop).

Several cranial nerves may be encountered in the operative field, including IX, X, XI, XII, and the marginal mandibular branch of VII, and these must be carefully protected from injury. Aneyrysm growth may have distorted the nerves' usual anatomic courses, and they may be densely adherent to the aneurysm or other structures. Use of bipolar cautery is an important adjunct when working close to these nerves. Exposure of the more distal portion of the internal carotid artery requires uncommon maneuvers, such as division of the digastric muscle, removal of the sternocleidomastoid muscle from its insertion on the mastoid, elevation of the parotid gland, and excision of the styloid process. If anticipated in advance, distal carotid exposure is facilitated by the use of nasotracheal rather than orotracheal intubation and subluxation of the mandible. Control of backbleeding from the distal internal carotid artery can be achieved with an

intraluminal balloon catheter (or shunt) rather than a cross clamp. However, if still more distal exposure is necessary to permit arterial reconstruction, portions of the mastoid and petrous portion of the temporal bones can be removed. Participation of an otolaryngologist or neurosurgeon experienced in skull-base surgery is recommended for these maneuvers. The difficulties and morbidity with this type of distal exposure favor an endovascular approach whenever possible.

Open reconstructive options include ligation, resection with patch closure, or resection with restoration of arterial continuity using conduits. Ligation is the oldest form of therapy and technically the least demanding. It may be the only option for high lesions for which distal access to and control of the internal carotid artery cannot be achieved in spite of the maneuvers described or for rapid control when there is exsanguination from rupture or trauma. Unfortunately, ligation is associated with a high risk of stroke and mortality (30% to 60%).

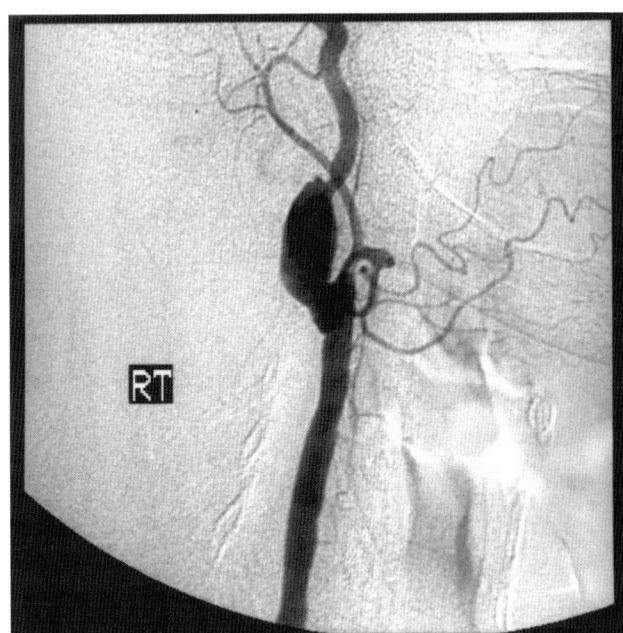

FIGURE 2 Digital subtraction angiogram showing atherosclerotic aneurysm of internal carotid artery.

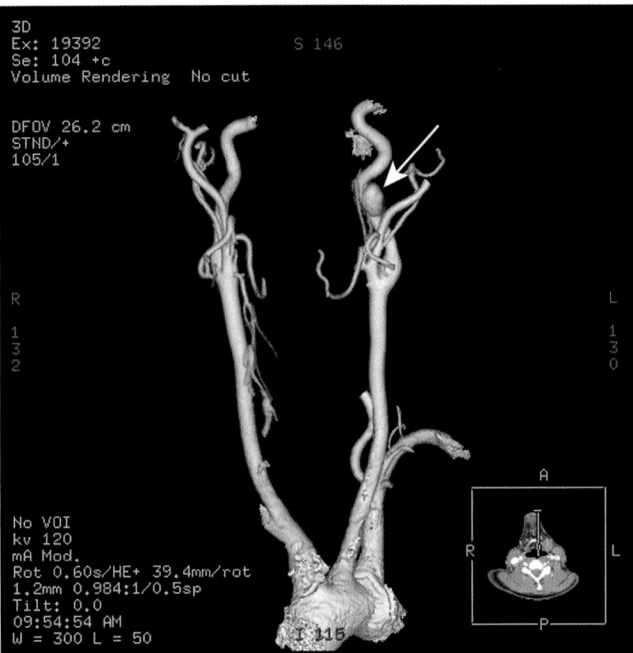

FIGURE 4 CT angiogram showing traumatic pseudoaneurysm (*arrow*) of mid-distal internal carotid artery caused by fractured mandible.

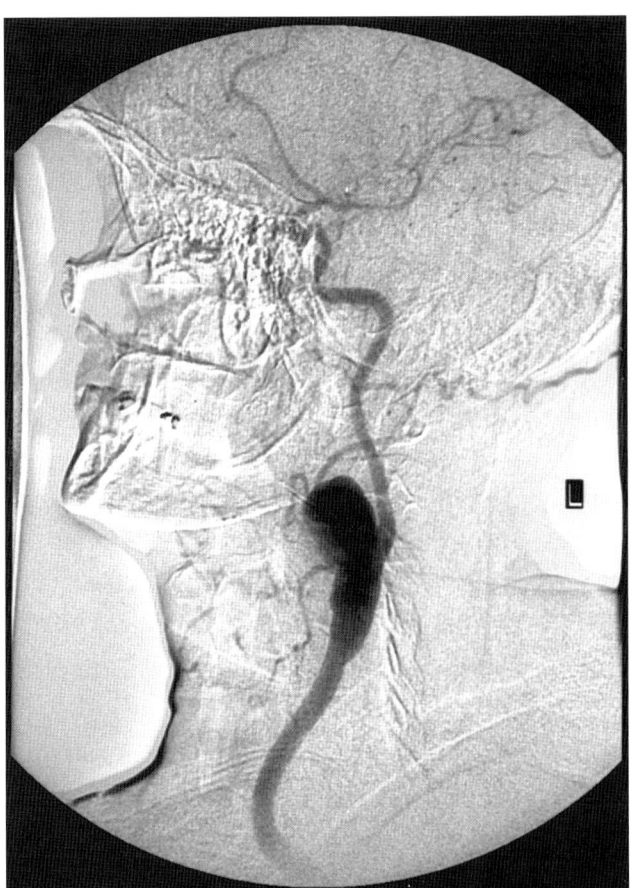

FIGURE 3 Digital subtraction angiogram showing pseudoaneurysm of left carotid bifurcation at site of previous carotid endarterectomy.

Identification of patients who will tolerate carotid ligation can be accomplished preoperatively by performing a balloon occlusion test at the time of cerebral angiography. After heparinization, a balloon is inflated in the internal carotid artery to stop antegrade cerebral flow for approximately 30 minutes while monitoring the patient's neurologic status for changes. Carotid back pressures of 70 mm Hg or greater are usually associated with freedom from neurologic symptoms and indicate collateral cerebral perfusion that is adequate to permit carotid ligation when necessary. Intraoperatively measured carotid back pressure at the same level can be used for the same purpose, but under conditions of general anesthesia, there is no way to monitor cerebral function. When this is done, maintenance of the patient's baseline blood pressure is essential. Postprocedure anticoagulation should be maintained for 6 to 12 weeks to prevent propagation and downstream embolization of thrombus off the static column of the ligated internal carotid artery. Patients who cannot tolerate carotid ligation due to low back pressure and symptoms with trial occlusion should be considered for extracranial-intracranial (EC-IC) bypass, an effective but infrequently performed procedure, before aneurysm ligation.

Aneurysm resection and patch repair of the ICA is appropriate for small-necked, saccular aneurysms or noninfected pseudoaneurysms. Use of autologous vein (usually the greater saphenous vein from the groin), bovine pericardium, and prosthetic material for patches have all been described. We have used bovine pericardium as a patch almost exclusively in recent years, even in infected fields. Prosthetic material should not be used as either a patch or conduit if the possibility of infection exists as the etiology of the aneurysm.

Complete resection of the aneurysm with restoration of arterial continuity is the preferred technique for fusiform or wide-mouthed aneurysms. If there is redundancy of the internal carotid, it is sometimes possible to mobilize enough vessel to be able to perform an end-to-end anastomosis or perform an anastomosis to the external carotid artery if it is intact. Interposition grafting can be performed using greater saphenous vein or prosthetic (Figure 5). If the field is infected and no autologous vein is available, an arterial autograft can be obtained from the superficial femoral artery, and that artery can be replaced with a prosthetic conduit in a noninfected field. In a few

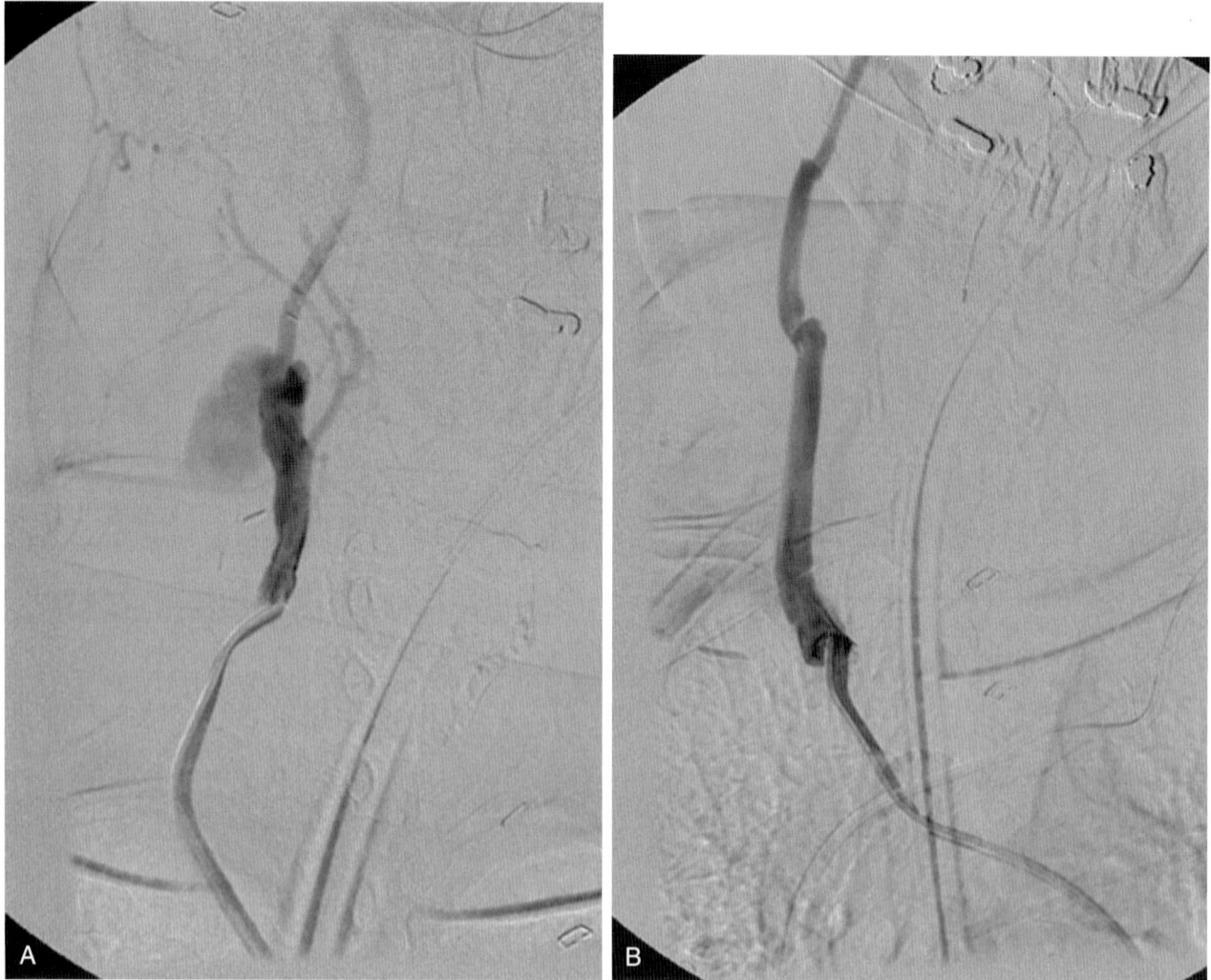

FIGURE 5   Digital subtraction angiogram of carotid aneurysm before (**A**) and after (**B**) repair with interposition vein graft. *(Courtesy of Wei Zhou, MD, Baylor College of Medicine.)*

cases, we have even used a segment of endarterectomized, occluded superficial femoral artery. Use of a shunt is facilitated by threading the shunt through the graft while the distal anastomosis is being completed and then removing it just before completion of the proximal anastomosis. For cases that are infectious in nature, culture-specific or broad spectrum antibiotics should be administered before the operation begins and continued for several weeks postoperatively. Intraoperative cultures are important for proper antibiotic selection. This process is especially important if methicillin-resistant *Staphylococcus aureus* is known or suspected of being the causative organism. All nonviable and infected tissues should be thoroughly débrided, and the arterial reconstruction should be covered with healthy vascularized tissue, ideally the sternocleidomastoid muscle. For some cases, particularly those with previous treatment for head and neck cancer, a myocutaneous flap may have to be created to ensure adequate vessel coverage.

Endovascular treatment of carotid artery aneurysms has become more common along with the advances in endovascular devices and the growing experience with the endoluminal treatment of carotid occlusive disease. Endovascular treatment avoids the need for the often difficult dissections, especially for high cervical exposure. The risks of bleeding and cranial nerve injury are markedly reduced. Multiple case reports populate the literature, and although 70% of cases in a 2006 report were treated endovascularly, no large series have been reported. Even more recent publications from 2010 and

2012 had only 0 of 19 and 3 of 30 aneurysms, respectively, treated with stents. Endovascular treatment requires an experienced staff, a modern imaging suite, and appropriate equipment and devices, including carotid-specific stents and embolic protection devices. Suitable patients must have aortic arch anatomy that can accommodate stable, selective catheterization of the common carotid artery with a large-caliber, long sheath over a supportive wire. Endovascular treatment should be preferentially considered for surgically inaccessible lesions, when there is a hostile operative field (prior radiation or cervical surgery), or for patients deemed unfit for a lengthy general anesthetic.

Although treatment techniques have mostly used a transfemoral approach, both transaxillary and transcarotid approaches have been described. Following systemic heparinization and selective catheterization of the common carotid artery with the long sheath, an embolic protection device is deployed in the internal carotid artery distal to the aneurysm. Bare metal stents, double stents, vein-covered stents, and prosthetic-covered stents have all been successfully used. Covered stents are most frequently used, but they require larger sheaths and delivery systems. The covered stent (stent-graft) can then be deployed across the aneurysm to exclude it from the circulation, thereby preventing expansion and rupture as well as emboli entering the flow channel. Accurate sizing of the proximal and distal landing zones is necessary to ensure adequate seal. The stent may occlude side-branch flow—that is, the external carotid artery—but this is usually well tolerated. Bare metal stents can be used to tack down a dissection entry point (flap) or even to cover a small aneurysm neck sufficient to impede flow and cause aneurysm sac thrombosis. Thrombogenic materials, such as microcoils, detachable balloons, synthetic particles, or glue, can be injected directly into the aneurysm sac through the interstices of a noncovered stent to induce thrombosis. However, extreme care must be taken to prevent the escape of such materials into the parent artery, which could cause thrombosis or distal embolization. Postprocedure antiplatelet therapy should be administered as with carotid stenting for occlusive disease.

Results

There are no randomized or controlled trial data available for analysis of the treatment of extracranial carotid artery aneurysms. Proximal lesions and those associated with a very tortuous internal carotid are probably best managed with open surgical repair, whereas large aneurysms and those involving the distal one third of the internal carotid are safer managed with endovascular techniques. The results of observation alone, with or without anticoagulation, parallel the natural history of the disease with 50% to 70% morbidity and mortality rates. Ligation also results in a high rate of stroke and death ranging from 30% to 60%, but careful patient selection can reduce this risk substantially, as shown in one recent report of a 12% stroke and death rate. Results of open surgical treatment with arterial reconstruction are much better and appear to vary with the size, location, and etiology of the lesion. In the report from the Texas Heart Institute, which included data from 13 single-center series that were reviewed in that paper, combined stroke and mortality was just 10%. The average rate of cranial nerve injury, which is more frequent in repairs involving the distal internal carotid artery, is much higher at approximately 30%. Fortunately, many of these cranial nerve deficits are temporary. Long-term results also seem to be generally favorable, with most deaths occurring from other cardiovascular diseases or diagnoses not related to the carotid aneurysm repair. In patients who have had postprocedure imaging studies, most arterial reconstructions have been reported as patent, and those that were not usually were not associated with symptoms.

Initial technical success rates with endovascular treatment are high, with acceptably low periprocedural stroke and death rates, but all reported series are small. Cranial nerve injuries, access site complications, and hospital length of stay are all reported to be much lower when compared to open repair. Short-term and midterm results of up to 4.5 years after treatment are encouraging with persistent exclusion of the aneurysm and patency of the parent vessel. It is somewhat surprising that there are not more long-term data published about this subject.

VERTEBRAL ARTERY ANEURYSMS

Extracranial carotid aneurysms are rare, but vertebral aneurysms are extremely rare. Most are caused by blunt and penetrating trauma, resulting in pseudoaneurysm formation or true aneurysmal dilatation following intimal dissection. Spontaneous dissection has been the most frequent etiology in several recent reports. Forceful head turning from trauma or iatrogenic manipulation (chiropractic), vascular catheterization, arterial dysplasia, prior radiation, and collagen vascular disease have all been described as causes of vertebral artery aneurysm.

The most frequent manifestations are headache and neck pain or symptoms of vertebrobasilar territory ischemia. If the intracranial portion of the vertebral artery is involved, rupture can cause subarachnoid hemorrhage. Palpation of a pulsatile neck mass is less frequent than with carotid aneurysms. Duplex ultrasound is not very useful for evaluation of vertebral arterial pathology other than the determination of the presence of flow and flow direction. The best

diagnostic imaging modality in the past has been contrast angiography, but CTA and MRA are now favored because they are quicker to obtain and provide important anatomic information about the vessels and adjacent structures that may influence the interventional approach. More than 80% of vertebral dissections resolve spontaneously, and for this reason, most patients can be managed nonoperatively with anticoagulation and close follow-up with repeat imaging. However, in patients with hemorrhage (i.e., rupture), continued neurologic symptoms, aneurysmal enlargement or absence, or impaired flow in the contralateral vertebral artery, intervention may provide the best outcome.

Surgical exposure of the vertebral artery can be challenging due to its anatomic position, arising from the subclavian artery (V1 segment) deep in the neck and then running within the transverse processes of the cervical vertebrae emerging at the level of C-2 (V2 segment), where it courses around the transverse process (V3 segment) and enters the foramen magnum (V4 segment). Exposure of the proximal vertebral artery from its origin off the subclavian to where it enters the vertebral foramen of C-6 is achieved through a transverse supraclavicular incision. Repair options here include ligation, resection with repair, transposition onto the common carotid artery, or bypass from the subclavian. All of these are challenging due to the small working space and the short segment of artery available. If the contralateral vertebral artery is normal, it is safer in most cases to simply ligate the affected artery. However, this does not always solve the problem of bleeding because of backflow from the contralateral vertebral artery, so distal ligation or balloon occlusion is also required.

Surgical repair of the vertebral artery in its intraosseous location can be especially challenging due to bony structures and the luxuriant venous plexus that accompanies the artery at this location. The more distal portions of the vertebral artery at C-2 and above also provide challenges to exposure because most vascular surgeons have little experience working in this area. A posterior cervical approach may be necessary, and repair is accomplished by bypass from the carotid or subclavian arteries to the distal vertebral or transposition of the vertebral to the carotid circulation. Because of these technical challenges, there has been widespread adoption of endovascular treatment. Endovascular access and repair using covered stents, detachable coils, or balloons have been reported for lesions at all levels of the vertebral artery and may be especially useful for surgically inaccessible areas. Both ligation and endovascular occlusion of the vertebral artery are well tolerated in the presence of a normal contralateral vertebral artery. With both methods, trapping the aneurysmal segment of artery both proximally and distally may be necessary to control bleeding or aneurysm expansion. An aneurysm involving a dominant or single vertebral artery is best treated by a method designed to maintain its patency and prevent distal embolization. Both intraluminal stents and bypass with aneurysm exclusion have been used successfully with good results.

SUGGESTED READINGS

Bush RL, Lin PH, Dodson TF, et al: Endoluminal stent placement and coil embolization for the management of carotid artery pseudoaneurysms, *J Endovasc Ther* 8:53–61, 2001.

El-Sabrout R, Cooley DA: Extracranial carotid aneurysms: Texas Heart Institute Experience, *J Vasc Surg* 31:702–712, 2000.

Garg K, Rockman CB, Lee V, et al: Presentation and management of carotid artery aneurysms and pseudoaneurysms, *J Vasc Surg* 55:1618–1622, 2012.

Kai Y, Nishi T, Watanabe M, Morioka M, et al: Strategy for treating unruptured vertebral artery dissecting aneurysms, *Neurosurgery* 65:1085–1091, 2011.

Kurata A, Yamada M, Ohmomo T, et al: The efficacy of coil embolization at the dissection site of ruptured dissecting vertebral aneurysms, *Interv Neurorad* 7(suppl 1):73–82, 2001.

Longo GM, Kibbe M: Aneurysms of the carotid artery, *Sem Vasc Surg* 18:178–185, 2005.

Padayachy V, Robbs JV: Carotid artery aneurysms in patients with human immunodeficiency virus, *J Vasc Surg* 55:331–337, 2012.

Rosset E, Albertini JN, et al: Surgical treatment of extracranial internal carotid aneurysms, *J Vasc Surg* 31:713–723, 2000.

Rothstein J, Goldstone J: Carotid artery aneurysms. In Cronenwett JL, Rutherford RB, editors: *Decision making in vascular surgery*, Orlando, FL, 2001, WB Saunders, p 54.

Strivastava SD, Eagleton MJ, O'Hara P, et al: Surgical repair of carotid artery aneurysms: A 10-year, single-center experience, *Ann Vasc Surg* 24:100–105, 2010.

Winslow N: Extracranial aneurysms of the internal carotid artery: History and analysis of the cases registered up to August 1, 1925, *Arch Surg* 13:689–729, 1926.

Zhou W, Lin PH, Bush RL, et al: Carotid artery aneurysms: evolution of management over two decades, *J Vasc Surg* 43:493–497, 2006.

BRACHIOCEPHALIC RECONSTRUCTION

Gregory J. Pearl, MD

INTRODUCTION

The most common anatomic configuration of the brachiocephalic vessels off the transverse aortic arch is three separate and discreet branches: the innominate artery, the left common carotid artery, and the left subclavian artery. The innominate artery gives rise to the right subclavian and right common carotid artery. The most common variant of arch anatomy is the bovine arch in which the left common carotid artery shares a common origin with the innominate artery off the arch or that arises directly off the innominate artery. Other variants include the left vertebral artery arising directly off the arch between the left common carotid and the left subclavian arteries and the aberrant right subclavian artery that arises just distal and posterior to the left subclavian artery, coursing across the midline between the esophagus and anterior spinal ligament to the right upper extremity (Figure 1).

The brachiocephalic vessels supply the upper extremities as well as the brain, so any disease entity that affects these vessels, either as a result of flow limiting stenosis or as a source of embolization, may produce serious symptoms that are difficult to correct surgically (Figure 2). The underlying lesions affecting the great vessels may be a result of, and associated with, disease arising in the aortic arch or may be secondary to lesions intrinsic to the brachiocephalic vessels themselves. The pathologic entities include atherosclerotic disease, inflammatory arteritides, blunt or penetrating trauma, or a pathologic process involving the ascending or transverse aortic arch such as aortic dissection or aneurysm. Additionally, occlusive or aneurysmal lesions of the subclavian arteries may be associated with arterial thoracic outlet syndrome. Debranching procedures of the brachiocephalic vessels have also become an important adjunct in the endovascular treatment of aortic dissections or aortic aneurysmal disease involving the transverse arch or proximal descending thoracic aorta.

CLINICAL PRESENTATION

The clinical manifestations of lesions involving the brachiocephalic arteries are in large part dependent on the underlying pathogenesis and extent of vessel involvement, such as single-vessel versus multivessel disease, as well as the anatomic location of the culprit lesions. In Berguer's report on brachiocephalic revascularization, he identified an approximately 40% incidence of multivessel involvement of the brachiocephalic arteries.

Atherosclerotic disease involving the arch vessels is not uncommon and in most instances is asymptomatic. Symptoms caused by occlusive lesions involving the brachiocephalic vessels may be those typical of carotid artery distribution transient ischemic attack (TIA) or stroke, vertebrobasilar events, or upper-extremity ischemia such as arm fatigue or digital ischemia. Multivessel occlusive lesions, as seen in patients with advanced atherosclerotic disease or Takayasu arteritis, may produce nonlateralizing neurologic symptoms such as dizziness and visual disturbances secondary to cerebral hypoperfusion. Patients presenting with classic lateralizing hemispheric neurologic events that cannot be attributed to cervical or intracranial carotid disease should undergo aggressive interrogation of the brachiocephalic vessels as a potential source of these symptoms.

Severe occlusive disease in the proximal subclavian arteries may produce reversal of flow in the ipsilateral vertebral artery, leading to the condition known as subclavian steal syndrome. Reversal of flow in the vertebral artery noted on duplex ultrasound examination of the neck is not an uncommon finding and is frequently asymptomatic. However, in the classic clinical picture of subclavian steal, the patient will experience typical symptoms of vertebrobasilar insufficiency associated with arm exercise. Complaints of arm fatigue secondary to proximal subclavian atherosclerotic occlusive disease are uncommon due to the extensive capacity of collateral flow to the upper extremity combined with the decreased physical demands inherent in the atherosclerotic age group and therefore rarely require intervention. However, findings of unilateral digital ischemia as a result of microembolization should lead to a high index of suspicion for the culprit lesion to be located in the proximal subclavian or brachiocephalic vessels. Interrogation for the source lesion in this setting should not be delayed and should be pursued aggressively because ongoing embolization could potentially lead to extensive distal tissue loss and consequent severe functional impairment.

DIAGNOSTIC EVALUATION

A thorough history and physical examination are paramount in the initial evaluation of these patients. Careful palpation of the carotid and upper-extremity pulses in conjunction with auscultation of the neck, including the parasternal and paraclavicular areas, for the presence of bruits is necessary. Bilateral upper-extremity blood pressure measurements may easily and quickly be performed and yield useful information if a significant discrepancy is discovered. Any significant alteration in the comparison of the quality of pulses, the presence or absence of bruits, or significant upper-extremity blood pressure discrepancies of greater than 20 mm Hg is highly suggestive of hemodynamically significant subclavian or brachiocephalic disease. Of note, a significant blood pressure discrepancy in the upper extremity in an asymptomatic elderly patient is not uncommon and does not necessarily warrant additional investigation in the absence of symptoms or worrisome physical findings of digital ischemia.

Duplex ultrasound is extremely useful and sensitive in the interrogation of the cervical portion of the carotid arteries; however, it is of more limited use in the assessment of the brachiocephalic vessels

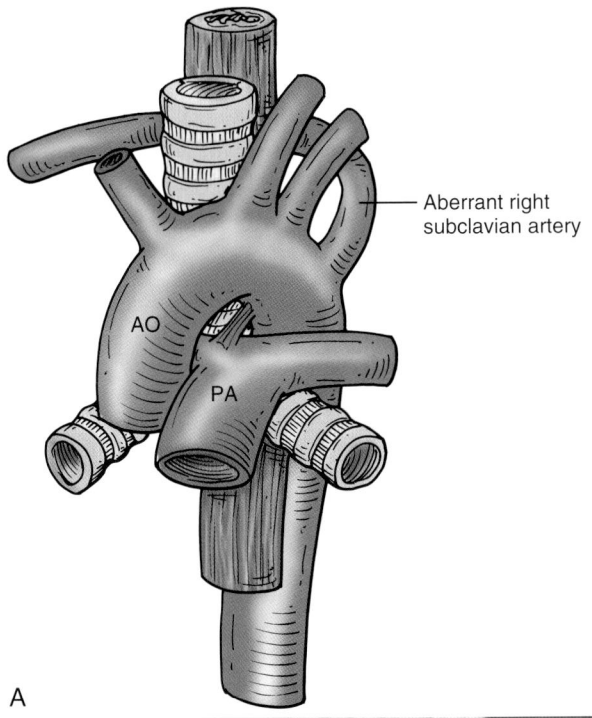

Aberrant right
subclavian artery

AO

PA

A

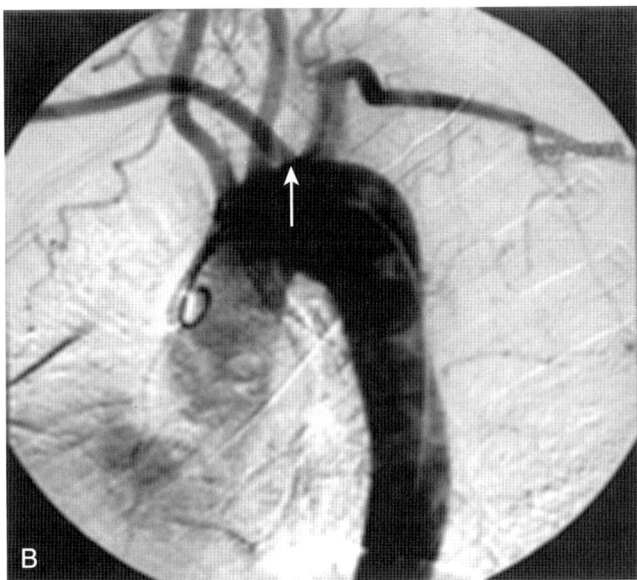

B

FIGURE 1 Drawing and digital subtraction arteriogram
demonstrating the anatomic configuration of aberrant right subclavian
artery (*arrow*).

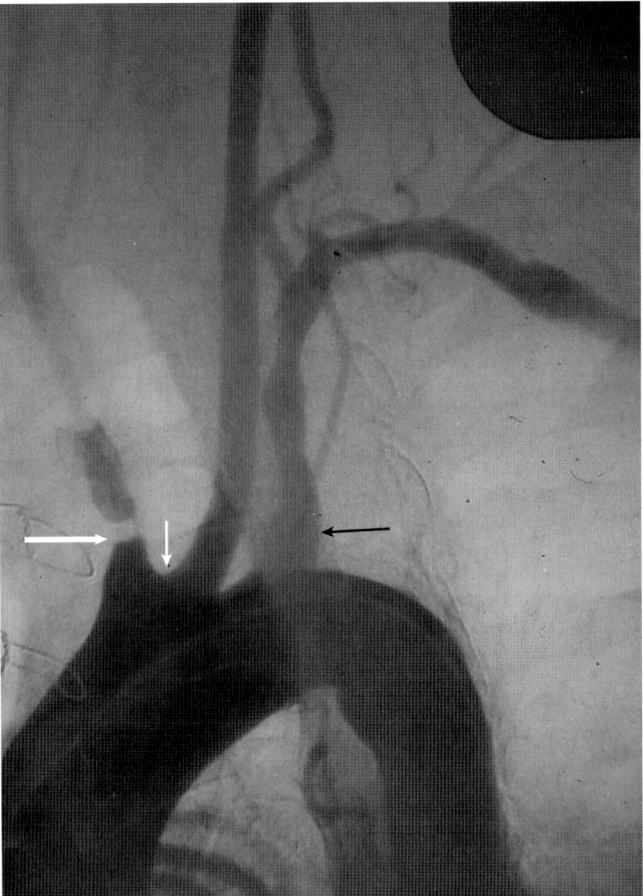

FIGURE 2 Digital subtraction angiogram showing multivessel
atherosclerosis involving brachiocephalic (*bold horizontal arrow*), left
common carotid (*short arrow*), and left subclavian (*thin black arrow*)
arteries.

due to their intrathoracic location. A diminished carotid pulse noted
on palpation in conjunction with altered low velocity and dampened
waveforms in the carotid artery at the base of the neck may be indirectly indicative of a hemodynamically significant proximal occlusive
lesion that may mandate further investigation depending on the
clinical setting. As described previously, duplex ultrasound can easily
detect reversal of flow in the cervical part of the vertebral artery suggestive of proximal subclavian occlusive disease. Magnetic resonance
angiograms (MRA) and computed tomographic angiography (CTA)
are additional noninvasive imaging modalities that are useful in the
assessment of the aortic arch and brachiocephalic vessels. Both
modalities require intravenous contrast administration for adequate
imaging of these vascular structures. In our experience, MRA tends
to be fraught with motion artifact related to the underlying cardiac
cycle and respiratory variation and also tends to overestimate the
degree of stenosis of the occlusive lesions. CTA seems to be better
tolerated by the patients due to the much shorter time required to
complete the study and obviates the problems associated with claustrophobia seen in many patients undergoing MRA. Multiplanar
digital subtraction angiography remains the gold standard imaging
modality, and despite its more invasive nature, it remains particularly
appropriate in those patients for whom potential endovascular treatment of the brachiocephalic disease is being considered.

TREATMENT

Indication for Treatment

The most frequent indication for the treatment of brachiocephalic
disease includes patients with the location and severity of disease
appropriate to their symptoms and clinical presentation. The symptoms may include lateralizing neurologic hemispheric symptoms,
vertebrobasilar insufficiency, or upper-extremity ischemic symptoms. One would expect to identify significant lesions in the common
carotid, subclavian, or innominate artery compatible with the lateralizing neurologic clinical presentation of the patient. In patients with
nonlateralizing symptoms related to global hypoperfusion, multivessel brachiocephalic involvement, bilateral carotid disease, or tandem
lesions should be suspected and confirmed on thorough workup.
Classic subclavian steal syndrome with onset of vertebrobasilar

symptoms with arm exercise would indicate a need for treatment as well. There is a paucity of natural history data to direct decision making in patients with asymptomatic brachiocephalic disease. The rich data from retrospective analyses and, subsequently, prospective analysis of the risks inherent in severe asymptomatic carotid bifurcation disease do not exist for asymptomatic brachiocephalic disease. General agreement exists that asymptomatic subclavian artery occlusive disease need not be treated other than in the occasional patient that requires normalization of subclavian artery flow in order to support the use of an internal mammary bypass graft for coronary artery revascularization or in the difficult hemodialysis patient requiring placement of dialysis access in the extremity supplied by the stenotic subclavian artery. In the patient with asymptomatic severe proximal common carotid artery occlusive disease, it seems intuitive that intervention should be considered for a preocclusive or critical stenosis at its origin in order to preserve patency of the common carotid artery and consequently reduce long-term risk for stroke.

Prior to the routine use of endovascular techniques in the cerebrovascular circulation, treatment of tandem carotid disease presented a quandary for the treating physician. In the symptomatic patient, it was often unclear whether the symptoms were related to a carotid bifurcation lesion or to a more proximally located common carotid or innominate lesion. Prioritization of which lesion to treat first could be quite problematic. The currently favored strategy involves a combined approach with open carotid endarterectomy and retrograde angioplasty and stenting of the proximal common carotid artery or innominate lesion. To be clear, the proximal disease need only be intervened upon for a severe, flow-limiting stenosis. Mild or moderate proximal lesions need not be treated concomitant to carotid endarterectomy and should simply be observed prospectively. In patients with nonatherosclerotic conditions affecting the brachiocephalic vessels, again, the indications for treatment should be reserved for the symptomatic patient. In the patient with inflammatory arteritis such as Takayasu's arteritis, the acute inflammatory phase should be treated medically to quiescence, and intervention should be reserved for resultant fibrotic stenosis in the affected vessels based on symptoms and severity as is done with atherosclerotic lesions (Figure 3).

Treatment Options

A number of therapeutic modalities are currently available for the treatment of brachiocephalic disease. The treatment options are categorized into two groups: open surgical reconstruction or endovascular intervention. These two general approaches are not mutually exclusive, and as mentioned previously, certain clinical situations may require combined treatment with both modalities to best treat more complex disease. Open surgical approaches may be further categorized as direct, or anatomic, reconstruction and indirect, or extraanatomic, reconstruction. The direct approach requires a median sternotomy for treatment of innominate or left common carotid artery lesions or a left posterior lateral thoracotomy for treatment of proximal left subclavian disease. The anatomic reconstruction maintains antegrade laminar flow accomplished through a bypass arising from the ascending aorta to the innominate and/or left common carotid artery. In the setting of isolated focal lesions localized to the innominate artery alone, endarterectomy may provide a suitable treatment option. Open repair may be preferred in suitable risk patients with extensive severe calcific atherosclerotic disease at the origin of the vessel to be treated. If severe brachiocephalic disease is identified in a patient being considered for coronary artery bypass grafting, the coronary revascularization may be performed concomitant with the brachiocephalic revascularization safely.

In patients with severe calcific disease in the ascending aorta and aortic arch, where cross-clamping the aorta would be impossible or extremely hazardous and construction of a graft anastomosis would be difficult, or in patients deemed to be poor candidates for median sternotomy due to advanced age, prior sternotomy or mediastinal radiotherapy, or multiple comorbidities, the indirect approach is preferable. This procedure is performed through supraclavicular or cervical incisions and involves bypass grafting or arterial transposition. Extraanatomic procedures are very well tolerated, with inherently low morbidity and mortality rates, and excellent long-term patency rates have been reported. The choice between performing a direct or indirect vascular procedure for brachiocephalic disease is also dependent on a number of other anatomic/pathologic factors, including the number of vessels involved, the location and distribution of the occlusive lesions in the involved vessel, the underlying pathogenesis and nature of the symptoms (embolic vs hypoperfusion), and the status of the other vessels supplying the brain not requiring or amendable to intervention, such as total internal carotid artery occlusion.

Advances in guide wire, angioplasty balloon, and stent design, as well as the availability of covered stent grafts, have broadened the applicability of endovascular treatment of severe brachiocephalic disease. As the experience and skill of the interventionalist have grown with the technological advances and improved device availability, endovascular treatment of fairly complex brachiocephalic disease has gained wider acceptance and use. With appropriate careful technique, excellent outcomes have been achieved with low associated morbidity. As is true for intervention in any vascular bed,

FIGURE 3 Axial images from CT angiogram **(A)** and 3-D reconstructed MRA **(B)** of a young woman with Takayasu's arteritis. Note the lucency surrounding the proximal brachiocephalic vessels on the CTA and the double contour of the ascending and descending thoracic aorta demonstrating wall thickening and inflammation.

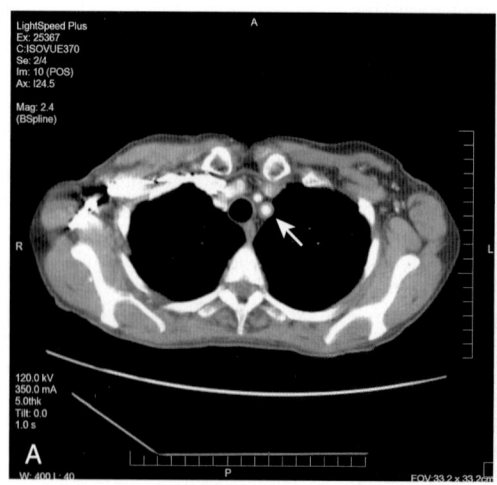
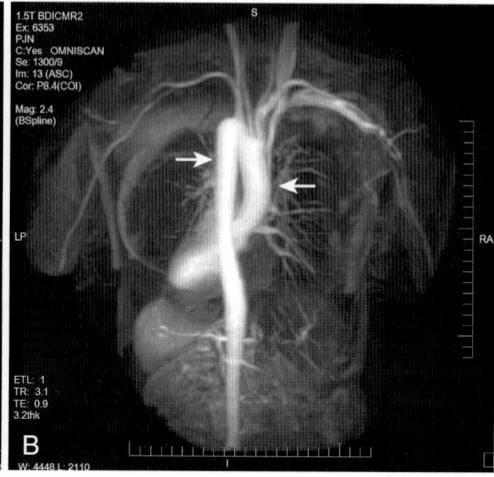

close follow-up and regular surveillance is mandatory regardless of the type of intervention performed in the treatment of brachiocephalic disease.

ANATOMIC (DIRECT) REVASCULARIZATION

Endarterectomy

Endarterectomy may be considered for focal atherosclerotic lesions in the innominate artery. It should not be attempted in patients in whom the lesion is located at the ostium of the vessel because these lesions are an extension of severe atherosclerotic disease in the aortic arch. The calcific atherosclerotic disease involving the aortic arch could make placing a side-biting clamp on the arch just proximal to the takeoff of the innominate artery quite hazardous, and achieving a satisfactory end point of the endarterectomy into the aortic arch would be difficult with the associated risks for embolization, residual flap formation, or dissection. Additionally, innominate artery endarterectomy should not be considered in patients possessing a bovine configuration because this would require temporary disruption of flow into the right and left carotid systems simultaneously. Accomplishing a satisfactory end point in the left common carotid artery may also prove difficult with this anatomy.

Proper endarterectomy for innominate arterial atherosclerotic lesions requires placement of a side-biting clamp across the aortic arch at the level of the takeoff of the innominate artery. This allows extension of the endarterectomy proximally onto the aortic arch itself to remove all of the plaque that arises from the aorta. The endarterectomy is performed through a longitudinal arteriotomy that typically does not require patch closure due to the large caliber of the vessel. Distribution of plaque into the right subclavian and right common carotid artery may require extension of the median sternotomy incision up into the right side of the neck along the anterior border of the sternocleidomastoid. Again, achievement of satisfactory end points with this extent of disease may prove difficult, and bypass from the ascending aorta in these situations is probably more prudent.

Endarterectomy for isolated atherosclerotic lesions in the proximal left common carotid artery and left subclavian artery may be performed; however, these procedures require a median sternotomy in the case of the left common carotid lesions and left thoracotomy in the setting of left subclavian origin disease and are more appropriately treated with extraanatomic approaches, which have proven to be better tolerated with excellent patency rates. Endovascular approach to these lesions either through an antegrade transfemoral approach or a retrograde cervical approach for the left common carotid artery lesions or retrograde left brachial approach for the left subclavian lesions has been successfully performed with excellent technical success and patency rates. These techniques are discussed more fully in a later section.

Bypass Graft

Bypass grafts constructed in an antegrade configuration are performed through a median sternotomy incision, with the origin of the bypass graft arising from the anterolateral aspect of the ascending aorta. Careful palpation of the ascending aorta should be performed to avoid placement of the partially occluding side-biting clamp in an area of significant atherosclerotic disease. Careful sizing and positioning of the graft is mandatory to avoid kinking or graft compression in the retrosternal space when the sternum is closed. Additionally, the grafts are tunneled posterior to the innominate vein. A bulky graft may cause compression of the innominate vein, leading to left brachiocephalic vein occlusion and left arm swelling post procedure.

Therefore, in the clinical setting where both the innominate artery and the left common carotid artery are to be bypassed, use of a bifurcated graft should be avoided due to the large volume and bulky nature of these grafts in this limited space.

Following systemic heparinization, a partially occluding clamp is applied on the ascending aorta as previously described and a 10- to 12-mm woven Dacron tube graft is anastomosed to the ascending aorta in an end-to-side fashion with 4-0 Prolene (Ethicon, Piscataway, NJ). suture. The graft is then clamped and distended with blood to assess hemostasis of the suture line and proper length of the graft prior to trimming. The distal anastomosis to the innominate artery is then performed either in an end-to-end or end-to-side fashion, depending on the clinical situation. When concomitant bypass to the left common carotid artery is required, an 8-mm knitted Dacron graft is taken off the innominate bypass graft in an end-to-side fashion above the thoracic inlet and left brachiocephalic vein to avoid graft kinking or compression. The distal anastomosis to the left common carotid artery may then be performed in an end-to-end or end-to-side configuration with 5-0 Prolene suture—again, depending on the clinical situation. Proximal occlusive lesions of the left subclavian artery are rarely symptomatic, and therefore, a "triple bypass" of all three brachiocephalic vessels is rarely, if ever, indicated. As noted previously, isolated left subclavian disease, when symptomatic, is best treated with endovascular treatment or extraanatomic bypass.

Brachiocephalic reconstruction may be performed safely with excellent outcomes. Multiple series have historically reported 30-day mortality rates of 4% to 7%, perioperative stroke rates ranging from 2% to 5%, and 5-year and 10-year patency rates exceeding 90%. As in the case of patients undergoing carotid endarterectomy, these patients must be followed closely with annual physical exam and surveillance duplex ultrasound for assessment of graft patency.

EXTRAANATOMIC (INDIRECT) REVASCULARIZATION

Isolated unilateral proximal common carotid artery or proximal subclavian artery lesions are readily treatable with extraanatomic reconstructions. These indirect methods of revascularization are performed through supraclavicular and/or cervical incisions and are better tolerated, with less perioperative morbidity and mortality, and they achieve patency rates similar to those of direct reconstruction. The most common form of revascularization is for construction of a prosthetic bypass between the ipsilateral carotid and subclavian arteries. The prosthetic graft utilized is usually a 7-mm or 8-mm knitted Dacron or polytetrafluoroethylene (PTFE) conduit. For treatment of proximal lesions, the procedure is performed through a single transverse supraclavicular incision at the base of the neck. The clavicular head of the sternocleidomastoid muscle is divided, and the scalene fat pad is reflected cephalad, taking care to identify and protect the phrenic nerve coursing anterior to the anterior scalene muscle. The anterior scalene muscle is then transected off its insertion to the first rib, exposing the underlying subclavian artery. The internal jugular vein is identified at the medial aspect of the supraclavicular incision and is mobilized laterally, exposing the underlying common carotid artery at the base of the neck. Care is taken to identify and protect the vagus nerve, which should be gently retracted laterally with the internal jugular vein. A short tunnel through the scalene fat pad is then made carefully behind the internal jugular vein and the vagus nerve. On the left side, great care should also be taken to avoid injury to the thoracic duct. In this exposure, a short bypass graft is constructed between the proximal common carotid artery and midsubclavian artery in end-to-side fashion with 5-0 or 6-0 Prolene sutures. It is not necessary to consider placement of a shunt during cross-clamping of the common carotid artery for performance of a carotid to subclavian bypass, and obviously a shunt is not necessary for a subclavian to common carotid artery revascularization.

In the performance of a subclavian to carotid bypass, it may at times be necessary to perform a concomitant carotid endarterectomy. In this setting, the procedure is performed through a supraclavicular incision at the base of the neck, as well as an additional incision higher up the neck along the anterior border of the sternocleidomastoid muscle, as is typically performed in standard carotid exposure for endarterectomy. End-to-side anastomosis to the subclavian artery is constructed, and the bypass graft is then tunneled and brought up distally to the carotid bifurcation to the endarterectomy arteriotomy site with the distal subclavian to carotid anastomosis serving as a patch closure. This type of reconstruction is particularly required in situations where the entire common carotid artery is occluded up to the level of the carotid bifurcation and internal carotid artery patency has been preserved via retrograde filling through the external carotid artery and its branches. Our current preference in the treatment of coexistent focal hemodynamically significant stenosis of the proximal carotid artery with severe carotid bifurcation disease is performance of retrograde angioplasty and stenting of the proximal common carotid lesion with open carotid endarterectomy and patch angioplasty. The technique for retrograde angioplasty is discussed in a later section.

In settings for which the subclavian artery is not suitable for use, as in flow for ipsilateral subclavian to carotid bypass, a carotid to carotid bypass may be considered. The contralateral carotid artery is used as the inflow vessel for revascularization. The common carotid arteries are exposed through longitudinal incisions at the base of the neck along the anterior border of the sternocleidomastoid muscle. The common carotid arteries are then dissected free and exposed in a standard fashion, and the pharynx is identified medially. A short retropharyngeal tunnel is then made between the pharynx and the anterior spinal ligament with a combination of sharp and blunt digital dissection. It is helpful to have a nasopharyngeal tube or temperature probe in place to facilitate palpitation of the pharynx and ensure dissection in the proper plane. The retropharyngeal tunneling facilitates a shorter bypass graft and avoids the possibilities of skin erosion and the feeling of strangulation that sometimes occur with subcutaneous tunneling of these grafts in the anterior neck. The grafts also pose a cosmetic issue in patients with a very slender neck when tunneled anteriorly. The prosthetic graft utilized is a 7- or 8-mm knitted Dacron or PTFE graft anastomosed in end-to-side fashion at both common carotid arteries with 5-0 and 6-0 Prolene sutures. The common carotid arteries are not cross-clamped simultaneously, and therefore placement of a shunt is typically not required.

In rare instances, subclavian-subclavian or axillary-axillary bypasses have been utilized to restore pulsatile flow into the subclavian and vertebral arteries for symptomatic vertebral basilar disease, or in the presence of a total occlusion of the innominate artery, they may restore pulsatile flow to the right common carotid artery as well. The subclavian arteries are approached through supraclavicular incisions as described previously. The grafts are constructed in end-to-side fashion and are tunneled across the suprasternal notch. The axillary-axillary bypass grafts are constructed through bilateral infraclavicular incisions. The pectoralis major muscle is split along the length of its fibers, and the clavipectoral fascia is incised. The axillary vein will be encountered initially during the dissection with the axillary artery located just posterior and slightly superior to the vein. The axillary vein is completely mobilized with ligation and division of side branches to facilitate exposure to the axillary artery. The prosthetic graft is then anastomosed in an end-to-side fashion to the axillary artery and is tunneled subcutaneously across the front of the manubrium sterni. The subclavian-subclavian and axillary-axillary grafts are utilized in high-risk patients, usually those with hostile anatomy that would be encountered with the more standard direct or extraanatomic procedures.

ARTERIAL TRANSPOSITION

Subclavian-carotid or carotid-subclavian transposition has the advantage of avoiding prosthetic material and the small attendant risk of infection. The transposition procedure is more technically challenging than utilization of a bypass due to the requirement of a more extensive dissection and mobilization of the vessels. The dissection requires more retrosternal exposure of the proximal portion of the vessels, and particular attention must be paid to visualization and exposure of the internal mammary and vertebral arteries for transposition of the subclavian artery. The procedures are performed through a transverse supraclavicular incision. The dissection then proceeds along the anterior border or between the heads of the sternocleidomastoid muscle down to the internal jugular vein. The internal jugular vein and vagus nerve are then mobilized and gently retracted, laterally exposing the proximal common carotid artery. The subclavian artery is then exposed after identification and ligation/ division of the vertebral vein. The subclavian artery is carefully dissected sharply, with dissection carried proximal to the takeoff of the internal mammary and vertebral artery. In the subclavian to carotid transposition, the proximal subclavian artery is clamped with a Cooley-Darra clamp, transected, and carefully sutured. Great care must be taken to avoid loss of control of this proximal stump because the stump is placed with tension to facilitate exposure in the upper mediastinum, and loss of this stump into the thoracic cavity prior to satisfactory suture ligation would be disastrous. The common carotid artery is then cross-clamped proximally and distally, and the subclavian artery is transposed and sewn in an end-to-side fashion with 5-0 or 6-0 Prolene suture. Care is taken to avoid kinking of the vertebral artery with the transposition. The indication and clinical situation requiring a carotid to subclavian transposition is much less common but is performed in a nearly identical fashion with the transection and suturing of the common carotid artery in the upper mediastinum and transposition of the common carotid artery to the subclavian artery just beyond the takeoff of the vertebral and internal mammary arteries. Subclavian to carotid transposition is our preferred technique in the event that debranching is required in the performance of thoracic aortic endograft treatment for aneurysm or dissection (Figure 4).

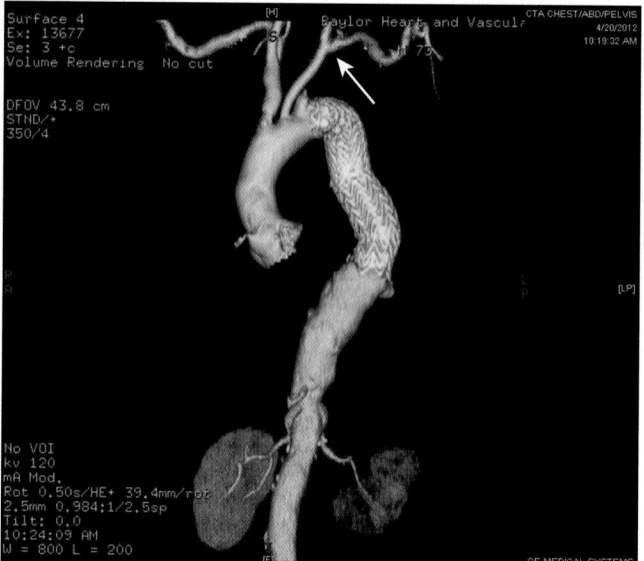

FIGURE 4   CTA of follow-up surveillance endovascular thoracic aneurysm repair in which debranching of the left subclavian artery with subclavian to left common carotid artery transposition *(arrow)* had been performed preoperatively.

Outcomes for extraanatomic brachiocephalic reconstructions are excellent. Multiple series have shown low incidences of paraprocedural stroke, and 30-day mortality is less than 3%. Five-year and 10-year patency rates exceed 90% in most series, and the patency rates of arterial transposition approach 100%.

ENDOVASCULAR TREATMENT

Numerous reports have demonstrated excellent results with open surgical revascularization in the setting of brachiocephalic disease with acceptably low 30-day mortality, stroke, perioperative stroke, and achievement of superb long-term patency of the reconstruction. However, as is true for all vascular beds, pursuit of minimally invasive procedures to treat brachiocephalic disease has been inevitable. Early reports of endovascular intervention in the arch vessels consisted mainly of lesions treated with angioplasty alone, and follow-up was limited. These studies revealed that endovascular intervention was feasible, and, as expected, utilization of endovascular techniques has increased with improvements in balloon and stent technology and maturation of technical skills in the treatment of cerebrovascular disease. In skilled hands, excellent outcomes with low morbidity and acceptable patency rates have been demonstrated.

Anatomic considerations are important in the planning of any treatment of brachiocephalic disease, but especially so if endovascular therapy is being considered. The anatomic characteristics of the lesions to be treated are key in the assessment for feasibility of treatment with catheter-based therapy. Endovascular intervention is preferable for stenosis rather than total occlusion and for nonostial, nonulcerative, and minimally calcified concentric lesions. Endovascular treatment is less favorable for severely eccentric lesions and lesions that extend contiguous to or into a major branch vessel, such as the vertebral artery arising off the subclavian artery, the left common carotid artery arising off the innominate artery in the Bovine configuration, or minimal separation of the origins of the innominate and left common carotid artery off the arch. These configurations carry the added risk of the compromise of the origin of one vessel in the treatment of another. Additionally, rotation of the vessel origin around the arch downward toward the ascending aorta for severe atherosclerotic disease affecting the aortic arch may make access and intervention of the brachiocephalic vessels much more challenging, and in these instances, open surgical treatment may be preferable.

INNOMINATE ARTERY INTERVENTIONS

Endovascular treatment of innominate lesions exposes the patient to potential embolization to both the right carotid and right vertebral artery distributions and therefore must be performed with great precision. Documentation of the position of the origins of the right common carotid and right subclavian artery branches in relation to the disease process is imperative. A kissing balloon technique is necessary to treat innominate lesions that extend directly proximate to or into the primary branches and to ensure proper distal stent placement. It is also important to ensure that the origin of the left common carotid is not compromised by angioplasty and stenting of a proximal calcific lesion in the innominate artery (Figure 5).

The innominate artery has the most challenging angulation extending off the aortic arch for cannulation through an antegrade transfemoral approach. Prolonged attempts at cannulation should not be pursued from this approach due to the risk of trauma and consequent embolization from the associated atherosclerotic disease in the aorta. In this situation, a retrograde brachial access may be performed and safe traversal of the innominate lesion accomplished. The innominate lesion may then be treated over the wire placed from

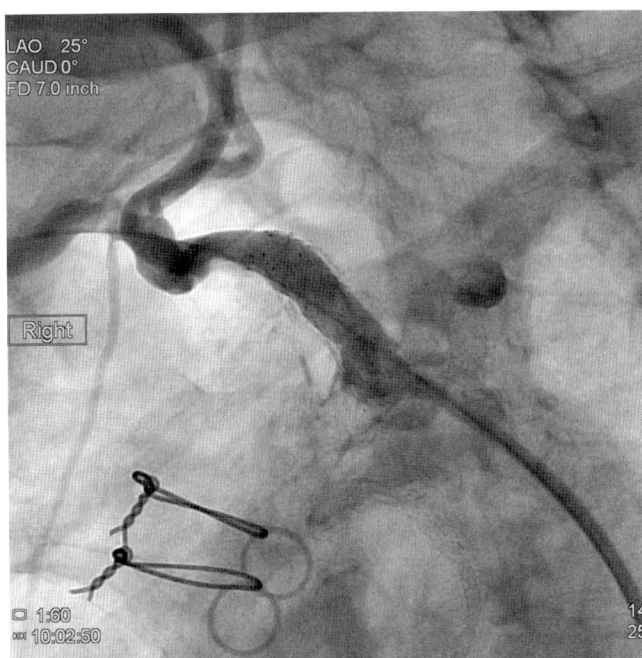

FIGURE 5 Innominate artery following PTA and stenting. Note sternal wires from previous coronary artery bypass which would have made an open innominate artery revascularization technically challenging.

the retrograde brachial approach, or the retrograde brachial wire can be snared from below and brought down with a through-and-through technique for greater stability for passage of the sheath and angioplasty system.

For ostial lesions, 1 to 2 mm of the stent should protrude into the aortic lumen. If the angioplasty and stent are being performed through the retrograde right brachial approach, it may be difficult to inject adequate contrast to visualize the exact position of the innominate orifice relative to the aortic arch. It is helpful to have an angiographic pigtail catheter in place for arteriography and facilitation of better imaging. The transfemoral guide wire or angiographic catheter itself can act as a marker as it curves around the arch abutting the innominate orifice. With the brachial approach, the guide wire should be directed into the ascending aorta rather than making the sharp curve into the descending thoracic aorta because this facilitates in-line alignment for deployment of the stent.

The risk of embolization with primary angioplasty and stenting of innominate lesions appears to be low, and therefore the requirement for cerebral protection in these procedures remains unclear. In most instances, the simplest, most straightforward approach without protection is best unless a "high-risk" lesion with a worrisome potential for embolization is to be treated.

Left Common Carotid Artery

Endovascular treatment of left common carotid artery lesions at the level of the arch is feasible and safe and may be performed in an antegrade transfemoral approach similar to that described with the innominate artery intervention. In the situation of an angulated takeoff of the left common carotid artery from the arch and when better stability of the angioplasty system is required, a "buddy wire" may be positioned in the external carotid artery to facilitate maintenance of the guide wire and sheath position at the origin of the vessel, as is done in the treatment of more distal carotid disease. A protection device is frequently used with the antegrade transfemoral approach for endovascular interventions on "high-risk" lesions.

Again, when transfemoral access to the origin of the vessel proves difficult, a retrograde approach from the distal common carotid artery may be performed, particularly in situations where a concomitant ipsilateral carotid endarterectomy is to be performed. The carotid branches are thus readily controlled with application of a distal clamp, and cerebral protection is ensured.

Left Subclavian Artery

Antegrade transfemoral access to the left subclavian artery off the arch is the easiest of the three vessels to obtain. After accessing the origin of the vessel, a 0.035 guide wire is passed across the lesion into the distal subclavian artery. The guide wire may then be exchanged for a stiffer wire if deemed necessary. A long 6 French or 7 French sheath is then positioned just across the origin of the vessel at the level of disease. Predilatation with a 4-mm angioplasty balloon may be necessary to facilitate passage of the stent. Correct sizing of the stent is essential to ensure that the area of disease is covered fully and that the vertebral artery origin is not "jailed." For ostial lesions, the stent should extend 1 to 2 mm into the aorticlumen (Figure 6).

If the subclavian lesion approaches the origin of the vertebral artery, it may be important to protect the vertebral artery origin. This may be accomplished after placement of a larger sheath into the origin of the subclavian artery and exchange of the 0.035 wire for two separate 0.014 wires, one placed antegrade out into the axillary artery and the other placed antegrade in the vertebral artery. A balloon expandable stent may be accurately placed over both 0.014 wires immediately at the takeoff of the vertebral artery. In another approach where both antegrade transfemoral access and retrograde brachial access into the subclavian artery are obtained, the 0.014 wire is placed through the retrograde transbrachial sheath into the vertebral artery, and the angioplasty and stenting are performed across the 0.035 wire from the antegrade transfemoral approach. The retrograde transbrachial sheath also facilitates the imaging of the vertebral artery at the time of the intervention. Embolic protection of the vertebral artery has been described, but its routine use cannot be advocated due to the exceedingly low risk of emboli to the vertebral basilar system during subclavian artery intervention, as well as the risk of dissection of the vertebral artery with instrumentation. Again, for emphasis, the simplest, most straightforward approach with the least guide wire and catheter manipulation is generally best.

SUMMARY

The treatment of symptomatic disease affecting the brachiocephalic vessels is safe, effective, and durable. Younger, low-risk patients are suitable candidates for direct anatomic reconstruction performed through a median sternotomy, particularly those patients with multivessel involvement. The direct anatomic reconstructions include a bypass arising from the ascending aorta or innominate arterial endarterectomy. Older patients with multiple comorbidities or those individuals with prior median sternotomies or a hostile mediastinum due to other reasons are better treated with an indirect extraanatomic approach or should be considered for endovascular intervention. Extraanatomic surgical reconstructions are performed with various types of prosthetic bypasses or arterial transposition. Endovascular therapy is performed via an antegrade transfemoral approach, a retrograde brachial approach, or, at times, a combination of both. Selection of the mode of treatment in each individual patient is based on various patient, anatomic, or pathologic factors in which one approach may be safer and more effective than another. The requirements for brachiocephalic reconstruction have increased with the ever-expanding treatment of aortic aneurysmal disease and aortic dissection for the purposes of debranching and expansion of the applicability and appropriateness for endovascular treatment of aortic arch and descending thoracic aortic disease.

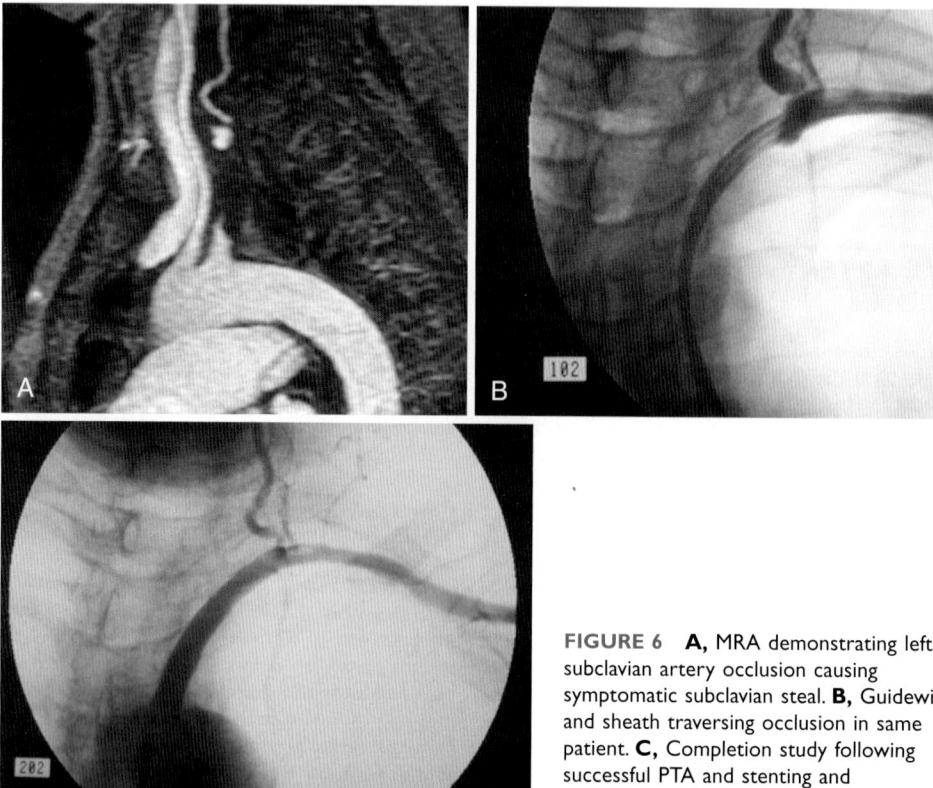

FIGURE 6   A, MRA demonstrating left subclavian artery occlusion causing symptomatic subclavian steal. **B,** Guidewire and sheath traversing occlusion in same patient. **C,** Completion study following successful PTA and stenting and re-established antegrade flow in vertebral artery.

SELECTED READINGS

Byrne J, Darling RC, Roddy SP, et al: Long-term outcome for extra-anatomic arch reconstruction, analysis of 143 procedures, *Eur J Vasc Endovasc Surg* 234(4):444–450, 2007.

Fields CF, Bower TC, Cooper LT, et al: Takayasu's arteritis: operative results and influence of disease activity, *J Vasc Surg* 43:64–71, 2006.

Sullivan TM, Gray BH, Bacharrach JM, et al: Angioplasty and primary stenting of the subclavian, innominate and common carotid arteries in 83 patients, *J Vasc Surg* 28:1059–1065, 1998.

Takach TJ, Reul GJ, Cooley DA, et al: Brachiocephalic reconstruction: operative and long-term results for complex disease, *J Vasc Surg* 42(1):47–54, 2005.

Tracci MC, Cherry KJ: Surgical treatment of great vessel occlusive disease, *Surg Clin North Am* 89(4):821–836, 2009.

Usman AA, Resnick SA, Benzuly KH, et al: Late stent fractures after endoluminal treatment of ostial supraaortic trunk arterial occlusive lesions, *J Vasc Interv Radiol* 21(9):1364–1369, 2010.

Vogt DP, Hertzer NR, O'Hara PJ, et al: Brachiocephalic arterial reconstruction, *Annals of Surgery* 196(5):541–542, 1982.

UPPER EXTREMITY ARTERIAL OCCLUSIVE DISEASE

**Virginia L. Wong, MD, FACS, and
Vikram S. Kashyap, MD, FACS**

OVERVIEW

Upper extremity arterial occlusive disease and ischemia is much less common than in the lower extremity and can be caused by a wide variety of etiologies, including systemic inflammatory conditions. Due to extensive collateralization around the shoulder and elbow, patients may remain asymptomatic despite significant chronic obstruction. However, once ischemic symptoms manifest, they are poorly tolerated and result in significant disability. Therefore, diagnosis and management of upper extremity ischemia can be considerably more challenging than for lower extremity disease.

ETIOLOGY

The causes of upper extremity ischemia are listed in (Box 1). Atherosclerosis and inflammatory arteritides tend to affect larger, more proximal arteries. Digital and small vessel disease is commonly seen with diabetes, chronic renal failure, and connective tissue disorders. The brachial artery is most commonly affected by embolism and trauma. Iatrogenic manipulation, such as for catheterization or hemoaccess procedures, may exacerbate the effects of underlying arterial disease and lead to new ischemic symptoms.

Systemic Disease

In the United States, atherosclerosis is the most common cause of subclavian artery obstruction, more commonly affecting the left side. Patients have risk factors typically associated with atherosclerosis (e.g., hypertension, hyperlipidemia, diabetes, smoking) and/or manifestations of the disease in other arterial beds (e.g., coronary artery disease, peripheral arterial disease). Takayasu's arteritis, typically described in young Asian females, frequently affects the supraaortic trunk vessels. Temporal (giant cell) arteritis, generally found in patients older than 60 years, affects the axillary to brachial arteries, as well as superficial temporal and ophthalmic arteries. Both diseases are associated with an initial inflammatory stage, characterized by fever, fatigue, myalgias, arthralgias, and elevated erythrocyte sedimentation rate. Both produce characteristic smooth, tapering arterial stenoses that differ in angiographic appearance from typical atherosclerotic disease (Figure 1). Superficial temporal artery biopsy may provide definitive diagnosis in cases of giant cell arteritis.

Occlusive disease of the more distal upper extremity arteries is associated with a number of autoimmune, inflammatory, and rheumatologic conditions. Scleroderma, CREST syndrome (calcinosis,

---

BOX 1: Causes of upper extremity ischemia

Vasospasm
Raynaud disease
Medication-induced vasopressors, β-blockers
Ergot poisoning

Intrinsic Arterial Disease
Atherosclerosis
Radiation arteritis
Azotemic arteriopathy
Spontaneous dissection
Fibromuscular dysplasia

Inflammatory Diseases
Connective tissue disorders
Buerger disease
Takayasu's arteritis
Temporal (giant cell) arteritis
Hypersensitivity angiitis

Noninflammatory Medical Disease
Thrombophilic states
Myeloproliferative disorders
Cold injury
Hepatitis-associated vasculitis
Cryoglobulinemia
Vinyl chloride exposure

Embolism
Cardiac (most common)
Proximal aneurysm
Arterial thoracic outlet syndrome
Atheroembolism
Paradoxic embolus (with accompanying septal defect)

Trauma
Iatrogenic
Blunt arterial injury
Penetrating arterial injury
Hypothenar hammer syndrome
Vibration

Raynaud's phenomenon, esophageal dysmotility, sclerodactyly, and telangiectasia), lupus, and rheumatoid arthritis are associated with small vessel disease, affecting palmar and digital arteries (Figure 2). Thromboangiitis obliterans (Buerger's disease) affects small distal arteries and is strongly associated with ongoing tobacco exposure.

Embolism

Embolism is a frequent cause of acute upper extremity ischemia. Cardiac emboli secondary to arrhythmia are most common, with the majority of these lodging in the brachial artery terminus or more proximally at the deep brachial artery origin (Figure 3). Other sources include proximal arterial aneurysm, ulcerated atherosclerotic plaque, and paradoxical embolus from deep venous thrombosis through a septal defect. Multiple emboli (embolic shower) affecting smaller, more distal arteries should prompt a search for a proximal arterial source, particularly in the absence of arrhythmia. Subclavian artery aneurysm or ulcerative lesion secondary to thoracic outlet obstruction is the most common scenario (Figure 4). Repetitive compression of the subclavian artery by myofascial and/or osseous structures at the thoracic outlet leads to poststenotic dilatation and embolization of mural thrombus. Posttraumatic and infectious aneurysms can also cause embolization.

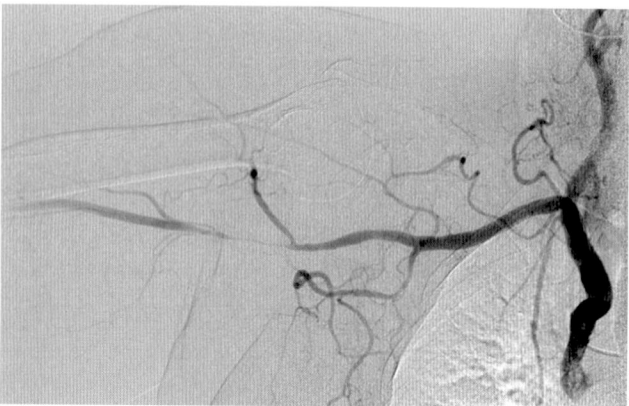

FIGURE 1   Right upper extremity angiogram of a 57-year-old woman with temporal arteritis showing a classic, smooth, tapering stenosis in the proximal brachial artery. The patient's primary presenting complaint was forearm effort fatigue.

Trauma

Blunt and penetrating trauma involving the upper extremity can cause ischemia by arterial transection, intimal dissection, and thrombosis. Iatrogenic pseudoaneurysm and thrombosis after brachial artery manipulation (arterial lines, interventional procedures) are complications that may not be immediately recognized, due to rich collateral supply around the elbow. Effort fatigue in the hand and forearm may develop later.

Repetitive trauma can also cause arterial injury. Hypothenar hammer syndrome, which affects the terminal portion of the ulnar artery in Guyon's tunnel (formed by the pisiform, the hook of hamate, and the transverse carpal ligament), results from repeatedly striking objects with the base of the palm. Segmental ulnar artery occlusion or aneurysm formation with digital artery embolism can occur (Figure 5). Vibration-induced digital artery injury is associated with prolonged use of pneumatic tools (e.g., jackhammer) and chain saws.

EVALUATION

History and Physical Examination

A detailed history and physical examination are essential for diagnosing the correct etiology of upper extremity arterial disease. Symptoms may include color changes, coolness, numbness, weakness, effort-induced fatigue ("arm claudication"), rest pain, and tissue loss. Raynaud's phenomenon may represent benign vasospasm, but it can also manifest from fixed occlusive lesions, which must be ruled out. Effort-induced fatigue generally results from proximal or large vessel disease, while hand symptoms suggest involvement of small vessel disease as well. Digital tissue loss is nearly always associated with small vessel disease, with or without more proximal involvement. Posterior circulation symptoms (e.g., dizziness, ataxia, diplopia) or angina following coronary revascularization with right or left internal mammary artery (RIMA or LIMA) suggest occlusion of the subclavian or innominate artery proximal to the internal mammary and vertebral artery origins (subclavian steal syndrome). Atherosclerotic risk factors, occupational activities, personal and family history of autoimmune or connective tissue disorders, and history of upper extremity arterial intervention or trauma should be investigated. Renal failure and vascular procedures for hemodialysis access should be noted.

A complete examination of the neck and upper extremities should be performed, documenting pulses at superficial temporal, common carotid, subclavian, axillary, brachial, radial, and ulnar

FIGURE 2   Left-hand angiogram of a patient with scleroderma and small artery occlusive disease, producing multiple occlusions of the distal forearm, palmar, and digital arteries. The patient presented with severe Raynaud's syndrome and nonhealing fingertip ulcerations.

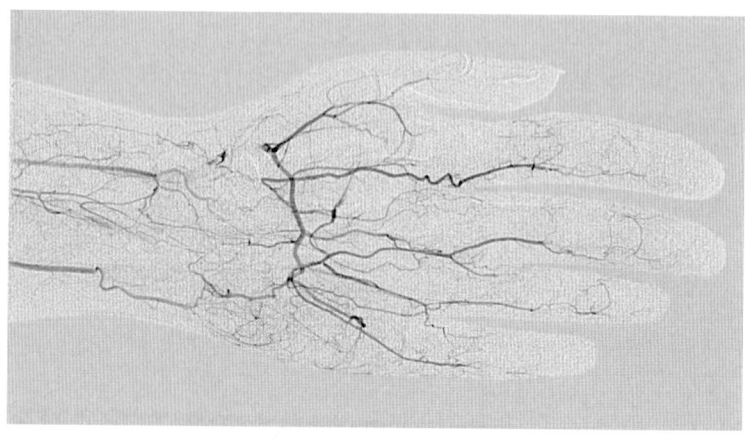

locations on both sides. Diminished or absent pulses indicate significant stenosis or occlusion proximal to that location; symmetric disease may suggest a systemic condition. Auscultation over the proximal arteries for bruit and inspection of hands and digits for color, temperature, trophic changes, and tissue loss are important. Electrocardiogram and echocardiogram evaluate for arrhythmia and atrioventricular thrombus, which predispose to cardioembolism. Chest and cervical spine radiographs evaluate for cervical ribs or osseous anomaly causing thoracic outlet obstruction. Computed tomographic scan or magnetic resonance imaging may be necessary to identify myofascial or ligamentous entrapment. Serum evaluation for erythrocyte sedimentation rate, connective tissue disorder (rheumatoid factor, antinuclear antibody, complement levels), hypercoagulable disorder (factor V Leiden, prothrombin gene mutation, antithrombin III, protein C and S deficiencies, antiphospholipid antibody, and hyperhomocysteinemia) may be helpful.

Noninvasive Vascular Evaluation

Segmental arterial pressures, wrist-brachial index (WBI), absolute digit pressures, digital plethysmography, and arterial duplex are useful for evaluating upper extremity arterial disease and ischemia. Normal WBI with digital waveform dampening induced by cold exposure is helpful in diagnosing Raynaud's phenomenon and for ruling out more proximal fixed arterial lesions. Brachial artery pressure difference greater than 20 mm Hg between right and left sides suggests unilateral axillosubclavian arterial disease. Diminishment greater than 15 mm Hg between ipsilateral arm segments suggests intervening hemodynamically significant disease. Absolute digit pressure less than 50 mm Hg suggests significant ischemia. Arterial calcification due to diabetes or longstanding renal failure may falsely elevate pressures. Duplex provides detailed anatomic information but is less useful for evaluation of intrathoracic arterial lesions, due to lack of sufficient visualization.

Computed tomographic angiography (CTA) and magnetic resonance angiography (MRA) are important noninvasive modalities for evaluating upper extremity arterial supply. Visualization of aortic arch and large proximal arteries is superb, and three-dimensional reconstruction and other postprocessing techniques are valuable for identification of thoracic outlet obstruction and planning surgical release and revascularization of these lesions (Figure 6). Imaging of smaller forearm and hand arteries is less useful with these modalities,

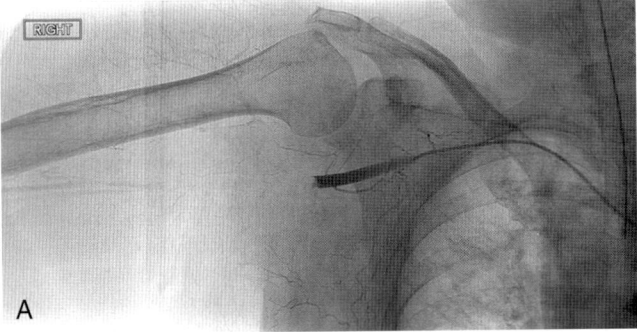

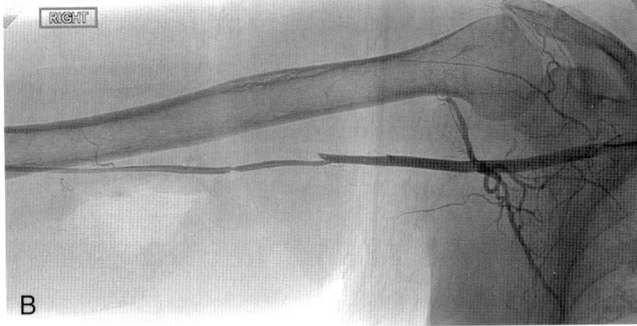

FIGURE 3 **A,** Embolic occlusion of right axillobrachial artery secondary to atrial fibrillation. **B,** Completion angiogram following surgical embolectomy.

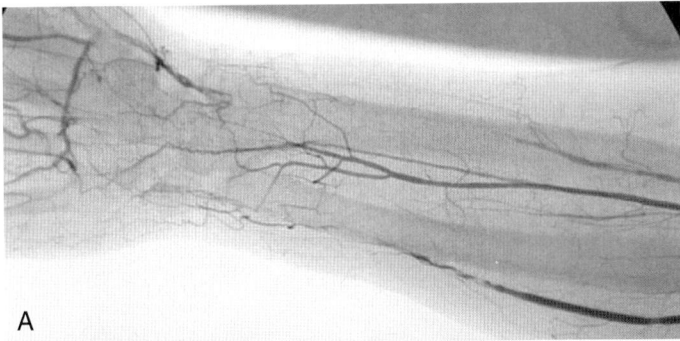

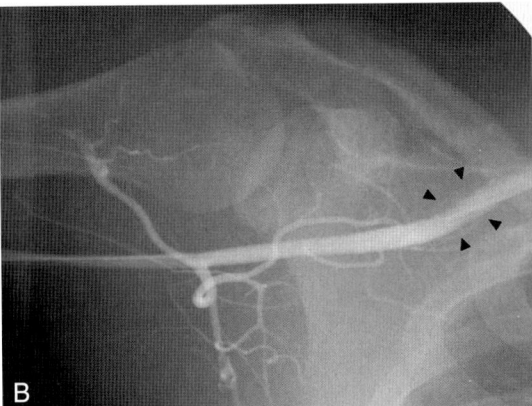

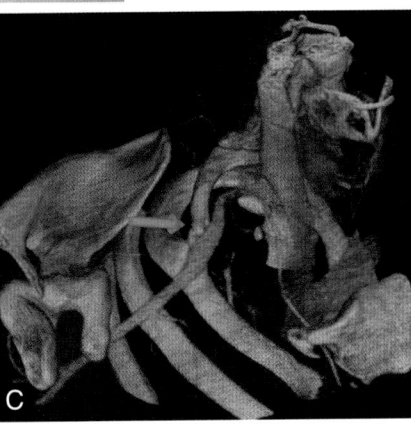

FIGURE 4 **A,** Right upper extremity angiogram in a 28-year-old, showing embolic shower to right forearm and hand arteries. **B,** Right subclavian artery aneurysm with mural thrombus (arrowheads). **C,** Three-dimensional reconstruction of CT angiogram showing right subclavian artery pressed downward by overlying clavicle (removed from image for arterial visualization) onto bony exostosis between first and second ribs (arrow).

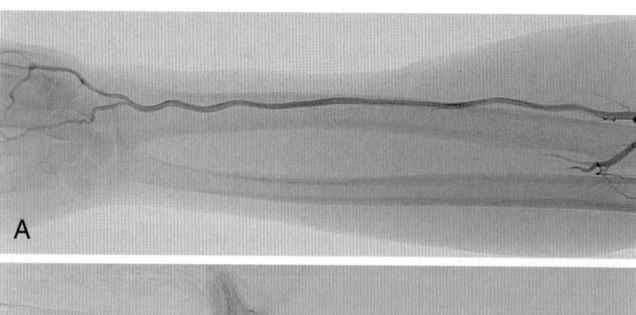

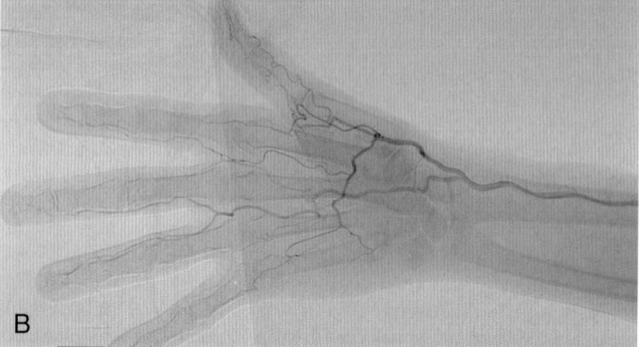

FIGURE 5 **A** and **B**, Angiogram showing right ulnar artery occlusion in a 59-year-old retired millwright. Palmar and digital arterial supply is from the radial distribution (**B**). Hypothenar hammer syndrome is suspected.

although advances in equipment and imaging techniques are providing more and more detailed distal evaluation. Artifact from heavy arterial calcification, metallic stents, or orthopedic hardware may obscure detail. Risk of contrast-induced nephropathy must be considered with CTA in patients with severe renal dysfunction. Risk of nephrogenic systemic fibrosis in end-stage renal disease (ESRD) patients may preclude use of MRA.

Catheter angiography remains a standard diagnostic imaging modality that may also offer the opportunity for endovascular treatment of selected upper extremity arterial lesions. Higher-quality images of smaller forearm and palmar arteries can be obtained with selective administration of contrast into the distal brachial artery. Provocative or diagnostic maneuvers such as catheter-directed vasodilator administration, pull-back intraarterial pressure measurement, and compression of flow through a patent ipsilateral arteriovenous access (e.g., during evaluation for arterial steal) can be performed for diagnosis and better visualization of distal arteries. Evaluation of the aorta and proximal upper extremity arteries requires aortic arch catheterization, usually from a transfemoral approach, while focal evaluation of distal brachial and forearm arteries can be accomplished via a transfemoral approach or by antegrade/retrograde brachial arterial catheterization above the level of disease involvement.

MANAGEMENT

Medical therapy represents the first line of treatment for many patients with upper extremity arterial disease and is the preferred management during the acute phase of inflammatory arteritides. Interventional treatment is generally reserved for patients with acute traumatic or embolic disease, or those with debilitating symptoms or significant ischemia. Endovascular techniques provide an opportunity for less invasive revascularization and have become the preferred option for treatment of focal proximal lesions that would otherwise require thoracotomy or sternotomy for proximal vascular control. Catheter directed thrombolysis may be more effective than surgical techniques, particularly for acute small vessel occlusion.

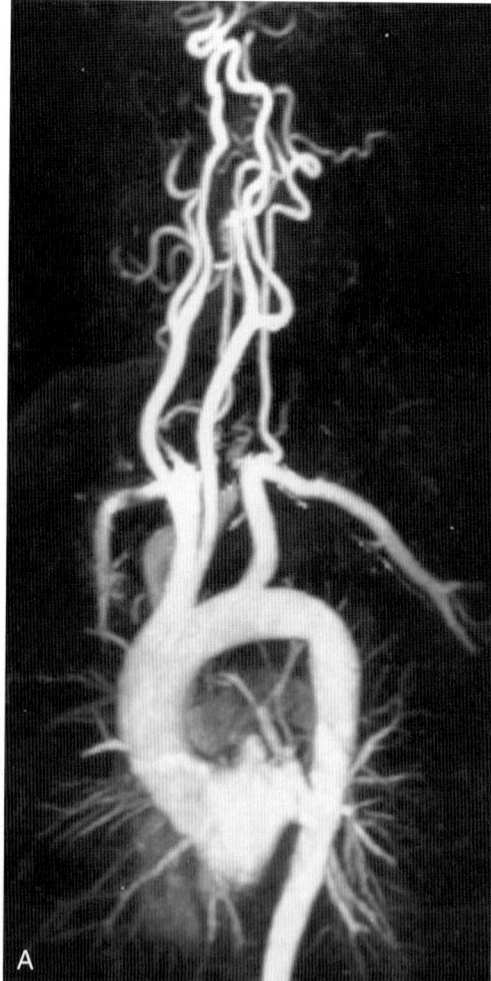

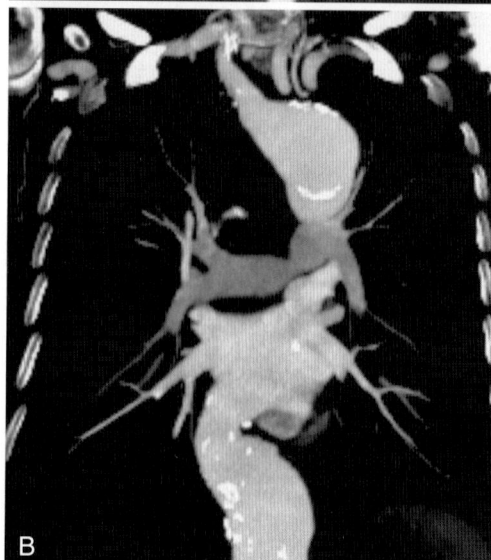

FIGURE 6 **A,** MRA of the aortic arch and supraaortic vessels. **B,** Coronal reconstruction CT angiogram demonstrating aberrant right subclavian artery origin from distal posterior aortic arch, beyond innominate and left common carotid artery origins.

However, the utility and durability of endovascular treatment is limited for more extensive and more distal arterial lesions, where surgical reconstruction is preferred.

Medical Therapy

Risk factor modification, including abstinence from tobacco and the use of lipid-lowering and antiplatelet therapy, is indicated for atherosclerotic disease. Cold avoidance and calcium channel blockade with nifedipine may be useful for treatment of Raynaud's symptoms. The acute inflammatory stage of Takayasu's and giant cell arteritis is treated with corticosteroids or other antiinflammatory agents such as cyclophosphamide, methotrexate, azathioprine, infliximab, or mycophenolate mofetil. Intervention on these lesions with endovascular or surgical techniques should be avoided during the acute inflammatory stage, due to poor results and high restenosis rates.

Endovascular Therapy

Endovascular techniques are particularly suited for short, focal obstructive lesions in the innominate, subclavian, and axillobrachial arteries. A transfemoral approach allows antegrade aortography and selective angiography through a long, supportive sheath. Retrograde access from the ipsilateral brachial artery affords the most direct access to orificial supraaortic trunk lesions, but passage of large sheaths and device delivery profiles may be limited by brachial artery diameter or may require cutdown and surgical repair to prevent access site complications. Anticoagulation during the procedure and monitoring afterward for hand ischemia and median nerve compression symptoms from brachial sheath hematoma are routine.

Once wire access across the lesion has been achieved, balloon angioplasty alone may provide sufficient treatment. Self-expanding bare metal stents are used for significant residual stenosis (>20% luminal diameter or persistent pressure gradient >20 mm Hg), immediate elastic recoil, or dissection following angioplasty. Balloon-expandable stents are useful for treatment of calcific focal lesions at the innominate, carotid, or left subclavian artery orifice, where obstruction is due to spillover aortic plaque, requiring higher radial force and precise stent deployment for treatment (Figure 7). Covered stents can be used for traumatic arterial pseudoaneurysm or for rupture following balloon angioplasty. Deployment of stents in the subclavian artery at the thoracic outlet should be considered with care, as repeated compression during arm movement can crush or fracture them. Endovascular treatment of lesions in this area may be considered following surgical decompression of underlying thoracic outlet obstruction.

For patients with severe, acute ischemia due to thrombosis or embolism, surgical catheter embolectomy provides the most rapid restoration of inflow, but access to smaller arteries of the hand and digits is not possible in this manner. Catheter-directed thrombolysis can be very useful for involvement of distal forearm, palmar, and digital arteries. The transfemoral approach using a long, supportive sheath is preferred for delivery of thrombolytic agent via an infusion wire or catheter advanced into thrombus, or positioned to allow the agent access to affected vessels. Continuous thrombolytic infusion is continued for 24 to 72 hours, monitoring for signs of hemorrhage and for a decrease in the serum fibrinogen level. Angiography through the existing catheter takes place at regular intervals during therapy to assess thrombolytic progress or adjust catheter position for maximum gain. Return to angiography occurs 12 to 24 hours following initial catheter placement, and then every 12 to 24 hours thereafter. Therapy is complete when an acceptable clinical or angiographic result is obtained or is terminated when no further progress is made or if bleeding or a critical drop in the serum fibrinogen level occurs. Risk of bleeding complications increases with duration of therapy and total amount of lytic agent delivered. Forearm or hand fasciotomy may be required for release of compartment syndrome following revascularization in patients with severe ischemia lasting more than 6 hours or in those who exhibit compromised neuromotor function.

AbuRahma and colleagues (AbuRahma A, et al., 2007) compared results of subclavian artery balloon angioplasty/stent with carotid-subclavian bypass for symptomatic lesions. Over a 10-year period, 121 patients were treated with balloon angioplasty/stent, while 51 patients were treated with bypass. There was no difference in survival between the two groups. Primary patency at 1 year was 93% for angioplasty/stent and 100% for bypass. Superior primary patency was noted at 5 years in the surgery group (96%), compared to the endovascular group (70%).

Surgical Therapy

Exposure techniques, revascularization options, and procedural success vary depending on the etiology and extent of arterial disease, as well as anatomic location of the lesion.

Operative Exposure of the Subclavian Artery

Due to the oblique and posterior course of the aortic arch, access to proximal right and left subclavian arteries requires different approaches. The origin of the right subclavian artery is best exposed through median sternotomy. Mobilization of the left brachiocephalic vein allows complete visualization of the innominate artery and its bifurcation into right subclavian and common carotid arteries. Cervical extension of the incision allows access to the right carotid sheath. Care must be taken to avoid injury to the right recurrent

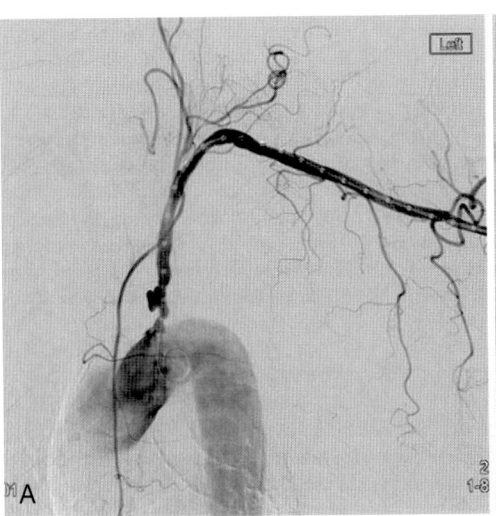
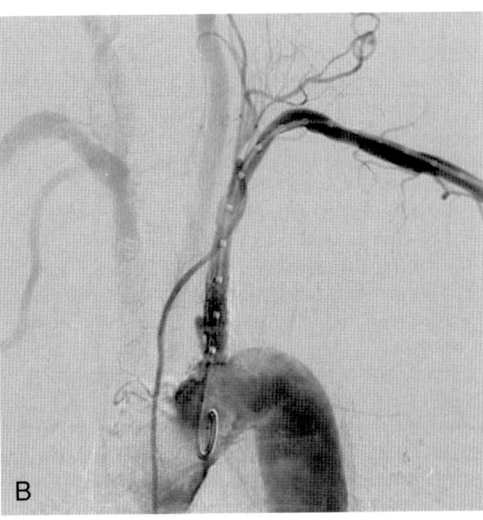

FIGURE 7 A, Aortogram from retrograde left brachial artery approach showing orificial subclavian artery stenosis. **B,** Aortogram following deployment of a balloon-expandable bare metal stent across the lesion.

laryngeal nerve, which courses inferiorly around the proximal right subclavian artery and ascends medially between the esophagus and trachea. The preferred approach to the more posteriorly positioned left subclavian artery origin is through left lateral thoracotomy, sited between the fourth and fifth ribs. Following entry into the pleural cavity, inferior retraction of the left upper lobe will reveal the aortic arch, visible through the mediastinal pleura. The vagus nerve passes anterolateral to the left subclavian artery, and the thoracic duct lies posteromedial to the artery. Care must be taken to avoid injury to either of these important structures. Limited exposure of either right or left proximal subclavian artery can be achieved via supraclavicular cervical incision, as described below.

Surgical Reconstruction for Proximal Subclavian Artery Lesions

Carotid-subclavian artery bypass and subclavian artery transposition have both been described extensively for operative treatment of proximal subclavian artery obstruction, with 75% to 90% patency at 5 years and acceptable morbidity. Preoperative evaluation should include carotid duplex to determine whether common carotid and/ or bifurcation disease also requires treatment and to evaluate the vertebral arteries. Advantages of transposition include completely autogenous reconstruction and the need to perform only one anastomosis. Bypass avoids the need to obtain very proximal subclavian artery control deep in the incision, and it is better suited for extensive lesions beyond the orifice. Bypass is also preferred for preservation of a patent internal mammary artery to coronary artery bypass graft.

Subclavian Artery Transposition

The patient is positioned supine, with the head turned away from the operative side. A small roll placed under the shoulders helps provide better neck extension. A short, transverse cervical incision is made 2 cm above the clavicle and parallel to it, from the sternoclavicular joint toward midclavicle. The platysma is divided, and then the clavicular head of the sternocleidomastoid muscle is divided for better visualization. The scalene fat pad is mobilized superiorly, exposing the anterior scalene. The phrenic nerve, which runs from lateral to medial across the anterior scalene on its way into the chest, must be identified and preserved. The anterior scalene is divided from its attachment to the first rib. The internal jugular vein is mobilized and retracted laterally to allow access to the common carotid artery. The vagus nerve should be identified and preserved. On the left, the thoracic duct may require ligation; inadvertent injury will cause serious lymphatic leak. The subclavian artery is skeletonized, obtaining control of the thyrocervical trunk, vertebral, and internal mammary arteries. Following heparinization, branch vessels are occluded first to prevent embolism. The subclavian artery is clamped and divided as far proximal as safely possible. The proximal arterial stump is oversewn immediately with stay sutures to prevent retraction of the artery back into the chest before secure closure. The common carotid artery is clamped; shunting is usually not required as long as the carotid bifurcation remains open. The common carotid artery is opened longitudinally on its posterolateral surface, and end-to-side anastomosis is performed between the transected subclavian artery and the common carotid artery (Figure 8). If the subclavian artery is too short to reach, mobilization of the common carotid artery may bring it farther laterally. Division of the internal mammary artery may provide more length as well. The incision is closed over a closed suction drain, left in place for 24 hours, and removed when sanguinous and/or lymphatic drainage has diminished.

Carotid-Subclavian Bypass

Patient positioning and initial exposure is as above for subclavian artery transposition. For bypass, only a short segment of the

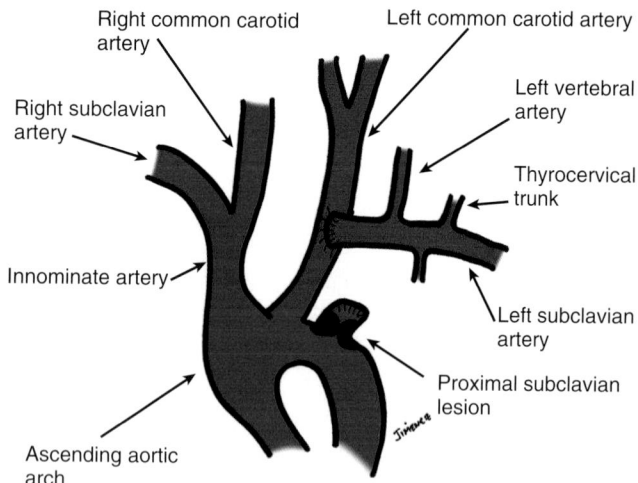

FIGURE 8   Left subclavian transition.

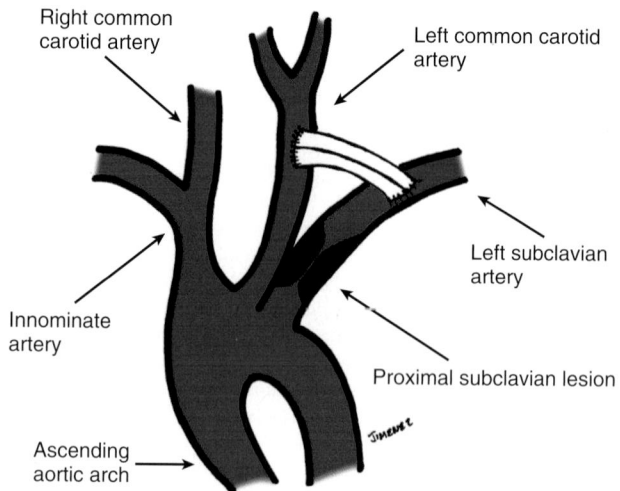

FIGURE 9   Carotid-subclavian bypass.

subclavian artery need be exposed. The usual site is just distal to the thyrocervical trunk. As such, most of the dissection takes place lateral to the clavicular head of the sternocleidomastoid muscle. Phrenic nerve injury is more common during this more lateral approach. A short polytetrafluoroethylene (PTFE) graft is tunneled beneath the internal jugular vein, and an end-to-side anastomosis is performed to the common carotid and subclavian arteries (Figure 9). Beveling the carotid end of the graft 20 to 30 degrees is necessary to direct the bypass graft downward toward the subclavian artery.

Ziomek and colleagues reported that prosthetic graft is the conduit of choice for these short-length carotid-subclavian bypasses, with superior long-term patency than for autogenous vein bypass (94% vs 58% at 5 years). However, they and others conclude that subclavian transposition may yield slightly better results. Systematic review by Cina and colleagues (Cina C, et al., 2002) suggests higher mean 1-year patency and symptomatic freedom rates with subclavian transposition (98% and 99%) compared to carotid-subclavian bypass (84% and 88%).

Axillary Artery

Occlusive lesions of the axillary artery are rare. Exposure may be required for trauma or for proximal anastomosis of axillofemoral bypass. The ipsilateral arm is abducted onto an arm board. An infraclavicular incision is made two fingerbreadths below the midclavicle and extended to the deltopectoral groove. Fibers of the pectoralis major muscle are split, and the underlying clavipectoral fascia is opened. The pectoralis minor muscle is divided near its tendinous insertion onto the acromion for better visualization. The axillary vein lies slightly anterior and inferior to the artery; overlying venous branches may require division for full exposure of the artery. Care must be taken to avoid transection of the lateral pectoral nerves, which may cause postoperative pectoralis muscle atrophy.

Surgical revascularization of the axillary artery for occlusive disease is required infrequently. Carotid-axillary, carotid-brachial, subclavian-brachial, and axillobrachial bypasses have been described and may be required for extensive subclavian artery lesions, trauma, or revascularization of failed, less-extensive bypasses. Autogenous vein appears to be the preferred conduit in this location, likely due to the length of graft required for revascularization.

Brachial Artery

The ipsilateral arm is abducted onto an arm board or table. Exposure can be achieved through a longitudinal incision anywhere along the bicipital groove, medially between the biceps and triceps muscles. The basilic vein will be medial and superficial to the brachial sheath. The median nerve lies immediately adjacent to the brachial artery and is usually encountered first upon opening the brachial sheath. Great care must be taken with the use of cautery to avoid injury to this large sensorimotor nerve. Mobilization over several centimeters will allow enough slack for gentle vessel loop retraction of the nerve away from the underlying brachial artery. Crossing branches from paired brachial veins may require division for full exposure of the artery. Exposure of the terminal brachial artery and its bifurcation into radial and common ulnar interosseus arteries can be achieved by extension of the incision onto the anterior forearm in "lazy S" fashion so as to avoid longitudinal scar contracture across the antecubital crease. Division of the bicipital aponeurosis will allow contiguous exposure of the artery across the antecubital space. In 15% of patients, a separate and high takeoff of the radial artery will be identified (brachioradial artery variant). Its origin may be located anywhere between the axillary artery and the brachial artery terminus. This artery is usually encountered as a smaller-caliber, more superficial artery, not in immediate proximity to the median nerve. It is the most commonly identified upper extremity arterial variation, and it is distinct from the rare superficial brachial artery or truly duplicated brachial artery variations. Definitive identification of the high radial artery requires either extensive proximal exposure or angiography, but the persistence of the radial pulse at the wrist following brachial artery cross-clamp should confirm the anatomy.

For localized brachial artery trauma or for catheter retrieval of embolus, exposure and mobilization of a relatively short distance of the brachial artery will suffice. Control of uninvolved proximal and distal artery should be obtained. Primary suture repair or anastomosis can be considered if adequate length and sufficient vessel circumference remain after débridement of devitalized tissue. Patch angioplasty or interposition graft may be required for repair or bypass of more extensive lesions. Saphenous vein is the preferred conduit for brachial artery bypass, due to size match and improved patency over PTFE. Prosthetic material should be avoided in contaminated traumatic fields. Penetrating or extensive blunt trauma may also be associated with nerve injury; detailed sensory and motor exam should be performed before and after revascularization.

Radial and Ulnar Arteries

Exposure of the radial artery in the forearm is achieved via a longitudinal incision oriented along a line extending from the antecubital crease to the styloid process of the radius. The fascia is opened along the medial border of the brachioradialis muscle. Proximally, the artery lies beneath the muscle. More distally, the artery lies deep to the antebrachial fascia, between the brachioradialis and flexor carpi

radialis tendons. At the wrist, the radial artery is quite superficial, lying just beneath the antebrachial fascia and medial to the radius. Exposure of the ulnar artery in the forearm is achieved by following a plane between the flexor carpi ulnaris and flexor digitorum superficialis muscles. In the midforearm, the artery lies beneath the flexor carpi ulnaris muscle and adjacent to the ulnar nerve. Distally, the artery lies just beneath the antebrachial fascia.

Bypass to the forearm arteries is rarely used and is most often required for trauma or neglected embolic occlusion. Mesh and colleagues (Mesh C, et al., 1993) performed 95 upper extremity arterial bypass procedures over a 15-year period. Overall 5-year patency was 63%, with autogenous conduit demonstrating superior patency at all anatomic sites compared with prosthetic material (71% vs 38%). All far distal forearm prosthetic grafts failed within 1 year. A series by Spinelli and colleagues (Spinelli F, et al., 2009) reported on 23 upper extremity bypasses performed over a 10-year period in patients primarily with critical limb ischemia. They achieved 83% primary 3-year patency, using autogenous conduit in 83% of cases. Thus, the surgical literature supports using arterial bypass with autogenous conduit for upper extremity arterial disease, with acceptable patency rates.

Angioaccess-Induced Arterial Steal Syndrome

Hand ischemia following creation of ipsilateral arteriovenous (AV) access for hemodialysis is an infrequent, but potentially debilitating, complication. Given the increasing incidence of renal failure requiring dialysis in the United States, AV access–induced steal may be the most common hand ischemia syndrome seen by most practitioners. Distal ischemia results from an imbalance in perfusion hemodynamics, where arterial occlusive disease proximal or distal to the AV anastomosis restricts supply to the hand or where high-volume flow through the AV anastomosis literally steals blood from the distal supply, reversing direction of arterial flow in the parent artery distal to the AV anastomosis. Predicting which patients will develop steal is challenging. Several factors may increase the risk of steal, including diabetes, advanced age, female sex, and use of proximal (brachioaxillary) inflow rather than forearm (radial) inflow. Symptoms of arterial steal may be mild, moderate, or severe and include persistent digital numbness, tingling, pallor, hand and finger motor weakness, and digital ulceration or gangrene. Many patients develop transient symptoms immediately following AV access creation, possibly due to local sensory neuropraxia after surgical manipulation or until arterial collateral accommodation takes place. Persistent mild symptoms that are well tolerated may be observed. More severe symptoms that affect daily activities, particularly in the dominant hand, require further evaluation and treatment. Rapidly progressive or severe ischemia and tissue loss mandate prompt evaluation and treatment to avoid limb loss or permanent devastating disability.

Arterial steal is diagnosed by a combination of clinical examination, duplex ultrasound and plethysmography, and catheter angiography. Arterial occlusive disease located proximal or distal to the AV anastomosis must be identified and addressed, if present; these can often be treated with balloon angioplasty during angiographic evaluation. In severely ischemic patients, or in those who are poor surgical candidates, simple ligation and sacrifice of the AV access are definitive and acceptable treatments for limb salvage. High-flow steal can be treated by operative flow-restriction techniques, such as fistula banding or plication. However, therapeutic failure and access thrombosis rates are high with these procedures, due to inability to accurately determine intraoperatively how severely to restrict flow for optimal results. Revascularization for relief of steal symptoms while preserving a functioning AV access can be considered in patients who are good surgical candidates.

The distal revascularization with interval ligation (DRIL) procedure is effective, with acceptable results. Arterial bypass, preferably saphenous vein, is routed around the AV anastomosis, from the proximal brachial or axillary artery to the distal brachial, radial, or ulnar artery. The proximal bypass anastomosis is placed at least 6 cm proximal to the AV anastomosis, and the interval brachial artery is ligated just beyond the AV anastomosis, eliminating reversal of flow (Figure 10). The major disadvantage of DRIL is ligation of the native brachial artery, which eliminates some brachial collateral flow to the forearm and hand and could place the hand in jeopardy, should the DRIL bypass fail. However, devastating ischemic consequences of failed DRIL bypass are seldom reported, possibly due to the relatively short life expectancy in this patient population. Huber and colleagues reported 64 DRIL procedures, where operative mortality was 3% and complication rate was 22% (14% of which were wound complications). Bypass patency at 5 years was 71%. While the majority of patients (78%) experienced relief of ischemic symptoms, 5-year mortality was 33%, reflecting the severity of comorbid conditions in this subset of dialysis patients. These results are similar to other reported series.

Revision of inflow into the AV access can be achieved using proximalization of arterial inflow (PAI procedure, described by Zanow, 2006) or revision using distal inflow (RUDI procedure, described by Minion, 2005). PAI uses a small-diameter PTFE feeder conduit (4 or 5 mm) from a large proximal artery (usually axillary) to supply the AV access (Figure 11). The more proximal artery has higher perfusion pressure and is better able to collateralize, providing better perfusion to both the AV access and the distal extremity. RUDI achieves inflow restriction to the AV access by bringing an extension conduit from a smaller forearm artery, usually the proximal radial or ulnar artery

(Figure 12). This alters the perfusion imbalance and improves distal extremity supply. In either case, severe flow restriction to the AV access can result in access loss. However, unlike DRIL, both PAI and RUDI preserve continuity of flow through the native brachial artery, avoiding the need to ligate an axial artery. Failure of revascularization places only the AV access in jeopardy. Thermann and colleagues (Thermann F, et al., 2010) reported results of 40 PAI procedures over a 5-year period. High clinical success was achieved, with primary patency 62% at 1 year and secondary patency 75% at 18 months.

SUMMARY

Upper extremity arterial occlusive disease and ischemia are less common than in the lower extremity, but when symptomatic, they cause significant disability. The etiology is diverse and may include systemic conditions, necessitating a thorough clinical evaluation before deciding upon treatment strategy. Medical management is useful for optimizing and controlling systemic disease. Endovascular therapy is emerging as an effective, less invasive treatment option, particularly for less extensive or intrathoracic lesions. Surgical revascularization remains the standard therapy for more extensive and distal lesions, with acceptable results for most upper extremity bypass procedures. Hand ischemia caused by AV access–induced arterial steal syndrome is a potentially devastating condition. Surgical revascularization in appropriate patients may offer symptom relief while preserving access function in these very challenging patients.

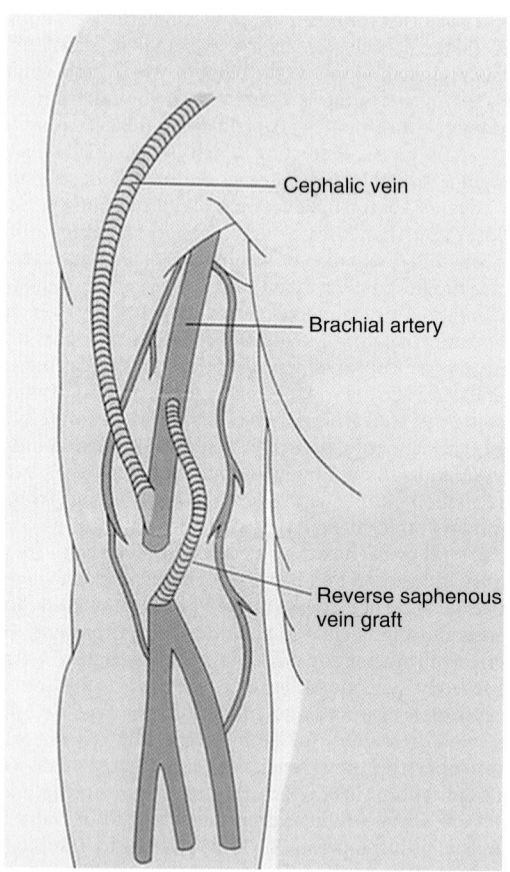

FIGURE 10 Distal revascularization with interval ligation (DRIL) procedure. *(Modified from Knox R, Berman S, Hughes J, et al.: Distal revascularization-interval ligation: a durable and effective treatment for ischemic steal syndrome after hemodialysis access. J Vasc Surg 362:250-256, 2002.)*

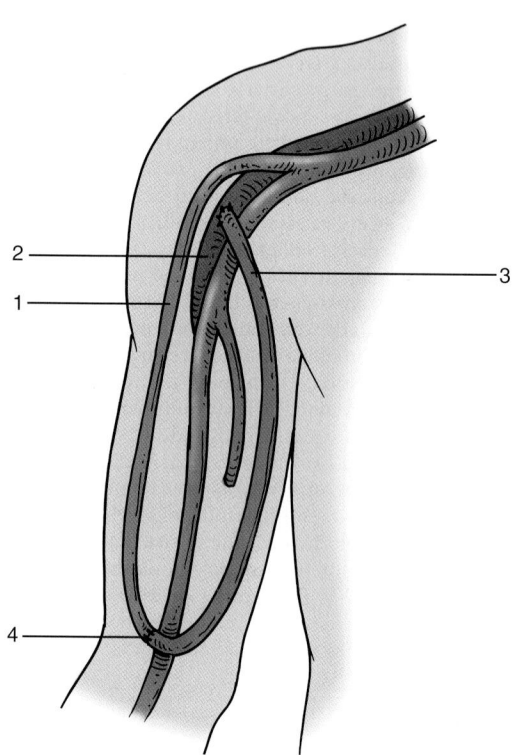

FIGURE 11 Proximalization of arterial inflow (PAI) reconstruction. *1,* Cephalic vein arteriovenous fistula (AVF); *2,* Axillary artery; *3,* PTFE feeder conduit; *4,* New anastomosis between AVF and PTFE conduit. *(From Annals of Vascular Surgery, Volume 23, Issue 4, July-August 2009, pp. 485-490, Fig. 1.)*

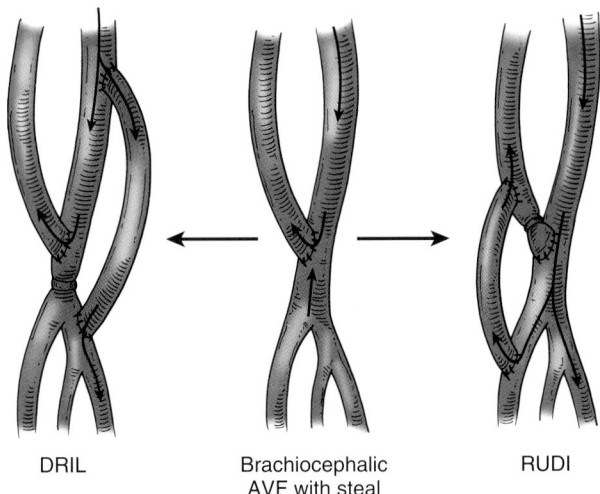

DRIL   Brachiocephalic   RUDI
              AVF with steal

FIGURE 12   Revision using distal inflow (RUDI) reconstruction. Original brachiocephalic arteriovenous (AV) anastomosis to distal brachial artery has been ligated. Interposition graft has been constructed from proximal radial artery to the flow-proximal aspect of the AV access. *AVF,* Arteriovenous fistula; *DRIL,* distal revascularization with interval ligation. *(From Scali ST, Huber TS: Treatment strategies for access-related hand ischemia, Seminars in Vascular Surgery, 24(2):128-136, 2011, Fig. 6. Reprinted from Minion DJ, Moore E, Endean E: Revision using distal inflow: a novel approach to dialysis-associated steal syndrome. Ann Vasc Surg 19:625-628, 2005, with permission.)*

SUGGESTED READINGS

AbuRahma AF, Bates MC, Stone PA, et al: Angioplasty and stenting versus carotid-subclavian bypass for the treatment of isolated subclavian artery disease, *Endovasc Ther* 14:698–704, 2007.

Cina CS, Safar HA, Lagana A, et al: Subclavian carotid transposition and bypass grafting: consecutive cohort study and systematic review, *J Vasc Surg* 35:422–429, 2002.

Mesh CL, McCarthy WJ, Pearce WH, et al: Upper extremity bypass grafting: a 15-year experience, *Arch Surg* 128:795–801, 1993.

Minion DJ, Moore E, Endean E: Revision using distal inflow: a novel approach to dialysis-associated steal syndrome, *Ann Vasc Surg* 19(5):625–628, 2005.

Regalado S, Navuluri R, Vikingstad E: Distal revascularizaion and interval ligation: a primer for the vascular and interventional radiologist, *Semin Intervent Radiol* 26:125–129, 2009.

Spinelli F, Benedetto F, Passari G, et al: Bypass surgery for the treatment of upper limb chronic ischaemia, *Eur J Vasc Endovasc Surg* 39:165–170, 2009.

Thermann F, Wollert U, Ukkat J, Dralle H: Proximalization of the arterial inflow (PAI) in patients with dialysis access-induced ischemic syndrome: first report on long-term clinical results, *J Vasc Access* 11:143–149, 2010.

Zanow J, Kruger U, Scholz H: Proximalization of the arterial inflow: A new technique to treat access-related ischemia, *J Vasc Surg* 43:1216–1221, 2006.

AORTOILIAC OCCLUSIVE DISEASE

Shant M. Vartanian, MD, and Michael S. Conte, MD

INTRODUCTION

Aortoiliac occlusive disease (AIOD) is a common cause of lower extremity ischemia. The spectrum of clinical presentations is broad—from asymptomatic peripheral arterial disease (PAD) to limb-threatening critical limb ischemia (CLI). Even moderate ischemia, which manifests as intermittent claudication (IC), can be significantly disabling. By limiting the patients' ability to perform their primary occupation or carry out activities of daily living, IC can have a profoundly negative impact on quality of life. Because the risk of progression from claudication to major limb amputation is low—5% over 5 years—and the overall mortality is close to 20% over that same time period, the indication for intervention in IC is to improve the quality of life. In contrast, CLI should generally be treated with revascularization to reduce ischemic pain, heal wounds, and avoid major limb amputation.

INITIAL EVALUATION AND INDICATIONS FOR INTERVENTION

The initial evaluation for all patients with PAD starts with a detailed history and physical examination. Symptomatic patients with AIOD often present with claudication symptoms that involve the proximal muscles of the thigh, hip, buttocks, and calf. Depending on the location of the occlusive disease, pelvic ischemia can present with buttock claudication and erectile dysfunction. The syndrome of IC, impotence in males, and reduced femoral pulses due to AIOD was first recognized by the French surgeon René Leriche and bears his name. CLI symptoms manifest in the lower leg or foot with ischemic rest pain, nonhealing wounds, or gangrenous changes.

AIOD can be well collateralized with reconstitution of the infrainguinal circulation from the upper torso through the inferior epigastric artery and through the abdomen via mesenteric, retroperitoneal, and pelvic collaterals. Many patients have palpable femoral pulses, even in the setting of significant occlusive disease. In contrast, patients that present with rest pain or tissue loss often have extensive occlusions or multilevel disease. Diminished femoral pulses can be confirmed with noninvasive vascular lab studies, which should be performed as part of the initial evaluation. Segmental Doppler pressures or pulse volume recordings are useful for demonstrating the physiologic significance of disease and can help to localize hemodynamically significant lesions or suggest the presence of multilevel disease.

There are distinct anatomic patterns of AIOD. Typically, focal lesions present with lower extremity claudication. AIOD secondary to atherosclerosis is largely a disease of smokers, although advanced age, hypercholesterolemia, hypertension, and diabetes are also common risk factors. Ethnic variation in the anatomic pattern of AIOD has also been noted. Arteriopathies other than atherosclerosis can also involve the aortoiliac system, such as Takayasu's disease and radiation arteritis. Because of the unique pathophysiology of these entities, these nonatherosclerotic etiologies require alternative management approaches that are not further considered here.

The goals of therapy for patients with IC are secondary prevention of cardiovascular events and improvement in walking ability. Initial interventions should include management of risk factors, such as smoking cessation, hypertension, and glycemic control, and it should be coupled with a 3- to 6-month trial of exercise. There is mounting evidence that exercise therapy may be as effective as revascularization procedures in some patients with IC. The CLEVER trial, a randomized controlled study comparing supervised exercise therapy versus endovascular treatment of aortoiliac occlusive disease, showed greater objective short-term improvements in walking performance for the exercise therapy group but higher patient-reported satisfaction outcomes for iliac stenting. Similar results have been reported from randomized trials comparing exercise therapy to endovascular treatment of infrainguinal occlusive disease. Therefore, vascular interventions for IC, either open or endovascular, should be reserved for patients with disabling symptoms despite optimal medical therapy, for whom the risk to benefit ratio is low and a durable result is expected.

The treatment algorithm is altered for patients presenting with CLI. Though these patients have a shorter life expectancy than patients with IC, they are also at much higher risk for major amputation. The goal of therapy in CLI is healing of wounds, relief of pain, and prevention of limb loss. Revascularization, whether through direct surgical or endovascular means, is more aggressively pursued because medical management alone is in general a poor option.

In patients who are candidates for intervention, imaging studies are paramount for developing a treatment strategy. Though ultrasound can identify areas of stenosis, its utility in the setting of AIOD is limited by the presence of bowel gas, the patient's habitus, and heavily calcified vessels. Computed tomographic (CT) or magnetic resonance (MR) angiography are excellent at evaluating the aortoiliac segment, and the CTA in particular informs the operator about the location and distribution of calcified lesions, which is an important consideration in operative planning (Figure 1). The optimal and most cost-effective approach to imaging is debatable. Whereas in the past diagnostic angiography was a routine part of the workup, unless the patient is a candidate for an endovascular intervention, surgeons can often proceed directly to open surgical revascularization with the quality of the imaging seen on contemporary CT and MR angiograms. However, diagnostic catheter-based angiography may still be preferred in some cases, such as in the presence of prior stenting or spine hardware artifact, which can render CT or MR less accurate. In some cases, when the physical exam and noninvasive studies point to a high likelihood of an endovascular intervention and access appears straightforward, the value of a preliminary CT in terms of both cost and contrast exposure is questionable. However, our preferred approach is to obtain a cross-sectional imaging study to outline the options and to develop the strategy for intervention.

The patient's comorbid conditions, functional status, and life expectancy help frame the risks of intervention, but the underlying anatomic pattern of disease is supremely important in determining the safety, benefit, and durability of the procedure. The most commonly used anatomic classification system was presented by a multidisciplinary, multisociety consensus statement in 2000 and revised in 2007: the Trans-Atlantic Inter-Society Consensus (TASC) guidelines (Figure 2). Because endovascular interventions have a comparatively lower procedural morbidity than open surgical revascularization for AIOD, it is generally agreed upon that claudicants with focal and

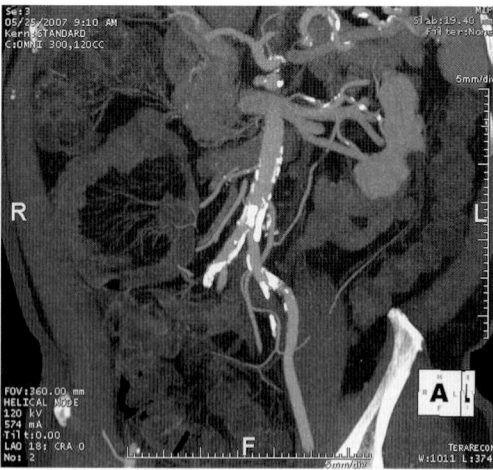

FIGURE 1 Preprocedure imaging. Computed tomographic (CT) angiography is an excellent imaging modality for evaluating aortoiliac occlusive disease. Not only is it informative regarding the degree and length of stenosis or occlusions, but the location and distribution of calcified atheroma are also revealed. Understanding both is important in selecting the appropriate revascularization strategy. In this maximum intensity projection, heavy calcification of the aortoiliac segment is evident, with occlusion of the right external iliac artery.

discrete lesions (TASC A or B) should be preferentially treated with endovascular interventions first. More advanced patterns of disease (TASC D) should be treated with surgical revascularization, unless the operative risk is prohibitive. In either case, immediate procedural success is high, but optimal management should carefully consider the long-term implications of the intervention because the disease is chronic and frequently progressive.

DIRECT SURGICAL REVASCULARIZATION

Direct surgical revascularization of AIOD is considered the "gold standard" treatment for durable vascular interventions. Ten-year patency rates of 85% for both aortofemoral bypass and aortoiliac endarterectomy are unmatched by endovascular procedures (Figure 3). For those patients with unilateral disease, the 3-year patency rate for iliofemoral bypasses exceeds 90% in most reports. Despite advances in patient selection, anesthetic care, and postoperative management—all of which have made the conduct of the operation much safer—direct revascularization today is reserved for patients with advanced aortoiliac occlusive disease for whom the risks of surgery are low and a durable result is expected.

The degree and distribution of atherosclerosis helps dictate which revascularization strategy will be most successful. The TASC II aortoiliac classification scheme helps serve as a framework for stratifying which patterns of disease are more likely to respond well to endovascular interventions (Types A and B) and which are more likely to have a durable result with direct revascularization (Type D). Examples of disease patterns that are served well with direct surgical revascularization include diffuse aortic or bilateral iliac disease, long segment chronic total occlusions, concordant aneurysmal disease of the aorta, patients with early and aggressive recurrence after a previous endovascular intervention, or those that have had atheroembolic events related to aortoiliac atheroma.

In patients with extensive comorbid conditions, such as uncorrectable coronary artery disease, poor ventricular function, advanced pulmonary disease, renal failure, or hostile abdominal anatomy, the increased risks of open surgery may make direct revascularization prohibitive, even in the setting of Type D lesions. Aggressive

Type A lesions

- Unilateral or bilateral stenoses of CIA
- Unilateral or bilateral single short (≤3 cm) stenosis of EIA

Type B lesions

- Short (≤3 cm) stenosis of infrarenal aorta
- Unilateral CIA occlusion
- Single or multiple stenosis totaling 3-10 cm involving the EIA not extending into the CFA
- Unilateral EIA occlusion not involving the origins of internal iliac of CFA

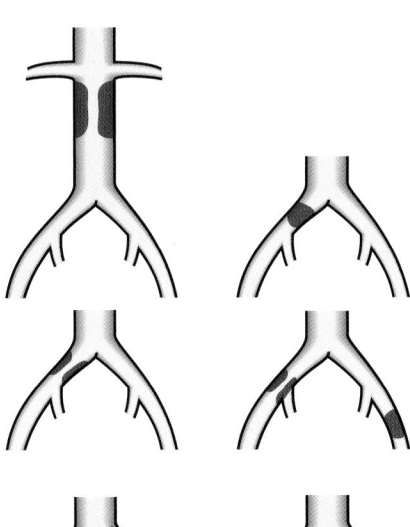

Type C lesions

- Bilateral CIA occlusions
- Bilateral EIA stenoses 3-10 cm long not extending into the CFA
- Unilateral EIA stenosis extending into the CFA
- Unilateral EIA occlusion that involves the origins of internal iliac and/or CFA
- Heavily calcified unilateral EIA occlusion with or without involvement of origins of internal iliac and/or CFA

Type D lesions

- Infrarenal aortoiliac occlusion
- Diffuse disease involving the aorta and both iliac arteries requiring treatment
- Diffuse multiple stenoses involving the unilateral CIA, EIA, and CFA
- Unilateral occlusions of both CIA and EIA
- Bilateral occlusion of EIA
- Iliac stenoses in patients with AAA requiring treatment and not amenable to endograft placement or other lesions requiring open aortic or iliac surgery

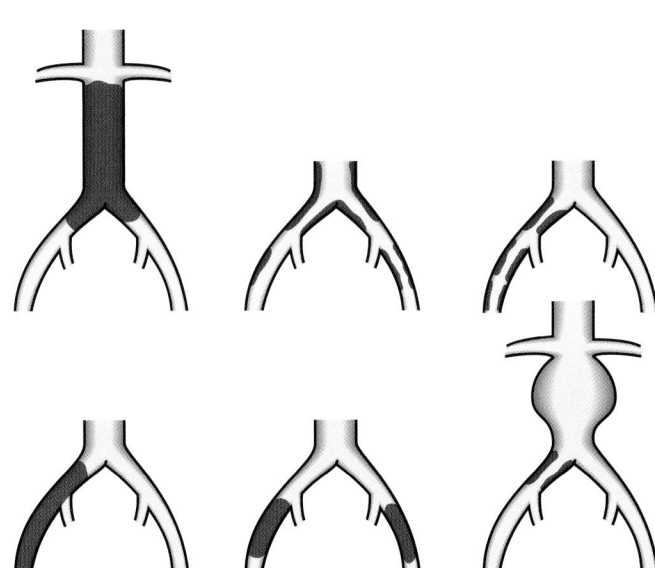

FIGURE 2   TASC II classification of aortoiliac occlusive disease. The TASC II classification scheme characterizes the location and morphology of aortoiliac occlusive disease. Anatomy alone does not dictate surgical approach, but rather the synthesis of surgical risk, comorbid conditions, functional status, and life expectancy help weigh the risks and benefits of each intervention. *(Norgren L, Hiatt WR, Dormandy JA, et al: Inter-society consensus for the management of peripheral arterial disease (TASC II). TASC II working group, Eur J Vasc Endovasc Surg 33 (Suppl 1):S1-S75, 2007.)*

endovascular techniques, which can achieve high levels of technical success in experienced centers, may be appropriate despite the absence of long-term outcome data. Conversely, extraanatomic bypasses are an alternative approach in such patients, particularly when the indication for intervention is limb-threatening ischemia.

In addition to direct and extraanatomic bypass options in treating bilateral AIOD, unilateral iliac occlusive disease presents additional revascularization options, including the unilateral aortofemoral bypass, the iliofemoral bypass, the femoral-femoral bypass, and the axillary-femoral bypass. Choosing between an aortofemoral bypass

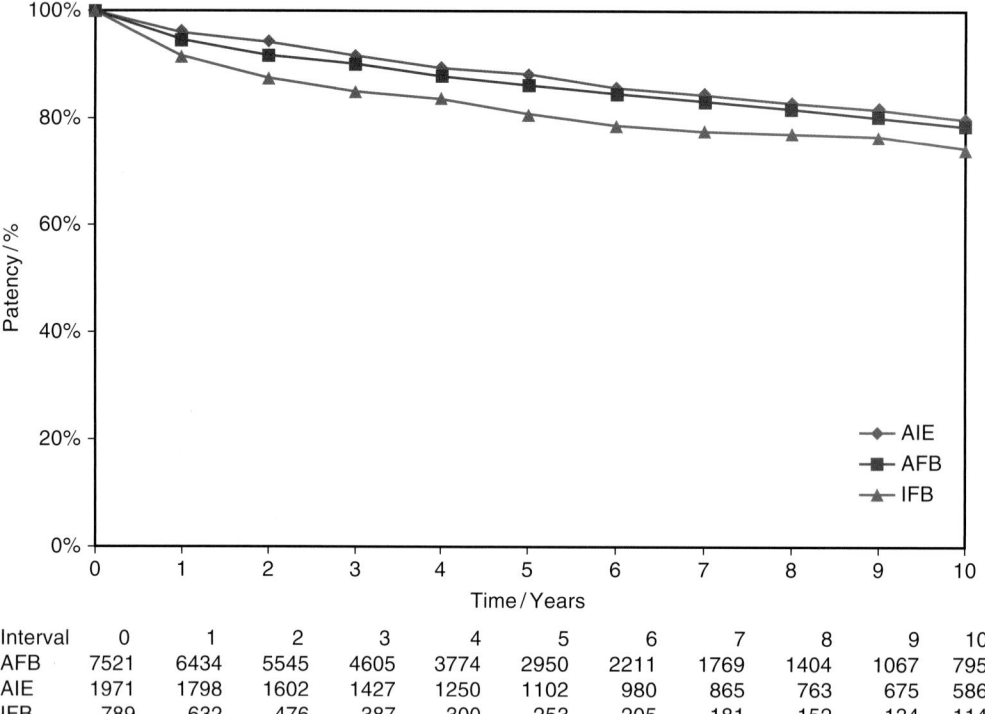

FIGURE 3 Long-term patency for direct revascularization. A review of 51 studies of direct surgical revascularization spanning 4 decades of compiled long-term patency data from **8006** patients. Durability of each type of procedure was excellent. *AIE*, aortoiliac endarterectomy; *AFB*, aortofemoral bypass; *IFB*, iliofemoral bypass. *(Adapted from Chiu KW, Davies RS, Nightingale PG, et al: Review of direct anatomical open surgical management of atherosclerotic aorto-iliac occlusive disease, Eur J Vasc Endovasc Surg 39(4):460-471, 2010.)*

Interval	0	1	2	3	4	5	6	7	8	9	10
AFB	7521	6434	5545	4605	3774	2950	2211	1769	1404	1067	795
AIE	1971	1798	1602	1427	1250	1102	980	865	763	675	586
IFB	789	632	476	387	300	253	205	181	152	134	114

and an iliofemoral bypass is largely dependent on the distribution of atherosclerosis and whether the inflow artery can be safely controlled and the graft anastomosed at the level of the common iliac or distal aorta. Cross-sectional imaging is particularly helpful for examining the degree of calcification in these vessels, which may preclude this approach if extensive. Progression of atherosclerosis in the nonaffected limb is possible, but concern about future obstructive disease should not preclude a unilateral bypass. By basing the graft distally on the aorta and not mobilizing the infrarenal aorta extensively, the option to return for direct revascularization of the contralateral side remains viable. Crossover femoral-femoral bypass grafts are a useful approach in unilateral disease, particularly for patients who are higher risk, have had extensive prior abdominal surgeries, or have had failure of a prior graft limb. Unilateral axillary-femoral grafts are rarely indicated in elective scenarios, as the long-term results are inferior to direct revascularization or axillary-bifemoral bypasses. Clinical scenarios that may warrant such a reconstruction include presentation with acute or subacute ischemia with absent femoral pulses in a high-risk patient or when the contralateral groin is either septic or has soft tissue compromise in a patient that otherwise needs an extraanatomic bypass.

Although the long-term outcomes for direct revascularization with aortobifemoral or iliofemoral bypasses set the mark for durable outcomes, certain demographic features bear careful consideration. Female patients consistently have lower patency rates, in part due to the smaller size of their native vessels. Patients with multilevel disease also have worse long-term outcomes. A particular note of caution concerns the young patient (age <50) with AIOD, as several reports have highlighted markedly inferior outcomes in these patients with premature PAD. This likely reflects the presence of poorly controlled risk factors, particularly smoking, or an aggressive vascular disease phenotype. Even a seemingly straightforward endovascular procedure in these patients can have reduced durability and can accelerate the progression of disease toward complex reconstruction at an early age. We strongly advocate conservative management for the majority of younger patients and reserve intervention for severely progressive or limb-threatening symptoms.

The most common cause of failure of surgical reconstructions for AIOD is progression of atherosclerosis or neointimal hyperplasia at the distal anastomosis. Appropriate management of femoral disease at the time of the index operation is the key to maximizing the benefit and durability of any revascularization for AIOD. Unobstructed outflow through the profunda femoris is adequate runoff to maintain graft patency. A careful inspection of the profunda orifice following femoral arteriotomy should always be performed, and if there is any suspicion of obstructive disease at this level, a femoral endarterectomy with or without a formal profundaplasty should follow. Specific details on managing the femoral artery can be found in the section on aortofemoral bypass that follows.

AORTOBIFEMORAL BYPASS

Careful preoperative planning is essential in direct aortoiliac reconstruction. Body habitus, prior surgical history, presence of stomas, and skin conditions are important factors to consider in choosing an approach. Vascular imaging studies are critical for determining the level of aortic and iliac artery control, presence of concomitant renal or visceral artery disease, extent of common femoral and outflow disease, and the presence of concomitant aneurysmal degeneration of the aorta or iliac arteries. The location of the left renal vein should also be identified on cross-sectional imaging, as a retroaortic renal vein is not uncommon and may be inadvertently damaged during aortic mobilization or clamping if not anticipated.

Determining the level and configuration of the proximal and distal anastomoses is central to the preoperative strategy and should include careful consideration of the pelvic circulation. The proximal anastomosis to the aorta may be created in either an end-to-end or end-to-side fashion, with the former being preferred in most cases. With the end-to-end anastomosis, pelvic perfusion is maintained via retrograde flow from the external iliac arteries and proximal lumbar and mesenteric collaterals. In the presence of severe bilateral external iliac artery disease, an end-to-side configuration may be preferred. Alternatively, reimplantation of a patent inferior mesenteric artery may be performed regardless of the proximal configuration, particularly if there is suggestion of significant superior mesenteric artery disease or both hypogastric arteries are either occluded or will be excluded. An absolute indication for end-to-end reconstruction is the presence of concomitant aneurysmal degeneration of the abdominal aorta, which must then be fully excluded. Because the end-to-side aortic anastomosis requires a longer disease-free segment of infrarenal aorta, extensive atherosclerotic changes may also preclude it. In general, the immediate infrarenal aorta is more disease free and less likely to progress over time, which is an important reason to favor the end-to-end configuration.

The aortobifemoral bypass (AFB) procedure begins with exposing the femoral arteries. Minimizing the duration of time the abdomen is open limits insensible fluid losses, hypothermia, and inevitably blood loss. The common femoral artery is exposed through a longitudinal incision in standard fashion. The extent of exposure is predicated upon the extent of disease within the femoral artery. Proximally, exposure of the external iliac just above the inguinal ligament is often necessary to identify a soft, disease-free segment of artery that is amenable to clamping. The ligament may either be mobilized and retracted or partially divided to achieve the appropriate exposure. The inferior epigastric artery and circumflex iliac arteries should be identified and controlled because these are major collateral pathways in the setting of aortoiliac occlusive disease. Uncontrolled, these arteries will be a source of formidable back bleeding into the surgical field. The overlying deep circumflex iliac vein, which traverses anterior to the external iliac artery, deep to the inguinal ligament, should also be divided. Tunnels for the graft limbs are initiated from the groin by gentle finger dissection in the plane just anterior to the external iliac artery. Inadvertent injury to the crossing veins is avoided by ligating the vein before developing the tunnel.

The distal extent of exposure depends on whether an adjunctive femoral endarterectomy or profundaplasty is necessary. In all cases, the proximal superficial and deep femoral arteries are exposed for at least 2 to 3 cm beyond their origins. Assessment of these vessels by direct palpation, in addition to the preoperative imaging, is important to determine if they can be safely clamped or whether more extensive disease should be addressed by endarterectomy or patch angioplasty. This determination is most critical for the profunda femoris artery (PFA), the critical collateral pathway for the entire lower limb. If disease is present in the proximal PFA, more distal exposure of the secondary branches of the artery is necessary, and this often requires division of the overlying lateral circumflex femoral vein. After completing the groin exposures, these incisions are packed with antibiotic-soaked gauze sponges, and attention is turned to the abdomen.

The abdominal aorta is usually exposed via a transperitoneal approach through a midline incision. Though transverse exposures allow for generous access to the abdominal aorta, this incision requires division of the inferior epigastric arteries, which are major collateral pathways in the setting of AIOD. In the event of graft thrombosis, preserving the native collateral circulation can protect against the development of severe ischemia. The retroperitoneal approach via a left flank or a left paramedian incision may be desirable in select cases, such as those patients with "hostile" abdomens; however, it is slightly more challenging to develop the tunnel for the right limb of the bypass graft.

For transabdominal exposures, after exploring the abdomen and ensuring the appropriate placement of the nasogastric tube, an inframesocolic approach is used to enter the retroperitoneum. The ligament of Trietz is taken down, mobilizing the duodenum to the patient's right, until the vena cava is visualized. The anterior surface of the aorta is exposed from the inferior mesenteric artery up to the renal vein. Numerous lymphatics are encountered during this portion of the exposure, and they should be ligated to prevent a postoperative chyle leak. The renal vein is then mobilized from the vena cava medially to the adrenal and gonadal branches laterally. With adequate mobilization, including ligating the adrenal and lumbar branches, it is generally unnecessary to divide the renal vein, even if a suprarenal clamp is planned. If an aortic or renal artery endarterectomy is anticipated, or suprarenal clamping of the aorta is necessary for control, the renal arteries should be individually controlled. If an end-to-side anastomosis is planned, more extensive aortic mobilization is required to control or ligate lumbar arteries that would otherwise back bleed.

The distal extent of exposure is predicated upon the location of atheromatous disease. Palpation of the distal aorta, common iliac, and external iliac arteries will help identify a soft spot that is amenable to clamping. The peritoneum overlying the segment of artery is incised and the artery is exposed. Circumferential control is not necessary, and limiting dissection can minimize the chance of adjacent iliac vein injury. When exposing sites of distal control, be mindful of the location of the hypogastric plexus and the presacral nerves, which course anterior to the aorta and travel caudally over the aortic bifurcation. Injury to the plexus, which controls the autonomic functions of the pelvis, can result in impotence and retrograde ejaculation in men. To avoid this complication, approach the common iliac arteries laterally, and sweep up the peritoneum and the underlying nervous plexus toward the midline.

Deciding how and where to clamp the aorta is not trivial. Heavily calcified atheroma can be incompressible, or its irregular contour may prevent adequate hemostasis. The aorta is carefully palpated to identify a soft spot that is compressible. Atraumatic vascular clamps are applied in either a side-to-side or front-to-back fashion to ensure adequate apposition of the aortic walls. Clamping calcified atheroma can result in intimal tears, and the resulting clamp site injury can be a formidable challenge from which to recover. Side-biting or partial occlusion clamps are not recommended for an end-to-side anastomosis, as occasionally an endarterectomy of the aortic arteriotomy is necessary, and the partial occlusion clamps prevent adequate exposure and visualization of the lumen.

Tunnels for the graft limbs are then completed from the abdomen with careful blunt dissection directly over the external iliac artery. The graft limbs should be tunneled posterior to the ureter under direct visualization to prevent late upper urinary tract obstruction (Figure 4). Working from both the peritoneal cavity and the femoral exposure, a length of plasma tubing or a Penrose drain is passed with a curved aortic clamp to mark the tunnel. On the patient's left side, the tunnel is created deep to the mesentery of the sigmoid colon.

A bifurcated graft is selected—typically a collagen-coated or presealed knitted Dacron prosthesis. Generally, the graft is sized according the diameter of the aortic cuff. However, it may be advantageous to err in favor of a larger size if the graft limbs appear too small to maintain adequate outflow (i.e., <7 mm). Heparin sodium is then given as a bolus dose of 70 mg/kg and allowed to circulate for 3 minutes. Maintaining an activated clotting time of 250 to 300 seconds prevents lower extremity thrombus formation. Because atheromatous or thrombotic debris may break free and embolize in the process of applying vascular clamps, the distal clamps are applied first.

As noted previously, although there are advantages and disadvantages of each approach, most proximal anastomosis should be fashioned end-to-end. The in-line flow patterns result in less turbulent flow than an end-to-side anastomosis. After excising a portion of the aorta, the graft lies flat in the retroperitoneum, making for closure of the retroperitoneum over the graft simpler and theoretically resulting in a lower incidence of enteric erosions and graft infections (Figure 5). If planning an end-to-end anastomosis, the aorta is transected 2 cm distal to the proximal aortic clamp. Excising a short segment of aorta (2-4 cm), stopping short of the IMA, gives the main body of the graft space to lie within the retroperitoneum and allows for retrograde flow to perfuse the IMA if patent. The distal segment of aorta is oversewn or stapled, and if heavily diseased, it may require an endarterectomy first.

The proximal aortic cuff may also require an endarterectomy or may be lined with laminar thrombus or loose plaque that should be

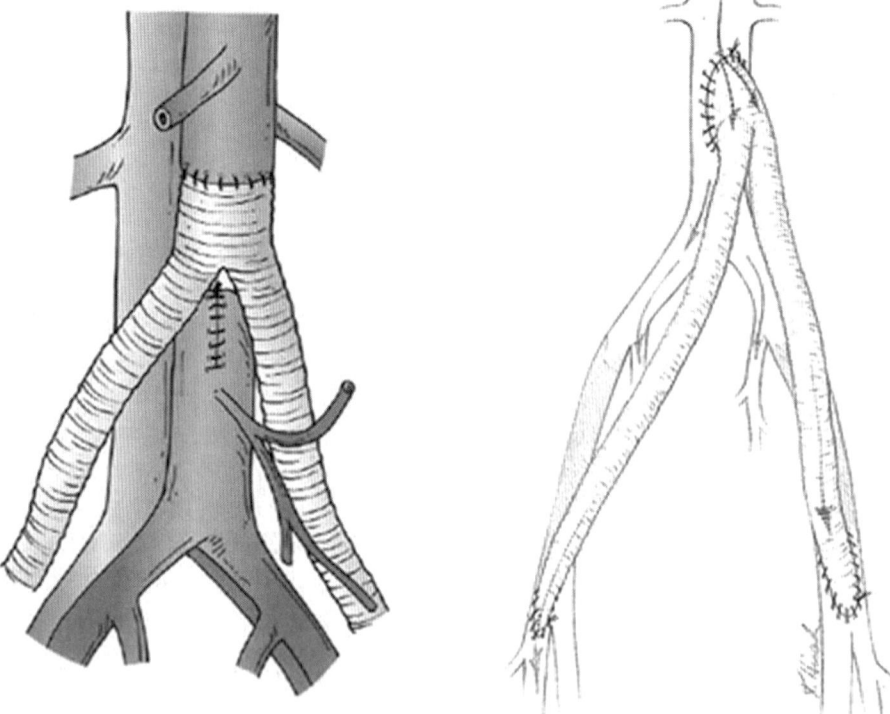

FIGURE 4 The proximal anastomosis. By resecting a short segment of aorta, the end-to-end proximal anastomosis lies flat along the retroperitoneum. This configuration ensures nonturbulent flow at the proximal anastomosis and simplifies the retroperitoneal closure at the completion of the reconstruction. In situations where antegrade flow to the pelvis needs to be preserved, an end-to-side anastomosis is favored. *(Adapted from Cronenwett JL, Johnston, KW: Rutherford's vascular surgery, ed 7, Philadelphia, 2010, Saunders; and from Zarins CK, Gewertz BL: Atlas of vascular surgery, St. Louis, 2005, Elsevier.)*

cleared prior to fashioning the anastomosis. This should be done with great care as to limit debris entering the lumen of the renal arteries or inadvertently developing a deep endarterectomy plane with resulting thin adventitia that may tear easily during suturing. If this is anticipated, the proximal anastomosis should be buttressed with a felt strip or sewn with interrupted pledgeted mattress sutures. The body of the graft is then shortened to less than 4 cm in length so the graft limbs straddle the oversewn aortic stump rather than lie over them. The proximal aorta is flushed to clear remaining debris, and the anastomosis is then created with 3-0 monofilament polypropylene suture. The graft limbs are then individually flushed, rinsed with heparinized saline, clamped, and then passed through the previously made tunnel with a curved aortic clamp.

One key to maintaining durability of the AFB graft is ensuring adequate outflow. In some cases, AIOD exists without significant femoral or infrainguinal occlusive disease. In these situations a simple end-to-side anastomosis to the common femoral artery is adequate. Very rarely, as in the case of truly isolated Type I disease, the distal anastomosis may be to the intraabdominal external iliac artery. However, due to the high frequency of disease progression in the external iliac and common femoral arteries, this should be done cautiously. The graft limb is beveled and sewn to the distal artery with continuous 5-0 monofilament polypropylene suture.

More commonly, however, multilevel or common femoral disease is also present. Unobstructed flow into PFA is sufficient outflow to maintain graft patency. Even in the setting of a complete SFA occlusion, a well-collateralized profunda system is adequate runoff for an AFB graft and will often alone result in significant hemodynamic improvement of the limb distally. After creating the longitudinal arteriotomy, the orifice of the profunda should be visually inspected and interrogated with a series of dilators, and it should easily accommodate at least a 4-mm probe.

When orificial disease of the PFA is present, a limited endarterectomy is indicated, and the arteriotomy can be extended onto the profunda so a profundaplasty is created with the hood of the graft (Figure 6). When more extensive PFA disease is present, a longer endarterectomy and patch angioplasty may be required. If the distal endpoint of the endarterectomy is not firmly secure, it should be reinforced with interrupted sutures. The arteriotomy and patch closure should be extended to just beyond this transition zone. The graft limb is then flushed, the arteries are back bled, and the clamps are released sequentially so that residual debris preferentially flows into the pelvis. The anesthetist should be advised prior to unclamping that significant hypotension may result from perfusing the ischemic limb.

With appropriately managed outflow disease, a sequential bypass to the lower extremity is rarely needed. These adjunctive procedures add to blood loss and operating time, and they expose the patient to the complications of infrainguinal bypass without necessarily improving the long-term patency of the AFB. They are largely reserved for limbs with severe limb-threatening ischemia, such as those with extensive tissue loss in the setting of complete SFA occlusion, which cannot wait for a staged infrainguinal procedure.

After completion, an assessment of distal perfusion is made by palpating the artery in the field and by listening with Doppler intonation to both the target artery and the pedal arteries. When outflow is limited to the PFA, improvement in pedal Doppler signals may not be immediately appreciated in the operating room due to the patient's hemodynamic status and peripheral vasoconstriction. If content with the technical result, hemostasis is achieved, and the retroperitoneum overlying the graft is closed with absorbable suture. Inadequate coverage of the graft may lead to a graft-enteric fistula. In the setting of end-to-side anastomosis, it may not be possible to close the retroperitoneum over the graft directly. In these situations, a tongue of omentum can be mobilized and secured to the retroperitoneum between the graft and the overlying bowel.

ILIOFEMORAL BYPASS

Just as in the AFB, the iliofemoral bypass (IFB) procedure begins with the femoral exposure. There are no significant differences in the conduct of this portion of the operation. The degree of exposure is

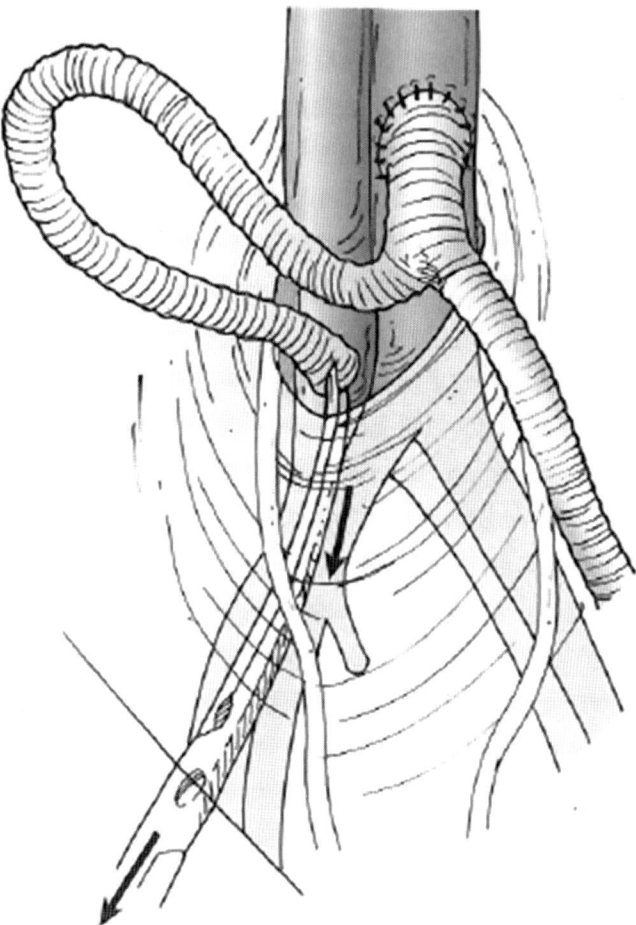

FIGURE 5 Tunneling of the graft limbs. The retroperitoneal tunnel is developed by blunt manual dissection under direct vision, taking care to establish a plane posterior to the ureter. After completion of the proximal anastomosis, the graft limb is passed through the tunnel with a curved aortic clamp. *(Adapted from Cronenwett JL, Johnston, KW: Rutherford's vascular surgery, ed 7, Philadelphia, 2010, Saunders.)*

a function of the extent of atherosclerotic disease in the femoral artery. If anticipating a femoral endarterectomy, generous exposure of the profunda femoris artery should be performed.

Unlike in AFB, where a transperitoneal or retroperitoneal exposure to the abdominal aorta is an option, in treating unilateral disease, the retroperitoneal exposure is particularly suitable. Advantages include avoiding potential trauma to the hypogastric plexus and presacral nerves, avoiding adhesions if the patient has had previous abdominal surgery, and theoretically minimizing the postoperative ileus because the peritoneal space is not entered. Either an oblique lower abdominal or a paramedian incision may be used for iliac artery exposure. Regardless, the surgical field extends from the costal margins to the knees in case more proximal exposure is required.

The location of the inflow is dependent on the distribution of atherosclerotic disease. Anticipate the need for extending the arteriotomy or performing a local endarterectomy when choosing a location for the vascular clamps. Often, this means being prepared to clamp the distal abdominal aorta and contralateral iliac artery even though the surgical plan calls for a common iliac artery anastomosis. Just as in the AFB, the prosthetic graft is then passed through the tunnel, and the remainder of the operation is completed.

EXTRAANATOMIC BYPASS

Although direct reconstruction of aortoiliac disease can be done with low morbidity and mortality in well-selected patients, those with significant coexistent cardiac and pulmonary disease—who are at high risk for open aortic surgery due to either physiologic or anatomic constraints—would be better served with extraanatomic reconstruction. These techniques, such as the femorofemoral bypass or the axillobifemoral bypass, limit the morbidity associated with major vascular surgery but come at the price of limited durability. These techniques are usually reserved for patients with critical limb ischemia and are generally not performed for intermittent claudication.

FEMOROFEMORAL BYPASS

The principle advantage of femorofemoral bypass (FFB) is that it can be done under local or regional anesthesia, minimizing pulmonary complications associated with direct reconstruction of the abdominal aorta. This procedure is well suited for patients who have iliac occlusive disease limited to one iliac system and a contralateral side that is free from hemodynamically significant stenosis. However, even this principle is in evolution. Multiple groups have reported satisfactory outcomes with hybrid procedures, where focal iliac lesions of the donor iliac system are treated first with endovascular techniques, before completion of the femorofemoral bypass graft.

The technique is performed through bilateral longitudinal incisions exposing the femoral arteries. Oblique incisions, though common when placing cross-femoral grafts during endovascular treatment of aortic aneurysms, are less versatile when treating occlusive disease. However, it may be advantageous in obese patients to help reduce the risk of wound complications related to crossing skin folds. Following adequate exposure of the inflow and outflow arteries, the graft tunnel is made in the subcutaneous tissue directly overlying the pubis, immediately anterior to the fascia of the abdominal wall, by blunt finger dissection or with the assistance of a curved clamp. The choice of graft material, whether supported or unsupported PTFE or polyester, has been well studied and does not appear to have significant effect on outcomes. Multiple configurations of the graft have been described, but the most common is the inverted C orientation. Following heparinization and clamping, an end-to-side anastomosis is fashioned with the beveled end of the graft to the common femoral artery at a slightly oblique angle, oriented from medial to lateral. In obese patients, the inguinal ligament can descend significantly when the patient moves from the supine to the standing position. Grafts sewn too proximally on the common femoral artery may undergo kinking at the heel of the graft. To avoid this complication, place the graft distally on the common femoral artery. The graft is then passed through the tunnel, ensuring that the course the graft takes is a gentle turn into the contralateral groin. The graft is then distended to ensure accurate measurement of length, trimmed to size, and then sewn end-to-side to the target femoral artery.

AXILLOBIFEMORAL BYPASS

The axillobifemoral bypass (AxBF) graft is well suited for frail patients with aortic or proximal iliac occlusive disease with advanced lower extremity ischemia, such as tissue loss or rest pain. Other indications are patients with a "hostile" abdomen, including previous radiation therapy, intestinal stomas, or intraabdominal sepsis. Unlike the FFB, the AxBF usually requires general anesthesia (though the original report describes the procedure under local anesthesia). Due to the limited inflow the axillary artery can provide, the procedure is typically reserved for patients with limb-threatening ischemia, not IC alone.

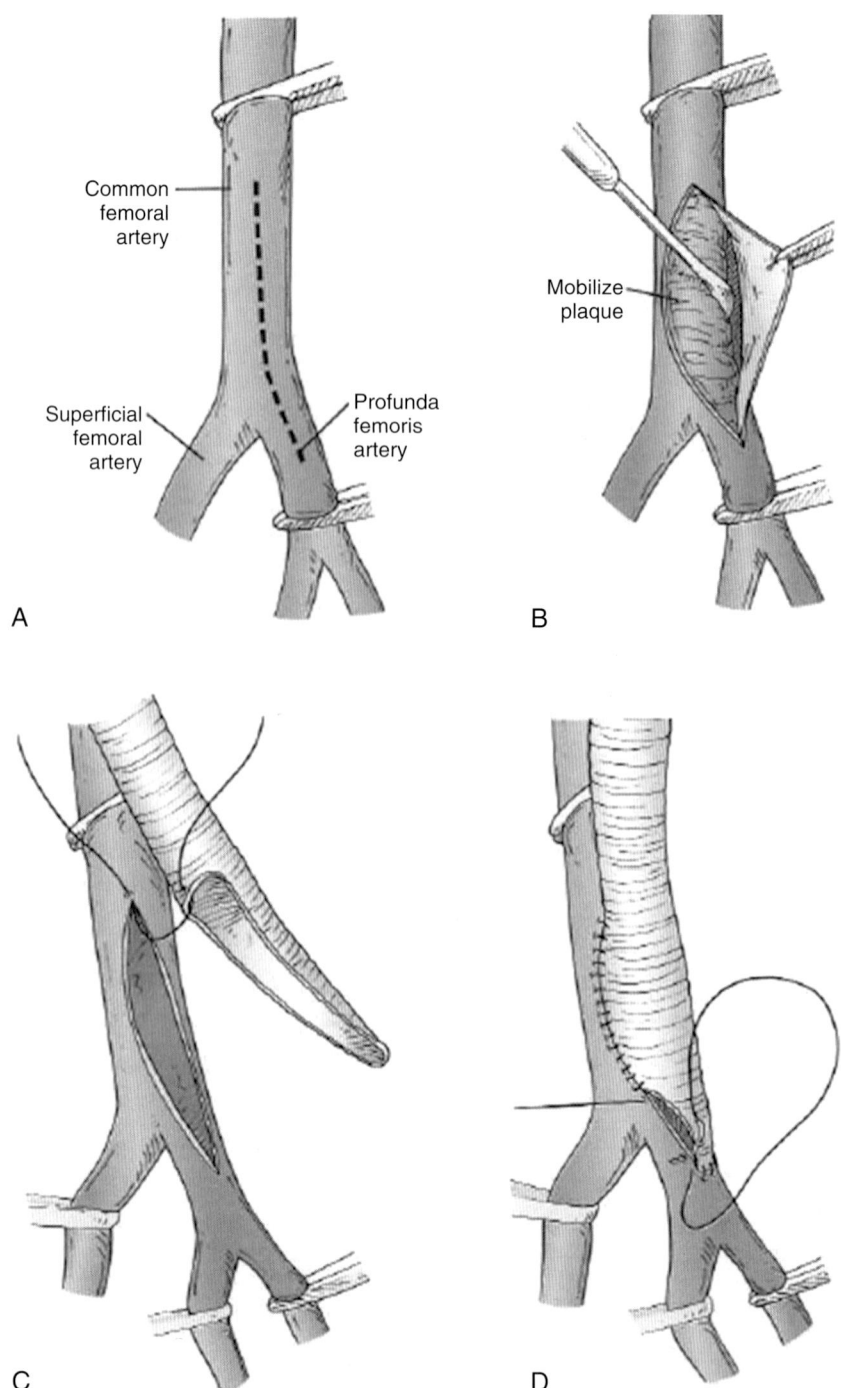

Common
femoral
artery

Superficial
femoral
artery

Profunda
femoris
artery

A

Mobilize
plaque

B

C

D

FIGURE 6 Adjunctive profundaplasty. Graft patency is optimized by maximizing the graft limb outflow. Concomitant disease of the profunda femoris orifice should be treated with limited endarterectomy and a profundaplasty using the toe of the aortofemoral graft limb. *(Adapted from Cronenwett JL, Johnston, KW: Rutherford's vascular surgery, ed 7, Philadelphia, 2010, Saunders.)*

Outflow plays a particularly important role in the midterm durability of this procedure. A long prosthetic bypass graft based upon the axillary artery is at risk for thrombosis. Providing outflow via both femoral arteries rather than upon the ipsilateral femoral artery alone has been shown to increase flow within the graft at the axillary artery and improve the long-term patency of the bypass. Preoperatively, blood pressure measurements in both arms dictate whether to use the right or left side for inflow. Typically, the left subclavian artery is atheroprone, and the right axillary artery is the source of inflow. The patient is positioned supine on the operating table, a shoulder roll is placed behind the patient, and the arm is tucked to the side. The skin is prepped widely, and the patient is draped low to the bed

should there develop the need for a counterincision or if there is a mishap during the tunneling of the graft.

An infraclavicular incision overlying the insertion of pectoralis minor is used to expose the axillary artery. The clavipectoral fascia is divided, and a muscle-splitting technique is used to dissect through the pectoralis major into the deep pectoral fascia. The pectoralis minor is divided to expose the second portion of the axillary artery. The axillary artery is fragile in comparison to the femoral artery and should be handled with care to prevent inadvertent laceration or dissection. Mobilizing a generous length of artery without traumatizing the closely associated brachial plexus allows for delivering the artery up into the surgical field, simplifying the anastomosis.

This maneuver is facilitated by dividing the deep thoracic artery (Figure 7).

The femoral exposure is performed as in FFB—a longitudinal incision to expose the common femoral artery—and the cross-femoral graft is tunneled in a similar manner. The graft tunnel from the axillary artery to the femoral artery should traverse anterior to the anterior superior iliac spine, along the fascia of the abdominal wall, posterior to the breast in women, and deep to the pectoralis major. An externally supported prosthetic graft (i.e., ringed PTFE) is used, because the graft can be compressed and will thrombose while the patient lies on his or her side while sleeping. The graft should be trimmed with the artery in its native position, with enough redundancy to allow for shoulder abduction postoperatively without placing tension on the anastomosis. Following heparinization and clamping, the beveled graft is anastomosed end-to-side along the anteroinferior portion of the axillary artery to minimize the possibility of graft kinking as it passes into the tunnel.

A variety of configurations for the distal anastomoses have been described. As in the femorofemoral graft, we prefer an inverted C orientation, with the cross-femoral graft based upon the axillofemoral graft rather than the native artery. Inverted S configurations, graft flow dividers, or other manipulations to limit competitive flow in the iliac artery have been described but do not appear to significantly affect the quality of the procedure.

OTHER SURGICAL REVASCULARIZATION OPTIONS

Prior to the popularization of prosthetic grafts, the standard treatment for aortoiliac occlusive disease was the endarterectomy. The open, eversion, and semiclosed methods have all been described with excellent patency. The advantage of the endarterectomy is avoidance of complications related to prosthetics grafts (infection, pseudoaneurysm formation, etc.) and potentially improved inflow into the hypogastric arteries. However, the excellent result with AFB and endovascular techniques has limited the number of patients who are candidates for this type of intervention. Currently, the ideal candidate for endarterectomy is the younger patient who has focal (e.g., Type I) disease in a large-caliber vessel, who is not better served with endovascular interventions. The high success rates of angioplasty and stenting for these more limited disease patterns have essentially rendered aortoiliac endarterectomy obsolete in current practice.

Rarely, there will be patients who are candidates for direct surgical revascularization but may not have an accessible abdominal aorta. This may be because of abdominal radiation, proximal aortic disease above the renal arteries that prevent aortic clamp application, or a failed previous aortic operation. In these cases, an alternative source of inflow is the distal thoracic aorta. This requires exposure through either a lateral thoracotomy, high retroperitoneal or thoracoretroperitoneal approach. The latter simplifies tunneling of the graft limbs through the retroperitoneum, posterior to the kidney. A transperitoneal approach with medial visceral rotation may also be used, though more commonly this is necessary when the initial plan for an infrarenal anastomosis is abandoned due to unanticipated disease severity or calcification. The durability of this procedure rivals that of the AFB.

COMPLICATIONS OF SURGICAL REVASCULARIZATION

Aortobifemoral grafting is considered the "gold standard" for durable AIOD treatment. Improvements in patient selection, intraoperative anesthetic care, surgical proficiency, and postoperative management have made the procedure safe for most. In multiple contemporary series, AFB can be performed with a less than 1% in-hospital mortality (Table 1). The overall morbidity rate approaches 20% to 35% when using a composite endpoint that includes both major and minor complications. Postoperative cardiac events occur in less than 5% of patients and can be minimized with appropriate use of medications such as beta-blockers, aspirin, and statins in accordance with current practice guidelines. Pulmonary complications are not infrequent, occurring in up to 7% of patients. Adequate pain control with

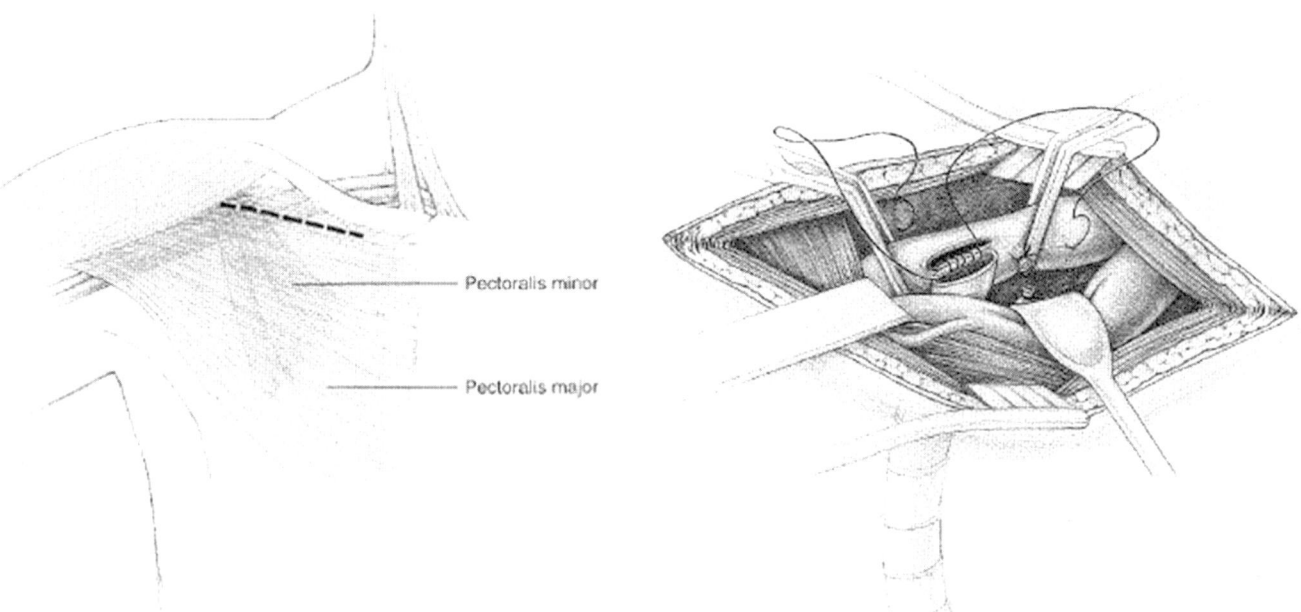

FIGURE 7 Axillofemoral bypass. An infraclavicular incision overlying the insertion of pectoralis minor is used to expose the axillary artery. The pectoralis minor is divided, exposing the second portion of the axillary artery. Dividing the deep thoracic artery allows for a generous mobilization and helps deliver the artery up into the surgical field, simplifying the anastomosis. *(Adapted from Zarins CK, Gewertz BL: Atlas of vascular surgery, St. Louis, 2005, Elsevier.)*

TABLE 1: Results of direct surgical revascularization

Procedure	5-year patency	Perioperative morbidity	Operative mortality
Aortofemoral bypass	80% to 95%	10% to 30%	2% to 4%
Iliofemoral bypass	80% to 90%	10% to 25%	1% to 3%
Femorofemoral bypass	55% to 85%	10% to 25%	1% to 3%
Axillobifemoral bypass	50% to 75%	10% to 40%	1% to 4%
Axillofemoral bypass	45% to 70%	10% to 40%	1% to 4%
Iliac endarterectomy	80% to 90%	10% to 20%	1% to 3%

epidural anesthesia to facilitate pulmonary toilet and avoidance of volume overload can help prevent these complications. Atheroemboli can be liberated during the procedure, manifesting as end organ ischemia in the skin, pelvis, spinal cord, and bowel. Attention to detail during clamping and flushing can minimize this complication. Ischemic colitis and pelvic ischemia are rare and can be avoided by planning a procedure that maintains pelvic perfusion. Other complications include renal failure from ischemia secondary to prolonged clamp times or embolization during aortic cuff endarterectomy; wound complications, particularly in the groin (lymphocele, lymphocutaneous fistula, wound infections); and postoperative hemorrhage.

The most frequent late complication of the aortobifemoral bypass graft is thrombosis, typically involving a single graft limb. The 10-year patency of this bypass is approximately 85%. A classic mistake is to base the graft too far distal on the abdominal aorta. Disease progression proximal to the graft presents as bilateral limb thrombosis. Unilateral graft limb thrombosis is invariably a result of outflow obstruction from either neointimal hyperplasia in the anastomotic area or progression of native disease in the femoral artery. This can be managed with a thrombectomy through a femoral exposure and revision of the distal anastomosis.

Pseudoaneurysm formation secondary to material fatigue or suture fracture is not as frequent as it once was and may also result from either degeneration of the native femoral artery or occult graft infection. Nonvirulent species of bacteria can present with a pseudoaneurysm long after the index procedure. An index of suspicion for infection should be maintained when treating all pseudoaneurysms. Graft infection remains an uncommon but dreaded complication of AFB. Less subtle signs of a graft infection at the level of the groin include a draining sinus tract or evidence of cellulitis or induration. Infections involving the intraabdominal portion of the graft can present with abdominal tenderness with or without an ileus, sepsis, or a gastrointestinal bleed. Infrequently, a graft enteric fistula may develop when a loop of bowel, typically but not always the duodenum, erodes into the graft. This challenging complication is minimized by carefully closing the retroperitoneum over the graft or interposing a tongue of omentum at the time of the index operation.

Complications related to extraanatomic bypasses are similar to those of arterial surgery in general. There are risks of hemorrhage, wound complications, hematoma, graft infection, and pseudoaneurysm formation. Specific to the cross-femoral graft, complications of tunneling subfascial with subsequent bowel and bladder perforation have been reported. Specific to the axillary graft, trauma to the brachial plexus, atheroemboli to the hand, or graft avulsion have been reported. This last complication can be minimized by planning enough redundancy of the graft to allow for comfortable shoulder abduction postoperatively.

RESULTS OF SURGICAL REVASCULARIZATION

AFB grafting is the "gold standard" for treating aortoiliac occlusive disease. Irrespective of the surgical indication—be it claudication or critical limb ischemia—graft patency at 5 years is nearly 90% and at 10 years is about 85% (see Table 1). Although gender may affect the outcomes, transperitoneal or retroperitoneal exposure and end-to-end or end-to-side anastomosis do not appreciably alter the results. Results of IFB for unilateral disease are generally at least as good as AFB in reported series.

Extraanatomic bypasses do not fare as well but have acceptable midterm results. Though these interventions are typically reserved for patients with coexistent comorbid conditions that are not candidates for direct revascularization, and therefore have a higher expected mortality over the long term, many series have reported 5-year patency rates averaging approximately 70%. The long-term results with AxBF are more muddled. Often, these patients have shortened life expectancy, and survivors with less burden of disease bias long-term outcome data. Even so, stratifying results by indication shows results are inferior to aortobifemoral grafting, with an estimated 5-year patency of 50% to 70%.

ENDOVASCULAR INTERVENTIONS

Just as in open surgery, preprocedure planning sets the stage for a successful endovascular intervention. Noninvasive imaging, in particular with CT angiography, delineates the location and extent of disease, as well as the degree of calcification. It also helps assess the quality of the access vessels and whether an ipsilateral retrograde, contralateral antegrade, brachial approach, or concomitant open femoral exposure will be necessary. In general, CIA disease is treated through an ipsilateral retrograde approach, and EIA disease is treated with a contralateral antegrade approach. If the CIA is occluded, bilateral punctures of the femoral arteries will be necessary to perform an aortogram proximal to the lesion.

Access is gained in the CFA using the Seldinger technique under ultrasound guidance. Inspection of the anterior surface of the CFA not only identifies segments of artery that are disease free and likely to be receptive to puncture but also a segment of artery that is favorable for maintaining hemostasis during sheath removal. This maneuver can circumvent common complications related to endovascular interventions, such as retroperitoneal hematomas, pseudoaneurysm formation, and iatrogenic arteriovenous fistulas.

In situations where there is significant femoral disease but limited AIOD (i.e., TASC A or B), a hybrid approach utilizing an open femoral endarterectomy with endovascular treatment of the aortoiliac system is preferred. In these cases, carefully weigh the option of a formal AFB versus the reduced morbidity and durability of the hybrid procedure. The hybrid approach can be executed in a number of ways. We favor performing the endarterectomy first, as it allows for the possibility of stenting the external iliac artery right down to, or even into, the endarterectomy site without having to achieve inflow occlusion of the stent. After endarterectomy and patch angioplasty, the patch can be punctured directly, or the sheath can be introduced between the patch suture line prior to tying down the patch. It can sometimes be difficult to stay out of the dissection plane when passing the wire retrograde. Securing the proximal edge of the endarterectomy with suture minimizes this risk. Alternatively, puncturing the artery and leaving the wire across the true lumen of the iliac artery during the endarterectomy eliminates problems with wire passage. However, even with soft insert clamps, bleeding around the wire may be a persistent nuisance. Otherwise, an "up-and-over" wire can be passed from a contralateral antegrade approach into the surgical field.

With either technique, a 5 French sheath is used at the access site, and a hydrophilic guidewire with an angled tip catheter is used to access the aorta. The patient is heparinized to maintain an activated clotting time of 250 to 300 seconds, and a power injector is used to perform flush aortography with a multisidehole catheter (Figure 8). The AP projection is ideal for evaluating the aortic bifurcation, and oblique views of the pelvis are needed to open the iliac bifurcation. In general, a 50% stenosis is considered hemodynamically significant. If the significance of the lesion is in doubt, direct pressure measurements or intravascular ultrasound can be used to more accurately estimate the degree of stenosis. A resting pressure gradient of over 10 mm Hg when pulling back an end-hole catheter through the lesion or an enhanced gradient of over 20 mm Hg when infusing a vasodilator distally (e.g., nitroglycerin or tolazoline) is considered hemodynamically significant.

Stenosis can usually be crossed with a hydrophilic guidewire and catheter combination with relative ease. Chronic total occlusions are technically more challenging. Finding a serviceable plane depends on plaque morphology. Crossing occlusions retrograde has the mechanical advantage of "push ability," as the wire and catheter combination is not working around a curve. However, it can be difficult to precisely reenter the lumen once subintimal, and this can be particularly problematic if inadvertently extending the plane up along the aorta. Reentry catheters have been developed to facilitate this process. The antegrade approach from the contralateral iliac artery eliminates worries about reentry into the aorta, but it can be difficult to engage a subintimal plane because push ability is lost at the bifurcation. This is particularly true with flush iliac occlusions. The brachial approach is another option, but larger sheath sizes needed for iliac stenting typically mean starting with an open brachial exposure. In addition, a long catheter passed around the aortic arch also has its own set of mechanical disadvantages.

Lesion length, location, and degree of calcification dictate whether angioplasty alone, a balloon-expanding stent, or a self-expanding stent should be used. Occlusive disease of the terminal aorta, or orificial disease of the common iliac artery, should be treated with balloon-expanding "kissing" stents (Figure 9). Balloon-expanding stents can be deployed accurately and have greater radial strength. Theoretically, treating only one iliac artery orifice can result in plaque shift during angioplasty, obstructing the contralateral lumen. Treating both sides simultaneously avoids this complication. Covered balloon-expanding stents may have improved patency in long-term follow-up because covered stents prevent the development of neointimal hyperplasia through the interstices of the stent. They may also be safer in the setting of small, heavily calcified, or tortuous iliac arteries that are more prone to rupture with balloon inflation.

The external iliac artery is more mobile than the common iliac artery, and as such, the treatment algorithm is slightly different. Balloon angioplasty alone is reasonable for TASC A and B lesions in the external iliac artery. Based upon the degree of recoil or the presence of a dissection flap, the external iliac artery is selectively treated with self-expanding stents. As these devices tend to be more flexible than the stiff balloon-expanding stents, they handle the mobility of the external iliac artery better and are less likely to get crushed if deployed in close proximity to the inguinal ligament. As noted above, heavily calcified lesions that are likely to rupture should be treated with covered self-expanding stents so that aggressive angioplasty does not result in rupture with active extravasation into the retroperitoneum.

Complications of Endovascular Interventions

In appropriately selected patients, the procedural complication rate for endovascular intervention in AIOD is low. Access site complications are the most common and total less than 2% in most series. Pseudoaneurysms, retroperitoneal bleeding, dissection, and atheroembolism can be avoided by using ultrasound guidance to access the femoral artery. A femoral angiogram will inform the operator if an inadvertently high puncture was performed. Though percutaneous closure devices have not been shown to unequivocally decrease access site complication rates, this is one situation where they may be useful.

The most serious intraoperative complication is arterial rupture during angioplasty. In the presence of active extravasation, quickly reinflating the balloon can maintain hemodynamic control until an appropriately sized stent graft can be deployed to cover the disruption. Other intraoperative complications include dissection, vessel spasm, thrombosis, and atheroembolism. Another common postprocedure complication includes contrast-induced nephropathy, particularly in patients with preexisting renal insufficiency. Though there are no absolute contraindications for endovascular interventions, patients with renal insufficiency should be pretreated with hydration to minimize the effect of contrast exposure. In patients who are at risk for contrast-induced nephropathy, contrast should be used sparingly, and consideration should be given to CO_2 angiography, which works reasonably well within the aortoiliac segment.

RESULTS OF ENDOVASCULAR INTERVENTIONS

The technical success rate of iliac angioplasty and stenting is quite high, on the order of 98% in many reports. Though this translates into hemodynamic improvement, maintaining long-term patency

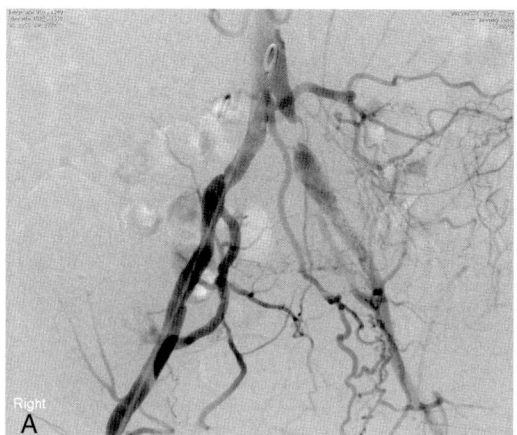
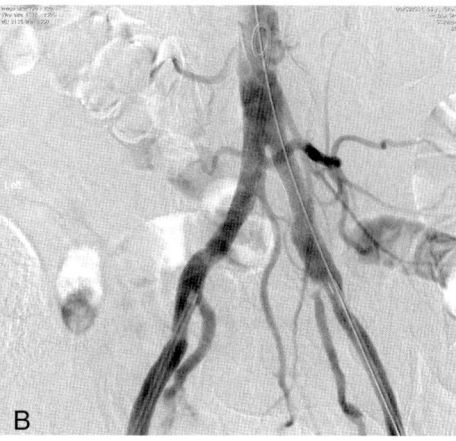

FIGURE 8 Diagnostic angiography and percutaneous intervention. A diagnostic angiogram shows a left common iliac stenosis, with extensive collateralization from the middle sacral and segmental lumbar arteries. **A,** Focal lesions, are excellent candidates for endovascular interventions. **B,** Note the absence of collateralized vessels after the left common iliac lesion is treated with a stent.

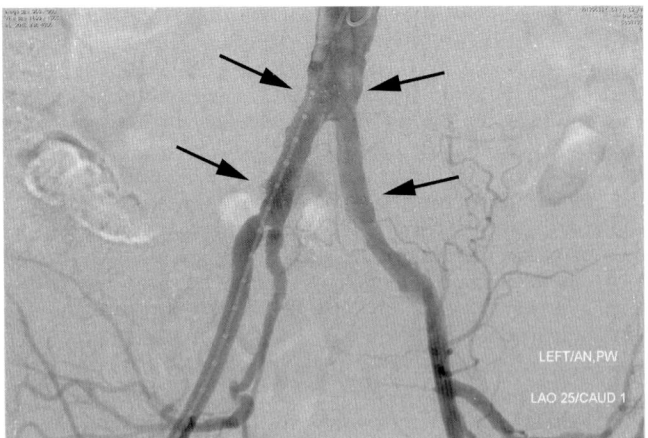

FIGURE 9 "Kissing" stents. Endovascular treatment of bilateral common iliac disease originating at or near the aortic bifurcation requires "kissing" stents. Simultaneous deployment of balloon-expanding stents avoids complications related to plaque shift during angioplasty. Well-positioned and appropriately sized stents do not encroach upon the distal abdominal aorta or the contralateral limb.

requires dedication to surveillance and often requires multiple reinterventions (Figure 10). Most lesions will need to be treated with primary stenting, but in lesions amenable to angioplasty alone, primary stenting is less likely to have an early recurrence or need reintervention, and it may be more cost effective to treat with primary stenting at the index procedure. Surveillance with ankle brachial indices, and possibly ultrasound if the patient's habitus is amenable, is necessary because as a group, the primary patency of iliac stenting is approximately 70% at 5 years (Table 2). Maintaining patency with reinterventions can improve this rate to about 85%. All patients should be maintained on antiplatelet therapy indefinitely. Although there is little literature addressing this specifically for iliac angioplasty and stenting, extrapolating from the experience of percutaneous cardiac interventions, antiplatelet therapy will help prevent early thrombosis.

Although a variety of factors that affect outcomes have been reported, including renal failure, diabetes, and the diameter of the treated vessel, the most important determinant of long-term outcomes is the underlying burden of disease. The TASC classification captures this relatively well, and long-term outcomes are far better with TASC A or B lesions than with TASC C or D lesions. As it currently stands, the TASC working group has recommended endovascular interventions for TASC A and B lesions and direct surgical revascularization for TASC D lesions. Treatment of TASC C lesions is individualized for each patient, though given the high degrees of technical success, endovascular interventions are often opted for first.

FIGURE 10 Long-term patency of endovascular interventions A retrospective review of 413 patients with aortoiliac occlusive disease treated with primary stenting was performed. Cumulative primary patency was 83% at 5 years. Long-term primary patency lessens with advancing patterns of disease. (Adapted from Ichihashi S, Higashiura W, Itoh H, et al.: Long-term outcomes for systematic primary stent placement in complex iliac artery occlusive disease classified according to Trans-Atlantic Inter-Society Consensus (TASC)-II, J Vasc Surg 53(4):992-999, 2011.)

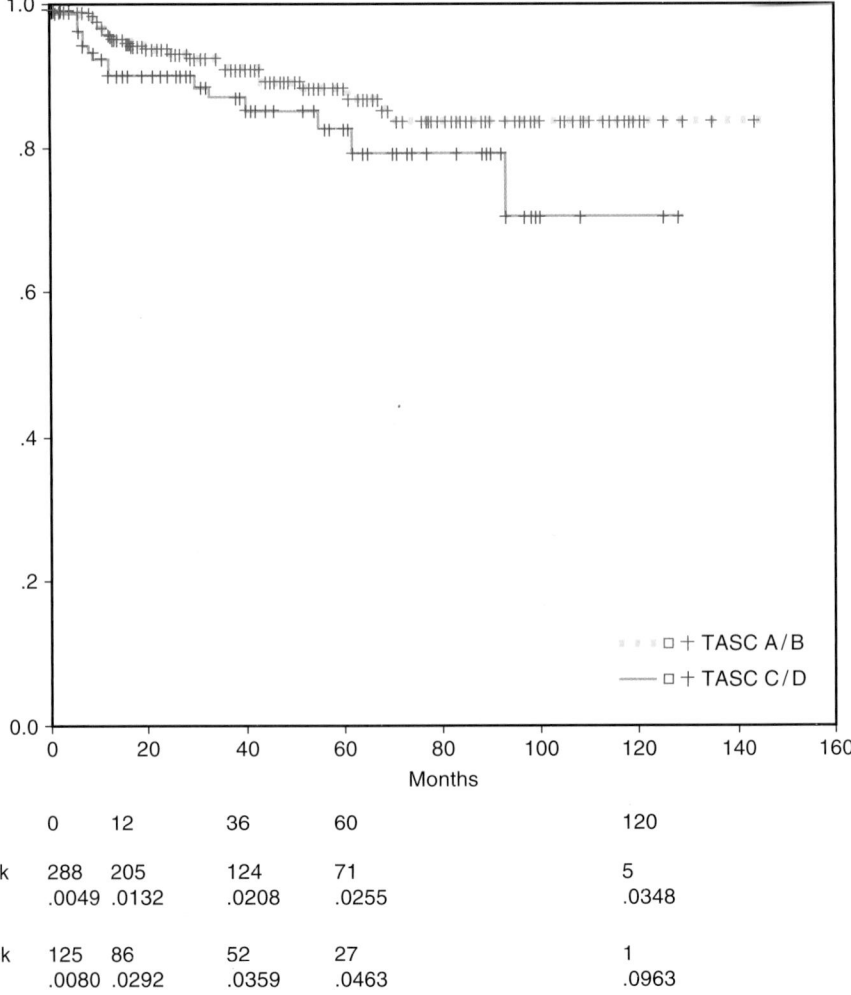

	0	12	36	60	120
A/B					
At risk	288	205	124	71	5
S.E.	.0049	.0132	.0208	.0255	.0348
C/D					
At risk	125	86	52	27	1
S.E.	.0080	.0292	.0359	.0463	.0963

TABLE 2: Results of endovascular interventions

TASC II classification	Technical success	Procedural complications	5-Year patency
TASC A or B	98%	5% to 10%	80%
TASC C	95%	5% to 10%	65%
TASC D	90%	5% to 10%	65%

TASC, Trans-Atlantic Inter-Society Consensus.

those with localized disease. However, direct surgical revascularization still plays an important role in treating patients with a more advanced burden of disease and also serves as a means of salvaging failed endovascular interventions. Even in high-risk patients, extraanatomic bypass procedures can prove useful to treating lower extremity ischemia in AIOD. As with all vascular interventions, long-term outcomes are optimized by aggressive postprocedural medical management, risk factor reduction, and surveillance.

SUMMARY

AIOD is a common cause of lower extremity ischemia syndromes. For claudicants, the decision to intervene must include a careful assessment of procedural risks and expected benefits. The success, safety, and reasonable durability of endovascular interventions have made the application of this technique the intervention of choice for

SUGGESTED READINGS

Chiu KW, Davies RS, Nightingale PG, et al: Review of direct anatomical open surgical management of atherosclerotic aorto-iliac occlusive disease, *Eur J Vasc Endovasc Surg* 39(4):460–471, 2010.

LoGerfo FW, et al: A comparison of the late patency rates of axillobilateral femoral and axillounilateral femoral grafts, *Surgery* 81(1):33–38; discussion 38–40, 1977.

Norgren L, et al: Inter-Society Consensus for the Management of Peripheral Arterial Disease (TASC II), *Eur J Vasc Endovasc Surg* 33(Suppl 1):S1–75, 2007.

Sharafuddin MJ, et al: Kissing stent reconstruction of the aortoiliac bifurcation, *Perspect Vasc Surg Endovasc Ther* 20(1):50–60, 2008.

FEMOROPOPLITEAL OCCLUSIVE DISEASE

**Natalia O. Glebova, MD, PhD, and
Thomas Reifsnyder, MD, FACS**

INTRODUCTION

Peripheral arterial disease (PAD) has a prevalence rate of up to 10% in the general population and of nearly 20% in people over the age of 70 years. With the aging population and the increasing prevalence of PAD risk factors such as diabetes mellitus, hypertension, and dyslipidemia, the societal burden of PAD continues to grow. Vascular surgeons need to be knowledgeable and proficient with the wide variety of treatment modalities. As a subset of PAD, femoropopliteal occlusive disease affects the vasculature between the inguinal ligament and the tibial vessels and is a pattern of disease frequently seen in cigarette smokers. The most frequently obstructed vessels are the superficial femoral (SFA) and popliteal arteries. The decreased blood flow leads to tissue ischemia of the calf and foot. Atherosclerosis is the culprit in the overwhelming majority of patients, although occasional patients with fibromuscular dysplasia, giant cell arteritis, Takayasu's arteritis, or other arteriopathies may present similarly.

EVALUATION

Patient evaluation begins with a history and physical examination. The identification and modification of risk factors such as cigarette smoking, diabetes, hypertension, dyslipidemia, and dietary habits is paramount. The patient's symptom complex combined with a thorough pulse examination usually reveals the level of the arterial lesion and guides the subsequent treatment regimen.

Patients with femoropopliteal occlusive disease present in one of three ways: incidentally found asymptomatic disease, intermittent claudication, or limb-threatening ischemia. Claudication (from the Latin *claudicare* meaning "to limp") manifests as crampy achy calf pain with walking that occurs at a reproducible distance and is relieved with rest. Although it is a strong risk factor for other atherosclerotic problems, the natural history of intermittent claudication is relatively benign with less than 3% of patients needing a major amputation within 5 years. However, patients with significant claudication have functional limitations that affect lifestyle and employment. In these patients and in those who present with limb-threatening ischemia, further workup and revascularization are warranted.

The noninvasive vascular laboratory is a useful tool; however, its indiscriminate use should be discouraged, particularly as a screening method. The most common tests are the ankle-brachial index (ABI) and color duplex scan. The former is determined with calculation of the ratio of the higher systolic pressure at the ankle (either at the dorsalis pedis or posterior tibial artery) to the higher systolic brachial pressure in either arm. In general, an ABI greater than 0.97 is considered normal, and values less than 0.4 are often associated with critical limb ischemia. The best use of the ABI is to discriminate between vasculogenic and neurogenic claudication. Only in patients with vasculogenic claudication does the ABI drop significantly when the patient walks to the point of calf pain (this test requires a treadmill in the vascular laboratory). The presence of femoropopliteal occlusive disease usually can be determined with physical examination, so unless there is a diagnostic dilemma, confirmation of the presence of disease with a vascular laboratory ABI is not warranted. Not infrequently, ABIs cannot be calculated because of the incompressibility of diabetic calcified vessels. Noninvasive alternatives include digital or toe pressures, pulse volume recordings, or transcutaneous oxygen measurements.

Duplex ultrasound scan arterial mapping is also available from the vascular laboratory. In this era of endovascular intervention, distinguishing patients that have TASC II (see subsequent) A and B lesions from C and D lesions helps with decision making. If the patient is not a good open surgery candidate, preintervention duplex scan arterial mapping can minimize the number of patients who undergo purely diagnostic arteriography.

After the decision is made for invasive treatment of femoropopliteal occlusive disease, the next step is digital subtraction angiography with possible synchronous angioplasty or stenting. Angiography also allows the identification and treatment of an unsuspected inflow problem, and the delineation of the best outflow option. Although surgical decisions can be based on computed tomographic angiography (CTA) or magnetic resonance angiography (MRA), contrast arteriography remains the gold standard.

TREATMENT

Treatment of femoropopliteal occlusive disease is based on a careful weighing of the patient's symptoms, intervention required, expected durability of the intervention, and the risks of the procedure.

Medical

Patients with mild claudication should be treated nonoperatively with medical optimization and an exercise program. This includes risk factor modification: cessation of cigarette smoking, dietary and pharmacologic (statin) reduction in low-density lipoprotein (LDL) cholesterol and triglyceride levels, treatment of hypertension with thiazide diuretics and angiotensin-converting enzyme (ACE) inhibitors, and control of diabetes. All patients with demonstrable PAD should take aspirin to reduce the risk of cardiovascular morbidity and mortality. Although technically cilostazol (Pletal, which is expensive) and pentoxifylline (Trental, which requires thrice daily dosing) have been shown to statistically improve walking distance, the authors have not found them to be particularly effective.

A crucial part of nonoperative management of PAD is a walking regimen. Although supervised programs work the best, these frequently are not available. Instead, an explicit instruction sheet outlining how to do a walking program should be given to the patient. This structured program consists of at least 3 weekly walking sessions of 30 minutes. Patients walk until they experience calf pain; they then stop and rest until the pain goes away and then repeat until the half hour is over. The old adage "no pain, no gain" does not apply to claudication, and patients should be advised not to try and push through the pain. If strictly followed, such exercise programs along with risk factor modification and medical optimization usually improve walking distance to the point of patient satisfaction.

For patients with critical limb ischemia, noninterventional treatment is not the first line of therapy, although risk factor modification is mandatory for the patient's overall health.

Interventional

Many options are available for treatment of femoropopliteal occlusive disease, but few high-quality clinical trials are available to guide decision making. For intermittent claudication, the goal of treatment is symptom relief and improvement in patient's functional status. For critical limb ischemia, interventions aim at relief of pain and prevention of limb loss.

Endovascular treatment options include plain or cutting balloon angioplasty, stenting, and atherectomy. Surgical options are autogenous or synthetic bypass grafts, profundaplasty, and endarterectomy. Hybrid procedures may be used. Bear in mind that there must be adequate inflow before any interventional treatment of infrainguinal occlusive disease.

A classification of arterial lesions established by the Trans-Atlantic Inter-Society Consensus for the Management of Peripheral Arterial Disease (TASC II) is helpful in choosing the right treatment option (Figure 1). Type A lesions are short and in general are successfully treated with endovascular means. Type B lesions are intermediate in length and complexity; endovascular techniques are thought to provide excellent results and should be used, unless open revascularization is indicated for other associated lesions. The treatment of type C lesions is evolving. At the time TASC II was published, type C lesions were thought to be best treated with open revascularization, with endovascular methods recommended only for patients with a prohibitive risk to open surgery (Figure 2). With improved endovascular techniques, the treatment of type C lesions really depends on the skill set of the surgeon. Type D lesions are long complex lesions that are best treated with surgical bypass.

Endovascular Treatment

Endovascular treatment of short isolated infrainguinal lesions has a high technical success rate. The optimal lesions for percutaneous interventions are located in proximal larger caliber arteries, are stenotic rather than occlusive, are short in length and focal rather than multiple, have good runoff, and are in the absence of multilevel disease. Results are better if the indication for endovascular intervention is claudication rather than critical limb ischemia.

The fundamental steps are: obtaining arterial access, identifying the lesion with diagnostic angiography, crossing the lesion with a guidewire, treating the lesion with balloon angioplasty or stent placement, and performing completion angiography to evaluate the result. Arterial access is usually obtained via the contralateral common femoral artery (CFA). Alternatively, in thin patients, the ipsilateral CFA may be used for antegrade access. The brachial artery may be used if the patient has had a prior aortobifemoral bypass. Next, a sheath is placed, and a catheter is used to perform an angiogram and delineate the lesion. The lesion is then crossed with a guidewire, and a balloon is placed over the wire, centered on the lesion, and inflated. The size of the balloon depends on the residual lumen size of the nearby more normal artery. Completion angiography is then performed. If a more than 30% residual stenosis exists or if the angioplasty has created a local dissection, then a self-expanding stent should be placed across the lesion. The authors do not advocate stenting in the popliteal artery because mechanical trauma from artery flexion may lead to stent occlusion. Heparin (~80 units/kg) is administered intravenously at the start of the procedure, and if stent placement is deemed likely, prophylactic antibiotics are given. All patients should already be on an aspirin regimen; after intervention, clopidogrel (Plavix) is prescribed for 6 weeks. Follow-up is routine. After a single postprocedure ABI, the patient is followed symptomatically. If symptoms recur, then a duplex scan is performed to see whether there is in-stent restenosis or a new lesion.

Stent placement should be strongly considered in percutaneous interventions for femoropopliteal occlusive disease because restenosis rates after angioplasty are high, especially for longer lesions. For

Type A lesions
- Single stenosis ≤10 cm in length
- Single occlusion ≤5 cm in length

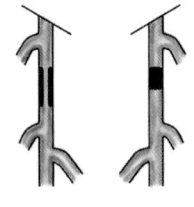

Type B lesions
- Multiple lesions (stenoses or occlusions, each ≤5 cm)
- Single stenosis or occlusion ≤15 cm not involving the infrageniculate popliteal artery
- Single or multiple lesions in the absence of continuous tibial vessels to improve inflow for a distal bypass
- Heavily calcified occlusion ≤5 cm in length
- Single popliteal stenosis

Type C lesions
- Multiple stenosis or occlusions totaling >15 cm with or without heavy calcification
- Recurrent stenoses or occlusions that need treatment after two endovascular interventions

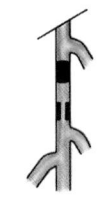

Type D lesions
- Chronic total occlusions of CFA or SFA (>20 cm, involving the popliteal artery)
- Chronic total occlusion of popliteal artery and proximal trifurcation vessels

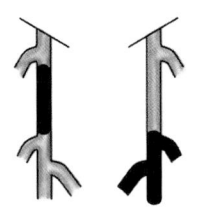

FIGURE 1 Trans-Atlantic Inter-Society Consensus (TASC) classification of femoral popliteal lesions. *CFA,* Common femoral artery; *SFA,* superficial femoral artery. *(From Norgren L, Hiatt WR, Dormandy JA, et al: Inter-Society Consensus for the Management of Peripheral Arterial Disease [TASC II], J Vasc Surg 45[Suppl 1]:S5-S67, 2007.)*

example, the ABSOLUTE trial is a randomized prospective trial that compared implantation of self-expanding nitinol stents with angioplasty in 10-cm SFA stenotic lesions. At 6 months, the rate of restenosis was 24% in the stent group and 43% in the angioplasty group ($P = 0.05$); at 12 months, the rates were 37% and 63%, respectively ($P = 0.01$). At 2 years, restenosis rates were 46% versus 69% in favor of primary stenting compared with balloon angioplasty, with optional secondary stenting with an intention-to-treat analysis ($P = 0.031$). Consistently, stenting (whether primary or secondary) was superior to plain balloon angioplasty in this study.

As technology develops, endovascular options for treatment of femoropopliteal occlusive disease will undoubtedly improve. Drug eluting and absorbable stents are currently being evaluated.

Surgical Treatment

Surgery for femoropopliteal occlusive disease usually entails a bypass operation and occasionally endarterectomy of calcified CFA lesions. Long-term patency rates are superior to those of endovascular interventions. Infrainguinal bypass requires the presence of adequate inflow and outflow. The distal target should be the least diseased artery with the best continuous runoff to the foot. Grafts constructed with autogenous vein have superior patency to those made of prosthetic material. The bypass may originate from the common, deep, or superficial femoral arteries, although use of the proximal SFA in a patient with femoropopliteal occlusive disease should be done with caution. The distal target site may be the above-knee or below-knee popliteal or tibial vessels.

Other than surgeon skill, the major determinant of bypass patency is the conduit. Autogenous vein has always been and continues to be the superior conduit for all infrainguinal bypasses. The greater saphenous vein is the preferred conduit and should be evaluated and mapped with a preoperative duplex scan. Lesser saphenous, contralateral greater saphenous, basilic, and cephalic arm veins are other possible conduits. Nondiseased vein at least 3 mm in diameter can be used; if the bypass is for claudication, smaller veins may be flow limiting and only partially relieve symptoms. Vein bypasses may be placed in a reversed, nonreversed, or in situ configuration. If used in a reversed fashion, the vein should be of similar size throughout. The in situ technique should be reserved for bypasses distal to the knee joint. Cryopreserved vein and human umbilical vein have patency rates similar to prosthetic grafts but are more expensive. However, they can be helpful in situations where infection is present. Prosthetic conduit options are Dacron, expanded polytetrafluoroethylene (ePTFE), and ePTFE bonded with heparin. No clear superiority of one prosthetic over another has been shown.

The conduct of a bypass operation begins with planning the incisions. Unless the bypass is combined with an extensive groin reconstruction, the incisions should not cross the groin crease. Exposure of the common femoral artery is through an oblique skin line incision several centimeters above the crease (Figure 3). If a CFA endarterectomy/profundaplasty may be necessary, one may start with a vertical incision, but kept above the groin crease and only extended distally if necessary. Exposures of the popliteal, posterior tibial, and peroneal arteries are through the medial leg incision used to harvest the greater saphenous vein.

The greater saphenous vein harvest begins just below the groin crease (see Figure 3). The incision is then extended distally along the path delineated and marked at the time of preoperative vein mapping. Alternatively, the vein is marked at the beginning of the case with a bedside ultrasound scan machine. Before the incision is made, use the backside of a #15 scalpel to crosshatch the incision. This makes reapproximating the skin much easier at the time of closure (see

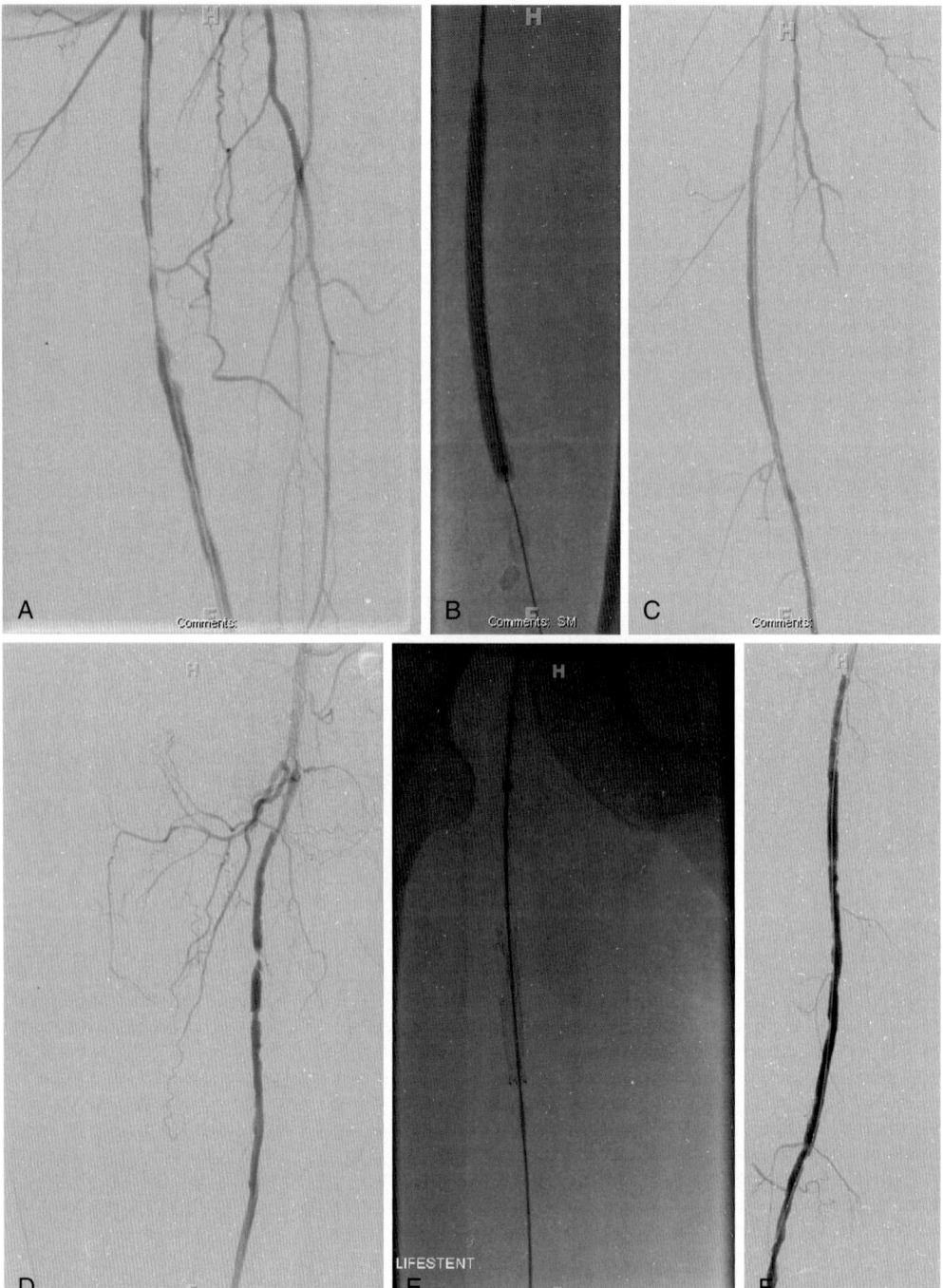

FIGURE 2 Endovascular treatment of Trans-Atlantic Inter-Society Consensus (TASC) A lesions with percutaneous transluminal angioplasty/stent. **A,** Occlusive disease in superficial femoral artery (SFA) of a patient with claudication. **B,** Balloon angioplasty of SFA lesion. **C,** Postangioplasty angiogram showing resolution of lesion. **D,** Another example of occlusive SFA disease in a different patient with claudication. **E,** Stent deployment. **F,** Poststent angiogram showing improvement in flow.

Figure 3). Meticulous technique must be used to avoid damage to the vein. Use a vessel loop around the vein to retract it side to side while dissecting. Ligate all side branches 1 to 2 mm away from the vein so when the vein is distended the ties do not bind. Although veins may be harvested endoscopically or through small interrupted incisions, the authors believe that a long continuous incision affords the best opportunity to harvest an undamaged vein. Lastly, it is always better to have an extra inch of vein than to fall an inch short.

Once the vein is removed, gently distend it with heparinized saline solution. After the administration of systemic heparin, a longitudinal arteriotomy is made in the inflow artery. A local endarterectomy of the posterior plaque is always tempting, but this should be avoided

unless a formal endarterectomy/profundaplasty is planned. The end of the vein is spatulated, and if a nonreversed or in situ configuration is to be used, the most proximal valve is excised with direct vision. Alternatively, Leather Karmody valve scissors (Medline Industries, Inc., Mundelein, Ill) can be used to cut the first valve or two. The end-to-side anastomosis is created with a running 5-0 or 6-0 polypropylene suture. Flow is then restored into the bypass and native circulation. With arterial pressure distending the vein, a valvotome (the authors prefer the Mills retrograde valvulotome; Pilling) is inserted from the distal end. The remaining valves are then gently cut. If an in situ technique is used, then the valvotome is inserted through side branches. Once all the valves have been cut, there should

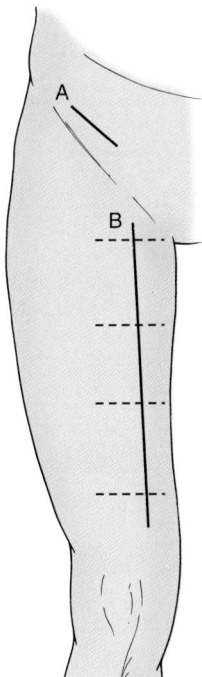

FIGURE 3 Incisions for exposure of common femoral artery *(solid line A)* and greater saphenous vein *(solid line B)*. Crosshatch markings are indicated with *dashed lines*.

be strong continuous flow from the distal end of the bypass. Alternative valvotomes (LeMaitre) may be used, but because of cost concerns, the authors prefer the easy to use and reusable Mills.

Unless the bypass is in situ, it is now tunneled anatomically to the distal anastomotic site. The authors have found that the Jenkner (Aesculap) tunneler is easy to use. For an above-knee bypass, the tunneler is passed just deep to the sartorius muscle and superficial to the SFA. Care must be taken not to pass the tunneler through some of the sartorius fibers. For the below-knee popliteal artery, pass the graft to the above-knee area. With the index fingers from above and below the knee, create a tunnel between the heads of the gastrocnemius muscle and gently pass an aortic clamp from distal to proximal. Gently grasp the end of the vein graft and pull it to the below-knee position.

After each step, check that the bypass is not twisted and that there is still strong continuous blood flow. Mark the distal end of the vein to help maintain orientation and then perform an end-to-side distal anastomosis. If one of the tibial vessels is the distal target, use a pneumatic tourniquet instead of clamps to control bleeding.

After completion of the bypass, confirm bypass patency with palpation of distal pulses. In addition, augmentation of flow distal to the distal anastomosis should be found when checked with a continuous wave Doppler scan. Completion contrast angiography or intraoperative duplex imaging should be used liberally if there is any question concerning the technical result. The most important part of the operation begins once the bypass is in place. Most bypass operations involve lengthy incisions, and closure must be meticulous and not left to the intern. The groin is closed with multiple layers of absorbable 2-0 suture in the femoral sheath, fascia, and subcutaneous layers. The skin closure depends on the incision. If the incision is a skin line, then absorbable 4-0 subcuticular closure may be used. If the incision is vertical, then the skin should be closed with interrupted 3-0 nylon vertical mattress sutures. The long saphenous vein harvest incision is closed with a single layer of running 2-0 absorbable suture in the fascia. The skin is closed with vertical mattress 3-0 nylon sutures, making sure to reapproximate the hash marks made

at the beginning of the case. There is no place for stapled closures during lower extremity bypass.

Although solid data confirming its benefit are lacking, the authors start dextran-40 at 25 mL/h during the operation and continue it until a total of 500 mL has been infused. After surgery, the patients are managed in a regular surgical unit. Home medications, particularly beta blockers, statin, and aspirin, are administered. On postoperative day 1, either a soft cast or compression garment is applied from the knee down. The physical therapy department then evaluates the patient, and ambulation is begun. Once patients are off parenteral narcotics, can void, and can ambulate safely, they are discharged to home. In uncomplicated cases, discharge is on postoperative day 2 or 3.

Strong evidence shows that a graft surveillance program leads to higher assisted primary patency. If a nonspliced greater saphenous vein was used as conduit, the first follow-up duplex scan is at the time of suture removal. If the bypass is normal, then the patient should be rechecked every 4 to 6 months for 24 months and then yearly thereafter. If the bypass was constructed of alternative autogenous vein or spliced vein or an abnormality is found on the initial scan, then surveillance should be more rigorous.

DISCUSSION

The treatment of femoropopliteal occlusive disease is evolving, with many available options but a dearth of high-quality evidence to guide the physician. Clearly, should a bypass operation be performed, every effort should be made to use autogenous vein and not prosthetic for the conduit. Patency rates up to 90% at 5 years for saphenous vein femoropopliteal bypasses can be attained. Graft patency is superior for autogenous vein conduits as compared with prosthetic materials (Table 1).

The debate of open versus endovascular for femoropopliteal occlusive disease has no easy answer. The TASC II guidelines are helpful, but presenting symptoms, patient characteristics, and surgeon training and skill outweigh the guidelines.

Two recent studies compared bypass operations with endovascular treatments, one for claudication and one for critical limb ischemia. Siracuse and colleagues in 2012 made a retrospective comparison of bypass operations with percutaneous transluminal angioplasty with and without stent (PTA/S) as first-time intervention for claudication from SFA occlusive disease. This study showed that PTA/S resulted in significantly higher rates of restenosis and recurrent symptoms when compared with bypass. Operations were associated with a greater length of stay and an increased wound infection rate. Stratified by TASC class, no significant differences were found in restenosis between PTA/S and bypass in TASC A and B lesions. However, C and D lesions had a significantly lower restenosis rate with bypass versus PTA/S. Incidentally, statins also improved freedom from restenosis and symptom recurrence. The study does have the limitation of being retrospective.

The Bypass versus Angioplasty in Severe Ischaemia of the Leg (BASIL) trial is the only randomized controlled trial that compared open surgical bypass with endovascular therapy as the initial treatment strategy for severe limb ischemia. At 2 years, the main clinical outcomes of overall survival and amputation-free survival were similar between the two arms of the trial. An extended analysis showed that beyond 2 years, patients who were initially randomized to bypass had improved overall survival and amputation-free survival rates. Patients who received a prosthetic bypass had worse outcomes than those who received a vein bypass. In addition, patients who underwent bypass after failed angioplasty had worse outcomes than those who underwent a bypass first. The overall conclusion of this trial is that patients with severe leg ischemia should preferably undergo a bypass operation with vein as the initial procedure. Endovascular treatment in these patients comes with a higher risk of failure and a subsequent increased risk of failure with bypass surgery.

TABLE 1: Graft patency, aggregate of multiple studies

Type of bypass	Suprageniculate femoropopliteal bypass			Infrageniculate femoropopliteal bypass			Femorotibial bypass		
	1 y	3 y	5 y	1 y	3 y	5 y	1 y	3 y	5 y
Saphenous Vein									
Primary patency	86%	79%	75%	86%	83%	71%	82%	72%	69%
Secondary patency	89%	83%	80%	82%	87%	83%	88%	79%	79%
Limb salvage	82%	80%	81%				94%	87%	89%
Survival	86%	81%	70%		68%	74%	85%	69%	60%
PTFE									
Primary patency	80%	58%	53%	74%	53%	44%	60%	40%	24%
Secondary patency	87%	65%	70%	69%	48%	46%	65%	47%	28%
Limb salvage	86%	79%	72%	74%	71%	63%	75%	69%	57%
Survival	86%	81%	70%			42%	74%	55%	40%
Dacron									
Primary patency	79%	67%	62%	74%	46%	51%			
Secondary patency	88%	75%	75%						
Limb salvage		94%							
Survival	87%	77%	77%	86%		60%			

PTFE, Polytetrafluoroethylene.
Modified from Ziegler KR, Muto A, Eghbalieh SD, et al: Basic data underlying clinical decision-making in endovascular therapy, Ann Vasc Surg 25:413-422, 2011.

The BASIL trial questions the argument for a percutaneous first approach proposed by some. According to that philosophy, patients who should undergo open bypass are those with failed endovascular therapy. In fact, it strongly argues that for severe limb ischemia, the best treatment is a bypass operation with autogenous vein.

SUMMARY

Femoropopliteal occlusive disease is a subset of peripheral arterial disease that involves the vasculature below the inguinal ligament and above the tibial vessels. Patients may present with symptoms of intermittent claudication, critical limb ischemia, or nonhealing wounds. Evaluation begins with a history and physical examination, and non-invasive studies such as ankle-brachial indices, toe pressures, and pulse volume recordings are used as adjuncts for diagnosis. Medical treatment and life style management should be the first line of treatment for mild claudication. Interventional therapy should be used for severe claudication that affects the patient's function and for critical limb ischemia. Endovascular therapy is probably best reserved for claudication with discrete stenoses or occlusions. For patients with severe limb ischemia, operative bypass with autogenous vein is preferred. Lastly, prosthetic grafts should be avoided if at all possible.

SUGGESTED READINGS

Bradbury AW, Adam DJ, Bell J, et al: Bypass versus Angioplasty in Severe Ischaemia of the Leg (BASIL) trial: an intention-to-treat analysis of amputation-free and overall survival in patients randomized to a bypass surgery-first or a balloon angioplasty-first revascularization strategy, *J Vasc Surg* 51(5 Suppl):5S–17S, 2010.

Norgren L, Hiatt WR, Dormandy JA, et al, for the TASC II Working Group: Inter-Society Consensus for the Management of Peripheral Arterial Disease (TASC II), *J Vasc Surg* 45(Suppl S):S5–S67, 2007.

Schillinger M, Sabeti S, Loewe C, et al: Balloon angioplasty versus implantation of nitinol stents in the superficial femoral artery (ABSOLUTE trial), *N Engl J Med* 354:1879–1888, 2006.

Siracuse JJ, Giles KA, Pomposelli FB, et al: Results for primary bypass versus primary angioplasty/stent for intermittent claudication due to superficial femoral artery occlusive disease, *J Vasc Surg* 55(4):1001–1007, 2012.

Tibioperoneal Arterial Occlusive Disease

Hari Kumar, MD, Raghu Motaganahalli, MD, FACS, and
Michael Patrick Murphy, MD

It has been estimated that 8 to 10 million people suffer from peripheral arterial disease (PAD); this prevalence approximates the prevalence of coronary artery disease in the United States. PAD is a systemic inflammatory process that affects the entire arterial tree; however, anatomic patterns of distribution are associated with specific patient demographics, medical risk factors, and symptoms. Symptoms of PAD are caused by ischemia of the skeletal muscle bed distal to the more proximal location of the flow-limiting arterial lesion. *Claudication* is defined as pain in the thigh or calf muscles with exercise that remits with rest and is indicative of disease in the iliac or femoral arteries, respectively. Critical limb ischemia (CLI) results from insufficient blood flow to meet the metabolic demands of the tissue in the leg and is characterized by pain at rest, ulceration, or gangrene, all heralding signs of eventual limb loss. Patients with a predominant distribution of atheroocclusive disease in the tibial and peroneal arteries are more likely to initially present with signs and symptoms of CLI than are patients with proximal femoropopliteal disease caused by absence of collateral vessel flow to the foot. In addition to recognized risk factors, patients with PAD and tibioperoneal occlusive disease (TPOD) have a higher frequency (>60%) of diabetes mellitus and renal insufficiency. These patients are also at significant risk for vascular disease of the coronary, cerebral, and renal arteries; thus when an intervention is planned, the vascular surgeon must consider these risk factors and always prioritize life before limb.

PATIENT ASSESSMENT

In the assessment of a patient with TPOD, a complete history and physical examination are critical for planning treatment. This evaluation should include an assessment of the patient's functional status with regard to current ability to ambulate, the patient's expectations of therapy, and risk stratification for major adverse cardiac events, with planning for possible intervention. Patients who are physically active, do not have cardiac symptoms, and have normal electrocardiographic findings do not need further workup. Patients with limited physical reserve (are unable to climb a flight of stairs), have had a recent myocardial infarction, or report symptoms consistent with exertional angina should undergo a myocardial stress test. Patients with claudication should be managed conservatively with risk factor modification that focuses on cessation of tobacco use and glycemic control, as fewer than 5% of such patients progress to CLI. A supervised exercise program and treatment with cilostazol have demonstrated efficacy in improving exercise tolerance in claudicants.

A thorough examination of the leg and foot helps determine the likelihood of functional salvage. The examiner should note the patient's ability to walk, evidence of flexion contractures, or other neuromuscular disabilities that may affect ambulation. The presence of local infection, soft tissue edema, venous disease, and prior surgical incisions influence the choice of intervention. The physical examination should also focus on arterial perfusion of the symptomatic limb; the examiner should note presence and quality of the femoral, popliteal, posterior tibial, and dorsalis pedal pulses. The quality of the femoral pulses is a crucial aspect of the examination because it reveals whether there is concomitant suprainguinal vascular disease and whether the common femoral artery (CFA) is suitable for a bypass graft to restore inflow. Inflow disease involving the common and external iliac arteries should be addressed before or during distal revascularization, as discussed elsewhere. Likewise, an atherosclerotic CFA can be reconstructed with endarterectomy at the time of bypass. A palpable pulse in the popliteal artery, felt in the posterior fossa of the knee, usually indicates absence of flow-limiting proximal stenosis or occlusion in the femoral artery and is a common finding in young diabetic patients who have disease predominantly in the tibial and peroneal arteries. Dorsalis pedis and posterior tibial pulses are often not palpable in patients with TPOD, and Doppler assessment with a handheld probe is most helpful. Triphasic signals indicate normal arterial wall transduction of systolic and diastolic pressures; transduction signals become attenuated to a biphasic pattern with mild to moderate disease and monophasic with severe disease. Absence of hair and shiny tone of the skin on the lower leg reflect chronic arterial insufficiency, and evidence of ulceration is a sign of severe ischemia and potential limb loss. A full set of laboratory tests is conducted, with particular attention to renal function, in anticipation of imaging studies with contrast materials that may be nephrotoxic.

In the vascular laboratory, arterial perfusion is estimated from absolute pressures measured at the upper thigh, midthigh, calf, and ankle. A pressure change greater than 20 to 30 mm Hg between each segment indicates intervening flow-limiting disease. Critical levels of ischemia are evidenced by (1) ankle pressures lower than 50 mm Hg for rest pain and lower than 70 mm Hg for tissue loss or (2) toe pressures lower than 30 mm Hg for rest pain and lower than 50 mm Hg for tissue loss. If a venous conduit is to be used for surgical bypass, the authors routinely use duplex ultrasonography to ensure that the proposed vein is adequate, with a diameter of at least 3.5 mm throughout its length. Preoperative marking of the venous conduit is also performed because incisions can be directly placed without creation of a flap, to avoid postoperative wound problems.

Once a patient is determined to have CLI, it is imperative to plan a revascularization procedure with endovascular techniques or surgical bypass because the risk of limb loss within a year of diagnosis is 40%. Although the perception that amputation is a less morbid procedure in the patient with CLI who is at high risk, current data reveal that the 30-day mortality rates for endovascular intervention (2% to 8%) and surgical bypass (2% to 6%) in CLI are similar, whereas the rate is generally higher for primary amputation (6% to 12%). High-resolution imaging is essential for planning revascularization, regardless of whether a surgical or endovascular approach is being considered, and digital subtraction angiography (DSA) with iodinated contrast material delivered via an intraarterial catheter is considered the "gold standard." DSA image quality is not compromised by calcification of the arterial wall, and selective catheter placement in the external iliac or femoral arteries can provide high-quality images of the tibial and peroneal arteries in the lower leg in the presence of multilevel disease. In diabetic patients and patients with renal insufficiency, nephrotoxicity of iodinated contrast material can be minimized with preprocedure and postprocedure hydration with normal saline, administration of acetylcysteine, and selection of a non-ionic contrast agent. Carbon dioxide gas can be used as a contrast agent; it produces excellent resolution and avoids any risk of renal injury.

Multiple-slice spiral computed tomographic angiography (CTA) is a noninvasive technique for imaging the entire arterial tree from the abdominal aorta to the level of the foot; it provides superb spatial and temporal resolution with a single-bolus infusion of contrast agent. The accuracy of CTA in visualizing lumen patency is restricted by calcification in the vessel wall, a frequent occurrence in the infrapopliteal arteries of diabetic patients. Gadolinium-enhanced magnetic resonance angiography is highly accurate for detection of stenosis greater than 50% or occlusion within the entire lower extremity arterial tree. However, it is difficult to estimate luminal patency with calcifications, and gadolinium cannot be used in patients with renal failure because of the risk of nephrogenic systemic fibrosis. Time-resolved imaging of contrast kinetics is used to image the infrapopliteal vessels with greater accuracy, comparable with that of DSA.

In the initial planning for intervention in the patient with TPOD, the arterial tree should be imaged from the diaphragmatic hiatus of the abdominal aorta with continuous image acquisition through the lower extremities, with multiple dedicated views of the ankle and foot. In the setting of impending limb loss in a patient with renal insufficiency in whom duplex ultrasonography demonstrates no evidence of hemodynamically significant suprainguinal disease, selective imaging of the ischemic limb with DSA and adjunctive renal protective measures or CO_2 angiography should be performed immediately, with the intent to treat in the same setting. Furthermore, extensive calcification of the tibial arteries may preclude an accurate assessment of the infrapopliteal arteries; in this situation, DSA should be performed. In the planning of surgical bypass, the tibial or peroneal artery chosen for the distal anastomosis should have continuous unimpeded flow to the plantar arches of the foot, especially in patients with tissue loss. In many diabetic patients, the peroneal artery is the only remaining patent artery below the knee; however, either the anterior branch to the dorsalis pedal artery or the posterior branch to the posterior tibial artery (ideally both) must be intact to provide perfusion to the foot as the artery terminates above the ankle. In patients with occlusion of the tibial and peroneal arteries throughout the lower leg, the plantar and tarsal arteries should be examined as possible sites of a distal anastomosis for limb salvage.

SELECTION OF INTERVENTION

The primary objectives in treating patients with TPOD are to relieve pain, promote healing of ulcers, preserve a functional limb, and restore or maintain the ability to ambulate. These objectives must be tempered by the patient's general medical condition, current ambulatory status, and previous operations. In general, the success of surgical bypass is the availability of a single segment of autogenous vein of suitable diameter, whereas success of endovascular treatment is determined by extent of atherosclerotic disease, as quantified by the Trans-Atlantic Inter-Society Consensus (TASC) I Working Group in 2000. Infrapopliteal lesions are categorized in severity from classes A to D (Table 1). The Bypass versus Angioplasty in Severe Ischaemia of the Leg (BASIL) trial is the only randomized trial (452 patients) in which outcomes of surgical bypass and percutaneous transluminal angioplasty (PTA) were compared and provides level 1 evidence in the field. At 1 year, the amputation-free survival (AFS) rates were equivalent; however, at 2 years, AFS rates were better among the

patients undergoing bypass. The BASIL authors concluded that bypass with autogenous vein is the best treatment for patients with severe limb ischemia expected to survive more than 2 years and that bypass with prosthetic grafts in patients without sufficient autogenous vein are associated with poor results. Thus endovascular interventions are the preferred option for TASC classes A, B, and single-level C lesions, whereas surgical bypass is recommended for multilevel TASC classes C and D lesions in a surgical patient with average risk. Bypass is the first choice with significant tissue loss (ulcer larger than 1 cm or gangrene involving the foot; Figure 1). The surgeon should be both flexible and creative. A patient with an open wound over the anticipated distal anastomosis site or without adequate single segment vein would best be served with PTA.

SURGICAL BYPASS

All patients are maintained on an aspirin regimen before the surgical procedure. Unless it is contraindicated, warfarin (Coumadin) and clopidogrel therapy is stopped several days before elective open operations. However, if limb ischemia is acute, patients are admitted and undergo system anticoagulation with intravenous heparin. Patients are provided Hibiclens towelettes for a total body wash the evening before and the morning of surgery for same-day admissions to minimize risk of wound infections.

Anesthesia and Positioning

Options for anesthesia include local, epidural, and general anesthesia, and selection should be based on the patient's relative risk. Patients with chronic obstructive pulmonary disease and coronary artery disease are best served with local and epidural anesthetics; otherwise the authors prefer general anesthesia for patient comfort, as most surgical bypasses to the tibial or peroneal arteries require 4 to 6 hours. The patient is placed supine on the operating table, and any open wounds are covered with Ioban drape. Hair is clipped from the groin and over the area anticipated for exposure of the greater saphenous vein (GSV)—the authors leave the vein course marked on the skin with duplex ultrasonography before surgery—and the distal anastomosis. The skin of the lower abdomen, both sides of the groin, legs, and feet are painted with ChloraPrep. If the patient has evidence of methicillin-resistant *Staphylococcus aureus* colonization or infection, Hibiclens scrub is used. The authors prepare both legs in case the GSV in the ipsilateral leg is inadequate or inadvertently injured beyond repair during its harvest. Disposable paper drapes are placed to leave both sides of the groin exposed, and then the groin is covered

TABLE 1: Trans-Atlantic Inter-Society Consensus (TASC) classification for infrapopliteal lesions

Class	Lesion characteristics
A	Single stenosis <1 cm long
B	Multiple focal stenoses <1 cm long or one or two stenoses <1 cm involving the trifurcation
C	Stenoses 1 to 4 cm long, occlusion 1 to 2 cm long, or extensive stenosis involving the trifurcation
D	Occlusion >2 cm long or diffuse disease

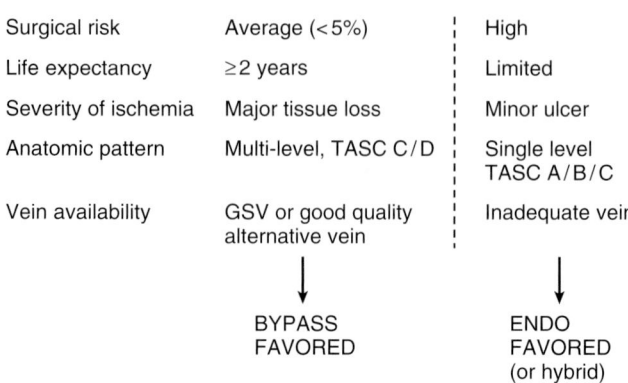

Surgical risk	Average (<5%)	High
Life expectancy	≥2 years	Limited
Severity of ischemia	Major tissue loss	Minor ulcer
Anatomic pattern	Multi-level, TASC C/D	Single level TASC A/B/C
Vein availability	GSV or good quality alternative vein	Inadequate vein
	↓	↓
	BYPASS FAVORED	ENDO FAVORED (or hybrid)

FIGURE 1 Schema for bypass or endovascular treatment (ENDO). *GSV,* Greater saphenous vein; *TASC,* Trans-Atlantic Inter-Society Consensus (class). *(From Conte MS: Critical appraisal of surgical revascularization for critical limb ischemia, J Vasc Surg 57:2, 2013.)*

with Ioban drape pressed into the creases of the skin. Two Bovie electrocautery devices are used to enable simultaneous exposure of the inflow and outflow arteries.

Operative Exposures

Inflow Vessels

The CFA is the artery most commonly used for the proximal anastomosis and is easily exposed with either a tangential incision in the groin crease or a longitudinal incision centered over the femoral pulse. The tangential incision is used if preoperative imaging demonstrates a disease-free CFA and profunda femoral artery (PFA) and has fewer wound complications than the longitudinal incision. The authors use a longitudinal incision if concomitant disease in the CFA or PFA necessitates reconstruction with endarterectomy or patch angioplasty. This incision is started at the inferior border of the inguinal ligament and is extended distally for approximately 6 to 8 cm. The proximal CFA, PFA, and superficial femoral arteries (SFA) are circumferentially controlled with vessel loops. If there are no flow-limiting lesions in the SFA, alternative inflow sites for the proximal anastomosis include the middle and distal SFA at the adductor hiatus and the popliteal artery above and below the knee, which are invaluable when the length of the GSV is limited.

Outflow Vessels

The anterior or posterior tibial arteries are the first choice for the distal outflow anastomosis because they are more accessible and are in direct continuity with the arterial arches of the foot. The peroneal artery is selected if the anterior tibial and posterior tibial arteries are diffusely diseased. The target for the distal anastomosis must be free of calcified plaque because this may lead to dissection of the intima and compromise graft patency. If at the time of exposure the posterior tibial artery is found to have concentric calcifications throughout its length not seen on preoperative imaging, the authors expose the anterior tibial artery and use it, if it is less diseased, and vice versa.

Proximal Posterior Tibial and Peroneal Arteries

To expose the tibioperoneal trunk and the proximal segments of the posterior tibial and peroneal arteries, an incision is made approximately 2 cm posterior to the medial edge of the tibia, starting just proximal to the knee joint and extending distally as needed. If the ipsilateral GSV is being used as conduit, the authors make the incision directly over the course of the vein, which is marked on the skin preoperatively. The fascia of the gastrocnemius muscle is incised, and the medial head is retracted posteriorly with a Weitlaner retractor with dull prongs. The popliteal fossa is entered, and the popliteal vein is encountered medial and anterior to the artery and usually has several large tributary branches at the level of the tibioperoneal trunk that should be ligated and divided. The popliteal vein is then mobilized with sharp dissection and retracted posteriorly with a vessel loop, which exposes the distal popliteal artery. The soleus muscle is detached as close as possible to the tibia to prevent obstruction of view, and a second Weitlaner retractor is placed. Meticulous dissection with Metzenbaum scissors exposes the distal popliteal artery and is continued distally to expose the tibioperoneal trunk and then subsequently the proximal portions of the posterior tibial and peroneal arteries. Care must be taken because there are multiple vein branches that tear easily; thus these should be ligated and divided when encountered to avoid bleeding as the transected vein will retract into the muscle if inadvertently torn. The two concomitant veins that run parallel to each artery are equally friable and send branches that cross the arteries at frequent points that should be ligated as well.

The middle and distal portions of the posterior tibial artery are exposed with a longitudinal incision approximately 1 cm posterior to the medial edge of the tibia (Figure 2, *A*). The fascia is incised longitudinally, and the plane between the flexor digitorum longus muscle and posterior tibialis muscle is entered and expanded bluntly with the surgeon's fingers. The posterior tibial artery can be tracked between the two muscles by following the small muscular arterial branches in a retrograde direction. A Weitlaner retractor is placed for posterior retraction of the flexor digitorum longus (FDL) and gastrocnemius muscles, and the periadventitial fascia overlying the artery is opened with Metzenbaum scissors, again with care to ligate and divide venous branches that cross the artery anteriorly (see Figure 2, *B*). The surgeon exposes the bifurcation of the posterior tibial artery into the medial and lateral arteries by dividing the flexor retinaculum distally. The medial plantar branch continues in a straight course from the bifurcation along the medial portion of the sole of the foot. Division of the abductor hallucis muscle is usually necessary to facilitate exposure. The lateral plantar artery takes a slightly more inferior course to the medial plantar artery and is often larger. Usually a segment suitable for bypass can be exposed before it courses laterally across the sole of the foot.

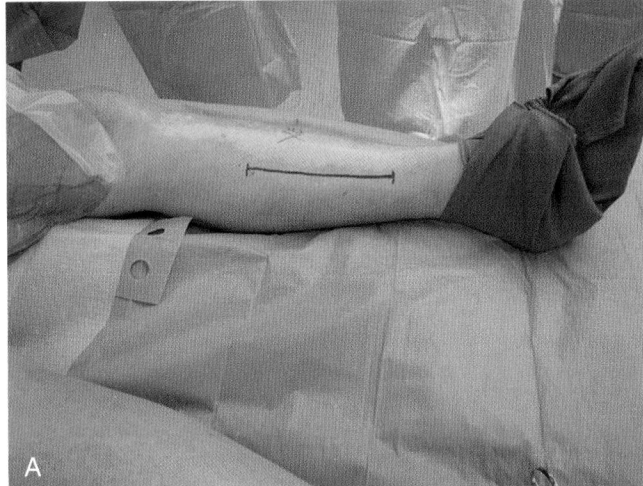

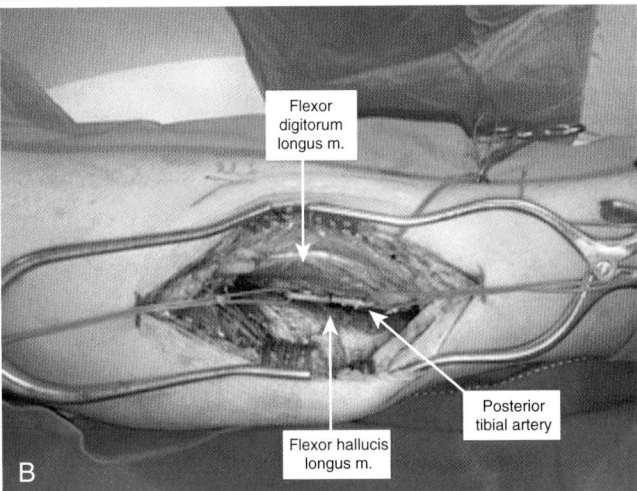

Flexor digitorum longus m.

Flexor hallucis longus m.

Posterior tibial artery

FIGURE 2 Exposure of the posterior tibial artery. **A,** An incision is made on the middle third of the medial portion of the leg. **B,** The posterior tibial artery lies between the flexor digitorum longus and flexor hallucis longus muscles, which are separated with sharp and blunt dissection.

The middle segment of the peroneal artery can be exposed through the same incision used to expose the posterior tibial artery, and the plane of dissection is carried more deeply. The tibial nerve is retracted anteriorly and the flexor hallucis longus muscle posteriorly to expose the peroneal artery and its terminal branches. The distal peroneal artery is exposed with an incision placed laterally over the fibula, and the bone is cleared of all muscular and tendinous attachments (Figure 3, *A* and *B*). The bone is then gently resected for a distance of at least 8 cm, and the peroneal artery lies medially on the flexor hallucis longus muscle (see Figure 3, *C* and *D*).

Anterior Tibial Artery and Dorsalis Pedis Artery

The anterior tibial artery is exposed through a longitudinal incision placed lateral to the anterior border of the tibia (Figure 4, *A*). The fascia overlying the tibialis anterior and the extensor digitorum longus muscles is opened, and the groove between the these two muscles is separated (see Figure 4, *B*), which exposes the anterior tibial artery, its concomitant veins, and the deep peroneal nerve (see Figure 4, *C*).The dorsalis pedal artery is the continuation of the anterior tibial artery onto the dorsum of the foot and is exposed by

an incision made just lateral to the extensor hallucis longus tendon and not directly overlying the artery. Division of the inferior extensor retinaculum exposes the proximal dorsalis pedal artery and its lateral tarsal branch.

Conduit

For patients with TPOD, bypass grafting with single-segment GSV remains the "gold standard" of revascularization; 1-year and 5-year limb salvage rates exceed 90% and 80%, respectively. If the ipsilateral portion of the GSV is inadequate or previously used for bypass, then the GSV from the contralateral leg should be used. If the contralateral leg has extensive PAD that will eventually necessitate bypass, then an endovascular approach should be used in the ipsilateral limb. If no GSV is available and endovascular attempts for revascularization are unsuccessful, then the lesser saphenous vein or the basilic and cephalic veins from the arms are second options, if they are of adequate diameter. The basilic and cephalic veins, if not damaged by repeated venipuncture, can be harvested as a single continuous graft of significant length. In a retrospective analysis, heparin-bonded expanded polytetrafluoroethylene (ePTFE) bypass to the tibial

FIGURE 3 Lateral exposure of the peroneal artery. **A,** The incision is made longitudinally over the fibula.
B, Cross-section view of the lower leg, illustrating the lateral approach with fibula resection.
C, The muscle and fascia are stripped from the fibula, and an 8-cm section is removed. **D,** The peroneal artery is exposed and seen to lie on the surface of the hallucis longus muscle. *(Copyright Herbert Dardik, 2001.)*

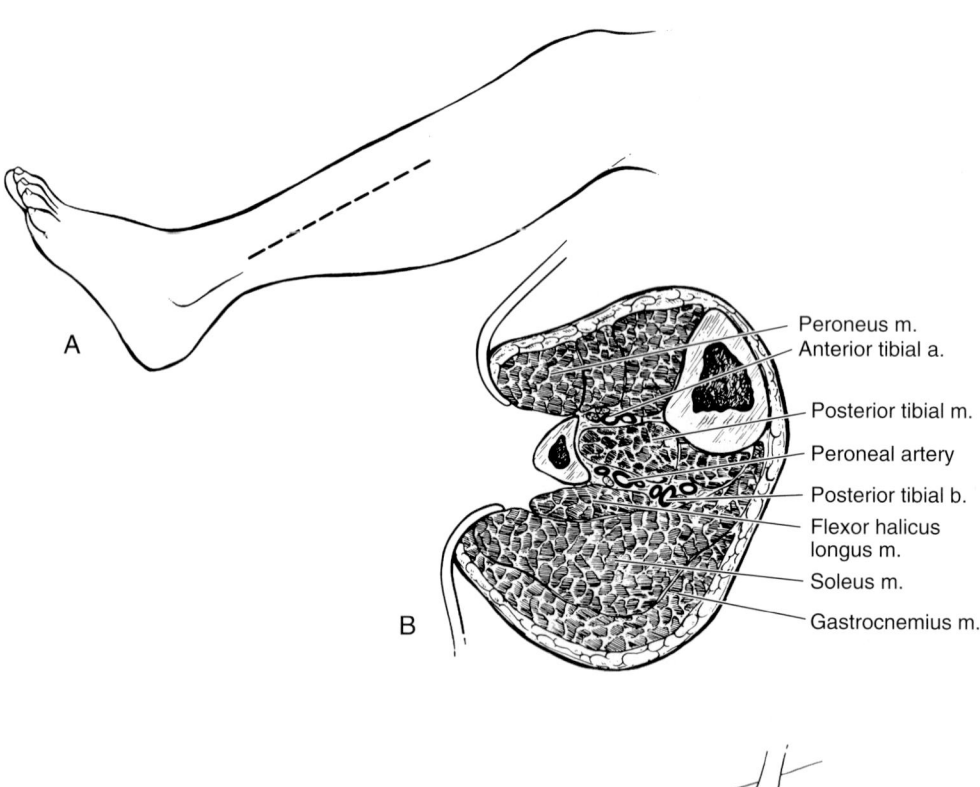

Peroneus m.
Anterior tibial a.
Posterior tibial m.
Peroneal artery
Posterior tibial b.
Flexor halicus longus m.
Soleus m.
Gastrocnemius m.

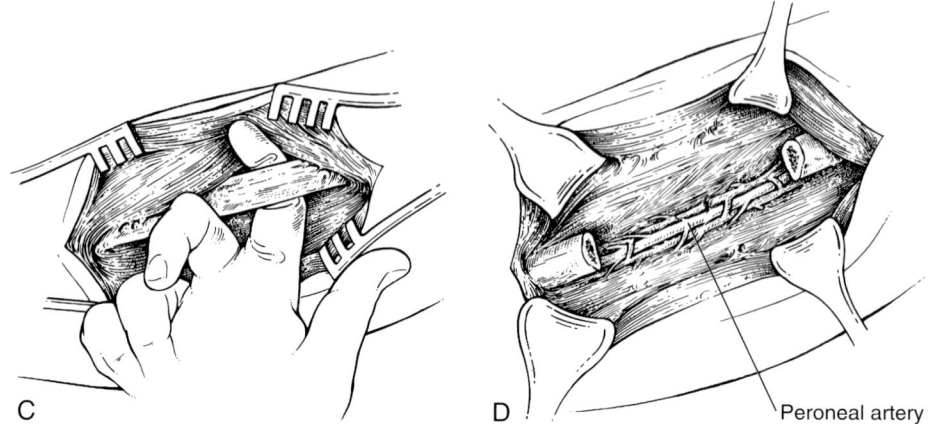

Peroneal artery

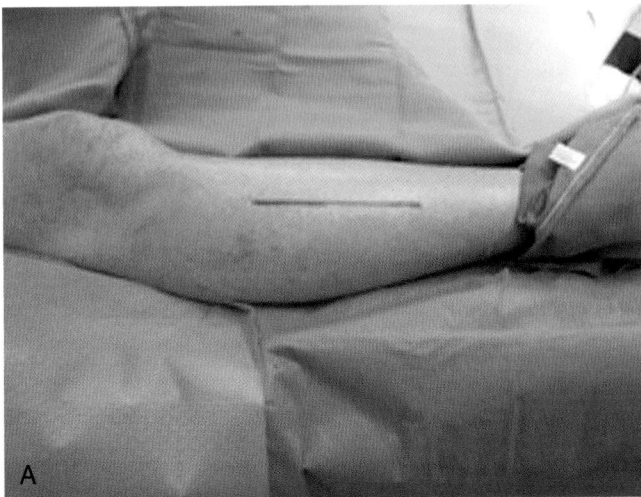

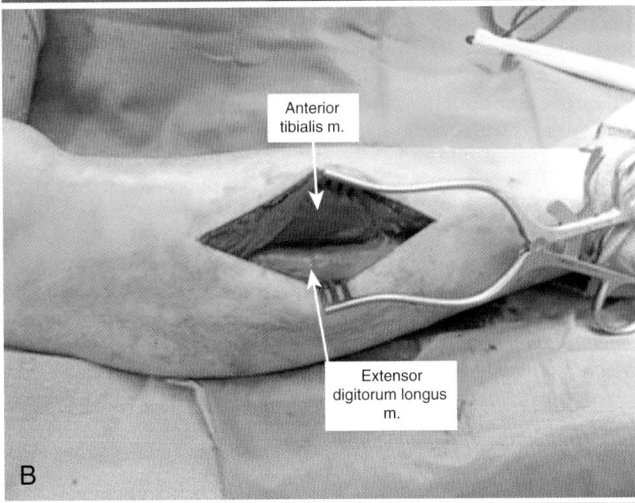

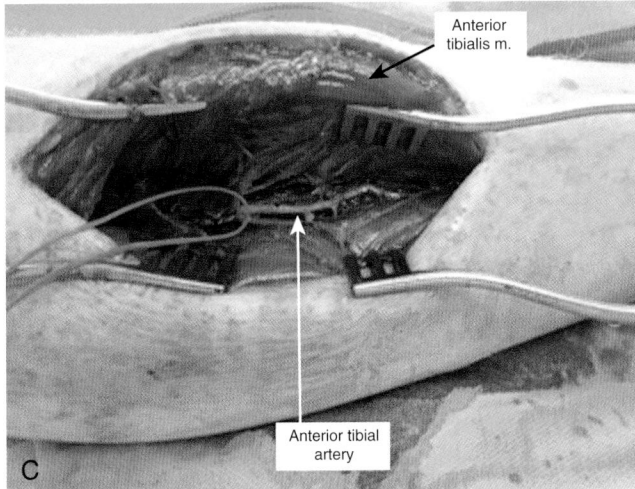

FIGURE 4 Exposure of the anterior tibial artery. **A,** A longitudinal incision is placed lateral to the anterior border of the tibia. **B,** The groove between the tibialis anterior and the extensor digitorum longus muscles is separated. **C,** The anterior tibial artery is exposed.

arteries had a 1-year primary patency rate of 75.4% and is thus an option in an otherwise young, previously active patient without infected wounds. Less optimal choices are composite segments of arm and leg veins and cryopreserved vein allografts; however, all are equivalent to prosthetic conduit in terms of graft patency and limb

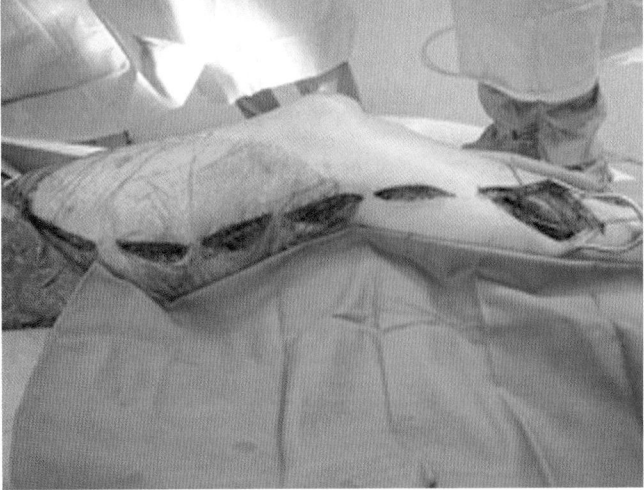

FIGURE 5 The greater saphenous vein is exposed with a series of incisions along its course on the medial aspect of the leg. Skin bridges are left in place to minimize tension on the incision closure and prevent wound dehiscence.

salvage but should be considered when a leg with a contaminated wound is treated.

The GSV can be procured with either open or endoscopic techniques; patency rates and wound complication rates are equivalent. It is crucial that the GSV be exposed and extracted with meticulous technique because injury and repair may compromise patency. The authors use a series of skip incisions with 2- to 3-cm skin bridges to expose the vein (Figure 5), which provides adequate exposure of tributary branches and fewer wound complications than does a continuous incision. The authors ligate branches approximately 1 to 2 mm distal to their origin from the GSV to prevent crimping and luminal narrowing of the GSV. The authors begin harvesting after exposure of the proximal and distal arterial targets, which allows estimation of the length of conduit necessary and helps minimize ischemia of the vein. The GSV can be used in a reversed, nonreversed, or in situ manner. In the authors' experience with bypass to the tibial or peroneal arteries, the best lumen size match is with a nonreversed GSV. For the proximal anastomosis, the authors select the most disease-free segment of CFA and often must sew it to the distal external iliac artery if necessary; thus leaving the vein in situ compromises the ability to reach this far proximally.

Inflow Anastomosis

The distal external iliac artery, CFA, PFA, and SFA are exposed as previously described. Tunnels for the bypass graft are created, and the patient undergoes systemic anticoagulation with heparin at an initial dose of 80 to 100 U/kg, followed by periodic boluses of 1 to 2000 U of heparin to maintain an activated clotting time of 250 to 300 seconds throughout the operation. The CFA is palpated to determine the site that is most free of atherosclerosis. Atraumatic clamps are placed on the SFA, PFA, and proximal portion of the CFA, and an arteriotomy is created with a No. 11 scalpel blade. The arteriotomy is expanded to 25 to 35 mm, depending on the diameter of the GSV. The proximal portion of the GSV is cut with tenotomy scissors in a beveled manner, and the anastomosis is created with 5-0 monofilament suture in a continuous manner. In patients without flow-limiting lesions (<50%) in the proximal SFA, more distal sites can be used for the proximal anastomosis that include the SFA just proximal to the sartorius muscle.

Tunnels for Bypass Grafts

Before the patient receives heparin for the proximal anastomosis, tunnels for the bypass graft are created by advancing a Gore tunneling device or a large aortic clamp beneath the sartorius muscle from an incision at the level of the adductor hiatus, usually one already made for GSV harvest. Once the proximal anastomosis is completed, the vein graft is clamped distally and inflated with blood. The anterior aspect of the vein is marked longitudinally on its anterior surface to prevent twisting, and the distal aspect of the vein is dragged through the tunnel. To reach the proximal third of the posterior tibial and peroneal arteries, the graft is tunneled from the adductor hiatus thorough the popliteal fossa to maintain a straight path. To reach the distal segments of the posterior tibial and peroneal arteries, the vein graft is tunneled subcutaneously and medial to the knee. For the anterior tibial artery, the vein graft is tunneled on the lateral aspect of the leg subcutaneously. This approach avoids acute turns in the graft that occur with a medial path and is especially useful when the patient has had prior bypass surgery.

Outflow Anastomosis

Creation of the outflow anastomosis requires adherence to meticulous technique and gentle manipulation of arteries, many of which are calcified. Loupe magnification is essential. The vessels can be controlled with constricting vessel loops, vascular clamps, or a proximally placed pneumatic tourniquet. An arteriotomy is initiated with a No. 11 scalpel blade, with care not to lacerate the posterior wall of the artery. In general, the arteriotomy should be approximately 1.5 times the diameter of the vein graft because longer anastomoses tend to flatten the hood of the vein and create a sharp angle at the heel, which lead to flow turbulence and consequently a nidus for intimal hyperplasia. Monofilament suture (7 0) is used to create a running sutures line from the heel forward to a point two thirds from the toe. At this point, the authors use interrupted sutures beginning at the toe and proceeding in a retrograde direction, placing five to seven sutures (Figure 6) and tying the last to the running suture line. This technique allows direct visualization of the arterial lumen and precise placement of sutures at the most critical area of the anastomosis, the toe, with regard to flow into the distal artery. Furthermore, the series of interrupted sutures prevents constriction of the anastomosis, as

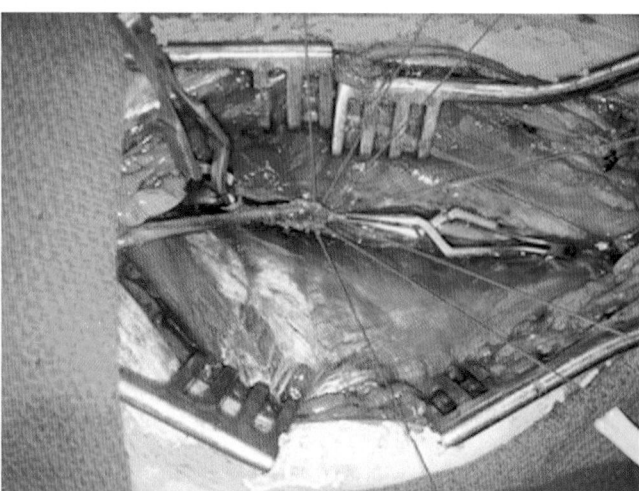

FIGURE 6 The distal anastomosis is created with a running suture of 7-0 monofilament, beginning at the heel and running continuously to the middle of the anastomosis. Interrupted sutures are then placed beginning at the toe and proceed back towards the running sutures. The interrupted sutures are not tied until after placement is complete, to enable visualization of the arterial lumen.

may occur with a running suture line. When the surgeon encounters a patent but diffusely calcified artery, the creation of a distal arteriovenous fistula with vein patch, as described by Neville, may improve bypass graft patency. A common ostium is created between the tibial or peroneal artery and an adjacent vein. A section of GSV is used to place a patch over the common ostium, and the vein graft is then anastomosed to the patch.

ENDOVASCULAR REVASCULARIZATION

Indications for Intervention

With lower rates of perioperative morbidity and mortality, high rates of technical success, and equivalent rates of limb salvage, PTA of the tibial and peroneal arteries is a critical skill of the vascular surgeon. Evidence of long-term efficacy was provided by the Beth Israel Deaconess Medical Center, which demonstrates that PTA of the tibial and peroneal arteries results in 1- and 5-year primary patency rates of 57% and 38% and limb salvage rates of 84% and 81%, respectively. Although some authorities advocate PTA as the first line of therapy in all patients with symptomatic TPOD, the authors advocate its use for patients who do not have a continuous single segment of GSV, those with significant comorbid conditions that increase the risk of problems with general anesthesia and a long operation, and those with a limited life expectancy. According to the TASC I classification for infrapopliteal lesions (TASC II did not include an anatomic classification of tibial disease), PTA is recommended for TASC classes A, B, and single-level C lesions in the tibial or peroneal arteries. In general, lesions that are more amenable to successful endovascular interventions are stenoses narrower than 4 cm or segments of occlusion narrower than 2 cm. Extensive disease that involves the trifurcation, numerous stenoses, a diffusely diseased tibioperoneal artery, or long occlusions are best treated with surgical bypass. In these situations, endovascular therapies may be employed as an adjunct to open surgical bypass to improve inflow or outflow during bypass procedures or for patients who are poor candidates for open surgical bypass because of either a lack of conduit or significant medical comorbid conditions.

Vascular Access and Imaging

Preprocedure imaging with CTA is most helpful in planning the point of arterial access and locations of critical stenoses and occlusions. For tibioperoneal interventions, the contralateral CFA is the preferred access site. If this is not a suitable option, either because of extensive atherosclerosis or because of the presence of an aortobifemoral graft, then the left brachial artery or ipsilateral CFA can be accessed with an antegrade approach. These alternatives are less ideal because of the increased level of difficulty and complication rate. The contralateral CFA is accessed with a 21-gauge needle. The Seldinger technique is used, and under continuous fluoroscopic guidance, a short 5F or 6F sheath is placed in the artery. The patient then receives systemic heparin, with an initial dose of 80 to 100 U/kg, followed by periodic boluses to maintain an activated clotting time of 250 to 300 seconds.

A diagnostic catheter is advanced into the abdominal aorta and exchanged for a pigtail catheter in order to cross the aortic bifurcation and guide a wire into the ipsilateral iliac artery. As with open surgical bypass, inflow and outflow must be considered in maintaining perfusion throughout the infrapopliteal system. The advantage of contralateral retrograde access is that it allows for access to the aortoiliac and femoropopliteal regions; stenoses in this area can be addressed at the same time as the infrapopliteal intervention in many cases. Once the aortic bifurcation is crossed, the short sheath is then exchanged for a longer and stiffer sheath that is parked at the ipsilateral femoral or distal external iliac artery. This allows for stable access to support the various devices and catheters used in infrapopliteal interventions. Additional support sheaths (e.g., tibial shuttle sheath, Cook Medical, Bloomington, Ind) in association with a crossing catheter is used to provide adequate support to cross the tibial arterial occlusions. The authors also use 0.014-inch or 0.018-inch wires with added weight at the tip, which provide enough "pushability" to cross the infrapopliteal lesions. If this route is unsuccessful, the pedal arteries can be cannulated under ultrasound guidance, and a wire can be advanced in a retrograde direction. A snare device can then be employed to grasp the proximal wire and navigate it through the tibioperoneal arteries (Figure 7, A to D). Although these techniques are intuitive, they require significant operator experience as well as adequate imaging tools.

Precise mapping of infrapopliteal anatomy is crucial for proper intervention. In more proximal arterial imaging, diluted contrast material or carbon dioxide can be used to reduce the contrast load. However, for imaging below the knee, full-strength contrast material allows for the best resolution. Imaging of the trifurcation is usually performed with a zero-degree anterior-posterior view. A 30-degree ipsilateral oblique or 90-degree true lateral view may be utilized to properly detail the anterior and posterior tibial arteries. While the tibial vessels are imaged, the catheter should be positioned at the distal popliteal artery.

Balloon Angioplasty and Stent Placement

The mainstay of endovascular treatment of the tibioperoneal vessels has been PTA. Balloons suitable for these interventions range from 1.5 to 4 mm in diameter and are up to 20 cm in length. Currently available tibial arterial balloons are delivered into shaft lengths of up to 170 cm. It is better to use a balloon length that will cross the entire lesion in a single pass. These balloons are noncompliant and low profile, and a long inflation time of 1 to 3 minutes reduces the risk of dissection of the artery. If disease is still present, then the balloon can be inflated for 3 to 4 minutes, or a cutting balloon can be utilized.

The use of stents has previously been as a "bailout" technique after PTA if there was residual stenosis of more than 30% or a flow-limiting dissection after balloon inflation. The stents used in these situations were classically bare metal, and the restenosis rate was approximately 50% at 6 months. There has been a growing trend toward placement of drug-eluting stents (DES) in hopes of improving patency rates similar to those observed with the use of DES in coronary revascularization. Because of the comparable caliber of coronary and tibioperoneal arteries, researchers in several case series have employed coronary DES in the infrapopliteal arteries and have shown that restenosis rates decreased to nearly 10% at 6 months. Randomized trials are currently under way to see whether there is a benefit to routine use of DES comparison with PTA alone. At the completion of the procedure, various commercial closure devices can be used to seal the arteriotomy at the access site. This reduces the amount of time spent on manual compression. Protamine can be administered at the physician's discretion to reverse the anticoagulation.

OTHER TECHNOLOGIES

Mechanical atherectomy devices, both rotational and directional, can be used to remove a portion of the atheromatous plaque from the luminal surface. The advantage of this method is an actual decrease in the plaque burden in comparison with PTA and stent placement; however, the concern is for distal embolization of plaque. Other interventions include laser atherectomy devices, cryo-balloon angioplasty, and drug-covered balloon angioplasty. Industry-sponsored trials are currently underway to determine the role of these devices in endovascular interventions.

POSTINTERVENTION MANAGEMENT AND SURVEILLANCE

After intervention, all patients are placed in a monitored setting in which pulses are routinely checked every 1 to 2 hours. Patients who received an endovascular intervention with percutaneous access to the groin are kept on strict bed rest with the hip in a neutral position for 6 hours. Patients in whom access to the groin was open are kept on bed rest for at least 24 hours in order to decrease the incidence of lymph leak. After a period of observation of 6 hours and if no hematoma is present at the access site, discharge may be considered for patient who underwent percutaneous endovascular intervention. Those who underwent open surgical bypass are kept in a monitored setting for approximately 72 hours to assess for hemodynamic stability and fluid shifts. After this period of time, the focus can then shift to physical therapy and mobility. All patients should be maintained on aspirin regimens after their intervention. Dual antiplatelet therapy of aspirin and clopidogrel is prescribed to all endovascular therapy recipients; strong consideration is given to patients who underwent open surgical bypass as well. Patients who underwent open surgical bypass are started on routine thromboembolism prophylaxis after 24 hours. Patients with a synthetic conduit are started on a therapeutic heparin regimen, with eventual conversion to warfarin (Coumadin). Medical therapy should include beta-blockade to maintain a heart rate of 80 to 100 beats per minute and tight glucose control. Statin therapy has been shown to improve the patency rate in bypass recipients, and this is routinely started if a patient is not already receiving it.

Patients who have undergone bypass grafting are monitored by duplex ultrasonography of the bypass along with measurement of the ankle-brachial index (ABI) before discharge and then again at 1 month, 3 months, 6 months, and 1 year. Increasing focal velocities within the bypass or at the anastomoses or a decrease in the ABI of more than 0.15 should prompt further investigation with angiography (CTA, magnetic resonance angiography, or catheter-based angiography) in order to prevent graft failure. Patients with endovascular interventions are monitored at similar intervals, although reintervention is based on symptoms of CLI rather than on numeric values.

COMPLICATIONS

Immediate complications include hemorrhage or graft thrombosis and necessitate reoperation. Hemorrhage manifests as an expanding hematoma in the groin or leg and possibly hemodynamic instability. Affected patients should be taken back to the operating room for exploration and evacuation of the hematoma in order to prevent shock, infection, or formation of a pseudoaneurysm. Early graft thrombosis is almost always the result of a technical complication but can arise from compression of the graft or an undiagnosed hypercoagulable state. Affected patients should undergo thrombectomy and arteriography to examine for issues related to anastomosis, twisting of the graft, an intimal flap, or inadequate outflow.

Late complications include infection, pseudoaneurysm formation, and graft thrombosis. Graft thrombosis during the period of 1 to 24 months after the initial operation probably results from neointimal hyperplasia, whereas those that occur after this period are typically caused by recurrent atherosclerotic disease.

FUTURE TREATMENT: CELL-BASED THERAPIES

Although revascularization with either surgical bypass or endovascular techniques can result in exceptional improvements in AFS with

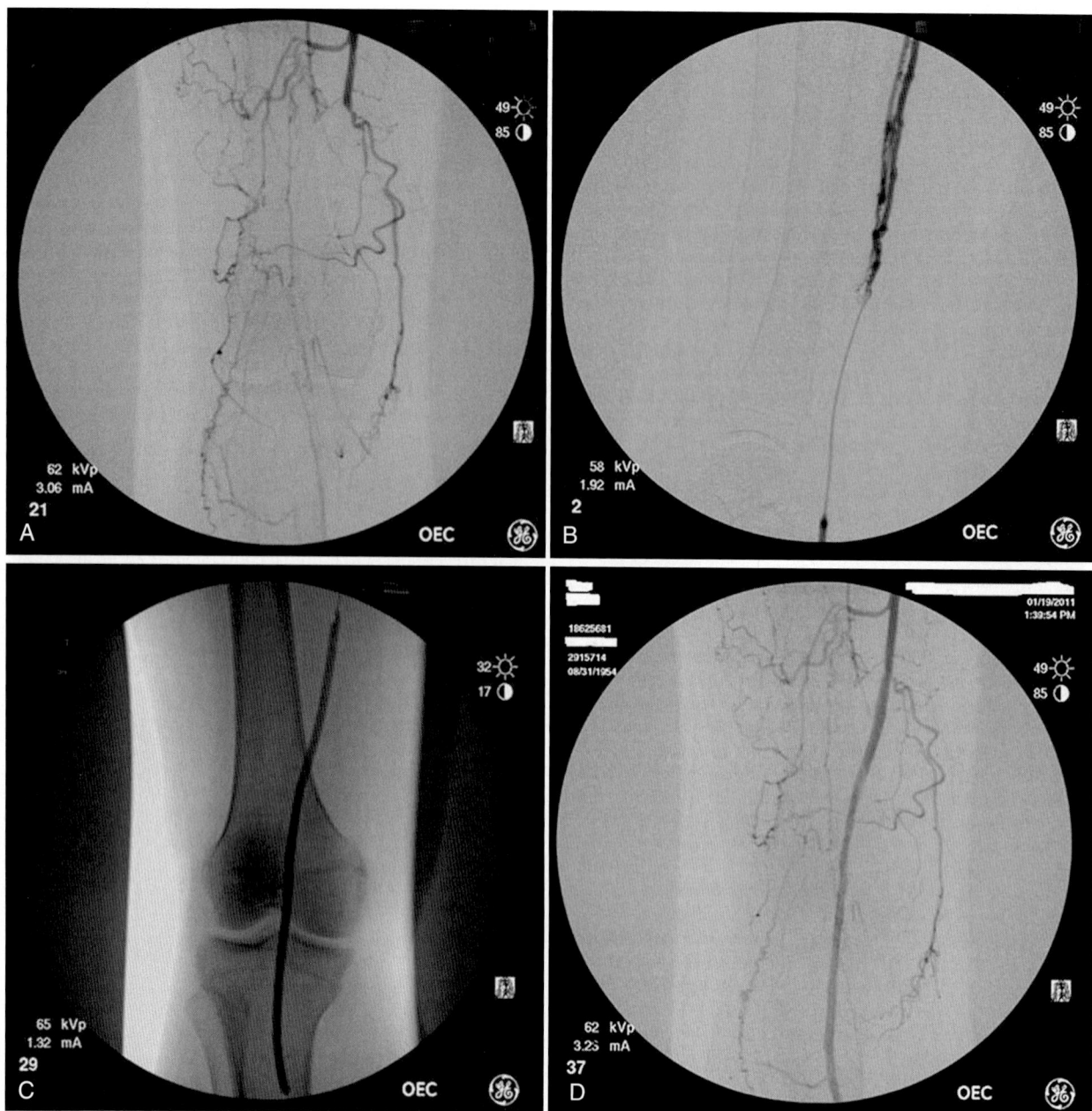

FIGURE 7 Retrograde access of the posterior tibial artery in a patient with critical limb ischemia and previously harvested great saphenous vein. **A,** Chronic total occlusion that could not be traversed with subintimal dissection with a guide wire. **B,** Retrograde access of the posterior tibial artery with a 0.014-inch guidewire and Quick-Cross catheter that is snared from the ipsilateral common femoral artery (CFA) acccess. **C,** Inflation of 3 mm × 20 cm balloon placed in an antegrade manner after wire exchange. **D,** Completion arteriogram, demonstrating unrestricted flow to the ankle. *(Courtesy George A. Akingba, MD, PhD.)*

acceptably low rates of morbidity and mortality, approximately 20% to 40% of patients with CLI are not candidates for these interventions because of lack of conduits or because of extensive disease within the outflow tibioperoneal vessels. For these patients with historically unsalvageable disease, stem cell therapies are emerging as a potential option.

The authors completed the first Food and Drug Administration–approved cell-based trial for PAD within the United States. In this phase I/II trial, the researchers utilized intramuscularly injected autologous bone marrow mononuclear cells (ABMNCs) in patients who were not candidates for revascularization. The AFS was 86.3%

at 1 year; 33% to 50% of patients had clinically significant improvements in arterial perfusion (TBI or ABI > 0.15); and 33% of ulcers healed completely.

These results are encouraging but must be tempered by the fact that the study's patient population excluded those with renal failure or a hemoglobin A_{1C} level higher than 8.5%. Any conclusions regarding cell-based therapies for CLI await the results of a much broader, randomized study. The authors are currently conducting a phase III randomized, double-blind study to test the concept that ABMNCs can affect AFS in patients with CLI with no other options.

CONCLUSION

The management of TPOD should be focused on promoting amputation-free survival. Claudication should be dealt with through medication management and lifestyle modification, and intervention should be reserved for patients who present with CLI. Open surgical bypass and endovascular therapies are available treatment options. There is significant enthusiasm for endovascular therapy because of its decreased morbidity and mortality rates and shortened hospital stay. However, in cases of severe disease, the open surgical bypass is the preferred procedure if the patient is an appropriate surgical candidate and has adequate conduit. Endovascular therapies are increasingly used in the management of CLI, and the role of drug-eluting stents and balloons is now recognized in the management of these complex lesions. Cell-based therapies are an intriguing option for patients who do not qualify for surgical or endovascular intervention, but this therapy is only in the preliminary stages of research.

SUGGESTED READINGS

Adam DJ, Beard JD, Cleveland T, et al: Bypass versus Angioplasty in Severe Ischaemia of the Leg (BASIL): multicentre, randomised controlled trial, *Lancet* 366(9501):1925–1934, 2005.

Beard JD: Which is the best revascularization for critical limb ischemia: endovascular or open surgery? *J Vasc Surg* 48(6 Suppl):11S–16S, 2008.

Conte MS: Critical appraisal of surgical revascularization for critical limb ischemia, *J Vasc Surg* 57:8S–13S, 2013.

Lo RC, Darling J, Bensley RP, et al: Outcomes following infrapopliteal angioplasty for critical limb ischemia, *J Vasc Surg* 57(6):1455–1463, 2013.

Trans-Atlantic Inter-Society Consensus Working Group: Management of peripheral arterial disease: Trans-Atlantic Inter-Society Consensus, *J Vasc Surg* 31(Part 2):S54–S75, 2000.

Trans-Atlantic Inter-Society Consensus Working Group II: Inter-Society Consensus for the Management of Peripheral Arterial Disease (TASC II), *J Vasc Surg* 45(Suppl S):S5–S67, 2007.

Valentine RJ, Wind GG: *Anatomic exposures in vascular surgery*, Philadelphia, 2003, Lippincott Williams & Wilkins.

PROFUNDA FEMORIS RECONSTRUCTION

Tod M. Hanover, MD, Mark P. Androes, MD, and Spence M. Taylor, MD

PROFUNDA FEMORIS ARTERY

The profunda femoris artery (PFA), or deep femoral artery, is critical to the viability of the lower extremity because it is the primary source of blood flow to the muscles of the thigh. In addition, it provides rich collateral flow to the tibial arteries in the event of significant superficial femoral or popliteal artery disease. The PFA also provides collateral flow to the pelvis in the event of common iliac or internal iliac artery occlusion.

BASIC ANATOMY

The common femoral artery (CFA) bifurcates into the profunda femoral artery and the superficial femoral artery (SFA) 3 to 5 cm distal to the inguinal ligament. The profunda femoral artery arises from the posterolateral surface of the common femoral artery and travels in a posterior direction deep to the superficial femoral artery. The medial and lateral circumflex femoral arteries that provide collateral supply to the tibial and pelvic vessels usually arise directly from the profunda femoral artery. They do, however, originate directly from the common femoral artery 14% to 20% of the time. The PFA continues distally to give off three perforating branches to supply the muscles of the thigh before terminating in the distal thigh. The lateral circumflex femoral vein crosses anterior to the profunda femoral artery near the latter's origin. Anatomically, the profunda femoris artery may be divided into three zones. The proximal zone (zone 1) begins at the origin of the artery and extends to the lateral circumflex femoral artery (LCFA). The middle zone (zone 2) begins at the LCFA and extends to the second perforating branch. The distal zone (zone 3) continues beyond the second perforating branch and lies deep to the adductor longus muscle. An oblique line from the anterior superior iliac crest to the medial knee corresponds to the course of the sartorius muscle and serves as a useful landmark (Figures 1 to 3).

OPERATIVE ROLE

The profunda femoris artery offers a variety of uses to the operating surgeon. It can provide inflow as an origin vessel, for infrainguinal procedures such as femoropopliteal bypass or femorotibial artery bypass. It can also serve as an outflow, or target vessel, for suprainguinal procedures such as aortofemoral bypass, axillofemoral bypass, femoral-femoral bypass, and iliofemoral obturator bypass. Finally, in certain situations, localized surgery on the PFA may be indicated (i.e., profundaplasty).

Profunda Femoris as an Inflow Vessel

Indications for use of the profunda femoris as a graft origin include inadequate available vein length, the need for concomitant extended profundaplasty, occlusion or stenosis of the superficial femoral or popliteal arteries (thereby precluding their use as an inflow vessel), and avoidance of groin scar from previous surgical reconstruction or wound infection. The profunda femoris artery tends to be spared of significant atherosclerotic occlusive disease, and when present, the disease tends to be confined to the origin or proximal portion of the PFA, especially in the patient without diabetes (Figure 4).

The route for access to the PFA as an inflow source is dictated by the specific indication for operation and is tailored to the individual patient. Recognized surgical approaches include the standard anterior incision, an anterolateral and anteromedial incision, a posteromedial incision (previously called the posterior incision), and the true posterior incision. If exposure of the CFA is performed to treat occlusive disease within the CFA or proximal PFA as an addition to an infrainguinal bypass, the standard anterior approach through an extended anterior groin incision should be used. For these, the PFA is traced from its origin far enough distally to obtain suitable length for a proximal anastomosis. If the patient needs both prosthetic inflow graft revision and outflow bypass, sufficient PFA should be dissected distally to permit anastomosis of the infrainguinal vein graft to native PFA. This should be done in preference to anastomosis of the proximal vein graft to a prosthetic inflow graft.

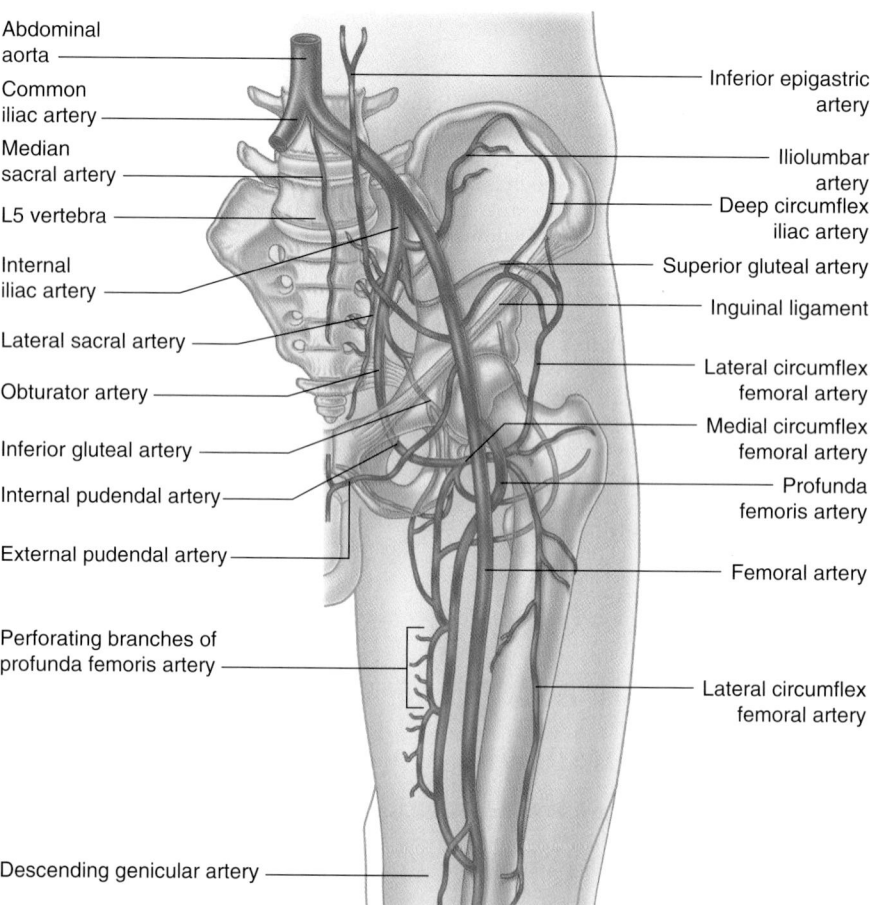

Abdominal aorta

Common iliac artery

Median sacral artery

L5 vertebra

Internal iliac artery

Lateral sacral artery

Obturator artery

Inferior gluteal artery

Internal pudendal artery

External pudendal artery

Perforating branches of profunda femoris artery

Descending genicular artery

Inferior epigastric artery

Iliolumbar artery

Deep circumflex iliac artery

Superior gluteal artery

Inguinal ligament

Lateral circumflex femoral artery

Medial circumflex femoral artery

Profunda femoris artery

Femoral artery

Lateral circumflex femoral artery

FIGURE I Vascular anatomy of the thigh depicting the rich collateral network between the internal iliac artery, profunda femoris artery, and popliteal artery.

Outflow

The profunda femoral artery is well suited as a critical outflow source for suprainguinal bypasses such as aortofemoral, axillofemoral, and femorofemoral bypasses. Often the profunda femoral artery outflow is crucial for maintenance of inflow graft patency. If progressive stenosis or occlusion of the superficial femoral artery occurs, the profunda femoral flow is usually adequate to support aortofemoral bypass graft outflow and maintain limb viability. Although not validated with prospective studies, intraoperative evaluation of a PFA that accepts a 4-mm probe and then allows passage of a soft catheter for 20 to 25 cm implies significant runoff in the presence of SFA occlusion and proves to be adequate for patency of an aortofemoral, axillofemoral, or femorofemoral bypass (Brewster and colleagues, 1987). If the PFA does not reliably serve as the only outflow, then a synchronous distal bypass (such as PFA to popliteal artery or profunda femoral to tibial artery bypass) may be necessary. In patients with tissue loss, synchronous infrainguinal bypass with vein is preferred for in-line pulsatile flow to the foot.

In some situations, a proximal groin incision is to be avoided in a femoral outflow procedure. If the groin is infected or scarred from previous operations or arteriography reveals the profunda target to be more distal, an alternative incision should be chosen.

ISOLATED PROFUNDAPLASTY

Although the role of isolated profundaplasty is limited it can be an effective alternative to more extensive surgery and is an important adjunct when performing concomitant infrainguinal bypass.

Profundaplasty may prove useful in removal of an infected prosthetic graft from the groin, in salvage of a nonhealing above-knee or below-knee amputation, and in improvement of the clinical status of constant rest pain to intermittent claudication with limited bypass or endovascular options. It is not recommended for the treatment of tissue loss unless concomitant distal bypass is performed to provide pulsatile in-line flow to the foot.

The success of an isolated profundaplasty at improvement of distal flow can be estimated with the profunda popliteal collateral index (PPCI):

$$PPCI = AKSP - BKSP/AKSP$$

with AKSP for above-knee segmental pressure and BKSP for below-knee segmental pressure.

A PPCI of more than 0.5 indicates poor collateral development and likely failure of a stand-alone profundaplasty. A PPCI of less than 0.19 represents significant collateral development and an expected good response to isolated profundaplasty (Boran and associates, 1980).

OPERATIVE APPROACHES

Standard Anterior Approach

The standard anterior approach is useful for access to the common femoral artery and the proximal profunda and superficial femoral arteries. It is by far the most common incision used for the

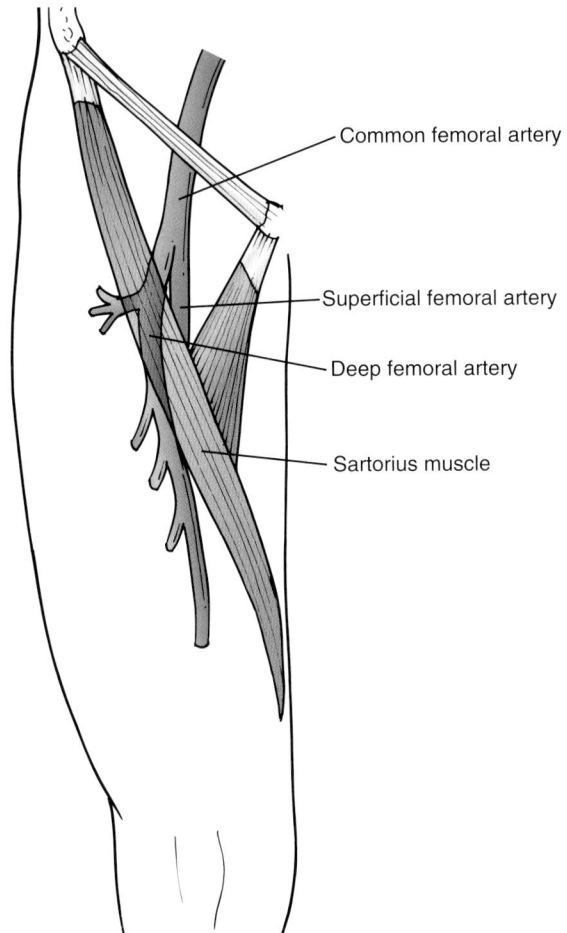

FIGURE 2 The course of the sartorius muscle is represented in relation to the profunda femoris artery.

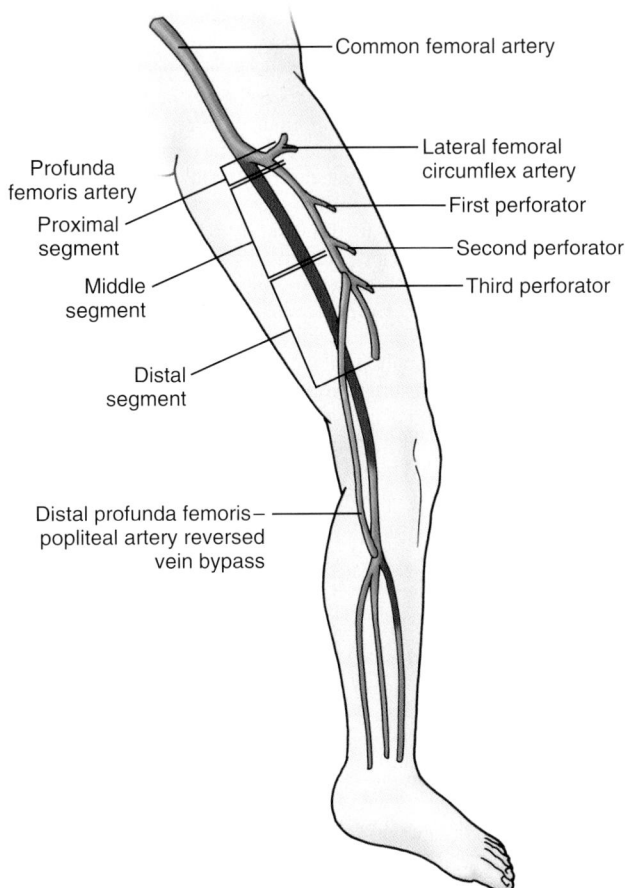

FIGURE 4 Schematic of the profunda femoris artery used as an inflow source for an infrainguinal bypass.

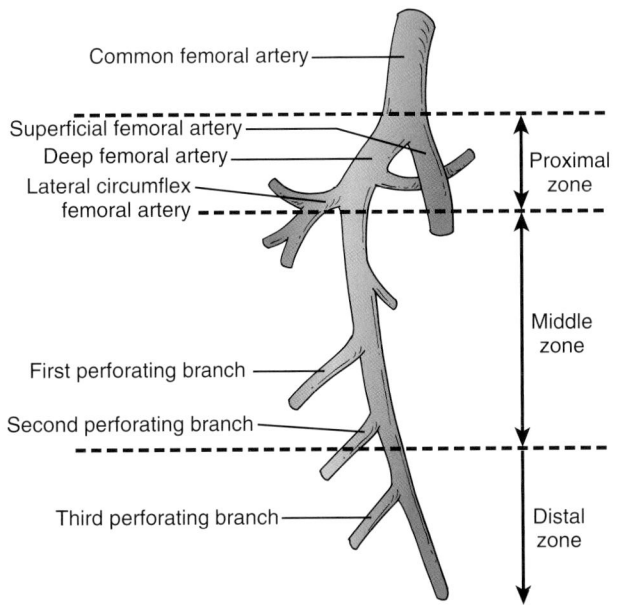

FIGURE 3 The branches and zones of the profunda femoris artery.

aortobifemoral bypass and for infrainguinal bypasses arising from the common femoral artery.

This incision is begun over the femoral pulse or, if the pulse is absent, two fingers breadth lateral to the pubic tubercle and extended distally for 5 cm. The subcutaneous tissue is divided, with ligation of any visible nodal tissue or small veins and the superficial circumflex iliac vein if needed. Dissection is continued to the femoral sheath, which is then opened to gain access to the CFA and proximal profunda femoral and superficial femoral arteries. If the common femoral artery is pulseless, it often can be identified with palpation of its calcifications. Dissection should continue close to the vessel in a relatively avascular loose areolar plain. Occasionally dissection is more difficult because of the inflammatory nature of atherosclerotic disease.

Vessel loops around the CFA assist with more distal dissection. Progressing distally, a visible decrease is seen in the diameter of the CFA. At this point, the PFA branches off in a posterolateral direction. Dissection continues along the lateral aspect of the CFA at the diameter change to expose the PFA. If needed, PFA dissection can be aided with either medial or lateral traction on vessel loops placed on the CFA and SFA.

The PFA is a soft, thin-walled artery, and care should be taken not to avulse any of its branches. The medial and lateral circumflex femoral arteries usually arise from the PFA but as noted previously may come directly from the CFA. Their control needs to be obtained (Figure 5).

Standard Anterior Approach for Extended Profundaplasty

The required length of dissection of the PFA depends on extent of disease and indication for the operation. Extent of disease is judged with palpation of the artery combined with review of previously obtained imaging studies. A single view arteriogram without pull-back pressures can be misleading and may underestimate significant disease layering on the posterior wall.

The profunda femoris is identified at its origin as in the standard anterior approach. Further dissection distally on the PFA requires division of the lateral circumflex femoral vein where it crosses anterior to the proximal PFA. Care must be taken to remain close to the profunda femoris artery to avoid injuring femoral nerve fibers. Dissection is continued distally until past any significant disease. In the mid thigh, the adductor longus muscle must be partially divided for distal profunda exposure.

The patient undergoes systemic anticoagulation with heparin. Vessels loops are pulled taunt to occlude any inflow or outflow.

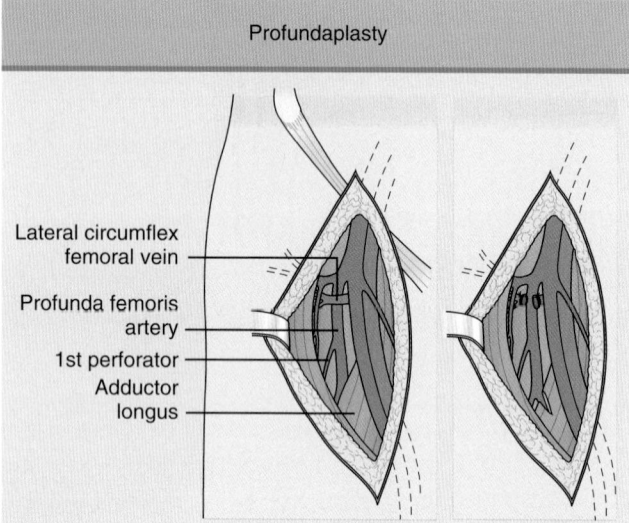

Profundaplasty

Lateral circumflex femoral vein

Profunda femoris artery

1st perforator

Adductor longus

FIGURE 5 Standard anterior approach to the profunda femoris artery.

FIGURE 6 Profundaplasty. **A,** Endarterectomy of the profunda femoris artery. **B,** Tacking sutures placed on distal endpoint. **C,** Vein patch angioplasty.

Profunda clamps are shaped to provide distal PFA occlusion without being cumbersome or intrusive. Because clamps do not put longitudinal tension on the vessel, the arterial back wall is not pulled close to the front wall and thus visualization of the lumen is enhanced. Arteriotomy is begun in the common femoral artery with a #11 blade and extended onto the profunda with Potts scissors until past gross disease.

With significant atherosclerosis, an endarterectomy is then indicated. Proximally, in the CFA, a deep media plane is entered with an elevator, the plaque is divided, and the elevator is used to continue the endarterectomy into the PFA. Ideally, the endarterectomy is continued to the distal extent of disease where a thin, feathered endpoint is often reached. If this feathered endpoint is not seen, then the plaque is sharply divided and its endpoint tacked down with interrupted 7-0 polypropylene sutures. In the authors' experience, tacking sutures are usually needed to prevent distal arterial flap formation and should be used liberally. Remaining medial fibers are removed with fine forceps in a radial fashion.

The extended arteriotomy is closed with a vein patch. If vein is not available, a piece of occluded superficial femoral artery can be used as an autogenous patch. The needed length of this occluded artery is removed and opened longitudinally. A complete endarterectomy of the scavenged artery makes it a durable patch (Figure 6).

Anteromedial and Anterolateral Approach

The anteromedial and anterolateral approaches are quite similar. The anteromedial allows access to the proximal and mid zones. The anterolateral gives access to the mid and distal zones. These incisions are commonly used when groin infection or intense scarring precludes the standard anterior approach. Both incisions are parallel to the sartorius muscle and are begun along the medial or lateral border, respectively, of the sartorius muscle, dependent on the approach chosen. The sartorius is retracted medially for the lateral route and correspondingly laterally for the medial approach. Dissection is continued deep to the SFA neurovascular bundle. The PFA is found lying between the vastus medialis and adductor longus muscle. A dense connective tissue membrane, or raphe, overlying the PFA must be incised to expose the artery. If used as an inflow vessel, a pulse may be palpable through the raphe. If used for outflow, a pulse may not be palpable and continuous wave Doppler scan then aids in identifying its location (Figures 7 and 8).

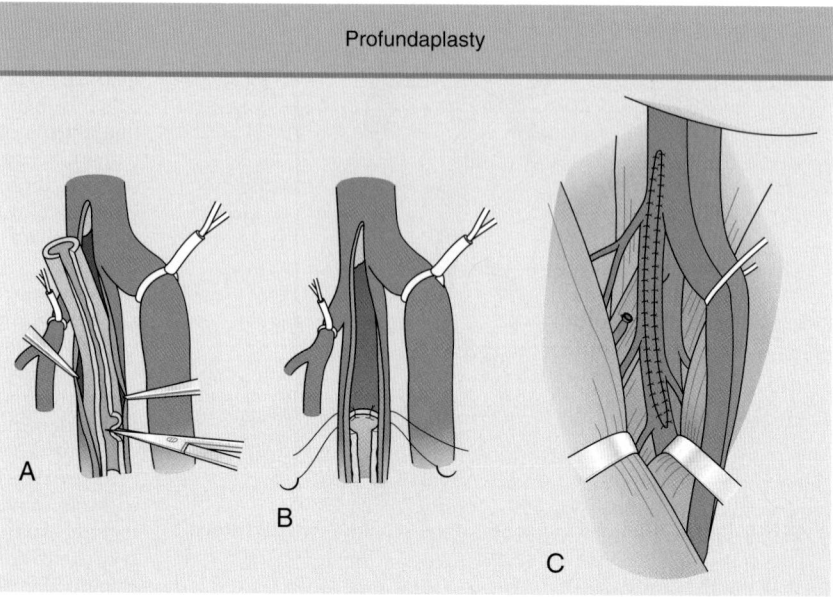

Profundaplasty

A

B

C

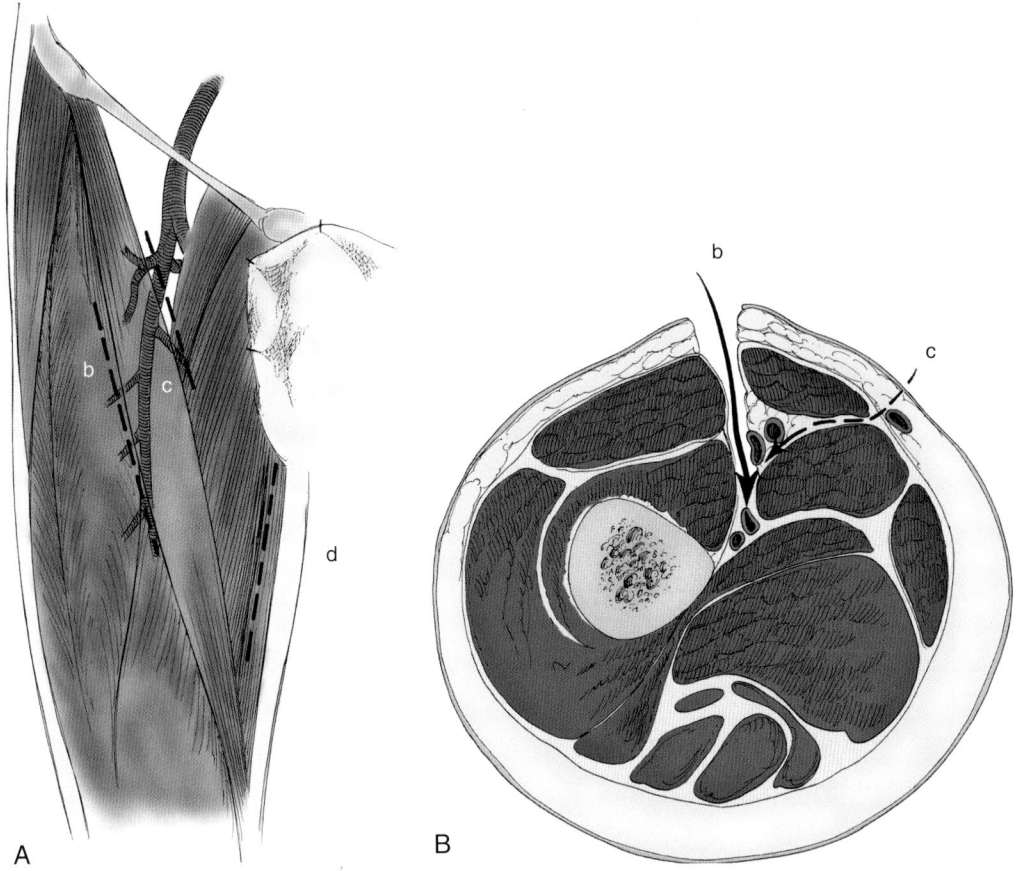

FIGURE 7   **A,** Incisions to expose middle and distal profunda femoris artery *(b)* arterolateral approach, *(c)* arteromedial approach, *(d)* posteromedial approach; **B,** Cross sectional view of the right thigh *(b)* arterolateral approach, *(c)* arteromedial approach.

Posteromedial Approach

The posteromedial approach has previously been referred to as the posterior approach. However, posteromedial characterization is more accurate and less confusing because there is a true posterior approach. The posteromedial approach is best used for situations in which standard groin incision is contraindicated (infection or scar), SFA occlusion is present, or an extraanatomic bypass target is required, such as in the case of an iliofemoral obturator bypass. The distal zone can be reached with this approach and allows access to the profunda femoris artery without encroachment into the subsartorial plane. With the knee flexed and the hip externally rotated, a longitudinal incision is placed on the medial thigh. The deep fascia is opened, and dissection is continued posterior to the adductor longus muscle. The profunda femoris artery is located between the deep portion of adductor longus and the adductor brevis (see Figure 7; Figure 9).

Posterior Approach

The true posterior approach is rarely needed, although it may be the best choice if other approaches are unsuitable because of trauma, infection, scarring, or radiation. Computed tomographic angiography may be helpful for anatomic definition in this approach. The patient is placed in the prone position. A vertical incision is placed to extend one third proximally and two thirds distally to the gluteal crease. The sciatic nerve must be identified. A plane can be developed between the biceps femoris muscle retracted medially and the vastus lateralis muscle laterally. The adductor magnus and adductor brevis are separated from the linea aspera of the femur and then retracted medially. The profunda femoris is thereby exposed.

ENDOVASCULAR THERAPY

Although endovascular treatment of PFA stenosis historically has been infrequently used, it is used more frequently as surgeons have become increasingly familiar with percutaneous interventional techniques. In general, PFA angioplasty is reserved for cases where severe systemic patient morbidity or intense local scarring of the groin precludes open reconstruction. Most disease in the PFA is near the artery origin and thus lends itself to endovascular treatment techniques. When the native common and external iliac and common femoral arteries are patent, a contralateral retrograde endovascular approach to the CFA is used. After heparinization, a sheath is passed over the aortic bifurcation for access to the target lesion. Angioplasty can then be performed in the standard fashion. The use of stents as a bailout procedure in the case of dissection, recoil, rupture, or significant residual stenosis remains controversial at this time.

With a history of aortobifemoral bypass, passing of a sheath from the contralateral CFA across the prosthetic bifurcation seldom is feasible because of the acute angle of the prosthetic bifurcation. In the case of outflow stenosis in the PFA, a left brachial artery endovascular access is preferred. The left brachial approach allows access to either lower extremity without crossing the aortic arch and accordingly should decrease associated complications. With newer, low-profile balloons, access through the brachial artery can be performed with a long 4F sheath (Figure 10).

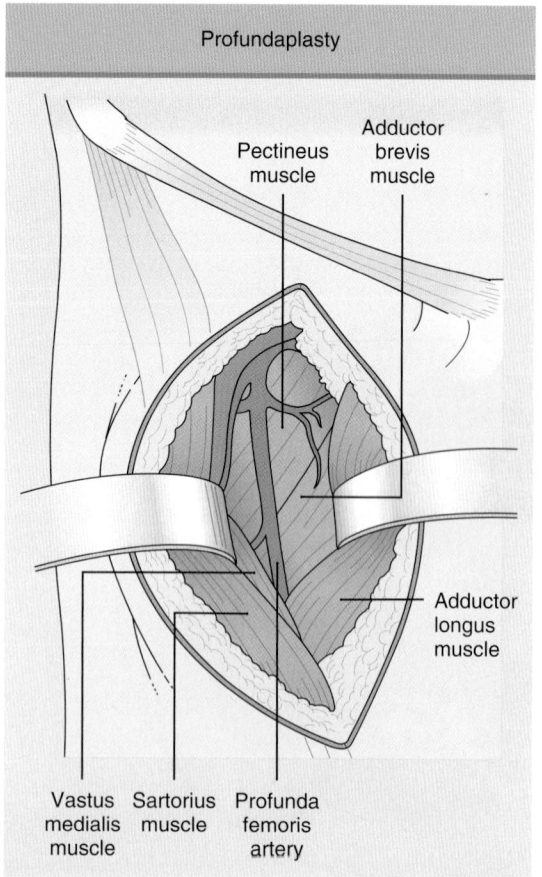

FIGURE 8   Schematic depicting a view of profunda femoris artery through the anteromedial approach.

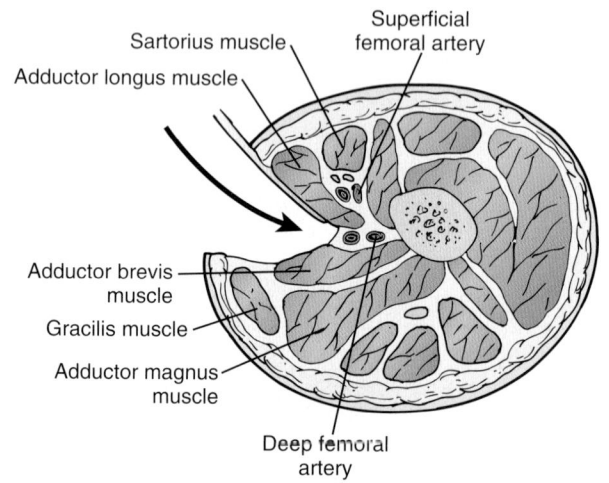

FIGURE 9   Schematic depicting posteromedial approach to the left PFA.

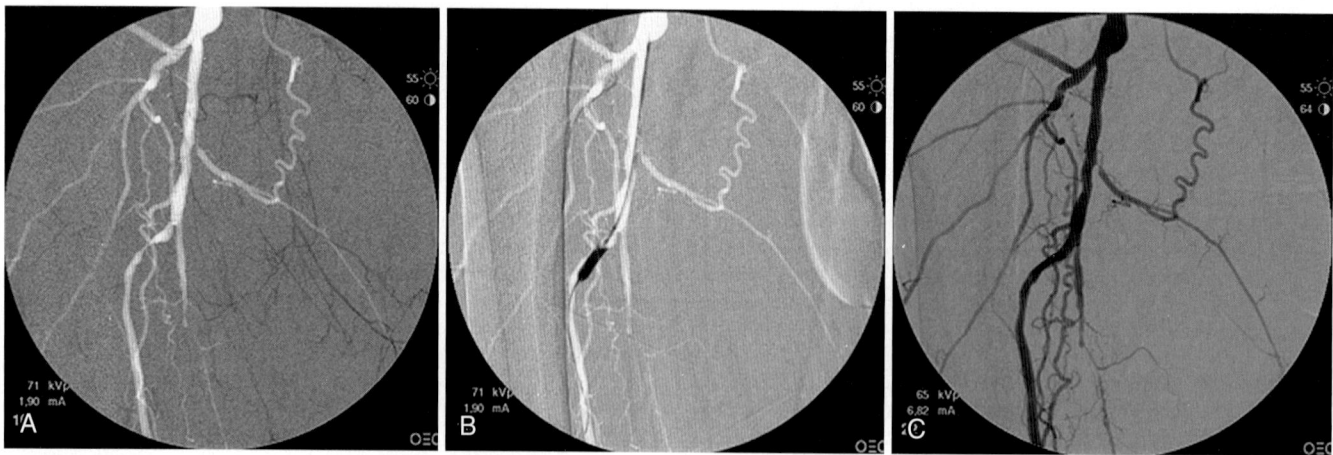

FIGURE 10   Arteriogram. **A,** Profunda femoris artery stenosis. **B,** Angioplasty of profunda femoris artery stenosis. **C,** Profunda femoris artery after angioplasty.

CONCLUSION

The PFA plays an important role in maintaining viability of the lower extremity in the presence of superficial femoral or popliteal artery occlusive disease. It is a versatile vessel that serves as an outflow target for suprainguinal bypass or as an inflow source for infrainguinal bypass. Isolated profundaplasty may be useful in selected cases that do not involve tissue loss. Although controversial, the use of endovascular therapy is increasing and may become more applicable in the future as technology advances.

SUGGESTED READINGS

Bonvini RF, Rastan A, Sixt S, et al: Endovascular treatment of common femoral artery disease: medium-term outcomes of 360 consecutive procedures, *J Am Coll Cardiol* 58(8):792–798, 2011.

Boran CH, Towne JB, Bernhard VM, et al: Profundapopliteal collateral index: a guide to successful profundaplasty, *Arch Surg* 115:1366–1372, 1980.

Brewster DC, Meier GH, Darling RC, et al: Reoperation for aortofemoral graft limb occlusion: optimal methods and long-term results, *J Vasc Surg* 5:363–374, 1987.

Mills JL, Taylor SM, Fujitani RM: The role of the deep femoral artery as an inflow site for infrainguinal revascularization, *J Vasc Surg* 18(3):416–423, 1993.

Nunez AA, Veith F J, Collier P, et al: Direct approaches to the distal portions of the deep femoral artery for limb salvage bypasses, *J Vasc Surg* 8:576–581, 1988.

FEMORAL AND POPLITEAL ARTERY ANEURYSMS

James L. Guzzo, MD, and Ying Wei Lum, MD

OVERVIEW

Peripheral arterial aneurysms in the lower extremity are the second most common type of arterial aneurysm after abdominal aortic aneurysms (AAAs). However, unlike AAAs, the natural history of (true degenerative) extremity arterial aneurysms is not one of expansion and rupture but of thromboembolism. This is particularly true of popliteal aneurysms, which are encountered more frequently than true femoral aneurysms.

True femoral and popliteal aneurysms are typically degenerative aneurysms that occur as a result of atherosclerosis, whereas false aneurysms, or pseudoaneurysms, are frequently the result of access site complications after vascular sheath removal for endovascular procedures. In clinical practice, femoral pseudoaneurysms are more frequently encountered than any other lower extremity aneurysm.

Both femoral and popliteal aneurysms are strongly associated with contralateral extremity arterial aneurysms, and as much as 50% of patients with a femoropopliteal aneurysm also have a coexistent infrarenal abdominal aortic aneurysm. Hence, the diagnosis of a femoral or popliteal aneurysm mandates routine imaging evaluation to rule out concomitant disease of the contralateral extremity and the abdominal aorta before any operative intervention is planned. If indeed multiple aneurysms are identified, sequential treatment of the lesions is preferable, with the more symptomatic or threatening lesion addressed first.

DEGENERATIVE FEMORAL ANEURYSMS

Introduction

True degenerative aneurysms (involving all three layers of the arterial wall) must be distinguished from false aneurysms (pseudoaneurysms) because of differing treatment principles. Although most popliteal aneurysms are true degenerative aneurysms, most femoral "aneurysms" encountered in current clinical practice are usually pseudoaneurysms (see discussion in the next section). In fact, true degenerative femoral aneurysms of the common femoral artery are rather rare. Aneurysms limited to just the deep femoral artery and superficial femoral artery are even less common.

Clinical Presentation and Diagnosis

Femoral artery aneurysms are frequently asymptomatic and can often be discovered incidentally as a pulsatile mass. However, some present with local pain or with distal ischemia as a result of thromboembolic events. Rupture and bleeding is rarely encountered. Once the aneurysms are discovered, patients should be evaluated with duplex ultrasound scan or contrast-enhanced computed tomographic (CT) scan with the objective of identification of other concurrent aneurysms and the extent of the femoral aneurysm. Contrast angiography and magnetic resonance angiography (MRA) are also useful adjuncts that can provide further precise information regarding patency of the distal outflow if concern exists for thromboembolic events.

Treatment

All symptomatic femoral aneurysms, regardless of etiology, should be repaired. Asymptomatic (true) aneurysms larger than 2.5 cm at presentation should also warrant consideration for surgical intervention. Aneurysms less than 2.5 cm typically have a more benign natural history and can be followed serially with duplex ultrasound scan on an annual basis.

Open surgical repair for aneurysms limited to the common femoral artery remains the gold standard management with excellent early and long-term outcomes. Endovascular options are generally not recommended in this location because of the flexion crease in the groin, which subjects the endovascular prostheses to potential kinking, migration, and metal fatigue. Surgical reconstruction for common femoral artery aneurysms is dependent on the extent of the aneurysm, the patency of the femoropopliteal segment, and the patency of the aneurysm itself. Aneurysms that are limited to the proximal common femoral artery (type I) can be repaired with an interposition graft (Figure 1), whereas aneurysms that involve the origin of the deep femoral artery (type II) typically require more complex reconstructions that involve revascularization of both the superficial femoral artery and the deep femoral artery (Figure 2).

Prosthetic grafts (8-mm to 10-mm polyester or expanded polytetrafluoroethylene [ePTFE]) can be used for most cases, although reversed saphenous vein graft should be used if concern exists for an infected or mycotic aneurysm.

The principles for repair of deep femoral artery aneurysms are similar, with the primary goal of aneurysm exclusion and maintenance of distal arterial perfusion. A vertical groin incision is preferred with adequate exposure of the common femoral artery for proximal control and medial retraction of the superficial femoral artery. Overlying venous branches off the deep femoral vein need to be carefully ligated to obtain adequate exposure of the deep femoral artery. Balloon occlusion catheters can be useful adjuncts in obtaining distal control. Although surgical reconstruction to maintain distal arterial perfusion is generally preferred, simple ligation may

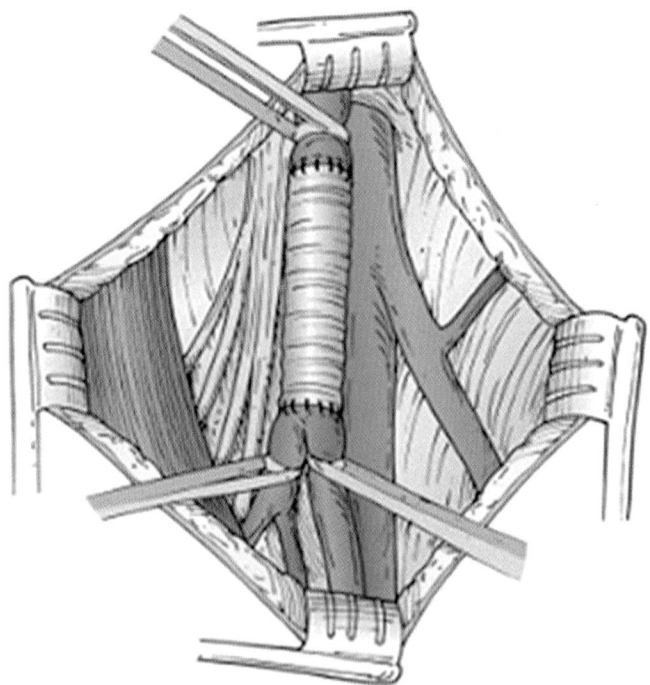

FIGURE 1   Interposition graft for type I common femoral artery aneurysm repair. *(From Ouriel K, Rutherford RB, editors: Atlas of vascular surgery, Philadelphia, 1998, Saunders.)*

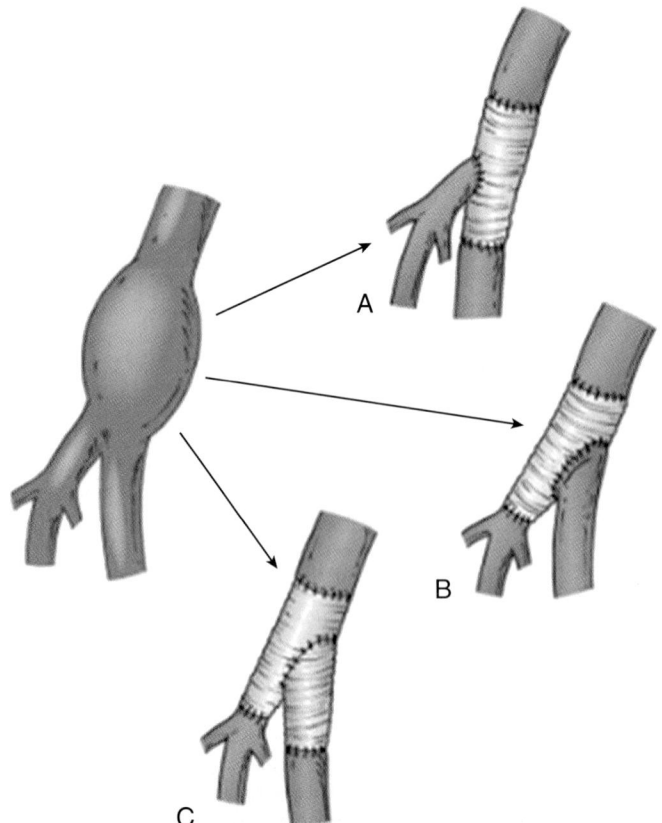

FIGURE 2   Reconstruction options for type II common femoral artery aneurysm repair. **A,** Interposition graft with deep femoral artery implanted in end-side configuration. **B,** Interposition graft with superficial femoral artery implanted in end-side configuration. **C,** Reconstruction to proximal portions of both the deep femoral artery and superficial femoral artery. *(From O'Hara P: Treatment of femoral and popliteal artery aneurysms. In Zelenock GB, Huber TS, Messina LM, et al, editors: Mastery of vascular and endovascular surgery, Philadelphia, 2006, Lippincott Williams & Wilkins.)*

also be used, particularly in patients who present with rupture or when the aneurysm is located in the deeper branches of the deep femoral artery. Alternatively, aneurysms that are located in the deeper branches of the deep femoral artery have also been treated endovascularly with transcatheter coil embolization. This technique can be used safely in selected patients when no disease is found in the common femoral artery and the origin of the profunda femoral artery.

Surgical treatment options for aneurysms in the superficial femoral artery depend on location. Open surgical techniques include direct repair with interposition graft (prosthetic or saphenous vein, depending on size match with the proximal and distal ends of normal caliber artery). Alternatively, arterial bypass in conjunction with proximal and distal ligation is also another option. Although open repair remains the gold standard, a few case reports have used endovascular stent grafts for aneurysm exclusion. This is in contrast to aneurysms located in the common femoral artery, which are less suitable for endovascular repair. Self-expanding nitinol stent grafts covered with expanded polytetrafluoroethylene are typically used and can be deployed either via the ipsilateral common femoral artery or across the aortic bifurcation from the contralateral common femoral artery. Device profiles for such endovascular prostheses have improved in the last decade, and these procedures can be done entirely percutaneously with a closure device or via a common femoral artery cut down, depending on individual surgeon experience.

Results

Published results from individual institutions have reported 5-year patency rates of up to 85% for open surgical common femoral artery aneurysm repairs. Choice of conduit does not seem to affect results. Deep femoral artery and superficial femoral artery aneurysms are rarer; not many case series with long-term results have been reported. Endovascular repairs (particularly for superficial

femoral artery aneurysms) have only recently been reported with satisfactory short-term patency rates. Long-term outcomes remain to be determined. Of early failures recognized after endovascular repair, the lack of adequate distal outflow appears to be a negative prognostic factor.

IATROGENIC FEMORAL PSEUDOANEURYSMS

Introduction

Iatrogenic femoral pseudoaneurysms are well-recognized complications of arterial catheterization that occur in 0.2% to 6% of interventional procedures. They are formed as a result of a direct defect in the arterial wall after arterial cannulation and subsequent sheath removal. The pseudoaneurysm is formed as a result of this persistent communication between the arterial lumen and the hematoma. The risk of pseudoaneurysm formation has been correlated with the use of anticoagulant, antiplatelet, and thrombolytic therapy. Other technical factors associated include inadequate manual compression for hemostasis after sheath removal, larger diameter sheath sizes, and duration of procedure.

Clinical Presentation and Diagnosis

The spectrum of clinical presentation for iatrogenic femoral pseudoaneurysms can range widely. Quite commonly, they are identified incidentally during physical examination with the presence of a femoral bruit, on the day after the endovascular procedure. Another classic presentation is a painful pulsatile mass in the groin associated with hematoma and overlying ecchymosis. Fortunately, presentation with rupture and hemorrhagic exsanguination is less common. Such cases are usually associated with "high sticks" in which the puncture site is along the external iliac artery where manual compression against the femoral head is less effective.

Treatment

The treatment algorithm for iatrogenic femoral pseudoaneurysm is dependent on several factors and is summarized in Figure 3.

In patients not receiving any form of anticoagulation therapy with an iatrogenic femoral pseudoaneurysm less than 2 cm in diameter, several studies have shown that a vast majority (90%) of these lesions thrombose and resolve on their own within 2 months. On the contrary, prompt treatment is usually warranted for pseudoaneurysms greater than 2 cm or pseudoaneurysms that develop in patients undergoing anticoagulation, antiplatelet, or thrombolytic therapy.

The treatment principles differ greatly for pseudoaneurysms versus true aneurysms. Surgical repair was previously the mainstay of treatment, but other methods such as ultrasound scan–guided compression therapy and direct thrombin injection into the pseudoaneurysm cavity have now emerged to be safe and effective first-line therapy. Ultrasound scan–guided compression allows visual

confirmation that flow within the pseudoaneurysm is being compressed while flow is maintained in the common femoral artery. Compression should be performed for 10 to 20 minutes and may be repeated again if flow persists after the first try.

Alternatively, direct thrombin injection can be performed with ultrasound scan guidance. Duplex ultrasound scan should be performed first to evaluate the anatomy of the pseudoaneurysm in relation to the femoral artery (Figure 4). The characteristics of the neck, including its visualization, length, and width, should be taken into consideration because short wide necks have the highest risk for distal thromboembolism as a complication from thrombin injection. After infiltration with local anesthetic, the authors prefer to puncture the pseudoaneurysm cavity with a 22-gauge spinal needle. The tip of the needle may be scored with a sterile scalpel to increase echogenicity and assist with visualization with ultrasound scan. Once the needle is visualized with ultrasound scan and centered in the middle of the pseudoaneurysm cavity, topical recombinant thrombin (1000 IU/mL) is infused percutaneously through the spinal needle with color Doppler visualization. Typically less than 1 mL is required to cause complete thrombosis of the pseudoaneurysm almost instantaneously (Figure 5). Repeat duplex scan examination is then performed to evaluate flow in the femoral artery and vein.

In both ultrasound scan–guided compression and direct thrombin injection, patients are required to remain on bed rest for 6 hours after the procedure, and a repeat duplex examination is performed 24 hours later to confirm thrombosis of the pseudoaneurysm.

Open surgical repair is indicated in patients in whom previously mentioned therapies have failed and in patients whom present with hemorrhage, expanding hematoma, unsuitable pseudoaneurysm neck anatomy, ischemic necrosis of the overlying skin, and compression neuropathy of the femoral nerve. The surgical dissection can

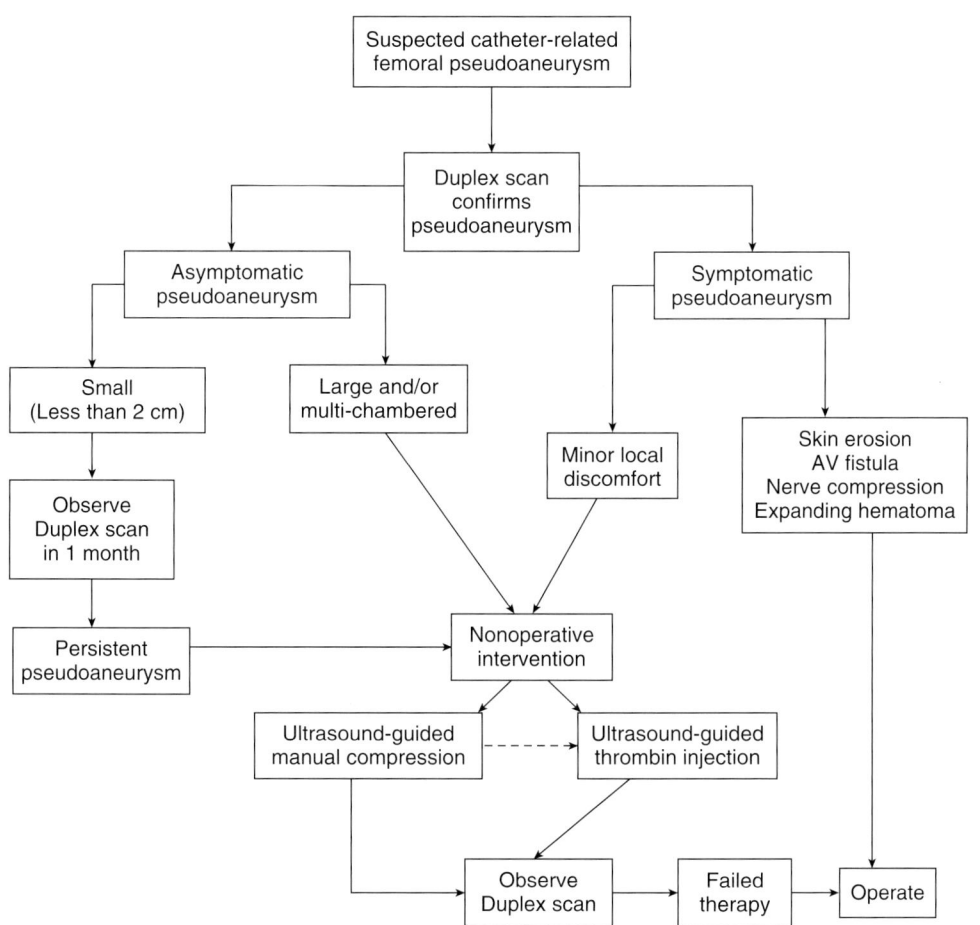

FIGURE 3 Algorithm for treatment of iatrogenic femoral artery pseudoaneurysms. *(Hirsch AT, Haskal ZJ, Hertzer NR, et al: Peripheral arterial disease: ACC/AHA 2005 guidelines for the management of patients with peripheral arterial disease [lower extremity, renal, mesenteric, and abdominal aortic]. J Am Coll Cardiol 47:1239-1312, 2006.)*

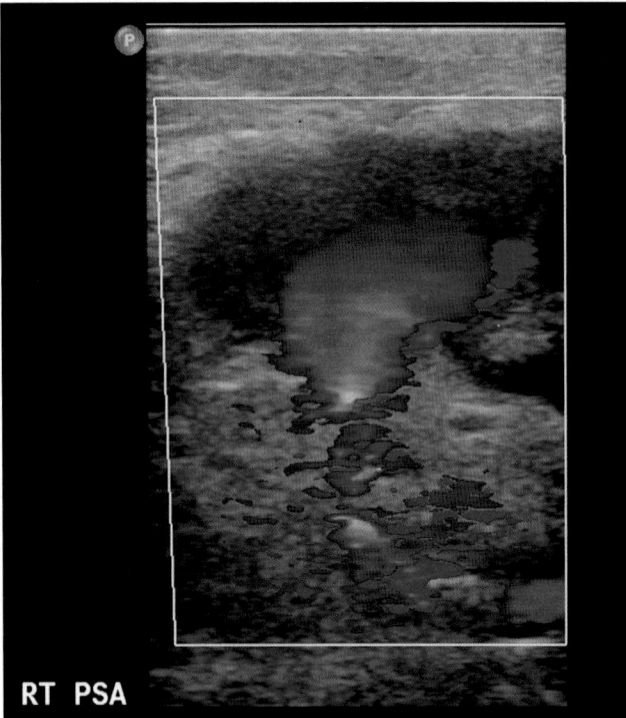

FIGURE 4   Color duplex ultrasound scan shows a pseudoaneurysm coming off the common femoral artery with some surrounding hematoma.

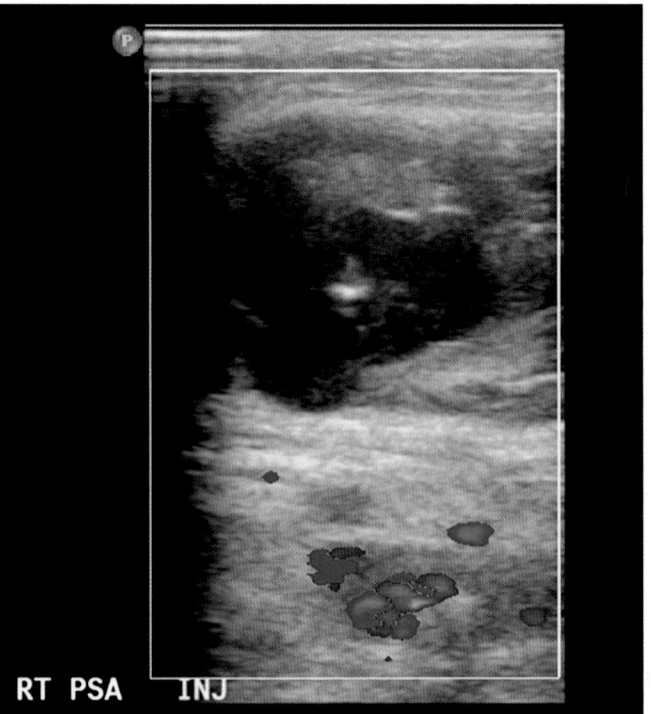

FIGURE 5   Color duplex ultrasound scan shows thrombosed femoral artery pseudoaneurysm with needle in the middle of the cavity *(horizontal axis)*.

occasionally be troublesome given the presence of the overlying pseudoaneurysm above the femoral vessels that bleed profusely once it is encountered. A peanut sponge is often useful and can be placed over the underlying arterial puncture site to assist in controlling hemorrhage while proximal and distal control is obtained. A distal retroperitoneal dissection may sometimes be necessary to obtain more proximal control of the distal external iliac artery in difficult circumstances. Simple surgical repair with horizontal stitches is usually sufficient once the arterial puncture site is clearly visualized and dissected free from the surrounding femoral sheath. The femoral sheath should be closed together in the event of a wound breakdown that can occur, particularly in cases with extensive undermining of the skin from the hematoma cavity. A closed-suction drain should be left in place in these circumstances. In some instances in which extensive skin necrosis is present, wide débridement followed by placement of a wound vacuum device has been used with success.

Results

Although ultrasound scan–guided compression is relatively safe and effective, it has several limitations. From a practical standpoint, this method imposes considerable constraint on the resources and availability of the vascular laboratory. It can be particularly uncomfortable for the patient as well. Furthermore, the results in patients who are undergoing concurrent anticoagulation therapy have considerably lower success rates (<40%). Consequently, direct thrombin injection with ultrasound scan guidance is frequently more favorable. Several studies have reported success rates of 92% to 100% with a periprocedural complication of distal arterial thromboembolism in less than 2% of cases. The recurrence rate after injection is approximately 5% after an initial injection, but repeat attempts of thrombin injection may be attempted safely. The major morbidity of open surgical repair of iatrogenic femoral pseudoaneurysms is related to wound healing issues, particularly in patients who are obese.

POPLITEAL ANEURYSMS

Introduction

Popliteal aneurysms account for nearly 70% of all lower extremity arterial aneurysms and are most commonly true degenerative aneurysms. Similar to degenerative aneurysms of the femoral artery, other coexistent aneurysms are frequently discovered. Popliteal aneurysms are bilateral in up to 50% of patients, and 30% to 60% harbor aneurysms in the aortoiliac location as well. As such, a thorough physical examination is indeed important to ensure all potential aneurysm sites are investigated.

Clinical Presentation and Diagnosis

Popliteal aneurysms are frequently asymptomatic at presentation. However, when they are symptomatic, they can present with a constellation of symptoms that range from compressive phenomena, thromboembolism and acute limb threat, intermittent claudication, ischemic rest pain, and rarely, rupture. When aneurysm size approaches or eclipses 3 cm, compressive symptoms may occur. Symptoms include posterior knee fullness or decreased range of motion, painless pulsatile mass, nerve related pain (paresthesias, foot drop), and congestive venous symptoms of distal swelling and deep vein thrombosis. The absence of foot pulses can be a harbinger of poor outcome because this finding is seen in patients with the highest rate of progression to ischemic complications.

Depending on the manner of presentation (incidental examination finding, acute or chronic ischemic symptoms), a number of modalities can be helpful with an accurate diagnosis that supports physical examination findings and assists operative reconstruction planning. Given that outcomes are best if popliteal aneurysms are treated in the elective setting with reconstruction before acute limb ischemia, imaging the lesions becomes a critical step. The vascular laboratory can be helpful in diagnosis of popliteal aneurysms with duplex ultrasound scan; in evaluation of size, presence of mural thrombus, and velocity through the vessel; and in objective documentation of overall leg perfusion with ankle-brachial indices. CT angiogram can be particularly useful in the elective setting not only for identification of the lesion of interest but also for evaluation of the entire aortic tree to ensure all potentially occult aneurysms are identified. MRA yields information similar to CT angiogram, and both offer three-dimensional reconstructions that greatly aid operative planning. Contrast angiography alone generally is limited by showing only luminal flow through the aneurysm, but it is useful in assessing distal outflow, particularly in cases in which distal thromboembolism is suspected or in which endovascular intervention is being considered.

Treatment

Patients who present with symptomatic popliteal aneurysms should undergo prompt operative repair. Those that present with acute thrombosis or distal embolization have a significantly lower rate of limb salvage. Hence, identification of patients at risk of such complications before occurrence is important. Elective repair is often recommended in asymptomatic patients once an aneurysm diameter greater than 2 cm is discovered. Patient-specific variables, such as medical comorbidities, ambulation and functional status, and life expectancy, should be taken into account in consideration of elective repair.

After delineation of lower extremity arterial anatomy and anastomotic targets with contrast angiography or MRA, elective repair can be accomplished with two open reconstruction options via two different exposures. The medial approach affords the vascular surgeon with two arterial exposures that are very familiar: the above-knee and below-knee popliteal artery segments. Nontunneled reversed or nonreversed saphenous vein grafts with ligation of the artery between the anastomoses bypass the aneurysmal segment and interrupt flow via ligation. Surgeons who champion this approach note the familiarity with the exposures and the ease of harvesting the greater saphenous vein. However, genicular branches may still feed the aneurysm sac between ligation points, and endotension similar to endovascular aneurysm repair has been reported during follow-up, prompting secondary procedures. The posterior approach with the patient in a prone position via a lazy S-curve incision in the popliteal fossa allows the surgeon to perform aneurysmorrhaphy and also allows ligation of geniculate vessels and other tributaries in a manner similar to treatment of lumbar vessels in abdominal aortic aneurysm repair. Proponents of this approach report complete aneurysm excision, ligation of all branches, and relief of any compression symptoms by larger aneurysms. This approach, however, places the tibial nerve at risk, and the surgeon must be sure the aneurysm can be safely controlled proximally and distally from within this space. In addition, vein harvest, if necessary, is more challenging in the prone patient position.

Endovascular repair has become an attractive option for patients with suitable anatomy and outflow vessels (Figure 6). It may have an important role in the treatment of patients with extensive major medical comorbidity as well. The standard considerations for any endograft apply, requiring healthy proximal and distal landing zones and freedom from excessive calcification, thrombus, or tortuosity. CT angiogram is pivotal before any endovascular procedure to appropriately measure for the diameter, length, and number of stent grafts needed to exclude the aneurysm. Percutaneous access is an option for patients with normal-sized proximal and distal superficial femoral or popliteal artery landing zones and can usually be accommodated with a 6F or 7F sheath. For patients with arteriomegaly and larger landing zones that necessitate larger diameter devices, a larger

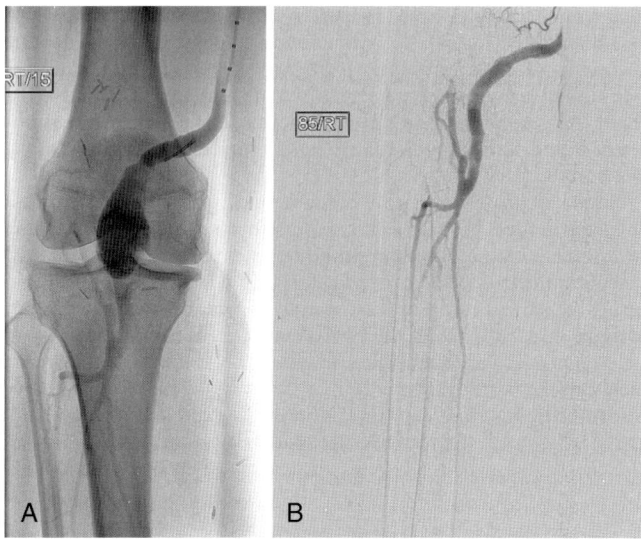

FIGURE 6   A, Arteriogram shows popliteal artery aneurysm with three vessel run-off. **B,** Arteriogram shows endovascular exclusion of popliteal artery aneurysm with two covered stent grafts, with preservation of three vessel runoff.

introducer sheath may be necessary and an open femoral cut down may be preferred.

With regards to deployment of the stent graft, remember that although traversing the knee joint with any endovascular device may not seem appealing, studies have suggested that graft slippage and kinking can be minimized if areas of flexion are appropriately overlapped. In particular, the most proximal position of the stent-graft deployment should be generous and allowed to span widely. This is because the distal superficial femoral artery/proximal popliteal artery is most flexible and where graft migration is most likely to occur if insufficient stent graft is deployed proximally. After endovascular repair, patients should be continued on dual antiplatelet therapy (aspirin and clopidogrel) lifelong. Close follow-up with ultrasound scan or CT angiogram is recommended.

In patients who present with acute ischemia from popliteal aneurysm thrombosis or distal embolism, catheter-directed thrombolysis or mechanical thrombectomy is recommended to restore distal runoff and resolve emboli. Catheter-directed therapy is more likely to be successful if the thrombotic event is recent. If severe limb ischemia is present at the time of diagnosis, then endovascular therapy should not be considered given the longer duration of time necessary to establish reperfusion. Surgical mechanical thrombectomy should be recommended instead in such instances.

If catheter-directed thrombolytic therapy is indicated and initiated, repeat angiogram should be performed at 12 to 24 hours to assess progress and potentially identify a suitable distal reconstruction target. In addition, thrombolysis can treat the microvascular circulation and reperfuse the infragenicular vessels in a less traumatic manner compared with open mechanical thrombectomy. When targets are identified after lysis, arterial reconstruction should be planned expeditiously as described previously. This paradigm has seen improvement in limb salvage rates. However, if no suitable outflow vessel target appears, thrombolysis beyond 24 hours is unhelpful, bypass is not indicated, and full anticoagulation therapy should be continued. Unfortunately, these patients ultimately need amputation.

Results

At the present time, open operative therapy remains the gold standard for elective repair of popliteal artery aneurysms. Several long-term case series have reported limb salvage rates of up to 90% at 10 years for repair of asymptomatic popliteal aneurysms. The success rates are significantly less when surgery is performed for symptomatic aneurysms, particularly acute limb ischemia. There is a trend to suggest that long-term patency is affected by the choice of conduit, with autogenous saphenous vein conduit associated with the best results.

Endovascular repair with covered stent grafts has become an attractive option for repair in select patient populations. The main determinate of successful surgical outcome remains the number of patent outflow vessels. Current data have shown favorable short-term results in patients with at least two vessel outflow who are able to tolerate dual antiplatelet therapy. Most studies that compare open with endovascular approaches reveal that endovascular therapy yields similar early and midterm patency as open repair but frequently requires secondary interventions to maintain patency. Nevertheless, several studies have suggested that endovascular repairs perform at least as well as prosthetic graft reconstructions for popliteal aneurysms. As always, surgeon familiarity with the chosen procedure and patient selection remain critical for successful and durable outcomes.

SUGGESTED READINGS

Hirsch AT, Haskal ZJ, Hertzer NR, et al: Peripheral arterial disease: ACC/AHA 2005 guidelines for the management of patients with peripheral arterial disease (Lower Extremity, Renal, Mesenteric, and Abdominal Aortic), *J Am Coll Cardiol* 47:1239–1312, 2006.

Cina CS: Endovascular repair of popliteal artery aneurysms: evidence summary, *J Vasc Surg* 51:1056–1060, 2010.

Lovegrove RE, Javid M, Galland RB: Endovascular and open approaches to non-thrombosed popliteal aneurysm repair: a meta-analysis, *Eur J Endovasc Surg* 36:96–100, 2008.

Piffaretti G, Mariscalco G, Tozzi M, et al: Twenty-year experience of femoral artery aneurysms, *J Vasc Surg* 53:1230–1236, 2011.

THE TREATMENT OF CLAUDICATION

Neal R. Barshes, MD, MPH, and C. Keith Ozaki, MD, FACS

With the aging population and the rising prevalence of diabetes and the metabolic syndrome, peripheral arterial disease is increasingly common. Among patients with peripheral arterial disease, up to half, including 6% to 8% of the general U.S. population over the age of 65 years, may have exertional leg pains consistent with vasculogenic claudication. Although claudication is not a limb-threatening problem, the symptoms associated with it can be disabling. Furthermore, atherosclerotic disease in the lower extremities stands as a marker for generalized atherosclerosis and an increased risk of cerebrovascular and coronary events.

This chapter focuses on the standard management of lower extremity arterial claudication from atherosclerosis. Recommendations for management are based on consensus guidelines and high-quality clinical data where available. The lifestyle, symptoms, medical comorbidities, and anatomic heterogeneity present with claudication necessitate that decision making be tailored to each patient, but fundamental principles do exist. Attentive management of patients with claudication not only diminishes or relieves the discomfort associated with walking but also lessens the chance of stroke, myocardial infarct, progression to critical limb ischemia, and premature death.

THE INITIAL EVALUATION OF THE PATIENT WITH SUSPECTED CLAUDICATION

The initial evaluation of a patient with exertional lower extremity pain must be thorough. The first objective is to elicit the quality of the pain, location, inciting and relieving factors, consistency and progression of symptoms, and other related characteristics. Typical claudication symptoms occur in a muscular area of the limb (calf, thigh, or buttock) with onset at a relatively fixed distance, are relieved with rest, and have developed gradually over the course of several years. Electric-like "shooting" pains, especially those that began suddenly or after exertion, should raise suspicion for radiculopathy, and pain that is relieved only with sitting or leaning over may be the result of spinal stenosis (neurogenic claudication). Pains that are located at a joint, are worse in the mornings or after inactivity, and are variable in intensity ("good days" and "bad days," especially when dependent on the weather) may be more suspicious for osteoarthritis or rheumatoid arthritis.

In addition to the quality of the symptoms, the impact of these symptoms on a patient's daily life should be assessed. Impact ranges from the mere presence of symptoms with no functional impairment to symptoms that limit some vigorous activities (e.g., unloading a truck at work) to symptoms that are truly disabling and impair even activities of daily living (e.g., walking from the bedroom to the kitchen or from the front door to the mailbox). The severity of typical claudication symptoms is often quantified by pain-free walking distance, but the correlation between this and impact on daily function is imperfect. Claudication at 300 ft may have no impact on an 80-year-old man who lives with his son but may prevent a 55-year-old man from fulfilling his responsibilities on the job.

Evaluation is important for rest pain or nonhealing wounds of the foot, both of which represent limb-threatening problems that may be present in patients with claudication. Rest pain of a vascular etiology may range from cramping pains that awaken the patient at night and are relieved with standing or putting the leg in a dependent position to severe pains present throughout the day and night. Any history of foot ulceration, digital gangrene, toe amputation, or other nonhealing wounds should also be elicited.

Other history of relevance includes risk factors for atherosclerotic disease (e.g., diabetes, hypertension, chronic kidney disease, dyslipidemia, and hyperhomocystinemia) and other comorbidities that may influence functional status, procedural risk, or long-term mortality (e.g., chronic obstructive pulmonary disease, congestive heart failure, cerebrovascular disease, and significant coronary artery disease). Finally, a thorough history related to tobacco use is important. This should include current smoking status, smoking history (measured in pack-years), previous attempts at smoking cessation, and current interest in smoking cessation.

The focused physical examination of the patient with claudication consists of palpation for pulses (specifically femoral, popliteal, and pedal). Pulses should be quantified as normal (2+), weak (1+), or absent (0). Conversely, the presence of a large-amplitude, wide popliteal pulse is suspicious for the presence of a popliteal aneurysm. The feet should be inspected for ulcers or evidence of thromboembolism.

The systemic blood pressure, as measured with an arm cuff, is relevant as well.

Ankle-brachial indices (ABIs), either done informally in the clinic or formally in the noninvasive vascular laboratory, are of utility for objective documentation of resting arterial hemodynamics. Patients with claudication typically have an ABI of less than 0.9 at rest, and most with moderate to severe symptoms have ABIs in the range of 0.6 to 0.8. Some active patients, however, may have normal ABIs at rest (i.e., >0.9). In such patients, ABIs done after treadmill testing can unmask subcritical stenosis, show an abnormal ABI with activity, and better quantify walking distance. Anatomic imaging is generally *not* needed for the diagnosis of claudication and should be reserved until the decision to treat invasively has been made (see subsequent discussion).

Laboratory testing is not necessary for the diagnosis of claudication but may help manage associated risk factors. Specifically, a complete blood count, serum creatinine, fasting blood glucose or hemoglobin A1C, fasting lipid profile, serum homocystine level, and urinalysis (for microalbuminuria) may help identify or manage diabetes, hyperlipidemia, hyperhomocysteinemia, and chronic kidney disease.

Finally, some consideration may be given to other testing to further rule out or rule in nonvascular etiologies that may be causing or contributing to exertional leg symptoms. Although rare, some consideration should be given to other nonatherosclerotic vascular causes of exertional leg pain, including popliteal artery entrapment, chronic compartment syndrome, thromboembolic complications from arterial aneurysmal disease, arterial dissections, arteritis, adventitial cysts, radiation, iliac artery compression syndrome (endofibrosis; e.g., in avid cyclists), or vascular injury from previous trauma.

INITIAL MANAGEMENT OF THE PATIENT WITH CLAUDICATION: MANAGEMENT OF LIMB SYMPTOMS

After the diagnosis of claudication is made, two important objectives exist for the initial management of all patients: (1) amelioration of the exertional limb symptoms and (2) modification of risk factors to minimize the mortality from coronary and cerebrovascular events and to reduce the risk of progression to critical (limb-threatening) ischemia. These objectives refer to the management of patients with claudication alone and do not apply to patients with rest pain or nonhealing foot wounds.

Exercise therapy has been the first-line treatment for patients with claudication for decades. It is a level 1, grade B recommendation in multiple multispecialty consensus guidelines for the management of claudication. Specifically, multiple randomized trials have shown that consistent participation in an exercise regimen doubles the pain-free walking distance of patients with claudication. This improvement is likely the result of biologic changes in the affected muscle groups. Exercise does not improve macrovascular arterial circulation and thus should not be expected to improve ABIs. The vast majority of patients with claudication can safely participate in exercise therapy. Patients with mild to moderate chronic obstructive pulmonary disease, congestive heart failure, and coronary artery disease (without angina) can participate, and data suggest that this may also help lung and cardiac symptoms.

Exercise therapy has most thoroughly been studied in the context of supervised regimens and should be used in practice environments in which a formal (i.e., supervised) exercise program or cardiac rehabilitation is available. In practice environments without access to supervised exercise programs, a home-based exercise regimen can serve as an alternative. Although the adherence to home-based regimens is lower than adherence to supervised programs, home-based programs can have comparable effectiveness and, because of the negligible costs, may represent a cost-effective alternative.

Asking a patient to initiate a home-based regimen is more than simple advice to "go out and walk," however. Specifically, the authors recommend that patients with claudication start by walking at least 3 times per week for 30 minutes initially, working up to 60 minutes per walking session and as many days per week the patient is willing to do. Patients are instructed to walk until symptoms appear, to stop walking and remain standing until symptoms resolve, and then to start walking again to repeat this cycle. A route near the patient's home is recommended because it is more accessible and because a consistent route can be used to track progress. In warm climates, indoor shopping malls serve as a comfortable venue. Several investigators have shown that pedometers improve patient adherence to walking regimens, and patients should be asked to log their efforts in a journal to document compliance and further track progress. Finally, walking is generally the best form of exercise because of the ease and accessibility to this modality, but other forms of cardiovascular activity such as bicycling, stationary bicycle riding, or swimming may suffice. Regardless of the exercise modality chosen, adherence to and improvement with the exercise program should be assessed with frequent follow-up, either through return clinic visits or telephone calls.

In addition, reducing obesity can help reduce claudication symptoms, as the increased metabolic demand of walking with an obese body habitus can be lessened by simple weight loss. Obviously, an exercise regimen may help in this regard, but obese patients with claudication should specifically be counseled on the benefits of weight loss for both amelioration of limb symptoms and risk factor modification (see subsequent discussion).

Two medications are approved by the U.S. Food and Drug Administration (FDA) for intermittent claudication treatment. Consensus guidelines recommend a trial of cilostazol for *all* patients with lifestyle-limiting claudication without congestive heart failure (level A evidence). Cilostazol is a reversible phosphodiesterase inhibitor and is thought to improve symptoms by acting as a vasodilator. In eight randomized clinical trials, patients with claudication given cilostazol had a 67% improvement in pain-free walking distance. Pentoxifylline, a xanthine derivative that enhances red blood cell deformability, has also been extensively studied in the context of claudication. Multiple randomized clinical trials suggest a statistically significant benefit, but the clinical improvement in absolute walking distance with pentoxifylline appears to be small if any.

Data from several small randomized clinical trials suggest that the over-the-counter supplements ginkgo biloba, propionyl-L-carnitine, and L-arginine may all improve walking distance among patients with claudication who participate in an exercise regimen. Although the results from many of these studies reached statistical significance, whether the benefits from these supplements translate to meaningful clinical benefits is not clear. Likewise, some small randomized clinical trials have suggested that simvastatin may improve pain-free walking distance among patients with claudication, but its role has yet to be defined.

INITIAL MANAGEMENT OF THE PATIENT WITH CLAUDICATION: MANAGEMENT OF GENERALIZED ATHEROSCLEROSIS

In addition to addressing the limb symptoms, the clinician must educate the patient on the generalized nature of atherosclerosis and address modifiable risk factors (this should also be done for patients without claudication symptoms who are found through ABIs or other testing to have asymptomatic peripheral arterial disease). The simplest way for surgeons to remember the critical elements of risk-factor modification is by recalling the ABC(D)s: *A*spirin, *B*eta-blockers/management of hypertension, *C*holesterol management, and *D*iabetes management. Antiplatelet therapy reduces overall cerebrovascular and coronary event rates by 25% and is recommended in all patients with peripheral arterial disease. Beta-blockers or other antihypertensives (including angiotensin-converting enzyme [ACE] inhibitors or thiazide diuretics) should be considered for all patients with peripheral arterial disease and for systolic blood pressure above the goal of 130 mm Hg for patients with diabetes or 140 mm Hg for patients without diabetes. The identification and management of dyslipidemia is also important in reducing the risk of cerebrovascular and coronary events. Among patients with peripheral arterial disease, the goal low-density lipoprotein (LDL) is less than 100 mg/dL. This goal can be achieved through statin therapy if diet modification alone does not suffice. Patients with diabetes with peripheral arterial disease should be urged to work with their primary care providers to achieve tight control of glucose because this too has been shown to reduce the risk of cardiovascular mortality.

Smoking cessation is critical and should be urged to all patients with peripheral arterial disease who remain active smokers. Smoking cessation has clear benefit in reducing cerebrovascular and coronary events, and patients with claudication who smoke should be reminded that it is never too late in life to derive health benefits from smoking cessation. Interest in smoking cessation should be assessed, and smokers should be counseled in strategies to succeed at smoking cessation efforts and be offered pharmacologic adjuncts (including nicotine replacement therapies, bupropion, or varenicline). In addition to the clear decrease in risk of cerebrovascular and coronary events and the decreased risk of cancer, data suggest that smoking cessation among patients with claudication can decrease the likelihood of progression to rest pain.

Patients with peripheral arterial disease, especially those with diabetic sensory neuropathy, should be taught the importance of daily inspection of their feet and shoes. Patients and their families should also be educated on the signs and symptoms of critical limb ischemia (rest pain and nonhealing ulcers) and be instructed to return for reevaluation should these develop.

FOLLOW-UP AFTER INITIATION OF MEDICAL MANAGEMENT AND SELECTION OF PATIENTS FOR INTERVENTION

An exercise regimen has remained the first-line therapy for the exertional limb symptoms of claudication because it is safe, effective, durable, and low cost. Patients should not be expected to successfully implement an exercise regimen, however, after a single clinic visit. Multiple follow-up appointments should be planned to verify interest and readiness, identify obstacles, and assess adherence to exercise regimens. Once patients are compliant with risk-factor modification and exercise therapy and have had a good response, follow-up appointments can be decreased in frequency. Some form of follow-up, either with the physician, with associated providers, or with the patient's primary care provider, should continue to ensure long-term compliance.

Invasive intervention, in the form of surgical or endovascular procedures, is not warranted for most patients with claudication. Multiple randomized clinical trials that have compared percutaneous endovascular interventions (angioplasty and stenting) with exercise therapy have failed to show a consistent benefit to endovascular intervention. In addition, claudication is *not* a limb-threatening problem (associated with a 1% to 2% risk of limb loss per year). Intervention, when performed, is done purely to ameliorate limb symptoms and is therefore purely discretionary.

In spite of a lack of an evidence-based benefit, however, the utilization of percutaneous endovascular interventions has doubled over the past decade in the United States. In addition to an increase in the frequency of interventions, there has been a growth in the number of specialties involved in the management of claudication, both invasive and noninvasive, and this has likely added to the heterogeneity in management strategies.

This being said, there continues to be some role for invasive treatment in the care of the patient with claudication. Traditionally, these interventions have been reserved for patients with "disabling" claudication with failed medical management. To date, no unified attempts to clarify what constitutes "disabling" or "failure" of medical management have been seen. Regardless, the following characteristics are often considered reasons to consider invasive intervention:

- Short-distance (<300 ft) claudication
- Claudication that impairs or prevents employment or prevents performance of all necessary job duties
- Claudication that impairs the patient's ability to perform important activities of daily living.

Additional consideration can also be given to patients with severe claudication and unilateral disease because intervention may be more straightforward and improve the patient's condition to a highly functional baseline. Also, patients with claudication with an ABI of less than 0.4, toe pressures of less than 40 mm Hg, or dependent rubor do merit more frequent clinic visits and a lower threshold for triage to procedural revascularization because they have a higher incidence of limb-threatening problems.

When a patient does meet criteria for invasive intervention and the decision has been made to pursue this, the physician has two preparatory tasks: (1) evaluation and optimization of the patient's cardiopulmonary status and (2) completion of imaging to delineate vascular anatomy and make a detailed plan for revascularization options. First, patients should be evaluated with the American Heart Association/American College of Cardiology guidelines for preprocedural cardiac optimization. History of unstable angina, severe or decompensated heart failure, recent myocardial infarction, severe valvular disease, or ventricular dysrhythmias merits further evaluation. Evidence from several good-quality observational studies suggests that perioperative use of beta-blockers can lower the incidence of cardiac complications, but at least one randomized trial has shown that preemptive coronary revascularization for all but the patients at highest risk may not significantly lower the rate of cardiac events.

Multiple imaging approaches have been used in patients with claudication to define anatomy before interventions, and the combination of physical examination with multilevel segmental blood pressures and renal function assessment is best to identify the most proximal level of disease and select the proper imaging modality. In general, patients with claudication with weak or nonpalpable femoral pulses and patients with high thigh pressures that are equal to or lower than brachial pressures should be suspected of having aortoiliac or common femoral artery disease. In these patients, computed tomographic angiography (CTA) or magnetic resonance angiography (MRA) can serve as the initial imaging modality to delineate anatomy when baseline renal function is not impaired (i.e., estimated glomerular function [eGFR] >60 mL/min) (Figure 1). In patients with suspected aortoiliac or common femoral artery disease and impaired renal function (eGFR <60 mL/min), an aortogram with pelvic runoff from contralateral femoral access or brachial access is probably the best initial imaging modality to limit contrast exposure.

Patients with claudication with palpable femoral pulses but impaired ABIs and suspected infrainguinal (femoropopliteal or tibial level) disease should probably undergo digital subtraction angiography (DSA) to further delineate anatomy (see Figure 1) because this provides the opportunity to treat patients with claudication with good baseline renal function and lesions that are amenable to percutaneous endovascular intervention in a single setting (see subsequent discussion).

Duplex ultrasound scan can identify the location of arterial lesions, but the examination is often time consuming and technician dependent. This modality holds the most utility for determination of the anatomy of vein conduit available for surgical reconstructions. Like duplex ultrasound scan, MRA with gadolinium avoids ionizing radiation, but it requires post image acquisition processing for useful

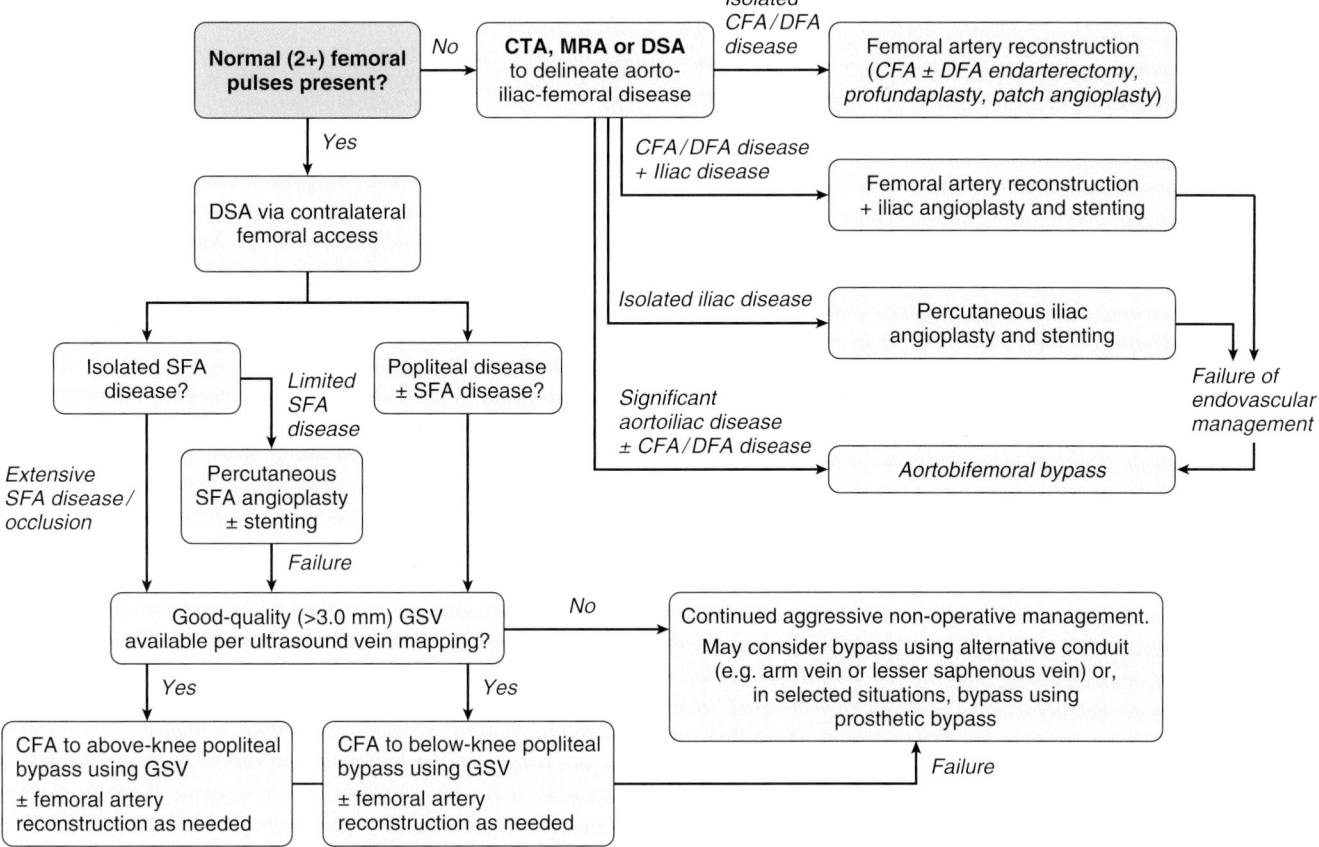

FIGURE 1 General decision-making algorithm for patients with lifestyle-limiting claudication and failed nonoperative therapy, assuming medical fitness for intervention. *CFA,* Common femoral artery; *CTA,* computed tomographic angiography; *DFA,* deep femoral artery; *DSA,* digital subtraction angiography; *GSV,* greater saphenous vein; *MRA,* magnetic resonance angiography; *SFA,* superficial femoral artery.

evaluation. Furthermore, the use of gadolinium in patients with severe renal insufficiency can cause the debilitating side effect of nephrogenic systemic fibrosis.

Regardless of the imaging modality that is selected, profunda femoris (deep femoral) artery disease should also aggressively be sought and treated. It usually occurs at the origin with at least some degree of common femoral disease or iliac disease, so it is uncommon that patients with significant profunda disease have normal high-thigh ABIs. However, CTA or DSA might be worth considering to evaluate for common femoral/profunda femoris disease in thigh claudication and normal high-thigh ABIs.

TREATMENT OF THE ARTERIAL OCCLUSIVE LESIONS THAT CAUSE CLAUDICATION

When formulating interventional strategies for patients with claudication, the objectives should be either optimizing inflow to the deep femoral (profunda femoris) artery in patients with aortoiliac disease or establishing durable perfusion to the popliteal artery in patients with isolated femoropopliteal artery disease. Vascular imaging may show multilevel atherosclerotic disease (i.e., aortoiliac and femoropopliteal disease) in many patients with claudication. However, in contrast to the management of multilevel disease in the context of nonhealing wounds or rest pain, *the symptoms of claudication generally resolve or are greatly improved with treatment*

of aortoiliac disease alone if the profunda is of good quality or reconstructed.

Aortobifemoral bypass has been the mainstay of treatment for patients with aortoiliac occlusive disease. Although this operation does offer excellent long-term patency rates, it also has a nonnegligible rate of morbidity, including groin lymphocele formation (9%), surgical site or other infection (23%), and need for emergent reoperations (6%). As an alternative, the first-line therapy for most patients with aortoiliac occlusive disease is now angioplasty and stenting. The patency rates for iliac artery angioplasty and stenting approach those of aortobifemoral bypass and with lower morbidity rates. Once reserved for patients with stenotic but nonoccluded iliac vessels, clinicians with endovascular skills can now often recanalize completely occluded iliac arteries with long-term patency rates that are comparable with those of stenotic nonoccluded arteries (see Figure 1).

Disease isolated to the common and proximal deep femoral arteries can be effectively treated with common femoral endarterectomy, profundaplasty, and patch angioplasty (typically done with either autogenous or prosthetic patch material) or iliofemoral bypass (usually prosthetic conduit). When aortoiliac disease occurs in conjunction with common femoral disease, the combination of common femoral endarterectomy, profundaplasty, and patch angioplasty plus iliac stenting is a good treatment option (see Figure 1). Again, patients with multilevel disease should undergo treatment of aortoiliac disease first because this alone (i.e., without anything to address femoropopliteal disease) suffices to resolve or greatly diminish claudication symptoms in most patients with claudication.

Femoral-femoral bypass and axillofemoral bypass are alternative options to establish inflow in the context of aortoiliac occlusive disease, but because of the relatively low patency of these options in the context of occlusive disease, they should not be routinely considered for patients with claudication. Patients who are deemed too ill for either aortobifemoral or ileofemoral bypass or iliac artery angioplasty and stenting and have claudication only are generally best managed with medical management alone.

Patients with either isolated superficial femoral artery disease or those who have severe symptoms in spite of having had inflow addressed may merit treatment of this segment. As with iliac lesions, endovascular intervention is becoming first-line therapy for selected superficial femoral artery lesions, albeit with less good-quality data to support this practice. Furthermore, endovascular intervention of femoropopliteal disease should be limited to the treatment of disease in the superficial femoral artery only; popliteal angioplasty and especially popliteal stenting is generally not recommended, especially for claudication, because the durability is poor and it constrains further treatment options.

In patients whose anatomy is not amenable to angioplasty with or without stenting or in patients in whom this treatment fails, bypass may be considered. Perhaps the most important determination of whether this is a good option is the availability of good-caliber, single-segment saphenous vein because this leads to the best long-term outcome, regardless of level. Patients who do not have good-caliber, single-segment saphenous vein should probably be largely managed with medical therapy. Whereas occluded vein graft bypasses only infrequently cause limb-threatening ischemia, occluded prosthetic grafts frequently do. When this does occur, a patient with claudication, a disease whose natural history is benign and *not* limb-threatening, may find the viability of the limb in jeopardy. So although some patients may explicitly ask for an intervention for symptoms that they see as very bothersome, infrainguinal bypass for claudication with prosthetic grafts should only be done with a detailed, informed discussion between the physician and the patient about the long-term potential risks. In addition, patients who continue to smoke have a threefold to sixfold higher risk of graft occlusion, so putting prosthetic infrainguinal bypasses in a patient with claudication who continues to smoke should be especially discouraged. Finally, biologic conduits such as cryopreserved cadaveric vein and artery are expensive and have dismal long-term patency and therefore are not generally helpful in the setting of claudication.

Other treatment strategies are being investigated. Intermittent pneumatic compression, angiogenesis (TRAFFIC [The Rapeutic Angiogenesis with recombinant Fibroblast growth Factor-2 for Intermittent Claudication]), and cell-based therapies are emerging techniques to enhance lower limb perfusion, but none of these approaches currently have sufficient supporting evidence for recommendation as a first-line therapy.

SUMMARY

Claudication is an increasingly common problem that is not limb threatening but may impair quality-of-life or daily functioning. The systemic nature of atherosclerotic disease does put patients with claudication at high risk for mortality from coronary and cerebrovascular events.

Initial management for all patients with claudication includes efforts to ameliorate limb symptoms and modification of atherosclerotic risk factors. Exercise therapy is the mainstay of medical management for claudication; cilostazol and loss of excess body weight may also help ameliorate exertional limb pains. Risk factor modification with antiplatelet agents; control of obesity, hypertension, and hyperlipidemia; and diabetes management are important to decrease the risk of death from cerebrovascular and coronary events.

Interventions (percutaneous endovascular procedures, open surgical reconstructions, or combination "hybrid" procedures) are considered for severe, lifestyle-limiting symptoms that have not improved with the patient compliant to medical therapy. Interventions done for patients with claudication should focus on establishing inflow to the deep femoral artery. Highly selected patients with isolated femoropopliteal artery disease may benefit from intervention for this segment.

Finally, although general algorithms for patient care are offered, the field of lower extremity arterial peripheral vascular disease is ripe for further investigation to better define best practice approaches for individual patients.

SUGGESTED READINGS

Jackson MR, Belott TP, Dickason T, et al: The consequences of a failed femoropopliteal bypass grafting: comparison of saphenous vein and PTFE grafts, *J Vasc Surg* 32:498–504, 2000.

Muluk SC, Muluk VS, Kelley ME, et al: Outcome events in patients with claudication: a 15-year study in 2777 patients, *J Vasc Surg* 33:251–257, 2001.

Norgren L, Hiatt WR, Dormandy JA, et al: Inter-Society Consensus for the Management of Peripheral Arterial Disease (TASC II), *J Vasc Surg* 45(Suppl S):S5–S67, 2007.

Olin JW, Allie DE, Belkin M, et al: ACCF/AHA/ACR/SCAI/SIR/SVM/SVN/SVS 2010 performance measures for adults with peripheral artery disease: a report of the American College of Cardiology Foundation/American Heart Association Task Force on performance measures, the American College of Radiology, the Society for Cardiac Angiography and Interventions, the Society for Interventional Radiology, the Society for Vascular Medicine, the Society for Vascular Nursing, and the Society for Vascular Surgery (Writing Committee to Develop Clinical Performance Measures for Peripheral Artery Disease), *Circulation* 122:2583–2618, 2010.

Spronk S, Bosch JL, den Hoed PT, et al: Intermittent claudication: clinical effectiveness of endovascular revascularization versus supervised hospital-based exercise training: randomized controlled trial, *Radiology* 250:586–595, 2009.

Pseudoaneurysms and Arteriovenous Fistulas

Phong T. Dargon, MD, and Erica L. Mitchell, MD

PSEUDOANEURYSMS

Definitions

Pseudoaneurysms (PSAs), or false aneurysms, are the result of a contained arterial wall rupture. PSAs usually result from injury to the arterial wall but can result from other etiologies (Table 1). Injury to the arterial wall results in pulsatile flow into the perivascular space, dissection into surrounding tissues, and hematoma formation. Luminal recanalization of the injury site results in a flow channel, or neck, that leads into a false lumen, or sac. PSAs, unlike true aneurysms, lack all three normal elements of the arterial wall and are therefore at risk of rupture. Rupture of the PSA can lead to catastrophic bleeding. Postcatheterization femoral artery PSAs are the focus of this section.

Risk Factors

PSAs most commonly result from complications related to arterial access. The common femoral artery (CFA) is the most common access site for catheter-based interventions. The incidence of femoral artery PSA is increased when the puncture site is not in the CFA but rather in the external iliac artery (EIA) or superficial femoral artery (SFA) or profunda femoral artery (PFA). Risk factors for the development of iatrogenic PSA associated with arterial access procedures are listed in Table 2 and can be divided into procedural contributing factors and patient contributing factors. Complexity of intraarterial interventions has been shown to increase the risk of vascular complications, and therapeutic interventions, such as arterial angioplasty and stenting, atherectomy, and intraprocedural thrombolytic therapy, have a higher rate of PSA formation (2% to 8%) than diagnostic procedures (0.05% to 2%). The diameter of the catheter used to access the artery also correlates with PSA development, and larger catheters and sheaths result in higher rates of PSA formation. Other procedure-related factors include simultaneous arterial and venous puncture, the use of arterial puncture closure devices, and insufficient duration of compression of the puncture site after the sheath is removed. PSA formation is less common when ultrasound scan guidance or fluoroscopic localization of the femoral head is used for femoral artery (FA) puncture. Patient-related risk factors that contribute to PSA formation include those listed in Table 2.

Diagnosis

The presence of pain or swelling in the groin after catheterization is the most common presentation of a PSA. Mass effect of a hematoma or large PSA may result in skin necrosis (Figure 1) or compression of nerves and vessels in the groin. Any patient who experiences pain disproportionate to that expected after a percutaneous procedure should undergo evaluation to exclude PSA. Examination should include a thorough peripheral pulse examination, documentation of

ankle-brachial index (ABI) and limited ultrasound scan of the vasculature in the affected groin.

The diagnostic examination of choice is duplex ultrasound scan (DUS; 5-MHz to 7-MHz linear transducer). Because B-mode imaging alone is unable to differentiate PSA from hematoma, color Doppler scan should be used to enhance the diagnostic accuracy of ultrasound scan (sensitivity, 94%; specificity, 97%) as it allows for identification of pulsatile flow within the sac. The typical appearance of a PSA on DUS is shown in Figures 2 and 3. The PSA size and the length and width of the PSA neck should be measured with DUS because they are important for determination of treatment options. If an arterial duplex examination cannot be performed or the results are equivocal, computed tomographic (CT) imaging (with intravenous contrast) can be used to make the diagnosis of PSA (Figure 4).

Treatment

A number of treatment options for iatrogenic femoral PSA exist, depending on the PSA size, neck characteristics, and patient symptoms. Treatment options include observation, ultrasound scan (US)–guided compression, percutaneous US-guided thrombin injection, and open surgical repair.

Observation

Studies have shown that most small PSAs (<2 cm) thrombose spontaneously within 4 weeks. Conservative management, or a watch-and-wait policy, has been advocated for small asymptomatic PSAs. Spontaneous resolution, however, can be unpredictable; therefore, patients with small PSAs need surveillance with DUS. The disadvantage of this watch-and-wait policy is that patients undergoing surveillance may have activity restrictions, discomfort with serial DUS, and prolonged hospital stays.

Ultrasound Scan–Guided Compression

Ultrasound scan–guided compression (USGC) therapy has been shown to be a safe and noninvasive method for treatment of PSA, with success rates ranging between 73% and 93%. US is used to identify the PSA sac and neck of the PSA. The ultrasound transducer is positioned over the PSA neck, and pressure is applied. Compression of the PSA neck and obstruction of flow into the sac is maintained while flow in the native artery is preserved. Direct US visualization confirms cessation of flow into the PSA sac. Compression is usually held for increments of 10 to 15 minutes. This process is repeated until successful PSA sac thrombosis or until a discretionary failure time is met. Compression times average 33 minutes for acute PSAs and 51 minutes for more chronic PSAs (>14 days).

Successful USGC can be limited by patient and operator factors. The procedure is generally restricted to lower extremity peripheral arterial PSAs. Suprainguinal PSA compression is generally not recommended because it may result in PSA rupture and inability to quickly control bleeding. Brachial artery PSAs usually require operative decompression because of concomitant nerve compression symptoms. Unfortunately, PSA neck compression can be time consuming and is often not tolerated by patients, despite conscious sedation. Compression can also be technically challenging and tiring in the morbidly obese patient. Predictors of poor outcome include concomitant anticoagulation therapy, large PSA size (>4 cm), and patient obesity. Patients with these negative predictors generally have lower technical success rates (25% to 35%), higher recurrence rates (20%), and greater complication rates (3.6%) than patients without these

TABLE 1: Etiologies of pseudoaneurysm formation

Acquired	Iatrogenic	Spontaneous
Trauma		
Penetrating:		
Gunshot wound	Vascular access	Vasculitis:
Stab wound		Behçet's disease
Blunt:		Polyarteritis nodosa
Proximity injury		
Stretch injury		
Infection		
Drug abuse		
Contamination		
Bacterial seeding		

TABLE 2: Risk factors for pseudoaneurysm formation

Procedural factors	Patient factors
Therapeutic > diagnostic procedures:	Advanced age
Complex procedures	Female gender
Large sheath size (>8F)	Obesity
Prolonged procedure	Hypertension
Simultaneous artery and vein cannulation	Hemodialysis-dependent end-stage renal disease
Use of closure device	Concurrent anticoagulation therapy
Poor technique:	Calcified vessels
Low (SFA or PFA) or high (EIA) puncture sites	Steroid use
Inadequate compression of puncture site	

EIA, External iliac artery; *PFA,* profunda femoral artery; *SFA,* superficial femoral artery.

factors. Complications and contraindications to USGC are listed in Table 3.

Ultrasound Scan–Guided Thrombin Injection

Ultrasound scan–guided thrombin injection (UGTI) has become the treatment of choice for postcatheterization PSA. Thrombin is injected into the PSA sac for immediate thrombosis of the PSA (Figure 5 and Box 1). This is off-label use of thrombin; thrombin is approved by the U.S. Food and Drug Administration (FDA) "for topical use only." UGTI is contraindicated in the setting of lower extremity ischemia, infection, arteriovenous fistula, and pregnancy.

UGTI has many advantages over USGC therapy for the treatment of PSA. Procedural times are shorter, and the procedure is better tolerated by patients. It achieves greater technical success (>96%) and can be used effectively in the setting of concomitant anticoagulation

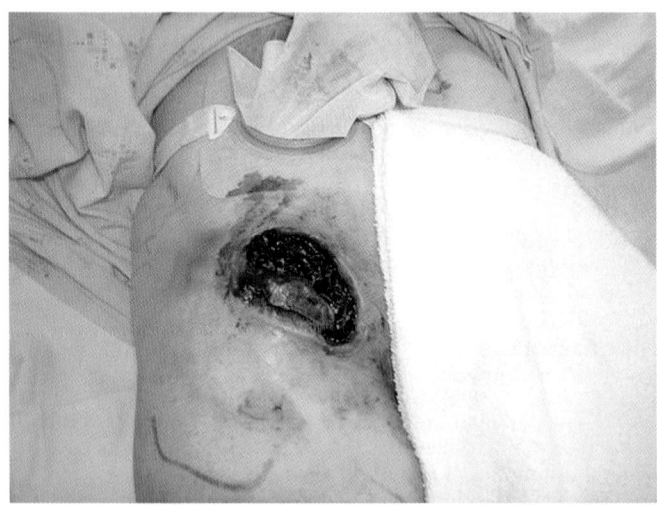

FIGURE 1 Pseudoaneurysms can cause mass effect with resultant tissue and skin necrosis as depicted in this photograph. Patients with tissue and skin necrosis need operative débridement and surgical pseudoaneurysm repair with or without hematoma evacuation.

FIGURE 2 Duplex ultrasound scan (DUS) revealing a pseudoaneurysm *(PSA)*. DUS findings of a PSA include a fluid collection adjacent to the femoral artery (FA), high velocity jet through the FA wall, and a neck or communication with the FA.

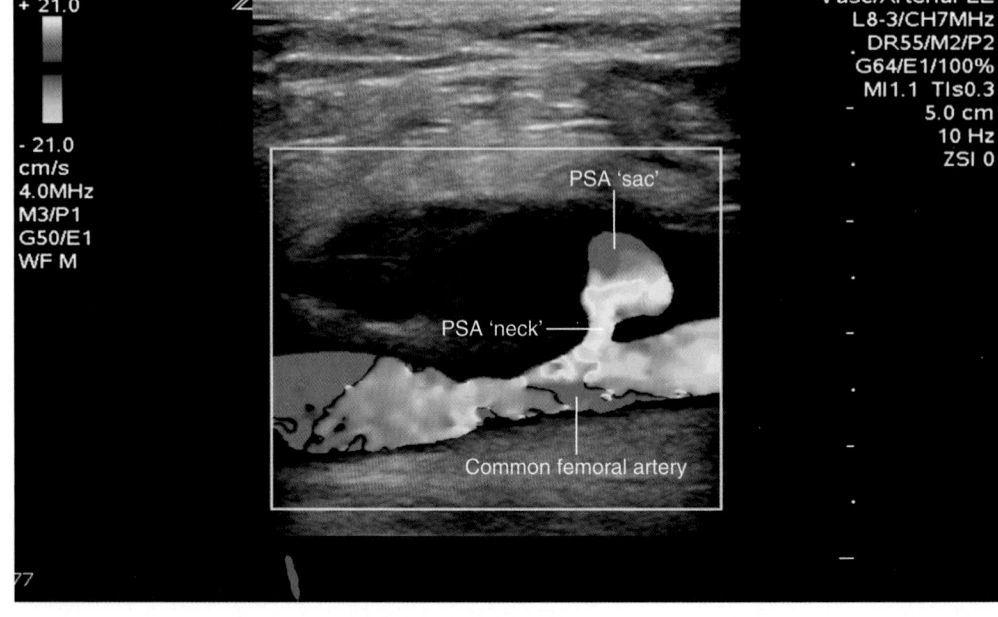

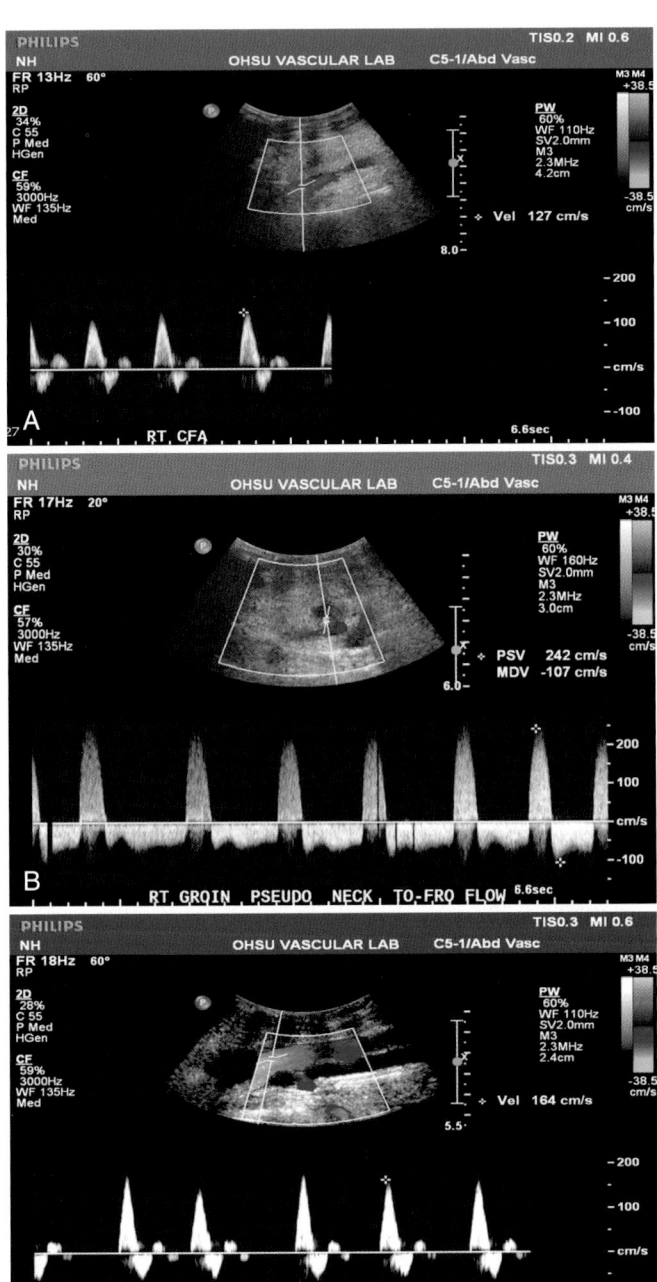

FIGURE 3 Duplex ultrasound scan of right common femoral artery (CFA) pseudoaneurysm (PSA). Images show: **A,** normal flow and peak systolic velocities (PSVs) in the proximal CFA; **B,** PSA arising off of the distal CFA with abnormal "to and fro" flow in the PSA neck; and **C,** normal flow and PSVs in the superficial femoral artery (SFA).

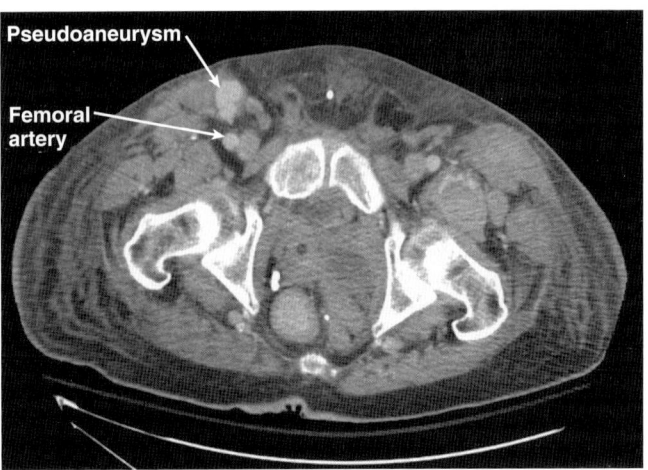

FIGURE 4 Computed tomographic scan image of femoral pseudoaneurysm. The scan was performed to exclude the diagnosis of a retroperitoneal hematoma; however, this femoral pseudoaneurysm was identified.

TABLE 3: Complications and contraindications of pseudoaneurysm ultrasound scan–guided compression therapy

Complications	Contraindications
Skin necrosis	Peripheral ischemia
Distal embolization	Cutaneous ischemia
Venous thrombosis	Infection
Rapid enlargement of PSA sac	Suprainguinal PSA
PSA rupture	Anastomotic PSA Brachial artery PSA with compressive symptoms

PSA, Pseudoaneurysm.

Endovascular Repair

Covered stents have been widely used in the treatment of aneurysms, but their use in femoral PSA is limited. Current barriers include high cost, lower patency rates, the need for larger delivery systems, and the lack of long-term data. Endovascular repair is not recommended if treatment of the PSA requires placement of a stent across the groin crease or across the origin of the PFA. Complications unique to covered stents include infection, migration, and thrombosis. Duplex surveillance is required after the procedure to monitor for in-stent restenosis and stent patency.

Open Surgical Repair

Noninfected Pseudoaneurysms

Open surgical repair is indicated for patients with contraindications to nonoperative management (i.e., peripheral or cutaneous ischemia, infection, surgical graft, large suprainguinal PSA) and those who present with complications (i.e., rapid enlargement, skin necrosis, distal embolization, rupture). Suprainguinal PSAs require access to the retroperitoneum to achieve proximal control of the iliac vessels. Repair of the arterial defect with simple, interrupted polypropylene suture is usually sufficient to repair the vessel. The back wall of the

therapy or for suprainguinal PSAs. The ability to perform this procedure in the outpatient setting or at the bedside also reduces the relative cost. Complications for UGTI include intraarterial thrombosis (<2%), PSA rupture, and allergic response to bovine thrombin. Arterial thrombosis has been associated with the treatment of small PSAs (<2.5 cm) but appears not to be related to short neck length (<5 mm). Exposure to bovine factor V may cause some patients to form antibodies that cross react with human factor V and induce coagulopathy.

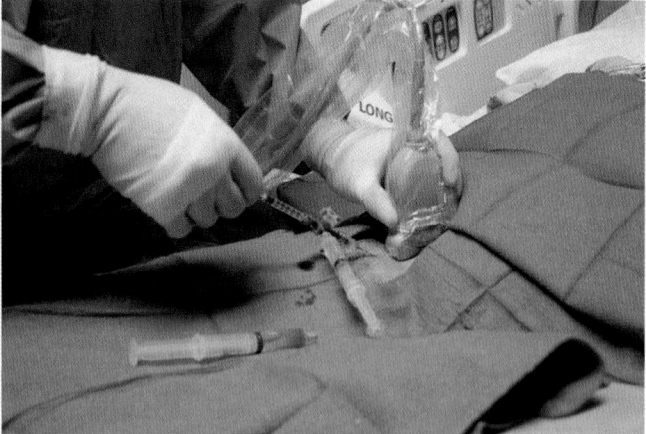

FIGURE 5   Technique of ultrasound scan (US)–guided thrombin injection. A 1-mL syringe containing bovine thrombin (1000 units/mL) and a 5-mL syringe with sterile normal saline solution flush are connected to a 3-way stopcock fitted with a 22-gauge needle (40-mm or 70-mm). If the pseudoaneurysm (PSA) is deeper than 3.75 cm, then a 21-gauge × 9-cm Echotip needle (Cook Medical, Bloomington, Ind) can be used. The PSA sac is visualized in transverse and longitudinal views on US. The thrombin port is placed in the "off" position, and the saline port is placed in the "on" position. US imaging is used to guide the needle into the PSA sac superficially and far from the PSA tract. Needle placement is confirmed with aspiration of blood, and a small injection of saline solution produces a flash of color on US. The thrombin port is placed in the "on" position, and the saline port is placed in the "off" position. Thrombin is then injected into the PSA sac in 0.2-mL aliquots until there is cessation of blood flow in the PSA sac and tract. This is usually achieved in seconds. The tract should never be directly injected because of associated risk of thrombosis of the native artery. An average of 300 units (0.3 mL) of thrombin (range, 50 to 1000 units) is necessary to thrombose the PSA sac. Arterial duplex scan should be repeated 24 hours after the procedure to check for recurrence (0 to 9%) and to rule out postprocedure complications.

BOX 1: Three-way stopcock technique of ultrasound scan–guided thrombin injection

1. The patient's groin is prepped and draped in the usual sterile fashion.
2. The distance from the skin to the most superficial portion of the pseudoaneurysm (PSA) sac and the distance to the PSA tract are measured.
3. The skin and subcutaneous tissue are infiltrated with 1% to 2% lidocaine.
4. A three-way stopcock is prepared as described in Figure 6.
5. The needle is advanced with ultrasound scan (US) guidance to the depth measured in step 2, and the PSA sac is entered superficially. Entry into the PSA sac is confirmed with aspiration of blood, and proper placement of the needle tip is confirmed with saline solution injection on US. The needle must be in the PSA sac and *not* in the tract, artery, or vein.
6. The thrombin port is turned "on," and the saline port is turned "off." Thrombin is injected gently in 0.2-mL aliquots until the PSA sac and tract are thrombosed or until 1.0 mL of thrombin is used.
7. If there are two or more PSA sacs, then the most superficial sac is injected first.
8. If the tract persists, do *not* inject directly into the tract. Follow the patient as the tract normally thromboses within 24 hours.
9. An arterial duplex scan is repeated 24 hours after the procedure to check for recurrence (0 to 9%), to confirm continued PSA thrombosis, and to rule out postprocedure complications such as arterial or venous thrombosis.
10. This procedure may be performed on an outpatient basis with the patient discharged immediately after injection.
11. A PSA that recanalizes after thrombin injection may be reinjected on follow-up visit.

artery should also be inspected to ensure no other arterial injury exists. Patch angioplasty or interposition bypass may be necessary if the arterial wall is significantly damaged or if there is luminal narrowing of the artery with primary repair. Hematoma evacuation and drainage may also be necessary. Complications associated with open surgical repair include wound infection, bleeding, lymphocele, radiculopathy, perioperative myocardial infarction, and death.

Infected Pseudoaneurysms

Infected PSAs should be managed aggressively with appropriate antibiotic coverage, débridement of infected tissue, and arterial repair or replacement with autogenous vein graft. Arterial ligation without revascularization is reserved for aggressive bacterial infection and may be associated with intermittent claudication or limb loss.

Anastomotic Pseudoaneurysms

Anastomotic PSAs are an infrequent but important late complication of prosthetic arterial reconstruction (Figure 6). The FA anastomosis is the most common site for an anastomotic PSA (13.6%). The presence of an anastomotic PSA should raise suspicion of a graft infection, and treatment should be performed with this in mind. Typically, an anastomotic PSA is composed of a fibrous pseudocapsule that surrounds the area of occult graft infection or arterial degeneration in a previously endarterectomized artery. Because anastomotic PSAs

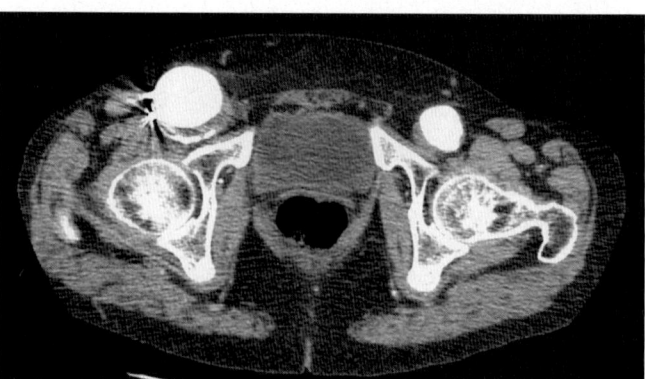

FIGURE 6   Bilateral femoral anastomotic pseudoaneurysms. This patient underwent bilateral common femoral endarterectomies and an aortobifemoral bypass for aortoiliac occlusive disease 15 years before presentation. There are no fluid collections or edematous streaks within the tissue surrounding the pseudoaneurysms, which suggests no evidence of infection. On physical examination and laboratory testing, no clinical evidence of infection was found.

are unpredictable and are associated with a high incidence of rupture, they should be treated early and aggressively.

Observation is recommended only for patients with very small PSAs, prohibitive operative risk, or short life expectancy; operative repair is generally recommended for all groin anastomotic PSAs greater than 3 to 4 cm in diameter. Arterial replacement is usually necessary, with an interposition graft replacing the degenerative aneurysmal portion of the existing graft, providing there is no sign of ongoing infection. If the graft is infected, then removal and replacement of all infected graft and tissue is necessary. Revascularization may require extraanatomic bypass grafting in a noninfected field or replacement of the infected conduit with autogenous femoral vein. Grossly infected arterial beds may require coverage with sartorius or rectus femoris muscle flaps. Endovascular repair of FA anastomotic PSA has been reported; however, it is generally not recommended in the setting of infection or when stenting would result in occlusion of the PFA origin.

ARTERIOVENOUS FISTULA

An arteriovenous fistula (AVF) is described as an abnormal communication between an artery and a vein. The communication can be congenital but is frequently of an iatrogenic or traumatic etiology. Femoral AVFs almost always develop from penetrating injuries and percutaneous vascular interventions. The incidence rate of postcatheterization femoral AVF is 0.2% to 2%. Patient-related risk factors include female gender, hypertension, and ongoing anticoagulation therapy. Age and morbid obesity have not been identified as risk factors. Procedure-related risk factors include left-sided groin punctures and intense levels of anticoagulation therapy (>12,500 units of heparin). Postcatheterization femoral AVFs are the focus of this section.

Diagnosis

The diagnosis of an AVF in the extremities can be made with history and physical examination. Physical examination may reveal a loud bruit on auscultation and thrill on palpation. A to-and-fro holosystolic/diastolic bruit at the puncture site is diagnostic and pathognomonic for an AVF. The intensity of the sounds on auscultation typically correlates with the size of the fistula. Traumatic AVFs may also present as unilateral limb swelling, mild to severe limb ischemia (claudication or tissue loss), or heart failure. When the characteristic physical examination findings are not present but an AVF is suspected, DUS can be a useful tool in diagnosis of AVF (Figure 7). AVFs are characterized by high arterial peak systolic velocities (PSVs) proximal to the fistula because of low resistance at the fistula site (see Figure 7, A). Reduced arterial flow is seen distal to the fistula as a result of shunting (see Figure 7, B), and bidirectional or turbulent flow is seen at the fistula site (see Figure 7, C). Flow in the venous side of the AVF is characterized by elevated and pulsatile venous outflow PSVs that result from mixing of arterial and venous flows (see Figure 7, D).

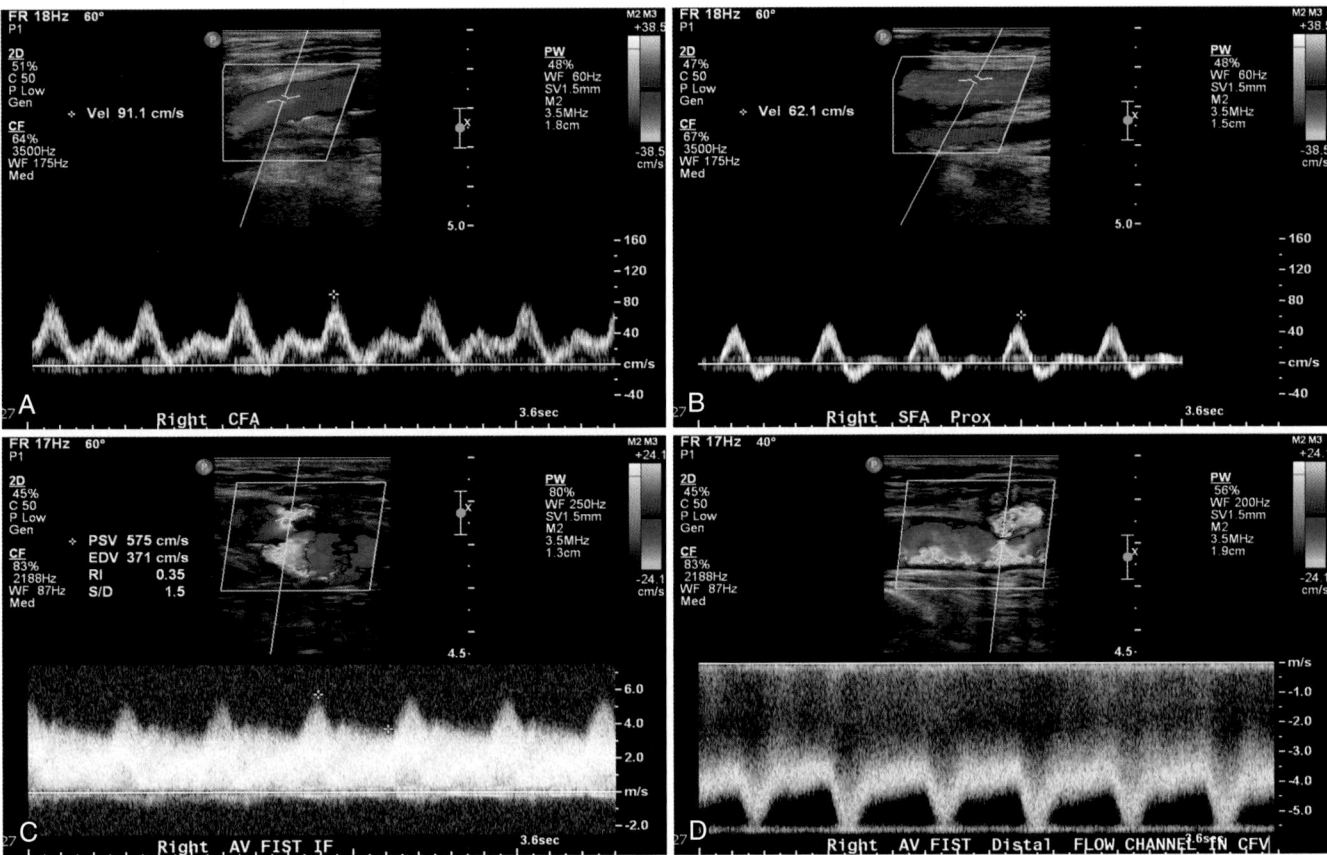

FIGURE 7 Duplex ultrasound scan examination of a traumatic arteriovenous fistula between the common femoral artery and common femoral vein (CFV). **A,** The arterial inflow is characterized by high peak systolic velocities. **B,** Reduced flow in the distal artery is caused by shunting at the fistula. **C,** Turbulent flow is seen at the fistula site. **D,** Mixing of arterial and venous flows causes elevated and pulsatile venous flow in the CFV.

Treatment

Iatrogenic AVFs, unlike traumatic AVFs, may close spontaneously. Studies have shown that 50% to 66% of iatrogenic postcatheterization femoral AVFs resolve spontaneously. Iatrogenic AVFs, however, are more likely to persist in patients with chronic renal insufficiency or concomitant steroid use. AVF repair is indicated for all symptomatic patients.

Open Surgical Repair

Surgical repair is the established method for treatment of femoral AVF and is associated with morbidity and mortality rates of 25% and 8%, respectively. Because AVF can result in significant enlargement of venous structures, operative repair can be associated with significant blood loss. Preoperative placement of arterial or venous balloons for intraoperative occlusion may help decrease blood loss during the repair, and cell-saver and rapid-infusion devices can be used when large volumes of blood loss are anticipated. Surgical repair requires obliterating the fistula and restoring normal arterial and venous blood flow. Therefore, repair of the fistula tract usually requires proximal and distal control of both the artery and the vein. Repair can be achieved with primary closure of the fistula tract. Vein patch angioplasty or interposition bypass grafts may be necessary for large AVF repair.

Endovascular Repair

Endovascular treatment of iatrogenic or traumatic femoral AVFs is becoming more commonplace. Catheter-based interventions are indicated for patients at high surgical risk or for those who present with "hostile" anatomy such as morbid obesity, previous femoral interventions, or groin surgery, and with obvious massive enlargement of venous collaterals. Patients who are not candidates for endovascular repair are those in whom endovascular stenting will obliterate the PFA or cross the groin crease. Intraarterial covered stents are required to obliterate the fistula connection with the vein. Venous stents are usually reserved for iliac vein or vena caval AVF occlusion after unsuccessful intraarterial stent placement. SFA stent grafts for iatrogenic femoral AVFs have reported 1-year and 4-year primary patency rates of 76% and 55%, respectively, and a 4-year secondary patency rate of 80%.

SUGGESTED READINGS

Ahmad F, Turner SA, Torrie P, et al: Iatrogenic femoral artery pseudoaneurysms: a review of current methods of diagnosis and treatment, *Clin Radiol* 63:1310–1316, 2008.

Perings SM, Kelm M, Jax T, et al: A prospective study on incidence and risk factors of arteriovenous fistulae following transfemoral cardiac catheterization, *Int J Cardiol* 88:223–228, 2003.

Thalhammer C, Kirchherr AS, Uhlich F, et al: Postcatheterization pseudoaneurysms and arteriovenous fistulas: repair with percutaneous implantation of endovascular covered stents, *Radiology* 214:127–131, 2000.

Tisi PV, Callam MJ: Treatment for femoral pseudoaneurysms, *Cochrane Database Syst Rev* (2):CD004981, 2009.

Toursarkissian B, Allen BT, Petrinec D, et al: Spontaneous closure of selected iatrogenic pseudoaneurysms and arteriovenous fistulae, *J Vasc Surg* 25:803–808, 1997.

AXILLOFEMORAL BYPASS

Jennifer A. Stableford, MD, and Evan C. Lipsitz, MD

INTRODUCTION

Although atherosclerosis is a diffuse process, distinct patterns of arterial occlusive disease can be identified. One such pattern is disease within the aortoiliac segment. Classic symptoms of aortoiliac occlusive disease include thigh and/or buttock claudication as well as impotence in male patients. This constellation of symptoms is known as Leriche syndrome. Aortoiliac occlusive disease can be seen in isolation, or in combination with infrainguinal occlusive disease. In patients with multilevel disease, the clinical presentation is more severe. The diagnosis of aortoiliac occlusive disease can be made on the basis of history and physical exam. Patients often have an extensive smoking history. Physical exam will reveal diminished or absent femoral pulses.

The diagnosis can be confirmed with a number of diagnostic tests. Pulse-volume recordings, a plethysmographic evaluation of lower-extremity arterial circulation, will show decreased waveforms in all segments. This is in distinct contrast to infrainguinal occlusive disease, which will have normal thigh tracings and diminished waveforms in the calf and ankle segments. Arterial duplex mapping can be used to estimate the degree of stenosis or occlusion within the aortoiliac segment, as well as identify any infrainguinal disease. Traditional angiography provides detailed anatomic information of the abdomen, pelvis, and lower-extremity arterial tree. In addition, it can identify patterns of collateral flow around obstructions. If warranted, intervention can be performed at the time of the diagnostic procedure. In the setting of aortoiliac occlusive disease, femoral artery access may be difficult or impossible, and the use of alternative access sites, such as the brachial artery, may be required. Computed tomographic (CT) angiography is another useful imaging modality for defining aortoiliac anatomy and planning intervention. CT angiography has the added advantage of delineating the extent of calcification within the aortoiliac segment, which assists in operative planning. A potential limitation of CT angiography is its ability to evaluate the extent of disease in the tibial vessels in the case of concomitant infrainguinal disease. Magnetic resonance angiography can also be useful in the evaluation of aortoiliac and lower-extremity disease; however, it, too, may be limited in the evaluation of distal circulation and does not provide information on the extent of calcification.

Axillofemoral bypass was first introduced in the early 1960s as an alternative to direct aortoiliac reconstruction with an aortoiliac or aortofemoral bypass. Axillofemoral bypass is considered an extra-anatomic bypass as it does not course along the normal anatomic path of the vessels being bypassed (Figure 1). The grafts are tunneled subcutaneously, avoiding a midline laparotomy and aortic cross-clamping, which significantly reduces the operative stresses, making this a favorable choice for reconstruction in patients at high risk (Figure 2).

INDICATIONS

Axillofemoral bypass is typically performed in patients with chronic arterial insufficiency and symptoms of critical limb ischemia, such as disabling claudication, rest pain, ischemic ulceration, or gangrene.

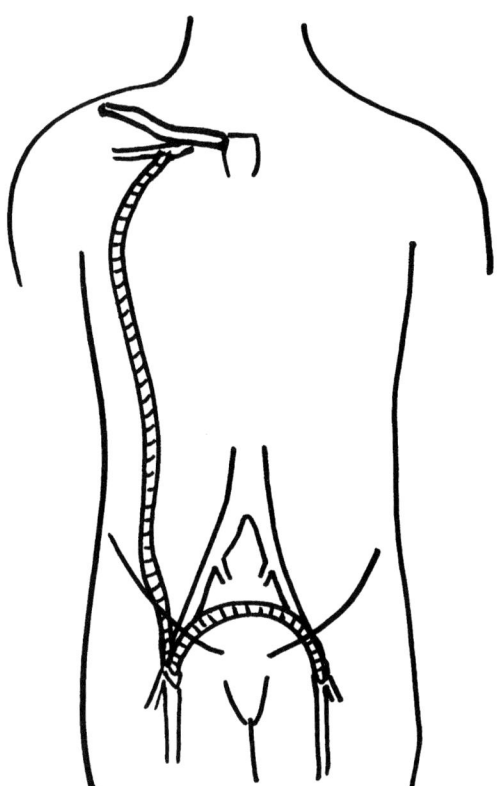

FIGURE 1 Typical configuration of a right axillobifemoral bypass.

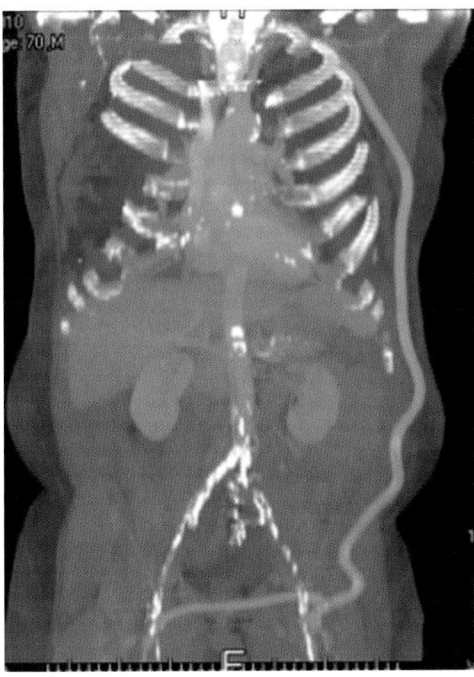

FIGURE 2 A three-dimensional reconstruction of a computed tomographic angiogram in a patient with a left axillobifemoral bypass.

Occasionally it may be performed in the setting of acute occlusion or aortic dissection resulting in acute lower limb ischemia. The timing of intervention depends on the indication for the operation as well as the overall health status of the patient. The primary indication for axillofemoral bypass is a patient with severe aortoiliac disease, who is unable to undergo aortofemoral bypass. Aortofemoral

<table>
<tr><td colspan="2">

BOX 1: Indications for axillofemoral bypass

Anatomic
Heavy aortic calcification
Hostile abdomen
   Previous surgery
   Extensive scarring
   Pelvic irradiation
Peritoneal dialysis

Comorbid Conditions
Severe cardiopulmonary disease
Severe renal or hepatic disease
Otherwise unfit for major surgery

Infectious
Infected intraabdominal graft
Other intraabdominal infection
Mycotic aneurysm
Aortoenteric fistula

Temporary
Need for temporary visceral and renal perfusion during major
   aortic reconstruction
</td></tr>
</table>

bypass may be deemed unfavorable on the basis of anatomic considerations such as a heavily calcified aorta; a hostile abdomen or the need for peritoneal dialysis; medical comorbidities such as severe cardiopulmonary, renal, or hepatic disease; or the presence of intraabdominal infection (Box 1). Another indication is the temporary placement of axillofemoral bypass in order to maintain visceral and renal artery perfusion during complex thoracoabdominal aortic reconstruction.

The development and advancement of endovascular therapies has altered, and will continue to alter, the treatment of aortoiliac disease. In the early 1990s, reports demonstrating the efficacy and relative durability of angioplasty and stenting of focal stenoses (Trans-Atlantic Inter-Society Consensus [TASC] A and B lesions) led many patients to undergo endovascular treatment as their primary mode of therapy, reducing the number of aortofemoral reconstructions performed. Since the mid-1990s, advancements for crossing total occlusions (TASC C and D lesions), including the development of subintimal angioplasty, have made the treatment of an even greater number of patients with endovascular methods possible. As a result, many of the patients who ultimately require surgical repair are older, have more significant comorbidities, and are thus not candidates for direct aortic reconstruction, therefore requiring axillofemoral bypass.

A small subset of patients presenting with aortoiliac occlusive disease will also have associated abdominal aortic aneurysms, and axillofemoral bypass is not the preferred treatment for this group. These patients require aortofemoral bypass to address the aneurysmal component of the disease process, unless the aneurysms are particularly small or the patient is believed to be a prohibitive surgical risk.

For those patients in whom the abdominal aorta is unsuitable for inflow, an alternative is to use the supraceliac or distal thoracic aorta for inflow, gaining access through a transperitoneal incision with medial visceral rotation, a retroperitoneal incision, or a thoracotomy. When the common femoral artery is occluded, an alternative outflow artery must be selected, such as the profunda femoral artery, superficial femoral artery, or popliteal artery.

In patients with combined aortoiliac and infrainguinal occlusive disease requiring intervention, decisions regarding the extent of reconstruction are based on the patient's clinical status. In patients with claudication, rest pain, or minor tissue lesions, it is preferable to first address the proximal aortoiliac segment. Restoration of inflow

AXILLOFEMORAL BYPASS

to the femoral level alone should be sufficient to relieve symptoms and the infrainguinal component treated subsequently only if needed. In cases of severe limb-threatening ischemia, concomitant axillofemoral and infrainguinal reconstruction may be required.

PREOPERATIVE EVALUATION

Patients should undergo a thorough preoperative evaluation. Many patients are selected for axillofemoral bypass on the basis of their comorbid conditions and therefore should be medically optimized to the greatest degree possible prior to surgery.

The choice of donor axillary artery depends on a number of factors. The axillary arteries may be evaluated by a number of invasive and noninvasive methods. Most simply, blood pressure measurements are taken in both arms and compared. If there is a significant gradient between the two sides (>20–30 mm Hg), the arm with the higher pressure is chosen as the inflow artery. The presence of such a gradient in the upper extremities may itself prompt further evaluation. Upper-extremity pulse-volume recordings and Doppler waveforms are useful in guiding therapy. Direct duplex of the subclavian arteries can be used to identify proximal stenoses. In addition, the inflow arteries may be evaluated with CT angiography or magnetic resonance angiography. Finally, digital subtraction angiography provides detailed anatomic information on the upper-extremity circulation. Full evaluation should include views of the aortic arch and great vessels. Although an invasive procedure, digital subtraction angiography provides the opportunity to address any lesion with angioplasty and stenting prior to the bypass procedure.

In cases with no notable disease on either side, the right axillary artery is typically selected for inflow because of the somewhat higher propensity for the left subclavian artery to develop a stenosis. This choice is made despite the fact that most patients are right-handed. Some authors advocate choosing the axillary artery ipsilateral to the lower extremity with the more severe symptoms. Grafts should not be based off an upper extremity with significant distal ischemia or where dialysis access is present. Additional anatomic considerations include the presence of thoracic outlet syndrome, breast cancer, or the presence of an ostomy, abdominal hernia, or previous surgery, which may complicate graft positioning. Finally, in patients undergoing axillofemoral bypass for reasons such as intraabdominal sepsis, who in the future may be candidates for aortic reconstruction via left retroperitoneal approach, the right axillary artery should be used to avoid interference with the retroperitoneal approach by a left-sided graft.

TECHNIQUES

Although this procedure can be performed under local anesthesia with sedation, general anesthesia is preferred because of the large volume of local anesthetic required to cover the extensive area, including all incisions and the subcutaneous tunnels. The room should be kept warm to prevent hypothermia, given the large body surface area that is exposed. The patient is positioned supine on a fluoroscopy-compatible table with the donor arm abducted to 90 degrees. A rolled towel is placed between the scapulae to facilitate exposure of the medial-most portion of the axillary artery. This also facilitates exposure of the lateral body wall for creation of the subcutaneous tunnel. The chest, abdomen, pelvis, and upper thighs are prepared and covered with impervious, sterile, plastic dressing. This permits wide exposure in the event that a thoracotomy or celiotomy is required. The donor arm is prepared, and an impervious stocking is placed to the level of the mid upper arm. This allows the operator to move the arm during the procedure to ensure that undue tension has not been placed on the axillary anastomosis.

A transverse, infraclavicular incision is made approximately one fingerbreadth below the lateral third of the clavicle, and

the dissection is carried down through the clavipectoral fascia. The pectoralis major muscle fibers are split in the horizontal plane, exposing the deep fascia with the investing fat of the axillary artery, vein, and brachial plexus below. The pectoralis minor may be retracted laterally to enhance exposure of the first portion of the axillary artery; however, in most cases, it is preferable to divide the pectoralis minor. This both improves exposure and reduces the risk of graft kinking. The axillary vein is first identified, then isolated and retracted caudally. Frequently this requires ligation of venous tributaries. The axillary artery is then exposed and encircled with silicon vessel loops. Branches of the axillary artery are either controlled with silicone vessel loops under gentle tension or with removable microclips. Division of these arteries is rarely required. Because of the proximity to the brachial plexus, it is best to avoid excessive use of electrocautery in the vicinity of the vessels (Figure 3).

The femoral arteries are exposed through longitudinal groin incisions. This approach allows flexibility in the placement of the femoral anastomoses and facilitates the performance of any adjunctive procedures, which may be required, such as femoral endarterectomy. Oblique incisions may be used but can limit the ability to perform adjunctive procedures in the femoral vessels. If such incisions are used, the location of the femoral bifurcation should be identified preoperatively. The anastomoses are generally placed in the distal common femoral artery over the takeoff of the profunda femoris artery. In cases with a concomitant superficial femoral artery occlusion, the anastomosis can still be placed onto the common femoral artery, provided there is no stenosis of the profunda femoris artery. If there is an orificial stenosis, the distal anastomosis can be used to perform a profundaplasty, with the heel of the anastomosis over the common femoral artery and the toe onto the profunda femoral artery. Direct anastomosis to the profunda femoris may also be performed. If the common, superficial, and deep femoral arteries are all occluded, direct reconstruction to the popliteal artery may be required.

Once the vessels are exposed, a long, standard tunneling device is used to create a tunnel between the axilla and the groin. The graft must initially take a lateral course under the pectoralis major and

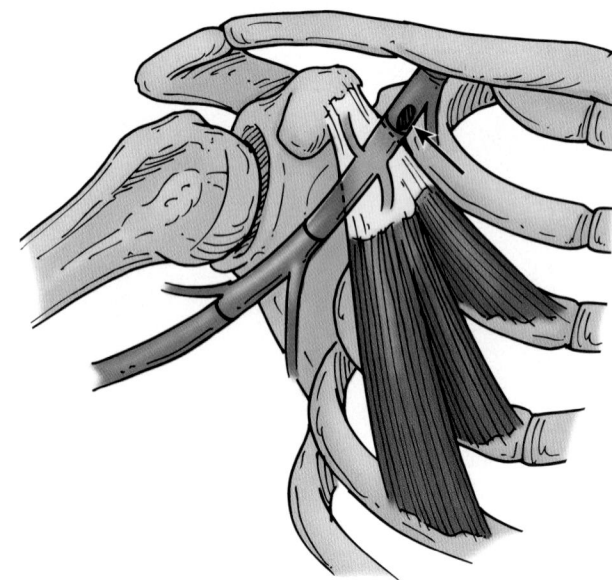

FIGURE 3 Following division of the pectoralis major, the approximate position of the axillary anastomosis at the distal portion of the first segment of the axillary artery is shown *(arrow)*. The divided pectoralis minor is indicated by the *dashed lines* and overlies the second portion of the axillary artery.

away from the axillary anastomosis before heading caudally in the subcutaneous tissue along the midaxillary line. It then courses anteromedially over the iliac crest and inguinal ligament to the groin. The use of a counter incision below the inferior aspect of the pectoralis major on the chest wall facilitates tunneling along the abdominal wall, thereby avoiding inadvertent injury to the abdominal contents. In the cases when a bifemoral bypass is being performed, a suprapubic tunnel for the crossover bypass is made in the subcutaneous space over the inguinal ligaments with either a tunneling device or large aortic clamp.

An externally supported polytetrafluoroethylene (PTFE) or Dacron graft is used for conduit. An 8-mm graft is preferred, but a 6-mm graft may be used in patients with small arteries without compromising patency. The graft is passed through the tunnels, and the patient is systemically heparinized. The graft is then cut to the appropriate length. It is essential that the graft not be made too short to avoid undue tension on the anastomoses, as well as not too long to prevent redundancy and possible kinking of the graft. We prefer to leave external ring supports to within 1 cm of the anastomosis as a further protection against kinking.

The axillary anastomosis is fashioned so that the graft takes an acute angle relative to the artery as it travels laterally to the abdominal sidewall (Figure 4). This is essential to reduce tension on the anastomosis and avoid graft dehiscence. It is sewn with a 5-0 or 6-0 polypropylene suture. The axillary artery is generally soft and delicate, so it should be handled with care when dissecting or suturing to avoid tearing of the vessel. The anastomosis can be constructed either in standard fashion from heel and toe toward the center of the arteriotomy, or the suture can be initiated at the midpoint of the posterior aspect of the anastomosis and run toward the heel and toe. In either case, it is essential to ensure that the posterior suture line is secure and without gaps because this area is difficult if not impossible to repair after the suture line is completed. The femoral anastomosis is sewn in standard fashion, beginning with the heel and proximal half of the anastomosis, then completing the distal anastomosis with the toe suture.

Confirmation of the patient's pulse status in both upper and lower extremities should be performed prior to reversal of heparin and closure. The incisions are closed in layers using absorbable polypropylene sutures. We prefer to use a subcuticular closure for all skin incisions, as staples and exposed sutures can catch clothing, requiring dressings until removed.

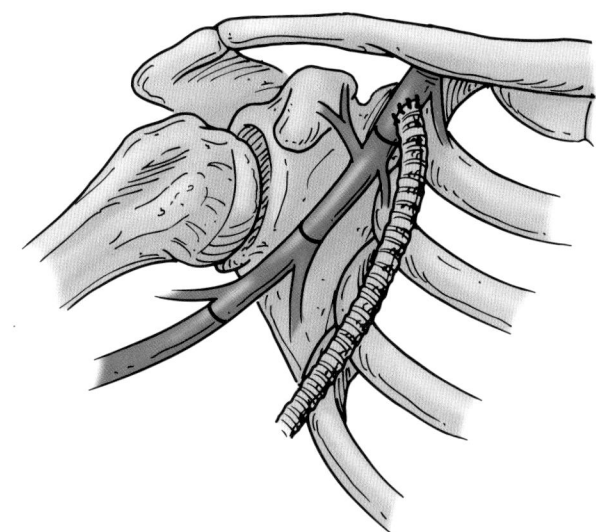

FIGURE 4 The course of the graft at the proximal anastomosis with the axillary artery.

GRAFT CONFIGURATIONS

Multiple possible graft configurations can be used when constructing the axillofemoral bypass, depending on the surgeon's preference and the patient's anatomy (Figure 5). There are now preformed grafts available with the femorofemoral graft fastened to the long axillary graft. Using such grafts reduces the total number of anastomoses from four to three, thereby reducing operative time. The order of anastomosis completion depends on the surgeon's preference as well as the number of operators. It is advantageous to have two teams so that anastomoses can be performed simultaneously, reducing operative and total anesthesia time.

RESULTS

The overall 5-year patency for axillobifemoral grafts, once as low as 30% to 40%, is now as high 60% to 80% since the introduction of externally supported grafts. These external rings prevent compression of the graft when the patients lie on their sides. Although this effect has not been proven by direct comparison, the use of externally supported grafts has been widely adopted on the basis of these theoretical advantages. There does not appear to be any difference in externally supported Dacron versus PTFE. The actual patency rates achieved vary widely according to the indication for surgery, patient selection, and extent of disease. Patients undergoing axillobifemoral bypass for infected abdominal grafts originally placed for aneurysmal disease, without concomitant occlusive disease, can be expected to have better patency than patients for whom the grafts were placed for severe occlusive disease. Axillobifemoral bypass grafts have better 5-year patency than the axillounifemoral grafts, presumably because of the increased flow rate in the axillary limb.

In the event of graft thrombosis, patency can frequently be reestablished with thrombectomy performed under local anesthesia. We prefer to perform these procedures under direct fluoroscopic guidance for several reasons. First, the chance of injury to the native vessel is reduced by preventing overdistention of the balloon-thrombectomy catheters. Second, it allows the surgeon to identify and possibly treat any underlying inflow or outflow lesions with an endovascular approach. Finally, should a revision be required, an angiogram defining the patient's anatomy can be obtained.

When comparing reports in the literature regarding axillofemoral bypass grafts, it is important to note that there is considerable variability in the techniques used and the outcome measures defined (e.g., primary versus secondary patency). In addition, it must be noted whether graft components are considered separately in patency calculations, as some authors may consider the axillofemoral and the femorofemoral components as distinct grafts.

COMPLICATIONS

Potential complications of this procedure include the standard risks of bleeding and wound infection common to all surgical procedures. The risk of graft infection is especially problematic because the majority of patients undergoing these procedures already have limited reconstructive options and significant medical comorbidities. Another potential complication is injury to intrathoracic or intraabdominal contents during tunneling of the graft. As noted earlier, care must be taken to avoid injury to other neurovascular structures, such as the axillary vein or brachial plexus.

POSTOPERATIVE MANAGEMENT

Patients are placed on an antiplatelet agent if not already on one preoperatively. Anticoagulation with warfarin is reserved for patients with a known hypercoagulable state, or in whom a secondary

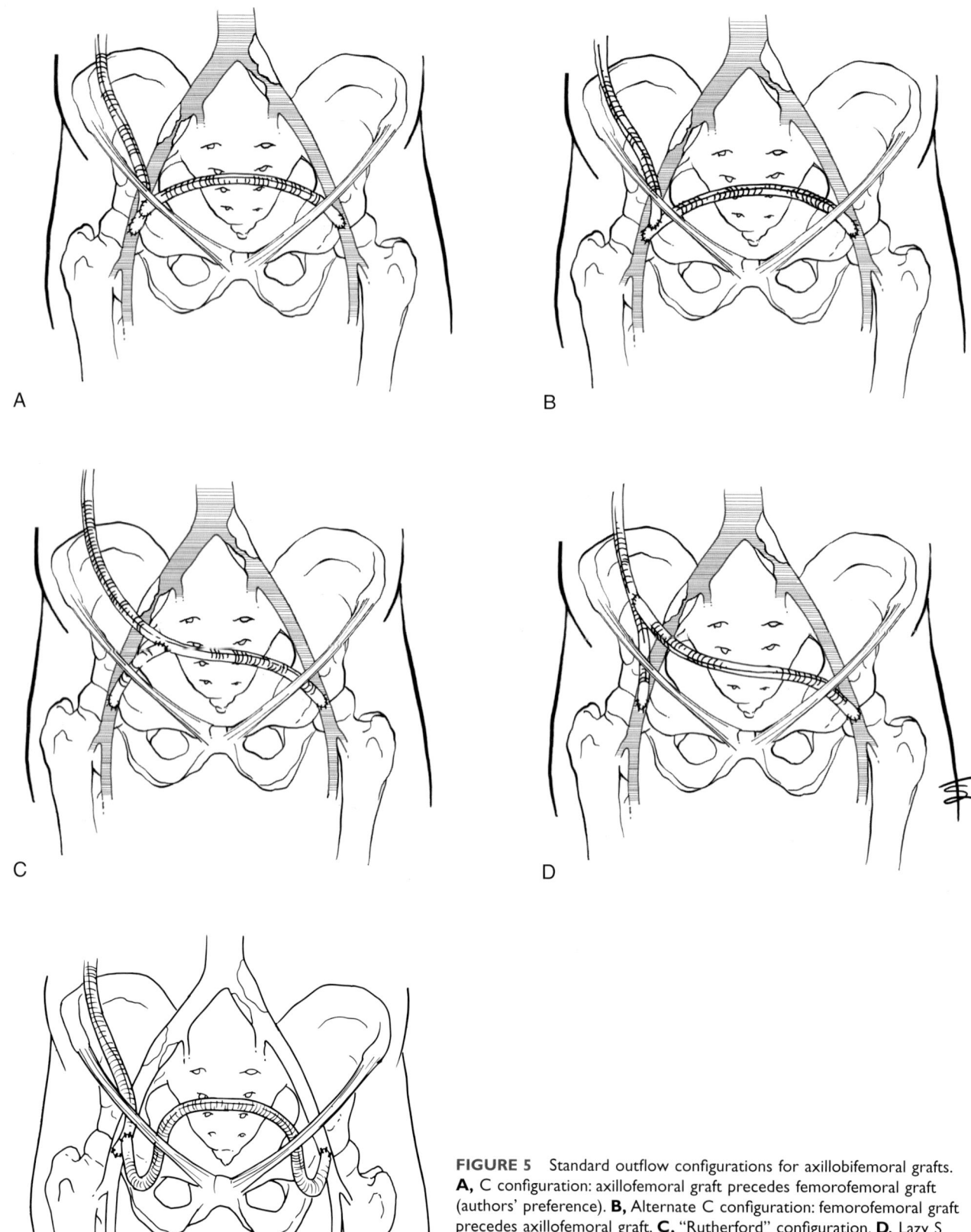

FIGURE 5 Standard outflow configurations for axillobifemoral grafts. **A,** C configuration: axillofemoral graft precedes femorofemoral graft (authors' preference). **B,** Alternate C configuration: femorofemoral graft precedes axillofemoral graft. **C,** "Rutherford" configuration. **D,** Lazy S configuration. **E,** Ram's horn configuration: stress is displaced from the anastomosis to the inferior curve of the graft, reducing the risk of disruption (preferred in obese patients). Can be used with either the C or alternative C configuration.

procedure was required to reestablish patency. As in all patients with peripheral artery disease, the use of a statin is recommended. Graft surveillance is performed every 3 months for the first year, every 6 months for the second year, and yearly thereafter. The need for a subsequent intervention or other abnormal findings on duplex may necessitate more frequent surveillance.

CONCLUSIONS

Axillofemoral bypass is an important and valuable option in the treatment of patients with aortoiliac occlusive disease. For many reasons, it is the preferred or only viable option for patients with significant anatomic or medical comorbidities, which preclude standard bypass options. Axillofemoral bypass can be performed with acceptable morbidity, mortality, and long-term results, even in patients at high risk. For these reasons, surgeons should be familiar with the indications and application of this technique.

SUGGESTED READINGS

Johnson WC, Lee KK: Comparative evaluation of externally supported Dacron and polytetrafluoroethylene prosthetic bypasses for femoral-femoral and axillofemoral arterial reconstructions, *J Vasc Surg* 30:1077–1083, 1999.

Landry GL, Moneta GI, Taylor LM Jr, et al: Axillofemoral bypass, *J Vasc Surg* 14:296–305, 2000.

Musicant SE, Giswold ME, Olson CJ, et al: Postoperative duplex scan surveillance of axillofemoral bypass grafts, *J Vasc Surg* 37:54–61, 2003.

Schneider JR, Golan JF: The role of extraanatomic bypass in the management of bilateral aortoiliac occlusive disease, *Sem Vasc Surg* 7:35–44, 1994.

Seeger JM, Preetus HA, Wellborn MB, et al: Long-term outcome of treatment of aortic graft infection with staged extra-anatomic bypass grafting and aortic graft removal, *J Vasc Surg* 32:451–459, 2000.

THE MANAGEMENT OF PERIPHERAL ARTERIAL EMBOLI

Tze-Woei Tan, MD, and Alik Farber, MD, FACS

OVERVIEW

Embolus, derived from the Greek word *embolos* or plug, refers to intravascular material that originates in one location and travels to a remote site. When an embolus lodges in a distal artery or arteriole, it causes interruption of blood flow to downstream tissue. In the case of peripheral arteries, this often leads to acute limb ischemia (ALI). ALI presents a challenge for the surgeon because of both the consequences of potential tissue injury and the associated medical comorbidities inherent to this patient population. Diagnosis of ALI that results from embolism can often be successfully made with a comprehensive history and physical examination and selective use of diagnostic imaging studies. The goals of management of peripheral arterial embolism include immediate anticoagulation therapy to prevent thrombus propagation, expeditious restoration of arterial circulation with open or endovascular techniques, and identification and appropriate management of the source of embolism. Introduction of the Fogarty balloon embolectomy catheter in 1969 simplified surgical intervention by allowing an embolectomy to be performed from a remote surgical access site. Development and optimization of percutaneous endovascular techniques such as mechanical thrombectomy and pharmacologic thrombolysis have broadened minimally invasive approaches for treatment of peripheral arterial embolism.

CLASSIFICATION, SITE, AND SOURCE OF EMBOLISM

Peripheral arterial embolism can be classified according to the size of embolus (macro or micro), the site of embolism (extremity,

visceral, or cerebral), and the source of embolism (cardiac or noncardiac; Table 1).

The heart is the most common source of macroembolism, whereas microembolism is typically associated with a noncardiac etiology. Embolism can affect the peripheral arterial (lower and upper extremity), visceral, or cerebral circulation. In the lower extremity, the most commonly affected site is the bifurcation of the common femoral artery, followed by the aortoiliac arterial segment and the popliteal artery. In the upper extremity, the most common location is the brachial artery at the bifurcation of the radial and ulnar arteries, followed by the axillary artery at the take-off of the deep brachial artery (see Table 1). Embolism is the most common cause of upper extremity ALI. Conversely, arterial embolization is second to in situ thrombosis as a cause of ALI in the lower extremity because of the higher predilection of arterial occlusive disease in the lower extremity.

The heart is the most frequent source of peripheral embolism; it accounts for approximately 80% of all cases. Although rheumatic heart disease used to be the most common cause of cardiogenic embolism, over the past several decades, atrial fibrillation has replaced it in frequency. Stagnant blood flow in a dilated left atrium of patients with atrial fibrillation predisposes to formation of thrombus that can lead to peripheral embolization. Similar conditions can occur in a dyskinetic left ventricle or ventricular aneurysm of a patient who has had a myocardial infarction. Less commonly, valvular abnormalities associated with rheumatic heart disease, infected vegetations associated with bacterial endocarditis, thrombus generated on prosthetic heart valves, and atrial myxoma can give rise to distal embolization (Figure 1).

Noncardiac sources account for 15% to 20% of peripheral arterial emboli. A discrete aortic ulcerative plaque can lead to microembolization of intraplaque debris or facilitate formation of associated aortic thrombus that may embolize to the periphery (Figure 2). Diffuse aortoiliac atheromatous plaque ("shaggy aorta") and ulcerative lower extremity plaque are less common causes for microembolization. Other sources of peripheral embolization include aneurysms, most commonly involving the aorta and popliteal artery. In some cases, embolization can be significant and can lead to complete obliteration of outflow vessels (Figure 3). Arterial thoracic outlet syndrome with associated subclavian artery aneurysm can also cause embolism and is the most common etiology of nontraumatic upper limb ischemia in young patients. Finally, paradoxic embolization, a less frequent cause of peripheral artery embolism, can occur

TABLE 1: Classification and frequency of extremity arterial embolism

Classification	Approximate frequency
Site of Emboli	
1. Lower Extremity	**84%**
Aortoiliac	25.7%
Common femoral	34%
Superficial femoral	4.5%
Popliteal	14.2%
Tibial	5.6%
2. Upper Extremity	**16%**
Brachial	9.1%
Axillary	4.5%
Radial and ulnar	2.4%
Origin of Emboli	
1. Cardiac Source	**80%**
Atrial fibrillation	
Mural thrombus	
Ventricular aneurysm	
Rheumatic heart disease	
Valvular prosthesis	
Infectious endocarditis	
Atrial myxoma	
2. Noncardiac Source	**15%**
Aortic mural thrombus	
Ulcerative plaque	
"Shaggy aorta"	
Aortic aneurysm	
Peripheral arterial aneurysm	
Paradoxic embolus	
Iatrogenic	
Foreign body	
3. Unknown	**5%**

in patients with a deep venous thrombosis and a right to left cardiac shunt usually caused by a patent foramen ovale.

PATHOPHYSIOLOGY

Macroemboli are usually composed of organized thrombus. They tend to lodge at arterial bifurcations where branching arteries decrease in caliber. Acute limb ischemia may ensue; its severity depends on the size and proximity of the vessel involved and the presence and extent of preexisting collateral circulation. Embolism to a normal artery leads to sudden onset of severe ischemia from absence of collateral circulation. In comparison, occlusion of a vessel with underlying atherosclerotic disease may provoke mild or even absent clinical symptoms as a result of preservation of distal perfusion through preexisting collateral pathways. Propagation of thrombus with subsequent occlusion of collateral vessels or fragmentation of an embolus with more distal embolization may aggravate limb ischemia.

The pathophysiologic basis of tissue injury from peripheral macroembolization is ischemia and reperfusion. Tissue hypoperfusion causes cellular hypoxia and local accumulation of toxic metabolites, including potassium and lactic acid, which lead to necrosis. Reperfusion, brought on by revascularization or embolus autolysis, provokes release of free oxygen radicals that further injure ischemic tissue. Locally, limb reperfusion and associated muscle edema can cause compartment syndrome. Systemic effects of reperfusion include hyperkalemia, metabolic acidosis, myoglobinuria, and acute renal failure. Limb ischemia and reperfusion in patients with ALI are associated with significant morbidity and mortality. Nerve is the most sensitive tissue to limb ischemia, and ischemic injury to peripheral nerves often leads to debilitating functional outcomes such as foot drop or Volkmann's contracture. Although irreversible nerve injury begins after 6 to 8 hours of ischemia, individual vascular limb anatomy and physiology may significantly increase this interval. Skeletal muscle, skin, and bone are less sensitive to ischemia and are able to tolerate longer delays in revascularization.

Microemboli are typically composed of platelet aggregates or cholesterol crystals that originate from atherosclerotic plaque. They can occur spontaneously as a result of plaque rupture or as a result of plaque disruption caused by arterial instrumentation during the course of a percutaneous endovascular procedure. Embolization of such debris into small arterioles induces an acute inflammatory response that is initially characterized by infiltration of polymorphonuclear cells and eosinophils. This process transitions into a chronic inflammatory state notable for endothelial and fibrous tissue proliferation that leads to luminal occlusion. Microembolization characteristically causes transient focal ischemia without major tissue loss; however, degree of injury correlates with the aggregate volume of embolus and can be extensive.

CLINICAL PRESENTATION

Patients with acute peripheral embolism usually present with ALI. The classic signs and symptoms of ALI, traditionally described as the six Ps, include *p*ain, *p*allor, *p*oikilothermia (coolness), *p*ulselessness, *p*aresthesias, and *p*aralysis. Pain is acute in onset, severe, and constant and is typically the main reason patients seek medical attention. It usually afflicts the distal limb; however, in the setting of proximal arterial occlusion, the entire limb may be affected. Skin pallor and coolness, or temperature level, usually occur at least one joint distal to the embolic occlusion and correlate with the extent of collateral flow. A careful pulse examination is important to the diagnosis of ALI and the relative location of arterial occlusion. Along with the patient's medical history, the pulse examination can help differentiate an embolic from a thrombotic arterial occlusion; normal palpable pulses in the contralateral limb, for example, may imply an embolic process. Conversely, a history of chronic ischemic symptoms and absence of palpable pulses in the contralateral extremity is highly suggestive of in situ thrombosis. An important note is that proximal to an embolic occlusion, a pulse may have a "water-hammer" quality and thereby can feel paradoxically augmented.

In some patients, sensory changes (numbness and paresthesias) in the distal extremity, rather than pain, can be the initial presenting symptom. Complete sensory loss, however, along with a motor deficit

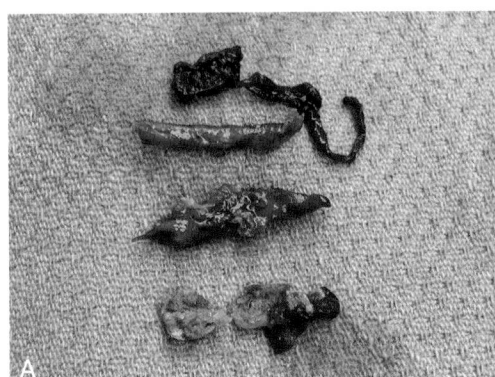

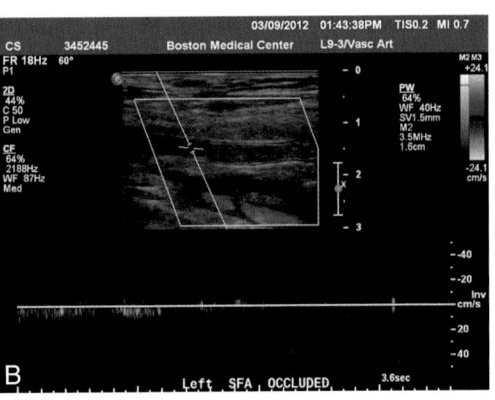

FIGURE 1 **A,** Intraoperative embolectomy specimens from a patient with acute limb ischemia from bacterial endocarditis. **B,** Preoperative duplex ultrasound scan of same patient reveals embolic occlusion of left superficial femoral artery.

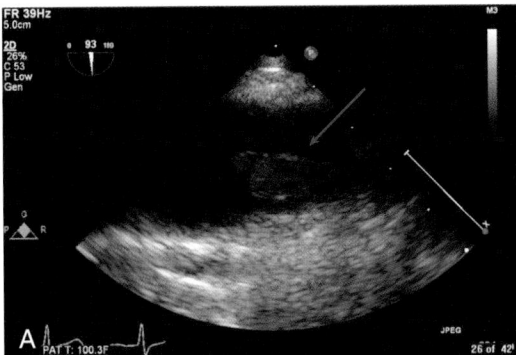

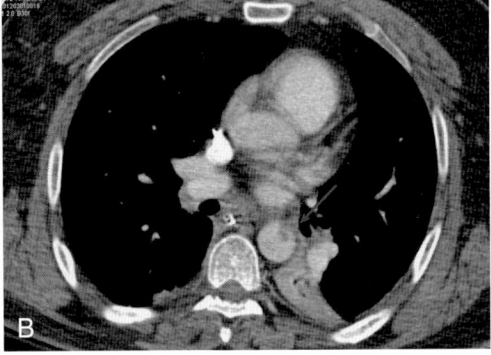

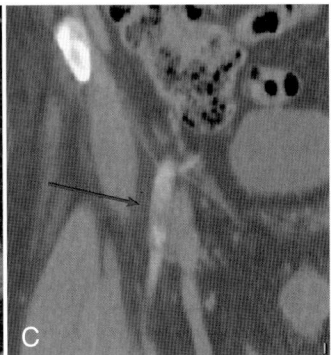

FIGURE 2 **A,** Chest computed tomographic angiography and **B,** transesophageal echocardiogram show a pedunculated, mobile thrombus *(arrow)* in the descending thoracic aorta of a patient who presented with peripheral embolization and right lower extremity acute limb ischemia. **C,** The embolus in the right common femoral artery is noted on computed tomographic angiography.

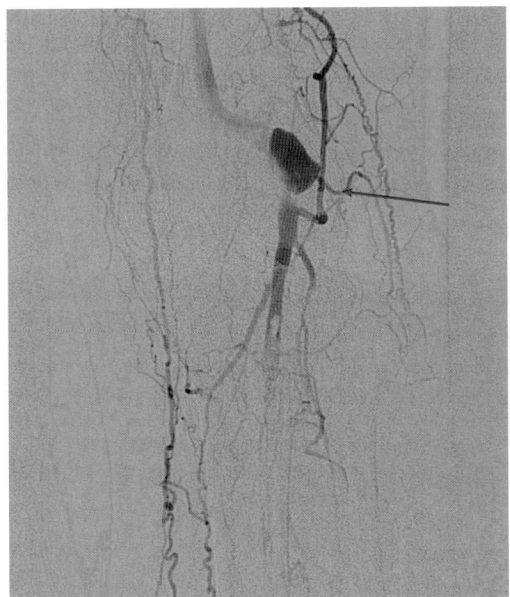

FIGURE 3 This popliteal artery aneurysm *(arrow)* caused embolic obliteration of all tibial outflow vessels.

represents advanced ischemia. Distal muscle weakness is strongly associated with ischemia severity and duration and, as such, is the most important factor in determination of both the urgency of revascularization and functional limb salvage. Continuous-wave Doppler scan is an important adjunct to the physical examination as the quality and presence of arterial Doppler flow correlates with degree of ischemia. Although a high clinical suspicion of ALI is important in patients who present with acute onset of limb pain, the differential diagnosis of this entity includes other clinical conditions, such as infection and deep venous thrombosis.

Acute limb ischemia is categorized based on the neurologic and vascular examination of the affected limb. The current Society for Vascular Surgery classification provides guidance with respect to the timing and the type of intervention and correlates with limb-related outcomes (Table 2). Class I, or viable, ALI defines patients with no continuing ischemic rest pain, no neurologic deficit, adequate skin capillary circulation, and clearly audible Doppler arterial signals in a pedal artery. Class II ALI refers to a limb with threatened viability and implies reversible ischemia in an extremity that is potentially salvageable with expeditious revascularization. This category further divides ischemic limbs into those that are marginally threatened (IIa) and immediately threatened (IIb). Patients with class IIa ALI may experience ischemic pain and have mild to moderate sensory loss. There is no muscle weakness, and venous Doppler signals are present. Patients with class IIb ALI have persistent ischemic rest pain and persistent lack of sensation in toes and have an associated loss of motor function. Lastly, patients with class III, or irreversible ischemia, have profound sensory and motor loss that extends above the foot, with evidence of advanced ischemia including muscle rigor or skin marbling. In these patients, thrombosis of the venous circulation from stagnant blood flow is often observed. For optimized limb salvage, patients with class I ALI need semiurgent (24 to 48 hours) intervention and patients with class IIa ALI need urgent (within 24 hours) intervention. Those with class IIb ischemia require emergent (within 2 to 4 hours) revascularization. Finally, patients with class III ischemia are best served with limb amputation rather than revascularization.

TABLE 2: Clinical categories of acute limb ischemia

Category	Description/prognosis	Findings		Doppler Signals	
		Sensory loss	Muscle weakness	Arterial	Venous
I. Viable	Not immediately threatening	None	None	Audible	Audible
II. Threatened					
a. Marginally	Salvageable if promptly treated	Minimal(toes)/none	None	Absent	Audible
b. Immediately	Salvageable with immediate revascularization	More than toes, associated rest pain	Mild, moderate	Absent	Audible
III. Irreversible	Major tissue loss or permanent neurologic damage	Profound, anesthetic	Profound, paralysis (rigors)	Absent	Absent

Modified from Rutherford RB, Baker JD, Ernst C, et al: Recommended standards for reports dealing with lower extremity ischemia: revised version, J Vasc Surg 26:517-538, 1997.

TABLE 3: Differences in clinical presentation of acute peripheral artery embolism and in situ arterial thrombosis

	Arterial embolism	In situ thrombosis
History	Acute onset No history of PAD Arrhythmia, MI, valvular abnormalities may be present	Acute or gradual onset History of PAD usually present Arrhythmia, MI, valvular abnormalities usually absent
Physical examination	Pulses in contralateral leg usually normal Extremity signs suggestive of chronic ischemia (hair loss, shiny skin, hypertrophic nails, wounds) usually absent	Pulses in contralateral leg may be absent Extremity signs suggestive of chronic ischemia (hair loss, shiny skin, hypertrophic nails, wounds) may be present

MI, Myocardial infarct; *PAD,* peripheral artery disease.

When considering ALI, differentiation between peripheral arterial embolism and in situ vessel thrombosis is important (Table 3) because this can affect both choice of treatment approach and patient outcomes. Although such differentiation can be challenging, a careful history and physical examination is invaluable. Patients with peripheral embolism present with acute onset of leg pain without preexisting symptoms of peripheral arterial disease (PAD). They can usually pinpoint the exact onset of symptoms, and their degree of limb ischemia is usually more severe because of lack of collateral circulation. Cardiac history such as atrial fibrillation, myocardial infarction (MI), or valvular disease may be present. These patients may have a known history of aneurysm. On examination, pedal pulses on the unaffected leg are usually normal. As noted previously, patients with acute in situ thrombosis usually have preexisting symptoms of PAD, such as intermittent claudication, rest pain, or tissue loss. A history of previous percutaneous or open limb revascularization may be seen. Risk factors for PAD including hypertension, hyperlipidemia, diabetes, smoking, and a history of associated coronary or cerebrovascular atherosclerosis may be manifest. Because PAD is usually a diffuse and symmetric process, the contralateral leg may have nonpalpable pedal pulses.

Peripheral microembolism typically presents with localized toe or finger pain. It is more common in the lower rather than upper extremity. Patients with lower extremity embolization or "blue toe syndrome" have a painful and discolored toe. This process can involve multiple toes and, when extensive, is referred to as "trash foot." Depending on the degree of embolization, patients with diffuse toe ischemia may have palpable pedal pulses. Involvement of toes on *both* feet suggests that the culprit lesion is proximal to the aortic bifurcation. Livedo reticularis, or netlike mottling of the skin, can occur in the feet, thighs, and buttocks and reflects diffuse microembolization. Other potential skin manifestations include petechiae, purpura, and splinter hemorrhages. Palpation of the abdomen, popliteal fossa, and groin is important because it may reveal culprit aortic, popliteal, or femoral aneurysm.

DIAGNOSTIC EXAMINATION

Patients with peripheral arterial embolization may need diagnostic imaging for assessment of the degree of limb ischemia and identification of the embolic source. Although the diagnosis is usually made based on a careful history and physical examination, arterial noninvasive tests, such as an ankle-brachial index (ABI), pulse volume recording (PVR), or tibial Doppler waveform scan, may be confirmatory. Duplex ultrasound scan can be used to corroborate the site of embolic occlusion (see Figure 1, *B*). These studies can be performed at the bedside, and their use should be relegated to cases in which the diagnosis is not clear or the ischemia is not severe. In the setting of class IIb ALI and an immediately threatened limb, care must be taken to avoid tests that add little to the diagnosis and potentially delay definitive treatment.

Cross-sectional imaging studies such as computed tomographic angiography (CTA) or magnetic resonance angiography (MRA) of the aorta and extremity arteries can be used to diagnose the location of an embolus but are more useful in the determination of an embolic source (see Figures 2, B and C). These studies can be used to visualize culprit ulcerative plaque or aneurysms and can evaluate for other causes of ALI such as aortic dissection and trauma.

Electrocardiogram can assess for cardiac dysrhythmias, ischemia, or prior infarct. Echocardiography is used to assess the heart when a cardiogenic embolism is suspected. Transthoracic echocardiography (TTE) is noninvasive and is performed first. An enlarged atrium, wall motion abnormality, intracardiac thrombus, and tumors may be identified. Transesophageal echocardiography (TEE) is more sensitive and should be ordered when TTE is negative yet suspicion for a cardiac source is high. A TEE with bubble study can identify a cardiac defect and lead to the diagnosis of paradoxic embolism.

Conventional angiography is performed when the diagnosis of peripheral embolism is unclear and significant preexisting atherosclerotic vascular disease is present or when an endovascular therapeutic approach is planned. Typical angiographic appearance of an embolus is that of an abrupt vessel occlusion associated with a meniscus sign. Minimal contrast filling is observed distal to the occlusion as a result of minimal collateral development (Figure 4). Intraoperative completion angiography may be necessary if concern regarding adequate revascularization persists or if distal extremity runoff needs to be visualized.

Laboratory evaluation should include complete blood count, electrolytes, creatinine, prothrombin time (PT), and activated partial thromboplastin time (PTT). In the setting of prolonged ischemia, lactate, creatinine phosphokinase (CPK), and urine myoglobin levels may be ordered to identify patients who need aggressive medical management to prevent nephrotoxicity. A hypercoagulable profile may be indicated in patients with a suspected hypercoagulable state.

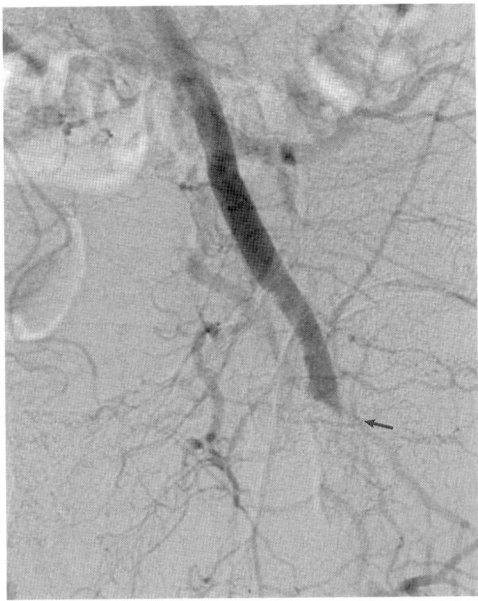

FIGURE 4 Angiogram shows an abrupt cutoff of the left common femoral artery consistent with the appearance of an embolus *(arrow)*.

MANAGEMENT

Medical Management

On diagnosis of peripheral embolization and ALI, systemic anticoagulation therapy is administered as long as no contraindication exists. Unfractionated heparin is given as an initial bolus of 80 to 100 unit/kg, and an 18 to 20 unit/kg/h continuous infusion is started. Anticoagulation therapy prevents propagation of thrombus and thus mitigates against worsening of limb ischemia. For patients who need emergent intervention, anticoagulation therapy should be continued up to the time of the procedure. Degree of anticoagulation therapy should be carefully monitored with intermittent measurement of PTT with a goal of 60 to 80 seconds. In patients with history of heparin-induced thrombocytopenia, a direct thrombin inhibitor such as argatroban or lepirudin is used.

Patients with peripheral embolism usually have significant medical comorbidities that may require careful optimization before intervention. Tachyarrhythmias, dehydration, and electrolyte and metabolic abnormalities need to be appropriately corrected. In the setting of class IIb ALI, such interventions may need to be performed in the operating room. After reperfusion, care is taken to avoid or treat hyperkalemia and myoglobinuria. Myoglobinuria can cause acute renal failure; therefore, hydration and urine alkalinization with bicarbonate may be needed in patients with significant tissue damage and rising CPK values.

Surgical Management

Open embolectomy is the surgical approach of choice for management of embolic ALI during which thrombus is extracted from an artery though an arteriotomy. This procedure is performed with a Fogarty balloon embolectomy catheter that allows for extraction of thrombus distal and proximal to the arteriotomy site.

The choice of arteriotomy depends on several factors, including anticipated location of emboli, convenience of vascular exposure, and ease of arteriotomy closure. For iliac, femoral, and popliteal emboli, the common femoral artery (CFA) is the access artery of choice because of its ease of exposure and relatively large diameter. The below-knee popliteal artery can be used in the case of popliteal or tibial thrombus. Bilateral CFA access is necessary for embolectomy of a saddle embolus at the aortic bifurcation. The distal brachial artery, at its bifurcation, is usually accessed during upper extremity embolectomy. Smaller arteries, at the ankle or wrist, can also be accessed directly in selected cases where other approaches are not fruitful.

With exposure of the CFA, a horizontal or longitudinal skin incision is made at the groin below the inguinal ligament. This procedure can be performed with local anesthesia if general anesthesia is considered too high risk. The common, superficial, and deep femoral arteries are encircled with vessels loops for vascular control to prevent excessive blood loss during embolectomy. Before arteriotomy, systemic heparin is administered, with its dose dependent on the elapsed time since heparin cessation. The decision to perform a transverse or longitudinal arteriotomy depends on the quality of the CFA or the potential need to use the femoral arteriotomy as inflow to an infrainguinal bypass. The arteriotomy is made at the arterial bifurcation to allow intraluminal access to both the superficial and the deep femoral arteries. A transverse arteriotomy at the CFA bifurcation is used when the artery is normal and the need for a potential concomitant bypass is unlikely. In case of a diseased artery, a longitudinal arteriotomy is made to facilitate a potential endarterectomy or bypass if necessary. Such longitudinal arteriotomy allows for exposure of more proximal or distal artery if needed; however, it often requires closure with a patch. Although vein, polytetrafluoroethylene, polyester, and bovine pericardium can be used, the latter material has the advantage of being "off the shelf" and having a lower risk of infection. The same principles with regard to arteriotomy choice apply to the popliteal, brachial, calf, and forearm arteries. The popliteal or brachial artery arteriotomy is made over the takeoff of the anterior tibial artery or the bifurcation of the brachial artery, respectively.

The Fogarty balloon embolectomy catheter is carefully inserted through the arteriotomy site with appropriate vessel loop vascular control. The catheter is advanced beyond the embolus, and the balloon is gently inflated while the catheter is slowly withdrawn. Inflation is only performed during slow withdrawal of the catheter to establish the appropriate amount of tension between the inflated balloon and the intimal surface of the artery. Overinflation is avoided because it can cause severe intimal injury. Although saline solution is used by some to fill the balloon, the authors believe that use of air allows for better sense of appropriate degree of balloon inflation. The catheter is retracted as thrombus is withdrawn from the artery. This maneuver is repeated multiple times proximal and distal to the arteriotomy until no further thrombus can be retrieved. Adequate proximal inflow and distal back bleeding suggest a successful result. The arteriotomy is then closed, and the affected limb is examined for evidence of restored perfusion. Completion angiogram is performed if the limb remains inadequately perfused and there is need to delineate arterial anatomy so as to locate residual thrombus. Adjuvant intraoperative recombinant tissue plasminogen activator (rTPA) can be injected intraarterially (5 to 10 mg) if adequate runoff cannot be established with embolectomy.

The Fogarty balloon embolectomy catheter is available in a variety of sizes: 2F catheters are reserved for the smallest pedal, tibial or forearm arteries; 3F-4F catheters are used in the femoral, popliteal, and brachial arteries; 4F-5F catheters are usually used in femoral and iliac arteries. When inserted through the CFA, the catheter usually takes a straight path into the peroneal artery. Insertion of the catheter into other tibial vessels can be facilitated by bending the catheter tip. If blind insertion is unsuccessful, other options include the use of the over-the-wire Fogarty balloon catheter with fluoroscopic guidance or open embolectomy through the distal below-knee popliteal artery.

Endovascular Approach

Minimally invasive approaches for treatment of peripheral artery embolism include percutaneous pharmacologic thrombolysis and mechanical thrombectomy. Multiple trials performed in the 1980s, including the Rochester study, STILE (Thrombolysis for Ischemia of the Lower Extremity) trial, and Thrombolysis or Peripheral Arterial Surgery (TOPAS) trial, showed that pharmacologic thrombolysis is a safe and effective treatment of ALI of less than 14 days duration. Thrombolysis with a lytic medication such as rTPA can be beneficial in the setting of class I or IIa ALI and in patients at medically high risk. Little role for this procedure is found in the setting of class IIb ALI. The theoretic benefits of thrombolysis are avoidance of general anesthesia that may be necessary for an open surgical procedure, gentle revascularization of an ischemic limb, and the ability to dissolve thrombus in smaller size vessels that would otherwise be difficult to treat with open embolectomy. In the case of thromboembolism associated with a popliteal artery aneurysm, if time permits, establishment of the distal peripheral circulation with thrombolysis is the first choice of therapy. The downsides of thrombolysis are the relatively longer time periods required to achieve tissue reperfusion and the risk of potential bleeding complications. Thrombolysis appears to work best on acute as opposed to subacute or chronic thrombus; therefore, thrombolytic agents have little effect on organized macroemboli. Embolic occlusion is, in general, less likely to respond to thrombolysis than in situ thrombosis.

The first step in percutaneous thrombolysis is to obtain vascular access and insert a vascular sheath. Angiography is performed to identify both the location of emboli and the remaining runoff vessels.

A wire is inserted across the thrombus and exchanged for a multiple-hole infusion catheter. A thrombolytic agent is then delivered into the thrombus. Thrombolysis can be performed over 30 to 60 minutes (pulse-spray) or continued for 12 to 24 hours (infusion). In the setting of infusion thrombolysis, with use of rTPA, a rate of 1 mg/h is typically chosen. Heparin infusion (500 U/h) is administered concurrently to prevent sheath thrombosis. The patient is monitored closely in the intensive care unit for signs of bleeding or coagulation factor depletion. Rate of lysis is adjusted accordingly, and at a designated time, the patient is returned to the angiography suite to assess for successful recanalization. If persistent thrombus is present, the catheter may be advanced distally and the infusion continued for another period of time.

Percutaneous mechanical thrombectomy (PMT) is an evolving technique in the management of peripheral arterial embolism. Available devices include aspiration thrombectomy catheters and automated PMT devices such as Angiojet (Possis Medical, Minneapolis, Minn). After angiography is performed to identify the location of the embolus, the aspiration thrombectomy catheter is advanced to the area of embolus and syringe suction is used to aspirate the embolus. With Angiojet, the device is advanced across the embolus multiple times as thrombectomy is performed through the Venturi effect created by the negative pressure at the tip of the catheter. Pharmacologic thrombolysis with rTPA can be concurrently administered to treat residual thrombus. Although mechanical thrombectomy has the advantage of increasing the rate of thrombus breakdown, it is associated with a risk of distal embolization and hemolysis.

Compartment Syndrome

Compartment syndrome can develop during reperfusion as previously ischemic tissue swells within a confined fascial space of the calf or forearm. The incidence of compartment syndrome correlates with length and severity of ischemia. Severe pain is common, and neurologic changes portend a bad outcome. Distal pulses may be normal. Loss of sensation over the first web space is an early sign of a progressing compartment syndrome as the common peroneal nerve is compressed in the anterior compartment of the calf which is most sensitive to ischemia.

The diagnosis of compartment syndrome is made on clinical grounds, although compartment pressures may be helpful in guiding treatment. Fasciotomies are warranted if the difference between the diastolic pressure and the intercompartmental pressure is less than 10 mm Hg. During fasciotomy, care is taken to release every compartment and to open the skin over its entire length. The wound is kept open until muscle edema resolves. Incomplete skin release and attempts at early closure are to be avoided because they may lead to muscle necrosis. Delayed closure with split-thickness skin graft may be necessary. Delayed recognition and management of compartment syndrome has devastating consequences and can lead to both limb loss and mortality. An aggressive posture toward early, complete fasciotomy improves outcomes.

Postoperative Management

After successful embolectomy, patients with peripheral macroembolism should undergo anticoagulation therapy with heparin and conversion to warfarin as the risk of recurrent peripheral arterial embolism approaches 30%. Patients are maintained on lifelong anticoagulation therapy in the setting of cardiogenic embolism or when the source of embolism cannot be identified. Patients with microembolization caused by atherosclerotic plaque rupture benefit from antiplatelet agents that are purported to stabilize ulcerative plaque. In addition, evidence shows a benefit for use of antiinflammatory nonsteroidal agents to reduce local inflammation associated with microemboli.

After successful revascularization, workup to evaluate for the source of arterial embolism ensues. Transthoracic echocardiography, TEE, and CTA of the thoracic and abdominal aorta are performed. In cases of lower extremity embolization, and when no source is identified, a CTA or angiogram of the affected limb may identify a culprit atherosclerotic plaque. If a discrete noncardiogenic source is identified, it is addressed as long as the risk of the procedure is acceptable. Stent grafts have been used in the thoracic and abdominal aorta to treat both aneurysms and ulcerative plaque responsible for embolization. Aortobifemoral bypass and infrainguinal bypass have also been used. Atherosclerotic lesions in the arch of the aorta are difficult to address and therefore tend to be treated conservatively.

OUTCOMES/RESULTS

Patients with acute peripheral arterial emboli are usually elderly and have multiple associated medical comorbidities. Management of these patients is challenging, and operative mortality with open embolectomy is reported to be between 20% and 30%. The mortality rate has not changed significantly over the last decade, despite overall improvement in medical care. Limb salvage for survivors, however, is excellent, with rates approaching 80%. Limb salvage among patients with in situ thrombosis tends to be significantly lower. Depending on the source, recurrent emboli can occur in up 20% to 30% of patients despite appropriate anticoagulation therapy.

SUGGESTED READINGS

Abbott WM, Maloney RD, McCabe CC, et al: Arterial embolism: a 44-year perspective, *Arch Surg* 143:460–464, 1982.
Alonso-Coello P, Bellmunt S, McGorrian C, et al: Antithrombotic therapy in peripheral artery disease: antithrombotic therapy and prevention of thrombosis, 9th ed: American College of Chest Physicians evidence-based clinical practice guidelines, *Chest* 141:e669S–e690S, 2012.
Cambria RP, Abbott WM: Acute arterial thrombosis of the lower extremity: its natural history contrasted with arterial embolism, *Arch Surg* 119:784–787, 1984.
Eliason JL, Wainess RM, Proctor MC, et al: A national and single institutional experience in the contemporary treatment of acute lower extremity ischemia, *Ann Surg* 238(3):382–389, 2003.
Rutherford RB, Baker JD, Ernst C, et al: Recommended standards for reports dealing with lower extremity ischemia: revised version, *J Vasc Surg* 26:517–538, 1997; erratum in *J Vasc Surg* 33(4):805, 2001.

ACUTE PERIPHERAL ARTERIAL AND BYPASS GRAFT OCCLUSION: THROMBOLYTIC THERAPY

Gregory J. Landry, MD

OVERVIEW

Acute lower extremity arterial occlusion remains one of the most challenging clinical conditions encountered by vascular surgeons. Early recognition is critical in maximizing clinical outcomes. Options for treatment include both surgical and endovascular techniques. Despite significant technologic advances in this area, particularly in endovascular technology, morbidity—in particular, limb loss—and mortality remain high in this patient group. In this chapter, the current status of endovascular management of acute lower extremity arterial and graft occlusion is summarized.

PATIENT PRESENTATION AND WORKUP

History and Physical Exam

Prompt recognition of acute limb ischemia is critical for treatment success. In this regard, the six P's (*p*ain, *p*ulselessness, *p*allor, *p*oikilothermia, *p*aresthesias, and *p*aralysis) remain important clinical signs, either alone or in combination. It is important to note that patients with significant motor or sensory dysfunction have advanced ischemia with limited time for revascularization and high risk of limb loss. Given the time required for complete endovascular intervention, prompt surgical revascularization should be considered in this patient cohort. Patients with intact motor and sensory function are more appropriately considered for endovascular revascularization.

Acute native arterial occlusion is generally either embolic or thrombotic in nature. Embolic occlusion is most frequently (>80%) cardiac in origin, so history of arrhythmia, congestive heart failure, coronary artery disease, or valvular disease should be elicited. Non-cardiac sources of emboli include atheroemboli from a proximal atherosclerotic lesion or mural thrombus from proximal aneurysmal disease.

Thrombotic occlusion tends to occur in the setting of underlying native atherosclerotic disease. While both may be of abrupt onset, embolic disease tends to be more severe symptomatically, as opposed to thrombosis of an underlying diseased artery in which some degree of native arterial collateralization may have already occurred. Acute thrombotic occlusion can also occur in association with hypercoagulable states.

Likewise, in cases of lower extremity bypass graft occlusion, the degree of presenting symptomatology may vary. Autogenous graft occlusion tends to occur in the face of antecedent vein graft stenosis, detectable with duplex surveillance, and tends to result only in occlusion of the graft itself. As such, patients tend to present with recurrence of their prebypass symptoms—that is, claudication or rest pain. In contrast, prosthetic graft occlusion often occurs without duplex-detected stenosis and frequently results not only in graft occlusion but also occlusion of native arterial outflow. As such, presenting symptoms may be worse than those present prior to the initial bypass.

In addition to examination of the affected extremity, examination of the contralateral extremity can give important clues as to the nature of the ipsilateral occlusion. Normal pulses throughout the contralateral extremity, in particular in a patient without other atherosclerotic risk factors, suggest an embolic process, whereas diminished pulses or reduced ankle:brachial index in the contralateral extremity suggest the presence of underlying atherosclerotic disease. However, the possibility of bilateral emboli must also be considered.

After the initial assessment, patients should be classified according to the Society for Vascular Surgery/International Society for Cardiovascular Surgery (SVS/ISCVS) system, with category I: viable, not immediately threatened; category IIa: marginally threatened, salvageable if promptly treated; category IIb: immediately threatened, salvageable with immediate revascularization; and category III: irreversible, major tissue loss or permanent nerve damage inevitable.

Patients for whom thrombolysis is most appropriate are those in category I and possibly IIa, with category IIb requiring a more immediate attempt at surgical revascularization.

Imaging

Duplex ultrasound is generally the most readily available diagnostic imaging modality. Abrupt arterial occlusion with "water hammer" pulse in the proximal patent artery is seen in embolic occlusion. In thrombotic occlusion, atherosclerotic arterial wall abnormalities are seen, often with extensive collateralization around the area of occlusion. Computed tomographic (CT) and magnetic resonance (MR) angiography can give accurate anatomic information regarding the nature and location of arterial occlusion, but in most cases, they are not necessary. If contrast arteriography is planned, CT angiography has the disadvantage of increasing exposure to both iodinated contrast and radiation. It does, however, provide a rapid assessment as opposed to magnetic resonance imaging (MRI), which requires a longer acquisition time and also carries the potential risk of nephrogenic systemic fibrosis in patients with renal dysfunction.

Arteriography remains the gold standard for diagnosis with the additional benefit of allowing simultaneous percutaneous access for thrombolysis. As such, arterial access for arteriography should be chosen with this possibility in mind.

Medical Management

Regardless of etiology or therapy chosen, initial medical management should consist of intravenous hydration, supplemental oxygen, antiplatelet therapy (aspirin 81-325 mg orally) if the patient is not already taking it, and initiation of a continuous intravenous heparin infusion, with an initial bolus of at least 100 U/kg followed by a continuous infusion of at least 10 U/kg/hr, with a goal of maintaining the partial thromboplastin time at least twice normal.

Catheter Directed Thrombolysis

The indications for performing catheter-directed thrombolysis are relative and subject to debate. The most frequently accepted indication for thrombolysis is acute thrombosis (<14 days) of a native artery or bypass graft in patients of Rutherford class I or IIa. In Rutherford class IIa and IIb patients, adjunctive mechanical thrombectomy should be considered to reduce treatment and, thus,

ischemic times. The surgeon's judgment is necessary to determine which patients should undergo direct surgical revascularization. Additional indications for thrombolysis include acute arterial embolus not accessible with embolectomy, acute popliteal artery aneurysm occlusion without identifiable runoff (in which thrombolytic therapy may reestablish runoff for subsequent surgical therapy), or in patients who are felt to be too high risk for surgery. Both absolute and relative contraindications for catheter-directed thrombolysis exist and are listed in Box 1.

Results of Thrombolysis

Three large randomized controlled trials comparing surgical with thrombolytic therapy in acute limb ischemia were performed in the 1990s and remain the only such trials in the medical literature: the Rochester (1994), Surgery Versus Thrombolysis for Ischemia of the Lower Extremity (STILE) (1996), and Thrombolysis or Peripheral Arterial Surger (TOPAS) (1996, 1998) trials. Results of these trials are summarized in Table 1.

In the Rochester trial, 114 patients with ischemia duration of less than 1 week were equally randomized to surgery or thrombolysis

---

BOX 1: Contraindications to catheter-directed thrombolysis

Absolute
Active bleeding
Gastrointestinal bleeding within 10 days
Stroke/TIA within 2 months
Neurosurgical intervention or intracranial trauma within 3 months

Relative
Cardiopulmonary resuscitation within 10 days
Major surgery or trauma within 10 days
Hypertension (SBP >180 mm Hg, DBP >110 mm Hg)
Intracranial tumor or arteriovenous malformation
Recent eye surgery
Diabetic hemorrhagic retinopathy
Intracranial tumor
Hepatic failure
Bacterial endocarditis
Pregnancy

TABLE 1: Results of randomized trials of thrombolysis

Trial	Number of patients	Length of follow-up (months)	Limb salvage—thrombolysis (%)	Limb salvage—surgery (%)	Survival—thrombolysis (%)	Survival—surgery (%)
Rochester (1994)	114	12	82	82	84	58
STILE (1994) overall	393	6	88	87	93	91
STILE (1994) ≤14 days ischemia	112	6	89	70	94	90
STILE (1994) >14 days ischemia	275	6	88	97	93	92
STILE (1996) native artery	237	12	90	100	89	85
STILE (1996) bypass graft	124	12	82	70	94	100
TOPAS (1998)	544	12	65	70	80	83

STILE, Surgery Versus Thrombolysis for Ischemia of the Lower Extremity; *TOPAS,* Thrombolysis or Peripheral Arterial Surger.

with urokinase. A significant survival advantage at 12 months was noted in the thrombolysis group (84% vs 58%, $P = 0.01$), which was largely due to increased cardiovascular morbidity and mortality in the surgery group. No difference in limb salvage was noted. Interestingly, the increase in cardiovascular mortality was not substantiated in the subsequent larger TOPAS trial.

The STILE trial was stopped early by the Safety Monitoring Committee due to a higher number of adverse outcomes in the group randomized to thrombolytic therapy, likely due to enrollment of patients with ischemia out to 6 months. In post hoc subgroup analysis, patients with duration of ischemia greater than 14 days had significantly improved amputation rates with surgery compared to the thrombolytic group at 6 months (3% vs 12%), but lower amputation rates were noted in the thrombolytic group if the duration of ischemia was less than 14 days (11% vs 30%). In the thrombolysis group for those with native artery ischemia, there was also a significant reduction in the level of surgical procedure performed—that is, initial thrombolysis reduced the magnitude of the subsequent surgical procedure required for revascularization. Subgroup analysis for bypass grafts similarly showed improved amputation rates for those with bypass graft occlusion less than 14 days treated with thrombolysis. Among patients with bypass grafts, greater morbidity was encountered in those with prosthetic grafts compared with autogenous grafts. It should be noted, though, that over 80% of the patients in the trial had an ischemia duration of over 14 days, so the subgroup analysis of the less than 14 days group has relatively small numbers.

The TOPAS trial was the largest of the three randomized trials, with 544 patients enrolled with an ischemia time of less than 14 days. Patients with all forms of ischemia (native artery thrombosis, prosthetic and vein graft thrombosis) were included. One-year limb salvage and mortality were not significantly different between the surgical and thrombolysis groups. The need for open surgical procedures was significantly reduced in the thrombolytic group (54% vs 91%, $P > 0.001$), which is not surprising given the study design.

A subsequent meta-analysis of the randomized trials showed no significant differences in limb salvage or mortality at 30 days, 6 months, and 12 months between patients treated with thrombolysis or surgery. While patients undergoing thrombolysis have a less severe degree of surgical intervention (odds ratio [OR] 5.4, 95% confidence interval [CI] 4.0-7.2), they also experience a higher rate of stroke, hemorrhage, and distal embolization. These findings have been substantiated in a number of large nonrandomized registries and clinical trials. Given these findings, thrombolysis for acute limb ischemia is appropriate for selected patients but does not supplant the need for open surgical revascularization, particularly in those with a longer duration or more severe presentation of ischemia.

Techniques of Thrombolysis

Competency in basic catheter and guidewire skills is essential to successfully perform peripheral thrombolysis. Access for thrombolysis is typically "up and over" from the contralateral side. Antegrade ipsilateral access can also be used, but this is less optimal for long-term infusion, particularly in patients with an abdominal pannus in which the catheter may be prone to kinking. Upper extremity access is suboptimal because the catheter would cross the vertebral artery origin. To minimize the risk of multiple punctures, posterior wall puncture, side wall puncture, or high (external iliac) or low (superficial or profunda femoral) puncture, ultrasound-guided access using a micropuncture (21-gauge) needle is preferred. Up and over access can be achieved with any standard curved catheter depending on the operator's choice. Guidewire placement into the contralateral external iliac or common femoral artery facilitates catheter placement over the aortic bifurcation. The initial starter wire can then be exchanged for a stiff wire, over which a sheath can be placed. Most thrombolytic infusion catheters can be placed through a 5 French (F)

sheath, whereas mechanical thrombectomy devices may require a 6 to 8 F sheath.

Arteriography performed through a diagnostic catheter or through the sheath will show the site of arterial occlusion and will also give additional information about the nature of the occlusive process, showing abrupt occlusion with little collateralization in embolic occlusions and evidence of atherosclerotic disease (luminal irregularity, collateralization) in thrombotic occlusion. In a vein graft occlusion, knowledge of the site of origin of the graft is critical in locating the proximal graft. Often a small stump of patent graft will be present, but flush occlusion is also possible. Multiple oblique projections may be necessary to determine the optimal site of access of the occluded graft.

The next step is traversal of the occluded segment. Fresh thrombus is generally easy to traverse with standard 5 F catheters and 0.035-inch wires. A good catheter/guidewire combination to use in this setting is a catheter with a straight or slightly curved tip in association with either a straight or curved hydrophilic wire. In the presence of more chronic atherosclerotic disease, microcatheters (3 F) and wires (0.014-inch or 0.018-inch) may be necessary. In the acute setting, reentry into the patent native artery is rarely difficult. Reentry devices such as the Outback or Pioneer catheters may occasionally be necessary, but they are more typically used in the chronic setting. Once crossed with a guidewire, a catheter should be placed distal to the site of occlusion and contrast injected to ensure intraluminal placement.

A multisidehole infusion catheter is used for the lytic infusion. The infusion length of most multisidehole catheters ranges from 5 to 20 cm. The infusion length should ideally equal the length of occlusion, with all of the sideholes embedded in the thrombus. Sideholes outside of the thrombus are less effective in facilitating lysis because the agent generally washes out through collaterals. For longer occlusions, an infusion wire can be placed through the catheter, with lytic infusion administered simultaneously through both the catheter and the wire.

Proper securing of the sheath and catheter is critical to prevent dislodgement or movement of the devices. The sheath should be sutured to the skin and a sterile occlusive dressing placed over the sheath/catheter/infusion wire system.

Lytic Agents

Currently used lytic agents include urokinase (UK) and recombinant tissue plasminogen activator (rt-PA). Both act indirectly by converting plasminogen to plasmin, which, in turn, cleaves fibrin, leading to clot resolution. The safety and efficacy of these agents appear equal in studies to date, although there is some evidence that clot resolution occurs more quickly with rt-PA. Alfimeprase is a direct thrombolytic agent that has also been shown to be efficacious, although not studied as extensively as UK and rt-PA. Streptokinase is mainly of historical interest because it is less efficacious and more antigenic than the other agents.

A number of techniques can be used for lytic infusion. The most frequently used is the "pulse-spray" technique, in which an initial forced infusion bolus is followed by a continuous infusion. Urokinase is typically given as a 240,000-U bolus, followed by an infusion of 60,000 U/hr. Tissue plasminogen activator bolus and infusion rates vary, with a typical initial bolus of 1 to 5 mg, followed by an infusion rate of 0.125 to 2 mg/h. Simultaneous infusion of heparin, 500 U/hr, through the sheath is recommended to prevent thrombus formation on the catheter. The lytic agent and heparin should not be infused through the same catheter because precipitation can occur.

After initiation of therapy, patients should be monitored in an intensive care unit for potential complications of thrombolysis. Minor bleeding occurs in 15% of patients, with major bleeding in roughly 5% and intracranial bleeding in 1% to 2.3%. Distal embolization is occasionally encountered as thrombus dissolution occurs, occurring in 1% to 20% of cases, depending on the series. This typically manifests as an increase in pain distal to the site of infusion. This is typically transient and resolves with continuation of therapy or catheter repositioning. Reperfusion may also be associated with compartment syndrome or rhabdomyolysis. In general, the risk of complications correlates with duration of therapy, with an overall complication rate of 4% at 8 hours and 34% at 40 hours. Examples of successful thrombolysis are shown if Figure 1 (occluded bypass graft) and Figure 2 (native artery occlusion).

Mechanical Thrombolysis

A number of devices are available as adjuncts to chemical thrombolysis (Table 2). Mechanical thrombolysis has the theoretical advantage of reducing the overall length of time required for catheter-directed thrombolysis. Many devices are approved only for use in thrombosed dialysis access, but some are also appropriate for use in the periphery. A general classification of mechanical thrombectomy devices includes suction thrombectomy, hemodynamic (rheolytic) devices, rotational devices, and ultrasonic devices.

Suction Thrombectomy

Simple aspiration catheters can be used to manually extract thrombus. The catheters are connected to a stopcock and large syringe, which creates a vacuum for clot removal. This is a low-cost technique because ancillary capital equipment is not required, but it does carry the risk of vessel wall injury during clot extraction. An additional use for suction thrombectomy catheters is the removal of distal embolic debris during percutaneous catheter-based procedures. Examples of suction thrombectomy devices include Pronto, Xpress, and Export catheters.

Rheolytic Devices

Rheolytic thrombectomy devices work by creating negative pressure at the catheter tip (Venturi effect) through saline pumps. Because the

method of extraction is not through direct mechanical forces but rather through negative pressure at the catheter tip, risk of vessel wall damage is less than with the aspiration devices. Examples of such devices include the AngioJet, Hydrolyzer, Oasis, and ThromCat systems, of which only the AngioJet is currently FDA approved for use in the periphery. The device is most frequently used as an adjunct to pharmacologic thrombolysis, allowing reduced overall procedure time, but it can potentially be used as a stand-alone device in cases where pharmacologic thrombolysis is contraindicated.

Of all the mechanical thrombectomy devices currently available, the largest clinical experience has been with the AngioJet device. Technical success rates range from 56% to 95%, with distal embolization rates up to 10%. Another potential complication is hemolysis with associated renal dysfunction, so a treatment time of less than 10 minutes is advised by the manufacturer.

Rotational/Infusion Devices

The Trellis catheter has gained popularity for use in acute limb ischemia. This device combines rotational dynamics with drug infusion. A multisidehole sinusoidal infusion catheter is positioned between two balloons. After catheter positioning, the balloons are inflated to isolate the site of occlusion and to minimize the risk of distal embolization. When the catheter is activated, lytic agent is infused as the catheter oscillates, causing both clot fragmentation and dissolution. After 10 minutes of treatment, the proximal balloon is deflated, and the thrombus is aspirated through an 8 F sheath prior to deflating the distal balloon. In small series, technical success rates of up to 90% have been reported, although distal embolization occurs in up to 11% of cases.

Ultrasonographic

The EKOS device uses ultrasonic waves to augment chemical thrombus dissolution. The device combines a multisidehole infusion catheter with a coaxial ultrasonic core. Saline coolant and the lytic agent can be infused simultaneously when the catheter is activated. Thrombus deformation by the ultrasonic wave increases the surface area

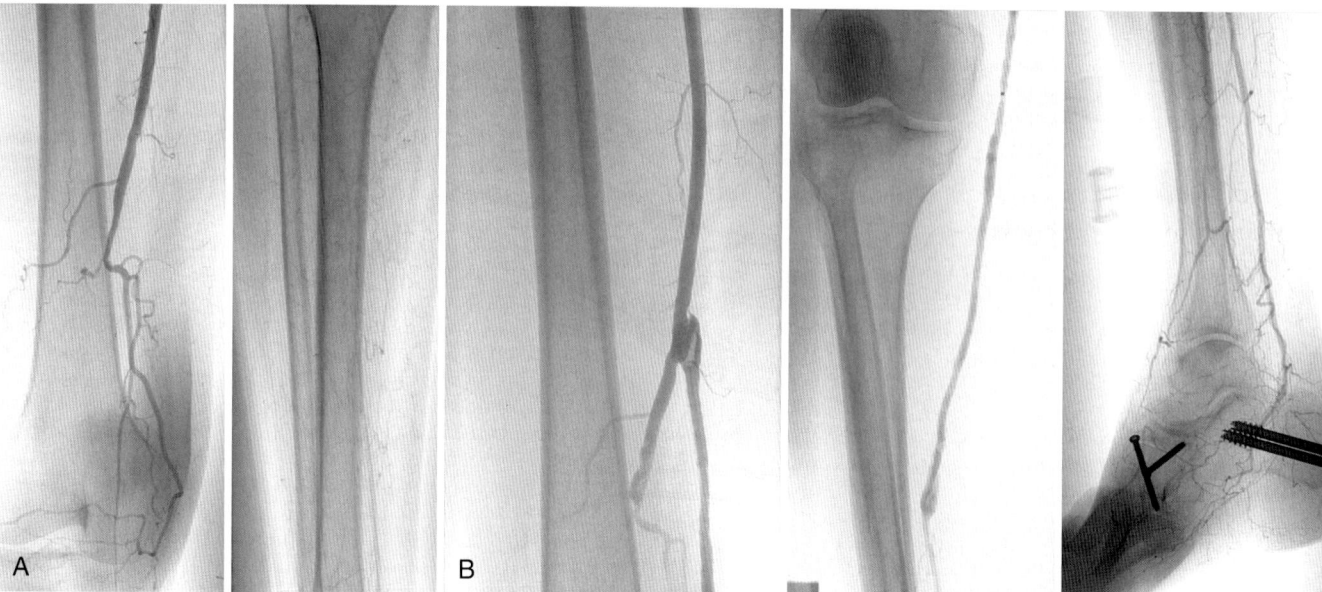

FIGURE 1 **A,** Angiogram demonstrating occlusion of superficial femoral to posterior tibial reversed saphenous vein graft. Minimal distal collateralization with weak reconstitution of distal posterior tibial artery. **B,** Postinfusion arteriogram at 24 hours demonstrating patency of graft with residual chronic thrombus present in proximal anastomosis. Markedly improved posterior tibial runoff. Patient subsequently underwent open revision of vein graft with removal of chronic thrombus from proximal hood of graft.

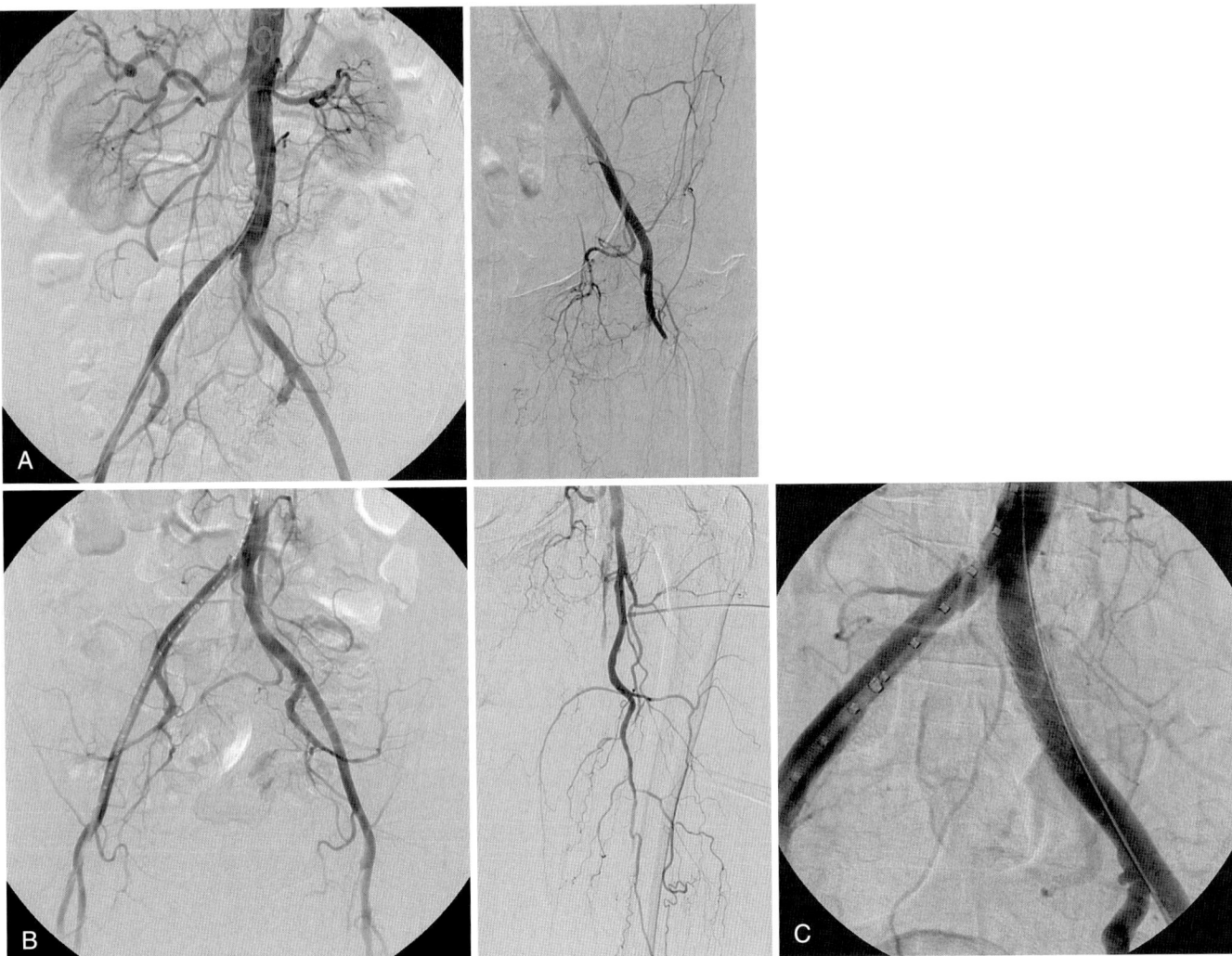

FIGURE 2   A, Arteriogram demonstrating acute thrombus in left common iliac artery, and occlusion of left internal iliac artery and left superficial and profunda femoral arteries. **B,** Postinfusion arteriogram at 24 hours showing resolution of thrombus in common and internal iliac and profunda femoral arteries. Superficial femoral artery found to be chronically occluded. Distal leg perfusion was present through internal iliac and profunda femoral collaterals, resulting in limb salvage. **C,** Left common iliac artery stenosis treated with balloon expandable stent with no residual stenosis.

TABLE 2: Mechanical thrombectomy devices

Mechanism	Name, manufacturer	Sheath size (French)	Guidewire (inches)	Working length (cm)
Suction thrombectomy	Pronto, Vascular Solutions	5.5-10	0.014-0.035	115-140
	Xpress, Atrium	6-7	0.014	140
	Export, Medtronic	6-7	0.014	140-145
Rheolytic devices	AngioJet, Possis/Medrad	4-6	0.014-0.035	50-145
	Hydrolyser, Cordis	7	0.025	65-100
	Oasis, Boston Scientific	6	0.014	65-100
	ThromCat, Spectranetics	6	0.014	150
Rotational infusion devices	Trellis, Covidien	6-8	0.035	80-120
Ultrasound devices	EkoSonic Endovascular System, EKOS Corporation	6	0.035	106-135
	OmniWave, Cybersonics	7	0.018	100

exposure for the lytic agent. In small, uncontrolled series, treatment times have been shown to be significantly reduced with ultrasound augmentation.

CONCLUSION

Since its initial use over 30 years ago, catheter-directed thrombolysis for acute arterial and bypass graft occlusion has grown and now can be considered the procedure of choice in some patients, particularly those with minimal or no symptoms and with ischemia duration of less than 14 days. While previously in the purview of interventional radiology, the acquisition of advanced catheter and guidewire skills among vascular surgeons has led to this technique becoming an important component of the vascular surgical armamentarium. While still associated with significant morbidity and mortality, technical advances continue to reduce treatment times and associated risks.

SUGGESTED READINGS

Ansel GM, Botti CF, Silver MJ: Treatment of acute limb ischemia with a percutaneous mechanical thrombectomy-based endovascular approach, *Catheter and Cardiovasc Intervent* 72:325–330, 2008.

Berridge DC, Kessel DO, Robertson I: Surgery versus thrombolysis for initial management of acute limb ischaemia, *Cochrane Database of Systematic Reviews* 2002, Issue 1. Art No.: CD002784. DOI: 10.1002/14651858. CD002784.

Earnshaw JJ, Whitman B, Foy C: National audit of thrombolysis for acute leg ischemia (NATALI): clinical factors associated with early outcome, *J Vasc Surg* 39:1018–1025, 2004.

Hynes BG, Margey RJ, Ruggiero N, et al: Endovascular management of acute limb ischemia, *Ann Vasc Surg* 26:110–124, 2012.

Karnabatidis D, Spiliopoulos S, Tsetis D, et al: Quality improvement guidelines for percutaneous catheter-directed intra-arterial thrombolysis and mechanical thrombectomy for acute lower-limb ischemia, *Cardiovasc Intervent Radiol* 34:1123–1136, 2011.

Kashyap VS, Gilani R, Bena JF, et al: Endovascular therapy for acute limb ischemia, *J Vasc Surg* 53:340–346, 2011.

Kessel DO, Berridge DC, Robertson I: Infusion techniques for peripheral arterial thrombolysis, *Cochrane Database of Systematic Reviews* 2004, Issue 1. Art. No. CD000985. DOI: 10.1002/14651858. CD000985.pub2.

Ochoa C, Weaver FA: Basic data related to thrombolytic therapy for acute arterial thrombosis, *Ann Vasc Surg* 26:292–297, 2012.

Van den Berg JC: Thrombolysis for acute arterial occlusion, *J Vasc Surg* 52:512–515, 2010.

ATHEROSCLEROTIC RENAL ARTERY DISEASE

Francis J. Caputo, MD, and Gregorio A. Sicard, MD

INTRODUCTION

Twenty to thirty percent of the population in the United States is hypertensive. Approximately 5% of patients with hypertension will have renovascular hypertension. While renal artery disease includes many different pathophysiologies, this chapter focuses on atherosclerotic renal artery stenosis (RAS), the most common cause of RAS. Atherosclerotic RAS has been implicated as a major contributor to systemic hypertension as well as impaired renal function. However, rarely is RAS the sole contributor to these two multifactorial clinical pathologies. Although the incidence of RAS may be as high as 45% in high-risk groups, no data are available to justify prophylactic treatment of patients with asymptomatic disease. In fact, the majority of patients with symptomatic RAS will be medically managed, and revascularization will be unwarranted.

INCIDENCE

Ninety percent of RAS is due to atherosclerosis. Autopsy reports found increased prevalence of significant RAS with increasing age: 6% in patients younger than 55 years, 18% in patients 65 to 74 years of age, and 40% in patients older than 75, with the proximal renal artery being the most common location. The prevalence of unsuspected renal artery stenosis in 5194 consecutive autopsies found RAS greater than 50% in 4.3% of the patient population, with 73% of these patients having had a history of hypertension. The prevalence of RAS increases as a population becomes more high risk (Table 1).

NATURAL HISTORY OF RENAL ARTERY STENOSIS

Anatomic Progression

While RAS is often implicated as a cause of hypertension and worsening renal function, frequently RAS is an incidental finding either through a screening test or while undergoing intraabdominal imaging, computed tomographic angiography (CTA), magnetic resonance angiography (MRA), or arteriography for other reasons. Although

TABLE 1: Prevalence of renal artery stenosis in high-risk populations

Population	Prevalence
All commers	0.1%
Hypertensive	4.0%
Hypertensive and coronary artery disease	30%
Malignant hypertension	20% to 30%
Renal insufficiency and malignant hypertension	30% to 40%

the severity of RAS is an independent predictor of mortality (Table 2), it is uncertain as to whether RAS is a direct cause or just a marker of decreased survival. Thus, the importance of treating "silent lesions" remains to be fully understood. In angiographic studies, the percentage of patients showing progression of renal artery atherosclerosis ranged from 11% to 44%, and approximately 10% to 16% progressed to complete occlusion in arteries that previously had severe stenosis. Interestingly, only 3% had loss of a previously reconstructible renal artery. Duplex ultrasound has also been used in surveillance of RAS. Zierler and colleagues performed serial duplex ultrasounds on 90 patients diagnosed with renovascular hypertension. The patients' arteries were classified as normal, less than 60% stenosis, or greater than 60% stenosis. At the 3-year follow-up, 8% of normal arteries and 43% of arteries with less than 60% stenosis had progressed to greater than 60% stenosis. Seven percent of arteries surveyed progressed to complete occlusion, but this only occurred in arteries with a preexisting lesion that was less than 60%.

Functional Progression

The implication of RAS on functional end points has been studied using ultrasound surveillance. Dean and colleagues found that 46% of patients ($n = 41$) being treated with medical therapy showed a significant rise in serum creatinine, and 37% of patients had lost more than 10% of renal length. At a 33-month follow-up, Caps and colleagues observed renal atrophy (loss of 1 cm length) of 5.5%, 11.7%, and 20.8% in renal arteries classified as normal, less than 60% stenotic, and greater than 60% stenotic, respectively. Other factors correlated with renal atrophy include elevated creatinine, systolic blood pressure of greater than 180 mm Hg, peak systolic velocity of greater than 400 cm/sec, and an end diastolic velocity of less than 5 cm/sec. Schrieber and colleagues showed that a large number of patients with greater than 60% RAS had increased creatinine.

TREATMENT

Patient Selection

Although RAS is a negative predictor for cardiovascular morbidity and mortality, no consensus statement has been made regarding treatment of RAS. Furthermore, no level 1 data show that revascularization of asymptomatic RAS leads to better outcomes and survival as compared to medical management. Therefore, we reserve revascularization of patients with RAS for those patients with renovascular hypertension nonresponsive to maximal medical therapy and for those patients with renovascular hypertension and concomitant worsening of excretory renal function. Flash pulmonary edema is an uncommon manifestation of RAS—in particular, bilateral RAS or high-grade RAS in a single kidney. These patients often benefit from revascularization.

TABLE 2: Renal artery stenosis–independent predictor of mortality

Severity of renal artery stenosis	4-year survival
50%	70%
75%	68%
>95%	48%

Medical Therapy

As mentioned before, patients with RAS, even if asymptomatic, are at increased risk of cardiac mortality and morbidity. Therefore, all patients with diagnosed RAS should be treated for hypertension and risk factors associated with progression of atherosclerosis. Goals of therapy include aggressive treatment of hypertension, smoking cessation, aggressive lipid-lowering strategies, and antiplatelet therapy.

Hypertension Control

Control of hypertension remains a key component in patients with RAS. While there are several classes of medication to control blood pressure, particular interest has been given to angiotensin converting enzyme inhibitors (ACEI) and angiotensin receptor blockers (ARBs). Since a leading mechanism of hypertension due to RAS is secondary to the effects of the increased renin-angiotensin pathway, it makes sense that inhibiting this pathway would prove to be a favorable therapeutic maneuver. Furthermore, several studies have suggested that in patients with preexisting cardiovascular disease, treatment with ACEI leads to reduction in total mortality and adverse cardiovascular events, as well as being renoprotective in patients with nephropathy. ACEI/ARBs have been associated with renal failure in patients with severe RAS, most often in patients with bilateral severe RAS or high-grade RAS in a single kidney. Although physicians are hesitant to use ACEI or ARBs in patients with bilateral RAS due to the potential of acute deterioration of renal function, this is uncommon. While ARBs/ACEI should be the initial treatment of hypertension in patients with renovascular hypertension, additional medications may be needed when blood pressure is difficult to control.

Lipid-Lowering Agents

Statins remain the cornerstone of treating hypercholesterolemia in patients with atherosclerosis and its associated morbidities. It has been shown that statins prevent coronary artery disease, decrease myocardial infarction rates, prevent progression of atherosclerosis, and decrease cardiovascular death. While few studies have correlated statin use with outcomes of patients with RAS, Cheung and colleagues showed a reduction of 72% in risk for angiographic progression of patients with RAS. Statins have been shown to decrease progression of disease in carotid artery stenosis as well as peripheral vascular disease.

Antiplatelet Therapy

While aspirin or clopidogrel has not been shown to directly affect RAS, antiplatelet therapy has been shown to be important in the decrease of adverse cardiovascular events and mortality in patients with significant atherosclerotic burden. Also, antiplatelet therapy is an important adjunct when endovascular revascularization is employed for RAS. Typically patients are loaded with clopidogrel either preoperatively or immediately postoperatively after percutaneous revascularization. Antiplatelet therapy presumably decreases immediate thrombotic events as well as helps prevent progression of restenosis.

Other Risk Modifications

It is recommended, as in other high-risk populations, that patients should be counseled in smoking cessation. Smoking has been implicated in endothelial cell damage, increased low-density lipoprotein (LDL) cholesterol, increased platelet aggregation, and a source of oxidative stress. Furthermore, smoking leads to increased vasoconstriction, increased heart rate, and increased blood pressure. Smoking cessation has shown to improve survival in patients with peripheral arterial disease (PAD) as well as coronary artery disease (CAD). In fact, patients who quit smoking have a 13% decreased reduction in risk for all-cause mortality.

Additionally, patients with documented diabetes and concomitant atherosclerosis are at increased risk of progression of disease. While intensive glycemic control has not been shown to decrease cardiovascular events, good glycemic control (hemoglobin A1c <7.0%) does help prevent microvascular complications.

Surgical Therapy

We reserve surgical intervention, whether endovascular or open, to patients with refractory hypertension despite maximal medical therapy as well as patients with hypertension and concomitant progressive decreasing renal function. While endovascular revascularization is technically feasible and early-patency is excellent, increased restenosis rates as well as lack of long-term patency data lead us to prefer open surgical revascularization when the patient is a good candidate.

Unilateral Renal Artery Stenosis

In patients with unilateral RAS, we prefer a retroperitoneal approach to renal revascularization. While direct aortorenal bypass is possible through this exposure, we prefer ileorenal bypass if the common iliac is free of plaque and calcific disease. With the patient in the lateral decubitus position, a curvilinear incision is performed extending from just lateral to the rectus muscle and sheath to the 12th rib (Figure 1). This incision is carried down through the subcutaneous tissue and fascia. The anterior sheath is divided, and the 12th rib is excised. The internal oblique and transversalis muscles are divided, and the retroperitoneum is entered just lateral to the junction of the rectus sheath in the lateral abdominal wall muscles. The peritoneum is then mobilized medially and cephalad. Once the peritoneum is mobilized, the ureter is identified and gently dissected down to the level of the distal common iliac artery inferiorly and superiorly to the level of the renal pelvis. If the dissection is being performed on the left side, it is often necessary to identify and ligate the gonadal

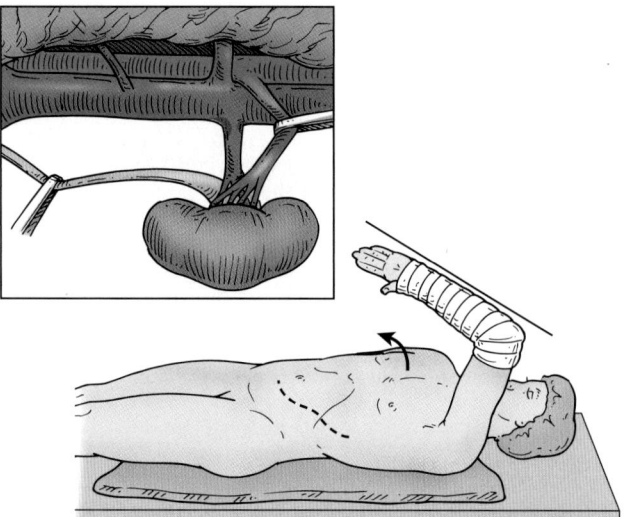

FIGURE 1 Proper positioning of patient for retroperitoneal dissection includes right lateral decubitus, with flexion of bed and elevated kidney rest. Dashed line shows planned incision from 12th rib to umbilicus. *(Inset)* Left renal vein is fully mobilized with ligated left gonadal vein. Ureter is dissected from surrounding tissue, and disease is shown at ostium of left renal artery.

vein as well as the inferior lumbar branch of the left renal vein. Once the ureter is mobilized, Gerota's fascia is entered, and the kidney is circumferentially mobilized. The renal artery is identified and dissected to its junction with the aorta. At this point, the patient is systematically heparinized, the common iliac artery is clamped, and an end-to-side anastomosis is performed to our conduit. We prefer to use saphenous vein, but if deemed unsuitable (<3 mm, sclerotic), PTFE is used. Once the iliac anastomosis is performed, the renal artery is mobilized proximally and doubly ligated with silk suture. Iced slush is applied over the kidney to decrease its temperature, and an end-to-end anastomosis is performed between the conduit and the renal artery in a running or interrupted fashion, depending on the size of the renal artery. Doppler signals confirm flow in the renal artery and the renal parenchyma. In patients with right-sided RAS (Figure 2), it is important to circumferentially mobilize the right renal vein at the lateral border of the inferior vena cava in order to fully dissect the right renal artery. In instances where two small diseased renal arteries are identified (Figure 2, *A*), it may be necessary to surgically combine the two arteries into one larger orifice to facilitate revascularization (Figure 2,*B*).

Bilateral Renal Artery Stenosis

In patients with bilateral RAS, often the renal artery plaque is an extension of aortic wall atherosclerosis. In this situation, bilateral renal endarterectomy is the procedure of choice. While transaortic endarterectomy has been described, transrenal endarterectomy (Figure 3) allows direct visualization of distal end points and permits tacking sutures if necessary. A midline incision is made from the xiphoid process to the symphysis pubis. The linea alba is incised and the peritoneal cavity is entered. It is necessary to extend the incision superior along one side of the xiphoid process to allow full abdominal wall mobilization. The posterior peritoneum overlying the aorta is incised, the ligament of Treitz is sharply dissected, and the duodenum is mobilized. The small bowel is eviscerated and retracted to the right. The aorta is identified and dissected in a cephalad direction until the renal vein is identified. Circumferential dissection of the renal vein is necessary, as is dissection of the immediate inferior vena cava superiorly and inferiorly 2 cm. Usually, the gonadal and adrenal veins must be ligated, as well as the inferior lumbar branch of the left renal vein. This allows full visualization of both renal arteries. Once both renal arteries are fully mobilized, the patient is systemically heparinized, the aorta is clamped above and below the renal arteries, and a transverse incision is made across both renal arteries (Figure 3). An endarterectomy is performed using a dural elevator, and any concerning flaps at the distal end point are tacked with 6-0 Prolene suture. A Dacron patch closure (Figure 3,*B*) is then used to close the aortotomy and prevent narrowing.

Other Surgical Options

Other surgical techniques, including splanchnorenal bypass and renal artery transposition, have been described. This may be necessary in situations where the aorta or iliac is of inadequate quality to provide inflow for revascularizations. Situations may include ectatic vessels as well as severe calcification.

Open Surgical Results

Open renal artery carries an approximate mortality of 0.8% for isolated renal artery repair and 1.6% for bilateral renal artery revascularization. While perioperative morbidity can be as high as 20%, patients who ended up on permanent dialysis within 30 days of their revascularization were less than 1%. The majority of patients (85%) exhibit improved hypertension, and more than 50% of patients have improved renal function. Open repair of RAS has a patency of greater than 95% at 2 years as surveilled by duplex ultrasonography.

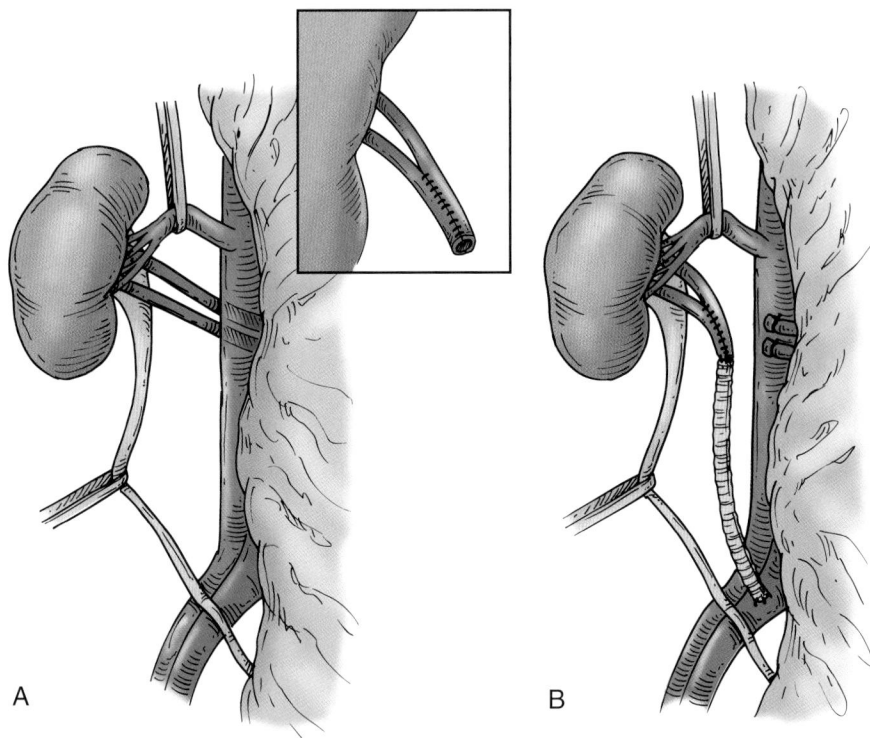

FIGURE 2   A, Right retroperitoneal dissection is shown, with kidney having two small diseased arteries. A circumferentially dissected left renal vein is retracted cephalad. The two arteries are surgically combined into one main trunk. **B,** Completed right ileorenal bypass with PTFE is shown.

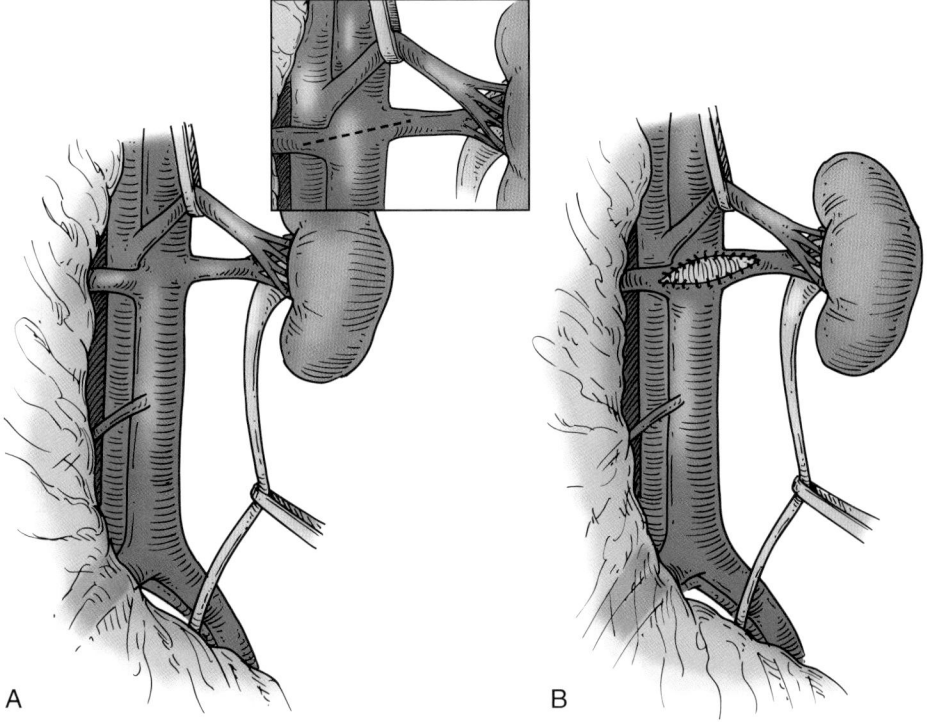

FIGURE 3   A, Exposure of the juxtarenal aorta and bilateral diseased renal arteries. Dashed line shows path of transrenal arteriotomy in preparation for endarterectomy. **B,** Completed patch angioplasty after endarterectomy is shown.

Endovascular Revascularization

While open surgical revascularization has excellent results in terms of outcomes and patency, there is a significant morbidity associated with repair. Also, many patients with advanced hypertension and progressive renal failure have concomitant comorbidities that preclude them from being open surgical candidates. Therefore, an alternative to open revascularization is percutaneous angioplasty and stenting (PTAS). While PTAS has excellent short-term results, restenosis rates can be as high as 60%. Contributors to increased rates of

restenosis include small vessels, female gender, multiple lesions, and diffuse aortic atherosclerotic disease. Optimal renal artery size for stenting is greater than 5 mm with a single focal ostial lesion.

Renal Artery Stenting

The key to renal artery stenting is understanding that in most instances, renal artery lesions are ostial and are extensions from the aorta. Thus, the stent needs to be placed just outside the ostium in order to provide a lumen from the encroaching aortic plaque. We use a 6F system. Once a diagnostic aortogram is performed using a pigtail catheter, the anatomy is assessed in order to see if the lesion is amenable to PTAS (size, length, accessibility). The patient is systemically heparinized, the renal artery is cannulated, and the lesion is crossed using a 0.018-inch wire and various catheters. Once the artery has been cannulated, the catheter is advanced into the renal artery and the 0.018-inch wire is exchanged for a stiffer, less traumatic J-wire. A sheath is then exchanged over the guidewire into the renal ostium, and a renal angiogram is performed to characterize the RAS, as well as perform measurements for PTAS. If deemed amenable to PTAS, the long sheath is advanced over the wire and through the lesion. The selected balloon-expandable stent is brought over the wire and placed in the appropriate location, making sure to extend slightly into the aorta. The sheath is retracted and the stent is deployed. Occasionally, predilation using a smaller balloon is necessary. The patient is started on antiplatelet therapy—namely, clopidogrel for 30 days—and aspirin is continued indefinitely.

Endovascular Results

Renal artery stents have a high technical success (>95%) in most series. Mortality and morbidity are low, but response to treatment has yet to be fully elucidated. While it does appear in some series to have some beneficial effects on hypertension, there is very little evidence that renal artery stenting prevents renal dysfunction in the face of unimpaired baseline renal function. Furthermore, PTAS has been implicated in worsening of renal function postprocedure. In fact, some series report that an equivalent number of patients have worsened renal function compared with those with improved renal function. Combining this with the high rate of restenosis (>10%) should dissuade practitioners from performing prophylactic renal artery stents in patients with angiographic lesions that are functionally silent.

SUMMARY

While frequently diagnosed, RAS is often treated in the modern era medically. Patients whose hypertension cannot be controlled and in the setting of worsening renal function may benefit from revascularization, but the "gold standard" remains open surgical techniques. Endovascular techniques should be reserved for patients who are unfit surgical candidates. Treatment of angiographic lesions without a functional component should not be performed because no current level 1 evidence suggests there is an improvement in outcomes compared with medical therapy.

SUGGESTED READINGS

Astral Investigators: Revascularization versus medical therapy for renal-artery stenosis, N Engl J Med 361:1953–1962, 2009.
Cherr GS, Hansen KJ, Craven TE, et al: Surgical management of atherosclerotic renovascular disease, J Vasc Surg 35:236–245, 2002.
Edwards MS, Corriere MA: Contemporary management of atherosclerotic renovascular disease, J Vasc Surg 50:1197–1210, 2009.

RAYNAUD'S SYNDROME

Andy M. Lee, MD, and Elliot L. Chaikof, MD, PhD

OVERVIEW

Raynaud's syndrome (RS) is a condition that typifies an exaggerated vasoconstrictive response in extremities triggered by cold or emotional stimuli. First observed by Maurice Raynaud in 1862, characteristically, a triphasic color progression is observed in fingers and toes that is described as digital pallor due to arterial spasm, cyanosis as a consequence of reduced venous flow and pooling of deoxygenated blood, and a hyperemic response from warming reperfusion (Figure 1). This abnormal vascular response can also affect other sites, such as the tongue, nose, and cheeks, and can range in severity and presentation. Raynaud's is referred to as *primary Raynaud's syndrome* if an underlying disease process cannot be identified and is classified as *Raynaud's disease* or *secondary Raynaud's syndrome* if an associated underlying disease, such as systemic sclerosis or mixed connective tissue disease, is identified.

The distribution of RS is worldwide and its incidence varies from 3% to 14% in men and 3% to 20% in women. Populations in colder regions have greater prevalence of Raynaud's, which also contributes to a higher frequency of attacks. Raynaud's phenomenon can occur at any age, but onset typically begins at a younger age. Many risk factors have been suggested to contribute to primary and secondary forms of Raynaud's. However, definitive therapy is lacking and remains an area of evolving research.

Primary Raynaud's syndrome (PRS) is the most prevalent form in the general population, follows a benign course, and is characteristically a self-limited functional vascular defect with intervention seldom needed. Secondary Raynaud's syndrome (SRS) is rarer, is associated with an immunologically mediated systemic disease, and is characterized by episodes of intense pain with eventual progression in most patients to ischemic ulceration and gangrenous digits. SRS is associated with microvascular occlusive disease and the lack of a compensatory vasodilatory response. Because of the presence of more severe symptoms, patients that suffer from SRS will often need medical treatment and may require surgical intervention (Table 1).

PATHOGENESIS

The pathogenesis of Raynaud's is unclear. The disruption between vasoconstrictive and vasodilatory responses is associated with systemic, neural, and local structural vascular abnormalities. For instance, impaired endothelial production of nitric oxide and prostacyclin, as well as endothelin-1 and angiotensin II, have been postulated to contribute to impaired vasodilatory and vasoconstrictive responses, respectively. Abnormal expression of endothelial cytokines and growth factors is thought to elicit an inflammatory process leading to structural changes, including intimal fibrosis. Alternatively, impaired smooth muscle cell responses leading to abnormal production of the vasodilator, calcitonin-related peptide, or activation of the alpha-2 adrenergic receptor can also contribute to Raynaud's. Unopposed sympathetic vascular tone has also been proposed as a contributing factor. Lastly, hypercoagulable states, activated platelets and leukocytes, as well as diminished fibrinolysis, have been observed in both primary and secondary RS.

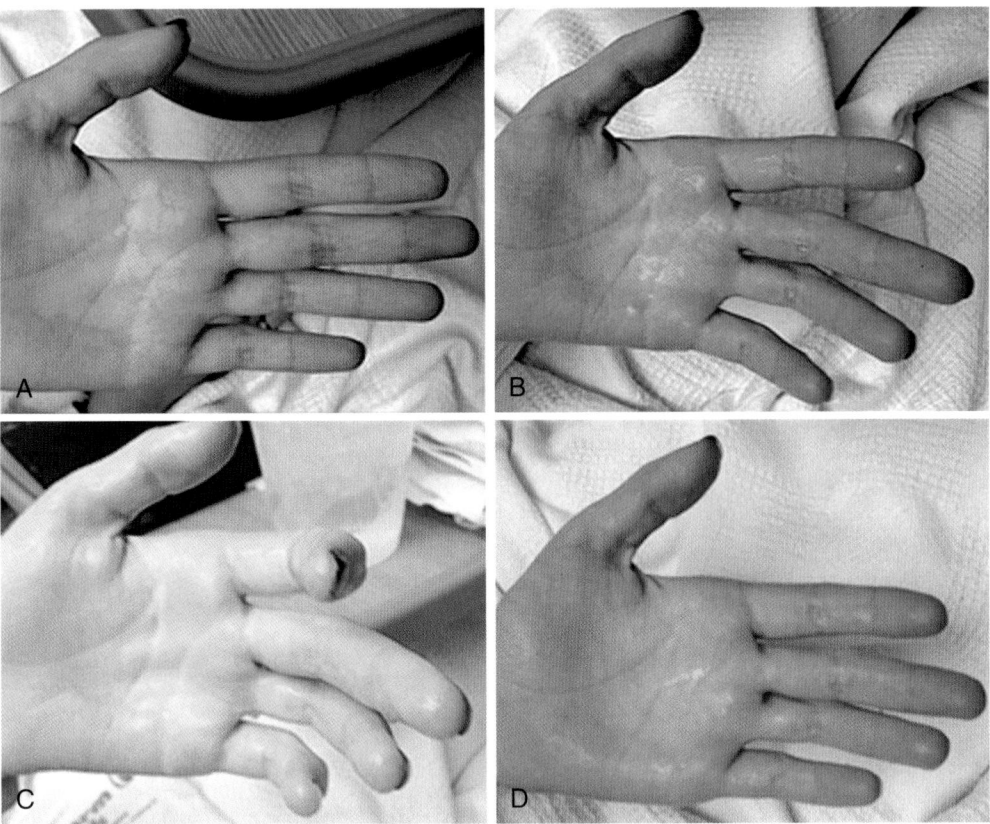

FIGURE 1 Raynaud's syndrome in patient with Ehlers-Danlos syndrome to illustrate the color changes associated with stressful stimuli. **A,** Normal appearing hand. **B,** After cold stimuli, the pallor from vasoconstriction can be seen. **C,** After 30 seconds, the hyperemic red appears in fingers with blood reperfusion. **D,** Hand after 3 minutes exposed to stimuli.

DIAGNOSIS AND PRESENTATION

The diagnosis of RS is based on history, including episodes of pain with notable color variation. It is important that triggers related to the onset of symptoms are noted. To exclude secondary causes, an occupational history, drug and medication use, family history, and current smoking status should be obtained (Box 1). A thorough vascular exam should exclude underlying symptomatic aneurysmal or atherosclerotic arterial occlusive disease that could mimic the presentation of RS. Thoracic outlet obstruction could produce unilateral upper extremity symptoms that could be mistaken for RS. The presence of pitting scars or healed digital ulceration should be noted, as well as flexion deformities, joint effusions, skin pigmentation, or ulcers that may be associated with scleroderma or systemic lupus erythematosus.

Routine blood work should include a complete blood count, immunologic and inflammatory markers for autoantibodies, antinuclear antibodies, Sjögren factors (SS-A and SS-B), rheumatoid factor, thyroid hormone levels, and an erythrocyte sedimentation rate. Specialized diagnostic tools can be used to assess the digital vascular response. Temperature-dependent digital plethysmography is obtainable in most noninvasive vascular laboratories. Infrared thermography and nailfold videocapillaroscopy may also be helpful in confirming the diagnosis of RS.

Angiography should be considered in the presence of severe hand ischemia or gangrene, primarily to exclude multilevel atherosclerotic occlusive disease or an embolic source due to a proximal aneurysm in the subclavian artery or distal ulnar artery aneurysm observed in hypothenar hammer syndrome. Comprehensive evaluation of the arterial supply of the hand, including the radial and ulnar arteries, as well as the palmar arch and digital vessels, can facilitate surgical planning to prevent further tissue loss.

Nailfold video capillaroscopy is performed with an ophthalmoscope or dermatoscope to assess capillary changes in the nail bed.

Capillaries appear normal in PRS, whereas distorted, hemorrhagic, enlarged, and avascular capillary loops are characteristic of patients with scleroderma. If available, capillaroscopy is recommended for diagnosing scleroderma.

TREATMENT

The distinction between primary and secondary forms of Raynaud's is important in deciding on treatment. In PRS, episodes are self-limited and respond to supportive measures, changes in lifestyle, and avoidance of factors that can trigger symptoms. In SRS, treating any underlying disease, in addition to conservative measures and pharmacologic therapy, is often required. In the presence of digital ulceration and gangrene, local wound care and surgery may be needed to prevent further ischemic progression and avoid amputation. Severity of disease will dictate treatment and need for pharmacologic or surgical intervention (Table 2).

Conservative Treatment

Through avoidance of cold exposure and other triggers, milder Raynaud symptoms can be effectively controlled, minimizing the frequency and severity of attacks. The entire body should be covered and well insulated to protect exposed skin. Discontinuation of smoking is also recommended to reduce the severity of symptoms. Medication with vasoconstrictive potential, such as beta-blockers, sumatriptan, and ephedrine, should be avoided. Other substances with vasospastic properties include caffeine, decongestants, cocaine, and amphetamines.

Patients are advised to reduce stress with coping and relaxation techniques. Although biofeedback has been reported to minimize

TABLE 1: Characteristics of primary and secondary Raynaud's syndrome

	Primary	Secondary
Age	Younger (<30 years)	Older (>30 years)
Gender preference	Female	Male (depending on secondary cause)
Incidence	Most common	Less common
Familial predisposition	Yes	Yes
Combination with other disease	No, idiopathic	Associated with systemic disease
Vascular defect	Functional dysregulation of autonomic nervous system	Structural changes in connective tissue and/or vessels
Associated signs	None	Arthritis, sclerodactyly, cardiopulmonary abnormality, rash
Frequency	Precipitated by stimuli	Periodic and stimuli trigger
Severity of symptoms	Long history of mild attacks	Severe and disabling pain
Distribution	Symmetric	Asymmetric
Duration	Self-limited	Need for additional treatment (pharmacologic/surgery)
Critical complications	None	Ischemia and ulcers
Capillaroscopy	Normal (symmetric, thin, and uniform)	Abnormal (dilated, irregular, elongated, and tortuous vessel)
Vascular exam	Normal pulses	Abnormal pulses
ESR	Normal	Elevated
Serologic studies	Negative	Antinuclear antibody, autoantibodies
C-reactive protein	Normal	Elevated

ESR, Erythrocyte sedimentation rate.

symptom severity, a meta-analysis by Malenfant and colleagues (2009) of five randomized controlled trials showed no difference in severity, frequency, or symptom duration. Use of vibration-proof tools may also decrease the occurrence of RS.

Pharmacologic

Calcium Channel Blockers

For symptoms that are not responsive to conservative methods, calcium channel blockers are the drug of choice in the medical management of RS. Nifedipine has been studied most extensively and reduces vascular tone through an effect on the voltage gated calcium channel. Dihydropyridine-derived calcium channel blockers, including amlodipine, nicardipine, and felodipine, are currently favored because of their selectivity for peripheral vascular smooth muscle cells. Treatment is initiated at a low dose that is slowly increased to avoid hypotension, reflex tachycardia, headache, and flushing. In several meta-analyses of randomized control trials, Thompson and colleagues (2001) and Thompson and Pope (2005) noted that nifedipine decreased the frequency and severity of attacks (35%). Sustained release preparations are better tolerated and exhibit longer acting effects.

Prostaglandins

Prostaglandins (PGEs) have several beneficial effects for both primary and secondary forms of Raynaud's, including vasodilatory and antiproliferative effects in smooth muscle cells and the capacity to inhibit platelet aggregation. PGEs are used in the absence of a response to other vasodilators. Iloprost, an intravenous prostacyclin analogue, has been used in severe RS. In a multicentered randomized trial, Wigley and colleagues (1994) demonstrated that 5-day administration of iloprost decreased the frequency of attacks and healed 50% more lesions compared with placebo. In a randomized study of 30 patients, Milio and colleagues (2006) administered iloprost therapy over 3 to 18 months, which led to a reduction in the duration and frequency of attacks with improved quality of life. Compared to nifedipine, iloprost demonstrated improved long-term skin and functional scores. Adverse effects of iloprost include headache, flushing, and nausea. PGEs should be used with caution in patients with congestive heart failure because of the risk of exacerbating pulmonary edema. Controversial results exist for oral PGE analogues, and currently only the intravenous formulation is recommended in severe cases.

Alpha-2 Adrenoreceptor Blockers

The alpha-2 adrenergic pathway regulates sympathetic peripheral vascular tone. In a randomized, double-blinded, placebo controlled

BOX 1: Secondary causes of Raynaud's syndrome

Rheumatologic
Systemic sclerosis (CREST syndrome)
Sjögren's syndrome
Systemic lupus erythematosus
Ehlers-Danlos syndrome
Rheumatoid arthritis
Dermatomyositis
Polymyositis
Mixed connective tissue disease

Autoimmune
Reiter's syndrome
Vasculitis (polyarteritis nodosa, Henoch-Schönlein purpura)
Antiphospholipid syndrome
Primary pulmonary hypertension

Endocrine
Hypothyroidism
Pheochromocytoma
Carcinoid

Infectious
Hepatitis B and C infection
Mycoplasma pneumonia

Medications
Cyclosporine
Ergotamine
Beta-blockers
Cytotoxic (bleomycin, cisplatin, vinblastine)
Bromocriptine
Nicotine
Cocaine
Sulfasalazine
Interferon alpha and beta

Clonidine
Sympathomimetics
Estrogen in oral contraceptives
Caffeine

Occlusive Vascular
Arteriosclerosis
Vascular trauma (hypothenar hammer syndrome)
Buerger's disease
Thoracic outlet syndrome
Thromboembolism

Hematologic/Proliferative
Leukemia
Lymphoma
Polycythemia vera
Multiple myeloma
Disseminated intravascular coagulation
Cryoglobulinemia
Cold agglutinin disease

Neurologic
Migraines
Carpal tunnel syndrome
Polyneuropathy

Environmental
Emotional stress
Frostbite
Repetitive trauma or injuries to hand

Malignancy
Lung, stomach, small bowel
Paraneoplastic syndrome
Neurofibromatosis

study of 24 patients with RS, Wollersheim and colleagues (1986) observed a reduction in frequency and duration of attacks. Pope and colleagues (2000a) have demonstrated that prazosin was effective in treating Raynaud's secondary to scleroderma. Side effects of alpha-adrenoreceptor blockers include nausea, dizziness, headache, and hypotension. Drug resistance may occur with prolonged use. Despite some evidence of utility in Raynaud's, at this time sympatholytic agents cannot be recommended as first-line agents.

Angiotensin-Converting Enzyme Inhibitors and Angiotensin Receptor Blockers

Angiotensin-converting enzyme (ACE) inhibitors inhibit the synthesis of angiotensin II and prevent the degradation of bradykinin, which is a potent vasodilator. Nonetheless, ACE inhibitors have a limited role in RS. In a randomized controlled study of losartan and nifedipine, Dziadzio and colleagues (1999) observed that losartan decreased symptoms and the severity of attacks. In contrast, Gliddon and colleagues (2007) treated patients who had Raynaud's with quinapril for 2 to 3 years and noted no change in symptom frequency or severity or occurrence of digital ulcers. Although angiotensin inhibitors have an acceptable side effect profile, there is insufficient evidence for their clinical use in RS.

Phosphodiesterase Inhibitors

Phosphodiesterase inhibitors increase cyclic guanosine monophosphate (cGMP) in circulation that decreases vascular smooth muscle

tone. In several randomized trials, these inhibitors decreased the frequency and severity of attacks in primary and secondary RS and had a favorable effect on ulcer healing. In a randomized double-blinded trial, Fries and colleagues (2005) reported that a 4-week regimen of sildenafil reduced attacks and improved ulcer healing, but recurrence was observed when treatment was halted. Similar results were observed by Shenoy and colleagues (2010) in a 6-week trial of tadalafil. Common side effects include headache and nasal congestion. As these drugs are well tolerated, phosphodiesterase inhibitors represent a promising therapy for Raynaud's.

Endothelin-1 Receptor Antagonist

Endothelin-1 is a vasoconstrictor found at increased levels in patients with systemic sclerosis. Recent studies indicate a role for endothelin-1 receptor antagonist in patients who have severe RS with ulceration not responding to other therapies. Endothelin-1 receptors are found in both endothelial (ETa) and smooth muscle (ETb) cells with distinct receptors mainly responsible for vasoconstriction (ETa) and vasodilation (ETb). Bosentan is a competitive antagonist to both receptors and is currently approved for clinical use in Europe. Korn and colleagues (2004) assessed the effects of bosentan in treating digital ulcers in 122 patients with systemic sclerosis. Bosentan showed a 48% reduction in the mean number of new ulcers but had no effect on ulcer healing. Likewise, in another randomized trial of 188 patients, after 20 to 32 weeks, bosentan decreased the number of new ulcers by 30% without affecting ulcer healing. Endothelin-1 has pro-fibrotic activity, and two case reports suggest that bosentan may be

TABLE 2: Available treatment options for Raynaud's syndrome

Treatment	Indications		Comments
Conservative	First-line therapy with mild symptoms		Smoking cessation; avoiding stress, cold, vasoconstrictive stimulants and medications; biofeedback

Pharmacologic treatment	Indications	Common adverse effects	Comments
Calcium channel blockers (CCBs)	Conservative therapy ineffective	Hypotension, reflex tachycardia, flushing, headache	Nifedipine most studied; sustained long-acting CCB (amlodipine, nicardipine, and felodipine) gaining popularity
ACE inhibitors and ARBs	When CCBs ineffective, can substitute or add	Cough	Losartan preferred based on clinical data; quinapril provided no benefit based on randomized controlled trials
PDE inhibitors (sildenafil)	Severe ischemia and ulcer healing	Flushing, hypotension, dyspepsia	Used when not responding to other medical therapy; sildenafil and tadalafil benefit noted after 4 and 6 weeks, respectively
Alpha-adrenergic blockers	When CCBs ineffective, can substitute or add	Nausea, dizziness, headache, palpitations, hypotension	Pharmacologic tolerance; better tolerated for those sensitive to vasodilator side effects; prazosin effective in Raynaud's secondary to scleroderma
Endothelin receptor antagonist (bosentan)	Ulcer healing and prevention	Increased liver enzymes	Approved for clinical use in Europe
Prostaglandin analogue (prostacyclin, iloprost)	Ulcer healing and critical ischemia	Dose-dependent, headache, flushing, nausea; use with caution in patients with CHF	Intravenous form for severe Raynaud's; antiplatelet therapy required for procoagulant tendency in SRS; iloprost used in severe RS and with healing potential
Serotonin reuptake inhibitor	When CCB ineffective, can substitute or add	Nausea, gastrointestinal upset	Tolerated for those sensitive to vasodilator side effects

Interventional treatment	Indications	Complications	Comments
Débridement	Necrotic tissue, complicated wounds		Use with antibiotics and analgesia
Amputation	Gangrene		Careful assessment of vascular and infection status
Regional sympathectomy (cervicothoracic or lumbar)	Painful ulcers	Pneumothorax, Horner syndrome, anhidrosis with hyperhidrosis, denervation supersensitivity	Endoscopic sympathectomy better tolerated; can also perform radiofrequency ablation; durability not yet fully validated
Botulinum A injection	Severe ischemia	Hyperhidrosis	Case series demonstrate benefit
Digital sympathectomy	Painful ulcers	Anhidrosis, denervation supersensitivity	Periarterial sympathectomy, decompression (excise fibrosis); randomized control trials lacking

ACE, Angiotensin-converting enzyme; *ARB,* angiotensin receptor blocker; *CHF,* congestive heart failure; *PDE,* phosphodiesterase; *RS,* Raynaud's syndrome; *SRS,* secondary Raynaud's syndrome.

effective even in the presence of underlying structural damage to small vessels. Clinical trials showed no benefit when bosentan was used to treat individuals with milder forms of Raynaud's disease. Bosentan may lead to liver injury.

Selective Serotonin Reuptake Inhibitors

Platelets release serotonin, which is a vasoconstrictor, but the mechanism of action in RS is unclear. Selective serotonin reuptake inhibitors (SSRIs) may cause nausea, insomnia, and tremors. In a randomized study, fluoxetine (an SSRI) reduced severity and frequency of attacks compared with nifedipine in patients with PRS. However, in a prospective trial, sarpogrelate (SSRI) administered over 4 to 8 weeks showed marked symptom improvement in 32 patients with SRS. However, in a meta-analysis, Pope and colleagues (2000b) reported limited benefit in patients with scleroderma. Currently, there are insufficient data to support routine use of SSRIs to treat patients with RS.

Surgical Intervention

Surgery is generally reserved for patients with severe and disabling symptoms that have not improved after pharmacologic intervention. Progression to critical ischemia or digital ulceration requires hospitalization and surgical evaluation, and patients typically have an underlying systemic disease. On admission, intravenous PGE (prostanoid) should be considered and antibiotics administered in the presence of a concurrent infection. Analgesia should be provided and local wound care instituted. Débridement and amputation may be necessary. An abnormal pulse exam may suggest the presence of a large vessel arterial lesion, which may necessitate initiation of anticoagulation with subsequent surgical revascularization.

Sympathectomy, which may be temporary or permanent, eliminates sympathetic tone to improve blood flow and reduce ischemic pain, improve oxygenation, and prevent further tissue damage. Temporary sympathectomy can be produced by injecting a regional anesthetic near the appropriate cervical or lumbar sympathetic ganglia or, more distally, in the course of a digital or wrist block. Interdigital injections of botulinum toxin have been shown to be effective in decreasing pain, healing digital ulcers, and improving blood flow in patients with primary and secondary Raynaud's. Van Beek (2007) noted immediate pain relief within 48 hours in 11 patients who received perivascular injections of botulinum toxin A, and these patients remained symptom free for several months. Nine of 11 patients also demonstrated improved ulcer healing. Neumeister (2010) observed that botulinum toxin A (50 to 100 units) improved pain and perfusion in 28 out of 33 patients.

Surgical sympathectomy has been reserved for refractory patients with digital ulceration, with more favorable outcomes found in patients who have primary RS. Various methods have been described, including chemical ablation, resection, clipping, and stripping of the thoracic sympathetic chain. Cervicothoracic sympathectomy via supraclavicular, transaxillary, or thoracoscopic approaches is associated with an attendant risk of Horner's syndrome, pneumothorax, compensatory truncal sweating, persistent neuralgia, or phrenic nerve injury. de Trafford (1988) surveyed 140 patients who underwent sympathectomy and observed that only 18.6% claimed lasting benefit. Matsumoto and colleagues (2002) performed 54 endoscopic sympathectomy procedures without major complications and reported an initial improvement in 93% of patients but recurrence in 82% within 60 months. Similarly, Coveliers and colleagues (2011) performed a review of available studies and noted long-term benefit after endoscopic sympathectomy for only 58% with PRS.

Digital or palmar sympathectomy was first described in 1980 and does not have the major side effects associated with either a thoracotomy or thoracoscopy. The periarterial adventitia is stripped off the digital arteries of the involved finger. Depending on the appearance of the artery, especially in vessels with structural damage from scleroderma, open decompression with resection of the fibrotic layer is needed to remove the external compression and may be extended to include the radial and ulnar arteries of the wrist. Several case studies report successful outcomes, but randomized controlled trials are not available. In a retrospective review of six patients, Tomaino (2000) noted that five patients claimed significant improvement in quality of life after 6 months, including reduced ischemic digital pain and moderate improvement in cold intolerance. In a systematic review of 16 different retrospective and prospective studies that included 156 patients, Kotsis and Chung (2003) observed that 14% of patients eventually required amputation and 18% of ulcers failed to heal despite digital sympathectomy. Likewise, in a prospective study, Hartzell and colleagues (2009) reported that after 90 to 113 months, 26% of digits with an underlying autoimmune disorder and 59% of digits with associated atherosclerosis ultimately required amputation. This approach provides early symptomatic relief and may enhance ulcer healing, but additional studies to assess long-term benefit are needed.

CONCLUSIONS

Raynaud's is a challenging condition with an ill-defined pathogenesis. Distinguishing between primary and secondary forms is critical to formulating appropriate management. Presentations are similar in both forms, but critical ischemia with tissue loss is most common in secondary Raynaud's. Diagnosis is suggested by history and thorough physical exam to exclude other pathologies; digital plethysmography, nailfold capillaroscopy, and serologic testing are helpful in differentiating between primary and secondary forms.

Mild Raynaud's symptoms can be managed by conservative lifestyle changes such as avoiding stimuli that exacerbate symptoms and wearing appropriate protective garments. However, pharmacologic treatment may be necessary, and calcium channel blockers are the initial agent recommended. Depending on the progression of symptoms, other medications, including PGE, phosphodiesterase inhibitors, ACE inhibitors, or SSRIs, may be considered, although clinical studies have shown variable results. For those with severe vasospastic ischemia and ulcers that fail to respond to medical and conservative measures, sympathectomy may be appropriate although long-term effectiveness has not been confirmed.

SUGGESTED READINGS

Coveliers HM, Hoexum F, Nederhoed JH, et al: Thoracic sympathectomy for digital ischemia: a summary of evidence, *J Vasc Surg* 54(1):273–277, 2011.
Cutolo M, Sulli A, Smith V: Assessing microvascular changes in systemic sclerosis diagnosis and management, *Nat Rev Rheumatol* 6(10):578–587, 2010.
de Trafford JC, Lafferty K, Potter CE, et al: An epidemiological survey of Raynaud's phenomenon, *Eur J Vasc Surg* 2(3):167–170, 1988.
Dziadzio M, Denton CP, Smith R, et al: Losartan therapy for Raynaud's phenomenon and scleroderma: Clinical and biochemical findings in a fifteen-week, randomized, parallel-group, controlled trial, *Arthritis Rheum* 42(12):2646–2655, 1999.
Fries R, Shariat K, von Wilmowsky H, et al: Sildenafil in the treatment of Raynaud's phenomenon resistant to vasodilatory therapy, *Circulation* 112(19):2980–2985, 2005.
Gliddon AE, Doré CJ, Black CM, et al: Prevention of vascular damage in scleroderma and autoimmune Raynaud's phenomenon: a multicenter, randomized, double-blind, placebo-controlled trial of the angiotensin-converting enzyme inhibitor quinapril, *Arthritis Rheum* 56(11):3837–3846, 2007.
Hartzell TL, Makhni EC, Sampson C: Long-term results of periarterial sympathectomy, *J Hand Surg Am* 34(8):1454–1460, 2009.
Herrick AL: The pathogenesis, diagnosis and treatment of Raynaud phenomenon, *Nat Rev Rheumatol* 8:469–479, 2012.
Korn JH, Mayes M, Matucci Cerinic M, et al: Digital ulcers in systemic sclerosis: Prevention by treatment with bosentan, an oral endothelin receptor antagonist, *Arthritis Rheum* 50(12):3985–3993, 2004.
Kotsis SV, Chung KC: A systematic review of the outcomes of digital sympathectomy for treatment of chronic digital ischemia, *J Rheumatol* 30(8):1788–1792, 2003.
Malenfant D, Catton M, Pope JE: The efficacy of complementary and alternative medicine in the treatment of Raynaud's phenomenon: a literature review and meta-analysis, *Rheumatology (Oxford)* 48(7):791–795, 2009.
Matsumoto Y, Ueyama T, Endo M, et al: Endoscopic thoracic sympathicotomy for Raynaud's phenomenon, *J Vasc Surg* 36(1):57–61, 2002.
Milio G, Corrado E, Genova C, et al: Iloprost treatment in patients with Raynaud's phenomenon secondary to systemic sclerosis and the quality of life: a new therapeutic protocol, *Rheumatology (Oxford)* 45(8):999–1004, 2006.
Neumeister MW: Botulinum toxin type A in the treatment of Raynaud's phenomenon, *J Hand Surg Am* 35(12):2085–2092, 2010.
Pope J, Fenlon D, Thompson A, et al: Prazosin for Raynaud's phenomenon in progressive systemic sclerosis, *Cochrane Database Syst Rev* (2):CD000956, 2000a.
Pope J, Fenlon D, Thompson A, et al: Ketanserin for Raynaud's phenomenon in progressive systemic sclerosis, *Cochrane Database Syst Rev* (2):CD000954, 2000b.

Shenoy PD, Kumar S, Jha LK, et al: Efficacy of tadalafil in secondary Raynaud's phenomenon resistant to vasodilator therapy: a double-blind randomized cross-over trial, *Rheumatology (Oxford)* 49(12):2420–2428, 2010.

Thompson AE, Pope JE: Calcium channel blockers for primary Raynaud's phenomenon: A meta-analysis, *Rheumatology (Oxford)* 44(2):145–150, 2005.

Thompson AE, Shea B, Welch V, et al: Calcium-channel blockers for Raynaud's phenomenon in systemic sclerosis, *Arthritis Rheum* 44(8):1841–1847, 2001.

Tomaino MM: Digital arterial occlusion in scleroderma: is there a role for digital arterial reconstruction? *J Hand Surg Br* 25(6):611–613, 2000.

Van Beek AL, Lim PK, Gear AJ, et al: Management of vasospastic disorders with botulinum toxin A, *Plast Reconstr Surg* 119(1):217–226, 2007.

Wigley FM, Wise RA, Seibold JR, et al: Intravenous iloprost infusion in patients with Raynaud phenomenon secondary to systemic sclerosis. A multicenter, placebo-controlled, double-blind study, *Ann Intern Med* 120(3):199–206, 1994.

Wollersheim H, Thien T, Fennis J, et al: Double-blind, placebo-controlled study of prazosin in Raynaud's phenomenon, *Clin Pharmacol Ther* 40(2):219–225, 1986.

THORACIC OUTLET SYNDROMES

Brandon W. Propper, MD, and
Julie A. Freischlag, MD

OVERVIEW

Thoracic outlet syndrome (TOS) refers to the anatomic compression of one or more of the neurovascular structures as they exit the chest. Classically, each syndrome is described by the neurovascular structure that is compressed: subclavian vein TOS (vTOS), subclavian artery TOS (aTOS), and nerve root TOS (nTOS). Although controversy exists with regard to diagnosis, careful evaluation and clinical workup can help to identify those patients most likely to benefit from surgical treatment.

ANATOMY OF THE THORACIC OUTLET

Comprehensive treatment relies on a solid understanding of the thoracic outlet and the surrounding structures. Think of the thoracic outlet as a triangle with the apex facing the manubrium. The lower and upper edges are defined by the first rib and clavicle, respectively (Figure 1). Moving anterior medial to posterior lateral, the first structure encountered is the subclavius muscle. The tendon from the subclavius inserts onto the superior portion of the first rib, and the muscle hugs the inferior surface of the clavicle. The subclavian vein lies next to the subclavius tendon and can often be partially compressed. Separating the subclavian vein and artery is the anterior scalene. The relationship between the subclavian vessels and the anterior scalene is key to a safe surgical treatment. Posterior lateral to the subclavian artery are the nerve roots of the brachial plexus, then the middle scalene muscle.

Special anatomic consideration should be given to patients with cervical ribs. Previous autopsy data revealed that about 0.5% of the population has a cervical rib; furthermore, the rib can be fully formed or partially developed. When present, a bony or a fibrous connection exists between the cervical rib and the first rib (Figure 2). The presence of cervical ribs in the TOS population is reported between 10% and 65%. If a cervical rib is causing compression of the neurovascular structures, the cervical rib and fibrous connections should be removed during resection. The structure at greatest risk is the subclavian artery, which lies closest to the cervical rib attachments. In the authors' practice, all patients with TOS are screened for a cervical rib with routine chest radiographs.

ARTERIAL COMPRESSION

Subclavian artery compression is the least common of the three syndromes. Repeated compression over time can lead to a wide array of presentations. These patients are often young and are involved in activities or work that require repeated motion. The presenting symptoms can be subtle, including hand fatigue, mild edema, or temperature sensitivity. More obvious presentations include color changes from embolic events and digital ischemia. Repeated compression on the artery can lead to intraarterial scarring or wall weakening and development of a subclavian artery aneurysm. On physical examination, patients may display diminished radial pulses or disparate blood pressures in the upper extremities. Aneurysmal changes may be apparent on examination as a pulsatile mass in the clavicular region. More advanced testing has been advocated, including elevated arm stress testing (EAST) and abduction and external rotation test (Adson's). Both are noninvasive and are useful to perform during physical examination, but the examiner must be aware that neither test is diagnostic because multiple other disease processes can produce a positive test.

Arterial compression is relatively uncommon; as such, there is no standard complement of testing. The authors suggest further

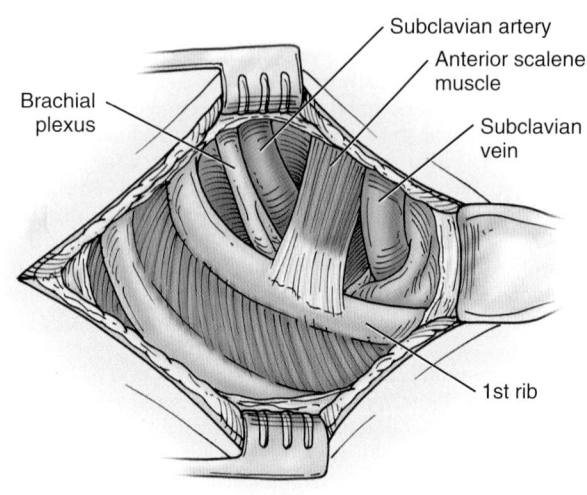

FIGURE 1 Anatomy of the thoracic outlet.

evaluation with imaging. At a minimum, standard chest radiographs should be done to evaluate for cervical ribs or other bony abnormalities. Dynamic ultrasound scan is a reasonable second step because flow changes in the subclavian artery can be seen with abduction and adduction of the arm. In addition, ultrasound scan can illustrate whether aneurysmal development has occurred. Computed tomographic (CT) scan is another imaging modality that can give clear visualization of arterial anatomy with regard to the proximal subclavian artery. It is not the authors' standard practice to use CT scan with most patients; however, if concern exists for proximal arterial disease or aneurysmal change, this modality is used. Finally, arteriography is helpful when the diagnosis is unclear. Dynamic imaging with the arm in abduction and adduction can elucidate arterial compression; however, it is rare that this modality is required when true arterial compression is present.

Treatment of aTOS depends on the clinical presentation and attributed symptoms. Compression without concomitant aneurysm formation can be treated with transaxillary rib resection; however, for those patients that need arteriotomy and reconstruction, the supraclavicular approach is favored. When complex reconstruction is necessary, an infraclavicular incision can be added for more distal exposure.

VENOUS COMPRESSION (PAGET-SCHROETTER SYNDROME)

Venous compression is the second most common form of TOS. Presentation is often in young healthy patients with a history of repetitive motion (swimming, pitching, manual labor) or an active lifestyle. These patients present with a painful swollen extremity and distinct color changes (rubor or cyanosis). Color change may be confused with infection, which can delay diagnosis. Edema of the arm into the fingers is substantial and often triggers patients to seek early medical attention. A history of arm fatigue or a feeling of heaviness may precede dramatic swelling but is usually unnoticed until advanced axillosubclavian compromise is present. Long-standing disease may also reveal multiple collateral veins around the upper arm and shoulder. In younger patients, the surgeon must always consider an underlying hypercoagulable state; however, in the authors' series of patients with vTOS, only 8% were shown to have a prothrombotic disorder.

On presentation, treatment should not be delayed, and anticoagulation therapy should be initiated. Admission begins with 24-hour to 48-hour intravenous heparin therapy and arm elevation. Chest radiographs and dynamic duplex ultrasound scan are recommended to evaluate for venous compression. Findings on ultrasound scan include: (1) decrease in venous velocity by 50% with abduction; (2) presence of venous thickening suggestive of deep venous thrombosis (DVT); and (3) presence of acute or chronic thrombus. Patients are transitioned to low molecular-weight heparin and warfarin for discharge and scheduled for first rib resection and scalenectomy. Initial reporting advocated for a 3-month interval of anticoagulation therapy before surgery. Multiple reports have shown that earlier resection is safe with excellent outcomes. Some large centers advocate for urgent resection performed during the initial hospital admission. The authors' practice is to schedule surgery between 2 and 4 weeks after hospital discharge. Before surgery, the authors prefer arm swelling to have resolved; this short delay allows for venous remodeling and a decrease in swelling. Furthermore, it affords patients a chance to plan for surgery without any compromise in long-term outcome. Inpatient venography, venoplasty, and thrombolysis have been advocated previously and are still performed routinely in some institutions. A stronger argument can be made for thrombolysis for those patients who present with acute upper extremity thrombosis. The authors' practice has moved away from venography and thrombolysis in the preoperative setting because no benefit has been found in long-term patency when compared with initiation of low molecular-weight heparin. Furthermore, regardless of treatment, more than 90% of patients had a patent subclavian vein at the 16-month follow-up.

For definitive treatment, the first rib and anterior scalene are removed via the transaxillary approach. This technique is discussed subsequently in the chapter, but vTOS also requires cutting of the subclavius tendon located at the apex of the thoracic outlet. Other institutions advocate for a supraclavicular approach for surgical treatment. The surgery is more extensive and consists of full mobilization of the subclavian vein, venotomy, and patch venoplasty with saphenous vein. Specific centers have reported good long-term patency with this approach.

After the transaxillary approach, patients are admitted for 1 night, and systemic anticoagulation therapy is held for 3 days and then resumed. The authors schedule all patients with vTOS for venogram 2 weeks after surgery. Venogram serves to identify those patients in whom anticoagulation therapy can be stopped. At venogram, the subclavian vein has recanalized in half of the patients. Fifty percent have a flow lumen amendable to venoplasty and are continued on anticoagulation therapy until follow-up at 1 month. In a small subset, wire access cannot be gained through the subclavian vein and these patients are continued on anticoagulation therapy without subsequent venogram. Figure 3 shows the treatment algorithm for vTOS at the authors' institution.

Fully formed   Partially developed

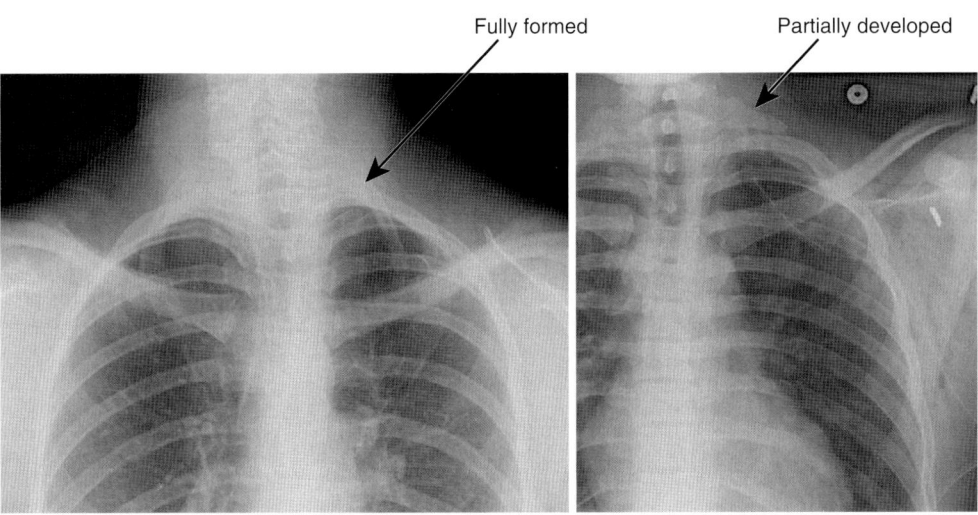

FIGURE 2 Radiographs show both a fully formed and a partially developed cervical rib.

Johns Hopkins protocol for venous TOS

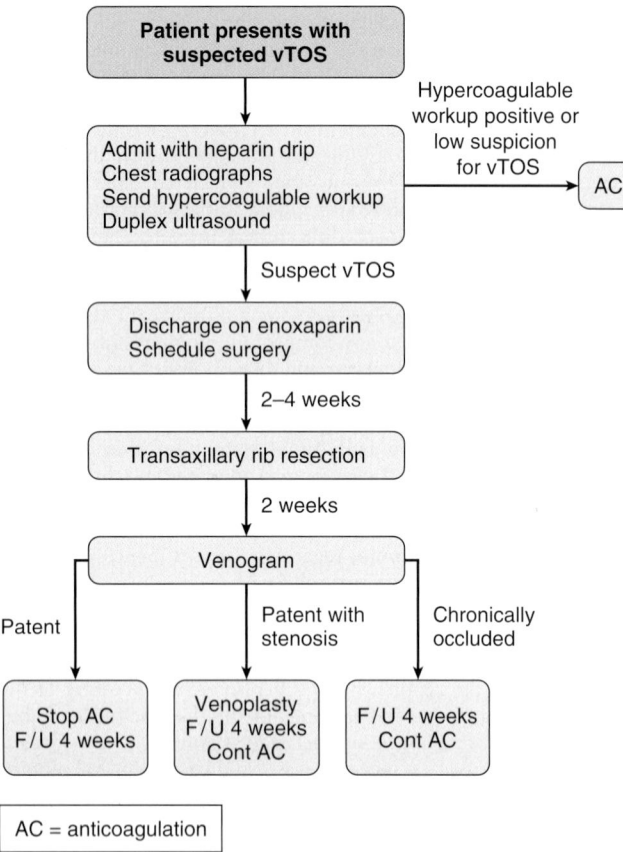

FIGURE 3 The Johns Hopkins algorithm for subclavian vein thoracic outlet syndrome (*vTOS*). *AC*, Anticoagulation; *F/U*, follow-up.

NERVE COMPRESSION

Nerve compression remains the most common form of TOS, although this is also the most controversial. Patients can present with a wide array of symptoms, including pain (back, arm, and shoulder) and headaches. However, the most common presenting symptom, which is present in 90% of patients, is arm paresthesias. Often the symptoms follow a traumatic event such as a motor vehicle crash or are found in patients who engage in repetitive upper extremity activity.

On physical examination, subtle findings of muscle atrophy or a winged scapula may be present. Tenderness with palpation over the anterior scalene may be present; palpation of this region may reproduce arm paresthesia or pain. As with aTOS, EAST and Adson's test may reproduce symptoms but should not be used as diagnostic for nTOS.

Patient selection and further evaluation are highly recommended in the nTOS population. All patients should undergo a period of observation and physical therapy to see whether symptoms can be alleviated without surgery. In addition, patient age should be taken into consideration. Recent data have illustrated that patients less than 40 years of age are more likely to have pain relief after rib resection and scalenectomy. Scalene injection or scalene block should be considered in patients over 40 years of age. Those over 40 years who experience pain relief with scalene block are more likely to benefit from surgical resection. Botulinum toxin injection continues to be a controversial topic. Although many patients experience temporary pain relief, current literature suggests no benefit over placebo

TABLE 1: Preferred surgical approach for thoracic outlet syndrome

TOS syndrome	Surgical approach
aTOS	Supraclavicular
vTOS	Transaxillary
nTOS	Transaxillary
Recurrent disease	Supraclavicular or posterior high thoracoplasty

aTOS, Subclavian artery thoracic outlet syndrome; *nTOS*, nerve root thoracic outlet syndrome; *TOS*, thoracic outlet syndrome; *vTOS*, subclavian vein thoracic outlet syndrome.

injection. Ongoing studies are in progress, but no current evidence suggests long-term benefit from botulinum toxin injection. In patients who are deemed suitable for rib resection, resection is carried out via the transaxillary approach.

TRANSAXILLARY APPROACH

Table 1 illustrates the authors' preference for surgical approach based on underlying pathology.

Preparation and Position

Before the procedure, a discussion with the anesthesia team is appropriate to ensure that the operative arm is free from intravenous lines and that no long-term paralytic agents are used. General anesthesia is induced, and once complete, the patient is positioned and clipped free of hair. A suction beanbag is preferred to help maintain the lateral positioning. In addition, an axillary pad should be placed between the patient's chest wall and the bed to protect the contralateral axilla. Once positioned, the chest wall, axilla, and arm are prepped into the sterile field. The arm is flexed at the elbow and secured into the Machleder retractor (Koros, USA, Inc.) with elastic wrap. It is important to protect the ipsilateral arm and pad the retractor (Figure 4). Use of at least one lighted retractor is recommended, and the operating surgeon should wear a headlight.

Operative Approach

Once positioned, the border of the pectoralis major and latissimus dorsi are identified and marked as the anterior and posterior border. A line between these marks is made as the inferior edge of the hair baring area. This line is used for the incision. Dissection is carried out down to the level of the chest wall, with care taken to stay superior to the axillary fat. Potential structures encountered include the intercostal brachial nerve, which should be preserved if possible but can be sacrificed if necessary. Once the chest wall is indentified, palpation of the first and second rib can be achieved. Typically, the second rib protrudes further and is easily palpable. The first rib is flat and more difficult to identify. At this point, the Machleder retractor is raised to open the axillary space. Loose areolar tissue often can be bluntly dissected while the surgeon identifies the subclavian vein and artery. For patients with vTOS, the vein may be thrombosed and difficult to identify. Once the artery and vein are identified, the anterior scalene muscle is visualized and bluntly dissected free from the vein and artery. Sharp dissection is cautioned against because injury to the vein or artery is difficult to repair. The inferior border of the first rib is cleared of muscular tissue with a combination of blunt

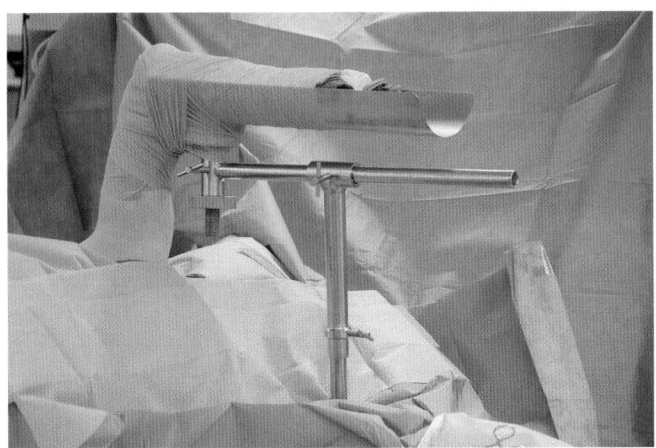

FIGURE 4   Operative photograph of setup.

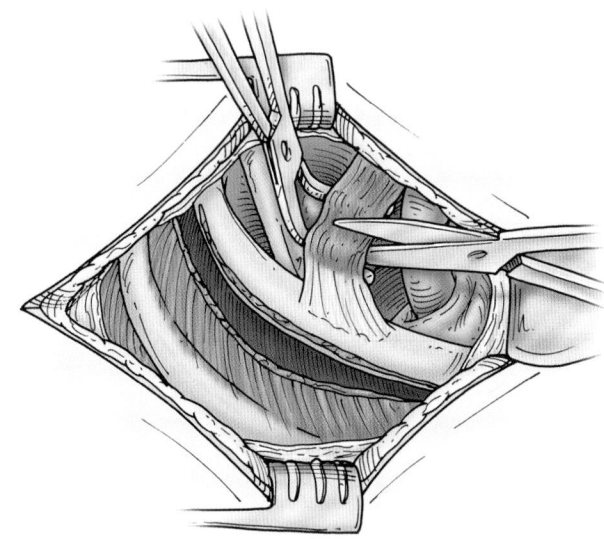

FIGURE 6   Transection of the anterior scalene muscle with a right angle clamp and scissors.

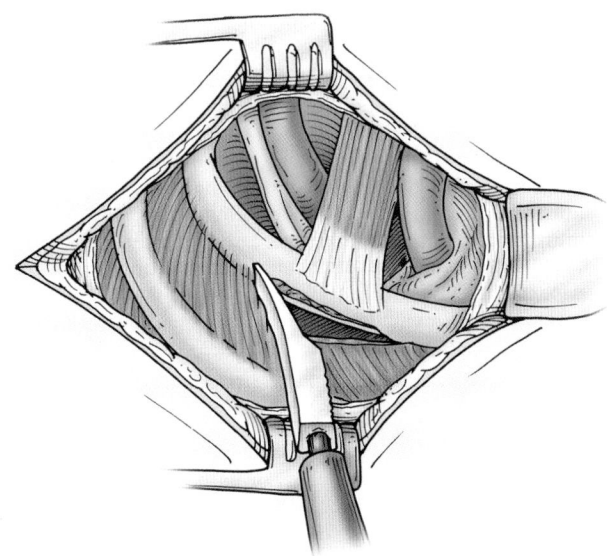

FIGURE 5   Use of the periosteal elevator to remove tissue from the first rib.

Subsequent dissection of additional muscle fibers helps to facilitate posterior rib transection. Posteriorly, the rib should initially be cut anterior to the nerve root. The rib specimen can be removed from the field. Rongeurs can be used to remove additional post anterior to the vein and posterior to the nerve root. Once complete, irrigation is instilled into the field, and Valsalva's maneuver is used to check for a pneumothorax. If pneumothorax is present, a small chest tube is placed.

SUGGESTED READINGS

Angle N, Gelabert HA, Farooq MM, et al: Safety and efficacy of early surgical decompression of the thoracic outlet for Paget-Schroetter syndrome, *Ann Vasc Surg* 15:37–42, 2001.

Brooke BS, Freischlag JA: Contemporary management of thoracic outlet syndrome, *Curr Opin Cardiol* 25(6):535–540, 2010.

Caparrelli DJ, Fresichlag JA: A unifed approach to axillosubclavian venous thrombosis in a single hospital admission, *Semin Vasc Surg* 18:153–157, 2005.

Guzzo JL, Chang K, Demos J, et al: Preoperative thrombolysis and venoplasty affords no benefit in patency following first rib resection and scalenectomy for subacute and chronic subclavian vein thrombosis, *J Vasc Surg* 52(3):658–662, 2010.

Lum YW, Brooke BS, Likes K, et al: Impact of anterior scalene lidocaine blocks on predicting surgical success in older patients with neurogenic thoracic outlet syndrome, *J Vasc Surg* 55(5):1370–1375, 2012.

Schneider DB, Dimuzio PJ, Martin ND, et al: Combination treatment of venous thoracic outlet syndrome: open surgical decompression and intrapoerative angioplasty, *J Vasc Surg* 40:599–603, 2004.

Urschel HC, Razzuk MA: Paget-Schroetter syndrome: what is the best management, *Ann Thorac Surg* 69:1663–1669, 2000.

dissection and a periosteal elevator (Figure 5). The dissection of the first rib includes removal of all muscle tissue from the rib surfaces. This maneuver often causes bleeding of the dissected muscle, and periodic packing and lowering of the Machleder retractor are recommended for hemostasis. The surgeon should isolate the anterior scalene with a right angle instrument, while the assistant sharply divides the muscle fibers (Figure 6). Once the anterior scalene is divided, the rib can be divided with bone cutters. The anterior side should be cut first, with care taken not to damage the subclavian vein.

THE DIABETIC FOOT

Gilbert Aidinian, MD, FACS, RPVI,
Patrick R. Cook, DO, FACS, RPVI, and
Todd E. Rasmussen, MD, FACS

INTRODUCTION

The prevalence of diabetes mellitus worldwide has reached epidemic proportions and the myriad of complications that result from this disease cannot be overstated. In the United States alone, the diabetic population continues to grow exponentially, affecting an estimated 24 million people. Approximately 15% of patients with this disease will develop some form of foot complication and despite ongoing improvements in care, the annual cost associated with diabetic foot infections, tissue loss, and amputations exceeds $10 billion.

Up to 10% of patients with diabetes will develop a foot ulcer or tissue loss on the foot in their lifetime. In those patients who have other specific risk factors, such as peripheral arterial occlusive disease and altered foot architecture, the percentage rises to nearly 30%. The ideal management of patients with diabetes involves preemptive education and an awareness of the clinical manifestations of diabetes as well as routine surveillance of the foot surfaces. Patients at high risk for development of foot pathology are best cared for in a multidisciplinary setting that includes medicine, surgery, wound care, and rehabilitation specialists. Should a patient with diabetes mellitus experience a break in the integument of the skin, referral to a surgical specialist for evaluation is appropriate for optimal results.

PATHOPHYSIOLOGY

There are three categories of foot ulcers that can occur in those with diabetes mellitus: neuropathic, ischemic, and those that arise from mixed neuropathic and ischemic components. Understanding these categories and recognizing the etiology of a given ulcer is necessary for efficient and effective management. Conversely, failure to understand and recognize the categories of foot ulceration may lead to unnecessary tests and procedures or delays in recognition and treatment.

The first category is a result of diabetic peripheral neuropathy affecting the surfaces of the toes and feet of patients with long-standing diabetes. Even in the setting of normal arterial perfusion, diabetic neuropathy represents a frequent cause of foot injury, infection, and subsequent tissue loss. Neuropathic ulcers are also referred to as traumatic and originate because of abnormal or absent sensation to the toes and feet. In the setting of neuropathy, activity or injury that would otherwise be uncomfortable and prompt examination, behavioral adjustment, or treatment goes unnoticed or neglected. An example is repetitive irritation or abrasion from poor fitting shoes, which may go unrecognized in patients with neuropathy until the trauma results in a break of the skin integument and initiation of an ulcer. Similarly, a puncture wound or laceration to the foot, which would normally prompt examination and medical attention, may go unnoticed in patients with diabetic neuropathy. In addition to abnormal sensation, chronic diabetic neuropathy may lead to malformation of the joints of the foot and toes, which, in turn, leads to a condition termed *neuropathic arthropathy* or *Charcot's foot* (Figure 1). In this condition, joints and surfaces of the foot not otherwise prone to injury become abnormally positioned and exposed to surface trauma and ulceration. Finally, chronic diabetic neuropathy affects autonomic innervation of the skin of the foot and toes, which leads to abnormally dry surfaces. Dry skin associated with chronic neuropathy leads to scaling, cracking, or other breaks in the integument and predisposition to ulceration, infection, or both.

Chronic lower extremity ischemia from arterial occlusive disease may also affect those with diabetes who have normal sensation to the surfaces of the foot and toes. In these instances, the ulceration is referred to as *ischemic tissue loss* or *ischemic ulceration*. Ischemic ulcers of the foot or toes arise from multilevel arterial occlusive disease, meaning that more than one arterial level between the aorta and the foot is affected by significant stenosis or occlusion. Most commonly, patients with chronic diabetes have severe occlusive disease of one or more of the tibial arteries in combination with aortoiliac occlusive disease, femoral-popliteal artery occlusive disease, or both (Figure 2). Finally, depending on the duration and severity of diabetes, patients may have foot or toe ulcerations that are of a mixed neuropathic and ischemic component. These cases are typically the most severe and prone to significant tissue loss that leads to amputation.

From the standpoint of pathophysiology, it is important to keep in mind that a common pathway to ulceration and infection in diabetic patients is reduced local and systemic immune defense. This phenomenon increases significantly the propensity for any breaks in the skin integument, whether due to trauma or ischemia, to progress to complications. The abnormal local inflammatory response in patients with diabetes is due to alterations at the cellular level, including thickening of the endothelial basement membrane of the microvessels of the foot. Thickening of the basement membrane impairs leukocyte migration to the site of injury and the local cellular capability to defend against pathogens. Diabetes mellitus also impairs the function of circulating inflammatory cells through variations in blood glucose levels and as a result of chronic insulin administration, which interacts with circulating hormones (e.g., growth hormone) to negatively affect the immune response.

PRESENTATION

Whether from neuropathy, ischemia, or both, skin breakdown typically occurs on the pressure-bearing surfaces of the foot, such as hard calluses or bony prominences. The chronicity of any foot ulceration is important to discern, as is the history of other healing or nonhealing ulcers on the same foot. These factors often provide insight as to whether or not there is a significant ischemic component to the situation at hand. For example, a patient who presents with a chronic nonhealing ulcer that has been stagnant or indolent over a number of weeks or months is less likely to have a profound ischemic component. Likewise, a patient with a recurrent ulcer or a new ulcer on a foot on which healing has occurred in the recent past is less likely to have severe ischemia. In these cases, the fact that the ulcer has not progressed or may have healed in the past suggests that there is adequate blood flow to support tissue stabilization and ward off gangrene. In these scenarios, the ulcer most likely is caused by recurrent trauma to an area of surface pressure or injury. In contrast, first-time foot ulcers that show significant necrosis, deep space infection, or both, are more likely to have a significant ischemic component with or without neuropathy.

The presentation of foot ulcerations range from superficial blisters or chronic wounds to painful, erythematous or necrotic ulcerations with deep space infection. As mentioned previously, the intrinsic muscles of the foot may atrophy as a result of chronic neuropathy, resulting in a condition known as neuropathic arthropathy or Charcot's foot. This condition is recognized easily on examination and creates abnormal pressure points on the foot. The degenerative arthropathy associated with Charcot's foot also leads to loss of normal foot architecture and collapse of the arch, also referred to as a "rocker bottom" deformity. Examination of the foot frequently reveals dry and cracked skin and forefoot; erythema, edema, or tenderness is suggestive of a more extensive deep space infection. Of particular importance in this patient population is the presence of unexplained hyperglycemia. Elevation in circulating blood glucose levels in patients with diabetes, and especially those with foot ulceration, should prompt an aggressive search for infection. In these instances, one should suspect undrained fluid collections or osteomyelitis or deep space forefoot infections.

The contribution of ischemia to a foot ulcer can be gauged quickly by performing an assessment of perfusion to the extremity, beginning with an assessment of peripheral pulses. This aspect of the physical exam begins with palpation of the femoral pulse, which may be compared in strength to that of the pulse in the opposite groin. Similarly, palpation for the popliteal and pedal pulses should be performed comparing their strength with those in the opposite extremity. Completing the pulse exam is most useful in determining the ischemic component to a foot ulcer at the two ends of the clinical spectrum: normal versus severe ischemia. A patient who has normal palpable pulses throughout an extremity, including the foot, on the initial examination is much more likely to have an isolated neuropathic ulcer. Conversely, a patient who has absent femoral, popliteal, and pedal pulses on the initial exam has an ischemic component and should be managed accordingly. Patients in whom the pulse exam is difficult or equivocal require further noninvasive testing, beginning with use of the continuous wave Doppler.

Continuous wave Doppler is an extension of the physical exam and used to determine the presence and quality of arterial signals in the foot. Normal signals are strong and biphasic, whereas weak monophasic signals are indicative of arterial occlusive disease and ischemia. The ankle brachial index (ABI) is the ratio of the occlusion pressure of the arterial signal at the ankle or foot compared with that in the arm. This aspect of the exam is performed using a manual blood pressure cuff and a continuous wave Doppler to assess the pressure at which the signals of the dorsalis pedis and posterior tibial arteries of the foot and the brachial artery of the arm occlude as the cuff is inflated. The normal index is 0.9 or greater while an index of 0.4 or less is diagnostic of critical limb ischemia.

It is important to note that chronic diabetes may result in medial calcinosis of the tibial arteries, also referred to as *Monckeberg's arteriosclerosis*. In patients with this condition, occlusion of the tibial vessels with the cuff is not possible, even at high pressures; thus, it is impossible to measure ABI. Noncompressible ABI occurs mostly in patients with long-standing, insulin-dependent diabetes, and this condition necessitates other types of noninvasive vascular testing to assess perfusion.

One test that is similar to ABI and that can be used to assess perfusion to the foot in the diabetic patient is the toe brachial index (TBI). Interestingly, the digital vessels of the toes are spared from medial calcinosis and are therefore compressible with small specialized cuffs and a form of plethysmography. While the upper values do not correlate well with ABI, a TBI of less than 0.4 is indicative of critical limb ischemia. Whether it is ABI or TBI, measured values of less than 0.4 is indicative of severe ischemia. Patients with indices of 0.4 or less are unlikely to heal a foot or toe ulceration or any débridement of the affected area.

TREATMENT

Treatment of the diabetic foot ulcer and any associated infection should be accomplished with a multidisciplinary approach. An important initial step that should not be overlooked is blood glucose control with an hemoglobin A_{1c} target level of less than 6.5% to 7.0%. Local infection control is also paramount and requires débridement of nonviable tissue and opening of any deep space or forefoot infection. In the case of toe ulceration with gangrene or infection, amputation of the digit with or without proximal extension to include the metatarsal head (i.e., Ray amputation) may be necessary. If more than one toe is affected or there is suspicion for a more extensive forefoot infection, a transmetatarsal amputation may be required. In cases involving digit, Ray, or transmetatarsal amputations, we favor starting the incision distally at the infected ulcer and extending proximally with the goal of exposing all of the relevant plantar spaces. The surrounding tissues should be carefully palpated for unrecognized and undrained abscess, especially along tendon sheaths, which can disguise and facilitate spread of infection (Figure 3).

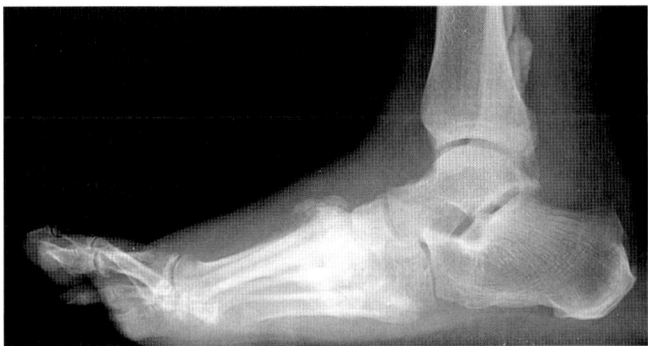

FIGURE I Lateral foot film demonstrating loss of foot architecture resulting in classic neuropathic arthropathy.

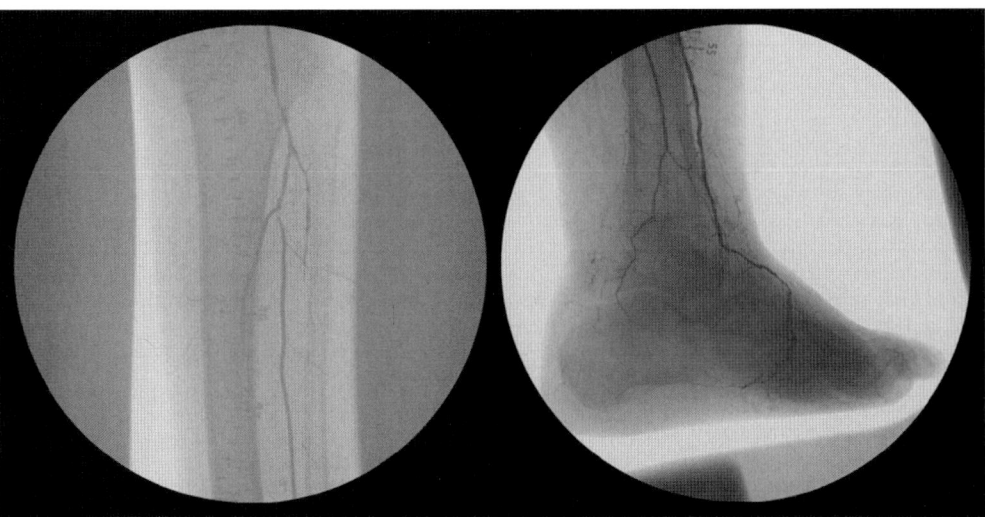

FIGURE 2 Tibial occlusive disease showing proximal anterior tibial artery and posterior tibial artery occlusion with peroneal artery runoff. At the level of the ankle, the anterior tibial artery reconstitutes and retrograde fills via perforating branch of the peroneal artery.

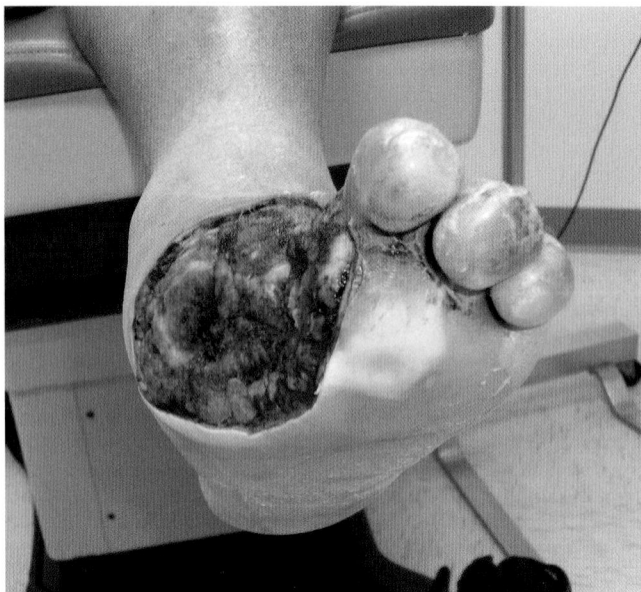

FIGURE 3 Left medial forefoot deep space infection necessitating wide débridement with first and second toe amputation.

Chronic or indolent ulcers without soft tissue or deep space infection can be treated without an extensive operation. These ulcers may have elements of surrounding cellulitis and often have necrotic tissue with polymicrobial colonization. In these cases, initial antibiotic therapy should be broad-spectrum, based on institutional culture and sensitivities and include coverage for methicillin-resistant *Staphylococcus aureus*. The antibiotic regimen should be modified and focused based on the results of the cultures obtained during the initial evaluation and débridement. Antibiotic therapy for chronic ulcers is continued until the cellulitis or superficial infection is resolved (7-10 days) and is not necessary until the wound is healed. Long-term intravenous antibiotic therapy is no longer recommended for diabetic foot ulcers with osteomyelitis given the high recurrence rate in this patient population.

Offloading of or minimizing trauma to the affected area of the foot is also paramount. This strategy may include bed rest, foot elevation, and restricted weight bearing to decrease edema and prevent further mechanical damage of tenuous tissue. Specialized orthotics are available to assist the provider and patient in this strategy, including custom-fit shoes for neuropathic or malformed feet. Although offloading and surface protection should be started during the initial evaluation of any foot ulcer, this strategy should be approached in combination with comprehensive foot care measures as a life-long requirement for patients with diabetes mellitus.

Correction of arterial ischemia will be required for ulcers that fail to heal despite conservative and local wound care and for those with critical ischemia (i.e., ABI or TBI <0.4). Diabetic patients with nonhealing ischemic foot ulcers should be evaluated first for the merit of limb salvage, as some already immobile or debilitated patients may be better served with a primary amputation. This overall assessment for limb salvage should be made in patients with acutely septic ulcers as well as those with more chronic or indolent, nonhealing ulcers.

If a patient is deemed a candidate for limb salvage, a vascular operation should be undertaken after control of associated foot infection and performance of vascular imaging. Revascularization for ischemic ulceration or tissue loss should be undertaken with the goal of restoring in-line or pulsatile flow to the foot. In other words, direct arterial flow is required, through recanalization of an existing artery or with a bypass conduit, to a tibial artery below the extent of occlusion. The arterial target in these cases is free of distal stenosis or occlusion and therefore provides direct flow to the affected foot. In

most cases, distal bypass or recanalization for ischemic tissue loss is performed to the anterior or posterior tibial artery, either of which provides direct flow to the plantar arch of the foot. In contrast, the peroneal artery ends at the ankle and provides perfusion to the foot only through collateral branches. While collateral perfusion to the leg and foot may be adequate to relieve claudication or even ischemic rest pain, in-line pulsatile flow is typically required to meet the metabolic demands needed to heal an ischemic foot ulcer.

Lower extremity revascularization options can be considered in two categories: open surgical and endovascular. Regardless of the chosen approach, revascularization must begin with assuring or establishing adequate inflow to the extremity at the level of the common and deep femoral arteries. Options to establish flow from the femoral artery level to the foot will depend on the extent of occlusive disease. As previously discussed, nearly all diabetic patients with ischemic foot ulcers have multilevel arterial occlusive disease that includes the tibial vessels. Because endovascular procedures are yet to be established as effective or durable in the tibial vessels, bypass to a reconstituted tibial artery is most common in this scenario. In most instances, this is performed using autologous saphenous vein as the conduit and either the common femoral or popliteal artery as the inflow vessel. Prosthetic grafts (i.e., expanded polytetrafluoroethylene) can be used for conduit in distal bypass procedures, but they have not been shown to be as durable as saphenous vein. Although distal bypass with saphenous vein as a conduit is superior to endovascular therapy in terms of primary and secondary patency, there is no difference in limb savage rates between the two modalities. In some cases, endovascular therapy and bypass surgery are complementary techniques (i.e., hybrid procedures) for the treatment of ischemic, nonhealing diabetic foot ulcers.

Numerous adjunctive methods are available to aid healing of diabetic ulcers. These methods include hyperbaric oxygen therapy, which has been shown to facilitate wound granulation, contraction, and healing but has not been shown to be cost-effective given the lack of evidence for optimal duration of therapy. One adjunct that has been shown to result in faster rates of wound healing in diabetic patients with adequate perfusion is the negative pressure wound therapy device or VAC. Appropriately applied, closed negative pressure wound therapy results in fewer dressing changes and outpatient wound care visits and improved quality of life. The vacuum-assisted wound closure (VAC) dressing adjunct has also been shown to improve local wound oxygenation, granulation, and contraction.

One of the most difficult decisions in managing a chronic, nonhealing, or septic diabetic foot ulcer is whether to use leg amputation as the primary procedure. Certain patients will not be candidates for staged surgical revascularization and attempted limb salvage because of their preexisting immobility or severe comorbidities. In general, bedridden and wheelchair-bound patients with little potential for ambulation should have an amputation as the initial procedure to reduce complications and speed any chance for recovery. Patients with significant medical comorbidities such as advanced chronic kidney disease may also benefit from primary amputation instead of revascularization and attempted limb salvage. Finally, it should be noted that diabetic foot ulcers heal at a slow rate, even after revascularization. Ulcers over the calcaneus are particularly slow to contract and close because of a relatively lower arterial perfusion and their exposure to pressure or trauma. On average, only one quarter of foot ulcers treated with revascularization are healed within 6 months of surgery. Two thirds of such ulcers are healed within a year of operation, and freedom from amputation ranges from 80% at 1 year to 70% at 3 years.

CONCLUSION

The number of people with diabetes mellitus has reached epidemic proportions, and therefore a firm understanding of the etiology, presentation, and management of foot ulcers is increasingly important.

If present, gangrene or forefoot infection must be débrided or drained in the acute setting along with pursuit of tight glucose control. Chronic or indolent diabetic foot ulcers may be managed more conservatively initially, although failure to heal should prompt a detailed examination of arterial perfusion. The presence of critical limb ischemia will press a decision on the merits of limb salvage, including the potential for revascularization or preference for primary leg amputation.

DISCLAIMER

The views expressed in this chapter are those of the authors and do not reflect official policy of the Department of Defense.

SUGGESTED READINGS

Hobizal KB, Wukich DK: Diabetic foot infections: current concept review, *Diabet Foot Ankle* 2012;3. doi: 10.3402/dfa.v3i0.18409. Epub 2012 May 8.

Lipsky BA, Berendt AR, Cornia PB, et al: 2012 Infectious Diseases Society of America clinical practice guidelines for the diagnosis and treatment of diabetic foot infections, *J Am Podiatr Med Assoc* 103(1):2–7, 2013.

Malhotra S, Bello E, Kominsky S: Diabetic foot ulcerations: biomechanics, Charcot foot, and total contact cast, *Semin Vasc Surg* 25(2):66–69, 2012.

Pinzur MS: Diabetic peripheral neuropathy, *Foot Ankle Clin* 16(2):345–349, 2011.

Zgonis T, Stapleton JJ, Roukis TS: A stepwise approach to the surgical management of severe diabetic foot infections, *Foot Ankle Spec* 1(1):46–53, 2008.

GANGRENE OF THE FOOT

Louis Lewandowski, MD, Joseph Caruso, MD, and Mark E. Fleming, DO, MC(FS/FMF), USN

OVERVIEW

Critical limb ischemia can lead to gangrene, which in turn can lead to localized coagulative or liquefactive necrosis. This process is further complicated by superimposed bacterial infection and subsequent accelerated tissue decay. Gangrene can affect any part of the body, most commonly the distal extremities; however, when present in a location such as the perineum (Fournier's gangrene), the rates of associated mortality and morbidity are dramatically increased.

Gangrene is classified as either "dry" or "wet." Both disease processes are based on arterial occlusion and loss of perfusion. Dry gangrene occurs in the absence of bacterial infection and is characterized by mummification and desiccation of the necrotic tissue (Figure 1, *A*). In these cases, emergency amputation is not indicated; the natural course of the disease will result in autoamputation. Autoamputation is the process of spontaneous detachment of the desiccated necrotic tissue. Wet gangrene (Figure 1, *B*), however is associated with superimposed bacterial infection that can lead to overwhelming sepsis and multisystem organ failure. Patients presenting with gangrene with a superimposed infection need to be evaluated on an emergency basis for adequate infection control, through either amputation and aggressive débridement or revascularization procedure.

RISK FACTORS AND EPIDEMIOLOGY

Critical limb ischemia is estimated to affect 2 million patients in the United States, and that number is predicted to grow to 2.8 million by 2020. The number of patients with diabetes—a known risk factor for critical limb ischemia—is estimated to expand from 16.8 million currently to more than 24.5 million in the next 10 years; hence the prevalence of critical limb ischemia could be closer to 3.5 million by 2020.

Fortunately, the number of patients with diabetes who require lower extremity amputation has been nearly halved to 4.6 per 1000 within the last decade. Despite these improvements, the mortality rate remains as high as 30% at 1 month after amputation and 50% at 1 year after amputation, according to a study of 96 patients who underwent non–trauma-related amputations of the lower extremity. It is also estimated that more than 60% of nontraumatic lower amputations of the extremity are a result of diabetic complications; 25% of diabetic patients with foot infections require amputation.

Smoking continues to be an important risk factor for the development of peripheral artery disease and its progression to critical limb ischemia. In the TransAtlantic Inter-Society Consensus report, smoking was recognized as a greater risk factor for the development and progression of peripheral artery disease than for coronary artery disease. Heavy smokers with intermittent claudication are statistically more likely to require revascularization procedures and major amputations than are nonsmokers.

Gangrene is traditionally viewed as a unilateral phenomenon because of the conditions just described. In critically ill patients, however, disseminated intravascular coagulation can lead to symmetric gangrene. Other conditions leading to peripheral gangrene in critically ill patients include hypercoagulable states and use of vasoactive drugs. The mortality rate associated with symmetric peripheral gangrene is estimated to be approximately 35%; almost half of affected patients require amputation of at least one lower extremity. In the absence of ischemic arterial disease, other conditions that cause arterial occlusion and thereby lead to peripheral ischemia and gangrene include myeloproliferative disorders and vasculitides or vasospastic conditions such as Raynaud's syndrome.

EVALUATION

Clinical Presentation

The patient's evaluation begins as always with a thorough history and physical examination. The physician should look for risk factors and preexisting comorbid conditions that can complicate medical and surgical management of the patient. In patients with superimposed infection, it is of the utmost importance to determine the extent of the infection. Patients with sepsis have significant metabolic abnormalities and hemodynamic instability that necessitate immediate surgical and intensive care management.

The level of the amputation required can be approximated empirically by a thorough physical examination and through the clinical judgment of an experienced surgeon. Physical examination findings of critical limb ischemia include changes in skin temperature, loss of hair, muscle atrophy, presence of arterial bruit, and diminished pulses. Strong palpable pulses proximal to the anticipated level of

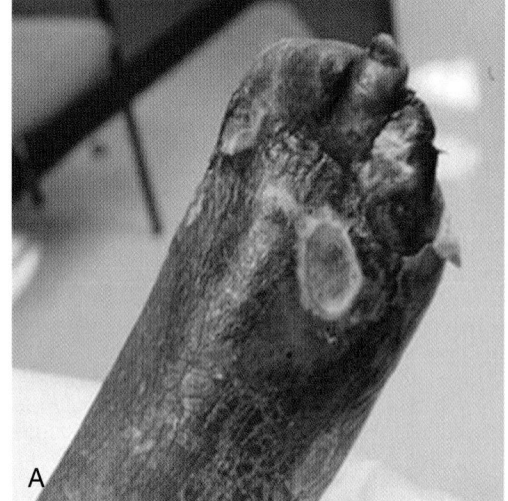
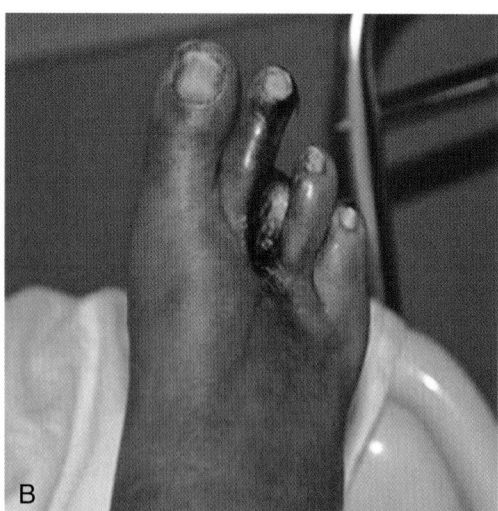

FIGURE I Dry and wet gangrene. **A,** Dry gangrene with evidence of autoamputation. **B,** Acute wet gangrene.

amputation are a good indicator of healthy wound healing. Numerous noninvasive tests provide valuable data for the adequacy of tissue perfusion and oxygenation to further determine the patient's ability to heal.

Diagnostics

The evaluation should proceed with noninvasive vascular studies to confirm the clinical diagnosis and further define the level and extent of arterial disease. Various noninvasive examinations help assess presence and severity of arterial disease, defining both the adequacy of inflow from large vessels and the quality of microcirculation. Physiologic tests include calculation of pressure index values (e.g., ankle-brachial index [ABI], toe-brachial index, blood pressures in segmental limbs) and measurement of transcutaneous partial pressure of oxygen (TcPO$_2$). Imaging can be used to determine whether a lesion is amenable to revascularization and to assist with decisions on surgical approach (e.g., endovascular versus open, choice of conduit). Ultrasonography is the mainstay of vascular imaging with each mode, providing specific and useful information. Other frequently employed techniques include computed tomographic scan and magnetic resonance imaging. Contrast arteriography (digital subtraction arteriography) is the "gold standard" of imaging tests and can be the primary imaging modality because it enables intervention if the anatomy is amenable.

Ankle-Brachial Index

The ABI is the ratio of the systolic blood pressure in the dorsalis pedis or posterior tibial artery to that in the brachial artery. Continuous-wave Doppler mode is used to listen to the arterial signal, and a manual blood pressure cuff is inflated until the sound disappears. The pressure at which the sound returns is recorded. The higher of the two pressures from the dorsalis pedis or posterior tibial artery is used. An ABI of 0.9 or lower is diagnostic of occlusive arterial disease; a value below 0.4 suggests multilevel disease and is predictive of poor wound healing. ABI values above 1.3 suggest calcification of vessels and the need for additional vascular studies.

Toe-Brachial Index

The toe-brachial index is a more reliable indicator of limb perfusion, particularly in patients with diabetes, because the small vessels of the toe are usually spared of calcifications. A photoelectrode is used to obtain an arterial waveform with infrared light. As in ABI

measurement, the toe cuff is inflated until the arterial waveform flattens. The cuff is then deflated until the baseline waveform returns. A pressure gradient of 20 to 30 mm Hg is normal between the toe and the ankle, and so a normal toe-brachial index is 0.7 to 0.8. An absolute pressure of more than 30 mm Hg is favorable for wound healing, but pressures higher than 45 to 55 may be required for healing in patients with diabetes.

Segmental Limb Pressures

Segmental limb pressures are obtained with a series of four cuffs on the lower extremity: proximal and distal thigh, calf, and ankle. Pressures at each level are compared with the brachial pressure. With these comparisons, the level of arterial occlusion can be localized. A 20–mm Hg reduction in pressure between segments in the same leg or in comparison with the same level in the opposite leg is abnormal and suggests a significant lesion.

Transcutaneous Oxygen Measurement

TcPO$_2$ measurements can provide supplemental information regarding local tissue perfusion. Electrodes are placed on the chest wall and legs or feet. The absolute value of the oxygen tension in a location, or a ratio of that value to the chest wall, can be used. A normal value at the foot is 60 mm Hg, and a normal chest/foot ratio is 0.9. Local edema, skin temperature, inflammation, and pharmacologic agents can limit the accuracy of this test, and so the level of TcPO$_2$ that portends poor tissue healing remains controversial. A value of 40 mm Hg is generally accepted as adequate for healing (in the absence of edema or diabetes). Values lower than 20 mm Hg indicate severe ischemia, and revascularization is needed for wound healing. A meta-analysis of four studies revealed more than a threefold risk of healing complication in patients with a TcPO$_2$ below a threshold of 20 to 30 mm Hg (odds ratio, 3.26; 95% confidence interval: 1.07 to 9.69).

Duplex Ultrasonography

In real-time ultrasonography, reflected sound waves are used to produce images and assess blood velocity. *Duplex* refers to the use of two modes: B-mode (brightness) and Doppler mode. Ultrasonography does not require intravenous contrast or ionizing radiation and can provide precise anatomic location and accurate grading of lesion severity. It is, however, highly operator dependent.

Multidetector Computed Tomographic Angiography

Multidetector computed tomographic angiography (MDCTA) allows rapid acquisition of high-resolution, contrast agent–enhanced arterial images. It is more expensive than ultrasonography and involves the use of ionizing radiation and contrast agent. According to a meta-analysis of 20 studies in which MDCTA was compared with digital subtraction angiography, the sensitivity and specificity of MDCTA in detecting stenosis of more than 50% were 95% and 96%, respectively.

Magnetic Resonance Angiography

In magnetic resonance angiography, rapid three-dimensional imaging sequences are obtained with gadolinium contrast agents. This method is becoming a more time-efficient and cost-effective means for evaluation of arterial disease in the lower extremity. It has the advantage of employing nonionizing radiation, but it lacks the small vessel spatial resolution of MDCTA. Gadolinium, however, is contraindicated in patients with renal insufficiency.

Assessment of Metabolic Status

Evaluations of a patient's serum glucose and hemoglobin A_{1C} levels provide a starting point for a laboratory evaluation of diabetic control. It is also important to ensure that the total serum protein level is higher than 6.2 g/dL and that the serum albumin level is higher than 3.5g/dL to predict a patient's ability to heal. A total lymphocyte count higher than 1500/mm³ is also a predictor of healing potential.

MANAGEMENT

Antibiotics and Medical Management

Current recommendations from the infectious disease literature warn against the use of empiric antibiotics before optimal wound cultures are obtained. Proper cultures should be obtained after initial débridement of deep tissue through biopsy or curettage, not by swab specimens, to increase accuracy of results. Antibiotic-resistant organisms continue to proliferate, especially methicillin-resistant *Staphylococcus aureus;* highly resistant *Pseudomonas* organisms and extended-spectrum β-lactamase bacilli are also increasingly isolated. With this rising risk of resistant organisms, tailored antibiotic regimens are increasingly important for clearing infections.

The choice of therapy is based largely on the severity of the infection; severe and some moderate infections necessitate parenteral therapy. However, highly bioavailable oral antibiotics alone are sufficient in most mild and many moderate infections. The length of antibiotic therapy is based on the extent of the infection: for mild soft tissue infections, treatment must continue for approximately 2 weeks, and for moderate to severe infections, 3 weeks.

Débridement

Débridement is the key step in the treatment of moderate to severe infection, with the removal of devitalized tissue that provides a substrate for bacteria. Devitalized tissue is poorly vascularized and therefore is not penetrated appropriately by systemic antibiotics. The most commonly used method of débridement is a sharp, surgical procedure. Sharp débridement can be augmented in the operation room with the addition of hydrodébridement devices to help débride non-viable tissue while maintaining healthy tissue. Techniques that continue the effects of surgical débridement between procedures are mechanical or pharmacologic, involving wet-to-dry dressings or topical enzymes. Negative-pressure wound therapy can also be used between débridements to decrease contamination of the wounds, remove wound debris, and promote granulation and microvascular ingrowth. Protease scavengers and biologic wound matrices will also aid in wound healing between operative interventions. In conjunction with local wound care, these agents have been shown to reduce healing times and increase overall healing rates, which lead to reduced amputation rates.

Revascularization

In patients with an ulcer caused by arterial insufficiency, intervention is necessary to optimize the potential for the wound to heal or, at the very least, to optimize the healing potential of an amputation wound. Arterial lesions are graded from A to D on the basis of complexity; type A ulcers are the simplest lesions, and type D ulcers are the most complex. Endovascular therapy is the treatment of choice for type A lesions and preferred for type B lesions. Open surgery is the treatment of choice for type D lesions and preferred for type C lesions. Nonetheless, technological advancements allow increasingly complex lesions to be addressed in endovascular approaches, which gives patients who are otherwise poor surgical candidates an opportunity for limb salvage.

For patients of an acceptable surgical risk, controversy exists as to the best initial approach. In the Bypass versus Angioplasty in Severe Ischemia of the Leg (BASIL) trial, investigators compared a surgery-first approach (with autogenous vein) with an angioplasty-first approach for infrainguinal disease. There was no difference between the two procedures in the rate of amputation-free survival 1 year after the procedure or at the end of follow-up. There was no difference in overall survival at 30 days or by the end of the study (mean follow-up period, 3.7 years). However, for patients surviving at 2 years after the procedure, the surgery-first approach was associated with a lower subsequent mortality rate, with a hazard ratio of 0.61 (95% confidence interval: 0.50 to 0.75). In view of this outcome, current American College of Cardiology/American Heart Association guidelines recommend endovascular intervention for patients if life expectancy is less than 2 years and bypass for patients expected to live longer than 2 years (provided that an autogenous vein is available).

Improvements in endovascular techniques have allowed for increases in attempted limb salvage in patients at high risk for limb loss who would have otherwise been candidates only for primary amputations. With these improvements, there have been decreasing rates of primary amputation; however, the incidence of limb loss despite patent revascularization is increasing in this patient population. Patients at high risk for limb loss after revascularization are those with diabetes, renal insufficiency, and gangrene. In such patients, inability to control primary or recurrent infection and inability to reverse ischemia are major factors contributing to limb loss despite intervention. Even with improved techniques and early intervention, a number of studies have demonstrated that the clinical durability of limb salvage in the setting of significant soft tissue infection is often limited.

Amputations

The initial goal in the treatment of severe infections of the lower extremity is the thorough débridement of all devitalized tissue and infectious material. The viability of muscle is determined according to its ability to contract when stimulated, capacity to bleed when débrided, color, and consistency. In order to ensure débridement is adequate, the wound can often be left open with a negative-pressure wound dressing in order to return to the operating room for a second-look procedure. Once the surgeon is satisfied with the débridement, the goal is preservation of the greatest amount of viable tissue for reconstruction. It is important to note the increased energy requirements for ambulation that are associated with lower extremity amputation because these requirements, combined with the patient's preexisting comorbid conditions, dramatically decrease postoperative ambulation.

Although some authorities advocate the use of a proximal tourniquet when amputation of an infected hyperemic limb is required, no trials have yielded supportive evidence of improved healing rates with intraoperative tourniquet use. A tourniquet may be used to control blood loss while the affected limb is removed, but it should be released later to ensure adequate perfusion and viability of the skin flaps. One important consideration in applying a pneumatic tourniquet for any lower extremity amputation is the presence of an underlying vascular graft.

Wound closure in dysvascular amputations is arguably the most important component of the procedure. Careful attention should be paid to ensure that wounds are not closed under tension in order to ensure the greatest perfusion of the skin flaps. Also, monofilament suture should be used whenever possible to decrease infection risk; antibiotic sutures can also be used. For distal amputation, full-thickness flaps can be closed with nonabsorbable 2-0 or 3-0 suture. Major lower extremity amputation should be closed in layers with #0 nonabsorbable sutures to approximate deep fascia, augmented with 2-0 absorbable suture. All cutaneous sutures should be placed in a mattress or Allgower-Donati style to ensure placement of the knot on the proximal flap.

Postoperative dressing of the residual limbs should account for the decreased vascularity of these extremities. Either incisional negative-pressure dressings or fluffed gauze should be held in place with loosely wrapped elastic dressings. Tight compression wraps, although traditionally used in traumatic amputations, should be avoided because they can increase the risk of wound dehiscence.

Toe Amputation

Gangrene that is limited to the middle or distal phalanges, not involving the metatarsal head, is often amenable to simple toe disarticulation. This provides adequate treatment of the infection without affecting the patient's ambulation. Digit amputation should not be performed if ischemia of the forefoot is present or if infection involves the metatarsal head.

Great Toe Amputation

If amputation of the great toe is required, it is advantageous to preserve the base of the proximal phalanx rather than perform a complete metatarsophalangeal disarticulation. The first metatarsal head is important for balance and gait, and preservation of the proximal phalanx allows for better distribution of weight and pressure. This is particularly important in diabetic patients, who are susceptible to development of mal perforans ulcers. A curvilinear incision at the base of the toe is carried down to the level of the bone in a circumferential manner. Skin incisions can be created in a fish-mouth configuration, which involves the use of dorsoplantar or mediolateral skin flaps, or in a racquet-like manner. The choice of incision is based on viable tissue that is available to cover the remaining end of the proximal phalanx. An oscillating power saw is used to transect the distal phalanx, and the proximal phalanx (at least 1 cm) is preserved. Bone edges are smoothed to a bevel with a saw, rasp, or rongeur. Finally, full-thickness skin flaps are approximated.

Lesser Toe Amputations

The metatarsophalangeal joint is identified by flexing and extending the toe. A circumferential racquet-like or fish-mouth incision is made at the midpoint of the proximal phalanx (Figure 2). The incision is carried down to the level of the bone, and the joint capsule is opened. Resection of the cartilage at this time is not recommended; however, if viable skin flaps are present, cartilage ischemia is rarely a problem.

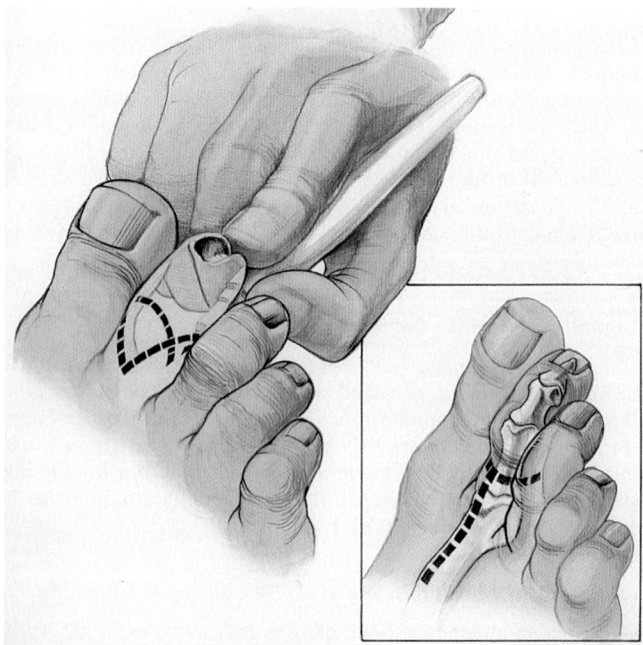

FIGURE 2   Ray amputation. Skin incision for a ray amputation is made with equal sagittal or dorsal and plantar flaps to ensure adequate blood supply. A racquet-like incision encircles the base of the toe and extends proximally over the dorsum of the metatarsal head. *(Modified from Barnes RW, Cox B: Amputations: an illustrated manual, Philadelphia, 2000, Hanley & Belfus, p 17.)*

The distal end of the affected phalanx is resected with the use of an oscillating power saw.

Ray Amputation

Ray amputations involve complete resection of the phalanx and partial resection of the corresponding metatarsal. Ray amputations are indicated when there is not enough viable tissue to provide coverage for a disarticulation as described previously. First and fifth ray amputations are often referred to as *border amputations* and are the easiest to perform. However, ray amputation to remove two adjacent toes is also possible.

For border ray amputations, a racquet-like incision is carried out in a circumferential manner and extended onto the dorsal aspect of the foot. For amputation of the second, third, or fourth toe, a racquet-like incision that extends over the metatarsal is also used (see Figure 2). Nerves and tendons are resected under tension, and the distal aspect of the metatarsal is transected with an oscillating saw; the metatarsal head is left intact.

Transmetatarsal Amputation

Transmetatarsal amputation is indicated for gangrene that results in significant forefoot tissue loss. A slightly curved dorsal skin incision is made in a mediolateral direction (Figure 3). The medial and lateral aspects of the dorsal skin excision are extended distally to ensure adequate skin coverage over the bone ends. The corresponding plantar flap is created slightly longer than the dorsal flap, and the tendons are resected under tension to the proximal edge of the wound and are allowed to retract.

Next, the metatarsals are resected with the use of a power saw with a 15-degree bevel in relation to the transverse axis. Each metatarsal should be cut successively shorter than the adjacent metatarsal in a mediolateral fashion. Next, the amputated forefoot is resected away from the plantar flap. Before approximation of the plantar and dorsal

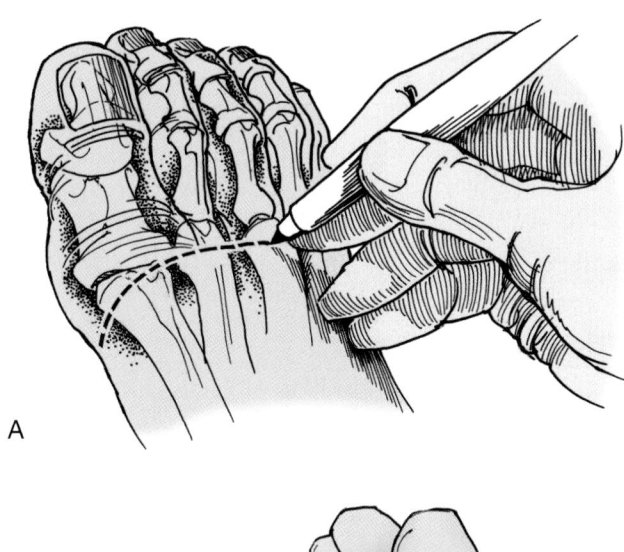

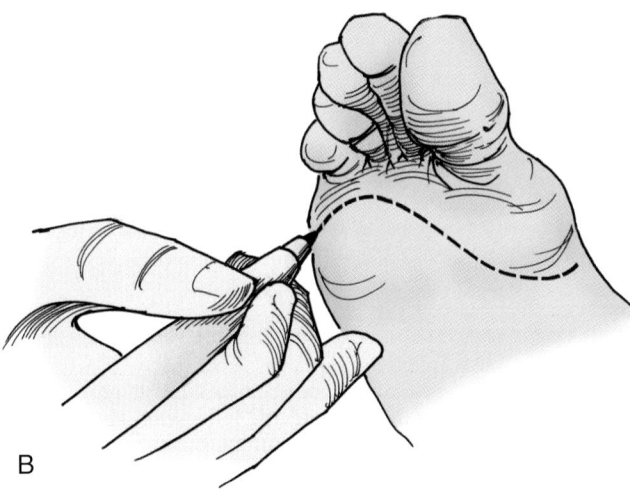

FIGURE 3 Transmetatarsal amputation. A transverse dorsal incision is made proximal to the metatarsal heads **(A),** and a curvilinear plantar incision is made at the base of the toes **(B)** to create a long plantar flap. *(Modified from Barnes RW, Cox B: Amputations: an illustrated manual, Philadelphia, 2000, Hanley & Belfus, p 39.)*

skin flaps, the plantar flap often requires thinning to avoid undue tension on the closure, which threatens viability.

Syme Amputation

The chief indication for a Syme amputation is forefoot necrosis not amenable to a transmetatarsal amputation with a healthy, viable heel pad. The Syme amputation allows for preservation of limb length and a partially weight-bearing residual limb. The sole vascular supply to the heel pad is the posterior tibial vessels, which should be carefully preserved. A transverse anterior incision that connects the anterior points of each malleolus is carried down to the bone. The corresponding dorsal incision is made down to the level of the calcaneus. The anterior tendons are identified and dissected under tension and allowed to retract (Figure 4).

The anterior tibial artery is identified and ligated, and the collateral ligamentous attachments of the talus are divided. After the medial neurovascular bundle is identified, the calcaneus is dissected away from the surrounding soft tissues, while traction is applied on the talus to facilitate dissection. During this aspect of the dissection, careful attention must be paid to avoid any injury to the subcutaneous attachment of the Achilles tendon, which would compromise the integrity of the heel pad and cause the amputation to fail. Subperiosteal dissection is carried out until the calcaneus is completely free from the soft tissue. Next, the malleoli are dissected flush with the joint surface, and the remaining bones are trimmed to avoid potential pressure points. The remaining soft tissue envelope is reapproximated with a three-layer closure. The plantar and deep fascias are approximated over the anterior portion of the tibia, followed by closure of the subcutaneous tissue and skin.

Transtibial Amputation

In patients whose necrotic tissue is not amenable to foot salvage, a transtibial amputation is indicated. An important consideration in major lower extremity amputations is what constitutes adequate débridement of necrotic tissue with maximal soft tissue preservation. Care should be taken to avoid creation of inadequate tissue flaps; such flaps may mandate a more proximal amputation than originally planned. Also, as a result of a guillotine-style amputation for the initial procedure, the residual limb may need to be shortened in order to provide adequate soft tissue coverage.

In the most commonly performed procedure for transtibial amputation, a longer posterior flap technique is used. The risk in using a true long posterior flap in patients with critical limb ischemia is poor perfusion of this distal flap, which needs to be monitored closely. If the extent of limb ischemia or gangrenous tissue precludes

FIGURE 4 Syme amputation. *(Modified from Barnes RW, Cox B: Amputations: an illustrated manual, Philadelphia, 2000, Hanley & Belfus, p 53.)*

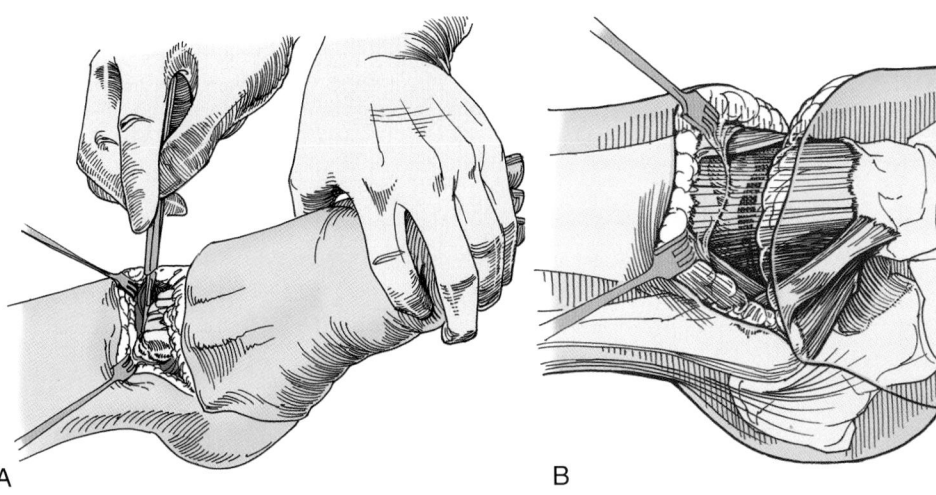

creation of a viable long posterior flap, numerous alternative techniques can be employed, including equal anteroposterior flaps, unequal anteroposterior flaps, and sagittal flaps. The anterior skin incision to create a long posterior flap is made approximately 10 cm distal to the tibial tuberosity and extended medially and laterally approximately two thirds of the way across the circumference of the calf (Figure 5). The incision is extended distally to create a posterior flap that extends 9 to 13 cm beyond the anterior flap. The distal aspects of the medial and lateral incisions are created in a curved manner and joined on the posterior surface of the calf, and the skin incision is carried down to the level of the fascia.

Next, the muscles of the anterior compartment are dissected sharply with a scalpel or electrocautery. As the muscle is further divided, the anterior tibial artery and vein are often encountered in the more posterior aspect of the anterior compartment; these vessels should be ligated and transected. The tibia and fibula are circumferentially cleared of the periosteum and are transected with an oscillating power saw. The anterior tibia is beveled approximately 1 cm proximal to the skin incision, and the fibula is transected 1 cm proximal to the tibia. A bone hook is used to apply traction on the tibia, and the muscles of the posterior compartment are carefully divided until the posterior tibial and peroneal neurovascular bundles are encountered; these bundles are then suture ligated and divided. The remaining muscles in the deep and superficial posterior compartment are divided, and the crural fascia is left in place with the posterior flap. At this time, the thickness of the posterior flap is evaluated and debulked as necessary to achieve a tension-free closure when it is approximated to the anterior flap.

Transfemoral Amputation

A transfemoral amputation is indicated for patients with ischemic limbs that are nonreconstructable or with extensive infection that precludes healing at a more distal amputation site. In addition, patients with a fixed knee contracture or a nonfunctional distal limb should also be considered for transfemoral amputation. In these patients, the postoperative energy cost of ambulation increases 60% to 100%, in comparison with 30% to 60% in patients who have undergone transtibial amputation. Increased energy costs have been shown to reduce postoperative ambulation to approximately 40% in patients with diabetes and occlusive arterial disease.

A suprapatellar fish-mouth incision is carried down to the level of the deep subcutaneous fascia to create equal-sized anterior and posterior skin flaps. The skin and subcutaneous tissue are retracted in a proximal manner, and the deep muscle fascia is sharply incised. After division of the quadriceps muscle, proximal traction is placed on all mobilized skin, subcutaneous tissue, and muscle to allow for periosteal elevation of the femur 2 to 3 cm proximal to the skin incision. The femur is transected with an oscillating or manual saw at the proximal level of the periosteum and is then beveled. The transected femur is retracted anteriorly, and the posterior muscle bundle is sharply divided. As major vessels and nerves are encountered, they should be clamped, transected, and ligated with an absorbable 2-0 suture. Wound closure is performed in multiple layers by

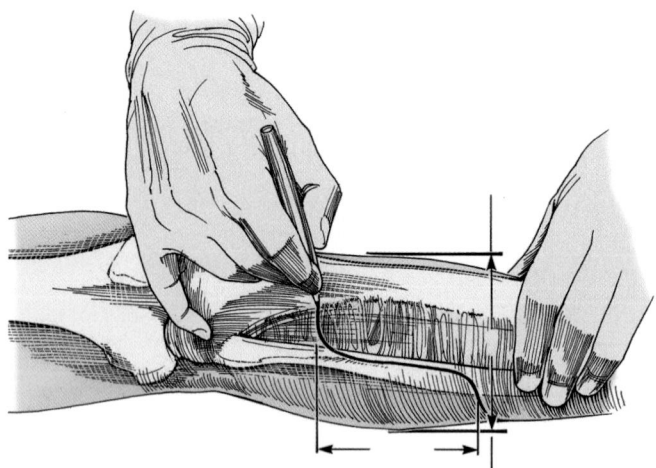

FIGURE 5 Below-the-knee amputation. The anterior skin incision is made at the level of maximal girth of the calf, approximately 3 to 4 fingerbreadths distal to the tibial tuberosity. *(Modified from Barnes RW, Cox B:* Amputations: an illustrated manual, *Philadelphia, 2000, Hanley & Belfus, p 68.)*

approximating the anterior and posterior deep subcutaneous and muscle fascia to a cuff of periosteum. This myoplasty effectively stabilizes the anterior and posterior muscle bundles.

SUMMARY

Lower extremity gangrene is a devastating disease process that accounts for a majority of nontraumatic lower limb amputations. The rates of morbidity and mortality from gangrene can best be reduced through a multidisciplinary approach and early treatment, beginning with local wound care and infection control. Vascular assessment and possible repair are critical for preoperative planning and attempted limb salvage, when suitable.

SUGGESTED READINGS

Barnes RW, Cox B: *Amputations: an illustrated manual,* Philadelphia, 2000, Hanley & Belfus.

Ernst CB, Stanley JC, Ahn SS: *Current therapy in vascular surgery,* ed 4, Hamilton, Ontario, 2001, BC Decker.

Lipsky, BA, Berendt AR, Cornia PB, et al: 2012 Infectious Diseases Society of America clinical practice guideline for the diagnosis and treatment of diabetic foot infections, *Clin Infect Dis* 54(12):e132–e173, 2012.

Lumsden AB, Davies MG, Peden EK: Medical and endovascular management of critical limb ischemia, *J Endovasc Ther* 16(Suppl. II):II31–II62, 2009.

Zelenock GB: *Mastery of vascular and endovascular surgery,* Philadelphia, 2006, Lippincott Williams & Wilkins.

Zgonis T, Stapleton JJ, Girard-Powell VA, et al: Surgical management of diabetic foot infections and amputations, *AORN J* 87(5):935–946, 2008.

Buerger's Disease (Thromboangiitis Obliterans)

Carl Magnus Wahlgren, MD, PhD, and
Bruce L. Gewertz, MD

INTRODUCTION

Thromboangiitis obliterans (TAO), or Buerger's disease, is a nonatherosclerotic, segmental, inflammatory disease that affects the small- and medium-sized arteries and veins of the extremities. Patients are mostly young male tobacco smokers who present with distal extremity ischemia, ischemic ulcers, or gangrene. Buerger's disease has a worldwide distribution, but it is more prevalent in the Mediterranean, the Middle East, and Asia. Recently, the prevalence of disease seems to have declined in the United States and Europe. In the United States, an eightfold decrease was found in the prevalence rate of disease between 1947 and 1986 (104 to 12.6 cases per 100,000 patient registrations). The disease also decreased in Japan between 2000 and 2006. Whether this represents a true decline attributed to the decline in smoking or an adoption of more uniform stricter diagnostic criteria is unclear. An increase has been seen in the incidence in women, who now constitute up to 20% of patients in certain series. This relative rise in incidence in women is undoubtedly a result of the increase in cigarette smoking among women.

Although the etiology of Buerger's disease is unknown, the condition is strongly associated with heavy tobacco use. Smoking is considered by most to be an absolute requirement for diagnosis, and progression is closely linked to continued use. However, a causal relationship has not been conclusively shown. Reports have been made of the presence of TAO in cigar smokers and in users of smokeless tobacco, such as chewing tobacco and snuff. The disease is classified pathologically as a vasculitis. Features that distinguish TAO from other types of vasculitis include highly inflammatory thrombus with relative sparing of the blood vessel wall, normal acute phase reactants, and no serum markers of immunoactivation.

CLINICAL PRESENTATION

Buerger's disease typically begins with involvement of the distal small arteries and veins. More proximal arteries may be involved when the disease progresses, but involvement of large arteries is unusual. The onset of symptoms usually occurs before the age of 40 to 45 years. Patients may present with claudication of the feet, legs, hands, or arms. Two or more limbs are always involved; all four limbs are affected in about 40% of patients. Intermittent symptoms are initially localized to the forefoot or the arch of the foot because of the distal nature of the disease, as opposed to patients with peripheral atherosclerotic disease who first experience symptoms located to the calves. Progression of the inflammatory disease leads to development of ischemic rest pain and ulcerations in the distal portion of toes or fingers. In most series, about three fourths of patients present with ischemic ulcers. Raynaud's phenomenon and superficial migratory thrombophlebitis are manifestations that are commonly encountered.

Although Buerger's disease predominantly affects the vessels of the extremities, a few instances of aortic, cerebral, coronary, mesenteric, pulmonary, and renal involvement have been reported in the literature. Mesenteric Buerger's disease is extremely rare and is associated with a poor prognosis. For this reason, patients with known Buerger's disease who present with gastrointestinal manifestations should be urgently evaluated for bowel ischemia; early surgical intervention is recommended.

DIAGNOSIS

Several criteria have been proposed for the diagnosis of TAO. The common clinical criteria can be summarized as:

- Age younger than 45 years
- Current or recent history of tobacco use
- Distal extremity ischemia documented with noninvasive vascular testing
- Findings suggestive of TAO on conventional angiography or magnetic resonance imaging.
- Exclusion of autoimmune disease, hypercoagulable states, diabetes mellitus, proximal source of emboli, trauma, and local lesions (popliteal entrapment syndromes, adventitial cystic disease)

The physical examination often reveals cyanotic and erythematous extremities. Sensory abnormalities (burning, hypoesthesia, numbness, and tingling) as a result of ischemic neuropathy are common as is cold sensitivity that may be related to ischemia or to increased muscle sympathetic nerve activity. Absent distal pulses in the presence of normal proximal pulses are typical in patients with the disease. Ankle-brachial indices should be included in the vascular examination. Involvement of both the upper and the lower extremities is common. Dry punctate ischemic lesions are often seen on both the hands and the feet. Although nonspecific, a positive Allen's test in a young smoker with digital ischemia is strongly suggestive of the disease.

A definitive diagnosis of TAO can only be made with a vessel biopsy that shows cellular thrombus and the classic acute phase lesion, but the physical examination and history are often classic. As a consequence, biopsies are rarely needed unless a patient presents with unusual characteristics, such as large artery involvement or an age of more than 45 years.

No specific laboratory tests confirm the diagnosis, but several serologic tests should be included in the workup to rule out other diseases that mimic TAO, including scleroderma, calcinosis, Raynaud's phenomenon, esophageal dysmotility, sclerodactyly, and telangiectasia (CREST) syndrome, mixed connective tissue disease, systemic lupus erythematosus, and hypercoagulability disorders. A complete blood count is routinely obtained with differential, electrolyte, renal and liver function tests, fasting blood glucose, urinalysis, sedimentation rate/C-reactive protein, and a complete hypercoagulability screen, including antiphospholipid antibodies. Serologic markers that should be obtained are antinuclear antibody, rheumatoid factor, complement measurements, and serologic markers for CREST syndrome and scleroderma (SCL-70 and anticentromere antibody). Patients with giant cell arteritis or Takayasu's arteritis usually present with more proximal vascular involvement and more frequently have elevations of acute phase reactants.

Standard arteriography is not essential for the diagnosis. Noninvasive imaging methods such as magnetic resonance angiography (MRA) and computed tomographic angiography (CTA) are good alternatives. Four-limb segmental arterial pressures and digital plethysmography (waveform or digital pressure measurement) are useful to document distal occlusive disease. When suggested by unilateral involvement, a proximal source of emboli should be excluded with echocardiography or CTA/MRA.

Arteriography should be performed in those patients with threatened limb loss. Although a number of angiographic findings are highly suggestive of TAO, there are no pathognomonic findings (Box 1 and Figures 1 and 2). The angiographic appearance of TAO may be identical to other types of small vessel vasculitis or toxic arterial responses related to amphetamine, cannabis, or cocaine abuse. If a nonsmoking patient presents with signs consistent with Buerger's disease, a toxicology screen for the previously mentioned drugs is advisable.

Because of the relatively young age of most patients, the possibility of popliteal artery entrapment syndrome, cystic adventitial disease, or popliteal artery aneurysm should be considered in patients with lower extremity symptoms. The presence of diabetes mellitus, end-stage renal disease, or significant risk factors for atherosclerosis argues against a diagnosis of Buerger's disease.

BOX 1: Angiographic findings in thromboangiitis obliterans (Buerger's disease)

- Involvement of small and medium-sized vessels
- Palmar, plantar, tibial, peroneal, radial, and ulnar arteries and digital arteries of fingers and toes (see Figure 1)
- Normal extremity arteries proximal to the popliteal and distal brachial levels
- Absence of proximal atherosclerosis and vascular calcification
- No source of thrombus
- Abrupt transition from a normal and smooth proximal artery to an area of occlusion
- Symmetric and segmental arterial involvement
- Tortuous "corkscrew" collaterals that are suggestive, but not pathognomonic, of Buerger's disease (see Figure 2)

TREATMENT

The main and most effective treatment for Buerger's disease is the total abstinence from tobacco products. Smoking is closely related to exacerbation and remission of the disease. Even a few cigarettes a day or use of smokeless tobacco or nicotine replacement may keep the disease active. Smoking cessation was initially thought to not be possible in patients with Buerger's disease. The authors' experience and that of others suggest that this is unduly pessimistic; up to one third of the authors' patients have successfully discontinued tobacco use with proper counseling and support.

A correlation is found between continued smoking and limb amputation. If patients discontinue tobacco use, they can be reassured that the disease often remits and that amputation can be avoided as long as ischemic ulcers have not already occurred. That said, patients with already significant occluded arterial segments may continue to experience intermittent claudication or Raynaud's phenomenon.

In patients with disease progression despite smoking cessation, effective therapeutic options are limited (Box 2). Initial enthusiasm for infusion of the prostaglandin analogue iloprost has not been borne out by further trials or experience. Anticoagulants, antiplatelet drugs, and rheologic agents seem to be ineffective. Calcium channel blockers are only helpful if significant vasospasm is present. Intraarterial thrombolytic therapy is not effective and has not been used in the authors' practice. Therapeutic angiogenesis, including intramuscular gene transfer of vascular endothelial growth factor and bone marrow–derived stem cell therapy, seems promising and beneficial, although further studies are needed to evaluate safety and efficacy.

Unfortunately, arterial reconstruction is usually not an attractive option because of the diffuse segmental involvement and distal nature of the disease. Also, the concomitant inflammatory venous

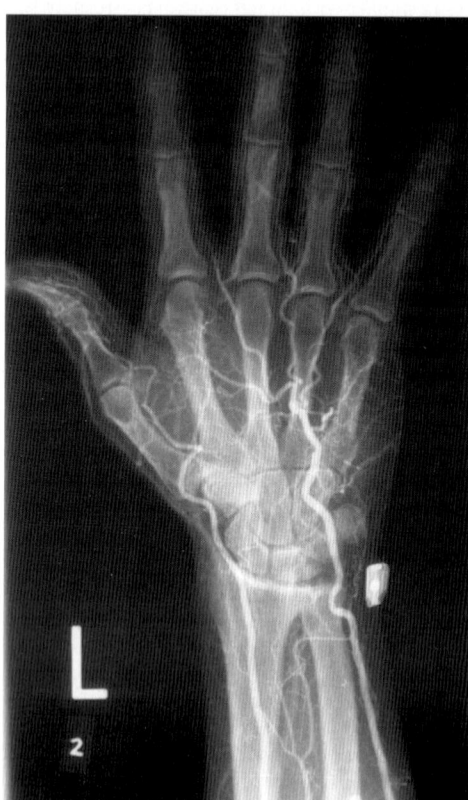

FIGURE 1 Hand angiogram of a patient with Buerger's disease showing involvement of the digital arteries with several occlusions and collaterals.

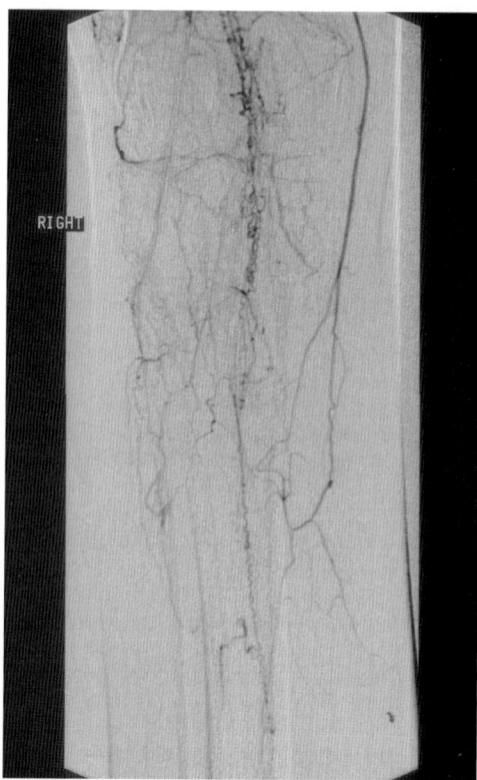

FIGURE 2 Lower extremity angiography of a patient with Buerger's disease showing multiple occlusions and "corkscrew" collaterals.

BOX 2: Treatment options in thromboangiitis obliterans (Buerger's disease)

1. Cessation of tobacco products
2. Local wound care
3. Arterial reconstruction with vein graft or endovascular therapy
4. Therapeutic options
    a. Prostaglandin analogue iloprost or treprostinil sodium
    b. Cilostazol
    c. Hyperbaric oxygen therapy
    d. Calcium channel blockers (i.e., amlodipine or nifedipine), if vasospasm
    e. Intermittent pneumatic compression pump
    f. Implantable spinal cord stimulator
    g. Therapeutic angiogenesis with gene-based or cell-based therapies
5. Amputation

disease often renders the saphenous veins unsatisfactory for use as conduits. However, if conservative treatment fails in patients with severe ischemia and nonhealing ischemic ulcers of the lower extremities, revascularization should be considered. The distal arteries must be thoroughly evaluated with arteriography for optimal preoperative planning. If surgical exploration reveals a diminutive receiving vessel, bypass should be abandoned.

Although less invasive endovascular approaches might be attractive in this population, the diffuse, distal, and segmental involvement of the lesions confounds available catheter-based techniques, and their role is likely to be similar to that of surgery. Extended endovascular interventions down to the foot have shown to be technically feasible in a limited number of patients with TAO, but long-term data are lacking. More proximal femoropopliteal lesions in patients with advanced disease should be addressed to maximize inflow to collateral vessels.

As with many interventions for occlusive vascular disease, limb salvage rates usually exceed graft patency rates. Although the patency rate for distal bypass is no more than 50% even in the small number of patients with Buerger's disease who can undergo bypass, limb salvage rates frequently exceed 75%. In these well-selected patients, even limited periods of revascularization provide a sufficient interval to heal ischemic ulcers in the feet.

Sympathectomy as a primary or adjunctive treatment option has been tried in a large number of patients with Buerger's disease without encouraging results. This lack of success reinforces the obstructive rather then vasospastic nature of the disease. Still, in some patients, spinal cord stimulation can have a salutary effect through pain reduction.

Amputations are inevitable in patients with extensive gangrene or sepsis. The goal is to remove all nonviable tissue, preserve optimal residual function, and minimize surgical morbidity. Application of these principles may result in unconventional amputation levels with a preponderance of multiple digital or distal amputations.

PROGNOSIS

In general, the prognosis for many patients with Buerger's disease is surprisingly good and depends largely on the ability to discontinue tobacco use. Despite the considerable morbidity, life expectancy for patients approaches that of an age-matched population. This could possibly be explained by the young age of presentation and the lack of coronary involvement in the disease process.

Even though ischemic ulcers are already present in most patients presenting for medical care, the overall limb amputation rate is less than 50%. It seems that occurrence of necrotic lesions subsides in patients older than 60 years. Still, follow-up of patients with TAO shows frequent hospitalization and surgical procedures. Major amputation and prolonged hospitalization markedly influence quality of life, with many patients losing any opportunity for productive employment.

SUMMARY

Thromboangiitis obliterans or Buerger's disease is a nonatherosclerotic, segmental, and inflammatory disease. It is characterized by the development of segmental thrombotic occlusions of the medium-size and small arteries and veins of the extremities.

It occurs in young smokers who present with distal extremity ischemia, ulcers, or gangrene. The most important diseases to exclude are atherosclerosis, emboli, and autoimmune diseases. The only effective treatment is complete and permanent abstinence from tobacco products. Several medical, endovascular, and surgical therapies are palliative.

SUGGESTED READINGS

Dargon PT, Landry GJ: Buerger's disease, *Ann Vasc Surg* 26:871–880, 2012.
Malecki R, Zdrojowy K, Adamiec R: Thromboangiitis obliterans in the 21st century: a new face of disease, *Atherosclerosis* 206:328–334, 2009.
Mills JL Sr: Buerger's disease in the 21st century: diagnosis, clinical features, and therapy, *Semin Vasc Surg* 16:179–189, 2003.
Olin JW: Thromboangiitis obliterans (Buerger's disease), *N Engl J Med* 343:864–869, 2000.
Olin JW, Shih A: Thromboangiitis obliterans (Buerger's disease), *Curr Opin Rheumatol* 18:18–24, 2006.
Piazza G, Creager MA: Thromboangiitis obliterans, *Circulation* 121:1858–1861, 2010.

ACUTE MESENTERIC ISCHEMIA

Charlie C. Cheng, MD, Lorraine Choi, MD,
Zulfiqar Cheema, MD, and Michael B. Silva, Jr., MD

OVERVIEW

Acute mesenteric ischemia is a relatively uncommon condition that can potentially have fatal outcomes. Despite advances in diagnostic imaging, perioperative management, and treatment modalities, mesenteric ischemia remains a challenging clinical dilemma. It is estimated that about 1 per every 1000 hospital admissions in the United States is for mesenteric ischemia. The 30-day mortality rate remains high, at 32% to 80%, because of delay in diagnosis and treatment. The prevalence is likely to increase because the population is aging and because of the comorbid conditions of elderly patients. A high index of suspicion with early diagnosis and treatment is essential for improving outcomes.

ANATOMY AND COLLATERALIZATION

The arterial perfusion to the gastrointestinal system is provided by three branches of the abdominal aorta: the celiac artery (CA), the superior mesenteric artery (SMA), and the inferior mesenteric artery (IMA; Figure 1). The CA originates from the ventral surface of the aorta near the level of T12 to L1. It provides arterial circulation to the foregut (distal esophagus to duodenum), spleen, and the hepatobiliary system. The SMA originates just distal to the CA near the level of L1 to L2 and supplies the midgut from the jejunum to midcolon. The IMA originates from the left lateral surface of the aorta near the L3 level, about 10 cm distal to the SMA. It supplies the hindgut from the midcolon to the rectum.

There is rich collateral circulation between these mesenteric arteries (Figure 2). Chronic mesenteric ischemia from the occlusion of one or even two mesenteric arteries is usually well tolerated if time is allowed for enlargement and development of these uninvolved mesenteric collateral circulations. In acute mesenteric ischemia, however, there may be profound ischemia as a result of the lack of these collateral networks. The collateral circulation between the CA and the SMA is via the superior and inferior pancreaticoduodenal arteries from the gastroduodenal artery. The communication between the SMA and the IMA is via the arch of Riolan centrally and the marginal arteries of Drummond near the periphery of the colon. There is also important collateralization between the IMA and the internal iliac artery to supply the hindgut.

PATHOPHYSIOLOGY

There are four primary causes of acute mesenteric ischemia. The most common cause is embolization to the SMA (Figure 3), which accounts for approximately 50% of all cases. Most emboli originate from left atrial or ventricular mural thrombi or from valvular lesions. The emboli then travel to the SMA preferentially because its course is a nearly parallel course to the aorta and because of its high flow rate. Most emboli lodge 3 to 10 cm distal to the SMA origin, in the tapered segment just past the branching of the middle colic artery. The result is that the proximal midjejunum is spared from ischemia.

Mesenteric thrombosis accounts for about 20% of cases of acute ischemia and is located at the origin of the vessel in a preexisting

atherosclerotic lesion (Figure 4). Because of this preexisting lesion, most affected patients have a history of symptoms of chronic mesenteric ischemia that include postprandial pain and "food fear," which leads to weight loss. The thrombosis occurs at the origin flush with the aorta. If the SMA is involved, the result is ischemia of the entire midgut.

Nonocclusive mesenteric ischemia accounts for about 20% of cases and is caused by a low-flow state resulting from any type of shock or the use of vasoconstrictors. The underlying medical condition and delay in diagnosis result in high rates of mortality, regardless of treatment.

Mesenteric venous thrombosis accounts for about 10% of cases and is caused by thrombosis of the veins draining the intestine (Figure 5). These veins include the inferior mesenteric, superior mesenteric, splenic, and portal veins. Venous thrombosis leads to decreased venous outflow, edema, distension, and decreased mesenteric perfusion. The thrombus is located in the superior mesenteric vein in 70% of patients, and in the portal and inferior mesenteric veins in approximately 30%. Risk factors include hypercoagulable syndromes, such as protein C and S deficiency, and hypercoagulable states, such as cancer.

Regardless of the cause, decreased perfusion leads to anaerobic metabolism and acidosis. If these states are persistent, there is mucosal compromise, with release of intracellular toxin and influx of toxin from the bowel lumen into the splanchnic and systemic circulation. With advanced ischemia, there is full-thickness necrosis with resulting bowel perforation and peritonitis. If blood flow is restored, reperfusion injury may develop, and the inflammatory cascade may result in systemic effects, with cardiac, pulmonary, or renal dysfunction.

CLINICAL PRESENTATION AND DIAGNOSIS

The classic manifestation of acute mesenteric ischemia is sudden abdominal pain out of proportion to the physical examination. This

FIGURE 1 Mesenteric circulation, showing the celiac, superior mesenteric, and inferior mesenteric arteries.

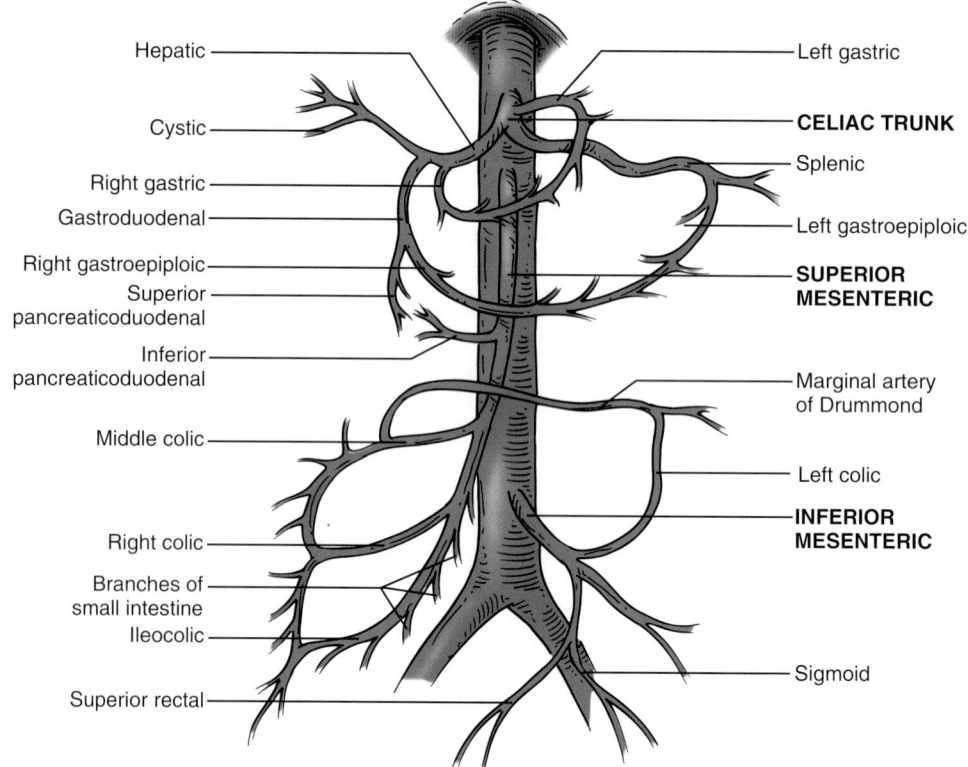

Hepatic

Cystic

Right gastric

Gastroduodenal

Right gastroepiploic

Superior pancreaticoduodenal

Inferior pancreaticoduodenal

Middle colic

Right colic

Branches of small intestine

Ileocolic

Superior rectal

Left gastric

CELIAC TRUNK

Splenic

Left gastroepiploic

SUPERIOR MESENTERIC

Marginal artery of Drummond

Left colic

INFERIOR MESENTERIC

Sigmoid

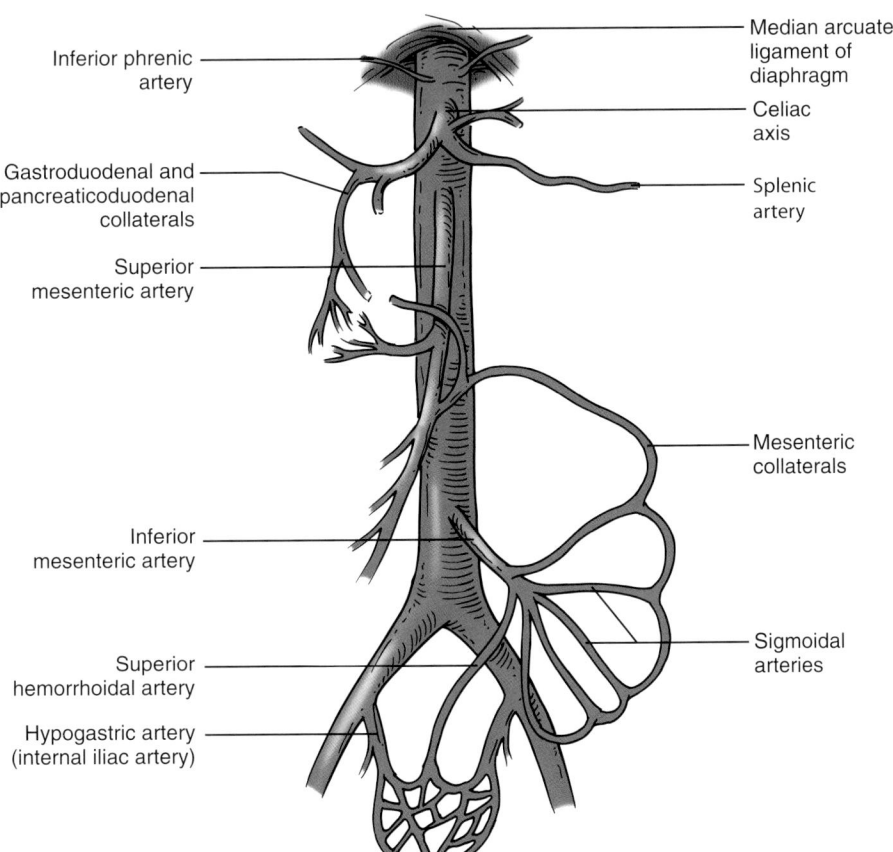

Inferior phrenic artery

Gastroduodenal and pancreaticoduodenal collaterals

Superior mesenteric artery

Inferior mesenteric artery

Superior hemorrhoidal artery

Hypogastric artery (internal iliac artery)

Median arcuate ligament of diaphragm

Celiac axis

Splenic artery

Mesenteric collaterals

Sigmoidal arteries

FIGURE 2 Collateral circulation between the three mesenteric arteries.

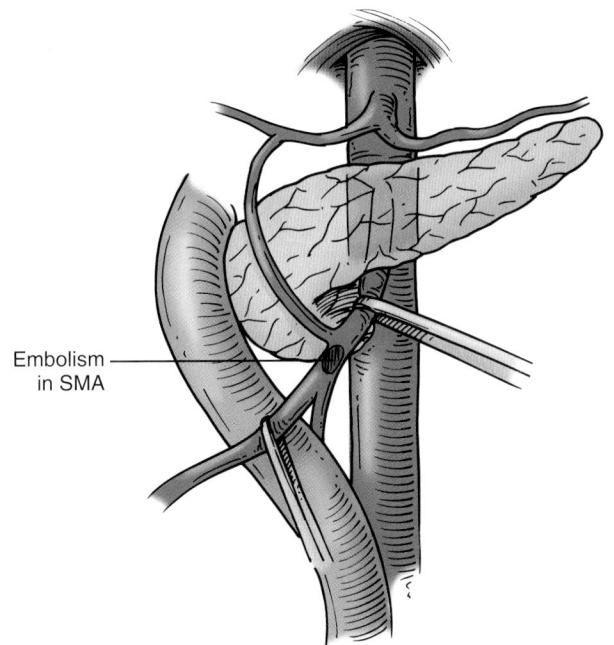

Embolism in SMA

FIGURE 3 Embolization of the superior mesenteric artery (SMA).

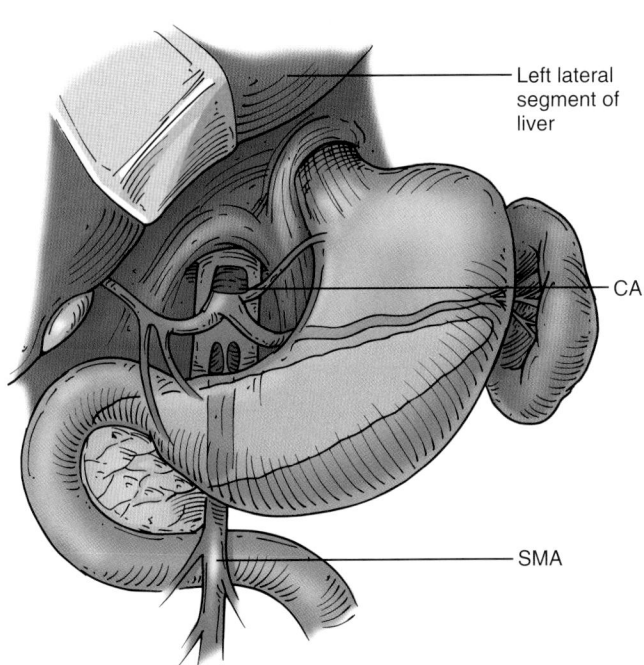

Left lateral segment of liver

CA

SMA

FIGURE 4 Mesenteric thrombosis. This usually occurs at the origin of the celiac artery (CA) or superior mesenteric artery (SMA).

occurs frequently after an embolic event in patients with a history of cardiac arrhythmia or recent myocardial infraction. The abdominal pain is often followed by bloody diarrhea with progression of mucosal sloughing. Common nonspecific symptoms also include fever, nausea, vomiting, and abdominal distension. Patients may present with either (1) acute mesenteric ischemia or (2) chronic mesenteric ischemia and a history of abdominal angina, food intolerance, and weight loss. The subacute presentation is characterized by a more gradual development of abdominal pain. In nonocclusive mesenteric ischemia, there may be severe pain that varies in intensity and location. If abdominal pain is absent or if the patient in the intensive care unit is unresponsive, there is progressive abdominal distension with acidosis. There should be a high index of suspicion in elderly patients with a recent history of cardiogenic, hypovolemic, hemorrhagic, or septic shock.

No laboratory evaluation is specific for mesenteric ischemia. Complete blood cell count may show hemoconcentration with increased hemoglobin and hematocrit. There is also a leukocytosis with "left shift." With advanced ischemia and bowel necrosis, metabolic acidosis occurs, and amylase, lactic dehydrogenase, and alkaline phosphatase levels are elevated. Plain abdominal radiographs are used to exclude other causes of abdominal pain, such as perforation or intestinal obstruction. With bowel infarction in advanced ischemia, there may be pneumatosis intestinalis, portal venous gas, and pneumoperitoneum. Color Doppler ultrasonography can show stenosis or occlusion in the CA or SMA and is more specific than clinical evaluation. However, this tool may be difficult in patients with acute ischemia when bowels are dilated and filled with air. Computed tomographic scan of the abdomen and pelvis is helpful in diagnosing ischemia in patients with subacute symptoms, showing focal or segmental bowel wall thickening. In the mesenteric or portal veins, the appearance of thrombus or lack of contrast opacification indicates mesenteric or portal venous thrombosis. Upper endoscopy and colonoscopy do not provide any useful information, and barium contrast evaluation is contraindicated. The intraluminal barium can limit visualization of the mesenteric arteries during angiography.

The definitive diagnostic study for mesenteric ischemia is angiography (Figure 6). Angiography with multiple views is needed for adequate evaluation. The lateral views are used to assess the origin of the CA and the SMA, whereas the circulation of the distal CA and SMA is best evaluated with the anteroposterior views. In most cases, the IMA has been occluded by aortic atherosclerotic disease. Selective catheterizations of the CA and the SMA are also needed for complete visualization of the anatomy and to define the pathophysiologic process. In mesenteric embolization (usually in the SMA), the emboli that lodge at branch points create a "meniscus sign," with an abrupt occlusion of a normal proximal SMA several centimeters from its origin. In contrast, with mesenteric thrombosis, the lesion occurs near the origin and tapers off 1 to 2 cm distally. Usually, patients with thrombosis have a history of chronic mesenteric ischemia, and collateral circulations such as the arch of Riolan and the marginal arteries of Drummond can be visualized. In nonocclusive mesenteric ischemia, angiography shows a normal-appearing SMA with segments of vasospasm.

TREATMENT

Initial Management

The goal of treatment is to restore mesenteric blood flow to alleviate the mesenteric ischemia and to prevent bowel necrosis. Initial

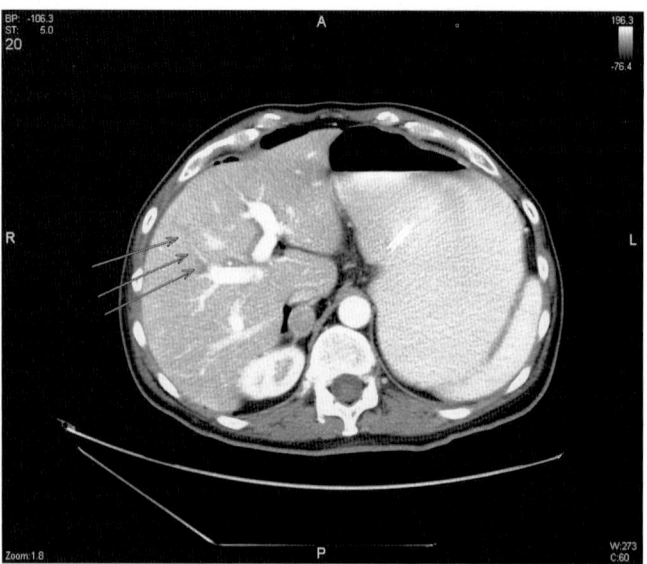

FIGURE 5 Computed tomographic scan showing mesenteric thrombosis *(arrows)* of the right hepatic vein.

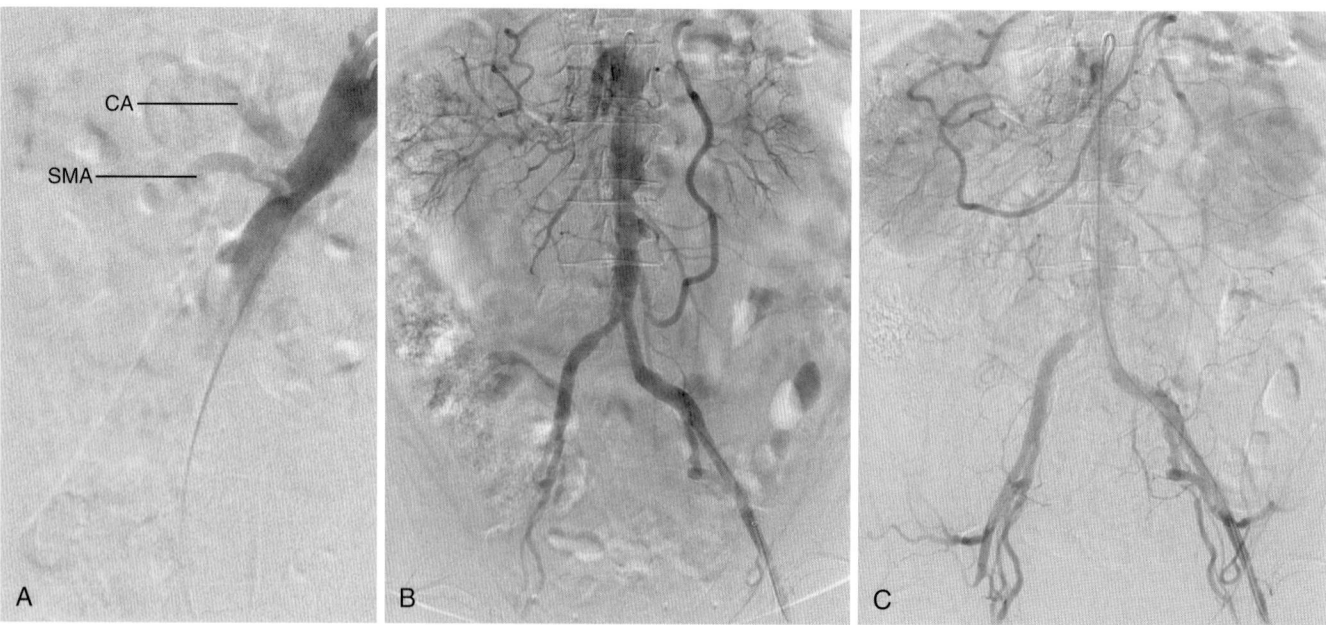

FIGURE 6 Angiography for mesenteric ischemia. **A,** Stenosis of the celiac artery (CA) and superior mesenteric artery (SMA). **B,** Retrograde filling of the SMA from the inferior mesenteric artery (IMA) via collateral vessels in the same patient. **C,** Delayed angiography showing retrograde filling of CA from the SMA.

treatment includes fluid resuscitation, correction of metabolic acidosis with sodium bicarbonate, and administration of antibiotics. Anticoagulation with heparin is used to prevent further propagation of thrombus. A central venous catheter, a peripheral arterial catheter, and a Foley catheter are placed to monitor volume and hemodynamic status. Mesenteric angiography is performed immediately to confirm the diagnosis and to plan for appropriate intervention according to the cause of the ischemia.

Embolism of Mesenteric Artery

In acute embolic mesenteric ischemia, the treatment is surgical removal of the embolus to restore arterial blood flow. As mentioned previously, the majority of the emboli are lodged in the SMA. A midline incision is made, and the extent of the mesenteric ischemia and bowel necrosis is assessed. There is usually variable bowel ischemia from the midjejunum to the transverse colon (Figure 7). Bowel resection is usually delayed until revascularization of the mesenteric artery. To expose the SMA, the transverse colon is reflected superiorly and the small bowel is retracted to the right upper quadrant. The ligament of Treitz is divided to mobilize the fourth portion of the duodenum. The SMA is palpated at the root of the mesentery over the junction of the third and fourth portions of the duodenum. Proximal and distal vascular control of the proximal SMA segment is obtained in the standard manner. A longitudinal arteriotomy is made, and an embolectomy balloon catheter is passed proximally and distally to ensure complete removal of the embolus. When proximal inflow and distal back flow are adequate, a vein or synthetic (polyester [Dacron] or polytetrafluoroethylene [PTFE]) patch is used for closure of the arteriotomy. If embolectomy is unsuccessful in reestablishing blood flow, this longitudinal arteriotomy can be used for distal anastomoses of the bypass graft. A longitudinal arteriotomy is recommended over a transverse arteriotomy (Figure 8).

After restoration of mesenteric blood flow, the viability of the bowel is assessed. Segments of bowel whose viability was equivocal previously may improve after revascularization. Intravenous fluorescein injection followed by Wood lamp inspection and Doppler imaging can assist in assessing the viability of the bowel. If bowel viability remains questionable, a second-look operation can be performed in 24 to 36 hours. This allows for bowel resection to be limited and to ensure that bowel anastomoses are performed with viable bowel.

Thrombosis of Mesenteric Artery

The management of mesenteric thrombosis is more challenging and differs from that of mesenteric embolism. The mesenteric artery is usually normal in mesenteric embolism. In mesenteric thrombosis, in contrast, there is disease progression from atherosclerosis that usually involves multiple mesenteric artery branches at their origins (Figure 9). Mesenteric bypass to a distal, uninvolved segment is needed for definitive revascularization. Single-vessel or two-vessel revascularization may be performed. The donor vessel for the mesenteric bypass can be the supraceliac abdominal aorta in antegrade bypass or the infrarenal aorta or the iliac artery in retrograde bypass. Advantages of antegrade bypass include the use of supraceliac aorta, which is usually free of atherosclerotic disease, and the use of a short bypass graft that avoids kinking when the bowel is returned to its anatomic position after revascularization. However, this bypass requires supraceliac aortic occlusion and the aortic exposure is more difficult, especially in obese patients. Advantages of retrograde bypass include the ease of infrarenal aortic or iliac exposure. However, there is higher risk for bypass graft kinking in retrograde bypass, and this requires the use of donor vessels that frequently are involved in atherosclerotic disease.

The graft material of choice is the saphenous vein. Prosthetic graft should be avoided in patients with nonviable bowel or in patients requiring bowel resection. In situations in which a prosthetic graft

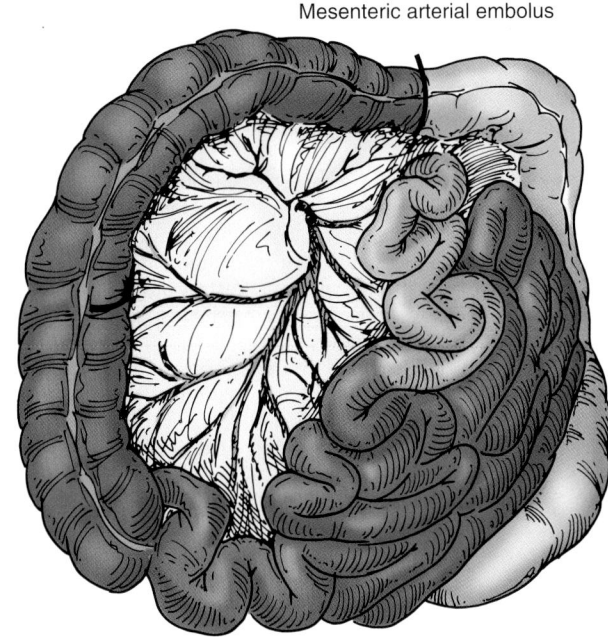

Mesenteric arterial embolus

FIGURE 7 Embolization of superior mesenteric artery. There is usually viable proximal small bowel with variable bowel ischemia from the midjejunum to the transverse colon. *(From Rutherford RB: Rutherford vascular surgery, ed 6, Philadelphia, 2005, WB Saunders.)*

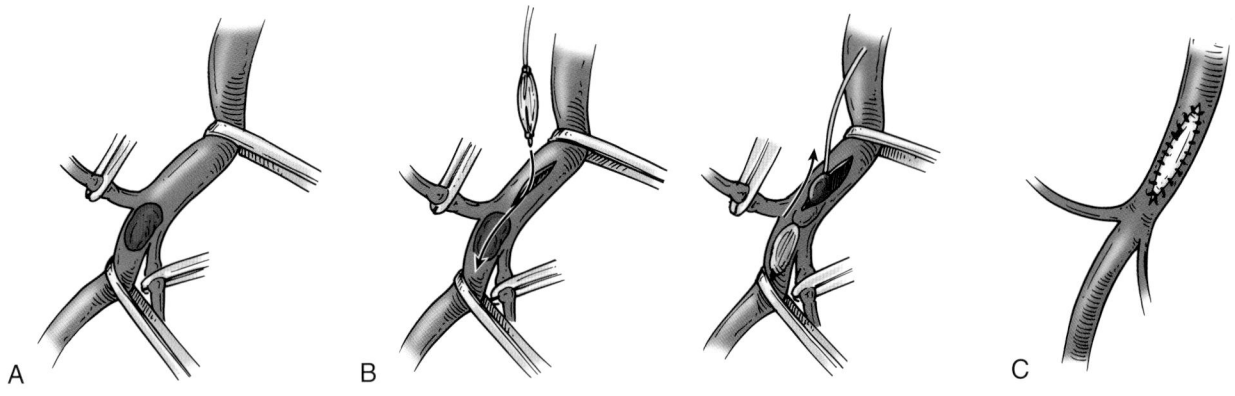

A   B   C

FIGURE 8 Technique of superior mesenteric artery (SMA) embolectomy.

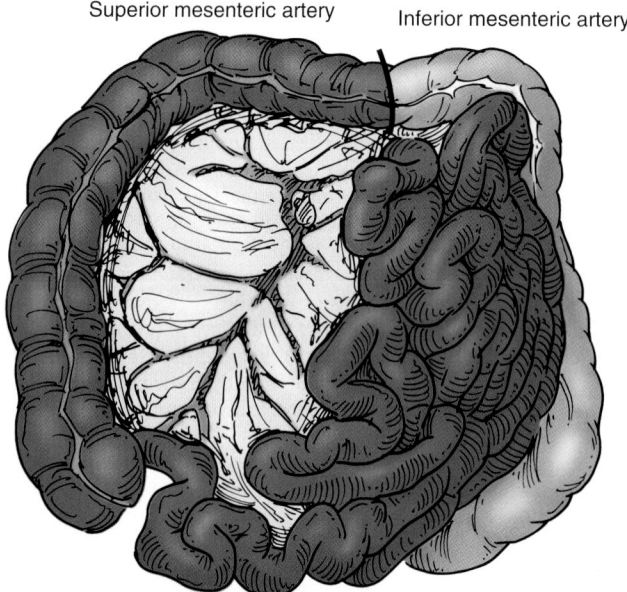

Superior mesenteric artery   Inferior mesenteric artery

FIGURE 9   Mesenteric thrombosis. The disease involves the origin of the mesenteric arteries, resulting in extensive bowel ischemia. *(From Rutherford RB: Rutherford vascular surgery, 6th ed. Philadelphia, 2005, WB Saunders.)*

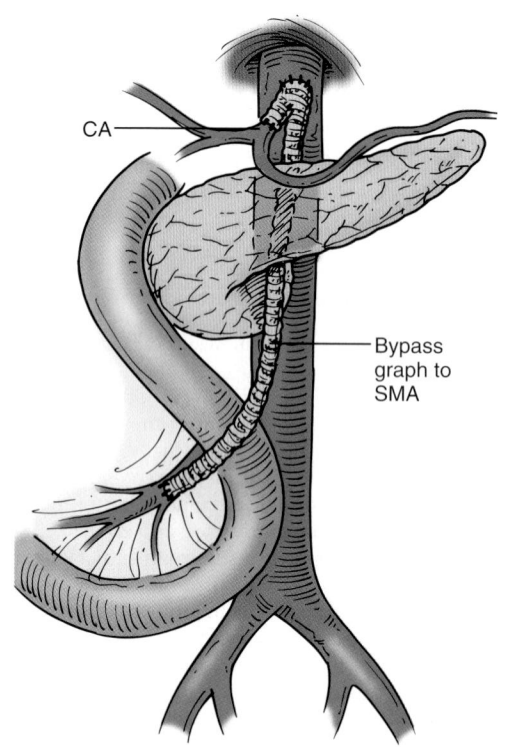

CA

Bypass graph to SMA

FIGURE 10   Antegrade bypass with the use of a bifurcated graft to the celiac artery (CA) and superior mesenteric artery (SMA).

can be used, a small-diameter woven or PTFE graft is used for single-vessel revascularization. For two-vessel revascularization, a bifurcated graft may be used to bypass to the CA and SMA.

In antegrade bypass, initial exposure is accomplished by dividing the gastrohepatic ligament and mobilizing the left lobe of the liver. The esophagus is retracted to the left, and division of the diaphragmatic crura and median arcuate ligament provides exposure of the distal 10 cm of thoracic aorta without division of the diaphragm. The origin of the CA has already been dissected during exposure of the aorta, and dissection is continued distally until a soft, patent distal target is reached. The SMA is dissected at the root of the mesentery as described previously. The vein graft is bypassed first to the CA and then sequentially to the SMA via a tunnel behind the pancreas. In patients without bowel ischemia or infarct, a synthetic graft can be used. If a bifurcated graft is used, the proximal aortic graft is beveled and sutured to the supraceliac aorta. The limbs are cut into appropriate lengths and anastomosed to the CA and the SMA (Figure 10).

In retrograde bypass, the most proximal SMA segment that is patent is exposed as it exits from behind the pancreas. This decreases the risk of kinking in the bypass graft. This anastomosis is completed first, and the bowel is returned to its anatomic position. The bypass graft is pulled and placed adjacent to the aorta. A soft spot on the infrarenal aorta or the iliac artery is located and used for the proximal anastomosis. Tension is maintained on the vein graft during anastomosis to avoid graft laxity and kinking (Figure 11, *A*). Revascularization to the CA is usually performed via the common hepatic artery (see Figure 11, *B*) or, less commonly, via the splenic artery. The distal anastomosis is again performed first, and the graft is pulled taut behind the duodenum and the head of pancreas. The graft is tunneled behind the tail of the pancreas, and if the distal anastomosis is to the splenic artery, anterior to the left renal vein.

Nonocclusive Mesenteric Ischemia

The primary treatment of nonocclusive mesenteric ischemia is catheter-directed infusion of vasodilatory agents. A catheter is placed into the CA and the SMA for selective mesenteric angiography, and a diagnosis is made when segments of vasospasm are seen in a

normal-appearing mesenteric artery. A vasodilatory agent such as papaverine is directly infused into the mesenteric artery via the catheter at a dose of 30 to 60 mg/hour. System anticoagulation is achieved with heparin, given via peripheral intravenous catheter, to prevent thrombosis in the catheterized vessels. Vasoconstricting agents should also be stopped. The hemodynamic status of the patient is monitored for any hypotension that may signify systemic infusion of the vasodilator with migration of the infusion catheter into the aorta.

The patient's response and clinical status are observed closely. If abdominal symptoms improve, mesenteric angiography is repeated to ensure resolution of the vasospasm and perfusion of the bowel. If the patient develops acute peritonitis with rebound tenderness and involuntary guarding, there is continued bowel ischemia or infarction, and surgical exploration is needed to assess bowel viability. The room temperature is elevated, and the bowel is wrapped in warm, moist laparotomy pads to minimize vasoconstriction. Papaverine is continued perioperatively, and any nonviable bowel is resected. A second-look operation can be performed in 24 to 36 hours if bowel viability is questionable.

Mesenteric Venous Thrombosis

In addition to the initial management as described previously with fluid resuscitation and anticoagulation, patients need to be evaluated for hypercoagulopathies and hypercoagulable states such as cancer. Surgical exploration is indicated in a patient with signs of bowel ischemia and infarction. Surgery should be limited to bowel resection because venous thrombectomy has not been shown to be effective. Bowel resection is generous, and repeated surgical explorations may be necessary to ensure adequate bowel resection.

In patients who do not have peritonitis but continue to have abdominal pain despite resuscitation and anticoagulation, catheter-directed thrombolytic therapy is potentially useful. The thrombolytic agent is delivered to the mesenteric venous circulation via catheter-directed infusion of the splenic artery and the SMA (Figure 12). Bilateral common femoral arterial access is obtained for

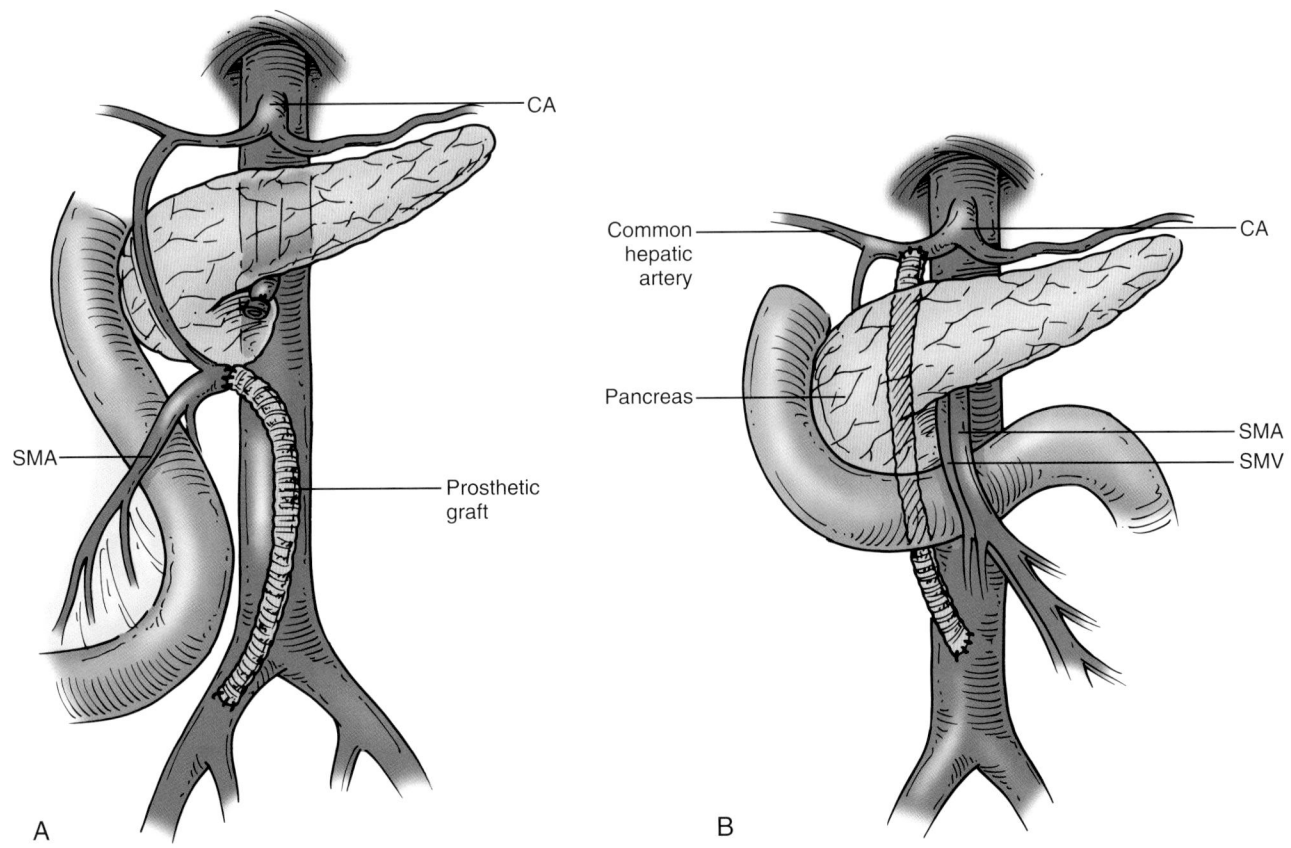

FIGURE 11 **A,** Retrograde bypass to the superior mesenteric artery (SMA). **B,** Retrograde bypass to the celiac artery (CA) via the common hepatic artery. *SMV,* Superior mesenteric vein.

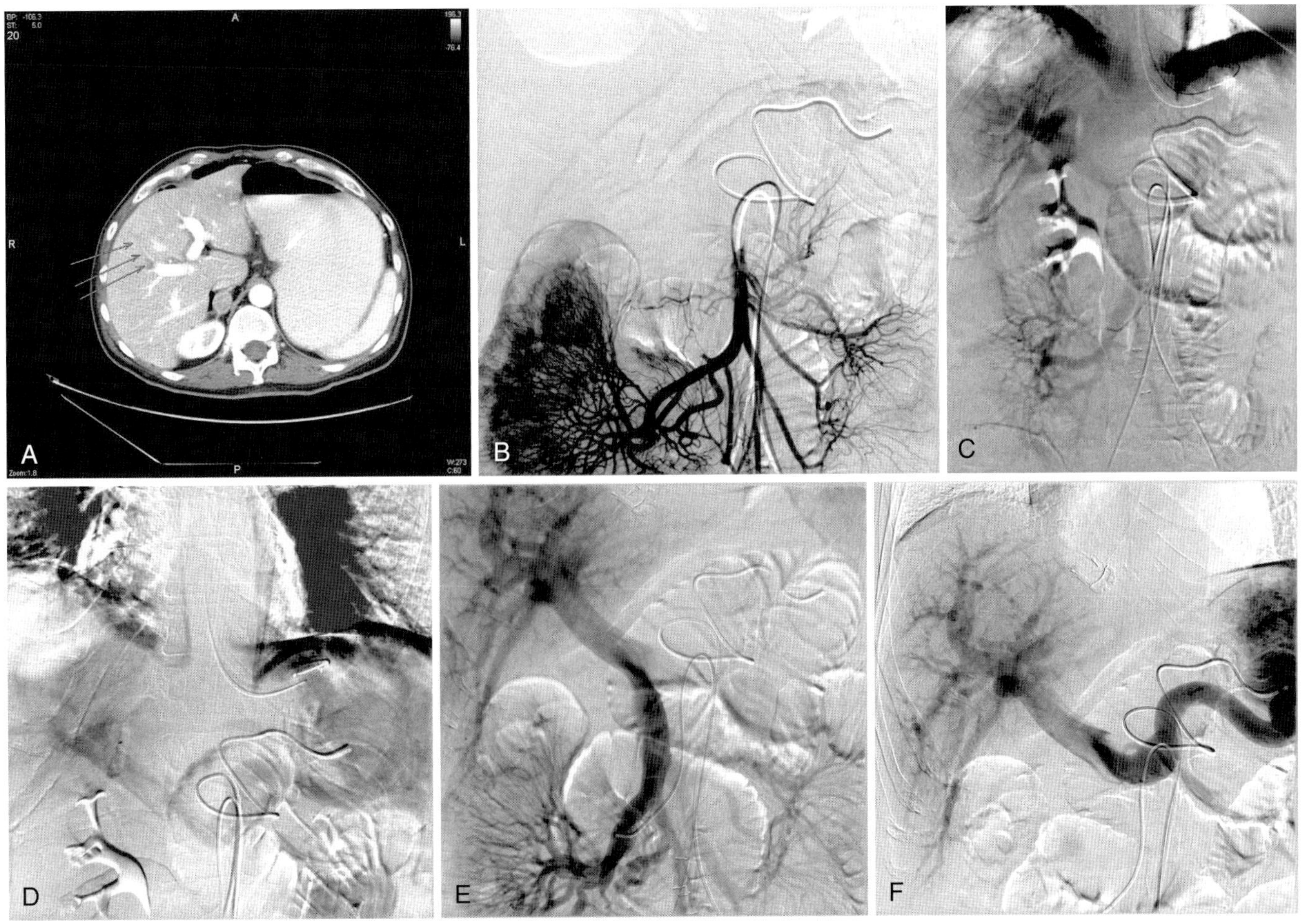

FIGURE 12 Hepatic venous thrombosis. **A,** CT scan showing thrombus. **B,** Angiogram of superior mesenteric artery (SMA). **C,** Catheter in SMA, delayed imaging showed patent mesenteric venous outflow. **D,** Catheter in splenic artery, delayed imaging showed patent splenic and portal veins, with poor visualization of hepatic veins. **E,** After thrombolytic therapy, angiogram from SMA catheter showed patent mesenteric and hepatic veins. **F,** Angiogram from splenic catheter showed patent splenic, portal and hepatic veins.

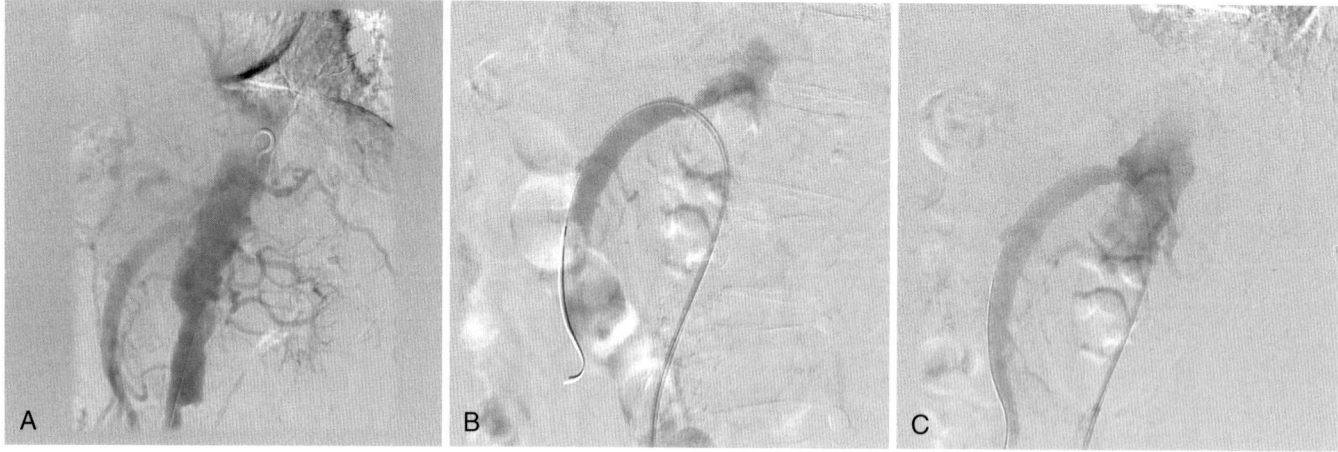

FIGURE 13   Endovascular treatment with stent placement in the stenosed superior mesenteric artery (SMA).

placement of two catheters for infusion of the two mesenteric arteries. The thrombolytic agent is infused slowly overnight, and angiography is repeated in 24 hours to assess for progress of lytic therapy. If there is residual thrombus, slow thrombolytic therapy is continued for another 24 hours. After a maximum of 48 hours of lytic therapy, sheaths and catheters are removed, and the patient is continued on anticoagulants. The patient's response and clinical status are monitored closely. Any signs of bowel ischemia or infarction necessitate surgical exploration to assess for bowel viability.

Endovascular Treatment

Mesenteric angiography used for the diagnosis of mesenteric ischemia can also be used for therapeutic interventions. Endovascular therapy involving catheter-directed delivery of pharmacologic agents was described previously for nonocclusive mesenteric ischemia and mesenteric venous thrombosis. This treatment modality can also be used for short-segment stenosis or occlusion, recurrent disease, or anastomotic stenosis from prior mesenteric intervention (Figure 13). In patients with medical comorbid conditions who are at high risk for open surgical interventions, endovascular therapy is a useful, less invasive treatment modality.

Arterial access is obtained in a common femoral artery. Left brachial arterial access may be needed in mesenteric arteries that branch in an acute angle from the aorta. A diagnostic catheter is placed in the proximal abdominal aorta below the diaphragm. Lateral aortography is used to assess the origin of the CA and SMA, and anteroposterior mesenteric angiography is used to assess the distal mesenteric circulation. An angled catheter is used to catheterize the CA and SMA, and selective mesenteric angiography is performed. When the location of the lesion is identified, a 6F working sheath is placed with the tip at the origin of the mesenteric artery, and the lesion is crossed with a wire. For occlusive lesions, a trial of lytic therapy is undertaken, whereby a thrombolytic agent is given via an infusion catheter that is placed across the length of the occlusive arterial segment. Any residual stenotic lesion identified on angiography can be treated with balloon angioplasty. Postangioplasty angiography is performed to assess for evidence of possible suboptimal angioplasty results such as dissection or residual stenosis. This is best treated with placement of a stent across the lesion. Stent placement should also be considered for mesenteric thrombosis because the lesion at the origin is caused by atherosclerotic disease in the aorta. It is important to maintain the wire across the lesion until the result appears satisfactory on completion angiography.

CONCLUSION

Long-term outcomes in patients with acute mesenteric ischemia are dependent on early diagnosis and prompt treatment. The prevalence is likely to increase among the aging population with multiple medical comorbid conditions. It is important to have a high index of suspicion in patients who present with abdominal pain and who have risk factors for mesenteric ischemia. With advances in treatment modalities involving less invasive endovascular revascularization, outcomes may improve in patients with acute mesenteric ischemia.

SUGGESTED READINGS

Arthurs ZM, Titus J, Bannazadeh M, et al: A comparison of endovascular revascularization with traditional therapy for the treatment of acute mesenteric ischemia, *J Vasc Surg* 53(3):698–704, 2011; discussion 704–705. doi: 10.1016/j.jvs.2010.09.049. Epub 2011 Jan 14.

Kougias P, Lau D, El Sayed HF, et al: Determinants of mortality and treatment outcome following surgical interventions for acute mesenteric ischemia, *J Vasc Surg* 46(3):467–474, 2007. Epub 2007 Jul 30.

Moore WS: *Vascular and endovascular surgery, a comprehensive review*, ed 7, Philadelphia, 2006, Saunders Elsevier, pp 603–616.

Tallarita T, Oderich GS, Gloviczki P, et al: Patient survival after open and endovascular mesenteric revascularization for chronic mesenteric ischemia, *J Vasc Surg* 57(3):747–755, 2013; discussion 754–755. doi: 10.1016/j.jvs.2012.09.047. Epub 2013 Jan 17.

Valentine RJ, Wind GG: *Anatomic exposures in vascular surgery*, Philadelphia, 2003, Lippincott Williams & Wilkins, pp 267–288.

Wyers MC: Acute mesenteric ischemia: diagnostic approach and surgical treatment, *Semin Vasc Surg* 23(1):9–20, 2010. doi: 10.1053/j.semvascsurg.2009.12.002. Review.

Zelenock GB, Huber TS, Messina LM, et al: *Mastery of vascular and endovascular surgery*, Philadelphia, 2006, Lippincott Williams & Wilkins, pp 293–311.

The Management of Chronic Mesenteric Ischemia

Linda M. Reilly, MD

Chronic mesenteric ischemia (CMI) results from inadequate arterial perfusion of the abdominal viscera. The postprandial pain that is the hallmark of symptomatic CMI prevents adequate nutrition, causing progressive and ultimately life-threatening weight loss. CMI is also believed to be a precursor to intestinal infarction, usually a lethal event because of the extent of viscera involved. Therefore, the goals of treatment are to restore normal tissue perfusion, to provide durable protection against visceral infarction, and to provide durable relief of pain so that normal nutrition can be maintained. Like most disorders of perfusion, visceral blood flow may be impeded by arterial obstruction, venous obstruction, or systemic conditions with a global effect on perfusion. Venous obstruction or systemic conditions that reduce mesenteric perfusion produce *acute* mesenteric ischemia, which is not discussed in this chapter.

ARTERIAL DISEASE

The most common cause of chronic visceral ischemia is atherosclerotic arterial occlusive disease. Arteritis may also cause CMI but is less common. The frequent observation of asymptomatic stenosis or even occlusion of a visceral artery in adults older than 65 years (about 20% of cases of CMI), and the abundant potential routes of collateral flow to the viscera have led to the belief that flow must be impaired through at least two of the three main visceral arteries in order to reduce perfusion sufficiently to cause symptom development. Although it is clear that compromise of flow in both the celiac artery and the superior mesenteric artery (SMA) can produce CMI, it is less predictable whether compromise of inferior mesenteric artery (IMA) flow and either celiac artery or SMA flow will produce symptoms of visceral ischemia. In the author's experience, all but one or two patients had involvement of both the celiac axis and the SMA. None of the author's patients developed symptoms with involvement of only the IMA and either the celiac artery or SMA. The pattern of the flow-reducing lesions is also important in the development of symptoms. The more diffuse the distribution of lesions, the more likely it is that all potential collateral routes are affected and that the patient will have symptoms.

Occlusion of the visceral arteries has three patterns: lesions involving the orifices of the visceral arteries, lesions involving long segments of the main visceral artery trunks (with or without orifice involvement), and lesions involving the branches of the visceral arteries (with or without proximal trunk/orifice involvement). These patterns of disease determine which treatment method is applicable, as well as the prognosis for a successful and durable reconstruction. The importance of establishing the arterial pathologic process is not so much in knowing the diagnosis as it is in understanding the implication of a given process for successful treatment. For example, typical visceral atherosclerotic lesions are located at the vessel origins; thus they actually represent aortic lesions that spill into the visceral artery orifice. The involvement of the visceral artery is usually limited to the 1 to 2 cm of the main trunk. The lesions of early-onset atherosclerosis more often involve longer segments of the main visceral arteries and may not have as much association with aortic disease. In contrast, unusual pathologic processes involving the visceral arteries, such as an arteritis, generally affect long segments of the arteries, involving both the main trunk and primary branches.

RECONSTRUCTION OPTIONS

Reconstruction options for visceral arterial occlusive disease take three forms: endovascular techniques (consisting of angioplasty with or without stents, either bare metal or covered stents), endarterectomy, and bypass.

Endovascular Techniques

As is the case with all atherosclerotic occlusive disease, intraluminal techniques are most suitable for the treatment of focal arterial lesions (Figure 1, *A* and *B*). Unfortunately, visceral occlusive lesions are rarely truly focal, and thus the effectiveness of endoluminal treatment is limited. As mentioned previously, typical atherosclerotic lesions represent aortic disease that extends into the mesenteric artery origins. Although the visceral involvement in this pattern of disease is focal, the aortic involvement is not. In general, orificial lesions are less optimally treated by angioplasty or stent placement, but the common approach of extending the visceral stent a few millimeters into the aortic lumen (Figure 2, *A*) and flaring the intra-aortic end of the stent (Figure 2, *B* and *C*) is successful in treating disease involving the visceral orifice. In addition, the very dense median arcuate ligament surrounding the celiac axis and (to a lesser extent) the SMA can be a mechanical barrier to achieving and maintaining an adequate lumen with endovascular treatment, even if adjunctive stents are placed. Extrinsic compression may be effectively managed by placement of one stent inside the other, so as to create a rigid artery (rifle-barrel) with a reasonable likelihood of resisting compression by the ligament (Figure 3). Nonetheless, stent fracture commonly results from extrinsic compression. These approaches have improved at least the initial success of endovascular treatment of orificial visceral lesions; however, when the lesions extend through long segments of the main trunk or into the branches (the other two patterns of visceral occlusive disease), even initial success is less likely.

Several key technical points are pertinent to endovascular treatment of visceral arterial occlusive disease. First is the choice of access site: femoral versus brachial. The femoral access site is more familiar to vascular interventionalists, but entry into the visceral artery involves at best a right angle and more commonly an acute backwards turn, resulting in unfavorable force vectors. In contrast, brachial access, although less familiar and carrying a slightly greater risk, provides an optimal angle of approach, as well as the support that might be needed to cross tightly stenotic lesions, heavily calcified lesions, or total occlusions. In fact, a parallel brachiofemoral wire may be necessary in some cases to provide sufficient sheath stabilization to allow the considerable pushing needed to cross a difficult stenosis or an occlusion. The risk of embolization during the treatment of visceral occlusive disease, particularly when total occlusions are recanalized, has prompted a gradual increase in the use of distal embolic protection devices (filters) to catch fractured plaque fragments or thrombus. This increases technical complexity, but it may improve procedural safety.

Because of the orificial nature of the lesions, the common finding of heavy calcification, and the likelihood of some extrinsic ligament compression, simple balloon angioplasty of the mesenteric arteries is rarely sufficient. Stent placement is necessary to treat the stenosis effectively, and balloon-expandable stents are almost always used because they exert greater radial force. Balloon-expandable covered stents have become the device of choice. The covered stent provides

947

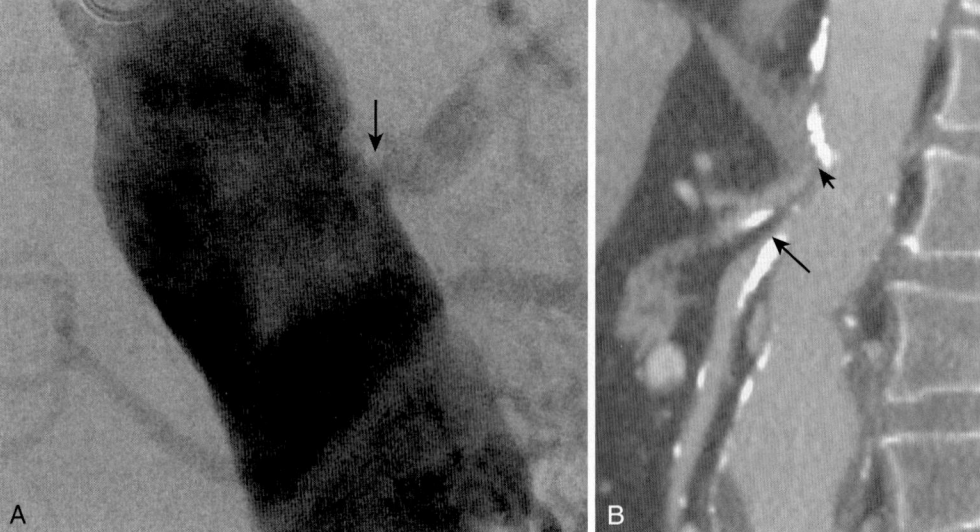

FIGURE 1 Focal stenosis in visceral arteries. **A,** Focal high-grade stenosis of the celiac axis *(arrow)* with poststenotic dilation. **B,** Focal stenosis of the celiac axis *(short arrow)* and superior mesenteric artery *(long arrow).*

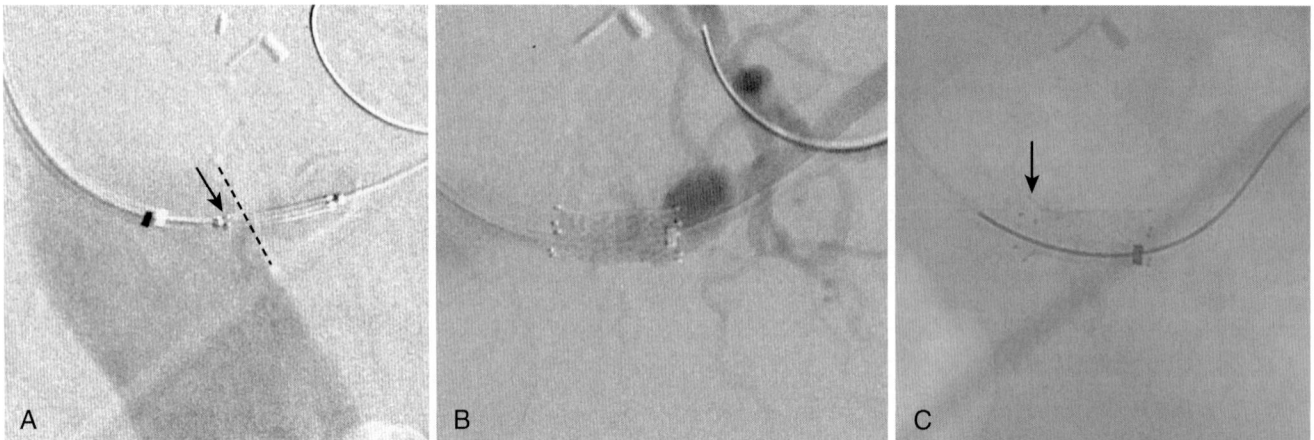

FIGURE 2 Placement of stents in a visceral artery. **A,** Intraprocedural angiographic image demonstrating optimal position of the celiac stent, extending a few millimeters into the aortic lumen. The *arrow* represents the proximal end of the stent; the *dotted line* represents the aortic wall. **B,** Angiographic image of the celiac stent after pressure-monitored balloon inflation and stent deployment. **C,** Angiographic image of deployed celiac stent, showing the flared proximal end *(arrow).* The slight "waist" represents the location of the aortic wall.

some protection against inadvertent visceral branch or aortic injury from the high pressures that may be necessary to efface the stenosis. In addition, the covered stent traps plaque, protecting against distal embolization that might occur if an uncovered stent was used. The visceral arteries are also unique in the difference between the orifice segment and the rest of the artery. As described previously, the orificial visceral segments tend to be fixed, involved by dense, heavily calcified plaque and possibly extrinsically compressed, all features that necessitate stents with high radial force (balloon-expandable). The more distal celiac artery and SMA segments, however, are quite flexible and mobile, and thus a flexible (self-expanding) stent with lower radial force is a better choice.

In spite of the challenges associated with endovascular treatment of visceral arterial occlusive disease, technical success rates approach 100%, anatomic results are good, and initial clinical outcomes are comparable with or better than open surgical treatment (Table 1). However, the lower rates of mortality and morbidity and high rate of technical success come at the price of less durability. Outcomes from reviews of large data samples (meta-analyses, National Inpatient Sample) consistently show primary patency rates well below that achieved with open surgical mesenteric revascularization.

Durability is therefore the issue to be resolved with endovascular treatment of the visceral arteries.

The author's experience with endovascular treatment of visceral occlusive disease is also favorable, with only one death among approximately 30 patients who underwent celiac or SMA angioplasty (or both) and stent placement. The single death resulted from a shower of atheroemboli in a patient with SMA occlusion and celiac stenosis. That patient had experienced a relatively recent symptom change, which, in retrospect, probably indicated progression of SMA stenosis to complete occlusion. At the time of intervention, this subacute occlusion probably contained thrombus, which embolized during placement of an uncovered stent. Whether this outcome would have been different if embolic protection or a covered stent were used is unknown, but the case highlights a critical factor in successful endovascular outcome: the potential for plaque or thrombus embolization.

The appeal of an endovascular approach to treating CMI is obvious. Patients with CMI are always nutritionally impaired and commonly have significant comorbid conditions. Endovascular procedures, even if a brachial approach is used, can be performed while the patient is under local anesthesia, which reduces procedural risk.

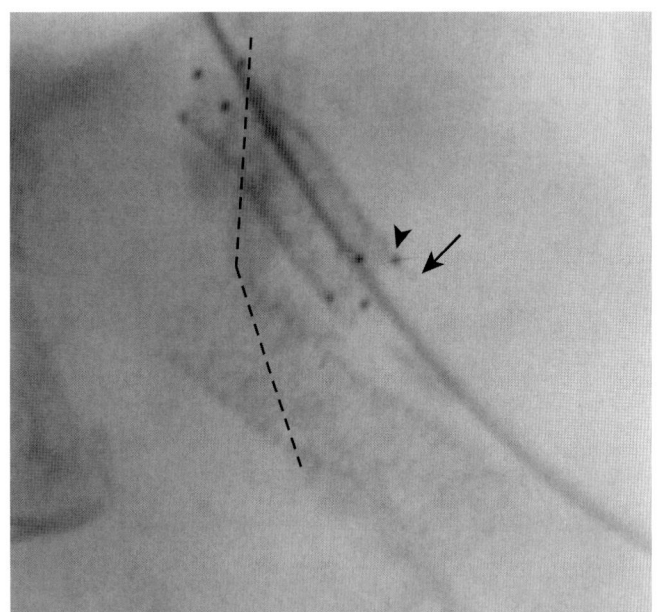

FIGURE 3 Angiogram obtained after placement of a balloon-expandable, covered stent into the celiac axis, lined with a balloon-expandable uncovered stent. The *arrow* indicates the distal end of the covered stent; the *arrowhead* indicates the distal end of the lining uncovered stent; and the *dotted line* indicates the aortic wall. Note complete resolution of the stenosis and slight extension of the stent into the aortic lumen.

Relief of symptoms is immediate, and patients can begin nutritional repletion without the additional interval of negative balance associated with open surgery. Many authorities now regard endovascular treatment of mesenteric occlusive disease to be the first choice for treatment, particularly for high-risk patient. Endovascular treatment can also serve as a bridge that allows nutritional repletion and optimization of comorbid conditions before definitive open operative repair. Because the price for a lower risk procedure is less durability, however, patients must be monitored regularly and indefinitely with appropriate imaging studies (duplex arterial imaging or computed tomographic angiography) to ensure continued patency and prevent catastrophic occlusion. Many authorities have reported that endovascular reintervention also has low mortality and morbidity rates, if performed electively.

Endarterectomy

Endarterectomy was the earliest operative technique applied to visceral artery occlusive disease. However, in the initial procedures, the transarterial retrograde approach, through either the celiac artery or SMA, or both, was used to remove the obstructing lesion. The use of this approach indicates the early failure to recognize the significance of the aortic involvement and was unsuccessful because it did not allow complete removal of the aortic portion of the lesion. Endarterectomy is currently performed through the aorta, and the lesions extending into the visceral artery orifices are extracted by eversion endarterectomy.

Aortic exposure is achieved through a transabdominal approach with medial rotation of the viscera from the left. Either a full-length

TABLE 1: Treatment of visceral arterial occlusive disease

Study	No. of patients/ No. of vessels	Mortality	Morbidity	Symptom relief	Primary patency
Endovascular Treatment					
Aburahma et al. (2013)	83/105	2.0%	2.0%	65% (5 yr)	68% (1 yr)
Tallarita et al. (2013)	156/173	2.6%			
Pecoraro et al. (2013)	786/1007	3.6%	13.2%		49.1% (5 yr)
Turba et al. (2012)	166				
Tallarita et al. (2011)	157/170				
Schoch et al. (2011)	107/130	0.0%	7.0%	54.0%	44% (1 yr)
Gupta et al. (2010)	776/1018	3.1%-4.1%	4%-14%	53%-88% (2 yr)	79%-89% (3 yr)
Oderich et al. (2009)	409	6.0%	15.0%	75.0%	74% (1 yr)
Schermerhorn et al. (2009)	3455	3.7%	20.2%		
Open Surgical Treatment					
Tallarita et al. (2013)	187/327	2.7%			
Pecoraro et al. (2013)	1009/1593	7.2%	33.1%		80.9% (5 yr)
Davenport et al. (2012)	156	7.7%	40.0%		
Ryer et al. (2011)	116/203	2.6%	50.0%		80.5% (5 yr)
Gupta et al. (2010)	1163/1995	4.5%-7.5%	29-35%	83-88% (5 yr)	78-80% (5 yr)
Oderich et al. (2009)	992	11.0%	47.0%	93.0%	89% (1 yr)
Schermerhorn et al. (2009)	2128	15.4%	39.7%		

midline incision or a bilateral subcostal incision may be used; the author prefers the latter and to leave the left kidney in its anatomic position, while the plane behind the left colon, spleen, pancreas, and stomach is developed to allow displacement of these structures toward the midline (Figure 4). If necessary, the entire aorta, from the distal thoracic level to the bifurcation, can be completely exposed with this technique. During complete aortic occlusion, including control of any intervening intercostal branches, a U-shaped trapdoor aortotomy circumscribes the orifices of the celiac and superior mesenteric arteries, and an endarterectomy is performed to remove the aortic lesion and the extensions into the visceral orifices. In many cases, the significant aortic atheroma is confined to the ventral surface of the aorta immediately around the celiac artery and SMA orifices, and the aortic endarterectomy can be limited to the trapdoor segment itself. However, more diffuse aortic disease, frequently in the setting of associated renal artery occlusive lesions, necessitates extension of the aortotomy caudally to allow sleeve aortic endarterectomy and bilateral or unilateral renal artery endarterectomy. In this circumstance, the aortotomy takes the shape of a hockey stick rather than a trapdoor. After completion of the endarterectomy, the aortotomy is closed with a running suture or with a patch. If the disease extends well out into the visceral branches, it may be necessary to use a separate longitudinal arteriotomy in the visceral artery itself to allow complete removal of the disease. This visceral arteriotomy is then closed with a patch.

Endarterectomy is perhaps the most elegant approach to visceral artery occlusive disease, but surgeons must be aware of its limitations. It is most applicable to visceral artery lesions that are limited to the first 1 to 2 cm of the artery. Longer lesions may be successfully treated with transaortic endarterectomy; in the author's experience, however, endarterectomy in that setting is less durable. Endarterectomy is not applicable to lesions extending into branches of the visceral arteries. Transmural calcification of the involved portions of the aorta or visceral artery should generally be considered a contraindication to endarterectomy. Transmural lesions force the use of a very deep endarterectomy plane, which usually results in inadequate integrity of the adventitia. Attempting endarterectomy in this setting usually results in extensive bleeding through the porous adventitia and prolonged visceral ischemia as a consequence of attempts to repair the

bleeding artery—an invariably fatal combination. Endarterectomy is particularly appealing when occlusive disease involves the renal arteries, because it is much faster than individual bypasses to all four arteries (celiac artery, SMA, and both renal arteries). If multiple renal arteries are present, endarterectomy is even more attractive. Endarterectomy is often the most appropriate technique for occlusive disease involving the IMA. Because of the smaller size of this artery and the less predictable location of the endpoint, however, the author favors a longitudinal incision that extends past the IMA to a disease-free segment. After the endarterectomy is completed, the arteriotomy is closed with a patch. In this location, the author prefers a vein patch.

Visceral flow must be restored—endarterectomy completed and the aorta closed—within 40 to 45 minutes. Longer intervals of total visceral ischemia, particularly hepatic ischemia, lead to coagulopathy that is usually impossible to reverse. In the author's experience, visceral flow was restored in 30.5 ± 15.5 minutes.

Bypass

At least theoretically, bypass is the only reconstruction technique applicable to all patterns of arterial visceral occlusive disease. Practically, the more extensive the disease and the more distal the branch involvement, the less feasible bypass becomes. Bypass to the mesenteric arteries may originate from the supraceliac portion of the aorta (antegrade bypass) or from the infrarenal portion of the aorta or iliac arteries (retrograde bypass).

Antegrade Bypass

Aortic exposure for antegrade bypass can be achieved through a transabdominal, transcrural approach (Figure 5) or medial visceral rotation from the left (as described previously). The transcrural approach is appealing because it is a less extensive exposure. Either an upper vertical midline incision or a bilateral subcostal incision can be used. The upper vertical midline incision yields a relatively small operative field, which may make creation of the aortic anastomosis awkward because both visibility and movement may be restricted. The author prefers to use a bilateral subcostal incision and, if the costal margin angle is narrow, to add a short superior midline extension. Graft length and alignment are easy to determine with the transcrural approach, but a retropancreatic tunnel may be needed for the SMA graft (Figure 6), depending on the extent of disease in the SMA. Medial visceral rotation provides a much larger operative field but at the cost of a larger operation. Graft length and alignment are more difficult to determine with medial rotation of the viscera because the viscera are retracted to the right. Prosthetic conduits are almost always used.

Regardless of the exposure, the proximal anastomosis of the antegrade bypass is placed in the disease-free supraceliac or distal thoracic portion of the aorta. The author prefers total aortic occlusion of the aortic segment for this anastomosis. When a partial aortic occlusion clamp is used, most of the time it occludes the aorta almost completely. Preserving a minimal amount of aortic flow does not warrant the disadvantages of limited visibility, increased technical difficulty, and longer periods of visceral ischemia. Circumferential supraceliac aortic mobilization is not routinely performed unless there is an intervening pair of intercostal arteries that need to be controlled. Historically, the author used a small, bifurcated prosthetic graft (12 mm × 6 mm) and excised a small, obliquely oriented ellipse of aorta at the site of the proximal anastomosis (see Figure 6). However, to reduce the risk of kinking, the graft must assume a low profile along the front of the aorta. This requires a lengthy graft bevel and a lengthy matching aortotomy. In many cases there is simply not enough disease-free aortic tissue to allow such a long aortotomy. Consequently, the author now creates a bifurcated graft from two limbs of smaller diameter (Figure 7). With this technique, less normal aortic tissue is required for the proximal anastomosis because the

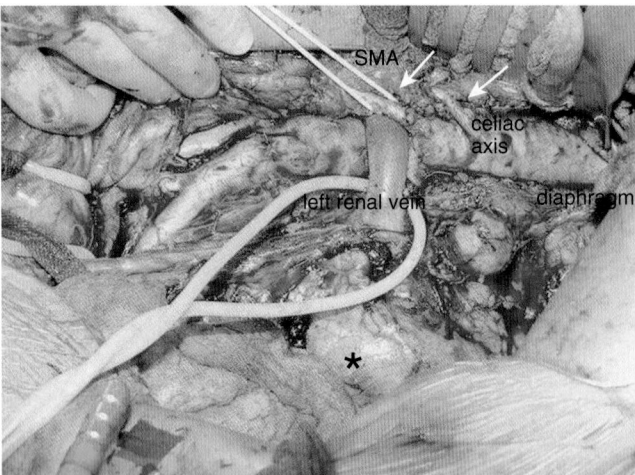

FIGURE 4 Aortic exposure provided by transabdominal approach with medial rotation of the viscera from the left. Note that the entire abdominal aorta from the diaphragm (under the narrow retractor blades at the right) to the bifurcation of the iliac arteries can be exposed. Note that the left kidney (*asterisk*) remains in its anatomic position. The large vessel loop encircles the left renal vein, which can usually be left intact. *SMA,* Superior mesenteric artery.

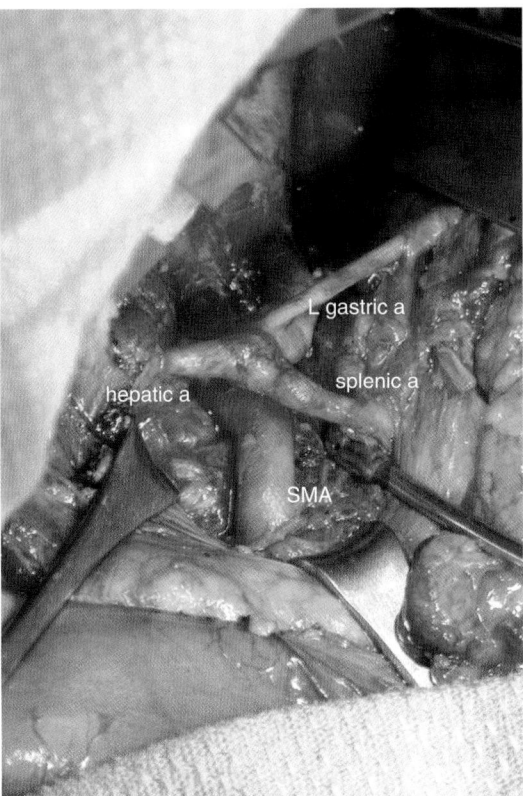

FIGURE 5 Transcrural exposure of the celiac axis and its branches (left gastric, hepatic, and splenic arteries) and the superior mesenteric artery (SMA). Note the caudal retraction of the stomach and pancreas. Note also the complete division of the median arcuate ligament and the complete removal of the celiac ganglion and plexus from around the anterior surface of the aorta and the proximal trunks of the celiac axis and the SMA.

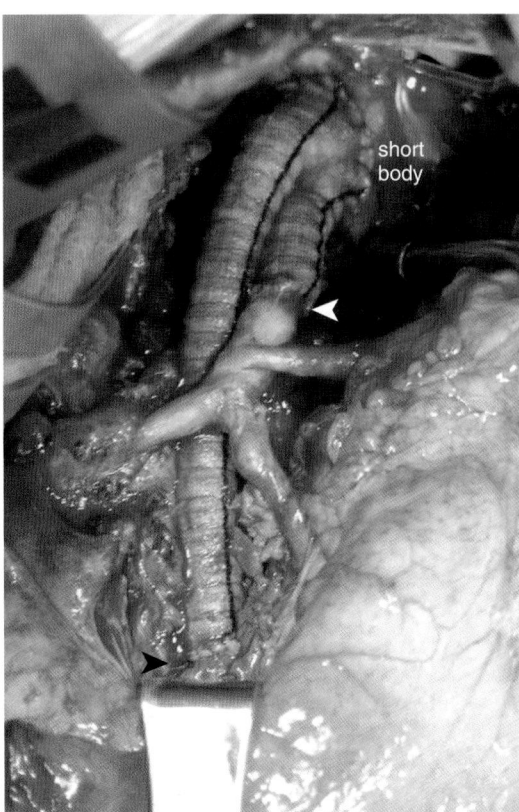

FIGURE 6 Completed antegrade bypass to the celiac axis and superior mesenteric artery. Note the very short body portion of the graft and, again, the inferior retraction of the stomach and pancreas. Note also that the orientation of the graft limbs prevents either limb from compressing the other. The *white arrowhead* indicates the celiac artery anastomosis; the *black arrowhead* indicates the superior mesenteric artery anastomosis.

aortotomy for the proximal anastomosis is shorter, and it is easier to ensure a low profile for the graft. After completion of the proximal anastomosis, aortic flow is restored, and an occluding clamp is placed on the graft. In the author's experience, this anastomosis can be performed and aortic flow restored in 26.0 ± 15.8 minutes. Operative times are shorter when the surgeon-created bifurcated graft is used.

If the transcrural exposure is used, the celiac axis and SMA are exposed above and behind the pancreas; this exposure requires careful and complete dissection of the visceral arteries from the surrounding celiac ganglion tissue and the median arcuate ligament (see Figure 5). Usually the left graft limb is anastomosed to the celiac axis and the right graft limb to the SMA (see Figure 6). However, it is always wise to check the relative positions of the two visceral arteries before committing to this arrangement. When the medial rotation of the viscera exposure is used, it may be better to perform the anastomosis to the SMA *first*. Usually the anastomosis to the SMA is performed more distally on that artery than the anastomosis to the celiac axis. This is particularly so when the SMA lesion is longer. As a consequence, the SMA anastomosis may actually lie *under* the graft limb to the celiac axis. Performing the SMA anastomosis first improves exposure and avoids the need for significant retraction on the celiac graft. The distal anastomoses can be performed either end to end or end to side, as determined by the disease pattern.

Retrograde Bypass

The infrarenal portion of the aorta, iliac artery, or a previously placed prosthetic aortic or aortoiliac graft can all serve as inflow conduits

to the visceral arteries. For exposure of the aorta, the standard infracolic approach is used. Both the inflow (aortic, iliac, or graft) and outflow (visceral branch) anastomoses are performed end to side. If the SMA is the revascularization target, it is exposed beyond the diseased areas in the root of the mesentery. The celiac axis itself is rarely the target for a retrograde bypass, partly because it is too short to accommodate an end-to-side anastomosis and partly because the graft alignment would be awkward. More commonly, the bypass is anastomosed to a branch of the celiac artery, usually the hepatic artery, because hepatic and gastric perfusion are more important than splenic flow. Positioning and alignment are more difficult with retrograde conduits, and as a consequence they are more susceptible to twisting, kinking, and compression. Some authorities recommend that the conduit be constructed in the shape of a long, gentle backwards C-shaped curve. This orientation allows antegrade flow at both the proximal and the distal anastomoses, although flow through the conduit itself is still retrograde. The advantages of retrograde bypass are simpler exposure, no supraceliac aortic occlusion, and sometimes no aortic occlusion at all.

EXTENT OF VISCERAL ARTERY RECONSTRUCTION

Although it is generally agreed that at least two visceral arteries must be involved by the occlusive process to produce symptoms, there is more debate regarding the number of visceral arteries that need to

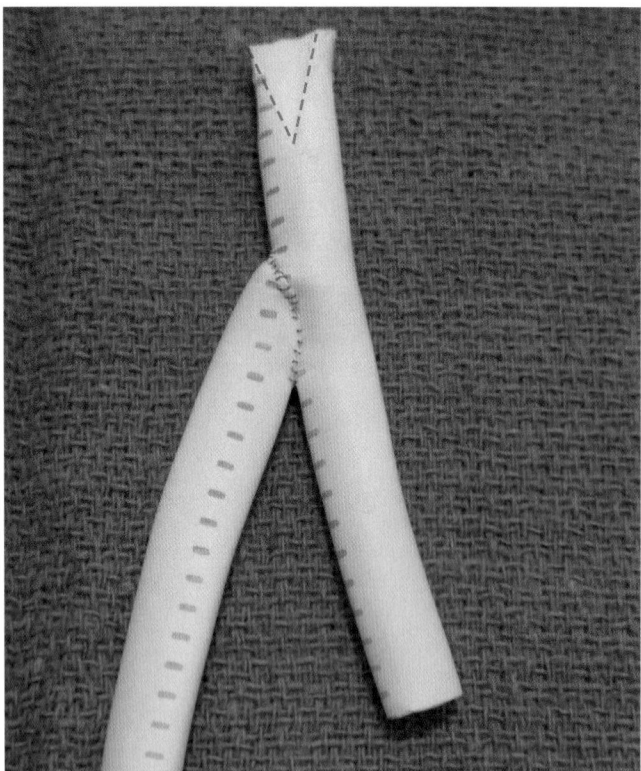

FIGURE 7 Bifurcated graft created for visceral revascularization. The *dotted line* indicates the much shorter flange for the proximal anastomosis, in comparison with a manufactured bifurcated graft. The length of each limb can be customized. Polyester (Dacron) can also be used.

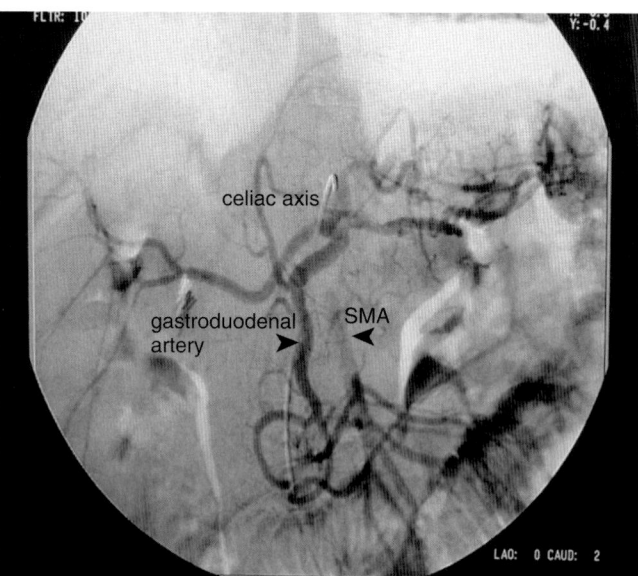

FIGURE 8 Selective injection into the celiac axis results in opacification of the superior mesenteric artery (SMA) via a very large gastroduodenal artery. In this case, reconstruction of either the celiac axis or the SMA provides perfusion to the entire visceral circulation.

be reconstructed to provide durable symptom relief and protection against visceral infarction. Some authorities have reported a correlation between durable symptom relief and "complete" visceral revascularization, whereas others have reported equivalent results with single-vessel revascularization. Among those who believe that single-vessel reconstruction is adequate, there is further debate about the optimal choice of the single vessel. In fact, if all of the collateral pathways between the three main visceral arteries are intact, revascularization of any single visceral artery should be sufficient for relief of symptoms (see Figure 7). Practically speaking, if single-vessel reconstruction is chosen, either the celiac artery or the SMA should be the target artery as long as this is technically feasible (Figure 8). Single-vessel reconstruction to the IMA should be performed only if neither the celiac artery nor the SMA can be repaired.

OUTCOME OF OPEN REVASCULARIZATION

Since 1990, the author and colleagues have performed open visceral reconstruction in more than 100 patients with an overall perioperative mortality rate of approximately 20%. The mortality rate in the last half of this time interval has been about half that experienced in the early half of the time interval. The author and colleagues attribute this improvement to the increasing proportion of patients managed with antegrade bypass, as well as to the routine performance of transaortic endarterectomy through an abdominal approach, rather than through a thoracoretroperitoneal approach. In general, the perioperative outcome achieved with the two standard open reconstruction options—transaortic endarterectomy and antegrade bypass—are equivalent.

Furthermore, in the author's experience, the long-term relief of symptoms is the same whether it is achieved with transaortic endarterectomy or with antegrade bypass. Approximately 80% of patients undergoing one of the two standard open operative treatments have remained symptom free. Factors that are correlated with increased probability of recurrent symptoms include very early age at first diagnosis, greater weight loss at the time of initial presentation, and intraoperative modification of the planned reconstruction technique. These factors are probably indicative of a more aggressive and extensive arterial process.

Of equal interest is the fact that two thirds of patients with recurrent symptoms can be rendered symptom free again by repeat visceral revascularization. This result is also durable, inasmuch as these patients have remained symptom free during an average further follow-up of 6 to 7 years. Thus, during this extensive follow-up interval, fatal recurrent visceral ischemia has occurred in only approximately 5% of patients.

Published results from the literature (see Table 1) also show improvement in comparison to earlier experiences. These series also demonstrate the better durability associated with open surgical visceral revascularization, in comparison to the durability of endovascular techniques.

SUGGESTED READINGS

Aburahma AF, Campbell JE, Stone PA, et al: Perioperative and late clinical outcomes of percutaneous transluminal stentings of the celiac and superior mesenteric arteries over the past decade, *J Vasc Surg* 57(4):1052–1061, 2013.

Cunningham CG, Reilly LM, Rapp JH, et al: Chronic intestinal ischemia: three decades of surgical progress, *Ann Surg* 214:276–288, 1991.

Davenport DL, Shivazad A, Endean ED: Short-term outcomes for open revascularization of chronic mesenteric ischemia, *Ann Vasc Surg* 26:447–453, 2012.

Foley MI, Moneta GL, Abou-Zamzam AM Jr, et al: Revascularization of the superior mesenteric artery alone for treatment of intestinal ischemia, *J Vasc Surg* 32:37–47, 2000.

Gupta PK, Horan SM, Turaga KK, et al: Chronic mesenteric ischemia: endovascular versus open revascularization, *J Endovasc Ther* 17:540–549, 2010.

Oderich GS, Malgor RD, Ricotta JJ II: Open and endovascular revascularization for chronic mesenteric ischemia: tabular review of the literature, *Ann Vasc Surg* 23:700–712, 2009.

Oderich GS, Tallarita T, Gloviczki P, et al: Mesenteric artery complications during angioplasty and stent placement for atherosclerotic chronic mesenteric ischemia, *J Vasc Surg* 55(4):1063–1071, 2012.

Pecoraro F, Rancic Z, Lachat M, et al: Chronic mesenteric ischemia; critical review and guidelines for management, *Ann Vasc Surg* 27(1):113–122, 2013.

Rapp JH, Reilly LM, Qvarfordt PG, et al: Durability of endarterectomy and antegrade bypass in the treatment of chronic visceral ischemia, *J Vasc Surg* 3:799–806, 1986.

Ryer EJ, Oderich GS, Bower TC, et al: Differences in anatomy and outcomes in patients treated with open mesenteric revascularization before and after the endovascular era, *J Vasc Surg* 53:1611–1618, 2011.

Schermerhorn ML, Giles KA, Hamdan AD, et al: Mesenteric revasculariation: management and outcomes in the United States, 1988–2006, *J Vasc Surg* 50:341–348, 2009.

Schneider DB, Schneider PA, Reilly LM, et al: Reoperation for the patient with recurrent chronic visceral ischemia, *J Vasc Surg* 27:276–286, 1998.

Schoch DM, LeSar CJ, Joels CS, et al: Management of chronic mesenteric vascular insufficiency: An endovascular approach, *J Am Coll Surg* 212:668–677, 2011.

Staniloae CS: The new state of the art in endovascular treatment of chronic mesenteric ischemia, *J Endovasc Ther* 19:495–496, 2012.

Tallarita T, Oderich GS, Gloviczki P, et al: Patient survival after open and endovascular mesenteric revascularization for chronic mesenteric ischemia, *J Vasc Surg* 57:47–55, 2013.

Tallarita T, Oderich GS, Macedo TA, et al: Reinterventions for stent restenosis in patients treated for atherosclerotic mesenteric artery disease, *J Vasc Surg* 54(5):1422–1429, 2011.

Turba UC, Saad WE, Arslan B, et al: Chronic mesenteric ischemia: a 28-year experience of endovascular treatment, *Eur Radiol* 22(6):1372–1384, 2012.

HEMODIALYSIS ACCESS SURGERY

Bonnie E. Lonze, MD, PhD, and
Thomas Reifsnyder, MD, FACS

INTRODUCTION

For the past decade, the overall prevalence of end-stage renal disease in the United States has increased at a rate of approximately 2% per year. In 2009, 116,395 patients initiated dialysis, and the overall number of Americans living on dialysis grew to exceed 397,000. For the vast majority of these patients hemodialysis is the preferred mode of renal replacement therapy. The ability to deliver this lifesaving therapy is dependent on the creation and maintenance of adequate vascular access.

HISTORICAL NOTES

Over the course of approximately a century, end-stage renal failure went from a universally fatal disease to a tolerable chronic illness with reasonable long-term survival. In the United States, a series of events involving science, medicine, and politics led to universally available and undeniable renal replacement therapy.

The concept of dialysis was introduced by the Scottish physical chemist Thomas Graham, whose experiments in the 1850s characterized the movement of water across semipermeable membranes and led to an understanding of the principle of osmosis. It was in fact Graham himself who first applied the term *dialysis* to describe the phenomenon of exploiting osmotic gradients to move solutes across a membrane separating two solutions.

Fifty years later, John Jacob Abel, a pharmacologist at Johns Hopkins Hospital, first explored the application of dialysis in a clinical setting. Abel, working with Leonard Rowntree and B. B. Turner, described in 1914 the construction of the "artificial kidney," an apparatus that consisted of 32 tubes connected in series and encased in a large glass container filled with a dialysate solution. Using hirudin as an anticoagulant to prevent clotting in the tubes, they tested the invention on anesthetized animals. Using arterial cannulae to channel blood into the narrow tubes of the circuit, they demonstrated that indeed blood could be dialyzed.

The first successful human use of dialysis is credited to Willem Kolff, a Dutch physician who had studied Abel's work. During the German occupation of the Netherlands in the 1940s, he designed and built, mainly from household items, a dialysis device he named the "rotating drum kidney." This device consisted of a large drum, covered with thin tubing that sat partly submerged in a large tank of dialysate. Blood passed through the series of tubes affixed to the drum that then rotated within the tank, facilitating dialysis of the blood across the tubing. Kolff's first surviving patient was a 67-year-old woman with acute renal failure secondary to sepsis. She endured an 11-hour dialysis session in which a measured 60 grams of urea were removed. He foresaw many possible applications of hemodialysis and was astutely aware that its implementation for chronic renal failure would require durable vascular access.

The first solution to the access problem was developed by Belding Scribner at the University of Washington. Having been introduced to a newly engineered material called polytetrafluoroethylene, or PTFE (Teflon; DuPont, Wilmington Del.), and recognizing its inert and noninflammatory properties, he conceived of using a U-shaped Teflon tube to create an external arteriovenous connection that could be accessed for dialysis. On March 9, 1960, the first dialysis by way of the "Scribner shunt" was performed. While this did establish an important proof of principle, Scribner shunts had unacceptably high rates of infection, thrombosis, and hemorrhage, and their functional patency rarely exceeded a few months. Seeking to improve upon this, James Cimino and Michael Brescia invented the radiocephalic arteriovenous fistula and described the technique in their landmark *New England Journal of Medicine* manuscript in 1966.

With safe and reliable vascular access technically feasible, widespread availability of hemodialysis had a final major obstacle: its prohibitive cost. Lobbying at local and national levels resulted in government funding for improvements in dialysis machine technology and the construction of more dialysis units. However, due to its cost, most people believed that without federal government support, access would remain limited to the privileged few. In November 1971, a chronic dialysis patient named Shep Glazer and his nephrologist demonstrated a dialysis session before a congressional committee in Washington, D.C. This had a tremendous impact on both the committee members and the press, leading Congress to take action. In October 1972, President Richard Nixon signed into law a bill authorizing Medicare coverage of dialysis.

In this chapter, we review and summarize our current practices for the evaluation, placement, and maintenance of hemodialysis access. In 2002, the Society for Vascular Surgery and the American Association for Vascular Surgery published recommendations for standardized reporting of dialysis access techniques, procedures, and configurations. For purposes of brevity, however, we preferentially utilize common nomenclature throughout our discussion.

NATIONAL PRACTICES AND GUIDELINES

In 2009, the End-Stage Renal Disease Program alone consumed 6% of the overall Medicare budget—a total of $29 billion—and this staggering sum is rising annually. As health care cost containment has become a major national focus, there has been great motivation within the dialysis community to identify best practices that minimize costs and maximize patient benefit. Until recently, the majority of arm accesses placed had been prosthetic grafts. Certainly some of these grafts were placed out of necessity. Unfortunately, convenience, lack of surgeon experience, and the higher reimbursement rate for prosthetic grafts undoubtedly played a role in their preferential placement. Specifically, in 1990, ePTFE grafts were placed twice as frequently as autogenous arteriovenous fistulae. According to the Centers for Disease Control, in 1995, just over 20% of patients on dialysis were utilizing autogenous access. Clear evidence has since emerged that autogenous fistulae are associated both with better outcomes and lower costs, and this has drawn attention to the unacceptably low proportion of patients in the United States dialyzing through autogenous accesses. The disproportionate and often inappropriate use of prosthetic grafts fueled the National Kidney Foundation's Kidney Disease Outcomes and Quality Initiative (KDOQI). This is a comprehensive analysis of the best practices with regard to the management of end-stage renal disease. An offspring of KDOQI was the Centers for Medicare and Medicaid Services' Fistula First Breakthrough Initiative, which aimed to promote awareness among patients and physicians of the superiority of autogenous access. The current national goal is to place autogenous access in at least 65% of new dialysis patients.

Currently, the three main avenues for hemodialysis access are tunneled central venous catheters, arteriovenous prosthetic grafts, and autogenous arteriovenous fistulae. Clearly, the worst outcomes are associated with catheter usage, and therefore every effort should be made to avoid them. To this end, current KDOQI guidelines stipulate that all patients should be referred to a surgeon for the placement of autogenous access when they reach stage 4 chronic kidney disease (glomerular filtration rate [GFR] $<30\,\text{mL/min}/1.73\,\text{m}^2$). This allows sufficient time for fistula placement and maturation prior to the commencement of dialysis. The caveat to this scenario is that not all patients have a suitable vein for autogenous fistula creation. Only those with a suitable vein should have their access placed far in advance of the initiation of dialysis, and this access should be an autogenous fistula. The most common cause of prosthetic graft failure is stenosis at the venous anastomosis due to neointimal hyperplasia. This worsens with time, so if a prosthetic graft is required, it should only be placed when dialysis is imminent or has already begun.

The options for dialysis access are frequently impacted by treatment options instituted years before the patient reaches end-stage renal disease. Patients and physicians alike must be aware that for those with any degree of renal dysfunction, subclavian vein central lines and ports, PICC (peripherally inserted central catheter) lines, and even forearm intravenous catheters (intern's vein or distal cephalic vein) should be avoided whenever possible. PICC lines are the curse of the dialysis access surgeon. Not only do they frequently ruin a normally good access vein—the basilic vein—but they are also associated with rates of central venous stenosis or thrombosis estimated up to 85%, which renders the arm unusable for dialysis access of any type.

The algorithm for selecting which fistula to place is fairly straightforward. One should begin distally and work proximally in the nondominant arm: radiocephalic (Figure 1), brachiocephalic, and then upper-arm basilic transposition. We believe that the benefits of autogenous access are so great that many exceptions to the standard algorithm are permitted. Although use of the nondominant arm is preferable, frequently the veins are better in the more active dominant arm. In this circumstance, the dominant arm is used without hesitation for fistula placement. If a patient has no suitable vein for autogenous access, then a prosthetic graft may be used. A good prosthetic graft is better than a bad vein. Although prosthetic grafts may be placed between any artery with sufficient flow and any suitable vein with unobstructed outflow, it is best to begin as far distally as possible and reserve more proximal sites for the future. For example, we would consider these configurations in the following order: distal radial artery to brachial vein straight graft, distal brachial artery to distal brachial vein forearm loop graft, and finally, distal brachial artery to proximal brachial vein or distal axillary vein straight graft. With education and careful attention to best practices, autogenous accesses can be preferentially placed, and the use of prosthetic grafts can and should be limited.

PREOPERATIVE EVALUATION

End-stage renal disease is rarely an entity that exists in isolation, and dialysis patients have a higher incidence of significant comorbid conditions. According to the United States Renal Data System, among the cohort of new dialysis patients who were registered in 2006-2009, 84% had hypertension, 21% had coronary artery disease, 32% had congestive heart failure, 35% had insulin-dependent diabetes, 14% had peripheral vascular disease, 9% had a history of previous stroke or transient ischemic attack, and 7% were unable to ambulate. Briefly stated, these patients are poor operative candidates. The preoperative evaluation revolves around assessing cardiopulmonary reserve and selecting the anesthetic with the least risk.

Aside from a history of events relevant to cardiopulmonary status and prior dialysis access attempts, it is imperative to inquire as to all previous venous access procedures, including dialysis catheters, subclavian lines or ports, PICC lines, pacemakers, and defibrillators. Prior trauma to the upper extremities or clavicles should be noted. The physical exam should include auscultation of the heart and lungs and an evaluation of the extremities to determine the patient's best option for dialysis access. The radial, ulnar, and brachial pulses should be palpated bilaterally. Uncommonly, a radial pulse is present with an occluded brachial artery. An Allen's test to confirm adequacy of ulnar flow to the hand should be performed if a radiocephalic

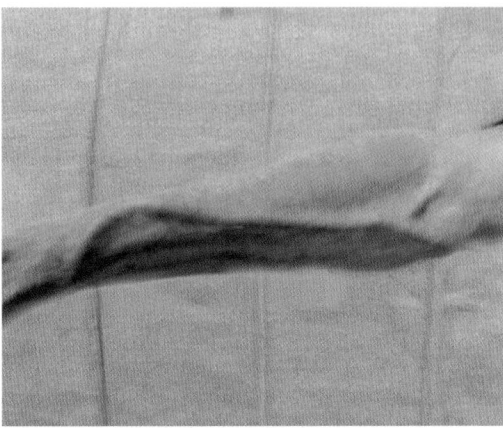

FIGURE 1   Mature radiocephalic arteriovenous fistula 6 weeks postoperatively.

fistula is contemplated. It cannot be overemphasized that the preoperative physical examination is incomplete unless a venous tourniquet is used to assess the superficial veins. To end up with a successful radiocephalic fistula, the forearm cephalic vein should be palpable from the wrist to the antecubital fossa. Otherwise, attention should be directed to the upper-arm veins.

Duplex ultrasound–based vein mapping prior to dialysis access surgery was essentially mandated by the KDOQI guidelines. We strongly disagree with this blanket recommendation. Although vein mapping at times may be helpful for operative planning, it is frequently unnecessary, adds cost, and may not always give valid information. In patients already on dialysis via a catheter, we rarely request a vein map. If no suitable vein is found at surgery (see operative techniques below), then the patient will require a prosthetic graft. In patients referred prior to the initiation of dialysis, vein mapping may be helpful in those who are obese, are intravenous drug abusers, or have had prior PICC lines. It may also be helpful in patients with normal-sized arms where neither an adequate basilic nor cephalic vein is palpable with a tourniquet in place. Lastly, with the ubiquity of portable ultrasound machines, surgeon-performed vein mapping in the preoperative area or intraoperatively is becoming more routine, and this option generally obviates the need for a formal vein mapping study.

Venography is an important component of successful dialysis access surgery. Its primary use is not to road map the arm veins but rather to confirm central vein patency. Our practice is to use it liberally in any patient with a history of arm swelling or prior central venous cannulation on the side of proposed access. In predialysis patients, carbon dioxide may be used as a contrast agent, thereby avoiding the risks of iodinated contrast-induced nephrotoxicity. If a hybrid endovascular operative suite is available, the venogram may be done at the beginning of the access case, allowing for a combined procedure that is more convenient for the patient. Lastly, for the safety of the surgical team, any patient with a history of intravenous drug use should have a plain radiograph of the upper extremity to evaluate for the presence of foreign bodies.

Prior to surgery, standard blood chemistries and a complete blood count are all that are necessary. The surgeon can assume that uremic platelet dysfunction will always be present, and we have found no utility in checking bleeding times preoperatively. Uncommonly, DDAVP (arginine vasopressin) at a dose of 0.3 µg/kg will be needed intraoperatively to control oozing. Additionally, aspirin use does not seem to impact bleeding significantly, and considering the cardiovascular risk profile of these patients, we routinely administer a dose of 81 mg in the preoperative area. Clopidogrel does seem to increase oozing in some patients, so this should be held for 5 to 7 days unless the patient has recently undergone coronary artery stenting. Many patients are also on warfarin. In general, we do not advocate holding warfarin and feel comfortable proceeding with access surgery with an international normalized ratio (INR) up to 2.5.

OPERATIVE TECHNIQUES

The best option for anesthesia depends on the patient's comorbid conditions, the anesthesiologist, and the proposed surgery. While local anesthesia is a viable option for many patients, it works best for patients undergoing radiocephalic or nontransposed brachiocephalic fistulas. While we have used it successfully for upper-arm basilic transpositions, it tends to be somewhat less than ideal for both patient and surgeon due to the relatively large area that must be anesthetized. More recently we have used infraclavicular regional nerve blocks. The blocks are placed in the preoperative area by a dedicated block team while the preceding case is underway. This helps to maximize efficiency and shorten turnover time. If the skin incision approaches the deltopectoral groove or the axilla, supplementation of the regional block with local anesthetic will be necessary. Our experience with supraclavicular blocks has been less

satisfactory. Over the last year, three cases were canceled due to shortness of breath secondary to phrenic nerve paresis following this more proximal nerve block.

Autogenous Arm Fistulae

The patient is positioned supine, with the shoulder of the operative side near the edge of the bed. The arm board should be positioned such that the arm rests in the center of the board. A standard skin preparation including the shoulder and axilla is performed. If available, an arm board drape is most convenient, but an extremity drape will suffice.

Radiocephalic Fistula

A 3-cm to 4-cm incision is placed just proximal to the wrist along the lateral or radial aspect of the arm. Once the skin is incised, the surgeon and assistant both lift the skin with Adson forceps, facilitating easy identification of the cephalic vein after some gentle blunt dissection. The vein is encircled with a vessel loop and then sharply dissected out, tying all branches with 4-0 or 5-0 ties. The radial artery is dissected out circumferentially in a standard fashion and controlled with vessel loops. Any side branches are tied but not divided, which helps to maintain its orientation. The cephalic vein is divided distally, gently dilated with sequential coronary dilators, and then flushed with heparinized saline. After flushing the radial artery, a spatulated end-to-side anastomosis is performed using 6-0 or 7-0 polypropylene suture. Any large proximal vein branches are ligated through separate 1-cm incisions. Closure consists of 3-0 interrupted absorbable dermal sutures and a 4-0 running absorbable subcuticular suture.

Upper-Arm Fistula

If there is a potentially good cephalic vein, then a transverse incision is made in the antecubital crease (Figure 2, *A*), and the cephalic vein is identified (Figure 2, *B*). If the vein is of suitable size, it is dissected out to its confluence with the median cubital vein, ligated distally, and divided. Sequential coronary dilators are gently passed cephalad and should easily pass if there is no intraluminal scarring. Although a sufficient length of vein can be mobilized at this point to easily reach the brachial artery, we frequently convert the incision into a hockey stick–shaped incision (with the handle of the stick along the cephalic vein; Figure 2, *C*) and mobilize 10 to 15 cm or more of the vein (Figure 2, *D* and *E*). Not only does this allow ligation of the accessory cephalic vein and other small branches, but it also allows superficial tunneling of the vein (Figure 2, *F*), which is necessary in all but the thinnest of arms. With the vein transposed, accessing the fistula can be performed earlier (as soon as 4 weeks, depending on vein size), easier, and more consistently, enabling earlier removal of dialysis catheters.

Dissection of the distal brachial artery through the medial aspect of the antecubital incision is done in a standard fashion, with control obtained with vessel loops. If the brachial artery appears smaller than expected, the patient most likely has a high brachial bifurcation. In these cases, the more suitable donor artery almost always is the deeper of the two vessels and should be evaluated before proceeding with the anastomosis. The vein is tunneled just beneath the skin, making sure there is no kink or twist at the most proximal site of mobilization (Figure 2, *G*). Once an arteriotomy is made and the artery is flushed with heparinized saline, the vessel loops are replaced with baby bulldog clamps. This eliminates any vessel stretching and makes the end-to-side anastomosis easier to perform. Closure consists of 2-0 absorbable sutures in the subcutaneous tissue and 3-0 nylon vertical mattress skin sutures (Figure 2, *H*). In our experience,

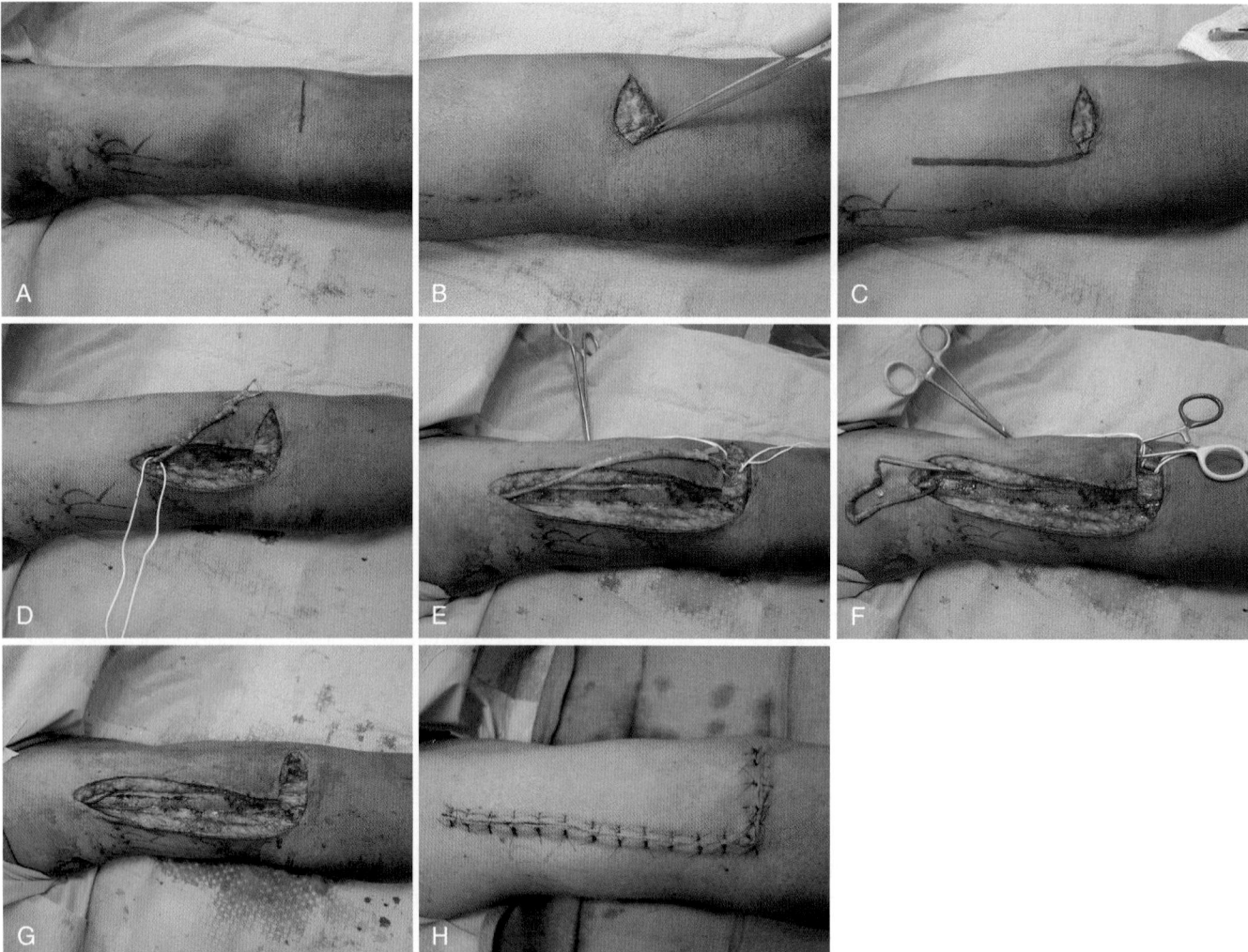

FIGURE 2 Brachiocephalic arteriovenous fistula creation. **A,** Antecubital incision. **B,** Identification of cephalic vein in antecubital fossa. **C,** Hockey stick incision. **D,** Proximal dissection of cephalic vein. **E,** Ligation of cephalic vein branches, dissection of brachial artery in antecubital fossa. **F,** Superficial tunneling of mobilized cephalic vein. **G,** Completed arteriovenous anastomosis. **H,** Closure of skin with vertical mattress nylon sutures.

subcuticular closures in the upper arm have been associated with postoperative wound problems much more frequently than with interrupted nylon closures. In addition, patients are much more apt to keep their follow-up appointment if they have sutures that need to be removed. If the cephalic vein is not of adequate size or quality, then the median cubital vein is identified near the medial aspect of the incision. If the median cubital vein is adequate, it is ligated distally, divided, and flushed with heparinized saline. We then extend the medial end of our skin incision in a hockey stick fashion along the medial aspect of the arm nearly to the axilla. The vein is dissected circumferentially over its course toward the axilla as it joins the basilic vein, which subsequently joins the proximal brachial vein. If the median cubital vein is not adequate, then the basilic vein is used. In this instance we place two surgical towels under the upper arm to improve positioning and then make a new incision just anterior to the medial epicondyle of the humerus. Once the basilic vein is identified and found to be of appropriate size and quality, the incision is extended proximal and distally until enough vein for a transposition has been exposed. The brachial artery is then dissected out at the antecubital fossa either through a separate incision or through the medial aspect of the antecubital incision if that incision had already been made to inspect the cephalic vein. The vein is then tunneled and the anastomosis prepared and performed as described above. The

fascia and subcutaneous layers are reapproximated with running 2-0 absorbable sutures. The skin is closed with interrupted 3-0 nylon vertical mattress sutures. At the end of the case, there should be a palpable thrill in the fistula. If there is not, then there is a technical problem and the incision should be reopened.

Prosthetic Arteriovenous Grafts

If there is no suitable vein, then a prosthetic graft must be placed. Although the most commonly used graft is 6-mm ePTFE, bovine carotid artery and polyurethane-urea (Vectra; Bard, Tempe Ariz.) grafts may also be used. A transverse incision is made over the brachial artery in the antecubital fossa. The brachial artery and vein (if at least 5 mm in diameter) are isolated and encircled with vessel loops. The vein should be generously dissected out to allow a long venous anastomosis. A second, smaller counterincision is made on the volar surface of the midforearm on the radial side. Placement of the counterincision in this fashion skews the graft toward the radial aspect of the forearm, and this affords the most comfortable arm positioning during dialysis. The venous anastomosis is performed first, particularly if the graft has a premade flared end. The graft is tunneled in a gentle arc to the counterincision and then back to the antecubital fossa. Tunneling is best accomplished with a Kelly-Wick tunneler (IMPRA; Bard, Tempe Ariz.), although an aortic clamp may be used. The arterial anastomosis is then performed, and the incisions are closed. If the brachial vein is too small at the antecubital fossa, then a second incision is made on the proximal medial aspect of the upper arm, and the proximal brachial or distal axillary vein is used for the venous outflow. While this describes the two most common graft configurations, in reality any suitable artery and vein may be used. We strongly believe in fistula first and therefore do not agree with the use of forearm grafts to help mature upper-arm cephalic or basilic veins.

Special Considerations

Not uncommonly, patients present for dialysis access after many months of catheter usage and already have upper extremity central vein occlusion or stenosis. The thigh prosthetic graft is the next best access in most circumstances. Although we have extensive experience utilizing femoral vein and find it particularly useful for home hemodialysis patients who have no useful upper extremity veins, its use for a thigh fistula should be carefully planned and works best in thin legs. Saphenous vein may also be used as a thigh fistula (tunneled anteriorly as a straight fistula and anastomosed to the distal superficial femoral artery), but if the vein is not generous in size (at least 5 mm) at the time of surgery, failure to mature into a useful access is common. For a prosthetic thigh graft, an oblique skin line incision is made just distal to the groin crease, and either the deep femoral or proximal superficial femoral artery is used for arterial inflow. Through the medial aspect of that incision the proximal saphenous vein or saphenofemoral junction is preferentially used for venous outflow. The proximal femoral vein may be used, but the dissection is somewhat more difficult.

COMPLICATIONS AND MANAGEMENT

Infection is the most frequent complication of hemodialysis access and is a major cause of morbidity and mortality in the dialysis population (Table 1). Up to 30% of all deaths in dialysis patients are due to infections, and most come from vascular access sites. Compared to autogenous fistulae, the relative risk of infection-related death is 1.8 times greater in those dialyzing through catheters and 1.3 times greater in those dialyzing through prosthetic grafts. The cumulative probability of developing a catheter-related infection is over 50% after 2 months of dialysis through a catheter. Diabetes and human immunodeficiency virus (HIV) are also independent risk factors for greater infection rates among all access types. Staphylococcal species

are the most frequently isolated organisms. Access-derived infections often lead to systemic complications, including bacterial endocarditis, osteomyelitis, septic emboli, and septic arthritis. For catheter-related bacteremia, management consists of culture-directed parenteral antibiotics and removal or exchange of the infected catheter. For infected ePTFE grafts, management must be guided by an attempt to balance the benefits of preserving a functioning access with the severity of infection. Some local infections can be successfully treated with aggressive intravenous antibiotic therapy combined with resection and replacement of a portion of the graft, though recurrent infection is not uncommon. Abscess formation, purulent drainage from the graft site, or the development of infected pseudoaneurysms all mandate removal of the infected portion or the entirety of the graft.

The risk of access failure due to thrombosis is more common in prosthetic grafts than in autogenous fistulae. Early failure is generally due to technical factors but can also be related to hypercoagulability, low flow states, or use of inadequate vein. In mature accesses, most problems will be detected by the dialysis unit. High venous pressures, poor arterial inflow, recirculation, and diminishing effectiveness of the dialysis all indicate access problems. The anatomic location of the problem usually can be ascertained by physical examination. The lack of bruit and thrill indicates thrombosis. A weak thrill or bruit suggests inflow problems. Pulsatility in a fistula generally indicates an outflow problem. Early intervention can often salvage an otherwise threatened fistula or graft. A duplex scan can further pinpoint the area of the problem, but it is frequently unnecessary. Generally, the diagnostic test of choice is a fistulogram, at which time therapeutic interventions, such as thrombectomy, angioplasty, and stenting, can be carried out. Occasionally open revision is necessary, with many options available to improve either arterial inflow or to relieve venous outflow obstructions.

Almost all arm accesses create a steal syndrome, but significant steal occurs less than 15% of the time, with brachial artery–based accesses presenting the highest risk. Loss of a palpable distal pulse at the time of fistula creation indicates that a significant steal syndrome could develop. Manual compression of the fistula should result in restoration of the distal pulse. Options for improving distal perfusion include ligation, plication, banding, proximalization of the arterial inflow, and the distal revascularization with internal ligation (DRIL) procedure. The DRIL has the benefit of leaving the functioning fistula undisturbed and eliminates the physiologic pathway for the steal and restores downstream perfusion.

Other complications that occur with varying frequencies and degrees of morbidity include edema due to venous hypertension, seromas, wound problems, and carpal tunnel syndrome. Aneurysmal dilatation of mature grafts or fistulae generally does not need to be addressed operatively unless there is overlying skin breakdown. In general, having a low threshold to investigate and intervene on a fistula that is not performing optimally will minimize the need for repeated access surgeries.

CONCLUSIONS

1. Assume dialysis is forever, so when performing access surgery, do not jeopardize future options.
2. Try to avoid all catheters and, if possible, prosthetic materials—in other words, fistula first.
3. Fistula dysfunction mandates prompt investigation and intervention to maximize chances of fistula salvage.
4. Dialysis access preformed properly will be rewarding for the patient as well as the surgeon.

SELECTED READINGS

Fistula First: National Vascular Access Improvement Initiative, Available at www.fistulafirst.org. Accessed September 1, 2012.

TABLE 1: Frequency of dialysis access–derived infections in a study of 1574 surgery patients

Overall incidence of infection, n (%)	132 (8.3%)
Category of Infection	
Dialysis center–derived infection (>30 days after surgery)	66 (50%)
Spontaneous infection in nonfunctional graft	30 (22.7%)
Infection in remaining stump of partly excised graft	22 (16.7%)
Operative site infection (<30 days after surgery)	6 (6.1%)
Postinterventional radiology thrombectomy	6 (4.5%)

Gottschalk CW, Feiner SK: History of the science of dialysis, *Am J Nephrol* 17:289–298, 1997.

KDOQI Clinical Practice Guidelines and Clinical Practice Recommendations for Diabetes and Chronic Kidney Disease, *Am J Kidney Dis* 49(2 Suppl 2):S12–S154, 2007.

Konner K: History of vascular access for hemodialysis, *Nephrol Dial Transplant* 20:2629–2635, 2005.

Nassar GM, Ayus JC: Infectious complications of the hemodialysis access, *Kidney Int* 60:1–13, 2001.

Schild AF, Simon S, Preito J, et al: Single-center review of infections associated with 1,574 consecutive vascular access procedures, *Vasc Endovasc Surg* 37(1):27–31, 2003.

Sidawy AN, Gray R, Besarab A, et al: Recommended standards for reports dealing with arteriovenous hemodialysis accesses, *J Vasc Surg* 35(3):603–610, 2002.

Sidawy AN, Spergel LM, Besarab A, et al: The Society for Vascular Surgery: clinical practice guidelines for the surgical placement and maintenance of arteriovenous hemodialysis access, *J Vasc Surg* 48(5 Suppl):S2–S25, 2008.

VENOUS THROMBOEMBOLISM: PREVENTION, DIAGNOSIS, AND TREATMENT

Catherine G. Velopulos, MD, MHS, and
Elliott R. Haut, MD, FACS

INTRODUCTION

Venous thromboembolism (VTE) disease, which encompasses deep vein thrombosis (DVT) and pulmonary embolism (PE), has become an increasingly recognized source of morbidity and mortality, particularly in surgical cases. The Agency for Healthcare Research and Quality (AHRQ) has suggested that appropriate VTE prophylaxis is the number one patient safety initiative that can be undertaken to prevent in-hospital death. In 2008, the Surgeon General issued "A Call to Action to Prevent Deep Venous Thrombosis and Pulmonary Embolism," and the U.S. Congress designated March as DVT Awareness Month in an effort to raise awareness for this disease that kills more than 100,000 and is diagnosed in more than 600,000 Americans per year.

In the setting of this potentially preventable disease, it is important to recognize the scope and impact of the problem, the risk factor profile of each patient, prophylaxis and prevention strategies, and appropriate screening and diagnosis. In patients who are identified as having disease, optimal treatment algorithms must be used to reduce morbidity and mortality.

IMPACT

Multiple patient populations treated by surgeons are particularly vulnerable because of physiologic derangements in the perioperative period. VTE is more prevalent, and more deadly, in patients with malignant disease; patients with gastrointestinal, pancreatic, and colorectal cancer are at highest risk. VTE is one of the most common and deadly complications among trauma patients, with reported rates as high as 50%. Patients who undergo orthopedic surgery (particularly hip or knee joint replacement) have been shown to be at a tenfold increased risk for VTE. Intensive care unit (ICU) admission is an independent risk factor for VTE, although this is often difficult to differentiate from other risk factors present in the same patients. Studies of patients on mechanical ventilation show an incidence rate of up to 25% for DVT and greater than 10% for PE even in patients who were given appropriate prophylaxis.

Economic evaluations have reported a doubling in the length of stay and hospital costs for patients with VTE, with estimated per patient added costs of $15,000 to $25,000, and increased hospital readmission rates. In the era of pay for performance and decreased reimbursements for preventable events, VTE prevention represents an area of significant potential improvement, particularly in the arena of patient safety and quality.

RISK FACTORS

Any disease process that augments Virchow's triad of venous stasis, endothelial injury, and hypercoagulability increases the risk of VTE. Factors such as trauma that leads to immobilization, paralysis (i.e., spinal cord injury, stroke, or pharmacologic event during surgery), indwelling venous catheters, and insufflation for laparoscopic surgery contribute to venous stasis. Any type of venous injury leads to endothelial damage and release of factors, whether traumatic or iatrogenic (i.e., central venous catheter placement). Disease states such as trauma, neoplasm, congestive heart failure, congenital disorders, and obesity, along with pregnancy and treatments such as hormone therapy and chemotherapy, contribute to a hypercoagulable state. Some of the commonly accepted risk factors for VTE are included in Box 1.

PREVENTION AND PROPHYLAXIS

In the years before routine VTE prophylaxis was adopted, general surgery patients who were untreated had rates of DVT and PE of 19.1% and 1.6%, respectively, with a remarkably high fatal PE rate of 0.87%. Even in the current era in which prophylaxis is more frequently used, VTE rates of more than 2% to 3% are reported after some major general surgery and surgical oncology cases. Numbers such as these should remind clinicians of the importance of VTE prevention.

All surgical patients should be evaluated for VTE risk factors and be offered appropriate prophylaxis, with the vast majority warranting pharmacologic prophylaxis. Well-researched evidence-based guidelines are routinely published by national societies to aid clinicians in determining the ideal prophylaxis for their patients. The American College of Chest Physicians (ACCP) updates their guidelines approximately every 4 years and is thought by many to be the definitive resource on VTE prevention. Other groups, such as The Eastern Association for the Surgery of Trauma (EAST) and The American Academy of Orthopedic Surgeons (AAOS) have guidelines for specific patient subgroups as well.

Nearly all surgical patients have at least some risk factors that warrant pharmacologic prophylaxis in the perioperative period. Specific regimens should be selected based on individual patient risk

BOX 1: Risk factors for venous thromboembolism

Major VTE Risk Factors
Previous VTE
Cancer
Thrombophilia
Prolonged surgical procedure (>2 h)
Major general surgery
Major trauma
Fracture of hip or leg
Hip or knee replacement
Spinal cord injury
NYHA class III/IV heart failure
Respiratory failure requiring mechanical ventilation
Acute stroke with paresis (<3 mo)
Pregnancy/postpartum (up to 6 wk)

Minor VTE Risk Factors
Acute infection/sepsis
Bed rest
Immobility from prolonged sitting (e.g., travel)
Central venous catheter
Increasing age
Laparoscopic surgery
Estrogens/selective estrogen receptor modulators (e.g., tamoxifen)
Inflammatory bowel disease
Obesity
Pregnancy/antepartum
Varicose veins, arteriovenous malformations

NYHA, New York Heart Association; *VTE*, venous thromboembolism.

factors and the type of surgery being performed. Most protocols use subcutaneous injections of unfractionated heparin or low molecular-weight heparin (LMWH) after surgery. A preoperative dose 1 to 2 hours before surgery has shown some benefit and is used in many protocols. There is no definitive recommendation for which pharmacologic agent is used in most surgical patients, although the trauma and orthopedic literature suggest an advantage of LMWH over unfractionated heparin. The duration of prophylaxis is still a subject of debate, and it is routinely stopped at hospital discharge. However, excellent data in orthopedic surgery mandate extended, outpatient use, which is frequently prescribed. Similarly, data and guidelines suggest this extended prophylaxis be ordered for many patients undergoing major cancer or abdominal-pelvic surgery, although this is not routinely done.

An example schema of one published VTE prophylaxis algorithm for general surgery inpatients is shown in Figure 1. This algorithm places patients with major VTE risk factors and older patients (>60 years of age) with any risk factors into a "very high risk" category. Patients between the ages of 40 and 60 years, in the absence of major risk factors, are placed in the "high risk" category. The remainder of all other surgical patients is at "moderate risk." No surgical inpatients are truly at "low risk," although some patients undergoing short/minor, ambulatory, outpatient procedures warrant no specific recommendations for pharmacologic VTE prophylaxis.

Patients capable of ambulation should have their activity advanced as soon as feasible because this remains an effective adjunct (although it should not be routinely relied on as the sole VTE prevention measure). Additional mechanical prophylaxis approaches include graduated compression stockings, sequential compression devices, and intermittent pneumatic compression devices. Their efficacy is well proven, and they are often ordered as adjunctive measures in addition to pharmacologic prophylaxis. However, their effectiveness is hampered by poor compliance in routine practice (<50% of patients have working devices on in some studies) and contraindications in certain patients with lower extremity wounds, casts, immobilizers, or external fixation devices.

The use of inferior vena cava (IVC) filters for primary prophylaxis against PE (in the absence of documented DVT) is currently the object of some study and much controversy and debate and is discussed later in this chapter.

Despite evidence that VTE prophylaxis is effective, routine use of adequate prophylaxis is remarkably low. Published compliance rates hover around 50% to 60% in many studies of surgical patients across the United States and around the globe. Many approaches to improve this poor guideline adherence and improve quality of care have been attempted, often with little success.

Simple electronic reminders to use VTE prophylaxis in surgical patients have been shown to increase ordering of prophylaxis but had no change in VTE outcomes. A targeted electronic alert that tells ordering physicians that their patients are not being given prophylaxis has shown some improvement in adherence; however, this approach is reactive and does not instruct providers to use best practice VTE prevention from the beginning. The authors have recently published multiple papers that show significant benefits of a mandatory computerized clinical decision support (CDS) tool embedded within the hospital's computerized provider order entry (CPOE) system. This approach dramatically improves documentation of risk status, increases compliance with evidence-based guidelines for VTE prophylaxis, and decreases preventable harm from VTE events.

DIAGNOSIS

Diagnosis of VTE must always be considered and aggressively pursued when indicated in patients with clinical suspicion for DVT or PE. Historically, DVT has been confirmed with invasive contrast venography, but it now is diagnosed almost exclusively with duplex ultrasound scan. DVT can also be seen on contrast-enhanced computed tomographic (CT) scan or magnetic resonance imaging (MRI), although these tests are only rarely ordered for this indication specifically.

Similar changes in diagnostic testing for PE have occurred, and PE is now primarily diagnosed with contrast-enhanced CT angiogram of the chest. Improved techniques and capabilities of the current multidetector helical scanners allow for diagnosis of increasingly smaller PEs at the subsegmental level, the clinical significance of which is yet to be fully determined. Although CT scan is the current test of choice, other modalities must be considered in certain patient populations. Ventilation/perfusion (V/Q) scanning, a nuclear medicine test, can be used in patients who cannot receive contrast dye because of renal insufficiency or allergy, but this test must be interpreted in combination with the pretest probability of PE to be clinically useful. Critically ill patients in the ICU whose conditions are too unstable for transport to CT scan can be evaluated with transthoracic or transesophageal echocardiogram. Findings of right heart failure or pulmonary hypertension are highly suggestive of PE, and clot can sometimes be visualized directly with echocardiography. In combination with classic echocardiographic results suggestive of right heart strain, this is fairly specific for PE. Serum testing of D-dimer levels is quite helpful in the outpatient and emergency department settings to both rule in and rule out VTE. This laboratory test is less useful in perioperative surgical inpatients because D-dimer is often elevated in this patient population; however, it should still be routinely ordered because a normal test definitively rules out clinically important VTE. In patients in whom VTE is highly suspected and anticoagulation therapy is not contraindicated, empiric treatment should be rapidly initiated even before definitive diagnosis has been confirmed.

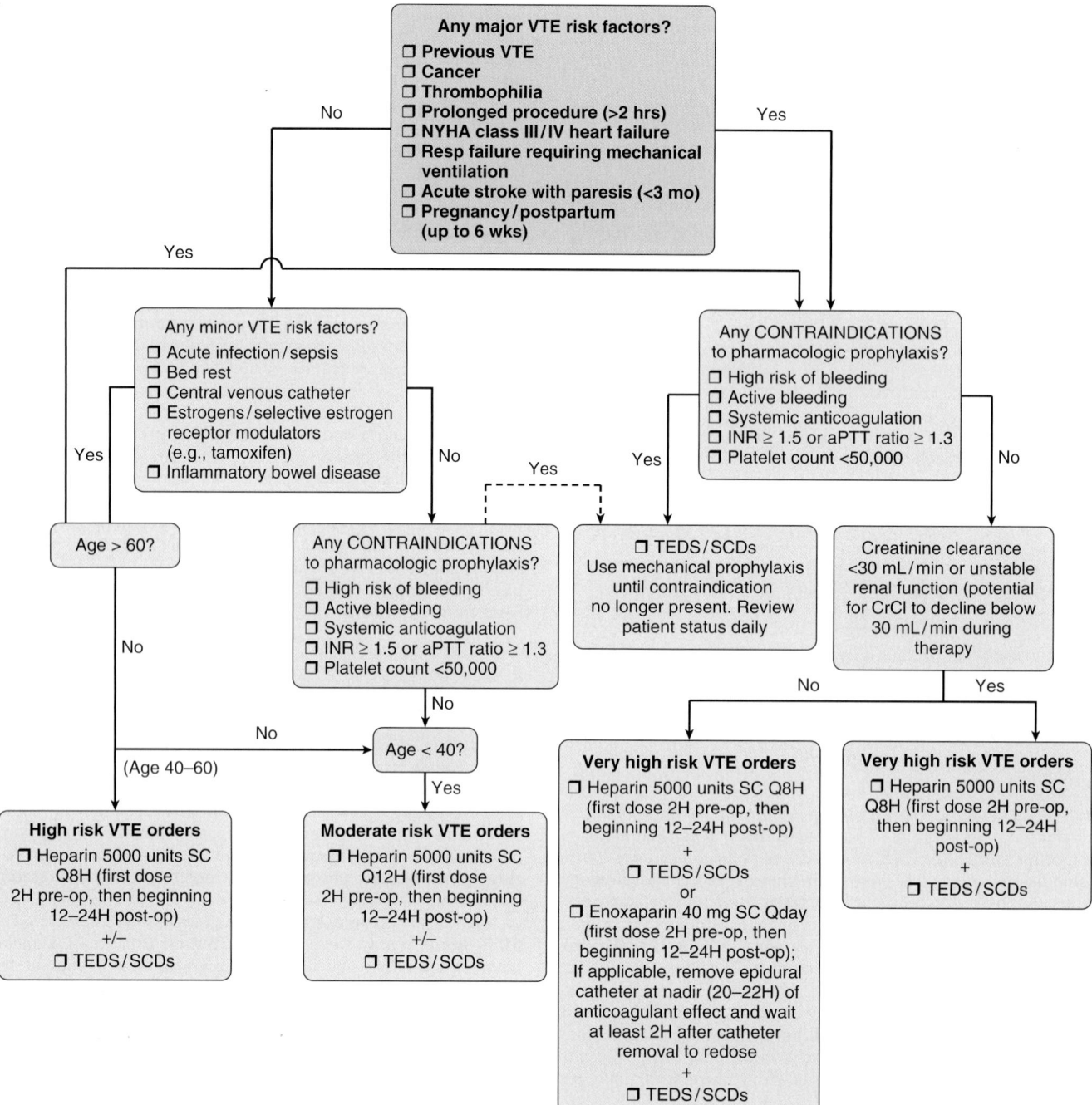

FIGURE 1   General surgery venous thromboembolism *(VTE)* prophylaxis schema. *aPTT,* Activated partial thomboplastin time; *CrCl,* creatinine clearance; *INR,* international normalized ratio; *NYHA,* New York Heart Association; *Q8H,* every 8 hours; *Q12H,* every 12 hours; *SC,* subcutaneous; *SCDs,* sequential compression devices; *TEDS,* thromboembolism-deterrent stockings.

SCREENING OF ASYMPTOMATIC PATIENTS

Screening of asymptomatic patients for DVT remains controversial. Proponents of screening see benefit in performing a relatively inexpensive, noninvasive, nonradiation–based test (duplex ultrasound scan) to identify and treat DVT early, before progression to larger symptomatic DVT or conversion to PE. Opponents raise concerns about the direct financial costs of increased medical testing. In addition, identification of clots that never would have become clinically significant puts patients at risk by committing them to months of potentially dangerous anticoagulation therapy.

The largest body of literature on the topic of screening patients at high risk for DVT is in trauma surgery. Wide practice variation exists, primarily because studies have yet to show any definite improvement in patient outcomes with this strategy, particularly in patients who have been given adequate prophylaxis. Disagreement is found among guideline developers as well. The ACCP guidelines state that screening should not be performed, and the EAST guidelines suggest that it may benefit certain trauma patients at high risk.

Surveillance bias (the idea of "the more you look, the more you find") remains a primary concern, as studies have shown a direct correlation between increasing screening and increasing DVT rates. This issue is a timely and important problem because DVT rates have

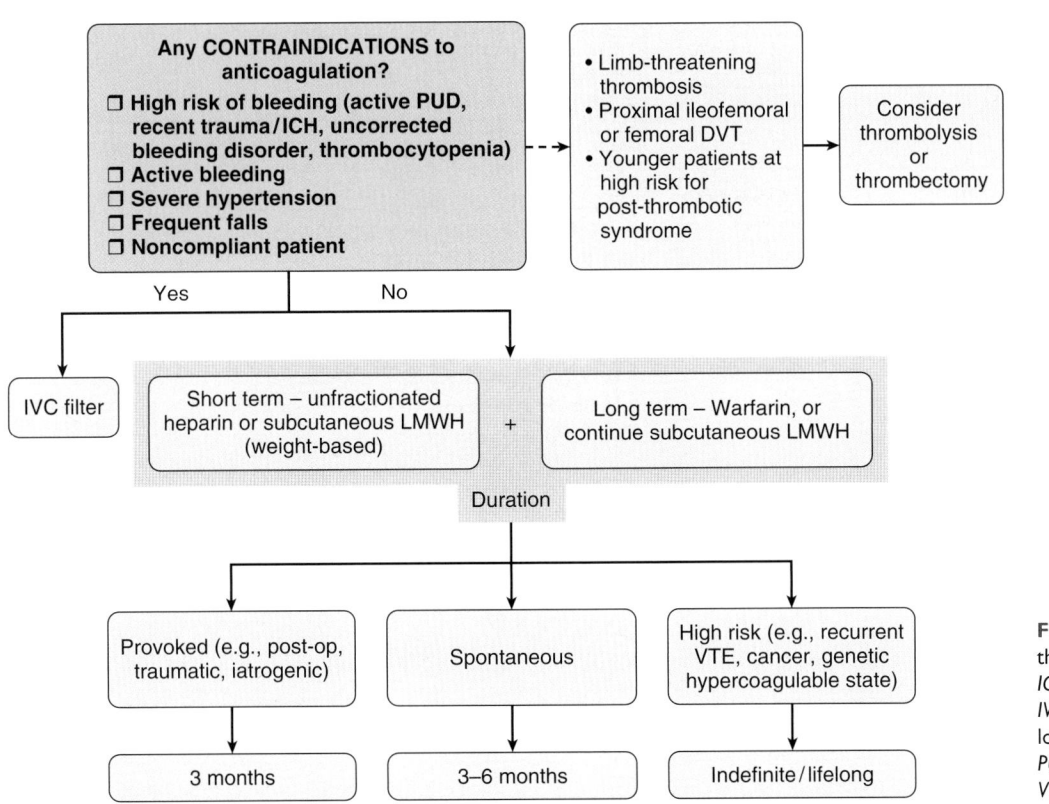

FIGURE 2 Deep vein thrombosis *(DVT)* treatment. *ICH,* Intracranial hemorrhage; *IVC,* inferior vena cava; *LMWH,* low-molecular-weight heparin; *PUD,* peptic ulcer disease; *VTE,* venous thromboembolism.

been proposed as a quality outcome measure and may be publicly reported in the near future. Comparison of a hospital (or trauma center) that screens many patients and identifies many DVT events with one that does many fewer duplex ultrasound scans gives biased information on quality of medical care. The increasing frequency of performing higher resolution CT scan may lead to similar problems. These CT scans are identifying increasing numbers of incidentally noted PEs, presenting a dilemma for how these patients should be treated and how these adverse event rates are used to study and report complications and outcomes and quality of care.

TREATMENT

Deep Venous Thrombosis

Treatment for DVT is largely medical and primarily based on anticoagulation therapy. Most protocols involve the rapid initiation of heparin, either weight-based intravenous unfractionated heparin or subcutaneous LMWH. One such protocol is shown in Figure 2. Long-term anticoagulation therapy can use either warfarin or ongoing weight-based LMWH. Duration of therapy is dependent on the particular circumstances surrounding the VTE event and individual patient characteristics. In general, recommendations suggest 3 months for provoked DVT (e.g., postoperative, trauma-related, or iatrogenic), 3 to 6 months for spontaneous DVT, and indefinite or lifelong therapy in patients at high risk (e.g., recurrent VTE, cancer diagnosis, inherited hypercoagulable states). Some clinicians routinely perform repeat duplex ultrasound scan to ensure the clot is gone and use these data to decide on how long therapy is needed.

Although the vast majority of patients with DVT are treated with anticoagulation therapy alone, other treatments for specific subpopulations exist. Some patients with isolated below-knee DVT who are at low risk of propagation (i.e., mobile outpatients without

underlying predisposing factors) can be treated with compression stockings. In this case, repeat duplex scan (at approximately 2 weeks) is used to ensure the clot has resolved. Propagation above the knee should prompt a change to anticoagulation therapy. In patients with a contraindication to anticoagulation therapy, an IVC filter should be placed instead to prevent embolization of the DVT as it becomes a PE. Patients with limb-threatening thrombosis such as phlegmasia cerulea dolens or phlegmasia alba dolens may need open surgical or catheter-based thrombectomy in an attempt at limb salvage.

The role of thrombolysis in treatment of DVT has undergone much scrutiny. This therapy has been suggested for patients with proximal iliofemoral or femoral DVT, younger patients with long life expectancy and good physiologic reserve, and those with limb-threatening thrombosis. Early studies have shown a decreased incidence of postthrombotic syndrome, but this benefit was offset by higher rates of bleeding complications, primarily because systemic thrombolytics were used. Newer catheter-based techniques, involving catheter-directed mechanical or pharmacologic thrombolysis with much smaller doses of thrombolytics, have the potential to change the DVT treatment algorithm. An ongoing large, National Institutes of Health (NIH)–funded, multicenter, randomized, clinical trial named ATTRACT (Acute Venous Thrombosis: Thrombus Removal with Adjunctive Catheter-Directed Thrombolysis) is currently examining the role of this modality in a prospective fashion. This study is examining the safety, efficacy, cost effectiveness, and long-term outcomes (including postthrombotic syndrome and quality of life) when catheter-based therapy is compared with standard therapy alone.

Pulmonary Embolism

Treatment of PE depends first on the clinical cardiopulmonary stability of the patient. One potential algorithm is shown in Figure 3. In patients with hemodynamically stable conditions, the initial treatment algorithm is similar to that for DVT. Most protocols involve the

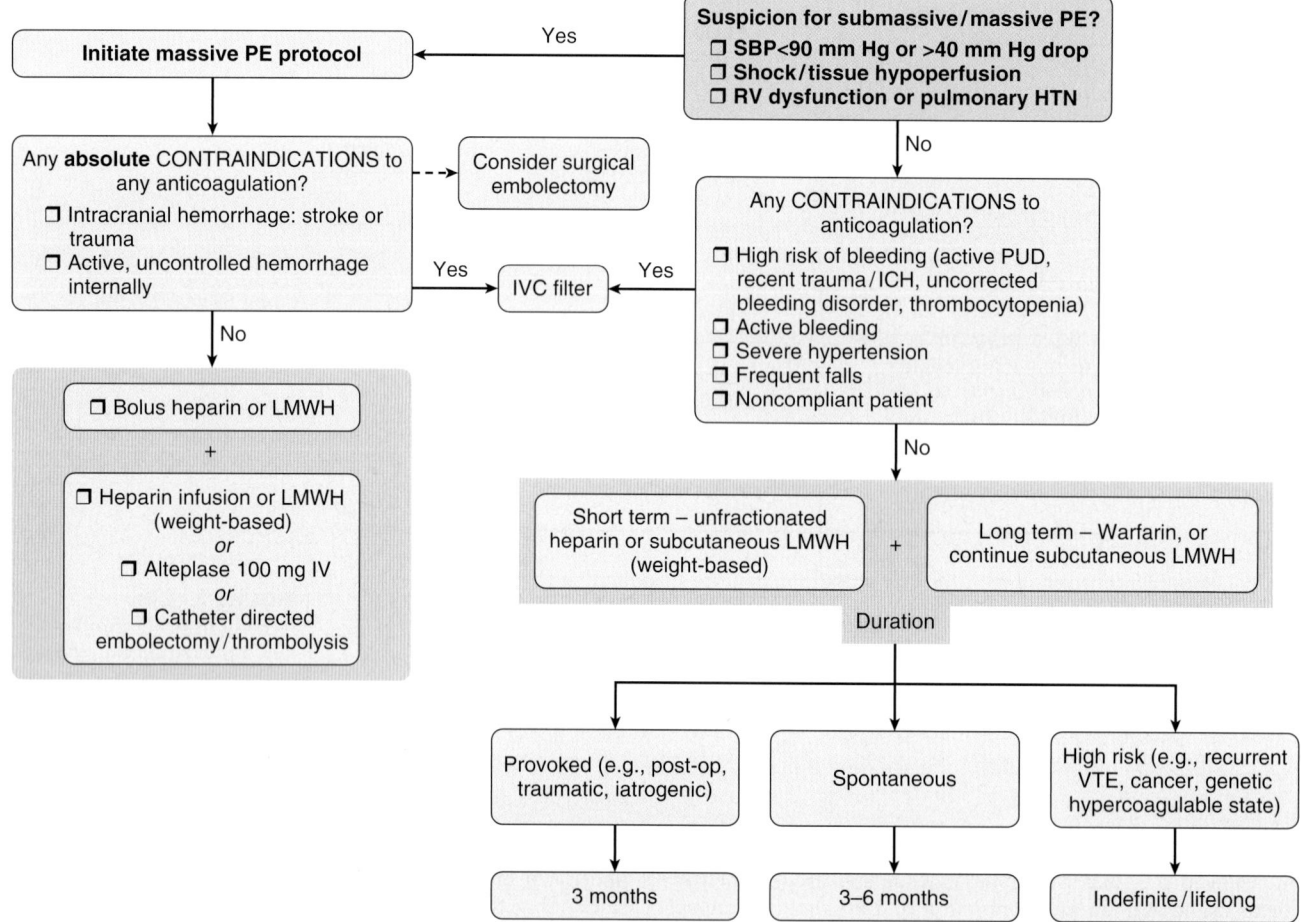

FIGURE 3   Pulmonary embolism *(PE)* treatment. *HTN,* Hypertension; *ICH,* intracranial hemorrhage; *IV,* intravenous; *IVC,* inferior vena cava; *LMWH,* low-molecular-weight heparin; *RV,* right ventricle; *SBP,* systolic blood pressure; *VTE,* venous thromboembolism.

initiation of heparin, either unfractionated or LMWH, with conversion to long-term anticoagulation therapy, with either warfarin or continuation of weight-based dosing of LMWH. Bilateral lower extremity duplex scan is suggested by some to assess for further risk of clot burden, although most of the time, this is negative once the PE is identified. Other clinicians do not perform this study as the presence or absence of DVT does not change therapy. In patients with a contraindication to anticoagulation therapy, an IVC filter should be placed to prevent embolization of more DVT into pulmonary emboli.

Patients with submassive or massive PE, defined as actual or impending cardiopulmonary collapse or progression to right heart failure and shock, should be treated more aggressively. A "Scientific Statement from the American Heart Association" (Jaff et. al.) gives excellent guidance on therapy in these patients (and others with certain subsets of VTE). Patients with massive PE should be treated with systemic fibrinolysis (i.e., alteplase 100 mg intravenously [IV]), assuming they have no definite contraindication and have acceptable bleeding risk. In patients unable to receive systemic fibrinolysis, surgical embolectomy (Trendelenburg's procedure) and catheter-based embolectomy or fragmentation are appropriate options, depending on locally available expertise and resources.

Inferior Vena Cava Filters

Although introduced decades ago, the use of IVC filters has recently been on a rapid upswing. The ease with which these devices can be placed and the technology of removable (also known as optional) IVC filters have likely driven this upward trend of their use. Filters are now routinely placed by many specialists, including interventional radiologists and invasive cardiologists, and trauma, general, and vascular surgeons in operating rooms, interventional suites, and intensive care units. This can be done with the familiar technique of fluoroscopic imaging, although this is no longer necessary as filters are now routinely inserted with intravascular ultrasound scan (IVUS) to guide placement.

Indications for IVC filter placement fall into three main groups. They include absolute and relative indications (both for proven VTE) and prophylactic indications (patients without VTE). In recent years, a consensus has been reached regarding this, and a multidisciplinary study involving representatives from interventional radiology, cardiology, hematology, general surgery, and vascular surgery outlined these indications in detail as seen in Box 2. Although the primary treatment for VTE is acknowledged to be pharmacologic, filters are indicated in certain specific patients. Consideration should be made from the outset as to whether the patient has a limited period of risk, such as in major surgery and trauma, or whether underlying mechanisms dictate a lifelong need for filter. In patients with a contraindication to anticoagulation in whom a filter is placed, anticoagulation therapy should be reconsidered and started as soon as feasible.

The advent of newer retrievable filters that can be removed once the period of highest PE risk has passed has driven the interest in prophylactic filters. However, issues of poor follow-up and nonremoval remain significant. No consensus exists in the literature regarding the prophylactic use of filters. The greatest push has been

---

BOX 2: Indications for inferior vena cava filter

Absolute Indications
Recurrent VTE on adequate anticoagulation therapy
Absolute contraindication to anticoagulation therapy
Complications from anticoagulation therapy
Pulmonary hypertension in setting of chronic PE
Immobile trauma patients with ICH

Relative Indications
Iliocaval DVT
After thrombolysis for iliocaval DVT
Large, free-floating thrombus
Difficulty reaching therapeutic levels of anticoagulation or poor
   compliance
VTE in patients with poor cardiopulmonary reserve
Propagating DVT in setting of adequate anticoagulation therapy
After surgical or mechanical pulmonary embolectomy
After catheter-directed thrombolysis for PE
After surgical or mechanical ileofemoral thrombectomy
Recurrent PE with filter in place
High risk of complications from anticoagulation therapy (e.g.,
   ataxia, movement disorders, frequent falls)

Prophylactic Indications: Primary
Prophylaxis Not Feasible
Multitrauma patients with long bone or pelvic fractures and
   contraindication to pharmacologic prophylaxis other than
   ICH (e.g., solid organ injury)
Patients with cancer undergoing extensive resection with high
   risk for VTE and for postoperative hemorrhage
Other surgical patients or those with medical conditions with
   high risk for VTE

DVT, Deep vein thrombosis; *ICH*, intracranial hemorrhage; *IVC*, inferior vena cava; *PE*, pulmonary embolism; *VTE*, venous thromboembolism.
Adapted from Kaufman JA, Kinney TB, Streiff MB, et al: Guidelines for the use of retrievable and convertible vena cava filters: report from the Society of Interventional Radiology multidisciplinary consensus conference, J Vasc Interv Radiol *17:449-459, 2006, www.sirweb.org/misc/Guidelines_filters.pdf.*

in trauma patients at high risk, specifically those with contraindications to pharmacologic prophylaxis (i.e., head injury, solid organ injury). Other suggested uses for prophylactic IVC filters are in bariatric, oncologic, and spine reconstruction surgery.

CONCLUSION

VTE remains a common source of morbidity and mortality in surgical practice, despite increased awareness. Prevention of these events requires diligent prophylaxis, which must be considered for all surgical patients. Early recognition and treatment of VTE is crucial to prevent immediate mortality and long-term morbidity in surgical patients. New technology promises to improve the way in which this disease is prevented and treated; however, the basic premises of giving appropriate prophylaxis and monitoring closely for clinical events should remain a key component of surgical training and practice.

SUGGESTED READINGS

Agnelli G, Becattini C: Acute pulmonary embolism, *N Engl J Med* 363:266–274, 2010.

Guyatt GH, Akl EA, Crowther M, et al, American College of Chest Physicians Antithrombotic Therapy and Prevention of Thrombosis Panel: executive summary: antithrombotic therapy and prevention of thrombosis, 9th ed: American college of chest physicians evidence-based clinical practice guidelines, *Chest* 141:7S–47S, 2012.

Haut ER, Lau BD: Prevention of venous thromboembolism: brief update review. In *Making Health Care Safer II: An Updated Critical Analysis of the Evidence for Patient Safety Practices*, Rockville, MD, 2013, Agency for Healthcare Research and Quality. http://www.ahrq.gov/research/findings/evidence-based-reports/ptsafetyuptp.html.

Haut ER, Lau BD, Kraenzlin FS, et al: Improved prophylaxis and decreased rates of preventable harm with the use of a mandatory computerized clinical decision support tool for prophylaxis for venous thromboembolism in trauma, *Arch Surg* 147(10):901–907, 2012.

Haut ER, Lau BD, Kraenzlin FS, et al: Improved prophylaxis and decreased rates of preventable harm with the use of a mandatory computerized clinical decision support tool for prophylaxis for venous thromboembolism in trauma, *Arch Surg.* 147(10):901–9073, 2012.

Haut ER, Pronovost PJ: Surveillance bias in outcomes reporting, *JAMA* 305(23):2462–2463, 2011.

Jaff MR, McMurtry MS, Archer SL, et al, on behalf of the American Heart Association Council on Cardiopulmonary, Critical Care, Perioperative and Resuscitation, Council on Peripheral Vascular Disease, and Council on Arteriosclerosis, Thrombosis and Vascular Biology: Management of massive and submassive pulmonary embolism, iliofemoral deep vein thrombosis, and chronic thromboembolic pulmonary hypertension: a scientific statement from the American Heart Association, *Circulation* 123(16):1788–1830, 2011.

Rogers FB, Cipolle MD, Velmahos G, et al: Practice management guidelines for the prevention of venous thromboembolism in trauma patients: the EAST practice management guidelines work group, *J Trauma* 53:142–164, 2006.

Streiff MB, Carolan HT, Hobson DB, et al: Lessons from the Johns Hopkins Multi-Disciplinary Venous Thromboembolism (VTE) Prevention Collaborative, *Br Med J* 344:e3935, 2012.

U.S. Department of Health and Human Services: The Surgeon General's call to action to prevent deep vein thrombosis and pulmonary embolism, (website). www.surgeongeneral.gov/library/calls/deepvein/. Accessed September 14, 2012.

DEEP VENOUS THROMBOSIS

Mun Jye Poi, MD, and Peter H. Lin, MD

V enous thromboembolism (VTE) consists of two related conditions including deep venous thrombosis (DVT) and pulmonary embolism. Clinical consequences associated with DVT remain a major clinical problem despite advances in the modern health care system. It is estimated that DVT affects more than 3 million people in the United States annually. Among them, more than 120,000 patients suffer fatal outcomes as a result of pulmonary embolism. The clinical presentation of DVT commonly involves extremity swelling and pain, which is easily recognized by most physicians. The primary treatment strategy for DVT involves systemic anticoagulation, which is to prevent both worsening of acute symptoms and VTE-associated sequelae, including pulmonary embolism, recurrent thromboembolism, and postthrombotic syndrome. Although surgical interventions are typically not considered a first-line treatment strategy for VTE, it is important for surgeons to be familiar with the diagnostic process and therapeutic strategies of this condition because they can often affect patients undergoing surgery and influence surgical treatment outcomes.

RISK FACTORS

The basic mechanisms resulting in VTE were described by Virchow, which include vascular endothelial damage, stasis of blood flow, and blood hypercoagulability. The most frequent risk factors for DVT include major surgery, trauma, hip fracture, lower extremity paralysis, previous VTE, advanced age, cardiac or respiratory failure, prolonged immobility, presence of central catheters, and hypercoagulable conditions.

DVT occurring in the setting of a known risk factor is defined as secondary, whereas that occurring in the absence of a known risk factor is termed *primary* or *idiopathic.* Men have a higher risk of recurrent VTE than do women, with a relative risk of 3.6 after an initial episode of unprovoked VTE. The recurrence rate reported in Hispanic and black women was also significantly higher than that of white women (3.1% per year vs 1.8% per year). The incidence of DVT increases with age. The influence of age on the incidence of DVT is probably multifactorial. DVT in children is almost always associated with recognized thrombotic risk factors. DVT is more common among pediatric patients in the intensive care unit and those with spinal cord injury, orthopedic immobilization, infection, trauma, or congenital thrombophilia. The prevalence of lower extremity DVT is parallel with the duration of bed rest; the incidence is increased among patients with prolonged bed rest and patients with paralysis. Prolonged immobilization in trauma and surgical patients is known to increase the risk of DVT.

Approximately 20% of all first-time VTE events are associated with malignancy. In older patients with primary DVT, the occurrence may be the first manifestation of a hidden malignancy. The mechanisms contributing to venous thrombosis in patients with malignancy are the hypercoagulable state and venous compression secondary to tumor growth. The risk is further increased by chemotherapy and metastasis. The role of other molecular thrombophilia as a risk factor for recurrent DVT has also been recognized. Abnormalities of the inhibitors of coagulation (antithrombin, protein C, and protein S), gene polymorphisms (factor V Leiden and prothrombin 20210A), elevated levels of coagulation factors (factor VIII), elevated levels of homocysteine, and circulating antiphospholipid antibodies have all been indicated as risk factors for thrombosis. Pregnancy and estrogen have also been associated with increased risk of DVT. Obesity is another independent predictor of VTE recurrence.

DIAGNOSIS

Multiple strategies have been developed to diagnose DVT. These include combinations of clinical risk stratification, measurement of D-dimer levels, venous ultrasound imaging, and contrast medium–enhanced venography. Duplex ultrasonography is the diagnostic test of choice for DVT. The hallmark of acute DVT is noncompressibility with venous distension and a hypoechoic lumen. Duplex ultrasonography has a mean sensitivity and specificity of 97% and 94%, respectively, with mean positive and negative predictive values of 97% and 98%, respectively, for symptomatic proximal DVT. Other noninvasive imaging includes computed tomographic venography (CTV) and magnetic resonance venography (MRV). If iliofemoral thrombus is identified, contrast medium–enhanced venography should be performed in anticipation of intervention.

Fibrin D-dimer is the final product of the plasmin-mediated degradation of crosslinked fibrin. Its plasma concentration is dependent on fibrin generation and subsequent degradation by the endogenous fibrinolytic system. D-Dimer levels are typically elevated in patients

with acute venous thrombosis. As the result, the sensitivity of an elevated D-dimer concentration for VTE is very high. On the other hand, D-dimer levels can be elevated in other clinical conditions that are associated with enhanced fibrin production, including malignancy, trauma, increased age, disseminated intravascular coagulation, inflammation, infection, sepsis, postoperative states, and preeclampsia. Consequently, the specificity of an elevated D-dimer level for acute thrombosis is rather poor. Thus the diagnostic strength of D-dimer tests lies in ruling out DVT or pulmonary embolism.

Venous duplex ultrasonography, which combines B-mode imaging and Doppler signal analysis, is the first-line imaging modality for patients with clinically suspected DVT. The femoral and popliteal veins are directly visualized and subsequently assessed for their compressibility. Noncompressible femoral or popliteal vein, or both, is diagnostic for a first episode of acute proximal DVT in patients suspected of having clinically manifested DVT. In general, venous duplex ultrasonography is a cost-effective, accurate, and noninvasive diagnostic tool and serves as a first choice of imaging modality in patients with clinically suspected DVT of the lower extremities.

Historically, contrast medium–enhanced venography has been the diagnostic modality for lower extremity DVT. The diagnosis of DVT is confirmed when a constant intraluminal filling defect is identified on at least two views angiographically after intravenous administration of contrast material. Contrast medium–enhanced venography is contraindicated in pregnant women to avoid exposure of the fetus to radiation. Administration requires an invasive approach and can often lead to allergic reaction. Consequently, this invasive and costly diagnostic modality is seldom used today.

Computed tomographic scan (CT) and magnetic resonance imaging (MRI) may serve as alternative or complementary imaging tools to duplex ultrasonography. However, in comparison with duplex ultrasonography, both modalities have not been as well evaluated. The majority of clinical studies of the diagnostic accuracy of CT were performed in patients with suspected pulmonary embolism without symptoms or signs of lower extremity venous thrombosis, for whom the CT scan was subsequently extended to the legs. MRV can be performed with or without intravenously administered gadolinium. Although numerous studies have demonstrated that the sensitivity and specificity of CTV and MRV are comparable with those of duplex ultrasonography, the safety of withholding anticoagulant treatment on the basis of normal findings on CTV or MRV has not been evaluated. Consequently, these imaging modalities cannot be recommended as first-line imaging approaches. CTV or MRV could be useful in patients with a suspected DVT in whom duplex ultrasonography cannot be performed or is less reliable, such as patients with morbid obesity or casts and patients with a suspected DVT in the iliac or inferior cava vein or suspected venous anomaly.

THERAPY

The latest guidelines of the American College of Chest Physicians recommend treatment with a full-dose of unfractionated heparin (UFH), low-molecular-weight heparin (LMWH), fondaparinux, vitamin K antagonist (VKA), or thrombolysis for most patients with objectively confirmed VTE. However, to prevent life-threatening pulmonary embolism (PE) in patients with VTE and contraindications to anticoagulant treatment, such as bleeding complications during antithrombotic treatment or VTE recurrences despite optimal anticoagulation, interruption of the inferior vena cava (IVC) with a filter should be considered. Likewise, catheter-guided thrombolysis and mechanical thrombectomy are interventional modalities that can be considered in selected patients. The efficacy and safety of these therapeutic approaches and the appropriate indications are discussed herein.

Anticoagulation

Patients with acute DVT should be treated with parenteral anticoagulant therapy, followed by VKA therapy, for 3 months. The duration depends on the risk of recurrence, as determined by the presence or absence of an inciting event and the presence of hypercoagulable states. Anticoagulation, however, only prevents clot propagation; the patient's own fibrinolytic system must open occluded segments to restore patency and preserve valvular function. The anatomic location of DVT can influence the risk of VTE recurrence. The more proximal the upper limit of the initial clot, the higher the risk of recurrence. In comparison with patients with femoral or popliteal DVT, patients with iliofemoral DVT have a significantly higher risk of recurrence. Isolated distal DVT could be safely treated with 6 weeks of anticoagulant therapy, especially when the event was triggered by a transient risk factor. In patients with acute isolated distal DVT of the leg and without severe symptoms or risk factors for extension, serial imaging of the deep veins for 2 weeks is an acceptable alternative to initial anticoagulation, especially in patients with high risk of bleeding. Anticoagulation should be started if the thrombus extends. Proximal DVT should be treated for 3 months. If the DVT is unprovoked, extended therapy is given if bleeding risk is low or moderate. When DVT is associated with active cancer, extended therapy with LMWH is recommended over VKA, and is given as long as the cancer remains active.

Surgical Thrombectomy

Enthusiasm for surgical thrombectomy for DVT in the United States was initially high and has fallen with subsequent reports of poor results. Serial reports of the European results have rekindled interest. In a series of reports, Plate described surgical therapy for acute iliofemoral DVT. These reports detailed the experience of patients randomly assigned to undergo anticoagulation versus surgical thrombectomy with creation of a temporary arteriovenous fistula who were monitored for 5 and then 10 years. The numbers of those completing follow-up were small, which reduced the ability to produce statistical significance. Radionuclide venous study showed patency of the iliac vein in 83% of patients with surgical treatment, in comparison with 41% of patients with anticoagulation; this difference was significant. Surgical thrombectomy can be considered if thrombolytic therapy is contraindicated. Surgical thrombectomy can be performed with a Fogarty balloon to remove thrombus through a groin incision for proximal and distal thrombus removal. A temporary arteriovenous fistula is sometimes created to reduce early rethrombosis.

Thrombolytic Therapy

In light of the morbidity of postthrombotic syndrome, more aggressive treatment regimens of DVTs have been proposed. The early reports of surgical thrombectomy and its effect on postthrombotic syndrome encouraged development of nonsurgical methods to remove clots and achieve the same goals with minimally invasive means. Thrombolysis of DVTs offers the potential to rapidly clear thrombus from the obstructed segments and reduce the chance of subsequent obstruction and reflux. There are various means of achieving thrombolysis of occluded venous segments. The basic options are pharmacological thrombolysis, administered directly into the thrombus via an infusion catheter; mechanical thrombectomy; and the combination of the two, termed *pharmacomechanical thrombolysis*. These various options of thrombolytic therapy are discussed as follows.

Catheter-Directed Thrombolytic Therapy

Routine use of systemic thrombolysis for acute DVT is discouraged because of the high rate of incomplete thrombolysis and bleeding complications. Because of inconsistent results, long treatment times, and high complication rates reported with systemic infusions, attention has turned to catheter-directed thrombolysis. Mewissen and colleagues (1999) published a multicenter registry experience of catheter-directed urokinase infusion that included a total of 287 patients who underwent catheter-directed thrombolysis for lower extremity DVT. In this series, complete lysis was noted in 31% of patients; in another 52%, more than 50% lysis was achieved. The degree of lysis was found to be correlated with patency at 1 year. The DVTs in the iliofemoral segment responded better, with 64% patency at 1 year, in comparison with 47% in the femoral popliteal segment. Major bleeding complications occurred in 11% of patients, the majority being puncture site hematomas. There was one intracranial hemorrhage, which was fatal, and one subdural hematoma, which was sustained after a fall. There were PEs in 2% of patients, which was within the expected incidence among patients with proximal DVTs.

Multiple authors have found that catheter-directed therapy is more effective than systemic infusion of thrombolytic agents for treatment of DVTs. Although the numbers are small and the trial was nonrandomized, the data reported by Laiho and colleagues provide a comparison between systemic and catheter-directed thrombolysis for iliofemoral DVTs. Using a hospital registry, they identified 32 patients with iliofemoral DVTs. Equal numbers of patients received catheter-directed and systemic thrombolysis. Catheter-directed thrombolysis proved superior, with a deep system competence of 56% in comparison with 19% in patients with systemic thrombolysis. Paralleling the incidence of deep system reflux was a significantly higher incidence of postthrombotic syndrome in the systemic therapy group. In a review, Baldwin documented the experience in the literature of more than 600 patients with catheter-directed thrombolysis and found decreased rates of postthrombotic syndrome, improved quality of life, and some evidence for reduced incidence of recurrent DVT. The pooled risk of intracranial hemorrhage was noted to be 0.2%.

Mechanical Thrombectomy

Although a detailed discussion of mechanical thrombectomy in DVT is beyond the main focus of this section, this therapeutic modality has become important in the management of thrombotic occlusion, particularly when a mechanical thrombectomy device can be used in conjunction with pharmacological thrombolysis. One of the percutaneous mechanical thrombectomy (PMT) systems that has been shown to be effective in the removal of acute DVT is the AngioJet (Medrad, Minneapolis, Minn.) system. The principle of this device is based on the Venturi effect, which creates rapidly flowing saline jets that are directed backward from the tip of the device to outflow channels in a coaxial manner. This generates a vacuum force that draws the thrombus into the catheter. One major advantage of this treatment modality is that the thrombectomy catheter can be delivered through a small-bore introducer sheath, which reduces access site trauma and avoids operative exposure required with conventional Fogarty thromboembolectomy. A clinical study in which researchers evaluated the efficacy of the AngioJet system demonstrated that such a mechanical thrombectomy system is effective in thrombus removal, venous patency restoration and maintenance, and symptom relief. The Angiojet rheolytic thrombectomy system is designed to produce an area of extremely low pressure at the catheter tip by controlled high-velocity saline jets. Through this mechanism, thrombus surrounding the catheter tip is macerated and rapidly evacuated via an effluent lumen into a collection chamber. In this study, only 4 (23.5%) patients achieved more than 90% thrombus clearance with PMT alone. Adjunctive thrombolytic agents were used in 9 of 17 patients, in whom a lesser amount of clot was extracted with the use of the PMT catheter. Often the thrombolytic catheter was left in place, and the average duration of lytic therapy was 20.2

hours. Clinical symptomatic improvement was seen in 82% over a follow-up time frame of 11 months.

Permanent Inferior Vena Cava Filters

Decousus and colleagues conducted a randomized study to evaluate the efficacy of permanent IVC filter in the prevention of PE. These authors randomly assigned 400 patients with proximal DVT and at risk for PE to receive an IVC filter (200 patients) or no IVC filter (200 patients), in addition to standard anticoagulant therapy. The authors noted that there were no significant differences in mortality or other outcomes at 24 months. The authors therefore concluded that in patients with proximal DVT at high risk, the initial beneficial effect of IVC filters for the prevention of PE was counterbalanced by an excess of recurrent DVT, without any difference in mortality. In a Cochrane review, researchers evaluated all existing published controlled clinical trials and randomized clinical trials in which investigators examined the efficacy of filters in preventing PE. The authors concluded that no recommendations could be made with regard to the use of permanent IVC filter in prevention of pulmonary embolism. Because of the lack of strong evidence in the literature, the most recent guidelines of the American College of Chest Physicians (ACCP) recommend against the routine use of an IVC filter in addition to anticoagulants in patients with DVT; the placement of an IVC filter is suggested only for patients with acute proximal DVT or PE and a contraindication to anticoagulation because of bleeding risk.

Retrievable Inferior Vena Cava Filters

Nonpermanent filters are classified as temporary or retrievable devices. Temporary filters remain attached to a wire or catheter that exits the skin; they are often difficult to manage and are accompanied by frequent complications such as thrombosis, infections, or migrations. They must be removed within a few days of placement, which is often not enough time to solve the clinical problem that had led to their placement. Retrievable filters are a new generation of IVC filters and may represent a more attractive option because they may be either left in place permanently or safely retrieved after a quite long period when they become unnecessary. This optimism must be tempered by important unresolved issues, including the appropriate maximum implantation time, the possibility of safely and efficaciously removing the filters without compromise by entrapped clots, and the use of anticoagulants during the implantation period and at the time of removal.

SPECIAL CONSIDERATIONS

Phlegmasia Alba Dolens and Phlegmasia Cerulea Dolens

Phlegmasia alba dolens, also known as *milk leg* or *white leg syndrome,* is part of a spectrum of clinical syndromes associated with extensive iliofemoral thrombosis. In phlegmasia alba dolens, the iliac vein is occluded, but the hypogastric and collateral veins remain patent. Affected patients have severe swelling and leg tenderness but no ischemia. Management is anticoagulation with or without catheter-directed thrombolysis. Phlegmasia cerulea dolens is characterized by massive swelling, cyanosis, and pain. Pedal pulses remain palpable in 50% of affected patients. Massive fluid sequestration may lead to hypovolemia and hypotension. Sixty percent of affected patients progress to venous gangrene. Anticoagulation alone is ineffective in the treatment of phlegmasia cerulea dolens. Catheter-directed pharmacomechanical thrombolysis is strongly recommended for impending venous gangrene in the presence of iliofemoral thrombosis.

External Compression of Deep Veins

Venous occlusion may result from external compression by retroperitoneal fibrosis, tumor, cyst, aneurysm, abnormal muscle insertion (popliteal vein entrapment), fibrous band of ligament (soleal arch syndrome and femoral vein compression by inguinal ligament), left iliac vein compression by right iliac artery (May-Thurner syndrome) and compression of the subclavian vein by cervical ribs, clavicular anomalies, and musculofascial bands ("effort thrombosis," thoracic outlet syndrome, or Paget-Schroetter disease). The treatment of DVT caused by external compression should include removal of the source of external compression if possible, such as first rib resection and scalenectomy for thoracic outlet syndrome. Percutaneous endovascular stent placement has emerged as the method of choice for treatment of May-Thurner syndrome. Open venous reconstruction is usually performed only in selected cases of failed stent procedures or occlusion of the stent.

Internal Jugular Vein/Axillosubclavian Vein Thrombosis

In the general population, the majority of DVTs occur in the lower extremity. Upper extremity DVTs constitute only 4% of all DVTs. Upper extremity DVT has become more common as a result of increased intravenous catheterization and transvenous pacer placement. Treatment of internal jugular and subclavian vein thrombosis consists of one of the following elements: rest, elevation, external compression, anticoagulation, catheter removal, thrombolytic therapy, surgical decompression of the thoracic outlet, or open or endovascular venous reconstruction. The treatment options depend on the location of the thrombosis; severity of symptoms; the patient's age, level of activity, and general medical condition; the presence of central venous catheter and whether it can be removed; and any contraindications to anticoagulation, thrombolysis, or surgical treatment. Patients with mild symptoms or who are debilitated with significant comorbid conditions tend to have acceptable results with anticoagulation alone. For those with catheter-associated central venous thrombosis, the catheter should be removed if possible. For patients with nonreversible risk factors, such as malignancy and the presence of catheters or pacemaker that cannot be removed, a longer course of anticoagulation (3 to 6 months) is indicated.

Catheter-directed thrombolysis should be considered in patients with axillosubclavian DVT who present with extensive swelling and functional impairment of the arm and who are at low risk for bleeding complications. Affected patients who are young and active with vigorous exercise often have persistent arm swelling and pain exacerbated by upper extremity exercise because the venous outflow from collateralized central venous occlusion often cannot keep up with the arterial inflow. Thrombolytic therapy is more likely to be successful for acute thrombus that has been present less than 1 week. Patients in whom provocative arm positioning elicits extrinsic compression should be considered for a thoracic outlet decompression procedure. Patients with intrinsic venous compromise caused by residual scar or thrombus can be treated with balloon angioplasty with or without stent placement or venous repair in conjunction with thoracic outlet surgery.

Superficial Vein Thrombosis

The majority of the superficial vein thromboses are associated with intravenous catheter placement or related to varicose veins and involve the great saphenous vein (GSV). Such thromboses are treated with rest and nonsteroidal antiinflammatory medication. When the GSV is involved, follow-up ultrasonography should be performed. If the thrombus propagates to the saphenofemoral junction, anticoagulation should be started. Extensive superficial vein thrombosis should be treated with a prophylactic dose of fondaparinux or LMWH.

SUGGESTED READINGS

Bauersachs RM: Clinical presentation of deep vein thrombosis and pulmonary embolism, *Best Pract Res Clin Haematol* 25(3):243–251, 2012.
Casey ET, Murad MH, Zumaeta-Garcia M, et al: Treatment of acute iliofemoral deep vein thrombosis, *J Vasc Surg* 55(5):1463–1473, 2012.
Guyatt GH, Eikelboom JW, Gould MK, et al: Approach to outcome measurement in the prevention of thrombosis in surgical and medical patients: *Antithrombotic therapy and prevention of thrombosis, 9th ed: American College of Chest Physicians evidence-based clinical practice guidelines.* American College of Chest Physicians, *Chest* 141(2 Suppl): e185S–e194S, 2012.
Hogg K, Wells PS, Gandara E: The diagnosis of venous thromboembolism, *Semin Thromb Hemost* 38(7):691–701, 2012.
Imberti D, Ageno W, Manfredini R, et al: Interventional treatment of venous thromboembolism: a review, *Thromb Res* 129:418–425, 2012.
Wilbur J, Shian B: Diagnosis of deep venous thrombosis and pulmonary embolism, *Am Fam Physician* 86(10):913–919, 2012.

VENA CAVA FILTERS

**Christos S. Georgiades, MD, PhD, FSIR, and
Todd Schlachter, MD**

INTRODUCTION

The rationale for inferior vena cava (IVC) interruption by means of filter placement is prevention of clinically significant pulmonary embolism (PE) with trapping of venous emboli that originate in the deep veins of the pelvis or the lower extremities. Deep venous thrombosis (DVT) is a major cause of morbidity and mortality in the United States, with an annual incidence of approximately 2,000,000. The incidence of clinically significant PE in the United States is reportedly between 150,000 and 600,000, with 25% to 40% of patients presenting with sudden death. The remaining patients are treated with either systemic anticoagulation therapy or placement of IVC filter, and rarely with surgical or catheter-directed thrombectomy or thrombolysis. Venous thromboembolic disease (VTE) constitutes a clinical spectrum that includes both DVT and PE.

The history of IVC interruption for the prevention of PE was born from the work of Virchow, Trousseau, and Bottini in the mid to late 1800s. Mechanical prevention of pulmonary embolus has evolved from open surgical ligation of the IVC to the percutaneous endovascular filters used today. Since the advent of a percutaneous approach by Greenfield in 1983, the use of IVC filters has drastically increased. From 1980 to 2000, the number of filters placed increased from 2000 to about 50,000 per year. The first IVC filter was marketed in the late 1960s. Before that, surgical ligation of the IVC, first described by Armand Trousseau in 1865, was the only option for prevention of PE in patients at high risk. In 2007, almost 167,000 filters were implanted, with an estimated 259,000 IVC filters to be deployed in 2012. With the increasing market demand for filters came a diversity of filter designs and capabilities including, most notably, the ability for retrieval.

The standard treatment of acute DVT or PE is nearly always immediate, full pharmacologic anticoagulation therapy. IVC filters are indicated when a patient has VTE and contraindications to or complications from anticoagulation, or recurrent embolism while on adequate therapy. IVC filters may also be used as PE prophylaxis in patients deemed at high risk for clinically significant PE. Although filters are accepted as safe devices, there are still filter-associated risks. Therefore, the indications for filter placement and the choice of the appropriate filter must be carefully followed. Figure 1 shows the 10 filter types (13 different filters) available in the United States, and Table 1 showcases their features.

INDICATIONS AND CONTRAINDICATIONS FOR INFERIOR VENA CAVA FILTER PLACEMENT AND RETRIEVAL

Table 2 summarizes the indications for IVC filter placement. Most IVC filters are placed in patients with DVT who have a contraindication to anticoagulation (56%) or in patients at high risk for prophylaxis (27%) or in patients with recurrent PE despite anticoagulation therapy (15%). Patients may have a preexisting contraindication to anticoagulation because they are at high risk for bleeding complications. Such conditions include intracranial neoplasm, vascular neoplasm in critical locations, recent myocardial infarction (MI), and recent surgery or trauma. Other patients may "declare" themselves as high risk with a recent history of gastrointestinal (GI) hemorrhage, intracranial hemorrhage (ICH), or other hemorrhage. Combined, this group represents the majority of patients (56%) who receive an IVC filter.

Trauma-related severe multiorgan injury is a major risk factor for DVT and PE. When these patients have a PE, their mortality risk is much higher compared with patients with non-trauma–related PE. PE is thought to contribute to or be the direct cause of death in at least 85% of trauma patients with PE. Therefore, prevention is crucial for a positive outcome. In some patients with major trauma, the associated bleeding risk precludes effective anticoagulation therapy, leaving IVC filters as the only option to prevent PE from DVT.

Major surgery raises the risk for VTE for many reasons. Prolonged immobilization of the patient is common, especially after major abdominal, neurologic (especially), and orthopedic surgeries. The risk of VTE is increased, albeit less, even in minor surgeries. Transient dehydration is another factor that predisposes patients to the formation of clot, as is surgery-associated vascular injury or extrinsic compression. All patients undergoing surgery should receive some form of prophylaxis for VTE. In most cases, pneumatic compression stockings are adequate because recovery from surgery is relatively short. When recovery is prolonged and the risk of DVT is high, pharmacologic anticoagulation therapy has been shown to reduce the risk of VTE. However, many patients are not candidates for anticoagulation therapy after surgery. Until recently, placement of an IVC filter in these patients was avoided because of the transient nature of the risk for VTE. Since the advent of retrievable filters, however, their use in the perioperative period has increased because they can be removed after the risk normalizes. In particular, preoperative placement of an IVC filter reduces the risk of pulmonary embolus and perioperative mortality in patients undergoing open gastric bypass for morbid obesity with a body mass index (BMI) of more than 55 kg/m².

A smaller percentage of patients (15%) receive an IVC filter because of recurrent PE during anticoagulation therapy. An important note is that PE during anticoagulation therapy does not

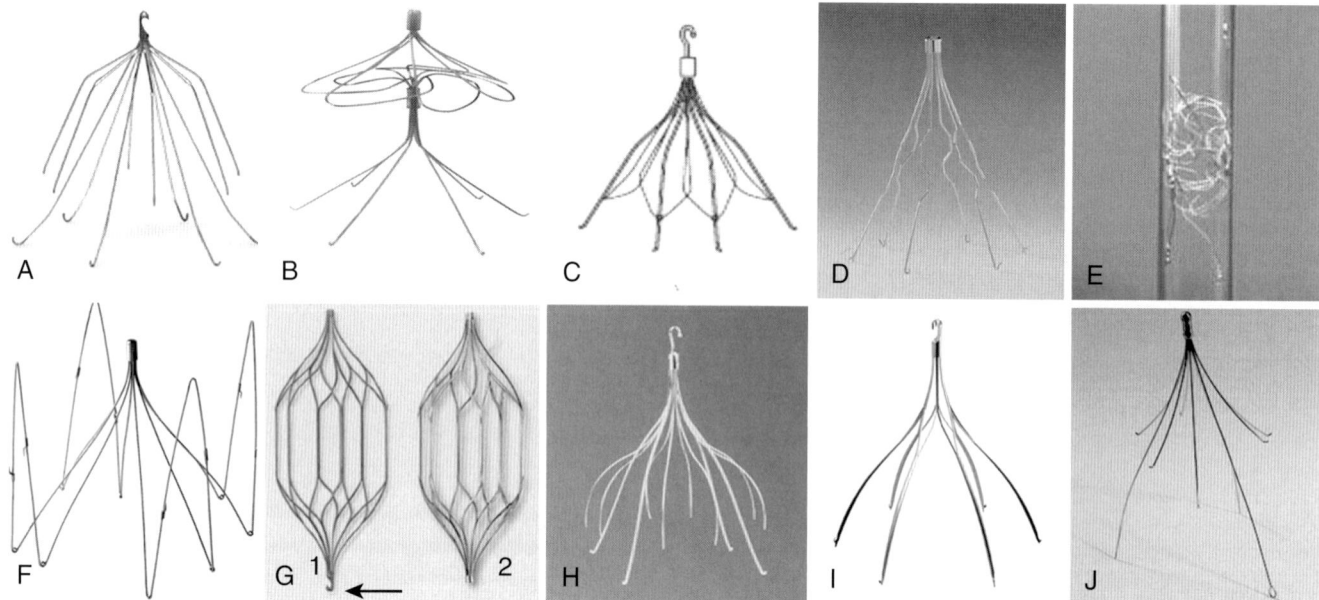

FIGURE 1   The filters available in the United States. **A,** The Bard family of filters that includes the original G2, the newest Meridien, and the (electropolished) Eclipse (Bard, Tempe, Ariz). **B,** Simon Nitinol (Bard, Tempe, Ariz). **C,** Gunther-Tulip (Cook Medical, Bloomington, Ind). **D,** Greenfield (Boston Scientific, Natick, Mass). **E,** Bird's Nest (Cook Medical, Bloominton, Ind). **F,** Vena-Tech (B-Braun Medical, Bethlehem, Penn). **G,** Optease (*1*; with retrievability hook in bottom) and Trapease (*2;* Cordis , Bridgewater, NJ). **H,** Celect (Cook Medical, Bloominton, Ind). **I,** Option (Argon/Rex Medical, Plano, Tex). **J,** ALN (ALN, Miami, Fla).

represent failure of anticoagulation. One must ensure that the measure of the efficacy of anticoagulation (international normalized ratio [INR] for warfarin; activated partial thromboplastin time ratio [aPTTr] for heparin) was within the therapeutic range when the PE occurred. If not, the dose should be adjusted so that the outcome measure is within therapeutic range. Only then should a filter be considered. The risk of PE recurrence for patients during therapeutic anticoagulation is 5% to 10%.

Free-floating clot in the IVC or iliofemoral veins is extremely rare. If clot is identified incidentally, then a prophylactic filter is indicated as is anticoagulation therapy. Free-floating clots are usually fresh clots and thus vulnerable to anticoagulation. If the patient does not need long-term prophylaxis with a filter, then a retrievable one is indicated; it is removed when the clot resolves. Chronic pulmonary hypertension with limited pulmonary reserve is a rare condition of unknown cause, although chronic thromboembolic events have been postulated to be the main culprit. Along with etiology, treatment is controversial. It does not present a serious medical problem from an epidemiologic standpoint because only 500 to 2500 new cases are reported each year. However, given the limited pulmonary reserve in these patients, prevention of further embolic events is crucial for survival. Although no prospective, randomized study exists to show any benefit from routine IVC filter placement in such patients, most centers that treat such patients recommend routine IVC filter placement for the prevention of new embolic events. Even without anticoagulation therapy, patients who receive an IVC filter alone show a significantly reduced PE-related mortality.

A smaller percentage of patients who receive a filter (19% to 27%) do so because they are considered at high risk for development of DVT and therefore sustaining a life-threatening PE. This category includes patients with multiple risk factors that when combined place them at significant risk for VTE.

Both acquired and congenital thrombotic risk factors are additive for each patient presentation. Acquired risk factors include the following: age, surgery or major trauma, cancer, human immunodeficiency virus (HIV), antiphospholipid syndrome, pregnancy/ postpartum, immobility, oral contraceptives, smoking, travel, and infections. Patients may be immobilized because of major trauma, central nervous system (CNS) injury or deficit, or intensive care unit (ICU) level of care. Congenital hypercoagulable states include antithrombin III deficiency, protein C or S deficiency, factor V Leiden mutation, prothrombin 20210A, sickle cell disease, and hyperhomocysteinemia, most commonly.

These patients are very common in clinical practice and present a difficult therapeutic challenge. On one hand, the underlying disease predisposes the patient to DVT and thus an increased risk for PE; on the other hand, the filter itself may be the cause of focal clot formation and subsequent IVC thrombosis. Even in patients with contraindication to anticoagulation, filter placement should be considered carefully and only with input from the hematology service. Patients who despite their hypercoagulable state do not have a DVT or PE should in general not receive a filter. At the other end of the spectrum are patients with DVT and recurrent PE who cannot receive anticoagulation and should receive a filter. The gray zone in between is more common, and the decision to place a filter should be based on a careful multidisciplinary risk–benefit analysis. For example, asymptomatic DVTs have been reported in 60% to 80% of patients with permanent spinal cord injury, whereas symptomatic DVT is reported in less than 20%. Therefore, IVC filter placement in patients with paraplegia or tetraplegia should not be routine but reserved in patients with documented, symptomatic DVT or in those who cannot or will not receive lifelong systemic anticoagulation therapy.

FILTER SELECTION

No study exists that compares the efficacy and safety of the available filter types in a rigorous manner. Therefore, the choice of filter should depend on technical factors (i.e., size of IVC) and operator experience.

TABLE 1: Profiles of the 13 filters available in the United States

Filter (company)	Sheath size	Max IVC diameter	MRI compatibility	Retrievability	Notes
G2, Meridien, Eclipse (Bard, Tempe, Ariz)	10F	28 mm	Conditional (up to 3 T)	Yes	
Simon-Nitinol (Bard, Tempe, Ariz)	7F	28 mm	Safe	No	If general anesthesia within 2 wk, maximal IVC diameter is 24 mm
Gunther-Tulip (Cook Medical, Bloomington, Ind)	8.5F	30 mm	Conditional (up to 1.5 T)	Yes	
Greenfield Meditech, Boston Scientific Corp., Natick, Mass	12F	28 mm	Conditional	No	(Titanium Greenfield system, Steel not available)
Bird's Nest (Cook Medical, Bloomington, Ind)	11F	40 mm	Conditional (up to 1.5 T)	No	(7-cm footprint)
Vena-Tech (B-Braun Medical, Bethlehem, Penn)	9F	28 mm	Safe	No	
Optease (Cordis, Bridgewater, NJ)	6F	30 mm	Conditional (up to 3 T)	Yes (up to 23 d)	
Trapease (Cordis, Bridgewater, NJ)	6F	30 mm	Conditional (up to 3 T)	No	
Celect (Cook Medical, Bloomington, Ind)	8.5F	30 mm	Conditional (up to 3 T)	Yes	
Option (Argon/Rex Medical, Plano, Tex)	6.5F	30 mm	Conditional (up to 3 T)	Yes	
ALN (ALN, Miami, Fla)	7F	28 mm	Compatible (limited data)	Yes	

IVC, Inferior vena cava; *MRI,* magnetic resonance imaging.
(Three successive generations of Bard filters are included in first row). All current filters are MRI safe or conditional, meaning they are safe for immediate MRI use up to 1.5 to 3.0 T. For IVC diameters above 30 mm, only the Bird's Nest can be deployed. Retrievability is another major determinant of filter choice.

TABLE 2:   Current indications for inferior vena cava filter placement

DVT with high risk for bleeding (i.e. recent major trauma, surgery including cardiopulmonary resuscitation)	56%
Hemorrhage on or failure of anticoagulation (i.e., recurrent PE, patient non-compliance)	15%
Extreme risk of morbidity/mortality from next PE (i.e., limited cardiopulmonary reserve, large/free floating thrombus, chronic PE with pulmonary HTN)	2%
High risk despite anticoagulation (i.e., severe trauma with prolonged immobilization, paraplegia, quadriplegia, multiple/severe bone fractures, surgery in patients with BMI >55 Kg/m^2	27%
Total	100%

BMI, Body mass index; *CNS,* central nervous system; *DVT,* deep vein thrombosis; *HTN,* hypertension; *PE,* pulmonary embolism.

Special Considerations: Suprarenal Inferior Vena Cava Filter

The ideal location of any IVC filter is properly centered (not skewed) in the IVC with its cephalad tip at or just below the lowermost renal vein. Placement of the filter too low may result in a higher rate of IVC thrombosis related to filter-induced turbulent flow. Placement of the filter above the renal veins may result in renal failure if the filter thromboses and the resulting clot obstructs the renal vein drainage, although this is an extremely rare complication. At times, placement of a filter in a suprarenal location is necessary despite this higher risk. Such indications include pregnancy, duplicated IVC, and thrombosis of the infrarenal IVC. Whatever the indication, if feasible, any suprarenal IVC filter should be removed as soon as the risk of PE returns to baseline. Therefore, retrievable filters are preferred in this location.

Special Considerations: Superior Vena Cava Filters

There is little indication that superior vena cava (SVC) filters offer any VTE protection. In addition, a higher risk of complications is found, especially of filter migration or embolization, and retrieval may be more challenging. Therefore, the insertion of an SVC filter should be reserved for well-selected cases of significant risk of life-threatening PE from the upper extremities.

Contraindications for Placement of Inferior Vena Cava Filter

Contraindications for IVC filter placement are both technical and clinical. Technical reasons include a thrombosed or occluded IVC, clot in the intrahepatic IVC, and no available venous access. Clinical contraindications include severe uncorrectable coagulopathy, severe prothrombotic state, and active bacteremia. Although active bacteremia is a contraindication to filter placement, the risk of seeding a filter is probably extremely low. If a filter is necessary in a patient with active bacteremia, then a retrievable one may be placed; it should be removed as soon as not needed or replaced as soon as bacteremia resolves. A prothrombotic state increases the risk for in situ filter clot formation. It should not prevent filter placement if

protection against potentially lethal PE is necessary. Hematology input is important to screen these patients and have a plan of action related to type of filter used, duration of protection, retrieval, and possibly concurrent systemic anticoagulation therapy.

TECHNIQUE

Optimum performance requires catheter expertise, proper venous access selection, appropriate filter type, and proper location and orientation of the deployed filter. First, the clinical indication for IVC filter placement should be scrutinized and confirmed. Next, informed consent must be obtained from the patient. Then, review of imaging studies and physical examination of the patient dictate appropriate venous access selection.

The basic steps of filter insertion are:

1. Selection of appropriate venous access. Left common femoral vein access has the advantage of showing clearly the presence (or absence) of a duplicated or left-sided IVC. Of course, the location of DVT may confound site selection. Right common femoral, right jugular, and left jugular vein accesses are also available. If a long enough sheath or filter is available, antecubital of popliteal vein access is also possible.
2. IVC venogram. This necessary step is used to measure the diameter of the IVC, exclude clot in the IVC, and delineate any aberrant anatomy (i.e., retroaortic or duplicated renal veins).
3. Deployment of filter. Ideal location is with its cephalad tip being bathed by the renal vein inflow to mitigate the filter's thrombogenicity.
4. A post deployment venogram or plain view to ensure proper filter positioning.

For patients with a duplicated IVC, the filter may be placed in both inferior cavae, or a suprarenal filter may be considered when technically feasible. If the vena cava diameter is greater than 28 to 30 mm ("mega cava"), an appropriate filter must be selected. Currently, the only available filter for a mega cava is the Bird's Nest filter (Cook Medical, Bloomington, Ind). Up to 2% of patients have a mega cava. Although a Bird's Nest filter expands to 40 mm, it requires a 7-cm infrarenal footprint. Alternatively, bilateral common iliac vein filters may be deployed. Once all diagnostic imaging has been reviewed, final filter selection may occur. Figure 2 shows the critical aspects of IVC filter deployment.

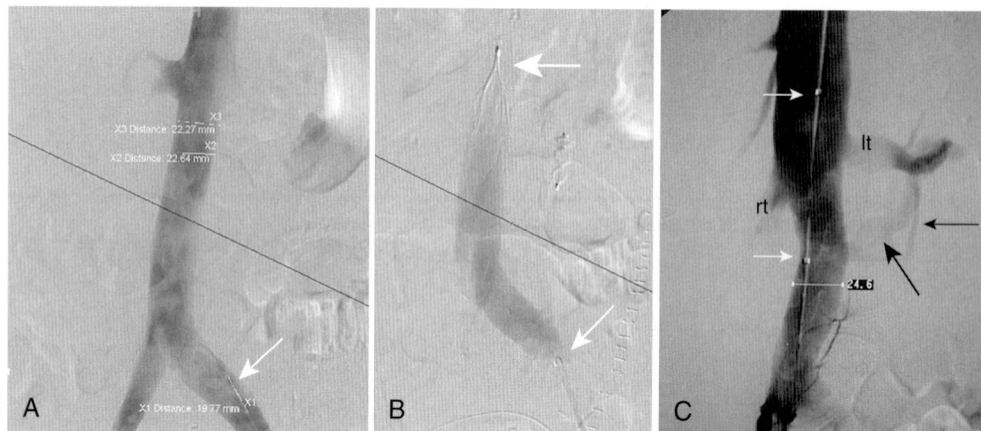

FIGURE 2 Steps during filter deployment. **A,** Inferior vena cava (IVC) venogram performed via a left common femoral vein access *(black arrow)* shows a single IVC, no obstructive clot, and no aberrant venous anatomy. The diameter of the IVC is measured at the level of the filter hook implantation at 23 mm. **B,** Postdeployment venogram in a different patient shows the filter properly centered and with its tip bathed by the renal vein inflow, the optimum location. **C,** Predeployment IVC venogram in a different patient uncovers a left retroaortic renal vein *(large black arrow)* next to a normal gonadal vein *(small black arrow)*. To prevent PE via the retroaortic renal vein, the filter must be deployed below that vein's origin.

FILTER RETRIEVAL

Any filter that can be retrieved and is no longer needed or effective should be removed as soon as possible. If the patient's underlying risk factors for PE are low or if the patient has become a candidate for anticoagulation therapy, the filter should be removed. If the filter itself is ineffective (migrated, kinked, fractured), it should be removed and, if necessary, replaced. In patients with active bacteremia when no other source is isolated, the possibly of an infected filter should be considered and the filter removed or replaced. Regarding retrievable filters, the U.S. Food and Drug Administration (FDA) issued the following statement: "implanting physicians and clinicians responsible for the ongoing care of patients with retrievable IVC filters consider removing the filter as soon as protection form PE is no longer needed."

Filter retrieval is more challenging and requires more extensive skills; however, in experienced hands, filter retrieval is successful greater than 90% on the time. Filter endothelialization is thought to start to occur around 3 weeks; therefore, the less time a filter has been in place, the higher the retrieval success rate. A venogram is required to exclude residual clot within the filter before removal. A filter with a large volume of clot cannot be removed for fear of causing PE during removal. Thus, many filters that are labeled as retrievable become permanent ones. If a small amount of clot is present, bringing the patient back in 6 weeks for reevaluation may show resolution of clot from endogenous lyses. Another contraindication to filter removal is persistent clot in the pelvic or lower extremity veins, unless the patient can now undergo anticoagulation therapy. Unless the risk for PE normalizes and if the patient is still not a candidate for anticoagulation therapy, the filter cannot be removed.

Proper access depends on the type of filter used. The Celect (Cook Medical, Bloomington, Ind), G2 (Bard, Tempe, Ariz), and Günther-Tulip filters (COOK Medical, Bloomington, Ind) are removed via a jugular approach, whereas the Optease (Cordis, Bridgewater, NJ) is removed via a femoral approach. Figure 3 shows the steps for filter removal for a G2 filter.

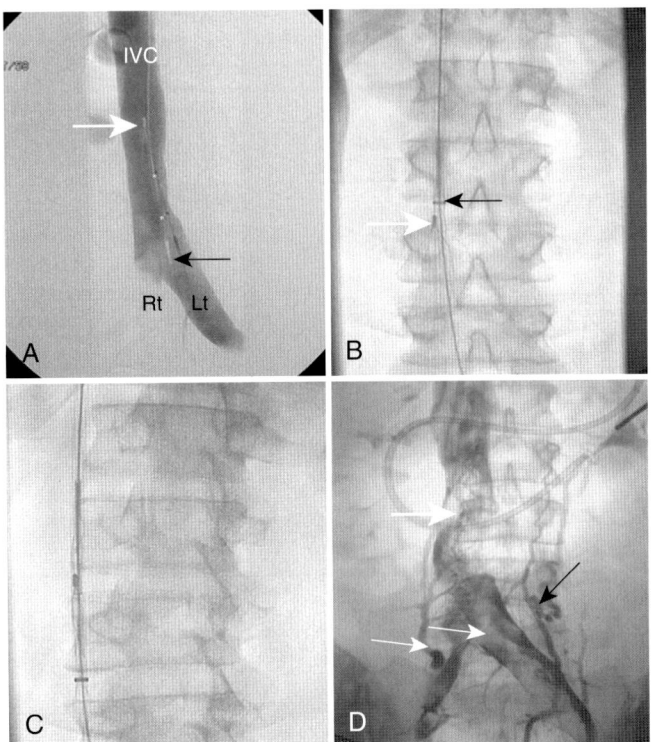

FIGURE 3   Retrieval of a G2 filter. **A,** A preretrieval venogram performed via the jugular-placed catheter *(black arrow)* excludes clot in the right, left common iliac veins, and inferior vena cava (IVC). Filter tip is indicated with *white arrow.* **B,** Then, the sheath is advanced over the conical retrieval system *(black arrow)* and grabs the cephalad tip of the filter *(white arrow).* **C,** The filter is pulled into the sheath and is then removed en bloc. **D,** Preretrieval IVC venogram in a different patient shows a large burden of clot in filter *(large white arrow),* iliac vein *(white arrows),* and collateral drainage *(black arrow)* precluding filter removal.

COMPLICATIONS

Complications related to IVC filters are periprocedural or delayed. Periprocedural complications include filter malpositioning, migration, iatrogenic pulmonary embolism, groin hematoma, and infection. All of these complications can be avoided with experience and proper patient preparation. Meticulous technique and experience can prevent malpositioning, choice of appropriate filter can prevent migration, and proper technique and patient care can prevent hematoma and infection. The rates of these complications are listed in Table 3 and range between 0 and 6%. The most feared complication of IVC filters is filter thrombosis with subsequent IVC occlusion and possible PE. Long-term IVC thrombosis after filter placement is reportedly between 2% and 19%, and the risk increases with indwelling time.

DISCUSSION

The standard of treatment for VTE is systemic anticoagulation therapy. A major misconception is that systemic anticoagulation therapy with warfarin, heparin, low molecular-weights heparin (LMWH), or argatroban treats existing thrombus. The goal of systemic anticoagulation therapy is to prevent extension of existing clot and recurrence of DVT or PE. A 6-month systemic anticoagulation therapy reduces the 2-year risk of recurrent DVT or PE by 50%, from 18% to 9%. However, not all patients have the same risk for development of thromboembolic disease nor do all patients have the same pulmonary reserve. Therefore, treatment should be tailored according to individual risk and ability to sustain a thromboembolic event. Patients with first-time DVT or PE with idiopathic disease and normal pulmonary reserve should be treated with systemic anticoagulation therapy alone. This group represents the majority of patients. However, a large number of patients for a variety of reasons cannot receive anticoagulation and still others have comorbid conditions that increase their risk of recurrence, limit their tolerance to another event, or altogether prevent them from undergoing anticoagulation therapy. These are the patients that should be considered for an IVC filter.

An explosive increase in IVC filter utilization has been seen in the last decade with the advent of more versatile filters and increased incidence of VTE. IVC filters reduce the risk of PE without affecting all-cause mortality and have increased rates of rethrombosis at 8 years. Breakthrough pulmonary emboli are reported to occur in 1% to 6% of patients; however, recurrent fatal PE is less than 1%. Most worrisome is the possibility that IVC filters may confer a risk of postthrombotic syndrome. It is therefore prudent to properly select the patients and ensure placement of an IVC filter is truly indicated. The clinical scenario for each patient is different and affects the choice of filter, retrievability, location, duration, and associated risks. When unsure about the duration of required protection, a retrievable filter should be selected. Any filter that is no longer providing its intended benefit, whether because the underlying risk for PE has returned to baseline or the filter is ineffective, should be removed as soon as possible. The longer a filter remains in a patient, the more likely it will become permanent because of clot formation or

TABLE 3: List of periprocedural and long-term complications of filter deployment

Complication	Reported rates (%)
Death	0.1
Access site thrombosis	3-10
Deployment outside target area	1-9
Iatrogenic pulmonary embolism	1
Filter movement	0-18
Filter embolization	0.1
Filter fracture	2-10
IVC penetration	<1
IVC occlusion	2-30 (long-term)

IVC, Inferior vena cava.

The herein reported rates of access site thrombosis (up to 10%) and filter movement (up to 18%) are extremely high and should approach 0 with experience and proper technique.

Complications from IVC filter placement can be procedure related (groin hematoma, infection, or iatrogenic pulmonary embolism [PE]) or delayed (migration, IVC thrombosis). With the exception of in situ filter thrombosis, the associated risks are minimal (1% to 6%). However, IVC thrombosis can lead to considerable morbidity, including PE and symptoms of lower extremity venous stasis. Long-term follow-up of patients with filters is limited, and the true risk of IVC thrombosis is unknown. Removal of a filter that is no longer needed or is ineffective (kinked, fractured, source of PE upper extremities) is indicated to minimize this risk.

BOX 1: Take-home messages

1. IVC filters may reduce mortality from PE, but only in well-selected patients.
2. IVC filters reduce risk for symptomatic PE.
3. Permanent IVC filters increase risk of future DVT.
4. Err on side of retrievable filters.
5. Remove filter as soon as indicated.
6. Incidence of symptomatic PE in United States is 160,000 to 600,000.
7. 260,000 filters will be deployed in 2012.

DVT, Deep vein thrombosis; *IVC,* inferior vena cava; *PE,* pulmonary embolism.

endothelialization. The main take-home messages of this chapter are summarized in Box 1.

SUGGESTED READINGS

Caplin DM, Nikolic B, Kalva SP, et al: Quality improvement guidelines for the performance of inferior vena cava filter placement for the prevention of pulmonary embolism, *J Vasc Interv Radiol* 22:1499, 2011.
Kaufman JA, Kinney TB, Streiff MB, et al: Guidelines for the use of retrievable and convertible vena cava filters: report from the Society of Interventional Radiology multidisciplinary consensus conference, *J Vasc Interv Radiol* 17(3):449–459, 2006.
Kinney TB: Update on inferior vena cava filters, *J Vasc Interv Radiol* 14:425–440, 2003.
PREPIC study group: Eight-year follow-up of patients with permanent vena cava filters in the prevention of pulmonary embolism: the PREPIC randomized study, *Circulation* 112:416, 2005.

THE PREVENTION OF VENOUS THROMBOEMBOLISM

Eric J. Turney, MD, and Sean P. Lyden, MD

EPIDEMIOLOGY

Venous thromboembolism (VTE) is defined as deep vein thrombosis (DVT), pulmonary embolism (PE), or both. Two thirds of the patients with VTE present with DVT, and the remaining one third present with PE. DVT can occur in the setting of an inciting event or be idiopathic. According to the Centers for Disease Control and Prevention, VTE affects 300,000 to 600,000 individuals in the United States each year and causes significant morbidity. Up to one third of patients with VTE have a recurrence within 10 years, and the mortality rate from pulmonary embolism can be as high as 30%. VTE may account for 100,000 deaths per year and is the leading cause of preventable hospital death. Unfortunately, fewer than 40,000 deaths associated with VTE are recorded each year in vital records. One half of lower extremity DVT patients have development of chronic venous insufficiency and postthrombotic syndrome.

Both hospitalized medical and surgical patients routinely have multiple risk factors for VTE, and pharmacologic methods to prevent VTE are safe, effective, and cost effective and advocated by authoritative guidelines. Despite the nearly universal risk of VTE among inpatients, large prospective studies continue to show that preventative measures are significantly underutilized. In the era of changing healthcare and pay for performance, the Centers for Medicare and Medicaid Services is considering the inclusion of hospital-acquired DVT and PE in its list of events for which hospitals will no longer be reimbursed. The need for understanding of risk factors, appropriate use of preventative measures, and use of algorithms to treat VTE has never been more important.

RISK FACTORS

Rudolph Virchow first proposed in 1884 that thrombosis was the result of at least one of the following etiologic factors: vascular endothelial damage, stasis of blood flow, and hypercoagulability of blood. In the last century, we have recognized that all VTE risk factors (Table 1) reflect these underlying processes, and convincing evidence shows that risk increases in proportion to the number of predisposing factors. Strong risk factors for VTE (odds ratio, >10) include hip or leg fracture, hip or knee replacement, major general surgery, major

TABLE 1: Identified risk factors for venous thromboembolism

Genetic	Acquired	Transient acquired
Family history	Advanced age	Pregnancy
Factor V Leiden	Antiphospholipid antibodies	Oral contraceptives/hormone therapy
Prothrombin G20210A	Cancer	Central venous lines
Protein C deficiency	Chronic disease	Hospitalization
Protein S deficiency	Obesity	Surgery
Antithrombin deficiency	Congestive heart failure	Trauma
Sickle cell trait	Stroke	Immobilization

TABLE 2: Risk of deep vein thrombosis in hospitalized patients with no prophylaxis and routine objective screening

Patient group	DVT incidence rate (%)
Medical patients	10-26
Major gynecologic, urologic, or general surgery	15-40
Neurosurgery	15-40
Stroke	11-75
Hip or knee surgery	40-60
Major trauma	40-80
Spinal cord injury	60-80
Critical care patients	15-80

DVT, Deep vein thrombosis.

TABLE 3: Contraindications and other conditions to consider with pharmacologic venous thromboembolism prophylaxis

Absolute	Relative	Other conditions
Active hemorrhage Severe trauma to head or spinal cord with hemorrhage in the last 4 wk	Intracranial hemorrhage within last year Craniotomy within 2 wk Intraocular surgery within 2 wk Gastrointestinal, genitourinary hemorrhage within last month Thrombocytopenia (<50K) or coagulopathy (prothrombin time, >18 s) End-stage liver disease Active intracranial lesions/neoplasms Hypertensive urgency/emergency Postoperative bleeding concerns	Immune-mediated heparin-induced thrombocytopenia Epidural analgesia with spinal catheter (current or planned)

trauma, and spinal cord injury. Moderate risk factors for VTE (odds ratio, 2 to 9) include arthroscopic knee surgery, central venous lines, chemotherapy, congestive heart failure, respiratory failure, hormone replacement therapy, malignancy disease, oral contraceptive therapy, paralytic stroke, postpartum pregnancy state, previous venous thromboembolism, and thrombophilia. Weak risk factors for VTE (odds ratio, <2) include bed rest for longer than 3 days, immobility from sitting (prolonged car or air travel), increasing age, laparoscopic surgery, obesity, antepartum pregnancy state, and varicose veins.

Without proper prophylactic measures, the risk of DVT can be quite high in surgical patients, with specific factors such as age, type of surgery, immobility, infection or inflammatory state, central venous access, and history of cancer or previous thrombosis playing an important role (Table 2). Major general surgery is a risk, and the term is generally used for patients undergoing abdominal or thoracic surgical operations that require general anesthesia lasting longer than 30 minutes. Advanced cancers, especially cancers of the breast, lung, brain, pelvis, rectum, pancreas, and gastrointestinal tract, are associated with a high risk of VTE. The administration of chemotherapy for cancer also increases VTE risk.

VENOUS THROMBOEMBOLISM PROPHYLAXIS

A VTE prophylaxis protocol is the best way to ensure all hospital patients are treated. An ideal VTE protocol should be well integrated into all admission, transfer, and postoperative orders. A properly constructed protocol should give the provider the option of using, or not using, the decision support elements. The protocol should define what appropriate prophylaxis is for patients of varied risk. A VTE prophylaxis tool should also offer decision support for contraindications to pharmacologic or heparin prophylaxis (Table 3). Ideally, the best protocols are easy to access and simple to use and fit into the normal workflow of orders as a default action. Multiple VTE risk assessment protocols exist, and no single VTE risk assessment has been prospectively validated as superior to others.

Primary VTE prophylaxis is accomplished by either mechanical or pharmacologic means, or with a combination of the two. Mechanical prophylaxis includes use of intermittent pneumatic compression

(IPC) or graduated compression stockings and early ambulation. Pneumatic compression works by both reduction in venous stasis and reduction of plasminogen activator inhibitor-1, which results in stimulation of intrinsic fibrinolytic processes. Mechanical prophylaxis is appropriate for surgical patients in the low-risk category and can also be valuable when bleeding risk prohibits pharmacologic methods. Barriers to successful mechanical prophylaxis include noncompliance and presence of extremity surgical procedures or fractures.

Pharmacologic prophylaxis has been shown to be the most effective method for VTE prevention, and multiple agents are available. Low-dose unfractionated heparin (UFH), 5000 units injected subcutaneously every 8 or 12 hours, has been shown to decrease the risk of fatal PE from 0.7% to 0.1%, with negligible risk of bleeding. It is easily administered and inexpensive, and no monitoring is required for the level of anticoagulation. There is a risk of heparin-induced thrombocytopenia (HIT), so platelet levels should be checked every 3 days.

Low molecular-weight heparin (LMWH; dalteparin, enoxaparin), administered subcutaneously once or twice daily, is an alternative that has been shown to be effective in preventing VTE. In the general surgery population, it has been shown to be noninferior to UFH, with a similar risk of bleeding and a slightly decreased risk of HIT. In the trauma and oncologic populations, LMWH has been found to be superior to unfractionated heparin with a similar risk profile.

Fondaparinux, a synthetic pentasaccharide factor Xa inhibitor, has mixed data when compared with LMWH. Several studies suggest it is superior to both dalteparin and enoxaparin, particularly in oncology patients, with similar bleeding profiles, and other studies with an alternative dose of LMWH did not reach the same conclusion.

New oral anticoagulants, rivaroxaban (factor Xa inhibitor) and dabigatran etexilate (factor IIa inhibitor), are two products currently under review in the United States for use in VTE prophylaxis. Pooled data from both phase III trials and randomized control trials suggest that both are more effective than enoxaparin with a similar bleeding risk.

Instances of clear superiority or inferiority do exist among prophylaxis options but only for just a few select patient groups. In medical patients, fondaparinux and the LMWHs enoxaparin and dalteparin have efficacy comparable with heparin given three times a day subcutaneously but offer lower complication rates. In certain higher risk patient groups (e.g., hip and knee replacement, trauma, and spinal cord injury), LMWH has shown superiority over subcutaneous heparin. In certain patient groups (e.g., hip replacement, surgery for cancer, and possibly medical patients with reduced mobility), extending prophylaxis with LMWH to approximately 5 weeks is more effective than providing it for 1 week. In certain patient groups, such as medical inpatients, the adequacy of heparin given twice a day subcutaneously has not been proven. High-quality randomized trials showing relative equivalence of LMWH to UFH all used a 5000-unit, three times a day dosing of UFH. In very high-risk patient groups, the addition of mechanical prophylaxis to a pharmacologic regimen may offer an added benefit. Certain patient groups should not receive certain pharmacologic agents or doses or should receive smaller doses (e.g., LMWH if creatinine clearance less than 30 mL/min, and UFH and LMWH if patient has HIT). Certain patient groups should receive pharmacologic doses in close coordination with other events (e.g., surgery or neuroaxial blockade).

For patients with contraindications to pharmacologic prophylaxis, an alternative approach to decrease the risk of clinically significant VTE is secondary prevention. This consists of screening ultrasound scans at a regular interval aimed at early detection of subclinical venous thrombi. Screening ultrasound scan often is used in conjunction with mechanical prophylaxis measures in the high-risk population.

VENOUS THROMBOEMBOLISM DIAGNOSIS

Any patient with new unilateral extremity swelling or unexplained pain should raise suspicion for DVT. Pain on passive dorsiflexion (Homans' sign) is not reliably present, and any clinical suspicion should prompt venous duplex imaging. For the ambulatory patient, a D-dimer assay is an exceptionally sensitive test (as high as 95%) when the goal is to rule out presence of venous thrombosis.

New-onset shortness of breath, hypoxia, anxiety, or congestive heart failure should prompt concerns for pulmonary embolism. Computed tomographic (CT) angiography of the chest with imaging timed to highlight the pulmonary veins has supplanted ventilation/perfusion scans in the diagnosis of PE. Clinically significant PE is detected with this method with nearly 100% sensitivity.

The gold standard for evaluation for presence of extremity deep venous thrombosis is venous duplex scan. Venous duplex examination is highly sensitive and specific, noninvasive, and poses no risk to the patient. In quality noninvasive vascular laboratories, the evaluation of the infrapopliteal veins is also easily accomplished, as are upper extremity/neck veins. With utilization of Doppler flow characteristics, thrombosis of veins within the abdomen and chest can also be detected, although not always visually confirmed. Duplex scan can determine whether DVT is acute or chronic. Acute clot is hypoechoic, with distended noncompressible veins. Respiratory phasic flow is lost, and flow does not augment with compression. Chronic clot is hyperechoic, and the vein is contracted or nondilated. With chronic clot, the vein remains noncompressible or partially compressible.

Other means of diagnosing DVT include contrast-enhanced venous phase CT scan, magnetic resonance venographic (MRV) imaging, and contrast venography. CT scan and MRV also evaluate surrounding structures and can identify potential sources of extrinsic compression or etiologies for venous obstruction.

VENOUS THROMBOEMBOLISM TREATMENT

Systemic anticoagulation therapy is the primary treatment modality in VTE as it both helps prevent pulmonary embolism and reduces local clot propagation and helps minimize risk or recurrence. Therapeutic levels of anticoagulation should be achieved as soon as possible, which reduces the risk of recurrence fourfold. This can be done with weight-based dosing of LMWH or intravenous unfractionated heparin. LMWH has the advantage that it does not require monitoring and has a lower risk of bleeding as a result of a more predictable anticoagulation level. Unfractionated heparin is titrated to an activated partial thromboplastin time (aPTT) of 2 to 2.5 times normal. Once adequate anticoagulation therapy is achieved, patients are typically bridged to oral therapy. Warfarin is most commonly used for long-term anticoagulation therapy. Overlap of heparin or LMWH therapy with warfarin is important because protein C and S are the first factors to be inhibited, leading to a transient hypercoagulable state.

Long-term anticoagulation therapy can also be done with LMWH. It has also been shown to be superior to warfarin for patients with malignancy disease. Fondaparinux can be used to bridge to warfarin and as an alternative long-term therapeutic option. Dabigatran etexilate is currently indicated for anticoagulation therapy for stroke prevention for patients with atrial fibrillation but has not yet been approved for VTE therapy in the United States.

Duration of anticoagulation therapy is highly variable, and specific patient factors must be taken into account. The initial occurrence of a femoral-popliteal DVT without other predisposing risk factors should be treated for at least 3 months with systemic anticoagulation therapy, whereas an infrapopliteal DVT can be treated for 6 to 12 weeks. For those with calf vein thrombosis, either 3 months of anticoagulation therapy or ambulation and repeat weekly imaging to ensure no further propagation is reasonable.

Recurrent or unprovoked VTE necessitates prolonged anticoagulation therapy for 12 months or longer and consideration of evaluation for a hypercoagulable state and occult malignancy disease. Individuals with homozygous factor V Leiden, prothrombin 20210A mutation, protein C or protein S deficiency, antithrombin deficiency, antiphospholipid antibodies, and active malignancy disease should be considered for long-term anticoagulation therapy. In addition, patients with a substantial pulmonary embolism at initial presentation are also considered for prolonged anticoagulation therapy.

For patients undergoing surgical intervention within the period of required anticoagulation therapy after an acute VTE, bridging with UFH or LMWH can be performed perioperatively. For those individuals who are at high risk for PE, a removable inferior vena cava (IVC) filter should be considered.

Venous compression stocking therapy (30 to 40 mm Hg) is an important component of therapy for the treatment of patients with DVT that is commonly overlooked. Pain, swelling, and chronic venous insufficiency (CVI) lead to lifelong postphlebitic limb issues. Use of stockings has been shown to reduce the risk of chronic venous ulceration by 50%. There is no curative therapy for chronic venous insufficiency from chronic DVT. Compression stockings play a critical role in the management of CVI. Stockings reduce limb edema and ambulatory venous hypertension, thus reducing the risk of skin breakdown.

INFERIOR VENA CAVA FILTER

Inferior vena cava interruption with percutaneously placed filters is indicated for patients with a contraindication to anticoagulation or recurrent or propagated VTE despite therapeutic anticoagulation. Multiple approved devices are on the market, all with similar efficacy and risk profile. In individuals with an enlarged IVC (>28 mm), most permanent filters are too small to anchor in place, so either bilateral iliac vein filters or a Birds Nest filter (Cook Inc., Bloomington, Ind) can be used. Protection from PE (>95%) with IVC filters is equivalent to that of properly managed systemic anticoagulation therapy, with no increased benefit when both are used concurrently. For those patients with a limited period of time in which anticoagulation is contraindicated, removable filters are available. The importance of removal of temporary filters after the period of risk of hemorrhage has passed cannot be emphasized enough because IVC filters do pose some long-term risk of fracture, embolization, perforation, and caval thrombosis.

CATHETER-DIRECTED THROMBOLYTIC THERAPY

Extensive iliofemoral deep venous thrombosis predisposes the most significant risk of long-term sequelae from chronic venous insufficiency. Patients with limb-threatening venous outflow obstruction (phlegmasia cerulea dolens or venous gangrene) also benefit from rapid recanalization. In this population, active treatment with percutaneous pharmacomechanical thrombectomy or catheter-directed lysis can substantially reduce the thrombus burden and restore valvular function. When followed by systemic anticoagulation therapy, these percutaneous therapies have reduced long-term sequelae. Technical success is greater when intervention is performed with 14 days of thrombotic event, and long-term success correlates with the amount of thrombus clearance.

SYSTEMIC THROMBOLYSIS

Patients with a large pulmonary embolism and hemodynamic compromise are candidates for systemic thrombolytic therapy, if it is initiated within 48 hours of onset. Right ventricular strain and dysfunction on echocardiography can be seen as the sequelae of massive PE. Ultrasound scan–enhanced catheter-directed pharmacologic thrombolysis of PE has also shown to be beneficial for patients with hemodynamic compromise. In the short term, hemodynamic improvement is more rapid with lytic therapy, but long-term outcomes are not necessarily superior to anticoagulation-based therapy alone. In patients with failed lytic therapy and ongoing hemodynamic instability, surgical embolectomy remains an option.

COMPLICATIONS

Major bleeding is the most common complication of long-term anticoagulation therapy, occurring between 2% and 6% per year in those with an international normalized ratio (INR) of 2 to 3. Major bleeding is defined as intracranial hemorrhage, significant gastrointestinal bleeding, or deep tissue bleeding, such as retroperitoneal. Reversal of anticoagulation, protamine for unfractionated heparin and vitamin K/fresh frozen plasma for warfarin, should be performed immediately, and a vena cava filter should be placed as indicated. An unfortunate consequence of LMWH and some of the novel anticoagulants is that there is no reversal available, so supportive management and transfusion as necessary are all that can be done.

A second complication specific to heparinoids is heparin-induced thrombocytopenia. This can occur both with prophylactic and therapeutic dose unfractionated and low molecular-weight heparin. Immune-mediated thrombocytopenia most often occurs within 3 to 5 days after exposure, and the incidence increases with serial exposures. HIT should be suspected with an acute drop in platelet count by 50% or to below 100,000. A platelet factor-4 enzyme-linked immunosorbent assay (ELISA) is the initial test performed; it may be confirmed with a serotonin release assay. The morbidity of HIT comes from the small vessel thrombosis that occurs, so cessation of heparin exposure is followed by anticoagulation therapy with direct thrombin inhibitors.

Inferior vena cava filter complications can be categorized as those that involve the implantation and long-term complications. Short-term complications include access site (hematoma, arteriovenous fistula, hemorrhage, access site thrombosis), treatment site (improper position, tilt, vessel perforation), and systemic (dye allergy, contrast-induced nephropathy) issues. Most conical filters retain protection from PE even with tilt angles of up to 30 degrees.

Long-term complications of filter placement include PE around the filter, filter fracture, and migration. Inferior vena cava thrombosis can lead to impaired venous return, hemodynamic compromise, and massive lower extremity edema. Filter strut perforation (intact or fractured) into adjacent structures such as the aorta or small bowel can lead to substantial morbidity and mortality.

SUMMARY

Venous thromboembolic disease is a major source of preventable morbidity and mortality in both medical and surgical patients. With accurate assessment of risk factors and proper application of prophylactic measures, this risk can be reduced significantly. Diagnosis is best made with duplex ultrasound scan. Furthermore, timely diagnosis before clinical consequences and prompt initiation of anticoagulation therapy is important for improved outcomes. Therapeutic anticoagulation therapy for 3 months for uncomplicated situations is the minimum, but longer duration treatment may be necessary. Long-term anticoagulation is achieved with LMWH or warfarin and with novel agents. Use of 30-mm Hg to 40-mm Hg elastic compression stockings is important in reducing the risk of late chronic venous ulceration. In cases of iliofemoral thrombosis, pharmacomechanical thrombolysis should be considered. When anticoagulation therapy is contraindicated, vena cava interruption is an alternative to protect against PE but not the sequelae of DVT.

SUGGESTED READINGS

Caprini JA: Identification of patient venous thromboembolism risk across the continuum of care, *Clin Appl Thromb Hemost* 17(6):590–599, 2011.
Casey ET, Murad MH, Zumaeta-Garcia M, et al: Treatment of acute iliofemoral deep vein thrombosis, *J Vasc Surg* 55(5):1463–1473, 2012.
Fowkes FJ, Price JF, Fowkes FG: Incidence of diagnosed deep vein thrombosis in the general population: systematic review, *Eur J Vasc Endovasc Surg* 25(1):1–5, 2003.
Gangireddy C, Rectenwald JR, Upchurch GR, et al: Risk factors and clinical impact of postoperative symptomatic venous thromboembolism, *J Vasc Surg* 45(2):335–342, 2007.
Guyatt GH, Akl EA, Crowther M, et al: Executive summary: antithrombotic therapy and prevention of thrombosis, 9th ed: American College of Chest Physicians evidence-based clinical practice guidelines, *Chest* 141 (2 Suppl):7S–47S , 2012.
Meissner MH, Gloviczki P, Comerota AJ, et al: Early thrombus removal strategies for acute deep venous thrombosis: clinical practice guidelines of the Society for Vascular Surgery and the American Venous Forum, *J Vasc Surg* 55(5):1449–1462, 2012.

LYMPHEDEMA

**Natalia O. Glebova, MD, PhD, and
Jennifer Heller, MD**

Lymphedema is a condition characterized by the interstitial accumulation of protein-rich fluid as a result of impaired lymphatic drainage. Whereas the venous capillary system is responsible for 90% of the return of interstitial fluid into circulation, the lymphatic system handles the return of the largest macromolecules and their associated fluid. Reduced lymphatic uptake capacity causes a net increase in the amount of interstitial proteins and fluid.

As the condition progresses, increasing dilation of the remaining functional lymphatics causes valvular incompetence and reversal of flow. Lymphatic walls then undergo fibrosis, and fibrinoid thrombi ultimately obliterate the remaining patent channels. Stasis of interstitial proteins leads to an inflammatory response, with macrophages and fibroblasts replacing supple, elastic interstitium with fibrosclerotic, thickened, congested tissues. Soft, pitting edema gives way to induration, hypertrophy of adipose deposits, acanthosis, hyperkeratosis, and skin breakdown. Infectious complications often ensue, with recurrent bouts of cellulitis and lymphangitis. Rarely, chronic lymphedema degenerates into a highly aggressive lymphangiosarcoma, known as *Stewart-Treves syndrome*. A consensus on the staging of lymphedema has been published by the International Society of Lymphology (Box 1).

Lymphedema may be either primary or secondary. *Primary lymphedema* is the result of a developmental abnormality, although often with delayed manifestations. *Secondary lymphedema* is acquired and results from disease, trauma, or iatrogenic causes.

Primary lymphedema is further subclassified on the basis of inheritance (familial versus sporadic) and time of onset (congenital, praecox, or tarda). Women are predominantly affected by all forms of primary lymphedema. *Congenital lymphedema*, or Milroy's disease, includes all forms that present within the first 2 years of life, representing 10% to 25% of all primary cases. It typically involves bilateral lower extremities, is not progressive, and may improve spontaneously with age. *Lymphedema praecox*, or Meige's disease, typically presents at puberty (by definition before age 35 years) and represents 65% to 85% of primary lymphedema cases. Unilateral lower extremity involvement is usual. *Lymphedema tarda* presents spontaneously after the age of 35 years and is the rarest form of primary lymphedema. Table 1 describes demographics and typical presentations of the three forms of primary lymphedema.

Secondary lymphedema represents an acquired dysfunction of normally developed lymphatics. Worldwide, the most common cause is infection by the nematode *Wuchereria bancrofti*, spread by mosquitoes. Adult filarial worms reside in and obstruct lymphatic channels, causing irreversible scarring and fibrosis and often massive edema. In the United States and other developed nations, nearly all causes of secondary lymphedema are related to malignancies and their therapies. Mainstays of cancer treatment, such as tumor resection, radiation therapy, and lymphadenectomy, are related to higher rates of lymphedema. Lymphadenectomies are often performed to stage and treat malignant disease, including superficial and deep inguinal lymph node dissections for extremity melanoma and other tumors and axillary dissections commonly done during breast cancer treatment. Other risk factors including trauma, infection, and obesity are considered to contribute to secondary lymphedema (Figure 1).

DIAGNOSIS

The workup for lymphedema starts with a thorough history and physical examination. Other causes for edema must be ruled out, including cardiac, venous, renal, and hepatic etiologies and

---

BOX 1: Lymphedema staging

Stage 0: Latent
- Impaired lymphatic function
- No evident edema; subclinical
- May last months or years before progression

Stage I: Spontaneously Reversible
- Early accumulation of protein-rich fluid
- Pitting edema
- Subsides with elevation

Stage II: Spontaneously Irreversible
- Accumulation of protein-rich fluid
- Pitting edema progresses to fibrosis
- Does not resolve with elevation alone

Stage III: Lymphostatic Elephantiasis
- Nonpitting
- Significant fibrosis
- Trophic skin changes

From International Society of Lymphology: The diagnosis and treatment of peripheral edema: 2009 consensus document of the International Society of Lymphology, Lymphology 42(2):51-60, 2009.

TABLE 1: Primary lymphedema classifications

Classification	Age of onset	Gender predilection	Presentation	Genetics
Congenital (Milroy's disease)	Birth to 2 y	Female:male = 2:1	Predominantly lower extremity involvement, usually bilateral May involve gastrointesinal tract, intestinal lymphangiectasias, cholestasis Anaplastic lymphatic trunks	Autosomal dominant inheritance FLT4, tyrosine receptor kinase signaling pathway in lymphatics
Praecox (Meige's disease)	15 to 35 y	Female:male = 4:1	Predominantly lower extremity involvement, usually unilateral Associated anomalies may include vertebral defects, cerebrovascular malformations, distichiasis, yellow nails, sensorineural hearing loss, cleft palate Hypoplastic peripheral lymphatics	Autosomal-dominant inheritance FOXC2, involved in adipocyte metabolism FLT4
Tarda	>35 y	Female > male	Spontaneous onset Typically lower extremity involvement Hyperplastic histologic pattern, large tortuous lymphatics with absent or incompetent valves	FOXC2

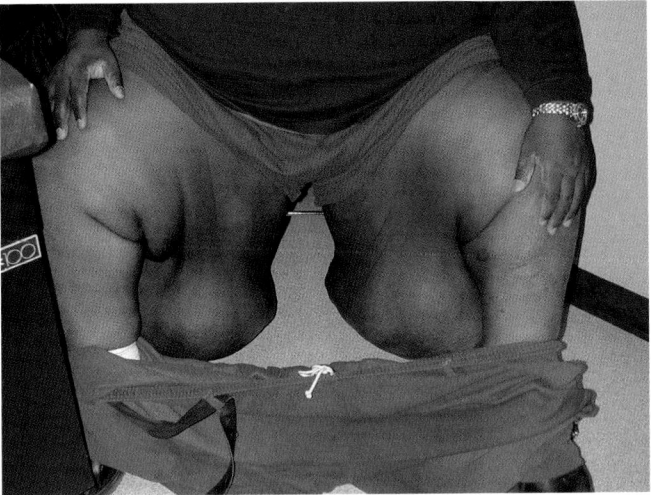

FIGURE 1   Bilateral lower extremity edema in the setting of morbid obesity.

TABLE 2: Differential diagnosis of peripheral edema

Etiology	Characteristics
Lymphedema	Asymmetric, painless, dorsum of foot involvement, Kaposi-Stemmer sign, hyperkeratosis
Cardiac	Symmetric, heart failure signs (jugular venous distention, lung crackles)
Hepatic	Symmetric, presence of ascites
Venous insufficiency	Asymmetric, pitting, aching, presence of varicosities, brawny hemosiderin deposits
Postthrombotic syndrome	Asymmetric, pitting, aching

compressive or occlusive vascular syndromes (Table 2). Physical examination characteristics include pitting edema that decreases with limb elevation, thickened skin, hyperkeratosis, and dermatitis. Lymphangioscintigraphy is currently the imaging gold standard for patients in whom these secondary etiologies are not suspected. This technique uses radioactively labeled macromolecules that are too large to enter systemic capillaries, such as Technetium-labeled human serum albumin. After a subcutaneous or intradermal injection into the interstitium (usually into a web space of hand or foot), the path of the tracer is visualized with a gamma camera. Quantitation can be achieved after correction for the decay of the tracer. This technique is somewhat limited by resolution and can be nondiagnostic with suboptimal injection but is low risk. Magnetic resonance imaging and computed tomographic scan are also useful in lymphatic visualization and may help to rule out associated malignant disease. Contrast magnetic resonance lymphangiography with gadobenate dimeglumine is a fast, less invasive diagnostic test for evaluation of lymphedema. Although imaging studies may be of some value, most patients can be diagnosed without additional confirmatory testing.

TREATMENT

Nonoperative Management

Nonoperative management is the mainstay of treatment for lymphedema. Public health measures to reduce vector transmission of W. bancrofti with diethylcarbamazine plus ivermectin can have significant effects on secondary lymphedema caused by the parasite.

The goal of nonoperative therapy is reduction of proteinaceous interstitial fluid, with the hope of stemming the cycle of edema, inflammation, and fibrosis. Modalities include hygiene management, compression and elevation, physical therapy, and long-term compliance. Treatments are often time intensive and inconvenient, and patient compliance is a necessary component of any regimen.

Basic lifestyle modifications are essential in managing the sequelae of lymphedema. Skin hygiene is important to reduce skin breakdown and resulting infection. Patients should be encouraged to lose weight if obese, to address minor skin traumas and breakdown appropriately, and to avoid constrictive clothing.

Compression therapies range widely and include graduated compression garments, multilayered inelastic bandaging, and controlled compression therapy. Compression garments are refitted as swelling decreases. These methods reduce the volume of excess edema by approximately 30% to 45%. External sequential compressive devices have also been used with variable success. Compression therapies are typically combined with elevation of the affected extremity whenever feasible.

Physical therapy, specifically decongestive lymphatic therapy, is a more time-intensive treatment strategy. This modality emphasizes manual lymphatic drainage via massage, compressive garments, and exercise. Numerous protocols exist for such therapies, which operate on the belief that these methods reduce edema by augmenting lymphatic contractility and increasing lymphatic flow. Studies vary as to whether lymphatic massage therapy leads to improved outcomes as compared with compression garments or bandaging alone.

The success of nonoperative strategies varies widely, in part because of differences among patient populations and individual patients. However, patient compliance plays a significant role; discomfort or embarrassment associated with compression garments or the inconvenience of physical therapy may limit outcomes.

Pharmacologically, antibiotics are used to treat recurrent infections that range from superficial infections to more serious cases of cellulitis or lymphangitis. Beyond antibiotics, however, pharmacologic therapies play a limited role in the management of lymphedema. Benzopyrenes are thought to increase lymphatic uptake of peptides through proteolysis of interstitial proteins, facilitating absorption into the bloodstream. Literature shows conflicting results with respect to benzopyrene usage, and documented hepatotoxicity limits long-term therapy (published trials are no longer than 3 to 6 months in duration). Diuretics have been used historically, but with only limited benefit, and they may actually lead to increased interstitial protein accumulation and fibrosis. Studies that examine the use of nutritional supplements, such as sodium selenite or vitamin E with pentoxifylline, have not shown any significant benefit in patients with lymphedema.

Operative Treatment

Surgery is an adjunct to primary conservative therapy in refractory cases, but the surgical indications for lymphedema are not absolute. Surgery is usually reserved for moderate to severe lymphedema, and its goal is long-term remission and improvement in quality of life. A number of variables are taken into account during assessment. Relative indications include size and weight of the patient, extent of lymphedema, recurrent lymphangitis, lymphorrhagia, abscess, fistula, diminished quality of life, worsening comorbidities, and most importantly, failure of nonoperative management.

The two general categories of surgical therapy are *debulking* and *physiologic procedures*. Nonoperative therapies such as lifestyle modifications, proper hygiene, and compressive therapies should be continued immediately after any surgical procedures because these surgical procedures are adjuncts to the previously mentioned therapies.

Debulking Procedures

The Charles procedure (1912), a radical excision technique, removes all skin and subcutaneous tissue down to the muscle fascia. Excised skin is used for grafting on the fascia (Box 2). The Van der Walt modification allows for negative-pressure dressing with grafting done in a delayed fashion. The operation is indicated for severe cases and carries a high risk of complications, including but not limited to infection, ulceration, hyperpigmentation, dermatitis, and a severe altered aesthetic outcome (Figure 2).

The Sistrunk procedure (1918) is a planned, staged excision of affected subcutaneous tissues. This technique has been modified over

---

BOX 2: Charles procedure

1. Mark the lymphedematous area proximally and distally.
2. Make an incision medially and laterally down to the muscle fascia.
3. Excise all the tissue superficial to this plane.
4. Remove the skin of the affected area with a dermatome for a split-thickness graft or with a knife for a full-thickness graft. If a full-thickness graft is used, be sure to remove all the fat from the skin.
5. Use this graft to cover the exposed area.
6. Apply petroleum gauze or other nonadherent dressing over the graft.
7. Apply a pressure dressing via a vacuum-assisted device, bolster, or cotton.
8. Splint the extremity in the proper anatomic position.
9. Remove dressing after 3 to 5 days for a split-thickness graft or after 7 to 12 days for a full-thickness graft.

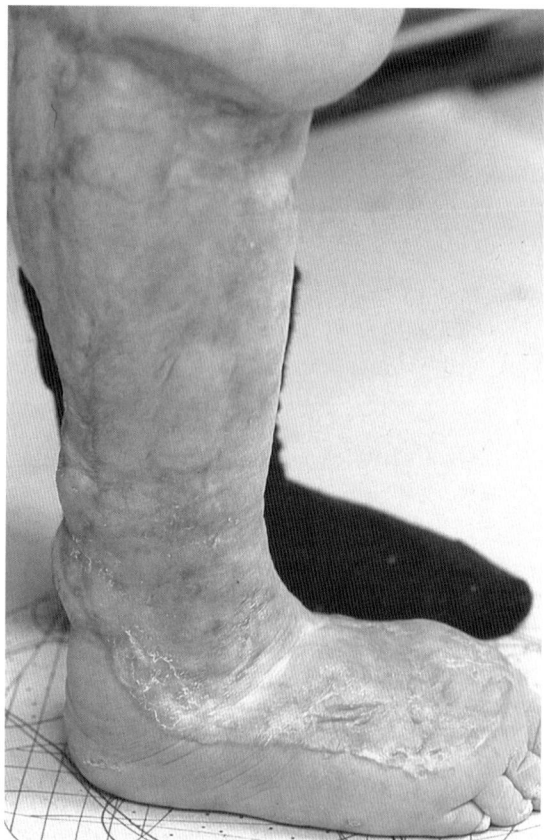

FIGURE 2   Lower extremity after Charles procedure.

the last 80 years and incorporates burying of dermal flaps within the skin flaps (Box 3). Long-term results can achieve a reduction of at least half of the affected tissue in 75% of patients. It is safe, reliable, and predictable. Complications include nerve damage in the affected area, epidermolysis from poor blood supply, wound dehiscence, and infection.

Liposuction was first used for brachial lymphedema in 1987 and was refined in 1993; it is now a useful adjunct for treatment (Box 4). Liposuction is safe, quick, and allows for an immediate decrease in

BOX 3: Sistrunk procedure

1. Mark out the affected area.
2. Plan to excise and debulk sufficient tissue, leaving dermal flaps to bury beneath the skin in the closure. A variation of this is carried out in the Thompson procedure, in which dermal flaps are buried beneath the muscle.
3. Close the incision over drains.
4. Allow 12 weeks to heal before the next serial excision.

BOX 4: Liposuction

1. Mark out affected area and 2 cm beyond.
2. Choose port sites to effectively reach all areas, both proximally and distally.
3. Inject tumescent solution (1 L Ringer's lactate mixed with 1 mL ampule of epinephrine 1:1000 and 30 mL of 1% lidocaine) until blanching is achieved and a moderate amount of turgor is seen.
4. Wait 30 to 45 minutes.
5. Suction with a 4-mm to 6-mm cannula in a deep plane in all areas, followed by a 2-mm to 3-mm cannula in a more superficial plane for a smoother contour.
6. Close port sites with absorbable suture.
7. Apply sterile dressings and a pressure garment.
8. Advise the patient not to shower or remove the pressure garment for 72 hours, and encourage the patient to walk at least 3 times a day.
9. After 3 days, the patient can shower daily and may begin massaging the affected areas.
10. The pressure garment should be worn for 6 to 10 weeks.

BOX 5: Microsurgical lymphovenous shunt

1. Begin with lymphatic and venous scintigraphy.
2. Inject lymphazurin into the web space in the distal extremity.
3. Take postobstruction dissection down to venous and lymphatic channels.
4. Use microsurgical connection to reestablish lymph flow directly or use a vein graft.
5. Insert a Penrose nonsuction drain.
6. Evaluate postoperative flow and imaging studies.

BOX 6: Vascularized nodal transplantation

1. Palpate femoral pulse and design skin paddle lateral to pulse, inferior and parallel to the inguinal ligament.
2. Take dissection of the flap from distal to proximal, harvesting the superficial fibronodal tissue with the superficial circumflex iliac vessels.
3. Make a transverse incision on the wrist, and perform microvascular anastomosis to the radial artery and vein.
4. Use a skin paddle for monitoring.

volume and pressure of the lymph fluid, promoting better lymphatic flow. Brorson of Sweden reports a complete reduction with no recurrence in his 15-year experience. Risks include lidocaine toxicity, thrombotic and fat emboli, hematoma, seroma, and contour irregularities. It has been used alone and in addition to other debulking procedures.

Physiologic Procedures

The main aim of physiologic procedures is to improve lymphatic flow and drainage. Omental flaps, enteromesenteric bridging, dermal flaps, and lymphangioplasty have all been attempted with minimal to no success. More recently, operations have been devised to construct connections between the lymphatic system and the venous system in the periphery. Lymphatic vessel and small veins have been used as grafts to reestablish lymphatic flow (prosthetic grafts have been investigated and determined to have abysmal patency). Microvascular lymphovenous shunts and nodal transplantation are new therapies that are showing promising results.

Microvascular lymphovenous shunts were first introduced in 1953 by Sherman and colleagues. Over the decades, microsurgery has evolved and is now used more to relieve postobstructive lymphedema (Box 5). A more recent study describes Campisi's experience in treating more than 800 patients with failed previous nonoperative therapies, with an average follow-up of 7 years. More than 80% of patients undergoing microsurgical lymphovenous shunting experienced significant reduction of excess volume (67% on average), with an even

greater reduction in the incidence of cellulitis. Results were stable with both volumetric assessment and lymphoscintigraphy.

Vascular nodal transplantation has had several successful animal studies, those in rats by Shesol in 1979 and again by Chen in 1990. This technique harvests vascularized fat and nodal tissue from the groin and transplants it to the distal upper extremity via microvascular anastomoses to the radial artery and vein (Box 6). This technique shows improvements that include decreased size, increased skin elasticity, decreased infection, increased lymphatic flow, increased lymphatic pathways toward the flap site, and most importantly, discontinued use of physiotherapy.

SUMMARY

Lymphedema remains a challenging clinical problem with significant morbidities. Treatment includes early implementation of long-term nonoperative measures along with surgical procedures for more difficult cases. Patient commitment and lifestyle modifications are central to the success of any therapeutic regimen.

SUGGESTED READINGS

Badger C, Preston N, Seers K, et al: Benzopyrones for reducing and controlling lymphoedema of the limbs, *Cochrane Database Syst Rev* (2):CD003140, 2004.

Becker C, Assouad J, Riquet M, et al: Postmastectomy lymphedema: long-term results following microsurgical lymph node transplantation, *Ann Surg* 243(3):313–315, 2006.

Brorson H, Ohlin K, Olsson G, et al: Controlled compression and liposuction treatment for lower extremity lymphedema, *Lymphology* 41(2):52–63, 2008.

Campisi C, Davini D, Bellini C, et al: Lymphatic microsurgery for the treatment of lymphedema, *Microsurgery* 26(1):65–69, 2006.

International Society of Lymphology: The diagnosis and treatment of peripheral lymphedema: 2009 consensus document of the International Society of Lymphology, *Lymphology* 42(2):51–60, 2009.

Karakousis CP: Surgical procedures and lymphedema of the upper and lower extremity, *J Surg Oncol* 92(2):87–91, 2006.

Liu NF, Lu Q, Jiang ZH, et al: Anatomic and functional evaluation of the lymphatics and lymph nodes in diagnosis and lymphatic circulation disorders with contrast magnetic resonance lymphangiography, *J Vasc Surg* 49(4):980–987, 2009.

Moseley AL, Carati CJ, Piller NB: A systematic review of common conservative therapies for arm lymphoedema secondary to breast cancer treatment, *Ann Oncol* 18(4):639–646, 2007.

Walter WH, Witte CL, Witte MH, et al: Radionuclide lymphangioscintigraphy in the evaluation of peripheral lymphedema, *Clin Nucl Med* 25(6):451–464, 2000.

Warren AG, Brorson H, Borud LJ, et al: Lymphedema: a comprehensive review, *Ann Plast Surg* 59(4):464–472, 2007.

INITIAL ASSESSMENT AND RESUSCITATION OF THE TRAUMA PATIENT

Gregory Peck, DO, and Timothy G. Buchman, PhD, MD, FACS, FCCP, MCCM

INITIAL ASSESSMENT AND RESUSCITATION OF THE TRAUMA PATIENT

The purpose of this chapter is to provide the practicing surgeon with a framework for assessment and resuscitation of the acutely injured patient. The principles and their implementation reflect the experience of the worldwide trauma community and the clinical practice of the authors. Effective surgical care depends on collaborative practice with prehospital providers, emergency and critical care physicians, radiology and operating room teams, and consultant specialty surgeons. A "shared mental model" of care fosters close collaboration, effective integration, and ultimately better outcomes for patients. The authors therefore recommend this chapter be shared among those providers, discussed, and then modified as needed to best suit local needs and established care patterns. The existence of a standard practice is more important than any specific component.

Stop the Harm and Do No (Further) Harm

The Hippocratic Oath includes a promise "to abstain from doing harm." The acutely injured patient has already been harmed, and therefore, the immediate goal of the surgeon must be to stop the result of the initial harm and take action to minimize the possibility of well-intended interventions to cause additional harm. The general approach requires that a team of providers agree on and practice a structured system of care that simultaneously identifies and addresses immediate life-threatening injury, initiates general resuscitative measures, inventories all injuries, and then prioritizes the treatment of injuries towards a patient-specific, comprehensive plan of care.

One framework for that general approach is contained within the Advanced Trauma Life Support (ATLS) Program of the American College of Surgeons that is currently taught in more than 60 countries and can therefore be considered a global standard. This chapter reflects that framework.

Preparation of the Team and Resuscitation Area

Successful assessment and resuscitation require that all team members know their role and can fulfill that role within the resuscitation area. Prior planning and mock resuscitations help to ensure that team members are cross-trained in the various roles and are familiar with the location and operation of essential equipment (such as physiologic monitors, oxygen sources, and airway adjuncts).

When a trauma patient is announced (either by information from prehospital providers or through the unexpected appearance of the patient), the team leader should assign tasks as described subsequently and, whenever possible, supervise and coordinate others in those roles. Often, one team member may have to assume more than one task, but all tasks must be fulfilled. The team leader is always responsible for ensuring completion of all tasks. The team leader is also responsible for the safety of the team and therefore must ensure that standard precautions, including appropriate personal protective equipment (gowns, gloves, and masks), are maintained throughout the resuscitation.

PRIMARY SURVEY

To stop the harm, the team must identify the immediate threats to life and address them in the order they are identified. The urgency of the tasks is self evident. Thus, the primary survey seeks to support three core physiologic functions (namely, ventilation, oxygenation, and perfusion) while verifying the integrity of neurologic, pulmonary, and cardiovascular systems. To simplify and coordinate these tasks, an alphabet sequence is recommended: A, B, C, D, E, and F, which represent Airway, Breathing, Circulation, Disability, Exposure, and FAST (Focused Assessment with Sonography for Trauma).

Airway (With Cervical Spine Control)

Looking and listening often verify that the patient has a patent airway. Observation of a speaking, screaming, or crying patient is sufficient to establish the airway at least temporarily patent. Conversely, patients who struggle to sit up, especially those with facial or cervical trauma, often do so because of imminent loss of the (natural) airway. Hoarseness and stridor are audible signs of impending airway loss. Although suction can clear secretions and a jaw thrust can displace the tongue to open the pharynx, trauma patients with a compromised airway nearly always need an artificial airway. Most often this involves endotracheal intubation with a translaryngeal tube with a sedative-amnestic (such as etomidate) and a short-acting neuromuscular blocking drug (such as succinylcholine). In every case, the team must ensure that all airway manipulations are performed with the cervical spine kept neutrally positioned until a cervical spine injury can be reasonably excluded. In every case, the surgeon must be prepared to provide a surgical airway via cricothyrotomy in the event that a translaryngeal tube cannot be safely and expeditiously inserted. Assessment and verification of the airway should always be followed by supply of 100% oxygen.

Breathing

Looking and listening is important for verification of normal ventilation. The trachea should be midline; deviation to one side suggests either ipsilateral atelectasis or contralateral tension pneumothorax. The chest should expand symmetrically. During the primary survey, with the patient typically supine, auscultation through the chest wall of the axilla is the most reliable way to verify ventilation of peripheral lung. Auscultation at this location minimizes both intervening tissue and the chance that tracheobronchial air movement is confused with peripheral ventilation. Any abnormality of tracheal position, chest expansion, or breath sounds (asymmetry or absence) must immediately be followed by three steps: reassess presence of an adequate airway; palpation of the chest to detect crepitus, fracture, or a flail segment; and percussion of the chest to identify a potential pneumothorax. Clinical suspicion of a tension pneumothorax is sufficient justification to decompress the hemithorax before chest radiography; whether a needle is used before tube thoracostomy is less important than securing adequate drainage, typically via the fourth intercostal space in the anterior-midaxillary line connecting the tube to −20-cm water suction to accelerate decompression.

Circulation (With Hemorrhage Control)

Obvious bleeding should be controlled with direct pressure. If the blood is from an extremity where a blood pressure cuff can be applied proximally, inflation of that cuff in excess of systolic pressure is sufficient to temporarily control that blood loss. Otherwise, the assessment of circulation relies on the palpation of carotid, femoral, and radial pulses along with compression and release of a nail bed for qualitative assessment. The carotid pulse is the last to be lost, disappearing when the systolic pressure falls below 60 mm Hg. Initial support typically consists of infusion of 30 mL/kg balanced salt solution (normal saline solution or lactated Ringer's solution) via two peripheral intravenous cannulas, size 16-gauge or larger. Palpable pulse asymmetry speaks either to underlying vascular disease (common in the older trauma victim) or focal acute injury. Absent pulses at every point of palpation speaks either to a systolic blood pressure below 60 mm Hg or absence of mechanical cardiac function, both of which demand immediate action.

At this point in the care of the patient, the team leader should *explicitly assess and announce* that oxygenation, ventilation, and perfusion are adequate, recovering, or unresponsive. The two key assessment tools are pulse oximetry (which provides evidence of perfusion and oxygenation) and capnometry (which provides evidence of perfusion and ventilation, especially in patients on mechanical ventilation). Electrocardiographic (ECG) tracing confirms electrical activity of the heart, but this can be uncoupled from perfusion by cardiac tamponade, tension pneumothorax, or exsanguinations and should not be taken as independent evidence of perfusion.

Defects in oxygenation are the result of defective delivery to the lungs, defective diffusion across the lung tissue, or defective perfusion. Check that the oxygen source is connected to and flowing into whatever device is supplying the patient, including the fractional concentration of oxygen in inspired gas (FiO_2) setting on the ventilator. If delivery to the lungs is adequate, a significant lung injury or a perfusion compromise is likely.

Defects in ventilation are typically mechanical: the patient cannot self ventilate or something is interfering with mechanical ventilation. Disconnecting the patient from mechanical ventilation and "handbagging" the patient with a bag-valve device (AMBU bag) quickly

establishes whether gas flows easily into and out of the lungs. If ventilation is easy, falling or absent end-tidal CO_2 is often evidence of a serious perfusion problem.

Defects in perfusion are common. The most common cause of underperfusion is hypovolemia as a result of hemorrhage. Although the initial balanced salt solution is infusing, perfusion failure from arrhythmia, cardiac tamponade, or tension hemopneumothorax should be reconsidered, especially in the absence of an obvious bleeding point or cavity. The quickest way to exclude these three as cause of the perfusion defect may be ultrasound scan, which can display mechanical cardiac function, visualize pericardial fluid, and confirm that neither fluid nor gas lie between the chest wall and the lung parenchyma (extended FAST examination). If bleeding is the suspected or is the obvious cause of severe hypoperfusion, transfusion with the constituents of whole blood (red blood cells, fresh frozen plasma, and platelets transfused at a ratio of 1:1:1) is necessary. The hemorrhage, depending on the severity and location, is expeditiously halted with operative intervention. Vasopressor and inotrope treatment may be appropriate for some causes of perfusion compromise but should be recognized as adjuncts to volume return and search with reversal of the cause is underway. Vasopressor and inotropes are not the treatment for hemorrhagic shock but are instead indicated in perfusion compromise from neurogenic or cardiogenic shock.

Disability (Neurologic Assessment)

This evaluation is meant to be brief and aims to determine level of consciousness and any lateralizing signs. Operationally, this means a determination of the Glasgow coma score, an inspection of the pupils, and a command to "wiggle" fingers and toes. The responsive patient who has sustained a fall, direct blow to the neck or head, rapid deceleration, torque, or an axial load should also be asked about transient loss of consciousness and transient hemiplegia or quadriplegia. Positive responses dictate advanced imaging, particularly computed tomographic (CT) angioplasty or magnetic resonance imaging (MRI), to seek evidence of vascular dissection or cord impingement, respectively. The unresponsive patient with a Glasgow coma score of less than 9 should have the airway secured with an endotracheal tube before a CT scan or MRI. Unresponsive patients with asymmetric pupils constitute a neurosurgical emergency; immediate neurosurgical consultation and intervention is necessary, treatment with osmotic diuretics or hypertonic saline solution should be initiated, and plans should be made for immediate CT scan to define the lesion.

Exposure (With Environmental Control)

The patient must be completely undressed, and all surfaces are inspected. "Logrolling" with attention to maintaining spine neutrality is important to assess focal level of spine pain or deformity, all dependent on the level of a patient's consciousness. The posterior skin and the perineum and axillae should be inspected for lacerations, punctures, and hematomas. If penetrating injuries are found, clinical impressions should be formed as to likely trajectories, particularly if there is a likely violation of key anatomic zones (such as the central chest or abdominal vascular). Obvious traverse of the thoracic cavity and abdomen accompanied by hypotension suggests a life-threatening thoracic or intra-abdominal injury that necessitates immediate transfer to the operating room for exploration.

Palpation should assess for masses, fluid collections, crepitus, and obvious fracture, including the spine and pelvis. Constrictions (rings, bracelets, and circumferential eschar in burn cases) should be relieved if circulation or ventilation is threatened.

The importance of environmental control cannot be overstated. Injured patients often have defects in thermoregulation that are amplified in the setting of hemorrhage or directly by wet clothes or bed sheets. Patients with spinal cord injuries have no vasoconstriction in response to cooling and become poikilothermic. The resuscitation bay should therefore be kept uncomfortably (with respect to the gowned resuscitation team) warm. Environmental control also requires attention to mitigation of pressure points, especially in the unconscious patient.

Focused Assessment With Sonography for Trauma

Ultrasound scan is now a standard tool for initial assessment of the injured patient. Four conditions dictate its immediate use during the primary survey: hypotension, abdominal trauma, impaired consciousness, and pulseless electrical activity. Four views are obtained, including the pericardium and heart, the perihepatic spaces, the perisplenic space, and the pelvis. If no cardiac motion is seen, then the patient is clinically dead and the team can determine whether sufficient reason exists to attempt resuscitative thoracotomy. Otherwise, the purpose of the FAST examination is to detect fluid that would compromise perfusion, either tamponade around the heart or frank blood loss into the abdomen leading to hypovolemia. Furthermore, lateral thoracic and parasternal views to assess for hemothorax or pneumothorax, respectively, are used routinely depending on user experience.

RESUSCITATION AND MONITORING

The next phase of care is resuscitative. The team leader should revisit the components of the primary survey and reverify that the patient is oxygenated and ventilated and that fluids are infusing if indicated. Four key decisions follow. First, is additional fluid necessary? Second, if additional fluid is necessary, is colloid indicated? Third, is a medication or procedure immediately necessary to resuscitate the patient? Finally, does the procedure need to be performed in the resuscitation area? Here, some judgment is needed to tailor the resuscitation.

The resuscitation target is often a systolic pressure of 90 mm Hg and definitive control of any site of hemorrhage. If fluids beyond 2 L are necessary, blood products are required and plans should be made to promptly control the bleeding either via the interventional radiology route or operatively. Newer concepts are damage control resuscitation, introducing the concept of frontloading resuscitative efforts with permissive hypotension, minimization of crystalloids, use of hypertonic saline solution, and early transfusion of packed red blood cells or whole blood, fresh frozen plasma, and specific coagulation cascade factors if massive hemorrhage is present. Hypotension is never neurologic in origin, with one notable exception: patients with cervical spinal cord transection can require both a vasoconstrictor and a cardiac accelerator to overcome the traumatic sympathectomy and thereby augment blood pressure (dopamine or low-dose epinephrine conveniently combines both effects).

Thoracotomy performed in the resuscitation area (resuscitative thoracotomy) is successful only in a very narrowly selected patient population. The strongest indication is penetrating thoracic trauma leading to loss of signs of life either in front of the team or within 5 minutes of arrival to the trauma center. Reported success rates are more favorable in penetrating injury than in blunt, and in knife wounds better than in gunshot.

Monitoring of the patient should already be underway with pulse oximetry, capnometry (if mechanical ventilation is being used), and display of the ECG. Blood sampling should be performed by protocol and include (at a minimum) type and screen, a hemogram, a basic metabolic panel, and base deficit with lactate determination. Coagulation studies are often useful as a baseline determination because it is a comprehensive metabolic panel if there is a chance of major intra-abdominal injury. Patients who are ventilated and those with burn with potential inhalation injury (including CO poisoning)

require arterial blood gas analysis. In all but the most minor trauma, a bladder catheter should be inserted after the absence of blood at the urethral meatus is verified. The urine should be inspected for gross blood or microscopic hematuria to exclude genitourinary injury. The Foley system should have an urimeter to record subsequent urine output.

Adequately resuscitated patients should make 0.5 to 1 mL/kg/h of urine and have lactate levels that trend to below 2.5 mmol/L. Persisting oliguria or metabolic acidosis should prompt a search for a perfusion defect.

If an oxygenation, ventilation, or perfusion defect persists at this point, a chest radiograph must be performed to exclude an undetected thoracic injury or a hemodynamically compromising pelvic fracture. Otherwise, imaging strategies depend on local custom. The time-honored recommendation that every patient undergo plain radiography of the cervical spine (three views), chest (anteroposterior view), and pelvis remains valid and appropriate for smaller hospitals where CT scan equipment is often located some distance from the emergency department or not available 24 hours a day. Many major trauma centers have installed close-by scanners and have operationally shifted to the rapid use of comprehensive CT scan that includes the brain and cervical spine, followed by infusion of intravenous contrast with the scan continued caudally through the chest, abdomen, and pelvis. Such a sequence can be performed with current generation scanners in less than 10 minutes and yield far more comprehensive information than conventional plain films. Again, assessment and clinical suspicion determine the indication for each anatomic area to be surveyed.

SECONDARY SURVEY

The secondary survey, which must be completed before the patient leaves the trauma resuscitation area for additional imaging, is simply a head-to-toe physical examination that includes a finger or tube in every natural orifice in patients who are unconscious and therefore cannot describe their symptoms. (In such cases, the stomach should be drained with a nasal or oral gastric tube. The rectum should be checked for injury. The vagina should be inspected for injury, and any foreign body [tampon] should be removed.) The purpose of the secondary survey is to complete an inventory of the evident injuries and direct additional imaging as necessary (e.g., a skeletal radiograph at the site of a deformity, pain, or extremity hematoma). The secondary survey is also the time to at least temporarily stabilize obvious fractures with splints, traction apparatus, and pelvic compression for unstable pelvic fractures.

NEXT STEPS

Details of further care depend on the injury pattern. Experience suggests a few points that can help the surgeon avoid common pitfalls.

1. Some member of the team should be assigned to document the resuscitation. This might be a nurse or nonphysician provider. Whoever it is should not have any other responsibilities, except to take a brief focused history from the patient or personal representative. The key elements include allergies, medications, significant history, time of the last oral intake, and the events leading up to the trauma. (The mnemonic here is AMPLE.)

2. Patients with unstable conditions belong in a treatment area, such as the operating room or the interventional radiology suite. The trauma bay in the emergency department is a place to initiate resuscitation while defining a treatment plan. It is not a place to execute a treatment plan.

3. A head CT scan is tempting to obtain in patients with unstable conditions with multiple injuries. Experience suggests that

patients with serious isolated head injuries are rarely hemodynamically unstable. The question arises in the patient who has multiple injuries, including a head injury, and is poorly responsive to the initial resuscitation—to scan or to explore? If the source of bleeding is known, it should be controlled and the blood pressure normalized. This is by far the best treatment for the injured brain, which can be scanned as soon as temporary control of the hemorrhage is obtained or simultaneously addressed in the operating room by neurosurgery. The situation is harder when FAST and plain films fail to show a bleeding source or explanation for the instability. In such cases, a CT scan can be considered as one of a collection of bad options, if mechanism suggests a devastating head injury.

4. Pouring blood into a patient who is bleeding is most helpful after bleeding is controlled surgically. Attempting to resuscitate a patient to normal hemodynamics before the offending vessels are clamped wastes time and blood, both of which are costly to the patient.

5. After initial treatment (operative, interventional, or merely supportive) and the patient's return to the intensive care unit or to the ward, someone must conduct a tertiary survey. It is best performed when the patient can communicate but should always be done within the first postinjury day. The tertiary trauma survey is a comprehensive review of the medical record with emphasis on the mechanism of injury and pertinent comorbid factors, such as age. It includes the repetition of the primary and secondary surveys, a review of all laboratory data, and a review of images and their official interpretation. New physical findings are quite common and require further studies to exclude missed injuries.

SUGGESTED READINGS

ATLS: *Advanced trauma life support for doctors (student course manual)*, ed 9, Chicago, 2012, American College of Surgeons.

Dente CJ, Shaz BH, Nicholas JM, et al: Improvements in early mortality and coagulopathy are sustained better in patients with blunt trauma after institution of a massive transfusion protocol in a civilian level one trauma center, *J Trauma* 66(6):1616, 2009.

Duchesne JC, McSwain NE, Cotton BA, et al: Damage control resuscitation: the new face of damage control, *J Trauma* 69(4):976, 2010.

Holcomb JB, Wade CE, Michalek JE, et al: Increased plasma and platelet to red blood cell ratios improves outcome in 466 massively transfused civilian trauma patients, *Ann Surg* 248:447–458, 2008.

Rozycki GS, Ochsner MG, Jaffin JH, et al: Prospective evaluation of surgeons' use of ultrasound in trauma patients, *J Trauma* 34:516, 1993.

AIRWAY MANAGEMENT IN THE TRAUMA PATIENT

Samuel M. Galvagno, Jr., DO, PhD, and
Thomas M. Scalea, MD

Airway management is the first step in the management of the trauma patient to prevent hypoxia and cellular hypoperfusion. Cervical spine instability, brain injury, hemodynamic instability, lack of patient cooperation, risk of aspiration, time pressure, and facial injuries can make this more challenging. Techniques for rapid establishment and maintenance of a patent airway, with emphasis on the importance of adequate oxygenation and ventilation throughout all phases of airway management, are described.

INITIAL AIRWAY ASSESSMENT AND THERAPY

A patient who is alert, oriented, and speaking normally without injuries to the head or neck has an adequate airway. Any change in voice, report of a sore throat, dyspnea, tachypnea, use of accessory muscles, noisy breathing (snoring or stridor), or unexplained agitation may be a sign of imminent airway compromise.

A systematic approach to airway assessment should predict a potentially difficult airway. This should follow the line of sight of the provider from the upper incisors to the vocal cords, with a focus on the inside of the mouth and pharynx, and conclude with examination of the mandibular space, neck, and chest. Figure 1 and Boxes 1 and 2 describe clinical tests that can be used to determine whether one is likely to have a poor view of the vocal cords during direct laryngoscopy.

Oxygen therapy helps maintain pulse oximetry (SpO_2) above 92%. A nonrebreathing mask provides a fractional concentration of oxygen in inspired gas (FiO_2) of more than 90% and should be the initial choice. Oxygen therapy can be modified later to a simple face mask (FiO_2, 35% to 55%), a Venturi mask (FiO_2, 24% to 60%), or a nasal cannula (FiO_2, 24% to 44%).

If the airway is compromised and the patient is not ventilating and oxygenating adequately, noninvasive interventions can maintain oxygenation during preparation for definitive airway. Bag-valve mask ventilation with 15 L/min of oxygen should be initiated (FiO_2, 90% to 100%). Independent risk factors that predict an inability to perform bag-mask ventilation include male gender, a history of sleep apnea, Mallampati 3 or 4 status, and the presence of a beard. The spinal cord must be protected until spinal cord injury has been excluded.

Oropharyngeal or nasopharyngeal airways alleviate airway obstruction by the tongue. Oral airway size can be gauged with measurement of the airway from the corner of the patient's mouth to the external auditory canal. Nasopharyngeal airways should not be used if the patient has a suspected craniofacial injury for fear of inserting the devices through an injured cribriform plate into the brain. The chin-lift method gently lifts the mandible without hyperextension of the neck and may open the airway. The jaw-thrust maneuver can help by displacing the mandible forward while applying pressure to both angles of the mandible. Either can be performed during in-line cervical stabilization.

RAPID SEQUENCE INDUCTION AND INTUBATION

In most trauma patients, rapid sequence induction and intubation (RSII) is used to establish a definitive airway. RSII is a highly organized sequence of events that starts with preoxygenation for at least 3 minutes. The "6 Ps" of RSII describe the recommended sequence (Table 1). During the preparatory stage, a suction catheter is prepared

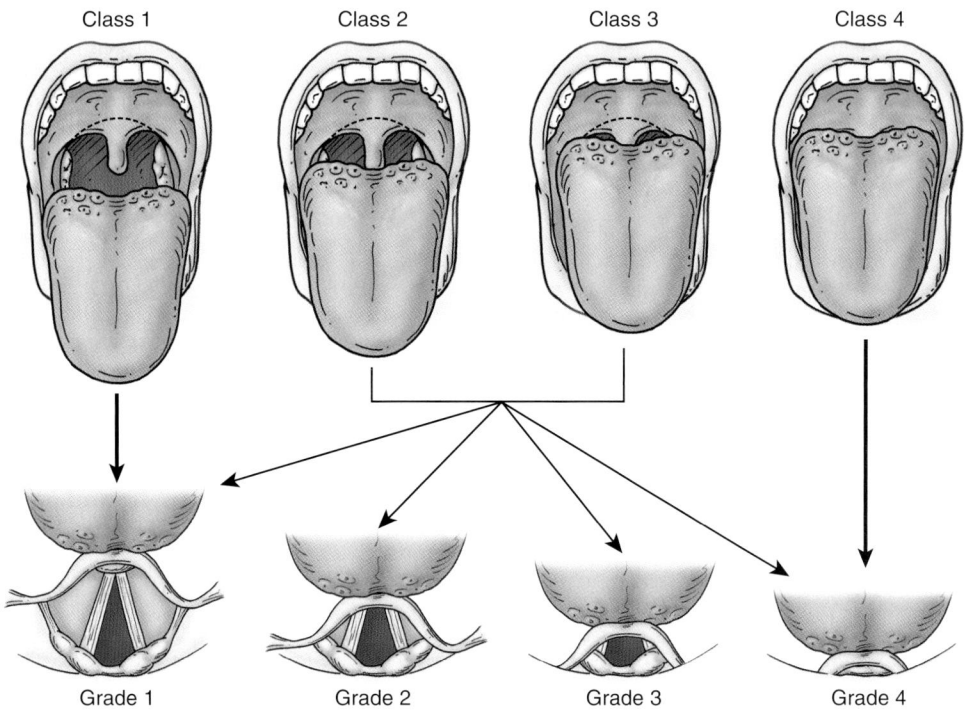

Class 1   Class 2   Class 3   Class 4

Grade 1   Grade 2   Grade 3   Grade 4

FIGURE 1 The Mallampati classification. The higher the class, the worse the Cormack-Lehane view of the vocal cords during direct laryngoscopy. *(From Lalwani AK, ed:* Current diagnosis and treatment in otolaryngology: head and neck surgery, *ed 2,* http://accessmedicine.com, *Accessed July 28, 2013.)*

BOX 1: Mandibular protrusion test

Class A
Lower incisors can be protruded anterior to the upper incisors.

Class B
The lower incisors can be brought edge to edge with upper incisors.

Class C
The lower incisors cannot be brought edge to edge with upper incisors.
The test assesses jaw mobility. Class A portends better vocal cord visualization during direct laryngoscopy than class B or C.

BOX 2: Indications of potentially difficult airway

Prominent incisors or abnormal dentition
Mandibular protrusion (see Box 1)
Mouth opening (>3 fingerbreadths or 5-6 cm is normal)
Mallampati classification (see Figure 1)
Thyromental distance (>3 fingerbreadths or 6 cm is normal)
Cervical range of motion (should *not* be tested in any patient with a suspected C-spine injury)
Anatomic abnormalities (masses, swelling)
Thickness of neck
Length of neck (shorter neck associated with difficult intubation)

TABLE 1: Sequence of steps for rapid sequence induction and intubation

RSII step	Time interval	Pharmacologic agents
Preoxygenation	0-3 min	Oxygen
Premedication	3 min	Induction agent ± fentanyl, lidocaine, atropine, defasciculation agents (vecuronium, rocuronium; usually 1/10 the induction dose)
Paralysis	3.5-5.5 min	Midazolam, ketamine, etomidate, propofol, or other induction agents *followed by* succinylcholine or rocuronium
Placement	6-6.5 min	Oxygen
Performance	7-7.5 min	Oxygen
Postintubation management	7.5 + min	Oxygen, sedatives, analgesics, etc.

RSII, Rapid sequence induction and intubation.

and tested, a source of oxygen is readied for connection, a pulse oximeter is attached to the patient, pharmacologic agents are prepared, and airway equipment is organized. RSII ideally requires at least four providers: one to apply cricoid pressure, one to maintain in-line cervical stabilization, one to ventilate with a bag-valve mask (BVM) and intubate, and one to administer drugs and assist with airway devices (Figure 2).

Many practitioners find that gentle mask ventilation (inspiratory pressure, <20 cm H_2O) is acceptable during the induction sequence and may help prevent hypoxemia in obese, pregnant, pediatric, and critically ill patients. This also tests for the adequacy of mask ventilation in the event that intubation attempts fail.

Before paralytics are given, an induction agent is administered (Table 2). Paralytics are recommended as part of RSII because omission of neuromuscular blockade results in suboptimal intubation conditions. Either succinylcholine (1 to 1.5 mg/kg) or rocuronium (0.8 to 1.2 mg/kg) is administered for paralysis. Succinylcholine can be administered intramuscularly if an intravenous line is not established, but an increased dose of 3 to 4 mg/kg is recommended for this route. Both succinylcholine and rocuronium provide optimal intubation conditions when dosed appropriately.

Priming doses of nondepolarizing agents are usually not used in trauma patients because these agents must be administered at least 3 minutes before the loading dose of muscle relaxant. In elderly or debilitated patients, pretreatment with a small dose of muscle relaxant may predispose to aspiration. Succinylcholine is contraindicated in patients with burns, open globe injuries, neuromuscular disorders, hyperkalemia, pseudocholinesterase deficiency, severe crush injuries, and chronic paralysis. Rocuronium, a nondepolarizing agent, is an alternative, but this agent cannot be administered intramuscularly and the duration of action is much longer (typically up to 45 minutes) than in succinylcholine (6 to 10 minutes).

Use of opioids may be considered during RSII. Fentanyl (2 µg/kg), alfentanil (20 to 30 µg/kg), or remifentanil (1 µg/kg) may help attenuate hemodynamic responses to intubation in unpremedicated cases. Opioids alone do not provide adequate amnesia and thus are usually not used as sole induction agents for RSII. Midazolam, a short-acting benzodiazepine with excellent amnestic properties, is often used. After preoxygenation, lidocaine may be given to attenuate increases in intracranial pressure, although a paucity of data exists to support this.

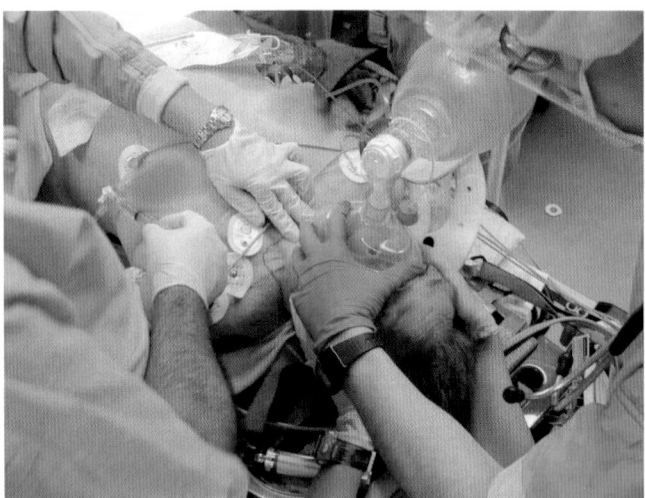

FIGURE 2 Four providers are recommended for securing the airway. Providers are assigned to: (1) ventilate with the bag-valve mask and intubate; (2) maintain in-line cervical stabilization; (3) administer cricoid pressure; and (4) push drugs and assist with airway devices.

ENDOTRACHEAL INTUBATION

Endotracheal intubation remains the first-line standard intervention for securing the airway in trauma patients. Cricoid pressure (backward and upward application of pressure to the cricoid cartilage) occludes the esophagus and prevents regurgitation. However, the technique is often incorrectly applied and may worsen laryngoscopic views. If the laryngoscopic view worsens with the technique, pressure can simply be released or adjusted as necessary.

Cervical immobilization is critical in any patients at risk for cervical spine injury. Manual in-line stabilization has been shown to be

TABLE 2: Properties of induction agents commonly used during airway management in trauma patients

Induction agent	Dose for RSII	Onset	Duration of action	Comment
Propofol	1-3 mg/kg	10-30 s	8-10 min	Dose usually reduced, sometimes by as much as 1/10 the recommended induction dose; causes decreased systemic vascular resistance and hypotension
Ketamine	1-2 mg/kg IV 2-4 mg/kg IM	30-60 s	5-20 min	Acceptable for use in patients with increased ICP; direct myocardial depressant but has indirect stimulatory effects (best avoided in patients with coronary artery disease)
Etomidate	0.2-0.3 mg/kg	30-45 s	10-20 min	A single dose causes adrenocortical suppression; recent evidence supports safety in septic shock
Remifentanil	1 µg/kg	30-60 s	<10 min	250 times more potent than morphine; may cause hypotension; not a reliable amnestic; does not accumulate; broken down by nonspecific esterases
Midazolam	0.3-0.6 mg/kg	2-3 min	20-30 min	When combined with opioids, can cause marked hypotension and respiratory depression

ICP, Intracranial pressure; *IM,* intramuscularly; *IV,* intravenously; *RSII,* rapid sequence induction and intubation.

superior for prevention of inadvertent movement of the cervical spine during intubation as compared with a cervical collar alone. During intubation, one provider is dedicated to maintain manual in-line stabilization.

A laryngoscope with a MacIntosh or McGill blade should be held in the left hand and inserted into the right side of the patient's mouth, displacing the tongue to the left. The airway structures are lifted into view, avoiding use of the blade as a fulcrum on the teeth. The epiglottis and vocal cords are visualized. The endotracheal tube should be gently inserted with the cuff past the vocal cords and inflated with enough air to provide a good seal (<30 cm H$_2$O). In general, intubation attempts should not take more than 30 seconds. Verification of tube placement is accomplished with auscultation of bilateral lung sounds, observation of chest rise, absence of epigastric/gastric gurgling or distension, and presence of end-tidal carbon dioxide with either a colorimetric device or continuous capnography. If a colorimetric device is used, the color indicator should change from purple to yellow, and at least six ventilations with an appropriate color change should be observed to avoid potential false-positive results. A chest radiograph confirms tube position.

In patients with a poor visualization of cords, a gum elastic bougie may used. The bougie is a flexible 60-cm 15F introducer with a Coude tip angled at 40 degrees, 3.5 cm from the distal end.

The bougie is lubricated and inserted with the Coude tip directed anteriorly and advanced until at the level of the tracheal rings. The endotracheal tube is then advanced over the bougie into the trachea. Videolaryngoscopy (VL) has evolved as a technology that allows direct visualization of the airway by all airway team members. VL can be used at all stages of intubation, including initial laryngoscopy.

SUPRAGLOTTIC AIRWAY DEVICES

A variety of supraglottic devices exist for use when attempts at endotracheal intubation or BVM ventilation fail. The laryngeal mask airway, multilumen esophageal airway (Combitube, Kendall-Sheridan Corporation, Argyle, NY).), and the laryngeal tube airway are three devices that can be placed without direct visualization of the glottis. Although these devices enable ventilation, either by providing a seal around the laryngeal inlet or occluding the esophagus, none of these devices represent a definitive airway. Each of these devices requires additional training, and all must eventually be replaced with a definitive airway.

AWAKE FIBEROPTIC INTUBATION

When patients are suspected of having cervical spinal cord injuries but do not need *emergent* intubation, awake fiberoptic intubation (AFOI) may be used to secure the airway. This method minimizes cervical spine movements, preventing neurologic impairment. Careful titration of sedation is mandatory for AFOI because spontaneous ventilation is needed with this technique. Oxygen is delivered via a nasal cannula. Patients are premedicated with glycopyrrolate (0.2 to 0.4 mg) to reduce secretions.

Sedation with opioids or benzodiazepines can be helpful. Opioids can cause synergistic respiratory depression when used with benzodiazepines. Opioids may be used instead of benzodiazepines, keeping in mind that opioids do not provide reliable amnesia. Lidocaine ointment is applied to the posterior tongue via a tongue depressor to anesthetize the glossopharyngeal nerve. Cotton balls (with strings attached to ensure easy retrieval from the airway) are soaked in 4% lidocaine. With either a Magill forceps or right angle tonsil holder, the cotton balls are gently introduced deep into the piriforms and held in place for 60 to 90 seconds on each side, effectively

anesthetizing both branches of the superior laryngeal nerve. Finally, an oral airway is inserted (to prevent biting of the fiberoptic scope), and the fiberoptic scope is introduced.

Once the vocal cords are visualized, 1 to 2 mL of 1% or 2% lidocaine is sprayed through the fiberoptic scope directly on the vocal cords, anesthetizing the recurrent laryngeal nerve. Once all three nerves are anesthetized, the endotracheal tube can safely be inserted with either a videolaryngoscope (i.e., "awake" video laryngoscopy) or over a fiberoptic bronchoscope. Careful attention must be paid to the amounts of lidocaine used because a dose greater than 5 mg/kg may result in anesthetic toxicity. The technique can be modified accordingly for nasotracheal intubation with use of topical vasoconstrictors and anesthetics to anesthetize and mitigate bleeding in the nasal passages.

AIRWAY MANAGEMENT DECISION MAKING

Figure 3 provides a decision algorithm for patients in need of an immediate airway. Initial priorities always include adequate preoxygenation and in-line cervical immobilization. In trauma patients, the option to wake the patient, as one would do for an elective surgical procedure, is not feasible. After a third failed attempt at intubation, an laryngeal mask airway (LMA) can be inserted to facilitate the transition to a definitive airway via fiberoptic intubation or intubation through the LMA. However, if the airway cannot be expeditiously secured after the third laryngoscopy attempt, a surgical airway is necessary. The rate of conversion to a surgical airway has been reported to range from 0.2% to 2%.

SURGICAL AIRWAY

Cricothyroidotomy is usually the surgical technique of choice (Figure 4). The patient is placed in the supine position with the neck in a neutral position. After the neck is prepped and draped, the thyroid notch, thyroid cartilage, cricothyroid membrane, cricoid cartilage, and trachea are identified with palpation. With the thyroid cartilage stabilized with one hand, a 2.0-cm to 2.5-cm vertical incision is made over the cricothyroid membrane with a #10 or #11 surgical blade. A hemostat or tracheal spreader is introduced into the incision and rotated 90 degrees to open the airway. Either a cuffed endotracheal tube (5.0 or 6.0 size) or tracheostomy tube is inserted through the cricothyroid membrane incision. The cuff is inflated, and placement of the tube is confirmed with the usual methods.

In the event of insufficient time to complete the dissection for a full cricothyroidotomy, a needle cricothyroidotomy can be performed. The anatomic landmarks are identified, and a 12-gauge or 14-gauge needle attached to a 5-mL to 10-mL syringe is used to puncture the skin in the midline directly over the cricothyroid membrane. A small incision with a #11 blade may enable passage of the needle through the skin. Once the needle has passed through the skin, the needle is angled 45 degrees caudally for insertion through the lower half of the cricothyroid membrane. Aspiration of air should be noted once the needle is in the airway, and the syringe is removed. The needle is then connected to a jet ventilation device. Alternatively, a 3-mL syringe can be connected to the needle and attached to a plastic endotracheal tube connector. This allows for connection to a BVM device. Ventilation via a needle cricothyroidotomy only maintains oxygenation for approximately 30 to 45 minutes; hypercarbia may quickly develop. For both needle and surgical cricothyroidotomies, the airway is typically converted to a formal tracheostomy by 24 to 48 hours.

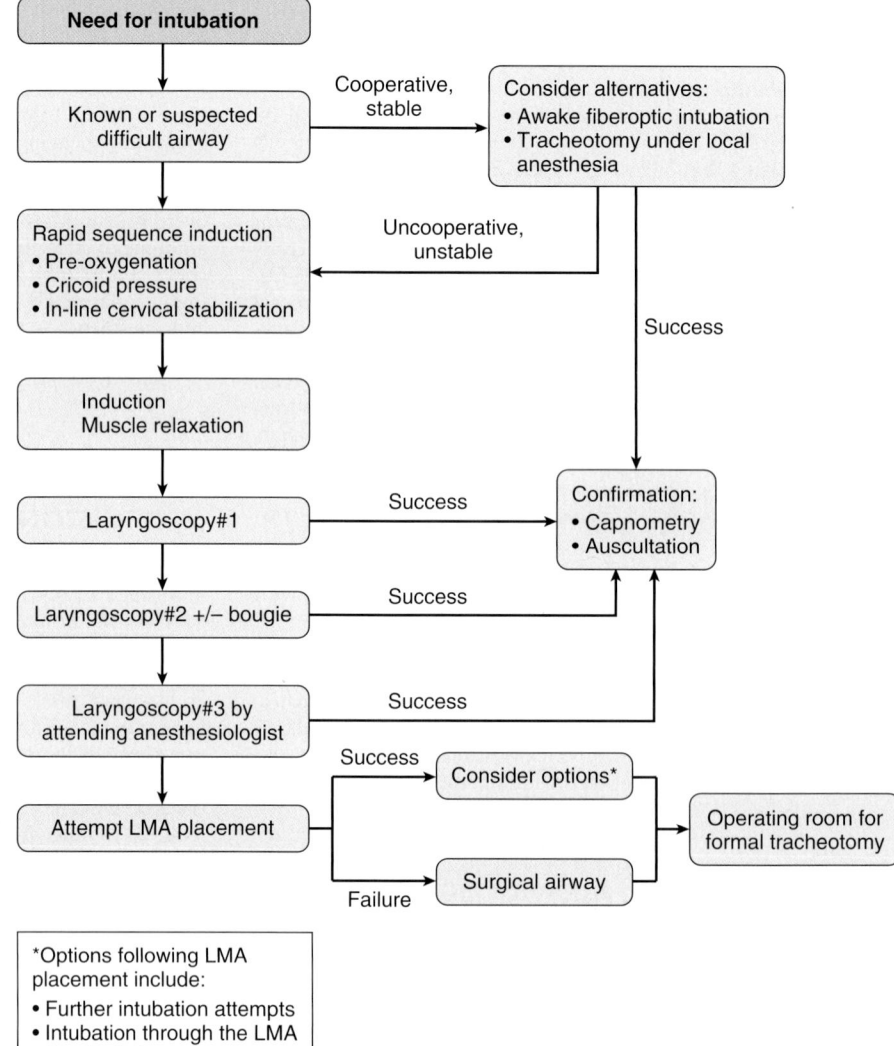

FIGURE 3 Airway management algorithm at the R Adams Cowley Shock Trauma Center. Laryngoscopy may include the use of a videolaryngoscope such as the GlideScope or Ranger (Verathon, Bothell, Wash) at multiple steps. *LMA*, laryngeal mask airway. *(From Stephens CT, Kahntroff S, Dutton RP et al: The success of emergency endotracheal intubation in trauma patients: a 10-year experience at a major adult trauma center, Anesth Analg 109:866-872, 2009.)*

When and Where to Intubate? Field Versus Emergency Department or Trauma Unit Endotracheal Intubation

Several reports over the past decade have described the potential risks associated with endotracheal intubation, and these data must be considered carefully before endotracheal intubation is used to secure the airway in the prehospital environment. Rates of successful endotracheal intubation by emergency medical services (EMS) providers vary widely by jurisdiction and have been reported to be less than 70% in some studies. One patient population that has been shown to benefit from early rapid sequence intubation is patients with traumatic brain injury (TBI); at least one randomized controlled trial has shown improved functional outcomes in adults with severe TBI. Nonetheless, in other studies, patients intubated in the field have been shown to have delays to definitive neurosurgical procedures, increased risk of pneumonia, worse functional outcomes, and higher mortality.

The American College of Emergency Physicians (ACEP), the American College of Surgeons Committee on Trauma (ACS-COT),

and the National Association of EMS Physicians (NAEMSP) endorse the use of drug-assisted endotracheal intubation by non-physician EMS providers, but only for providers who have adequate training and regular practice. EMS providers who perform drug-assisted endotracheal intubation must possess training, knowledge, and experience in the techniques and drugs used to perform endotracheal intubation. Robust medical direction, proper patient selection, ongoing airway management training, standardized intubation protocols, and quality assurance are essential components for any prehospital program that chooses to use drug-assisted intubation for trauma patients in the prehospital arena. Drug-assisted intubation should not be considered mandatory for all trauma patients, and each EMS system must evaluate whether there is a specific need for the procedure and adequate resources to develop and maintain a safe protocol. In systems where endotracheal intubation is not feasible and safe in the prehospital environment, the airway should be managed with airway adjuncts, supraglottic devices, and properly performed bag-valve mask ventilation until the patient arrives in the emergency department or trauma resuscitation unit.

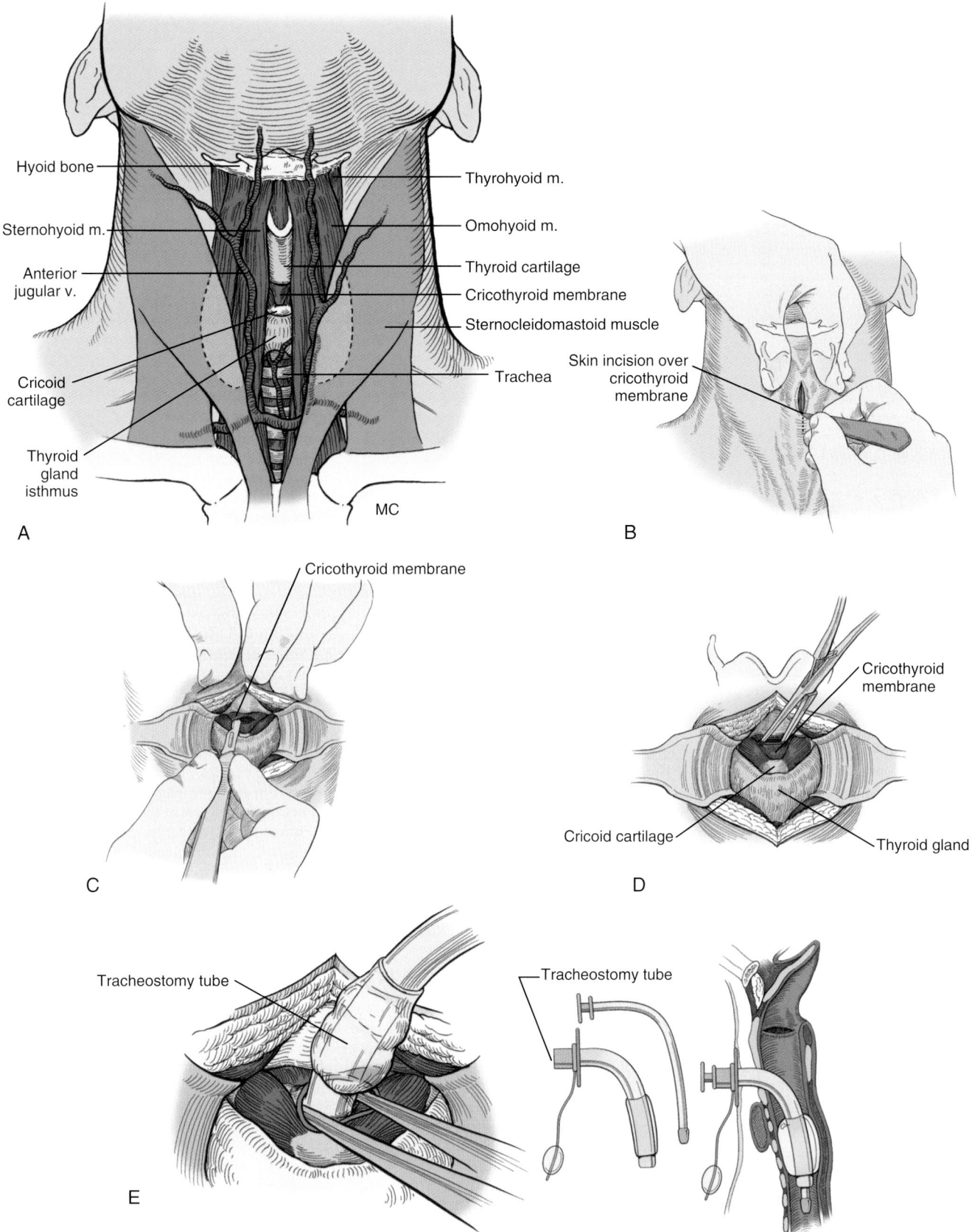

Hyoid bone

Sternohyoid m.

Anterior
jugular v.

Cricoid
cartilage

Thyroid
gland
isthmus

Thyrohyoid m.

Omohyoid m.

Thyroid cartilage

Cricothyroid membrane

Sternocleidomastoid muscle

Trachea

MC

A

Skin incision over
cricothyroid
membrane

B

Cricothyroid membrane

C

Cricothyroid
membrane

Cricoid cartilage

Thyroid gland

D

Tracheostomy tube

E

Tracheostomy tube

FIGURE 4 Cricothyroidotomy. **A,** The cricothyroid membrane is located between the thyroid cartilage above and the cricoid ring below. **B,** The operator's nondominant hand holds the thyroid cartilage, and the other hand performs the procedure. A vertical skin incision avoids the anterior jugular veins to minimize bleeding. **C,** The cricothyroid membrane is incised transversely. **D,** The opening is widened with a small hemostat. **E,** The tracheostomy tube is placed into the airway, and the cuff is inflated. *(From Haut ER: Evaluation and acute resuscitation of the trauma patient. In Evans SRT, editor:* Surgical pitfalls: prevention and management, *Philadelphia, 2009, Saunders Elsevier, pp 757-771.)*

SUGGESTED READINGS

American College of Surgeons: *Advanced trauma life support (ATLS)*, ed 8, Chicago, 2009, American College of Surgeons.

Bernard SA, Nguyen V, Cameron P, et al: Prehospital rapid sequence intubation improves functional outcome for patients with severe traumatic brain injury: a randomized controlled trial, *Ann Surg* 252(6):959–965, 2010.

Bochicchio, GV, Ilahi O, Joshi M, et al: Endotracheal intubation in the field does not improve outcome in trauma patients who present without an acutely lethal traumatic brain injury, *J Trauma* 54:307–311, 2003.

Bochiicchio GV, Scalea TM: Is field intubation useful? *Curr Opin Crit Care* 9(6):524–529, 2003.

Graham DB, Eastman AL, Aldy KN, et al: Outcomes and long term follow-up after emergent cricothyroidotomy: is routine conversion to tracheostomy necessary? *Am Surg* 77(12):1707–1711, 2011.

Kheterpal S, Han R, Tremper KK, et al: Incidence and predictors of difficult and impossible mask ventilation, *Anesthesiology* 105:885–891, 2006.

Mohammad E, Connolly LA: Rapid sequence induction and intubation: current controversy, *Anesth Analg* 110:1318–1325, 2010.

Patterson H: Emergency department intubation of trauma patients with undiagnosed cervical spine injury, *Emerg Med J* 21:302–305, 2004.

Pierre EJ, McNeer RR, Shamir MY, et al: Early management of the traumatized airway, *Anesthesiology Clin* 25:1–11, 2007.

Stephens CT, Kahntroff S, Dutton RP, et al: The success of emergency endotracheal intubation in trauma patients: a 10-year experience at a major adult trauma center, *Anesth Analg* 109:866–872, 2009.

THE SURGEON'S USE OF ULTRASOUND IN THORACOABDOMINAL TRAUMA

**Christopher J. Dente, MD, and
Grace S. Rozycki, MD, MBA**

For nearly 15 years, surgeons in American trauma centers have successfully performed, interpreted, and taught ultrasound examinations of patients who are injured or critically ill. Real-time imaging allows the surgeon to receive instantaneous information about the clinical condition of the patient and, therefore, helps to expedite the patient's management. In many trauma centers, ultrasound machines are owned by surgeons and are part of the standard equipment in the trauma resuscitation room. While diagnostic peritoneal lavage and computed tomographic (CT) scanning are still valuable diagnostic tests for the detection of intraabdominal injury in patients, ultrasound is faster, noninvasive, and painless. As such, it is an examination that is well tolerated not only by adults but also by children. Moreover, the portability of the ultrasound machine makes it useful not only in the hospital setting but also in more austere settings.

As an extension of the physical examination, surgeons routinely use ultrasound in the acute setting to determine the presence or absence of fluid in the peritoneal cavity, the pericardium, and the pleural cavities. Additional uses of this modality include the detection of pneumothoraces and sternal fractures. What follows is a discussion of the use of ultrasound in blunt and penetrating thoracoabdominal trauma, with an additional discussion of the use of ultrasound in forward settings and in space exploration.

FOCUSED ASSESSMENT FOR THE SONOGRAPHIC EVALUATION OF THE TRAUMA PATIENT

The *Focused Assessment for the Sonographic* evaluation of the *Trauma* (FAST) patient is a rapid diagnostic examination to assess patients with potential injuries to the thorax or abdomen. The test sequentially surveys for the presence or absence of fluid in the pericardial sac and in the dependent abdominal regions, including the Morison's pouch region of the right upper quadrant (RUQ), the left upper quadrant (LUQ) behind the spleen and between the spleen and kidney, and the pelvis including the area posterior to the bladder.

The FAST is performed in a specific sequence; the pericardial area is visualized first so that blood within the heart can be used as a standard to set the gain. Most modern ultrasound machines have presets so the gain does not need to be reset each time the machine is turned on. Occasionally, if multiple types of examinations are performed with different transducers, the gain should be checked to ensure that intracardiac blood appears anechoic. This maneuver ensures that hemoperitoneum will also appear anechoic and will be readily detected on the ultrasound image. The abdominal part of the FAST should begin with a survey of the RUQ, which is the location within the peritoneal cavity where blood most often accumulates and is most readily detected with the FAST. In a multicenter trial of 275 blunt and penetrating trauma patients, investigators found that regardless of the injured organ (with the exception of those patients who had an isolated perforated viscus), blood was most often identified on the RUQ image of the FAST. This can be a time-saving measure because when hemoperitoneum in the RUQ view is identified on the FAST examination of a hemodynamically unstable patient, then that image alone, in combination with the patient's clinical picture, is sufficient to justify an immediate abdominal operation. However in the hemodynamically stable patient, the examination of the RUQ is followed by the LUQ and pelvis as discussed later.

Technique

Ultrasound transmission gel is applied on four areas of the thoracoabdomen, and the examination is conducted in the following sequence: the pericardial area, RUQ, LUQ, and the pelvis (Figure 1). Abdominal structures are best imaged with a lower frequency transducer, which allows for deeper penetration into tissues (sacrificing some resolution). Most ultrasound probes are now capable of imaging in multiple frequencies, which allows achievement of the best balance of resolution (higher frequency) and tissue penetration (lower frequency) based on a patient's individual body habitus.

To begin the examination, a 3.5-MHz convex transducer is oriented for sagittal or longitudinal views and positioned in the subxiphoid region to identify the heart and to examine for blood in the pericardial sac. The normal and abnormal views of the pericardial area are shown in Figure 2. The subxiphoid image is usually not difficult to obtain, but a severe injury to the chest wall, a very narrow subcostal area, subcutaneous emphysema, or morbid obesity can prevent a satisfactory examination. Both of the latter conditions are associated with poor imaging because air and fat reflect the sound wave too strongly and prevent penetration into the target organ. If the subcostal pericardial image cannot be obtained or is suboptimal, a parasternal ultrasound view of the heart should be performed.

Next, the transducer is placed in the right anterior or midaxillary line between the 11th and 12th ribs to identify a sagittal section of the liver, kidney, and diaphragm (Figure 3). The presence or absence of blood is sought in Morison's pouch and in the right subphrenic space. Next, attention is turned to the LUQ and with the transducer positioned in the left posterior axillary line between the 10th and 11th ribs. The spleen and kidney are visualized and blood is sought in between the two organs and in the left subphrenic space (Figure 4). The splenic window is often the most difficult window, and the transducer should be placed more posterior (posterior axillary line) and superior (i.e., one to two rib spaces higher) than with the RUQ window.

Finally, the transducer is directed for a transverse view and placed about 4 cm superior to the symphysis pubis. It is swept inferiorly to obtain a coronal view of the full bladder and the pelvis, examining for the presence or absence of blood (Figure 5).

Accuracy of the FAST

Improper technique, inexperience of the examiner, and inappropriate use of ultrasound have long been known to adversely impact

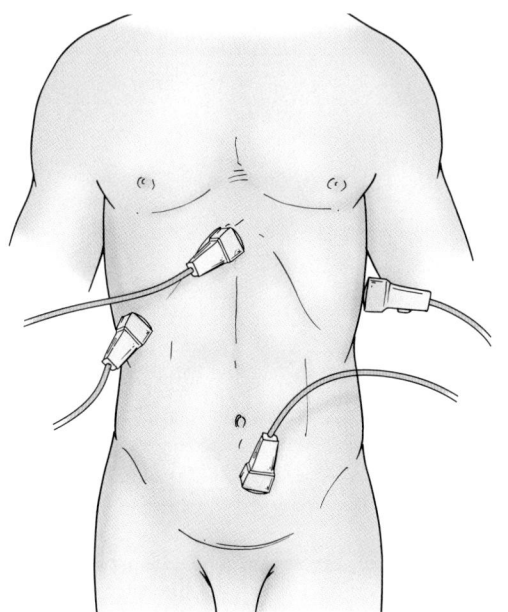

FIGURE 1 Transducer positions for FAST: pericardial, right upper quadrant, left upper quadrant, and pelvis.

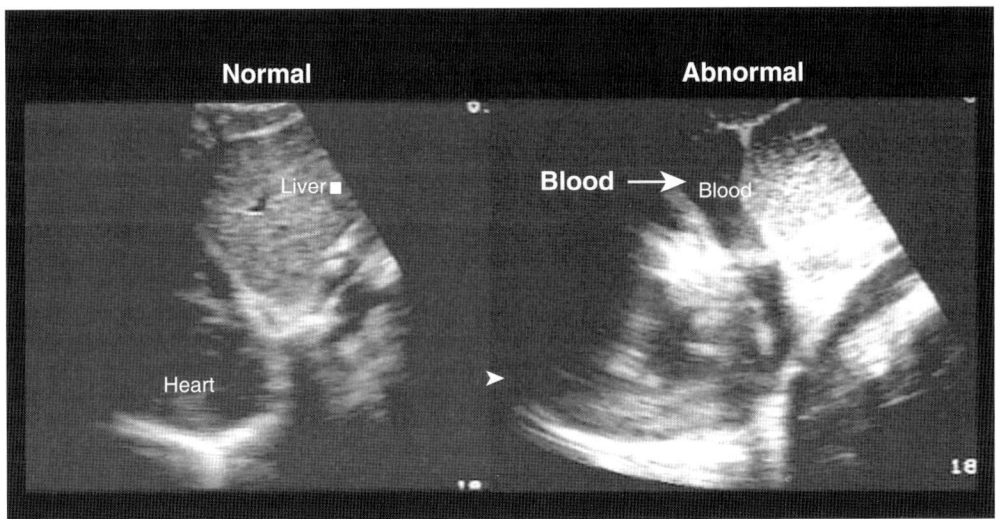

FIGURE 2 Normal sagittal view of pericardial area showing pericardium as single echogenic line *(left)*. Sagittal view of pericardial area showing separation of visceral and parietal areas of pericardium with blood *(arrow)* that appears anechoic *(right)*.

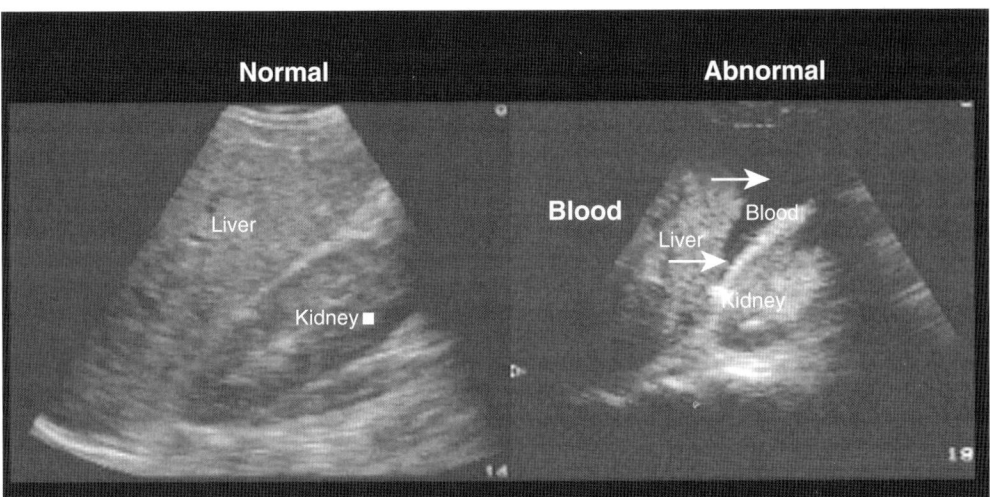

FIGURE 3 Normal sagittal view of liver, kidney, and diaphragm *(left)*. Note Gerota's fascia is hyperechoic. Abnormal sagittal view of liver, kidney, and diaphragm *(right)*. Note fluid (blood) in between liver and kidney *(arrows)*.

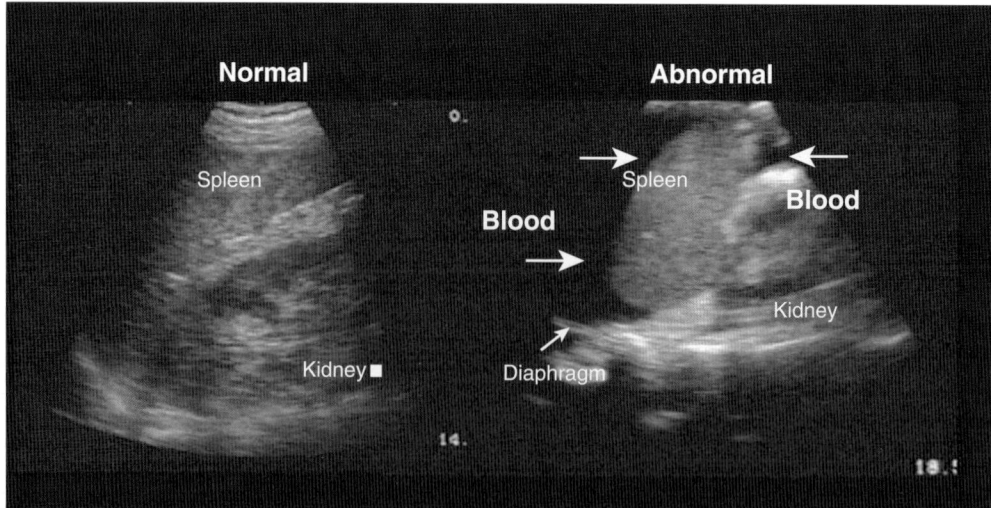

FIGURE 4 Normal sagittal view of spleen, kidney, and diaphragm *(left)*. Abnormal sagittal view of spleen, kidney, and diaphragm with fluid (blood) in between spleen and kidney and above the spleen in the subphrenic space *(right)*.

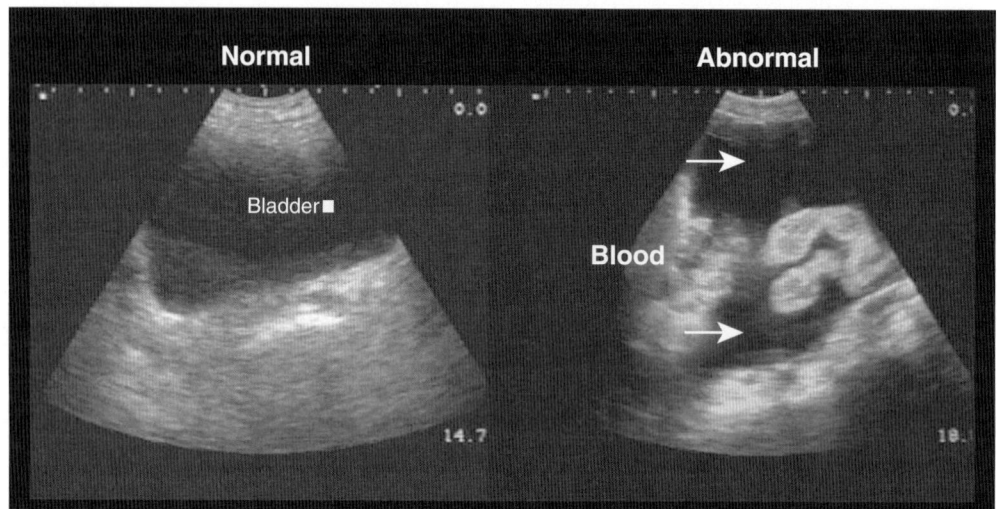

FIGURE 5 Normal transverse view of full urinary bladder *(left)*. Abnormal coronal view of full bladder with fluid in pelvis *(right)*. (Note the bowel floating in fluid.)

ultrasound imaging. The etiology of injury, the presence of hypotension on admission, and select associated injuries have also been shown to influence the accuracy of this modality. Failure to consider these factors has led to inaccurate assessments of the accuracy of the FAST by inappropriately comparing it to a CT scan and not recognizing its role in the evaluation of patients with penetrating torso trauma. Both false positive and negative pericardial ultrasound examinations have been reported to occur in the presence of a massive hemothorax or mediastinal blood. Repeating the FAST after the insertion of a tube thoracostomy improves the visualization of the pericardial area and decreases the number of false positive and false negative studies. Notwithstanding these circumstances in which false studies may occur, a rapid focused ultrasound survey of the subcostal pericardial area is a very accurate method to detect hemopericardium in most patients with penetrating wounds in the "cardiac box." In a large study of patients who sustained either blunt or penetrating injuries, the FAST was 100% sensitive and 99.3% specific for detecting hemopericardium in patients with precordial or transthoracic wounds. Furthermore, the use of pericardial ultrasound has been shown to be especially helpful in the evaluation of patients who have no overt signs of pericardial tamponade. This was highlighted in a study in which 10 of 22 patients with precordial wounds and hemopericardium on the ultrasound examinations had admission systolic blood pressures over 110 mm Hg and were relatively

asymptomatic. Based on these signs and the lack of symptoms, it is unlikely that the presence of cardiac wounds would have been strongly suspected in these patients, and therefore this rapid ultrasound examination provided an early diagnosis of hemopericardium before the patients underwent physiologic deterioration.

The FAST is a focused examination for the detection of fluid in dependent areas of the abdomen and designed to answer the simple question of "fluid or no fluid." Therefore, its results should not be compared to those of a CT scan because the FAST does not readily identify intraparenchymal or retroperitoneal injuries. Select patients considered to be at high risk for occult intraabdominal injury should undergo a CT scan of the abdomen regardless of the results of the FAST examination. These patients include those with fractures of the pelvis or thoracolumbar spine, major thoracic trauma especially pulmonary contusion and lower rib fractures, and hematuria.

Recent Advances and Organ Specificity

As surgeons have become more facile with ultrasound examinations and as technology has improved, extensions of the FAST examination have been described. Again, it is noted that the standard FAST examination is designed to accurately answer two simple questions: Is there fluid in the peritoneal cavity, and is their fluid in the pericardial sac?

The use of ultrasound for more complex diagnostic interventions is described below, but these areas are less well studied and beyond the purview of the traditional FAST examination.

A prospective, multicenter trial conducted by members of the Western Trauma Association reported on the use of ultrasound to serially evaluate patients with documented solid organ injuries (SOI) after trauma. The so-called "BOAST" examination, or the *B*edside *O*rgan *A*ssessment with *S*onography after *T*rauma, was performed by a limited number of experienced surgeon-sonographers in 126 patients with 135 SOI in 4 American trauma centers. This study, performed over nearly 2 years, was designed to be a more thorough abdominal ultrasound examination, with multiple views obtained of each solid organ (kidneys, liver, and spleen). Criteria for enrollment included normal hemodynamics, absence of peritonitis or other need for urgent laparotomy, and lack of excessive blood transfusion in the attending physician's judgment. All patients were victims of blunt trauma, with a mean injury severity score (ISS) of nearly 15.

Overall, only 34% of injuries to solid organs were seen with BOAST, yielding an error rate of 66%. None of the 34 Grade I injuries were identified, and only 13 (31%) of the Grade II injuries were identified. Sensitivities for Grades III and IV injuries ranged from 25% to 75%, and only one Grade V injury (to the liver) was examined and positively identified. It is noted, however, that 11 patients developed 16 intraabdominal complications (8 pseudoaneurysms, 4 bilomas, 3 abscesses, and 1 necrotic organ), and 13 (81%) were identified by the sonographers. This study emphasizes that ultrasound, in most surgeons' hands, should not be considered a reliable modality for diagnosis and grading of SOI, although it may be acceptably accurate in the diagnosis of posttraumatic abdominal complications in patients who undergo nonoperative management for solid organ injury.

In Europe, preliminary work using Power Doppler to identify specific organ injuries has been published in recent years. Many of these examinations include the use of a sonographic contrast agent injected peripherally during the scan. In one study, the authors were able to document contrast extravasation in 20 of 153 patients (13%). Extravasation was seen not only from the spleen, liver, and kidney after trauma but also in postoperative patients (aortic aneurysm repair, postsplenectomy) and in a patient with a ruptured aortic aneurysm. In 9 of 20 patients, CT scan was performed, and all 9 confirmed contrast extravasation. In the 133 patients without extravasation, the absence of active bleeding was inferred by a subsequent CT scan in 82 patients, surgical data in 13 patients, and clinical follow-up in 38 cases, with no cases of active bleeding missed by ultrasound. Thus, the addition of ultrasonic contrast agent and Power Doppler may be of some benefit in the diagnosis of specific injuries. It should be emphasized, that the FAST examination in most American trauma centers is used simply as a screening tool to identify the presence or absence of hemoperitoneum or hemopericardium in a trauma patient.

TRAUMATIC HEMOTHORAX

A focused thoracic ultrasound examination was developed by surgeons to rapidly detect the presence or absence of a traumatic hemothorax in patients during the American College of Surgeons Advanced Trauma Life Support (ATLS) secondary survey. This examination is worthwhile because it dramatically shortens the interval from the diagnosis of a hemothorax to the insertion of a thoracostomy tube.

Technique

The technique for this examination is similar to that used to interrogate the upper quadrants of the abdomen in the FAST and also uses the same type and frequency of transducer. It is performed one to two rib spaces higher than the RUQ and LUQ FAST views. Ultrasound transmission gel is applied to the right and left lower thoracic areas in the mid to posterior axillary lines between the 9th and 10th intercostal spaces (Figure 6). The transducer is slowly advanced cephalad to identify the hyperechoic diaphragm and to interrogate the supradiaphragmatic space for the presence or absence of fluid (Figure 7) that appears anechoic. In the positive thoracic ultrasound

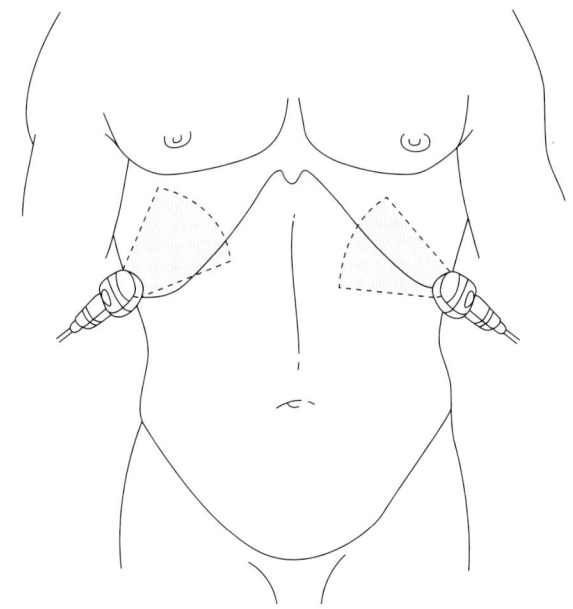

FIGURE 6 Transducer positions for thoracic ultrasound examination (detection of hemothorax).

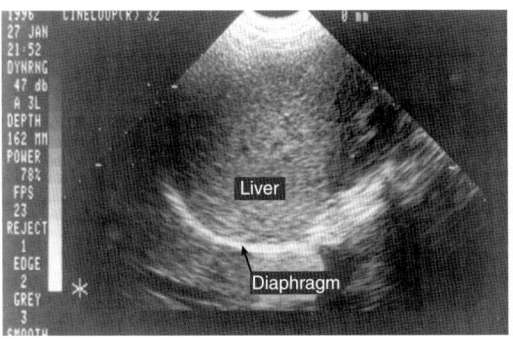

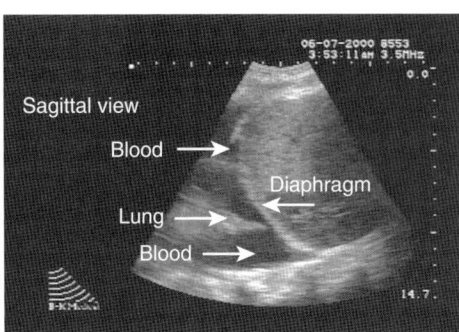

A   B

FIGURE 7 **A,** Sagittal view of liver, kidney, and diaphragm. Note supradiaphragmatic (lung) area but absence of pleural effusion. **B,** Sagittal view of right supradiaphragmatic space. The right hemothorax contains fluid (blood) that appears anechoic.

examination, the hypoechoic lung can be seen "floating" amidst the fluid. The same technique can be used to evaluate a critically ill patient for a pleural effusion.

Accuracy

Surgeons at Grady Memorial Hospital have examined the accuracy of this examination in 360 patients with blunt and penetrating torso injuries. They compared the time and accuracy of ultrasound with that of the supine portable chest x-ray and found both to be very similar: 97.4% sensitivity and 99.7% specificity observed for thoracic ultrasound versus 92.5% sensitivity and 99.7% specificity for the portable chest x-ray. Performance times, however, for the thoracic ultrasound examinations were statistically much faster ($P < 0.0001$) than those for the portable chest x-ray. Although it is not recommended that the thoracic ultrasound examination replace the chest x-ray, its use can expedite treatment in many patients and decrease the number of chest radiographs obtained.

PNEUMOTHORAX

Ultrasound examination is useful to the surgeon to evaluate a patient for a potential pneumothorax if (1) radiology equipment is not readily available; (2) inordinate delays for obtaining a chest x-ray are anticipated; or (3) numerous injured patients must be rapidly assessed and triaged. Although useful in the trauma resuscitation area, surgeons may also find this examination helpful to detect a pneumothorax in a critically ill patient after a thoracentesis procedure, or after discontinuing the suction on an underwater seal device.

Technique

A 5.0-MHz to 7.5-MHz linear array transducer is used to evaluate a patient for the presence of a pneumothorax. This higher frequency transducer allows for better resolution of superficial structures and the examination may be performed while the patient is in the erect or the supine position. Ultrasound transmission gel is applied to the right and left upper thoracic areas at about the 3rd to 4th intercostal space in the midclavicular line, and the presumed unaffected thoracic cavity is examined first. The transducer is oriented for longitudinal imaging, placed perpendicular to the ribs, and is slowly advanced medially toward the sternum and then laterally toward the anterior axillary line. The normal examination of the thoracic cavity identifies the rib (seen as black on the ultrasound image because it is a refraction artifact), pleural sliding, and a comet tail artifact. "Sliding" is the identification of the visceral and parietal layers of the pleura seen as hyperechoic superimposed pleural lines moving upon each other with respiration. When a pneumothorax is present, air becomes trapped between the visceral and parietal pleura and does not allow for the transmission of the ultrasound waves. Therefore, the visceral pleura is not imaged, and pleural sliding is not observed. The comet tail artifact is generated because of the interaction of two highly reflective opposing interfaces: air and pleura (Figure 8). When air separates the visceral and parietal pleura, the comet tail artifact is not visualized. If desired, the examination may be repeated with the transducer oriented for transverse views, and images obtained with the transducer parallel to the ribs.

Accuracy

Several studies have documented the sensitivity and specificity of ultrasound for the detection of a pneumothorax. Dulchavsky and colleagues from Detroit Receiving Hospital showed that ultrasound

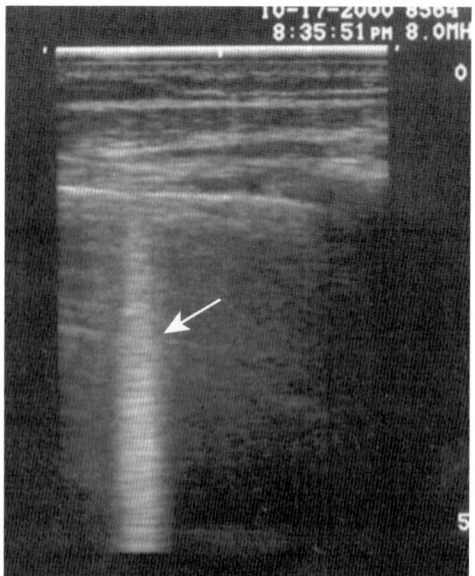

FIGURE 8   Comet tail artifact *(arrow).*

can be successfully used by surgeons to detect a pneumothorax in injured patients. Of the 364 patients (362 trauma; 18 spontaneous) evaluated with ultrasound, 39 had pneumothoraces, and ultrasound successfully detected 37 of them, yielding a 95% sensitivity. Pneumothoraces in two patients could not be detected because of the presence of significant subcutaneous emphysema. The authors recommended that when a portable chest x-ray cannot be readily obtained, the use of this bedside ultrasound examination for the identification of a pneumothorax can expedite the patient's management. In this authors' experiences, ultrasound is very sensitive for the detection of pneumothorax, and we have detected many that were seen only on subsequent thoracic CT scan. Thus, this test may be useful not only to rapidly diagnose a pneumothorax in a hemodynamically unstable patient but also to avoid an unnecessary chest tube in a patient who becomes hypotensive for unclear reasons.

STERNAL FRACTURE

Fractures of the sternum are visualized on a lateral x-ray view of the chest, but this film may be difficult to obtain in a multisystem injured patient. For this reason, an ultrasound examination of the sternum can rapidly detect a fracture while the patient is still in the supine position and, therefore, avoid the need to obtain an x-ray.

Technique

The ultrasound examination of the sternum is performed using a high-frequency linear array transducer that is oriented for sagittal or longitudinal views. Ultrasound transmission gel is applied over the sternal area while the patient is in the supine position. Beginning at the suprasternal notch, the transducer is slowly advanced in a caudad direction to interrogate the bone for a fracture, and then the examination is repeated with the transducer oriented for transverse views. The examination of the intact sternum is shown in Figure 9. A sternal fracture is identified on the ultrasound examination as a disruption of the cortical reflex (Figure 10). Investigators have found that the use of ultrasound for this diagnosis is as accurate as a lateral x-ray view of the chest.

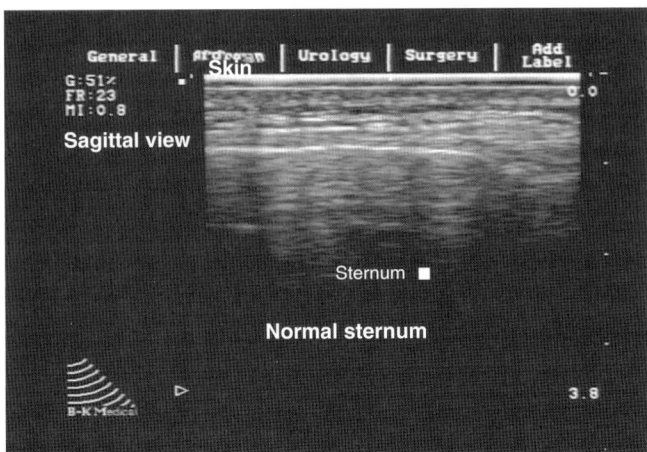

FIGURE 9 Sagittal view of sternum. Normal findings.

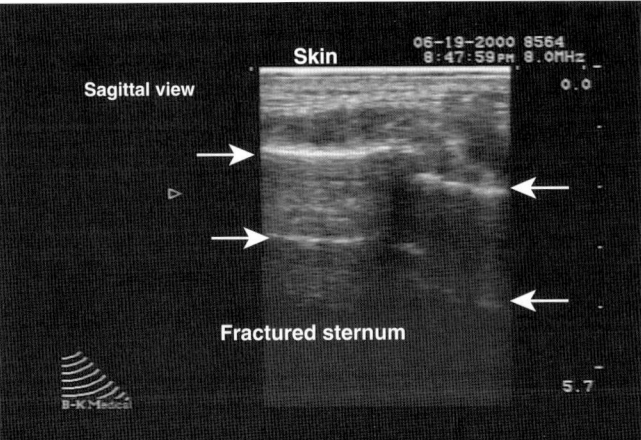

FIGURE 10 Sagittal view of sternum illustrating fracture (interruption of hyperechoic line).

SPECIAL SITUATIONS

Ultrasound in the Pregnant Trauma Patient

Ultrasound would seem to be an ideal method of evaluating a pregnant patient with suspected blunt abdominal trauma because it is portable, noninvasive, and free of ionizing radiation. The American College of Surgeons ATLS course teaches that unrecognized abdominal trauma is one of the leading causes of death in the pregnant trauma patient. Concerns over changes in abdominal anatomy leading to difficulty in obtaining ultrasound images of the pregnant patient have not borne out in objective evaluation. Goodwin and colleagues reported on their 8-year experience with the FAST examination used to evaluate 127 injured pregnant patients. Five of 6 patients with hemoperitoneum were found to have fluid on FAST examination, yielding a sensitivity of 83%. Of the 120 patients without abdominal injury, 117 had true negative results (specificity 98%) and there were 3 false positive examinations due to serous intraperitoneal fluid. Furthermore, Brown and colleagues reported their experience with a more extensive ultrasound examination in 101 hemodynamically stable, pregnant patients with suspected blunt abdominal trauma. The median gestational age was just over 24 weeks. Patients underwent a standard abdominal ultrasound examination as well as an examination of the fetus and placenta by a registered ultrasound technician. The sensitivity of the examination was

80% and untrasound identified injuries to the placenta, spleen, liver, and kidney. None of the 96 patients with a negative ultrasound examination had injuries discovered later in their hospital course (specificity 100%). Thus, it would seem that ultrasound remains a good screening tool for the pregnant patient with blunt abdominal trauma.

Ultrasound in Penetrating Trauma

Ultrasound as used to evaluate patients with penetrating trauma has been studied much less extensively than its use for blunt trauma. Several of the larger, well-known series have included patients with penetrating trauma, and, as stated previously, the ultrasound of the pericardium has been shown to be accurate for diagnosis of injury in patients with penetrating injury to the "cardiac box." In a study of 32 patients with penetrating anterior chest trauma, ultrasound was used to diagnose 8 pericardial effusions with a reported 100% accuracy (8 true positive and 24 true negative examinations). Eight other patients were noted to have intraperitoneal fluid and underwent therapeutic exploration, including repair of the diaphragm, liver, spleen, stomach, small bowel, and adrenal gland. No false positive or fast negative examinations of the abdomen were reported. Other studies have shown that the accuracy of FAST after penetrating trauma is somewhat less, with one study reporting sensitivity for the detection of abdominal injury after penetrating trauma as low as 67%.

A report by Murphy and colleagues looked at the utility of ultrasound to diagnose fascial penetration after anterior abdominal stab wounds. In this study, 35 patients underwent ultrasound evaluation of their anterior abdominal fascia with an 8.0-MHz linear array transducer followed by a local wound exploration. While ultrasound had only a 59% sensitivity (13 out of 22 patients), it did have a 100% specificity with no false positive studies. Thus, if fascial penetration is noted on ultrasound, a more invasive wound exploration is probably not needed; however, a negative ultrasound evaluation is less helpful and does not preclude peritoneal penetration.

Use of Ultrasound in Austere Settings

Ultrasound on Deployment

The portability of ultrasound makes it ideal for use in forward settings. In fact, training courses are in place to teach military surgeons the use of the FAST examination, and handheld ultrasound is now routinely deployed within the British Defence Medical Services. In a survey of surgeons reviewing potential preventable casualties in Vietnam, ultrasound was the fourth most commonly mentioned advancement in technology (behind modern ventilators, CT scanners, and modern antibiotics) that may have assisted in better patient salvage.

Although up to 90% of war wounds are penetrating, ultrasound may allow quicker, more accurate triage decisions because patients with penetrating abdominal trauma with no or minimal hemoperitoneum may be transferred to the next echelon of care, where the study may be repeated or additional diagnostic tests undertaken. In a study from the Croatian conflict in 1999, FAST was shown to have a sensitivity of 86%, a specificity of 100%, and an accuracy of 97% when applied to 94 casualties evaluated over a 72-hour period. This was comparable to the accuracy achieved by the authors in their civilian experience with FAST in more than 1000 patients over the 3 years prior to the conflict. In a small series, FAST was used with excellent results in a British military hospital in Iraq. Fifteen casualties were evaluated with serial FAST examinations, and 14 of them had negative examinations on admission and again at 6 hours. One patient underwent laparotomy based on missile trajectory alone and two small perforations were discovered in the cecum. The other

13 patients recovered without sequelae. One examination was positive and led to immediate laparotomy in a patient with a Grade V liver injury after a motor vehicle collision.

Because ultrasound is portable enough to use in active combat situations, research is ongoing to evaluate the best method to teletransmit images obtained in the field. Several different satellite transmission systems have been evaluated, and high-quality images were able to be obtained in the majority of cases, although the balance between the weight of the system and the minimum image quality has still not been completely achieved. It is noted, that images can be transmitted from up to 1500 feet from the antennae without significant degradation. As technology advances, one would expect imaging systems to continue to become smaller and lighter with improved image quality, making ultrasound even more appealing as a modality for use in the forward setting.

Ultrasound in Space

Many of the same qualities that make ultrasound appealing for use in combat make it equally appealing as a diagnostic modality in space, where an injury might require abortion of a multimillion-dollar mission. Indeed, ultrasound is one of the only feasible diagnostic modalities on space missions, given size and weight restrictions. Also, ultrasound examinations are easily taught, and images can be relayed with minimal delay to physicians on the ground. ATLS procedures are also feasible in space, and lifesaving procedures could be performed based on ultrasound findings.

Ultrasound has been used in space for several decades. It has been ultrasound technology that has taught us much about the physiologic effects of microgravity, especially the fluid shifts associated with space travel. As early as 1982, cardiac ultrasound was used to evaluate left ventricular systolic function and cardiac chamber size in cosmonauts. The first American ultrasound system in space was the American flight echograph from Advanced Technology Laboratories (Bothel, Wash) that first flew in 1984 and eventually was capable of three-dimensional images using a tilt frame device. Currently, the Human Research Facility aboard the International Space Station (ISS) is equipped with a state-of-the-art Philips HDI 5000 (Philips Medical, Bothel Wash).

Because surface tension and capillary action are the principal physical forces in space, scientists questioned whether images obtained on the standard FAST examination would be useful in microgravity. There are now several published studies of ultrasound examinations performed on parabolic flights onboard the NASA Microgravity Research Facility, a KC-135 aircraft. This aircraft can generate 25 to 30 intervals of weightlessness using serial parabolic trajectories. A porcine model of intraabdominal hemorrhage was created on the ground and studied during parabolic flights. Over 2000 ultrasound segments were recorded, with 80% of these considered feasible for diagnosis of the presence or absence of abdominal fluid. The sonographers determined the examination was no more difficult than one done on the ground as long as the sonographer and patient were adequately restrained. For the intraperitoneal portion of the examination, a fourth view (the midline "abdominal sweep") was added, and with this addition, the FAST examination was able to reliably detect even relatively small amounts of intraperitoneal fluid. The Morison's pouch view remained the most sensitive window for fluid detection. Further study using a similar model revealed that ultrasound can also reliably detect both hemothorax and pneumothorax in microgravity.

Recently, astronauts aboard the ISS performed FAST examinations that were transmitted with a 2-second satellite delay to directors on the ground, who provided instructions for transducer position and system adjustments. Examinations were able to be completed in roughly 5 minutes, with adequate images obtained in all views. Astronauts have also been able to perform comprehensive ocular ultrasound examinations aboard the ISS with similar feedback.

In summary, ultrasound fulfills all the necessary criteria for a diagnostic modality in space. It is sufficiently portable, teletransmittable, teachable, and accurate. It will likely continue to be the only feasible technology to evaluate patients on space missions in the near future.

USING ULTRASOUND TO ASSESS INTRAVASCULAR VOLUME STATUS AND CARDIAC FUNCTION

For several years, ultrasound has been used by specialists to assess a patient's intravascular volume status at the bedside. This focused examination is performed with the same transducer as that used for the FAST examination. The longitudinal view of the vena cava is identified in the subxiphoid view and then assessed for compressibility. A vena cava that is easily compressible indicates that the patient is hypovolemic, whereas a vena cava that is noncompressible or has a diameter greater than 2 cm indicates that the patient is euvolemic or hypervolemic. A study by Ferrada and colleagues showed that the focused examination was 100% sensitive relative to a change in the vena cava diameter with a fluid challenge. A multicenter prospective study is being conducted to confirm the accuracy of the examination to guide the patient's initial resuscitation and that during the intensive care stay.

The Focused Rapid Echocardiographic Examination, or FREE, is a transthoracic examination that was developed to assess the critically ill patient's volume and cardiac status. This point of care examination uses hemodynamic information from the ultrasound examination with the patient's clinical parameters to determine whether the patient needs volume, inotropes, or pressors. Surgeons have shown that its accuracy is high and that it can be performed accurately by trauma team members who have been trained in the basic principles of ultrasound.

SUMMARY

As the role of the general surgeon continues to evolve, the surgeon's use of ultrasound will surely influence practice patterns, particularly for the evaluation of patients in the acute setting. With the use of real-time imaging, the surgeon receives "instantaneous" information to augment the physical examination, narrow the differential diagnosis, or initiate an intervention. Algorithms for the suggested use of ultrasound in penetrating trauma and blunt abdominal trauma are included as Figure 11.

The advantages of ultrasound are easily seen in each of the following clinical scenarios. As a noninvasive, nonionizing radiation modality, ultrasound can be used to evaluate the injured pregnant patient and simultaneously identify the fetal heart so that its rate can be recorded. For the patient with multiple fractures who is in traction, the portable machine is wheeled to the patient's bedside, and the FAST is performed without having to move the patient. If hypotension or an unexpected decrease in hematocrit occurs, an ultrasound examination can be easily repeated to exclude hemoperitoneum as the source of hypotension. When several patients with penetrating thoracoabdominal injuries present simultaneously to the emergency department, a rapid FAST examination with thoracic views can assess for pericardial effusion, massive hemothorax, or hemoperitoneum within seconds. This information helps the surgeon to prioritize resources and triage patients. Finally, this painless, noninvasive modality is well accepted, even by children, because it is performed at the bedside and is not intimidating. As surgeons become more facile with ultrasound, it is anticipated that other uses will develop to further enhance its value for the assessment of patients in the acute setting.

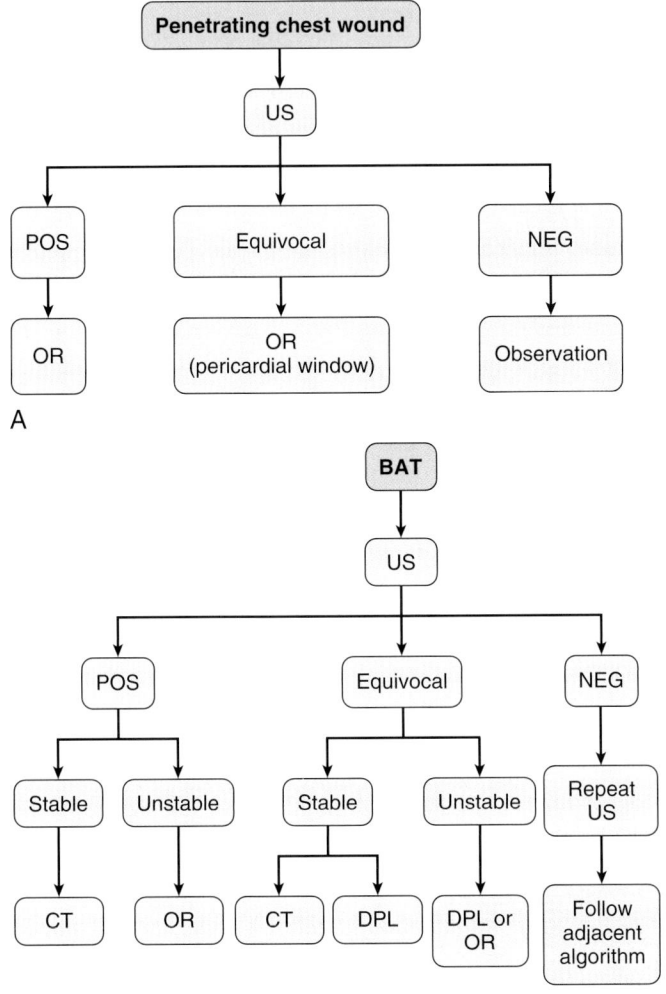

FIGURE 11   **A,** Algorithm for the use of ultrasound in patients with penetrating chest wounds. **B,** Algorithm for the use of ultrasound in patients with blunt abdominal trauma. *BAT,* Blunt abdominal tumors; *CT,* computed tomography; *DPL,* diagnostic peritoneal lavage; *NEG,* negative; *OR,* operating room; *POS,* positive; *US,* ultrasound.

NEW HORIZONS IN POINT OF CARE ULTRASOUND

Current reliance on computed tomographic scanning for the assessment of surgical patients, especially those who are injured, is a major source of radiation exposure. This is particularly concerning because long-term, cumulative doses of radiation have been shown to have potential adverse effects on the patient's physiology. In an effort to address this concern, the American Institute of Ultrasound in Medicine is launching *Ultrasound First,* an initiative designed to call attention to the safe, effective, and affordable advantages of ultrasound as an alternative to other imaging modalities that are more costly and/or emit radiation. Unfortunately, despite its many advantages, ultrasound as a first-line diagnostic test is underutilized in the assessment of surgical patients. *Ultrasound First* will focus on educating health care workers and stakeholders on the benefits of ultrasound in medical care. Further, to bolster its validity as a "first-line modality," the *Journal of Ultrasound in Medicine* has launched a special feature, the Sound Judgment Series, consisting of invited articles highlighting the clinical value of using ultrasound as the first test in select patients and diagnoses where it has shown to be at least comparable to other diagnostic modalities. The integration of ultrasound into medical education is an equally critical component for realizing the benefits of ultrasound in patient care. With these efforts and the growing body of physicians using bedside ultrasound, it is anticipated that the use of evidenced-based guidelines for this modality will continue to grow and become a critical part of medical education.

SELECTED READINGS

American Institute of Ultrasound in Medicine (AIUM): *Ultrasound First,* http://www.ultrasoundfirst.org/ultrasoundFirst/pages/news.aspx. Accessed November 1, 2012.

Ballard RB, Rozycki GS, Newman PG, et al: An algorithm to reduce the incidence of false-negative FAST examination in patients at high-risk for occult injury, *J Am Coll Surg* 189:145–151, 1999.

Brown MA, Sirlin CB, Farahmand N, et al: Screening sonography. In Pregnant patients with blunt abdominal trauma, *J Ultrasound Med* 24:175–181, 2005.

Dulchavsky SA, Schwarz KL, Kirkpatrick AW, et al: Prospective evaluation of thoracic ultrasound in the detection of pneumothorax, *J Trauma* 50:201–205, 2001.

Ferrada P, Anand RJ, Whelan J, et al: Qualitative assessment of the inferior vena cava: useful tool for the evaluation of fluid status in critically ill patients, *Am Surg* 78:468–470, 2012.

Ferrada P, Murthi S, Anand RJ, et al: Transthoracic focused rapid echocardiographic examination: real-time evaluation of fluid status in critically ill trauma patients, *J Trauma* 70:56–64, 2011.

Goodwin H, Holmes JF, Wisner DH: Abdominal ultrasound examination in pregnant blunt trauma patients, *J Trauma* 50:689–694, 2001.

Kirkpatrick AW, Hamilton DR, Nicolaou S, et al: Focused assessment with sonography for trauma in weightlessness: a feasibility study, *J Am Coll Surg* 196:833–844, 2003.

Murphy JT, Hall J, Provost D: Fascial ultrasound for evaluation of anterior abdominal stab wound injury, *J Trauma* 59(4):843–846, 2005.

Proceedings from AIUM ultrasound first forum reveal future agenda for ultrasound. (2013). Retrieved August 1, 2013, from http://www.ultrasoundfirst.org/ultrasoundFirst/pages/news.aspx.

Rozycki GS, Ballard RB, Feliciano DV, et al: Surgeon-performed ultrasound for the assessment of truncal injuries: lessons learned from 1,540 patients, *Ann Surg* 228:557–567, 1998.

Rozycki GS, Feliciano DV, Schmidt JA, et al: The role of surgeon-performed ultrasound in patients with possible cardiac wounds, *Ann Surg* 223:737–746, 1996.

Yanagawa Y, Sakamoto T, Okada Y: Hypovolemic shock evaluated by sonographic measurement of the inferior vena cava during resuscitation in trauma patients, *J Trauma* 63:1245–1248, 2007.

Zagzebski JA, editor: *Essentials of ultrasound physics,* St. Louis, Missouri, 1996, Mosby-Year Book, Inc.

Emergency Department Thoracotomy

Matthew V. Benns, MD, and
J. David Richardson, MD

OVERVIEW

Emergency department thoracotomy (EDT) following trauma has been used for a variety of indications since its introduction in the 1960s. Initial enthusiasm for the procedure was tempered by the reality of very poor overall meaningful survival. Results reported in the literature vary depending on the definition of EDT and the condition of the patients being treated. If the EDT is performed as a "resuscitative thoracotomy" on patients with a measurable arterial pressure, the results will likely be better than results following procedures performed on patients with signs of life only. The focus over the past several decades has been to better define the indications for effective use of EDT. Controversy still exists, however, with critics citing futility of care and potential dangers of exposure to healthcare workers. Nevertheless, EDT represents an immediate lifesaving intervention for a select group of patients. An understanding of the indications, pathophysiology, and techniques of EDT allows practitioners the best chance at achieving favorable outcomes.

INDICATIONS

EDT is a technique that can be employed rapidly to address a few basic injury patterns and assist with resuscitation. Specifically, EDT is performed for release of pericardial tamponade, control of cardiac or intrathoracic hemorrhage, correction of bronchovenous air embolism, open cardiac massage, or temporary occlusion of the descending thoracic aorta. It is ideally suited to address simple injuries within the thoracic cavity that are causing serious physiologic insult and impending death (Box 1). Unfortunately, the specific nature and severity of injuries are usually unknown until the EDT has been performed. Therefore, criteria have been developed to try to identify patients in whom EDT has the best chance of being beneficial. These criteria are broadly based on the patient's physiologic status, the mechanism of injury, and the timing of events prior to the patient's arrival to the emergency department.

Appropriate candidates for EDT uniformly present in *extremis*, but physiologic status is often discussed in terms of the presence of *vital signs* or *signs of life*. Vital signs include a measurable blood pressure, a palpable pulse, and spontaneous respiratory activity. Signs of life (SOL) include pupillary response, spontaneous respiratory effort, extremity movement, and cardiac electrical activity. The presence of SOL in the emergency department or within a known and short interval prior to arrival is a firm requirement for appropriate EDT. As a practical matter, judging if SOL were present prehospital and the length of time these have been absent is extremely difficult.

Defining absolute criteria for EDT is difficult, as aggressiveness must be balanced by real concerns regarding futility of care and the appropriate use of healthcare resources. In addition, there will always be an occasional outlier who survives EDT who is well beyond any established criteria for appropriate use of EDT. Box 2 lists the main indications and contraindications for EDT. It has been used successfully for patients with blunt and/or penetrating mechanisms of trauma, but outcomes are significantly better for penetrating thoracic injuries as the chances are greater of identifying a localized area of injury. Victims of blunt trauma who lose SOL often have significant associated multisystem injuries. Even if a blunt thoracic injury is discovered with EDT, the character of these injuries is often not amenable to simple and rapid control. Although there are many survivors reported in the literature, blunt mechanism remains controversial and should prompt a more rigid adherence to established guidelines.

Figure 1 shows a decision-making algorithm for EDT based on injury mechanism, SOL, and timing. Use of EDT is ultimately at the discretion of the clinician and will be heavily influenced by previous experience and clinical judgment.

PROCEDURAL TECHNIQUES

Initial Exposure

EDT is performed in the supine position. The patient's left arm is abducted to provide access to the left chest. A splash prep is performed, and an incision is made from the sternum and extending laterally to the mid-axillary line. The incision is located just inferior to the nipple in men and in the inframammary fold in women, which generally places it in the fourth or fifth intercostal space. The incision should curve gently along with the underlying ribs (Figure 2). The underlying soft tissue and intercostal musculature are rapidly divided with a scalpel or scissors, running along the top of the selected rib interspace to avoid the neurovascular bundle. The pleura is sharply incised to enter the chest and a Finochietto retractor is placed in the rib interspace. The handle of the retractor should be placed laterally (within the axilla) to facilitate extension of the EDT incision into a "clamshell" thoracotomy if needed. A clamshell thoracotomy involves dividing the sternum with a Lebsche knife or heavy shears and creating a matching thoracotomy incision on the patient's right side (Figure 3). The internal mammary arteries will be divided and must be controlled if circulation is restored. This type of incision provides unparalleled access to both thoracic cavities and the mediastinum.

Pericardotomy and Control of Cardiac Injuries

Pericardotomy is performed for release of pericardial tamponade and to evaluate any underlying myocardial injuries. Pericardial tamponade cannot be completely excluded based on visual inspection alone; thus, pericardotomy should always be performed during EDT. The pericardium is incised longitudinally from the aortic root to the apex. The incision should be made well anterior to the phrenic nerve to avoid inadvertent injury (Figure 4). Ideally, the pericardium should be grasped and pulled away from the heart when it is incised. In some situations of pericardial tamponade, the pericardium will be bulging and may prove difficult to grasp adequately. In these situations, a knife or single tine of scissors can be used to make an initial "stab" pericardotomy that is then extended. Extreme care must be undertaken to avoid injury to the underlying heart, but there will usually be a space buffer of underlying blood in these situations. Once the pericardium has been opened, all underlying blood and clot are evacuated and the myocardium is inspected. Injuries should be controlled rapidly with digital pressure or sutures. A skin stapler may also be used to quickly obtain temporary control of long myocardial lacerations. Any intervention performed in the emergency department should be simple and rapid to allow for restoration of vital signs and expeditious transport to the operating room for definitive repair.

Control of Intrathoracic Hemorrhage

Pulmonary or thoracic great vessel lacerations can lead to rapid exsanguination due to the lack of adjacent tissue tamponade within

BOX 1: Therapeutic maneuvers in emergency department thoracotomy

- Release of pericardial tamponade
- Control of intrathoracic or cardiac hemorrhage
- Performance of open cardiac massage
- Temporary occlusion of descending aorta
- Evacuation of bronchovenous air

BOX 2: Indications and contraindications for emergency department thoracotomy

Indications
- Penetrating injury with loss of vital signs in the ED, or with less than 15 minutes of prehospital CPR
- Blunt injury with loss of vital signs in the ED, or with less than 5 minutes of prehospital CPR

Contraindications
- No field SOL with penetrating or blunt injury
- Penetrating injury with greater than 15 minutes of prehospital CPR
- Blunt injury with greater than 5 minutes of prehospital CPR

CPR, Cardiopulmonary resuscitation; *ED,* emergency department; *SOL,* signs of life.

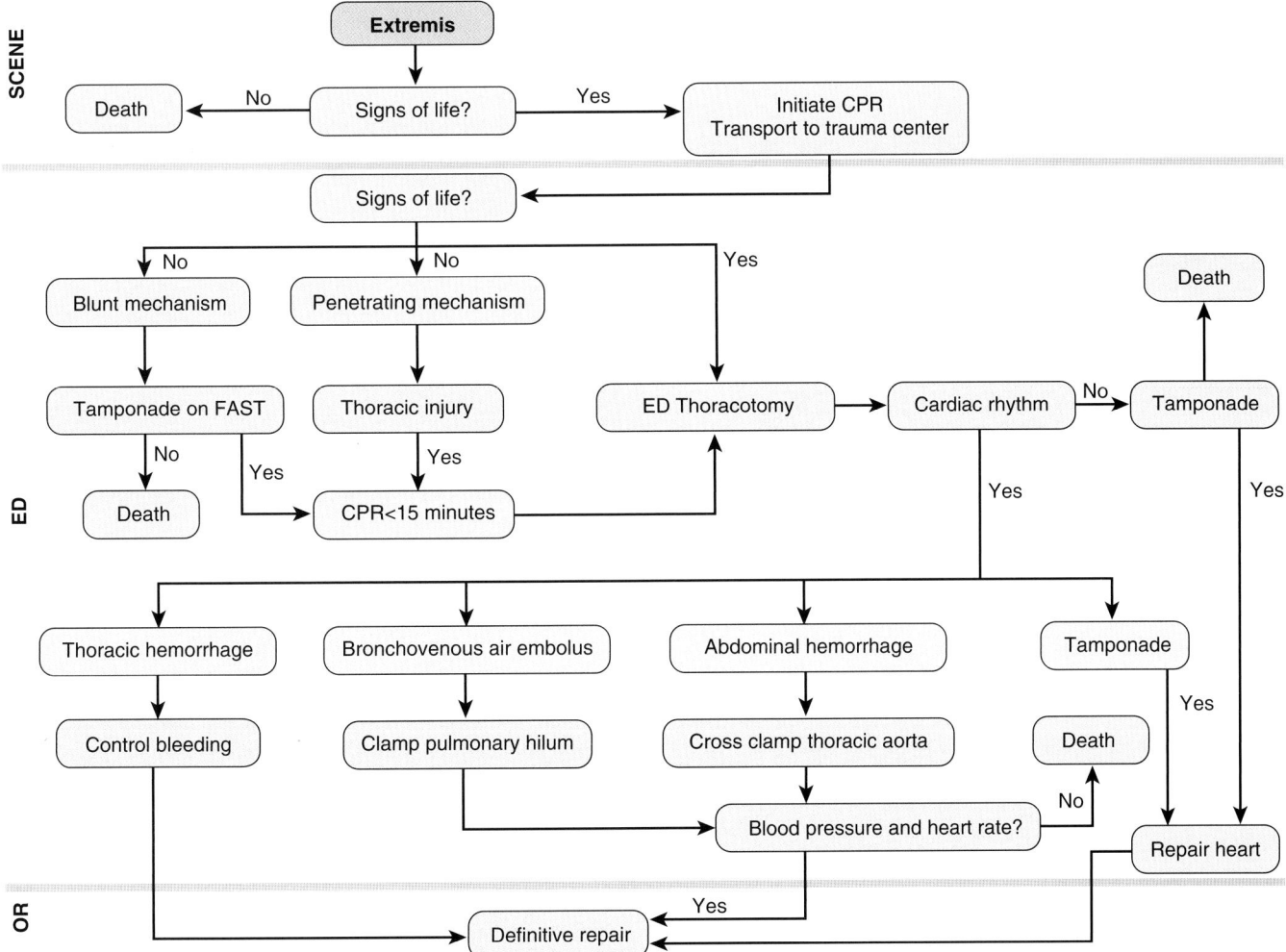

FIGURE 1   Decision-making algorithm for emergency department thoracotomy (EDT). *CPR,* Cardiopulmonary resuscitation; *ED,* emergency department; *FAST,* Focused Assessment with Sonography for Trauma; *OR,* operating room.

the chest. Injuries to smaller vessels such as the intercostals can also cause exsanguination if there is a delay in presentation. These injuries may be addressed with EDT. Digital pressure may be successful on a temporary basis for great vessel injuries if isolated. Straight or side-biting vascular clamps can also be used. Suture control in the emergency department may be appropriate for some injuries, but, in most cases, temporary control with formal repair in the operating room is the preferred approach. For major pulmonary vascular injuries, the pulmonary hilum can be clamped to provide temporary control. If an appropriate clamp is not available, the hilum can be twisted 180 degrees after release of the inferior pulmonary ligament. This maneuver generally will occlude hilar bleeding.

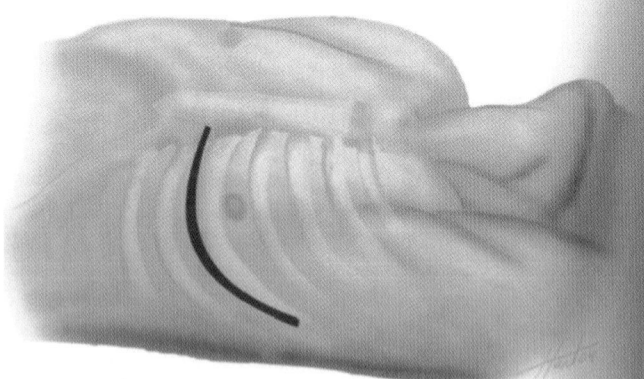

FIGURE 2 Incision for emergency department thoracotomy in the fourth or fifth intercostal space. The left arm is abducted and the incision is made just below the nipple in males or at the inframammary fold in females. The incision should follow the curvature of the ribs and be carried down to at least the mid-axillary line.

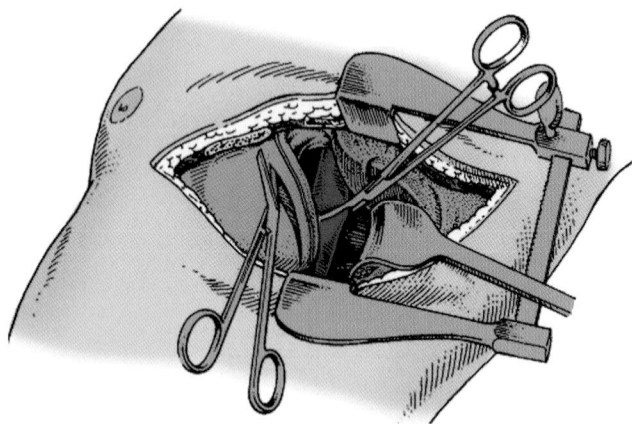

FIGURE 4 Pericardotomy and thoracic aortic cross clamping. The pericardium should be opened longitudinally and anterior to the phrenic nerve.

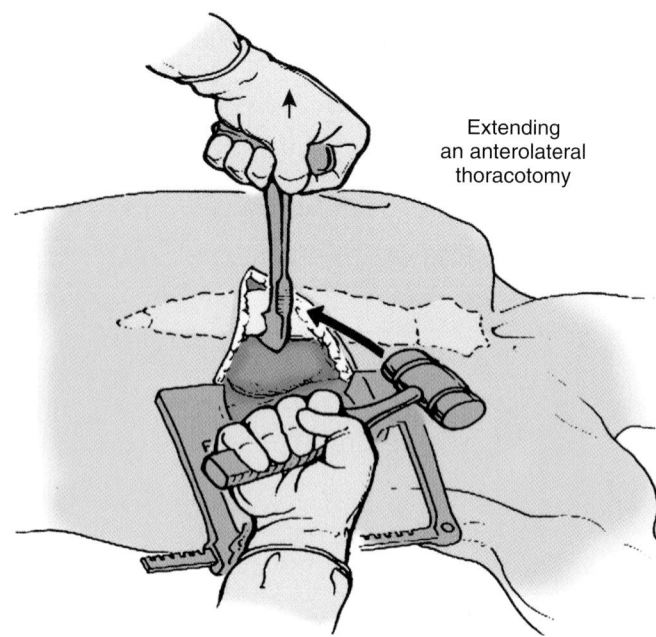

Extending an anterolateral thoracotomy

FIGURE 3 A left anterolateral thoracotomy can be extended easily into the right thoracic cavity to create a "clamshell" thoracotomy. A Lebsche knife and mallet or durable bandage scissors can be used to divide the sternum. The internal mammary vessels will be divided with this procedure and should be ligated. A clamshell thoracotomy provides wide exposure to both pleural cavities and the mediastinum.

Occlusion of the Descending Aorta

The primary rationale for aortic occlusion during EDT is that it redistributes the patient's limited blood volume to the heart and brain. In addition, patients with intraabdominal injuries (the extent of which are often unknown at the time of EDT) will experience less subdiaphragmatic blood loss. Visibility is generally poor during EDT, and this maneuver is often performed using tactile senses rather than visual ones (i.e., "done by feel"). The lung is retracted medially, and a hand is slid along the left lateral thoracic wall. The aorta is located as a tubular structure on the anterolateral portion of the vertebral body. It is usually readily palpable even in the absence of pulsations. Digital compression can be achieved quickly by pressure against the vertebral column. More effective control can be obtained using a vascular clamp, but this requires dissection of the overlying pleura off the aorta. This dissection can proceed either bluntly or sharply starting in the groove between the aorta and vertebral column. Failure to adequately expose the aorta can lead to ineffective cross clamping or complete slippage of the clamp. Care should be taken to avoid injury to the esophagus or intercostal arteries during this maneuver. Cross-clamp time should be carefully monitored and should not exceed 30 minutes if possible, as there is a substantial metabolic burden with prolonged ischemia. Additionally, there is a risk of spinal cord ischemia and subsequent paraplegia with

prolonged clamp times. We believe caution should be used in employing a thoracotomy to clamp the aorta for known intraabdominal injuries. Control of the hiatus can be achieved with a celiotomy and is our preferred method of aortic control. Although the transthoracic route may afford control slightly more quickly, it opens a second cavity, promotes more heat loss, and may potentiate coagulopathy.

Open Cardiac Massage

Patients who do not recover vital signs following initial EDT maneuvers require open cardiac massage. This maneuver provides better cardiac output than closed chest massage. It can be accomplished using a one- or two-handed (preferred) technique. In the one-handed technique, the heart is lifted and compressed against the underside of the sternum. In the two-handed technique, the heart is cupped between two hands opposed at the wrist. A gentle "clapping" motion is used to compress the heart from the apex toward the aortic root (Figure 5). In either technique, excessive fingertip pressure should be avoided to prevent injury to the heart. Internal cardiac defibrillation with 15 to 30 J of energy may also be utilized if clinically indicated.

Bronchovenous Air Embolism

Traumatic alveolovenous communications may produce air emboli that migrate and cause coronary artery or ventricular outflow obstruction. The typical scenario is that of a patient sustaining chest injury who develops profound hypotension or cardiac arrest following endotracheal intubation and positive-pressure ventilation. The combination of low intrinsic pulmonary venous pressure secondary to blood loss and high alveolar pressure from assisted positive-pressure ventilation increases the gradient for air emboli formation. Air embolism can be addressed by EDT by first isolating the injured lung and clamping the pulmonary hilum to prevent further

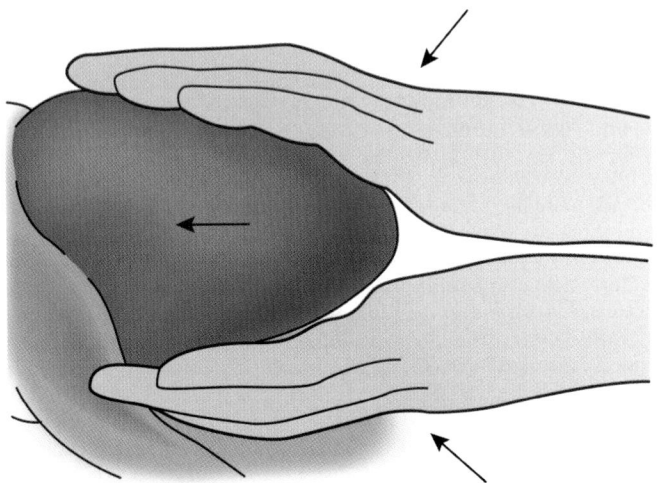

FIGURE 5 Bimanual cardiac massage. The two-handed technique provides better cardiac output and is the preferred method. The palmar surfaces of the fingers act in a clapping motion to compress the heart from the apex toward the aortic root. Fingertip pressure should be avoided at all times.

propagation of air. The inferior pulmonary ligament will usually need to be taken down to facilitate hilar isolation. Vigorous cardiac massage may promote dissolution of air present within the coronary arteries. The patient should then be placed in Trendelenburg position to trap air within the apex of the ventricle. Needle aspiration of the ventricle, atrium, or aortic root can then be performed as needed. If cardiac activity is achieved, the lung injury can be oversewn or stapled to prevent continued emboli formation.

OUTCOMES

Outcomes after EDT vary significantly depending on the mechanism, underlying injuries, and physiologic state at presentation. The highest overall survival rate is seen among patients with isolated cardiac injuries (3% to 35%), followed by victims of penetrating trauma (1% to 14%) and victims of blunt trauma (0% to 2%). A critical appraisal of EDT outcomes should consider "meaningful" survival, however. Many patients included in published series of EDT survivors have significant neurologic impairments as a result of prolonged hypotension and hypoxia.

SUGGESTED READINGS

Cothren C, Moore E: Emergency department thoracotomy for the critically injured patient: objectives, indications, and outcomes, *World J Emerg Surg* 24(1):4, 2006.
Moore EE, Knudson MM, Burlew CC, et al: Defining the limits of resuscitative emergency department thoracotomy: a contemporary Western Trauma Association perspective, *J Trauma* 70(2):334–339, 2011.
Passos EM, Engels PT, Doyle JD, et al: Societal costs of inappropriate emergency department thoracotomy, *J Am Coll Surg* 214(1):18–25, 2012.
Rhee PM, Acosta J, Bridgeman A, et al: Survival after emergency department thoracotomy: review of published data from the past 25 years, *J Am Coll Surg* 190(3):288–298, 2000.

THE MANAGEMENT OF TRAUMATIC BRAIN INJURY

Jon David Weingart, MD

The management of head injuries involves rapid evaluation of the extent of injury, followed by rapid intervention to halt ongoing injury and to prevent additional secondary injury. The overall goal of treatment is to maintain intracranial pressure (ICP) at a normal level. Elevated ICP results in decreased blood flow to the brain and subsequently leads to irreversible brain injury. Treatment includes surgical interventions to remove space-occupying mass lesions, primarily hematomas, and nonsurgical treatments to reduce brain tissue volume.

EVALUATION

The evaluation of a patient with a head injury is multidisciplinary. All patients must undergo a complete trauma evaluation because patients with severe head injuries secondary to nonpenetrating trauma are likely to have injuries to other systems. Assurance of cervical spine stability is an important aspect of the initial evaluation. The neck should be immobilized with a cervical collar until the stability of the cervical spine has been verified. A lateral cervical plain radiograph and an odontoid view plain radiograph are used to evaluate the cervical spine. The C7-T1 disk space must be visualized on the lateral image to verify stability of the cervical spine. If the C7-T1 disk space is not visualized, a computed tomographic (CT) scan through the C7-T1 disk space is obtained.

Ideally, the extent of the head injury is assessed before the patient is given any medications that will alter function of the central nervous system (CNS). When this is not possible because of cardiovascular instability or other unstable injuries, short-acting muscle relaxants should be used. The initial evaluation of the patient's CNS function is aimed at assessing for global brain dysfunction (i.e., level of consciousness) and for focal brain dysfunction (i.e., unilateral signs such as hemiparesis). The Glasgow Coma Scale (GCS) is an excellent, rapid way to evaluate for global or focal brain dysfunction. The GCS involves three parameters: eye opening, verbalization, and motor responses (Table 1). The GCS score is also reproducible and can be used to monitor a patient's neurologic status over time. Other aspects of the neurologic examination are papillary responses, corneal responses, and gag responses. These reflexes are used to evaluate brainstem function in an unresponsive patient with severe head injuries.

After the initial stabilization and evaluation are complete, the patient is taken as quickly as possible for a noncontrast brain CT scan. In the patient with a severe head injury, the brain CT scan should be obtained as quickly as possible because it helps determine whether a mass lesion, which necessitates surgical evacuation, is present. The CT scan should be evaluated for (1) presence of extra-axial or intraaxial blood, (2) mass effect or effacement of the lateral ventricle, (3) midline shift, and (4) presence or absence of cerebrospinal fluid in the basal cisterns. A patient with a mass lesion and a GCS score of 8 or less should undergo rapid surgical decompression.

TABLE 1: Glasgow coma scale

Parameters for evaluation of global or focal brain dysfunction	Points
Best Eye Opening	
Spontaneous	4
In response to speech	3
In response to pain	2
None	1
Best Verbal Response	
Oriented	5
Confused	4
Inappropriate	3
Incomprehensible	2
None	1
Best Motor Response	
Obeying	6
Localization to pain	5
Withdrawing in response to pain	4
Flexor response	3
Extensor response	2
None	1

SURGICAL TREATMENT

Acute Subdural Hematoma

Any patient with severe head injury (GCS score of 3 to 8) should be initially approached as if an acute subdural hematoma is causing increased ICP. The patient should be intubated and hyperventilated to achieve a partial pressure of carbon dioxide (Pco_2) of 28 to 30 mm Hg before the head CT scan is obtained. Mannitol, 1 g/kg, should be given intravenously over 15 minutes. Throughout this phase of the evaluation, intravascular volume should be maintained. Hypotension causes a decrease in cerebral perfusion and therefore should be treated if it occurs.

Early evacuation of acute subdural hematomas (within 4 hours of injury) has been shown to reduce the mortality rate. Patients with more than 1 cm of subdural blood in association with shift of the midline structures should be taken to the operating room immediately for evacuation. Patients with thin subdural hematomas (5 mm) and mild neurologic symptoms can be observed and treated medically because small subdural hematomas can resolve on their own. Such patients should be monitored with serial CT scans until the hematoma has resolved.

Patients with large subdural hematomas are taken directly from the CT scanner to the operating room. While the anesthesiologist is preparing the patient, the surgeon is positioning the patient's head. The head can be positioned on a donut or horseshoe cushion, but the author prefers to stabilize the head with head pins and the Mayfield skull clamp (SchaererMayfield USA, Cincinnati, Ohio). The entire half of the head is shaved. The location of the incision depends on the size of the subdural hematoma. The incision must be large enough to allow for the entire subdural space to be included in the craniotomy. For a subdural hematoma that is primarily frontal and temporal, a standard frontotemporal incision may be adequate. For a more posteriorly located subdural hematoma, a linear incision may be adequate. For a large subdural hematoma involving the frontal, temporal, and parietal areas, a large trauma or hemicraniotomy incision. The incision begins anteriorly in the midline and extends posteriorly to the lambdoidal suture, where it is curved forward to above the ear and around to the root of the zygoma.

After the area is prepared and draped, the incision is made quickly through the galea, with Raney clips placed on the skin edge to control bleeding. The temporalis muscle is incised with the cautery pen in line with the scalp incision. Cautery and periosteal elevators are used to dissect the pericranium off the skull with the skin flap. The skin and temporalis muscle are held back with towel clips or suture and a rubber band. The power perforator is used to quickly place burr holes in the temporal fossa at the root of the zygoma. If the dura seen through the burr hold appears blue, the dura should be opened at this point to allow for partial decompression. Several additional burr holes are placed frontally, along the midline, and posteriorly. The dura is stripped off the inner table, and a power craniotome is used to evaluate the craniotomy flap. At this point, several holes are placed in the flap and on the intact skull, through which size 0 Tevdek sutures (Deknatel, Mansfield, Mass) are passed. The Tevdek sutures are readied in case the bone flap must be replaced quickly, as in the case of malignant brain swelling. At this point, the dura is opened in a cruciate manner, allowing the hematoma to be extruded. Normal saline irrigation is used to wash the clot off the brain. At the edge of the dural opening, cotton strips are placed, and handheld brain spatulas are used to gently depress the brain. With use of irrigation again, the residual clot is washed off the cortex and evacuated. This is particularly important in the anterior frontal and temporal areas. Along the midline, the surgeon should be cautious when removing small clots, which may be causing tamponade in a torn bridging vein. While the hematoma is being washed out, any source of bleeding—from veins or arteries—is controlled with bipolar coagulation.

After evacuation of the convexity hematoma, the herniation in the medial temporal lobe and the uncal herniation over the tentorium should be relieved. This is accomplished by retracting and lifting the anterior temporal lobe off the floor of the middle fossa. If the anterior temporal lobe is contused and hemorrhagic, it can be resected, which will improve visualization. The brain spatula elevating the temporal lobe is advanced until the edge of the tentorium is identified. An attempt is made to lift the herniated medical temporal lobe back into the supratentorial space if the tissue looks viable. If the surgeon is unable to reduce the herniation or if the medial temporal lobe appears contused and nonviable, a subpial resection of the tissue should be carried out with suction and bipolar coagulation. Arachnoid attachments from the ambient cistern to the temporal lobe should be cut. A gush of cerebrospinal fluid is often seen when the temporal lobe has been reduced and the brainstem decompressed.

After the medial temporal lobe has been decompressed, the operative field is irrigated to check for any additional bleeding. The dura is closed in a primary manner if possible. If the closure appears to strangulate the brain because of brain swelling, a pericranial graft is used to cover the brain. Gelfoam (Pfizer, New York, NY) is placed in the epidural space, and the bone flap is attached with sutures or titanium plates.

At the end of the procedure, an ICP monitor should be placed on the opposite side. The ICP measurement is crucial for managing a patient with poor neurologic findings. Medical management is directed toward maintaining the ICP in a normal range. This ensures adequate blood flow to the brain and minimizes secondary injury. If

ICP increases rapidly while being monitored, head CT scanning should be repeated to look for development of a new hemorrhagic mass lesion.

All patients with acute subdural hematomas should have a follow-up head CT scan immediately after surgery and again 24 hours after surgery. It is not unusual for small remnants of the hematoma to remain or for a small amount of blood to reaccumulate. This baseline head CT scan is invaluable for interpreting follow-up head CT scans 2 to 5 days after surgery.

Two scenarios that can occur in the setting of a subdural hematoma are (1) the presence of a large intraparenchymal hematoma and (2) malignant brain edema. If a large intraparenchymal hematoma is present and is contributing to the mass effect in the brain, it should be decompressed. The hematomas usually come to the surface, and it is not difficult to enter them and to evacuate the blood clot. The goal is to decompress the brain and not to remove every small piece of hematoma. Intraparenchymal hematomas should be removed with irrigation and gentle suction. Aggressive removal of the clot in the wall of the hematoma cavity can produce bleeding that is difficult to stop. If this occurs, different hemostatic agents can be used to achieve hemostasis because bipolar cauterization is often ineffective. Hemostatic agents include cotton balls soaked in thrombin; thrombin-soaked Gelfoam; Avitene (fibrillar collagen; Davol, Cranston, RI); and, as a last resort, cotton balls soaked in half-strength hydrogen peroxide.

The second scenario to be aware of is the development of malignant brain edema and swelling, which occurs after the dura is open. When this occurs, the brain begins to swell out of the dural opening. This is a poor prognostic sign and probably reflects a severe diffuse brain injury. When met with this situation, the surgeon should quickly close. The dura can be reapproximated or left open. Similarly, the bone flap can be left off or replaced.

Epidural Hematoma

Epidural hematomas occur in the potential space between the dura and the inner table of the skull. Because the dura is strongly adherent to the cranial sutures, epidural hematomas typically do not cross the sutures. On a head CT scan, an epidural hematoma has a convex shape. Epidural hematomas usually occur in the setting of blunt trauma to the head and, in most cases, are associated with a skull fracture. The classic history of a patient with an epidural hematoma is a transient loss of consciousness after a head injury, followed by a lucid phase and then neurologic deterioration. Five different clinical courses have been described in patients with epidural hematomas: (1) unconscious-conscious-unconscious, (2) unconscious throughout, (3) conscious-unconscious, (4) unconscious-conscious, and (5) conscious throughout. On occasion, in a patient with an initial normal head CT scan, an epidural hematoma will develop, after some delay. Regardless of how the patient presents, the key issue for patients with epidural hematomas is that prompt treatment before loss of consciousness results in excellent outcomes. Because of the excellent prognosis with rapid treatment, all patients with impairment in consciousness after head trauma should have a head CT scan to rule out the presence of an epidural hematoma.

For an epidural hematoma that is causing alteration either in consciousness or in the patient's neurologic function, the treatment is evacuation of the hematoma. Patients can deteriorate quickly, so they should have surgery immediately. The general surgical approach involves adequate exposure of the hematoma and obliteration of the epidural space with dural tack-up sutures.

Patients can be positioned with the head on a horseshoe pad or in a three-point fixation head-holding device. The craniotomy should be large enough to completely expose the hematoma. Because epidural hematomas are commonly in the temporal area, a standard frontotemporal incision with or without posterior extension of the incision behind the ear is often used. As the burr holes are placed,

the epidural hematoma is encountered immediately beneath the burr hole, and a partial evacuation can be carried out quickly. After the bone flap is elevated, the hematoma is evacuated and the source of the bleeding, if found, is controlled. Middle meningeal and other dural branches are the most common cause of epidural hematomas. The dura around the craniotomy edge is tacked up to the skull. Similarly, multiple tack-up sutures serve to obliterate the epidural space and reduce or eliminate the risk of recurrence. If the head CT scan indicates the presence of a concomitant subdural hematoma, the subdural space is explored before the bone flap is replaced. Ultrasonography can also be used to assess for a subdural hematoma before the intradural compartment is explored. If the intradural space is to be explored, a linear dural incision is adequate. If a subdural hematoma is encountered, the dura can be opened widely to drain the hematoma. In patients with GCS scores of 8 or lower, an ICP monitor is placed at the end of the hematoma evacuation. Postoperative management of increased ICP is the same as in patients with an acute subdural hematoma.

Epidural hematomas near the midline or in the posterior fossa should be approached with a plan to control a hole or tear in a venous sinus. A skull fracture crossing the sinus is typically seen. As long as there is no concern for the patency of the venous sinus, the bone flap should extend up to the sinus but not across it. Any sinus bleeding can be controlled with tack-up sutures located along the sinus. Gelfoam and Avitene can be useful in controlling sinus bleeding.

Epidural hematomas that are small and exert no mass effect can be managed conservatively. These are often located in the high parietal area, where the risk of herniation is lower because of the falx tentorial junction, which offers some protection against herniation. If an epidural hematoma is to be monitored conservatively, then serial CT scans are obtained until it resolves.

Penetrating Injuries and Gunshot Wounds

Gunshot wounds to the head are evaluated and treated in the emergency department in the same way as blunt head trauma. The entrance site and, if present, an exit site should be identified on the scalp. Once stabilized, patients immediately undergo head CT scanning to evaluate the trajectory and the areas of brain affected by the missile. The two major issues in management of these types of injuries are (1) the presence of a hematoma, extraaxial or intraaxial, that causes mass effect and increased ICP and (2) the risk of infection because of the bone fragments and other debris carried into the brain by the force of the bullet. Hematomas that cause mass effect and neurologic compromise are unusual and should be surgically removed.

The standard treatment of gunshot wounds to the head remains controversial. Some surgeons believe that débridement of the bullet track in the brain leads to better outcomes. Bone chips, hair, and bullet fragments, along with necrotic brain tissue, are removed. The craniotomy is carried out with standard techniques to adequately expose the bullet entry point. The dura is opened in a cruciate manner, and the bullet track is débrided. All hemorrhagic and devitalized brain tissue should be removed until normal-appearing white matter is visible. Handheld brain spatulas or a speculum can be used to provide exposure to enable débridement of the bullet track. Irrigation flushed down the bullet track helps débride in the deeper portions of the bullet track. An attempt to remove all bone fragments should be made. Once the bullet track has been débrided and hemostasis achieved, the dura is closed in a watertight manner to prevent postoperative cerebrospinal fluid leaks and infections. A pericranial tissue graft is usually necessary to achieve dural closure. Both the bone and skin should also be débrided. In addition, closure of the scalp with healthy viable tissue is important. Postoperatively, patients are administered broad-spectrum antibiotics, although the most common pathogens are gram-positive *cocci*.

Most studies of the treatment of gunshot wounds have arisen out of wartime experiences. Because of the high incidence of infection in these series, débridement became the standard approach. However, more recent experiences have demonstrated that local débridement and closure of the entry site, followed by a regimen of intravenous antibiotics, are also effective at preventing infectious complications of the gunshot wound. Although this more conservative treatment course may not be appropriate for all patients, it is appropriate for patients with poor neurologic function and poor prognosis. Poor prognosis is associated with bullet wounds that cross the midline or pass through the ventricle.

In addition to antibiotics, anticonvulsants are given, and a tetanus toxoid shot is administered. Steroids are not indicated.

Decompressive Craniectomy

The role of decompressive craniectomy in the management of medically intractable intracranial hypertension remains controversial. Clinical studies to date demonstrate that ICP is better controlled after decompressive craniectomy, but outcomes are not improved, and complications may be increased. Patients with prolonged elevation of ICP despite maximal medical therapy are potential candidates for these procedures. The most common decompressive procedures are (1) hemicraniectomy with duraplasty and (2) bifrontal craniectomy. The bone can be removed in one or more pieces and is placed in the bone bank for later replacement. For the hemicraniectomy, the bone flap should extend back to the occipital region. The dura should be opened in a cruciate manner to allow the swollen brain to expand outward. Large pieces of bovine pericardium are used to cover the brain so that a plane of dissection exists between the galea and the brain when the bone is replaced at a later date.

The goal of these procedures is to limit the secondary damage caused by extended intracranial hypertension. There is some suggestion in the clinical studies available that these procedures have more effect on outcome when performed earlier in the course of the injury.

NONSURGICAL MANAGEMENT

The nonsurgical management of head injuries includes that in the postoperative period and that of patients for whom surgery was not indicated. The primary management issue is control of the ICP. By controlling ICP in a normal range, the clinician maintains adequate cerebral perfusion and oxygenation, and ongoing secondary injury is thus limited.

In 1993, a task force established by the Brain Trauma Foundation examined 12 issues related to the medical management of patients with severe head injures. Within each category, a treatment was designated as a *standard* when the treatment represented principles of patient management that reflect a high degree of clinical certainty; as a *guideline* when the treatment represented a particular strategy or range of management strategies that reflect moderate clinical certainty; and as an *option* for remaining management strategies that reflect low clinical certainty.

Of the 12 categories evaluated, only 3 met the standards criteria:

1. Chronic prolonged hyperventilation therapy (partial pressure of carbon dioxide [$Paco_2$]of 25 mm Hg) should be avoided after severe traumatic brain injury.
2. The use of glucocorticoids is not recommended to improve outcome or reduce ICP in patients with severe head injury.
3. Prophylactic use of phenytoin carbamazepine or phenobarbital is not recommended for preventing late posttraumatic seizures.

Medical Management of Increased Intracranial Pressure

Who Should Be Monitored?

Most of the 12 guidelines addressed by the task force involve decisions to monitor ICP and the interventions to take to reduce ICP when it is elevated. Although the indications to monitor ICP did not reach standard criteria, the data in the literature strongly support ICP monitoring in patients with a GCS score of 3 to 8 and an abnormal CT scan. This includes both patients who have undergone surgery and those who have not. These patients are at high risk for increased ICP, and intervention to lower ICP can prevent secondary brain injury.

In patients with GCS scores of 3 to 8 and normal head CT scans, the risk for increased ICP is lower. However, among such patients, it has been shown that if patients demonstrated two of three adverse features (age >40 years, unilateral or bilateral motor posturing, or systolic blood pressure <90 mm Hg), then the risk for increased ICP was similar to that in patients with abnormal head CT scans. Therefore, patients meeting these criteria should also be monitored.

How Should Patients Be Monitored?

The two ways to monitor ICP are with a ventriculostomy, which is placed into the cerebrospinal fluid ventricular space, or with a device that measures only pressure. The advantage of the ventriculostomy is that cerebrospinal fluid can be drained so as to decrease ICP. Therefore, in patients in whom monitoring is recommended, a ventriculostomy should be placed when possible.

What Intracranial Pressure Is Considered High?

An absolute threshold of ICP at which point treatment should be initiated does not exist; however, current data support 20 to 25 mm Hg as an upper threshold.

How Should Elevated Intracranial Pressure Be Treated?

Osmotic diuretics such as mannitol have been used over the years to reduce ICP. Mannitol has become the most commonly used osmotic diuretic. Although its exact mechanism is still debated, it is effective at decreasing ICP. Mannitol can be administered in a large bolus (1 g/kg) when ICP increases above a threshold such as 25 mm Hg, or it can be administered in smaller doses (0.25 g/kg) every few hours regardless of the ICP. Serum osmolarity should be monitored closely and kept below 320 mOsm. If mannitol is used for several days continuously, the patient must be weaned off slowly because abrupt cessation can lead to increased ICP.

An alternative, now more commonly used, is hypertonic saline; a solution of 7.5% given in a 30-mL bolus is effective at acutely decreasing ICP. Treating patients with continuous infusions of 3% saline also can control ICP. The goal of hypertonic saline is to raise the sodium levels to 155 to 160 mEq/L. One advantage of the hypertonic saline treatment is that the patient's intravascular volume is maintained at a normal level, which is advantageous for maintaining cerebral perfusion. As with mannitol, patients must be weaned off the hypertonic saline infusions slowly.

In patients with a ventriculostomy in place, ICP can be controlled with constant cerebrospinal fluid drainage. However, it is often not possible to place a ventriculostomy in cases of trauma because of the compression of the ventricular space secondary to the brain injury.

For patients in whom osmotic or hypertonic saline therapy is ineffective, barbiturates are the next option. Barbiturate therapy is an option in patients who are hemodynamically stable. A loading dose of pentobarbital is given as a bolus, 10 mg/kg over 30 minutes, followed by 5 mg/kg every hour for three doses. This is then followed by a maintenance infusion of 1 mg/kg/hr. The correlation between serum levels and therapeutic effect is poor. For this reason, all patients should have electroencephalographic monitoring with the goal of inducing a burst-suppression pattern; near-maximal reduction in cerebral metabolism and cerebral blood flow occurs when this pattern is present. After several days of pentobarbital coma, the drug is discontinued, and the effect allowed to wear off; this can take several days. When the pentobarbital has disappeared from the patient's system, the patient is reevaluated by a neurologic examination, ICP measurement, and head CT scan.

MANAGEMENT OF MILD TO MODERATE HEAD INJURIES

Many patients sustain head injuries that do not necessitate surgery and ICP monitoring. The extent of the injury can vary from alteration in neurologic function with normal head CT scan to abnormal head CT scan with the usual finding of subarachnoid blood or a brain contusion. Brain contusions caused by trauma are often located at the frontal and temporal poles. On the initial head CT scan, contusions appear to be of low density, often with punctate hemorrhages within the low density. These contusions can change over several days into large, consolidated hemorrhages, which can produce a mass effect. Neurologic deterioration may ensue when these contusions change into hematomas.

The management of such patients centers on close observation and frequent neurologic checks. Because these patients can be monitored with neurologic examinations, any changes occurring within the brain are reflected in the neurologic function of the patient. If a change in the patient's examination findings is noted, a head CT scan is obtained. If a new mass lesion has appeared, surgical evacuation may be indicated, depending on the size of the mass and its effect on the surrounding brain.

When admitted, patients with mild to moderate head injuries should be placed on two-thirds' maintenance fluid restriction. If intravenous fluids are given, normal saline should be used. The goal of this therapy is to increase the serum osmolality, which results in decreasing brain volume and ICP. Some patients may require an intensive care setting for observation and for receiving hypertonic saline or mannitol regularly over the first few days after the head injury. Steroids and anticonvulsants are not given routinely to these patients. If a patient has a seizure, anticonvulsants are started. All patients admitted with abnormal head CT scans after trauma should have undergo repeat head CT scanning 24 hours after the trauma. Patients with large contusions, especially temporal lobe contusions, should have several head CT scans over the first week while in the hospital in order to check for delayed development of an intraparenchymal hematoma.

Patients with mild head injuries can have persistent symptoms and cognitive dysfunction for many months after the injury despite imaging studies that yield unremarkable findings. Evaluation by experts in cognitive neurology and neuropsychology can be helpful.

COMMENTS

The prognosis for patients with severe head injuries is generally poor. The damage sustained at the moment of the trauma is irreversible. However, with rapid evaluation and treatment aimed at maintaining ICP in a normal range, ongoing and secondary injury can be halted and reversed.

SUGGESTED READINGS

Brain Trauma Foundation: *Guidelines for the management of severe traumatic head injury*, New York, 1995, Author.

Bullock MR, Chesnut R, Ghajar J, et al: Guidelines for the surgical management of traumatic brain injury, *Neurosurgery* 58(Suppl 3):S2–S6, 2006.

Chestnut DJ, Temkin N, Carney N, et al: A trial of intracranial-pressure monitoring in traumatic brain injury, *N Engl J Med* 367(26):2471–2481, 2012.

Cooper DJ, Rosenfeld JV, Murry L, et al: Decompressive craniectomy in diffuse traumatic brain injury, *N Engl J Med* 364(16):1493–1502, 2011.

Hofbauer M, et al: Predictive factors influencing the outcome after gunshot injuries to head—a retrospective cohort study, *J Trauma* 69(4):770–775, 2010.

Kaufman HH: Civilian gunshot wounds to the head, *Neurosurgery* 32:962–964, 1993.

Rahimi-Movaghar V, Jazayer SB, Alimi M, et al: Lessons learned from war: a comprehensive review of the published experiences of the Iranian neurosurgeons during the Iran-Iraq conflict and review of the related literature, *World Neurosurg* 79(2):346–358, 2013.

Ryu JH, Wakott BP, Kahle KT, et al: Induced and sustained hypernatremia for the prevention and treatment of cerebral edema following brain injury, *Neurocrit Care* 2013 [Epub].

Seelig JM, Becker DP, Miller JD, et al: Traumatic acute subdural hematoma: major mortality reduction in comatose patients treated within four hours, *N Engl J Med* 304(25):1511–1518, 1981.

Bur-Senj-Shu E, Figueiredo EG, Amorim RL, et al: Decompressive craniectomy: a meta-analysis of influences on intracranial pressur and cererebral perfusion pressure in the treatment of traumatic brain injury, *J Neurosurg* 117(3):589–596, 2012.

Wilberger JE, Harris M, Diamond DL: Acute subdural hematoma: morbidity, mortality, and operative timing, *J Neurosurg* 74(2):212–218, 1991.

CHEST WALL TRAUMA, HEMOTHORAX, AND PNEUMOTHORAX

**Raul Coimbra, MD, PhD, FACS, and
David B. Hoyt, MD, FACS**

Chest trauma is common. Data suggest that approximately 30% to 50% of all blunt trauma patients admitted to trauma centers have sustained chest trauma. Thoracic injuries account for 20% to 25% of all trauma-related deaths, and complications of chest trauma contribute to another 25% of all deaths. Early deaths in patients with chest trauma are caused primarily by major respiratory problems, such as tension pneumothorax and massive hemothorax. These clinical situations must be recognized and managed promptly. The most common injury in thoracic trauma is chest wall trauma. Because of the high prevalence of rib fractures and the associated pneumothorax and hemothorax, most thoracic injuries can be managed with simple procedures such as thoracentesis, respiratory support, and adequate analgesia. Only 15% of patients with chest trauma need a thoracotomy for definitive management of intrathoracic injuries.

In this chapter, the most current concepts of diagnosis and management of chest wall injuries, pneumothorax, and hemothorax are reviewed.

INITIAL EVALUATION

The physical examination of the chest is extremely important in identification of life-threatening situations that necessitate immediate attention. These situations include tension pneumothorax, massive hemothorax, open pneumothorax, flail chest, and cardiac tamponade.

Assessment of the chest begins with removal of all clothing and visual inspection of the anterior and posterior chest and axillae. A thorough inspection for lacerations, ecchymoses, open wounds, air bubbling from wounds, symmetry of chest rise, paradoxical motion of any portion of the chest, and use of accessory muscle for respiration should be performed. Pulse oximetry should be applied as soon as the patient arrives. The chest should be palpated for crepitus, tenderness, and instability of the sternum or ribs. Auscultation for presence and symmetry of breath sounds and dullness of cardiac or breath sounds is also performed. A chest x-ray should be performed as soon as is feasible for radiographic evaluation of the soft tissues, bones, lung parenchyma, and thoracic cavities. Throughout the assessment, high-flow oxygen should be administered to the patient. The chest x-ray is of the utmost importance in thoracic trauma; however, the life-threatening injuries mentioned previously preclude the necessity of a chest x-ray for diagnosis and should be identified clinically. In hemodynamically stable polytrauma cases, a chest computed tomographic (CT) scan with contrast (angiographic CT scan) may be useful in identification of injuries not seen on the initial chest x-ray (Figure 1).

SPECIFIC INJURIES

Rib Fractures

Blunt chest wall trauma varies from an isolated rib fracture to bilateral multiple rib fractures from crush mechanisms of injury that lead to significant respiratory distress from pneumothorax, hemothorax, or marked pulmonary contusion. Mortality rates after blunt chest wall trauma range from 4% to 20%.

Rib fractures are the most common injuries after blunt chest injuries, and ribs 4 through 10 are usually fractured. An isolated single rib fracture without lung involvement, pneumothorax, or hemothorax is usually treated on an outpatient basis. However, the ideal management of patients with multiple rib fractures

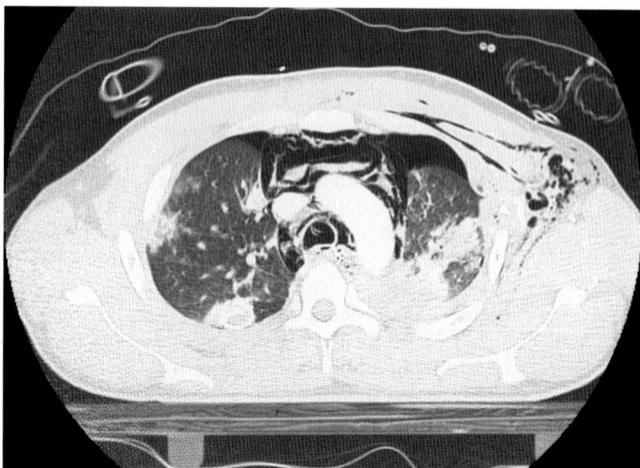

FIGURE 1 Computed tomographic scan of the chest shows deformity of chest wall, rib fractures, bilateral pulmonary contusions, subcutaneous emphysema, and bilateral pneumothoraces.

or significant chest wall trauma without life-threatening injuries is controversial. In the elderly population, decreased bone density, reduced chest wall compliance, and increased incidence of underlying parenchymal disease may cause rib fractures to lead to decreased ability to cough, reduced vital capacity, and increased incidence of infectious complications.

The primary clinical manifestation after rib fracture is pain. Other clinical signs associated with rib fracture include tenderness to palpation and crepitus. Rib fractures are confirmed with a chest x-ray or with chest CT scan. Approximately 55% of rib fractures are missed on routine chest radiographs. Special views, including an oblique view, may increase sensitivity but are not commonly used during the initial evaluation of a trauma patient. CT scans are the most sensitive study for diagnosis of rib fractures.

Multiple rib fractures are the hallmark of severe trauma from high-energy transfer. Patients with multiple rib fractures should undergo complete evaluation to rule out intrathoracic and abdominal injuries. Fractures of the lower ribs (9 to 12) are associated with increased incidence of solid organ injuries (liver and spleen), and fractures of the upper ribs (1 to 3), clavicle, or scapula are associated with major vascular injuries.

Poor pain control significantly contributes to complications after rib fractures, such as atelectasis and pneumonia. Pain control is attempted initially with oral or intravenous (IV) analgesics. Intercostal nerve blocks with bupivacaine are effective for pain control; however, bupivacaine is not feasible for multiple fractures, and it requires frequent injections. Epidural analgesia is adequate for patients with multiple or bilateral fractures; it provides adequate pain control and appropriate pulmonary toilet, decreasing the number of complications.

Flail Chest

A flail chest occurs when three or more contiguous ribs are broken in two places, creating a segment of bone and muscle that can move independently of the thoracic wall; however, it can also occur after costochondral separation. Fractures can be located in the anterior, lateral, or posterior chest wall. Flail chest occurs in 10% to 15% of patients with major chest trauma, and the chance of having an intrathoracic injury increases several fold. Closed traumatic brain injury is the most frequent associated extrathoracic injury; it contributes to higher morbidity and mortality rates. Isolated flail chest carries a low mortality rate in younger patients.

This independent segment of the chest wall moves paradoxically with spontaneous respirations, pulling inward with inspiration as a result of negative intrathoracic pressure. The paradoxical respiratory movement can cause significant pain to the patient and lead to a respiratory pattern characterized by rapid shallow breaths, which may lead to atelectasis and hypoxia. In addition, the force required to create a flail segment is excessive and usually also results in significant underlying pulmonary contusion, further increasing hypoxia. Sequential measurements of forced vital capacity, tidal volume, and inspiratory force are useful to predict which patients will need ventilatory support. The pathophysiologic effects may be present immediately or may progress over several hours and present as late respiratory decompensation. Lastly, the flail segment may be associated with a hemothorax or pneumothorax, which is treated with tube thoracostomy.

Treatment of the flail segment varies according to the patient's clinical presentation. If the patient's condition is stable from a respiratory standpoint, administration of supplemental oxygen, aggressive pulmonary toilet, and adequate analgesia is enough. Pain can be controlled with oral or intravenous analgesics, patient-controlled analgesia (PCA), intercostal nerve blocks, or catheters, which deliver a continuous stream of local anesthetic, or with epidural anesthesia. Evidence shows that epidural pain control is superior to other methods. In patients with development of respiratory distress, intubation and positive pressure ventilation is the treatment of choice. The intubation allows more aggressive pain management and sedation, and the positive-pressure ventilation can be used to recruit atelectatic lung and support contused lung to improve oxygenation. In addition, the positive-pressure ventilation splints the flail segment so that the paradoxical motion is halted and the entirety of the thoracic wall can move in synchrony, relieving pain and allowing healing of the soft tissue and bones.

Elderly trauma patients are particularly susceptible to deterioration after chest wall trauma. In this special patient population, pain control and aggressive pulmonary toilet should be implemented early, with a low threshold for intubation. Care should be taken to avoid fluid overload in these patients because it may further impair respiratory function. Pneumonia is the most frequent complication, particularly in the elderly; it aggravates chronic lung diseases, increases ventilator days, and significantly contributes to mortality.

Open reduction and internal fixation (ORIF) of sternal or rib fractures are rarely needed and remain controversial. No class 1 data exist to support the routine use of rib fracture ORIF. The indications for operative intervention in rib fractures are presented in Box 1. The proponents of rib fracture ORIF cite shorter recovery time, shorter intensive care unit (ICU) and hospital length of stay, decreased incidence of pneumonia, and shorter duration of mechanical ventilation after the procedure. In addition to the indications presented in Box 1, other clinical situations that may be taken into account in the decision to perform operative intervention in chest wall injuries include pain induced with deep breaths during spontaneous breathing trials, failure of obtaining adequate pain control with narcotics, intercostal nerve block or epidural analgesia, significant decrease in thoracic volume from chest crush injuries, marked chest wall deformity, fracture nonunion, and persistent paradoxical respiratory movement.

Sternal Fractures

Although rare, sternal fractures may occur after blunt mechanisms that include motor vehicle accidents and falls. The presence of a fractured sternum suggests a significant trauma to the anterior chest wall with high-energy transfer. Signs and symptoms include chest pain, particularly over the sternum, and crepitus. A hematoma over the sternum or across the chest may be seen, and it is a common occurrence after frontal car crashes in patients wearing a three-point seatbelt. A lateral x-ray should be obtained in these circumstances and usually confirms the diagnosis. Sternal fractures also constitute a marker for serious associated injuries, including myocardial contusion, myocardial rupture, esophageal perforation, airway injury, and thoracic aortic rupture.

Treatment of sternal fractures is usually conservative, although patients with significant chest wall instability may need open reduction and internal fixation.

Pneumothorax

A pneumothorax occurs when air from an injured lung or airway is trapped within the pleural cavity, increasing the normal negative intrapleural pressure. It may be caused by penetrating or blunt

mechanisms. After blunt trauma, pneumothorax is caused by rib fractures penetrating the lung parenchyma or by lung injuries without chest wall involvement. Deceleration injuries and sudden increases in intrathoracic pressure also may cause pneumothorax.

Clinical findings suggestive of a pneumothorax include decreased breath sounds, hyperresonance to percussion, and decreased expansion of the affected lung during inspiration. Pneumothoraces are classified according to the volume of lung loss or collapse identified on chest x-ray or according to respiratory and systemic signs. In a small pneumothorax, the volume loss is one third of the normal lung volume. In a large pneumothorax, the lung is completely collapsed, but no mediastinal shift or associated hypotension is found.

Tension pneumothorax is the most rapidly life threatening of all breathing problems. It occurs when air continuously enters the thoracic cavity from the lung, airway, or atmosphere and cannot escape. The pressure causes collapse of the lungs and prevents oxygenation and ventilation on the ipsilateral side and eventually causes deviation of the mediastinum to the opposite side. This causes compression of the superior and inferior vena cava, decreasing preload to the heart and resulting in hypotension. Tension pneumothorax should be recognized immediately with signs of air hunger, hypoxia, tachypnea, hyperresonance, unilateral absence of breath sounds, deviation of the trachea away from the affected side, distended neck veins, hypotension, and tachycardia. The tracheal deviation may be difficult to visualize and may be prevented from occurring if the patient is intubated. Distended neck veins may not be present if the patient is hypovolemic. Tension pneumothorax may be confused with pericardial tamponade because both result in distended neck veins, a feeling of impending doom or restlessness, and hypotension. However, tamponade results in muffled heart sounds and does not cause tracheal deviation or asymmetric breath sounds.

Tension pneumothorax is diagnosed clinically and constitutes a life-threatening emergency. Chest x-rays are not necessary to confirm the diagnosis, and delays to definitive treatment significantly increase the risk of circulatory collapse and cardiorespiratory arrest.

If tension pneumothorax is suspected, emergent decompression must be performed. Advanced Trauma Life Support (ATLS) recommends needle decompression with large-bore needles or angiocatheters placed in the second intercostal space in the midclavicular line. If the needle is properly placed, a rush of air should be observed with an immediate improvement in vital signs, as the tension pneumothorax is converted to a simple pneumothorax (Figure 2). This procedure should then be followed by the placement of a chest tube for more permanent decompression of the affected hemithorax and drainage of any blood that may be associated with the tension pneumothorax.

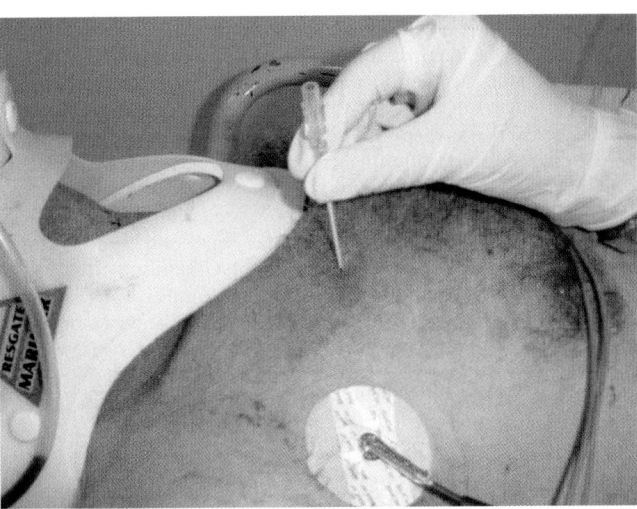

FIGURE 2 Needle decompression for tension pneumothorax.

BOX 1: Indications for open reduction and internal fixation of rib fractures

Crushed chest with marked deformity
Flail chest
Rib fracture nonunion with chest wall deformity
Open rib fracture

Occasionally, in the obese patient or in patients with significant soft tissue edema or hematomas, needle decompression may not be possible because the device may not be long enough to reach the thoracic cavity. In this situation, needle decompression may be skipped in favor of immediate chest tube placement. Reexpansion of the lung and reapproximation of the pleural surfaces usually seal the lung defect. All patients with a pneumothorax, regardless of its size, who will undergo positive-pressure ventilation should have a chest tube placed before the start of mechanical ventilation.

Open Pneumothorax

Open pneumothorax, also known as sucking chest wound, occurs when a significant defect in the chest wall (e.g., large-caliber gunshot wounds, traumatic thoracotomy) is large enough to exceed the laryngeal cross-sectional area, allowing the air to enter from the exterior into the pleural cavity and leading to lung collapse from a rapid equilibration between the intrathoracic pressure and the atmospheric pressure. The increased intrathoracic pressure also causes mediastinal shift and decreased venous return. Signs and symptoms include hypoxia, hypercarbia, hypotension, and respiratory and circulatory failure.

Management of open pneumothorax includes application of an occlusive dressing and placement of a chest tube before closure of the chest wall defect to avoid the development of a tension pneumothorax. When the initial assessment is completed and the patient's condition is stable, the wound should be cleansed, débrided, and closed in the operating room.

Occult Pneumothorax

Occult pneumothorax is defined by the presence of a pneumothorax seen on CT scan but not seen on conventional chest x-ray. The incidence rate of occult pneumothorax in trauma patients varies from 2% to 10%. The critical issues related to occult pneumothoraces are the question of clinical relevance; the identification of those with the potential to grow and cause problems, particularly in patients undergoing positive-pressure ventilation; and the question of preemptive treatment with tube thoracostomy. A recent multiinstitutional prospective observational study sponsored by the American Association for the Surgery of Trauma (AAST) was carried out to elucidate those issues. The objective of the study was evaluation of management strategies of occult pneumothoraces in an attempt to identify factors related to failure of observation to avoid unnecessary tube thoracentesis.

The authors analyzed 588 cases of occult pneumothoraces. Of those, 121 patients (21%) underwent immediate tube thoracostomy, and 448 (79%) were observed. Observation failure, defined by the need for tube thoracostomy after a period of observation, occurred in 27 (6%). The observation failure rate of patients undergoing positive-pressure ventilation was 14% (10 of 73). Increased hospital and ICU lengths of stay and ventilator days were observed in the failure of observation group. Univariate analysis identified size of the occult pneumothorax (7 mm), use of positive-pressure ventilation, progression of the occult pneumothorax (seen on subsequent chest x-ray films), respiratory distress, and the presence of a hemothorax as independent factors associated with failure of observation. Multivariate regression analysis identified only progression of the occult pneumothorax and respiratory distress as significant predictors of failed observation. Because no patients with failed observation had a tension pneumothorax develop or experienced any adverse events, the authors concluded that patients with occult pneumothorax can be carefully monitored and observed without tube thoracostomy.

Hemothorax

Blood may accumulate in the pleural cavity after blunt or penetrating injuries. Depending on the nature of the injury, bleeding may vary from minor to massive. Symptoms depend on the amount of blood accumulated in the pleural space. On physical examination, breath sounds may be decreased on the side of the injury. A chest x-ray obtained in the upright position may reveal accumulations of blood greater than 200 mL; however, a supine film may show a diffuse haziness or none at all. The pleural space can accumulate up to 3 L of blood.

Hemothoraces are initially treated with chest tube placement (36F tube); in approximately 85% of the cases, the bleeding stops as the lung is reexpanded as a result of the low pressure in the systemic circulation. A small number of cases have continued bleeding and need a thoracotomy. These cases are usually injuries in systemic arteries (intercostal arteries or internal mammary artery) or veins or major pulmonary vessels or are cardiac in origin.

Massive hemothorax is usually the result of major pulmonary vascular injury or major arterial wounds, and minor lung injuries cause small hemothoraces.

Massive hemothorax may present with tension physiology similar to tension pneumothorax. Hypotension may be a result of decreased preload from tension physiology or of massive blood loss (Figure 3). Treatment is immediate placement of a chest tube to the affected side. In contrast to tension pneumothorax, massive hemothorax rarely results in distended neck veins because of associated hypovolemia. Blood loss of greater than 1500 mL defines a massive hemothorax and is an indication for operative exploration. Additional indications for thoracotomy include massive continuous air leak that may indicate massive parenchymal lung injury or injury to a major airway and blood loss of 200 mL/h for greater than 4 hours (Box 2). Shed blood should be collected in a sterile fashion so that it may be autotransfused.

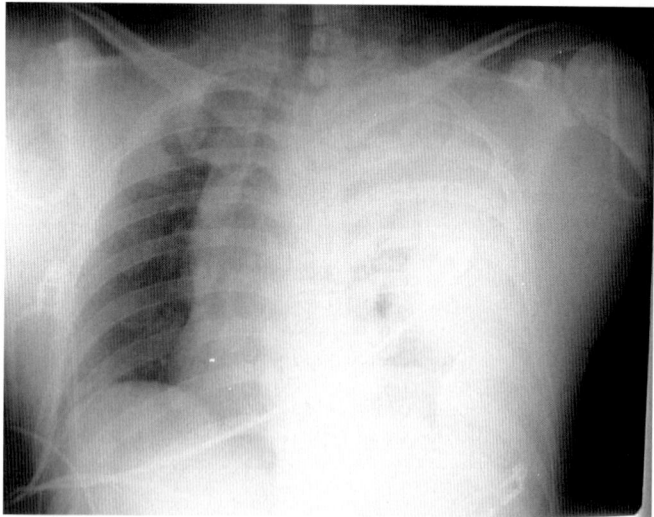

FIGURE 3 Massive hemothorax with tension component. Note the tracheal deviation to the right side and marked opacification of the left hemithorax.

BOX 2: Indications for thoracotomy after thoracentesis

Drainage of blood greater than 1500 mL on placement of chest tube
Persistent bloody drainage more than 200 mL/h
Persistent major airway leak
Suspicion of major airway injury with "flooding" of contralateral lung

Retained Hemothorax

Although retained hemothorax is common (approximately 10% of hemothoraces are treated with tube thoracostomy), the true incidence is unknown. Retained hemothorax is not only a complication of chest trauma and tube thoracentesis but is also recognized as a risk factor for the development of posttraumatic empyema and fibrothorax.

In modern trauma centers, the diagnosis of retained hemothorax is based on CT scan images of the chest because it seems to be a reliable method to characterize and quantify the volume of retained clot in the pleural cavity.

Treatment strategies include observation, image-guided drainage, thoracostomy, video-assisted thoracoscopy (VATS), intrapleural fibrinolytics, and thoracotomy. Although considered the gold standard, thoracotomy is associated with complications. In recent years, trauma surgeons have preferred to use less invasive modalities initially, leaving the open thoracotomy approach for cases that do not resolve with less invasive methods.

A recent AAST multiinstitutional prospective observational trial was carried out to determine current management strategies used in modern trauma centers in North America. The authors analyzed 328 cases of retained hemothorax from 20 centers over a 2-year period. Successful observation occurred in cases of hemothorax volume less than 300 mL. VATS was used in 33.5% of patients, and factors related to its success included hemothorax volume up to 900 mL, absence of a diaphragmatic injury, and use of periprocedural antibiotics for thoracostomy placement. Of note, several patients needed more than one, and sometimes more than two, VATS procedures to completely evacuate the pleural cavity of retained blood. Thoracotomy was necessary in 20.4%. The overall incidence rate of empyema was 26.8%.

TUBE THORACOSTOMY

Tube thoracostomy is the most common procedure performed in the management of thoracic trauma. In fact, 85% of the patients with chest injuries need only clinical observation or tube thoracostomy. A large-bore (36F to 40F) chest tube should be used in adolescents and adult patients. The chest tube should be placed in the midaxillary line in the fourth or fifth interspace at the level of the nipple in males and the inframammary fold in females. A small incision approximately 1.5 to 2 cm in length is made with a scalpel, and a clamp is used to bluntly dissect the subcutaneous tissue until the bony rib is felt. The clamp is then used to bluntly enter the thoracic cavity immediately over the top of the rib to avoid injury to the neurovascular bundle located beneath each rib. The index finger should be inserted into the pleural space before tube placement to ensure that the pleural cavity has been entered and is free of adhesions and that intraabdominal organs have not herniated through the diaphragm. The tube should be advanced posteriorly and superiorly in the pleural cavity. In most adults, insertion of 10 to 12 cm of the tube should be adequate to ensure the last side port is within the chest cavity. In all cases, further advancement of the tube should be stopped as soon as resistance is felt. The tube is then secured in place with a suture, and the insertion site is dressed with an occlusive dressing.

The end of the tube should then be connected to a closed drainage system. After insertion, the tube should be secured in the skin of the chest wall and connected to a collection system with suction. The procedure should be performed with universal precautions. A cap, mask, gown, and sterile gloves should be worn by the surgeon, and a cap and mask should be worn by everyone in the room. Chlorhexidine preparations are preferred because they have a decreased risk of surgical site infections. The site should be properly cleansed and anesthetized and completely draped to avoid contamination of the site, instruments, or chest tube. A single dose of preprocedure antibiotics with gram-positive coverage has proven as effective as a 24-hour course of periprocedure antibiotic prophylaxis.

A chest x-ray is usually obtained after chest tube insertion to confirm adequate placement and positioning. General criteria for chest tube removal include absence of air leak and less than 150 mL of fluid drainage over a 24-hour period.

Chest tubes in experienced hands can be placed fairly rapidly and efficiently. The most important step is entry of the thoracic cavity to allow escape of the air trapped there, which is accomplished even more rapidly and occurs once the thorax has been entered with blunt dissection. A rush of air or blood should be observed on entry into the pleural cavity, with immediate relieving of intrathoracic tension and improvement in the patient's vital signs.

SUGGESTED READINGS

Barrios C, Malinoski D, Dolich M, et al: Utility of thoracic computed tomography after blunt trauma: when is chest radiograph enough? *Am Surg* 75:966–969, 2009.

Battle CE, Hutchings H, Evans PA: Risk factors that predict mortality in patients with blunt chest wall trauma: a systematic review and meta-analysis, *Injury Int J Care Injured* 43:8–17, 2012.

Bulger EM, Edwards T, Klotz P, et al: Epidural analgesia improves outcome after multiple rib fractures, *Surgery* 136:426–430, 2004.

DuBose J, Inaba K, Demetriades D, et al: Management of post-traumatic retained hemothorax: a prospective, observational, multicenter AAST study, *J Trauma* 72:11–24, 2012.

Kaiser ML, Whealon MD, Barrios C Jr, et al: Risk factors for traumatic injury findings on thoracic computed tomography among patients with blunt trauma having a normal chest radiograph, *Arch Surg* 146(4):459–463, 2011.

Khandhar SJ, Johnson SB, Calhoon JH: Overview of thoracic trauma in the United States, *Thorac Surg Clin* 17:1–9, 2007.

Kiraly L, Schreiber M: Management of the crushed chest, *Crit Care Med* 38(Suppl):S469–S477, 2010.

Lafferty PM, Anavian J, Will RE, et al: Operative treatment of chest wall injuries: indications, technique, and outcomes, *J Bone Joint Surg Am* 93:97–110, 2011.

Mayberry JC, Ham LB, Schipper PH, et al: Surveyed opinion of American trauma, orthopedic, and thoracic surgeons on rib and sternal fracture repair, *J Trauma* 66:875–879, 2009.

Menger R, Telford G, Kim P, et al: Complications following thoracic trauma managed with tube thoracostomy, *Injury* 43:46–50, 2012.

Moore FO, Goslar PW, Coimbra R, et al: Blunt traumatic occult pneumothorax: is observation safe? Results of a prospective, AAST multicenter study, *J Trauma* 70:1019–1025, 2011.

Nirula R, Diaz JJ Jr, Trunkey DD, et al: Rib fracture repair: indications, technical issues, and future directions, *World J Surg* 33:14–22, 2009.

ABDOMINAL TRAUMA

LD Britt, MD, MPH, D.Sc (Hon), FACS, FCCM,
FRCSEng (Hon), FRCSEd (Hon), FWACS (Hon),
FRCSI (Hon), FCS(SA) (Hon)

INITIAL MANAGEMENT

Before focusing on the specific anatomic region of an obvious traumatic injury, an initial assessment of the entire patient is imperative.

The concept of initial assessment includes the following components: (1) rapid primary survey; (2) resuscitation; and (3) detailed secondary survey (evaluation) and reevaluation. Such an assessment is the cornerstone of the Advanced Trauma Life Support (ATLS) program. Integrated into primary and secondary surveys are specific adjuncts. Such adjuncts include the application of electrocardiographic monitoring and other monitoring modalities, such as arterial blood gas determination, pulse oximetry, measurement of ventilatory rate and blood pressure, and insertion of urinary or gastric catheters, and the incorporation of necessary x-rays and other diagnostic studies, when applicable, such as focused assessment with sonography for trauma (FAST) and plain radiography of the spine/chest/pelvis and computed tomographic (CT) scan.

The focus of the primary survey is both identification and expeditious address of immediate life-threatening injuries. Only after the primary survey is completed (including the initiation of resuscitation) and hemodynamic stability is addressed should the secondary survey be conducted; this survey entails a head-to-toe (and back-to-front) physical examination, along with a more detailed history.

Only the emergency care disciplines of medicine have this two-tier approach to their initial assessment of the patient, with primary and secondary surveys as integral components. As highlighted previously, the primary survey is designed to quickly detect life-threatening injuries. Therefore, a universal approach has been established with the following prioritization:

- Airway maintenance (with protection of the cervical spine);
- Breathing (ventilation);
- Circulation (including hemorrhage control);
- Disability (neurologic status);
- And exposure and environmental control.

Such a systematic and methodical approach (better known as the ABCDEs of the initial assessment) greatly assists the surgical or medical team in the timely management of those injuries that could result in a poor outcome.

A. Airway assessment management (along with cervical spine protection).

Because loss of a secure airway can be lethal within 4 minutes, airway assessment and management always has the highest priority during the primary survey of the initial assessment of any injured patient, irrespective of the mechanism of injury or the anatomic wound. The chin-lift and jaw-thrust maneuvers are occasionally helpful in attempting to secure a patent airway. However, in the trauma setting, the airway management of choice is often a translaryngeal, endotracheal intubation. If this cannot be achieved because of upper airway obstruction or some technical difficulty, a surgical airway (needle or surgical cricothyroidotomy) should be the alternative approach. No other management can take precedence over obtaining appropriate airway control. Until adequate and sustained oxygenation can be documented, administration of 100% oxygen is required.

B. Breathing (ventilation assessment).

An airway can be adequately established and optimal ventilation still not be achieved: for example, in the case of an associated tension pneumothorax (other examples include a tension hemothorax, open pneumothorax, or a large flail chest wall segment). Worsening oxygenation and an adverse outcome ensue unless such problems are expeditiously addressed. Therefore, assessment of breathing is imperative, even with an established and secure airway. A patent airway but poor gas exchange still results in a poor outcome. Tachypnea, absent breath sounds, percussion hyperresonance, distended neck veins, and tracheal deviation are all consistent with inadequate gas exchange. Decompression of the pleural space with a needle or chest tube insertion should be the initial intervention for a pneumothorax or hemothorax. A large flail chest, with underlying pulmonary contusion, likely requires endotracheal intubation and the administration of positive-pressure ventilation.

C. Circulation assessment (adequacy of perfusion management).

The most important initial step in determination of adequacy of circulatory perfusion is quick identification and control of any active source of bleeding, along with restoration of the patient's blood volume with crystalloid fluid resuscitation and blood products, if necessary. Decreased levels of consciousness, pale skin color, slow (or nonexistent) capillary refill, cool body temperature, tachycardia, and diminished urinary output are all suggestive of inadequate tissue perfusion. Optimal resuscitation requires the insertion of two large-bore intravenous lines and infusion of crystalloid fluids (warmed). Adult patients with severely compromised conditions need a fluid bolus (2 L of Ringer's lactate or saline solution). Children should receive a 20-mL/kg fluid bolus. Blood and blood products are administered as needed. Along with the initiation of fluid resuscitation, emphasis needs to remain on identifying the source of active bleeding and stopping the hemorrhage. For a patient in hemorrhagic shock, the source of blood loss is an open wound with profuse bleeding, or within the thoracic or abdominal cavity, or an associated pelvic fracture with venous or arterial injuries. Disposition (operating room, angiography suite, etc.) of the patient depends on the site of bleeding. For example, a FAST assessment that documents substantial blood loss in the abdominal cavity in a patient with a hemodynamically labile condition dictates an emergency celiotomy. However, if the quick diagnostic workup of a patient with a hemodynamically unstable condition who has sustained blunt trauma shows no blood loss in the abdomen or chest, then the source of hemorrhage could be from a pelvic injury that would likely necessitate angiography or embolization if external stabilization (e.g., a commercial wrap or binder) of the pelvic fracture fails to stop the bleeding. Profuse bleeding from open wounds can usually be addressed with application of direct pressure or occasionally with ligation of torn arterial vessels that can easily be identified and isolated.

D. Disability assessment and management.

Only a baseline neurologic examination is required when performing the primary survey to determine neurologic function deterioration that might necessitate surgical intervention. A detailed neurologic examination is inappropriate to attempt initially. Such a comprehensive examination should be done during the secondary survey or evaluation. This baseline neurologic assessment could be the determination of the Glasgow Coma Scale (GCS), with an emphasis on the best motor or verbal response and eye opening. An alternative approach for a rapid neurologic evaluation is the assessment of the pupillary size and reaction, along with establishing the patient's level of consciousness (alert, responds to visual stimuli, responds only to painful stimuli, or unresponsive to all stimuli). The caveat that must be highlighted is the fact that neurologic deterioration can occur rapidly and that a patient with a devastating injury can have a lucid interval (e.g., epidural hematoma). Because the leading causes of secondary brain injury are hypoxia and hypotension, adequate cerebral oxygenation and perfusion are essential in the management of a patient with neurologic injury.

E. Exposure and environmental control.

For a thorough examination, the patient must be completely undressed. This often requires cutting off the garments to safely expedite such exposure. However, care must be taken to keep the patient from becoming hypothermic. Adjusting the room temperature and infusing warmed intravenous fluids can help establish an optimal environment for the patient.

The secondary survey should not be done until the primary survey has been completed and resuscitation initiated, with some evidence of normalization of vital signs. This head-to-toe evaluation must be performed in a detailed manner to detect less obvious or occult injuries. This is particularly important in the unevaluable patient (e.g., with head injury or severely intoxicated). The physical examination should include a detailed assessment of every anatomic region, including the following:

- Head
- Maxillofacial region
- Neck (including cervical spine)
- Chest
- Abdomen
- Perineum (including the rectum and genital organs)
- Back (including the remaining spinal column)
- Extremities (musculoskeletal)

A full neurologic examination needs to be performed, along with an estimate of the GCS score if one was not done during the primary survey. The secondary survey and the utilization (when applicable) of the armamentarium of diagnostic adjuncts previously mentioned allow detection of more occult or subtle injuries that could, if not found, account for significant morbidity and mortality. When possible, the secondary survey should include a history of the mechanism of injury, along with vital information regarding allergies, medications, past illnesses, recent food intake, and pertinent events related to the injury.

It cannot be overemphasized that frequent reevaluation of the injured patient is necessary to detect any deterioration in the patient status. This sometimes requires repeating both the primary and the secondary surveys.

TOPOGRAPHY AND CLINICAL ANATOMY

The abdomen is often defined as a component of the torso that has for its superior boundary the left and right hemidiaphragm, which can ascend to the level of the nipples (fourth intercostal space) on the frontal aspect and to the tip of the scapula in the back. The inferior boundary of the abdomen is the pelvic floor. For clinical purposes, further division of the abdomen into four areas is helpful: (1) anterior abdomen (below the anterior costal margins to above the inguinal ligaments and anterior to the anterior axillary lines); (2) intrathoracic abdomen (from the nipple or the tips of the scapula to the inferior costal margins); (3) flank (inferior scapular tip to the iliac crest and between the posterior and anterior axillary lines); and (4) back (below the tips of the scapula to the iliac crest and between the posterior axillary lines). Most of the digestive system and urinary tract, along with a substantial network of vasculature and nerves, are contained within the abdominal cavity. A viscera-rich region, the abdomen can often be the harbinger for occult injuries as a result of

penetrating wounds, particularly in the unevaluable abdomen as the result of a patient's compromised sensorium.

PHYSICAL EXAMINATION

A complete and thorough physical examination of the entire body is essential in the management of abdominal injury. Some findings (Box 1) on physical examination are absolute indications for operative intervention. The components of the physical examination should include careful inspection, palpation, and auscultation.

With respect to penetrating abdominal trauma, inspection can sometimes determine the trajectory of the missile or other wounding agents and, consequently, guide management decisions. Often this can be determined by the location, extent, and number of wounds. For example, a patient with a documented, superficial tangential gunshot wound (low-velocity) with no other remarkable physical findings is likely to be managed expectantly (observation). However, if a penetrating abdominal injury results in a patient presenting with an evisceration, exploratory laparotomy is the management option of choice. Palpation enables the examiner to elicit abdominal tenderness or frank peritoneal signs and to detect abdominal distention and rigidity. On occasion, missiles can be palpated lodged in the soft tissue. Unless the setting is controlled and sterile, such as the operative theater, probing of a wound should be avoided. Auscultation is also an important component of the physical examination. It can help determine diminished or absent bowel sounds that could be suggestive of evolving peritonitis. Also, auscultation could detect a trauma-induced bruit, suggestive of a vascular injury.

The examiner has to be keenly aware of situations in which the abdominal examination is unreliable because of possible spinal cord injury or a patient's altered mental state.

DIAGNOSTIC STUDIES

The abdomen is notorious for hiding its secrets: occult injuries. Access to an extensive diagnostic armamentarium is imperative in the optimal management of these injuries. The mainstay diagnostic modality for evaluation of blunt abdominal trauma is CT scan. Although CT scan is beginning to have a more pivotal role in the assessment of penetrating abdominal injuries, there are diagnostic options strongly advocated by some for abdominal stab wounds. Local wound exploration, for example, has the advantage of allowing the patient to be discharged from the trauma bay or emergency department if surgical exploration of the wound fails to show penetration of the posterior fascia and peritoneum. However, if the patient has to go to the operating room for other injuries, the local wound exploration should be done in the surgical suite that has better lighting and a more sterile environment. A positive finding during local wound exploration dictates a formal laparotomy or laparoscopy. However, even with local wound exploration as a guide, the nontherapeutic laparotomy rate can be high, given that only a third of the patients with stab wounds to the anterior abdomen need therapeutic laparotomy. In the patient who has an evaluable abdomen,

---

BOX 1: Absolute indications for exploratory laparotomy in abdominal injuries

A. Peritonitis

B. Evisceration

C. Impaled object

D. Hemodynamic instability (documented or suspected intra-abdominal source)

E. Associated bleeding from natural orifice

serial abdominal examinations are an acceptable alternative to local wound exploration, to determine the need for operative intervention. Local would exploration should only be done for stab wounds to the anterior abdomen. Such an approach is potentially too hazardous for thoracoabdominal penetrating injuries and back or flank wounds. Plain radiography (abdomen/pelvis/chest) can be pivotal in documenting the presence of missiles and other foreign bodies and determining the trajectory of the injury tract, particularly for wounds from firearms. Also, the presence of free air might be confirmed with plain radiography. Unless concern exists about a retained broken blade or some other object, plain radiography has little utility for stab injuries. The diagnostic peritoneal lavage (DPL) developed by David Root in 1965 was a major advance in the care of the hemodynamically labile case of blunt trauma. With the advent of FAST and rapid CT scan, DPL has very limited utility. Diagnostic peritoneal lavage has never had a broad appeal in the diagnostic evaluation of penetrating abdominal wounds. Although some have advocated its use with tangential wounds of the abdominal wall, the technique has failed to receive widespread support. Its reliability in detection of clinically significant injuries sustained as a result of penetrating abdominal injuries has been a prevailing concern. The reported sensitivity and specificity of DPL for abdominal stab wounds are 59% to 96% and 78% to 98%, respectively. Also, DPL is a poor diagnostic modality for detection of diaphragmatic and retroperitoneal injuries.

Diagnostic imaging has had the greatest impact in changing the face of trauma management, with CT scan taking the lead in this area. Its ubiquitous presence in the management of blunt abdominal trauma is well established. As underscored previously, it is becoming an important diagnostic study in the evaluation of penetrating abdominal injuries. In addition to its excellent sensitivity in detection of pneumoperitoneum, free fluid, and abdominal wall/peritoneal penetration, CT scan is helpful in identification of the tract of the penetrating agent. Hauser and colleagues recommended the use of triple-contrast CT scan in the assessment of penetrating back and flank injuries. CT scan evaluation is an essential diagnostic tool in the increasing advocacy for selective management of abdominal gunshot wounds, obviating the need for mandatory surgical exploration. However, two major limitations of CT scan still remain: detection of an intestinal perforation and finding of a diaphragmatic injury.

Unless the injury is confined to the solid organ of the abdomen, such as the liver or spleen, the matrix of intestinal gas patterns makes detection of penetrating injuries difficult. Kristensen, Buemann, and Kuhl were one of the first teams to introduce the role of ultrasound scan as part of the diagnostic armamentarium in trauma management. Kimura and Otsuka endorsed use of ultrasound scan in the emergency room for evaluation of hemoperitoneum. FAST does not have the same broad application in the evaluation of penetrating trauma as it does in blunt trauma assessment. Rozycki, Ochsner, Schmidt, and associates reported on the expanded role of ultrasound scan as the "primary adjuvant modality" for the injured patient assessment. Rozychi also reported that FAST examination was the most accurate for detection of fluid within the pericardial sac. Such a finding is confirmatory for a cardiac injury and possible cardiac tamponade, given a mechanism of injury that could result in an injury to the heart.

As a diagnostic modality, laparoscopy is not a new innovation. Other specialists have used this operative intervention for several decades. However, it was formally introduced as a possible diagnostic procedure of choice for specific torso wounds when Ivatury and colleagues did a critical evaluation of laparoscopy on penetrating abdominal trauma. Fabian and associates also reported on the efficacy of diagnostic laparoscopy in a prospective analysis.

No conventional diagnostic tool can conclusively rule out a diaphragmatic laceration or rent, so diagnostic laparoscopy becomes the study of choice for penetrating thoracoabdominal injuries, particularly left thoracoabdominal wounds. Laparoscopy can also be used to determine peritoneal entry from a tangential penetrating injury.

PENETRATING ABDOMINAL INJURIES AND THE HEMODYNAMICALLY STABLE AND UNSTABLE CONDITION

The management principles in patients with penetrating abdominal injuries whose conditions remain hemodynamically stable depend on the mechanism and location of injury, along with the hemodynamic status of the patient. Irrespective of the patient's hemodynamic parameter, the ATLS protocol should be strictly followed on arrival of the patient to the trauma bay.

EXPLORATORY LAPAROTOMY IN TRAUMA

The operative theater should be large enough to accommodate more than one surgical team, in the event the patient might need simultaneous procedures. In addition, the room should have the capability of maintaining room temperature as high as the lower 80°F-plus range to avoid hypothermia in the patient. Also, a rapid transfusion device should be in the room to facilitate the delivery of large fluid volume and ensure that the fluid administration is appropriately warm.

Abdominal exploration for trauma has basically four imperatives: (1) hemorrhage control; (2) contamination control; (3) identification of the specific injury; and (4) repair or reconstruction. The abdomen is prepared with a topical antimicrobial from sternal notch to bilateral mid thighs and extended laterally to the side of the operating room table followed by wide draping of the patient. Such preparation allows for expeditious entry into the thorax if needed and possible vascular access or harvesting. Exploration is initiated with a midline vertical incision that should extend from the xiphoid to the symphysis pubis for optimal exposure.

The first priority on entering the abdomen is control of exsanguinating hemorrhage. Such control can usually be achieved with direct control of the lacerated site or with proximal vascular control. After major hemorrhage is controlled, blood and blood clots are removed. Abdominal packs (radiologically labeled) are used to tamponade any bleeding and allow for identification of any injury bleeding. The preferred approach to packing is to divide the falciform ligament and retract the anterior abdominal wall. This allows manual placement of the packs above the liver. Abdominal packs should also be placed below the liver. This arrangement of the packs on the liver creates a compressive tamponade effect. After manual evisceration of the small bowel out of the cavity, packs should be placed on the remaining three quadrants, with care taken to avoid an iatrogenic injury to the spleen. During the packing phase, after ongoing hemorrhage has been controlled, the surgeon should communicate with the anesthesia team that major hemorrhage has been controlled and that this is an optimal time to establish a resuscitative advantage with fluid, blood, or blood product administration.

The next priority should be control or containment of gross contamination. This begins with the removal of the packs from each quadrant, one quadrant at a time. Packs should be removed from the quadrants that are least suspected as the source for blood loss, followed by removal of the packs from the final quadrant, the one that is believed to be the area of concern.

After control of major hemorrhage has been achieved, any evidence of gross contamination must be addressed immediately. Obvious leakage from intestinal injury can be initially controlled with clamps (e.g., Babcock clamp), staples, or sutures. The entire abdominal gastrointestinal tract needs to be inspected, including the mesenteric and antimesenteric border of the small and large bowel, along with the entire mesentery. Rents in the diaphragm should also be closed to prevent contamination of the thoracic cavity.

Further identification of any and all intra-abdominal injuries should be initiated. Depending on the mechanism of injury and the estimated trajectory of wounding agent, a thorough and meticulous abdominal exploration should be performed, including entering the lesser sac to better inspect the pancreas and the associated vasculature. In addition, mobilization of the C-loop of the duodenum (Kocher's maneuver) might be necessary, along with medial rotation of the left or right colon for exposure of vital retroperitoneal structures.

The final component of a trauma laparotomy is definitive repair, if possible, of specific injuries. As highlighted subsequently in this chapter, the status of the patient dictates whether each of the components of a trauma laparotomy can be achieved at the index operation. A staged celiotomy ("damage control" laparotomy) might be necessary if the patient becomes acidotic, hypothermic, coagulopathic, or hemodynamically compromised.

Diaphragm

The diaphragm, a dome-shaped muscular structure with an aponeurotic sheath ("central tendon"), effectively separates the thoracic and abdominal cavities. It attaches to the first three lumbar vertebrae, the ribs, and the posterior aspect of the lower sternum. Because of the decussation of its crura and hiatal architecture, the diaphragm provides an avenue for many vital structures, including the aorta, esophagus, thoracic duct, vagi, azygos vein, and inferior vena cava. Physiologically, the wide excursion of the diaphragm during inspiration and expiration contributes to both respiratory function and venous return.

Blunt trauma accounts for up to 30% of traumatic diaphragmatic ruptures in the United States. Motor vehicle collisions and falls from heights are the most common mechanisms of injury. Diaphragmatic rupture occurs as a result of an acute increase in the intra-abdominal pressure. Probably because of the buttressing effect of the liver, right-sided diaphragmatic ruptures occur less frequently than those on the left.

In addition to ruling out a possible cardiac injury if the penetrating wound is more central, the paramount reason that the thoracoabdominal region (Figure 1) presents such a diagnostic challenge to the acute care surgeon is the possibility of an occult diaphragmatic injury. Patients who are hemodynamically labile or have peritoneal

signs need mandatory exploration. Patients with clinically stable conditions should undergo a more selective approach. Although the imaging armamentarium is quite vast, no conventional diagnostic modalities can consistently and conclusively make the definitive diagnosis of a diaphragmatic injury. The diagnosis of a diaphragmatic injury is important for two basic reasons. First, the presence of an acute injury to the diaphragm mandates abdominal exploration because of the potential of risk for an associated intra-abdominal injury. Second, both acute and long-term risks exist for diaphragmatic herniation and possible incarceration or strangulation. Even with chest x-ray (CXR), CT scan, FAST, DPL, magnetic resonance imaging (MRI), and fluoroscopy, this dilemma persists, because none of these diagnostic modalities reliably detect a diaphragmatic rent. Because of this diagnostic challenge, the thoracoabdominal region was correctly underscored as "the ultimate blind spot" in penetrating trauma. This ongoing challenge was attributed to the presence of the diaphragm in this region. Documentation of a diaphragmatic injury has been a difficult task since it was first described by Sennertus in 1541. Patients who present with indications for exploration (Box 2) need no essential diagnostic studies. Without any definitive way of determining diaphragmatic injury, even with no absolute indication for operative intervention, a celiotomy was often the management approach of choice for such injuries, particularly *left* penetrating thoracoabdominal injuries. An expectant approach (observation only) does not address potential for the presence of an injury to the diaphragm and its sequela, such as the increased risk for the development of a herniation of abdominal viscera. This potential complication is thought to be secondary to nonhealing of the injury site. Factors proposed that may contribute to hernia formation include: (1) relative thinness of the diaphragm; (2) constant motion; and (3) pressure difference across the diaphragm that favors movement of abdominal contents from the abdomen into the thoracic cavity. Although the injury occurs acutely, clinical signs of a hernia are usually lacking and a high index of suspicion is imperative to prompt optimum investigation. The time from injury to presentation of a symptomatic diaphragmatic hernia may vary from days to many years after injury. This has led to the development of a classification system for diaphragmatic hernias based on time of presentation. The acute phase occurs during or shortly after the time of injury. The next phase is the interval, or latent, phase. During this phase, the patient may have abdominal pain that greatly resembles that of common etiologies for upper abdominal pain. The final phase is the obstructive, or strangulation phase; the patient may present with signs and symptoms of bowel obstruction or even peritoneal signs as a result of necrosis of the incarcerated bowel. Patients who present in the obstructive phase with necrotic viscera are common and have a documented mortality rate of greater than 40%. This further emphasizes the importance of diagnosis and repair of these injuries in the acute setting, to avoid such complications.

Several diagnostic modalities have been used in the evaluation of thoracoabdominal trauma in both the blunt and the penetrating settings. Chest x-ray is the usual screening diagnostic modality.

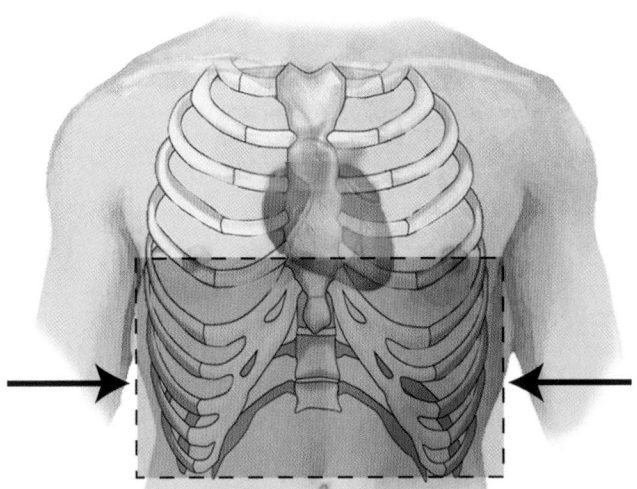

FIGURE I   Areas of concern for thoracoabdominal injuries.

BOX 2: Absolute indication for celiotomy

1. Hemodynamic lability
2. Peritoneal signs
3. Free air
4. Bleeding from an orifice
5. Massive hemothorax
   CT scan, >1500-mL initial output
   CT scan, >200 mL/h for more than 4 h
6. Impaled object

CT, Computed tomographic.

However, the diagnostic accuracy for diaphragmatic injuries ranges from as low as 13% to as high as 94% in the literature. Shah and associates looked at a collective series where CXR was diagnostic in 40.7% of cases reviewed. This approaches the 50% accuracy rate. They also found that the accuracy was increased when the study was repeated after the placement of a radiopaque nasogastric tube. However, the sensitivity of CT scan has been less than optimal. Shanmuganathan and colleagues looked retrospectively at CT scan as a diagnostic modality in thoracoabdominal injuries. Forty-one patients with both blunt and penetrating injuries were included. CT scan had a sensitivity of 63% and a specificity of 100% for diaphragmatic "rupture" in the blunt cases. CT scan failed to diagnose diaphragmatic injuries without associated visceral herniation. Patients with penetrating injuries are less likely to have visceral herniation; therefore, their injuries can easily be missed if CT scan is used as a mode of diagnosis. In the McQuay/Britt study, five patients would have fallen into this category. These and other radiologic studies are usually not accurate in the acute phase of penetrating injuries. This was the rationale for establishing a practice of mandatory exploration to evaluate better the integrity of the diaphragm and associated injuries.

The incidence rate of diaphragm injuries as a result of penetrating trauma ranges from 0.8% to 15%. Mandatory exploration of all penetrating thoracoabdominal injuries has been advocated for many years on the premise that it is the only way to assess definitively the diaphragm. The importance of adequate visualization cannot be underestimated, considering the increased morbidity and mortality as a result of a missed diaphragmatic injury.

Mandatory celiotomy for an injury with such a low incidence resulted in a high number of nontherapeutic explorations, prompting the need for an alternative approach. In 1992, Rao Ivatury and associates introduced for this cohort of patients diagnostic laparoscopy as the definitive modality for identification of diaphragmatic injuries in penetrating thoracoabdominal trauma. In the acute setting of penetrating thoracoabdominal injuries, few (if any) indications exists for performing diagnostic thoracoscopy to determine the integrity of the diaphragm. Such an intervention likely requires a double-lumen endotracheal tube insertion and lateral decubitus positioning of the patient. If a diaphragmatic through-and-through injury is actually confirmed (especially on the left side), the patient needs to be repositioned in the supine position and prepared and draped for a celiotomy. Therefore, a diagnostic laparoscopy is more appropriate and efficient management for these injuries.

Laparoscopy was introduced as a possible alternative for the evaluation of penetrating thoracoabdominal trauma. Fabian and colleagues studied 182 patients over a 19-month period. Laparoscopy revealed no peritoneal penetration in 55% of the patients reviewed. Of the remaining patients, 66% had therapeutic laparotomy, 17% had nontherapeutic laparotomy, and 17% had negative laparotomy. Ortega and colleagues studied 24 patients with penetrating thoracoabdominal injuries and reviewed their experience with diagnostic laparoscopy (DL). Their specificity and positive predictive values were 100% for lesions of the diaphragm, liver, spleen, and hollow viscus. Others have attempted to use DL not only to document peritoneal penetration but also to determine the extent and operative management of intra-abdominal injury. Zantut and associates looked at laparoscopy as both a diagnostic and a therapeutic modality. Retrospective data of 510 patients from 3 institutions were included. Laparotomy was avoided in 303 patients (59.4%) in whom laparoscopy was negative for peritoneal penetration. Livingston and colleagues prospectively evaluated 39 patients with hemodynamically normal conditions with penetrating thoracoabdominal injuries with DL. Laparoscopy correctly identified the presence of intra-abdominal injuries in 26 patients. The McQuay/Britt study revealed 22 unsuspected injuries, 17 of them with intra-abdominal organ injuries that necessitated operative repair.

The ability to adequately evaluate the diaphragm with the laparoscope provides an attractive diagnostic modality that benefits those patients with diaphragmatic injury and avoids an unnecessary celiotomy. As the technology and the laparoscopic skills of surgeons develop, diagnostic laparoscopy will become more of a therapeutic option.

In the acute setting, diaphragmatic injuries are preferentially repaired primarily in a two-layer fashion, with a heavy nonabsorbable suture. Although the implications are infrequent, a nonabsorbable mesh can be incorporated in the diaphragmatic closure where there is significant tissue destruction, which usually occurs in blunt trauma. In the unlikely event of a gross contamination, endogenous tissue can be used for a definitive repair. Such tissue includes a latissimus dorsi flap, tensor fascia lata, or omentum. Some practitioners advocate use of biologic tissue grafts, such as AlloDerm (human acellular tissue matrix; Life Cell Corporation). The durability of such a repair is questionable. Figure 2 is a treatment algorithm for generating thoracoabdominal injuries, the most common mechanism for diaphragmatic injuries.

Overall, the expected outcomes for diaphragmatic injuries are good (Table 1). Mortality and significant morbidity are related to associated organ injuries.

Stomach, Small Bowel, Colon, and Rectum

Stomach

The stomach is the second most common intraperitoneal hollow viscus injured. Its size and intraperitoneal location make this organ a vulnerable target, with size being affected by the intraluminal volume. Gastric injury from blunt trauma is quite infrequent. When it does occur, it is often the result of increased intraluminal pressure and distension. Seatbelt injuries and direct blows to the epigastrium are common causes of gastric injuries. With respect to penetrating wound of the stomach, a more frequent mechanism of injury, the anterior and posterior aspects of the stomach need to be meticulously inspected for accompanying through-in-through injuries. Penetrating injuries of the stomach should be repaired primarily after débridement of nonviable edges. The primary repair can be performed in either a single layer with nonabsorbable suture or as a double-layer closure with an absorbable suture (e.g., Vicryl, Ethicon, Inc., Somerville, NJ), with the first layer and the second layer closed with unabsorbable sutures (e.g., silk). This approach compromises the gastric lumen in only a very few penetrating injuries of the stomach. Fortunately, major resective procedures are not commonly necessary in gastric injuries. Because gross contamination is usually associated with stomach wounds, copious irrigation of the abdominal cavity is an essential component of the operative strategy.

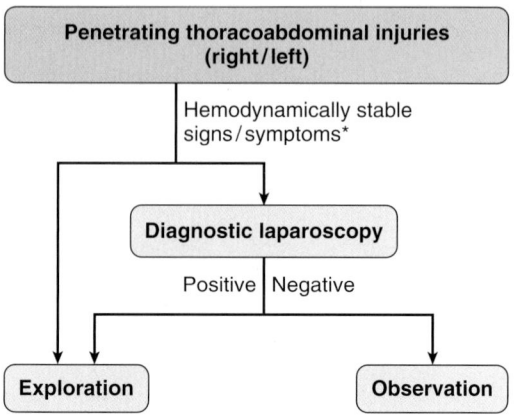

*Patients who have no absolute indication for exploration

FIGURE 2 Treatment algorithm.

TABLE 1: Diaphragmatic injuries

Organ	Incidence rate	Diagnosis	Specific management	Outcome

Diaphragm	6% of all intra-abdominal injuries that result from penetrating trauma	Physical examination
		• Chest pain and shortness of breath
		• Scaphoid abdomen
		• Bowel sounds on auscultation of the hemithorax
		Plain radiography
		• Hollow viscus noted in the left hemithorax
		  Nasogastric tube in the left hemithorax
		FAST examination
		• Unreliable
		DPL
		  • Inconclusive; high false-negative
		CT scan
		  • Inconclusive
		Laparoscopy, the diagnostic modality of choice
			Preoperative antibiotics
			Primary closure is the preferred definitive management
			With documentation of a diaphragmatic rent (laceration), exploratory laparotomy is necessary
				Associated injuries dictate morbidity and mortality

CT, Computed tomographic; *DPL,* diagnostic peritoneal lavage; *FAST,* focused assessment with sonography for trauma.

Small Intestine

Small bowel is the most common intraperitoneal hollow viscus injured. As with other hollow viscus injuries, nonoperative management has no place in a small bowel perforation or rupture. CT scan evaluation is usually not necessary with penetrating injuries, but it can be helpful in detection of a possible bowel injury. The two basic types of findings of bowel injury on CT scan are direct and indirect (Table 2). The management of injuries to the small intestine is well established, with control of bleeding and gross spillage being strategic mainstays. If bowel viability is questioned secondary to blunt or penetrating trauma, a segmental resection should be performed. Isolated small bowel enterotomies can be closed primarily with nonabsorbable sutures for a one-layer closure. If the edges of the enterotomy appear nonviable, they should be gently débrided before primary closure. However, multiple contiguous small bowel holes or an intestinal injury on the mesenteric border with associate mesenteric hematoma likely necessitate segmental resection and anastomosis of the remaining viable segments of the small bowel. The operative goal is always the reestablishment of intestinal continuity without substantial narrowing of the intestinal lumen, along with closure of any associated mesenteric defects. Application of noncrushing bowel clamps can contain ongoing contamination while the repair is being performed. Although a hand-sewn or stapler-assisted anastomosis is operator dependent, trauma laparotomies are time-sensitive interventions and expeditious management is imperative. In the immediate postoperative period, bowel decompression for 12 to 24 hours is prudent. As in most trauma laparotomies, antibiotics should be routinely given in only the perioperative period, unless an ensuing infectious complication occurs in the postoperative period.

Colon/Rectum

Penetrating trauma accounts for most of the colon and rectal injuries that occur in the civilian setting. Even today, a debate remains regarding the optimal treatment of colon injuries, with the preponderance of evidence supporting primary closure of the colonic wounds and segmental resection (with primary anastomosis) in most traumatic settings. Most colonic injuries are quickly diagnosed during the initial exploration and mobilization of the colon. With two thirds of the rectum being extraperitoneal and bordered by the bony pelvis, detection and direct management of a localized rectal injury is a challenge. Rectal injuries are usually a result of pelvic fractures and penetrating trauma. Oftentimes, rectal injuries are managed with

TABLE 2: Computed tomographic scan findings of blunt bowel injury

Direct	Indirect
Oral contrast extravasation	Mesenteric hematoma
Free air	Mesenteric blush
	Bowel wall edema
	Unexplained ascites
	Fat streaking
	Unopacified (vascular contrast media) bowel loops

proximal diversion. The segment of injured bowel should be thoroughly inspected for potential through-in-through enterotomies and associated mesenteric injuries. This requires adequate mobilization of the colon for visualization of the entire circumference of the bowel wall. As highlighted previously, initially controversial, an enterotomy (right-sided or left-sided injuries) of the colon can be closed primarily, irrespective of contamination or transient shock state. If the colon injury is so extensive that primary repair is not possible or would severely compromise the lumen, a segmental resection should be performed. Depending on the environmental setting, the remaining proximal segment can be anastomosed to the distal segment or a proximal ostomy and Hartmann's procedure can be performed. If the distal segment is long enough, a mucous fistula should be established. Documented rectal injuries below the peritoneal reflection should necessitate a diverting colostomy and presacral drainage (exiting from the perineum). Such drainage is, however, not universally endorsed.

A capsule summary of the incidence, diagnosis, management options, and related outcomes for injuries of the stomach, small intestine, colon, and rectum is depicted in Table 3.

Retroperitoneal Injury

The retroperitoneum is an anatomic bonanza because several of the most vital structures reside in this area, including portions of the duodenum, the pancreas, the kidneys and adrenals, and major vessels

TABLE 3: Injuries of the stomach, small intestine, colon, and rectum: incidence, diagnosis, management options, and outcomes

Organs	Incidence	Diagnosis	Specific management	Outcome
Stomach	More common injury in penetrating trauma than in blunt 10% of penetrating injuries of the abdomen	Physical examination • Epigastric tenderness • Peritoneal signs • Bloody gastric aspirate Plain radiography • Free air under the diaphragm FAST examination • Unreliable DPL • Lavage RBCs WBCs Gross contamination CT scan • Pneumoperitoneum Laparoscopy • Operator dependent	Preoperative antibiotics Débridement when necessary Primary closure (two layers)	Associated injuries dictate morbidity and mortality
Small bowel	Highest incidence rate of injury of the intra-abdominal organ	Physical examination • Cannot rely on tenderness or peritoneal signs in the early stage of injury Plain radiography FAST examination: free fluid with CT scan shows no solid organ injury CT scan • High false-negative rate • Pneumoperitoneum • Free fluid	Preoperative antibiotics Primary closure of simple lacerations Segmented resection of complex injuries with functional end-to-end tensionless anastomosis One-layer (or double-layer) closure/anastomosis or stapled anastomosis	Outcome is good Negligible leak rate even in contaminated field
Colon	Majority Stab wounds Gunshot wounds Instrumentation Blunt trauma, infrequent	Physical examination • Tenderness/peritoneal signs • Gross blood on rectal examination	Preoperative antibiotics Primary closure of simple injuries (avoid narrowing the lumen) Segmental resection and fecal diversion of complex colonic wounds	Overall, favorable outcome Complications • Low leak rate • Wound infection • Intraperitoneal abscess

CT, Computed tomographic; *DPL,* diagnostic peritoneal lavage; *FAST,* focused assessment with sonography for trauma; *RBCs,* red blood cell counts; *WBCs,* white blood cell counts.

(aorta, inferior vena cava, and other vasculature), along with other organs. The specific retroperitoneal injury is usually easily detected with advanced diagnostic imaging, such as CT scan. However, on occasion, such injuries are found during an abdominal exploration for blunt or penetrating trauma. In this setting, the only suggestion of an injury to a structure in this region might be discovery of a retroperitoneal hematoma.

Retroperitoneal Hematomas

The retroperitoneum, an organ-rich region, has several key structures that can be injured when its boundaries are penetrated. The retroperitoneal hematoma can be a major potential site for hemorrhage in patients with either penetrating or blunt trauma because of the substantial vascularity, along with bleeding, that can occur from an associated solid organ wound (e.g., kidney). In the central region (zone I) of the retroperitoneum resides the abdominal aorta, celiac axis, and the superior mesenteric artery, vena cava, and proximal renal vasculature. The lateral retroperitoneum (zone II) encompasses the proximal genitourinary system and its vasculature. The pelvic retroperitoneum (zone III) contains the iliac arteries, veins, and their tributaries. In addition to the vasculature and the kidneys (plus ureters) highlighted previously, the retroperitoneum contains the second, third, and fourth portion of the duodenum, along with the pancreas, the adrenals, and the intrapelvic portion of the colon and rectum. Table 4 underscores the management principles of traumatic retroperitoneal hematomas. Ideally, proximal (and when applicable, distal) control needs to be achieved before exploration of any retroperitoneal hematoma. For retroperitoneal hematomas in zone I, irrespective of a penetrating or blunt mechanism, mandatory exploration is required. Also, a retroperitoneal hematoma in any of the three zones requires exploration for all penetrating injuries. For zone II retroperitoneal hematomas that result from blunt trauma, all pulsatile or expanding hematomas should undergo exploration. Gross extravasation of urine also necessitates exploration. Zone III (pelvic

TABLE 4: The "Zones" of penetrating cervical injuries

Zone	Blunt	Penetrating
I (Central)	Explore	Explore
II (Perinephric)	Observe	Explore
III (Pelvic)	Observe	Explore

retroperitoneum) hematomas should be explored only for penetrating injuries to determine whether there is a specific intrapelvic colorectal, ureteral, or vascular injury. However, such an approach should not be taken for blunt trauma because the injury is likely venous and application of an external compression device is the preferred intervention. An arterial injury could be addressed with arteriography or embolization.

Specific Injuries

Table 5 provides an overview of specific injuries.

TABLE 5: Retroperitoneal

Organs	Incidence	Diagnosis	Specific management	Outcomes
Duodenum/ pancreas	Isolated injuries are uncommon High percentage of associated injuries	Physical examination • Abdominal tenderness • Peritoneal signs Plain radiography • Free air • Retroperitoneal air FAST DPL CT scan	Preoperative antibiotics Duodenal injury: operative armamentarium • Primary repair with gastrostomy retrograde • Jejunostomy: feeding • Jejunostomy • Pyloric exclusive Pancreatic injury: operative armamentarium • Drainage • Débridement • Partial resection • Pancreaticoduodenectomy	Highly lethal as a result of associated injuries Increased mortality with delayed diagnosis of duodenal injury
Kidney	20% of renal injuries result from penetrating trauma	Physical examination Penetrating wound or trajectory in close proximity to the kidney • Hematuria Plain radiography • Nonspecific FAST DPL CT scan (if peritoneal penetration not suspected in a gunshot wound) • Perinephric hematoma • Extravasation	Preoperative antibiotics Operative armamentarium Primary repair with viable tissue buttress • Partial nephrectomy • Nephrectomy	Mortality related to the associated injuries
Bladder	Usually an occult injury found during intraoperative abdominal exploration	Physical examination • Penetrating wound or trajectory in close proximity to the bladder • Hematuria Plain radiography • Nonspecific FAST DPL CT scan (if peritoneal penetration not suspected) Perinephric hematoma • Extravasation of contrast agent	Preoperative antibiotics Multilayer closure with absorbable sutures with indwelling bladder catheter	Excellent outcomes Morbidity and mortality relate to associated injuries
Ureter	Infrequent injury in penetrating trauma	Usually an intraoperative diagnosis	Preoperative antibiotics Management armamentarium Primary repair/stenting Delayed repair and suprapubic cystostomy Diverting nephrostomies	Good outcome if no major associated injuries

CT, Computed tomographic; *DPL,* diagnostic peritoneal lavage; *FAST,* focused assessment with sonography for trauma.

Duodenum and Pancreas

The most frequent retroperitoneal hollow viscus injury, particularly in blunt trauma, is the duodenum. Full-thickness duodenal wounds demand operative management.

Duodenal injuries can be repaired primarily in a one-layered or two-layered fashion if the penetration is less than half the circumference of the duodenum. However, for more complex duodenal injuries, an operative procedure is needed to divert gastric contents away from the site (where closure of the wound has been attempted). A pyloric exclusion with the establishment of a gastrojejunostomy is such a procedure.

Superficial or tangential penetrating wounds of the pancreas, in which there is no injury to the main pancreatic duct, can be externally drained. However, a penetrating injury that transects the pancreas, including the main pancreatic duct, requires extirpation of the distal pancreas (distal pancreatectomy), particularly if the transection site is to the left of the superior mesenteric vessels. A more proximal penetrating injury that involves the main pancreatic duct, with associated complex duodenal injury (e.g., injury to the ampulla) likely necessitates a pancreatoduodenectomy. Unfortunately, because of the rich vascular network that surrounds the pancreas, penetrating pancreatic wounds can be lethal injuries.

In blunt abdominal trauma, assessment of pancreatic injuries to determine whether surgery is required can be extremely challenging. Clinical symptoms, physical examination, and diagnostic imaging (e.g., CT scan) are all important parameters in making the correct decision regarding operative intervention. If a patient presents with abdominal pain and examination has associated abdominal tenderness, along with CT confirmation of pancreatic injury, then that patient needs to proceed to the operative theater for exploration. If the patient is relatively asymptomatic and CT scan findings are consistent with a likely pancreatic injury, endoscopic retrograde cholangiopancreatography (ERCP) can assist in determining whether there is a major ductal injury. Such a finding necessitates exploration for definitive management.

Genitourinary System

Less than 10% of patients with penetrating abdominal wounds sustain genitourinary tract injuries, with most of the injuries being renal. Penetrating injuries that result in a grade IV (cortical/calyceal injury and associated vascular injury with contained hemorrhage) or grade V (shattered kidney and vascular avulsion) invariably necessitate a nephrectomy, particularly if there is a viable contralateral kidney. Lacerations or more superficial wounds of the kidney might require renorrhaphy, with approximation of the disrupted capsule with pledgeted sutures or a prosthetic (mesh) wrap. Absorbable interrupted suture should be used, and all repairs should be drained. On occasion, the injury pattern dictates the need for a partial nephrectomy. Ureteral injuries can be extremely difficult to identify in penetrating wounds with an accompanying retroperitoneal hematoma. When possible, the ureter should be repaired primarily with interrupted absorbable suture over a double J stent. A complete transection of the ureter requires débridement of the nonviable edges, spatulation of the ends, and primary repair over a stent. All repair sites should be adequately drained. If the anastomosis cannot be performed in a tension-free fashion, a bladder flap (Buari's) could be surgically constructed, with implantation of the proximal segment of the transected ureter into the flap. A psoas "hitch" might be necessary if there is any tension on the flap and the tunneled ureter.

Penetrating injury to the intraperitoneal bladder requires surgical repair. After confirmation of no involvement of the trigone, the bladder should be closed with a two-layer closure with absorbable suture (the second layer incorporates Lembert sutures to imbricate the first layer). Suprapubic drainage should only be done selectively; however, a Foley catheter should be left in place.

Abdominal Vascular Injury

With no suggestion of an abdominal visceral injury, a patient who is hemodynamically labile with increasing abdominal distension has a vascular injury, either secondary to a mesenteric rent or specific vessel wound. Several major intra-abdominal vessels can, if injured, result in substantial bleeding. In the central area (zone I), these include the abdominal aorta, the celiac axis vessels, the superior mesenteric artery or vein, the portal vein, and the inferior vena cava. The perinephric region (zone II) encompasses the renal artery and vein, bilaterally. Zone III represents the pelvic region where the iliac arteries and veins and their tributaries lie. Although blunt trauma can result in mesenteric avulsions with associated bleeding, most vascular injuries occur from penetrating abdominal and transpelvic trauma.

The role of aggressive crystalloid resuscitation in the initial management of patients who are in shock from intra-abdominal hemorrhage is still being debated. However, less aggressive fluid resuscitation has been reported to have some benefit, particularly in situations in which the time between the prehospital setting and the definitive hospital management is relatively short. Also, some investigators advocate for performing an emergency thoracotomy, with cross clamping of the descending aorta, to sustain intracranial and coronary flow while decreasing arterial inflow into the abdomen to temporarily address ongoing intra-abdominal hemorrhage in a patient who is in profound shock. In the trauma bay, the quickest method of confirming intra-abdominal hemorrhage is by performing the FAST examination. Such an assessment can be done while the patient is undergoing expeditious ATLS protocol, with the establishment of an optimal airway and the insertion of large-bore intravenous catheters.

On entering the abdomen, free blood and clots should be removed followed with gauze (laparotomy pads) packing of each of the four quadrants. Areas of concern should be manually compressed as the pads are carefully removed from the other quadrants. Also, operative prioritization of intra-abdominal hemorrhage should be done, expeditiously, with identification and control of aortic and inferior vena caval injuries, followed by management of bleeding solid organs. Afterwards, contained retroperitoneal hematomas should be addressed. When appropriate, the fundamental principle of obtaining proximal and distal control of an injured vessel before repair remains the same. Definitive management of specific arterial and venous injuries is elucidated in Tables 6 and 7. Two fundamental maneuvers in gaining access to the central vasculature are medial mobilization of right-sided and left-sighted intra-abdominal viscera (Figures 3 and 4). In addition to having a prepared blood bank, a trauma surgeon encountering a major abdominal vascular injury should have certain adjuncts (e.g., conduits for establishment of temporary shunts and material for silo development in the open abdomen) to assist in the management of the injured patient.

Approximately 25% of patients with major abdominal injuries have significant vascular trauma. No other intra-abdominal presentation defines time-sensitive management like this cohort of injuries.

SUMMARY

Although the concept of standard-of-care management is broadly accepted and adamantly advocated, such care is at times institution dependent. Unfortunately, resource-rich trauma facilities and systems are *not* uniform throughout the country and regionalization has not been perfected nationwide.

However, the overarching mission remains the same: optimal management for everyone, irrespective of where the patient receives trauma care.

TABLE 6: Abdominal arterial injuries: exposure and management options

Site of abdominal vascular injury	Principle route of operative exposure	Preferred management options
Infrarenal aorta	Midline inframesocolic retroperitoneum	Lateral suture, patch repair, or interposition graft (rare) Ligation requires extraanatomic bypass reconstruction
Suprarenal aorta	Left-to-right medial visceral rotation (spleen, pancreas, and left colon)	Lateral suture or patch repair Interposition graft requires bypass to celiac, superior mesenteric, or renal arteries (rare) No ligation
Celiac axis	Left-to-right medial visceral rotation (spleen, pancreas, and left colon)	Lateral suture if feasible; ligation otherwise preferred; interposition graft if collaterals disrupted (rare)
Hepatic artery	Hepatoduodenal ligament	Lateral suture, interposition graft, or ligation (may require bypass graft)
Splenic artery	Through lesser sac	Ligation preferred
Superior mesenteric artery	Left-to-right medial visceral rotation (spleen, pancreas, and left colon); base of mesentery	Lateral suture, patch repair, or ligation and distal bypass
Inferior mesenteric artery	Midline inframesocolic retroperitoneum	Ligation preferred
Proximal renal arteries	Midline inframesocolic retroperitoneum, right-to-left medial visceral rotation (right colon and duodenum), or left-to-right medial visceral rotation	Lateral suture, patch repair, litigation and bypass, or nephrectomy
Distal renal arteries	Right-to-left medial visceral rotation (right colon and duodenum) on right; left-to-right medial visceral rotation on left	Lateral suture, patch repair, interposition graft or nephrectomy
Common and external iliac arteries	Midline pelvic retroperitoneum; medical reflection of sigmoid colon on left	Lateral suture, patch repair, interposition graft, or ligation with bypass to external iliac artery (may be extraanatomic)
Internal iliac arteries	Midline pelvic retroperitoneum	Ligation preferred

Adapted from Kokino, PG, Thompson RW: Abdominal vascular trauma. In Soper NJ, Thompson EC, editors: Problems in general surgery: abdominal trauma, vol 15, Philadelphia, 1998, Lippincott-Raven, p. 84.

TABLE 7: Abdominal venous injuries: exposure and management options

Site of abdominal vascular injury	Principal route of operative exposure	Preferred management options
Infrarenal inferior vena cava	Midline inframesocolic retroperitoneum or right-to-left medial visceral rotation (right colon)	Lateral suture, patch repair, or ligation
Renal veins	Right-to-left medial visceral rotation (right colon and duodenum) on right; midline inframesocolic retroperitoneum on left	Lateral suture or patch repair, ligation if collaterals intact on left; interposition vein graft on right or on left if no collaterals; nephrectomy
Juxtarenal inferior vena cava	Right-to-left medial visceral rotation (right colon and duodenum)	Lateral suture or patch repair
Retrohepatic inferior vena cava	Right-to-left medial visceral rotation (right colon, duodenum and right liver) with vascular exclusion of the liver (Pringle's maneuver and atriocaval shunt)	Lateral suture or patch repair

Continued

TABLE 7: Abdominal venous injuries: exposure and management options—cont'd

Site of abdominal vascular injury	Principal route of operative exposure	Preferred management options
Portal vein	Hepaduodenal ligament; right-to-left medial visceral rotation (right colon and duodenum); lesser sac and transpancreatic	Lateral suture, patch repair (vein), splenic vein bypass to superior mesenteric vein, or ligation
Iliac veins	Midline pelvic retroperitoneum; medial reflection of sigmoid colon on left; divide iliac artery (rare)	Lateral suture, patch repair, or ligation

Adapted from Kokino, PG, Thompson RW: Abdominal vascular trauma in problems in general surgery. In Soper NJ, Thompson EC, editors: Problems in general surgery: abdominal trauma, vol 15, Philadelphia, 1998, Lippincott-Raven, p. 85.

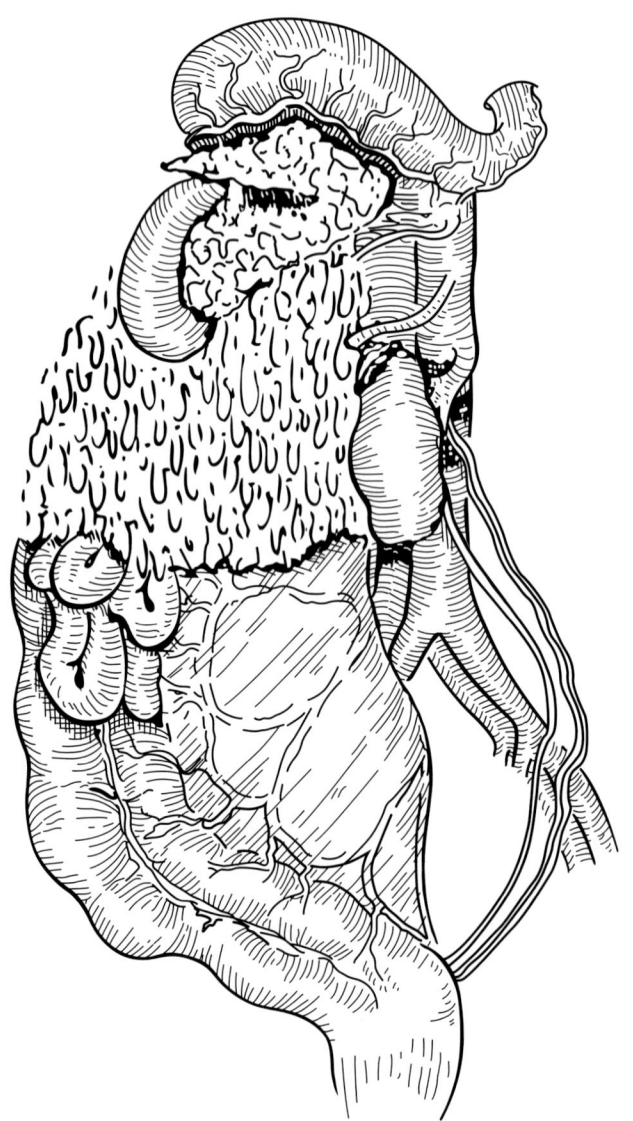

FIGURE 3 Medial rotation of the right-sided intraabdominal viscera. *(Adapted from Kokinos PG, Thompson RW: Abdominal vascular trauma. In Soper NJ, Thompson EC, editors: Problems in general surgery: abdominal trauma, vol 15, Philadelphia, 1998, Lippincott-Raven, p. 85.)*

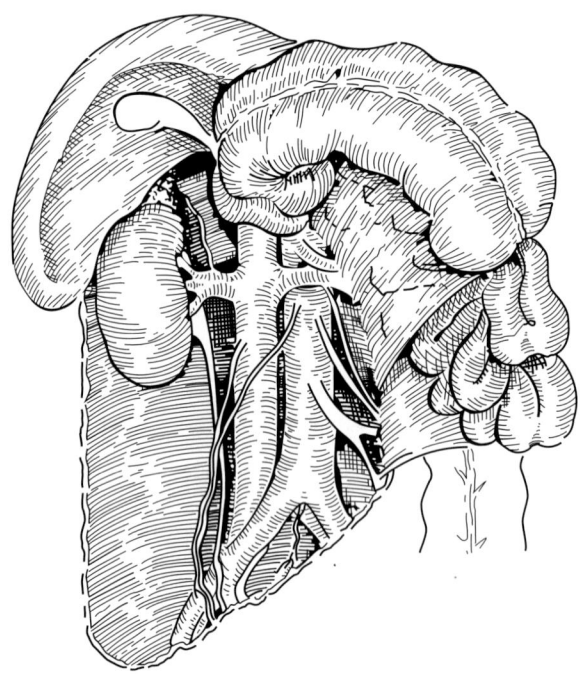

FIGURE 4 Medial rotation of the left-sided intraabdominal viscera. *(Adapted from Kokinos PG, Thompson RW: Abdominal vascular trauma. In Soper NJ, Thompson EC, editors: Problems in general surgery: abdominal trauma, vol 15, Philadelphia, 1998, Lippincott-Raven, p. 86.)*

SUGGESTED READINGS

American College of Surgeons Committee on Trauma: *Advanced trauma life support*, ed 6, Chicago, 1997, American College of Surgeons.

Asensio JA, Demetriades D, Chahwan S, et al: Approach to the management of complex hepatic injuries, *J Trauma* 48(1):66–69, 2000.

Asensio JA, Britt LD, Borzotta A, et al: Multiinstitutional experience with the management of superior mesenteric artery injuries, *J Am Coll Surg* 193:354, 2011.

Asensio JA, Feliciano DV, Britt LD: Management of duodenal injuries, *Curr Probl Surg* 30(11):1023, 1993.

Britt LD, McQuay N Jr: Laparoscopy in the evaluation of penetrating thoracoabdominal trauma, *Am Surg* 69(9):788–791, 2003.

Croce MA, Fabian TC, Menke PG, et al: Nonoperative management of blunt hepatic trauma is the treatment of choice for hemodynamically stable patients: results of a prospective trial, *Ann Surg* 221(6):744–755, 1995.

David Richardson J, Franklin GA, Lukan JK, et al: Evolution in the management of hepatic trauma: a 25-year perspective, *Ann Surg* 232(3):324–330, 2000.

Davis TP, Feliciano DV, Rozycki GS, et al: Results with abdominal vascular trauma in the modern era, *Am Surg* 67:565, 2001.

Demetriades D, Cahralambides D, Lakhoo M, et al: Gunshot wounds of the abdomen: the role of selective conservative management, *Br J Surg* 78:220, 1996.

Demetriades D, Murray JA, Chan L, et al: Penetrating colon injuries requiring resection: diversion or primary anastomosis? An AAST prospective multicenter study, *J Trauma* 50(5):765–775, 2001.

Fabian TC, Croce MA, Stewart RM, et al: A prospective analysis of diagnostic laparoscopy in trauma, *Ann Surg* 217:557, 1993.

Feliciano DV: Injuries to great vessels of the abdomen. In Holcroft JW, editor: *Scientific American surgery*, New York, 1998, Scientific American.

Flint LMJ, Brown A, Richardson JD, et al: Definitive control of bleeding from severe pelvic fractures, *Ann Surg* 189:709, 1979.

Hauser CJ, Huprich JE, Bosco P, et al: Triple contrast computed tomography in the evaluation of penetrating posterior abdominal injuries, *Arch Surg* 122:1112, 1987.

Ivatury RR, Simon RJ, Stahl WM: A critical evaluation of laparoscopy in penetrating abdominal trauma, *J Trauma* 34:822, 1993.

Jurkovich G, Carrico C: Management of pancreatic injuries, *Surg Clin North Am* 70(3):575–594, 1990.

Maxwell RA, Fabian TC: Current management of colon trauma, *World J Surg* 27(6):632–639, 2003.

Meredith JW, Young JS, Bowling J, et al: Nonoperative management of blunt hepatic trauma: the exception or the rule? *J Trauma* 36(4):529–535, 1994.

Pachter HL, Knudson MM, Esrig B, et al: Status of nonoperative management of blunt hepatic injuries in 1995: a multicenter experience with 404 patients, *J Trauma* 40(1):31–38, 1996.

Peitzman AB, Heil B, Rivera L, et al: Blunt splenic injury in adults: multi-institutional study of the Eastern Association for the Surgery of Trauma, *J Trauma* 49(2):177–189, 2000.

Root HD, Hauser CW, McKinley CR, et al: Dianostic peritoneal lavage, *Surgery* 57:633, 1965.

Rozychi GS, Ochsner MG, Schmidt JA, et al: A prospective study of surgeon-performed ultrasound as the primary adjuvant modality for injured patient assessment, *J Trauma* 39:492–498, 1995.

Shafton GW: Indications for operations in abdominal trauma, *Am J Surg* 99:657–662, 1960.

Shah R, Sabanathan S, Mearns AJ, et al: Traumatic rupture of the diaphragm, *Ann Thorac Surg* 60:1444–1449, 1995.

Shapiro MB, Jenkins DH, Schwab CW, et al: Damage control: collective review, *J Trauma* 49:969–978, 2000.

Smego DR, Richardson JD, Flint LM: Determinants of outcome in pancreatic trauma, *J Trauma* 25(8):771–776, 1985.

Stone HH, Fabian TC: Management of perforating colon trauma: randomization between primary closure and exteriorization, *Am Surg* 190:430, 1979.

PENETRATING ABDOMINAL TRAUMA

**Fredric M. Pieracci, MD, MPH, and
Gregory J. Jurkovich, MD**

Penetrating abdominal trauma may cause life-threatening injuries that can only be treated with emergent operative intervention. However, in some patients, a nonoperative approach of careful observation is both safe and cost-effective. The initial management of penetrating abdominal trauma is thus directed towards rapid identification of those who need immediate operative intervention, those who may be safely observed for the development of delayed signs of injury, and those who need no further therapy and may be discharged from the emergency department. Although various diagnostic modalities, discussed herein, aid in this decision, a thorough physical examination remains the cornerstone of this triage decision scheme.

HISTORICAL PERSPECTIVE

Nonoperative management of all penetrating abdominal trauma was the standard of care before the late 1800s. That dictum was initially challenged by the southern surgeon J. Marion Sims. Sims criticized the high mortality associated with a nonoperative approach to abdominal gunshot wounds (GSWs), which likely contributed to the death of many famous Americans, including President James Garfield. So began the era of mandatory exploration of all injuries, which remained in effect until G.W. Shaftman introduced the concept of "selective conservatism" in the 1960s. Selective conservatism was based primarily on Shaftman's observation that most penetrating abdominal trauma did not result in injuries that necessitated operative repair. Ignited by Shaftman's hypothesis, work by several traumatologists, including the Western Trauma Association Multicenter Trials Committee, has helped to better define the subset of patients with anterior abdominal stab wounds (AASWs) who may be managed

safely with nonoperative algorithms. Similarly, mandatory exploration of abdominal GSWs has been revisited by select high-volume trauma centers, particularly in those patients who are morbidly obese and in whom the trajectory appears tangential, or limited to the high right upper abdominal quadrant. Although this was initially met with skepticism, many trauma surgeons now agree that a selective nonoperative approach for abdominal GSWs may be instituted safely in certain situations and centers. Finally, the introduction of damage control surgery in the late 1970s has changed the conduct of laparotomies for patients with major vascular injuries from penetrating abdominal trauma. It is now recognized that the acidotic, hypothermic, and coagulopathic condition is better served by an abbreviated operation, in which major sources of bleeding and intestinal contamination are controlled, followed by a period of resuscitation before definitive injury repair. This damage control approach has saved innumerable lives compared with the prior strategy of initial definitive management of abdominal injuries in the face of worsening shock.

ANATOMIC DEFINITIONS

In development of management strategies for penetrating abdominal trauma, division of the abdomen into the following three regions is useful: anterior abdomen, flank and back, and thoracoabdomen (Figure 1).

Anterior abdomen: The anterior abdomen is bound by a transverse line through the inferior costal margins superiorly, the groin creases inferiorly, and the anterior axillary lines laterally. Penetrating wounds to the anterior abdominal wall have the highest incidence rate of intraperitoneal injury and are least amenable to a nonoperative approach. Furthermore, injury to intraperitoneal structures (as opposed to retroperitoneal structures) is usually apparent with both a competent clinical examination and a focused abdominal sonography for trauma (FAST) examination.

Flank and back: The flank is bounded superiorly by the inferior costal margin, anteriorly by the anterior axillary lines, posteriorly by the posterior axillary lines, and inferiorly by the anterior superior iliac spines. The back is bounded superiorly by a transverse line through the inferior scapular tips, laterally by the posterior axillary

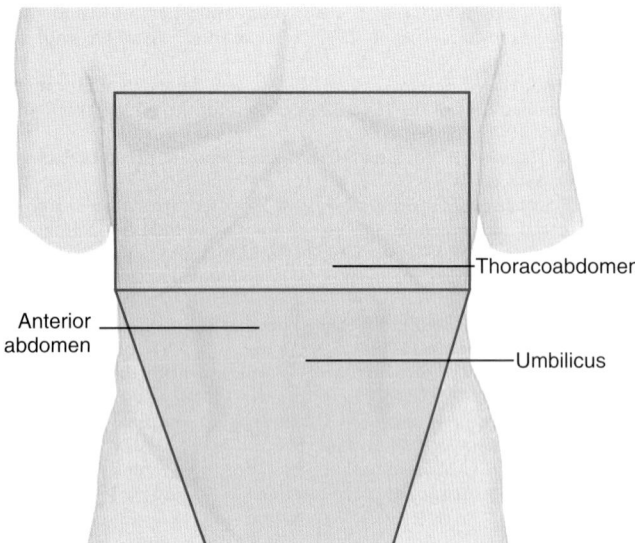

FIGURE 1 Anatomic boundaries of the anterior abdomen and thoracoabdomen.

lines, and inferiorly by a transverse line through the posterior superior iliac spines. Organs of specific concern in these locations include the retroperitoneal portion of the colon, the diaphragm, the kidney, the liver and spleen, and less commonly, the pancreas, duodenum, aorta, inferior vena cava, and ureters. Penetrating wounds to both the flank and the back are associated with a much lower incidence of injury that requires operative intervention as compared with anterior abdomen wounds. However, injury to retroperitoneal structures often eludes the diagnostic capabilities of both physical examination and FAST examination, and delayed diagnosis leads to severe morbidity and often mortality. For this reason, evaluation of these injuries often includes additional imaging methods, most commonly contrast-enhanced computed tomographic (CT) scan.

Thoracoabdomen: The thoracoabdominal region is bounded superiorly by a horizontal line through the nipples in men and inframammary fold in women, inferiorly by a transverse line crossing the inferior costal margins, and laterally by the anterior axillary lines. Management of penetrating wounds to the thoracoabdominal region deserves special consideration for the following reasons. First, with exsanguination, a decision must be made regarding the cavity responsible for the hemorrhage (thoracic, abdominal, or both). These potentially multiple sources of bleeding must then be prioritized vis-a-vis the operative approach. Physical examination, chest radiography, and FAST examination may be useful in this regard. Second, the diaphragm is particularly vulnerable to injury after penetrating thoracoabdominal trauma. Thoracoabdominal wounds that injure the diaphragm have the potential to result in delayed herniation of abdominal contents into the thoracic cavity. Incarceration and eventual strangulation may ensue. This is particularly germane for left-sided thoracoabdominal injuries because right-sided diaphragmatic injuries are extremely unlikely to result in bowel herniation as a result of coverage by the liver. Accordingly, diaphragmatic injury must be considered in all left-sided thoracoabdominal penetrating trauma. The rate of associated intraabdominal injury in patients with left-sided diaphragmatic injuries approaches 90%.

MECHANISM OF INJURY

The next important consideration beyond the location of the wound is the mechanism of injury. The mechanism of abdominal penetration is of relevance primarily with respect to the likelihood of associated intraabdominal injury requiring operative repair. Missile injuries

(most commonly as the result of GSWs) are associated with an approximately 90% incidence rate of abdominal injury requiring operative intervention. This relatively high proportion has led to the traditional recommendation of mandatory laparotomy for all patients with abdominal GSWs. However, further stratification is possible. Specifically, patients with a GSW to either the flank or the back have a much lower rate of abdominal injury requiring operative intervention (most series estimate 10% to 15%). Other clinical scenarios associated with a low incidence rate of significant abdominal injury (and thus need for immediate operative intervention) include isolated right upper quadrant GSWs and GSWs in the morbidly obese patient. In addition to a higher likelihood of direct intraabdominal injury compared with stab wounds, GSWs also carry the potential for significant blast effect to organs that are not in the immediate trajectory of the missile.

Shotgun blasts represent a subcategory of missile injuries that may lead to severe blast effect from the simultaneous impact of multiple pellets (buckshot). In general, the greater the distance between the shotgun and the patient, the greater the scatter and the lower the chance of intraabdominal injury requiring operative repair. This principle has been translated into the following classification schema for shotgun injuries: type I, >25 cm scatter; type II, 10 to 25 cm scatter; and type III, <10 cm scatter. A direct relationship is found between the scatter grade and the likelihood of intraabdominal injury; more than one third of patients with a type I injury do not need operative intervention.

In contrast to anterior abdominal GSWs, only 50% to 75% of AASWs enter the peritoneal cavity, and only 50% to 75% of these cause an injury that necessitates operative repair. Consequently, only a minority of stable, asymptomatic cases with AASWs (approximately 20%) need operative intervention. Similar to GSWs, the likelihood of intraabdominal injury after a stab wound is higher for the anterior abdominal region as compared with both the back and the flank.

INITIAL MANAGEMENT

The initial management of patients with penetrating abdominal trauma proceeds according to the guidelines espoused by the American College of Surgeon's Advanced Trauma Life Support. Evaluation begins with the primary survey, which includes assessment of airway, followed by breathing, followed by circulation (ABCs), and the establishment of intravenous assess and institution of resuscitative fluids. The primarily survey also includes a focused neurologic examination (D, disability) and complete exposure (E) of the patient. Patients in shock should receive immediate blood product transfusion. In general, lower extremity access points (e.g., femoral vein) should be avoided in patients with suspected abdominal vascular trauma because venous extravasation limits efficacy. Both nasogastric and urinary bladder tubes, and emergency room x-rays, are considered adjuncts to the primary survey. Insertion of these tubes may be both diagnostic (e.g., bleeding, diaphragm injury) and therapeutic. Abdominal injury does not preclude concomitant thoracic injury, particularly in the case of thoracoabdominal trauma. Thus, the search for immediately life-threatening injuries, such as tension pneumothorax, massive hemothorax, and cardiac tamponade, should be pursued aggressively with physical examination, FAST examination, and chest radiography. Results from each of these tests may be obtained rapidly and are invaluable with respect to ruling out extraabdominal sources of shock. Once these injuries have been ruled out, the patient with a hemodynamically unstable condition should be transported promptly to the operating room because the most likely source of hemorrhagic shock is a major vascular injury. Patients who are transient responders to resuscitation fluids may be further stratified by obtaining a marker of end-organ perfusion, such as a serum lactate concentration or base deficit. These rapid measurements may unmask occult hypoperfusion in the patient with relative hypotension and should preclude an unnecessary and potentially dangerous trip to radiology. Finally, patients with either agonal or absent vital signs may be candidates for emergency department resuscitative thoracotomy provided: (1) signs of life were at some point noted; and (2) a relatively short period of time has elapsed between arrest and presentation (e.g., less than 15 minutes).

DIAGNOSTIC ADJUNCTS

Patients with hemodynamic instability rarely need adjunctive testing before operation. Important exceptions are extraabdominal sources of shock such as tension pneumothorax and cardiac tamponade, in which both the FAST examination and chest radiograph are useful. The patient with an otherwise stable and hemodynamically normal condition should receive a complete secondary survey, with identification and marking of all wounds. Standard trauma laboratory panels, including a hemoglobin determination and type and cross matching of blood, are obtained routinely. Measurement of a baseline global marker of tissue perfusion, such as lactate or base deficit, is also useful in both detecting occult shock and tracking resuscitative efforts. In general, patients with missile injuries to the abdomen should undergo plain films of both the abdomen and one cavity in either direction (i.e., chest and pelvis films). All wounds should be marked with radiopaque markers (e.g., paper clip, electrocardiogram lead). A single missile wound with nonvisualization of a foreign body on radiograph is suggestive of bullet embolism. Differentiation of "entrance" from "exit" missile wounds is not recommended because this is often not possible and may hamper forensic investigations. The presence of two wounds may represent either a through-and-through missile injury or two separate missiles that remain intracorporeal.

Because of the relatively low incidence of intraabdominal injury from AASWs, local wound exploration (LWE) has emerged as the standard initial diagnostic maneuver in the patient with a hemodynamically normal and stable condition and AASW with a normal physical examination of the abdomen. The goal of the LWE is to assess fascial penetration; if the injury stopped short of the anterior fascia, there is virtually no chance of intraperitoneal injury and the patient may be discharged (negative LWE). In contrast, if the anterior fascia was penetrated, tracking the wound through the muscle is difficult; hence, peritoneal violation must be assumed (positive LWE), and the patient is carefully observed.

The technique of LWE involves administration of local anesthesia and extension of the wound such that adequate evaluation of the track and its distal extent is possible. In some cases, substantial lengthening of the skin incision is necessary, and at no time should wounds be probed blindly, lest a clot occluding a major vascular injury be dislodged. Although the exact definition of a positive LWE has been debated, a generally accepted one is penetration of the anterior fascia (either anterior rectus sheath or external oblique aponeurosis, depending on the location of the wound). When performed properly, LWE allows for approximately one half of asymptomatic, stable AASW cases to be discharged from the emergency department. Patients with positive examination results are observed with serial clinical assessments (discussed subsequently). Importantly, LWE may be nondiagnostic in certain situations, including morbidly obese patients and patients with long, tangential wound tracks. Furthermore, LWE may not be practical in patients with multiple (i.e., ≥3) stab wounds. In these patients, an alternative diagnostic modality, such as abdominal CT scan or laparoscopy, may be considered. Alternatively, if the pretest probability of an intraabdominal injury that necessitates operative repair is low, admission for serial clinical assessments may also be selected.

The FAST examination has now become a routine part of the emergency department evaluation of all trauma patients in many institutions. A "positive" abdominal FAST examination is defined as the presence of fluid on one or more of the three abdominal views (hepatorenal, splenorenal, pelvic). The utility of the FAST examination in the setting of penetrating abdominal trauma rests in three main areas: (1) delineation of an abdominal source of hemorrhagic shock in patients with an unstable condition with multiple possible sources of bleeding (e.g., multiple bullet wounds spanning multiple body cavities); (2) delineation of peritoneal penetration, and thus diaphragm injury, in patients with a thoracoabdominal stab wound; and (3), delineation of peritoneal penetration in patients with AASWs. A positive abdominal FAST examination thus obviates the need for LWE because the peritoneal cavity must have been entered to cause the accumulation of fluid. Importantly, a negative abdominal FAST examination does not rule out intraabdominal injury that necessitates operative repair. The negative predictive value in this setting is approximately 70%; hence, a nonpositive FAST should be called "nondiagnostic" and not "negative." Conversely, the positive predictive value of abdominal FAST examination for detection of intraabdominal injury that necessitates operative repair in the stable case is only 50%. Patients explored solely based on FAST examination findings thus incur an unacceptably high rate of nontherapeutic laparotomy, and FAST examination findings alone should not be the sole deciding factor in the decision to operate on patients with penetrating abdominal trauma.

Diagnostic peritoneal lavage (DPL) involves an infraumbilical incision and passage of a catheter into the peritoneal cavity with local anesthesia, saline solution infusion, withdrawal of the effluent, and testing for blood, enzymes, and foreign material. Once widely applied in the evaluation of abdominal injuries of all mechanisms, this technique has largely been supplanted by CT scan and FAST examination. However, great utility remains for the diagnostic peritoneal aspirate (DPA), the initial step after insertion of the catheter into the peritoneal cavity. If the initial aspirate contains more than 10 mL of gross blood, bile, succus entericus, or food, it is considered positive, and laparotomy is undertaken. If not, 1 L of warm normal saline solution is instilled and recovered with gravity siphonage, and the lavage effluent is sent for biochemical analysis. Generally accepted criteria for a positive DPL include more than 100,000 red blood cells (RBCs)/mm³, more than 500 white blood cells/mm³, or elevated amylase, alkaline phosphatase, or bilirubin values in the lavage effluent. Important limitations to the DPL technique include the time necessary to perform the procedure and analyze the effluent, the inability to evaluate for retroperitoneal injury, and the potential for iatrogenic complications.

DPL remains a useful technique in the patient with a hemodynamically normal and stable condition with a benign abdominal examination in whom massive intraabdominal fluid is observed on FAST examination. In this case, DPA is useful in documenting the etiology of the fluid, which is likely preexisting ascites in the aforementioned scenario. The second involves evaluation of the unexaminable, hemodynamically normal, stable case with intraabdominal fluid in the absence of a solid organ injury (as determined with abdominal CT scan). Because solid organ injury is likely to cause at least some amount of hemoperitoneum, the finding of intraabdominal fluid in association with a solid organ injury is expected. In contrast, patients with intraabdominal fluid and without solid organ injury must be considered to have a hollow viscus or mesenteric injury until proven otherwise. In general, the physical examination is used to monitor the patient for signs of bowel injury. However, the inability to examine the patient's abdomen (most commonly because of intoxication, concomitant brain injury, or prolonged exposure to general anesthesia for associated injuries) necessitates an additional diagnostic modality. In this case, DPL can rapidly rule out a bowel injury with high sensitivity and according to the aforementioned criteria.

The final contemporary application of DPL relates to thoracoabdominal wounds in the presence of a normal chest x-ray (CXR) and FAST examination. In this setting, a DPL RBC value below threshold may effectively rule out a diaphragmatic injury and obviate the need for costly additional procedures such as laparoscopy or laparotomy. In this specific setting, the RBC threshold above which further investigation should proceed has been debated and generally ranges from 1000 to 10,000 RBCs/mm^3. The authors' group currently uses a threshold of 5000 RBCs/mm^3; patients with cell counts below this are observed, whereas those above the threshold undergo laparoscopy with the intent of diagnosis and repair of a diaphragm injury.

Although abdominal CT scan may provide valuable information, it stands out as the only diagnostic modality that involves transport of the patient from the relatively controlled setting of the emergency department. Thus, the hemodynamic integrity of the patient must be ensured before embarking on a journey to radiology, which may involve fatal misadventures, such as inadvertent endotracheal tube dislodgement, loss of intravenous access, and failure to closely monitor and respond to changes in vital signs. Despite this admonition, the ease of obtaining CT imaging, the breadth of information it provides, and the avoidance of direct physician involvement in this diagnostic study are all seductions reminiscent of the Greek mythologic sirens. Abdominal CT scan should thus be relegated to the hemodynamically stable and normal case and has limited utility even within this subgroup. Data from the Western Trauma Association studies indicate a 47% positive predictive value and 91% negative predictive value for intraabdominal injury that necessitates operative repair among hemodynamically stable cases of AASWs. Most false-negative results relate to either hollow viscus or diaphragmatic injuries, both of which are notoriously elusive on CT scan. As a result of this nonspecificity, abdominal CT scan is used primarily to evaluate penetrating trauma to either the back or flank, as retroperitoneal structures are well visualized by this modality and may evade detection with both physical examination and FAST examination. Although patients were traditionally given triple contrast (oral, intravenous, and rectal), rectal contrast is of primary value in left-sided back and flank stab wounds because adequate colonic contrast to the right side of the colon is difficult and uncomfortable for the patient.

Abdominal CT scan has been used to determine the wound track in morbidly obese patients. Contemporary scanners usually provide adequate resolution to determine peritoneal violation and avoid hospitalization in such patients with a low pretest probability of intraabdominal injury. One final scenario in which abdominal CT scan is useful relates to isolated right upper quadrant GSWs in the patient with a hemodynamically stable condition without peritonitis. Documentation of a bullet track isolated to the liver may assist in successful nonoperative management of these patients, although the risk of a missed injury, delayed bile leak, and even hemobilia are consequences that must be anticipated.

The role of laparoscopy in the management of penetrating abdominal trauma continues to evolve. Select situations in which laparoscopy may be beneficial include determination of peritoneal penetration in the setting of a nondiagnostic LWE (e.g., morbidly obese patient, oblique wound track, multiple wounds) and determination of a diaphragm injury in patients with left-sided thoracoabdominal wounds, normal CXR, and normal FAST examination. Although routine laparoscopy in patients with thoracoabdominal wounds is accurate in ruling out diaphragmatic injury, it is not cost effective. The role of laparoscopy may evolve further to include complete abdominal exploration as both surgical skill and technology improve.

INDICATIONS FOR OPERATIVE INTERVENTION AND PRACTICAL ALGORITHMS

Indications for operative intervention in patients with penetrating abdominal trauma may be divided into immediate and delayed. Absolute indications for immediate operative intervention are listed in Box 1. Patients in shock, and those with peritonitis, evisceration, impalement, or blood from a natural orifice, should be explored, regardless of anatomic region or mechanism of injury.

BOX 1: Indications for immediate laparotomy after penetrating abdominal trauma

Shock
Peritonitis
Evisceration
Impalement
Bleeding from any nature orifice

The distinction between omental and bowel evisceration has been entertained with respect to the need for exploration. The observation that as many as one third of patients with omental evisceration do not have an intraabdominal injury that necessitates repair has led some authorities to recommend against mandatory exploration. However, the authors believe that because the patient has, at the very least, a symptomatic hernia, it should be repaired, and given the relatively high likelihood of finding an associated intraabdominal injury, it should be repaired in the operating room rather than the emergency department.

The remaining discussion of specific injury patterns assumes that the aforementioned indications for mandatory exploration are absent. Most patients with GSWs to the anterior abdomen should be explored. A selective nonoperative approach in patients with stable conditions with either isolated right upper quadrant GSWs as documented with abdominal CT scan or in morbidly obese patients without evidence of peritoneal penetration on abdominal CT scan should be undertaken with caution and in the presence of adequate resource for frequent reexamination. Patients with stable conditions with GSWs to the flank and back should undergo abdominal CT scan to delineate the bullet track and diagnose associated injuries. Patients with GSWs to the left thoracoabdomen should undergo abdominal exploration. Both chest radiography and FAST examination should precede laparotomy to rule out concomitant thoracic trauma. Patients with either massive hemothorax or uncontrolled air leak should in general undergo anterior thoracotomy before laparotomy. However, preparation must be made for rapid laparotomy because intrathoracic blood may originate from an abdominal source via a diaphragmatic laceration.

Patients with stable and hemodynamically normal conditions with AASWs should undergo FAST examination. If results are positive, patients are admitted for serial clinical assessments or laparotomy with any change in a physical examination or vital signs. If FAST examination results are nondiagnostic (negative), LWE is performed. Patients with positive LWE results are also admitted for serial clinical assessments. Patients with negative FAST and negative LWE results are discharged from the emergency department, assuming no other injuries require investigation. Patients with nondiagnostic LWE results are either observed with serial clinical assessments or undergo further diagnostic modalities, including abdominal CT scan or laparoscopy, depending on the pretest probability of intraabdominal injury.

Serial clinical assessments involve the repeated determination of vital signs, hemoglobin concentration, leukocyte concentration, and abdominal examination. Although many algorithms for serial clinical assessments exist, the authors' algorithm involves reassessment of vital signs, complete blood count, and abdominal examination every 8 hours for a total of 24 hours. If results are normal, the patient is fed and discharged if food is tolerated. With this protocol, approximately 15% of patients in the Western Trauma Association studies underwent laparotomy during the 24-hour period of observation, each within 8 hours of presentation. The vast majority underwent exploration for the development of peritonitis and harbored bowel injuries. No complications were found among this group, and hospital length of stay did not differ significantly from patients who were managed with immediate laparotomy. The seemingly equivalent morbidity in the "delayed" laparotomy group has been used to justify a routine strategy of serial clinical examination for stable AASW cases with positive LWEs. Importantly, this course differs markedly from that of blunt small bowel injuries, in which relatively minor delays in diagnosis translate into increased morbidity. Successful implementation of serial clinical assessments is contingent on both adequate resources and a cooperative coherent patient. Although most intoxicated patients retain the ability to manifest abdominal tenderness, caution must be exercised in interpretation of the abdominal examination of an obtunded, confused, or drug-altered patient. If the reliability of the abdominal examination is in question, alternative diagnostic modalities, such as DPL, laparoscopy, or laparotomy, must be used.

In summary, patients with stable AASW with negative LWEs may be discharged from the emergency department. Patients with stable AASW with positive LWEs may be observed for occult intraabdominal injury via serial vital sign, hemoglobin, and leukocyte determination and abdominal examination. Approximately 15% of these patients need laparotomy, which should be manifest and acted on within 8 hours of initial presentation to avoid undue morbidity. The most common reason for progression to laparotomy is the development of peritonitis, underscoring the importance of serial thorough abdominal examinations. The authors' algorithm for the management of AASW is shown in Figure 2.

Stable cases of flank or back stab wounds should undergo abdominal CT scan with contrast to delineate the track and diagnose any associated injuries. Patients with left-sided thoracoabdominal stab wounds should undergo chest radiography and FAST examination (Figure 3). If both results are normal, a DPL is performed with a RBC threshold of 5000/mm³. A positive DPL mandates laparoscopy or laparotomy. If a hemothorax or pneumothorax is found with a negative FAST examination, thoracoscopy is performed. Because the patient already needs tube thoracostomy, this adds little additional morbidity. If a diaphragm injury is found (as expected in approximately 25% of patients), laparotomy is performed to exclude injury below the diaphragm. Finally, with positive FAST examination results, laparotomy is necessary because diaphragmatic penetration is assumed.

OPERATING ROOM CONDUCT AND MANAGEMENT OF SPECIFIC INJURIES

As soon as the decision to operate is made, blood should be made available and the operating room warmed. If major vascular injury is suspected, a massive transfusion protocol should be activated. Intravenous access should be ensured. The patient is placed supine on the operating table, prepped, and draped from the neck to the knees, allowing for maximal exposure and harvesting of the saphenous vein should it become necessary for a vascular repair. Access to the chest allows for extension into a sternotomy or anterolateral thoracotomy incision. A long midline incision is made and carried through the fascia with the scalpel blade. With the exception of patients with agonal conditions, release of tamponade with incision of the peritoneum should proceed only after adequate intravenous access is obtained and blood products are available. After the abdomen is opened, blood and clot are removed only to the extent that exposure is obtained. The four abdominal quadrants are packed with laparotomy pads, and a systematic exploration for bleeding is undertaken. If the peritoneal cavity is filled with blood, the location of clots is often a clue as to the source of hemorrhage. Immediately life-threatening injuries include solid organ injuries and injuries to major abdominal vessels. With few exceptions, bleeding from the liver and spleen may be transiently controlled with a combination of packing and manual compression of the hilar structures. After this, the retroperitoneal zones are examined for evidence of bleeding: central (zone I), paracolic gutters (zone II), and pelvis (zone III). Although distinction by zones is made for blunt retroperitoneal

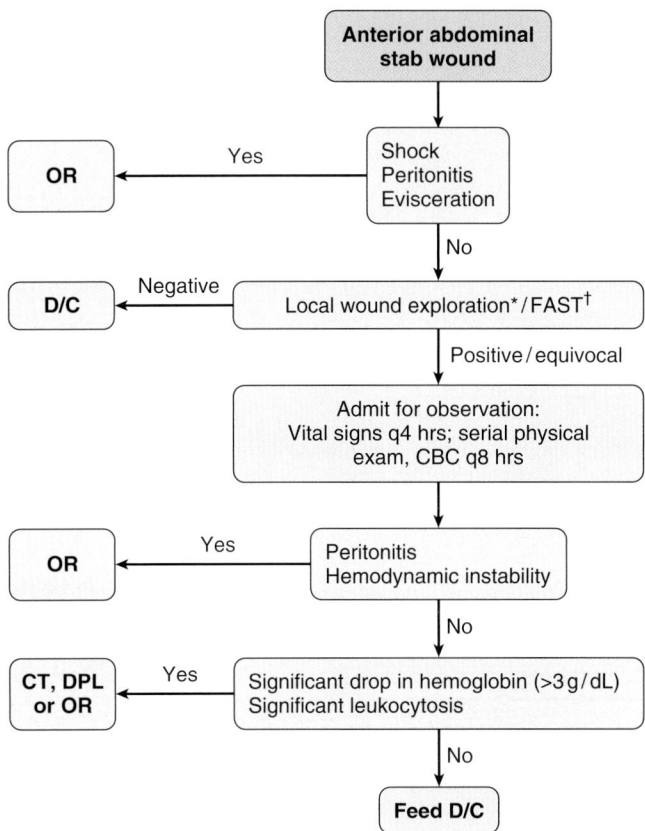

FIGURE 2 Clinical pathway for patients with anterior abdominal stab wounds. *CBC,* Complete blood count; *CT,* computed tomographic scan; *D/C,* discharge; *DPL,* diagnostic peritoneal lavage; *FAST,* focused abdominal sonography for trauma; *OR,* operating room; *WBC,* white blood cells.
*Consider CT scan or laparoscopy if patient is morbidly obese (body mass index, >40), wound tract is long and tangential, or multiple stab wounds preclude local wounds exploration.
†FAST examination shows hemoperitoneum may be used as evidence of peritoneal penetration, obviating the need for local wound exploration. *(Reproduced with permission from Biffl WL, Kaups KL, Pham TN, et al: Validating the Western Trauma Association algorithm for managing patients with anterior abdominal stab wounds: a Western Trauma Association multicenter trial,* J Trauma *71:1494, 2001.)*

hematomas, all retroperitoneal hematomas from penetrating trauma should be explored. One notable exception includes a stable, nonpulsatile, retrohepatic hematoma. In this specific case, release of the tamponade effect on the retrohepatic caval or hepatic venous injury is ill advised and almost uniformly fatal. In contrast, expectant management is associated with a much higher survival rate from hemorrhage control through venous thrombosis.

Rapid exposure of major vessels is imperative in patients with exsanguinating hemorrhage. The general principal of proximal and distal vascular control should be used whenever possible. Exposure of a zone I retroperitoneal hematoma is dependent on location; supramesocolic hematomas usually involve injury to the proximal abdominal aorta and are best addressed via either supraceliac control at the diaphragmatic hiatus or a left-sided medial visceral rotation. The former approach is favored when exsanguination is imminent, the latter when time permits. Access to the inframesocolic aorta is obtained at the root of the transverse mesocolon, after evisceration of the small bowel to the patient's right and lifting of the transverse colon superiorly. Right-sided zone II hematomas usually represent either renal hilar or inferior vena caval injuries and are best

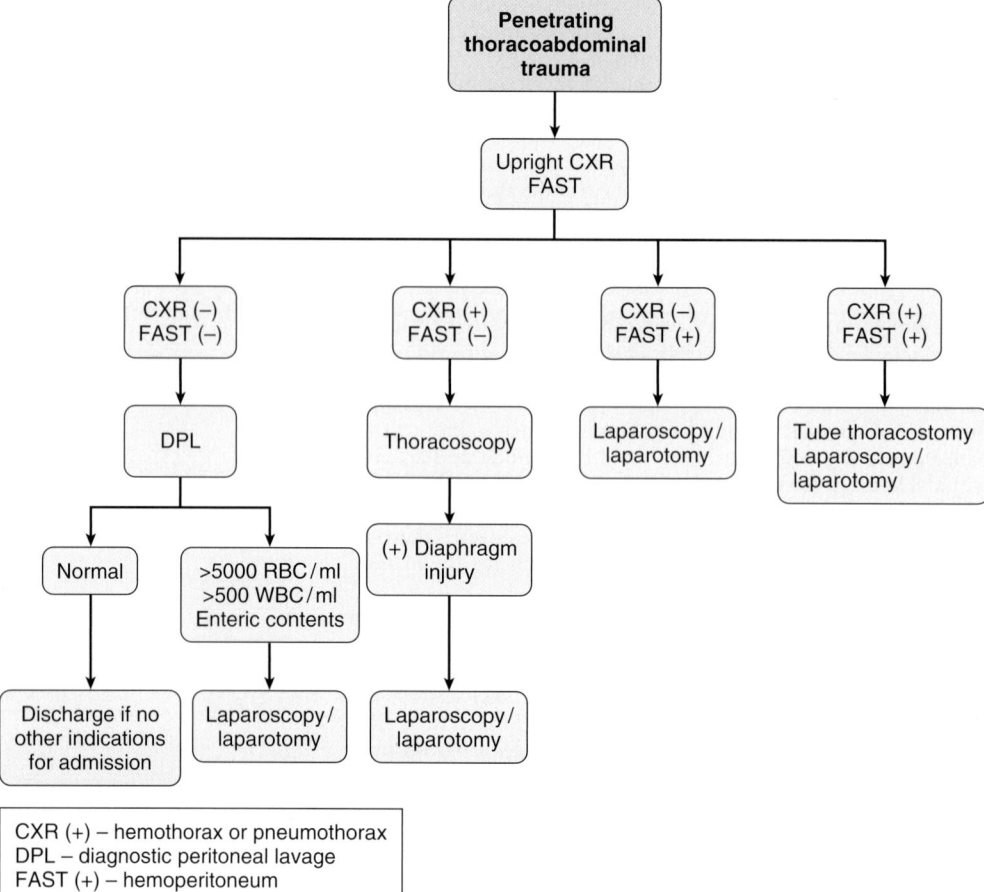

FIGURE 3 Management of patients with stable conditions with penetrating thoracoabdominal trauma. *CXR,* Chest x-ray; *DPL,* diagnostic peritoneal lavage; *FAST,* focused abdominal sonography for trauma; *RBC,* red blood cells; *WBC,* white blood cells. *(Reproduced with permission from Biffl WL, Moore EE: Management guidelines for penetrating abdominal trauma,* Curr Opin Crit Care *16:609, 2010.)*

approached via a right-sided medial visceral rotation, with the right kidney left in situ. Left-sided zone II hematomas are approached via a left-sided medial visceral rotation. Some authors recommend obtaining vascular control of the renal vessels through the posterior midline peritoneum before exploring left-sided zone II injuries. Zone III (pelvic) hematomas are approached by obtaining proximal aortic control at the root of the mesentery. Distal control of the external iliac arteries is then obtained near the femoral canal. Transection of the common iliac vessels may be necessary to obtain exposure to the proximal common iliac veins and their confluence. Finally, portal hematomas are approached initially via Pringle's maneuver (hilar occlusion), with subsequent isolation of the hepatic artery and portal vein. If hemodynamic embarrassment occurs at any time, the supraceliac aorta is occluded at the diaphragmatic hiatus. Once vascular control is obtained, resuscitation should proceed before attempts at further dissection or definitive repair. In patients with profoundly acidotic, coagulopathic conditions, intravascular shunts may be used to maintain perfusion during a period of resuscitation (damage control).

A detailed description of specific organ injuries and their management is presented elsewhere in this text. Some general guidelines follow. In the damage control scenario, all hollow viscus injuries are rapidly sutured to minimize subsequent contamination. In the patient with a stable condition, management ranges from simple repair to resection and exclusion, dependent on the severity of injury. Severe injuries to the duodenum are débrided and may be treated with either pyloric exclusion or Roux-en-Y jejunoduodenostomy. Distal pancreatic injuries may be treated with resection and drainage. Proximal injuries are treated in general with drainage alone with evaluation and possible endoscopic management of the ductal system

in the postoperative period. Gallbladder injuries are treated with cholecystectomy, and biliary ductal injuries with choledochoenterostomy. Liver and spleen injuries are treated based on the size and degree of hemorrhage, ranging from manual application of pressure to resection. Finally, primary closure or resection with primary anastomosis of simple, right-sided colon wounds results in acceptable postoperative morbidity. In contrast, left-sided colonic injury is best managed with fecal diversion. If bowel viability is in question, a second look laparotomy is planned.

SUMMARY

Effective management of penetrating abdominal trauma involves an early, systematic differentiation of patients who need immediate operation from those who may be safely observed with serial examinations. Although laboratory testing, FAST examination, DPL, abdominal CT scan, and laparoscopy all have their place in the management of these patients, thorough and serial physical examinations of the abdomen remain the cornerstone of diagnostic evaluations. The algorithms presented herein allow for the safe discharge from the emergency department of many patients with penetrating trauma and minimize the incidence of nontherapeutic laparotomy. However, there are many nuances to these and other similar algorithms for nonoperative management of penetrating abdominal trauma, and in unusual situations, one should err on the side of definitive abdominal exploration via laparotomy. The trauma surgeon should be prepared to rapidly expose and control all major sources of intraabdominal hemorrhage and be familiar with the indications for and technique of damage control surgery.

SUGGESTED READINGS

Biffl WL, Kaups KL, Pham TN, et al: Validating the Western Trauma Association algorithm for managing patients with anterior abdominal stab wounds: a Western Trauma Association multicenter trial, *J Trauma* 71:1494, 2011.
Hirshberg A, Wall MJ Jr, Allen MK, et al: Double jeopardy: thoracoabdominal injuries requiring surgical intervention in both chest and abdomen, *J Trauma* 39:225, 1995.

Lee JC, Peitzman AB: Damage control laparotomy, *Curr Opin Crit Care* 12:346, 2006.
Moore EE, Marx JA: Penetrating abdominal wounds: rationale for exploratory laparotomy, *JAMA* 253:2705–2708, 1985.
Navsaria PH, Nicol AJ, Krige JE, et al: Selective nonoperative management of liver gunshot injuries, *Ann Surg* 249:653, 2009.

DIAPHRAGMATIC INJURIES

Philip T. Ramsay, MD, and David V. Feliciano, MD

INTRODUCTION

Diaphragmatic injuries have always been a diagnostic challenge for the surgeon. A high index of suspicion is necessary to avoid delays in diagnosis and missed injuries with resultant visceral herniation and strangulation. The objectives of this chapter are to review the incidence and mechanisms of diaphragmatic injury and the anatomy of the diaphragm as it pertains to surgical repair and to provide an approach to diagnosis and treatment.

EPIDEMIOLOGY

Diaphragmatic injuries are infrequent, but the true incidence is difficult to estimate because an unknown number are occult or overlooked. The reported incidence rate of acute diaphragmatic injury in the literature varies widely and ranges from 0.8% to 8% after thoracoabdominal trauma. The incidence rate of penetrating injury is higher than blunt injury with a ratio of 2 to 1.

The most common mechanisms for blunt injuries to the diaphragm are motor vehicle crashes and falls from a height. In these patients, a transfer of kinetic energy to the diaphragm occurs through an acute increase in intraabdominal pressure. Because blunt diaphragmatic injuries are more common on the left than the right in a ratio of 9 to 1, the general consensus is that the acute increase in intraabdominal pressure is absorbed by the liver, which protects the right hemidiaphragm. The liver also prevents herniation, which may lead to an underdiagnosis of this uncommon injury. Of interest, autopsy studies show an equal incidence of right and left injuries to the diaphragm after blunt trauma. In such patients, the most common associated intraabdominal injuries are to the spleen, liver, bowel, and kidney. Other associated injuries in patients with blunt rupture of the diaphragm are to the lung, ribs, thoracic aorta, brain, spinal cord, and pelvis.

The location of a diaphragmatic injury after penetrating trauma is dependent on the trajectory, but most injuries from stab wounds are to the left hemidiaphragm. This is believed to result from most assailants being right hand dominant. In contrast, gunshot wounds to the abdomen have an equal distribution between injuries to the right and left hemidiaphragms. Stab wounds to the thoracoabdominal area (nipple to costal margin medial to anterior axillary line) cause an injury to the diaphragm 15% of the time, and this increases to 45% when a gunshot wound is the mechanism of injury.

ANATOMY

The diaphragm is a dome-shaped musculotendinous partition that separates the abdominal cavity from the thoracic cavity (Figure 1). The muscle fibers of the diaphragm originate peripherally from the lower ribs, upper lumbar vertebrae, and sternum and insert into the central tendon. The diaphragm has separate hiatuses for the esophagus, aorta, and inferior vena cava. The aorta, thoracic duct, and azygous vein pass through the aortic hiatus. The esophagus and vagus nerves pass through the esophageal hiatus, and the only structure that passes through the caval hiatus is the inferior vena cava.

The arterial blood supply to the diaphragm comes from the phrenic arteries, branches of the abdominal aorta, and intercostal arteries, and venous drainage is to the inferior vena cava. Motor innervation to the diaphragm comes from the phrenic nerves. Sensory innervation to the central tendon and peritoneum is carried by the phrenic nerves as well, and sensory innervation to the periphery is carried by the intercostal nerves. The left and right phrenic nerves divide into a varying number of branches above the diaphragm (Figure 2). They most commonly branch anteriorly, posteromedially, and laterally. These branches enter the medial portion of the diaphragm and run obliquely, resulting in a pattern that is often described as a "double handcuff." Knowledge of this pattern is important because injury to the phrenic nerve should be avoided, if at all possible, during repair of the diaphragm.

DIAGNOSIS

The goal of early diagnosis of diaphragmatic injuries is to avoid the added morbidity and potential mortality of herniation of an abdominal viscus and strangulation. Diagnosis is especially difficult in patients without indications for an emergency laparotomy for other associated intraabdominal injuries. The mechanism of injury, and the location of impact, can raise the index of suspicion.

A diaphragmatic injury can cause thoracic or abdominal symptoms and signs. Thoracic symptoms include dyspnea, respiratory distress, orthopnea, chest pain, and referred pain to the ipsilateral shoulder, and thoracic signs include dullness to percussion, decreased breath sounds, bowel sounds in the chest, crepitus, and chest wall movement from associated rib fractures. Abdominal symptoms range from mild upper abdominal pain on one side of the abdomen to severe diffuse abdominal pain, and abdominal signs include tenderness and a scaphoid abdomen from herniated abdominal viscera.

The surgeon-performed focused assessment with sonography for trauma (FAST) examination with a 3.5-MHz ultrasound probe is the first screening test used in most adult patients with blunt trauma to the thorax or abdomen. A break in or the absence of the usual hyperechoic curved line characteristic of a hemidiaphragm above the liver or spleen is presumptive evidence that a large blunt rupture has occurred. The FAST examination usually does not detect small perforations that occur with stab or gunshot wounds.

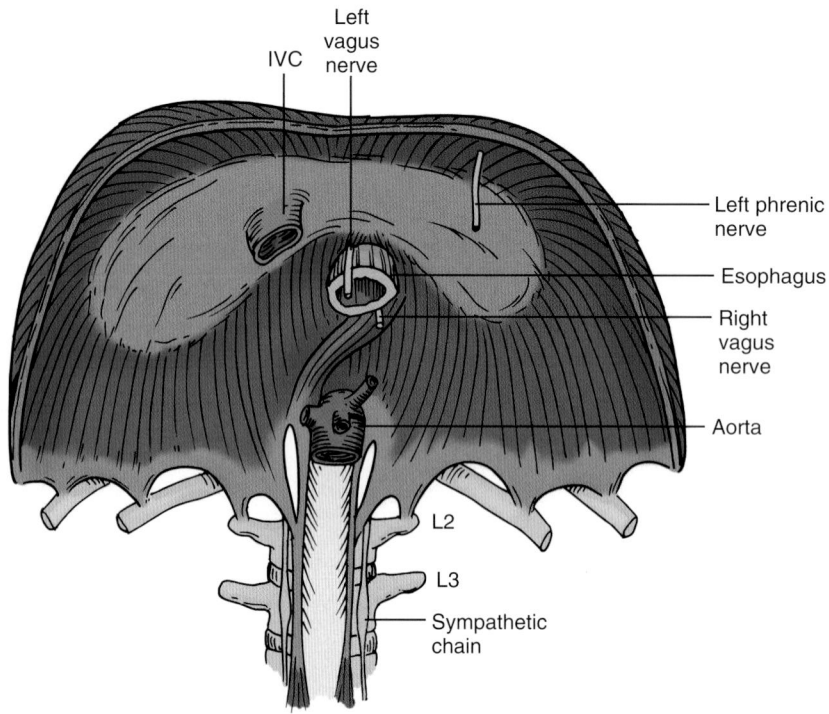

FIGURE 1 Anatomy of the diaphragm, including the central tendon and structures that pass through the three hiatuses. *IVC,* Inferior vena cava. *(With permission from Davis JW, Eghbalieh B: Injury to the diaphragms. In Feliciano DV, Mattox KL, Moore EE, editors: Trauma, ed 6, New York, 2008, McGraw-Hill, 624.)*

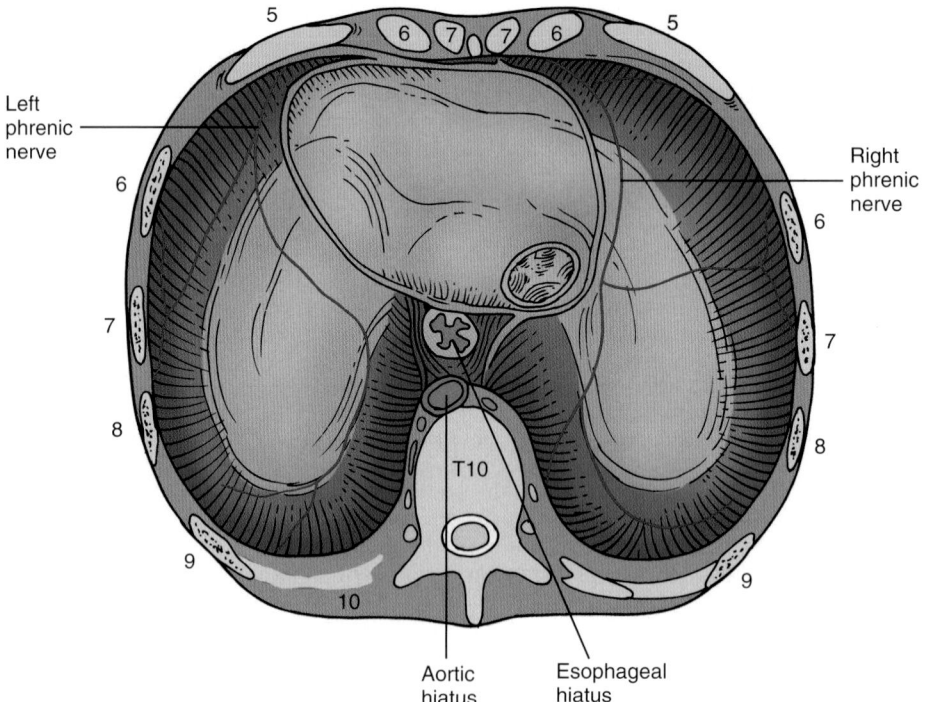

FIGURE 2 Anatomic distribution and branching pattern of the phrenic nerves. *(With permission from Davis JW, Eghbalieh B: Injury to the diaphragms. In Feliciano DV, Mattox KL, Moore EE, editors: Trauma, ed 6, New York, 2008, McGraw-Hill, 625.)*

A chest x-ray is part of the initial workup of the trauma patient and is the next screening modality used to detect injuries to the diaphragm; however, the initial study in the trauma room may be normal or inconclusive and miss 20% to 50% of diaphragmatic injuries. The accuracy of the chest x-ray is lower in penetrating injuries to the right hemidiaphragm as compared with the left because the liver may prevent herniation of abdominal contents into the right hemithorax through a small hole as previously noted. In contrast, the liver may herniate into the chest with a large blunt tear of the right hemidiaphragm (Figure 3). On the left side, gastric, small bowel, or colonic air fluid levels may be visualized in the thorax on the admission chest x-ray. Other findings on a chest x-ray include elevation of a hemidiaphragm, obscured diaphragmatic silhouette (Figure 4), failure of a hemothorax to clear after insertion of a thoracostomy tube, and associated rib and sternal fractures. In a patient with a "suspicious" chest x-ray, a nasogastric tube may be seen coiled in the

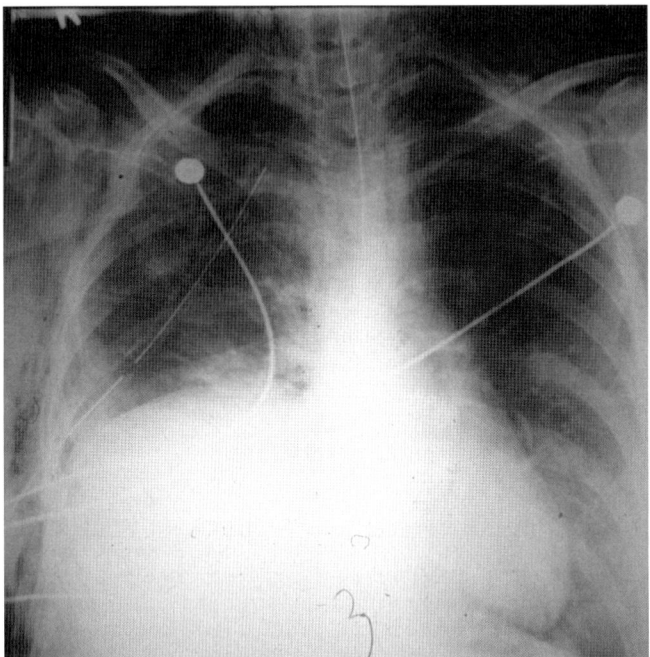

FIGURE 3 A suspicious admission chest x-ray of a 41-year-old woman who was a front-seat passenger in a lateral impact motor vehicle collision. Computed tomographic scan confirmed a large blunt rupture of the right hemidiaphragm.

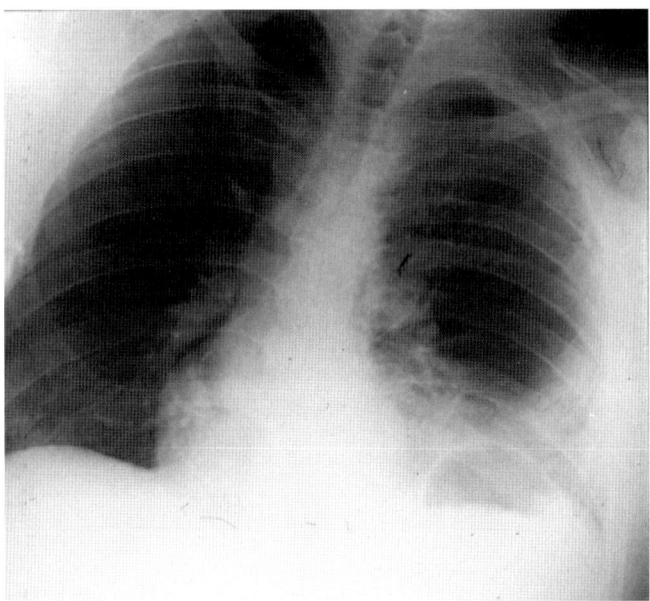

FIGURE 4 A 34-year-old man with a gunshot wound through the left diaphragm and gastric fundus had an abnormal chest x-ray on admission, but the diagnosis was delayed for 4 days. *(With permission from Feliciano DV, Cruse PA, Mattox KL, et al: Delayed diagnosis of injuries to the diaphragm after penetrating wounds, J Trauma 28:1135-1144, 1988.)*

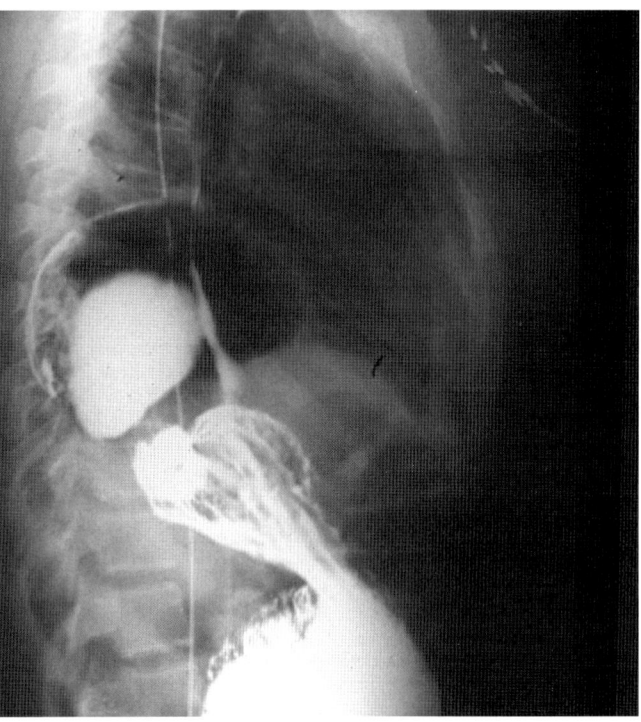

FIGURE 5 An 18-year-old woman with a left thoracoabdominal stab wound and herniation of the stomach into the left pleural cavity shown on an upper gastrointestinal x-ray series.

Contrast studies may be useful when the initial chest x-ray is suggestive of an injury to the diaphragm, but the position of the nasogastric tube is not diagnostic. An upper gastrointestinal series can document gastric herniation (Figure 5), and a barium enema can be used to diagnose colonic herniation. Computed tomographic (CT) scan has a low sensitivity for diaphragmatic injuries, and results are variable. The reported sensitivity and specificity of conventional CT scan in diagnosing of diaphragmatic rupture are 14% to 61% and 76% to 99%, respectively. Thick axial slices, respiratory motion, and poor reconstructions likely contribute to the low sensitivity. CT findings include discontinuity of the diaphragm and intrathoracic herniation of abdominal contents. The "collar sign" is a constriction of a herniated viscus through the diaphragmatic defect, and the "dependent viscera sign" is the abnormal dependent position of the viscera against the posterior ribs. With the introduction of helical CT scan, the accuracy has improved as a result of better quality images. Magnetic resonance imaging (MRI) is impractical in the acute setting but may be useful in the evaluation of a possible chronic diaphragmatic hernia.

Laparoscopy with general anesthesia in the operating room is indicated in patients in whom concern still exists about a possible diaphragmatic injury after the usual imaging studies. It is particularly indicated in patients whose conditions are hemodynamically stable with no other indications for laparotomy. The use of a 30-degree or 45-degree telescope aids in evaluation of the entire diaphragm; a risk of a tension pneumothorax exists when the pneumoperitoneum is introduced. If thoracoscopy is necessary to evacuate a clotted hemothorax, the ipsilateral hemidiaphragm should always be evaluated.

ACUTE MANAGEMENT

Diaphragmatic injuries are graded on a scale of I to V in the Organ Injury Scale developed by the American Association for the Surgery of Trauma in 1994 (Table 1). Injuries from blunt trauma tend to be of a higher grade (III to V) and occur in the posterolateral

left hemithorax on a repeat film. If the patient is intubated in the trauma room, positive airway pressure from mechanical ventilation may, however, prevent herniation. On rare occasions, an injury to a hemidiaphragm can be diagnosed with finger palpation during insertion of an ipsilateral chest tube.

TABLE 1: Organ injury scale

Grade	Injury description
I	Contusion
II	Laceration ≤ 2 cm
III	Laceration 2-10 cm
IV	Laceration > 10 cm with tissue loss ≤ 25 cm^2
V	Laceration with tissue loss > 25 cm^2

With permission from Moore EE, Malangoni MA, Cogbill TH, et al: Organ injury scaling. IV: Thoracic vascular, lung cardiac and diaphragm, J Trauma 36:299-300, 1994.

hemidiaphragm. Penetrating injuries are typically of a lower grade (I to II) and can occur anywhere in the diaphragm. Almost all diaphragmatic perforations and lacerations, regardless of size, should be repaired to reduce the risk of herniation of intraabdominal viscera and strangulation. The one exception is an isolated injury to the right hemidiaphragm from a penetrating wound where a subsequent CT scan documents that there is no bleeding from an associated hepatic or renal injury and no injury to the gastrointestinal tract.

Several operative approaches are used for the treatment of diaphragmatic injuries. The operative approach is determined by whether the diaphragmatic injury is acute or chronic (see subsequently), by the hemodynamic stability of the patient, the presence or absence of associated injuries, and by the surgeon's comfort level with the particular approach. For acute diaphragmatic injuries, laparotomy is the preferred method. After the patient is placed on the operating table in the supine position, the operative field is prepared and draped, with the chest included. A nasogastric or orogastric tube should be carefully placed to allow for decompression of the stomach, but this may be difficult in the patient with gastric herniation. A midline laparotomy incision is made, and after control of bleeding and contamination, the entire abdominal cavity should be explored. Any abdominal viscus that has herniated through a diaphragmatic defect should be carefully reduced. The thoracic cavity should be inspected through the diaphragmatic defect for any ongoing bleeding or contamination from spillage of gastrointestinal contents. If any thoracic contamination has occurred, the thoracic cavity should be thoroughly irrigated with normal saline solution containing antibiotics until returns through the suction device are clear. This often mandates enlargement of the diaphragmatic defect.

The left side of the diaphragm is fully exposed by mobilizing and retracting the spleen, splenic flexure of the colon, stomach, and left lobe of the liver inferiorly and medially. The left triangular ligament of the liver may need to be divided to allow for adequate exposure as well. The right side of the diaphragm is fully exposed by dividing the falciform ligament and the right triangular ligament and retracting the right lobe of the liver inferiorly and medially.

For most injuries, primary closure can be achieved. Long Allis clamps are placed on the edges of the perforation or laceration to allow for elevation of the defect and easier visualization. After nonviable tissue is débrided, #0 or #1 permanent suture is used in a continuous locking fashion or with interrupted simple or vertical mattress sutures to repair large defects. Interrupted simple or vertical mattress sutures can be used to repair small defects as well. Because the diaphragm is highly vascular, the repair is inspected at completion to rule out continuing hemorrhage. If contamination, a concomitant injury to the lung, or risk of a hemothorax is found, then a large ipsilateral thoracostomy tube should be placed. If no injury to the lung or a hemothorax is found, there is no need to place a tube. A catheter may be inserted through the diaphragmatic defect to

evacuate any air as anesthesia hyperventilates the patient just before the final suture is placed.

In patients undergoing a "damage control" trauma laparotomy, diaphragmatic repair is unnecessary. Any smaller defect can be covered with folded laparotomy pads used as packs. A larger defect can be covered with opened laparotomy pads held in place with staples or packs.

For acute diaphragmatic injuries in patients with a hemodynamically stable condition with no other indication for laparotomy, laparoscopy can be used. The decision is dependent on the individual surgeon's comfort level with laparoscopic techniques of suturing. The risk of a tension pneumothorax with laparoscopy is significant, as previously noted, and the patient must be carefully monitored.

SPECIAL SITUATIONS

Diaphragmatic Detachment From Chest Wall

In cases that involve detachment of the diaphragm from its posterolateral attachments, any devascularized diaphragmatic muscle is débrided. The diaphragm is reattached to the body wall with placement of interrupted #1 polypropylene sutures through the edge of the detached diaphragm, around the adjacent rib, and then through the edge of the diaphragm again before tying. Visualization is improved by placing all sutures before tying the knots.

Loss of Diaphragmatic Tissue

In cases of massive diaphragmatic destruction, the insertion of the remaining hemidiaphragm may be translocated to a more superior rib level to allow a tension-free repair. The technique involves dividing the anterior, lateral, and posterior attachments of the hemidiaphragm to the chest wall as needed to decrease tension as the hemidiaphragm is sutured around a more superior rib (Figure 6). In addition, nonporous synthetic mesh can be used as a bridge. In cases of contamination, a significant risk of infection exists if synthetic mesh is inserted, and biologic mesh may be used to provide temporary repair. Once the infection has been adequately treated, biologic mesh can be replaced by synthetic mesh if there is evidence of a diaphragmatic hernia on serial chest x-rays. Alternatively, autologous tissue such as omentum, tensor fascia lata, or a latissimus dorsi flap may be used.

Loss of Chest Wall

In patients with large open defects of the chest wall from a thoracoabdominal shotgun wound, any perforations of the hemidiaphragm are repaired before it is translocated to a more superior rib level. The defect in the chest wall is then essentially converted to an abdominal wall defect that can be managed with local wound care. This includes covering the defect with absorbable mesh, performing daily gauze dressing changes above this, and applying a split-thickness skin graft after granulation tissue appears.

Injury to the Central Tendon

Rupture of the central tendon involving the pericardium is a rare event. The heart may herniate inferiorly into the peritoneal cavity, or abdominal viscera may herniate superiorly into the pericardium and cause cardiac tamponade. The heart must be inspected for associated injuries, and careful attention must be given during suture repair of the rupture to avoid injury to the myocardium.

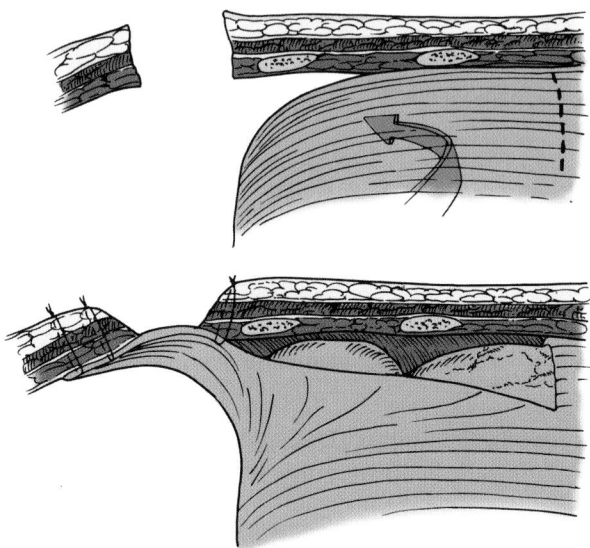

FIGURE 6 Immediate reconstruction of the chest wall after destructive types of injury may be accomplished by detaching the affected hemidiaphragm anteriorly, laterally, and posteriorly. The diaphragm is then resutured to the muscle of a higher intercostal space, thus effectively translocating it to a position above the full-thickness chest wall defect and converting such a defect functionally into an abdominal wall defect. The abdominal wall defect is then managed with local wound care in anticipation of further reconstruction with either split-thickness grafts or myocutaneous flaps at a later date. *(With permission from Asensio JA, Demetriades D.)*

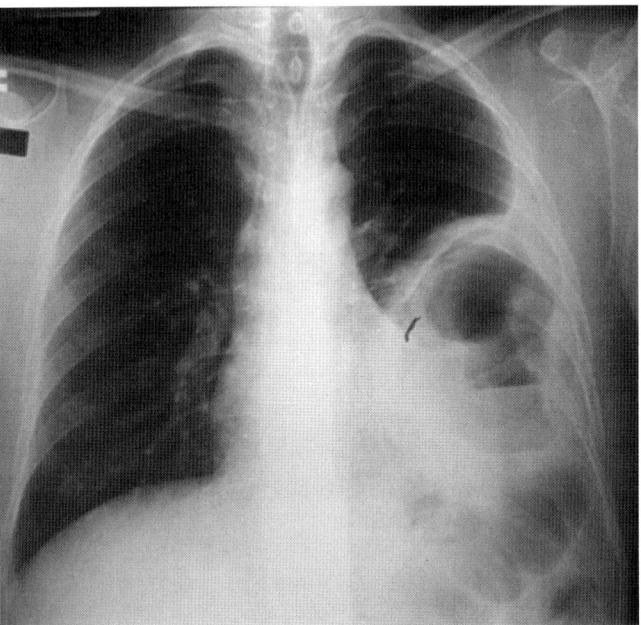

FIGURE 7 A 28-year-old man with a chronic posttraumatic diaphragmatic hernia 1 year after a stab wound to the left chest.

Injury to the Esophageal Hiatus

In cases of injury to the esophageal hiatus, the esophagus should be clearly visualized before suture repair is performed. If any concern exists that the repair may narrow the esophagus, a bougie should be passed down the esophagus to confirm that the lumen is patent.

MANAGEMENT OF THE CHRONIC POSTTRAUMATIC HERNIA

Missed diaphragmatic injuries can appear years after injury as chronic diaphragmatic hernias (Figure 7). Patients may be asymptomatic or report worsening respiratory compromise from progressive visceral herniation. Some patients may present with signs and symptoms of obstruction, strangulation, or perforation of the stomach or colon. All chronic posttraumatic hernias should be repaired in patients at reasonable risk to avoid these secondary gastrointestinal complications. With time, adhesions develop between the herniated abdominal viscera and the pleural cavity. Also, the diaphragm retracts and atrophies, making reduction of herniated viscera and repair more difficult. Therefore, a thoracic approach is preferred because this allows for easier division of chronic adhesions. The decision between thoracotomy and thoracoscopy is dependent on the individual surgeon's comfort level and experience with thoracoscopy. A small hernia into the pleural cavity, however, can still be approached through a laparotomy. In some patients, prosthetic mesh may be required to cover a chronic rigid defect (see previous). Occasionally, reduction of a giant chronic hernia has the potential to cause a secondary abdominal compartment syndrome from loss of abdominal domain. The technique of creating and gradually increasing a pneumoperitoneum before surgery is appropriate in such a patient. If the surgeon is unwilling or uncomfortable to use this

uncommon approach, insertion of a permanent prosthesis into the abdominal wall may be necessary at the time of the reduction and repair to expand the volume of the peritoneal cavity.

MORBIDITY AND MORTALITY

The morbidity and mortality from diaphragmatic injury depends on several factors, including the mechanism of injury, the severity of injury to the diaphragm itself, the presence or absence of associated injuries, and the extent of surgery required to repair the injury and associated injuries. Most complications and deaths are caused by injuries to other organs. The reported mortality rate has ranged from 4.3% to 41%, with a higher mortality rate in patients with blunt injuries as opposed to those with penetrating trauma. Early complications from repair of the diaphragm include breakdown of the repair, paralysis of the hemidiaphragm from injury to the phrenic nerve, and respiratory embarrassment.

On rare occasions, a patient with a penetrating wound to the right lower lobe of the lung, right hemidiaphragm, and liver has a bronchobiliary fistula develop. This results from a biliary fistula eroding through the repair of the diaphragm and connecting to the hole in the lung. The patient has respiratory distress, may cough up bile, and has a worsening appearance of the right lower lobe on chest x-ray. Any delay in transabdominal drainage of the biliary leak, repair or rerepair of the hemidiaphragm, and débridement of the right lower lobe leads to progressive necrosis of the lung.

As previously noted, patients with chronic posttraumatic diaphragmatic hernias can have complications develop from visceral obstruction, strangulation, and perforation. Delays in treatment can lead to postoperative empyema and subdiaphragmatic abscesses and sepsis and multiple organ failure.

SUGGESTED READINGS

Davis JW, Eghbalieh B: Injury to the diaphragm. In Feliciano DV, Mattox KL, Moore EE, editors: *Trauma*, ed 6, New York, 2008, McGraw-Hill, pp 623–635.
Duane TM, Ivatury RR, Aboutanos MB, et al: Injury to the diaphragm. In Flint L, Meredith JW, Schwab CW, et al, editors: *Trauma: contemporary*

principles and therapy, Philadelphia, 2008, Lippincott Williams & Wilkins, pp 383–389.

Feliciano DV, Cruse PA, Mattox KL, et al: Delayed diagnosis of injuries to the diaphragm after penetrating wounds, *J Trauma* 28:1135–1144, 1988.

Kemp CD, Yang SC: Thoracic trauma. In Sellke FW, del Nido PJ, Swanson SJ, editors: *Sabiston and Spencer: surgery of the chest*, ed 8, Philadelphia, 2010, Elsevier, pp 96–97, 103–105.

Lucas CE, Ledgerwood AM: Diaphragmatic injury. In Asensio JA, Trunkey DD, editors: *Current therapy of trauma and surgical critical care*, Philadelphia, 2008, Elsevier, pp 326–339.

Renz BM, Feliciano DV: Gunshot wounds to the right thoracoabdomen: a prospective study of nonoperative management, *J Trauma* 37:737–744, 1994.

THE MANAGEMENT OF LIVER INJURIES

Stephanie A. Savage, MD, MS, FACS, and Martin A. Croce, MD, FACS

INTRODUCTION

The liver, due to its size and location, which spans a large portion of the right thoracoabdominal region, is the most frequently injured abdominal organ. As a relatively low-pressure system, operative exploration is frequently unnecessary after blunt injury. Over the past 30 years, trauma surgeons have gradually abandoned most surgical exploration of hepatic trauma in hemodynamically stable patients suffering a blunt mechanism. Regardless, operative indications remain. The decrease in hepatic explorations has also resulted in decreased familiarity by trauma surgeons with the technically challenging management of devastating hepatic injuries. Careful nonoperative observation, the decision to proceed to the operating room, and techniques for the control of hemorrhage of the liver remain important skills in the trauma armamentarium.

Management of traumatic liver injuries begins with the arrival of the patient to the trauma bay. Advanced Trauma Life Support principles remain the foundation of care and will not be reiterated here. For critically injured patients, early efforts should be focused on avoiding the deadly triad of hypothermia, acidosis, and coagulopathy. Resuscitation should quickly transition to blood products in a 1-to-1 ratio, with active warming of the patient. A focused assessment with sonography for trauma (FAST) should occur early in the evaluation of the patient. FAST exam is notoriously unreliable for hemoperitoneum less than 300 to 600 cc and may be confounded by additional factors, including body habitus of the patient, operator skill, and the presence of associated injuries such as subcutaneous emphysema or pelvic fracture. A positive exam is a valuable piece of information which, when combined with the hemodynamic status of the patient, is instrumental in the decision making for or against operative exploration.

Computed tomographic (CT) scan may also play an invaluable role in patient assessment. Intravenous contrast is, of course, required to achieve maximum benefit from the exam. CT allows quantification of the degree of hepatic trauma. Lacerations may be categorized according to their severity grade (Figure 1). Though potentially all grades of liver injury may be candidates for nonoperative management (excluding grade VI), multiple studies have demonstrated that nonoperative management fails more frequently with increasing severity of liver injury. Perhaps up to two thirds of grade IV and V liver injuries will ultimately fail observation. Further, CT delineates the presence of pseudoaneurysm within the parenchyma of the liver, hemoperitoneum, and associated injuries (Figure 2). Obviously patients must be hemodynamically stable to travel to radiology for

this study. Finally, although not routinely used in penetrating trauma, CT may be useful in determining trajectory or peritoneal penetration in selected patients.

Ultimately, decision algorithms will vary somewhat depending on whether an injury is blunt or penetrating. Multiple algorithms have

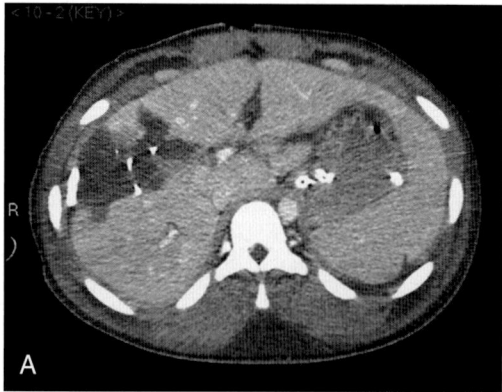
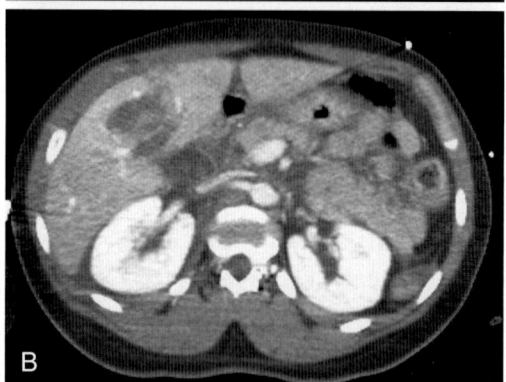
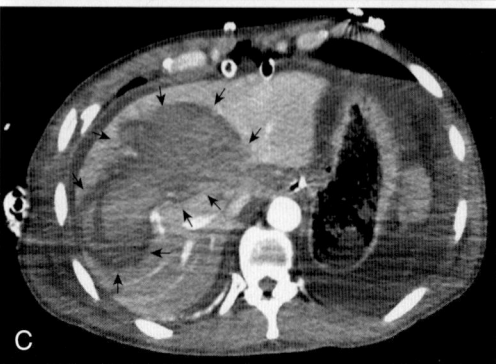

FIGURE 1   **A,** Grade III liver laceration with greater than 50% subcapsular hematoma or liver laceration of greater than 3 cm depth. **B,** Grade IV liver laceration with disruption of 25% to 75% of hepatic parenchyma. **C,** Grade V liver laceration with greater than 75% hepatic parenchyma disruption or major venous injury. The arrows mark the extent of the hepatic laceration.

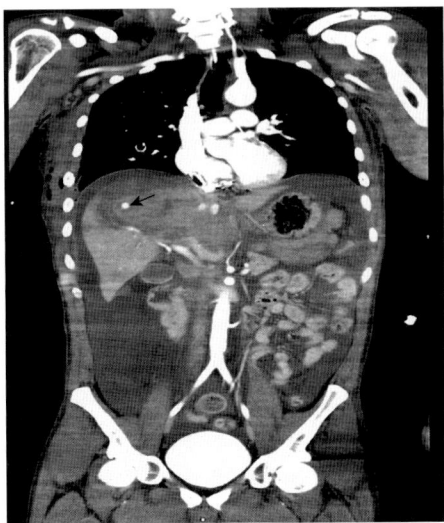

FIGURE 2 Hepatic laceration containing a pseudoaneurysm. Hepatic laceration containing a pseudoaneurysm, as marked by the arrow.

been published on the management of blunt hepatic trauma, with decision making focused on the degrees of hepatic injury and patient stability (Figure 3). Penetrating trauma has generally been taken directly to the operating room, though published series do exist regarding observational management of highly selected patients. Management decisions must be made with a focus on the particular physiology of the liver, in addition to patient status, mechanism, and associated injuries.

BLUNT HEPATIC TRAUMA

Evaluation of patients suffering a blunt mechanism of injury may be challenging, as the extent of the injury can be much greater and more difficult to define than seen in penetrating trauma. Initial assessment includes the evaluation of airway, breathing and circulation (the "ABC's"), as well as imaging techniques. The patient's progression will largely depend on hemodynamic status. In current practice, more than 80% of cases of isolated liver trauma will result in nonoperative management. Patients who are eligible for observation must be hemodynamically stable, must not require laparotomy for associated

Nonoperative management of blunt liver injury

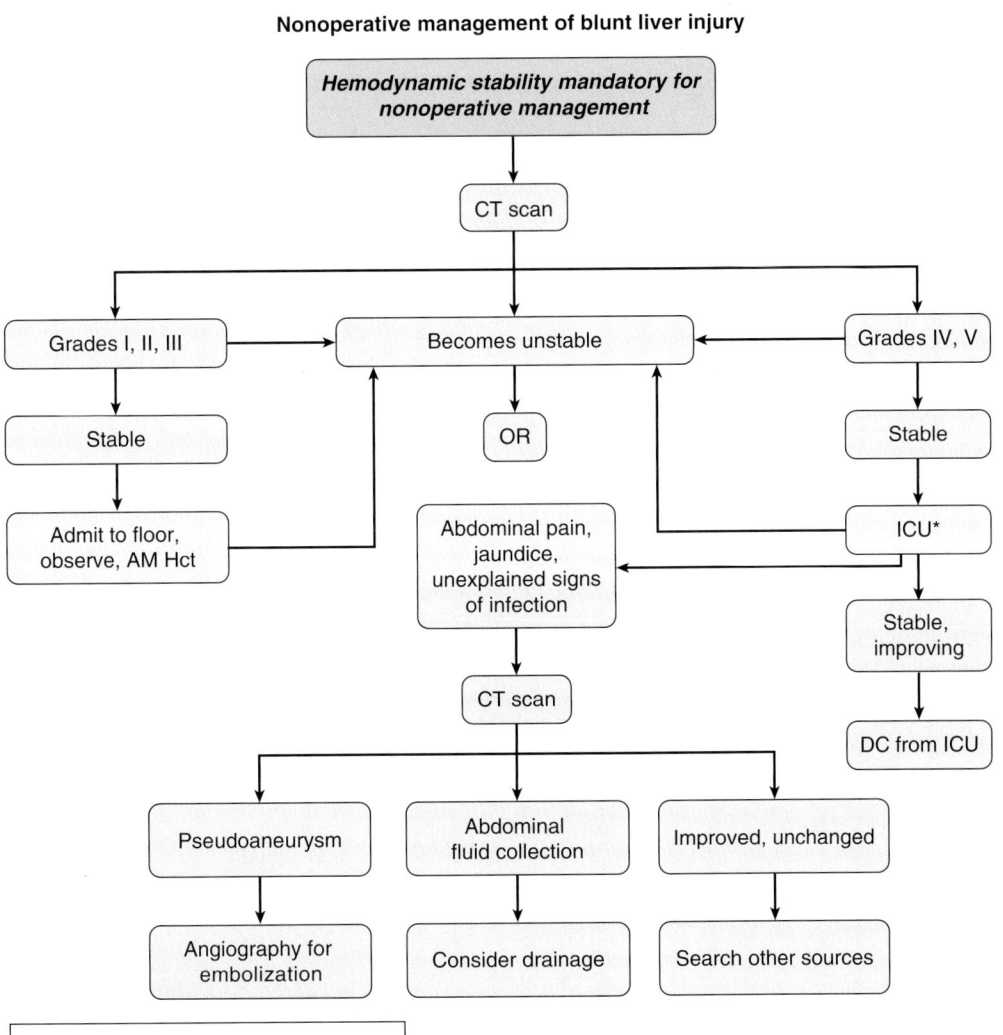

FIGURE 3 Memphis algorithm for the nonoperative management of blunt hepatic trauma. *CT,* Computed tomography; *DC,* discharge; *ICU,* intensive care unit; *OR,* operative therapy.

injuries, and should not have an ongoing unexplained transfusion requirement. The presence of a blush from the liver on contrasted CT scan or the presence of a moderate to large volume of hemoperitoneum is not an absolute indication for intervention. It is important to remember that bleeding from the liver differs greatly from active bleeding from that other oft-injured intra-abdominal solid organ: the spleen. In general, bleeding from the hepatic parenchyma is low pressure and will stop, whether spontaneously or secondary to compression by the hemoperitoneum (though this may not be true of bleeding from a lacerated hepatic artery). Therefore, even patients with these findings on CT may be observed if they meet other criteria.

The most important consideration in observational management of blunt hepatic injuries is that this modality can ultimately be more labor-intensive than surgical exploration. The patient must be admitted to a monitored setting so that any deterioration in hemodynamic status is immediately detected. Serial hemoglobin and hematocrit studies should be followed to assess for ongoing bleeding. Serial lactate levels, and the evaluation of base deficit, are also useful in trending the success of the resuscitation. Finally, it is mandatory for a surgeon to perform serial abdominal exams over the first 24 hours. Observation that results in a trip to the operating room immediately upon a change in status is successful observational management. Fortunately, most patients do well following nonoperative management.

INTERVENTIONAL RADIOLOGY

The scope and availability of interventional radiology (IR) has increased exponentially over the last 10 to 15 years. IR has been a key player in the growing success of nonoperative management of traumatic spleen injuries. The applicability of IR to hepatic trauma is somewhat more limited. The persistence of a pseudoaneurysm in the hepatic parenchyma may benefit from angioembolization. IR is also superior to evaluate patients who develop hemobilia with upper gastrointestinal bleeding following hepatic trauma. Access to IR should not be considered a crutch or a method to avoid operative intervention. As noted, for unstable patients with high-grade liver injuries, the appropriate setting for evaluation and management is the operative, not IR, suite. Mobilization of IR resources, even in the most responsive centers, typically takes more than 1 hour—time that bleeding patients may not be able to tolerate. It is also important to remember that IR suites are often remote from trauma care and intensive care unit (ICU) areas of the hospital and cannot provide the monitoring and resuscitative capabilities over the necessary 1 to 2 hours that these patients require. Further, for higher-grade liver injuries, even a successful embolization will not address the potential morbidity of a bile leak, thus necessitating a return trip to IR for a later percutaneous drain. Undoubtedly, avoidance of a laparotomy is beneficial for some patients. However, all these factors must be taken into consideration when opting for IR.

PENETRATING HEPATIC TRAUMA: CLINICAL DECISION MAKING

Decision for laparotomy in penetrating hepatic trauma is usually fairly straightforward. In most cases, the remainder of the abdominal cavity must be assessed for associated injuries. Clearly the right colon and duodenum are at significant risk, as are the biliary system and diaphragm. There are factors, however, that may delay or alter the decision for surgical therapy. Clearly, stab wounds have a more limited area of affect, and the trajectory is typically easier to define. In gunshot wounds or penetrating injuries from blasts (as seen in the military setting), the trajectory is much more difficult to anticipate. Transabdominal penetration or hemodynamic instability requires

exploration immediately. In stable patients for whom trajectory is unclear, imaging can be helpful. Plain AP and lateral abdominal films, in conjunction with site of missile entry, can suggest trajectory. CT scan is both more sensitive and specific, as subcutaneous air can demonstrate missile path, in addition to defining the extent of liver injury, the presence of hemoperitoneum, and evidence of hematoma at other sites. These modalities, however, may be misleading in low-velocity gunshots. If the missile is present in the abdominal cavity, trajectory is relatively unimportant, as the patient will need abdominal exploration.

In stable patients with minimal abdominal pain, injury may be limited solely to the liver. While exploration may still be required, a nontherapeutic laparotomy imposes significant morbidity burden on patients. In these cases, diagnostic laparoscopy is a reasonable compromise. The laparoscope allows evaluation of peritoneal penetration, volume of hemoperitoneum, inspection of the liver surface for signs of active bleeding or bile leak, and evaluation of other intra-abdominal organs. Hepatorrhaphy may be performed, if needed, and hemoperitoneum may be evacuated. If bleeding or bile leak is difficult to control, or if specific conditions prevent an adequate evaluation of associated structures, conversion to laparotomy is indicated.

OPERATIVE TECHNIQUES FOR HEPATIC TRAUMA

The initial operative approach to hepatic trauma is the same as any abdominal exploration. The patient should be widely prepped, with special care to include the thoracic cavity, lest sternotomy is necessary for intrapericardial inferior vena cava control. Broad-spectrum antibiotic prophylaxis should be chosen if there is a concern of a hollow viscus injury, but otherwise antibiotics may focus on coverage of skin flora. Even if the surgeon is aware of hepatic injury preoperatively, a midline incision is preferred over a right upper quadrant subcostal incision, as the former allows more complete exploration of the entire abdominal cavity. Adequate blood should be available to anesthesia in the event of ongoing hemorrhage; uncrossmatched blood is given if there is no time for a type and cross.

Upon entering the abdomen, it is important to evacuate the blood present in the peritoneal cavity in order to identify any bleeding vessels. Bleeding areas may then be packed with gauze laparotomy pads more effectively than random placement of packs in all four quadrants. The ligamentum teres is then clamped, divided, and ligated, and the falciform ligament is divided close to the abdominal wall back to the hepatic veins to allow better exposure of the liver. To completely mobilize the liver and thoroughly inspect the surface, the right and left triangular ligaments, as well as the coronary ligament, should be divided. This will allow nearly complete rotation of the liver for inspection and repair. Care should be taken if significant hematoma is contained within these ligaments, which may suggest hepatic venous injury. Injudicious entry into the hematoma may release physiologic tamponade, allowing potential exsanguination from a caval or hepatic vein injury. In these cases, the ligaments are best left undisturbed.

When the liver is unpacked, it must be inspected for injury. Superficial to moderate lacerations may respond well to compressive packing, and this may be the only therapy required. When hemorrhage from raw surfaces is controlled, the substance of the liver should be inspected to determine if small vessels or biliary tributaries require ligation. Persistent bleeding or a bile leak should always be addressed with suture ligature. In many cases, the involved lumen is located at the base of a laceration deep within the substance of the liver. In these cases, a finger-fracture or clamp-and-crush technique should be employed to allow adequate exposure to the area in question. In short, the obstructing parenchyma is crushed either between the surgeon's fingers or in a Kelly clamp (for finer control). This results in a separation of the substance of the liver to expose small branches of the hepatic artery or biliary tributaries. These small branches are then ligated and divided. If available, a harmonic device may perform all of these steps at once to more rapidly reach the injured region. Once at the level of injury, the bleeding vessel or bile duct may then be suture ligated for definitive control.

Whether or not finger-fracture is required, blunt lacerations or penetrating parenchymal wounds often leave exposed raw parenchyma and large empty spaces within the substance of the liver. These are prone to continued bleeding, persistent bile leak, and potential abscess formation. Ideally, if the patient's anatomy is amenable, a long tongue of omentum may be mobilized and packed into the hepatic wound. The parenchyma may then be closed over the "omental pack" with a running monofilament suture. The viable omental pedicle fills the dead space nicely, is hemostatic, and may allow better migration of immune mediators into the injury. In actual practice, however, the omentum is often inadequate or destroyed by the same mechanism that injured the liver. This leaves the trauma surgeon searching for some other option to fill the deadspace and achieve hemostasis. A nice alternative is the hemostatic tampon. Constructed of an absorbable gelatin-compressed sponge wrapped in woven hemostatic fabric, it can be constructed on the field, to any size, to fill bleeding cavities within the liver. Alternatively, if second-look laparotomies are planned for the future, the injury site may be packed with laparotomy sponges, which will afford hemostasis and allow for continued resuscitation.

Wounds that traverse the entire liver, such as a transhepatic gunshot wound, may be especially challenging. With a tendency to bleed vigorously, it is difficult to reach the vessels in question, and attempts to do so may disrupt healthy liver. A popularly described technique is construction of a balloon for tamponade. Utilizing a large Penrose drain and a red rubber catheter, the catheter is trimmed to create additional ports in the body of the device. The catheter is then passed through the Penrose, and the drain is secured at either end to the catheter with suture (the distal opening of the red rubber catheter must be occluded). The "balloon" is passed into the tract of the injury and inflated with a syringe until bleeding ceases. The balloon is left inflated until the second-look operation. It may be reinflated at that time, if needed.

The role of abbreviated laparotomy cannot be overstated in trauma surgery, especially in regards to liver injuries. Compression is a very effective therapy for most hepatic hemorrhage, and the role of packing is central to this. Except in cases of major arterial hemorrhage from the liver or noncompressible hemorrhage from sites such as the retrohepatic cava, packing in conjunction with an abbreviated laparotomy, consisting of an open abdomen and planned second look, is a reliable management choice. Second look should occur between 48 and 72 hours from the initial surgery, late enough to allow adequate resuscitation and stabilization but prior to increased risk of sepsis from retained packs. It is generally useful to place a tongue of sterile cassette cover or other nonadherent item between the packed liver and bowel contents, as adjacent bowel can quickly dry, become adherent to sponges, and be difficult to free without iatrogenic injury to large or small bowel. Once unpacked, the liver is examined, and any residual bleeding may be ligated or addressed with electrocautery or argon-beam cauterization. Omental packing at this point will stop minor bleeding. Persistent significant bleeding may warrant repacking and, in some cases, evaluation in the IR suite. An additional benefit of a second-look laparotomy is that nonviable parenchyma may be evaluated for the need for resection as well.

The role of hepatic resection in trauma is limited. Resection should never occur at the initial laparotomy when injuries are still being defined and the patient is undergoing active resuscitation and can poorly tolerate a prolonged, anatomic resection. Additionally, parenchyma that initially looks questionable may be viable upon second look, when the patient is stable and perfusion is better. Unless the substance of the liver is grossly macerated by the injury mechanism, the liver should be packed for hemostatic control. At second look, frankly necrotic liver may be debrided. A formal anatomic

resection will be needed in rare cases, and primarily in events where massive hemorrhage or injury necessitated ligation of vascular inflow. If the operative surgeon is not familiar with formal hepatectomy, an experienced hepatic surgeon should be consulted for assistance at the take-back procedure.

Torrential hepatic bleeding, uncontrolled by packing, may be encountered on laparotomy. True difficulty arises when the bleeding is too brisk to allow visualization and control. The classic method for control of hepatic bleeding is the Pringle maneuver, named after J. Hogarth Pringle. The lesser sac is entered, and rotation of the hand clockwise will access the Foramen of Winslow, leaving the structures of the porta hepatis in the surgeon's hand. Immediate manual compression is achieved, followed by placement of a Rommel tourniquet or vascular clamp to free the surgeon's hand and allow further access to the field. Some controversy exists as to the length of time the porta may be occluded before significant damage to the liver occurs, but most agree that occlusion for up to 60 minutes is safe. In some cases, primarily in incidences of juxtahepatic caval injury or damage to the suprahepatic veins, hepatic isolation may be required. In these circumstances, control of the distal inferior vena cava (IVC) is required, preferably above the renal veins. This is followed by control of the proximal IVC. No attempt should be made to control the proximal IVC from within the abdomen. A sternotomy must be performed with access to the IVC obtained within the pericardial sac. Escalation to total abdominal vascular exclusion is completed with cross-clamping of the supraceliac aorta.

Some recent case reports in the literature have advocated a multidisciplinary approach to these injuries, especially retrohepatic caval injuries, by trauma surgery and either IR or vascular surgery. Endovascular occlusion of the IVC above and below the injury is obtained, and, in some cases, stenting of the IVC may occur. This is only a viable option if the patient is stable and the injury is identified prior to laparotomy. The logistics of the multidisciplinary approach are unrealistic when the abdomen is open and torrential bleeding is in progress. Angioembolization may be a viable option for persistent arterial bleeding from a grade IV or V liver laceration discovered at laparotomy. If hemorrhage is controllable with packing, the patient may proceed to the IR suite for definitive control, rather than attempting surgical exposure and subsequent ligation in the face of ongoing hemorrhage.

Many of these patients will benefit from staged laparotomies. Second-look procedures provide the opportunity to ensure that bleeding is controlled and to debride any nonviable liver. At time of abdominal closure, it is important to leave close-suction drains for higher-order lacerations, as the postoperative rate of bile leak in these situations is significant.

MUSEUM PIECES

In particularly difficult cases of liver injury with hemorrhage, traditional techniques have at times proven inadequate to salvage patients. Extraordinary efforts at patient rescue have resulted in the development of aggressive techniques that are used rarely and have a poor success rate. The classic atriocaval shunt, as described by Schrock in 1968, involves introduction of a bypass (usually constructed from a thoracostomy tube) into the right atrium, to end at the level of the distal IVC. In theory, the shunt bypasses a presumed retrocaval or similar injury until the injury can be identified and repaired. In practice, survival following an atriocaval shunt is uniformly poor. Venovenous bypass is another option described for use in exsanguinating hemorrhage due to liver trauma or associated major vascular injury. Once the patient is placed on the bypass circuit, repair can proceed in a relatively bloodless field, while the heart and brain remain perfused. Though theoretically appealing, venovenous bypass requires some experience at cannula placement by the operative surgeon and immediate availability of a pump and technician. This option is not readily available in most level one trauma centers. Liver explantation with back-table repair and autotransplant has proven interesting in case reports but has little practical applicability. Finally, liver transplant has occurred in a small number of cases in which the liver has either been destroyed (grade VI injury) or has necrosed due to the requirement to ligate inflow to control hemorrhage. Transplantation is not a viable option for most trauma patients, due to limited donor availability over a very short time frame and the frequent presence of disqualifying related injuries in the recipient. The common variable among all these techniques is that, although they represent heroic measures to save the patient, they are resource intensive and impractical and should be abandoned in all but the most unusual cases.

CONCLUSION

While hepatic trauma is the most common intra-abdominal injury, the need for operative therapy is less common than in the past. Decision for surgical therapy rests upon mechanism of injury, patient status, and concern for associated injuries. Upon laparotomy, compression via packing is frequently all that is required for control of hemorrhage, and abbreviated laparotomy is an important component of this technique. Mobilization of the liver for further exposure, with finger-fracture when indicated, is often required to allow access and ligation of bleeding vessels and biliary tributaries. Hepatic

resection and vascular isolation are less commonly required, as is the assistance of interventional radiology both pre- and postoperatively. However, these options may be invaluable adjuncts in certain patients. More aggressive techniques have largely been abandoned due to poor success rates. Though infrequently requiring laparotomy on their own, the successful operative management of hepatic trauma is dependent on well-considered operative plans, cool judgment, and meticulous technique for success.

SUGGESTED READINGS

Croce MA, Fabian TC, Menke PG, et al: Nonoperative management of blunt hepatic trauma is the treatment of choice for hemodynamically stable patients. Results of a prospective trial, *Ann Surg* 221(6):744–755, 1995.

Delva E, Camus Y, Nordlinger B, et al: Vascular occlusions for liver resections. operative management and tolerance to hepatic ischemia: 142 cases, *Ann Surg* 209(2):211–218, 1989.

Pachter HL, Feliciano DV: Complex hepatic injuries, *Surg Clin North Am* 76(4):763–782, 1996.

Pringle JVH: Notes on the arrest of hepatic hemorrhage due to trauma, *Ann Surg* 48:541–549, 1908.

Stassen NA, Bhullar I, Cheng JD, et al: Nonoperative management of blunt hepatic injury: an eastern association for the surgery of trauma practice management guideline, *J Trauma Acute Care Surg* 73(5 Suppl 4):S288–S293, 2012.

PANCREATIC AND DUODENAL INJURIES AND CURRENT SURGICAL THERAPIES

Juan Carlos Duchesne, MD, FACS, FCCP, FCCM, Eric R. Simms, MD, and Norman McSwain, Jr., MD, FACS

injuries are usually associated with hemorrhage control because the vena cava, intestinal vessels, and aorta are in the anatomic region and are frequently injured concomitantly. Greater than 70% of mortality associated with pancreaticoduodenal trauma is attributable to hemorrhage, so the immediate focus should be on hemorrhage control with damage control strategies, if necessary.

The four management priorities based on life-threatening conditions for patients managed with damage control surgery for pancreaticoduodenal injuries are:

1. Control of hemorrhage from major vessel injuries.
2. Control of hemorrhage from solid organs.
3. Control of contamination or spillage from hollow organ injuries.
4. Stabilization of major bony injuries.

EPIDEMIOLOGY AND MANAGEMENT PRIORITIES

Overall, pancreatic and duodenal injuries are uncommon, representing less than 10% of patients admitted with blunt abdominal trauma or explored for penetrating trauma. The types of injuries to the duodenum and pancreas vary depending on the makeup of the various trauma center "clientele." Trauma centers with a high percentage of penetrating injuries are more likely to have severe injuries to the duodenum or pancreas than those with mainly blunt trauma; reported series vary from 1.5% to 6% of the population. Isolated duodenal or pancreatic injuries are relatively rare, with only 20% of blunt trauma patients having pancreatic injury with no other organ injury, and exceedingly rare in penetrating abdominal trauma. Because of their location, pancreatic and duodenal injuries are usually associated with concomitant injuries to the spleen, liver, stomach, or the vascular structures associated with these. Therapeutic strategies must include management of both organs and effective hemorrhage control. Management of duodenal and pancreatic

KINEMATICS (MECHANISM OF INJURY)

Blunt Trauma

Blunt trauma to the duodenum or pancreas is usually from direct compression. For example, in a frontal motor vehicle impact, the torso continues to move forward after the vehicle stops, and the continued motion of the posterior abdominal wall compresses the duodenum and pancreas against the spine. This is like placing the duodenum and pancreas on an anvil and hitting them with a hammer. The result is crushing of the bowel wall, rupture of the lumen, fracture-disruption of the pancreatic parenchyma and possibly the duct, and vascular injury to surrounding vessels. A common pediatric compressive injury is associated with a deceleration injury of the abdomen against bicycles handlebars, which traps the duodenum and pancreas against the vertebra.

Penetrating Trauma

At the time of operative exploration, the surgeon must assess the trajectory of the penetrating object to assess injury potential. The two components in the assessment of penetrating trauma injury potential are:

1. The anatomic structures in the vicinity of the penetrating object's trajectory
2. The energy exchanges into the tissue:
    a. Crush
    b. Cavitation

Diagnosis of pancreatic or duodenal injuries depends on mechanism of injury. For penetrating trauma, a surgeon must follow the trajectory of penetration during exploratory laparotomy, and all parts of the duodenum and pancreas must be inspected visually and manually. Blunt trauma, on the other hand, requires a high index of suspicion and a thorough understanding of the kinematics of blunt trauma at the time of impact. The pancreas and duodenum are located retroperitoneally, so physical examination in the first 24 hours after blunt trauma is difficult for discerning injuries to these organs. There are often no peritoneal signs in retroperitoneal organ injury, and hemorrhage from associated vascular structures may not be immediately evident because of retroperitoneal tamponade or a lack of abdominal distention. Focused assessment with sonography for trauma (FAST) scan is not suited for evaluation of retroperitoneal structures, and laboratory assays (including serum amylase levels) may be normal immediately after pancreatic injury. Because of this, most diagnoses of pancreatic injury after blunt trauma are made with contrast-enhanced computed tomographic (CT) scan, in particular in hemodynamically stable cases. Hemodynamic instability or penetrating trauma with clear intraperitoneal or retroperitoneal involvement warrants exploratory laparotomy, which reveals a pancreatic injury. The CT scan findings diagnostic of pancreatic injury are seen in Table 1.

TABLE 1: Contrast-enhanced computed tomographic scan findings suggestive and diagnostic of pancreatic injury

Suggestive findings	Diagnostic findings
Transverse mesocolon hematoma	Parenchymal laceration or hematoma
Fluid in the lesser sac/posterior to pancreas (between pancreas and splenic vein)	Transection of the parenchyma, with fluid in the lesser sac
Duodenal laceration or hematoma	Disruption of the head of the pancreas
Injury to left kidney, adrenal gland, or spleen	Diffuse swelling consistent with posttraumatic pancreatitis
Thickening of the left anterior renal fascia	
Lumbar spine transverse fracture (chance fracture)	

DUODENUM

Unfortunately, rupture of the duodenum does not produce abdominal pain, and it is often only when bacterial infections develop that an isolated duodenal injury is evident on physical examination. Other surrounding structures, such as the pancreas and vessels, can produce signs and symptoms of shock or peritoneal inflammation. Examination of the duodenum should always be performed during any abdominal exploration for blunt trauma. Because of the positioning of the duodenum and pancreas, laparoscopic assessment is extremely difficult and is not recommended for blunt or penetrating trauma evaluation with suspected pancreaticoduodenal injury.

In patients with minimal abdominal examination findings, contrast-enhanced CT scan assessment of the duodenum and pancreas is frequently not positive in the first 12 to 24 hours after injury. Evidence of abdominal inflammation such as fat stranding or even presence of free air or fluid in the abdominal cavity can be indicative of duodenal injury. Because the duodenum is only partially intra-abdominal, retroperitoneal air or fluid with associated inflammatory changes are extremely suggestive of duodenal perforation.

Anatomy

The unique anatomy and associated structures of the duodenum make usual assessment and management techniques for the duodenum quite different from the rest of the gastrointestinal (GI) tract. The duodenum is only partially covered by peritoneum, so the usual signs of peritoneal inflammation are usually not present. Because the peritoneum does not cover a significant portion of the duodenum, repair can likewise be challenging.

With the development of the Murphy button in the mid 18th century, we discovered that peritoneal closure in any anastomosis is critical to healing. Repair of injuries in the anterior first, second, and third portion of the duodenum are readily achieved because the peritoneum and serosa are present; however, the posterior parts of the duodenum are without the anastomotic protection of the peritoneum, so other considerations must be entertained. The duodenum is composed of four parts. The proximal (first) part begins at the pyloric valve and continues until the first bend of the duodenum around the head of the pancreas. Along the head of the pancreas is the second portion of the duodenum. The close association of the third portion of the duodenum to the pancreas is called the J portion because it turns medially around the head of the pancreas to traverse the posterior pancreas and proceed under the colon, finally entering the peritoneal cavity at the ligament of Treitz.

The blood supplies to the duodenum and head/body of the pancreas are continuous with each other. The anterior and posterior pancreaticoduodenal arteries are frequently in the groove between the pancreas and duodenum and supply both organs with multiple side branches. The pancreaticoduodenal arteries connect superiorly to the hepatic artery via the gastroduodenal artery and inferiorly connect to the superior mesenteric artery anterior to the superior mesenteric vein. The dual-source blood supply is critical to the management of duodenal trauma because either end of the pancreaticoduodenal artery can be tied off with adequate blood supply coming from the other end.

Because of the retroperitoneal, retrocolic position of the fourth portion of the duodenum and its blood supply associations with the pancreas, anastomoses of the fourth portion are fought with hazard. It is much better to remove the fourth portion and anastomose the jejunum to the second or third portion to maintain GI continuity for enteral feeding. An understanding of the details of the duodenal anatomy is critical in the management of patients with duodenal trauma.

Assessment

Assessment of the duodenum begins in the emergency department with a high index of suspicion based on the mechanism of injury. Especially with blunt trauma, a specific diagnosis of duodenal trauma is virtually impossible without radiographic or direct visual (operative) evidence. The first step should nonetheless be a detailed physical examination looking for signs of trauma anteriorly, such as tenderness to deep palpation, rebound tenderness, guarding, and the absence of bowel sounds. These are clear signs of peritoneal irritation, not specific signs related to the duodenum. CT scan can augment the physical examination, demonstrating free air or fluid in the abdomen and increasing suspicion for bowel perforation or injury.

Operative assessment of the duodenum begins with visualization of the entire first, second, and third portions of the duodenum. Kocher's maneuver may be used to assess the posterior aspects of the duodenum. A digital assessment of the length of the fourth portion of the duodenum is necessary from the beginning to the other side of the ligament of Treitz because visual evaluation of the fourth portion is frequently difficult. At the very minimum, the surgeon's left hand should traverse posteriorly toward the ligament of Treitz, and the right hand should carefully palpate from the ligament of Treitz toward the left hand until the fingers touch. The entire portion of the fourth part of the duodenum can then be felt, with the index finger or middle finger posterior to the duodenum and the thumbs of the right and left hand anterior to the duodenum.

Operative Management

Priorities in operative management for duodenal trauma are:

- Assessment is needed of the entire duodenum for integrity or perforation, intramural clots, and blood supply.
- Closure is performed of serosa-covered duodenum, usually with intestinal two-layer closure.
- Closure is performed of nonserosa components of the duodenum, closed in layers and assisted with a serosal patch when possible.
- Extraluminal drains increase the risk of intra-abdominal abscess and fistula formation.
- Intraluminal decompression (either antegrade, retrograde, or both) is critical when nonserosal duodenum has been closed or there is otherwise compromise or potential compromise of the anastomosis or closure.
- Duodenal cavity diversion with creation of a Bilroth II–type gastroenterostomy may be required for severe trauma or compromised anastomoses (see subsequent).
- Continued controversy exists as to the actual benefits of temporary duodenal diversion; only use it as a last resort.
- Assessment is needed if there is injury to the pancreas.

A simple repair of a duodenal injury is done the same way as repair of any serosa-covered GI tract injury: a two-layer closure (absorbable on the inside) with diagonal not longitudinal closure to prevent tension or stricture of the repair. When injury extends to the portions of the duodenum that do not have serosa or peritoneum exteriorly to facilitate healing, or if the injury is more than 50% of the circumference of the duodenum, other protective steps have to be taken. For a simple injury, an adequate closure can be obtained with two-layer repair and other steps to ensure sealing. This is similar to operative management of the esophagus, such as swinging of peritoneum over the nonperitonealized portion of the injury. Abdominal wall is a very good source of peritoneum on occasion, as the peritoneum from the peritoneal wall itself can be rotated around similarly to esophageal injuries or from another piece of small bowel that can be placed over the injury (Thal patch).

As injuries become more complex (e.g., greater than 50% of the duodenum affected, two or more adjacent injuries, etc.), a concern exists for pressure gradients between the intraluminal and extraluminal areas. The Bernoulli principle identifies the rate of leak as proportional to intraluminal pressure versus extraluminal pressure. Therefore, the intraluminal pressure needs to be reduced in the duodenum. An intraluminal drain, such as a nasogastric tube, passed through the pylorus into the duodenum, or a similar tube passed retrograde from the jejunum through fourth portion into the second portion of the duodenum, is an acceptable method. Placement of drains outside the lumen is not appropriate because this violates several surgical principles, including avoiding foreign bodies in the anastomotic regions to reduce extraluminal pressure relative to intraluminal pressure, forming connections between sterile abdomen and external environments, and avoiding other sources of potential contamination.

The theory behind protecting the nonperitoneal side of the duodenum includes the reduction of intraluminal pressure without addition of pressure of a foreign body to the extraluminal area, reduction of food passage through the injured and repaired areas, and sometimes total diversion (e.g., Roux-en-Y gastrojejunostomy with stapling across the duodenum at the pylorus). All of these techniques have proponents and adversaries; however, almost all research on duodenal injuries is anecdotal, and no single institution has developed a large enough sample size to perform adequately powered comparison studies. This leaves us at the mercy and discretion of the operating surgeon. Several years ago, diverticularization and exclusion were encouraged, and they may be coming back into favor. Since 1980, several studies (again anecdotal, with some retrospective reviews without controls) have questioned the usefulness of simply cross clamping or sewing up the pylorus. In most series, either stapling across the duodenum at the pylorus or sewing up the pylorus does not provide a permanent solution because most of these open up in 3 to 6 weeks. Some studies have even proposed that such surgical constructs become nonfunctional within a week. It is the experienced opinion of the author that with very extensive wounds of the first, second, or third portion of the duodenum, diverticularization is probably the correct approach. For lesser injuries, with only a short term of decreased functionality of the duodenum predicted, either cross clamping below the pylorus or sewing up the pylorus with diversion allows protection of the duodenum for up to 3 weeks. Both approaches, however, emphasize internal decompression as very important. Whichever approach the surgeon attempts, these rules apply. In summary, the duodenum is unfortunately not protected fully about its circumference or along its length by serosa, as are other parts of the small bowel. Therefore, extra attention is warranted to allow healing.

PANCREAS

Assessment

Assessment and classification of pancreatic injuries depends on the status of the duct and the site of the injury. Nonoperative assessment usually relies on trauma CT scan findings, although CT scan misses pancreatic injuries in approximately 31% of abdominal trauma cases. In penetrating trauma or with unstable blunt trauma, operative assessment involves the pancreas being completely exposed to assess it. Patients with hemodynamically unstable conditions, especially those with acidosis, coagulopathy, or hypothermia, should undergo damage control management. This includes immediate surgical exploration with control of major hemorrhage or contamination, packing or drainage, followed by intensive care unit (ICU) stabilization, and return to the operating room in 12 to 24 hours to definitively expose, assess, and repair the pancreas and associated injuries. Direct palpation and visualization of all parts of the pancreas should

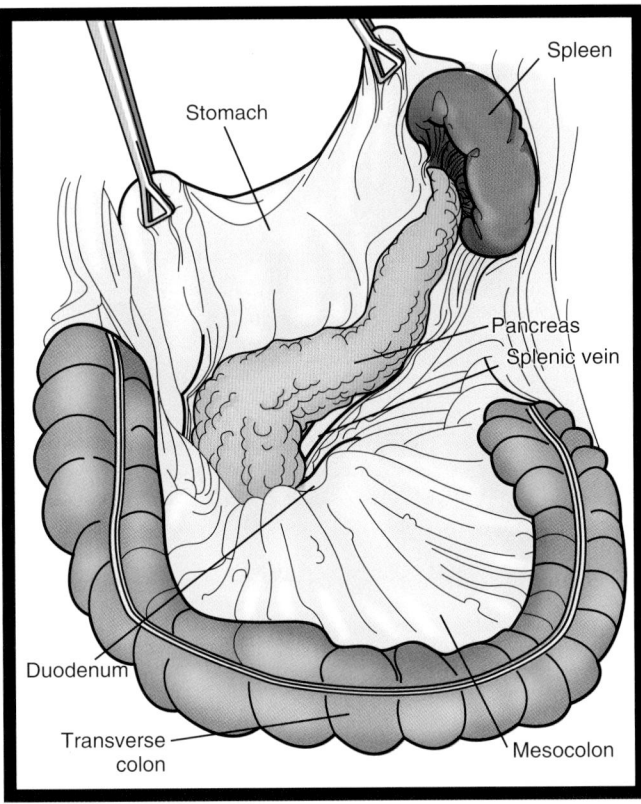

FIGURE 1   Exposure of the pancreas.

Eric R. Simms

TABLE 2: The American Association for the Surgery of Trauma pancreas organ injury scale

Grade*	Type of injury	Description of injury
I	Hematoma	Minor contusion without duct injury
	Laceration	Superficial laceration without duct injury
II	Hematoma	Major contusion without duct injury or tissue loss
	Laceration	Major laceration without duct injury or tissue loss
III	Laceration	Distal transection or parenchymal injury with duct injury
IV	Laceration	Proximal† transection or parenchymal injury involving ampulla
V	Laceration	Massive disruption of pancreatic head

*Advance one grade for multiple injuries up to grade III.
†Proximal pancreatic injuries are injuries to the patient's right of the superior mesenteric vein.

be possible with the following maneuvers but may be complicated by the amount of damage to surrounding structures:

1. Opening of the lesser sac through the gastrocolic ligament and omentum, below the gastroepiploic arteries.
2. Extension of this opening towards the splenic flexure and mobilization of the transverse colon, which can be retracted inferiorly as the stomach and spleen are gently retracted superiorly. This allows an approach to the body of the pancreas for circumferential palpation.
3. Performance of Kocher's maneuver to assess the pancreatic neck, head, and uncinate process.
4. Potential mobilization of the hepatic flexure to fully access the head and uncinate process.
5. Mobilization of the splenic flexure and spleen with freeing of the lateral peritoneal attachments, and any attachments between the kidney and spleen/pancreatic tail, and mobilization of the spleen and pancreatic tail medially and anteriorly. This allows for inspection of the distal body and tail of the pancreas (Figure 1).

The American Association for the Surgery of Trauma (AAST) Committee on Organ Injury Scaling works well, in coordination with the Abbreviated Injury Scale (AIS), for classification of pancreatic injury (Table 2), in a way meaningful to management decisions. Status of the duct and site of injury are the most important factors, with major ductal injuries treated differently than distal ductal injuries or parenchymal injuries. In general, grade I and II injuries can be managed nonoperatively or sometimes with external drainage; severe combined pancreaticoduodenal injuries are preferentially managed with trauma Whipple's procedure, or damage control strategies with interval Whipple's procedure; and extensive pancreatic parenchymal damage with or without major duct injury can be managed with external drainage based on the locus of injury.

Ductal Injury

Injuries to the major duct are present in 15% to 20% of pancreatic trauma. For penetrating trauma, most ductal injuries can be assessed with careful survey of the trajectory and path of the injury, after the aforementioned exposure techniques. If the status of the duct is not clear after direct evaluation, intraoperative pancreatography may be necessary in an otherwise stabilized case. A patient with an unstable condition may need damage control measures followed by postoperative endoscopic retrograde cholangiopancreatography (ERCP). For blunt trauma that warrants exploratory laparotomy, the extent of pancreatic disruption determines management. Minor lacerations or contusions may be managed just with placement of drains. In the rare instances when the major duct is transected without parenchymal, transection requires a high index of suspicion, meriting intraoperative pancreatography or postoperative ERCP. Needle cholecystocholangiopancreatography or postoperative ERCP remain preferable to duodenotomy with ampullary cannulation.

Operative and Nonoperative Management

Grade I and II Injuries

In patients without hemodynamic instability, peritoneal signs, or clear intraperitoneal or retroperitoneal penetrating trauma, contrast-enhanced CT scan may suggest only minor pancreatic parenchymal injury. Minor parenchymal lacerations or contusions (without extensive parenchymal decimation) in the absence of ductal injury can be managed nonoperatively, or with external drainage. Grade I pancreatic injuries (minor contusion, hematoma, or capsular laceration) represent about half of all pancreatic injuries. Grade II injuries (pancreatic lacerations without major tissue loss or ductal injury) represent another 25% of pancreatic injuries. Both of these injuries can be managed nonoperatively, even if peripancreatic fluid collection is noted on CT scan. Often a follow-up contrast-enhanced CT scan is prudent 5 to 7 days after injury, to reassess peripancreatic fluid collections, or in the presence of worsening laboratory findings, abdominal symptoms, or physical examination findings. If detected during exploratory laparotomy, they can be managed with external drainage alone, after careful exposure and inspection of the entire gland and hemostasis. Lacerations in the absence of major ductal injury are managed without surgical repair of the laceration because of the high risk of pseudocyst formation associated with these attempts. Closed-suction drains are preferred to Penrose drains or Davol sumps because of less skin excoriation and complications such as abscess. Drains are left in place until there is no longer evidence of pancreatic leak. Nutrition should focus on enteral feedings as soon as possible to improve outcomes.

Grade III Injuries

Distal pancreatic injuries (defined as distal to the level of the superior mesenteric vessels) with involvement of the major duct (grade III) are best managed with distal pancreatectomy. These injuries can be recognized via CT scan (if performed at least 4 hours after injury), or at the time of exploratory laparotomy, with or without the aid of pancreatography. Often mid-to-distal pancreatic duct injuries are associated with notable fat necrosis in the lesser sac and can be considered to be evidence of ductal injury, especially with evidence of local penetrating trauma.

As long as at least 20% of pancreatic tissue is left, there should be adequate endocrine and exocrine function after distal pancreatectomy. Usually, pancreatectomy at the level of the portal vein provides enough residual parenchyma to preserve endocrine and exocrine function, and resection at the level of the common bile duct does not. Nonoperative management for grade III injuries usually fails or has extensive complications, including repetitive drainage interventions, failed stenting or endoscopic management attempts, abscesses, pseudocysts, or persistent fistulas. If any doubt exists about the integrity of the proximal duct, intraoperative pancreatography should be performed with cannulation of the transected end of the proximal duct. Some experts recommend closing the remaining duct with a U stitch of nonabsorbable suture and approximating the pancreatic parenchyma with absorbable mattress sutures, with the belief that staplers crush excess parenchyma. TA (thoracoabdominal) staplers can be safely and effectively used to close the proximal pancreas, however, with fewer complications. Either technique often benefits from the use of an omental patch to buttress the distal end of the proximal remnant.

Grade III injuries in the pancreatic tail may have splenic involvement that necessitates splenorrhaphy or splenectomy. If splenectomy is not mandated by injuries, a splenic salvage may be attempted. To accomplish this, the spleen and pancreas must both be very well mobilized. 3-0 or 4-0 silk or Vicryl ties (Ethicon, Somerville, NJ) may be used to ligate small pancreatic vessels on the side of the splenic artery and vein, with clips used on the pancreatic vessels near the segment to be resected. Difficulties include avoiding damage to the splenic artery or vein while ligating the small pancreatic branches off of each and splenic vein thrombosis. Splenic salvage requires an average of 50 additional minutes of operative time, so it should only be attempted in patients without signs of acidosis, coagulopathy, or hypothermia. If pancreatectomy/splenectomy is performed, the splenic artery should be suture ligated with 4-0 polypropylene approximately 2 cm proximal to the pancreatic segment to be resected. Similar ligation should then be performed for the splenic vein. The vessels may also be covered by an omental patch after resection of the pancreatic segment and spleen, to protect them against pancreatic enzymatic erosion (Figure 2).

Grade IV and V Injuries

Injuries to the pancreatic head are the most difficult to manage, especially if there is parenchymal transection or injury to the proximal duct. Immediate management priorities are control of hemorrhage and limiting of gross spillage or contamination. This may be

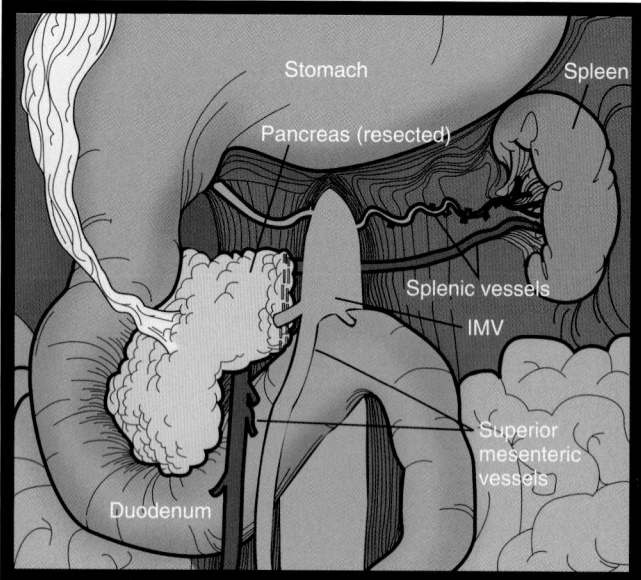

Eric R. Simms

FIGURE 2 Distal pancreatectomy with splenic salvage. *IMV*, Inferior mesenteric vein.

accomplished with damage control methods (for hemodynamically unstable cases with present or worsening acidosis, coagulopathy, or hypothermia), with ICU stabilization and subsequent return to the operating room for definitive repair, or definitive repair at the time of original operation if the patient's condition is otherwise stable. Before any definitive management, the anatomy must be clearly defined to assess the extent of injury. The duct status can usually be discerned with careful direct inspection after appropriate mobilization techniques previously described. If the integrity of the main duct cannot be clearly determined with local operative exploration, intraoperative pancreatography must be considered, either via needle cholecystocholangiopancreatography or external drainage followed by postoperative ERCP. In rare instances when the proximal duct is injured in the absence of concomitant duodenal/ampullary injury, extended distal (subtotal) pancreatectomy or Roux-en-Y pancreaticojejunostomy (tail-sparing) may be performed. Subtotal pancreatectomy should be performed with external drain placement for control of leaks from the transected edge and ultimately results in the small portion of residual proximal gland draining into the duodenum. If the residual amount of pancreas is likely insufficient for endocrine and exocrine function (e.g., proximal to the plane of the superior mesenteric vessels), distal Roux-en-Y pancreaticojejunostomy (end-to-end or end-to-side) may be performed to preserve pancreas distal to the injury. To perform this, after débridement of devitalized tissue, the pancreas is divided at the site of injury, and the proximal duct and parenchyma closed via TA stapler or U stitch. The distal duct opening is anastomosed to the Roux-en-Y jejunal limb, as a cuff-type pancreaticojejunostomy. A tube stent may be placed through the anastomosis to decrease the possibility of pancreatic fistula formation (Figure 3).

Combined Pancreatic and Duodenal Injury

Combined pancreaticoduodenal injuries are rare and are usually the result of penetrating trauma. These injuries are usually associated with multiple other intra-abdominal trunk injuries, and mortality from pancreaticoduodenal injury is usually the result of associated vascular injuries. Immediate damage control techniques are mandatory to control hemorrhage and contamination, especially in the face

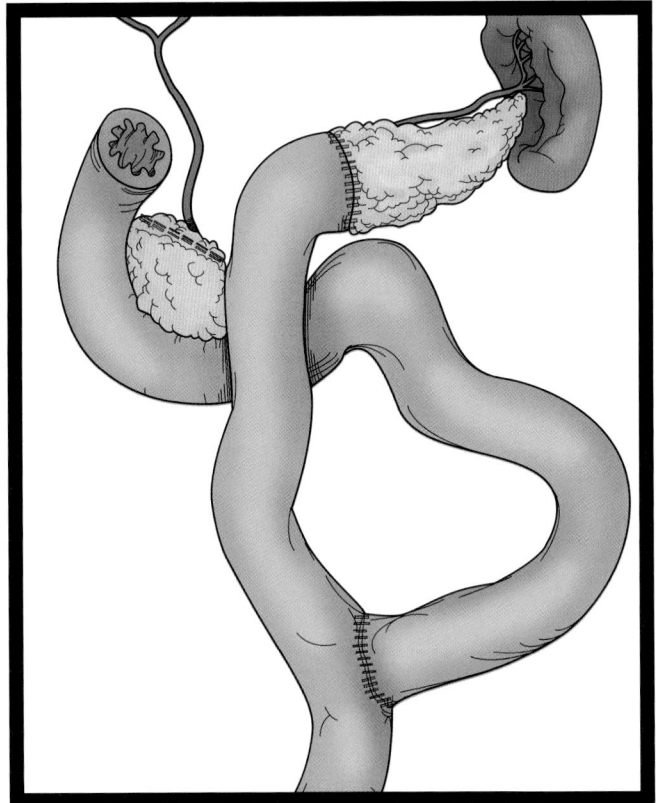

Eric R. Simms

FIGURE 3   Roux-en-Y pancreaticojejunostomy.

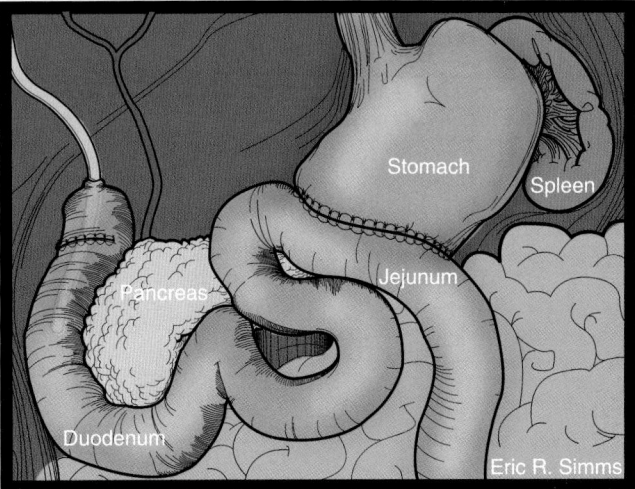

FIGURE 4   Duodenal diverticularization.

decimated, complete resection of one often results in ischemia of the other because of their intimately associated vasculature. Some surgeons may opt to control hemorrhage/contamination and perform the resections for Whipple's procedure at the initial operation and then return after stabilization for reconstruction (staged Whipple's). If pancreaticoduodenectomy is not mandated by injury, it is often necessary to divert gastric and biliary contents from the repaired duodenum. One technique for this is duodenal diverticularization, wherein the duodenal injury is closed primarily, and antrectomy/vagotomy performed with end-to-side gastrojejunostomy (Figure 4). The common bile duct is decompressed with T-tube drainage, and duodenal fistulization is controlled by duodenostomy tube. Enteral nutrition is then performed through the gastrojejunostomy. Even if this technique is not used, a Witzel jejunostomy should be performed for all patients undergoing Whipple's procedure for pancreatic or pancreaticoduodenal trauma, to provide enteral feeding access.

SUGGESTED READINGS

Asensio JA, Feliciano DV, Britt LD, et al: Management of duodenal injuries, *Curr Probl Surg* 30:1021–1100, 1993.
Asensio JA, Petrone P, Roldan G, et al: Pancreaticoduodenectomy: a rare procedure for the management of complex pancreaticoduodenal injuries, *JACS* 197(6):937–942, 2003.
Jurkovich GJ: Injuries to the pancreas and duodenum, *ACS Surgery: Principles and Practice*, 2008.

of hemodynamic instability or metabolic/coagulation derangements. If a patient is stabilized (in the ICU after damage control surgery, or rarely, at the time of initial operation), the status of the common bile duct, main pancreatic duct, and ampulla must be assessed via intraoperative cholangiogram/pancreatogram, or postoperative ERCP, to determine the best definitive management. Most cases have an intact ampulla and common duct, so the duodenal injury can be primarily repaired and the pancreatic duct injury managed as previously described.

If the pancreatic head and duodenum are devitalized or not amenable to primary repair (e.g., common bile duct, pancreatic duct, and ampullary injury), Whipple's procedure (pancreaticoduodenectomy) can be used. Even if only the duodenum or only the pancreas are

INJURIES TO THE SMALL AND LARGE BOWEL

Syed Nabeel Zafar, MB, BS, MPH, and Edward E. Cornwell, III, MD, FACS, FCCM

Small and large bowel injuries are infrequent but potentially morbid sequelae of abdominal trauma. Of the 2.5 million patients in the National Trauma Databank, years 2007 to 2010, full-thickness small and large bowel injuries occured in approximately 0.3% and 0.4%, respectively (Table 1). Of these injuries, approximately 92% are secondary to penetrating trauma, particularly from gunshot wounds and stab wounds. Mortality rates are significant—9.7% for small bowel injuries and 9.2% for large bowel injuries—and death results largely from associated injuries. Mean lengths of hospital stays are 11% and 14 days, respectively. In 2003, the Eastern Association for the Surgery of Trauma published results of a multiinstitutional survey of hollow viscus injuries, collecting data from 95 participating centers between the years 1998 and 1999. The incidences of perforating small and large bowel injuries were 0.3% and 0.2% of all trauma admissions. However, the mortality rates were significantly higher than the death rates reported by the recent National Trauma Databank: 15%

TABLE 1: Small and large bowel injuries reported by the National Trauma Data Bank, 2007 to 2010

	Small bowel injury (N = 7558)	Large bowel injury (N = 11,164)
Blunt injury	480 (6.4%)	656 (5.9%)
Gunshot wound	4597 (60.8%)	8290 (74.3%)
Stab wound	2340 (30.9%)	2005 (17.9%)
Mortality	691 (9.7%)	981 (9.2%)
Mean length of hospital stay (in days with standard deviations)	11.2 (±15.8)	14.3 (±18.5)

for small bowel injuries and 19% for colorectal injuries. The marked improvement in mortality rates since then can be attributed to advances in diagnosis and management of traumatic injuries overall. This chapter reviews the mechanisms, the diagnosis, and the surgical management of traumatic small and large bowel injuries.

MECHANISM OF INJURY

Any penetrating wound between the nipples and the groin should raise the suspicion of bowel injury. The actual incidence of bowel injury varies according to factors such as length of knife, velocity and type of bullet, location and trajectory of the penetrating injury, and body habitus of the victim. For example, the index of suspicion would be high for a gunshot wound to the anterior abdomen with an exit wound through the back in a lean victim, and it would be lower for a pocket knife stab wound through the flank of an obese individual.

Blunt trauma, in contrast, poses an ongoing challenge to the clinician. Such bowel injuries are not as clinically obvious as in the case of penetrating injuries, and the incidence of bowel injury after blunt trauma is low. However, delays in diagnosis can lead to significant morbidity and mortality. Motor vehicle crashes and impact injuries in pedestrians have been shown to produce a higher incidence of bowel injuries than do falls and other modes of blunt trauma. Mechanisms of bowel injury include shearing of the bowel from its mesentery secondary to sudden deceleration, and "blow-out" of a loop of bowel as a result of a sudden increase in intraluminal pressure. The latter occasionally occurs when a high-riding automobile lap-belt squeezes a loop of bowel against the retroperitoneum or spine. The degree of suspicion for this type of injury should be high when the so called seatbelt sign—a transverse ecchymosis visible on the lower abdominal wall, corresponding to the position of the seatbelt on the patient—is present. The presence of a seatbelt sign alone is associated with a markedly increased risk of a bowel injury.

DIAGNOSIS

Because the overwhelming majority of small and large bowel injuries are caused by penetrating trauma, they are most commonly discovered during trauma laparotomy. This is performed on the basis of the clinical presentation of patients with abdominal gunshot or stab wounds: hemodynamic instability, omental or visceral evisceration, and peritoneal signs or tenderness away from the entry wound. For selected patients in stable condition with stab wounds or even gunshot wounds to the abdomen, nonoperative management may be pursued in the appropriate setting. Selective nonoperative management should be undertaken only if the following two conditions are met: (1) the patient is hemodynamically stable with no signs of evisceration, peritonitis, or intra-abdominal hemorrhage and (2) the clinical decision occurs in a setting with 24-hour availability of a surgeon, in which the patient can be monitored continuously and serial abdominal examinations are routinely performed.

Frequently, physical examination findings are not reliable because the patient is affected by alcohol or drug intoxication, head injuries, heavy sedation, or neurologic deficit. In these circumstances, other adjunct tests are helpful. An upright chest radiograph may show air under the diaphragm or a Chance fracture of the lumbar vertebral body. Chance fractures have been associated with bowel injuries and are caused by decelerating mechanisms, as with high-riding automobile seatbelts in high-speed motor vehicle crashes. Another useful tool is the focused assessment with sonography for trauma (FAST) examination, which may identify free fluid in the abdominal cavity.

Computed tomographic (CT) scanning has become the standard diagnostic tool for occult abdominal injuries. Because of advances in technology and availability, its use has become widespread. Helical CT scanners have been shown to have a high accuracy in detecting gastrointestinal injuries, with sensitivities ranging from 83% to 94% for bowel injuries. Although opinions vary on the use of oral contrast material in detecting gastrointestinal injuries, it is not used in the authors' trauma center. It causes unnecessary delays in diagnosis, increases risk of aspiration, and has not conclusively been demonstrated to increase the accuracy of scans. CT findings suggestive of small or large bowel injury include pneumoperitoneum, intraperitoneal fluid not associated with solid organ injury, bowel wall thickening, mesenteric fat streaking, mesenteric hematoma, and extravasation of luminal content. If free fluid is the only CT finding in a hemodynamically stable patient, then the surgeon either can continue to observe the patient if the patient is able to cooperate with serial clinical examinations or can perform diagnostic laparoscopy or even exploratory laparotomy.

Preparation for diagnostic laparoscopy must always include preparation for a possible exploratory laparotomy. The technique for a diagnostic laparoscopy varies, depending on the surgeon. In general, the patient is administered a general anesthetic and placed in the Trendelenburg position. A single umbilical port or single left upper quadrant port may be placed to advance the laparoscope. At any signs of peritoneal penetration or intraperitoneal injury, many surgeons convert the procedure to exploratory laparotomy. Others, depending on skill and experience, place three ports, explore all intraperitoneal organs and quadrants for signs of injury, and investigate the entire length of bowel with the use of graspers.

The "gold standard" for diagnosing bowel injuries remains the exploratory laparotomy. However, this procedure can also produce morbidity. Thus the resultant challenge is the need to combine the aforementioned adjunct diagnostic tests to create a composite sensitivity of 100% for detecting bowel injuries, balanced by the importance of minimizing nontherapeutic laparotomies. Once detected, bowel injuries are managed surgically.

SURGICAL MANAGEMENT

Perioperative Care

All patients should receive perioperative antibiotics for 24 hours; the first dose should be administered immediately when the need for surgery is recognized. A broad-spectrum third-generation cephalosporin has been proven effective. As with all major operations, early ambulation, chemical and mechanical prophylaxis for deep venous thrombosis, incentive spirometry, appropriate wound care, and early diet advancement are recommended.

Although variations exist in technical management, a few general principles are recognized and hold true for both small and large bowel injuries. These principles are described in Box 1.

Small Bowel

In general small bowel injures are primarily repaired. If the perforation is less than 50% of the circumference of the bowel (grade II injury), then the defect can be repaired transversely with absorbable running sutures. A second interrupted nonabsorbable seromuscular layer may be placed. However, if the perforation is greater than 50% of the circumference (grade III and worse injuries), then resection and primary anastomosis are recommended. If multiple injuries are present in close proximity, then all of these can be managed by a single resection and anastomosis (Figure 1). Another option is to perform stapled anastomoses. Although the role of gastrointestinal staplers is established in an elective setting, the use of staplers in patients with traumatic injuries is somewhat controversial. Retrospective analysis suggests a higher incidence of complications and anastomotic leaks when staples are used; this analysis does not adequately account for the tendency to use this time-saving device in the more challenging setting with multiple injuries. No randomized controlled trials have yet been conducted to compare these techniques. If stapled anastomoses are performed, however, care must be taken to use appropriate sized staples and to account for bowel edema secondary to resuscitation. The surgeon should always pause between locking and firing the stapler to allow edema around the staple line to dissipate. The skin can be closed in cases of small bowel injury, unless for some reason surgery is delayed and there is gross contamination with succus or purulent material, in which case the fascia are closed and the skin is left open to heal by secondary intention.

In general, any mesenteric hematoma that extends to the bowel wall or is enlarging must be explored and any hemorrhage controlled. In the setting of damage control surgery, in which the objective is to stop the bleeding and control the contamination in the shortest amount of time as possible, many surgeons staple both ends of the bowel and leave it in discontinuity. After the patient is resuscitated and organ function is restored, the anastomosis can be made during the second definitive operation. The authors' preference is to perform a stapled anastomosis of the two bowel segments, even in the damage control setting, so as to avoid adding a closed loop obstruction to the challenges of a patient in physiologic extremis. The time required to perform a stapled anastomosis is minimal, and the anastomosis can be revised during the second, definitive operation.

Complications such as anastomotic leaks, intra-abdominal abscesses, and enterocutaneous fistulas occur in up to 10% of patients after repair of a small bowel injury. There is no conclusive evidence on the association between rate of complications and surgical technique. However, damage control procedures and the presence of associated injuries such as pancreaticoduodenal injuries have been associated with higher rates of complications.

Large Bowel

There is now significant level 1 and level 2 evidence supporting primary repair or resection and anastomosis of colon injuries in the vast majority of cases. As a result, resection and anastomosis are recommended for patients in stable condition with penetrating wounds and minimal associated injuries or comorbid conditions. The prior practice of routine colostomy formation is not recommended and should be practiced only in very specific settings (to be described). Simple lacerations can be débrided and repaired with hand-sewn sutures in single or double layers, as previously described. Care must be taken to débride the area of perforation. Most destructive colon injuries can be resected, and primary anastomosis can be performed with side-to-side or end-to-side techniques. There is no difference in the leakage rates between hand-sewn and stapled anastomoses, and the choice of technique is left to the surgeon's discretion. The authors utilize a running absorbable full-thickness suture for the inner layer and an outer seromuscular layer of interrupted 3-0 silk.

Consideration of colostomy creation is reserved for "high risk" patients with destructive injuries; such patients are defined as those with a high penetrating abdominal trauma index score ($\geq$25), those with high transfusion requirements (greater than six units), and those in whom surgery is delayed. Another area in which colostomy formation is still strongly considered is with extraperitoneal rectal injuries.

Diversion of the fecal stream away from colon injuries can be achieved by an end colostomy (Hartmann's procedure), end colostomy with creation of a mucous fistula, loop colostomy with closure or occlusion of the distal limb, or loop colostomy alone. Each of these techniques has been shown to be effective in the management of penetrating injury to the colon in the civilian population. Although purists have long advocated Hartmann's procedure or end colostomy and mucous fistula for complete fecal diversion, Rambeau and associates demonstrated that this can also be achieved with a properly constructed loop colostomy. Keys to this technique include (1) maintenance of the posterior wall above the level of the skin with a rod or red Robinson rubber catheter that occludes the distal lumen and is secured to the skin; (2) an anterior wall colotomy; and (3) maturation of the colon edges to the skin (with a 4-0 absorbable suture on a cutting needle). A "rosebud" appearance is created by passing the suture through full-thickness colon edge, then through a more proximal seromuscular bite, and finally through the dermis (Figure 2). A loop colostomy created in this manner has the advantage of allowing colostomy closure through a paracolostomy incision, as opposed to reentering the midline laparotomy wound. It also prevents the challenge of dissecting out the distal stump under what are often challenging conditions. The authors are so impressed with these advantages that even with destructive rectal injuries and associated risk factors, it is their practice to perform resection, primary anastomosis, and proximal fecal diversion with a loop colostomy.

Although the authors recognize the existing variation in opinion, the era of popularized running fascial closures has enhanced their commitment to leaving the skin incision open after repair of traumatic colon injuries. Even thin patients with minimal gross fecal spill receive "sleeper stitches" in the skin with large air knots placed in 3-0 nylon suture, allowing for wet-to-dry gauze dressing changes. Because the overwhelming majority of patients with gunshot wounds to the colon are still in the hospital at day 5, the appearance of a granulating base in the wound would prompt the authors to cut the air knot and achieve secondary skin approximation by tying the suture. This is a bedside procedure that is accomplished without so much as local anesthesia. This pathway avoids the scenario of a primarily closed

---

BOX 1: Operative principles for managing small and large bowel injuries

1. Completely define all injuries with proper dissection.
2. Grade injuries according to severity.
3. Decide on type of repair: simple repair or resection and repair.
4. Débride all devitalized tissue.
5. Resect bowel that has any evidence of ischemia.
6. Establish clean bowel edges in the area of repair.
7. Use absorbable suture if a stapling technique is not employed. A second interrupted seromuscular layer may be added.
8. Repair lacerations transversely to avoid strictures.
9. Close mesenteric defects.
10. Irrigate peritoneal cavity with warm saline solution.

FIGURE I Small bowel injury necessitating resection. **A,** The bowel is clamped proximally and distally to the perforation while dividing the mesentery. **B,** The injured segment of bowel is resected. **C,** A single-layered anastomosis is performed with a running absorbable 3-0 using the Lembert suture technique, inverting the posterior wall. **D,** Then completing the suture on the anterior surface. **E,** The mesentery is then reapproximated. (Modified from Thal ER, Weigelt JA, Carrico CJ, editors: Operative trauma management, an atlas, ed 2, New York, 2001, McGraw-Hill, p. 207. Reproduced with permission from the McGraw-Hill Companies.)

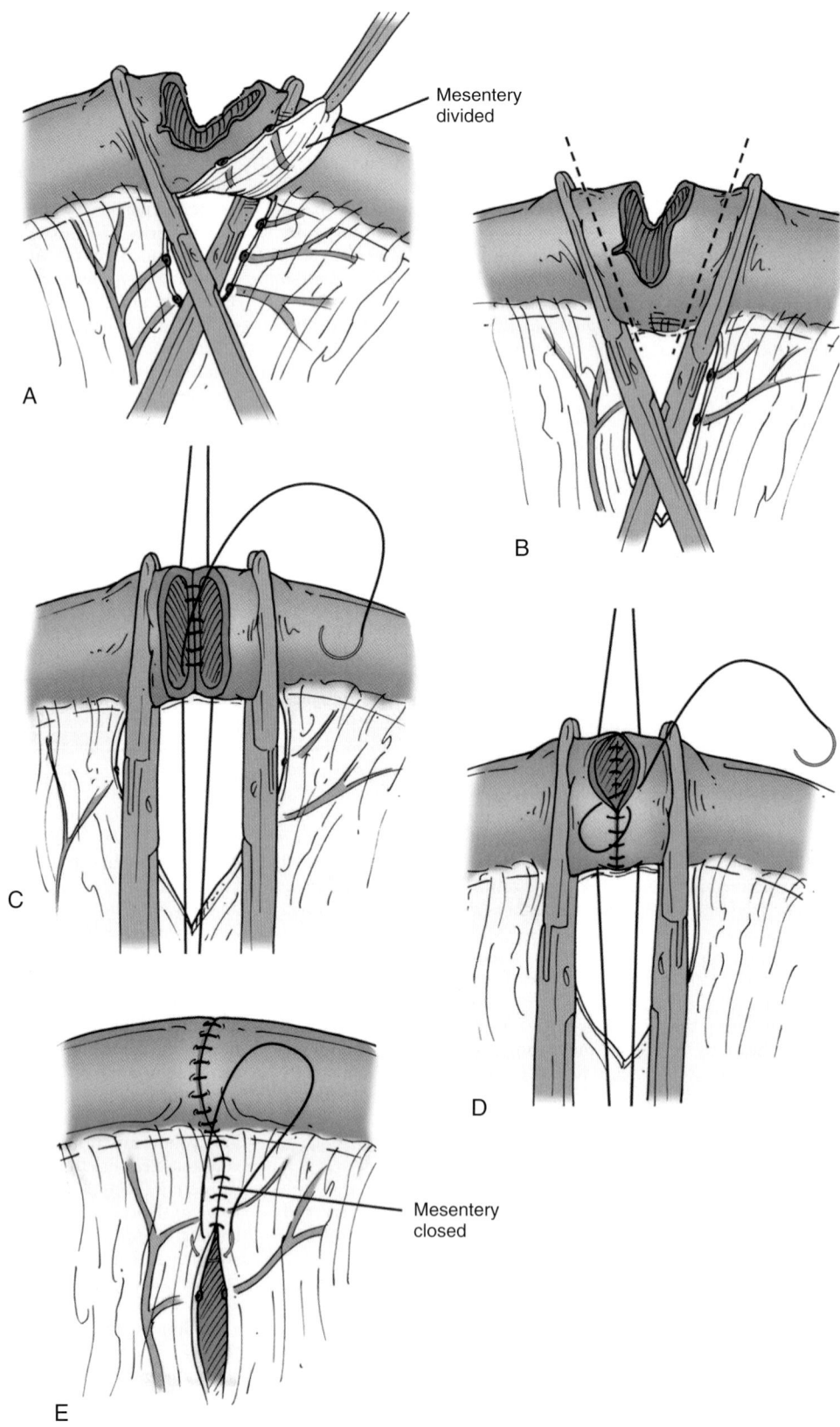

Mesentery divided

Mesentery closed

skin incision after a case of contamination in which subcutaneous wound infection and signs of inflammation may escape early detection in an obese patient or one with a dark complexion. A delay in detection of subcutaneous space infection, combined with a running fascial closure, is a recipe for regional fascial necrosis and subsequent fascial dehiscence.

In the damage control setting, as with small bowel injuries, the authors recommend performing a primary anastomosis instead of leaving the bowel in discontinuity. At the time of the primary operation, the formation of a colostomy is not recommended.

Complications after colon repair remain an important concern. The most common complication includes anastomotic leaks or suture line failure. The rate of these complications is fortunately low (between 2% and 9% of cases). Colon leaks can result in intra-abdominal abscesses, fecal fistulas, and in some cases severe intra-abdominal sepsis that leads to death. Fistulas and abscesses can be managed nonoperatively by appropriate diet and antibiotic treatment. Intra-abdominal sepsis may necessitate reoperation and possible proximal diversion. The overall mortality rate after colonic anastomotic leaks is about 0.1%. Ostomy formation carries its own complications, including necrosis, infection, retraction, prolapse, parastomal abscesses and hernias, skin irritation, and significant emotional trauma. Severe or early minor complications have been reported in up to 22% of cases and late complications in about 3% of cases.

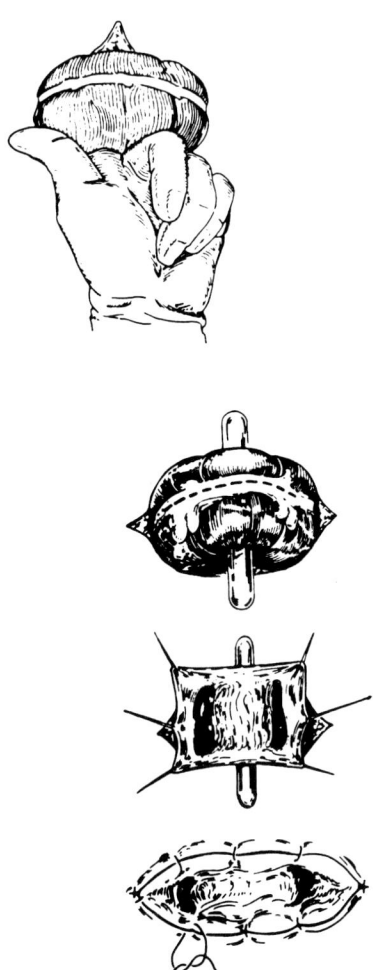

FIGURE 2   Formation of a loop colostomy. A segment of large bowel is eviscerated through a defect in the abdominal wall. The posterior wall is maintained above the level of the skin with the benefit of a red rubber catheter. Securing the catheter to the skin an angle towards the distal lumen achieves luminal occlusion and functional diversion. The colon edges are approximated to the skin by first passing the suture through the full thickness of the colon, then a more proximal seromuscular bite, and finally through the dermis.

SUGGESTED READINGS

Brownstein MR, Bunting T, Meyer AA, et al: Diagnosis and management of blunt small bowel injury: a survey of the membership of the American Association for the Surgery of Trauma, *J Trauma* 48(3):402–407, 2000.

Committee on Trauma, American College of Surgeons: *National Trauma Data Bank: Admission years 2007–2010, User Manual*, Chicago, 2011.

Cornwell EE 3rd, Velmahos GC, Berne TV, et al: The fate of colonic suture lines in high-risk trauma patients: a prospective analysis, *J Am Coll Surg* 187(1):58–63, 1998.

Demetriades D: Colon injuries: new perspectives, *Injury* 35(3):217–222, 2004.

Demetriades D, Velmahos G, Cornwell E 3rd, et al: Selective nonoperative management of gunshot wounds of the anterior abdomen, *Arch Surg* 132(2):178–183, 1997.

Watts DD, Fakhry SM, EAST Multi-Institutional Hollow Viscus Injury Research Group: incidence of hollow viscus injury in blunt trauma: an analysis from 275,557 trauma admissions from the EAST multi-institutional trial, *J Trauma* 54(2):289–294, 2003 [erratum, in: *J Trauma* 54(4):749, 2003].

THE MANAGEMENT OF RECTAL INJURIES

David J. Ciesla, MD, and John Y. Cha, MD

OVERVIEW

Surgical management of colon and rectal injuries has evolved dramatically since World War II. Accepted treatment at that time generally consisted of resection and end colostomy based on experience with battlefield casualties. Although a difference between civilian and military injuries was recognized, the treatment by civilian trauma surgeons paralleled that of their military counterparts. In the most recent decades, treatment based on anatomic level of rectal injury has replaced mandatory colostomy as the sole approach. Similarly, adjuncts to repair, such as presacral drainage and distal rectal irrigation, have been used selectively to good effect.

Mechanisms of rectal injuries can be classified as direct penetration of the bowel wall by a foreign body, high-pressure blowout of the bowel wall as occurs in blunt trauma, and rarely, a devascularization injury from avulsion of the supporting mesentery. Approximately 80% of rectal injuries are caused by firearms, 10% by blunt trauma, 6% by transanal or impalement injuries, and 3% by trans-abdominal stab wounds.

DIAGNOSIS

The approach to diagnosis of rectal injuries is determined by the injury mechanism and index of suspicion. Patients with pelvic fractures, truncal gunshot and stab wounds, or impalements of the lower abdomen, buttocks, perineum, or upper thighs and any patient with a history of anal manipulation and lower abdominal or pelvic pain are at risk and should be suspected of having a rectal injury. The incidence rate of rectal injury in patients with pelvic fractures sustained during high-energy transfer mechanisms can be as high as 1%. Evaluation begins with a digital rectal examination in which the presence of gross blood should trigger further investigation. However, a negative digital rectal examination does not rule out a rectal injury. Although an organ-specific diagnosis is rarely made before surgery in the setting of an acute abdomen, free intraperitoneal air may occasionally be seen on chest x-ray or abdominal computed tomographic (CT) scan. Suspicion of enteric injury should be raised in all patients with evidence of fever, tachycardia, peritonitis, and leukocytosis.

In the preoperative setting, rigid proctosigmoidoscopy should be performed in all patients with suspected rectal injury. Transanal palpation or visualization of a perforation is diagnostic. Occasionally, intraluminal blood or submucosal hematoma is the only evidence of rectal injury. Therefore, these patients should be treated in the same manner as patients with confirmed rectal injuries. Suspicion of intraperitoneal involvement warrants abdominal exploration. Diagnostic laparoscopy has been proposed to evaluate peritoneal violation in patients with stable conditions with low-velocity transpelvic gunshot and stab wounds with conversion to celiotomy on identification of intraperitoneal injury. In any case, determination of the anatomic location of rectal injury is important because it is a key factor in choosing the appropriate therapeutic strategy.

Most rectal injuries are discovered during abdominal exploration after an abdominal gunshot wound. As such, a thorough evaluation of the pelvis during a systematic abdominal exploration is important immediately after control of life-threatening hemorrhage. Superior displacement of the small bowel exposes the structures of the pelvis. This is best accomplished with cephalad retraction of the viscera and mesentery, with only the distal colon and rectum left in the pelvis. Blood and enteric contents are then evacuated with laparotomy pads, and the peritoneal surfaces are inspected for violation or underlying hematoma. Although penetrating rectal injuries to the extraperitoneal rectum are usually obvious, missed injuries are often the result of small-caliber gunshot wounds or stab wounds to areas that are difficult to examine, such as the rectosigmoid junction and the proximal retroperitoneal rectum. Opening of the peritoneum and mobilization of the proximal retroperitoneal rectum can easily be accomplished. However, proceeding more distally simply for diagnosis is not recommended because of the potential for iatrogenic, vascular, urologic, neurologic, or additional rectal injury. When necessary for hemorrhage control, the presacral space is developed with blunt dissection posterior to the rectum in the sacral hollow. Most presacral bleeding is effectively managed with packing with laparotomy pads and can be supplemented with topical clotting adjuncts, such as a slurry of particulate gel foam suspended in activated thrombin. Patients who have undergone laparotomy for hemorrhage control with a suspicion of distal penetrating rectal injury should have the abdomen temporarily closed and be repositioned for proctoscopy.

ANATOMIC LOCATION OF INJURY AND INJURY GRADING

The rectum begins at the rectosigmoid junction and ends at the dentate line in the anal canal. Blood is supplied by the superior hemorrhoidal branch of the inferior mesenteric artery and the middle and inferior hemorrhoidal branches of the internal iliac or internal pudendal arteries. Venous drainage of the rectum follows the arteries, with the superior hemorrhoidal vein draining into the portal system and the middle and inferior hemorrhoidal veins draining via the internal iliac veins. The rectum can be further divided into intraperitoneal and extraperitoneal zones that help guide surgical decision making (Figure 1). The Organ Injury Scaling Committee of the American Association of the Surgery of Trauma (AAST) has developed a rectal injury scale (RIS) that facilitates comparison of injuries between patients and facilities and helps identify patients at high risk for postoperative complications (Table 1).

SURGICAL MANAGEMENT

The anatomic level, degree of injury, and physiologic state of the patient governs the surgical management of rectal injuries. Nondestructive injuries to the proximal intraperitoneal and extraperitoneal rectum that do not require resection based on intraoperative

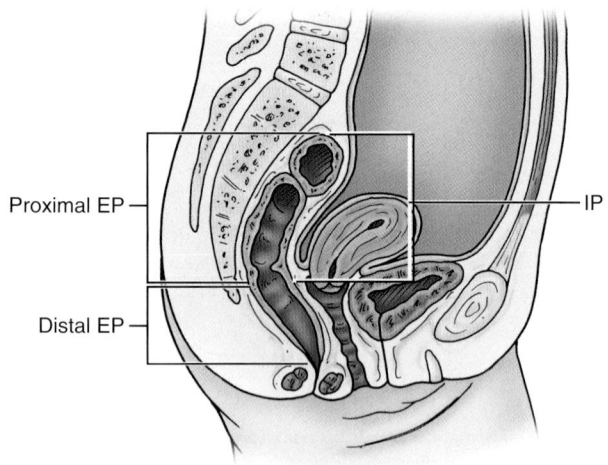

FIGURE I The intraperitoneal *(IP)* and extraperitoneal *(EP)* divisions of the rectum. *(From Weinberg JA, Fabian TC, Magnotti LJ, et al: Penetrating rectal trauma: management by anatomic distinction improves outcome,* J Trauma 60[3]:508-514, 2006.)

TABLE 1: American Association of the Surgery of Trauma rectal injury grading

	Grade	Injury description
I	Hematoma	Contusion or hematoma without devascularization
	Laceration	Partial thickness, no perforation
II	Laceration	Laceration < 50% of circumference
III	Laceration	Laceration > 50% of circumference
IV	Laceration	Full-thickness laceration with extension into perineum
V	Vascular	Devascularized segment

Note: Advance one grade for multiple injuries to the same organ.
Modified from Organ Injury Scaling Committee of the American Association of the Surgery of Trauma. Moore EE, Cogbill TH, Malangoni MA, et al: Organ injury scaling II: pancreas, duodenum, small bowel, colon and rectum, J Trauma 30:1427, 1990.

evaluation (AAST RIS I to III) are repaired primarily. These injuries are generally lacerations with minimal surrounding tissue destruction that are easily exposed after mobilization of the proximal rectum and sutured. A running single layer of 3-0 absorbable monofilament suture is used. With repair of rectal gunshot wounds, débridement of the devitalized edges of the wound back to healthy bleeding bowel wall is important before suture repair. Placement of drains in the pelvis after primary repair of proximal rectal injuries is not necessary and may increase the risk of fistula.

Proximal rectal injuries with extensive loss of the rectal wall or devascularization (AAST RIS IV and V) are generally treated with resection distal to the injury and proximal end colostomy followed by delayed reconstruction. If necessary, the rectum can be divided within a few centimeters of the anal verge with the aid of a thoracoabdominal (TA) stapler after mobilization of the distal rectum. In addition, the advent of the end-to-end circular stapling device has facilitated elective colostomy closure. This has proved to be a much safer approach to destructive colon injuries than primary repair. Select patients with minimal coincident injuries, minimal contamination, and normal physiology are candidates for resection and immediate primary colorectal anastomosis. Patients with extensive abdominal injuries, significant contamination, or persistent shock should undergo resection and proximal diversion. A damage control posture should be adopted in patients with a persistent base excess of −10 or less, a temperature less than 33°C, and refractory nonsurgical bleeding. After surgical control of hemorrhage, fecal contamination can be controlled with stapled division or resection of the injured segment of rectum followed by temporary abdominal closure, resuscitation, and return to the operating room once the acidosis, hypothermia, and coagulopathy are corrected.

Wounds to the distal extraperitoneal rectum are generally treated with proximal diverting colostomy. As mentioned previously, extensive dissection to definitively visualize distal rectal injuries offers no advantage and should be avoided because of the potential for vascular, urologic, neurologic, or iatrogenic rectal injury. Although several methods for open and laparoscopically assisted proximal diversion are described, the chosen technique must completely divert the fecal stream from the rectal injury. The authors use a loop colostomy located in the patient's left lower quadrant with the sigmoid colon (Figure 2). The critical technical elements to ensure complete

diversion are creation of a longitudinal colotomy, maintenance of the common wall or spur between the afferent and efferent limbs above the level of the skin, and maturation of the stoma to the skin immediately. A loop colostomy created in this manner completely diverts the fecal stream. Same admission colostomy closure can be considered 7 to 10 days after injury in select patients with radiographic (contrast enema) evidence of rectal wound healing. Successful nonoperative management of isolated nondestructive distal rectal injuries without proximal diversion has been reported. Candidates for treatment without diversion are limited to those in whom intraperitoneal rectal injury and bladder injury have been excluded.

Distal rectal washout has been advocated as a means to reduce the septic complications associated with rectal injuries based on military experience but has not consistently been associated with improved outcome in the civilian setting. The authors use a selective approach based on the level of injury and the chosen repair. In general, the rectal contents are removed during diagnostic proctosigmoidoscopy, either before or during the main operation. Patients with proximal nondestructive rectal injuries are generally repaired primarily without distal rectal washout unless the stool burden is large. In such cases, the injury is repaired and the washout is performed with transanal irrigation and manual expulsion of rectal contents with the aid of rigid proctosigmoidoscopy. The repair is always reinspected after expulsion of stool to ensure its integrity. Patients with destructive proximal rectal injuries undergoing resection and anastomosis or proximal diversion generally receive transanal distal rectal irrigation with the aid of rigid proctosigmoidoscopy of the rectal stump. The authors do not routinely perform distal rectal washout of patients with distal rectal injuries that are not repaired, whether or not a proximal diverting loop colostomy is created.

Presacral drainage has long been considered an integral component of treatment of distal rectal injures. The principal is to drain the presacral space of perirectal contamination resulting from violation of the bowel and avoid the potential for pelvic sepsis. Several authors have reported successful management of distal rectal injuries without presacral drainage in both the presence and the absence of proximal diversion. Nonetheless, many still advocate its use, reasoning that the minimal morbidity of presacral drainage is outweighed by the risk of pelvic sepsis and its attendant morbidity and mortality. For destructive injuries with contamination, proceeding with presacral drainage seems most prudent. A curved incision is made posterior to the anus, and the presacral space is developed bluntly to the level of the sacral hollow (see Figure 2). Ideally, Penrose drains are placed in proximity but not in contact with the injury. The drains are secured to the skin with silk sutures for better patient comfort and usually removed between 4 and 7 days after placement.

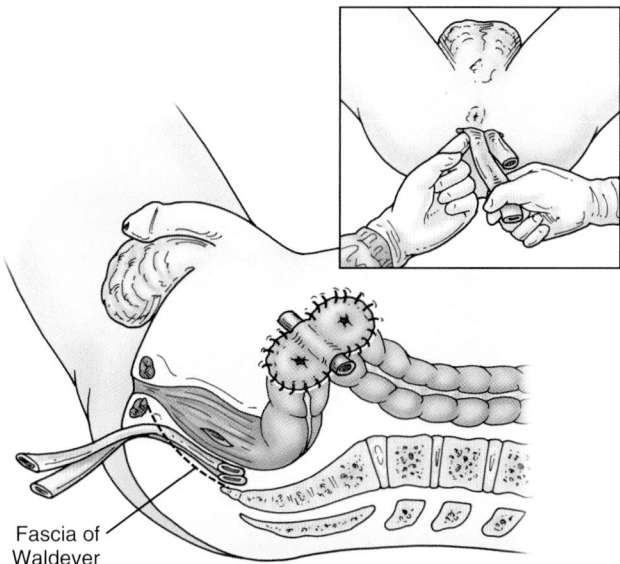

FIGURE 2 Technique for presacral drainage and proximal diversion for treatment of occult or unrepaired distal colon injuries. *(Courtesy Baylor College of Medicine.)*

Fascia of Waldeyer

MORBIDITY AND COMPLICATIONS MANAGEMENT

Intra-abdominal abscess is the most frequent septic complication after rectal injury. Small abscesses of less than 2 cm often respond to intravenous antibiotic therapy and do not require drainage. Many intra-abdominal abscesses can be managed with image-guided percutaneous drainage. Occasionally, percutaneous drainage reveals an underlying fistula. In such cases when the patient has no evidence of sepsis, the percutaneous drain is left in place until imaging shows obliteration of the abscess cavity. Once this occurs, the drain is slowly removed. Larger intra-abdominal abscesses that are inaccessible to percutaneous drainage and those associated with sepsis require operative drainage.

Suture line failure and fecal fistula are observed in 1% to 8% of patients. Fistulas that extend to the incision are often associated with intra-abdominal abscesses and evidence of sepsis. A fistulogram should also be performed to determine whether there is

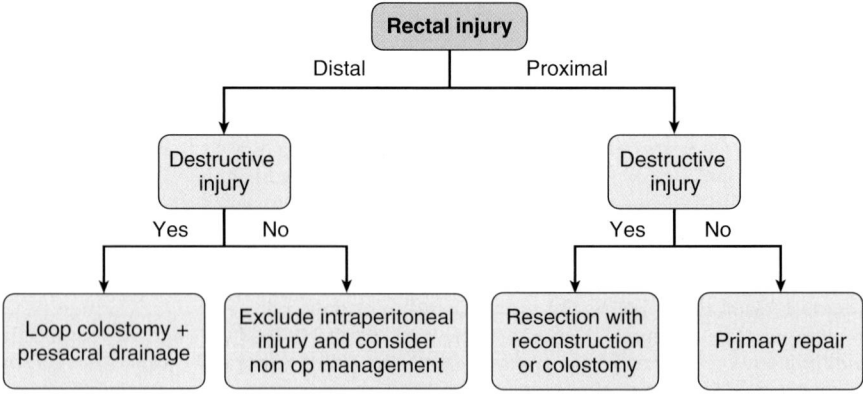

FIGURE 3 Algorithm for the management rectal injuries.

diffuse leakage throughout the abdominal cavity, and an abdominal CT scan is obtained to look for intra-abdominal abscesses. A controlled fistula can be managed nonoperatively, but the wound must be carefully inspected for evidence of necrotizing fasciitis. Uncontrolled fistulae require operative intervention and are usually treated with resection and proximal diversion with an end colostomy.

Wound infections occur in up to 50% of patients with colon or rectal injuries but should not be considered a complication of the repair. Virtually all wound infections can be avoided by leaving the wound open at the time of abdominal closure. Closure of the wound during the initial operation should be reserved for the patient with few associated injuries, minimal subcutaneous fat, and little contamination and without prolonged shock.

CONCLUSION AND ALGORITHM

As with colon injuries, the management of rectal injuries has progressed from near universal treatment with diversion to selective management according to injury characteristics and risk of complications. Prompt recognition, hemorrhage control, and control of enteric spillage are the immediate management priorities, followed by repair or diversion. Although more severe injuries in patients with compromised conditions are still best treated with repair or resection, proximal diversion, and presacral drainage, it is recognized that some patients with limited injuries can be successfully treated with a less invasive approach. With these considerations, the authors have adopted an approach to injuries outlined in Figure 3. The critical decision-making points are level of injury, the extent of tissue destruction, and the metabolic state of the patient.

The first consideration is the location of the injury. Nondestructive intraperitoneal and proximal extraperitoneal injuries are repaired primarily, and destructive injuries are resected. Reconstruction via

colocolostomy is preferred for patients with minimal additional injuries and an appropriate physiologic condition. Resection and proximal diversion is performed in patients with more extensive injuries and persistent shock. Destructive distal rectal injuries are treated with proximal diversion and presacral drainage. Isolated nondestructive distal injuries are considered for nonoperative management. In cases that are unclear, a more aggressive traditional approach of diversion and drainage is favored.

SUGGESTED READINGS

Burch JM, Feliciano DV, Mattox KL: Colostomy and drainage for civilian rectal injuries: is that all? *Ann Surg* 209(5):600–611, 1989.

Gonzalez RP, Falimirsky ME, Holevar MR: The role of presacral drainage in the management of penetrating rectal injuries, *J Trauma* 45(4):656–661, 1998.

Gonzalez RP, Phelan H, Hassan M, et al: Is fecal diversion necessary for non-destructive penetrating extraperitoneal rectal injuries? *J Trauma* 61:815–819, 2006.

Ivatury RR, Licata J, Gunduz Y, et al: Management options in penetrating rectal injuries, *Am Surg* 57(1):50–55, 1991.

Moore EE, Cogbill TH, Malangoni MA, et al: Organ injury scaling: II: pancreas, duodenum, small bowel, colon, and rectum, *J Trauma* 30(11):1427–1429, 1990.

Navsaria P, Edu S, Nicol AJ: Civilian extraperitoneal rectal gunshot wounds: surgical management made simpler, *World J Surg* 31:1345–1351, 2007.

Renz BM, Feliciano DV, Sherman R: Same admission colostomy closure (SACC): a new approach to rectal wounds: a prospective study, *Ann Surg* 218(3):279–293, 1993.

Rombeau JL, Wilk PJ, Turnbull RB Jr, et al: Total fecal diversion by the temporary skin-level loop transverse colostomy, *Dis Colon Rectum* 21(4):223–226, 1978.

Vitale GC, Richardson JD, Flint LM: Successful management of injuries to the extraperitoneal rectum, *Am Surg* 49(3):159–162, 1983.

Weinberg JA, Fabian TC, Magnotti LJ, et al: Penetrating rectal trauma: management by anatomic distinction improves outcome, *J Trauma* 60(3):508–514, 2006.

INJURY TO THE SPLEEN

Ho Phan, MD, and
Christine S. Cocanour, MD, FACS, FCCM

OVERVIEW

The spleen is the most commonly injured organ in blunt abdominal trauma. The management of splenic injury has fluctuated over the past century from observation and expectant management in the early twentieth century to primarily operative management for all injuries, and now to the current practice of selective nonoperative management (NOM). The shift in treatment is a result of our changing technology and understanding of the spleen's role in immunologic function.

The spleen's role in immunologic response was demonstrated in a publication by Morris and Bullock in 1919, revealing an increase in mortality in postsplenectomized rats challenged with *Bacterium enteritidis* compared to controls. The risk of postsplenectomy infection was not demonstrated in humans until 1952 in a landmark paper by King and Shumacker. In this case series, the authors described death due to sepsis in two of five infants who had undergone splenectomy for congenital hemolytic anemia. Subsequently, several authors noted this increased rate of overwhelming sepsis in adults. The reported rate of postsplenectomy overwhelming sepsis varies depending on the age at splenectomy and indications, with the highest risk in very young children and in patients undergoing splenectomy for hematologic disorders. Although the rate of sepsis after splenectomy is low, it is a lifelong risk for these patients. This knowledge led to an increased emphasis on splenic preservation.

Initially attempted in children, comfort grew with NOM of splenic injury in adults as computed tomography (CT) became more widely available and with the realization that negative laparotomies carry significant morbidity. As angioembolization techniques become more refined, it is increasingly used as an adjunct to NOM, with improvement in NOM success.

DIAGNOSIS

The initial management of all trauma patients should follow the guidelines of the American College of Surgeons Advanced Trauma Life Support. Trauma patients often have multiple confounding injuries that make physical examination unreliable. Therefore, the diagnosis of splenic injury relies on a high index of suspicion. Factors that should increase the index of suspicion include hypotension, abdominal ecchymosis, abdominal pain or tenderness, presence of lower left rib fractures, and presence of pelvic fractures. It is important to point out that the presence of acute hemoperitoneum does not always lead to abdominal pain and tenderness, especially in the absence of clot lysis. Referred left shoulder pain (Kehr sign) is not reliably present, but even if present, it is often confounded by multiple injuries.

Diagnostic and management decisions in patients with blunt splenic injury rely heavily on the presence or absence of hemodynamic stability and the response to resuscitation. The initial evaluation and management of patients with blunt splenic injury is summarized in Figure 1. During the initial assessment, blood should be drawn for laboratory testing, including hemoglobin, electrolytes, markers of metabolic stress (base deficit or lactate), coagulation profile, and blood typing. Intravenous access should be obtained for resuscitation and potential intravenous contrast administration. A hypotensive, patient who does not respond to fluid resuscitation or who only transiently responds to fluid administration should undergo a focused assessment with sonography for trauma (FAST) examination. A positive FAST examination indicates presence of peritoneal fluid and, in the case of a trauma patient, hemoperitoneum until proven otherwise. An emergent laparotomy is indicated in these patients. For patients who are unstable and have a negative FAST examination, intra-abdominal hemorrhage is not reliably excluded. FAST may be repeated in 15 to 30 minutes or a diagnostic peritoneal aspirate (DPA) or lavage (DPL) should be considered as the next step to rule out intra-abdominal hemorrhage. Other alternative causes of hemorrhagic shock, such as thoracic injuries, pelvic injuries, external blood loss, or other types of shock, should be considered. For patients without a clear source of hemorrhage and who remain unstable despite resuscitation, immediate laparotomy should be considered.

The FAST examination evaluates three areas of the abdomen for the presence of intra-abdominal fluid: the hepatorenal fossa (Morrison's pouch), the splenorenal fossa, and the area around the bladder. A fourth view evaluates the pericardium for pericardial fluid. The presence of fluid in any of these locations indicates a positive examination. Like other sonographic studies, the accuracy of FAST is operator dependent and limited by the patient's body habitus and presence of subcutaneous emphysema. FAST only allows determination of the presence of fluid within the abdominal cavity. It does not provide the source of the fluid or evaluation of the retroperitoneum. The reported sensitivity of FAST varies. Generally, FAST has a sensitivity of 80% and specificity of 96%; however, at some large trauma institutions, the sensitivity may be as low as 50%. The false negative rate for FAST is higher in the setting of pelvic trauma, thoracolumbar spine fracture, hematuria, and rib fractures.

When FAST is negative, the suspicion for intra-abdominal hemorrhage remains high, and the patient remains too unstable to be safely taken to the CT scanner, DPA may quickly provide an answer. It is the aspiration portion of the diagnostic peritoneal lavage without the lavage. When performed percutaneously, DPA is rapid and safe, and it does not have the high sensitivity of DPL. In a small prospective, observational trial, DPA had a sensitivity of 89% and a specificity of 100%.

For patients deemed hemodynamically stable, intravenous contrast-enhanced CT scan of the abdomen and pelvis is the study of choice for diagnosis of splenic injury. It allows for the grading of splenic injuries as developed by the American Association of the Surgery of Trauma (Table 1). When a single-phase CT scan identifies contrast extravasation outside the splenic parenchyma, it usually indicates active splenic hemorrhage, whereas a focal accumulation of contrast within the parenchyma is often a contained vascular injury. Contrast extravasation or "blush" has been used in the past to predict failure of NOM, guide selection for angioembolization, or even laparotomy. With the introduction of multidetector row CT systems in 1998, CT scanning is more rapid and has better spatial resolution, which has led to a greater sensitivity in detecting "blush." However, with the greater sensitivity, it is not unusual to find no active bleeding on angiography in patients identified with a contrast "blush" on CT scan. Only 5% to 7% of all patients with blunt splenic injury have been found to have extravasation of contrast requiring angioembolization.

NONOPERATIVE MANAGEMENT

Selective nonoperative management is the standard of care for the hemodynamically stable patient with a blunt splenic injury in the absence of peritonitis. NOM should only be considered in environments that have the capability of monitoring and providing serial clinical exams and that have an operating room available for emergent laparotomy. Original exclusions for NOM in adults suggested

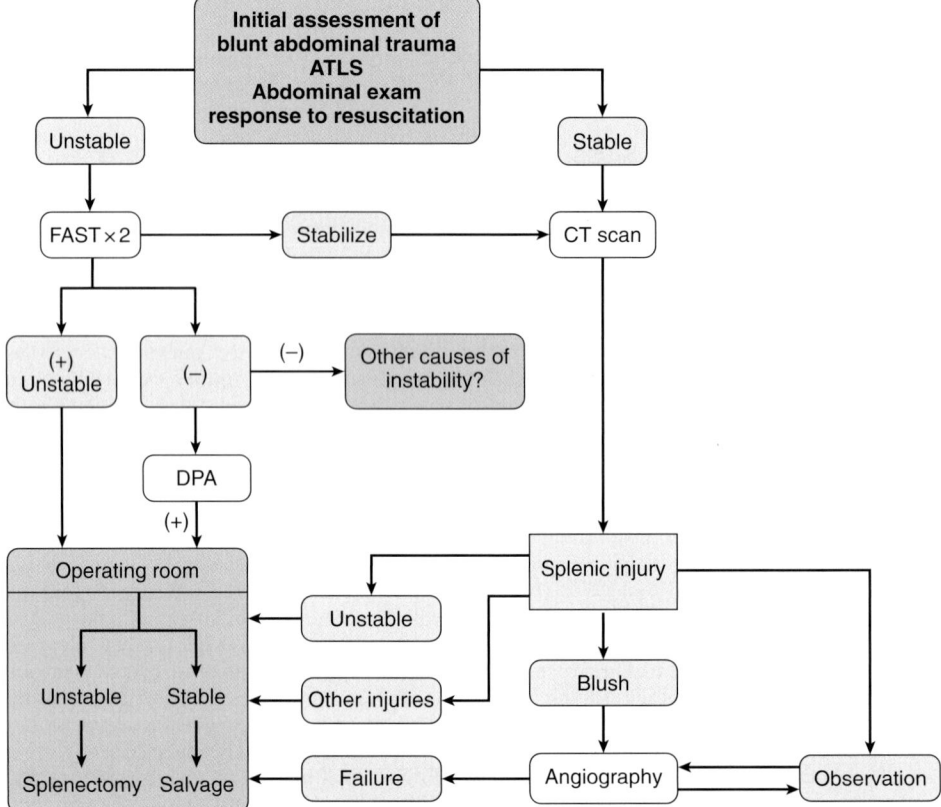

FIGURE 1 Algorithm for management of blunt splenic injury. *ATLS,* Advanced trauma life support; *CT,* computerized tomography; *DPA,* diagnostic peritoneal aspiration; *FAST,* focused abdominal sonography for trauma. *(Adapted from Moore FA, Davis JW, Moore EE, et al: Western Trauma Association (WTA) Critical decisions in trauma: management of adult blunt splenic trauma, J Trauma 65:1007-1011, 2008.)*

TABLE 1: Spleen injury scale

Grade	Injury	Description
I	Hematoma	Subcapsular, >10% surface area
	Laceration	Capsular tear, <1 cm parenchymal depth
II	Hematoma	Subcapsular, 10% to 50% surface area, intraparenchymal, <5 cm in diameter
	Laceration	1-3 cm parenchymal depth that does not involve a trabecular vessel
III	Hematoma	Subcapsular, >50% surface area or expanding; ruptured subcapsular or parenchymal hematoma
	Laceration	>3 cm parenchymal depth or involving trabecular vessels
IV	Laceration	Laceration involving segmental or hilar vessels producing major devascularization (>25% of spleen)
V	Laceration	Completely shattered spleen
	Vascular	Hilar vascular injury that devascularizes spleen

Modified from Moore EE, Cogbill TH, Jurkovich GJ, et al: Organ injury scaling: spleen and liver (1994 revision), J Trauma 38:323-324, 1995.

that a high grade of injury, head trauma, quantity of hemoperitoneum, age greater than 55, contrast "blush," and a large number of associated injuries precluded the ability to offer NOM. However, more recent literature has shown that the severity of splenic injury (by either grade or amount of hemoperitoneum), age greater than 55, neurologic injury, presence of contrast "blush," and associated injuries should no longer be considered as absolute contraindications to NOM. Although found in only 0.3% of all blunt trauma admissions, hollow viscous injury as suggested by peritonitis, increasing abdominal pain, or suspicion for hollow viscous injury mandates exploration.

Angiography and embolization are controversial adjuncts to NOM. First described by Sclafani in 1996, embolization allows an improved splenic salvage rate, especially for grades III to V. Its success and acceptance are most likely tempered by the availability and skill of the interventionalist. Indications for angiography with embolization in blunt splenic trauma include contrast "blush" on CT with evidence of ongoing hemorrhage, pseudoaneurysm, AAST grades IV and V, moderate hemoperitoneum, or clinical evidence of continued hemorrhage. Multiple studies have shown improved success of NOM with its use. A NOM failure rate of 13% to 15% dropped to as low as 2% with embolization.

There is concern that the small increase in splenic salvage rate is not worth the 19% risk of major complications and 23% risk of minor complications reported in early studies. Major, potentially life-threatening complications include continued hemorrhage, total splenic infarction, splenic abscess, contrast-induced nephropathy, pancreatitis, and pneumonia. Minor, non–life-threatening complications include fever, pleural effusion, partial splenic infarction, pain, coil migration, and puncture site injuries. Bleeding is the most common complication and has been reported in 5% to 24% of those undergoing embolization. Minor complications such as fever are seen in over 50% of patients undergoing embolization. Centers where angiography and embolization for splenic injury are common often report low numbers of complications.

Controversy exists over embolization techniques. In experienced hands there is no difference in outcome when main splenic coil embolization is compared to distal or combined proximal and distal embolization. Although there is concern that embolization leads to splenic necrosis and negates the advantage of splenic salvage, recent studies have shown that splenic embolization does not impact immune function.

Roughly 85% of patients with blunt splenic injury are managed nonoperatively with over a 90% success rate. Patients with high-grade injury, large hemoperitoneum, vascular blush, pseudoaneurysm, and arteriovenous fistula are all at high risk of failure of NOM. Velmahos and colleagues found that of 40% of patients with grade IV splenic injuries treated nonoperatively, 65.5% were successful. Sixteen percent of patients with grade V injuries were treated nonoperatively, and 40% were successful. Of those patients who do fail, approximately 75% will fail within 48 hours of injury, 88% within 5 days, and 93% within 1 week of injury. In a review of a statewide discharge database, the 180-day risk of splenectomy following NOM and discharge home was 1.4%. Patients must be given specific discharge instructions about what symptoms may indicate a need for rapid return to the hospital.

Controversy continues to reign over the hospital management of a patient with blunt splenic injury treated nonoperatively. The frequency of serial hemoglobins, abdominal exams, and monitoring; determining when an oral diet should be started; deciding whether to use bed rest; determining the optimum length of stay in both the intensive care unit (ICU) and the hospital; determining the necessity of repeat imaging; and setting limitations on activities after discharge are all questions in which definitive data are lacking. As resources have become more limited, recent studies have attempted to address the optimal care of the patient with blunt splenic injury without sacrificing safety. A retrospective study found that early mobilization did not alter the risk of delayed hemorrhage and that bed rest was unnecessary. Recently published protocols suggest that grade I splenic injuries can be discharged as early as 1 to 2 days after injury if their hemoglobin is stable and vital signs remain normal. Grade II and higher injuries differ between published protocols. Most will discharge grade II injuries when the hemoglobin is stable and vital signs are normal. Grade III injuries and above are admitted to the ICU and had a minimum overall length of stay of at least 3 days. Figure 2 is a suggested management guideline for patients chosen for NOM. Each institution will need to modify this depending on its resources and patient population.

Repeat imaging in patients managed nonoperatively is controversial. Most repeat CT scans did not change patient management. An Eastern Association for the Surgery of Trauma survey found that only 14.5% of surveyed surgeons routinely obtain follow-up CT scans. Those physicians who routinely reimage splenic injuries with CT scans and angioembolize as indicated believe that their aggressive approach greatly contributes to their high NOM success rate. Currently, there is not enough evidence to recommend routine follow-up CT scans.

Clinical judgment is the predominant factor in determining a return to activity, including contact sports for patients with blunt splenic injuries treated nonoperatively. Restrictions may be recommended for less than 6 weeks for grades I and II injuries and longer than 6 months for grades IV and V injuries. The American Pediatric Surgical Association published management guidelines in 2000 for return to unrestricted activity that included "normal" age-appropriate activities that suggested 3 to 6 weeks for grades I to IV, respectively. Return to full-contact, competitive sports was left at the discretion of the pediatric surgeon.

PENETRATING SPLENIC INJURY

Penetrating abdominal injuries due to gunshot wounds are usually managed by laparotomy. Isolated stab wounds to the spleen may undergo a trial of NOM. However, splenic injuries from penetrating trauma are often accompanied by injuries to the bowel. Penetrating injuries to the spleen tend to violate intraparenchymal anatomic planes, and as a consequence, arterial injury and subsequent pseudoaneurysm formation are common. Because of the risk of delayed bleeding, splenectomy should be considered at the initial exploration. If it is an isolated splenic pole injury that can be treated by resection of the injured segment of the spleen, splenorrhaphy may be considered in the absence of accompanying bowel injury.

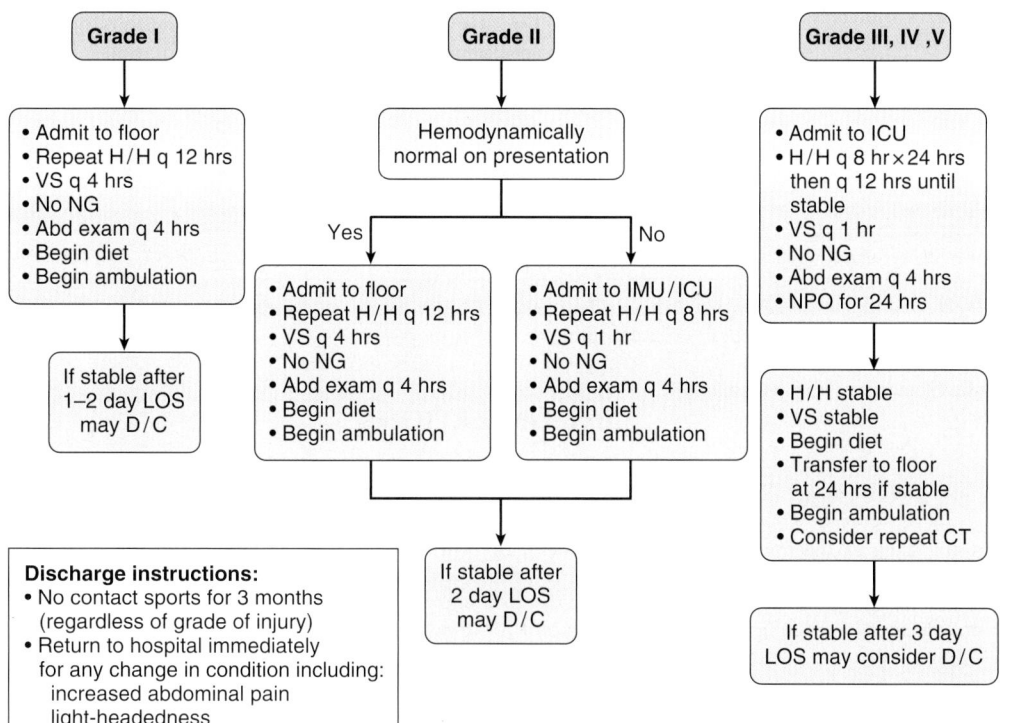

FIGURE 2 Suggested management guidelines for those patients chosen for nonoperative management (NOM). A "stable" hemoglobin is defined as a decline of 0.5 g or less. *D/C,* Discharge; *H/H,* hemoglobin/hematocrit; *LOS,* length of stay; *Abd,* abdominal; *NG,* nasogastric tube; *VS,* vital signs. *(Adapted from Cocanour CS: Blunt splenic injury,* Curr Opin Crit Care *16:575-581, 2010.)*

OPERATIVE MANAGEMENT

When it is determined that the patient with blunt splenic injury requires operative management, preparation for trauma laparotomy is essential. Blood is sent for crossmatch, and preoperative antibiotics are given. The patient should be placed in a supine position and is induced under general anesthesia. The patient's chest, abdomen, pelvis, and midthighs are prepped and sterilely draped. All measures to prevent hypothermia should be instituted, including using only warm intravenous (IV) fluids.

A midline incision is made that extends from the xyphoid to the pubic symphysis. Upon entering the abdomen, blood and clots are rapidly evacuated, and the abdomen is packed in all four quadrants to control hemorrhage. The priority should be given to hemorrhage control first followed by control of gastrointestinal contamination. The presence of clots in a particular quadrant should provide a clue as to where the source of hemorrhage may be. Active hemorrhage should first be controlled, and then the rest of the abdomen should be inspected systematically.

To adequately evaluate the injured spleen, it must be completely mobilized from all of its attachments and brought to the midline. Splenic attachments are shown in Figure 3. The left costal margin is retracted laterally and superiorly to facilitate exposure. The surgeon's hand is placed posterior to the spleen, and the spleen is rotated medially to expose the lienophrenic and lienorenal ligaments. By compressing the spleen against the spine medially with the surgeon's hand, bleeding from the spleen can be temporarily controlled. The lienophrenic and lienorenal ligaments are generally avascular and can be divided either with cautery or Metzenbaum scissors. Sometimes, these ligaments have to be divided by feel with scissors because exposure is not always adequate. The surgeon's index finger is inserted under the cut lienorenal ligament, and with a combination of blunt and sharp dissection, the spleen is freed from Gerota's capsule and the diaphragm. In the same plane, the surgeon's hand slides to the posterior surface of the tail of the pancreas, and both the spleen and the tail of the pancreas are elevated to the midline incision. It is helpful at this point to place a few laparotomy pads in the splenic fossa to help elevate the spleen. The lienocolic ligament is then divided, freeing the spleen from the omentum and colon. This ligament generally contains small vessels that require ligation. The short gastric vessels are then ligated and divided at this time, freeing the spleen from the stomach. Care should be taken during this step to ligate the short gastric vessels far from the stomach to prevent entrapment of the stomach wall. A nasogastric tube in the stomach can be used as traction, which helps expose the short gastric vessels for ligation.

At this point the spleen is mobile on its vascular pedicle and can be adequately inspected. If splenectomy is required, the splenic artery and vein are suture ligated close to the spleen to avoid injury to the tail of the pancreas. The splenic bed is then inspected to ensure hemostasis. Using a rolled-up laparotomy pad in the deepest part of the fossa and slowly rolling the pad anteriorly and medially allow systematic inspection of the fossa. The tail of the pancreas should be inspected for injury. If injury to the tail of the pancreas is suspected, a closed-suction drain should be placed near the tail of the pancreas. Routine use of drains after splenectomy is not recommended because it is associated with increased incidence of subphrenic abscess.

Most patients with splenic injuries are taken to the operating room for hemodynamic instability. Therefore, the most prudent operation is splenectomy. Splenic salvage should be considered only in hemodynamically stable patients who are not coagulopathic or hypothermic. Grades I and II injuries can be controlled with electrocautery, argon beam coagulation, and application of topical hemostatic agents. Sutures buttressed with omentum, Teflon, absorbable mesh, and oxidized regenerated cellulose (Surgicel; Ethicon, Inc., Somerville, NJ) have been described for higher-grade

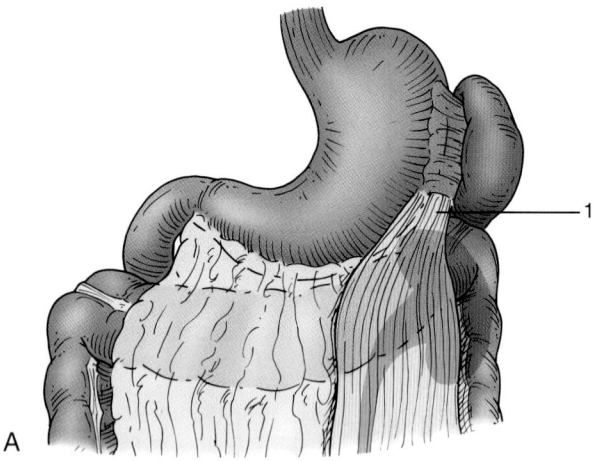

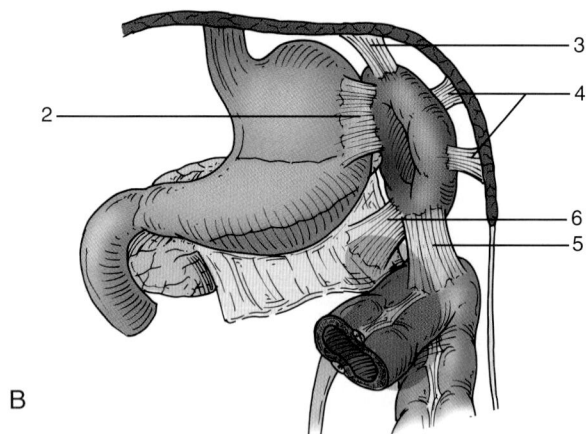

FIGURE 3 Splenic attachments encountered when completely mobilizing the spleen. **A,** Lieno-omental peritoneal band *(1)*. **B,** Lienogastric ligament *(2)*, lienophrenic ligament *(3)*, lateral perisplenic adhesions *(4)*, lienocolic ligament *(5)*, and lienorenal ligament *(6)*. *(Adapted from Cooper CS, Cohen MB, Donovan JF, Jr: Splenectomy complicating left nephrectomy, J Urol 155:30-36, 1996.)*

injuries. If simple hemostatic methods do not work, splenectomy should be considered. More aggressive approaches to splenorrhaphy could be considered in very young children who are hemodynamically stable.

IMMUNIZATIONS

The Surgical Infection Society guidelines recommend that patients undergoing splenectomy should receive pneumococcal vaccine and meningococcal vaccine, and for high-risk patients, *Haemophilus influenza* vaccine. The optimal time for vaccinations for patients undergoing splenectomy for trauma is 14 days postoperatively. However, due to concern for lack of follow-up, many institutions give vaccinations prior to discharge. Pneumococcal vaccination should be repeated 5 years after the first dose.

SUGGESTED READINGS

Cocanour CS: Blunt splenic injury, *Curr Opin Crit Care* 16:575–581, 2010.

Moore FA, Davis JW, Moore EE Jr, et al: Western Trauma Association (WTA) critical decisions in trauma: management of adult blunt splenic trauma, *J Trauma* 65:1007–1011, 2008.

Stassen NA, Bhullar I, Cheng JD, et al: Selective nonoperative management of blunt splenic injury: an Eastern Association for the Surgery of Trauma practice management guideline, *J Trauma Acute Care Surg* 73:S294–S300, 2012.

Stylianos and the APSA Trauma Committee: Evidence-based guidelines for resource utilization in children with isolated spleen or liver injury, *J Pediatr Surg* 35:164–169, 2000.

Velmahos GC, Zacharias N, Emhoff TA, et al: Management of the most severely injured spleen, *Arch Surg* 2145:456–460, 2010.

RETROPERITONEAL INJURIES: KIDNEY AND URETER

**Benjamin N. Breyer, MD, MAS, and
Jack W. McAninch, MD, FACS**

KIDNEY

Overview

The kidney is the most common genitourinary organ injured from external trauma, occurring in 1% to 5% of all injuries. The vast majority of kidney injuries can be successfully managed nonoperatively. Blunt traumas are more frequent than penetrating (around an 80:20 ratio). Penetrating trauma is more common in urban areas, is commonly caused by gunshot or stab wounds, and more commonly requires exploration. Blunt trauma results from falls from heights, motor vehicle and motorcycle crashes, or blunt assaults. An estimated 2% of blunt injuries require exploration as opposed to over 50% of penetrating injuries.

Similar to other solid organ injuries such as spleen and liver, advances in staging techniques (computed tomographic scan) have helped promote nonoperative management of renal injuries. Nevertheless, certain severely injured kidneys require exploration and reconstruction or, rarely, removal. Advances in embolization techniques have produced a useful adjunct treatment modality for renal trauma. Ultimately, the objective of managing these patients is to stem life-threatening bleeding while retaining enough nephron mass to avoid end-stage renal disease.

Initial Evaluation

The initial evaluation begins with the American College of Surgeons Acute Life Support Program algorithm of airway, breathing, circulation (external bleeding control), disability (neurologic status), and exposure (undress)/environment (temperature control). Subsequently, one should perform a history and physical examination, including blood pressure measurements to assess for shock (systolic blood pressure [SBP] <90 mm Hg) and an examination for gross or microscopic hematuria. Microhematuria is commonly defined as greater than three red blood cells per high-powered field on urine microscopy. Hematuria is a common sign of penetrating and blunt trauma, but the presence and degree of hematuria do not correlate

with injury location and severity. This is particularly true for penetrating injuries where no hematuria may be present. The first void should be observed and analyzed because hematuria may clear quickly in the setting of aggressive fluid resuscitation. Hematuria helps guide whether imaging is needed.

Blunt Trauma

The suspected blunt renal trauma algorithm is shown in Figure 1. The mechanism of trauma should be documented. For motor vehicle collisions, the speed and angle of impact and whether the patient was restrained or ejected on impact are important history to gather. One should record the height from which the patient fell, whether a significant deceleration injury occurred, or where on the body a blunt assault was perpetrated.

Signs of renal injury on physical exam include flank ecchymoses, rib fractures, and transverse spinal process fractures. Minor trauma can cause significant damage to congenitally abnormal kidneys such as horseshoe or pelvic kidneys that are less protected from external trauma.

Penetrating Trauma

The suspected penetrating renal trauma algorithm is shown in Figure 2. Understanding the mechanism of injury is again important. If a knife was used, noting the size of the blade can help with determining the depth of penetration. If a firearm was used, knowledge of the type of bullet (high-velocity vs low-velocity) can provide information about injury extent. High-velocity bullets cause blast effects and will often produce delayed tissue necrosis. Low-velocity missiles are less devastating.

Stab wounds or bullet entry locations should be noted. Abdominal stab wounds anterior to the anterior axillary line (a vertical line that runs along the anterior axillary fold or armpit crease) that injured the kidney are often associated with current commitment abdominal injuries. Renal injuries posterior to this line may injure the ascending or descending colon but are less likely to injure intra-abdominal contents.

Children

Children under 16 require increased suspicion for renal injury because of anatomic and physiologic differences from adults. They have relatively large kidneys, underdeveloped Gerota's fascia and less perirenal fat, incomplete ossification of the lower ribs, and kidneys that are located in the abdomen and are less protected by the ribs. Shock is an unreliable indicator of injury extent in children because they can have a robust catecholamine response to stress that can mask severe blood loss.

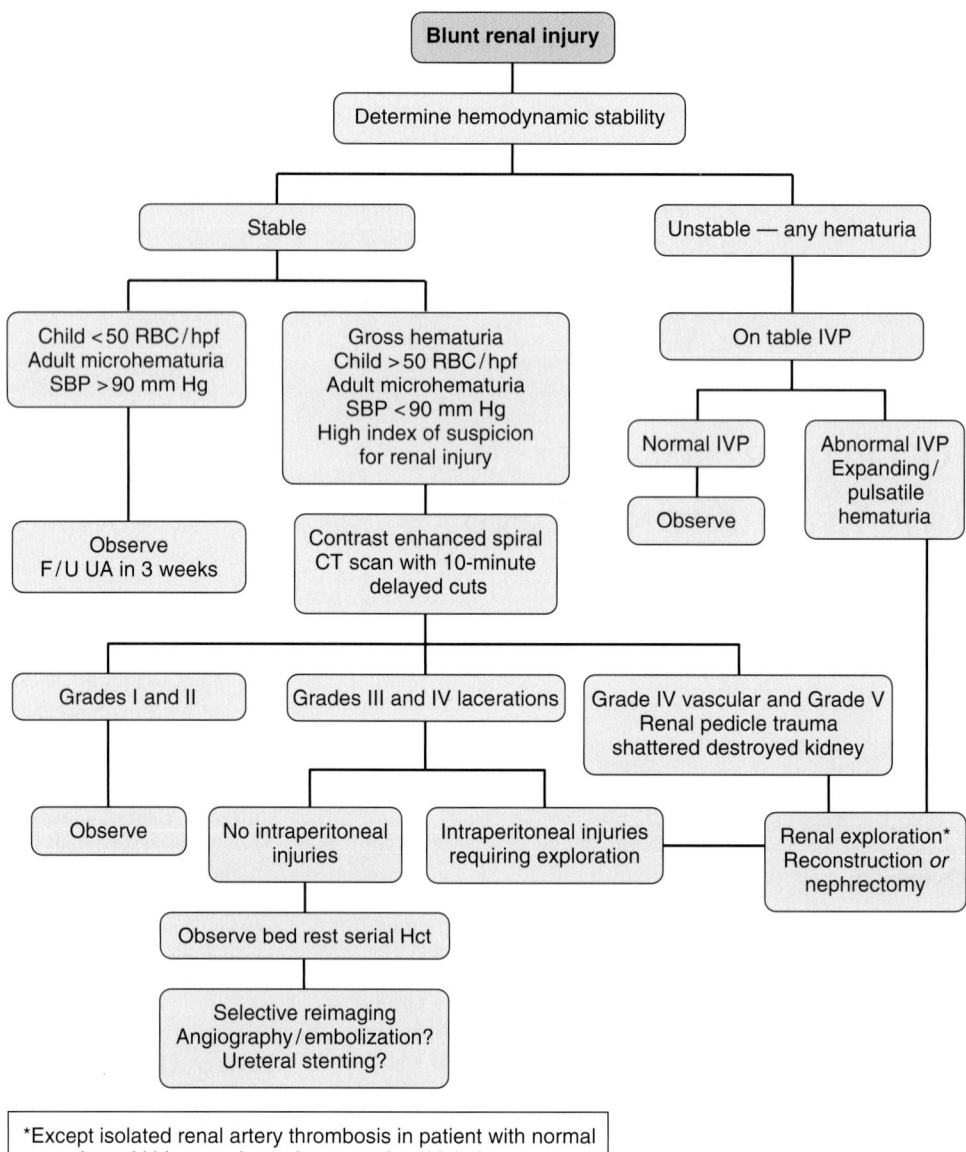

FIGURE 1   Blunt renal trauma algorithm. *CT,* Computed tomography; *F/U,* follow up; *Hct,* hematocrit, *hpf,* high-power field; *IVP,* intravenous pyelogram; *RBC,* red blood count; *SBP,* systolic blood pressure; *UA,* urinalysis. *(From Santucci RA, Wessells H, Bartsch G, et al: Evaluation and management of renal injuries: consensus statement of the renal trauma subcommittee,* BJU Int *93:937, 2004.)*

Indications for Renal Imaging

Decisions regarding whether to image are predicated on mechanism (blunt/penetrating), presence of hematuria (gross/microscopic), and shock (blood pressure of less than 90 mm Hg). In adults, blunt trauma with gross hematuria should prompt imaging, as should blunt trauma with microscopic hematuria and shock. In adults with blunt trauma, microscopic hematuria without shock has not been associated with significant injury and does not call for imaging. Major acceleration or deceleration injuries such as a fall from a great height or a high-speed motor vehicle accident should prompt imaging.

In adults with penetrating injuries, any degree of hematuria or injury location suspicious for renal injury should prompt imaging. Lower thresholds to image children exist given their anatomic differences. Any pediatric trauma (younger than 16 years) with any degree of significant hematuria (greater than 50 red blood cells per high-powered field) should be imaged.

Imaging Studies

Computed Tomography

Contrast enhanced computed tomographic (CT) scan with additional 10-minute delay scans is the gold standard imaging modality to stage the stable renal trauma patient and is both sensitive and specific for renal injuries. Expert opinion contends that no delays are required if the kidneys are uninjured and no perinephric, retroperitoneal pelvic or perivesical fluid is present. CT helps to delineate concurrent abdominal solid organ and vascular injuries. With CT imaging, one can determine the size and location of perinephric hematomas, the degree of parenchymal laceration, collecting system injuries, differential contrast uptake and excretion indicative of arterial injury or obstruction, a cortical rim sign indicating an arterial injury, and the degree of devitalized tissue. A renal vein injury can be subtle and marked by a hematoma medial to the renal artery and vein, while medial arterial contrast excretion represents a major

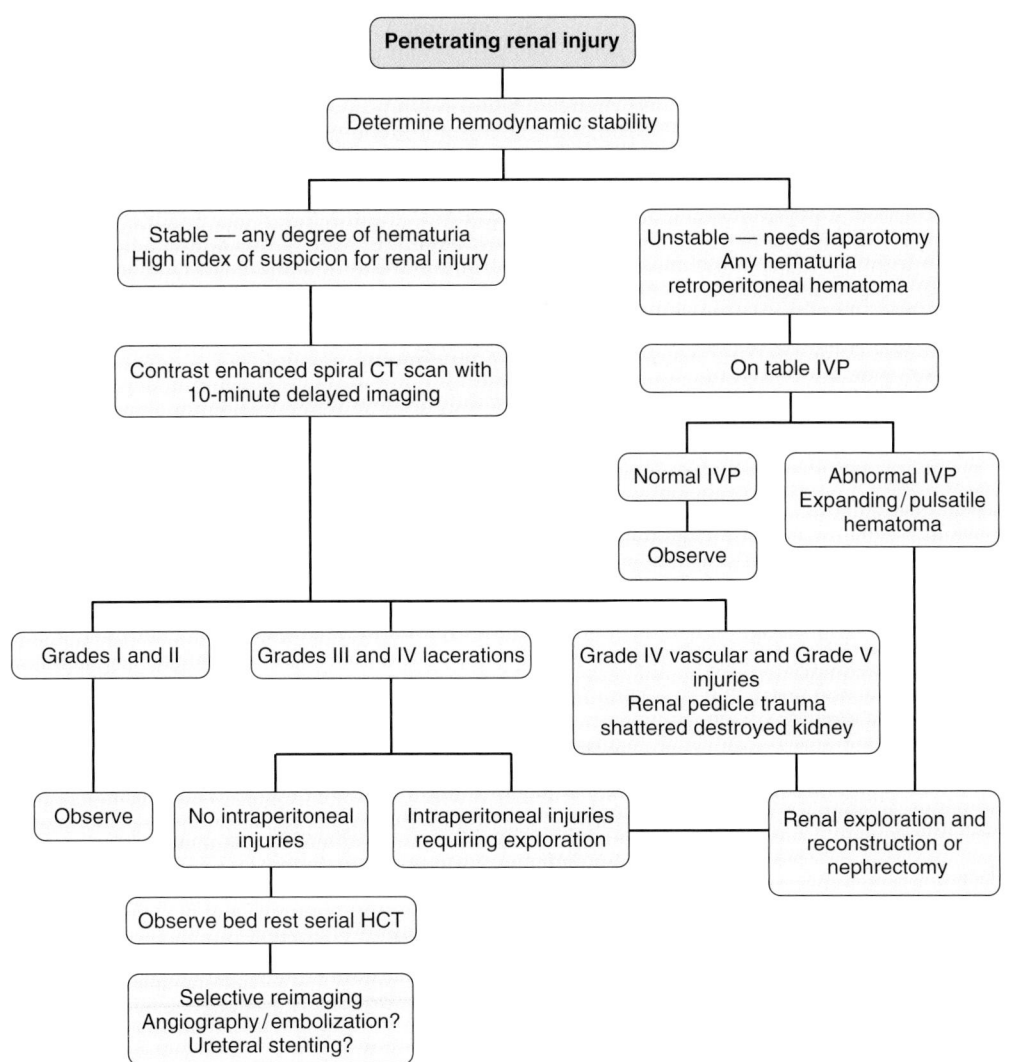

FIGURE 2 Penetrating renal trauma algorithm. *CT,* Computed tomography; *Hct,* hematocrit; *IVP,* intravenous pyelogram. *(From Santucci RA, Wessells H, Bartsch G, et al: Evaluation and management of renal injuries: consensus statement of the renal trauma subcommittee, BJU Int 93:937, 2004.)*

arterial injury. Medial urinary contrast excretion may indicate a major tear in the ureteropelvic junction, while this finding teamed with a lack of distal contrast excretion suggests ureteropelvic junction avulsion.

Ultrasound

While ultrasound (US) is a widely used imaging tool in the assessment of the abdominal trauma patient, it is not an effective modality to image acute kidney injuries. The kidney is bound by Gerota's fascia, and unless there are tears in the fascia, retroperitoneal bleeding will not be visualized. Ultrasound cannot reliably differentiate urine and blood. US can provide rapid, inexpensive, and noninvasive imaging of the abdomen. The focused assessment with sonography for trauma (FAST) is frequently used to identify intra-abdominal fluid and abdominal injuries.

Intravenous Pyelogram

While CT scan has replaced intravenous pyelogram (IVP) as the imaging modality of choice for the traumatized urinary system, IVP still plays a role in genitourinary trauma staging. In patients directly taken to the operating suite without CT staging of their kidney or ureteral injury, a one-shot IVP can help indicate the presence of a contralateral functioning kidney and indicate possible collecting system or ureteral injury. An IVP may demonstrate an abnormal renal outline, loss of the psoas margin, or displacement of the bowel or ureter suggestive of a hematoma. Patients found to have a solitary functioning kidney require every attempt possible to save the kidney, as even a portion of a solitary kidney can keep someone off dialysis. Opponents of the one-shot IVP contend it causes unneeded delays during critical moments in the trauma suite. While opponents advocate simple palpation to verify the contralateral kidney, the surgeon can be fooled by a prominent psoas muscle. The one-shot IVP is performed by administering 2 mL/kg body weight of contrast medium followed by a plain film x-ray of the kidneys, ureters, and bladder (KUB) 10 minutes later. IVP should only be employed in normotensive patients, as the timing of imaging in hypotensive patients is difficult when the kidneys are poorly perfused.

Angiography

Angiography and subsequent super-selective embolization therapy for renal trauma have evolved and have a place in the treatment armamentarium of renal trauma patients. Super-selective coil embolization provides an effective and minimally invasive means to stop bleeding. Given that the majority of the renal injuries can be managed conservatively, care should be taken to avoid needless embolizations. The kidney is an end arterial organ that lacks significant collateral arterial blood supply, and as such, embolization will cause nephron death in addition to causing bleeding cessation.

Injury Scale for the Kidney

The American Association for the Surgery of Trauma renal organ injury scale is shown in Table 1. Grading is important clinically to help guide management and for outcomes research. The renal injury classification is one of the few classifications schemes that have been prospectively validated and found to correlate directly with the need for surgical intervention. Grades I and II injuries are minor, Grade III injuries are intermediate, and Grades IV and V injuries are severe. Grade I injuries include subcapsular nonexpanding hematomas without parenchymal laceration. Grade II injuries include lacerations in the parenchyma less than 1 cm. Grade III is a laceration greater than 1 cm that does not extend into the collecting system. Grade IV includes parenchymal lacerations extending into the collecting system and main vascular injuries with contained hemorrhage. Grade V includes shattered or avulsed kidneys.

Management

Nonoperative Management

The vast majority of renal injuries can be managed nonoperatively. Improvements in the reliability of staging imaging have resulted in increased nonoperative management. In addition, as surgeons have increasingly managed other solid organ injuries such as spleen and liver nonoperatively, there has been a rise in the nonoperative management of kidney injuries.

After appropriate staging, patients are typically managed with bed rest, hemodynamic monitoring, and serial hematocrits. Some evidence suggests that bed rest can be avoided unless hematuria increases

or resumes after ambulation. Transfusions should be given as needed, but when more than 6 units are needed or hemodynamic instability develops, repeat imaging and possible embolization or surgical exploration may be needed.

Conservatively managed kidneys with collecting system injuries should be reimaged 3 to 5 days later to evaluate persistent urine leak or urinoma formation. Patients with large leaks are typically managed with indwelling stents, while large or infected urinomas are drained percutaneously. For patients with a urine leak, Foley catheter drainage is used to decompress the urinary system, and antibiotic therapy is used to prevent infected urinomas.

Indications for Embolization

Angiography and embolization are recommended for (1) patients with persistent bleeding from a segmental renal artery, (2) unstable patients with a Grade III or IV renal injury, (3) treating a pseudoaneurysm or arteriovenous malformation, (4) cases of persistent gross hematuria, and (5) a rapidly declining hematocrit requiring 2 units of blood.

Indications for Renal Exploration

Absolute indications for renal exploration include expanding, pulsatile, uncontained retroperitoneal hematomas; renal pedicle avulsion; persistent, life-threatening hemorrhage or shock; and ureteropelvic junction disruption.

Relative indications for renal exploration include urinary extravasation with nonviable tissue; concurrent colon/pancreas/trauma exploration with incomplete staging or Grade III or greater concurrent renal injury; renovascular hypertension; and failed embolization.

Surgical Management

Retroperitoneal Exploration

Controversy exists regarding whether to obtain proximal vascular control for every operative renal injury. Some advocate a lateral approach by medializing the overlying colon and approaching the vasculature after dissecting the kidney from Gerota's fascia, dissecting lateral to medial with respect to the great vessels. Manual compression or a Satinsky clamp can be used to stop bleeding, and the kidney can then be repaired. Proponents of this method argue that it takes less time, and, particularly for lateral parenchymal injuries, isolating each vessel for possible clamping is overkill.

We contend that early vascular control can decrease the nephrectomy rate. Unplanned nephrectomy in a trauma setting results from uncontrolled hemorrhage. If approached in a systematic fashion, vascular control can be done quickly and efficiently.

The approach to the injured kidney is made through a standard trauma laparotomy midline incision from the pubic symphysis to the xiphoid process. The incision should be extended to the xiphoid if not already done so to gain exposure to the renal hilum. A fixed retractor such as the Bookwalter may be employed, but more typically the surgical assistants will perform manual retraction.

The transverse colon is wrapped in a moist laparotomy sponge and placed on the chest. The small intestine can be placed in a bowel bag or protected with moist lap sponges and retracted superiorly and placed on the chest to the right. This maneuver exposes the root of the mesentery, the ligament of Treitz, and the underlying great vessels. The retroperitoneum is incised over the aorta superior to the inferior mesenteric artery, and the incision is extended to the ligament of Treitz. Occasionally, a retroperitoneal hematoma can prevent distinct palpation of the aorta. An incision can be made medial to the inferior mesenteric vein because it runs a few centimeters to the

TABLE 1: American Association for the Surgery of Trauma: injury scale for the kidney

Grade*	Type	Description
I	Contusion	Microscopic or gross hematuria, urologic studies normal
	Hematoma	Subcapsular, nonexpanding, and without parenchymal laceration
II	Hematoma	Nonexpanding perirenal hematoma confirmed to renal retroperitoneum
	Laceration	<1 cm parenchymal depth of renal cortex without urinary extravasation
III	Laceration	<1 cm parenchymal depth of renal cortex without collecting-system rupture or urinary extravasation
IV	Laceration	Parenchymal laceration extending through renal cortex, medulla, and collecting system
	Vascular	Main renal artery or vein injury with contained hemorrhage
V	Laceration	Completely shattered kidney
	Vascular	Avulsion of renal hilum, which devascularizes kidney

*Advance one grade for bilateral injuries up to Grade III.
Modified from Moore EE, Shackford SR, Pachter HL, et al: Organ injury scaling: spleen, liver, and kidney, J Trauma 29:1664-1666, 1989.

left of the aorta and is easily identifiable. March along the anterior surface of the aorta until the left renal vein is encountered at its crossing. Rarely (less than 5% of the time), the left renal vein will be retro-aortic. A vessel loop should be placed around the left renal vein, and this vessel can be used as a guide to help find the remaining renal vasculature, each of which is then encircled with a vessel loop but not clamped. The vast majority of bleeding can be controlled during repair with manual compression of the kidney; rarely will vessel occlusion be necessary (Figure 3).

After vascular control has been achieved, the injured kidney is exposed by mobilizing the ipsilateral colon along the white line of Toldt and reflecting it medially. Gerota's fascia is then incised along its lateral aspect. A lateral incision is important because it avoids accidentally dissecting the kidney subcapsularly, avoids ureter injury, and preserves perinephric fat for reconstruction. Preserving the renal capsule is important because this fascia is a strength layer needed during reconstruction and tearing it can result in more bleeding.

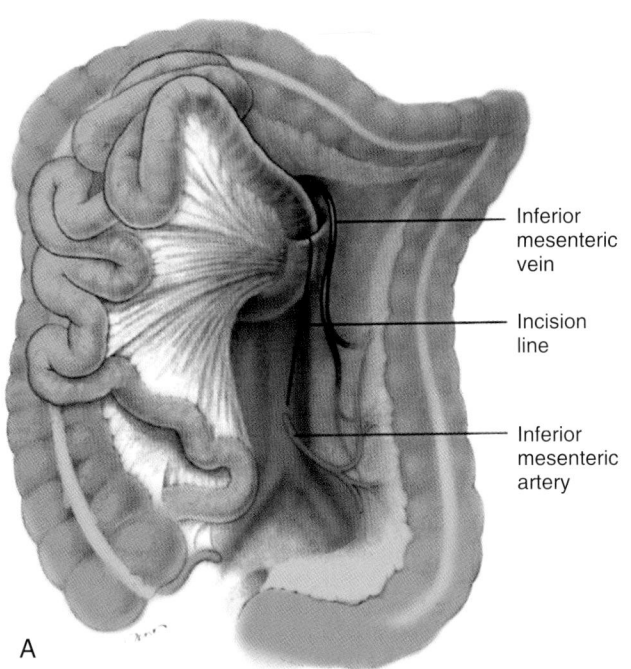

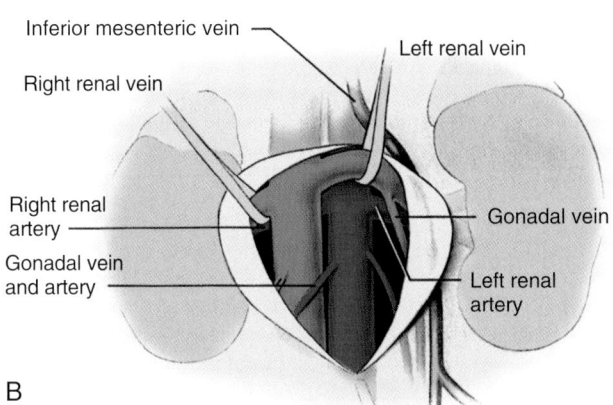

FIGURE 3 Technique to obtain vascular control. **A,** Exposure of the major vessels. **B,** Relationship of renal vasculature after incision of the posterior peritoneum over the aorta. *(From McAninch JW: Surgery for renal trauma. In Novick AC, Streem SB, Pontes JE, editors:* Stewart's operative urology, *Baltimore, 1989, Williams & Wilkins.)*

Renovascular Injuries

In contrast to parenchymal injuries, renovascular injuries are frequently irreparable and often result in nephrectomy. In cases where vascular injury is suspected, proximal vascular control is critical. Main renal vein injuries can result in significant hemorrhage and may require ligation. A partially lacerated vein may be repaired after it is controlled, clamped, and sutured with a 5-0 Prolene. Segmental and duplicated veins can be ligated given the extensive renal venous collateral circulation.

Arterial thrombosis or dissection in the setting of a normal contralateral kidney and no concurrent hemorrhage can be managed conservatively. A subset of these cases of nonperfusion of the kidney results from the spasm secondary to stretch injury. Follow-up imaging may demonstrate reperfusion of the kidney without intervention. In cases where these injuries are explored, efforts to perform a thrombectomy and débridement of the damaged arterial segment are often unsuccessful. Endovascular stents have been used to treat arterial thrombosis. Issues related to postoperative anticoagulation have limited their use. The ultimate outcome of attempted renal artery reconstruction is time dependent. Segmental arteries can be ligated safely. Partially lacerated segmental arteries can be repaired with 5-0 Prolene.

Renal Reconstruction

In a hemodynamically stable patient who is not coagulopathic, renal reconstruction should be employed. Heroic measures should be used in patients with solitary kidneys. The typical renal injury reconstruction is analogous in many ways to the repair performed during a partial nephrectomy for cancer. First, excellent exposure of the kidney should be provided. Bleeding should be limited either by manual compression or, in severe cases, vascular occlusion. Perform sharp excision of all nonviable parenchyma. Obtain meticulous hemostasis of individual bleeding vessels with stitches, cautery, or an argon beam. The collecting system should be closed in a watertight fashion. An antegrade ureteral stent can be placed for significant collecting system reconstructions. Parenchymal defects will be reconstructed by approximating capsular edges over a hemostatic dissolvable bolster such as Surgicel or thrombin-soaked Gelfoam. Omental interposition can be used to separate the injured kidney from concurrently injured abdominal organs (Figures 4 and 5).

Damage Control

In situations where the patient is unstable and the kidney is shattered or major vascular injury with hemorrhages is present, an expeditious nephrectomy can be lifesaving. Occasionally, it will be necessary after exsanguinating hemorrhage is controlled to pack the retroperitoneum, resuscitate the patient, and complete the repair later.

Complications

Complications after renal trauma are rare. They usually occur within the first month after trauma.

Early Complications

Urinoma formation and prolonged urinary extravasation are the most common complications and result from collecting system injury. When urinomas become infected, an abscess may form. Large urinomas or abscesses require percutaneous drainage. Prolonged urinary extravasation can typically be managed with a ureteral stent.

Late Complications

Late complications include delayed bleeding, abscess formation, urinary fistula, hypertension, and hydronephrosis. Delayed bleeding

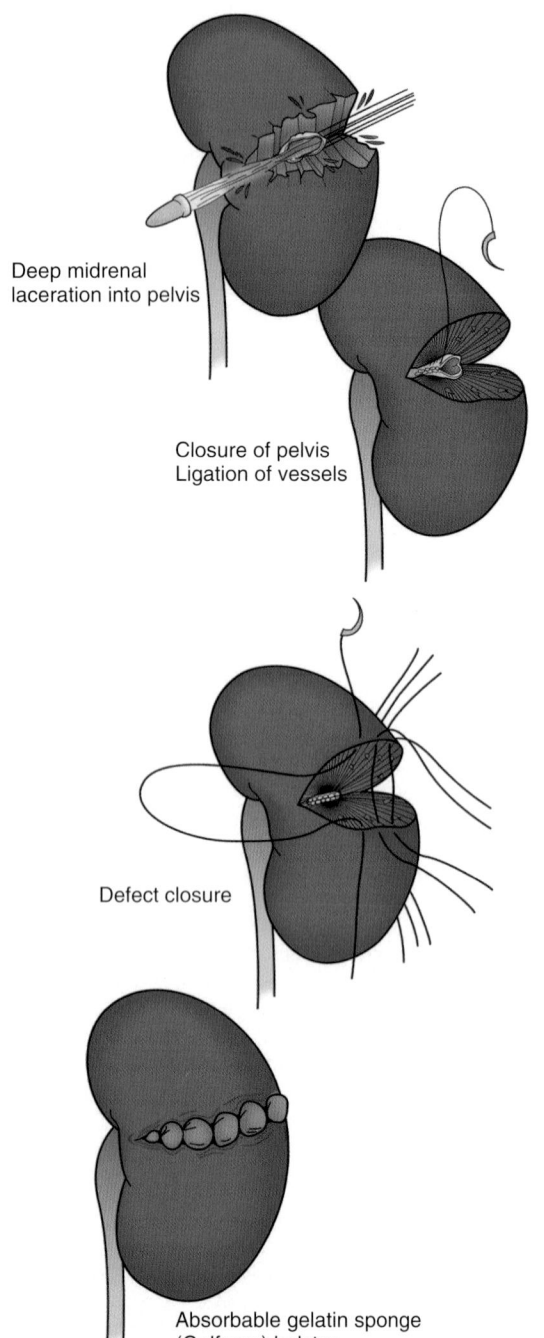

Deep midrenal
laceration into pelvis

Closure of pelvis
Ligation of vessels

Defect closure

Absorbable gelatin sponge
(Gelfoam) bolster

FIGURE 4 Example of renal repair after penetrating trauma. *(From Armenakas NA, McAninch JW: Genitourinary tract. In Ivatury RR, Cayten CG, editors: The textbook of penetrating trauma, Media, Penn, 1996, Williams & Wilkins.)*

is typically caused by a pseudoaneurysm or arteriovenous fistula, either from the initial injury or the repair, and presents 2 to 4 weeks after surgery. This can be effectively treated with coil embolization. Abscess formation is treated by percutaneous drainage and systemic antibiotics.

A delayed urinary fistula should be evaluated to determine its location. Concurrent ureteral stricture or injury may be discovered. An indwelling stent and/or percutaneous drainage of the kidney should be used with a delayed definitive repair 3 to 6 months later. Hypertension is a rare, long-term complication that results from either parenchyma compression (Page kidney) or arterial stenosis

(Goldblatt kidney) and chronic upregulation of the renin/angiotensin axis. Hypertension is usually controlled medically, although severe renal compression secondary to a hematoma detected in the postoperative period may benefit from immediate surgical decompression. Hydronephrosis may develop after perinephric fibrosis that involves injuries to the ureteropelvic junction or lower pole of the kidney. Interposition of the omentum or perinephric fat between the injured kidney and the ureter is recommended to prevent such a complication.

URETER

Overview

Most ureteral injuries are iatrogenic, with the most common cause being from abdominal hysterectomy. Ureteral injuries constitute less than 1% of genitourinary trauma. The ureter is protected by the vertebral column and major muscle groups. Typically, ureteral injury caused by external trauma results in severe concurrent injuries with a high mortality, including bowel perforations and renal and bladder injuries.

Initial Evaluation

External Trauma

Penetrating injuries to the ureter are infrequent, and blunt injuries are even more rare. As such, the appropriate diagnosis and treatment of ureteral injuries require a high index of suspicion and an in-depth knowledge of ureteral anatomy and its relation to adjacent structures. High-velocity projectiles can cause direct transection and also blast injury, compromise of intramural blood supply, and subsequent delayed necrosis. Damage can extend up to 2 cm from the site of transection, which often results in underestimation of tissue destruction. Débridement should be taken to the bleeding edge of the ureter. Blunt trauma such as a significant fall from a great height or a high-speed motor vehicle collision that results in extreme force applied over the body can result in ureteral injury. Fracture of the lumbar processes and thoracolumbar spinal dislocation can cause ureteral injury. This can result from hyperextension of the back, particularly in children, who are more flexible and more limber. In addition, rapid deceleration causes ureteral injury at fixed locations such as the ureteropelvic junction or the uretero vesical junction.

Iatrogenic

The most common iatrogenic injuries occur during urologic (ureteroscopy, radical prostatectomy), gynecologic (transabdominal hysterectomy, salpingo-oophorectomy, cystocele repair), colorectal, and vascular surgeries. Risk factors include uncontrolled hemorrhage and reoperative surgery.

Diagnosis of Ureteral Injury

A high index of suspicion is required for successful management of ureteral injuries. Intraoperative direct inspection is the most effective means of injury detection, although retroperitoneal hemorrhage can make detection more difficult. When a blast injury is suspected and no clear tissue destruction is identified, a small incision can be made in the ureter to verify adequate perfusion. Simple peristalsis of the suspect segment is not sufficient. With a small butterfly needle, methylene blue or indigo carmine dye can be injected into the collecting system or ureter to look for injury. If a concurrent bladder rupture repair is being performed, an exchange catheter or feeding tube can

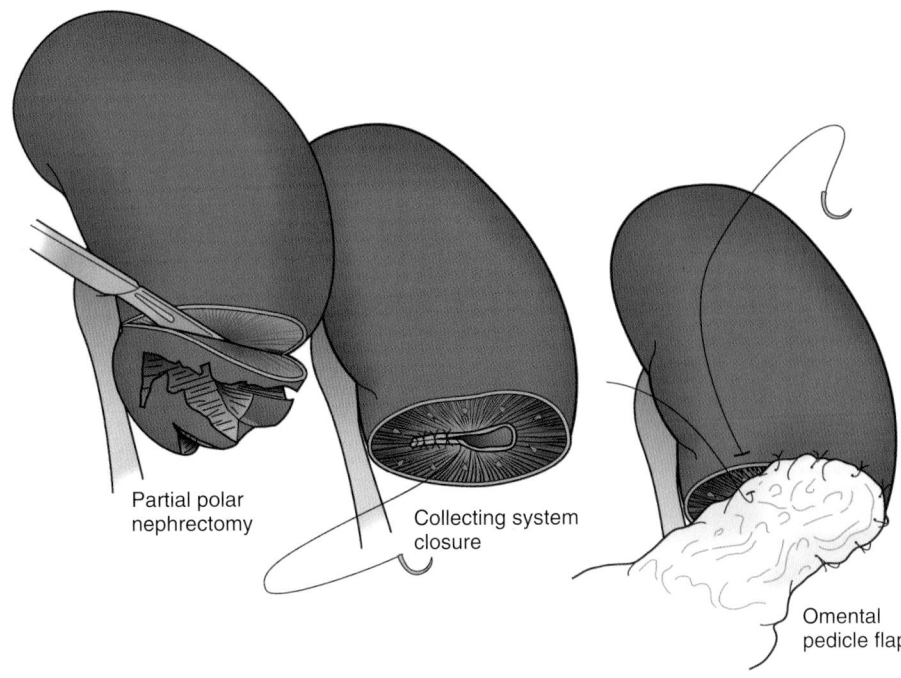

Partial polar nephrectomy

Collecting system closure

Omental pedicle flap

FIGURE 5 Lower pole injury requiring partial nephrectomy with omental patch. *(From Armenakas NA, McAninch JW: Genitourinary tract. In Ivatury RR, Cayten CG, editors: The textbook of penetrating trauma, Media, Penn, 1996, Williams & Wilkins.)*

be inserted into the ureter and dye injected in a retrograde fashion. Frank extravasation of dye or tissue staining at the injured level will aid identification.

Missed ureteral injuries may present days later with serious complications. While yellow drainage with an elevated creatinine from an abdominal drain post injury can be a telltale sign, often the signs are less clear. Prolonged ileus, a palpable abdominal or renal mass, urinary obstruction, abscess, sepsis, and flank and abdominal pain can all result from a missed ureteral injury. Depending on the time elapsed from injury to diagnosis, a nephrostomy tube should be placed to drain the kidney, as well as a drain in any fluid collection that has accumulated.

Imaging

Intravenous Urography

CT scan has replaced intravenous urography as the imaging modality of choice for appropriate staging of ureteral injuries. Occasionally in the unstaged patient in an acute trauma setting, an intravenous urogram can provide data suggestive of a ureteral injury such as incomplete visualization of the ureter, ureteral dilation, or urinary extravasation. Given the sensitivity, specificity, and variability of intravenous urography, these findings do not obviate the need for direct inspection.

Computed Tomography

High-resolution CT scan with delayed views provides excellent anatomic detail of the traumatized ureter. Medial extravasation of contrast from the hilum is the most common finding of renal ureteropelvic junction injury. In the setting of complete avulsion, the ipsilateral ureter will not fill, while a partial tear will likely show distal ureteral filling. The presence of a hematoma on axial imaging may indicate the site of ureteral injury.

Retrograde Pyelography

Given the need for time-consuming fluoroscopy, retrograde pyelography is not performed in the acute trauma setting. For delayed

injuries, retrograde pyelography can help define injury location and extent.

Injury Scale for the Ureter

Table 2 shows the American Association for the Surgery of Trauma injury scale for the ureter. Injury severity is defined by degree of transection and length of devitalized tissue.

Management

When deciding how to manage a ureteral injury in the acute setting, one must take into account the location and length of the injury and the patient's stability. In the damage control setting, a temporary cutaneous ureterostomy over a single-J ureteral stent can be performed. Alternatively, the ureter can be tied off proximal to the injury and a percutaneous nephrostomy tube can be placed. Definitive repair can be made at a later time.

Bruising or contusion of the ureteral wall should prompt treatment because it could lead to necrosis and subsequent fistula or stricture formation. Minimal contusion can be treated with a ureteral stent, while severe contusion should be débrided and reanastomosed, and a drain inserted (Figure 6).

All ureteral injuries where débridement and reanastomosis are required follow the same reconstructive principles:

1. Ureteral dissection that preserves the supporting adventitia and does not skin the ureter, which can lead to vascular compromise and stricture, is required.
2. Appropriate ureteral débridement to a bleeding edge must be performed. High-velocity projectiles can result in blast injury and ischemia, which can produce occult injury up to 2 cm away from the transection.
3. The repair should be a tension-free, watertight, spatulated, mucosa-to-mucosa anastomosis.
4. A ureteral stent should be employed.
5. Wrapping the ureter with omentum or local tissue flaps helps support the ureter and isolate it from adjacent organs.
6. To prevent urinoma, a drain adjacent to the repair, but not overlaying it, should be left.

TABLE 2: American Association for the Surgery of Trauma: injury scale for the ureter

Grade*	Type	Description
I	Hematoma	Contusion or hematoma without devascularization
II	Laceration	Transection <50%
III	Laceration	Transection <50%
IV	Laceration	Complete transection with <2 cm of devascularization
V	Laceration	Avulsion with >2 cm of devascularization

Note: Injury severity is defined by degree of transection and length of devitalized tissue.

*Advance one grade for bilateral up to Grade III.

Modified from Moore EE, Shackford SR, Pachter HL, et al: Organ injury scaling: spleen, liver, and kidney, J Trauma 29:1664-1668, 1989.

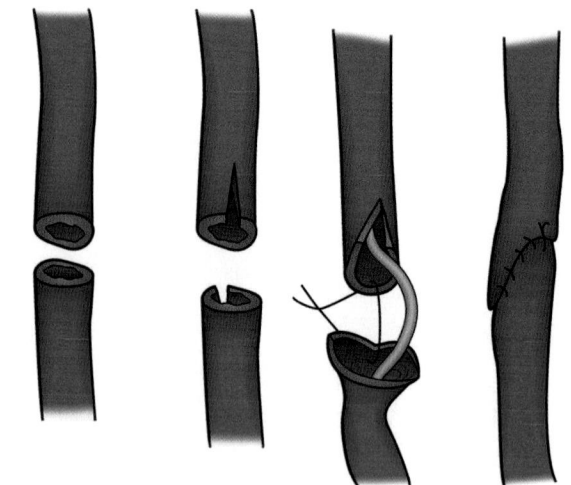

FIGURE 6 Ureteroureterostomy with débridement, spatulation, stenting, and anastomosis. *(From Peterson NE: Genitourinary trauma. In Feliciano DV, Moore EE, Mattox KL, editors: Trauma, ed 3, Stamford, Conn, 1996, Appleton & Lange.)*

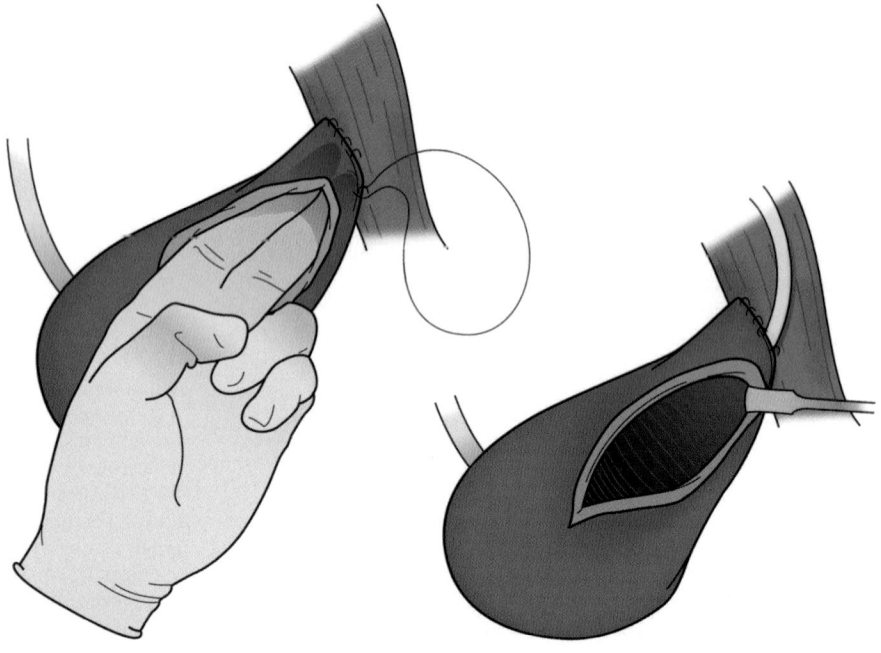

FIGURE 7 Use of the psoas hitch for treatment of distal ureteral injuries. *(From Peterson NE: Genitourinary trauma. In Feliciano DV, Moore EE, Mattox KL, editors: Trauma, ed 3, Stamford, Conn, 1996, Appleton & Lange.)*

Lower Ureteral Injuries

Ureteral injuries near the bladder are the most straightforward to treat. Many can be repaired by simple débridement and creating a refluxing ureteral reimplantation into an adjacent area on the bladder, either the posterior wall or the dome. A stent should be left for 3 to 6 weeks. Tunneled nonrefluxing repairs in adults are not needed and are associated with stenosis.

Psoas Hitch and Boari Flap

When the injury is more proximal than adjacent to the bladder, the bladder can be mobilized and brought to the ureter. The psoas hitch procedure is performed by suturing the bladder to the ipsilateral psoas minor tendon. Sutures should be placed in the tendon/muscle parallel to the course of its fibers to avoid entrapment of the genitofemoral nerve, which can lead to chronic pain. The contralateral

supravesical pedicle should be ligated to help mobilize the bladder. A ureteral stent and Foley catheter are left in place. Typically, a cystogram is obtained prior to removing the Foley (Figure 7). The vast majority of lower ureteral injuries can be treated this way. Rarely, for longer injuries, a Boari flap is required. Here, a flap of bladder tissue is tubularized to make up the distance. The bladder is also pexed to the psoas to relieve tension.

Midureteral Injuries

Most midureteral transections can be repaired by primary ureteroureterostomy. The repair should be tension-free, watertight, and spatulated over a double-J stent. In situations where the ureter loss is more significant, a transureteroureterostomy may be performed. This is rarely utilized during the trauma setting given its complexity.

Traditionally, a transureteroureterostomy should be avoided in patients with a history of nephrolithiasis, urothelial cancer, genitourinary tuberculosis, or retroperitoneal fibrosis. More commonly, when a large segment of ureter is not salvageable, a damage control approach should be employed by temporarily diverting the urine over a ureteral stent to the abdominal wall. Definitive reconstruction of the damaged segment can be undertaken in the future. Large-segment ureteral loss can be treated by autotransplant, ileal interposition, or some type of conduit or neobladder procedure at a later time.

Upper Ureteral Injuries

Ureteropelvic junction injuries typically occur after blunt or penetrating trauma. Complete disruptions/avulsions require acute surgical management. A primary anastomotic repair can be performed. Similar to other locations, a stent and a retroperitoneal drain should be utilized.

Complications

Over 50% of ureteral injuries are missed on initial presentation and discovered later. Patients may develop hydronephrosis, urinoma formation, fistula, abscess, and systemic infection. Unnoticed chronic obstruction can lead to kidney damage. Complication management depends on time elapsed after injury, but typically large fluid collections should be drained percutaneously and the ureteral obstruction bypassed.

Delayed Treatment

Injuries diagnosed 1 to 2 weeks after the insult should be explored and repaired. During this time, suture ligatures around the ureter can be excised and the ureter can be stented. In situations where the abdomen is hostile or the injury detected after 2 weeks, a temporizing nephrostomy tube should be placed and the reconstruction delayed for a few months.

SUGGESTED READINGS

Alsikafi NF, McAninch JW, Elliott SP, et al: Nonoperative management outcomes of isolated urinary extravasation following renal lacerations due to external trauma, *J Urol* 176:2494, 2006.
Breyer BN, McAninch JW, Elliott SP, et al: Minimally invasive endovascular techniques to treat acute renal hemorrhage, *J Urol* 179:2248, 2008.
Buckley JC, McAninch JW: Selective management of isolated and nonisolated grade IV renal injuries, *J Urol* 176:2498, 2006.
Dugi DD 3rd, Morey AF, Gupta A, et al: American Association for the Surgery of Trauma grade 4 renal injury substratification into grades 4a (low risk) and 4b (high risk), *J Urol* 183:592, 2010.
Elliott SP, Olweny EO, McAninch JW: Renal arterial injuries: a single center analysis of management strategies and outcomes, *J Urol* 178:2451, 2007.
Santucci RA, Wessells H, Bartsch G, et al: Evaluation and management of renal injuries: consensus statement of the renal trauma subcommittee, *BJU Int* 93:937, 2004.

DAMAGE CONTROL OPERATION

Caitlin W. Hicks, MD, MS, and
Adil Haider, MD, MPH, FACS

BASIC PRINCIPLES

Damage control operation (DCO) refers to the strategy of limiting the initial operation to lifesaving aspects of surgery, and delaying definitive surgical management in critically ill or injured patients, until they are physiologically capable of tolerating a prolonged procedure. The primary operation consists of an abbreviated procedure that focuses on obtaining surgical control of hemorrhage, restoring blood flow to critical vessels, and eliminating intracompartmental contamination as efficiently as possible. This is followed by temporary wound closure until the patient can be stabilized enough to undergo a definitive procedure.

The concept of DCO has a military origin. The expression "damage control" was first coined by the U.S. Navy in World War II, in reference to procedures employed to maintain function of a damaged warship. On the battlefield, DCO was developed as a means to minimize hemorrhagic morbidity with the fewest resources in the least amount of time possible. It was adopted for civilian trauma in

the early 1990s with a shift in focus to minimize operative time in the setting of physiologic derangement. As opposed to the traditional surgical approach of complete surgical repair immediately following injury, DCO uses a staged operative approach in an attempt to improve patient outcomes by normalizing physiology as soon as possible, optimizing perioperative physiology, and restoring homeostasis prior to definitive surgical repair. Although originally developed for major abdominal trauma, DCO has since been extended for use in thoracic, vascular, and orthopedic procedures as well.

DCO can be divided into three phases: (1) initial operation, (2) resuscitation, and (3) definitive surgical management. In the first phase, hemodynamically unstable patients are taken to the operating room (OR) for an initial, rapid lifesaving or limb-saving operation. The majority of operative repairs employ temporary stabilizing techniques; however, any major bleeding vessels must be controlled and perfusion to critical structures needs to be established. In phase 2, the patient is resuscitated in the intensive care unit (ICU) and physiologic parameters are restored. Once stabilized, the patient is then taken back to the OR for definitive procedures—reconstruction and closure of the abdomen or other cavity being operated on (phase 3). If, on return to the OR, the patient is not ready for completion of phase 3, then the patient can be returned to the ICU with a temporary closure and phase 2 and 3 are repeated.

PHYSIOLOGY AND INDICATIONS

Severely injured and critically ill patients are at risk of developing a "lethal triad" of hypothermia, acidosis, and coagulopathy. In the setting of trauma, hypothermia may be caused by hemorrhage, evaporative and conductive heat loss, peripheral vasoconstriction, and massive transfusion of cold fluids and blood products. Acidosis occurs secondary to hypoperfusion due to hemorrhage and impaired myocardial function, as well as massive transfusion, vasopressors, and impaired oxygen use. In turn, these lead to coagulopathy, which is further worsened as a result of hemodilution and consumption of clotting factors in the setting of acute hemorrhage and inflammation. Hypoperfusion may also result in the activation of protein C and systemic hyperfibrinolysis. Each of the three factors in the cycle exacerbates the others, leading to a self-perpetuating downward spiral that becomes lethal (usually in the form of a fatal arrhythmia) if not identified and treated early in the process.

The driving concept of DCO is to break the cycle of the lethal triad early in its course, and it has been shown to improve morbidity and mortality following severe trauma. Some parameters have been developed to help identify those patients most at risk of deterioration during an acute or emergent procedure (Table 1). It must be kept in mind that the results of many of these measurements may take too long to come back in the setting of hemodynamic instability, and thus the decision to proceed with DCO is ultimately a clinical one.

PHASE 1: INITIAL OPERATION ON THE ABDOMEN OR OTHER BODY CAVITIES

Damage Control Laparotomy

The primary components of a phase 1 DCO for major abdominal injury include rapid laparotomy, hemorrhagic control, containment of gastrointestinal spillage, and temporary abdominal closure. Rather than grossly packing the abdominal cavity to prevent hemorrhage, blood and clots should be evacuated for aid in rapid exploration, the identification and containment of specific injuries, and targeted packing.

Liver

In general, liver hemorrhage should be managed with packing to pressure tamponade the injury. Packing should be placed concentrically around, but never inside, the site of the wound to reapproximate tissue edges using pressure control.

Large retrohepatic injuries should be assessed visually for active bleeding and left unexplored, if under control, to prevent the possible unroofing of a contained inferior vena cava or hepatic vein injury.

Packing placed anterior to the liver should provide sufficient compression to temporarily control further retrohepatic hemorrhage, but one must be careful about impeding venous return to the heart as a result of excessive inferior vena cava compression. A couple of rolled-up towels placed on the underside of the liver can be used to prevent this occurrence, but the towels should be applied with caution to prevent dislodgement of the retrohepatic hematoma.

Penetrating liver wounds may be controlled best with an intrahepatic balloon tamponade. In the case of more shallow lacerations, including translobular injuries, a red rubber catheter can be inserted into a 1-inch Penrose drain, placed in the injury, and inflated with saline until bleeding is controlled. For deeper penetrating hepatic injuries, such as gunshot injuries, a Foley catheter with 30-mL balloon can be employed in similar fashion. Multiple inflations and repositioning may be necessary with this technique before bleeding is under sufficient control to allow for hematoma formation (Figure 1).

Simple hepatorrhaphy using 0-0 chromic catgut for deep horizontal mattress sutures and packing may also be effective for shallow penetrating liver wounds and superficial hepatic lacerations. Sutures should be placed away from the edges of the injury to prevent tearing and worsening the hemorrhage. Where indicated, finger fracture and identification of bleeding hepatic arterial vessels can be performed and vessels suture ligated. Patients should be observed for signs of hepatic necrosis, intrahepatic abscess, and hemobilia with this technique, all of which can usually be managed through secondary operations or minimally invasive techniques.

Biliary Tract

Simple bile duct injuries can be definitively repaired by primary closure during the initial operation. More complex repairs, including lacerations greater than 50% the circumference of the duct, will eventually need definitive repair with choledochojejunostomy or hepaticojejunostomy. During the initial DCO, these complex injuries should be managed temporarily by ductal ligation with T-tube or cholecystostomy placement.

Solid Organs

Injuries to solid organs such as the spleen or a single kidney should be managed with removal. Repair procedures to stem blood loss and preserve function are not indicated in DCO, as patients may not be able to tolerate the attempt at primary repair or a secondary insult in the ICU if the repair unravels.

A rapid nephrectomy can be performed by entering Gerota's fascia and manually compressing the kidney while controlling the

TABLE 1: Indications for damage control operation

Vital signs	Laboratory indications	Clinical indications
Core temperature ≤ 35° C	Arterial pH ≤ 7.2	Estimated blood loss ≥ 4 L
Systolic blood pressure persistently ≤ 80 mm Hg	Base deficit > 14 mmol/L	Blood transfusion ≥ 10 units
*Revised trauma score ≤ 5	INR > 50% of normal PTT > 50% of normal	Fluid replacement ≥ 10 L Life-threatening traumatic injury in two or more anatomic locations Vascular injuries in inaccessible locations Inability to close abdomen due to visceral edema Persistent nonsurgical bleeding

*Based on Glasgow Coma Scale, systolic blood pressure, and respiratory rate.
INR, International normalized ratio; *mm Hg,* millimeters of mercury; *mmol/L,* millimole per liter; *PTT,* partial thromboplastin time.

hilar vessels and the ureter. Prior to nephrectomy, the contralateral kidney should be assessed for size, location, and assessment of injury. In cases where ureteral damage is possible, an indigo carmine dye test can be used to ensure proper outflow of the undamaged kidney. If deemed normal, renal function tests are not necessary prior to removal of the damaged kidney. Ureteral injuries without kidney damage can be managed with ureterostomy, where a tube is inserted into the damaged ureter and exteriorized through the skin. If both kidneys are injured, then the lesser damaged organ should be assessed for salvage. Before removing the kidney and committing the patient to dialysis and a future kidney transplant, risks of repair must be balanced against the potential for further bleeding and hemodynamic instability.

Splenectomy should be performed for major injuries to the spleen, splenic artery, and distal pancreas. The splenic hilum can be clamped to control bleeding, and the spleen removed quickly to allow for visualization and exploration of the operative field. It should be noted that perioperative immunization and antibiotic prophylaxis are essential in the asplenic patient, especially in cases of polytrauma when the risk of infection is high. In our practice, we administer these when the patient is being discharged from the hospital or at 2 weeks after definitive repair.

Pancreas

During a DCO, pancreatic injuries should be managed with drainage and packing regardless of the location or extent of injury. Ductal exploration should be postponed until a definitive repair can be made. A distal pancreatectomy with splenectomy for severe hemorrhagic distal pancreatic injuries may be considered by an experienced surgeon, but proximal pancreatic injuries necessitating pancreaticoduodenectomy are rarely indicated during the initial operation. Once the patient has been resuscitated, reconstruction procedures are much easier.

Hollow Viscera

Aside from controlling hemorrhage, an effective DCO also limits gastrointestinal spillage. On initial identification, atraumatic clamps (e.g., Babcock clamps) can be used to control hollow visceral perforations. Following exploration for further injuries, small bowel hollow viscera perforations can be controlled through primary repair with sutures or staplers. Larger duodenal perforations (>50% circumference) can be controlled by closing the injury around a large-bore drainage tube or with a serosal patch, duodenojejunostomy, or pyloric exclusion procedure if the patient is relatively stable. Larger jejunal, ileal, and colonic injuries should be treated with resection using a gastrointestinal anastomosis (GIA) stapler. Bowel reanastomosis and stoma formation should be delayed until definitive repair. In the rare case where anastomosis is deemed most appropriate, hand sewing with two running sutures placed in opposing directions has similar outcomes to staplers. A generous amount of warm irrigation fluid should be used to wash out the abdomen in all four quadrants prior to temporary closure.

Abdominal Closure

In damage control laparotomies, the abdomen is left open following the initial operation to facilitate reoperation and obviate the risk of abdominal compartment syndrome. Although temporary abdominal closure techniques vary, the most effective are those that employ negative-pressure therapy (NPT). NPT allows for the removal of reperfusion-related ascites, including associated bacteria, toxins, and/or inflammatory cytokines. It also allows for easy access during reoperation and is associated with a high rate of definitive closure with minimal morbidity.

The three-layer vacuum-packed technique is the general NPT standard for temporary closure of the abdomen. If a commercially available device is unavailable, a fenestrated drape is placed in the

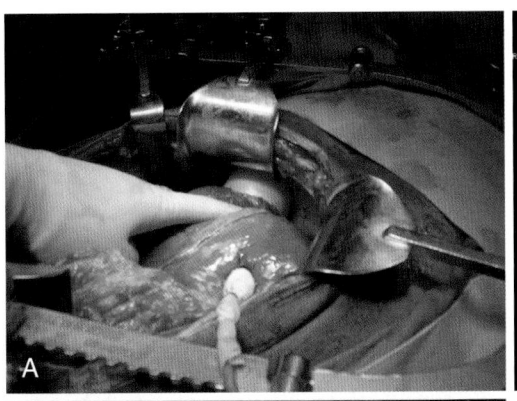
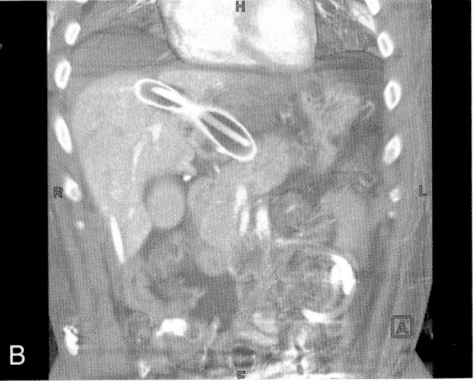
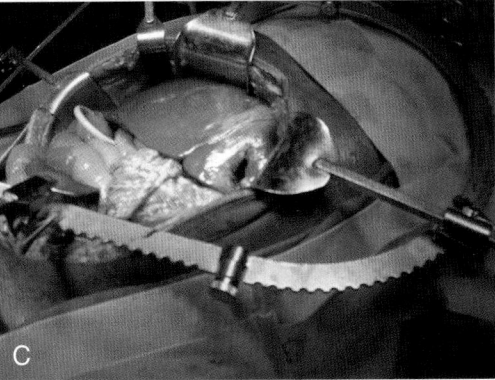

FIGURE 1 Use of a balloon tamponade device to control a gunshot wound across the liver. **A,** Insertion of balloon tamponade device into the liver tract that was bleeding during phase 1 damage control operation (DCO). **B,** Computed tomography scan showing how the tamponade device appears in the liver; taken when the patient was in the intensive care unit and in phase 2 DCO. **C,** Complete resolution of bleeding after removal of the device during phase 3 of DCO. *(Courtesy of Elliott Haut, MD, Department of Surgery, Johns Hopkins Hospital, Baltimore, Md.)*

subfascial space and covered with moist towels or gauze. Two large drains are placed along the fascial edges, and an antimicrobial iodophor-impregnated surgical incise drape is laid on top. The drains are placed to a closed suction canister at 100 to 150 mm Hg to remove and quantify developing ascites. The vacuum-assisted closure system (V.A.C. Abdominal Dressing System, KCI Inc, San Antonio, Tex) and other commercial NPT systems have similar setups that use a polyurethane foam dressing and tubing connected to a computerized suction pump to generate negative pressure.

Abdominal closure using skin approximation with towel clips or running suture should be avoided because of the high risk of abdominal compartment syndrome. Other methods of closure, such as Bogota bags, silo closure, and synthetic mesh, are not recommended because they do not allow for monitoring and removal of reperfusion-related ascites and, in the case of nonabsorbable mesh, are associated with a high risk of enteric fistula.

Damage Control Thoracotomy

DCO for chest injuries should focus on controlling hemorrhage and identifying and containing any air leaks. Patients should be placed in the supine position, as lateral positioning may waste time and provides only limited access. If necessary, a clamshell extension of an anterior thoracotomy may be performed to gain access to all structures. Patients should be intubated using a simple single-lumen endotracheal tube, and the chest is commonly entered through a left anterolateral incision, unless it is clear that the major hemorrhage is emanating from the right thorax. Whatever side is entered first, a chest tube should also be placed in the contralateral hemithorax to assess hemorrhage. If necessary, the incision can be extended to the other side to allow adequate exposure. If the patient is able to tolerate a bronchial blocker, one may be used as needed to exclude a single lung.

Heart

Assessment of cardiac injury should be achieved by anteriorly opening the pericardium parallel to the phrenic nerve. Superficial injuries to the heart may be repaired with skin staples or a running suture with 3-0 nonabsorbable polypropylene. Larger penetrating injuries can be controlled by a Foley catheter tamponade or direct, simple, finger occlusion to allow for visualization and simple suture repair with 2-0 nonabsorbable suture on a large needle (such as a V26) with pledgets. If finger compression is used, the suture bites need to be wide enough to come around the width of the surgeon's finger. During this procedure, one must be cognizant of the location of cardiac vessels, as incorporating these in the repair may cause irreparable cardiac ischemia. In cases of severe cardiac hemorrhage, injury visualization and repair may be possible only by stopping the heart from actively beating. Temporary cardiac arrest can be achieved through compression of the superior and inferior venae cavae. This approach should be used with caution and only for short periods of time. The heart can be restarted, following repair, through manual compression or electric shock.

Hemodynamically unstable patients with difficult venous access and an open thorax can be infused fluids through an intraatrial Foley catheter. The catheter should be secured with a purse-string suture and can be used for fluid resuscitation until alternate venous access is achieved.

Lungs

Acute pulmonary hemorrhage can be controlled to allow for exploration by clamping the lung parenchyma or hilum with a Satinsky clamp, or by twisting the lung 180 degrees in a "hilar twist" to occlude blood flow.

Pulmonary injuries involving the apices or costophrenic angles can often be managed with packing. When packing fails, or for blunt pulmonary injuries in other locations, a nonanatomic wedge resection using a GIA or thoracoabdominal stapler is the procedure of choice. In the case of continued uncontrollable parenchymal bleeding, a complete lobectomy can be performed by firing a stapler twice along the hilar structures en masse.

Penetrating pulmonary injuries should be approached with pulmonary tractotomy. The lung parenchyma is divided with a GIA stapler or a transaction/anastomosis stapler applied through the injury, which allows for visualization and access of injured bronchi or vessels. Bronchial and small vessel injuries should be controlled and repaired with individual ligation using 3-0 nonabsorbable or slow-absorbing suture. The access tract should be left open until definitive repair can be completed to allow for reexploration and ease of further pulmonary resection.

Tracheobronchial and Esophageal Injuries

All tracheal and most bronchial injuries should be initially treated with débridement and primary repair if the patient is stable enough. An endotracheal tube may be used to stent across an injured trachea until a formal repair is possible. Larger bronchial injuries may require a quick, stapled lobectomy to ensure air leak control.

Esophageal injuries should be diverted with wide drainage during the initial operation. Early antibiotic therapy is essential to minimize infectious morbidity.

Thoracic Wall Injury and Closure

Thoracic wall injuries should be treated with packing to control hemorrhage, although it is often difficult to achieve effective compression against the bony structure of the ribs. Obvious vessel injuries can be repaired with simple ligation followed by packing to improve control.

Similar to a DCO laparotomy, the thorax should be left open following phase 1 of a DCO thoracotomy. Although it is unclear whether the benefits of this practice prevent thoracic compartment syndrome, an open thorax allows for expedited reoperation and access during definitive surgical management. Temporary closure can be accomplished by placing a blue towel above the ribs, followed by an occlusive plastic dressing over the wound to seal it closed. Alternatively, the wound can be closed using a simple mass closure of the skin and muscle. In both cases, the chest must be drained with thoracostomy tubes to prevent development of a pneumothorax and to remove hemorrhage or monitor further acute hemorrhage. NPT and vacuum closure devices are not indicated.

Damage Control Vascular Surgery

The primary goal of DCO is to control hemorrhage without causing end-organ ischemia. Vasculature injuries should be managed with simple repairs whenever possible, including lateral repair, ligation, and temporary shunts. Destructive injury to the celiac artery can be managed with ligation. In extreme circumstances, the portal vein can be ligated as well. Injuries to the superior mesenteric artery, external iliac arteries, and infrainguinal arteries should be managed with a temporary intravascular shunt to maintain blood flow. With the exception of the suprarenal inferior vena cava, and popliteal veins, which also require shunt repair to maintain blood flow, most venous injuries can be ligated to achieve hemorrhagic control. Severe aortic injuries should be repaired with a polytetrafluoroethylene graft. Heparinization is probably unnecessary in patients with shunts and grafts because of the temporary nature of the implant and the patients' presumed coagulopathic state.

Fasciotomy with delayed closure is advised in patients with severe traumatic vascular injuries to prevent compartment syndrome.

When ligated, the infrarenal inferior vena cava and iliac veins are particularly prone to temporary edema and may require fasciotomy with eventual in situ reconstruction or extraanatomic bypass. Fasciotomy closure should be delayed even beyond the definitive repair of vascular injuries to prevent the formation of late compartment syndrome and limb ischemia.

Damage Control Orthopedics

Although open fractures are traditionally treated in urgent fashion, orthopedic injuries associated with severe head wounds or pulmonary contusions are often cited as an indication to perform a DCO rather than definitive repair. DCO can be used to prevent exsanguination from vascular injuries in the chest, abdomen, pelvis, or long bones, and to explore and control potential multi-cavity injuries. Hemodynamically unstable patients with severe orthopedic injuries should be treated with splinting or traction early to control hemorrhage and reduce the risk of fat embolism before transfer to the OR. Patients who are more stable may be candidates for angioembolization, either before or after the initial DCO procedure.

Long Bones

Long bone fractures can be treated temporarily with external fixation and traction in patients with severe associated traumatic injuries. During the DCO, open fractures should be carefully inspected for the presence of foreign material and fully débrided to remove all particulate matter and dead tissue. Wound washout and débridement within 6 hours of injury are recommended to prevent infection and potential osteomyelitis, which can have devastating long-term consequences. Open reduction and internal fixation should be delayed until the patient is stable enough to withstand the physiologic stress of a definitive procedure. The use of external fixators allows optimization of definitive repair with minimal long-term functional consequences.

With all severe extremity injuries, one must be particularly vigilant about monitoring the patient for compartment syndrome. A lack of pulses, change in color, and/or change in temperature necessitates immediate fasciotomy to prevent limb ischemia and death.

Pelvis

Patients with unstable pelvic fractures, particularly those presenting after high energy injuries, are at extremely high risk of mortality. Along with the use of a pelvic binder, angiography is an excellent mode to stem hemorrhage associated with open book or other severe pelvic fractures. The main stems of both internal iliac arteries can be embolized using gelatin sponge particle injections. Compared with selective coil embolization, this method is much faster, promotes clotting, and allows for some continued blood to ensure distal organ perfusion. Alternatively, pelvic hemorrhage can be controlled with extraperitoneal packing through a lower midline or Pfannenstiel incision. Intraperitoneal packing is less effective because the vasculature compression is difficult against the bony prominences of the pelvis.

Following packing, a damage control laparotomy is commonly indicated to assess associated intraabdominal injuries. The laparotomy incision should be made discontinuously from the pelvic incision to keep the retroperitoneal space separate from the intraperitoneal cavity. It is important that the pelvic binder be left in place at all times, as extraperitoneal packing is only effective in the setting of external stabilization. Once major hemorrhage has been controlled in all body parts, an external fixator can be placed on the pelvis during DCO, as this will help with restoring physiologic normalcy in phase 2 of damage control.

PHASE 2: RESUSCITATION

Following the first stage of a DCO, the patient is brought to the ICU for resuscitative management and prevention or correction of the lethal triad of acidosis, coagulopathy, and hypothermia (Figure 2). Low body temperature should be managed with active rewarming (including use of warm ambient temperatures, warm blankets, infusion of warm fluids, and forced warm-air devices) to a core temperature of 37°C. Coagulopathy should be treated with fresh frozen plasma, platelets, cryoprecipitate, vitamin K, and calcium to achieve the following values: international normalized ratio (INR) <1.2, prothrombin time (PT) <15 seconds, fibrinogen >100 mg/dL, and platelets >100,000/mm³. Acidosis is managed best through reversal of hypothermia and coagulopathy and continued fluid resuscitation.

Damage control resuscitation (DCR) as described by the military should be continued throughout this phase as well as during the initial DCO. The principles of DCR include (1) use of permissive hypotension until hemorrhage control has been achieved (this should be achieved prior to entering the phase 2 resuscitative phase), (2) judicious use of crystalloid resuscitation, and (3) early and increased transfusion of plasma and platelets. The rationale behind DCR is that aggressive preoperative crystalloid resuscitation may be detrimental to the severely injured patient by causing a dilutional coagulopathy, dislodging unstable clots to worsen hemorrhage, exacerbating hypothermia (in the case of unwarmed fluids), worsening acidosis as a result of the high chloride content, and increasing the intraabdominal pressure. Patients requiring massive blood transfusions are particularly appropriate candidates for this approach and should be transfused with a ratio of fresh frozen plasma to platelets to packed red blood cells of 1:1:1. DCR is credited with significant improvements in mortality rates and is thought to be one of the most important lessons learned in the resuscitation of causalities of the recent Iraq and Afghanistan conflicts. Adjunct studies can also be employed in phase 2 of DCO. Computed tomographic scans may be useful for planning definitive procedures, and radiographic studies should be obtained to evaluate for missed indolent orthopedic injuries. Hemodynamically stable patients with continued postoperative bleeding may be appropriate for angiographic intervention (e.g., those with a liver laceration that may benefit from unilateral hepatic arterial embolization), either as a temporary reprieve to delay returning to the OR or as definitive vascular management. Most patients will continue to have some amount of bleeding following the initial DCO procedure, so a balance between when to intervene and when to maintain the patient's hemodynamic status through the transfusion of blood products must be achieved. If a patient truly has developed a disseminated intravascular coagulopathy, he or she will not benefit from a return to the OR and will require resuscitation and correction of coagulopathy. On the other hand, if postoperative bleeding is severe, patients may need a second abbreviated laparotomy to gain surgical control of the hemorrhage and allow for continued resuscitation before definitive operative management is attempted.

PHASE 3: DEFINITIVE SURGICAL MANAGEMENT

Definitive management of DCO patients' injuries should wait until their physiologic parameters return to normal, meaning that hypothermia is corrected, acidosis is reversed, and coagulopathy is resolved. In many patients, definitive surgical management may require multiple reoperations. The staging and timing of these return trips to the OR should be planned according to patient stability and clinical condition, the extent of surgical repair required, and surgeon experience.

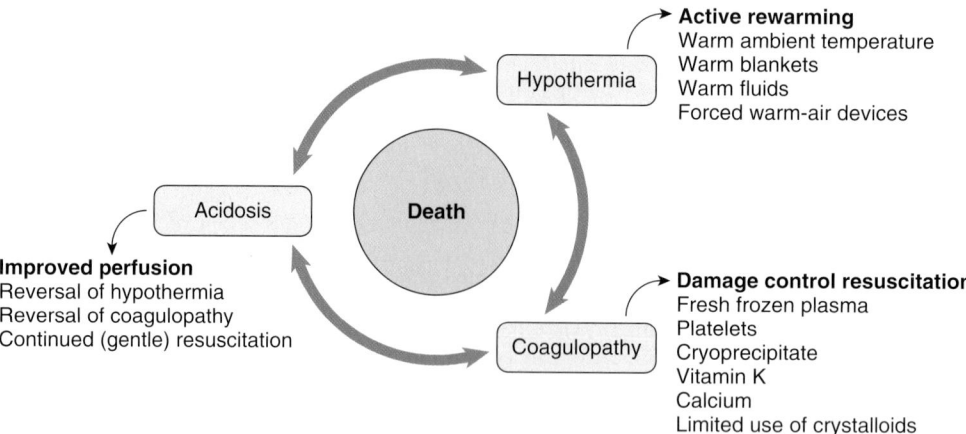

FIGURE 2 The lethal triad. Severely injured and critically ill patients are at risk of developing a "lethal triad" of hypothermia, acidosis, and coagulopathy, which is associated with a high rate of mortality. Phase 2 of a damage control operation is aimed at halting the progression of the triad, and should be approached using the strategies outlined in section on Phase 2.

In most cases, reoperation and definitive surgical care can be attempted within 24 to 48 hours of the initial operation. Definitive management following thoracic DCO procedures should be as early as possible (ideally less than 12 hours) because of the high risk of decreasing pulmonary compliance that can lead to difficulties with patient ventilation. In contrast, there is some evidence to suggest that definitive orthopedic repairs should occur within 24 hours or up to 5 days following injury to prevent pulmonary complications.

During phase 3, all packing should be removed, and the patient should be thoroughly reexplored for any injuries that may have been missed during the initial operation. Once exploration is complete, definitive surgical repair can proceed as necessary depending on the patient's specific injuries (e.g., bowel reanastomosis with diversion for hollow viscous injuries, definitive thoracic closure for thoracic injuries, reconstruction or extraanatomic bypass with insertion of permanent graft for vascular injuries, etc). Following completion of definitive repair, if the patient is stable and not at risk for abdominal compartment syndrome, the abdomen can be closed. However, if there is any potential for its development, or if definitive repairs cannot be completed, then the abdomen should be left open (using one of the mechanisms described previously) and the patient should be returned to phase 2 of DCO.

EVIDENCE FOR EFFECTIVENESS OF DCO

DCO in patients with major abdominal trauma has been shown to reduce rates of morbidity and mortality compared with immediate definitive surgery in a number of descriptive and retrospective series. By reducing operative time and allowing for focused perioperative resuscitation in physiologically unstable patients, the potential insults of a complex definitive repair are thought to be decreased. However, there is limited prospective evidence from randomized clinical trials on the subject and minimal data of any kind versus immediate definitive surgery in the setting of severe nonabdominal injuries. In addition, a DCO approach tends to be more costly than immediate surgical repair, and multiple return trips to the OR may increase the risk of some surgical morbidities, including intraabdominal abscess, bile leak, enteric fistula, and wound infection (Table 2). As a result, there is some controversy among experts regarding its appropriate use in trauma, and concerns regarding its overuse are now arising.

Currently, the general consensus is that DCO should be employed when a longer procedure may cause risk of clinical deterioration, particularly in the setting of multiple and/or complex organ injuries.

TABLE 2: Estimated incidence of morbidity and mortality following abdominal damage control operation versus traditional single-stage procedure

Measured outcome		Damage control operation	Single-stage procedure
Prevalence of procedure in trauma*		30%	70%
Mortality†		44%	63%
Morbidity‡	Sepsis	42%	3%
	Intraabdominal abscess	18%	4%
	Enteric fistula	18%	2%
	Recurrent hemorrhage	6%	0%
	Wound infection	6%	2%

*Hatch QM, Osterhout LM, Ashraf A, et al: Current use of damage-control laparotomy, closure rates, and predictors of early fascial closure at the first take-back. *J Trauma* 70(6):1429-1436, 2011.
†Stawicki SP, Brooks A, Bilski T, et al: The concept of damage control: extending the paradigm to emergency general surgery. *Injury* 39(1):93-101, 2008.
‡Nicholas JM, Rix EP, Easley KA, et al: Changing patterns in the management of penetrating abdominal trauma: the more things change, the more they stay the same. *J Trauma* 55(6):1095-1108; discussion 1108-1110, 2003.

Recent estimates demonstrate that DCO is used in as many as 30% of trauma patients undergoing emergent laparotomy, which may suggest an overuse of the technique. There is some evidence that, particularly in older patients, certain characteristics such as chronic congestive heart failure or acute renal insufficiency may be correlated with an increased risk of death following DCO. Thus, individual patient history, both chronic and acute, must be considered when making the decision to proceed with DCO. Future studies will help differentiate those patients most likely to benefit from a staged operative approach and help delineate specific indications for abdominal, thoracic, vascular, and orthopedic injuries.

SUGGESTED READINGS

Cirocchi R, Abraha I, Montedori A, et al: Damage control surgery for abdominal trauma, *Cochrane Database Syst Rev* 1(1):CD007438, 2010.

Cotton, BA, Reddy N, Hatch QM, et al: Damage control resuscitation is associated with a reduction in resuscitation volumes and improvement in survival in 390 damage control laparotomy patients, *Ann Surg* 254(4):598–605, 2011.

Rotondo MF, Schwab CW, McGonigal MD, et al: Damage control: An approach for improved survival in exsanguinating penetrating abdominal injury, *J Trauma* 35(3):375–382; discussion 382–383, 1993.

Shapiro MB, Jenkins DH, Schwab CW, et al: Damage control: collective review, *J Trauma* 49(5):969–978, 2000.

UROLOGIC COMPLICATIONS OF PELVIC FRACTURE

Hunter Wessells, MD, FACS

It is the urologist who will have to share with the patient, the burden of any residual disability when thoracic, abdominal, and even the orthopedic aspects are long forgotten.

– Richard Turner Warwick

Pelvic injuries cause a significant disease burden in the United States, representing 7.5% of all traumatic injuries. It is estimated that more than 110,000 pelvic injuries occur every year with direct costs exceeding $1.1 billion. Patients with pelvic trauma are severely injured, the majority having injury severity scores exceeding 16. There is significant mortality due to associated head injury, but the genitourinary and gastrointestinal complications can be morbid and life threatening as well.

Pelvic trauma has a male preponderance, with approximately two thirds of injuries occurring in men and one third in women. Conventional wisdom states that 5% of patients with a pelvic fracture will have an associated bladder injury and that a subset of these will have urethral injury. More recent data suggest that the proportion of patients with a urethral injury will be higher, with 3% of males with pelvic fracture demonstrating a urethral disruption, and many will not have bladder injury. Urethral and bladder neck injuries occurred in 6.8% of female pelvic fractures. Notably, these figures represent rates of injury at large trauma centers and may not be representative of the experience in community hospitals or centers without trauma designation.

BLADDER INJURY

Identification of pelvic fracture–associated bladder injury requires a detailed history, physical examination, urinalysis, and appropriate imaging. Ninety-five percent of patients with a bladder rupture will have gross hematuria, and the remaining few with microhematuria can be detected, with appropriate algorithms, during the initial trauma evaluation. There is no clinical prediction rule to identify patients requiring cystography after pelvic fracture other than the degree of hematuria. Recent studies suggest that patients with microscopic hematuria are unlikely to suffer bladder injury. Thus, criteria for imaging the bladder include any blunt trauma with gross hematuria; blunt trauma with a pelvic fracture and greater than 30 red

blood cells per high-power field; and penetrating trauma with any degree of hematuria and an injury to the pelvis. Fracture patterns associated with bladder and urethral injuries are similar, namely, diastasis of the pubis and obturator ring fractures. The greater the displacement of these fractures is, the more likely a genitourinary injury will happen.

Imaging is important because failure to recognize a bladder injury can lead to significant complications, including urinary ascites, infection of pelvic hematoma, chronic bladder dysfunction, and sepsis. A spiral computed tomographic (CT) scan with 5-mm cuts obtained after complete filling of the bladder will delineate all intra- and extraperitoneal bladder injuries. The degree of bladder filling is important and, in responsive patients, should be as much as they can tolerate. In unresponsive patients, the contrast is hung at 40 cm of water and a volume of 350 mL infused. With a CT cystogram, there is no need for scout or postevacuation imaging because the cross-sectional nature of the imaging identifies both anterior and posterior leaks. Conversely, with plain film cystography, scout and postevacuation films are required. Because of these differences, CT cystogram is more expedient and is now the standard in most trauma centers.

The classic intraperitoneal bladder rupture, whether identified by CT or plain film cystography, will outline loops of bowel consistent with intraperitoneal location. Extraperitoneal bladder ruptures lead to extravasation of contrast in the retroperitoneum, including the space of Retzius, the lateral colic region, and into the groin and thigh. Typically, the direct defect in the bladder wall can be visualized with a CT cystogram (Figure 1). Combined intra- and extraperitoneal bladder ruptures can be missed when a large injury in one location makes it difficult to distend the bladder.

The sensitivity and specificity of computed tomography and cystography has been determined for blunt trauma and is 95% and 100%, respectively, based on operative findings as a gold standard. Intraperitoneal rupture has a lesser degree of sensitivity, possibly because of the aforementioned confounding that is due to multiple sites of rupture. Importantly, no such data exist for penetrating injuries, and although these may be delineated with a CT scan, caution must be exercised when considering a nonoperative approach. In cases of penetrating injury, additional imaging to delineate vascular and gastrointestinal injuries should be coordinated.

Management of bladder injuries can be nonoperative with catheter drainage as long as the rupture is extraperitoneal and does not involve open pelvic fractures, urinary infection, bony fragments, or foreign body in the bladder. Use of an appropriate-sized catheter is essential to avoid obstruction by clots and poor bladder drainage. Absolute indications for bladder repair include a bladder neck injury (Figure 2), concomitant rectal injury, major vaginal laceration, and the previously mentioned caveats.

Operative management of bladder rupture requires differing exposure depending on whether the lesion is felt to be intra- or extraperitoneal. With extraperitoneal bladder rupture, a lower midline or transverse Pfannenstiel-type incision provides access to the bladder and allows primary closure of injuries. For intraperitoneal bladder ruptures, which tend to be stellate in nature, and large,

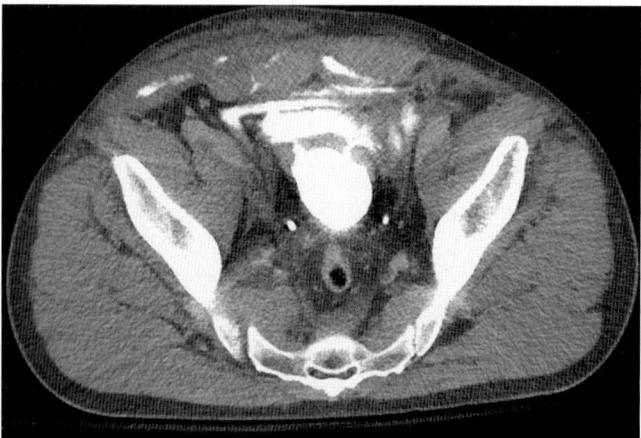

FIGURE 1 Computed tomographic cystogram showing extraperitoneal bladder rupture with two defects in the anterior bladder wall.

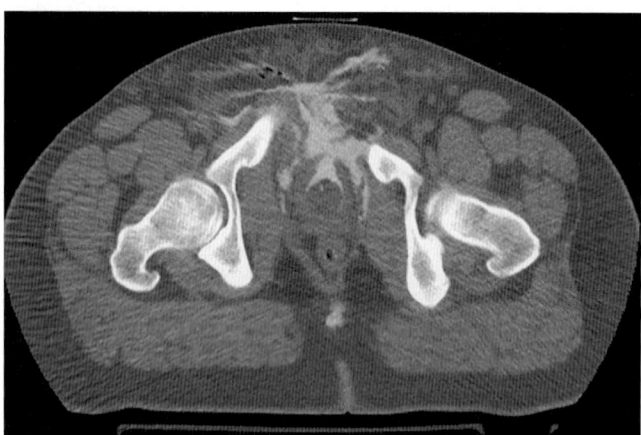

FIGURE 2 Computed tomographic cystogram showing extravasation at level of catheter balloon consistent with a bladder neck injury.

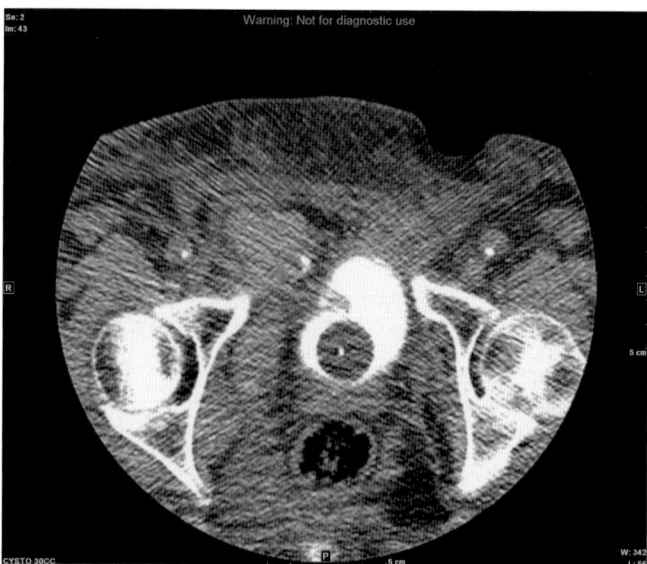

FIGURE 3 Computed tomographic cystogram showing bony spicule in bladder lumen in a patient with unrecognized bladder injury treated nonoperatively.

a midline incision slightly higher on the abdominal wall gives good access to the dome of the bladder.

In performing bladder exploration, it is important to identify associated injuries to the genitourinary tract. Although ureteral injury is very uncommon in pelvic fractures, when the bladder is open, as long as visualization is adequate, assessment of the ureteral orifices is mandatory. This can be performed by observing a jet of clear urine out of each orifice, intubation of the orifice with a feeding tube or other small 5F catheter, or by the administration of intravenous indigo carmine and observation of blue dye excreted in the urine. The bladder neck should also be assessed, by visual inspection, palpation, or endoscopic evaluation.

Bladder lacerations should be repaired in a standard two-layer closure with running slowly absorbable suture such as 2-0 polyglycolic acid. The first layer incorporates the mucosa and the muscularis. The second layer incorporates the muscularis and overlying serosa. In the region of the bladder neck, where access to the urinary tract behind the pubic bone may be difficult, a single layer of well-placed interrupted absorbable sutures is sufficient to allow appropriate healing. In patients with multiple bladder lacerations, smaller lacerations can be fixed from within the bladder with a single layer of slowly absorbable suture. A closed suction drain is placed adjacent to the bladder to prevent collections. Urinary drainage after bladder repair may be carried out either with suprapubic cystostomy or, in most cases, with urethral catheter drainage alone. There is no evidence that

suprapubic cystostomy leads to improved outcomes compared with urethral catheterization alone.

Follow-up imaging is required after nonoperative management by catheter drainage is selected, and after operative repair. Cystography should be carried out 10 to 14 days after injury in order to assess the healing process for nonoperative management (Figure 3) or to confirm appropriate healing after operative repair. Once bladder integrity has been confirmed, the catheter can then be removed based on the patient's other injury status and mobility. If extravasation persists, repeat cystography is recommended at appropriate intervals until healing occurs. Overall, only a very small subset of patients with bladder injury will require reoperation or delayed closure.

URETHRAL INJURY

Pelvic fracture urethral injury is a rare but significant injury and is associated with potential genitourinary morbidity, including urethral stricture, urinary incontinence, sexual dysfunction, and chronic pain. The signs and symptoms of these injuries are nonspecific and include blood at the urethral meatus, difficulty or inability to void, a palpable bladder, butterfly perineal hematoma, high-riding prostate on digital prostate examination, fracture of the pubic symphysis, pelvic hematoma, or associated bladder injury.

These injuries are suspected in cases of pubic diastasis or fracture of the inferior pubic ramus. Such "straddle fractures" lead to significantly greater odds of injury. Urethral injuries are classified according to American Association for the Surgery of Trauma (AAST) grades I through V. Grades I and II injuries (contusions and stretch injuries, respectively) need only urethral catheter drainage until the patient recovers from other injuries. Grade III injuries (partial disruptions) are best managed with realignment, whereas grades IV and V (complete disruptions with or without extensive separation or involvement of the prostate or vagina) may be treated with early endoscopic realignment or suprapubic cystostomy. There is debate as to the benefit of early endoscopic realignment, and suprapubic cystostomy remains the most commonly elected treatment nationwide.

Male urethral injuries after pelvic fracture are best delineated with retrograde urethrogram (Figure 4). However, when patients have blood at the urethral meatus and immediate catheter drainage is required, a single attempt at urethral catheterization may be

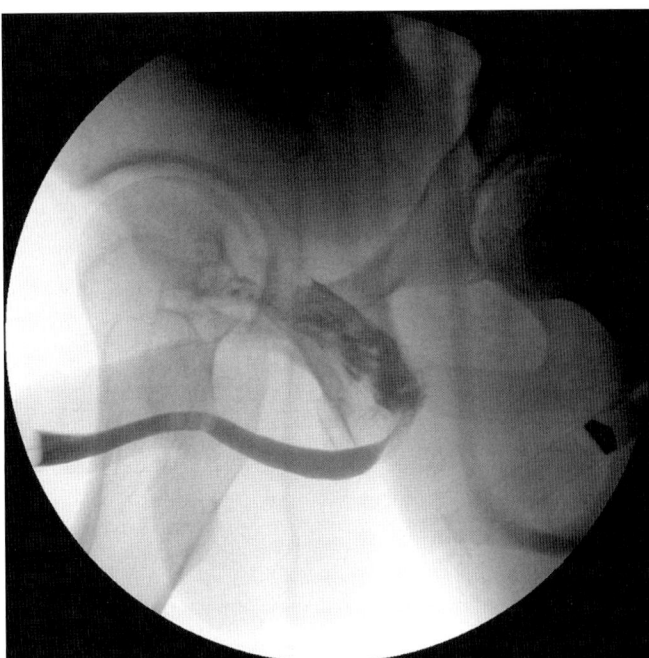

FIGURE 4   Retrograde urethrogram showing complete urethral disruption with extravasation of contrast and no filling of the proximal urethra or bladder (grade IV injury).

considered. There is no strong evidence to suggest that this maneuver will convert a partial urethral injury to a complete injury. Nevertheless, in stable patients without immediate need for catheter drainage, retrograde urethrogram is still the primary diagnostic modality. Cystoscopy can provide additional information and may be performed in the emergency department, but overall it is not favored as a primary diagnostic modality. Female urethral and bladder neck injuries are more difficult to identify and diagnose when compared with male injuries. These injuries may only be identified with intraoperative physical examination or incidentally in the intraoperative setting (40% of injuries). Thus, with all such patients, a thorough history and physical examination, laboratory studies, and imaging as indicated remain important. The decision whether to perform suprapubic cystostomy or urethral realignment depends on the patient's stability and associated injury status. When patients are unstable, suprapubic cystostomy urinary diversion is appropriate as the initial step in the emergency department. Indications for realignment include a stable patient with complete or partial urethral disruption. Other rare but considerable factors include a concomitant bladder rupture, rectal and vaginal laceration, bladder neck injury, severe bladder displacement ("pie in the sky"), and open reduction and internal fixation with the placement of orthopedic hardware.

Stricture rates will be higher after suprapubic cystostomy compared with primary urethral realignment; realignment allows healing without strictures in 40% to 50% of patients versus less than 5% with suprapubic diversion. The standard approach for realignment uses flexible endoscopes inserted per urethra and per suprapubic tract. This can be performed when the patient is stable. Typically, this requires two urologists skilled in flexible endoscopy, fluoroscopy, and,

in many cases, coordination with orthopedic procedures. As long as suprapubic cystostomy can temporize urinary drainage, realignment can be performed in an elective or semi-elective fashion when appropriate resources can be brought to bear, up to a week after injury.

After urethral realignment, pericatheter retrograde urethrogram is recommended at 6 weeks after injury to assess for persisting leak. If leaks persist, repeat imaging is required until healing. Aggressive treatment of the complications of these injuries requires close vigilance to detect urethral strictures and urinary incontinence.

CONCLUSIONS

Immediate identification of acute genitourinary injuries and appropriate urinary drainage is essential to prevent early septic complications and to ensure subsequent normal organ function. Coordination with the trauma team allows appropriate operative repair or nonoperative management based on the injury severity and presence of associated injuries. Close follow-up is required to identify fistulae, strictures, urinary incontinence, and sexual dysfunction resulting from injury to the bladder, urethra, and pelvic vascular structures. Even in the absence of overt genitourinary organ injury, soft tissue and vascular damage may lead to delayed complications, including urinary and sexual dysfunction, and cause significant impairment of quality of life.

SUGGESTED READINGS

Avey G, Blackmore CC, Wessells H, et al: Radiographic and clinical predictors of bladder rupture in blunt trauma patients with pelvic fracture, *Acad Radiol* 13(5):573–579, 2006.

Basta A, Blackmore CG, Wessells H: Predicting urethral injury from pelvic fracture patterns in male patients with blunt trauma, *J Urol* 177(2):571–575, 2007.

Bjurlin MA, Fantus RJ, Mellett MM, et al: Genitourinary injuries in pelvic fracture morbidity and mortality using the National Trauma Data Bank, *J Trauma* 67(5):1033–1039, 2009.

Black P, Miller E, Porter JR, et al: Urethral and bladder neck injury associated with pelvic fracture in 25 female patients, *J Urol* 175(6):2140–2144; discussion 2144, 2006.

Chapple C, Barbagli G, Jordan B, et al: Consensus statement on urethral trauma, *BJU Int* 93(9):1195–1202, 2004.

Deck AJ, Shaves S, Talner L, et al: Computerized tomography cystography for the diagnosis of traumatic bladder rupture, *J Urol* 164(1):43–46, 2000.

Hadjizacharia P, Inaba K, Teixeira PG, et al: Evaluation of immediate endoscopic realignment as a treatment modality for traumatic urethral injuries, *J Trauma* 64(6):1443–1449; discussion 1449–1450. doi: 10.1097/TA.0b013e318174f126, 2008.

Kielb SJ, Voeltz ZL, Wolf JS: Evaluation and management of traumatic posterior urethral disruption with flexible cystourethroscopy, *J Trauma* 50(1):36–40, 2001.

Leddy L, Vanni A, Wessells H, et al: Outcomes of endoscopic realignment of pelvic fracture associated urethral injuries at a level 1 trauma center, *J Urol* 188(1):174–178, 2012.

Turner-Warwick R: Prevention of complications resulting from pelvic fracture urethral injuries–and from their surgical management, *Urol Clin North Am* 16(2):335–358. Review, 1989.

Vanni A, Wessells H: Injuries to the urogenital tract. In Souba WW, Fink MP, Jurkovich GJ, et al, editors: *ACS Surgery*, New York, 2012, WEBMD.

Wright JL, Nathens AB, Rivara FP, et al: Specific fracture configurations predict sexual and excretory dysfunction in men and women 1 year after pelvic fracture, *J Urol* 176(4):1540–1545, 2006.

Facial Trauma: Evaluation and Management

John J. Chi, MD, and Daniel S. Alam, MD, FACS

OVERVIEW

Facial trauma evaluation and management remains an unfortunate necessity in our contemporary society. Although most patients who present with facial trauma can be safely assessed and stabilized by the trauma surgery and emergency department teams, complex injuries often result in consultation with a facial plastic surgeon, plastic surgeon, otolaryngologist, or oral maxillofacial surgeon for definitive management. The complex interplay between the aesthetics and the function of the maxillofacial region requires a consideration for anatomy and mechanics that is generally not necessary in traumatic injuries outside of the head and neck. This chapter provides a general overview of the critical aspects of the evaluation and management of facial trauma.

EMERGENT TREATMENT AND EVALUATION

Emergent Treatment of Facial Trauma

The evaluation of any patient who presents with a traumatic injury begins with the Advanced Trauma Life Support (ATLS) protocol. An assessment of the ABCs (airway, breathing, and circulation) must be made judiciously before evaluation of the facial injuries. Airway evaluation is of particular importance because of the myriad head and neck injuries that can cause airway compromise (i.e., larynx trauma, mandible fractures, neck hematoma, etc.). Acute airway management may require direct laryngoscopy with intubation, fiberoptic intubation, or a surgical airway (cricothyrotomy or emergent tracheotomy). Because of the vascular nature of the head and neck region, traumatic injuries may present with hemorrhage that needs to be urgently addressed. The acute management of hemorrhage in the head and neck is vital as a result of the potential for airway compromise, from extraluminal compression (neck hematoma, bilateral mandible fracture), intraluminal obstruction (epistaxis, oral cavity/oropharyngeal bleeding), or airway luminal separation (laryngotracheal injury). Hemorrhage from most branches of the external carotid artery can be addressed with pressure, surgical ligation, or embolization. For example, severe epistaxis can be managed with nasal packing, endoscopic blood vessel ligation, or angiography with embolization. Hemorrhage from the internal carotid, subclavian, or vertebral arteries, however, usually requires endovascular management because of the difficulty with open surgical control of the proximal and distal ends of these vessels (Burgess, 2012; Kesser, 2009). The management of penetrating neck trauma is dictated by patient presentation, symptomatology, and the location of the injury within the neck. A diagram of the zones of the neck is shown in Figure 1. Zone 1 and 3 injuries are initially managed with angiography (computed tomographic [CT] or conventional). Definitive treatment with endovascular management or neck exploration is contingent on patient presentation and imaging studies. These injuries are usually treated with an endovascular approach because of the

difficulty with surgical access to the blood vessels in these regions. Zone 2 injuries are initially treated with neck exploration or angiography based on patient presentation. Although historically these injuries were all treated with neck exploration, recent studies suggest that neck exploration may be reserved for selected cases (Tisherman, 2008; Burgess, 2012; Kesser, 2009). In general, neck exploration is recommended for patients with unstable or symptomatic conditions. Contrast gastrointestinal studies and aerodigestive endoscopy should also be performed on a selective basis depending on the level of concern for airway or gastrointestinal injury. On completion of the primary survey, attention can then be placed on specific body systems and injuries during the secondary survey.

Evaluation of Facial Trauma

After immediate life-threatening conditions are ruled out or stabilized, attention can be focused on a comprehensive assessment of facial injuries. The physical examination of the head and neck is a critical aspect of the evaluation of patients with facial trauma. This examination should begin by carefully cleaning the head and neck of debris and blood to allow a thorough visual inspection. These patients are often intubated and present for evaluation with a cervical collar placed by first responders in the field. Without confirmation of cervical spine stability, the trauma patient must be maintained in inline stabilization. Radiographic evaluation should be a precursor to removal of the immobilizer.

The examination of the face should proceed in thirds: upper face, mid face, and lower face. Evaluate each third of the face for neurovascular integrity, bony factures, and lacerations. A systematic assessment of sensation and voluntary facial movement should be performed in each third of the face. Unique structures in each region require special assessment. For example, in the upper face, integrity of the frontal bone overlying the frontal sinuses should be assessed. The midface assessment should include a thorough assessment of the eyes, including pupillary light reflex, extraocular movements, globe position, and visual acuity. An evaluation of the bony structures should include palpation of the inferior and lateral orbital rim, bony nasal dorsum, zygomatic arch, palate, and maxillary dentition. An intranasal examination should also be performed to rule out a septal hematoma. The lower face assessment should include palpation of the mandible and mandibular dentition as well as assessment of the floor of mouth, tongue, and oral airway. Special attention should also be given to the patient's occlusion, bite abnormalities (open bite, cross bite, early contact) and dental wear facets.

Once the facial examination is complete, the examination of the scalp, ears, and neck completes the head and neck examination. The hair-bearing scalp should be carefully assessed for lacerations and foreign bodies. The ears are assessed for lacerations, auricular hematoma, otorrhea, and hemotympanum. The neck is assessed for crepitus, lacerations, foreign bodies, and hematomas. Special attention should be given to the palpation of the larynx to assess for occult injuries and fractures.

Several imaging modalities are useful in the evaluation of facial trauma. The selection of the imaging modality depends on the primary survey, the mechanism of injury (blunt versus blast versus penetrating), and the suspected injuries. CT scan is the primary radiographic study used for the evaluation of facial fractures. Intravenous contrast is usually not necessary for this evaluation. Three-dimensional reconstruction of axial and coronal CT scan images can also be obtained and may provide the additional advantage of helping in the planning of any surgical repair. In the absence of three-dimensional reconstruction, a panoramic tomographic view, or panorex, of the mandible may allow improved characterization of fractures, specifically, ramus and subcondylar fractures. An example is show in Figure 2. If embedded foreign bodies are suspected, then

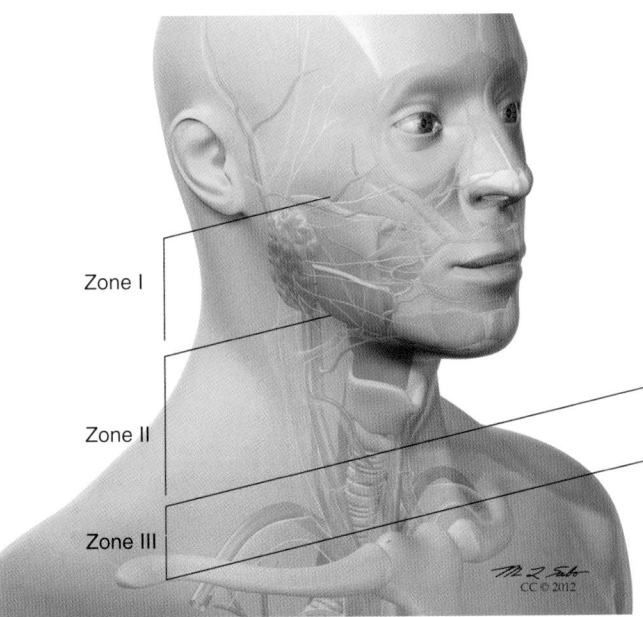

FIGURE 1   The zones of the neck. Zone 1 extends from the clavicle to cricoid cartilage. Zone 2 extends from the cricoid cartilage to the angle of the mandible. Zone 3 extends from the angle of the mandible to the skull base. *(Reprinted with permission from Cleveland Clinic Center for Medical Art & Photography, 2012. All rights reserved.)*

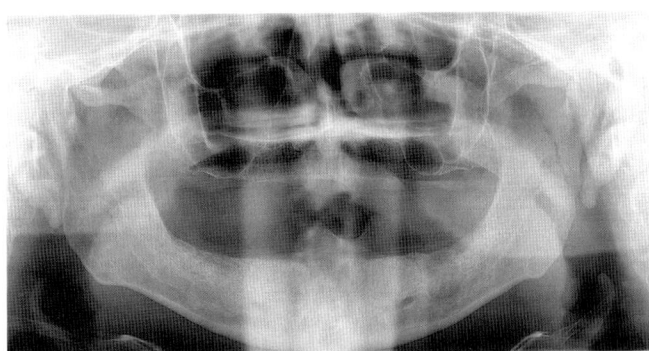

FIGURE 2   Panorex of a nondisplaced left mandibular ramus fracture.

imaging should be tailored to the investigation. CT scans and plain film x-rays can be used for the detection of glass and metal. Magnetic resonance imaging (MRI) can be used for the detection of wood and organic foreign bodies. If a vascular injury is suspected, as is the case with penetrating injuries to zone 1 and zone 3 of the neck, then CT angiography or conventional angiography is recommended.

SOFT TISSUE INJURIES AND MANAGEMENT

Lacerations and Avulsions

The initial assessment of soft tissue injuries of the head and neck begins with cleaning of the area of interest. Blood, clot, and debris should be cleared to allow for a thorough inspection of all lacerations. The wounds should be irrigated liberally with copious amounts of sterile saline solution with gentle pressure to remove debris. Failure to remove debris, especially dark foreign matter, can lead to

traumatic dermal tattooing. When possible, documentation of the size, depth, and extent (skin/mucosa, subcutaneous tissue, muscle, bone, nerve) of any wound is appropriate. Clean wounds should be closed primarily either in the trauma bay or, if necessary, in the operating room. Débridement of frayed, tattered, and nonviable skin and tissues may be necessary for effective wound closure. Deeper injuries and injuries communicating with a mucosal surface may require a multilayered closure or a passive drain. Large soft tissue defects that are not amenable to early primary closure should be dressed with saline solution–soaked gauze or a wound vacuum-assisted closure (VAC) dressing to promote wound closure with secondary intent healing. Avulsed soft tissue may be returned to its native site. If the tissue is viable, then it provides the best functional and aesthetic outcome. If the avulsed tissue is not viable, then it at least serves as a temporary biologic dressing. After closure, the wounds should be maintained with a thin moisture layer, such as petroleum jelly or water-based ointment, applied twice daily for 1 to 2 weeks. Sutures should be removed within approximately 5 to 7 days. Aesthetically unacceptable scars can be revised in 6 to 9 months.

The Facial Nerve and Parotid Duct

The assessment of facial nerve function is critical. The decision to explore, decompress, or repair the facial nerve is based on the level of function, the mechanism of trauma, and the temporal onset of the paralysis in relation to the injury. A quick assessment of facial nerve function should document normal movement, incomplete paralysis (paresis), or complete paralysis in the tasks of eyebrow raising, eye closure, smile and snarl, and lower lip depression. Attention should be paid to any asymmetry and its location. An anatomic diagram of the facial nerve branches is shown in Figure 3. However, even in the awake patient, assessment may be difficult and limited to the observation of facial expressions in response to the pain of the injuries, as in the obtunded patient. In addition, time should be allowed for the clearance of any local or general anesthetic before a facial nerve examination.

The mechanism of trauma (blunt versus blast versus penetrating) is an important factor in determination of clinical intervention in facial nerve paralysis. Most penetrating injuries in the distribution of the facial nerve with incomplete facial paralysis can be managed conservatively with observation. The presence of some function implies some neuronal and axonal integrity. In contrast, lateral penetrating injuries with complete facial paralysis are generally explored for possible repair of the facial nerve. The location of the facial injury influences the decision to explore. Exploration is necessary for penetrating trauma lateral to the lateral canthus of the eye. If the injury is medial to the lateral canthus, the facial nerve has been shown to have significant arborization, which allows for greater recovery potential, particularly in the midface region. These medial injuries may be observed. Blunt and blast injuries with associated facial paralysis should also involve an investigation of the temporal bones as a possible etiology of the facial paralysis.

Facial lacerations with facial nerve paralysis that warrant exploration should be explored within 72 hours of injury. During this clinical window, the distal nerve can be identified with probing with electrical stimulation. Once this period has temporally passed, wallerian degeneration prevents this clinical evaluation, and the identification of the nerve endings, which are often less than a millimeter in diameter, becomes much more difficult.

If a transection is identified, the proximal and distal ends of the nerves should be minimally mobilized to allow for a tension-free epineural repair. This should ideally be performed with magnification to avoid inadvertent axonal injury and align the epineurium optimally. Nerve interposition grafts should be placed wherever there is a missing segment of facial nerve. In addition, care must be taken to maintain separate and distinct branches of the facial nerve when facial nerve repair is performed to avoid synkinesis.

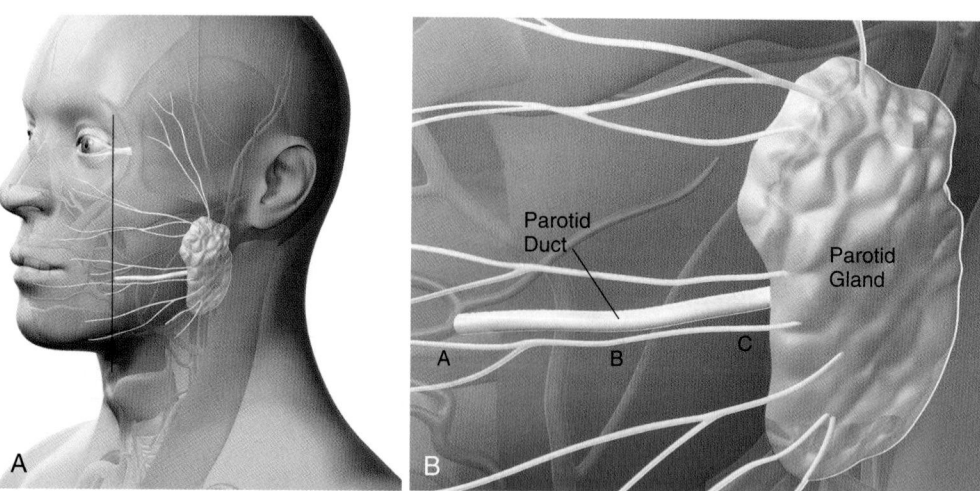

FIGURE 3 A, Facial nerve branches with vertical line demarcating lateral canthus and region for nerve exploration. **B,** Inset of parotid gland and duct: *point A,* distal near papilla; *point B,* midparotid duct; *point C,* proximal near parotid gland. *(Reprinted with permission from Cleveland Clinic Center for Medical Art & Photography, 2012. All rights reserved.)*

Facial lacerations in the vicinity of the parotid duct (Stenson's duct) or blood at the orifice of the parotid duct warrant evaluation with cannulation with a lacrimal probe to identify injuries to the duct. A diagram of the parotid gland and duct is shown in Figure 3, *B.* Injuries to the parotid duct should be repaired primarily whenever possible and ideally in the operating room. The cannulation of the duct can aid in performing this repair. A silicone elastomer stent is cannulated into the orifice of the parotid duct intraorally and passed proximally across the transected segment of the parotid duct and then into the proximal parotid duct segment. The transected parotid duct is then closed over the silicone elastomer stent. The stent may be left in place for several weeks to divert saliva and prevent stenosis of the parotid duct during its healing. Injuries to the more distal aspect of the duct with a reasonable length of viable parotid duct present should be reimplanted either into the papilla (Figure 3, *point A)* or into the buccal mucosa at a more posterior location in the oral cavity (Figure 3, *point B).* Injuries to the very proximal aspect of the parotid duct near the parotid gland without hope for primary repair are usually best treated with parotid duct ligation (Figure 3, *point C).* A drain should be placed in the wound bed to evacuate residual blood and saliva and prevent sialocele formation.

Bites: Human and Canine

Approximately 44,000 facial dog bite injuries occur annually according to the Centers for Disease Control (Karlson, 1984). Traditionally, the approach to management of a dog bite injury was washout, débridement, and then delayed closure or healing with secondary intention (Callahan, 1980). However, some studies suggest that primary repair of a facial injury carries no greater risk of infection and allows the best chance for a superior functional and aesthetic outcome (Javaid, 1998). Consideration should be given to a primary closure, if the wound has not suffered a significant loss of soft tissue. In addition, antibiotics should be administered for coverage against the flora present in a dog's mouth, *Staphylococcus aureus, Streptococci, Pasteurella multocida,* and anaerobes. Finally, the rabies status of the animal should be determined early in the evaluation to allow for appropriate treatment.

Human bite injuries are the third most common bite injury of the face, after dogs and cats. The basic tenets of initial wound care are similar to those described previously for dog bite injuries. Additional consideration should be given to the increased pathogenicity and potential for transmission of infection with human bites. Hepatitis B and C, herpes simplex virus, syphilis, tuberculosis, tetanus, and human immunodeficiency virus (HIV) are transmissible through human bite injuries (Harrison, 2009). In addition, antibiotic

coverage for human bites should include coverage for *Eikenella corrodens* and *Corynebacterium* species, both known causes of delayed abscesses after human bites. In contrast to human bites outside of the head and neck, bites to the face that are not grossly infected at the time of presentation should be closed primarily to achieve the best functional and aesthetic outcome. Human bites to the face are less likely to result in infection because of the vascularity of the facial region. Consideration for a delayed repair should be made with infected wounds and ear injuries with exposed cartilage (Ambro, 2010).

Most facial soft tissue injuries from canine or human bites can be addressed primarily at the bedside with local anesthesia with or without intravenous sedation. Antibiotics and continued local wound care, especially for delayed healing wounds, are critical to the achievement of satisfactory functional and aesthetic outcomes.

BONY INJURIES AND MANAGEMENT

Overview

The facial skeleton can be divided into two major structural components: the vertical and the horizontal buttresses. The vertical buttresses include the vertical portion of the mandible, nasomaxillary buttress, zygomaticomaxillary buttress, and the pterygomaxillary buttress. Their primary functional role is with mastication, so they are strong and well developed to withstand these compressive forces. The horizontal buttresses include the frontal bar, inferior orbital rim, and hard palate. These support structures act as an interconnected framework to stabilize the vertical buttresses. A diagram of the facial skeleton is shown in Figure 4.

Mandibular Fractures

Types

Mandibular fractures are the second most common facial fracture (Allareddy, 2011). Mandibular fractures are classified according to the location of the fracture: symphysis/parasymphysis, body, angle, ramus, coronoid process, and condyle. Figure 5 illustrates common fracture locations along with relative frequency. The most common sites of fracture are the angle and body, followed by the symphysis/parasymphysis (Ogundare, 2003). Assessment should include palpation of the mandible, inspection of the quality of the mandibular dentition, inspection of dental wear facets, and mental nerve

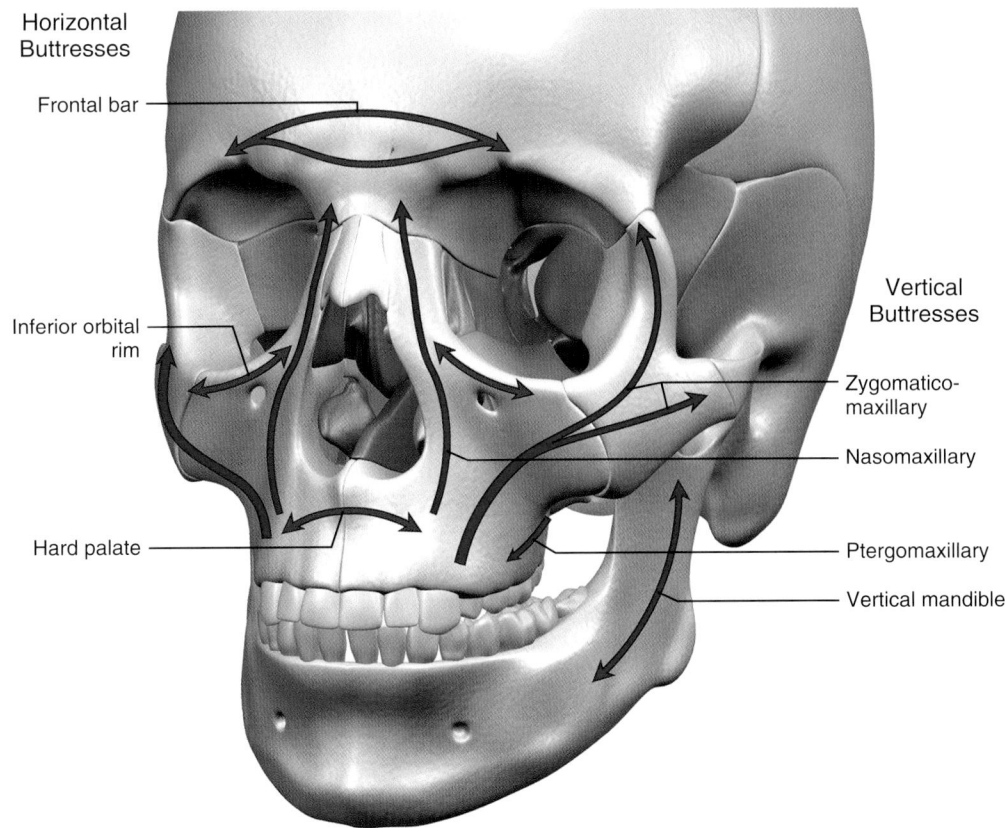

FIGURE 4 Facial skeleton with buttresses. *(Reprinted with permission from Cleveland Clinic Center for Medical Art & Photography, 2012. All rights reserved.)*

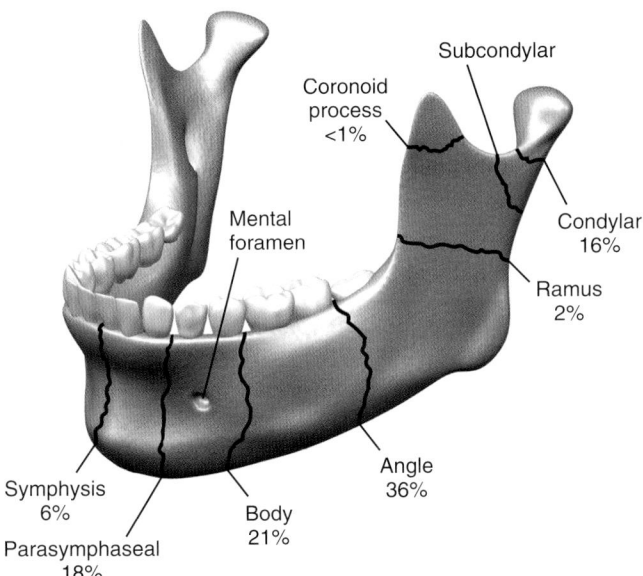

FIGURE 5 Common mandible fracture locations and relative frequency shown in percentages. *(Reprinted with permission from Cleveland Clinic Center for Medical Art & Photography, 2012. All rights reserved.)*

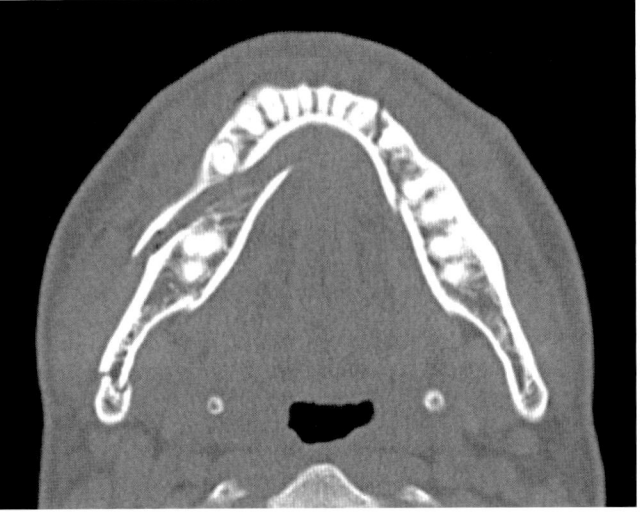

FIGURE 6 Axial computed tomographic scan image without contrast showing right ramus, right body, and left parasymphyseal fractures of the mandible.

function. CT scan of the facial bones and mandible is necessary to evaluate the extent of injury. An example is shown in Figure 6. When possible, evaluation of the patient's occlusion and mouth opening should be made. Presenting signs and symptoms include trismus, malocclusion, numbness, and loose or missing teeth. A discussion of the patient's preinjury occlusion can also be helpful.

Treatment

The ultimate goals of mandibular fracture management are restoration of the preinjury occlusion, bony union after reduction of fracture segments, and preservation of facial contour and facial height. The location and type of mandibular fracture (greenstick, displaced/nondisplaced, comminuted/noncomminuted) dictate the surgical approach, the hardware used, and the nature of postoperative rehabilitation. Greenstick fractures can be treated with closed reduction

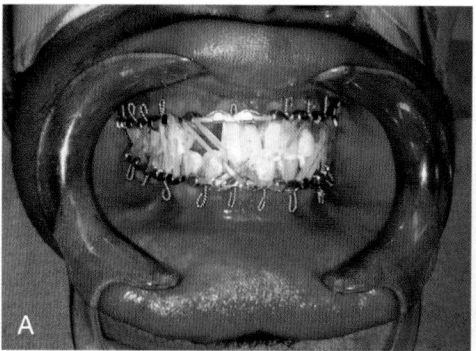
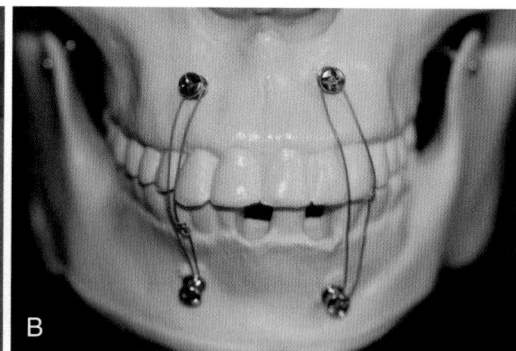

FIGURE 7 **A,** Maxillomandibular fixation with arch bars and elastic rubber bands. **B,** Maxillomandibular fixation with intermaxillary fixation screws and wires.

without fixation and maintenance of a soft diet. Maxillomandibular fixation (MMF) can be used to achieve closed reduction in patients who cannot spontaneously bring their teeth to their preinjury occlusion. Steel arch bars are applied to the maxillary and mandibular gingiva and tightly secured to the underlying dentition with loops of 24-gauge wire. The maxillary arch bar is then fastened to the mandibular arch bar, locking the patient into rigid fixation and ideally the preinjury occlusion. Examples are illustrated in Figure 7. If MMF is chosen as the definitive treatment for a mandibular fracture, then it should be maintained for approximately 6 weeks. MMF should be used with caution in patients with questionable mental status, mental retardation, seizure history, or substance abuse history. These patients may not be capable of removing their MMF in the event of emesis, which can lead to aspiration and potentially life-threatening airway compromise. Beyond the airway risks, MMF has significant morbidity associated with its use. Poor dental hygiene and enamel loss, discomfort, and speech and articulation difficulties are common reports of patients in intermaxillary fixation. The inability to chew and the lack of solid food consumption for 6 weeks can result in difficulty maintaining nutritional balance, with resultant weight loss during the fixation. Adult patients may lose up to 20 lbs during this period. These prolonged and significant morbidities have led to the increased use of open approaches with permanent rigid internal fixation as the primary mode of treatment for the vast majority of operative mandibular fractures.

Advances in plating systems have improved outcomes over the last few decades. Displaced fractures of the angle, body, and symphysis/parasymphysis can be managed with open reduction and rigid internal fixation with plates and screws via a transoral or transcervical approach. Figure 8 shows a compression plate and tension band. The use of dynamic compression plates allows a force vector to be created across the fracture line to optimize bone healing and reduce callus formation. The incorporation of lower profile hardware, superiorly based tension bands, and occlusal splints has reduced the morbidity of rigid fixation and improved outcomes.

Condylar fractures are unique because of the complexities with surgical approach and the difficulties with plating at this location. They can be managed closed (with or without MMF) or open (Zide, 1983; Palmieri, 1999; De Riu, 2001). The closed approach without MMF can be used in patients with good spontaneous occlusion. These patients are encouraged to exercise a full range of motion while maintaining a soft diet. The closed approach with MMF can also be used, but a greater concern exists for subsequent temporomandibular joint (TMJ) dysfunction because of the inflammatory response at the TMJ in condylar fractures. The open approach, either transoral or transcervical, involves plating across the fractured condylar segments with or without the assistance of endoscopic instrumentation. The indications for open repair of condylar fractures are displacement into the middle cranial fossa, poor occlusion with closed reduction, lateral extracapsular displacement of the condyle, presence of a foreign body, and open fracture with potential for fibrosis (Zide, 1989).

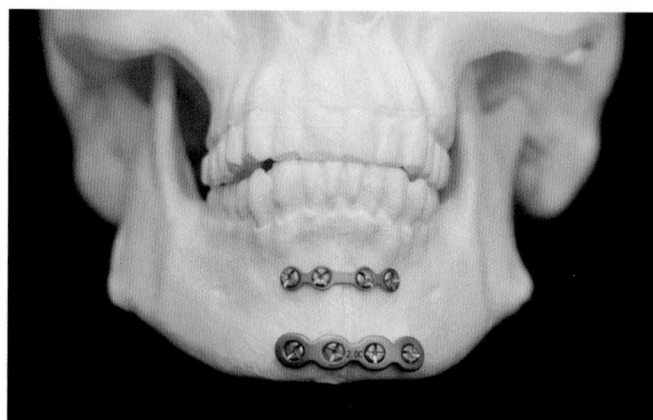

FIGURE 8 Compression plate and tension band at the symphysis.

Most high ramus and nondisplaced angle fractures do not warrant the morbidity of an open approach and can be treated with a closed approach with or without MMF. Isolated coronoid process fractures are rare and usually do not require treatment.

Complications

The major complications of mandibular fractures are infection, malunion, nonunion, malocclusion, and TMJ dysfunction. Antibiotics in the perioperative period have not been associated with a decrease in infection risk (Furr, 2006). The risk of TMJ ankylosis can be reduced with shorter periods of MMF (<3 weeks) and physiotherapy, such as range of motion exercises.

Special Considerations

Patients often present with more than one site of fracture (Allareddy, 2011; Ogundare, 2003). Unstable bilateral mandible fractures can lead to airway compromise through hemorrhage or edema followed by prolapse of the base of the tongue or fractured segments of mandible. Urgent airway intervention may be necessary in these cases. Edentulous mandibles present additional challenges in their management because of the atrophic nature of the mandible. The patient's dentures may need to be used for MMF, and a more aggressive open reduction internal fixation approach with load-bearing plates may be considered to minimize postoperative complications. Comminuted fractures can be difficult because of the mobility of the small mandible fragments. These patients should be placed into MMF; the smaller fracture segments are realigned with miniplates, and then the larger fracture segments are spanned by a more durable load-bearing plate.

Nasal Fractures

Types

Nasal bone fractures are the most common facial fracture (Allareddy, 2011). Nasal bone fractures can be unilateral, bilateral, nondisplaced, and displaced and with variable involvement of the septum. Assessment should include palpation of the nasal bones, nasal dorsum, and intranasal examination for septal hematoma or fracture. Radiographic imaging is usually not necessary in isolated nasal bone fractures but may be warranted depending on the comorbid injuries. Figure 9 illustrates a nasal bone fracture. Presenting signs and symptoms include epistaxis, nasal airway obstruction, alterations in smell, and cosmetic deformity. A review of the patient's preinjury nasal breathing and appearance can be helpful.

Treatment

The goals of nasal fracture management are to reestablish the preinjury nasal airway and restore the nasal contour. Nasal fractures can be treated with closed reduction or open reduction with osteotomy of the nasal bones. Closed reduction involves the mobilization of displaced nasal bones and cartilages with or without the use of a blunt elevating instrument inserted into the nose. Rapid spontaneous healing of these fractures requires acute intervention within 10 days of the injury. Even with early intervention, however, unsatisfactory cosmesis may still necessitate an open reduction procedure in the future. If the fractures are not managed within the acute time frame, then it is generally advisable to wait at least 3 months for adequate bone healing and overall nasal structural stabilization before performing an open reduction with osteotomy of the nasal bones. After reduction of the nasal fracture, external fixation should be applied with a nasal splint. If necessary for nasal breathing, a septoplasty may be performed in the operating room to correct any septal deviation or fracture. A septal hematoma should be drained as soon as possible to prevent septal cartilage necrosis, septal perforation, and potential saddle nose deformity.

Special Considerations

Although most cases of traumatic epistaxis can be managed conservatively with topical nasal decongestants, digital pressure, or blood pressure control, severe epistaxis may necessitate nasal packing, endoscopic blood vessel ligation, or angiography with embolization. Clear nasal drainage in the patient with facial trauma may also warrant an investigation for cerebrospinal fluid (CSF) rhinorrhea from a skull base fracture. Patients often note a salty or metallic taste

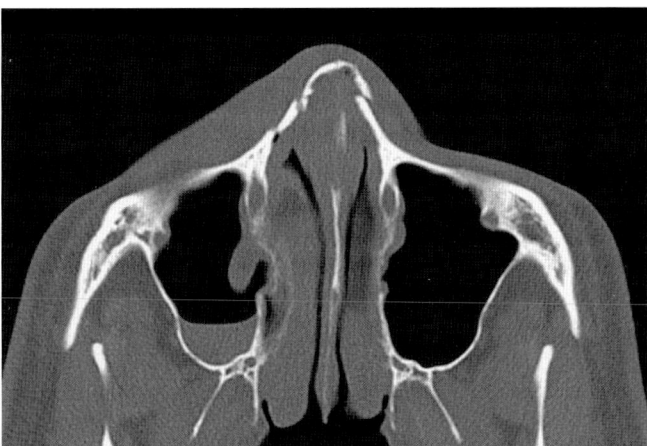

FIGURE 9 Axial computed tomographic scan image without contrast showing bilateral nasal bone fractures.

if a CSF leak is present. The halo sign, from differential capillary action of CSF and blood on a white cloth or tissue can also suggest the diagnosis. Collection of adequate sample volume to do this test is often not possible. It is primarily of historical significance. The advent of beta 2 transferrin testing allows accurate diagnosis with minimal sample collection and has become the standard of care to confirm the diagnosis.

Complications

The major complications of nasal fractures include nasal airway obstruction, unsatisfactory cosmesis, epistaxis, and septal perforation from septal hematoma.

Nasoorbitoethmoidal Fractures

Types

Nasoorbitoethmoidal (NOE) fractures are usually the result of a high-impact blunt trauma to the mid face. They can occur in isolation but usually present as part of a panfacial fracture. NOE fractures are classified according to the extent of bony fracture and condition of the medial canthal tendon. Figure 10 illustrates the classification scheme for NOE fractures. Assessment should include palpation of the nasal bones, visual acuity check, evaluation of eyelid and globe condition and position, and intranasal examination. CT scan of the facial bones is necessary to evaluate the extent of injury. Presenting signs and symptoms include telecanthus, enophthalmos, epiphora, nasal airway obstruction, and epistaxis.

Treatment

The goals of NOE fracture management are to restore nasal contour and intercanthal and interpupillary distance by reestablishing the medial orbital rim and attachment of the medial canthal tendon to the frontal process of the maxilla. An open approach through an existing laceration or a facial incision, such as coronal, Lynch, midface degloving, or gull wing, is necessary to ensure adequate reduction and fixation. NOE fractures are often severely comminuted. Fractured segments of bone can be sutured, wired, or screwed with miniplates into fixation. The complex comminuted nature of these fractures often precludes plate fixation of the bone with medial canthal tendon attachment. In these cases, the detached medial canthal tendon must be secured to the frontal process of the maxilla via a transnasal canthopexy to restore the preinjury intercanthal distance. Type 2 and 3 NOE fractures may require bone grafts to reconstruct the medial orbit and the nasal dorsum.

Special Considerations

NOE fractures may have concomitant injury to the nasolacrimal system. However, routine exploration of the lacrimal apparatus or a dacryocystorhinostomy in the acute settings is not indicated unless obvious injury is noted.

Complications

The major complications of NOE fractures include epiphora, telecanthus, enophthalmos, midface retrusion, and saddle nose.

Frontal Fractures

Types

The frontal bone is the strongest of the facial bones, but its superior anatomic location also makes the area prone to traumatic injury in

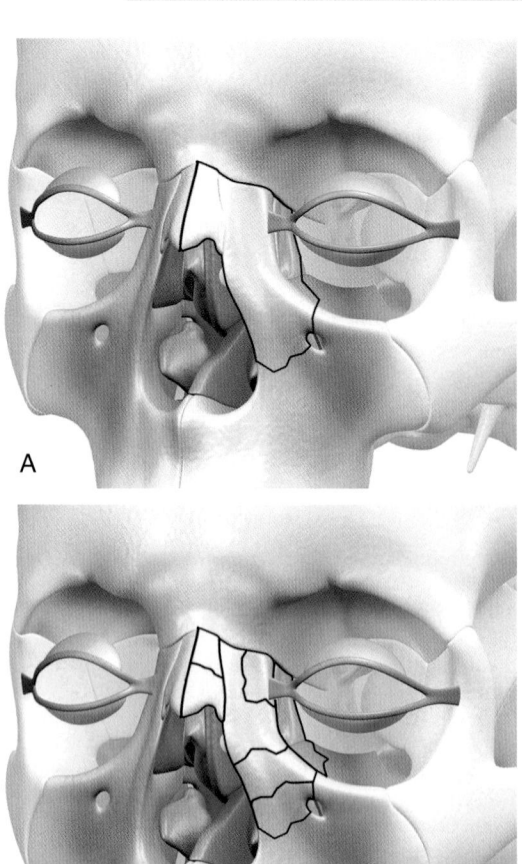

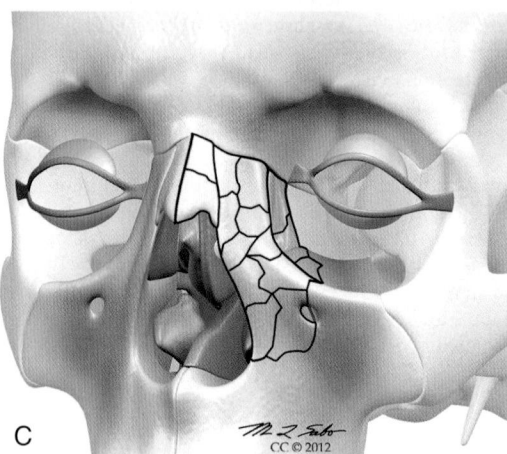

FIGURE 10 Nasoorbitoethmoidal (NOE) fracture classification scheme: **A,** type 1 NOE; **B,** type 2 NOE; **C,** type 3 NOE. *(Reprinted with permission from Cleveland Clinic Center for Medical Art & Photography, 2012. All rights reserved.)*

vehicular injuries and falls. Fractures in the region are therefore not uncommon. Frontal sinus fractures can be displaced, nondisplaced, comminuted, and noncomminuted. Figure 11 illustrates a frontal sinus fracture. Assessment should include palpation of the frontal bar, evaluation of forehead sensation, visual acuity check, and intranasal examination. CT scan of the facial bones and sinuses is a critical portion of the assessment of frontal sinus fractures. Presenting signs and symptoms include forehead lacerations and numbness, epistaxis, and rhinorrhea. Any posterior table fracture should be examined with a high suspicion for possible CSF leak.

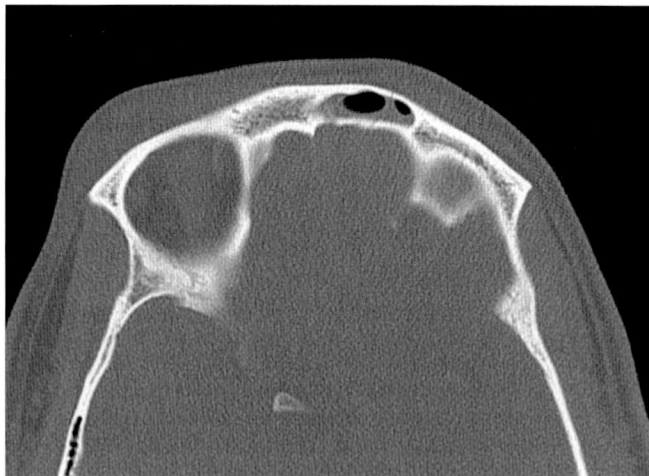

FIGURE 11 Axial computed tomographic scan image without contrast showing nondisplaced anterior and posterior table frontal sinus fractures.

Treatment

The goals of frontal sinus fracture management are to restore the aesthetic appearance of the frontal region and maintain the drainage and aeration of the frontal sinus system. The management of frontal sinus fractures is dependent on the condition of the anterior and posterior tables of the frontal sinus, the nasofrontal duct, and the anterior cranial fossa. Nondisplaced anterior table fractures do not require intervention. Displaced anterior table fractures require intervention if there are cosmetic concerns or if the fracture interferes with the frontal sinus drainage via the nasofrontal duct. Frontal sinus obliteration is used for fractures that involve the nasofrontal duct. Posterior table fractures that are nondisplaced do not require immediate intervention but should be followed with serial CT scans to evaluate the sinus. Posterior table fractures that are displaced or comminuted or present with pneumocephalus should be explored. Frontal sinus obliteration should be reserved for cases where the frontal sinus floor is not comminuted and the posterior table bone is largely intact. Frontal sinus cranialization is the treatment of choice for posterior table fractures with severe comminution or displacement of bone.

Special Considerations

Intracranial morbidity is a primary short-term concern with frontal sinus fractures. CSF leak through an anterior skull base injury can be both an early and a late complication. Delayed mucocele formation is another complication that warrants long-term follow-up with serial CT scans of the sinuses and anterior skull base.

Complications

The major complications of frontal sinus fractures include obstruction of the frontal sinus drainage pathway with resultant sinusitis, mucocele, or intracranial extension of infection.

Zygomaticomaxillary Complex Fractures

Types

Anatomically, zygomaticomaxillary complex (ZMC) fractures involve four suture lines: zygomaticofrontal, zygomaticomaxillary, zygomaticotemporal, and zygomaticosphenoid. Figure 12 illustrates a ZMC

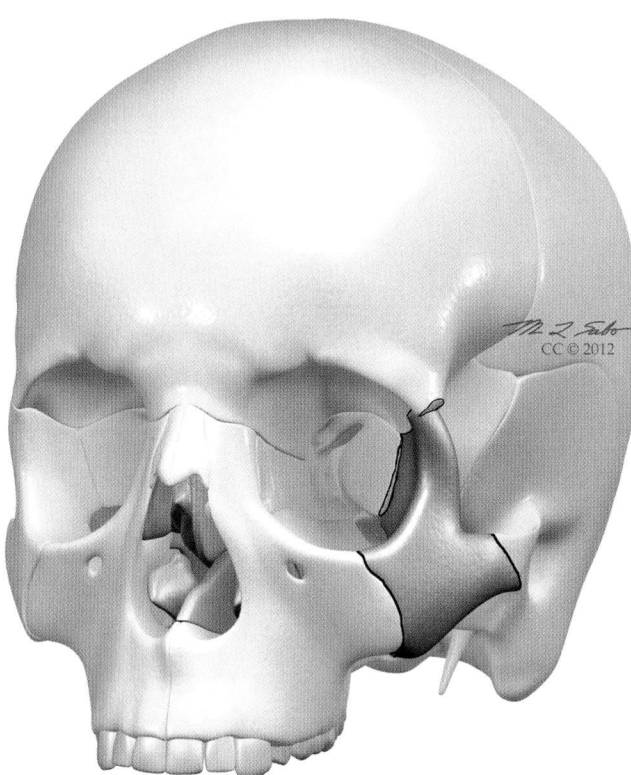

FIGURE 12 A typical displaced zygomaticomaxillary complex fracture. *(Reprinted with permission from Cleveland Clinic Center for Medical Art & Photography, 2012. All rights reserved.)*

fracture. Radiographically, ZMC fractures usually involve fractures of the lateral orbital wall, orbital floor/inferior orbital rim, anterior maxillary sinus wall, lateral maxillary sinus wall, and zygomatic arch. ZMC fractures can lead to significant aesthetic disturbances because the malar eminence of the zygoma is the most anterior projection of the lateral mid face and the zygomatic arch is the most lateral projection of the mid face. Assessment should include palpation of the zygoma, intraoral and intranasal examination, mouth opening, visual acuity check with extraocular muscle function, and midface sensation. Ophthalmologic consultation should be considered for any vision symptoms or significant orbital injury. CT scan of the facial bones and sinuses is a critical portion of the assessment of ZMC fractures. Presenting signs and symptoms include epistaxis, vision changes, midface and dental numbness, malar depression, enophthalmos, trismus, and malocclusion.

Treatment

The goals of ZMC fracture management are restoration of the height, width, and projection of the malar eminence; reestablishment of the buttresses of the mid face; restoration of orbital volume; and adequate reduction of the fractures. Fractures can be approached with a combination of surgical incisions: upper gingivobuccal (sublabial), lateral upper blepharoplasty, transconjunctival, subciliary, or Gilles. After exposure and adequate reduction of the fractures, forced duction testing should be performed to rule out extraocular muscle entrapment during fracture reduction. Confirmation of continuity of the orbital floor after fracture reduction should also be considered. Fixation should be done at a minimum of two fracture points with plates and screws. Isolated zygomatic arch fractures may need to be reduced if the fracture produces a depression over the lateral face or if the fracture segments impinge on the temporalis muscle, leading

to trismus or masticatory dysfunction. Maxillary sinus fractures in isolation without other associated ZMC fractures rarely require intervention. Patient counseling regarding the risks of facial and orbital cellulitis and swelling with future episodes of sinusitis is advisable when appropriate.

Special Considerations

Given the intimate relationship between the ZMC and the orbit, preoperative and postoperative ophthalmologic evaluation may be warranted in certain circumstances.

Complications

The major complications of zygomaticomaxillary complex fractures include maxillary nerve anesthesia, trismus, globe malposition, vision changes, ectropion, and malar depression.

Le Fort Fractures

Types

The Le Fort fracture classification scheme is used to describe midface fracture patterns with separation of the tooth-bearing bone and cranium. Figure 13 illustrates the Le Fort fracture classification scheme. All Le Fort fractures have bilateral pterygoid plate fractures. Le Fort type 1 is a horizontal fracture through the maxilla superior to the maxillary dentition. Type 2 is a pyramidal fracture through the maxilla and orbit, outlining the nose. Type 3 is a fracture of the facial bones from the skull, a complete craniofacial separation. These fracture patterns are suggestive of a high-impact trauma.

Assessment should include manipulation of the hard palate relative to the skull, facial sensation, visual acuity check with extraocular muscle function, and intraoral and intranasal examination. CT scan of the facial bones and sinuses is a critical portion of the assessment of Le Fort fractures. Presenting signs and symptoms include facial anesthesia, epistaxis, vision changes, and malocclusion.

Treatment

The goals of Le Fort fracture management are restoration of the continuity of the facial bones with the cranium and reduction of fractures with the goal of returning the patient to the preinjury occlusion. Putting the patient into MMF ensures satisfactory occlusion and provides a stable foundation for the remainder of the repair. Type 1 injuries can be approached through an upper gingivobuccal (sublabial) incision. Type 2 and 3 injuries usually require the addition of eyelid incisions or a coronal approach. The details of the management of Le Fort fractures are analogous to the management of ZMC fractures discussed previously.

Special Considerations

Multiple Le Fort fracture patterns can be present in the same patient. For example, a complex type 3 fracture may have a concomitant fracture at the Le Fort 1 level (horizontal fracture through the maxilla superior to the maxillary dentition). For complex Le Fort fractures, a top-down approach is used to reduce the complexity of the overall fracture pattern as the fractures are sequentially reduced.

Complications

The major complications of Le Fort fractures include facial anesthesia, malocclusion, trismus, globe malposition, vision changes, ectropion, midfacial distortion, and nasal obstruction.

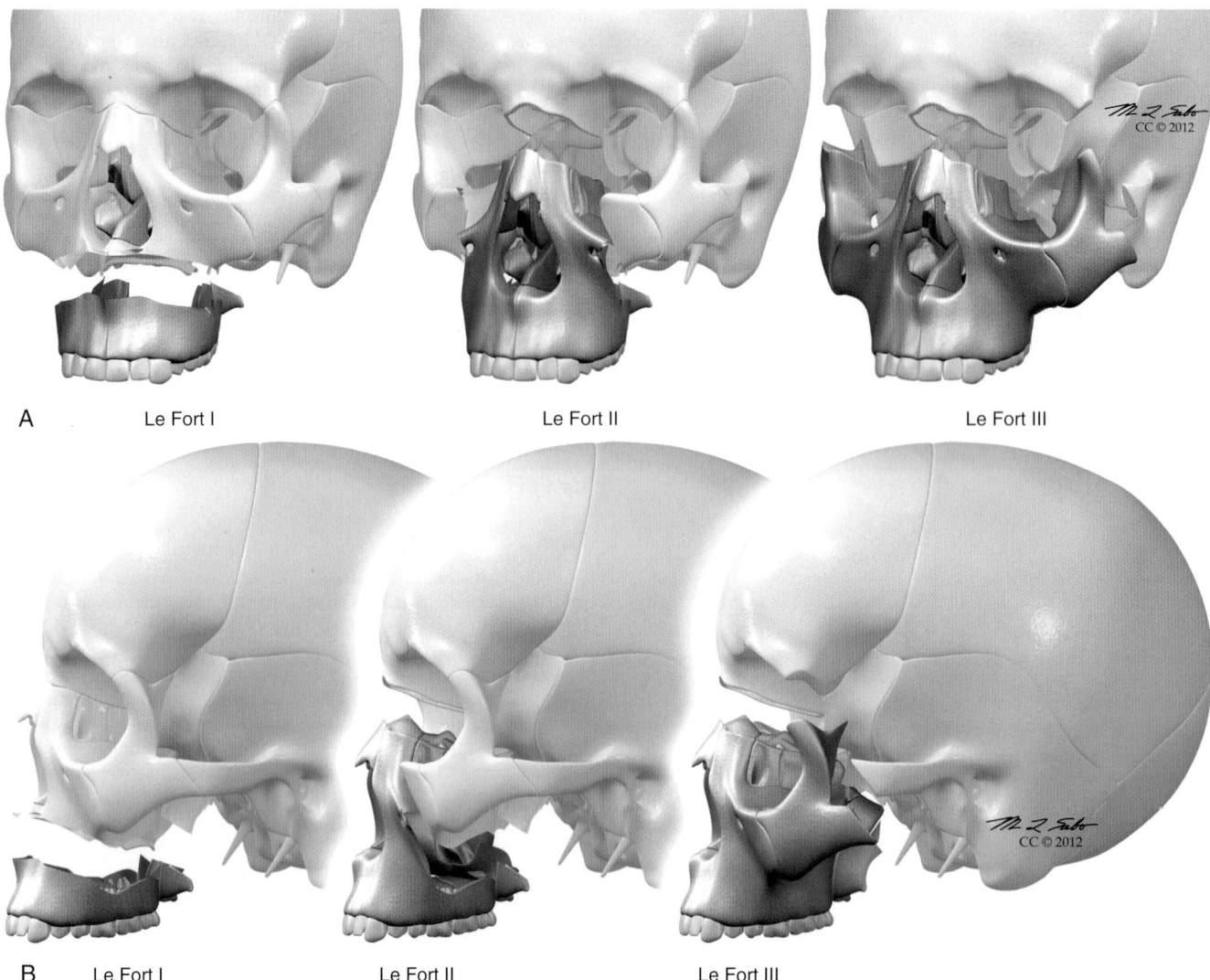

FIGURE 13 Le Fort fracture classification. **A,** Anterior view. **B,** Lateral view. *(Reprinted with permission from Cleveland Clinic Center for Medical Art & Photography, 2012. All rights reserved.)*

Panfacial Fractures

Types

Panfacial fractures involve fractures of the mandible, mid face, and frontal bones. These complex fractures may present with any of the signs and symptoms of the aforementioned facial fractures. For the purposes of panfacial fractures, the Le Fort type 1 fracture is used to delineate the facial skeleton into an upper and lower segment (Manson, 1999). CT scan of the facial bones and sinuses is imperative to the correct diagnosis and treatment of these injuries.

Treatment

The goals of panfacial fracture management are to restore the upper and lower facial skeleton in continuity with the cranium. Both the upper and the lower facial fractures should be secured to adjacent nonfractured bony landmarks. The upper facial skeleton (superior to the Le Fort type 1 fracture line) should be reduced and fixated to the frontal bone and cranium. The lower facial skeleton (inferior to the Le Fort type 1 fracture line) should be reduced

and fixated to the mandible, which via the TMJ is secured in continuity with the cranium. Although the sequence of fracture reduction and fixation is not critical, it should allow for flexibility in the management of the multiplicity of fractures. Manson and colleagues suggest the following: for the upper facial skeleton, reduce the frontal bones, then the NOE complex, followed by the ZMC; and for the lower facial skeleton, reduce the palate, then the vertical mandible (condyle, ramus, proximal angle), followed by the horizontal mandible (distal angle, body, symphysis/parasymphysis; Manson, 1999). The lower facial skeleton should be put into MMF to ensure proper occlusion and allow another point of fixation. After both the upper and the lower face are reconstructed in their proper alignment relative to the cranium, the two units are then fixated at the Le Fort 1 fracture line.

Special Considerations

Although initially a daunting task, the reconstruction of panfacial fractures can be simplified to smaller component fractures. In addition, the best chance for satisfactory functional and aesthetic outcome is with early reconstruction of soft tissue and bony injuries.

Complications

These complex fractures may present with any of the complications of the aforementioned facial fractures.

Orbital Fractures

Types

Orbital fractures can involve the inferior orbital rim, the lateral orbital rim, the medial orbital wall, the orbital floor, and rarely, the superior orbital rim. The isolated orbital floor fracture is commonly known as an orbital blowout fracture. These fractures can present with a trapdoor pattern with associated extraocular muscle entrapment seemingly outside of the orbital confines, especially in children. Assessment should include palpation of the orbital rims, evaluation of eyelid and globe condition and position, visual acuity check with extraocular muscle function, and evaluation of forehead and midface sensation. Ophthalmologic consultation should be considered for any vision symptoms or for significant orbital injury. CT scan of the facial bones and sinuses is a critical portion of the assessment of orbital fractures. Figures 14 and 15 illustrate orbital floor fractures. Presenting signs and symptoms include vision changes, forehead and midface numbness, enophthalmos, dystopia, chemosis, hyphema, and subconjunctival hemorrhage.

Treatment

The goals of orbital fracture management are restoration of orbital structure and volume. Orbital fractures are unique from other facial fractures in that the goal of treatment is not the healing of fractured bone but the reconstruction of violated orbital walls to restore volume. For correction and prevention of enophthalmos, dystopia, and diplopia, the orbital volume and globe position of the injured eye must be comparable with that of the uninjured eye. For reconstruction of the injured orbit, the surgeon must have an understanding of the complex anatomy of the orbit. Critically important is recognition of the S shape of the orbital floor as it extends posteriorly toward the orbital apex. Reconstruction of this complex floor is critical to achieving a satisfactory outcome. Orbital fractures can usually be approached through upper and lower eyelid, upper gingivobuccal, and coronal incisions. Isolated orbital floor fractures medial to the infraorbital nerve may be amenable to transmaxillary endoscopic repair. Isolated medial orbital wall fractures without extraocular muscle entrapment or significant orbital volume distortion do not require intervention. After adequate exposure of the orbital fracture is gained, the primary focus becomes restoration of the orbital volume. First, the orbital contents (extraocular muscles, fat, periorbita) are deposited back into the confines of the orbit. Next, the orbital wall defects are reconstructed with autogenous grafts (split calvarial bone, septal cartilage), absorbable alloplastic implants (polydioxanone, polyglycolide), or nonabsorbable alloplastic implants (titanium, silicone, polytetrafluoroethylene [PTFE], porous polyethylene).

Special Considerations

Appropriate consultation with ophthalmology and oculoplastic surgery should be initiated with significant globe or eyelid injuries or vision symptoms.

Complications

The major complications of orbital fractures include vision loss and changes, forehead and midface anesthesia, and eyelid and globe malposition.

EXTENSIVE INJURIES AND MANAGEMENT

Gunshot Wounds and Blast Injuries

Gunshot wounds cause tissue injury through three mechanisms: direct tissue injury, cavitation, and blast injury after entry. The management of gunshot wounds requires knowledge of the weapon used.

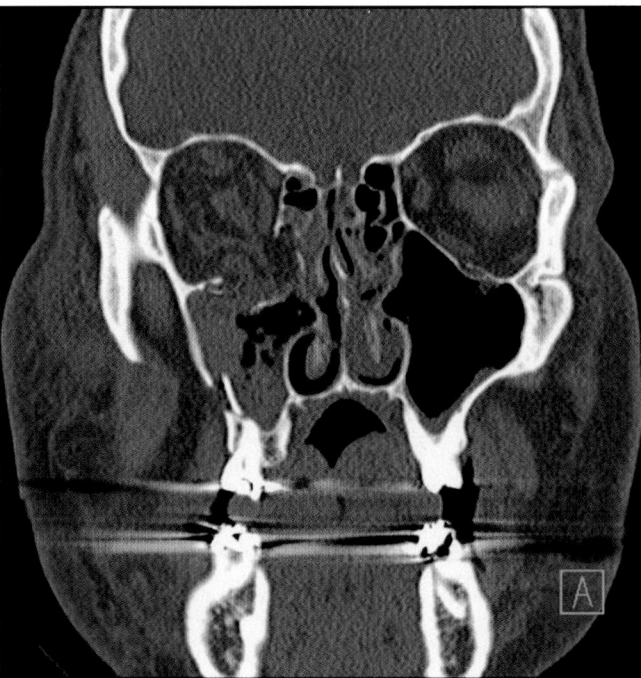

FIGURE 14 Coronal computed tomographic scan image without contrast showing displaced right orbital floor fracture with associated right lateral maxillary sinus wall fracture

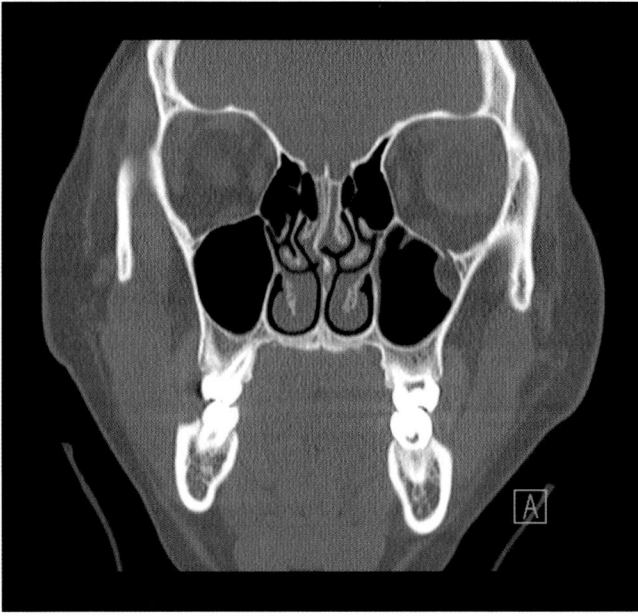

FIGURE 15 Coronal computed tomographic scan image without contrast showing minimally displaced left orbital floor fracture.

The weapon's muzzle velocity and ballistics of the penetrating missile dictate the survivability and extent of injury. The tissue damage caused by a gunshot wound depends on four characteristics of the projectile: kinetic energy, yaw, deformation, and fragmentation. The kinetic energy that is transferred from the missile to the body in a gunshot wound is dependent on the velocity and mass of the projectile (kinetic energy $= \frac{1}{2}$ mass $\times$ velocity^2). Yaw is the amount of movement about the axis with which the projectile is traveling. Deformation is the change in shape or size of the projectile during its flight. Fragmentation is the separation of the missile into multiple smaller projectiles.

Handguns generally fire smaller caliber missiles at a lower muzzle velocity, and hunting and military rifles fire larger caliber missiles at higher muzzle velocity. Rifles also often implement missiles that deform in flight or fragment on entry, creating greater tissue damage. Shotgun missiles tend to have high velocity at close range but decrease rapidly as they travel through the air.

Blast injuries are commonly classified into four categories: primary, secondary, tertiary, and quaternary. Primary blast injuries result from the direct interaction of the blast wave with the body. Secondary blast injuries are caused by objects propelled by the blast. Tertiary blast injuries are the result of displacement of the body by the blast wind. Quaternary blast injuries encompass all other injuries (psychologic, thermal, crush, respiratory, etc.) related to exposure to the blast.

Management

The initial assessment and management of ballistic trauma to the head and neck follow the same algorithm for treatment outlined previously in Emergent Treatment and Evaluation. After initial treatment and stabilization, the patient should be taken to the operating room for a thorough examination of the extent of injuries, washout, and débridement of nonviable tissues. An attempt should be made to preserve and stent the facial soft tissue envelope and all orifices. Fractures that can be reduced and fixated should be repaired. Tracheotomy may need to be performed. Planning for a staged definitive repair should be done at this time.

Facial injuries from ballistic trauma differ from other types of traumatic facial injuries. The restoration of bony landmarks and closure of soft tissue wounds are often not possible because of the loss of viable soft tissue and bone. In addition, the inherently poor vascularity of the severely traumatized tissues that remain and the associated evolving tissue necrosis and infection make a challenging situation worse. Primary repair of the injured tissues is rarely feasible because adequate viable tissue is no longer present locally. The paradigm must shift from the classic conceptions of injury repair to rebuilding. Successful restoration of form and function can only be achieved by recruiting tissues to rebuild the deficient structures of the face.

The treatment approach for extensive traumatic head and neck injuries has shifted away from delayed repair to early repair with local tissue and free tissue transfer reconstructions. Staged early definitive reconstruction allows for fewer surgeries and shorter hospitalizations (Doctor, 2007). The initial repair may involve some elements of healing with secondary intention or primary closure but usually requires early recruitment of healthy tissue into the face via local tissue rearrangement, pedicled regional flap, or free tissue transfer (anterolateral thigh flap, osteocutaneous fibula flap). Local tissue advancement with a cervicofacial flap can be used to reduce the soft tissue deficit and provide skin coverage. Although this flap brings healthier adjacent tissue into the defect, it is a randomly based flap and susceptible to vascular compromise and distal flap necrosis. Pedicled regional flaps (paramedian forehead flap, deltopectoral flap, latissimus dorsi flap) are supplied by a vascular pedicle, allowing for greater tissue viability and versatility. The paramedian forehead flap

can be used for nasal reconstruction. The deltopectoral flap and latissimus dorsi flap can be used to reconstruct large skin defects of the neck, lateral face, and scalp.

The evolving success and reliability of microvascular surgery has led to the early use of healthy vascularized free tissue transfer for trauma reconstruction. The advantages of recruiting nontraumatized naive tissue for the reconstruction include a more physiologic restoration of function and a reduction in scar contracture. Free tissue transfer also allows for the reconstruction of varying tissue defects (mucosa, bone, skin) with comparable vascularized tissue. The anterolateral thigh flap can be used to reconstruct large skin and soft tissue defects. The osteocutaneous fibula flap can be used to reconstruct orbitomaxillary and mandibular defects. The ultimate evolution of this concept is the use of allograft flaps. Face transplants have been used to reconstruct severe facial trauma injuries where massive loss of facial structures exist (Alam, 2009). Figure 16 illustrates the skeletal deficit from a face transplant recipient. Although technically more challenging than the typical free tissue transfer and requiring lifelong immunosuppression for the recipient, face transplants allow a composite transfer of varying soft tissue and bone that replaces the lost tissue with an exact anatomic match. With the development and success of face transplant programs, this once implausible surgery may soon become just another tool in the facial trauma surgeon's toolbox.

CONCLUSION

The importance of the face goes beyond its function, form, or aesthetics. An individual's membership and participation in society is contingent on the face. Although the trauma patient may present with many life-threatening and severe injuries, few are more damaging to an individual's existence than a significant trauma to a person's face.

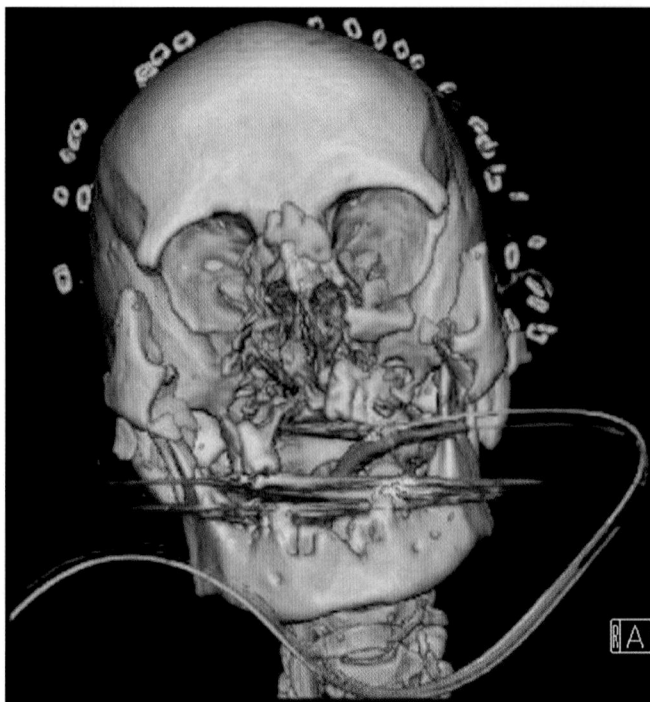

FIGURE 16 Three-dimensional reconstruction of the skeletal deficit in a face transplant recipient.

SUGGESTED READINGS

Alam DS, Papay F, Djohan R, et al: The technical and anatomical aspects of the world's first near-total human face and maxilla transplant, *Arch Facial Plast Surg* 11(6):369–377, 2009.

Allareddy V, Allareddy V, Nallia RP: Epidemiology of facial fractures, *J Oral Maxillofac Surg* 69(10):2613–2618, 2011.

Ambro BT, Wright RJ, Heffelfinger RN: Management of bite wounds in the head and neck, *Facial Plast Surg* 26(6):456–463, 2010.

Burgess CA, Dale OT, Almeyda R, et al: An evidence based review of the assessment and management of penetrating neck trauma, *Clin Otolaryngol* 37(1):44–52, 2012.

Callahan M: Dog bite wounds, *JAMA* 244:2327–2328, 1980.

De Riu G, Gamba U, Anghinoni M, et al: A comparison of open and closed treatment of condylar fractures: a change in philosophy, *Int J Oral Maxillofac Surg* 30(5):384–389, 2001.

Doctor V, Farwell G: Gunshot wounds to the head and neck, *Curr Opin Otolaryngol Head Neck Surg* 15(4):213–218, 2007.

Furr A, Schweinfurth J, May W: Factors associated with long-term complications after repair of mandibular fractures, *Laryngoscope* 116:427–430, 2006.

Harrison M: A 4-year review of human bite injuries presenting to emergency medicine and proposed evidence-based guidelines, *Injury* 40(8):826–830, 2009.

Javaid M, Feldberg L, Gipson M: Primary repair of dog bites to the face: 40 cases, *J R Soc Med* 91:414–416, 1998.

Karlson TA: The incidence of facial injuries from dog bites, *JAMA* 252:3265, 1984.

Kesser BW, Chance E, Kleiner D, et al: Contemporary management of penetrating neck trauma, *Am Surg* 75(1):1–10, 2009.

Manson PN, Clark N, Robertson B, et al: Subunit principles in midface fractures: the importance of sagittal buttresses, soft-tissue reductions, and sequencing treatment of segmental fractures, *Plast Reconstr Surg* 103(4):1287–1307, 1999.

Ogundare BO, Bonnick A, Bayley N: Pattern of mandibular fractures in an urban major trauma center, *J Oral Maxillofac Surg* 61(6):713–718, 2003.

Palmieri C, Ellis E III, Throckmorton G: Mandibular motion after closed and open treatment of unilateral mandibular condylar process fractures, *J Oral Maxillofac Surg* 57(7):764–776, 1999.

Tisherman SA, Bokhari F, Collier B, et al: Clinical practice guideline: penetrating zone II neck trauma, *J Trauma* 64(5):1392–1405, 2008.

Zide MF: Open reduction of mandibular condyle fractures: indications and technique, *Clin Plast Surg* 16:69, 1989.

Zide MF, Kent JN: Indications for open reduction of mandibular condyle fractures, *J Oral Maxillofac Surg* 41(2):89–98, 1983.

PENETRATING NECK TRAUMA

**Ronald V. Maier, MD, FACS, and
Deborah Lane Marquardt, MD**

INTRODUCTION

Penetrating neck injuries represent approximately 5% to 10% of traumatic incidents in adults. Though this is a small portion of the total traumatic events nationally, it is a particularly important topic given the number of significant structures located within the small space of the neck. It is critical to understand the anatomic relationships of the neck and to have a clear approach to the evaluation and management of penetrating neck injuries.

ANATOMY

The neck has classically been divided into both triangles and zones. The borders of the posterior triangle are the sternocleidomastoid muscle anteriorly, the trapezius muscle posteriorly, and the clavicle inferiorly. Within this triangle lie the spine and the vertebral arteries. The borders of the anterior triangle are the midline anteriorly, the sternocleidomastoid posteriorly, and the lower edge of the mandible superiorly. It contains many vital structures, including the carotid artery, jugular vein, trachea, esophagus, and recurrent laryngeal nerve (Figure 1). From inferior to superior, the neck is divided into zones that help direct investigation. Zone I refers to the thoracic inlet and the structures lying below the level of the cricoid cartilage. Zone II lies between the cricoid cartilage and the angle of the mandible, and Zone III includes structures above the angle of the mandible to the base of the skull (Figure 2). In considering the evaluation and

management of penetrating trauma to the neck, the zones are the most useful because they divide the anterior triangles where the vast majority of critical structures reside and can help direct the pathway for evaluation and management (see Figures 1 and 2).

INITIAL EVALUATION/MANAGEMENT

As with all traumatic injuries, the first step in the evaluation and management of penetrating neck trauma is addressing the ABCs. Ensuring a secure airway is paramount. However, even in the setting of tracheal injury, the vast majority of patients may be managed either without an artificial airway or via standard endotracheal intubation. Only rarely will emergent cricothyrotomy or tracheostomy be necessary. Once a secure airway is in place, a chest x-ray and lateral c-spine films are recommended. It is critical to evaluate for the presence of a pneumothorax or hemothorax, which can come from an injury to Zone I or if more than one zone is involved. A lateral c-spine film can be useful to outline the presence of foreign bodies and subcutaneous air and to further evaluate the anatomy of the airway. C-spine immobilization is an area of some controversy. Though significant vertebral injuries or ligamentous disruption is uncommon in the vast majority of penetrating neck injuries, it is judicious to proceed with immobilization if there are any signs of neurologic deficits, if the patient cannot be examined, or if the mechanism of injury is from a high energy source such as a gunshot wound.

Zone I and III Injuries

The thoracic inlet and submandibular regions of Zones I and III, respectively, represent areas less easily managed operatively due to limited access due to restrictive anatomy. In Zone I, this consists of the sternum, rib cage, and clavicle. One or more of these must be divided for full visualization of the underlying structures. In Zone III, surgical access is particularly limited due to the proximity to the skull base and relatively fixed mandible and the narrow space between them. In patients without signs of life-threatening hemorrhage, the

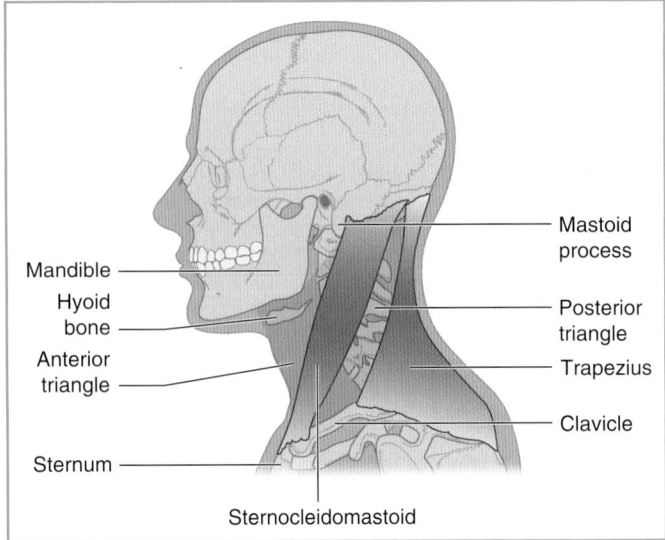

A

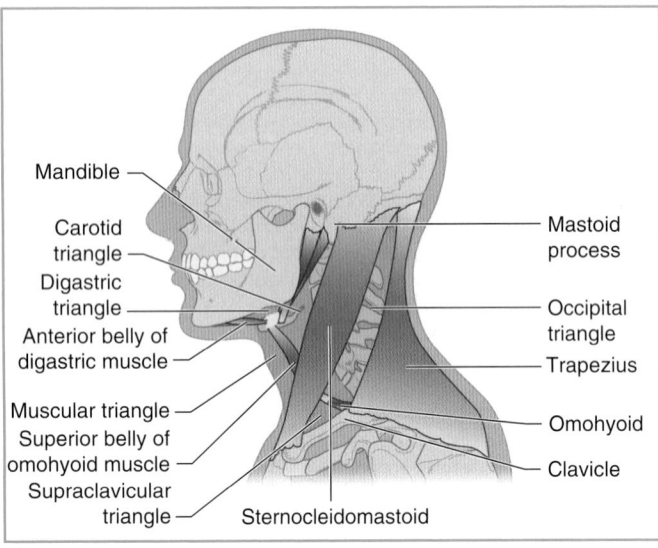

B

FIGURE I Anatomic triangles of the neck. **A,** The sternocleidomastoid muscle divides the main anterior and posterior triangles. **B,** Subdivision of the triangles further defines the structures at risk of injury. (*From Bogart BI: Elsevier's* Integrated anatomy and embryology, *Philadelphia, 2007, Elsevier, pp 10-26.*)

initial approach to both of these zones is to proceed with imaging studies to evaluate for significant injury. Computed tomographic (CT) angiography is the most commonly used imaging modality for penetrating neck trauma. It provides high-resolution images that can outline the path of the penetrating injury, which may help to identify injuries to pertinent structures, identify that key structures are distant from any signs of injury, and assist in planning the operative approach. Angiography remains the gold standard for evaluation of the vasculature, though it is infrequently utilized as the initial diagnostic modality today. It is most appropriate for use in a confirmatory diagnostic manner when debris or a foreign body causes artifact that distorts CT images, and it may also be used therapeutically for definitive intervention such as embolization, balloon occlusion, or endovascular stent placement to control vascular injury.

With signs of life-threatening hemorrhage and penetrating injury to Zone I of the neck, the most versatile surgical approach is a median sternotomy. This will provide access to the origin of the right subclavian, innominate, and left carotid arteries. This incision may be extended into the neck along the anterior boarder of the sternocleidomastoid muscle if more distal vascular control is necessary. To expose and manage distal subclavian vascular injuries, a supraclavicular extension of the median sternotomy may be performed on the ipsilateral side. In the process of accessing the subclavian vessels in this manner, initial control for hemorrhage from a supraclavicular wound can often be obtained using a finger or inflating a urinary catheter balloon within the tract behind the clavicle to tamponade bleeding. For proximal left subclavian injuries, a left anterolateral thoracotomy in the third interspace is the preferred additional incision for operative exposure. However, creation of the classic "open book" exposure is time-consuming, difficult, and highly morbid, and is thus rarely utilized (Figure 3). If a subclavian artery injury is noted during angiography, a proximal occlusion balloon may be placed to control hemorrhage prior to definitive surgical repair. Additionally, consideration should be given to endovascular stent placement to bridge an injury in the midportion of the vessel as definitive therapy (see Figure 3).

Zone III injuries are particularly difficult in that they offer limited operative accessibility due to the hardened structures of the mandible and the base of the skull. Superior posterior extension of an anterior sternocleidomastoid incision across the origin of the sternocleidomastoid with dislocation of the temporal mandibular joint and forward mobilization of the mandible has been described but rarely utilized. More commonly, division of the omohyoid will assist with exposure. Care must be taken to avoid injury to the glossopharyngeal (CN IX) nerve in this process because it lies just below the angle of the mandible parallel to the omohyoid muscle. Currently, injuries to the internal carotid artery in this location are frequently managed via angiography and endovascular stent placement or via ligation dependent on the extent and duration of any neurologic deficit.

Zone II

The definition of a penetrating neck injury is that which extends deep to the platysma muscle fascia. Zone II penetrating injuries that present with hard signs of significant injury mandate surgical exploration (Box 1). The most common surgical approach is via an incision along the ipsilateral anterior border of the sternocleidomastoid muscle. This will provide excellent exposure of the internal and external carotid arteries, internal jugular vein, trachea, esophagus, and larynx. If bilateral injury is encountered, this incision may be extended to include a transverse collar incision above the sternal notch, as well as a contralateral anterior sternocleidomastoid incision.

Treatment of Zone II injuries that penetrate the platysma but are not associated with any hard signs of significant injury is an area of ongoing debate and local tradition. The most definitive approach is to proceed with mandatory surgical exploration for all such injuries. Advocates of this approach cite overall low morbidity and early discharge after surgical neck exploration and high morbidity and potential mortality associated with missed injuries, particularly to the esophagus. However, in multiple series it has been noted that there is a 40% to 60% negative exploration rate with this approach. The least invasive approach is to utilize physical exam alone in patients with no signs or symptoms of deep injury. This may be appropriate in some cases, but it mandates that the patient be admitted for a minimum of 24 hours for observation and having the local resources available to manage injuries operatively or with angiography should they become apparent during the period of observation. Between these two extremes of approach is perhaps the most common approach to management of patients with either soft signs of injury or who are asymptomatic, which includes a hybrid of physical

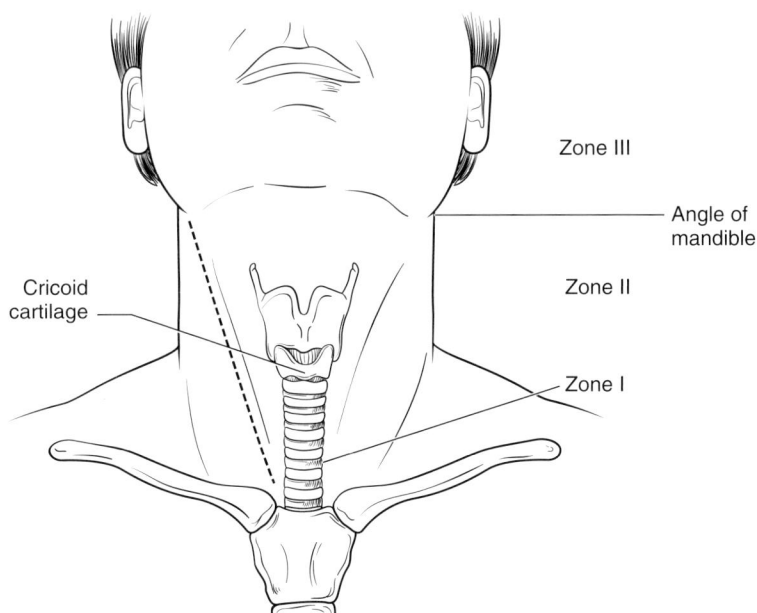

FIGURE 2   Zones of the neck. *(From Townsend CM, Evers BM:* Atlas of general surgical techniques, *Philadelphia, 2010, Saunders.)*

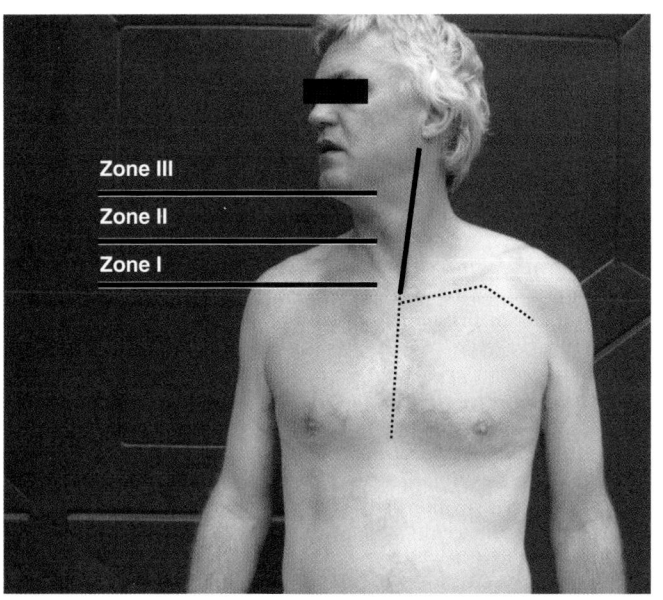

FIGURE 3   Neck exploration incisions.

BOX 1: Hard signs of significant injury

Shock
Large, expanding, or pulsatile hematoma
Active bleeding
Subcutaneous emphysema
Dyspnea or stridor
Hemoptysis/hematemesis
Focal or lateralizing neurologic deficit

examination, imaging, laryngobronchoscopy, and esophagography/ esophagoscopy (Box 2). It is important to remember that vascular and aerodigestive injuries may be present in the absence of any significant symptoms on initial presentation, so a high index of suspicion is always warranted with any penetrating neck injury (see Boxes 1 and 2).

BOX 2: Soft signs of significant injury

Dysphonia or voice change
Cough
Hoarseness
Dysphagia or odynophagia

As with Zone I and III injuries, Zone II penetrating injuries without hard signs mandating immediate operative intervention are most commonly initially evaluated with CT angiography. This technology is readily available in most hospitals and provides for an expeditious means to evaluate key structures for injury. As noted above, formal angiography or operative intervention will be necessary if artifact from foreign bodies obscures the carotid vessels on CT angiography. Additionally, laryngobronchoscopy can be utilized to further evaluate the upper and lower airways when injury is suspected on CT imaging. There is debate over the use of esophagography versus esophagoscopy to further evaluate for esophageal injury. Though neither study has proved 100% successful alone at identifying all injuries, in combination they are nearly 100% successful. In most circumstances, local resources and the degree of clinical indications should dictate the use of such modalities or need for transfer to a higher-level facility.

Operative Exposure

As noted above, most injuries to structures in Zone II may be managed via an incision anterior to the sternocleidomastoid muscle. Dissection is carried through the platysma. Bridging veins are ligated to facilitate exposure. The trachea and thyroid may be retracted medially and anteriorly to better expose the carotid sheath and its contents, as well as the tracheoesophageal groove. If esophageal injury is suspected, further dissection can be undertaken both anterior and posterior to the esophagus. For tracheal injuries at the level of the thyroid, the injury may provide the dissection needed for exposure. Additionally the thyroid isthmus may be divided to further facilitate visualization and repair. The proximal vertebral artery may be accessed by retracting the carotid sheath anterosuperiorly or posteroinferiorly to expose the prevertebral space and beginning of the intravertebral canal.

MANAGEMENT OF SPECIFIC INJURIES

Venous Injuries

Venous injuries are the most common cause of non–life-threatening bleeding in penetrating neck injuries. Small veins can and should be ligated without concern for significant sequelae. The internal jugular vein may be repaired with fine monofilament suture for unilateral injuries involving less than 50% of the circumference of the vessel. For larger or through-and-through injuries, ligation may be performed. Unilateral ligation of the internal jugular vein is very well tolerated. Bilateral ligation should be avoided because this significantly limits venous drainage of the brain and can predispose to intracerebral hypertension and significant facial swelling.

Arterial Injuries

Obtaining proximal and distal control is the key step in managing any major arterial injury. This may be done bluntly with a finger, particularly in areas adjacent to major nerve trunks, while dissection proceeds to allow proper clamp placement proximal and distal to the area of injury. Isolated arterial injuries without significant contusion or vessel loss may be primarily repaired with 5-0 or 6-0 permanent monofilament suture. For larger or through-and-through injuries, segmental resection should be considered. For resection or vessel loss of less than or equal to 1 cm in length, mobilization and potential repair can be undertaken by a primary anastomosis. When this is not possible, the use of reversed saphenous vein autograft is recommended. If no vein is available, prosthetic graft or a bovine patch graft may be used, but they carry higher risks for infection and graft failure. Additionally, the distal external carotid artery may be ligated and the proximal limb used as an in-continuity bypass graft for injury to the proximal internal carotid artery. The injured external carotid artery may be ligated if successful repair or reimplantation is not possible or if the patient is otherwise too systemically ill to tolerate the time required for such a repair. For the injured internal carotid artery, a shunt may be used as a temporizing measure in the setting of systemic extremis and higher treatment priorities overall. Additionally, a carotid shunt should be considered intraoperatively at the time of internal carotid repair if there is minimal backbleeding from the distal segment. Systemic heparinization is not necessary. Instead, instillation of a heparin solution proximal and distal into the vessels is recommended in the setting of acute traumatic injury.

In patients with a neurologic deficit and concomitant carotid injury, there is debate as to whether the internal carotid should be repaired or ligated due to fear of converting an ischemic stroke into a hemorrhagic one. Despite this concern, the best data to date suggest that repair of the artery provides for the best chances of a favorable outcome unless the neurologic deficit has been present for a prolonged period of time. Strict postoperative blood pressure control is indicated in all such circumstances.

Vertebral arterial injury is very uncommon in penetrating neck trauma due to its protected location within the vertebral column. Injury is most commonly identified during imaging via CT or formal angiography and less commonly via hemorrhage originating posteriorly during neck exploration. Acute hemorrhage, pseudoaneurysm, and arteriovenous fistula formation of the vertebral vessels warrant intervention. This is most commonly managed via angiographic embolization or permanent balloon occlusion. Operative ligation at the time of neck exploration may be accomplished via exposure of the prevertebral fascia as described above followed by blind hemoclip or bone wax placement between the transverse processes, behind the longus colli muscle at the level of C6 to C7. Proximal ligation may also be accomplished at the vertebral artery origin off of the subclavian artery via a supraclavicular approach with transection of the sternal head of the sternocleidomastoid muscle.

Tracheal Injuries

The trachea is easily visualized via the anterior sternocleidomastoid incision. Blunt dissection posterior to the trachea will allow for mobilization and visualization of its posterior aspect. As above, the thyroid may be divided along the isthmus to facilitate anterior visualization. For injuries to the trachea through significant portions of the thyroid gland, resection of the affected thyroid tissue is recommended.

The trachea is best repaired with a single-layer 3-0 absorbable suture, being sure to tie all knots on the outside. Sutures may need to be placed in the innerspace above and below the adjacent tracheal rings to provide stability. If necessary, up to one or two cartilaginous rings may be resected while still maintaining the ability to perform a primary anastomosis. For significant injuries that involve near to full loss of a ring level, placement of a tracheostomy is indicated to ensure a secure airway. Locating the tracheostomy at the level of the second cartilaginous ring is still preferred, even if this is above the level of the injury. For injury to the arytenoids, reattachment and mucosal repair with absorbable suture are required.

When concomitant esophageal and tracheal injuries are present, a vascularized muscle flap from the omohyoid or sternocleidomastoid should be placed between the repairs to promote healing and decrease the chance of fistulization or leak.

Esophageal Injuries

The esophagus may be bluntly dissected free anteriorly in the tracheoesophageal groove and posterior from the prevertebral fascia. Having a nasogastric tube placed facilitates identification and dissection of the esophagus. Once the injuries are fully visualized and evaluated, repair should be performed in two layers. The first is a full-thickness closure using 4-0 absorbable suture, taking care to include the inner mucosal layer with the outer muscular layer. The outer layer of sutures should be interrupted through the muscular layer using 4-0 permanent suture. Because of the high rate of temporary leakage from esophageal repairs, a drain should be left in place after esophageal repair, and a contrast swallow study is recommended a week after repair prior to oral feeding. Maintaining an nasogastric tube (NGT) post repair can allow for prompt feeding into the stomach or upper small bowel. Devastating injuries involving large-volume tissue loss may necessitate distal ligation and creating a proximal esophagostomy by bringing the proximal limb out via the left side of the neck. In this setting, a jejunal feeding tube should be placed to facilitate feeding.

Thoracic Duct Injury

Thoracic duct injuries can occur with penetrating injury to Zone I or II on the left side. They are rare and represent less than 1% of all penetrating neck injuries. If identified at the time of surgical exploration by visualizing leaking or welling of milky fluid, ligation is recommended to prevent progression to chylothorax. Most injuries that present later in the form of a chylothorax may be managed with a chest tube and a low-fat diet without the need for surgical ligation.

SUGGESTED READINGS

Asensio JA, Chahwan S, Forno W, et al: Penetrating esophageal injuries: multicenter study of the American Association for the Surgery of Trauma, *J Trauma* 50:289–296, 2001.

Barkana Y, Stein M, Scope AM, et al: Prehospital stabilization of the cervical spine for penetrating injuries of the neck—is it necessary? *Injury* 31:305, 2000.

Inaba K, Branco BC, Menaker J, et al: Evaluation of multidetector computed tomography for penetrating neck injury: a prospective multicenter study, *J Trauma* 72(3):576–584, 2012.

Inaba K, Munera F, McKenney M, et al: Prospective evaluation of screening multislice helical computed tomographic angiography in the initial evaluation of penetrating neck injuries, *J Trauma* 61:144–149, 2006.

Stanley RB Jr, Armstrong WB, Fetterman BL, et al: Management of external penetrating injuries into the hypopharyngeal-cervical esophageal funnel, *J Trauma* 42:675–679, 1997.

Woo K, Magner DP, Wilson MT, et al: CT angiography in penetrating neck trauma reduces the need for operative neck exploration, *Am Surg* 71:754, 2005.

Blunt Cardiac Injury

Ashish Shah, MD, and Keki R. Balsara, MD

INTRODUCTION

Blunt cardiac injury (BCI) is the general term for injury resulting from blunt trauma to the heart. The spectrum of injury that can result is broad and ranges from asymptomatic to sudden death from ventricular wall rupture. Cardiac injury is subclassified based on the nature of the injury and the resultant symptoms; these symptoms include (1) complex arrhythmia, (2) minor electrocardiogram (ECG) or enzyme abnormalities, (3) pump failure, (4) coronary artery thrombosis or dissection, and (5) septal or free wall rupture.

INCIDENCE

Because BCI includes a wide spectrum of injury, the true incidence of BCI in those who have sustained chest or abdominal trauma remains unknown. Many patients with BCI die in the field from either their cardiac or other traumatic injuries; thus, the total number of individuals affected may be underestimated. Moreover, there is little consensus on the appropriate workup for patients with suspected BCI, and this influences the reported incidence in the literature. A review of the current literature suggests an incidence between 8% and 71% for all individuals who sustain blunt thoracoabdominal trauma.

Schultz and colleagues found that the most common BCI identified in clinical studies is myocardial contusion (60% to 100%), followed by right ventricular injury (17% to 32%) and right atrial injury (8% to 65%) because of the anatomic positioning in the chest.

The left heart is less commonly involved with left ventricular injury (8% to15%) and left atrial injury (0 to 31%) being somewhat less common. Injuries to the coronary arteries and valves as the result of blunt trauma are found only as a series of case reports in the literature suggesting that their incidence is quite low. Autopsy series have demonstrated an incidence of 3% to 5% of such injuries in patients following blunt trauma.

The largest autopsy series, published by Parmley and colleagues, reviewed nearly 208,000 cases from the Armed Forces Institute of Pathology. The study showed a 0.1% incidence of BCI. The most common chamber injured was the right ventricle (66 cases), followed by the left ventricle (59 cases), right atrium (41 cases), and left atrium (26 cases). Of these, 106 cases had combined chamber rupture and 80 had an associated aortic injury.

MECHANISM OF INJURY

The heart is well protected by the bony thoracic cavity. A significant amount of force, usually associated with polytrauma, is necessary to impart serious injury to the heart. Historically, motor vehicle accidents had the greatest incidence of BCI. Increasingly, blast injuries, assault, and sports-related injuries are recognized as causative agents. Due to its varied presentation, blunt cardiac trauma requires a high degree of clinical suspicion before it is properly diagnosed. Physical exam findings, including thoracic bruising, fractured sternum, murmur, jugular venous distention, and hemodynamic shock, should all raise the possibility of cardiac injury.

Myocardial contusion is the most common injury in those patients who arrive in the emergency room following blunt thoracic trauma. Although myocardial contusion remains a poorly defined entity, the presentation is typically one with stable cardiac arrhythmias. Additional problems include valvular rupture, thromboembolism, ventricular aneurysm, and constrictive pericarditis. The initial workup includes an ECG. There is little use for serial cardiac enzymes. Patients with persistent rhythm disturbances, ECG changes, or hemodynamic lability should undergo a transthoracic echocardiogram to exclude functional or structural abnormalities. Traditionally, the prognosis of patients with myocardial contusion is excellent.

Valvular injuries, while rare, most commonly involve the aortic valve, followed by the tricuspid and mitral valves. This usually presents with a new systolic murmur. Most patients present with a tear of the noncoronary leaflet. These injuries can usually be managed conservatively and present for elective repair. Symptoms suggesting acute aortic insufficiency, including dyspnea, arrhythmia, and heart failure, mandate urgent surgical intervention. Rarely can the valve be salvaged, and most patients undergo valve replacement.

Cardiac rupture is perhaps the most dramatic presentation of BCI. Free rupture at the time of initial trauma is usually not survivable, and many of those patients die in the field. Those who survive to the emergency room often show evidence of pericardial tamponade and, less commonly, of hemothorax. In decreasing order of frequency, survivors sustain injury to the right atrium, left atrium, right ventricle, and left ventricle. The key to survival is rapid diagnosis and resuscitation. Operative repair is mandated and most effectively achieved via median sternotomy. Cardiopulmonary bypass can be used, but this is rarely needed for most injuries. Most injuries can be repaired primarily.

Ventricular aneurysms most commonly occur along the anterolateral wall of the left ventricle. They usually occur in a delayed fashion and are the result of myocardial injury with resultant necrosis and scarring. Findings of recurrent arrhythmias, heart failure, or embolic events may occur months to years after initial injury. Treatment includes surgical resection and/or plication of the aneurismal segment of the ventricular wall.

Coronary artery injury from blunt chest trauma is exceedingly rare. The vessel most commonly injured is the left anterior descending artery. Most commonly, intimal disruption and dissection results in a thrombosed vessel with distal ischemia. Laceration or rupture of the coronaries with resultant tamponade has also been reported. Asymptomatic patients can be managed conservatively. Many proximal injuries can be managed in the catheterization lab with balloon angioplasty or stent deployment; those that cannot often proceed to coronary artery bypass grafting.

More than 75% of patients with BCI will have associated thoracic injuries, including rib and sternal fractures, pulmonary contusions, pneumothorax, hemothorax, and great vessel injury. Moreover, extrathoracic injury is commonly encountered in patients with BCI, including closed head injury (20% to 73%), extremity injury (20% to 66%), solid abdominal organ injury (5% to 43%), and spinal injury (10% to 20%).

The American Association for the Surgery of Trauma (AAST) Organ Injury Scale for cardiac injuries describes six injury grades, from minor ECG abnormalities to avulsion of the heart (Table 1).

TABLE 1: American Association for the Surgery of Trauma organ injury scale: cardiac injuries

Grade*	Cardiac injury
I	Blunt cardiac injury with minor ECG abnormality (nonspecific ST-wave or T-wave changes, premature atrial or ventricular contraction, or persistent sinus tachycardia) Blunt or penetrating pericardial wound without cardiac injury, cardiac tamponade, or cardiac herniation
II	Blunt cardiac injury with heart block or ischemic changes without cardiac failure Penetrating tangential cardiac wound, up to but not extending through endocardium, without tamponade
III	Blunt cardiac injury with sustained or multifocal ventricular contractions Blunt or penetrating cardiac injury with septal rupture, pulmonary or tricuspid incompetence, papillary muscle dysfunction, or distal coronary artery occlusion without cardiac failure Blunt pericardial laceration with cardiac herniation Blunt cardiac injury with cardiac failure Penetrating tangential myocardial wound, up to but not through endocardium, with tamponade
IV	Blunt or penetrating cardiac injury with septal rupture, pulmonary or tricuspid incompetence, papillary muscle dysfunction, or distal coronary artery occlusion producing cardiac failure Blunt or penetrating cardiac injury with aortic or mitral incompetence Blunt or penetrating cardiac injury of the right ventricle, right or left atrium
V	Blunt or penetrating cardiac injury with proximal coronary artery occlusion Blunt or penetrating left ventricular perforation Stellate injuries, less than 50% tissue loss of the right ventricle, right or left atrium
VI	Blunt avulsion of the heart Penetrating wound producing more than 50% tissue loss of a chamber

ECG, Electrocardiogram.
*Advance one grade with multiple penetrating wounds to a single chamber or multiple chamber involvement.
From Moore EE, Malangoni MA, Cogbill TH, et al: Organ injury scaling. IV: thoracic vascular, lung, cardiac, and diaphragm, J Trauma 36(3):299–300, 1994.

DIAGNOSIS

There is no gold standard test to diagnose BCI. Initial evaluation should include a thorough physical examination and trauma resuscitation as defined by the American College of Surgeons Advanced Trauma Life Support (ATLS) program. ECG should be the first screening tool to rule out evidence of arrhythmia or ischemia. In the resuscitation bay in experienced hands, focused assessment with sonography for trauma (FAST) can aid in diagnosis and risk stratification for patients. It can quickly aid in the diagnosis of tamponade and give some idea about ventricular function. If an abnormality is suspected, a formal transthoracic echocardiogram should be obtained.

The Eastern Association for the Surgery of Trauma established practice guidelines for blunt cardiac trauma after an extensive literature review (Box 1). It encourages the use of ECG as an initial screening tool for suspected BCI. Further workup, including transthoracic echocardiogram and admission with continuous cardiac monitoring, should be reserved for those individuals with demonstrated ECG abnormalities. Their recommendations also argue against serial cardiac enzymes, nuclear medicine studies, and the like, as they have never been shown to alter management or change outcomes.

BOX 1: EAST practice management guidelines for blunt cardiac injury workup

Recommendation Level I
1. An admission ECG should be performed on all patients in whom a BCI is suspected.

Recommendation Level II
1. If the admission ECG is abnormal (arrhythmia, ST changes, ischemia, heart block, unexplained ST changes), the patient should be admitted for continuous ECG monitoring for 24 to 48 hours. Conversely, if the admission ECG is normal, the risk of having a BCI that requires treatment is insignificant, and the pursuit of diagnosis should be terminated.
2. If the patient is hemodynamically unstable, an imaging study (echocardiogram) should be obtained. If an optimal transthoracic echocardiogram cannot be performed, the patient should have a transesophageal ECG.
3. Nuclear medicine studies add little when compared with ECG; thus, they are not useful if an ECG has been performed.

Recommendation Level III
1. Elderly patients with known cardiac disease, unstable patients, and those with an abnormal admission ECG can be safely operated on provided they are appropriately monitored. Consideration should be given to placement of a pulmonary artery catheter in such cases.
2. The presence of a sternal fracture does not predict the presence of BCI and thus does not necessarily indicate that monitoring should be performed.
3. Neither creatinine phosphokinase with isoenzyme analysis nor measurement of circulating cardiac troponin T is useful in predicting which patients have or will have complications related to BCI.

BCI, Blunt cardiac injury; *EAST*, Eastern Association for the Surgery of Trauma; *ECG*, electrocardiogram.
From Pasquale, MD, Nagy K, Clarke J: Practice management guidelines for screening of blunt cardiac injury, J Trauma 44:941–956, 1998.

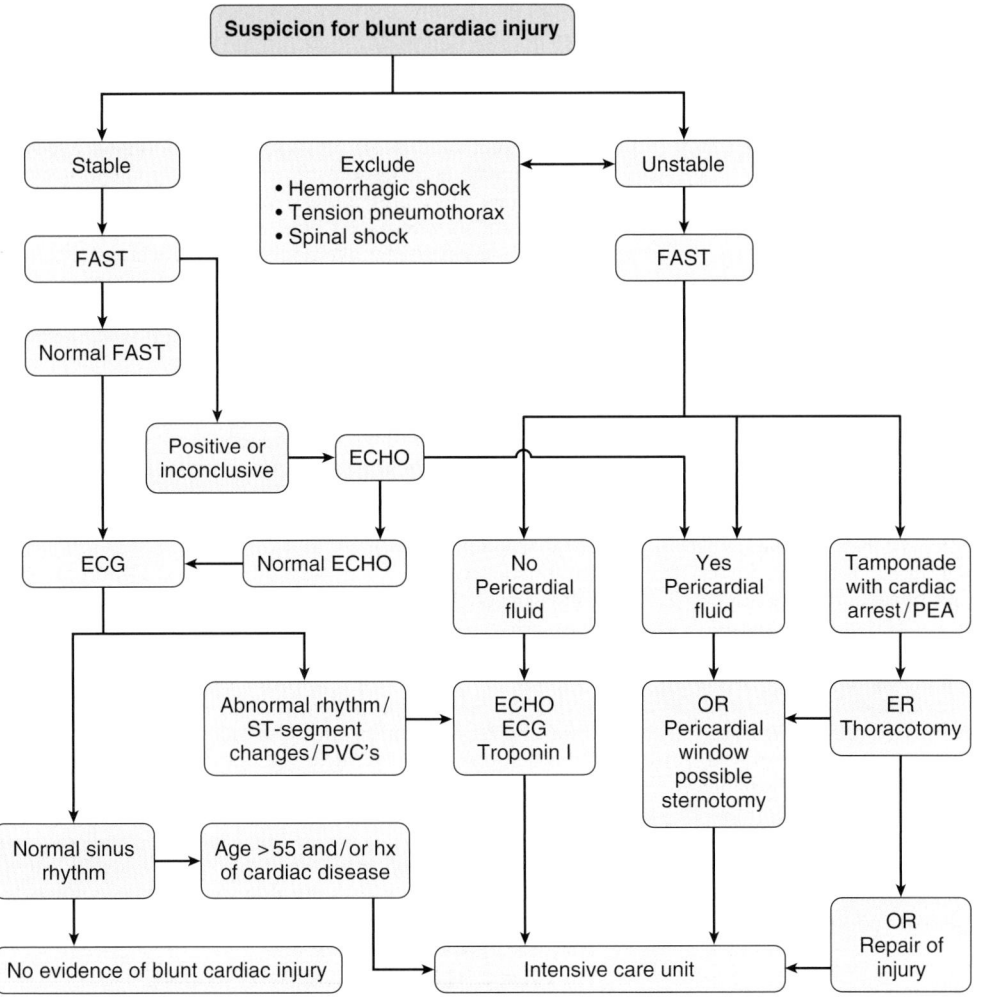

FIGURE 1 Algorithm for blunt cardiac injury. *ECG,* Electrocardiogram; *ECHO,* echocardiogram; *ER,* emergency room; *FAST,* Focused Assessment with Sonography for Trauma; *hx,* history; *OR,* operating room; *PEA,* pulseless electrical activity; *PVC,* premature ventricular contraction.

TREATMENT

The treatment of BCI is dictated by the presumptive injury and the hemodynamic status of the patient (Figure 1). Unstable patients need immediate resuscitation with treatment of the underlying problem, whether it is shock, pneumothorax, tamponade, or other. In cases of hemodynamic stability with evidence of pericardial effusion, pericardiocentesis should be attempted until definitive management with operative window/sternotomy can be undertaken. For patients who are hemodynamically unstable and undergo witnessed cardiac arrest, some centers advocate resuscitative thoracotomy with a left anterolateral approach. The goal is to evacuate pericardial fluid, clamp the aorta, and temporize any injury until definitive surgical intervention can be undertaken. Survival is rare. In cases of prehospital cardiac arrest, resuscitative thoracotomy has never been shown to improve outcomes and thus is strongly discouraged. Complex valvular or coronary injuries should be repaired in the operating room through median sternotomy with the assistance of cardiopulmonary bypass.

Patients who are hemodynamically stable and present only with ECG changes or dysrhythmias should be monitored with continuous telemetry for at least 24 hours. A small subset of this population is at risk for lethal ventricular arrhythmias, usually in the form of ventricular fibrillation. Immediate defibrillation is the treatment of choice and has been shown to be lifesaving in nearly 25% of patients if performed expeditiously.

The long-term outcome of BCI has not been adequately studied, and longitudinal studies do not exist. In the acute setting, patients with isolated rhythm problems usually recover fully with no residual long-term effects. Those who undergo surgical intervention, provided their other injuries are non–life-threatening, enjoy good long-term survival anecdotally. Ultimately, it appears, patient survival and discharge to home are directly related to accuracy of diagnosis and rapid, definitive intervention.

SUGGESTED READINGS

Becker A, Elias M, Mizrahi H, et al: Blunt heart trauma, *J Trauma* 71(1):261, 2011.

Berg RJ, Okoye O, Teixeira PG, et al: The double jeopardy of blunt thoracoabdominal trauma, *Arch Surg* 147(6):498–504, 2012.

Bernardin B, Troquet JM: Initial management of resuscitation of severe chest trauma, *Emerg Med Clin North Am* 30(2):377–400, 2012.

Moore EE, Malangoni MA, Cogbill TH, et al: Organ injury scaling. IV: thoracic vascular, lung, cardiac, and diaphragm, *J Trauma* 36(3):299–300, 1994.

Pasquale MD, Nagy K, Clarke J: Practice management guidelines for screening of blunt cardiac injury, *J Trauma* 44:941–956, 1998.

Schultz JM, Trunkey DD: Blunt cardiac injury, *Crit Care Clin* 20(1):57–70, 2004.

Abdominal Compartment Syndrome and Management of the Open Abdomen

Nathan T. Mowery, MD, FACS, Preston R. Miller, MD, FACS, Michael C. Chang, MD, FACS, and J. Wayne Meredith, MD, FACS

Understanding the pathophysiology of abdominal compartment syndrome (ACS) and the management of the subsequent open abdomen has proven to be a lifesaving advance in acute care surgery. Patients with a variety of abdominal and nonabdominal pathology are at risk for the development of ACS. The syndrome produces significant cardiopulmonary and renal derangements. The bleeding or edema that mandates decompressive laparotomy in the face of ACS may also make abdominal closure untenable for days to weeks. The care of patients with ACS requires three critical judgments: early recognition and intervention for ACS, timing and location of subsequent operations, and techniques to be used in closure of the patient. The formulation of a plan to address these branch points ultimately determines the mortality of the patient and can significantly impact the morbidity associated with the ACS. From the moment the surgeon decides to pursue decompressive laparotomy, a plan must be formulated that includes definitive repair and closure of the patient.

PATHOPHYSIOLOGY OF ABDOMINAL HYPERTENSION

Abdominal hypertension develops on a scale with increasing extraabdominal manifestations as the pressure increases. The detrimental effects of increased intraabdominal pressure (IAP) have been well described in several populations of surgical patients. The relationship between oliguria, acute renal failure, and increased IAP has also been well characterized. Increased IAP has been shown to compromise blood flow to both the portal and the splanchnic circulatory systems. The development of increased IAP in surgical patients thus has profound detrimental effects on virtually all important organ systems and therefore dramatic effects on outcome. This syndrome of the adverse physiologic consequences that occur as a result of acute increases in IAP has been called the abdominal compartment syndrome.

It is important to recognize that intraabdominal hypertension (IAH) and ultimately ACS come from visceral and retroperitoneal edema from poor or late source control of bleeding, dead or injured tissue, or infection. Overadministration of any type fluid, in the absence of poor source control, does not result in ACS (Box 1).

RECOGNITION OF ABDOMINAL COMPARTMENT SYNDROME

The early recognition and treatment of ACS is the most critical step in the dealing with this pathology. Early identification of ACS can avoid many of the late complications that result from avoiding the perfusion/reperfusion injuries. Abdominal hypertension decreases venous return, increases systemic vascular resistance and intrathoracic pressure, and therefore reduces cardiac output. These physiologic responses to increased intraabdominal pressure lead to some of the earliest signs of ACS.

Physical examination is the first hallmark of abdominal hypertension. Patients with large resuscitations with development of significant abdominal girth or tightness must be considered for ACS. Conversely patients who have a pliable abdomen do not have ACS and should be evaluated for alternative causes of clinical deterioration. ACS was initially described as a cause of respiratory failure. Patients with rising ventilator peak airway pressures (or falling volumes on pressure-control ventilation) should be considered for ACS. Unexpected response to resuscitation is another indication of ACS. Because there is restriction of cardiac output, patients with ACS are often misdiagnosed as hypovolemic and given more fluid. This has the possibility of worsening the abdominal hypertension. Unfortunately, intraabdominal hypertension has a profound effect on measured values of preload, such as right ventricular end-diastolic volume, pulmonary artery wedge pressure, and central venous pressure. Also, blood flow to the liver and kidney may be reduced, resulting in functional impairment of both organs. Identification of abdominal hypertension from low urine output means warning signs that have been present for some time have been missed.

Another important facet of the treatment of ACS is the recognition for the potential for development. Surgical intervention can often mark the beginning of patient's resuscitation with the potential for bowel and retroperitoneal edema to follow. Surgeons must consider the tension created by definitive closure and anticipate the potential resuscitation that follows. Patients with hypotensive conditions that require vasopressors at the end of the initial laparotomy must be carefully considered for staged surgery. The best treatment for ACS is avoidance.

MEASUREMENT OF INTRAABDOMINAL PRESSURE

IAP can be measured with direct and indirect methods. Direct measurements are relegated to laboratory studies currently. Multiple means for indirect measurement have been used, but the most common is urinary bladder pressure. This simple minimally invasive method can be easily performed at the bedside because the bladder behaves as a passive diaphragm when its volume is between 50 and 100 mL. Pressure measurements in animals recorded simultaneously through a urinary bladder catheter and directly via peritoneal catheters were equal for pressures ranging from 5 to 70 mm Hg. Evidence has shown that instilling the bladder with 50 mL of sterile water creates pressures where intraabdominal pressure is closest to intravesicular pressure. The Foley catheter is then clamped, and the pressure is transduced via the port of the Foley catheter. The manner with which abdominal pressure is measured can be either intermittent or continuous. Some evidence shows that continuous, or at least more frequent intervals (every 1 hour) of, monitoring in high-risk groups can lead to earlier recognition of abdominal hypertension. The effect that this earlier recognition has on outcome is still being determined. Consideration should be given to prophylactic bladder pressures in a group of patients at high risk (Box 2).

TREATMENT OF ABDOMINAL COMPARTMENT SYNDROME

The surgeon must take in the entire clinical picture before deciding when to intervene for abdominal hypertension. In general, 20 mm Hg is used as a number where physiologic changes occur that require consideration for decompression. If patients have exceeded that number and are beginning to manifest other symptoms of ACS, then

BOX 1: Grades of severity

Mild abdominal hypertension: Acute sustained elevation of intraabdominal pressure above 10 to 20 mm Hg. Physiologic effects are generally well compensated and usually clinically nonsignificant. Nonoperative therapy may be required.
Moderate hypertension: Sustained elevation of 21 to 35 mm Hg. Therapy is generally necessary. Surgical abdominal decompression may be critical.
Severe hypertension or *abdominal compartment syndrome:* Sustained elevation above 35 mm Hg. Operative decompression is almost always indicated.

BOX 2: Factors that put patients at high risk for development of abdominal compartment syndrome

1. More than 10 units of blood products or 10 L of crystalloid resuscitation needed.
2. Pelvic fracture with retroperitoneal hematoma.
3. More than 30% burns.
4. Pancreatitis.

decompression should be strongly considered. This number is not an absolute though. There is no role for mandatory decompression in patients with otherwise stable conditions that reach the 20 mm Hg threshold. One must examine all the data available, such as physical examination, respiratory status, vital signs, and fluid responsiveness. If all those data point toward ACS, then decompression should follow.

Although the recognition of ACS can have subtle variances, the treatment is straightforward. Decompression laparotomy is the gold standard for patients with ACS. Decompression has been shown to improve preload, pulmonary function, and visceral perfusion in patients with ACS. The lack of a recent laparotomy should not influence the decision to proceed with decompression. It is well documented that patients without primary abdominal pathology can have ACS develop. Decompression should follow the diagnosis of ACS with or without recent surgery.

Less invasive means have been described, such as paralysis, percutaneous drainage of ascites, and diuresis. These interventions should only be used in low-grade abdominal hypertension or when extreme circumstances exist. Such circumstances might be in patients whose conditions are so frail that the family does not wish to pursue more aggressive interventions.

Decompression requires a full-length midline laparotomy incision. Lesser incisions may not adequately decompress the abdomen, leaving the question of persistent compression lingering. Unfortunately, the decompression surgery is usually the least technically challenging portion of operative interventions for this population. The sequential interventions that follow in an attempt to close the patient can test a surgeon's operative and clinical skills.

UNPLANNED REOPERATION

When the goals of the first phase of ACS treatment (recognition and decompression) fail, the surgeon must consider reexploration. Attending surgeons and house staff can be given a false sense of security with an open abdomen that the risk of ACS is not present. Often after decompression, patients require significant ongoing resuscitation that puts them at risk for tertiary compartment syndrome. If a patient's clinical picture remains consistent with compartment syndrome, then the surgeon must consider the decompression inadequate or the means of temporary abdominal closure too effective.

TEMPORARY ABDOMINAL WALL CLOSURES

Once the patient has undergone adequate decompression, an immediate plan for the eventual closure must begin to be formulated. A variety of temporary closure techniques have been advocated over time. Some simply contain the abdominal viscera and protect them from further injury. Other techniques have the advantage of preserving abdominal domain while still allowing room for expansion if required. Finally, some techniques allow for the recruitment of domain as the patient's physiology allows. The authors use the abdominal vacuum dressing for that very reason. Not only does it protect the viscera, but as the edema resolves, the vacuum can shrink to continually recover lost abdominal domain. Other dressings (Whitman's patch, Bogata bag) can also be adjusted to regain domain but necessitate physician intervention on a regular basis. Whatever dressing is chosen, it must not recreate the abdominal hypertension that was just released.

ABDOMINAL WALL RECONSTRUCTION

During reoperation, the surgeon should consider each time whether the patient can be safely closed. This is predicated on the determination of the amount of tension on the abdominal wall. A variety of ways can be used to determine whether the amount of tension created will be excessive and lead to complications. The key is to make use of all information that is readily available in the operating room or at the bedside. Although no technique has been validated with research, many surgeons use the change in the patients peak airway pressure (PAP) as a means of determining tension. Most anesthesia machines and bedside ventilators report a constant PAP, and if the change is greater than 10 mm Hg in approximation of the fascia, too much tension exists to proceed with closure. If undue tension is created with approximation, then a temporary method of closure must be applied again.

Planned Reexploration

The timing of reexploration is important. Traditional thinking was usually that a time period of 3 to 5 days should elapse before reexploration, with the thought that correction of physiology was not possible in less time. The timing can be tailored for each individual patient. Patients whose conditions are still physiologically altered may benefit from space between interventions and the minimized stress on the patient. Other patients who recover quickly do not have to wait for 3 days to pass before going back to the operating room (OR). Recognition of these patients should be based on the patient's current clinical picture. The degree of initial injury is not always predictive of a patient's physiologic derangement.

Control of contamination is another cornerstone of open abdomen management. Each time the abdomen is explored, an attempt to irrigate to decrease bacterial counts should be made. The surgeon should use these windows into the abdomen to evaluate contamination, hemostasis, and degree of inflammation, all of which play key roles in determining progression to the next stage of the plan, reconstruction.

Surgeons should balance the desire to see all portions of the bowel with avoidance of injury to the bowel at the time of surgery. Once the bowel becomes adherent to itself, there should be an effort to minimize disruption of these new adhesions. This is especially true when anastomosis is present. Serosal injuries and traction injuries can occur at anastomosis and have the potential to lead to fistula, which significantly complicates any open abdomen.

Where Should Abdominal Washouts Occur?

The location chosen to perform bedside washout is highly dependent on the resources available to the surgeon. In patients in whom definitive closure is clearly not possible, a bedside washout can be faster, place less stress on the patient, and protect vital OR time. These benefits must be weighed with the intensive care unit (ICU) resources and the fact that each intervention should provide the patient with the best opportunity to work toward definitive closure. If the bedside intervention will inhibit the ability to adequately place a partial closure or adequate dressing, then it should not be considered. Bedside intervention can only be done if bedside laparotomy protocols have been developed and practiced in advance. Issues that may necessitate bedside reexploration include high ventilatory requirements, hemodynamic instability that precludes transport, and unstable intracranial hypertension. Bedside surgery has the following limitations: inadequate lighting, a substerile environment, absence of trained personnel, and limited surgical instruments. In the end there lacks a defined criteria which preclude patient transport the decision falls on clinical judgment to guide the surgeon, but they should feel confident that bedside laparotomy is proven technique that is commonly practiced at a variety of centers.

When to Abandon Attempts at Definitive Closure?

Patients should undergo assessment at the time of each abdominal exploration, with the goal of working toward expedited primary facial closure. Miller and associates were able to show a marked increase in the risk of associated complications if the abdomen was unable to be closed within 8 days. Twenty-two of 185 patients (12%) in whom the fascia closed in 8 days or less had a complication develop, whereas 47 of 91 patients (52%) with closure after 8 days had a complication develop.

A variety of factors impacts this 8-day goal and affects the long-term success of the closure. Early recognition of ACS can lead to better long-term outcomes. Addressing abdominal hypertension before physiologic exhaustion helps to avoid the perfusion-reperfusion injuries that lead to bowel edema that inhibits definitive abdominal wall closure during the hospital stay.

Preservation of the integrity of the fascia is important leading up to the time of closure. In the evolution of damage control surgery, a variety of techniques have been used for temporary closure of the abdomen. Many of these techniques involved direct suturing or fastening of material to the patient's fascia. Although these techniques met the short-term needs of maintaining abdominal domain, the repeated manipulation of the fascia led to decreased strength and increased morbidity.

Some authors have used this increase in complications in late closure to advocate that attempts at definitive closure should be abandoned at that time and closure with a planned hernia proceed. Although an increase in complications may be seen after 8 days, the authors advocate that one should still continue trying to work toward abdominal closure after that time has passed. With the use of negative-pressure vacuum dressings, success has occurred with late closure, up to 49 days. Complications usually associated with late closure, such as hernia and fistula development, are low, and the complications with a second intervention are avoided. At the authors' institution, an adaptation of the negative-pressure dressing described by Barker and colleagues is used. A sponge vacuum is substituted for the towels, and the skin is closed over top of it. The system preserves the abdominal domain. The authors' own institutional experience has shown an abdominal closure rate in patients undergoing vacuum-assisted closure of 88%, with a mean time to closure of 9.5 days.

Vacuum-Assisted Closure Technique

With this method, the polyethylene sheet is perforated, placed over the viscera, and tucked under the wound edges (Figure 1). The surgeon should make every attempt to place the sheet into the gutters of the abdomen to allow the anterior abdominal wall complete mobility to "slide" to the midline. The polyurethane sponge is then placed over the plastic sheet, pushing the viscera down, and tightly laced into place with 1-0 nylon suture on the skin edges (Figure 2). The surgeon should pass the needle from the inside out, rather than use a normal baseball stitch, to avoid sewing toward the bowel. After the sponge is assured to be in contact with the full thickness of the wound edges, the surrounding skin is coated with benzoin, and suction tubing and adhesive dressing (Ioban, 3M) are applied. After an occlusive seal is obtained, suction is applied (Figure 3). This causes the sponge to apply tension to the full thickness of the wound edges, including the abdominal fascia. After suction is applied, the sutures no longer have tension on them.

Vacuum-assisted fascial closure differs from these and other techniques in that it prevents both fascial retraction and visceral adherence, allowing for continuing attempts at abdominal closure several weeks after laparotomy. This is an extension of the standard vacuum pack technique and has two important components that allow for later closure. The first is the perforated polyethylene sheet placed over the bowel. This must be tucked under the fascial edges to prevent adherence. The second is the thick polyurethane sponge, as opposed to the surgical towel used in the original technique. This provides suction to the cross section of the abdominal wall, preventing fascial retraction by creating constant medial tension on the fascia without injuring it, as some similar techniques with suture might. These two features likely account for the higher closure rate seen with this technique and reduce the need for future hernia repair (Figures 4 and 5).

Adjuvants to Late Closure

Also important is the need to supplement the patient's nutrition to prevent a catabolic state from developing in an already stressed patient. Traditionally, patients with an open abdomen were fed via a parenteral route because physicians assumed decreased bowel

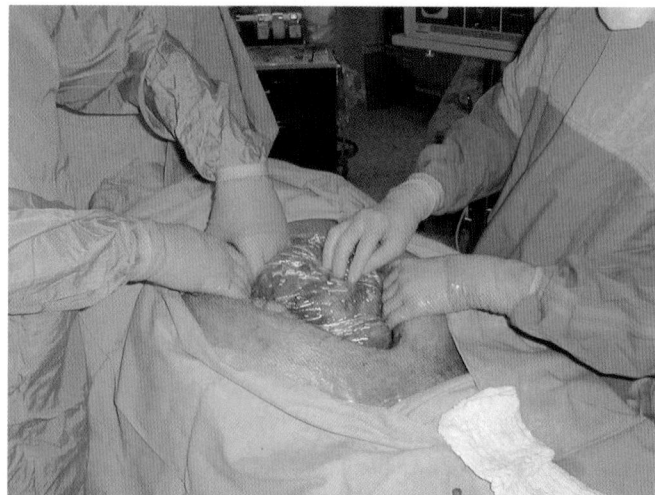

FIGURE 1   Polyethylene sheet being tucked under fascial edges. *(From Miller PR, Thompson JT, Faler BJ, et al: Late fascial closure in lieu of ventral hernia: the next step in open abdomen management, J Trauma 53(5):843-849, 2002.)*

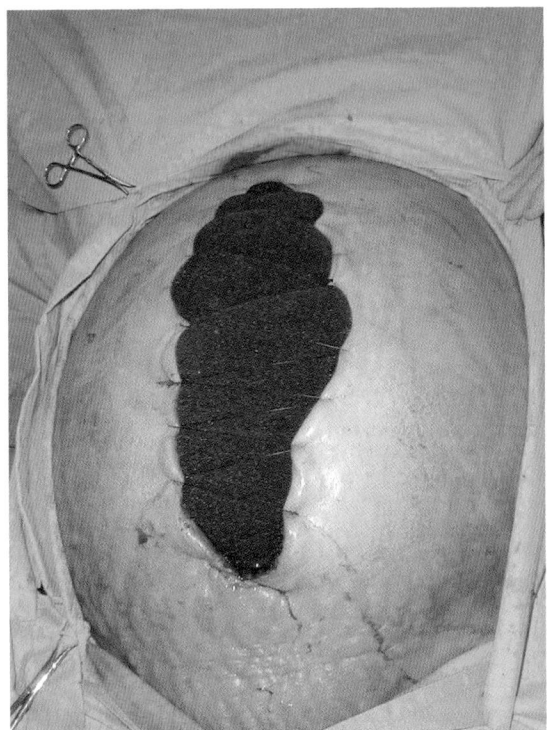

FIGURE 2 Sponge laced into position. *(From Miller PR, Thompson JT, Faler BJ, et al: Late fascial closure in lieu of ventral hernia: the next step in open abdomen management,* J Trauma *53(5):843-849, 2002.)*

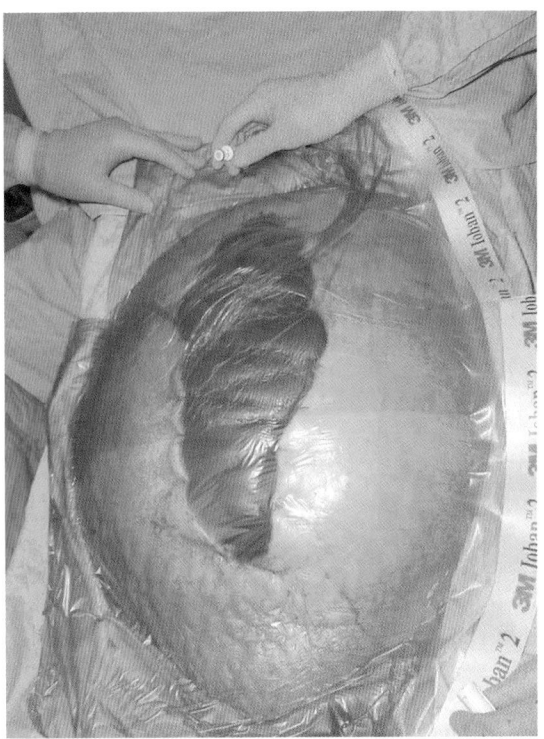

FIGURE 3 Vacuum application after adhesive dressing placement. *(From Miller PR, Thompson JT, Faler BJ, et al: Late fascial closure in lieu of ventral hernia: the next step in open abdomen management,* J Trauma *53(5):843-849, 2002.)*

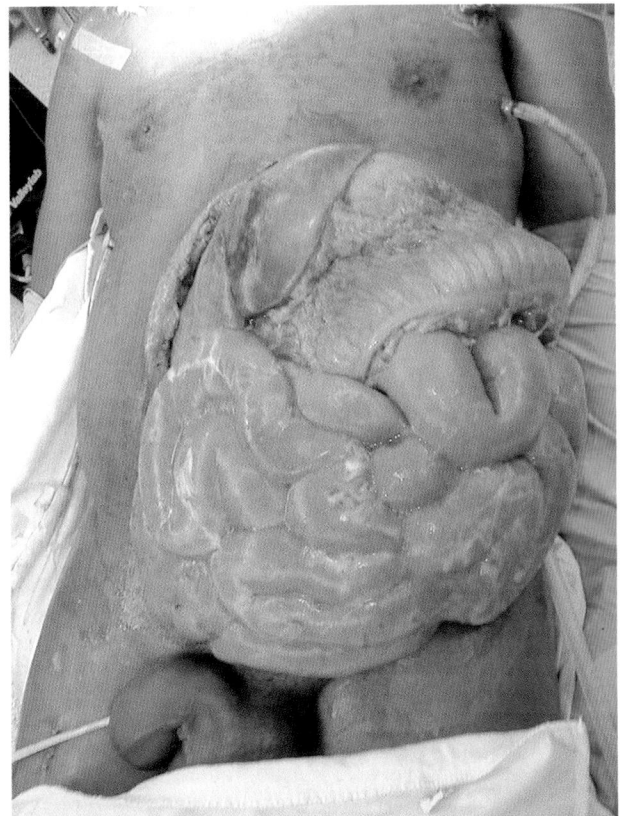

FIGURE 4 Severe visceral edema in a blunt trauma victim shortly after admission. *(From Miller PR, Thompson JT, Faler BJ, et al: Late fascial closure in lieu of ventral hernia: the next step in open abdomen management,* J Trauma *53(5):843-849, 2002.)*

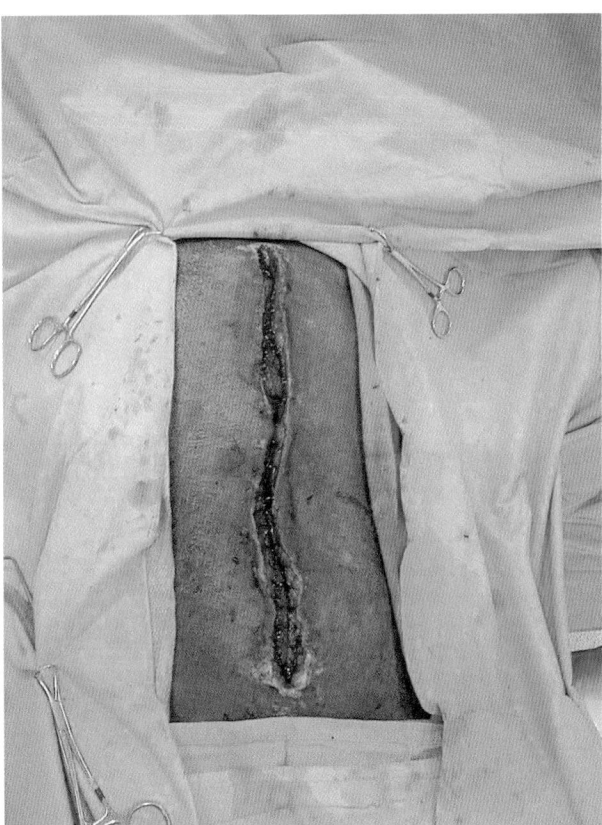

FIGURE 5 Abdomen closed on postinjury day 21 with vacuum-assisted closure. *(From Miller PR, Thompson JT, Faler BJ, et al: Late fascial closure in lieu of ventral hernia: the next step in open abdomen management,* J Trauma *53(5):843-849, 2002.)*

motility and absorption would be present with an open abdomen. Collier and associates were able to show that enteral feedings with an open abdomen were safe and could lead to decreased bowel wall edema and early closure of the abdomen.

Also paramount to the ability to close the patient is the overall fluid status of the patient. Although the appropriate means of resuscitation of a trauma patient are outside the bounds of this chapter, careful balancing of the patient's fluid status can greatly affect the success rate of closure. Early resuscitation efforts based on invasive hemodynamic monitoring have been shown to result in earlier correction of acidosis, coagulopathy, and hypothermia and in improved mortality. This could result in less interstitial edema and in higher success rates of abdominal closure.

Other authors have explored the concept that active diuresis can increase the success of closure. Diuresis has been said to be aided by the addition of albumin in the classic "push/pull" method. This combination has shown to be successful in removal of fluid in other populations (ARDS) but has not been validated in the open abdomen population.

The patient's physiology often dictates the rate of transfusions, but evidence shows that a more restrictive transfusion strategy can lead to increased success in early abdominal closure. Transfusion of blood and blood products and crystalloid resuscitation are known causative factors in the development of the abdominal compartment syndrome. Patients must be given the appropriate resuscitation to maintain perfusion, but care must be taken to tailor the amount given to address the patient's current needs.

Another means to attempt to preserve abdominal domain has been the practice of maintaining chemical paralysis in between subsequent trips to the operating room with open abdomens. This practice stems from the belief that persistent contraction of the abdominal musculature in the nonparalyzed patient can lead to retraction of the fascia and abdominal musculature. No good evidence has been shown to support the standard use of paralytics, and often in this complex patient population, the usage may subject these patients to additional risks of hypercoagulability, positioning, and long-term polyneuropathy.

In the end, the ability to close these patients falls on the shoulders of the surgeon. No amount of monitoring or strategy can substitute for an attentive surgeon who is constantly reassessing the patient and asking the question of whether the patient is ready for definitive closure. Although a variety of objective means can be applied, they only augment the physician in developing a plan for closure that both meets the patient's current needs and looks to avoid possible pitfalls that may develop in the patient's course, with adaptations when they do develop.

FAILURE TO ACHIEVE PRIMARY CLOSURE

There is no definitive maximal time for closure of a patient. The morbidity of a planned hernia should not be assumed lightly. A second operation at a remote date carries its own complications and disruption to patient recovery. Conversely, the serial "take backs" cannot continue indefinitely. The patient's progress often dictates the upper limit of when delayed primary closure will be attempted. When a patient's condition has progressed to the point that the sole reason for reintubation and continued critical care is the open abdomen, it is time to find an alternative means of closure. This allows patients to continue to progress in their recovery. Alternative closure may take many forms, such as native tissue, biosynthetic meshed implants, and absorbable mesh. Each of these closure methods has positive and negative aspects. Surgeons who frequently deal with this patient population should be experienced with multiple methods to allow tailoring of each patient's care.

TYPES OF DEFINITIVE ABDOMINAL CLOSURES

Modified Component Separation

Component separation (CS) uses a sliding myofascial flap to provide tension-free closure of large abdominal wounds without implantation of mesh. This allows for a vascularized tissue to be brought together with little or no tension. Care must be taken with this option because of the large scope of the operation.

Permanent Mesh (Polypropylene Mesh, Polytetrafluoroethylene)

Authors have argued that polypropylene mesh placement is an effective alternative for abdominal closure after emergency laparotomy, even when intraabdominal sepsis is present. Fistula rates as low as 7.1% have been reported. However, more commonly, authors have argued that polypropylene mesh use in this setting has resulted in an unacceptably high complication rate that includes fistula rates up to 50%. Some authors have used polytetrafluoroethylene (PTFE) mesh as a temporary patch to prevent evisceration and allow for the development of granulation tissue to serve as a bed for STSG. Its advantages are that it is relatively poorly incorporated, allowing for easier removal if the need arises. All permanent meshes can become infected and create a catabolic drain that can brew in an indolent manner for months. Although the short-term goal of abdominal closure is obtained, the long-term wound complications make the use of permanent mesh in this setting unacceptable when alternatives exist.

Polyglycolic Acid Mesh (Vicryl)/Split-Thickness Skin Graft

Most patients in the literature who cannot be primarily closed undergo abdominal closure with polyglycolic acid mesh with subsequent split-thickness skin grafting before leaving the hospital. Healthy granulation tissue occurs within about 7 to 10 days of insertion. However, the mesh itself usually is not incorporated tightly. Recent studies on abdominal closure in the open abdomen in trauma report an overall enterocutaneous fistula rate of 7% to 8%.

Biosynthetic Reconstruction

New biosynthetic meshes available on the market now have the advantage of the ability to be placed in the contaminated wound. Authors have shown success with only minor superficial wound infections in the early application of biosynthetic meshes to open abdomens when closure is not possible. Some questions have arisen about the long-term durability of this type of mesh. Some degree of bulge is accepted if the mesh is used to span a gap in the fascia. As long-term data continue to accumulate for the use of this biosynthetic mesh, its applications and its efficacy continue to be more accurately described. Cost also plays an important role. Some risk is assumed with placement of such an expensive option in a wound that may not be suitable for definitive closure.

A word of caution is warranted. Although a definitive closure is appealing, the patient's physiologic status must weigh heavily on the decision-making process. A catabolic patient with poor nutrition is not a good candidate for wound healing, regardless of the technique used. Patients must be ready to undergo the scope of operation and healing of the wound after surgery. If a patient is not metabolically ready for such a large scale intervention, a smaller less definitive solution may be the safer and more economic choice.

SPECIAL SITUATIONS IN DAMAGE CONTROL SURGERY

Fistulas in the Open Abdomen

Despite attention to detail and vigilant surveillance, situations arise in staged surgery, including fistula formation. The best plan for dealing with fistula formation is prevention of development. Techniques that can decrease the rate of formation include early closure, protection of the bowel, avoidance of permanent mesh, and burying of the anastomosis.

Early closure has been shown to decrease fistula formation. Measures to protect the bowel include use of bowel bag and decreased manipulation of the bowel on subsequent washouts. Also, the type of closure technique can have a dramatic impact on fistula rate. Studies have shown that use of absorbable mesh as discussed previously can reduce the fistula rate when compared with permanent mesh. The risk for fistulas occurs whenever a nondynamic mesh material is sewn to dynamic abdominal wall. This creates mechanical stress where sewn together, and if the bowel is stuck underneath (as it almost always is), then this increases risk for fistula.

The treatment of fistulas in the open abdomen follows the same tenants of surgery in other situations. The primary goal is to isolate the output and decrease the flow through the output. Isolation can be complicated by the fact that repeated washouts and dressing changes can disturb the body's attempt to wall off the collection. Also, the fact that these abdomens often progress to a "cocooned" appearance can make intervention problematic. Fortunately, the best plan is usually the simplest, meaning simple drainage. Attempts to resect or repair fistula in the hyperinflammatory setting usually lead to worsening of the problem, unless attempts are made very early in the process.

Ostomy in the Open Abdomen

In a variety of illnesses, surgeons are faced with dealing with both an open abdomen and an ostomy. Although ostomies can make dressing changes and care a challenge, they often are the safest option for the patient. The ostomy itself can sometimes be an obstruction to sequential closure. The ostomy can fix the underlying viscera to the abdominal wall, which restricts the medial slide of the abdominal wall necessary for delayed primary closure. When creating ostomies in patients with a planned hernia, surgeons should consider a more lateral placement of the ostomy. Although it increases the chances of a peristomal hernia, placement of the ostomy lateral to the rectus sheath preserves important planes, making component separation more efficacious.

CONCLUSION

The management of the open abdomen does not stop once the initial life-saving decompression occurs, but this marks the beginning of what often becomes the most complex portion of the patient's care. The postoperative decisions have a dramatic impact on the morbidity and mortality of the patient. Although algorithms and advice can help guide the surgeon in making decisions, nothing can replace a vigilant surgeon's reassessment of the patient and adaptation to changes in the patient's physiology and presentation. When an individually tailored approach is taken, this patient population can be safely navigated through the course with improved outcomes without long-term morbidity. Although this surgical approach is associated with a significant complication and readmission rate, its long-term survival and benefit are indisputable.

SUGGESTED READINGS

Barker DE, Kaufman HJ, Smith LA, et al: Vacuum pack technique of temporary abdominal closure: a seven year experience with 112 patients, *J Trauma* 48:201–207, 2000.

Chang MC, Miller PR, D'Agostino R, et al: Effects of abdominal decompression on cardiopulmonary function and visceral perfusion in patients with intra-abdominal hypertension, *J Trauma* 44:440–445, 1998.

Miller PR, Meredith JW, Johnson JC, et al: Prospective evaluation of vacuum-assisted fascial closure after open abdomen: planned ventral hernia rate is substantially reduced, *Ann Surg* 239(5):608–616, 2004.

Miller PR, Thompson JT, Faler BJ, et al: Late fascial closure in lieu of ventral hernia: the next step in open abdomen management, *J Trauma* 53(5):843–849, 2002.

BLOOD TRANSFUSION THERAPY IN TRAUMA

Terence O'Keeffe, MD, FACS, and
Peter Rhee, MD, MPH, FACS, FCCM

INTRODUCTION

Many of the advancements in trauma surgery can be linked to periods of conflict, such as World War II and the Vietnam War. The past decade has seen similarly rapid changes that have taken hold in transfusion therapy—changes related, at least partly, to the treatment of casualties from Middle East conflicts. The concept of so-called 1:1:1 blood transfusion, where each unit of red cells is accompanied by a unit of plasma and a unit of platelets, has rapidly diffused from military practice into civilian hospitals. This concept has gone by many names, but it is now commonly referred to as "hemostatic" or "damage control" resuscitation, and includes the following tenets:

1. permissive hypotension,
2. early use of blood and blood products,
3. minimization of crystalloids,
4. use of hypertonic saline,
5. use of drugs such as tranexamic acid, factor 7 or 9, and
6. the use of whole blood if available.

Its application has been associated with improved mortality and morbidity rates, as well as with decreased resource utilization. Such benefits have been the subject of intense research activity, yielding some evidence on which to base these therapies; however, given the often retrospective nature of the data, the issue of survivor bias remains ever-present.

BLOOD COMPONENTS

Current civilian practice is to fractionate blood into its component parts. Doing so enables clinicians to target specific defects within an individual patient's hematologic profile, thus maximizing the potential benefit from a single donated unit of whole blood. However, for trauma patients, this practice is less than ideal.

In the recent Middle East conflicts, fresh whole blood has been used successfully by the U.S. Military because of the military's ability to access a "walking blood bank" (i.e., obtaining fresh donations from a previously screened group of individuals whose blood type is already known). Use of this fresh whole blood has been credited with helping reduce the incidence of mortality from the serious penetrating injuries that have been characteristic of these conflicts. Whole blood is rarely used in civilian settings, especially because refrigeration inactivates the platelets but also because data providing the effectiveness of refrigerated whole blood is currently lacking. Although a feasibility study of the use of whole blood in civilian trauma patients was recently completed, the results are not yet available.

Predominant practice in most blood banks involves fractionating a unit of blood into packed red blood cells (PRBCs); plasma, which is subsequently frozen and designated as fresh frozen plasma (FFP); platelets; and cryoprecipitate (Figure 1). Specific-component therapy can be highly useful. For example, most patients with anemia do not have a coagulopathy and therefore can be treated with PRBCs alone. Conversely, coagulopathic patients, such as those with a warfarin overdose, do not require PRBCs but rather need to be treated with FFP alone. Patients with hematopoietic disorders such as leukemia frequently have thrombocytopenia, and this can be treated with specific-component therapy with platelet transfusion alone.

Stored in a variety of citrated buffers, PRBCs have a shelf life of either 35 days if citrate-phosphate-dextrose-adenine solution is used or 42 days if additive solution is used. Transfusion of PRBCs is indicated for patients with ongoing, acute blood losses and for patients symptomatic from their anemia. The average unit of PRBCs has a hematocrit of about 80%, which will usually raise the hemoglobin level by 1 g/dL or the hematocrit by 3%. The decision for transfusion should NEVER be based on a number from a blood test alone.

Stored frozen at −18°C, FFP can be kept this way for up to a year. It contains varying amounts of fibrinogen, von Willebrand factor, and coagulation factors I, VII, VIII, IX, X, and XIII. FFP is indicated for the reversal of either acquired or congenital coagulation defects, as well as for the reversal of anticoagulant agents. For stable, nonbleeding patients, FFP should never be used to correct abnormal coagulation tests alone (e.g., per the international normalized ratio [INR]).

Stored at room temperature on a gentle shaker, platelets have a shelf life of only 5 days and are tested daily for bacterial contamination. They are a precious commodity and should be used extremely judiciously. They may be collected in two ways: (1) from random donors, yielding a volume of about 50 mL, that is, 5×10^{10} platelets; or (2) from a single donor by apheresis, yielding a volume of 200 to 250 mL, equivalent to 5 to 8 random units, that is, a minimum of 3×10^{11} platelets. Accepted transfusion triggers for platelet transfusion are shown in Table 1.

Cryoprecipitate is so named because it is the cold-insoluble portion of FFP that precipitates out of solution when FFP is slowly thawed at 1°C to 6°C. It contains clotting factors from a single donor that are then suspended in 10 to 15 mL of plasma. Each unit contains a minimum of 80 IU of factor VIII and at least 150 mg of fibrinogen, in addition to significant amounts of von Willebrand factor, factor XIII, and fibronectin. It is stored frozen at −18°C until needed; it is then stored at room temperature after thawing. It has a short shelf life: it must be transfused within 6 hours of thawing and 4 hours of pooling, if pooling is performed.

Cryoprecipitate is available in prepooled concentrates of five units. Each unit from a separate donor is suspended in 15 mL plasma prior to pooling. Cryoprecipitate is indicated for bleeding or immediately prior to an invasive procedure in patients with significant hypofibrinogenemia (<100 mg/dL). It has been used in some massive transfusion protocols, but this is by no means universally accepted.

In most U.S. blood banks, although it remains controversial, leukoreduction has become the standard of care. It has been extensively studied but with contradictory results regarding its benefit to patients. Leukoreduction refers to an extra process that PRBCs go through to wash out and specifically remove any white blood cells. Doing so is thought to reduce the risk of complications to transfusion recipients by decreasing their exposure to the donors' humoral immune system.

Similarly, concerns have been raised about the use of older banked blood, especially considering the storage issues that occur with prolonged storage of PRBCs. Some storage problems, such as loss of 2,3-diphosphoglycerate (2,3-DPG) and loss of adenosine triphosphate (ATP), are rapidly corrected after transfusion back into a patient, whereas others, such as loss of membrane lipids, are irreversible and lead to decreased survival of the transfused PRBCs (Figure 2). These concerns have led to recommendations (not universally adopted) that patients with critical conditions, such as hypoxia, receive only "fresh" blood (i.e., <7 days old).

Trauma patients who need blood transfusions must be clearly separated into two groups: (1) those who are actively bleeding and (2) those who are no longer bleeding but remain critically ill in the intensive care unit (ICU). For patients who are actively bleeding, hemostatic resuscitation is critically important. We will cover the concept of massive transfusion, or hemostatic resuscitation, in more detail later in the chapter.

For ICU patients who are no longer bleeding, transfusing less blood appears to be better. That idea was first promulgated in 1999 with the Transfusion Requirements in Critical Care (TRICC) trial, which compared a restrictive transfusion strategy (maintaining

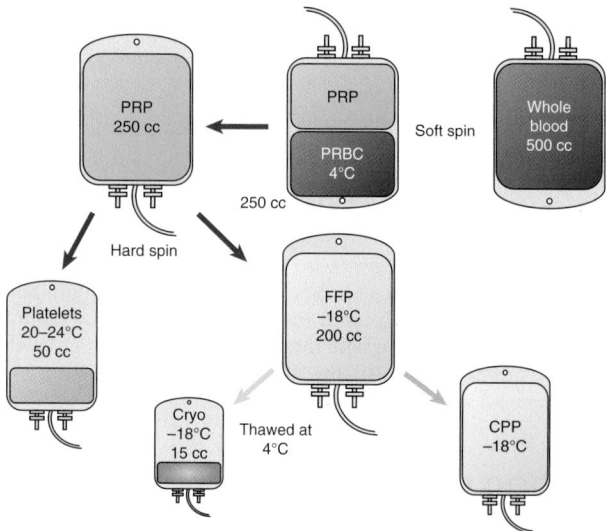

FIGURE I Fractionation of whole blood into its components for storage. *CPP,* Cryoprecipitate-poor plasma; *FFP,* fresh frozen plasma; *PRBC,* packed red blood cell; *PRP,* platelet-rich plasma. *(Courtesy of Dr. Ravi Sarode, Blood Bank Director, Department of Pathology, UT Southwestern Medical Center, Dallas, Tex..)*

TABLE I: Platelet transfusion triggers

Clinical condition	Platelet count per microliter
Stable heme/oncology	10,000
Complicated oncology	>20,000
Minor surgery	25-50,000
Major surgery	>50,000
Neurosurgery	100,000
Platelet dysfunction: congenital or acquired	As clinically indicated

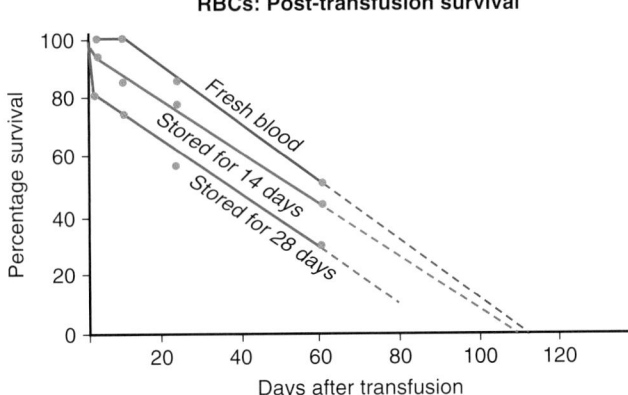

FIGURE 2 Fate of transfused red blood cells (RBCs) based on the age of transfused blood. *(Courtesy of Dr. Ravi Sarode.)*

TABLE 2: Massive transfusion protocol example

MTP cooler	PRBCs (units)	FFP (units)	Platelets (units)
1	6	6	1
2	6	6	1
3	6	6	—
4	6	6	1
5	6	6	—
6	6	6	1

FFP, Fresh frozen plasma; *MTP,* massive transfusion protocol; *PRBCs,* packed red blood cells.
Note: Each platelet unit is an apheresis pack—equivalent to 5 to 6 random donor platelets.

hemoglobin levels between 7 and 9 g/dL) to a more liberal strategy (10 to 12 g/dL). According to that trial's results, the two strategies were equivalent in terms of survival rates, although better survival rates were found in younger patients (<55 years old) and in patients with lower Acute Physiology and Chronic Health Evaluation-II (APACHE II) scores (<20). The finding of similar survival rates with restrictive and liberal strategies has led to a lowering of the transfusion trigger in most institutions and to a general abandonment of the essentially arbitrary 10/30 rule (i.e., transfusing patients to 10 g/dL or to a hematocrit of 30%).

More recent studies looking at restrictive transfusion strategies in patients with cardiac risk factors who were anemic after hip surgery, or in patients with gastrointestinal bleeding, have confirmed the TRICC trial's findings. Healthcare organizations, in general, are moving toward controlling transfusions where clear evidence of benefit is lacking, thus helping alleviate blood supply concerns and decreasing the risk of complications.

AUTOLOGOUS BLOOD TRANSFUSIONS

Autologous blood transfusions once comprised as many as 6% of the units of blood transfused, but this practice has largely fallen out of favor. Reasons include the difficulties associated with storage and the need to ultimately discard many of these units. Moreover, autologous blood transfusions are of limited use in trauma patients, for whom the need for transfusions is usually unpredictable.

ACUTE COAGULOPATHY

Many studies have demonstrated that up to a third of trauma patients arrive at the hospital with an established coagulopathy, which significantly increases both the mortality rate (by up to 4 times) and the morbidity rate. Many patients were not receiving enough coagulation factors to be adequately treated for coagulopathy. Mathematic modeling has been used to ascertain the perfect "ratio" of FFP to PRBCs: the ideal ratio appears to be about 1 to 1.5 units of FFP to each unit of PRBCs. Multiple retrospective studies appear to corroborate that low ratios of FFP to PRBCs are detrimental, even though the exact ideal ratio remains controversial.

MASSIVE TRANSFUSION AND MASSIVE TRANSFUSION PROTOCOLS

In patients who are bleeding, delays in obtaining the results of coagulation testing can lead to undertreatment, so most massive

transfusion protocols use fixed ratios of blood products and do not include coagulation testing. Massive transfusion has been variously defined, but the two most common and useful definitions are as follows: a transfusion requirement of 10 or more units of PRBCs in a 24-hour period *or* the replacement by transfusion of the patient's entire circulating blood volume within 24 hours. Both definitions have been criticized as arbitrary and retrospective. Other triggers have been proposed, such as a critical administration threshold of the transfusion of 3 units of PRBCs within 1 hour. Notwithstanding the way that massive transfusion is defined, this subgroup of severely injured patients clearly represents a separate clinical entity from the vast majority of trauma patients. The incidence of patients requiring a massive transfusion varies from 1% to 3% of the trauma patient population, depending on the institution and the frequency of penetrating trauma.

Again, much of the impetus for the 1:1:1 ratio came from data from the military, which pioneered work on massive transfusions because of the massive injuries sustained by combatants in Afghanistan and Iraq. The preponderance of explosive injuries with multiple amputations and severe blood loss led to implementation of both the fresh whole blood and the massive transfusion protocol. With the return of many of the U.S. Army surgeons to civilian centers, the pendulum swung toward the use of massive transfusion protocols in the most severely injured civilian patients throughout the United States. It is fair to say that this is one of the most avidly researched areas in trauma currently, in both civilian and military arenas.

The essential components of a massive transfusion protocol are as follows: (1) its automaticity (i.e., blood products are prepared without being specifically requested); (2) its ability to be activated 24 hours a day, 7 days a week, and in locations as diverse as the emergency department, ICU, operating room, and angiography suite; (3) its lack of requirements for blood testing; (4) its delivery of blood products in predefined ratios; and (5) its automatic continuation until halted by a physician. The protocol's precise form, components, ratio, and timing depend on the individual institution, although the vast majority of level I and level II trauma centers now have some type of massive transfusion protocol. An example is given in Table 2. A further refinement is noted in Figure 3, where each blood component unit is sequentially numbered, so that the surgeon and/or anesthesiologist has a visual aid (not only showing the number of units transfused but also allowing quick calculation of the PRBCs-to-FFP ratio).

A thawed plasma protocol can be an adjunct to a massive transfusion protocol. Once FFP is thawed, it can be kept refrigerated for up to 5 days with minimal loss (roughly 20%) of functional activity. Keeping thawed plasma in stock can rapidly reduce the amount of time taken to get it to the bedside. With careful attention to the stock, thawed plasma can also be used for nontrauma purposes, in essence recycling it and preventing waste—a useful and cost-effective practice at many institutions.

Not all civilian authorities are convinced of the efficacy of the 1:1:1 fresh whole blood protocol. In fact, some have suggested that the increased dosage of FFP can lead to the development of transfusion-related acute lung injury (TRALI) and to multiple-organ dysfunction syndrome (MODS). Some studies have demonstrated that early transfusion of plasma is associated with MODS, with the greatest effect in patients who received less than 6 units of PRBCs. These troubling associations make the necessity of prospective randomized trials even greater. The best prospective data that we have currently come from the U.S. Department of Defense's PRospective Observational Multicenter Major Trauma Transfusion (PROMMTT) study. This study enrolled patients who received early initial transfusions and required at least 3 units of PRBCs in the first 24 hours. The trial showed that higher plasma-to-platelet ratios were associated with decreased mortality rates, without causing an increase in late deaths.

We hope that the ongoing randomized clinical trial now being conducted at 12 clinical sites across the United States and Canada—the Pragmatic, Randomized Optimal Platelet and Plasma Ratios (PROPPR) trial—will definitively answer this question, but results are unlikely to be available until 2014.

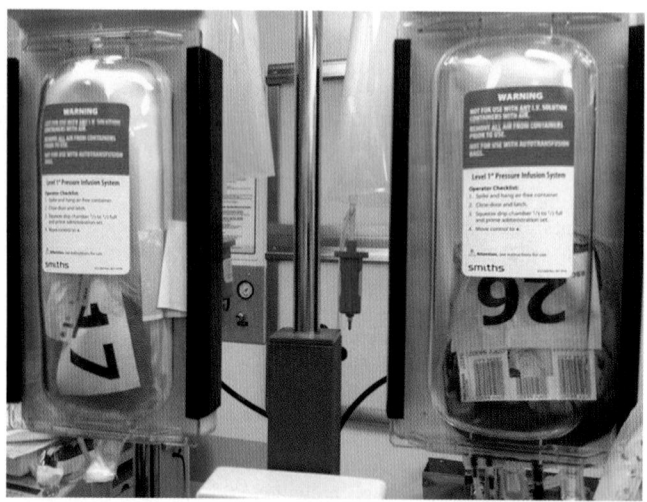

FIGURE 3 Labeling of blood and fresh frozen plasma (FFP) bags during a massive transfusion.

COAGULATION TESTING IN THE TRAUMA PATIENT

Trauma patients hemorrhage whole blood and therefore lose not only red blood cells (RBCs) but also platelets and coagulation factors. It is becoming increasingly clear that the results of current coagulation tests, such as prothrombin time (PT), INR, and partial thromboplastin time (PTT), are poor reflections of the rapidly changing blood profile in trauma patients, particularly those who are receiving multiple transfusions. Furthermore, most laboratory tests have a lag time of 40 to 60 minutes before results are available to clinicians, making interpretation even more difficult.

The thromboelastogram (TEG), although not as easy to interpret as a simple number such as the INR, is proving its utility both in research studies and in the clinical arena. Figure 4 shows an example of a TEG tracing. The TEG helps assess multiple different arms of the clotting cascade, including platelet function, and therefore may represent the true in vivo clotting profile more completely than, say, the INR. Its downsides include the necessity for dedicated equipment, which is fairly sensitive, and the requirement of frequent and careful calibration. Rapid TEG testing can be incorporated, rather simply, into clinical practice, but full thromboelastography suffers from the same drawback as coagulation profiles, namely, a significant time delay from testing to results.

Newer technology (e.g., VerifyNow; Accumeterics, San Diego, Calif) has been developed that looks more narrowly at just platelet function, but these machines have not been widely introduced into clinical practice. They may have more of a role in assessing the impact of antiplatelet therapy instead of the coagulopathy of trauma. But with the aging of the trauma population, clinicians are seeing larger and larger numbers of geriatric trauma patients who are on anticoagulants of various types.

HEMOSTATIC ADJUNCTS

Factor VIIa generated much interest as an adjunct for bleeding trauma patients in the early 2000s, but clinical trials did not reveal a significant benefit, certainly not enough of a benefit to justify its considerable expense. Whereas this drug has fallen out of favor, there have been others that have come to the forefront, such as prothrombin complex concentrates (PCCs) and, more recently, tranexamic acid (TXA).

A heterogenous class of plasma-derived compounds, PCCs were initially developed to treat hemophilia B. They have been used with some success to treat congenital or acquired deficiency of vitamin K–dependent clotting factors, especially in trauma patients. Containing varying amounts of primarily factor VIII or IX, they have been used, mostly, to reverse excessive coagulopathy related to warfarin

FIGURE 4 Sample thromboelastography tracing.

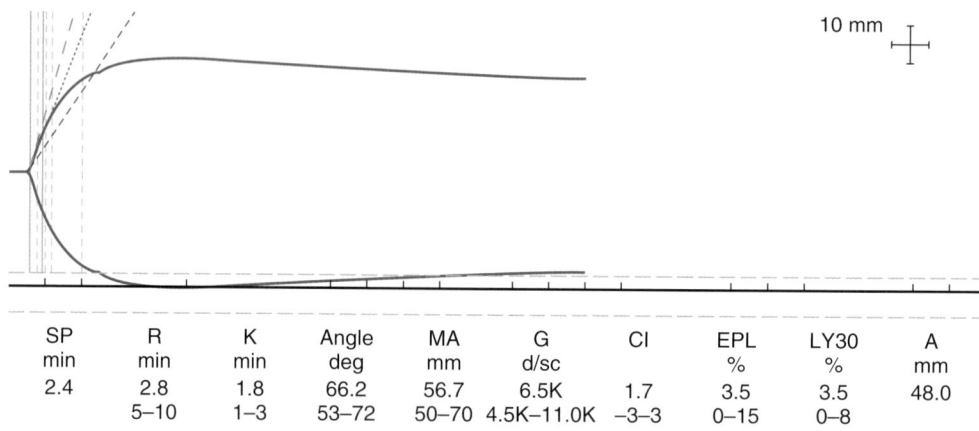

SP min	R min	K min	Angle deg	MA mm	G d/sc	CI	EPL %	LY30 %	A mm
2.4	2.8	1.8	66.2	56.7	6.5K	1.7	3.5	3.5	48.0
	5–10	1–3	53–72	50–70	4.5K–11.0K	−3–3	0–15	0–8	

10 mm

and, increasingly, to treat coagulopathy in trauma patients. But the reports on PCCs are largely uncontrolled case series, so until the availability of better data, it is difficult to separate out their effect from that of concurrently used therapies.

In contrast, level I evidence exists for the use of TXA in trauma patients, namely, the Clinical Randomisation of an Antifibrinolytic in Significant Haemorrhage (CRASH-2) trial results. That trial randomized 17,000 patients in 40 countries to receive either TXA or placebo. TXA resulted in a significant drop in the mortality rate from 16% to 14.5%. Interestingly, a prespecified subgroup analysis showed a *worse* mortality rate in patients given TXA 3 or more hours after injury. In addition, some emerging military data are concordant with the CRASH-2 trial results, and a civilian U.S. clinical trial is planned for the near future. Many U.S. trauma centers have already created guidelines on the use of TXA in trauma patients, with most centers restricting it to the first 3 hours after injury.

COMPLICATIONS FROM TRANSFUSION THERAPY

While this is not intended as an exhaustive discussion of the risks and complications associated with blood transfusion, clinicians should be aware of a number of complications, in particular the following.

Transfusion-Related Acute Lung Injury

The highest number of transfusion-related deaths are now, most likely, caused by TRALI, with an incidence of 1 death per 1700 to 5000 patients. Its onset is within 6 hours after the transfusion (Box 1). Clinical findings include tachypnea, dyspnea, tachycardia, hypotension, cyanosis, and fever. In intubated patients, froth may be noted in the endotracheal tube. The mechanism is thought to be human leukocyte antigen–specific or neutrophil-specific antibodies that exist in donors' plasma—antibodies that cause neutrophil aggregation and complement activation with subsequent endothelial damage, capillary leaks, and the release of inflammatory cytokines. Treatment includes oxygen supplementation and, if necessary, vasopressor support.

Of patients who develop TRALI, 80% will survive with normal lung function, and it does not affect the ability to receive blood

transfusions in the future. The risk of TRALI is highest among recipients of FFP (Figure 5), particularly from multiparous women, but other blood products are also culpable. It is of utmost importance to inform the blood bank of any case of TRALI, so that both the donor and the recipient can be tested; if the donor has a significant number of antibodies, he or she can be deferred as a donor in the future. In the United Kingdom, blood bank authorities have moved to collect plasma only from males, and some U.S. blood banks are adopting a similar approach, particularly in light of data showing that such a policy can reduce the incidence of TRALI; however this is not universal, in part due to shortage in supply of AB or "universal" plasma.

Transfusion-Associated Circulatory Overload

A new name for a long-standing problem, transfusion-associated circulatory overload (TACO) is thought to be precipitated when a patient's circulatory system is overcome by either the volume or the speed of a transfusion of blood products. Clinically underrecognized, TACO has a reported incidence of only 1 out of 700 patients. But its true incidence may be as high as 8%, taking into account all blood products; in fact, it may be responsible for as many as 20% of all reported transfusion-related deaths. TACO is characterized by an acute onset of tachypnea, dyspnea, hypertension, and tachycardia. It is difficult to distinguish from TRALI. Usually, in TACO patients

---

BOX 1: Criteria for transfusion-related acute lung injury

- Acute onset: during, or within 6 hours of, transfusion
- Hypoxemia
  - O_2 saturation < 90% at room air
  - Ratio of PaO_2/FiO_2 < 300 mm Hg
- Bilateral infiltrates on chest x-ray
- No evidence of left atrial hypertension
- No preexisting acute lung injury prior to transfusion
- No temporal relationship to alternative risks for acute lung injury

---

FIGURE 5 Risk of developing TRALI based on specific blood component transfusion. *FFP,* Fresh frozen plasma; *RBC,* red blood cell; *TRALI,* transfusion-related acute lung injury. *(From Food and Drug Administration Vaccines, Blood and Biologics website: http://www.fda.gov/BiologicsBloodVaccines/default.htm.)*

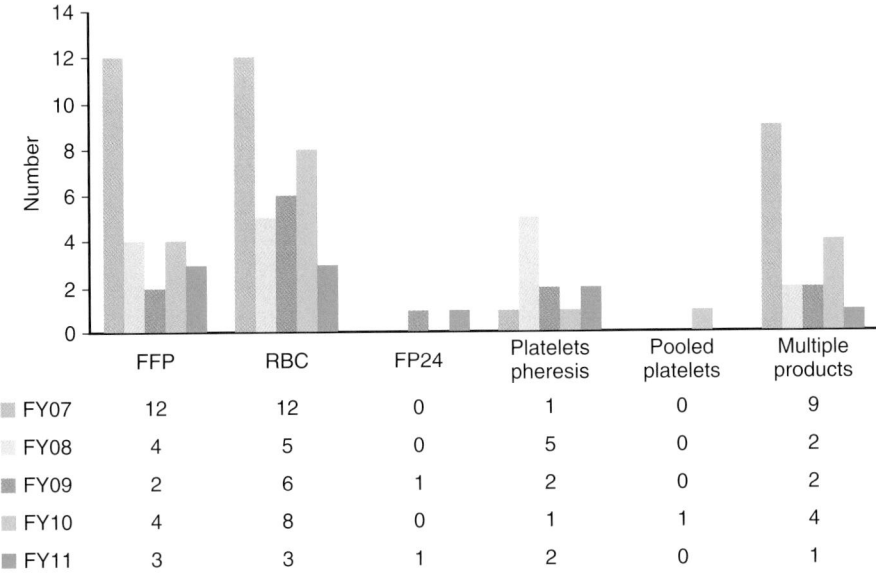

	FFP	RBC	FP24	Platelets pheresis	Pooled platelets	Multiple products
FY07	12	12	0	1	0	9
FY08	4	5	0	5	0	2
FY09	2	6	1	2	0	2
FY10	4	8	0	1	1	4
FY11	3	3	1	2	0	1

Blood product

(unlike in TRALI patients), serum brain natriuretic peptide levels are significantly elevated above baseline.

It is not surprising that TACO is more common in older patients with poor cardiopulmonary reserve and/or those with renal insufficiency. TACO increases ICU and hospital length of stay as well as morbidity and mortality rates. Treatment is limited to supportive care (e.g., oxygen therapy, diuresis, mechanical ventilation if necessary). The best strategy is prevention by only the judicious administration of blood products.

Fever and Allergic Reactions

About 1 out of 100 to 200 patients will develop a fever or have an allergic reaction after a transfusion of a blood product. Nontoxic, circulating, immune complexes are thought to be responsible. Usually, fevers and allergic reactions can be safely treated with Tylenol and Benadryl. In addition, it is prudent to discontinue the transfusion and report the complication to the blood bank, in the event that it may be an early sign of a more serious hemolytic reaction.

Hemolytic Reactions

Hemolytic reactions can be either acute or delayed. Patients can develop different symptomatic patterns, depending on the timing of the presentation of the reaction. Acute hemolytic reactions typically occur within 24 hours after a transfusion with intravascular symptoms; delayed hemolytic reactions more commonly occur 1 to 10 days after a transfusion with extravascular manifestations (Table 3). The incidence is 1 out of 12,000 to 25,000 patients, but the mortality rate is as low as 1 out of 650,000 patients.

Reactions are caused by the immune-mediated lysis of RBCs. Acute hemolytic reactions are usually related to preformed antibodies. The transfusion should be immediately halted and the reaction reported to the blood bank. Treatment consists of supportive care and fluid resuscitation, with an emphasis on preventing acute kidney injury. To confirm the diagnosis, the patient's workup should include a direct Coombs test.

Electrolyte Disturbances

RBCs gradually leak potassium into the supernatant in which they are suspended, putting patients who receive multiple units of PRBCs at risk for hyperkalemia. In clinical practice, this is rarely an issue in patients with normal renal function. Even in patients who undergo massive transfusions, recent data have suggested that the potassium level rarely rises high enough to be a problem.

A more significant concern is the hypocalcemia associated with multiple transfusions: it can lead to cardiac depression because of the citrate contained in the buffer storage solutions, which chelates the Ca^{2+} ions. Patients who undergo multiple transfusions should have their ionized calcium level checked regularly; if it is low, supplementation should be aggressive.

Infectious Risks

Since the mid-1990s, transfusion-related infectious risks have decreased dramatically and are now extremely rare. Estimates of the current incidence of various infections are shown in Table 4. These numbers represent the risk of exposure; actual seroconversion is also related to multiple host factors. Bacterial contamination is obviously much more common from transfusions of platelets, whose storage requirements are ideal for bacterial growth.

Hypothermia

Inattention to detail, especially in patients undergoing multiple transfusions, can lead to fairly profound hypothermia, with deleterious consequences for enzymatic functioning of the entire body. A number of commercially available warming devices (e.g., Level 1 and Hotline, Smiths Medical, Rockland, Mass; Belmont, Belmont Instrument, Billerica, Mass; enFlow, Vital Signs, Totowa, NJ) can be used to allow for the warming of fluids (usually to 40°C). Such devices should be used whenever more than 1 or 2 units of blood products are to be transfused.

NOVEL ANTICOAGULANTS

Increasing problems with novel anticoagulants have recently emerged in our older trauma population with numerous comorbidities. As clinicians, we are well aware of the problems associated with antiplatelet therapy or warfarin in trauma patients, but new medications

TABLE 3: Incidence of symptoms in hemolytic reactions

Symptom	Acute (intravascular)	Delayed (extravascular)
Fever, chills	80%	55%
Renal failure	35%	5%
Pain	15%	2.5%
Nausea, vomiting	10%	—
Hypotension, tachycardia	12%	—
Disseminated intravascular coagulation	10%	5%
Jaundice	—	10%

TABLE 4: Risk of exposure to an infectious agent per unit of blood component therapy

Infectious agent	Risk per unit
HIV	1:1,860,000
Hepatitis B	1:365,000
Hepatitis C	1:1,650,000
HTLV	1:3,390,000
Bacterial contamination	1:1000 to 1:100,000 for platelets 1:100,000 to 1:1,000,000 for red blood cells
NvCJD	Unknown, not yet described
Rabies	Unknown
Dengue, West Nile virus	Possible, risk unknown

HIV, Human immunodeficiency virus; *HTLV*, human T-cell lymphotrophic virus; *NvCJD*, new variant Creutzfeldt-Jakob disease.

such as the direct thrombin inhibitor argatroban pose fresh challenges. Licensed for use in patients with nonvalvular atrial fibrillation, argatroban currently has no specific "antidote" per se, although up to 72% of its activity can be removed via hemodialysis. In the case of massive hemorrhage, manufacturers of argatroban suggest the use of PRBCs, FFP, and even factor VIIa, but with minimal human data to support the recommendation.

The anticoagulant effects of a similar drug, rivaroxaban, were completely and immediately reversed by the administration of PCCs, according to a study of healthy human volunteers. PCCs were ineffective, however, in reversing the anticoagulant effect of yet another new drug, dabigatran. Other new anticoagulant drugs also exist that are not yet currently available in the United States, which may pose even more challenges.

NEW DIRECTIONS

The largest randomized clinical trial ever performed on blood management in trauma patients is currently enrolling patients. It was specifically designed to determine the most effective ratio of plasma to PRBCs in the civilian arena. Its two randomization strategies are a 1:1:1 ratio versus a 1:1:2 ratio of PRBCs to platelets to FFP. The trial will likely be completed in 2014. It is hoped that the trial will help answer, once and for all in civilian patients, whether the higher ratio leads to improved outcomes or to increased complications.

We are also rediscovering some of the lessons of the past, as recent work has highlighted a technique that the U.S. Navy incorporated into its practice many decades ago, namely, the use of cryopreserved deglycerolized blood. Initially described in 1950, this practice allows blood to be stored for up to 10 years when frozen at −80°C. Although this seems to be counterintuitive to the usual adage that older blood is worse for patients, a pilot study published in 2013 by Fabricant and colleagues suggests that results are at least equivalent to, and possibly better than, results obtained in trauma patients requiring transfusion. Further work needs to be done to confirm these preliminary findings.

Blood substitutes continue to be the holy grail of transfusion therapy in trauma patients. Theoretically, such substitutes would provide the benefits of transfusions with few, if any, of the infectious risks; would obviate the need for blood donation; and would, ideally, cost less. To date, however, none of these substitutes have made it out of clinical trials, and interest in them has waned, especially after the well-publicized and unfortunate negative results of the Hemoglobin-Based Oxygen Carrier (HBOC) trial.

In contrast, the use of lyophilized, freeze-dried plasma continues to garner significant interest, in both civilian and military arenas. At least one phase 1 human safety trial has been completed, and phase 2 human trials in trauma patients will begin soon. The U.S. Department of Defense has identified such work as a top research priority and has awarded millions of dollars to help develop this resurgent field.

SUGGESTED READINGS

Eder AF, Dy BA, Perez JM, et al: The residual risk of transfusion-related acute lung injury at the American Red Cross (2008-2011): limitations of a predominantly male-donor plasma mitigation strategy, *Transfusion* 2012 Nov 1. [Epub ahead of print]
Fabricant L, Kiraly L, Wiles C, et al: Cryopreserved deglycerolized blood is safe and achieves superior tissue oxygenation compared with refrigerated red blood cells: a prospective randomized pilot study, *J Trauma Acute Care Surg* 74(2):371–376; discussion 376–377, 2013.
Fatalities Reported to FDA Following Blood Collection and Transfusion: Annual Summary for Fiscal Year 2010. Accessed March 2013. http://www.fda.gov/biologicsbloodvaccines/safetyavailability/reportaproblem/transfusiondonationfatalities/ucm254802.htm
Hébert PC, Wells G, Blajchman MA, et al: A multicenter, randomized, controlled clinical trial of transfusion requirements in critical care. Transfusion Requirements in Critical Care Investigators, Canadian Critical Care Trials Group, *N Engl J Med* 340(6):409–417, 1999.
Neal MD, Marsh A, Marino R, et al: Massive transfusion: an evidence-based review of recent developments, *Arch Surg* 147(6):563–571, 2012.
Teixeira PG, Inaba K, Shulman I, et al: Impact of plasma transfusion in massively transfused trauma patients, *J Trauma* 66(3):693–697, 2009.
Wang D, Sun J, Solomon SB, et al: Transfusion of older stored blood and risk of death: a meta-analysis, *Transfusion* 52(6):1184–1195, 2012.

COAGULATION ISSUES AND THE TRAUMA PATIENT

Jeffry L. Kashuk, MD, FACS, and
Reuven Rabinovici, MD, FACS

OVERVIEW

Postinjury coagulopathy accounts for more than half of trauma-related deaths globally. Despite improvements in surgical techniques and critical care, including advances in damage control surgery, the death rate associated with this condition has changed little over the past 25 years. Furthermore, the exact relationship between trauma-induced coagulopathy and death has not yet been established.

Previous studies have shown that in patients presenting with massive hemorrhage after injury, refractory coagulopathy ultimately leads to death even when surgical control of the wound has been accomplished, a phenomenon termed "the bloody vicious cycle." Furthermore, survivors of the hemorrhagic insult are at increased risk of late death associated with multiple organ failure.

Although the bloody vicious cycle has been recognized for more than 35 years, its pathogenesis is still obscure, and improved understanding of the coagulation issues associated with the trauma patient has evolved only recently. This understanding resulted primarily from knowledge gained in three principle areas: (1) evolution of the cell-based model of coagulation; (2) improved analyses via rapid, point-of-care determination of whole blood coagulation (thromboelastography [TEG] or thromboelastometry [ROTEM]); and (3) clinical experience gained in recent international military conflicts (hemostatic resuscitation).

ETIOLOGY AND NATURAL HISTORY

Traditionally, clotting factor depletion, dilution from crystalloid administration, hypothermia, acidosis, and hypocalcemia were considered the primary factors that fuel postinjury coagulopathy. Indeed, multiple protocols were developed to carefully address these issues during the resuscitation of the injured patient.

Clotting Factor Depletion and Dilution With Fluid Resuscitation

Recent evidence suggests that traditional Advanced Trauma Life Support (ATLS)–guided crystalloid resuscitation for the patient in shock may be detrimental. Frequently, excess fluid administration in patients with hypotensive conditions results in cyclical swings in blood pressure, which necessitate additional fluid administration. Consequently, intravascular volume is increased and clotting factors are diluted. This dilutional coagulopathy, combined with clotting factor depletion from blood loss, exacerbates the bleeding and shock state. In response to this deterioration, more fluids are administered, and this vicious cycle perpetuates. Recent reports suggest that the procoagulants fibrinogen, factor V, and factor VIII are particularly important and can be restored to adequate levels (>20%) to promote timely hemostasis in the injured patient. In addition, platelet counts have been shown to be slower to fall compared with red blood cell counts or coagulation factors, likely because approximately one third of the platelets are trapped in the spleen or attached to the vascular endothelium. Specifically, platelet counts of less than 50,000/mL are uncommon in patients who need less than 20 units of packed red blood cells (pRBC).

Hypothermia

Severely injured trauma patients are at substantial risk for hypothermia, which is a known independent risk factor for death in this group. Hypothermia has direct detrimental effects on the coagulation enzymatic cascade, including fibrinogen cross linking and platelet adhesion and function. Recent data suggest that although hypothermia compromises the activity of procoagulant plasma proteins, it exerts a more significant effect on platelet activation through traction on the glycoprotein Ib/IX/V complex by von Willebrand's factor. This important phase of platelet activation is completely inhibited in 50% of patients with hypothermia at 30°C. Accordingly, major efforts to control the environment of the injured patient should be accomplished as soon as the patient presents to the trauma center. These efforts should include the use of the Baer Hugger device (Arizant, Inc., Eden Prairie, Minn), warm resuscitation agents, and warm irrigating solutions during surgery.

Acidosis

Acidosis develops in injured patients with shock, hypoperfusion, and concomitant anaerobic metabolism. This condition has been shown to affect multiple aspects of coagulation. Recent reports have clearly established that acidosis is a highly reliable indicator of hypoperfusion and shock, is associated with an increased risk of death, and is best corrected with appropriate resuscitation with restoration of oxygen delivery to the tissues. Because the coagulation pathway is dependent on multiple enzymatic reactions eventuating in a stable clot, completion of these reactions is an essential aspect of hemostasis. Accordingly, acute alteration in pH impedes the process, mainly through compromising fibrinogen cross linking, platelet aggregation, and thrombin generation. In addition, acidosis has been shown to accelerate fibrinogen consumption with no effect on fibrinogen production, resulting in a deficit in fibrinogen availability. Lastly, acidosis prevents the congregation of procoagulant complexes in which calcium and negatively charged phospholipids interact. For example, a pH of 7.2 decreases the activity of the Xa/Va/prothrombinase complex by 50%, and a pH to 6.8 turns the complex off.

Hypocalcemia

Hypocalcemia frequently occurs in the patient who undergoes massive transfusion, conceivably through chelation by the citrate used to preserve banked blood (each unit of pRBC contains approximately 3 g of citrate). Because this electrolyte is a key cofactor to many procoagulation proteins, it likely plays an inhibitory role in the evolution of trauma-related coagulopathy. Indeed, some studies suggest that ionized calcium concentrations of less than 0.6 to 0.7 mmol/L could lead to coagulation defects and recommend maintaining a concentration of at least 0.9 mmol/L. In contrast, other reports suggested that hypocalcemia per se does not clinically affect coagulation but rather induces hypotension and tetany in the patient with massive transfusion.

Anticoagulants

Anticoagulants may contribute to the coagulopathic state and may complicate the management of trauma patients taking such medications. Thus, injured patients need a careful history to ascertain whether preexisting antiplatelet or anticoagulant agents have been administered. Current evidence suggests that empiric protocols for reversal of these agents reduce mortality and improve functional outcomes, particularly in elderly patients with intracranial hemorrhage. One study showed that the activation of a warfarin protocol consisting of fresh frozen plasma (FFP) improved functional survival in patients who sustained intracranial hemorrhage. Other reports support the use of factor VIIa to reverse coagulopathy in patients with an international normalized ratio (INR) of more than 1.4 and traumatic brain injury (Glasgow coma scale [GCS], <14). Because many of these patients are elderly with cardiac comorbidities, recombinant factor VIIa (rFVIIa) also prevents the fluid overload associated with large volumes of FFP, otherwise necessary to reverse coagulopathy.

More injured patients increasingly arrive in the trauma room taking a new variety of direct thrombin inhibitors, such as Pradaxa (dabigatran) (Boehringer Ingelheim Pharma GmbH & Co., Ingelheim, Germany). Because no established reversal agent exists for these novel anticoagulants, current protocols have suggested that activated charcoal or dialysis may be helpful to clear the drug from the body. Both techniques are of little use in the patient with acute bleeding, so direct thrombin inhibitors remain a challenge to the trauma surgeon. Accordingly, current protocols continue to emphasize all traditional methods of support, including FFP, blood, and specific factor replacements, although no current evidence supports such use.

CURRENT CONCEPTS OF COAGULATION

Several new concepts regarding trauma-related coagulopathy have evolved recently. The first suggests that coagulopathy occurs very early after trauma independently of clotting factor or platelet deficiency. Because this condition, termed "acute endogenous coagulopathy," occurs in the presence of normal concentrations of coagulation factors and platelets, it is unresponsive to factor replacement therapy. Experience from the U.S. military conflicts in Iraq and Afghanistan and civilian data suggest that nearly 30% of severely injured patients arriving at the hospital have coagulopathy (based on conventional coagulation testing) despite the absence or deficiency of clotting factors. In a recent trial of hemoglobin-based oxygen carriers, such early coagulopathy was noted in 29% of patients based on field blood obtained within 15 minutes of injury. Of note, this subset of patients was shown to have a substantially increased risk of multiple organ failure and death. Furthermore, a 2012 prospective study of 101 trauma patients showed clinically relevant platelet dysfunction measured with multiple electrode impedance aggregometry in the presence of normal platelet count. Although conventional coagulation tests are still most commonly used to evaluate for the presence of coagulopathy, a true definition of the entity is not clear because most reports use varied and arbitrary thresholds such as prothrombin time

(PT) more than 18 seconds, activated partial thromboplastin time (aPTT) more than 60 seconds, and INR more than 1.5. All of these commonly used assays have substantial limitations for evaluation of the patient with acute bleeding. They are static tests, have buffers added, and are plasma based, meaning that the contribution of the platelet and associated thrombin generation to clot strength cannot be appreciated. In addition, they are performed at normal pH and 37°C, which may not accurately reflect the in vivo status of coagulation in the bleeding trauma patient.

Another evolving concept in trauma-related coagulopathy is the introduction of a new cell-based model of coagulation. This concept, which challenges the traditional paradigm of intrinsic and extrinsic pathways, emanates from in vivo studies that highlight protein and other cellular components in the presence of an active vessel wall. According to this paradigm, tissue injury/ischemia, exposed tissue factor, inflammatory mechanisms, hypoperfusion, and hyperfibrinolysis combine to drive the initial process. Later, as factor and platelet deficiency from blood loss and dilution occurs, systemic coagulopathy evolves. The model defines initiation, amplification, and propagation as three distinct activation phases. The initiation of primary hemostasis, which includes clot formation through adherence of platelets to the injured endothelium, occurs via thrombin generation induced by interactions of tissue factor expression at the endothelial level under the influence of activated factors VII (VIIa), X, and Va. This process has been shown to involve significant "cross talk" with inflammatory mechanisms, and current research suggests that the complement system may represent a common pathway linking inflammation and coagulation. Secondary hemostasis is initiated by thrombin generation via the coagulation cascade, resulting in deposition and cross linking of fibrin. The net result of platelet aggregation, fibrin deposition, and fibrin cross linking should be a stable clot. On the basis of this new cell-based model, it is apparent that burst thrombin generation is a central event for hemostasis because it triggers platelet activation and subsequent cleavage of soluble fibrinogen into fibrin. Interestingly, experimental studies have shown that the inception of clot propagation occurs with only minute amounts of thrombin being present, accounting for less than 5% of the total amount generated. After clot initiation and achievement of maximum clot strength, the process of fibrinolysis is initiated. Thus, this lytic process allows for a global assessment of the duration and strength of the clotting factors. Current understanding of fibrinolysis suggests that the beta globulin plasminogen is converted to a physiologically activated form via tissue plasminogen activator (t-PA), although the process of fibrinolysis may be initiated via several mechanisms, including activation of streptokinase or kallikrein, which directly activates plasminogen. Of particular current interest, protein C is believed to stimulate release of t-PA from the endothelium after injury, resulting in plasminogen activation. These processes result in breakdown of fibrin and fibrinogen with generation of fibrin split products, which are often measured in the clinical scenario.

Unfortunately, most currently used tests to assess coagulopathy do not address the events identified by the cell-based model of coagulation. Furthermore, they are too nonspecific or time-consuming for use in the trauma setting. Accordingly, two new clinical approaches have evolved. First, growing evidence suggests the empiric use of antifibrinolytic therapy in patients at risk for postinjury coagulopathy. Second, viscoelastic tests, such as TEG or ROTEM, to identify the hyperfibrinolytic state were developed and implemented in clinical use (see subsequent).

TREATMENT OF THE BLEEDING TRAUMA PATIENT: OPTIMAL USE OF COMPONENT THERAPY

Warm whole blood appears to be the ideal resuscitation method for the patient with acute bleeding, but this product is rarely available in the civilian setting, except for the occasional use of autotransfused intracavitary blood (cell saver). This technique is not commonly used for several reasons. First, it can be applied only in the absence of contamination. Second, it requires citrate addition to prevent coagulation in the collection device. And third, its logistics often cannot be accommodated because of the emergent nature of the traumatic injury. Thus, the current techniques of component transfusion therapy remain the mainstay of treatment. Unfortunately, refrigeration and storage result in multiple changes in blood products, including decrease in factors V and VII concentration and rapid deterioration of red blood cell and platelet function. Interestingly, recent clinical evidence suggests that platelet dysfunction is the earliest defect that should be treated because endogenous bursts of circulating clotting factors during the hyperacute phase seem to maintain procoagulant effect.

Fresh Frozen Plasma

FFP remains the major source of clotting factors for component transfusion in the United States. FFP is prepared by isolating the plasma from the cellular components via centrifugation of whole blood within 6 to 8 hours of collection. With most systems, the hemostatic activity of the various coagulation factors can be maintained for long periods of time when frozen, although on thawing, the factor concentrations begin to rapidly decrease. Thawed FFP contains excellent concentrations of the various coagulation factors, including up to 400 mg of fibrinogen. Accordingly, FFP should be maintained until a rapid need is present, at which time thawing can be initiated via warming baths in the blood bank. Several busy trauma centers, where larger volumes of plasma are anticipated for use, have initiated the use of prethawed plasma, which is cycled for less than 24 hours to allow for optimal levels of coagulation factors. This plasma (primarily type O or A) may be readily available in the emergency room without the need for waiting the additional 15 to 20 minutes for the thawing process.

The exact dosing and timing of FFP administration is one of the most widely debated topics in trauma. Current evidence from both civilian and military data suggests that early preemptive administration of FFP combined with minimal crystalloids infusion and permissive hypotension improves survival and reduces risks for complications, such as multiple organ failure and abdominal compartment syndrome. Most up-to-date clinical practice suggests that an initial resuscitation transfusion ratio of FFP to red blood cell (RBC) in the range of 1:2 appears to result in optimal survival thresholds. The need for ongoing transfusions, however, may be best determined based on the clinical course of the patient, surgical hemorrhage control, the need for damage control procedures, and the clinical assessment of clot strength, which may be best ascertained via point of care viscoelastic testing.

Platelets

Platelet concentrates were traditionally prepared from pooled platelets obtained from centrifugation of individual units of whole blood. Nevertheless, apheresis or single donor collections, which result in fewer donor exposures for a given dose of platelets, are used in most centers. Transfusion of 1 unit of apheresis platelets, which contains approximately 3×10^{11} platelets in 200 to 250 mL of donor plasma, increases platelet count by 30 to 50 K/mm^3. Although the classic threshold for platelet transfusion has been 50 K/mm^3, a higher target level of 100 K/mm^3 has been suggested for those patients at risk for postinjury coagulopathy. Similar to plasma and packed red cell administration, platelet transfusion has been associated with immunologic complications, with a reported incidence rate of more than 200 per 100,000 transfused patients. Because the cell-based model of coagulation emphasizes the central role of the platelet towards thrombin generation, it is likely that platelet function rather than any absolute threshold of platelet count should be the focus of future therapies. Lastly, current evidence supporting routine prophylactic platelet administration in the patient who has been injured and is at risk for coagulopathy seems less convincing than that for plasma, and the risks of transfusion-related complications may be significant.

Cryoprecipitate

Cryoprecipitate is the cold insoluble fraction formed when FFP is thawed at 4°C. "Cryo" is rich in factors VIII and XIII, von Willebrand's factor, and fibrinogen. Generally, fibrinogen levels greater than 50 mg/dL have been considered sufficient to support hemostasis. Although current evidence suggests that fibrinogen should be replaced early in trauma patients at risk for coagulopathy, this can usually be accomplished via administration of FFP. Further, many guidelines recommend a replacement threshold for plasma fibrinogen levels of less than 100 mg/dL (1 g/L), with either fibrinogen concentrate, which is used increasingly in Europe (3 to 4 g), or cryoprecipitate (50 mg/kg, or 15 to 20 units). It is often underappreciated, however, that FFP, pooled platelets, and even some pRBCs contain fibrinogen (Table 1). Current recommendations, therefore, call for evaluation of plasma fibrinogen levels after administration of component FFP or platelets during massive transfusion with supplementation of cryoprecipitate as necessary based on such testing. Currently, no clinical evidence supports routine preemptive administration of cryoprecipitate in patients at risk for coagulopathy.

Aminocaproic Acid, Aprotinin, and Tranexamic Acid

Although shock has long been recognized to induce fibrinolysis, the contribution of this process to reduced clot strength in the injured patient has been poorly understood and difficult to identify in the clinical setting. Growing clinical evidence, however, suggests that patients with significant trauma with associated blood loss and coagulopathy likely have hyperfibrinolysis develop as an integral aspect of their pathophysiology. Furthermore, patients with development of this state, as identified with viscoelastic testing, likely need antifibrinolytic therapy to reverse this process, which has been associated with the highest mortality in this cohort. Accordingly, the most common agent administered in the United States is epsilon aminocaproic acid (Amicar), a lysine analogue that binds reversibly to plasminogen, preventing its activation to plasmin. Other agents available include aprotinin and tranexamic acid, which is being extensively used in Europe. The authors' preliminary experiences suggest that in the face of suspected or proven hyperfibrinolysis, Amicar (5 to 10 g/20 mL) should be administered as necessary to reverse the lytic process and restore hemostasis.

Recombinant Factor VIIa

rFVIIa is approved by the U.S. Food and Drug Administration (FDA) for the treatment of hemophilia with inhibitory antibodies. However, because factor VII is thought to play a key role in local hemostasis at the site of injury, it was targeted as a potential therapeutic agent for the bleeding trauma patient. In spite of extensive efforts to show efficacy, including several randomized placebo-controlled double-blind clinical trials, no clear evidence shows that rFVIIa alone or as an adjunct to standard resuscitation improves mortality in exsanguinating trauma cases. Unfortunately, the last such study (the CONTROL study), which included 150 centers in 26 countries, was prematurely discontinued after enrolling 573 patients because of unexpected low mortality prompted by futility analysis and difficulties consenting and enrolling sicker patients. Nevertheless, several observations regarding the use of rFVIIa in trauma patients emerged based on the best available data. First, rFVIIa seems to be safe with no increased risk for thromboembolic complications compared with placebo. Second, the administration of rFVIIa, as a single therapeutic agent, is unlikely to be efficacious. Third, rFVIIa possibly decreases blood transfusion requirements in blunt, but not penetrating, trauma cases. Fourth, the administration of rFVIIa in patients with coagulopathic conditions with traumatic brain injury seems to be cost effective, reduces time to surgery, and is efficacious. Given the previous observations, many trauma centers use rFVIIa off label to control massive bleeding, although its efficacy as a general hemostatic drug has not been confirmed. This practice may lose popularity with the evolution of the new principles guiding damage control resuscitation.

Massive Transfusion Protocol

Current evidence suggests that an institutional massive transfusion protocol, which allows for preemptive administration of readily available blood products in a "push" rather than "pull" system, can improve management of postinjury coagulopathy and result in improved survival of the injured patient. Although only 3% to 5% of civilian patients who present to the trauma center need a massive transfusion, it is precisely this cohort that maximally consumes costly hospital resources. Of paramount importance, the protocol, which defines an initial automatic blood bank response to the exsanguinating patient, should be tailored to the individual hospital's local support system, with particular attention to establishing cooperation between the trauma department, anesthesiology department, and laboratory or blood bank. This facilitates a smoothly functioning mechanism that is reliably activated when required to instantly address the needs of the trauma patient with massive bleeding. Although no class 1 data prove that such protocols save lives, it is doubtful that such studies will ever be performed because of wide variability of transfusion and institutional protocols. Despite this, most protocols allow for early, preemptive administration of high-ratio FFP:RBC (approximately 1:2), with the addition of platelets and cryoprecipitate depending on ongoing blood losses. Many

TABLE 1: Composition of various component blood products

Component	Fibrinogen (mg)	Clotting factors
Fresh frozen plasma (4 units)	1600	1 mL contains 1 unit of each coagulation factor*
Cryoprecipitate (10 pack)	1200-1500	VIII/VWF: 800-1000 units
Apheresis platelets (6-10 pack)	300	>3 × 10 platelets/apheresis unit 200-250 mL of plasma equivalent†
Packed red blood cells	50-300‡	None

*Thawed plasma (day 1-5) has a 230% decrease in factors V and VIII.
†As a result of room temperature platelet stroage, factors V and VIII are decreased in the plasma portion.
‡Most red blood cells preservations via Adsol (Fenwal, Inc., Lake Zurich, Ill) have low fibrinogen levels, whereas preservations with CPDA (citrate-phosphate-dextrose-adenine) have higher fibrinogen concentrations.
From Kashuk JL, Moore EE, Sawyer M: Postinjury coagulopathy management: goal directed resuscitation via POC thrombelastography, Ann Surg 251(4):604-614, 2010.

trauma centers use a predetermined amount of blood products sent to the trauma room, operating room, or surgical intensive care unit immediately on activation. This usually consists of 2 to 3 trauma packs, each including 8 to 10 units of group O blood (either O-positive or O-negative, based on patient age and gender), 4 to 6 units of thawed type AB plasma, and 1 unit of single donor platelets. Additional support beyond these packs is discussed between the trauma attending and the blood bank. Other hospitals have developed protocols that rely on the frequent (every 30 minutes, if needed) assessment of laboratory coagulation function and point-of-care TEG. Conventional coagulation tests include PT, usually via the INR; aPTT; platelet count; and fibrinogen level. Clinical evidence suggests that ongoing coagulopathy occurs in the face of an INR more than 1.5, PTT more than 1.5 normal, platelet count less than 100 K, and fibrinogen less than 100 mg/dL. A growing number of trauma centers base their massive transfusion on TEG readings, as described subsequently.

Viscoelastic Testing

The viscoelastic test is the only currently available method with which thrombosis and lysis may be simultaneously evaluated in the injured patient. Although the PT is limited as a measure of only the extrinsic clotting system (factors VIIa, Xa, and IIa), and the PTT is limited by the reactions of the intrinsic system (factors XIIa, XIa, IXa, and IIa), TEG allows the evaluation of the whole system and of platelet function and thrombolysis in whole blood. Rapid TEG is a technique that involves addition of tissue factor to the whole blood specimen, resulting in an even more rapid reaction, particularly suited for the trauma patient. In brief, TEG is a graphic representation of the evolving blood clot (Figure 1) generated via a transducer, which senses the resistance to motion of a microprobe inserted into a small vial of whole blood that is under motion to generate the clot. The resulting tracing is then computer generated and reflects component deficits in the plasma, fibrinogen, platelets, or fibrinolysis. In addition, this methodology assesses clot initiation, maximal clot strength, and rates of subsequent lysis. These capabilities allow for component-specific treatment of traumatic coagulopathy, as described subsequently.

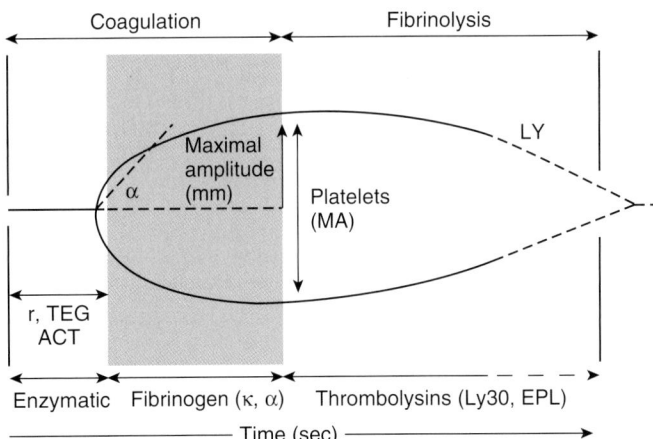

FIGURE 1   Graphic representation of clot formation in rapid thromboelastography (r TEG). The r value (TEG-ACT [activated clotting time] in r TEG) represents initial thrombin generation and is a reflection of enzymatic clotting activation. κ value is the interval measured from the r (TEG-ACT in r TEG) to a fixed level of clot firmness or the point that the amplitude of the tracing reaches 20 mm; this reflects thrombin's ability to cleave soluble fibrinogen. The α angle is the angle between the tangent line drawn from the base horizontal line to the beginning of the cross-linking process, measured in degrees, and is affected primarily by the rate of thrombin generation. Thus, the α angle represents clot rapidity; a higher angle indicates an increased rate of clot formation. The maximal amplitude (MA), measures the end result of maximal platelet-fibrin interaction, reflecting the formation of the platelet plug and thus, the clot strength. The final reading of the tracing is the estimated percent lysis (EPL), also expressed as the LY30, or degree of lysis at 30 minutes of the tracing. An EPL of greater than 15% reflects significant hyperfibrinolysis. In addition, the TEG can measure the clot strength (G), which is a computer-derived value, suggested to be the best measure of clot strength because it reflects components of both the enzymatic and the platelet components of hemostasis.

Goal-Directed Therapy of Trauma-Induced Coagulopathy

Transfusion therapy guided by viscoelastic testing has become an integral part of resuscitation strategy in many institutions in the United States (TEG) and Europe (ROTEM). Because of the rapidity of results and point-of-care, this technology has allowed for evolution of goal-directed therapy of specific coagulation deficits identified during massive resuscitation. Such an approach has allowed for accurate, stepwise correction of coagulation dysfunction with comparative analysis of various tracings generated (Figure 2).

Institutional experience with these techniques is growing despite a significant learning curve for all providers, and TEG and ROTEM–guided therapy is gaining popularity. The potential benefits of such an approach could result in reduced transfusion requirements, earlier correction of coagulation deficits, and ultimately improved survival in this critically ill cohort.

MILITARY EXPERIENCE

The recent Iraq-Afghanistan conflicts have significantly advanced our knowledge and understanding of thrombosis and hemostasis in the injured patient. The most significant progress has been the recognition that decreased crystalloid administration combined with the principles of hemostatic/damage control resuscitation is

beneficial. Although the military demonstrated impressive advantages to the use of warm whole blood for shock resuscitation, this product has not been available in the civilian sector for more than 30 years because of cost concerns and quality control issues related to the transmission of blood-borne pathogens. Accordingly, the military showed that resuscitation strategies that attempt to mimic whole blood with use of component therapy in ratios approaching 1:1 FFP: RBC resulted in significant, often dramatic improvements in survival of patients at risk for postinjury coagulopathy. Some studies also advocated equal use of preemptive platelets. These concepts have been embraced over the past 5 years by the civilian sector as well. Although there are still no level one evidence studies, current civilian experience learned from the military has established the importance of preemptive plasma to RBC in ratios of at least 1:2 as being effective while maintaining a reduced risk of transfusion-related lung injury, multiple organ failure, and abdominal compartment syndrome. Thus, these military-derived resuscitation paradigms have led to a major shift in our approach to the injured patient at risk for coagulopathy.

SUMMARY

Postinjury coagulopathy is a multifactorial syndrome that demands meticulous attention in the acutely bleeding patient. Current approaches include early recognition of the patient at risk, with

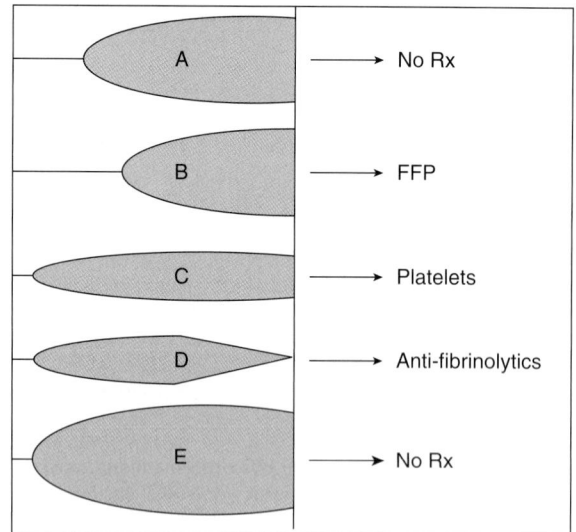

FIGURE 2 Thromboelastography (TEG) tracing patterns indicating specific coagulation deficits. *A*, Normal TEG graphic. *B*, Prolonged r value (TEG-ACT [activated clotting time] in rapid TEG), suggestive of the need for additional fresh frozen plasma *(FFP)* treatment. *C*, A narrowed maximal amplitude (MA), or decreased clot strength, is suggestive of the need for platelet therapy, and an increased MA and short r value may indicate a hypercoagulable state. *D*, Hyperfibrinolysis, which should prompt antifibrinolytic treatment. *E*, Decreased clotting and clotting formation time, elevated α-angle, and increased MA represent a hypercoagulable state. *(Reprinted with permission from Haemonetics Corp, Braintree, Mass.)*

prompt resuscitation techniques, which include early provision of blood component therapy, significantly reduced crystalloid administration, and particular attention to the effects of hypothermia, acidosis, and other associated factors. Because of the difficulty in estimating the massive transfusion needs of the injured patient, current evidence suggests that an established massive transfusion protocol with preemptive blood product availability significantly assists in the successful resuscitation of the injured patient. Finally, growing experience with viscoelastic testing suggests that this technology may offer great promise for the continuing management of these patients.

SUGGESTED READINGS

Hoffman M, Monroe D III: A cell-based model of hemostasis, *Thromb Haemost* 85:958–965, 2001.

Kashuk J, Moore EE, Sawyer M, et al: Primary fibrinolysis is integral in the pathogenesis of postinjury coagulopathy, *Ann Surg* 252(3):434–444, 2010.

Kashuk JL, Moore EE, Sawyer M: Postinjury coagulopathy management: goal directed resuscitation via POC thrombelastography, *Ann Surg* 251(4):604–614, 2010.

Williams-Johnson JA, McDonald AH, Strachan GG, et al: Effects of tranexamic acid on death, vascular occlusive events, and blood transfusion in trauma patients with significant haemorrhage (CRASH-2): a randomized, placebo-controlled trial The CRASH-2 Collaborators, *Lancet* 376(9734): 23–32, 2010.

THE ABDOMEN THAT WILL NOT CLOSE

Jordan A. Weinberg, MD, and
Timothy C. Fabian, MD

The appreciation of abdominal compartment syndrome (ACS) in the 1980s ultimately led to a fundamental change in the management of the laparotomy wound. The "open abdomen" has become the standard treatment both for the management of ACS, by decompressive laparotomy, and for the prevention of ACS, by leaving the abdomen open after operations in the setting of shock. Although the open abdomen has contributed to the salvage of patients who may otherwise have died, the surgeon is then faced with the subsequent management of this open wound, with its inherent acute and chronic challenges. The acute challenge involves prevention of potential collateral damage, including the disastrous complication of intestinal fistulae. The chronic challenge created by the successful avoidance or treatment of ACS is that of definitive reconstruction of the large abdominal wall defect in the patients who recover from the acute insult. At the authors' institution, a fairly standardized staged approach for managing the abdominal wound has developed. The three stages are (1) prosthetic insertion and attempt at delayed primary closure, (2) staged split-thickness skin grafting for planned

ventral hernia, and (3) definitive reconstruction with a modification of the components separation technique (Figure 1).

STAGE 1: PROSTHETIC INSERTION AND ATTEMPT AT DELAYED PRIMARY CLOSURE

Ideally, temporary wound closure should allow for containment and protection of the bowel from mechanical injury, prevention of adherence of the viscera to the closure materials and the abdominal wall, minimization of fascial injury, protection against abdominal compartment syndrome, and minimization of the loss of abdominal domain. Multiple methods and techniques have been advocated, and all optimize some of the characteristics described at the expense of others. It is also important to consider the time course of the open abdomen because techniques that optimize protection against abdominal compartment syndrome should be employed immediately after initial laparotomy, whereas techniques that limit fascial retraction my be indicated once the risk for abdominal compartment syndrome has waned and the primary goal becomes abdominal closure.

The authors' institutional approach to stage 1 is as follows. After the initial laparotomy, the authors favor the vacuum pack technique as described by Brock and coworkers in 1995 (Figure 2). A plastic drape is inserted in the peritoneal cavity covering the viscera, and on top of this is placed a surgical towel along with two sump drains

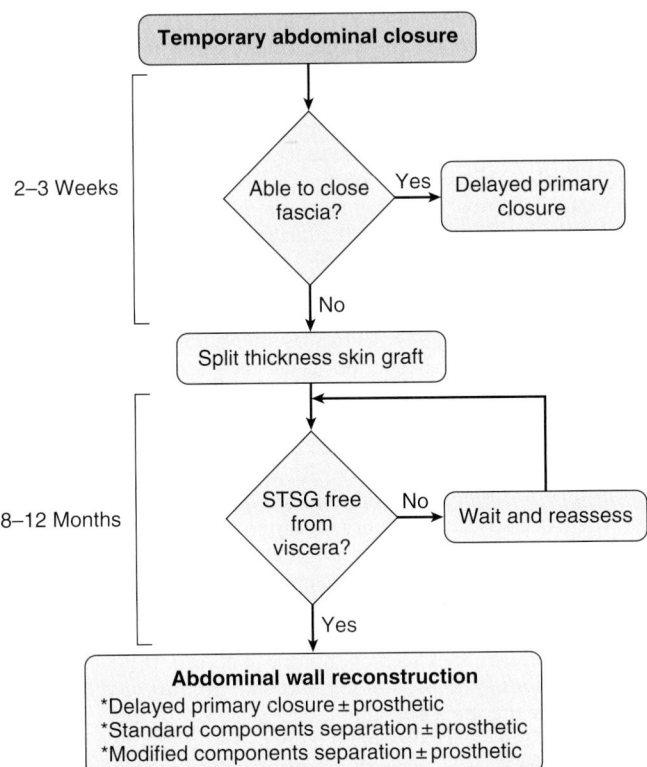

FIGURE 1   Flow diagram representing three-staged approach to management of the open abdomen. *STSG,* Split-thickness skin graft.

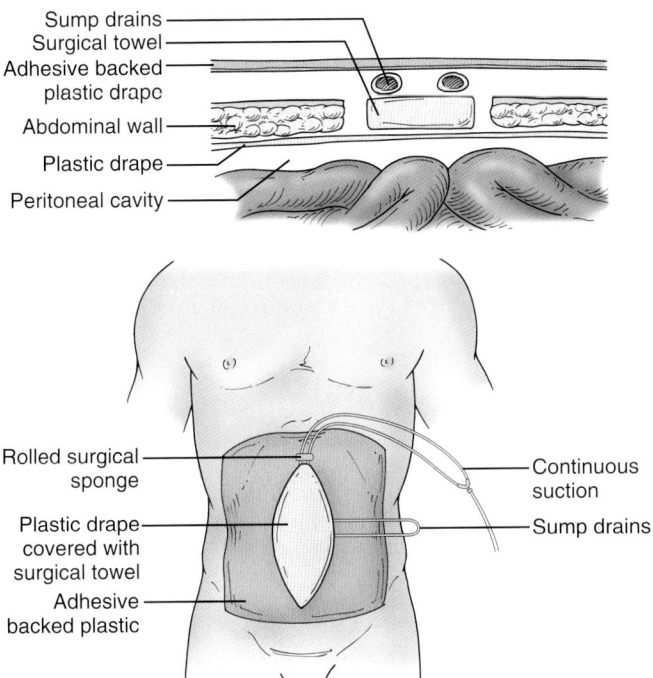

FIGURE 2   Vacuum pack technique for temporary abdominal closure.

covered with an adhesive-backed plastic drape attached to the patient's skin. The sump drains are placed on continuous suction. The advantages of using this technique after initial laparotomy are that it can be rapidly completed, it prevents abdominal compartment syndrome, and the material is easily removed at subsequent abdominal exploration for pack removal or bowel anastomosis. The authors

have also found proprietary negative-pressure appliances designed for the open abdomen to be similarly efficacious. In cases of exceptional bowel and retroperitoneal edema in which the viscera protrude well above the level of the skin incision, the authors utilize a modification of the Bogota bag, whereby an x-ray cassette cover is fashioned as a silo and sewn to the skin with running heavy nylon suture.

The second phase of stage 1 is the attempt at delayed fascial closure. Once the resuscitative phase after initial laparotomy is completed and the patient has returned to the operating room for pack removal or definitive management of hollow viscus injuries, or both, delayed fascial closure may be possible, but often closure at this time would place too much tension on the fascia with risk for subsequent fascial necrosis and dehiscence. It is at this point that a technique that emphasizes minimization of fascial retraction should be employed. The preference at the authors' institution is to bridge the fascial wound gap with woven polyglactin 910 mesh, secured circumferentially to the fascia with running suture. Patients either recover and mobilize fluids over the next several days, which allows for gradual closure of the abdomen, or develop varying degrees of multiple organ dysfunction or sepsis. In the latter group, it is often not possible to close the fascia by progressive approximation. In that circumstance, the viscera granulate and adhere to the abdominal wall laterally and to the prosthesis, and the patient's wound is managed according to the principles of stage 2 (described next). If, however, the patient's hemodynamic status recovers and tissue edema begins to resolve, attempts are made at the bedside to pleat the mesh gradually with suture, with the goal of maintaining midline tension to attain a potential secondary fascial closure. If it becomes apparent that secondary fascial closure is feasible, as manifested by laxity in the mesh and physiologic improvement in the patient, the patient can be taken back to the operating room for mesh removal and fascial closure.

It has been the authors' experience, however, that the minority of open abdomens achieve delayed primary closure. In their reported experience from a randomized trial in which the authors compared polyglactin 910 mesh with vacuum-assisted closure utilized up to postoperative day 9, the authors found that closure rates were low, regardless of the technique employed (31% for vacuum-assisted closure, 26% for mesh). Other researchers, however, have reported much higher rates of fascial closure in single-institution case series, on the order of 70% to 100 % with the utilization of vacuum-assisted closure or other techniques that limit fascial retraction, such as the Velcro-like Wittmann patch. The challenge in accounting for these disparate results lies in the fact that the indications for utilizing the open abdomen are not uniform and in fact vary from center to center and from surgeon to surgeon. Institutions that err toward leaving abdomens open after laparotomy for trauma probably have a much higher rate of closure than do institutions that utilize the open abdomen less liberally, and in fact, there is growing concern that the open abdomen is being overutilized. In the authors' institutional experience, approximately 15% of trauma laparotomies are left open after initial operation.

STAGE 2: STAGED SPLIT-THICKNESS SKIN GRAFTING FOR PLANNED VENTRAL HERNIA

Should delayed fascial closure prove to be unattainable, a more permanent solution is required for the large ventral defect. The goal at this stage is to create a planned ventral hernia, whereby the absorbable mesh protecting the viscera is exchanged for split-thickness skin graft.

Although conventional wisdom suggests that absorbable mesh would be absorbed completely and not have to be removed, that has not been the authors' experience with the woven variety of polyglactin 910. Usually within 2 to 3 weeks, granulation occurs and a suppurative interface between mesh and viscera develops, which begins to separate the two. At this point of healthy granulation, the viscera are stuck together and circumferentially to the abdominal wall, and patients are taken to the operating room. The mesh is removed easily because of the suppurative interface. After removal of the mesh, a pulsatile pressure irrigation system is used to reduce colonization of the granulation tissue, and a split-thickness skin graft is harvested and applied to the granulating viscera. The authors routinely mesh the graft 2:1 with a Brennan meshing device and secure the graft to the skin edges with staples or absorbable suture, depending on the surgeon's preference. For relatively large defects, multiple grafts may need to be secured together with absorbable suture in the manner of a quilt, and the authors have found it useful to additionally secure the graft with the application of aerosolized fibrin glue, which can also be applied to the donor site for hemostasis. A nonadherent dressing is then placed over the graft, and a Wound Vac sponge is placed on top, with negative pressure set at 75 mm Hg. On postoperative day 4, the Wound Vac sponge is removed, and the graft is covered with nonadherent dressings until healed. The final result is demonstrated in Figure 3.

Prevention and Management of Fistula

During the interval between mesh coverage and skin graft placement, development of fistulas is of concern. The authors analyzed their experience with fistulas in the open abdomen setting in 380 trauma patients managed over a 10-year period. The fistula rate in this group of patients was 8%, and the majority (65%) arose from the small bowel. Most fistulas formed during the interval of mesh coverage (nearly 70%), and patients in whom fistulas formed were more likely to have had mesh coverage for a significantly longer time than the patients who did not develop this complication (27 vs 18 days). It is therefore important to perform the skin graft relatively early rather than late because the longer the wound is left to granulate without coverage of the bowel, the more likely the bowel wall is to erode through the granulation tissue and instigate fistula formation. It appears as if a skin graft would not necessarily give much support to the wound and that this sort of coverage would not necessarily prevent a fistula. In the authors' experience, however, skin grafting does stabilize the wound significantly. Skin coverage of the open granulating wound also helps to decrease the proteinaceous losses through the wound, similar to the benefit of early grafting of large surface burns, as these large open wounds produce a tremendous ongoing catabolic drain.

If a fistula ultimately does occur, it may range in severity from a relatively minor nuisance to a life-threatening catastrophe. Should a low-output fistula develop on the lateral aspect of the wound, there is a reasonable chance for spontaneous closure as the wound granulates and contracts over the fistula. Small fistulas that do not close can be handled as semiformal ostomies with bags placed over them until definitive repair is performed.

Fistulas that occur away from the lateral wall, in the midportion of the wound, are problematic (and have been dubbed "enteroatmospheric"). For relatively low-output fistulas that occur in this area, the authors' approach is to apply a skin graft on the entire wound around the fistula. After the graft adheres and heals, a bag can usually be fixed to the abdominal wall, effectively converting the fistula to a controlled ostomy. Although not always successful, this approach works better than might be anticipated. In contrast, midwound proximal, high-output small bowel fistulas have significant rates of morbidity and mortality. The authors' usual approach is to operate early to prevent the complications secondary to metabolic derangements and nutritional depletion. Surgery consists of sharply incising the granulation tissue right at the ostium of the fistula. In general, a relatively normal serosa is identified. Once the serosa is identified, the bowel loop is isolated gradually and resected back to nonindurated, nonedematous tissue. A primary anastomosis generally is performed. After anastomosis, an attempt is made to bury the anastomosis as deeply as possible in the abdomen beneath other bowel loops to minimize the likelihood of fistula recurrence. Following this, the large open wound is managed with the replacement of absorbable mesh to maintain the viscera within the abdomen. If the viscera are relatively "stuck," the authors perform skin grafting at this time in lieu of replacing the absorbable mesh. Resection of these fistulas is an arduous task that takes many hours. We believe, however, that patients do better with this early approach rather than waiting several weeks to months and having their nutritional status and overall recovery continue to erode while they are receiving total parenteral nutrition.

STAGE 3: DEFINITIVE RECONSTRUCTION WITH A MODIFICATION OF THE COMPONENTS SEPARATION TECHNIQUE

The appropriate timing for abdominal wall reconstruction is of paramount importance. If performed too early, dense adhesions make split-thickness skin graft removal difficult, often leading to multiple enterotomies or significant bowel deserosalization. When reconstruction is delayed for an excessive amount of time, the musculature of the abdominal wall tends to contract with a progressive

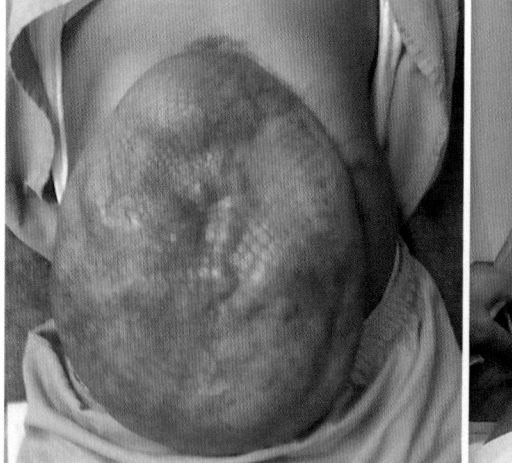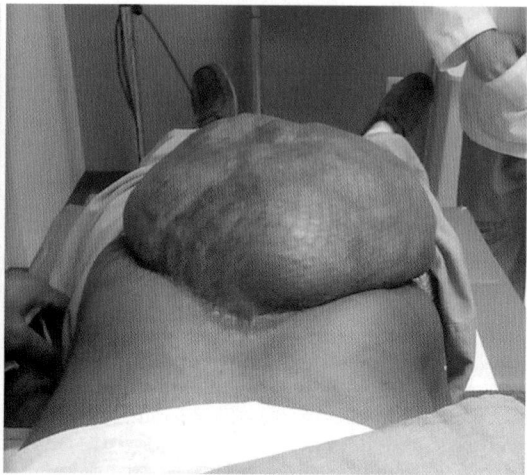

FIGURE 3 Well-healed planned ventral hernia with split-thickness skin graft.

loss of domain, which makes reconstruction considerably more difficult. The authors generally proceed with the operation when the intra-abdominal adhesion process has matured to the point that flimsy adhesions develop between loops of bowel and skin graft. This can be ascertained simply by pinching the skin graft between the fingers, and, if the bowel falls away, it is time for reconstruction. If the loops of bowel seem to be densely adhered to the skin graft, reconstruction should be delayed. The authors' experience suggests that most patients develop these flimsy adhesions in the 6- to 12-month interval after hospital discharge. Beyond 12 months, it is unlikely for the graft to become any less adherent, and deferring reconstruction any longer increases the patient's risk for ongoing loss of domain.

The authors' own modification of the component separation technique described by Ramirez and colleagues is the preferred method of reconstruction in the majority of these cases. The original component separation technique consisted of local myocutaneous flap advancement after extensive relaxing incisions in the abdominal wall. It provides autologous continuity with dynamic support of the abdominal wall. The original technique provided for 3 to 5 cm of mobilization on each side. These large abdominal wall defects, however, usually cannot be repaired with this amount of mobilization. After recognizing this drawback of limited mobilization, the authors added a modification of Ramirez and colleagues' component separation technique, outlined as follows.

Modified Component Separation

Step 1: Removal of Skin Graft

The skin graft is grasped between the fingers or with tissue forceps and sharply incised in an area that is obviously free of underlying bowel. Once the incision is made, the skin graft is divided in its midportion from top to bottom. After this, adhesions of small bowel to the skin graft are mobilized bilaterally, and dissection extends a few centimeters beyond the lateral edge of the rectus abdominis muscles bilaterally.

Step 2: Raising of Full-Thickness Skin Flaps

Full-thickness skin and subcutaneous fat are mobilized on each side of the wound, just superficial to the fascia. Musculocutaneous perforator vessels will be encountered and should be preserved when possible. In general, each flap is raised laterally beyond the anterior axillary line, always several centimeters beyond the lateral border of the rectus sheath. The skin edges should now be free enough to be pulled together in the midline. If additional distance is required, further lateral mobilization of the flaps is performed.

Step 3: Release of External Oblique Component of Anterior Rectus Fascia

The rectus abdominis muscle is grasped in the palm of the hand with the thumb on top and the fingers inside the abdominal cavity. The external oblique fascia is divided approximately 1 cm lateral to the rectus abdominis muscle with use of a hemostat to dissect the external oblique freely from the internal oblique component. The external oblique fascia then is divided superiorly and inferiorly, over the lower costal region superiorly and down to the pubic symphysis inferiorly (Figure 4).

Step 4: Dissection of Posterior Rectus Sheath

The medial border of the rectus sheath is incised for the entire length of the muscle. This exposes the anterior and posterior fascia and rectus muscle as three distinct layers (Figure 5). The posterior sheath should then be freed from the rectus muscle, from the superior aspect of the wound to the level of the arcuate line (inferior to this level, the posterior component comprises only peritoneum).

FIGURE 4 The external oblique release is extended cephalad over the costal margin and caudally to the pubic symphysis.

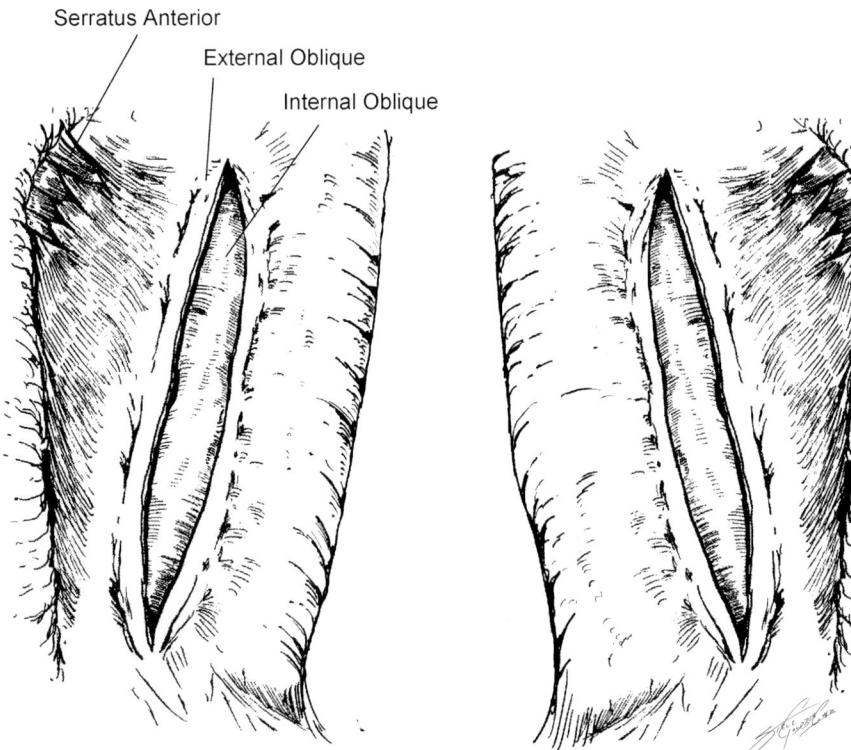

Serratus Anterior

External Oblique

Internal Oblique

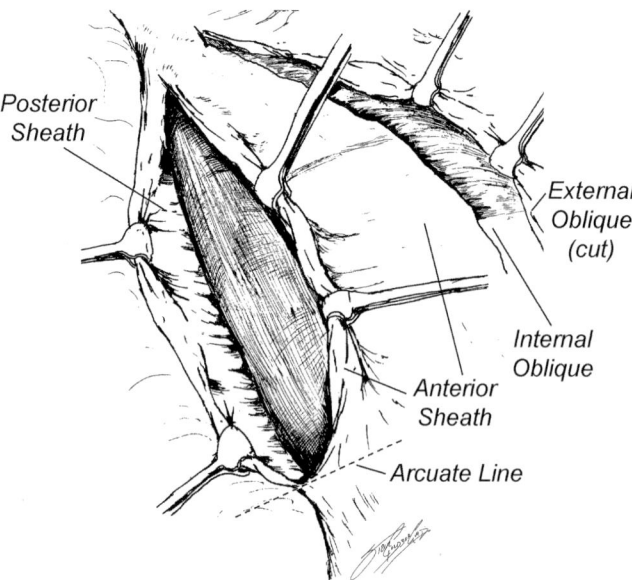

FIGURE 5   The medial edge of rectus sheath is divided, and the posterior sheath is freed from the overlying rectus muscle.

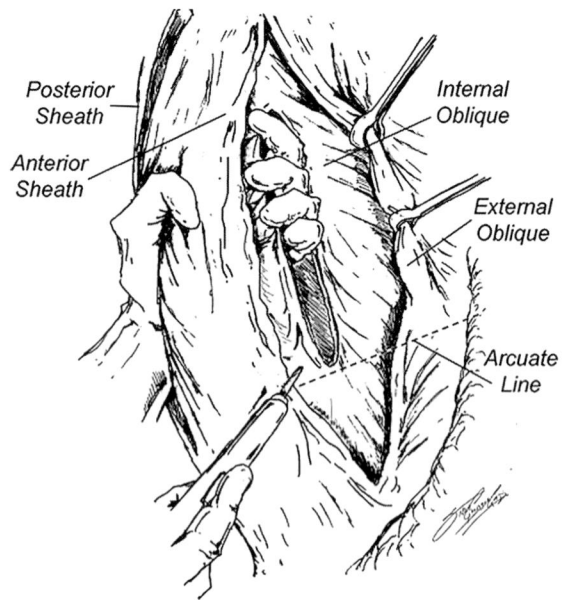

FIGURE 6   Release of internal oblique component. The dorsum of the surgeon's hand is lying on the posterior sheath as the palmar surface cups the rectus muscle. The incision is made over the surgeon's finger to ensure that only the anterior component is divided.

Step 5: Release of Internal Oblique Component of Anterior Rectus Fascia

This step constitutes the Memphis modification of Ramirez and colleagues' components separation. The internal oblique component of the anterior rectus sheath is divided. This is done by sharply incising the anterior fascia approximately 1 cm lateral to the rectus muscle (Figure 6). This opening is then extended for the length of the rectus muscle from the costal border, down to the level of the arcuate line. It is imperative that the incision be stopped at the arcuate line. If the internal oblique component of the anterior rectus sheath is divided below this point, a large hernia will develop because there is no posterior fascia below the arcuate line. At this point in the procedure, the anterior rectus sheaths (with adherent rectus muscle) have been freed medially and laterally.

Step 6: Translocation of Anterior Fascia and Midline Closure

The medial aspect of the posterior sheath is sutured to the lateral aspect of the anterior sheath, typically with running monofilament suture. The abdominal wall is then closed by suturing the medial components of the anterior rectus fascia. The appearance of the completed fascial reconstruction is depicted in Figure 7. Four flat closed suction drains then are inserted to drain the skin flaps, two superiorly and two inferiorly bilaterally. The skin then is approximated in the midline to complete the procedure.

The procedure as just described provides approximately 10 cm of medial advancement in the epigastrium, 20 cm in the midabdomen, and 8 cm in the lower abdomen. The authors have found that when this mobilization is sufficient for fascial closure, the incidence of hernia after reconstruction is low (5% over a 15-year experience). Some patients, however, have a remaining fascial gap despite performance of the reconstruction as described, which necessitates the use of a prosthetic to complete the procedure. It has become the authors' preference to use biologic prosthetics in this scenario because of the possibility of serosal tears (and in some cases, ostomy reversal may have been performed concomitantly). The preferred technique is an underlay with at least 2 cm of overlap with healthy fascia. The underlay technique is used selectively to buttress the repair when the quality of the fascia is questionable or appears attenuated, even when

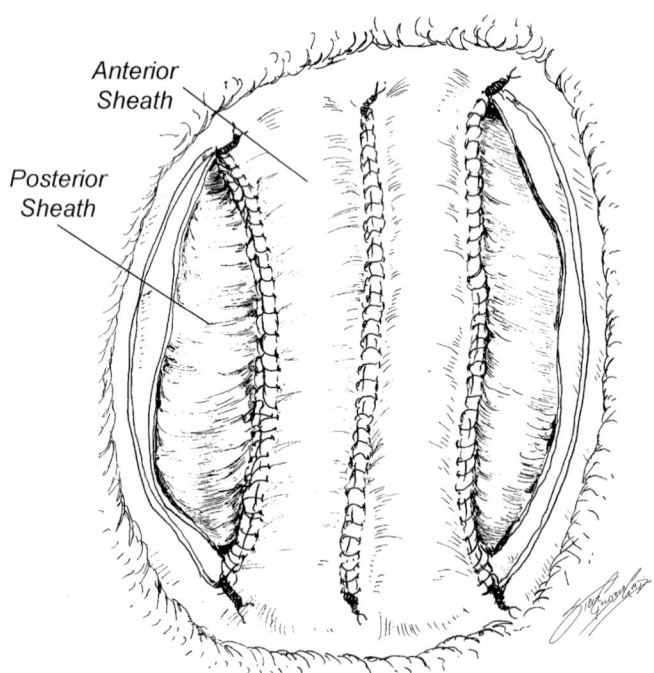

FIGURE 7   Final fascial closure with three suture lines.

able to close the fascia without a prosthetic. Not surprisingly, patients who require adjunctive prosthetics are at greater risk for recurrence (20% in the authors' experience) but have improved outcomes in comparison with patients who undergo standard components separation (i.e., without the Memphis modification) with prosthetic (44% recurrence rate). Thus the additional releases required for the Memphis technique are preferable to using a larger prosthetic.

Suggested Readings

Bee TK, Croce MA, Magnotti LJ, et al: Temporary abdominal closure techniques: a prospective randomized trial comparing polyglactin 910 mesh and vacuum-assisted closure, *J Trauma* 65:337–344, 2008.

Brock WB, Barker DE, Burns RP: Temporary closure of open abdominal wounds: the vacuum pack, *Am Surg* 61:30–35, 1995.

DiCocco JM, Fabian TC, Emmett KP, et al: Components separation for abdominal wall reconstruction: the Memphis modification, *Surgery* 151:118–125, 2012.

DiCocco JM, Magnotti LJ, Emmett KP, et al: Long-term follow-up of abdominal wall reconstruction after planned ventral hernia: a 15-year experience, *J Am Coll Surg* 210:686–698, 2010.

Fischer PE, Fabian TC, Magnotti LJ, et al: A ten-year review of enterocutaneous fistulas after laparotomy for trauma, *J Trauma* 67:924–928, 2009.

Ramirez OM, Ruas E, Dellon AL: "Components separation" method for closure of abdominal wall defects: An anatomic and clinical study, *Plast Reconstr Surg* 86:519–526, 1990.

The Management of Vascular Injuries

K. Shad Pharaon, MD, and Donald D. Trunkey, MD

OVERVIEW

Vascular injuries are associated with high morbidity and mortality. Management is transitioning from open surgery to endovascular repair for many of these injuries. Unstable patients still need to proceed to the operating room without delay, and the operation will be directed based on the clinical exam performed in the emergency department. If the patient is stable after the initial resuscitation, then assessment of vascular injury by computed tomographic angiography (CTA) should occur. In patients with contrast allergy, magnetic resonance angiography (MRA) is an option. The contrast media used for MRA is usually less toxic than those used for CTA and catheter-based angiography, with fewer people having any risk of allergy. MRA is typically more expensive, takes longer, and is unsafe in patients with metal such as a pacemaker. Duplex ultrasonography can be used to diagnose vascular trauma, but subcutaneous air, fragments, and hematomas make ultrasound less reliable.

After undergoing high-quality imaging, the patient is often taken to a hybrid operating room to undergo endovascular repair with the option of an open procedure. In recent years, endovascular repair of certain injuries has become the norm and often has better outcomes. Numerous small studies have documented the successful management of traumatic arterial injuries with endografts. This chapter will describe the treatment options of vascular injury to the neck, chest, abdomen, pelvis, and extremities.

INITIAL EVALUATION AND MANAGEMENT

Vascular injuries can be caused by blunt forces, deceleration forces, or penetrating injuries due to knives, gunshot wounds, or impalement. Thorough prehospital assessment of these patients—including measurement of vital signs and determination of the presence or absence of shock, as well as early resuscitation—is now standard practice. This prehospital resuscitation starts in the field, continues with transport, and carries through to the emergency department. The use of tourniquets for vascular injury to extremities has seen resurgence. Bleeding is the leading cause of potentially preventable death on the battlefield, and the availability of tourniquets has

increased among military medics. This has carried over into the civilian population. Although tourniquets have been used for many years, their safety and efficacy have recently been looked at more closely, and their availability as a commercial device has increased. Debates will continue on the best tourniquet design, duration, and inflation pressure.

If the patient has a systolic blood pressure of 80 mm Hg, pushing fluids is not necessary to achieve a normal blood pressure. Fluid management should not contribute to the bleeding process. In hemorrhaging patients without traumatic brain injury, permissive hypotension is acceptable in the short term. A blood pressure of 80 mm Hg achieves cerebral perfusion and minimizes excessive hemorrhage. It must be emphasized that the grossly unstable patient with a systolic blood pressure less than 80 mm Hg should go immediately to the operating room and bypass the CT scanner. The body cavity that needs to be opened so that the source of bleeding can be found will be dependent on the surgeon's physical examination and assessment of entry and exit wounds. In unstable patients with blunt trauma, a chest x-ray and focused assessment with sonography for trauma (FAST) are the only imaging that is needed prior to the operating room. If the patient can be stabilized, a pan CT scan with CTA for suspected vascular injury can be invaluable for identifying the location of injury as well as planning the repair. Increasingly, Level 1 and some Level 2 trauma hospitals are developing endovascular hybrid operating rooms, allowing the surgeon to bring a trauma patient directly to the room and perform endovascular repair, endovascular adjunctive care, or an open operation. In those that are unstable who undergo an open operation, the objective is to obtain proximal and distal control of the bleeding vessel. The surgeon must quickly develop a strategy of repair, bypass, or ligation. For all patients, the proximal thighs should be prepared and included in the operative field for potential vein conduit. A longitudinal incision over the lateral portion of the sartorius muscle exposes the superficial femoral-popliteal vein (SFPV). The SFPV has been used in the reconstruction of the innominate artery, common carotid artery, inferior vena cava (IVC), and portal vein.

BODY REGIONS AND TYPICAL VASCULAR INJURIES

Neck

All neck injuries require a neck and chest x-ray to look for fractures, missiles, associated hemopneumothorax, widened mediastinum, and subcutaneous emphysema. Unstable patients with a penetrating neck injury are taken directly to the operating room. If the patient has stable vital signs, CTA of the neck and upper chest is the best initial screening tool for a penetrating neck injury. It gives a sense of the trajectory of the bullet, associated cervical spine fractures, involvement of the spinal cord, fragments, and hematomas. If the CTA images have excessive scatter from metallic fragments or excessive air, conventional four-vessel angiography might be useful. If the patient has neurologic deficits, a brain CT scan without contrast is needed. CTA of the neck is also performed on patients with suspected blunt carotid injury. Although MRA is impractical in an unstable trauma patient with multiple injuries, it is an attractive noninvasive modality, particularly to assess the intracranial architecture for signs of stroke. The mainstay of treatment for blunt carotid injury is antithrombotic therapy.

The neck is divided into three zones. Zone 1 is the base of the neck below the cricoid cartilage. Zone 2 extends from the cricoid cartilage to the angle of the mandible. Zone 3 extends from the angle of the mandible to the base of the skull (Figure 1). Zone 1 and zone 3 injuries are more difficult to expose than zone 2 injuries. Zone 1 requires proximal intrathoracic control, often with a median sternotomy. Exposure of zone 3 is difficult because of the retromandibular position of the carotid artery. Exposure of this area may require manipulation of the mandible. Zone 2 injuries are readily accessible surgically.

The approach to zone 1 injuries is through an incision along the sternocleidomastoid muscle and occasionally extended inferiorly into a median sternotomy when more proximal control is needed. The innominate veins (brachiocephalic) can be seen deep to the thymus. Retraction or division of innominate veins will expose the aortic arch. Dissection along the arch will reveal the origin of the innominate, left common carotid artery, and perhaps a portion of the proximal left subclavian artery. Due to its posterior location, most of the left subclavian artery is difficult to isolate from this incision, and a high anterolateral thoracotomy may be needed. The origin of the common carotid is identified and encircled with vessel loops or a vascular clamp. Before clamping, identify the vagus nerve. The preferable approach to these injuries, if a simple laceration cannot be repaired, is resection and either primary anastomosis or replacement with an interposition graft, preferably of autogenous tissue.

Zone 2 exposure is best approached using an incision along the sternocleidomastoid muscle. When bilateral structures of the neck are potentially injured, a collar incision may be preferable. The facial vein is divided to obtain better exposure of the carotid artery bifurcation, which is located deep to the vein. On rare occasions, a clean laceration to the carotid may be amendable to simple lateral repair or end-to-end anastomosis. Shunts should be used in patients already at risk for cerebral hypoperfusion secondary to shock and to injuries of the internal carotid artery. Heparin should be given before clamps

are placed on the vessel. Most external carotid injuries may be ligated without consequence. Ligation of the common or internal carotid artery should be avoided because it can result in devastating neurologic sequelae. The great saphenous vein is a good size match with the internal carotid artery and can be used as an interposition graft with excellent patency and limited risk of infection. Vein does take more time to harvest and prepare. The external carotid artery is an ideal conduit for interposition grafting in injuries to the internal carotid artery near the areas of the bifurcation. Transposition of the mobilized external carotid to connect it to the internal carotid artery is also an option. Polytetrafluoroethylene (PTFE) can also be used to reconstruct the common or internal carotid arteries, but in the setting of an esophageal injury, autogenous conduit should be used. The injured vessel is débrided and a 5-0 polypropylene suture is used for the anastomosis. Intraoperative duplex ultrasonography should be considered after the repair to confirm flow and to look for an intimal flap. Patients who undergo carotid artery repair are prescribed lifetime daily aspirin.

The retromandibular position of the distal carotid artery makes zone 3 a challenging operative exposure. Exposure often requires subluxation of the mandible or mandibular osteotomy. The latter adds risk to the marginal mandibular and inferior alveolar nerves. Anterior subluxation usually requires that the patient be nasotracheally intubated so that the mandible can be wired to the maxilla to hold exposure. The digastric muscle is divided, the styloid process may be excised, and injury to the glossopharyngeal, hypoglossal, and facial nerves is possible.

Operative exposure of the vertebral artery is problematic. The vertebral artery can be divided into four anatomic zones. The first portion of the vertebral artery (V-1) extends from the origin of the vertebral artery off the subclavian to the foramen of the transverse process of C6. The second portion (V-2) is the interosseous portion ascending from C6 to C2. The third portion (V-3) is that portion from C2 to the base of the skull. The fourth portion (V-4) extends from the base of the skull to the confluence of the right and left vertebral arteries, which forms the basilar artery. One option for rapid control of the proximal vertebral artery is to approach it where it comes off the subclavian artery. However, even after clamping, there may be continued backbleeding from the circle of Willis. Insertion of a Fogarty balloon catheter (Edwards Lifesciences, Irvine, Calif) may achieve temporary control of bleeding. As the vertebral artery ascends through the transverse foramina toward the base of the skull, access becomes very difficult. Bleeding from this area may be better served with packing of bone wax into the hole until an endovascular approach is possible. Embolization of the vertebral artery is preferred, and the collaterals are usually sufficient to avoid an ischemic stroke.

Chest

Most patients with blunt injury to the descending thoracic aorta die immediately at the scene from exsanguination. The injury to the descending thoracic aorta usually occurs at the isthmus, just distal to the left subclavian artery. The patients that do survive the initial aortic injury may have other injuries that are a more immediate threat to their lives. If the patient has a stable thoracic hematoma and concomitant abdominal injury, laparotomy should be the initial procedure. If the patient has a rapidly expanding hematoma around his or her aorta, the chest should be addressed expeditiously. The lesion that is most likely causing the exsanguination should be addressed first.

In rare cases, a patient with blunt aortic injury (BAI) makes it to the hospital in extremis. This patient should be resuscitated and should undergo an anterolateral thoracotomy through the fourth intercostal space on the side of injury. On the left, this provides rapid access to the pericardium, pulmonary hilum, and aorta. If further exposure is needed, a clamshell is performed by transecting the

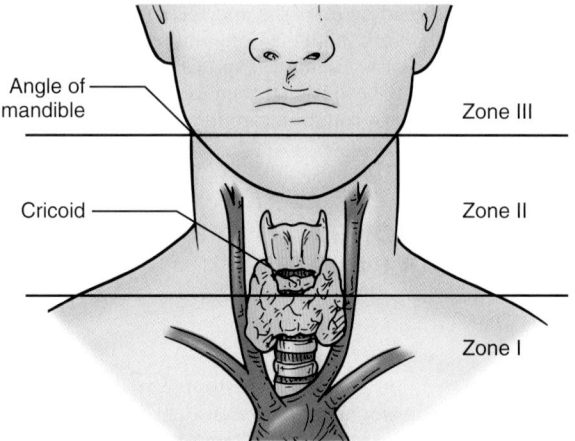

FIGURE 1 Definition of the three anatomic zones used in neck trauma. Zone I is base of neck to cricoid cartilage. Zone II is cricoid cartilage to angle of mandible. Zone III extends from angle of mandible to base of skull.

sternum and extending the incision to include a right thoracotomy. Ligation of both sides of the internal mammary arteries should occur if a clamshell is performed; otherwise, delayed bleeding is likely to occur. The lung is mobilized by dividing the inferior pulmonary ligament. The pericardium is opened anterior to the phrenic nerve to rule out a tamponade. The descending thoracic aorta, particularly in the hypotensive patient, is flaccid and pulseless. The aorta can be manually compressed against the spine until an aortic clamp can be placed. A small window through the parietal pleura on either side of the aorta assists in getting a vascular clamp securely on the vessel. Clamping of the thoracic aorta is a double-edged sword. It may improve circulation to the brain and the heart, but if the patient becomes hypertensive, the left ventricle can become overdistended and result in demise of the patient. Previously, injury to the descending thoracic aorta was repaired with clamping and direct reconstruction. The most feared complication of this technique is paraplegia. Ischemic bowel and renal failure may also result from prolonged clamping. Lower mortality and almost nonexistent paraplegia now make the use of thoracic endovascular aortic repair (TEVAR) for BAI very compelling.

For the patients that survive BAI, the usual presentation is one with normal hemodynamics and with multiple other injuries. The tendency is to focus on the aorta and overlook the other injuries. Recent evidence suggests that some BAIs do not need repair at all. There is a new way of classifying BAIs based on the absence (intimal tears and large intimal flaps) or presence (pseudoaneurysms and ruptures) of external contour abnormalities of the aorta. Intimal tears can be managed nonoperatively. Patients with large intimal flaps do well, and most are treated with a stent graft. If a pseudoaneurysm is going to rupture, it does so early. Most pseudoaneurysms and ruptures are now treated with endovascular repair, within 1 week, if the patient has a reasonable likelihood of survival. Hypotensive patients with hematoma around their aorta may benefit from earlier repair. Patients who undergo endovascular repair should be monitored with CT imaging at 1 month, 6 months, 1 year, and every other year thereafter. For penetrating injury to the descending thoracic aorta, lateral suture repair is usually possible in those who survive because the trauma is limited frequently to lacerations. Of course, larger arterial wounds are not compatible with survival.

Median sternotomy provides access to the superior mediastinum. Dividing the left innominate vein improves exposure and gives the surgeon access to the aortic arch and its branches. Repair of the aortic arch often requires cardiopulmonary bypass. Occasionally, minor injuries to the innominate artery can be repaired primarily. More often, injuries to the innominate artery require repair via the bypass exclusion technique (Figure 2). A piece of synthetic interposition graft is sewn from the ascending aorta to the distal innominate artery. The proximal innominate artery is oversewn. With transection of the left common carotid artery, a bypass to the aorta using PTFE is preferred over end-to-end anastomosis. The SFPV has been used in the reconstruction of the innominate artery and common carotid artery.

The right and left subclavian arteries are exposed differently depending on the location of injury with respect to the vertebral artery. For right-sided injury distal to the vertebral, the preferred method is to start with a right supraclavicular incision. This incision starts at the sternoclavicular junction and extends over the length of the clavicle (Figure 3, A). Should additional exposure be needed, such as those with injury proximal to the vertebral, median sternotomy is performed (Figure 3, B).

The choice of surgical incision for left-sided injury is more difficult because of the orientation of the aorta and the very posterior origin of the left subclavian artery. There are three ways to expose the left subclavian artery—a supraclavicular incision with clavicle resection, a left anterolateral thoracotomy, and a sternoclavicular flap (trap door). The supraclavicular incision is made one fingerbreadth above and parallel to the clavicle, extending from the sternal notch to the lateral end of the clavicle (Figure 4). Once the clavicle has been cut and removed, the underlying scalene fat pad is removed and the phrenic nerve identified. This is a key anatomic landmark that must be preserved. The nerve courses lateral to medial along the anterior scalene muscle. The nerve can be isolated with a vessel loop and gently retracted out of the way. The anterior scalene muscle should be cut as low as possible, and the subclavian artery can be found behind it. A supraclavicular incision is adequate if the injury is proximal to the vertebral.

When a supraclavicular incision is inadequate, such as in those patients with injury of the left subclavian artery distal to the vertebral, an anterolateral thoracotomy is used. A high anterolateral thoracotomy through the third intercostal space will provide access to the origin of the subclavian (Figure 5). A posterolateral thoracotomy will give even better exposure to the distal subclavian artery, but the patient will need to be in right lateral decubitus position. The preferred sequence of steps to obtain control of the left subclavian artery in an injury that has not been identified preoperatively is to begin with a supraclavicular incision and quickly move to a thoracotomy if the necessary exposure is not obtained. If exposure is still inadequate, as a last resort, the supraclavicular and thoracotomy incisions can be connected with a median sternotomy, completing the trap

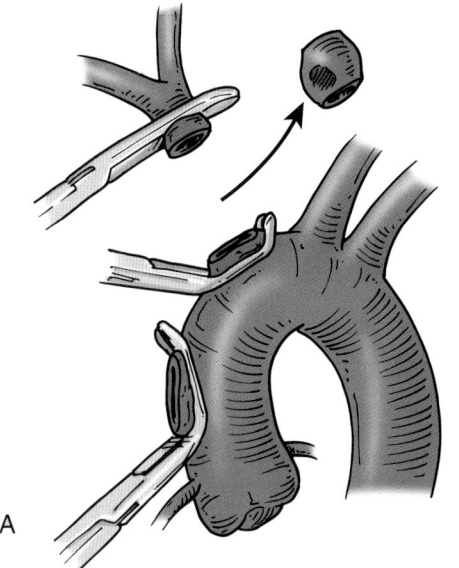 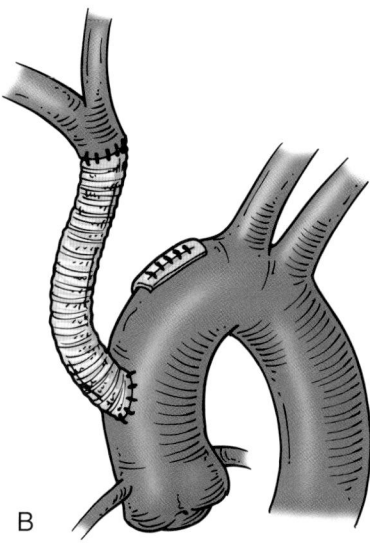

FIGURE 2 A, Injuries to the innominate artery require repair via the bypass exclusion technique. **B,** The stump is oversewn, and bypass grafting is from the ascending aorta to the distal innominate artery.

A   B

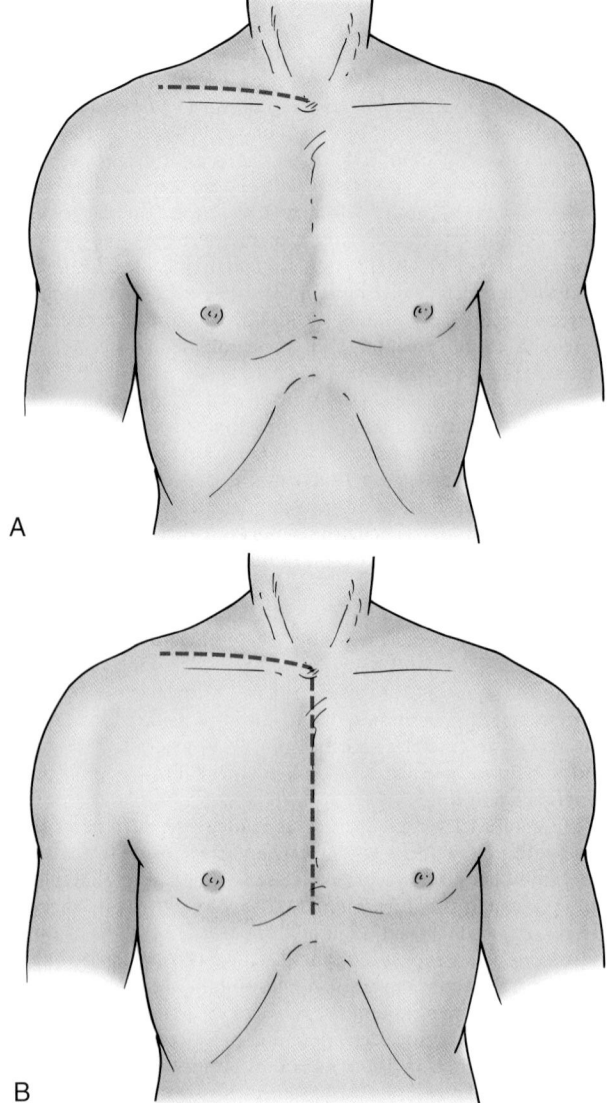

FIGURE 3   A, The right supraclavicular incision provides exposure to the right subclavian artery. **B,** In some instances, a median sternotomy is added to obtain more proximal control.

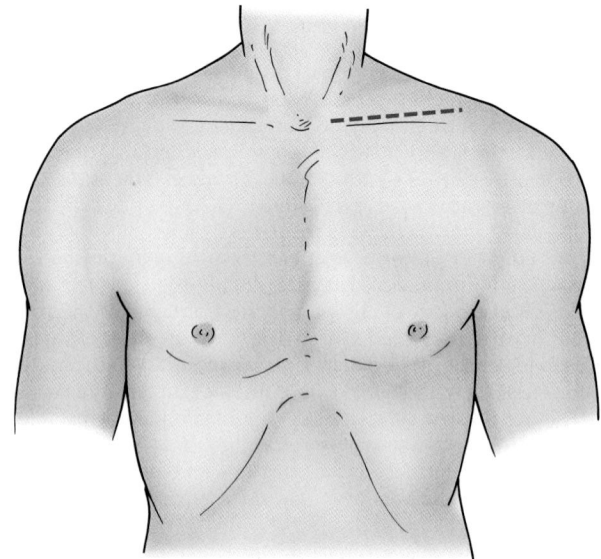

FIGURE 4   The left supraclavicular incision will provide exposure to a portion of the left subclavian artery. Resection of the medial clavicle will improve exposure.

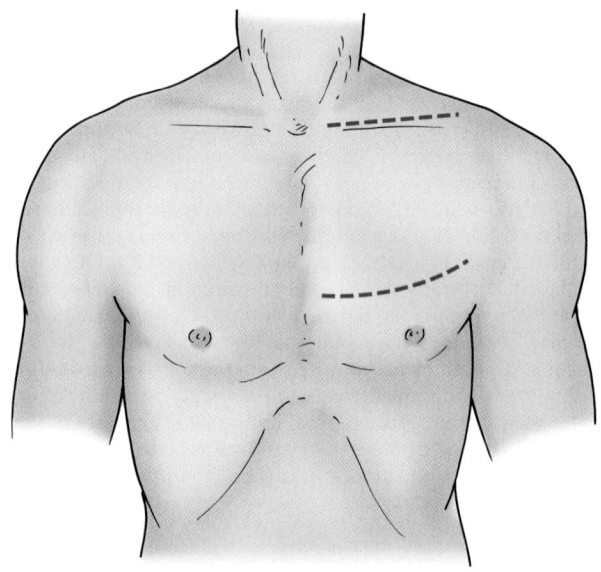

FIGURE 5   A high anterolateral thoracotomy through the third intercostal space will provide access to the proximal left subclavian artery.

door (Figure 6). This incision has a high rate of postoperative morbidity.

A small laceration in the subclavian artery may be repaired primarily, but usually the injury requires an interposition graft. For extensive injuries, an interposition graft should be performed using vein or PTFE. A proximal and distal Fogarty thrombectomy is performed, and the artery is repaired with saphenous vein from the leg. Vein is preferred, particularly in an infected field. If the patient is unstable and time does not permit vein harvest, then PTFE is acceptable. A completion angiogram should be performed. Attempting to mobilize the soft and friable subclavian artery to gain enough length for an end-to-end repair is rarely successful.

Although subclavian artery injuries should be repaired if possible, there are some patients who will need damage control. For the patient in extremis, the subclavian artery can be ligated. If possible, ligation of the subclavian artery proximal to the vertebral artery is preferred because this allows for retrograde flow to the extremity through the vertebral and collateral circulation of the shoulder. At the first suspicion of ischemia after subclavian artery ligation, the patient should

undergo heparinization followed by prompt arterial reconstruction, and if necessary, fasciotomy.

A few individuals with injuries to the chest will arrive at the hospital with no obvious clinical signs of vascular compromise. These patients are best served with a CTA of the chest. The patient with blunt injury to the descending thoracic aorta is typically hemodynamically stable and has a contained hematoma. Endovascular treatment offers an effective alternative to operative repair of these injuries. The long-term effects of having an endograft in the aorta for 50 or more years has yet to be determined. As a person ages, the shape of the aorta changes, which may result in future incidences of endoleaks. For subclavian artery injuries, endovascular options, including balloon tamponade and stent grafting, can be life and limb saving. Arterial access is commonly approached percutaneously through the femoral artery. The size of the stent graft to be implanted

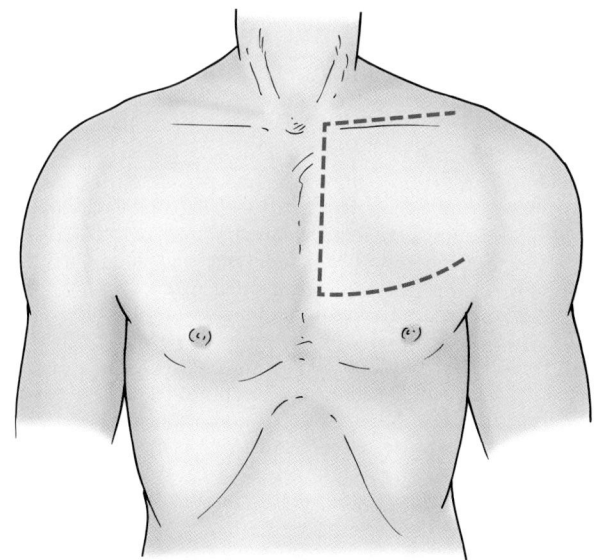

FIGURE 6 The trap door. Connecting the supraclavicular and anterolateral thoracotomy with a median sternotomy. This incision has a high postoperative morbidity rate and should be used as a last resort.

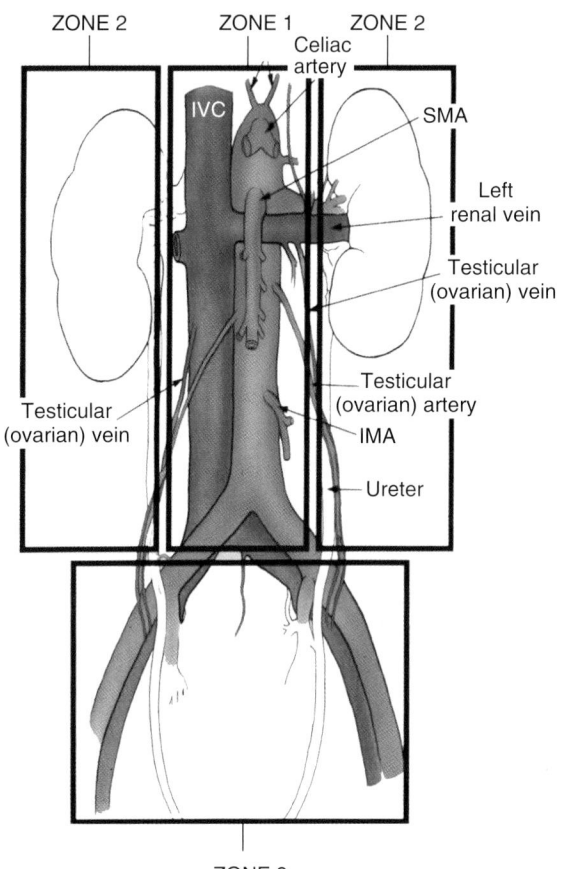

FIGURE 7 The retroperitoneal zones. Zone 1 is central. Zone 2 is lateral. Zone 3 is pelvic. *IMA,* Inferior mesenteric artery; *IVC,* inferior vena cava; *SMA,* superior mesenteric artery.

is determined with intravascular balloons of known length and diameter.

Abdomen

Major abdominal vascular injuries result more commonly from penetrating trauma rather than blunt trauma. Patients with penetrating abdominal wounds who do not respond adequately to initial resuscitation are considered to have a major vascular injury until proven otherwise. These injuries are very challenging for surgeons. Even for the experienced surgeon, it is sometimes difficult to determine which cavity to enter first. There may be bleeding from the chest and abdomen. If the patient arrives profoundly hypotensive or experiences cardiopulmonary arrest in the operating room, an immediate left anterolateral thoracotomy with aortic cross-clamping, pericardiotomy, and open cardiopulmonary resuscitation should be performed before proceeding with the laparotomy. A midline incision is made from the xiphoid to the pubic symphysis. With free intraperitoneal bleeding, the first maneuver is to pack all four quadrants. Solid organ injuries with active bleeding are best managed with packing until definitive control can be obtained. For patients who decompensate during laparotomy, the abdominal aorta can be controlled by cross-clamping at the aortic hiatus. Retroperitoneal hematomas are classified according to their location: zone 1 (central), zone 2 (lateral), and zone 3 (pelvic). This classification helps with surgical planning (Figure 7). All zone 1, some penetrating zone 2, and all penetrating zone 3 should be explored. Blunt zone 2 and blunt zone 3 hematomas should not be explored unless they are ruptured, pulsatile, or rapidly expanding.

If a hematoma or hemorrhage is above the transverse mesocolon, injury to the suprarenal aorta, celiac axis, superior mesenteric artery, or renal artery should be suspected. Injuries to the suprarenal aorta are difficult to access. To obtain proximal control of the aorta at the hiatus of the diaphragm, a left-sided medial visceral rotation is best. This is performed by taking down the left colon, kidney, spleen, tail of the pancreas, and fundus of the stomach to the midline (Figure 8). One alternative is to leave the left kidney in place while the rest of the viscera are mobilized. Either way, the end result will be exposure of the aorta from the diaphragm to the aortic bifurcation. In our experience, the injured aorta in the suprarenal position seems to have a higher survivability than those below the renal arteries. This may be due to the celiac and superior mesenteric ganglia that are very fibrous and tend to control the bleeding. The most devastating wounds are those caused by shotgun blasts, high-velocity missiles, and large-caliber missiles. Most survivable injuries are those that can be closed with sutures. Injuries to the infrarenal aorta can be approached from the left side of the abdomen as noted earlier, or a right-sided medial visceral rotation can be performed for injuries to the right renal artery or the right common iliac artery and vein (Figure 9).

Injury to the celiac axis is extraordinarily rare, and ligation is the treatment of choice. Very few successful complex repairs of the celiac axis have been reported. If the splenic artery is transected or has a partial tear, it is prudent to remove the spleen and possibly the tail of the pancreas in order to get rapid control. Splenic and left gastric artery injuries are best treated with ligation. Hepatic artery injuries can be ligated if they are proximal to the gastroduodenal branch, but repair should be performed if possible.

The superior mesenteric artery (SMA) is similar to the subclavian artery in that it has very little elastic tissue. Sharp partial transections of the SMA can be managed with lateral arteriorrhaphy using 6-0 polypropylene suture. Because mobilization of the SMA is restricted, it is rarely repaired by end-to-end anastomosis, particularly if it is under tension. It may be better to do an aorto-SMA bypass with saphenous vein graft or PTFE. Autogenous tissue is preferred if there is small bowel or fecal contamination. SMA ligation is associated with ischemia to the small bowel and right colon. In the hemodynamically unstable patient with hypothermia, acidosis, and coagulopathy, the

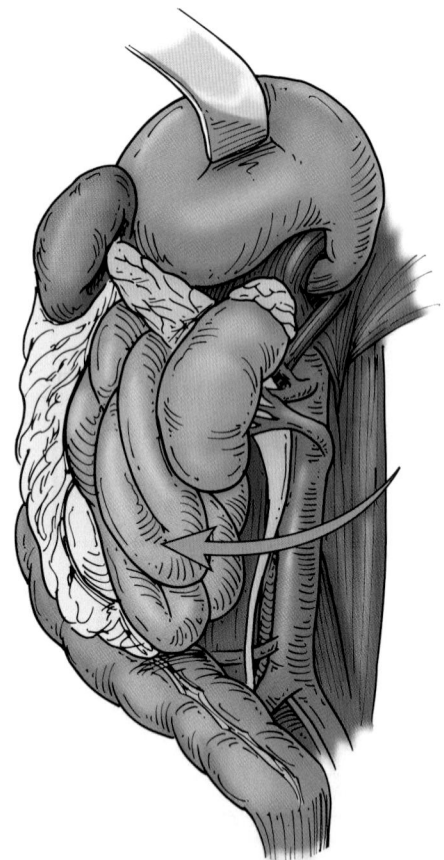

FIGURE 8   Medial rotation of left-sided viscera. This will expose the aorta from the diaphragm to the aortic bifurcation.

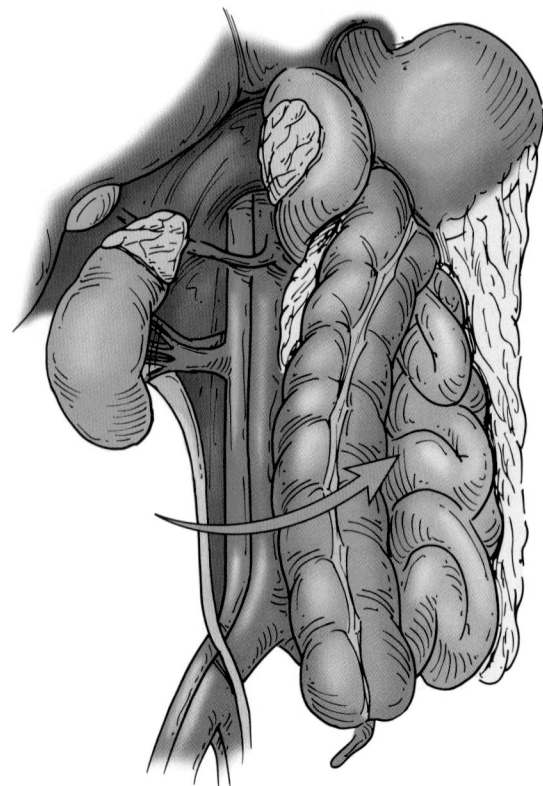

FIGURE 9   Medial rotation of right-sided viscera. This will expose the right renal artery, right common iliac artery and vein, and inferior vena cava.

insertion of a temporary intraluminal shunt into the débrided ends of the SME is appropriate.

The kidney does not tolerate prolonged ischemia. In some cases, small perforations of the artery can be repaired, but, in most cases, nephrectomy is a better choice. Arterial repairs of the renal artery have a high incidence of thrombosis. The surgeon should perform intraoperative palpation, an intravenous pyelogram, or both, to confirm a functioning contralateral kidney. Those patients with bilateral renal artery injury or solitary kidney should be considered for revascularization. When dealing with an ischemic kidney after blunt trauma in a stable patient, an endovascular repair is optimal treatment since it can be placed rapidly, minimizing the effect of ischemia on the kidney.

If the iliac artery requires only a simple lateral repair, then this can be done primarily. If definitive repair is not possible, iliac artery injuries can have a temporary shunt placed. Extensive injury to the common or external iliac artery in the presence of significant fecal contamination is a serious problem. End-to-end anastomosis or insertion of a synthetic conduit in a contaminated field often leads to postoperative pseudoaneurysm formation and potentially a blowout of the anastomosis. A safe treatment of these injuries is ligation of the common iliac artery, closure of the abdomen with appropriate washout and drainage, and an extraanatomic femorofemoral bypass graft. The external iliac artery also needs to be repaired when possible. If it cannot be repaired, a femorofemoral bypass graft using a synthetic conduit can be performed. The internal iliac artery can be ligated with impunity. Definitive repair is not necessary unless it is a small wound that can be repaired with simple sutures. Most arterial pelvic bleeding is best treated with embolization.

Pelvis

Pelvic fractures are quite common after blunt trauma. Pelvic vascular injury and hemorrhage are responsible for many deaths. The appropriate use of a pelvic binder, along with the recent evolution of earlier pelvic stabilization with external fixation, angiographic embolization, and preperitoneal pelvic packing, has decreased some of these deaths. Packing has been an important part of damage control in Europe for many years and was reintroduced in the United States recently. The procedure involves opening the anterior fascia beneath the umbilicus, retracting the rectus muscles laterally, and placing three laparotomy sponges on each side of the bladder deep in the pelvis without opening the peritoneum (Figure 10). This technique may be useful in a patient with pelvic bleeding who is too unstable to transport to the angiography suite or if an angiography suite is not present in your hospital. In a hypotensive patient with negative FAST results and pelvic fracture, embolization should be considered. A hemodynamically labile patient with a contrast blush is best served in the angiography suite. The superior gluteal artery is the most commonly injured artery after a pelvic fracture. There is an extensive network of veins in the pelvis that is often destroyed with a pelvic fracture, and bleeding from these veins is more frequent than arterial bleeding. Venous bleeding can be controlled by external fixation.

Extremity

Any hard sign of vascular injury, such as active or pulsatile hemorrhage, expanding hematoma, or absent pulse, warrants surgical exploration, ideally in a hybrid operating room so that an on-table arteriogram can be performed. Although an open operation is still the preferred treatment for many extremity vascular injuries, endovascular stenting of extremities is becoming more common. Injury to vessels in the upper extremity can result from shoulder dislocation, elbow fractures and dislocations, lacerations, and gunshot wounds. Reducing the fracture or dislocation should precede any repair to the vessel. The axillary artery is usually disrupted by blunt trauma when

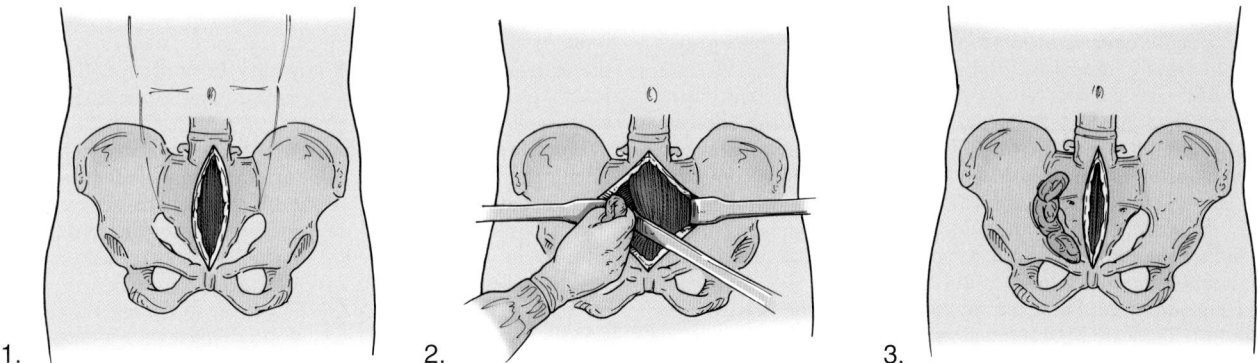

1.   2.   3.

FIGURE 10 Preperitoneal packing. This involves packing three lap sponges in the preperitoneal space on each side to contain pelvic bleeding. Useful in those patients who are too unstable to go to an angiography suite or if angiography is not available. *(From Cothren CC, Osborn PM, Moore EE, et al: Preperitoneal pelvic packing for hemodynamically unstable pelvic fractures: a paradigm shift,* J Trauma *62:834–839, 2007.)*

there is tearing of the shoulder girdle. The axillary artery can sometimes be repaired with a simple suture, but it may require a saphenous vein interposition graft. If there is damage to the brachial plexus, repair of the axillary artery may not be indicated, but this is difficult to assess in the acute setting. If the expertise to repair the vessel is not available, a damage control option is shunt insertion. Only in rare circumstances are ligation and fasciotomy needed. Although collateral circulation usually prevents critical ischemia in axillary artery injury, reconstruction is the preferred treatment. The brachial artery is frequently injured. It can be exposed with an incision in the groove between the biceps and triceps muscles. The median nerve should be identified and protected. Like the axillary artery, the brachial artery can be ligated in some settings, but the preferred treatment is simple suture, if possible, or a saphenous vein interposition graft. If injured separately, the radial artery and ulnar artery do not need to be repaired since there is excellent collateral circulation in the hand. If both are injured, at least one must be repaired.

The common femoral artery should be repaired if possible. Exposure is with a vertical incision over the inguinal ligament halfway between the anterior superior iliac spine and the pubic tubercle. Approximately one third of the incision should be above the groin crease. The use of a temporary arterial shunt is an acceptable option until the patient can get to a center that can provide definitive arterial reconstruction. If bypass is needed, saphenous vein or PTFE can be used. It is rarely necessary to do a repair of the profundus artery. Most of the time the profunda will do well with ligation since there is adequate collateral blood supply around the upper hip.

The superficial femoral artery should also be repaired. In contrast to arteriosclerosis of the femoral artery, the injured femoral artery has not had time to establish collaterals. The superficial femoral artery can be exposed by the slight flexion and external rotation of the leg. An incision over the anterior border of the sartorius muscle allows retraction of the muscle and identification of the fascia directly underneath. This is Hunter's canal. Opening of the canal reveals the superficial femoral artery. Although simple repair may be possible, most require an interposition graft. Reversed autologous saphenous vein from the uninjured leg should be used if possible. If the superficial femoral vein cannot be easily repaired, then ligation should occur. Fasciotomy of the lower leg after superficial femoral artery repair should be considered. Orthopedic surgeons often perform bone alignment before definitive repair of the vessel to avoid disruption of arterial reconstruction, although occasionally the arterial injury is completed first.

The popliteal artery is injured following posterior dislocation of the knee or penetrating injuries of the leg. The collateral flow around the knee is poor. Popliteal artery injury should be repaired in a timely manner or there will be a high incidence of amputation. Fasciotomy

is strongly encouraged after popliteal repair. A posterior knee dislocation merits a CTA of the leg, even if distal pulses are present. The popliteal artery can be exposed from either the medial or posterior approach. The medial approach occurs by making an incision along the medial leg between the vastus medialis and sartorius muscles. The popliteal artery will be adjacent to the posterior aspect of the femur. The popliteal artery is repaired by harvesting a piece of reversed saphenous vein from the other thigh and inserting it as an interposition graft between the proximal and distal popliteal artery, excluding the injured segment. PTFE has been used when autologous conduit is not available, but it has a high late failure rate. Endovascular repair of popliteal aneurysms has been used successfully, particularly in patients with no available conduit. To avoid an open operation in a high-risk patient, a popliteal artery injury could be treated with an endovascular approach.

Injury to one infrapopliteal artery rarely results in limb ischemia. The foot remains viable as long as there is adequate flow through the remaining vessels. When in doubt, an intraoperative arteriogram should be obtained. The anterior tibial and posterior tibial arteries may be repaired in stable patients without other significant injuries. The best reconstructive option is a size-matched reversed saphenous vein. Severely injured patients are best treated with ligation of single vessel injuries distal to the popliteal artery. The peroneal artery rarely requires repair, except in the elderly or diabetic with poor collateral circulation. Patients who undergo repair to their extremities should have a completion angiogram, be maintained on aspirin, and be followed long-term for postoperative surveillance.

Veins

Venous injuries are a common cause of bleeding from penetrating neck wounds. Small veins and the external jugular vein are best treated with ligation. Simple lacerations of the internal jugular vein may be repaired, but, if extensive, they can be ligated without consequences. The facial vein can be ligated if injured and should be ligated when an attempt is made to expose the carotid bifurcation beneath it.

The innominate and azygous vein may be ligated without consequence. For subclavian vein injuries, thrombosis often results from the low-pressure venous system. These injuries are repaired only if the patient remains stable and repair can be done without producing stenosis and without the need for an interposition graft. If this is not possible, ligation of the subclavian vein should be performed. Besides transient edema, no significant long-term complications result from its ligation.

In many ways, IVC injuries are potentially more lethal than abdominal aortic injuries. In theory, one can ligate any injury below the renal veins; however, there is an approximately 30% morbidity rate from venous hypertension in the lower extremities. The infrarenal IVC has several lumbar veins that are posterior on the IVC, and rotation of the IVC during repair can be problematic. Initial control is another issue and can be achieved with a side-biting Satinsky clamp; however, this must be carefully handled to avoid torsion and iatrogenic tear of the thin and friable IVC. Our personal recommendation is to use sponge sticks initially to control the bleeding. Alternatively, the surgeon's index and middle finger can be placed on the hole, and a running stitch of 3-0 polypropylene can be started with gentle traction to avoid stenosis of the vessel.

The portion of the IVC from the renal veins to the heart can be treacherous. There are 12 to 15 small veins that enter the cava directly from segment 1 of the liver. In some instances of deceleration injury, all of these veins are avulsed from the superior surface of the cava, giving the appearance of a laceration. This can be a real challenge to control. Proximal control of the IVC should be attempted where it pierces the diaphragm. In some instances, it can be done superior to the liver as the IVC goes through the diaphragm. This has to be done carefully since both the right and left hepatic veins join the anterior portion of the cava at this juncture. Alternatively, the IVC can also be identified in the right chest, and supradiaphragmatic control can be achieved with a Rummel tourniquet. The final alternative is a sternotomy in which the pericardium is opened longitudinally and the IVC can be dissected inside the pericardium as it joins the right atrial portion of the heart. Again, a Rummel tourniquet can be placed around this portion of the vessel.

Branches of the superior mesenteric vein can usually be ligated if they are injured since there are adequate collaterals within the mesentery. A portion of the superior mesenteric vein as it exits through the mesentery joins with the splenic vein to form the portal vein. Ligation of the superior mesenteric vein may lead to postoperative edema of the mesentery and small bowel. This edema resolves with time, and there are usually no sequelae. A few days of vigorous postoperative fluid resuscitation in these patients helps with the transient peripheral hypovolemia that occurs.

Avulsion of the renal vein can occur following deceleration injury. Gunshot and stab wounds can cause penetrating injury to

the renal vein. Both can lead to exsanguination. Venorrhaphy remains the preferred technique. If extensive damage to the hilum of the kidney occurs, nephrectomy may be indicated. The surgeon must verify that the kidney on the other side is present and functional.

Portal vein injuries can be very difficult to manage since there are often other associated arterial injuries. These include injuries to the SMA, splenic artery, or the right and left hepatic arteries. Surgical transection of the neck of the pancreas exposes the retropancreatic portal vein. Injury to the portal vein should be primarily repaired whenever possible. If portions of the vein are under tension or are retracted or severely injured, it is possible to harvest the saphenous vein and do an end-to-end repair. Alternatively, the jugular vein can also be used as a conduit for repair. If the patient is acidotic, hypothermic, and coagulopathic, the portal vein can be ligated. One of the authors has experience with portal vein injuries in San Francisco, and the postoperative mortality rate was approximately 25%. Two patients had their portal vein injuries ligated and, although both survived, the patients experience splanchnic hypervolemia and systemic hypovolemia.

Trauma to the confluence of the common iliac veins is particularly difficult to control because of its location. This confluence of iliac veins lies just behind the right common iliac artery. The right common iliac artery can be divided between clamps in order to give access to the confluence of veins (Figure 11). The divided right common iliac artery should be repaired when the venous repair is complete. Injuries to the iliac veins, in most instances, can be achieved with simple sutures. If this is not possible because of loss of tissue, ligation is an option, as it has been well tolerated. There may be postoperative swelling of the leg.

Almost all extremity veins can be ligated if necessary. Ligation of the superficial femoral and popliteal veins has some disadvantages. In the absence of near exsanguination and sequelae of shock, these two vessels ideally should be repaired. With venous congestion, there is a risk of affecting arterial inflow. The patient may also develop chronic edema of the leg. If there are extensive injuries to these veins, however, ligating them is an option, as it has been well tolerated in young trauma patients.

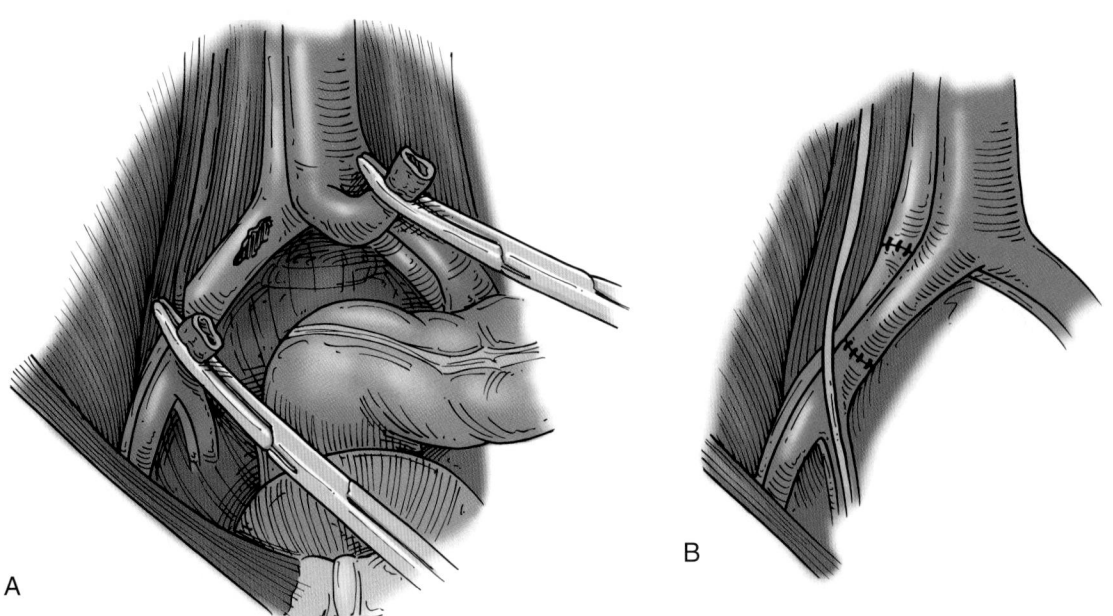

A

B

FIGURE 11 **A,** Deliberate division of the right common iliac artery to repair an injury to the right common iliac vein. **B,** Once the vein has been repaired, the artery can be reanastamosed. *(From Salam AA, Stewart MT: New approach to wounds of the aortic bifurcation and inferior vena cava, Surgery 98:105–108, 1985.)*

SUMMARY

Vascular injuries are associated with high morbidity and mortality rates depending on the vessels injured. Although the unstable patient with a vascular injury still needs an open operation, many stable patients are being evaluated with CTA to assess the injury and are being revascularized with an endovascular approach. All stable patients with penetrating and blunt neck injuries should get a CTA. There are some injuries to the neck that are difficult to expose and may be better served with an endovascular approach. Injuries to the great vessels are usually fatal. For most individuals who suffer an aortic injury, the result is death. Those who survive are assessed for all other potential life-threatening injuries before they undergo endograft repair of their aorta. There are a few patients who present in extremis and undergo a thoracotomy with open repair, but these are extremely rare cases. Open repair of descending aortic injuries in stable patients is now occurring largely when endovascular repair is not technically feasible. The right and left subclavian arteries are exposed differently depending on the location of injury. The left subclavian artery is usually more difficult to expose, and the choice of incision is more controversial. Many subclavian artery injuries are treated with endovascular stents. Deciding if hemorrhage is coming from the chest or abdomen is sometimes difficult, and occasionally it is coming from both. To access either the suprarenal aorta or the infrarenal aorta, alternate techniques of mobilization are used. Extensive iliac injury with fecal contamination is best treated with extraanatomic bypass. Bleeding in the pelvis is common after pelvic fracture. Most of this bleeding is venous and will stop with external fixation. Arterial bleeding in the pelvis is best treated with embolization. Definitive open repair of extremity artery injuries is more common, but endovascular treatment is increasing. If definitive repair is not possible, a temporary shunt can be placed. Most veins can be ligated without long-term sequelae. Superior mesenteric vein ligation is an option, but hypovolemia is a common occurrence. Portal vein and IVC injuries should be repaired. The retrohepatic IVC is particularly difficult to access and is often a lethal injury. To repair the confluence of the iliac veins, the right iliac artery must be divided and repaired after the vein has been repaired.

SUGGESTED READINGS

Cothren CC, Osborn PM, Moore EE, et al: Preperitoneal pelvic packing for hemodynamically unstable pelvic fractures: a paradigm shift, *J Trauma* 62:834–839, 2007.
DuBose JJ, Rajani R, Gilani R, et al: Endovascular management of axillo-subclavian arterial injury: a review of published experience, *Injury* 43(11):1785–1792, 2012.
Hagino RT, Bengtson TD, Fosdick DA, et al: Venous reconstructions using the superficial femoral-popliteal vein, *J Vasc Surg* 26(5):829–837, 1997.
Hoyt DB, Coimbra R, Potenza BM, et al: Anatomic exposures for vascular injuries, *Surg Clin North Am* 81(6):1299–1330, 2001.
Lee WA, Matsumura JS, Mitchell RS, et al: Endovascular repair of traumatic thoracic aortic injury: clinical practice guidelines of the Society of Vascular Surgery, *J Vasc Surg* 53(1):187–192, 2011.
Sinha S, Patterson BO, Ma J, et al: Systematic review and meta-analysis of open surgical and endovascular management of thoracic outlet vascular injuries, *J Vasc Surg* 57(2):547–567, 2013.
Starnes BW, Lundgren RS, Gunn M, et al: A new classification scheme for treating blunt aortic injury, *J Vasc Surg* 55(1):47–54, 2012.
Stone PA, Jagannath P, Thompson SN, et al: Evolving treatment of popliteal artery aneurysms, *J Vasc Surg* 57(5):13-16-1310, 2013.
Vaughan GD, Mattox KL, Feliciano DV, et al: Surgical experience with expanded polytetrafluoroethylene (PTFE) as a replacement graft for traumatized vessels, *J Trauma* 19(6):403–408, 1979.
Von Oppell UO, Dunne TT, et al: Traumatic aortic rupture: twenty-year metaanalysis of mortality and risk of paraplegia, *Ann Thorac Surg* 58(2):585–593, 1994.

ENDOVASCULAR MANAGEMENT OF ARTERIAL INJURY

Nyali Taylor, MD, and Joseph V. Lombardi, MD, FACS

Endovascular interventions have been described in the vascular surgical literature since the 1980s and debuts in the trauma literature for vascular repair in the early 1990s. Since that time, with the improvement and implementation of newer endovascular technology, the application of endovascular therapies to iatrogenic and traumatic vascular injuries has expanded significantly. Operators can have a diagnostic or therapeutic modality to intervene on lesions from the extracranial cerebrovascular arteries to the extremities. Adjunctive endovascular measures have been utilized in open procedures as well, which have aided in delineating injuries and controlling hemorrhage. These "hybrid" approaches have now become very commonplace in the management of patients with multiple injuries among high-volume centers. This chapter discusses some of the endovascular techniques employed to repair arterial injuries in the cerebrovascular, upper extremity, aortic, pelvic, and lower extremity vascular trees.

There are several generic points to be aware of when planning an endovascular therapeutic intervention: patient preparation, operating room (or interventional suite) equipment, staffing, endovascular instrumentation, and available medications. Once it has been determined that the surgeon is going to perform an endovascular intervention or adjunct, the correct operating room or interventional suite should be booked. It needs to contain a fluoroscopy-compatible bed. The side rails need to be removed for compatible armboards to be inserted if the upper extremity or cerebrovascular region is the area of interest. As part of planning, knowing the necessary access sites and having the patient adequately exposed is the key because your first choice of access is not always going to work. Depending on the institution, you may need to have fluoroscopy technologists called in to assist if the case is done in the operating room. Make sure the available staff has a working knowledge of the sheaths, catheters, wires, and medications that will be requested.

Once prepped and draped for the planned procedure, you will need to gain either percutaneous access via a 21-gauge micropuncture needle and 0.018-inch Mandril wire or cutdown for open exposure and employ an appropriate-gauge needle (19-gauge introducer for femoral or common carotid, 21-gauge for upper extremity or infrageniculate vessels). We would suggest utilizing ultrasound guidance for percutaneous access because it reduces the number of attempts and likelihood of complications. Utilize a basic braided 0.035-inch wire to maintain access, and exchange for the smallest-circumference introducer sheath that is appropriate for the chosen access site. Prior to insertion of large-circumference, near-occlusive sheaths, or any intervention (other than embolization), approximately 5000 units (or 80 units/kg) of heparin should be given, unless contraindicated. In the event that a contraindication exists, the surgeon can decide if she or he is comfortable with heparinized saline flushes of the access vessel for local anticoagulation. If there will be any carotid sinus manipulation, consider the use of prophylactic atropine. Atropine (0.5-1.0 mg) is given prophylactically at our institution. It may be prudent to have several medications on hand: vasodilator of the operator's choice, tissue plasminogen activator, and protamine. Completion imaging should be obtained for documentation of the adequacy of the intervention. In the following sections, we discuss the major anatomic regions' indications for repair, the basic techniques, and outcomes.

EXTRACRANIAL CEREBROVASCULAR INJURY

No system is infallible, and even in the era of ultrasound-guided access, there is a less than 1% incidence of iatrogenic trauma to the carotid or subclavian arteries during percutaneous central venous catheter insertion, and specifically arterial dilation with catheters 7 Fr circumference and larger. These patients may endure significant sequelae of this injury—hematomas, pseudoaneurysms (PSA), or stroke—so rapid identification and intervention are important. If immediate repair is not possible, anticoagulation must be initiated to prevent thrombus formation and potential embolus. The literature does not support the pull and compression method if a large-bore needle or dilator was inserted because the morbidity appears to be significantly greater than repair. Guilbert and colleagues (2008) have suggested a treatment algorithm that recommends percutaneous intervention in poorly accessible areas. Employing the use of covered or overlapping bare metal stents in the carotid arteries has been described. It is important to image patients who had a pull and hold technique to assess for PSAs or arteriovenous fistulae (AVF) as late as 2 weeks post event.

Technique

Before the endovascular repair of a carotid lesion is undertaken, either computed tomography angiography (CTA) or magnetic resonance angiography with three-dimensional reconstruction should be obtained to assess the arch anatomy: type, variants, tortuosity of great vessels, and preexisting disease. To begin with a percutaneous approach, the patient is placed in the supine position with both arms tucked at the sides for femoral access or with the left arm extended for brachial access. For open access, a standard longitudinal incision anterior to the sternocleidomastoid muscle will provide exposure to the carotid sheath. Expose and control each of the vessels, taking care to preserve the vagus nerve.

Once access is obtained, advance an appropriate length 0.035-inch wire into the aorta. If the approach was retrograde from the femoral artery, allow the wire to retroflex off of the aortic valve. Advance a 6Fr guide catheter proximal to the innominate artery. Using an angiographic flush catheter, a digital subtraction arteriogram (DSA) of the arch should be taken in 30 to 45 degrees anterior oblique (AO) orientation. Use the guide catheter to engage the common CA (CCA). The guide catheter will be advanced over a stiff angled guidewire into the mid-CCA if the lesion is in the internal or external carotid. For lesions in the CCA, the sheath should be placed proximal to the lesion. At this point, a 0.014-inch wire can be exchanged for the guidewire and advanced past the lesion into the petrous portion of the internal CA or into the external CA. Once the wire is in place, advancement of an embolic protection device (EPD) is dependent on the type of injury and concomitant disease. Select an appropriately oversized (10% to 15%) covered stent based on the normal artery, and deploy this across the lesion. Postdilate the stent with a nominal-diameter balloon. Retrieve the EPD, and remove all sheaths and wires. One should document anterior cerebral circulation *both* preintervention and postintervention. Note that this technique can help balloon occlude a hostile injury to assist open repair or be an option for repair alone (Figures 1 and 2).

UPPER EXTREMITY INJURY

As with the iatrogenic carotid arterial injury, subclavian arterial (SCA) injuries can occur via traumatic or iatrogenic mechanisms as well. The algorithm for repair would be the same as for carotid arterial injuries, discussed previously. The SCA is a prime vessel for endovascular repair due to its difficult exposure behind the clavicle and very straightforward endovascular access via the brachial artery.

Trauma to the subclavian and axillary arteries occurs in 5% to 10% of arterial trauma, most often by a penetrating mechanism and

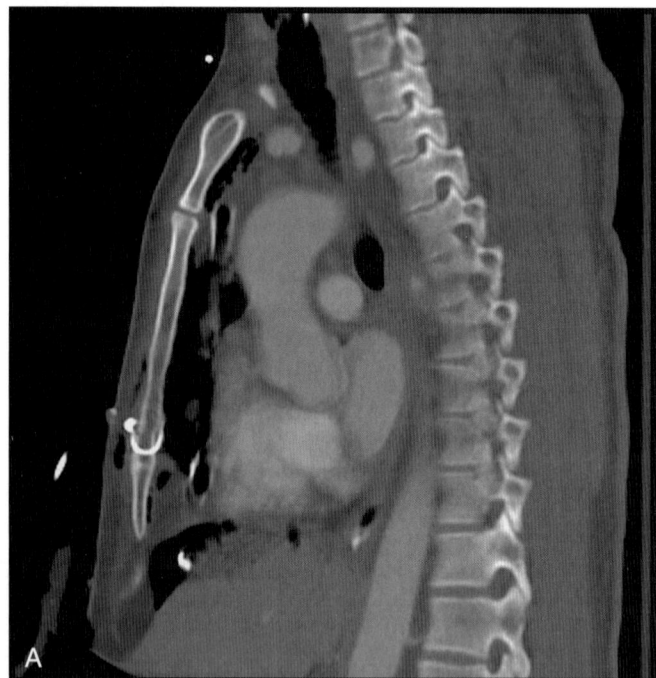

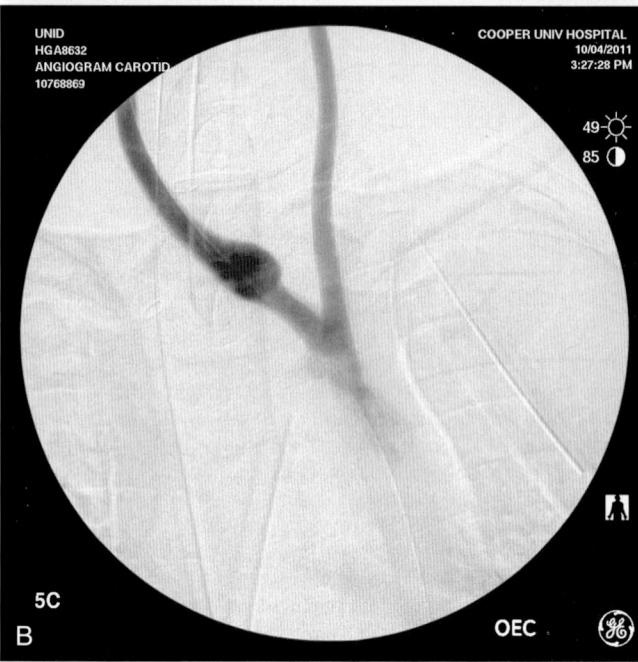

FIGURE 1 **A,** A sagittal reconstruction of the CT arteriogram image demonstrates a right common carotid pseudoaneurysm after a gunshot to the chest. **B,** The follow up digital subtracted arteriogram in AP orientation confirming the right common carotid pseudoaneurysm prior to endovascular repair.

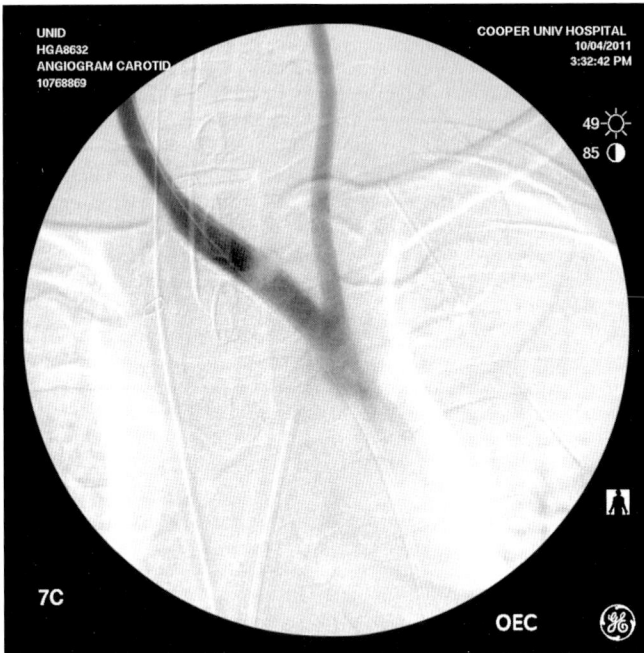

FIGURE 2 Repair of right common carotid pseudoaneurysm with a covered stent from a retrograde open carotid approach.

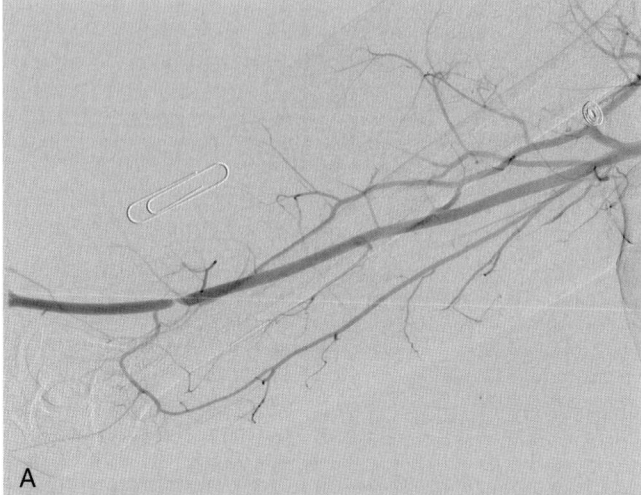

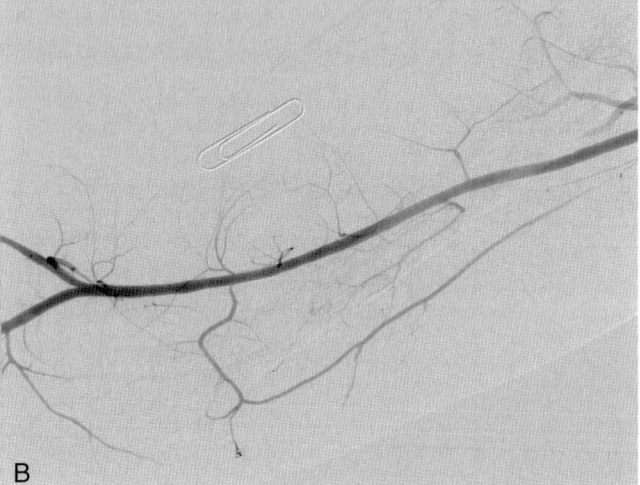

FIGURE 3 **A,** A focal intimal flap in the distal right brachial artery after gunshot to the right arm. **B,** An arteriogram after angioplasty of the lesion shows no evidence of residual defect and contrast in the radial and ulnar vessels.

frequently forming PSAs and AVFs. These patients may have multiple associated injuries, and the associated mortality is 5% to 39%. There are several considerations when selecting the appropriate candidates: lesion length, ability to cross the lesion, brachial plexus injury, and other concomitant injuries. The appropriate types of lesions for treatment are PSAs, focal lacerations, AVFs, avulsions, or dissections. The lesion should be focal, and a guidewire must be able to cross it or an intervention cannot be performed. At the very least, if a lesion cannot be traversed, insufflate a balloon catheter to control hemorrhage when arriving from the inflow vessel. The location of the injury is also important. For instance, one must consider the possibility of compressing a rigid stent as it passes through the thoracic outlet. Also, one must preserve the vertebral and internal mammary arteries when there is a proximal injury. Overtly avulsed first- or second-order branches can be controlled via balloon occlusion and/or embolization.

One feasibility study found that nearly 50% of these injuries should be amenable to endovascular repair. In an underpowered study, short-term results from retrospective reviews show patency at 1 year. Du Toit reports long-term results that noted that 5% of patients had early (<30 days) endograft occlusion, whereas 12% and 20% developed late occlusions and significant stenoses, respectively. There were no amputations in the cohort followed over 4 years. Although further investigation needs to be done with this subgroup, the data suggest that endovascular intervention is safe with reasonable long-term patency.

Technique

The patient is placed in the supine position with the ipsilateral arm abducted. Percutaneous common femoral arterial access and the DSA imaging of the aortic arch and branch selection should be obtained utilizing a similar wire and catheter combination as described in the prior section. After characterization of the lesion, decide what type of intervention is indicated: stent, embolization, or balloon tamponade. If the injury is in the distal SCA or axillary arteries, advance the catheter into the mid-SCA and obtain another image in an anteroposterior (AP) orientation. Size the vessel and choose the

correct type and size of balloon, stent, or coil for the given intervention. If embolizing branch vessels, consider the use of a microcatheter system.

Retrograde brachial arterial access is useful in the setting of an SCA occlusion. We would suggest the use of ultrasound guidance. Access the brachial artery no more than 1 to 2 cm proximal to the antecubital fossa with a 21-gauge micropuncture needle. Obtain access with a sheath that is not greater than 6 Fr in circumference. Vessel selection and intervention will be accomplished in the same manner as previously described (Figures 3 and 4).

AORTOILIAC INJURY

Descending Thoracic Aorta

Traumatic injury of the thoracic aorta has been a growing area of interest since Parodi reported endovascular repair in 1991. Open repair was the standard at that time, and it continues to have significant associated morbidity and mortality. Thoracic endovascular aortic repair (TEVAR) in the current literature has been shown to have a mortality rate from 5% to 20% in some series. The reported

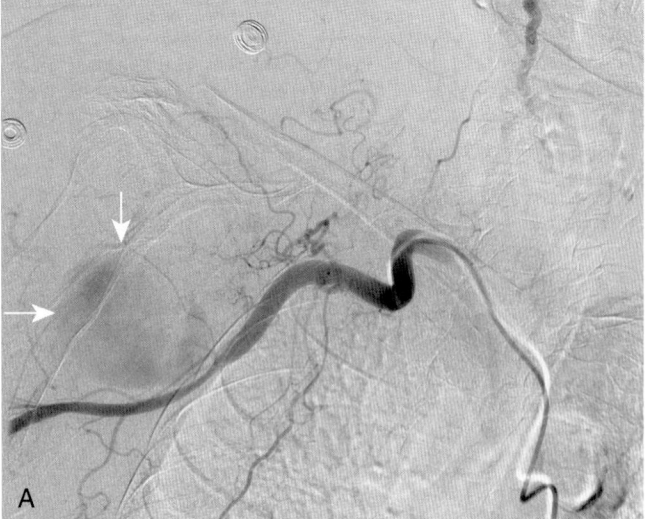

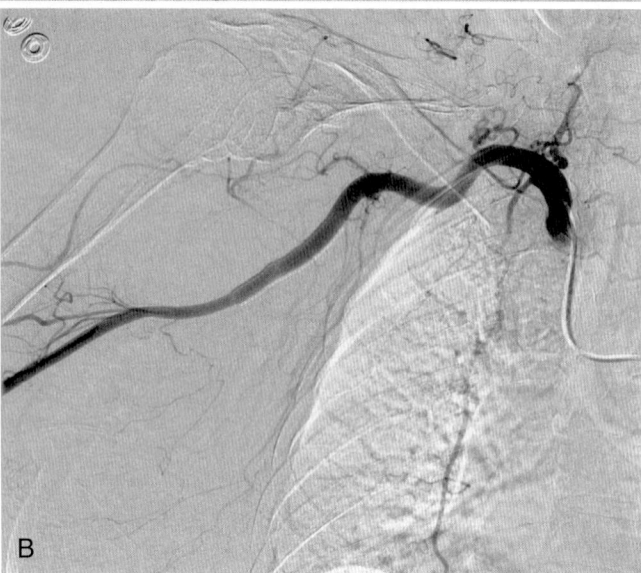

FIGURE 4 **A,** A selective arteriogram of the right axillary artery after a gunshot injury. The arrows highlight extravasation from the artery. **B,** A selective arteriogram of the right axillary artery after treatment with a covered stent. There is good opacification of the distal vessel without extravasation of contrast.

morbidity is also significantly less when compared to open repair. Interestingly, many series report no paraplegia and low rates of endoleak. The Society for Vascular Surgery (SVS) clinical practice guidelines support the urgent repair of traumatic aortic injury after stabilization of other injuries without routine use of spinal drainage. Commonly seen injuries are PSAs, dissection, and transaction occurring at the ligamentum arteriosum. Penetrating injuries with a contained process also provide an opportunity for these techniques. Coverage of the left SCA is acceptable with selective revascularization based on clinical symptoms, except in the cases of left internal mammary artery (IMA) bypass, stenotic or occluded right vertebral artery, left vertebral arising from the arch, or left vertebral terminating in the posterior inferior cerebellar artery. Important caveats to understand are related to the arch anatomy and variants as mentioned above; appropriate device selection for a small-diameter aorta to prevent stent collapse (oversize no more than 10%); and utilizing retroperitoneal exposure of the common iliac artery (CIA) for difficult access or for a short device.

Technique

The patient is placed in the supine position with arms abducted over the patient's head in an AP orientation or tucked at the patient's sides. General anesthesia is preferred in order to control respirations for clear imaging. The access vessel (femoral or iliac) is exposed surgically, and a 19-gauge introducer needle is utilized to puncture the vessel under direct visualization. Exchange the access wire for a stiff wire, advancing it until it retroflexes off the aortic valve. Percutaneous access will be obtained on the contralateral side as previously described. A marker flush catheter can be advanced through the contralateral side, and a DSA of the arch employing 30 to 60 degrees of left anterior oblique (LAO) can be obtained proximal to the innominate artery. Imaging of the vertebral anatomy must be documented (either by CTA or on-table DSA). Once the anatomy has been adequately delineated and decisions made regarding coverage of the left SCA, then the device can be deployed per the specific instructions for use. Molding balloons in this setting are optional. A completion arteriogram must be obtained to evaluate for patency of the great vessels and endoleak. Repair the access vessels with 5.0 Prolene suture in a standard fashion (Figure 5).

ABDOMINAL AORTA AND ILIAC VASCULATURE

Penetrating injuries of the abdominal aorta or the visceral vessels are unlikely to be repaired in an endovascular fashion because the patients undergo laparotomy for exploration in the current practice algorithm. There are sparse case reports that discuss the use of endovascular management in this setting. Where the endovascular interventions may become important are for missed injuries in a stable patient identified at a point remote from the time of injury. For the purposes of this chapter, we focus here on blunt injuries for which there is a small body of evidence.

Although blunt abdominal aortic injury (BAAI) is a rare entity, endovascular intervention lends itself to the types of injuries sustained (PSA, AVF, acute occlusion, intimal flap +/− dissection). These injuries occur most often as a result of motor vehicle collisions. A review of the National Trauma Data Bank found that 10% of those with BAAI underwent surgical repair, and 69% of that subgroup were treated endoluminally. Recently, Shalhub characterized BAAI in a retrospective review, describing the most common site of injury as Zone III (infrarenal aorta to the aortic bifurcation), with the morphology of injury ranging from intimal tears (21%) to free rupture (29%.) Twenty-one percent of the patients were repaired via endovascular methods, with mortality approaching 32% overall. Small intimal tears appear to remain stable or resolve with medical management. Data across multiple sources demonstrate that the patients with free rupture have 100% mortality. Therefore, the lesions to consider for repair in the hemodynamically stable patient are a PSA or large intimal tear, symptomatic dissection, or extension of dissection.

Technique

The technique will be altered depending on whether the surgeon is using an aortic cuff or bifurcated stent graft. In both cases, the patient is placed in the supine position with arms tucked at the sides. General anesthesia is preferred but not required. For a bifurcated stent graft, bilateral (or ipsilateral external iliac artery with a conduit) femoral arteries are exposed surgically. The access wires are exchanged for stiff wires. Advance a marker flush catheter on the contralateral side to obtain a DSA of the abdominal aorta in an AP orientation. Once the anatomy has been adequately delineated and the injury distinguished, the device can be deployed. Deploy the stent graft in a stepwise fashion, ensuring its position below the level

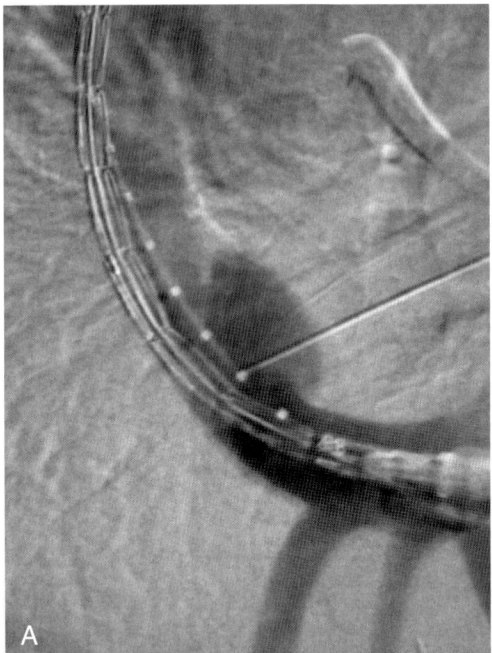

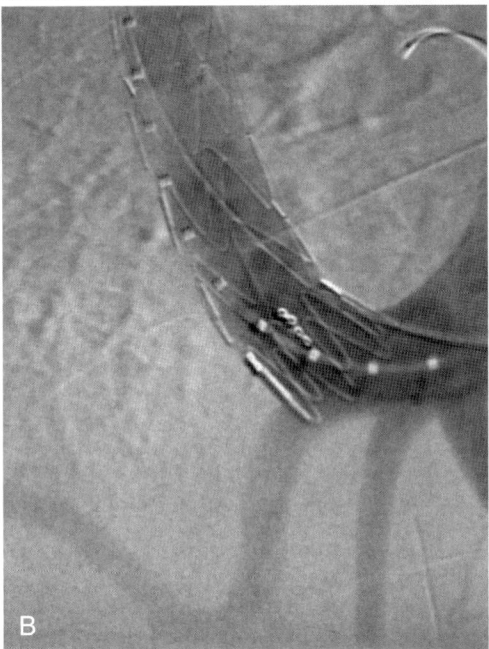

FIGURE 5   A, An arteriogram of the thoracic aorta in a patient with blunt thoracic aortic injury (BTAI) caused by a motor vehicle collision. There is a large pseudoaneurysm distal to the left subclavian artery. **B,** An arteriogram of the aorta after deployment of an aortic stent graft across the injury, successfully excluded the pseudoaneurysm. The left subclavian artery is preserved.

of the renal arteries. For an aortic cuff, the ipsilateral vessel is exposed surgically. Percutaneous access will be obtained on the contralateral side as previously described in other sections. A third option may be to employ an aorto-uni iliac device with contralateral iliac occlusion in conjunction with a femoral-to-femoral bypass. In a stable patient this is rarely preferred. After successful device deployment, repair the access vessels with 5.0 Prolene suture in a standard fashion. If images of the abdominal visceral vessels are needed, advance the flush catheter to T12-L1 to opacify them. Due to the more anterior takeoff of the celiac and superior mesenteric

artery (SMA) axis, it will be useful to place the image intensifier in a lateral orientation (Figure 6).

ILIAC ARTERIES

In an era in which endovascular intervention is employed for a broad scope of medical comorbidities, the iliac vessels will inevitably sustain iatrogenic injuries. These lesions can range from dissections to perforation. Fernandez defines the incidence of iliac arterial rupture during endovascular aortic repair (EVAR) as 4% overall. When the group is subdivided into EVAR and TEVAR interventions, the rupture rates are 3% and 9%, respectively. The injury was typically sustained distal to the origin of the hypogastric artery and identified from extravasation during the arteriogram. Most injuries were successfully repaired with stent grafts in 94% of patients with primary and primary-assisted patency of 88% and 94%, respectively, after a median follow-up of 40 months.

There are other mechanisms that include the misplacement of femoral intravascular catheters and orthopedic and spine procedures. Based on the National Surgical Quality Improvement Program (NSQIP) database, the incidence of injury associated with orthopedic procedures is less than 1%. In a small series of patients who had undergone lumbar spine surgery, the lesions were characterized as lacerations, AVFs, and PSA, which were successfully treated. The patients had no morbidity or mortality and 100% patency at a median follow-up time of 9 years.

In terms of traumatic injuries, iliac arterial injuries are uncommon. During laparotomy for penetrating mechanisms 2% to 10% of patients will have an iliac arterial injury. A retrospective review of the National Trauma Database (NTDB) demonstrated that of the injuries repaired, 45% were penetrating and 55% were blunt. Injury associated with blunt trauma is rare and usually affects branches of the hypogastric artery. Limb-threatening ischemia is an unusual presentation, so the repair can often be managed in a more elective fashion. The outcome data are limited in this subgroup.

Technique

Percutaneous, open, antegrade, or retrograde access can be obtained as previously described. The iliac arteries and pelvic collateral vasculature can be visualized by bringing a flush catheter down to L4-L5 and obtaining a DSA in an AP orientation.

Advance a guidewire across the injured segment into healthy artery. Choose a stent, stent graft, or coils, depending on the goals of the therapy. Balloon-expandable stents are appropriate for the proximal common iliac artery where precision placement is required. Self-expanding stents will be better able to accommodate tortuosity. If there is a flush occlusion of the iliac, an endovascular approach may not be possible (Figures 7 and 8).

LOWER EXTREMITY INJURY

Iatrogenic injuries of femoropopliteal arteries are not uncommon. With the vast number of percutaneous procedures undertaken, complications are encountered in as many as 5% of all patients. Arteriovenous fistulae, PSAs, dissections, and intimal flaps are all injuries that are incurred. Danetz and collegues (2005) note the incidence of AVF and PSA to be 0.1% and 0.5%, respectively. These injuries are typically managed at the time of injury with balloon angioplasty or stenting, depending on the complication.

In the trauma literature, the NTDB was queried and found to have a penetrating mechanism in 66% and blunt mechanism in 33% of lower extremity injuries. Lesions were characterized as occlusions, transection, laceration, or dissection/intimal injury. The popliteal artery and superficial femora artery (SFA) were the most frequently

FIGURE 6   A, An intra-operative arteriogram demonstrates a contained AAA rupture. The arrow highlights the region of rupture along the lateral wall. The left renal artery is patent. **B,** An arteriogram showing the deployed stent graft excluding the aneurysm sac. There is no active extravasation of contrast or evidence of endoleak. The left renal artery is preserved.

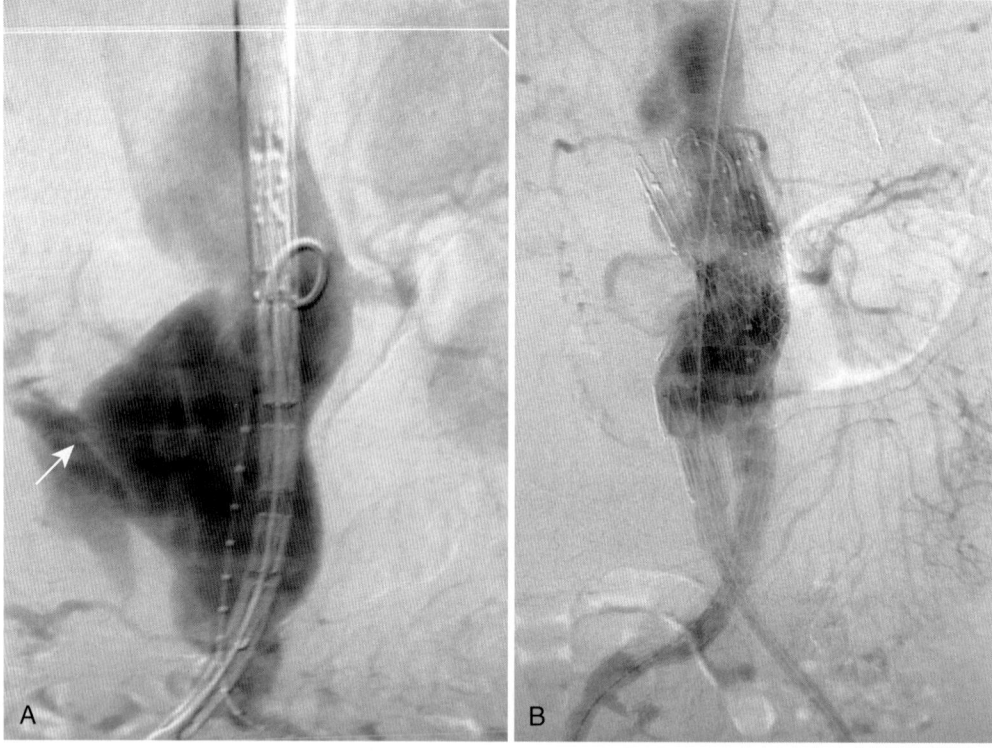

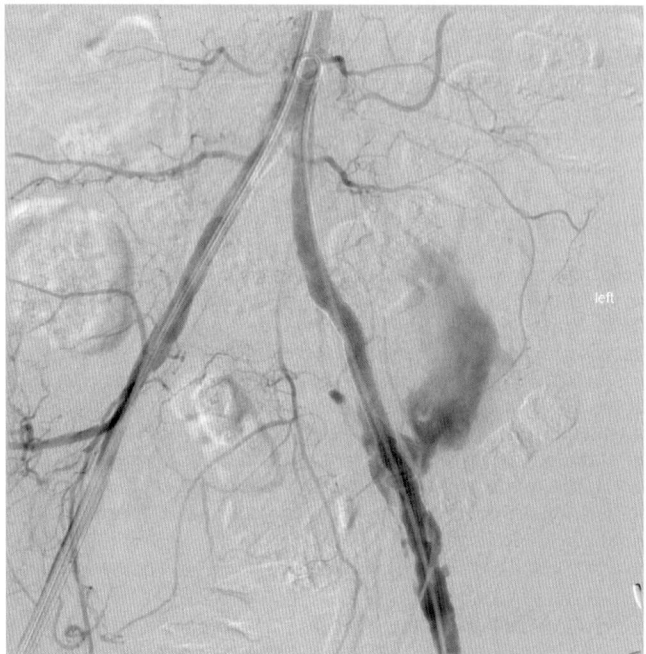

FIGURE 7 Iatrogenic perforation of the left external iliac artery with extravasation of contrast into the retroperitoneum.

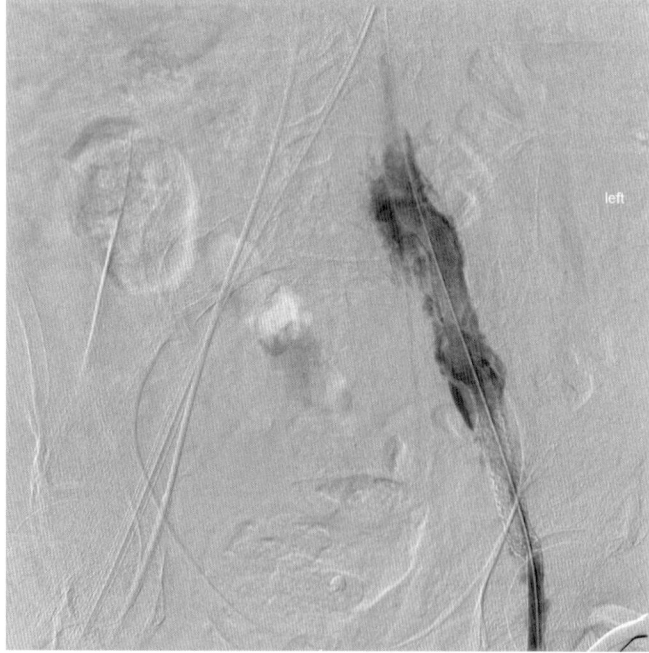

FIGURE 8 Repair of the injury with a nitinol, self-expanding stent. Residual contrast is present without active extravasation.

affected (16% to 35% and 24% to 28%, respectively). Mortality was 3% overall but was greatest within the common femoral artery (CFA) subgroup. Amputation occurred in 8% of popliteal/tibial arterial injuries, and 9% of injuries occurred by a blunt mechanism. In one small series, endovascular stent grafts and coil embolization had been utilized to manage 7% of femoral injuries. The literature points to the need for intervention in both blunt and penetrating injuries. Endovascular intervention may be best if there are soft signs present and an ankle-brachial index of less than 0.9, suggesting a potential major injury.

Technique

The technique is the same as described for iliac arterial access. Once the wire and catheter traverse the level of the injury, obtain a DSA in 25 degrees of anterior oblique angled to the ipsilateral proximal femoral trifurcation. For the remainder of the evaluation, the image intensifier can remain in an AP orientation. If accessing tibial vessels, exchange for an 0.018-inch or 0.014-inch wire. Utilize a self-expanding stent or stent graft, or embolize as indicated for the injury (Figures 9 and 10).

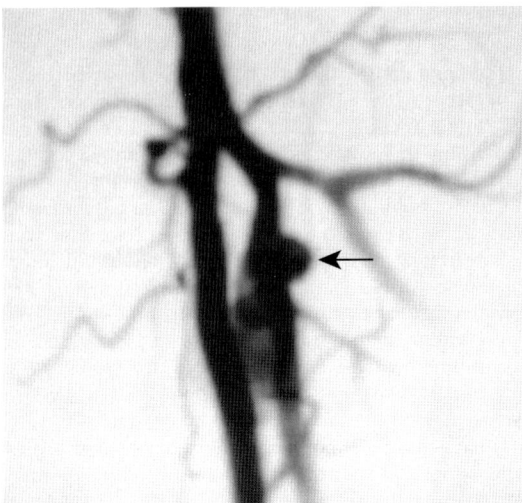

FIGURE 9 Gunshot to the left profunda femoris artery, creating a pseudoaneurysm with contrast extravasation (arrow).

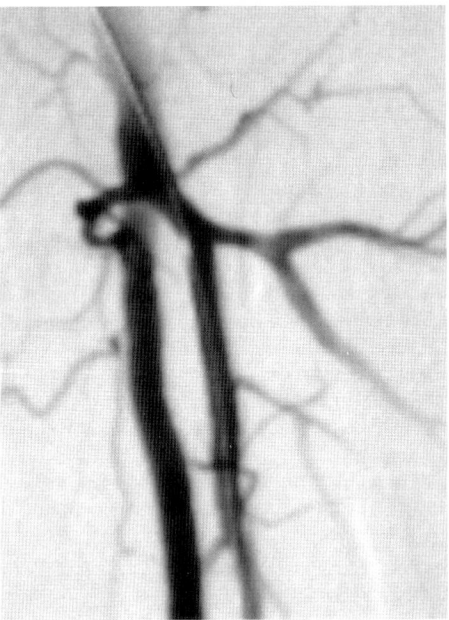

FIGURE 10 Completion arteriogram demonstrating the pseudoaneurysm repaired with a covered stent. No contrast extravasation is present.

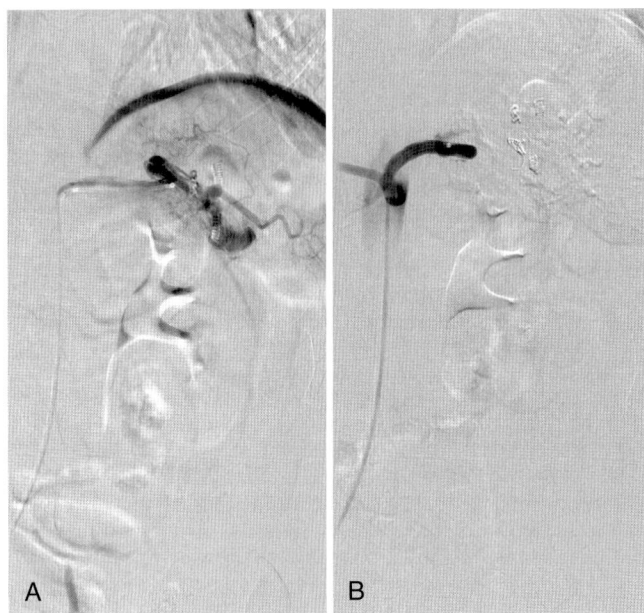

FIGURE 11 **A,** A selective arteriogram of the splenic artery demonstrates extravasation of contrast at the hilum. **B,** After embolization, endovascular coils are present at the splenic hilum with no evidence of contrast in the distal vessel or any further extravasation.

Access is obtained according to the vessel to be embolized (see the previous sections). Caution should be taken to select appropriate-sized coils and wire as recommended by the manufacturer in order to reduce the risk of distal embolization or faulty deployment. Once the vessel of interest is selected, obtain a DSA to confirm the presence and level of the injury. Position the delivery catheter distal to the injured segment. Deploy enough coils to fill the lumen and demonstrate minimal retrograde flow. Withdraw the catheter proximal to the injured segment and repeat deployment. Complete a DSA to evaluate for minimal contrast extravasation and continued patency of named or collateral vasculature (Figure 11).

Balloon Tamponade/Inflation

With wire access obtained across the vessel of interest (as previously described), choose a balloon circumference with a balloon-to-arterial ratio of 1.2 : 1. Serial inflations should be performed with the balloon below the nominal pressure. Maintain each inflation for 2 to 3 minutes. Obtain an angiographic image between inflations to determine whether hemostasis has been achieved. If hemostasis cannot be attained or if there is hemodynamic instability that cannot be corrected, the balloon can be used to occlude the vessel temporarily until the patient is stabilized and definitive care instituted.

ADJUNCTIVE TECHNIQUES

Two endovascular techniques are discussed briefly here because they are useful adjuncts either to open repair, as a bridge to definitive repair, or as the definitive repair itself to manage hemorrhage in stable or unstable patients. Serial balloon inflations can also be employed for flow-limiting antegrade dissections at locations for which stents may have a relative contraindication.

Embolization

In 1985, Panetta and colleagues described the usefulness of embolization in different anatomic locations, determining that it was a superior method to control hemorrhage over open surgery in the pelvis. In the past 25 years, this has become a standard maneuver for controlling hemorrhage in a multitude of regions that are difficult to access, such as intercostal arteries.

SUGGESTED READINGS

Danetz JS, Cassabo AD, Stoner MC, et al: Feasibility of endovascular repair in penetrating axillosubclavian injuries: a retrospective review, *J Vasc Surg* 41:246–254, 2005.

Farber MA, Mendes RR: Endovascular repair of blunt thoracic aortic injury: techniques and tips, *J Vasc Surg* 50(3):683–686, 2009.

Guilbert MC, Elkouri S, Bracco D, et al: Arterial trauma during central venous catheter insertion: case series, review and proposed algorithm, *J Vasc Surg* 48:918–925, 2008.

Li W, D'Ayala M, Hirshberg A, et al: Comparison of conservative and operative treatment for blunt carotid injuries: analysis of the National Trauma Data Bank, *J Vasc Surg* 51:593–599, 2010.

Yadav JS, Casserly IP, Sachar R: *Manual of peripheral vascular intervention*, Philadelphia, 2005, Lippincott Williams & Wilkins.

THE MANAGEMENT OF EXTREMITY COMPARTMENT SYNDROME

Anna M. Ledgerwood, MD, and
Charles E. Lucas, MD

An extremity compartment syndrome develops from swelling of muscle in a confined space. This swelling may increase the tissue pressure within an anatomically contained space above capillary hydrostatic pressure, thereby compromising arteriolar inflow and leading to muscle and nerve ischemia and ultimately necrosis.

PATHOPHYSIOLOGY

Recognition of compartment syndrome began with Bywaters and Beall's (1941) descriptions of the crush syndrome in World War II. They reported on a small number of patients who were entrapped by collapsing buildings during the London Blitz. After extrication by their neighborhood civil defense workers and delivery by horse-drawn vehicles to the nearest hospitals, these initially stable and oriented patients deteriorated. The subsequent life-threatening events included hypotension from extravasation of fluid into the crushed limb, ischemia of the crushed limb as a result of high tissue pressure, rhabdomyolysis with myoglobinemia, renal failure, and death from inadequate volume replacement. Prevention of this fatal outcome requires an understanding of the pathophysiology of each step of this lethal sequence. Regardless of whether the increased tissue swelling and tissue pressure results from increased interstitial and intracellular fluid from reperfusion or crush injury or from external compression from a cast or a tourniquet, the subsequent pathophysiology of the compartment hypertension is comparable (Box 1).

The venous system is the primary egress for the extremity. When tissue pressure rises, venous outflow is impaired. This compromises the lymphatic flow, which empties locally into small veins leading to larger veins. The resultant rise in the interstitial fluid space (IFS) causes an elevation of the pressure in the intracellular fluid (ICF) spaces. Cellular hypertension compromises the nutrient flow from the capillaries through the IFS to the cells, which impairs cellular perfusion and leads to cell swelling as a result of intracellular sodium and water retention. The combination of increased pressure in the IFS and ICF shuts off transcapillary movement. The resultant cellular ischemia leads to acidosis and muscle necrosis with myoglobinemia, which is exacerbated when the restriction causing the compartment syndrome is corrected. When the insult is prolonged, extensive tissue injury and necrosis of entire muscles results, so that alleviation of the compartment syndrome must be followed by extensive débridement and occasionally amputation to remove dead tissue in order to salvage life.

ETIOLOGY

There are myriad conditions that can lead to an extremity compartment syndrome (Box 2). Tightly placed plaster casts or bandage wraps placed soon after injury can cause external compartment compression and fail to allow normal soft tissue swelling. Likewise, a circumferential third-degree burn with eschar decreases the volume of the underlying compartment and prevents the expected swelling that would occur with burn resuscitation.

Most compartment syndromes result from an internal compartment expansion that causes increased tissue pressure. The classic example is ischemia with reperfusion. Arterial occlusion from injury, thrombosis, or prolonged application of a tourniquet leads to cellular ischemia, with extensive cellular swelling once flow is restored. Patients with injury involving the femoral artery trifurcation or the popliteal artery are especially prone to severe ischemia of the leg muscles when reconstruction is delayed beyond 6 hours. The likelihood for compartment syndrome increases when the ischemic insult is combined with severe soft tissue injury, typically associated with long bone fractures and venous injury that necessitates ligation. Extensive combined injuries of bone, vessels, and soft tissues are seen after pedestrian/motor vehicle collisions and high-velocity rifle wounds. Arterial shunting, external fixation of fractures, rapid vascular reconstruction, and extensive fascia decompression are usually needed to salvage the involved limb. Burns without eschar and swelling caused by frostbite and generalized sepsis rarely increase muscle tissue pressure to the point that it impedes capillary flow. Internal compartment expansion may occur from a direct cellular insult with subsequent swelling. Classic examples include crush injury, most commonly seen today from mechanical compression of the extremity in an industrial accident. Other causes include excessive exertion or exercise and direct cellular insult from an electrical injury.

Accumulation of blood and edema with soft tissue injury are common features of fractures, particularly in the lower extremity. Alternatively, blood could accumulate spontaneously from minor trauma in a patient with a coagulopathy such as hemophilia or with the use of anticoagulants. Venous occlusion caused by iliofemoral thrombosis or venous return impaired by external pressure may lead to compartment syndrome. In the latter case, it may occur when an intoxicated patient lies on the extremity for a prolonged period of time. Miscellaneous causes of compartment syndrome include intramuscular injection of illicit drugs into the muscular compartment, which causes infection with subsequent abscess formation, cellulitis, and tissue ischemia. In rare cases, infiltrations of intravenous fluids cause compartment syndrome, inasmuch as these are usually in the subcutaneous tissue and not the muscle compartment.

DIAGNOSIS

Documenting a history of any of the many conditions that may lead to a compartment syndrome requires a careful examination of the involved extremity. An alert and cooperative patient should be assessed for the six Ps associated with compartment syndrome (Box 3). Pain is the first and most important symptom and is usually described as a deep throbbing, unrelenting pressure. *Pain* out of proportion to physical findings is common. *Pressure* is the earliest and only truly objective finding of a compartment syndrome and is manifested as swelling, hardness, and tenderness of a muscle. This is most commonly appreciated in the anterior compartment of the lower extremity. *Pain with stretch* of the involved muscles is common but difficult to assess if there is a fracture or contusion. *Paresis,* or weakness of the muscle, is also difficult to interpret and may be secondary to nerve involvement or guarding secondary to pain. *Paresthesia* is the most reliable physical finding. Each compartment of the forearm and leg has at least one nerve coursing through it, and so careful sensory examination of the hand or foot may help confirm the compartment involved. For example, the deep peroneal nerve is located in the anterior compartment and innervates the web space of the great toe. Decreased sensation in this area is indicative of an anterior compartment syndrome. The *presence of pulses* does not exclude a compartment syndrome. The increased compartment

BOX 1: Pathophysiology of compartment syndrome

1. Increased tissue pressure
2. Venous hypertension
3. Lymphatic blockade
4. Interstitial space hypertension
5. Intracellular hypertension
6. Reduced capillary perfusion
7. Tissue ischemia
8. Tissue death

BOX 2: Etiology of compartment syndrome

External Compartmental Compression
Cast/ACE wrap
Military antishock garments
Burn eschar

Internal Compartment Expansion
Ischemia and reperfusion
   Arterial injury, thrombosis, tourniquet
   Burns, frostbite
Cellular insult and swelling
   Crush injury
   Exercise/exertion
   Electrical injury
Blood accumulation and edema
   Fractures
   Hemophilia
   Anticoagulants
   Venous occlusion
Miscellaneous
   Intravenous infiltration
   Drug injection

BOX 3: The six _Ps_ of compartment syndrome

Pain	Paresis
Pressure	Paresthesia
Pain with stretch	Pulses present

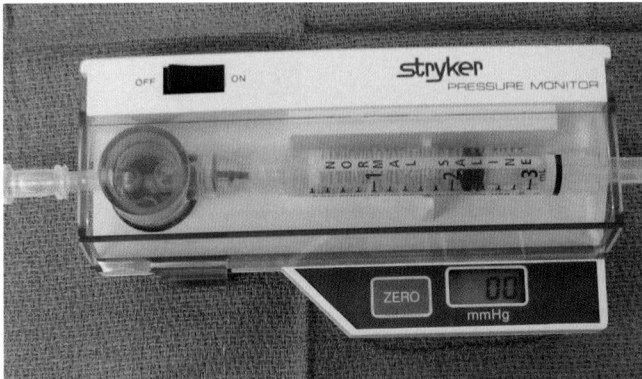

FIGURE 1 The Stryker pressure monitor is a handheld solid-state transducer device that can be used to directly measure muscle tissue pressure. The syringe and manometer are housed in a special chamber, and the directions for use are engraved on the back of the chamber.

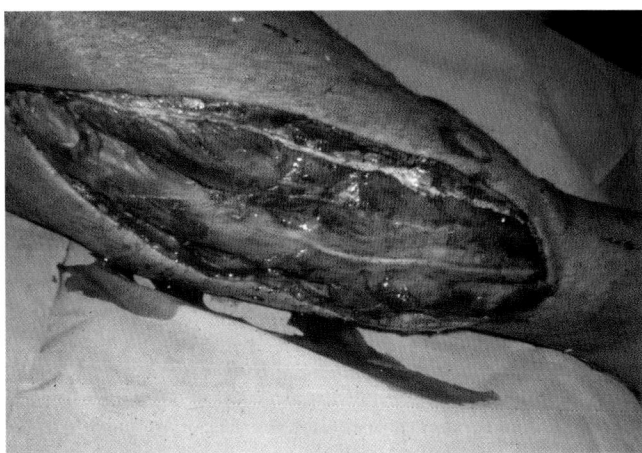

FIGURE 2 A fasciotomy was performed for muscle ischemia of the calf after repair of a popliteal artery injury with ligation of the injured vein. There are areas of ischemia of the muscle that are allowed to demarcate with superficial débridement at 2 to 3 weeks. Early débridement leads to loss of muscle that probably would have survived.

pressure may cause muscle and nerve ischemia, but rarely is it elevated sufficiently to occlude a major artery.

Objective confirmation of a compartment syndrome requires direct monitoring of tissue pressure. Compartment decompression may be performed on the basis of clinical examination findings and does not require monitoring of tissue pressure. However, certain patients cannot be assessed clinically, such as those under anesthesia, those inhibited by alcohol or street drugs, or those suffering a head injury. There are a number of techniques available to monitor tissue pressure or, more specifically, intramuscular pressure. The direct needle puncture with a handheld solid-state transducer device (STIC catheter; Stryker Surgical, Kalamazoo, Mich) allows for repeated pressure measurements and is the technique most commonly used to measure tissue pressure (Figure 1). Alternatively, the authors have used a central venous pressure manometer, which is filled with sterile saline and attached to an extension tube, and a regular 18-gauge needle, which is inserted directly into the muscle compartment. The manometer is set so that its top is level with or slightly below the compartment, and the stopcock is opened. The manometer is gradually raised until the meniscus is seen to fall. The measurement is

expressed in centimeters of water or divided by 1.4 to equal millimeters of mercury. Muscle compartmental pressure is normally less than 20 mm Hg. The authors tend to perform compartment decompression in a patient with suspected compartment syndrome whose muscle compartment pressure is greater than 35 mm Hg.

TREATMENT: COMPARTMENT DECOMPRESSION

The definitive treatment of compartment syndrome is release of the constricting tissue. Nonoperative therapies have no role in the treatment of compartment syndrome. Release of the constricting tissues almost always requires a long incision that involves the skin, subcutaneous tissues, and underlying fascia. Subcutaneous fasciotomy is best avoided. Débridement of ischemic muscle should be conservative because many segments of muscle that appear necrotic actually survive, and the negative or detrimental systemic effects of ischemic muscle are avoided once the compartment is decompressed and the products of dead muscle escape onto the dressing (Figure 2).

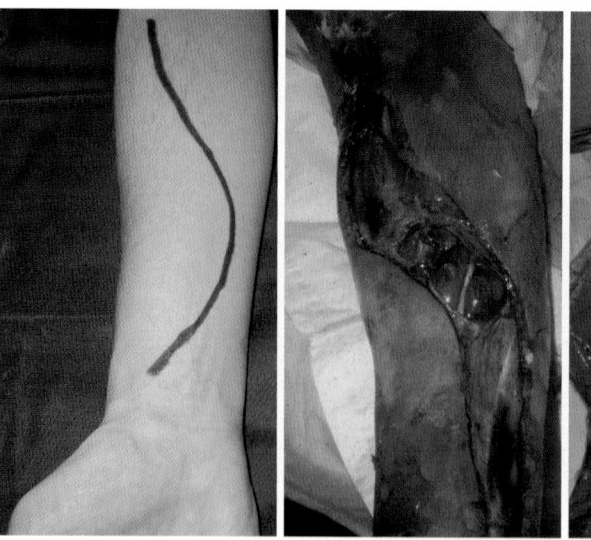
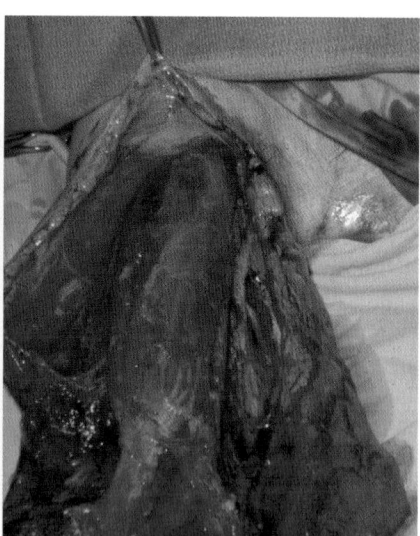

FIGURE 3 Street drugs were injected inadvertently into the subcutaneous plane of the forearm, and the extensive soft tissue necrosis and fasciitis that developed led to compartment syndrome. Extension of the forearm fasciotomy incision up to involve the anterior compartment of the arm, followed by extensive soft-tissue débridement *(left)* resulted in limb salvage and reasonable function.

The upper extremity, or arm, has two compartments containing primarily the deltoid and biceps brachii muscles anteriorly and the triceps muscle posteriorly. Anterior compartment syndrome of the arm may occur after the inadvertent subcutaneous injection of street drugs such as heroin when the intended vein is missed. The resultant extensive cellulitis compromises perfusion, necessitating a long incision beginning just distal to the deltoid to just above the elbow, staying lateral to the brachial artery and median nerve.

A compartment hypertension of both the anterior and posterior arm compartments is more likely to occur with crush injury or as a result of long-term venous occlusion caused by the patient's sleeping on the arm while intoxicated. The posterior incision extends over the triceps muscle in the midline to approximately 3 cm above the elbow. If necessary, decompression of the deltoid muscle can be achieved by extending the anterior incision proximally to the rotator cuff.

Forearm Compartment Syndrome

The forearm has three muscular compartments. The volar compartment contains the flexors of the wrist while the dorsal compartment contains the extensors to the wrist. The lateral compartment contains the brachial radialis and the extensor carpi radialis longus and extensor carpi radialis brevis. Isolated volar compartment syndrome of the forearm occurs after subcutaneous injection of street drugs, extravasation of intravenous infusions, insect bites, or crush injury. Decompression of the volar compartment is achieved through an incision that begins laterally near the elbow and descends medially in a curved manner for the first proximal half of the forearm and then curves laterally down to just above the wrist (Figure 3). This incision also decompresses the lateral compartment.

When all three forearm compartments are compromised—whether after severe burns or as a result of extensive trauma with long bone fractures and ischemia that necessitate vascular reconstruction—a posterior decompression should be added. This incision extends just distal to the radial head to the midportion of the wrist.

Above-the-Knee Compartment Syndrome

A thigh compartment syndrome is rare but may result from crush injury, venous outflow occlusion, or extensive bone and soft tissue disruptions caused by explosions, mines, or high-velocity rifle

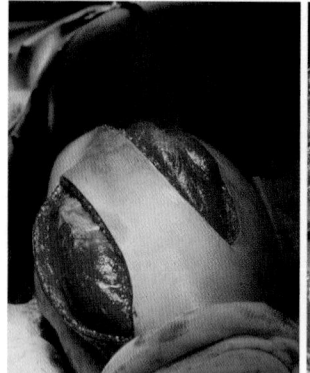
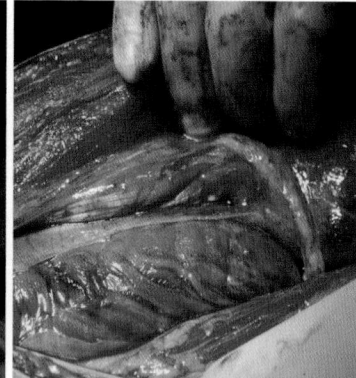

FIGURE 4 A patient who was admitted for a drug overdose was seen in consultation in the medical intensive care unit for a swollen right thigh. The thigh was hard and tense, and the patient excreted 40 mL of black urine. Medial and lateral thigh fasciotomies revealed pale muscles *(right)*. In spite of aggressive resuscitation, he developed oliguric acute renal failure and required dialysis for 3 weeks before urine output recovered. All muscle groups survived, and the wounds were treated with split-thickness skin grafting.

wounds (Figure 4). Compartment syndrome of the thigh is likely to involve all three compartments and to necessitate total decompression. The thigh has three compartments. The anterior compartment contains the sartorius and the quadriceps femoris muscles; the medial compartment contains the gracilis and three adductor muscles; and the posterior compartment contains the biceps femoris, semitendinosus, and semimembranosus muscles. Decompression of the anterior and posterior compartments can be achieved with an incision that extends from the greater trochanter posterior laterally to just above the knee. The fascia overlying the vastus lateralis muscle is identified so that the anterior compartment can be exposed throughout the length of the incision by an incision in the intramuscular septum separating the anterior and posterior compartments. The fascia from the vastus lateralis and its attachments on the femur are divided, thereby giving access to the lateral muscle fibers of the posterior compartment. Decompression of the medial compartment is achieved by a medial incision that stays posterior to Hunter's canal and opens the fascia of the gracilis and adductor muscles, including the adductor longus, brevis, and magnus.

Below-the-Knee Compartment Syndrome

Most compartment syndromes occur in the lower leg, or calf, and are caused by ischemic reperfusion injury associated with elective or emergency vascular reconstruction or with crush injuries involving fractures and soft tissue injury.

The lower leg has four compartments. The anterior compartment contains the tibialis anterior, the extensor hallucis longus, the extensor digitorum longus, and a portion of the peroneus tertius muscles. The lateral compartment contains the peroneus longus and peroneus brevis muscles, and the posterior compartment contains the soleus, gastrocnemius, and plantaris muscles. The deep posterior compartment contains the flexor hallicis longus, tibialis posterior, flexor digitorum longus, and popliteus muscles. Although the lateral compartment contains the peroneal nerve, the peroneal artery runs deep in the posterior compartment along with the posterior tibial artery. The deep peroneal nerve runs in the anterior compartment, whereas the superficial peroneal nerve is in the lateral compartment.

Anterior Compartment Syndrome

An unusual entity is the stress-induced anterior compartment syndrome. Affected patients uniformly have a history of increased physical activity and exercise for an extended time. The patients state that the anterior calf tightened and became extremely painful; massage did not help. The severe constant pain is localized to the anterior compartment. The diagnosis is made clinically by noting that the anterior compartment is very hard. This is a surgical emergency, and immediate anterior compartment decompression as described previously is required.

Four-Compartment Syndrome

Patients presenting with ischemic reperfusion injury or severe trauma with concomitant injury to bone and muscle are more likely to have a four-compartment syndrome. The most common way of decompressing the four compartments is to use bilateral incisions (Figure 5). The medial incision is made just distal to the medial tibial condyle and extends inferiorly between the superficial posterior muscle group and the posterior ridge of the tibia. This incision should be approximately 1 cm posterior to the tibia and then carried through the superficial fascia. This decompresses the superficial posterior compartment. In order to decompress the deep posterior compartment, the fibers of the soleus muscle must be detached from the posterior tibial attachments (Figure 6). The lateral and anterior compartments are decompressed by a lateral skin incision along the anterior margin of the fibula between the muscle fibers of the lateral compartment and the lateral portion of the anterior compartment. The skin must be retracted anteriorly to expose the fascia of the anterior compartment muscles and then inferiorly to expose the fascia of the lateral compartment, both of which are incised the full length of the earlier incision (see Figure 6). Care must be taken to be certain the lateral incision includes the anterior compartment muscles. Likewise, the soleus muscle must be taken off the tibia if the deep posterior compartment is to be decompressed. On occasion, decompression of three compartments lowers the pressure in the deep posterior compartment. Tissue pressures can be obtained after a three-compartment fasciotomy; if the deep posterior compartment pressures are below 25 mm Hg, no further decompression is needed.

POSTOPERATIVE MANAGEMENT

The extremities are dressed with dry gauze and a soft wrap and elevated. A vacuum-assisted closure device can be applied if drainage is extensive. A posterior splint of the lower extremity is strongly recommended to prevent footdrop. Some fasciotomy incisions can be closed in 5 to 7 days with closure of the skin. The fascial incision should be left open because closure will lead to recurrences of compartment syndrome. If extensive muscle bulging precludes skin approximation, full-thickness skin grafts can be performed. Sometimes there is a delay to compartment decompression, which leads to superficial muscle ischemia. The superficial layer of muscle may appear necrotic. In most cases, the underlying muscle is compromised but does survive. A superficial layer of necrotic muscle can be débrided at 2 to 3 weeks (see Figure 2). The patient is monitored for

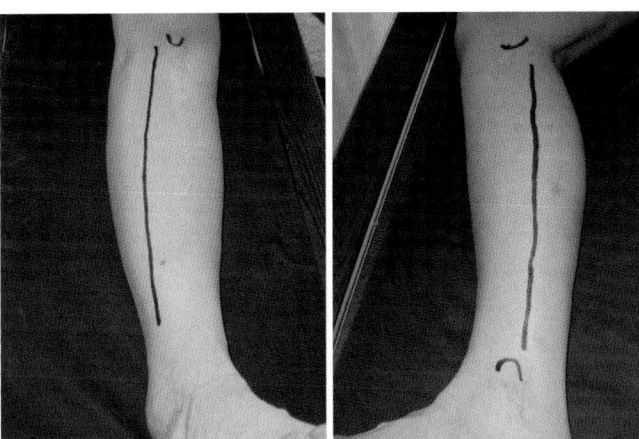

FIGURE 5 Four-compartment fasciotomy of the calf is made by a lateral skin and fascial incision made along the anterior margin of the fibula between the muscle fibers of the lateral compartment and the lateral portion of the anterior compartment. The medial incision is made just distal to the medial tibial condyle and extends inferiorly between the superficial posterior muscle group and the posterior ridge of the tibia.

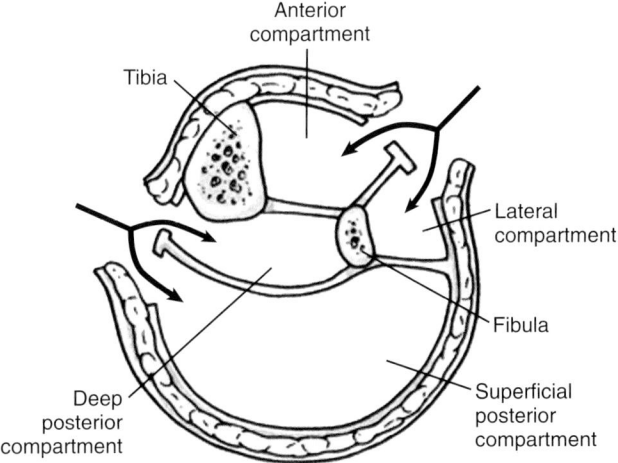

FIGURE 6 To decompress the anterior compartment, it is crucial that the skin of the lateral incision be retracted anteriorly and the fascia of the anterior compartment muscles be exposed and incised. Likewise, to decompress the deep posterior compartment, the gastrocnemius muscle needs to be retracted inferiorly in the medial wound and the soleus muscle taken off the posterior tibia. Unless the soleus muscle is taken down from the tibia, only a three-compartment fasciotomy has been performed.

myoglobinuria and, if it is present, treated with alkalinization of the urine and hydration.

SUGGESTED READINGS

Bywaters EGL, Beall D: Crush injuries with impairment of renal function, *BMJ* 1:427–432, 1941.
Ledgerwood AM, Lucas CE: Massive thigh injuries with vascular disruption: role of porcine skin grafting of exposed arterial vein grafts, *Arch Surg* 107:201–207, 1973.
Mubarak SJ, Hargens AR: Acute compartment syndrome, *Surg Clin North Am* 63:539–565, 1983.
Trunkey D: Changes in combat casualty care, *J Am Coll Surg* 214:879–891, 2012.
Williams AB, Luchette FA, Papaconstantinou HT, et al: The effect of early versus late fasciotomy in the management of extremity trauma, *Surgery* 122:861–866, 1997.

BURN WOUND MANAGEMENT

Stephen M. Milner, MBBS, BDS, DSc (Hon), FRCS (Ed), FACS, and Malachy E. Asuku, MBBS, FWACS

OVERVIEW

Although the etiology and mechanism that lead to burn injury remain diverse, the common pathway to tissue damage involves sustained exposure to temperatures outside the physiologic range. The resultant injury is dependent on the magnitude of the temperature and the duration of the exposure. Whereas the cellular damage induced by heat and ischemia is localized in minor burns, large surface area burns induce additional systemic effects mediated by inflammatory cytokines that cause generalized capillary endothelial dysfunction. The severity of the ensuing metabolic and endocrine disturbance is determined by the percentage total body surface area (TBSA) burn and the patient's age. Concomitant injuries, such as inhalation injury and patient comorbidities, have equally been shown to contribute to the overall outcome.

The strategy in the management of the burn patient as enshrined in the mission statements directs attention to life-threatening concerns before focus on the burn wound (Box 1). Therapy demands prompt attention to Advanced Trauma Life Support (ATLS) workup, fluid resuscitation, pain control, prevention of wound infection, and pharmacomodulation of the hypermetabolic state. Nutritional support by way of supplemental tube feeds has been shown to enhance epithelialization, granulation tissue formation, and immunocompetence. The consolidation of the multidisciplinary resource in the modern burn center incorporating invasive continuous cardiac monitoring, ventilator support, and renal replacement therapy (RRT) has led to improved survival in the last few decades. However, it is the preponderance of early burn wound excision and closure with skin graft that has contributed most to survival of the burn patient (Figure 1).

THE BURN WOUND

The effective treatment and ultimate healing of the burn wound remains the sine qua non of successful treatment of the burn patient. Survival with good quality of life is contingent on complete closure of the burn wound, a feat that requires adequate understanding of the peculiar pathophysiology of the burn wound. The local effect of burn injury is depicted by the three-dimensional Jacksonian model of three concentric zones. The zone of necrosis, which is in the center, is the part exposed to the highest intensity of insult. The tissue is irreversibly damaged as the cellular protein is denatured by intense heat or cold. In the periphery lies the zone of inflammation, where injury is minimal as it is most remote from the inciting agent. The tissue is expected to make complete recovery within 7 to 10 days. In the middle is the zone of ischemia, where massive release of inflammatory cytokines lead to increased capillary permeability (Figure 2). This injured tissue has a tendency to progress to a deeper wound within 24 to 48 hours in a process described as conversion.

BOX 1: Mission statement in the management of burns

Mission Statement in the Management of Burns: The Big Picture at a Glance

1. Institution of adequate airway and breathing
2. Prevention and treatment of burn shock
3. Prevention and treatment of infection
4. Provision of permanent and durable skin cover
5. Correction of functional disabilities
6. Correction of cosmetic concerns
7. Rehabilitation and reintegration into society

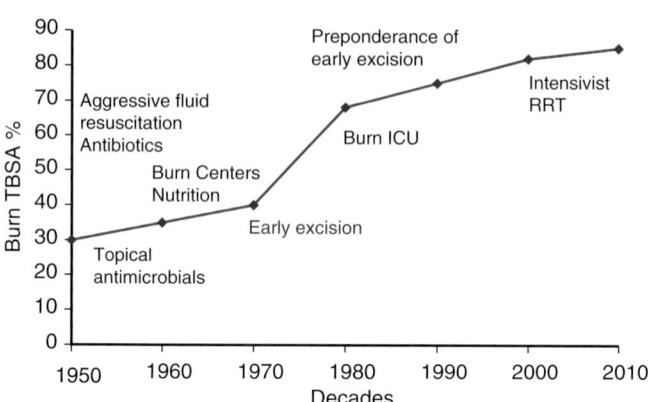

FIGURE 1 Line graph depicting burn lethal total body surface area (TBSA). *ICU,* Intensive care unit; *RRT,* renal replacement therapy. *(From Kasten KR, Makley AT, Kagan RJ: Update on the critical care management of severe burns,* J Intensive Care Med *26(4):223-236.)*

The objectives of treatment of the burn wound are therefore to rescue the tissue in the zone of ischemia, hasten the recovery of tissue in the zone of inflammation, and surgically facilitate removal of eschar in the zone of necrosis. Clinically, this translates into burn wound excision, wound dressing to provide moisture and prevent infection, and the resurfacing of epithelial defects with skin grafts where indicated. The depth of burn injury is the most important variable in determining the degree of complexity necessary in its management (Table 1). This places a high premium on the accurate assessment of burn depth, a science that has remained an enigma. Sophisticated techniques for determination of burn depth have included color temperature mapping, injection of vital dyes such as India ink and fluorescein, and ultrasound scan. The laser Doppler imaging that uses a color-coded map dependent on tissue perfusion may be the most reliable technique at this time. For the most part, however, the judgment remains a clinical one that requires a measure of experience.

The principles of the reconstructive ladder may be effectively applied to the management of the burn wound. Superficial burns have minimal requirements; provision of moisture and protection against infection allow spontaneous reepithelialization within 14 to 21 days. Topical antimicrobial ointments or other occlusive dressings have been used with great success. In deeper burns, healing is accelerated with excision and split-thickness skin graft coverage of the excised wound bed. However, composite tissue losses may necessitate the use of full-thickness skin grafts, flap coverage including free flaps, use of synthetic skin substitutes, tissue expansion, and interval use of negative-pressure therapy to facilitate granulation tissue formation preparatory to skin grafting.

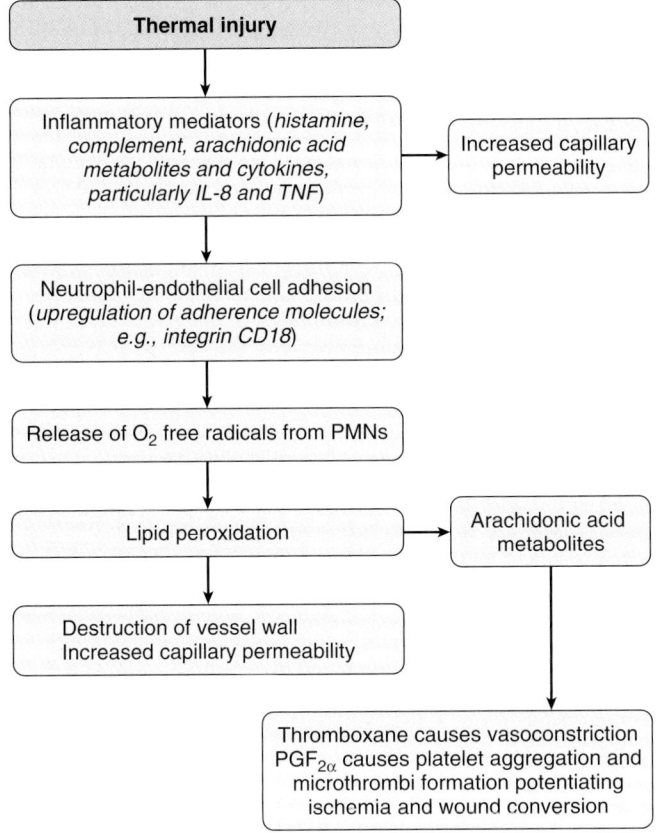

FIGURE 2 Algorithm showing the systemic effect of burns. *CD18,* Integrin beta-2; *IL-8,* interleukin-8; *PGF$_{2\alpha}$,* prostaglandin F-2 alpha; *PMN,* polymorphonuclear leucocytes; *TNF,* tumor necrosis factor.

MANAGEMENT OF SUPERFICIAL BURNS

Débridement of the burn wound facilitates assessment of extent of injury and serves as the first step in wound care. Intravenous narcotic analgesia provides adequate pain control and allays patient's anxiety. The core body temperature must be maintained above 36°C in patients with large surface area burns. The exposure of limited areas at a time, use of warm cleansing solution, and use of an overhead heating shield have been helpful in this regard. The wound surface is cleansed with an antiseptic solution such as 5% chlorhexidine. Nonviable tissue and blisters are excised with sharp dissection to rid the body of proinflammatory cytokines contained in blister fluid. Furthermore, débridement accords topical antimicrobial agents adequate contact with the wound bed.

Topical antimicrobial ointments have continued to play a role, albeit nominal, in the management of superficial burns. Silver sulfadiazine, marketed under different trade names across the globe (Silvadene, [Monarch Pharmaceuticals Inc., Bristol, Tenn]; Dermazene, [Silvestre Laboratorios Quimica and Farmaceutica, Brazil]; Thermazene, [Kendall Healthcare Products, Mansfield, Mass]; and Flamazine [Smith and Nephew Pharmaceuticals Ltd., Hull, UK]), remains the most widely used of these agents. Its antimicrobial properties include bactericidal activity against gram-positive and gram-negative organisms including *Pseudomonas* species and yeast. It is readily available, painless, and easy to apply. Drawbacks include infrequent hypersensitivity in individuals with sulfa allergy, transient neutropenia with prolonged use over large surface areas, and the formation of pseudoeschar capable of interfering with assessment of burn depth. Other widely used antimicrobial creams and ointments in the care of superficial burn wounds include Bacitracin (E. Fougera & Co., a division of Nycomed U.S. Inc., Melville, NY), Neosporin (Johnson and Johnson Consumer Co., Inc., NJ), and Polymyxin B

TABLE 1: Classification of burn wounds: superficial versus deep burns

Depth	Traditional	Characteristics	Significance
Superficial	1st and 2nd degrees. Superficial partial-thickness burn.	Wet, pink, blistered; blanches with pressure; and painful.	Sufficient epithelial appendages to allow healing within 3 weeks. Scarring is minimal.
Deep	3rd degree. Deep partial and full-thickness burns.	Ranges from cherry red, mottled, white, and nonblanching to leathery brown and insensate.	Insufficient epithelial appendages; healing is slow with resultant unstable scar, scar hypertrophy, and contractures. Best treated with excision and skin grafting.

Asuku ME, Milner SM: Burn surgery. In Granick MS, Teot L, editors: Surgical wound healing and management, *ed 2, New York, 2012, Informa Healthcare, pp 49-57.*

(Cayman Chemical Co., Ann Arbor, Mich). In Europe and other parts of the world, fine meshed fabric described as tulle is widely used as dressing for superficial burns. The fabric is usually impregnated with Vaseline (Tulle gras, Smith and Nephew Healthcare Ltd., Hull, UK), chlorhexidene acetate (Bactigras; Smith and Nephew Healthcare Ltd., Hull, UK), or framycetin sulfate (Sofra- tulle; Hoechst Marion Russel Ltd., Uxbridge, England). The ideal dressing remains one that is inexpensive and comfortable and requires minimal dressing changes. It should provide a suitable environment for reepithelialization and protect against microbial colonization.

MANAGEMENT OF DEEP BURNS

Full-thickness circumferential extremity and trunk burns in which eschar constitutes a leathery nonyielding band are indications for escharotomy. Early recognition of the need for escharotomy or fasciotomy on an injured extremity is vital to prevention of loss of limb. Close surveillance must be extended to circumferential partial-thickness burns and full-thickness noncircumferential extremity burns in patients who need large volumes of fluid for resuscitation. Excruciating pain on passive movement and palpable firmness of the compartment precede the ominous signs of distal neurovascular compromise, such as pallor and loss of pulse. Direct measurement of compartmental pressures with the need for escharotomy established at a threshold of 30 mm Hg with a wick catheter technique has been widely adopted.

Escharotomy may be performed by the patient's bedside with minimal doses of analgesics and anxiolytics. Electrocautery is preferred to the use of scalpel blade because this minimizes bleeding. It is safe practice to outline and carry out incisions with the limbs in anatomic positions to avoid damage to neurovascular structures (Figure 3). The longitudinal decompressing incisions must traverse the depth of the eschar until the subcutaneous tissue spouts and should extend to nonburned tissue proximally and distally. It is vital to immediately ascertain the adequacy of an escharotomy by demonstrating softness of previously firm compartments and improved distal perfusion. The absence of these signs should be considered an indication for fasciotomy, which is best performed in the operating room with general anesthesia. This procedure is aimed at relieving of pressure within the well-defined fascioosseous compartments of the limbs. High-voltage electrical burn injury is a frequent cause of extremity compartment syndrome that necessitates fasciotomy. The high incidence of limb amputations associated with this injury is indicative of a need for higher index of suspicion for compartment syndrome at presentation. It is customary to explore all the fascial compartments of a limb and allow the skin incision to heal by secondary intention or delayed primary closure with split-thickness skin graft.

EXCISION OF BURN WOUNDS

Basic science and clinical research have shown that early excision of burned tissue that serves as nidus for bacterial proliferation and invasive burn wound sepsis attenuates the systemic inflammatory response in patients with major burn injury. The pioneering work of Zora Janzekovic and other researchers has proven that early burn wound excision and closure improve survival, shorten length of hospital stay, improve the quality of scarring, and enhance early return to work. Tangential excision entails serial layered excisions of the burned tissue until punctate capillary bleeding indicative of healthy bed is encountered. The handheld Weck knife mounted with a Goulian guard is most suited for this purpose. Availability of the guard in sizes ranging from 8 to 12 (representing 1/1000 of an inch) allows caution and precision at excision to be tailored to the thickness of the skin in different parts of the body. The Humby knife and the powered dermatome have also been used in the excision of larger burn surfaces. Tangential excision is associated with significant blood loss in the magnitude of 0.75 to 1 mL/ cm^2 excised. Proponents of immediate excision of burn wounds argue that the blood loss is reduced to 0.40 mL/cm^2 if excision is done within the first 24 hours of injury. Strategies aimed at minimization of blood loss include use of nonadherent Telfa pads (Telfa AMD, Covidien, Mansfield, Mass) soaked in epinephrine 1:10,000 to 1:50,000 solution applied for 7 to 10 minutes, use of topical thrombin solutions, preexcision tumescence with 1:500,000 epinephrine solution, and limb elevation/suspension from the ceiling. The use of tourniquets inflated above the systolic pressure after exsanguination is most effective in controlling blood loss in extremity excisions; however, experience is required to determine viable versus nonviable tissue in this setting.

Fascial excision, which refers to the excision of burned skin along with the underlying subcutaneous tissue with preservation of the deep fascia, is reserved for patients with limited donor skin as a result of full-thickness large surface areas burns. It is also suitable in elderly patients with multiple comorbidities in whom reducing operative time and blood loss and obtaining early wound closure are most desirable. The procedure that is undertaken with the aid of electrocautery is faster and entails less blood loss compared with tangential excision. However, the major disadvantages include long-term contour deformity as a result of loss of subcutaneous tissue.

CLOSURE OF EXCISED BURN WOUNDS

Split-thickness autograft coverage of the burn wound is the ultimate goal in the management of the burn wound. The benefits of early excision are realized only when the excised wound is covered with skin or its substitute. For the burn patient, closure of the wound with durable skin represents a major landmark on the way to recovery. Favored donor sites include the thighs, the buttocks, the back, and the scalp. Donor skin is harvested with either the powered dermatome or the handheld dermatomes such as the Humby knife. The usual thickness of split-thickness skin graft is 10/1000 to 12/1000 of an inch. The donor site is usually covered with a protective dressing to minimize pain and facilitate reepithelialization. Meshing the graft to ratios of 1:1, 2:1, 3:1, and 4:1 permits egress of blood and serum and allows coverage of larger surface areas at the expense of durability and cosmetic appearance. Survival of widely meshed autograft (3:1 and 4:1) and healing of the wide interstices is enhanced by an allograft overlay in a sandwich technique. In patients with inadequate donor skin, recropping previously harvested skin may become necessary. The interval to recropping is dependent on the thickness of the

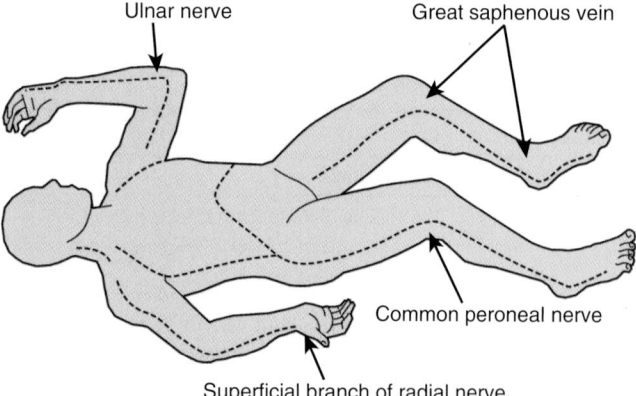

FIGURE 3 Escharotomy incision sites and neurovascular structures at risk of injury.

Ulnar nerve

Great saphenous vein

Common peroneal nerve

Superficial branch of radial nerve

residual dermis, which determines the rate and quality of donor site healing. Generally, a minimum of about 3 weeks may be necessary, and usual practice is to harvest thinner grafts, such as 10/1000 of an inch, when recropping skin.

Several options are available for dressing the grafted wound bed. The ideal is a comfortable dressing that provides moisture to keep the graft alive, adequate pressure to prevent collection under the graft, and immobilization to prevent shearing. Revascularization of the split-thickness skin graft is achieved through the processes of plasmatic imbibition, inosculation, and neovascularization. Reattachment, however, depends on fibrin clot on the wound bed providing the scaffold for the deposition of collagen to form fibrous adhesions. The use of full-thickness skin grafts and flaps in the coverage of acute burn wounds is limited to very small deep burns and such procedures as early correction of ectropion. Aside from being limited in supply, the full-thickness skin graft has more stringent requirements for survival. The graft is harvested with the scalpel blade, and the donor site is usually closed primarily.

Cultured epithelial autograft (CEA), which provides sheets of in vitro cultured keratinocytes, is an additional means of obtaining skin cover in patients with limited donor skin. The inadequacy of use of an epidermal component to replace full-thickness skin loss has been a major drawback to this technique. Attempts at enhancing the durability of CEA have included engrafting the cultured cells over widely meshed autograft or vascularized allogeneic dermis obtained by excising the epidermis and upper dermis of engrafted allograft. The expense, stringent requirements, and suboptimal outcome of CEA are generally accepted to only be justified by an overwhelming burn wound size in which options are limited.

Cadaver allograft represents the best option for temporary burn wound coverage. Its immediate "take" sterilizes the wound bed and prepares it for autograft placement. Allograft serves as an expendable bridge in patients with hemodynamically unstable conditions in which vasopressors known to jeopardize graft take may be necessary. It is also useful in tangentially excised wounds where the adequacy of excision is questionable. It is, however, best substituted before the onset of the process of rejection, which may set in as early as in the third week. Several cycles of allograft coverage may be required while waiting for autograft to become available. Allograft is usually meshed to a ratio of 2 : 1 or 1 : 1, depending on the site to be covered. It may be used as a sheet graft in the temporary coverage of facial and hand excisions where bleeding precludes the immediate use of autograft.

Integra (Life Sciences Laboratory Corp., Plainsboro, NJ) is a bilaminar dermal regeneration template approved by the U.S. Food and Drug Administration (FDA) for use in patients with limited donor sites as a result of massive life-threatening burns. Its outer layer is an impermeable polymeric silicon sheet, and the dermal component is a highly porous matrix composed of cross-linked coprecipitate of bovine collagen and chondroitin-6-sulphate derived from shark cartilage. Within 3 weeks of grafting, the dermal template is incorporated into the recipient bed, forming a neodermis at which stage the polymeric silicon layer is replaced by an ultrathin autograft. Integra has been found most useful in resurfacing the hands and face where it restores normal texture and elasticity. It has also shown success in the coverage of small relatively devascularized areas, such as exposed tendons and bone. Its major disadvantage remains its prohibitive cost and its limited ability to engraft in the presence of wound colonization and infection.

The negative-pressure wound therapy (NPWT) device has since its introduction continued to feature prominently in burn wound management. Its ability to splint skin grafts while allowing range of motion exercises of adjacent joints has been most useful in the patient with large surface area burns. With its control of drainage, it has been shown to equally contribute to bacteriologic control and enhance skin graft take even in areas of unfavorable contours such as the axilla and groin. Although it is not a panacea for inadequate surgery, the technique has led to significant reduction in length of hospital stay.

COMPLICATIONS OF BURN WOUND HEALING

Despite concerted efforts, a scientific tool capable of accurately determining burn depth and directing decisions on the need for surgery or otherwise has continued to evade the burn community. Consequently, complications that result from protracted healing of the burn wound abound. These complications include burn scar hypertrophy, burn scar contractures and unstable scars, and chronic wounds with their long-term potential for malignant transformation into Marjolin's ulcers. The management of these complications constitutes the bulk of the work in the realm of burn reconstruction and rehabilitation.

SUGGESTED READINGS

Asuku ME, Milner SM: Burn surgery. In Granick MS, Teot L, editors: *Surgical wound healing and management*, ed 2, New York, 2012, Informa Healthcare, pp 49–57.

Janzekovic Z: A new concept in the early excision and immediate grafting of burns, *J Trauma* 10:1103, 1970.

Klein MB, Heimbach D, Gibran N: Management of the burn wound. In Wiley WS, Douglas WW, Mitchell PF, et al, editors: *ACS surgery online: principles and practice*, New York, 2004, WebMD, available at http://www .acssurgery.com.

Mosier MJ, Gibran NS: Surgical excision of the burn wound, *Clin Plastic Surg* 36(4):617–625, 2009.

Saffle JR. Closure of excised burn wound: temporary skin substitutes, *Clin Plastic Surg* 36(4):627–641, 2009.

PRACTICAL MANAGEMENT OF THE BURN PATIENT

Rob Sheridan, MD

INTRODUCTION

The outlook for burn patients continues to improve both for survival and for quality of life. Current expectations include eventual return to community, school, family, and work for the large majority. Realization of these results in patients with serious injuries requires a coordinated response by a multidisciplinary group over an interval of time that can span years. This care strategy has four overlapping phases (Table 1). The initial evaluation and resuscitation phase begins at presentation and generally is complete by 48 hours. This first phase includes an accurate fluid resuscitation and through evaluation for nonburn injuries and comorbid conditions. The initial wound excision and biologic closure phase begins during or immediately after and is ideally completed in 5 to 7 days. This second phase is characterized by a series of staged operations in which deep burns are identified and excised and the resulting viable wounds are biologically closed. The definitive wound closure phase immediately follows. This third phase varies in duration with donor skin availability and involves replacement of temporary wound membranes

TABLE 1: Phases of burn care

Phase and rough time course	Objectives
One: Initial evaluation and resuscitation Injury through about 72 hours	Complete evaluation for injuries and comorbid conditions Accurate fluid resuscitation
Two: Initial wound excision and biologic closure Days 1 through 7	Identification and excision of all deep wounds Achievement of permanent or temporary biologic closure
Three: Definitive wound closure Days 1 through acute discharge (depending on donor availability)	Replacement of all temporary membranes with permanent closure Refined functional closure of face, hands, feet, and genitalia
Four: Rehabilitation and reconstruction Day 1 through first year (depending on injury severity)	Independence in activities of daily living Return to family, work, school, and community

with autografts and acute reconstruction of areas of small surface but high complexity (particularly the face and hands). The rehabilitation phase blends into the prior phase and also varies with injury severity. This fourth phase focuses on rehabilitation, reconstruction, and reintegration. In individuals with severe burns, this phase can last for years, with staged interventions, timed to minimally interfere with recovery.

PHYSIOLOGIC CHANGES WITH BURN INJURY

Like major trauma, burn injury induces a stereotypical sequence of physiologic changes that increase in magnitude and duration with injury severity and concomitant complications. A variety of efforts to modify potentially harmful elements of this physiology has been trialed but not been widely adopted. Fortunately, purposeful support of these changes is reliably successful.

Hypodynamic Phase

Postburn physiologic changes are biphasic and follow a predictable time course. Support requirements are different for each phase, as are the complications associated with inadequate support. From injury to approximately 72 hours is a hypodynamic phase, "ebb phase" or "burn shock," that is characterized by hypoperfusion and a diffuse capillary leak that roughly increases with injury size and depth. The diffuse capillary leak is assumed to be to the result of wound-released mediators and causes extravascular extravasation of fluids, electrolytes, and moderate-sized colloid molecules. Support of this phase requires individualized fluid resuscitation, which is detailed subsequently. Consequences of inadequate support include splanchnic ischemia, acute tubular necrosis, and other consequences of systemic hypoperfusion. Adverse sequelae result from overresuscitation as well, including compartment syndromes, intra-abdominal hypertension, and pulmonary edema. A timely and accurate individualized resuscitation minimizes the adverse consequences of this early postburn physiology.

Hyperdynamic Phase

In patients who have been successfully resuscitated, the early hypodynamic period is followed by a protracted phase of hyperdynamic physiology. Volume requirements fall to between 100% and 150% of a calculated maintenance rate, and cardiac output gradually increases. This physiology is characterized by fever and increased protein catabolism and is thought to be a consequence of released inflammatory mediators, cortisol, catecholamines, and glucagon. Bacterial colonization and infection exacerbate this hyperdynamic catabolic state. Support of this hyperdynamic physiology includes accurate fluid repletion, provision of adequate quantity and quality of substrate, control of environmental temperature, removal of eschar before infection, wound closure, and control of pain and anxiety.

PHASE ONE MANAGEMENT: INITIAL EVALUATION AND RESUSCITATION

The initial management of a patient with serious burns should be structured similar to that of a patient with complex trauma. In addition to the trauma considerations, a number of common pitfalls should be avoided. This is often called the burn-specific secondary survey and occurs in conjunction with fluid resuscitation.

Burn-Specific Secondary Survey

A detailed burn-specific secondary survey begins with a history. Important points include injury mechanism, initial neurologic status, extrication time, and tetanus immune status. These findings often drive subsequent imaging and management decisions.

Progressive mucosal edema can compromise airway patency over the first few postinjury hours, particularly in small children. Semiemergent intubation is indicated in the presence of worrisome facial edema, stridor, or progressive hoarseness. The presence of inhalation injury is not an absolute indication for intubation in the absence of looming airway obstruction or respiratory failure. Many patients with inhalation injury and small surface burns can be managed without intubation. Patients with coincident nonburn trauma or a large surface burn are likely to have edema develop; this should be considered in the decision for early intubation. Unplanned extubation in the patient with a burned face can be life-threatening and is best avoided though careful attention to tube security.

The head and face should be inspected for nonburn trauma. The globes should be inspected before the development of facial edema that can limit adequate examination. Burns of the globe usually impart a clouded appearance to the cornea; subtle injuries are detectable with fluorescein staining. Acute tarsorrhaphy is virtually never indicated because edema ensures globe coverage initially in the vast majority of patients, even in the presence of periocular burns. Rarely, decompression of the orbit is needed for intraocular hypertension pressures secondary to intraocular edema; this is easily effected by lateral canthotomy. Ear burns are noted, and pressure is avoided while topical mafenide acetate is applied to minimize the development of subsequent chondritis. Signs of inhalation injury should be sought, including carbonaceous oral debris and singed nasal hairs.

Neurologic status is accessed with history and examination. Imaging of the head and spine generally depends on the mechanism of injury. Pain and anxiety should be managed judiciously with small repeated intravenous doses of opiates and benzodiazepines. Obtunded patients with inhalation injury should be assessed for carbon monoxide exposure and treated with 6 hours of 100% normobaric oxygen or hyperbaric oxygen.

The chest should be assessed for symmetric air movement and compliance. Small children exposed to irritating smokes can have significant bronchospasm develop. Deep eschar should be sectioned if it interferes with ventilation.

Burned extremities must be assessed for nonburn trauma and monitored for turgor and perfusion. Tense extremities should be decompressed with escharotomy or fasciotomy. Imaging may be necessary for diagnosis of some fractures in obtunded patients. Fractured and burned extremities are initially stabilized with external splints. Progressive edema during resuscitation can result in the late development of profound limb ischemia, as a result of swelling within circumferential eschar or inelastic muscle compartments. Extremity perfusion should be monitored throughout the resuscitation period.

The burn wounds should be assessed roughly for size with the "rule-of-nines" or a Lund-Browder chart, for depth generally with physical examination, and for the presence of near-circumferential components that may require decompression (Figure 1).

Very few laboratory or imaging studies are useful initially. Carboxyhemoglobin and arterial blood gas determinations are helpful in patients with respiratory issues or inhalation injury. Chest radiographs are appropriate to ensure proper placement of lines and the

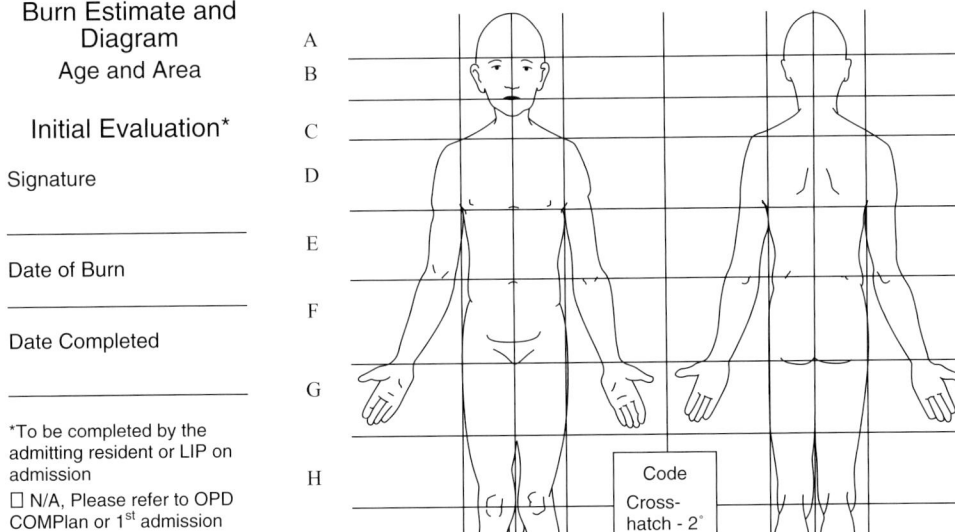

Burn Estimate and Diagram
Age and Area

Initial Evaluation*

Signature

_____

Date of Burn

_____

Date Completed

_____

*To be completed by the admitting resident or LIP on admission
☐ N/A, Please refer to OPD COMPlan or 1st admission burn diagram

This is a working burn estimate diagram only, and is not as accurate as photography.

Code
Cross-hatch - 2°
Solid - 3°

FIGURE 1 Age-adjusted charts and tables are available to help quantify burn size over a broad range of ages.

Area	Birth-1 yr.	1-4 yrs	5-9 yrs	10-14 yrs	15 yrs	Adult	2°	3°	Total
Head	19	17	13	11	9	7			
Neck	2	2	2	2	2	2			
Anterior Trunk	13	13	13	13	13	13			
Posterior Trunk	13	13	13	13	13	13			
Right Buttock	2.5	2.5	2.5	2.5	2.5	2.5			
Left Buttock	2.5	2.5	2.5	2.5	2.5	2.5			
Genitalia	1	1	1	1	1	1			
Right Upper Arm	4	4	4	4	4	4			
Left Upper Arm	4	4	4	4	4	4			
Right Lower Arm	3	3	3	3	3	3			
Left Lower Arm	3	3	3	3	3	3			
Right Hand	2.5	2.5	2.5	2.5	2.5	2.5			
Left Hand	2.5	2.5	2.5	2.5	2.5	2.5			
Right Thigh	5.5	6.5	8	8.5	9	9.5			
Left Thigh	5.5	6.5	8	8.5	9	9.5			
Right Lower Leg	5	5	5.5	6	6.5	7			
Left Lower Leg	5	5	5.5	6	6.5	7			
Right Foot	3.5	3.5	3.5	3.5	3.5	3.5			
Left Foot	3.5	3.5	3.5	3.5	3.5	3.5			
** Only 2° and 3° burns are included in the total TBSA burn percent Total									

endotracheal tube and the absence of chest trauma. The mechanism of injury dictates the need for other radiographs and laboratory studies.

All patients should be screened for abuse. In many studies, up to 20% of burns in young children are reported to state authorities for investigation, but abuse occurs in all age groups. Careful documentation of the history and injury, ideally photographic, is useful (Figure 2).

Fluid Resuscitation

In the first hour or two after even large burns, patients experience little change in intravascular volume, which explains the common observation that patients can be quite alert for the first couple of hours after injury. However, as wound-released mediators and pain-triggered hormones are absorbed, a diffuse loss of capillary integrity occurs that results in the extravasation of fluid and electrolytes. For unknown reasons, this leak abates between 18 and 24 hours later in well-resuscitated patients. Increased leakage is routinely seen in patients whose resuscitations are delayed and in those with inhalation injury, possibly contributed to by a whole-body ischemia-reperfusion reaction.

A variety of body and burn size adjusted burn fluid resuscitation formulas have been promulgated over the past 50 years. None are universally accurate in light of the inherent variability of burn wounds and patients. A common consensus is based on the modified Brooke formula, which recommends administration of 2 to 4 mL/kg/percent burn of Ringer's lactate solution over the first 24 postinjury hours (half in the first 8 postinjury hours) and a small dose of colloid (5% albumin solution) from hour 24 to hour 48 (Table 2). However, numerous publications have described the widely varying individual needs of burn patients. No formula is accurate enough to be relied on in actual practice. Quality resuscitation requires an hourly reevaluation of physiologic endpoints with adjustment of infusions accordingly. Markers of adequate resuscitation include normal vital signs, urine output, and peripheral perfusion (Box 1).

The role of colloid in burn resuscitation is increasingly controversial. The trauma literature shows that many practitioners use colloid early during resuscitation. This author's routine practice is to administer a maintenance rate of 5% albumin to most patients with burns in excess of 30% from the beginning of resuscitation, subtracting this from the calculated crystalloid rate. The crystalloid rate is weaned as tolerated based on serial measurement of resuscitation endpoints. In small children, a maintenance rate of 5% dextrose in lactated Ringer's solution substitutes for an equal portion of calculated Ringer's lactate solution. The practice of early colloid administration seems to be associated with reduced overall fluid requirements and a reduced incidence of morbidity related to edema. Patients with burns smaller than 15% generally do not need a calculated resuscitation; they are well managed with 150% of maintenance needs and careful clinical monitoring of hydration.

TABLE 2: Consensus resuscitation formula

First 24 Hours

Adults and children >20 kg

Ringer's lactate solution: 2-4 mL/kg/% burn/24 h (first half in first 8 h)

Colloid: None*

Children <20 kg

Ringer's lactate solution: 2-3 mL/kg/% burn/24 h (first half in first 8 h)

Ringer's lactate solution with 5% dextrose: maintenance rate (approximately 4 mL/kg/h for the first 10 kg, 2 mL/kg/h for the next 10 kg; and 1 mL/kg/h for weight >20 kg)

Colloid: None*

Second 24 Hours

All patients

Crystalloid: To maintain urine output. If silver nitrate is used, sodium leeching mandates continued isotonic crystalloid. If other topical is used, free water requirement is significant. Serum sodium should be monitored closely. Nutritional support should begin, ideally via the enteral route. Total input generally approximately 140% maintenance, depending on injury severity.

Colloid* (5% albumin in Ringer's lactate solution):

0-30% burn:	None
30%-50% burn:	0.3 mL/kg/% burn/24 h
50%-70% burn:	0.4 mL/kg/% burn/24 h
70%-100% burn:	0.5 mL/kg/% burn/24 h

*An increasing body of clinical practice favors earlier institution of colloid. This author routinely substitutes 100% maintenance rate of calculated Ringer's lactate solution with equal volume of 5% albumin beginning at start of resuscitation in patients with larger injuries.

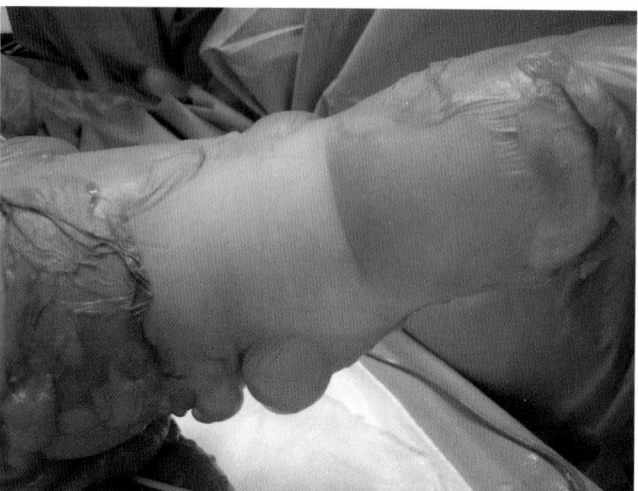

FIGURE 2 Flexor sparing suggests possible immersion of a flexed body part and is seen here in the popliteal fossa.

BOX 1: Burn resuscitation endpoints

Sensorium: Arousable and comfortable
Digital temperature: Warm peripherally
Systolic blood pressure: For infants, 60 mm Hg systolic; for older children, 70 to 90, plus 2× age in years, mm Hg; for adults, mean arterial pressure over 60 mm Hg
Pulse: 80-180 per minute (age-dependent)
Urine output: 0.5-1 mL/kg/h (glucose-negative)
Base deficit: <2

PHASE TWO MANAGEMENT: WOUND EXCISION AND BIOLOGIC CLOSURE

If fluid resuscitation reduces morbidity and mortality from otherwise inevitable burn shock, early wound excision and closure reduces morbidity and mortality from otherwise inevitable burn wound sepsis. "Early" has been variably defined but implies excision is complete before heavy wound colonization and infection has occurred, generally within the first few days after injury. The definition of "early" varies with the severity of the wound, the stability of the patient, and the resources available for surgery and critical care support. Although conceptually logical, a relative paucity of data remains to support the strategy. Serial physical examination by an experienced surgeon remains the most reliable method of determination of need for wound excision. When carefully planned, appropriately staged, and expeditiously performed with hemostatic techniques, these operations are well tolerated by most patients.

Determination of the Need, Timing, and Extent of Operation

Burn size and depth drive the need for and timing of burn wound excision. Patients with small superficial burns rarely have systemic sepsis develop and can be safely treated with topical therapy, with only grafting of small nonhealed areas subsequently. Very deep dermal and full-thickness burns are best identified early and excised and grafted promptly, to minimize septic morbidity, patient suffering, hypertrophic scarring, and hospital length of stay.

Patients with large injuries benefit from a more aggressive surgical approach because the injury size alone presents a physiologic threat. The objective of operation is to identify, excise, and achieve biologic closure of all full-thickness components. When the wounds are very large, this may necessitate staged procedures. If autograft is temporarily exhausted or if patient conditions are not stable, temporary biologic closure of excised wounds can be achieved with human allograft Integra (Integra Life Sciences, Plainsboro, NJ), or other temporary wound closure materials.

Techniques of Burn Wound Excision

Wounds that are superficial require no excision and are simply cleansed and treated with topical medications or temporary biologic dressings. Middermal wounds can be similarly addressed. Topical proteolytic enzymes can be useful in such wounds but have not been widely adopted because currently available formulations débride over days rather than hours. Very deep dermal wounds are often excised and grafted because healing is generally quite prolonged with a high incidence of hypertrophic scarring. Deep dermal excisions should only be done when they quite clearly will give better results than those obtained with protracted topical care. Full-thickness wounds are ideally excised with a layered technique to viable subcutaneous fat to optimize function and contour. It is important to conform grafts to the small irregularities of such wound beds and to prevent exposure and desiccation of subcutaneous fat because this results in compromised engraftment.

Fascial excisions are much less frequently done today than in prior decades because they may exacerbate aesthetic and functional deformities. However, they are still indicated if burns involve subcutaneous fat or if patients have massive full-thickness burns and the risk of graft loss on extensive wounds excised to subcutaneous fat is life threatening. Fascial excisions can be hemostatically performed with coagulating electrocautery, which provides excellent hemostasis and a clear viable plane that reliably accepts autograft. The plume from these excisions can be controlled with a high-efficiency suction device. Subfascial excisions are infrequently necessary in high-voltage electrical injuries or remarkably deep thermal burns. Exploration of muscle compartments can readily be done through decompressive fasciotomy incisions. Definitive closure may require delayed grafting, local flaps, or free tissue transfer.

Hemostatic Excision Techniques

Historically, burn wound excision was associated with substantial blood loss because free capillary bleeding was used to ensure tissue viability. Several very simple maneuvers, when practiced, minimize blood loss during these operations. Careful planning before excision reduces operating time, which itself can markedly reduce blood loss. Performing extremity excisions after inflation of a pneumatic tourniquet and wrapping the extremity in a hemostatic dressing before tourniquet deflation reduce blood loss. Layered torso excisions and donor skin procurement after dilute epinephrine clysis is very effective in reducing bleeding. Use of coagulating cautery to perform fascial excisions keeps these fields dry. Tissue viability can be determined with the practiced eye looking for bright moist yellow fat, patent small blood vessels, the absence of thrombosis of small vessels, and the absence of extravascular hemoglobin. Maintaining patient euthermia enhances innate coagulation mechanisms and is best done through operating room heating. Minimized blood loss in burn excision is an essential element in successful management of large wounds.

BURN CRITICAL CARE

Critical care is an integral component of all aspects of burn care, but it is a particularly prominent component of the period of wound excision and closure. An imbedded or seamlessly integrated critical care unit is an essential element of a successful burn program. Although many burn patients need additional temperature support and wound care, they can be well managed in trauma or general surgical intensive care units with the proper coordination.

Inhalation Injury

Inhalation injury complicates care of those injured in structural fires; it causes variable degrees of upper airway edema from direct thermal injury, bronchospasm from aerosolized irritants, small airway occlusion from sloughed endobronchial debris and loss of the ciliary clearance mechanism, increased dead space and intrapulmonary shunting from alveolar flooding, decreased lung and chest wall compliance from interstitial and alveolar edema and swelling or burn of the chest wall, and secondary infection of the denuded tracheobronchial tree (tracheobronchitis) or pulmonary parenchyma (pneumonia). The diagnosis of inhalation injury is usually clinical, based on a history of closed space exposure, burns of the face or nasal hairs, and carbonaceous debris in the mouth or sputum. Routine early diagnostic or therapeutic bronchoscopy has no clearly demonstrated value. Patients with inhalation injury usually have 2 to 5 days of relatively normal gas exchange before endobronchial slough with associated infection and respiratory compromise. Use of this window of relatively normal pulmonary function to effect large initial excisions is important.

Carbon monoxide (CO) binds avidly to heme-containing enzymes, most notably hemoglobin and mitochondrial cytochromes, interfering with oxygen delivery and utilization, respectively. Such patients can be treated with 6 hours of normobaric 100% oxygen. If patients have stable conditions and have no contraindications (particularly mucous plugging or bronchospasm), hyperbaric oxygen may diminish a small incidence of long-term neurologic sequelae. However, these treatments are not without risk, and not all studies support the efficacy of hyperbaric oxygen in this regard.

Pneumonia, tracheobronchitis, and respiratory failure occur in approximately 30% of those with inhalation injury, as a result of loss of the ciliary clearance mechanism and sloughed endobronchial debris. Antibiotic therapy is directed by sputum gram stain and cultures and should not be prolonged beyond a 7-day to 10-day therapeutic course. Vigorous pulmonary toilet is an important component of therapy. When gas exchange failure requires mechanical support, patients should be managed with the same low-volume strategy widely practiced in general surgical intensive care units today. Tracheostomy is useful if prolonged ventilation or difficult weaning is anticipated. It is ideal if neck edema has subsided so that the procedure is not technically difficult. Tracheostomy in small children may be associated with a higher incidence of prolonged cannulation and long-term complications and is ideally avoided when possible.

Neurologic Issues

Peripheral neuropathies develop in about 5% of patients with serious burns. These are secondary to direct thermal injury, metabolic derangements, compartment syndromes, or pressure. Some may be avoided with tight control of electrolyte disturbances, prompt decompression of ischemic extremities, and attention to the fitting of splints and intraoperative position.

Multidisciplinary management of treatment-related burn pain and anxiety enhances short-term and long-term outcomes. Opiate and benzodiazepine synergy facilitates good control with modest drug doses. Newer agents, such as dexmedetomidine, can further help control symptoms while minimizing morbidity related to higher opiate and benzodiazepine dosing. Nonpharmacologic interventions and wound membranes are playing an increasing role in control of the inevitable treatment-related burn pain and anxiety.

Postresuscitation Hemodynamic and Electrolyte Issues

After resuscitation, burn patients predictably have hyperdynamic hemodynamics develop, with a high cardiac output and low peripheral resistance. This physiology is exacerbated by wound colonization and sepsis. Intravascular volume is best judged with serial physical examination, intravascular pressures, urine output, serum osmolality, base deficit, and serum sodium concentration.

Cerebral edema and seizures have been reported with rapid development of hyponatremia during burn resuscitation with hypotonic fluids. Overly rapid correction of hyponatremia is associated with demyelination. Many patients have development of derangements of serum potassium, magnesium, and phosphate. These issues are best avoided through careful control of serum electrolytes. Patients with large open wounds are at particular risk because evaporative free water loss and transeschar electrolyte flux are impossible to predict with accuracy.

Most patients with large burns require protracted central vascular access. Rotation of catheters to diminish the incidence of catheter sepsis is variably practiced. The author is convinced that a weekly rotation of catheters is a reasonable compromise that minimizes both catheter-related sepsis and the mechanical complications. If antiseptic catheters are used, durations out to 2 weeks seem safe.

Nutritional Support

The hypermetabolic response to burns is characterized by fever, increased metabolic rate, increased minute ventilation, increased cardiac output, decreased afterload, increased gluconeogenesis, insulin resistance, and increased skeletal and visceral muscle catabolism. Patients remain hypermetabolic for a variable period after

wound closure. Modification of the catabolic component of the response is desirable and may be aided with anabolic steroids or beta-blockade. Most patients do very well if the physiology is supported through accurate nutritional support. Overfeeding is associated with hepatic steatosis, dysfunction, and increased CO_2 production. Underfeeding results in inanition and poor wound healing.

Basal metabolic rate can be calculated with a number of formulas. Resting energy expenditure can be roughly measured with expired gas indirect calorimetry. Most authors advocate provision of 150% of basal energy needs for burn patients managed with prompt wound excision and closure. Protein administration of 2.5 g/kg/d adequately supports the needs of most burn patients. Most patients can be supported enterally, beginning coincident with resuscitation. This author generally begins with nasogastric sump tubes because these tubes facilitate assessment of gastric residuals. These are subsequently changed to a soft enteral feeding tube. Occasional patients with very large wounds or septic complications do not tolerate enteral feedings; supplemental parenteral nutrition is a safe and useful adjunct.

Septic Complications and Multiple Organ Failure

Burn patients have immunosuppression, compromised epithelial barriers, and multiple invasive devices. They are prone to a host of septic complications until wound closure is complete. Infection control measures should be rigorously followed to prevent cross contamination. Multiple organ dysfunction is a manifestation of uncontrolled systemic inflammation, infection, or tissue hypoxia. Successful management requires identification and treatment of any septic foci, including excision of infected eschar, hemodynamic support, and management of failing organ systems.

PHASE THREE MANAGEMENT: DEFINITIVE WOUND CLOSURE

Phase three involves replacement of temporary membranes and completion of closure of physiologically small but functionally important areas, such as the face and hands. At this point, most patients are extubated and have bulk physiologic wound closure and hemodynamically stable conditions.

Skin Substitutes

Most deep burn wounds are best closed as quickly as possible with split-thickness autograft. Currently available skin substitutes are designed to be temporary or permanent. A large number of temporary membranes are designed to provide a vapor and bacterial barrier and enhance pain control as underlying wounds epithelialize. These membranes minimize the need for dressing changes and are particularly useful in the outpatient setting. A very limited number of membranes are designed to become incorporated into the wound as permanent dermal or epidermal elements. For now, these membranes are useful only in a very small minority of patients with massive injuries. When a practical permanent skin replacement becomes available, it will profoundly change the nature of acute and reconstructive burn care.

Face and Head

Burns of the face are physiologically small but aesthetically and functionally critical. Patients with larger burns are ideally approached in a thoughtful manner after bulk wound closure has been achieved and conditions are stable. Skin of the nose and central face is thick and rich in sweat and sebaceous glands; even deep second-degree burns often heal with quite a nice result when they are managed with good topical wound care. Anatomy of the skin in this area makes a conservative initial approach physiologically sound. No topical or membrane is clearly superior to another for facial burn management. Common practice is to apply petroleum-based ointments containing antibiotics on superficial burns and silver sulphadiazine on deeper wounds. Burns around the eyes can be dressed with topical ophthalmic antibiotic ointments. Those facial wounds that need to be grafted should be resurfaced with thick split-thickness grafts of optimal color match in cosmetic units as long as this does not require the sacrifice of significant areas of healed burn or unburned skin (Figure 3). Excisions are done in a layered fashion. The operations can be bloody, but subeschar dilute epinephrine clysis and elevation of the head of the operating table reduce blood loss. After the grafts have vascularized, massage and pressure therapy should begin.

External ear burns are best managed with avoidance of pressure on the burned auricle and prevention of auricular chondritis with application of topical mafenide acetate, which penetrates the cartilage. Subsequent management is based on depth of injury. Wounds generated by débridement of necrotic skin and cartilage can generally be closed with thin split-thickness grafts with good aesthetic results.

If eyelid burns are present, globe protection from edema is generally good for the first 1 to 2 weeks. An acute tarsorrhaphy is almost never necessary. This can be followed by contraction and globe exposure. When this is relatively mild, no intervention beyond globe lubrication and monitoring is necessary. Should exposure keratitis occur, early lid release should be performed to prevent corneal desiccation, ulceration, and infection (Figure 4).

Hands and Feet

During the first 72 hours, hand perfusion should be optimized with escharotomy and fasciotomy as needed and hemodynamic support. Seriously burned hands should be ranged twice daily and at other times elevated and splinted in a position of function. Deep dermal

and full-thickness burns should undergo excision and grafting as soon as practical and splinted; ranging can generally commence a few days later. Burns of the feet are managed similarly. Neutral ankle position is important to maintain in bedridden patients.

PHASE FOUR MANAGEMENT: RECONSTRUCTION AND REINTEGRATION

Expectations for the quality of burn recovery are now high. Patients are surviving serious burns more routinely. These facts have quietly increased the need for and complexity of burn rehabilitation and reconstruction. High-quality functional and aesthetic outcomes are most effectively delivered by a coordinated burn aftercare program, rather than isolated physical therapists and surgeons.

Burn Rehabilitation

Attention to this issue should start early during the acute hospitalization. Ranging and antideformity positioning and splinting minimize the otherwise inevitable capsular contraction and shortening of tendon and muscle groups, which complicate later rehabilitation efforts (Table 3). As the patient with serious burns is weaned from the critical care environment, rehabilitation efforts begin to focus on active ranging and strengthening, reduction of edema, and activities of daily living. A good program of passive ranging during critical illness pays great dividends here.

In the outpatient setting, the rehabilitation focus moves toward strengthening, work-hardening, postoperative therapy after reconstructive operations, and scar management. The number of tools available to manage scar maturation has increased in recent years. Pruritus, discomfort, contraction, and thickening are not inevitable. In wounds destined to become hypertrophic, a marked increase in neovessel formation and erythema is seen 2 or 3 months after healing. Optimally, these areas are identified and become the focus of efforts to modulate scar development. Available methods include scar massage, compression garments, topical silicone, steroid injections, serial casting, tunable dye and fractional carbon dioxide lasers, and surgery. No one of these tools is usually successful alone. They must be applied within a multimodality program, best coordinated in a burn aftercare program.

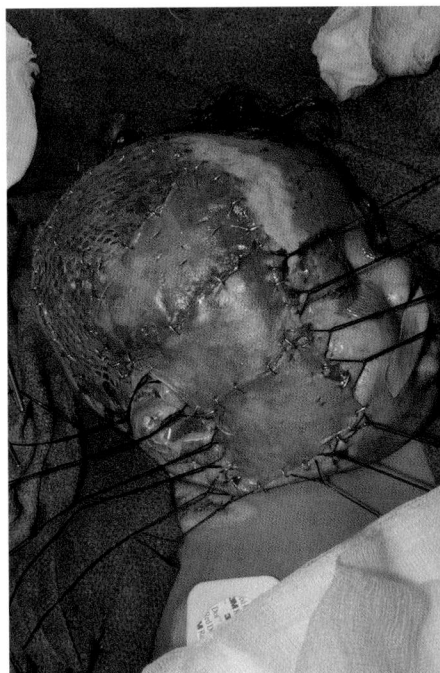

FIGURE 3 Facial grafting does not require sacrifice of well-healed wounds or unburned skin to complete aesthetic units.

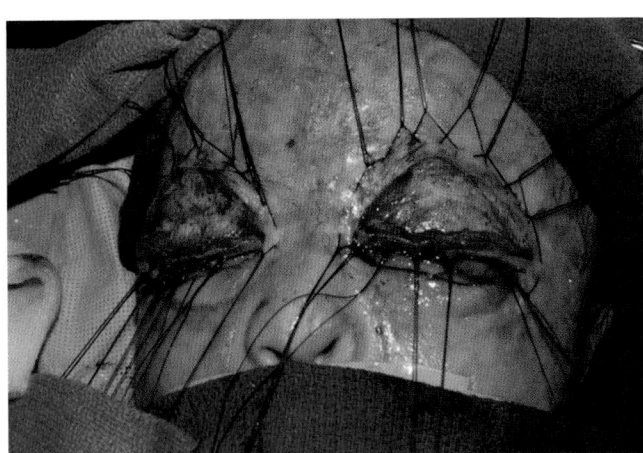

FIGURE 4 If lid contracture leads to exposure keratitis, early lid release should be performed to prevent corneal desiccation, ulceration, and infection.

TABLE 3: Common burn unit contractures and prevention strategies

Common contracture	Splinting and positioning strategy
Neck flexion	Daily ranging and extension splinting and conformers, split mattress
Shoulder adduction	Daily ranging and abduction splinting with axillary splints or troughs
Elbow flexion and extension	Daily ranging and alternating extension and flexion splints
Wrist flexion and extension	Daily ranging and splinting in functional position (20 degrees of extension)
Metacarpophalangeal (MCP) joint extension	Daily ranging and splinting in functional position (MCP joints at 70-90 degrees with interphalangeal joints in extension)
Hip flexion	Daily ranging and extension splints and prone positioning (if tolerated)
Knee flexion	Daily ranging and knee splints and knee immobilizers
Ankle extension	Daily ranging and neutral splints
Metatarsophalangeal joint extension	Daily ranging and splinting in functional position, rocker bottom shoes

Early Burn Reconstruction

A plan of acute burn reconstruction should be made collaboratively with the patient, family, therapists, and surgeon. A list of surgical needs should be balanced with the patient's reintegration plans. Woven into the plan should be ongoing scar management and rehabilitation efforts. Early facial reconstruction primarily involves function. Lip eversion, microstomia, thickened nasolabial bands, canthal webs, and obstruction or distortion of the nares may develop, depending on the severity of the initial burn and efficacy of initial treatment. Hand and upper extremity deformities should also be addressed on presentation if they significantly limit function. Most common are dorsal hand and web spaces. Burn boutonniere deformities are difficult to treat if they become established and should also be addressed early. On occasion, heterotopic ossification develops early, most commonly forming in the soft tissues around the triceps tendon of deeply burned elbows. This may resolve with resolution of systemic inflammation; but when it is severe, it usually requires surgery. Axillary contractures are usually amendable to simple reconstruction and should be addressed if they limit activities of daily living. Lower extremity contractures that limit ambulation and sitting should also be addressed in the early postacute period. The most common issues are dorsal foot, popliteal, and flexion hip contractures. All are generally amenable to simple stellate release and graft reconstruction.

Outpatient Burn Care

Most burn patients can be managed as outpatients. Those who need hospitalization receive major parts of the overall care in the outpatient setting. Ideally, a seamless interface occurs between the inpatient and the outpatient setting. Quality outpatient burn care is neither simple nor easy, and if done poorly, it results in significant pain and morbidity. Key components of a successful program are elaborated in Table 3 and include prudent patient selection, caregiver identification and teaching, simple wound hygiene and topical care, judicious pain management, specific hospitalization and follow-up teaching, and long-term follow-up.

CONCLUSION

A number of other issues, including high-voltage electrical injuries, chemical and tar burns, cold injuries, toxic epidermal necrolysis, and soft tissue infections, are commonly managed in burn programs and are addressed in other chapters. The burn unit offers a critical care and wound management resource useful for many of these patients. Patients with burns or complex wound needs are best managed in an organized program of care that seamlessly spans the continuum from resuscitation through reintegration. An increasing body of data supports the efficacy and cost effectiveness of this concept. Ultimately, it is the happiness and success of our patients that provides the most important endorsement.

SUGGESTED READINGS

Cancio LC, Lundy JB, Sheridan RL: Evolving changes in the management of burns and environmental injuries, *Surg Clin North Am* 92(4):959–986, 2012.

Caruso TJ, Janik LS, Fuzaylov G: Airway management of recovered pediatric patients with severe head and neck burns: a review, *Paediatr Anaesth* 22(5):462–468, 2012.

Donelan MB, Parrett BM, Sheridan R: Pulsed dye laser therapy and z-plasty for facial burn scars: the alternative to excision, *Ann Plast Surg* 60(5):480–486, 2008.

Sheridan R: Closure of the excised burn wound: autografts, semipermanent skin substitutes, and permanent skin substitutes, *Clin Plast Surg* 36(4):643–651, 2009.

Sheridan RL: Comprehensive treatment of burns, *Curr Probl Surg* 38(9):657–756, 2001.

Sheridan RL: Burn care: results of technical and organizational progress, *JAMA* 290(6):719–722, 2003.

Sterling JP, Heimbach DM: Hemostasis in burn surgery: a review, *Burns* 37(4):559–565, 2011.

Williams FN, Pham TN, Klein MB, et al: What, how, and how much should burn patients be fed? *Surg Clin North Am* 91(3):609–629, 2011.

COLD INJURY, FROSTBITE, AND HYPOTHERMIA

Colleen M. Ryan, MD, and Philip H. Chang, MD

OVERVIEW

Localized cold injuries can be classified according to the temperatures that produce them, either freezing or nonfreezing temperatures. Trench foot, immersion hand and foot, and chilblains (pernio) are all produced by exposure to nonfreezing temperatures. Freezing temperatures produce frostbite. Generalized cold injury presents as hypothermia. Hypothermia can be from environmental exposure or can be medically induced for treatment of anoxic conditions.

NONFREEZING COLD INJURIES

Trench Foot, Immersion Foot (Cold)

Prolonged exposure (as little as 13 hours) to nonfreezing cold temperatures (32°F to 60°F) in the presence of moisture can result in trench foot. Cold immersion foot (or hand) is seen after prolonged exposure to cold but not freezing water. Trench foot was a significant public health issue during World War I, when soldiers spent days in the wet mud of the war trenches in ill-fitting shoes. It resulted in tremendous suffering and often required amputation for gangrene. These injuries involve alternating arterial vasospasm and vasodilation, with the affected tissue first cold and numb. After 24 to 48 hours of exposure, hyperemia occurs, accompanied by dysesthesias and severe burning pain. Tissue damage is evidenced by edema, blistering, redness, ecchymosis, and ulceration. Complications include cellulitis and gangrene. Late findings can include tissue cyanosis with increased sensitivity to cold. Pain, paresthesias, and nerve paralysis can be seen after all types of cold injuries.

Prevention consists of keeping feet warm and dry and prevention and management of hyperhidrosis. In World War I, the requirement for soldiers to carry extra pairs of socks and the pairing of soldiers to inspect each other's feet prevented trench foot. Treatment consists of immediate removal of the extremity from the cold wet environment and exposure of the feet (or hands) to warm dry air. The extremity should be elevated to minimize edema and protected from pressure injuries from ill-fitting shoes. Local and occasionally systemic measures to combat infection are indicated. Massage, soaking of the feet, and rapid rewarming are not indicated. Demyelination of nerves, muscle atrophy, fallen arches, and osteoporosis may all present as long-term complications, and a tendency toward marked vasospasm during subsequent exposure to cold develops in some patients.

Chilblains (Pernio)

Repetitive exposure to cold and damp, but not freezing temperatures, can result in chilblains, also known as pernio, perniosis, or blain. These terms are descriptive for the consequences of local cold injury. Acute chilblains is characterized by pruritic red-purple papules, macules, plaques, or nodules on the skin, usually the face, the anterior surface of the tibia, or the dorsum of the hands and feet, and can occur within hours of the exposure. Chronic chilblains can also occur

and persist long after the cold exposure. The lesions can blister and ulcerate, making them susceptible to secondary infection. Women, infants, and the elderly are at risk. Medical conditions such as chronic myelomonocytic leukemia, lupus, and anorexia nervosa can be associated with chilblains.

Treatment consists of sheltering the patient, elevating the affected part, and allowing gradual rewarming at room temperature. Rubbing and massage are contraindicated because they can cause further damage and secondary infection. Severe itching can be treated with topical steroids, and open lesions with topical antibiotics. Nifedipine promotes faster healing and prevents recurrence. Lesions usually subside in 2 to 3 weeks, but hypersensitivity can persist. Depigmentation and scarring can result.

FREEZING COLD INJURIES

Frostnip

Frostnip occurs with brief exposures to freezing temperatures when ice crystals, appearing as a frost, form on the surface of the skin, usually on the exposed skin of the face. An intense local vasoconstriction occurs, which results in numbness and pallor. By definition, ice crystals do not form in the tissue nor does tissue loss occur in frostnip. The numbness and pallor resolve quickly with rewarming, and no long-term damage occurs. The appearance of frostnip signals conditions favorable for frostbite, and appropriate action should be undertaken immediately to prevent injury.

Frostbite

Tissue injury from freezing temperatures, frostbite, evolves through four overlapping processes. First, during the prefreeze stage, vasoconstriction and ischemia occur devoid of ice crystallization. Paresthesias and pain are associated with neuronal cooling. Second, ice crystals form intracellularly (during a more rapid-onset freezing injury) or extracellularly (during a slower freeze) during the freeze-thaw stage. This causes alteration in proteins, lipids, and intracellular electrolytes, resulting in intracellular dehydration, membrane disruption, and cell death. The thawing process brings ischemia-reperfusion injury and inflammation. Third, a vascular stasis stage occurs in which blood vessels constrict and dilate. Blood coagulates within the vessels or leaks into the tissues. Fourth and finally, the late ischemic phase results from progressive tissue ischemia, infarction, and inflammation from continued reperfusion injury, microemboli, and thrombus formation. The microcirculation is destroyed, resulting in further cell death.

CLASSIFICATION OF FROSTBITE

Frostbite has been historically classified into degrees of injury depending on the depth of damage, paralleling the classification of burn injuries. Often, several degrees of injury are seen in the same extremity. These classifications are based on the physical examination after rewarming.

First-degree frostbite is a superficial skin injury that is characterized by numbness, edema, and erythema. A white or yellow firm, slightly raised plaque develops in the area of injury. The injury heals spontaneously, usually within 1 to 2 weeks. Superficial desquamation can occur (Figure 1).

Second-degree frostbite injury results in numbness, edema, erythema, and vesiculation. Blisters can contain a clear or milky fluid and are surrounded by erythema and edema (Figure 2). This partial

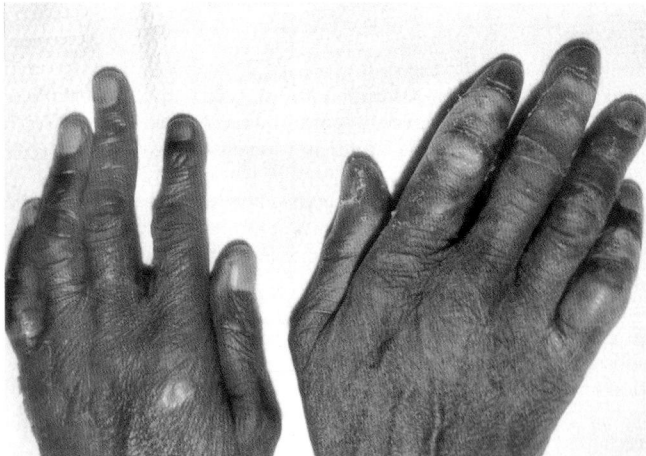

FIGURE 1 First-degree and second-degree frostbite. Epidermal skin loss and peeling are seen.

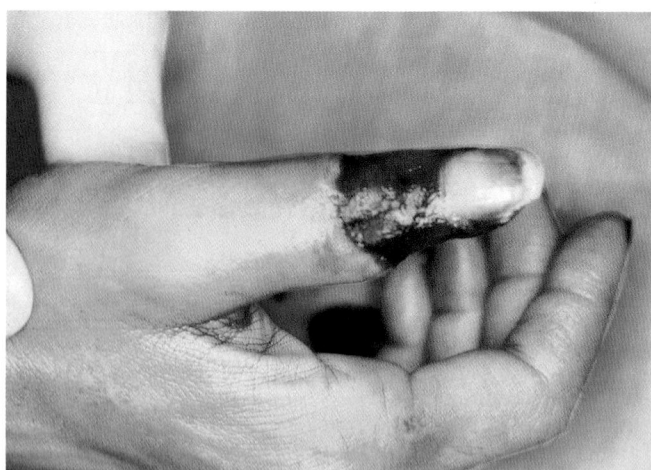

FIGURE 3 Third-degree and fourth-degree frostbite with tissue death; note demarcation beyond the interphalangeal joint.

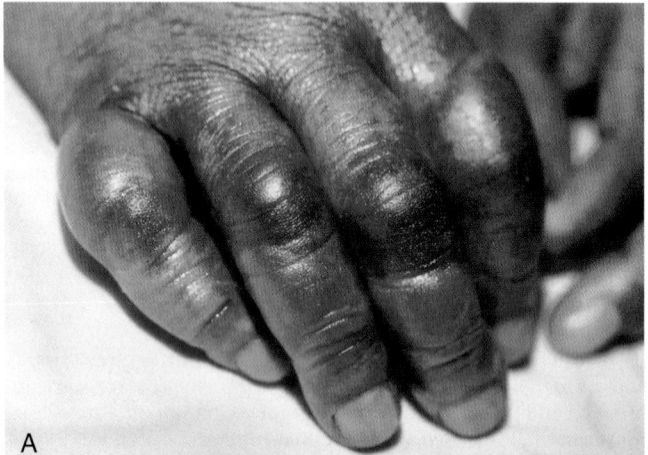

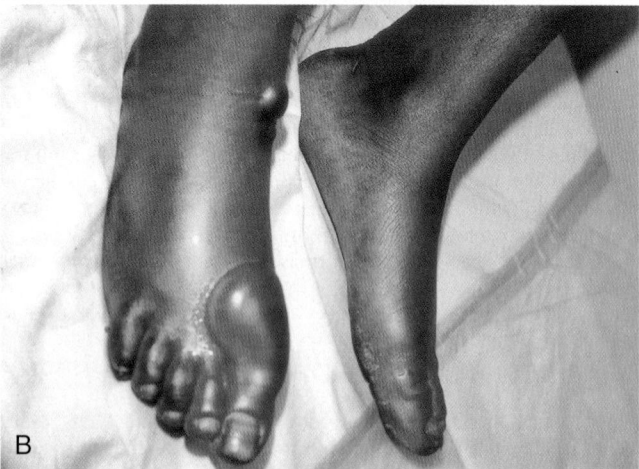

FIGURE 2 **A,** Second-degree frostbite in the fingers. Vesicles and swelling are seen. **B,** Second-degree frostbite in the feet. Vesicles and swelling are seen.

thickness injury heals in 2 to 4 weeks. The healed skin is atrophic and has a reduced number of skin appendages.

Third-degree frostbite creates deeper hemorrhagic blisters, which indicate full-thickness loss. Nonviable skin can present initially as a gray-blue patch, or death of the skin may follow an initial period of

reactive hyperemia after 24 to 72 hours. Eventually, a black eschar forms and generally separates slowly in 1 to 3 months (Figure 3).

Fourth-degree frostbite injury results in necrosis that extends completely through the dermis and into muscle and to the level of bone. The black, mummified tissues are present with the initial episode. If infection develops, the mummified tissue softens and adjacent viable margin becomes swollen and macerated.

A simpler classification scheme is used in the field and before rewarming. Superficial injuries have no anticipated tissue loss (corresponding to first-degree and second-degree injuries), and deep injuries have anticipated tissue loss (corresponding to third-degree and fourth-degree injuries).

PREVENTION OF FROSTBITE

Frostbite is typically preventable. The risk of frostbite is related to underlying medical problems, and prevention must address both the environmental and the medical issues that put the person at risk. When tissue heat loss exceeds the ability of local tissue perfusion to maintain the temperature of the tissues above freezing, frostbite occurs. Environmental conditions below –15°C, even with low wind speeds, increase the risk of frostbite.

Key elements to prevent frostbite include maintenance of core temperature and hydration, minimization of effects of drugs and diseases that decrease perfusion, maintenance of covering on skin and scalp, minimization of restrictive clothing, and maintenance of exercise to encourage peripheral vasodilation. Skin should be protected from moisture and wind, and clothing should be layered. The ability to respond appropriately to changing environmental conditions is often compromised by alcohol, drugs, or anoxia.

INITIAL FIELD TREATMENT OF FROSTBITE

Treatment of hypothermia or serious trauma is the first priority if present. No specific studies examine concurrent hypothermia and frostbite. Hypothermia frequently accompanies frostbite and causes peripheral vasoconstriction that impairs blood flow to the extremities. Mild hypothermia may be treated concurrently with the frostbite injury. Moderate and severe hypothermia should be treated effectively *before* treatment of the frostbite injury.

If a body part is frozen in the field, the frozen tissue should be protected from further damage. Jewelry should be removed. The affected area should be rapidly rewarmed in water heated and maintained between 37°C and 39°C (98.6°F and 102.2°F) until the area becomes soft and pliable to the touch (approximately 30 minutes). Rapid rewarming is preferred; however, if it is not available and repeat freezing is not expected, the affected area should be allowed to thaw spontaneously. Refreezing can exacerbate the injury by recycling through the freeze-thaw stage, increasing inflammatory mediators, vasoconstriction, and thrombosis.

Rewarming is painful, and opiates should be administered as needed. The affected area should be air dried, wrapped in dry bulky dressings, and elevated if possible. Topical aloe vera cream or gel can be used if available. Further trauma to the affected part should be avoided. Hydration should be administered as available.

MEDICAL THERAPY

Treatment of trauma and hypothermia remains a priority once the patient reaches the hospital. The patient should be hydrated. Rapid rewarming of the part should be undertaken as previously described unless already done in the field.

Clear or cloudy blisters contain prostaglandins and thromboxanes that may damage underlying tissue. Hemorrhagic blisters are thought to signify deeper tissue damage into the dermal vascular plexus. Common practice is to selectively drain clear blisters (e.g., with needle aspiration) and leave hemorrhagic blisters intact. Although this selective débridement is recommended by many authorities, comparative studies have not been performed and data are insufficient to make absolute recommendations. Some authors argue that unroofing blisters may lead to the desiccation of exposed tissue and that blisters should only be removed if they are tense, likely to be infected, or interfere with the patient's range of motion. Débridement or aspiration of clear, cloudy, or tense blisters may be at the discretion of the treating provider, with consideration of patient circumstances, until better evidence is available.

Wounds should be dressed with dry sterile dressings. Topical aloe vera cream or gel can be applied to the thawed tissue with each dressing change. Extremities should be splinted in positions of function, and pressure areas should be avoided. Ambulation should be initially avoided in lower extremity injuries unless it is limited to the toes. Systemic antibiotics are not indicated unless there are signs of cellulitis or sepsis. Tetanus prophylaxis should be administered according to standard guidelines.

Ibuprofen is recommended at a lower dose of 12 mg/kg divided twice daily (to inhibit harmful prostaglandins but remain safer on the gastrointestinal system) until the frostbite wound is healed or surgical management occurs (typically 4 to 6 weeks).

THROMBOLYTIC, VASODILATOR, AND PROSTACYCLIN THERAPY

The goal of thrombolytic therapy in frostbite injury is to address microvascular thrombosis. Thrombolytic therapy should be reserved for deep frostbite injuries and should be administered in settings with resources for intensive care unit (ICU) care and experienced surgical assessment. For deep frostbite injury with potential significant morbidity, angiography and use of either intravenous (IV) or intraarterial tissue plasminogen activator (t-PA) within 24 hours of thawing may salvage some or all tissue at risk. The potential risks of t-PA include systemic and catheter-site bleeding, compartment syndrome, and failure to salvage tissue. The long-term functional consequences of digit salvage with t-PA have also not been evaluated. Use of t-PA in the field setting is not recommended because detection and treatment of bleeding complications may be impossible. Published protocols include the use of heparin in conjunction with thrombolytic therapy to prevent recurrent local thrombosis, and heparin is recommended in this circumstance as adjunctive therapy. Angiography or pyrophosphate scanning should be used to evaluate the initial injury and monitor progress after t-PA administration as directed by local protocol and resources (angiography scanning for intraarterial, and pyrophosphate scanning for IV).

No evidence supports the use of low molecular-weight heparin or unfractionated heparin as a monotherapy for initial management of frostbite in the field or hospital. Vasodilators, such as prostaglandin E1 (PGE1), the prostacyclin analogue iloprost, nitroglycerin, pentoxifylline, phenoxybenzamine, nifedipine, reserpine, and buflomedil, have been used as primary and adjunctive therapies in the treatment of frostbite injuries. In addition to vasodilation, some of these agents may also prevent platelet aggregation and microvascular occlusion that occur after frostbite. Intraarterial infusion of nitroglycerin during angiography, before t-PA infusion, has been recommended. Pentoxifylline, a methylxanthine-derived phosphodiesterase inhibitor, has yielded some promising results in animal and human frostbite. Controlled-release pentoxifylline, one 400-mg tablet 3 times a day with meals, is continued for 2 to 6 weeks after injury. However, controlled studies of pentoxifylline in the management of frostbite have yet to be performed. Buflomedil is an alpha adrenolytic agent that is used widely in Europe with some preliminary and anecdotal evidence of good results; however, animal models have not replicated these findings. In addition, the medication is not approved by the U.S. Food and Drug Administration. Intraarterial reserpine has been studied in a case–control study and found not to be effective.

Certain vasodilators have the potential to improve outcomes and can be used with minimal risk. However, as discussed previously, the data that show benefit are limited. Iloprost is the only vasodilator with reasonable scientific evidence supporting its use, although it is currently not available in many countries, including the United States.

Other postthaw medical therapies, including hyperbaric oxygen, hydrotherapy, sympathectomy, and IV guanethidine, have insufficient data to support their use.

SURGICAL INTERVENTION

Significant swelling should prompt an evaluation for compartment syndrome. Thawing reperfuses ischemic tissue that, in turn, can result in the development of elevated pressures within a closed soft tissue compartment. Compartment syndrome is clinically manifest by tense, painful distension with reduction in movement and sensation. Urgent attention and consultation are necessary to evaluate compartment pressures. If elevated compartment pressures are present, urgent surgical decompression is indicated for limb salvage. After frostbite occurs, complete demarcation of tissue necrosis may take 1 to 3 months. Angiography, technetium-99 bone scan, and magnetic resonance imaging may be used to assist determination of surgical margins in conjunction with clinical findings. If the patient has signs and symptoms of sepsis attributed to infected frostbitten tissue, amputation should be performed expeditiously. Otherwise, amputation should be delayed until definitive demarcation occurs, a process that may take weeks to months. The affected limb is often insensate. Consequently, an approach that addresses both protective footwear and orthotics to provide optimal function is essential. The authors' experience has shown that early involvement of a multidisciplinary rehabilitation team produces better long-term functional results. Telemedicine or electronic consultation with a surgical frostbite expert to guide local surgeons should be considered when no local expert is available. Because significant morbidity may result from unnecessary or premature surgical intervention, a surgeon with experience evaluating and treating frostbite should assess the need for and the timing of any amputations.

CHRONIC CHANGES OF FROSTBITE

Patients with the chronic sequelae of frostbite may benefit from sympathectomy in that sympathetic overactivity (hyperhidrosis and vasoconstriction) and cold sensitivity are reduced. The symptoms represent diminished circulation and reflect pallor, vasospasm, and pain symptoms. Lubrication of atrophic skin and protection from extreme temperatures are important. The parts affected must be prevented from further cold exposure because they are more susceptible to cold injury. Degenerative joint disease may be seen in severe cases, and stiff painful joints with fibrosis may be a consequence of moderately severe frostbite. Intrinsic muscle atrophy and fibrosis has also been described as a long-term outcome of severe frostbite, and these changes might be attenuated with proper physiotherapy, splinting, and appropriate exercise. In children, even mild frostbite can cause injury to epiphyseal growth centers, resulting in short digits, deviated digits, or osteoarthritis. Parents should be advised that these sequelae are possible despite appropriate therapy of frostbite during the acute phase of injury.

ACCIDENTAL HYPOTHERMIA

Hypothermia is defined as a core body temperature less than 35°C (95°F). Primary hypothermia occurs when heat production in a healthy person is overwhelmed by the stress of excessive cold. Secondary hypothermia can occur in warmer environments when an underlying illness interferes with the body's ability to regulate temperature. Hypothermia is often seen as a result of environmental exposure from military situations, recreational activities, homelessness, or substance abuse. In healthcare settings, hypothermia can occur in surgical patients under anesthesia and lead to coagulopathy. Trauma patients may present with hypothermia, especially in the presence of brain injury. The risk of death from cardiac arrest increases significantly at a body temperature of 28°C.

CLASSIFICATION OF HYPOTHERMIA AND SYMPTOMS

Traditional classification of hypothermia includes mild, moderate, severe, and profound. Mild hypothermia (core temperature, 90°F to 94°F) is symptomatic with shivering, reports of being cold, and mild mental confusion, but the patient maintains a normal blood pressure. In moderate hypothermia (84°F to 89°F), the patient becomes more confused and is often agitated, delirious, or combative. The shivering ceases. Muscle spasticity, dilated pupils, and slow respirations are present. At this stage, atrial fibrillation and other arrhythmias commonly develop. In severe hypothermia (70°F to 84°F), the patient becomes comatose, has a flaccid paralysis, and begins to develop apnea. Eventually, this progresses to ventricular fibrillation and death. Patients with profound hypothermia (<70°F) manifest cessation of cardiac electromechanical activity with electroencephalogram (EEG) silencing and typically present with complete loss of vital signs. The lowest adult accidental hypothermia survival reported was with a core temperature of 56.7°F.

The Swiss staging system of Durrer (stages HT 1 to HT IV) is useful when the temperature cannot measured. This system classifies based on symptoms (stage HT I, conscious and shivering; stage HT II, impaired consciousness and no shivering; HT III, unconscious, not shivering, but vital signs present; and stage IV, no vital signs).

PHYSIOLOGIC EFFECTS OF HYPOTHERMIA

Basal heat production usually ranges between 40 and 60 kcal/m²/h, which is roughly equivalent to the heat of a 100-watt incandescent light bulb. The body responds physiologically to lowered temperatures by increasing cardiac output with tachycardia. Hypotension then follows with apnea and bradycardia. Peripheral vascular resistance increases with decreased cardiac output, and then, mean arterial pressure increases. Cardiac arrhythmias and sudden death occur in this sequence after ventricular ectopy and atrial fibrillation. Cardiac standstill occurs with a body temperature of less than 21°C (70°F). The blood becomes more viscous with each drop in temperature, and hemoconcentration is seen related to cold diuresis. Cold diuresis is renal water loss from cold-induced vasoconstriction and decreased antidiuretic hormone release. Sludging occurs in the peripheral vessels. Respiratory depression follows. A decrease in the ability to clear bronchial secretions is seen, along with a diminished cough reflex that results in cold bronchorrhea. Metabolic acidosis and pulmonary edema occur with rewarming, and cold diuresis results in hypovolemia.

DIAGNOSIS AND TREATMENT

Diagnosis may be made based on history of cold exposure and measurement of core temperature. Most standard clinical thermometers lack the ability to measure the low range of temperatures seen with severe hypothermia, and peripheral vasoconstriction and low cardiac output can interfere with measurements. Jugular venous bulb and pulmonary artery catheters are the gold standard for continuous temperature monitoring. Proximal esophageal probes can be falsely high from warmed ventilation, bladder temperatures can be influenced by peritoneal lavage, and rectal temperatures can lag during rewarming. Thermister probes in contact with the tympanic membrane accurately measure brain temperature if properly insulated. When accurate measurement is not feasible, management may be based on clinical symptoms correlating with the severity of the hypothermia. Electrocardiographic (ECG) findings of dangerous hypothermia include a prolonged QRS interval and Osborn waves, positive deflections that occur at the junction between the QRS complex and the ST segment.

When the victim is identified in the prehospital setting, removal of wet clothing and replacement with dry clothing should be performed. No massage, friction rubbing, or manipulation should be performed. For HT stage I, active movement should be encouraged if possible. Patients with HT stage I can be triaged to local hospitals if they are unable to be rewarmed in the field, and any patient with mental status changes warrants transport to a hospital. Patients with HT stage II can be rewarmed with minimally invasive techniques, including thermal packs or blankets (electrical, forced hot air, or chemical) and warm IV fluids (38°C to 42°C, or 100°F to 108°F). The volume of crystalloid administered should account for fluids lost from cold diuresis plus intravascular replacement for vasodilation. Standard resuscitation markers (volume status, electrolytes, glucose, pH, and lactate measurements) should be assessed for each individual patient, and fluid infusions adjusted. In patients with hemodynamically unstable conditions, pressors should be used cautiously because of the risk of cardiac arrhythmias and the risks associated with peripheral vasoconstriction if concurrent frostbite has occurred. In patients with mental status changes, cardiac instability, or a temperature of 28°C (82°F), transport to a tertiary center with advanced invasive rewarming capabilities (cardiac bypass, dialysis, or extracorporeal membrane oxygenation [ECMO]) is warranted if possible. If ECMO or cardiopulmonary bypass is not available, such as a situation with other pressing traumatic injuries, thoracic lavage of the left pleural space with two chest tubes is an alternative method of rewarming that should be considered.

Patients who have had cardiopulmonary arrest should undergo resuscitation according to standard protocols because patients survived after rewarming with long periods of CPR. If asystole persists in a patient with hypothermia despite rewarming to 32°C, survival is unlikely. If the serum potassium level is higher than 12 mmol/L, CPR is likely to be futile.

During transport of the patient with significant hypothermia or during therapeutic interventions such as central lines or radiologic workups, care must be taken not to precipitate cardiac arrhythmias with manipulations, sustain further cooling, or allow the patient to succumb to hypovolemic shock.

INTRAOPERATIVE HYPOTHERMIA

Surgeons should be especially cognizant of the risks of hypothermia in patients in the intraoperative setting. A slight drop in body temperature during surgery is associated with an increased incidence of postoperative respiratory failure, infections, and delays in postanesthesia recovery. Severe hypothermia can result in impaired coagulation and lead to increased blood loss. A few examples of patients at high risk of intraoperative hypothermia include patients with large burns, prolonged abdominal cavity exposure, and large blood losses. The elderly and very young are also at risk. Trauma patients also experience heat loss in the emergency department with extensive radiologic workups, and temperatures should be monitored during this process. Prevention measures include but are not limited to manipulating the room temperature, limiting exposure of the patient with use of a more selective operative field, use of reflective coverings and warming blankets, and warm fluid. Monitoring temperature during the procedure and truncating the procedure when necessary are important steps.

THERAPEUTIC HYPOTHERMIA

Therapeutic hypothermia is used to reduce mortality and neurologic complications after out-of-hospital ventricular fibrillation cardiac arrest (class Ia recommendation) and in-hospital and other rhythm cardiac arrests (class Ib recommendation). Studies are ongoing to assess efficacy in other indications, including spinal cord injury and traumatic brain injury. The American Heart Association recommends the performance of therapeutic hypothermia in a complete ICU setting with intubation, central temperature monitoring, arterial and central lines, cardiac monitoring, and EEG monitoring if available. Standard protocols are implemented rapidly for the induction of hypothermia. Length and depth of hypothermia vary depending on the indication. For mild hypothermia, these protocols might include infusion of 2 L of cold (4°C) normal saline solution and wrapping the body in cooling equipment to reach a temperature of 32°C to 34°C within 4 hours. The mild hypothermia is maintained at this temperature for 12 to 24 hours. Induced paralysis with train of four (TOF) monitoring may be indicated to prevent shivering. Angiograms and cardiac interventions have been safely performed during this period.

Rewarming occurs slowly at less than 0.5°C/h. Potassium, magnesium, glucose, and phosphorus might require attention during the process. Normal side effects of mild therapeutic hypothermia include tachycardia then bradycardia when temperature is less than 35°C, vasoconstriction with increased blood pressure, and increased central venous pressure (CVP) from venoconstriction (but decreased blood pressure from cold diuresis may also be present). Mottling of the skin is seen. Arrhythmias are rare if temperature is maintained at more than 30°C. The mild hypothermia results in a shifting of the oxyhemoglobin curve to the left, decreased metabolic rate, hyperglycemia, and changes in metabolism of some drugs. Contraindications to institution of therapeutic hypothermia include Glasgow coma scale of less than 6, other reasons for coma than sudden cardiac arrest, uncontrolled bleeding or cardiac arrhythmias, hemodynamic instability, multiple organ dysfunction syndrome (MODS) or septic state, comfort care code status before arrest, or prearrest impaired cognition. Indications in prolonged arrest (>60 minutes) or pregnancy are unclear. One of the risks of the cutaneous contact systems used to produce therapeutic hypothermia is cold injury to the skin. Treatment of such injuries is the same as for injuries detailed previously.

SUGGESTED READINGS

Bruen KJ, Ballard JR, Morris SE, et al: Reduction of the incidence of amputation in frostbite injury with thrombolytic therapy, *Arch Surg* 142:546–551, 2007.

Cauchy E, Chetaille E, Marchand V, et al: Retrospective study of 70 cases of severe frostbite lesions: a proposed new classification scheme, *Wilderness Environ Med* 12:248–255, 2001.

Cauchy E, Cheguillaume B, Chetaille E: A controlled trial of a prostacyclin and rt-PA in the treatment of severe frostbite, *N Engl J Med* 364:189–190, 2011.

Brown DJ, Brugger H, Boyd J, et al: Current concepts: accidental hypothermia, *N Engl J Med* 367:1930–1938, 2012.

Durrer B, Brugger H, Syme D: The medical on-site treatment of hypothermia: ICAR-MEDCOM recommendation, *High Alt Med Biol* 4:99–103, 2003.

McIntosh SE, Hamonko M, Freer L, et al: Wilderness Medical Society practice guidelines for the prevention and treatment of frostbite, *Wilderness Environ Med* 22(2):156–166, 2011.

Twomey JA, Peltier GL, Zera RT: An open-label study to evaluate the safety and efficacy of tissue plasminogen activator in treatment of severe frostbite, *J Trauma* 59:1350–1354, 2005.

ELECTRICAL AND LIGHTNING INJURY

Laurie Anne Loiacono, MD, FCCP and
Leigh Ann Price, MD

Electrical injury is one of the most destructive and disfiguring traumatic events a human can sustain. The injury complex is typically a combination of electrical shock, thermal injury, and blunt trauma, involving potentially devastating associated multisystem damage with high morbidity and mortality rates. Overall incidence of these injuries is low compared with other multisystem trauma injuries in the United States. Because of this, most healthcare teams have limited experience with this mechanism of injury, adding to the complexity of developing an effective medical and surgical care plan.

Optimal management of electrical and lightning injury victims necessitates: (1) a basic understanding of electrical injury mechanisms and their associated patterns of disease, (2) timely and appropriate resuscitation, (3) aggressive surgical and critical care medical management, and (4) implementation of coordinated multidisciplinary care for these patients from onset of injury through injury recovery and rehabilitation.

EPIDEMIOLOGY

Electrical burns and lightning injuries result in approximately 6000 injuries per year in the United States. Electrical burn survivors make up approximately 5% of total admissions to major burn centers, and a bimodal distribution exists with respect to age. In the majority of cases, non–lightning-related electrical injuries to children are accidental in nature and occur in the home; similar injuries to adults generally occur in the workplace. About two thirds of all non–lightning-related electrical injuries occur in the workplace; the majority of the rest occur in the home.

Electrical injuries account for 2% to 3% of all burns in children. The majority of electrical injuries in children are associated with transient, low-voltage exposure to household electrical and extension cords and wall outlets. Older children are exposed to life-threatening high-voltage injury through climbing activities. More than 200 household-related electrocutions (i.e., death by electricity) occur annually and are typically associated with consumer product misuse or malfunction.

The majority of construction and utility worker electrical injuries are related to brief, high-voltage exposure. Up to 40% of serious electrical injuries are fatal (56% of these deaths occur in the workplace). Electrical injuries represent 5% to 6% of all work-related traumatic deaths and account for an excess of 500 deaths per year. They are the second leading cause of occupation-related deaths in the United States. Short- and long-term morbidity in many electrical injury survivors is related to significant musculoskeletal and neurologic disability.

ELECTRICITY BASICS

Current

Electricity is defined as the flow of electrons through a conductor. *Electrical current* (I) is the volume of electrons between these points per second. Current exists in two forms: *alternating current* (AC) and *direct current* (DC). High-voltage utility power lines may be either AC (most common, commercial) or DC.

Alternating Current

AC is the directional flow of current in a circuit that is constantly being reversed back and forth in a repetitive pattern and is a more efficient way of generating and distributing electricity than DC current. Standard household current is AC at a rate of 60 Hz (cycles per second) and is supported by 100 to 250 amperes (A). AC can be much more dangerous than DC in certain circumstances because it causes tetanic muscle contractions that prevent a victim from releasing the electrical source. This is known as the "let-go" threshold. The bidirectional flow of AC produces cutaneous burns know as contact points; this is in contrast to the entrance and exit wounds from DC current. The "let-go" current intensity varies from 3 to 9 milliamperes (mA) depending on body size; tetany occurs at 16 to 20 mA. Although AC current is generally lower voltage and produces less direct tissue injury, prolonged contact can alter the cardiac cycle, causing arrhythmias and cardiac arrest. Ventricular fibrillation occurs at 50 to 100 mA and asystole occurs at more than 2 A. Keep in mind that although most providers speak about voltage, it is the amperage that kills.

Direct Current

DC means that the direction of electrical current remains constant. It is found in automobile electrical systems, railway tracks, batteries, and lightning. DC provides a vector directionality to the electrical current exposure, hence the typical "entrance and exit" point cutaneous wounds that identify potential current pathway. High-voltage DC injury often produces smaller, cutaneous "entrance and exit" wounds but much more significant deep tissue injury in addition to the electrical current tissue effects. DC does not produce the same contraction of the muscles that is found with AC. Although low-voltage DC current is not as dangerous as the corresponding AC current, contact with high-voltage DC is more apt to be fatal than contact with AC of the same voltage.

Voltage and Resistance

Voltage

The force that drives current (I) across the potential difference is the voltage (V), which contributes critically to the intensity of the electrical injury. Electrical injuries are classified as either high voltage (>1000 V) or low voltage (<1000 V). Typical voltage delivered to homes in the United States and Canada is 120/240 V, providing 240 V for appliances requiring high power and 120 V for general use. Low-voltage injuries tend to occur indoors and are almost exclusively AC. The AC power system in the United States and Canada operates at 60 Hz, causing the current to reverse polarity 120 times a second. Based on this fact, the terms *entrance* and *exit* should be abandoned and the resultant wounds from AC should be referred to as *contact points*. Voltage in high-tension power lines tends to exceed 100,000 V and is most commonly AC in developed areas. High-voltage mortality and amputation rates typically exceed low-voltage rates twofold to threefold.

Resistance

Resistance (R) is the hindrance to current flow and is measured in ohms. Resistance creates heat according to Joule's law. *Joule heating* is energy transfer that occurs when charged particles meet resistance and lose energy to tissues in the form of heat.

Joule's law:

$$\text{Power (J, Joule)} = I^2 \text{ (Current)} \times R \text{ (Resistance)}$$

Materials that are the best conductors (meaning they facilitate current flow) have the least resistance. With increasing resistance, more energy is expended in the form of heat and results in thermal tissue damage.

Different tissues have innately different resistances (Figure 1), and resistances will vary under different conditions. Overall resistance of a tissue depends on the surface area of contact, the tissues in the current's pathway, pressure applied, duration of exposure, magnitude of current flow, and absence or presence of moisture. For example, dry skin has a much greater resistance (approximately 100,000 ohms) than moist skin (<2500 ohms).

The relationship between the previously defined forces is described by *Ohm's law:*

$$I = V/R$$

where the current (I) is directly proportional to the voltage (V) and inversely proportional to resistance (R).

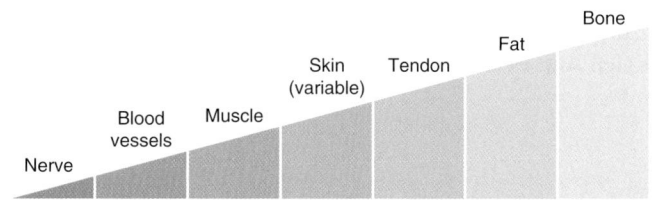

FIGURE 1 The magnitude of average electrical resistance across body tissues.

PHYSICS AND PATHOPHYSIOLOGY OF ELECTRICAL INJURY

All electrical injury involves both direct and indirect mechanisms. The direct damage is caused by the actual effect of electrical current on the body tissues or organs (e.g., brain or heart) or by the conversion of electrical to thermal energy resulting in burns. Indirect injuries are the result of associated tissue injury from severe muscle contraction, blunt trauma from falls or ejection, or associated multiorgan system dysfunction (e.g., renal failure from rhabdomyolysis).

Direct Injury (Electrical and Lightning)

The severity of direct electrical injury is determined by several critical factors:

1. Voltage (high or low)
2. Type of current (alternating or direct)
3. Intensity of current (amperage)
4. Pathway of the current through the body (vertical, horizontal, peripheral)
5. Duration of current exposure
6. Area of contact on the body
7. Resistance of the body tissues involved

Injury to the affected tissue predominantly depends on the intensity and duration of electrical exposure. For example, brief exposure to current will conduct rapidly across low resistance tissues (Ohm's law) with less heat production and structural tissue damage, but more electrophysiologic derailment of end organs (i.e., heart, central nervous system [CNS], and muscle). Hence, lightning causes little, if any, direct tissue injury.

If contact time is brief, nonthermal direct electrical damage to tissue occurs as the current disrupts the microelectrical gradient across cell membranes via electroporation and conformational changes in membrane proteins. Electroporation results in a significant increase in the electrical conductivity and cell plasma membrane permeability leading to tissue edema and possible cell injury. Muscle fibers and nerves are the most susceptible. Electroporation can induce cell necrosis or permanently, partially, or reversibly affect cell membrane function in the absence of joule heating. Damage will be relatively localized to the involved tissue cell membranes and result in functional disruption of those end organs dependent on coordinated electrical activity such as heart, brain, spinal cord, and muscle (Table 1). These cell membrane effects may progress over time and

partially explain some of the delayed clinical symptoms observed following electrical injury, such as vascular thrombosis and rupture, cognitive dysfunction, and late-appearing spinal cord deficits (Table 2).

Lightning, a form of DC current, is one of the most dramatic examples of high-voltage direct electrical injury. Its injuries are a small subset of electrical injuries, but DC is responsible for an average of 300 injuries and 100 deaths per year in the United States. Estimated fatality from lightning is 30%, and 70% to 80% of survivors may have permanent disabilities. Lightning discharges can be either positively or negatively charged (Table 3).

Lightning injury can be minor, moderate, or severe.

1. Minor: often awake and alert, may have confusion or amnesia, dysesthesia, hearing or vision changes. Physical findings may be temporary, and complete recovery can occur.
2. Moderate: disorientation, combativeness, unconsciousness, paralysis, skin mottling, hypotension, respiratory failure, secondary cardiac arrest. Physical symptoms may resolve over time. Long-term sequelae, such as cognitive and sleep disorders, weakness, dysesthesias and peripheral neuropathy, can develop.
3. Severe: Serious injury or death occurs in 30% of victims. Injuries include blunt trauma, contusion from the shock wave, cardiac dysrhythmias, cardiac arrest (primary or secondary), and CNS dysfunction. Asystole may be transient and spontaneous rhythm may recover as a result of cardiac automaticity. Hypoxia related to central apnea may lead to secondary cardiac arrest. Long-term sequelae such as cognitive and sleep

TABLE 2: Examples of late electrical injury organ tissue dysfunction

Tissue	Late effect
Heart	Patchy cardiac tissue necrosis (myocardium, nodal tissue, conduction pathways, coronary arteries); late arrhythmias are rare
CNS	Cognitive deficits, spinal cord and peripheral nerve dysfunction, cataracts
Muscle	Weakness, arthropathy, nonspecific myopathy/fibrosis, limitation of joint function
Vascular	Venous thrombosis, arterial rupture

CNS, Central nervous system.

TABLE 1: Examples of acute, direct electrical organ tissue dysfunction

Tissue	Acute effect
Heart	Asystole, arrhythmia, cardiac tissue necrosis (myocardium, nodal tissue, conduction pathways, coronary arteries)
CNS	Brain stem dysfunction: central apnea, loss of consciousness, seizure, confusion, amnesia, cranial nerve deficits, paralysis, spinal cord transection, visual and hearing disturbances
Muscle	Tetany (rhabdomyolysis, lactic acidosis, bone stress fracture, "locking-on" phenomenon)

CNS, Central nervous system.

TABLE 3: Different patterns of lightning strikes

Type	Pattern
Direct strike	Lightning directly strikes victim
Splash strike	Lightning hits another object and "splashes" onto the victim
Side flash	Individual is inside a building and exposure to current occurs through a conductive source within the structure (e.g., metal object or landline telephone)
Step voltage	Lightning strikes the ground and the current is conducted along the ground to an adjacent victim

disorders, weakness, dysesthesias, and peripheral neuropathy can develop without direct evidence of initial direct anatomic brain injury.

The two most common causes of death are (1) cardiopulmonary arrest due to an interruption of the cardiac cycle by the direct current, resulting in asystole; and (2) apnea from the direct current's interference with the brain's respiratory center, which, if left untreated, will result in hypoxia, arrhythmia, and secondary cardiac arrest. There is an estimated morbidity rate of 5 to 10 times higher than the rate of casualties of non–lightning-related electrical injury (Table 4). A pathognomonic fernlike pattern called keraunographic markings or Lichtenberg figure (Figure 2) may appear on the skin of victims of lightning strike. This is not a burn and often disappears within 24 hours.

Direct Injury (Thermal)

When contact time is prolonged, heat damage will dominate as the whole cell in the pathway is compromised. Thermal burn injury caused by electricity may be classified into three categories:

- Joule heat: This is the direct effect of electrical current on tissue resistance causing heating of tissue, resulting in deep and superficial burns. The extent of specific tissue injury depends on the current path, Joule's law, and the duration of exposure.

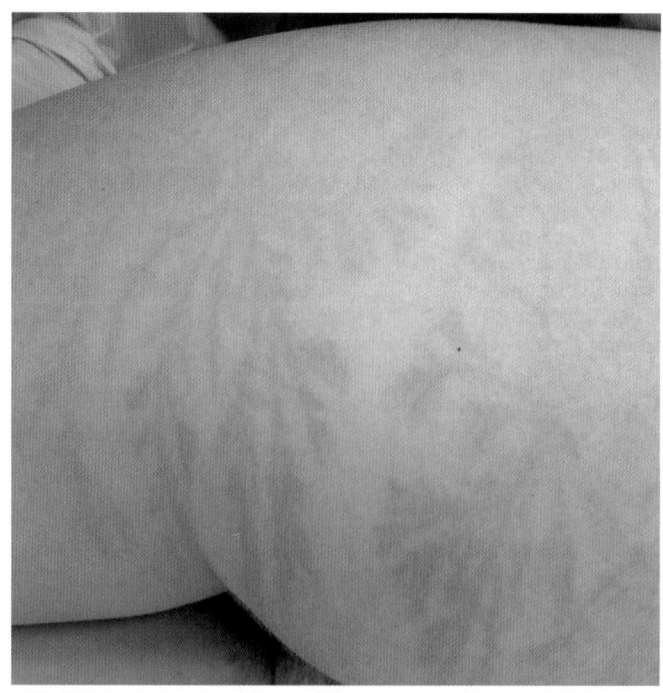

FIGURE 2   Lichtenberg figure. *(Photo courtesy of Andrew R. Doben, MD, FACS.)*

TABLE 4: Comparison between lightning, high-voltage, and low-voltage electrical injuries

	Lightning	High-voltage	Low-voltage
Voltage (V)	$>30 \times 10^6$	>1000	<1000
Current (A)	>200,000	Variable	240
Duration	Instantaneous	Brief	Prolonged
Type of current	DC	DC or AC	Mostly AC
Cardiac effect	Arrest: asystole	Arrest: ventricular fibrillation	Arrest: ventricular fibrillation
Respiratory effect	Respiratory arrest: direct CNS injury	Respiratory arrest: indirect trauma or tetanic contractions of respiratory muscles	Respiratory arrest: tetanic contractions of respiratory muscles
Muscle effect	Single	Contraction: DC: single AC: tetanic	Contraction: tetanic
CNS effect	Early and delayed brain injury, coma, seizures, blindness, deafness, aphasia, cerebral vein thrombosis, late spinal cord deficits, cataracts	Early and delayed brain injury, coma, seizures, blindness, deafness, aphasia, cerebral vein thrombosis, late spinal cord deficits, cataracts	Paresthesias, transient neuropathy
Burns	Rare: superficial ("flashover" diverts current around the body)	Common: superficial (less) and deep (most)	Usually superficial, can be full-thickness
Rhabdomyolysis	Uncommon	Very common	Common
Blunt injury	Blast effect, shock wave	Muscle contraction, fall	Fall (uncommon)
Mortality rate (early)	Very high (about 30%)	Moderate (about 5%-15%)	Low

AC, Alternating current; *CNS,* central nervous system; *DC,* direct current.

■ Arc: Direct thermal injury from arcing is caused by high-voltage current passing through the air. These injuries are most commonly seen in electricians working with metal objects close to an electrical source. These injuries occur without actual current flowing *through* tissue. Electricity arcs at a temperature up to 4000°C to 5000°C generating a "flash" type injury.

■ Flame: Thermal burns result from ignited clothes or surroundings and are managed as conventional flame burns.

Most direct injuries are a combination of both electrical current conduction and heat transfer to tissues (Figure 3). Both mechanisms should be expected and fully explored in the course of the electrically injured patient's evaluation.

Importance of Current Pathways

Identification of "contact points" often helps establish the path current has taken. A path parallel or "vertical" to the axis of the body (craniocaudal) is most dangerous because it may affect all the vital organs. A "horizontal path" for example, from hand to hand, may spare the brain but may still be fatal from its effect on the heart and respiratory muscles. A path with contact points confined to a single extremity may cause extensive local damage but not be lethal (Figure 4).

Immediate cardiac arrest and life-threatening arrhythmias may occur with the conduction of current across the heart. AC current tends to cause ventricular fibrillation, whereas DC current tends to cause asystole. Actual injury to the heart or the metabolic effects from injury elsewhere in the body (e.g., hyperkalemia and rhabdomyolysis) may result in delayed cardiac arrhythmias and acute renal failure. Paralysis of the muscles of respiration can result in apnea. Effects on the spinal cord and brain can lead to immediate death or long-term neurologic abnormalities.

Indirect Injury

Additional tissue and organ injury not directly caused by, but clearly related to, the electrical insult is a significant contribution to morbidity and mortality of these patients. Many electrically injured patients fall from a height or are thrown or ejected following a blast or arc. These patients should receive a full multitrauma assessment on initial evaluation, including full spine and airway stabilization.

Respiratory failure can result from direct, blunt, or electrical lung injury; smoke or chemical inhalation; pulmonary edema; or acute lung injury. Many victims who develop muscle injury from tetany, direct electrical injury, or blunt trauma develop early acute kidney injury secondary to rhabdomyolysis or shock. CNS abnormalities can be transient, permanent, or delayed based on gross and histologic anatomic structure injury.

MANAGEMENT

The development of guidelines and outcome-based benchmarks requires established standards of practice; however, no specific guidelines exist at this time for electrical injuries. Due to the traumatic, multisystem nature of electrical injury (including potential associated blunt or penetrating trauma injuries), these patients should be managed according to both trauma and burn reconstruction guidelines for care and include the following.

1. Establish safe access to the electrically injured patient.
2. Rapidly assess the patient's airway, breathing, circulation, and disability (rapid neurologic assessment) and provide in-line immobilization of the entire spine (primary survey).
3. Treat life-threatening findings immediately. Control threatened airway and/or ventilation, decompress a tension pneumothorax or pericardial tamponade, control external hemorrhage, expose patient, and manage potential core-temperature heat loss (hypothermia).
4. Establish intravenous (IV; or interosseous, if in the field) access and continuous vital signs (including temperature), neurologic exam, pulse oximetry, respiratory function, electrocardiogram (ECG), and urine output monitoring (urinary catheter); central venous pressure.

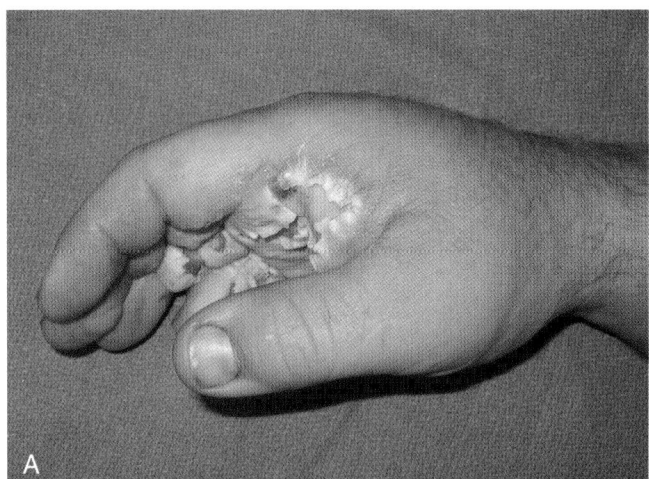
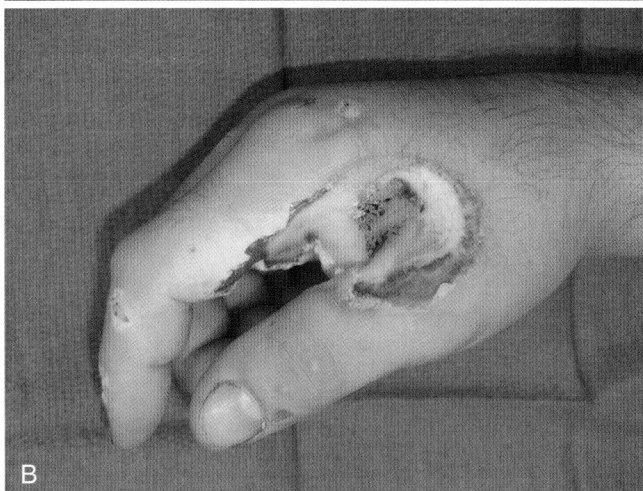

FIGURE 4 **A,** A farmer working in the field came in direct contact with a low hanging wire (7000 V). **B,** An electrician grabbed a cable (270 V, alternating current) overhead to avoid falling into a ditch.

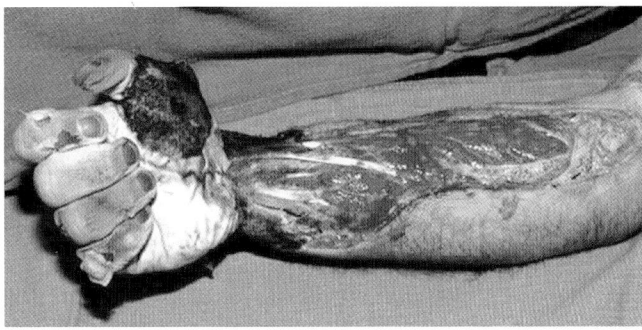

FIGURE 3 High-voltage electrical injury.

5. Expose and cover thermal burn sites with clean, dry sheets or towels; then use appropriate topical dressing when at the hospital. Keep in mind the need for escharotomy or fasciotomy.
6. Initiate fluid resuscitation with warmed, isotonic crystalloid IV fluids (Parkland formula suggests Ringer's lactate for the burned patient) to a target urinary output (UO) of 0.5 mL/kg/hr if the patient is at low risk for rhabdomyolysis (>1.0 mL/kg/hr if at high risk for rhabdomyolysis).
7. Closely monitor physiologic response to initiated therapies, if deterioration occurs.
8. Initiate aggressive surgical and critical care medical management.
9. Implement coordinated multidisciplinary care for these patients from onset of injury through injury recovery and rehabilitation.

Prehospital Management and Special Considerations

Access to the Victim and Scene Safety

The scene of an electrical injury is unique compared to other trauma sites. The rescuer can easily become another victim.

Be aware of the following:

■ Victim's existing contact with the current source. "DO NOT TOUCH," specialized nonconductive equipment is necessary to safely recover these victims.
■ Active live electrical sources and confirm disconnection.
■ Environment conductors to avoid (i.e., puddles of liquid, exposed metals and wires).

Victims of lightning injury may be treated immediately.

Critical Care Management

Early, goal-directed resuscitation and aggressive surgical management are cornerstones for optimal patient outcome. Targeted multi-organ system assessment and support are critical in the first hour following injury (Table 5).

Optimal surgical treatment will vary with the severity and etiology of electrical injury and the specific location of the injury site.

Multidisciplinary, System-Based Critical Care Management of the Electrical Injury Patient

Neurologic

Serial neurologic assessments, spine clearance (within 24 hours) for mobilization, pain management, early mobilization, aggressive physical and occupational therapy, cognitive/vision/hearing assessments, and rehabilitation plan.

Complications

Neurologic complications are common sequelae of electrical injuries and can affect both the central and the peripheral nervous system. Early manifestations include varying levels of unconsciousness (including coma), sensory dysfunction, memory disturbances, autonomic dysfunction, respiratory paralysis, and motor dysfunction. Deficits may be "patchy" with sensory deficits not coinciding with the motor findings. Clinical manifestations of neurologic injury may be delayed for days or even months and are not consistent with the size or location of the injury.

Cardiac

Continuous ECG monitoring for the first 24 hours. If no acute cardiac issues or arrhythmia occur, continuous monitoring can be stopped, Avoid hypotension and tachycardia. Check an echocardiogram if hypotension occurs or if acute myocardial injury is suggested based on cardiac enzyme levels.

Complications

Ventricular fibrillation is the most common fatal arrhythmia, occurring in up to 60% of patients in whom the current has taken a horizontal pathway. However, virtually any cardiac dysrhythmia can be precipitated by any electrical injury. The overall estimate of arrhythmia following electrical injury is up to 15%; most of these are benign and occur within the first few hours of hospital admission. Recent studies have shown that new onset atrial fibrillation is the most common dysrhythmia seen in survivors; it can be managed easily with medical treatment. ECG should be performed in all patients who sustain electrical injuries, whether low or high voltage. Duration of cardiac monitoring needed is generally between 24 and 48 hours, but it should continue if any underlying cardiac injury has not been completely ruled out.

Direct myocardial injury is uncommon, but it can present as a traumatic cardiac contusion. Myocardial infarction is rare.

Respiratory

Extubated patients: incentive spirometry, cough and deep breathing, early mobilization, oxygen (O_2) as needed to maintain arterial oxygen saturation level (SaO_2) above 92%.

Intubated patients: use a "lung protective" ventilator strategy, develop a weaning plan, consider the value of early tracheostomy, maintain head of bed at 30 degrees or higher, provide venous thromboembolism and ulcer prophylaxes, perform a daily sedation holiday.

Gastrointestinal

Early enteral feedings, twice-weekly acute phase protein assessment, daily bowel assessment and regimen.

Renal

Goal UO is O.5 mL/kg/hr (adjusted goal for rhabdomyolysis: UO > 1.0 mL/kg/hr).

Complications

Massive tissue necrosis associated with electrical injury can result in rhabdomyolysis and subsequent pigment-induced acute kidney injury from myoglobinuria. Mechanisms of myoglobin-induced acute renal failure include (1) renal constriction and ischemia from hypovolemia due to extravascular extravasation of fluid, (2) direct cytotoxic action of myoglobin on the proximal convoluted tubules due to tissue and muscle breakdown, and (3) myoglobin cast formation in the distal convoluted tubules.

It is essential to manage rhabdomyolysis with aggressive fluid resuscitation and increased urine output goals targeting UO at 1-2 mL/kg/hr. Osmotic diuresis with mannitol and alkalinization of urine has been proposed as adjunct strategies but are not currently supported by level I evidence.

Infectious Disease

Tetanus administration should be considered where appropriate. Systemic inflammatory response syndrome (SIRS) criteria should be monitored for sepsis for needed workup.

TABLE 5: Critical care management of patients with electrical injury (first hour)

Concern	Action	Goal
Airway (PRIORITY) Assess for • Airway patency • Altered mental status • Facial injuries • Airway obstruction • Aspiration	1. Provide manual airway support as needed (e.g., clear airway, bag-valve-mask [BVM]). 2. Intubate EARLY. Edema and multisystem organ dysfunction will progress quickly (surgical airway may be necessary). 3. Clinically confirm placement with exam and end-tidal CO_2 monitor; secure endotracheal tube in place. 4. Immobilize cervical/thoracic/lumbar/sacral spine immediately. 5. Initiate pulse oximetry.	• Secure airway
Breathing Assess for • Spontaneous effort • Pneumothorax • Hemothorax • Chest wall compromise (musculoskeletal or burn) • Smoke inhalation (if associated material ignition)	1. Treat pneumothorax immediately. 2. Initiate mechanical ventilation if needed. 3. Correct hypoxia with supplemental O_2 (start with 100% FiO_2). 4. Check ABGs. 5. CXR (confirm tube placement, identify injury). 6. Perform early escharotomy if needed.	• AVOID hypoxia. • SaO_2 >92% • PCO_2 35-45 mm Hg • Plateau pressure <30 mm Hg
Circulation Assess for • Cardiac tamponade • Distended neck veins • Shock • Cardiac arrhythmia • Cardiac dysfunction • Hemorrhage • Peripheral pulses	1. Treat cardiac tamponade immediately. 2. Establish adequate IV access. Edema and multisystem organ dysfunction will progress quickly. 3. Infuse isotonic IV fluids toward target goals. 4. Ensure continuous ECG and blood pressure monitoring. 5. Place urinary catheter. 6. Perform FAST exam and/or abdominal and pelvic CT scan. 7. Consider central venous access for resuscitation monitoring. 8. Perform early fasciotomy. 9. Complete blood count, type & cross, cardiac enzymes, lactate.	• MAP ≥ 60 mm Hg • UO ≥ 0.5 mL/kg/hr (if suspect rhabdomyolysis: UO >1.0 mL/kg/hr) • SvO_2 60-65 mm Hg • Lactic acid <2.0 • Closely monitor for development of pulmonary edema.
Disability Assess for • Acute brain injury • Acute spine injury • Musculoskeletal deformity	1. Assess consciousness, pupillary size and response, lateralizing signs, and level of spinal cord injury. 2. Assess GCS score. 3. Assess spine pain and gross function. 4. Do a full neurologic exam when possible. 5. Perform head and spine CT scan as needed.	
Exposure Assess for • Core temperature • Cutaneous injury	1. Warm IV fluids. 2. Warm room. 3. Provide insulating covers (if needed). 4. Assess the burn wound area. 5. Cover burn sites with dry, clean linen (pending definitive burn care). 6. Splint unstable fracture sites to avoid neurovascular compromise. 7. Make serial, focused neurovascular checks.	AVOID hypothermia. Core temp 98.6° F (37° C)
Comprehensive Evaluation Assess for • Efficacy of current treatment • Additional or missed injuries; identify and treat them.	1. Perform Secondary and Tertiary Surveys per ACS Trauma (ATLS) Protocol. 2. Order pertinent additional lab and radiologic studies. 3. Consider transfer to burn center.	

ABGs, Arterial blood gases; *ACS*, American College of Surgeons; *ATLS*, Advanced trauma life support; *CT*, computed tomographic; *CXR*, chest x-ray; *ECG*, electrocardiogram; *FAST*, focused assessment with sonography for trauma; *FiO₂*, fractional inspired oxygen; *GCS*, Glasgow Coma Scale; *IV*, intravenous, *MAP*, mean arterial pressure; *SvO₂*, mixed venous saturation; *UO*, urinary output.

Musculoskeletal

Radiologic studies of suspicious areas are necessary to evaluate for fractures, frequent neurovascular checks to affected extremities are necessary to monitor for evolving tissue injury, early fasciotomy is required for compartment syndrome, early carpal tunnel release may be necessary for clinical signs of tissue entrapment, and performance of early aggressive débridement of nonviable tissue should be done, including splinting the affected extremity in its position of function.

Musculoskeletal Complications

Bone has the highest resistance of any body tissue, thus generating the greatest amount of heat when exposed to an electrical current. This then causes the greatest amount of thermal damage to tissue adjacent to long bone structures and manifests as periosteal burns and possible osteonecrosis. Tetanic muscular contractions induced by AC may result in fractures or dislocation of bone or joint.

In addition, traumatic injuries resulting in fractures from blast injuries, falls, or repetitive forceful muscle contractions have also been reported. Patients with significant electrical injuries or altered mental status should have imaging studies of their cervical spine to rule out any evolving pathology.

Unfortunately, escharotomy is not of much use in patients with electrical burn because of the depth of the injury. Fasciotomies and/or carpal tunnel releases should be performed in the operating room immediately when circulation is presumed to be impaired. Initial fasciotomy should be performed in the areas of contact and conduction; for instance, the carpal tunnel may be released if the injury occurs in the wrist. The injury may be confined to the digits, the hand, or both, but if the patient has a considerable amount of pain, it may be advisable to complete a carpal tunnel release as the canal may become narrow as a result of the recent trauma and deep tissue injury, which may cause swelling leading to early signs of compression. Fasciotomy plays a major role in the early management of electrical burns and can dramatically improve the salvage of tissue, including the limb. Splinting extremities in positions of function must be accomplished for preservation of joint use in the extremities.

Skin Complications

By far, the most common manifestations of electrical injuries can be attributed to the thermal damage caused to exposed skin. Although surgeons often refer to entrance (more tissue damage) and exit wounds, with AC there is no such thing as the current entering or leaving. Instead, injuries are labeled as contact points.

Superficial, partial-thickness, and full-thickness burns can occur from any electrical injury. Estimates have shown that exposure to only 20 to 35 mA per mm^2 of skin surface for 20 seconds raises the skin temperature to 50° C, causing denaturing of protein, which leads to blistering and swelling. A crucial point to remember is that the degree of external injury cannot be used to determine the extent of the internal damage, regardless of voltage. Minor superficial burns may coexist with massive muscle coagulation and necrosis.

Of note, the incidence of superficial surface burns is high in victims of lightning injury, but deep burns are uncommon.

Surgical Management

Low-Voltage Injury Management

Low-voltage injuries (<1000 V) (see Figure 4, *B*; also see Figure 4, *A* although considered a high-voltage injury) are less devastating but can remain just as debilitating. These injuries often require close monitoring for the first few hours of admission in order to rule out

evolving vascular sequelae to the limb or potential complications of myoglobin clearance. The first elective operative procedure is sharp excision of the eschar, often completed using a tourniquet, followed by initial placement of meshed allograft. The allograft is placed during the first excision even if the wound bed appears healthy and completely viable; this allows metabolic changes to alter the tissue beneath. In general, after the second débridement, sheet (non-meshed) autograft is then applied to those wounds on the face, neck, and hands; otherwise, meshed autograft can be used at the surgeon's discretion. Again, splinting the extremity in its position of function must be accomplished for preservation of joint(s) use in the extremity. Early intervention by a rehabilitation therapist (giving occupational therapy and physical therapy) will optimize patient outcome and advance function with better range of motion and strengthening. It is considered good practice to educate patients that in the distant future they may require additional surgical therapy for burn contracture release, which may include placement of a full-thickness skin graft.

High-Voltage Injury Management

Most electrical injuries cause damage to limb tissue by generation of heat causing thermal insult and by endothelial damage with progressive tissue necrosis. These injuries are often associated with limb loss via amputation at various levels and carry a high rate of morbidity. Limb salvage and appropriate, aggressive initial resuscitation are challenging from the moment these injuries are first encountered. The American Burn Association referral criteria recommend that patients with high-voltage electrical trauma to the upper extremity be referred to specialized burn centers experienced with these injuries.

Most high-voltage (>1000 V) injuries are associated with deep tissue injury that is often underappreciated and more extensive than initially apparent. The initial management of the limb involves immediate (first 6 to 8 hours after injury has occurred) surgical exploration and decompressive fasciotomies. Fasciotomy plays a major role in the early management of electrical burns and can dramatically improve the salvage of tissue, including the limb. Escharotomy alone (incision is made into the subcutaneous fat just beyond the eschar) is of limited benefit. Although escharotomies may often be performed at the bedside, fasciotomies and carpal tunnel release should be performed in the operating room.

Indications for surgical decompression include progressive neurologic dysfunction, vascular compromise, increased compartment pressure, and systemic clinical deterioration from suspected ongoing myonecrosis. Decompression includes forearm fasciotomy and assessment of muscle compartment integrity. The decision to include a carpal tunnel release should be made on a case-by-case basis. Initial fasciotomy should be performed in the areas of contact and conduction; for instance, the carpal tunnel may be released if the injury occurs in the wrist. However, if the injury is confined to the digits, the hand, or both, and if the patient has a considerable amount of pain, it may be advisable to complete a carpal tunnel release as the canal can become narrow as the result of the recent trauma and deep tissue injury and there may be resultant swelling leading to early signs of compression. Delayed exploration and decompression in the compromised extremity may result in increased amputation rates along with increased organ failure and mortality. To date, no definitive data exist to illustrate that immediate surgical decompression reduces the need for amputation in any series.

As in Figure 3, lack of opportunity for limb salvage may be obvious early, regardless of the number of surgical débridements, because of the extent of devitalized tissue noted on presentation. However, one important consideration regarding amputation is the length of tissue able to be retained and the remaining length required to fit a prosthesis. Do not confuse nonviable tissue with minimally bleeding tissue. As a general surgical principle, surgeons are not trained to "leave behind" nonviable tissue as there is risk for infection, but there is evidence that supports keeping some (minimally bleeding) tissue in question with multiple serial débridements and a watchful eye. Always start with débridement of devitalized tissue and continue every other day until sustainably viable tissue is apparent and the source is controlled. Leaving tendon intact that lacks its peritenon may be of use in long-term limb salvage, as there may be regeneration along the intact, viable tissue. Serial débridements can then be performed and continued in preparation for definitive reconstruction or formal amputation. Splinting the extremity in position of function must be accomplished for preservation of joint use in the extremity, and this should be commenced even prior to the first surgery.

Significant advances in extremity reconstruction have been made through the development of high-quality, functional prostheses and new advances in tissue engineering such as vascularized composite allotransplantation (VCA). VCA is an option held in reserve after all other attempts have been exhausted and the patient has survived the initial injury, as the immunosuppression necessary for graft survival can harm the patient in the acute phase prior to chimerism.

In addition to basic general surgical principles—such as débridement of nonviable tissue, protection of tissue perfusion, nutritional optimization, and control of infection—reconstructive surgery follows basic principles of the reconstructive ladder: healing by secondary intention, primary closure, delayed primary closure, grafts (split-thickness, full-thickness), tissue expansion, flaps (random, axial, and free). This organizational ladder provides a systematic approach to wound closure from the emphasis of simple to complex techniques based on local wound requirements and complexity.

In burn surgery, rarely are the first few rungs of the ladder helpful due to the nature of the injury; surgeons often jump to the rung of grafting secondary to tissue loss. There must be a healthy, vascularized wound bed for a split-thickness graft to take (i.e., if the peritenon or periosteum is lacking, the graft will not take). Allograft versus autograft is a very important tissue choice and ultimately the decision of the surgeon (keep in mind that if the allograft does not adhere, neither will the autograft). Use of allografting preserves the patient's tissue until the wound bed is ready and allows the surgeon to return to the operating room for re-débridement of areas where microscopic changes at the cellular level are noted.

Full-thickness skin grafting is often susceptible to infection if nonviable tissue is left behind as a result of the lack of adequate vascular blood supply. Rarely is tissue expansion considered in patients with acute burn injuries. Random and axial flaps are used when appropriate and are often the preferred method of reconstruction, especially in the acutely injured. However, the operating surgeon must keep in mind that during an electrical injury, significant vessel damage may occur to the media or endothelium of the vessel in which the flap is based.

Other vascular abnormalities, such as vascular occlusions, arteritis and aneurysm formation, thrombosis and segmental narrowing of major extremity vessels, and a marked decrease in the density of small nutrient vessels, have been described after electrical injuries. As a rule of thumb, the ideal tissue to be used is outside of the zone of injury; this principle should also be respected and strongly adhered to during free tissue transfer. Although free flap reconstruction is rarely indicated in patients with acute burn injuries, as the versatility and variability of the free flaps have evolved, so has their applicability to tissue reconstruction. Timing of the reconstructive procedure in relation to the injury, the age of patient, existing medical comorbidities, the length of the operative procedure, and extent of the zone of injury all have a significant impact on the success rate of a free flap reconstruction. The importance of these issues should not be minimized, as free flap coverage may be necessary for coverage of exposed joint, bone, vessels, and tendons. The failure rate of free tissue transplantation post injury is well documented as ranging from postoperative day 5 up to 6 weeks. Therefore, it is critical to optimize the

burn patient's treatment from its onset, as the outcomes of these types of injuries will be life-altering.

Commissure Injuries

The American College of Surgeons has recommended that all facial burns be triaged to an American Burn Association burn center. Commissure burns typically occur in the young patient and commonly result from biting or teething on a household appliance cord. Although considered a relatively low-voltage (120 to 240 V) injury, this soft tissue injury can be devastating and lead to significant tissue loss (Figure 5). The burn is a result of the saliva permitting the local conduction and arcing of electricity. The electrical energy is generally concentrated to the oral commissure and the anterior tongue. As with any trauma, the initial management, according to the Advanced Trauma Life Support guidelines, involves a thorough assessment from head to toe. Rarely do these isolated injuries require intubation.

The contact burn wound, often a grayish-white eschar, should be cleaned gently and dressed with an ointment of choice. On examination of the vestibule of mouth, digital palpation may reveal a "woody," indurated buccal mucosa as far posterior as the tonsillar pillars. Early surgical intervention can lead to loss of potentially salvageable tissue that may be necessary for the reconstructive surgery and thus should be avoided. The goal is to maintain a clean, moist environment that allows the tissue to heal. The child should be encouraged to continue to eat and drink. Involvement of a speech pathologist can be of significant help from the onset. The use of a custom-made splint can help reduce scar formation and should be initiated between 10 and 14 days after the injury has occurred. The eschar will continue to demarcate and slough within 7 to 21 days. Based on the proximity of the labial artery to the oral commissure, vessel rupture can be expected to occur in approximately 10% of the patients. Parents and caregivers should be educated that should labial artery rupture bleeding occur, compression of the site between the index finger and thumb should be performed to minimize the hemorrhage, and they should immediately return to the hospital. Seldom do these need surgical intervention for ligation.

The continued healing from the burn can result in tissue scarring and contracture. Contracture can interfere with normal vocalization, facial expression, eating, oral hygiene (including dental care), not to mention the psychologic sequelae of the trauma. Long-term burns to the mouth can be associated with microstomia. Contracture of the angle of the mouth is generally treated approximately 1 year after the burn injury has occurred, as it takes at least 1 year for the burn to

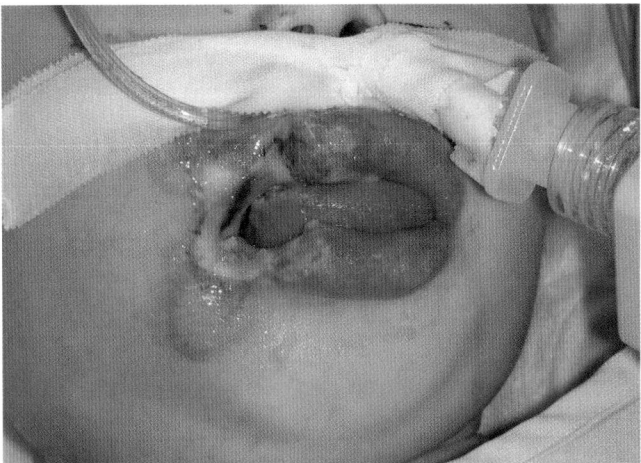

FIGURE 5 Oral commissure burn due to contact with a household electrical wire. Associated complication: labial artery rupture may occur 7 days post burn.

become stable because of the sphincteral action of the orbicularis oris muscle. Late effects of burn reconstructive surgery may include Z-plasty, tongue advancement flap, or commissuroplasty. Of note, the tongue advancement flap, often the only choice based on initial injury, may give a less aesthetically pleasing appearance, as the tongue papilla are transferred to the external orifice.

Late Complications

A multitude of late complications from electrical injuries include cataracts, increased cholelithiasis causing cholecystitis, delayed hemorrhage from blood vessel rupture, skeletal complications of fibrosis, and limitation of joint function.

Although there have been significant advances in both burn and the critical care management of these very specialized patients, prevention and safety remain the best ways to avoid or minimize the occurrence and severity of electrical injury. With the exception of lightning, electrical injuries are almost always preventable.

SUGGESTED READINGS

Arnoldo BD, Purdue GF, Kowalske K, et al: Electrical injuries: A 20-year review, *J Burn Care Rehabil* 25:479–484, 2004.

Hunt JL, Mason AD, Masterson TS, Pruitt BA: The pathophysiology of acute electric burns, *J Trauma* 16:335–340, 1976.

Koumbourlis AC: Electrical injuries, *Crit Care Med* 30:S424–S430, 2002.

Lee R: Injury by electrical forces: pathophysiology, manifestations and therapy, *Curr Prob Surg* 34:677–764, 1997.

Purdue GF, Arnoldo BD, Hunt JL: Electrical injuries. In Herndon D, editor: *Total Burn Care*, ed 3, 2007, Saunders Elsevier.

PREOPERATIVE AND POSTOPERATIVE CARE

FLUIDS AND ELECTROLYTES

Seth Goldstein, MD, Bellal Joseph, MD, and Albert Chi, MD

INTRODUCTION

Surgical diseases affect the body's equilibrium of water and electrolytes. Surgeons must understand changes in fluid and electrolyte balance caused by different disease processes at the cellular level. This chapter discusses the normal anatomic distribution of fluid and electrolytes, resuscitation fluids, and corrective therapies for correction of fluid and electrolyte abnormalities.

FLUID COMPARTMENTS AND OSMOLALITY

Approximately 50% to 60% of an individual's total body weight is made up of water, referred to as total body water (TBW). Because the water content of muscle exceeds that of fat, TBW as a percentage of body weight is lower in obese individuals. Males, on average, have greater muscle mass than females. TBW is approximately 60% of total body weight in males and 50% to 55% of total body weight in females.

Body fluid in a healthy subject is generally contained in one of multiple compartments as shown in Figure 1. Two thirds of the body's TBW is intracellular, and one third is extracellular, which is further divided into interstitial and intravascular or plasma compartments. Three fourths of the extravascular fluid is found within the interstitium and one fourth in the plasma. Thus, a 70-kg man is predicted to have a TBW of 42 L (60% TBW). The intracellular TBW volume is 28 L, and 14 L are extracellular, of which 4 L is the estimated intravascular plasma volume.

Osmotic equilibration occurs when water moves across membranes from areas of lower to areas of higher osmolality. The membranes that separate the intracellular and extracellular compartments are freely permeable to water, resulting in equal osmolality of intracellular, interstitial, and intravascular spaces. In contrast, there are different permeabilities for various solutes, and those that cannot traverse a given membrane have the capacity to exert an osmotic force that directs water movement across that membrane; such solutes are known as effective osmoles. Such movement occurs either through intercellular junctions or via a transcellular route. Water

crosses the lipid-rich cell membrane by simple diffusion, or alternatively, it passes through fenestrations and water channels known as aquaporins that are embedded in the cell membrane.

Capillary membranes are permeable to most small solutes, including sodium, potassium, glucose, and small molecular-weight proteins (less than 50,000 kDa). These small solutes have no role as effective osmoles; rather, movement of water across capillary membranes is directed by the osmotic pressure generated by plasma proteins that are too large to cross the capillary wall and by the hydrostatic pressure from blood flow. This force that is generated is known as oncotic pressure. Taken together, the oncotic and hydrostatic pressures are known as Starling's forces, and their effect on transcapillary movement can be described by Starling's law, which states that net filtration is the difference between the hydrostatic pressure and the oncotic pressure of both the capillary and interstitial fluids. The plasma proteins are effective osmoles that hold water in the intravascular space and generate oncotic pressure. This opposes the hydrostatic pressure of the plasma, which tends to force fluid into the interstitium. At the arteriolar end of the capillary, intravascular hydrostatic pressure exceeds oncotic pressure, and fluid moves out. With the net efflux of fluid along the length of the capillary, the situation is reversed at the venous end, and fluid is drawn from the interstitium back into the intravascular space.

Although small solutes do not contribute to water movement across capillary membranes, they do act as effective osmoles that direct water movement between the intracellular and extracellular spaces across cell membranes. Sodium (Na^+) and potassium (K^+) are the principal determinants of extracellular and intracellular osmolality, respectively; they are unable to diffuse passively across the lipid-rich cell membrane. The imbalance between the intracellular and extracellular concentrations of these two solutes is generated and maintained by the Na^+K^+ adenosine triphosphatase mechanism. This transmembrane transporter exchanges three Na^+ molecules for two of K^+ and generates a net negative cell membrane potential. Were the concentration of either of these ions to change, water would be forced to move from the compartment with lower osmolality to the compartment with higher osmolality to reestablish equilibrium. For example, if hypotonic saline solution (e.g., 0.45% NaCl normal saline solution) is administered, the extracellular osmolality is lowered, and water moves from the extracellular to intracellular space, causing cellular swelling. In contrast, with administration of hypertonic saline solution (e.g., 3% NaCl normal saline solution), the extracellular osmolality increases, and water moves from the intracellular to the extracellular space, causing cellular dehydration. Serum osmolality is maintained in a narrow range by the process of osmoregulation and is calculated with the following formula:

$$mOsm/kg = 2 \times (Na + K) + (BUN/2.8) + (glucose/18)$$

where *BUN* is blood urea nitrogen and *mOsm/kg* is serum osmolality. Normal serum osmolality is 275 to 290 mOsm/kg, and variations of only 1% to 2% stimulate mechanisms to restore the normal level, a

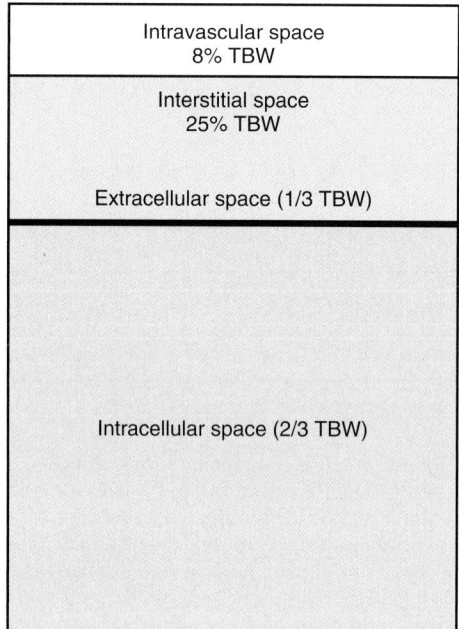

FIGURE 1   Body fluid distribution. *TBW,* Total body water.

TABLE 1: Maintenance fluid requirements

Body mass (kg)	Fluid volume (mL/kg/h)	Fluid volume (mL/kg/d)
First 10 kg	4	100
Second 10 kg (10 to 20 kg)	2	50
Each kg >20 kg	1	20
60 kg	100	2300

The rate of maintenance fluid administration for both pediatric and adult patients can be calculated for a 24-hour period by the 100-50-20 rule or hourly by the 4-2-1 rule (Table 1). The electrolyte composition of maintenance fluids is based on daily losses. Daily sodium requirement in the postoperative period is 1 to 2 mEq/kg/d, and potassium requirement is 0.5 to 1 mEq/kg/d. Postoperative maintenance fluids may also include dextrose to maintain plasma osmolality and reduce short-term proteolysis. Specific electrolyte and carbohydrate requirements may vary with the clinical situation and should be monitored closely in all critically ill patients. The usual postoperative maintenance fluid for an adult is composed of dextrose 5% (D5) in isotonic, half-normal saline solution (0.45% NaCl) with 20 mEq/L KCl. Children older than 2 years can receive the same maintenance fluids as an adult, but younger children are usually given D5 quarter-normal saline solution (0.22% NaCl) with 20 mEq KCl. Until age 2 years, the kidney has a glomerular filtration rate (GFR) that is one quarter the adult level, and the distal nephrons are unable to effectively concentrate the urine, leading to a difficulty in excreting high sodium loads.

process known as osmoregulation. Osmoreceptors in the hypothalamus detect high plasma osmolality and stimulate the thirst mechanism and antidiuretic hormone (ADH) secretion by the posterior pituitary gland. ADH then upregulates aquaporins in the distal collecting tubules of the kidney to reabsorb free water. As a result, adult urine osmolality has a wide range that can vary from 100 to 1200 mOsm/kg depending on the serum osmolality. On average, patients with a high serum osmolality and intact renal function have a urine osmolality greater than 500 mOsm/kg. Circulatory baroreceptors also stimulate ADH secretion based on detection of plasma volume, although volume is a less potent stimulus than osmolality.

Hormones that influence total body sodium content are the principal mediators of volume regulation. These include the renin-angiotensin-aldosterone axis and atrial natriuretic peptide (ANP). Renin is secreted by the juxtaglomerular cells in response to renal hypoperfusion or low sodium concentration in the macula densa region of the distal tubule. Renin secretion leads to activation of angiotensin and release of aldosterone, which both promote sodium reabsorption. ANP is a systemic hormone released in response to cardiac atrial stretch and enhances renal blood flow while inhibiting sodium reabsorption in the kidney.

DAILY REQUIREMENTS AND CHOICE OF MAINTENANCE FLUIDS

Maintenance fluids replace normal sensible and insensible losses. Replacement fluids replace abnormal or excess losses and correct for any water or electrolyte deficits. Sensible water losses can be quantified and occur primarily in urine and stool. Insensible losses cannot be measured and include evaporative losses from the skin (75%) and the upper respiratory tract (25%). Normal daily sensible losses include 800 to 1500 mL in urine and 250 mL in stool, and insensible losses are approximately 8 to 12 mL/kg/d. The insensible losses increase in various physiologic and pathologic conditions, including fever, hyperventilation, burns, tachycardia, and other hypermetabolic states. Cutaneous insensible losses increase by 10% per day for every 1°C increase in body temperature above 37°C. During a thoracotomy or laparotomy, insensible losses from the operative field can approach 1 L/h.

ASSESSMENT OF FLUID STATUS AND CHOICE OF REPLACEMENT FLUIDS

In the immediate postoperative period, patients may have fluid deficits that result from preoperative or intraoperative fluid losses. During the extended postoperative period, continued excess fluid losses in the urine, skin, and gastrointestinal (GI) tract are common. Fluid management in the postoperative period requires a close assessment of fluid status and selection of an appropriate type and rate of fluid replacement. Importantly, in an inflammatory state, it is common to have low intravascular volume despite overall positive fluid balance.

Common signs and symptoms of low effective circulatory volume include abnormal mentation, excessive thirst, dry mucous membranes, poor skin turgor, tachycardia, hypotension, orthostatic changes in heart rate and blood pressure, and oliguria. In addition to clinical signs and symptoms, daily weights, serum and urine electrolyte levels, acid-base balance, and invasive monitoring can be used to measure volume status and assess the adequacy of resuscitation. Urine output is an excellent measure of volume status and should be at least 0.5 mL/kg/h for adults and 1 to 2 mL/kg/h in children. Urine output may be an inaccurate measure if the patient has renal insufficiency, is receiving diuretics, or is hyperglycemic.

Increases in either serum or urine osmolality suggest intravascular hypovolemia. Other indicators of intravascular depletion include an elevated hematocrit value, low serum bicarbonate level with a base deficit, a BUN/creatinine (Cr) ratio of greater than 20:1 (prerenal azotemia), and a fractional excretion of sodium (FeNa) of less than 1%.

$$FeNa = ([urine\ Na] \times [plasma\ Cr]/[plasma\ Na] \times [urine\ Cr]) \times 100$$

TABLE 2: Electrolyte composition (mEq) of parenteral fluids

Fluid	Na⁺	K⁺	Cl⁻	Ca²⁺	HCO₃⁻	Dextrose	pH
Extracellular fluid	142	4	103	5	27	0	7.4
Ringer's lactate solution	130	4	109	2.7	28	0	6.5
Normal saline solution (0.9% NaCl)	154	0	154	0	0	0	4.5
1/4 Normal saline solution (0.45% NaCl)	77	0	77	0	0	0	4.5
1/4 Normal saline solution (0.2% NaCl)	34	0	34	0	0	0	4.5
3% Saline solution	513	0	513	0	0	0	4.5
5% Dextrose in water	0	0	0	0	0	50 g	4.5
5% Albumin	145	0	0	0	0	0	7.4

As in the case of urine output, the FeNa is altered and is not a useful indicator of volume status if the patient has underlying renal dysfunction or is receiving diuretics, most commonly furosemide.

The rate of replacement fluid administration is determined by the severity of the existing deficit, presence of ongoing losses, and comorbidities. Severe fluid losses that result in hemodynamic instability should be replaced with intravenous (IV) fluid boluses of 0.9% NaCl (normal saline solution [NS]) or lactated Ringer's solution (LR) at volumes of 10 to 20 mL/kg, with boluses repeated until an adequate resuscitation is reached.

The composition of various replacement fluids is shown in Table 2. NS and LR are most commonly used for replacement because they best approach the composition of extracellular fluid. LR contains 28 mEq of HCO₃⁻, whereas NS does not contain any HCO₃⁻ but has a greater concentration of Na⁺ and Cl⁻ (154 mEq). Thus, NS is used preferentially in patients with a metabolic alkalosis but can cause a hyperchloremic metabolic acidosis. Colloid solutions, such as 5% albumin, are theoretically useful in restoring intravascular volume because of the oncotic pressure afforded by the protein content. However, liberal use of colloid solutions has not been consistently shown to improve patient outcomes in randomized studies.

The electrolyte compositions of different GI fluids are listed in Table 3. The optimal replacement for gastric losses is D5 half NS with 20 mEq/L KCl; for pancreatic, biliary, or small intestinal losses, LR; and for large intestinal losses, LR with 20 mEq/L KCl. If GI losses are substantial or persistent, they should be replaced on a milliliter-for-milliliter basis with the correct fluid.

DIAGNOSIS AND TREATMENT OF ELECTROLYTE DISORDERS

Sodium

Sodium is the principal determinant of serum osmolality and free-water balance. The normal range of serum sodium concentration is 135 to 145 mEq/L. Sodium is an effective osmole that stimulates free-water movement across membranes because the cell wall is impermeable to sodium.

Hypernatremia is defined as a serum sodium concentration greater than 145 mEq/L. In moderate cases, the serum sodium is 145 to 159 mmol/L; in severe cases, it is greater than 160 mEq/L. Severe hypernatremia, or acute increases in serum sodium levels, can result in central pontine myelinolysis (CPM). Other symptoms of severe hypernatremia include muscle weakness, restlessness, insomnia, lethargy, and coma.

TABLE 3: Electrolyte composition (mEq) of gastrointestinal fluids

Source	Daily loss (mL)	Na⁺	K⁺	Cl⁻	HCO₃⁻
Saliva	1000	30-80	20	70	30
Gastric	1000-2000	60-80	15	100	0
Pancreas	1000	140	5-10	60-90	40-100
Bile	1000	140	5-10	100	40
Small bowel	2000-5000	140	20	100	25-50
Large bowel	200-1500	75	30	30	0

Hypernatremia is always associated with hypertonicity and can occur in the context of hypovolemia, euvolemia, or hypervolemia. Hypovolemic hypernatremia is most often seen in dehydrated patients with limited free water intake and uncontrolled fluid losses, such as infants, the elderly, and patients with mental impairments. Patients with high GI losses from nasogastric suction, vomiting, or diarrhea are also at risk. Euvolemic hypernatremia occurs with excess loss of urinary free water in patients with neurogenic or nephrogenic diabetes insipidus. These states of low ADH secretion are characterized by low urine osmolality with hypernatremia and are differentiated by observing response to desmopressin, an ADH analog that lacks a vasoconstrictive effect. Nephrogenic diabetes insipidus results from an impaired ability of the renal tubules to respond to ADH and therefore is unresponsive to exogenous desmopressin administration. Lastly, hypervolemic hypernatremia is usually iatrogenic, the result of fluid resuscitation with hypertonic solutions or states of mineralocorticoid excess such as Conn's or Cushing's syndrome.

Treatment of hypernatremia begins with calculation of the free water deficit.

$$\text{Free water deficit (L)} = [(\text{Serum Na} - 140)/140] \times 0.6 \times \text{weight (kg)}$$

Patients with severe (>160 mEq/L) or symptomatic hypernatremia should receive D5 water, and patients with mild or moderate hypernatremia can be given isotonic half NS. The first half of the free water deficit should be corrected over the first 24 hours, and the second half subsequently. Serum sodium levels should be frequently checked, and serum Na$^+$ concentration should not be reduced more than 0.5 mEq/L/h to avoid cerebral edema.

Hyponatremia is defined as a serum sodium concentration below 135 mEq/L and is classified as mild (130 to 135 mEq/L), moderate (120 to 130 mEq/L), or severe (<120 mEq/L). Hyponatremia most often occurs in association with low serum osmolality (hypotonic hyponatremia). Similar to hypernatremia, assessment of volume status is important in establishing cause, and hypotonic hyponatremia can be further categorized as hypervolemic, euvolemic, or hypovolemic.

The notable exception to the association with low serum osmolality is hypertonic hyponatremia, which occurs when BUN or glucose levels are elevated, thus increasing oncotic pressure and causing water to shift from the intracellular to the extracellular space. For each 100 mg/dL increase in glucose over normal, 2 mEq/L should be added to the reported sodium level for a truly representative value. Isotonic hyponatremia, or pseudohyponatremia, occurs when elements that do not contribute to the serum osmolality are elevated, such as triglycerides and proteins. Most laboratories now correct the sodium level for these artifacts and have eliminated cases of pseudohyponatremia.

In hypervolemic hypotonic hyponatremia, the extracellular fluid (ECF) and interstitium are expanded, but plasma volume is contracted, thus stimulating ADH release. Common clinical circumstances include congestive heart failure, chronic renal insufficiency, nephrotic syndrome, cirrhosis, and hypoalbuminemia. Hypervolemic hyponatremia is uncommon in the perioperative period and most often results from iatrogenic excessive administration of hypotonic fluids. It may occur in patients with advanced cirrhosis with development of hepatorenal syndrome or with renal insufficiency that occurs as a result of a low effective circulatory volume and renal blood flow. Patients with hypervolemic hypotonic hyponatremia are most effectively managed with a low-sodium diet (1500 to 2000 mg/d) and fluid restriction (1 L/d). In addition, spironolactone or amiloride can be added to promote a negative sodium balance.

Euvolemic hyponatremia can result from the syndrome of inappropriate ADH secretion (SIADH), hypothyroidism, or excessive water intake (psychogenic polydipsia). Increased ADH secretion occurs transiently in the early postoperative period, after trauma or with severe burns, but it can also occur with pulmonary malignancies, including carcinoid tumors and small-cell lung cancers, lung infections, and central nervous system (CNS) injuries and infections. Euvolemic hyponatremia is the most common presentation of acquired immune deficiency syndrome (AIDS)-related CNS infections. SIADH can be diagnosed by the presence of high urine osmolality (>150 mmol/kg) and high urine sodium (>20 mmol/L); it must be differentiated from adrenal insufficiency, which is accompanied by hypokalemia. SIADH is treated with fluid restriction (<1 L/d). Isotonic fluids actually worsen the hyponatremia because sodium is filtered in the glomerulus and free water is reabsorbed in the distal tubule.

Hypovolemic hypotonic hyponatremia is the most common form of hyponatremia in postoperative cases. If urine sodium is greater than 20 mmol/L, the sodium loss is primarily renal in origin. If urine sodium is less than 20 mmol/L, the sodium deficit is primarily from sequestration of isotonic fluids in the extravascular (third) space or loss from the GI tract or skin or from bleeding. Treatment of hypovolemic hyponatremia differs from euvolemic or hypervolemic cases because fluid restriction only worsens the clinical picture. Mild to moderate cases are best managed with slow correction with isotonic saline solution.

Severe cases of hyponatremia or acute changes in serum sodium concentration can result in cellular edema and cerebral swelling and produce symptoms that include headache, lethargy, seizures, and coma (Tables 4 and 5). Because of the other determinants of serum osmolality, primarily BUN and glucose, hyponatremia can occur with high, normal, or low serum osmolarity. Regardless of the serum osmolality, patients with severe or symptomatic hyponatremia should be aggressively treated with 3% NaCl hypertonic saline solution. Before treatment, it is important to calculate the sodium deficit, which is directly proportional to the TBW.

$$Na \text{ deficit} = (140 - serum\ Na) \times TBW$$

TBW can be estimated at 0.6 times total body weight for males and 0.55 times total body weight for females.

Rapid correction of hyponatremia with hypertonic saline solution can lead to CPM, with potential for permanent spastic quadriparesis and pseudobulbar palsy. Therefore, serum sodium should not be corrected more rapidly than 0.25 mEq/L/h or 8 mEq/kg/d. Hypertonic saline solution (3% NaCl) should be given in 250-mL aliquots at a rate of 50 mL/h, with frequent serum sodium level measurements. Furosemide can also be used to minimize the volume of resuscitation and aids in correcting the hyponatremia, as furosemide-induced diuresis is osmotically equivalent to administration of half NS.

Potassium

Serum potassium is maintained in a narrow range from 3.5 to 5 mmol/L, and variations in either direction from this range have potentially significant morbidity. Of total body potassium, 98% resides in the intracellular fluid compartment. Serum potassium is tightly regulated by the renin-angiotensin-aldosterone axis. Aldosterone causes secretion of potassium in the distal renal tubule.

Hyperkalemia, defined as K$^+$ above 5.5 mEq/L, is cardiotoxic and can lead to ventricular arrhythmias. Electrocardiographic (ECG) findings include, in order of progression, peaked T waves, QRS widening, shortened QT intervals, and ventricular ectopy. Chronic K$^+$ elevations in patients with chronic renal failure are well tolerated, but acute changes are not. Acute causes of hyperkalemia include acute renal failure, acidosis, rhabdomyolysis, cell lysis, and insulin deficiency. Pseudohyperkalemia occurs when red blood cells lyse in the collection tube; if this is suspected, the K$^+$ level should be rechecked.

Hypokalemia, defined as serum K$^+$ below 3.5 mEq/L, is encountered commonly in the postoperative period. Signs and symptoms of hypokalemia include generalized fatigue and weakness, atrial arrhythmias, ileus, and acute renal insufficiency. Flat T or U waves are seen on ECG. Causes of hypokalemia include large losses from the kidney or GI tract via nasogastric suctioning, vomiting, or diarrhea; alkalosis; catecholamine secretion; and insulin administration. Because most of the K$^+$ is stored intracellularly, small changes in serum K$^+$ reflect large changes in body stores. Low K$^+$ is frequently associated with hypomagnesemia and acidemia. Magnesium must first be replenished before K$^+$ corrects in response to exogenous administration. In patients who are both hypokalemic and acidemic, K$^+$ administration should precede correction of acidemia with bicarbonate, to avoid a precipitous drop in serum K$^+$ as the pH increases. Potassium can be replenished orally or via IV administration. For treatment of mild hypokalemia, oral replacement with KCl is recommended. Because the oral form is well absorbed, IV administration should be reserved for patients who do not tolerate the oral form or for those who have severe hypokalemia.

The ischemia-reperfusion cycle poses great risk of hyperkalemia in patients who undergo reperfusion of an ischemic extremity. Severe systemic hyperkalemia may occur in response to revascularization with at least 4 to 6 hours of ischemia. The authors routinely administer prophylactic bicarbonate before reperfusion. Another cause of hyperkalemia is succinylcholine, a depolarizing paralytic agent, particularly in patients with disuse atrophy usually from prolonged bed rest, neurologic denervation syndromes, severe burns, or muscle trauma.

Hyperkalemia must be identified and treated immediately. Patients should receive at least 1 ampule of prophylactic calcium gluconate to antagonize the K$^+$ depolarization effect on cardiac

TABLE 4: Signs and symptoms of electrolyte disorders

Disorder	Neurologic	Cardiovascular	Gastrointestinal	Renal	Other
Hyponatremia	Confusion, seizures, coma	Hypotension, hypertension	Salivation	Oliguria	
Hypernatremia	Confusion, seizures, coma	Fluid overload (edema)	Thirst		Tachypnea
Hypokalemia	Fatigue, weakness	Atrial arrhythmias, flat T wave, U waves	Ileus	Nephrotoxicity	
Hyperkalemia	Confusion, paralysis, areflexia	Ventricular arrhythmias, peaked T wave, prolonged PR interval, wide QRS complex	Nausea, vomiting, abdominal pain		
Hypocalcemia	Paresthesia, perioral tingling, carpopedal spasm, Chvostek's sign	Ventricular arrhythmias, prolonged QT interval			Laryngospasm
Hypercalcemia	Confusion, fatigue, coma	Shortened QT interval	Abdominal pain	Renal stones, nephrogenic diabetes insipidus (long-term)	
Hypomagnesemia	Weakness, cramping, hyperreflexia	Atrial ventricular arrhythmias (torsades des pointes)	Dysphagia		Refractory hypokalemia, hypocalcemia
Hypermagnesemia	Sedation, paralysis, areflexia	Atrial, ventricular arrhythmias	Diarrhea		
Hypophosphatemia	Confusion, seizures, weakness	Heart failure, respiratory failure			Bone pain
Hyperphosphatemia	Symptoms of hypocalcemia				

myocytes. Treatment strategies to decrease the serum K^+ include shifting the K^+ intracellularly or eliminating it from the body altogether. Intracellular shift is promoted by administering 10 U of insulin along with 1 ampule of D50 to prevent hypoglycemia or giving 1 ampule of $NaHCO_3$. Potassium excretion in urine or stool is promoted with administration of a loop diuretic, such as furosemide or bumetanide, or a sodium-potassium exchange resin, such as kayexalate, either orally or as a retention enema with sorbitol. With the exchange resin, 1 mEq of K^+ is taken up in exchange for 2 mEq Na^+, and an osmotic diarrhea ensues. The retention enema should not be given to patients with immunosuppression because it can cause rectal perforation. If these measures are unsuccessful, hemodialysis may be used as a last resort.

Calcium

Calcium is the most abundant electrolyte in the body. The normal range of serum calcium is 8.5 to 10.5 mg/dL, with 99% stored in bone. Approximately 50% of calcium circulates as the biologically active ionized form, and the other 50% as the biologically inactive bound form. As most of the nonionized form is bound to albumin, the serum calcium level must be adjusted for the serum albumin level in patients who are malnourished; calcium falls 0.8 mEq/dL for every 1 g/dL reduction in serum albumin. Serum calcium concentrations

are regulated by parathyroid hormone (PTH) and vitamin D. Conditions that alter PTH and vitamin D levels also indirectly alter calcium levels.

Hypocalcemia is defined as total serum concentration below 8.4 mg/dL or ionized calcium concentration below 4.5 mg/dL. Common causes of hypocalcemia include hypoparathyroidism and vitamin D deficiency. Less common causes include hyperphosphatemia, hypomagnesemia, acute pancreatitis, malnutrition, rhabdomyolysis, infusion of large volumes of fluid, and acute alkalosis from hypoventilation.

Acute hypocalcemia in the postoperative period can occur in response to rapid blood transfusions and hypoparathyroidism. In the past, stored blood contained a higher concentration of citrate, which binds to and chelates serum calcium. Now that citrate has been eliminated from blood-banking techniques, this is rarely seen. Patients who undergo thyroidectomy or parathyroidectomy may have hypocalcemia develop after surgery.

Symptoms of hypocalcemia include perioral numbness and tingling, hyperreflexia on stimulation of the facial nerve (Chvostek's sign), and spasm of muscles of the hand and forearm with inflation of a blood pressure cuff (Trousseau's sign). Prolonged QT intervals and arrhythmias may also been seen.

Hypocalcemia should be treated in symptomatic patients and also in patients with total serum calcium below 7.0 mg/dL or ionized calcium below 3.0 mg/dL. Calcium may be given orally, or

TABLE 5: Treatment options for electrolyte disorders

Disorder	Therapy
Hyponatremia	Fluid restrictions 0.9% NaCl Hypertonic saline solution ± diuretic
Hypernatremia	Free water 0.45% NaCl
Hypokalemia	Oral/IV potassium
Hyperkalemia	IV insulin + 50% dextrose 10% calcium gluconate
Hypocalcemia	IV calcium gluconate 1,25 Dihydroxyvitamin D_3
Hypercalcemia	IV 0.9% NaCl Furosemide
Hypomagnesemia	IV magnesium Magnesium sulfate
Hypermagnesemia	Sodium or potassium phosphate
Hyperphosphatemia	IV 0.9% NaCl Diuretics Acetazolamide

IV, Intravenous.

intravenously, in the form of calcium gluconate or calcium chloride. Severe hypocalcemia and symptoms such as overt tetany, laryngospasm, and seizures are indicative of IV calcium replacement. Calcium gluconate has 9 mg of elemental Ca^{2+} per mL, whereas $CaCl_2$ contains 27 mEq of Ca^{2+} per mL; hence, $CaCl_2$ contains three times more elemental Ca. $CaCl_2$ must be administered via central access and in a monitored setting to avoid associated bradycardia or hypotension. Concurrent hypomagnesemia or hyperphosphatemia must be corrected first for the calcium supplementation to be effective.

Calcium salts available for oral use include calcium carbonate and calcium gluconate. When hypocalcemia is resistant or severe, calcium salts should be supplemented with vitamin D_3.

Hypercalcemia is defined as serum calcium concentration greater than 10.4 mg/dL or ionized concentration greater than 5.6 mg/dL. It occurs most commonly with malignant diseases in hospitalized patients and with hyperparathyroidism in the general population. Breast cancer is the most common malignant cause. Other causes include vitamin A and D overdose, thyrotoxicosis, immobilization, excess exogenous calcium intake, granulomatous diseases, familial hypocalciuric hypercalcemia, and medications such as thiazide diuretics and lithium.

Symptoms of hypercalcemia include nausea, vomiting, altered mental status, constipation, depression, lethargy, myalgias, arthralgias, polyuria, headache, abdominal and flank pain (renal stones), and coma. Patients with symptoms or serum calcium above 14 mg/dL should be treated to avoid a hypercalcemic crisis. Goals of treatment include expansion of intravascular volume with normal saline solution to dilute circulating calcium and increase filtration of calcium in the kidneys. Furosemide should be administered via IV to increase renal calcium excretion and offset fluid administration.

Mild hypercalcemia (Ca < 12 mg/dL) can be managed with restriction in calcium intake and treatment of the underlying etiology. Hypercalcemic crisis usually occurs with serum calcium levels in excess of 14 mg/dL, and it requires aggressive treatment with bisphosphonates or calcitonin in addition to fluids and diuretics. Bisphosphonates, such as pamidronate (60 to 90 mg IV), inhibit osteoclast-induced bone resorption with onset of action between 24 and 48 hours. Bisphosphonates are the best choice for long-term calcium control and for hypercalcemia from enhanced bone resorption. Calcitonin (4 U/kg subcutaneously every 12 hours) inhibits bone resorption and decreases renal tubular resorption of calcium, with a shorter onset of action than bisphosphonates; therefore, it is the better choice for short-term control of calcium.

Magnesium

Magnesium is essential for energy metabolism, protein synthesis, cell division, and calcium homeostasis. Normal serum magnesium level is 1.4 to 2.0 mEq/L. Magnesium is primarily intracellular, with less than 1% of body stores in the extracellular fluid.

Hypomagnesemia is defined as serum concentration below 1.6 mg/dL; it often is seen after surgery because of dilution. Alternatively, hypomagnesemia may occur as a result of poor intake or GI losses, including diarrhea and biliary and enteric fistulas. Signs and symptoms rarely occur unless serum levels are below 1.0 mEq/dL. Serum magnesium levels must be monitored after surgery because severe hypomagnesemia may cause ventricular arrhythmias such as torsades des points. Oral magnesium oxide is the agent of choice for correction of mild to moderate hypomagnesemia. IV therapy with $MgSO_4$ is reserved for severe hypomagnesemia associated with arrhythmias.

Magnesium is easily replenished with oral or IV magnesium sulfate. IV replacement is usually reserved for patients with serum magnesium levels below 1.2 mg/dL. Patients with development of ventricular arrhythmias are treated acutely with bolus doses of IV magnesium sulfate, 1 to 2 g over 3 to 5 minutes.

Hypermagnesemia is a rare disorder that usually is seen with burns, trauma, or long-term hemodialysis. Hypermagnesemia is defined as serum concentration above 2.8 mg/dL. Symptoms are uncommon until the serum magnesium reaches 4.0 mg/dL, at which point patients become lethargic. Treatment is similar to that for hypercalcemia. Calcium is given to stabilize cardiac myocytes, NS is given to expand the plasma volume, and loop diuretics are used to induce renal excretion. Severe hypermagnesemia is treated with IV calcium gluconate 10% (10 to 20 mL over 10 minutes).

Phosphorus

Similar to calcium, 80% of phosphorus is stored in bone, with less than 1% of total body phosphorus in the intravascular space. Normal serum phosphate ranges from 2.2 to 4.7 mg/dL.

Hypophosphatemia is defined as serum concentration below 2.5 mg/dL; symptoms include respiratory and cardiac failure. Hypophosphatemia is frequently encountered in the postoperative period. Common causes include decreased intake and intestinal malabsorption from vitamin D deficiency, increased renal excretion from diuretics, alkalosis, hyperparathyroidism and hungry bone syndrome, major hepatic resection, rhabdomyolysis, and refeeding syndrome. Refeeding syndrome occurs in nutritionally depleted patients who are given carbohydrates; the resultant insulin surge causes the already depleted phosphate pool to redistribute into cells. Phosphate is an essential component for the adenosine triphosphatase backbone and should be replenished when serum concentration falls below 2.0 mg/dL. Phosphorous replacement should begin with intravascular therapy in patients with mild or severe hypophosphatemia. Five to 7 days of IV fluids may be required to replenish serum phosphorous levels. Once the serum phosphorous levels exceed 2 mg/dL, patients can be switched to oral therapy.

Hyperphosphatemia is defined as serum phosphate concentration greater than 5.0 mg/dL. Patients with renal insufficiency can have hypophosphatemia develop primarily because of decreased 1,25 dihydroxy–vitamin D production. Hyperphosphatemia is also a common feature of postoperative hypoparathyroidism. Patients with hyperphosphatemia primarily have symptoms that result from hypocalcemia. Hypocalcemia occurs because of precipitation of calcium with excess phosphate ions in the serum. Treatment includes expanding the plasma volume with NS and then stimulating renal excretion with acetazolamide. Acute cases of severe refractory hyperphosphatemia can be treated with hemodialysis. Patients in renal failure with chronic hyperphosphatemia are maintained on phosphate binders such as aluminum hydroxide or sevelamer.

SUGGESTED READINGS

Adrogue HJ, Madias NE: Hypernatremia, *N Engl J Med* 18:342:1493–1499, 2000.
Adrogue HJ, Madias NE: Hyponatremia, *N Engl J Med* 25:342:1581–1589, 2000.
Adrogue HJ, Madias NE: Management of life-threatening acid-base disorders, *N Engl J Med* 338:26–34, 107–111, 1998.
Jacob M, Chappell D, Rehm M: Clinical update: perioperative fluid management, *Lancet* 369:1984–1986, 2007.

PREOPERATIVE ASSESSMENT OF THE OLDER PATIENT: FRAILTY

**Mara McAdams-DeMarco, PhD, and
Dorry Segev, MD, PhD**

OVERVIEW

Approximately half of all operations in the United States are performed in older patients over the age of 65 years, and this number is rapidly growing. Surgical risk prediction and treatment decision-making in this population are challenging because of the heterogeneity of health status in older adults. For many years, it has been recognized, anecdotally and intuitively, that some older patients might not have the physiologic reserve to withstand surgery, but standardized measures of physiologic reserve have, until recently, been limited. Current research is focused on developing measures of frailty that improve prediction of adverse surgical outcomes in older adults; much of this work is already helping to guide clinical practice.

The purpose of this chapter is to: (1) describe the frailty phenotype; (2) review surgical risk prediction based on frailty; (3) relate frailty to disability and comorbidity; (4) describe the role of frailty in the preoperative assessment of older patients; and (5) explore sarcopenia as a potential measure of frailty.

OLDER SURGICAL PATIENTS

Approximately half of all surgical patients in the United States are over 65 years old. Recent population projections suggest that the average volume of a surgical practice will increase by 14% to 47% from the year 2000 to 2020 as a result of the increasing population of older adults. As the population of the United States ages, tools from the gerontology literature may prove critical in guiding clinical decision-making for older surgical patients.

Older surgical patients have a unique physiologic vulnerability that requires assessment beyond the standard preoperative evaluation to identify those at risk for postoperative complications. Older adults undergoing surgery are at increased risk for morbidity, mortality, and postoperative complications even after accounting for differences in comorbidity and disability. Older patients may experience a functional decline after major surgery, and 20% to 44% of older patients are discharged to a skilled nursing facility or other institutional care.

Surgical indications in younger patients are not necessarily generalizable to older patients because physiologic changes from aging can alter the risk-benefit balance by increasing the risk or reducing the benefit. Medical care for older patients must be based not only on the patient's long-term prognosis but also on the patient's personal goals. For older patients, survival may not be as relevant as other outcomes, including physical function, quality of life, and institutionalization. Traditional preoperative evaluation strategies identify risk based on a single domain; this approach does not capture the unique vulnerability of older patients. However, newly emerging research suggests that novel metrics from gerontology can provide insights into more accurate vulnerability assessment. Additional information that is not typically part of the surgical evaluation of younger patients may improve the accuracy of predictions during the preoperative assessment and thus help patients make more informed and personal treatment choices.

FRAILTY

Frailty is increasingly recognized as a unique domain of health status, separate from comorbidity and disability. Frailty is a global phenotype of physiologic reserve, resistance to stressors, and vulnerability in older patients. Although the concept of frailty may initially appear abstract, recent work helps to quantify this "foot of the bed" judgment of an experienced clinician in a generalizable, repeatable manner. Our goal is to move from the intuitive concept of frailty to the validated quantifiable measure of frailty.

Frailty is the composite of individual components of physiologic decline. These components can be measured in the preoperative clinic, usually in less than 5 to 10 minutes by trained personnel of various backgrounds, to generate a frailty score. This score can then be used to predict adverse surgical outcomes, which are directly related to the number of frailty components present. In general, each increase in the number of components of frailty is associated with an increase vulnerability to a surgical stressor and decreased physiologic reserve to withstand the operative stress.

Although many definitions of frailty are found in the gerontology literature, the definition of frailty by Fried and colleagues is one of the most cited; this definition is measured with a validated scoring system of five components and is widely used in both research and clinical settings. The five components in Fried's scoring system include shrinking, weakness, exhaustion, low physical activity, and slowed walking speed (Table 1). These components have been found to have good validity and reliability.

Each component yields a score of 0 or 1 based on the criteria listed. The raw frailty score is the sum of the number of components (range, 0 to 5) and is usually categorized as frail or nonfrail—or frail, intermediately frail, or nonfrail—based on the distribution of the component score in the population of interest. For example, Makary and associates found that in surgical patients, those with a score of 4 or 5 were frail, of 2 or 3 were intermediately frail, and of 0 or 1 were nonfrail. Both intermediately frail and frail patients were predisposed to adverse outcomes; however, the risk was higher in those who were frail versus those who were intermediately frail.

The frailty phenotype was first described in the Cardiovascular Health Study, a cohort study of community-dwelling older adults. Frail participants had 2.24-fold higher risk (95% confidence interval [CI], 1.51 to 3.33) of mortality than their nonfrail counterparts, even after accounting for differences in comorbidity and disability. In nonsurgical populations, frailty has been associated with mortality, morbidity, falls, cardiovascular disease, insulin resistance, venous thromboembolism, and hospitalizations. The research identifying the consequences of frailty supports the hypothesis that frailty is the capacity to adapt to stressors.

It appears that the physiology underlying frailty is complex; evidence is accumulating that immune system dysregulation may play a leading role, resulting in heightened inflammation and alteration in innate and adaptive immune systems. The frailty phenotype has been associated with dysregulation of multiple physiologic systems, including not only a generalized inflammatory state but also dysregulated cortisol, altered heart rate variability, changes in hormonal status, and decreased immune function. It has been posited that each component of this phenotype is related in a vicious cycle of dysregulation, a cycle that spirals downward with decreasing adaptive capacity. The physiologic consequences of this dysregulation are easily recognizable in older surgical patients.

FRAILTY, COMORBIDITY, AND DISABILITY

Frailty is considered to be a phenotype that is independent of, but sometimes associated with, disability and comorbidity (Figure 1). Although older frail surgical patients are likely to have comorbidities and disability, some older patients are frail but do not have comorbidities or disability; likewise, some older patients have comorbidities or disability but not frailty.

In the formative studies of frailty, disability was defined as dependence in one or more activities of daily living (ADL) with the Katz activity of daily living score. ADLs describe six tasks necessary for independent living: bathing, dressing, transferring, walking, using a toilet, and feeding. In older patients undergoing surgery, disability has emerged as an important risk factor for mortality, postoperative institutionalization, and higher healthcare costs. In one study by Robinson in 2009, older surgical patients with ADL disability had 13.9-fold higher odds (95% CI, 2.99 to 65.49) of 6-month mortality compared with those with no ADL disability; ADL disability was the strongest predictor of mortality in this study. In another study by the same group, ADL disability was associated with 5.66-fold higher odds (95% CI, 2.37 to 13.52) of discharge to institutional care.

TABLE 1: Components of frailty

Component	Definition and measurement
Shrinking	Shrinking is defined as unintentional weight loss ≥10 lb in the past year.
Weakness	Weakness is assessed by grip strength and is measured directly with a hand-held Jamar dynamometer. Three serial tests of maximal grip strength with the dominant hand are performed, and a mean of the three values is adjusted by gender and BMI. Weakness is defined as an adjusted grip strength in the lowest 20th percentile of a community-dwelling population of adults 65 years of age and older. Men meet the criteria for weakness if BMI and grip strength are ≤24 and ≤29 kg; 24.1-26 and ≤30 kg; 26.1-28 and ≤31 kg; >28 and ≤32 kg, respectively. Women meet the criteria for weakness if BMI and grip strength are ≤23 and ≤17 kg; 23.1-26 and ≤17.3 kg; 26.1-29 and ≤18 kg; and <29 and ≤21 kg, respectively.
Exhaustion	Exhaustion is measured by responses to the following two statements from the modified 10-item Center for Epidemiological Studies depression scale: "I felt that everything I did was an effort" and "I could not get going." Patients are asked, "How often in the last week did you feel this way?" Potential responses were: 0, rarely or none of the time (<1 day); 1, some or a little of the time (1-2 days); 2, a moderate amount of the time (3-4 days); and 3, most of the time. Patients who answer either statement with response 2 or 3 meet the criteria for exhaustion.
Low physical activity	Physical activities are ascertained for the 2 weeks before this assessment with the short version of the Minnesota Leisure Time Activities Questionnaire and include frequency and duration. Weekly tasks are converted to equivalent kilocalories of expenditure, and individuals who report a weekly kilocalorie expenditure in the lowest 20th percentile for their gender (men, <383 kcal/wk; women, <270 kcal/wk) are classified as having low physical activity.
Slowed walking speed	Slowness is measured by averaging three trials of walking 15 ft at a normal pace. Individuals with a walking speed < 20th percentile, adjusted for gender and height, are scored as having slow walking speed. Men meet criteria if height and walk time are ≤173 cm and ≥7 seconds, or >173 cm and ≥6 seconds, respectively. Women meet criteria if height and walk time are ≤159 cm and ≥7 seconds, or >159 cm and ≥6 seconds, respectively.

BMI, Body mass index.

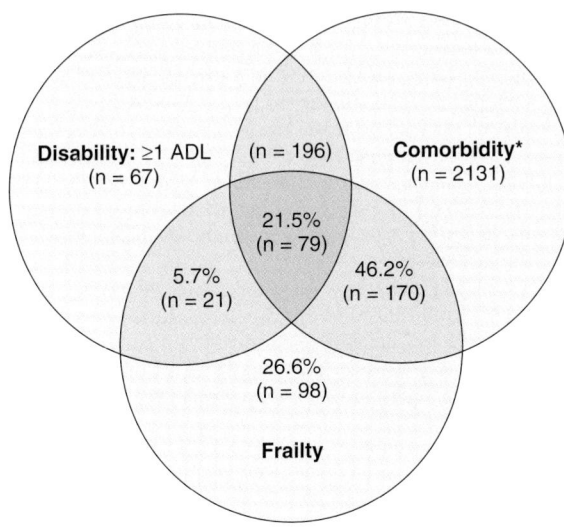

FIGURE 1 Overlap of frailty with disability and comorbidity in older adults participating in the Cardiovascular Health Study. *ADL,* Activities of daily living. *Two or more out of the following nine diseases: myocardial infarction, angina, congestive heart failure, claudication, arthritis, cancer, diabetes, hypertension, chronic obstructive pulmonary disease (COPD). *(From Fried LP, Tangen CM, Walston J, et al, Cardiovascular Health Study Collaborative Research Group: Frailty in older adults: evidence for a phenotype, Gerontol A Biol Sci Med Sci 56(3):M146-M156, 2001.)*

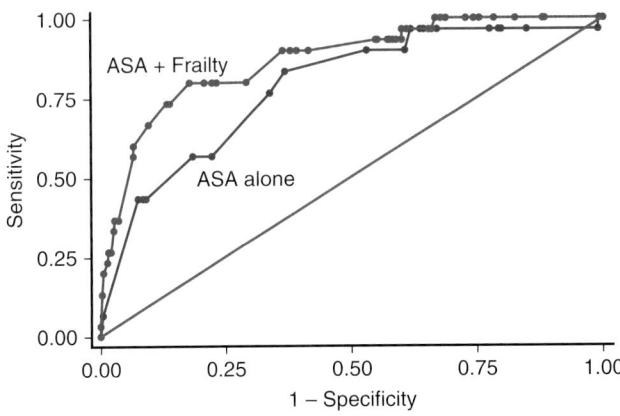

Area under ROC curve = 0.8694

FIGURE 2 Example of nested receiver operator characteristic (ROC) curves that show the ability of frailty to predict surgical complications beyond established risk scores. *ASA,* American Society of Anesthesiologists. *(From Makary MA, Segev DL, Pronovost PJ, et al: Frailty as a predictor of surgical outcomes in older patients, J Am Coll Surg 210(6):901-908, 2010.)*

In addition, in the formative studies of frailty, comorbidity was defined as the presence of two or more chronic diseases. Two thirds of individuals in the United States 65 years and older have two or more chronic diseases, and half of them have four or more chronic diseases. Multiple measures of comorbidity are available for preoperative assessment. Some measures of comorbidity are as simple as counting the number of chronic conditions. Others, such as the Charlson comorbidity index, are summary scores of chronic conditions. In the Charlson index, each chronic condition is given a score based on its particular risk of mortality, and the summary score represents the burden of comorbidities.

FRAILTY AND SURGICAL RISK PREDICTION

Numerous predictors of postoperative complications are commonly used, such as the Lee and Eagle criteria and the American Society of Anesthesiologists (ASA) score. However, these predictors have substantial limitations when used in older adults and do not account well for the physiologic reserve specific to this population. In older surgical patients, frailty improves risk prediction because a measure of physiologic reserve quantifies the resilience of an older adult to recover from an operation.

Frailty has been shown to predict operative risk in older surgical patients beyond that which is predicted with the Lee and Eagle or ASA scores. Makary and colleagues prospectively studied frailty as a predictor of surgical outcomes in older adults. At the time of surgery, 10.4% of the older patients were frail and 31.3% were intermediately frail. After a minor surgical procedure, 11.4% of the frail patients, 7.3% of the intermediately frail patients, and 3.9% of the nonfrail patients experienced a complication as defined by the American College of Surgeons National Surgical Quality Improvement Program (NSQIP). After adjusting for the Lee and Eagle and ASA scores, frailty was independently associated with increased risk of surgical complications; patients who were intermediately frail had 2.06-fold higher

adjusted odds (95% CI, 1.18 to 3.60) of complications, and frail patients had 2.54-fold higher adjusted odds (95% CI, 1.12 to 5.77) of complications when compared with nonfrail patients. Furthermore, frailty predicted length of stay and discharge to an assisted or skilled nursing facility. When added to the best available surgical risk scores, frailty improved the ability to predict which older adults would experience a postoperative complication (improvement in area under the receiver operating characteristic curve [AUC] by frailty for each risk score: Lee, 0.05; Eagle, 0.04; ASA, 0.07) and which would be discharged to an assisted or skilled nursing facility (Lee, 0.13; Eagle, 0.10; ASA, 0.10; Figure 2).

Recent data suggest that frailty also improves risk prediction for patients undergoing kidney transplantation; interestingly, this risk prediction is relevant for patients of all ages undergoing this procedure, rather than just older adults, consistent with the conceptual framework that dialysis creates an "accelerated aging" of sorts and that patients on chronic dialysis react to stressors more like older adults than like their otherwise-healthy contemporaries. Among a cohort of kidney transplant recipients of all ages, 25% were found to be frail; this was about threefold higher than the rate of frailty in community-dwelling older adults. The adjusted risk of early allograft dysfunction, as measured by need for dialysis in the first week after transplant, was 1.94-fold higher for frail patients (95% CI, 1.13 to 3.36) compared with nonfrail patients. Frailty improved standard risk prediction in this study (the AUC improved from 0.67 to 0.73); in fact, frailty was the strongest predictor among recipient factors.

These studies show how preoperative characterization of frailty can predict surgical outcomes and augment other risk assessment tools. Frailty captures a quantifiable domain of surgical risk not previously measured in older adults. The measurement of frailty in the preoperative assessment could aid in predicting which older adults are at high risk of surgical complications and improve decision making for older surgical patients.

ALTERNATIVE MEASURES OF FRAILTY AND SURGICAL OUTCOMES

In addition to the validated Fried criteria for frailty, other definitions of frailty have been evaluated. Alternative definitions of frailty include components such as functional decline, low cognition, poor nutrition, high chronic disease burden, perceived poor health, depression, medication issues, incontinence, low social support, mobility difficulties, and the presence of the "geriatric syndrome."

Robinson and colleagues in 2009 measured frailty with an alternative definition in older patients undergoing elective surgery and found that this alternative definition was associated with increased risk of 6-month mortality. In addition, patients who were classified as frail were more likely to be discharged to institutional care (59% vs 0%; *P* value, <0.001) and readmitted to the hospital (32% vs 4%; *P* value, 0.04). This research group also showed that, with increasing number of alternative frailty components, there was an increase in hospital ($76,363 vs $27,731; *P* value, <0.001) and postoperative ($110,702 vs $33,453; *P* value, <0.001) costs.

Although there are multiple definitions of frailty, physiologic reserve is an important predictor of surgical outcomes; until comparative data are available, the choice of frailty measure to be used in clinical practice might be best made based on experience of the provider or hospital.

SARCOPENIA AND SURGERY

Two of the components of frailty, walking speed and grip strength, represent muscle wasting and sarcopenia. As such, an alternate way to measure physiologic reserve is to measure sarcopenia directly with radiographic imaging. Englesbe and colleagues have studied sarcopenia as an objective and reproducible measure of frailty. Sarcopenia is not only considered to be part of the aging process but is also accelerated by chronic illness. However, sarcopenia is not altered by acute illness and thus is a good measure of overall health. Sarcopenia is easily quantified with a preoperative computed tomographic (CT) scan to measure the size of the psoas muscle, a core muscle of the trunk that is susceptible to changes in chronically ill patients.

Englesbe and colleagues in 2010 found a correlation between cross-sectional psoas area and model for end-stage liver disease (MELD) score (i.e., the probability that the patient would die in the next 90 days) in patients undergoing liver transplantation. Not surprisingly, increased total psoas area was associated with a decrease in 1-year mortality (hazard ratio, 0.27; 95% CI, 0.14 to 0.53), even after accounting for pertinent patient and donor factors. The same research group has shown that in elective general surgery, vascular abdominal surgery, and abdominal aortic aneurysm repair, psoas area is associated with mortality; in major, elective general, and vascular surgery, the 1-year survival rate was 87% versus 95% for those with smaller psoas area. In addition, the cost increased by $10,110 for every 1000-mm² decrease in core muscle size. This work suggests that sarcopenia is a clinical measure of risk in older surgical patients and may be a useful objective measure for clinical decision making.

LOGISITICS OF PREOPERATIVE MEASUREMENT OF FRAILTY

The growing literature on frailty and adverse surgical outcomes in older patients supports the clinical utility of measuring frailty as part of the preoperative assessment. Implementing a frailty scoring system during a preoperative assessment to identify vulnerable older patients who are considering surgery is feasible and may aid in clinical decision-making.

A preoperative screening for frailty can easily be implemented into clinical practice. For example, the frailty assessment outlined in Table 1 can be performed in every older preoperative patient by, for example, the person who obtains vital signs. Frailty assessment takes no more than 5 to 10 minutes and can be completed before the physician encounter. A template to record frailty components could be incorporated into the electronic health system to allow for quick calculations of the frailty score and longitudinal measurement. The frailty score can provide prognostic information about older patients during the preoperative consultation, during which a decision regarding surgical intervention might take place. If a patient is identified as frail, the implications of this can be integrated into the discussions of the risks and benefits of surgical intervention. The clinical assessment of frailty used for preoperative decision making should be viewed as a supplement to, but not replacement of, the traditional risk assessment.

As more studies establish frailty as an important phenotype in surgery, growing evidence shows that patients might benefit from interventions to reduce frailty, such as preoperative conditioning (sometimes referred to as "prehabilitation"). In the postoperative period, it might be possible to decrease the risk of complications in frail patients through closer monitoring, attention to nutrition and mobility, and aggressive physical and occupational therapy. Anticipation of which older adults are at risk for surgical complications and which will need discharge to an institutional care facility after a major operation is important for preoperative counseling of expected outcomes and preoperative care planning for older patients and their caregivers.

CONCLUSION

Frailty is a well-established phenotype that was developed in gerontology and is directly applicable to older surgical patients. Older patients who are frail are at increased risk for adverse surgical outcomes, including complications, longer length of stay, discharge to institutional care, and mortality. Although patients who are frail are likely to also have disability and comorbidities, frailty is a distinct phenotype and provides information and risk prediction above and beyond the other two domains. Sarcopenia is an objective measure of frailty, and novel research is exploring risk prediction based on radiographic measures of muscle mass. In conclusion, frailty is a clinically useful predictor of adverse surgical outcomes that can be incorporated into the preoperative assessment of older adults.

SUGGESTED READINGS

Englesbe MJ, Patel SP, He K, et al: Sarcopenia and mortality after liver transplantation, *J Am Coll Surg* 211(2):271–278, 2010.

Fried LP, Tangen CM, Walston J, et al: Cardiovascular Health Study Collaborative Research Group: frailty in older adults: evidence for a phenotype, *Gerontol A Biol Sci Med Sci* 56(3):M146–M156, 2001.

Garonzik-Wang JM, Govindan P, Grinnan JW, et al: Frailty and delayed graft function in kidney transplant recipients, *Arch Surg* 147(2):190–193, 2012.

Makary MA, Segev DL, Pronovost PJ, et al: Frailty as a predictor of surgical outcomes in older patients, *J Am Coll Surg* 210(6):901–908, 2010.

Robinson TN, Eiseman B, Wallace JI, et al: Redefining geriatric preoperative assessment using frailty, disability, and co-morbidity, *Ann Surg* 250(3):449–455, 2009.

Preoperative Preparation of the Surgical Patient

Kristine E. W. Breyer, MD, and
Michael A. Gropper, MD, PhD

INTRODUCTION

The patient population undergoing surgery is becoming increasingly complex from a medical standpoint. At the same time, there is increasing pressure to provide cost-effective care. In order to improve outcomes, understanding the patient's medical history and optimizing comorbidities prior to surgery are essential. The preoperative preparation of the surgical patient serves to evaluate and optimize comorbidities in order to minimize morbidity and mortality during and immediately following the surgical procedure.

Many patients ask, "What are my risks from anesthesia?" This is a complicated question, which depends not only on the type of anesthesia administered but also on the type of surgical procedure planned and the patients' comorbidities. Generally, anesthesia has become incredibly safe over the past several decades. Major perioperative events are rare, but they can be devastating and can include myocardial infarction, stroke, renal failure, airway compromise, and death. The American Society of Anesthesia (ASA) classifies patients according to the number of comorbidities and the severity of illness called the ASA class (Table 1). This classification system is well validated, and the risk of a major adverse event during anesthesia increases with increasing ASA class.

Preoperative preparation varies by institution and practices, depending on what preoperative services are available. Large institutions often have preoperative clinics staffed by members from the anesthesia department to which surgeons can refer patients for history and physical examination. Some surgical practices will not have this luxury, and the surgeon may have the burden of collecting and ordering preoperative tests to ensure his or her patient is prepared for surgery. Although the availability of specific surgical preoperative services varies greatly, the goal is always the same: to minimize as many risks as possible to ensure that the patient goes through surgery as safely as possible. This chapter outlines the major and most common risks, testing, and medication recommendations.

Generally, a healthy ASA I or II patient undergoing low- to intermediate-risk surgery should not require evaluation by a preoperative clinic or primary care physician. However, for patients who are ASA III or greater or undergoing high-risk surgery, evaluation by a preoperative clinic or primary care physician prior to surgery is important (Figure 1).

ORAL INTAKE GUIDELINES

The ASA recently revised guidelines for fasting prior to anesthesia. These recommendations include fasting before administration of anesthesia regardless of type of anesthetic—general, regional, or monitored anesthesia care. Adult and pediatric patients should fast from intake of clear liquids at least two hours prior to the start of anesthesia. The guidelines state that the type of liquid is more important than the specific volume and therefore do not give specific recommendations on volume. A clear liquid includes water, coffee, or tea without dairy; clear fruit juice without pulp; and clear carbonated beverages. Pediatric patients should fast from human breast milk for 4 hours and from infant formula for 6 hours prior to the start of anesthesia.

All patients should fast from solid food and nonhuman milk for a minimum of 6 hours prior to the start of anesthesia. The guidelines do make note that a large meal or a fatty meal may benefit from a longer duration of fasting and recommend 8 hours of fasting in these cases.

PREOPERATIVE TESTING

In recent years there has been momentum to move away from routinely testing every patient. Selective testing is recommended when tests may change perioperative management. Changes in perioperative management include medical optimization, changes to intra- and postoperative monitoring, and preoperative coronary revascularization, to name a few. Unnecessary testing can burden patients, increase expenses, and even cause delays over unanticipated nonspecific test results. However, the decision not to order certain tests must be weighed against possible surgical delays if a test was not ordered that is needed. Of course, ultimately the preoperative testing required for a particular patient will need to be determined by both the surgeon and the anesthesiologist.

Electrocardiograms and Other Cardiac Testing

The ASA, American College of Cardiology (ACC), and the American Heart Association (AHA) all agree that resting electrocardiograms (ECGs) for asymptomatic patients undergoing low-risk surgery are unnecessary. The ACC and AHA recommend cardiac evaluation based on the Lee Revised Cardiac Risk Index (RCRI) and surgical risk (Box 1 and Table 2). According to the 2007 ACC/AHA Guidelines and 2009 update, ECGs are recommended for patients with at least one RCRI risk factor who are undergoing vascular surgery. Resting ECGs are also recommended for all patients with known coronary artery disease, peripheral vascular disease, or cerebral vascular disease who are undergoing intermediate- or higher-risk surgery. The guidelines also state that it is "reasonable" to obtain resting ECGs in patients undergoing vascular surgery or in any patient undergoing at least intermediate-risk surgery who also have one or more RCRI risk factors.

Further cardiac evaluation may be indicated for patients with cardiac risk factors or active cardiac disease, depending on the surgical risk (Figure 2). In patients with known cardiac disease or severe pulmonary disease, an echocardiogram can be helpful in delineating systolic and diastolic dysfunction and pulmonary artery hypertension. This in turn may inform intraoperative monitoring plans.

Chest Radiographs

The ASA does not offer specific recommendations on preoperative chest radiographs (CXRs). The ASA does not recommend routine CXRs but does recommend consideration for obtaining CXRs in patients who are smokers, have had recent upper respiratory tract infections, have chronic obstructive pulmonary disease (COPD), and have heart disease. The CXR is more likely to provide useful information in patients with less stable pulmonary disease and also in patients with heart failure.

Blood Tests

Routine blood testing is not recommended, but blood testing is reasonable in ASA III or greater patients and should be considered in all patients undergoing high-risk surgery. Hematocrit, or hemoglobin, is specifically recommended in higher-risk patients for more invasive procedures, patients with liver disease, patients with a history of bleeding or anemia, and patients at extremes of age. Coagulation studies are specifically recommended by the ASA for patients with dysfunctional bleeding, renal disease, and liver disease.

BOX 1: Revised cardiac risk index

1. Heart failure
2. Cerebrovascular disease
3. Ischemic heart disease
4. Diabetes
5. Creatinine >2.0 mg/dL

Adapted from Fleisher LA: Cardiac risk stratification for noncardiac surgery: update from the American College of Cardiology/American Heart Association 2007 guidelines, Cleve Clin J Med 76 Suppl(4):S9-S15, 2009; and Lee TH, et al.: Derivation and prospective validation of a simple index for prediction of cardiac risk of major noncardiac surgery, Circulation 100(10):1043-1049, 1999.

TABLE 1: American Society of Anesthesia classification system

ASA class	
I	Healthy patient
II	Mild/well-controlled disease
III	Severe/multiple systemic disease(s)
IV	Life-threatening disease
V	Severely ill patient who may not survive without operation
VI	Brain-dead patient for organ procurement

From American Society of Anesthesia (ASA) Classification System.

TABLE 2: Risk of perioperative cardiac morbidity for noncardiac surgery

Risk category	Surgical procedure	Cardiac morbidity risk
High	Vascular	>5%
Intermediate	Carotid, neurosurgery, ears/nose/throat, abdominal, thoracic, urologic (excluding endoscopic), and orthopedic	1% to 5%
Low	Superficial, cataract, endoscopic, and breast	<1%

Adapted from ACC/AHA 2007 guidelines for noncardiac surgery.

FIGURE 1 Preoperative evaluation algorithm. All patients will have at least a day of surgery. History and physical performed with the anesthesiologist. *COPD*, Chronic obstructive pulmonary disease; *ESRD*, end stage renal disease, *H&P*, history and physical; *h/o*, history of; *HTN*, hypertension; *ILD*, interstitial lung disease; *PFO*, patent foramen ovale; *RA*, rheumatoid arthritis; *VSD*, ventricular septal defect. *(Adapted from UCSF preoperative stepwise approach to determining the timing and nature of the preoperative assessment for elective noncardiac surgery [2013]).*

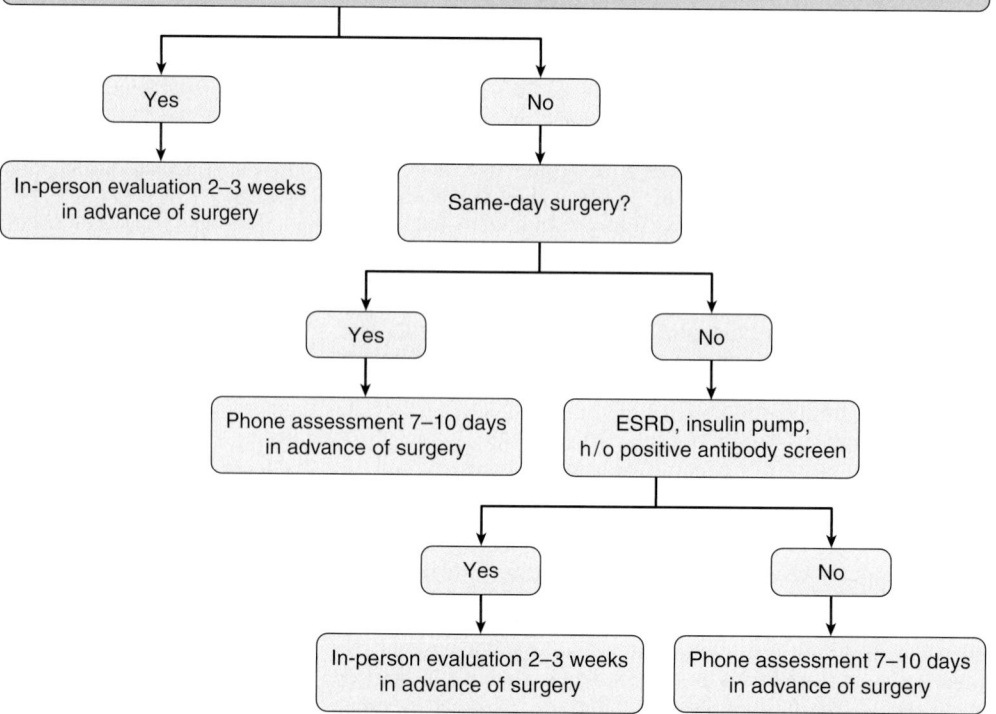

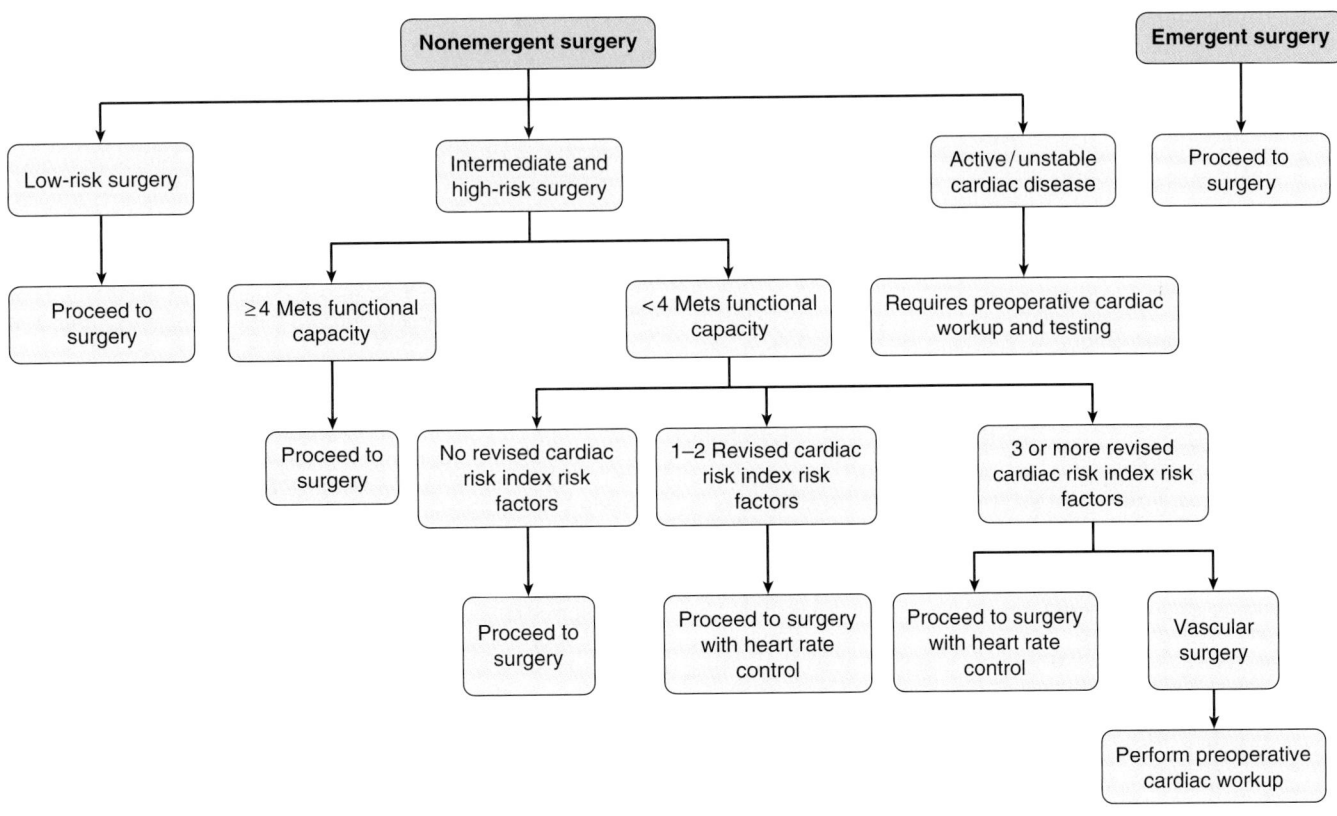

FIGURE 2   Algorithm for preoperative cardiac testing. Note this algorithm refers to the need for additional specific cardiac testing only. Depending on the patient's comorbidities and planned surgery, preoperative testing and evaluation may still be required. *(Adapted from Fleisher LA, et al: ACC/AHA 2007 guidelines on perioperative cardiovascular evaluation and care for noncardiac surgery. Executive summary: a report of the American College of Cardiology/American Heart Association Task Force on practice guidelines [writing committee to revise the 2002 guidelines on perioperative cardiovascular evaluation for noncardiac surgery] developed in collaboration with the American Society of Echocardiography, American Society of Nuclear Cardiology, Heart Rhythm Society, Society of Cardiovascular Anesthesiologists, Society for Cardiovascular Angiography and Interventions, Society for Vascular Medicine and Biology, and Society for Vascular Surgery, J Am Coll Cardiol 50(17):1707-1732, 2007.)*

Urine Testing

Urinalysis is specifically recommended by the ASA for patients scheduled for prosthetic implantation, patients with urinary tract infection symptoms, and some urologic procedures. Pregnancy testing should be obtained in any female of childbearing age.

COMORBIDITIES

Chronic comorbidities are common in the surgical patient, and many patients often have multiple comorbidities. The most important principles in managing chronic disease in the preoperative setting are to optimize and stabilize patients' diseases as much as possible. It's always preferable to delay operation, whenever possible, in the setting of an acute or recent exacerbation of any chronic state. Communication among the surgeon, anesthesiologist, primary care physicians, and specialists is essential. Usually, patients with stable chronic disease who receive normal follow-up for their disease will not require additional testing prior to surgery.

Cardiac Disease

Ischemic heart disease, heart failure, and valvular abnormalities represent the most common cardiac conditions encountered in the perioperative period. Surgery should be delayed in any patient with unstable angina, with unstable heart failure, or who otherwise meets

criteria for further cardiac workup until that workup is completed (see Box 1 and Figure 2). A recent echocardiogram should be available in patients with moderate to severe valvular disease and heart failure.

If surgery is emergent and a necessary workup cannot be completed, then obtaining an ECG, CXR, and a full set of labs may be helpful. Many institutions can provide transthoracic echocardiography on an emergent basis, and this is likely the single most useful evaluation.

Ischemia and Stents

Following placement of coronary artery stents, dual antiplatelet therapy with aspirin and glycoprotein IIb/IIIa inhibitors is critical to prevent major adverse cardiac events from stent thrombosis. Discontinuation of this therapy places the patient at risk for in-stent thrombosis. Bare-metal stents require a minimum of 1 month of dual antiplatelet therapy, whereas drug-eluting stents require a minimum of 3 months of dual antiplatelet therapy for Sirolimus stents and 6 months of minimum therapy for Paclitaxel stents. One year of therapy is strongly recommended for all stent placements. In-stent thrombosis rates of up to 25% to 30% have been reported in patients when dual antiplatelet therapy was prematurely discontinued.

Whenever possible, all elective surgical procedures should be deferred until the patient is out of this initial 1-year window following stent placement. If semielective or urgent surgery is necessary, it is preferred to delay the procedure until a patient with a bare-metal stent is 1 month out from stent placement and a patient with a drug-eluting stent is 3 months out from stent placement. The American College of Chest Physicians advocates waiting 6 weeks after bare-metal stent placement and 6 months after drug-eluting stent placement. Aspirin should be continued if possible. Close communication with the patient's cardiologist is critical for perioperative management recommendations and to determine whether ASA can be continued perioperatively.

Pacemakers and Defibrillators

Pacemakers and defibrillators are becoming more common in the surgical patient. The increasing variety and complexity of these devices can make perioperative care challenging. Device firing and malfunction are a risk with most surgical procedures. For example, some pacemakers may sense electrocautery discharges as abnormal heartbeats and therefore suppress discharges. This is particularly problematic in pacemaker-dependent patients. An internal defibrillator may sense the same electrocautery discharges as an arrhythmia, causing the defibrillator to attempt cardioversion.

Historically, a magnet was placed over the electric cardiovascular device during surgery. However, with the current generation of devices, the response to magnet placement is not always predictable. Some defibrillators turn off when a magnet is placed over them and do not turn back on until the magnet is removed and replaced over the device again. Some pacemakers enter a no-sense pacing mode when a magnet is placed over them, whereas other pacemakers may reprogram with magnet placement. Pacemaker-defibrillator combination devices are also common with unpredictable magnet responses. The guidelines for preoperative management were organized in a 2011 consensus statement by the Heart Rhythm Society and the American Society of Anesthesiologists.

Find out the type of cardiovascular implantable device and the indication for the device. If the patient does not know, try to obtain this information from the patient's primary caregiver or cardiologist. Pacemakers should be interrogated every 12 months and defibrillators interrogated every 6 months at a minimum in stable patients. Obtain information about the last interrogation, pacemaker dependency, underlying rhythm, battery longevity, and magnet response. Patients are also given wallet-size cards with their device name and serial number. These cards will have the phone number of the company that manufactured the device, which can be contacted for information and advice. Companies keep records of the patients, their devices, indications, and programming. Representatives will be able to tell you what the implanted device does and its response to magnets. This is particularly useful in the case of emergent surgical procedures where outside records are not easily accessible. It is also recommended that the devices be interrogated at the conclusion of the procedure to be sure they are functioning as intended.

Pulmonary Disease

Pulmonary diseases can increase the risk of both pulmonary and nonpulmonary perioperative complications. Asthma does not increase the risk of postoperative pulmonary complications but does increase the risk of intraoperative pulmonary complications, such as bronchospasm with intubation. COPD and obstructive sleep apnea (OSA) both increase the risk of intraoperative and postoperative pulmonary complications. A diagnosis of COPD confers the highest risk of postoperative pulmonary complications. OSA increases the risk for airway management problems in the perioperative period. Extremes of age and higher ASA status have been shown to be independent predictors of increased postoperative pulmonary complications. Thoracic, major abdominal, open abdominal aortic aneurysm repair, and surgical procedures lasting more than 3 hours all increase the risk of postoperative pulmonary complications. However,

additional testing is usually not necessary prior to surgery for these patients.

Specific questions to ask your patient include ascertaining the severity of their illness, exercise tolerance, baseline symptoms, recent exacerbations, and medications. Generally, regular medications, such as inhaled bronchodilators and corticosteroids, should be continued through the perioperative period. Patients taking oral corticosteroids should continue their corticosteroid medications and may require a perioperative burst dose. Smoking cessation should be encouraged. Smoking does increase the risk of postoperative pulmonary complications. Carbon monoxide levels from smoking within 12 hours of cessation and sputum production will begin to decrease within 1 to 2 months.

Routine spirometry testing is usually not indicated. Spirometry may be indicated in patients undergoing specific thoracic procedures, especially lobectomy and pneumonectomy. Low serum albumin is an independent predictor of postoperative pulmonary complications, as well as a predictor of increased postoperative morbidity and mortality.

For patients with high risk of intraoperative and postoperative pulmonary complications, the anesthesiologist may recommend peripheral or neuraxial nerve blockade versus general anesthesia where appropriate. For patients undergoing thoracotomy, epidural analgesia is particularly useful for postoperative pain management because it can spare large doses of opiates that cause respiratory depression.

Liver Disease

Liver disease is common in the surgical patient. Alcohol, viral hepatitis, and now nonalcoholic fatty liver disease are the most common causes of cirrhosis in the United States. Patients with liver disease are at significantly increased risk for perioperative morbidity and mortality. Classically, the Childs-Pugh score has been used to predict postoperative mortality. The Model for End Stage Liver Disease Score is now used more frequently to confer the severity of liver disease and perioperative risk.

All patients with liver disease should have complete blood counts, coagulation studies, complete metabolic panels, and albumin levels tested preoperatively. In fact, patients with unexplained thrombocytopenia should be investigated for possible liver disease. Hepatosplenomegaly, ascites, and signs of portal hypertension should all be sought on physical exam. Up to 30% of patients with cirrhosis have evidence of hepatopulmonary syndrome leading to hypoxemia. Low oxygen saturation, peripheral cyanosis, or clubbing should prompt investigation with arterial blood gases and possible echocardiography with bubble study to identify intrapulmonary or extrapulmonary shunting.

Diabetes

Diabetes is prevalent in the United States, and complications from diabetes affect multiple organ systems. Managing glucose perioperatively is essential but difficult. Hyperglycemia is associated with increased surgical site infections, whereas hypoglycemia can be devastating to the patient.

Patients with insulin pumps should continue their basal insulin rate unchanged. The only exception to this is if the patient has been hypoglycemic on his or her basal infusion, indicating that the basal infusion is too high. In this case, the basal rate should be decreased. Patients taking long-acting insulins such as glargine should continue to take it, but the preoperative dose should be 75% of normal. Patients taking NPH insulin can take their full dose of NPH the evening prior to surgery but decrease any morning dose by 50% on the day of surgery. Oral hypoglycemic agents can be taken the day prior to surgery but discontinued on the day of surgery. Metformin is an exception and should be discontinued the night prior to surgery. Of course, all diabetic preoperative patients should carefully monitor their glucose levels to avoid hypoglycemia or extreme hyperglycemia.

Diabetic patients are at risk for electrolyte abnormalities, as well as heart, vascular, kidney, and neuropathic disease and should be screened accordingly preoperatively. Obtain an ECG, complete blood count, and chemistry panel.

Renal Disease

Chronic kidney disease, defined as 3 months or greater with a glomerular filtration rate of less than 60 mL/min/1.73 m^2 or pathologic evidence of kidney damage, is estimated to affect over 26 million Americans. Diabetes and hypertension are common comorbidities that can make these patients challenging to manage perioperatively. In fact, kidney disease is an independent risk factor for cardiac disease (see Box 1). Additionally, the perioperative period marks a vulnerable time for chronic kidney patients who are not on dialysis. These patients are extremely susceptible to further kidney impairment, which often does not return to baseline.

Patients with chronic kidney disease requiring hemodialysis should receive dialysis as scheduled preoperatively, with laboratory studies checked following dialysis. Patients not on dialysis should be at their baseline creatinine preoperatively whenever possible. Chronic kidney disease patients are prone to volume shifts, electrolyte abnormalities, and anemia. Obtain a preoperative ECG, a chemistry panel, and complete blood counts preoperatively.

Obesity

Obesity is a growing epidemic in the United States and most developed countries. The obesity syndrome is often complicated by many of the comorbidities already mentioned. However, it is important to note that obesity itself represents an additional risk during surgery and anesthesia. Obese patients have a higher risk of surgical site infection and thromboembolic complications. Obese patients are also more likely to present airway management challenges for the anesthesiologist. Obstructive sleep apnea is a common comorbidity that may benefit from additional postoperative monitoring, such as continuous pulse oximetry or a more highly monitored bed. Obese patients are also more prone to positioning injuries and can have difficult intravenous access leading to infiltrated lines and may require central line placement. Optimizing as many of the associated comorbidities as possible in your obese patients prior to surgery is critical. Educating patients about these specific risks is important as well.

Obstructive sleep apnea is exacerbated postoperatively due to residual anesthetic and analgesic medications. If your patient does have obstructive sleep apnea, instruct him or her to bring their continuous positive airway pressure (CPAP) machine with them to the hospital for use in the recovery room and postoperative ward. If your patient does have OSA but does not have a CPAP machine, consider requesting one for use in-house. Use of a CPAP machine may require a ward with a higher level of care, depending on your institution. Requesting critical care or step-down care ahead of time will help to set patient expectations and reduce delays after surgery.

MEDICATION MANAGEMENT

Angiotensin Converting Enzyme Inhibitors

Angiotensin converting enzyme inhibitors (ACE-inhibitors) and angiotensin receptor blockers (ARBs) are common antihypertensive

agents. These agents have shown specific mortality benefit post myocardial infarction and in systolic heart failure. Intraoperative hypotension is a major side effect of ACE-inhibitors and ARBs. Intraoperative hypotension can be refractory, sometimes requiring vasopressin infusions. Common practice is to hold the ACE-inhibitor/ARB the morning of surgery. New studies are emerging showing a possible trend toward an increased number of postoperative cardiovascular events in patients where an ACE-inhibitor/ARB was held. Randomized controlled trials are needed to fully investigate this question. Given the known risk of refractory intraoperative hypotension, we recommend holding ACE-inhibitors/ARBs the morning of surgery and restarting this therapy as soon as the surgical patient is stable postoperatively.

Anticoagulants

Over 250,000 patients in North America are currently taking either a vitamin K antagonist (VKA) or antiplatelet drugs. The American College of Chest Physicians developed guidelines to inform decision making with regards to antithrombotic management in the perioperative period. Management should take into account the patient's risk for a thromboembolic event and the patient's risk of bleeding during the procedure.

Patients who require temporary interruption of VKAs for surgery should stop taking the VKA 5 days prior to surgery and resume taking the VKA 12 to 24 hours after surgery, providing adequate hemostasis. Patients with mechanical heart valves, history of venous thromboembolism, or atrial fibrillation at low risk for thromboembolism do not need bridging anticoagulation therapy. Those at high risk for thromboembolism do require bridging therapy (Table 3).

Patients undergoing minor dental procedures, dermatologic procedures, or cataract surgery should continue VKA therapy uninterrupted. Consider stopping VKA 2 to 3 days prior to dental procedure if the procedure is higher risk for bleeding or difficult hemostasis.

Direct thrombin inhibitors (DTIs) are an emerging drug class that can be used as an alternative to VKAs. The four most common DTIs are apixaban, dagibatran, edoxaban, and rivaroxaban. Clinically these drugs differ from VKAs in several ways. Therapeutic anticoagulation is achieved within hours of starting a DTI versus days for VKAs. DTIs affect INR, but the INR does not accurately reflect the level of anticoagulation. Currently, we do not have a readily available standardized laboratory test to monitor DTI anticoagulation levels. Importantly, there are no specific reversal agents for DTIs. This is particularly important to be aware of perioperatively. Activated factor VIIa is a nonspecific agent that can be used to promote hemostasis.

DTIs should be managed similarly to VKAs preoperatively with regards to risk stratification of venous thromboembolism and risk of surgical bleeding. One reasonable management scheme includes stopping the DTI 5 days prior to surgery and, when necessary, briding the patient with heparin (low molecular weight or unfractionated).

Aspirin should be continued for patients on aspirin therapy at high risk for cardiovascular events undergoing noncardiac surgery. If the patient is at low risk for cardiovascular events, aspirin can be discontinued 7 to 10 days prior to noncardiac surgery. Aspirin should be continued prior to cardiac surgery. Cardiac surgery patients on dual antiplatelet therapy should stop the antiplatelet drug prior to cardiac surgery but continue their aspirin. New antiplatelet drugs require different discontinuation times prior to surgery. Clopidogrel should be discontinued 5 days prior to surgery when appropriate. Other antiplatelet agents may require different stop times depending on their pharmacology.

Bridging therapy with unfractionated heparin drips should be discontinued 4 to 6 hours prior to surgery. Therapeutic enoxaprin should be discontinued 24 hours prior to the start of surgery and resumed 48 to 72 hours after surgery.

TABLE 3: Risk stratification for perioperative thromboembolism

Risk	Mechanical heart valve	Atrial fibrillation	Venous thromboembolism (VTE)
High (>10% annual risk)	Any mitral valve prosthesis Mechanical aortic valve prosthesis Stroke or TIA <6 months	CHADS₂ 5-6 Stroke or TIA <3 months Rheumatic heart disease	VTE <3 months Thrombophilia
Moderate (5% to 10% annual risk)	Bileaflet aortic valve prosthesis + (1 of the following): Atrial fibrillation Prior stroke/TIA HTN DM CHF >75 years old	CHADS₂ 3-4	VTE 3 to 12 months Factor V Leiden Recurrent VTE Active cancer
Low (<5% annual risk)	Bileaflet aortic valve prosthesis *without* additional risk factor	CHADS₂ 0-2	VTE > 12 months prior

Perioperative thromboembolism risk stratification. CHADS₂, Congestive heart failure (1 point); Hypertension (1 point); Age ≥ 75 years old (1 point); Diabetes (1 point); and VTE/stroke/TIA (2 points).
Adapted from Douketis JD, Spyropoulos AC, Spencer FA, et al: Perioperative management of antithrombotic therapy: antithrombotic therapy and prevention of thrombosis, *ed 9, American College of Chest Physicians Evidence-Based Clinical Practice Guidelines. Chest 141(2 Suppl): e326S-350S, 2012.*

Beta-Blockers

Recently, several large randomized control trials have investigated the benefit of beta-blockers in the perioperative setting. Early studies pointed to a decrease in perioperative myocardial ischemia and even decreased long-term postoperative mortality. More recent studies have elucidated some of the risks of beta-blocker therapy, most noticeably an increased risk for stroke in some beta-blocked surgical patients or increased postoperative mortality, particularly with high-dose untitrated beta-blockade.

The AHA has released new guidelines for beta-blocker therapy in the surgical patient. Patients who are currently taking beta-blockers should continue to take their beta-blocker perioperatively. Patients whose beta-blocker is taken twice daily should take their morning dose of the medication on the day of surgery. Beta-blockers are recommended for patients with signs of ischemia on preoperative testing or with known coronary artery disease who are undergoing vascular surgery. Initiation of beta-blockers is reasonable in patients undergoing vascular surgery, patients at risk for coronary artery disease, or patients at high cardiac risk who are undergoing intermediate risk surgery. Any patient initiated on beta-blocker therapy needs to be closely monitored and the beta-blocker started and titrated prior to surgery.

Herbal Medications

Herbal medications are becoming increasingly popular. Herbal medications are considered dietary supplements and therefore are not regulated for safety or efficacy. Many patients do not consider herbs and vitamins as medications and may not disclose them with their medication lists. Herbal medications have a wide range of possible clinical implications from garlic's antiplatelet properties to St. John's wart's inhibition of serotonin, norepinephrine, and dopamine reuptake.

Given the expanse of herbal medications available, some with known and some with unknown medical implications, we conservatively recommend discontinuing herbal medications for 7 to 10 days prior to surgery.

Opiates

Many surgical patients take opiates chronically. These patients can be challenging to manage perioperatively. An important aspect to keep in mind is that the pain medications the patient takes on a daily basis represent that patient's baseline opiate requirements. Obtaining an accurate history as to the actual opiate consumption preoperatively is crucial. The chronic pain patient will require pain medications in addition to this baseline requirement postoperatively. Therefore, we recommend that these patients take their scheduled opiates even on the day of surgery. Patients also taking as-needed opiates should continue to take those opiates if needed on the day of surgery.

Proton Pump Inhibitors and Histamine-2 Blockers

Patients routinely taking proton pump inhibitors or histamine-2 blockers should continue taking these medications throughout the perioperative period. Patients should take their daily dose of this medication on the morning of their surgical procedure.

SUMMARY

As our medical capabilities and knowledge expand, our surgical population grows more complex. Today our perioperative patients have more comorbidities than ever before. Similarly, the preoperative preparation of our patients is more important than ever. Our common goal is to safely get these patients into and out of the operating room. This chapter summarizes some of the common surgical comorbidities, testing, and medication strategies. No preoperative test will ever take the place of the thoughtful history and physical examination, and robust communication between the anesthesia and surgical teams provides the framework for optimal outcomes.

Suggested Readings

Apfelbaum JL, Connis RT, Nickinovich DG, et al: Practice advisory for pre-anesthesia evaluation: an updated report by the American Society of Anesthesiologists Task Force on Preanesthesia Evaluation, *Anesthesiology* 116(3):522–538, 2012.

Crossley GH, Poole JS, Rozner MA, et al: The Heart Rhythm Society (HRS)/American Society of Anesthesiologists (ASA) Expert Consensus Statement on the perioperative management of patients with implantable defibrillators, pacemakers and arrhythmia monitors: facilities and patient management: executive summary this document was developed as a joint project with the American Society of Anesthesiologists (ASA), and in collaboration with the American Heart Association (AHA), and the Society of Thoracic Surgeons (STS), *Heart Rhythm* 8(7):e1–e18, 2011.

Douketis JD, Spyropoulos AC, Spencer FA, et al: Perioperative management of antithrombotic therapy: Antithrombotic Therapy and Prevention of Thrombosis, 9th ed: American College of Chest Physicians Evidence-Based Clinical Practice Guidelines, *Chest* 141(2 Suppl):e326S–e350S, 2012.

Eilers H, Liu KD, Gruber A, et al: Chronic kidney disease: implications for the perioperative period, *Minerva Anestesiol* 76(9):725–736, 2010.

Fleischmann KE, Beckman JA, Buller CE, et al: 2009 ACCF/AHA focused update on perioperative beta blockade, *J Am Coll Cardiol* 54(22):2102–2128, 2009.

Fleisher LA, Beckman JA, Brown JA, et al: ACC/AHA 2007 Guidelines on Perioperative Cardiovascular Evaluation and Care for Noncardiac Surgery: Executive Summary: A Report of the American College of Cardiology/American Heart Association Task Force on Practice Guidelines (Writing Committee to Revise the 2002 Guidelines on Perioperative Cardiovascular Evaluation for Noncardiac Surgery) Developed in Collaboration With the American Society of Echocardiography, American Society of Nuclear Cardiology, Heart Rhythm Society, Society of Cardiovascular Anesthesiologists, Society for Cardiovascular Angiography and Interventions, Society for Vascular Medicine and Biology, and Society for Vascular Surgery, *J Am Coll Cardiol* 50(17):1707–1732, 2007.

Grines CL, Bonow RO, Casey DE Jr, et al: Prevention of premature discontinuation of dual antiplatelet therapy in patients with coronary artery stents: a science advisory from the American Heart Association, American College of Cardiology, Society for Cardiovascular Angiography and Interventions, American College of Surgeons, and American Dental Association, with representation from the American College of Physicians, *J Am Coll Cardiol* 49(6):734–739, 2007.

Qaseem A, Snow V, Fitteman N, et al: Risk assessment for and strategies to reduce perioperative pulmonary complications for patients undergoing noncardiothoracic surgery: a guideline from the American College of Physicians, *Ann Intern Med* 144(8):575–580, 2006.

Is a Nasogastric Tube Necessary After Alimentary Tract Surgery?

Jordan E. Fishman, MD, MPH, and
Adrian Barbul, MD, FACS

Nasogastric (NG) tubes have long been a mainstay in the surgical armamentarium and remain a well-established method for both gastrointestinal decompression and the provision of enteral nutrition. Routine postoperative placement of NG tubes entered clinical practice in the 1930s. Guided by both early clinical evidence and an understanding of the relevant gastrointestinal physiology, widespread adaption soon followed. So revered was NG tube placement that W.J. Mayo once remarked that he "would rather have a resident with a nasogastric tube in his pocket than a stethoscope." With the introduction of evidence-based medicine, many tenets long associated with surgical dogma have been evaluated in a prospective randomized controlled trial format; routine placement of NG tubes after alimentary tract surgery is no exception.

Some historical controversy surrounds the origin of NG tube usage. Many attribute the first NG tube to renowned anatomist and Italian surgeon Hieronymus Fabricius (Fabricus ab Aquapendente, 1537-1619) who described the insertion of a silver tube into a patient to provide enteral feeds. Others credit John Hunter with the first reported use of a NG tube based on a 1790 publication of the Transactions of a Society for the Improvement of Medical and Chirugical Knowledge. In it, Hunter describes the insertion of a tube composed of eel skin stretched over a whale bone into a patient who was unable to feed himself after a cerebrovascular accident. Although NG tube gastric lavage was reported in the early 19th century, it remained a largely ignored footnote. Adolph Kussmaul is credited with the first use of a NG tube for gastric decompression in 1884. The introduction of a flexible rubber tube (the Levin tube) in 1921 and McIver's theory published 5 years later that postoperative abdominal distention is caused by swallowed air and could be prevented with use of the Levin tube set the groundwork for mainstream application of NG tubes. McIver's theory was tested in 1933 by Wangensteen and Paine who proposed NG tube decompression for small bowel obstruction as an alternative to surgical intervention. This therapy was so successful that widespread adaptation of this practice soon followed, and prophylactic placement of a NG tube after abdominal surgery became de rigueur. This belief was further codified in 1971 by the American College of Surgeons manual of preoperative and postoperative care, which explicitly stated that "intestinal decompression is required after resection and reanastomosis of gastrointestinal tract."

Currently, two distinct purposes exist for the continuation of NG tubes after alimentary tract surgery: provision of enteral nutrition and decompression of the gastrointestinal tract. Although the specific route of enteral feeds (i.e., NG vs oral gastric vs percutaneous gastric, etc.) has not been explicitly addressed in a prospective randomized controlled trial, the superiority of enteral nutrition to both parenteral nutrition and nil per os (NPO) status after surgery has been addressed. Multiple prospective randomized controlled trials and subsequent meta-analyses have shown a reduction in overall mortality, postoperative infectious complications, length of hospital stay, and even decreased gastrointestinal anastomosis breakdown in patients who were fed enterally soon after surgery. Although a more thorough review of enteral feeding after gastrointestinal surgery is beyond the scope of this chapter, it can be reasonably surmised that in patients who are not expected to able to feed themselves after surgery, the placement and maintenance of a NG tube for the specific purpose of enteral nutrition is in keeping with best current surgical practice.

Unlike the placement of a NG tube specifically for enteral nutrition, the role of postoperative NG tube placement for gastrointestinal decompression has been well studied. Early proponents for NG tube placement after surgery believed that gastrointestinal decompression would decrease patient discomfort, reduce postoperative nausea and vomiting, and speed the recovery from postoperative ileus. It was also believed that decompression would decrease the intraluminal pressure of the gastrointestinal tract and thereby protect the newly created anastomosis from excessive tension and subsequent break-down. Furthermore, NG tube decompression was postulated to reduce tension on the abdominal wound and thereby reduce the rates of wound infection, wound failure, and hernia formation. NG tube usage was also thought to provide the surgeon insight into potential intraluminal complications such as postoperative leaks and hemorrhage.

The first to challenge the necessity of NG tube decompression after surgery was Gerber in 1958. In a nonrandomized study of 600 patients with paralytic ileus, half of the patients received a NG tube, and the other half did not. Patients who did not receive nasogastric decompression had less mortality and morbidity than those who did. NG tube decompression was also associated with a higher incidence of respiratory tract complications. After this publication, many case series and nonrandomized trials showing the safety of gastrointestinal surgery without the use of NG tube decompression were published throughout the 1960s and 1970s. Although these publications began to erode the belief in the necessity of gastrointestinal decompression, a greater understanding of the anatomy and physiology of the gastrointestinal tract was necessary before further changes in practice could be accepted.

The belief that postoperative ileus was a gastrointestinal problem was specifically challenged by Woods and colleagues in 1978. Previous work by Smith and associates showed that small bowel motility returns soon after surgery. Woods and colleagues, however, evaluated the entire gastrointestinal tract. With use of an animal model of laparotomy, the postoperative electromechanical activity of the gastric antrum, small bowel, right colon, and sigmoid colon were recorded. They noted that the electromechanical activity of the gastric antrum and the small bowel were affected by surgery but that they returned to normal levels almost immediately. This was in stark contrast to the electromechanical activity of the right colon, which was significantly decreased for a 24-hour period, and that of the sigmoid colon. The decrease in the electromechanical activity of the sigmoid colon was both more profound than that of any other segment and found to last for much longer, namely, 72 hours. Thus, postoperative ileus was cast as a dysfunction of the colon, not a dysfunction of the stomach or the small bowel, and therefore was unlikely amenable to decompression of the stomach or small intestine.

The first study to specifically address this issue in a prospective randomized controlled trial format was published by Reasbeck and associates in 1984. Patients with an operation that resulted in an enteric suture line were divided into two groups: one group received a prophylactic NG tube, and the other group did not. The outcomes studied were differences in postoperative complication rates. This study is notable for its broad inclusion of surgical anastomoses, ranging from the biliary-enteric to the colocolonic. No statistical difference in postoperative complication was noted between the two arms of the study. Unfortunately, because of the large range of surgical procedures and the relatively small sample size, a large number of the same type of cases was not included in the study.

In 1985, Bauer and colleagues examined the role of prophylactic postoperative NG tube placement in a prospective randomized control trial format in a study involving 200 patients. One hundred patients received a NG tube that was placed during surgery and remained in place until the passage of flatus; 100 other patients underwent NG tube placement during surgery and removal at the conclusion of the procedure. Although most cases in this study involved an anastomosis, the authors included a number of additional intraabdominal procedures that did not (splenectomy, cholecystecomy, etc.). Five patients who were randomized to the nasogastric decompression group had a NG tube reinserted after removal; six patients who were not subjected to postoperative NG tube decompression subsequently needed NG tube insertion. Indications for NG insertion or reinsertion included vomiting, gross distention, or overt obstruction in the postoperative period. No statistical difference was found in frequency or type of postoperative pulmonary complication

(pneumonia or atelectasis). In addition, no statistical difference was seen between wound dehiscence, anastomotic leak, or wound infection.

Although these studies were effective in establishing the general concept that routine NG tube decompression after alimentary tract surgery is unnecessary, many surgeons believed that they were inadequately powered to change management for specific operations. Given the large clinical interest in this subject, further prospective randomized control trials followed. Some of these trials showed that prophylactic postoperative nasogastric decompression via NG tube increased subsequent complications, and others reported no statistical difference in the overall complication rate. By the mid 1990s, a sufficient number of publications showed some diversity of opinion to support a meta-analysis.

Cheatham and associates published the first large scale meta-analysis of the use of prophylactic postoperative NG tubes in 1995 and included publications from 1955 through 1993. Both randomized and nonrandomized trials were included in the meta-analysis, encompassing a total of 26 trials, which brought the study population to 3964. Specific postoperative complications investigated included: death, pneumonia, atelectasis, aspiration, fever, nausea, vomiting, abdominal distention, wound dehiscence, wound infection, anastomotic leak, oral feeding, and hospital length of stay. In all measured outcomes, no advantage was found to routine use of postoperative NG tube placement. A statistically significant reduction was seen in the overall complication rate for patients who were not treated with routine placement of a NG tube. This was manifest as a statistically significant decreased rate of postoperative pneumonia, atelectasis, and fever. Although a trend towards significance in increased postoperative vomiting and abdominal distention was found, especially when six less rigorous clinical trials were excluded from the meta-analysis, this did not increase the incidence of serious or nonserious postoperative complications. This meta-analysis included a wide variety of intraabdominal surgical procedures, but it is notable for its inclusion of 20 nonrandomized trials and relative paucity of emergency cases. Additional research was needed to further resolve this issue.

Nelson and associates conducted an additional large-scale meta-analysis that was subsequently published in 2005 and supported the nonsuperiority of prophylactic NG tube placement. Several more followed, many including earlier studies (Table 1). In none of these analyses was any detrimental effect associated with the avoidance of routine NG tube placement.

Although there is a preponderance of high-quality research evaluating the issue of routine prophylactic nasogastric decompression, many surgeons still practice this treatment modality on the belief that it will hasten the return of bowel function, ease respiration or aspiration of gastric contents by emptying the stomach, increase patient comfort, protect intestinal anastomoses, and shorten hospital stay. In addition, many surgeons believe the complications of NG tube intubation are so rare and infrequent that it is essentially a risk-free procedure. In their 1985 article, Bauer and colleagues reported that 70% of patients found the NG tube to be a source of significant discomfort. Essenhigh and associates describe how 70% of patients found NG tube intubation either "distressing" or "unpleasant." One study that examined NG tube complications found these to occur in 63% of patients studied. Although many of these complications were minor, such as vomiting, nasopharyngeal soreness, cough, wheezing, or sinusitis, the result is nonetheless compelling. Reported complication rates for NG tube intubation vary from 0.2% to 7.6%. The most common complication, malposition, occurs between 1.3% and 2.4% and can result in both pneumonia and pneumothorax. Other reported serious complications include esophageal perforations, tracheoesophageal fistulas, gastric perforations, sinusitis, epistaxis, and intracranial placement. These complications are infrequent, but they serve to dispel the myth that NG tube intubation is entirely benign.

NG tube insertion should be undertaken with great care and with an understanding of the relevant anatomy involved. Numerous

TABLE 1: Summary of meta-analyses that address nasogastric tube placement

Author	No. of patients/no. of included studies	Outcomes evaluated	Benefits noted
Cheatham	3964/26	Death, pneumonia, atelectasis, aspiration, fever, nausea, vomiting, distension, wound dehiscence, SSI, leaks, time to oral feeds, hospital LOS	Decreased pneumonia, atelectasis, and fever
Nelson (2005)	4194/28	Time to flatus, pulmonary complications, SSI, ventral hernia, leaks, LOS, nausea/vomiting	Earlier return of bowel function
Nelson (2007)	5240/33	Time to flatus, pulmonary complications, fever, SSI, wound dehiscence, leaks, LOS, incisional hernia, nausea/vomiting, tube complications	Earlier return of bowel function, decrease in pulmonary complications
Yang	717/5	All gastrectomy: time to flatus, time to oral intake, leaks, pulmonary complications, LOS, morbidity, mortality	Decrease in time to starting oral diet
Verma	5711/37	Time to flatus, pulmonary complications, SSI, leak, incisional hernia, LOS, gastric upsets	Decrease pulmonary complications, earlier return bowel function

LOS, Length of stay; *SSI*, surgical site infection.

reports are found of NG tube passage into both the cranial vault, via the cribriform plate, and the mediastinum, through a perforated esophagus. Therefore, NG intubation should be undertaken with extreme caution, if at all, in patients with maxillofacial trauma. In addition, care must be taken in patients who have ingested caustic material, have a history of esophageal strictures, or have had recent esophageal surgery to avoid esophageal perforation.

Placement of the NG tube can be facilitated with application of topical anesthetics to the nasal and oral mucosa with viscous lidocaine jelly, or preferably, aerosolized benzocaine. Once the patient has been adequately anesthetized and the procedure has been adequately explained, the passage depth needed is approximated with measurement of the distance between the nostrils through the angle of the mandible to the xiphoid process. This position should be marked on the tube. Ask patients to sit up and place their chin to their chest to help facilitate esophageal placement. The tip of the NG tube is then lubricated with surgical jelly and advanced into the nares, with aiming posteriorly and inferiorly. Many patients gag as the tube approaches the laryngeal apparatus. Instruct the patient to swallow and time further tube advancement to occur during active swallowing. The NG tube is advanced in this fashion until the previously measured mark is reached. Rapid but imprecise confirmation of tube placement can be done with aspiration of gastric contents or audible gastric sounds with tube insufflation. Proper placement, however, should always be confirmed radiologically with visualization of the NG tube tip below the diaphragm. An excellent video tutorial describing NG tube placement is available online.

Since the advent of the Levin tube, nasogastric decompression has revolutionized the treatment of bowel obstruction. In fact, it remains the treatment of choice for temporizing bowel obstructions, often allowing for successful nonoperative management. There are also clear indications for the use of NG tubes for gastrointestinal decompression after gastrointestinal surgery (e.g., persistent vomiting and bowel obstruction). In addition, NG tube intubation is an easy solution for patients who need enteral nutrition or medication that

cannot be delivered orally. However, despite these specific indications for use, current evidence clearly shows that the routine placement of NG tubes after alimentary tract surgery does not benefit the patient and possibly causes an increase in detrimental outcomes and discomfort. In summary, the authors do not recommend routine or prophylactic NG tube usage after gastrointestinal surgery.

SUGGESTED READINGS

Bauer JJ, Gelernt IM, Salky BA, et al: Is routine postoperative nasogastric decompression really necessary? *Ann Surg* 201:233–236, 1985.

Cheatham ML, Chapman WC, Key SP, et al: A meta-analysis of selective versus routine nasogastric decompression after elective laparotomy, *Ann Surg* 221:469–476, 1995.

Metheny N, Meert K, Clouse R: Complications related to feeding tube placement, *Curr Opin Gastroenterol* 23:178–182, 2007.

Nelson R, Edwards S, Tse B: Prophylactic nasogastric decompression after abdominal surgery, *Cochrane Database Syst Rev* CD004929, 2005.

Nelson R, Edwards S, Tse B: Prophylactic nasogastric decompression after abdominal surgery, *Cochrane Database Syst Rev* CD004929, 2007.

Phillips N: Nasogastric tubes: an historical context, *Medsurg Nurs* 15:84–88, 2006.

Sorokin R, Gottlieb J: Enhancing patients safety during feeding-tube insertion: a review of more than 2000 insertions, *J Parenter Enteral Nutr* 30:440–445, 2006.

Stein IF, Lans HS: Abdominal surgery without gastrointestinal suction, *Arch Surg* 92:35–38, 1966.

Tanguy M, Seguin P, Malledant Y: Bench-to-bedside review: routine postoperative use of the nasogastric tube: utility or futility? *Crit Care* 11:201–207, 2007.

Thomsen TW, Shaffler RW, Setnik GS: Nasogastric intubation, *N Engl J Med* 354:e16, 2006.

Verma R, Nelson RL: Prophylactic nasogastric decompression after abdominal surgery (review), *Cochrane Database Syst Rev* 3, 2010.

Yang Z, Zheng Q, Wang Z: Meta-analysis of the need for nasogastric or nasojejunal decompression after gastrectomy for gastric cancer, *Br J Surg* 95:809–816, 2008.

SURGICAL SITE INFECTIONS

Laura H. Rosenberger, MD, MS, and
Robert G. Sawyer, MD

OVERVIEW

Surgical site infections (SSIs) are a common surgical complication that affects between 2% and 5% of the 30 to 40 million operations that occur in the United States per year. SSIs are the most common nosocomial infection among surgical patients and are consistently the second most common healthcare-associated infection overall. Mortality rates after SSI are markedly higher when compared with patients without an SSI, as are the patient's length of stay (mean, 7 days), hospital readmission rates, and direct patient costs ($500 to $3000 per infection).

DEFINITION

Controversy and ambiguity continue to exist in the definition of an SSI. Experts may disagree about the appearance of an incision in regards to SSI, particularly in the presence of surrounding cellulitis or wound drainage. In 1970, the Centers for Disease Control and Prevention (CDC) established the National Nosocomial Infections Surveillance (NNIS) system (now part of the National Healthcare Safety Network [NHSN]) in part to create criteria defining SSI and to standardize the definition for accurate surveillance and reporting. Currently, it is the national standard by which medical personnel and researchers consistently define SSI.

By definition, SSIs occur within the first 30 days after the operation if no implant is placed or within 1 year if an implant remains. The classification scheme defines the following two categories of SSI based on location: incisional SSI (subdivided into superficial and deep) and organ/space SSI (Figure 1). Specific criteria for defining each of the categories of SSI infection can be found in the CDC's Guidelines for Prevention of Surgical Site Infection.

RISK FACTORS

Development of an SSI requires microorganism contamination at the surgical site. During an operative procedure in which skin is incised, endogenous skin flora, the most common source of pathogens, are introduced into the exposed tissue. Additional sources of bacteria include patient colonization, mucous membrane or hollow viscous pathogens encountered during the operation, surgical personnel, operative instruments, and the operating room environment.

An accepted surrogate for bacterial contamination at the surgical site is the wound classification. The risk of SSI increases with the degree of contamination and higher wound classifications. Wounds are classically defined as clean, clean-contaminated, contaminated, or dirty/infected, as seen in Table 1. Numerous additional characteristics contribute to the risk of SSI development, including patient factors, environmental factors, and treatment factors, as seen in Table 2.

The NHSN developed a risk index by which the risk of an SSI can be predicted based on three major criteria: wound classification, American Society of Anesthesiologists (ASA) score, and duration of the operation. The SSI risk category is based on the number of factors present at the time of operation, including a wound class of 3

(contaminated) or 4 (dirty), an ASA class of 3 or greater, and an operation lasting longer than the 75th percentile of the duration of the specific operation. Each independent factor is given a single point if present, which determines the NHSN risk index category (0 to 3). As seen in Table 3, the risk of SSI increases with progressive wound classifications and with progressive NHSN score.

The laparoscopic approach to an operation has been associated with a decreased risk of SSI as a result of small wound size, limited use of cautery, and decreased inflammatory response to tissue injury. This decrease in SSI risk has led to a modification of the risk classification. For laparoscopic biliary, gastric, or colon operations, a –1 is applied, essentially subtracting one risk factor when the operation is completed via a laparoscope.

PREVENTION

Patient Preparation

Prevention of SSIs should start as early as the preoperative clinic visit. Patient factors that may be modified before surgery should be corrected when possible. This includes clearing of remote site infections; initiation of an active smoking cessation program; optimization of nutritional status, including potential supplemental enteric feeding; weight loss for obese patients; whole body showering with a chlorhexidine antimicrobial solution; and prohibition of shaving just before the operation. Although not all of these interventions have proven benefits, they are simple inexpensive interventions that involve patients in their own medical care, an invaluable contribution to SSI prevention.

Immediate Preoperative Prevention

In response to inconsistent compliance with *proven* infection prevention measures, the Centers for Medicare and Medicaid Services (CMS) collaborated with the CDC on the Surgical Infection Prevention (SIP) project in 2002. This project developed quality improvement measures including the timeliness, selection, and duration of prophylactic antibiotics. In 2006, the Surgical Care Improvement Project (SCIP) developed out of the SIP and its process measures. The SCIP initiatives were published in the Specifications Manual for National Inpatient Quality Measures (Specifications Manual) and provided a standard form of quality measures to document and track standards of care (available online at www.qualitynet.org). The manual outlined seven infection-related process measures applicable to the perioperative period (Table 4). The initiatives that are outlined in SCIP infection measures (INF) 1 to 4, 6, and 10 highlight important process measures to prevent SSIs.

Prophylactic Antibiotics (SCIP INF 1 to 3)

Numerous studies have shown that provision of antimicrobial prophylaxis within 1 hour before the surgical incision allows blood and tissue concentrations adequate to prevent SSIs. A number of studies revealed enhanced compliance with antibiotic timing significantly reduced postoperative infectious complications, including SSIs. One notable prospective multicenter study attempted to define the optimal timing for antimicrobial prophylaxis and found 0 to 30 minutes to be associated with the fewest SSIs (1.6%). They found the infection risk increased with an extended interval between administration of antimicrobials and incision and with antimicrobial prophylaxis given after incision (Table 5).

Prophylactic antimicrobials should provide coverage for the pathogens most likely to be encountered during the operation, have pharmacokinetics that ensure adequate serum and tissue concentrations, have demonstrated safety, and be cost effective. The class of antibiotics most commonly used for perioperative prophylaxis is the cephalosporins. They are effective against gram-positive and gram-negative pathogens commonly encountered in general surgery and meet other criteria for appropriate prophylactic antimicrobials. Cefazolin is generally the agent of choice for clean and many clean-contaminated cases; a second-generation cephalosporin such as cefoxitin is commonly selected for colon operations for additional anaerobic coverage. For specific classes of operations such as cardiac or orthopedic operations, the antibiotic selection becomes more complex. The SCIP released a pocket card (October 2010) to guide the selection of appropriate antimicrobials based on operative location, class, and potential allergies (Table 6). The authors recommend the surgeon consult a pathogen reference table to determine prophylaxis based on operative type and most likely pathogens encountered (Mangram and colleagues).

The discontinuation of prophylactic antimicrobials is also important in terms of infection control and outcomes regarding SSIs. Significant evidence shows no additional benefit to lengthening the course of prophylactic antimicrobials beyond 24 hours. This is consistent with the rationale that perioperative antibiotics are not meant to sterilize the tissue but rather to reduce the bacterial burden to an inoculum that may be controlled by the patient's defenses. Extending the length of prophylaxis increases the risk of drug resistance and secondary infections, such as *Clostridium difficile*–related disease; therefore, the authors recommend the discontinuation of prophylactic antibiotics after 24 hours.

Appropriate Hair Removal (SCIP INF 6)

The method of hair removal in the preoperative period has been related to the incidence of SSIs. A large prospective trial randomized 2000 patients to either electrical clipping or manual shaving with a razor for hair removal before open heart surgery. The patients who were electrically clipped had a significantly lower rate of mediastinitis compared with the manually shaved group $(P = 0.024)$. A Cochrane systematic review confirmed these findings, revealing three randomized trials that compared shaving with clipping. Statistically more SSIs occurred with shaving than with clipping. Shaving with a blade is now considered an inappropriate method of hair removal in the preoperative period and should not be done.

Postoperative Normoglycemia (SCIP INF 4)

Appropriate glucose control in the perioperative period has been shown to reduce the incidence of SSIs. Hyperglycemia impairs the immune system, increases the risk of infection, and worsens the outcomes in sepsis. Studies have shown that tight intraoperative glucose control by anesthesia personnel significantly decreases the risk of SSIs, as does implementation of a postoperative intravenous insulin therapy protocol, continuous insulin infusions (as compared with subcutaneous injections), and maintenance of a mean capillary glucose concentration below 200 mg/dL for a minimum of 48 hours after surgery.

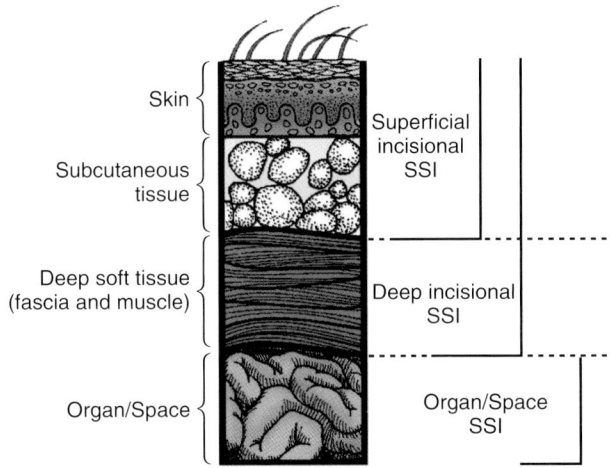

FIGURE 1 Cross section of abdominal wall depicting Centers for Disease Control classifications of surgical site infection *(SSI)*. *(From Mangram AJ, Horan TC, Pearson ML, et al: Guideline for prevention of surgical site infection,* Infect Control Hosp Epidemiol 20(4):247-278, 1999.)*

TABLE 1: Surgical wound classifications

Surgical wound classification	Description
Class I/clean	An uninfected operative wound in which no inflammation is encountered and the respiratory, alimentary, genital, or uninfected urinary tract is not entered. In addition, clean wounds are closed primarily and, if necessary, drained with closed drainage.
Class II/clean-contaminated	An operative wound in which the respiratory, alimentary, genital, or urinary tracts are entered under controlled conditions and without unusual contamination. Specifically, operations that involve the biliary tract, appendix, vagina, and oropharynx are included in this category, provided no evidence of infection or major break in technique is encountered.
Class III/contaminated	Open, fresh, accidental wounds. In addition, operations with major breaks in sterile technique (e.g., open cardiac massage) or gross spillage from the gastrointestinal tract and incisions in which acute, nonpurulent inflammation is encountered are included in this category.
Class IV/dirty, infected	Old traumatic wounds with retained devitalized tissue and those that involve existing clinical infection or perforated viscera. This definition suggests that the organisms that cause the postoperative infection were present in the operative field before the operation.

Modified from Mangram AJ, Horan TC, Pearson ML, et al: Guideline for prevention of surgical site infection, Infect Control Hosp Epidemiol 20(4):247-278, *1999.*

TABLE 2: Patient and operative characteristics that may influence the risk of surgical site infection development

Patient factors	Environmental factors	Treatment factors
Ascites	Contaminated medications	Emergency procedure
Chronic inflammation	Inadequate disinfection/sterilization	Failure to obliterate dead space
Coexistent remote infection	Inadequate skin antisepsis	Hypothermia
Colonization with microorganisms	Inadequate ventilation	Inadequate antibiotic prophylaxis
Corticosteroid therapy		Intraoperative blood transfusion
Diabetes		Oxygenation
Extended preoperative admission		Poor hemostasis
Hypocholesterolemia		Prolonged operative time
Hypoxemia		Surgical drains
Malnutrition		Tissue trauma
Obesity		
Peripheral vascular disease		
Perioperative anemia		
Preoperative shaving		
Prior site irradiation		
Recent operation		
Skin disease in the area of infection (e.g., psoriasis)		

Modified from the National Nosocomial Infections Surveillance (NNIS) system report: data summary from January 1992-June 2001, issued August 2001, Am J Infect Control 29:404-421, 2001; and from Mangram AJ, Horan TC, Pearson ML, et al: Guideline for prevention of surgical site infection, Infect Control Hosp Epidemiol 20(4):247-278, 1999.

TABLE 3: National Healthcare Safety Network (NHSN) risk index scoring

Wound class	NHSN risk index category*				
	NNIS 0	NNIS 1	NNIS 2	NNIS 3	All
I: Clean	1.0%	2.3%	5.4%	NA	2.1%
II: Clean-contaminated	2.1%	4.0%	9.5%	NA	3.3%
III: Contaminated	NA	3.4%	6.8%	13.2%	6.4%
IV: Dirty/infected	NA	3.1%	8.1%	12.8%	7.1%
All	1.5%	2.9%	6.8%	13.0%	2.8%

NA, Not applicable; NNIS, National Nosocomial Infections Surveillance system.
*NHSN risk index is based on three independent variables: American Society of Anesthesiologists (ASA) score > 2, contaminated or dirty/infected wound class, and length of operation above the 75th percentile for the operation being performed.
Modified from data presented in National Nosocomial Infections Surveillance (NNIS) system report: data summary from January 1992-June 2001, Am J Infect Control 29(6):404-421, 2001.

Although early data supported strict blood glucose control (<110 mg/dL) as a means to decrease morbidity and mortality in critically ill patients, recent data show higher rates of severe hypoglycemia and adverse events with intensive insulin protocols. The NICE-SUGAR study supported conventional (<180 mg/dL), as opposed to strict, insulin control with equivalent outcomes. This was not specific to SSI outcomes, but this target (180 mg/dL) is recommended as an appropriate glucose concentration level for surgical patients in the perioperative period.

Postoperative Normothermia (SCIP INF 10)

Postoperative hypothermia is a common problem and has been hypothesized to increase SSIs by peripheral vasoconstriction, reduced blood flow and oxygen tension at the tissue level, and impaired immune function in terms of decreased antibody production and reduced neutrophil function. A prospective randomized clinical trial found an active intraoperative warming protocol had significantly fewer SSIs when compared with a standard of care group (P = 0.009). Active warming protocols should be implemented in all surgical patients because this is a simple prevention strategy to reduce SSIs.

TABLE 4: Surgical Care Improvement Project (SCIP) performance measures applicable to the perioperative period

SCIP Infection (INF) measure designation	Performance measure title
INF 1	Prophylactic antibiotic received within 1 hour before surgical incision
INF 2	Prophylactic antibiotic selection for surgical patients
INF 3	Prophylactic antibiotics discontinued within 24 hours after surgery end time
INF 4	Cardiac surgery patients with controlled 6:00 AM postoperative blood glucose
INF 6	Surgery patients with appropriate hair removal
INF 9	Urinary catheter removed on postoperative day 1 or postoperative day 2 (with day of surgery being day 0)
INF 10	Surgery patients with perioperative temperature management

Modified from Rosenberger LH, Politano AD, Sawyer RG: The surgical care improvement project and prevention of post-operative infection, including surgical site infection, Surg Infect *12(3):163-168, 2011.*

TABLE 5: Association between timing and surgical site infections for antimicrobial prophylaxis, cephalosporins, or antimicrobials designated to be given within 60 minutes of incision

Timing of antimicrobial prophylaxis	Infections/no. of operations	Infection risk
>120 min before incision	4/96	4.7%
61-120 min before incision	12/489	2.4%
31-60 min before incision	38/1558	2.4%
0-30 min before incision	22/1339	1.6%
1-30 min after incision	4/100	4.0%
>30 min after incision	5/74	6.8%

Modified from Steinberg JP, Braun BI, Hellinger WC, et al: Timing of antimicrobial prophylaxis and the risk of surgical site infections, Ann Surg *250(1):10-16, 2009.*

Performance Measures

The SCIP quality measures have been implemented by CMS, and mandatory reporting of certain performance measures now helps determine hospital reimbursement. Numerous organizations endorse the notion that adherence to process measures serves as a valid assessment of surgical quality, and public reporting is intended to guide patients to quality centers for surgical care. The authors caution this

TABLE 6: Surgical Care Improvement Project (SCIP) pocket card: prophylactic antimicrobial regimen selection for surgery

Surgical procedure	Approved antibiotics
Coronary artery bypass grafting, other cardiac or vascular procedures	Cefazolin, cefuroxime, or vancomycin* If β-lactam allergy: Vancomycin[†] or clindamycin[†]
Hysterectomy	Cefotetan, cefaxolin, cefoxitin, cefuroxime, or ampicillin/sulbactam If β-lactam allergy: Clindamycin + aminoglycoside, or Clindamycin + quinolone, or Clindamycin + aztreonam or Metronidazole + aminoglycoside, or Metronidazole + quinolone
Hip/knee arthroplasty	Cefazolin or cefuroxime or vancomycin* If β-lactam allergy: Vancomycin[†] or clindamycin[†]
Colon operations	Cefotetan, cefoxitin, ampicillin/sulbactam, or ertapenem[‡] or Cefazolin or cefuroxime + metronidazole If β-lactam allergy: Clindamycin + aminoglycoside, or Clindamycin + quinolone, or Clindamycin + aztreonam or Metronidazole + aminoglycoside, or Metronidazole + quinolone

This table does not necessarily reflect Centers of Medicare and Medicaid Services policy.
*Vancomycin is acceptable with a physician, nurse practitioner, physician assistant, or pharmacist documented justification for its use.
[†]For cardiac, orthopedic, and vascular surgery, if the patient is allergic to β-lactam antibiotics, vancomycin and clindamycin are acceptable.
[‡]A single dose of ertapenem is recommended for colon procedures.
Modified from the Oklahoma Foundation of Medical Quality, the Quality Improvement Organization Support Center for Patient Safety, under contract with the Centers of Medicare & Medicaid Services (CMS), an agency of the U.S. Department of Health and Human Services: Surgical care improvement project pocket card, *October 2010.*

methodology because process measures often serve as poor proxies for overall quality of surgical care and a number of studies have revealed adherence to quality measures does not always result in improved outcomes. Overall, the authors encourage the implementation of performance measures to improve surgical outcomes; however, they do not support their use as quality metrics or reimbursement standards because limited data exist to prove adherence advances outcomes.

The inconsistent correlation between increased rates of adherence to these process measures (all based on previous positive trials) and decreased SSI rates has two other implications. First, even with total adherence to these measures, SSIs still occur, highlighting the fact that the pathophysiology of SSI is not completely understood. More research is needed to delineate the causes of SSI and to develop new technologies that can prevent them. Second, SSIs cannot, at this point in medical history, be considered "never events" and must not be considered so by regulating agencies.

Intraoperative and Postoperative Incision Management

Sound surgical technique must be used, including adequate hemostasis, conservation of blood supply when possible, atraumatic tissue handling, and a limited use of electrocautery. Clean and clean-contaminated incisions should be closed primarily and covered with a sterile dressing for 24 to 48 hours to allow sealing of the wound by epithelialization before dressing removal. Tissue adhesives or glue, such as Dermabond (Ethicon, Somerville, NJ), an octyl-cyanoacrylate, are alternatives to sterile dressings and provide an effective barrier to bacterial contamination of a sterile incision. Closing of the contaminated or dirty wound continues to be a dilemma for surgeons because the data are conflicting. One large prospective randomized study found greater wound failures and greater cost with closure of a contaminated abdominal incision as compared with delayed primary closure. In these conditions, delayed primary closure is frequently favored to minimize patient morbidity.

The use of drains for clean or clean-contaminated incisions is not supported because they provide a portal for pathogen entry and have been shown to increase the rate of SSI in these wound classes. When drains are used, they should be removed as soon as possible and should not justify concomitant antimicrobial therapy.

Special Considerations

Hand hygiene is an important topic within infection control practices. Preoperative surgeon hand antisepsis has transformed from the historic full 10-minute hand scrubbing to quicker protocols with various alcohol rubs. A large randomized clinical trial found a 1-minute nonantiseptic hand wash followed by an aqueous alcohol-based hand rub was equivalent to the traditional hand-scrubbing protocol. Numerous additional studies have found alcohol-based rubs are as effective as aqueous scrubbing procedures in SSI prevention.

Controversy certainly exists regarding the ideal preoperative skin antisepsis for the surgical site. The intent of skin preparation is to cleanse the skin of any microorganisms, the far leading source of pathogens for postoperative SSIs. Numerous skin preparations are available that use various combinations of chlorhexidine, povidone-iodine, iodine povacrylex, and isopropyl alcohol. The data are inconsistent, with the most recent large randomized trial concluding chlorhexidine-alcohol is superior to povidone-iodine, leaving the believers of isopropyl alcohol wondering whether the chlorhexidine matters. The authors conclude the routine use of a skin antiseptic should be undertaken with attention to the correct application protocol for the particular agent being used. Povidone-iodine alone, without alcohol, however, is probably inferior and should not be used. Differences between combinations of chlorhexidine or an iodophor with alcohol are perhaps minimal, and either approach is currently acceptable.

The pendulum continues to swing in terms of bowel preparation and enteric antibiotics for elective colorectal surgery. Traditional belief was that mechanical bowel preparation would reduce SSI and anastomotic leak. Recent data have revealed no statistically significant evidence that patients benefit from bowel preps or enemas in terms of wound infection or anastomotic leak. Antimicrobials, however, have been shown to reduce postoperative infectious complications substantially. Data reveal antibiotics covering aerobic and anaerobic organisms should be given both orally and intravenously before colorectal surgery. Some expert opinion continues to recommend mechanical bowel preparation before enteric antibiotics for

improved efficacy; however, data are conflicting. Currently, mechanical bowel preparation is only clearly indicated when intraoperative colonoscopy is either planned or likely, and its use at other times is based on surgeon preference, not evidence.

TREATMENT

All clearly infected wounds should be opened, irrigated, débrided, and treated with basic wound care. Most superficial and deep incisional SSIs can be managed with these techniques. The wound should be opened sufficiently for adequate visualization of the underlying tissue to ensure no additional processes are occurring, such as fascial dehiscence, drainage from an organ/space SSI, or enteric fistula.

Infected incisional wounds should be irrigated with an isotonic solution such as a saline solution to remove loose dead tissue and exudate, and mechanical débridement may be indicated to remove devitalized tissue. Wounds should be packed in a "wet to dry" fashion, with moistened gauze against the wound bed covered by layers of dry gauze. Daily dressing changes assist in débridement as the wet gauze removes residual necrotic tissue and exudate. Once the wound has stabilized and most of the devitalized tissue has been removed, consideration can be given to placement of a negative-pressure wound therapy device ("wound vac"). Although the overall outcome may not change, placement of such a device generally speeds closure and may be particularly helpful in larger wounds and those in which dressing changes are difficult, such as with the distal extremities.

The need for antimicrobial therapy is determined by magnitude of the infection, evidence of systemic involvement, presence of prosthetics, and status of the patient, including comorbidities. Uncomplicated SSIs that have been managed with incision and drainage can usually be managed without antibiotics. Topical antibiotics and additional agents such as antiseptics (hydrogen peroxide, povidone-iodine) have an unclear role in the management of infected wounds. Traditionally, many antiseptics have been applied to wounds, including iodine-containing solutions and sodium hypochlorite (Dakin's solution). These compounds can inhibit fibroblast growth in vitro and are only used for a relatively short period of time. Topical antibiotics, as opposed to antiseptics, probably have no role in the management of infected wounds. In resource-poor areas, both honey and granulated sugar have been used to treat open wounds, and their effectiveness may be based on their hypertonicity. Enzymatic débridement of wounds may be beneficial where aggressive wide surgical débridement is impossible.

For moderate to severe SSIs, including those associated with systemic toxicity, significant cellulitis (>2 cm beyond the incision), purulent drainage, fascial dehiscence, and deep drainage, antibiotics should be administered empirically. Initial selection should cover gram-positive organisms and likely infecting organisms based on colonization status, operative location, and recent infections. For wounds associated with operations on the gastrointestinal or genitourinary tracts, gram-negative coverage should also be provided. Source control is imperative for organ/space SSIs, including intraabdominal abscess, and requires either percutaneous or operative drainage.

Culture of wounds is at the discretion of the surgeon. Straightforward uncomplicated incisional SSIs without significant cellulitis that do not require antimicrobial therapy do not need to be cultured. On the other hand, all organ/space SSIs should be cultured because the role of antibiotics is greater in this instance. For other cases, cultures should only be sent when antibiotics are planned, the culture results will be used to guide antibiotic choice, and the patient is at high risk of having resistant pathogens. Patient characteristics that suggest culture might be indicated include recent receipt of therapeutic antibiotics, immunosuppression, care in an intensive care unit, and an unusually aggressive infection. Ideally cultures should be sterile aspirations or tissue, but swabs are useful if cautious interpretation of the results is used.

SUMMARY

SSIs are a common surgical complication and represent the most common nosocomial infection among surgical patients. These infections cause significant morbidity and increase costs, making them the focus of discussion and regulation at various levels. A number of process measures have been identified to reduce the risk of SSIs, and evidence-based standards should be incorporated into all surgeons' practices.

SUGGESTED READINGS

Alexander JW, Solomkin JS, Edwards MJ: Updated recommendations for control of surgical site infections, *Ann Surg* 253(6):1082–1093, 2011.

Barie PS, Eachempati SR: Surgical site infections, *Surg Clin North Am* 85(6):1115–1135, 2005.

Cohn SM, Giannotti G, Ong AW, et al: Prospective randomized trial of two wound management strategies for dirty abdominal wounds, *Ann Surg* 233(3):409–413, 2001.

Darouiche RO, Wall MJ Jr, Itani KM, et al: Chlorhexidine-alcohol versus povidone-iodine for surgical-site antisepsis, *N Engl J Med* 362(1):18–26, 2010.

Furnary AP, Zerr KJ, Grunkemeier GL, et al: Continuous intravenous insulin infusion reduces the incidence of deep sternal wound infection in diabetic patients after cardiac surgical procedures, *Ann Thorac Surg* 67(2):352–360, 1999.

Guenaga KF, Matos D, Wille-Jorgensen P: Mechanical bowel preparation for elective colorectal surgery, *Cochrane Database Syst Rev* (9):CD001544, 2010.

Hawn MT, Vick CC, Richman J, et al: Surgical site infection prevention: time to move beyond the surgical care improvement program, *Ann Surg* 254(3):494–501, 2011.

Hranjec T, Swenson BR, Sawyer RG: Surgical site infection prevention: how we do it, *Surgical Infections* 11(3):289–294, 2010.

Kurz A, Sessler DI, Lenhardt RA: Perioperative normothermia to reduce the incidence of surgical-wound infection and shorten hospitalization: study of wound infections and temperature group, *N Engl J Med* 334(19):1209–1215, 1996.

Mangram AJ, Horan TC, Pearson ML, et al: Guideline for prevention of surgical site infection, 1999: Hospital Infection Control Practices Advisory Committee, *Infect Control Hosp Epidemiol* 20(4):250–278, 1999.

McDonald M, Grabsch E, Marshall C, et al: Single- versus multiple-dose antimicrobial prophylaxis for major surgery: a systematic review, *Aust N Z J Surg* 68:388–396, 1998.

National Nosocomial Infections Surveillance (NNIS) system report: data summary from January 1992-June 2001, *Am J Infect Control* 29(6):404–421, 2001.

Nelson RL, Glenny AM, Song F: Antimicrobial prophylaxis for colorectal surgery, *Cochrane Database Syst Rev* (1):CD001181, 2009.

Parienti JJ, Thibon P, Heller R, et al: Hand-rubbing with an aqueous alcoholic solution vs traditional surgical hand-scrubbing and 30-day surgical site infection rates: a randomized equivalence study, *JAMA* 288(6):722–727, 2002.

Rosenberger LH, Politano AD, Sawyer RG: The surgical care improvement project and prevention of post-operative infection, including surgical site infection, *Surgical Infections* 12(3):163–168, 2011.

Steinberg JP, Braun BI, Hellinger WC, et al: Timing of antimicrobial prophylaxis and the risk of surgical site infections, *Ann Surg* 250(1):10–16, 2009.

Swenson BR, Hedrick TL, Metzger R, et al: Effects of preoperative skin preparation on postoperative wound infection rates: a prospective study of 3 skin preparation protocols, *Infect Control Hosp Epidemiol* 30(10):964–971, 2009.

Tanner J, Woodings D, Moncaster K: Peroperative hair removal to reduce surgical site infection, *Cochrane Database Syst Rev* (2):CD004122, 2006.

Zerr KJ, Furnary AP, Grunkemeier GL, et al: Glucose control lowers the risk of wound infection in diabetics after open heart operations, *Ann Thorac Surg* 63(2):356–361, 1997.

The Management of Intra-abdominal Infections

Adam D. Fox, DPM, DO, FACS, and
David H. Livingston, MD, FACS

INTRODUCTION

With intra-abdominal infection being one of the most common reasons for surgical consultation, understanding the evaluation and management of these processes becomes paramount in the day-to-day practice of the surgeon. The very broad nature of who is affected coupled with the interplay of patient comorbidities and their medications make dealing with intra-abdominal infections a challenge.

As with most complex problems in medicine, it is often useful to break them down into simpler and smaller parts. One useful way to categorize intra-abdominal infections is to divide them into those originating from previous abdominal trauma or operations and those presenting in a "virgin" abdomen. The latter group most commonly includes those patients presenting with specific organ-based infectious processes such as appendicitis, cholecystitis, or diverticulitis. These individual diseases are covered extensively in other chapters and are discussed only superficially in this chapter. The former are those patients who have sustained intra-abdominal trauma or have undergone previous abdominal interventions and are not recovering in the usual expected course. It is this group that taxes diagnostic and clinical skills and may require the most complex medical decision making.

DEFINITIONS

Intra-abdominal infections are a broad range of processes that result from bacterial invasiveness and growth in the abdominal cavity. There are several ways these types of infections have been defined or classified. One schema categorizes the infectious process into uncomplicated and complicated. The uncomplicated process is, in general, confined to the involved organ system. Examples of this include acute nonperforated appendicitis or localized acute diverticulitis. Many of these just require administration of appropriate antibiotics. Complicated intra-abdominal infections are those that extend beyond the normal confines of the organ system and diffusely invade the peritoneum. In addition to antibiotics, these infections usually require an invasive procedure in order to obtain source control.

When speaking of a complicated infection, the diffuse nature usually implies a degree of peritonitis. Peritonitis itself can be divided into primary, secondary, and tertiary. Primary peritonitis is an infection that develops in the absence of a distinct break in the structural integrity of the gastrointestinal (GI) tract. It is usually the result of bacterial translocation, hematogenous spread, or lymphatic seeding. The resulting infection is often monomicrobial, commonly gram-negative Enterbacteriaceae species or streptococci. Secondary peritonitis results from a break in the continuity of the GI tract. It is a polymicrobial infection often with both aerobic and anaerobic enteric bacteria. Tertiary peritonitis is often seen in immunosuppressed patients and results from failure of treatment of a secondary peritonitis. The flora seen with these types of infections are often nosocomial and include resistant gram-negative bacilli, enterococcus, staphylococcus, and yeast. This classification is somewhat more useful because primary peritonitis is treated by antimicrobial therapy alone compared to secondary and tertiary peritonitis, which almost always require some type of interventional procedures.

DIAGNOSTICS

The approach to each patient should begin with the standard history and physical, with a focus on signs of systemic illness and abdominal processes. Early recognition of systemic inflammatory response syndrome (SIRS) criteria (Box 1), especially in patients who are not in the early postoperative or posttrauma period, combined with abdominal findings such as pain, nausea, vomiting, and anorexia, are highly suggestive of a complicated intra-abdominal infection. An adequate history and physical examination in the awake patient will provide the information necessary to make a diagnosis in many cases. The severity of the illness should dictate what, if any, laboratory studies are needed. In the patient with a simple intra-abdominal process without hemodynamic or physiologic derangement, a white blood cell count with differential is sufficient. In those patients presenting with a more in-depth process, thought should be given to obtaining a complete blood count, electrolyte panel, arterial or venous blood gas, lactate, and blood cultures.

While hard to believe in today's modern imaging world, a percentage of these patients require little if any further diagnostic studies. However, many patients with intra-abdominal infections may present with physiologic derangements, including an altered mental status that precludes a complete history or physical exam. In this patient population or those in which more information is needed, further diagnostic studies are required. Standard radiography has a limited role, but the upright chest radiograph or lateral decubitus film remains very useful to help identify free air. Although ultrasound has been shown to have some utility in diagnosing acute appendicitis, with some studies reporting over 80% sensitivity and 90% specificity, it remains operator dependent, and its use has not been fully evaluated for other forms of intra-abdominal infection.

Computed tomographic (CT) scanning with oral and intravenous contrast has become the "gold standard" of diagnosing intra-abdominal infection. In fact, it is the rare patient who makes it from the emergency department to the operating room without a CT scan. While abdominal CT scanning is extraordinarily useful in identifying the breadth of intra-abdominal pathology, there remain situations where it is unnecessary or unhelpful. An example of the former is the patient with free air on a chest x-ray. Examples of the latter are those

patients imaged soon after an abdominal operation. Even with newer high-resolution CT technology, it remains almost impossible to differentiate infected versus noninfected fluid collections before postoperative day 5. The accuracy of CT is also dependent on technique. While the utility and added benefit of oral contrast has been questioned, the use of intravenous contrast markedly improves diagnostic accuracy. Thus, noncontrast CT scans are of limited usefulness and should be used to investigate possible intra-abdominal infections sparingly, if at all. Because new contrast agents are less nephrotoxic and allergenic, given the risk to benefit ratio, it is a rare patient who cannot tolerate one dose of intravenous contrast. Lastly, in this digital age of remote imaging and interpretation, routine direct communication between surgeons and radiologists has been often lost. In patients who have undergone complicated operations, it is incumbent on the operating surgeon to personally discuss the case with the radiologist, including what has been done and what is being searched for, so the proper study and interpretation are possible.

INTRA-ABDOMINAL INFECTIONS FOLLOWING ABDOMINAL TRAUMA OR SURGERY

The recovery from abdominal trauma or abdominal operation is similar with most patients, progressing in a standardized manner. Quite often, even patients who were desperately ill preoperatively "look great" on postoperative day 1 or 2. Physiologic derangements such as tachycardia, fever, and even pressor requirements are often improved, and the abdominal pain of peritonitis is often replaced by surgically induced incisional pain. It is the astute clinician who recognizes the plateauing of improvement on postoperative days 3 and 4, the slight increase in abdominal distension, and the failure to regain full bowel function. Unless one "thinks bad thoughts," one will never contemplate that something might be amiss. While a small fever at this time and a change in leukocyte count might be a urinary tract infection or phlebitis from an old intravenous site, the failure to entertain the possibility of an anastamotic leak following a colon resection for diverticulitis or a missed bowel injury following a thoracoabdominal gun shot wound will result in disastrous outcomes (Figure 1). One must be aware of the possibilities that can befall a patient following abdominal trauma or operative intervention. Nowhere in general surgery is the aphorism that *"good clinical*

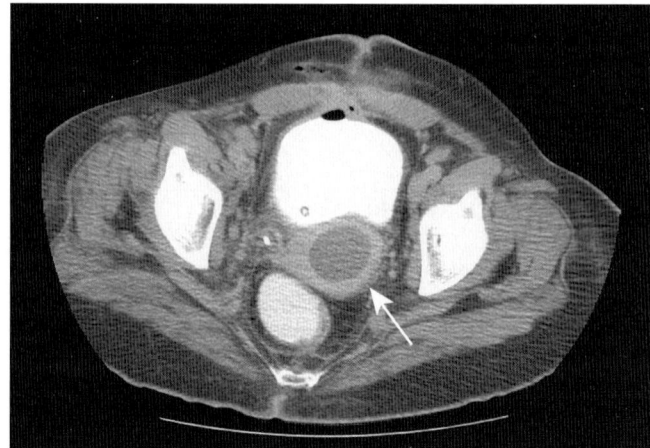

FIGURE 1 Pelvic abscess following multiple bowel resections secondary to a gunshot wound to the abdomen. Note the thick wall and contrast enhancement (*arrow*) that are classic for an abscess. The unilocular presentation and the abscess location make it ideal for percutaneous drainage.

BOX 1: Systemic inflammatory response syndrome criteria

Temperature: <36°C (96.8°F) or >38°C (100.4°F)
Heart rate: >90 beats per minute
Respiratory rate: >20 breaths per minute, or a $PaCO_2$ <4.3 kPa (32 mm Hg)
White blood cell count: <4000 cells/mm³ (4×10^9 cells/L), or >12,000 cells/mm³ (12×10^9 cells/L), or the presence of >10% immature neutrophils (band forms)

judgment comes from experience and experience comes from bad judgment" more true than dealing with postoperative or posttraumatic abdominal infection. In addition, CT imaging, especially early after operation or injury, may be difficult to interpret or frankly misleading. In these cases, an astute surgeon must look at the CT as either positive or "not positive" rather than negative, and if no other explanation for the infection is identified, the surgeon should urgently reexplore the patient. Waiting until the patient shows signs of organ dysfunction will markedly increase mortality.

It is in the elective surgical population where the presence of an intra-abdominal infection can be most easily diagnosed and treated. These patients are commonly optimized prior to surgery, are not malnourished, and have a typical and well-known course. As outlined, the use of radiographic imaging with CT scanning is often unhelpful prior to postoperative day 5, so clinical judgment is required to ascertain which patients are not progressing in the expected manner. The wound should be examined by experienced individuals at least once daily, if not more frequently. While many superficial wound infections are in fact just that, not uncommonly a wound infection is the tip of the iceberg of a subfascial or intra-abdominal infection. Although with attention to surgical care improvement project (SCIP) guidelines, there has been improvement in the delivery of appropriate prophylactic antibiotics, these interventions have been less uniformly successful in decreasing overall wound infection rates. More importantly one needs to remember that these interventions are not designed to decrease intra-abdominal infections.

Bariatric surgical patients now comprise an increasing number of routine elective cases on the surgical schedule. The presentation of an intra-abdominal catastrophe in this group can be quite subtle, often limited to an unexplained mild tachycardia without abdominal pain. The usual postoperative care of these patients involves defined care plans of early mobilization and oral intake. Deviation from the normal progression, especially in the presence of tachycardia, should prompt rapid investigation for leaks or compromised bowel. Rapid reexploration in the absence of diagnostics before physiologic deterioration will be lifesaving in this group.

MANAGEMENT OF INTRA-ABDOMINAL INFECTIONS

Several factors should come into play once suspicion for an intra-abdominal infection is entertained. These include resuscitation, antibiotic usage, and source control itself. Patients who present with either a suspected or diagnosed intra-abdominal infection should have some form of volume resuscitation. Even without hypotension, there are several reasons why these patients might be volume depleted. These include nausea and vomiting, fluid sequestration within the abdominal cavity or lumen of the bowel, and poor oral intake. As the process progresses, the patient may develop tachypnea, which results in an evaporative fluid loss. By this time, one can often elicit orthostatic hypotension in most patients. Fluid resuscitation should begin with the administration of isotonic crystalloid and in general be guided by evidence of end organ perfusion (adequate mental status, urine output, correction of acidosis). There is no utility-using colloid such as albumin or hetastarch in these circumstances, and some data suggest a worse outcome. Should the patient present with hypotension or evidence of poor perfusion, a more aggressive approach to volume resuscitation should be employed. Our recommendation is to follow the current surviving sepsis guidelines, which include fluid challenges, monitoring/assessment of filling pressures, and the potential use of pressors and steroids.

Early administration of appropriate antibiotics in the course of an infection reduces mortality in the septic patient and should be initiated as soon as a diagnosis of intra-abdominal infection is suspected. While the absolute duration of antibiotic administration is a matter of debate, this therapy should be maintained during the

interventions needed to achieve source control. As noted above, there are commonly encountered flora that will depend on the type of peritonitis as well as the presumed location of the infection in the GI tract. This can help dictate antimicrobial therapy. As one moves from the stomach, where gram-positive cocci (streptococci or lactobacilli) predominate, the number and type of bacteria change. The mid- to distal small bowel will still house gram-positive cocci, but enteric gram-negative aerobic and facultative anaerobic bacilli begin to increase in number. The colon will have large numbers of obligate anaerobes. The most common bacteria found in intra-abdominal infections are *E. coli*, *Klebsiella sp.*, *Enterobacter sp.*, *Streptococci* (mostly viridans), *Enterococcus sp.*, and *Bacteroides sp.* It is worth noting that the "expected flora" is altered in patients with previous antibiotic administration or those coming from other health care environments such as nursing homes. In this patient population, the upper GI tract should be considered to have a higher bacterial count that includes Enterobacteriaceae, *Pseudomonas*, and yeast, along with a potential for antimicrobial resistance.

Recommended antimicrobial regimens for mild to moderate community acquired intra-abdominal infections include ticarcillin-clavulanate, cefoxitin, ertapenim, or moxifloxacin as single-agent drugs or combination regimens with metronidazole and cefazolin, cefuroxime, ceftriaxone, levofloxacin, or ciprofloxacin. In those with a high-severity community-acquired infection (i.e., acute physiology and chronic health evaluation [APACHE] >15), and especially those patients who have previously been treated with antibiotics, one should avoid quinolones (high resistance) and think about using single agents such as meropenem, imipenem-cilastin, piperacillin-tazobactam, or ceftazidime or cefepime in combination with metronidazole. These broad-spectrum antibiotics should be tailored once culture and sensitivity reports become available. The duration of antibiotics should be limited to 4 to 7 days unless achieving source control had been difficult. Bowel injuries attributable to trauma that have been repaired in a timely fashion should be treated for no more than 24 hours.

SOURCE CONTROL: OPERATION VERSUS PERCUTANEOUS DRAINAGE ALONE

Source control, the single or multiple interventional processes by which one attains control or elimination of an infection, can potentially be achieved through a nonoperative or operative approach depending on the nature of the disease. There is little if any literature offering Level 1 advice as to the optimum technique under all circumstances. Globally, then, we recommend an appropriate source-control procedure based on the principles of control of ongoing peritoneal contamination, draining infection, and providing restoration of anatomic and physiologic parameters. This procedure can include resection/débridement of nonviable tissue, drainage, diversion, or a combination of each. As detailed below, intervention will then depend on the extent of the underlying process, how sick the patient presents, and resources available. The risk of failure for source control increases in the elderly (>70 years), higher illness severity (APACHE ≥15), delays to intervention, comorbidities, poor nutritional status, and extent of peritoneal involvement.

Once a need for intervention has been established, time to intervention becomes critical. Source control should proceed without delay. While many patients require at least some resuscitation, this should not delay intervention for more than a short time. Patients with severely altered physiology will likely never be resuscitated to "normal" values without source control. In these patients, operative source control may be the only way to halt an ongoing process, and resuscitation should be concomitant with the procedure.

The introduction of image-guided percutaneous drainage of intra-abdominal abscesses in the 1980s revolutionized the treatment of that disease to the point that it is now the standard of care and the first and best option for many infections. Despite three decades of improvements in imaging technology, the general guidelines for successful drainage have not changed. Absolute necessities include a window in which to drain the collection and material that can be drained though a catheter. Well-localized collections, especially in those patients without diffuse peritonitis, can be managed with a percutaneous drain and appropriate antibiotics. This can even include those with small amounts of localized free air. Examples of infections that are usually amenable and well handled by percutaneous drainage include subphrenic abscesses after splenectomy, pelvic abscess following perforated appendicitis, and diverticulitis with localized abscess (Hinchey class 1b or 2) (Figure 2). Loculated or multiple abscesses are not necessarily contraindications to percutaneous drainage, but these authors have observed patients being treated with three and four and more percutaneous drainages over several weeks when one open operation would have taken care of the problem easier, more expeditiously, and at a lower cost. Patients with poorly localized or diffuse collections, necrotic tissue, or inaccessible collections require open operative intervention. Those patients with diffuse peritonitis or massive amounts of free air require immediate surgery.

The operation performed should be based on the extent of the infection, the organs involved, and the patient's physiologic status. Despite the myriad possibilities in treating intra-abdominal infection, there are several concepts that apply across all diagnoses. The first is that complete identification of the pathology is an absolute necessity to affect proper therapy. It does no one any good to drain the abscess only to miss the necrotic piece of intestine or anastomotic disruption. The groups of patients that require operative intervention are often sicker and more complicated. These cases can be exceedingly challenging, and even senior surgeons can often benefit from another experienced pair of hands in the operating room. Consultation and collaboration with senior partners can also help in the overall intraoperative decision making. Once the anatomic problem is completely identified, the goal is now to achieve source control. As in the severely injured trauma patient, the extent and breadth of the procedure should be dictated by the patient's physiologic status.

In patients with intra-abdominal infection without an obvious GI perforation, unroofing of all abscess cavities and collections is all that is required. Intraoperative cultures should be performed and transported to the laboratory with some expedience. It is always unfortunate to perform these procedures in the middle of the night only to find out that the "negative cultures" of obvious purulence did not make it to the microbiology laboratory until the next day. In patients without any definable residual abscess cavities, there is no need for drains. In fact, drains in this situation are more often associated with subsequent infection than no drainage. In our estimation, the quantity of drains placed often far outweighs the quality of their use. What

we mean by this is that because almost all drains are of the closed suction variety, little thought is often given to drain placement, assuming that the suction will allow for proper drainage in all circumstances. While it may be true in concept, it is not always accurate in practice. Bulbs get filled, resulting in a loss of suction; tubing may be kinked by patient positioning or even the dressing.

Additionally, consideration should be given to how the drain is brought out through the abdomen. One must always remember that the drain exit site will ultimately end up several inches more medial when the abdomen is eventually closed. This can result in a loss of the "direct" path of the drain and can decrease efficacy. We believe and teach that placement of drains in a more "gravity-friendly" fashion with more lateral exit tracts will result in shorter and more direct drain paths and can even aid closed suction drainage. In addition, we do not advocate large sump-type drains. These drains often come with filters that are quickly clogged with serum and particulate matter, rendering the sump feature of the drains nonfunctional. If the material is too thick to be drained through a closed suction drain, it is also likely to clog a sump drain. In these circumstances, if sump drainage is employed, we have utilized a short course of continuous irrigation either through one of the sump ports or through a second drain. Lastly, all current drains on the market are made from silicone or a similar nonreactive material. As such, they induce little or no inflammation, and they will not form a tract. While in most cases this is beneficial, there are times where one is relying on the inflammation induced by a latex or rubber drain to "seal the area" and control the infection.

When the genesis of the infection is related to a break in the GI tract, source control involves eliminating or controlling the ongoing contamination. The two overriding concepts in these circumstances are not to make the hole bigger and not to create any new (unnecessary) holes. While on the surface these concepts appear obvious, the compulsion to put "just one stitch" in a leaking anastomosis in the face of gross peritonitis can sometimes be irresistible. The success of this is negligible and will most assuredly lead to further breakdown, a larger hole, and a bigger problem. The complexity of entry into the abdomen itself along with the actual dissection toward the primary pathology should not be underestimated. Creation of inadvertent enterotomies can occur but need to be recognized and treated. The care needed to do these cases cannot be underestimated. In addition, when enterotomies are created, one must critically decide how they should be handled, similarly to the primary pathology.

In most cases, intestinal perforation in the face of peritonitis should be handled by resection. One exception to this is perforated duodenal ulcers, which are treated by graham patch. Perforation in the body of the stomach can be closed primarily followed by imbrication using Lembert sutures because there is abundant gastric tissue to cover a suture line. In the proximal small bowel, resection is usually followed by anastomosis, whereas in the distal small bowel and colon,

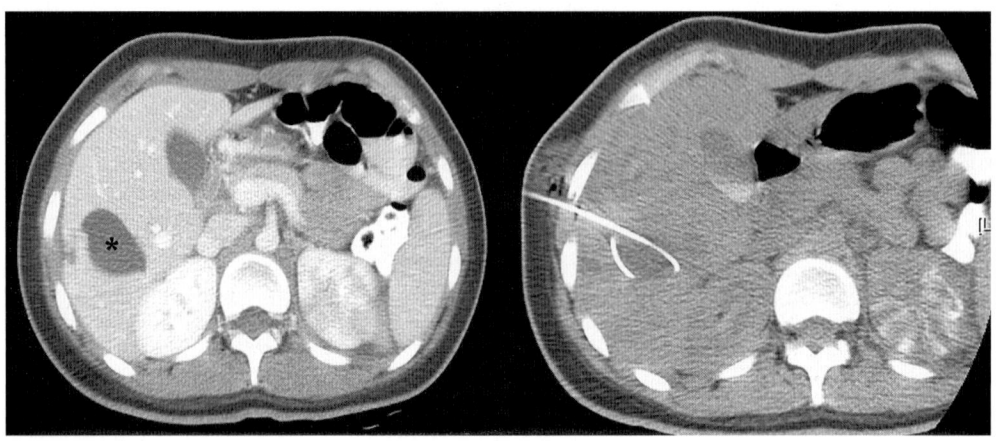

FIGURE 2 Liver abscess (*) following a stab wound to the liver *(left)*. The abscess was successfully percutaneously drained *(right)*.

one must consider the risk to benefit ratio of performing an anastomosis against creation of a stoma. If one chooses to restore intestinal continuity, it is necessary to use bowel that is not involved in the inflammatory process.

While there have been many studies showing equivalence between stapled and hand-sewn anastomosis in elective procedures, there is some suggestion in emergent surgery, and in multiple trauma especially, to suggest that hand-sewn anastomosis may be superior. In any event, when faced with peritonitis and bowel edema, it is our preference to perform only hand-sewn anastomosis. The decision to perform an anastomosis must also take into account the patient's physiologic status and the risk of failing to achieve source control. There is a surgical truism that the anastomosis that is never created will never leak. While a stoma commits the patient to a subsequent operation, surviving intra-abdominal infection and sepsis should be considered a success and an acceptable trade-off. In those patients with gross peritonitis, pressor requirements, and hemodynamic instability, a truncated procedure (i.e., damage control) should be employed. This allows the surgeon to eliminate the source of infection and provide ongoing resuscitation in a more controlled environment such as the intensive care department. During the subsequent operations, hopefully in a much less hostile abdomen, one can plan a more definitive approach to control infection and restore intestinal continuity.

There are also circumstances where a bowel resection or revision of an anastomosis is not possible. Some examples include duodenal stump blowouts, associated phlegmons compromising surrounding vascular structures, or pancreatico-intestinal anastomotic leaks. In these types of cases, the goal is controlling the effluent to create a controlled fistula while allowing the inflammatory and fibrotic process to "scar" over the problem. An important part of the management is the use of latex or red rubber drains placed in the lumen of the intestine. This both allows drainage and enhances the inflammatory process. T-tubes can be particularly useful because they are not prone to inadvertent removal. Liberal use of suction drains in proximity to these processes and placed as outlined above will further capture the effluent not coming through the latex drains. This drain strategy combined with appropriate nutritional support will lead to a controlled fistula that will often allow the clinician to remove the latex drains at much later time when the infection and inflammation has subsided.

SUGGESTED READINGS

Barie PS: Modern surgical antibiotic prophylaxis and therapy less is more, *Surg Infect* 1:23–29, 2000.

Lee MJ: Non traumatic abdominal emergencies: imaging and intervention in sepsis, *Eur Radiol* 12:2172–2179, 2002.

Malangoni MA, Shumate CR, Thomas HA, et al: Factors influencing the treatment of intra-abdominal abscesses, *Am J Surg* 159:167–171, 1990.

Solomkin JS, Mazuski JE, Bradley JS: Diagnosis and management of complicated intra-abdominal infection in adults and children, *Clin Infect Dis* 50:133–164, 2010.

Theisen J, Bartels H, Weiss W: Current concepts of percutaneous abscess drainage in post-operative retention, *J Gastrointest Surg* 9:280–283, 2005.

OCCUPATIONAL EXPOSURE TO HUMAN IMMUNODEFICIENCY VIRUS AND OTHER BLOODBORNE PATHOGENS

John G. Bartlett, MD

The treatment of human immunodeficiency virus (HIV) has undergone great progress since the introduction of highly active antiretroviral therapy (HAART) in 1996. This has totally changed the prognosis for this disease. At present, HAART has added an average of 43 years to the life of HIV-infected patients; for those who have achieved virologic control, the benefit could be a normal life span. Thus, these patients are likely to have the common medical problems that are found in the general population, such as complications associated with aging, including conditions necessitating surgical intervention. On the basis of the treatments that are currently available to patients with HIV infection, current projections are that patients will soon be in two categories: those who have good virologic control and live a relatively normal life and those whose infections are discovered late or who do not adhere to the medical regimen and have the pre-1996 complications. This chapter reviews some of the progress that has had such a dramatic effect, but the main emphasis is on the management of bloodborne exposures, which is the component that is perhaps most important to surgeons.

PROGRESS IN THE FIELD

Acquired immunodeficiency syndrome (AIDS) was first described in 1981, the putative agent (HIV) was described in 1983, serologic testing became available in 1985, and the effective therapy was established as zidovudine (AZT) in a trial that was completed in 1986. AZT was effective, but the results were temporary as a result of the rapid development of virologic failure and resistance. The beginning of effective therapy was HAART with protease inhibitors, introduced in 1996. Since then, new drugs, concepts of treatment, and simplification of regimens have evolved continuously, and at least 20 large cohorts have been studied to document population-based progress in the field. An assessment in 2012 is that virtually all patients with HIV infection should receive HAART: most commonly with three drugs, usually consisting of two nucleosides and a "third drug" that is either a nucleoside reverse transcriptase inhibitor (NRTI) or a nonnucleoside reverse transcriptase inhibitor, a protease inhibitor, or an integrase inhibitor. The HIV viral load averages 50,000 to 100,000 copies/mL (one copy equals one virion) at baseline; with this therapy, the viral load is expected to decrease to a level below the limits of detection with the standard assay (<50 copies/mL) within 4 to 8 weeks and remain "undetectable" on standard tests if the patient adheres to the regimen. There is good evidence that this level of viral control actually indicates a total shutdown of the virus, which means no replication and consequently no sequence evolution with development of resistance. The result is total virologic control with clinical stability and immune recovery. The problem associated with this ideal response is that the virus is still present in multiple reservoirs, so that HIV viremia recurs rapidly if therapy is discontinued. Furthermore, such a lapse in treatment is often associated with viral resistance, which necessitates medication changes and fewer future options. The relevance of this outcome to surgical practice is twofold. First, discontinuation of HAART for a surgical procedure increases these risks if caution is not taken, usually with the expert guidance of the HIV healthcare provider. Second, the risk of HIV transmission with occupational exposure is directly correlated with the level of HIV viremia, which is usually high in patients in whom the infection is undiagnosed or untreated or in whom treatment fails.

This information provides an optimistic view of HIV infection and the progress in management. Nevertheless, this is an infection that has not been cured, and researchers seem unlikely to achieve that goal with the drugs currently available and those in development. Another failure has been the ability to prevent transmission of HIV. Thus in the United States (prevalence, 0.3%), there have been an estimated 40,000 new cases every year since 1990. It is now estimated that approximately 1.1 million people live with HIV infection in the United States, and that number is anticipated to increase by approximately 25,000 per year with the dramatic decrease in HIV-related mortality and the continued rates of HIV transmission of about 10,000 per year in the United States. Thus the epidemic seems destined to grow, but patients who are treated have a good chance for a near-normal life expectancy.

Infection with hepatitis B virus (HBV) is also treatable and incurable. Contemporary treatment to reduce HBV viral load includes drugs such as lamivudine, tenofovir, and entecavir. For hepatitis C virus (HCV) infection, the field is rapidly changing, with a large number of new drugs that will substantially change the course of this disease. Unlike HBV and HIV infections, HCV infection can often be cured, and the new drugs are likely to change the epidemiology of this disease completely by 2014.

OCCUPATIONAL EXPOSURE TO BLOODBORNE PATHOGENS

Three pathogens of major concern include HIV, HBV, and HCV. All three are viremic and can be transmitted by sex or blood exposure. Substantial data document the relative risk of transmission from an infected host with blood exposure in healthcare workers, usually by needlestick injury but also, to a much less extent, with mucous membrane and skin exposure. The relative risk per exposure with sharps injury and the prevalence of each of these three viruses in the general population are noted in Table 1.

The prevalences of these infections in the general population do not necessarily represent their prevalences in hospitals; all three should be substantially higher in hospitals. Furthermore, with regard to hepatitis B, the data refer to the risk of an unvaccinated healthcare worker—a population that, it is hoped, is small.

Occupational Exposure to Human Immunodeficiency Virus

Risk

Analysis of 23 studies of needlestick injuries to healthcare workers from an HIV-infected source patient showed that the rate of HIV transmission in the pre-HAART era was 20 (0.33%) per 6135. With

TABLE 1: Risk of viral transmission with sharps exposure to bloodborne pathogens

Virus	Prevalence (U.S. general population)	Risk of exposure (per 1000)
Human immunodeficiency virus (HIV)	0.3%	3%
MSM	7%	
IDU		
Hepatitis B virus (HBV; HBsAg)	0.1%-0.2%	
MSM	6%-17%	
IDU	7%-10%	
Immigrants from high-risk areas	13%	
HIV-infected patients	7%-10%	
HBeAg positive		22%-30%
HBeAg negative		11%-6%
Hepatitis C virus (HCV)	1.8%	1.9%
People born 1945-1965	3.3%	
MSM	2%-8%	
IDU	60%-90%;	

HBeAg, Hepatitis B "e" antigen; *HBsAg,* hepatitis B surface antigen; *IDU,* injection drug use; *MSM,* men who have sex with men.

mucosal membrane exposure, the rate was 1 (0.69%) per 143 exposures, and there were no transmissions with 2712 skin exposures.

Through June 2010, there were 57 documented cases of occupationally acquired HIV infection in healthcare workers in the United States. The last report of such a case was in 1999, and there were none that the author is aware of since then. This reporting refers to individuals who had a defined exposure with subsequent seroconversion. There were also 138 cases of "possible occupational transmission" in which the healthcare worker had otherwise unexplained HIV infection. For obvious reasons, the best data are for those with documented exposure and seroconversion. In terms of the injuries that accounted for the 56 cases with available data, 48 resulted from parenteral exposure alone, 5 from mucosal injuries alone, 2 individuals from both, and 1 from an unknown source of exposure. With regard to needlestick injuries, all transmissions have been with a hollowbore needle; there is no record of HIV transmission with a suture needle, although the Centers for Disease Control and Prevention (CDC) recommend similar management of exposure with either needle type. No HIV transmissions to surgeons have been documented, and the great majority of exposures have occurred in nurses or laboratory technicians.

Analysis of cases with transmission reveals the following exposure-related factors that were correlated with the probability of HIV transmission:

- The depth or severity of the exposure
- The presence of visible blood on the device
- The history that the device had previously been used in the infected patient's vein or artery
- The fact that the source patient died within 60 days of the healthcare worker's exposure

A fifth factor that increased risk was the absence of prophylaxis with antiviral agents. The data were collected in the early phase of the HIV epidemic; progress in managing patients with HIV infection and managing exposures presumably explains the 10-year absence of seroconversions in the more recent experience.

Efficacy of Zidovudine

Several lines of investigation support the role of AZT for exposure to HIV infection. This agent is antiquated, but it is the best studied for the period with the most transmissions.

1. Retrospective analyses of cases show a risk reduction of approximately 80% when standardized for the four variables noted earlier.
2. The effectiveness of AZT in preventing HIV transmission has precedent, according to the early studies of perinatal transmission. The famous AIDS Clinical Trial Group (ACTG) study 076 showed that AZT reduced vertical transmission of HIV by 67%. These data have been substantiated by multiple studies that show consistent results with reductions in perinatal transmission rates from 27% in the absence of antiviral agents to less than 2% when there is virologic control in the maternal source at the time of exposure at birth.
3. There are supporting data from animal models in which both AZT and tenofovir were administered for 1 month, starting either before exposure or up to 24 to 48 hours after exposure.
4. Substantial data show that virologic suppression of HIV virtually eliminates the risk of transmission by sexual contact.

Despite these promising data on the effectiveness of postexposure prophylaxis (PEP), there are at least six cases in which PEP was not successful despite initiation of the treatment within 2 hours of exposure, with regimens that were generally advocated in the pre-HAART era. Moreover, the number of occupationally acquired infections in the United States since 1996 has been reduced to none to two per year.

Management of an Exposure

The first response must be decontamination as quickly as possible. Cutaneous injuries should be washed with soap and water. A visible defect such as an incision wound should be irrigated with saline or a disinfectant. Mucosal surfaces such as the mouth or nose should be flushed with copious amounts of water. Ocular exposures should be irrigated with saline or water. For decontamination, the use of bleach, peroxide, iodophors, or other disinfectants with immediate wound care is satisfactory but not viewed as necessarily an important priority.

Testing the Source

In the absence of recent positive test results, the source should be tested for all three bloodborne pathogens: HIV, HBV with hepatitis B virus surface antigen (HBsAg), and HCV (with anti-HCV). For HIV, the standard is rapid testing, which can detect HIV antibody within 20 minutes. In some patients with very early infection, the HIV viral load is high and seroconversion has not taken place. This means the source patient is antibody negative and has a high viral load. This window is only about 3 to 4 weeks, but it is the period of greatest transmission risk. Contemporary testing options include viral load testing, which requires 2 to 3 days, but newer tests (called fourth-generation tests for both antigen and antibody) provide results in less than 1 hour. These tests have a sensitivity and specificity of approximately 99%. Positive results may be verified with a Western blot test for purposes of HIV management of the source patient, but the early results can be presumed accurate for HIV prophylaxis. In the great majority of cases, negative test results nearly exclude this diagnosis. None of this screening is necessary in a patient known to have HIV infection. In that case, the review should note the recent viral load tests, resistance test results, and the medication record because these may alter drug decisions for antiviral prophylaxis.

The standard practice has been to acquire signed informed consent for testing the source patient. This may be problematic for patients who cannot give informed consent because of concurrent medical conditions. Some states have made allowances to permit obtaining blood from the source patient for HIV testing if the source patient is unable to provide it in the context of occupational exposure, but some states have no such legislation. The CDC and nearly all states have advocated "opt-out testing," which would treat HIV much like other tests, meaning that the patient has the opportunity to decline the test, as with any test or procedure, but there is no requirement for the signed informed consent with counseling. Thus the method of obtaining blood from the source patient for HIV serologic testing may vary substantially on the basis of individual state policy. The occupational health departments of hospitals clearly know the local rules.

Counseling

Healthcare workers must be informed about the risks involved in exposure to HIV, including the facts that (1) the odds of HIV transmission from an HIV-infected source patient are approximately 3 per 1000; (2) if the source patient is not receiving therapy, the healthcare worker does not accept antiretroviral therapy, and (3) the percutaneous injury is "average." With the average type of needlestick exposure to a source patient who is receiving therapy and has a viral load below the limits of detection (i.e., <50 copies/mL), the risk is probably vanishingly small—but it is not zero. This was demonstrated in the studies of perinatal transmission, which also showed a direct correlation between the probability of transmission and the viral load, but some transmission occurred even from women who had very low viral loads. Furthermore, PEP has documented benefit. AZT seems to reduce the probability of seroconversion by 80%, but the current recommendation is for a far more potent regimen; thus the prophylaxis is now expected to be substantially more effective. However, the additional benefit cannot be quantitated.

Timing of Initiation of Antiretroviral Drugs

Studies in macaques show that the earlier treatment is initiated, the more likely it is to be effective. The goal of PEP is to initiate treatment as quickly as possible, preferably within 1 to 2 hours of exposure. According to the CDC guidelines, the allowable window is 36 hours after exposure, but consensus is that earlier is better. In a review of 435 healthcare workers with HIV exposure, the median time from exposure to treatment was 1.8 hours. Even when the source patient's HIV status is unknown, rapid HIV tests enable treatment to begin within the time frame of test results to verify potential exposure. Standard serologic tests usually take 3 to 7 days to analyze, although a negative result of an enzyme immunoassay screening is usually available within 24 to 48 hours and is adequate for the decision to discontinue PEP when a rapid test is not available.

Healthcare Worker Counseling

Healthcare workers should be informed about the following:

1. The risk of transmission according to the data provided earlier, including the risk of seroconversion and the potential effect of PEP, which reduces risk by at least 80%.
2. The effect of time delays on PEP efficacy.
3. Methods to minimize the risk of secondary transmission, meaning "safe sex" or abstention until serologic test results are negative 6 months after exposure. The risk of transmission is greatest in the first 6 to 12 weeks, and many authorities recommend these precautions only through the 3-month test.
4. Description of the PEP regimens and the side effects of the drugs likely to be used.

5. Regardless of the PEP drug decision, there must be follow-up serologic testing at 6 weeks, 3 months, and 6 months. The current recommendation is to repeat serologic testing at 12 months in the healthcare worker who has also acquired HCV with the injury because this may delay the time of HIV seroconversion. Some occupational health departments perform a test at 1 year on all exposed healthcare workers because at least three seroconverted between 6 and 12 months.

6. Female healthcare workers who are not pregnant and have childbearing capacity must be advised that the agents used for HIV prevention are considered safe for use in pregnancy. The only drug that has been traditionally contraindicated is efavirenz, a drug that is not advocated for PEP. In terms of safety of other drugs, the pregnancy registry (*http://www.apregistry.com*) indicates birth defects in 110 of 4391 live births among HIV-infected women receiving antiretroviral drugs during pregnancy. This rate of 2.5/100 is not significantly different from the CDC population-based birth defects surveillance system, which indicates 3.1/100 live births.

Antiretroviral Regimens

Antiretroviral drug recommendations and policies for occupational exposure provided here are based on 2012 guidelines of the New York State AIDS Institute and are as follows:

1. The evaluation is considered urgent with the goal for initiate HAART within 2 hours.
2. If the source patient has a negative result of a test for HIV antibody but is at risk for HIV infection within 6 weeks of the testing, plasma HIV RNA (antigen) and PEP should be given to the healthcare worker within 2 hours of exposure if HIV test results are delayed.
3. The initial regimen should be tenofovir/emtricitabine (Truvada) plus raltegravir. The specific regimen is Truvada (1/day) plus raltegravir (400 mg/day orally) for 28 days. (AZT is no longer recommended because of poor tolerance.)
4. Alternative regimens:
   - If the exposed healthcare worker has renal disease with creatinine clearance rate lower than 50 mL/min, tenofovir disoproxil fumarate (TDF) is contraindicated; an alternative NRTI combination is AZT/lamivudine.
   - If resistance data are available from the source patient, these data should be used in the regimen selection.
   - Poor tolerance is a reason to change regimens. Other agents to consider are atazanavir/ritonavir (ATV/r), darunavir/ritonavir (DRV/r), fosamprenavir/ritonavir (FPV/r), and lopinavir/ritonavir (LPV/r).
   - There needs to be attention to drug interactions.
5. Follow-up monitoring of the exposed healthcare worker, with or without acceptance of HAART prophylaxis, should include HIV testing at 4 and 12 weeks.
6. Potential sources of HIV transmission include not only blood but also semen, vaginal secretions, breast milk, and cerebrospinal, pleural, pericardial and amniotic fluid. (Saliva, sweat, tears, nonbloody urine, and stool are not considered HIV sources).
7. The risk of HIV transmission from an HIV infected source patient in the absence of prophylaxis is estimated at 3 per 1000 with a needlestick exposure and 0.9 per 1000 with a mucocutaneous exposure. Prophylactic AZT reduced these risks by an estimated 80%.
8. The "window" of effective prophylaxis is considered probably closed at 36 hours after exposure. Decisions to start PEP after 36 hours are made a case-by-case basis.

Management of the Injury Site

Sites of skin exposure should be cleaned immediately with soap and water; sites of exposure at mucous membranes, with water flushing.

Source Testing

If HIV status of the source patient is unknown, the following measures should be taken: (1) obtain consent for the HIV test if consent is required according to institutional policy, and (2) use a rapid test if possible. (State laws vary with regard to testing when the source patient refuses or is unable to consent). The rapid test is preferred. If recent HIV acquisition is suspected (within 6 weeks), testing for antigen should be done if the antibody test result is negative (or both should be done simultaneously). Confirmatory tests should be performed if results are positive, but this should not delay prophylaxis. If HAART is given pending testing, it should be stopped when HIV in the source patient is ruled out.

Monitoring the Exposed Healthcare Worker

Baseline: Perform HIV test, (pregnancy test), and obtain chemistry profile and complete blood cell count (CBC).
Day 3: Assess adherence to and tolerance of the treatment regimen.
Week 1: Assess adherence and tolerance.*
Week 2: Assess adherence and tolerance,* and obtain a chemistry profile and CBC.
Week 3: Assess adherence and tolerance.*
Week 4: Assess adherence and tolerance*; obtain a chemistry profile and CBC; and perform an HIV test.
Week 12: Perform an HIV test.

Expert advice is available at the National Clinicians Center PEP Line: 888-448-4911. *Telephone contact or clinic visit.

Expert Opinion

The field of HIV infection has become extremely complicated with the rapid advances since 1995. Many hospitals do not have the available expertise within the occupational medicine department to deal with the complexities of issues and timeliness. Therefore, a CDC recommendation is frequently to seek expert consultation or use of the National Clinicians Center PEP line, which is operational from 9 AM to 2 AM Eastern Standard Time at 888-448-4911. Some common queries include the following situations:

- A delay in exposure report or a decision for PEP after the 24- to 36-hour window of opportunity
- Unknown source of a sharps injury, which must be reviewed on a case-by-case basis
- Use of PEP regimens in patients who are pregnant, potentially pregnant, or breastfeeding
- Resistance of the source virus to antiretroviral drugs
- Toxicity of the PEP regimen in terms of symptom management or decision for different drug regimens

Occupational Exposure to Hepatitis B

The risk of transmission is dependent on the vaccine status of the healthcare worker and the presence or absence of HBV e-antigen (HBeAg) in a patient with HBsAg (see Table 1). Recommendations for PEP are summarized in Table 2. Unvaccinated healthcare workers are highly vulnerable, as indicated in Table 1, and, when the source patient is HBeAg positive, exceptionally so. It is hoped that all healthcare workers, including all surgeons, will have been vaccinated, but rates of protection are somewhat variable. Response to the vaccine is age related; it is 95% for persons vaccinated at 20 to 30 years of age, 86% vaccinated at 40 to 50 years of age, and 45% for those vaccinated when older than 60 years of age. Titers of antibody decrease an average of 10% per year, but prior responders who had a

TABLE 2: Postexposure prophylaxis for hepatitis B*

Antibody status of healthcare worker	Vaccine or source patient status		
	HBsAg positive	**HBsAg negative**	**Unknown**
Not immune	HBIG × 1 + vaccine	HBV vaccine	HBV vaccine
Vaccinated responder	No Rx	No Rx	No Rx
Vaccinated nonresponder	HBIG × 1 + vaccine *or* HBIG × 2	No Rx	No Rx; if source patient is at high risk, treat as if HBsAg positive
Vaccinated response unknown	Vaccine booster dose	No Rx	Same as for vaccinated nonresponder
Ongoing vaccination	HBIG × 1 Complete series	Complete series	Complete series

*Adapted from New York State AIDS Institute Guidelines (*http://www.hivguidelines.org*), October 2012.
HBIG, Hepatitis B immune globulin; *HBsAg*, hepatitis B virus surface antigen; *HBV*, hepatitis B virus; *Rx*, treatment.

demonstrated response with an antibody titer exceeding 10 U/mL are probably protected as a result of cell-mediated immunity. It is now common practice to measure antibody response at 1 to 6 months after completion of the three-dose series, but many programs did not do this when the healthcare vaccination programs were initially launched. Currently, for nonresponders, the recommendation is to repeat the vaccination series, and nonresponders have a 55% probability of response with revaccination. The vaccine efficacy is approximately 80% to 95% for all vaccine recipients and 99% for those who have had a documented response.

On the basis of these data, healthcare workers are considered protected if they have been vaccinated and have documented antibody response at any time. If response was never measured, it should be measured in the context of exposure as the basis of subsequent decisions. If the antibody levels are greater than 10 U/mL, the healthcare worker is considered protected. If antibody levels were never measured and are now less than the stated threshold, the healthcare worker must be managed as a "nonresponder." Subsequent management recommendations are provided in Table 2.

Occupational Exposure to Hepatitis C

A review of 25 published studies from 1991 to 2002 indicated that the rate of HCV transmission after a sharps injury from an HCV-infected source patient was 44 (1.9%) per 2357. Cutaneous exposure on intact skin with blood from a contaminated source patient does not appear to confer risk. When a healthcare worker has an exposure to blood or body fluid from a source patient, the institution should follow these guidelines:

1. Wash exposed wounds with soap and water, and flush exposed mucous membranes with water.
2. Evaluate the source patient for HCV infection with HCV antibody.
3. If the source patient is HCV positive, test the source patient for HCV virus with HCV RNA or recombinant immunoblot assay (RIBA), and test the exposed healthcare worker's liver function and HCV antibody level; if the latter result is positive, test for the presence of HCV RNA.

Management guidelines are summarized in Table 3.

Healthcare Worker with Hepatitis C Virus RNA

Refer to a clinician experienced in HCV management.

TABLE 3: Guidelines for hepatitis C exposure

Source patient/healthcare worker	Follow-up
Source patient negative for HCV antibody	No further follow-up
Source patient not available for testing	Exposed healthcare worker: HCV antibody test at 3 and 6 months
Source patient HCV antibody positive and HCV RNA positive	Manage healthcare worker as exposed*
Healthcare worker – HCV negative	Manage healthcare worker as exposed*
Healthcare worker – HCV antibody and HCV RNA positive	Manage healthcare worker as infected

*Postexposure HCV testing in exposed healthcare worker is as follows: In week 4, HCV RNA and liver panel; in week 12, HCV RNA and liver panel; and in week 24, liver panel and HCV antibody testing. If alanine aminotransferase level is elevated at any time, the HCV RNA assay should be repeated, in addition to testing for acute HCV.

SUGGESTED READINGS

Ayoub WS, Keeffe EB, et al: Review article: current antiviral therapy of chronic hepatitis, *Ailment Pharmacol Ther* 34:1145, 2011.
Cardo DM, Culver DH, Ciesielski CA, et al: A case-control study of HIV seroconversion in healthcare workers after percutaneous exposure, *N Engl J Med* 337:1485, 1997.
Centers for Disease Control and Prevention: *Surveillance of occupationally acquired HIV/AIDS in healthcare personnel, as of May 2011* (online article). http://www.cdc.gov/HAI/organisms/hiv/Surveillance-Occupationally-Acquired-HIV-AIDS.html. Accessed May 22, 2013.
Connor EM, Sperling RS, Gelber R, et al: Reduction of maternal-infant transmission of human immunodeficiency virus type 1 with zidovudine treatment. Pediatric AIDS Clinical Trials Group Protocol 076 Study Group, *N Engl J Med* 331:1173, 1994.

De Carli G, Puro V, Scognamiglio P, et al: Infection with hepatitis C virus transmitted by accidental needlesticks, *Clin Infect Dis* 37:1718, 2003.

Durlach R, Laugas S, Freuler CB, et al: Ten-year persistence of antibody to hepatitis B surface antigen in healthcare workers vaccinated against hepatitis B virus, and response to booster vaccination, *Infect Control Hosp Epidemiol* 24:773, 2003.

European Association of the Study of the Liver: 2011 European Association of the Study of the Liver hepatitis C virus clinical practice guidelines, *Liver Int* 32(Suppl. 1):2–8, 2012.

Gerberding JL: Clinical practice. Occupational exposure to HIV in health care settings, *N Engl J Med* 348:826, 2003.

Ghany MG, Strader DB, Thomas DL, et al: Diagnosis, management and treatment of hepatitis C: An update, *Hepatology* 49:1335, 2009.

Henderson DK: Management of needlestick injuries: a house officer who has a needlestick, *JAMA* 307:75, 2012.

Henderson DK, Fahey BJ, Willy M, et al: Risk for occupational transmission of human immunodeficiency virus type 1 (HIV-1) associated with clinical exposures. A prospective evaluation, *Ann Intern Med* 13:740, 1990.

Landovitz RJ, Currier JS: Clinical practice. Postexposure prophylaxis for HIV infection, *N Engl J Med* 361:1768, 2009.

Mayer KH, Mimiaga MJ, Gelman M, et al: Raltegravir, tenofovir DF, and emtricitabine for post-exposure prophylaxis to prevent sexual transmission of HIV: safety, tolerability, and adherence, *J Acquir Immune Defic Syndr* 59:354, 2012.

Quinn TC, Wawer MJ, Sewankambo N, et al: Viral load and heterosexual transmission of human immunodeficiency virus type 1. Rakai Project Study Group, *N Engl J Med* 342:921, 2000.

Sulkowski MS, Ray SC, Thomas DL: Needlestick transmission of hepatitis C, *JAMA* 287:2406, 2002.

US Public Health Service: Updated U.S. Public Health Service Guidelines for the Management of Occupational Exposures to HBV, HCV and HIV and Recommendations for Postexposure Prophylaxis, *MMWR Recomm Rep* 50(RR-11):1–52, 2001.

Weinbaum CM, Williams I, Mast EE, et al: Recommendations for identification and public health management of persons with chronic hepatitis B virus infection, *MMWR Recomm Rep* 57:1, 2008.

ANTIFUNGAL THERAPY IN THE SURGICAL PATIENT

Kieren A. Marr, MD, and Shmuel Shoham, MD

INTRODUCTION

Fungal infections are a major problem in hospitalized surgical patients. The most important infections are invasive and superficial candidiasis and, to a lesser extent, aspergillosis and mucormycosis. Treatment of these infections is the main focus of this chapter. Whereas superficial fungal infections are rarely dangerous, invasive fungal infections continue to be associated with suboptimal outcomes. The reasons for this are related to both host and fungal factors. Patients at risk for developing invasive fungal infections tend to have multiple comorbid conditions and are often critically ill. Moreover, diagnosis of infection can be difficult, and institution of appropriate antifungal therapy is often delayed. With the advent of improved diagnostic modalities and safer antifungal therapy, outcomes are improving (Table 1).

In addition to antifungal chemotherapy, there is often a critical role for surgical management of invasive fungal infections. For example, removal of a potentially infected vascular catheter is frequently necessary in patients with candidemia. Moreover, drainage and/or débridement are often needed in cases of infected fluid collections and invasive tissue disease. In cases of filamentous fungal infections, debridement or excision of infected and necrotic tissue is frequently required in order to control the infection.

Coccidioidomycosis, blastomycosis, histoplasmosis, and cryptococcosis are important fungal diseases. Occasionally, lesions caused by *Coccidioides* and *Blastomyces* require surgical débridement, and patients with high cerebrospinal fluid pressure due to cryptococcosis may need placement of a spinal drain for intracranial pressure management. Because these infections are not typically encountered in a surgical practice, their medical management is not covered in this chapter.

ANTIFUNGAL AGENTS

Polyenes

The polyene class of antifungal agents consists of nystatin and the various formulations of amphotericin B (AmB). These agents work by disrupting the fungal cell membrane and are active against a broad range of clinically important fungi. Neither is absorbed orally. Nystatin is used topically as a solution, powder, or cream for a range of superficial infections such as oropharyngeal, cutaneous, and vulvovaginal candidiasis. AmB is principally used intravenously for systemic infections, but it may be used topically for oropharyngeal and bladder infections and as aerosolized inhalational treatment for prevention of lung infections.

Amphotericin B

AmB is active against a broad array of fungi, including *Candida*, *Aspergillus*, and the Zygomycetes (agents of mucormycosis). AmB is the principal therapy for mucormycosis and as empiric therapy for a suspected disseminated fungal infection when the etiology is unclear. Various formulations are available, including deoxycholate AmB (dAmB), AmB lipid complex (ABLC), and liposomal AmB (L-AmB). Dosing is usually 0.5 to 1.0 mg/kg/d for dAmB and 3 to 6 mg/kg/d for lipid formulations. Higher doses are sometimes used in cases of mucormycosis and for other difficult to treat filamentous fungal infection. AmB may be ineffective due to resistance in infections caused by *Candida lusitaniae*, *Aspergillus terreus*, *Fusarium*, *Scedosporium prolificans*, and *Trichosporon*.

The main drawbacks to AmB are its side effects, which are principally infusion-related reactions and nephrotoxicity. These are less common with the lipid formulations, and we therefore recommend their use over dAmB. Infusion-related toxicities include fevers, chills, myalgias, arthralgias, and occasionally hypotension. These can be prevented or reduced by slowing down the infusion rate and premedicating with acetaminophen. In many patients infusion-related reactions tend to resolve after a few doses. Manifestations of AmB nephrotoxicity include azotemia, hypokalemia, and hypomagnesemia. These are more common with higher cumulative doses of AmB and in patients with preexisting renal disease and/or concomitant

TABLE 1: Patient types and treatment options for adults with fungal infections

Infection	Patient type	Primary treatment/alternative treatment	Length of treatment	Comments
Candidemia	Critically ill, abdominal surgery, cancer chemotherapy, vascular access, burns, parenteral nutrition	**Primary** Caspofungin 70 mg × 1, then 50 mg/d IV Anidulafungin 200 mg × 1, then 100 mg/d IV Micafungin 100 mg/d IV Fluconazole 800 × 1, then 400 mg/d **Alternative** Deoxycholate AmB 0.7-1.0 mg/kg/d IV Lipid AmB 3-6 mg/kg/d IV Voriconazole 6 mg/kg BID × 2 doses, then 3 mg/kg BID	14 days after clearance of blood cultures. Longer if ocular involvement. If possible can switch to oral agent to complete therapy once patient has stabilized.	Remove vascular access devices if possible Do not use fluconazole for patients with neutropenia Evaluate for ocular involvement with fundoscopic examination
Candiduria/UTI	Urinary catheter, diabetes mellitus, kidney transplant recipients	**Primary** Fluconazole 200-400 mg/d **Alternative** Deoxycholate AmB 0.3-0.6 mg/kg/d IV	14 days 7-14 days	Patients with asymptomatic candiduria do not routinely need to be treated. Exceptions are neutropenia or planned instrumentation
Oropharyngeal candidiasis	Immunocompromised, radiotherapy, ill-fitting dentures	**Primary** Clotrimazole 10 mg 5/d PO Nystatin QID PO Fluconazole 100-200 mg/d PO **Alternative** Itraconazole solution 200 mg/d PO Posaconazole 400 mg BID PO Voriconazole 200 mg BID PO Caspofungin 70 mg × 1, then 50 mg/d IV Anidulafungin 200 mg × 1, then 100 mg/d IV Micafungin 100 mg/d IV	7-14 days	Use topical therapy for mild disease; relapses more common with echinocandins
Esophageal candidiasis	Immunocompromised (e.g., advanced HIV)	**Primary** Fluconazole 200-400 mg/d (IV or oral) **Alternative** Echinocandins, itraconazole, or posaconazole (see above for doses)	14-21 days	Relapses may be more common with echinocandins
Vulvovaginal candidiasis	Antibacterial therapy, diabetes mellitus	Topical therapy (e.g., clotrimazole, nystatin, miconazole) Fluconazole 150 mg × 1 PO	Schedules vary by agent	Vulvovaginal candidiasis, even if recurrent, is usually *not* due to an immunocompromised state

Continued

TABLE 1: Patient types and treatment options for adults with fungal infections—cont'd

Infection	Patient type	Primary treatment/alternative treatment	Length of treatment	Comments
Aspergillosis	Abnormalities of neutrophil number or function, structural lung abnormalities, burns	**Primary** Voriconazole 6 mg/kg BID × 2, then 4 mg/kg/d +/− echinocandin **Alternative** Lipid AmB 5 mg/kg/d Caspofungin, anidulafungin (see above for doses), micafungin 100-150 mg/d Posaconazole 800 mg/d in 2-4 divided doses	Length of Rx not clear	Consider monitoring voriconazole and posaconazole levels to help guide therapy
Mucormycosis	Systemic immunosuppression, burns, trauma, near drowning, uncontrolled DM, deferoxamine use	**Primary** Lipid AmB 5-7.5 mg/kg/d +/− echinocandin	Length of Rx not clear	Débridement and excision are often needed If patient is stable, consider switching to posaconazole after 3 weeks AmB

nephrotoxic processes. Giving prophylactic normal saline (0.9% NaCl) at 10 to 15 ml/kg/d and avoiding concomitant administration of nephrotoxic agents can reduce the chance of nephrotoxicity.

Azoles

The azoles are an extremely important class of antifungal agents with activity against a broad range of fungi. These drugs inhibit ergosterol biosynthesis, thereby impairing formation of the fungal cell membrane. Depending on the specific drug, the azoles are available as oral, intravenous, or topical therapy. These agents have the potential for multiple drug interactions via the cytochrome P450 system, and care must be taken when coadministered with other drugs metabolized by these isoenzymes. Important examples include elevation of warfarin, calcineurin inhibitors, and sirolimus levels with concomitant administration of an azole antifungal.

Fluconazole

Fluconazole is the most important azole for surgical patients. It is effective against most species of *Candida*, available in oral and intravenous formulations, and is generally well tolerated. Fluconazole continues to have excellent activity against *C. albicans*, but has variable activity against *C. glabrata*, which can account for up to 25% of candidiasis. It is inactive against *C. krusei*. Fluconazole is a first-line agent for oropharyngeal (100 to 200 mg/d) and esophageal candidiasis (200 to 400 mg/d) and is useful in cases of invasive candidiasis (400 to 800 mg/d; 6 to 12 mg/kg/d) in moderately ill, nonneutropenic patients. Fluconazole is also widely used for prevention of candidiasis in high-risk patients. Dose adjustment is required with renal dysfunction. Fluconazole occasionally causes liver toxicity, gastrointestinal (GI) upset, and rashes and is associated with multiple drug interactions as indicated above.

Voriconazole

Voriconazole is effective against *Aspergillus*, most species of *Candida*, and multiple other filamentous fungi. It is available in oral and intravenous (IV) formulations. Voriconazole is first-line treatment for invasive aspergillosis and can be used in cases of invasive candidiasis. It has excellent bioavailability, allowing for oral administration, but steady-state levels are reached more rapidly with IV loading doses of 6 mg/kg every 12 hours × 2 doses. This is followed by 4 mg/kg twice daily. Oral dosing for most adults is 200 to 300 mg twice daily. Renal adjustment is not necessary, but caution should be used when giving the IV solution in patients with decreased kidney function because the cyclodextrin carrier used in the IV formulation might damage the kidneys.

Voriconazole is associated with multiple adverse reactions, including changes in visual perception, vivid dreams, psychosis, hepatotoxicity, and phototoxicity. Drug levels can vary widely among patients, and this may impact efficacy and toxicity. Therapeutic drug monitoring is increasingly used to ensure that levels are in the acceptable range (troughs of approximately 2 to 5 mg/L). Adverse events are more likely to occur when serum levels exceed 5.5 mg/L. Voriconazole is associated with multiple drug interactions as indicated above.

Posaconazole

Posaconazole is effective against a broad range of fungi, including most species of *Candida*, *Aspergillus*, and many filamentous fungi, including the Zygomycetes. It is currently only available as an oral suspension, and attainment of steady-state levels can take a week or longer. For this reason it is generally not recommended as first-line therapy for established infections. The dose for invasive fungal infection is 800 mg/d in 2 to 4 divided doses. Total daily doses above 800 mg are poorly absorbed. A new formulation of posaconazole as a tablet and an IV solution are expected to have improved pharmacokinetic parameters and are currently in advanced clinical trials. The most common side effects of posaconazole are GI upset and hepatotoxicity. Posaconazole is also associated with multiple drug interactions as indicated above.

Itraconazole

Itraconazole is of limited importance in surgical patients. It is available as oral tablets and as a cyclodextrin oral solution, which results in better drug absorption. In some countries itraconazole is also available for IV therapy. The spectrum of activity is similar to fluconazole, but it is also active against some filamentous fungi, including *Aspergillus*. Several factors limit its use, including erratic gut absorption, need for drug-level monitoring, GI upset (particularly with the cyclodextrin solution), hepatic toxicity, and negative inotropic cardiac effects.

Echinocandins

The echinocandins (caspofungin, micafungin, and anidulafungin) are an important class of antifungal agents. They act by inhibition of fungal cell wall formation and have fungicidal activity against almost all *Candida* species (Figure 1). Treatment failures have been reported with *C. parapsilosis*, which has some innate resistance to the echinocandins. Under selective pressure, other species of *Candida* can also become resistant due to mutations. The echinocandins can also inhibit growth of *Aspergillus*, but they do not kill the organism. The echinocandins are extremely well tolerated and have very few drug interactions. They are only available via the IV route. Echinocandins are first-line therapy against invasive candidiasis and may also be used, but are not ideal, for cases of oropharyngeal and esophageal candidiasis. For adults with invasive candidiasis, dosing is micafungin, 100 mg/d; caspofungin, 70 mg loading dose, followed by 50 mg/d; and anidulafungin, 200 mg loading dose, followed by 100 mg/d.

SPECIFIC INFECTIONS

Candidiasis

Candida species are the most important fungal pathogens in surgical patients. These fungi are commensals of the human GI and genital tracts and of the skin. Infections are almost always of endogenous origin, but cross-contamination between colonized patients and/or from health care workers' hands can occur. Invasion occurs when host defenses break down or are breached. *C. albicans* is the most common colonizing and infecting species. The other important species include *C. parapsilosis, C. glabrata, C. tropicalis,* and *C. krusei.* Exposure to antifungal agents and transfer of the yeast among patients via health care workers' hands can alter fungal colonization patterns and subsequent infecting species.

Infection can be broadly divided into mucosal and systemic disease. Oropharyngeal candidiasis tends to occur in patients with abnormal cell-mediated immunity (as in those with advanced human immunodeficiency virus [HIV] and in recipients of corticosteroids). Cutaneous and vulvovaginal candidiasis are sometimes triggered by antimicrobial use and poor glycemic control but also can occur spontaneously. The majority of women with candidal vaginitis are not immunocompromised. Invasive candidiasis tends to occur in those with breached anatomic barriers due to surgery, cytotoxic chemotherapy, or vascular access catheters, and in patients with abnormalities in neutrophil number or function.

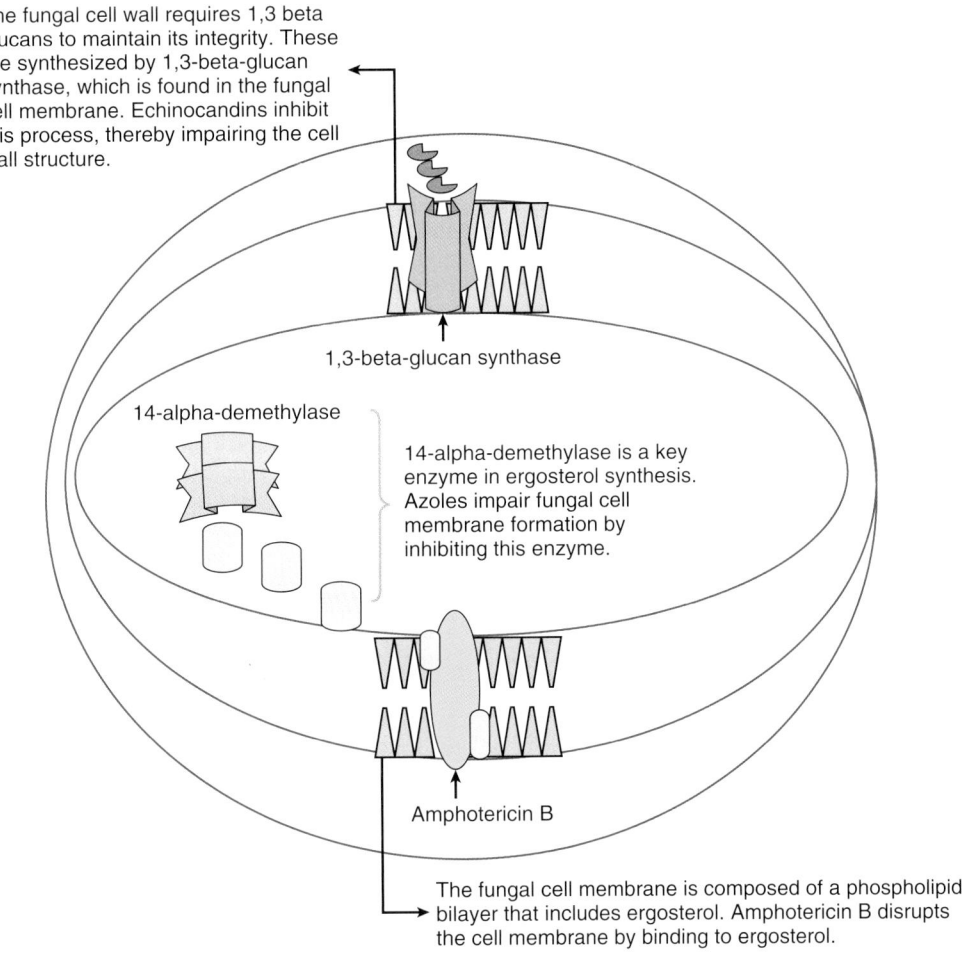

The fungal cell wall requires 1,3 beta glucans to maintain its integrity. These are synthesized by 1,3-beta-glucan synthase, which is found in the fungal cell membrane. Echinocandins inhibit this process, thereby impairing the cell wall structure.

1,3-beta-glucan synthase

14-alpha-demethylase

14-alpha-demethylase is a key enzyme in ergosterol synthesis. Azoles impair fungal cell membrane formation by inhibiting this enzyme.

Amphotericin B

The fungal cell membrane is composed of a phospholipid bilayer that includes ergosterol. Amphotericin B disrupts the cell membrane by binding to ergosterol.

FIGURE 1   Mechanisms of action.

Mucocutaneous Disease

Mucocutaneous fungal infections are very common, and their risk factors (e.g., diabetes mellitus, antibiotic exposure, corticosteroids) frequently overlap with those seen in surgical patients. These infections can cause significant discomfort but are rarely dangerous. Typical sites of infection include the oropharynx (thrush), esophagus, skin, and genitalia. Patients with symptomatic superficial infection should be treated, but because *Candida* species are normal commensals, simply culturing the organism from a superficial surface is not an indication for treatment.

Cutaneous Candidiasis

Cutaneous infections typically involve occluded areas and sites of large skin folds. Candidal intertrigo is a common infection at sites of warm, moist, and macerated skin, such as inframammary and large abdominal folds, the axillae, or groin. Diabetes mellitus, obesity, receipt of antibiotics or steroids, and inflammatory skin diseases are risk factors for such infections. The affected area may be itchy, red, and moist. The skin can be eroded with whitish scaling at the borders. Satellite lesions just beyond the main area's border are common. Diagnosis is generally based on clinical appearance. Superficial candidiasis can be treated with topical therapy. For moist macerated skin, an antifungal powder formulation may be preferable. Nystatin (100,000 units/g) and miconazole (2%) are available as either a powder or cream. A variety of other antifungal creams are also available, including econazole (1%), clotrimazole (1%), butenafine (1%), terbinafine (1%), tolnaftate (1%), and ketoconazole (2%).

Vulvovaginal Candidiasis

Candidal vulvovaginitis is extraordinarily common, and most women will have at least one attack during their lifetime. Risk factors include antibiotics, diabetes mellitus, and pregnancy. Vulvovaginitis may present with local irritation, itching, erythema, vaginal discharge, dysuria, and dyspareunia. Patients will often make a self-diagnosis of "yeast" vaginitis. This can be confirmed by identifying candidal elements (pseudohyphae and blastoconidia) on microscopic evaluation of a 10% KOH treated sample. In cases of vulvovaginal candidiasis, there are multiple intravaginal treatment options, including nystatin tablets (100,000 units/tablet), various azole creams (e.g., daily miconazole 2%, butoconazole 2%, clotrimazole 1%, and terconazole 0.4% and 0.8%), tioconazole 6.5% ointment, miconazole suppositories at 100 and 200 mg, and oral fluconazole 150 mg as a single dose. Some patients with recurrent vulvovaginal candidiasis require long term treatment with oral fluconazole 150 mg weekly or topical clotrimazole twice weekly. Boric acid vaginal suppositories (600 mg twice daily) are an option in recalcitrant cases.

Oropharyngeal and Esophageal Candidiasis

Oropharyngeal candidiasis is mainly a problem in immunosuppressed patients, and particularly in those with advanced HIV. Additional risk factors include extremes in age, poorly controlled diabetes mellitus, nutritional deficiencies, inadequately fitting dentures, systemic or inhaled steroids, radiotherapy, and cytotoxic chemotherapy. Clinical manifestations include thrush, which is characterized by curdlike, white patches on multiple surfaces of the oral mucosa, and erythematous candidiasis (acute atrophic candidiasis), which occurs by itself or in association with the white patches. Symptoms include local pain, burning, and changes in taste perception. Oropharyngeal candidiasis is almost always caused by *C. albicans* and can be treated with topical or systemic therapy. For mild disease, topical therapy tends to suffice. Options include nystatin suspension (100,000 units/mL) 4 to 6 mL four times daily, nystatin pastilles (200,000 units) 1 to 2 pastilles four times daily, or clotrimazole 10 mg troches five times daily. More severe disease may require fluconazole 100 to 200 mg daily. Treatment is typically for 7 to 14 days but may need to be extended, depending on response to therapy.

Esophageal candidiasis is usually associated with high levels of immunosuppression, as in advanced HIV and transplant recipients. Additional risk factors include advanced liver disease, receipt of proton pump inhibitors, and inhaled steroids. Symptoms are usually odynophagia, dysphagia, and retrosternal pain. Concurrent oropharyngeal candidiasis is common but may be absent. Infection is generally limited to the mucosa, but complications include volume depletion and malnutrition due to poor oral intake, esophageal strictures, and even esophageal perforation. Treatment is with oral fluconazole at 200 to 400 mg daily. In cases where the patient is unable to tolerate oral therapy, intravenous fluconazole can be given. Length of therapy is typically 14 to 21 days, depending on response to therapy.

Oropharyngeal and esophageal candidiasis refractory to fluconazole can occasionally develop in highly immunosuppressed and/or azole-experienced patients. This is an unusual situation in a surgical practice. Alternative oral options include itraconazole solution 200 mg/d, voriconazole 200 mg BID, and posaconazole 400 mg BID. These regimens are costlier and potentially more toxic than fluconazole. Furthermore, they may be ineffective due to resistance across the entire azole class. IV antifungal therapy with an echinocandin (micafungin 100 mg daily; caspofungin 70 mg loading dose, then 50 mg daily; and anidulafungin 200 mg loading dose, followed by 100 mg daily) can be effective, but some data suggest higher recurrence rates compared to treatment with an azole. Systemic AmB formulations are another option but can be associated with substantial toxicity.

Patients at significant risk for oropharyngeal candidiasis, such as those receiving cytotoxic chemotherapy, high-intensity immunosuppression, or who have advanced HIV, should be considered for prophylaxis. Topical agents such as nystatin or clotrimazole are generally effective. Systemic fluconazole 100 to 200 mg thrice weekly may also be effective as suppressive therapy in cases of recurrent infection.

Invasive Candidiasis

Invasive candidiasis is the most common serious fungal infection in the surgical population. Infections usually involve the bloodstream and/or intra-abdominal sites, although other organs (e.g., bones, joints, central nervous system) can be involved. Even with intense *Candida* colonization, host defenses must be breached for invasive infection to occur. The main lines of defense are intact GI and skin barriers and effective innate immune responses. Conditions that impact these include gut injury, surgical procedures, severe pancreatitis, thermal injury, vascular access catheterization (particularly if used for parenteral nutrition or hemodialysis), renal failure, corticosteroid use, and neutropenia.

The decision to treat is straightforward in patients with proven established infections. For invasive infection this generally means clinical signs and symptoms compatible with such an infection and material from a normally sterile source (e.g., blood, deep tissue, peritoneal fluid) showing culture or histopathologic evidence for fungal infection. One should never withhold therapy in patients with positive blood cultures because this can be associated with poor outcomes and increased secondary complications. Because symptoms can be nonspecific and blood cultures may be insensitive for detection of invasive candidiasis, treatment is often empiric. Development of prediction rules for invasive candidiasis and the emergence of nonculture techniques, such as serum beta-glucan measurements, are helping to guide initiation of antifungal therapy.

An additional challenge is interpreting the relevance of *Candida* growth in cultures from nonsterile sites. The presence of *Candida* in sputum, skin, and stool cultures suggests yeast colonization, but it does not indicate infection at those sites. Growth of *Candida* species from urinary catheter and abdominal drain cultures may indicate infection but may simply reflect colonization of the medical device.

Colonization with *Candida* at multiple sites in a critically ill patient suggests a high risk for invasive candidiasis. Discerning whether patients with signs and symptoms of sepsis and multiple sites of colonization have fungal infections can be difficult, and empiric therapy should be considered in such situations.

The choice of antifungal therapy depends on the site of infection, patient status, and antifungal susceptibility patterns. The echinocandins (caspofungin, micafungin, and anidulafungin) are the most effective agents for the treatment of candidemia. These agents are fungicidal against most *Candida* species and have an excellent safety profile. The doses are micafungin 100 mg/d; caspofungin 70 mg × 1, then 50 mg daily; and anidulafungin 200 mg × 1, then 100 mg daily. Fluconazole 800 mg (12 mg/kg) × 1, followed by 400 mg (6 mg/kg) daily is another option. Fluconazole should not be used for invasive candidiasis in patients who are neutropenic, unstable, or in whom azole resistance is a possibility. Other options include AmB formulations and voriconazole, but these are associated with more side effects than the echinocandins and fluconazole. Once the *Candida* species has been identified, treatment can be more focused. For infections due to *C. parapsilosis*, fluconazole is recommended because treatment failures can occur with the echinocandins. Fluconazole is active against most *Candida* species, with the exception of many *C. glabrata* and all *C. krusei* isolates. Fluconazole is generally less costly than the echinocandins and available as an oral agent. Patients who are stable and have an isolate that is likely to be susceptible to fluconazole may be transitioned to oral therapy to complete their course of treatment.

Duration of therapy depends on site of infection. Treatment of candidemia should be continued for 2 weeks after clearance of blood cultures and clinical resolution of infection because sites of microabscesses are frequent and not usually symptomatic. Patients with candidemia should be evaluated for dissemination to the eye with a fundoscopic exam, and if there is evidence for chorioretinitis, treatment should be extended to resolution of findings. In cases of endophthalmitis, a vitrectomy and intraocular instillation of an antifungal agent may be needed. The length of therapy for noncandidemic forms of invasive candidiasis is less clear. Treatment of intraabdominal infections is generally for 2 weeks but may be longer, depending on whether control of the infectious source has been attained. Infections such as osteomyelitis (e.g., poststernotomy *Candida* mediastinitis) and endocarditis generally require surgical management and many months of antifungal therapy.

Candida bloodstream infections often occur in patients with central venous catheters. Obviously infected catheters should be removed. However, it is not always possible to determine whether the catheter served as the primary source of infection, became secondarily infected, or is not infected at all. As a general rule, catheters should be removed. Retention of the catheter can be considered in patients with implanted access devices and candidemia in the setting of cytotoxic chemotherapy and neutropenia. In such patients, the catheter might not be infected.

Candiduria is a common finding in hospitalized surgical patients. Not all patients require treatment, and removal or exchange of a urinary catheter is effective in many cases. Indications for treatment include neutropenia, upcoming urinary instrumentation, and symptomatic disease. Fluconazole at 200 to 400 mg/d may be effective. Treatment of fluconazole-resistant isolates can be challenging because the urinary penetration of voriconazole and the echinocandins is suboptimal. Treatment with systemic or topical AmB is an option, but both are associated with side effects. The echinocandins do not penetrate well into urine but may be effective in cases of renal parenchymal disease.

Antifungal drugs are increasingly used for prevention of invasive candidiasis in high-risk surgical patients such liver, pancreas, small intestine, and lung transplant recipients. The role of antifungal prophylaxis in critically ill adults is evolving. Indications for prophylaxis in this population likely include patients with recurrent gastrointestinal perforations or anastomotic leakages and patients requiring prolonged intensive care unit (ICU) support who possess multiple risk factors for invasive candidiasis.

Filamentous Fungi

Infections due to filamentous fungi such as *Aspergillus*—and to a lesser extent the Zygomycetes *Fusarium, Scedosporium,* and the dark molds—may be encountered in surgical settings. These fungi are present in the environment, and infection can develop after inhalation or direct inoculation from external sources. Patients with abnormal lung anatomy or function may be chronically colonized with *Aspergillus* or other molds, which can then progress to invasive or saprophytic (e.g., fungal ball) disease. Aspergillosis, scedosporiosis, and mucormycosis may be encountered in patients with traumatic injury and in near-drowning victims.

Aspergillosis

Invasive aspergillosis is an increasingly important problem in surgical patients. Risk factors include prolonged and profound neutrophil dysfunction and use of corticosteroids and other immunosuppressive drugs. Because the respiratory tract is the main site of contact with *Aspergillus* spores, patients with significant abnormalities of respiratory tract structure and function, such as those with cystic fibrosis, chronic lung diseases, lung transplantation, and prolonged mechanical ventilation, are also at risk for aspergillosis. Rarely, infection occurs due to direct inoculation of a surgical site or following traumatic injury.

Treatment options for invasive aspergillosis have dramatically expanded in the past decade. Voriconazole at 6 mg/kg every 12 hours × 2 doses, followed by 4 mg/kg twice daily is the treatment of choice. Typically, treatment is initiated with IV voriconazole so as to rapidly achieve therapeutic drug levels. This is then quickly followed by transition to oral voriconazole for ease of administration. Monitoring of voriconazole levels is likely helpful for optimizing care, but its exact role is evolving. Adding an echinocandin to voriconazole may improve outcomes in invasive aspergillosis and has little downside. Treatment with AmB is another option. Prior to the introduction of voriconazole, this was the treatment of choice. This drug remains effective against most clinically relevant species of *Aspergillus*, but it is associated with substantial infusion-related and renal toxicities. Posaconazole is another option, but its role in treatment of invasive aspergillosis is not yet fully defined. Itraconazole has historically been used for mild to moderate cases of aspergillosis, but it use has been mainly supplanted by the newer azoles.

Zygomycetes

Mucormycosis typically affects immunocompromised patients but may also be seen following traumatic injury and near drowning in otherwise normal hosts. Additional risk factors for infections include uncontrolled diabetes mellitus and treatment with the iron chelator deferoxamine. Common sites of infection include the respiratory tract, sinuses, and skin. The infection is angioinvasive and may extend locally to involve adjacent structures (e.g., orbits, brain) and to cause extensive tissue destruction.

Management of mucormycosis generally requires a multidisciplinary approach. This includes correction of metabolic abnormalities (e.g., treatment of diabetic ketoacidosis, discontinuation of deferoxamine), reduction of immunosuppression, and surgical excision or débridement of infected material. This is particularly important if there is angioinvasion or necrosis. A lipid formulation of AmB (e.g., liposomal AmB) at 5 to 7.5 mg/kg/d is the treatment of choice. The addition of an echinocandin can be considered, but data to support this are sparse. Posaconazole may be considered for salvage therapy in patients intolerant to or failing AmB but should not be used as first-line treatment. Posaconazole may also have a role as maintenance therapy once the patient has received several weeks of AmB and infection is under better control.

CONCLUSIONS

Fungal infections are increasingly encountered in the surgical and critical care settings. Physicians now have unprecedented treatment options for patients with such infections. An understanding of the role of older agents such as fluconazole and AmB and the newer antifungals (e.g., voriconazole, posaconazole, and the echinocandins) is important for successfully managing these patients.

SUGGESTED READINGS

Nucci M, Marr KA: Emerging fungal diseases, *Clin Infect Dis* 15;41(4):521–526, 2005.
Pappas PG, Kauffman CA, Andres D, et al: Clinical Practice Guidelines for the Management of Candidiasis: 2009 Update by the Infectious Diseases Society of America, *Clin Infect Dis* 48:503–535, 2009.
Shoham S, Marwaha S: Invasive fungal infections in the ICU, *J Intensive Care Med* 25(2):78–92, 2010.

MEASURING OUTCOMES IN SURGERY

Caprice C. Greenberg, MD, MPH

INTRODUCTION

In the past two decades, an unprecedented focus on the need to measure outcomes in healthcare has resulted from two developments. First, in 1999, the Institute of Medicine (IOM) published its landmark report "To Err is Human" followed closely by "Crossing the Quality Chasm" in 2001. These two IOM reports catapulted the quality and safety issues in the U.S. healthcare system to the forefront of modern day healthcare issues. To improve quality, we must be able to accurately and efficiently measure it; the existing metrics for measuring outcomes, primarily morbidity and mortality, clearly were inadequate, and the required methodologies were underdeveloped.

The second reason for the increasing focus on measurement of outcomes in healthcare is the marked expansion and availability of electronic health information. Increasing numbers of institutions are adopting electronic medical records, and the sophistication of analyses with claims and other administrative data continues to improve. Taken together, the IOM reports and the increasing availability of electronic data have led to an increasing demand from healthcare consumers for the measuring and reporting of outcomes.

DONABEDIAN MODEL OF QUALITY

Although this chapter focuses on measurement of outcomes, the theoretic framework of Avedis Donabedian is important to point out. He believed that in evaluation of quality, structure and process measures must be considered in addition to outcomes. Structure refers to the fixed attributes of a system in which care is provided, such as the facilities, personnel, and policies of a given hospital. Perhaps the most widely recognized structural measure in surgery is volume. Volume is easy to measure, and decades of research document the relationship between higher volume and better outcome. The problem, however, is that the correlation between volume and outcomes is far from perfect. Use of volume to discriminate quality unjustly punishes high-performing, low-volume hospitals and rewards high-volume hospitals regardless of quality. Development of policy to operationalize volume-based referrals has also proven

difficult. For example, a volume threshold must be identified to instate volume-based referrals, and the studies that document the volume-outcome relationship have not reported a threshold. The critical ramifications that the value of a volume threshold has for individual hospitals have been shown.

A more direct measure of quality can be achieved with examination of the processes of care. Process measures document whether or not the right thing was done for the right patient at the right time with examination of the proportion of patients who receive a course of treatment that has been associated with improved outcomes. Process measures tend to be more reliable because they are not subject to variations in the risk profile of patients. If a surgeon gives antibiotics to a patient but a surgical site infection (SSI) develops because of uncontrolled diabetes, the surgeon "gets credit" with a process measure based on antibiotic administration but not in an outcome measure of the rate of SSI. Process measures are not without their limitations, however. Determination of the appropriate denominator can be difficult because not all patients should receive all treatments. Process measures also tend to be more difficult to quantify than outcome measures, and access to the required data can be challenging. For example, the required details of care are rarely available in large multiinstitutional data sets. Finally, there is often a lack of high level research to support the link between process measures and improved outcomes, especially those in surgery, which limits the number of process measures that are available.

Figure 1 depicts the relationship between structure, process, and outcome. Structural measures may directly relate to outcomes or may act through their relationship with processes of care. For example, the introduction of bar coding medications (structure measure) has a direct impact on the rate of medication errors (outcome). Increased nurse staffing ratios (structure) on the other hand cannot directly decrease the rate of SSI, but a mechanism can be identified by which an increased nurse to patient ratio (structure) leads to increased compliance with postoperative antibiotic administration (process measure) and ultimately a decrease in the SSI rate (outcome). Figure 2 depicts Birkmeyer's suggestion for the appropriate use of structure, process, and outcome measures based on mortality rate and volume.

Outcomes are the end result of the care that is received and ultimately the quality measures that are the easiest to measure and those that consumers most care about. Outcomes are an especially attractive approach to quality measurement in surgery. An operation is a distinct easily identified intervention and short-term outcomes, including in-hospital measures, are meaningful. For example, complications following a colectomy are much easier to identify in the short term than following a change in a patient's diabetic medication. For these reasons, outcome measures are the focus of the remainder of this chapter.

VARIATION IN OUTCOMES

Surgical outcomes may vary for three important reasons: chance, case mix, and quality of care. The goal in outcome measurement is to isolate the quality of care component, control for case mix, and minimize the influence of chance. Outcomes such as mortality tend to be rare events that can lead to imprecise measures and differences that are that result from chance rather than quality of care. A number

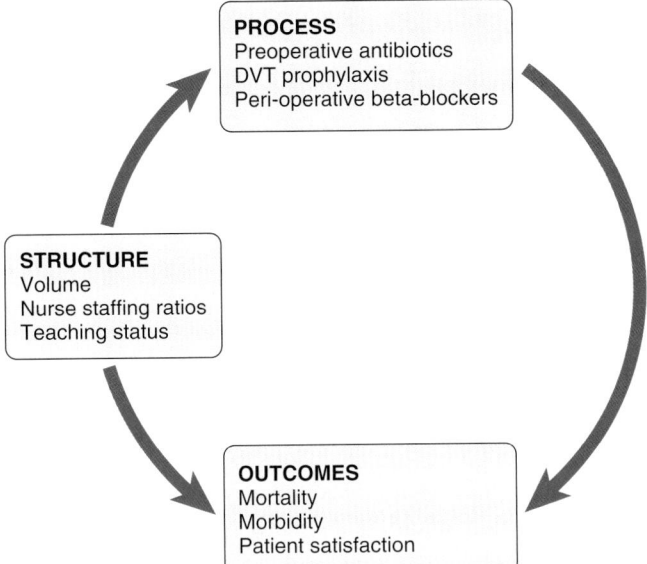

FIGURE 1 The relationship between structure, process, and outcomes. Structure and process measures are dependent on evidence of an impact on outcome. *DVT,* Deep vein thrombosis.

of publications have described the issues related to small sample size. Although outcomes tend to be easier to measure and compare than process measures, they are subject to many confounders, such as comorbidity or severity of illness, that can influence how well a patient tolerates surgery. It is important to use statistical techniques that can adjust for these variations in risk in any outcomes analysis to avoid penalizing surgeons or institutions that treat sicker, higher risk cases. Our ability to risk adjust is limited to those characteristics that can be measured and cannot account for unmeasured confounding.

CURRENT MEASURES OF OUTCOMES

Mortality

The most common outcome measure is mortality. Mortality is an unambiguous binary outcome that does not require further definition or clarification. It is easily available in most datasets, including a variety of administrative data sources. It is, however, particularly subject to the two limitations described previously: namely, confounding with the need for case mix adjustment and being a rare event with the associated imprecision in estimates. Most quality reporting that is based on mortality includes techniques for risk adjustment. For example, that National Surgical Quality Improvement Program (NSQIP) collects hundreds of data points per case, including preoperative, intraoperative, and postoperative variables that allow for comprehensive risk adjustment. Figure 3 depicts the impact of risk adjustment on ranking by mortality rate. Because mortality is such a rare event, few institutions have a large enough sample size to reliably use mortality to measure quality. Dimick and colleagues have shown that only coronary artery bypass grafting (CABG) has sufficient volume to reliably use mortality to measure quality. Despite this fact, many reporting systems are moving forward

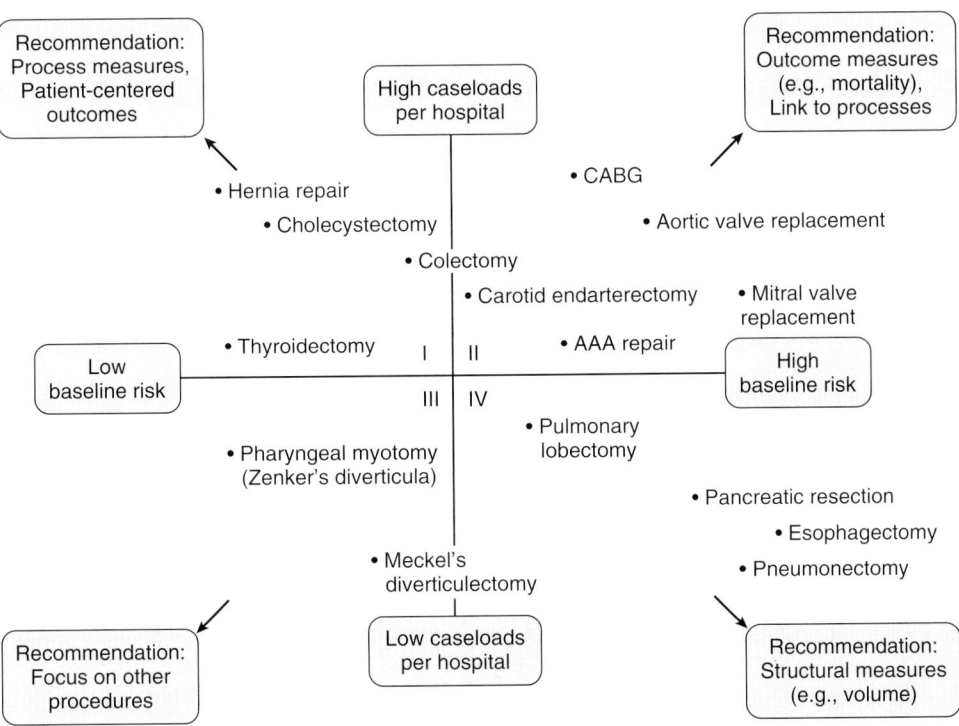

FIGURE 2 Recommendations for appropriate use of structure, process, and outcome measures. *AAA,* Abdominal aortic aneurysm; *CABG,* coronary artery bypass grafting. *(Reproduced from Birkmeyer JD, Dimick JB, Birkmeyer NJO: Measuring the quality of surgical care: structure, process, or outcomes, JACS 198(4):626, 2004.)*

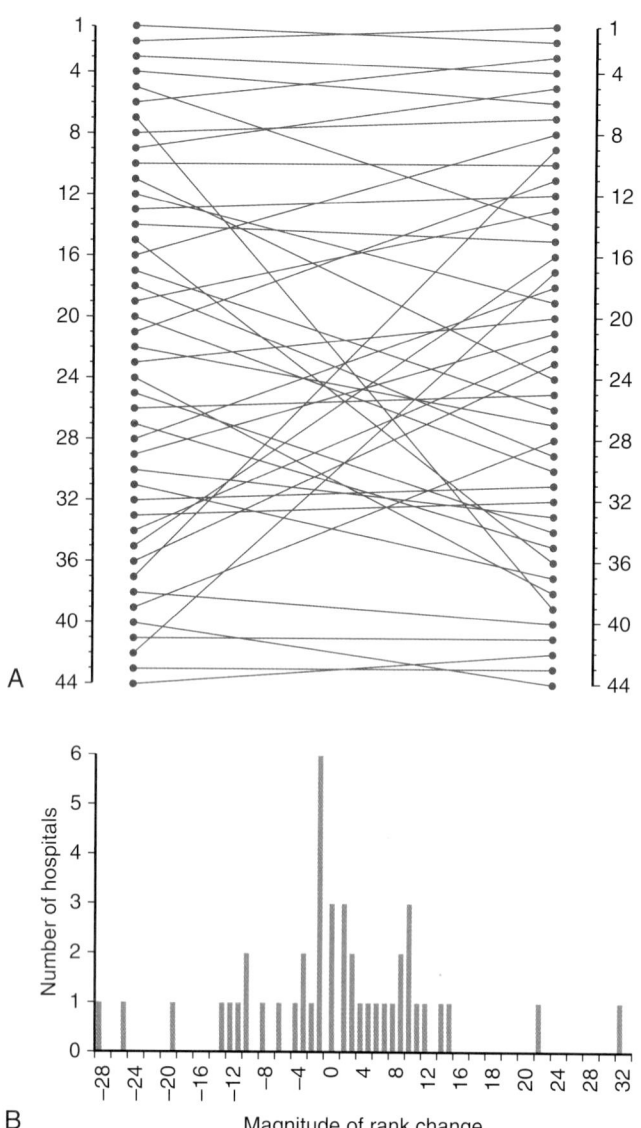

A

B   Magnitude of rank change

FIGURE 3 The impact of risk-adjustment on rank for mortality measures. **A,** Rankings of 44 hospitals participating in the Department of Veterans Affairs Surgical Risk Study (NVASRS; which became National Surgical Quality Improvement Program [NSQIP]) before (left-hand side) and after (right-hand side) risk adjustment. **B,** The magnitude of the change in rank induced by risk adjustment. *(Reproduced from Khuri SF, Daley J, Henderson W, et al: Risk adjustment of the postoperative mortality rate for the comparative assessment of the quality of surgical care: results of the National Veterans Affairs Surgical Risk Study, JACS 185(4):315, 1997; and Fink AS: Adjusted or unadjusted outcomes, Am J Surg 198(Suppl):S28, 2009.)*

with public reporting of risk-adjusted mortality rates without addressing this critical issue.

Morbidity

NSQIP also reports on risk-adjusted measures of morbidity, including overall and specific complication rates. The advantage of this type of outcome reporting is that it tends to be more actionable than

mortality rate. Providers can identify the processes of care that influence a given complication rate and design interventions to improve these processes of care. This is especially true for procedure-specific complication rates. For example, if a hospital has a higher than expected rate of SSI after colectomy, several points in the system can be identified for potential intervention. These include the approach to bowel preparation, administration of preoperative antibiotics, management of postoperative antibiotics, temperature regulation in the operating room, glucose control, and sterile technique. Once an aberrant process is identified (i.e., poor compliance with hair removal technique in Surgical Care Improvement Project [SCIP]), an intervention can be devised to improve performance and decrease the complication rate.

Composite Measures

Composite measures have been developed in an attempt to account for the limitations of individual quality measures as discussed previously. A composite measure based on mortality and volume has been proposed by Dimick and colleagues. An observed outcome, such as mortality, is clearly superior to a proxy measure, such as volume, but only to the extent that it is reliable. An ideal measure then uses observed data to the extent that it is reliable and proxy measures only to the extent necessary. Because the reliability of a measure of mortality is primarily determined by case volume, a statistical approach can be used to weight an institution's mortality rate by case volume and then determine the rest of the composite measure by volume. The weight assigned to volume and mortality is individualized for each hospital and each procedure, ensuring that the composite measure is optimized to predict future performance.

Patient-Centered Outcomes

Another approach to improvement of quality measurement is centered on expanding the available measures and focusing on outcomes that are most important to patients. Although morbidity and mortality measures are clearly important, quality of care goes beyond whether the patient lives or dies and whether a complication occurs or not. Surgical treatment can impact many aspects of a patient's life, and these patient-centered outcomes are becoming increasingly important. Patient centeredness was included as one of the six constructs that constitute quality healthcare according to the IOM definition. Patient-centered outcomes research (PCOR) is the study of the relationship between the health outcome and the treatment provided in the context of the patient experience.

A number of patient-centered outcomes can be considered. *Patient satisfaction* is the emotional or cognitive evaluation of a health encounter by patients as defined by their experience. This may include satisfaction with the clinical or technical skill of providers, interactions and communication with providers, accessibility and convenience, and aspects of the setting in which care is provided. Although subjective, patient satisfaction is increasingly used to assess measure performance and is one of the few measures to be collected at the individual surgeon level. In addition, this measure underscores the fact that patients are consumers of healthcare. *Decision regret* is an especially pertinent outcome given the recent increase in shared decision making and preference sensitive care. As patients take a more active role in determining their treatment course, they must remain confident in those decisions and it is important to evaluate remorse or a realization that one should have acted differently. *Health-related quality of life* (HRQL) measures different domains of health such as physical, emotional or social functioning, and can be influenced by both disease and treatment processes. Many previously validated instruments are available, both generic and disease-specific, to measure these patient-centered outcomes.

INTEGRATING OUTCOME MEASUREMENT INTO THE CURRENT PRACTICE OF SURGERY

Benchmarking and Performance Feedback

One of the goals of outcome measurement is to provide a metric to identify areas for improvement and monitor progress. To do this, a given provider or institution must be given a framework in which to interpret the data that are provided. This is often achieved by comparing an individual's performance with the anonymous performance of peers. The difficulty with this is that given the statistical "noise" or unreliability of estimates for outcome measures, most individuals fall within the margin of error. For example, NSQIP provides results as the ratio of the observed to the expected ratio (O/E) of a given outcome (Figure 4). The expected rate is derived with a regression model based on case mix and provides for risk adjustment. If a hospital performs as expected, therefore, the O/E ratio should be 1. If they perform better than expected, the O/E is less than 1; and if they perform worse than expected, it is greater than 1. They also provide 95% confidence intervals; the confidence intervals that are provided must be considered in quality measurement.

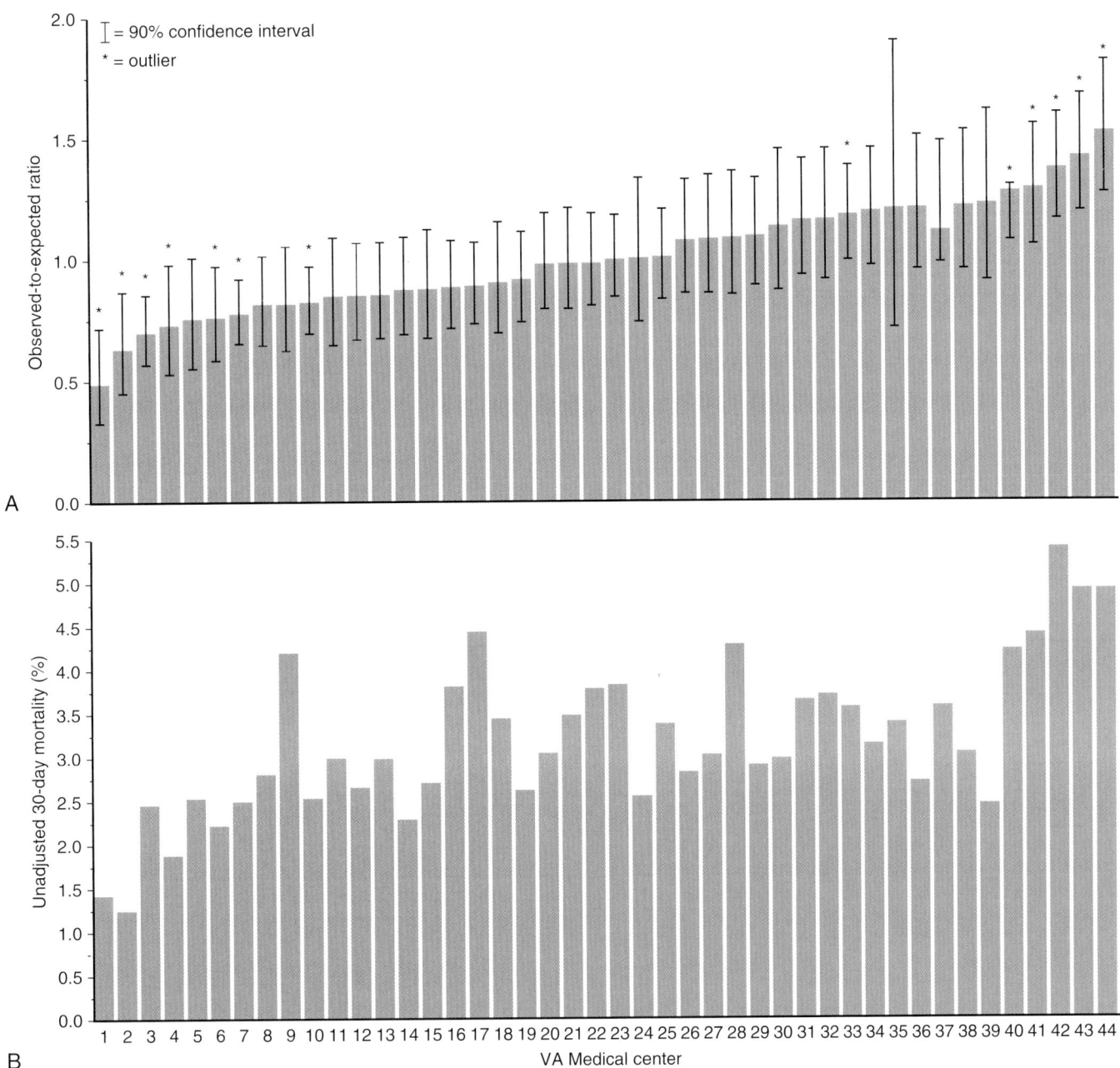

FIGURE 4 Results of the Department of Veterans Affairs *(VA)* Surgical Risk Study (NVASRS; which became National Surgical Quality Improvement Program [NSQIP]). **A,** The importance of considering the 90% confidence interval when interpreting performance. Only the *starred* institutions performed significantly differently than their expected mortality rate. *(Reproduced from Khuri SF, Daley J, Henderson W, et al: Risk adjustment of the postoperative mortality rate for the comparative assessment of the quality of surgical care: results of the National Veterans Affairs Surgical Risk Study, JACS 185(4):315, 1997.)*

For most hospitals, the confidence intervals cross 1, signifying that their performance falls within the margin of error regardless of where the point estimate lies. However, for high outliers or poor performers, these reports can provide motivation and an estimate of how much improvement is necessary. Another approach is to provide a benchmark based on either national guideline recommendations or the top performers. Although guideline recommendations can provide an objective measure that is stable over time, they are often based on expert opinion and may or may not be achievable. Benchmarks based on top performers can provide a reasonable goal with which individual performance can be compared. For example, SCIP calculates adherence rates for the top 10% of performers in each measure for use as a benchmark.

Quality Collaboratives

Outcome reporting as described previously is an important first step, but it falls short of providing participants with tools to improve performance. To meet this need, a number of regional quality collaboratives have developed across the country. The goal of these collaboratives is not only to share data about outcomes but also to share best practices and provide a forum for learning from other institutions so that performance can be improved. They are usually organized at the state or regional level to allow for regular in-person meetings. Tables 1 and 2 were published in a recent article in the Journal of the American College of Surgeons article that described the success of the Tennessee Surgical Quality Collaborative, which uses NSQIP data. Such significant improvements in outcomes and financial savings have been consistently reported by these collaboratives.

Maintenance of Certification

The American Board of Surgery currently requires that diplomats who certify or recertify after July 1, 2005, participate in Maintenance of Certification (MOC). One of the four core components of MOC is the ability to demonstrate evaluation of performance in practice. Such practice assessment can include participation in a national regional or local surgical outcomes database or quality assessment program, including those sponsored by specialty societies, the American College of Surgeons, regional collaboratives, or other quality improvement programs. For this reason, all practicing surgeons must be familiar with the approaches to outcome and other quality measures, and the limitations to each approach. Because this

TABLE 1: Surgical site infections: change in surgical site infections (SSIs) during the first year of the Tennessee Surgical Quality Collaborative

	Postoperative occurrences per 10,000 procedures		Relative risk (95% confidence interval)
	2009	2010	2010 Compared with 2009
Deep incisional SSIs	93.6	76.5	0.82 (0.63-1.06)
Organ/space SSIs	157.7	181.2	1.15 (0.96-1.38)
Superficial incisional SSIs	357.6	289.9	0.81 (0.71-0.92)
All SSIs	603.3	546.9	0.91 (0.82-0.99)

Reproduced from Guillamondegui OD, Gunter OL, Hines L, et al: Using the National Surgical Quality Improvement Program and the Tennessee Surgical Quality Collaborative to improve surgical outcomes, JACS 214(4):709, 2012.

TABLE 2: Financial model: savings realized during the first year of the Tennessee Surgical Quality Collaborative

	Postoperative occurrences per 10,000 procedures		Unit costs	Net savings per 10,000 procedures
	2009	2010		
Acute renal failure	75.3	56.4	$28,359	$535,985
Graft/prosthesis/flap failure	45.8	18.1	$14,851	$411,373
On ventilator > 48 h	293.6	250.3	$27,654	$1,197,418
Superficial incisional surgical site infection	357.6	289.9	$27,631	$1,870,619
Wound disruption	90.8	59.7	$14,827	$461,120
Full year 2010 savings				$4,476,515
Full year 2010 costs				$2,278,972
Net savings				**$2,197,543**

Reproduced from Guillamondegui OD, Gunter OL, Hines L, et al: Using the National Surgical Quality Improvement Program and the Tennessee Surgical Quality Collaborative to improve surgical outcomes, JACS 214(4):709, 2012.

is a requirement for board certification, surgeons may as well choose to participate in the outcome measurement and quality improvement programs with the greatest potential to improve their practice.

THE IMPORTANCE OF OUTCOME MEASUREMENT IN RESEARCH

Healthcare is supposed to be evidence based but frequently falls short of this ideal. There is often a lack of data available to inform many healthcare decisions, and the data that do exist are frequently limited in quality. In addition, the high-quality data that do exist may not be applicable to all patients; extrapolation from the select population of participants in a given clinical trial to the heterogenous population in everyday practice is often not possible. Finally, this evidence is often slow to disseminate to practitioners and to be implemented into and change practice. Comparative effectiveness research (CER) and PCOR are gaining traction as new research disciplines that aim to bridge these gaps. The federal government has recently committed significant funds for this type of research because of the potential immediate impact on care. For this reason, practicing surgeons must be familiar with the terms.

Comparative Effectiveness Research

CER compares the outcomes of two alternative approaches to care, either of which has the potential to be best practice, in real world settings. Comparative effectiveness research can be either retrospective or prospective and can include clinical trials as long as they meet the previous considerations. A clinical trial in CER does not contain a placebo arm and has few, if any, exclusion criteria. These types of trials are often referred to as pragmatic or effectiveness trials. The goal of comparative effectiveness research is to increase the evidence available to support healthcare decision making and to streamline the integration of new evidence into everyday practice. By providing increased evidence, CER has the potential to improve our approaches to quality measurement, for example, by providing new process measures.

Patient-Centered Outcomes Research

PCOR is a related discipline. In fact, CER can be considered as one type of PCOR. The Patient-Centered Outcomes Research Institute (POCRI) has developed the following definition: "Patient-Centered Outcomes Research (PCOR) helps people and their caregivers communicate and make informed health care decisions, allowing their voices to be heard in assessing the value of health care options. This research answers patient-centered questions such as:

1. 'Given my personal characteristics, conditions and preferences, what should I expect will happen to me?'
2. 'What are my options and what are the potential benefits and harms of those options?'

3. 'What can I do to improve the outcomes that are most important to me?'
4. 'How can clinicians and the care delivery systems they work in help me make the best decisions about my health and healthcare?'"

One of the goals of PCOR is to engage patients and other stakeholders in the research process and, in particular, in determination of appropriate outcomes. Often in research, we set intermediate outcomes that are easy to measure and compare but that do not have any impact directly on patient care. The goal in PCOR is to ensure that the outcomes of all studies are meaningful and important to patients, including the development of new patient-centered outcome measures.

CONCLUSION

The first step to improving healthcare is to determine what constitutes high-quality care and how best to measure it. In this chapter, the current approaches to quality measurement have been reviewed, with a focus on outcome measures. Although we have come a long way, much still remains to be done. The recent focus on patient-centered outcomes research suggests that there may be political will to support an improved approach to quality measurement. Much of the data required for clinically meaningful measures are currently difficult to capture. As a result, current measures often focus on what can be measured rather than what is most likely to improve quality of care, either because it reflects quality or because it is actionable. Quality measurement in healthcare is still in its infancy. As our ability to handle large amounts of electronic health data continues to improve, as our statistical methodologies become increasingly sophisticated, and as researchers identify new links between the care we provide and the outcomes that are observed, the field of quality measurement will continue to mature. Surgeons must recognize the impact of quality and outcome measurement on their practices and remain abreast of the developments in this important field.

SUGGESTED READINGS

Birkmeyer JD, Dimick JB, Birkmeyer NJO: Measuring the quality of surgical care: structure, process, or outcomes, *JACS* 198(4):626, 2004.
Christian CK, Gustafson ML, Betensky RA, et al: The Leapfrog volume criteria may fall short in identifying high-quality surgical centers, *Ann Surg* 238(4):447, 2003.
Dimick JB, Staiger DO, Baser O, et al: Composite measures for predicting surgical mortality in the hospital, *Health Affairs* 28(14):1189, 2009.
Guillamondegui OD, Gunter OL, Hines L, et al: Using the National Surgical Quality Improvement Program and the Tennessee Surgical Quality Collaborative to improve surgical outcomes, *JACS* 214(4):709, 2012.
Khuri SF, Daley J, Henderson W, et al: Risk adjustment of the postoperative mortality rate for the comparative assessment of the quality of surgical care: results of the National Veterans Affairs Surgical Risk Study, *JACS* 185(4):315, 1997.
Oliver A, Greenberg CC: Measuring outcomes in oncology treatment: the importance of patient-centered outcomes, *Surg Clin North Am* 89(1):17, 2009.

COMPARATIVE EFFECTIVENESS RESEARCH IN SURGERY

Hugh G. Auchincloss, MD, MPH, and
Matthew M. Hutter, MD, MPH

INTRODUCTION

The field of comparative effectiveness research (CER) has experienced unparalleled growth in recent years. This growth represents both an appreciation for the intrinsic value of evidence-based medicine and an acceptance of present and future economic realities. In short, patients deserve to know which treatments are most effective for them, and the healthcare system cannot afford to pay for those that are not. Surgery in particular stands to benefit from CER, and surgeons are positioned to become leaders in this field. Surgery is full of new treatments, techniques, and technology but little guidance as to how and when to adopt them. The result is wide variation in surgical practice among regions, hospitals, providers, and patient populations. Surgeons individually and as a whole must take an active role in grounding the practice of surgery in a solid evidence base. CER is a powerful tool to that end.

WHAT IS COMPARATIVE EFFECTIVENESS RESEARCH?

Two government agencies define CER in a way that illustrates both its breadth and its depth. The Institute of Medicine (IOM) focuses on the expansive mission of CER:

"CER is the generation and synthesis of evidence that compares the benefits and harms of alternative methods to prevent, diagnose, treat, and monitor a clinical condition or to improve the delivery of care. The purpose of comparative effectiveness research is to assist consumers, clinicians, purchasers, and policy makers to make informed decisions that will improve health care at both the individual and population level."

The Congressional Budget Office (CBO) provides a more technical definition that speaks to the depth of CER:

"As applied in the health care sector, analysis of comparative effectiveness is simply a rigorous evaluation of the impact of different options that are available for treating a given medical condition for a particular set of patients. Such a study may compare similar treatments, such as competing drugs, or it may analyze very different approaches, such as surgery and drug therapy. The analysis may focus only on the relative medical benefits and risks of each option, or it may also weigh both the costs and the benefits of those options. In some cases, a given treatment may prove to be more effective clinically or more cost-effective for a broad range of patients, but frequently a key issue is determining which specific types of patients would benefit most from it."

CER seeks to determine *which treatment* done on *which patient* is *most effective* at producing *an outcome*. The addition of "and at what cost" to the previous sentence, consistent with the CBO definition of CER, is appropriate but has proven controversial in the United States for reasons to be discussed subsequently. CER can be understood by looking at each of these components individually.

EFFECTIVENESS VERSUS EFFICACY

Efficacy is a measure of the ability of a treatment to produce results under experimental conditions. Effectiveness, in contrast, measures the performance of a treatment in the real world. Not infrequently, efficacy and effectiveness research yield surprisingly different results. For example, tight glucose control in critically ill patients was thought to decrease mortality based on the results of efficacy studies but failed to yield the same results when studied in actual intensive care units.

Both efficacy and effectiveness research have strengths and limitations. Efficacy studies, by virtue of the controlled environment in which they are performed, usually provide clear results and explanations. This clarity, though, comes at the price of generalizability. Practicing clinicians may not believe that the results of such studies are applicable to the conditions in which they practice. In contrast, effectiveness studies tend to produce more ambiguous results. The inherent complexity of the real-world conditions under which these studies are done may make understanding causal mechanisms challenging. However, clinicians may find the results of these studies more immediately relevant to their own practice.

WHICH TREATMENT?

Generally speaking, CER is a head-to-head comparison of two or more alternative treatment strategies. Treatment strategy in this context may mean comparison of a new drug or procedure with standard of care, a medical treatment with a surgical one, or different conditions of healthcare delivery. When the treatment strategies compared are similar, CER tends to produce results that are easy to accept, at least from a statistical standpoint. As the differences between treatments grow, research methods must become more rigorous to generate valid conclusions.

In its simplest form, CER in surgery compares two similar procedures or protocols. An example is comparison of open with laparoscopic repair of primary unilateral inguinal hernia (as with Neumayer in the *New England Journal of Medicine* in 2004) or albumin with saline solution for the resuscitation of critically ill patients (as in the Saline versus Albumin Fluid Evaluation [SAFE] study from 2004).

Pitting a medical therapy against a surgical one is more complex. For example, a 2012 *New England Journal of Medicine* study conducted jointly by the Society of Thoracic Surgeons (STS) and the American College of Cardiology Foundation (ACCF) found that older patients with multivessel coronary disease who underwent coronary artery bypass grafting had a long-term survival benefit compared with those who underwent percutaneous catheter-based intervention. The methodologic debate sparked by this study is perhaps a cover for a more passionate political debate occurring behind the scenes, which serves as a reminder that CER can create a minefield when professional interests are at stake.

CER may also compare the setting in which treatment occurs. Birkmeyer and colleagues have shown that certain high-risk operations like esophagectomy and pancreaticoduodenectomy are performed with lower overall mortality at high-volume institutions compared with low-volume institutions. Similar studies have compared outcomes based on hospital resources, surgeon age, individual surgeon volume, and involvement of surgical trainees. All of these studies fall under the umbrella of CER.

WHICH PATIENTS?

The characteristics of individual patients are important to CER in two fundamental ways. First, because of the real-world nature of CER studies, they often feature groups of patients who differ in significant ways. Statistical methods must be used to balance these differences and minimize their impact on the outcome. Second, the outcome of a treatment strategy depends in part on the group of patients to which it is applied. Studies often seek either by design or in retrospect to identify subgroups in which a treatment is particularly beneficial or harmful.

Balancing two or more groups of patients with dissimilar characteristics is one of the foremost challenges of CER. Patients may differ in age, demographics, diagnosis, comorbidities, severity or stage of illness, or concurrent procedures. When these differences impact the outcome independently of the treatment studied, they are known as confounders. Randomization, as in a prospective clinical trial, balances known and unknown confounders evenly between treatment arms. In an observational study, a researcher can only hope to acknowledge the uneven distribution of known confounders and adjust for them with statistical methods. Multiple such methods exist, including stratification, multiple regression modeling, and the use of propensity scores.

Stratification is the simplest method of balancing known confounders. If the study population is large enough, it can be divided into blocks based on known confounders, and the analysis can be conducted within each block. For example, the population could be divided into three blocks based on age group and then further divided into six blocks based on patient gender. The resulting analysis would compare young women only with young women, and so on. This method yields results that are easy to interpret, but its usefulness is limited to large populations with few confounders. With small populations or multiple confounders, stratification leads to inadequate power (i.e., the ability of a study to detect a difference when one really is present).

Multiple regression modeling is a more sophisticated and commonly used method of adjusting for confounders. Multiple regression modeling is a three-step process. First, the researcher determines which factors other than the treatment in question contribute to the outcome. Second, a statistical model is constructed that describes the outcome as a function of those factors and the treatment. Lastly, the model is used to adjust for the effect of the other factors, leaving behind only the effect of the treatment. Multiple regression models can be used to adjust for multiple confounders simultaneously without a significant loss of power. Most statistical software programs are equipped with a model-building function that makes this method accessible to researchers with a basic knowledge of statistics.

The use of propensity scores and propensity matching is an alternative to multiple regression modeling that has recently experienced an exponential growth in popularity. This method is based on two assumptions: first, in an observational study, a patient is more likely to have received one treatment versus another based on that patient's characteristics; and second, random chance explains why two patients with similar baseline characteristics may undergo different treatments. A propensity score is a measure of the likelihood of a patient receiving a specific treatment. It is the product of a multiple regression model that uses patient characteristics as predictors and treatment strategy as the outcome. Propensity scores can be used in a variety of ways but are most commonly used to match patients who underwent different treatments but, based on having the same propensity score, can be said to have similar baseline characteristics. Propensity matching is often advertised as a method of creating a randomized trial out of observational data. In reality, it suffers from the same limitations as multiple regression modeling, namely an inability to control for unknown confounders.

At first glance, these methods of adjustment appear to be formulaic and objective. In fact, the process is highly subjective. The researcher chooses which of the methods to use. Beyond this, the researcher chooses which confounders need to be adjusted for and what form those confounders should take. For example, most surgeons agree that a study comparing two types of hernia repair should be adjusted for patient weight. Is it sufficient to divide patients into obese versus nonobese? Or should body mass index (BMI) be retained in the model in continuous numeric form? Is the difference between a BMI of 25 and a BMI of 30 the same as that between 30 and 35 or that between 60 and 65? And what should be done with underweight patients? The answers to these questions are determined by the researcher and can have profound impact on the results of the study. Ideally, the plan for adjustment is made in prospective fashion based on previous studies, sound clinical judgment, and preliminary sense of the architecture of the data. However, even with experienced and thoughtful researchers, the results of observational studies should be examined critically for residual confounding.

CER can also identify groups of patients who, based on their characteristics, may benefit from a treatment strategy. These may be discovered during subgroup analysis of a larger study or, indirectly, through studies designed to determine which factors predict a certain outcome after a treatment. For example, the National Emphysema Treatment Trial (NETT), published in the *New England Journal of Medicine* in 2003, was a randomized controlled trial to evaluate lung volume reduction surgery in patients with chronic obstructive pulmonary disease (COPD). As a secondary goal, the study sought to identify patient characteristics that were associated with a good outcome after lung volume reduction surgery (LVRS). Indeed, although the overall benefit of LVRS remains unclear, in patients with predominantly upper lobe emphysema and low exercise tolerance, it appears to confer a significant improvement in survival and quality of life. Studies that look for predictors of an outcome after treatment indirectly address a similar question. The NETT protocol, for example, was informed by a series of earlier studies that showed upper lobe emphysema to be a predictor of good functional outcome after lung volume reduction surgery. Although these studies do not directly compare one treatment with another, they provide the foundation for future studies that do.

WHICH OUTCOME?

The effectiveness of one treatment versus another is measured in its ability to generate a desirable outcome, avoid an undesirable one, or some combination of the two. There are many such outcomes to choose from, including morbidity and mortality, freedom from disease or symptoms, cost, and quality of life. The choice of which to use depends on a combination of clinical relevance and practical considerations.

Mortality is an obvious choice. Death as an outcome has inherent face validity (everyone usually agrees it is something to be avoided). Its measurement is unambiguous. It is accurately recorded, and when it is unrecorded, it is frequently obtainable through publicly available resources like death certificates. Mortality, though, is an insensitive measure of effectiveness, particularly in surgery. Because mortality associated with most surgeries is thankfully quite low, it is seldom a useful method for discriminating one treatment strategy from another. Short-term mortality as an outcome in CER is therefore limited to studies regarding high-risk procedures or studies focusing on the delivery of healthcare at the hospital or regional level. Long-term survival and disease-specific survival may be more useful but are harder to reliably measure.

Morbidity, in contrast, is a frequent occurrence after most procedures and so is commonly used as an outcome in CER. Measures of morbidity, though, are more subjective than mortality. Even straightforward events like postoperative urinary tract infection may be defined in multiple ways. In addition, although some postoperative events clearly are worse than others, less clear is how to incorporate this subjective ranking into objective data. Composite measures of morbidity may help to address some of these inherent deficiencies.

Procedure-specific outcomes such as recurrence after hernia repair or continence after ileorectal anastomosis are favored by surgical researchers because of their clinical relevance. Measurement of these outcomes can be a subjective and resource-intensive process. Years may be needed to observe a difference in graft patency after two competing methods of lower extremity revascularization, for example. In addition, more often than not, the success of a procedure cannot be determined with one outcome measure alone. The success of bariatric surgery is a function not just of weight loss but of also of improvement in comorbidities and quality of life. Quantifying these outcome measures in a universally accepted fashion is challenging.

Specific groups of researchers tend to have outcomes that are of particular interest to them. Hospital administrators and insurance companies may focus on outcomes of efficiency such as length of stay, use of resources, or readmission rates. Health economics research deals in constructs such as the incremental cost effectiveness ratio. Countless other measures exist that may be relevant in certain contexts.

Lastly, patient-centered outcomes have assumed a prominent position in CER. Broadly speaking, these are outcomes that are important to patients but, because of the difficulty of quantifying and measuring them, have historically received little attention. Despite the challenges associated with comparing treatments based on constructs such as quality of life, improved functionality, and patient experience, this is likely to be an area of significant growth for CER in surgery in the future.

HOW IS COMPARATIVE EFFECTIVENESS RESEARCH DONE?

CER can take many forms, including reviews of the existing literature, observational studies, or randomized controlled trials. Each has strengths and weaknesses with regard to feasibility, relevance, and quality of evidence produced. (In simplified terms, evidence is often classified into several levels, with level I reserved for randomized controlled trials, level II for observational studies, level III for case studies and literature review, and level IV for expert opinion. These levels remain in common usage, although the most recent recommendation of the U.S. Preventative Services Task Force [USPSTF] is to classify evidence as "good," "fair," and "poor." These levels are distinct from the USPSTF's "grades," which are for use by clinicians regarding clinical practices; Tables 1 to 3).

The simplest method of CER is review of the existing literature. This may take the form of a meta-analysis or a literature review. The primary advantage of a review of existing literature is that it is cheap and can be done relatively quickly. The drawbacks are numerous. No studies regarding the effectiveness of many treatments exist. When these studies do exist, reconciling differences in their methodology can be challenging. Finally, there is the possibility of publication bias (i.e., the tendency of journals to publish positive studies but not negative ones). Despite these limitations, a comprehensive review of existing literature should be the initial step in all CER.

Observational studies are the most common form of CER. These vary greatly in size and complexity, ranging from case reports and case series to massive cohort studies and large national database projects. Observational studies are limited by the inability to control for unknown confounders. However, they have the advantage of being both relatively easy to perform and immediately applicable to clinical practice. The ability to perform high-quality observational studies in surgery has been aided greatly by the growing availability of large administrative and clinical databases. Administrative databases, including Medicare claims data and national registries such as the Healthcare Cost and Utilization Project Nationwide Inpatient

TABLE 1: Levels of evidence

Level	Type of evidence
Ia	Evidence from meta-analysis of randomized controlled trials
Ib	Evidence from at least one randomized controlled trial
IIa	Evidence from at least one controlled study without randomization
IIb	Evidence from at least one other type of quasiexperimental study
III	Evidence from nonexperimental descriptive studies, such as comparative studies, correlation studies, and case-control studies
IV	Evidence from expert committee reports or opinions or clinical experience of respected authorities

Adapted from Agency for Healthcare Research and Quality 1992 guidelines.

TABLE 2: Quality of evidence

Quality of evidence	Definition
Good	Evidence includes consistent results from well-designed, well-conducted studies in representative populations that directly assess effects on health outcomes
Fair	Evidence is insufficient to assess the effects on health outcomes because of limited number of power of studies, important flaws in their design or conduct, gaps in the chain of evidence, or lack of information on important health outcomes
Poor	Evidence is insufficient to assess the effects on health outcomes because of limited number or power of studies, important flaws in their design or conduct, gaps in the chain or evidence, or lack of information on important health outcomes

From U.S. Preventive Services Task Force's Guide to clinical preventive services, 2010-2011. http://www.ahrg.gov/clinic/pocketgd.htm.

Sample (HCUP-NIS), are publically available and contain millions of patient records. They can be a robust source of information for researchers skilled in navigating their complexity. However, administrative data, which exist primarily for the purpose of billing, can be highly variable depending on the provider or the hospital in which they are recorded. Moreover, they lack the rich clinical context that can be found in databases like the American College of Surgeons National Surgical Quality Improvement Project (ACS-NSQIP), the Metabolic and Bariatric Surgery Accreditation and Quality Improvement Program (MBSAQIP), the American College of Surgeons National Trauma Data Bank (ACS-NTDB), the Society of Thoracic Surgeons (STS) Adult Cardiac Surgery, Congenital Heart Surgery, and General Thoracic Surgery Databases, and the Scientific Registry of Transplant Recipients (SRTR). These databases have been developed on the initiative of surgeons and provide a unique opportunity to examine clinical questions on a national scale.

TABLE 3: Grade for practice recommendations

Grade	Definition	Suggestions for practice
A	The USPSTF recommends the service. There is high certainty that the net benefit is substantial.	Offer or provide this service.
B	The USPSTF recommends the service. There is high certainty that the net benefit is moderate, or there is moderate certainty that the net benefit is moderate to substantial.	Offer or provide this service
C	*Note: The following statement is undergoing revision.* Clinicians may provide this service to selected patients depending on individual circumstances. However, for most individual without signs or symptoms, there is likely to be only a small benefit from this service.	Offer or provide this service only if other considerations support the offering or provide the service in an individual patient.
D	The USPSTF recommends against the service. There is moderate or high certainty that the service has no net benefit or that the harms outweigh the benefits.	Discourage the use of this service.
I Statement	The USPSTF concludes that the current evidence is insufficient to assess the balance of benefits and harms of the service. Evidence is lacking, of poor quality, or conflicting, and the balance of benefits and harms cannot be determined.	Read the clinical considerations section of the USPSTF Recommendation Statement. If the service is offered, patients should understand the uncertainty about the balance of benefits and harms.

USPSTF, U.S. Preventative Services Task Force.
From U.S. Preventive Services Task Force, Grade definitions, updated July 2012, http://www.uspreventiveservicetaskforce.org/uspstf/grades.htm.

Randomized controlled trials (RCTs) have typically been thought of as efficacy rather than effectiveness research as described previously, which has led some researchers to suggest a new emphasis on "practical" clinical trials. These trials would retain the methodologic rigor of classic RCTs but accrue patients in liberal fashion and compare treatments in the form that clinicians are likely to encounter them, making their results more readily applicable to clinical practice.

COMPARATIVE EFFECTIVENESS RESEARCH IN THE NATIONAL AND INTERNATIONAL SPOTLIGHT

In the past decade, CER has become a national priority in the United States. This interest has been sparked by patients as they become increasingly savvy consumers of healthcare, clinicians who recognize the need to provide the highest quality care, and policymakers who see CER as a way to rescue the healthcare system from the staggering cost of unproven or ineffective treatments. Federal funding for CER is at its highest point ever.

The modern era of federally funded CER began in 2003 with the Medicare Modernization Act. This authorized the Agency for Healthcare Research and Quality (AHRQ; established in 1989 as a branch of the Department of Health and Human Services) to spend $50 million per year on research with focus on "outcomes, comparative clinical effectiveness, and appropriateness of health care items and services." In 2005, AHRQ used that funding to establish the Effective Health Care Program (EHC). EHC is tasked with providing systematic reviews of the existing literature regarding the clinical effectiveness of treatments. When that evidence does not exist, two related programs, Developing Evidence to Inform Decisions about Effectiveness (DEcIDE) and the Centers for Education and Research on Therapeutics (CERTS), perform original studies. AHRQ received additional funding for CER through the American Recovery and Reinvestment Act of 2009. In 2010, the Patient Protection and Affordable Care Act established the Patient-Centered Outcomes Research Institute (PCORI). PCORI's mission is to sponsor CER with a focus on patient-centered outcomes. Federal funding for CER has come with strings attached, though: PCORI and AHQR are expressly forbidden from sponsoring or conducting research regarding cost effectiveness. The bill includes the following: "The [PCORI] ... shall not develop or employ a dollars per-quality adjusted life year (or similar measure that discounts the value of a life because of an individual's disability) as a threshold to establish what type of health care is cost effective or recommended. The Secretary shall not utilize such an adjusted life year (or such a similar measure) as a threshold to determine coverage, reimbursement, or incentive programs ..." This underscores the unease that many policymakers, clinicians, and patients feel regarding the potential misuses of CER.

By European standards, federal involvement in CER in the United States remains superficial. In the United Kingdom, the National Institute for Health and Clinical Effectiveness (NICE) has existed as a branch of the National Health Service (NHS) since 1999 and is explicitly involved in CER, including cost effectiveness. NICE conducts CER on all treatments covered by the NHS. The results are presented in terms of cost versus potential benefit, and the findings directly influence coverage decisions by the NHS. Likewise, the Insitut Für Qualitat und Wirtschaftlichkeit im Gesndheitswesen (IQWiG) is officially an independent institution, but its sole contractor is the German government. Since 2004, it has been conducting CER, including cost effectiveness, and its recommendations frequently inform coverage decision. In France, the Haute Autorié de Santé (HAS) was established in 2004 to determine the cost versus benefit implications of emerging treatments. Like IQWiG, it is an independent body, but its recommendations are usually accepted.

CONTROVERSY

Critics of CER argue that the growing national obsession with comparative effectiveness stifles innovation and prevents personalized medicine. They reason that every advance in medical therapy goes through an experimental period. Submission of a new treatment to the rigors of CER before it is has found a proper application and been mastered by a number of clinicians ensures that the deck is always stacked in favor of the status quo. In addition, critics fear certain treatments that produce disappointing results on a large scale will never be given the chance to connect with the small subgroup of patients in which they are effective. Supporters counter that CER provides a context in which innovations that are truly effective are able to gain immediate traction and that identification of subgroups of patients in which treatments are effective is one of its chief strengths.

Always, though, the debate returns to the issue of cost. Those opposed to active government involvement in CER cite both an existential fear of government interference in the healthcare decisions of individuals and the pragmatic fear of healthcare rationing. These views were well articulated by Newt Gingrich during a debate with Sir Michael Rawlins, the chairman of NICE, in the pages of *The Economist*: "What happens when a drug is more effective than another but costs three times as much? To make this decision, government must weigh the cost it will bear with your quality of life. Do you want government to decide that the more expensive drug isn't worth the cost for you to have less pain and suffering?" For those on the other side of the debate, the issue is not whether healthcare resources should be rationed but how. Healthcare dollars are a finite resource, and CER provides a context for rationally allocating them. Rawlins responds to Gingrich's query with one of his own: "On what basis should nations use their resources to treat ill-health in a manner that is fair to all?" CER, he suggests, is the answer. The paradox of the 2010 Affordable Care Act, which draws what many believe is an artificial distinction between comparative effectiveness and cost effectiveness, reflects that this debate is far from over.

FUTURE DIRECTIONS

The role of CER is expanding in two directions. At the top, it is becoming an increasingly important part of the debate about the future of healthcare. Surgeons as a group need to be well versed in its methods, strengths, and limitations if they want to maintain control over their profession. The real strength of CER, though, is in the way in which it comes to strengthen the most fundamental element of medicine: the patient-doctor relationship. The future of surgery is one in which surgeon and patient together are able to make informed decisions about which treatment strategy to pursue based on the surgeon's expertise and the patient's profile, disease process, and expectations. CER provides the context for that clinical encounter.

SUGGESTED READINGS

Birkmeyer JD, Dimick JB, Birkmeyer NJ: Measuring the quality of surgical care: structure, process or outcomes? *Am Coll Surg* 198:828–832, 2004.

Bland KI, Hoyt DB, Polk HC Jr, et al: Comparative effectiveness research: relative and efficient outcomes in surgery patients, *Ann Surg* 254(4):550–557, 2011.

Economist debates: health care, *The Economist*, 2009, available at www.economist.com/debate/days/view/394. 2009.

Hoyt DB: Looking forward: comparative effectiveness, *Bull Am Coll Surg* 96(7):4–6, 2011.

Research on the comparative effectiveness of medical treatments: issues and options for an expanded federal role, 2007, Congressional Budget Office.

What is comparative effectiveness research? 2012, Agency for Healthcare Research and Quality, available at http://effectivehealthcare.ahrq.gov/index.cfm/what-is-comparative-effectiveness-research1/. 2012.

SURGICAL CRITICAL CARE

SURGICAL PALLIATIVE CARE

Geoffrey P. Dunn, MD, FACS

Surgical palliative care is the treatment of suffering and the promotion of quality of life for seriously or terminally ill patients under surgical care. The conceptual framework for surgical palliation has antecedents in the history of surgery and the hospice concept of care introduced by the late Dr. Cicely Saunders. The hospice concept she introduced in the 1960s was subsequently modified and expanded to apply to individuals with longer term prognoses, including those choosing to continue disease-directed treatment.

Several core values of surgical culture, including nonabandonment and preservation of hope, are consistent with the essence of palliative care as it has developed around the globe as a standard of care for advanced and terminal illness. The indication for palliative care in surgical practice is based on the patient and the patient's family's desire for relief of distress in any of its forms and the wish to improve the quality and promise of life regardless of diagnosis or prognosis. The choice of therapy is based on the ability of the treatment to meet the agreed upon goals of care, not its impact on the underlying disease process.

In 2005, The American College of Surgeons' Board of Regents endorsed the *Statement of Principles of Palliative Care* drafted by its Task Force on Surgical Palliative Care and Committee on Ethics (Box 1). In 2006, the National Quality Forum (NQF) established its *National Framework and Preferred Practices for Palliative and Hospice Care* based on consensus guidelines submitted by the leading five hospice and palliative care organizations. In 2009, the Accreditation Council for Graduate Medical Education (ACGME) recognized hospice and palliative medicine as a subspecialty of 11 parent boards, including the American Board of Surgery.

The primary target for palliative intervention is distress, not disease. To consistently dissect out this target, a conceptual model for pain and suffering is necessary. Useful models of pain and suffering widely recognized in clinical palliative care are Cicely Saunders's model of "Total Pain" and Eric Cassell's concept of suffering. Saunders's model outlines four cardinal dimensions of pain (physical, social/economic, psychologic, and spiritual) that in aggregate are referred to as "total pain" and that contribute to suffering. Cassell described suffering as the feeling that arises from a threat to integrity (wholeness) of the person. The elements of personhood include an individual's past, present, and future; social role; private life; and a transcendent dimension. Suffering is not relieved until the threat to personhood has passed or is diminished.

Principles of communication with individuals receiving palliative care are analogous to the right conduct of an operation: creation of the right physical and social context, assessment of the individual's preparedness, permission to proceed, definitive action, acknowledgment of the impact of the action on the recipient, closure, and follow-up.

Surgical palliative care assessment includes identification of previous illness and treatments, sources of pain in all dimensions, sources of personal strength, liabilities, and individual values and wishes (Table 1). Decision-making capacity, surrogacy, and advance medical directives are addressed at this time. *Relief of pressing symptoms should be done before or concurrently with assessment.* Patient's goals of care that emerge from this discussion set the parameters for the surgeon's involvement. In cases in which operative intervention is anticipated, preoperative anesthesiology consultation is helpful in planning of intraoperative and perioperative analgesia (especially if use of an epidural catheter is desired), in review of patient goals of care in light of what anesthesia expertise can offer, and in reconsideration of existing "do not resuscitate" (DNR) orders.

As a general rule, physical symptom relief takes immediate priority of action over intervention for nonphysical distress, even if nonphysical issues are ultimately more important to the patient. Symptom management is the work of palliative care and requires an interdisciplinary approach. A strong liaison with clinical pharmacists is particularly helpful because of the effectiveness of pharmacotherapy for the most common symptoms and the frequency of adverse drug reactions, including costs, that add to total symptom burden. Tables 2, 3, and 4 show medications and their conversions commonly used for control of major symptoms encountered during palliative care in the hospital setting. For nonphysical symptoms, the surgeon's role is to identify, triage, and refer appropriately and promptly.

The importance of collegiality with individuals entrusted with spiritual care of the individual cannot be overemphasized, particularly if spiritual anguish is the predominating form of the patient's distress. Despite differences in faith and values, "moral friendship," a concept proposed by clergyman and surgeon Daniel Hall, between surgeon and patient is *usually* possible and remains one of the worthiest goals of care. One can conceive of situations in which the moral perspectives of physician and patient are sufficiently opposed that a mutual accommodation might not be possible in the setting of the clinical relationship. Table 5 outlines specific ethical concerns frequently encountered in surgical palliative care.

Palliative care service consultation should be sought out to complement surgical expertise, especially when the nonphysical symptom burden is high and clarification of goals is difficult in the face of rapidly progressing or critical illness. Palliative care consultation services, which are increasingly available in the United States, have been shown to improve symptom control, enhance patient and family satisfaction, lower costs, and even improve survival. Surgeons should be mindful of the option of hospice referral for patients with an estimated survival of 6 months or less if the illness pursues its usual

BOX 1: Statement of principles of palliative care

- Respect the dignity and autonomy of patients, patient surrogates, and caregivers.
- Honor the right of the competent patient or surrogate to choose among treatments, including those that may or may not prolong life.
- Communicate effectively and empathically with patients, their families, and caregivers.
- Identify the primary goals of care from the patient's perspective, and address how the surgeon's care can achieve the patient's objectives.
- Strive to alleviate pain and other burdensome physical and nonphysical symptoms.
- Recognize, assess, discuss, and offer access to services for psychologic, social, and spiritual issues.
- Provide access to therapeutic support, encompassing the spectrum from life-prolonging treatments through hospice care, when they can realistically be expected to improve the quality of life as perceived by the patient.
- Recognize the physician's responsibility to discourage treatments that are unlikely to achieve the patient's goals, and encourage patients and families to consider hospice care when the prognosis for survival is likely to be less than half a year.
- Arrange for continuity of care by the patient's primary or specialist physician, alleviating the sense of abandonment patients may feel when "curative" therapies are no longer useful.
- Maintain a collegial and supportive attitude toward others entrusted with care of the patient.

From Task Force on Surgical Palliative care: Statement of principles of palliative care, Bull Am Coll Surg 90(8):34-35, 2005.

BOX 2: Prognostic indicators

General Indicators of Poor Prognosis
- Functional ability: single most important predictive factor
- Median survival of 3 mo: Karnofsky ≤ 50 or ECOG ≥ 3
- Additional evidence: unintentional progressive weight loss, >10% over prior 6 months; serum albumin, <2.5 g/dL (not to be used in isolation from other factors)

Cancer-Related Indicators of Poor Prognosis
- Patients with solid tumors typically lose 70% of functional ability in last 3 mo of life
- If >50% of time is spent sleeping or lying down and is increasing, median survival is 3 mo, less with increasing symptoms, especially dyspnea
- Most solid tumors that progress through 2 rounds of chemotherapy: <6 mo
- Hypercalcemia: 8 wk (except newly diagnosed myeloma or breast cancer)
- Pericardial effusion: 8 wk
- Carcinomatous meningitis: 8-12 wk
- Multiple brain metastases: 1-2 mo without radiation; 3-6 mo with radiation
- Malignant ascites or pleural effusion: <6 mo
- Most metastatic solid cancers, acute leukemias, high-grade lymphomas not on chemotherapy: <6 mo

ECOG, Eastern Cooperative Oncology Group.

course without further attempts to reverse it. Referral can follow operative palliation of symptoms but should not be made until the patient or surrogate has had a chance to become aware of a prognosis of 6 months or less. (Boxes 2 and 3 and show estimates for prognosis and referral criteria for palliative care and hospice services.)

Palliative surgery is currently moving away from its earlier definition of noncurative intervention to the more affirmative concept of deliberate symptom control and restoration of quality of life. This transition has been guided by increased emphasis on determination of personal relevance for symptom relief (patient-centered), minimization of morbidity, improvement in nonphysical domains, and durability of symptom relief.

Considerations for palliative surgery include the expected course of the disease, the psychology of the patient, the effectiveness of the given operation, and the capacities of the surgeon/surgical team. Therapeutic benefit from palliative surgery must achieve symptom control, durability of symptom control, and symptom control with minimal morbidity (including social morbidity of hospitalization of an individual during the last weeks of life). Major operative complications dramatically worsen the prospects of achieving durable symptom relief up to the time of death.

Although life expectancy of less than 2 months has been suggested as a contraindication for palliative surgery, prognostication by physicians is notoriously inaccurate, especially if the symptom is the reason for loss of function rather than progression of disease.

For major palliative intra-abdominal procedures, such as malignant bowel obstruction, generally agreed upon relative contraindications include diffuse intraperitoneal carcinomatosis, palpable multiple intra-abdominal masses, multiple liver metastases, extraabdominal metastases, pleural effusions, multiple sites of partial

BOX 3: Palliative care consultation indications and Medicare Hospice Benefit eligibility

Palliative Care Consultation
- Patient has an illness typified by progressive deterioration and worsening symptoms, often ending fatally.
- Patient has limiting/threatening conditions with declining functional status, mental or cognitive function.
- Suboptimal control of pain or other distressing symptoms.
- Patient/family would benefit from clarification of goals and plan of care, or resolution of ethical dilemmas.
- Patient/surrogate declines further invasive or curative procedures, preferring comfort-oriented symptom management only.
- Patients on medical/surgical or critical care units who are expected to die imminently or shortly after hospital discharge.
- Bereavement support of hospital workers, particularly after the death of a colleague under care.

Eligibility for Medicare Hospice Benefit
- Patient is eligible for Medicare Part A.
- Two physicians must certify that patient has a condition with a prognosis that is associated with a survival of 6 months or less if the illness pursues its natural course.
- Patient (surrogate if patient not competent) must sign form electing hospice benefit.
- Hospice care must be provided by a Medicare-certified hospice program.

Courtesy of Robert A. Milch, MD, FACS, Buffalo, NY.

TABLE 1: Palliative care staging

Domain	Assessment questions to ask the patient	Domain	Assessment questions to ask the patient
Illness/ treatment summary	Tell me what you know about your illness. Could you give me an account about your illness and treatment you have had until now? Tell me what stands out in your memory (about your illness, about treatment to date). I will review (have reviewed) your medical history in your chart, but I am really interested in hearing about it from your point of view.		Have you ever had problems with depression, alcohol, or other psychologic difficulties before your illness? Did you ever have treatment for these? Are you afraid we won't be there when you need us?
Physical symptoms	How long have you had (symptom)? Are you having this (symptom) all the time or on and off? How would you describe what you are feeling? Is the (symptom) staying the same, getting better, or getting worse? On a scale (provide a scale), what is the lowest you have been in the past day? The highest? Where are you now? In which number range would you be satisfied? Do you notice any change depending on what you are doing? Does anything make the (symptom) better? Worse? Is it (symptom) keeping you from sleeping (etc)? To what extent does the (symptom) interfere with what you want to do? Is the (symptom) causing problems in your relations to others? Have any treatments helped your (symptom)? How much? What do you think is causing it (symptom)? What does it (symptom) make you think about? Does it (symptom) frighten you? Why?	Spiritual issues	Do you consider yourself a religious or spiritual person? How important is your faith or belief in your life? Do you belong to a community of faith? Is there a group of people particularly important to you? What sustains your hope? Do you have religious or spiritual beliefs that help you through difficulty? What gives your life meaning? Does your faith influence your feelings about your illness? Your surgery? Do you see any possible conflicts between your healthcare and your beliefs? Do you have any specific observances or rituals we should be mindful of during your care (here)?
		Social context	Can you tell me about other people in your everyday life, at work, at home, etc?
		Communication preferences	Is it your preference to be alone or have someone close to you present when we discuss important matters? Is there anyone with whom you would like me to discuss your care? If I am approached by family members with questions about your situation, do I have your permission to discuss it? To what extent? Would an interpreter be helpful? (Professional interpreters, not family or friends, and definitely not children, are recommended.)
Psychologic symptoms	Does everything happening make any sense to you? What do you think will happen next? How has your illness affected your life? How would you describe your mood? What do you see as the biggest problem facing you now? What frightens you most about your illness? How well do you think you are coping now? Do you feel depressed? Have you ever thought of taking your life? Do you have a plan? Have you been sad? Frightened? Anxious? Are you afraid of being a burden to others? How have you handled tough times in your life previously? Who do you turn to for support in tough times?	Decision making	Who will make decisions about your medical care if (when) you are not able to?
		Practical concerns	When you are ready for home, will your home be ready for you?
		Anticipatory planning	Have you given any thought of what comes after your hospitalization? What plans have you made for your future? Are there things you need to know right now for planning for the future? Would it be helpful for us to schedule a meeting with us and your family to plan your future treatment and care?

From Nine dimensions of palliative care assessment identified in EPEC, American Medical Association's Education for Physicians on End-of-life Care, 1999.

TABLE 2: Pharmacopoeia for management of persistent pain

Symptom	Medication and usual starting doses (adults)
Mild persistent pain, VAS 1-3	Acetaminophen: 325-650 mg PO qid • Maximum dose: *3000 mg/24 h; use less (<2400 mg) with concomitant use of alcohol or other hepatotoxic drugs (cytochrome P450 inducers). Care must be taken to identify total daily intake of acetaminophen in other prescription and nonprescription preparations. Aspirin: 600-1500 mg PO qid • Gastropathy, decreased platelet aggregation. Choline magnesium trisalicylate (Trilisate): 750-1500 mg PO bid • Little effect on platelet aggregation. Ibuprofen (Advil, Motrin): 200-400 mg PO qid • Maximum dose: 3200 mg/24 h. Gastropathy, nephropathy, decreased platelet aggregation. Naproxen (Naprosyn): 250 mg PO bid • Usual adult dose: 500-1000 mg/24 h (maximal: 1300 mg/24 h). • Nonsteroidal antiinflammatory drugs are most useful with an inflammatory component of pain and can be used concomitantly with opioids that exploit this property. All of these agents have a maximal therapeutic dose, unlike opioids. They are not benign drugs, particularly for the elderly, and may be less safe than the use of opioids. Patients at increased risk of NSAID-induced renal dysfunction include the elderly and those with preexisting renal dysfunction, congestive heart failure, hepatic dysfunction, hypovolemia, and concomitant nephrotoxic drug use. Good hydration and dose reduction minimizes risk. • Major complications are not necessarily preceded by minor ones. Naproxen and ibuprofen have the safest cardiovascular risk.
Moderate to severe persistent pain, VAS 4-10; VAS 7-10 is a *pain emergency*	Hydrocodone (Vicodin, Lortab): 5-10 mg PO q3-4h • Hydrocodone in tablet form is only available compounded with acetaminophen or ibuprofen. Caution is used with escalating because of ceiling dose of acetaminophen and ibuprofen. Oxycodone: 5-10 mg PO q3-4h (moderate pain); 10-30 mg PO q4h (severe pain) • Compounded form (Percocet, Tylox) used only for moderate cancer pain because of dose-limiting toxicities of acetaminophen and aspirin (Percodan). Single-entity oxycodone can be used for moderate and severe cancer pain because it has no ceiling dose. • Available in immediate-release (Roxicodone) and controlled-release (OxyContin) forms. • Immediate release forms include a solution, concentrate (20 mg/mL), and tablet. IV form is not available. • Slow-release form can be given rectally. Slow-release preparations should never be crushed or cut. Morphine: 15-30 mg PO q3-4h; 10 mg IV q3-4h • The gold standard. Most flexible opioid for dosing forms. • Caution with use in elderly patients and patients with renal insufficiency. • Controlled release forms (MS Contin, Oramorph, Kadian) available and can be given rectally. Kadian can be opened and given via a PEG tube. Avinza capsules can be opened and the pellets sprinkled on applesauce, swallowed whole without chewing. Hydromorphone: 4-8 mg PO q3-4h; 1.5 mg IV q3-4h • Useful in patients with renal failure and for subcutaneous infusions. Fentanyl, transdermal: 12 µg/h patch q72h • Not for acute pain management. Should not use more than 12 µg patch in opioid-naive cases. Prolonged duration of effect may require close monitoring for up to 12-24 h once patch is removed if patient has excessive dose. Methadone: 5-20 mg PO q4-8h; 2.5-10 mg IV q4-8h • Not a first-line agent, although very effective, especially for pain with a neuropathic component. Very inexpensive. Flexible: can be given PO, IV, SQ, PR, SL, and vaginally. • Its long half-life makes dosing more difficult than with alternative opioids, and close monitoring is required when initiating and when making dosage adjustments. • Numerous medications, alcohol, and cigarette smoking can alter its serum levels. • Physicians who write methadone prescriptions *for pain* should specify this indication. Methadone use for drug withdrawal treatment requires special licensure. • Consultation with pain management, clinical pharmacists, or palliative care/hospice services skilled in methadone use is recommended for surgeons inexperienced with methadone.

TABLE 2: Pharmacopoeia for management of persistent pain—cont'd

Symptom	Medication and usual starting doses (adults)
	General comments:
	• Opioid analgesics are the agents of choice for severe cancer-related pain. Oral administration is the preferred route. There is no reason to use the painful and occasionally morbid intramuscular route.
	• Respiratory depression is most likely to occur in opioid-naive cases with significant pulmonary disease or obstructive or central sleep apnea. It is always preceded by sedation. Reversal with naloxone should be reserved for life-threatening respiratory depression or hypotension, not sedation or confusion. Sedation is a common side effect when initiating opioid therapy. Tolerance to this usually develops within a few days.
	• Initiate bowel stimulant prophylaxis for constipation when prescribing opioids unless contraindicated.
	• Management of moderate to severe persistent pain requires familiarity with approximate equivalent doses of differing opioids. See Table 4 (e.g., morphine 30 mg orally is equianalgesic to hydromorphone 7.5 mg orally) and the conversion between parenteral and oral dosing (e.g., morphine 30 mg PO is equianalgesic to 10 mg IV, IM, or SQ).
	• Adjuvant or coanalgesic agents are drugs that enhance analgesic efficacy of opioids, treat concurrent symptoms that exacerbate pain, or provide independent analgesia for specific types of pain (e.g., a tricyclic antidepressant [secondary amine; i.e., desimipramine]) for treatment of neuropathic pain. Coanalgesics can be initiated for persistent pain at any VAS level. Gabapentin is commonly used as an initial agent for neuropathic pain.
	• There is no place for meperidine (Demerol), propoxyphene, or mixed agonist-antagonist agents (Stadol, Talwin) in management of persistent pain.
	• Codeine is of limited use for persistent pain because of increasing untoward side effects for doses above 65 mg with plateau of analgesic effect. 7% of white patients genetically lack the capacity to convert codeine to morphine, which accounts for most of its analgesic effect. Compounding with acetaminophen imposes a ceiling for use, unlike uncompounded opioids.
	• Invasive techniques (axial analgesia, neurolytic blocks) should be considered at the outset of pain management in pain emergencies (VAS 9-10).
Constipation prophylaxis	Docusate sodium (Colace): 100 mg PO q d
	• Stool softener. Give with stimulant laxative and titrate up PRN. Increasing opioid dosage requires up titration.
	Sennosides (Sennakot): 15 mg PO q d
	• Combination products with docusate and sennosides are available (Senekot-S, Peri-Colace).
	Bisacodyl: 2 tabs PO q d or 1-2 suppositories q d
	Sorbitol 70% solution: 15 mL PO or PR q d
	• Use for exacerbations of constipation in patients already on bowel regimen.
	General
	• Avoid bulk-forming laxatives because of their propensity to form bowel concretions in underhydrated, debilitated patients.
	• Nausea and anorexia are frequent presentations of opioid-induced constipation.

bid, Twice a day; *IV*, intravenous; *NSAID*, nonsteroidal antiinflammatory drug; *PEG*, percutaneous gastrostomy tube; *PO*, orally; *PR*, per rectum; *PRN*, as needed; *qh*, every hour; *qid*, four times daily; *SL*, sublingual; *SQ*, subcutaneously; *VAS*, visual analogue scale.

*American Liver Foundation.

The medications listed are meant to give the surgeon a rough idea of the commonly used medications and their usual starting doses. These are not recommendations for specific patients. Considerable variability of response requires individualizing dosing and titration to effect.

Dosing recommendations from Miaskowski C, Cleary J, Burney R, et al: Guideline for the management of cancer pain in adults and children, APS Clinical Practice guidelines series, no. 3, Glenview, IL, 2005, American Pain Society, pp. 51-68.

TABLE 3: Approximate opioid equivalences for management of moderate to severe pain

Analgesic	IM, SQ, IV route (mg)	Oral route (mg)
Morphine	10	30
Hydromorphone	1.5	7.5
Oxycodone	Not available	20
Fentanyl	10 µg IV ≈ 1 mg IV morphine 25 µg/h patch q72h ≈ 50 mg oral morphine/24 h	
Methadone	Ratios relative to methadone depend on the dose of the previous opioid	<1000 mg daily oral morphine equivalent *and* <65 years old: 10:1 ratio (oral morphine:oral methadone). <1000 mg daily oral morphine equivalent *but* ≥65 years old OR >1000 mg but less than 2000 mg daily oral morphine equivalent regardless of age: 20:1 ratio (oral morphine:oral methadone). >2000 mg daily oral morphine equivalent regardless of age: consider higher ratio such as 30:1 (oral morphine:oral methadone). Methadone has a variable and long half-life. Dosing interval every 8-12 h.

IM, Intramuscular; *IV,* intravenous; *SQ,* subcutaneously.

These are not recommendations for specific patients. The interindividual and intraindividual variability to opioids requires individualizing dosing and titration to effect.

From Friedman LL, Rodgers PE: Pain management in palliative care, Clin Fam Pract 6:371-393, 2004.

TABLE 4: Pharmacopoeia for management of selected nonpain symptoms

Dyspnea	Hydrocodone (Vicodin, Lortab): 5 mg PO q4h

Hydrocodone (Vicodin, Lortab): 5 mg PO q4h
- Use in opioid-naïve patient for mild dyspnea.
- May use an equivalent dose every 1-2 h for breakthrough dyspnea.
- Syrup preparations of hydrocodone without acetaminophen (Hycodan) are available. Hydrocodone compounded with acetaminophen limits its dosing because of acetaminophen's ceiling.
- Useful agent if cough accompanies dyspnea.

Morphine: 5 mg PO q4h; 1.5 mg IV q4h
- Use in opioid-naïve patient with severe dyspnea.
- May use an equivalent dose every 1-2 h for breakthrough dyspnea.
- When 24-h requirements are determined and condition is stable, conversion to a controlled-release formulation is possible.

Oxycodone: 5 mg PO q4h
- Use in opioid-naïve patient with severe dyspnea.
- May use an equivalent dose every 1-2 h for breakthrough dyspnea.
- When 24-h requirements are determined and condition is stable, conversion to a controlled-release formulation is possible.

Hydromorphone: 1 mg PO q4h; 0.2 mg IV q4h
- Use in opioid-naïve patient with severe dyspnea.
- May use an equivalent dose every 1-2 h for breakthrough dyspnea.

General comments:
- Doses can be titrated up 50%-100% every 24 h as needed.
- For patients already receiving opioids, increase baseline opioid dose by 25%-50% and titrate as with opioid-naïve patients.
- In severe pulmonary disease, start with half of the previous doses and up titrate no more than 25% every 24 h.
- Extreme caution should be used with use along with anxiolytics for dyspnea because of additive sedating effect and potential for respiratory depression. Anxiety accompanying dyspnea often resolves with effective relief of dyspnea using opioids.
- Hypoxemia ≠ dyspnea. In situations in which life prolongation is not desired, oxygen supplementation is not needed in nondyspneic hypoxemic patients. Oxygen saturations and arterial blood gases are not needed under these circumstances and confuse the goals of care. Oxygen supplementation should be given only if it relieves symptoms.

TABLE 4: Pharmacopoeia for management of selected nonpain symptoms—cont'd

Nausea/vomiting	Prochlorperazine (Compazine): 5-10 mg PO/IV/PR qid Promethazine (Phenergan): 0.25-1 mg/kg PO/IV/PR q4h • Avoid: very sedating, increased risk of respiratory depression with other CNS depressants. Can cause dystonia. Metoclopropamide (Reglan): • Contraindicated in bowel obstruction. May be useful in reversing early, partial malignant bowel obstruction when used with other agents. • Avoid use with other agents with potential extrapyramidal side effects. Haloperidol (Haldol): 0.5 mg PO q8h; 0.25 mg IV/SQ q8h • Can cause dystonia. For dystonia, use diphenhydramine. (Benadryl): 1 mg/kg PO/IV; or benztropine (Cogentin): 0.02-0.05 mg/kg PO up to 4 mg • IV dosing can cause hypotension, although haloperidol is generally well tolerated by the infirm. • Can cause prolongation of QT interval on ECG. Ondansetron (Zofran): 0.15 mg/kg/dose PO/IV q6h (maximal, 8 mg) • Specific for chemotherapy-induced nausea. No evidence that its efficacy exceeds other antiemetics for other etiologies of nausea. Dexamethasone: 4-10 mg PO/SQ/IV, loading; then 2-4 mg bid • Useful for nausea from elevated intracranial pressure and has appetite-stimulating properties. Also helpful for reducing pain from hepatic capsular distention. • Can be used as adjunct to pharmacologic management of malignant bowel obstruction. • Side effects (mood swings, GI hemorrhage, myopathy) should not be overlooked, even in patients with very limited prognosis. Olanzapine: 2.5-5 mg PO/SL q12h and 2.5-5 mg SL q6h PRN up to 20 mg/d • Can be used for nausea and vomiting unresponsive to haloperidol. • Side effects: somnolence, postural hypotension, constipation, dizziness, restlessness, and weight gain. Scopolamine: 0.5 mg per transdermal patch changed q72h; 0.006 mg/kg/dose q6h IV/SQ • Useful for nausea and vomiting triggered by vestibular stimulation (motion sickness) or hypovolemia. • Helpful for reducing terminal secretions (i.e., "death rattle") • Anticipate dry mouth and, occasionally, confusion.
Malignant bowel obstruction "Pharmacologic nasogastric tube"	Antisecretory agent (glycopyrrolate, scopolamine, octreotide); Centrally acting antiemetic (haloperidol, chlorpromazine); Opioid (morphine, hydromorphone): • This combination of agents can be given to control the symptoms associated with inoperable MBO without nasogastric suctioning. For intractable symptoms on combination therapy, consider placement of PEG. Octreotide, which is expensive, is reserved for high-volume emeses and should be initiated only when opioid and a centrally acting antiemetic fail to control obstructive symptoms. Dexamethasone: • May reverse early, incomplete MBO in conjunction with a peristaltic agent (metoclopropamide, amidotrizoate).
Anxiety/restlessness	Lorazepam (Ativan): 0.5 mg PO q4h PO/SL/PR
Delirium, moderate	Haloperidol (Haldol): start at 1-2 mg PO/SQ qh until calmer, then 1-2 mg PO/SQ qid or bid Chlorpromazine (Thorazine): 25-50 mg PO/IV/PR qh until calmer, then 25-50 mg PO/IV/PR qid or bid • Benzodiazepines (diazepam, lorazepam) can worsen delirium. • Address and treat reversible causes of delirium (i.e., hypercalcemia, dehydration with opioid metabolite accumulation).
Delirium, severe, agitated	Haloperidol: combined with midazolam as an hourly infusion • Requires monitoring. Lorazepam: 1-2 mg PO/SL/IV qh Chlorpromazine: 100 mg qh PO/IV/PR Propofol (Diprivan): highly effective sedation, although its use is limited to closely monitored settings

Continued

TABLE 4: Pharmacopoeia for management of selected nonpain symptoms—cont'd

General:
- Sedation may worsen mental clouding seen in delirium but should be mentioned as the necessary cost of preventing bodily injury from thrashing or psychologic distress of the patient and caretakers.
- In very rare cases of refractory severe symptoms in the last hours/days of life, deliberate sedation to the point of unconsciousness (palliative sedation) can be considered in consultation with medical ethics and palliative care specialist.

bid, Twice a day; *CNS*, central nervous system; *ECG*, electrocardiogram; *GI*, gastrointestinal; *IV*, intravenous; *MBO*, malignant bowel obstruction; *PEG*, percutaneous gastrostomy tube; *PO*, orally; *PR*, per rectum; *PRN*, as needed; *qh*, every hour; *qid*, four times daily; *SL*, sublingual; *SQ*, subcutaneously. The medications listed are meant to give the surgeon a rough idea of the commonly used medications and their usual starting doses. These are not recommendations for specific patients. Considerable variability of response requires individualizing dosing and titration to effect.
The author acknowledges the assistance of James B. Ray, PharmD, University of Virginia, in the preparation of the pharmacologic tables.
Dosing recommendations from Storey P, Knight CF: UNIPAC four: management of selected non-pain symptoms in the terminally ill, ed 2, New York, 2003, Mary Ann Liebert, Inc, Publishers, p. 40-51.

TABLE 5: Common ethical issues in surgical palliative care

Issue	Commentary
Disclosure of bad news	Broad legal and ethical consensus supporting disclosure of bad news *when permitted* by patient or surrogate. No evidence that disclosure of bad news "takes away hope" if conveyed gently and in the spirit of nonabandonment. Empathic truth telling fosters trust that is the basis of hope.
Perioperative DNR orders	The American College of Surgeons, the Association of Operating Room Nurses, and the American Society of Anesthesiologists position papers condemn policies requiring automatic cancellation of existing DNR orders for patient undergoing anesthesia based on the principle of patient autonomy. All recommend preoperative discussion ("required reconsideration") during which patient or surrogate confirms patient's treatment goals and limits of care, including revision or implementation of a DNR order, risks of patient's care plan, and recommendations by anesthesiologist and surgeon. During this discussion, the anesthesiologist and patient can set the parameters for resuscitation for the procedure itself and in the recovery room.
Withhold/withdraw life support	The withholding and withdrawal of medical treatments are considered legally and ethically equivalent and are based on the right to bodily integrity. It is generally more difficult to withdraw a life-supporting treatment once it has been started than to not initiate it at all. A surrogate's persistent reluctance to consider termination of life support is usually related to the fear that of "killing the patient" or fear that withdrawing life support causes suffering. Legally and ethically, termination of undesired medical treatment of the properly informed and uncoerced patient/surrogate is not considered homicide or suicide.
Aggressive symptom management	Aggressive symptom management of unbearable symptoms is a moral imperative if effective treatment is available, even at the risk of hastening or causing death, as long as causing death is not the intention of treatment. The risk of hastening death is present with any surgical treatment for serious illness, including attempts to cure. In situations in which rapid escalation of dosing is necessary to relieve intractable severe symptoms (pain, dyspnea, agitated delirium) in the imminently dying patient, the Rule of Double Effect, broadly accepted by ethicists, is invoked. RDE is comprised of these elements: • The act must be good or morally neutral. • Bad effects are foreseen but not intended. • A good end cannot justify a bad means. • The risk/benefit ratio must be reasonable.
Terminal sedation	Rarely indicated in palliative care. Reserved for severe, intractable symptoms when death is imminent. The goal of palliative sedation is to use the minimal amount of sedation necessary to relieve severe physical symptoms to the point of unconsciousness, if necessary, not deliberate induction of coma or hastening of death. Consultation with ethics committee, neuropsychiatric consultant (to determine competency), and palliative care specialist are recommended.

DNR, Do not resuscitate; *RDE*, Rule of Double Effect.

obstruction or prolonged transit time of contrast on intestinal radiographs, ascites, cachexia or hypoalbuminemia, advanced age, poor performance status, recurrence after recent laparotomy for malignant obstruction, previous abdominal radiation therapy, and disease refractory to chemotherapy.

The availability of stenting, minimally invasive procedures, laparoscopic approaches, and improved adjuvant chemoradiation and radiation therapies have increased flexibility in relieving symptoms related to obstruction, pain, bleeding, fistula, and contaminated wounds. Many of the principles and interventions useful for the palliation of malignant disease can be applied to nonneoplastic disorders encountered in surgical practice, such as chronic pancreatitis, congestive heart failure, and chronic liver failure.

Patient self report is the gold standard for outcomes measurement after palliative treatment. Numerous validated measuring instruments exist, some of which offer multiple languages and disease-specific modules with ongoing updates. Some of the more commonly used questionnaires include the Functional Assessment of Cancer–General Version (FACT-G), the European Organization for Research and Treatment of Cancer Quality of Life Questionnaire-Core 30 (EORTC QLQ-C30), and the McGill Quality of Life Questionnaire (MQOL).

Access to bereavement services is a critical component of surgical palliative care, not only for patients and families but also for hospital caregivers. Hospital-based bereavement services, including pastoral care departments and family support services, have been shown to affect long-term psychosocial functioning of surviving family members and decisions about organ donation. Surgeons may also benefit from these services as they seek the balance between aloofness and overwhelming emotion in response to serial losses. Recognition that one's status as a surgeon does not inure the surgeon from the impact of loss is crucial for adapting to the responsibilities of surgical palliative care.

SUGGESTED READINGS

Dunn GP, Johnson AG, editors: *Surgical palliative care,* Chicago, 2004, Oxford University Press.

Dunn GP, editor: Surgical palliative care: recent trends and developments,, *Surg Clin North Am* 91(2):277–292, 2011.

Dunn GP, Martensen R, Weissman D: *Surgical palliative care: a resident's guide,* Chicago, 2009, American College of Surgeons.

McPhee SJ, Winker MA, Rabow MW, et al: *Care at the close of life: evidence and experience,* New York, 2011, McGraw-Hill Companies, Inc.

CARDIOVASCULAR PHARMACOLOGY

Jay G. Shake, MD, MS, FACS, and David P. Ciceri, MD

OVERVIEW

An understanding of the pharmacologic means of manipulating the cardiovascular system is essential for all of those involved in the care of surgical patients. Many patients who present for elective noncardiac surgery have significant cardiovascular comorbidities, especially ischemic heart disease and hypertension, which need careful perioperative management. Dysrhythmias are common, particularly in patients who have undergone thoracic surgery or are critically ill. Many patients with low cardiac output states and shock need support with vasoactive medications with inotropic or vasopressor activity.

TACHYARRHYTHMIAS

Narrow QRS Dysrhythmias

Narrow QRS dysrhythmias are common in patients after noncardiac surgery. They are particularly common after thoracic surgery and in hemodynamically unstable conditions. In addition, patients frequently have development of sinus tachycardia, which can increase risk in patients with ischemic heart disease and compromise cardiac function in patients with stenotic valvular heart disease or severe systolic or diastolic dysfunction. The first perioperative priority in a patient with sinus tachycardia is to ensure an adequate circulating blood volume and optimal analgesia. Agents to control the elevated heart rate may be considered in patients at increased cardiac risk once the patient's volume status has been assessed and pain is relieved.

After surgery, the patient may have a variety of narrow QRS tachydysrhythmias that include atrial fibrillation, accelerated junctional rhythms, and paroxysmal supraventricular tachycardia, but the most common is atrial fibrillation. The first critical step in management of a patient with atrial fibrillation is to assess whether the ventricular rate response and loss of atrial contribution to ventricular filling is causing significant hemodynamic compromise or severe cardiopulmonary symptoms (ischemic chest pain, dyspnea, etc.). If the patient's condition is severely compromised, the patient needs prompt treatment with electrical cardioversion. The patient with an unstable condition should undergo light sedation if the cardiac and pulmonary status allows. Some patients' clinical conditions do not tolerate sedation. The patient should undergo synchronized cardioversion at 120 to 200 J with a biphasic waveform defibrillator. The practitioner should ensure that synch is selected before each attempt at cardioversion because the defibrillator defaults back to the defibrillation mode after each electrical discharge. Unfortunately, many patients with hyperadrenergic postoperative conditions who develop atrial fibrillation and are hemodynamically unstable do not respond to synchronized cardioversion. These patients need to be supported with additional volume (if necessary) and the administration of an alpha-adrenergic vasopressor like norepinephrine or phenylephrine. The authors' opinion is that once blood pressure has stabilized, patients should receive intravenous (IV) amiodarone while electrolyte disturbances such as hypokalemia, hypomagnesemia, and any evidence of myocardial ischemia are corrected.

Patients with more stable conditions with atrial fibrillation should be treated in a stepwise fashion. The ventricular rate should be controlled with a parenteral beta-blocker (metoprolol, atenolol, or esmolol) or the calcium channel blocker diltiazem. A beta-blocker is preferred if patients have ischemic heart disease, particularly if they were on a beta-blocker in the preoperative period. On occasion, digoxin may be useful as a second additional agent in a patient with inadequate rate control with either a beta-blocker or diltiazem. The digoxin loading dose should be decreased by a third to a half if the patient is going to receive amiodarone (discussed subsequently) because amiodarone increases the serum digoxin level.

The second clinical question in a patient with atrial fibrillation after rate control has been achieved is whether to attempt to restore sinus rhythm. In ambulatory patients, the trend over the past few years has been to concentrate more on rate control and anticoagulation therapy rather than repeated attempts at electrical or chemical cardioversion. The authors' practice is to be more aggressive at attempting to restore sinus rhythm in patients in the immediate postoperative period. Many of these patients with even more stable conditions have some adverse hemodynamic effects from atrial fibrillation, and restoration of sinus rhythm in less than 24 to 48 hours avoids the issue of systemic anticoagulation therapy to avoid stroke in patients who have recently undergone surgery.

Beta-blockade can be effective as a postoperative prophylactic therapy in patients at high risk for atrial fibrillation. The beta-blocker needs to be given continuously (esmolol) or on a scheduled basis (metoprolol up to 15 mg IV every 4 to 5 hours) as tolerated, and it should be administered parenterally in patients with uncertain gastrointestinal function. Amiodarone is usually the preferred antiarrhythmic agent once atrial fibrillation has occurred. The conventional loading dose is 150 mg IV over 10 minutes. Critically ill patients frequently need higher loading doses, and the authors administer up to 450 mg IV over 45 minutes in sequential boluses if the patient does not convert to sinus rhythm. The patient then receives a continuous infusion of amiodarone at 1 mg/min for 6 hours followed by an infusion of 0.5 mg/min. The amiodarone infusion can be converted to the enteral route once gastrointestinal function is ensured. Nowadays, administration of any other antidysrhythmic agent to acutely ill patients with atrial fibrillation is uncommon, unless under the specific direction of a consultant. If the patient with a more stable postoperative condition persists in atrial fibrillation for 12 or more hours, despite amiodarone and correction of electrolyte abnormalities, electrical cardioversion should at least be considered. Systemic anticoagulation therapy to prevent stroke needs to be considered in patients who persist in atrial fibrillation for longer than 48 hours. The potential benefit of anticoagulation therapy has to be weighed against the bleeding risk in each individual patient.

Wide QRS Dysrhythmias

Wide QRS dysrhythmias are much less common in patients after surgery. The most common is monomorphic ventricular tachycardia, but patients may also have torsades de pointes, one form of polymorphic ventricular tachycardia. Other possibilities include a wide QRS in patients with preexisting conduction disturbances or a rate-dependent bundle branch block. The appropriate first therapy for a patient with a hemodynamically unstable condition with ventricular tachycardia is synchronized cardioversion with 100 to 200 J with a biphasic waveform defibrillator. If the defibrillator does not synchronize, the patient should receive 200 J in the defibrillation mode. The patient should receive a loading dose and infusion of amiodarone as described previously for atrial fibrillation with a hemodynamically stable condition despite the monomorphic wide QRS tachycardia or after successful cardioversion. If the patient is pulseless, a 300 mg amiodarone bolus should be administered during attempts at resuscitation. On occasion, lidocaine is administered to a patient with monomorphic ventricular tachycardia with failure to respond to amiodarone. The treatment of a patient with a hemodynamically stable condition with torsades de pointes is different and deserves special mention. Any precipitating drugs are discontinued first. The patient is treated with parenteral magnesium (1 to 2 g over 30 to 60 seconds; may be repeated in 3 to 5 minutes) even with normal serum magnesium levels. The patient should be watched closely for signs of weakness because hypermagnesemia can depress neuromuscular function. If torsades persists, the heart rate between bursts of torsades should be increased to 90 to 110 bpm because that shortens the QTc

interval and suppresses the rhythm disturbance. This is most frequently accomplished by pacing.

BRADYDYSRHYTHMIAS

Bradydysrhythmias can occur after surgery, but they are less common. In a patient who is not severely hypoxemic, bradycardia frequently results from medications. All agents that have negative chronotropic activity or that block conduction through the atrioventricular (AV) node need to be temporarily held and later, if still indicated, cautiously resumed. The first agent that should be given to treat symptomatic bradycardia is atropine. The dose is 0.5 mg IV repeated as needed every 3 to 5 minutes to a maximum of 3 mg. If atropine is ineffective, the patient should receive an infusion of either dopamine (2 to 10 µg/kg/min) or epinephrine (0.03 µg/kg/min starting dose). Pacing is also an excellent therapeutic option for patients with symptomatic bradycardia. The different options for pacing a patient after surgery include transcutaneous, transvenous, epicardial (cardiac surgery), and esophageal (intubated) pacing.

CONTROL OF CARDIAC AND SYSTEMIC VASCULAR PERFORMANCE

Control of Preload

Restoration and maintenance of an adequate intravascular volume to ensure optimal filling of the left and right ventricle is essential to the care of all ill patients. Surgical patients present and have a wide array of disturbances of hypovolemia from ongoing bleeding, ongoing loss of asanguineous fluid, vasodilation, and altered vascular permeability. The fluids that should be administered differ from patient to patient based on the clinical setting but most frequently consist of some combination of isotonic crystalloids, 5% albumin, and, when necessary, blood products. Historically used pressure parameters such as the central venous pressure (CVP) and pulmonary capillary wedge pressure (PCWP) have been repeatedly shown to be not useful in prediction of intravascular volume or response to a subsequent fluid bolus. Fortunately, the use of dynamic parameters (pulse pressure variation, stroke volume variation, etc.) and dynamic parameters shown with ultrasound scan (echocardiography) have been shown to be excellent predictors of fluid responsiveness in many clinical settings. An important caveat to remember is that 50% of all patients with unstable conditions in the intensive care unit (ICU) respond to fluid therapy alone. It is also essential to recognize when additional fluid administration is no longer helping and may even be harming the patient and to redirect efforts to resuscitate the patient.

Control of Myocardial Contractility

Assessing and optimizing intrinsic myocardial performance never occurs in a clinical vacuum. Each patient may have significant alterations in rate, rhythm, atrioventricular synchrony, preload, and systemic and pulmonary vascular resistance that need to be addressed. These dynamic abnormalities need to be continuously reassessed and acted on.

Left Ventricular Failure

Both acute and chronic systolic left ventricular dysfunction and failure are common in the most ill of surgical patients. Many patients presenting for elective or urgent surgery have moderate or severe chronic systolic heart failure and are on a complex medical regimen that can include angiotensin-converting enzyme inhibitor, angiotensin receptor blocker, beta-blockers, diuretics, and aldosterone receptor antagonists. Some of these medications need to be administered intravenously during the perioperative period, be held at times, and have the dose frequently adjusted.

Chronic Systolic Heart Failure

Beta blockade should be cautiously maintained during the perioperative period in patients with heart failure on chronic beta-blocker therapy, particularly if the patient is hypotensive or is suspected of having a compromised cardiac output. Use of a low dose of parenteral medications (esmolol, 50 to 100 µg/kg/min; metoprolol, 5 to 10 mg IV every 4 to 6 hours) may be necessary in patients in whom the gastrointestinal route is unavailable or unreliable. Beta blockade needs to be held in patients with hypotension, with ongoing severe problems with hypovolemia, or with decompensated heart failure. They should be cautiously reintroduced at very low doses once the patient's condition has stabilized.

Although it is still an area of controversy, the preoperative administration of either angiotensin-converting enzyme inhibitors or angiotensin receptor blockers may result in significant hypotension after the induction of general anesthesia. These medications are commonly held the morning of surgery in many practices for this reason. If hypotension does occur, the administration of vasopressin IV at a dose of 0.03 to 0.04 units/min may be very effective at restoring the blood pressure to normal levels. These medications need to be resumed after surgery, however, at reduced doses and cautiously in patients who have experienced any hemodynamic difficulties. Parenteral enalaprilat can be useful in patients who cannot receive enteral mediations. A reasonable starting dose is 0.625 mg IV every 6 hours. The dose is increased if tolerated every third or fourth dose to a maximum of 2.5 mg IV every 6 hours. Combination therapy with intravenous hydralazine and nitrates can be used instead of resuming an angiotensin-converting enzyme inhibitor or angiotensin receptor blocker in patients with development of renal insufficiency in the perioperative period.

Fluid and diuretic therapy in patients with severe systolic left ventricular failure who undergo major surgery can be very challenging. These patients need similar amounts of volume and blood component therapy during the initial perioperative period compared to their healthier counterparts. The left ventricle with systolic dysfunction does not continue to increase stroke volume in response to progressive fluid challenges as in patients with normal ventricular function. Furthermore, a patient with poor ventricular function has rapid decompensation with hypovolemia resulting in an inadequate preload. One must anticipate the need for diuretics the second or third postoperative day in the patient with heart failure to clear the sodium and fluid administered during the initial perioperative period. Mobilization of fluids and the need for diuresis may be delayed if the patient has had significant hemodynamic instability. The authors' practice is to initially use intravenous loop diuretics because of the wide range in oral bioavailability seen in patients with these agents. The initial dose should be at least what the patient's chronic prehospital dose had been and may need to be increased if there has been a decline in renal function. A continuous infusion of a loop diuretic (furosemide 0.1 mg/kg/h, increased every 2 hours to a maximum of 0.4 mg/kg/h if necessary) after a loading dose (typically 0.1 mg/kg bolus) may be needed if the patient does not respond to intermittent dosing. Higher doses of furosemide, in association with severe fluid overload in the setting of acute kidney injury or end-stage renal disease, may prompt one to consider use of another form of volume removal such as ultrafiltration. As always, one must ensure an adequate circulating blood volume, cardiac output, and blood pressure before attempting diuresis in an ill patient.

Acute Systolic Heart Failure

Acute systolic heart failure occurs most commonly as a result of decompensation of preexisting severe heart failure or because of a myocardial ischemic event. When acute systolic heart failure occurs in the perioperative setting, it is essential to ensure an optimal intravascular volume and to maintain or restore sinus rhythm and atrioventricular synchrony whenever possible. Echocardiography is desirable to exclude a previously unrecognized valvular abnormality or less common pathology such as hypertrophic cardiomyopathy and to assess the severity of left ventricular dysfunction. Depending on the clinical situation or new finding, the input of a consultant service such as a cardiologist may be advisable.

Vasoactive agents (Table 1) need to be used in patients in whom hypotension or inadequate perfusion persists despite an adequate blood volume and sinus rhythm. Although no proven outcome benefit is found in this setting, the authors routinely use hemodynamic monitoring in these patients to allow logical selection of agents and their titration to achieve reasonable hemodynamic goals. Fortunately, a number of minimally invasive hemodynamic monitors can be rapidly put into use to guide therapy along with echocardiography. On occasion, a pulmonary artery catheter may also be placed to guide therapy.

The goals of the vasoactive agents (Table 2) are to improve myocardial contractility enough to achieve an adequate stroke volume and cardiac output and to avoid provoking myocardial ischemia and to minimize increases in heart rate. At the same time, an adequate

TABLE 1: Commonly used inotropic and vasopressor medications

Medication	Dose range	Mechanism	Indications
Norepinephrine	1-20 µg/min	$\alpha_1, \alpha_2, \beta_1$	Inotrope and vasoconstrictor
Epinephrine	1-20 µg/min	$\alpha_1, \alpha_2, \beta_1, \beta_2$	Inotrope and vasoconstrictor
Dopamine	1-20 µg/kg/min	$\alpha_1, \alpha_2, \beta_1, \beta_2$, dopamine	Inotrope and vasoconstrictor
Dobutamine	2-20 µg/kg/min	β_1, β_2	Inotrope and vasodilator
Phenylephrine	20-200 µg/min	α_1	Vasoconstrictor
Isoproterenol	1-20 µg/min	β_1, β_2	Inotrope and chronotrope
Milrinone	0.25-0.75 µg/kg/min	Phosphodiesterase 3 inhibitor	Inotrope and vasodilator
Vasopressin	0.01-0.04 U/min	Vasopressin V_1 and V_2 receptors	Vasoconstrictor in catecholamine-resistant shock

TABLE 2: Effects of adrenergic and vasopressin receptor subtypes on cardiovascular system

Receptor	Location	Effect
α_1	Systemic arterioles (abdominal viscera, coronary, skin, skeletal muscle), veins, pulmonary arterioles	Vasoconstriction
α_2	Presynaptic and postsynaptic sympathetic nerve terminals, central nervous system	Vasodilation
β_1	Heart	Inotropy, chronotropy, dromotropy
β_2	Systemic arterioles (abdominal viscera, coronary, skeletal muscle), veins, pulmonary arterioles	Vasodilation
Dopamine	Systemic arterioles (abdominal viscera, renal, coronary)	Vasodilation
V_1	Vascular smooth muscle	Vasoconstriction
V_2	Renal distal convoluted tubule and collecting duct	Antidiuresis

blood pressure needs to be restored (mean arterial pressure, ≥65 mm Hg) and unnecessary increases in afterload, which impair left ventricular function with systolic dysfunction, avoided.

Dobutamine (5 to 15 µg/kg/min) is the agent most commonly used to enhance myocardial contractility in the setting of an adequate or normal blood pressure and low stroke volume in patients with systolic dysfunction. It is a moderately potent beta 1 agonist and has variable and usually modest effects on vascular tone, although significant hypotension can occur, particularly in patients with unrecognized hypovolemia. The tendency for dobutamine to cause increases in heart rate and provoke tachyarrhythmias is probably less than other agents in most clinical settings. Dopamine (5 to 20 µg/kg/min) has been the agent that has historically been used in the setting of hypotension and low stroke volume from systolic heart failure. In older studies, dopamine has been shown to worsen myocardial ischemia; it can cause increases in heart rate and tachyarrhythmias, but it can achieve the immediate hemodynamic goals in many patients. Many practitioners consider the addition of dobutamine to dopamine for additional inotropic support if necessary once an adequate blood pressure has been restored. The SOAP II trial was a large multicenter trial of patients in shock randomized to receive either dopamine or norepinephrine for hemodynamic support. Overall, no difference was found in mortality, but the patients who received dopamine had a twofold increase in the rate of development of atrial fibrillation (22% vs 11%). Of concern, in the a priori subgroup analysis of patients with cardiogenic shock, patients who received dopamine had a higher mortality than did those who received norepinephrine. Dopamine may still be the agent initially used in many practices in these patients, but the authors more commonly use the combination of norepinephrine and dobutamine. The substitution of epinephrine may be needed for severe tachycardia or tachyarrhythmias from dopamine or the hypotension associated with dobutamine use.

Another class of agents that may be beneficial in patients with systolic heart failure is the parenteral phosphodiesterase inhibitors. These agents are potent inodilators that cause both significant increases in myocardial contractility and vasodilation in the systemic and pulmonary vascular beds. Milrinone is the agent most commonly used, with a loading dose of 50 µg/kg over 10 minutes followed by an infusion of 0.125 to 0.75 µg/kg/min (standard starting dose, 0.375 µg/kg/min). Many times, it is best to omit the loading dose or to fractionate it and administer it much more slowly in patients with marginal hemodynamics. Milrinone may result in significant hemodynamic improvement in euvolemic or hypervolemic conditions with systolic dysfunction. Administration of a beta adrenergic agonist, like dobutamine or epinephrine, which acts by increasing cyclic adenosine monophosphate (cAMP) production, to a patient receiving milrinone can result in a synergistic increase in contractility. Disadvantages of milrinone are its relatively long half-life (2½ hours in patients with congestive heart failure [CHF]) and its accumulation in patients with renal insufficiency. Support of excessive vasodilation with an agent like norepinephrine for a period of time is not uncommon.

Acute Myocardial Ischemia

The hemodynamic management of patients with left ventricular systolic failure from acute myocardial ischemia is similar to that outlined previously. Minimization of increases in heart rate and myocardial oxygen demand to as great an extent as possible is of paramount importance. These patients should receive an aspirin and a statin (HMG-CoA reductase inhibitor) as soon as possible. Beta-blockade should be considered once patients have been weaned from inotropic and vasopressor support. An unfractionated heparin infusion or other anticoagulant therapy may be considered in some patients, with the potential benefit always weighed against the risk of surgical bleeding. Cardiology consultation should be obtained, and angiography should be considered for those patients with a large area of the left ventricle at risk, hemodynamic instability, and recurring or unremitting symptoms.

Right Ventricular Failure

Successful management of the patient with severe right ventricular failure can be tremendously challenging. One of the first critical aspects is determination of whether a significant contribution from an elevated pulmonary vascular resistance can dramatically worsen right ventricular function. If biventricular failure is being driven by a failing left ventricle, then initial efforts should be directed at restoring left ventricular function. If elevated pulmonary pressures and right ventricular failure are found and left ventricular function appears adequate, then therapy to decrease elevated pulmonary artery pressures can cause significant improvement. Initial attempts should be made to correct hypercapnia, hypoxemia, and severe acidosis because all cause an increase in pulmonary artery pressure. Also, excessively high tidal volumes and unnecessary levels of positive end-expiratory pressures (PEEP) should be avoided. Systemic administration of vasodilators may lower pulmonary artery pressures but can result in significant systemic vasodilation and profound hypotension. Inhaled vasodilators, such as nitric oxide, prostacyclin, or prostaglandin E1 (PGE1), can cause significant decreases in elevated pulmonary artery pressures with minimal or no adverse systemic hemodynamic effects. One needs to be vigilant so that the inhaled vasodilator therapy is not inadvertently interrupted, especially during patient transport, which may result in rapid deterioration in right ventricular function. Right ventricular function should also be supported with judicious fluid administration and vasoactive support. Adequate systemic blood pressure (mean arterial pressure [MAP], ≥65 mm Hg) and right ventricular perfusion pressure have to be maintained to allow right ventricular function, and the use of a vasopressor like norepinephrine may be necessary. Right ventricular preload has to be adequate, but overdistension causes right ventricular function to decline precipitously. Assessment of right ventricular preload is challenging because neither CVP nor the assessment of right ventricular area with echocardiography accurately predicts right ventricular preload or fluid responsiveness. Once an adequate systemic blood pressure has been restored, addition of dobutamine, epinephrine, or milrinone to improve right ventricular contractility may be beneficial.

Left Ventricular Diastolic Dysfunction

Patients with significant left ventricular diastolic dysfunction, even in an ambulatory outpatient setting, can be challenging. Very little definitive data are available to help guide management, even though it is a very common clinical problem. These patients are commonly treated with diuretics to manage symptoms, and at times, patients may be on a combination of angiotensin-converting enzyme inhibitors, angiotensin receptor blockers, beta-blockers, and calcium channel blockers, despite the lack of good outcome data. In the perioperative setting, one can anticipate that the patient will poorly tolerate hypovolemia and reduced preload but also be at risk of volume overload and pulmonary edema. Expert perioperative fluid management is extremely important, and once again, the need to administer diuretics to these patients on postoperative day 2 or 3 should be anticipated. These patients benefit significantly from maintaining or restoring sinus rhythm and atrioventricular synchrony. Beta-blockers and negative chronotropic calcium channel blockers like diltiazem may be helpful in some patients.

Control of Afterload

The most common condition in the surgical patient associated with an abnormal vascular resistance is vasodilated shock, which is most commonly caused by sepsis (septic shock). Although not as common, spinal cord injury, hepatic failure, adrenal insufficiency, anaphylaxis, postcardiotomy hypotension, and severe inflammation in the absence of infection are other causes of vasodilated shock seen in surgical patients. Fortunately, besides the obvious differences in etiology, many of the principles of hemodynamic management are similar. First, vasodilation occurs in both the arteriolar resistance and the venous capacitance vessels. The potential blood volume expands significantly and needs to be aggressively restored. Isotonic crystalloids, 5% albumin, and if necessary, in a bleeding or extremely anemic patient, blood products should be used for fluid therapy in septic patients. Hydroxyethyl starch preparations and hyperoncotic albumin should not be given to septic patients. Second, septic patients in particular have alterations in permeability and the function of the interstitium, which cause continued loss of intravascular fluid until the inflammation begins to abate.

The use of vasoactive medications is necessary to support many patients with septic shock. The two agents that have been used most commonly in this setting are dopamine and norepinephrine. The SOAP II trial, which compared the use of these two agents in almost 1000 patients in septic shock, found no difference in mortality but a twofold greater incidence of atrial fibrillation in patients given dopamine infusions. In addition, several systematic reviews, published after that landmark trial, suggest a higher mortality in patients treated with dopamine. Norepinephrine (starting dose, 0.03 µg/kg/min) should be the initial vasoactive agent used in most patients with septic or vasodilated shock while an adequate intravascular volume is ensured. Considerable research has been done in the past 15 years and has shown that a large number of patients with vasodilated shock from septic shock or after cardiopulmonary bypass have a relative vasopressin deficiency state. Administration of vasopressin to these

patients in physiologic replacement doses (0.03 to 0.04 units/min) allows a significant lowering of the doses of other vasoactive medication and a reduction in duration of vasoactive drug administration. The VASST trial was a large multicenter trial that looked at the outcomes of patients with septic shock who had initially responded well to moderate doses of norepinephrine. The patients were randomized to then receive vasopressin or placebo in addition to norepinephrine. The required dose of norepinephrine was decreased in those patients who received vasopressin, but no difference in mortality or other outcomes was found. The authors usually only consider adding vasopressin to patients in septic shock after reaching modest to high doses of norepinephrine (>0.1 µg/kg/min).

There has been growing recognition over the past decades that significant myocardial dysfunction is very common in patients with septic shock. At least one third of adults with septic shock have low or low normal cardiac outputs despite restoration and maintenance of an adequate intravascular volume. Common practice is administration of dobutamine (5 to 15 µg/kg/min) in addition to norepinephrine to improve cardiac performance to patients with severe myocardial depression. This approach has been consistently associated with improved survival rates in moderately sized studies compared with historical controls. One recent study looked at effects on outcome in 300 patients with septic shock randomized to receive norepinephrine plus dobutamine or epinephrine. They found a small increase in serum lactate levels in patients randomized to receive epinephrine, which resolved after 24 hours despite continued therapy, and no differences in mortality or other outcomes. Epinephrine should probably be considered a viable second-line agent in patients who are not responding adequately to norepinephrine or who have significant myocardial dysfunction.

Problems with excessive afterload can occur in surgical patients with hypertension (discussed subsequently) or, on occasion, low cardiac output states because of left ventricular systolic dysfunction and normal or elevated systemic blood pressure. In these patients, a vasodilator or inodilator may be an elegant choice to reduce vascular resistance and improve stroke volume and cardiac output without increasing myocardial oxygen demand. Sodium nitroprusside may be a good first choice for these patients because of its very short half-life (2 minutes), which makes it easy to titrate or discontinue. After an adequate preload is ensured, the initial dose used in these patients should be low (0.3 µg/kg/min) and very slowly increased. Once the patient has shown a good response and a stabilized condition, they can be transitioned gradually to a different regimen of scheduled vasodilator medications. Milrinone may be an acceptable initial choice in similar patients.

TREATMENT OF SYSTEMIC HYPERTENSION

Many useful medications can be successfully used to control systemic hypertension in the perioperative setting. One of the first principles is to avoid placing patients at risk from intentional or inadvertent discontinuation of chronic antihypertensive medications (frequently from continuing enteral medication with gastrointestinal tract dysfunction or ileus). The most critical of these medications are beta-blockers, especially in patients with known or at risk for ischemic heart disease. Perioperative beta-blockade for reduction of cardiac risk (discussed subsequently) is a topic in evolution, but all available data indicate that chronic beta-blocker therapy should not be discontinued. As previously mentioned, the major exception is in the setting of severe hemodynamic compromise and hypotension. All other patients should receive their chronic beta-blocker therapy as tolerated. If gastrointestinal function is not certain, then the patient should receive scheduled intravenous beta-blocker therapy. A reasonable goal is to target a heart rate of less than 80 bpm and avoid any hypotension. Failure to continue chronic beta-blocker therapy exposes the patient to a significant risk of a perioperative myocardial ischemic event or dysrhythmia, especially atrial fibrillation. Patients should be transitioned to their chronic enteral antihypertensive medication regimens as their gastrointestinal tract function improves.

Labetalol is a mixed alpha and beta adrenergic agent that has been used very successfully in many perioperative settings. No data are available to suggest that it should be used in patients on chronic beta-blocker therapy in the perioperative setting, however. Labetalol has been used successfully in beta-blocker naïve patients, particularly in patients who have neurotrauma or who have undergone neurosurgery because it does not cause cerebral vasodilation. Initial doses should be low (10 to 20 mg IV) and can be increased as tolerated. Patients with euvolemic, hemodynamically stable conditions with severe hypertension may be treated with more conventional doses of labetalol (test dose, 20 mg; followed by 40 and 80 mg boluses every 10 minutes to a maximum of 300 mg).

Vasodilator medications can be useful antihypertensive medications in the perioperative setting. Parenteral medications that are administered with a continuous infusion include nitroglycerin, sodium nitroprusside, nicardipine, clevidipine, and fenoldopam. Nitroglycerin and sodium nitroprusside are both cerebral vasodilators and should not be used in patients at risk for intracranial hypertension in the absence of an intact neurologic examination or intracranial pressure monitoring. Nitroglycerin is a fairly ineffective antihypertensive agent in most patients and is commonly used primarily for its antiischemic effects. Sodium nitroprusside is an effective antihypertensive agent, but it exposes the patient to the risk of cyanide toxicity because each molecule of nitroprusside disassociates to release 5 molecules of cyanide. The authors always mix thiosulfate with nitroprusside (100 mg thiosulfate to 1000 mg nitroprusside). Thiosulfate is a sulfur donor that is needed by the enzyme rhodanase to metabolize cyanide. Thiosulfate administration significantly reduces the risk of cyanide accumulation.

Nicardipine and clevidipine are parenteral dihydropyridine calcium channel blockers that have been used in the perioperative setting. Nicardipine (initial dose, 5 mg/h; titrated to maximal dose, 15 mg/h) has been shown to be effective in hypertensive emergencies and in a number of perioperative settings, particularly in neurosurgical cases. Nicardipine's half-life with infusions of usual duration is approximately 45 minutes, so there is a somewhat greater need to anticipate the change in blood pressure and adjust the dose accordingly than with agents with a very short half-life such as nitroprusside. Nicardipine can then be transitioned to its oral formulation. Nicardipine and labetalol alone or in combination are the current preferred agents in neurosurgical and neurotrauma cases. Very little published data look at clevidipine in noncardiac surgery patients at this time; for that reason, this agent is not routinely used in postoperative patients yet, despite its promise.

Fenoldopam is a dopaminergic 1 receptor agonist that is an effective parenteral antihypertensive agent and that has been investigated in multiple cardiac and noncardiac studies. In clinical trials, doses from 0.01 to 1.6 µg/kg/min have been used. In addition, multiple studies have examined the effect of fenoldopam on perioperative renal injury in cardiac surgery, aortic, major vascular, and transplant surgery cases. Benefit is suggested in current systematic reviews, but the benefit may be small and there is no consistently demonstrated effect on renal replacement therapy or survival. Large, multicenter, and appropriately powered trials are needed to confirm or refute this potential benefit.

Other antihypertensive agents used in the perioperative setting are angiotensin-converting enzyme inhibitors (discussed previously), which are available in a parenteral formulation; intravenous hydralazine; and transcutaneous and oral clonidine. Intravenous hydralazine is inexpensive and moderately effective. Its utility is limited by its variable onset to peak effect, antihypertensive efficacy, and duration of action. A reasonable starting regimen is 10 to 20 mg every 4 to 6 hours, which can be increased incrementally to

a maximum of 40 mg every 4 hours. One situation in which hydralazine may be particularly useful in combination with nitrates is in patients with CHF from systolic left ventricular dysfunction and renal insufficiency who cannot be treated with angiotensin-converting enzyme inhibitors or angiotensin receptor blockers. Clonidine is used primarily in the perioperative setting in those patients who are taking the medication chronically to prevent clonidine withdrawal syndrome and severe hypertension. Clonidine can also be used as an adjunct in the treatment of several different withdrawal syndromes.

Diuretics can play a role in the management of the patient with perioperative hypertension. Patients on chronic diuretic therapy need to have diuretic therapy resumed after the initial recovery period. This may need to occur sooner in patients with evidence of volume overload or pulmonary edema.

PHARMACOLOGIC REDUCTION OF PERIOPERATIVE CARDIAC RISK

Pharmacologic approaches to reduce perioperative cardiac risk, in patients with known or suspected ischemic heart disease, have been an area of intense investigation for the past 15 years. The enthusiasm for widespread use of perioperative beta-blockade based on initial studies in patients at high risk has been tempered by the recognition that this therapy may cause harm as well as benefit. In patients at lower risk, perioperative beta-blockade may still slightly decrease perioperative cardiac risk, but at the cost of a greater number of strokes and overall higher mortality. In brief, careful patient selection is of paramount importance when considering use of perioperative beta-blocker therapy. First, patients on chronic beta-blocker therapy with known or at significant risk for ischemic heart disease should not have beta-blockers withdrawn during the perioperative period. Second, patients undergoing major or moderate surgery should undergo an evaluation of cardiac risk. Multiple tools are available, but a simple tool that has been well validated is the revised cardiac risk index. It consists of six factors: high-risk surgical procedures (intraperitoneal, intrathoracic, or suprainguinal vascular), history of ischemic heart disease, history of congestive heart failure, history of cerebrovascular disease, diabetes requiring preoperative treatment with insulin, and a preoperative serum creatinine value of more than 2.0 mg/dL. Perioperative beta-blockade should be considered in patients with two or more cardiac risk factors who are undergoing major surgery. Patients with one or no cardiac risk factor who have not chronically been treated with beta-blockers should not be treated with perioperative beta-blockade. The beta-blocker therapy should ideally be initiated 2 weeks before surgery and titrated at a heart rate of 60 bpm with an acceptable blood pressure and then continued with parenteral agents, if necessary, in the immediate postoperative period. The beta-blocker therapy should be continued at least until hospital discharge and preferably to a follow-up appointment with the patient's primary care provider because of increased cardiac risk. If a patient has multiple revised cardiac index risk factors but has not been placed on outpatient beta-blocker therapy, the authors consider initiating parenteral beta-blockers carefully just before surgery and continuing that therapy throughout the perioperative period. In this circumstance, the authors attempt to maintain a heart rate of less than 80 and avoid any instance of hypotension.

Growing evidence shows that therapy with statins is associated with improved cardiovascular outcomes and that statin therapy should not be withdrawn in the perioperative settings. Statin therapy should be continued until the time of surgery and resumed as quickly as possible after surgery. Patients need to be on statin therapy for a minimum of 2 weeks before surgery to accrue benefit. This is an active area of research, and newer data and recommendations continue to emerge.

SUGGESTED READINGS

Annane D, Vignon P, Renault A, et al: Norepinpehrine plus dobutamine versus epinephrine alone for managemnt of septic shock: a randomized trial, *Lancet* 370:676–684, 2007.

De Backer D, Biston P, Devriendt J, et al: Comparison on dopamine and norepinephrine in the treatment of shock, *N Engl J Med* 362:779–789, 2010.

Fleisher L, Beckman J, Brown K, et al: ACC/AHA 2007 guidelines on perioperative cardiovascular evaluation and care from noncardiac surgery, *JACC* 50:e159–e241, 2007.

Fleisher L, Beckman J, Brown K, et al: 2009 ACC/AHA focused update on perioperative beta blockade incorporated into the ACC/AHA 2007 guidelines on perioperative cardiovascular evaluation and care for noncardiac surgery, *Circulation* 120:e1–e108, 2009.

Perner A, Haase N, Guttormsen A, et al: Hydroxyethyl starch 130/0.42 versus Ringer's acetate in severe sepsis, *N Engl J Med* 367:124–134, 2012.

Poise Study Group: Effects of extended-release metoprolol succinate in patients undergoing non-cardiac surgery (POISE trial): a randomised controlled trial, *Lancet* 371:1839–1847, 2008.

Reinhart K, Perner A, Spring C, et al: Consensus statement of the ESICM task force on colloid volume therapy in critically ill patients, *Intens Care Med* 38:368–383, 2012.

The SAFE Study Investigators: A comparison of albumin and saline for fluid resuscitation in the intensive care unit, *N Engl J Med* 350:2247–2256, 2004.

Vasu TS, Cavallazzi R, Hirani A, et al: Norepinephrine or dopamine for septic shock: a systemic review of randomized clinical trials, *Intens Care Med* 27(3):172–178, 2012.

GLUCOSE CONTROL IN THE POSTOPERATIVE PERIOD

Raminder Nirula, MD, and Meghan Lewis, MD

INTRODUCTION

Glycemic control has been a goal in postoperative care since the realization that diabetes mellitus was associated with postoperative complications. Although this association is presumably the result of perioperative hyperglycemia, the long-term effects of hyperglycemia lead to comorbidities such as coronary artery and peripheral vascular disease, which contribute to suboptimal postoperative outcomes. Postoperative hyperglycemia in patients without diabetes has also been linked to poor postoperative outcomes and may represent the body's stress response altering carbohydrate metabolism. Hemorrhage and tissue injury cause increased glucose production and impaired insulin sensitivity mediated largely through the release of adrenalin, although the exact mechanisms are numerous and complex. In addition, the perioperative administration of adrenergics or steroids confounds the relationship between hyperglycemia and outcome. Hyperglycemia, in turn, increases both infections and inflammatory mediators and alters wound healing and repair. Perioperative glycemic control, therefore, carries the potential to affect patient outcome and hospital resource utilization.

INDICATIONS

The association between postoperative hyperglycemia and poor outcomes has been well studied after cardiac surgery, hepatectomy, colectomy, and other general and vascular surgeries. This relationship has also been reported in septic, critically ill, and trauma patients. Tight glucose control then intuitively seems to be indicated for all of these patient populations. Indeed, tight glucose control has shown benefits in these populations; however, hypoglycemia has been reported from overly zealous hyperglycemia protocols.

Tight glucose control is indisputably indicated after cardiovascular surgery. The cardiac literature has reported improved outcomes with tight postoperative glucose control since the 1990s. Patients with tighter glucose control have been shown to have lower rates of superficial and deep wound infections, among other complications, after surgery. In 2011, a meta-analysis of randomized controlled trials comparing tight glucose control with conventional glucose control after cardiac surgery showed that tight glucose control reduced intensive care unit (ICU) mortality, incidence of atrial fibrillation, need for epicardial pacing, duration of mechanical ventilation, and ICU length of stay.

Other critically ill surgical patients have benefited from tight glucose control. A landmark randomized controlled trial in 2001 reported a statistically significant reduction in morbidity and mortality (4.6% compared with 8%; $P = 0.04$) in surgical intensive care unit (SICU) patients treated with strict maintenance of a normal blood glucose (defined as 80 to 110 mg/dL instead of 180 and 200 mg/dL in the control group). Reduced morbidity in the tight glucose control group was attributed to a reduction in bloodstream infection, acute renal failure, red cell transfusion, incidence of critical illness polyneuropathy, and need for mechanical ventilation.

Postoperative euglycema may be indicated in all postoperative patients. In 2008, a retrospective review of the National Surgical Quality Improvement Program (NSQIP) data of nearly 1000 patients who underwent general or vascular surgery identified elevated postoperative glucose as a strong independent predictor of postoperative pneumonia, wound infection, urinary tract infection, and sepsis within 30 days of surgery. In 2012, another retrospective analysis of the Veterans Affairs Surgical Quality Improvement Program (VASQIP) data determined that patients with postoperative hyperglycemia after elective colectomy had an increased risk for surgical site infections, respiratory complications, operative reintervention, myocardial infarction, cardiac arrest, venous thromboembolism, and mortality. Although hyperglycemia was linked to worse outcomes in these studies, one cannot assume, based on these studies alone, that glucose homeostasis necessarily translates into a reduction in these infectious complications, as the hyperglycemia may be a marker of the severity of illness or the magnitude of the surgical insult rather than a direct contributor to the postoperative complications.

Hyperglycemia from parenteral nutrition, particularly during the initiation period when the body has yet to adapt to the intravenous glucose infusion, requires correction. A randomized controlled trial of 248 gastrectomy patients who needed parental nutrition showed a significantly reduced overall postoperative complication rate with intensive glucose control (13.6% compared with 25.2%; $P = 0.024$).

TECHNIQUES

Because of the multifactoral and complex nature of postoperative hyperglycemia, tight glucose control during this time period can be an extremely difficult task. Intravenous insulin infusion is perhaps the most precise way to quickly adjust blood glucose levels after surgery because of its rapid action. A continuous insulin infusion, however, requires frequent blood glucose measurements and close monitoring, which leads to increased costs and use of resources. For this reason, the alternative of a sliding scale of subcutaneously administered insulin is the most common method used after surgery. This method, however, frequently achieves suboptimal glucose control. Alternative strategies for improved postoperative glucose control are an important area of current research.

Long-acting insulin for improved glucose control has been evaluated after surgery, specifically in patients with a preoperative diagnosis of diabetes mellitus. In a randomized controlled trial of 100 patients with diabetes, those treated with basal bolus glargine (supplemented with glulisine given before meals) had better glucose control than those treated with a conventional sliding scale. As predicted, the patients receiving glargine were also found to have a lower number of postoperative complications, such as wound infections. Regarding the complications of this therapy, the authors reported a higher incidence of hypoglycemia in the glargine group; however, no significant difference was found in severe hypoglycemia episodes between the two groups (blood glucose levels, <40 mg/dL).

Glucose and insulin administration with maintenance of normoglycemia (GIN therapy) is an alternative to the standard titratable insulin infusion. This is a technique of perioperative glucose control where insulin is infused at a preemptive constant rate and dextrose is titrated to a goal serum glucose concentration. The technique has been advocated by some and has shown acceptable safety and efficacy in small trials. The goal of this therapy is complete suppression of endogenous insulin production with a constant infusion of insulin. This allows easier maintenance of blood glucose levels because the dextrose infusion rate can be adjusted to exactly match the patient's glucose utilization rate (removing the variable of insulin resistance).

Another proposed mechanism for tight control of postoperative glucose levels is an artificial pancreas. These devices measure blood glucose levels and automatically infuse regular insulin into the bloodstream to maintain glucose control. In 2012, a prospective randomized study reported superior glucose control in 17 patients with the artificial pancreas compared with 15 patients using a conventional sliding scale after elective pancreatic resection. Devices such as these appear effective; however, widespread utilization may be cost prohibitive.

One final consideration for control of postoperative glucose levels is avoidance of excessive intravenous glucose infusion. This can be accomplished with the use of enteral feeds, preferentially whenever possible. Patients fed parenterally have poorer glycemic control and associated worse outcomes. The addition of even small amounts of ("trophic") enteral feeds for patients receiving parenteral nutrition after surgery has shown numerous benefits, including reduced blood glucose concentrations and reduced insulin resistance.

RESULTS

As evidence of improved outcomes with tight postoperative glucose control has become more compelling, postoperative glucose management protocols have been implemented. Protocols can help improve compliance and render results of new therapies more easily measurable. Standard insulin infusion protocols are now ubiquitous; however, newer insulin-resistance-guided (IRG) protocols may be preferred. These IRG protocols have shown superior glucose control in patients after cardiovascular surgery, including increased time in the normoglycemic range, reduced time to the first glucose measurement in the target range, and decreased episodes of both hyperglycemia and hypoglycemia. IRG protocols are created from a collection of insulin titration curves. Each patient is assigned to one of several columns and then treated with a protocol based on the patient's own predicted level of insulin resistance. The column for the patient is then adjusted as needed based on both planned treatments and the patient's response.

The ideal target range for blood glucose levels after surgery is yet to be determined. Strict glucose control (80 to 110 mg/dL) was strongly advocated after van den Berghe's study in 2001 showed a benefit for this level of glycemic control. Since that time, however, a number of studies refuted this recommendation based on the consequences (hypoglycemia) associated with strict glucose control. The NICE-SUGAR trial, published in the *New England Journal of Medicine* in 2009, challenged the notion of tight postoperative glucose control. This international randomized controlled trial of 6104 patients showed *increased* mortality in patients managed with tight glucose control (target blood glucose range, 81 to 108 mg/dL) compared with more conventional control (≤180 mg/dL). Although the authors were not able to definitively identify the cause of increased mortality, significantly more episodes of severe hypoglycemia (<40 mg/dL) occurred in the tight glucose control group compared with the conventional group (6.8% versus 0.5%; $P < 0.001$). The conclusion was a caution against controlling postoperative glucose levels too tightly.

SUMMARY

Patients are at risk for hyperglycemia after surgery because of the body's response to the stress of surgery. Postoperative hyperglycemia has been associated with increased morbidity and mortality in numerous surgical subpopulations, likely as a result of infectious and inflammatory effects. Tight glucose control has shown benefit after surgery; however, it must be balanced against the costs and consequences of such therapy. The ideal target blood glucose range, and the best method for glucose control, is yet to be determined.

SUGGESTED READINGS

Caddell KA, Komanapalli CB, Slater MS, et al: Patient-specific insulin-resistance-guided infusion improves glycemic control in cardiac surgery, *Ann Thorac Surg* 90(6):1818–1823, 2010.

Jackson R, Amdur R, White J, et al: Hyperglycemia is associated with increased risk of morbidity and mortality after colectomy for cancer, *J Am Coll Surg* 214(1):68–80, 2012.

The NICE-SUGAR Study Investigators, Finfer S, Chittock DR, et al: Intensive versus conventional glucose control in critically ill patients, *N Engl J Med* 360(13):1283–1297, 2009.

van den Berghe G, Wouters P, Weekers F, et al: Intensive insulin therapy in critically ill patients, *N Engl J Med* 345(19):1359–1367, 2001.

POSTOPERATIVE RESPIRATORY FAILURE

Lena M. Napolitano, MD, FACS, FCCP, FCCM

INTRODUCTION

Postoperative pulmonary complications (PPCs), particularly postoperative pneumonia and acute respiratory failure, are a significant cause of morbidity and mortality in surgical patients. Every effort should be made to prevent PPCs; therefore, surgeons must be acutely aware of patient-related, procedure-related, and laboratory test risk factors in the preoperative period (Table 1).

If these PPC risk factors are identified preoperatively, then all efforts to provide specific interventions to reduce the risk for PPCs should be implemented (Table 2). Preoperative efforts include smoking cessation at least 8 weeks prior to surgery and optimization of chronic pulmonary diseases, including asthma and chronic obstructive pulmonary disease. Intraoperative strategies to reduce the risk for PPCs include using a laparoscopic approach if possible, consideration of regional anesthesia and analgesia, and use of short-acting neuromuscular blockade. Postoperative strategies for PPC prevention focus on adequacy of pain control, increasing lung volume, pulmonary toilet, and preventing aspiration using selective gastric decompression. Lung expansion interventions via deep-breathing exercises, incentive spirometry, and positive pressure strategies have shown variable benefit in reducing the occurrence of PPCs.

ACUTE RESPIRATORY FAILURE

Acute respiratory failure (ARF) is respiratory system failure or dysfunction resulting in abnormalities of gas exchange, including oxygenation and/or carbon dioxide elimination. Common etiologies in surgical patients include pneumonia, atelectasis, aspiration, pulmonary edema, and acute respiratory distress syndrome (ARDS) and pulmonary embolus (Table 3 and Figure 1). Mechanical ventilation and noninvasive ventilation are the primary therapies for treatment of ARF.

CLASSIFICATION AND EPIDEMIOLOGY

ARF is classified as either hypoxemic or hypercapnic. Severe hypoxemic ARF should raise concern for possible ARDS.

- *Hypoxemic respiratory failure* (type I), defined as arterial partial pressure of oxygen (PaO_2) <60 mm Hg on room air, is the most common form of respiratory failure, and hypoxemia is a major immediate threat to organ function.
- *Hypercapnic respiratory failure* (type II) is defined as arterial partial pressure of carbon dioxide ($PaCO_2$) of >50 mm Hg on room air.
- *Acute lung injury (ALI) and ARDS* (see definitions in Table 4) are syndromes of acute hypoxemic respiratory failure that arise from *direct* (pulmonary) or *indirect* (extrapulmonary) insults (Table 5) that induce pulmonary inflammation, damage the cells of the alveolar-capillary membrane, and lead to severe ARF. A new definition for ARDS (Berlin definition)

has been recently proposed (Table 6), which classifies ARDS into mild, moderate, and severe categories and includes specific amounts of positive end-expiratory pressure (PEEP) at which the ratio of PaO_2 to fraction of inspired oxygen (FiO_2) is calculated.

ARDS and ALI are associated with pathologic changes in the lung with diffuse alveolar damage that includes alveolar flooding, characteristic hyaline membranes, resulting in the loss of the gas exchange and barrier functions of the lung as a result of injury to the endothelial and epithelial layers of the alveolar-capillary membrane. Parenchymal injury is not a truly "diffuse" process and has significant regionalization of the inflammation, injury, and subsequent mechanical abnormalities. This heterogeneity can have significant impact on a mechanical ventilation strategy since there is preferential delivery of ventilatory breaths to pulmonary regions with higher compliance and lower resistance (i.e., the more normal regions) rather than to diseased parenchyma resulting in potential regional overdistension. ARDS stages include exudative, proliferative, and fibrotic phases.

ARF TREATMENT: NONINVASIVE VENTILATION

Noninvasive ventilation (NIV) provides positive pressure ventilator support without the need for an invasive airway. NIV should be considered first-line therapy in ARF due to chronic obstructive pulmonary disease exacerbation, since it is associated with decreased mortality rates, decreased need for intubation, decreased complications, and reduced length of hospital stay. Similarly, NIV is an effective and safe treatment for adult patients with ARF due to acute cardiogenic pulmonary edema; a systematic review of 21 studies documented that NIV was associated with reduced hospital mortality and endotracheal intubation and reduced length of stay in the intensive care unit (ICU).

NIV as a weaning strategy for intubated patients with ARF uses early extubation with immediate application of NIV. A recent systematic review of 12 trials documented that NIV significantly decreased mortality, ventilator-associated pneumonia, ICU and hospital length of stay, and total duration of mechanical ventilation. The role of NIV for treatment of ARF due to severe exacerbations of asthma is less clear; thus, NIV should be used with caution and with careful monitoring for need for intubation. NIV can also be used to treat ARF caused by other conditions, such as severe pneumonia or obesity hypoventilation, and to improve respiratory outcome in postsurgical patients.

ARF TREATMENT: INTUBATION

- Endotracheal intubation is required, and the orotracheal route is recommended with direct laryngoscopy or the GlideScope (Verathon, Bothell, Wash) versus awake fiberoptic intubation for patients with potential difficult airway. Short-acting sedative/hypnotics with neuromuscular blockade are required in awake patients. Caution should be used with propofol (which can cause significant hypotension) and etomidate (which is associated with adrenal insufficiency), particularly in elderly patients and patients with hypotension or hemodynamic instability.
- Chest radiograph should be obtained to confirm position. The endotracheal tube should be inserted to approximately 23 cm in men and 21 cm in women (measured at the incisor). Cuff pressures should be monitored and closed-circuit suction catheters used.

TABLE 1: Patient-related, procedure-related, and laboratory risk factors for postoperative pulmonary complications

Factor	Strength of recommendation*	Odds ratio	Factor	Strength of recommendation*	Odds ratio
Patient-Related Risk Factor			**Procedure-Related Risk Factor**		
Advanced age	A	2.09-3.04	Aortic aneurysm repair	A	6.90
ASA Class ≥ II	A	2.55-4.87	Thoracic surgery	A	4.24
CHF	A	2.93	Abdominal surgery	A	3.01
Functionally dependent	A	1.65-2.51	Upper abdominal surgery	A	2.91
COPD	B	1.79	Neurosurgery	A	2.53
Weight loss	B	1.62	Prolonged surgery	A	2.26
Impaired sensorium	B	1.39	Head and neck surgery	A	2.21
Cigarette use	B	1.26	Emergency surgery	A	2.21
Alcohol use	B	1.21	Vascular surgery	A	2.10
Abnormal findings on chest exam	B	NA	General anesthesia	A	1.83
Diabetes	C		Perioperative blood transfusion	B	1.47
Obesity	D		Hip surgery	D	
Asthma	D		Gynecologic or urologic surgery	D	
Obstructive sleep apnea	I		Esophageal surgery	I	
Corticosteroid use	I		**Laboratory Test Risk Factor**		
HIV infection	I		Albumin level < 3.5 g/dL	A	2.53
Arrhythmia	I		Chest radiography	B	4.81
Poor exercise capacity	I		BUN > 21 mg/dL	B	NA
			Spirometry	I	

*A, Good evidence to support the particular risk factor or laboratory predictor; B, at least fair evidence to support the particular risk factor or laboratory predictor; C, at least fair evidence to suggest that the particular risk factor is not a risk factor or laboratory predictor does not predict risk; D, good evidence to suggest that the particular risk factor is not a risk factor or the laboratory predictor does not predict risk; I, insufficient evidence to determine whether the factor increases risk or whether the laboratory test predicts risk, and evidence is lacking, of poor quality, or is conflicting.

ASA, American Society of Anesthesiologists; *BUN*, blood urea nitrogen; *CHF*, congestive heart failure; *COPD*, chronic obstructive pulmonary disease; *HIV*, human immunodeficiency virus; *NA*, not available.

From Smetana GW, Lawrence VA, Cornell JE: Preoperative pulmonary risk stratification for noncardiothoracic surgery: systematic review for the American College of Physicians. Ann Intern Med 144:581–595, 2006.

■ Sedation is required for endotracheal tube and mechanical ventilation tolerance, and intravenous infusions of short-acting narcotics and sedatives are used most commonly. A sedation scale should be used to reduce sedation to the least amount required. As soon as gastrointestinal tract function is confirmed, a transition to enteral narcotics and sedatives can be made. Emerging data document that benzodiazepines are associated with increased delirium; thus, caution should be used with these agents, particularly in the elderly and in those critically ill patients with organ dysfunction or failure.

TREATMENT: VAP PREVENTION

■ All efforts to prevent ventilator-associated pneumonia (VAP) should be implemented immediately after intubation and initiation of mechanical ventilation. The key components of the ventilator bundle for VAP prevention are the following:
  ■ Elevation of the head of the bed
  ■ Daily "sedation vacations" and assessment of readiness to extubate (spontaneous awakening trial and spontaneous breathing trial [SAT/SBT])

TABLE 2: Specific interventions to reduce the risk for postoperative pulmonary complications (PPCs)

Risk reduction strategy	Strength of evidence*	Type of complication
Postoperative lung expansion modalities	A	Atelectasis, pneumonia, bronchitis, severe hypoxemia
Selective postoperative nasogastric decompression	B	Atelectasis, pneumonia, aspiration
Short-acting neuromuscular blockade	B	Atelectasis, pneumonia
Laparoscopic (vs open) operation	C	Spirometry, atelectasis, pneumonia, overall respiratory complications
Smoking cessation	I	Postoperative ventilator support
Intraoperative neuraxial blockade	I	Pneumonia, postoperative hypoxia, respiratory failure
Postoperative epidural analgesia	I	Atelectasis, pneumonia, respiratory failure
Immunonutrition	I	Overall infectious complications, pneumonia, respiratory failure
Routine total parenteral or enteral nutrition†	D	Atelectasis, pneumonia, empyema, respiratory failure
Right heart catheterization	D	Pneumonia

*A, good evidence that the strategy reduces the risk for PPCs and benefit outweighs harm; B, at least fair evidence that the strategy reduces the risk for PPCs and benefit outweighs harm; C, at least fair evidence that the strategy may reduce the risk for PPCs, but the balance between benefit and harm is too close to justify a general recommendation; D, at least fair evidence that the strategy does not reduce the risk for PPCs or harm outweighs benefit; I, evidence of effectiveness of the strategy to reduce the risk for PPCs is conflicting, of poor quality, lacking, or insufficient or the balance between benefit and harm cannot be determined.

†Evidence remains uncertain (strength of evidence I) for severely malnourished patients or when a protracted time of inadequate nutritional intake is anticipated.

From Lawrence VA, Cornell JE, Smetana GW: Strategies to reduce postoperative pulmonary complications after noncardiothoracic surgery: systematic review for the American College of Physicians. Ann Intern Med 144:596–608, 2006.

TABLE 3: Common etiologies of acute respiratory failure and indications for mechanical ventilation

Etiologies of respiratory failure	Indications for mechanical ventilation
• Exacerbation of chronic obstructive pulmonary disease • Respiratory muscle fatigue • Neuromuscular diseases • Obtundation or coma • Pneumonia • Sepsis • Acute respiratory distress syndrome (ARDS)	• Apnea or respiratory arrest • Tachypnea (respiratory rate >30 breaths per minute) or bradypnea • Vital capacity <15 mL/kg, <1.0 L or <30% predicted • Minute ventilation >10 L/min • Hypoxemia • Hypercarbia

- ■ Daily oral care with chlorhexidine gluconate
- ■ Peptic ulcer disease prophylaxis
- ■ Deep venous thrombosis prophylaxis
- ■ Weaning of mechanical ventilation should be initiated to allow spontaneous breathing as soon as possible. A paired SAT/SBT should be performed in all patients on mechanical ventilation since it is associated with improved outcomes with reduced mortality rates, increased ventilator-free days, and reduced ICU and hospital lengths of stay.
- ■ Other evidence-based strategies for VAP prevention can be considered in ICUs with a high prevalence of VAP, including continuous aspiration of subglottic secretion tubes, the use of silver-coated endotracheal tubes, and selective oral decontamination or digestive tract decontamination.

TREATMENT: MECHANICAL VENTILATION

- ■ Effective strategies in mechanical ventilation must ensure adequate oxygenation and alveolar ventilation and reduce work of breathing without ventilator-induced lung injury (VILI).
- ■ The treatment for hypoxemic ARF (type I) is to improve oxygenation and reverse or prevent tissue hypoxia by achieving adequate oxygen delivery to tissues with a goal of arterial oxygen saturations higher than 90% on the lowest FiO_2 concentration possible. The treatment of failure to ventilate—that is, hypercapnic ARF (type II)—is to increase alveolar ventilation by achieving adequate minute ventilation.

Causes of Respiratory Failure

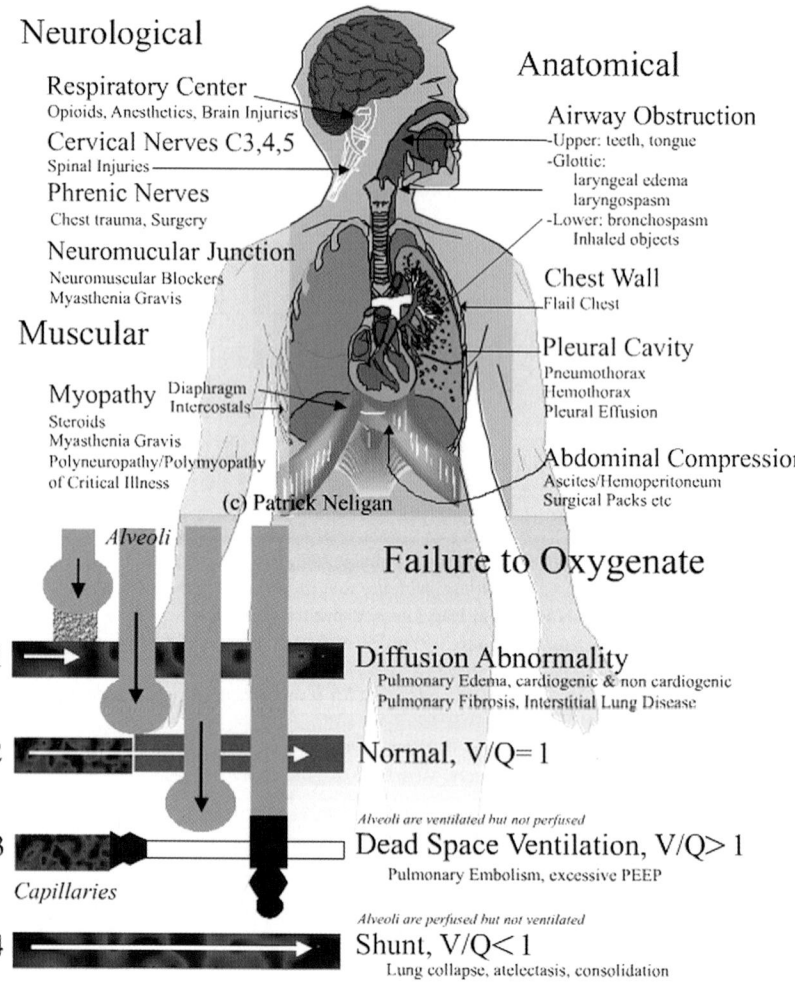

FIGURE 1 Causes of acute respiratory failure. *PEEP,* Positive end-expiratory pressure. *(From Sachdev G, Napolitano LM: Postoperative pulmonary complications: pneumonia and acute respiratory failure. Surg Clin North Am 92(2):321–344, 2012.)*

TABLE 4: The American-European Consensus Conference (AECC) definition of ALI and ARDS developed in 1994

ALI Criteria	Timing: acute onset Oxygenation: $PaO_2/FiO_2 \leq 300$ mm Hg (regardless of PEEP level) Chest radiograph: bilateral infiltrates seen on frontal chest radiograph Pulmonary artery wedge: ≤ 18 mm Hg when measured or no clinical evidence of left atrial hypertension
ARDS Criteria	Same as ALI except: Oxygenation: $PaO_2/FiO_2 \leq 200$ mm Hg (regardless of PEEP level)

ALI, Acute lung injury; *ARDS,* acute respiratory distress syndrome; *FiO_2,* fraction of inspired oxygen; *PaO_2,* arterial partial pressure of oxygen; *PEEP,* positive end-expiratory pressure.

TABLE 5: Clinical disorders associated with the development of ARDS

Direct insult pulmonary	Indirect insult extrapulmonary
Common	**Common**
Aspiration pneumonia	Sepsis
Pneumonia	Severe trauma
	Shock
Less Common	**Less Common**
Inhalation injury	Acute pancreatitis
Pulmonary contusions	Cardiopulmonary bypass
Fat emboli	Transfusion-related acute lung injury (TRALI)
Near-drowning	Disseminated intravascular coagulation
Reperfusion injury	Burns
	Traumatic brain injury
	Drug overdose

TABLE 6: New acute respiratory distress syndrome "Berlin" definition 2012

Acute respiratory distress	Syndrome (ARDS)
Timing	Within 1 week of a known clinical insult or new or worsening respiratory symptoms *(New addition, AECC stated "acute onset" with no definition)*
Chest imaging	Bilateral opacities on chest radiograph or chest computed tomographic scan *(No change from AECC definition)*
Origin of edema	Respiratory failure not fully explained by cardiac failure or fluid overload *(No change from AECC definition, but removed pulmonary artery wedge pressure criterion from definition given declining use of PA catheters)*
Oxygenation	
Mild	PaO_2/FiO_2 ratio 201-300 mm Hg with PEEP or CPAP $\geq$ 5 cm H_2O *(The term "acute lung injury, ALI" in AECC definition was removed, and added a minimum level of PEEP)*
Moderate	PaO_2/FiO_2 ratio 101-200 mm Hg with PEEP $\geq$ 5 cm H_2O
Severe	PaO_2/FiO_2 ratio $\leq$ 100 mm Hg with PEEP $\geq$ 5 cm H_2O

AECC, American-European Consensus Conference; *CPAP*, continuous positive airway pressure; *FiO_2*, fraction of inspired oxygen; *PA*, pulmonary artery catheter; *PaO_2*, partial pressure of arterial oxygen; *PEEP*, positive end-expiratory pressure.
Adapted from: The ARDS Definition Task Force, Ranieri VM, Rubenfeld GD, et al: Acute respiratory distress syndrome: the Berlin definition. JAMA (23):2526-2533, 2012:doi:10.1001/jama.2012.5669.

- Mechanical ventilation can lead to additional lung injury, that is, VILI. VILI mechanisms include barotrauma, diffuse alveolar injury resulting from overdistension (volutrauma), injury caused by repeated cycles of recruitment/derecruitment (atelectrauma; Figure 2), and the most subtle form of injury related to the release of local mediators in the lung (biotrauma).
- Variables that can be adjusted for mechanical ventilation include the following:
  - Mode of ventilation
  - Tidal volume (Vt)
  - Respiratory rate (RR)
  - Supplemental oxygen (FiO_2)
  - Inspiration/expiration ratio (I:E)
  - Inspiratory flow rate
  - Positive end-expiratory pressure (PEEP)
  - Trigger sensitivity (effort required to trigger the ventilator to deliver a breath)
  - Rise time (determines speed of rise of flow or pressure in each breath)
  - Temperature and humidity of inspired air
- Oxygen uptake via the lungs is dependent on both PaO_2 (FiO_2, alveolar pressure) and ventilation-perfusion matching (reversing atelectasis, reducing intrapulmonary shunting). To improve oxygenation, three main strategies are utilized:
  - Increase FiO_2. High levels (>50%) have been associated with oxygen toxicity, absorptive atelectasis, and other issues.
  - Increase mean alveolar pressure by increasing mean airway pressure (increase PEEP or increase I:E ratio, increase inspiratory time).
  - Recruitment maneuver with PEEP (i.e., 30 cm H_2O PEEP for 30 seconds, 40 cm H_2O PEEP for 40 seconds, or pressure control RM with high PEEP 40, low PEEP 20, respiratory rate 10-20, I:E 1:1, with mean airway pressure 30 for 2 minutes)
- Ventilation describes carbon dioxide elimination via the lungs and is largely dependent on alveolar ventilation. Alveolar ventilation = respiratory rate $\times$ (tidal volume − dead space). To improve CO_2 elimination:
  - Increase minute ventilation (increasing tidal volume or respiratory rate).

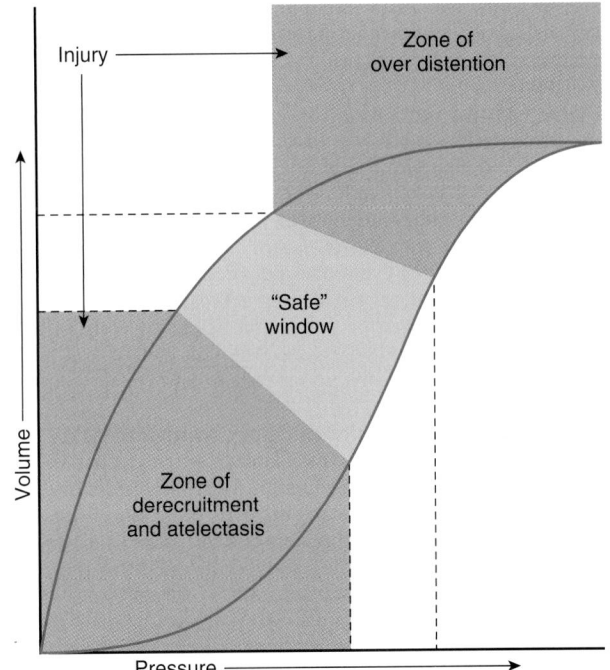

FIGURE 2 Pressure-volume curve of a moderately diseased lung, such as in ARDS. Two hazard zones exist: overdistension and derecruitment/atelectasis. Higher end-expiratory pressures and small tidal volumes are needed to stay in the "Safe" window. High-frequency oscillatory ventilation may have a larger margin of safety in keeping the lung open within the desired target range and avoiding alveolar overdistension. *ARDS*, Acute respiratory distress syndrome. *(Reprinted with permission from Imai Y, Slutsky AS: High-frequency oscillatory ventilation and ventilator-induced lung injury. Crit Care Med 33(3 Suppl):S129–S134, 2005.)*

MODES OF MECHANICAL VENTILATION

- Controlled mechanical ventilation is commonly used initially to ensure adequate alveolar ventilation and arterial oxygenation and reduce work of breathing and further lung damage. Recent studies suggest a benefit when early conversion to spontaneous breathing modalities during mechanical ventilation is employed. Therefore, spontaneous breathing is desired whenever possible.
- Mechanical positive pressure ventilation can be delivered via a volume or pressure target.
- No single mode of mechanical ventilation for ARF is superior in terms of clinical outcomes.

Volume Modes

Tidal volume is set and airway pressure is variable. The airway pressure will be variable based on the rate of delivery of the tidal volume, pulmonary compliance (plateau pressure), and airway resistance (peak pressure). This variability in airway pressure may result in barotrauma if high peak airway pressures occur.

Controlled Mechanical Ventilation (CMV): Set respiratory rate and tidal volume to achieve an exact minute ventilation; does not allow patient interaction. CMV may result in diaphragmatic inactivity, promoting atrophy and contractility dysfunction in this important inspiratory muscle, so it is not commonly used.

Assist-Control Ventilation (ACV): A commonly used mode of mechanical ventilation that is patient-triggered or time-triggered, flow-limited, and volume-cycled. The tidal volume of each delivered breath is the same, whether triggered by the ventilator or the patient. The ventilator delivers breaths in coordination with the respiratory effort of the patient. If a patient triggering event does not occur in a set time interval, then the ventilator will deliver a breath similar to control mode. This allows for patient participation with regard to breath initiation. ACV is associated with low work of breathing, as every breath is supported and tidal volume is guaranteed.

Synchronous Intermittent Mandatory Ventilation (SIMV): The ventilator delivers both mandatory (set rate, tidal volume) breaths delivered in coordination with the respiratory effort of the patient and pressure support (set pressure) breaths to support spontaneous breathing. Most SIMV modes will default to a control-mode setting in the event that the patient does not trigger the ventilator in a certain time window around the preset respiratory rate. Synchronization of the tidal volume delivery with the patient's inspiratory effort attempts to limit barotrauma that may occur with nonsynchronized intermittent mandatory ventilation when a preset breath could be delivered to a patient who is already maximally inhaling (breath stacking) or is forcefully exhaling.

Pressure Modes

Airway pressure is set and tidal volume is variable. The tidal volume will be affected by any factor that changes the airway pressure, including thoracic compliance and pulmonary resistance, and by the inspiratory time. As the lung inflates, the inspiratory flow tapers; this results in a more homogenous gas distribution throughout the lungs. Since tidal volume is variable in pressure control modes, a sudden decrease in pulmonary compliance can cause a rapid reduction in tidal volume and minute ventilation, resulting in acute respiratory acidosis. This mode necessitates close monitoring of the minute ventilation and possible intrinsic PEEP or auto-PEEP (Figure 3).

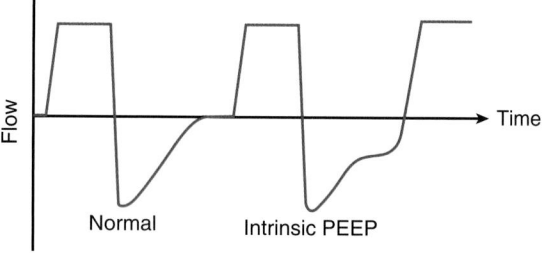

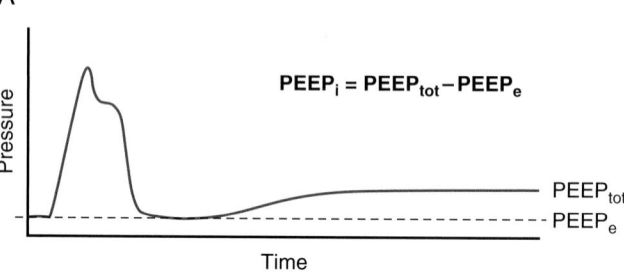

$$PEEP_i = PEEP_{tot} - PEEP_e$$

FIGURE 3 Intrinsic PEEP or auto-PEEP. **A,** Examination of the flow-time curve from the ventilator gives an indication that there is intrinsic PEEP but does not give an indication of the magnitude. The patient does not need to be apneic. **B,** A quantitative measurement of intrinsic PEEP can be obtained in an apneic patient by using the expiratory pause hold control on the ventilator. This allows equilibration of pressures between the alveoli and the ventilator, allowing the total PEEP to be measured. The value for total PEEP can be read from the PEEP display. Intrinsic PEEP = Total PEEP—Set PEEP. *PEEP,* Positive end-expiratory pressure.

Pressure Control Ventilation (PCV): Set an inspiratory pressure and inspiratory time rather than tidal volume and inspiratory flow rate. Tidal volume is dependent on set pressure, inspiratory time, and patient's compliance or resistance. In patients with hypoxemic ARF or ARDS, changing from a volume control mode to a pressure control mode may result in lower peak airway pressures.

Pressure Support Ventilation (PSV): Breaths are assisted by a set inspiratory pressure, which is delivered until inspiratory flow drops below a predetermined threshold (e.g., 25% of peak flow). Respiratory rate and tidal volume are determined by the patient. PSV can be a stand-alone mode or can function with SIMV (PSV only with spontaneous breaths). Apnea alarms are required to ensure patient safety. Some ventilators may have a set backup intermittent mechanical ventilation rate in case spontaneous respirations cease. PSV has been advocated to limit barotrauma and decrease the work of breathing. PSV is also used at low levels (5 cm H_2O) during spontaneous breathing trials.

Pressure-Regulated Volume Control (PRVC) or Volume Control Plus (VC+): Automatically adjusts inspiratory pressure in response to dynamic changes in patient mechanics to guarantee a set tidal volume in a pressure-control breath. Constant pressure is applied throughout inspiration (like pressure control), but the ventilator will adjust the inspiratory pressure with each breath (compensating for changes in airway resistance and compliance) to deliver a set tidal volume. PRVC is a patient-triggered or time-triggered, pressure-limited, time-cycled mode.

Airway Pressure Release Ventilation (APRV): This is an inverse-ratio pressure mode of mechanical ventilation that alternates between high PEEP (generally set between 25 and 30 cm H_2O) and low PEEP (usually 0 cm H_2O), with a longer inspiratory time (time-high), I : E commonly 7 : 1 to 10 : 1, and a very short expiratory time or "release" (time-low). APRV is an excellent treatment for severe hypoxemia as it achieves high mean airway pressures, resulting in improved alveolar recruitment without high plateau pressures. Tidal volume is determined by the difference between high PEEP and low PEEP. Spontaneous breathing can occur, and APRV is well tolerated hemodynamically and in terms of patient comfort with minimal sedation.

Bilevel or Biphasic Ventilation: Similar to APRV, mandatory breaths are pressure controlled, and spontaneous breathing can occur at time-high or time-low (Figure 4). Spontaneous breaths may be pressure supported. Compared to APRV, bilevel time-low is generally longer, which allows for more spontaneous breaths during time-low.

ADVANCED MODES OF MECHANICAL VENTILATION IN THE ICU

Newer modes of mechanical ventilation are focused on improving the patient-ventilator interface, resulting in decreased ventilator dyssynchrony and improved patient comfort, allowing greater time in spontaneous breathing.

Proportional Assist Ventilation (PAV): During PAV, the airway pressure is proportional to the instantaneous effort of the patient and is amplified according to the patient respiratory mechanics (pulmonary compliance and airway resistance) and the chosen level of assistance (0% to 100%) for the respiratory muscles. A recent advance is the development of PAV+, a mode that provides intermittent automated measurements of the patient's compliance and resistance, which are used by the ventilator to adjust the specific support for the patient. No studies have yet documented improved outcome using PAV.

Adaptive Support Ventilation (ASV): This mode can deliver both controlled (similar to pressure-control) and assisted (similar to pressure support) pressure cycles related to a minute ventilation target set by the clinician and based on automated measurements of the patient's respiratory mechanics.

Neurally Adjusted Ventilatory Assist (NAVA): Like PAV, with NAVA, the level of ventilator assistance is proportional to the patient's effort, but the signal is a diaphragmatic electromyogram signal from diaphragmatic contraction obtained from electrodes on an esophageal catheter. A significant benefit of NAVA is improvement in patient-ventilator synchrony and reduced work of breathing by ensuring the respiratory muscles are supported throughout inspiration when compared with other commonly used mechanical ventilation modes. NAVA is not yet in widespread use, and the patient groups most likely to benefit have not yet been defined.

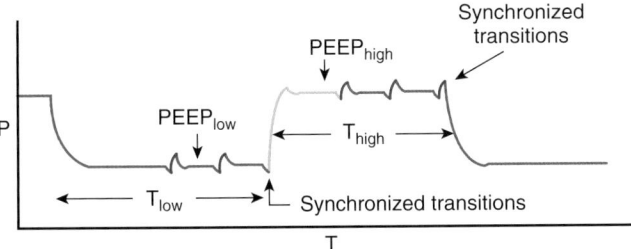

FIGURE 4   Bilevel ventilation uses two pressure levels (PEEP-low and PEEP-high) for two time periods (time-low and time-high), with spontaneous breathing at PEEP-low or PEEP-high. *PEEP,* Positive end-expiratory pressure.

SmartCare (Dräger Medical, Lübeck, Germany): This closed loop system provides automated adaptation of the level of PSV and initiates an automated weaning protocol to decrease the level of PSV and initiate SBTs when a low level of PSV is attained. The first multicenter study comparing automated weaning to standard of care ($n = 144$) documented that automated weaning reduced the total duration of mechanical ventilation and weaning duration, and the proportion of patients requiring NIV after extubation. Additional clinical trials are under way.

MECHANICAL VENTILATION STRATEGIES FOR ALI AND ARDS

Many recent advances have been made in developing protective mechanical ventilation strategies for patients with ARDS. These include low tidal volume ventilation, permissive hypercapnia, open lung strategy, and high-frequency oscillatory ventilation. The initial strategy for management of ALI/ARDS should include the use of low tidal volume ventilation (6 mL/kg) with adequate PEEP.

Low Tidal Volume Ventilation: Alveolar stretch from high tidal volumes can result in VILI through stimulation of an exaggerated alveolar and systemic inflammatory response. High tidal volumes are associated with high plateau pressures, which are associated with increased mortality. The ARDS-Network landmark ARMA multicenter, randomized controlled trial documented that low tidal volume (6 mL/kg) versus high tidal volume (12 mL/kg) ventilation in patients with ARDS was associated with a significantly lower mortality rate (31% vs 40%; $P = 0.007$) in the low tidal volume group. Ventilator-free days and number of days without non–pulmonary organ system failures were also decreased in the low tidal volume group. The incidence of barotrauma was similar: 10% versus 11%. The *Guidelines for Mechanical Ventilation of the Trauma Patient* from the participants of the Inflammation and Host Response to Injury, a large-scale collaborative research project, standardized clinical management in trauma patients to ensure that a low tidal volume, lung-protective strategy is used for patients with ALI or ARDS. This also provides guidelines for the PEEP and weaning of mechanical ventilation (Box 1).

Permissive Hypercapnia: Low tidal volume ventilation to reduce volutrauma can result in decreased minute ventilation leading to hypercapnia and acute respiratory acidosis. Permissive hypercapnia accepts deliberate hypoventilation in order to reduce alveolar overdistension and pressures in ARDS patients with severe hypoxemia. Resultant hypercarbia and respiratory acidosis are managed medically. Hypercapnia may worsen intracranial pressure and should be avoided in patients with traumatic brain injury. Tidal volume is gradually reduced to allow a slow increase in $PaCO_2$. Alkali therapy with sodium bicarbonate or tromethamine can be used to treat the acute respiratory acidosis.

Open Lung Strategy: Combining the use of low-volume tidal volume strategies, with the application of PEEP at levels above the lower inflection point, and permissive hypercapnia has been termed the "open-lung approach." Depletion of surfactant and low levels of PEEP lead to cyclic atelectasis with repeated collapsing and opening of the remaining function alveoli in patients with ARDS. Cyclic opening and closing of alveoli can lead to leukocyte activation, VILI, and loss of functional residual lung capacity. Increased levels of PEEP lead to recruitment of collapsed alveoli, reduced ventilation-perfusion mismatch, improved arterial oxygenation, and increased functional residual lung capacity. By maintaining end-expiratory pressure, alveoli that are unstable and prone to collapse will

BOX 1: Pocket card summary of mechanical ventilation of the trauma patient

Mechanical Ventilation Protocol: Inflammation and the Host Response to Injury

In patients with ALI or established ARDS ($PaO_2/FiO_2 \leq 300$ or $PaO_2/FiO_2 \leq 200$, respectively, with bilateral pulmonary infiltrates), aim for the following within 24 hours of meeting criteria.

1. Initial tidal volumes may be set at 8 mL/kg predicted body weight (PBW); tidal volumes should be reduced by 1 mL/kg at intervals of <2 hours until the tidal volume = 6 mL/kg. Tidal volume calculations are based on predicted body weight as follows:

   For Males: PBW (kg) = 50 + 2.3 {height (inches) − 60}
   For Females: PBW (kg)= 45.5 + 2.3 {height (inches) − 60}

2. PaO_2 55-80 mm Hg or SpO_2 88%-95%. FiO_2/PEEP ratio should be ≤ 5 and PEEP must be ≤ 35 cm H_2O.

3. Arterial pH 7.25-7.45 with RR <35 and $PaCO_2 \geq 25$. HCO_3 infusion may be given if necessary. If pH <7.15, then Vt may be increased by 1 mL/kg to pH ≥7.15 and target plateau pressures (see number 4) may be exceeded.

4. Plateau pressures (Pplat) ≤ 30 cm H_2O. Reduce Vt to no less than 4 mL/kg. If Vt <6 mL/kg and Pplat <25, then increase Vt until Pplat = 25-30 or Vt = 6 mL/kg.

Patients not meeting ALI/ARDS criteria can be ventilated using the mode, rate, and tidal volume chosen at the treating physician's discretion.

Patients should undergo a daily assessment of their readiness for a spontaneous breathing trial (SBT):

(a) resolution or stabilization of the underlying disease process; (b) no residual effects of neuromuscular blockade; (c) exhibiting respiratory efforts; (d) hemodynamically stable; (e) $FiO_2 \leq 0.5$ and PEEP ≤ 8 cm H_2O; (f) PaO_2 >70 mm Hg; (g) Ve <15 L/min; (h) Arterial pH between 7.30-7.50; (i) ICP <20 cm H_2O. If not ready for an SBT, then return to a comfortable, nonfatiguing mode of ventilator support and reassess daily.

If ready, then the patient should receive **a trial of spontaneous breathing (SBT) on CPAP for 30-90 minutes. Criteria for failure of a SBT:**

(a) RR >35 for ≥ 5 min; (b) SpO_2 <90% for ≥ 30 seconds; (c) HR >140 or increase or decrease of 20% from baseline; (d) SBP >180 mm Hg or <90 mm Hg; (e) sustained evidence of respiratory distress; (f) cardiac instability or dysrhythmias; (g) arterial pH ≤ 7.32; (h) ICP ≥ 20 cm H_2O. If any criteria are met, the CPAP trial is terminated and patient returned to a nonfatiguing mode of support and rested overnight. Repeat CPAP in the morning.

If patient completes CPAP trial, the following criteria should be assessed to determine readiness for extubation and patient should be extubated if possible:

(a) does not require suctioning more than every 4 hours; (b) good spontaneous cough; (c) endotracheal tube cuff leak; (d) no recent upper airway obstruction or stridor; (e) no recent reintubation for bronchial hygiene.

ALI, Acute lung injury; *ARDS,* acute respiratory distress syndrome; *CPAP,* continuous positive airway pressure; *FiO2,* fraction of inspired oxygen; *HCO3,* bicarbonate; *ICP,* intracranial pressure; *PaO2,* arterial partial pressure of oxygen; *PEEP,* positive end-expiratory pressure; *RR,* respiratory rate; *SBT,* spontaneous breathing trial; *SpO2,* saturation of peripheral oxygen; *Ve,* minute ventilation; *Vt,* tidal volume.

From Nathens AB, et al: Inflammation and the host response to injury, a large-scale collaborative project: patient-oriented research core—standard operating procedures for clinical care. I. Guidelines for mechanical ventilation of the trauma patient. J Trauma 59(3):764–769, 2005.

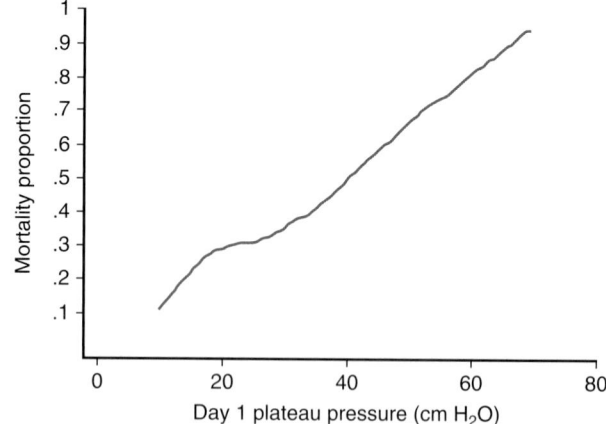

FIGURE 5 Relationship between mortality and day 1 plateau pressures. *(Reprinted with permission from Hager DN, et al: Tidal volume reduction in patients with acute lung injury when plateau pressures are not high. Am J Respir Crit Care Med Nov 15;172(10):1241–1245, 2005.)*

remain open. The optimal PEEP level is difficult to determine, but evidence suggests that maximal recruitment and lung volume maintenance occurs when the PEEP is set at a level just above the inflection point (Pflex) on the pressure-volume curve in patients with ARDS. A recent meta-analysis confirmed that higher versus lower levels of PEEP was associated with improved an survival rate among patients with ARDS. Despite the use of increased PEEP, it has been shown that decreasing plateau pressures (Pplat) results in a lower mortality rate in patients with ARDS (Figure 5). The study does not reveal a safe threshold for Pplat in ALI/ARDS patients. A bivariate analysis also showed that lower Pplat quartiles were associated with reduced mortality compared with higher Pplat quartiles ($P = 0.039$) suggesting that tidal volume reduction benefits patients even when Pplat is already less than 30 to 35 cm H_2O.

High-Frequency Oscillatory Ventilation (HFOV): HFOV delivers small tidal volumes at frequencies of 3 to 15 Hz to maintain adequate minute ventilation. Oxygenation is manipulated by adjusting mean airway pressure similar to the use of PEEP in conventional mechanical ventilation. Ventilation and carbon dioxide elimination are controlled by changing the tidal volume, by amplitude or power, or by adjusting the frequency. Increasing the amplitude or decreasing the frequency will cause an increase in carbon dioxide elimination. Amplitude or power is set to achieve appropriate chest wall movement and adequate CO_2 elimination. HFOV is used as a rescue strategy when other modes of mechanical ventilation fail. It is also used in patients with bronchopleural fistulae or tracheo-bronchial injuries to maintain low mean airway pressures in an effort to resolve air leaks within the tracheobronchial system.

Two randomized trials—the Oscillation for ARDS Treated Early (OSCILLATE) Trial by the Canadian Critical Care Trials Group and the High-Frequency Oscillation in ARDS (OSCAR) Trial in the United Kingdom—showed that in adults with moderate-to-severe ARDS, early application of HFOV, as compared with a ventilation strategy of low tidal volume and high PEEP, did not reduce in-hospital mortality rates.

Although the exact severity threshold at which to initiate a trial of HFOV remains unclear, an emerging approach includes the following severity criteria:

- $FiO_2 > 0.6$ and $SpO_2 < 88\%$ on CMV with PEEP > 15 cm H_2O, or
- Plateau pressures > 30 cm H_2O, or

■ Mean airway pressure 24 cm H_2O, or APRV with high pressure 35 cm H_2O

Airway Pressure-Release Ventilation (APRV): APRV is a pressure-limited, time-cycled mode of mechanical ventilation that allows the patient unrestricted spontaneous breathing during application of continuous positive airway pressure (CPAP) with a very short release time, resulting in open lung mechanical ventilation. APRV has two settings of pressure. The high pressure setting allows spontaneous breathing and accounts for 80% to 95% of the cycle time creating an open lung. The remainder of the cycle allows for a periodic pressure release to the low pressure setting to allow for ventilation and carbon dioxide clearance while preventing alveolar collapse. APRV is used when patients are able to spontaneously breathe, yet high mean airway pressure is required for alveolar recruitment for severe hypoxemia.

ADJUNCTS TO MECHANICAL VENTILATION IN PATIENTS WITH ARDS AND SEVERE HYPOXEMIA

In patients with severe life-threatening hypoxemia, a number of strategies are used, including fluid management, recruitment maneuvers, neuromuscular blockade, prone position, inhaled nitric oxide, and extracorporeal membrane oxygenation.

Recruitment Maneuvers: Alveolar recruitment is aimed at improving pulmonary gas exchange and preventing VILI, atelectasis, and atelectrauma. Recruitment maneuvers (RMs) can increase alveolar functional residual lung capacity, and PEEP can then maintain the alveoli to prevent collapse. Recruitment refers to the dynamic process of reopening unstable airless alveoli through an intentional transient increase in transpulmonary pressure, accomplished via many methods. A common method for RMs is to provide sustained inflation with 30 cm H_2O PEEP for 30 seconds or 40 cm H_2O PEEP for 40 seconds; alternatively, the use of a pressure control RM with high PEEP 40, low PEEP 20, I : E 1 : 1 for 2 minutes is effective. The optimal methods of RMs (sustained inflation vs incremental PEEP) and optimal pressure, duration, and frequency of RMs have not been tested in large clinical trials. A recent systematic review concluded that RMs were associated with a significant increase in oxygenation with few serious adverse events. Transient hypotension and desaturation during RMs is common but is self-limited without sequelae. Given the uncertain benefit and lack of information regarding impact on clinical outcomes, RMs should be considered for use only in patients with life-threatening hypoxemia.

Fluid Management: A conservative fluid management strategy was superior to a liberal strategy in ALI/ARDS patients; outcomes included improved lung function and oxygenation and decreased duration of mechanical ventilation and ICU stay but no difference in 60-day mortality. Diuretic therapy should be considered in severe hypoxemia (PaO_2/FiO_2 ratio < 100). A careful assessment of adequacy of perfusion and cardiac performance should be completed before initiation of diuretic therapy. Reassessment should be continued while diuresis is ongoing.

Neuromuscular Blockade: A multicenter, double-blind trial of 340 patients with severe ARDS confirmed that early administration of a neuromuscular blocking agent (cisatracurium) improved 90-day survival and increased time off mechanical ventilation without increasing muscle weakness compared to placebo. Enthusiasm for this approach must be tempered with concern for critical illness polyneuropathy.

Inhaled Nitric Oxide: Nitric oxide is a selective pulmonary vasodilator leading to decreased pulmonary vascular resistance,

pulmonary arterial pressure, and right ventricular afterload. Low-dose inhaled nitric oxide has shown improved short-term oxygenation in ALI and ARDS patients without affecting duration of mechanical ventilatory support or mortality rate. Inhaled nitric oxide may be considered a salvage therapy in patients who continue to have life-threatening hypoxemia despite optimization of all other treatment strategies.

Prone Positioning: Changes in patient positioning can have a dramatic effect on oxygenation and ventilation in patients with severe ARDS and severe hypoxemia. Prone position can improve the distribution of perfusion to ventilated lung regions, decreasing intrapulmonary shunt and improving oxygenation. The use of intermittent or extended prone positioning can significantly improve oxygenation in 60% to 70% of patients. Prone positioning can be performed safely by trained and dedicated nursing staff who are aware of its potential benefits in critically ill patients with severe hypoxemia. Prone positioning is a useful tool for treatment of severe hypoxemia. Recent meta-analyses in patients with ARDS documented a significantly decreased mortality rate with prone positioning, with an absolute mortality reduction rate of 10% in severely hypoxemic ARDS patients.

Extracorporeal Membrane Oxygenation (ECMO): ECMO is considered in patients with severe ARDS and hypoxemia with reversible lung disease who have failed other rescue strategies. ECMO provides oxygenation, provides ventilation with total extracorporeal CO_2 clearance, minimizes barotrauma with complete lung rest, and is accomplished via venovenous ECMO support, until the patient's endogenous lung function improves. Substantial progress in ECMO has been achieved. Potential complications resulting from the use of ECMO include bleeding (including intracranial hemorrhage), coagulopathy, thrombosis, and mechanical complications. Of 1473 adults with severe ARDS, ECMO was associated with a 50% survival to discharge. Patients with severe ARDS and hypoxemia should be referred to an ARDS center with ECMO experience to achieve the best outcomes possible. Adult patients are cannulated percutaneously with large 21F to 31F venous catheters for drainage of deoxygenated blood and infusion and oxygenated blood. Anticoagulation is necessary, and heparin continuous infusion is common, and monitored with ACT or PTT studies.

The CESAR trial (Conventional Ventilation or ECMO for Severe Adult Respiratory Failure) was a prospective randomized trial ($n = 180$) in the United Kingdom. Of the 90 patients assigned to ECMO treatment, only 68 received ECMO; others were managed with mechanical ventilation and rescue strategies. Sixty-three percent of patients transferred to an ECMO center survived to 6 months without disability versus 47% in the conventional management group (RR 0.69, CI 0.05-0.97, $P = 0.03$). A criticism of this study is that the conventional cohort was not managed with low tidal volume, low plateau pressure, open lung protective mechanical ventilation. Another multicenter ECMO clinical trial, ECMO to Rescue Lung Injury in Severe ARDS (EOLIA), is being initiated in France to address this issue.

INCREMENTAL APPROACH TO THE MANAGEMENT OF SEVERE ARDS

■ Development of ICU protocols reduces undesirable variability, mandates best evidence practice, promotes action and timeliness, and facilitates multidisciplinary communication.

■ At the University of Michigan, we have developed an algorithm (Figure 6) for management of critically ill patients with severe ARDS/severe hypoxemia to provide evidence-based care.

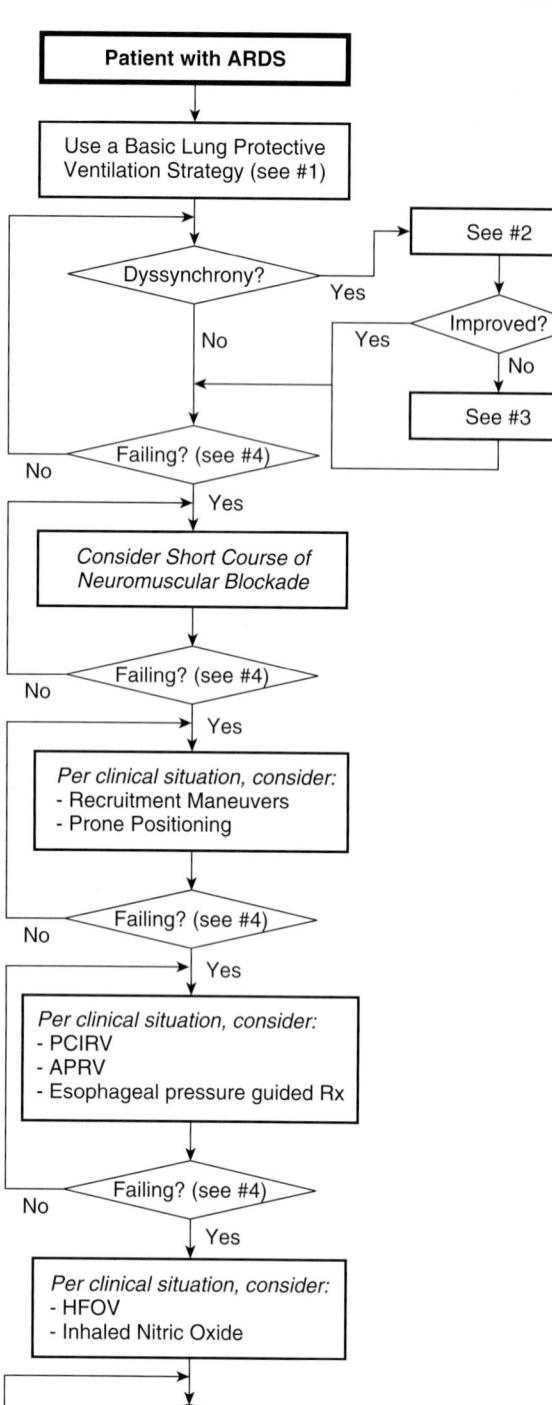

1: Basic LPVS
- ARDS Network ventilation strategy:
  a. Using VCV or PCV and targeting VT 4-6 mL/kg PBW
  b. Maintain Pplat ≤30 cm H_2O
  c. PEEP/FiO_2 per table

2: Pt-Vent Dyssynchrony, Step 1
- Initial strategy should be to:
  a. Assess potential to treat with pharmacologic agents (e.g., sedation, NMB agents), and
  b. Consider minor ventilator adjustments (e.g., flow rate & pattern, inspiratory pause)
- If above does not work, consider increasing VT 1 mL/kg (max 8 mL/kg), provided Pplat ≤28-30 cm H_2O

3: Pt-Vent Dyssynchrony, Step 2
- Consider a variable flow pressure breath mode of ventilation:
  a. Volume Control+
  b. Pressure Control Ventilation

4: Criteria for Failing LPVS
- PaO_2 <55 torr on FiO_2 =1.0 and Pplat >30 cm H_2O on VT =4 mL/kg PBW

Neuromuscular Blockade
* Short course (48 hrs) associated with mortality benefit in RCT

Recruitment Maneuvers
* Use: 35-45 cm H_2O x 20 sec, or PCV with 40/20 for 2 minutes

Prone Positioning
* Use unit specific rotation frequency, but evidence suggests majority of day (>17 hrs) in prone position, if tolerated
* Recommend a 48 hr trial, stop if no improvement, as evidenced by:
  - Reduced FiO_2 by 0.10
  - Increased PaO_2/FiO_2 by 30

Pressure Control Inversed Ratio (PCIRV) Ventilation
* Lengthen Ti to increase Pmean
* Observe exp flow graphic; stop when auto-PEEP present, regardless of I:E ratio

Airway Pressure Release Ventilation (APRV)
Refer to Respiratory Care policy

Esophageal Pressure (Pes) Guided Therapy
* Requires switch to AVEA ventilator & placement of Pes catheter
* Informs of transpulmonary end-inspiratory (Ptp-plat) and end-expiratory (Ptp-PEEP) pressures

High Frequency Oscillatory Ventilation (HFOV)
Refer to Respiratory Care policy (policy follows Oscillate protocol)

Inhaled Nitric Oxide (iNO)
* iNO Test
  - 20-60 minute test on 40 ppm
  - Positive response: increase in PaO_2/FiO_2 of >10
* If positive response, titrate and consider iloprost, per Respiratory Care Policy
* If no response, discuss with team to consider stopping
Note: iNO is a very costly drug compared to alternatives

Extracorporeal Membrane Oxygenation (ECMO)
* Absolute contraindications: irreversible pulmonary process and inability to anticoagulate
* Evaluate, but lower survival if on vent 7-10 days pre-ECMO

FIGURE 6   ARDS mechanical ventilation algorithm, including rescue strategies, used at the University of Michigan. (AVEA ventilator; CareFusion, San Diego, Calif.) *ARDS,* Acute respiratory distress syndrome; *FiO₂,* fraction of inspired oxygen; *LPVS,* lung protection ventilation strategy; *NMB,* neuromuscular-blocking; *PaO₂,* arterial partial pressure of oxygen; *PBW,* predicted body weight; *PCV,* pressure control ventilation; *PEEP,* positive end-expiratory pressure; *RCT,* randomized controlled trial; *VCV,* volume controlled ventilation; *Vt,* tidal volume.

- In patients with ARDS, initial low tidal volume ventilation should be initiated, set at 6 to 8 mL/kg of predicted body weight (PBW); tidal volumes should be reduced by 1 mL/kg at intervals of 2 hours until the tidal volume is set at 6 mL/kg. Goal: SpO_2 88% to 95%, PaO_2 55 to 80 mm Hg, plateau pressures < 30 cm H_2O while using lowest FiO_2 possible.
- If no improvement is made, recruitment maneuvers should be considered. If oxygenation improves during recruitment maneuvers, the PEEP should be increased until optimal PEEP is achieved.
- If no improvement, evaluation for a possible intracardiac shunt and/or pulmonary hypertension should be initiated. Diagnostic strategies include pulmonary artery catheter placement and/or transthoracic or transesophageal echocardiogram. Inhaled nitric oxide should be considered as a therapeutic strategy to improve oxygenation. If there is still no improvement in oxygenation, prone positioning should be considered.
- At this point, for a patient with persistent severe hypoxemia, transfer of the patient to an ARDS Referral Center with experience in other ARDS treatment modalities, including rescue strategies, APRV, HFOV, and ECMO should be considered (Figure 7).

WEANING AND LIBERATION FROM MECHANICAL VENTILATION

- Mechanical ventilation has significant potential risks such that efforts should be focused on liberation from mechanical ventilation once adequate lung recovery has occurred.
- Nearly half of the time spent with mechanical ventilation is spent weaning the patient.
- A daily SAT followed by an SBT should be performed in all patients on mechanical ventilation. A randomized multicenter trial that compared this "wake up and breathe" protocol

(paired SAT/SBT) versus usual care plus a daily SBT in the control cohort confirmed that SAT/SBT resulted in improved outcomes with reduced mortality rate, increased number of ventilator-free days, and reduced ICU and hospital length of stay.

- Continuous protocols for weaning from mechanical ventilation directed by respiratory therapists are associated with shorter duration of ventilation and shorter ICU length of stay. Patients who fail an SAT/SBT trial are returned to their previous ventilator settings and rescreened for another SAT/SBT trial in 24 hours. The patient must be carefully evaluated to determine the cause of the SAT/SBT failure. The patient must be assessed for anxiety, pain, secretions, muscle weakness, atelectasis, hypoxemia, hypercarbia, and all other potential causes for lack of resolution of ARF.
- Patients who complete a paired SAT/SBT trial (CPAP with low pressure support [5 cm H_2O] or automatic tube compensation, or T piece) should be assessed to determine readiness for extubation. At the completion of the SAT/SBT trial, the rapid shallow breathing index (RSBI), the ratio of respiratory frequency to tidal volume (f/Vt, respiratory rate × tidal volumes in liters), is calculated and an arterial blood gas is obtained to evaluate for hypercarbia. For example, a patient who has a respiratory rate of 25 breaths/min and a tidal volume of 250 mL/breath has an RSBI of (25 breaths/min)/(0.25 L) = 100 breaths/min/L. RSBI less than 105 is associated with 80% wean success; RSBI that is 105 or higher is associated with 95% wean failure.
- Prior to considering extubation, additional assessment includes the following: (a) does not require tracheal suctioning more than every 4 hours; (b) good spontaneous cough; (c) endotracheal tube cuff leak; (d) no recent upper airway obstruction or stridor; (e) no recent reintubation for bronchial hygiene.
- If failure to wean and/or extubate persists despite maximal and repeated efforts to achieve these endpoints, other steps may be required prior to successfully liberating the patient from

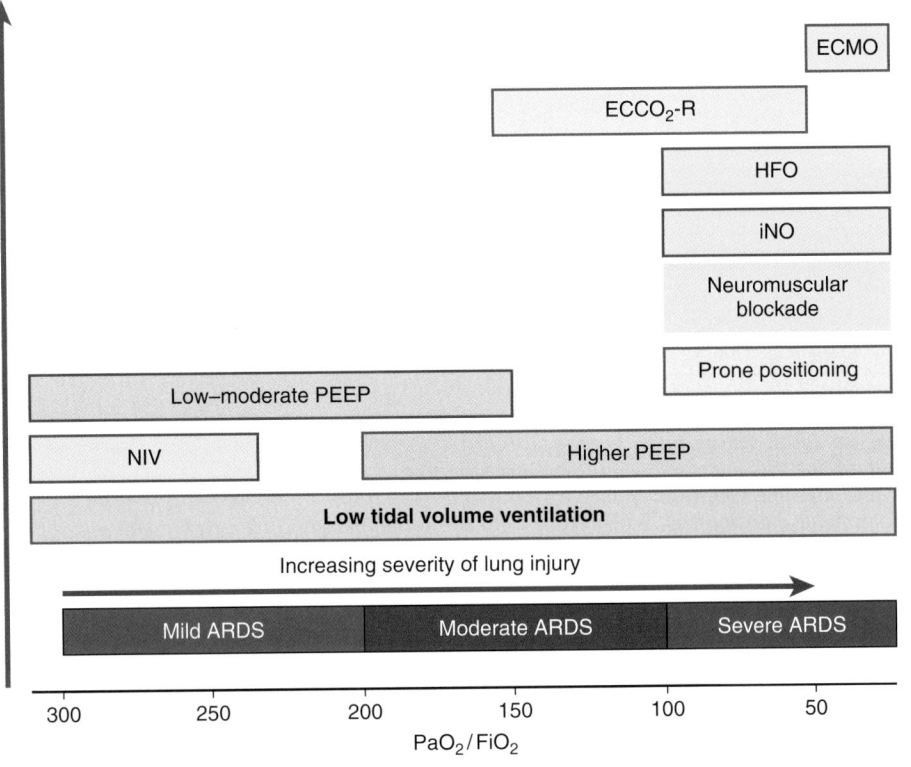

FIGURE 7 Increasing intensity of treatment intervention for increasing severity of ARDS, with all treatment strategies available at ARDS Referral Center, including ECMO. *ARDS*, Acute respiratory distress syndrome; *ECCO₂-R*, extracorporeal carbon dioxide removal; *ECMO*, extracorporeal membrane oxygenation; *FiO₂*, fraction of inspired oxygen; *HFO*, high-frequency oscillation; *iNO*, inhaled nitric oxide; *PaO₂*, arterial partial pressure of oxygen; *PEEP*, positive end-expiratory pressure. *(From Thompson BT: Problems with ARDS trials: Time for more splitting and less lumping? Critical Care Canada Forum 2011. Available at: http://www.criticalcarecanada.com/presentations/2011/ards_trials_time_for_more_splitting_and_less_lumping.pdf)*

mechanical ventilation. Some patients require prolonged and more gradual ventilator weaning, which may be best facilitated by tracheostomy placement. In addition, data from observational studies show that up to 60% of ventilator-dependent patients who are discharged from the ICU can be successfully weaned when they are transferred to specialized units dedicated to ventilator weaning.

TRACHEOSTOMY

- Some patients benefit from early tracheostomy, including those with traumatic brain injury and ARF for airway protection, and those who will require prolonged mechanical ventilation (i.e., patients with ARDS) for patient comfort.
- Previous studies suggested that tracheostomy was superior to prolonged intubation for VAP prevention. However, two recent, large, prospective, randomized clinical trials have found no difference in VAP or any other outcomes measures in comparing early (6-8 days) with late (13-15 days) tracheostomy in 419 patients or comparing early (4 days) with late (after 10 days) tracheostomy in 909 patients in the TracMan trial. Early tracheostomy should not be performed for VAP prevention but may be considered for other reasons, such as difficult airway and difficult-to-wean patients, particularly for patient comfort.

SUGGESTED READINGS

The Acute Respiratory Distress Syndrome Network: Ventilation with lower tidal volumes as compared with traditional tidal volumes for acute lung injury and the acute respiratory distress syndrome, *N Engl J Med* 342:1301–1308, 2000.

Briel M, Meade M, Mercat A, et al: Higher vs lower positive end-expiratory pressure in patients with acute lung injury and acute respiratory distress syndrome: systematic review and meta-analysis, *JAMA* 303(9):865–873, 2010.

Dickinson S, Park PK, Napolitano LM: Prone-positioning therapy in ARDS, *Crit Care Clin* 27(3):511–523, 2011.

Ferguson ND, Cook DJ, Guyatt GH, et al: High-frequency oscillation in early acute respiratory distress syndrome, *N Engl J Med* 2013.

Girard TD, Kress JP, Fuchs BD, et al: Efficacy and safety of a paired sedation and ventilator weaning protocol for mechanically ventilated patients in intensive care (Awakening and Breathing Controlled trial): a randomised controlled trial, *Lancet* 371(9607):126–134, 2008.

Hemmila MR, Napolitano LM: Severe respiratory failure: Advanced treatment options, *Crit Care Med* 34(Suppl 9):S278–S290, 2006.

Muscedere J, Dodek P, Keenan S, et al; VAP Guidelines Committee and the Canadian Critical Care Trials Group: comprehensive evidence-based clinical practice guidelines for ventilator-associated pneumonia: prevention, *J Crit Care* 23(1):126–137, 2008.

Napolitano LM, Park PK, Raghavendran K, et al: Nonventilatory strategies for patients with life-threatening 2009 H1N1 influenza and severe respiratory failure, *Crit Care Med* 38(4 Suppl):e74–90, 2010.

Nathens AB, Johnson JL, Minei JP, et al: Inflammation and the Host Response to Injury, a large-scale collaborative project: patient-Oriented Research Core—standard operating procedures for clinical care. I. Guidelines for mechanical ventilation of the trauma patient, *J Trauma* 59(3):764–769, 2005.

Park PK, Napolitano LM, Bartlett RH: Extracorporeal membrane oxygenation in adult acute respiratory distress syndrome, *Crit Care Clin* 27(3):627–646, 2011.

Raghavendran K, Napolitano LM: ALI and ARDS: challenges and advances, *Crit Care Clin* 27(3):xiii–xiv, 2011.

Raghavendran K, Napolitano LM: Definition of ALI/ARDS, *Crit Care Clin* 27(3):429–437, 2011.

Sachdev G, Napolitano LM: Postoperative pulmonary complications: pneumonia and acute respiratory failure, *Surg Clin North Am* 92(2):321–344, 2012.

Ware LB, Matthay MA: The acute respiratory distress syndrome, *N Engl J Med* 342(18):1334–1349, 2000.

Young D, Lamb SE, Shah S, et al: High-frequency oscillation for acute respiratory distress syndrome, *N Engl J Med* 2013.

VENTILATOR-ASSOCIATED PNEUMONIA

Amy Rushing, MD

INTRODUCTION

Pneumonia, the most common nosocomial infection, remains a postoperative complication that prolongs hospital stay and increases mortality. Clinicians categorize pneumonia into multiple subtypes: community-acquired pneumonia (CAP), hospital-acquired pneumonia (HAP), and ventilator-associated pneumonia (VAP). Each condition has its own group of common bacterial pathogens; the latter two share multidrug-resistant organisms. This chapter focuses on ventilator-associated pneumonia, defined as pneumonia that develops 48 hours after endotracheal intubation. The incidence of VAP ranges from 9% to 27%, with the rate of occurrence at 1% to 3% per ventilator day. The mortality rate approaches 50% depending on an individual patient's clinical circumstances. In spite of the evolving sophistication of critical care medicine, VAP can be difficult to diagnose, leading to a delay in treatment of a potentially fatal infection. This, in addition to the ongoing antimicrobial resistance that pervades the intensive care unit (ICU), warrants a review of how to recognize and treat VAP, with special attention to selecting appropriate empiric antibiotic therapy and tailoring subsequent therapy to available culture data. The latter task is particularly important in prevention of further spread of multidrug-resistant bacteria, such as methicillin-resistant *Staphylococcus aureus* (MRSA) and the gram-negative organisms, *Pseudomonas aeruginosa* and *Acinetobacter baumannii*.

DIAGNOSIS

Diagnosis of VAP in the intensive care unit remains a challenge for clinicians because the classic signs and symptoms are nonspecific in nature. At present, the only modality that provides an absolute diagnosis is a lung biopsy that shows microbial invasion with inflammatory changes. Because this procedure is invasive and carries a high risk of potential complications, intensivists rely alternatively on a combination of findings and clinical acumen to obtain a diagnosis. Patients with development of new onset hypoxia, purulent sputum, and fever with leukocytosis or infiltrates on chest radiograph should be evaluated for pneumonia. Some of these manifestations may occur with other conditions (acute lung injury, congestive heart failure, pulmonary embolus, and tracheobronchitis), so careful assessment of the patient with a high index of suspicion is important so as not to delay collecting cultures and starting empiric antibiotic therapy.

Culture collection remains a key element in the diagnosis and appropriate treatment of VAP. Some debate exists as to what method yields the most accurate microbiologic data that differentiate simple colonization from an actual infection. For some time, fiberoptic bronchoscopy with quantitative analysis of bronchoalveolar lavage (BAL) was thought to be one of the best techniques for diagnosis of pneumonia. Mueller and colleagues found that the preliminary culture results obtained from a BAL correlated well with final culture data when the quantitative threshold was defined as 10^5 cfu/mL or more. A separate study performed by Wood and colleagues compared this invasive technique with blind bronchial brushings and blind endotracheal aspirates and found no statistically significant differences in the reliability of culture data and each technique's ability to detect clinically relevant pathogens. The study's findings were substantiated by a Cochrane review that showed similar results where nonquantitative, transbronchial aspirates yielded similar results to quantitative, directed culture collection with similar clinical outcomes. With these data in mind, the clinician should consider patient tolerance for and patient comfort with a selected collection technique. The caveat to this concept is that directed quantitative cultures may be appropriate for patients who have already received antibiotic therapy during a prolonged ICU stay or who have immunosuppression.

With recognition of VAP as a diagnostic dilemma, Pugin and colleagues developed the Clinical Pulmonary Infection Score (CPIS) to aid clinicians in making a timely diagnosis. The score includes several clinical factors that can be determined at the bedside (Table 1). A CPIS of 6 or higher has been shown to predict significant pulmonary infection with a high sensitivity and specificity of 100% and 93%, respectively. The advantage of this system lies in the relative ease and rapidity of determining a score based on traditional signs and symptoms of VAP. CPIS has been endorsed by the American Thoracic Society and the Infectious Diseases Society of America as an aid to not only initiating empiric antibiotic therapy in patients with suspected VAP but also to determining initial clinical response to such therapy. Currently, a level I recommendation is that those patients who maintain a CPIS score of 6 or less after 72 hours of empiric

antibiotic therapy should be evaluated for early discontinuation of such therapy. Although there is validity to this scheme, some have shown that it carries a much lower specificity and sensitivity and may not apply to certain patient populations. Parks and colleagues recently studied the value of the CPIS among a trauma population and found that it was inconsistent in determining resolution of VAP based on the threshold score of 6 or less. Specifically, they found the sensitivity and specificity of CPIS were 72% and 53%, respectively, among trauma patients who contracted hospital-acquired pneumonia. This work cautions clinicians that CPIS, although a potentially useful aid for bedside diagnosis, may not apply to patients who have sustained significant chest trauma or subsequent hypoxemia from transfusion-related acute lung injury (TRALI).

TREATMENT

After the diagnosis of VAP is made, the next step lies in appropriate treatment of suspected organisms. Empiric antibiotic therapy is recommended to start as soon as VAP is clinically suspected, followed by rapid deescalation of therapy once the specific microorganism has been identified. Empiric therapy is determined based on the patient's ventilator length of stay (LOS). Patients who have had a ventilator LOS less than 4 days typically yield pathogens native to nasopharyngeal flora: methicillin-sensitive *S. aureus* (MSSA), *Haemophilus influenzae*, and *Streptococcus pneumoniae*. Late-onset VAP, defined as VAP that occurs in those with a ventilator LOS greater than 4 days, yields gram-negative and multidrug-resistant organisms: *P. aeruginosa*, *A. baumanii*, and *Stenotrophomonas maltophilia*. Representing approximately 25% of pathogens implicated in VAP, *S. aureus* remains the most common microorganism, with one half of the isolates expressing methicillin resistance. On the basis of these data, the American Thoracic Society published antibiotic recommendations for empiric treatment of VAP (Table 2). The initial treatment includes initiation of an antipseudomonal cephalosporin, carbapenem, or beta-lactam/beta-lactamase inhibitor in addition to an antipseudomonal fluoroquinolone or aminoglycoside and vancomycin or linezolid to cover MRSA. The combination of antibiotics should continue until a specific organism with its sensitivity has been identified or interval evaluation at 72 hours reveals a CPIS score of 6 or less.

Once the culpable pathogen has been identified, the duration of treatment can be determined. Historically, acceptable practice was treatment of VAP for 14 to 21 days. This concept, however, has changed with evidence that a shorter duration of antibiotic therapy provides ample treatment with less incidence of recurrent infection by multidrug-resistant organisms. A Cochrane review of studies

TABLE 1: Clinical pulmonary infection score

Diagnostic feature	0	1	2
Tracheal secretions	Rare	Abundant	Abundant and purulent
CXR infiltrate	None	Diffuse	Localized
Temperature (°C)	≥36.5 and ≤38.4	≥38.5 and ≤38.9	≥39.0 or ≤36.5
White blood cells (× 10^9/L)	≥4.0 and ≤11.0	<4.0 or >11.0	<4.0 or >11.0 + bands ≥0.5
PaO₂/FiO₂ (mm Hg)	>240 or ARDS	—	<240 or no ARDS

ARDS, Adult respiratory distress syndrome; *CXR*, chest x-ray; *PaO₂/FiO₂*, partial pressure of oxygen in arterial blood/fractional concentration of oxygen in inspired gas.
From Pugin J: Clinical signs and scores for the diagnosis of ventilator-associated pneumonia, Minerva Anestesiol 68:261-265, 2002.

TABLE 2: Empiric antibiotic therapy for ventilator-associated pneumonia

Early onset VAP defined as ventilator LOS <4 d	Ceftriaxone, fluoroquinolone, ampicillin-sulbactam, or ertapenem ± macrolide
Late onset VAP defined as ventilator LOS >4 d	Antipseudomonal cephalosporin or antipseudomonal carbapenem or beta-lactam/beta-lactamase inhibitor + antipseudomonal fluoroquinolone or aminoglycoside + linezolid or vancomycin

LOS, Length of stay; *VAP*, ventilator-associated pneumonia.
From American Thoracic Society and Infectious Diseases Society of America: Guidelines for the management of adults with hospital-acquired, ventilator-associated, and healthcare-associated pneumonia, Am J Respir Crit Care Med 171:389-416, 2005.

looking at 1700 patients found that a limited 7-day to 8-day course of directed antibiotic therapy resulted in an increased number of antibiotic-free days and decreased the incidence of recurrent VAP by multidrug-resistant organisms when compared with a longer 10-day to 15-day course. The exception to these findings was noted among patients who were diagnosed with VAP resulting from nonfermenting gram-negative bacilli (NF-GNB). This particular subset of patients had a greater recurrence of VAP after a shorter antibiotic course. Thus, patients with development of VAP as a result of NF-GNB likely benefit from a longer course of therapy up to 2 weeks in duration. This conclusion was further validated by Magnotti and colleagues when looking at antibiotic duration based on interval quantitative BAL. Surveillance culture data collected during directed antibiotic therapy revealed that longer treatment courses were required for *P. aeruginosa* and MRSA and *A. baumannii*. Thus, clinicians should not only consider the patient's clinical progress but also the isolated microorganism when determining the duration of VAP treatment.

One NF-GNB that has emerged as one of the most challenging pathogens in VAP is *A. baumannii*. In the last decade, *A. baumannii* has developed multidrug-resistant isolates that have limited therapeutic options. In particular, carbapenem-resistant strains have led to the treatment of this pathogen with second-line agents that include polymyxin E (colistin) and tigecycline, an antimicrobial initially approved for complicated intraabdominal and soft tissue infections. Multiple studies have examined the efficacy of these two drugs, specifically aerosolized regimens of colistin that limit its known nephrotoxicity. Arnold and colleagues examined the use of adjunctive aerosolized colistin in the treatment of multidrug-resistant *A. baumannii* and found patients had a survival advantage despite a greater severity of illness. Further studies are needed to develop novel approaches to treat *A. baumannii* pneumonia given that current therapeutic interventions are limited and this robust organism carries a more significant mortality risk compared with other nosocomial pathogens.

One other pathogen that warrants discussion is MRSA. As previously mentioned, it is the most common isolate in VAP and carries a significant morbidity and mortality. Currently, two primary antibiotic options exist for the treatment of MRSA VAP: vancomycin and linezolid. Several trials have compared clinical efficacy of these drugs, and overall, the results vary. A meta-analysis of seven randomized trials performed by Kalil and colleagues showed no significant difference in clinical cure rates between the two antibiotics. Linezolid was associated with an increased risk of thrombocytopenia and adverse gastrointestinal effects. A more recent randomized double-blind trial performed by Wunderink and colleagues showed greater eradication of MRSA pneumonia with linezolid compared with vancomycin based on clinical and microbiologic endpoints. In spite of these findings, they found no difference in all-cause 60-day mortality between the two groups. At present, the recommendation endorsed by the American Thoracic Society is that either antibiotic may be prescribed to treat MRSA pneumonia and the choice is ultimately made at the clinician's discretion.

SUMMARY

Although VAP is quite common in the ICU setting, it still remains a clinical challenge to diagnose and treat. A high index of suspicion should lead to early culture collection and initiation of empiric antibiotic therapy because early treatment reduces mortality. Considering the patient's hospital LOS and one's own institutional antibiogram, empiric therapy should cover potential multidrug-resistant organisms with plans to stop certain antibiotics once culture data have been elucidated. Careful management of broad-spectrum antibiotics helps to slow the evolution of multidrug-resistant pathogens, as does limiting the duration of treatment to a 7-day to 8-day course for organisms other than NF-GNB. Although *A. baumannii* and MRSA continue to pose serious risks to patients in the ICU, clinicians can help limit further development of multidrug-resistant pathogens by following evidence-based guidelines in antibiotic administration.

SUGGESTED READINGS

American Thoracic Society and Infectious Diseases Society of America: Guidelines for the management of adults with hospital-acquired, ventilator-associated, and healthcare-associated pneumonia, *Am J Respir Crit Care Med* 171:389–416, 2005.

American Thoracic Society: Hospital-acquired pneumonia in adults: diagnosis, assessment of severity, initial antimicrobial therapy, and preventive strategies (consensus statement), *Am J Respir Crit Care Med* 153:1711–1725, 1996.

Arnold HM, Sawyer AM, Kollef MH: Use of adjunctive aerosolized antimicrobial therapy in the treatment of Pseudomonas aeruginosa and Acinetobacter baumannii ventilator-associated pneumonia, *Resp Care* 57(8):1226–1233, 2012.

Bassetti M, Taramasso L, Roberto D, et al: Management of ventilator-associated pneumonia: epidemiology, diagnosis, and antimicrobial therapy, *Expert Rev Anti Infect Ther* 10(5):585, 2012.

Kalil AC, Murthy MH, Hermsen ED, et al: Linezolid versus vancomycin or teicoplanin for nosocomial pneumonia: a systematic review and meta-analysis, *Crit Care Med* 38:1802, 2010.

Magnotti LJ, Croce MA, Zarzaur BL, et al: Causative pathogen dictates optimal duration of antimicrobial therapy for ventilator-associated pneumonia in trauma patients, *J Am Coll Surg* 212(4):476–484, 2011.

Mueller EW, Wood GC, Kelley MS et al: The predictive value of preliminary bacterial colony counts from bronchoalveolar lavage in critically ill trauma patients, *Am Surg* 69(9):749–755, 2003.

Parks NA, Magnotti LJ, Weinberg JA, et al: Use of the clinical pulmonary infection score to guide therapy for ventilator-associated pneumonia risks antibiotic overexposure in patients with trauma, *J Trauma Acute Care Surg* 73(1):52–59, 2012.

Pugh R, Grant C, Cooke RPD, Dempsey G: Short-course versus prolonged-course antibiotic therapy for hospital-acquired pneumonia in critically-ill adults (review), *The Cochrane Collaboration* 2:1–25, 2012.

Pugin J, Auckenthaler R, Mili N, et al: Diagnosis of ventilator-associated pneumonia by bacteriologic analysis of bronchoscopic and nonbronchoscopic 'blind' bronchoalveolar lavage fluid, *Am Rev Respir Dis* 143:1121–1129, 1991.

Sachdev G, Napolitano L: Postoperative pulmonary complications: pneumonia and acute respiratory failure, *Surg Clin North Am* 92:321–344, 2012.

Wood AY, Davit AJ, Ciraulo DL, et al: A prospective assessment of diagnostic efficacy of blind bronchial brushings compared to bronchoscopic-assisted lavage, bronchoscope-directed brushings, and blind endotracheal aspirates in ventilator-associated pneumonia, *J Trauma* 55(5):825–834, 2003.

Wunderink RG, Niederman MS, Kollef MH, et al: Linezolid in methicillin-resistant Staphylococcus aureus nosocomial pneumonia: a randomized, controlled study, *Clin Infect Dis* 54:621, 2012.

EXTRACORPOREAL MEMBRANE OXYGENATION FOR RESPIRATORY FAILURE IN ADULTS

Robert J. Moraca, MD, and
George J. Magovern, MD

INTRODUCTION

Acute respiratory distress syndrome (ARDS), first described nearly in 1967, continues to be a major contributor to morbidity and mortality, as well as an important component of resource consumption, in the intensive care unit. The syndrome is the most serious manifestation of acute lung injury, which can develop from a wide range of direct pulmonary (aspiration, toxic inhalation, infection, near drowning) or extrapulmonary (disseminated sepsis, thoracic trauma, circulatory shock) sources. Ventilator management focuses on minimization of barotrauma and prevention of increasing levels of CO_2 retention. Standard ventilator strategies to limit development of pulmonary distention and promote recruitment of atelectatic alveoli include pressure-controlled ventilation, inverse-ratio ventilation, and low-frequency ventilation. Current mortality rates remain high and range between 40% and 100% in published reports, and the long-term pulmonary morbidity from ventilator-induced lung injury secondary to barotrauma is underreported. Veno-veno extracorporeal membrane oxygenation (VV ECMO) removes deoxygenated blood from the venous circulation, removes carbon dioxide, and oxygenates the blood and returns it to the right atrium and ventricle. Theoretically, VV ECMO is a logical approach to broker the competing problems of lung protection and effective gas exchange in ARDS because it separates these processes and allows control over the degree of native lung function. The use of VV ECMO has significantly increased since 2007 with the improvement in techniques and outcomes (Figure 1).

THE EXTRACORPOREAL MEMBRANE OXYGENATION SYSTEM

A typical ECMO system comprises a membrane oxygenator, heat exchanger, roller or centrifugal pump, circuit tubing, and catheters appropriate to the mode of access. A parallel circuit containing a second pump and oxygenator may be used to ensure efficient CO_2 removal at low-flow rates or to increase oxygenation at higher flow rates. In some systems a parallel circuit is included to minimize the effects of oxygenator complications and to facilitate oxygenator exchange. Heparin-bonded components are utilized where possible to decrease anticoagulation requirements and reduce the systemic inflammatory response to the circuit. Most systems maintain the circulating blood at normothermic temperatures, but slight hypothermia has been suggested to reduce oxygen consumption requirements with high metabolic demand or concern for cerebral injury.

Indications

VV ECMO should be considered in any adult patient suffering from acute onset and potentially reversible severe respiratory failure with significant hypoxia or hypercarbia despite maximal ventilator management. Although there are many causes of respiratory failure in adults, including pulmonary embolism, acute cardiogenic pulmonary edema, and hypercarbic respiratory failure, the most common etiology is ARDS. Although variations in the clinical definition of ARDS are common, the criteria established by the American-European Conference on ARDS are the accepted standard (Box 1). Several methods for grading the severity of ARDS have been developed, but the most commonly used is the Murray Score, which assesses four factors: extent of infiltration on chest film, degree of hypoxemia, level of positive end expiratory pressure (PEEP) required for oxygenation, and respiratory system compliance. A Murray Score of higher than 3 is generally accepted as an indication for consideration of VV ECMO in severe ARDS.

Contraindications

VV ECMO can be a life-saving tool for severe refractory respiratory failure when appropriate patients are selected. Absolute contraindications for VV ECMO include active intracranial hemorrhage, prolonged high pressure, FiO_2 ventilation greater than 10 days, metastatic malignancy with a short life expectancy, and severe baseline advanced respiratory failure without potential treatment options such as lung transplantation or lung volume reduction surgery. Premorbid conditions in patients considered for VV ECMO are very common, so each patient should be evaluated on a case-by-case basis, with attention to baseline function and comorbidities, duration of current illness, number of organ system failures, and overall prognosis. Young patients with few to no medical problems and isolated pulmonary system failure tend to have the best outcomes. In addition, daily multidisciplinary assessment for medical futility should be measured by the progression of illness, subsequent organ failure(s), and complications that may become a contraindication for continuing VV ECMO support.

Technique

The following are the well-accepted percutaneous approaches for the insertion of VV ECMO for respiratory failure:

1. Right femoral vein to the right internal jugular vein (Figure 2)
2. Right internal jugular vein and inferior vena cava (IVC) into right atrium with a three-port Avalon cannula (Maquet, Wayne, NJ) (Figure 3)

The goals of both of these approaches are to take deoxygenated blood from the IVC (see Figure 2) or IVC and superior vena cava (SVC) (see Figure 3), pass it through an oxygenator, and return it to the right atrium and right ventricle. Prior to placing VV ECMO, patients should have a central line in the left internal jugular or left subclavian vein as well as an arterial line. Telemetry monitoring during insertion is important, as multiple wires inserted into the right atrium in a hypoxic patient are prone to inducing arrhythmias. In the supine position, both groins to the knees bilaterally and the neck from the tragus to the sternal notch are prepped with an antiseptic. It is important to use sterile drapes that extend from the patient's feet to avoid contamination of the long wires used during insertion. It is our preference to access the right femoral vein, as the left femoral vein crosses behind the left common iliac artery, making insertion more difficult. Using ultrasound guidance, we identify and access both the right femoral vein and right internal jugular vein with a 0.038-inch × 210-cm guidewire and 0.038-inch × 100-cm guidewire, respectively. Once both wires, have been placed, a bolus 100 units/kg of heparin is given intravenously. The right internal jugular vein is serially dilated with 8F, 12F, and 16F dilators prior to insertion of 18F

ECLS Registry Report
International Summary
January, 2013

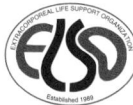

Extracorporeal Life Support Organization
2800 Plymouth Road
Building 300, Room 303
Ann Arbor, MI 48109

Overall Outcomes

	Total Patients	Survived ECLS		Survived to DC or Transfer	
Neonatal					
Respiratory	26205	22145	85%	19559	75%
Cardiac	4987	3058	61%	2010	40%
ECPR	851	540	63%	331	39%
Pediatric					
Respiratory	5656	3692	65%	3183	56%
Cardiac	6225	4034	65%	3054	49%
ECPR	1745	948	54%	708	41%
Adult					
Respiratory	3761	2400	64%	2084	55%
Cardiac	2884	1581	55%	1132	39%
ECPR	876	325	37%	241	28%
Total	53190	38723	73%	32302	61%

Centers

Centers by Year

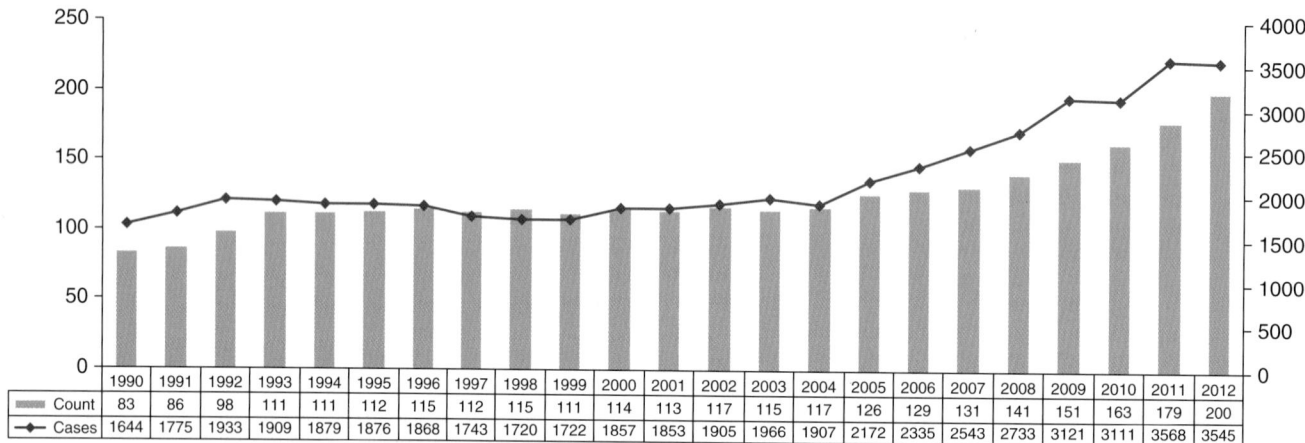

	1990	1991	1992	1993	1994	1995	1996	1997	1998	1999	2000	2001	2002	2003	2004	2005	2006	2007	2008	2009	2010	2011	2012
Count	83	86	98	111	111	112	115	112	115	111	114	113	117	115	117	126	129	131	141	151	163	179	200
Cases	1644	1775	1933	1909	1879	1876	1868	1743	1720	1722	1857	1853	1905	1966	1907	2172	2335	2543	2733	3121	3111	3568	3545

FIGURE I   ECLS Registry Report, International Summary.

BOX I: Criteria for acute respiratory distress syndrome

1. Acute onset
2. PaO_2/FiO_2 of less than 200 mm Hg
3. Bilateral infiltrates on chest radiography
4. Pulmonary capillary wedge pressure less than 18 mm Hg and no clinical evidence of left ventricular dysfunction

Fem-Flex II femoral arterial cannula (Edwards, Irvine, Calif). Once inserted, the wire and dilators are removed, and the cannula is clamped. Either simultaneously or sequentially, the right femoral vein, accessed with a 0.038-inch × 210-cm guidewire, is serially dilated with 8F, 12F, and 16F dilators prior to inserting the 24F Fem Trak multiport femoral venous cannula (Edwards, Irvine, Calif). The wire and dilators are removed, and the cannula is clamped. The long venous cannula is premeasured to have the metal tip lie just below the right costal margin in the IVC. The VV ECMO lines are then brought onto the field and connected to the circuit. It is critical to ensure that no air bubbles are in the tubing during connection. Communication with the perfusionist is paramount to ensure that the *inflow* from the patient to the circuit is the femoral cannula and the *outflow* with oxygenated blood into the patient is through the right internal jugular vein into the right atrium (see Figure 2). Cannulas are secured in position with zero silk sutures at the insertion point and Foley catheter holders along the leg and behind the ear onto the chest. Transient desaturation after the institution of VV ECMO commonly occurs due to the transfer of pump prime into the circulation and should resolve within 1 to 2 minutes. Most patients will flow between 3.5 and 5 L/min with 2200 to 2800 revolutions per minute. The maximum inflow flow negative pressures should not exceed −100 mm Hg, and the maximum outflow pressures should not exceed −150 mm Hg. Initial ECMO settings are the oxygenator at 100%, and the sweep is set at 4 L/min. A chest and abdominal

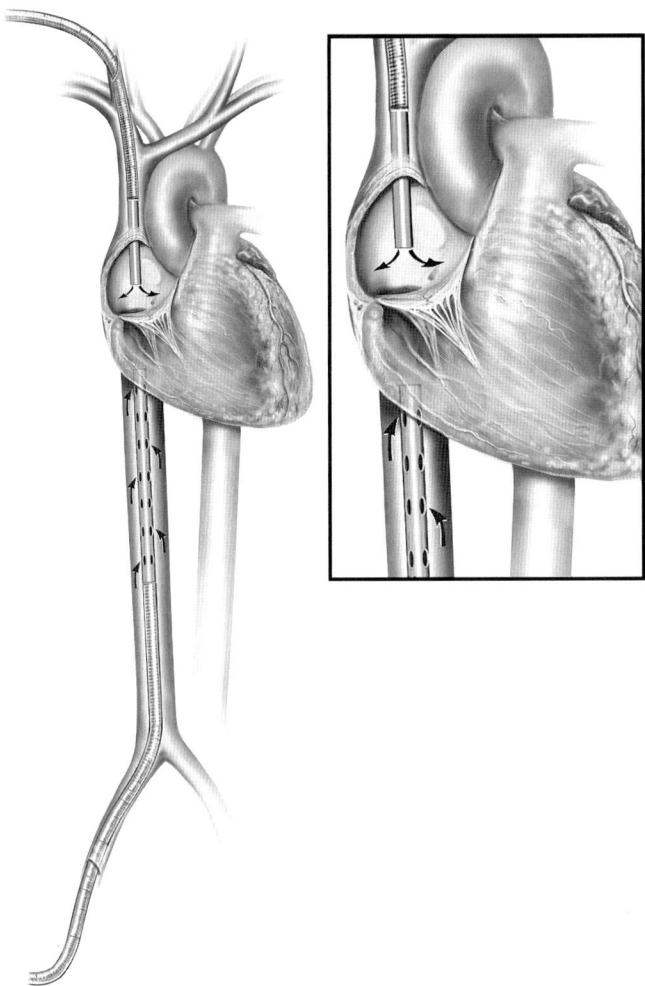

FIGURE 2 Right femoral venous to right internal jugular venous cannulation for veno-veno extracorporeal membrane oxygenation (ECMO). Inflow of deoxygenated blood through the inferior vena cava to the ECMO circuit, and the oxygenated blood is then returned into the right atrium.

radiograph are obtained to confirm cannula position, and a heparin infusion is begun to maintain partial thromboplastin time (PTT) between 40 and 50 seconds.

The Avalon cannula is a multiport single cannula placed in the right internal jugular vein with two ports: one for patient *inflow* from the IVC and SVC and the second for *outflow* from the right atrium (see Figure 3). Using ultrasound guidance, identify and access the right internal jugular artery with a 0.038-inch × 100-cm guidewire and serially dilated with 10F, 12F, and 16F dilators prior to inserting the cannula. It is imperative during insertion of the Avalon cannula that echocardiographic or fluoroscopic guidance is used to ensure that the introducer wire is in the IVC and not the right ventricle, as there have been several case reports of improper wire position and subsequent cannula insertion through the free wall of the right ventricle, with frequently fatal consequences. Once inserted, the wire and dilators are removed, and the cannula is clamped and connected to the VV ECMO circuit. The patient has *inflow* to the circuit from the IVC and SVC and *outflow* with oxygenated blood to the right atrium (see Figure 3). The cannula comes in multiple sizes ranging from 13F to 31F and should be selected based upon patient size and desired VV ECMO flow. The Avalon cannula has the advantage of an avoiding groin access with the rare potential for patient extubation and ambulation while on VV ECMO.

MANAGEMENT

A critical care nurse and an ECMO specialist (typically a perfusionist, respiratory therapist, or physician) should be assigned to provide 24-hour monitoring and care for the ECMO system and the patient on support. It is imperative that individual institutions develop their own protocols and certification of the team, including nurses, critical care physicians, and surgeons for ECMO circuit management.

Ventilator Management

The goal of VV ECMO is to minimize both barotrauma from hyperinflation and high airway pressure and to limit pulmonary oxygen toxicity. Following stabilization on VV ECMO, we typically set ventilators to assist control, tidal volume (TV) of 4 to 6 cc/kg, a maximum peak inspiratory pressure (PIP) of 30 cm H_2O, and a PEEP of 5 cm H_2O, oxygenation set at 100%, with a ventilator rate of 10. The ventilator FiO_2 is then weaned to maintain a PaO_2 greater than 60. In some circumstances, when the respiratory failure is severe, we will use pressure control ventilation. Baseline lung compliance is calculated (Compliance = TV/PIP-PEEP) and then measured daily to assess improvements in the respiratory system. VV ECMO flow rates are titrated to produce venous blood saturation of 80% to 85% and arterial saturation of greater than 90%. To optimize the oxygenation-carrying capacity in patients, we maintain hemoglobin greater than 10 to 12 g/dL. The sweep gas flow rate is adjusted to produce pCO_2 at 40 mm Hg. Patients with primary hypercarbic respiratory failure are maintained on low-flow ECMO (15-30 mL/kg/min) to effect carbon dioxide removal while providing maximum lung rest. It is our practice to wean the ventilator to normal settings and achieve a compliance of greater than 50 prior to VV ECMO weaning.

Systemic Anticoagulation

Systemic anticoagulation is maintained with continuous infusion of heparin to produce PTT of 40 to 50 seconds to reduce aggregation on the VV ECMO tubing and deposition on the membrane oxygenator. Aggressive correction of coagulopathy and prompt surgical response to bleeding sites can reduce bleeding complications to manageable levels in most patients. In patients with refractory bleeding and other contraindications for anticoagulation, we have successfully managed VV ECMO patients without anticoagulation.

Sedatives and Analgesia

The use of sedation and paralysis is based on patient requirements. In situations where agitation significantly elevates O_2 demand and movement impairs ventilation, reduces venous return, or risks accidental decannulation, both may be needed. Clinical assessments of sedation are made every 4 hours and documented, and sedation is adjusted as indicated. It has been our experience that significantly higher doses of sedation are needed due to reduced drug bioavailability from sequestration in the circuit, interaction with the PVC tubing, and loss of blood volume from the VV ECMO prime. Standard critical care protocols of daily sedation weaning are important to limit the prolonged use of high sedatives and especially paralytics in the ICU, which can have deleterious consequences.

Renal

An attempt should be made to aggressively diurese the patient to dry weight or less to reduce and minimize the interstitial edema. In situations where renal function is compromised, the early use of continuous veno-veno hemofiltration (CVVH) is utilized to remove volume. This will help to reduce overall body edema and improve pulmonary compliance to facilitate lung recovery and VV ECMO weaning.

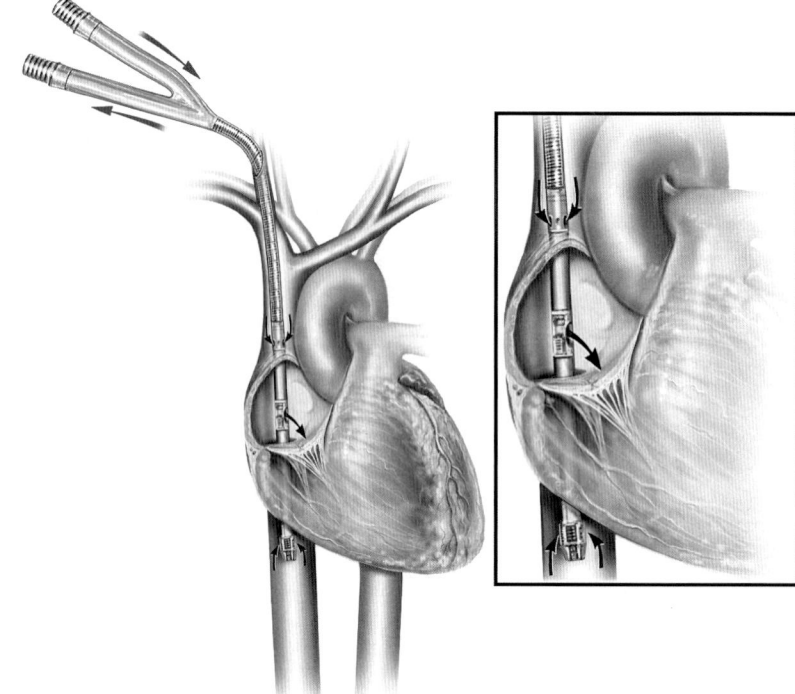

FIGURE 3 Avalon cannulation for veno-veno extracorporeal membrane oxygenation (ECMO). Inflow of deoxygenated blood through the inferior vena cava and the right internal jugular vein to the ECMO circuit, and the oxygenated blood is then returned into the right atrium.

Infection

Prophylactic antibiotics are given prior to insertion and discontinued within 24 hours, with further antibiotic or antifungal therapy directed to the underlying infectious illness. White blood cell count, C-reactive protein, and systemic vascular resistance are good predictors of ongoing infection. However, temperature may be unreliable while on VV ECMO because a significant amount of passive cooling occurs. Therefore, cultures are routinely performed while on VV ECMO. Activated protein C has a demonstrated survival benefit in severe sepsis, but its use with VV ECMO poses a serious bleeding risk.

TROUBLESHOOTING THE ECMO

Recirculation

Recirculation is a phenomenon that occurs when the inflow and outflow cannulas are too close together. Although not inherently dangerous, it reduces the efficiency of the VV ECMO circuit and may be a cause for persistent hypoxia. This can be assessed by visually examining the cannulas for appropriate color differential (the *inflow* to the circuit should be dark red and the *outflow* back to the patient should be bright red) and radiographic location of the cannulas (the metal tip of the femoral venous cannula on chest x-ray should be below the diaphragm). In addition, the PaO_2 of the *inflow* cannula should not be higher than the systemic PaO_2. When this does occur, repositioning the cannulas farther apart will solve the problem.

Superior Vena Cava Syndrome

SVC syndrome can occur in patients on VV ECMO due to mechanical obstruction of the SVC, typically with the right internal jugular VV ECMO cannula. It may occur rapidly after insertion or insidiously over the first several hours. Once it occurs, it is best managed

by downsizing and exchanging the SVC cannula. Manipulation of the patient position to head-up is only a temporary measure. SVC syndrome is typically seen in smaller patients with a body surface area (BSA) less than 1.6 and in patients with significant hardware already lying in the SVC (pacemaker leads, indwelling dialysis catheters). It is important to obtain an echocardiogram and chest x-ray to ensure that cardiac misadventure with subsequent tamponade or pneumothorax is not the etiology.

Persistent Hypoxia

Some patients with severe respiratory failure may require maximal ventilator support in addition to maximal VV ECMO support for several days to weeks before any sign of recovery is seen. After ensuring proper ventilator and oxygenator function, strategies to address persistent hypoxia include systemic cooling to 33° F (to reduce metabolic demand), increasing hemoglobin to greater than 14 g/dL, and adding a second oxygenator in parallel.

Hemolysis

Heparin-bonded circuits and centrifugal pumps have greatly reduced the incidence of hemolysis to approximately 6% of patients, as reported in registry data. This complication is manifested by refractory anemia and elevated bilirubin and confirmed by elevated serum plasma free hemoglobin, lactate dehydrogenase, and decreased haptoglobin.

Thrombocytopenia

Thombocytopenia is a common problem with VV ECMO and is rarely caused by heparin-induced thrombocytopenia (HIT). Unless documented on serotonin release assay, direct thrombin inhibitors

International summary — January 2013

Adult respiratory runs by diagnosis

	Total runs	Avg run time	Longest run time	Survived	% Survived
Viral pneumonia	152	282	1357	100	66%
Bacterial pneumonia	644	240	1973	393	61%
Aspiration pneumonia	92	195	1663	58	63%
ARDS, postop/trauma	277	245	1656	151	55%
ARDS, not postop/trauma	452	302	5014	224	50%
Acute resp failure, non-ARDS	317	223	1317	167	53%
Other	1924	213	3018	1031	54%

Run time in hours. Survived = survival to discharge or transfer based on number of runs

Adult respiratory support mode

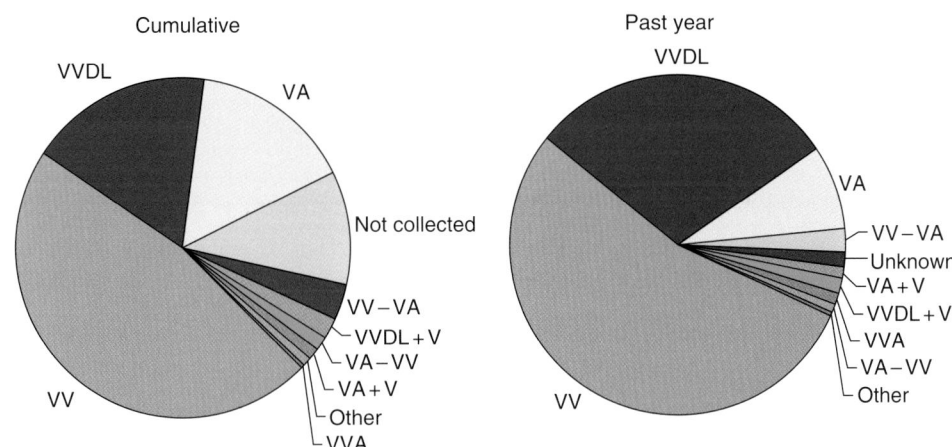

Adult respiratory support mode details

	Total runs	Avg run time	Longest run time	Survived	% Survived
VV	1813	235	5014	1062	59%
VVDL	679	245	2245	451	66%
VA	601	164	2554	253	42%
Not collected	418	226	1357	210	50%
VV–VA	135	444	3018	37	27%
VVDL+V	74	312	990	51	69%
VA–VV	47	288	976	23	49%
VA+V	45	169	1200	20	44%
Other	33	209	791	16	48%
VVA	13	331	888	1	8%

Run time in hours. Survived = survival to discharge or transfer based on number of runs

FIGURE 4 Etiologies for acute respiratory distress syndrome requiring veno-veno extracorporeal membrane oxygenation.

are not routinely used. Patients with bleeding complications or persistent thrombocytopenia may be managed safely without heparin. Platelets are transfused as necessary to maintain the platelet count at higher than 25,000.

WEANING AND LUNG RECOVERY

The return of lung function is signaled by improving PaO_2 with the ability to wean the ventilator FiO_2, improving lung compliance, and reducing peak airway pressures. The ventilator is set to a TV of 7 to 8 cc/kg with PIP less than 35 mm Hg and a FiO_2 less than 60%. Then VV ECMO FiO_2 is weaned slowly over several days to maintain a systemic PaO_2 greater than 70. The FiO_2 of 21% is maintained for 24

hours with PaO_2 greater than 70, the heparin infusion is stopped, and the VV ECMO cannulas are clamped and removed at the bedside. Hemostasis is achieved with direct pressure for at least 30 to 45 minutes. In our experience, open surgical repair of the venous access site is rarely needed, even in cannulas that have been in for 4 to 6 weeks. The patient is maintained on the ventilator until a standard ventilator weaning process is instituted.

DISCUSSION

ECMO was first used successfully over 30 years ago and has become the standard of care for refractory respiratory failure in neonates and older children. Adult ARDS carries a mortality rate that can approach

100% in patients who are failing conventional treatment, and the care of these patients is expensive and resource intensive. Theoretically, VV ECMO support melds well with the needs of the ARDS patient: it provides excellent CO_2 removal, while reducing barotrauma and oxygenation demands on the potentially recoverable native lung. ECMO support is associated with significant comorbidity, particularly related to anticoagulation and bleeding, but these complications are usually manageable and occur at a rate that can be reconciled with the high mortality seen in untreated patients.

Etiologies for ARDS requiring VV ECMO are quite diverse (Figure 4). VV ECMO is rarely evaluated in a cohort consistent for diagnosis because these niche populations are usually too small for timely recruitment. Nevertheless, over the last decade, survival to discharge following VV ECMO appears to be stabilizing at around 50% for patients with respiratory failure without concomitant cardiac failure (see Figure 1). This appears to be related to the development of improved oxygenators and cannulas and the use of veno-veno rather than veno-arterial cannulation when cardiac support is not necessary. Use of heparin-bonded components in the ECMO circuit has not eliminated serious bleeding but has reduced the level of heparin infusion required to maintain an acceptable anticoagulation status.

Recognition of the role of ventilator-induced barotrauma in limiting the efficacy of mechanical ventilation has led to the development of less traumatic ventilator management approaches such as pressure-controlled and inverse-ratio ventilation. When used as a component of a standardized protocol, these methods can increase the number of patients who recover without transition to ECMO support and may also increase the recovery potential of the native lung in patients who progress to ECMO.

In summary, although the results of a robust randomized clinical trial in a well-defined patient population are awaited, there is evidence that VV ECMO can increase survival in patients with ARDS refractory to conventional therapy. Use of this technique, however, is appropriate only in conjunction with a well-constructed respiratory management protocol that is initiated at the time of ARDS diagnosis.

SUGGESTED READINGS

Bartlett RH, Roloff DW, Custer JR, et al: Extracorporeal life support: the University of Michigan experience, *JAMA* 283:904, 2000.

ECMO Extracoporeal Cardiopulmonary Support in Critical Care 4th Edition. In Annich GM, Lynch WR, MacLaren G, et al, editors: 2012, Extracorporeal Life Support Organization (ELSO).

Kolla S, Awad SS, Rich PB, et al: Extracorporeal life support for 100 adult patients with severe respiratory failure, *Ann Surg* 226:544, 1997.

Magovern GJ Jr, Simpson KA: Extracorporeal life support following open-heart surgery. In Zwischenberger JB, Steinhorn RH, Bartlett RH editors: *ECMO: Extracorporeal cardiopulmonary support in critical care*, ed 2, 2000, Extracorporeal Life Support Organization (ELSO).

TRACHEOSTOMY

William D. Tobler, Jr., MD, and
Suresh "Mitu" Agarwal, MD

INTRODUCTION

Tracheostomy is a commonly performed procedure by trauma/critical care surgeons, otolaryngologists, and pulmonologists. The term *tracheostomy* and *tracheotomy* are often used interchangeably. However, *tracheostomy* denotes the formation of a stoma, whereas *tracheotomy* defines the act of creating an opening in the trachea.

The first reports of open tracheostomies date back to Egypt circa 3600 BC, with the first elective procedures described by Asclepiades of Bithynia in 124 AD. Modern-day procedures were not specified until Chevalier Jackson provided a detailed description in 1909. In particular, he emphasized a long incision, good exposure, division of the thyroid isthmus, and avoidance of an incision near the first and second tracheal rings. Since that time, the advent of respiratory ventilators and further advances in the medical care of critically ill patients have increased the incidence of those undergoing tracheostomy.

In the 1980s, Pasquale Ciaglia popularized the percutaneous tracheostomy, which was first described in 1957. This technique is an alternative approach performed via sequential dilatation. This can be readily performed at the bedside, which prevents risks associated with transporting patients and concomitantly limits resources required to run an operating room.

INDICATIONS AND CONTRAINDICATIONS

The indications to perform a tracheostomy are many but include most commonly ventilator dependence, followed by airway obstruction, and to assist with pulmonary toilet (Table 1). The two absolute contraindications to performing a tracheostomy are a significant skin or soft tissue infection and conditions leading to distorted anatomy.

Timing

The appropriate timing to perform a tracheostomy remains an issue of debate. Some advocate performing a tracheostomy after 3 days of intubation, while others support waiting up to 3 weeks of ventilator dependence. When deciding to perform a tracheostomy, the most important, yet often most challenging, factor to determine is the expected length of time a patient will require ventilator support. The advantages of a stoma include improved patient comfort, decreased nursing care, lessened oropharyngeal ulceration, and better patient communication. Tracheostomy has also been shown to decrease the need for ventilator dependence in certain patient populations. In contrast, prolonged laryngeal intubation increases the risk of subglottic stenosis and should be avoided. At this current time there are no large prospective randomized trials that show improved long-term outcomes with early tracheostomy. The authors recommend performing tracheostomy within 7 days when the need for ventilator support is expected to be greater than 2 weeks.

TABLE I: Indications for tracheostomy or cricothyroidotomy

Ventilator dependence	Facilitation of ventilation support Prolonged intubation
Airway obstruction	Anatomic abnormalities Angioedema Burns Failed intubation Infection leading to obstruction Laryngeal dysfunction Neck irradiation Neoplasm Neurologic dysfunction or injury Obstructive sleep apnea Postoperative Traumatic obstruction
Pulmonary toilet	Aspiration Excessive bronchopulmonary secretions

Open Tracheostomy

Elective open tracheostomies are usually performed under general anesthesia, but they can be completed with local anesthesia if a patient cannot be intubated. This is executed in the operating room under most circumstances but can also be performed safely at the bedside if adequate resources are available. When performed in the intensive care unit, the surgeon should make every effort to replicate the utilities of an operating room such as appropriate lighting, an open tracheostomy tray, and electrocautery.

The patient is placed in the supine position, and a shoulder roll is utilized for neck extension if cervical immobilization is not an issue. Next, the patient is prepped and draped from the nipple line to above the thyroid cartilage. Some advocate prepping inferiorly to below the xiphoid in preparation for the unlikely scenario of an emergent sternotomy. A 3-cm horizontal incision is made using a scalpel 2 cm above the sternal notch. A horizontal incision is recommended in elective cases because it follows Langer's lines and leaves a cosmetically appealing incision after decannulation. A vertical incision can also be performed, which transverses tension lines but also avoids injury to the anterior jugular veins. After incision, the subcutaneous tissue and platysma muscle are dissected bluntly with electrocautery. The sternohyoid and sternothyroid muscles are then encountered and retracted laterally with an incision made vertically through the linea alba. The next structure deep to the strap muscles is the thyroid isthmus. This can either be ligated using electrocautery or suture ligation. Once the thyroid isthmus is retracted, the pretracheal fascia should be cleared using sharp dissection. At this time, the important landmarks of the airway should be identified. Superiorly, the cricoid cartilage provides a marker for the first tracheal ring, which lies immediately caudad.

A cricoid hook is then employed to elevate the tracheal rings. Using a #11 blade, the surgeon makes a horizontal incision between the second and third tracheal rings. Placement superior to this increases the risk of subglottic stenosis, whereas inferior placement increases the risk for tracheoinominate fistula formation. Per surgeon preference, stay sutures can be placed on each ring above and below the incision. These allow identification of the tracheotomy in the event of an unanticipated decannulation. Similarly, a Bjork flap can be created by an H-type incision in the trachea and subsequently suturing the inferior tracheal mucosa to the skin. This flap is rarely

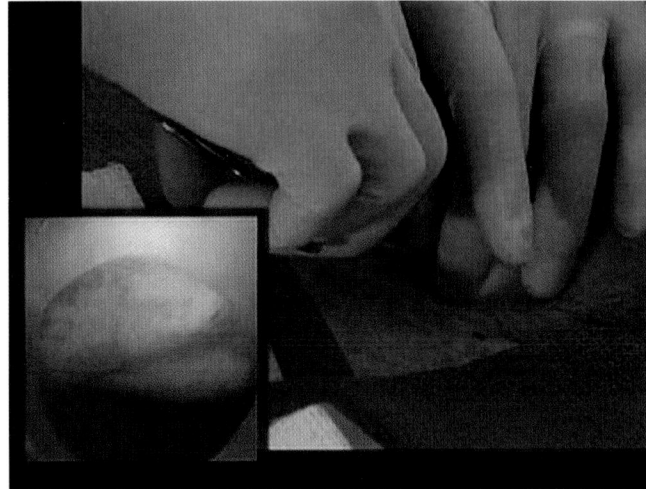

FIGURE I Palpation of the tracheal wall is visualized bronchoscopically to identify optimal placement.

created because it has been seen to result in delayed cutaneous closure of the stoma after decannulation.

At this point, the anesthesiologist retracts the endotracheal tube, and a Trousseau dilator is used to open the tracheal incision. The surgeon then places the tracheostomy into the airway under direct visualization. The cuff is inflated, and the ventilator is connected to the tracheostomy cannula. Similar to intubation, proper placement is verified by chest rise, bilateral breath sounds, and CO_2 confirmation. Lastly, the four corners of the tracheostomy neck plate are secured using 3-0 prolene sutures, and a tracheostomy tube tie is placed.

Percutaneous Dilatational Tracheostomy

Percutaneous dilatational tracheostomy utilizes the Seldinger technique to perform a minimally invasive approach that can be easily performed at the bedside. This requires two trained physicians: one who performs the tracheostomy and one who does a simultaneous bronchoscopy. The procedure is safe and successful, but an open tracheostomy kit should always be available at the bedside.

The patient is positioned, prepped, and draped as mentioned above for the open technique. The surgeon at the head of the bed performs a continuous bronchoscopy to visualize the airway and endotracheal (ET) tube placement (Figure 1). Occasionally, the ET tube needs to be retracted a few centimeters. A 1.5-cm incision is then made in the skin 2 cm above the sternal notch. Blunt dissection is performed through the subcutaneous tissue. The bronchoscope is then used for transcutaneous illumination to verify anticipated placement of the tracheostomy. At this point, a 14-gauge needle is inserted through anterior tracheal tissue into the tracheal lumen after the endotracheal tube has been pulled back to the level of the vocal cords (Figure 2). Once visualization of the needle is confirmed in the airway by bronchoscopy, a guidewire is placed through the catheter inferiorly toward the carina (Figure 3). The insertion needle is removed over the guidewire, and a series of well-lubricated dilators are passed to create a sufficient tracheotomy. There are several modifications of this system ranging from one tapered dilator to a series of multiple graduated dilatations (Figure 4). Recently a technique that allows for balloon dilatation of the trachea has been developed. Once adequate dilation is performed, the tracheostomy tube is threaded over the dilator and into the airway under direct visualization (Figure 5). Next, the bronchoscope is cannulated into the tracheostomy to confirm placement of the tracheostomy tip in the airway 3 to 5 cm above the carina. Once this is achieved,

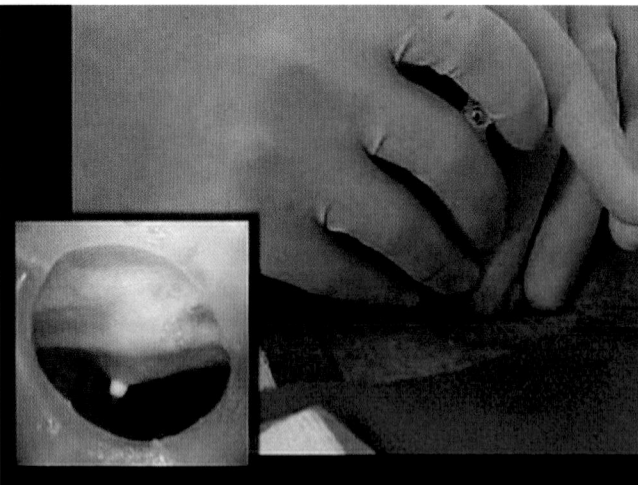

FIGURE 2 A 14-gauge angiocatheter is introduced into the tracheal lumen to place a guidewire.

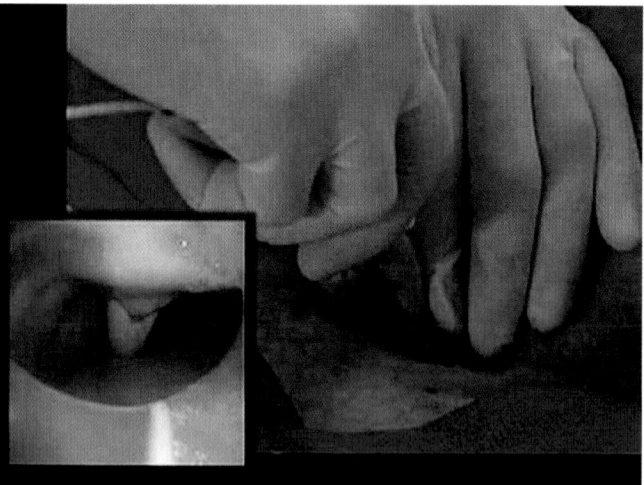

FIGURE 4 After a small punch is used to facilitate dilation, a single tapered dilator is introduced over the guidewire until the stoma is dilated to an aperture of 36 French.

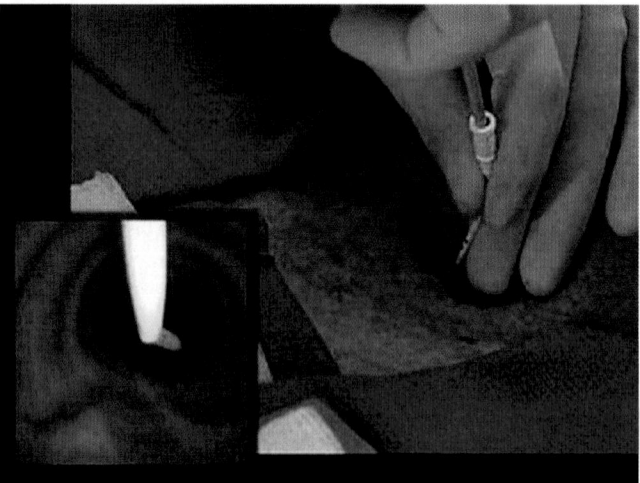

FIGURE 3 A guidewire is passed through the angiocatheter, and the angiocatheter is removed.

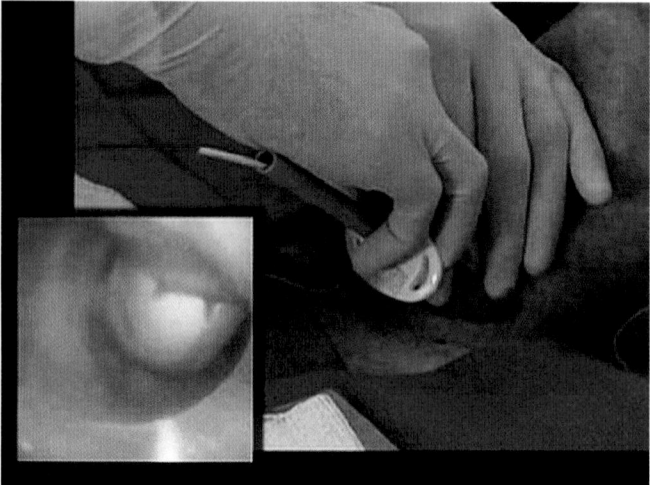

FIGURE 5 The tracheostomy tube is inserted over the guidewire.

the ventilator is connected and the ET tube is removed. A formal bronchoscopy may be necessary to remove blood, secretions, or debris. Tracheostomy placement is then confirmed and secured as described above.

Emergent Cricothyroidotomy

In the event that an airway must be obtained immediately and ET tube intubation has failed, an emergent cricothyroidotomy should be performed. In this situation, the cricothyroid membrane is identified between the thyroid and the cricoid cartilage. A scalpel is used to make a generous incision superficial to this area in a vertical fashion to avoid the anterior jugular veins. The soft tissue is then bluntly dissected. Once the cricothyroid membrane is identified, a horizontal incision is made through the membrane into the airway lumen. The back handle of the scalpel can assist to circumferentially dilate the opening. Once this is achieved, a tracheostomy tube or ET tube is placed directly into the airway. Confirmation is obtained by the measures stated above and the airway is secured with sutures. This is only a temporary measure if airway protection is still indicated. A formal conversion to tracheostomy should be performed once the patient has stabilized. Emergent tracheostomy is more difficult than

cricothyroidotomy and should only be performed if the cricothyroidotomy will worsen the patient's condition (i.e., laryngeal fracture). See Figure 4 in the chapter on "Airway Management in the Trauma Patient."

Complications

Complications of tracheostomy are divided into early and late subsets. In the past, routine postoperative chest x-ray was recommended for surveillance, but this has largely been abandoned. Currently, chest x-ray is only indicated after technically difficult procedures or if the patient experiences clinical deterioration unresponsive to ventilator modification.

Early Complications

Early complications encompass intraoperative and postoperative complications that occur within 7 days. These include hemorrhage, pneumothorax, pneumomediastinum, subcutaneous emphysema, infection, airway fire, loss of airway (accidental decannulation), and airway obstruction. Postoperative bleeding and pneumothorax are the most common early complications.

In order to avoid hemorrhage, all patients should have corrected coagulopathy before proceeding with tracheostomy. Minor bleeding occurs more frequently and is usually self-limited. If more substantial bleeding is encountered, then packing of the wound with hemostatic agents or suture ligation of superficial sources should be performed. The sources of this bleeding are most frequently from the skin incision, anterior jugular veins, thyroid isthmus, or thyroid ima artery. In the event that uncontrollable hemorrhage is encountered, the patient needs to be taken back to the operating room for a tracheostomy revision.

Pneumothorax can occur if the dome of the parietal pleura is penetrated. This can be managed by observation if the pneumothorax is small and the patient does not have respiratory failure. However, a chest tube thoracostomy will need to be inserted if the patient experiences acute respiratory failure or significant pneumothorax on chest x-ray. Pneumomediastinum and subcutaneous air usually resolve without intervention but should be monitored for improvement.

The remaining early complications occur infrequently. Avoiding electrocautery once the trachea is entered prevents airway fire. In the event of an airway fire, the procedure should be stopped and the ET tube replaced. Lastly, when the airway is compromised or obstructed, the source should be identified quickly. Airway obstruction often occurs from mucus plugging of the tracheostomy and malposition of the tube against the tracheal wall. Therefore, continued nursing care and caution when manipulating the tracheostomy are postoperative priorities. After accidental decannulation, the tracheostomy tube can be replaced through the stoma if the tract has epithelialized. However, if this proves difficult, then replacement through the stoma should be abandoned because of impending respiratory failure and the creation of false passages. The safest measure to take when dealing with airway compromise after decannulation or obstruction is to perform an oral-laryngeal reintubation.

Late Complications

Late complications occur after 7 days. These include laryngotracheal stenosis, fistula (tracheoinnominate and tracheoesophageal) formation, delayed stoma closure, tracheomalacia, and rarely vocal cord paralysis. Laryngotracheal stenosis results from infection and chondritis of the tracheal wall, leading to granulation tissue formation. This can be prevented by limiting incision size during the initial operation and postoperative tracheostomy care to prevent local infection and maintaining cuff pressures of less than 25 mm Hg. Stenosis can be treated with tracheal dilatation or surgical resection.

Fistula formation is a dreaded complication of tracheostomy placement. Tracheoinnominate fistula occurs by erosion of the tracheostomy tip through the tracheal wall and into the artery. Placing the tracheostomy above the fourth tracheal ring prevents this. If this complication is suspected, immediate pressure should be applied to the area, which can be achieved by hyperinflation of the cuff or by placing a finger directly through the skin incision inferiorly to compress the vessel against the sternum. Definitive repair needs to be performed in the operating room, but mortality remains extremely high. In addition, tracheoesophageal fistula occurs from direct injury to the posterior tracheal wall during the initial procedure or from erosion of the tracheostomy tube posteriorly. This can be stented but likely will require definitive operative repair.

The remaining complications are uncommon. Tracheomalacia and delayed stoma closure are the result of wound healing issues. Tracheomalacia occurs from ischemic insult to the tracheal wall and may require tracheoplasty if conservative measures fail. Delayed stoma closures occur when a patient has been decannulated after a prolonged period of time. If this is encountered, the tract can be surgically excised and closed primarily.

Tracheostomy Types, Postoperative Care, and Decannulation

In order to place a tracheostomy and take care of them in the postoperative period, it is important to know the various types of tracheostomy tubes because they come in various sizes and shapes. Today, most tracheostomies are made from synthetic plastic material, but in the past, they were made of metal. Initially, an 8-mm inner diameter tube with an 89-mm length should be inserted if patient anatomy permits. This allows for an open airway with minimal resistance and can be easily downsized when appropriate. Ideally the tip of the tube should be in the middle of the tracheal lumen 3 to 5 cm above the carina. Obese patients or patients with a longer neck may require an extended-length tube to prevent obstruction against the tracheal wall. Most tracheostomies are supplied with an inner cannula, which allows for easy removal in the event of mucus plugging or to block fenestrations before a patient is ready. Fenestrations are holes located on the tube of some tracheostomies. These allow air to pass around the tube in order to permit phonation. Because this affects air delivery to the lungs, patients should only have fenestrated tubes when stable and showing improvement in respiratory status. The last significant variable is the tracheostomy cuff. The cuff is an inflatable balloon that secures the tube within the airway, allows for positive pressure ventilation, and may prevent aspiration. Cuffs can cause necrosis of the surrounding tracheal wall, but this occurs less frequently when cuff pressure is less than 25 mm Hg. Once a patient is stable and respiratory status is improving, it is recommended to switch to an uncuffed tracheostomy tube.

In the postoperative period it is important to maintain a patent and clean tracheostomy with frequent nursing care. Suctioning can help decrease secretions, but there is a fine line between too much suctioning because this can cause trauma to the airway. Inner cannulas should be removed daily and cleaned, and the airway should be assessed for patency. The surrounding surgical site should also remain clean to prevent infection.

Patients can be considered ready for decannulation when safely off the ventilator for at least 48 hours and there are no future anticipated indications to be placed back on the ventilator. In addition, a patient must have few secretions before decannulation can proceed. Decannulation can occur at any time with any size tracheostomy. However, the usual course is to downsize the tracheostomy and trial a capped period of 24 to 48 hours. Downsizing and tracheostomy exchange can safely be performed after a stoma track is well formed—usually 7 to 10 days after the initial procedure.

SUMMARY

Tracheostomy is a common procedure, and the principles of placement and care should be in the armamentarium of any surgeon taking care of critically ill patients. Open and percutaneous tracheostomies have associated benefits and risks, so the performing surgeon should decide which to perform on a patient-by-patient basis. Tracheostomy is a safe procedure, but it has its own complications. Understanding the etiology of each complication will allow the surgeon to prevent their occurrences.

SUGGESTED READINGS

Cabrini L, Monti G, Landoni G, et al: Percutaneous tracheostomy, a systematic review, *Acta Anaesthesiol Scan* 56(3):270–281, 2012.
De Leyn P, Bedert L, Elcroix M, et al: Tracheotomy: clinical review and guidelines, *Eur J Cardiothorac Surg* 32(3):412–421, 2007.
Halum SL, ting JY, Plowman EK, et al: A multi-institutional analysis of tracheostomy complications, *Laryngoscope* 122(1):38–45, 2012.
Tobler WD Jr, Mella JR, Ng J, et al: Chest X-ray after tracheostomy is not necessary unless clinically indicated, *World J Surg* 36(2):266–269, 2012.

ACUTE KIDNEY FAILURE

Kenneth Waxman, MD, FACS

OVERVIEW

Alterations in renal function are common after surgical emergencies, trauma, and major operations. In these settings, successful recovery of renal function is dependent on prompt diagnosis and protective management strategies.

Acute kidney injury (AKI) is characterized by an acute decrease in glomerular filtration rate (GFR). The true incidence of AKI and acute renal failure (ARF) has been difficult to define, given the broad and various definitions used to quantify and study altered renal function. Relatively recent introduction of consensus definitions, such as RIFLE (risk, failure, loss, and end-stage renal failure) criteria and AKIN (Acute Kidney Injury Network) staging, have provided standard definitions to facilitate more uniform outcome reporting. With use of these definitions, recent studies suggest that AKI occurs in up to two thirds of patients in the intensive care unit (ICU). Moreover, increasing severity of AKI is associated with increasing mortality. AKI is also associated with increased morbidity, such as increased hospital length of stay and cost of care, and has been linked to other in-hospital complications, such as increased difficulty in weaning from mechanical ventilation. Preoperative risk factors for development of AKI include older age, emergent surgery, hepatic disease, obesity, high-risk surgery, vascular disease, and chronic obstructive pulmonary disease (COPD). Prompt recognition of AKI facilitates effective treatment. Although the incidence rate of AKI appears to be rising, overall outcomes from AKI are gradually improving.

DEFINITIONS

The RIFLE criteria (Table 1), defined in 2004 by the Acute Dialysis Quality Initiative (ADQI) Group, quantifies the severity of AKI. Studies by Hoste and colleagues and by Osterman and Chang found that mortality progressively increased with increasing RIFLE severity and that patients in all of the RIFLE classifications had higher mortality rates than those in the ICU without AKI.

In 2005, the AKIN also formulated consensus diagnostic criteria for AKI (Table 2). The AKIN definition of AKI is "an abrupt (within 48 hours) reduction in kidney function currently defined as an absolute increase in serum creatinine of either ≥0.3 mg/dL or a percentage increase of ≥50% (1.5-fold from baseline) or a reduction in urine output (documented oliguria of <0.5 mL/kg/hr for >6hrs)." These criteria can only be applied in the face of adequate fluid hydration. The AKIN staging system is arguably more inclusive than the RIFLE criteria. Chertow and associates found that an acute absolute change in creatinine of 0.3 or more was associated with increased mortality, length of stay, and cost of care. Barrantes and colleagues found that patients who met the AKIN definition of AKI were three times as likely to die during hospitalization.

In 2007, Coca and colleagues published a review and meta-analysis of eight studies that suggested that even smaller elevations in serum creatinine values than recommended in RIFLE and AKIN (on the order of 10% to 24%) were associated with a twofold risk of short-term death in several clinical settings; the Coca paper hypothesized that poor outcomes from AKI may in part result from delay in diagnosis caused by the lag time of serum creatinine testing.

DIAGNOSIS OF ACUTE KIDNEY INJURY

Comorbidities and potentially nephrotoxic medications should be identified. Identification of signs and symptoms suggestive of urinary tract obstruction is also important. Although physical examination in critically ill patients with AKI has been shown to be of limited accuracy, ascertaining clinical clues to patients' hemodynamic and volume statuses is essential.

Urinalysis with microscopy is useful in determination of the etiology of AKI. Presence of casts or other cells can suggest etiology. Red cell casts suggest glomerulonephritis or vasculitis, and white cell casts may raise the possibility of interstitial nephritis or pyelonephritis. "Muddy brown" casts and renal tubular epithelial cells are pathognomonic for acute tubular necrosis (ATN) and differentiate ATN from prerenal azotemia, which is characterized by normal sediment or occasional hyaline casts. Dark heme-positive urine without red blood cells (RBCs) on microscopy is diagnostic of rhabdomyolysis.

Distinguishing between prerenal azotemia and ATN, the two most common etiologies of AKI, is critical but not always simple. Aside from analysis of urine sediment, response to fluid repletion is frequently used in this distinction. Return to baseline of renal function in 24 to 72 hours after fluid repletion suggests prerenal etiology. Urine chemistries can also aid in the diagnosis. The fractional excretion of sodium (FeNa) measures the ratio of the sodium excreted to the sodium filtered by the formula:

$$FeNa = (urine\ sodium \times serum\ creatinine) / (serum\ sodium \times urine\ creatinine) \times 100$$

Prerenal azotemia is characterized by FeNa less than 1%, and FeNa more than 1% suggests ATN. However, FeNa may be spuriously low in patients with severe sepsis, heart failure, or cirrhosis, despite the presence of ATN. Conversely, FeNa may be falsely elevated in patients on diuretics, with glucosuria, or with preexisting renal insufficiency. In the case of diuretic use, the fractional excretion of urea (FEurea) has been shown to accurately distinguish between prerenal azotemia and ATN with the following formula:

$$FEurea = (urine\ urea\ nitrogen \times serum\ creatinine) / (BUN \times urine\ creatinine) \times 100$$

with BUN for blood urea nitrogen. Prerenal azotemia is indicated by FEurea less than 35% and ATN by FEurea more than 50%. Although of variable utility, other serum and urinary measures may also be used in aggregate to distinguish ATN from prerenal azotemia. These tests are summarized in Table 3, in order of general usefulness.

Serologic tests, such as antinuclear antibody, hepatitis B surface antigen, and antiglomerular basement membrane antibody, are useful for distinguishing the etiology of glomerular diseases. Elevated creatinine phosphokinase levels are seen with rhabdomyolysis.

BUN levels reflect the balance between urea production, metabolism, and excretion and frequently rise as renal function declines. Numerous nonrenal sources of BUN exist, including dietary protein intake, parenteral hyperalimentation therapy, catabolism of endogenous proteins, corticosteroid administration, and upper gastrointestinal bleeding. However, a recent study by Beier and colleagues suggests that elevation of BUN value is predictive of long-term mortality, independently of normal creatinine.

Most clinicians rely on changes in serum creatinine and BUN values as indicators of renal function because they are accessible and familiar. However, BUN and creatinine values can be misleading, as serum creatinine levels are influenced by nonrenal factors such as age, gender, race, body weight, muscle mass, protein intake, and drugs; accordingly, changes in creatinine values tend to lag behind actual alterations in GFR. BUN levels are influenced by nutritional intake and the degree of catabolism, independently of renal function. For

TABLE 1: RIFLE criteria

	S_Cr criteria	Urine output criteria
Risk	Increased 1.5×-2× baseline	<0.5 mL/kg/h for 6 h
Injury	Increased 2×-3× baseline	<0.5 mL/kg/h for 12 h
Failure	Increased >3× baseline *or* S_Cr >4.0 mg/dL with acute rise ≥0.5 mg/dL	<0.3 mL/kg/h for 24 h *or* Anuria for 12 h
Loss	Persistent renal failure for >4 wk	
ESRD	Persistent renal failure for >3 mo	

ESRD, End-stage renal failure; *RIFLE*, risk, injury, failure, loss, and end-stage renal disease; S_{Cr}, serum creatinine.

TABLE 2: Acute Kidney Injury Network staging system

Stage	S_Cr criteria	Urine output criteria
I	Absolute increase ≥0.3 mg/dL *or* Increased 1.5×-2× baseline	<0.5 mL/kg/h for 6 h
II	Increased 2×-3× baseline	<0.5 mL/kg/h for 12 h
III	Increased >3× baseline *or* S_Cr ≥4.0 mg/dL with absolute increase ≥0.5 mg/dL *or* Need for RRT	<0.3 mL/kg/h for 24 h *or* Anuria for 12 h

RRT, Renal replacement therapy; S_{Cr}, serum creatinine.

TABLE 3: Diagnostic indices that distinguish prerenal azotemia from acute tubular necrosis

Measurement	Prerenal azotemia	ATN
Urinalysis	Normal or hyaline casts	Muddy brown casts
Response to fluid repletion	Within 24-72 h	No response
FeNa	<1%	>1%
FEurea	<35%	>50%
BUN/creatinine ratio	20	10
Urine sodium (mEq/L)	<20	>30
Urine osmolality (mOsm/L)	>350	300

ATN, Acute tubular necrosis; *BUN*, blood urea nitrogen; *FeNa*, fractional excretion of sodium; *FEurea*, fractional excretion of urea.

these reasons, alternatives to serum creatinine and BUN values serve as more specific markers, earlier indicators, and better prognostic tools for kidney injury.

Belcher and associates reviewed one of the most promising of these markers, interleukin-18 (IL-18). A proinflammatory cytokine thought to be released by injured proximal renal tubules, IL-18 is both a mediator and biomarker of AKI and can be reliably measured in the urine. The authors cite research that identifies IL-18 as an early indicator of AKI, as a tool for distinguishing prerenal azotemia and hepatorenal syndrome (HRS) from ATN, and as a prognostic tool to predict mortality and viability of renal transplant.

Belcher and associates also discuss neutrophil gelatinase-associated lipocalin (NGAL), an acute-phase reactant indicative of inflammatory injury that is upregulated and released by proximal renal tubular cells within a few hours of tubular damage. Like IL-18, studies suggest that NGAL can be used as an early indicator, in the differential diagnosis, and as a prognostic tool for AKI.

Kidney injury molecule 1 (KIM-1) is a type 1 cell membrane glycoprotein only expressed by proximal tubular cells in response to injury. It is detectable in urine and has been shown to discriminate ATN from other causes of AKI and is also used as a prognostic tool, as it predicts outcomes.

Cystatin C is a cysteine protease inhibitor secreted by all nucleated cells and is freely filtered by the glomerulus. Although several studies suggest that serum cystatin C is superior to serum creatinine as a surrogate for GFR and thus better for the early detection of AKI, another study suggests urinary cystatin C may be better.

Liver-type fatty acid–binding protein (L-FABP) is an intracellular molecule found in the proximal renal tubules where it binds lipid peroxidation products. Although urinary levels of L-FABP may be affected by liver injury or systemic inflammation, they are largely determined by tubular injury.

RADIOLOGIC IMAGING

Renal ultrasound scan is an important test to differentiate the etiology of AKI. Use of ultrasound scan to determine kidney size and echogenicity, cortical thickness, and the presence or absence of hydronephrosis is convenient and noninvasive. The presence of a thin rim of decreased echogenicity ("renal sweat") may surround the kidneys in patients with kidney injury. The addition of color Doppler technology may also useful in the diagnosis of AKI. Measurement of the resistivity index (RI), an indicator of perfusion based on measurement of flow at the level of the arcuate or interlobar arteries, may help differentiate between prerenal azotemia (normal RI), ATN (reduced RI), and postrenal obstruction (elevated RI). Another promising ultrasound technique for the diagnosis of AKI is contrast-enhanced ultrasound scan, which makes use of microbubble-based contrast agents to help quantify renal blood flow, which is often decreased early in the progression of AKI. Ultrasound scan is critical for the diagnosis of hydronephrosis, in which it is more than 95% accurate in detecting dilation of the collecting systems and renal pelvis. A postrenal obstructive cause of AKI is suggested when hydronephrosis is present bilaterally. Assessment of bladder volume with ultrasound scan is important in the case of bilateral hydronephrosis. A postvoid residual volume greater than 150 mL is suggestive of bladder-outlet obstruction, and if it is observed in the presence of a urinary catheter, catheter malfunction should be considered. If ultrasound scan results are negative, computed tomographic (CT) scan may be necessary to elucidate the etiology of obstruction, such as obstructing stones or pelvic mass.

MEDICATION REVIEW

Thorough investigation of medications and ingestions is essential in determining the etiology of AKI. Certain medications can elevate serum creatinine levels without affecting GFR, leading to misdiagnosis of AKI. The drugs cimetidine and trimethoprim do this by blocking tubular creatinine secretion, and several drugs and substances interfere with the creatinine assay. The drug tenofovir disoproxil fumarate, used in the treatment of HIV/AIDS, has been shown to elevate serum creatinine levels without affecting measured GFR by an undefined mechanism.

A number of medications and substances can induce AKI (Table 4). The use of nephrotoxic agents should be limited when possible, especially in the presence of shock and decreased renal blood flow. If AKI is already present, medication doses must be adjusted to avoid toxicity.

DIFFERENTIAL DIAGNOSIS

Prerenal Azotemia

Prerenal azotemia is caused by decreased renal perfusion. This can occur as a result of decreased cardiac output for any reason, an absolute decrease in extracellular fluid volume (i.e., hemorrhage, gastrointestinal losses, burns), a decrease in the effective circulating volume (i.e., heart failure, portal hypertension), or shifting volume out of the intravascular space (i.e., third spacing). Prerenal azotemia is reversible if treated early and aggressively with fluid resuscitation, improvement in cardiac output, or correction of the third-space defect. If untreated, however, hypoperfusion of the kidney leads to tissue ischemia and cell death, resulting in progression to renal injury.

Abdominal compartment syndrome has increasingly been recognized as an important cause of prerenal azotemia. High intraabdominal pressures (>20 mm Hg bladder pressure) result in renal venous hypertension, which can lead to renal hypoperfusion and oliguria. If the condition is detected early, medical management with fluid resuscitation may be effective. However, early decompressive laparotomy is usually necessary for definitive reversal of abdominal compartment syndrome; immediate reversal of prerenal azotemia often results.

TABLE 4: Medications associated with direct and indirect nephrotoxicity

Direct nephrotoxicity				Indirect nephrotoxicity		
ATN	Osmotic Nephrosis	Interstitial Nephritis	Glomerular Injury	Decrease in Intrarenal Blood Flow		Volume Depletion
				Crystal Deposition (Intrarenal Obstruction)	Retroperitoneal Fibrosis (Ureteral Obstruction)	Diuretics (Loop, Mannitol, Thiazide)
Iodinated Contrast	Hypertonic Solutions	NSAIDs	NSAIDs			
Aminoglycosides	IVIG	Beta-lactams	Zoledronate	Indinavir	Ergotamine	
Amphotericin B		Quinolones	Pamidronate	Sulfadiazine	Sotalol	
Petamidine		Sulfonamides	Ticlopidine	Sulfamethoxazole	Propranolol	
Foscarnet		Phenytoin	Clopidogrel	Methotrexate	Bromocriptine	
Cisplatinum		Allopurinol	Cyclosporine	High-dose acyclovir		
Acetaminophen		Thiazide and loop diuretics	Gemcitabine			
Cidofovir		Indinavir				
Adefovir		PPIs				
Tenofovir		Vancomycin				
Melphalan						
IVIG						
Hetastarch						
Mannitol						

ATN, Acute tubular necrosis; *IVIG*, intravenous immunoglobulin; *NSAIDs*, nonsteriodal antiinflammatory drugs; *PPIs*, proton pump inhibitors.

Postrenal Azotemia

Postrenal azotemia occurs from obstruction of urinary flow at any point in the urinary tract from the renal collecting system to the level of the urethra. Increased backflow builds pressure and decreases filtration. This type of azotemia can be caused by prostatic disease, neurogenic bladder, obstruction of an in-dwelling urinary catheter, abdominal or pelvic tumors, adhesions from prior surgery or radiation, vesicoureteral reflux, ureteral or bladder stones, medications that cause crystals or fibrosis, or myeloma light chains (in multiple myeloma). The obstruction must be corrected to resolve the azotemia. Complications of postrenal azotemia include urinary tract infection from urinary stasis, hyperkalemia caused by impaired excretion, and rarely, postobstructive diuresis marked by significant diuresis that leads to hypotension.

Intrinsic Renal Disease

Intrinsic renal disease results from injury to the parenchyma of the kidney, including the glomeruli, the interstitium, and the renal tubules.

Glomerular Disease

Glomerular disease is classified as nephritic or nephrotic and can have an acute or insidious onset. Nephritic syndrome is characterized by hematuria, proteinuria, hypertension, and edema from pores in the glomeruli allowing leakage of red blood cells and protein into the urine. Etiologies include bacterial endocarditis, systemic lupus erythematosus (SLE), poststreptococcal glomerulonephritis, hepatitis B antigenemia, immunoglobulin A (IgA) nephropathy, and hepatorenal syndrome.

The hallmark of nephrotic syndrome is marked proteinuria with minimal hematuria and anasarca. Frequently, the diagnosis of nephrotic syndrome requires renal biopsy. Etiologies include minimal change disease (MCD), focal segmental glomerulosclerosis, and membranous nephropathy.

Interstitial Disease

Many conditions that affect the renal interstitium have been recognized, including allergic, drug-induced, infectious (bacterial, viral, fungal, parasitic), autoimmune (SLE, Sjögren's disease, Goodpasture syndrome), infiltrative (lymphoma, sarcoid), and idiopathic forms of disease. The most common etiology of acute interstitial nephritis (AIN) is a drug-induced disease; it is thought to underlie 60% to 70% of cases. Illicit drugs, penicillins, cephalosporins, sulfonamides, and nonsteroidal antiinflammatory drugs (NSAIDs) are some of the most common offenders. AIN can cause fever, rash, eosinophilia, and eosinophiluria; however, none of these are reliably diagnostic. Kidney biopsy is the gold standard of diagnosis but is rarely needed. Timely discontinuation of the offending agent is usually effective treatment. The use of steroids in drug-induced AIN is controversial, but a recent study suggests that early administration of steroids (within 2 weeks) may prevent long-term sequelae.

Hyperuricemia, hyperuricosuria, and hyperphosphatemia, seen in tumor lysis syndrome, can cause deposits of crystals in the renal interstitium and tubules, leading to AKI. Similarly, ingestion of oral sodium phosphate solutions in bowel preparations for colonoscopy has been recognized as a cause of AKI resulting from crystal deposition. Allopurinol and rasburicase have been used for the prevention and treatment of tumor lysis syndrome.

Tubular Disease

Acute tubular necrosis was originally thought to be caused by a period of ischemia followed by reperfusion causing extensive necrosis. More recently, investigators have clarified the role of endothelial dysfunction, systemic inflammatory mediators, and oxidative stress in causing AKI. With this in mind, the term ATN currently is more often used to describe a clinical situation with adequate renal perfusion to largely maintain tubular integrity but not enough to sustain glomerular filtration. This is particularly true in the case of sepsis and shock of any etiology.

ATN is also caused by toxins, most commonly the aminoglycoside antibiotics. Other toxins that cause ATN include platinum, antifungals, rhabdomyolysis, hemolysis, and radiographic contrast, to highlight a few (see Table 4). Risk factors for ATN include volume contraction, age, and concomitant use of other nephrotoxins. Prevention of ATN is focused on achieving euvolemia while maintaining renal perfusion and avoiding further renal insults.

Rhabdomyolysis is caused by massive breakdown of muscle, with release of myoglobin, which can result in ATN. Rhabdomyolysis can be precipitated by drugs (heroin, cocaine, statins, alcohol), multiple trauma, crush injuries, seizures, muscle compression, and extreme exertion.

Contrast-induced nephropathy (CIN) is an acute decline in renal function seen after administration of intravenous radiographic contrast, specifically, an increase in serum creatinine of 25% above baseline or absolute increase of 0.5 mg/dL within 48 hours after administration of parenteral contrast. Although not well understood, it is likely the result of several factors. Transient hypotension from osmotic diuresis, vasoconstriction of glomerular vessels, and direct cytotoxic effect have been hypothesized. CIN is the third most common cause of hospital-acquired renal injury and is most prevalent among those with underlying renal disease.

Nephrogenic systemic fibrosis (NSF) is a recently diagnosed disease that occurs in patients with preexisting stage IV and V chronic kidney disease or acute renal failure that has been linked to intravenous administration of gadolinium-based contrast media for magnetic resonance imaging (MRI). Shortly after exposure to gadolinium (2 to 12 weeks) patients have development of skin thickening and fibrosis, similar to scleroderma, and can have rapid progression to joint contractures and severe disability. Systemic involvement may occur, leading to cardiomyopathy, pulmonary fibrosis, pulmonary hypertension, diaphragmatic paralysis, and death. The pathophysiology of the disease still remains unclear, but recent studies have shown gadolinium deposits in tissues of patients diagnosed with nephrogenic systemic fibrosis. Currently, prevention of NSF entails avoidance of gadolinium administration in this population. Several treatment options (steroids, intravenous immunoglobulin [IVIG], ultraviolet light, renal transplant) have been studied and have some benefit, but the evidence is based on small case studies or case reports and further evaluation is needed.

RENAL PROTECTIVE STRATEGIES

Prevention of Contrast-Induced Nephropathy

Contrast-induced nephropathy has historically been a common cause of AKI. Low-volume nonionic low-osmolar or isoosmolar contrast media are now clearly associated with a significantly lower incidence of CIN than high-osmolar agents that were commonly used in the past. For this reason, older high-osmolar contrast agents should be avoided.

Volume expansion is the primary prevention of CIN. Patients who receive fluid administration before radiologic studies have a lower incidence of nephropathy. However, the optimal choice of fluid has been controversial. Several meta-analyses of isotonic sodium bicarbonate show benefit over isotonic saline solution; however, a recent randomized controlled trial (RCT) suggested no difference between the two fluids, both of which were beneficial in preventing CIN.

N-acetylcysteine (NAC) is a free radical scavenger that has been shown in some studies to decrease the incidence of CIN compared with both placebo and saline solution alone. However, more recent studies showed no benefit to NAC in the prevention of CIN. Despite an unproven benefit, because it is safe and inexpensive, NAC is often used as part of a preventive regimen, in addition to volume expansion.

Other Preventive Strategies

The most important priority in renal protection is to maintain renal perfusion. Fluid choice, specifically crystalloid or colloid, for this purpose has been controversial. The landmark SAFE (Saline versus Albumin Fluid Evaluation) study compared saline solution and albumin and found no differences in the need for dialysis or survival between the two groups.

The use of synthetic colloids for volume expansion has been questioned because of studies implicating an increased risk of renal dysfunction. An increased risk of AKI was shown by a recent systematic review of the use of hydroxyethyl starches in patients with sepsis.

When fluid resuscitation is administered in critically ill patients, the amount given is of paramount importance. In general, early and aggressive fluid resuscitation has been associated with a lower incidence of AKI and better survival, particularly after trauma and sepsis. However, an observational study in patients with AKI reported increased mortality associated with a positive fluid balance, and an RCT in patients with acute lung injury reported fewer ventilator days with conservative fluid management, which did not increase the need for renal replacement therapy (RRT). The likely explanation for these conflicting results is that the need for fluid therapy changes during the time course of shock, with aggressive fluid administration essential in early prevention and resuscitation and more measured fluid administration optimal later in the course of AKI.

Erythropoietin (EPO) has shown some promising nonerythropoietic properties, including tissue protection and antiapoptotic effect in animal models of brain, heart, and kidney. Despite preclinical data that show protective effects in AKI, the EARLYARF (early acute renal failure) RCT in humans did not show benefit in EPO administration. However, proponents of EPO cite the use of poorly validated biomarkers, among other flaws in study design that may have been responsible for the apparent failure.

The use of diuretics, such as mannitol and furosemide, in the prevention and treatment of AKI has not been found to shorten the duration of AKI, reduce the need for RRT, or improve overall outcomes. Mannitol has proven beneficial in preventing ATN in patients after renal transplant and after severe crush injury. In a recent study, high-dose furosemide showed a protective effect on mortality in patients with acute lung injury but no significant effect after adjustment for post-AKI fluid balance.

Atrial natriuretic peptide (ANP) dilates afferent glomerular arterioles and constricts efferent glomerular arterioles and may selectively increase GFR. It has also been reported to inhibit agents that reduce renal blood flow. Although a recent RCT shows promising results in reducing the need for dialysis in cardiac surgery patients, prior studies did not show any benefit of ANP. Further studies are needed before its use can be recommended.

Dopamine at low doses increases renal perfusion and GFR; for this reason, dopamine has been evaluated for its role in renal protective strategies. Despite numerous studies on this subject, none have yielded evidence to support the usefulness of dopamine in AKI.

Fenoldopam, a dopamine-1 receptor agonist used in hypertensive emergencies, has been shown at its lowest dose to increase renal blood flow. In a recent meta-analysis of 16 randomized trials in critically ill patients with AKI, fenoldopam appears to reduce both mortality and need for RRT.

A promising study by Heemskerk and associates reports a significant decrease in plasma creatinine after an infusion of alkaline phosphatase (AP) in patients in intensive care with severe sepsis or septic shock. The authors propose that exogenous AP attenuates production of nitric oxide (NO), a systemic vasodilator that causes compensatory renal vasoconstriction, by inhibiting inducible nitric oxide synthase (iNOS), an enzyme that catalyzes production of NO. Reduction in NO may protect renal function; however, larger trials are needed to determine the presence of morbidity or mortality benefit.

Other agents evaluated for potential use in prevention of CIN or ATN include theophylline and prostaglandin E1. Both have shown promising but conflicting results; further study is needed before their use is recommended.

TREATMENT

Both hyperglycemia and hypoglycemia during the perioperative period or during critical illness correlate with adverse renal outcomes. Several studies suggest that aggressive glucose control is associated with decreased incidence of AKI and reduced need for RRT and may be protective of renal function in critically ill surgical patients. However, the largest and most recent RCT that compared intensive insulin therapy with conventional glucose control found no difference in need for RRT. Lung protective ventilation has become a mainstay in the treatment of adult respiratory distress syndrome (ARDS) as a result of the ARDSnet trial, which also suggested that the low-volume ventilation may be beneficial for the kidney as well. High-volume and high-pressure ventilation have been reported to contribute to AKI.

Renal Replacement Therapy

RRT remains the mainstay for treatment of severe AKI. Approximately 4% of critically ill patients with development of AKI go on to need RRT. However, consensus on best practice in regards to initiation, dose, and modality of RRT has not been established.

Timing of Initiation of Renal Replacement Therapy

Accepted indications for initiation of dialysis include severe acidemia, severe hyperkalemia, ingestion of a dialyzable substance that causes renal injury, volume overload in the presence of oliguria, and clinically apparent signs of uremia. Evidence suggests that there is benefit to early initiation of RRT in AKI; however, the literature is confounded by variable definitions of early and late, and differing indications for initiation of RRT. Continued studies are needed to further define when RRT is best initiated.

Frequency and Rate of Renal Replacement Therapy

Currently, wide variations are found in clinical practice in the frequency of RRT. Current studies have conflicting conclusions. A multicenter trial that studied outcomes related to dose of renal support was the Acute Renal Failure Trial Network (ATN) Study. This study assigned patients with hemodynamically stable conditions to the intermittent hemodialysis (IHD) group and patients with hemodynamically unstable conditions to continuous renal replacement modalities. The intensive management strategy underwent IHD 6 times per week or continuous therapy at 35 mL/kg/h. The less intense management strategy underwent IHD 3 times per week or continuous therapy at 20 mL/kg/h. No significant differences were seen between treatment groups in 60-day survival or renal recovery. To date, studies have not defined best practice guidelines for the frequency of RRT.

Modalities for Renal Replacement Therapy

Peritoneal dialysis (PD) is a simple but limited method for clearance of solute and ultrafiltration. Patients must have intact peritoneal cavities for PD to be effective, which is often not the case in critically ill surgical patients. PD has the advantage of being well tolerated hemodynamically, but the dialysate fluid increases intraabdominal pressure and thus can compromise respiratory status. Nonetheless, PD remains a useful option for selected patients with AKI.

Ultrafiltration (UF) is a technique that allows rapid removal of volume without significant solute removal. The ability to regulate the rate of UF allows titration to maintain intravascular volume and therefore maintain hemodynamic stability. UF has the primary application of treating volume overload in the presence of oliguria.

IHD is the most frequently used method for RRT in the United States. This method uses a semipermeable biocompatible synthetic membrane and an electrochemical gradient maintained with continuous dialysate flow to remove solute. The major benefit of IHD is rapid removal of solute. However, intravascular volume removal is frequently limited by hypotension. Another frequent drawback is hypoxia during treatment.

Continuous renal replacement therapies (CRRTs) are the most common methods for RRT internationally but are used less frequently in the United States. Continuous therapies use hemofiltration, a technique that, like ultrafiltration, removes volume but also has equal removal of solute as a result of the high permeability of the membrane used. In this case, solute clearance is dependent on volume filtered, and because the volume filtered is substantial, replacement fluid is infused continuously to avoid hemodynamic instability. Hemodiafiltration adds a dialysate flow to supplement hemofiltration clearance. Whether this addition adds benefit to hemofiltration alone is unclear.

Continuous venovenous hemofiltration (CVVH) and continuous venovenous hemodiafiltration (CVVHDF) are two frequently used methods of CRRT that have been evaluated and compared with IHD. These continuous methods were initially thought to be safer for patients with hemodynamically unstable conditions and more physiologic and thus better for the critically ill. However, studies to determine the optimal method of RRT have yielded contradictory results. In a recent meta-analysis of nine randomized trials, Bagshaw and colleagues found no difference in mortality or renal recovery between continuous and intermittent modalities.

Hybrid therapies also exist but have not yet been evaluated by prospective randomized trials. The most common hybrid modality is slow low-efficiency dialysis (SLED). SLED is a technique that is based on the observation that slower flow and longer treatments of IHD improve hemodynamic stability. SLED is sometimes performed over 8 to 12 hours nightly, avoiding typical daytime interruptions (procedures, radiology, surgery) and allowing for daytime mobilization.

Currently, many questions regarding the optimal choices for RRT remain unanswered; there are no evidence-based best practice guidelines. However, RRT clearly plays an essential role in the support of patients with AKI. A variety of techniques are available, all of which appear to be effective. RRT therapy should currently be selected based on institutional experience and expertise, and individual patient tolerance.

PROGNOSIS

The reported mortality rate of AKI is 30% to 60%. If RRT is necessary, reported mortality rates are over 50%. The reason for such high mortality is that AKI now usually occurs as part of a spectrum of multiple organ failure, most often associated with severe sepsis or septic shock. The mortality in this setting is often determined by the underlying septic syndrome, rather than by complications of individual organ failure. Of surviving patients of AKI, a significant number have development of chronic renal insufficiency, which necessitates chronic dialysis. The precise rate of development of chronic renal failure varies greatly in the literature, depending on the patient populations. A recent review of AKI estimates that overall, the risk of necessary chronic dialysis is approximately 12%.

SUGGESTED READINGS

Barrantes F, Tian J, Vazquez R, et al: Acute kidney injury criteria predict outcomes of critically ill patients, *Crit Care Med* 36:1397–1403, 2008.

Cherry RA, Eachempati SR, Hydo L, et al: Accuracy of short-duration creatinine clearance determinations in predicting 24-hour creatinine clearance in critically ill and injured patients, *J Trauma* 53:267–271, 2002.

Eachempati SR, Wang JCL, Hydo LJ, et al: Acute renal failure in surgical patients: persistent lethality despite new modes of renal replacement therapy, *J Trauma* 63:987–993, 2007.

Kellum JA, Cerda J, Kaplan LJ, et al: Fluids for prevention and management of acute kidney injury, *Int J Artif Org* 31:96–110, 2008.

Kelly AM, Dwamena B, Cronin P, et al: Meta-analysis: effectiveness of drugs for preventing contrast-induced nephropathy, *Ann Intern Med* 148:284–294, 2008.

Kindgen-Milles D, Amman J, Kleinekofort W, et al: Treatment of metabolic alkalosis during continuous renal replacement therapy with regional citrate anticoagulation, *Int J Artif Organs* 31:363–366, 2008.

Osterman M, Chang R: Acute kidney injury in the intensive care unit according to RIFLE, *Crit Care Med* 35:1837–1843, 2007.

Palevsky P: Indications and timing of renal replacement therapy in acute kidney injury, *Crit Care Med* 36(Suppl):S224–S228, 2008.

Schrier RW, Wang W: Acute renal failure and sepsis, *N Engl J Med* 351:159–169, 2004.

Venkataraman R: Can we prevent acute kidney injury? *Crit Care Med* 36(Suppl):S166–S171, 2008.

ELECTROLYTE DISORDERS

Randall S. Friese, MD

OVERVIEW

A thorough understanding of fluid and electrolyte homeostasis is essential for the practitioner managing the surgical patient. The human body consists mostly of water. Body water composition is influenced by multiple factors, including age, gender, lean body mass, and degree of metabolic stress (trauma, surgery, and critical illness). Additionally, specific fluid and electrolyte concentrations are required to support normal cellular function. Neuronal impulse transmission, transmembrane action potential generation, skeletal muscle contraction, oxidative phosphorylation, and hormone release are examples of essential cellular mechanisms dependent on electrochemical gradients.

Fluid and electrolyte hemostasis is important in maintaining these electrochemical gradients, and this homeostasis can be perturbed by infection and injury, as well as excessive fluid losses or fluid administration. Most important, it should be recognized that abnormal fluid and electrolyte concentrations affect all organ systems simultaneously. Appropriate diagnosis and treatment of fluid and electrolyte imbalances are vital in the care of the surgical patient.

SODIUM

Homeostasis

The cell membrane plays an important role in determining the distribution of total body water (TBW) across the intracellular and extracellular compartments. Water within the cell constitutes the intracellular fluid (ICF) compartment. Water within the interstitial space and intravascular space (plasma) constitutes the extracellular fluid (ECF) compartment. Free water will distribute across these compartments based on its concentration gradient (osmosis), which in turn is dependent on the amount of solute in each compartment. In an adult, body water constitutes 50% to 70% of TBW; the remaining proportion is composed of lipid and other non–aqueous-based materials (Figure 1).

The sodium/potassium pump, a transmembrane protein, maintains a high extracellular sodium concentration (low intracellular sodium levels) and a high intracellular potassium concentration (low extracellular potassium levels; Table 1). Thus, by controlling solute distribution across these compartments, the sodium/potassium pump is essential in moderating the distribution of body water. Additionally, since sodium is the main solute in the extracellular compartment (interstitial space and plasma), it is the major determinant of tonicity and osmolality.

Measurements of osmolar concentration and osmotic activity are often expressed in osmolarity and osmolality. Osmolarity is a measure of the amount of solute per liter of solution. Since the volume of solution is altered by changes in temperature and pressure as well as by the amount of solute added, osmolarity is difficult to determine. Osmolality is a measure of the amount of solute per kilogram of solvent, commonly water. Since the amount of solvent will remain constant regardless of changes in temperature and pressure, osmolality is easier to evaluate and is more commonly used. Tonicity describes solutions' osmotic activity relative to each other. Based on the amount of dissolved solute, one solution is either hypotonic (less solute), isotonic (similar amount of solute), or hypertonic (more solute) relative to another.

Plasma osmolality, normally 275 to 290 milliosmole per kilogram of water (mOsm/kg H$_2$O), is regulated by tight control of water intake and output. Osmolality is measured by osmoreceptors located in the supraoptic and paraventricular nuclei of the hypothalamus. In an increased osmotic state (depleted ECF volume), free water leaves the cytosol and these cells shrink, stimulating the release of arginine vasopressin (antidiuretic hormone [ADH]) from the posterior pituitary. ADH results in an increased permeability of water in the renal collecting tubules, causing water retention and an increase in ECF volume. ADH will also stimulate thirst, thereby increasing water intake (and ECF volume) in the conscious patient. With this increase in ECF volume, the increased osmotic state is reversed. Conversely, in a decreased osmotic state (expanded ECF volume), ADH and thirst are suppressed; this results in decreased fluid intake and increased renal water loss.

Total body sodium levels are regulated by the kidney through the renin-angiotensin-aldosterone axis and circulating B-type natriuretic peptide. However, sodium concentration is determined by changes in TBW. Alterations in sodium levels occur to support and maintain plasma volume and tissue perfusion, not sodium concentration. Most disorders of sodium concentration are secondary to abnormal water balance; therefore, an assessment of circulating volume status is always one of the earliest steps in assessing serum sodium disorders.

Hyponatremia

Defined as a serum sodium level lower than 135 mEq/L, hyponatremia is very common in hospitalized patients, particularly the elderly, the critically ill, and patients with neurologic disease and traumatic brain injury. Additionally, hyponatremia is associated with a significantly increased risk of mortality. In the simplest of terms, hyponatremia implies a greater amount of plasma water relative to sodium. Although it can occur with any osmotic state (hypotonic, isotonic, hypertonic), hyponatremia is most commonly associated with the hypotonic state (Figure 2).

Isotonic (isoosmolar) hyponatremia indicates a low measured serum sodium level in the presence of a normal serum osmolality (275–290 mOsm/kg H$_2$O). This low measured serum sodium level occurs when significant hyperlipidemia or hyperproteinemia is present. Proteins and lipids in plasma usually occur in micromolar concentrations having minimal effect on osmolality. However, when large concentrations of proteins and lipids are present in plasma, a bias occurs to the apparent concentrations of plasma constituents that exclusively occupy the aqueous fraction, such as sodium. TBW and total body sodium levels are unchanged. This

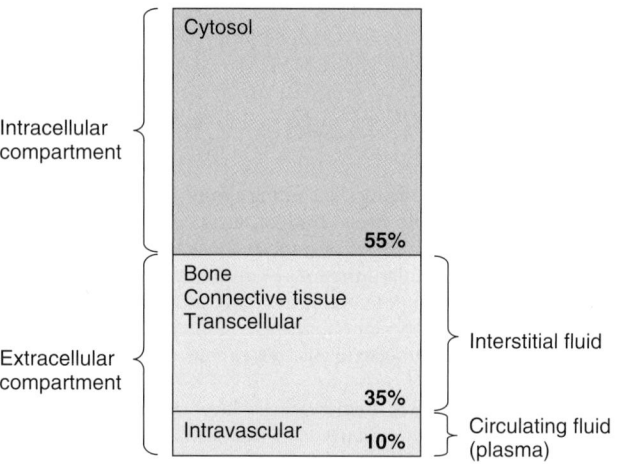

FIGURE 1 Distribution of total body water.

TABLE 1: Electrolyte composition of intracellular and extracellular compartments

	Intracellular compartment (mEq/L)	Extracellular compartment (mEq/L)	
		Plasma	Interstitial fluid
Sodium (Na$^+$)	10	140	145
Potassium (K$^+$)	150	4	4
Chloride (Cl$^-$)	0	103	114
Bicarbonate (HCO$_3^-$)	12	24	24
Magnesium (Mg^{2+})	40	3	2
Calcium (Ca^{2+})	0	5	3
Phosphorous (PO$_4^{3-}$)	120	2	2

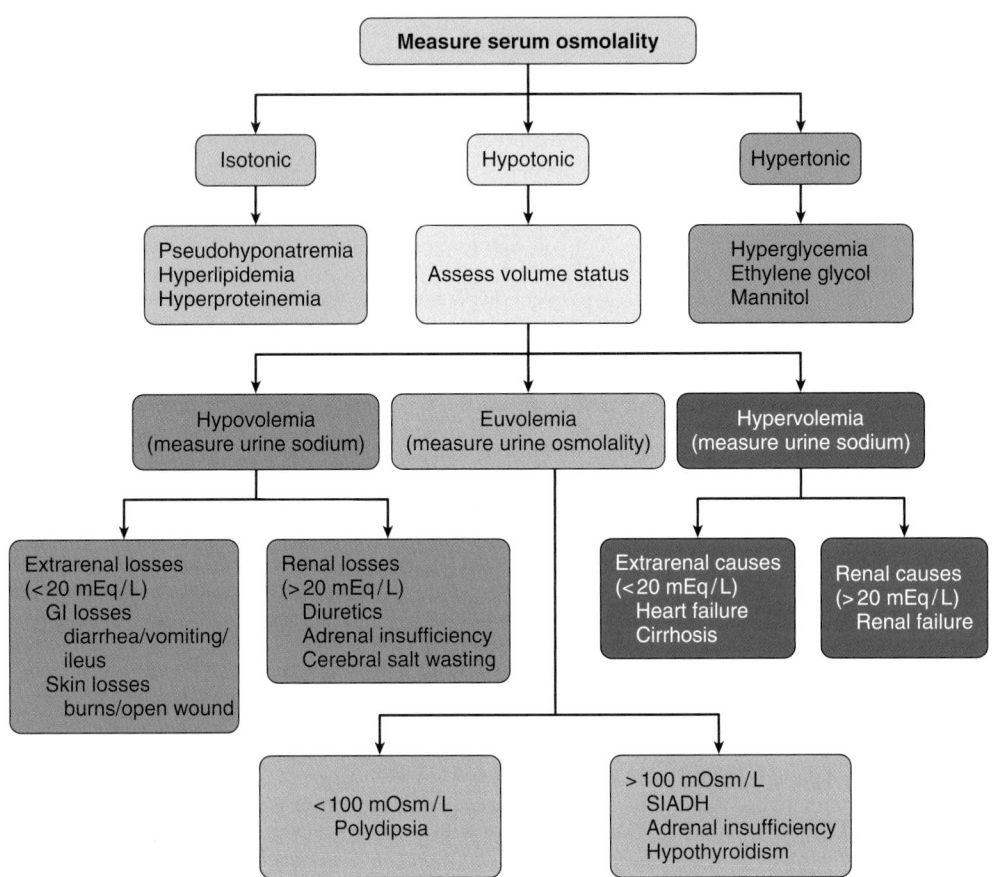

FIGURE 2 Hyponatremia algorithm. *GI,* Gastrointestinal; *SIADH,* syndrome of inappropriate antidiuretic hormone secretion.

type of hyponatremia is frequently referred to as pseudohyponatremia since it is secondary to a sampling error. By utilizing an analytic method that does not require a known volume of sample, such as a direct ion sensitive electrode, introducing bias into sodium measurements in the face of hyperlipidemia and hyperproteinemia can be avoided.

Hypertonic (hyperosmolar) hyponatremia indicates a low serum sodium level in the presence of high serum osmolality (>290 mOsm/kg H$_2$O). Because of the hyperosmolar state, a shift of water from the ICF compartment to the ECF compartment has occurred, resulting in a dilution of serum sodium. TBW and total body sodium levels are unchanged. Because this is a normal total body sodium state, something other than sodium is responsible for the increase in serum osmolality. Common causes include highly aqueous solutes, such as glucose, mannitol, glycerol, ethylene glycol, and glycine. Computation of an osmotic gap (OG), measured serum osmolality (MO) minus calculated osmolality (CO), can be helpful in identifying what compounds other than sodium are contributing to a hyperosmolar state.

$$CO = 2 \times (Na) + 1.15 \times (glucose/18) + BUN/2.8$$

$$OG = MO - CO \ (OG > 15 \text{ is indicative of unmeasured osmoles})$$

The relationship between hyperglycemia and measured sodium concentration is well described; for each 100 mg/dL increase in serum glucose, the measured sodium concentration will decrease by 1.6 mEq/L. For example, a patient with a serum glucose of 400 mg/dL should have 6.4 mEq/L (4 × 1.6 mEq/L) added to their measured serum sodium concentration in order to more correctly represent true sodium concentration. However, this relationship is nonlinear.

For serum glucose measurements less than 400 mg/dL, a correction factor of 1.6 is used for each 100 mg/dL increase. For serum glucose measurements greater than 400 mg/dL, a correction factor of 2.4 is used for each 100 mg/dL increase. Treatment of hypertonic hyponatremia is directed toward eliminating the additional offending osmotically active agent. In the setting of hyperglycemia, serum glucose should be decreased with insulin injection. Hemodialysis may be required to eliminate other offending osmoles.

The most common type of hyponatremia, hypotonic (hypoosmolar) hyponatremia, indicates a low serum level in the presence of low serum osmolality (<275 mOsm/kg H$_2$O). It is important to recognize that this type of hyponatremia can occur with any volume state (hypovolemia, euvolemia, or hypervolemia). In fact, determining ECF volume status will aid in identifying the cause of the hyponatremia (see Figure 2). However, measuring ECF volume is difficult. Frequently, assessments of circulating (plasma) volume are used to estimate ECF volume. Unfortunately, these estimates are notoriously inaccurate.

Hypovolemic hypotonic hyponatremia results from renal or extrarenal losses of sodium. Renal sodium losses may be secondary to diuresis (diuretics) or adrenal insufficiency. Extrarenal losses are from the gastrointestinal tract (diarrhea/vomiting). Renal sodium losses can be distinguished from extrarenal losses through examination of urine sodium levels (renal losses: urine sodium > 20 mEq/L; extrarenal losses: urine sodium <20 mEq/L). The effects of these sodium losses on hyponatremia are exacerbated by fluid replacement with free water (drinking). In general, the treatment of hypovolemic hypotonic hyponatremia requires replacement of the sodium deficit with isotonic fluid; however, if the hyponatremia is severe and symptomatic (i.e., seizures), judicious administration of hypertonic saline is warranted. Sodium deficit is estimated by calculating the product of TBW and the difference between the desired serum sodium concentration (140 mEq/L) and the current measured serum sodium concentration.

$$TBW = 0.6 \times \text{body weight in kg (TBW is roughly 60\%}$$
$$\text{of body weight)}$$

$$Na^+ \text{ deficit (mEq)} = TBW \times (140 - \text{current}[Na^+])$$

For example, a 70-kg patient has current measured serum sodium of 115 mEq/L. The estimated sodium deficit would be:

$$TBW = 0.6 \times 70 = 42 \text{ liters (L)}$$

$$Na^+ \text{ deficit (mEq)} = 42 \text{ L} \times (140 - 115) \text{ mEq/L} = 1050 \text{ mEq}$$

The concentration of the sodium solution used will determine the total volume required to replace the desired amount of sodium. If normal saline, which has 154 mEq sodium/L, is chosen as the sodium replacement fluid, then 6.8 L would be required. If 3% hypertonic saline, which has 513 mEq sodium/L, is chosen as the sodium replacement fluid, then 2.0 L would be required.

$$\text{Normal Saline: } 1050 \text{ mEq sodium} \div 154 \text{ mEq sodium/L} = 6.8 \text{ L}$$

$$\text{3\% hypertonic saline: } 1050 \text{ mEq sodium}$$
$$\div 513 \text{ mEq sodium/L} = 2.0 \text{ L}$$

Euvolemic hypotonic hyponatremia results from net increases in free water without clinical hypervolemia, most commonly resulting from inappropriate antidiuretic hormone secretion, glucocorticoid insufficiency, hypothyroidism, or psychogenic polydipsia. There are no associated sodium losses. Measurement of urine osmolality will help distinguish between water intoxication and an endocrine etiology. Since there are no sodium losses, the treatment is usually water restriction. However, there are now antagonists to vasopressin receptors (vaptans) that increase electrolyte-free water excretion and raise serum sodium concentration.

Hypervolemic hypotonic hyponatremia results from sodium and water gain (with free water gain exceeding sodium gain), most likely resulting from congestive heart failure, renal failure, or hepatic dysfunction (cirrhosis). Treatment requires sodium augmentation with isotonic fluid; however, if the hyponatremia is severe and symptomatic (i.e., seizures), judicious administration of hypertonic saline is warranted. Additionally, diuretics may be used to induce loss of free water.

Lastly, it should be noted that treatment of hypotonic (hypoosmolar) hyponatremia should also take into account the timing of the disease process. Acute hyponatremia is less common than chronic hyponatremia. Patients with acute hyponatremia, a decrease in serum sodium occurring over 48 hours or less, are at risk for brainstem herniation as sodium levels drop below 120 mEq/L. In patients with acute hyponatremia sodium levels should be corrected relatively quickly with sodium replacement (4 to 6 mEq/L over the first several hours) and free water restriction. Patients with chronic hyponatremia are at less risk of brain stem herniation, even with levels as low as 120 mEq/L. Sodium replacement in these patients should occur more slowly. Treatment in these patients with overly rapid sodium correction has been associated with osmotic demyelination syndrome (central pontine myelinolysis). In chronic hyponatremia, sodium should be replaced no faster than 0.5 mEq/L/h in order to avoid this demyelinating encephalopathy. For example, the previously referenced patient with a serum sodium of 115 mEq/L is down 25 mEq/L (140 − 115 = 25). To replace the sodium deficit of 1050 mEq no faster than 0.5 mEq/L/h, the sodium would need to be delivered over 50 hours.

$$25 \text{ mEq/L} \div 0.5 \text{ mEq/L/h} = 50 \text{ h}$$

Hypernatremia

Defined as a serum sodium level higher than 145 mEq/L, hypernatremia results from hypotonic fluid loss (most commonly) or hypertonic fluid gain and is frequently seen in extreme cases of dehydration. As ECF osmolality rises, ADH is released, the urine is concentrated, and thirst is stimulated. Hypernatremia is most commonly a disorder of free water imbalance, not sodium homeostasis. Thus, the high sodium concentration is usually secondary to a free water deficit. Unlike hyponatremia, where any osmotic state can be present (hypo, iso, or hyper), hypernatremia is always associated with a hyperosmotic state (serum osmolality > 290 mOsm/kg H_2O). Similar to hypotonic hyponatremia, hypernatremia can exist in conjunction with any volume state (hypovolemia, euvolemia, or hypervolemia). In fact, determining ECF volume status will aid in identifying the etiology of the hypernatremia (Figure 3). However, measuring ECF volume is difficult. Frequently, assessments of circulating (plasma) volume are used to estimate ECF volume. Unfortunately, these estimates are notoriously inaccurate.

Hypovolemic hypernatremia is secondary to a loss of hypotonic fluid, such as excessive diuresis, intractable vomiting, frequent diarrhea, or extreme sweating. Treatment focuses on correction of the free water deficit. However, in the presence of hypovolemia, circulating volume should be corrected with infusion of isotonic fluids prior to the correction of the free water deficit. Euvolemic hypernatremia results from a net loss of free water with normal circulating volume. Free water loss occurs commonly via the kidneys or as an increase in insensible fluid losses with poor water intake. A common cause of euvolemic hypernatremia is diabetes insipidus, either nephrogenic or central. Another common cause in hospitalized patients is excessive diuresis replaced by isotonic fluids. Treatment is focused on correction of the free water deficit. Hypervolemic hypernatremia is uncommon and usually secondary to iatrogenic sodium loading. This iatrogenic gain of hypertonic fluid is frequently secondary to hypertonic saline infusions or aggressive intravenous bicarbonate loading. Treatment for this uncommon type of hypernatremia focuses on free water replacement as well as diuretic use to enhance sodium excretion. Free water deficit is estimated by calculating the difference between normal TBW and current TBW. Current TBW is estimated based on normal TBW, desired serum sodium concentration (140 mEq/L), and the current measured serum sodium concentration.

$$\text{Current TBW} = \text{Normal TBW} \times (140/\text{current}[Na^+])$$

$$\text{Normal TBW} = 0.6 \times \text{body weight in kg (TBW is roughly 60\%}$$
$$\text{of body weight)}$$

$$\text{Free Water Deficit} = \text{Normal TBW} - \text{Current TBW}$$

For example, a 70-kg patient has current measured serum sodium of 160 mEq/L. The estimated free water deficit would be:

$$\text{Normal TBW} = 0.6 \times 70 = 42 \text{ L}$$

$$\text{Current TBW} = 42 \times (140/160) = 36.75 \text{ L}$$

$$\text{Free Water Deficit} = 42 - 36.75 = 5.25 \text{ L}$$

Similar to treatment for hyponatremia, treatment for hypernatremia should take into account the timing of the disease process. Acute hypernatremia, an increase in serum sodium occurring over 48 hours or less, may be corrected more rapidly (1-2 mEq/L/h) than chronic hypernatremia (0.5 mEq/L/h). In the presence of chronic hypernatremia, a slower correction, over 48 to 72 hours, is warranted because of the development of idiopathic osmoles, cytoplasmic proteins within neurons, during the period of hypernatremia. These cytoplasmic proteins limit neuronal dehydration during prolonged hypernatremia and must be allowed to degrade prior to free water repletion in order to prevent cerebral edema.

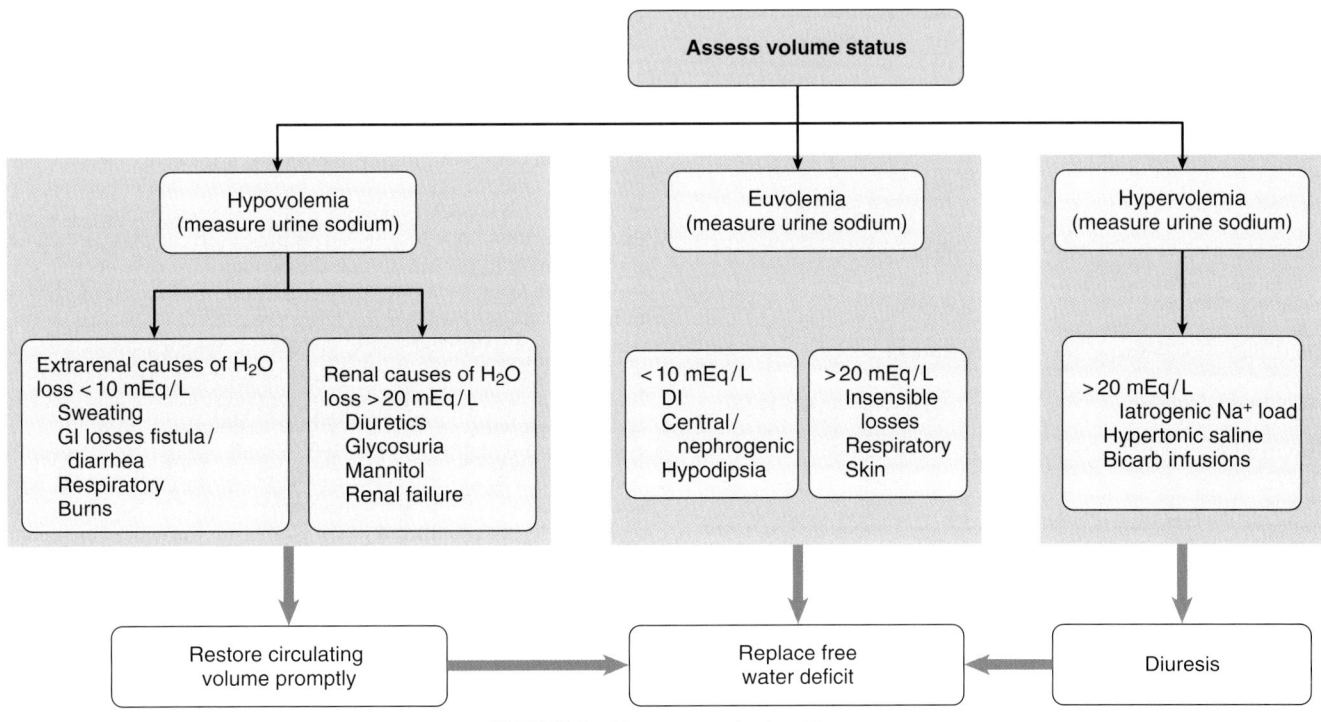

FIGURE 3   Hypernatremia algorithm.

POTASSIUM

Homeostasis

Potassium is the principle intracellular cation, with 98% of the body's potassium stores located within cells. The sodium/potassium pump, a transmembrane protein, actively maintains the concentration gradients of sodium and potassium across the cell membrane. The sodium and potassium electrochemical gradients across the cell membrane establish a resting membrane potential. An established resting membrane potential is essential for the normal function of nerve conduction, cardiac function and automaticity, and skeletal muscle contraction.

Homeostatic control of plasma and interstitial potassium concentration is critical. Within the ECF compartment, potassium concentration is maintained at a very narrow range (3.5-4.5 mEq/L). Potassium, as compared to other electrolytes, has the highest ratio of daily turnover and presents a significant homeostatic challenge. Potassium is efficiently cleared from the ECF compartment after intake; conversely, ECF potassium concentration is held constant even during times of poor potassium intake and fasting. The essential components of potassium homeostasis include sensing potassium intake through the gastrointestinal tract (normal dietary intake is 80 mEq/day), regulating potassium distribution between the ECF and ICF compartments, and regulating potassium excretion (stool 5 mEq/day; urine 75 mEq/day).

Hypokalemia

Hypokalemia, defined as a serum potassium level less than 3.5 mEq/L, is much more common than hyperkalemia in hospitalized patients; it occurs in up to 20% of that patient population. Because potassium homeostasis is essential to maintaining resting membrane potential, hypokalemia commonly presents as weakness, myalgias, and fatigability progressing to cramps, paresthesias, and tetany at levels below 2.5 mEq/L. Additionally, myocardial dysfunction, including

premature ventricular contractions, sinus bradycardia, and ventricular tachycardia/fibrillation, can occur. Severe hypokalemia can result in rhabdomyolysis, myoglobinuria, and ascending paralysis leading to respiratory arrest. Other pathologic sequelae include renal free water losses secondary to diminished urinary concentrating ability as well as metabolic alkalosis from enhanced renal production of NH_3 and NH_4^+ as hydrogen ion is excreted in exchanged for renal potassium perseveration.

In patients with normal renal function, hypokalemia is commonly related to decreased potassium intake or loop diuretic use. However, several other less common etiologies should be considered (Table 2). It is important to note that a measured plasma potassium deficit is not linearly related to the amount of potassium required to replenish ECF levels, particularly when the measured ECF potassium concentration is less than 3.0 mEq/L. Because of the large intracellular stores of potassium, extracellular deficits draw on this source to maintain homeostasis. Thus, a total body potassium deficit exists when plasma levels are less than 3.0 mEq/L, and patients generally require large amounts of potassium replacement to correct deficits of this magnitude.

Treatment of hypokalemia focuses primarily on potassium replacement. However, a search for, and correction of, potential ongoing potassium losses should be undertaken. In the presence of dysrhythmias, electrocardiogram changes, severe myopathy, or paralysis, rapid intravenous administration of potassium chloride is warranted and should precede diagnostic testing. Continuous cardiac monitoring is essential during rapid potassium replacement. In addition, serum potassium concentrations should be intermittently checked since the total body potassium deficit is likely profound. It is difficult to determine total body potassium deficit, and a precipitous rise in plasma potassium concentration can occur once intracellular stores have been reestablished.

Hyperkalemia

Defined as a serum potassium level higher than 5.0 mEq/L, hyperkalemia is frequently secondary to either impaired potassium excretion

TABLE 2: Potential etiologies for potassium disorders

Hypokalemia	Hyperkalemia
Inadequate K⁺ intake	Hemolysis
Increased K⁺ excretion	Impaired excretion
Diarrhea	Renal failure
Metabolic alkalosis	Acidosis
Mineralocorticoid excess	Succinylcholine
Magnesium depletion	Massive tissue destruction
Insulin administration	
Delirium tremens	

or an impaired ability to redistribute ECF potassium into the ICF compartment. Since the kidney is extremely capable of maintaining ECF potassium levels by adaptive excretion, the development of hyperkalemia suggests renal dysfunction (see Table 2). The degree of hyperkalemia will also be influenced by the administration of potassium supplementation, a common medical therapy. Although renal dysfunction is the most common cause of hyperkalemia in the hospitalized patient, life-threatening increases in potassium concentration are also associated with a sudden shift of intracellular potassium into the ECF space (plasma and interstitium). These large shifts occur with acute severe metabolic acidosis or massive tissue destruction secondary to ischemia or significant soft tissue crush injury.

Although classically asymptomatic, hyperkalemia can be fatal secondary to an alteration in the cellular transmembrane potential of the cells responsible for cardiac automaticity as well as the conducting system. Initial electrocardiogram changes include peaked T waves with a shortened QT interval. At higher levels of hyperkalemia, progressive lengthening of the PR interval and QRS duration occur. Ultimately, the QRS interval widens and ventricular tachycardia occurs. Ventricular tachycardia further progresses into ventricular fibrillation, and the electrocardiogram will eventually flatline as electrical activity ceases.

Therapy for hyperkalemia is multifaceted and focuses on three main goals: (1) reduction of plasma potassium concentration, (2) preservation of myocardial conduction and membrane stability, and (3) reduction of total body potassium levels. These goals are prioritized based on the degree of renal dysfunction present, the patient's ability to tolerate plasma volume expansion, and the severity of the hyperkalemia. Reduction in plasma potassium concentration is achieved by saline loading, given the patient can tolerate plasma volume expansion. In conjunction with volume expansion with normal saline or other isotonic crystalloid solutions, concomitant administration of a kaliuretic diuretic will aid in decreasing total body potassium levels. The amount of renal dysfunction present will influence the degree of kaliuresis induced by the diuretic. Preservation of myocardial conduction and membrane stability is attained by administration of supplemental magnesium and calcium as well as by the relocation of potassium from the ECF compartment (plasma and interstitium) into the ICF compartment (cytosol). Magnesium sulfate and calcium chloride are administered intravenously and have immediate bioactive availability. Insulin and glucose are given to drive plasma potassium into the cell, shifting the potassium load to the ICF compartment. Finally, reduction of total body potassium is attained by kaliuresis, the use of a cation-exchange resin (Kayexalate), and/or hemodialysis.

MAGNESIUM

Homeostasis

Magnesium is the second most abundant intracellular cation (after potassium) and the most abundant intracellular divalent cation. The majority of total body magnesium is complexed to bone, and less than 1% of total body magnesium is present in the plasma. Magnesium is similar to calcium in that the biologically active portion is in the ionized form. However, unlike calcium, ionized magnesium is difficult to measure and serum levels are used to assess magnesium concentration. Although most circulating magnesium is ionized, about 33% is protein bound. Magnesium serves many important functions. It is required for protein synthesis, nucleic acid stability, and neuromuscular excitability. Similar to potassium, serum magnesium levels are maintained in a very narrow range (1.5-2.5 mEq/L). Magnesium is absorbed from the gastrointestinal tract through both active and passive transport mechanisms. In the kidney, 80% of serum magnesium is filtered in the glomeruli, with 95% being reabsorbed along the nephron.

Hypomagnesemia

Hypomagnesemia, defined as less than 1.5 mEq/L, is ubiquitous in critical illness because of the use of magnesium-poor maintenance intravenous fluids and is commonly secondary to insufficient intake or enhanced gastrointestinal or renal losses. Symptoms of low magnesium levels are anorexia, nausea, vomiting, lethargy, weakness, paresthesias, confusion, tetany, seizures, and cardiac arrhythmias (including ventricular fibrillation, torsades de pointes, and cardiac arrest). Hypomagnesemia occurs commonly in conjunction with hypokalemia, and concomitant replacement therapy is the rule rather than the exception. Similar to treatment of hypokalemia, treatment of hypomagnesemia often requires large amounts of magnesium to restore normal serum magnesium levels.

Hypermagnesemia

Defined as serum levels higher than 2.5 mEq/L, hypermagnesemia is uncommon and occurs almost exclusively in patients with renal failure. Other causes of hypermagnesemia include rhabdomyolysis, adrenal insufficiency, and benign familial hypocalciuric hypercalcemia. Symptoms that do not occur until levels exceed 5.0 mEq/L and are primarily neuromuscular and cardiovascular. Early symptoms, such as nausea and facial paresthesias, progress to sedation, hypoventilation, decreased deep tendon reflexes, and muscle weakness. Severe symptoms and sequelae of hypotension, bradycardia, and coma are not observed until magnesium levels exceed 15 mEq/L. Magnesium toxicity is exacerbated by concomitant hyperkalemia, hypocalcemia, and uremia. The mainstay of therapy for hypermagnesemia is magnesium administration cessation, plasma volume expansion, and intravenous calcium administration. Similar to treatment of hyperkalemia, plasma magnesium levels will be diluted with saline hydration. The addition of loop diuretics will increase magnesium renal excretion, thereby decreasing total body magnesium levels.

CALCIUM AND PHOSPHATE

Homeostasis

Calcium and phosphate homeostases are mediated through coordinated efforts of the gastrointestinal tract, bone, and kidney, which are all influenced by circulating parathyroid hormone levels. Calcium is essential for neuromuscular function, coagulation, bone metabolism, as well as endocrine and exocrine secretion. Phosphorous is essential for bone metabolism, glucose utilization, and energy storage and utilization (adenosine triphosphate synthesis). Ninety-eight percent of total body calcium and phosphate are stored in bone. Plasma calcium occurs in three states: ionized (50%), protein bound (40%), and complexed (10%). The metabolically active form of plasma calcium is the ionized form. Total calcium concentration can be affected by serum albumin levels. Corrected serum calcium levels can be calculated based on circulating serum albumin levels using the following equation:

$$\text{Corrected}\,[Ca^{2+}] = \text{Measured}\,[Ca^{2+}] + 0.8(4 - [\text{Albumin}])$$

Due to its stabilizing effect on voltage-gated ion channels, plasma calcium concentration is tightly controlled. When calcium concentration is too low in the ECF space (hypocalcemia), voltage-gated channels start opening spontaneously, causing nerve and muscle cells to become hyperactive. This hyperactivity results in involuntary muscle spasms (hypocalcemic tetany). Conversely, when calcium concentration is too high in the ECF space (hypercalcemia), voltage-gated ion channels do not open as readily; this results in depressed nervous system function.

There are two important hormones for maintaining calcium and phosphate homeostasis; these are parathyroid hormone and 1,25-dihydroxycholecalciferol (calcitriol). Parathyroid hormone, part of a negative feedback loop, secretion is stimulated by hypocalcemia and counteracts this low calcium state by three modalities. First, parathyroid hormone secretion stimulates release of calcium from bone by inducing the generation of osteoclasts, which increase bone reabsorption. Second, urinary calcium losses are decreased by stimulation of renal tubular reabsorption of calcium. Third, parathyroid hormone indirectly increases calcium absorption by the small intestine by stimulating synthesis of calcitriol in the kidney (Figure 4). The synthesis of calcitriol involves several steps, including conversion of 7-dehydrocholesterol into vitamin D in the skin, the hydroxylation of vitamin D into 25-(OH)D in the liver and the final hydroxylation into 1,25-(OH)$_2$D, which occurs in the kidney.

Hypocalcemia

Hypocalcemia (calcium levels <8.4 mg/dL) is less common than hypercalcemia and is generally secondary to disorders of parathyroid hormone (decreased levels after surgical parathyroidectomy) or vitamin D (decreased synthesis in renal failure). Hypocalcemia is also commonly seen in critically ill patients with sepsis and burns. Clinical manifestations of hypocalcemia include perioral numbness, Trousseau sign (induction of carpopedal spasm with blood pressure cuff inflation), Chvostek sign (facial muscle spasm after facial nerve stimulation), muscle cramps, laryngeal spasm, and seizures. As hypocalcemia progresses, prolongation of the QT interval occurs and progression to malignant arrhythmias such as torsades de pointes or heart block may follow. Treatment of acute symptomatic

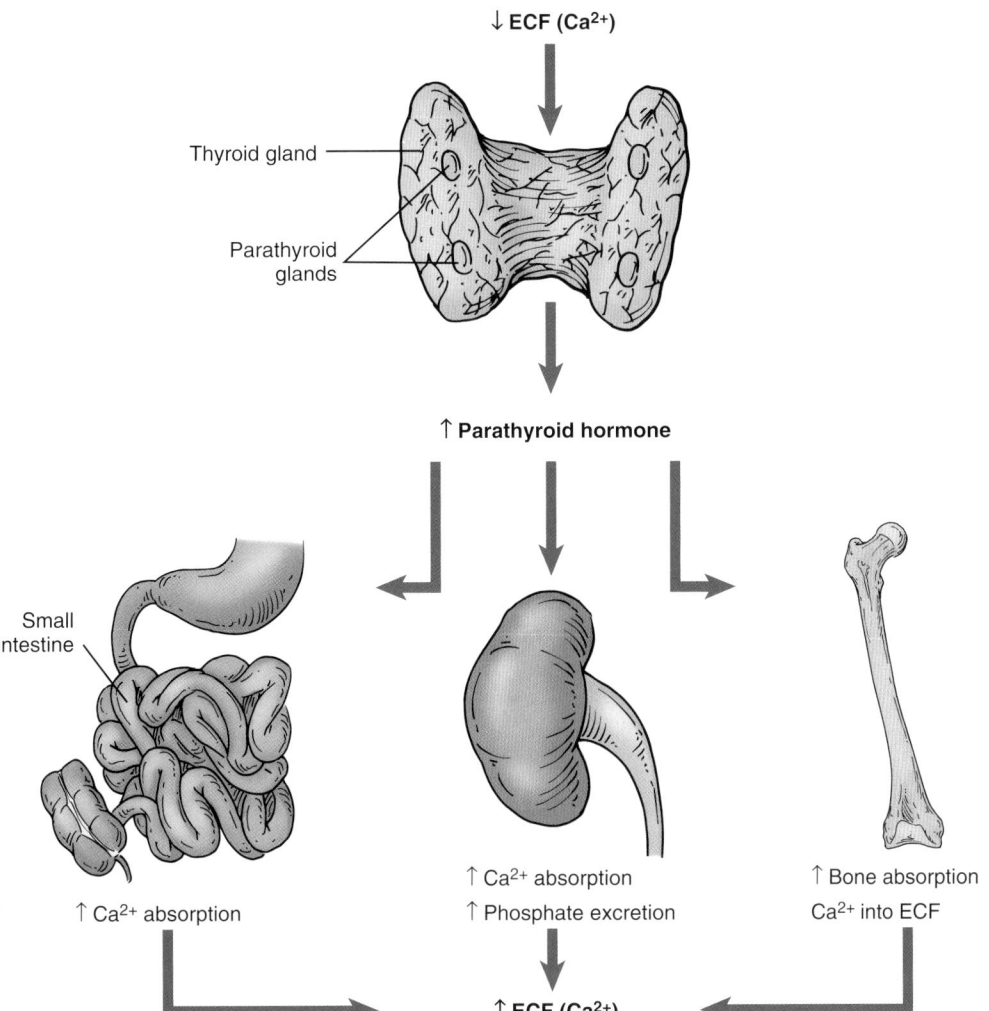

FIGURE 4 Calcium homeostasis. *ECF,* Extracellular fluid.

hypocalcemia should include administration of parenteral supplementation of calcium gluconate or calcium chloride. Cardiac monitoring and frequent reassessments of serum calcium levels should be carried out during calcium replacement.

Hypercalcemia

Hypercalcemia (calcium levels >10.4 mg/dL) is frequently due to either increased bone reabsorption or excessive calcium intake. Frequent symptoms are associated with renal (nephrolithiasis, nephrocalcinosis), musculoskeletal (weakness), intestinal (nausea, vomiting, constipation), neurologic (fatigue, depression, mental confusion), and cardiovascular (short QT interval, arrhythmias) manifestations. The most common etiology of clinically significant hypercalcemia is hyperparathyroidism. Non–parathyroid-mediated hypercalcemia can be due to malignancy, vitamin D intoxication, or granulomatous disease. Patients with asymptomatic hypercalcemia should be screened for hyperparathyroidism; urgent treatment is not required. Treatment of symptomatic or acute hypercalcemia is directed at increasing calcium excretion while minimizing bone reabsorption. These goals are attained with intravenous hydration and diuretic administration. The use of bisphosphonates can be added in the case of malignancy, but they work slowly. Glucocorticoids have been used as adjunctive agents for managing hypercalcemia associated with vitamin D intoxication, malignancy, and granulomatous disease. Hypercalcemic crisis (calcium levels >13 mg/dL) may require acute hemodialysis, especially in cases of renal dysfunction.

Hypophosphatemia

Hypophosphatemia (PO_4^{3-} levels <2.4 mg/dL) usually results from decreased gastrointestinal absorption, increased renal excretion, or may be secondary to a shift of serum phosphate into the ICF compartment. A significant intracellular shift of serum phosphate from plasma can occur after glucose loading in cases of malnutrition (refeeding syndrome), causing extreme hypophosphatemia. Most hypophosphatemia is asymptomatic; however, severe low levels can result in impaired cellular energy production resulting in rhabdomyolysis, cardiomyopathy, erythrocyte dysfunction, skeletal demineralization, muscle weakness, and respiratory dysfunction. Treatment is

focused on replacement. Parenteral replacement should be used in cases of severe deficiency.

Hyperphosphatemia

Hyperphosphatemia (PO_4^{3-} levels >5 mg/dL) is most likely secondary to decreased renal excretion. Although often asymptomatic, there is potential for metastatic calcification, particularly with a calcium-phosphorus product in excess of 70 mg/dL. Assessing urinary phosphorus excretion will aid in determining the cause of hyperphosphatemia. In the absence of renal dysfunction, elevated levels of urinary phosphorous (>1500 mg/dL) indicate either exogenous phosphate ingestion or cellular release of phosphates secondary to tumor lysis of rhabdomyolysis. When renal function is preserved, hydration is the mainstay of therapy because it increases renal excretion of phosphates. In patients with renal failure, all exogenous phosphate sources should be discontinued. Calcium carbonate, aluminum, and magnesium can be used to bind phosphorous in the gastrointestinal tract. Finally, hemodialysis may be required for adequate phosphate clearance in patients with symptomatic hyperphosphatemia.

SUMMARY

Electrolyte disorders can be complex in etiology and require a thoughtful and therapeutic plan of correction. Serial electrolyte measurements are imperative to assess response to therapy. These disorders are potentially life-threatening conditions that require rapid assessment coupled with diligent follow-up.

SUGGESTED READINGS

Felsenfeld AJ, Levine BS: Approach to treatment of hypophosphatemia, *Am J Kidney Dis* 60:655–661, 2012.

Friedman B, Cirulli J: Hyponatremia in critically ill patients: frequency, outcome, characteristics, and treatment, *J Crit Care* 28:219e.1–219e.12, 2013.

Piper GL, Kaplan LJ: Fluid and electrolyte management for the surgical patient, *Surg Clin North Am* 92:189–205, 2012.

Sam R, Feizi I: Understanding hypernatremia, *Am J Nephrol* 36:97–104, 2012.

Youn JH, McDonough AA: Recent advances in understanding integrative control of potassium homeostasis, *Annu Rev Physiol* 71:381–401, 2009.

ACID-BASE PROBLEMS

Glen Whitman, MD

A certain mystique exists in medicine today regarding the subject of acid-base balance. Research conducted among several test group physicians at teaching hospitals revealed that arterial blood gas (ABG) interpretations are correct only 40% of the time. More distressingly, management error occurred 33% of the time because of incorrect interpretation. As many as 90% of intensive care patients have an acid-base disorder; thus, understanding acid-base balance is

an essential component in the clinical management of critically ill patients.

NORMAL ACID-BASE METABOLISM

In general, the body attempts to maintain the pH of its fluids between 7.35 and 7.45, a pH that is associated with a H^+ ion concentration of 40 nmol/L. To put this concentration in perspective, the Na or K concentration in the body, which is expressed in mmol/L, is one million times more concentrated than the simple hydrogen ion H^+. Despite this minute concentration, H^+ is carefully regulated, as it has far-reaching effects and reacts readily with proteins and enzymes, which significantly alters the rates of reactions for which they are responsible.

Most of the daily acid production comes from the metabolism of fats and carbohydrates. This produces carbon dioxide that, when combined with water, produces carbonic acid, which is in equilibrium with hydrogen and bicarbonate:

1. $CO_2 + H_2O = H_2CO_3$
2. $H_2CO_3 = H^+$ and HCO_3

In addition, proteins and phosphates that are eaten contribute a small amount to this acid load.

The body maintains acid-base homeostasis in a variety of ways, but an important mechanism is the direct buffering of H^+ via intracellular and extracellular proteins, bone, and serum HCO_3. The kidneys also play a major role, specifically compensating for acidosis through the absorption of HCO_3^- in the proximal tubule and through H^+ excretion in the distal tubule.

By far, however, the most effective manner of maintenance of appropriate pH is through ventilation, with modulation of the elimination of CO_2 production. This is immediately apparent on viewing the Henderson-Hasselbalch equation, which points out the importance of partial pressure of CO_2 (pCO_2) and HCO_3^- as they relate to pH:

$$pH = 6.10 + \log(HCO_3)/0.03 \, pCO_2$$

One can see that pH is inversely related to pCO_2 and, of course, directly related to serum HCO_3^-.

Although normally minute ventilation is between 5 and 7 L, this can be increased by a factor of 10, thereby eliminating even a significantly abnormal quantity of CO_2 production through the lungs.

Arterial Blood Gas Interpretation

Most commonly, blood pH is measured with an arterial blood gas. In this type of analysis, the pH, pCO_2, and partial pressure of oxygen (pO_2) are directly measured. For the purposes of this chapter, a normal arterial blood gas has a pH of 7.40, a pCO_2 of 40, and a pO_2 of 100. For fluency in the discussion of acid-base issues, acidemia is the term used by convention when the pH is less than 7.4, and alkalemia is used when the pH is greater than 7.4 (e.g., the patient's condition is acidemic in the former case and alkalemic in the latter). But the measured pH, whether normal, acidemic, or alkalemic, is invariably the result of two or more processes that raise or lower the H ion concentration (e.g., hyperventilation, which lowers the H concentration, and uremia, which raises it). These individual processes are referred to as alkaloses and acidoses; depending on which is dominant, the patient experiences alkalemia or acidemia.

An unknown wag wrote that "human survival is a constant battle against the hydrogen ion," which emphasizes the point that death is invariably preceded by an acidosis. But to the extent that the process is caught early, intervention and reversal of the acidosis may be possible, and thus, a life may be saved. The key lies in early recognition.

What follows is a useful way to interpret a blood gas at the bedside, with the intent that the caregiver will have ample warning of an impending problem. To this end, the only two important values in a blood gas are the pH and the pCO_2. One needs to know both to determine the acid-base status of a patient. pO_2 has no relevance in this analysis. Hypoxia may be a cause of a metabolic acidosis, but knowledge of the patient's pO_2 does not help with determination of the presence or the degree of the acidosis (Figure 1).

On the basis of the Henderson-Hasselbalch equation, if the pCO_2 acutely drops 10 mm Hg, the pH rises 0.08 units, and vice versa. This assumes that there is no metabolic component to the patient's acid-base disorder. The serum bicarbonate concentration does change when the pCO_2 changes, because a change in dissolved CO_2 changes the HCO_3 concentration, but the change is only minimal. (To be

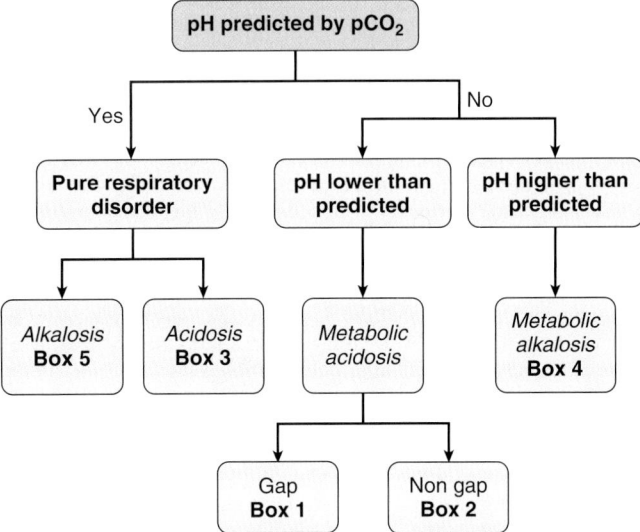

ABG - *only* pH & pCO_2 are necessary for acid base analysis
Using $\Delta \, pCO_2 \times 0.8 = \Delta \, pH$ (*opposite direction*)

FIGURE I   Algorithm for arterial blood gas *(ABG)* interpretation. One needs to know only the pH and the partial pressure of CO_2 *(pCO_2)* to determine the acid-base status of a patient; partial pressure of oxygen *(pO_2)* has no relevance in this analysis.

perfectly accurate, if the pCO_2 changes 10 mm Hg, the HCO_3 concentration changes 2 mEq/L, in the same direction.) Thus, if one assumes no metabolic component to the acid-base disturbance, when faced with the results of an ABG, immediately on looking at the pCO_2, one can predict what the pH should be. The rule of thumb is that when the pCO_2 drops 10 mm Hg, the pH rises 0.08 units. However, if the measured pH is higher than that which was predicted based on the pCO_2 alone, the patient has a metabolic alkalosis on top of the respiratory disturbance. If the pH is lower than what would have been predicted based on the pCO_2 alone, the patient has a metabolic acidosis.

One can take this analysis a step further and become more quantitative regarding the degree of the metabolic disturbance. The difference between the predicted pH, based on the pCO_2 alone, and the measured pH (multiply the predicted and actual pH by 100 to work with a whole number) gives one a measure of the degree of the metabolic acidosis or alkalosis present. Furthermore, multiplication of that difference by 2/3 yields a variable called the base excess (if the pH was higher than predicted) or the base deficit (if the pH was lower than predicted). In reality, the base deficit quantifies the absolute deficit (or excess) of total body bicarbonate, expressed in mEq/L. In general, the bicarbonate space can be assumed to be roughly 1/3 body weight. Consequently, a 90-kg person has a bicarbonate space of 30 L. A base deficit of 6 in such a person represents a total body bicarbonate deficit of 180 mEq (30 L bicarbonate space × base deficit of 6). By following the base deficit, one can determine the effectiveness of one's treatment of a metabolic disturbance (e.g., a lactic acidosis from cardiogenic shock). Successful therapy with improved cardiac output and oxygen delivery is associated with a decrease in anaerobic metabolism and a progressive amelioration of the base deficit.

METABOLIC ACIDOSIS

Metabolic acidosis is the most common acid-base disorder in medicine, a state characterized by excessive acid production (e.g., lactic acid), reduced acid excretion (e.g., renal failure), or the loss of whole body alkali (e.g., diarrhea). Many life-threatening conditions are associated with metabolic acidosis, thus raising the importance of its prompt diagnosis and treatment. A metabolic acidosis is diagnosed when the serum HCO_3 concentration is less than 22 mEq/L, which roughly corresponds to a base deficit of more than 2.

To determine the cause of metabolic acidosis, first determine the presence or absence of an anion gap, which is the calculated difference between the serum cations and anions obtained at the same time that the arterial blood gas was drawn. In serum, the sum of the commonly measured cations (e.g., sodium) outnumber the anions (e.g., HCO_3 and chloride), which is the "gap." The normal anion gap is between 8 and 12 mEq/L and is made up of unmeasured and therefore "hidden" anions. When these unmeasured gap anions are added to the Cl^- and HCO_3^-, the sum equals the Na^+ concentration, in keeping with the fact that the body maintains electrical neutrality. In normal conditions, these unmeasured anions consist mainly of albumin, phosphate, and sulfate. In the intensive care unit (ICU), where albumin concentrations are frequently low, an appropriate correction should be taken into account. Albumin is negatively charged, and when its concentration diminishes, Cl^- and HCO_3^- concentration increases to compensate, thus lowering the acceptable gap. Roughly, for every 1.0 g/dL decrease in serum albumin below 4.4 g/dL, the measured anion gap should decrease by 3 mmol/L.

Gap Acidosis

A large anion gap indicates the loss of HCO_3 ions without a concurrent increase in chloride. Electroneutrality is maintained by elevated levels of unmeasured anions, such as lactate, beta-hydroxybutyrate, acetoacetate, or abnormal quantities of PO_4, and SO_4, anions that do not normally make up the gap. A search for conditions that lead to these excess hidden anions and a widened gap should be undertaken (Box 1).

Methanol or Ethylene Glycol Toxicity

Both alcohols are toxic but are sweet and therefore are often ingested. Methanol is metabolized to formic acid, which inhibits oxidative phosphorylation-producing lactate, and ethylene glycol is converted to oxalic acid. In both cases, there is a widened osmolar gap (different from the anion gap) and an anion gap.

Diabetic Ketoacidosis

In uncontrolled diabetes, the increase in ketoacids is buffered by bicarbonate, diminishing its concentration, with a resultant gap acidosis. Once effective treatment with insulin has begun, the production of ketoacids ceases and the bicarbonate concentration rapidly normalizes.

Propylene Glycol

This substance is an additive for antifreeze, a solvent, and a moisturizer, among other uses. When ingested, it is converted to pyruvic acid, acetic acid, and then lactic acid, all of which cause an increased anion gap.

Isoniazid

Isoniazid (INH) is an antibiotic that is used in the treatment of *Mycobacterium tuberculosis*. In some cases, it can cause a significant diminution in gamma-aminobutyric acid, leading to seizures, and a lactic acidosis on that basis.

Lactic Acidosis

Although most commonly seen in hypoperfusion syndromes in which cells undergo anaerobic metabolism producing significant lactate, a lactic acidosis may also arise from defects in lactate clearance, pyruvate dehydrogenase, or thiamine deficiency.

Renal Failure

A drastic decrease in glomerular filtration leads to a decrease in the excretion of sulfates, phosphates, urate, and hippurate (all unmeasured anions), along with a decrease in HCO_3 reabsorption.

Ethylene Glycol

As stated previously, this sweet alcohol, prone to abuse, leads to formation of the unmeasured anions, glycolate and oxalate, which cause a gap acidosis. Both are primary renal toxins.

Rhabdomyolysis

Crush injuries or other causes of myocyte cell death release organic acids into the blood stream, leading to an increase in unmeasured anions.

Salicylate

Aspirin overingestion initially causes a respiratory alkalosis with a compensatory metabolic acidosis. However, at high concentrations, salicylates inhibit key enzymes in the Kreb's cycle, uncoupling oxidative phosphorylation and causing a lactic acidosis. A useful mnemonic used to recall the causes of a gap metabolic acidosis is MUDPILERS (see Box 1).

In all acidoses, when a net retention of hydrogen ion occurs, the body activates three compensatory responses, namely: (1) buffering; (2) increased ventilation; and (3) increased renal absorption and regeneration of HCO_3.

In the face of a metabolic acidosis, the drop in pH immediately stimulates the ventilatory drive, enhancing CO_2 elimination with a concomitant rise in the pH toward normal.

Treatment of a Gap Acidosis

Immediate recognition and treatment of a metabolic acidosis can be lifesaving. In all cases, the underlying cause must be addressed with simultaneous support of the patient. In the ICU, severe metabolic acidoses is frequently treated with bicarbonate. However, its use does not come without a price: fluid overload, hypernatremia, hypocalcemia, impairment of hemoglobin/oxygen dissociation, and an acute lowering of cerebrospinal fluid (CSF) pH, which can cause mental status changes. Nevertheless, although the etiology for the acidosis is being addressed, maintenance of pH above 7.3 with hyperventilation and bicarbonate administration provides a margin of safety.

Interestingly, a low pH itself does not independently lead to the hemodynamic collapse seen in the acidemic, critically ill patient. In fact, there is a striking discordance between the clinical course and the outcome of acidemias caused by respiratory failure as opposed to those that are metabolic in origin. As an example, lactate may play

---

BOX 1: Anion gap metabolic acidosis

M	Methanol (osmol gap, >10)
U	Uremia
D	Diabetic ketoacidosis
P	Propylene glycol (radiator fluid and preservative in diazepam and lorazepam)
I	Isoniazid
L	Lactic acid (sepsis, ischemia, propofol, short gut)
E	Ethylene glycol (osmol gap, >10)
R	Rhabdomyolysis
S	Salicylates

a key role in circulatory collapse, apart from the associated increase in H^+ concentration. Thus, although hemodynamic improvements are commonly observed after bicarbonate administration, given to buffer the acidosis, the truly pathologic molecule may not be addressed.

Nongap Acidosis

The causes of anion gap acidoses differ significantly from those of nongapped acidoses, most particularly in that none of the latter is primarily lethal. A nongap acidosis occurs when loss of HCO_3 is completely compensated for by an increase in Cl^- concentration and is perhaps better described as a hyperchloremic nongap acidosis. The two organs capable of contributing to this process are the gut and the kidney. A useful pneumonic for remembering its causes is FUSEDCARS (Box 2).

Gastrointestinal loss of HCO_3, as occurs in diarrhea, and renal losses, as seen in renal tubular acidoses, often part of longstanding diabetes, are typically seen in the ICU setting. When faced with a nongap hyperchloremic acidosis, the first step, therefore, is to determine whether the intestine or the kidney is the culprit. Urine pH is high or alkaline if the kidney is responsible but low if the intestine is the cause of bicarbonate loss. Physiologically, the normal kidney compensates for an acidosis both by reabsorbing bicarbonate in the proximal tubule and thick ascending limb, increasing proton secretion in the distal tubule, and by collecting duct and excreting protons as ammonium chloride (NH_4Cl). This process causes the urine pH to be low (<5) and implicates the intestine as the cause.

When the etiology is renal, the differential diagnosis can be narrowed down to a renal tubular acidosis, use of carbonic anhydrous inhibitors, spironolactone, early renal failure, or ureteral diversions. The loss of HCO_3 and impairment of H^+ secretion from the kidneys constitutes the renal tubular acidoses (RTA). With a proximal renal tubular acidosis, there is also a loss of HCO_3 absorption proximally, as opposed to a distal renal tubular acidosis in which there is dysfunction of the distal tubule and an inability to secrete protons.

Although the kidney and the intestine should be viewed as the primary causes, hyperchloremic acidosis is iatrogenically seen with the rapid administration of 0.9% NaCl resuscitation solution, a process that results in the loss of HCO_3, fully replaced by Cl^-.

RESPIRATORY ACIDOSIS

Respiratory acidosis (Box 3) occurs when ventilation fails to remove all of the CO_2 produced by the body's metabolism, with a resultant rise in pCO_2 above 40. Causes include loss of pulmonary elasticity as seen in idiopathic pulmonary fibrosis or sarcoid and long-standing chronic obstructive pulmonary disease (COPD) with gradual inability to eliminate CO_2. Both lead to a slow increase in CO_2 compensated for by the kidneys, which increase bicarbonate reabsorption.

However, an exacerbation of COPD and bronchiolar spasm as seen in an allergic reaction or asthma are acute causes of a respiratory acidosis frequently encountered in the surgical setting. But the

most common cause is central nervous system (CNS) depression from narcotics; benzodiazepines; stroke, which can cause either hypoventilation or hyperventilation; and chest wall muscle weakness from residual muscular paralysis after surgery.

Treatment

In all situations, the aim of the provider is to facilitate ventilation. In the case of bronchospasm, bronchodilators with beta agonists, anticholinergics, or steroids may be appropriate. For muscular weakness or even CNS depression, noninvasive pressure ventilation with pressure support and continuous positive airway pressure may obviate the need for intubation. It is important to address the adequate reversal of residual effects of neuromuscular blockade, with the administration of neostigmine, or the effects of narcotics or benzodiazepines, which can be neutralized with naloxone or flumazinal. However, if the rise in pCO_2 is poorly tolerated and associated with a change in mental status or hypoxia, then intubation and mechanical support are necessary. To a large degree, whenever a question exists regarding the effectiveness of noninvasive support, intubation is always appropriate. Hypoventilation is effectively treated with mechanical support, and given the ability to intubate atraumatically, allowing a patient to become hemodynamically compromised from hypoventilation, hypoxemia, and severe respiratory acidemia should almost never occur in the monitored setting.

METABOLIC ALKALOSES

In the ICU setting, a metabolic alkalosis (Box 4) is almost always the result of upper gastrointestinal losses or diuretic therapy. To occur, however, the alkalosis must be to some degree associated with intravascular volume depletion or hypokalemia; if not, the kidney simply excretes the excess bicarbonate.

Gastrointestinal Hydrogen Loss

As pointed out in the section on metabolic acidosis, loss of lower gastrointestinal secretions, as in diarrhea, causes an acidosis because these fluids are high in bicarbonate concentration. However, gastric secretions are high in hydrogen concentration, and gastric suctioning or vomiting leads to its loss and a concomitant alkalosis. In general, gastric acid, on entering the duodenum, causes pancreatic bicarbonate secretion, and the event is pH neutral. However, gastric suctioning prevents the secreted H^+ from reaching the duodenum,

---

BOX 2: Nongapped acidoses

F	Fistula, pancreatic
U	Ureteroenterostomy
S	Saline administration
E	Endocrine (hyperparathyroidism)
D	Diarrhea
C	Carbonic anhydrase inhibitors
A	Ammonium chloride
R	Renal tubular acidosis
S	Spironolactone

BOX 3: Respiratory acidosis

CNS depressants (sedatives, CNS disease, obesity hypoventilation syndrome)
Lung disease (COPD, bronchospasm)
Kyphoscoliosis
Guillain-Barré syndrome
Myasthenia gravis

CNS, Central nervous system; *COPD*, chronic obstructive pulmonary disease.

BOX 4: Metabolic alkalosis

Volume contraction (vomiting, overdiuresis, ascites)
Hypokalemia
Mechanical ventilation in a hypercapneic condition
Alkali ingestion (bicarbonate)
Excess glucocorticoids or mineralocorticoids

and consequently, no stimulation to pancreatic bicarbonate secretion occurs.

Diuretic Therapy

In the surgical setting, postoperative patients experience hyperaldosteronism, the result of stress-induced stimulation of the renin-angiotensin system. In this setting, when loop diuretics are used, increased Na^+ delivery to the distal tubule occurs. This increased Na delivery in the face of aldosterone leads to increased Na absorption in exchange for K^+ and H^+. The H^+ loss is exacerbated by hypokalemia which invariably occurs in this situation. To a degree, a shift of intracellular K^+ to the extracellular space to compensate, but to maintain electrical neutrality, H+ ion enters the cell. This increased H^+ concentration in the distal tubular cell leads to its preferential secretion in exchange for Na^+, exacerbating the resulting alkalosis. Similarly, any cause in an increased circulating mineralocorticoid can lead to an alkalosis, and it always is associated with hypokalemia, for the reasons stated previously.

Contraction Alkalosis

Significant losses of predominantly bicarbonate-free fluid cause a contraction alkalosis. This is most commonly seen in the edematous patient treated with diuretics who has a significant, rapid fluid loss. In this situation, loss of free water around a fixed quantity of bicarbonate leads to its increased concentration. Similarly, significant dehydration or sweating with free water and NaCl loss leads to a rise in bicarbonate concentration. But by far, in the hospital, diuretic therapy is the most common cause of this metabolic derangement.

Hypercapneic Alkalosis

Chronic hypercapnea and its associated respiratory acidosis lead to increased H^+ secretion by the kidney. The ensuing rise in bicarbonate concentration can compensate to a large degree for the primary respiratory acidosis. However, if in this setting, the pCO_2 is rapidly lowered, as might be the case with overzealous mechanical ventilation, the respiratory acidosis vanishes in the face of the ongoing metabolic alkalosis. This can be dangerous if the rise in pH is significant and sudden, as acute intracerebral alkalosis can lead to delirium, seizures, and even death.

Therapy

Most metabolic alkaloses are volume responsive. Adequate volume expansion inhibits the production of renin and decreases any hyper-aldosterone effect that may be contributing. Furthermore, NaCl administration replenishes the Cl^- ion, which is necessary for the adequate excretion of HCO_3^- in the collecting duct of the kidney. Finally, as mentioned previously, K^+ repletion is essential, or the kidney continue to excrete H^+ in exchange for Na^+ absorption, maintaining the alkalosis. Occasionally, acetazolamide is helpful to inhibit the carbonic anhydrase in the proximal tubular cells, preventing the absorption of bicarbonate in that portion of the kidney and allowing it to be excreted. However, this increases Na delivery to the distal tubule, which in the face of aldosterone activity leads to its resorption

---

BOX 5: Respiratory alkalosis
Catastrophic CNS event (CNS hemorrhage)
Drugs (salicylates, progesterone)
Pregnancy (especially the third trimester)
Decreased lung compliance (interstitial lung disease)
Liver cirrhosis
Anxiety

CNS, Central nervous system.

in exchange for K^+. Profound hypokalemia can result if this ion is not aggressively supplemented. Finally, if hypokalemia is allowed to continue in the face of acetazolamide therapy, Na reabsorption in exchange for hydrogen maintains the alkalosis, despite the prevention of bicarbonate resorption proximally.

RESPIRATORY ALKALOSIS

As discussed in the beginning of this chapter, a fall in CO_2 leads to a rise in pH. Clinically, this is the result of hyperventilation. Although frequently the result of anxiety or pain, the most important causes are primary CNS stimulation, hypoxemia, sepsis, and pulmonary embolus. In the critically ill, CNS stimulation can be the result of a stroke or an acute rise in intracranial pressure, hypoxemia from heart failure or an acute lung injury, or sepsis from a gram-negative organism. Pulmonary embolus causes hyperventilation from primary stimulation of lung receptors. An acute respiratory alkalosis, of course, can be the result of hyperventilation from overaggressive mechanical ventilation. Hyperventilation with its resultant alkalemia causes cerebral vasoconstriction, with a decrease in cerebral blood flow. Neurologic symptoms, such as dizziness, confusion, and paresthesias, classically numbness around the mouth, can result. This is in distinct contrast to a metabolic alkalosis, which rarely causes CNS changes, as the increase in serum bicarbonate concentration is reflected in the brain much more slowly because of the blood–brain barrier, and the pH change associated with a decrease in pCO_2 occurs immediately (Box 5).

Treatment

Apart from overzealous ventilation, which is easily and immediately correctable, the clinical settings associated with respiratory alkalosis can be life threatening. Considering that stroke, brain tumor, sepsis, and pulmonary embolism are diagnoses that must be entertained, this acid-base disturbance should create a sense of urgency on the part of the provider to make a diagnosis and provide treatment. Attributing hyperventilation to anxiety, stress, or pain should be a diagnosis by default.

SUGGESTED READINGS

Adrogué HJ, Madias NE: Management of life-threatening acid-base disorders, *N Engl J Med* 338:26–34, 1998.
Forsythe SM, Schmidt GA: Sodium bicarbonate for the treatment of lactic acidosis, *Chest* 117(1):260–267, 2000.
Gluck SL: Acid-base, *Lancet* 352(9126):474–479, 1998.

Central Line– Associated Bloodstream Infections

Anthony J. Baldea, Jr., MD, and
Christine S. Cocanour, MD, FACS, FCCM

INTRODUCTION

Central venous catheters (CVCs) are indispensible to the care of surgical patients. Fluid and blood product administration, hemodynamic monitoring, and dispensation of high-tonicity solutions such as antibiotics, vasopressors, and total parenteral nutrition are common indications for the approximately 7 million CVCs placed annually in the United States alone. One potential drawback associated with CVCs is that these indwelling devices provide a route for microorganisms to gain access to a patient's bloodstream. Bacteremia from colonization and subsequent infection from CVCs is termed catheter-related bloodstream infection (CRBSI). This diagnosis is problematic because whether the bloodstream infection (BSI) is from the central line or from another source can be difficult to establish; therefore, simpler definitions are used for surveillance. Central line–associated bloodstream infection (CLABSI) is the term used by the Centers for Disease Control's (CDC's) National Healthcare Safety Network and is defined as a BSI in a patient who had a central line within 48 hours before the development of the BSI and in whom no other source of infection is found. CLABSI is the most prevalent nosocomial infection, with an estimated 41,000 infections occurring in U.S. hospitals each year.

CLABSI is a significant burden on our healthcare system; it is associated with increased intensive care unit (ICU) and hospital length of stay (LOS) and higher mortality. A significant associated economic burden also exists, as each CLABSI is estimated to add an attributable cost of $5734 to $36,441 to the patient's hospitalization. Beginning October 1, 2008, the Center for Medicare and Medicaid Services (CMS) considers CLABSI to be a "never" event and refuses to pay for any associated additional healthcare costs. This has led to a heightened national focus on decreasing CLABSI, with significant progress being made. From 2001 to 2009, the incidence rate of CLABSI in ICU cases dropped 58%. With the continued emphasis on eliminating the adverse clinical sequelae and decreasing the financial burden that accrues from the development of nosocomial infections, the importance of understanding how to prevent, properly diagnose, and adequately treat CLABSI becomes paramount to surgical practice. This chapter focuses on the prevention and clinical management of CLABSI in short-term, nontunneled CVCs.

PREVENTION

Sixty-five percent to 70% of CLABSI cases are estimated to be preventable with the application of current evidence-based strategies. Many institutions have implemented "central line insertion and maintenance" bundles in an attempt to decrease CLABSI rates. The implementation of these catheter-care bundles has led to promising results, with a more than 50% reduction in CLABSI rates. These evidence-based bundles focus on basic concepts: maintenance of sterile conditions during insertion of CVCs, recommendations for site of insertion and catheter selection, optimization of postinsertion catheter care, appropriate catheter surveillance, and comprehensive education of the entire healthcare team. The following prevention guidelines are specifically of interest to the surgeon. For a complete set of recommendations, please see the CDC's 2011 Guidelines for the Prevention of Intravascular Catheter-Related Infections.

Hand Hygiene

Perhaps the most overlooked method of preventing CLABSI is also the simplest: hand washing with conventional soap and water or with alcohol-based foams or gels before the procedure. Despite the repeated emphasis in the literature and constant reminders from hospital administration, physicians consistently show poor compliance with basic hand hygiene, with an estimated 32% rate of appropriate hand-washing technique and frequency among physicians.

Skin Preparation

Minimization of CVC contamination at the time of catheter placement is critical. A key component of this process is skin preparation. Multiple studies have shown that the preferred agent for skin antisepsis is a greater than 0.5% chlorhexidine preparation with alcohol, which has an approximate 50% reduction in CLABSI rates when compared with the use of alcohol-based povidone-iodine solutions. The site should be scrubbed and allowed to dry for at least 30 seconds or according to the manufacturer's recommendation before proceeding with venipuncture.

Full Barrier Precautions

The placement of a CVC should entail the same sterile precautions that are followed in the operating room. The use of full barrier precautions (consisting of a mask, cap, sterile gloves, sterile gown, and a sterile full body drape) lowers CLABSI rates dramatically. The cost effectiveness of this strategy has been proven because the costs associated with purchasing these barrier supplies are more than offset by the savings accrued from CLABSI prevention.

Choice of Insertion Site

The subclavian, the internal jugular, and the femoral veins are the primary sites of CVC placement. In choice of a site, the benefits of use of that site must be weighed against the risk of infectious complications and the risk for mechanical complications such as pneumothorax, subclavian artery puncture, subclavian vein laceration, subclavian vein stenosis, hemothorax, thrombosis, air embolism, and catheter misplacement. CLABSI rates are lowest for short-term, nontunneled CVCs, when the chosen insertion site is the subclavian vein. Because the density of skin flora is a major risk factor for CRBSI, the femoral vein should be avoided in adults as it has a high colonization rate when compared with the internal jugular or subclavian vein. In addition, catheters placed in the femoral vein are associated with a higher risk of deep venous thrombosis.

The use of ultrasound scan guidance for the placement of CVCs is now recommended; its use substantially decreases mechanical complications and the number of attempts required for cannulation.

Catheter Selection

The choice of CVC has several potentially important implications on CLABSI rates. In general, one should select the CVC with the minimal number of lumens essential for patient management because infection rates increase with an increased number of catheter lumens. A chlorhexidine/silver sulfadiazine or minocycline/rifampin-impregnated catheter is recommended whenever the catheter is expected to be in place for more than 5 days; both have been shown to decrease CLABSI rates.

Catheter Care

Sterile gauze or a sterile, transparent, semipermeable dressing can be used to cover the CVC site to minimize colonization. If the dressing becomes damp, loosened, or soiled, it should be changed. Routine dressing changes for short-term CVCs should be performed every 2 days for gauze dressings or at least every 7 days for transparent dressings. The use of a chlorhexidine-impregnated sponge placed at the skin insertion site can further decrease the risk for CRBSI.

Topical and systemic antibiotics should not be used for the sole purpose of CLABSI prophylaxis because the former is associated with fungal overgrowth and both are associated with promoting antimicrobial resistance.

Daily skin cleansing with 2% chlorhexidine rather than bathing with soap and water significantly decreases CLABSI rates.

Daily Assessment of Central Venous Catheter Necessity

Because the risk of CLABSI rises the longer that the catheter is in place, CVCs that are no longer essential to patient care should be removed as soon as possible. To accomplish this goal, daily assessment of the necessity of the CVC should be made by the surgical team. Catheter tip cultures do not need to be routinely obtained on removal.

Replacement of Central Venous Catheters

The routine replacement of CVCs that are functioning and have no local or systemic signs of infection is not necessary. Although this practice has been advocated to decrease CLABSI rates in the very high-risk population of adult burn patients, the same results have not been replicated in other critically ill patients; in fact, routine replacement increases CLABSI rates.

Catheter insertion over a guidewire should only be performed in replacement of a malfunctioning catheter, in exchange of a pulmonary artery catheter for a CVC, or in someone with difficult access in which the risk of complications from a new puncture is greater than the risk of infection. This technique is associated with a significantly lower rate of mechanical complications. Guidewire exchange should not be performed in those patients with CRBSI because the source of infection is often colonization of the insertion tract.

DIAGNOSIS AND TREATMENT

The most sensitive clinical finding of CRBSI is fever; this, however, has very poor specificity. Purulence and inflammation around the catheter insertion site is more specific but has poor sensitivity. A definitive diagnosis of CRBSI requires that peripheral blood cultures grow the same organism as that grown from a catheter tip or from quantitative catheter and peripherally obtained cultures of differential time to positivity criteria. Given the lack of reliable clinical indicators, a high index of suspicion of CRBSI in the proper clinical scenario is mandatory to initiate the workup, confirm the diagnosis, and implement an appropriate treatment strategy.

Diagnostic Workup

The suspicion of CRBSI should prompt the collection of peripheral blood cultures before antimicrobial therapy is started. If sufficient suspicion exists that the CVC is the source of infection, it should be removed and the distal 5 cm of the catheter tip sent for culture. The preferred method of microbiologic analysis of short-term CVCs is the roll plate technique with semiquantitative culture. Growth of greater than 15 colony-forming units (CFUs) from this segment of catheter is indicative of catheter colonization. A CRBSI is present when the same organism grows from both the peripheral blood and the catheter tip. Clinical improvement within 24 hours of catheter removal suggests that the catheter was the source of infection, but without positive cultures, it is not proven.

When it is unclear whether the CVC is the source of infection, and its removal is not desirable, quantitative blood cultures should be obtained, one from a peripheral vein and one from the CVC. CRBSI is diagnosed if the bacterial count from the catheter-drawn blood is threefold greater than that from the peripheral blood. If the laboratory has the ability to perform differential time to positivity (DTP), a CRBSI is defined when the growth of microbes from the CVC-drawn blood occurs at least 2 hours before the growth of microbes from the peripherally drawn blood. The suspicion of CLABSI should be heightened in a patient with no other obvious source of infection and multiple positive blood cultures.

The organisms that most commonly cause CLABSI are: *Staphylococcus aureus*, coagulase-negative *Staphylococcus* species, *Candida* species, and enteric gram-negative bacilli. The presence of common skin flora on only one blood culture typically represents a contaminated specimen and does not necessarily mandate immediate treatment.

Catheter Removal

A dilemma arises when a patient with a CVC has clinical signs of infection but whether the CVC is the cause is not clear. The decision to remove the catheter is made based on the clinical status of the patient and the appearance of the catheter insertion site. If a patient with a CVC has development of severe hemodynamic decompensation or signs of end organ failure in the setting of no other identified source of infection, the most prudent strategy is to obtain blood cultures, remove the CVC, culture the catheter tip, and start empiric antibiotics. In patients with severe immunocompromise, the catheter should likewise be removed if a CRBSI is suspected. If the insertion site has purulent drainage or is severely inflamed, the catheter should be removed. If the patient does not have the aforementioned clinical signs and also has no identified source of infection, the catheter may be left in place while awaiting the results of the blood cultures as described previously. In a study by Rijnders and colleagues in 2004, this "watchful waiting" strategy led to a 62% reduction in unnecessary catheter removal, without any significant changes in hospital length of stay or mortality.

Empiric Antimicrobial Selection

In the setting of a patient with a septic or neutropenic condition with suspected CRBSI, prompt initiation of appropriate empiric antimicrobials and removal of the CVC are essential to improving outcomes. In most healthcare settings, vancomycin is the preferred empiric antibiotic because of the high incidence of methicillin-resistant *S. aureus* (MRSA). In institutions that have a high percentage of MRSA isolates with a vancomycin minimum inhibitory concentration (MIC) value of more than 2 µg/mL or when the use of vancomycin is contraindicated, an alternative antibiotic, such as daptomycin, should be selected. Empiric antibiotic coverage for multidrug-resistant gram-negative bacilli (such as *Pseudomonas aeruginosa)* should be added for patients with profound neutropenia, severely ill patients with sepsis, patients with femoral CVCs, and patients known to have colonization with these pathogens. To increase the likelihood of appropriate empiric antimicrobial therapy, the broad-spectrum antibiotic of choice in this setting should be selected based on the institution's unit-specific antibiogram and the susceptibility patterns of the organisms colonizing each individual patient. In addition, empiric therapy for suspected CRBSI from candidemia should be added if the patient has any of the following risk factors: prolonged use of broad-spectrum antibiotics, use of total parenteral nutrition, history of solid-organ or bone marrow transplant, presence of a femoral CVC, or use of total parenteral nutrition. To minimize the development of multidrug-resistant organisms, the cornerstone of treatment is to initiate broad-spectrum empiric antimicrobial coverage and promptly deescalate this therapy as soon as culture speciation and susceptibilities are known.

Therapy of Specific Pathogens

The diagnostic workup and management of a patient with a CRBSI depends on which specific pathogen is identified. The recommended duration of antimicrobial therapy varies depending on the pathogen, patient factors, and any associated complications from the bacteremia.

Coagulase-Negative Staphylococcus Species

Coagulase-negative *Staphylococcus* species commonly colonize the skin and represent the most common cause of CRBSI. Because the ubiquitous skin colonization with *Staphylococcus* species leads to high rates of contaminated blood cultures, whether a positive blood culture indicates a true CRBSI or contamination is difficult to tell. A high proportion of positive blood cultures drawn from multiple sites is indicative of a true coagulase-negative staphylococci CRBSI. Treatment for patients with an uncomplicated coagulase-negative staphylococci CRBSI consists of catheter removal and antibiotics given for 5 to 7 days. Vancomycin is the preferred antibiotic because most coagulase-negative staphylococci are methicillin resistant. Alternatively, in patients without intravascular or orthopedic hardware, the catheter is removed and the patient is observed without antibiotics. Additional blood cultures are obtained after catheter removal to confirm that bacteremia has resolved.

The presence of persistent bacteremia despite CVC removal should prompt further diagnostic investigation for other sources (such as endocarditis and septic thrombophlebitis). In the setting in which it is deemed clinically mandatory to keep the CVC in place and the patient has a suspected coagulase-negative *Staphylococcus* CLABSI, antibiotic catheter lock therapy is an option. This approach involves instillation of an antibiotic-heparin solution into the catheter lumen without removal of the CVC. This method, in conjunction with a longer course (10 to 14 days) of systemic antibiotic therapy, clears approximately 80% of coagulase-negative *Staphylococcus* infections without removal of the CVC. Failure of this approach to appropriately resolve the bacteremia should lead to CVC removal.

Staphylococcus Aureus

S. aureus bacteremia has a 25% to 30% risk of hematogenous complications, including infective endocarditis and other deep tissue infections. Failure to remove the CVC in the setting of *S. aureus* bacteremia and suspected CLABSI leads to delayed response to therapy, a higher relapse rate, and increased risk of complications. The treatment of uncomplicated *S. aureus* CRBSI is to remove the CVC and treat with systemic targeted antibiotic therapy for a course of at least 14 days. The strongest predictor of development of a complication from *S. aureus* CLABSI is failure of the bacteremia or fevers to resolve within 72 hours of instituting these measures. In this scenario, endocarditis should be suspected, and a transesophageal echocardiogram should be performed. Other diagnoses that should likewise be entertained are suppurative thrombophlebitis and osteomyelitis. In the situation of complicated *S. aureus* CLABSI, the duration of antibiotic therapy should be expanded to 4 to 6 weeks.

Gram-Negative Bacilli and Other Bacterial Species

Although the usual sources of gram-negative bacillary bacteremia are noncatheter sources (i.e., urinary tract infection, intraabdominal infection, pneumonia), the rate of gram-negative bacillus-related CLABSI appears to be increasing, representing a prevalence rate of up to 40% of all CLABSI in some series. This trend is thought to result from increased rates of solid organ transplants, improved care of chronically ill patients with immunocompromise, and changes in antibiotic utilization patterns. Catheter retention correlates with increased rates of treatment failure and risk of recurrent bacteremia, and CVC removal leads to a 1% risk of relapse. Thus, the current Infectious Disease Society of America (IDSA) recommendation in the setting of a gram-negative bacillus-related CLABSI is to remove the CVC and treat with systemic antibiotics for at least 7 days.

The treatment recommendations are similar for *Enterococcus* CLABSI, with ampicillin as the antibiotic of choice. Vancomycin may be used for *Enterococcus* species resistant to ampicillin, with an agent like daptomycin reserved for vancomycin-resistant *Enterococcus* species. For less-virulent bacterial species that are difficult to eradicate (i.e., *Bacillus*, Propionibacteria, *Corynebacterium*, *Micrococcus* species), the general recommendation (after contamination is ruled out with multiple positive blood cultures) is to likewise remove the CVC and treat with targeted systemic antibiotics for at least 7 days.

Candida Species

For patients with CLABSI and candidemia, prompt CVC removal has consistently been shown to decrease CLABSI-related mortality. The choice of antifungal agent depends on the species of *Candida*. Fluconazole is the agent of choice for most *Candida* species. It is preferred over amphotericin B because of an enhanced safety profile and equivalent treatment rates. In institutions with increased prevalence of fluconazole-resistant Candidal species, such as *Candida glabrata* and *Candida krusei*, the most efficacious and safest antifungal agent is an echinocandin (i.e., caspofungin). The current IDSA-approved treatment recommendation of uncomplicated catheter-related candidemia is to remove the CVC and initiate systemic antifungal therapy for at least 14 days after the first negative blood culture. In the setting of complicated candidemia, such as association with endocarditis or septic thrombophlebitis, the duration of antifungal treatment is extended to 4 to 6 weeks.

SUMMARY

Central venous catheters are commonly used instruments for complex, critically ill surgical patients. To minimize the negative sequelae associated with central line–associated bloodstream infections, strict adherence of all healthcare workers to simple, preventative measures is essential as is daily assessment of catheter necessity. A high index of suspicion regarding the identification of a central line–associated bloodstream infection is paramount because the signs and symptoms are generally nonspecific. Diagnosis is confirmed with the same organism harvested from multiple blood cultures and the catheter tip culture. The cornerstone of treatment of central line–associated bloodstream infection is timely diagnosis, catheter removal, prompt initiation of appropriate antimicrobial therapy, and deescalation of therapy once the susceptibility pattern of the offending organism is known.

SUGGESTED READINGS

Mermel LA, Allon M, Bouza E, et al: Clinical practice guidelines for the diagnosis and management of intravascular catheter-related infection: 2009 update by the Infectious Diseases Society of America, *Clin Infect Dis* 49(1):1–45, 2009.

O'Grady NP, Alexander M, Burns LA, et al: Healthcare Infection Control Practices Advisory Committee (HICPAC) (Appendix 1): summary of recommendations: guidelines for the prevention of intravascular catheter-related infections, *Clin Infect Dis* 52(9):1087–1099, 2011.

Raad I, Hanna H, Maki D: Intravascular catheter-related infections: advances in diagnosis, prevention, and management, *Lancet Infect Dis* 7(10):645–657, 2007.

Siempos II, Kopterides P, Tsangaris I, et al: Impact of catheter-related bloodstream infections on the mortality of critically ill patients: a meta-analysis, *Crit Care Med* 37(7):2283–2289, 2009.

Srinivasan A, Wise M, Bell M, et al: Vital signs: central line-associated blood stream infections: United States, 2001, 2008, and 2009: Centers for Disease Control and Prevention (CDC), *MMWR Morb Mortal Wkly Rep* 60(8):243–248, 2011.

THE SEPTIC RESPONSE

William G. Cioffi, Jr., MD, and Michael D. Connolly, MD

Sepsis is the dysregulated inflammatory response caused by infection. It is one of the most common causes of admission to an intensive care unit (ICU) and is a leading cause of death in patients in ICUs around the world. The incidence of sepsis continues to increase, and despite a significant amount of both clinical and basic science research, treatment of severe sepsis and septic shock remains a challenge for practitioners.

DEFINITION

Sepsis and the continuum of severe sepsis and septic shock were defined during a consensus conference in 1991, and the definitions were further revised during the International Sepsis Definitions Conference in 2001, sponsored by multiple international critical care and infection societies. These definitions were created to assist clinicians in recognizing sepsis at a patient's bedside and to more clearly define sepsis for future research:

- Systemic inflammatory response syndrome (SIRS) is the dysregulated inflammatory response to a variety of noninfectious stimuli, such as trauma, burns, pancreatitis, surgery, and autoimmune disorders. SIRS is considered present when two or more of the following conditions exist:
  1. Temperature greater than 38°C or less than 36°C
  2. Heart rate greater than 90 beats/minute
  3. Hyperventilation, demonstrated by respiratory rate of more than 20 breaths/min or partial pressure of carbon dioxide ($Paco_2$) lower than 32 mm Hg
  4. White blood cell count greater than 12,000 cells/mm³, fewer than 4,000 cells/mm³, or consisting of more than 10% immature (bands) forms
- Sepsis: the presence of systemic inflammation resulting from infection
- Severe sepsis: sepsis resulting in tissue hypoperfusion or organ dysfunction
- Septic shock: sepsis with persistent hypotension despite adequate fluid resuscitation

EPIDEMIOLOGY

The incidence of sepsis has increased dramatically over the last thirty years; the most recent data show that 1.66 million cases of sepsis are diagnosed annually in the United States. This increase is the result of improved diagnosis, but it also reflects an increasingly older population, multidrug-resistant organisms, and increased use of immunosuppressive drugs. Despite an aggressive campaign to diagnose and treat sepsis, the mortality rate still ranges from 20% to 50%; thus, sepsis is the eleventh leading cause of death in the United States.

Several risk factors for sepsis have been identified, including age of 65 years or older, belonging to certain racial and ethnic groups, and the presence of comorbid conditions. Heart disease, diabetes, renal failure, chronic obstructive pulmonary disease, malignancy, and chronic substance abuse also increase the risk for sepsis.

PATHOPHYSIOLOGY

The septic response occurs when the inflammatory process caused by an infection exceeds the body's ability to maintain a local response. The inflammatory process, usually triggered by the innate immune system, responds to the invasion of tissue by bacteria by initiating a cascade of proinflammatory and antiinflammatory mediators. Numerous proinflammatory cytokines have been described (tumor necrosis factor α, interleukin [IL]–1, IL-2, IL-6, IL-8, IL-10) and have been targeted as potential sites of therapy in the treatment of sepsis, unfortunately without much success at this time.

The inflammatory response is mediated by macrophages, monocytes, and neutrophils that secrete more cytokines, including leukotrienes, prostaglandins, and platelet-activating factor. When the proinflammatory cytokines exceed the homeostatic mechanisms of the inflammatory cytokines, the local environment is no longer able to contain the inflammatory process, and the inflammatory response becomes systemic. This systemic response leads to alterations in the microcirculation, tissue ischemia, apoptosis, and other destructive processes that result in organ dysfunction and failure.

DIAGNOSIS

The diagnosis of sepsis requires a high index of suspicion, thorough documentation of the history, and a careful physical examination to identify possible sites of infection. Laboratory and imaging studies are then ordered as appropriate to assess for evidence of infection or organ dysfunction. Laboratory testing should include complete blood cell count, serum electrolyte measurements, liver panel, lactate measurement, arterial blood gas measurements, blood cultures, urinalysis and urine culture, and culture of potential sites of infection when indicated. Radiographic imaging is often valuable in localizing the site of infection and usually includes plain radiography, ultrasonography, or computed tomographic scan.

Despite myriad potential indicators of sepsis, no single test guarantees a diagnosis of sepsis; therefore, clinician judgment and

TABLE 1: Clinical signs and symptoms of sepsis

Infection	General	Inflammatory	Hemodynamic	Tissue perfusion
Documented or suspected	Temperature: >38°C or <36°C Heart rate: >90 beats/min Respiratory rate: ≥20 breaths/min Altered mental status Hyperglycemia Third spacing of fluid	WBC count: <4000 or >12,000 cells/mcL or ≥10% bands Plasma C-reactive protein level: >2 SD above normal and plasma procalcitonin level: >2 SD above normal	Hypotension: systolic blood pressure < 90 mm Hg MAP: <70 mm Hg Svo₂: >70% CI: >3.5 L/min/m²	Hypoxemia: (PaO₂/FiO₂ <300) Acute oliguria (urine output <0.5 mL/kg/hr) Coagulopathy Abnormal LFT results Platelet count: <100,000 cells/mcL Lactic acidosis Skin mottling

CI, Cardiac index; *FiO₂*, fraction of inspired oxygen; *LFT*, liver function tests; *MAP*, mean arterial blood pressure; *PaO₂*, partial pressure of oxygen; *SD*, standard deviation; *SvO₂*, mixed venous oxygen saturation; *WBC*, white blood cell.

clinical evidence of systemic inflammation (Tables 1 and 2) are necessary to identify patients with sepsis. The use of biomarkers is being intensely investigated and may eventually improve this diagnostic accuracy.

TREATMENT

Early and aggressive treatment of patients is crucial to improving outcomes in patients with sepsis. Rivers and colleagues demonstrated that early goal-directed therapy (EGDT) could dramatically improve outcomes for patients presenting to the emergency department with evidence of sepsis. Patients should be quickly assessed for adequacy of the airway and breathing; appropriate intravenous access should be obtained; and fluids should be administered. Patients should be triaged to the appropriate level of care, which is frequently the ICU, but initial therapy should be started immediately and not reserved until the patient reaches the ICU (Tables 3 and 4).

Initial Resuscitation

Immediate resuscitation with isotonic fluid boluses should be started. In patients with evidence of hypoperfusion and hypovolemia, an initial fluid challenge of up to 30 mL/kg is recommended. After the initial fluid bolus, the patient's response to the fluid challenge is determined, and if the response is inadequate, further fluid boluses should be administered as needed. Adequacy of response is determined by both clinical factors and measured endpoints of resuscitation, if necessary. Initial goals should be for a mean arterial blood pressure of 65 mm Hg or higher or a urine output of 0.5 mL/kg/hr or higher. If the patient does not respond to the second fluid bolus, then the clinician should consider placing a central venous catheter to measure central venous pressure (CVP) and either superior vena cava oxygen saturation (ScvO₂) or mixed venous oxygen saturation (SvO₂). Resuscitation should then continue to achieve a CVP of 8 to 12 mm Hg and either ScvO₂ of 70% or SvO₂ of 65%. In patients in whom lactate levels are elevated as a result of tissue hypoperfusion, resuscitation to a normal lactate level may also be used as an adequate endpoint of resuscitation.

The fluid of choice during initial resuscitation should be an isotonic crystalloid. Hydroxyethyl starches should not be used because they have not been shown to improve mortality rates and have been shown to increase risk for acute kidney injury. In patients who require a large volume of resuscitative measures, albumin supplementation may be considered. Although the initial description of EGDT recommended transfusing to a hemoglobin level of 10 g/dL or higher, current recommendations support restricting blood transfusion to patients with a hemoglobin level lower than 7 g/dL.

TABLE 2: Signs of organ dysfunction and failure

Central nervous system	Encephalopathy Polyneuropathy/myopathy
Cardiac function	Tachycardia Tachyarrhythmias Myocardial depression
Pulmonary system	Acute respiratory failure Acute lung injury Acute respiratory distress syndrome
Renal function	Acute renal failure
Gastrointestinal system	Ileus/pseudo-obstruction Gastritis Acalculous cholecystitis Pancreatitis Gut ischemia
Liver	Cholestasis Ischemic hepatitis
Metabolic function	Hyperglycemia Hyperlipidemia
Hematologic function	Disseminated intravascular coagulation Thrombocytopenia
Immunologic function	Immune dysfunction
Endocrine system	Pituitary, adrenal, and thyroid dysfunction

Antimicrobial Therapy

Antimicrobial therapy targeting all likely pathogens should be administered as soon as possible, ideally within 1 hour, after the diagnosis of severe sepsis or septic shock. If possible, cultures of blood, urine, and other fluids, if necessary, should be obtained before administration of antibiotics, but the need for these specimens should not delay antibiotic therapy. Multiple studies have shown increased rates of mortality when antibiotic therapy is delayed in septic shock.

When selecting an appropriate antimicrobial regimen, practitioners must be aware of the antimicrobial resistance patterns at their

TABLE 3: Summary of recommendations and goals for care of the septic patient

Initial resuscitation diagnostics	MAP: >65 mm Hg CVP: 8-12 mm Hg UOP: >0.5 mL/kg/hr Hemoglobin: >10 g/dL History and physical examination, cultures, radiographic studies
Antibiotics	Broad-spectrum antibiotics against likely pathogens; adjust therapy when culture results are available
Source control	Surgical repair, resection or drainage of source of contamination, evacuation of infectious material
Vasopressors	MAP: >65; fluid resuscitation and arterial catheter required
Inotropes	Physiologic cardiac output; fluid resuscitation and PAC/echocardiography required
Steroids	For septic shock unresponsive to fluid resuscitation and vasopressors; may be beneficial in relative adrenal insufficiency
Blood transfusion	Hemoglobin of 10 g/dL for initial resuscitation for lactic acidosis, hemorrhage, and coronary ischemia; otherwise goal of 7–9 g/dL may be considered
Ventilation	Tidal volume of 6 mL/kg and plateau pressure <30 cm H_2O for ARDS
Glucose control	Serum glucose: 140-180 mg/dL; insulin infusion and frequent blood glucose monitoring may be required
Renal replacement	Intermittent hemodialysis for hemodynamically stable patients; consider continuous hemodialysis for hemodynamically unstable patients;
Prophylaxis	VTE: Mechanical compression devices and heparin or low-molecular-weight heparin; use cautiously in patients at risk for bleeding; consider inferior vena cava filter when heparin cannot be used Stress ulcer: histamine blocker or proton pump inhibitor VAP: Maintain head of bed >30 degrees in intubated patients

ARDS, Acute respiratory distress syndrome; *CVP*, central venous pressure; *MAP*, mean arterial blood pressure; *PAC*, pulmonary artery catheter; *UOP*, urine output; *VAP*, ventilator-associated pneumonia; *VTE*, venous thromboembolism.

institutions and the most likely causative organisms. Patients with prior exposure to antibiotics, prolonged history of hospitalization, or history of colonization or infection with resistant organisms are at the greatest risk for sepsis from resistant organisms. Empiric antifungal therapy should be started in immunocompromised patients, including those receiving chemotherapy, chronic steroids, or immunomodulators and those who have received organ transplants.

The antimicrobial regimen should be assessed daily to determine whether deescalation of therapy can safely be achieved. Deescalation limits organism resistance, reduces toxicity, and decreases the cost of therapy.

Hemodynamic Support

Vasopressor support should be instituted when patients continue to demonstrate hypotension or tissue hypoperfusion despite fluid resuscitation. The initial goal for mean arterial blood pressure should be at least 65 mm Hg because this pressure has been shown to preserve tissue perfusion. However, the optimal mean arterial blood pressure may then be individualized to the patient on the basis of response to resuscitation. Norepinephrine is the initial vasopressor of choice. In comparison with dopamine, norepinephrine causes fewer complications of tachycardia and may improve outcomes.

Vasopressin should be added as the second vasopressor when patients fail to respond adequately to norepinephrine. Patients with septic shock have been shown to have relatively low vasopressin levels, and the addition of vasopressin has been shown to improve blood pressure and decrease norepinephrine requirements. However, vasopressin should not be used as a single agent and should be used only at low doses (up to 0.03 U/min). Although vasopressin appears effective at supporting blood pressure in septic shock, studies have failed to show any survival benefit.

In patients with continued hypoperfusion despite adequate fluid resuscitation and blood pressure, the addition of an inotrope should be considered. Both dobutamine and milrinone can increase the cardiac output but have a high incidence of causing hypotension. Historically, inotropes were also used in an attempt to increase cardiac function to supranormal levels; however, this approach is no longer recommended.

Monitoring

In patients with severe sepsis and septic shock, vital signs and other markers of resuscitation must be monitored frequently. All patients should be monitored with simple noninvasive measures such as telemetry, pulse oximetry, and blood pressure cuff measurements. Depending on the patient's condition, a number of invasive monitors may be indicated and added in a stepwise manner as the patient's condition warrants.

A Foley catheter should be placed in all septic patients, except those who are anuric. Arterial catheterization should be performed in patients who require prolonged vasopressor therapy, in order to more accurately measure blood pressure. Although these two interventions carry risk for serious complications, their benefit outweighs their risk in the short term.

TABLE 4: Timeline of implementation of recommended diagnostic and therapeutic goals

Time	Resuscitation	Antimicrobials	Vasopressors/ inotropes	Monitoring	Specific therapy	Supportive therapy
1 hr	Initiate crystalloid fluid resuscitation (500 mL every 10-15 min)	Empiric, broad-spectrum, high-dose antimicrobials		Continuous ECG, arterial saturation, blood pressure and UOP		O$_2$; consider intubation and mechanical ventilation before overt respiratory distress
1–8 hr	Titrate fluid resuscitation to elimination of base deficit and normalization of serum lactate	Radiographic investigation for localization and delineation of infection source Source control if necessary	Norepinephrine if circulatory shock persists after adequate fluid resuscitation Inotropes if chloride level or SvO$_2$ is persistently decreased	ICU transfer with full monitoring support Arterial catheter assessment If shock persists with >2 L resuscitation, central venous line (goal: CVP ≥8 mm Hg)		Consider low-dose steroid therapy ± ACTH stimulation test
8–24 hr	Dynamic evaluation of resuscitative goals (on basis of clinical and invasive monitoring endpoints)		Consider vasopressin if shock is refractory to norepinephrine	If pressor dependence persists after 3-5 L crystalloid infusion and CVP ≥8 mm Hg is achieved, suspect intravascular volume depletion or limited cardiovascular reserves, echocardiography, or PAC placement (initial goal: PCWP, 12-15 mm Hg)	Consider initiation of drotrecogin alfa if single organ fails and APACHE II score ≥25, or two or more organ failures in absence of APACHE score	Initiate enteral feeding Consider intensive insulin therapy
>24 hr		Narrow antimicrobial regimen, depending on isolation of pathogenic organisms or clinical improvement Reassess necessity for or efficacy of source control		Consider PAC in vasopressor-dependent patients with progressive respiratory, renal, or multiple-organ dysfunction		Intensive hemodialysis therapy for renal failure Low-pressure, volume-limited ventilation for ARDS

Modified from Kumar A, Kumar A: Sepsis and septic shock. In Gabrielli A, Layon AJ, Yu M, editors: Critical care, ed 4, Philadelphia, 2009, Lippincott Williams & Wilkins.
ACTH, Adrenocorticotropin hormone; *APACHE*, Acute Physiology and Chronic Health Evaluation; *ARDS*, acute respiratory distress syndrome; *CVP*, central venous pressure; *ECG*, electrocardiography; *ICU*, intensive care unit; *PAC*, pulmonary artery catheter; *PCWP*, pulmonary capillary wedge pressure; *SvO$_2$*, mixed venous oxygen saturation; *UOP*, urine output.

EGDT and the guidelines for surviving sepsis advocate for placement of a central venous catheter as a protocol for resuscitation in patients with evidence of tissue hypoperfusion. This catheter is used to reach a target CVP of 8 to 12 mm Hg and a target ScvO$_2$ of 70% or higher. Unfortunately, the value of CVP measurements in determining a patient's intravascular volume status remains controversial.

A low CVP is probably indicative of a favorable response to volume resuscitation; however, in patients with normal to high CVP and in patients with abnormal cardiac function or pulmonary hypertension, CVP is likely to be an unreliable indicator of volume status. A pulmonary artery catheter is an even more invasive monitor that can provide more information about cardiac function than a central venous catheter. The use of a pulmonary artery catheter has not been shown to improve outcome in septic patients and, in fact, may worsen outcomes.

The use of more dynamic indices of resuscitation is becoming more common. Arterial waveform analysis can be useful in intubated patients in sinus rhythm. Ultrasonography has become ubiquitous in the ICU, and it can be useful in determining a patient's volume status and cardiac function. Ultrasonography has the advantage of being noninvasive, but it is a static measure, therefore necessitating serial imaging Interpreting images is prone to variability in user skill.

Source Control

Rapid diagnosis and treatment of septic patients is crucial for a good outcome, but early resuscitation and supportive therapy must be accompanied by early identification of the source of infection. Failure to quickly identify a surgically correctable source of sepsis frequently leads to worsening sepsis and death. Implanted devices that are the potential source of sepsis should be removed if this is feasible. Patients with surgically correctable sources of infection (e.g., necrotizing soft tissue infections, peritonitis) should be taken to the operating room as soon as possible for eradication of the infectious source. Other infections may be amenable to percutaneous or endoscopic therapies (abdominal abscess, cholangitis).

SUPPORTIVE CARE

Ventilatory Support

Patients with sepsis frequently require mechanical ventilation because the sepsis increases the work of breathing or because mental status changes caused by infection can compromise the airway. Septic patients are at risk for developing acute respiratory distress syndrome (ARDS); therefore, ventilation of septic patients should follow the volume- and pressure-limited strategies used in patients with ARDS. Patients should be ventilated with a low tidal volume (6 mL/kg) and peak plateau pressures of 30 cm H_2O or lower. Positive end-expiratory pressure should be maintained to minimize alveolar damage from alveolar collapse at the end of expiration. Sepsis frequently progresses to severe ARDS, which may necessitate additional strategies such as recruitment maneuvers, prone positioning, advanced ventilatory modes, and extracorporeal membrane oxygenation.

Blood Products

Red blood cell transfusions during active resuscitation for sepsis-induced hypoperfusion are still a consideration during EGDT, but a more restrictive approach to transfusion is required once hypoperfusion has been corrected. Transfusion should be reserved for patients with hemoglobin levels lower than 7.0 g/dL, with active cardiac ischemia, or with poor oxygen delivery. Large studies have demonstrated that with more restrictive transfusion practices, outcomes have been similar or improved, even in patients with a history of cardiac disease. The reasons for improved outcomes probably depend on the multiple complications associated with transfusions, such as immunosuppression, acute lung injury, and transfusion reactions.

Corticosteroids

The adrenal glands and cortisol production are vital to the patient's response to stress and critical illness. Multiple investigators have evaluated the use of glucocorticoid supplementation during sepsis with mixed results; however, patients who remain in shock despite adequate fluid resuscitation and vasopressors appear to be the best candidates for hydrocortisone therapy. The cosyntropin stimulation test is no longer recommended, and hydrocortisone therapy should be started in patients with septic shock refractory to fluids and vasopressors. The hydrocortisone dosage should be 200 mg/day. Corticosteroids are not recommended in septic patients who are not in shock.

Glycemic Control

Hyperglycemia is associated with poor outcomes in critically ill patients; however, tight glucose control does not improve mortality rates and results in increased episodes of hypoglycemia. Blood glucose levels of 140 to 180 mg/dL should be the current target of therapy, with insulin therapy started for blood glucose levels higher than 180 mg/dL.

Renal Replacement Therapy

The incidence of acute kidney injury and renal failure in patients with sepsis remains high. The timing and intensity of renal replacement therapy have not been consistently shown to affect patient outcome, but early, intensive renal replacement may be helpful. In addition, no clear benefit of continuous renal replacement over intermittent hemodialysis has been shown. Therefore, recommendations for acute renal replacement therapy in septic patients should be similar to the indications in nonseptic patients.

Nutrition

In patients without contraindications to enteral nutrition (bowel obstruction, ileus, peritonitis), feedings should be started within 48 hours of diagnosis. Enteral delivery is preferred to parenteral nutrition when possible to decrease the risk of infection. In adequately nourished patients, deliberate low-calorie delivery in the first week, with titration to full goal only as tolerated, decreases diarrhea and infectious complications.

Chemical Prophylaxis

Patients with sepsis are at high risk for thrombotic events as a result of the inflammatory response and immobility. Chemoprophylaxis should be administered with daily subcutaneous low-molecular-weight heparin and intermittent pneumatic compression devices. Patients with decreased creatinine clearance should receive unfractionated heparin in place of low-molecular-weight heparin.

Prophylaxis of stress ulcers in vulnerable patients in the ICU has been shown to decrease gastrointestinal bleeding; therefore, septic patients with coagulopathy-related need for mechanical ventilation longer than 48 hours, with traumatic brain or spinal cord injury, with burns, or with recent upper gastrointestinal bleeding should receive prophylaxis with a proton pump inhibitor.

Activated Protein C

Recombinant human activated protein C (rhAPC) was introduced in 2001 after a large trial showed decreased rates of mortality among septic patients. Previous guidelines had recommended rhAPC in patients with severe sepsis and organ failure. However, more recent trials have failed to show a mortality benefit, and the drug has been withdrawn from the market.

Goals of Care

Despite improvements in care for septic patients, the mortality rate remains high, especially among patients in septic shock. An early discussion with the patient and family is imperative for clarifying appropriate expectations and goals of care. Family care conferences improve communication, improve family satisfaction, and, when necessary, facilitate end-of-life decision making.

SUMMARY

Sepsis is a common problem in surgical patients, and its incidence continues to increase. An early, aggressive treatment plan is vital to limiting organ dysfunction and improving patient outcomes.

SUGGESTED READINGS

Dellinger RP, Levy MM, Rhodes A, et al: Surviving sepsis campaign; international guidelines for managment of severe sepsis and septic shock: 2012, *Crit Care Med* 41(2):580–637, 2013.

Hebert PC, Wells G, Blajchman MA, et al: A multicenter, randomized, controlled clinical trial of transfusion requirements in critical care. Transfusion Requirements in Critical Care Investigators, Canadian Critical Care Trials Group, *N Engl J Med* 340(6):409–417, 1999.

Kumar A, Roberts D, Wood KE, et al: Duration of hypotension before initiation of effective antimicrobial therapy is the critical determinant of survival in human septic shock, *Crit Care Med* 34(6):1589, 2006.

Rivers E, Nguyen B, Havstad S, et al: Early goal-directed therapy in the treatment of severe sepsis and septic shock, *NEJM* 345(19):1368, 2001.

MULTIPLE ORGAN DYSFUNCTION AND FAILURE

Anne C. Mosenthal, MD, FACS

Multiple organ dysfunction syndrome (MODS) has paralleled the advances of critical care. A disease that is the direct result of a major physiologic insult and its resuscitation, it remains the most common cause of death in surgical intensive care units (ICUs). It is characterized by organ injury and/or failure that is distant from the primary cause of illness or insult, with clinical features of inflammation and immune dysfunction. Essentially the sine qua non of surgical critical illness, the syndrome is an artifact of the invention of the ICU and artificial life support systems. As our ability to reverse previously lethal insults and support failing organs continues to advance, the sequelae of extending life as well as the treatments themselves inevitably precipitate organ dysfunction. Despite many advances in critical care since the first description of MODS, few treatments for multiple organ failure have been identified, and therapy remains primarily supportive. Research in the risk factors for MODS has yielded more promise in identifying *prevention* strategies that are clinically applicable; strong evidence exists that advances in resuscitation, nutrition, transfusion, and ventilatory support can prevent MODS, ameliorate MODS, or shorten its duration. In the last decade these have clearly changed the epidemiology, outcome, and prognosis of MODS should it occur, but none can be identified as direct therapy. Survival to hospital discharge is increasingly possible, even with severe multiple organ failure, but the long-term sequelae from the syndrome are now being recognized as significant, with major disability, functional impairments, and up to 50% delayed mortality at 1 year.

HISTORY AND PATHOPHYSIOLOGY

A syndrome of organ failure was first described in the 1960s, shortly after the creation of ICUs helped patients to survive serious physiologic injury or sepsis. Baue coined the term "multiple organ system failure" in a landmark editorial in 1975, when he described the phenomenon of death in the ICU as a failure of multiple organ systems, often with uncontrolled infection. It was soon realized that multiple organ system failure was the final pathway to death after sepsis, systemic inflammatory response syndrome, or trauma, even if no infection could be identified, suggesting that a derangement of inflammation and immunity was the driving force with the syndrome. The clinical syndrome was generally defined as failure of two or more organ systems—pulmonary, renal, hepatic, cardiovascular, neurologic, or hematologic—with failure of more than three organs carrying a high risk of mortality. For the next 25 years, many studied this vexing syndrome, which was responsible for the majority of deaths in surgical ICUs, particularly after trauma, sepsis, and seemingly life-saving surgery. Attempts to identify the mechanisms and pathophysiology of MODS seemed to parallel the advances of surgical critical care. Studies identified microvascular thrombosis and ischemia of end organs as the histopathologic features of MODS. This, coupled with advances in hemodynamic monitoring that provided evidence of diminished oxygen delivery, suggested that global and regional hypoperfusion in shock and sepsis could be the final common pathway to MODS.

Although the oxygen delivery hypothesis was based on pathophysiologic evidence, an intense focus on measuring and maximizing oxygen delivery to supranormal levels to prevent multiple organ dysfunction did not ultimately translate into the hoped-for clinical benefit. The "gut-origin hypothesis" as described by Deitch and others suggested that MODS was the result of regional mesenteric hypoperfusion, mucosal ischemia, and loss of gut barrier function, leading to systemic immune dysfunction and inflammation. This led to the development of gut-targeted therapies that might preserve gut barrier function, including early enteral nutrition, nutritional supplements, glutamine, and selective decontamination of the digestive tract, to prevent multiple organ dysfunction. The two-hit hypothesis suggested that ongoing or secondary cellular hypoxia following an episode of shock or sepsis might be responsible for the derangements in inflammation and immune regulation. Mechanistic studies found that cellular hypoxia leading to targeted cell death or apoptosis, dysregulated immune and inflammatory cells, cytokine derangements at the cellular and tissue level, and endothelial cell damage in organ beds might be the mediators of MODS. While these mechanisms have been well characterized, their translation into clinical therapies has proved disappointing; chemotherapeutics targeting cytokines, protein C, and other mediators of MODS have never translated into significant improvements in mortality or patient outcomes in critical illness. More recently, it has been recognized that ICU interventions themselves, while supporting organ function, can also precipitate MODS through barotrauma, endothelial injury, and predisposition to nosocomial infection. Currently, the mitochondrial dysfunction theory suggests that cellular hypoxia in shock or sepsis injures the mitochondrial cellular respiration process directly, leading to further derangements in oxidative metabolism, inflammation, and immunity.

CLINICAL PRESENTATION AND ORGAN SYSTEM MANAGEMENT

The clinical syndrome, while first described as multiple organ failure, has been redefined to multiple organ dysfunction, as the clinical presentation is now recognized to be a spectrum of organ derangements, from mild dysfunction to complete failure, the former of which can be reversible. Multiple scoring systems have been proposed in an effort to stratify the clinical severity, progression of disease, and prognosis. The most commonly used are the Marshall Multiple Organ Dysfunction Score (Table 1) and the Sequential Organ Failure Assessment (SOFA) score (Table 2). Each describes the clinical criteria across the spectrum for dysfunction to failure for six organ systems: pulmonary, renal, hepatic, central neurologic, cardiovascular, and hematologic. In addition, current understanding of each organ system dysfunction can be defined by organ-specific scoring systems, as exemplified by acute lung injury or acute kidney injury (Table 3). MODS also includes derangements of the endocrine system, metabolic system, immunologic system, and gastrointestinal system, which were not originally included in the description of the syndrome. These may present in a variety of ways that are clinically relevant, but they have not been systematically classified.

The clinical presentation of MODS begins at the time of physiologic insult and has an onset of organ dysfunction within 24 to 48 hours. The classic sequence of organ dysfunction typically begins with pulmonary dysfunction, followed by hepatic/gastrointestinal and then renal dysfunction, in that order. While it has long been held that once multiple organ failure has set in, high mortality is

TABLE 1: Multiple organ dysfunction (MOD) score

Organ system	Score				
	0	1	2	3	4
Respiratory PaO$_2$/FiO$_2$	>300	226-300	151-225	76-150	≤75
Renal creatinine (μmol/L)	≤100	101-200	201-350	251-500	>500
Hepatic bilirubin (μmol/L)	≤20	21-60	61-120	121-240	>240
Cardiovasc aPAR	<10.0	10.1-15	15.1-20.0	20.1-30.0	>30.0
Hematologic platelet count	>120	81-120	51-80	21-50	≤20
Neurologic Glasgow Coma Scale score	15	13-14	10-12	7-9	≤6

aPAR, Product of the heart rate and the ratio of the right atrial pressure to the mean arterial pressure; FiO$_2$, fractional inspired oxygen; PaO$_2$, arterial oxygen tension; PAR, pressure-adjusted heart rate.
Marshall JC, Cook DJ, Christou NV, et al: Multiple organ dysfunction score: a reliable descriptor of a complex clinical outcome. Crit Care Med 23:1638–1652, 1995.

TABLE 2: Sequential organ failure assessment (SOFA) score

Organ system	0	1	2	3	4
Cardiovascular* hypotension (mm Hg)	MAP >70 mm without vasopressors	MAP <70 without vasopressors	Dopamine ≤5 or dobutamine (any dose)	Dopamine >5 or epinephrine ≤0.1 or norepinephrine ≤0.1	Dopamine >15 or epinephrine >0.1 or norepinephrine >0.1
Respiratory, PaO$_2$/FiO$_2$ (mm Hg)	>400	<400	<300	<200 with respiratory support	<100 with respiratory support
Renal† creatinine (mg/dL)	<1.2	1.2-1.9	2.0-3.4	3.5-4.9	>5.0
Hematology, platelet count (×10^3/mm^3)	>150	<150	<100	<50	<20
Hepatic, bilirubin (mg/dL)	<1.2	1.2-1.9	2.0-5.9	6.0-11.9	>12.0

MAP, Mean arterial pressure.
*Adrenergic agents are administered for at least 1 hour (doses given are in μg/kg/min).
†Renal SOFA was modified to exclude urine output.

TABLE 3: Risk, injury, failure, loss, and end-stage kidney disease (RIFLE) classification

Class	Glomerular filtration rate criteria	Urine output criteria
Risk	Serum creatinine ×1.5 over baseline	<0.5 mL/kg/hr × 6 hr
Injury	Serum creatinine ×2 over baseline	<0.5 mL/kg/hr × 12 hr
Failure	Serum creatinine ×3, or serum creatinine ≥4 mg/dL with an acute rise >0.5 mg/dL	<0.3 mL/kg/hr × 24 hr, or anuria × 12 hr
Loss	Persistent acute renal failure = complete loss of kidney function for >4 weeks	
End-stage kidney disease	End-stage kidney disease for >3 months	

For conversion of creatinine expressed in conventional units to SI units, multiply by 88.4. RIFLE class is determined based on the worst of either glomerular filtration criteria or urine output criteria. Glomerular filtration criteria are calculated as an increase of serum creatinine above the baseline serum creatinine level. Acute kidney injury should be both abrupt (within 1 to 7 days) and sustained (more than 24 hours). When the baseline serum creatinine is not known and patients are without a history of chronic kidney insufficiency, it is recommend to calculate a baseline serum creatinine using the Modification of Diet in Renal Disease equation for assessment of kidney function, assuming a glomerular filtration rate of 75 mL/min/1.73 m². When the baseline serum creatinine is elevated, an abrupt rise of at least 0.5 mg/dL to more than 4 mg/dL is all that is required to achieve the Failure class.

inevitable, in the current decade the epidemiology has changed; judicious management of early organ dysfunction can prevent its progression, and some of the process is reversible. Mortality from severe acute lung injury (acute respiratory distress syndrome; ARDS) has been improved with changes in ventilator management, which appear to prevent progression to full multiple organ failure. These gains have not been seen when multiple organ failure includes acute renal failure; despite advances in renal replacement therapies, mortality remains as high as it was 20 years ago. Thus, the duration, progression, and prognosis of multiple organ dysfunction still are directly proportional to the management of the original insult. When sepsis is the inciting event, early source control with appropriate surgical débridement and drainage of infection, targeted empiric antibiotic coverage within 6 hours of sepsis, and adequate resuscitation to restore oxygen delivery are evidence-based strategies for ameliorating MODS. In the setting of acute traumatic injury with hemorrhage, immediate restoration of blood volume with a 1:1 to 1.5:1 ratio of red blood cells to plasma and minimal crystalloid resuscitation is now the standard of care to mitigate the development and progression of MODS to organ failure.

PULMONARY DYSFUNCTION—ACUTE LUNG INJURY

Acute lung injury is the most common element of MODS and usually the first to present. It is characterized by impaired gas exchange, primarily hypoxemia, and is stratified by the ratio of partial pressure of oxygen to the fraction of inspired oxygen (P:F ratio) regardless of the degree of ventilator support. Adult respiratory distress syndrome, the most severe acute lung injury, is defined by P:F less than 100.

Therapy is aimed at maintaining oxygen saturation of greater than 92%, optimizing oxygen delivery, while minimizing toxicity of oxygen, barotrauma, and volutrauma, and minimizing risk of ventilator-associated pneumonia. Ventilatory support that includes positive-end expiratory pressure (PEEP) with low tidal volumes between 6 and 8 mL/kg ideal body weight (IBW) is the standard of care to both prevent and support MODS. This strategy, coupled with maintenance of airway pressures of less than 30 cm H_2O, has significantly reduced mortality from acute lung injury and reduced progression to full-blown ARDS and multiple organ failure.

ACUTE KIDNEY INJURY

Previously labeled *acute renal failure* or *renal dysfunction*, the full spectrum of acute kidney injury is now described. This includes reversible mild to moderate dysfunction up to severe renal failure, which has a high mortality and risk of permanent end-stage renal disease. The degree of acute kidney injury is defined by serum creatinine levels and urine output based on the RIFLE classification (see Table 3).

Therapy for acute kidney injury is primarily focused on maintaining renal perfusion to prevent microvascular damage and tubular necrosis and to avoid nephrotoxic medications. Once severe AKI has set in, continuous renal replacement therapy (CRRT) is the primary mode of support, as it can be used in the hemodynamically unstable patient, without anticoagulation if necessary. CRRT can ameliorate or mitigate severity of MODS in sepsis, pancreatitis, or shock due to rapid clearance of inflammatory mediators. However, hopes that it would improve outcome and mortality have not been borne out in clinical trials. Nor has it been shown to be superior to intermittent hemodialysis. Despite these many advances in renal replacement therapy, the mortality from AKI in the surgical ICU remains as high as it was 25 years ago.

Cardiovascular Dysfunction

The cardiovascular abnormalities of MODS are essentially the vascular features of systemic inflammatory and hypermetabolic state. These include hyperdynamic circulation with decreased peripheral vascular resistance, decreased regional blood flow to organ beds, increased capillary permeability, right ventricular cardiac depression, and diminished heart rate variability. Therapy is primarily supportive with judicious use of pressors, inotropes, and fluids to support physiology such that aerobic metabolism is maintained. Pressors should include norepinephrine or vasopressin; it is unclear if vasopressin has improved outcomes in this situation. This should be monitored and titrated to physiologic parameters such as urine output, central venous pressure, mean arterial pressure, and aerobic metabolism parameters such as mixed venous oxygen saturation or lactate clearance. There is no evidence that achieving supranormal physiology improves or prevents MODS, or that invasive hemodynamic monitoring, such as pulmonary artery catheterization, improves outcomes. Use of bedside echocardiography for hemodynamic monitoring and titration of therapy holds significant promise, particularly in the setting of right heart failure, but the exact goals of therapy to improve outcome remain unclear. Marshall MODS score includes the PAR, or product of the heart rate times the ratio of atrial pressure to arterial pressure, as a measure of cardiovascular dysfunction, which can be used to monitor progression, but again, its use for prognosis and therapy has not been upheld.

HEPATIC DYSFUNCTION

The liver is classically the second organ system to fail after pulmonary dysfunction sets in. The pathophysiology is poorly understood, but again appears to be related to cellular hypoxia and ischemia, due to splanchnic vasoconstriction and hypoperfusion. Two syndromes are described: one, also known as "shock liver," is characterized by initial elevated transaminases, followed by hyperbilirubinemia, and then synthetic dysfunction with increased international normalized ration (INR). Depending on the severity of the initial insult, this can progress to severe hepatic failure. Treatment is entirely supportive and is focused on minimizing further hepatic damage by avoiding hepatotoxins, providing nutrition, and managing encephalopathy. A subtler form of hepatic dysfunction is more common and is characterized by mild hyperbilirubinemia, with or without cholestasis, but usually synthetic function is unaffected. In most cases, enteral nutrition is tolerated in patients with hepatic dysfunction, but if it is not, other causes of hyperbilirubinemia or jaundice should be sought. This includes biliary obstruction, acalculous cholecystitis, or pancreatitis.

CENTRAL NERVOUS SYSTEM DYSFUNCTION—DELIRIUM

It is now recognized that delirium and cognitive dysfunction in critical illness are the brain's manifestations of multiple organ dysfunction and are important markers of systemic illness and prognosis in MODS. While previously believed to be transient phenomena due primarily to medications, it is now clear from functional magnetic resonance imaging (MRI) studies that these are potentially permanent or long-lasting consequences of structural, physiologic, and functional changes in the brain that result from systemic injury, sepsis, and surgery. These dysfunctions are more likely and more severe if patients are elderly and have premorbid dementia, cognitive dysfunction, or substance abuse. The interaction of pain, anxiety, and sleeplessness, with the noisy environment of the ICU and the very medications used to address these issues, all clearly play a role in this complex syndrome. There are multiple strategies that can prevent or ameliorate brain dysfunction, but few have proven conclusively effective. These include pharmacologics such as atypical antipsychotics, minimizing exposure to benzodiazepines, and measures to promote sleep-wake cycles and early mobilization.

ENDOCRINE AND METABOLIC DYSFUNCTION

Derangements of the hypothalamic-pituitary axis and glucose and protein metabolism are common manifestations of MODS. Acute or chronic inflammation, injury, or surgery lead to hypermetabolism and a persistent catabolic state, which can last for months during and after critical illness. Despite this recognition, it is poorly understood whether these findings represent the driving force of MODS (and should be treated) or are merely side effects of underlying pathophysiology. The clinical presentation includes hyperglycemia, hypothyroidism, and hypoadrenocortical function. Laboratory studies will also reveal low growth hormone levels and testosterone levels. Therapeutic goals include maintaining glucose levels between 120 and 150 with insulin drip to minimize infectious complications, with the risk of hypoglycemia outweighing any benefits of tighter glucose control. Replacement of thyroid hormone and cortisol is of less clear benefit but should be entertained if a true hypothyroidism (low T3 or T4) is present. Replacement of growth hormone, testosterone, or androgens is not indicated in either physiologic or pharmacologic doses; in spite of abnormally low levels, replacement has been shown to be deleterious to patient outcomes.

THERAPEUTIC STRATEGIES— NUTRITION

Evidence-based treatments for MODS remain scarce. The mainstay of therapy is enteral nutrition for all patients, with organ-specific strategies such as low tidal volume ventilator management and a minimal transfusion strategy targeting hemoglobin of 7 gms/dL. Outcome of MODS is clearly improved by initiation of early (within 24 hours) enteral nutrition. Feeding the intestinal tract ameliorates the gut-driven inflammatory response in MODS. It is unclear if feeding the stomach is better or equivalent to feeding the small intestine. Enteral nutrition should provide 15 to 25 kcal/kg/day and 1.2 to 2 gram/kg/day protein, depending on the primary disease process, with sepsis and burns requiring higher calories and protein. Parenteral nutrition is second best, and while it provides calories and protein, it does not improve outcome in MODS in the same fashion, has increased infectious complications, and should be used only if enteral nutrition is not possible.

Specific nutrients provide immunotherapy beyond their basic nutritional functions and should be included in enteral formulae. Glutamine supports gut mucosa and improves outcome in MODS. Omega-3 fatty acids support immune function and decrease infectious complications in MODS, and they should be included in enteral nutrition. Supplementation of vitamins and minerals is important for wound healing, immune function, and support of the hypermetabolic state. This includes zinc, selenium, vitamin C, and folate. Some evidence suggests that pharmacologic doses of these vitamins are therapeutic as antioxidants and can prevent or ameliorate MODS, but this is not standard of care at this time.

PATIENT-CENTERED OUTCOMES AND PALLIATIVE CARE

Early goal-directed therapy, nutrition, and control of infection are the most important determinants of mortality outcome from MODS, although patient age and premorbid conditions also play a role. Despite many advances, mortality remains high, and long-term disability and poor quality of life are prevalent among survivors. Persistent MODS becomes chronic critical illness, requiring prolonged ICU stays or long-term care in skilled nursing facilities. Multiple studies have shown that patients with MODS have a very high symptom burden while in the ICU, including pain, anxiety, posttraumatic stress disorder, thirst, weakness, and fatigue. Evidence-based therapies directed at symptoms include continuous pharmacologic management of pain and anxiety with opioids, benzodiazepines, and management of procedural pain. Nonpharmacologic therapies are equally if not more important and include early mobilization with physical therapy, massage, maintenance of sleep-wake cycle with light therapy, and minimization of night stimulation.

While the mortality of MODS is high, predicting the outcome in any given patient is difficult, so discussions around goals of care and end-of-life decisions need to be started early with families. Strategies to improve communication among physicians, nurses, and family are beneficial for many outcomes. A first family meeting within 72 hours of admission to the surgical ICU, regardless of prognosis, is standard of care and will decrease the use of nonbeneficial life support at the end of life, decrease conflict in decisions, and improve family satisfaction and bereavement outcomes.

SUMMARY

MODS is a systemic disease of inflammatory response that continues to change as ICU care advances. Despite these advances, the outcome from MODS remains poor, with a high mortality and a high long-term disability for survivors. Its management ultimately requires global therapies that address these systemic disturbances, with additional organ targeted therapies to improve outcome. Currently, surgical therapy is aimed at prevention of MODS with goal-directed therapy for sepsis, trauma, and other conditions. Once MODS develops, management is primarily supportive, both for the patient as a whole and for maintenance of specific organ function. Outcomes can be improved with focus on nutrition, ventilator strategies, early mobilization, and symptom relief.

SUGGESTED READINGS

Baue AE: Multiple, progressive, or sequential systems failure, *Arch Surg* 110:779–781, 1975.

Deitch EA: Multiple organ failure. Pathophysiology and potential future therapy, *Ann Surg* 216:117–134, 1992.

Heyland DK, Cook DJ, King D, et al: Maximizing oxygen delivery in critically ill patients: a methodologic appraisal of the evidence, *Crit Care Med* 24:517–524, 1996.

Marshall JC, Cook DJ, Christou NV, et al: Multiple organ dysfunction score: a reliable descriptor of a complex clinical outcome, *Crit Care Med* 23:1638–1652, 1995.

Stewart TE, Meade MO, Cook DJ, et al: The Pressure- and Volume-Limited Ventilation Strategy Group. Evaluation of a ventilation strategy to prevent barotrauma in patients at high risk for acute respiratory distress syndrome, *N Engl J Med* 338:355–361, 1998.

Ulvik A, Kvale R, Wentzel-Larsen T, et al: Multiple organ failure after trauma affects even long-term survival and functional status, *Crit Care* 11:R95, 2007.

Vincent JL, Moreno R, Takala J, et al: The sepsis-related organ failure assessment (SOFA) score to describe organ dysfunction/failure, *Intens Care Med* 22:707–710, 1996.

ANTIBIOTICS FOR CRITICALLY ILL PATIENTS

Vanessa P. Ho, MD, MPH, and
Philip S. Barie, MD, MBA, FIDSA, FCCM, FACS

Critically ill surgical patients are at risk for a variety of complicated infections that may lead to morbidity and mortality. Traditionally, surgical infections are those that necessitate surgery for treatment, such as surgical site infections (SSIs), complicated intra-abdominal infections (cIAIs), and skin or soft tissue infections (SSTIs). However, critically ill surgical patients are vulnerable to a variety of other nosocomial infections, including central line–associated bloodstream infections (CLABSIs), urinary tract infections (UTIs), and hospital-acquired/ventilator-associated pneumonia (HAP/VAP).

Antibiotics are the cornerstone of treatment for infection, but dosing in this patient population can be challenging because of day-to-day variations in fluid status, renal function, and hepatic function. In intensive care units (ICUs), this challenge is complicated further when infection is caused by bacteria that are resistant to antibiotics used commonly. A vicious cycle develops in which increasingly broad-spectrum antibiotics must be prescribed empirically to ensure that initial antibiotic treatment is adequate and pathogens acquire more resistance subsequently. Clinicians must be vigilant, accurate, and precise about the diagnosis and proper treatment of these infections, not only to treat patient diseases but also to prevent further development of antibiotic resistance.

DIAGNOSIS OF INFECTION AND EMPIRIC THERAPY

Infection may manifest via a variety of clinical signs and symptoms, including hypotension, tachycardia, tachypnea, confusion, rigors, skin lesions, oliguria, lactic acidosis, leukocytosis or leukopenia, and thrombocytopenia. Fever is usually the trigger for workup of a potential infection, although the definition is variable and some infected patients do not manifest a febrile response; some patients may even be hypothermic in response to infection. Clouding the clinical picture further, fever in a surgical patient is often a manifestation of a non-infectious state of inflammation. In the first 72 hours after surgery (unless surgery was performed to treat an infection), fever is more likely to be a result of atelectasis, venous thromboembolism, tissue ischemia, or adrenal insufficiency than infection, although patients may present with a coincident community-acquired infection, such as pneumonia (CAP). Once more than 96 hours have passed, fever is more likely to represent infection.

When infection is suspected, a careful, thorough, and expeditious search for the source must be performed. Antibiotics should not be given until this evaluation has occurred, including the collection of specimens for culture. Therefore, the evaluation must be performed immediately, as delay in antibiotic administration is associated with an increased risk of death. Current guidelines recommend that initial empiric antibiotic treatment should be administered within 1 hour after the initial suspicion of sepsis.

The patient should be examined for clinically evident infections, including the removal of surgical dressings for examination of incisions. If an incision is opened, a culture specimen should be obtained from the deep wound space (not superficially) to minimize isolation of contaminants. A chest x-ray is optional unless the patient has been ventilated mechanically or exhibits signs or symptoms of a pulmonary infection, such as an abnormal physical examination, tachypnea, pulmonary secretions, or abnormal arterial blood gases. In patients who have been ventilated mechanically, a chest x-ray and lower respiratory cultures should be obtained. Pulmonary disease in the early setting may result from aspiration of gastric contents or CAP. Urinalysis or culture is not mandatory unless a UTI is suspected (e.g., genitourinary trauma, posturologic surgery, urinary catheterization).

Blood cultures should be obtained from patients with any clinical suspicion of infection. These should be obtained via venipuncture, and at least 10 mL/bottle should be collected from adults to ensure adequate sampling. Two to three sets of cultures (two bottles/set) should be performed from different sites, including one set from any indwelling vascular catheters. The cumulative yield of pathogens is optimized when three sets of blood cultures (10 to 15 mL blood/bottle) are drawn. Multiple sets of cultures allow differentiation between true pathogens and contaminants (e.g., if one of multiple cultures is positive for an organism found commonly on the skin, such as coagulase-negative *Staphylococcus* spp.), and a pathogen from a colonized catheter (i.e., if only the culture drawn from the catheter is positive, with negative peripheral [venipuncture] blood cultures). Fungal blood cultures should be obtained from patients who have received antibiotics recently or have immunosuppression or development of a hospital-acquired infection after a course of antimicrobial therapy.

Inappropriate initial therapy is associated with increased mortality, so empiric antibiotic therapy must be targeted appropriately and given in a dose sufficient to ensure bacterial killing. Deescalation to a narrower spectrum antibiotic should occur as soon as possible (if appropriate) on the basis of microbiologic data and clinical response. Pathogens that require empiric coverage depend on the suspected disease process, whether the infection is community-acquired or hospital-acquired, and whether the patient is likely to have multidrug-resistant (MDR) pathogens (defined as resistance to all agents of at least three classes; e.g., penicillins, cephalosporins, fluoroquinolones) present. Local antimicrobial resistance patterns must also be considered. A variety of agents are available for empiric therapy (Box 1); therapy should be chosen on the basis of clinical suspicion of the spectrum required (broad or targeted, gram-positive or gram-negative, antipseudomonal, antianaerobic) and knowledge of local patterns of susceptibility (antibiogram). Common nosocomial pathogens are presented in Table 1. If a nosocomial gram-positive pathogen is suspected (e.g., from an incision, central venous catheter, or VAP) or methicillin-resistant *Staphylococcus aureus* (MRSA) is endemic, empiric therapy with vancomycin or linezolid is warranted. Combination empiric therapy (e.g., double coverage for *Pseudomonas* pathogens) is recommended by some authorities, but evidence for efficacy is mixed. Some infections such as VAP or hospital-acquired cIAI require combination empiric therapy to cover both gram-positive and gram-negative pathogens. Specific considerations for the major antibiotic classes are shown in Table 2.

Duration of antimicrobial therapy continues to be debated because of the lack of class I evidence. If all cultures are negative, empiric antibiotic therapy should be stopped after 48 to 72 hours. Unnecessary antibiotic therapy increases the risk of future infection with MDR pathogens, so prolonged therapy in the absence of a pathogen is not recommended. If infection is evident, treatment is continued as indicated clinically. Every decision to start antibiotics should be accompanied by an a priori decision regarding duration of therapy; recommended treatment durations for various types of infection are given in Table 3. Clinical evidence of infection past the predetermined treatment endpoint could indicate new infection, development of resistance, or treatment failure with the current regimen. In cases such as these, the clinician should consider discontinuation of antibiotics and reevaluation for infection.

PRINCIPLES OF ANTIBIOTIC THERAPY

Antimicrobial therapy is a mainstay of infection management, but these drugs must be used correctly. An understanding of basic principles of pharmacokinetics (PK) and pharmacodynamics (PD) is essential because each medication has specific attributes that affect its interaction with the patient and the pathogen. PK describes the fate of the drug once administered to a patient, including absorption, distribution, metabolism, and excretion. Basic concepts of PK include bioavailability, half-life, clearance, and volume of distribution. *Bioavailability* is the percentage of drug that reaches the systemic circulation; intravenous antibiotics are 100% bioavailable, but oral bioavailability depends on absorption, intestinal transit time, and

---

BOX 1: Antibacterial agents for empiric use

Antipseudomonal
Piperacillin-tazobactam
Cefepime, ceftazidime
Imipenem-cilastatin, meropenem, doripenem
Ciprofloxacin, levofloxacin (depending on local susceptibility patterns)
Aminoglycosides
Polymyxins (polymyxin B, colistin [polymyxin E])

Targeted-Spectrum
Gram-positive
Glycopeptide (e.g., vancomycin, telavancin)
Lipopeptide (e.g., daptomycin; not for known/suspected pneumonia)
Oxazolidinone (e.g., linezolid)
Vancomycin
Gram-negative
Aminoglycoside
Third-generation cephalosporin (except ceftriaxone)
Monobactam
Polymyxins (polymyxin B, colistin [polymyxin E])
Antianaerobic
Metronidazole

Broad-Spectrum
Piperacillin-tazobactam
Carbapenems (not ertapenem)
Fluoroquinolones (depending on local susceptibility patterns)
Tigecycline (plus an antipseudomonal agent)

Antianaerobic
Metronidazole
Carbapenems
Beta-lactam/beta-lactamase combination agents
Tigecycline

Anti-MRSA
Ceftaroline
Daptomycin (not for use against pneumonia)
Minocycline (oral only)
Linezolid
Telavancin
Tigecycline (not in pregnancy or for children under the age of 8 y)
Vancomycin

MRSA, Methicillin-resistant *Staphylococcus aureus*.

---

hepatic metabolism. *Half-life* ($T_{1/2}$) is the time required for the serum drug concentration to reduce by one half. *Volume of distribution* (V_D) is the theoretic volume in which the total amount of drug needs to be distributed uniformly to produce the desired concentration of a drug. V_D can be increased by renal or liver failure and decreased in dehydration; reduced V_D causes a higher plasma drug concentration. *Clearance* is the volume of liquid from which drug is eliminated completely per unit of time, whether by tissue distribution or elimination via metabolism, excretion, or dialysis; knowledge of drug clearance is important for determining the dose of drug necessary to maintain a steady-state concentration. Hydrophilic antibiotics (e.g., aminoglycosides, beta-lactams, glycopeptides, and colistin [polymyxin E]) are affected by increased V_D and altered drug clearance. Lipophilic antibiotics (e.g., fluoroquinolones, macrolides, tigecycline, and lincosamides) are less susceptible to alterations in V_D but may have altered drug clearance in critically ill patients.

PD describes the effect of a drug on the patient or the pathogens and accounts for drug-patient, drug-microbe, and microbe-patient

TABLE 1: Common pathogens isolated from cases of healthcare-associated infections

Pathogen	Percentage	Most common site
Coagulase-negative Staphylococcus	15.3	Bloodstream
Staphylococcus aureus	14.5	Surgical site
Enterococcus spp.	12.1	Bloodstream
Candida spp.	10.7	Urinary tract
Escherichia coli	9.6	Urinary tract
Pseudomonas aeruginosa	7.9	Respiratory tract
Klebsiella pneumonia	5.8	Urinary tract
Enterobacter spp.	4.8	Respiratory tract
Acinetobacter baumannii	2.7	Respiratory tract
Klebsiella oxytoca	1.1	Respiratory tract
Other	15.6	

Reported to the National Healthcare Safety Network, U.S. Centers for Disease Control and Prevention, 2006-2007.

interactions; antimicrobial agents are unique medications because the most important interaction is not between the patient and the drug but rather the microbe and the drug. This interaction can be affected by inoculum size, microbial physiology, and resistance mechanisms. The most important PD parameter to consider is the *minimal inhibitory concentration* (MIC), which is the lowest serum drug concentration that inhibits bacterial growth. Dosing strategies with both PK and PD reflect how different antibiotics work. In addition, some antibiotics may suppress bacterial growth at subinhibitory concentrations (postantibiotic effect [PAE]), which can allow the dosing interval to be extended.

Time-dependent bacterial killing with antibiotics requires the concentration of antibiotic to exceed the MIC for a certain proportion of the dosing interval; this is denoted as fT>MIC (proportion of time the plasma concentration is above the MIC). Beta-lactams and carbapenems are examples of time-dependent antibiotics. Concentration-dependent bacterial killing with antibiotics requires the peak concentration to be more than tenfold higher than the MIC; examples include aminoglycosides and polymyxin B. Bacterial killing with time-dependent, concentration-enhanced antibiotics is described by the area of the plasma concentration-time curve above the MIC (AUC); examples include fluoroquinolones, vancomycin, and clindamycin. Table 4 outlines which strategies should be used with specific drug classes and tactics to maximize effectiveness.

SPECIFIC CONSIDERATIONS

Specific circumstances are particularly relevant in the critically ill patient population. Postoperative HAP/VAP, urinary tract infections, CLABSI, and infection from MDR organisms are worthy of consideration.

Postoperative Pneumonia

Critically ill surgical patients are particularly susceptible to HAP/VAP, particularly if they need mechanical ventilation. VAP is defined

as pneumonia that occurs at least 72 hours after intubation and is the most common infection that occurs in the ICU among surgical and trauma patients. The incidence of VAP increases with the duration of mechanical ventilation at a rate of 3% per day during the first 5 days, 2% per day during days 5 to 10, and 1% per day after that. Additional risk factors for VAP include age more than 60 years, acute respiratory distress syndrome, underlying pulmonary disease, impaired consciousness, poor nutrition, burn/trauma, blood transfusions, organ failure, supine positioning, large-volume gastric aspiration, sinusitis, and immune suppression.

Despite the high prevalence of VAP, the diagnosis is difficult to make because noninfectious processes may mimic pneumonia. As a result of the low specificity of clinical criteria, culture of the lower respiratory tract is mandatory in the ICU. The method of specimen collection (invasive or noninvasive) and specimen analysis (semi-quantitative or quantitative) is debated. Invasive methods (bronchoalveolar lavage [BAL] and protected specimen brush [PSB]) collect samples via bronchoscopy and allow examination of the airway but are expensive and resource intensive. Noninvasive techniques include endotracheal suction aspiration, blinded plugged telescoping catheter, blinded PSB, and mini-BAL. Commonly used thresholds for quantitative culture are 10^3 colony-forming units (CFU)/mL for PSB, 10^4 CFU/mL for BAL, and 10^5 CFU/mL for endotracheal aspirate. Any threshold should be lowered by one order of magnitude if a patient received antibiotics before sample acquisition.

Organisms that may be pathogens in VAP when recovered from the airway include Pseudomonas *aeruginosa*, Acinetobacter *calcoaceticus-baumannii* complex, Enterobacteriaceae, *S. aureus*, and *Haemophilus influenzae*. Enterococci, viridans streptococci, coagulase-negative staphylococci, and *Candida* spp. are rare causes of HAP/VAP. If a patient was started on empiric therapy for HAP/VAP and the culture is negative for growth, antimicrobial therapy should be discontinued as long as the patient has not had clinical deterioration. If a susceptible pathogen is identified and the patient's condition is improving, the antibiotic may be deescalated to a narrower spectrum agent. If the culture shows a MDR pathogen, the broad-spectrum agent may be continued, or therapy can be escalated if the initial agent was not active against the pathogen.

Once pathogen-specific therapy is underway, the duration of therapy must be planned. Clinical and radiographic parameters typically lag the eradication of infection. A randomized, multicenter trial by Chastre and colleagues of 401 patients (VAP proved with bronchoscopy and quantitative microbiology) showed that an 8-day course (vs 15-day) of initially appropriate antimicrobial therapy is effective, provided that the patient's condition is stable; the exception was that a 15-day course was superior if the pathogen was a nonfermenting gram-negative bacillus (i.e., *P. aeruginosa*, *Stenotrophomonas maltophilia*, *Acinetobacter* spp.).

Patients who do show a response to therapy pose a dilemma. Inadequate therapy, misdiagnosis, or a pneumonia-related complication (e.g., empyema, lung abscess) must be considered. The evaluation should be repeated, including repeat quantitative cultures. Broadened empiric antibiotic coverage should be reinstituted thereafter until new data become available.

Urinary Tract Infection

When clinical evaluation suggests the urinary tract as a possible source of fever, a urine specimen collected with sterile technique from the catheter sampling port should be evaluated with direct microscopy, gram stain, and quantitative culture. Urine should arrive in the laboratory promptly to prevent multiplication of bacteria within the transport container, which might lead to the misdiagnosis of infection. Routine monitoring or surveillance cultures have minimal utility. Rapid dipstick tests, which detect leukocyte esterase and nitrite, are unreliable in the setting of catheter-related UTI. The

TABLE 2: Drug classes and dosing considerations

Drug class	Dosing considerations	Adjustment

Aminoglycosides	Examples: gentamicin, tobramicin, amikacin
	Require a concentration peak:MIC ratio >10
	Loading dose is necessary
	Must check trough concentrations:
	  0.5-1 µg/mL recommended for gentamicin, tobramycin
	  5-10 µg/mL recommended for amikacin
	Not first-line because of toxicity
	Synergistic against *Pseudomonas*, *Enterococcus*, and MDR gram-negative pathogens
	Bactericidal
	Consider single daily-dose therapy to ensure high ratio (not validated in pregnant women, children, burn patients, elderly >70 y)
		Renal

Beta-lactams	Includes penicillins, cephalosporins, monobactam (aztreonam), and carbapenems Efficacious when fT>MIC is >40% of dosing interval Activity dependent on class: penicillins have little activity against gram-negatives; cephalosporins should not be used against MDR pathogens, with the exception of possibly cefepime (which is more resistant to hydrolysis by beta-lactamases) Carbapenems (imipenem-cilastatin, meropenem, ertapenem, and doripenem) have the widest clinical utility of any antibiotics, including against gram-positives, gram-negatives, and anaerobes; ertapenem is not useful against *Pseudomonas*, *Acinetobacter*, *Enterobacter*, or MRSA	Variable
Cyclic lipopeptides	Example: daptomycin Bactericidal Concentration-dependent killing Active against aerobic and anaerobic gram-positives 4 mg/kg/d for nonbacteremic infections 6 mg/kg/d for bacteremia Not to be used for pneumonia	Renal
Fluoroquinolones	Examples: ciprofloxaxin, levofloxacin, moxifloxacin Excellent oral absorption and bioavailability Bactericidal Efficacy reflected with the AUC Some activity against gram-negatives, although resistance is increasing Activity against gram-positives is variable (best with moxifloxacin) Moxifloxacin has some antianaerobic activity Can cause cartilage and tendon damage Caution with prolonged QT interval (can precipitate dangerous dysrhythmias [torsades de pointes]) and with patients on warfarin (will markedly increase the International Normalized Ratio)	

Lipoglycopeptides	Examples: Vancomycin, telavancin
	Active against gram-positives
	Efficacy reflected by the AUC
	For vancomycin:
	  Initial dose should be calculated as 15-20 mg/kg, not to exceed 2 g/dose; for patients with sepsis, meningitis, pneumonia, or endocarditis, a loading dose of 25-30 mg/kg may be considered
	  Dose adjustments should be based on trough serum concentrations, obtained before the 4th dose
	  For serious infections or MRSA, trough serum concentrations of 15-20 µg/mL are recommended
	For telavancin:
	  10 mg/kg over 60 min, given every 24 h
		Renal

Polymyxins	Examples: polymyxin B, colistin Bacteriostatic and bactericidal Concentration-dependent killing Activity only against gram-negative pathogens Dosed as 1.5-2.5 mg/kg daily in divided doses (polymyxin B) Clinical response rates for respiratory infections are lower than other sites of infection Nephrotoxic and neurotoxic	Renal

TABLE 2: Drug classes and dosing considerations—cont'd

Drug class	Dosing considerations	Adjustment
Oxazolidinones	Example: linezolid Bacteriostatic (except against pneumococci) Active against gram-positives, including MSSA, MRSA, VRE, and penicillin-resistant *S. pneumonia* No dose adjustment for renal mild-moderate hepatic disease Nearly 100% oral bioavailability	No adjustment needed
Sulfonamides	Example: trimethoprim-sulfamethoxazole Bacteriostatic Oral absorption rapid and bioavailability nearly 100% Widespread resistance Active against gram-positives, sensitive gram-negatives Treatment of choice for community-acquired MRSA Trimethoprim-sulfamethoxazole is treatment of choice for *S. maltophilia*	Renal

Tetracyclines	Examples: doxycycline, minocycline, tigecycline (a glycylcycline derivative of minocycline)
	Bacteriostatic
	Active against anaerobes
	Tigecycline has broad-spectrum activity
	   Covers MRSA, VRE, gram-negative pathogens including ESBL and MDR organisms
	   Does not cover *Pseudomonas* spp.
	   Not indicated for hospital-acquired pneumonia
	Active against anaerobes
		Hepatic adjustment for tigecycline

AUC, Area of the plasma concentration-time curve above the MIC; *ESBL,* extended-spectrum beta-lactamase; *fT>MIC,* the proportion of time the plasma concentration is above the MIC; *MDR,* multidrug-resistant; *MIC,* minimum inhibitory concentration; *MRSA,* methicillin-resistant *Staphylococcus aureus*; *MSSA,* methicillin-sensitive *Staphylococcus aureus*; *VRE,* vancomycin-resistant *Enterococcus.*

TABLE 3: Current recommendations for duration of therapy for selected serious infections

Bacterial Meningitis	
Gram-negative bacilli (e.g., postoperative)	21 d
Central Line–Associated Bloodstream Infection	
Coagulase-negative *Staphylococcus*	5-7 d
S. aureus	14 d-6 w (for persistent bacteremia)
Enterococcus	7-14 d
Gram-negative bacilli	7-14 d
Candida spp.	14 d after last positive culture
Complicated Intra-abdominal Infection	**4-7 d**
Pneumonia	
Community-acquired pneumonia	≤5 d
Ventilator-associated pneumonia	7 d
Nonfermenting gram-negative bacilli	14 d
Other bacteria	7 d

leukocyte esterase test correlates with the degree of pyuria, which may or may not be present in a catheter-related UTI. The nitrite test reflects Enterobacteriaceae, which convert nitrate to nitrite, and is therefore unreliable to screen for *Enterococcus* spp., *Candida* spp., and *Staphylococcus* spp.

Catheter-associated bacteriuria or candiduria usually represents colonization, is rarely symptomatic, and is an unlikely cause of fever or secondary bloodstream infection, even in patients with immunocompromise, unless there is urinary tract obstruction; a history of recent urologic manipulation, injury, or surgery; or neutropenia. Traditional signs and symptoms, (e.g., dysuria, urgency, pelvic or flank pain, fever, and chills) that correlate with bacteriuria in patients without catheterization are reported rarely in ICU patients with documented catheter-associated bacteriuria or candiduria ($>10^5$ CFU/mL). In the ICU, most UTIs are related to urinary catheters and are caused by MDR gram-negative bacilli. For confirmed nonbacteremic catheter-associated UTI, a 5-day to 7-day course of treatment is sufficient.

Central Line–Associated Bloodstream Infection

Critically ill patients often need central venous access, but these catheters are prone to infection. Strict adherence to infection control, proper insertion, and catheter care are crucial for prevention; in addition, the need for the catheter should be reassessed daily. Optimal technique for insertion includes chlorhexidine skin preparation and maximal barrier protection (full-bed drape and cap, mask, sterile gown, and gloves for the operator). Catheters placed in suboptimal conditions (e.g., during an emergency resuscitation) should be removed and replaced as soon as the patient's condition permits. Catheters inserted in the femoral vein pose the highest risk of infection; subclavian vein catheters have the lowest risk. Tunneled catheters and peripherally inserted central catheters have lower risk of

TABLE 4: Pharmacokinetics of bacterial killing: implications for antibiotic dosing

Characteristic	Drug	Therapeutic goal	Tactic
Time-dependent (no or minimal PAE) fT > MIC > 70% ideal	Carbapenems Cephalosporins Linezolid Penicillins	Maintain drug concentration	Maximize duration of exposure with prolonged or continuous infusion*
Time-dependent, concentration-enhanced (with PAE) AUC:MIC$_{24h}$ >125; AUC:MIC$_{24h}$ > 400 for MDR pathogens	Clindamycin Glycylcyclines Macrolides Streptogramins Tetracyclins Vancomycin	Maximize effectiveness of bacteriostatic/weak bactericidal antibiotics with prolonged PAEs PAE is concentration-dependent	Maximize drug dosage consistent with avoidance of toxicity†
Concentration-dependent (with PAE)	Aminoglycosides Daptomycin Fluoroquinolones Ketolides Metronidazole Polymixins	PAE is concentration-dependent Achieve Cmax ([peak]:MIC) > 10	Maximize peak concentration‡

AUC, Area under the concentration-time curve; *Cmax*, maximal drug concentration (peak concentration); *fT*, proportion of time; *MDR*, multidrug-resistant; *MIC*, minimum inhibitory concentration; *PAE*, postantibiotic effect.

*Continuous or prolonged infusion of linezolid is not recommended because efficacy has not been established.

†Examples of maximized drug dosages include clindamycin 900 mg every 8 h rather than 600 mg every 6 h and vancomycin 15 mg/kg every 8 to 12 h for patients with normal renal function. Larger doses of tigecycline (a glycylcycline) and streptogramins (e.g., quinupristin/dalfopristin) may be limited by increased toxicity.

‡Examples of dosing to achieve maximized peak drug concentrations include single daily-dose aminoglycoside therapy and metronidazole 1 g every 12 h rather than 500 mg every 8 h. Prolonging the dosing interval is not recommended for polymyxins because of a negligible PAE.

infection than central venous catheters inserted percutaneously. Abrupt signs and symptoms of sepsis or shock should prompt suspicion of infection. Blood cultures positive for staphylococci or *Candida* spp. strongly suggest infection of a vascular catheter, which should prompt removal and culture of the catheter. For febrile patients without other signs of infection, there is no immediate need to remove or change all indwelling catheters. Catheter removal is prudent in a patient with a prosthetic heart valve or a fresh arterial graft and recommended for severe sepsis or septic shock, peripheral embolization, disseminated intravascular coagulation, and acute respiratory distress syndrome. Patients with persistent *S. aureus* bacteremia, or fungemia, should have endocarditis excluded with echocardiography.

MULTIDRUG-RESISTANT ORGANISMS

Patients in the ICU characteristically have multiple risk factors for infections with MDR bacteria (Box 2). The most important factor is a patient's prior antibiotic exposure; even a single dose of antibiotic increases the risk of infection with an organism resistant to that antibiotic, in that person, for up to 1 year. Partial, incomplete, or inappropriate therapy from mistargeted initial therapy or underdosing of antimicrobial agents is also associated with emergence of resistance. Proper infection control practice, in particular hand hygiene, is the most important infection control tactic to control spread of MDR organisms; increased hand-washing compliance decreases rates of infection.

S. aureus evolved rapidly to become resistant to penicillin and methicillin (MRSA). This evolution occurred, concurrently, within and outside of hospitals and created two distinct strains: hospital-acquired MRSA and community-acquired MRSA (CA-MRSA). Increasing prevalence of CA-MRSA in the hospital suggests that the phenotypic differences between these strains will become less marked

BOX 2: Risk factors for acquisition of infection caused by multidrug-resistant pathogens

Chronic indwelling catheter (vascular or urinary)
Chronic renal replacement therapy (dialysis)
Colonization with an MDR pathogen (e.g., nasal colonization with MRSA, fecal colonization with VRE)
High total or cumulative antibiotic exposure
High severity of illness/care in an intensive care unit
Prolonged acute-care hospitalization
Prolonged endotracheal intubation/mechanical ventilation
Recent antibiotic therapy (within 3 mo)
Recent hospitalization (within 3 mo)
Recent surgery
Residence in a skilled-nursing or extended-care facility
Solid-organ or bone marrow transplantation

MDR, Multidrug-resistant; *MRSA*, methicillin-resistant *Staphylococcus aureus*; *VRE*, vancomycin-resistant *Enterococcus* spp.

over time. Vancomycin-resistant *S. aureus* remains rare, but treatment failures can occur with isolates that have intermediate sensitivity with MIC testing or susceptibility close to the MIC cut point (>1 µg/mL). High-dose vancomycin is recommended for MRSA infections; provided renal function is normal, a dose of 15 mg/kg intravenously (IV) every 8 to 12 hours is recommended to achieve a vancomycin trough concentration of ~15 µg/mL (measurement of peak concentration is unnecessary). Clinical failure with vancomycin or a MIC of more than 1 µg/mL should prompt treatment with a different antibiotic, such as high-dose daptomycin (alone or in combination therapy), linezolid, or ceftaroline.

Vancomycin-resistant *Enterococcus* (VRE) first emerged in 1987 and has become a common pathogen in hospitalized patients. Most strains of *Enterococcus faecalis* are inhibited (but not killed) with attainable concentrations of standard antienterococcal agents, but *E. faecium* is increasingly resistant to vancomycin. VRE can be treated with daptomycin, linezolid, or tigecycline.

P. aeruginosa is a highly prevalent nonfermenting gram-negative bacillus that is a opportunistic pathogen. *P. aeruginosa* acquires resistance by a variety of mechanisms and can develop resistance, even an MDR phenotype, during therapy. Serial cultures and susceptibility testing should be performed during therapy, even when prior cultures have shown susceptible isolates. *Acinetobacter* spp., especially *A. baumannii*, is an aerobic nonfermenting gram-negative coccobacillus that infects debilitated hospitalized patients. They can survive on inanimate surfaces and pose a high risk for spread within hospitals. *Acinetobacter* spp. are innately resistant to many classes of antibiotics, including penicillins, cholamphenicol, and often aminoglycosides; they can also develop resistance to fluoroquinolones during therapy. Carbapenems are the gold-standard therapy, but resistance is increasing worldwide as a result of the increasing prevalence of carbapenemases.

Of further concern are bacteria that produce extended-spectrum beta-lactamase (ESBL). These bacteria are often not detected with automated systems because there is no single definitive marker for production of ESBL, but the phenotype can be found most commonly in the Enterobacteriaceae family (e.g., *Escherichia coli, Klebsiella pneumoniae, Proteus mirabilis*) and other bacteria, including *P. aeruginosa* and *Acinetobacter* spp. In general, an isolate can be suspected to produce ESBL when it shows in vitro susceptibility to cephamycins (i.e., cefoxitin) but resistance to third-generation cephalosporins and aztreonam. In addition, one should be suspicious if treatment of a gram-negative infection results in clinical failure despite reported susceptibility in vitro. ESBL-producing bacteria may be treated with a carbapenem, tigecycline, an aminoglycoside, a polymixin, or combination therapy. Proposed combination therapy regimens for MDR infections are shown in Box 3.

Knowledge of administration tactics can be advantageous in treatment of these pathogens. An increasing body of literature has supported the use of prolonged-infusion or continuous-infusion beta-lactams and carbapenems. As these antibiotics exhibit time-dependent bacterial killing, prolonged infusion allows the serum concentration to exceed the MIC for a longer period of time, improving efficacy against difficult-to-treat pathogens. Aminoglycosides, which exhibit concentration-dependent bacterial killing, can be given with single-daily dosing to ensure a high peak concentration and minimized toxicity. Although polymyxins are also concentration-dependent, they should not be given with single-daily dosing because there is negligible PAE and bacteria may reemerge when the antibiotic is not present.

High-dose daptomycin (e.g., 10 to 12 mg/kg/d) can be used for recalcitrant non-VAP gram-positive infections, provided that the small possibility of myositis is monitored with serial determinations of creatine phosphokinase. Infections caused by MDR gram-negative bacilli pose a major problem, and there are few options for therapy. Carbapenems, aminoglycosides, tigecycline, and polymyxins have useful activity against ESBL-producing pathogens; cefepime and piperacillin/tazobactam are less successful. MDR nonfermenting gram-negative bacilli and carbapenemase-producing Enterobacteriaceae may require therapy with a polymyxin or combination therapy.

ANTIBIOTIC TOXICITIES

Beta-Lactam Allergy

Allergic reaction is the most common toxicity of β-lactam antibiotics. The incidence rate is approximately 7 to 40 per 1000 treatment courses of penicillin. Parenteral therapy is more likely to provoke an allergic reaction. Most serious reactions occur in patients with no

---

BOX 3: Combination therapy options for the treatment of recalcitrant or highly resistant multidrug-resistant infections

Management of Persistent MRSA Bacteremia or Vancomycin Treatment Failures
Search for and Eradicate Foci of Infection, Including Débridement or Surgical Drainage, with
High-dose daptomycin (10-12 mg/kg/d)*
 alone or in combination with:
Gentamicin 1 mg/kg/d IV, *or*
Rifampin 600 mg IV/PO daily *or* 300-450 mg IV/PO twice daily, *or*
Linezolid 600 mg IV/PO twice daily, *or*
Televancin 10 mg/kg IV once daily, *or*
Trimethoprim/sulfamethoxazole 5 mg/kg IV twice daily, *or*
A β-lactam antibiotic

If Reduced Susceptibility to Vancomycin or Daptomycin are Present[†]
Quinupristin/dalfopristin 7.5 mg/kg IV every 8 h, *or*
Linezolid 600 mg IV/PO twice daily, *or*
Televancin 10 mg/kg IV once daily, *or*
Trimethoprim/sulfamethoxazole 5 mg/kg IV twice daily

Management of MDR Gram-Negative Bacillary Infections When Effective Conventional Monotherapy is not Available Based on in Vitro Susceptibility Testing or is Contraindicated (e.g., Hypersensitivity)[‡]
High-dose, prolonged-infusion, or continuous-infusion carbapenem with or without a polymyxin or aminoglycoside
Dual carbapenem therapy
Aminoglycoside combined with a β-lactam agent (antipseudomonal cephalosporin or BLIC agent) or antipseudomonal fluoroquinolone, with or without rifampin
Aminoglycoside plus fosfomycin
Intravenous combined with inhalational aminoglycoside (for pneumonia)
Intravenous combined with inhalational polymyxin B plus a carbapenem, aminoglycoside, fluoroquinolone, or aztreonam (for pneumonia)
Antipseudomonal cephalosporin or BLIC agent combined with an antipseudomonal fluoroquinolone
Polymyxin combined with one or more of a carbapenem, aminoglycoside, fluoroquinolone, or β-lactam agent
Polymyxin or aminoglycoside plus tigecycline
Polymyxin combined with rifampin, an antipseudomonal carbapenem (or both), with or without azithromycin or doxycycline

BLIC, β-Lactamase inhibitor combination; *IV,* intravenous; *MDR,* multidrug-resistant; *MRSA,* methicillin-resistant *Staphylococcus aureus; PO,* oral.
*Assumes the organism is susceptible in vitro. Data from Liu C, Bayer A, Cosgrove SE, et al: Clinical practice guidelines by the Infectious Diseases Society of America for the treatment of methicillin resistant Staphylococcus aureus infections in adults and children, *Clin Infect Dis* 52:e8-e45, 2011.
†Agents may be given alone or in combination. Data from Liu C, Bayer A, Cosgrove SE, et al: Clinical practice guidelines by the Infectious Diseases Society of America for the treatment of methicillin-resistant Staphylococcus aureus infections in adults and children, *Clin Infect Dis* 52:e8-45, 2011.
‡Suggestions are derived from in vitro testing, animal studies, or case reports. No class I data or large class II studies are available.

history of penicillin allergy, simply because a history of penicillin allergy is sought commonly and reported by 5% to 20% of patients (far in excess of the true incidence rate). Patients with a prior reaction have a fourfold to sixfold increased risk of another reaction compared with the general population. However, this risk decreases with time, from 80% to 90% skin test reactivity at 2 months to 20% reactivity at 10 years. The risk of cross reactivity between penicillins and carbapenems and cephalosporins is ~5%, and there is negligible cross reactivity to monobactams.

Nephrotoxicity

Aminoglycosides cause nephrotoxicity as a result of ischemic toxicity to the renal proximal tubular cell (PTC). Ultimately, injury is manifested by necrosis of PTCs, reduction of the glomerular filtration rate, and decreased creatinine clearance, although this is usually reversible and progression to dialysis dependence is rare. Aminoglycoside nephrotoxicity is accentuated by frequent dosing, older age, sodium or volume depletion, acidemia, hypokalemia, hypomagnesemia, and coexistent liver disease. The risk of injury is ameliorated with single daily-dose therapy. The offending drug should be discontinued unless treatment is for a life-threatening infection.

Vancomycin nephrotoxicity is on the increase because of higher dosing and concurrent administration of other nephrotoxins. Nephrotoxicity of polymyxins may be an unavoidable consequence of the need to use an agent with known nephrotoxic potential to treat serious infections cause by MDR gram-negative bacilli when alternatives are few or none.

Ototoxicity

Aminoglycosides cause cochlear or vestibular toxicity that is usually irreversible and may develop after the cessation of therapy. Repeated exposures create cumulative risk. Most patients have development of either cochlear toxicity or a vestibular lesion; rarely are both organs injured. Few patients report hearing loss; yet when sought, the incidence rate of cochlear toxicity may be more than 60%. Clinical hearing loss may occur in 5% to 15% of patients. Ototoxicity caused directly by vancomycin is documented poorly in the literature. Hearing loss attributed to vancomycin is better described as neurotoxicity, manifesting as auditory nerve damage, tinnitus, and loss of acuity for high-frequency tones. Synergistic injury is possible with coadministration of other ototoxic drugs, especially aminoglycosides or furosemide. No correlation is found between ototoxicity and nephrotoxicity for drugs that cause both (e.g., aminoglycosides, vancomycin).

▮ AVOIDANCE OF TOXICITY: ADJUSTMENT OF ANTIBIOTIC DOSAGE

Hepatic Insufficiency

The liver metabolizes and eliminates drugs that are too lipophilic for renal excretion. Drug dosing in hepatic insufficiency is complicated by insensitivity of clinical assessments to quantify liver function and changing metabolism as the degree of impairment fluctuates (e.g., resolving cholestasis). Changes in renal function with progressive

hepatic impairment add considerable complexity. Renal blood flow is decreased in cirrhosis, and glomerular filtration is decreased in cirrhosis with ascites. Adverse drug reactions are more frequent with cirrhosis than with other forms of liver disease. The effect of liver disease on drug disposition is difficult to predict in individual patients; none of the usual tests of liver function can be used to guide dosage. Generally, a dosage reduction of up to 25% of the usual dose is considered if hepatic metabolism is 40% or less and renal function is normal. Greater dosage reductions (up to 50%) are advisable if the drug is administered chronically, there is a narrow therapeutic index, protein binding is low or reduced substantially (e.g., hypoalbuminemia), or the drug is excreted renally and renal function is impaired severely.

Renal Insufficiency

Renal drug elimination depends on glomerular filtration, tubular secretion, and reabsorption, any of which may be altered with renal dysfunction. Chronic kidney disease or acute kidney injury (AKI) may affect hepatic and renal drug metabolic pathways. Drugs with hepatic metabolism that is likely to be disrupted in renal failure include aztreonam, several cephalosporins, macrolides, and carbapenems. Accurate estimates of renal function are important in patients with mild-to-moderate renal dysfunction and should be measured when a patient's renal function is suspected to have changed. Critically ill patients with AKI who need renal replacement therapy pose a particular challenge because drug dosing can be difficult in the setting of fluctuating renal function and volume status. These patients may have increased V_D from capillary leakage and low protein binding and may need increased doses of antibiotics despite poor renal function; as the patient's condition improves and the volume is removed, doses may have to be adjusted again.

Administration of loading doses of antibiotics that will achieve the target serum concentration based on the expected V_D without adjustment for renal function is generally appropriate; subsequent doses should be based on available literature for specific antibiotics and renal therapy regimens. Doses and regimens should be reassessed frequently with serum concentrations whenever possible. The need to dose patients during or after a renal replacement therapy treatment must be borne in mind; during continuous renal replacement therapy, the estimated creatinine clearance is ~15 to 25 mL/min in addition to the patient's intrinsic clearance. Cefaclor, cefoperazone, ceftriaxone, chloramphenicol, clindamycin, cloxacillin and dicloxacillin, doxycycline, erythromycin, linezolid, methicillin/nafcillin/oxacillin, metronidazole, rifampin, and tigecycline do not require dosage reductions in renal failure.

SUGGESTED READINGS

Barie PS: Multidrug-resistant organisms and antibiotic management, *Surg Clin North Am* 92:345–391, ix-x, 2012.

Dellit TH, Owens RC, McGowan JE Jr, et al, Infectious Diseases Society of America and Society of Healthcare Epidemiology: Infectious Diseases Society of America and Society of Healthcare Epidemiology of America guidelines for developing an institutional program to enhance antimicrobial stewardship, *Clin Infect Dis* 44:159–177, 2007.

Liu C, Bayer A, Cosgrove SE, et al: Clinical practice guidelines by the Infectious Diseases Society of America for the treatment of methicillin-resistant Staphylococcus aureus infections in adults and children, *Clin Infect Dis* 52:e8–45, 2011.

Owens RC Jr, Shorr AF: Rational dosing of antimicrobial agents: pharmacokinetic and pharmacodynamic strategies, *Am J Health Syst Pharm* 66(12 Suppl 4):S23–S30, 2009.

ENDOCRINE CHANGES IN CRITICAL ILLNESS

Zvonimir Milas, MD, FACS,
Douglas F. Naylor, Jr., MD, FACS, FCCM, and
Kresimira Milas, MD, FACS

OVERVIEW

Critically ill patients treated either in surgical or medical intensive care units (ICUs) experience significant changes in endocrine system functions. All forms of critical illness, whether from injury, surgery, infection, or burns, are subject to these changes. Numerous hormones are released in the acute and prolonged phases of illness (Table 1) that shunt oxygen and substrates to crucial organs, affect the immune system, and lead to hypermetabolism and hypercatabolism that if excessive may exacerbate organ failure and death. This chapter focuses on the two most frequent clinical scenarios of endocrine imbalance with critical illness, adrenal insufficiency and hyperglycemia; highlights recent concepts of thyroid dysfunction as a marker of adverse prognosis in critically ill patients; and draws attention to iatrogenic or drug-induced endocrine disorders in the ICU setting.

ADRENAL INSUFFICIENCY

Adrenal insufficiency represents failure of the adrenal gland itself (primary adrenal insufficiency) or failure of the hypothalamus or pituitary gland to stimulate the adrenal cortex (secondary adrenal insufficiency). Other terms have also been applied to describe adrenal dysfunction in critically ill patients, including relative adrenal insufficiency (RAI) and critical illness–related corticosteroid insufficiency (CIRCI). Table 2 provides etiologies of adrenal insufficiency. Diseases that directly destroy adrenal function are rare; instead, conditions that induce severe stress can frequently precipitate adrenal failure. Adrenal insufficiency is difficult to recognize, and objective criteria of diagnosis have been notoriously difficult to establish. Many factors influence this: lack of pathognomonic features for hypoadrenalism, masking of presentation by other comorbidities, transient changes or treatments in the critical care setting, and inherent limitations to elicit symptoms and examination findings in critically ill patients. No universal, reliable, biochemical reference standard exists for diagnosis with plasma cortisol profiles. Thus, detection requires surgeons to think of the possibility of adrenal insufficiency, actively search for clues, and apply common sense towards management.

Normal function of the hypothalamic-pituitary-adrenal (HPA) axis is for the hypothalamus to secrete vasopressin and corticotrophin-releasing hormone (CRH), which in turn stimulate the anterior pituitary gland to release adrenal corticotrophic hormone (ACTH). Cortisol release from the adrenal is the primary effect of ACTH, as aldosterone and androgen secretion respond more to the renin-angiotensin system and pituitary gonadotropins than to ACTH. Cortisol secretion in normal conditions is pulsatile and has diurnal variation, with highest levels in the morning. Cortisol is not stored in the adrenal cortex. Rather, the HPA axis has a feedback loop in which hypercortisolism inhibits the axis and cortisol deficiency stimulates new cortisol production. The HPA axis activation is essential to normal physiologic responses to stress. The "flight or fight" response is the HPA axis diverting adrenal function from mineralocorticoid to glucocorticoid production. Extremes of stress, as encountered in the critical care setting and with sepsis, can alter all components of this process, including cortisol binding, diurnal variation of secretion, and the feedback loop. Mortality in the critical care setting is influenced both by very high and by very low levels of cortisol.

Primary adrenal insufficiency has the following clinical symptoms: weakness, anorexia, weight loss, depression, fatigue, nausea, vomiting, orthostatic hypotension, and craving for salt. Clinical signs include tachycardia, hypotension, fever, mental status change, amenorrhea, hypovolemia, and hyperpigmentation, which, as a result of ACTH elevation, is seen only with primary adrenal failure. Laboratory abnormalities include hyponatremia, hyperkalemia, hypoglycemia, eosinophilia, and normocytic normochromic anemia. Although similar in overall patterns, secondary adrenal insufficiency lacks hyperpigmentation and mineralocorticoid insufficiency, thus limiting losses of water, sodium, and chloride. The lack of volume and electrolyte disturbances may reduce gastrointestinal reported complaints but may present with hypoglycemia from alterations in glucocorticoid levels. As alluded to previously, classic findings may not always be present in the critically ill. Fever and hypotension may accompany many illnesses; treatments or comorbidities may mask other symptoms (e.g., aggressive electrolyte protocols may eliminate electrolyte laboratory abnormalities).

Most characteristics of adrenal insufficiency are hemodynamic instability and hyperinflammation despite fluid resuscitation and pressor support. Diagnosis is supported when hemodynamics improve on cortisol administration. Biochemical testing for the purposes of diagnosis can be difficult to interpret. For example, HPA reactivity is tested with measurement of a baseline random cortisol level, followed by administration of 250 mcg ACTH (cosyntropin) intravenously and assessment of cortisol levels at 30 and 60 minutes after infusion. The normal adrenal gland responds to stress by producing cortisol levels above 18 to 20 mcg/dL; this definition, however, is derived from high-dose ACTH stimulation or insulin-induced hypoglycemia in patients who are not stressed or critically ill. Another definition of 'normal' is derived from studies of factors correlating with poor outcomes in ICU patients: "normal" is when random serum cortisol levels exceed 25 mcg/dL or increase by more than 9 mcg/dL from baseline after stimulation. With this latter definition, 60% of patients with sepsis have inadequate adrenal responses. The varying definitions and uncertainty of diagnosis of adrenal insufficiency also account for widely different incidence rates reported in studies.

Significant variables still exist in assessment and management of adrenal insufficiency. The basic understanding of whether this is a transient, functional, or structural adrenal problem remains unknown. Differences are seen in sensitivity, accuracy, and reproducibility among commercially available cortisol assays, and factors such as protein binding, cortisol metabolism and clearance, and end-organ resistance can all affect cortisol measurements. High-dose 250-mcg ACTH is a supraphysiologic concentration that can cause normal cortisol response because it overcomes ACTH resistance in the adrenals without adequate functional reserves. But then, the adrenals may already be maximally stimulated at baseline in response to illness and are unable to show an increase of 9 mcg/dL. Outcomes of treatment protocols have varied with the use of high-dose (30 mg/kg) or moderate-dose (200-300 mg/d) glucocorticoid replacement.

A low-dose synthetic 1-mcg ACTH stimulation test may be more physiologic and sensitive for diagnosis. Another option is to test with this low-dose 1-mcg ACTH stimulation first and then use the high-dose 250-mcg ACTH only in patients without response. Data remain limited about the optimal method of biochemical confirmation of hypoadrenalism.

How should a surgeon logically approach this problem, given these limitations? Some generalizations are outlined in Figure 1 and can be supplemented with a review of the American College of Critical Care Medicine consensus statement on the diagnosis and

TABLE 1: Overview of the endocrine system response to acute and prolonged phase of critical illness and potential interventions

Hormone	Acute phase	Prolonged phase	Potential intervention
Sympathomimetic System			
Norepinephrine	++	+/=	May need vasopressor therapy if endogenous stores are inadequate
Epinephrine	++	+/=	
Somatotropic Axis			
Pulsatile GH release	+	−	
GHBP	−	+	
IGF-1	−	−	Exogenous GH administration associated with increased mortality rate
ALS	−	−	
IGFBP-3	−	−	
Hypothalamic-Pituitary-Thyroid Axis			
Pulsatile TSH release	+/=	−	
T4	+/=	−	No benefit of replacement and may prolong recovery to euthyroid state
T3	−	−	
rT3	+	+/=	
Hypothalamic-Pituitary and Lactotropic Axis			
Pulsatile LH release	+/=	−	
Testosterone	−	−	No benefit of replacement
Dehydroepiandrosterone	−	−	
Pulsatile prolactin release	+	−	
Hypothalamic-Pituitary-Adrenal Axis			
ACTH	+	−	Replace if biochemical evidence of relative insufficiency in septic shock
Cortisol	++	+/=	

ACTH, Adrenocorticotropic hormone; *ALS*, acid-labile subunit; *GH*, growth hormone; *GHBP*, growth hormone binding protein; *IGF-1*, insulin-like growth factor-1; *IGFBP-3*, insulin-like growth factor binding protein-3; *LH*, luteinizing hormone; *rT3*, reverse triiodothyronine; *T3*, triiodothyronine; *T4*, thyroxine; *TSH*, thyroid stimulating hormone.
+, Increase from baseline; −, decrease from baseline; =, no change from baseline.
Modified from Vanhorebeek I, Van den Berghe G: The neuroendocrine response to critical illness is a dynamic process, Crit Care Clin 22:1, 2006.

management of corticosteroid insufficiency and best practice parameters from the Endocrine Society.

Unexplained hemodynamic instability should raise suspicion of HPA dysfunction. Because administration of steroid therapy in the patient with refractory hypotension is a clinical decision, biochemical confirmation of adrenal failure may not always be required. Testing is recommended for patients with subtle signs of adrenal insufficiency. A random cortisol level of less than 25 mcg warrants high dose (250-mcg) ACTH testing. Failure of cortisol levels to increase by more than 9 mcg/dL over baseline after ACTH stimulation suggests adrenal insufficiency, and cortisol therapy should be implemented. A random cortisol level of less than 10 mcg/dL is also indicative of adrenal insufficiency and justifies glucocorticoid therapy.

If steroid replacement treatment is administered, whether immediately for a clinical decision of septic shock unresponsive to therapy or after testing, steroid therapy is given as follows. Patients with refractory hypotension should receive 200 to 300 mg/d of intravenous hydrocortisone in divided doses. Hydrocortisone should be continued for 7 days and then tapered slowly over the next 7 days. Mineralocorticoid supplementation with 50 mcg/d oral fludrocortisone is optional because the oral route may not be available and because there is sufficient mineralocorticoid activity with more than 50 mg/d hydrocortisone. Surgeons should have a low threshold to reinstitute steroids as needed if symptoms return after the taper.

It cannot be overstressed that hydrocortisone therapy is not warranted as an adjuvant therapy for sepsis without evidence of shock. Diagnostic testing and treatment should be started together in the patient with an unstable condition. Steroid therapy can be started after test results become available in the patient with a hemodynamically stable condition. Steroids are of no benefit in the treatment of sepsis without signs of shock or abnormal cortisol test results. Dexamethasone was once recommended as a bridge to treatment while

TABLE 2: Etiology of adrenal insufficiency in critical illness

Adrenal insufficiency	Etiology
Primary	Bilateral adrenal necrosis and hemorrhage caused by sepsis, hypotension, and hemorrhage
	Unmasking of chronic known or latent primary insufficiency
	Autoimmune adrenalitis in developed countries
	Tuberculous adrenalitis in developing countries
	Infectious diseases (fungal, viral, HIV)
Secondary	Irreversible anatomic damage to the hypothalamus or the pituitary gland
	Necrosis or hemorrhage in sepsis as a result of prolonged hypotension or coagulopathy
	Unmasking of chronic known or latent secondary adrenal insufficiency caused by sepsis
	Hypothalamic or pituitary tumors
	Chronic inflammation
	Congenital adrenocorticotropic hormone deficiency
	Drug therapy
	Inhibition of early increase in adrenocorticotropic hormone caused by high-dose diazepam and fentanyl administration
	Previous treatments with glucocorticoids including topical administration
	Inhibition of steroid genesis with a single dose of etomidate
	Accelerated metabolism of cortisol by ketoconazole and cyclosporine, clarithromycin, rifampicin, and antiepileptic drugs, such as phenytoin and phenobarbital

awaiting results; however, because it inhibits the HPA axis longer and can alter test or therapy outcomes, it is no longer advised. Similarly, a previous approach of use of a short course of high-dose steroids is now viewed as ineffective and possibly harmful. The currently recommended dose range (200 to 300 mg/d) of hydrocortisone seems to reduce time for reversal of septic shock, but effects on mortality remain unproven. Future guidelines may altogether abandon the use of steroids in septic shock.

HYPERGLYCEMIA

In critically ill patients, an acute sustained increase in serum glucose in response to stress is defined as hyperglycemia. Once the acute illness resolves, this "diabetes of injury" ends, and previously euglycemic patients return to their normal physiologic state. Hyperglycemia in this context was thought to be a compensatory response in coping with critical stress, but it also imposes significant adverse consequences: abnormal immune function, increased infection, hemodynamic and electromyocardial disturbances, increased insulin resistance, and higher insulin requirements. The degree of hyperglycemia also depends on an individual's capacity to meet the increased insulin demand. The finding of hyperglycemia during critical illness can unmask borderline diabetes in some patients. The American

Diabetes Association and American Association of Clinical Endocrinologists define stress hyperglycemia or hospital-related hyperglycemia as any blood glucose concentration of more than 140 mg/dL (7.8 mmol/L) without evidence of previous diabetes. Up to 60% of patients admitted with new stress hyperglycemia had confirmed diabetes 1 year later. Nearly 1 in 5 adult patients presenting with stress hyperglycemia had unrecognized diabetes identified by admission hemoglobin (Hb) A1c more than 6.1%.

Given the hypermetabolic changes in critically ill or septic patients, hyperglycemia is an understandable consequence. High catecholamine and glucocorticoid hormone levels produce hyperglycemia. Other hormones inhibit hepatic glycogenesis and peripheral glycolysis while promoting gluconeogenesis and lipolysis.

A direct relationship is found between the extent of stress hyperglycemia and mortality in critically ill patients. In a landmark study of surgical ICU patients, Van den Berghe and colleagues showed that intensive insulin therapy to achieve tight glycemic control (80 to 110 mg/dL) reduced in-hospital mortality by 34%, bloodstream infections by 46%, acute renal failure requiring dialysis by 41%, and transfusions by 50%. Patients were also less likely to need mechanical ventilation or intensive care. Other studies have shown that insulin treatment lowers short-term mortality by 15%. Similarly, in medical ICU patients, Van den Berghe and colleagues' study showed reduced morbidity and shorter ICU stay and hospitalization. Lower mortality was observed only for patients staying in the ICU longer than 3 days. Scalea and associates confirmed that hyperglycemia in trauma patients is similarly associated with numerous complications: infections, increased ventilator days/ICU and hospital days, and higher risk of mortality. Most significantly, they showed the importance of early glucose control; regardless of subsequent glucose levels, mortality remained high unless tight glucose control was achieved within the first week of injury.

How should a surgeon logically approach the issue of hyperglycemia in critically ill patients? First is recognition of preferred target glucose levels. Blood glucose levels of more than 180 mg/dL are unacceptable in critically ill patients. Hypoglycemic levels (<40 mg/dL) are likewise undesirable. The optimal target to aim for falls into two ranges: (1) a more conventional range of 140 to 180 mg/dL; and (2) a tighter glycemic range of 80 to 110 mg/dL. No significant differences in overall outcome were observed between these ranges in several large randomized trials, except perhaps that the tighter glycemic range was potentially more beneficial to trauma patients and cardiac surgical patients. The conventional range (140 to 180 mg/dL) remains the most preferred because it avoids the risks of severe hypoglycemia.

Next is the realization that optimal treatment of hyperglycemia in the critically ill population is administration of intravenous insulin. This is more predictable and effective than subcutaneous (SQ) insulin, the adsorption of which may be affected by changes in locoregional blood flow. Insulin infusions can be administered via defined protocols and allow rapid dosing but do require intensive monitoring and frequent glucose measurements (hourly until stable and then every 2 hours). Once a patient's condition stabilizes, transition to SQ insulin treatment can occur.

Finally, planning for glycemic management during the recovery phase of illness and on discharge is important. Measurement of HbA1C concentration during hospitalization can predict the need for insulin or oral antidiabetic agents after discharge. These are usually unnecessary in patients with HbA1C of less than 6.5%. This value can also help differentiate those patients with stress hyperglycemia that developed in the context of previously undiagnosed diabetes and those who need further evaluation and care.

THYROID DYSFUNCTION

Several thyroid abnormalities can develop in critically ill patients. Hypothyroxinemia occurs in the form of low thyroxine (T4) and

Adrenal Insufficiency in Critical Illness

Stressor

Hypothalamus

CRH

Secondary Adrenal Insufficiency: Chronic steroid use, hypothalamic or pituitary tumors, head trauma, HIV, sarcoidosis, cancer, sepsis, postpartum, ACTH resistance

Posterior Pituitary

Anterior Pituitary

ADH

ACTH

Classic signs and symptoms of adrenal insufficiency: hyponatremia, hyperkalemia, hypoglycemia, eosinophila, normocytic, normochromic anemia, anorexia, weight loss, nausea, vomiting, mental status changes, depression, orthostatic hypotension, tachycardia, fever, weakness, fatigue, craving for salt, hyperpigmentation (primary AI).

Signs and symptoms associated with adrenal insufficiency in critical illness: hypotension despite fluid resuscitation and pressor support, signs of hyperinflammation

Adrenal Cortex

Aldosterone

Cortisol

Primary Adrenal Insufficiency: autoimmune adrenalitis, adrenal hemorrhage (HIT, DIC, meningococcemia), infectious adrenalitis (HIV, CMV, TB, fungal), drug-induced adrenal failure (etomindate, ketoconazole, Mitotane), hypothermia, sepsis, peripheral resistance to cortisol

Recommendations for diagnosis and management of adrenal insufficiency in critical illness:

Refractory hypotension in the critically ill is highly suggestive of AI and should be treated with 200-300 mg/day IV hydrocortisone (moderate dose steroid) for 7 days.

Adrenal insufficiency in patients with potential symptoms is best diagnosed with high dose (250 mcg) synthetic ACTH testing and treatment is as above:

• Random total cortisol level < 25 mcg/dL should be tested
• Random total cortisol level < 10 mcg/dL suggests adrenal insufficiency
• A failure to increase baseline random total cortisol level > 9 mcg/dL after stimulation with HD synthetic ACTH indicates adrenal insufficiency

After 7 days, hydrocortisone should be tapered slowly and reinstituted if rebound effects occur.

Mineralocorticoid supplementation with oral fludrocortisone is not required, but may be helpful in patients who were previously on oral prednisone.

Dexamethasone is not recommended for treatment or during adrenal testing

Stress dose steroids are warranted in the endocrine challenged and those with a history of glucocorticoid use.

Metabolic actions: increases hepatic gluconeogenesis, activates lipolysis and proteolysis to release free fatty acids and amino acids, inhibits adipose glucose uptake
Immunologic actions: stimulates antiinflammatory cytokines and mediators, inhibits pro-inflammatory cytokine production and inflammatory mediator expression, inhibits inflammatory cell migration
Cardiovascular actions: increases cardiac contractility, vascular tone and blood pressure via cortisol mediated reactivity to angiotensin II, epinephrine and norepinephrine, inhibits nitric oxide synthesis

FIGURE 1 A summary of adrenal insufficiency in critical illness.

triiodothyronine (T3) levels in circulation. Because T3 decreases occur earliest and most uniformly during critical illness, the condition has been called the low T3 syndrome, the nonthyroidal illness syndrome (NTI), and euthyroid sick syndrome. Severe and prolonged illness also leads to declines in T4 levels and in pulsatile levels of thyroid-stimulating hormone (TSH; or thyrotropin). This is not a benign condition; hypothyroxinemia has recently been correlated to mortality in critically ill patients and those with surgical sepsis.

Understanding the nature of changes in thyroid axis function is useful. The normal thyroid gland produces T4 and T3 and stores these in large follicles bound to thyroglobulin. In healthy patients, the anterior pituitary secretes TSH in a pulsatile and diurnal fashion, causing thyroid hormones to be released into circulation, 90% as T4 and 10% as T3. Peripheral conversion of T4 to T3 supplies the remainder of T3. Both thyroid hormones are heavily bound to carrier proteins, and the amount of free hormone released is kept constant by matching to levels excreted by the thyroid gland. Free circulating

T4 and T3 are taken up by target cells in peripheral tissues, where enzymes of the iodothyronine deiodinase family (D1, D2, D3) convert T4 into T3, or into the inactive metabolite reverse T3 (rT3). Within the target cells, thyroid hormones bind nuclear receptors to accomplish organ-specific changes. The thyroid hormones form an autoregulatory loop by feedback inhibition at the levels of both the pituitary and hypothalamus to inhibit TSH secretion.

During critical illness or surgical stress, total T3 and free T3 levels in circulation decline during induction of anesthesia and remain low for the first few postoperative days. These levels normalize when a patient recovers but remain suppressed or decline even further with prolonged illness or sepsis. T4 follows a similar pattern that appears during the prolonged illness phase and is related to severity of illness. Random, single-sample TSH levels transiently rise in the first hours of acute illness but then normalize. TSH levels can actually become abnormally low during prolonged illness and, even if normal, lose nocturnal secretion surges and pulsatile fractions, thus exacerbating low states of T4 and T3. Recuperation stages often show elevated TSH levels.

The mechanisms that lead to these abnormalities are varied and may not be uniform among patients. They include variations in thyroid hormone uptake by peripheral tissues, altered metabolism of thyroid hormone by deiodinases, changes in thyroid hormone nuclear receptors in the target cells, set-point changes in the hypothalamic-pituitary axis, depletion of selenium that is required by several intrathyroidal enzymes and the deiodinases, and iatrogenic TSH suppression by drugs used in the ICU, notably dopamine and metoclopramide. Despite these diverse mechanisms, it is thought that the most likely driver of changes in serum T3 levels during critical illness is impaired thyroid hormone production.

When total serum T4 levels fall below 50 nmol/L and 25 nmol/L, mortality risks have been reported to rise up to 50% and even 80%, respectively. Most studies also favor the general concept that decreased thyroid function at baseline of the acute illness may be associated with worse outcomes from sepsis and septic shock, but it is unclear whether altered thyroid function actually participates in these adverse changes or is merely a predictor of poor outcome.

Also unclear are whether treatment to normalize thyroid function in critically ill patients is warranted and what combinations of pharmacologic agents (T4, T3, other novel compounds) are effective without producing harmful side effects. Only four small, randomized trials provide information, and none reveal a clear benefit of normalizing abnormal thyroid hormone parameters. These studies may have been underpowered to detect differences, and interest remains strong to elucidate this issue with future studies. More simple approaches are advocated, such as increasing awareness of iatrogenic side effects of ICU drugs (dopamine and metoclopramide, for example) that can affect thyroid function and modifying their use if appropriate. Currently, no evidence supports treatment of critically ill patients with exogenous thyroid hormone.

DRUG-INDUCED ENDOCRINE DISORDERS IN THE INTENSIVE CARE UNIT

Current emphasis in medicine focuses more so than ever on minimizing iatrogenic complications and avoiding errors. ICU settings are complex and require large numbers of different medications for therapy, some that may be essential for survival. These medications can also have important endocrine side effects. Table 3 summarizes the most common drug-induced changes according to components of the endocrine system that are affected. The surgeon is directed to the Suggested Readings to expand familiarity with these side effects, options in medication usage, and controversies that remain in this field. The crucial point that the authors wish to communicate by adding this topic in the chapter was that daily review of the patient's ICU medication list ought to consider the potential of such endocrine consequences.

TABLE 3: Drug-induced endocrine disorders in the intensive care unit

Endocrine system	Medications	Consequence
Pituitary/adrenal	Etomidate, azole antifungals	Inhibit cortisol synthesis
	Phenobarbital, phenytoin, rifampin	Induce cortisol metabolism
	Opioids, benzodiazepines	Suppress CRH and ACTH
	Glucocorticoids	Suppress CRH and ACTH
	Statins	Decrease cortisol substrate
	Heparin	Suppresses aldosterone
	All anticoagulants	Potential adrenal hemorrhage
	Metoclopramide	Suppresses TRH
Pancreas	ACE inhibitors	Increase peripheral insulin sensitivity
	Fluoroquinolones	Stimulate pancreatic insulin secretion
	Pentamidine, quinine, sulfonylurea, toxicity, salicylates	Increase insulin secretion
	Glucocorticoids	Increase gluconeogenesis and insulin resistance, decrease pancreatic insulin secretion
	Cyclosporine, tacrolimus	Decrease insulin biosynthesis/release
	Antipsychotics	Multifactorial glucose abnormalities
	Vasopressors	Activate glycogenolysis, increase hepatic gluconeogenesis, stimulate glucagon and cortisol

Continued

TABLE 3: Drug-induced endocrine disorders in the intensive care unit—cont'd

Endocrine system	Medications	Consequence
Thyroid	Dopamine, dobutamine, octreotide, corticosteroids	Reduce TSH concentration and T4 production
	Amiodarone, iodinated contrast dye	Increase thyroid hormone synthesis, may provoke hyperthyroidism
	Lithium	Decreased thyroid hormone synthesis
	Phenobarbital, phenytoin, rifampin, carbamazepine	Increase thyroid hormone metabolism
	Heparins	Transient increase in free T4 levels
	Furosemide	Displaces thyroid hormone from protein binding sites; in high doses, causes euthyroid sick syndrome
	Metoclopramide	Suppresses TRH

ACE, Angiotensin-converting enzyme; *ACTH,* adrenal corticotrophic hormone; *CRH,* corticotrophin-releasing hormone; *T4,* thyroxine; *TRH,* thyrotropin releasing hormone; *TSH,* thyrotropin or thyroid-stimulating hormone.
Modified from Thomas Z, Bandali F, McCowen K, et al: Drug-induced endocrine disorders in the intensive care unit, Crit Care Med *38(6 Suppl):S219-S230, 2010.*

SUGGESTED READINGS

Batzofin B, Sprung CL, Weiss YG: The use of steroids in the treatment of severe sepsis and septic shock, *Best Pract Res Clin Endocrinol Metab* 25(5):735–743, 2011.

Clark PM, Gordon K: Challenges for the endocrine laboratory in critical illness, *Best Pract Res Clin Endocrinol Metab* 25(5):847–859, 2011.

Farrokhi F, Smiley D, Umpierrez GE: Glycemic control in non-diabetic critically ill patients, *Best Pract Res Clin Endocrinol Metab* 25(5):813–824, 2011.

Marik PE: Mechanisms and clinical consequences of critical illness associated adrenal insufficiency, *Curr Opin Crit Care* 13(4):363–369, 2007.

Marik PE, Pastores SM, Annane D, et al: Recommendations for the diagnosis and management of corticosteroid insufficiency in critically ill adult patients: consensus statements from an international task force by the American College of Critical Care Medicine, *Crit Care Med* 36(6):1937–1949, 2008.

Mebis L, Van den Berghe G: Thyroid axis function and dysfunction in critical illness, *Best Pract Res Clin Endocrinol Metab* 25(5):745–757, 2011.

Pasricha PJ, Pehlivanov N, Sugumar A, et al: Drug insight: from disturbed motility to disordered movement: a review of the clinical benefits and medicolegal risks of metoclopramide, *Nature Clin Pract Gastroenterol Hepatol* 3(3):138–148, 2006.

Thomas Z, Bandali F, McCowen K, et al: Drug-induced endocrine disorders in the intensive care unit, *Crit Care Med* 38(6 Suppl):S219–S230, 2010.

Todd SR, Sim V, Moore LJ, et al: The identification of thyroid dysfunction in surgical sepsis, *J Trauma Acute Care Surg* 73(6):1455–1458, 2012.

van den Berge G, Wouters P, Weekers F, et al: Intensive insulin therapy in the critically ill patients, *N Engl J Med* 345:1359–1367, 2001.

Venkatesh B, Cohen J: Adrenocortical (dys)function in septic shock: a sick eudranal state, *Best Pract Res Clin Endocrinol Metab* 25(5):719–733, 2011.

NUTRITIONAL SUPPORT IN THE CRITICALLY ILL

Matthew D. Neal, MD, and Jason L. Sperry, MD

OVERVIEW

Critical illness is associated with a hypermetabolic and catabolic state that can result in significant energy expenditure and complicate the resuscitation and care of the patient in the intensive care unit (ICU). In recent years, an increasing appreciation for the morbidity and mortality associated with malnutrition in the hospitalized patient has emerged, and the concept of nutritional "support" has evolved into a more active practice of nutritional "therapy." As stated in the joint recommendations made by the Society for Critical Care Medicine (SCCM) and the American Society for Parenteral and Enteral Nutrition (ASPEN), the goals of nutritional support include preservation of immune function, avoidance of metabolic complications, and preservation of lean body mass. The new field of nutritional therapy focuses on favorable nutritional modification of the immune response and the attenuation of oxidative stress and cellular injury.

Despite the robust body of literature that has shown an increased morbidity and mortality associated with postoperative malnutrition, postoperative and acutely ill medical patients are still commonly subjected to prolonged periods of starvation. Although many patients tolerate this insult, those patients with preexisting malnutrition, advanced age, obesity, chronic disease, or extreme injury severity are particularly susceptible to the effects of acute malnutrition, which can impair recovery and contribute to a litany of complications.

Guidelines designed specifically to address nutritional support and therapy in the critically ill are targeted to those who have a planned ICU stay of greater than 2 to 3 days or an inability to return to normal enteral intake within 7 days of starvation. Although most of the evidence in the surgical and critical care literature addresses this cohort of patients, it is often difficult to predict the clinical course of these patients in advance, and thus, it is advisable that nutritional status be part of the initial evaluation of every critically ill or postoperative patient, with frequent reassessments to track progress toward clinical goals. Excellent evidence exists to support the use of feeding algorithms in the ICU, such as that found in Figure 1.

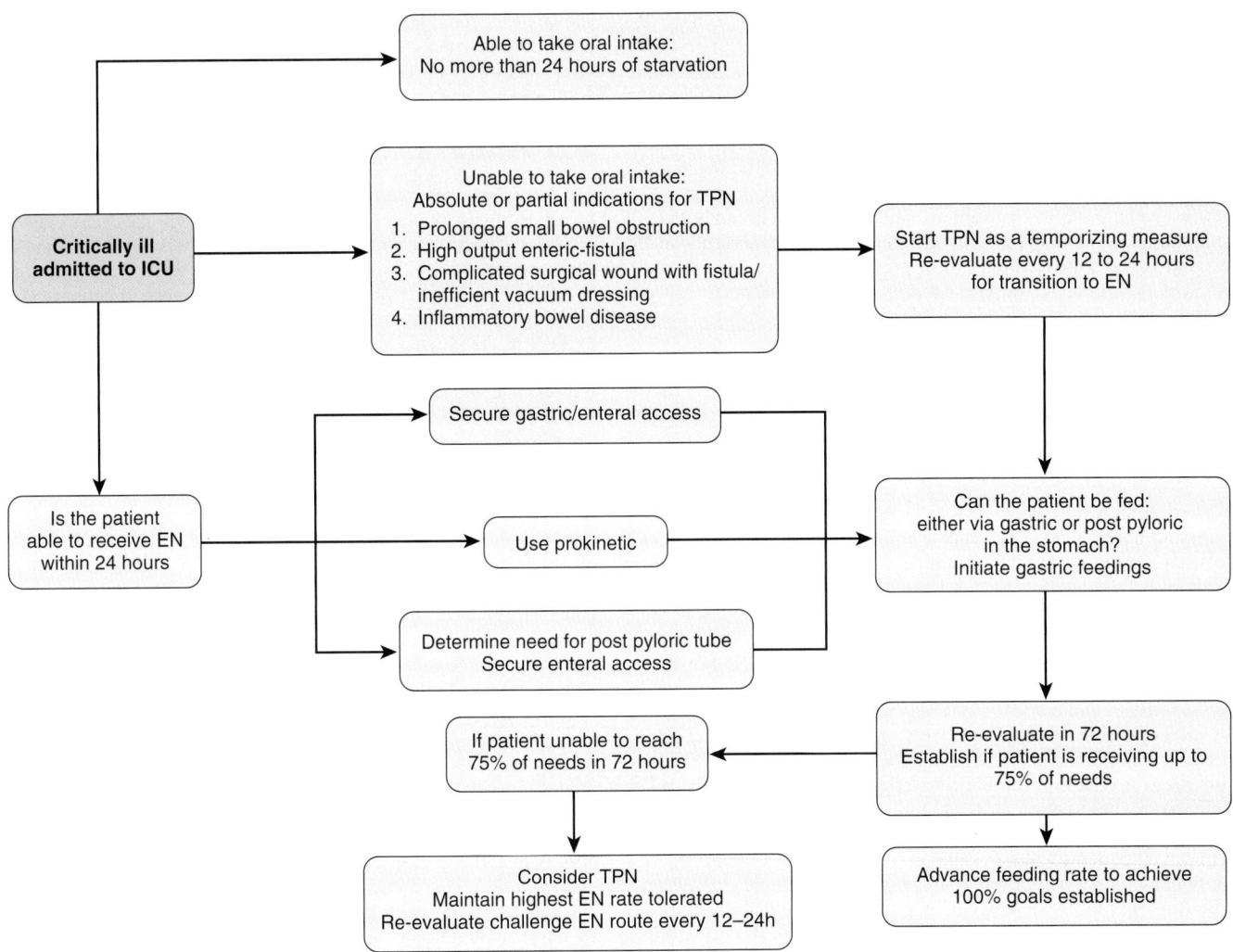

FIGURE 1 Algorithm to implement evidence-based feeding guidelines to improve nutrition practices and reduce mortality in the intensive care unit. *EN,* Enteral nutrition; *ICU,* intensive care unit; *TPN,* total parenteral nutrition. *(Data from Doig GS, Simpson F, Finfer S, et al: Effect of evidence-based feeding guidelines on mortality of critically ill adults: a cluster randomized controlled trial,* JAMA 300[23]:2731-2741, 2008.)

METABOLIC RESPONSE TO STRESS AND NUTRITIONAL REQUIREMENTS DURING CRITICAL ILLNESS

Multiple organ systems are affected by malnutrition, but the intestine is one of the earliest affected, with resultant mucosal atrophy and an inability to effectively absorb and process nutritional once it is initiated. Enteral nutrition supports the integrity of the intestinal mucosa by maintaining tight junctions and reducing gut barrier permeability. When intestinal epithelial integrity is compromised, as is the case when enteral nutrition is withheld for long intervals, the risks of systemic infection and multiple organ failure (MOF) increase substantially. The overwhelming catabolic state of critical illness also results in the loss of muscle and visceral mass from increased oxidative stress. This oxidative stress, which results from a relative deficiency of antioxidants, can lead to a proinflammatory state in multiple organs. Thus, malnutrition can lead to impaired wound healing, end organ injury, and increased rates of nosocomial infection through functional immunosuppression, which is explored in detail later in the chapter.

Most critically ill patients have in common an increased metabolic rate with an increase in energy requirements that ranges from 30% to 70% above normal; this rate can last for as long as 3 weeks after critical illness. The magnitude of this increase depends on the individual patient and the type and severity of illness. For this reason, it is impossible to assign a general number for caloric requirements in the ICU. Furthermore, the assessment of nutritional status with standard protein markers such as albumin and transferrin has not been validated in critically ill patients because of changes associated with the acute phase response. In general, a range of 20 to 40 kcal/kg/d is necessary, with a range of 1.2 to 2.0 g/kg/d of protein to address the hypercatabolic state and protein wasting. However, a number of predictive equations exist, including common formulas such as the Harris-Benedict, to aid in the assessment of caloric needs. These equations should be used with caution because they were not designed for the care of the modern critically ill patient and may be less accurate than indirect calorimetry, which is the most accurate form of energy expenditure assessment currently available. Unfortunately, indirect calorimetry is labor intensive, difficult to calculate, and not available at many institutions. Thus, the calculation of a nutritional goal is an imperfect science, and the ICU clinician should use a combination of existing tools and clinical assessment of injury severity, prehospital nutritional intake, and weight loss and possible consultation with dietary and nutrition service experts to assign a total caloric goal.

Once a goal is established, an effort to provide 50% to 65% of caloric goals should be made within the first week of hospitalization; this has been shown to improve clinical outcomes. Trophic feeding (also known as "trickle feeding" with 10 to 30 mL/h) does have the benefit of preventing mucosal atrophy but may not reach the clinical benefits seen with approaching 50% to 65% of caloric goals. Ongoing assessments of total caloric and protein needs should be made and altered as the clinical course dictates. Electrolyte levels should be monitored regularly to avoid abnormalities, and care should be taken to include calories delivered through intravenous supplements, such as dextrose or calories contained in propofol infusions, in the total count to avoid overfeeding. Quite possibly the most important aspect of the initial attempts to address nutritional needs is to use enteral feeding whenever possible.

EARLY ENTERAL NUTRITION

Level I evidence exists to support the use of enteral nutrition (EN) over parenteral nutrition (PN) in critically ill patients. Six meta-analyses exist to address this topic, with a consistent observation of reduced morbidity, especially in the form of reduced infectious complications. These studies cover a wide range of critically ill patients, from trauma to burns to pancreatitis, which advocates for the broad implementation of EN in the ICU. No significant reduction appears to exist in mortality associated with the use of EN over PN; however, various studies have documented decreased ICU stay, cost associated with nutrition, and noninfectious morbidity. Some studies do report an increased risk associated with EN, including rates of vomiting, need for nasogastric tube, and some observed increase in pulmonary complications. However, these risks appear to be significantly outweighed by the dramatic benefits outlined previously, and most, if not all, nutrition societies have endorsed the use of EN over PN in critically ill patients when possible.

EN has shown its greatest effectiveness when started early. Even with the significant heterogeneity among the published studies, early enteral nutrition (EEN) is defined as nutrition started within the first 24 to 72 hours of admission to the ICU. Table 1 presents the 10 randomized studies that compared EEN and delayed enteral nutrition (DEN) in critically ill patients. A clear reduction, which reaches significance in some studies and trends in others, in mortality and infectious complications has been shown for EEN. EEN should be initiated as soon as feasible on admission to the ICU, and no literature supports the need to wait for passage of stool/flatus or bowel sounds to initiate EN. One major contraindication to EN is significant hemodynamic compromise. Although some patients with low-dose vasopressor requirements may still tolerate EN, in general, significant hypotension or the need for significant hemodynamic support should be viewed as a contraindication to EN. The risk associated with EN in this population is largely attributed to intestinal ischemia caused by dysfunction of the intestinal microcirculation. When EN is used in patients with labile hemodynamics, they must be monitored closely for signs of intolerance, including distention, high residuals, changes in bowel function, and acidosis.

Multiple options exist for the route of feeding, including nasal, oral, and surgically placed enteral access tubes. The main distinction in the site of feeding is whether it is safe to feed the stomach or whether postpyloric feeding is necessary. In all cases, aspiration precautions should be strictly observed. Those patients with high gastric residuals or documented impaired gastric emptying or motility should have postpyloric tubes placed. Otherwise, multiple studies have shown no difference between gastric and small bowel feeding. Prokinetic agents may provide some benefit in patients with documented dysmotility, but no evidence supports their routine application. Tube feeding associated diarrhea is a common clinical problem that can be managed with well-studied algorithms such as

shown in Figure 2. Infectious etiologies, particularly *Clostridium difficile,* must be ruled out before diarrhea in the critically ill patient is attributed to the effects of tube feeding.

TOTAL PARENTERAL NUTRITION

The data reviewed previously lead to the conclusion that enteral nutrition is clearly preferred over total parenteral nutrition (TPN). However, clinical scenarios in which EN must be withheld or significantly delayed are quite common. In the past, TPN was hypothesized to confer a benefit over no nutrition support therapy in patients who could not tolerate or were not candidates for EN. The practice of use of TPN in the absence of preexisting malnutrition was a subject of great debate in the literature; however, two meta-analyses by Braunschweig and colleagues and Heyland and associates showed that the use of TPN was actually detrimental when compared with no nutrition support therapy in the acute setting. Both analyses showed trends towards higher levels of complications with TPN, and Heyland and associates' study showed an increase in mortality with the use of TPN.

Given the clear benefit of EN over TPN and the detrimental outcomes documented in nonmalnourished patients to whom TPN was administered in acute critical illness, the use of TPN has been progressively reduced. Nevertheless, it remains invaluable in the following very specific clinical circumstances: (1) a nonstressed patient who has severe protein-calorie malnutrition is scheduled to undergo surgery (a perfect example is the patient scheduled to undergo esophageal surgery because of obstruction); (2) a patient is malnourished, and TPN given 7 days before surgery is associated with a significant decrease in infection rates; (3) the patient has short gut, and indefinite survival is possible thanks to the use of TPN, which can be used for long-term management or as a bridge to intestinal transplantation; and (4) a patients has failure of oral or enteral nutrition. In fact, the authors of the two meta-analyses mentioned previously went on to document that after a certain duration of critical illness (controversy exists, but the window of time appears to be 7 to 14 days), withholding nutrition altogether begins to lose benefit when compared with TPN. Hospital length of stay and mortality increase in patients who receive no nutrition compared with TPN when duration of critical illness exceeds 7 to 10 days. Thus, the ASPEN and SCCM guidelines suggest that if EN is not feasible in the first 7 days of ICU admission, no nutrition support should be provided. However, in previously healthy patients (before ICU admission) without evidence of malnutrition, a potential benefit exists to the use of TPN when started after 7 days and when EN continues to be unavailable.

TPN should be implemented only after an adequate attempt at EN; however, the patient with complicated abdominal wounds that are clearly worsened by the presence of protracted fistulas that impair any healing may be a candidate for TPN, at least during the early phases of wound care. Often, the combined multidisciplinary care of these wounds and a period of enteral rest allow for the eventual reinitiation of full EN. Currently, no clear guidelines define "failure" of EN; however, it is clear that, at least early on, caloric goals are not necessary through the enteral route to see its benefits. Thus, there is little to no role for combined TPN and EN.

IMMUNONUTRITION

Recommendations regarding an exact composition or type of enteral formula are hard to make because of variations between manufacturers and heterogeneity in the studies that address their effects. However, conclusive and convincing evidence exists to support the use of immune-modulating enteral formulas in select populations. These formulas contain nutrients with pharmacologic properties that serve to enhance immune function and decrease inflammation.

TABLE 1: Randomized trials that assess early enteral nutrition versus delayed enteral nutrition

Study	Population	Study groups	ICU mortality	Infections*	LOS days (Mean ± SD)	Ventilator days (Mean ± SD)	Cost
Moore et al., 1986 Level II	Trauma (n = 43)	Early Delayed	1/32 (3%) 2/31 (6%)	3/32 (9%) 9/31 (29%)	NR	NR	$16,280 ± $2146 $19,636 ± $3396
Chiarelli et al., 1990 Level II	Burn (n = 20)	Early Delayed	0/10 (0) 0/10 (0)	3/10 (30%)† 7/10 (70%)	69.2 ± 10.4‡ Hosp 89.0 ± 18.9 Hosp	NR	NR
Eyer et al., 1993 Level II	SICU trauma (n = 52)	Early Delayed	2/19 (11%) 2/19 (11%)	29 per group 14 per group	11.8 ± 7.9 ICU 9.9 ± 6.7 ICU	10.2 ± 8.1 8.1 ± 6.8	NR
Chuntrasakul et al., 1996 Level II	SICU trauma (n = 38)	Early Delayed	1/21 (5%) 3/17 (18%)	NR	8.1 ± 6.3 ICU 8.4 ± 4.8 ICU	5.29 ± 6.3 6.12 ± 5.3	NR
Singh et al., 1998 Level II	Peritonitis (n = 43)	Early Delayed	4/21 (19%) 4/22 (18%)	7/21 (33%) 12/22 (55%)	14 ± 6.9 Hosp 13 ± 7.0 Hosp	NR	NR
Minard et al., 2000 Level II	Closed head injury (n = 27)	Early Delayed Early Delayed	1/12 (8%) 4/15(27%)	6/12 (50%) 7/15 (47%)	30 ± 14.7 Hosp 21.3 ± 13.7 Hosp 18.5 ± 8.8 ICU‡ 11.3 ± 6.1 ICU	15.1 ± 7.5 10.4 ± 6.1	NR
Kompan et al., 2004 Level II	SICU trauma (n = 52)	Early Delayed	0/27 (0) 1/25 (4%)	9/27 (33%) 16/25 (64%)	15.9 ± 9.7 ICU 20.6 ± 18.5 ICU	12.9 ± 8.1 15.6 ± 16.1	NR
Malhotra et al., 2004 Level I	Postoperative peritonitis (n = 200)	Early Delayed Early Delayed	12/100 (12%) 16/100 (16%)	54/100 (54%) 67/100 (67%)	10.6 Hosp 10.7 Hosp 1.6 ICU 2.1 ICU	NR	NR
Peck et al., 2004 Level II	Burn (n = 27)	Early Delayed Early Delayed	4/14 (29%) 5/13 (38%)	12/14 (86%) 11/13 (85%)	60 ± 44 Hosp 60 ± 38 Hosp 40 ± 32 ICU 37 ± 33 ICU	32 ± 27 23 ± 26	NR
Dvorak et al., 2004 Level II	Spinal cord injury (n = 17)	Early Delayed	0/7 (0) 0/10 (0)	2.4 ± 1.5/pt 1.7 ± 1.1/pt	53 ± 34.4 Hosp 37.9 ± 14.6 Hosp	31.8 ± 35.0 20.9 ± 14.4	NR

Hosp, Hospital; *ICU*, intensive care unit; *LOS*, length of stay; *NR*, not reported; *pt*, patient; *SD*, standard deviation; *SICU*, surgical intensive care unit.
*All infections represent number of patients per group with infection unless otherwise stated.
†Bacteremia.
‡$P \le 0.05$.
Adapted from McClave SA, Martindale RG, Vanek VW, et al: Guidelines for the provision and assessment of nutrition support therapy in the adult critically ill patient: Society of Critical Care Medicine (SCCM) and American Society for Parenteral and Enteral Nutrition (A.S.P.E.N.), JPEN J Parenter Enteral Nutr 33:277, 2009.

The most important task in deciding whether to use so-called immunonutrition is to determine whether the patient meets criteria for its use. Immunonutrition is generally more expensive than standard enteral formulas; so, although robust cost-benefit analyses have not been completed, it should likely be reserved for the patient populations that have been specifically studied. Fortunately, these include many of the patients seen in surgical critical care settings, including those who have undergone major gastrointestinal surgery; those with

trauma, burns (total body surface area, >30%), and head and neck cancer; and those who need mechanical ventilation. Patients with mild-moderate sepsis have also been shown to benefit from these formulations.

Three of the major components of studied and available immune-enhancing formulas included arginine, omega-3 fatty acids, and glutamine. The role of arginine and omega-3 fatty acids appears to be through the regulation of myeloid suppressor cells

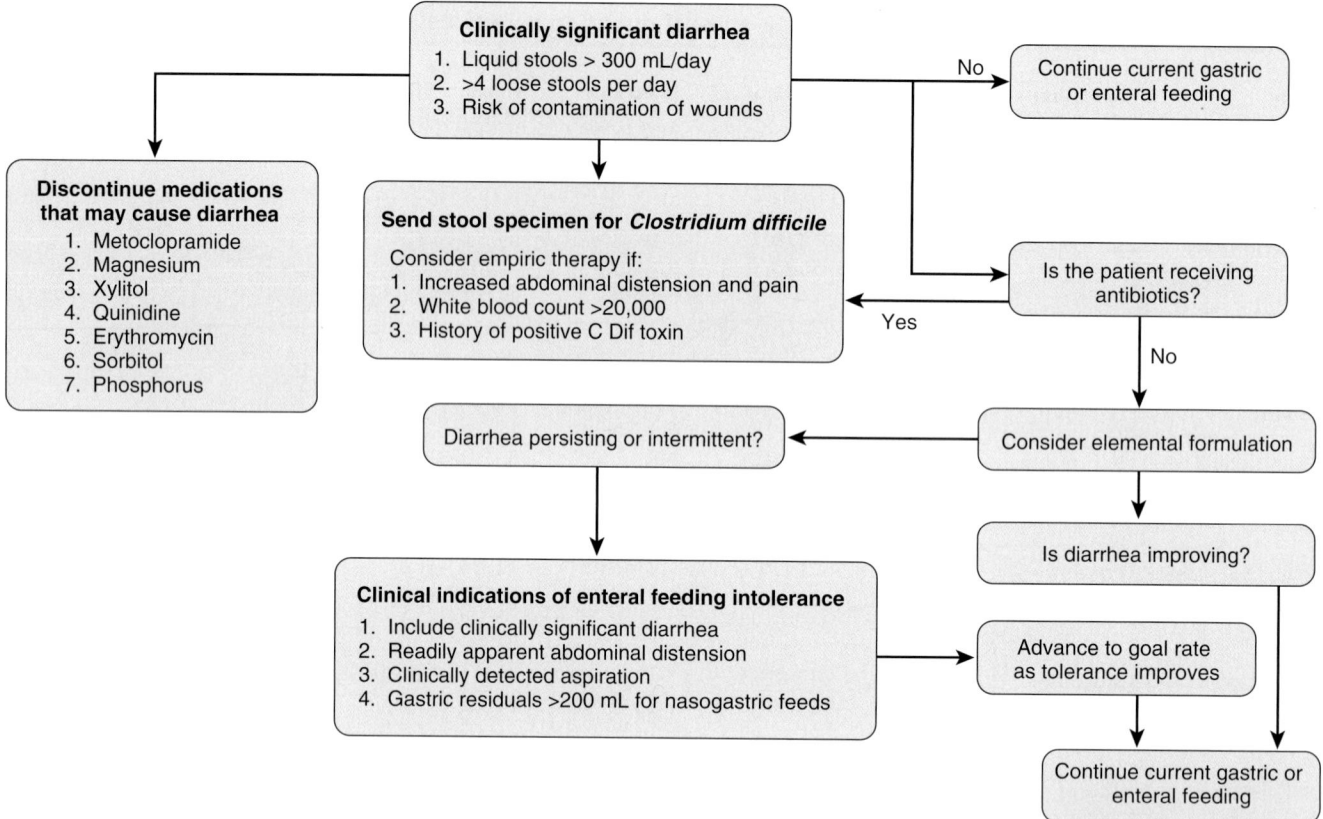

FIGURE 2 Management algorithm for patients with development of tube feeding–associated diarrhea. *(Data from Doig GS, Simpson F, Finfer S, et al: Effect of evidence-based feeding guidelines on mortality of critically ill adults: a cluster randomized controlled trial,* JAMA *300[23]:2731-2741, 2008.)*

through nitric oxide and combating T-cell suppression and decreasing neutrophil adhesion and subsequent inflammation. Glutamine is a key fuel for immune cells, increases human leukocyte antigen-DR expression on monocytes, enhances neutrophil phagocytosis, increases heat-shock protein expression, and serves as a precursor for the de novo production of arginine. Additional micronutrients, such as selenium, and antioxidants, such as vitamin C, are often added to immunonutrition to enhance the positive effects and have been shown to reduce mortality in systematic reviews and meta-analysis, including a recent meta-analysis by Visser and colleagues that reviewed 15 randomized controlled trials for their primary endpoint of mortality.

At least five meta-analyses have shown the benefits of immunonutrition over standard enteral formulas in selected patient populations. Although no benefit for mortality has been shown, multiple morbidities and hospital length of stay have been reduced with immunonutrition. These effects are most pronounced in surgical patients. The use of omega-3 fatty acids and antioxidants also has pronounced effects in patients with acute lung injury (ALI) and adult respiratory distress syndrome (ARDS). One clear limitation may be those patients with severe sepsis, in whom some evidence exists to suggest that the upregulation of nitric oxide seen with arginine supplementation may actually be detrimental. A summary of clinical practice recommendations for immune nutrients for specific patient populations is found in Table 2, which contains the recommendations for each of the four commonly used immune nutrients discussed previously (arginine, glutamine, omega-3 fatty acids, antioxidants) and the recommendations for each from the major nutrition societies: the Canadian Clinical Practice Guidelines (CCPG), the European Society for Parenteral and Enteral Nutrition (ESPEN), and the SCCM/ASPEN.

SPECIAL CIRCUMSTANCES: THE OBESE CRITICALLY ILL PATIENT

Because of the increasing incidence of obesity, especially in the United States and Western countries, and the numerous physiologic problems associated with obesity that complicate ICU care, special attention to the nutritional needs of these patients is warranted. Although randomized data to address the specific needs of the obese are limited, an evolving body of literature suggests that immunonutrition and specific supplements may be of significant benefit in this population. Multiple large clinical studies show that the obese critically ill patient has a higher risk of infectious complications, longer ICU stay, and need for mechanical ventilation. Importantly, multiple metabolic derangements found with obesity create a state of chronic inflammation and significantly increased levels of oxidative stress, at baseline and especially when challenged with an insult such as trauma, surgery, or infection. Recent studies of nutritional supplementation in obese critically ill patients have focused on offsetting this oxidative stress with pharmaconutrition. The use of antioxidants L-arginine, and L-citrulline appears to have positive effects in this patient population for many of the reasons previously outlined in this chapter. In addition, supplementation of L-leucine appears to be of some importance in critically ill obese patients to prevent the development of sarcopenia. One of the most frequent comorbidities associated with obesity is nonalcoholic fatty liver disease (NAFLD), which warrants special consideration in the nutrition regimen of these patients. A combination of basic science and clinical evidence suggests that the use of nutritional supplements rich in polyunsaturated fatty acids (PUFAs) can be of significant benefit through anti-inflammatory effects in patients receiving enteral nutrition. This benefit appears to be particularly enhanced in the setting of NAFLD.

TABLE 2: Immune nutrients for specific patient populations: summary of clinical practice recommendations

Nutrients	Elective surgery	General	Septic	Trauma	Burns	ALI/ARDS
Arginine*						
CCPG	No rec	No benefit	Harm	No benefit	No benefit	No benefit
ESPEN	Benefit (B)	No rec	Benefit (mild) (B) Harm (severe) (B)	Benefit (B)	No rec	No rec
SCCM/ASPEN	Benefit (A)	Poss benefit (A)	Poss benefit (mild/mod) (B) Poss harm (severe) (B)	Benefit (A)	Benefit (A)	No rec
Glutamine†						
CCPG	No rec	No rec	No rec	Poss benefit	Poss benefit	No rec
ESPEN	No rec	No rec	No rec	Benefit (A)	Benefit (A)	No rec
SCCM/ASPEN	No rec	Poss benefit (B)	No rec	Poss benefit (B)	Poss benefit (B)	No rec
Ω-3 fatty acids‡						
CCPG	No rec	No rec	No rec	No rec	No rec	Benefit
ESPEN	No rec	No rec	No rec	No rec	No rec	Benefit (B)
SCCM/ASPEN	No rec	No rec	No rec	No rec	No rec	Benefit (A)
Antioxidants§						
CCPG	No rec	Poss benefit	No rec	No rec	No rec	No rec
ESPEN	No rec	No rec	No rec	No rec	Benefit (A)	No rec
SCCM/ASPEN	No rec	Benefit (B)	Benefit (B)	Benefit (B)	Benefit (B)	Benefit (B)

ALI, Acute lung injury; *ARDS*, adult respiratory distress syndrome; *ASPEN*, American Society for Parenteral and Enteral Nutrition; *CCPG*, Canadian Clinical Practice Guidelines; *ESPEN*, European Society for Parenteral and Enteral Nutrition; *rec*, recommendation; *SCCM*, Society for Critical Care Medicine.
*Arginine administered in context of immune-enhancing diet that also contains fish oil, antioxidants, and nucleotides.
†Enteral glutamine added to enteral nutrition regimen.
‡Fish-oil-derived omega-3 fatty acids (EPA and DHA) administered in context of immune-enhancing diet that also contains borage oil and antioxidants.
§Antioxidant vitamins (including selenium) and trace elements.
From Mizock, BA: Immunonutrition and critical illness: an update, Nutrition 26(7-8):701-707, 2010.

However, at least one study suggests that PUFAs can be detrimental in the setting of alcoholic liver disease, where use of medium-chain triglycerides should be considered as an alternative fat source. Finally, limited evidence exists to suggest that a high-protein, hypocaloric nutritional regimen may result in reduced morbidity in obese critically ill patients. As the incidence of obesity and obesity-related comorbidities increases, close attention must be paid to the metabolic and nutritional needs of these patients, and the use of immunonutrition is highly recommended by many authors.

SUGGESTED READINGS

Doig GS, Simpson F, Finfer S, et al: Effect of evidence-based feeding guidelines on mortality of critically ill adults: a cluster randomized controlled trial, *JAMA* 300(23):2731–2741, 2008.

Hurt RT, Frazier TH, McClave SA, et al: Pharmaconutrition for the obese, critically ill patient, *JPEN J Parenter Enteral Nutr* 35(Suppl 5):S60–S72, 2011.

McClave SA, Martindale RG, Vanek VW, et al: Guidelines for the Provision and assessment of nutrition support therapy in the adult critically ill patient: Society of Critical Care Medicine (SCCM) and American Society for Parenteral and Enteral Nutrition (A.S.P.E.N.), *JPEN J Parenter Enteral Nutr* 33(3):277–316, 2009.

Mizock BA: Immunonutrition and critical illness: an update, *Nutrition* 26(7-8):701–707, 2010.

Ochoa JB, Caba D: Advances in surgical nutrition, *Surg Clin North Am* 86(6):1483–1493, 2006.

Visser J, Labadarios D, Blaauw R: Micronutrient supplementation for critically ill adults: a systematic review and meta-analysis, *Nutrition* 27(7-8):745–758, 2011.

COAGULOPATHY IN THE CRITICALLY ILL PATIENT

Nagamallika Jasti, MD, and Michael B. Streiff, MD

Bleeding and/or abnormal coagulation or platelet function test results are common among critically ill patients. Consequently, a working knowledge of the diagnostic evaluation and management of patients with hemostatic disorders is essential for physicians caring for critically ill patients. The purpose of this chapter is to review (1) a brief description of the hemostatic system, (2) a commonsense approach to critically ill patients with abnormal bleeding, and (3) an approach to the diagnosis and management of platelet, coagulation, and vascular disorders.

A MODEL OF HEMOSTASIS

Hemostasis is the end product of the coordinated and cooperative efforts of pro- and anticoagulant proteins, fibrinolytic proteins, platelets, and the vessel wall. Defects in any component can result in abnormal bleeding or thrombosis. The hemostatic mechanism springs into action when vascular damage exposes subendothelial collagen and tissue factor. Circulating platelets bind avidly to collagen via platelet membrane glycoproteins and von Willebrand factor to form a platelet monolayer at the site of injury. This event triggers platelet activation and the release of platelet granule components that activate surrounding platelets promoting platelet aggregation, formation of a multilayer platelet plug, and vasoconstriction. Defects in platelet adhesion, activation, or aggregation all lead to bleeding disorders of variable severity.

While the classic "waterfall" concept of the coagulation system does not accurately reflect what occurs in vivo, this model is very useful for interpreting coagulation test results (Figure 1). At the same time that platelet adhesion and activation are occurring, the coagulation cascade is activated by the exposure of subendothelial tissue factor that activates factor VII. The extrinsic pathway that consists of factor VII and tissue factor serves as the initiator pathway of hemostasis. The tissue factor-factor VII complex activates factor X, which leads to small amounts of thrombin formation that activates factor XI and VIII (intrinsic pathway) and factor V (common pathway cofactor for factor X). Activation of the intrinsic pathway by thrombin results in formation of large amounts of activated factor X and subsequently thrombin, which triggers fibrin formation and platelet activation. The end result is fibrin clot, which reinforces the platelet plug, stanching blood loss through the vascular defect. Thrombin also activates factor XIII, which catalyzes the formation of covalent crosslinks between fibrin monomers to ensure the formation of a fibrin clot that is resistant to fibrinolysis. The prothrombotic coagulation proteins are balanced by endogenous antithrombotic proteins such as antithrombin (III) (which inhibits thrombin—a reaction that is accelerated several thousand–fold by heparin), and the vitamin K-dependent protein C and protein S complex that inactivates the critical cofactor proteins, factor VIII, and factor V. The fibrinolytic proteins provide additional balance to the hemostatic mechanism by digesting and remodeling existing fibrin clot to focus clot formation at the site of vascular injury and to maintain vascular patency.

AN INITIAL APPROACH TO THE CRITICALLY ILL PATIENT WITH BLEEDING

Optimal management of the critically ill patient with bleeding requires prompt identification of the most likely cause of the bleeding. Bleeding can result from a coagulation factor deficiency, a disorder of platelet function or numbers, an abnormality of vessel walls, or combined defects in more than one of these systems. Identification of the defective system(s) is essential for targeted hemostatic therapy, which is more effective and preserves precious blood product resources that are always in short supply (Box 1). The patient's presentation can provide useful information about the cause of the bleeding. If the bleeding is localized to the operative/procedural site, and particularly if there is large-volume, rapid blood loss, then it is likely that an anatomic defect related to the recent procedure is responsible for the bleeding rather than a systemic hemostatic disorder. In this case, laboratory testing (e.g., complete blood count, including platelet count, prothrombin time (PT), activated partial thromboplastin time (aPTT), etc.) is appropriate to determine the current status of hemostasis, but surgical intervention is the most effective therapy. Conversely, bleeding from multiple locations, slow persistent oozing, and temporally delayed hemorrhage (from invasive procedures) generally indicate the presence of a systemic coagulopathy. Petechiae (small red spots—usually <3 mm in diameter—that do not blanche with pressure) indicate a defect in the number or function of platelets. Large hematomas or ecchymoses that elevate the skin surface or blood collections in deep tissue locations are characteristic of a coagulation factor defect.

If the patient has had a recent surgical procedure, the type of procedure should be considered in the evaluation. Patients returning from a cardiac bypass procedure can have residual heparin present following protamine reversal as a cause of bleeding and abnormal coagulation test results or acquired thrombocytopenia and platelet dysfunction due to the impact of cardiac bypass on platelet function and numbers. Therefore, the approach to these patients should focus on assessing the character of the bleeding (surgical versus coagulopathic) and the results of tests evaluating the patient for the presence of residual heparin or coagulation factor deficiencies (activated partial thromboplastin time, thrombin time, heparin neutralized thrombin time, Hepzyme), thrombocytopenia (complete blood count), and platelet dysfunction (platelet function analyzer 100, PFA-100, Dade-Behring, Inc. Deerfield, Ill).

It is also important to review the patient's medical and surgical history. Although preexisting hemostatic disorders are often identified preoperatively, occasionally coagulation or platelet disorders are not recognized prior to surgery. Therefore, a quick review of the patient's written history as well as questioning family members can be useful. Patients with renal or hepatic disorders often have abnormal hemostasis due to the impact of these disease processes on platelet function (uremic platelet defect) and numbers (cirrhosis) and coagulation factor levels (cirrhosis). Patients with platelet disorders typically suffer from bleeding that affects mucosal sites (history of menorrhagia, epistaxis, gum bleeding), while coagulation defects such as hemophilia typically trigger deep tissue bleeding or hemarthroses. Fibrinolytic defects and factor XIII deficiency typically result in delayed bleeding (days after surgery). Vessel wall disorders such as the connective tissue disease Ehlers-Danlos syndrome and amyloidosis can cause intraoperative or postoperative bleeding due to vascular/tissue fragility. It is also important to get an accurate list of a patient's prescription and nonprescription medications, including vitamins, supplements, and herbal remedies because these can significantly influence hemostasis. If these details are not available in the medical record, interviewing patients (if possible) or family members can be revealing.

1290

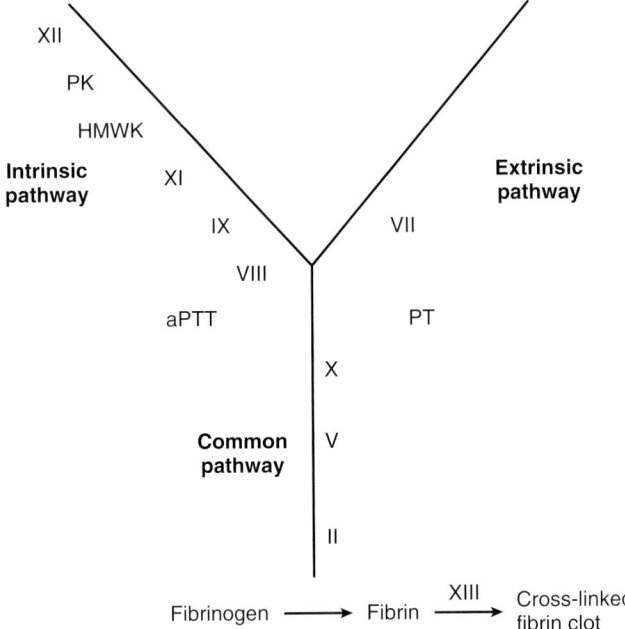

FIGURE 1   The coagulation cascade. *aPTT*, Activated partial thromboplastin time; *HMWK*, high-molecular-weight kininogen; *PK*, prekallikrein; *PT*, prothrombin time.

BOX 1: Evaluation of the bleeding patient

1. Assess character of bleeding: rapid, single location, multifocal, persistent oozing.

   Surgical bleeding: rapid blood loss, localized to surgical site, bright red blood, pulsatile blood loss.

   Coagulopathic bleeding: multifocal, persistent slow blood loss.

2. Send blood for hemoglobin, platelet count, PT, aPTT, TT, fibrinogen, D dimer, mixing studies, heparin contamination, thromboelastogram.

3. Review preoperative lab results (including liver and renal function).

4. Review patient's perioperative medications.

   Antiplatelet agents: aspirin, ticlopidine, clopidogrel, prasurgrel, NSAIDs such as ketorolac, glycoprotein IIb/IIIa inhibitors.

   Anticoagulants: UFH, LMWH, fondaparinux, lepirudin, argatroban, bivalirudin, desirudin, warfarin, rivaroxaban, dabigatran.

   Vitamins/dietary supplements/herbal remedies: vitamin E, omega-3 fatty acids, garlic, ginkgo biloba, ginger, willow bark, etc.

5. Review patient's medical/surgical and family history.

   Platelet-type bleeding: epistaxis, easy bruising, menorrhagia, oropharyngeal bleeding.

   Coagulation factor bleeding: hemarthrosis, hematomas, soft tissue bleeds.

   Vessel wall disorder: easy bruisability, joint laxity, poor wound healing.

6. Review compatibility of any intraoperative transfusions.

Basic screening coagulation tests and blood counts are essential to diagnosis of coagulation and platelet disorders. The basic coagulation tests include the aPTT, the PT, the thrombin time (TT), and a fibrinogen level. Platelet testing includes the platelet count (usually available as part of a CBC), the immature platelet fraction (a measure

of the percentage of young platelets in the circulation), the bleeding time, or the platelet function analyzer test (PFA-100, Dade-Behring Inc., Deerfield, Ill). Thromboelastography is being increasingly used in some patient settings (liver transplantation, cardiac bypass, major trauma) to assess patients' hemostatic systems, particularly for hyperfibrinolysis. Patient blood samples for hemostatic testing should be obtained, whenever possible, by a peripheral blood stick rather than through a central venous catheter to avoid the common pitfall of heparin contamination that can confuse diagnosis and lead to unnecessary blood product use. In the next sections we review the commonly used tests to assess hemostasis and then the clinical presentation and management of platelet, coagulation factor, and vascular wall disorders.

HEMOSTATIC TESTING IN THE CRITICALLY ILL PATIENT

Coagulation Tests

The most commonly used tests of coagulation are the aPTT, PT, TT, and a fibrinogen level. More specialized, but important coagulation tests to understand include the D dimer assay, mixing studies, coagulation factor assays, heparin contamination (Hepzyme) testing, and von Willebrand factor testing (Box 2). The aPTT measures the function of factors in the intrinsic pathway (factors XII, XI, IX, and VIII, as well as prekallikrein and high molecular weight kininogen) and the common pathway (see Figure 1). The aPTT is performed by adding phospholipid (an in vitro surrogate for activated platelet membranes) and an activator of factor XII, as well as calcium (to reverse the sodium citrate anticoagulant in the blood collection tube) and measuring the time to clot formation. The aPTT is useful for identifying hemophilia A (factor VIII deficiency), hemophilia B (factor IX deficiency of Christmas disease), factor XI deficiency (hemophilia C or Rosenthal's disease), as well as measuring unfractionated heparin and the direct thrombin inhibitors argatroban, bivalirudin, and lepirudin.

The PT measures the function of the extrinsic pathway (factor VII) and the common pathway (factors X and V, prothrombin, and fibrinogen) (see Figure 1). The PT is performed by adding a source of tissue factor and phospholipids (an in vitro surrogate for activated platelet membranes), also called thromboplastin and calcium (to reverse the sodium citrate anticoagulant in the blood collection tube) and measuring the time required for clot formation to occur. In addition to assessing the rare congenital deficiency states of factors VII, X, V, and prothrombin, the PT is also used to measure warfarin anticoagulation. For patients on warfarin, the results of the PT are usually expressed as an international normalized ratio (INR) value, which normalizes PT results for the sensitivity of the laboratory's thromboplastin to reductions in vitamin K–dependent factor levels (factor VII, X, and prothrombin are reflected in the PT) compared with an international reference standard. The INR is not designed for use to express the results of the PT for patients not on warfarin.

The TT is useful for assessing the functional status of fibrinogen, to which the PT and aPTT are much less sensitive. The TT is performed by adding thrombin and calcium to the citrated patient plasma sample and measuring the time to clot formation. The TT is exquisitely sensitive to heparin or direct thrombin inhibitors. Rare antibodies directed against thrombin (thrombin inhibitors) can also result in an abnormal thrombin time. The results of the thrombin time can be confirmed by obtaining a fibrinogen assay. This functional test of fibrinogen is performed by adding a large amount of thrombin to the patient plasma sample and measuring the time to clot formation. There is a linear relationship in this assay between the time to clot formation and the concentration of clottable fibrinogen. Fibrinogen assays are significantly less sensitive to the presence of heparin and direct thrombin inhibitors due to the increased

BOX 2: Laboratory tests of hemostasis

Activated Partial Thromboplastin Time (aPTT)
Used to identify deficiencies or inhibitors of factors in the intrinsic pathway (factors XII, XI, IX, and VIII; HMWK; and PK) and common pathway (factors X, V, and II [prothrombin] and fibrinogen)
Used to monitor unfractionated heparin and direct thrombin inhibitors (argatroban and bivalirudin)
Used to identify lupus inhibitors (antiphospholipid antibodies)

Prothrombin Time (PT)
Used to identify deficiencies or inhibitors of factors in the extrinsic pathway (factor VII) and common pathway (factors X, V, and II [prothrombin] and fibrinogen)
Used to monitor warfarin (use the INR)

Thrombin Time (TT)
Used to identify deficiency or dysfunction of fibrinogen or thrombin inhibitors
Used to identify the presence of unfractionated heparin

Fibrinogen
A sensitive test of fibrinogen function
Insensitive to heparin
Heparin contamination (Hepzyme)
Used to identify the presence of heparin by measuring aPTT before and after heparinase treatment of patient sample

Mixing Studies
Used to discriminate between deficiency states and inhibitors by assessing the correction of a prolonged PT or aPTT after addition of 1 part or 4 parts patient plasma to 1 part normal pooled plasma
Correction of abnormal assay = deficiency state
Failure to correct = factor inhibitor, lupus inhibitor, anticoagulant such as heparin

Factor Activity Assays
Used to determine the activity level of a specific factor using plasma deficient in the factor of interest and the PT or aPTT

D Dimer Assays
Used to detect D dimers, fragments of cross-linked fibrin that have been digested by plasmin—a marker of disseminated intravascular coagulation (DIC) or active thrombus formation.

Template Bleeding Time
Rough in vivo assessment of platelet function
Platelet function analyzer 100
An in vitro assay of platelet function

Platelet Aggregometry
Used to assess platelet aggregation and secretion in response to platelet agonists

Von Willebrand Antigen Assay
Used to measure the amount of von Willebrand protein

Ristocetin Cofactor Assay
Used to measure von Willebrand protein function

Thromboelastography (TEG/ROTEM)
Global tests of coagulation, platelet, and fibrinolytic function, particularly useful for identifying patients with hyperfibrinolysis

amount of thrombin used in the test. However, large concentrations of heparin or direct thrombin inhibitors will result in an abnormal fibrinogen result.

When a patient's coagulation test results are abnormal, it is important to determine whether the abnormal result is due to a deficiency state (such as hemophilia A) or an inhibitor (such as a factor VIII inhibitor). Deficiency states will respond to factor replacement therapy (factor concentrates, fresh frozen plasma, and cryoprecipitate), whereas inhibitors will not respond to this therapy. This distinction can be made in the laboratory by mixing the patient's plasma sample with normal pooled plasma. If a factor deficiency is responsible, then a 1:1 mix with normal pooled plasma will correct the abnormal clotting time. Conversely, if a specific factor inhibitor or a lupus inhibitor is present, then the addition of normal plasma will not correct the clotting time. Coagulation laboratories often perform 4:1 mixes of patient plasma and normal pooled plasma to detect low-titer inhibitors.

Specific factor levels are performed to identify the presence of particular factor deficiency states such as hemophilia A (factor VIII deficiency). These assays are performed by adding patient plasma to factor-deficient plasma. Consequently, the clotting time of such a mix is dependent solely on the patient sample's contribution of the particular factor of interest. If heparin contamination is suspected, a heparin contamination (Hepzyme) assay can be performed. The Hepzyme assay measures the aPTT of a plasma sample before and after the addition of heparinase, an enzyme that digests heparin. In the presence of significant heparin contamination, the aPTT after heparinase addition is significantly shorter than the baseline sample, confirming heparin contamination.

D dimers are a fragment of crosslinked fibrin that is produced by lysis of fibrin clot. It is a marker of clot formation that has been used as a sensitive test for the presence of disseminated intravascular coagulation and acute thrombosis. D dimer assays generally use antibodies directed against this fragment to measure its concentration in plasma by enzyme linked immunosorbent assays (ELISA) or antibody-coated bead agglutination.

Platelet Tests

Common tests of platelet function include platelet numbers as assessed in a complete blood count, the immature platelet fraction (a measure of the percentage of young platelets in the blood), the template bleeding time, the platelet function analyzer test (PFA-100, Dade Behring, Deerfield, Ill), and platelet aggregation studies (see Box 2). Blood cell analyzers can accurately assess the number and size of platelets in a volume of blood. The mean platelet volume is useful because a large mean platelet volume suggests the presence of a large number of immature platelets (young platelets are larger) such as might be seen in disorders associated with excessive platelet destruction. Another estimate of platelet production measured by some blood cell analyzers is the immature platelet fraction percentage (IPF %). The IPF % is assessed by staining platelets with a proprietary RNA avid fluorescent dye that can be measured with appropriately equipped automated hematology analyzers with flow cytometry. Similar to reticulocytes (young red cells), young platelets have higher concentrations of RNA that can be stained with RNA-avid fluorescent dyes. Patients with higher percentages of young RNA-rich (higher staining intensity) platelets have increased platelet production, which suggests the presence of a disorder causing platelet consumption/destruction.

The template bleeding time (TBT) is a rough guide of platelet function reflecting the importance of platelet function to primary hemostasis. The TBT is performed by making a standardized incision in the forearm with a razor blade–containing template device with a blood pressure cuff inflated proximally to 40 mm of mercury and measuring the time required for hemostasis to occur. Unfortunately, this result can be influenced by many factors other than platelet function, including operator technique and tissue vascularity. Therefore, the TBT is no longer widely used.

The shortcomings of the TBT led to the development of more standardized and convenient tests of platelet function, such as the platelet function analyzer test (PFA-100, Dade Behring, Deerfield, Ill). The PFA-100 assesses platelet function by aspirating whole blood at high shear rates through perforated membranes coated with the platelet agonists collagen and epinephrine or collagen and adenosine diphosphate (ADP). The time required for the aperture in the membrane to occlude correlates with platelet function. Both the TBT and the PFA-100 will be abnormal in patients with thrombocytopenia (platelet count <80-100,000/μL), so the results of these tests cannot be used to assess platelet function in patients with platelet counts at or below this level. The PFA-100 appears to be more sensitive and reproducible than the TBT, but neither test has proven useful in predicting surgical blood loss. Nevertheless, in a patient with ongoing bleeding, an abnormal PFA-100 in the absence of thrombocytopenia indicates an acquired (e.g., aspirin, bypass pump, uremia, etc.) or congenital platelet disorder (e.g., Bernard-Soulier syndrome, etc.).

Platelet aggregation studies assess platelet function by exposing platelet-rich plasma or whole blood to different platelet agonists such as thrombin, epinephrine, ADP, and ristocetin. Platelet aggregation is assessed by measuring the change in electrical impedance or light transmission through the sample after agonist addition. Platelet granule release can be assessed by measuring the amount of granule constituents such as ATP released into the test solution upon platelet activation. Thrombocytopenia (platelets <80,000/μL) will result in abnormal test results. Since platelet aggregation studies require considerable expertise to perform and interpret, they are not generally available at all medical centers or on an emergent basis. Nevertheless, platelet aggregation studies remain an invaluable test in the assessment of platelet function disorders.

Fibrinolytic Tests

The fibrinolytic system can be measured by assessing the amount and function of fibrinolytic proteins such as plasminogen, tissue plasminogen activator, alpha2-antiplasmin, and plasminogen activator 1 (PAI-1). Reductions in alpha2-antiplasmin and PAI-1, two proteins that negative regulate plasmin (the fibrinolytic enzyme) and tissue plasminogen activator (the primary plasminogen activator), respectively, can cause delayed bleeding after invasive procedures. In recent years, there has been a resurgence of interest in the use of thromboelastography (TEG) and rotational thromboelastometry (ROTEM) in the assessment of the total hemostatic mechanism. These tests can be used to assess global function of clotting proteins, platelets, and the fibrinolytic system. TEG and ROTEM have been used as point-of-care tests to identify patients with decreased coagulation or platelet function or hyperfibrinolysis during liver transplantation and cardiac surgery. Further investigation of TEG and ROTEM in the management of hemostatic disorders is warranted before broader application in clinical medicine.

PLATELET DISORDERS

Platelet disorders can be categorized as being quantitative (characterized by a reduced number of normally functioning platelets) or qualitative (characterized by the presence of dysfunctional platelets) (Table 1). Since platelets play an essential role in primary hemostasis, patients with platelet disorders often bleed during or soon after invasive procedures. Findings typical of platelet dysfunction include a history of mucosal bleeding (epistaxis, gingival bleeding, and menorrhagia) or easy bruisability and petechiae or purpura on physical examination. For most surgical or invasive procedures, a platelet count above 50,000/μL is adequate for hemostasis. For neurosurgery, spinal surgery, cardiac surgery, and prostatectomy, platelet counts in

excess of 100,000/μL are often preferred. In a patient without bleeding and no recent or planned invasive procedure, a platelet count transfusion trigger of 10,000/μL is often used to guide transfusion therapy. A higher target of 20,000/μL is used for febrile, infected patients, given their more rapid platelet turnover.

In patients with thrombocytopenia undergoing transfusion therapy, it is important to assess the platelet transfusion increment. The platelet transfusion increment is assessed by measuring the platelet count before transfusion and 1 hour posttransfusion. In the typical 70-kilogram patient, an increment of 5000/μL is expected for each random donor unit transfused. An increment of 30,000/μL is expected for each single donor apheresis unit transfused. If the platelet transfusion increment is less than calculated, then increased platelet destruction/consumption is present. In disorders characterized by platelet destruction, platelet increments in response to transfusion are negligible and/or short-lived. Identification of increased platelet consumption warrants consideration of platelet destructive disorders such as disseminated intravascular coagulation, platelet transfusion refractoriness due to human leukocyte antigen (HLA) alloimmune antibodies, or drug-dependent or independent immune mediated thrombocytopenia. Nevertheless, platelet transfusions should never be withheld due to poor platelet count increments in urgent situations associated with clinically significant bleeding due to thrombocytopenia.

Quantitative Platelet Disorders

Acquired Quantitative Platelet Disorders

Quantitative platelet disorders can be rapidly identified with a complete blood cell count. Quantitative platelet disorders can result from decreased production, increased destruction, splenic sequestration, or dilution associated with massive transfusions (see Table 1). While most laboratories confirm low platelet counts (platelets <50,000/μL) by visual inspection of a peripheral smear, it is essential for the clinician to make sure this procedure has been performed to avoid being misled by the entity of "pseudothrombocytopenia." Pseudothrombocytopenia is caused by antibodies that aggregate platelets in the presence of sodium ethylenediaminetetraacetic acid (EDTA) (the anticoagulant used in blood collection tubes for blood count measurement), resulting in significant platelet undercounting. This phenomenon is relatively common, occurring in 0.07% of hospitalized patients, so it is likely all clinicians will see this entity. If pseudothrombocytopenia is suspected, platelet counts should be performed simultaneously in sodium EDTA, sodium citrate, and heparin blood collection tubes, and a peripheral blood smear made from these tubes should be reviewed. Often platelet clumping will be significantly less in sodium citrate or heparin tubes, so these tubes can be used for platelet monitoring during the remainder of the hospital stay. Identification of this entity is important to avoid unnecessary transfusion and medical therapy for a laboratory artifact.

If true thrombocytopenia is present, identification of the primary etiology of the thrombocytopenia is essential to guide therapy. Decreased platelet production should be suspected when patients have thrombocytopenia and a normal or low immature platelet fraction and normal increments to platelet transfusions. Thrombocytopenia due to decreased production is typically associated with abnormalities in other counts (anemia or leukopenia) reflecting a diffuse disruption of normal marrow function. Disorders associated with decreased platelet production include acute leukemia, aplastic anemia, myelodysplastic syndrome, myelofibrosis, vitamin B_{12} or folate deficiency, liver disease, and exposure to myelotoxic substances such as chemotherapeutic agents and alcohol (see Table 1). Cell count abnormalities due to these disorders are typically evident to some degree on preoperative screening studies, although cytopenias may worsen in association with major surgery (results increased consumption of all three cell lines) and associated

TABLE 1: Platelet disorders

Quantitative (thrombocytopenia)	Qualitative (platelet dysfunction)
Decreased Production	**Congenital Platelet Dysfunction**
Vitamin deficiencies (vitamin B_{12}, folate deficiency)	Bernard-Soulier syndrome
Bone marrow disease (aplastic anemia, leukemia, myelodysplastic syndrome, etc.)	Glanzmann's thrombasthenia
Drugs (ethanol, chemotherapy)	Storage pool diseases (e.g., gray platelet syndrome)
Infection (human immunodeficiency virus [HIV], tuberculosis [TB])	Platelet-type von Willebrand disease
Liver failure	
Increased Destruction	**Acquired Platelet Dysfunction**
Immune thrombocytopenic purpura	Drugs (Aspirin, ticlopidine, clopidogrel, NSAIDs, etc.)
Infection	Uremia
Disseminated intravascular coagulation (DIC)	Liver disease
Drugs (heparin, quinine, glycoprotein IIb/IIIa inhibitors, etc.)	Post–cardiopulmonary bypass
Thrombotic thrombocytopenic purpura (TTP), hemolytic uremic syndrome (HUS)	Primary thrombocytosis (polycythemia rubra vera, essential thrombocythemia)
Posttransfusion purpura	
Catastrophic antiphospholipid syndrome	
Dilutional (massive transfusions)	
Sequestration (hypersplenism)	
Pseudothrombocytopenia	

disorders (e.g., infections) or treatments (blood or intravenous fluid associated dilutional cytopenias, cardiac bypass pump, intraaortic balloon pump). In patients with normal preoperative counts in whom thrombocytopenia associated with decreased production is suspected, infections or myelosuppressive medications should be investigated. Sepsis can result in decreases in platelet production as well as increased destruction. Antibiotics such as linezolid have been associated with myelosuppressive thrombocytopenia. A hematologist can be helpful in the investigation for possible causes of thrombocytopenia due to decreased production to assist in management. Treatment consists of platelet transfusions until definitive therapy targeted at the underlying defect can be initiated.

Dilutional thrombocytopenia can result when patients receive large volumes of blood during resuscitation. Thrombocytopenia and abnormal coagulation tests result because packed red cell units only retain small volumes of plasma (25 to 50 mL/unit) and platelets. This syndrome is most commonly seen in patients with massive gastrointestinal bleeding or trauma. One study found that 75% of patients who received 20 or more units of red cells within a 24-hour period developed significant thrombocytopenia (platelet counts <50,000/μL). No patients receiving less than 20 units of red cells developed platelet counts in this range. However, the use of prespecified triggers (e.g., 6 to 8 random donor platelet units or 1 plateletpheresis unit and 4 units of fresh frozen plasma (FFP) for every 10 units of blood transfused) for platelet and fresh frozen plasma transfusion should be avoided in most clinical situations, as bone marrow and hepatic function differ substantially between patients. Therefore, transfusion practice should be guided by regular measurement of platelet counts and screening coagulation studies and not formulas.

One exception to this rule is patients with massive trauma where formula-driven transfusion practice is essential to preservation of adequate hemostatic function and optimal outcomes. In other surgical populations where dilutional hemostatic disorders are less common, formula-driven transfusion practice is liable to result in excessive blood product utilization. Patients with platelet counts less than 50,000/μL and recent surgery or bleeding should be transfused with one to two aphaeresis (or three to six random donor) units of platelets. Routine measurement of the platelet count to assess response to transfusions and determine the need for additional blood products is essential, as many patients with dilutional thrombocytopenia due to massive bleeding also have reduced platelet survival. Platelet count triggers for transfusion therapy are shown in Table 2.

Consumptive thrombocytopenia is a much more common reason for thrombocytopenia in the critically ill patient. Common causes of consumptive thrombocytopenia are infections/sepsis, drug-induced immune thrombocytopenia, disseminated intravascular coagulation (DIC), and, less often, immune thrombocytopenic purpura (ITP). Review of the patient's medical history, medication lists, microbiology, and coagulation test results is useful in pinpointing the cause. Sepsis can be associated with rapid (within hours) dramatic reductions in platelet numbers that are coincident with clinical manifestations of bacteremia. Even in the absence of obvious signs of sepsis, it is important to consider infection as a cause of thrombocytopenia because ongoing, inadequately treated, or unrecognized infections are a common cause of consumptive and/or inadequate production thrombocytopenia. Therapy should focus on identification of the bacteria responsible, provision of broad-spectrum antibiotics directed at the most likely and serious pathogens, and blood product

TABLE 2: Recommended platelet transfusion thresholds

Indication	Platelet transfusion threshold
No recent surgery, afebrile	10,000/µL
No recent surgery, febrile	20,000/µL
Recent surgery or active bleeding	50,000/µL
Spinal anesthesia	50,000/µL
Massive transfusion	50,000/µL
Anticoagulation	50,000/µL
Disseminated intravascular coagulation (DIC)	50,000/µL
Eye surgery	100,000/µL
Multiple trauma/ central nervous system injury	100,000/µL
Cardiac surgery with cardiopulmonary bypass	100,000/µL
Neurosurgery or spinal surgery	100,000/µL

support. In severe cases of sepsis, particularly cases associated with gram-negative organisms and large amounts of lipopolysaccharide release, disseminated intravascular coagulation can occur, which is heralded by consumptive thrombocytopenia and coagulopathy accompanied by thrombocytopenia and abnormalities in screening coagulation tests (PT, aPTT, fibrinogen), as well as elevations of D dimer levels. Therapy should be multidimensionally directed at the proximate cause of disseminated intravascular coagulation and supportive to correct the thrombocytopenia and coagulopathy.

Drug-induced thrombocytopenia is an increasingly common cause of thrombocytopenia that must be considered in any critically ill patient developing thrombocytopenia. In general, drug-induced thrombocytopenia usually occurs within the first 2 weeks of drug exposure. Therefore, identification of possible agents should focus upon drugs started within the preceding 14 days. However, given the large number of medications that critically ill patients are exposed to, the list of potential suspects can be large. While laboratory testing to identify causative agents is available, it is generally time-consuming and only available through reference laboratories. Medications commonly associated with thrombocytopenia are presented in Table 3. The best approach to drug-induced thrombocytopenia is to eliminate potential suspects promptly. In severe cases, intravenous immunoglobulin (IVIG), anti-D immunoglobulin (Winrho SDF, Baxter Healthcare Corp., Deerfield, Ill), and, to a lesser extent, corticosteroids can be useful therapeutic maneuvers in severely affected patients. When using IVIG, it is important to use low-osmolality products, particularly in patients at heightened risk for renal toxicity (preexisting renal dysfunction, diabetic and elderly patients). Anti-D should be avoided in patients with concomitant autoimmune hemolytic anemia or positive direct antiglobulin testing.

Among causes of medication-associated thrombocytopenia, identification of heparin-induced thrombocytopenia (HIT) is particularly important. HIT is an antibody-mediated consumptive form of thrombocytopenia that occurs in 1% to 5% of patients most commonly after 4 to 14 days of heparin therapy and is associated with a substantial risk of thromboembolism (50% risk at 30 days). The diagnosis can be confirmed with laboratory testing for HIT antibodies (heparin-platelet factor 4 ELISA assay, serotonin-release assay).

Any patient suspected to have HIT should avoid all heparin (and low-molecular-weight heparin) exposure and be treated with a direct thrombin inhibitor (argatroban, bivalirudin, lepirudin). In the absence of bleeding, platelet transfusions should be avoided because they are generally ineffective and may precipitate thrombotic complications. The presence of subclinical thrombosis should be sought with routine screening duplex ultrasound on diagnosis because 50% of patients diagnosed with HIT have asymptomatic thrombosis, and the presence of thrombosis changes the duration of warfarin therapy. Since HIT is associated with a high incidence of thrombosis within 30 days of diagnosis, many recommend anticoagulation for at least a month in patients diagnosed with HIT. Warfarin should not be initiated until platelet counts have recovered to normal levels, as early warfarin therapy has been associated with extensive venous thrombosis/gangrene.

Immune thrombocytopenic purpura is caused by antibodies directed at platelet surface glycoproteins such as glycoprotein IIb/IIIa or Ib/IX. These antibodies precipitate platelet destruction in the reticuloendothelial system (spleen, liver, bone marrow). Generally, patients with ITP have thrombocytopenia of some degree noted on preoperative testing. Less commonly, immune thrombocytopenia will be triggered during the postoperative period. Patients with autoimmune disorders such as systemic lupus erythematosus or viral infections such as human immunodeficiency virus (HIV) or hepatitis C are at higher risk for ITP. Typically, ITP patients have significant thrombocytopenia (platelet counts <20,000/µL) but a normal hematocrit and white blood cell count. Direct platelet antibody testing demonstrates the presence of antiplatelet antibodies in many patients, and bone marrow examinations reveal normal numbers of platelet progenitor cells (megakaryocytes). Not surprisingly, platelet transfusions are generally ineffective but should not be withheld in the setting of life-threatening bleeding. Effective therapies include intravenous immunoglobulin or anti-D immunoglobulin (Winrho SDF, Baxter Healthcare Corp., Deerfield, Ill) or corticosteroids. Rituxamab (Rituxan, Genentech, Inc., San Francisco, Calif) and splenectomy are highly effective chronic therapy for persistent disease. More recently, thrombopoietin agonists such as eltrombopag and romiplostim have been shown to be very effective for ITP.

Rare consumptive causes of thrombocytopenia are thrombotic thrombocytopenic purpura (TTP), hemolytic uremic syndrome (HUS), posttransfusion purpura, and catastrophic antiphospholipid syndrome. TTP is caused by a deficiency of ADAMTS 13, an enzyme that processes large, highly adhesive von Willebrand factor (VWF) multimers into smaller, less adhesive fragments. In its absence, large von Willebrand factor multimers accumulate triggering the spontaneous formation of platelet aggregates that cause consumptive thrombocytopenia, a mechanical hemolytic anemia (from the physical cleavage of red cells as they traverse the microcirculation), and microvascular plugging/ischemia-induced renal and neurologic dysfunction. Diagnosis rests upon clinical recognition of these diagnostic features, confirmation of a microangiopathic picture on the peripheral smear, and laboratory testing confirming the absence of ADAMTS13 in the patient's plasma. Plasmapheresis is the most effective form of treatment. Platelet transfusions should be avoided except in the case of life-threatening bleeding because they can precipitate a dramatic worsening of the patient's clinical condition. HUS is most commonly caused by with calcineurin inhibitors (cyclosporine, tacrolimus), used for organ transplantation immunosuppression and, less commonly, with chemotherapeutic agents such as mitomycin C and gemcitabine (see Table 3). Calcineurin inhibitor–associated HUS usually responds to discontinuation of the offending agent.

Posttransfusion purpura (PTP) is a rare antibody-mediated consumptive form of thrombocytopenia that occurs in patients after transfusion with blood products. PTP is caused by alloantibodies-directed platelet glycoproteins. The vast majority of cases affect women because they are exposed to the causative antigen during childbirth. A typical presentation is the development of sudden,

TABLE 3: Drug-associated thrombocytopenia

Drug-associated immune thrombocytopenia	Drug-associated TTP/HUS
Unfractionated heparin	Ticlopidine
Low-molecular-weight heparin	Mitomycin C
Quinine/quinidine	Cyclosporin
Rifampin	Tacrolimus
Trimethoprim/sulfamethoxasole	Cisplatin
Acetamenophen	Gemcitabine
Digoxin	Quinine
Danazol	
Vancomycin	
Abciximab	
Eptifibatide	
Amiodarone	
Clopidogrel	
Ticlopidine	

TTP/HUS, Thrombotic thrombocytopenic purpura/hemolytic uremic syndrome.

Note: These lists include common causes of drug-associated thrombocytopenia but are by no means all-inclusive.

dramatic, and severe thrombocytopenia overnight, approximately a week after a blood product transfusion. Identification of antibodies directed against the causal antigen and typing the affected patient's platelets are diagnostic. Platelet transfusions are ineffective and can cause severe allergic reactions in affected individuals. IVIG has proven effective in shortening the course of thrombocytopenia.

Catastrophic antiphospholipid syndrome (CAS) is another uncommon cause of thrombocytopenia that can have devastating consequences. Affected patients typically have systemic lupus erythematosus or another autoimmune disorder associated with antiphospholipid antibodies or the primary form of antiphospholipid syndrome unassociated with another rheumatologic condition. Antiphospholipid syndrome is a hypercoagulable disorder associated with recurrent venous and/or arterial thromboembolism, recurrent pregnancy losses, and thrombocytopenia. CAS is typically triggered by discontinuation of anticoagulation or immunosuppressive medications for associated autoimmune disorders, severe infections, or major surgery. Clinical manifestations include disseminated microvascular thrombosis with evidence of peripheral ischemia, multiorgan dysfunction (including renal and neurologic dysfunction), and consumptive thrombocytopenia. Diagnosis is made based upon the characteristic clinical presentation and laboratory testing demonstrating the presence of antiphospholipid syndrome. Multimodality treatment is essential for optimal outcomes and includes anticoagulation, immunosuppression with high dose corticosteroids, and plasmapheresis.

Splenic Sequestration

Thrombocytopenia may also result from splenic sequestration of platelets in patients with significant splenomegaly. Normally, one third of the circulating platelet mass resides in the spleen. This proportion may grow substantially in patients with significant splenomegaly and result in moderately reduced platelet counts, as well as lower-than-expected responses to platelet transfusions. Splenic sequestration is commonly seen in patients with liver cirrhosis and hypersplenism due to hematologic disorders such as myelofibrosis. While splenectomy or operative portosystemic shunting may result in a reduction in the severity of thrombocytopenia, production defects also contribute to thrombocytopenia in these patients, so such major surgical procedures are rarely considered solely for treatment of thrombocytopenia due to splenic sequestration.

INHERITED QUANTITATIVE PLATELET DISORDERS

Inherited platelet disorders are a rare cause of bleeding in critically ill patients because these conditions are often identified prior to surgical procedures. Inherited aplastic anemia syndromes such as Fanconi's anemia, and inherited disorders affecting platelet production such as inherited amegakaryocytic thrombocytopenia, the thrombocytopenia with absent radius (TAR) syndrome, and Wiskott-Aldrich syndrome (WAS) result in chronic thrombocytopenia of varying severity. These patients can be identified by the presence of reduced peripheral blood counts and abnormal bone marrow examinations showing reductions in all three progenitor cell lines and hypersensitivity to DNA-damaging agents (Fanconi's anemia), or selective reductions in megakaryocytes, the platelet progenitor cells (inherited amegakaryocytic thrombocytopenia, TAR syndrome). The WAS is an X-linked disorder characterized by microthrombocytopenia—for example, the production of reduced numbers of small platelets, eczema, and immunodeficiency. Any male with thrombocytopenia and a small mean platelet volume on his complete blood count should be suspected of having WAS.

Qualitative Platelet Disorders

Acquired Platelet Dysfunction—Drug-Induced Platelet Dysfunction

Platelet dysfunction can also contribute to bleeding in critically ill patients. The most common qualitative disorders of platelet function are acquired (see Table 1). Use of medications or supplements with antiplatelet effects is a common cause of unanticipated surgical bleeding. Medications such as aspirin, clopidogrel, prasugrel, or ticlopidine should be discontinued 7 to 10 days prior to surgical procedures unless contraindicated by severe coronary artery disease or cardiac stents. It is always important to assess the indication for antiplatelet therapy prior to surgery, as inappropriate discontinuation can lead to fatal coronary thrombotic events. In patients with significant coronary artery disease or cardiac stents, it is advisable to discuss discontinuation of antiplatelet therapy with their cardiologist before surgery. Nonsteroidal antiinflammatory drugs (NSAIDs) can cause significant reversible platelet dysfunction, the duration of which varies by drug half-life. Ibuprofen, indomethacin, and ketoprofen have short half-lives (2 to 6 hours), so discontinuation 1 to 2 days preoperatively is sufficient. In contrast, naproxen and meloxicam have much longer half-lives (12 to 17 hours and 15 to 20 hours, respectively), so discontinuation 3 to 4 days preoperatively is warranted to avoid the presence of residual antiplatelet effects at the time of surgery. Dietary supplements and herbal remedies, particularly vitamin E and omega-3 fatty acids, are known to have antiplatelet effects. Exposure to these medications should be considered in any critically ill patient with bleeding. Although the TBT and the PFA-100 can measure the effects of antiplatelet medications, these tests should not be relied upon to identify patients at increased risk of bleeding with invasive procedures because these tests are not sensitive or specific enough for this purpose.

In patients with significant bleeding, platelet transfusions, and/or desmopressin (1-Desamino-8-D-Arginine Vasopressin or DDAVP), an arginine vasopressin analog that induces factor VIII and von Willebrand factor secretion can be used to improve hemostasis in the setting of antiplatelet therapy. In life-threatening bleeding, recombinant human factor VIIa (NovoSeven, Novo Nordisk, Inc., Princeton, NJ) has been used successfully to treat patients with acquired platelet dysfunction. Given the expense and prothrombotic risk associated with this agent, it should only be used for this purpose when conventional therapy has been ineffective.

Uremia/Myeloproliferative Disorders

Uremia is a common cause of platelet dysfunction among critically ill patients. The bleeding tendency in patients with renal insufficiency is multifactorial. Some contributing factors include increased production of the platelet inhibitory factors prostacyclin and nitric oxide by the endothelium, acquired defects in von Willebrand factor activity, decreases in platelet adhesive glycoproteins on the platelet surface, anemia (red cells serve as a sink for nitric oxide), and altered clearance of antithrombotic medications (heparin, low-molecular-weight heparin, aspirin, etc.). The TBT and/or the PFA-100 is usually prolonged in patients with uremic platelet dysfunction. Screening coagulation testing, including a PT and aPTT, should be included in any investigation of bleeding in a uremic patient to exclude the possibility of persistent heparinization associated with hemodialysis or acquired vitamin K deficiency. Bleeding in uremic patients can be improved by regular dialysis and increasing the hematocrit to 30% to 35% with transfusions or erythropoietin supplementation. Administration of DDAVP can also transiently improve hemostasis due to platelet dysfunction in dialysis patients by increasing the amount of von Willebrand factor available to assist in platelet adhesion/aggregation. Cryoprecipitate is also effective but carries a risk of transfusion-borne infectious illnesses and therefore should be avoided for this purpose. Conjugated estrogens produce slower but more durable responses at the cost of hormonal side effects.

Acquired platelet dysfunction is also common among patients with chronic myeloproliferative disorders such as polycythemia vera and essential thrombocythemia in association with markedly elevated platelet counts (typically exceeding 1,000,000/μL). Von Willebrand antigen levels (measures the amount of von Willebrand factor protein) and ristocetin cofactor activity (measures the function of von Willebrand factor) as well as TBT and the PFA-100 can be used to confirm the presence of this entity. Acute therapy for symptomatic patients includes administration of DDAVP or use of von Willebrand factor containing factor VIII concentrates or platelet transfusions. Cryoprecipitate should be avoided. Reduction of platelet counts with chemotherapeutic agents is often beneficial for long-term treatment.

INHERITED QUALITATIVE PLATELET DISORDERS

Inherited qualitative platelet disorders include the Bernard-Soulier syndrome, Glanzmann's thrombasthenia, and the platelet storage pool diseases such as Gray platelet syndrome. Patients with these conditions have platelet dysfunction that can vary from mild to severe. Common historical complaints include chronic epistaxis, gum bleeding, menorrhagia, easy bruisability, and excessive bleeding with invasive procedures, including dental extractions and minor surgery. The TBT and the PFA-100 are usually abnormal in these patients. In patients with severe Bernard-Soulier syndrome or Glanzmann's thrombasthenia, a TBT should probably be avoided if the diagnosis has been previously documented, as the TBT can be

extremely prolonged and lead to significant bleeding. Platelet aggregometry and platelet flow cytometry are invaluable in the diagnosis of inherited qualitative platelet disorders and thus should be ordered for definitive diagnosis. Platelet transfusions, DDAVP, and antifibrinolytic medications such as epsilon-amino caproic acid (Amicar, Wyeth-Ayerst, Collegeville, Penn) have all been used to achieve hemostasis in patients with these disorders. In general, platelet transfusions should be reserved for major surgery or serious bleeding in patients with platelet receptor disorders (Bernard-Soulier syndrome, Glanzmann's thrombasthenia), because these patients have a propensity to develop platelet alloantibodies, which can make them unresponsive to platelet transfusions in the future. Whenever possible, local hemostatic agents (e.g., fibrin sealants) should be employed. Preoperative hematology consultation is essential to achieve optimal surgical outcomes.

Coagulation Disorders

Five Basic Patterns of Coagulation Test Results

Coagulation factor disorders are a common cause of bleeding in the critically ill patient. Similar to platelet disorders, inherited and acquired coagulation factor disorders must be considered in the differential when approaching a bleeding patient. Rapid accurate interpretation of screening coagulation tests is key to identifying coagulation disorders. Five basic patterns of coagulation test results can be identified: a prolonged PT, a prolonged aPTT, a prolonged TT, a prolongation of the PT and the aPTT, and prolongation of all three screening tests.

An isolated prolonged PT occurs only in the presence of factor VII deficiency or a factor VII inhibitor. The most common cause of factor VII deficiency in the postoperative period is early vitamin K deficiency. Later vitamin K deficiency is characterized by reductions in factor IX, factor X, and prothrombin levels, which result in a prolonged aPTT and PT. If vitamin K deficiency is suspected, intravenous or oral vitamin K supplementation is the best initial management approach, as correction of the PT will likely take place before other diagnostic laboratory results return. If the PT fails to correct, then a factor VII activity assay can be used to confirm the presence of factor VII deficiency. Factor VII inhibitors are rarely seen except in patients with inherited factor VII deficiency. The presence of an inhibitor can be identified using mixing studies that demonstrate the failure of the PT to correct after the addition of normal pooled plasma.

An isolated prolonged aPTT can be seen in association with any deficiency state or factor inhibitor affecting one of the intrinsic pathway coagulation proteins (factors XII, XI, IX, VIII, prekallikrein, and high-molecular-weight kininogen). Specific factor assays can confirm the identity of the responsible factor. Knowledge of the incidence and clinical manifestations of coagulation disorders can help to prioritize factor testing. Factor VIII deficiency (hemophilia A) is the most common intrinsic factor deficiency disorder, followed by factor IX deficiency (hemophilia B) and factor XI deficiency (hemophilia C). Therefore, factor testing should proceed in this order in most patient populations. However, in patients of Ashkenazi Jewish ethnicity, factor XI testing should be considered early because the prevalence of heterozygous factor XI deficiency can be as high as 8%. Deficiencies of factor XII, prekallikrein, or high-molecular-weight kininogen are not associated with a clinical bleeding disorder, so factor assays for these coagulation disorders should be performed later.

The only deficiency state associated with a prolonged TT is a deficiency of fibrinogen. Confirmation of this result can be obtained by ordering a fibrinogen assay. Thrombin inhibitors develop rarely as a result of exposure to bovine thrombin. Combined prolongation of both the aPTT and the PT in the presence of a normal TT generally indicates that there is a deficiency of a common pathway factor (factor X, factor V, or prothrombin). Less commonly, this result is a consequence of factor deficiencies affecting both the extrinsic (factor VII) and intrinsic pathways (factors XII, XI, IX, and VIII; prekallikrein; and high-molecular-weight kininogen). Vitamin K deficiency can cause this clinical picture. Likewise, prolongation of the PT, aPTT, and TT generally represents severe fibrinogen deficiency or an inhibitor of thrombin (factor II inhibitor, heparin, etc.), although abnormalities in multiple factors could also generate this result.

INHERITED COAGULATION DISORDERS

The most common inherited factor deficiency states are the different hemophilias and von Willebrand disease (Table 4). Hemophilia A (factor VIII deficiency) is an X-linked recessive trait that affects 1 in 5000 male births. Disease severity correlates closely with factor levels. The normal range for factor VIII levels is generally 50% to 150%. Severe hemophilia A is characterized by factor VIII levels less than 1% and places affected individuals at high risk for spontaneous joint and soft tissue bleeds. Moderate hemophiliacs have factor VIII levels between 1% and 5% and usually bleed after trauma or invasive procedures. Minor hemophilia patients have factor levels greater than 5% and usually bleed only after significant trauma or surgical

TABLE 4: Coagulation disorders

Inherited coagulation disorder	Acquired coagulation disorders
Von Willebrand disease	Vitamin K deficiency
Hemophila A (factor VIII deficiency)	Liver disease
Hemophilia B (factor IX deficiency)	Anticoagulation-associated coagulopathy
Hemophilia C (factor XI deficiency)	Unfractionated heparin
Factor VII deficiency	Low molecular weight heparin
Factor X deficiency	Fondaparinux
A-, hypofibrinogenemia	Direct thrombin inhibitors
Factor V deficiency	Disseminated intravascular coagulation (DIC)
Factor II deficiency	Acquired factor inhibitors
Factor XII deficiency*	Factor V/thrombin inhibitors associated with bovine thrombin exposure
Factor XIII deficiency	Factor VIII inhibitors
High-molecular-weight kininogen deficiency*	Cardiac bypass coagulopathy Acquired von Willebrand disease (Heyde's syndrome) associated with severe aortic stenosis
Prekallikrein deficiency*	Dilutional coagulopathy (massive transfusions)

*Indicates disorders that can cause a markedly prolonged aPTT but do not cause clinical bleeding.

procedures. The diagnosis of hemophilia A can be confirmed with a factor VIII assay. Factor VIII inhibitors occur in approximately 15% to 25% of severe hemophiliacs, so mixing studies and factor VIII inhibitor assays should be assessed before surgical procedures and whenever a patient does not appear to respond appropriately to factor VIII replacement therapy. Plasma-derived and recombinant factor VIII concentrates are the principal treatment for patients with hemophilia A (Table 5 and Box 3). Although cryoprecipitate contains factor VIII, this product should not be used for treatment of hemophilia because it is a less concentrated source of factor VIII and is associated with a risk of transmission of blood-borne infectious diseases. Recombinant factor concentrates are generally preferred over plasma-derived concentrates for most patients because they are associated with a lower risk of transfusion-associated infections. DDAVP, which induces release of factor VIII and von Willebrand factor, can be used for hemostasis in mild hemophiliacs undergoing minor surgical procedures. When using DDAVP for treatment of mild hemophilia or von Willebrand disease, it is important to note that it is only effective for three or four doses, after which tachyphylaxis develops due to exhaustion of preformed stores of factor VIII and von Willebrand factor in the endothelium and liver. Antifibrinolytic medications such as epsilon aminocaproic acid (Amicar, Wyeth-Ayerst, Collegeville, Penn) are useful adjuvant hemostatic agents for hemophiliacs undergoing mild mucosal surgery.

For major surgery, factor VIII levels should be raised to 80% to 100% preoperatively and maintained there for the first 3 days and then maintained at 50% or more for 10 to 14 days. Daily trough factor VIII activity assays should be obtained to ensure that minimum factor VIII levels for hemostasis are maintained. For cardiac surgery and neurosurgery, trough levels should be maintained at 100% for the first 72 hours and then at 80% to 100% for the first week. Trough levels of 50% to 80% are adequate for days 8 to 14.

Factor IX deficiency (hemophilia B) is inherited in a X-linked recessive fashion and is about sevenfold less common than hemophilia A. Factor levels correlate with clinical severity similar to hemophilia A. Laboratory diagnosis relies upon factor IX assays, and plasma-derived and recombinant factor IX concentrates are used for therapy. The duration of therapy for surgery is similar to patients with factor VIII deficiency. Factor IX inhibitors are much less common, affecting only 2% of patients. Allergic reactions to factor IX concentrates often herald the development of a factor IX inhibitor.

Factor XI deficiency (hemophilia C) is an uncommon disorder except in patients of Ashkenazi Jewish descent, in whom as many as 8% carry one mutated allele. Fortunately, most individuals have mild to moderate deficiencies of factor XI, in whom bleeding symptoms are mild. Consequently, many individuals with factor XI deficiency are first identified on preoperative testing or after developing bleeding with invasive procedures. Unlike hemophilia A and B, very low factor XI levels do not always correlate with a bleeding tendency. Those patients who do bleed do so after significant trauma or major surgery. Factor XI inhibitors are rare except in patients with severe factor XI deficiency (<1%) who have been exposed to previous replacement therapy. Diagnosis is made by factor XI activity assays. Although factor XI concentrates are used in Europe, fresh frozen plasma is the only replacement product available in the United States. Generally, 15 mL/kg of plasma are transfused prior to invasive procedures. Factor XI levels of 20% to 25% are typically adequate for hemostasis. Daily assessment of factor XI levels and plasma replacement to maintain adequate factor levels for at least 3 to 5 days and 10 to 14 days are used to treat patients undergoing minor surgery and major surgery, respectively. Since factor XI is important in regulation of fibrinolysis, antifibrinolytic medications such as epsilon aminocaproic acid (Amicar, Wyeth-Ayerst, Collegeville, Penn) have been found to be useful for prevention of bleeding in patients with mild factor XI deficiency.

Von Willebrand disease (vWD) is caused by inherited autosomal deficiency of von Willebrand factor (vWF), a protein that plays a key

TABLE 5: Treatment of coagulation factor disorders

Bleeding disorder	Target factor level	Plasma product
Hemophilia A		
Minor surgery	>50% for 3-7 days	
Major surgery	>80% to 100% for 3 days, then >50% for next 7-11 days	Recombinant (preferred) or plasma-derived monoclonal factor VIII concentrates
Cardiovascular, prostate and neurosurgery	>100% for 3 days, then 80% to 100% for days 4-7 and >50% for days 8-14	
Hemophilia B		
Minor surgery	>50% for 3-7 days	
Major surgery	>80% to 100% for 3 days, then >50% for next 7-11 days	Recombinant or monoclonal plasma-derived factor IX concentrates
Cardiovascular, prostate and neurosurgery	>100% for 3 days, then 80% to 100% for day 4-7 and >50% for days 8-14	
Von Willebrand disease		
Minor surgery	>50% for 1-3 days	DDAVP or vWF-containing factor VIII concentrates (e.g., Humate P)
Major surgery	Keep 50% to 100% for 7-14 days	
Factor XI deficiency		
Minor surgery	>30% for 3-4 days	Fresh frozen plasma (FFP)
Major surgery	>45% for 7-10 days	
Factor VII deficiency		
Minor surgery	>15%	FFP or recombinant human factor VIIa
Major surgery	>25%	
Factor X deficiency		
Minor surgery	>15%	FFP or prothrombin
Major surgery	>50% perioperatively, then >30%	Complex concentrates
Factor V deficiency		
Minor surgery	>25%	FFP
Major surgery	>50% perioperatively, then >25%	
Prothrombin deficiency		
Minor surgery	20% to 40%	FFP or prothrombin complex concentrates
Major surgery	20% to 40%	
A-fibrinogenemia or hypofibrinogenemia		
Minor surgery	>50-100 mg/dL for 3 days	Cryoprecipitate or fibrinogen concentrate (Riastap)
Major surgery	>50-100 mg/dL for 2 weeks	
Factor XIII deficiency		
Minor surgery	>5%	FFP or cryoprecipitate
Major surgery	>5%	

role in platelet adhesion and serves as a carrier protein for factor VIII, protecting it from degradation by activated protein C. Reflecting its primary role in platelet function, vWD patients generally suffer mucosal bleeding (epistaxis, gum bleeding, menorrhagia, bleeding with dental surgery). The best laboratory assays for diagnosis of von Willebrand disease are the von Willebrand antigen assay, which measures the amount of vWF protein, and the ristocetin cofactor assay or the collagen-binding assay, both of which measure vWF protein function. Factor VIII levels are generally normal or only mildly reduced, so the aPTT is not a useful screening test for vWD.

Most patients with mild disease can be treated with DDAVP, but confirmation of DDAVP response preoperatively is important to avoid bleeding complications in nonresponders. In addition, it is important to remember that DDAVP cannot be used for extended

BOX 3: Hemostatic agents

Fresh Frozen Plasma (FFP)
Contains all coagulation factors in low concentrations
   (1 unit/mL)
Used for treatment of factor deficiency states without available
   factor concentrates
Used for treatment of coagulopathies associated with deficiency
   of multiple factors (e.g., liver disease, cardiac surgery,
   dilutional coagulopathy, etc.)

Cryoprecipitate
Contains factor VIII, von Willebrand factor, fibrinogen, factor
   XIII
Used for treatment of fibrinogen and factor XIII deficiency
Should *not* be used for treatment of factor VIII deficiency or von
   Willebrand disease *unless* factor VIII/von Willebrand–
   containing concentrates are not available
Factor VIII concentrates (recombinant, plasma derived)
Used for treatment of hemophilia A (factor VIII deficiency) and
   von Willebrand disease (e.g., Humate P and other von
   Willebrand factor containing factor VIII concentrates)
Factor IX concentrates (recombinant, plasma derived)
Used for treatment of hemophilia B (factor IX deficiency)

Prothrombin Complex Concentrate
Contains vitamin K–dependent factors II, IX, and X
Used for reversal of warfarin anticoagulation in patients with
   serious bleeding

Activated Prothrombin Complex Concentrates
Contain activated factors II, VII, IX, and X
Used for treatment for factor VIII inhibitors

Recombinant Human Factor VIIa (NovoSeven)
Licensed for treatment of factor VIII inhibitors (used off-label
   for treatment of bleeding in patients with inherited platelet
   dysfunction, cardiac surgery coagulopathy, etc.)

Fibrinogen Concentrate (Riastap, CSL Behring)
Licensed for treatment of A- or hypofibrinogenemia

Fibrin Sealants (e.g., Tisseel)
Contains fibrinogen, thrombin, factor XIII
Used as a local hemostatic agent

**Antifibrinolytic Agents (Epsilon Aminocaproic
Acid, Aprotinin)**
Inhibit the fibrinolysis by inhibiting plasmin activity or
   generation

Desmopressin (DDAVP)
Induces release of von Willebrand factor and factor VIII
Used for treatment of mild von Willebrand disease and factor
   VIII deficiency

replacement therapy (>72 hours) because of tachyphylaxis. Therefore, for extended therapy or treatment of patients with severe disease, vWF containing factor VIII concentrates should be used. Cryoprecipitate should not be used for treatment of vWD because of its greater risk of transfusion-transmitted infectious diseases. A functional measure of vWF, such as the ristocetin cofactor assay, should be used to monitor therapy.

Inherited deficiency states involving other factors are rare, affecting in general less than 1 in 500,000. Except for factor VII deficiency, for which recombinant human factor VIIa (NovoSeven, Novo Nordisk, Princeton, NJ) can be used, and fibrinogen deficiency, for which a plasma-derived fibrinogen concentrate (Riastap CSL, Behring, King of Prussia, Penn) is available, fresh frozen plasma is

the only available replacement product for these rare inherited deficiency states. The available plasma products for treatment of coagulation disorders and the appropriate doses and durations of therapy for bleeding and surgical procedures are listed in Table 5.

Fibrin sealants are a useful hemostatic adjunct to traditional blood products for critically ill patients with bleeding. Although fibrin sealants have traditionally been made in the operating room by adding bovine thrombin to cryoprecipitate, these "bedside" products are associated with the development of inhibitors against factor V and thrombin. More recently, human thrombin (Evithrom Ethicon, Summerville, NJ) and recombinant human thrombin (Recothrom, Zymogenetics, Seattle, Wash) have been developed that can be used with cryoprecipitate to make fibrin glue and are associated with a lower risk of coagulation factor inhibitors. Commercial fibrin sealants such as Tisseel VH (Baxter HealthCare, West Lake Village, Calif), which contain virally inactivated human fibrinogen and thrombin supplemented with aprotinin, an antifibrinolytic agent, are also effective local hemostatic agents and have not been associated with coagulation inhibitors. In addition, commercial fibrin sealants are pathogen-inactivated, so they are associated with a lower risk of transfusion-associated infections.

ACQUIRED COAGULATION DISORDERS

Acquired coagulation disorders are a common cause of coagulopathy in the critically ill patient (see Table 6). Among acquired coagulopathies, disseminated intravascular coagulation is among the most common and difficult to treat. Although there are a large number of stimuli that can trigger it (e.g., sepsis, snake venom, trauma, cancer, heparin-induced thrombocytopenia), disseminated intravascular coagulation ultimately, is a syndrome of excessive thrombin production. The end result is diffuse fibrin clot and platelet plug formation, consumption of fibrinogen, platelets and coagulation factors, and activation of the fibrinolytic system. Clinically, disseminated intravascular coagulation has at least three different presentations: diffuse microvascular thrombosis characterized by cool, cyanotic, or necrotic digits or extremities; diffuse hemorrhage manifested by bleeding from sites of previous invasive procedures; or asymptomatic. Clinical manifestations are dictated by the degree of activation of the coagulation cascade and the balance between clot formation and fibrinolysis. Laboratory markers of disseminated intravascular coagulation include thrombocytopenia; a prolonged aPTT, PT, or TT; elevations of D dimers or fibrin degradation products; and hypofibrinogenemia. Although rarely measured, antithrombin, protein C, and protein S levels are often reduced in disseminated intravascular coagulation as well. Although the aPTT and PT are the most commonly ordered tests when investigating patients for disseminated intravascular coagulation, D dimer levels are the most sensitive assay for this entity.

Therapy for disseminated intravascular coagulation should be directed principally against the underlying cause. Antibiotics and supportive therapy (intravenous fluids, vasoactive medications, blood products, etc.) should be employed in disseminated intravascular coagulation associated with infections. Aggressive blood product support is also reasonable for patients with disseminated intravascular coagulation and bleeding. While anticoagulation has generally not improved outcomes for most patients with thrombotic forms of disseminated intravascular coagulation, it is essential for patients with HIT and DIC or catastrophic antiphospholipid syndrome, and DIC as anticoagulation is essential to suppress the prothrombotic stimulus responsible for these forms of disseminated intravascular coagulation.

Vitamin K deficiency is a common cause of acquired coagulopathy in the intensive care unit, as critically ill patients often have limited vitamin K intake, exposure to broad-spectrum antibiotics, and disrupted hepatobiliary recirculation of vitamin K. The primary sources of vitamin K are green vegetables such as broccoli and spinach and supplemental vitamin K produced by intestinal flora. Therefore, patients who are not eating well and are being treated with broad-spectrum antibiotics are at high risk for this acquired coagulopathy. Several antibiotics containing the N-methyl-thiotetrazole side chain (e.g., cefamandole, cefotetan, cefoperazone, etc.) that inhibits vitamin K epoxide reductase, an enzyme in the vitamin K recycling pathway, place patients at particularly high risk of this complication. Vitamin K is essential to the production of functional forms of the coagulation factors prothrombin (factor II), factor VII, factor IX, and factor X, as well as the anticoagulant proteins, protein C, and protein S. Since factors such as factor VII have a half-life of 6 hours, prolongation of the PT can occur rapidly once vitamin K stores are depleted.

Clinically, vitamin K deficiency is manifested by the development of ecchymoses and bleeding from the site of blood draws or invasive procedures. Since factor VII has the shortest half-life of the vitamin K–dependent coagulation factors, the PT is the first test to become abnormal, followed by prolongation of the aPTT. Mixing studies will demonstrate complete correction of the laboratory abnormalities. Administration of vitamin K results in rapid correction of the coagulopathy. Since oral vitamin K_1 is as effective as subcutaneous vitamin K_1 in patients without biliary disease and poses no risk of anaphylaxis, this route should be used in patients without serious bleeding or biliary disease. Patients with serious or life-threatening bleeding should be treated with intravenous vitamin K_1 because it can result in substantial correction of the PT within 4 to 8 hours. Any time intravenous vitamin K_1 is administered to a patient, it should be given slowly (no more rapidly than 1 mg per minute), with close monitoring for evidence of anaphylaxis (estimated absolute risk 1 out of 3000). FFP should only be used for treatment of vitamin K deficiency in situations of life-threatening bleeding when rapid correction is necessary.

Anticoagulant-Associated Bleeding

Anticoagulants are an important cause of bleeding that should be investigated in any patient presenting with bleeding during anticoagulation. The most common anticoagulants in the inpatient environment are unfractionated heparin, low-molecular-weight heparin, and warfarin. Newer anticoagulants that are being used increasingly in inpatients are direct thrombin inhibitors such as argatroban (Novastan, GlaxoSmithKline, Research Triangle Park, NC) and bivalirudin (Angiomax, The Medicines Company, Parsippany, NJ), which are used for treatment of HIT, and desirudin (Iprivask, Canyon Pharmaceuticals, Hunt Valley, Md), which is approved for VTE prevention. Fondaparinux (Arixtra, GlaxoSmithKline, Research Triangle Park, NC), an indirect antithrombin-dependent parenteral factor Xa inhibitor, is approved for treatment and prevention of venous thromboembolism and acute coronary syndromes. More recently, dabigatran (Pradaxa, Boehringer Ingelheim, Ridgefield, Conn), the first oral direct thrombin inhibitor, and rivaroxaban (Xarelto, Janssen Pharmaceuticals, Titusville, NJ), the first oral direct factor Xa inhibitor, have been approved by the FDA for thromboprophylaxis in patients with nonvalvular atrial fibrillation (both medications) and in patients undergoing hip or knee arthroplasty (rivaroxaban only).

Unfractionated Heparin

Unfractionated heparin results in anticoagulation by virtue of its interaction with the endogenous anticoagulant protein antithrombin (III). Heparin accelerates the inhibitory interaction of antithrombin with thrombin and activated factors X, IX, and XI by several thousand–fold. Due to its broad spectrum of activity, unfractionated heparin results in a prolongation of the aPTT. The TT is also exquisitely sensitive to its effects. Definitive demonstration that heparin is responsible for a coagulopathy can be obtained by repeating the aPTT after exposing the patient's plasma to heparinase. A dramatic correction of the aPTT is conclusive evidence of heparin

contamination. The most frequent clinical situations when heparin is associated with clinical bleeding include patients immediately after cardiac bypass surgery, patients undergoing hemodialysis, and patients receiving heparin for venous thromboembolism prophylaxis or treatment. Protamine administered intravenously in a dose of 1 mg per 100 units of heparin can be used to reverse heparin-associated coagulopathy.

LOW-MOLECULAR-WEIGHT HEPARIN

Low-molecular-weight heparin (LMWH) can also precipitate bleeding complications. The three LMWHs available in the United States are dalteparin (Fragmin, Eisai, Inc., Woodcliff Lake, NJ), enoxaparin (Lovenox, Sanofi-Aventis, Bridgewater, NJ, and multiple generic enoxaparin manufacturers), and tinzaparin (Innohep, Celgene Corporation Boulder, Colo). LMWH-associated bleeding most commonly develops in patients receiving LMWH for treatment or prevention of VTE who develop worsening renal function or undergo unanticipated invasive procedures. LMWH exerts its anticoagulant effects by accelerating the antithrombotic effects of antithrombin (III), primarily against factor Xa and to a lesser extent thrombin. Since it has significantly less inhibitory activity toward thrombin, LMWH does not typically prolong the aPTT. LMWH concentrations can be measured using specialized assays measuring the activity of factor Xa. However, these assays are generally less rapidly available than routine assays such as the aPTT. Protamine can reverse a variable amount of LMWH activity (enoxaparin 54%, dalteparin 74%, tinzaparin 86%), depending on the agent used. The intravenous dose of protamine should be 1 mg per 100 units (of dalteparin or tinzaparin) or 1 mg per each mg of enoxaparin if the LMWH dose was given within 8 hours. If the LMWH was given more than 8 hours ago, then 0.5 mg of protamine should be given for each 100 units (of dalteparin or tinzaparin) or each mg of enoxaparin. If life-threatening bleeding is occurring and incomplete protamine reversal is a concern, recombinant human factor VIIa (NovoSeven, Novo Nordisk, Inc., Princeton, NJ) has been used successfully in this situation. However, the potential for prothrombotic effects associated with rhFVIIa should be weighed against the severity of bleeding.

WARFARIN

Millions of Americans are treated with warfarin each year for chronic anticoagulation. Warfarin results in anticoagulation by virtue of its inhibition of two enzymes in the vitamin K recycling pathway: vitamin K epoxide reductase and vitamin K reductase. The result is acquired vitamin K deficiency and significant reductions in the functional levels of the vitamin K–dependent coagulation factors prothrombin, factor VII, factor IX, and factor X, as well as protein C and protein S. The impact of warfarin on the coagulation cascade can be assessed using the PT/INR. In situations where rapid reversal is not needed, oral vitamin K can be used to reverse warfarin within 24 hours. If rapid reversal is needed, combined modality therapy with intravenous vitamin K and a prothrombin complex concentrate should be used. Prothrombin complex concentrates are plasma-derived factor concentrates that contain the vitamin K–dependent coagulation factors in high concentrations and can be prepared and administered within minutes. In contrast, plasma requires several hours to administer because it is often stored frozen and large volumes are required for PT/INR reversal.

DIRECT THROMBIN INHIBITORS

The available direct thrombin inhibitors (DTIs) include the parenteral medications argatroban (Novastan, GlaxoSmithKline, Research Triangle Park, NC), bivalirudin (Angiomax, The Medicines Company, Parsippany, NJ), desirudin (Iprivask, Canyon Pharmaceuticals, Hunt

Valley, Md), and the oral DTI dabigatran (Pradaxa, Boehringer Ingelheim, Ridgefield, Conn). Each of these agents directly binds and inhibits thrombin. Argatroban has a half-life of 45 minutes and is cleared by hepatic metabolism. Bivalirudin clearance is 80%, depending on plasma hydrolysis, and 20% renal clearance. It has a half-life of 25 minutes in patients with normal renal function. Desirudin has a half-life of 2 to 3 hours and undergoes renal elimination. Dabigatran has a half-life of 11 to 23 hours, depending on renal function.

The anticoagulant effects of argatroban, bivalirudin, and desirudin can be measured by the aPTT. Therapeutic concentrations of dabigatran can be detected using the aPTT, but it is best measured using a dilute thrombin time assay: the Hemoclot thrombin inhibition assay. No reversal agent is available for any of the DTI. Activated charcoal lavage can be used to prevent absorption of dabigatran in patients who have ingested the drug within the last 2 hours. Hemodialysis can be used to remove bivalirudin and dabigatran in the event of life-threatening bleeding. Argatroban clearance is not accelerated by hemodialysis. rhFVIIa (NovoSeven, Novo Nordisk, Inc., Princeton, NJ) and activated prothrombin complex concentrates (FEIBA NF, Baxter Healthcare Corp., Westlake Village, Calif) have been used with variable success for the reversal of the anticoagulant effects of DTI. Therefore, these reversal agents should be used only in cases of life-threatening bleeding because both agents are associated with an increased risk of thromboembolic complications. A specific reversal agent for dabigatran is in development.

Factor Xa Inhibitors

Fondaparinux (Arixtra, GlaxoSmithKline, Research Triangle Park, NC) is a parenteral indirect factor Xa inhibitor whose activity is mediated by accelerating antithrombin inactivation of factor Xa. It is used in the prevention and treatment of VTE and acute coronary syndromes. It is cleared renally and has a half-life of 17 to 21 hours in patients with normal renal function. It cannot be measured using the aPTT or PT. It should not be used in patients with compromised renal function (creatinine clearance less than 30 mL/min). There is no reversal agent available for fondaparinux, although rhFVIIa has been demonstrated to partially reverse its anticoagulant activity. Rivaroxaban (Xarelto, Janssen Pharmaceuticals, Titusville, NJ) is a direct oral factor Xa inhibitor. It has an elimination half life of 5 to 9 hours in young adults to age 45 years and 11 to 13 hours in older subjects. Rivaroxaban is cleared by hepatic metabolism and renal clearance. Rivaroxaban should be avoided in patients with severely reduced renal function (<15 mL/min) and moderate to severe hepatic function (Childs's class B and C hepatic dysfunction). There is no specific reversal agent for rivaroxaban, although activated prothrombin complex concentrates or rhFVIIa may have some utility in reducing its anticoagulant effects. Activated charcoal can be used to prevent absorption from the gastrointestinal tract in patients who have ingested rivaroxaban within the past 2 hours. Rivaroxaban is not dialyzable.

LIVER DISEASE

The liver is the principal synthetic organ for all of the coagulation factors except for von Willebrand factor and factor VIII and the main source of thrombopoietin, the platelet growth factor. In addition, the liver is responsible for clearance of activated coagulation factors, plasmin, fibrin split products, and D dimers, and it produces fibrinolytic inhibitors such as alpha2-antiplasmin and plasminogen activator −1. Consequently, patients with significant liver disease are at high risk for bleeding due to multiple acquired factor deficiencies, thrombocytopenia, platelet dysfunction due to the inhibitory effects of circulating fibrin split products, and a tendency toward hyperfibrinolysis. The PT, aPTT, and TT, as well as the fibrinogen level and platelet count, are useful parameters to assess the bleeding risk associated with liver disease. The thromboelastogram

or euglobulin lysis time can help to identify excessive fibrinolytic activity. D dimer levels will often be moderately elevated but do not indicate disseminated intravascular coagulation unless markedly elevated because the liver plays an important role in clearance of D dimers and fibrin split products.

Factor deficiencies associated with liver disease are amenable to FFP replacement. Factor replacement should be guided by clinical findings and coagulation test results. Generally, 15 mL of FFP per kg body weight is an adequate replacement dose. It is important not to strive to normalize the results of coagulation studies, particularly the PT, because factor VII has a short half-life, and attempting to achieve normal levels often results in fluid overload. Generally factor VII levels of 10% to 15% are adequate to stop bleeding. Factor VII levels of 15% to 20% are sufficient for surgical procedures. Often, reducing the PT and aPTT ratio to less than 1.5 is sufficient for most procedures.

If the fibrinogen level is less than 100 mg/dL, transfusion of cryoprecipitate or fibrinogen concentrate (Riastap, CSL Behring King of Prussia, Penn) is more efficient to achieve correction. In a 70-kg patient, each bag of cryoprecipitate will result in a 10 mg/dL increment in the fibrinogen level. On average 3 units of cryoprecipitate must be transfused on a daily basis to maintain fibrinogen levels above 100 mg/dL, but transfusions should be guided by fibrinogen levels. Fibrinogen concentrate is FDA-approved for congenital afibrinogenemia and hypofibrinogenemia, but its use for fibrinogen replacement in acquired fibrinogen deficiency would seem reasonable given its lower risk for transfusion-associated infectious diseases. The dose of fibrinogen concentrate is calculated using the following equation:

$$\text{Dose mg/kg body weight} = \text{Desired fibrinogen level (mg/dL)} - \text{Current fibrinogen level (mg/dL)}/1.7\ \text{mg/dL per mg/kg body weight}$$

$$\textit{Example}: 100\ \text{mg/dL} - 40\ \text{mg/dL}/1.7\ \text{mg/dL per mg/kg body weight} = 60/1.7 \times 70\ \text{kg} = 2470\ \text{mg of Riastap}$$

The target for fibrinogen replacement should be 100 mg/dL because excessive supplementation may result in a heightened risk of thrombosis. Platelet transfusions should be given to any afebrile patient with a platelet count less than 10,000/μL or a febrile patient with platelets less than 20,000/μL. Patients with active bleeding or planned surgery should have platelet counts increased to 50,000/μL. Table 2 provides the recommended platelet thresholds for different clinical situations.

To ensure that unsuspected vitamin K deficiency is not contributing to a patient's coagulopathy, all patients with liver disease and bleeding who do not have contraindications should be treated with vitamin K. Use of antifibrinolytic agents should be considered in any patient suspected of having primary fibrinolysis as a cause of bleeding. The presence of DIC or active thrombosis should be ruled out prior to initiating antifibrinolytic therapy because these medications can precipitate widespread microvascular thrombosis in patients with DIC. The dose of epsilon aminocaproic acid is a 5-g intravenous loading dose followed by 1 g/hr for 8 hours. The maximal daily dose is 30 g.

ACQUIRED FACTOR INHIBITORS

Factor V and Thrombin Inhibitors

Inhibitors to factor V and, less commonly, thrombin can develop in patients exposed to bovine thrombin. Most commonly this exposure occurs during cardiac surgery or neurosurgery when bovine thrombin is mixed with cryoprecipitate to make fibrin glue for topical hemostasis. Bovine thrombin is commonly contaminated with factor

V. Exposure, particularly repeated exposure, is associated with development of antibodies to bovine thrombin and factor V, which occasionally cross-react with human factor V and, less commonly, thrombin. These antibodies typically arise approximately a week postoperatively and occasionally have been associated with significant hemorrhagic consequences. Factor V and thrombin inhibitors should be considered in any patient who develops an abnormal PT and aPTT in the postoperative period. Thrombin times will be markedly prolonged in these patients, and mixing studies will demonstrate the presence of an inhibitor. Factor V and/or prothrombin levels can be reduced. In the absence of symptoms, patients should not be treated with blood products or immunosuppressant agents. In patients with bleeding, IVIG and corticosteroids have demonstrated utility in eliminating the inhibitor and reducing bleeding symptoms. Patients with life-threatening bleeding should receive multimodality therapy, including immunosuppression and plasmapheresis. Fortunately, bovine thrombin–associated factor inhibitors are transient, persisting for a mean of 2.3 months. The risk of factor V and thrombin inhibitors is less with newer bovine thrombin preparations. In addition, human thrombin (Evithrom, Ethicon, Summerville, NJ) and recombinant human thrombin (Recothrom, Zymogenetics, Seattle, Wash) and commercial fibrin sealants such as Tisseel VH (Baxter Health-Care, West Lake Village, Calif) appear to be much less likely to be associated with coagulation factor inhibitor development.

CARDIAC SURGERY–ASSOCIATED BLEEDING

Cardiac bypass is associated with significant perturbations of the hemostatic mechanism. Excessive bleeding, defined as a blood loss of greater than 1 liter, occurs in 5% of cardiac surgery patients. The reasons for post–cardiac surgery bleeding are multifactorial. Large doses of heparin are used to prevent thrombosis of the bypass circuit. Platelet number and function decline during and after cardiac bypass due to activation and consumption. Coagulation protein levels drop, and activation of the fibrinolytic system also occurs. Each of these abnormalities contributes to an increased risk of bleeding after cardiac surgery. The approach to bleeding after cardiac surgery depends on the rate of bleeding and the clinical status of the patient. Unstable patients with rapid blood loss ($\geq$500 mL/hr) should be resuscitated and surgically explored for a bleeding vessel. Since residual heparin may contribute to excessive bleeding, a second dose of protamine can be given to reverse any residual heparin present. If rapid access to point-of-care or conventional laboratory testing is available, the presence of residual heparin can be measured using an aPTT, thrombin time, or heparin neutralized thrombin time.

In stable patients with excessive bleeding, use of laboratory testing to guide therapy is appropriate. A heparin neutralized thrombin time; PT; aPTT; complete blood count, including platelet count; and fibrinogen should be measured. Patients with evidence of residual heparin (elevated thrombin time, aPTT, reversal with heparinase) should receive a second dose of protamine. Patients with platelet counts less than 50,000/μL should be transfused with platelets. Platelet counts in excess of 50,000/μL are generally not associated with excessive bleeding in the absence of platelet dysfunction. If other laboratory testing does not reveal an abnormality, platelet transfusions should be considered for patients with platelet counts less than 100,000/μL because cardiac bypass can result in dysfunctional spent platelets. Patients with hypofibrinogenemia (fibrinogen <100 mg/dL) should be treated with cryoprecipitate or a fibrinogen concentrate to achieve a fibrinogen level of greater than 100 mg/dL (each bag of cryoprecipitate will raise the fibrinogen level 10 mg/dL in a 70-kg patient). Patients with abnormal aPTT and PT test results unassociated with heparin or hypofibrinogenemia should be transfused with fresh frozen plasma (initial dose 10-15 mL/kg). Since hyperfibrinolysis can result after cardiac bypass, use of

antifibrinolytic agents such as epsilon-amino caproic acid or aprotinin should be considered for patients without significant thrombocytopenia (platelets >100,000/μL) and normal or minimally impaired PT and aPTT test results (PT and/or aPTT ratio <1.4). Thromboelastography can be useful in identifying patients with hyperfibrinolysis, although studies demonstrating superior outcomes with TEG-guided management are lacking. Occasional patients with severe aortic stenosis will develop acquired von Willebrand disease (Heyde's syndrome). Von Willebrand disease results from activation of ADAMTS13, resulting in excessive cleavage of vWF. Ristocetin cofactor and vWF antigen studies can be used to identify these patients. Preoperative identification is optimal because bleeding generally takes place during the operative procedure and the abnormality resolves after correction of aortic stenosis. vWF-containing factor VIII concentrates such as Humate P (CSL, Behring, Kankakee, Ill) can be used for replacement therapy.

DDAVP and rhFVIIa have been used to improve hemostasis in cardiac surgery patients. DDAVP, an analog of arginine vasopressin, is most useful as a hemostatic agent when applied to patients with platelet dysfunction. Case series of patients with critical bleeding after cardiac surgery suggest rhFVIIa may have utility in selected patients unresponsive to standard treatments. However, rhFVIIa should be used with caution for this indication given its association with thromboembolism.

VESSEL WALL DISORDERS

Disorders of vascular function are unusual causes for excessive surgical bleeding. Nevertheless, awareness of these disorders can be invaluable for the management of the occasional patient with a vessel wall disorder. Some of the inherited and acquired disorders of vascular function are presented in Table 6. Among the inherited disorders of vascular function, Ehlers Danlos syndrome is the most common to cause hemostatic difficulties. These patients have an inherited defect in collagen synthesis that results in a propensity to easy bruisability, skin and joint tissue laxity, arterial aneurysm formation, and poor wound healing. Some patients will display evidence of abnormal platelet function. A history of platelet-type bleeding is useful for identifying affected individuals in addition to the characteristic clinical findings. Generally, coagulation testing is normal. In patients with abnormal bleeding associated with surgical procedures, DDAVP has proven useful for improving hemostasis. Since patients with Ehlers-Danlos syndrome have poor wound healing, surgery should be undertaken only when absolutely necessary.

An unusual but important acquired cause of excessive surgical bleeding is amyloidosis. Amyloidosis is most often caused by a

TABLE 6: Vascular disorders

Inherited disorders	Acquired disorders
Hereditary hemorrhagic telangiectasia (Osler-Weber-Rendu syndrome)	Amyloidosis
Congenital hemangiomas	Hypercorticosteroidism (Cushing's syndrome, Cushing's disease)
Connective tissue disorders Ehlers-Danlos syndrome Loewy-Dietz syndrome Marfan syndrome Osteogenesis imperfecta Pseudoxanthoma elasticum	Vitamin C deficiency (scurvy)

monoclonal proliferation of plasma cells that produce light chains, a fragment of immunoglobulin that can collect in vessel walls and organs such as the kidney, liver, spleen, heart, and tongue. In addition to causing organ dysfunction, infiltration of the amyloid protein can cause vascular fragility and acquired factor X deficiency as a consequence of adsorption of factor X by exposed vessel wall amyloid fibrils. Patients with acquired factor X deficiency typically have a prolonged PT and aPTT and reduced factor X levels. Treatment with FFP is often associated with only transient increases in factor X levels because the amyloid fibrils avidly adsorb the transfused factor. RhFVIIa has also been used anecdotally to achieve hemostasis in these individuals. Patients with amyloidosis can be diagnosed by the presence of urinary monoclonal light chain proteins on urine protein electrophoresis and biopsy evidence of amyloid fibrils in skin or affected organs (kidney, heart, liver, bone marrow). Reduction of the amyloid protein with chemotherapy or, occasionally, splenectomy in patients with massive splenic amyloid deposits has been associated with amelioration of bleeding manifestations. Some additional acquired vascular disorders are listed in Table 6.

SUGGESTED READINGS

DeLoughery TG: Hemorrhagic and thrombotic disorders in the intensive care setting. In Kitchens CS, Alving BM, Kessler CM, editors: *Consultative Hemostasis and Thrombosis*, Philadelphia, 2002, W.B. Saunders Co., pp 493–514.

George JN, Raskob GE, Shah SR, et al: Drug-induced thrombocytopenia: a systematic review of published case reports, *Ann Intern Med* 129:886–890, 1998.

Kessler CM, Khokhar N, Liu M: A systematic approach to the bleeding patient: correlation of clinical symptoms and signs with laboratory testing. In Kitchens CS, Alving BM, Kessler CM, editors: *Consultative hemostasis and thrombosis*, Philadelphia, 2007, W.B. Saunders Co., pp 17–33.

Kitchens CS: Surgery and hemostasis. In Kitchens CS, Alving BM, Kessler CM, editors: *Consultative hemostasis and thrombosis*, Philadelphia, 2007, W.B. Saunders Co., pp 611–634.

Whitlock R, Crowther MA, Ng HJ: Bleeding in cardiac surgery: its prevention and treatment—an evidence-based review, *Crit Care Clin* 21:589–610, 2005.

MINIMALLY INVASIVE SURGERY

LAPAROSCOPIC CHOLECYSTECTOMY

L. Michael Brunt, MD

INTRODUCTION

Cholecystectomy is one of the most common operations performed by general surgeons; as many as 900,000 of these procedures are performed in the United States annually. Gallstones are also the most costly disorder of the gastrointestinal tract: approximately $5 billion annually. When laparoscopic cholecystectomy was first introduced into general surgery practice in the early 1990s, the advantages were obvious to patients and treating physicians alike, and it very quickly became the new "gold standard" for removal of the gallbladder. Today, few patients are not considered candidates for laparoscopic cholecystectomy, and alternative approaches such as single-incision techniques and natural orifice transluminal endoscopic surgery (NOTES) approaches have been developed and are under evaluation. Despite the maturation of this procedure in surgical practice and training, injuries to the common bile duct (CBD) continue to occur at a higher rate than in the open cholecystectomy era and remain the major disadvantage of this very common procedure. This chapter reviews the indications for and basic technique of laparoscopic cholecystectomy and intraoperative cholangiography, with a special emphasis on difficult cases and avoidance of biliary injury.

INDICATIONS FOR CHOLECYSTECTOMY

The indications for cholecystectomy are listed in Box 1. Large database analyses in the United States indicate that approximately 90% of all cholecystectomies are performed laparoscopically. The ability to remove the gallbladder laparoscopically with a high degree of success has probably resulted in a lowering of the decision threshold for operation. Despite this, of patients who are truly symptom free, 10% to 25% experience progression to symptoms, and prophylactic cholecystectomy is therefore not generally warranted unless the gallstone is large or there are associated medical conditions or related circumstances, such as candidacy for organ transplantation, the presence of hemolytic processes (sickle cell anemia, hemolytic anemias), and frequent travel to remote parts of the world. In a patient with asymptomatic gallstones, the presence of diabetes mellitus does not increase risk and is not an indication for cholecystectomy.

Biliary colic is the most common indication for cholecystectomy. The typical presentation is one of discrete episodes of epigastric/right upper quadrant abdominal pain that can last from several minutes to several hours. The pain may radiate around to the side, to the subscapular region, or to the substernal and lower chest area; in some patients, the pain prompts an initial cardiac evaluation to rule out a myocardial infarction. Episodes tend to be more frequent in the evening or nighttime because that is when most patients eat their largest meal of the day, and it is not unusual to be awakened at night with an attack. Because gallstones are so common in the population, patients with nonspecific symptoms of predominantly nausea, weight loss, or continuous abdominal pain should be considered for additional diagnostic evaluation with upper gastrointestinal endoscopy or other cross-sectional imaging such as computed tomographic (CT) scan, or both, before proceeding with cholecystectomy.

IMAGING DIAGNOSIS

Ultrasonography is the preferred imaging test for the evaluation of suspected cholelithiasis and is highly sensitive and specific (>95%) for the diagnosis (Figure 1). CT is less sensitive for detecting gallstones and should be reserved primarily for patients with acute abdominal pain in whom gallstones are less likely to be the cause and for patients with severe acute cholecystitis. Biliary scintigraphy is used primarily in patients without demonstrable stones in whom biliary colic is suspected, in order to evaluate gallbladder emptying, as discussed subsequently. In acute cholecystitis, the gallbladder is typically not visualized on scintigraphy; however, this modality is not often needed to establish the diagnosis if one or more gallstones are seen sonographically and the clinical presentation is appropriate. Endoscopic retrograde cholangiopancreatography (ERCP) should be reserved for patients with ongoing biliary obstruction, those in whom a CBD stone is visualized on ultrasonography, or postoperatively to remove CBD stones seen on cholangiography.

COMPLICATED GALLSTONE DISEASE

Complications of gallstones occur in a significant percentage of patients. The most common manifestation of complicated gallstone disease is acute cholecystitis, which accounts for approximately 20% of cases. The typical manifestation is of right upper quadrant pain with localized peritoneal signs, including tenderness with guarding, a positive Murphy's sign, and, in some cases, a palpable gallbladder. Many affected patients also have inflammatory signs of fever and an elevated white blood cell count, although neither is essential for the diagnosis. Ultrasonography may show a stone impacted in the neck of the gallbladder along with a thickened gallbladder wall, pericholecystic fluid and a distended gallbladder (Figure 2). Initial management of the patient with acute cholecystitis consists of nothing by

BOX 1: Indications for cholecystectomy

Symptomatic cholelithiasis (biliary colic)
Complicated gallstone disease
   Acute cholecystitis
   Gallstone pancreatitis
   Common bile duct stones
Asymptomatic cholelithiasis (large gallstone,
   immunosuppression, hemolytic anemias, impending remote
   travel)
Biliary dyskinesia (with typical biliary colic symptoms and low
   gallbladder ejection fraction)
Gallbladder polyps (>10 mm, enlarging, or symptomatic)

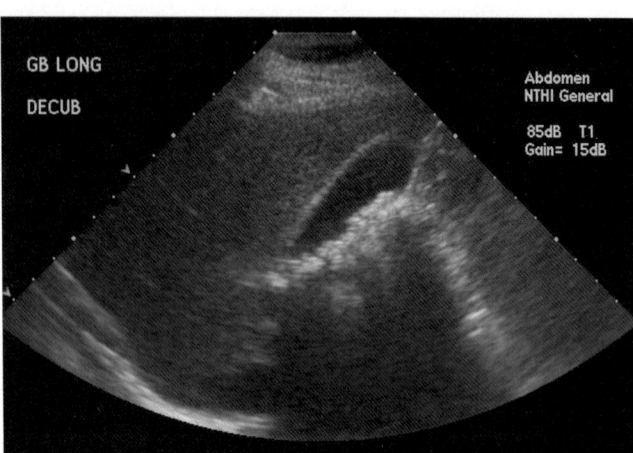

FIGURE 1 Ultrasound image of the gallbladder that shows multiple gallstones with posterior acoustic shadowing.

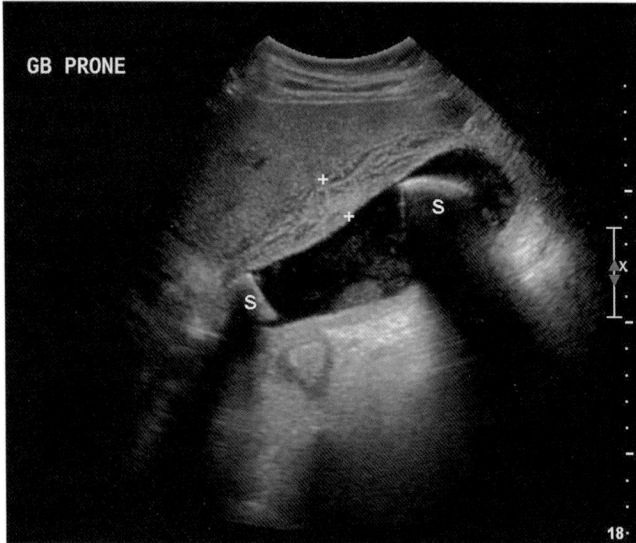

FIGURE 2 Gallbladder ultrasound image in a patient with acute cholecystitis that shows two large stones (S); the stone on the left is impacted in the neck of the gallbladder. The cursors demarcate the gallbladder wall, which is thickened.

mouth and intravenous antibiotics. The timing of surgery and other aspects of management of acute cholecystitis are discussed in further detail later.

About 10% of patients who have undergone cholecystectomy have or have had a CBD stone. In terms of pain, the presentation is much like that of an acute attack of biliary colic, although the presentation can be atypical, especially in elderly patients. In an acute presentation, there is often an associated elevation in liver enzymes, most notably the transaminases, whose levels become elevated before those of bilirubin and alkaline phosphatase. In any patient who presents with acute epigastric/right upper quadrant pain and laboratory values that show a threefold or higher elevation in the transaminase levels, a CBD stone should be suspected until proven otherwise. Initial ultrasound examination at that time may not show a dilated CBD or a stone in the duct. Most small stones pass spontaneously, but if the obstruction persists, the bilirubin and alkaline phosphatase levels increase, and biliary dilation becomes evident on ultrasonography. The majority of patients in whom a stone in the CBD is visible on ultrasonography are currently managed by preoperative ERCP and stone extraction. Patients with stones found at operation can be managed either by transcystic CBD exploration or by postoperative ERCP. Small stones can sometimes be flushed from the duct by administration of glucagon (1 mg intravenously), followed by saline irrigation of the duct.

An obstructing CBD stone can manifest as ascending cholangitis with fever, right upper quadrant pain, and jaundice (Charcot's triad). Affected patients should be treated conservatively, initially with intravenous antibiotics; ERCP with sphincterotomy and stone extraction should be carried out if clinical improvement is not rapid or if there is evidence of impending sepsis with hypotension and mental status changes.

Patients with gallstone pancreatitis often have midepigastric pain that penetrates to the back. In addition to elevated amylase and lipase levels, the transaminase enzyme levels are often elevated early in the presentation as a result of a distal obstructing CBD stone. In 10% to 25% of cases, the gallstone pancreatitis is severe, which may result in pancreatic necrosis, pseudocyst, or abscess. Most patients with mild gallstone pancreatitis can be managed with cholecystectomy during the index admission once their condition is stabilized and the symptoms and enzyme levels are improving. In one retrospective study, early laparoscopic cholecystectomy within 48 hours of admission was associated with a shorter length of hospital stay and lower rate of ERCP.

BILIARY DYSKINESIA/CHRONIC ACALCULOUS CHOLECYSTITIS

Up to 30% of cholecystectomies in recent years have been performed for biliary dyskinesia or chronic acalculous cholecystitis. For patients with typical symptoms and a reduced gallbladder ejection fraction, symptomatic outcome has been better after cholecystectomy than after medical treatment. However, in one retrospective review with a minimum follow-up of 6 months, 30% of patients had persistent symptoms after cholecystectomy. When pain symptoms are reproduced with administration of cholecystokinin, cholecystectomy has also been associated with symptomatic relief. Patients who have nontypical symptoms or a minimal decrease in gallbladder ejection fraction in comparison with normal should be managed cautiously and undergo a thorough gastrointestinal evaluation and treatment for other disorders such as irritable bowel syndrome before being subjected to surgery.

GALLBLADDER POLYPS

Most gallbladder polyps are benign cholesterol, inflammatory, or adenomatous hyperplastic polyps. Small (<10 mm) polyps should be monitored by periodic ultrasonography. In one series of 143 patients who had repeated ultrasonography follow-up, growth of the polyps was observed in only 9 (6% of cases). Indications for surgery include polyp growth during follow-up or large (>10 mm) polyps that are solitary. Because most gallbladder polyps are cholesterol in origin, the decision to perform cholecystectomy is often based on the presence or absence of typical symptoms.

The risk of gallbladder cancer in the setting of a porcelain gallbladder has been debated and appears to be less than 5%. If the patient's surgical risk is reasonable, it would be appropriate to proceed with laparoscopic cholecystectomy in this setting. Larger gallbladder masses that are suspect for gallbladder cancer should be approached using an open procedure.

LAPAROSCOPIC CHOLECYSTECTOMY TECHNIQUE

Initial Access

Initial laparoscopic access for laparoscopic cholecystectomy is most commonly achieved with an open Hasson cannula technique at the umbilicus. This approach also facilitates extraction of the gallbladder from the abdomen. If the patient has had previous abdominal surgery at the periumbilical midline, an alternative access site should be considered because of the potential for bowel to be adherent to the abdominal wall at that site. This procedure can be performed in either an open or closed manner. Preferably, access should be either closed (with the use of a Veress needle) in the right subcostal region, if that quadrant of the abdomen is expected to be free of adhesions, or open with an epigastric insertion site. The other ports are then placed under direct laparoscopic vision. Even in patients with multiple prior abdominal operations, a laparoscopic approach is usually possible if initial access can be gained and one ancillary port can be placed to start the adhesiolysis.

Basic Technique

Laparoscopic cholecystectomy is usually performed via four working ports. Only one of these need be 10 mm in diameter (for the clip applier and gallbladder extraction); the others can be 5 mm or smaller. The author's preference is to use a "mini" approach in uncomplicated cases with a 10-mm Hasson port at the umbilicus, a 5-mm epigastric port, and two 3-mm right subcostal ports, as shown in Figure 3. Adhesions to the gallbladder are first removed either by blunt stripping or with judicious application of monopolar electrosurgery (with a Bovie device). The fundus of the gallbladder should then be retracted cephalad and the infundibulum retracted laterally to expose the hepatocystic triangle. Cephalad retraction on the neck of the gallbladder should be avoided because it may tent the CBD and make it more vulnerable to injury. In cases in which the gallbladder is distended or tense with bile, contents should be aspirated before it is grasped (Figure 4) in order to avoid perforation of the wall and spillage of bile and stones, which also makes the subsequent visualization and dissection more difficult.

Critical View of Safety Method of Ductal Identification

The critical view of safety (CVS) as originally described by Strasberg has become the standard method of ductal identification during laparoscopic cholecystectomy. The CVS has three criteria: (1) the hepatocystic triangle should be cleared of fat and fibrous tissue; (2) the gallbladder should be dissected off the liver bed to the cystic plate; and (3) there should be only two structures entering the gallbladder, as illustrated in Figure 5. The CVS does not entail dissection or exposure down to the CBD.

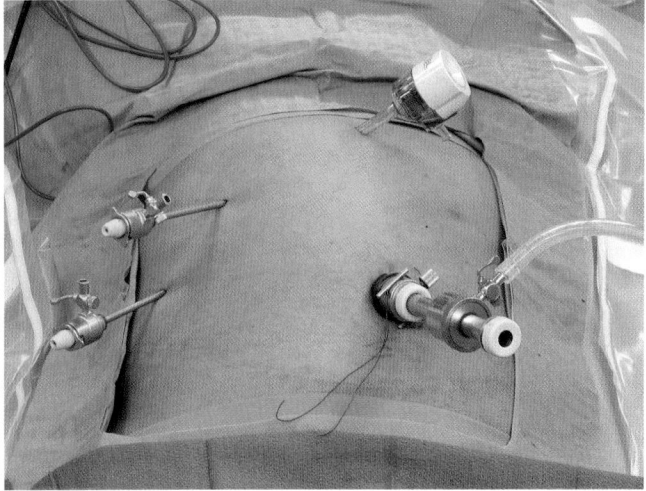

FIGURE 3 Port configuration for laparoscopic cholecystectomy. There is a 10-mm Hasson-type cannula at the umbilicus, a 5-mm epigastric port, and two 3-mm right subcostal ports.

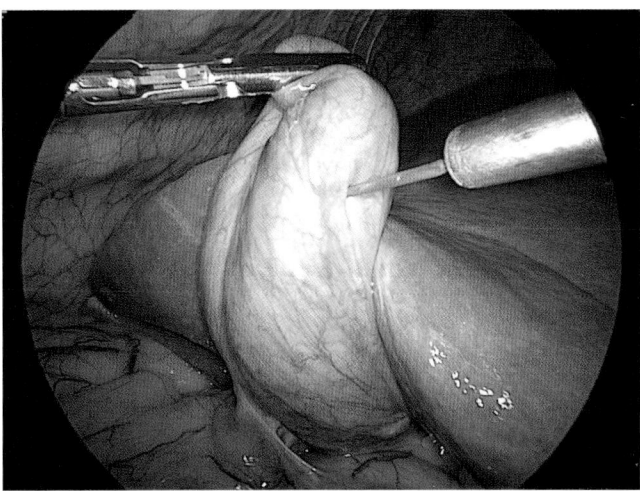

FIGURE 4 Technique of needle aspiration of a distended gallbladder. This approach is useful in the setting of a tense, distended gallbladder to avoid perforation from a grasper and spillage of bile and stones.

The rationale for the CVS is actually based on the ductal identification method that was and continues to be used for open cholecystectomy. The approach in open cholecystectomy entailed isolation of the cystic duct and cystic artery in the hepatocystic triangle. The gallbladder would then be dissected off the liver bed in its entirety, so that the only remaining attachments were the duct and artery entering the gallbladder. This approach is not feasible during laparoscopic cholecystectomy because of the greater difficulty in getting the entire gallbladder off the liver bed before the cystic structures are clipped.

The dissection to the CVS may be performed through a variety of techniques. In most cases, this involves a combination of (1) judicious use of electrosurgery with a hook device to elevate and divide the peritoneum over the gallbladder and the fat, fibrous tissue and small vessels and (2) blunt dissection with stripping of the fat and spreading between the duct and artery and between the artery and liver bed. The lowest possible electrosurgical power setting should be used (≤25-W setting), and the application should be in short bursts of no more than 2 to 3 seconds. Only small amounts of tissue should be divided at a time because of the risk of injuring an accessory biliary structure or blood vessel.

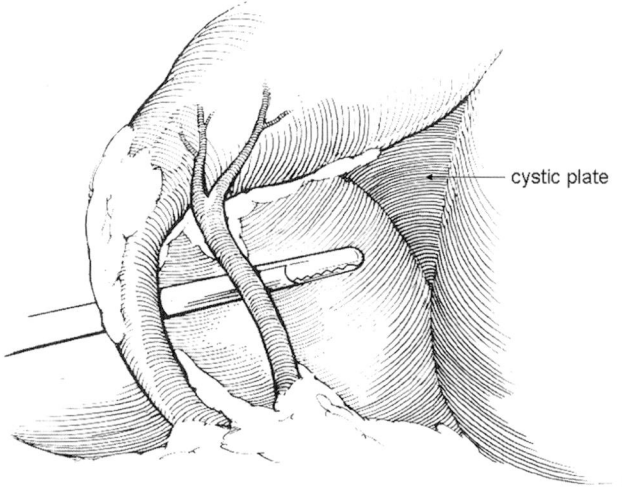

cystic plate

The critical view of safety

FIGURE 5   Schematic illustration of the critical view of safety. The hepatocystic triangle is clear of extraneous fat and fibrous tissue, only two structures are seen entering the gallbladder, and the gallbladder has been taken off the liver bed to the cystic plate. *(From Strasberg SM, Brunt LM: Rationale and use of the critical view of safety in laparoscopic cholecystectomy,* J Am Coll Surg *211:133, 2010, Figure 1.)*

Visual documentation of the CVS should be made both from the anterior and the dorsal or reverse Calot's view (Figure 6). The Dutch Society of Surgery has recommended routine photodocumentation of the CVS. Currently, no level I evidence exists to show a reduction in biliary injury with the CVS method. However, large retrospective reviews have shown lower-than-expected injury rates with this approach. It is still possible to injure a biliary structure in the attempt to dissect to the CVS, but once the CVS has been obtained, the risk of biliary injury should be essentially nil.

Intraoperative Cholangiography

Whether intraoperative cholangiography should be performed routinely or selectively has been widely debated in the surgical literature. The classic indications for performing cholangiography during cholecystectomy include a history of gallstone pancreatitis, abnormal liver function test results, and a dilated CBD seen either on preoperative ultrasonography or at operation. In addition, if a stone is found in the cystic duct at operation, then the patient should also undergo cholangiography because of the higher association with a CBD stone. Surgeons should also consider use of cholangiography routinely in the setting of the more difficult cholecystectomy, as with acute cholecystitis.

Cholangiography is performed typically after the CVS is obtained. A clip is placed on the neck of the gallbladder, and a small incision is made in the cystic duct. It may be necessary to open the valves within the cystic duct by spreading with fine scissors. A variety of cholangiographic catheters are available, including balloon-tipped catheters. The author's preference is to use a 4.0F ureteral catheter and a cholangiographic clamp device (Figure 7). Cholangiography is then performed under fluoroscopic imaging. With experience, this step in the operation can be performed routinely in 5 minutes.

Four arguments have been posited in favor of the use of routine over selective cholangiography: (1) routine use of cholangiography is essential for developing the expertise to perform it consistently and for proper interpretation of the findings on imaging; (2) cholangiography is a prerequisite for laparoscopic transcystic CBD exploration; (3) at the population level, routine use of intraoperative

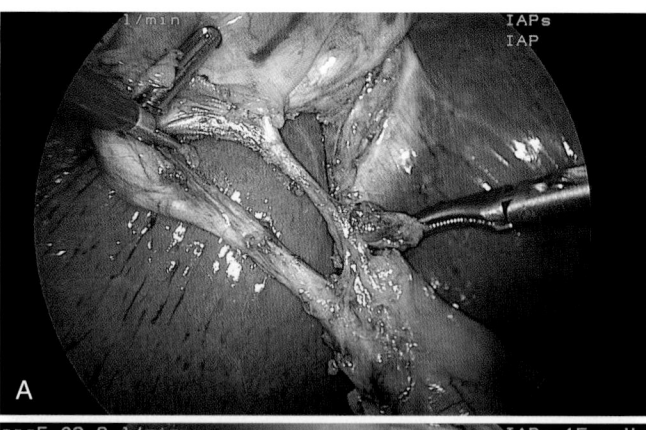

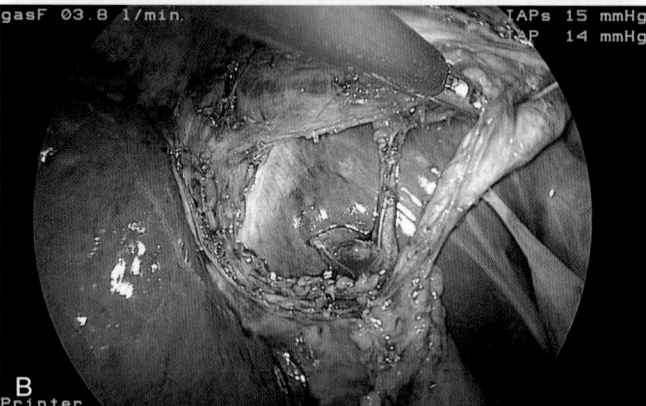

FIGURE 6   Operative photographs of the critical view of safety during laparoscopic cholecystectomy. **A,** Anterior view. **B,** Dorsolateral, or reverse Calot's, triangle view.

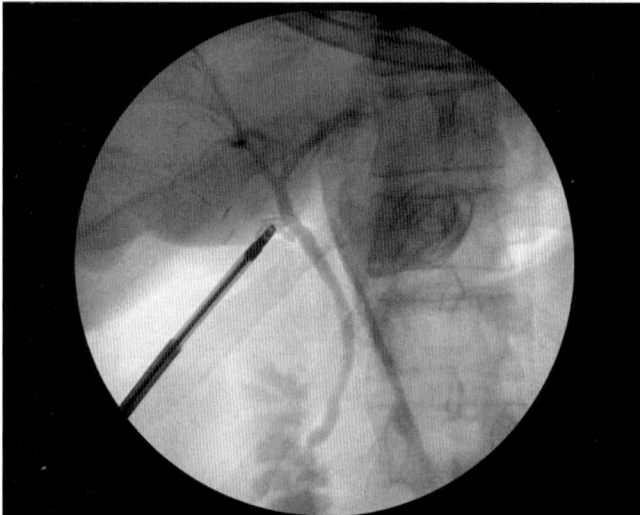

FIGURE 7   Intraoperative cholangiogram obtained during laparoscopic cholecystectomy. Intraoperative view of cholangiographic catheter being inserted within a locking cholangiographic clamp type of grasper.

cholangiography has been associated with a reduction in biliary injury by approximately 30% in studies across multiple continents; and (4) when findings are interpreted correctly, cholangiography should prevent higher level CBD injuries and also increase the chance of injury detection and timely repair. However, a limitation is that it may not always identify aberrant ducts.

THE DIFFICULT CHOLECYSTECTOMY

A number of risk factors have been identified to predict the difficulty of cholecystectomy and therefore the necessity for conversion to an open operation (listed in Box 2). Of these, acute cholecystitis is the most common condition associated with difficulty and conversion and is further discussed later. In addition, conversion rates are higher early in a surgeon's experience (first 50 cases). In a setting of elective laparoscopic cholecystectomy, conversion rates are typically low, less than 3% to 5%. The major risk factor in elective cholecystectomy is thickening of the gallbladder wall, especially in combination with thickening and contraction of the gallbladder, as in patients with repeated episodes of chronic cholecystitis. Patients should be counseled preoperatively about the risk of needing conversion to open cholecystectomy, and conversion should be viewed not as a complication but rather as good surgical judgment. In a patient who has undergone multiple prior abdominal procedures, the risk of needing enterotomy should also be discussed.

Obesity is the most common factor that can increase the difficulty of cholecystectomy. Because the umbilicus is displaced inferiorly, supraumbilical port site for the camera should be considered, in some cases several centimeters proximal to the umbilicus. Longer trocars may be necessary in some patients, and it may be necessary to add a fifth port to provide caudal retraction on the omentum and duodenum, particularly in obese men. The liver is often extensively infiltrated with fat in obese patients and can be difficult to elevate, thereby making the exposure more difficult. In addition, the gallbladder may be intrahepatic and have little if any associated mesentery for dissection from the liver bed.

Multiple Prior Abdominal Operations

In a patient who has undergone previous abdominal surgery at the periumbilical midline, an alternative access site should be considered. Any attempted access site in such a patient should be inspected for injury, especially if adhesions were encountered during access. Likewise, once the initial port has been placed, each subsequent port must be placed under direct laparoscopic vision. Surgeons should be extremely careful in retracting adherent bowel and should limit or avoid the use of electrosurgery or other energy devices for adhesiolysis.

Acute Cholecystitis

Acute cholecystitis is the most common presentation of complicated gallstone disease and accounts for up to 20% of cholecystectomies. Approximately 120,000 gallbladders are removed in the United States annually for acute cholecystitis. About 60% of these cases are in women, but the presentation tends to be more severe in men. Most affected patients have had prior episodes of biliary colic, and the incidence of this presentation may be falling somewhat as a result of earlier laparoscopic cholecystectomy and surgical intervention.

BOX 2: Patient risk factors for the need for conversion from laparoscopic to open cholecystectomy

Acute cholecystitis
History of acute cholecystitis
Multiple (>10) prior episodes of biliary colic
Morbid obesity
Male sex
Older age (>65 years)
Previous upper abdominal surgery
Portal hypertension or cirrhosis

The timing of early surgery versus conservative treatment has been addressed in a number of small, prospective randomized trials. Meta-analyses of these trials have shown that early cholecystectomy is associated with a shorter overall hospitalization. Approximately 20% of patients who undergo initial conservative treatment develop persistent or recurrent symptoms before surgical intervention. No differences in conversion rates, morbidity (including bile leaks), or mortality have been shown between early versus late surgery.

The current status of surgical treatment in the United States was reviewed with the use of a national hospital discharge sample of 1 million cholecystectomies for acute cholecystitis. In this study, 9.5% of the laparoscopic cholecystectomies were converted to open procedures, and open cholecystectomy was associated with a 1.3-fold increase in perioperative morbidity. In another multicenter trial from Belgium of 1089 patients, 93% of operations were performed laparoscopically and 6.8% open. The conversion rate from laparoscopic to open cholecystectomy was 11.4% and was twice as high in male patients (14.9%) as in female patients (7.5%). Complications occurred in 5.5% of patients, and the incidence of biliary injury was 1.2%, which is substantially higher than the 0.4% typically associated with elective operation. Of particular concern was the rate of biliary injury in the 116 patients whose procedure was started laparoscopically and then converted to open: The rate of CBD injury was 6.0%, the rate of biliary fistula was 7.7%, and the total incidence of biliary complications was 13.7%. Therefore, this study highlights both the risks and difficulty when a challenging laparoscopic cholecystectomy becomes a difficult open cholecystectomy, especially in view of the infrequent experience of today's trainees with the open approach.

Patients with acute cholecystitis who are at greatest risk for conversion or in whom the operation is predictably more difficult are those with a white blood cell count greater than $18,000/\mu L$, if the time from onset of symptoms is more than 72 hours, if the gallbladder is palpable, and if the patient is older and sicker. Other ultrasound features that may also predict difficulty are gangrenous changes with sloughing of the mucosa, emphysematous cholecystitis, and a gallbladder abscess or perforated gallbladder. Conservative measures, including percutaneous cholecystostomy and operation electively at 2 to 3 months, should be considered in this setting.

Percutaneous Cholecystostomy

Percutaneous cholecystostomy is associated with resolution of acute symptoms and inflammatory signs in more than 90% of cases. The tube must usually be left in until the cholecystectomy and, therefore, this is best reserved for patients at higher risk, especially elderly and critically ill patients. Laparoscopic cholecystectomy after percutaneous cholecystostomy is still a more difficult procedure, with conversion rates typically in the range of 10% to 15%. In one retrospective review in which percutaneous drains were compared with cholecystectomy from 2001 to 2010, patients who underwent percutaneous drainage were older, had higher white blood cell counts, and had more prolonged stays in the intensive care unit. They also experienced more complications per patient and had higher readmission rates (31.4% vs 13.3%). The authors concluded that percutaneous cholecystostomy should be reserved for patients who have a prohibitive surgical risk.

If during cholecystectomy a surgeon encounters severe inflammation in the area of the neck of the gallbladder and porta hepatis, the best strategy is to avoid entering that area because of the increased risk of an injury. Options include placing a cholecystostomy tube surgically or performing a partial or subtotal cholecystectomy. Lee and colleagues (2012) reviewed 10,872 gallbladder-damaged control cases from the National Inpatient Sample cohort from 2000 to 2008. About 50% of these patients had open partial cholecystectomies, 27% had laparoscopic partial cholecystectomies, and 25% had trocar cholecystostomies. Despite this approach, the CBD injury rate was 3.7%, and the overall total mortality rate was 7.4%. These observations emphasize the increased risk in this patient population and the extreme care required to avoid injury in this setting.

Portal Hypertension and Cirrhosis

The combination of portal hypertension and cirrhosis can be challenging, and affected patients are at much higher risk for the need for cholecystectomy. Consideration should be given to preoperative CT with portal phase contrast sequences to determine whether varices are present and where they are located. These may occur at the umbilicus through a recanalized umbilical vein, in the portal hepatis, and along the gallbladder bed. Surgeons should be especially careful with initial access in these patients because of the risk of injuring a large collateral vein at the umbilicus. Hepatic function should be optimized, and any coagulation deficits or ascites corrected. If there are collateral vessels around the gallbladder and liver bed, a subtotal or partial cholecystectomy should be considered. The use of advanced energy devices such as advanced bipolar or ultrasonic coagulation should also be considered in this setting.

ALTERNATIVE APPROACHES: SINGLE-INCISION LAPAROSCOPIC AND NOTES CHOLECYSTECTOMY

Single-incision laparoscopic cholecystectomy (SILC) and NOTES cholecystectomy have been promoted as potentially less invasive alternatives to conventional four-port laparoscopic cholecystectomy. NOTES cholecystectomy today is preferentially performed via a transvaginal access route. Although the NOTES technique is technically feasible, operative times are longer, and the advantages other than less visible scarring are unproven. Because NOTES cholecystectomy is technically challenging and the advantages are unproven, its performance in the United States has been limited primarily to centers participating in investigative trials.

The advantages of SILC are that it can be performed with conventional laparoscopic instrumentation and dissection techniques and a nearly scarless outcome can be achieved. However, disadvantages are the loss of triangulation, an in-line view of the operative field, and restricted freedom of movement of the instruments. The potential for more umbilical wound complications, including hernias, has also been voiced in view of the larger fascial incision at the umbilicus. A number of small, prospective randomized trials have been carried out to compare SILC with standard four-port laparoscopic cholecystectomy. Although the results of these trials have varied somewhat, most indicate that the single incision approach is associated with longer operative times and more postoperative pain but improved cosmesis. A robotic platform has been developed to facilitate single-incision approaches, but trials in which this is compared with conventional laparoscopic approaches are lacking. None of the SILC trials have been adequately powered to study the rate of CBD injury. However, one literature review of 45 published studies of more than 2600 patients showed a CBD injury rate with SILC of 0.72%, in comparison with 0.4% to 0.5% with multiple-port laparoscopic cholecystectomy. These data are of concern and, at a minimum, merit further trials to address this issue.

COMPLICATIONS

CBD injury continues to be the most feared complication of laparoscopic cholecystectomy, with reported injury rates of approximately 0.4% to 0.5%. Leaks from cystic duct stumps can also be a major source of morbidity after laparoscopic cholecystectomy. In one series, after more than 5751 laparoscopic cholecystectomies, 12 patients with such leaks were reported (incidence, 0.2%). These patients presented at a mean of 2.3 days postoperatively, and abdominal pain was the most common complaint. Most of these leaks can be managed with ERCP and stent placement, although some may also necessitate percutaneous drainage if fluid collection is significant. However, deaths have been reported after leaks from cystic duct stumps, and prevention is therefore the best strategy. Risk factors for leaks from cystic duct stumps include thickening of the cystic duct (which often occurs in acute cholecystitis), distal obstruction from a CBD stone, and a history of transcystic exploration. In the surgical setting, a pretied loop suture (ENDOLOOP; Ethicon Inc., Somerville, NJ) should be used to secure the cystic duct. Bile leaks after laparoscopic cholecystectomy may also arise from superficial ducts in the bed of the liver if the plane of the dissection has gone too deep. True leaks from the ducts of Luschka are rare, and most leaks from the liver bed are related to improper dissection plane.

Intestinal injury and enterotomy may occur during initial laparoscopic access, may result from adhesiolysis in patients with prior surgery, or may arise from the duodenum because of its closeness to the gallbladder. Trocars are the most common device named in medical malpractice injury claims associated with laparoscopic procedures, and cholecystectomy is the procedure most frequently associated with both fatal and nonfatal trocar injuries. Surgeons must also be wary of creating an injury out of the field of view by blind instrument insertion or as a result of untimely activation of the electrosurgical device (which is often controlled by a foot pedal on the floor) by the surgeon or another team member. The duodenum often adheres to or is close to the gallbladder. When working near the duodenum, surgical energy devices should be avoided. Surgeons must be cognizant of the adhesion with a narrow attachment to the duodenum because of the risk of concentrating the energy source at that site.

Any untoward or unexpected deviation from the usual postoperative course in a patient who has undergone laparoscopic cholecystectomy should be investigated immediately. Patients with severe or generalized abdominal pain or pain with nausea, vomiting, and fever should undergo prompt evaluation with laboratory testing and imaging to rule out a biliary injury or a missed enterotomy.

SUMMARY

Laparoscopic cholecystectomy has been the most significant advance in the management of symptomatic gallstones in several decades. This approach is associated with a high degree of success, low complication rates, and a rapid return to full physical health and activity. Every laparoscopic cholecystectomy should involve the CVS ductal identification method to minimize the risk of biliary injury and should be accompanied by the liberal use of intraoperative cholangiography. Strategies for managing the difficult cholecystectomy as outlined in this chapter may help reduce the rate of biliary injury and other complications.

Suggested Readings

Abi-Haidar Y, Sanchez V, Williams SA, et al: Revisiting percutaneous cholecystectomy for acute cholecystitis based on a 10 year experience, *Arch Surg* 147:416–422, 2012.

Csikesz N, Ricciardi R, Tseng J, et al: Current status of management of acute cholecystitis in the United States, *World J Surg* 32:2230–2236, 2008.

Duncan CB, Riall TS: Evidence-based current surgical practice: calculous gallbladder disease, *J Gastrointest Surg* 16:2011–2025, 2012.

Eisenstein S, Greenstein A, Kim U, et al: Cystic duct stump leaks: after the learning curve, *Arch Surg* 12:1178–1183, 2008.

Ingraham AM, Cohen ME, Ko CY, et al: A current profile and assessment of North American cholecystectomy: results from the American College of Surgeons National Surgical Quality Improvement Program, *J Am Coll Surg* 211:176–186, 2010.

Joseph M, Phillips MR, Farrell TM, et al: Single incision laparoscopic cholecystectomy is associated with a higher bile duct injury rate, *Ann Surg* 256(1):1–9, 2012.

Lee J, Miller P, Kermani R, et al: Gallbladder damage control: compromised procedure for compromised patients, *Surg Endosc* 26:2779–2783, 2012.

Massarweh NN, Flum DR: Role of intraoperative cholangiography in avoiding bile duct injury, *J Am Coll Surg* 204:656–664, 2007.

Navez B, Ungureanu F, Michiels M, et al: Surgical management of acute cholecystitis: results of a 2 year prospective multi-center survey in Belgium, *Surg Endosc* 26:2436–2445, 2012.

Singhal V, Szeto P, Norman H, et al: Biliary dyskinesia: how effective is cholecystectomy? *J Gastrointest Surg* 16:135–141, 2012.

Strasberg SM: Acute calculous cholecystitis, *N Engl J Med* 358:2804–2811, 2008.

Strasberg SM, Brunt LM: Rationale and use of the critical view of safety in laparoscopic cholecystectomy, *J Am Coll Surg* 211:132–137, 2010.

LAPAROSCOPIC COMMON BILE DUCT EXPLORATION

Yee Wong, MD, and Bipan Chand, MD, FACS, FASMBS, FASGE

INTRODUCTION

Every year, approximately 750,000 cholecystectomies are performed in the United States. Of these, approximately 10% to 15% are performed in patients who present with choledocholithiasis. The true incidence may be higher given that not all procedures involve ductal imaging. The probability of finding a common bile duct (CBD) stone may even increase to above 70% in patients who are elderly, those with an elevated bilirubin level, and those in whom a CBD appears dilated on abdominal ultrasonography. Patients who present with symptomatic cholelithiasis may not have signs or symptoms of CBD stones, and stones may be discovered only with preoperative imaging or intraoperatively. Preoperative diagnostic modalities used for detecting CBD stones include transabdominal ultrasonography, computed tomography, and magnetic resonance cholangiopancreatography (MRCP).

Transabdominal ultrasonography is most commonly used, and its sensitivity ranges from 55% to 91%. Dilation of the CBD to more than 6 mm is associated with an increased incidence of CBD stones. Advantages of transabdominal ultrasonography include its low cost, its noninvasive nature, and its availability at most centers; however, results are highly operator dependent. Abdominal computed tomography has sensitivity up to 95.5% for detecting CBD stones. However, it exposes the patient to radiation and also to the risk of contrast agent–induced nephropathy. It is not currently a standard diagnostic modality in the evaluation of acute cholecystitis and biliary calculi in the United States. In cases in which the findings on ultrasonography and computed tomography are inconclusive, MRCP may be used to detect CBD stones. Its accuracy is comparable with that of intraoperative cholangiography (IOC) and endoscopic retrograde cholangiopancreatography (ERCP), with sensitivity of 81% to 100% and specificity of 92% to 100%. MRCP is more expensive and may not be available at some centers.

Endoscopic modalities for use in biliary imaging include endoscopic ultrasonography and ERCP. Endoscopic ultrasonography has sensitivity of 88% to 97% and specificity of 96% to 100% in detecting CBD stones. It is less often used than MRCP because it is more invasive; however, it has similar accuracy. When choledocholithiasis is diagnosed preoperatively, most clinicians proceed with ERCP for stone extraction and then perform laparoscopic cholecystectomy. ERCP has the advantage of not only detecting CBD stones but also providing therapy with stone extraction or biliary drainage when patients present with jaundice or cholangitis secondary to ductal obstruction. With the advent of laparoscopic techniques and devices, laparoscopic CBD exploration is becoming utilized more frequently (Figure 1).

INTRAOPERATIVE EVALUATION OF COMMON BILE DUCT STONES

IOC remains the "gold standard" in detection of choledocholithiasis and can also assist in the identification of complex biliary ductal anatomy. Controversy remains about whether IOC should be performed routinely or selectively. In a systematic review from the United Kingdom, researchers compiled data from eight randomized controlled trials. This analysis failed to show a benefit of IOC in preventing retained CBD stones or bile duct injury. Nevertheless, IOC is necessary before CBD exploration. For selective IOC, indications include evidence of CBD dilatation to more than 7 mm on preoperative imaging, elevated results of cholestatic liver function tests, a history of gallstone pancreatitis, and jaundice. Surgeons who choose to perform IOC should be familiar with identifying different ductal anatomy and filling defects that may suggest presence of CBD stones or air bubbles within the biliary system (Figure 2).

Another option in the evaluation of CBD stones is laparoscopic ultrasonography (LUS), developed in 1990s after the introduction of laparoscopic cholecystectomy (see Figure 2). In this method, a 10-mm ultrasound probe is inserted through the subxyphoid port. After dissection of adhesions but before ductal dissection, bile ducts are scanned from the hepatic hilum to duodenum. Intrahepatic biliary ducts can also be evaluated by placement of the probe on the anterior surface of the liver. A review of 12 prospective studies in which LUS and IOC were compared showed that LUS is as accurate as IOC in diagnosing biliary calculi, with success rates ranging from 88% to 100% and a low false-positive rate. It requires less time (average, 4 to 10 minutes) to perform in comparison with IOC (10 to 17 minutes). Some advantages of LUS include its low cost, avoidance of radiation and exposure to contrast agents, and the potential for unlimited use. It also allows for imaging of surrounding structures and organs, such as the pancreas, hepatic artery, and portal vein. However, results are highly dependent on the surgeon's interpretation of images and experience in scanning techniques. Availability of LUS probes is also limited, and, unlike IOC, LUS cannot readily evaluate the flow of contrast material into the duodenum. As surgeons become better trained in laparoscopic techniques and resources become more readily available, LUS will be more commonly utilized as an intraoperative diagnostic tool for CBD stones.

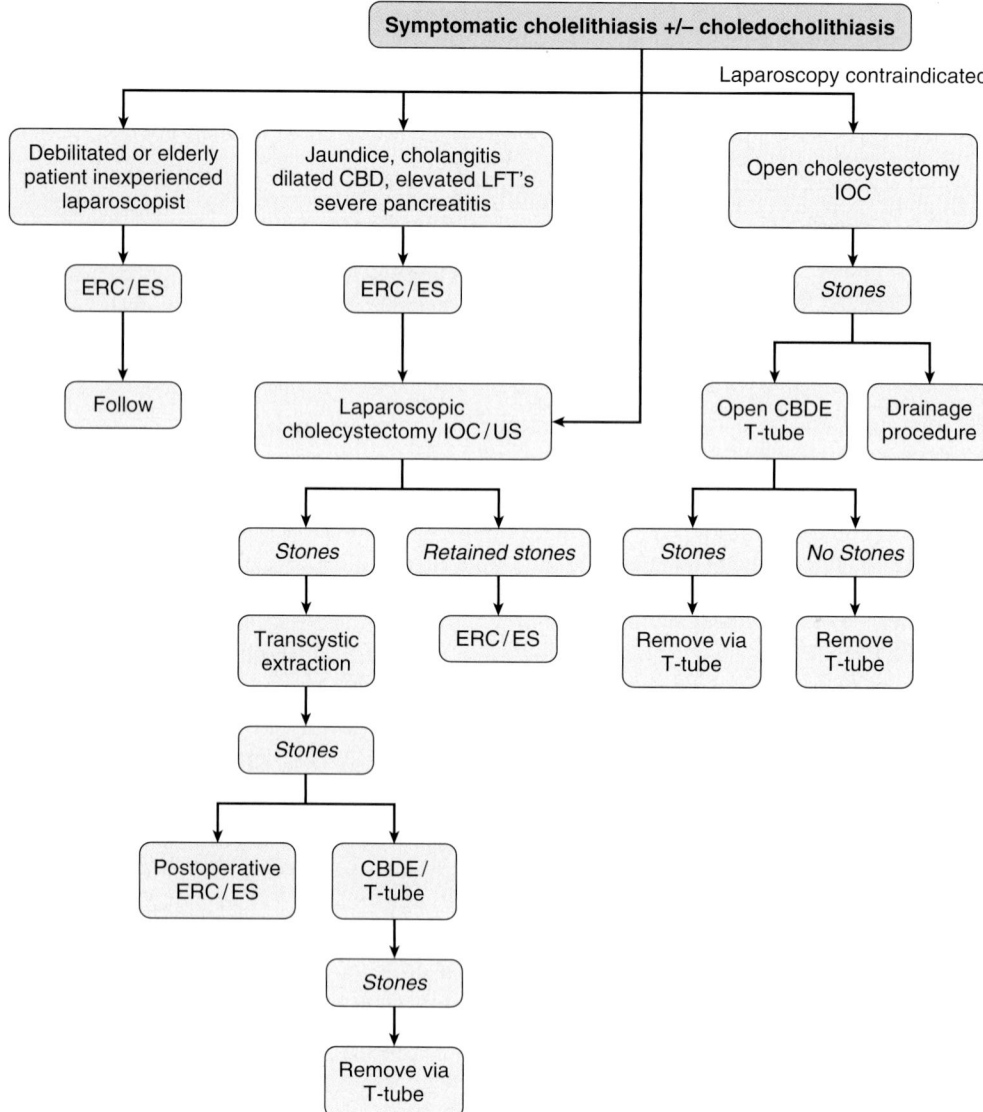

FIGURE 1   Flowchart detailing the management of symptomatic cholelithiasis with or without choledocholithiasis. *CBD,* Common bile duct; *CBDE,* common bile duct exploration; *ERC,* endoscopic retrograde cholangiopancreatography; *ES,* endoscopy; *IOC,* intraoperative cholangiography; *LFT,* liver function test (result); *US,* ultrasonography. *(From Hungness ES, Soper NJ: Management of common bile duct stones, J Gastrointest Surg 10(4):612–619, 2006.)*

TECHNIQUES

When CBD stones are identified during laparoscopic cholecystectomy, there are multiple different management options: open CBD exploration, laparoscopic CBD exploration, intraoperative ERCP, and postoperative ERCP. A decision to proceed with one option over another is usually based on the surgeon's experience with laparoscopic techniques, resource availability, and findings on IOC. Several factors that may influence the choice of management include the size, number, location, and characteristics of the stones. When stones are larger than 2 cm, the success rate of stone clearance with ERCP is decreased from 92% to 78%, with an increase in complications, including post-ERCP pancreatitis, papillae hemorrhage, biliary infection, and hypoxemia. ERCP has also been shown to be less effective in clearance than is laparoscopic CBD exploration for multiple or impacted stones, faceted stones, or ductal anatomy that renders cannulation difficult. Conversion from laparoscopic to open surgery is more likely to occur if stones are larger than 2 cm and if the clinician is less experienced in advanced laparoscopic skills. Location of stones can often present a challenge to the surgeon in the decision of management options. Intrahepatic stones are often difficult to clear by ERCP, and radiologic clearance or an open surgical approach may be

required. The preference of one laparoscopic technique over another may also be influenced by the size and number of stones, presence of biliary sludge, and diameter of CBD. Failure to clear the duct is higher in the transcystic approach when the CBD diameter is greater than 6 mm or the stone is larger than 5 mm. Rates of recurrence and inadequate clearance are also higher in this approach when more than three CBD stones and biliary sludge are present.

Two major techniques for laparoscopic CBD exploration have been employed: transcystic exploration and choledochotomy. In the transcystic approach, which is usually preferred by most surgeons, the common duct is accessed through the cystic duct close to its insertion (Figure 3). Stones can be irrigated out of the common duct with saline and the intravenous use of glucagon to relax the sphincter of Oddi. Glucagon facilitates the flow of stones into the duodenum. Dilation of the cystic duct may be necessary to allow passage of baskets or balloon catheters as well. Typically, a guidewire is advanced through the cystic duct into the CBD, and dilators are inserted over the wire. Serial dilations can be performed with balloon catheters or graduated bougies. Care should be taken to avoid dilating the cystic duct more than the diameter of the CBD. Helical stone baskets or balloon-tipped catheters can then be used to extract stones under fluoroscopic guidance. If the cystic duct is of adequate caliber, some

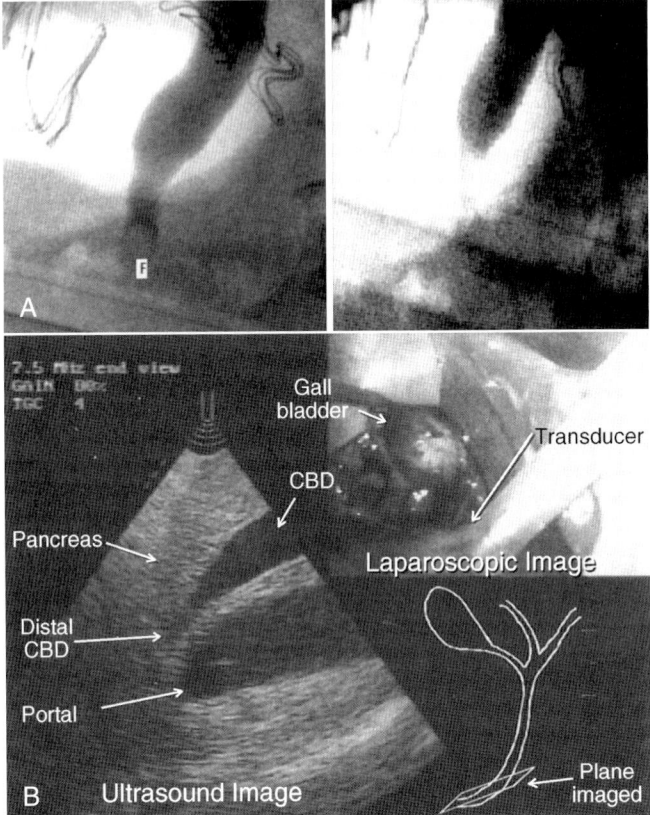

FIGURE 2   A, Intraoperative cholangiograms depicting dilated common bile duct with filling defect (*F*). **B,** Laparoscopic ultrasonography showing portal triad. *CBD,* Common bile duct. (**A** *From Luhmann A, Buter A, Abela JE: Haemobilia causing cholangitis in a patient on dual anti-platelet treatment suffering from acute acalculous cholecystitis,* Int J Surg Case Rep *4[4]:368–370, 2013.* **B** *From Berber E, Siperstein AE: Laparoscopic ultrasound,* Surg Clin North Am *84[4]:1061–1084, 2004.*)

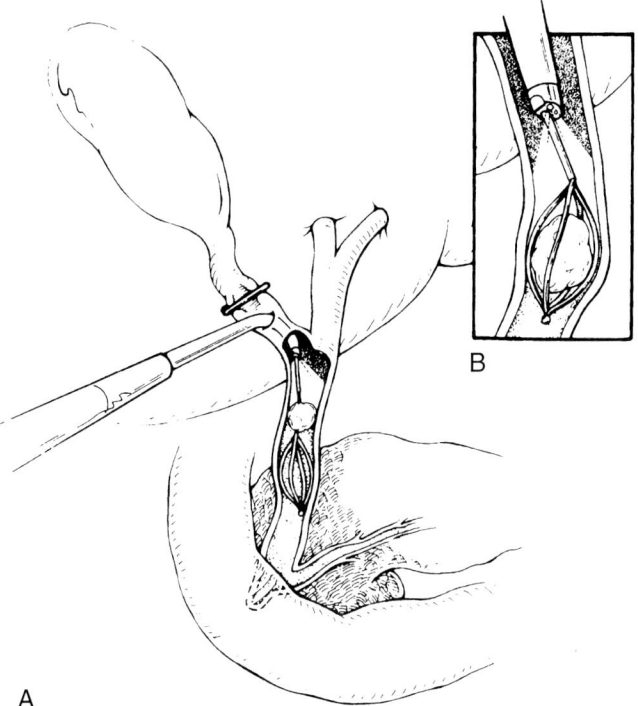

FIGURE 3   Laparoscopic common bile duct exploration. **A,** Transcystic approach. **B,** Stone extraction with wire basket. *(From Hungness ES, Soper NJ: Management of common bile duct stones,* J Gastrointest Surg *10[4]:612–619, 2006.)*

surgeons utilize a choledochoscope to increase the success rate of CBD exploration and verify clearance. Choledochoscopes are available in different sizes ranging from 3F to 10 F and have access channels to allow simultaneous use of baskets or balloon-tipped catheters. The choledochoscope can also be used to push stones into the duodenum and allows for visualization of common hepatic, right hepatic, and left hepatic ducts after stone removal. Using a choledochoscope often requires an additional 5-mm trocar and continuous irrigation of the ducts. However, in the extraction of CBD stones, its use increases the success rate from 77% to 97% in comparison with blind exploration. Completion cholangiography should be performed after transcystic exploration to ensure stone clearance.

The advantage of the transcystic approach is that it avoids choledochotomy, although when transcystic exploration is unsuccessful, choledochotomy may be necessary. However, it should be performed only when the CBD is dilated greater than 7 mm. Other factors that may influence a surgeon to proceed directly with choledochotomy include size of stones, presence of multiple stones, stones in the proximal duct, and faceted stones. This technique begins with a longitudinal incision along the anterior surface of the CBD to avoid the blood supply. The blood supply is often at the 3 and 9 o'clock positions on the CBD. Incision should be at least as long as the diameter of the largest stone. Stay sutures on either side of the incision may be used, as in open exploration. The duct should be irrigated initially to remove smaller stones. Larger stones can be extracted proximally through the choledochotomy with laparoscopic nontraumatic graspers. Biliary balloon-tipped catheters can also be used to sweep stones

out of the bile duct. As in the transcystic approach, choledochoscopes may be used for impacted stones to pass helical stone baskets and balloon catheters through the working channel (Figure 4). Again, completion cholangiography is necessary to evaluate for residual stones.

Once the stones are extracted through the choledochotomy, the CBD can be closed primarily or over a T-tube. Primary closure requires expertise in intracorporeal suturing. Absorbable sutures should be used to prevent ductal stenosis from a foreign body response. Studies demonstrate that primary closure by experienced surgeons is just as safe as closure with a T-tube. However, some authorities argue that the advantage of a T-tube is that it allows for confirmation that no residual stones remain. If a T-tube is left in place, cholangiography is performed 3 to 4 weeks after the initial surgery and before tube removal to confirm clearance. A T-tube may also prevent complications from primary closure such as bile duct leak, biloma, or abscess. However, placement of a T-tube is not without complications. Morbidity rates as high as 15% with complications of sepsis, tube dislodgment, bile leak, biliary peritonitis, biliary fistula, and delayed bile duct stricture have been reported with the use of T-tubes. The authors have tended not to use T-tubes in their practice when laparoscopic closure has been satisfactorily achieved.

In addition to a choledochotomy or transcystic approach, new techniques have been developed for difficult cases, including the presence of multiple CBD stones, common hepatic duct stones, and papillary stenosis. Laparoscopic antegrade sphincterotomy involves a combination of laparoscopic CBD exploration with sphincterotomy. It requires collaboration with an endoscopist to confirm correct position of the papillotome, which is passed from above through the cystic duct or CBD. In this scenario, the laparoscopist is performing the biliary cut. Another technique described as the *rendezvous technique* was first introduced by Cavina and associates (1998). Access to the papilla is made by passing a long wire, often used in ERCP, into

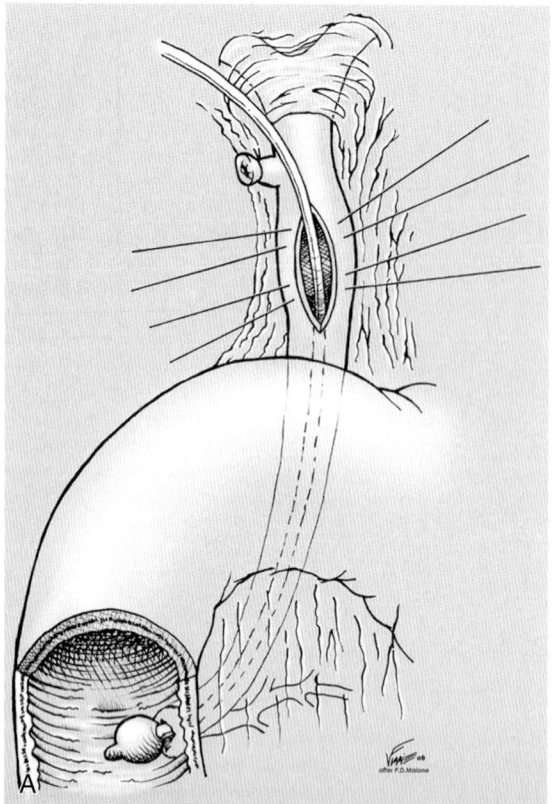

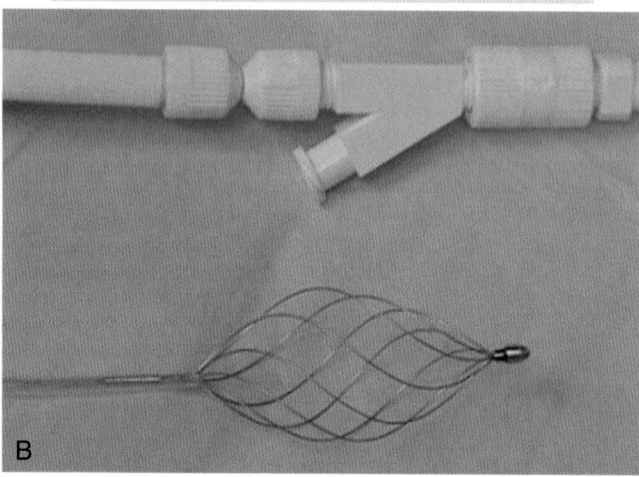

FIGURE 4   Laparoscopic common bile duct exploration. **A,** Stone extraction through a choledochotomy with a biliary balloon-tipped catheter. **B,** A helical stone basket can also be used. (**A** From Verbesey JE, Birkett DH: Common bile duct exploration for choledocholithiasis, Surg Clin North Am 88[6]:1315–1328, 2008. **B** From Chang S, Leung JW: Stone extraction. In Baron TH, Kozarek R, Carr-Locke DL [eds]: ERCP, Philadelphia, 2008, Saunders Elsevier, pp 119–128, Figure 13.7.)

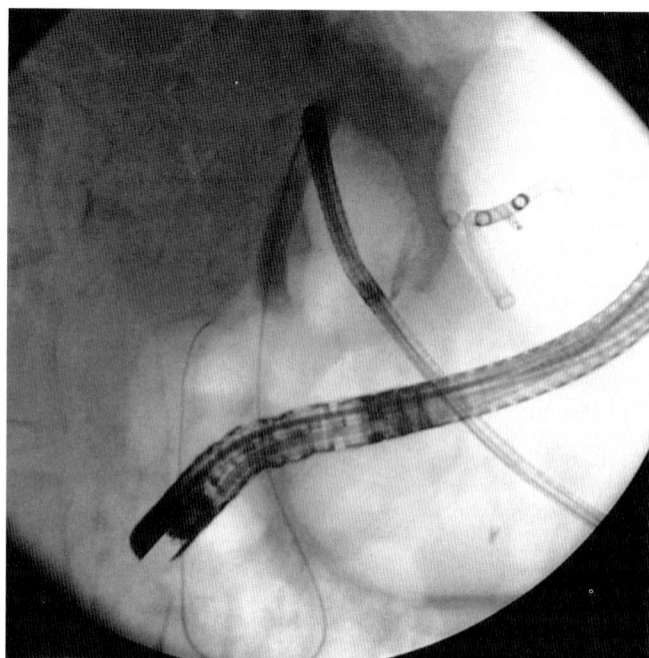

FIGURE 5   In the rendezvous technique, a long wire is inserted through the cystic duct into the duodenum. A duodenoscope is used to retrieve the wire and to perform a guided sphincterotomy. (From Bonin EA, Lopes TL, Baron TH: Percutaneous cholecystoscopy and internal rendezvous for removal of gallstones and common bile duct stones, Gastrointest Endosc 76(2):459–461, 2012.)

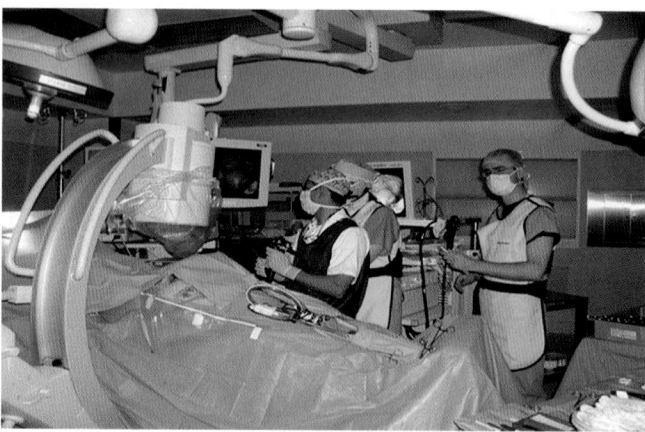

FIGURE 6   Intraoperative endoscopic retrograde cholangiopancreatography with endoscopy and stone extraction at the time of laparoscopic cholecystectomy.

the duodenum through the cystic duct. The endoscopist with a duodenoscope, positioned in the second portion of the duodenum, retrieves the wire through its working port and performs the sphincterotomy. In this scenario, the endoscopist performs the biliary cut (Figures 5 and 6). Cavina and associates reported a 100% cannulation rate in 15 patients. In a more recent randomized controlled trial, Tzovaras and colleagues compared the rendezvous technique with preoperative ERCP followed by laparoscopic cholecystectomy. They showed that hospital stays were significantly shorter with a single-

stage approach, and safety and efficacy were similar, in comparison with the two-stage approach.

Researchers in multiple studies who compared different techniques of laparoscopic CBD exploration have demonstrated similar effectiveness in removal of CBD stones, in comparison with open surgery; however, adoption of the laparoscopic technique has been slow. The success of the approach remains dependent on the surgeon's experience, the institution's resources, and availability of an endoscopist. Most centers today are still managing CBD stones with either preoperative or postoperative ERCP, depending on the timing of stone detection and presence of acute cholangitis or gallstone pancreatitis. ERCP has known morbid effects, including bleeding, post-ERCP pancreatitis from cannulation of pancreatic duct and contrast injection, duodenal perforation, papillary stenosis after sphincterotomy, cholangitis from reflux of duodenal content into CBD, and retained stones. Major morbidity and mortality rates are often quoted as 5% and 0.4%, respectively. Cannulation failure rates range from 4% to 18%. Therefore, with the advent of laparoscopic tools (often in standard commercially available kits) and standardized techniques, a single-stage approach is an attractive option in the treatment of choledocholithiasis.

AFTER CHOLECYSTECTOMY

In rare instances, patients present with retained CBD stones after cholecystectomy. Often ERCP is the initial treatment if stone disease is suspected. The timing of stone detection after operative intervention usually dictates therapy. If the time from operation to detection is more than 2 years, these stones may be considered primary. ERCP is still employed in most instances, and stone retrieval is successful. True primary CBD stones may be better treated with stone extraction and biliary-enteric bypass. For a laparoscopic choledochoduodenostomy, CBD must be dilated (at least 1.0 cm) and a surgeon must be technically competent to perform a complex anastomosis. The anastomosis can be either end-to-side or side-to-side, with the stoma being larger than 2 cm in order to prevent anastomotic stenosis. If performed by an experienced surgeon, this procedure is safe and produces good results for patients with retained biliary stones or recurrent choledocholithiasis.

EFFICACY OF LAPAROSCOPIC COMMON BILE DUCT EXPLORATION

Multiple comparisons of the safety and efficacy of single- and two-stage approaches to CBD management have been reported. In a systematic review published in 2006, data were compiled from 13 randomized controlled trials, and three approaches to the management of CBD stones were compared: ERCP versus open surgical clearance, preoperative ERCP versus laparoscopic bile duct clearance, and postoperative ERCP versus laparoscopic bile duct clearance. Results showed that ERCP was less effective in stone clearance than was an open approach and that laparoscopic CBD exploration was just as efficacious in stone removal as preoperative or postoperative ERCP, with no significant difference in morbidity and mortality. All laparoscopic trials demonstrated a shorter hospital stay in the comparison of surgery recipients. Results of a more recent prospective randomized trial in 2010 conducted by Rogers and associates echoed similar findings of the systematic review. Patients were randomly assigned to undergo either laparoscopic cholecystectomy with CBD exploration or preoperative ERCP with sphincterotomy followed by laparoscopic cholecystectomy. Rates of stone clearance were equivalent in both groups. However, hospital stays were significantly shorter for the patients who underwent laparoscopic CBD exploration, with an average of 55 hours in contrast to 98 hours for the ERCP recipients. Cost analysis was also studied; charges for the single-stage approach were significantly lower ($4820 vs $6139). Overall, surgical management of biliary duct stones at the time of laparoscopic cholecystectomy appears to be just as safe and effective as the "gold standard" of preoperative or postoperative ERCP. Advantages of laparoscopic CBD exploration are shorter hospital stay and perhaps lower cost; however, the skill sets are highly variable and are clearly related to morbidity and efficacy. Surgeon expertise and available resources may be the limiting factors in adoption of a laparoscopic approach to managing choledocholithiasis.

Because ERCP has become the "gold standard" in the management of bile duct stones, open CBD exploration has been used less frequently. Open surgery often entails an increased rate of morbidity, longer hospital stay, and increased postoperative pain. Nevertheless,

comparison between laparoscopic CBD exploration and open exploration has been evaluated in a randomized controlled trial in a single-center study. Patients were randomly assigned to undergo one of two procedures: laparoscopic CBD exploration and open CBD surgery. Diagnosis of choledocholithiasis was made preoperatively through ultrasonography, ERCP, or MRCP. The decision to use the transcystic approach or choledochotomy during laparoscopic CBD exploration was made intraoperatively on the basis of number, size, and location of stones and the anatomy of cystic ducts and CBDs. In comparison with open surgery, the laparoscopic approach again demonstrated significantly shorter length of hospital stay and less blood loss. The rates of complications such as intraabdominal bleeding, bile leak, intrahepatic abscess, reoperations, and morbidity were similar in the two groups, with the exception of wound infection, the rate of which was significantly higher in the patients who underwent the open procedure. Two different methods used for laparoscopic CBD exploration were also compared. Stone clearance via choledochotomy was more successful (94% vs 71%) but with the expense of longer operative time (90 minutes vs 62 minutes) and longer hospital stay (7.6 days vs 3.4 days) in comparison with the transcystic approach. The difference in operative time and length of stay may have been attributable to the presence of larger and multiple stones, which would make the transcystic approach unfeasible or more challenging. For single-stage laparoscopic or open management of choledocholithiasis, the less invasive approach is also just as efficacious and again has decreased hospital stay, blood loss, and rate of wound infection.

Even though laparoscopic management of CBD stones is associated with shorter hospital stay and is more cost effective, the rate of residual stones has ranged from 2.6% to 8%. Some of the reasons leading to failure of stone clearance in a transcystic approach may be the larger size of stones (>5 mm), the presence of multiple stones, and complex ductal anatomy. An impacted stone may also be a challenge in either a transcystic approach or a laparoscopic choledochotomy. Some authorities suggest that laparoscopic CBD exploration may be more difficult in patients with acute cholecystitis secondary to surrounding inflammation, which may contribute to a higher failure rate. The role of single-stage management in these patients remains controversial. Chiarugi and colleagues compared multiple outcome measures of laparoscopic transcystic exploration in patients with acute cholecystitis and those without inflammation of the gallbladder. Success rates in achieving stone clearance were 80% and 84%, respectively. Conversion rate, morbidity rate, mortality rate, length of hospital stays, readmission rate, and rate of residual stones were similar in both groups with the exception of significantly longer operative time in the group of patients with acute cholecystitis (175 minutes vs 141 minutes). Increases in operative times were probably caused by dissection of an inflamed gallbladder rather than bile duct exploration. The authors concluded that laparoscopic transcystic exploration in the setting of acute cholecystitis is just as safe and efficacious as when performed in elective laparoscopic cholecystectomy.

In addition to retained stones, other complications of laparoscopic CBD exploration include bile leak, biloma, intraabdominal hematoma, and biliary peritonitis. However, ERCP is not without its risks and significant morbidity. It is associated with a mortality rate of 0.4% and a postprocedure complication rate of 5.1%, mainly post-ERCP pancreatitis. Because single-stage management of CBD stones requires advanced laparoscopic skills, it is ultimately surgeons' decision to provide the safest approach for their patients according to their comfort level and experience.

ALTERNATIVE MANAGEMENT

In rare cases, patients present with intrahepatic stones or CBD stones larger than 1.5 cm. These stones may be difficult to remove via ERCP or laparoscopic exploration. The holmium laser was originally developed for management of renal calculi; however, it has been adapted for treatment of complex biliary stones. In this technique, a 200-μm laser fiber that generates 0.6 to 1.0 J at frequency of 6 to 10 Hz is used under video guidance with a flexible choledochoscope. Completion cholangiography is performed to confirm stone clearance. In a retrospective study published in 2007, the efficacy of this procedure was evaluated, and a 100% success rate in stone clearance in 13 patients was reported. The procedure required prolonged biliary access and multiple separate attempts to completely clear the calculi. This technique may also be combined with laparoscopic exploration in cases of impacted stones not removed by standard laparoscopic tools. Five patients who underwent this combined treatment in a retrospective review had successful clearance of impacted CBD stones.

SUMMARY

Advancements in techniques and devices enable the management of choledocholithiasis with multiple modalities, including laparoscopy, endoscopy, and combined approaches. The single-stage approach in treating CBD stones is comparable with two-stage management with preoperative or postoperative ERCP in terms of its safety profile and efficacy when performed by a surgeon with advanced laparoscopic training. Many studies demonstrated a shorter hospital stay and lower overall cost. Rates of mortality and morbidity are similar with the two approaches despite different complications. However, the requirement of expertise in laparoscopic skills contributes to the limited use of single-stage management. This issue will eventually resolve itself as more surgeons become proficient in minimally invasive procedures, and more institutions will probably provide the resources for laparoscopic CBD exploration.

SUGGESTED READINGS

Berthou JC, Dron B, Charbonneau P: Evaluation of laparoscopic treatment of common bile duct stones in a prospective series of 505 patients: indications and results, *Surg Endosc* 21:1970–1974, 2007.

Bove A, Bongarzoni G, Palone G, et al: Why is there recurrence after transcystic laparoscopic bile duct clearance? Risk factor analysis, *Surg Endosc* 23(7):1470–1475, 2009.

Cabada GT, Sarria Octavio de Toledo L, Martinez-Berganza Asensio MT, et al: Helical CT cholangiography in the evaluation of the biliary tract: application to the diagnosis of choledocholithiasis, *Abdom Imaging* 27:61–70, 2002.

Campagnacci R, Baldoni A, Baldarelli M, et al: Is laparoscopic fiberoptic choledochoscopy for common bile duct stones a fine option or a mandatory step? *Surg Endosc* 24(3):547–553, 2010.

Cavina E, Franceschi M, Sidoti F, et al: Laparo-endoscopic "rendezvous": a new technique in the choledocholithiasis treatment, *Hepatogastroenterology* 45(23):1430–1435, 1998.

Chander J, Mangla V, Vindal A, et al: Laparoscopic choledochoduodenostomy for biliary stone disease: a single-center 10-year experience, *J Laparoendosc Adv Surg Tech A* 22(1):81–84, 2012.

Chiarugi M, Galatioto C, Decanini L, et al: Laparoscopic transcystic exploration for single-stage management of common duct stones and acute cholecystitis, *Surg Endosc* 26(1):124–129, 2012.

Curet MJ, Pitcher DE, Martin DT, et al: Laparoscopic antegrade sphincterotomy. A new technique for the management of complex choledocholithiasis, *Ann Surg* 221(2):149–155, 1995.

DePaula AL, Hashiba K, Bafutto M, et al: Laparoscopic antegrade sphincterotomy, *Surg Laparosc Endosc* 3(3):157–160, 1993.

El-Geidie AA: Is the use of T-tube necessary after laparoscopic choledochotomy? *J Gastrointest Surg* 14(5):844–848, 2010.

Ford JA, Soop M, Du J, et al: Systematic review of intraoperative cholangiography in cholecystectomy, *Br J Surg* 99(2):160–167, 2012.

Freeman ML, Nelson DB, Sherman S, et al: Complications of endoscopic biliary sphincterotomy, *N Engl J Med* 335(13):909–918, 1996.

Grubnik W, Tkachenko AI, Ilyashenko W, et al: Laparoscopic common bile duct exploration versus open surgery: comparative prospective randomized trial, *Surg Endosc* 26(8):2165–2171, 2012.

Hallal AH, Amortegui JD, Jeroukhimov IM, et al: Magnetic resonance cholangiopancreatography accurately detects common bile duct stones in resolving gallstone pancreatitis, *J Am Coll Surg* 200:869–875, 2005.

Hazey JW, McCreary M, Guy G, et al: Efficacy of percutaneous treatment of biliary tract calculi using the holmium:YAG laser, *Surg Endosc* 21(7):1180–1183, 2007.

Liu TH, Consorti ET, Kawashima A, et al: Patient evaluation and management with selective use of magnetic resonance cholangiography and endoscopic retrograde cholangiopancreatography before laparoscopic cholecystectomy, *Ann Surg* 234:33–40, 2001.

Machi J, Tateishi T, Oishi AJ, et al: Laparoscopic ultrasonography versus operative cholangiography during laparoscopic cholecystectomy: review of the literature and a comparison with open intraoperative ultrasonography, *J Am Coll Surg* 188(4):360–367, 1999.

Martin DJ, Vernon DR, Toouli J: Surgical versus endoscopic treatment of bile duct stones, *Cochrane Database Syst Rev* (2):CD003327, 2006.

Moreaux J: Traditional surgical management of common bile duct stones: a prospective study during a 20 year experience, *Am J Surg* 169:220–226, 1995.

Norton SA, Alderson D: Prospective comparison of endoscopic ultrasonography and endoscopic retrograde cholangiopancreatography in the detection of bile duct stones, *Br J Surg* 84:1366–1369, 1997.

Paolo P, Nicoletta P, Carla M, et al: Ultrasonographic diagnosis of choledocholithiasis, *Acta Biomed Ateneo Parmense* 61:213–218, 1990.

Rogers SJ, Cello JP, Horn JK, et al: Prospective randomized trial of LC+LCBDE vs ERCP/S+LC for common bile duct stone disease, *Arch Surg* 145(1):28–33, 2010.

Shamamian P, Grasso M: Management of complex biliary tract calculi with a holmium laser, *J Gastrointest Surg* 8(2):191–199, 2004.

Stinton LM, Myers RP, Shaffer EA: Epidemiology of gallstones, *Gastroenterol Clin North Am* 39(2):157–169, vii, 2010.

Stromberg C, Nilsson M, Leijonmarck CE: Stone clearance and risk factors for failure in laparoscopic transcystic exploration of the common bile duct, *Surg Endosc* 22(5):1194–1199, 2008.

Tai CK, Tang CN, Ha JP, et al: Laparoscopic exploration of common bile duct in difficult choledocholithiasis, *Surg Endosc* 18(6):910–914, 2004.

Tzovaras G, Baloyiannis I, Zachari E, et al: Laparoendoscopic rendezvous versus preoperative ERCP and laparoscopic cholecystectomy for the management of cholecysto-choledocholithiasis: interim analysis of a controlled randomized trial, *Ann Surg* 255(3):435–439, 2012.

Varban O, Assimos D, Passman C, et al: Video. Laparoscopic common bile duct exploration and holmium laser lithotripsy: a novel approach to the management of common bile duct stones, *Surg Endosc* 24(7):1759–1764, 2010.

Wan XJ, Xu ZJ, Zhu F, et al: Success rate and complications of endoscopic extraction of common bile duct stones over 2 cm in diameter, *Hepatobiliary Pancreat Dis Int* 10(4):403–407, 2011.

Williams EJ, Green J, Beckingham I, et al: Guidelines on the management of common bile duct stones (CBDS), *Gut* 57(7):1004–1021, 2008.

Williams EJ, Taylor S, Fairclough P, et al: Are we meeting the standards set for endoscopy? Results of a large-scale prospective survey of endoscopic retrograde cholangio-pancreatograph practice, *Gut* 56(6):821–829, 2007.

Wills VL, Gibson K, Karihaloot C, et al: Complications of biliary T-tubes after choledochotomy, *Austral N Z J Surg* 72(3):177–180, 2002.

Zhang WJ, Xu GF, Wu GZ, et al: Laparoscopic exploration of common bile duct with primary closure versus T-tube drainage: a randomized clinical trial, *J Surg Res* 157(1):e1–e5, 2009.

Laparoscopic 360-Degree Fundoplication

**S. Scott Davis, Jr., MD, FACS, and
Rachel L. Medbery, MD**

BACKGROUND

Gastroesophageal reflux disease (GERD), which accounts for 4 to 5 million physician office visits per year, is one of the most commonly diagnosed medical conditions in the United States. The widely accepted definition of GERD is that of the 2008 Montreal consensus, which states it is a condition that develops when the reflux of stomach contents causes troublesome symptoms (those that adversely affect an individual's wellbeing) or complications for the patient. An estimated two thirds of all U.S. adults experience heartburn at least once in their lifetime. Among the 19 million Americans currently suffering from GERD, approximately 40% have symptoms 3 times a week, and 10% have symptoms daily.

SYMPTOMS AND COMPLICATIONS

Symptoms of GERD can be classified as either typical or atypical (Table 1). The most common symptom, heartburn, is reported by 80% of patients. Symptoms can often be difficult to elucidate from patients, and thus, a careful history is essential to diagnosis, in addition to consideration of other potential medical conditions. Left untreated, complications of GERD (both esophageal and extraesophageal) can lead to serious health problems (Table 2).

MEDICAL THERAPY

The appropriate first-line therapy for uncomplicated GERD is medical treatment with proton pump inhibitors (PPIs). Resolution of symptoms after initiation of medical therapy is considered confirmatory for the diagnosis of GERD. However, for patients with persistent symptoms or additional signs of complex disease, further workup may be necessary.

DIAGNOSTIC WORKUP

Endoscopy

In many cases, flexible esophagogastroduodenoscopy (EGD) can be used to diagnose GERD and rule out other conditions. For this reason, it should be the first test of choice to confirm the diagnosis of GERD (Table 3). Direct visualization of mucosal abnormalities (slough or erythema clearly demarcated from normal adjacent mucosa), ulcers, or stricture can be considered acceptable objective evidence of GERD in the appropriate clinical setting. All ulcers or strictures must be biopsied to rule out malignancy disease. Histologic evidence of Barrett's esophagus may also be considered objective proof for GERD.

Barium Swallow

Barium swallow (BS) is the second test that all patients should undergo before surgical intervention. Although BS is not necessary for diagnosis of GERD in and of itself, it is invaluable for definition of patient anatomy and for general characterization of gastric and esophageal motility. It is especially useful for ruling in or out large hiatal hernias and a shortened esophagus, which allows surgeons to better plan their operation.

pH Testing

When the diagnosis of GERD cannot be confirmed with EGD, esophageal pH testing should be the next testing modality pursued. Considered the gold standard for objective diagnosing of GERD, the test requires placement of a small pH sensor electrode 5 cm above the proximal border of the lower esophageal sphincter (LES). In the traditional 24-hour ambulatory test, a small transnasal catheter is attached to the pH sensor. Alternatively, the Bravo device (Medtronic, Inc., Shoreview, Minn) is a wireless radiotelemetric capsule that transmits pH data to a receiver on the patient's belt. In both methods, the frequency of reflux episodes, the number of episodes that last longer than 5 minutes, the duration of the longest reflux episode, and the cumulative time the esophageal pH is below 4 (both supine and upright) are all measured and reported. The transnasal catheter provides the added benefit of a second sensor located in the upper esophagus, which gives data to evaluate for possible laryngopharyngeal reflux disease (LPR).

Impedance Testing

Multichannel intraluminal impedance (MII) testing is a newer technology that allows for the detection of intraluminal bolus movement without the side effects of radiation. Multiple electrode pairs are used to detect changes in resistance to flow as a bolus moves across the electrode. The specific resistance can be used to interpret the nature of the bolus (liquid vs gas). MII can be combined with manometry to gather functional data, such as peristalsis and contractile pressures in the body of the esophagus, and the resting tone and relaxation of both the upper and the lower esophageal sphincters. Because esophageal manometry alone does not measure acid reflux, it cannot be used to diagnose GERD. However, it is a necessary preoperative tool for evaluation of patients with dysphagia or chest pain associated with GERD to exclude a primary esophageal motility disorder that may necessitate an alternate surgical plan. Furthermore, new technology allows for simultaneous MII and pH monitoring. Correlation of impedance data with pH measurements facilitates both the recording of acid and nonacid reflux episodes the proximal extent of the refluxate.

SURGICAL THERAPY

Reasons for Surgery

GERD is a mechanical disorder that results from one or more of the following: an incompetent LES (anatomically or functionally), impaired gastric emptying, or ineffective esophageal peristalsis. Although numerous treatment options exist for GERD, laparoscopic 360-degree fundoplication is the gold standard for reconstruction of a functioning LES. However, objective evidence of GERD is essential before any surgical intervention takes place. Once the diagnosis of GERD has been objectively confirmed, surgical intervention should be considered in the following circumstances: (1) the patient has failed medical management; (2) the patient opts for surgery despite successful medical management; (3) the patient has extraesophageal manifestations; or (4) the patient has complications such as Barrett's esophagus or peptic stricture.

TABLE 1: Symptoms of gastroesophageal reflux disease

Typical	Atypical
Heartburn	Asthma
Dysphagia	Hoarseness
Regurgitation	Cough
	Recurrent pneumonia
	Retrosternal chest pain
	Dental erosion
	Chronic sinusitis
	Anemia
	Weight loss

TABLE 2: Complications of gastroesophageal reflux disease

Esophageal	Extraesophageal
Esophagitis	Laryngitis
Esophageal ulcers	Laryngeal cancer
Peptic stricture	Laryngeal nodules
Barrett's esophagus	Globus
Adenocarcinoma	Chronic bronchitis
	Pulmonary fibrosis
	Pneumonitis

TABLE 3: Diagnostic workup

Test	Utility	When
Endoscopy	Diagnostic	First test in ALL patients
Modified barium swallow	Ancillary (*defines anatomy before surgery*)	ALL patients before surgery
24-hour pH monitoring	Diagnostic	Patients without objective evidence of GERD on endoscopy
Impedance/pH monitoring	Diagnostic	Patients without objective evidence of GERD on endoscopy
Impedance manometry	Ancillary (*rules out motility disorders*)	Patients with chest pain or dysphagia

GERD, Gastroesophageal reflux disease.

Patient Selection and Predictors of Success

Studies within the literature have shown that patient's symptomatic response to preoperative PPI treatment can be directly correlated with resolution of symptoms after fundoplication. Furthermore, patients who have poor compliance with preoperative PPI therapy are likely to have worse outcomes after surgery. Old age should not be considered a contraindication for surgical intervention, as long as the patient is otherwise an acceptable candidate for surgery. Outcomes in patients older than 65 years of age have been shown to be on par with those of younger patients. For patients with GERD and body mass index (BMI) of more than 35 kg/m², gastric bypass, not fundoplication, should be the procedure of choice. Not only does fundoplication have a high failure rate in morbidly obese patients, but the procedure does not adequately address the underlying problem (obesity) that causes GERD, nor does it address a number of other medical conditions related to obesity for which there is opportunity for resolution.

TECHNIQUE

The authors' center made a concerted effort to standardize the operating room setup and patient positioning amongst surgeons specializing in these procedures. Perioperative and postoperative care have also been standardized. These changes led to gains in operating room efficiency and improvement in surgical outcomes and rates of readmission.

Positioning

After induction of general anesthesia, the patient is placed in the supine position, with the arms extended and secured to arm boards. A foot board is placed on the bed to allow for significant reverse Trendelenburg's position. A Foley catheter is placed, and the patient is secured to the table. This positioning is less complicated and accomplished more expeditiously than with the use of split leg or stirrup table attachments. The surgeon stands on the patient's right side, and the assistant on the left. A pneumatic camera holder is used for the laparoscope. The clamp for fixating the liver retractor to the bed is placed under the patient's right arm.

Port Placement

Access is gained to the abdomen with an optically viewing trocar, inserted under the left subcostal margin 10 cm from the xiphoid process (Figure 1). The 10-mm camera port is then inserted just to the right of the midline, away from the falciform ligament, 15 cm

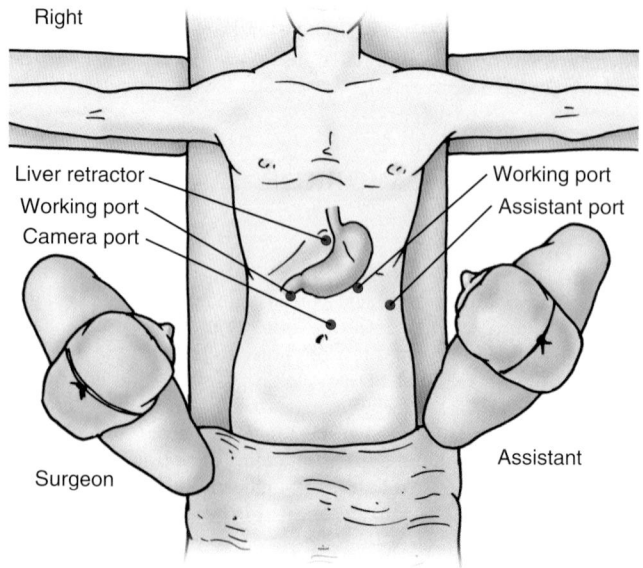

FIGURE 1 Port placement. (*Modified from Townsend CM, editor: Sabiston textbook of surgery, ed 18, Philadelphia, 2007, Saunders Fig. 2-6.*)

from the xiphoid process. Next, the assistant's port is inserted in the left abdomen along the left subcostal margin 10 cm further from the optically placed trocar. A subxiphoid incision is made as closely to the xiphoid process as reasonable for placement of a Nathonson-type liver retractor. The last working 5-mm port, the surgeon's left hand, is then placed for comfortable triangulation with the surgeon's right hand and below the caudal edge of the retracted liver, usually at the base of the falciform ligament. A 10-mm, 30-degree viewing scope is typically used. A 45-degree viewing scope is kept available for cases where the camera port is found to be too low for a good downward viewing angle to the hiatus, or where there is a large amount of visceral fat in lower aspect of the field of view.

The many alternatives to these port placements include the use of single port techniques, which can be used in selected settings but are beyond the scope of this discussion.

Early Gastric Mobilization

The dissection is begun along the greater curve of the stomach with division of the short gastric vessels with a bipolar sealing device (Figure 2). Most often, a posterior veil of the gastrosplenic ligament contains a few additional short gastric vessels near the gastroesophageal (GE) junction; division of this leads into the vessels that make up the most intimate part of the gastrosplenic ligament. Once these vessels are divided, the dissection plane leads to the left crura. If surgeons have difficulty seeing the left crura, they have most likely not completely divided the posterior veil of the gastrosplenic ligament. The peritoneum can now be incised at the angle of His (phrenoesophageal membrane), and the mediastinum entered (Figure 3). Here, the anterior mobilization of the esophagus should be straightforward. The most advantageous maneuver at this point is to complete the dissection of the peritoneum from the base of the left crura completely, mobilizing the esophagus medially. Completion of this now makes for a much easier creation of the retroesophageal window.

Left to Right Crural Dissection and Esophageal Mobilization

The dissection is then continued with the division of the gastrohepatic ligament. This is typically avascular. The only notable structure is the hepatic branch of the vagus nerve; on occasion, a replaced left hepatic artery may be present. These are typically preserved; however, they can be divided if they limit visualization of the hiatal dissection. A replaced left hepatic artery can be divided if needed, but this is usually not necessary. The right crus is dissected in the same manner as the left, with incision of the peritoneum and mobilization of the esophagus. Good tissue handling is critical, and this maneuver can be facilitated by the surgeon's left hand with a blunt grasper placed inside the crura with gentle medial retraction to serve as counter traction (Figure 4). In many cases, the mobilization of the esophagus can be accomplished with gentle blunt sweeps of the right-handed instrument away from this retraction. The dissection is completed to the base of the right crura (posteriorly) first, and this connects to the window that was previously made from the left side. This allows for the passage of a Penrose drain behind the esophagus, through the retroesophageal window, encircling the GE junction. The Penrose is held by the assistant who can now provide counter traction for the rest of the division of the phrenoesophageal membrane and mobilization of the esophagus. The anterior and posterior vagus nerves can be easily identified and preserved. Care must be taken by the assistant not to overly retract to avoid praxia or injury to the vagus nerves. The esophagus is mobilized widely to ensure ample intra-abdominal length, of which there should be a minimum of 3 to 4 cm without traction. This further ensures minimal risk of wrap migration.

Crural Closure

A dilating esophageal balloon is inserted into the esophagus with direct vision before closure of the crura (to minimize risk of esophageal injury proximal to the closure, which can be easily missed). Once

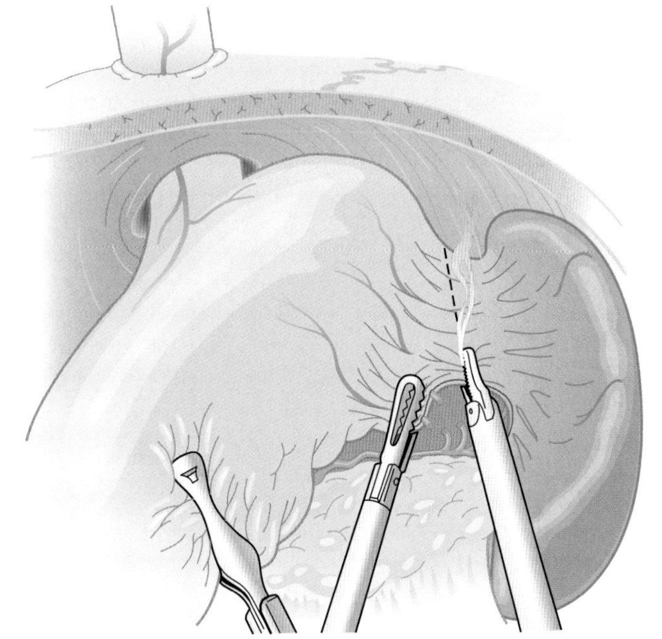

FIGURE 2 Early gastric mobilization. The dissection is begun along the greater curve of the stomach with division of the short gastric vessels with a bipolar sealing device. *(From Townsend CM, editor: Sabiston textbook of surgery, ed 18, Philadelphia, 2007, Saunders, Fig. 42-8.)*

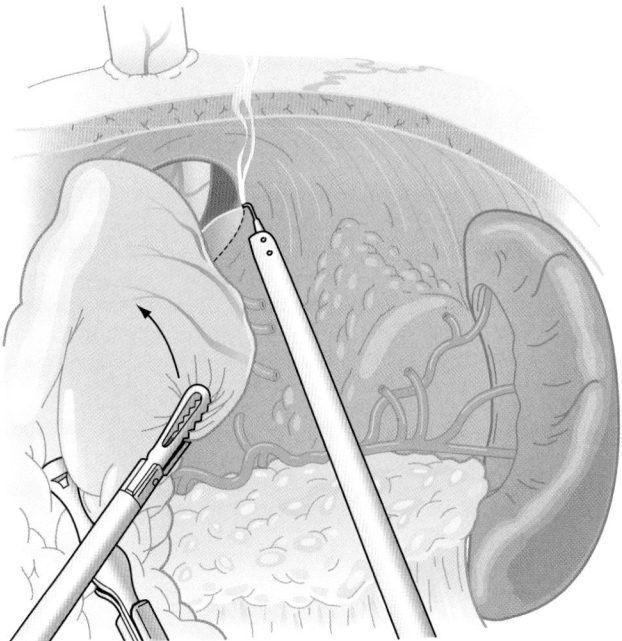

FIGURE 3 Mediastinal entry. The peritoneum is incised at the angle of His (phrenoesophageal membrane), and the mediastinum entered. *(From Townsend CM, editor: Sabiston textbook of surgery, ed 18, Philadelphia, 2007, Saunders, Fig. 42-9.)*

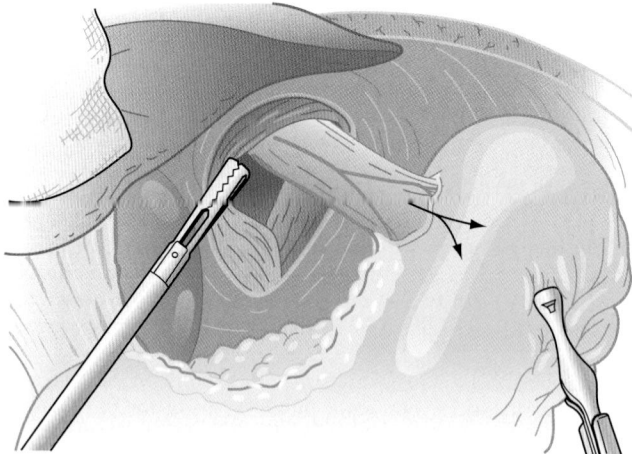

FIGURE 4 Esophageal mobilization. Gentle counter traction with a blunt grasper in the left hand is useful in assisting with dissection and mobilization. *(From Townsend CM, editor: Sabiston textbook of surgery, ed 18, Philadelphia, 2007, Saunders, Fig. 42-10.)*

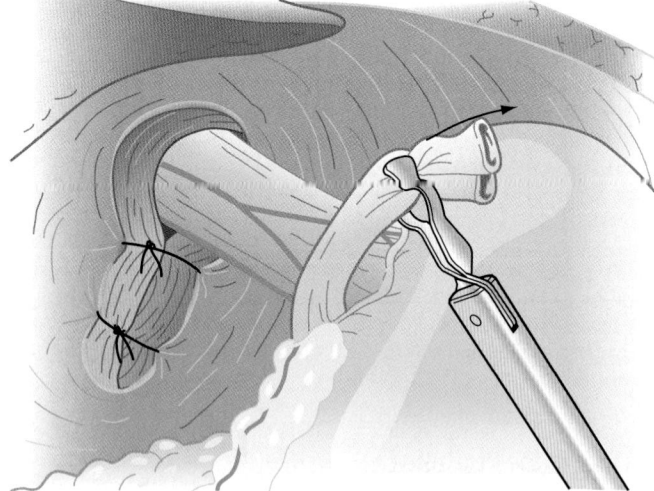

FIGURE 5 Crural closure. A Penrose drain encircles the gastroesophageal junction, and traction is used to provide adequate visualization for crural closure. *(From Townsend CM editor: Sabiston textbook of surgery, ed 18, Philadelphia, 2007, Saunders, Fig. 42-11.)*

placed, the crura are closed posteriorly, usually requiring two or three nonabsorbable sutures (Figure 5). Pledgets made of bioabsorbable material can be used to reinforce these sutures if the quality of the crura is deemed poor. However, they are not used routinely. Placement of prosthetic material at the hiatus is not recommended and not usually necessary. This is believed to increase the risk of rare, but potentially catastrophic, complications, such as prosthetic erosion into the esophagus. In most cases done for the indication of GERD in the absence of a hiatal hernia, esophageal length should not be an issue with wide mobilization, and crural closure without tension should be achievable.

Creation of Tension-free Fundoplication

The fundus is then brought through the retroesophageal window and should lie easily without retracting if the mobilization done initially is adequate and complete. Then, the esophageal balloon is inflated to 56F in the lumen of the esophagus. In some cases for large male patients, inflation to 60F is considered. The closure of the hiatus is then reexamined first to ensure that it is snug around the esophagus with the balloon inflated. Care is taken in orienting the fundus for the fundoplication. It is paramount to avoid twisting of the fundoplication, either at rest or functionally during a swallow. A slightly twisted wrap, on occasion, is exacerbated by a swallow, and a twisting action of the GE junction may be seen during endoscopy. This is prevented with three standard maneuvers: (1) ensuring that the posterior short gastric vessels are completely mobilized; (2) using a "shoe shine" technique to ensure the wrap is constructed with the same part of the fundus (Figure 6); and (3) placing sutures at or near the cut edge of the short gastric vessels on both the medial and the lateral sides of the fundoplication.

The fundoplication should be created without tension; this can be checked by the ease of passage of the grasper behind it along the stented esophagus. The wrap should be situated above the z-line and not on the cardia of the stomach to prevent slippage of the fundoplication. Typically, the wrap is created with three sutures placed 1 cm apart, for a total 2 cm length. The longitudinal outer fibers of the esophageal wall are incorporated in the first two sutures to fixate the wrap in the correct position, with care taken not to incorporate the anterior vagus nerve.

Endoscopy is routinely performed to assess the morphology of the fundoplication and to ensure there has been no occult perforation. The wrap should be further assessed with endoscopic

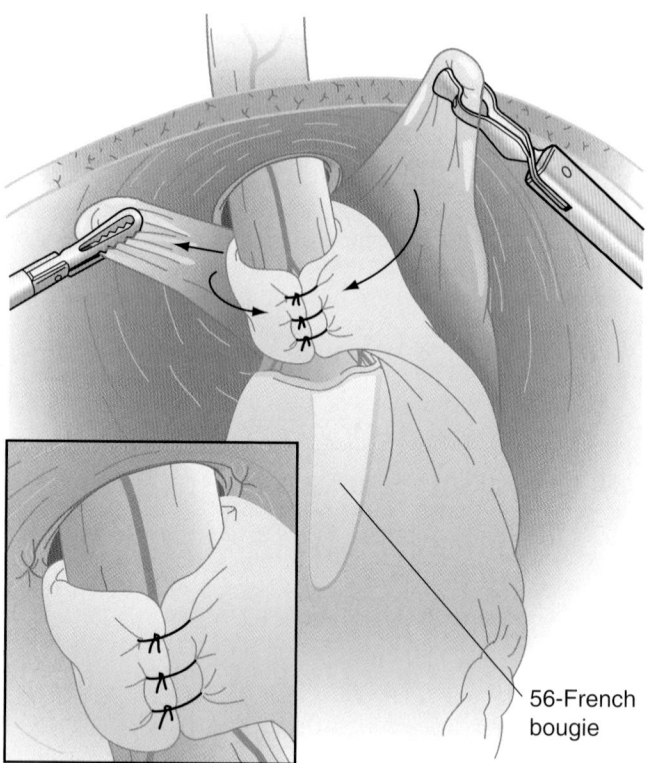

56-French bougie

FIGURE 6 Creation of tension-free fundoplication. The "shoe-shine" technique is used to create a wrap with the same portion of fundus. Wrap should be 2 cm in length, with sutures 1 cm apart. *(From Townsend CM editor: Sabiston textbook of surgery, ed 18, Philadelphia, 2007, Saunders, Fig. 42-12.)*

insufflation to ensure that the folds of the fundoplication do not twist into the GE junction. The folds should appear as a "stack of coins" going around the scope (Figure 7). Twisting into the GE junction around the scope indicate a malpositioned wrap. A gastropexy of the wrap to the diaphragm or crural closure is not routinely done.

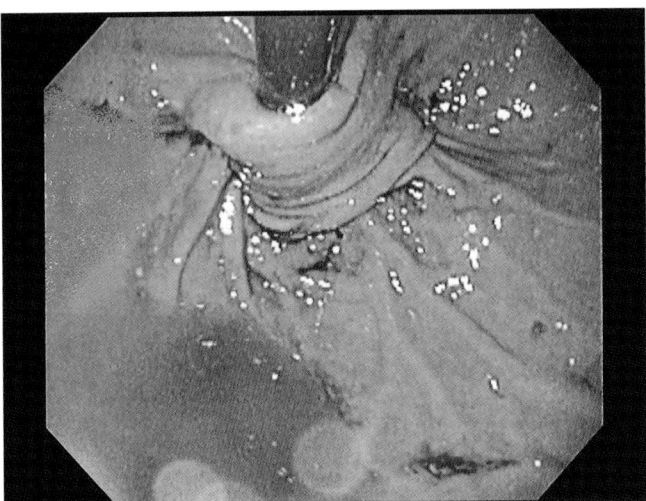

FIGURE 7 Stack of coins view. After completion of the wrap, the endoscope can be retroflexed within the lumen of the stomach to confirm proper wrap formation.

Additional Maneuvers and Controversy

Some recent publications advocate use of synthetic mesh to assist in closing the hiatus, typically as a posterior onlay reinforcement, with the argument that doing so decreases the likelihood of a postoperative hiatal hernia. This decrease in risk, however, can be associated with rare but significant complications, such as dysphagia, stricture, or esophageal erosion, which can necessitate a second operation—one that will be technically challenging because of the presence of incorporated mesh. In many of these cases, a major gastroesophageal resection may be required for remediation. As such, the authors believe the risk of routine mesh placement at the hiatus far outweighs the risk of a second operation for a hiatal hernia repair in which mesh was never placed. They only recommend the use of mesh in hiatal closure when it is impossible to approximate the tissue behind the esophagus or when the character of the crura is obviously poor. In such cases, a biologic material is chosen for buttress.

Similarly, some surgeons opt to secure the fundoplication via pexy to the diaphragm, advocating that anchoring sutures prevent wrap herniation into the chest. The authors advise against this technique for reasons similar to use of mesh at the hiatus. No available evidence shows that this practice decreases the incidence of wrap migration, the most common anatomic failure of this procedure. The authors have observed that revisions done after these sutures have been placed can be much more difficult because of dense scarring between the fundoplication and the diaphragm, and the benefit of these sutures is not clear.

POSTOPERATIVE CARE

This procedure is typically done with a planned overnight observation, although it can also be safely done on an outpatient basis. During this observation, the patient is on a clear liquid diet and is seen and counseled on the recommended dietary instruction by the nutritionist. If the procedure is done on an outpatient basis, this nutritional education can be done before surgery. The diet is then advanced to a full liquid diet on postoperative day 4, with a subsequent progression to a general diet after 3 weeks.

During the early postoperative period, unexpected increases in intra-abdominal pressure from excessive coughing, gagging, vomiting, or belching can predispose patients to early anatomic failure of the newly created fundoplication. Thus, to minimize the risk of wrap failure, patients are recommended to be placed on scheduled antiemetics for the first 24 to 48 hours.

COMPLICATIONS

Early postoperative complications after laparoscopic fundoplication are unusual, and mortality is rare. Conversion from a laparoscopic to an open approach occurs less than 2.4% of the time at high-volume centers. Gastric and esophageal perforation only occurs 0 to 4% of the time, with the highest rates seen in redo fundoplication cases. Aggressive dissection around the hiatus can lead to pneumothorax (0 to 1.5% of cases); however, because the injuries are usually to the pleura and not the lung parenchyma itself, very few are of clinical significance and they resolve without intervention.

Most notable complications from fundoplication occur in the longer term. Wrap migration is the most common form of anatomic recurrence and occurs in approximately 10% of cases. Other forms of anatomic failure include slippage of the wrap onto the cardia of the stomach or twisting of the wrap. Any of these can lead to recurrent symptoms, most notably recurrent reflux symptoms, dysphagia, or chest pain. Atypical symptoms may also occur. Studies show that as many as 60% of patients are again placed on PPIs in the long term, but in most cases, these treatments are not given based on objective evidence of recurrent reflux. In most of these patients, objective testing actually shows that pathologic reflux is not present.

Other symptoms such as post-Nissen syndrome (gas bloat) can occur and can be troublesome to treat. In most cases, these new gastrointestinal symptoms can be treated medically, and quality of life is much improved compared with preoperative measures. Approximately 3% to 4% of patients need revisional surgery to address these issues, and usually some type of anatomic failure is present.

OUTCOMES

Multiple series within the literature report equal efficacy between surgical and medical therapy for GERD, although surgery may in fact result in better symptom control and quality of life for the patient. After fundoplication, 80% to 85% of patients have complete resolution of typical GERD symptoms; atypical symptoms resolve 60% to 75% of the time. Mild dysphasia is not uncommon within the first 30 days of surgery. Only 4% of patients, however, continue to note dysphagia at 90-day follow-up. Most studies within the literature report postoperative use of acid-reducing medications to range from 30% to 60%. Among those patients who resume postoperative PPI therapy, however, only 25% to 30% have documented reflux recurrence on 24-hour pH testing. Long-term (>5 years after surgery) patient satisfaction rates range anywhere from 80% to 96%, with 81% to 95% of patients maintaining they would undergo surgery again.

CONCLUSION

The successful surgical treatment of GERD requires the combination of a meaningful elicitation of the patient's presenting symptoms, with appropriate preoperative workup to understand the underlying esophageal and gastric physiology and function, and practiced surgical technique. The authors' center too often treats patients with complications from surgeries done without adequate preoperative characterization of the disease process or in whom the procedure was not the best surgical choice. The surgeon must have an understanding of the nuances of the preoperative testing that is needed and other esophageal disorders to choose the most appropriate surgical therapy for any given patient.

SUGGESTED READINGS

Anvari M, Allen C, Marshall J, et al: A randomized controlled trial of laparoscopic Nissen fundoplication versus proton pump inhibitors for the treatment of patients with chronic gastoesophageal reflux disease (GERD): 3-year outcomes, *Surg Endosc* 25:2547–2554, 2011.

Ciovica R, Gadenstatter M, Klinger A, et al: Quality of life in GERD patients: medical treatment versus antireflux surgery, *J Gastrointest Surg* 10:934–939, 2006.

Evans SRT, Jackson PG, Czerniach DR, et al: A stepwise approach to laparoscopic Nissen fundoplication: avoiding technical pitfalls, *Arch Surg* 135:723–728, 2000.

Niebisch S, Fleming FJ, Galey KM, et al: Perioperative risk of laparoscopic fundoplication: safer that previously reported: analysis of the American Colleges of Surgeons National Quality Improvement Program 2005 to 2009, *J Am Coll Surg* 215(1):61–68, 2012; discussion 68-9. Epub 2012 May 10.

Stadlhuber RJ, Sherif AE, Mittal SK, et al: Mesh complications after prosthetic reinforcement of hiatal closure: a 28-case series, *Surg Endosc* 23(6):1219–1226, 2009.

Stefanidis D, Hope WW, Kohn GP, et al: *Guidelines for surgical treatment of gastroesophageal reflux disease: Society of American Gastrointestinal and Endoscopic Surgeons (SAGES), 2010 practice/clinical guidelines*, available online at http://www.sages.org/publications/guidelines/, accessed May 2012.

LAPAROSCOPIC APPENDECTOMY

**Brian R. Smith, MD, FACS, and
Ninh T. Nguyen, MD, FACS**

INTRODUCTION

Among the many disease processes and operations in general surgery, appendicitis and appendectomy remain not only the most common but arguably the most impactful form of surgical progress in the last two centuries. Since the mid 1700s, when Amyand performed the first appendectomy for trauma, and the late 1800s, when McBurney published the first series of appendectomy for acute appendicitis, this operation has become the most common operation performed annually worldwide and has saved countless millions of lives. More than 250,000 appendectomies are performed annually in the United States in both adults and children, and the procedure touches nearly 7% of the U.S. population annually.

PATHOPHYSIOLOGY

The pathophysiology of appendicitis is based on lumenal obstruction and visceral blood flow. The inside of the appendix is lined with gut mucosa-associated lymphoid tissue (MALT), which is more active in children and relatively quiescent in adults. In children, this MALT tissue can hypertrophy, causing lumenal obstruction along the length of the appendix. On doing so, ongoing mucous production from the appendiceal mucosa builds up distal to the obstruction, causing visceral distention and initiating visceral-type pain that is colicky, vague, and poorly localized. Along with most small intestinal visceral peritoneal distention, pain is typically periumbilical. As swelling increases distal to the obstruction, venous return from the appendix is initially compromised, followed later by arterial blood flow obstruction with eventual patches of necrosis of the appendiceal wall and subsequent perforation. In adults, firm pieces of stool serve to similarly obstruct the appendiceal lumen in the form of a fecalith. In elderly patients, tumors can occasionally serve a similar obstructive role that follows the same pathophysiology.

DIAGNOSIS

The classic presentation of appendicitis is the starting point from which clinicians should begin their evaluation, and progressive clinical deviation from this presentation warrants further investigation. Patients often present with acute onset of abdominal pain that typically precedes vomiting. Visceral distention usually results in anorexia from the time the pain starts. Pain is described as colicky and vague, initiating in the periumbilical region and difficult to localize initially. As the source of lumenal obstruction of the appendix persists, the localized inflammatory process on the serosal surface of the appendix eventually touches the parietal peritoneum. This causes pain that is well localized to the site of irritation and now migrates typically to the right lower quadrant overlying the inflamed appendix (McBurney's point tenderness). When a right lower quadrant appendicitis is nearby but not adjacent to the abdominal wall, it can be brought in close proximity with pressure or palpation in the left lower quadrant, which can elicit pain in the right lower quadrant (Rovsing's sign). Retrocecal and pelvic appendices may not have access to the parietal peritoneum and hence, may not manifest focal peritoneal symptoms. However, retrocecal appendicitis often approximates the psoas muscle, causing pain with active flexion of the hip (psoas sign). Similarly, pelvic appendicitis more closely approximates the parietal peritoneum when the pelvic space is closed down by passive adduction of the flexed hip (obturator sign). More advanced peritoneal irritation can occur and yield voluntary or involuntary guarding or rebound tenderness to palpation.

Other supportive evidence of appendicitis includes leukocytosis (>10K in 85% of patients), fever (present in 50%), anorexia (present in 75%), and absence of other obvious etiologies. The average appendicitis takes 72 hours to evolve from initial lumenal obstruction to perforation. On perforation, with the associated decompression of the appendiceal lumenal distention distal to the obstruction, patients often feel better transiently before generalized peritonitis sets in from lumenal content spillage. Therefore, patients with significantly longer periods of pain or pain that has failed to progressively worsen over several days should have other diagnoses entertained. In young healthy males, the differential diagnosis is relatively limited to terminal ileitis or colitis or Meckel's diverticulitis. In children, mesenteric adenitis, or diffuse lymph node swelling throughout the intestinal mesentery often as a result of a viral infection, can very closely mimic acute appendicitis and is highest on the differential. In women, pelvic inflammatory disease, adnexal cysts or torsion, and tuboovarian abscesses are all high on the differential and often require a pelvic examination to help delineate. Symptoms of vaginal discharge and a menstrual and sexual history often help provide insight into these differentials.

The further the clinical picture deviates from the previous classic presentation, the larger the differential diagnosis and hence, the greater the role imaging plays in securing the diagnosis. Right lower quadrant ultrasound scan can be helpful but is highly operator dependent and less sensitive and specific (~90% and 97%, respectively) than computed tomographic (CT) scanning (~95% and 98%, respectively). However, the value of ultrasound scan is high in children and pregnant females in whom radiation exposure from CT scanning is of concern. Indiscriminate use of imaging, particularly CT scanning, has been shown to increase cost and delay diagnosis and management of cases where appendicitis is clinically either obvious or unlikely.

INDICATIONS

For patients who present with acute nonperforated appendicitis, the appropriate treatment is timely appendectomy. Best evidence supports no increase in risk of perforation or postoperative complications if surgery is performed within 24 hours of presentation. Beyond 36 hours from time of symptom onset, the risk of appendiceal perforation goes up by 5% for every 12-hour period of delay, and most evidence supports increased postoperative morbidity beyond this period. Patients should ideally be started on antibiotics once the diagnosis is made and taken to surgery at the first feasible opportunity.

Benign and malignant tumors of the appendix are rare and most often manifest a clinical picture identical to that of acute appendicitis. As a result, preoperative diagnosis of these tumors is rare, and distinction is typically made by a pathologist. This group of tumors is composed of appendiceal carcinoid, adenocarcinoma, and mucocele. For the tumors that are diagnosed either on preoperative CT scan or after appendectomy, right hemicolectomy is indicated for tumors of more than 2 cm or the presence of any lymph node metastases. At the time of laparoscopic appendectomy for presumed appendicitis, obvious tumors larger than 2 cm or with clinically visible lymphadenopathy should be converted to either laparoscopic or open right hemicolectomy depending on surgeon skill level.

TECHNIQUES

The two fundamental and most often debated techniques for appendectomy are laparoscopic versus open. The open technique has been the dominant approach for well over a century. Yet in only the last 20 years, the laparoscopic approach has largely replaced the open approach at most institutions, despite ongoing debate about its true superiority. Regardless of which approach is used, all patients should be counseled about the risks and benefits of each and sign consent for both. Preoperative antibiotic prophylaxis should consist of gram-negative and anaerobic coverage. Patients should be placed under a general anesthetic, and a timeout should be performed by the entire surgical team to verify patient identification, correct operation and site, proper antibiotic prophylaxis, and presence of necessary equipment and review the need for blood products or special equipment. A Foley catheter should be placed for decompression of the bladder. Skin prep should ideally be with chlorhexidine solution, and the patient should be draped to expose the entire abdomen from nipples to the pubis and laterally to the midaxillary line.

For a laparoscopic approach, the patient's left arm should be tucked and arm board removed to facilitate both the camera operator and the surgeon standing on the patient's left side during surgery. The abdomen can be entered with Veress needle or Hassan technique per surgeon preference, and the abdomen is insufflated to 15 mm Hg with carbon dioxide gas. Preincisional infusion of local anesthetic at each trocar site has been shown to decrease postoperative pain. Ideal

trocar placement is one 5-mm trocar at the umbilicus to accommodate a 5-mm angled laparoscope and another in the midline just above the pubis under direct vision, with care taken to avoid bladder injury (temporary indwelling urinary catheter and bed positioning in Trendelenburg's position facilitate this; Figure 1). Initial insertion of the laparoscope should visualize the viscera and omentum beneath the entry site to ensure there are no signs of visceral injury during placement of the initial port. In the left lower quadrant (LLQ), centered vertically between the first two trocars and horizontally in the anterior axillary line, a 12-mm trocar is placed with direct vision, with care taken to avoid injury to the sigmoid colon (tilting the bed to the patient's right facilitates this). The bed is then tilted to the patient's left and in modest Trendelenburg's position to facilitate exposure of the right lower quadrant (RLQ) region.

A 5-mm atraumatic grasper is inserted in the suprapubic port and used by the left hand to grasp and retract the appendix. The appendix can always be located by following the tenia of the ascending colon to their termination at the appendiceal base. A Maryland dissector is placed through the 12-mm LLQ port and used by the right hand to dissect a window through the mesoappendix immediately adjacent to the base of the appendix (Figure 2). Care should be taken to stay against the appendiceal base when creating this window, as the appendiceal artery lies at the free (antimesenteric) margin of the mesoappendix and is less likely to be injured. Similarly, care must also be taken when creating this window to avoid injury to the cecum. Once the window is created, the Maryland dissector is replaced by a laparoscopic stapler; the mesoappendix is stapled first, and the

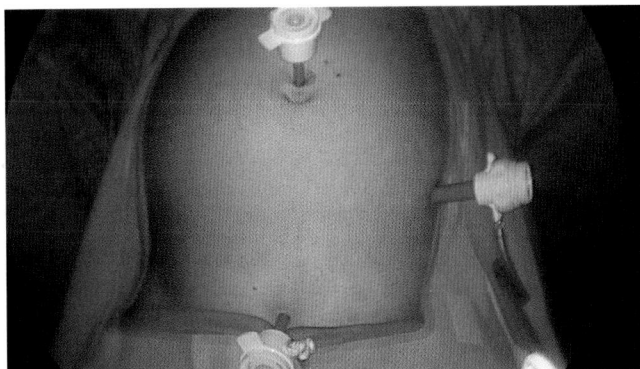

FIGURE 1   Trocar placement for laparoscopic appendectomy. The superior trocar is cephalad to the umbilicus.

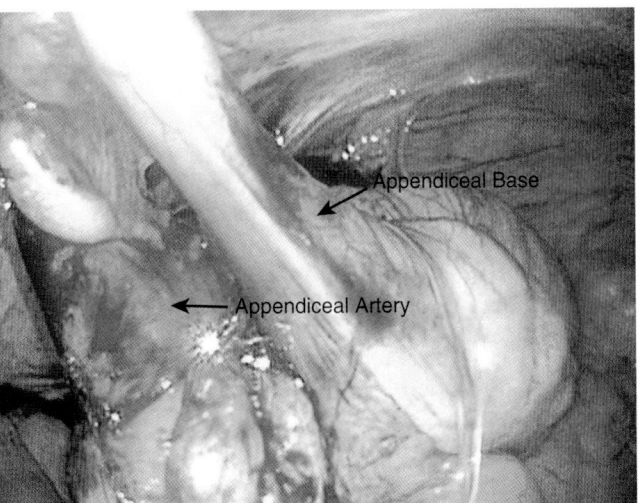

FIGURE 2   Laparoscopic view shows appendiceal artery separated away from appendix.

appendiceal base immediately adjacent to the cecum is stapled after (Figure 3). However, it is important to use a vascular staple load for the mesoappendix and medium bowel staple load for the appendiceal base, with great care taken to ensure all of the appendix is transected to avoid stump appendicitis in the future.

In the rare event that the cecum at the appendiceal base is inflamed or not healthy appearing, stapling in this region should be avoided in consideration of an alternative diagnosis of colitis. Once the appendix and mesoappendix are hemostatically stapled, the appendix should be placed inside of a protective bag and removed through the LLQ 12-mm port. Irrigation can then be undertaken as needed in the RLQ and pelvis until all purulent fluids are aspirated and hemostasis is ensured. Many surgeons prefer to close the 12-mm trocar fascial defect with absorbable suture, and again, bed tilt to the patient's right can minimize proximity of closure efforts to the colon. Skin is then reapproximated with absorbable subcutaneous sutures after irrigation of the port sites.

Open appendectomy is performed with the patient supine and both arms out on arm boards. A 4-cm to 5-cm transverse RLQ (Rocky-Davis) or oblique (McBurney's) incision is made approximately one third the distance from the umbilicus to the anterior superior iliac spine, centered over the midclavicular line. This incision is carried down through Scarpa's fascia to the external oblique, which is also incised transversely. The internal oblique and transversalis muscles are then separated with muscle-splitting and progressive dissection down to the peritoneum, which is opened sharply in a transverse fashion. The appendix is then palpated digitally and finger-dissected free from surrounding structures and delivered out through the wound with a Babcock clamp. A window in the mesoappendix is created, and the base of the mesoappendix ligated. The base of the appendix is then purse-stringed with a 2-0 absorbable suture. The base is then clamped, and the base is transected and specimen passed off the field. The base is then suture ligated and inverted into the cecum before the purse-string suture is tied, effectively inverting the appendiceal stump into the cecum. The surrounding area is then copiously irrigated until clear, and local purulence is removed. The peritoneum is then reapproximated with 3-0 running absorbable suture, followed by reapproximation of the external oblique fascia with a 2-0 absorbable suture. The wound is then copiously irrigated, and skin is closed with either clips or absorbable subcutaneous sutures. Routine drain placement is not indicated after appendectomy unless the presence of a clear abscess cavity may benefit from short-interval drainage.

For patients with nonperforated appendicitis, continuation of prophylactic antibiotics beyond 24 hours after surgery has shown no

documented benefit. For patients with perforated appendicitis or more serious intraabdominal sepsis, best evidence supports antibiotic therapy until the patient has been afebrile for 24 hours and with a normalization of leukocytosis. Dietary progression should be guided by overall clinical picture, presence of ileus, severity of intraabdominal sepsis, and patient's desire to eat. Most patients with nonperforated appendicitis can safely start a bland diet immediately after surgery. Like most operations, patients should ambulate as soon as possible after surgery, have their urinary catheter removed by postoperative day 1 unless otherwise indicated, aggressively use their incentive spirometer 10 times per hour every hour that they are awake, and undergo chemoprophylaxis against deep venous thrombosis (DVT) within 24 hours of surgery unless otherwise contraindicated or discharged home. Many patients with nonperforated appendicitis who undergo timely appendectomy can also be discharged the same day or within 24 hours of surgery if they are tolerating diet and are pain-controlled.

RESULTS

Despite extensive analysis of the outcomes of laparoscopic versus open appendectomy, very little level I data exist to document the superiority of one approach over the other. In addition, the laparoscopic approach is currently estimated to account for more than 80% (and growing) of all appendectomies done in the United States, which makes the ongoing debate over what may ultimately be small differences increasingly futile. However, some generalizations of the outcomes can be made based on large database analyses of both approaches.

Laparoscopic appendectomy has been definitively shown to be safe in all subgroups of patients, including children, pregnancy, complicated appendicitis, and the elderly. The laparoscopic approach has also been shown to modestly decrease postoperative pain, hospital stay, and recovery time when compared with open appendectomy. Laparoscopic appendectomy most consistently decreases wound complications when compared with the open approach but in many studies has a rate of intraabdominal/organ space infection that is higher than that of open appendectomy. Given the inconsistency in superiority of these two approaches, and true differences being relatively small, the value of the debate has decreasing clinical value.

SPECIAL CONSIDERATIONS

Pregnancy

Pregnant patients pose a considerable diagnostic and therapeutic dilemma. With modern diagnostic techniques and improved critical care, prior concerns about maternal mortality from complicated appendicitis have been largely replaced by concerns for preterm delivery and fetal loss. A study by McGory and colleagues in 2007 evaluated more than 3000 pregnant patients operated on for appendicitis, and found 30% of patients already had complicated appendicitis at presentation. Complicated appendicitis during pregnancy resulted in higher early delivery rates (11% vs 4%) and higher fetal loss rates (6% vs 2%) when compared with patients with uncomplicated appendicitis. Pregnant patients also have higher rates of negative appendectomy compared with nonpregnant counterparts (23% vs 18%, respectively). However, a negative appendectomy during pregnancy still holds rates of early delivery and fetal loss of 10% and 4%, respectively. Given these relatively high rates of early delivery and fetal loss in all groups of pregnant patients operated on for appendicitis, the ideal solution is timely diagnosis and operation for appendicitis before perforation. Use of ultrasound scan has been shown to lower negative appendectomy rates from 54% to 32% with examination alone. CT scanning can further lower negative appendectomy

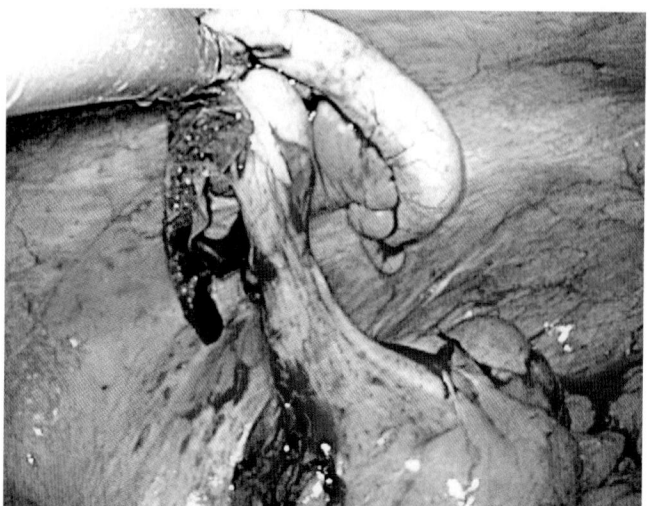

FIGURE 3   Laparoscopic view shows appendiceal vessels already divided with appendiceal base clearly seen.

rates to 8% but must be balanced with the yet unclear detriment of modern CT scanning during pregnancy, particularly during the first trimester. Patients must be counseled about all of these statistics and provided with thorough informed consent.

Incorrect Diagnosis

A negative appendix at laparoscopic evaluation provides a unique opportunity for global abdominal evaluation for an alternative diagnosis. In women, pelvic reproductive organs can be evaluated as they are high on the differential. The gallbladder can be easily evaluated, and a diligent search for a Meckel's diverticulum can also be performed. In addition, the colon and small bowel can be carefully evaluated for signs of inflammatory bowel disease. It is the view of these authors that, given the low morbidity of a completion appendectomy once laparoscopy has been established, a planned appendectomy should be carried out in all cases except when the cecum at the base of the appendix is inflamed, as the risk of postoperative leak from the appendiceal stump increases in this circumstance.

Complicated Appendicitis

Those patients who present with complicated appendicitis pose a much more difficult and debated therapeutic challenge. Traditional approach of surgery for all, regardless of perforation, revealed that patients often had prolonged hospital courses and significant morbidity after appendectomy for perforated appendicitis. This led to an era of antibiotic management without surgery for cases of documented or suspected perforated appendicitis. From these two periods, a complex debate has arisen over optimal management of these patients. To further plague the debate, very little high-quality evidence exists to point the clinician in the optimal direction. A recent meta-analysis that evaluated more than 1500 patients, while conceding overall suboptimal quality of the data, found patients who underwent initial nonoperative management for perforated appendicitis had overall lower rates of complications, particularly wound complications.

Interval Appendectomy After Nonoperative Management

For those patients who undergo initial nonoperative management of complicated appendicitis, indications for and optimal timing of interval appendectomy remain debated. Studies that follow patients for clinical recurrence show an incidence rate of 25% at 6 months from initial perforated episode, concluding little benefit to interval appendectomy in most patients. Others that follow histologic persistence/recurrence after interval appendectomy show a nearly 85% incidence rate of ongoing inflammatory changes seen at interval appendectomy and hence, justify routine performance. Overall, no high-quality data guide the management of patients initially treated nonoperatively, and this decision remains at the discretion of the surgeon. Regardless of the decision towards interval appendectomy, patients should undergo routine colonoscopy approximately 6 weeks after resolution of perforated appendicitis to rule out an oncologic source.

SUMMARY

The centuries-old approach to diagnosis of appendicitis has become simplified with the use of modern imaging. Despite these advances, many patients can still be diagnosed based on history and physical examination alone. The choice of surgical approach to appendectomy remains at the discretion of the surgeon, with numerous small benefits conferred to the laparoscopic approach, which continues to evolve as the clear dominate choice among modern surgeons for every patient group.

SUGGESTED READINGS

Faiz O, Clark J, Brown T, et al: Traditional and laparoscopic appendectomy in adults: outcomes in English NHS hospitals between 1996 and 2006, *Ann Surg* 248(5):800–806, 2008.

Fleming FJ, Kim MJ, Messing S, et al: Balancing the risk of postoperative surgical infections: a multivariate analysis of factors associated with laparoscopic appendectomy from the NSQIP database, *Ann Surg* 252(6):895–900, 2010.

Hemmila MR, Birkmeyer NJ, Arbabi S, et al: Introduction to propensity scores: a case study on the comparative effectiveness of laparoscopic vs open appendectomy, *Arch Surg* 145(10):939–945, 2010.

Korndorffer JR Jr, Fellinger E, Reed W: SAGES guideline for laparoscopic appendectomy, *Surg Endosc* 24(4):757–761, 2010; epub 2009.

McGory ML, Zingmond DS, Tillou A, et al: Negative appendectomy in pregnant women is associated with a substantial risk of fetal loss, *J Am Coll Surg* 205(4):534–540, 2007; epub 2007.

LAPAROSCOPIC INGUINAL HERNIORRHAPHY

Hien T. Nguyen, MD, FACS

OVERVIEW

Inguinal herniorrhaphy is the most common general surgery procedure performed, with 750,000 cases yearly in the United States. The lifetime risk of developing inguinal hernias is 27% in men and 3% in women, with direct annual costs at $2.5 billion. There are multiple contributing factors that lead to the development of inguinal hernias, including strain, collagen diseases, and hereditary factors. These stressors create a laxity of the muscles within the inguinal region, allowing progressive patency. Indirect hernias occur most commonly and result from the congenital invagination and eventual dilatation of a peritoneal sac running through the internal inguinal ring along the cord structures in men and round ligament in women. Direct hernias are the result of a weakened transversalis fascia lateral to the rectus muscles and above the inguinal ligament. Femoral hernias occur within the femoral canal medial to the femoral vein and are more commonly found in women with a high risk of incarceration.

The definitive treatment for inguinal hernias is surgery. The advantage of the laparoscopic approach is the ability to evaluate the entire myopectineal orifice and address all possible hernias originating from the inguinal region. The posterior approach of laparoscopic repair allows the lightweight mesh to be placed in an inlay fashion as opposed to the anterior onlay technique of open repair. There is a steeper learning curve for the laparoscopic approach compared to the open repair, as well as potentially longer operative times and higher costs. However, the benefits of the laparoscopic endeavor include less postoperative pain, shorter convalescence, and equivocal or lower recurrence rates compared to the open technique. However, complication rates for the laparoscopic approach may be higher than open until the surgeon performs up to 250 cases. Recurrence rates are lower than 6% and are commonly caused by incomplete reduction of the hernia sac, insufficient overlap of mesh over the defect, or missed small indirect hernias and cord lipomas. A common comment about laparoscopic inguinal herniorrhaphy is higher cost compared to open. The LEVEL-Trial by Langeveld and colleagues comparing laparoscopic and Lichtenstein inguinal hernia repair showed that operative costs were higher for the laparoscopic approach, mainly due to disposables and surgical equipment, but social costs were higher for the Lichtenstein approach due to more sick leave time needed. Overall, total costs were comparable between laparoscopic and Lichtenstein inguinal hernia repair, making the laparoscopic approach a worthwhile investment from the patient and societal perspectives due to decreased postoperative pain and shorter convalescence, allowing earlier return to work.

EVALUATING THE PATIENT

Patients with symptomatic inguinal hernias are candidates for surgical repair unless they have comorbidities that outweigh their risk of strangulation. According to Fitzgibbons and colleagues, minimally symptomatic men should have the option of postponing surgery with minimal risk of acute incarceration, but they have a 23% chance of requiring surgical repair within 2 years, mostly due to pain.

The patient is asked about any pressure or bulging sensation over the inguinal site, which is commonly associated with activities that increase intraabdominal pressure such as lifting or straining. Any acute onset of severe inguinal pain associated with obstructive symptoms such as nausea or vomiting suggests bowel incarceration or strangulation, which may require acute surgical intervention. Patients should also have risk factors for complications addressed such as smoking, chronic cough, constipation, and obesity.

Physical examination includes assessing for the amount of tenderness to palpation, hernia size, reducibility, and for a contralateral defect. The external inguinal ring is palpated by invaginating the scrotum with the index finger toward the pubic tubercle while the patient is standing. A defect descending into the scrotum is likely an indirect hernia, while a bulge at the external inguinal ring is a direct hernia. Femoral hernias are most commonly found in women and can be palpated below the inguinal ligament medial to the femoral vessels. Patients are asked to perform a valsalva maneuver such as coughing to palpate the impulse of a small defect and to evaluate for a subtle contralateral hernia. Griffin and colleagues found that up to 22% of patients with unilateral inguinal hernias may have an occult contralateral defect not detected on physical exam. Therefore, most patients are consented for laparoscopic evaluation for bilateral inguinal hernias.

RELEVANT ANATOMY

The preperitoneum is the space between the peritoneum and the bilaminar transversalis fascia. Both the totally extraperitoneal (TEP) and transabdominal preperitoneal (TAPP) procedures require entering this space. The anterior layer of the trasversalis fascia is attached to the rectus abdominus muscle, while the posterior transversalis fascial layer envelopes the cord structures and the bladder. Dissection of the peritoneal hernia sac off the cord structures should not disrupt

the translucent posterior transversalis fascial layer to minimize dissection injury and potential mesh irritation to the cord structures. The retropubic space of Retzius lies anterior to the bladder between the medial umbilical ligaments. The space of Bogros extends laterally from the space of Retzius toward the anterior superior iliac spine (ASIS). These spaces need to be developed to allow adequate room for repair of the inguinal hernia and mesh placement.

The pubic symphysis is the cartilaginous joint between the superior pubic rami and denotes the midline. Cooper's ligament, also known as the pectineal ligament, is a lateral extension of the lacunar ligament and forms the periosteum of the superior pubic rami.

The oval-shaped myopectineal orifice of Fruchaud is the origin of all inguinal hernias. It is bound medially by the edge of the rectus muscle, laterally by the iliopsoas muscle, superiorly by the arch of the transversus abdominus and internal oblique muscles, and inferiorly by Cooper's ligament. The iliopubic tract is a thickened fold of transversalis fascia that extends from the pubic ramus to the ASIS and divides the myopectineal orifice into a superior and inferior portion. Below this tract is the femoral canal medially and external iliac vessels laterally. The Triangle of Doom contains the external iliac artery and vein, and it is bordered medially by the ductus deferens and laterally by the spermatic vessels (Figure 1). The Triangle of Pain contains the lateral femoral cutaneous nerve, the femoral branch of the genitofemoral nerve, and the anterior branch of the femoral nerve. It is bound medially by the spermatic vessels and superolaterally by the iliopubic tract. The lateral femoral cutaneous nerve is most commonly injured and results in pain or numbness in the lateral upper portion of the thigh.

Hesselbach's triangle is bordered superolaterally by the inferior epigastric vessels, medially by the rectus muscles, and inferiorly by Cooper's ligament from the laparoscopic posterior perspective. Direct hernias protrude through Hesselbach's triangle medial to the inferior epigastric vessels, while indirect hernias enter the internal inguinal ring lateral to the epigastric vessels (Figure 2).

The inferior epigastric vessels arise from the external iliac vessels and ascend medially toward the rectus muscle between the two layers of the transversalis fascia. In 20% of patients, a large pubic branch of the inferior epigastric artery courses inferiorly across Cooper's ligament and anastomoses to the obturator artery. This aberrant vessel is called the Corona Mortis, and it can potentially be injured while dissecting areolar tissue laterally on Cooper's ligament toward the femoral canal, leading to brisk bleeding. There is also a network of veins within the lower subinguinal Space of Bogros branching from the exterial iliac, coursing underneath Cooper's ligament and along the lower lateral fibers of the rectus muscles and iliopubic tract that may be injured with dissection. Collectively, this variable deep venous circle is called the circulation of Bendavid and is composed of the suprapubic, retropubic, deep inferior epigastric, and rectusial veins (see Figure 2).

INDICATIONS AND CONTRAINDICATIONS

The laparoscopic approach is ideal for patients who are obese, have recurrence from a prior open approach, have bilateral hernias, or require an operation that may result in a shorter convalescence (Table 1). All laparoscopic inguinal hernia repairs require placing mesh in the preperitoneal space to reinforce the myopectineal orifice. This was initially performed with a TAPP approach requiring initial entry into the abdominal cavity followed by division of the peritoneum and subsequent entry into the preperitoneal space. TAPP is preferred for patients with a large hernia or a prior infraumbilical abdominal incision because the contents of a large hernia can be assessed and reduced from the abdominal cavity, and scar tissue from a prior midline incision makes TEP entry more difficult due to adhesions. However, TAPP requires a transfascial incision into the abdominal

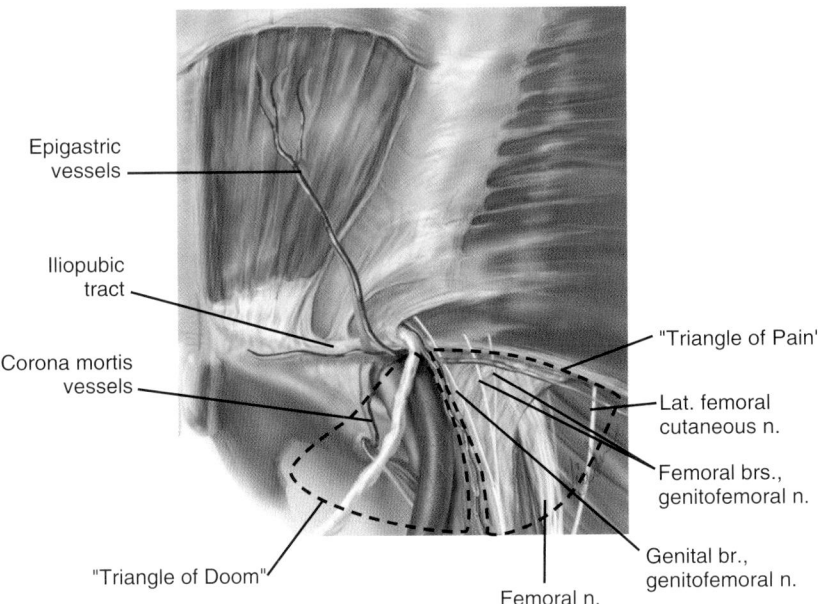

FIGURE I Triangle of doom and triangle of pain. *(Courtesy Anne Erickson, CMI.)*

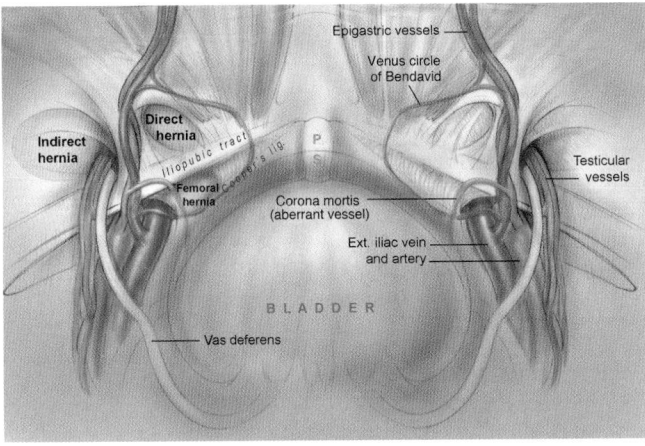

FIGURE 2 Hesselbach's triangle. *(Illustration from Cameron JL, Sandone C: Atlas of gastrointestinal surgery, ed 2, vol II (in press); used with permission from PMPH-USA, Shelton, CT.)*

TABLE I: Patient assessment for transabdominal preperitoneal versus totally extraperitoneal

Attributes	TAPP	TEP
Typical surgical candidates	Bilateral inguinal hernia	Bilateral inguinal hernia
	Recurrence from prior open inguinal hernia surgery	Recurrence from prior open inguinal hernia surgery
	Prior midline abdominal surgery	Smaller, fully reducible defect
	Prior preperitoneal surgery	
	Large, partially reducible defect	
	Morbidly obese patient	
Common complications	Bowel injury	Bleeding from injured epigastric vessels
	Port site hernia	Incomplete hernia reduction
	Mesh exposure to bowel	Higher risk of recurrence

cavity, which can lead to port site hernias and intestinal injury. TAPP also requires the divided peritoneum to be reattached to cover the mesh, which adds time to the operation. To address these issues, the TEP approach enters the preperitoneal space directly by staying above the posterior rectus sheath and peritoneal layer and never entering the abdominal cavity. TEP has a longer learning curve than TAPP due to a more limited operative field. However, TEP is associated with shorter operative time, fewer bowel injuries, and port site hernias, making it the preferred approach.

Absolute contraindications include severe illness, coagulopathy, and active severe infection. Acutely incarcerated hernias have a higher risk of bowel injury with laparoscopic manipulation and should undergo open repair. Although there are reports of laparoscopic inguinal herniorrhaphy being performed with spinal anesthesia, patients who cannot tolerate general anesthesia should undergo open repair. Relative contraindications include prior surgery in the retropubic space, sliding hernias, large chronic incarcerated hernias, and ascites.

PREPARING THE PATIENT

The patient is placed supine with video monitors at the feet, and bilateral sequential compression devices are placed on the lower extremities (Figure 3). The effectiveness of antibiotic prophylaxis is not clear. A randomized, double-blind study by Perez and colleagues looking at tension-free herniorrhaphy of 360 patients did not show a marked decrease in infections in the patient population receiving antibiotics.

After general endotracheal anesthesia is performed, the patient is positioned supine with both arms firmly tucked to the patient's side.

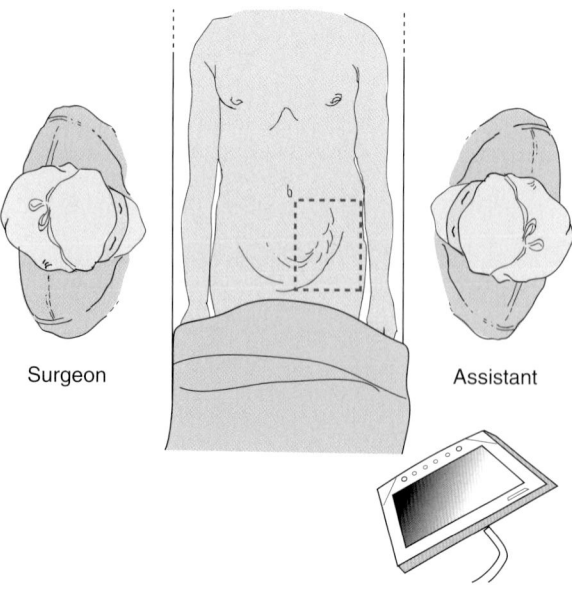

Surgeon   Assistant

FIGURE 3   Positioning of the patient and surgical team. *(Courtesy Anne Erickson, CMI.)*

A Foley is not placed to minimize the risk of postoperative urinary retention and urinary tract infections unless the patient has had prior inguinal or pelvic surgery. The patient is placed in mild Trendelenburg, and the hernia is manually reduced as much as possible.

The hair on the abdomen and groin are clipped, and the area is widely prepped with a chlorhexidine/isopropyl alcohol solution. The operative field is draped to allow for a TAPP, TEP, or open procedure using an iodophor adhesive sterile drape to keep the synthetic mesh from contacting skin.

TOTALLY EXTRAPERITONEAL

The surgeon stands on the contralateral side of the inguinal hernia. A 1-cm incision is made below the umbilicus, and blunt dissection continues past the thick orange Scarpa's fascia to the fibrous linea alba running between the rectus muscles (Figure 4). The linea alba is pulled up, and a 1-cm horizontal incision is made slightly laterally from the linea alba through the anterior rectus sheath extending toward the side with the hernia. The linea alba at midline is adherent to the peritoneum, so a deep incision will create a fascial defect communicating into the abdominal cavity. If this occurs, the defect is closed and the contralateral side can be incised to reattempt a preperitoneal approach, or a TAPP can be performed. The medial edge of the rectus muscle is visualized, and the fascial incision should be large enough to allow a finger to sweep behind the rectus muscle above the firm posterior rectus sheath (Figure 5). The rectus muscle is retracted laterally to visualize the white posterior rectus sheath. At this point, either the laparoscope or a dissecting balloon is used to bluntly dissect the preperitoneal space of Retzius. The use of the laparoscope as a blunt dissecting instrument begins with placing the scope below the rectus muscle and advancing toward the bony pubic symphysis while staying in the areolar space. Once below the arcuate ligament, the thick posterior rectus sheath is replaced by thin peritoneum. Blunt dissection is performed by moving the scope laterally within the preperitoneal plane to create enough space between the inferior epigastric vessels to allow 5-mm trocars to be placed.

The dissecting balloon can create a similar space in the preperitoneal plane (Figure 6). The balloon is placed below the rectus muscles and directed inferiorly toward the pubic symphysis. The dissecting balloon needs to be advanced with minimal effort, or either the balloon was placed too anteriorly or the incision was too

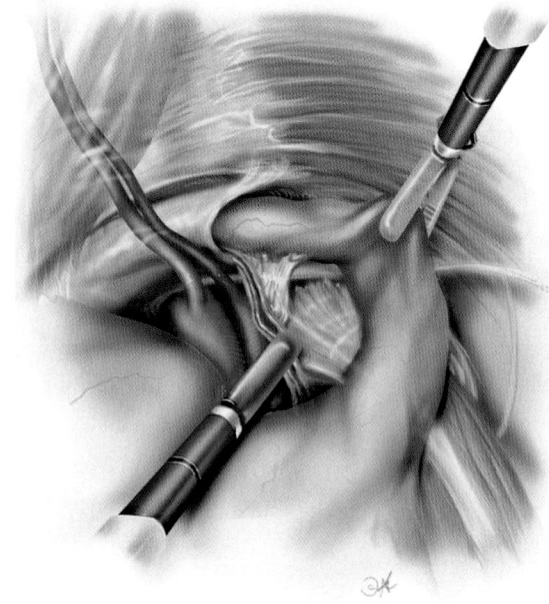

A

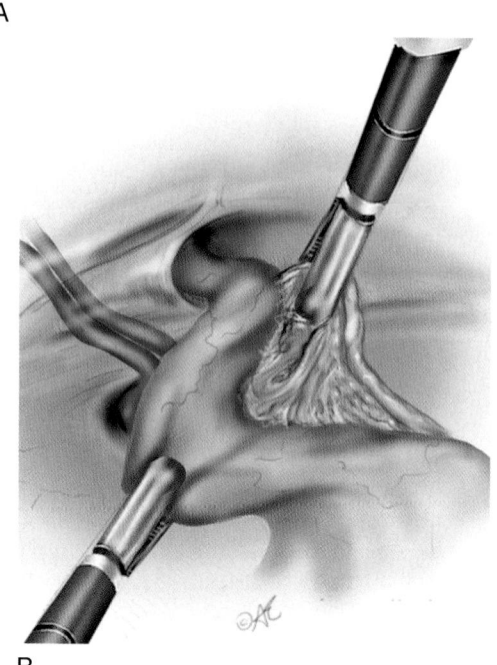

B

FIGURE 4   **A,** First maneuver in dissection of an indirect hernia sac. **B,** Second maneuver in dissection of an indirect hernia sac. *(Courtesy Anne Erickson, CMI.)*

small to accommodate the device. After the tip of the balloon touches the pubic symphysis, a 10-mm angled laparoscope is placed into the lumen of the balloon as it is inflated. Visualization of bowel or omentum means that the peritoneum is torn and the balloon is now in the abdominal cavity. If this happens, the operation can proceed as a TAPP or be converted to an open approach. Next, the inferior epigastric vessels should be seen anteriorly. Use of a dissecting balloon is associated with a higher incidence of vessel injury due to dissection between the inferior epigastric vessels and the rectus muscles. If the balloon was placed too anteriorly, insufflation should stop, and the balloon is repositioned more posteriorly to the epigastric vessels. These vessels may be subtle to visualize in obese patients and are best found by looking toward the internal inguinal ring and finding a purple-white stripe that can be traced superiorly. The

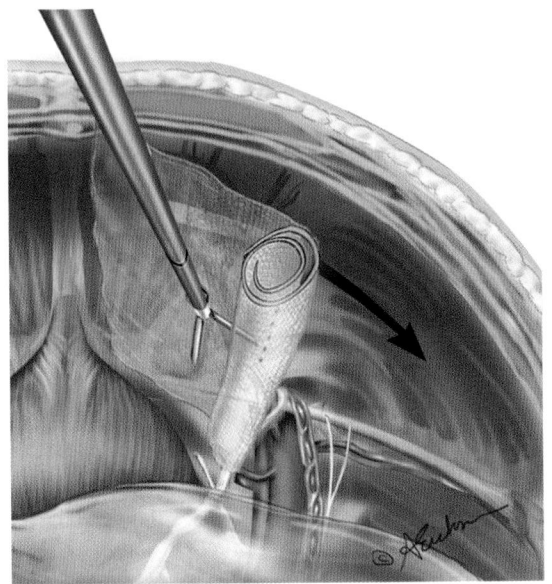

FIGURE 5 Insertion of mesh into preperitoneal space. *(Courtesy Anne Erickson, CMI.)*

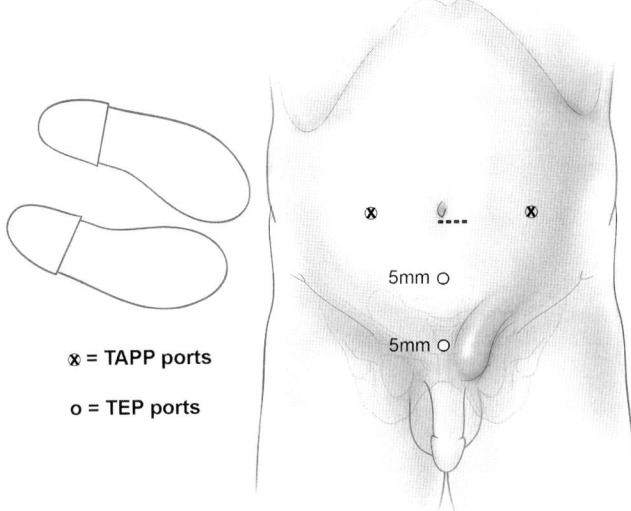

⊗ = TAPP ports

o = TEP ports

5mm ○

5mm ○

FIGURE 6 Dissecting balloon. *(Illustration from Cameron JL, Sandone C: Atlas of gastrointestinal surgery, ed 2, vol II [in press]; used with permission from PMPH-USA, Shelton, CT.)*

balloon is insufflated until a portion of the white edge of Cooper's ligament is seen. If there is minor bleeding from the dissection, the balloon is kept inflated to allow tamponade of the bleeding. Afterward, the scope and dissecting balloon are removed from this preperitoneal space and a 10-mm trocar is placed with insufflation set at 12 mm Hg to minimize subcutaneous emphysema.

The 5-mm trocars are placed inferiorly to the umbilicus through the linea alba, where space has been created to minimize the risk of tearing the peritoneum. The first 5-mm trocar is placed three fingerbreadths above the pubic symphysis to allow adequate space for mesh placement, and the second trocar is placed at the midpoint between the pubic symphysis and the umbilicus. The patient can be placed in further Trendelenburg to optimize visualization.

Dissection begins by palpating the bony pubic symphysis. The areolar space is bluntly separated to reveal Cooper's ligament as dissection continues laterally toward the femoral canal, looking for the aberrant Corona Mortis. Injury of this vessel can be prevented with gentle blunt dissection of the lateral portion of Cooper's ligament. If injury occurs, the Corona Mortis is grasped quickly to prevent posterior retraction and further bleeding, followed by clipping. Brisk bleeding can quickly obscure the injured vessel, which lies very close to the external iliac vein.

Dissection continues laterally by next identifying the inferior epigastric vessels and bluntly dissecting through the areolar tissue posterior to these vessels, with the intention of creating space toward the transversus abdominus arch and ASIS laterally. After the muscle striations of the transversus abdominus are seen laterally, dissection is continued superiorly past the ASIS to allow adequate space for mesh placement. In creating this space, the anterior-superior portion of the cord structure has been identified.

A direct hernia is encountered medially to the inferior epigastric vessels and is reduced by retracting the herniated contents posteriorly until the white edge of the weakened transversalis fascia is seen. The edge of this pseudosac is circumferentially peeled anteriorly as the herniated fatty tissue continues to be pulled posteriorly and reduced completely. The lateral edge of the defect can involve portions of the inferior epigastric vessel. If the direct defect is large, the redundant transversalis fascia can then be pulled into the preperitoneal space and tacked above Cooper's ligament medially to minimize seroma formation.

The cord structure needs to be separated from the iliac vessels to allow adequate space for the safe reduction of the indirect hernia sac. This is done most easily adjacent to the internal inguinal ring, which is identified by following the epigastric vessels inferiorly to the external iliacs. The internal inguinal ring and cord structure is directly lateral to the inferior epigastrics at this point. The cord structure spreads out in a triangular configuration proximally, with the ductus deferens being the medial border of the triangle. Loose fatty tissue overlying the cord is bluntly swept off. Once seen, the ductus is pushed anteriorly and laterally with the rest of the cord structure as gentle blunt dissection allows further separation between the cord structures and iliac vessels. The indirect sac is the thin blue-white peritoneum attached to the cord structure. Dissection adjacent to the internal inguinal ring allows identification and separation of the sac from the cord structures. The sac is often densely adherent to the cord structure and requires steady retraction to separate it from the cord structures. Blunt dissection is used to sweep the adherent tissue off the medial and lateral sides of the sac as the edge is isolated and peeled off the cord structure (Figure 7). Branches of the delicate pampiniform plexus may be adherent to the hernia sac and should be carefully handled to minimize the risk of venous thrombosis leading to testicular ischemia. Once separation between the sac and the cord structure is established, steady retraction and separation of the sac from the cord structure will allow it to be pulled out of the internal inguinal ring until the tip of the distal edge comes into view. The tip of the sac is peeled back to the psoas muscle, allowing mesh placement that will completely exclude the sac. If tearing of the sac occurs, a vessel loop or clipping is used to close the peritoneum to prevent bowel exposure to mesh and to minimize insufflation of the abdominal cavity. If necessary, veress decompression can be performed in the left upper abdominal quadrant. If the sac is large and cannot be completely separated from the cord structure, then a high ligation can be performed. After complete division, the distal sac can be seen retracting into the inguinal canal, and the proximal sac is closed with a vessel loop.

Often a large cord lipoma is identified running lateral to the cord structures into the internal inguinal ring. These lipomas can create a sizeable bulge that is clinically relevant to the patient and must be reduced from the inguinal ring. The fatty composition of the cord lipoma is slightly different from the cord fatty tissue, and the larger fat globules can be easily reduced from the inguinal canal with steady pressure, making sure that there are no vessels encased in the lipoma. Similar to a hernia sac, the cord lipoma is bluntly separated from the cord structures and reduced back from the internal inguinal ring to allow complete exclusion after the mesh is placed.

If clinically indicated, femoral hernias can be reduced by first identifying the external iliac vessels by tracing the inferior epigastrics caudally. After clearing the fatty tissue medial to the iliac vessels, the femoral canal is found below the iliopubic tract and above Cooper's ligament. The hernia is reduced with circumferential blunt

dissection. Lymphatics in the areolar tissue and large adjacent vessels require dissection directly over the hernia sac to minimize injury. If the hernia is too densely adherent or incarcerated, the operation should be converted to open to minimize catastrophic injury to the external iliac vessels.

Intraoperative evaluation of an occult contralateral hernia does not require additional skin incisions and should take less than 15 additional minutes to perform. Easy detection and repair of a contralateral hernia is a known advantage of the minimally invasive approach and saves the patient from a subsequent operation through a larger open incision or through scarred preperitoneal tissue.

After evaluation for a contralateral hernia, the operative field should have ample space from the pubic symphysis to the ASIS bilaterally. A lightweight 10×15-cm mesh can adequately cover and reinforce the myopectineal orifice on each side. The corners of the mesh are trimmed to allow ease of placement. Creating a slit in the mesh to allow the cord structures to pass may increase the risk of reherniation or chronic pain and is not done. There is commercially available mesh with a preformed notch to allow placement over the cord structures. The mesh is inserted through the 10-mm trocar and should lie flat, with the medial edge at midline over the pubic symphysis and the lateral edge at the palpable ASIS. The inferior edge of the mesh should extend 3 to 4 cm past Cooper's ligament inferiorly, leaving adequate mesh to cover the potential direct, indirect and femoral defects (Figure 8).

There is a growing body of evidence, such as studies by Messaris and colleagues, that show that hernia repair without mesh fixation does not lead to early recurrence. Furthermore, fibrin glue has also gained popularity as a way to fixate mesh with lower risk of complications from tacking such as inguinodynia. In performing a study evaluation comparing stapling versus fibrin glue fixation, we found that fibrin glue fixation achieves similar recurrence rates compared to staple fixation, but with a decreased incidence of chronic inguinal pain, and may be the preferred fixation technique. If tacking is to be performed, care must be taken to minimize risk of bleeding and bladder and nerve injury. Typically, the mesh is tacked above

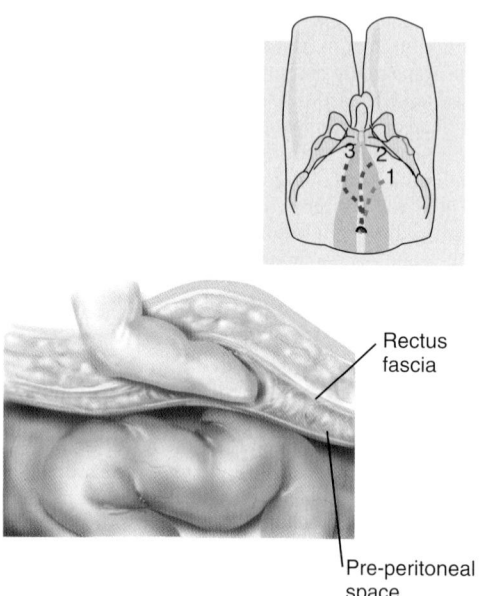

Rectus fascia

Pre-peritoneal space

FIGURE 7 Developing the preperitoneal space in the midline. *(Courtesy Anne Erickson, CMI.)*

FIGURE 8 The extraperitoneal fascial layer. *(Courtesy Anne Erickson, CMI.)*

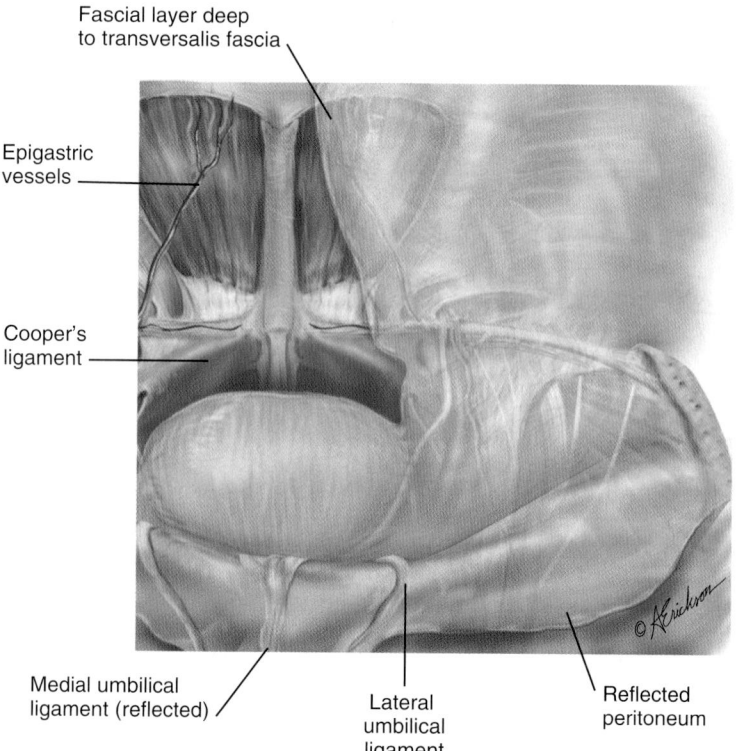

Fascial layer deep to transversalis fascia

Epigastric vessels

Cooper's ligament

Medial umbilical ligament (reflected)

Lateral umbilical ligament

Reflected peritoneum

Cooper's ligament and rectus abdominus medially, avoiding the circulation of Bendavid. The mesh is never tacked below the bony ligaments to prevent injury to the bladder. Laterally, the ASIS is palpated externally with the nondominant hand to ensure the mesh is tacked into the transversus abdominus muscle above the iliopubic tract to minimize injury to the nerves within the Triangle of Pain. A contralateral hernia is fixed similarly with a separate piece of mesh that should slightly overlap at midline.

Afterward, the operative field is evaluated for bleeding or peritoneal tears. At completion, the 5-mm trocars are removed under direct vision to check for port site bleeding. All trocars are then removed, and the preperitoneum is allowed to desufflate. Any persistent abdominal tympany means that the abdominal cavity was inadvertently insufflated due to a peritoneal tear. A Veress needle can be used to decompress the abdominal insufflation. The anterior rectus sheath incision is then closed with 0-gauge absorbable suture. Local anesthesia is injected, and the skin is reapproximated. The scrotum is checked for swelling caused by insufflation as well as a retracted testicle.

TRANSABDOMINAL PREPERITONEAL

Patient position and prepping is the same as TEP. The first incision is infraumbilical, and the abdominal cavity is entered with a Hasson technique and insufflated to 15 mm Hg. After initial laparoscopic evaluation of the abdominal cavity for overt pathology, two 5-mm trocars are then placed, each laterally from the umbilicus at the edge of the rectus muscle (see Figure 4). The patient is placed in further Trendelenberg, and the inferior epigastric vessels are followed caudally toward the external iliacs to identify the internal inguinal ring laterally and Cooper's ligament medially. A deep peritoneal indentation lateral to the inferior epigastrics at this point suggests the presence of an indirect hernia, while a broad indentation medial to the inferior epigastrics suggests a direct hernia. A punctate indentation medial to the external iliac vessels is consistent with a femoral hernia.

Herniated tissue through the defect is carefully reduced as adhesions to the pelvic peritoneum are sharply divided. The peritoneum is divided using cauterization starting laterally at the palpable ASIS and continues in an upward arc formation medially with 3 to 4 cm distance from the edge of the hernia past the medial umbilical ligament. The peritoneum is pulled away from the epigastric vessels to minimize risk of injury. The medial umbilical ligament may have a patent umbilical vessel and is clipped and divided to allow adequate access to the preperitoneal space. Once in the preperitoneal plane, blunt dissection proceeds in a manner similar to the TEP technique and continues inferiorly through the alveolar tissue toward the pubic symphysis (Figure 9). Cooper's ligament is then cleared of areolar tissue, extending toward the femoral canal.

Dissection continues laterally toward the transversus abdominus muscle between the inferior epigastric vessels and the cord structures, which are then followed into the internal inguinal ring. The entire myopectineal orifice should be visible. A direct hernia is reduced by peeling the transversalis fascia anteriorly and reducing the herniated fatty tissue back into the preperitoneal space. The transversalis fascia of a large pseudosac can then be tacked to the rectus muscle to minimize postoperative seroma formation. From within the abdominal cavity, the peritoneum of indirect hernia sac can be separated from the cord structures. The ductus deferens and adherent testicular vessels are bluntly separated from the sac, which can be completely reduced back to the psoas. Once separated from the cord structures, the sac can also be ligated if the distal tip is too firmly adherent and cannot be reduced from the inguinal canal. A femoral hernia is bluntly separated from the external iliac vessels and gently reduced. A 10 × 15-cm lightweight mesh is placed transversely in the preperitoneal space to completely reinforce the myopectineal orifice from the ASIS to the pubic symphysis, extending 3 cm inferiorly past Cooper's ligament. The edge of the mesh is cut and tucked anteriorly to the peritoneum, and the divided peritoneal edge is reapproximated to completely cover the mesh. The peritoneum can either be sutured or tacked back together with gaps less than 1 cm to prevent bowel herniation into the gaps (Figure 10). Tacks are placed flush with the

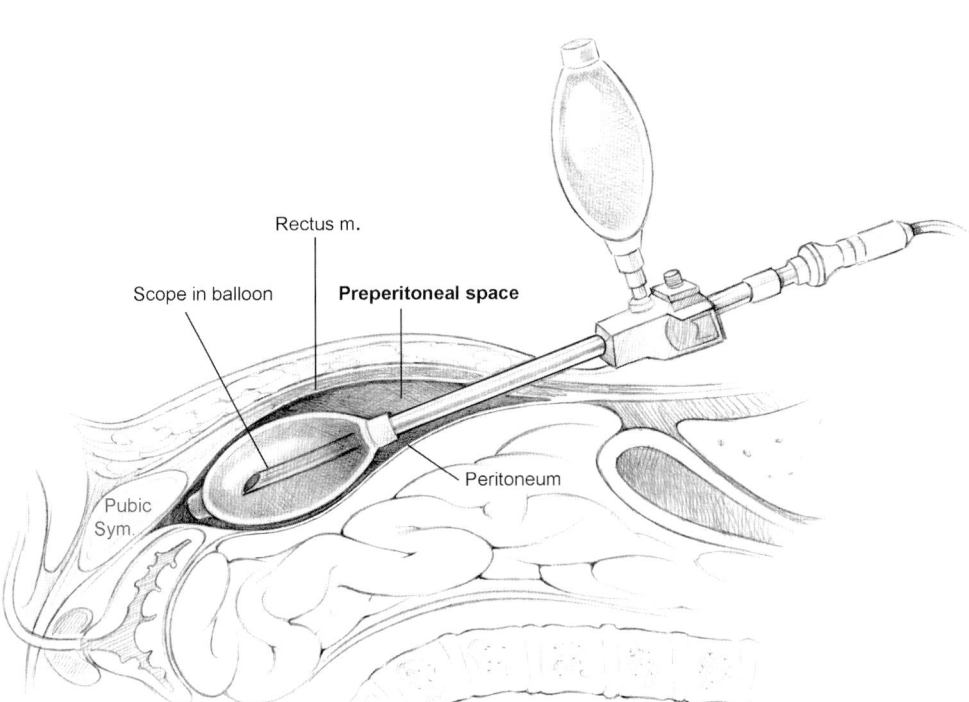

FIGURE 9 Transabdominal Ppreperitoneal (TAPP). *(Illustration from Cameron JL, Sandone C: Atlas of gastrointestinal surgery, ed 2, vol II [in press]; used with permission from PMPH-USA, Shelton, CT.)*

Rectus m.
Scope in balloon
Preperitoneal space
Peritoneum
Pubic Sym.

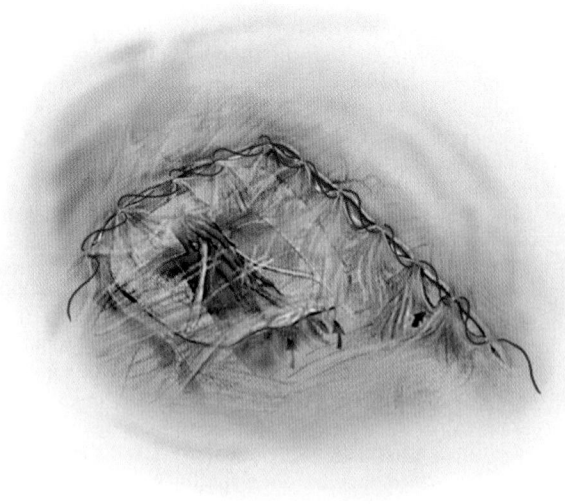

FIGURE 10 Closure of the peritoneal flap. *(Courtesy Anne Erickson, CMI.)*

abdominal wall along the edge of the divided peritoneum. A reduced hernia sac may allow the redundant peritoneum to be more mobile and allow overlap of the edges. Peritoneal tears away from the edge should be closed with vessel loops and not tacked to prevent potential injury of critical preperitoneal structures. Often the omentum can be pulled down to further insulate the operative field from the bowel. After evaluation of the contralateral side for an occult hernia, a final evaluation for bowel injury is performed. The trocars are then removed under direct vision to look for bleeding, and the abdominal cavity is desufflated. The infraumbilical fascial defect is closed with 0-gauge absorbable suture, followed by local anesthesia and skin incision closure. The scrotum and testicles are then checked for swelling and retraction, respectively.

MANAGEMENT OF COMPLICATED HERNIA

Reoperations for recurrent hernias comprise up to 17% of inguinal hernia repairs. They are typically performed laparoscopically if the prior attempt was an open approach to allow dissection within a plane with minimal scarring. Studies such as the ones by Kouhia and colleagues find that laparoscopic repair of recurrent inguinal hernia is superior to open mesh repair in several important clinical aspects, including less incidence of chronic pain and earlier return to work. Both TEP and TAPP approaches are acceptable methods with lower rerecurrence rates as compared to a reattempted repair with an open approach. The presence of prior mesh may cause the hernia sac to be more adherent and difficult to completely reduce and may require high ligation.

With large pantaloon hernias the direct and indirect defects may make dissection difficult in the TEP procedure. A TAPP approach allows more space for evaluation and reduction of the herniated contents and the hernia sac. A large direct component of the pantaloon hernia can sometimes obscure the inferior epigastric vessels. Therefore, it is reduced first to allow space for reduction of the indirect defect. A large patulous internal inguinal ring may be encountered, and the reduction of a cord lipoma first will allow easier identification and reduction of the indirect hernia sac. For large chronic hernias, high ligation may be necessary.

Incarcerated hernias are difficult to repair laparoscopically. The best approach is TAPP, where the herniated contents are visualized and potentially reduced. Placing the patient in steep Trendelenburg and applying taxis to the hernia may aid with reduction of herniated contents back into the abdominal cavity. Herniated omentum can be grasped and reduced with steady pressure, but laparoscopic reduction of incarcerated bowel can easily lead to injury, and the bowel must be inspected carefully.

Inguinal hernias are commonly found concomitantly in patients undergoing prostatectomies. Concerns regarding infection are raised with implantation of prosthetic mesh adjacent to newly formed bladder-urethral anastomosis. However, mesh infections have been shown to be low in studies such as the one published by Allaf and colleagues, prompting more patients to undergo simultaneous laparoscopic prostatectomy and inguinal herniorrhaphies with acceptable outcomes.

Laparoscopic inguinal hernia surgery after prior preperitoneal surgery can lead to a higher rate of bleeding and bladder injury. The dissection balloon of the TEP approach may cause excessive bleeding, so the TAPP approach is used because it allows controlled dissection into the adherent preperitoneal plane. If it is safe to proceed, then blunt dissection is used to find the landmarks discussed above. Mild oozing can be temporized with pressure from the endo-kuttners, and bipolar electrocauterization is judiciously used in the severely adhesed plane. The bladder can be adherent above Cooper's ligament, and a Foley catheter is used to minimize the risk of bladder injury.

AFTER SURGERY

Patients are typically discharged the same day of surgery if they have minimal discomfort, are able to ambulate, and can adequately urinate. Once discharged, patients are encouraged to remain active. Over-the-counter analgesics and compresses prior to prescription medications are encouraged for pain control. A weight restriction of 15 pounds for 1 to 2 weeks is imposed, and patients can return to their normal activities after 2 to 3 weeks. Patients follow up 2 weeks postsurgery.

COMPLICATIONS

Postoperative urinary retention is treated with catheterization. Wound infections are aggressively treated to minimize the risk of mesh infections. Seromas can occur after repair of a large direct hernia and can be clinically differentiated from hernia recurrence by palpation. Typically a recurrent hernia can be partially reduced, while a seroma is a nonreducible, firm, fluid-filled sac that causes minimal discomfort for the patient. Seromas can take 3 to 6 months to completely resolve, and aspiration is seldom required unless the patient is severely symptomatic. If necessary, aspiration is performed with sterile technique to minimize the risk of mesh infection.

According to Ferzli and colleagues, postoperative chronic inguinodynia can range from 9.7% to 34%, and occurs more commonly in obese patients and those with significant preoperative pain (Table 2). Mild postoperative discomfort can be explained by nerve irritation from extensive dissections and should be transient. Antiinflammatory treatment and compresses should provide relief. Severe immediate postoperative pain of the inguinal region is usually due to nerve entrapment by a lateral tack. Use of fibrin glue or positioning of the tacker above the ASIS should minimize nerve injury, but a small percentage of patients have aberrant nerves found above the iliopubic tract that can potentially be injured despite appropriate technique. These patients are taken back to the operating room, and the lateral tacks are removed. Although the risk of testicular infarction is low with laparoscopic inguinal hernia, patients presenting 2 to 3 days after surgery with severe testicular pain and swelling should undergo Doppler sonography to evaluate the testicular blood flow.

Bowel injury should lead to conversion to open, at which time the bowel is thoroughly assessed and repaired. In the setting of contamination, synthetic mesh should not be used due to the high risk of mesh infection. The inguinal hernia can then be repaired with either a biologic mesh or a nonmesh technique such as a Bassini or a McVay procedure. The long-term efficacy with the use of biologic mesh for inguinal herniorrhaphy is not known.

Bleeding from injury to the inferior epigastric vessels can be controlled in many ways, including clipping, ligation with a suture-passer, or use of a 5-mm energy ligation device. The epigastric vessels are fed caudally from the external iliacs, so controlling the caudal side first will slow the bleeding more substantially. Injury to the iliac vessels requires immediate action after recognition. The site of injury to the iliac vessel needs to be grasped, and pressure is held to minimize the bleeding as the case is converted to open. This is done expeditiously because iliac vein injury has the additional risk of air embolism.

SUMMARY

The laparoscopic inguinal herniorrhaphy can be performed safely and with good outcomes. Advantages include smaller wounds, shorter convalescence, and the ability to assess both sides. Earlier in the learning curve, surgeons should be comfortable with TAPP prior to attempting TEP and have a low threshold for conversion to open. Most of the operation can be performed with blunt dissection (Table 3).

ACKNOWLEDGMENT

The author would like to thank the following people for their help with this chapter: Mike Rosen, Bruce Ramshaw, Michael Schweitzer, Thomas Magnuson, Mark Duncan, Fatima Khambaty, Jenny Hong, Josh Grimm, and James Harris.

TABLE 2: Postherniorrhaphy pain

Types	Examples
Neuropathic factors	Nerve entrapment
	Nerve irritation due to aggressive dissection
	Neuroma formation
Postsurgical factors	Osteitis pubis
	Hernia recurrence
	Mesh irritation
Visceral factors	Cord irritation
	Ischemic orchitis

TABLE 3: Comparison of TAPP and TEP: steps of surgery

	TAPP	TEP
Entry	Hasson entry into abdominal cavity first Peritoneum divided to enter preperitoneal space	Division of infraumbilical anterior rectus sheath Blunt dissection of preperitoneal space and abdominal cavity is never entered
Insufflation pressure	15 mm Hg	12 mm Hg
Port placement	Lateral to rectus muscles at level of umbilicus	Through linea alba below umbilicus
Dissection	Pubic symphysis identified Dissection laterally over Cooper's ligament Dissection of space inferior to epigastric vessels toward transversus abdominus	Pubic symphysis identified Dissection laterally over Cooper's ligament Dissection of space inferior to epigastric vessels toward transversus abdominus Dissection of space between cord structures and iliac vessels
Hernia reduction	Herniated contents viewed from abdominal cavity and can be gently reduced Direct hernia contents reduced posteriorly and transversalis fascia pseudosac peeled off anteriorly Indirect hernia sac visualized from abdominal cavity and can be bluntly dissected off cord structures	Herniated contents never visualized unless peritoneum is torn Direct hernia contents reduced posteriorly and transversalis fascia pseudosac peeled off anteriorly Indirect hernia sac bluntly dissected off cord structures
Mesh placement	Must cover entire myopectineal orifice Spans from pubic symphysis to ASIS, extending 3 cm inferiorly past Cooper's ligament Tack vs fibrin glue vs free positioning of mesh Edge must be completely covered by reapproximated peritoneum	Must cover entire myopectineal orifice Spans from pubic symphysis to ASIS, extending 3 cm inferiorly past Cooper's ligament Tack vs fibrin glue vs free positioning of mesh
Closure	Peritoneal edges sutured together or tacked with 1-cm gaps Mesh must be completely covered by peritoneum Infraumbilical transfascial incision closed	Infraumbilical anterior rectus sheath closed

SUGGESTED READINGS

Eklund A, Montgomery A, Bergkvist L, et al: Swedish Multicentre Trial of Inguinal Hernia Repair by Laparoscopy (SMIL) study group: chronic pain 5 years after randomized comparison of laparoscopic and Lichtenstein inguinal hernia repair, *Br J Surg* 97(4):600–608, 2010.

Matthews RD, Neumayer L: Inguinal hernia in the 21st century: an evidence-based review, *Curr Probl Surg* 45(4):261–312, 2008.

Rosenberger R, Loeweneck H, Meyer G: The cutaneous nerves encountered during laparoscopic repair of inguinal: new anatomical findings for the surgeon, *Surg Endosc* (8):731–735, 2000.

Shah NR, Mikami DJ, Cook C, et al: A comparison of outcomes between open and laparoscopic surgical repair of recurrent inguinal hernias, *Surg Endosc* 25(7):2330–2337, 2011.

LAPAROSCOPIC REPAIR OF RECURRENT INGUINAL HERNIAS

Amir H. Fathi, MD, and Yuri W. Novitsky, MD

OVERVIEW

The first evidence of operative repair of a groin hernia dates to the first century AD. In the late 1880s, Bassini revolutionized the surgical repair of inguinal hernias with his novel anatomic dissection and low recurrence rates. However, in the 1990s, the tension-free Lichtenstein (anterior) mesh hernioplasty essentially became the operation of choice. Subsequently, technique modifications included the use of cone shape meshes "plugs" for groin hernia repairs. Recently, inguinal hernia repair has undergone another transformation with the advent of laparoscopic surgery. Two main laparoscopic (posterior) approaches have been described: totally extraperitoneal (TEP) and transabdominal preperitoneal (TAPP) repairs. Sixteen randomized, controlled trials and meta-analyses that compared laparoscopic and open techniques demonstrated that laparoscopic repair has a definite and likely beneficial role in modern surgery.

Beyond doubt, the traditional benefits of minimal access are pertinent for laparoscopic inguinal hernia repairs. It has been shown that the laparoscopic approach is associated with less postoperative pain, shorter hospital stays, decreased chronic pain, and increased patient satisfaction. The ultimate measure of success in hernia surgery is the rate of recurrence, regardless of the technique of repair. Although other procedure-related events are important and have been shown to affect health-related quality-of-life parameters, recurrence is one of the most difficult and frustrating issues facing both patients and surgeons. From the surgeon's perspective, repair of a recurrent inguinal hernia is technically more challenging because of prior mesh placement and scar tissue within dissected planes. For the patient, the initial physical and mental investment in the operation has failed, and subsequent operations carry fewer guarantees for success, more risks for serious complications, and the prospect of additional pain and recovery time. Currently, surgical repair of recurrent inguinal hernias account for 8% to 17% of more than 700,000 repairs performed each year in the United States. Although much has been published about primary repair of inguinal hernias, less is known about the best approach to address recurrent inguinal hernias.

INDICATIONS AND CHOICE OF THE REPAIR

The signs and symptoms of a recurrent inguinal hernia are usually similar to the initial herniation. However, only minimal pain and/or bulging is often present. Interestingly, most patients with recurrence are familiar with how their hernia "felt" the first time and will seek medical care if and when their symptoms recur. In fact, in our experience, most patients can even pinpoint the time their recurrence began to develop.

One of the important considerations in evaluating for a recurrent inguinal hernia is a missed femoral hernia, especially in women. In 2005, a large prospective analysis of inguinal hernia repair data from the Swedish Hernia registry showed at the time of reoperation, more than 40% of women previously reported to have inguinal hernias were found to have femoral defects. We found that patients with misdiagnosed femoral hernias will often report persistent discomfort and even bulging following the original operation. High index of suspicion, especially in elderly females, is mandatory to avoid missing a femoral defect when an anterior approach is undertaken.

The choice of repair of a recurrent inguinal hernia depends on a number of patient factors; however, the technique of the original operation is largely the main determinant of the surgical approach to be chosen (Figure 1). Initial repairs can consist of primary (no mesh) tissue-based repairs, such as Bassini, McVay, or Shouldice repairs. If a mesh was used, the plane of mesh placement as well as the type/shape of a prosthetic varies greatly. Primary anterior mesh repair, such as Lichtenstein, employs a flat mesh placed ventral to the floor of the inguinal canal. Posterior repairs, including retromuscular Stoppa and Kugel repairs, as well as the traditional laparoscopic repairs, involve a prosthetic placed dorsal to the floor of the inguinal canal. Finally, repairs with plugs or two-layered meshes (such as the Prolene Hernia System; Ethicon, Inc., Cincinnati, Ohio) violate both anterior and posterior planes, and failures of those repairs may present additional challenges for subsequent herniorrhaphies.

A vigilant review of previous operative reports is paramount in guiding the ensuing repair technique. In addition to patient factors, the choice of the procedure should be adjusted according to the surgeon's personal experience and the degree of laparoscopic skill/expertise. In certain cases, however, a referral to a more experienced surgeon may be warranted to minimize performing a necessary but less familiar operation. Multiple recurrent inguinal hernias with failed both anterior and posterior repairs represent a very formidable challenge, even in experienced hands.

Although we favor the laparoscopic approach to patients with failed open tissue–based repairs, either open anterior or open posterior approach is quite acceptable. However, if the initial anterior repair involved mesh placement, we recommend favoring an approach

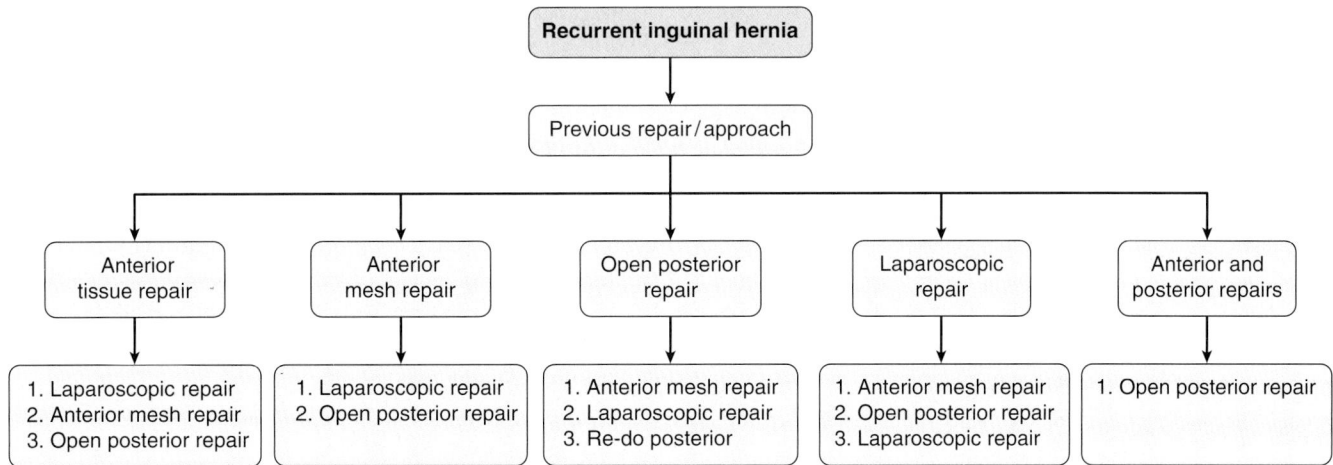

FIGURE 1   Recurrent inguinal hernia surgical repair/approach.

utilizing the space in which the tissue planes have not been violated previously (see Figure 1). A posterior approach including laparoscopic techniques is clearly the best choice after failed anterior repair. In our practice we utilize laparoscopy for failed anterior repairs in all cases except for patients with significant scrotal herniations and those with previous abdominopelvic procedures. The latter group is better served by an open posterior retromuscular or preperitoneal Stoppa repair.

Laparoscopic Repair of Recurrent Inguinal Hernias

Laparoscopic inguinal hernia repair affords the benefit of a panoramic view of the entire myopectineal orifice of Fruchaud. Therefore, all the potential hernia spaces, such as direct and indirect inguinal, femoral, and obturator defects, can be diligently evaluated. The laparoscopic approach for recurrent inguinal hernias after anterior repairs not only provides the technical advantage of operating through unscarred tissue but still carries the added advantages of a minimally invasive procedure. Without a doubt, failed anterior repairs are best approached laparoscopically. We strongly believe that those patients should be referred to centers where laparoscopic expertise is available.

The laparoscopic approach to failed laparoscopic repairs represents a significant technical challenge. In select cases, previously placed mesh may have been undersized or may have shrunk, making a redo laparoscopic repair fairly routine. However, the majority of those patients have extensive scarring of the preperitoneal plane, with the old mesh creating a major impediment to the dissection. Only surgeons with significant expertise in laparoscopy and laparoscopic inguinal hernia repairs should attempt to redo laparoscopic/posterior failures laparoscopically.

TEP Versus TAPP

There is a paucity of reliable data comparing TAPP and TEP, with no prospective randomized trials investigating repair efficacy. Recently, Bittner and colleagues published guidelines for TAPP and TEP repairs of inguinal hernia based on the Cochrane database review. They concluded that there was no statistically significant difference regarding postoperative complications, recurrence rates, and chronic groin pain. We have adopted TAPP as our approach of choice for both routine and recurrent inguinal hernias. We found that our approach allows for a reliable and reproducible dissection of the entire myopectineal orifice and allows for identification of both ipsilateral and contralateral herniations. In addition, surgeons who prefer the TEP approach must still be versed in TAPP to minimize the need for open conversions in cases of significant peritoneal tears.

Operative Considerations

As mentioned above, careful review of the antecedent operative report is of utmost importance, especially in cases of recurrence and associated groin pain. Review of the size, type, and shape of the mesh used, as well as the fixation method employed, is paramount for successful operative planning. If significant discomfort is present, we plan for the old mesh removal during reoperation. Preoperative counseling should include discussion of risks of visceral injuries, bleeding, vas deferens injury, chronic groin pain, and recurrence.

The patient is positioned supine with both arms tucked in the adducted position. The patient should be prepped widely to include the entire abdomen and both groin regions to midthigh. In contrast to our standard laparoscopic approach for initial inguinal hernias, patients with recurrent hernias routinely have a urinary catheter placed. This not only facilitates identification of the bladder by allowing for its distention (if necessary) but also allows for prompt identification of an inadvertent bladder injury during Cooper ligament dissection.

Once safe access to the peritoneal cavity is obtained, we perform a diagnostic laparoscopy to confirm the diagnosis. It is important to point out that the mechanism of recurrence varies depending on the original choice of the repair. Anterior repairs usually fail medially, and posterior recurrences usually occur inferiorly. At times, laparoscopic repairs fail because of inadequately sized mesh or cases of significant prosthetic migration or shrinkage. In those circumstances, the recurrence pattern may mimic the anterior failures.

We initiate our dissection just below the arcuate line. A preperitoneal plane is entered. We try to avoid dissecting in the pretransversalis fascia plane to minimize bleeding from the inferior epigastric vessels and easier dissection of the Cooper's ligament and myopectineal orifice. In cases of failed posterior or plug repairs, previous prosthetic may significantly complicate this dissection. In addition, those meshes often encase the inferior epigastric vessels. In those circumstances, we tend to control inferior epigastric vessels with clips both proximal and distal to the mesh to minimize bleeding. In addition, the meshes in these instances may extend very close to the iliac vessels, and thorough knowledge and understanding of anatomy are critical to avoid major vascular injuries. Similarly, the vas deferens may be closely adherent to the mesh and may need to be sacrificed during this dissection. Furthermore, a portion of the old mesh could be left behind if its dissection from the iliac vessels is difficult and/or deemed too risky.

Subsequent dissection is carried out to expose the inferior aspect of the myopectineal orifice and distal 2 to 3 cm of the psoas muscle. This extent is necessary to prevent recurrences along the inferior edge of the mesh due to inadequate mesh coverage. Once again, thorough knowledge of anatomic landmarks is critical to avoid neurovascular injuries.

Once the mesh is placed, we utilize tackers to fixate the mesh at Cooper's ligament as well as anterior-medially and anterior-laterally. No tacks are placed below the inguinal ligament or near any areas of neurovascular structures. We favor absorbable tacks, although there is no solid scientific evidence that supports such practice. Often, fibrin glue is used to fixate the inferior aspect of the mesh. Finally, the peritoneum is reclosed with tacks. In cases of significant peritoneal tears due to a difficult dissection or removal of the old mesh, we advocate the use of coated meshes with an antiadhesion barrier while leaving the peritoneal flap open. This approach will minimize the risks of intestinal obstruction in a peritoneal fenestration or avoid

bowel exposure to the uncoated synthetic mesh. We advocate against the use of biologic or bioabsorbable meshes during laparoscopic repair of recurrent inguinal hernias.

OUTCOMES

To date, contrary to primary inguinal hernias, there is no ample body of literature comparing laparoscopic approaches to open techniques for recurrent inguinal hernias. The results from large randomized studies have demonstrated that the Lichtenstein repair carries a low recurrence rate. However, a number of meta-analyses that have compared laparoscopic and open hernioplasty techniques have indicated that patients undergoing laparoscopic hernia repair experience less pain in the early postoperative period, have lower analgesic and narcotic requirements, return to their normal activities sooner, and have better cosmetic outcomes (Table 1). Eklund and colleagues from the Swedish Multicenter Trial of Inguinal Hernia Repair by Laparoscopy (SMIL) published a randomized trial and compared TAPP and

TABLE 1: Studies comparing open to laparoscopic recurrent inguinal hernia repair

First author	Type of repair	Type of study	Number of points	Findings
Yang (2012)	Lap (TAPP & TEP) versus open (mesh and nonmesh)	Meta-analysis	427	Recurrence, wound hematoma, urinary retention: No difference. Chronic pain, wound infection: Significantly less in lap group.
Demetrashvili (2011)	Open verus TAPP	Randomized controlled trials, single center	52	Recurrence, wound hematoma, urinary retention: No difference. Chronic pain, wound infection: Significantly less in lap group.
Karthikesalingam (2009)	Lap (TAPP & TEP) versus open (mesh and nonmesh)	Meta-analysis	404	Recurrence, wound hematoma: No difference. Chronic pain, return to daily activity, wound infection: Significantly less in lap group.
Kouhia (2009)	Open versus TEP (mesh)	Randomized controlled trials, single center	96	Recurrence, wound hematoma: No difference. Chronic pain, return to daily activity, wound infection: Significantly less in lap group.
Eklund (2007)	Open versus TAPP (Mesh)	Randomized controlled trials, multi center	147	Recurrence, wound hematoma, urinary retention: No difference. Chronic pain, return to daily activity, wound infection: Significantly less in lap group.
Feliu (2004)	Open versus TEP (mesh)	Prospective controlled study, single center	235	Less overall postoperative complication rate in TEP recurrence: No difference.
Dedemadi (2006)	Open versus TEP and TAPP (mesh)	Randomized controlled trials, single center	82	Recurrence, wound hematoma, urinary retention: No difference. Chronic pain, return to daily activity, wound infection: Significantly less in lap group.
Kumar (1999)	Open versus TEP (mesh)	Randomized controlled trials, single center	50	Recurrence, wound hematoma, urinary retention: No difference. Chronic pain: Significantly less in lap group
Beets(1999)	Open versus TAPP (mesh)	Randomized controlled trials, single center	79	Recurrence, wound hematoma: No difference. Chronic pain, return to daily activity, wound infection: Significantly less in lap group

TEP, Totally extraperitoneal; *TAPP*, transabdominal preperitoneal.

Lichtenstein repairs for recurrent inguinal hernias. They concluded that the short-term advantage for patients undergoing laparoscopic technique is less postoperative pain and shorter convalescence. In the long term, no differences were observed in the chronic pain or recurrence rate. In a recent prospective randomized trial, Sanna and colleagues showed the TEP technique to be superior to the Lichtenstein hernioplasty in treating recurrent inguinal hernias with regards to chronic pain, impaired sensibility in the inguinal region, and accelerated return to normal activity. However, it is important to point out that in our experience, the laparoscopic approach to failed posterior repairs is usually associated with prolonged dissection as well as frequent peritoneal tears. As a result, the major benefit of laparoscopy with regards to decreased pain and fast recovery is typically lost or minimized.

With recent advances in surgical techniques and equipment, increasing numbers of surgeons are using laparoscopic procedures for the management of recurrent inguinal hernias. However, the cost-effectiveness, patient satisfaction, and recurrence rates associated with laparoscopic repair are currently under investigation at our institution.

SUGGESTED READINGS

Bignell M, Partridge G, Mahon D, et al: Prospective randomized trial of laparoscopic (TAPP) versus open (mesh) repair for bilateral and recurrent inguinal hernia: incidence of chronic groin pain and impact on quality of life: results of 10 year follow-up, *Hernia* 16(6):635–640, 2012.

Bittner R, Arregui ME, Bisgaard T, et al: Guidelines for laparoscopic (TAPP) and endoscopic (TEP) treatment of inguinal hernia [International Endohernia Society (IEHS)], *Surg Endosc* 25(9):2773–2843, 2011.

Eklund A, Rudberg C, Leijonmarck C-E, et al: Recurrent inguinal hernia: randomized multicenter trial comparing laparoscopic and Lichtenstein repair, *Surg Endosc* 21:634–640, 2007.

Karthikesalingam A, Markar SR, Holt PJE, et al: Meta-analysis of randomized controlled trials comparing laparoscopic with open mesh repair of recurrent inguinal hernias, *Br J Surg* 97(1):4–11, 2010.

LAPAROSCOPIC VENTRAL HERNIA REPAIR

Michael J. Rosen, MD, FACS

INTRODUCTION

Ventral hernia repair is one of the most common procedures performed by general surgeons. Ventral hernias can be defined as primary or acquired. Primary hernias include epigastric, umbilical, spigelian (lateral), and rare hypogastric hernias. Acquired hernias can occur after traumatic events but most commonly are related to a prior surgical incision. The incidence rate of incisional hernia formation after a midline laparotomy is estimated at 10% to 20%, depending on the patient population at risk. With almost 2 million laparotomies performed annually, somewhere between 100,000 and 200,000 ventral hernia repairs are performed annually in the United States. Despite the prevalence of this disease, no universally accepted classification system exists. As a result, there is a wide spectrum of patients that development of ventral hernias, and significant variability is found in the complexity of ventral hernia defects. This spectrum includes those patients with small asymptomatic defects up to patients with massive hernias, loss of domain, and concomitant contamination present during repair. As a result of this diversity, no single repair technique is likely to take care of all patients with ventral hernias. Therefore, surgeons repairing abdominal wall defects should be familiar with both laparoscopic and open approaches to ventral hernias to offer the patient the most appropriate repair technique on the basis of unique patient factors and hernia defect characteristics (Table 1).

The laparoscopic approach to ventral/incisional hernia repair has gained widespread acceptance by the surgical community as a safe and effective approach. It borrows from the principles of abdominal wall reconstruction espoused by Rives and Stoppa of placement of a large sublay prosthetic deep to the hernia defect to provide wide coverage. Unlike the open counterpart, the laparoscopic approach requires the mesh to be placed within the peritoneal cavity. This mandates the use of appropriate tissue-separating prosthetics with a visceral side that prevents bowel ingrowth and an abdominal side that promotes tissue integration. The prosthetic should be fixed with full-thickness transfascial fixation sutures and spiral tacks. Given the absence of subcutaneous soft tissue dissection, a predictably lower rate of wound and mesh infections is seen, which is a major advantage of the laparoscopic approach. The laparoscopic repair also allows for full visualization of the entire anterior abdominal wall to avoid missing small Swiss cheese–type defects.

INDICATIONS

The natural history of an asymptomatic ventral/incisional hernia is largely unknown. Because surgical teaching has always suggested that these hernias pose significant risk for bowel incarceration or strangulation, most surgeons advocate repair on diagnosis of an incisional hernia. No large cohort of patients who have undergone nonoperative management is available, so the natural history remains largely unknown. However, given the increases in intraabdominal pressures with activities of daily living, a ventral hernia tends to grow over time, which makes repair increasing difficult once the hernias become very large. Incisional hernias can also result in unsightly bulges that impact quality of life. In addition, the thin skin overlying a large hernia can become ischemic, ulcerate, and even result in an ascitic leak. The three general indications for operation are: (1) a hernia that is symptomatic and causes pain, discomfort, surrounding cutaneous ulcerations, or changes in bowel habits; (2) a hernia that results in an unsightly bulge and affects the patient's quality of life; and (3) a hernia that poses a significant risk of bowel obstruction (e.g., a large hernia with a narrow neck). In consideration of operative intervention, an individualized approach is important, with patient comorbidities, defect characteristics, and the presence of contamination taken into account. Because a wide spectrum of patients develop a variety of hernias, one single technique is not able to address all patients. Few absolute contraindications are found for a laparoscopic ventral hernia repair, other than inability to tolerate general anesthesia or the presence of active contamination. However, several relative contraindications deserve mention. The ability to perform safe adhesiolysis is paramount to a successful laparoscopic ventral hernia repair; therefore, patients at risk for severe adhesions should likely not undergo a laparoscopic approach. Examples include patients

TABLE 1: Results of prospective randomized studies that compare laparoscopic with open ventral hernia repairs

Study	No. of patients	Mesh used	Complication rate	Recurrence rate
Itani (2010)				
Laparoscopic	73	PTFE	32%	13%
Open	73	Polypropylene	48%	8%
Olmi (2007)				
Laparoscopic	85	Polyester/collagen	17%	2%
Open	85	Polypropylene	29%	4%
Pring (2008)				
Laparoscopic	31	PTFE	33%	3%
Open	27	PTFE	49%	4%
Asencio (2009)				
Laparoscopic	45	PTFE/polypropylene	5%	10%
Open	39	Polypropylene	33%	8%

PTFE, Polytetrafluoroethylene.

with multiple reoperative abdomens, in particular with multiple intraperitoneal prosthetic meshes. Patients who have undergone prior intraperitoneal dialysis are at high risk for an obliterated peritoneal cavity. Patients with massive defects and loss of domain can be successfully completed laparoscopically but an advanced laparoscopic skill set is needed, which generally involves multiple pieces of mesh sewn together and a poor functional and cosmetic result. Patients with excessive scars that need revision should undergo an open repair. Patients with inflammatory bowel disease, in particular, Crohn's disease, should likely not have intraperitoneal mesh placed given the likelihood of reoperations and potential fistulas. Patients with larger defects of more than 10 to 12 cm in width are better served with an open formal abdominal wall reconstruction. The ideal candidate for a laparoscopic ventral hernia repair is an obese or elderly patient with a small to medium-sized defect. Thin, active, manual laborer patients are offered a formal abdominal wall reconstruction either laparoscopically with defect closure as described subsequently or open.

PREOPERATIVE WORKUP

A complete history and physical examination is important in ventral hernia cases. These patients often have significant comorbidities, and consideration of optimizing preoperative glucose control, nutritional parameters, smoking cessation, and weight reduction is key to a successful outcome. In addition, particular attention should be paid to the anterior abdominal wall skin for ulcerations or nonhealing wounds that might preclude a laparoscopic approach. Incarcerated hernias that cannot be reduced can be difficult laparoscopically and should be discerned before surgery. Locations of all prior surgical incisions are noted, and all prior operative reports are reviewed. Important information as to the type and location of prior prosthetic mesh and the history of upper quadrant surgery that could alter the initial access port is critical. A computed tomographic (CT) scan of the abdomen is performed in all but the smallest hernias in the author's practice. This image can provide valuable information as to the size of the defect, the contents of the hernia sac, the presence of occult hernias that might not be palpable in an obese patient, and the presence of prior synthetic mesh. In addition, the integrity of the rectus muscles and lateral abdominal wall musculature can be assessed for reconstructive options. Preoperative counseling is also

important for patients undergoing laparoscopic ventral hernia repair. Despite the minimally invasive nature of laparoscopic ventral hernia repair, postoperative pain is often similar to the open procedure. Because the hernia sac is often not excised, a postoperative seroma is almost universally present and the patient should be aware. The possibility of an enterotomy and the appropriate management, including the need to convert to an open procedure, should be clarified.

OPERATIVE TECHNIQUE

Patient Positioning

For patients with midline incisional hernias, patients are placed in the supine position with their arms tucked to the sides. Having the arms tucked facilitates the surgeon standing on the same side of the table as the camera operator (Figure 1). An iodine-impregnated adhesive drape is applied to the skin to protect the mesh from skin flora and facilitate marking the patient during mesh placement. A first generation cephalosporin is given, orogastric tube is placed, and a three-way Foley catheter is placed for any defect below the umbilicus to aid in identification of the bladder during dissection. Pneumatic compression devices are applied, and subcutaneous heparin is administered before surgery.

Access of the Reoperative Abdomen and Trocar Positioning

Gaining access to the reoperative abdomen can be the most treacherous step of a laparoscopic ventral hernia repair. Typically, the upper quadrants are free of adhesions, and the tip of the 11th rib provides a good access point. Attention to prior surgical incisions and intraabdominal procedures can provide clues as to the most appropriate side. For instance, patients who have had their splenic flexure mobilized should be approached through the right upper quadrant. Several methods have been described for access, including an open cut down approach, utilization of optical viewing trocars, and the use of a Veress needle. In skilled hands, each of these approaches is safe and effective and can be used. In general, this access point should be

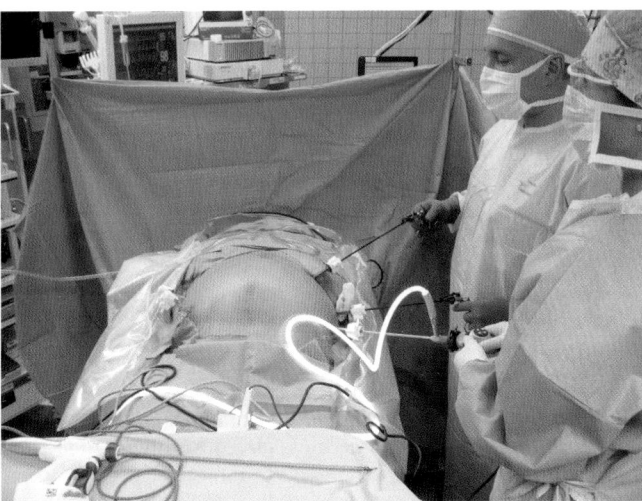

FIGURE 1   Intraoperative view of surgeon and camera operator standing on the same side of patient for adhesiolysis. Patient's arms are abducted and an iodine impregnated drape covers the abdomen.

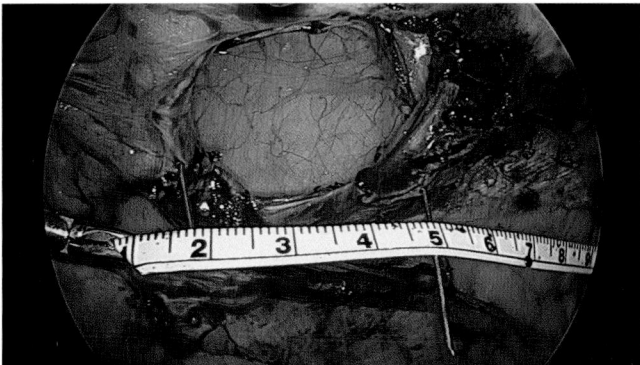

FIGURE 2   Intraperitoneal view of spinal needles placed at the edge of the defect and measured with a 15-cm plastic ruler.

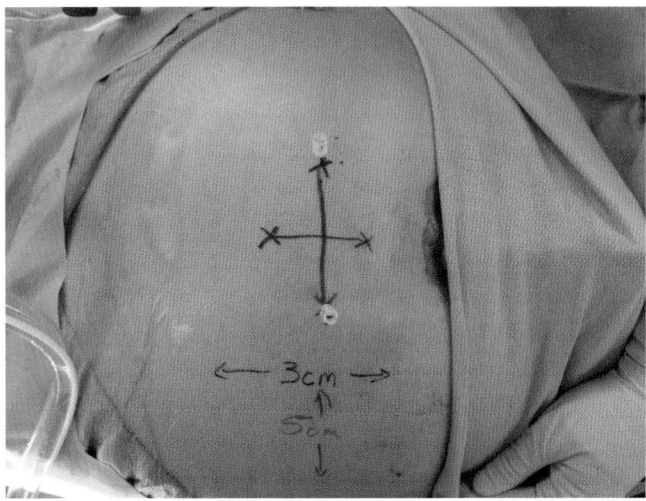

FIGURE 3   External lines mark maximal width and length of hernia defect measured internally with spinal needles.

as far lateral as possible to avoid being covered during mesh placement. Once the abdomen is accessed and insufflated, two additional 5-mm ports are placed ipsilateral to this trocar. This facilitates two-handed technique during adhesiolysis and avoids working in reverse to the camera during dissection. Once the adhesions are completely lysed, at least 1 or 2 additional 5-mm ports are placed on the contralateral side to position and secure the mesh. A 5-mm 30-degree laparoscope is helpful to allow placement through any of the trocars during adhesiolysis, and the angled scope provides superior vision around adhesions and up to the anterior abdominal wall.

Adhesiolysis

The most dangerous part of a laparoscopic ventral hernia repair is safe adhesiolysis. This can be the most time-consuming portion of the case and requires patience and meticulous technique. In general, no electrocautery should be used during adhesiolysis. In particular, vessel-sealing devices such as the ultrasonic dissector or Ligasure (Covidien, Boulder, Colo) should be avoided because they can create a sealed full-thickness injury to the bowel wall that does not leak for several days. If bleeding occurs, liberal use of 5-mm clips is warranted, or the surgeon should convert to an open approach. If prior intraperitoneal mesh is present, avoid blunt sweeping movements because the bowel will likely give way before the mesh. In cases in which the mesh is densely adherent to the intestines, the surgeon can perform a small incision and complete the adhesiolysis open and place the mesh laparoscopically, or rarely remove the mesh off the abdominal wall and leave some adherent to the bowel if no obstruction or fistula was present before surgery. In cases of serve adhesions to mesh, an open bowel resection can be necessary. In obese patients with incarcerated hernias, bimanual palpation of the abdominal wall can help identify the dissection plane during adhesiolysis. It is imperative to clear the entire anterior abdominal wall of adhesions all the way to the pericolic gutters. This avoids missing occult Swiss cheese–type defects and allows a large prosthetic mesh to be placed. Hernias above the umbilicus often require division of the falciform ligament to adequately adhere the mesh to the abdominal wall.

Sizing the Hernia Defect

An accurate measurement of the hernia defect is critical to appropriately size the mesh for adequate overlap and position the mesh for

maximal coverage of the defect. Oversizing of the mesh can result in significant technical challenges in accurate positioning of the prosthetic without buckling. In obese patients, external palpation of the hernia defects can be difficult and inaccurate. The author prefers to use a 3.5-inch, 20-gauge spinal needle to appropriate localize the hernia defect. Intracorporeal measurement of the defect is important because that is the location of the mesh. In obese patients with excessive subcutaneous tissue, a significant discrepancy between internal and external measurement can result in oversizing the hernia defect.

Two spinal needles are placed at the cranial and caudal limits of the hernia (Figure 2). In Swiss cheese defects, the maximal distance is used. A 15-cm plastic ruler is placed intracorporeally, and the distance between the spinal needles is recorded. The location of the spinal needles is also marked externally with a line. Next, the maximal width of the hernia defect is localized with spinal needles and measured internally and marked externally (Figure 3). Once the maximal width and length are calculated, 8 cm (4 cm of overlap on each side) is added to appropriately size the prosthetic material. Multiple different prosthetics are available for intraperitoneal placement. However, the author does advocate use of a tissue-separating mesh of some type.

Because all hernias are not perfect circles, identification of the center of the hernia is important to adequately center the mesh. The center point of the hernia can be identified externally. The surgeon measures the distance of the prior lines marked on the patient that indicate the length of the hernia. A transverse line is drawn across the patient at this point to indicate the x axis. Next, the middle of the line marking the maximal width of the hernia is measured, and a longitudinal line is drawn across the patient's abdomen to indicate the y axis. Where these two lines intersect is the center point of the hernia (Figure 4). In preparation of the mesh, the prosthetic is folded in half lengthwise, and a line is drawn, and in half along the width as well. Transfascial sutures are secured to the mesh at the edge of each of these lines. If done correctly, these sutures are retrieved on the labeled x axis and y axis on the patient to appropriately center the mesh (Figure 5).

Mesh Positioning

The four cardinal sutures are tucked into the mesh, and it is rolled tightly to fit through a trocar. Larger sheets of mesh sometimes require removal of the trocar. This can be facilitated by passing a 5-mm grasper across the abdomen, out the larger trocar; the trocar is removed, and the mesh is grasped and pulled into the abdomen.

Once inside the abdomen, the mesh is unfurled and the sutures are identified.

The initial cardinal suture should be brought up at the site with the least amount of potential coverage. This might be near the xiphoid or above the pubis. Regardless of how the mesh is measured, some excess mesh is common; to keep the mesh taut, more overlap might be necessary. The area at the edge of the hernia defect is localized on the prior y axis line drawn on the patient with a spinal needle. With a grasper used for measurements, the next spinal needle is placed on the y axis line 4 cm past the original spinal needle (Figure 6). A small incision is made, and a suture passer is used to retrieve each tail through separate fascial punctures. These sutures are tagged and left untied.

The lateral suture furthest from the camera is retrieved next. Again, a spinal needle is placed at the edge of the hernia defect on the prior externally marked x axis. With use of a grasper, 4 cm is measured, and another spinal needle is placed. Another stab incision is made, and the two tails are retrieved (Figure 7). In laparoscopic ventral hernia repair, the mesh is placed under insufflation, and it is important to be taut. If the mesh is not taut, the prosthetic buckles once the abdomen is desufflated and prolapses into the hernia sac. To avoid this problem, the two sutures that were placed before are pulled tightly by an assistant, while the surgeon grasps the mesh with a Maryland grasper near the remaining longitudinal knot and pulls

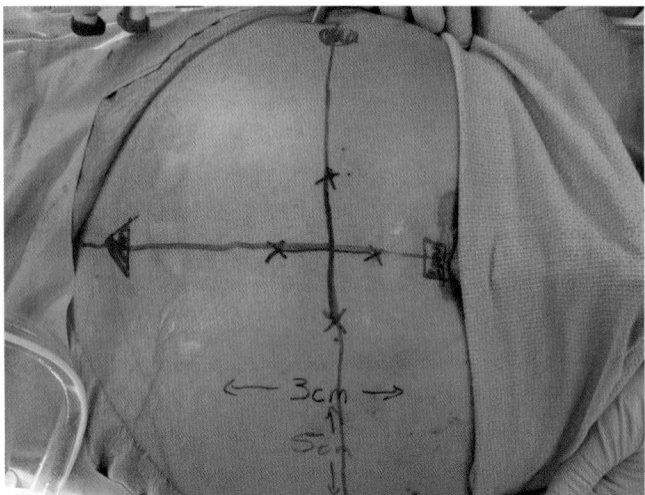

FIGURE 4   Center point of the lines marked externally is measured, which correlates to the center point of the hernia defect.

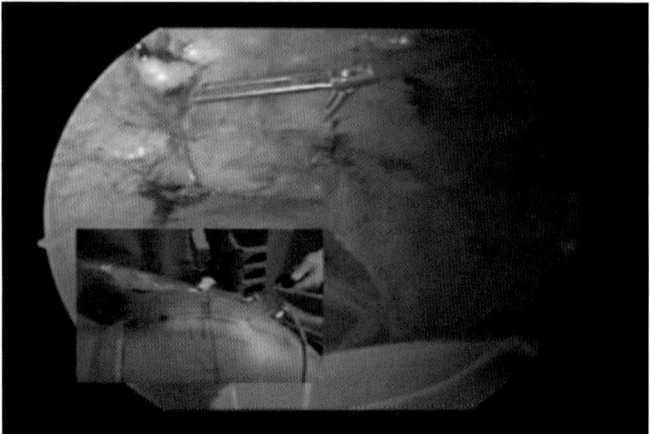

FIGURE 6   A spinal needle is placed at the edge of the defect on the external center line, and a 4-cm grasper is used to measure the overlap of the mesh and marked with another spinal needle. The skin is incised, and the transfascial suture retrieved at this site.

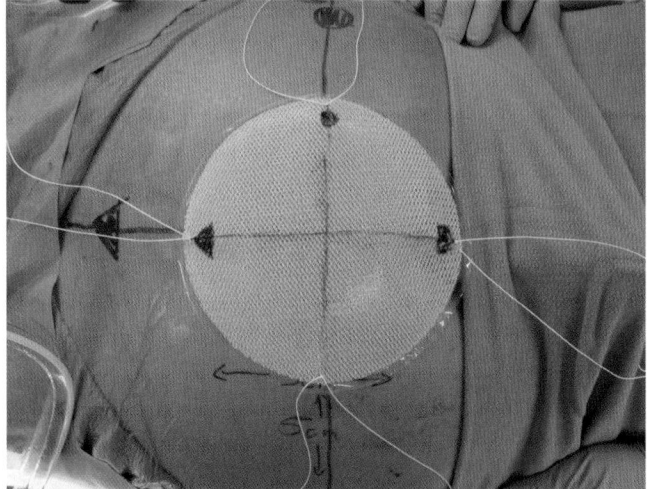

FIGURE 5   Center point of the mesh is identified, and four transfascial sutures are placed on these lines that correlate with the external center point lines previously measured.

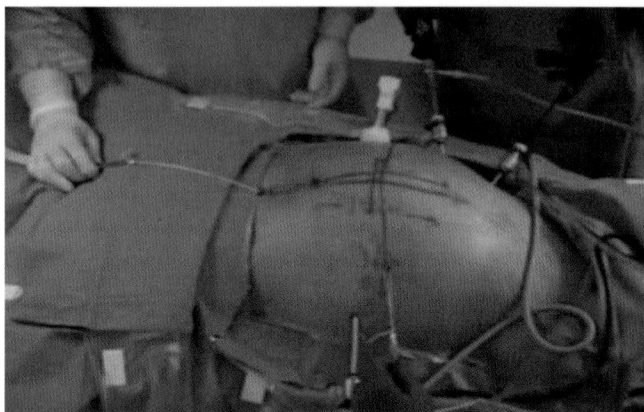

FIGURE 7   Cephalad and lateral suture retrieved through prior center point lines drawn externally on patient's abdomen.

the mesh along the externally marked y axis. Once the mesh is taut, the point on the y axis is marked with a spinal needle. A skin incision is made, and the tails are retrieved. The three sutures are then secured. The final transfascial suture is then pulled taut, the point on the x axis is identified with a spinal needle, and the tails are retrieved. The four sutures are secured, and the mesh is then secured to the remainder of the peritoneum with a tacking device (Figure 8). Multiple varieties of tacking devices are available, of both a permanent and an absorbable variety. No data are found to suggest the superiority of one tacking device over another at this time. These tacks do not provide strength to the repair. However, they do prevent bowel from slipping above the mesh for the first few weeks until the mesh is reperitonealized. The integrity of the repair is maintained by the transfascial sutures. The exact number of transfascial sutures required for a durable repair is unknown. The author uses an individualized approach. In patients with small defects or Swiss cheese–type defects, a large mesh with four sutures is sufficient. However, in obese patients, or those with large defects, 12 transfascial sutures are typically used. All ports over 5-mm should have the fascia closed particularly in hernia cases.

POSTOPERATIVE CARE

In highly selected cases, laparoscopic ventral hernia repair can be performed on an outpatient basis. However, postoperative discomfort can be significant, and most patients benefit from at least overnight observation and a patient-controlled analgesic device. Routine administration of ketorolac or muscle relaxants can also be helpful. Patients who need extensive adhesiolysis are kept on nothing by mouth (NPO) status until flatus. Routine hospital admission can also aid in detection of a missed enterotomy. This can be a life-threatening complication if diagnosis is delayed. Although radiographic evaluation can occasionally be helpful in the early postoperative period, if unexplained tachycardia or signs of sepsis persist, the patient should return to the operating room for a diagnostic laparoscopy.

SPECIAL CIRCUMSTANCES

Subxiphoid Hernia

Subxiphoid hernias are common after median sternotomies. They present particular challenges because the close proximity of body structures (ribs, costal margin) and major vascular structures (heart, aorta) can limit mesh fixation options. The procedure is carried out similar to a standard laparoscopic ventral hernia repair, although the falciform ligament must be taken down completely. The defect is

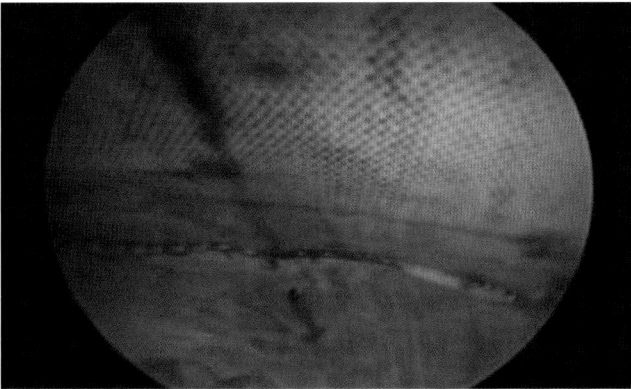

FIGURE 8   Final view of mesh taut across the abdominal cavity with tacks and transfascial sutures in place.

measured as previously described, and the mesh is sized appropriately. However, the most cranial suture is backed off at least 4 to 5 cm from the edge of the mesh. This suture can be retrieved at the xiphoid process, and the mesh is allowed to drape over the diaphragm and pericardium. To prevent buckling, the mesh can be fixated to the diaphragm with fibrin sealant. Tacking devices should not be used above the costal margin or xiphoid process to avoid injury to the pericardium.

Suprapubic Hernia

Suprapubic hernias pose challenges in obtaining adequate overlap while avoiding the bladder and major neurovascular structures. In reoperative cases, accurate identification of the superior extent of the bladder can be difficult. To facilitate identification, a three-way Foley catheter is helpful. After fully mobilizing the intraabdominal adhesions, the Foley catheter is clamped and 300 mL of normal saline solution is instilled through the irrigation port. With the bladder clearly visible, it is mobilized to expose the pubis and space of Retzius. The inferior sutures are backed off the edge of the mesh for several centimeters. These sutures can be retrieved at the pubis or Cooper's ligament, and the tail of the mesh can be tucked into the space of Retzius to maximize overlap. With placement of tacks to secure the periphery of the mesh, the tip of the tacker must be palpated externally. Like a laparoscopic inguinal hernia repair, if the tacker is below the iliopubic tract, major vascular and neurologic injuries can occur.

Defect Closure

With renewed interest in creation of a functional dynamic abdominal wall, some surgeons advocate closure of defects laparoscopically. The theoretic advantage of closing the defect is that it restores the abdominal wall integrity, may equalize pressure across the abdominal wall and mesh, reduces seroma rates, and might refunctionalize the abdominal wall. Several techniques have been described. The basic approach involves the use of a suture passing device, placed through a small stab incision over the hernia defect. A suture is brought into the abdomen through one side of the fascia, and the device is then placed through the opposite fascia and the suture retrieved through the same skin incision. This can be repeated to form a figure of 8 suture. This is the same technique used to close laparoscopic port sites. Once these sutures are placed, they can be tied, and the mesh is secured in a similar fashion. The mesh must be sized as if the defect were open, so if the midline repair were to break down, the hernia would not recur. Although this approach has an intuitive advantage, no comparative data at this time suggest it results in a superior outcome to a standard laparoscopic ventral hernia repair. In addition, it should be limited to defects less than 8 to 10 cm in maximal width because excessive tension can result.

COMPLICATIONS

Nearly all patients who undergo laparoscopic ventral hernia repair have development of a seroma. These seromas are mostly clinically insignificant and resolve without interventions. Patients must be counseled as to the likelihood of having an early persistent bulge, so as to avoid confusing it with a recurrence. Indications for aspiration are limited and include significant symptoms, impending skin ischemia, and failure to resolve after 6 months. The risk of contaminating the mesh must be weighed against the advantage of removing the fluid.

An enterotomy during laparoscopic ventral hernia repair is a serious potentially life-threatening complication if not dealt with appropriately. No steadfast rule exists for management of an enterotomy during laparoscopic ventral hernia repair, but some basic surgery principles can be applied. Most importantly, this complication must be recognized when it occurs. If surgeons identify an enterotomy, they must realize that this has the potential to be life threatening. Although several authors have described unique approaches to laparoscopic repair of the enterotomy and fixing the hernia with a biologic graft, or returning to the operating room in 3 to 5 days, this approach is not advocated by the author's group. Instead, if this complication occurs, at a minimum, the segment of bowel is exteriorized through a small incision and adequate repair is confirmed. At that time, the hernia can be left alone, with a return several months later for another attempt at repair. Alternatively, the procedure can be converted to open, with either primary closure of the defect or use of a biologic mesh to repair the hernia. Regardless of which approach is chosen, one should not let being a minimally invasive surgeon get in the way of the right operation for the patient. All patients should clearly understand what will happen if an enterotomy is encountered and that they may wake up with their stoma.

Unlike most laparoscopic procedures, laparoscopic ventral hernia can result in significant postoperative discomfort. The exact etiology of postoperative discomfort is likely multifactorial and includes peritoneal irritation from tacks, mesh, and transfascial sutures. Persistent pain beyond 6 weeks is rare and is often related to a transfascial sutures. These can be successfully managed with percutaneous injection of 30 mL of bupivacaine in most cases. Rarely, the offending suture must be removed.

The major advantage of a laparoscopic ventral hernia repair is that mesh infections are extremely rare. In fact, if the surgeon suspects a mesh infection after a laparoscopic ventral hernia repair, serious consideration should be given to an unrecognized bowel injury. Occasionally, laparoscopic mesh can become contaminated with skin flora during introduction into the abdomen. These patients present with erythema overlying the seroma cavity. The seroma should be aspirated and cultured. Rare cases of mesh salvage with percutaneous drainage, antibiotic irrigation, and lifetime suppression with antibiotics have been described. However, most patients need excision of the mesh and reconstruction.

OUTCOMES

Laparoscopic ventral hernia repair has gained widespread acceptance. Several prospective randomized trials have shown the safety and efficacy of laparoscopic ventral hernia repair when compared with open ventral hernia repair. The one common finding of all series is a significant reduction in wound-related morbidity associated with the laparoscopic repair. Most of these series have included a highly selected group of patients with relatively small defects, and whether the laparoscopic approach is appropriate for larger more complex hernias is unclear. In summary, the laparoscopic repair of ventral hernias is a valuable approach for the repair of abdominal wall defects. In skilled hands, performed appropriately with safe adhesiolysis and adequate mesh placement, excellent long-term results are possible.

SUGGESTED READINGS

Asencio F, Aguiló J, Peiró S, et al: Open randomized clinical trial of laparoscopic versus open incisional hernia repair, *Surg Endosc* 23(7):1441–1448, 2009.
Itani KM, Hur K, Kim LT, et al: Comparison of laparoscopic and open repair with mesh for the treatment of ventral incisional hernia: a randomized trial, *Arch Surg* 145(4):322–328, 2010.
Olmi, S, Scaubu A, Cesana GC, et al: Laparoscopic versus open incisional hernia repair: an open randomized controlled study, *Surg Endosc* 21(4):555–559, 2007.
Orenstein SB, Dumeer JL, Monteagudo J, et al: Outcomes of laparoscopic ventral hernia repair with routine defect closure using "shoelacing" technique, *Surg Endosc* 25(5):1452–1457, 2011.
Pring CM, Tran V, O'Rourke N, et al: Laparoscopic versus open ventral hernia repair: a randomized controlled trial, *ANZ J Surg* 78(10):903–906, 2008.
Rosen MJ, Fatima J, Sarr MG: Repair of abdominal wall hernias with restoration of abdominal wall function, *J Gastrointest Surg* 14(1):175–185, 2010.

LAPAROSCOPIC REPAIR OF PERISTOMAL HERNIAS

David E. Beck, MD, FACS, FASCRS

BACKGROUND

Approximately 100,000 enterostomies are created each year, with an estimated 40% being permanent. The artificial defect created in the abdominal wall fascia produces a weakness that contributes to hernia formation. Previous experience suggests that some degree of herniation around stomas is inevitable. However, little prospective data are available. Factors thought to contribute to hernia formation include age, chronic obstructive pulmonary disease, obesity, malnutrition, steroid use, malignancy, infection, and emergency surgery.

Most hernias occur within the first 2 years following stomal creation, but the risk of herniation continues throughout the life of the patient. Previous results of parastomal hernia repair have been unsatisfactory, and many providers avoid repairs until complications occur.

INDICATIONS AND CONTRAINDICATIONS

Indications for repair include bowel obstruction, incarceration, or enlargement of the hernia to the point where it interferes with appliance wear or the hernia is unsightly. Laparoscopic repair is suitable when the patient's stoma is appropriately sited, the patient lacks a history of extensive adhesions, and the hernia is not too large. Excessive large peristomal hernias are often more appropriately repaired with an open technique. Obtaining good results with underlay mesh usually requires a mesh with at least a 3-cm to 5-cm overlap of the mesh beyond the edges of the hernia. This is difficult to accomplish laparoscopically with large hernias. Another relative contraindication is the need for an associated open procedure. Both ileostomies and colostomies are suitable for laparoscopic procedures, and several techniques of repair have been described. These include various underlay techniques. One type of repair is similar to an open technique described by Sugarbaker in 1980. A second option is a "keyhole" technique of mesh placement. Other variations also include primary closure of the hernia defect with mesh reinforcement or repair with mesh alone.

PREOPERATIVE PLANNING

Preoperative Preparation

Standard bowel preparation is not mandatory. However, because the empty colon handles better than a stool-filled colon, it is the author's preference to have patients who can tolerate a preparation ingest a limited isotonic lavage prep (e.g., one fourth to one half gallon of a polyethylene glycol solution). Patients are instructed to take only clear liquids the day prior to surgery. Oral antibiotics are not prescribed, but standard intravenous broad-spectrum antibiotics are given within 1 hour of skin incision. Deep-vein prophylaxis is also ordered. Informed consent should include the potential for conversion to an open procedure.

SURGERY

Patient Positioning and Preparation

After induction of general anesthesia, an orogastric tube and indwelling urinary bladder catheter are placed. The patient is then placed in modified lithotomy position with the thighs even with the hips and pressure points appropriately padded. One or both arms may be tucked to facilitate securing the patient for the extremes of positioning used during laparoscopy. If only one arm is tucked, it should be on the side opposite the side of the hernia and stoma. The patient is then secured to the table, usually with tape. If one or both arms are kept out, the tape is placed in a "cross your heart" manner. The skin is prepped with antiseptic solution, and draping is done in a fashion to provide for lateral exposure for ports, especially on the side opposite the hernia and stoma. One author has suggested covering the abdominal wall with an adhesive drape to limit potential contamination of the mesh.

Instrument/Monitor Positioning

The primary surgeon will usually stand on the patient's side opposite the stoma or between the patient's legs (Figure 1). The primary monitor is placed on the patient's side that contains the stoma near

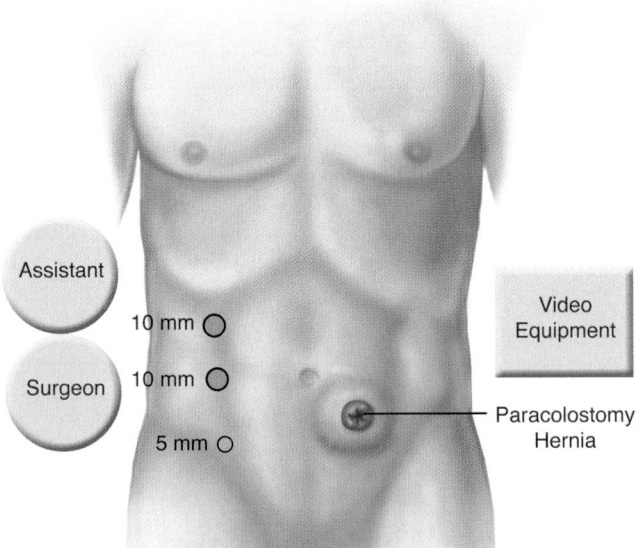

Assistant

10 mm ○

10 mm ○

Surgeon

5 mm ○

Video Equipment

— Paracolostomy Hernia

FIGURE 1 Positioning and port placement for laparoscopic assisted colostomy.

the level of the patient's hip. A secondary monitor can be placed at the patient's shoulder or at an alternate site viewable by the assistant or surgical technician. Insufflation tubing, suction tubing, cautery power cord, laparoscopy camera wiring, and a laparoscope light cord are brought off the patient's side. A 10-mm laparoscope with a 30-degree lens is preferred.

Port Selection and Placement

A 10/11-mm port with a balloon is placed using an open (modified Hasson) technique in the lateral abdomen on the side opposite the ostomy and hernia. A vertical skin incision with a scalpel is followed by dissection down to the fascia. If a balloon trocar is not used, a purse-string of 2-0 polyglycolic acid suture is placed, and the fascia is incised inside this suture. Muscles are split, and the peritoneum is opened sharply. Once entry into the peritoneal cavity is obtained, a 10/11 trocar is inserted, and the purse-string is tightened. Laparoscopic inspection of the peritoneal cavity rules out unsuspected pathology and identifies the patient with dense extensive adhesions that would make a laparoscopic approach problematic. If the abdomen is suitable, additional ports are placed under laparoscopic visualization at the locations described in Figure 1. Unless a quality 5-mm camera and mesh fixation device (tacker) are available, one of the other ports needs to be at least 10 mm in diameter. The remaining ports can be 5-mm trocars. The exact location will vary depending on adhesions and the location and size of the hernia. In general they are placed a hand's width apart and on the side of the abdomen opposite the hernia (see Figure 1, left-sided stoma). If the stoma is located on the right side of the abdomen, the trocar placement locations are reversed.

OPERATIVE TECHNIQUE

Division of Adhesions and Reduction of Hernia

Adhesions to the anterior abdominal wall are divided with sharp dissection and traction. This can often be tedious and has the potential for bowel injury. This is especially true if previous repairs have used mesh. Extensive dense adhesions may require conversion to an open technique. Bowel loops are gently reduced from the hernia using traction and careful division of adhesions. Alternate energy sources, such as Enseal (Ethicon Endosurgery, Cincinnati, Ohio), may be helpful for some vascular adhesions, but they are not a substitute for careful dissection. When all of the bowel has been reduced, the bowel leading to the stoma will remain. The peritoneal sac is left in place. The underlay techniques require that the bowel have adequate laxity to allow the bowel to track between the mesh and the abdominal wall. Reduction of the hernia will usually provide adequate laxity. If that does not, additional mobilization of the bowel may be necessary to allow adequate lateralization of the bowel. The ostomy bowel is pulled intra-abdominally to reduce any prolapse. The ostomy bowel is then pulled to the lateral or superior edge of the hernia defect. Some surgeons will then suture the ostomy bowel serosa to the peritoneum with absorbable sutures at the edge of the defect. The abdominal wall is also inspected for additional hernias that need repair.

A piece of mesh is selected that will cover the hernia defect with a 5-cm overlap. It is often helpful to compare the mesh on the abdominal wall, but to minimize the risk of contamination, the mesh should not touch the stoma itself, and contact with the skin should be avoided. Several types of mesh have been used, including nonabsorbable, absorbable, partly absorbable, and acellular collagen matrix meshes. Early authors used a polypropylene mesh. Subsequently, composite meshes were used, and more recent authors have expressed a preference for biologic meshes. Whatever mesh is chosen, it must be thin enough to allow tacking of the mesh to the posterior abdominal wall.

If peripheral tacking sutures will be used, they are placed at the edges of the mesh. The mesh is then tightly rolled and inserted through one of the larger trocars into the abdomen. Here it is unrolled and moved toward the stoma and hernia and oriented. After orienting the mesh, the traction sutures are extracted with a "suture passer" technique through small separate skin incisions. The sutures are tied down to the anterior abdominal fascia, creating transabdominal fixation. Authors have used a variable number of these traction/fixation sutures, ranging from a suture every 5 cm to just 4 sutures. As tacking devices have improved, the number of traction/fixation sutures has been reduced or eliminated. The author currently uses four sutures. After the traction/fixation sutures are secured, further fixation is done with a mechanical fixation device (e.g., SorbaFix or ProTack) at the margin of the mesh and along the bowel tract and edge of the fascial defect. Care is taken to produce appropriate tension on the mesh and to avoid putting the tackers into the ostomy bowel or mesentary and to allow enough laxity for the ostomy bowel to exit the mesh. After mesh fixation, the bowel is again inspected to exclude any unsuspected injury or bowel compression.

Another technique uses a keyhole piece of mesh. Mesh of appropriate size is cut with a central or slightly offcenter opening and a slit (Figure 2). The size of the mesh and location of the "central" opening should again allow a 5-cm overlap from the edges of the hernia. The central opening should be large enough to accommodate the bowel. If nonbiologic mesh is used, most authors have made the opening large enough that the mesh edges are not in direct contact with the bowel wall. With this technique, less laxity of the bowel leading to the stoma is required. After cutting the mesh, it is inserted into the abdomen as described previously and maneuvered into place. The four traction sutures are placed through the abdominal wall and secured. The edges of the mesh are tacked to the fascia as described previously (Figure 3). The fascia of larger trocar sites is closed with absorbable sutures, and the sites are infiltrated with local anesthetic (bupivacaine or bupivacaine liposome injectable suspension).

POSTOPERATIVE MANAGEMENT

The orogastric tube is removed prior to extubation, and the Foley catheter is removed later in the day or the next morning. Patients are supported with intravenous fluids and offered liquids when they are hungry. Solid food is started when flatus is expressed from the stoma. Pain management is usually provided by patient-controlled analgesia supplemented with acetaminophen, ibuprofen, or ketorolac. The patient is switched to oral pain medication when he or she is taking fluids and early ambulation is encouraged. Patients are ready for discharge when they can care for their stoma, are tolerating a diet, and have evidence of bowel function. Because the bowel is not detached from its skin attachment and stomal education is not required, recovery is usually rapid.

COMPLICATIONS

Early complications include unsuspected bowel injury, infection, or obstruction of the colon. Longer-term complications include hernia recurrence, bowel erosion, and, rarely, pain.

RESULTS

A number of small series have been published with short follow-up. Pooling four nonrandomized studies resulted in 7 recurrences out of 72 repairs. A laparoscopic technique is not feasible in all patients, and in one study, 15% of 55 patients had to be converted to an open procedure. Craft and colleagues described 27 consecutive patients repaired with a nonslit ePTFE mesh (Sugarbaker technique). There were a number of complications but no conversions, and mean length of stay was 6 days (ranging from 2 to 14 days). With a mean follow-up of 32 months, there was a 5% recurrence rate. In two studies of 59 patients, bowel injury occurred in 22% of patients. In another study of 47 patients in which ePTFE mesh was used, 9% had to have the mesh removed due to infection.

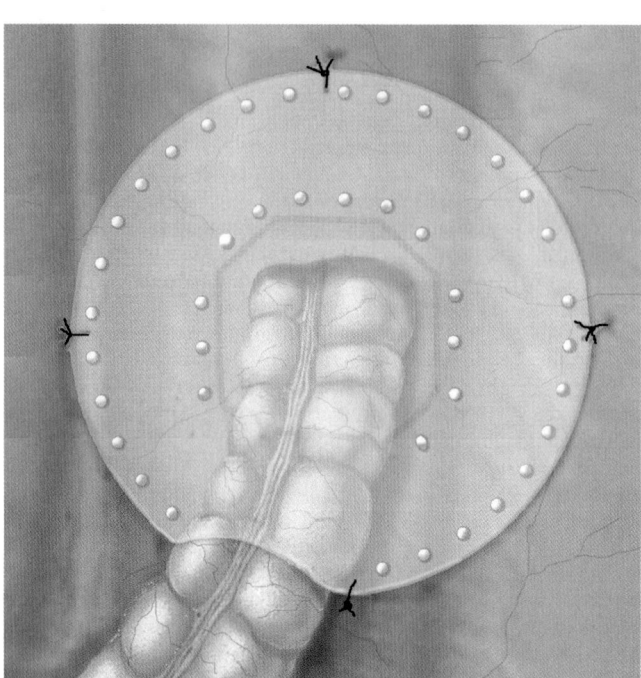

FIGURE 2   Fixation of mesh in a laparoscopic hernia repair.

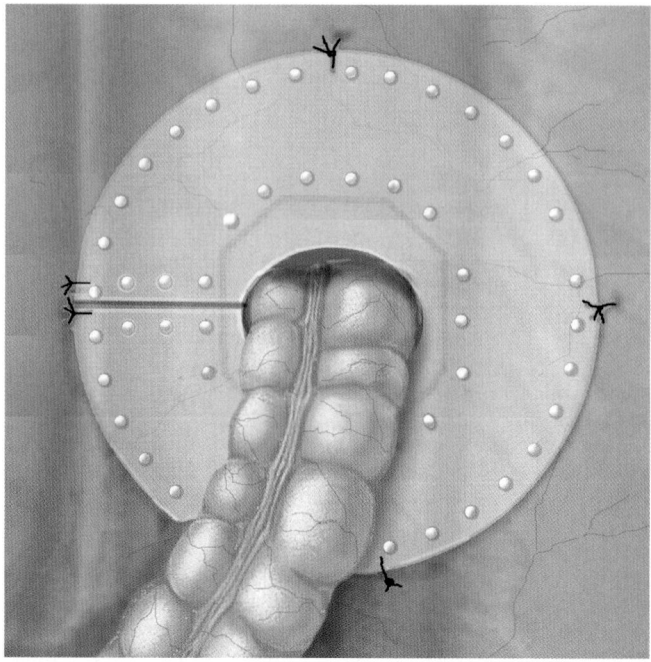

FIGURE 3   Keyhole mesh.

Most authors have not directly closed the hernia defect. This can leave a small bulge at the hernia site that can be displeasing to some patients.

CONCLUSIONS

Parastomal hernia repair is feasible as well as safe. Increasing experience and randomized prospective studies will be needed to define the optimal technique of repair. Until such information is available, laparoscopic repair with an underlay technique is a viable option in selected patients.

SUGGESTED READINGS

Craft RO, Huguet KL, McLemore EC, et al: Laparoscopic parastomal hernia repair, *Hernia* 12(2):137–140, 2008.

Mancini GJ, McClusky DA 3rd, Khaitan L, et al: Laparoscopic parastomal hernia repair using a nonslit mesh technique, *Surg Endosc* 21(9):1487–1491, 2007.

McLemore EC, Harold KL, Efron JE, Laxa BU, et al: Parastomal hernia: short-term outcome after laparoscopic and conventional repairs, *Surg Innov* 14(3):199–204, 2007.

Muysoms F: Laparoscopic Repair of parastomal hernias with a modified sugarbaker technique, *Acta Chir Belg* 107:476–480, 2007.

Serra-Aracil X, Bombardo-Junca J, Moreno-Matias J, et al: Randomized, controlled, prospective trial of the use of a mesh to prevent parastomal hernia, *Ann Surg* 201:344, 2009.

Sugarbaker PH: Prosthetic mesh repair of large hernias at the site of colonic stomas, *Surg Gynecol Obstet* 150(4):576–578, 1980.

LAPAROSCOPIC SPLENECTOMY

**Michael J. Lee, MD, and
Edward H. Phillips, MD, FACS**

OVERVIEW

Perhaps the earliest reference to splenectomy is an anecdotal description by C. Pliny (23-79 AD) in which incising the body to remove the spleen was believed to remove what hindered a man's running ability. As the spleen's function and the consequences of its removal became further elucidated, surgeons developed effective techniques for safe removal. Just as the laparoscopic approach has gained popularity for most abdominal surgical procedures, laparoscopic splenectomy has become the preferred method for elective splenectomy compared with conventional splenectomy because of the advantages that include decreased postoperative pain, shorter hospitalization, earlier return to normal activity, and improved cosmesis.

INDICATIONS AND CONTRAINDICATIONS

Laparoscopy is generally reserved for elective splenectomy for hematologic disorders, storage diseases, infiltrative disorders, and other benign disorders that benefit from splenectomy. Idiopathic thrombocytopenic purpura (ITP) is the most frequent indication for elective laparoscopic splenectomy. Depending on the surgeon's skill and experience, malignancy, splenomegaly, portal hypertension, pregnancy, and morbid obesity are not absolute contraindications for the laparoscopic approach. A hand-assisted port may even be useful for patients with splenomegaly and for cases that are difficult because of body habitus or inflammation from splenic infarction.

Laparoscopy is, however, contraindicated in emergent situations, such as splenic trauma or rupture with hemorrhagic shock, because of the impracticality of setting up laparoscopic equipment and the inability to pack the abdomen for vascular control if necessary. The inability to tolerate pneumoperitoneum is another absolute contraindication.

PREOPERATIVE PREPARATION

All patients must give informed consent, and the possibility of conversion to an open approach should be explained. In addition, the risk of overwhelming postsplenectomy sepsis should always be explained, with preoperative vaccination against meningococcus, pneumococcus, and *Haemophilus influenza* at least 2 weeks before. Postoperative vaccinations are administered generally on the last day of admission if not given before surgery. Prophylactic antibiotics covering skin flora administered within 30 minutes of incision should be strongly considered for patients with diabetes, morbid obesity, and immunocompromise. If available, preoperative imaging should be reviewed for accessory spleens.

Additional preoperative preparation is specific to the disease being treated. In ITP, intravenous immune globulin (IVIG) or plasmapheresis may help to elevate the platelet count and may benefit the patient with spontaneous bleeding or ecchymosis. Platelets should be available for transfusion after ligation of the splenic artery. Preoperative chemotherapy for splenomegaly from chronic myeloid leukemia may result in a 20% to 50% reduction in size within weeks of treatment. Portal or splenic vein thrombosis is also associated with splenomegaly but rarely with normal-sized spleens.

For patients with massive splenomegaly below the level of the iliac crest, splenic artery embolization on the morning of surgery followed by laparoscopic splenectomy may help to reduce the size of the spleen with manageable pain and ischemic complications. To ensure adequate hemostasis, the surgeon must be aware of the metal coils and avoid them during stapling of vasculature.

TECHNIQUES

Laparoscopic splenectomy has become the preferred approach for idiopathic thrombocytopenic purpura and other diseases with normal-sized spleens. The right lateral decubitus approach, also known as the "hanging spleen" technique, has become the preferred method for most surgeons because of availability of natural ligaments and gravity to lower the viscera to help maintain exposure.

The supine position was once used originally and may be necessary in combined cases but has fallen out of favor because of the easier exposure provided with a right lateral approach.

Regardless of the approach, the basic principles of achieving exposure, dividing the ligamentous attachments, and controlling the vascular supply, remain essential. Regard for anatomic relationships is always critical, and the surgeon should be aware of the attachments and the relationship of the spleen to the stomach, pancreas, left kidney, colon, and diaphragm. The two main attachments include the gastrosplenic and the splenorenal ligaments, which contain the short gastric and gastroepiploic vessels, respectively. The remaining ligaments, including the splenocolic and splenophrenic, are avascular, unless diseased from portal hypertension or myeloid metaplasia. Prior splenic infarction may result in dense inflammation in the splenophrenic ligament, necessitating a hand port, open conversion, or chest tube placement if the diaphragm is injured during dissection. The surgeon should also be aware that the vasculature of the spleen is variable with distributive and magistral patterns (Figures 1 and 2). Also important is awareness that the tail of the pancreas is usually within a centimeter of the splenic hilum and can also be in direct contact with the spleen in one third of all patients.

RIGHT LATERAL APPROACH

After the endotracheal tube is secured, an orogastric tube is placed, and a Foley catheter is placed at the discretion of the surgeon. Bilateral sequential compression devices should be applied to the lower extremities in the preoperative holding area. The patient is then positioned and padded on a taped beanbag in the right lateral position. Positioning should allow the point between the iliac crest and the lateral costal margin to rest at the central break of the table. The left arm is positioned in a semiflexed position on a pillow. An axillary gel foam roll is used, and the hips and legs are gently flexed and padded between pillows and secured to the bed with wide silk tape.

The patient is also placed at a 45-degree tilt to maximize exposure exploited by the natural ligaments and gravity (Figure 3). This also facilitates exploration in the abdomen in search for accessory spleens. Lateral positional beams attached to the rails may add to the lateral stability and help to reinforce the beanbag to maintain the 45-degree tilt. Egg crate foam pads should be generously used and added to the surface area to prevent slipping. Once meticulous positioning is complete, the table is then fully tilted in all practical directions to ensure that the patient can safely tolerate it during the operation because proper positional manipulation is key to this approach. The patient is then widely prepped from the nipple line to the hips for possible hand port placement, chest tube placement, or open conversion. The monitor should be placed at the head of the table at an ergonomic height and angle. Suction should be available and ready for use, as should a hook electrocautery device. An ultrasonic dissector should be available as well.

The surgeon stands on the patient's right side and directs the assistant (also standing on the patient's right side) who can drive the camera with the left and assist with the right hand. The patient is tilted to left side up to perform the operation but is tilted left side down such as in a supine position to provide for initial entry of trocars (Figure 4). Because of close proximity to the colon and necessity for specimen extraction, an initial 12-mm Hasson's trocar is the preferred technique in the anterior axillary line opposite the 11th or 12th rib. Once pneumoperitoneum is obtained, a 5-mm port is placed in the subxiphoid location for the surgeon's left hand. A 5-mm port is placed midway between the subxiphoid trocar and the Hasson's port. The most lateral trocar is a 12-mm one placed in the left axillary line between the costal margin and the iliac crest, with care taken to "open" the hip so an endovascular cutter can be inserted (Figure 5).

Initial inspection should begin with a search for accessory spleens in the splenic hilum, the splenic ligaments, the omentum, the small bowel mesentery, and the pelvis. Careful inspection at the start of the case avoids staining from dissection and disrupting small blood vessels and allows for better visualization.

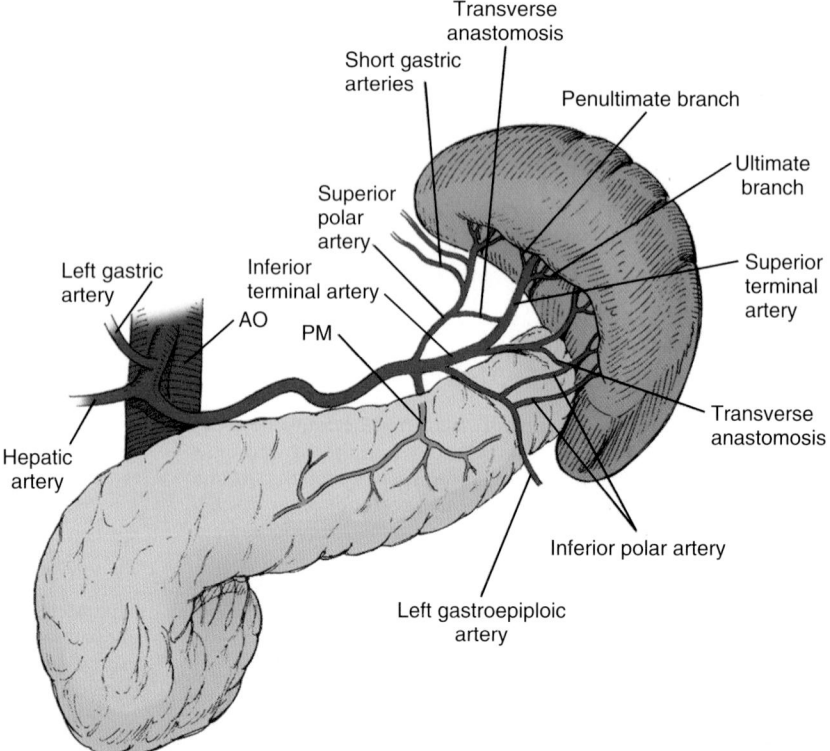

FIGURE 1 Distributed vascularization. By definition, the splenic trunk is short, and many long branches (6 to 12) enter over three fourths of the medial surface of the spleen. The branches originate between 3 to 13 cm from the hilum. Outside the spleen, the arteries also present frequent transverse anastomoses with each other, which according to Testud arise at a right angle between the involved arteries, as with most collaterals. Thus, the application of hemostatic clips or the embolization of coils occluding a branch of the splenic artery before such an anastomosis may fail to devascularize the corresponding splenic segment. AO, Aorta; PM, pancreatic magna. (From Poulin EC, Thibault C: The anatomical basis for laparoscopic splenectomy, Can J Surg 36[5]:485-488, 1993.)

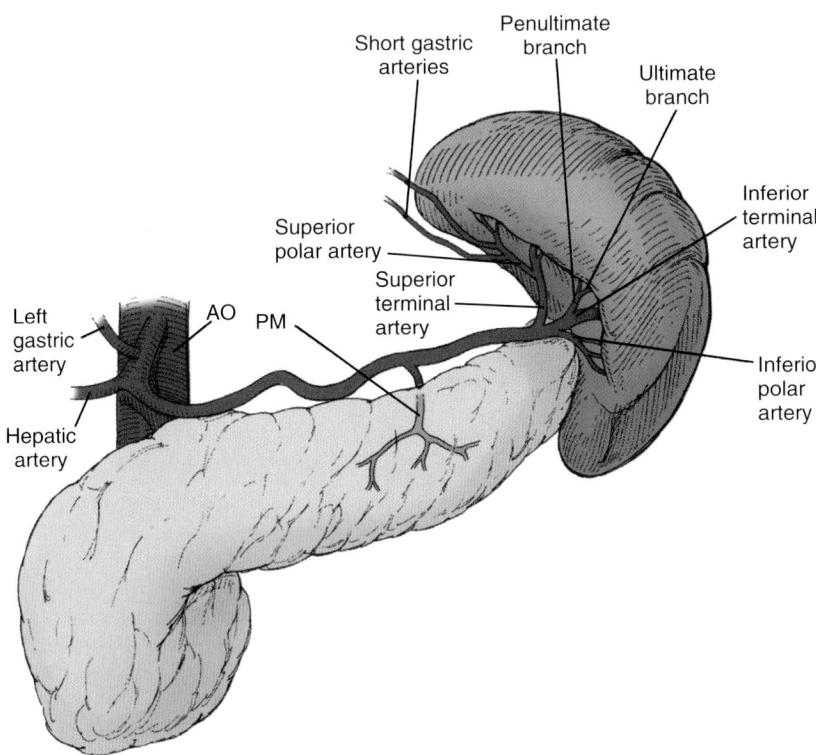

Penultimate branch
Short gastric arteries
Ultimate branch
Superior polar artery
Superior terminal artery
Inferior terminal artery
Left gastric artery
AO   PM
Hepatic artery
Inferior polar artery

FIGURE 2 Bundled (magistral) vascularization. The bundle type is characterized by the presence of a long main splenic artery that divides into short terminal branches near the hilum. In this type, the splenic branches enter over only a fourth to a third of the medial surface of the spleen. These branches are large, few (3 to 4), originate 3.5 cm on average from the spleen, and reach the center of the organ as a compact bundle. *AO,* Aorta, *PM,* pancreatic magna. *(From Poulin EC, Thibault C: The anatomical basis for laparoscopic splenectomy,* Can J Surg *36[5]:485-488, 1993.)*

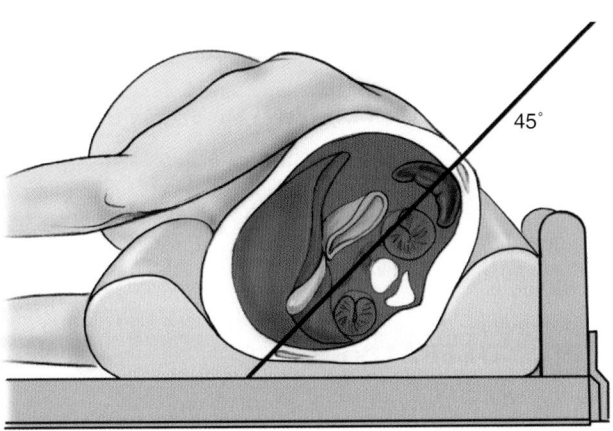

45°

FIGURE 3 The "leaning spleen" technique requires a 45-degree tilt with a beanbag or jelly roll positioning pad. *(Reprinted with permission from Hunter JG, editor:* The atlas of minimally invasive surgical operations, *New York, McGraw-Hill.)*

The safest course to approach splenectomy in cases of splenomegaly consists of ligating the splenic artery in the lesser sac because hemorrhage during hilar dissection can possibly occur. The lesser sac is entered through the gastrocolic ligament, and the pancreas is identified and retracted posteriorly and inferiorly to visualize the splenic artery or its pulsation slightly superior to the pancreas. The visceral peritoneum should be dissected with scissors, and clips should occlude the artery without dividing it. The clips should be carefully placed in a low position to later accommodate the linear cutting stapler.

The table should then be tilted to the right to facilitate division of the splenocolic ligament. The hook electrocautery or ultrasonic dissector is used to divide the ligament so that the inferior pole is

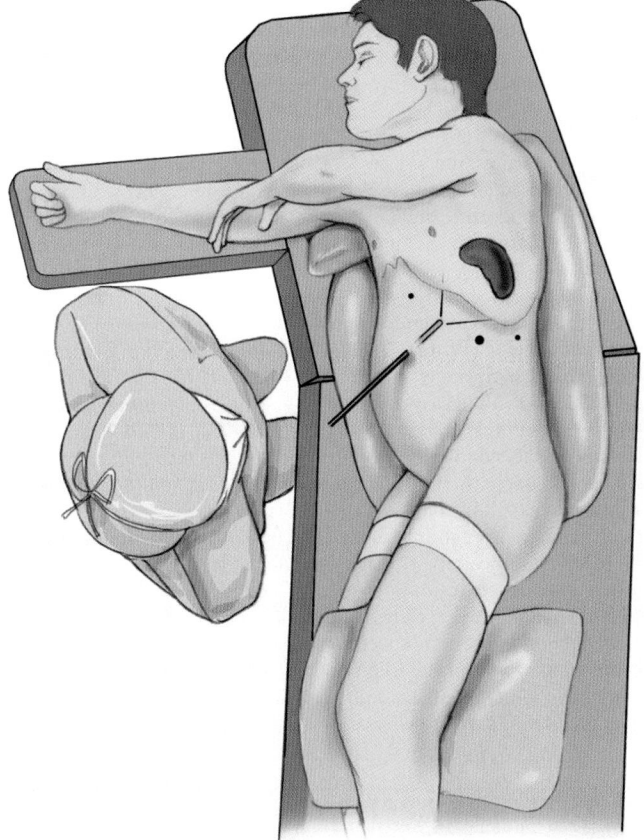

FIGURE 4 Patient, port, and laparoscope positions for the "leaning spleen" technique. *(Reprinted with permission from Hunter JG, editor:* The atlas of minimally invasive surgical operations, *New York, McGraw-Hill.)*

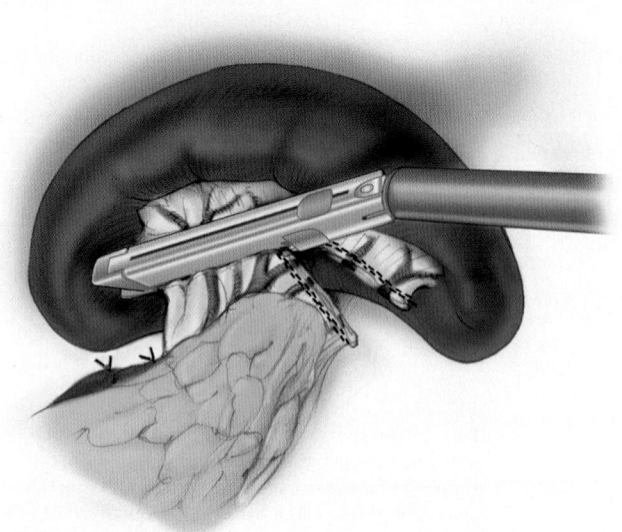

FIGURE 5 The splenic blood supply is controlled in the splenic hilum with a linear cutting stapler. *(Reprinted with permission from Hunter JG, editor: The atlas of minimally invasive surgical operations, New York, McGraw-Hill.)*

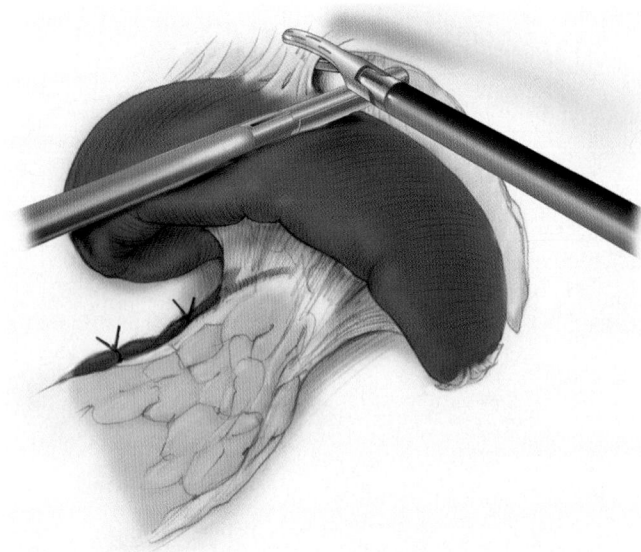

FIGURE 6 The spleen is released by dividing the peritoneal reflection with the Harmonic scalpel (Johnson & Johnson Gateway, Piscataway, NJ). *(Reprinted with permission from Hunter JG, editor: The atlas of minimally invasive surgical operations, New York, McGraw-Hill.)*

completely visible. The small tributaries of the left gastroepiploic vein are divided. The splenorenal ligament is then divided, and the dissection proceeds from the inferior pole cephalad to reach the splenophrenic ligament (Figure 6). The short gastric vessels are also divided, and the vascular pattern supplying the spleen should now be apparent. The distributed pattern is most common and present in 70% and is characterized by a short splenic trunk with many long branches (see Figure 1). The magistral type is characterized by a long dominant splenic artery with short terminal branches that enter the medial surface of the spleen (see Figure 2). The hilum should be widely exposed and searched again for accessory spleens. The endoscopic linear cutting stapler can be used to safely and efficiently divide the large vessels at the hilum, offsetting cost by the time savings.

Once the spleen is detached, the inferior pole peritoneal attachment may be grasped and pointed toward the diaphragm and held at three points (6, 10, and 12 o'clock) and then placed in a sturdy bag for extraction through the 12-mm fascial defect of the Hasson's working port. Alternatively, a sterile heavy duty commercial freezer bag may be useful for very large spleens. The bag is then grasped and partially removed into the wound. The spleen is morcellated to allow for extraction with ring forceps while avoiding spilling fragments, which may result in splenosis and recurrent disease. If concern exists that the diagnosis cannot be obtained from a morcellated specimen, direct communication with the pathologist before the procedure is important to decide whether to add a hand port or make a lower midline incision for specimen extraction. Traction provided by the assistant upwards on the specimen bag during morcellation can help avoid spilling of spleen fragments. A 19F closed suction drain is placed if concern exists for injury of the pancreas. All fascial defects greater than 10 mm are closed.

ANTERIOR APPROACH

The anterior approach has been largely replaced by the right lateral technique, but it should be considered in certain cases when the spleen size is normal and patients are undergoing concomitant procedures, such as laparoscopic cholecystectomy or laparoscopic distal pancreatectomy. In the anterior approach, the surgeon stands between the legs, which are placed in low lithotomy, or alternatively on the patient's right side with the patient supine. The dissection is carried similarly in the manner as the right lateral approach.

LAPAROSCOPIC HAND-ASSISTED

As mentioned previously, a hand port may help in cases with massive spleens or in cases with dense scar tissue between the diaphragm and spleen. In addition, if the specimen needs to be removed intact to aid in pathologic diagnosis, a hand port can be very helpful to avoid traumatizing the specimen.

POSTOPERATIVE CARE

After laparoscopic splenectomy, the postoperative care is routine. In addition, the surgeon should also be aware that if the patient was receiving steroids, a taper with oral steroids may be necessary. Patients are usually discharged home the next day when criteria are met.

COMPLICATIONS

Although rare in incidence (3.2%), overwhelming postsplenectomy sepsis carries an extremely high mortality rate reported up to 50%. Patients have the highest risk in the first 2 years after splenectomy but also carry a lifetime increase in risk; vaccination against meningococcus, pneumococcus, and *H. influenza* type B is important.

Portal or splenic vein thrombosis may occur in patients with hypercoagulable myeloproliferative disorders, hematologic malignancy, and massive splenomegaly.

Because of the close proximity, the tail of the pancreas is at risk for injury during dissection at the splenic hilum. If injured, any major duct should be repaired; a 19F closed suction drain should be placed in the vicinity and checked for amylase, and the patient should be placed on a low-fat diet.

RESULTS

No prospective randomized trial has compared laparoscopic with open splenectomy. Similar to the results for other laparoscopic approaches, the results of two meta-analyses show improvement in overall complication rates (9% to 15% vs 12% to 26%), mortality rates (0.2% to 0.6% vs 1.0% to 1.1%), and length of stay (3.6 vs 7.2 days), but at the expense of more than an hour of additional operative time (180 vs 114 minutes) with the laparoscopic approach. Operative times were significantly reduced by an average of 40 minutes (135 vs 177 minutes) by the addition of a hand-assisted port in patients with large spleens greater than 700 g in a comparative analysis of 56 patients.

SUMMARY

Laparoscopic splenectomy should be considered in the stable elective case. In certain situations, a hand port may facilitate dissection and specimen extraction for massive spleens and decrease operative time. The right lateral approach maximizes exposure with natural attachments for retraction and gravity to lower the viscera. Careful meticulous positioning and intraoperative manipulation in table positioning greatly helps. The laparoscopic advantages include lower complication rates, lower mortality rates, shorter hospitalization, and improved cosmesis.

SUGGESTED READINGS

Craryl SE, Buchanan GR: Vascular complications after splenectomy for hematologic disorders, *Blood* 114(14):2861–2868, 2009.

Di Sabatino A, Carsetti R, Corazza GR: Post-splenectomy and hyposplenic states, *Lancet* 378:86–97, 2011.

Ikeda M, Sekimoto M, Takiguchi S, et al: High incidence of thrombosis of the portal venous system after laparoscopic splenectomy: a prospective study with contrast-enhanced CT scan, *Ann Surg* 241(2):208–216, 2005.

Kojouri K, Vesely S, Terrell D, et al: Splenectomy for adult patients with idiopathic thrombocytopenia purpura, *Blood* 104(9):2623–2634, 2004.

Phillips EH, Korman JE, Friedman R: Laparoscopic splenectomy, *Surg Dis Spleen* 211–232, 1997.

Targarona EM, Balague C, Cerdan G, et al: Hand assisted laparoscopic splenectomy in cases of splenomegaly, *Surg Endosc* 16:426–430, 2002.

Winslow ER, Brunt LM: Perioperative outcomes of laparoscopic verus open splenectomy: a meta-analysis with an emphasis on complications, *Surgery* 134(4):647–653, 2003.

LAPAROSCOPIC GASTRIC SURGERY

Han-Kwang Yang, MD, PhD, FACS, and
Sebastianus Kwon, MBBS, FRACS

OVERVIEW

Laparoscopic surgery is now considered the standard of care in the surgical management of a number of benign esophagogastric conditions, such as acid reflux, as well as in bariatric surgery. However, application of laparoscopy in the treatment of early gastric cancer is still relatively new and its practice is not standardized around the world. This chapter will focus on laparoscopic surgery for gastric cancer: its rationale, indications, and technical aspects.

In the past two decades, there has been a rapid increase in the application of laparoscopic or laparoscopic-assisted gastrectomy for the treatment of gastric adenocarcinoma in Asia, particularly Japan and Korea, where currently, more than half of all gastrectomies are being performed laparoscopically at many leading centers. The move toward minimally invasive surgery is a result of multiple factors, not the least of which is the high incidence of gastric cancer and the high proportion of early gastric cancer—confined to the mucosa (T1a) or submucosa (T1b)—in Japan and Korea. Also, there is now a growing body of evidence suggesting oncologic feasibility of laparoscopic-assisted gastrectomy in early gastric cancers. In addition, surgeons have made concerted efforts to standardize surgical procedures and enable reproducibility of results. In comparison, in the West, gastric cancer is much less common and rarely diagnosed at an early stage. As such, the clinical application of laparoscopic-assisted gastrectomy has remained limited to a handful of referral centers and has included locally advanced gastric cancers. Clinical trials from the West are similarly limited in number, have small sample sizes, and include tumors of all stages.

INDICATIONS AND RATIONALE FOR LAPAROSCOPIC GASTRECTOMY

There is ample evidence supporting the technical feasibility and various short-term benefits of laparoscopic gastrectomy compared with conventional open surgery. A meta-analysis of randomized controlled trials (RCTs), conducted by Kodera and colleagues (2010), showed a reduction in overall morbidity rates among patients who underwent laparoscopic-assisted distal gastrectomy (LADG), compared with patients who underwent open surgery, but equivalent mortality rates across groups. A significant reduction in estimated blood loss was also observed in the LADG group at the expense of longer operating time. However, Level I evidence supporting the oncologic safety of laparoscopic gastrectomy is still lacking. To date, the evidence is limited to one small Western RCT by Huscher and colleagues (2005; n = 59), and numerous retrospective and phase II trials, mainly from Japan and Korea. At present, two notable RCTs assessing long-term outcomes of LADG for clinical stage I disease are in progress, namely the KLASS-01 study by the Korean Laparoscopic Gastrointestinal Surgery Study (KLASS) Group and the JCOG0912 study by the Japanese Clinical Oncology Group. The former study completed its targeted accrual of 1415 patients in 2010 and its 5-year survival data are expected to provide the first Level I evidence on oncologic safety of LADG for clinical stage I disease. For now, other than in the setting of clinical trials, the majority of surgeons in the East restrict laparoscopic gastrectomy to clinical T1N0 disease that falls outside of indications for endoscopic resection, although some centers have expanded their indication to more advanced stages. Another trial by KLASS group, the KLASS-02 study, which is aimed at assessing technical feasibility and oncologic safety of LADG for advanced gastric cancer, is currently in the recruitment phase. Similar studies are ongoing in Japan by groups led by Kitano. Until there are robust data to support its clinical use, laparoscopic gastrectomy for cancer ought to be considered investigational treatment.

Even greater caution is advised when considering the application of a laparoscopic approach for total gastrectomy, as the lymph node (LN) dissection, and particularly the reconstruction for a laparoscopic total gastrectomy (LTG), are technically more demanding compared with an LADG, and an anastomotic leakage is more consequential. To address this issue, the KLASS group has just commenced the KLASS-03 study, a phase II study, aimed at assessment of technical safety of various reconstructive techniques after total gastrectomy.

CONTRAINDICATIONS

The consideration of contraindications to laparoscopic gastric surgery should take into account the individual surgeon's experience in advanced laparoscopic surgery, stage of the disease, the patient's ability to tolerate prolonged pneumoperitoneum, and patient history of previous abdominal surgery.

PREOPERATIVE WORKUP AND PREPARATION

Accurate preoperative staging by means of endoscopy, endoscopic ultrasound, and abdominopelvic computed tomographic (CT) scan is critical in deciding on the optimal treatment modality (endoscopic or surgery) and the preferred surgical approach. Vascular anomalies, particularly an accessory or replaced left hepatic artery arising from the left gastric artery and a common or right hepatic artery arising from the superior mesenteric artery, should be actively sought on the arterial phase of the CT scan. Preoperative understanding of any variations in the course of the splenic artery can be helpful during LN dissection around it. Also, a three-dimensional arterial phase reconstruction can provide more intuitive information. Positron emission tomography (PET)-CT scan is performed selectively to exclude distant metastatic disease when suspected. In addition to guiding preoperative decisions on the extent of gastrectomy (distal or total, or pylorus-preserving gastrectomy), precise endoscopic localization of the tumor is critical to ensure negative resection margins, particularly for early or nonpalpable cancers. Endoscopic clips placed proximal and distal to the lesion preoperatively are used for this purpose. Other important preoperative considerations include the method of reconstruction (Billroth I, Billroth II, or Roux-en-Y) and its approach (extracorporeally through a mini-laparotomy or intracorporeally).

SURGICAL PRINCIPLES FOR LAPAROSCOPIC GASTRECTOMY

The principles of a laparoscopic gastrectomy for potentially curable disease are identical to those of an open gastrectomy: offering the best chance of cure by a R0 resection and adequate LN dissection, and minimizing surgical insult and complications. A thorough understanding of the anatomy of the LN stations (Figure 1) is a necessity, and the extent of the dissection should be identical to that of an open procedure. Also, the surgical team should be mindful of the risk of cancer cell dissemination from direct handling of tumor, spillage of intragastric content, and disruption of lymphatic vessels or metastatic LNs themselves.

In addition, the following surgical principles are considered essential in minimizing intraoperative complications during a laparoscopic gastrectomy. Setting up optimal exposure of the dissection field prior to dissection at each step is crucial. The importance of

identifying and staying in the correct surgical plane cannot be overemphasized. Also, safe techniques for using energy devices such as ultrasonic coagulating shears (UCS) should be adopted. For example, it is recommended that the active blade of UCS be kept visible during and immediately after its activation. Use of the insulated or inactive blade, which has a thinner tip profile, is recommended for blunt dissection and finding the correct tissue plane prior to instrument activation. Finally, surgeons should have a low threshold for converting to an open procedure or extending a mini-laparotomy until they have gained sufficient experience performing laparoscopic gastrectomies.

PITFALLS DURING A LAPAROSCOPIC GASTRECTOMY

A laparoscopic gastrectomy for cancer is a technically challenging procedure with a steep learning curve reported to extend to approximately 50 cases. Gastrectomy requires a large extent of LN dissection, much of it in the immediate vicinity of major blood vessels that need to be preserved. As such, many of intraoperative pitfalls relate to injury to either major blood vessels or bleeding from their branches or tributaries that impair vision and subsequently lead to other major complications. During the early phase of introduction of laparoscopic gastrectomy, there were reports of delayed rupture of a splenic artery pseudoaneurysm, which is unusual in the open setting. Blind attempts to control bleeding immediately after it occurs can invite more serious injury. Most minor bleeding will stop spontaneously with application of gauze alone. Other pitfalls relate to thermal injury to adjacent organs, particularly to the transverse colon, pancreas, duodenum, and esophagus, and steps of reconstruction, which is more difficult by the minimally invasive approach.

EXTENT OF LYMPHADENECTOMY

D2 dissection has long been the standard of care in Japan and Korea, and survival advantage of D2 dissection over D1 dissection has only recently been shown using Western data for the first time. The third English version of *Japanese Gastric Cancer Treatment Guidelines* (2010) recommends a D2 dissection for clinical T2-4b tumor or T1 tumor with suspicion of nodal involvement (Figure 2). Most gastric surgeons in Japan and Korea accept D1+ dissection as a safe alternative in cT1N0 disease. Oncologic safety of laparoscopic D2 dissection remains a topic of debate, as mentioned earlier. The extent of lymphadenectomy is now defined according to the type of gastrectomy indicated and not the location of the lesion (Figure 3).

OMENTECTOMY AND BURSECTOMY

Although there is lack of conclusive evidence regarding the optimal extent of omentectomy in gastrectomy, a partial omentectomy is generally performed for cT1 disease and a total omentectomy for cT2 or above. Results of RCTs in progress to assess the role of bursectomy, albeit in the open setting, are being awaited.

TECHNIQUE OF LAPAROSCOPIC GASTRECTOMY

The authors' standard technique for a LADG with partial omentectomy for an extracorporeal Billroth I anastomosis using a circular stapler is described in this section.

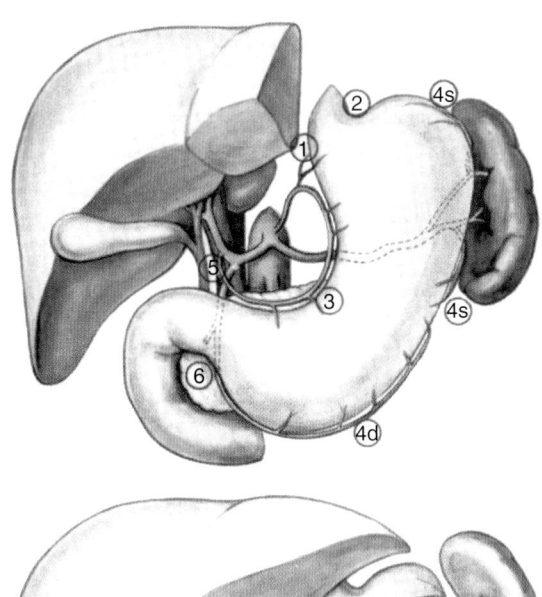

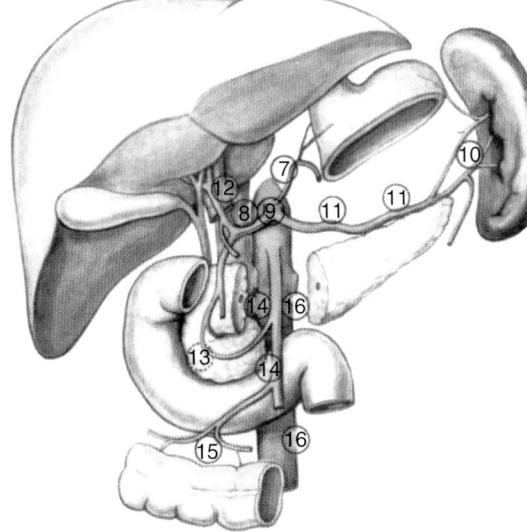

FIGURE 1 Lymph node stations surrounding the stomach. *1*, right cardial nodes; *2*, left cardial nodes; *3*, nodes along the lesser curvature; *4*, nodes along the greater curvature; *5*, suprapyloric nodes; *6*, infrapyloric nodes; *7*, nodes along the left gastric artery; *8*, nodes along the common hepatic artery; *9*, nodes around the coeliac axis; *10*, nodes at the splenic hilus; *11*, nodes along the splenic artery; *12*, nodes in the hepatodoudenal ligament; *13*, nodes at the posterior aspect of the pancreas head; *14*, nodes at the root of the mesenterium; *15*, nodes in the mesocolon of the tranverse colon; *4s*, nodes along the short gastric and left gastroepiploic vessels; *4d*, nodes along the right gastroepiploic vessels; *16*, para-aortic nodes. *(From Peeters KC, van de Velde CJ: Quality assurance of surgery in gastric and rectal cancer,* Crit Rev Oncol Hematol *51(2):105–119, Fig 1, 2004.)*

Room Setup and Patient Position

The patient is placed supine with arms extended out. A nasogastric tube and an in-dwelling urinary catheter are placed after general anesthesia. The patient is secured onto the bed using leg and arm straps. The operator sits or stands on the right side of the patient and the assistant on the left side throughout the procedure. The scopist sits or stands on the right side, next to the operator. A video monitor is placed above each of the patient's shoulders (Figure 4).

Placement of Ports

An infraumbilical 11-mm port is placed using open technique through which a 30-degree angled scope is introduced and

pneumoperitoneum to 12 mm Hg established. The peritoneal cavity is inspected for any evidence of tumor spread (Figure 6, *A*). The table is tilted 20 degrees in reverse Trendelenburg position. Three 5-mm ports and one 12-mm port are then placed under direct vision (Figure 5). The right subcostal port is placed aimed at the first part of the duodenum. Correct placement of the 12-mm port is critical. Placed roughly equidistant between the subcostal and the umbilical ports but the outside linea semilunaris, it should be low enough to allow adequate working space for the right side of the greater curvature mobilization and infrapyloric dissection but high and medial enough to allow safe access for the suprapancreatic LN dissection, particularly the proximal splenic artery (No. 11p) LN dissection. The two left-sided ports for the assistant roughly mirror those on the right.

Dissection of Greater Omentum and Left Gastroepiploic Vessels (Nos. 4d and 4sb Lymph Nodes)

Key points: Entry into the lesser sac, dissection between gastro-epiploic arcade and transverse colon, ligation of the root of left gastroepiploic vessels.

Potential pitfalls: Injury to middle colic vessels, thermal injury to transverse colon, hemorrhage from left gastroepiploic vessels, capsular tear of the spleen, inadvertent division of short gastric vessels (resulting in delayed infarction of remnant stomach), omental infarction (rare).

The greater omentum is lifted up anteriorly against gravity and spread out by grasping it just inside the gastroepiploic arcade (Figure 6, *B*). The gastrocolic ligament is divided with UCS, staying 3 to 4 cm outside of the arcade, and the lesser sac is laid open. Anteromedial retraction of the posterior wall of the stomach with the assistant's right-hand instrument facilitates the latter part of the dissection. Toward the lower pole of the spleen, the transverse colon is more closely related to the gastroepiploic arcade, and thermal injury to the colon is avoided by checking both sides of the gastro-colic and splenocolic ligaments for its location (Figure 6, *C*). The endpoint of station 4sb dissection is division of left gastroepiploic vessels, as close to their origin as safely possible. The origin can be difficult to find, particularly in obese individuals. The key to obtaining good exposure is to apply adequate traction along the gastro-splenic ligament. This ligament connects the hilum of the spleen and the tail of the pancreas to the greater curvature of the stomach and carries the left gastroepiploic and short gastric vessels. The vascular origins can be found between the tail of the pancreas and the lower pole of the spleen. The vessels are double-clipped and then divided with UCS, just distal to the main omental branch although this is often difficult to directly visualize (Figure 6, *D–F*). The dissection is then carried directly onto the greater curvature of the stomach to avoid inadvertent division of the short gastric vessels, which will be the sole blood supply to the remnant stomach. Finally a portion of the greater curvature of the stomach is prepared for later transection (Figure 6, *G,H*).

Dissection of Greater Omentum and Right Gastroepiploic Arcade (No. 4d Lymph Nodes)

Key points: Completion of mobilization of transverse colon with exposure of second part of duodenum and head of pancreas.

Potential pitfalls: Inadvertent division of transverse mesocolon, injury to superior mesenteric vein, thermal injury to duodenum or head of pancreas.

First, the right side ports are pulled as far back as possible to maximize the working space. Then, the previous line of dissection in

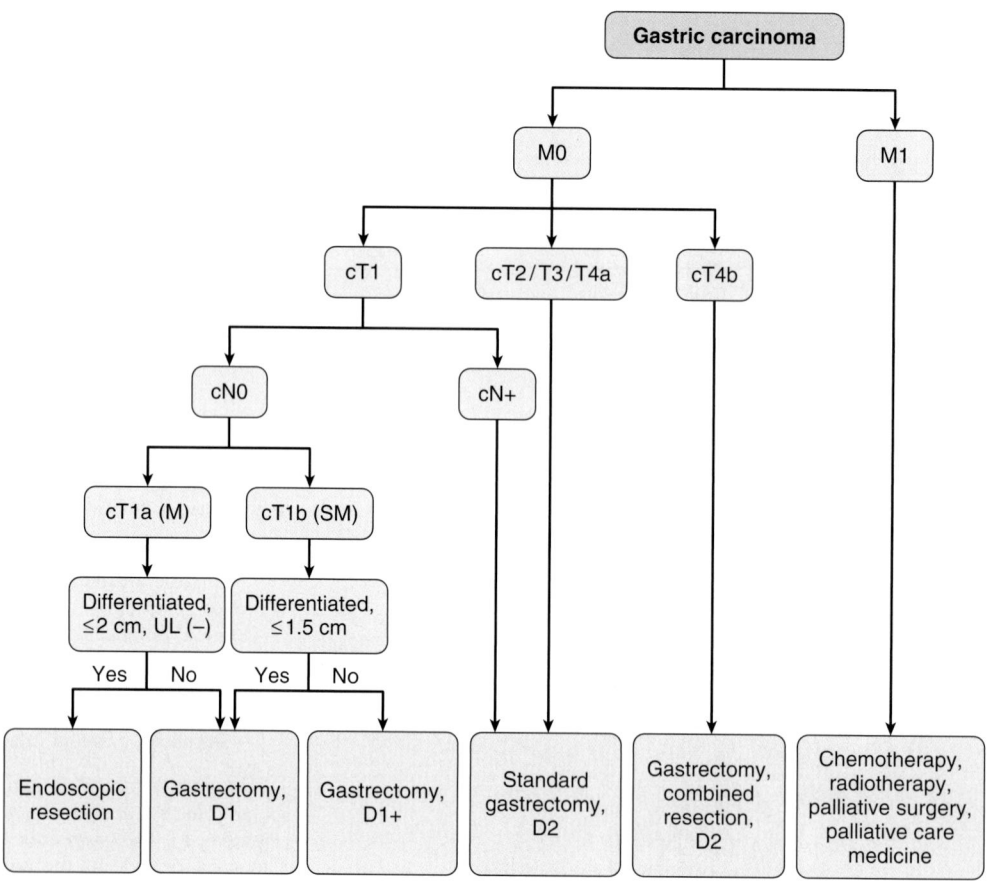

FIGURE 2 Recommended treatment algorithm. *(From Japanese Gastric Cancer Association: Japanese classification of gastric carcinoma: 3rd English edition, Gastric Cancer 14:101–112, 2011.)*

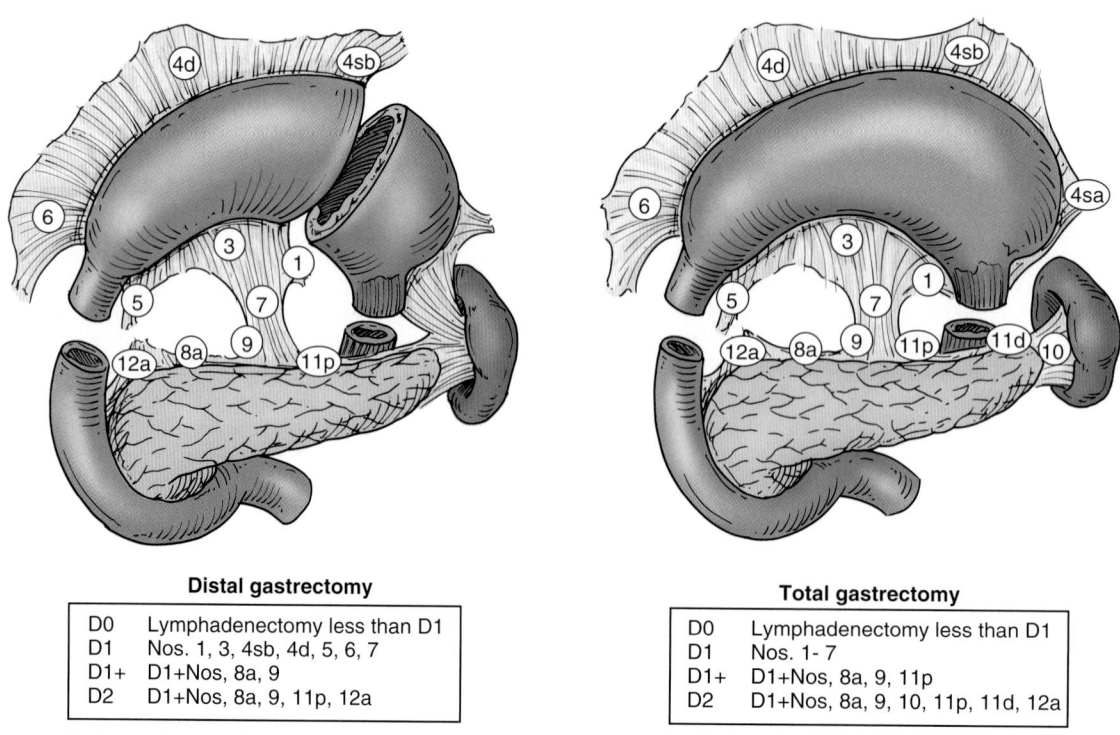

Distal gastrectomy

D0	Lymphadenectomy less than D1
D1	Nos. 1, 3, 4sb, 4d, 5, 6, 7
D1+	D1+Nos, 8a, 9
D2	D1+Nos, 8a, 9, 11p, 12a

Total gastrectomy

D0	Lymphadenectomy less than D1
D1	Nos. 1- 7
D1+	D1+Nos, 8a, 9, 11p
D2	D1+Nos, 8a, 9, 10, 11p, 11d, 12a

FIGURE 3 Extent of lymph node dissection in distal and total gastrectomies. *(From Japanese Gastric Cancer Association: Japanese classification of gastric carcinoma: 3rd English edition, Gastric Cancer 14:101–112, 2011.)*

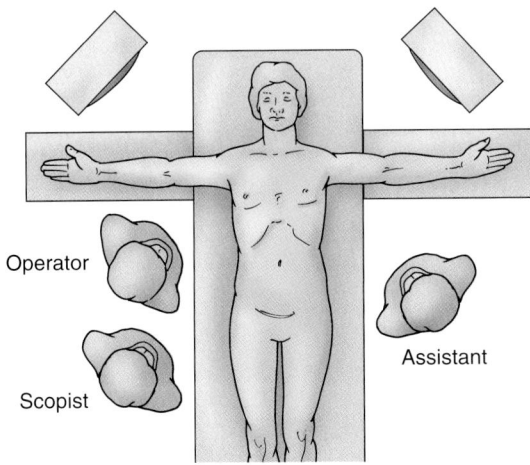

FIGURE 4 Room setup.

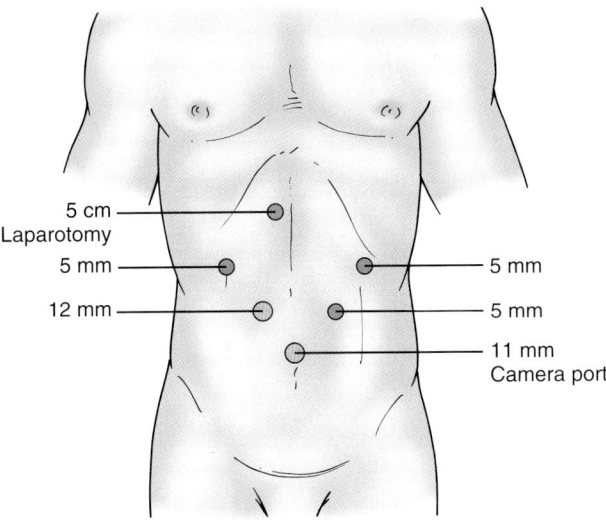

FIGURE 5 Port positions. The position of the right lower (12-mm) port is critical for lymph node dissection. Another 12-mm port for a liver retractor is placed at the medial end of where a 5-cm mini-laparotomy is planned (just to the right of the midline and overlying the pylorus).

the gastrocolic ligament is followed to the hepatic flexure, aiming for the gallbladder, and the dissection is deepened along the embryologic plane between the gastrocolic ligament and the anterior sheath of the transverse mesocolon, staying just anterior to transverse mesocolic vessels (Figure 7, A–D). Superior traction on the posterior wall of the antrum with the assistant's right-hand instrument and downward traction on the transverse mesocolon with the assistant's left-hand instrument facilitate this dissection. The endpoint of this dissection is exposure of the second part of the duodenum and the head of the pancreas.

Infrapyloric Dissection (No. 6 Lymph Nodes)

Key points: Division of origins of right gastroepiploic vein (RGEV), then right gastroepiploic artery (RGEA), clearing of first part of duodenum for a gastroduodenostomy.
Pitfalls: Bleeding (frequent), devascularization or perforation of the duodenum from excessive dissection.

The anterosuperior pancreaticoduodenal vein (ASPDV) runs across the anterior surface of the head of the pancreas and is a key landmark during this dissection and also marks the inferior border of LN station 6. It joins the RGEV at the level of the inferior border of the body of the pancreas. Within 1 to 2 cm of this confluence, the RGEV joins the accessory middle colic vein or, less frequently, the middle colic vein to form the gastrocolic trunk of Henle, which in turn drains into the superior mesenteric vein (SMV). The gastroduodenal artery (GDA) divides into two terminal branches—the RGEA and the anterosuperior pancreaticoduodenal artery (ASPDA)—at a significantly higher level compared with its venous counterpart, which divides closer to the superior border of the body of the pancreas.

Dissection is continued carefully along the same embryologic plane to reveal the origins of RGEV and ASPDV, and the gastrocolic trunk of Henle. During this dissection, downward traction on the transverse mesocolon is best achieved with a piece of gauze in the assistant's left-hand instrument, which helps to spread tension and prevent slippage. Further deeper dissection reveals the SMV; however, dissection of SMV (No. 14v) LNs is considered optional. The RGEV and ASPDV are dissected further and RGEV clipped and divided across its root. Then, LN tissues lying on the anterior surface of the head of the pancreas are carefully dissected until the dissection meets the lateral aspect of RGEA. On the opposite side of this vessel, the posterior wall of the antrum and the first part of the duodenum are dissected free from the neck of the pancreas, and the RGEA can be seen as a continuation of GDA. After confirming that the ASPDA has not been inadvertently elevated, the RGEA is double-clipped and divided on the surface of the pancreas. The infrapyloric dissection is completed by division of small branches of GDA to the first part of the duodenum and clearing the duodenum of any attached greater omentum in preparation for the gastroduodenostomy. At this point, perforation of the duodenal wall is a potential hazard.

Suprapyloric Dissection of Right Gastric Artery and Proper Hepatic Artery (Nos. 5 and 12a Lymph Nodes)

Key points: Sufficient infraduodenal dissection, fenestration of hepatoduodenal ligament, division of root of right gastric artery (RGA).
Pitfalls: Bleeding during suprapyloric fenestration, inadvertent injury to major vessels or common bile duct during dissection of hepatoduodenal ligament.

The RGA usually originates from the anteromedial aspect of the hepatic artery proper (HAP) midway up the hepatoduodenal ligament or, less frequently, from the GDA. The RGA gives rise to one or more suprapyloric branches. Suprapyloric branches and the supraduodenal artery from the GDA supply the pylorus and adjacent parts of the stomach and the duodenum.

Suprapyloric dissection is carried out in two portions: infraduodenal and supraduodenal. Adequate infraduodenal dissection makes the supraduodenal portion much safer. The infraduodenal portion of the dissection is a continuation of the infrapyloric dissection. Dissection is continued along the GDA with division of infrapyloric branches to the duodenum and antrum, to expose the junction between the GDA, common hepatic artery (CHA), and HAP (Figure 8, A). The CHA is partially dissected at this stage and its associated lymphatic tissues elevated. These are separated from the suprapyloric (No. 5) LNs using UCS, which helps to elevate the hepatoduodenal ligament away from the CHA and GDA for a safer supraduodenal dissection. Similarly, the left side of HAP can also be dissected and sometimes the origin of RGA itself visualized from below. Lastly, a piece of gauze is packed in the space created between the GDA and RGA to widen the space between the RGA and the first portion of the duodenum and to protect underlying vessels from injury during the fenestration of the gastroduodenal ligament (Figure 8, B–E).

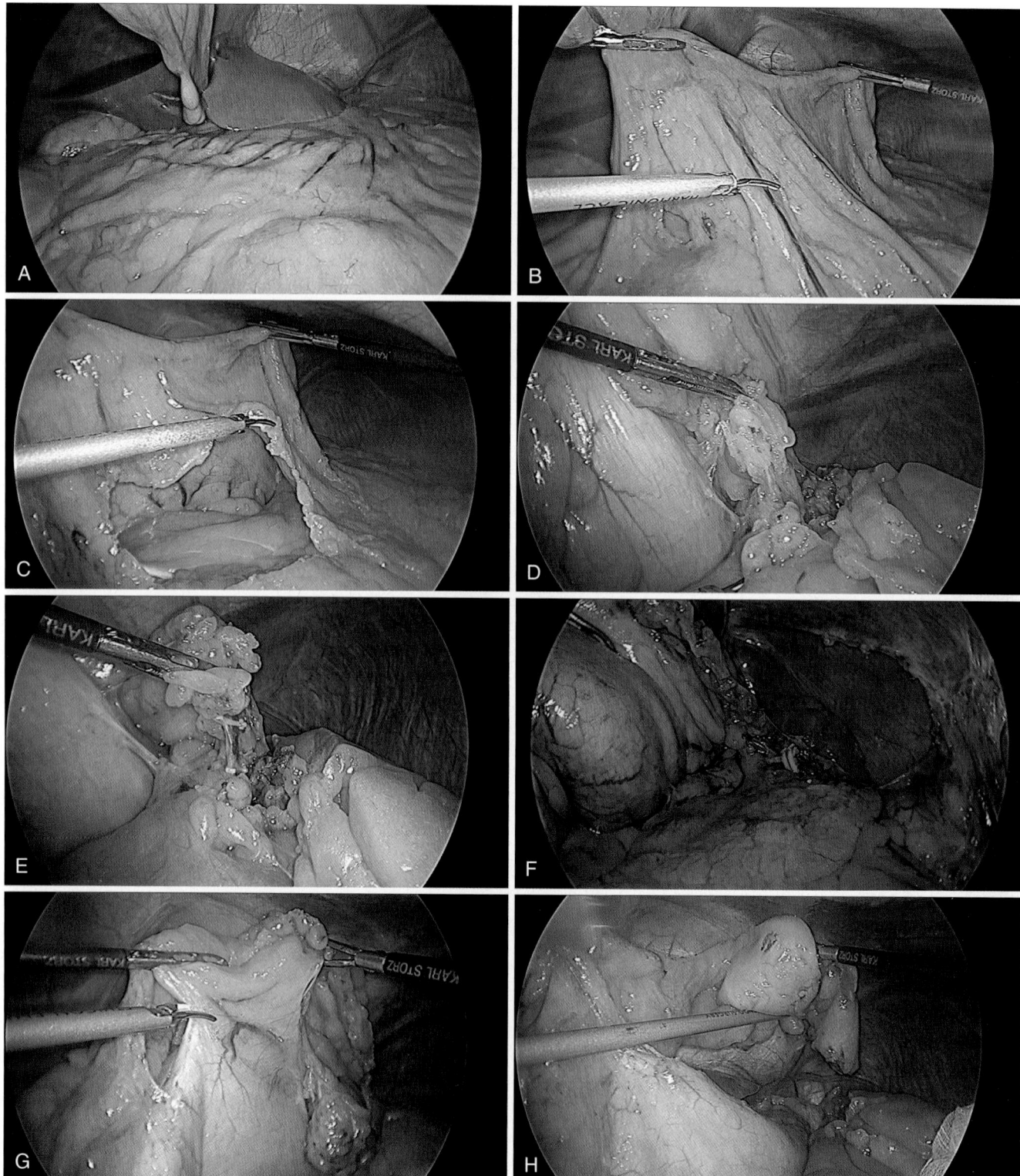

FIGURE 6 Dissection of greater omentum and left gastroepiploic vessels. **A–D,** Partial omentectomy; gastrocolic ligament is divided 3 to 4 cm outside the gastroepiploic arcade. Inspection of the posterior surface of the gastrocolic ligament helps to prevent injury to the transverse colon. **E,** Approaching the root of left gastroepiploic vessels. **F,** Ligation of transection of left gastroepiploic vessels. **G,H,** Clearing of greater curvature (No 4d).

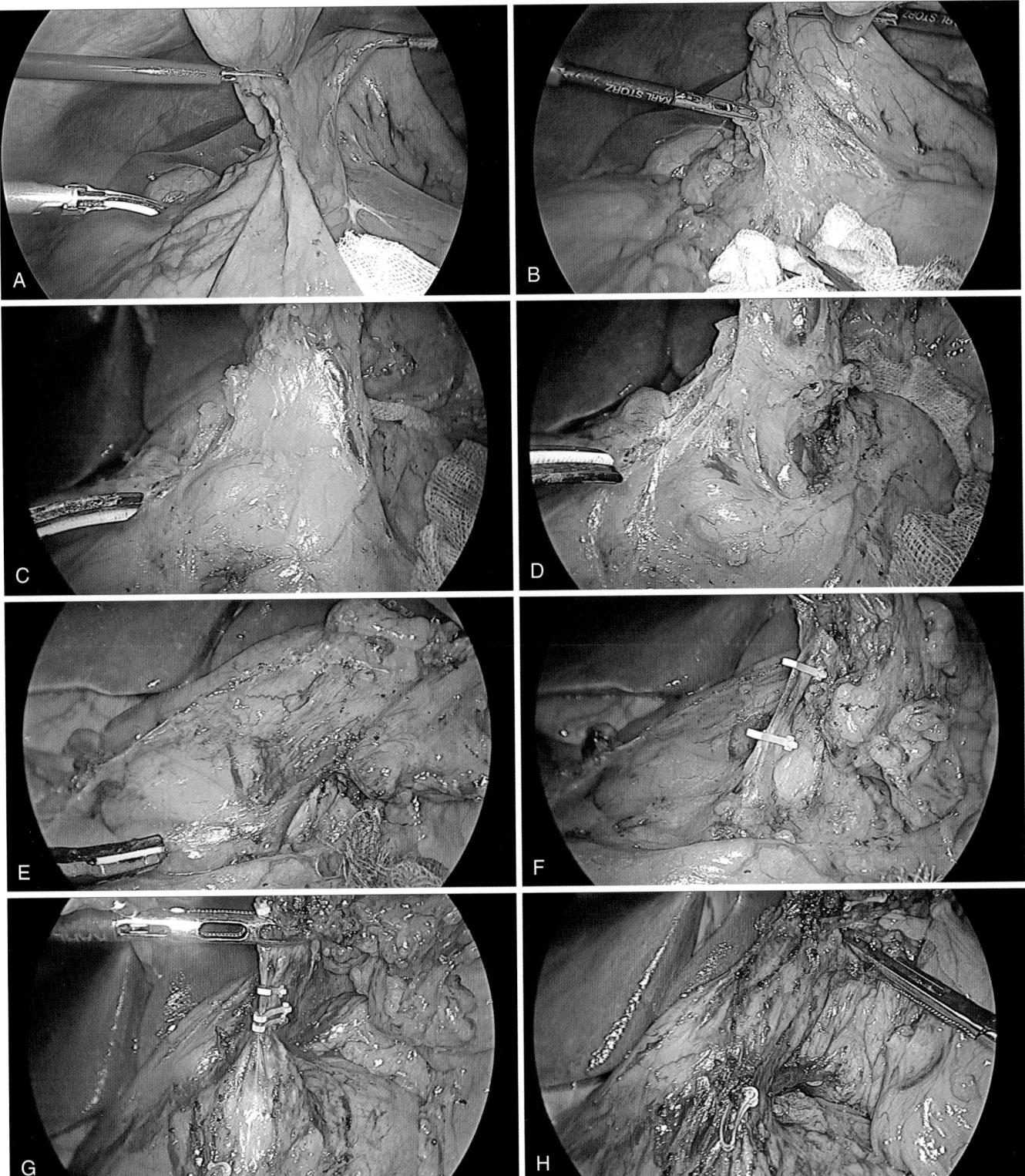

FIGURE 7   Infrapyloric dissection. **A–D,** Correct dissection plane for the infrapyloric dissection lies along the embryologic plane between the transverse mesocolon and the greater omentum. **E,** Completed infrapyloric dissection. **F,** RGEV is ligated. **G,** RGEA is ligated. **H,** Completed infrapyloric area. *RGEA,* Right gastroepiploic artery; *RGEV,* right gastroepiploic vein.

For the supraduodenal dissection, the left lobe of the liver is first retracted. The authors' preferred technique involves using a fan retractor introduced through a 12-mm port placed where a 5-cm long transverse mini-laparotomy is planned (see Figure 5). The mini-laparotomy will be placed to the right of the midline and directly overlying the duodenum. The fan retractor is secured in position with two nylon tapes around the ports to mimic a self-retaining retractor. The dissection starts with fenestration of gastroduodenal ligament. The optimal operative field is set up by splaying out the hepatoduodenal ligament between the surgeon's left-hand instrument and the assistant's right-hand instrument, and rolling down the pylorus with the assistant's left-hand instrument (Figure 8, B). Once a small window is created onto the gauze strip placed from below, the dissection is carried along the superior border of the antrum (about 1 cm) and duodenum (about 2 cm; Figure 8, C–E). Then the dissection is continued along the hepatoduodenal ligament in line with HAP and the root of RGA is identified, clipped, and divided, together with the right gastric vein (Figure 8, F,G). Dissection of HAP lymph nodes along the hepatoduodenal ligament (No. 12a LN) is included in a D2 dissection and involves dissection further cephalad along the hepatoduodenal ligament and more posteriorly onto the left border of the portal vein (Figure 9, A,B). Finally, the lesser omentum is divided close to its attachment to the left lobe of the liver until the dissection meets the apex of the right diaphragmatic crus. (The hepatic branch of anterior vagal trunk is preserved if a pylorus-preserving gastrectomy is planned.)

Suprapancreatic Dissection of Left Gastric, Common Hepatic, Celiac Trunk, and Proximal Splenic Artery Lymph Nodes (Nos. 7, 8a, 9, and 11p Lymph Nodes)

Key points: Rolling down of pancreas to obtain adequate exposure, entry into the retroperitoneal space at the superior border of the pancreas, division of left gastric artery (LGA) and coronary vein at their origins.

Pitfalls: Injury to the splenic artery and vein (may necessitate a conversion to a total gastrectomy), injury to the pancreas (leading to pancreatitis or pancreatic fistula) or the aorta.

The celiac trunk and its branches are partially covered by the superior border of the pancreas, particularly so when viewed with a laparoscope through the umbilicus. The pancreaticogastric fold connects the retroperitoneum to the lesser curvature of the stomach and carries the LGA and the coronary vein. The coronary vein usually runs behind and perpendicular to the superior border of the pancreas to drain into the splenic vein; however, when it drains into the portal vein, it is found running down obliquely further onto the right. The tortuosity of the splenic artery and its close relationship to the splenic vein (immediately posterior to it) makes station 11p dissection particularly hazardous. The posterior gastric artery originates from the midpoint of the splenic artery in close proximity to the posterior fundic wall. It is present in only half of all individuals.

The suprapancreatic dissection is one of the most technically challenging and hazardous steps during a laparoscopic gastrectomy. Maintaining an adequate exposure is critical. This can be achieved by applying upward traction on the pancreaticogastric fold (left gastric vessels) with the assistant's right-hand grasper while continually rolling down the superior border of the pancreas with a piece of gauze in the assistant's left-hand grasper as the dissection progresses (see Figure 8, H). The suprapancreatic dissection can be approached either with the stomach retracted superiorly (providing a wide view of the lesser sac) or with it resting down (more convenient for dissection to the right of the LGA). The first step of the suprapancreatic dissection is division of the pancreatic capsule along its superior

border, from right to left. Then, en bloc dissection is performed, first along the already partly dissected CHA onto its root and then along the splenic artery. The coronary vein lies superficial to the LGA in the pancreaticogastric ligament in this approach, and it is divided between clips, close to the superior border of the pancreas. The proximal splenic artery (No. 11p) LN station is bounded laterally by the posterior gastric artery, which is preserved. Complete 11p dissection is recommended in a LADG for cT2 or greater tumors and in a total gastrectomy. Surgeons tend to include a portion of 11p dissection in all distal gastrectomies, even for early gastric cancer, as this ensures exposure of the origins of the splenic artery and the LGA. After confirming the origins of all three branches of the celiac trunk, the LGA is double-clipped and divided across its root. Then both sides of the celiac trunk are dissected and the diaphragmatic crura exposed to complete station 9 and 11p dissection. Extreme caution is advised, particularly for the lateral extent of station 11p dissection to avoid injury to the splenic artery or vein (Figure 9, C–F).

Dissection Along Lesser Curvature of Stomach (Nos. 1 and 3 Lymph Nodes)

Key points: Splaying out and alignment of the stomach wall parallel to the energy device.

Pitfalls: Injury to the fundus of the stomach during station 1 dissection or to the lesser curvature of the stomach during station 3 LN dissection; inadequate dissection, especially on the posterior wall of the lesser curvature.

The right paracardial (No. 1) LN station includes LNs in the pericardial fat pad to the right of the longitudinal axis of the esophagus as well as LNs along the first branch of the ascending limb of the LGA (Figure 9, G,H). The lesser curvature (No. 3) LN station includes LNs along the LGA as well as those along the RGA from its second branch.

In preparation of this dissection, the lymphatic tissue attached to the lesser curvature is dissected completely free from the diaphragmatic crura up to the esophagogastric junction. The dissection starts at the top and is progressed distally. The authors' preferred direction of station 3 LN dissection is from the posterior gastric wall to the anterior wall. The key to a safe dissection here is to splay out and orient the gastric wall parallel to the blades of the UCS by applying adequate longitudinal traction along the lesser curvature with the assistant's left-hand instrument while continually rolling out the lesser curvature soft tissues toward the left upper quadrant with the assistant's right hand. Since the correct dissection plane lies just outside of the muscularis propria, a large area of muscle fibers along the lesser curvature will be exposed at the end of this dissection (Figure 9, I). When there is a replacing left hepatic artery originated from left gastric artery, we can preserve that replacing left hepatic artery during the dissection of station 7 LN for early gastric cancer (Figure 9, J). Lesser curvature dissection is continued distal to the proposed line of gastric transection. This completes the LN dissection for an LADG.

TECHNIQUES OF RECONSTRUCTION

The Billroth I anastomosis (gastroduodenostomy) is a favored method of reconstruction following a distal gastrectomy for cancer at many centers in Japan and Korea. This is in stark contrast to the West, where either Billroth II or Roux-en-Y reconstructions are being used almost exclusively. This section discusses the techniques and pitfalls of three commonly used approaches for a Billroth I reconstruction. Aspects of Billroth II and Roux-en-Y reconstructions that are relevant to laparoscopic distal gastrectomies are also briefly discussed.

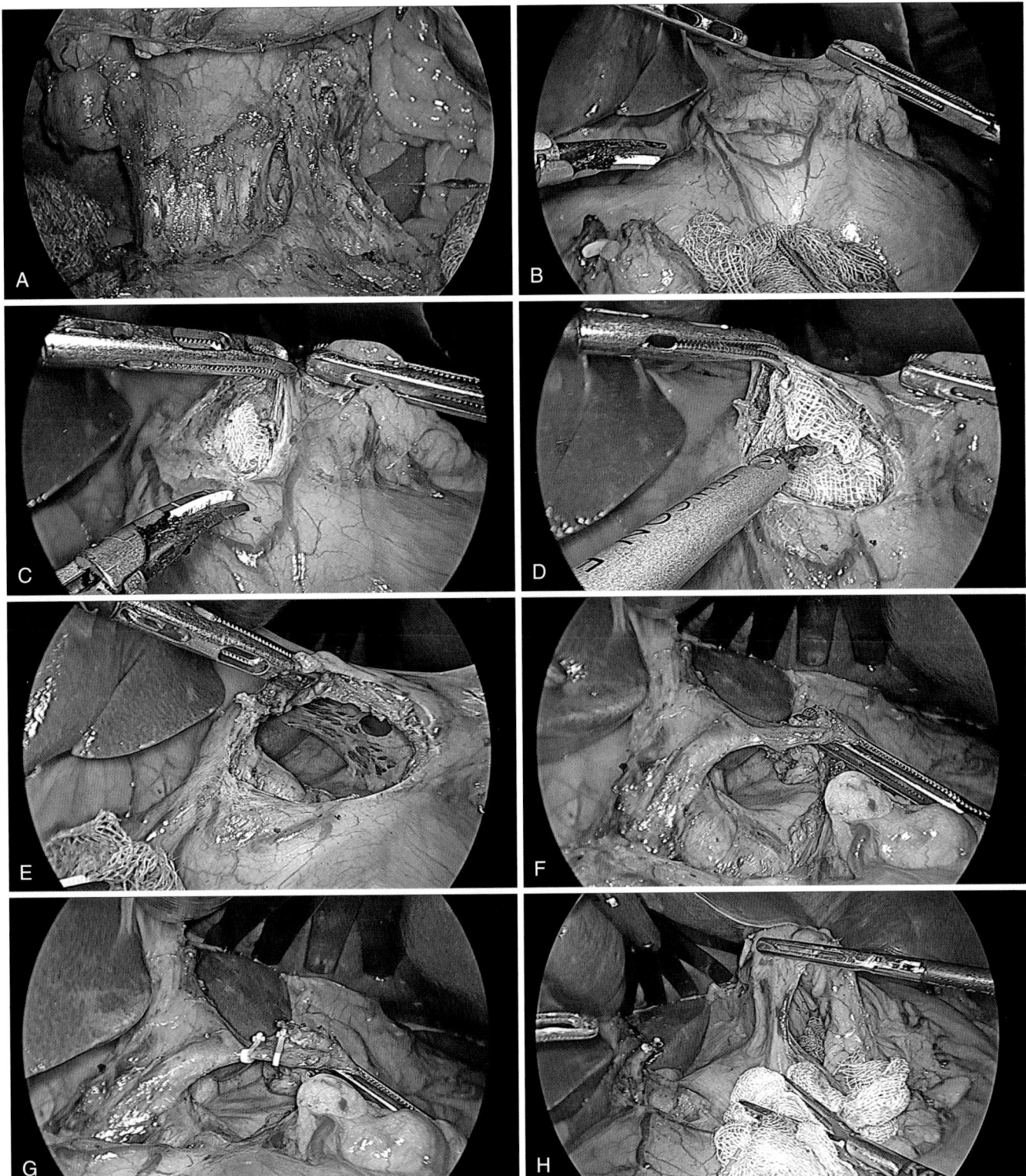

FIGURE 8 Dissection along GDA. **A,** Setup for suprapyloric dissection. **B,** Correct dissection. **C–E,** Opening space between RGA and duodenum. **F,G,** RGA dissected and ligated. **H,** set up for suprapancreatic dissection. *GDA,* Gastroduodenal artery; *RGA,* right gastric artery.

Techniques of Billroth I Anastomosis

An extracorporeal Billroth I anastomosis is commonly performed in one of two ways: modified double-stapled circular anastomosis (favored by the authors) and a side-to-end circular anastomosis through the posterior gastric wall.

Extracorporeal Modified Double-Stapled Circular End-to-End Gastroduodenostomy

A 5-cm transverse mini-laparotomy in the epigastrium is used to perform an extracorporeal anastomosis and to remove the specimen (see Figure 5). The distal stomach and proximal duodenum, as well as dissected LN stations, are first retrieved from the abdomen (Figure 10, B). A size 0 Prolene (Ethicon, Somerville, NJ) purse-string suture is applied to the proximal duodenum with a purse-string clamp, and the duodenum is transected just distal to the pylorus (Figure 10, C). The anvil of a 28-mm or 31-mm circular stapler is secured into the duodenal stump (Figure 10, D). The proximal resection line is determined by palpating the clips or sometimes the tumor itself. A gastrotomy is made, on the specimen side, between two stay sutures on the side opposite to the tumor; direct visualization of the clips or tumor confirms its location (Figure 10, E). The stomach is then partially transected, beginning at the greater curvature (Figure 10, F). During this first firing of a 60-mm linear stapler, it is imperative that the line of transection be as perpendicular to the greater curvature as possible and that enough of a gap is left medially for passage of the circular stapler. The circular stapler is introduced through the gastrotomy and into the proximal stomach (Figure 10, G and Figure 11, A). The stapler shaft and the distal stomach are rotated 180 degrees clockwise, and the trocar is advanced so as to penetrate the very corner of the staple line at the greater curvature of the remnant stomach, which is the longest part of the remnant stomach Figure 10, H-J and Figure 10, B. Rotation and downward angulation of the stapler then allows engagement of the trocar to the previously secured anvil (Figure 10, K). Prior to firing of the stapler, the linear staple line should be maneuvered to a 9 o'clock position, forming the new lesser curvature (Figure 10, L). Finally, using a 100-mm linear stapler, the

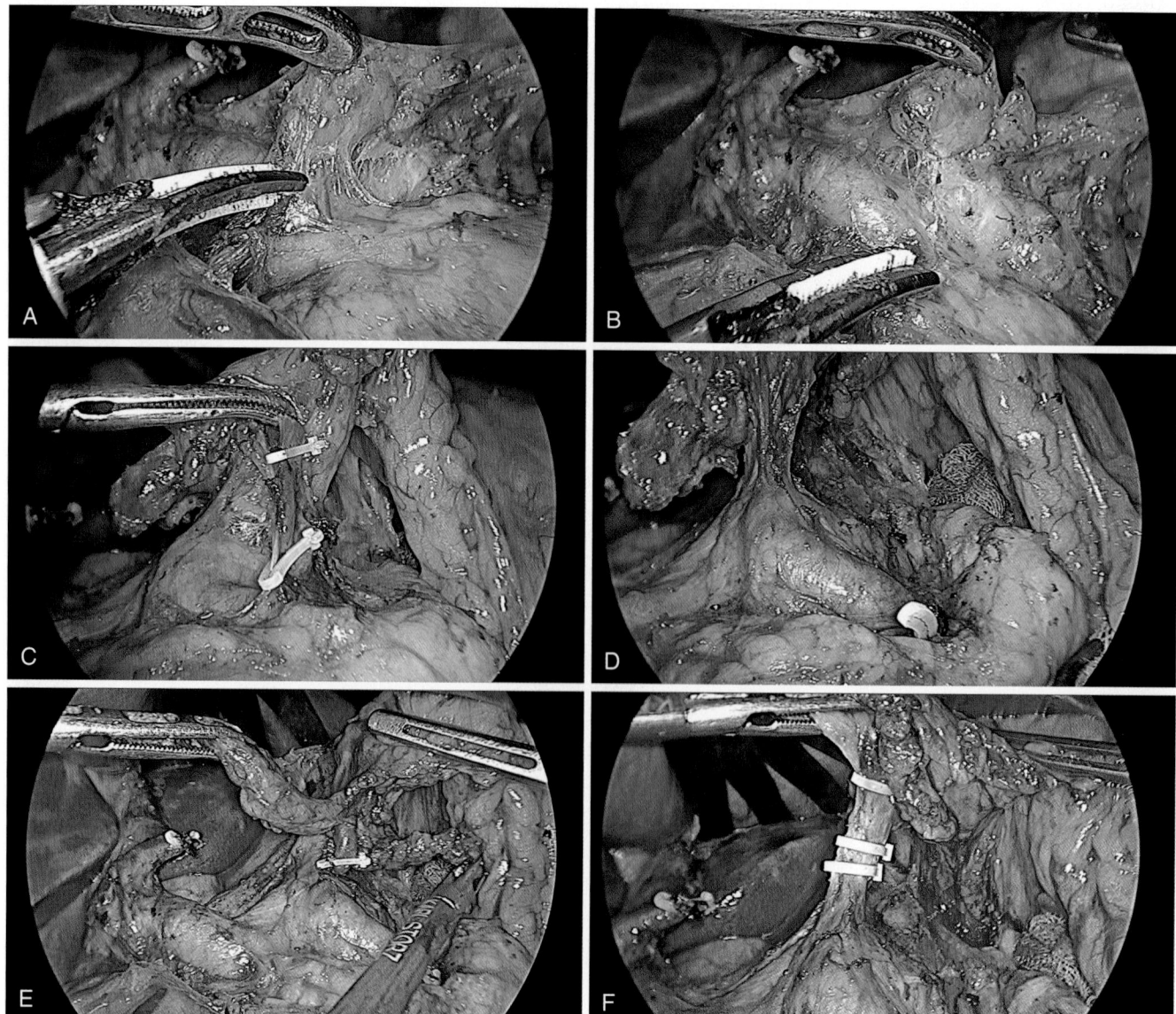

FIGURE 9 **A, B,** Correct dissection plane along CHA. Note the parallel approach of ultrasonic shears along CHA. **C–D,** Coronary vein and proximal part of splenic artery. **E,** Lifted lymph nodes from CHA and SA. **F,** Ligated LGA.

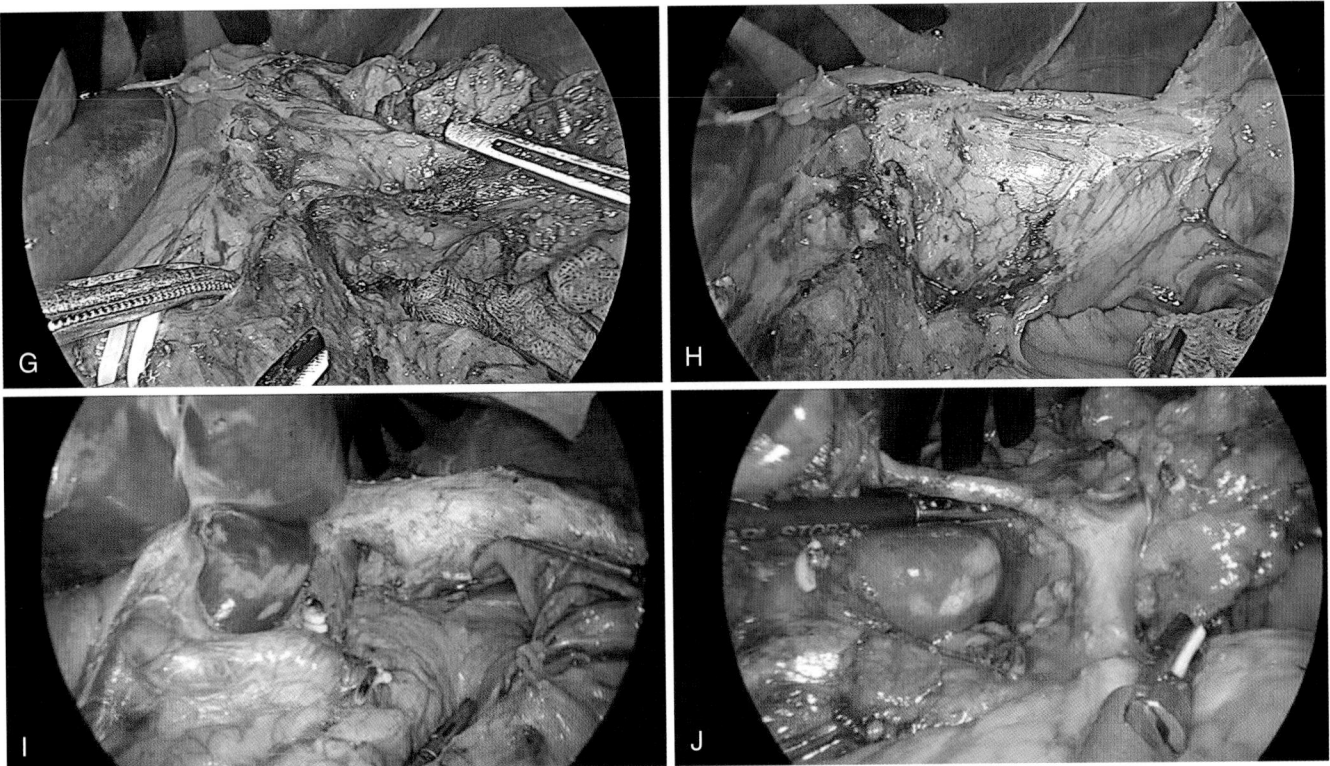

FIGURE 9, cont'd   G,H, Along the cardia and lesser curvature. **I,** Completed LN dissection. **J,** Preserved replacing left hepatic artery originating from LGA. *CHA,* Common hepatic artery; *SA,* splenic artery; *LGA,* left gastric artery.

lesser curvature side of the proximal stomach is transected toward the gastroesophageal junction with inclusion of the apex of the initial linear staple line into the specimen (Figure 10, *M* and Figure 11, *C* and *D*). The specimen is processed on a back table to assess resection margins. Margins are sent for frozen section routinely. Pneumoperitoneum is reestablished with a glove over a wound protector. After hemostasis has been established, the peritoneal cavity is irrigated and a closed suction drain is placed prior to closure (Figure 10, *N*).

Extracorporeal Side-to-End Circular Gastroduodenostomy

In this method, the duodenal stump is prepared in the same way as it is in the extracorporeal modified double-stapled method. The stomach is then partially transected from the greater curvature side between two clamps, and the transection is completed on the medial side of the stomach with a linear stapler, leaving a transverse gastrotomy laterally. The specimen is checked for adequacy of resection margins on a back table. The circular stapler is then introduced through the gastrotomy and a side-to-end gastroduodenostomy created between the posterior wall of the stomach and the duodenum. The anastomosis should be located close to the greater curvature to reduce tension as much as possible. A gap of around 1 to 2 cm between the two staple lines is ensured to avoid an ischemic bridge of stomach wall. The initial gastrotomy is closed with a linear stapler. This technique is simpler to perform; however, it has greater potential for creating tension in the anastomosis, as the anastomosis is naturally placed slightly more proximally.

Intracorporeal Delta-Shaped Gastroduodenostomy

The stated advantages of an intracorporeal anastomosis include less pain (no upper abdominal mini-laparotomy), improved exposure during the anastomosis (especially in obese individuals), and better cosmesis. However, it is technically more challenging, with numerous potential pitfalls, and requires more firings of the stapler (at least six). Because of the absence of a mini-laparotomy, intraoperative tumor localization poses another challenge. Therefore, this modality is usually limited to distal antral lesions unless an alternative method of intraoperative localization (such as intraoperative gastroscope or intraoperative simple abdomen with metal clips applied near the preoperative clips at the margin of the tumor) is employed. There is also greater potential for uncontrolled spillage of intragastric fluid in a totally laparoscopic approach. The authors' study demonstrated that intragastric luminal cytology was positive even in early gastric cancer and that this positivity increased after surgical maneuver.

For this technique, the duodenum and the stomach are transected with 60-mm linear staplers introduced through a 12-mm assistant's left-hand port. The specimen is removed, with a large plastic bag, through an extended umbilical incision. There are two key points in avoiding anastomosis-related complications. One is to transect the duodenum from the posterior wall to the anterior wall, instead of in the usual craniocaudal direction. This is important in preserving the vascularity of the duodenal stump as well as adequate duodenal cuff for the anastomosis. The other key point is to ensure wide-enough angles between staple lines when performing the gastroduodenostomy (with a 45-mm stapler) by everting the first two staple lines. A safe fallback option in the event of a major intraoperative mishap is conversion to either a Billroth II or a Roux-en-Y gastrojejunostomy.

Billroth II Reconstruction

There are several aspects to be considered when performing a gastrojejunostomy in an LADG. It can be performed extracorporeally (via an upper midline mini-laparotomy) or intracorporeally. An extracorporeal anastomosis may be sutured or stapled with a linear stapler. The antecolic route is easier and generally recommended. The

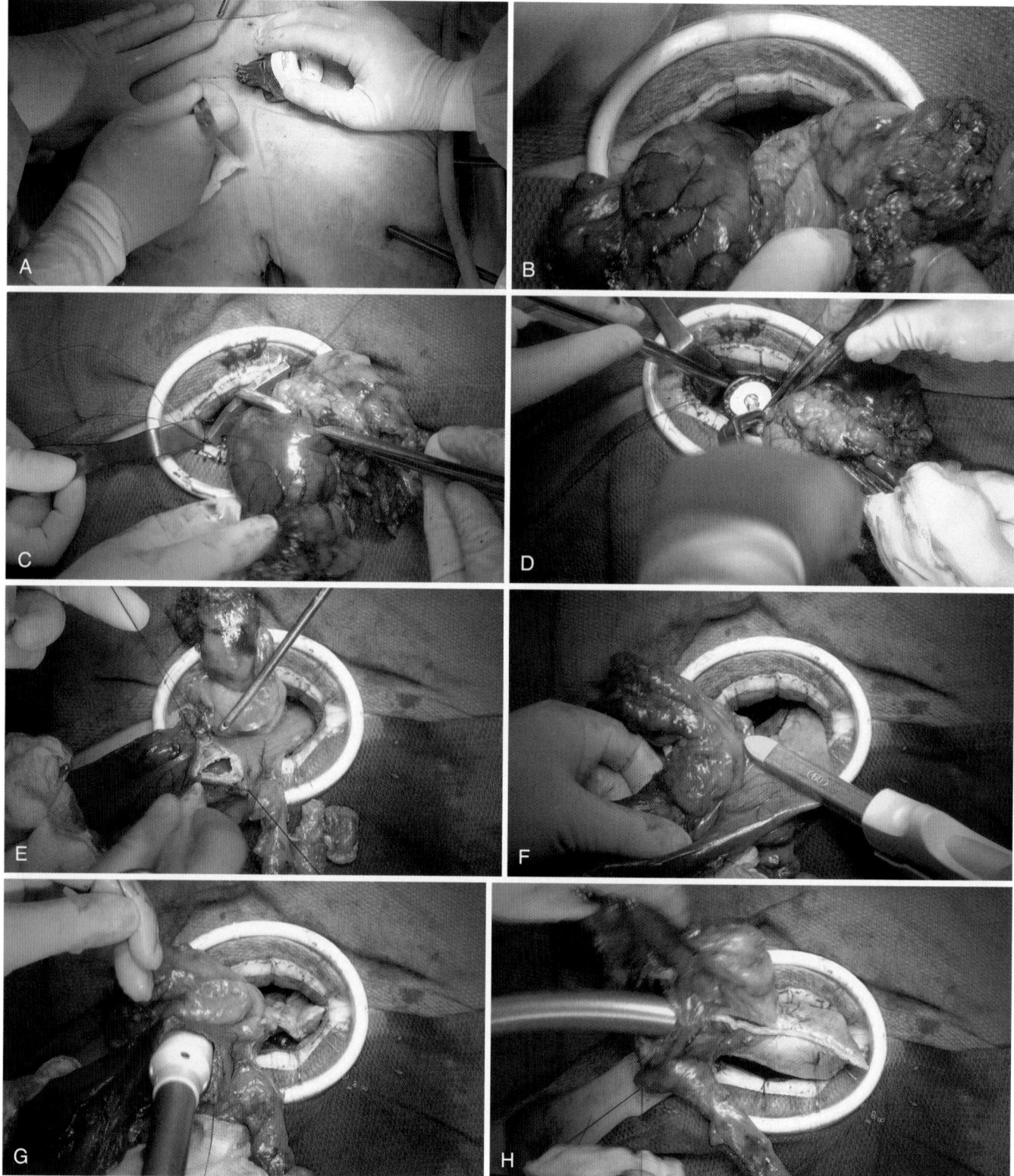

FIGURE 10 Extracorporeal modified double-stapled Billroth I anastomosis.

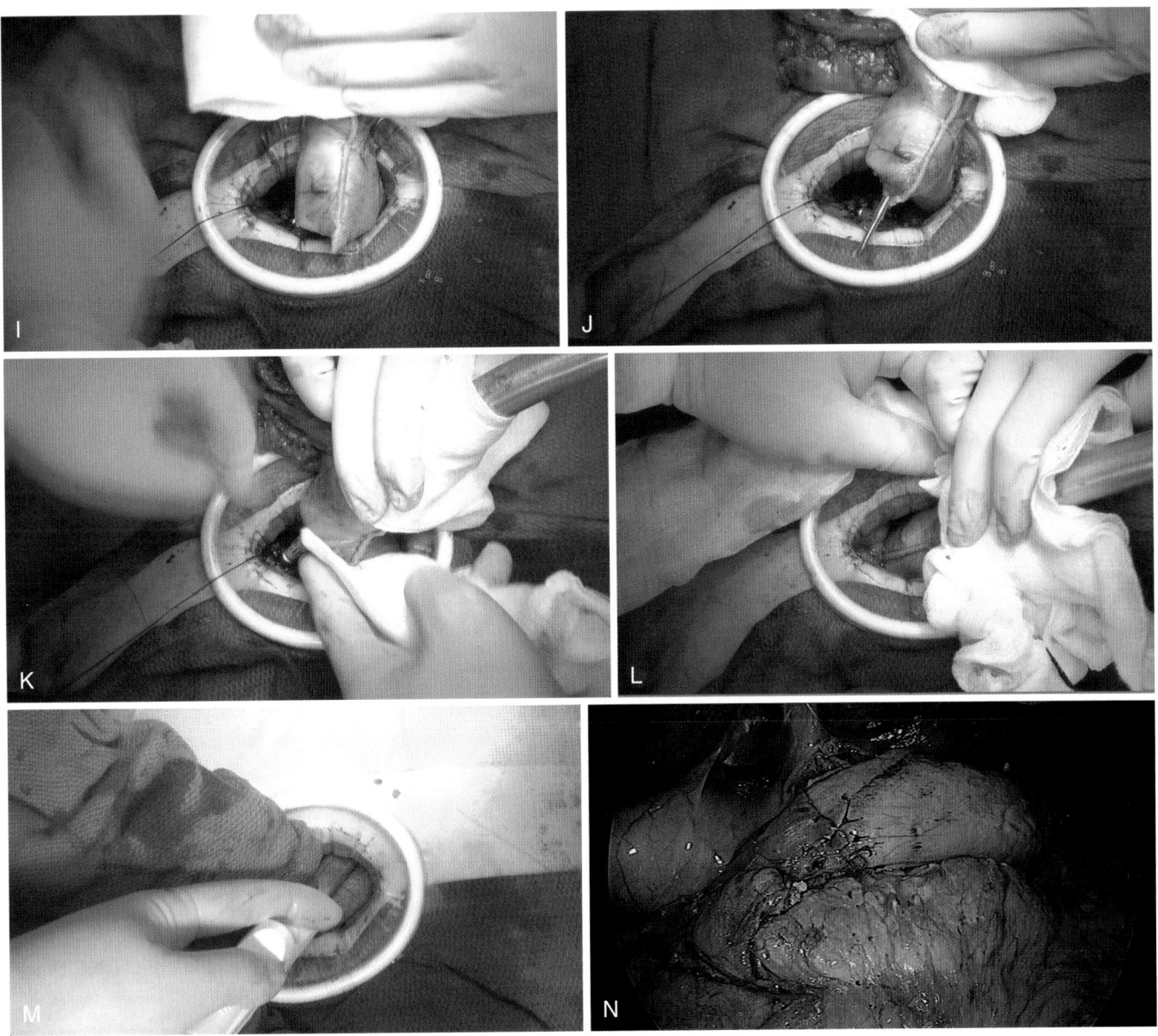

FIGURE 10, cont'd

posterior gastric wall adjacent to the greater curvature is the authors' preferred site for a stapled anastomosis. The jejunal loop can be aligned in either an isoperistaltic or an antiperistaltic manner. If the remnant stomach is small, a Braun anastomosis (a side-to-side jejunojejunostomy connecting the afferent and efferent limbs) can be added to decrease the incidence of bile reflux gastritis.

With a stapler to close the common entry hole in a stapled isoperistaltic anastomosis, the efferent limb can potentially be narrowed, especially if the staple is fired in a longitudinal manner. To avoid this problem, the initial enterotomy should be made as small as possible and the common entry should preferably be sutured close or else stapled in a transverse manner. Minor narrowing of the afferent limb in an antiperistaltic reconstruction may be inconsequential; however, significant narrowing can lead to a duodenal stump leak. If the remnant stomach is very small, a Roux-en-Y reconstruction is preferred, as this minimizes tension at the anastomosis and reduces the incidence of bile reflux esophagitis.

Roux-en-Y Reconstruction

Many of the discussions for a Billroth II reconstruction also apply to the Roux-en-Y reconstruction. For example, a Roux-en-Y reconstruction may be performed entirely laparoscopically or via a mini-laparotomy (upper midline or a left upper quadrant transverse), and the gastrojejunostomy can be similarly stapled or sutured, usually in an antecolic and isoperistaltic manner. Additional considerations include length of the Roux limb (25 to 30 cm is considered ideal for a distal gastrectomy to minimize both bile reflux and Roux limb stasis syndrome); potential to mistake the alimentary limb for the biliopancreatic limb; and potential for future internal herniation.

A Roux-en-Y reconstruction via a mini-laparotomy is described briefly, covering salient points. As in a Billroth II reconstruction, the duodenum is divided prior to the suprapancreatic dissection, which significantly improves the exposure. Following completion of LN dissection, in a Trendelenburg position, the proximal jejunum is

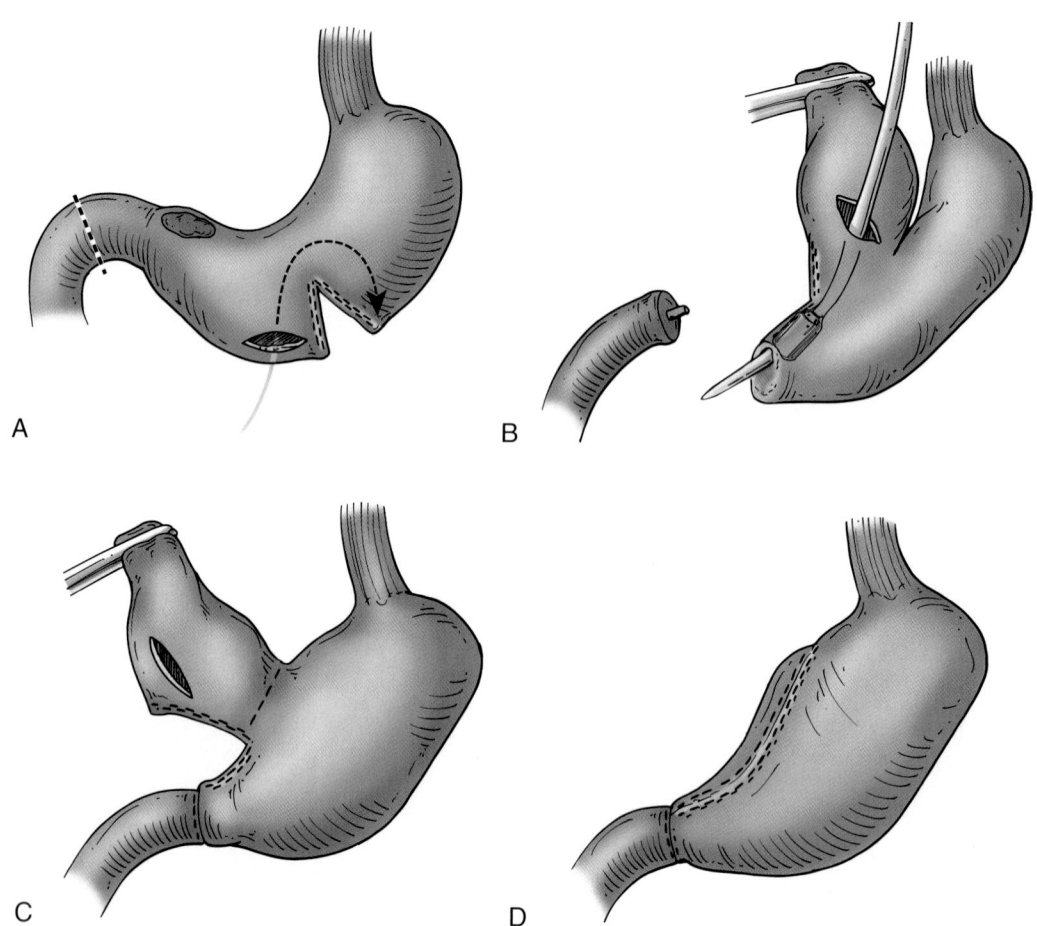

FIGURE 11 Schematic diagram of modified double-stapled Billroth I anastomosis. *(From Yang HK, et al: Safety of modified double-stapled end-to-end gastroduodenostomy in distal subtotal gastrectomy. J Surg Oncol 96:624–629, 2007).*

oriented with respect to the ligament of Treitz, and a loop with adequate mesenteric length to reach the remnant stomach is selected. Following orientation marking of the jejunal loop with either ink or a suture and with the loop held between two graspers by the assistant, an upper midline mini-laparotomy is made. The jejunal loop is delivered and stay sutures placed. The stomach is divided with adequate proximal margin, which is confirmed by frozen section. The jejunum is then divided with a linear stapler. A formal mesenteric division is usually not necessary in a distal gastrectomy and is difficult to achieve safely through the mini-laparotomy. A side-to-side jejunojejunostomy is created, either hand-sewn or stapled, and the mesenteric defect is closed. A stapled side-to-side gastrojejunostomy, again using the posterior gastric wall close to the greater curvature, with preservation of the short gastric vessels, completes the reconstruction. Closure of Peterson's space is recommended and is best achieved laparoscopically following reestablishment of pneumoperitoneum.

SPECIAL CONSIDERATIONS

Laparoscopic Total Gastrectomy

Currently, the authors' clinical indications for a LTG include early gastric cancer located in or extending into proximal stomach where a distal or subtotal gastrectomy is not possible. Compared to laparoscopic distal gastrectomy (LDG), data on the feasibility and oncologic safety of LTG are so far lacking. A LTG is technically more demanding—particularly the reconstruction, which has not been standardized.

Many reconstructive methods for esophagojejunostomy are used, including end-to-side circular stapler and linear side-to-side (overlap) methods. One of the main difficulties of the circular stapling method is how to apply purse-string sutures for esophageal stump with anvil. Different laparoscopic purse-string suture clamps are being developed; transorally inserted anvil, OrVil (Covidien, Mansfield, Mass) is another option. Because of high morbidity after laparoscopic esophagojejunostomy, a phase II study (KLASS-03) has started in South Korea.

Total Omentectomy

Total omentectomy is indicated in advanced gastric cancer but is time consuming and technically difficult. Care must be taken to avoid thermal injury to the transverse colon, especially when diverticular disease is suspected. Tilting the table in the Trendelenburg position can help in cephalad retraction of the greater omentum during its dissection. After omentectomy, it is difficult to lift the stomach with the omentum. The hanging method, that is, pulling the stomach with wrapped gauzes around the antrum and the lower body, including the omentum, is effective.

Robot-Assisted Gastrectomy

Despite initial enthusiasm and widespread use, robot-assisted gastrectomy has not been shown to have significant additional benefit when compared with standard laparoscopic gastrectomy in terms of patient outcomes or cost-effectiveness. Articulating energy devices may provide benefit compared with a standard laparoscopic approach.

SUGGESTED READINGS

Hayashi H, Ochiai T, Shimada H, et al: Prospective randomized study of open versus laparoscopy-assisted distal gastrectomy with extraperigastric lymph node dissection for early gastric cancer, *Surg Endosc* 19:1172–1176, 2005.

Huscher CG, Mingoli A, Sgarzini G, et al: Laparoscopic versus open subtotal gastrectomy for distal gastric cancer: five-year results of a randomized prospective trial, *Ann Surg* 241:232–237, 2005.

Japanese Gastric Cancer Association: Japanese classification of gastric carcinoma: 3rd English edition, *Gastric Cancer* 14:101–112, 2011.

Japanese Gastric Cancer Association: Japanese gastric cancer treatment guidelines 2010 (ver. 3), *Gastric Cancer* 14: 113–123, 2011.

Jiang L, Yang KH, Guan QL, et al: Laparoscopy-assisted gastrectomy versus open gastrectomy for resectable gastric cancer: an update meta-analysis based on randomized controlled trials, *Surg Endosc* 27:2466–2480, 2013 DOI: 10.1007/s00464-012-2758-6.

Kanaya S, Kawamura Y, Kawada H, et al: The delta-shaped anastomosis in laparoscopic distal gastrectomy: analysis of the initial 100 consecutive procedures of intracorporeal gastroduodenostomy, *Gastric Cancer* 14:365–371, 2011.

Kim HH, Hyung WJ, Cho GS, et al: Morbidity and mortality of laparoscopic gastrectomy versus open gastrectomy for gastric cancer: an interim report-a phase III multicenter, prospective, randomized Trial (KLASS Trial), *Ann Surg* 251:417–420, 2010.

Kim W, Song KY, Lee HJ, et al: The impact of comorbidity on surgical outcomes in laparoscopy-assisted distal gastrectomy: a retrospective analysis of multicenter results, *Ann Surg* 248:793–799, 2008.

Kim YW, Baik YH, Yun YH, et al: Improved quality of life outcomes after laparoscopy-assisted distal gastrectomy for early gastric cancer: results of a prospective randomized clinical trial, *Ann Surg* 248:721–727, 2008.

Kitano S, Yang HK, editors: *Laparoscopic gastrectomy for cancer—standard techniques and clinical evidences.* Tokyo, 2012, Springer.

Kodera Y, Fujiwara M, Ohashi N, et al: Laparoscopic surgery for gastric cancer: a collective review with meta-analysis of randomized trials, *J Am Coll Surg* 211:677–686, 2010.

Lee HJ, Kim HH, Kim MC, et al: The impact of a high body mass index on laparoscopy assisted gastrectomy for gastric cancer, *Surg Endosc* 23:2473–2479, 2009.

Lee HJ, Shiraishi N, Kim HH, et al: Standard of practice on laparoscopic gastric cancer surgery in Korea and Japan: experts' survey, *Asian J Endosc Surg* 5:5–11, 2012.

Nagai E, Ohuchida K, Nakata K, et al: Feasibility and safety of intracorporeal esophagojejunostomy after laparoscopic total gastrectomy: inverted T-shaped anastomosis using linear staplers, *Surgery* 153:732–738, 2013. DOI: pii: S0039-S6060(12)00630-7.

Noshiro H, Shimizu S, Nagai E, et al: Laparoscopy-assisted distal gastrectomy for early gastric cancer: is it beneficial for patients of heavier weight? *Ann Surg* 238:680–685, 2003.

Sakuramoto S, Kikuchi S, Futawatari N, et al: Technique of esophagojejunostomy using transoral placement of the pretilted anvil head after laparoscopic gastrectomy for gastric cancer, *Surgery* 147:742–747, 2010.

Shim JH, Yoo HM, Oh SI, et al: Various types of intracorporeal esophagojejunostomy after laparoscopic total gastrectomy for gastric cancer, *Gastric Cancer* 16:420–427, 2013. DOI: 10.1007/s10120-012-0207-9.

Song J, Oh SJ, Kang WH, et al: Robot-assisted gastrectomy with lymph node dissection for gastric cancer: lessons learned from an initial 100 consecutive procedures, *Ann Surg* 249:927–932, 2009.

Viñuela EF, Gonen M, Brennan MF, et al: Laparoscopic versus open distal gastrectomy for gastric cancer: a meta-analysis of randomized controlled trials and high-quality nonrandomized studies, *Ann Surg* 255:446–456, 2012.

Wall J, Marescaux J: Robotic gastrectomy is safe and feasible, but real benefits remain elusive, *Arch Surg* 146:1092, 2011.

Yang HK, Suh YS, Lee HJ: Minimally invasive approaches for gastric cancer—Korean experience, *J Surg Oncol* 107:277–281, 2013.

LAPAROSCOPIC MANAGEMENT OF CROHN'S DISEASE

Alessandro Fichera, MD, FACS, FASCRS, and Konstantin Umanskiy, MD, FACS

OVERVIEW

Despite significant advances in medical management of Crohn's disease (CD) with the introduction of immunomodulators and biologic agents in the late 1990s, patients with CD are still frequently referred for surgery; the lifelong need for surgery has been reported to be as prevalent as 82%. Patients with CD have traditionally been considered poor laparoscopic candidates because of the panintestinal nature of the disease, with "skip" lesions, inflammatory complications, and the use of aggressive and often medical management that increases the risk of postoperative complications. However, minimally invasive approaches have been developed for CD since 1990, and in single-institution retrospective small studies have been shown to improve cosmetic results and potentially reduce postoperative ileus and hospital stay. The impact of laparoscopy on short- and long-term recurrence rates has been poorly studied, and although small, single-institution studies, including the authors', have shown recurrence rates similar to those after open surgery, definitive large prospective studies to adequately answer this important question are lacking.

Modern principles of surgical management dictate that intestinal resections should be limited, without wide margins of normal tissue. Greater understanding of the clinical course of CD has led to a more conservative strategy, with surgery reserved for the treatment of complications of the disease and bowel-sparing approaches advocated. The indications for laparoscopic surgery for CD do not, and should not, differ from those for conventional open surgery (Figure 1). Relative contraindications to a laparoscopic approach include inability of critically ill patients to tolerate pneumoperitoneum because of

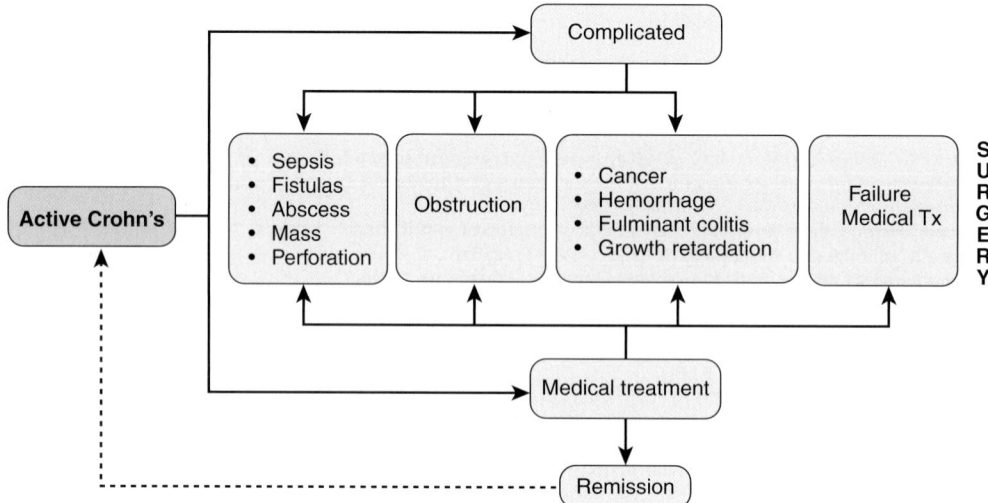

FIGURE 1 Indications for surgery in Crohn's disease. (© 2009 University of Chicago.)

hypotension or hypercarbia; the presence of dense adhesions or extensive intra-abdominal sepsis (abscess, free perforation, complex fistula); and difficulty in identifying the anatomy (previous surgery, obesity, adhesions). Because CD is commonly categorized according to the affected intestinal site, this chapter discusses the indications for surgery, surgical technique, and results as they pertain to the specific segment of the gastrointestinal tract.

STOMACH AND DUODENUM

Gastroduodenal involvement in CD is reported in only 2% to 4% of cases and is rarely confined to only the gastroduodenal segment, and 96% of patients have disease elsewhere. About one third of patients affected by gastroduodenal CD will require surgical intervention in their lifetime, most commonly for obstruction resulting from stenotic disease. Options for surgical management of complicated gastroduodenal CD include bypass, stricturoplasty, and, less frequently, resection. Although complex stricturoplasties and resections should be approached through a laparotomy, laparoscopy is a viable alternative in patients in need of a bypass. Traditionally, the "gold standard" for treating obstruction of the duodenum has been to bypass the duodenum via a gastrojejunostomy. An associated highly selective vagotomy is preferred over a truncal vagotomy to reduce the incidence of vagotomy-related diarrhea.

Operative Technique: Laparoscopic Gastrojejunostomy

Gastrojejunostomy can be performed in either an antecolic or a retrocolic fashion with a stapled anastomosis. If the colon is not involved, most surgeons prefer a side-to-side retrocolic approach, in which a window is made in the avascular plane of the transverse mesocolon to expose the posterior wall of the stomach. Care is taken to identify the middle colic artery to avoid injuring it. The most proximal loop of jejunum that lies tension free next to the greater curvature of the stomach is selected. Two stay sutures are placed to hold the stomach and bowel together, an enterotomy and gastrotomy are made, and the linear stapler is inserted and fired. The gastrotomy and enterotomy are closed with one or two layers of interrupted 3-0 sutures or with an additional firing of a laparoscopic stapler.

Outcomes

Although the available studies are very small, a more favorable experience with duodenal stricturoplasty, in comparison with bypass surgery for the treatment of duodenal CD, has been reported in terms of reoperation for recurrence and complications. However, if the duodenal stricture is lengthy, multiple strictures are present, or the tissues around the stricture are too rigid or unyielding, a stricturoplasty should not be performed, and an intestinal bypass procedure should be undertaken instead.

SMALL BOWEL

The small bowel is the most frequently affected gastrointestinal site in CD. Although any portion of the small bowel may be diseased, the terminal ileum is most commonly involved. Ninety percent of patients with CD of the small bowel experience symptoms resulting from obstructive or septic complications. A complete assessment of the gastrointestinal tract is mandatory prior to surgery to evaluate the full extent of disease and any associated complications that may require management before surgical intervention. Small bowel follow-through or enteroclysis can adequately assess the entire small intestine. CD is a relative contraindication for capsule endoscopy because of the high incidence of strictures. If the patient is seen initially with a fever or an abdominal mass, a CT scan should be obtained to assess for the presence of an intra-abdominal abscess amenable to percutaneous drainage.

Operative Technique: Laparoscopy-Assisted Small Bowel Resection

A planned small bowel resection is preceded by exploration of all four abdominal quadrants and the entire small bowel for evidence of coexisting CD, because up to 15% of patients will present with skip lesions. If areas of stenosis are suspected on serosal inspection, these should be marked with either an intracorporeal suture or a clip for subsequent identification upon exteriorization of the specimen. Matted loops of small bowel or omentum are often found adjacent to the diseased segment, especially if the terminal ileum is involved. Care must be taken to adequately mobilize the affected areas, and often mobilization of the ascending colon is needed. The matted loops of bowel can then be separated with a combination of blunt and sharp dissection, and the area to be resected can be inspected extracorporeally.

Division of the thickened mesentery of the involved small bowel is often the most challenging aspect of the procedure. The introduction of hand-activated advanced bipolar laparoscopic devices that allow for safe control of vessels up to 7 mm in diameter has dramatically improved surgeons' ability to complete these operations laparoscopically. Although the anastomosis could be completed intracorporeally, the authors prefer to exteriorize the specimen to construct the anastomosis extracorporeally. The bowel may be anastomosed in an end-to-end, end-to-side, or side-to-side fashion with a handsewn or a stapled technique. In the authors' practice, the bowel is anastomosed in a double-layered, handsewn, either end-to-end or side-to-side fashion. Clinical data have not demonstrated a significant clinical benefit of one configuration over another.

Nonresectional options such as stricturoplasty have gained popularity as an alternative to lengthy resections in the treatment of stricturing CD of the small intestine. Laparoscopy-assisted stricturoplasty is particularly advantageous when it is associated with a bowel resection, usually an ileocolic resection. The diseased area or areas can be marked with intracorporeal stitches or clips, exteriorized through a small abdominal incision needed for removal of the resected specimen, and the stricturoplasty is performed extracorporeally in a standard fashion.

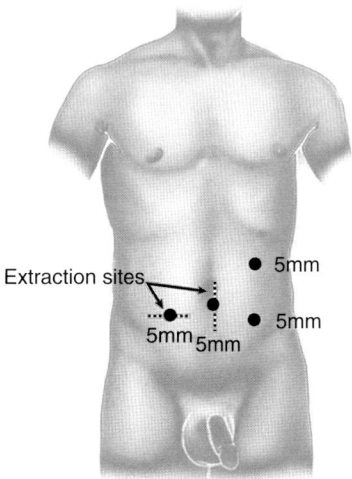

© 2007 University of Chicago

FIGURE 2   Trocar placement (on patient's left) and specimen extraction sites for ileocolic resection. *(Reprinted from Fichera A, Peng SL, Elisseou, NM, et al: Laparoscopic vs. open surgery in patients with ileocolonic Crohn's disease: a prospective comparative study, Surgery 142[4]:566–571, 2007. © 2007 University of Chicago.)*

Operative Technique: Laparoscopy-Assisted Ileocolic Resection

Laparoscopy-assisted ileocolic resection is currently the most commonly performed laparoscopic procedure for CD. The patient is placed on the operating table in the modified lithotomy position. Every operation for CD, whether open or laparoscopic, should start with a complete examination of the entire gastrointestinal tract, starting from the ligament of Treitz. The patient is in the reverse Trendelenburg position and right lateral decubitus, with the assistant standing on the patient's left side, retracting the transverse colon into the upper quadrants, and the surgeon standing between the patient's legs, evaluating the intestine from the ligament of Treitz all the way to the ileocecal valve. This maneuver is facilitated by progressively rotating the patient from the reverse Trendelenburg to a full Trendelenburg position and left lateral decubitus.

Skip areas of involvement from CD are marked intracorporeally with sutures or clips to facilitate retrieval of the diseased segments when the specimen is exteriorized. A technique employing four 5-mm trocars is utilized (Figure 2). After the bowel has been evaluated in its entirety, the surgeon moves to the left side of the patient (Figure 3), and the assistant places the ileocolic pedicle under tension. The surgeon dissects the mesentery and divides the ileocolic vessels (Figure 4). The ascending colon is mobilized in a medial-to-lateral fashion in the submesenteric plane to the hepatic flexure (Figure 5), and the assistant lifts the colon to allow clear visualization of the submesenteric plane.

When the submesenteric mobilization is complete, the lateral peritoneal reflection is divided to the hepatic flexure (Figure 6). The terminal ileum is completely mobilized by dividing the peritoneum at the level of the pelvic rim to allow a tension-free anastomosis through a small incision. It is often necessary to completely mobilize the hepatic flexure to facilitate exteriorization of the specimen (Figure 7). The instruments are removed, and the umbilical port site or, occasionally, the right lower quadrant port site is enlarged for exteriorization of the specimen. In the presence of skip areas of disease marked intracorporeally, either a resection or a stricturoplasty is performed. In the presence of isolated disease of the terminal ileum, an ileocolic resection is performed with an extracorporeal anastomosis.

Outcomes

Several studies have now confirmed the short-term benefit of a minimally invasive approach in well-selected CD patients with elective, complex, and even recurrent small bowel and terminal ileal disease. The faster postoperative recovery in laparoscopic patients is due in part to the decreased use of intravenous narcotic pain medications. Resection with primary anastomosis can usually be performed with a high degree of safety, and small bowel anastomotic dehiscence rates can be kept to less than 1%. In spite of the technical challenges posed by the hyperemic and thickened mesentery, the risk of postoperative bleeding requiring surgical intervention remains very low.

COLON AND RECTUM

The indications for surgery for colonic CD should not differ between laparoscopic and conventional open surgery (see Figure 1). In the presence of multiple sites of colonic involvement, the decision to perform an ileorectal anastomosis or total proctocolectomy with an end ileostomy is determined by the degree of involvement of the distal sigmoid and rectum. Restorative procedures such as ileal pouch–anal anastomoses are typically not performed in patients with CD because of the high pouch failure rates. However, a small subset of patients—those with disease limited to the colon and rectum without any history of small bowel or perineal involvement—may be considered candidates for a restorative proctocolectomy with a J-pouch ileoanal anastomosis. In this highly selected group of patients, restorative proctocolectomy with ileal pouch–anal anastomosis has been performed with acceptable results.

Operative Technique: Laparoscopy-Assisted Total Abdominal Colectomy

The patient is placed in a modified lithotomy position, which is preferable to the supine position because it allows the surgeon to access the perineum and to stand between the patient's legs during the mobilization of the transverse colon. Both upper extremities are tucked along the side of the body with a draw sheet. The hand-assisted technique through Pfannenstiel's incision is the authors'

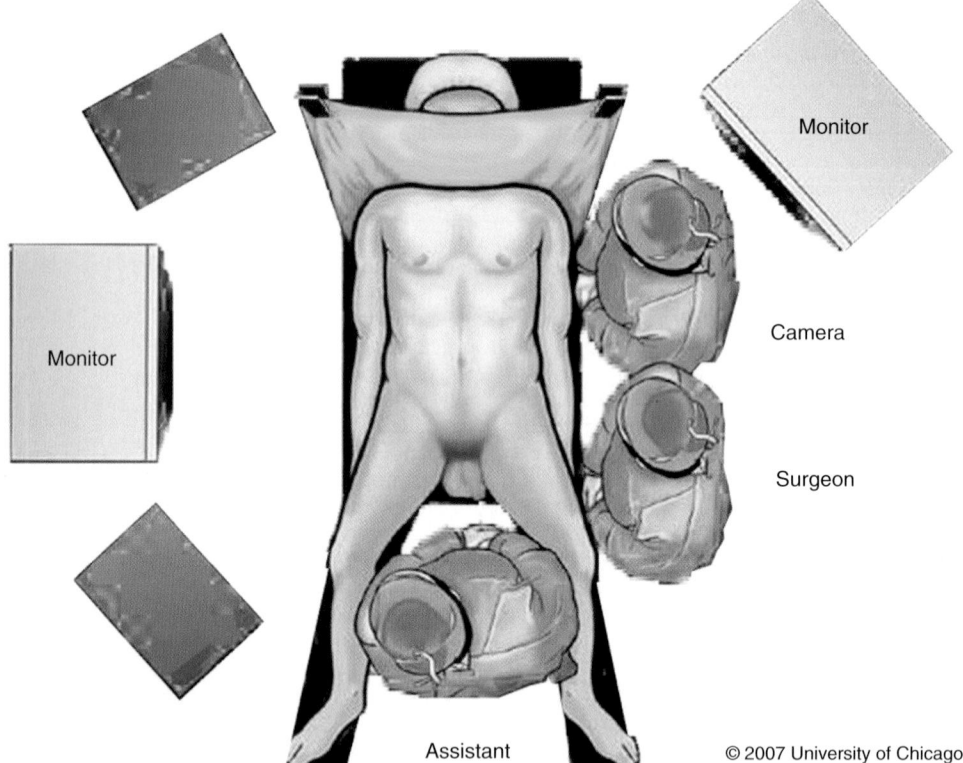

FIGURE 3   Operating room setup for ileocolic resection. *(Reprinted from Michelassi F, Hurst RD, Fichera A: Crohn's disease. In Zinner MJ, Ashley SW [eds]: Maingot's abdominal operations, ed 11, New York, 2007, McGraw-Hill, pp 521–550. © 2007 University of Chicago.)*

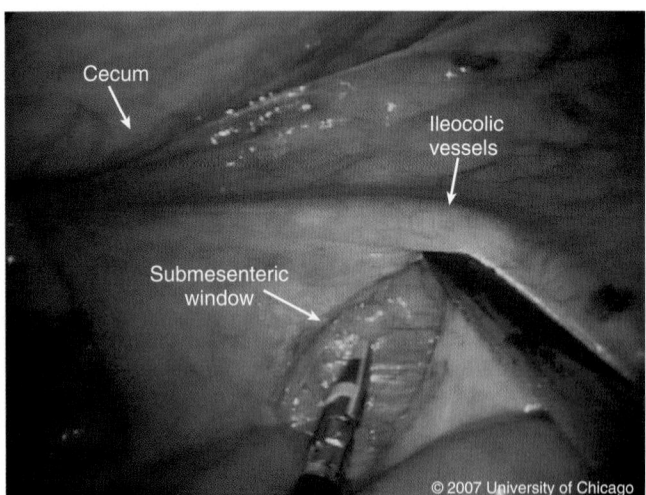

FIGURE 4   Dissection of the ileocolic vessels. *(Reprinted from Michelassi F, Hurst RD, Fichera A: Crohn's disease. In Zinner MJ, Ashley SW [eds]: Maingot's abdominal operations, ed 11, New York, 2007, McGraw-Hill, pp 521–550. © 2007 University of Chicago.)*

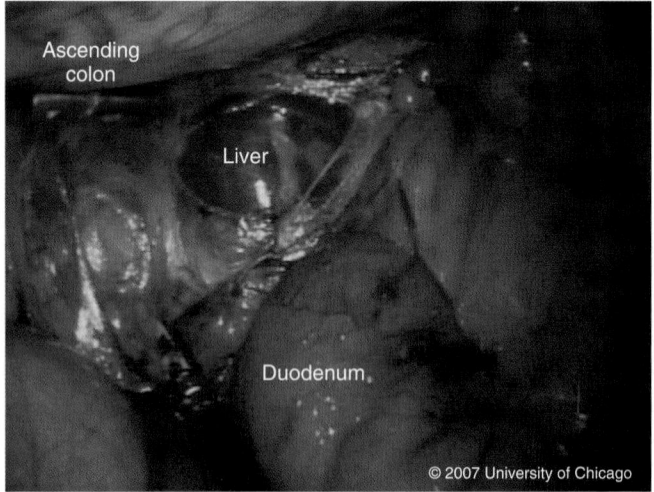

FIGURE 5   Submesenteric mobilization of the ascending colon to the hepatic flexure. *(Reprinted from Michelassi F, Hurst RD, Fichera A: Crohn's disease. In Zinner MJ, Ashley SW [eds]: Maingot's abdominal operations, ed 11, New York, 2007, McGraw-Hill, pp 521–550. © 2007 University of Chicago.)*

preferred approach. The presence of the surgeon's hand is particularly helpful in manipulating markedly inflamed or distended colon. Pfannenstiel's incision allows direct access to the pelvis for dissection, rectal transection, and anastomosis. If an end ileostomy is planned, the authors start with an incision at the ileostomy site and insert a 12-mm trocar, followed by a 5-mm camera port, at the umbilicus; a 5-mm trocar is inserted in the left lower quadrant. Otherwise the authors place a 5-mm camera port inferior to the umbilicus as the starting port for insufflation, followed by two additional 5-mm ports in the left lower and right lower quadrants.

Once pneumoperitoneum has been established, the feasibility of a laparoscopic approach is evaluated, and a hand-port device is placed in the suprapubic area (Figure 8). The small bowel is evaluated from the ligament of Treitz to the ileocecal valve to rule out small bowel involvement, and the right colon is mobilized as previously described. The mobilization of the transverse colon is facilitated significantly by use of the hand, but care must be taken to avoid injury to the duodenum and small bowel mesentery. Placing the greater curvature of the stomach under anterior and cephalad traction

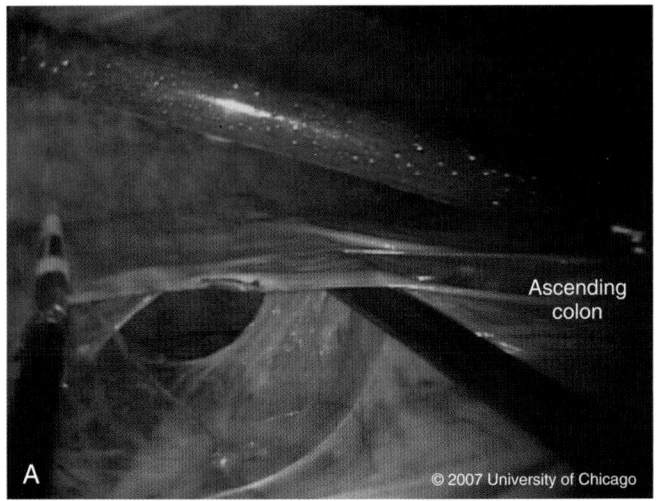

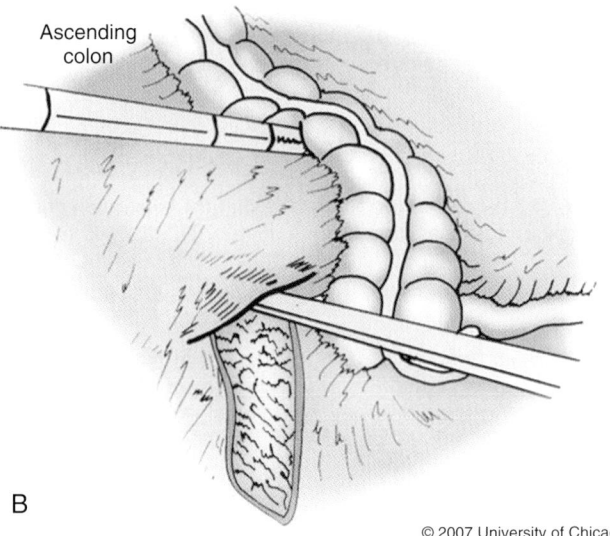

FIGURE 6 Division of the lateral attachments of the ascending colon. *(Reprinted from Michelassi F, Hurst RD, Fichera A: Crohn's disease. In Zinner MJ, Ashley SW [eds]: Maingot's abdominal operations, ed 11, New York, 2007, McGraw-Hill, pp 521–550. © 2007 University of Chicago.)*

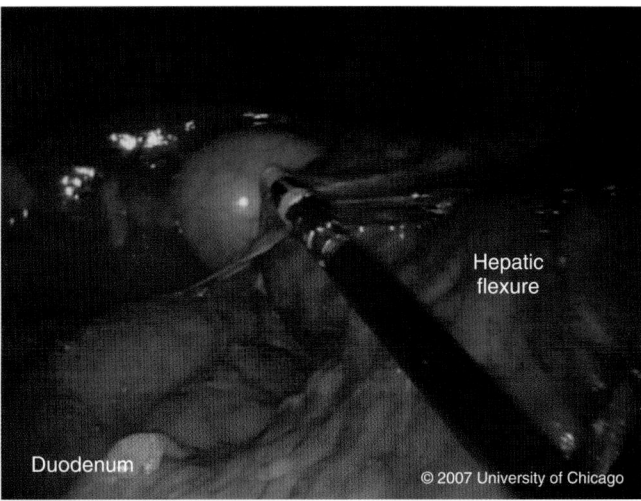

FIGURE 7 Final mobilization of the hepatic flexure. *(Reprinted from Michelassi F, Hurst RD, Fichera A: Crohn's disease. In Zinner MJ, Ashley SW [eds]: Maingot's abdominal operations, ed 11, New York, 2007, McGraw-Hill, pp 521–550. © 2007 University of Chicago.)*

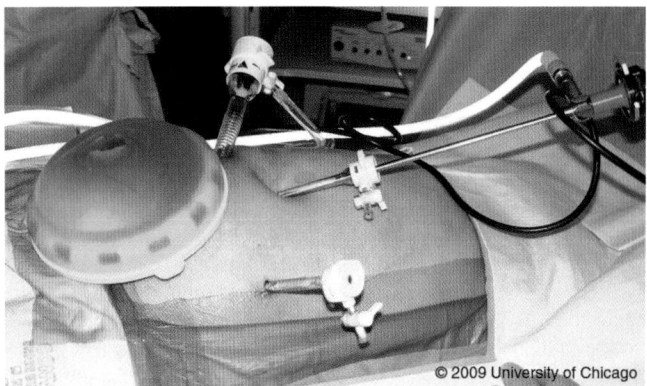

FIGURE 8 Port placement for hand-assisted total abdominal colectomy. *(© 2009 University of Chicago.)*

facilitates exposure of the gastrocolic ligament and entry into the lesser sac. The authors prefer to divide the greater omentum with the specimen, 3 to 4 cm away from the greater curvature of the stomach, taking care not to injure the gastroepiploic artery.

Next, the transverse mesocolon is divided with a bipolar vessel-sealing device after division of the greater omentum and exposure of the lesser sac; the mesocolon division proceeds from the hepatic to the splenic flexure. Chronically inflamed colon can become intimately attached to the inferior pole of the spleen, as the splenocolic ligament becomes foreshortened by inflammation. Traction on the colon or omentum could result in avulsion of the splenic capsule and result in troublesome bleeding that may require splenectomy.

It is imperative to keep the field as dry as possible with the use of a bipolar vessel-sealing device and precise and meticulous dissection. If necessary, the splenic flexure can be approached, so that the dissection alternates between the transverse colon moving distally and the descending colon moving proximally, thus minimizing traction on the spleen and the inflamed colon. The descending colon is then mobilized by division of its lateral attachments along the white line of Toldt and the mesentery.

Once the dissection reaches the level of the pelvic brim, the colon and terminal ileum are exteriorized through Pfannenstiel's incision. When a rectal-sparing technique is used, patients with diffuse colitis are candidates for a side-to-end ileorectal anastomosis, either stapled or handsewn, provided a close endoscopic examination confirms that the rectum is truly free of disease, fecal continence is satisfactory, and the patient does not have perineal complications. On the other hand, malnourished patients and those who are acutely ill should instead undergo an end ileostomy. A rectal tube is typically placed at the completion of the case for decompression of the rectal stump.

Operative Technique: Totally Laparoscopic Total Proctocolectomy

Extensive involvement of the colon and rectum or presence of dysplasia on surveillance colonoscopy requires a total proctocolectomy with permanent ileostomy. A totally laparoscopic approach virtually eliminates the risk of wound complication while providing the benefits of a minimally invasive approach.

The patient is placed in a modified lithotomy position, a 12-mm trocar is inserted at the ileostomy site, and four more 5-mm trocars are placed, as shown in Figure 9. The colon is mobilized

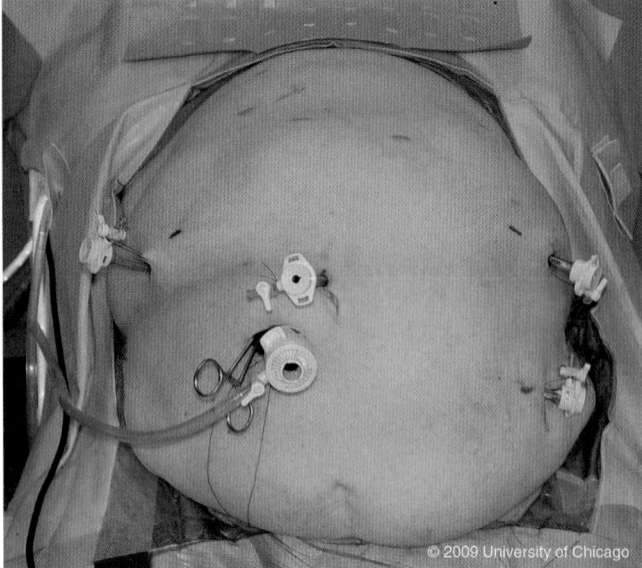

FIGURE 9 Port placement for a totally laparoscopic total proctocolectomy. The patient pictured has had a previous laparoscopic gastric bypass for obesity. The trocar sites in the upper quadrants are from the previous operation. (© 2009 University of Chicago.)

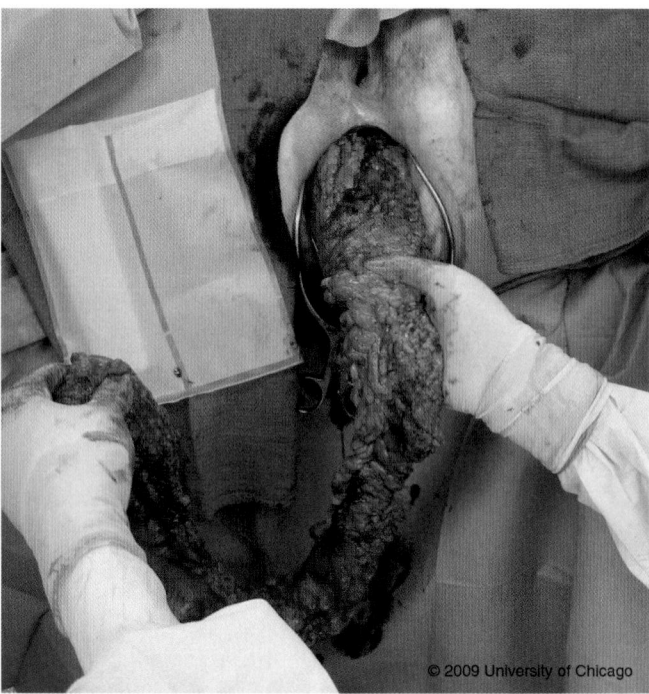

FIGURE 10 Perineal specimen extraction at the completion of a totally laparoscopic total proctocolectomy. (© 2009 University of Chicago.)

laparoscopically in a fashion similar to the hand-assisted approach described previously. The terminal ileum is intracorporeally divided and delivered through the ileostomy site. The superior hemorrhoidal pedicle is divided, after identification of the left ureter and gonadal vessels, and a totally laparoscopic proctectomy is performed in the avascular presacral space. The operating surgeon and the assistant holding the laparoscope stand on the patient's right, with the second assistant on the opposite side. The rectum is mobilized to the level of the levators, and identification of the pelvic sympathetic and para-sympathetic nerves is indicated to avoid postoperative urinary and sexual dysfunction. An intersphincteric dissection is completed through the perineum, the specimen is extracted (Figure 10), and the perineal wound is closed in layers with absorbable sutures.

Outcomes

Adopted rather slowly, laparoscopic colectomy in CD is nevertheless welcomed by patients who are generally young and would prefer an operation that involves minimal scarring and prompt recovery. Furthermore, patients probably require operations over a lifetime, and so a minimally invasive approach is more appealing, as it results in minimal intra-abdominal adhesion formation. In the authors' own series of 55 laparoscopic colectomies for colonic CD, they found potential benefits in favor of laparoscopy with regard to operative blood loss and length of stay, in addition to obvious benefits of improved cosmesis and decreased risk of incisional hernia.

PERINEUM

The goal of surgery in anorectal CD is control of sepsis and relief of symptoms with preservation of continence. The initial approach involves a combination of drainage, seton placement, and intensive medical therapy. In selected patients, to achieve complete healing and control of sepsis, a temporary ileostomy should be considered. Another scenario for consideration of fecal diversion is the presence of active anorectal disease; although it puts the patient in need for proctectomy, it precludes definitive procedure, thus requiring

creation of an end colostomy to control the sepsis prior to proctectomy.

When a temporary diversion is indicated, the authors prefer a diverting-loop ileostomy. An end-loop (Prasad) ileostomy can also be constructed, if diversion is likely to be required long term. An end-loop stoma allows for better pouching, as it is similar to the end ileostomy and can be reversed without the need for laparotomy. On the basis of the extent of disease, a permanent stoma could be either a colostomy or an ileostomy. Laparoscopy is currently the authors' preferred technique for fecal diversion with minimal morbidity. Moreover, laparoscopy provides useful information on the extent of disease. An initial incision at the stoma site is used to establish pneumoperitoneum and evaluate the abdomen. With the exception of emergency cases, every patient should undergo preoperative education and stoma marking by an enterostomal therapist.

Operative Technique: Laparoscopic Fecal Diversion

The authors start similarly for both colostomy and ileostomy. The patient is placed in a modified lithotomy position, and the stoma incision is made at the previously marked site. A 12-mm port is inserted, and a purse-string suture is used to cinch the anterior sheath around the port. Laparoscopic exploration is performed next to determine the feasibility of a laparoscopic operation and to determine the extent of disease. For a colostomy, the authors place two additional 5-mm trocars in the right lower and right upper quadrants, and a 5-mm infraumbilical port is placed for the 5-mm, 30-degree camera. The lateral attachments of the sigmoid and descending colon are taken down along the white line of Toldt, and the colon is mobilized to reach the abdominal wall at the stoma opening. Evacuation of pneumoperitoneum will add additional 3 to 4 cm of bowel length sufficient to help the stoma mature.

In the presence of a redundant sigmoid colon, very limited mobilization may be required. A very redundant sigmoid colon or the presence of adhesions could present a potential challenge in orienting the distal and proximal limbs. Sigmoidoscopy and insufflation with carbon dioxide, which is absorbed rapidly, can aid proper orientation. If an end stoma is planned, the colon is transected intracorporeally, and the transected proximal end is delivered through the stoma opening. Proper orientation must be maintained; when oriented correctly, the mesocolon is caudad. The abdomen is then reinsufflated, and correct orientation is confirmed with the laparoscope. The colostomy is completed in the standard fashion with slight Brooke eversion to allow better pouching.

Conversely, for an ileostomy the authors start at the stoma site as previously described and place two additional 5-mm trocars in the left lower and left upper quadrants, and a 5-mm infraumbilical port is placed for the 5-mm, 30-degree camera. The terminal ileum is identified by the visualization of the antimesenteric fat, the fold of Treves, and its connection to the cecum. It is essential to positively identify the terminal ileum to ensure correct orientation of the bowel. The ileum is then run proximally for at least 20 cm to ensure that an adequate length of healthy bowel is available. No mobilization of the ileum is usually required, as it almost always easily reaches the stoma site.

Once the bowel is correctly oriented, the loop of bowel is delivered through the ileostomy site. The authors orient the bowel so that the proximal limb is located cephalad and the distal limb is caudad. The abdomen is then reinsufflated, and correct orientation is confirmed with the laparoscope. Some authors advocate minimizing the number of ports used for laparoscopic diverting stoma, particularly for laparoscopic ileostomy. Although this approach can be quite tempting, establishing proper orientation of the bowel can be difficult, unless adequate visualization is achieved. The authors find it very helpful to place two 5-mm working ports on the opposite side of the abdomen to allow precise tissue handling and improved exposure, which results in an accurate orientation of the bowel. These benefits outweigh the minimal morbidity and cosmetic considerations of the 5-mm incisions.

Outcomes

The safety and efficacy of the laparoscopic approach for diverting ileostomy or colostomy is now well established. It is the authors' preferred method for fecal diversion.

SUMMARY

Although significant advancements have been made in the medical management of CD, surgical intervention is still required in the vast majority of patients to treat complications and palliate symptoms. Although CD has varying clinical manifestations that necessitate individualized treatment, the main goal of surgery in all individuals is to adequately relieve symptoms while avoiding excessive loss of bowel function or body disfigurement.

SUGGESTED READINGS

da Luz Moreira A, Stocchi L, Remzi FH, et al: Laparoscopic surgery for patients with Crohn's colitis: a case-matched study, *J Gastrointest Surg* 11(11):1529–1533, 2007.

Fichera A, Peng SL, Elisseou NM, et al: Laparoscopy or conventional open surgery for patients with ileocolonic Crohn's disease? A prospective study, *Surgery* 142(4):566–571, 2007.

Maartense S, Dunker MS, Slors JF, et al: Laparoscopic-assisted versus open ileocolic resection for Crohn's disease: a randomized trial, *Ann Surg* 243(2):143–149, 2006.

Milsom JW, Hammerhofer KA, Bohm B, et al: Prospective, randomized trial comparing laparoscopic vs. conventional surgery for refractory ileocolic Crohn's disease, *Dis Colon Rectum* 44(1):1–8, 2001.

Rosman AS, Melis M, Fichera A: Metaanalysis of trials comparing laparoscopic and open surgery for Crohn's disease, *Surg Endosc* 19(12):1549–1555, 2005.

LAPAROSCOPIC COLON AND RECTAL SURGERY

James W. Fleshman, MD, FACS, FASCRS

BACKGROUND

Even though a laparoscopic colectomy has been performed since 1990, some skepticism about its applicability to colorectal diseases still remains. This reticence is found most commonly in the community practice of colorectal surgery. Patients have not been demanding laparoscopic techniques as they had cholecystectomy and other procedures such as hernia repair. The use of the minimally invasive techniques in colorectal surgery is continuing to increase, but these techniques have not been universally adopted. In fact, in a 2011 survey of 123 expert colorectal surgeons, there was a wide variation in the use of laparoscopic techniques. Only 82% of the expert

surgeons surveyed from in the United States professed to using laparoscopy as a primary technique, and only 66% of the experts in colorectal surgery outside of the United States advocated laparoscopy. The percentage of cases in which laparoscopic colectomy was performed increased from 2.2% in the National Inpatient Sample (an administrative database covering private hospitals) in 1996 to 31% in 2009. The increase in adoption of laparoscopic colectomy seemed to coincide in 2004 with the publication of data from the Clinical Outcomes of Surgical Therapy (COST) trial, in which laparoscopic and open colectomy for colon cancer were compared. Laparoscopic colectomy is being adopted most rapidly in urban teaching institutions that serve a highly insured population.

As training programs began adopting the laparoscopic technique, the finishing residents have taken their skills with them to the community hospitals and other teaching programs. As a result, laparoscopic colectomy has descended into the general surgery residency training program as standard of care and is no longer considered a fellow-level procedure. This adoption should continue to increase the utilization of laparoscopic colectomy. Stamos at the University of California, Irvine, in looking at the National Inpatient Sample of 117,177 patients, in 2009 showed an increase in the prevalence of laparoscopic colectomies to 42.6% of cases. This may actually be a result of the publication of *the International Classification of Diseases,* 9th edition, which facilitated identifying the laparoscopic cases with a new code in 2008.

Reports of numerous randomized controlled trials of laparoscopic colectomy for cancer have improved the visibility of laparoscopic colectomy. The knowledge that laparoscopic techniques are safe, oncologically appropriate, and equivalent in outcome to open colectomy may have improved the surgical community's acceptance of and confidence in colectomy for cancer. The majority of colon cancers are still treated with open operation in nonacademic hospitals and by general surgeons across the country. Obtaining the skills verified by credentialed surgeons in controlled trials is possible at numerous training courses around the country. Most of these are based on cadaveric models. As these newly trained individuals adopt these techniques and perform this procedure on patients with colon cancer, it may become of benefit in treating other diseases. Oncologic outcome after laparoscopic colectomy for cancer is equivalent to that after open technique, but there is an improvement in short-term outcomes. The original concern over an increase in trocar site implantation is no longer valid if an appropriate technique is utilized. Decreased length of hospital stay, decreased pain, and fewer early complications (surgical site infections) are all benefits. Over the long term, the risk of small bowel obstruction and abdominal incision hernia decreased after laparoscopic surgery.

OPERATIVE PRINCIPLES AND TECHNICAL PEARLS

The approach to a colectomy is not always standard and, depending on the disease process, the surgeon may require comfort or experience with different approaches to remove a portion of the intestine. In severe inflammation or extensive cancer with regional progression, a combination of approaches may be required. A simplified classification of these approaches includes a medial-to-lateral approach, a lateral-to-medial approach, superior-to-inferior and inferior-to-superior approaches, and a posterior approach. Each of these approaches can be used in an open procedure to allow exposure of the point of maximum disease at the end of dissection in order to prevent tumor spill or contamination from the inflammatory process. Learning all of these approaches allows the surgeon to address more advanced disease and facilitates curative (R0) resection of cancer and appropriate cancer care for the patient.

The laparoscopic medial-to-lateral approach in the right colectomy can be performed either from a posterior aspect or from a transmesenteric approach. The posterior approach requires incising the peritoneum along the anterior surface of the right iliac vessels and entering the avascular retroperitoneal plane. This areolar tissue plane extends anterior to the ureter and major vessels and all the way behind the right colon, over the anterior surface of the kidney, outside the area curve of the second portion of the duodenum, and up to the level of the liver (Figure 1).

The posterior medial-to-lateral approach begins with the simple act of lifting the base of the cecum towards the anterior abdominal wall and incising along the right common iliac artery from the bifurcation of the aorta to the apex of the mesenteric attachment to the right lower quadrant retroperitoneum. This provides a safe reproducible view, or "critical view," for a right colectomy. The ureter, vessels, and duodenum can be protected and the dissection carried out in a bloodless plane, which limits the amount of energy needed for blood vessel control. Releasing the colon from the retroperitoneum allows the vessels to be identified and divided at the base of the right colon mesentery along the superior mesenteric artery. Appropriate mesenteric resection (total mesocolic excision) for cancer requires division of the feeder vessel at its origin (Figure 2).

The true medial-to-lateral approach begins by lifting of the ileocolic pedicle to facilitate the dissection at the base of the right colon mesentery along the superior mesenteric artery. The retroperitoneal

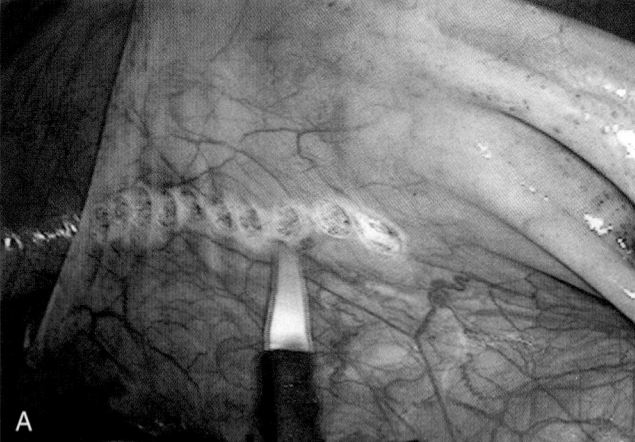
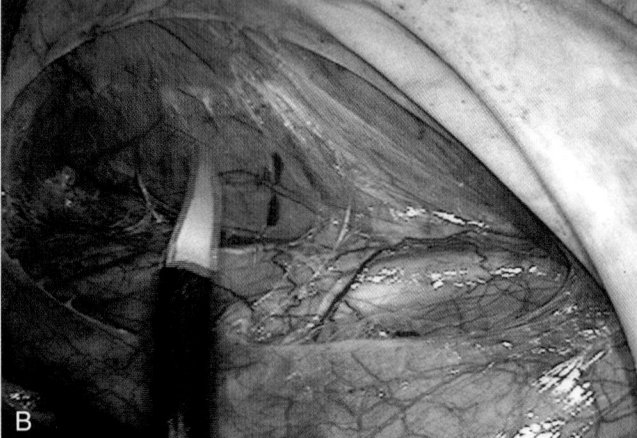

FIGURE 1 A and **B,** Laparoscopic medial to lateral approach to the right colectomy: operative images. *(From Fleshman JW, Birnbaum EH, Hunt SR, et al [eds]: Atlas of surgical techniques for colon, rectum, and anus, Philadelphia, 2012, WB Saunders.)*

avascular plane is entered after the peritoneal surface is incised along the superior mesenteric artery. This may violate the intact mesocolic envelope of the right colon if not performed exactly along the anterior surface of superior mesenteric artery distal to the origin of the ileocolic artery. Once again, the ileocolic pedicle is ligated at its origin in the patient being treated for cancer.

The lateral-to-medial approach is sometimes needed when the tumor has spread down to the base of the mesentery of the right colon along the superior mesenteric artery and when the ileocolic origin is initially difficult to identify or the tumor grows into the retroperitoneal tissue. A lateral-to-medial approach begins with an incision along the right gutter to lift the right colon up toward the midline. The retroperitoneal plane is entered laterally, and the mesenteric envelope is preserved. This approach facilitates a release of the colon from the right side of the abdomen when the posterior aspect of the colon is adherent to the midline structures. The retroperitoneal plane must be uninvolved and free along the side wall abdomen. Unfortunately, the lateral-to-medial approach pulls the bowel towards the camera, which enters through an umbilical part, and the view may be obscured as tissue is pulled toward the midline. This approach may require moving the camera to the suprapubic site, with a view toward the liver, and the dissection is performed with the surgeon standing between the patient's legs. The tissue is pulled toward the left side of the abdomen, and the working instrumentation originates through the suprapubic trocar site. The point of vascular ligation will need to be adjusted, in these situations, to allow complete removal of mesenteric disease. This may necessitate wider mesenteric resection and additional bowel removal as a result.

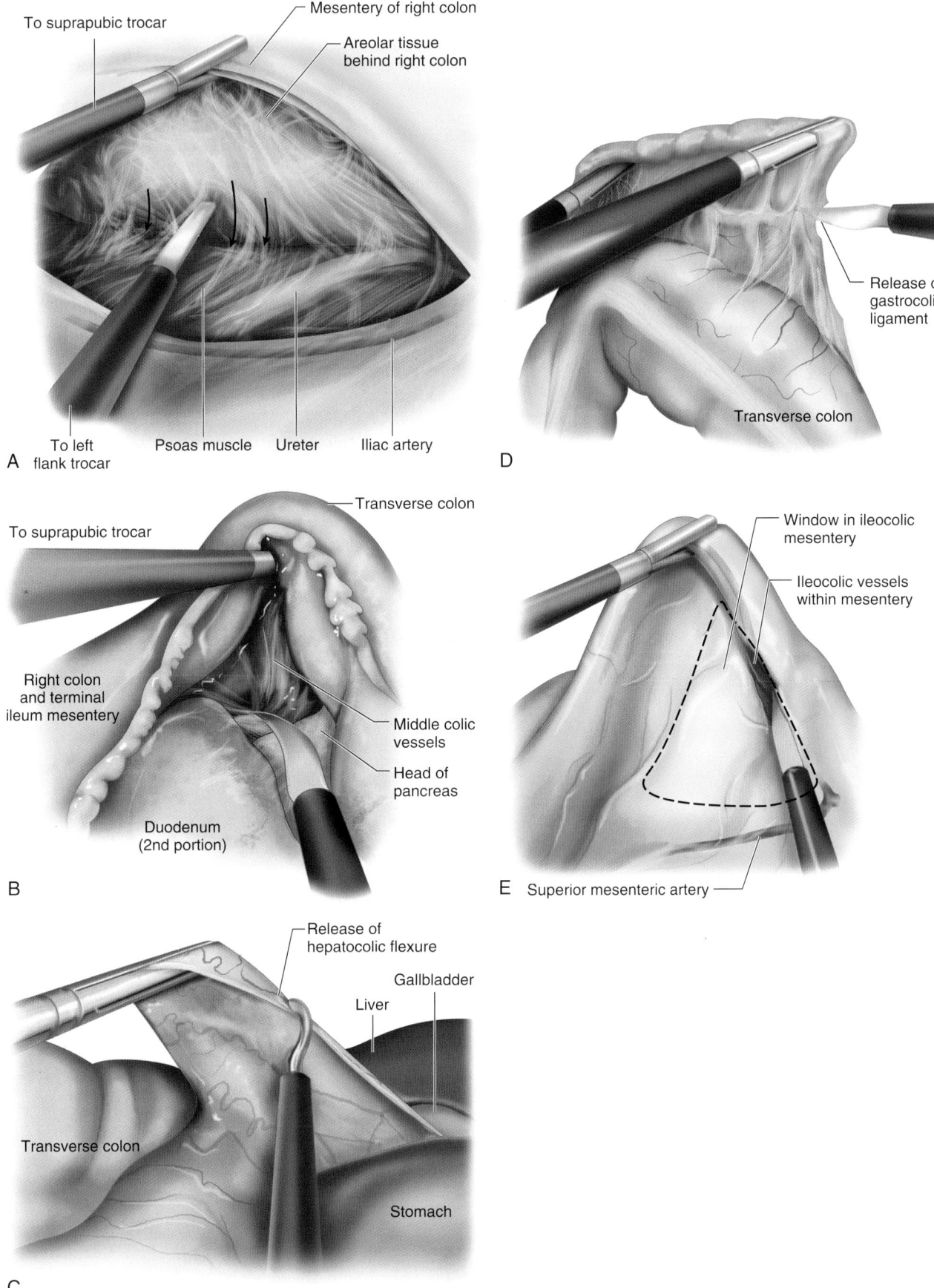

FIGURE 2 **A** to **E,** Laparoscopic posterior medial-to-lateral approach in the right colectomy: schematic views. *(From Fleshman JW, Birnbaum EH, Hunt SR, et al [eds]: Atlas of surgical techniques for colon, rectum, and anus, Philadelphia, 2012, WB Saunders.)*

The superior (not necessarily better) approach to the right colon is best suited for patients who have tumors or inflammatory process within the area of the cecum adherent to the pelvic brim, which precludes the posterior, lateral-to-medial, or the medial-to-lateral approach. The superior approach usually requires that the patient be placed in the steep reverse Trendelenburg position while still maintaining the left airplane position. The colon can be pulled from underneath the liver and released from the lateral side wall of the abdomen as tissue falls toward the midline. This maneuver has the advantage of lifting the right colon at the hepatic flexure off of the duodenum, pancreas, kidney, and retroperitoneum, leaving only the attachments at the pelvic brim. Once the ileocolic vessel is identified at its origin, it can be divided from the lateral approach, on the anatomic posterior aspect of the superior mesenteric artery. The attachments of the tumor and inflammatory process are dissected as the final maneuver.

Management of the mesenteric vessels of the right colon usually requires only division of the ileocolic vessel and possibly of a right colic vessel. The extraction of the right colon, with terminal ileum and hepatic flexure, through the abdominal wall allows selective division of the vessels at the extremes of the specimen appropriate to the disease process. It is not necessary to divide all of the blood vessels intracorporeally. Preferred extraction sites include midline at the umbilicus, transverse right upper quadrant, or right lower quadrant as needed. The standard approach, however, is usually to use the umbilical extraction site because the site is almost always positioned over the base of the middle colic and superior mesenteric arteries.

The approach to the left side of the colon can involve a medial-to-lateral, lateral-to-medial, and superior or inferior approach. The medial-to-lateral approach for a left colectomy is the same as that for a low anterior resection (Figure 3). An incision behind the superior hemorrhoidal artery at the level of the sacral promontory allows

FIGURE 3 Laparoscopic left colectomy to isolate and legate inferior mesenteric artery. **A,** Operating room setup. **B,** Illustration of procedure. *(From Fleshman JW, Birnbaum EH, Hunt SR, et al [eds]: Atlas of surgical techniques for colon, rectum, and anus, Philadelphia, 2012, WB Saunders.)*

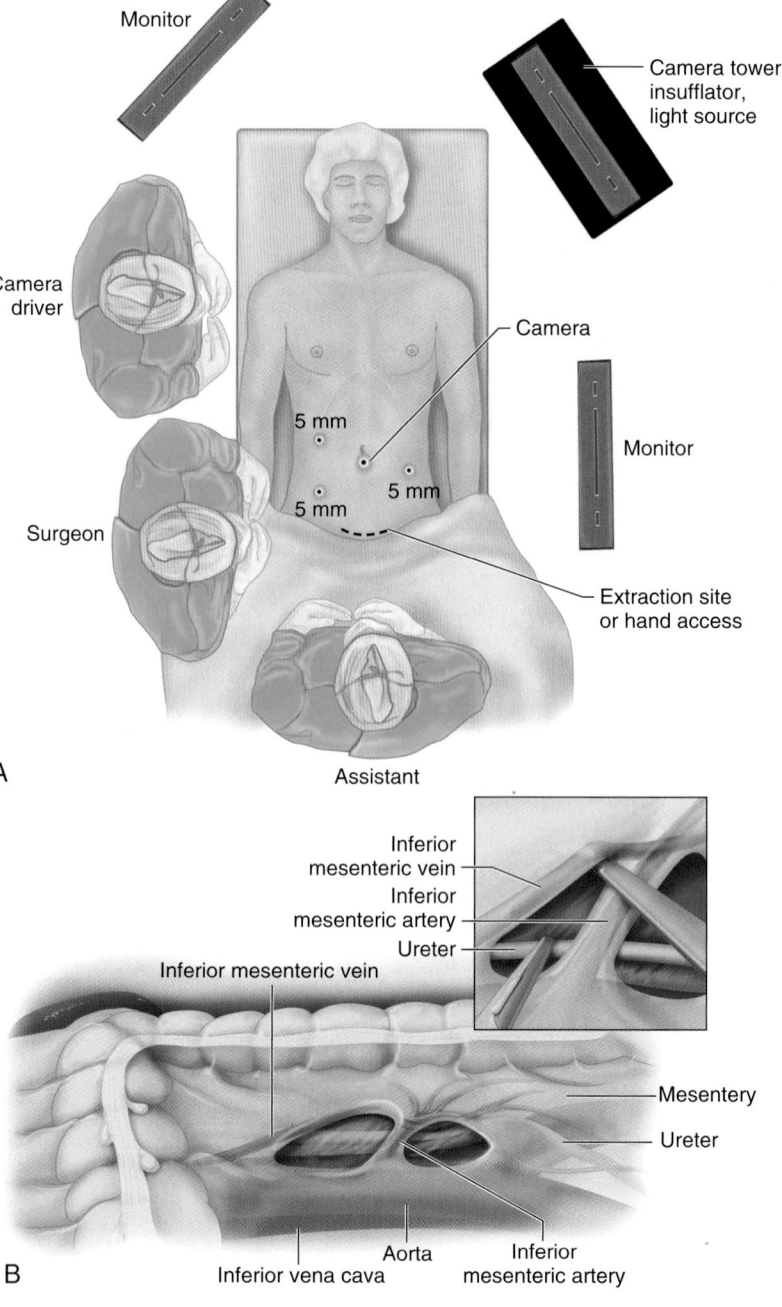

entry into an avascular plane over the retroperitoneum, which will protect the left ureter, the left common iliac vessel, and the gonadal vessels in that area. Dividing the inferior mesenteric artery at its origin with a sealing device or stapler can immediately release the left colic and sigmoid mesentery from the retroperitoneum. Blunt dissection in this plane all the way to the lateral side wall and up to the pancreas is possible because the embryologic plane has few blood vessels. The patient is positioned in steep Trendelenburg and airplane position to the right to allow gravity to remove the small intestine from the base of the left colon mesentery. The surgeon must remember to dissect in an "upward slope" direction to avoid digging into the retroperitoneal structures. As the dissection is continued toward the duodenum, the inferior mesenteric vein is found along the base of the mesentery. The inferior mesenteric vein is divided proximally at the portion of the vein, which dives behind the pancreas. The vein is transected just below the lower edge of the pancreas along the tail of the pancreas. Sealing or stapling of this vein then releases all of the left colon mesentery from the retroperitoneum. The advantage of the medial-to-lateral approach and dividing the inferior mesenteric vessels at their origin is that it also provides a medial approach to the lesser sac through the peritoneal membrane over the top of the pancreatic tail to create a window behind the stomach. The left colon and splenic flexure are then totally free from the retroperitoneum. The final attachments along the left side wall of the abdomen, which have been supporting the colon and providing countertraction, and the mesenteric attachments over the kidney are easily divided to release the entire colon to the midline.

The lateral-to-medial approach to a left colectomy results in the tissue's falling toward the camera and making it difficult to actually see behind the tissue as the colon is released, similar to the situation with a right colectomy. In circumstances in which an inflammatory process or a large tumor deposit with matted lymph nodes is present at the base of the mesentery, a lateral-to-medial approach may be appropriate. This dissection within uninvolved planes allows the surgeon to attack the worst areas of disease during the very last portion of the procedure and increases safety. The ability to utilize a combination of approaches is critical for the safety of the procedure.

The "superior" approach to the left colon begins with the patient in reverse Trendelenburg position, the release of the omentum from the antimesenteric surface of the transverse colon, and release of the splenic flexure from the attachments to the spleen, kidney, and pancreas (Figure 4). This then allows a lateral-to-medial approach or a medial-to-lateral approach to the base of the left colon mesentery, depending on whether a process prevents early management of the vessels or release of the mesentery from the retroperitoneum. This approach may also be preferred in patients with portal hypertension because collateral vessels around the splenic flexure and large collateral vessels along the omentum must be controlled early during the procedure to provide the safest approach in these patients.

Several techniques should be utilized to increase the safety of any laparoscopic colectomy. General safety maneuvers that should be applicable in all laparoscopic colectomy cases include the following:

1. Avoid grasping the bowel during retraction. Use only closed, blunt-tipped instruments to lift, sweep, push, or suspend it.
2. Always know what is behind the incision that is being made. Blind pushing or cutting is never safe unless the camera can show a clear space or anatomic consistency allows assumption of nonthreatening territory.
3. Never divide a vessel unless it can be immediately controlled if the sealing device fails. Place a grasper at the ready and in the camera field.

Fixation of a beanbag or a foam pad to the operating table, which cradles the patient on the table without risking pressure point nerve injury, is essential. The table is at extreme positions in Trendelenburg or airplane position in either direction and allows gravity to be

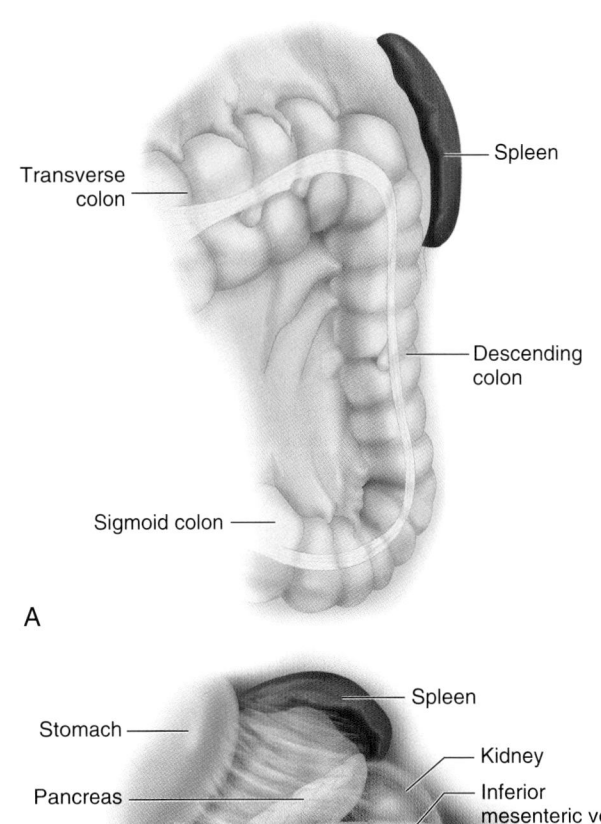

A

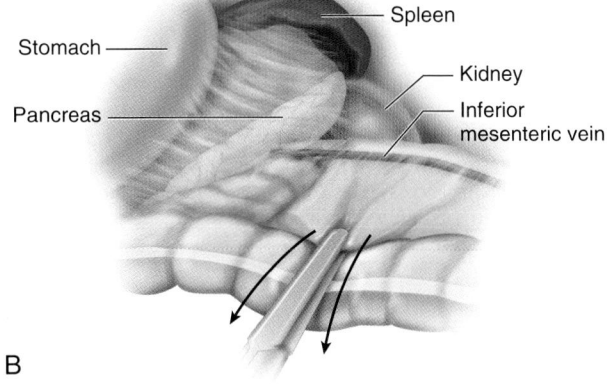

B

FIGURE 4 Exposure of the kidney. **A,** Anatomic relationships of the splenic flexure of the colon before mobilization. **B,** View of the splenic flexure area after release of the colon from the stomach and spleen. *(From Fleshman JW, Birnbaum EH, Hunt SR, et al [eds]: Atlas of surgical techniques for colon, rectum, and anus, Philadelphia, 2012, WB Saunders.)*

utilized as the primary retraction mechanism during a colectomy. Reliance on instrumentation for grasping and displacement of intestine can potentially result in damage to portions of the intestine. A flexible-tip laparoscope allows visualization over the top, behind, or underneath structures and provides a view of tissue that would be potentially damaged if the posterior view were obscured. The ideal would be three-dimensional with a flexible tip to improve the depth perception of the operating surgeon. A smoke evacuator or an insufflator system, which functions at a high enough volume, is essential to remove the plume generated by energy devices. Radiofrequency sealing devices, harmonic energy, or mechanical vessel control are all appropriate and should be part of the armamentarium of the surgeon. Because not all devices do everything, familiarity with specific advantages and disadvantages of each is key to maintaining safety during these difficult cases. Instruments at least 45 cm long are preferred, especially if splenic flexure mobilization is a standard part of the technique. The distance of mobilization from the right lower quadrant all the way up to the hepatic flexure and from the pelvic

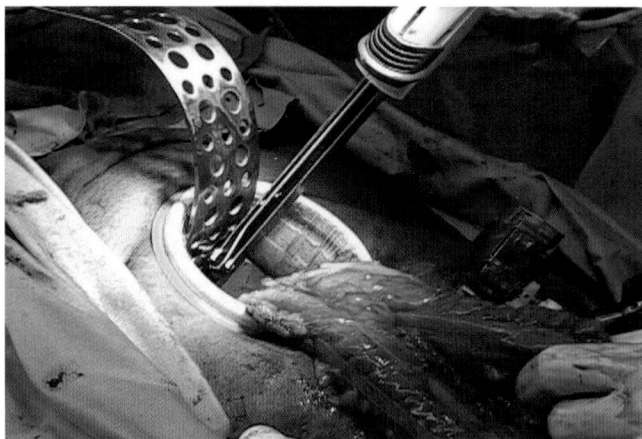

FIGURE 5 The rectosigmoid is transected through the access site at the level of the sacral promontory. *(From Fleshman JW, Birnbaum EH, Hunt SR, et al [eds]: Atlas of surgical techniques for colon, rectum, and anus, Philadelphia, 2012, WB Saunders.)*

brim up to the splenic flexure is sometimes very large in a male patient. The tips of instruments should be atraumatic and blunt; the wavy Raptor grasper is the most suitable. A Babcock tip is also preferred over a Kelly clamp–type instrument, which damages tissue with pressure.

At the extraction site of the specimen, a wound protector is recommended to prevent surgical site infection and to stretch the opening to its maximum without damaging the surrounding tissue (Figure 5). It is possible to insert small sponges through the extraction sites or hand access ports to improve visualization. Care must always be taken to remove each sponge before inserting another, rather than allowing them to accumulate in the abdominal cavity.

The use of robotics for colectomy has not been definitely shown to provide any advantage or safety over laparoscopy. The use of single-incision laparoscopic surgery (SILS), however, may have some advantage over multiport laparoscopy: SILS is very difficult to perform, requires a higher skill level, and requires longer operating times. Robotic SILS may be an answer to these technical difficulties. Time will tell.

Tattooing the disease site with India ink during colonoscopy for neoplasm has become the standard of care, even before laparoscopic colectomy. This is especially helpful in the setting of small lesions to be able to identify the site of the disease externally. A small nonpalpable cancer or polyp, which is identified colonoscopically, may not always be in the area reported by the endoscopist because of the telescoping of the bowel over the endoscope and the numerous twists and turns, which may result in overestimation of distance.

Hand-assisted laparoscopic surgery (HALS) is useful for addressing more complex disease processes and to help nonlaparoscopic surgeons to get started on minimally invasive surgery. The GelPort (Applied Medical, Rancho Santa Margarita, Calif) may be used to reduce the learning curve for surgeons who are not accomplished laparoscopic specialists. The use of HALS can be helpful to reduce the rate of conversion to an open procedure in the approach to more extensive disease, even by experienced laparoscopic surgeons. The short-term outcomes of HALS techniques have been shown to be equivalent to those of total laparoscopic approaches. However, limitation of the incision size on the abdominal wall or achieving a totally laparoscopic approach is the best way to achieve maximal benefit from a minimally invasive technique. HALS should be part of every surgeon's skill set to complete a laparoscopic case successfully.

Rectal dissection requires attention to anatomic detail to maintain dissection in the posterior avascular plane, outside the mesorectum as the preferred line of dissection (Figure 6). The embryologic avascular plane, which begins at the sacral promontory behind the

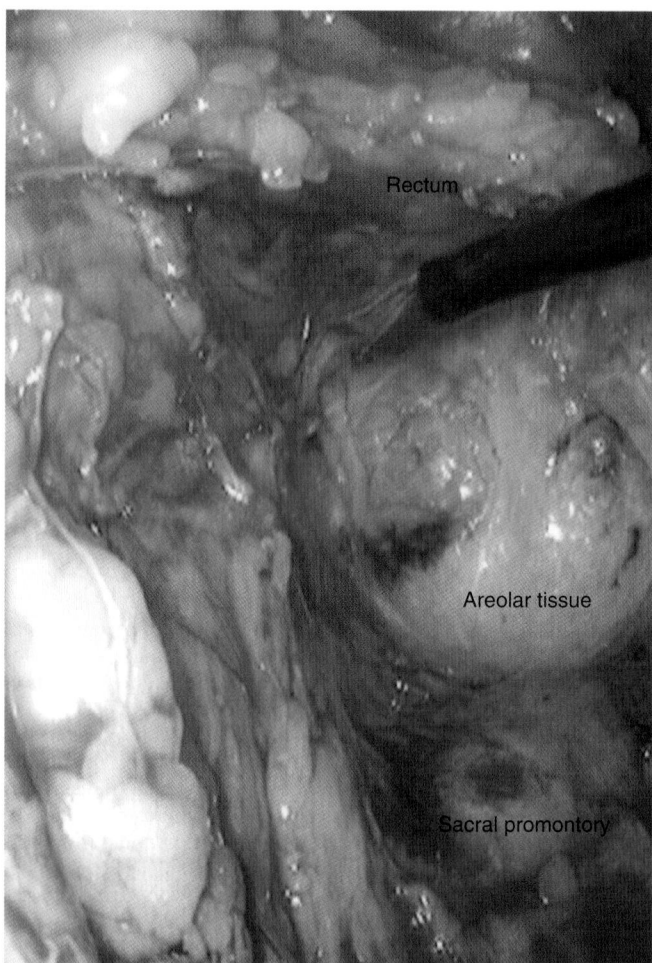

FIGURE 6 Laparoscopic low anterior resection. The dissection is carried further into the pelvis, all the way down to the pelvic floor posteriorly, to release the mesentery up and away from the sacral curve. *(From Fleshman JW, Birnbaum EH, Hunt SR, et al [eds]: Atlas of surgical techniques for colon, rectum, and anus, Philadelphia, 2012, WB Saunders.)*

superior hemorrhoidal vessels, extends all the way down to the pelvic floor. Waldeyer's fascia is the reflection of the presacral fascia onto the posterior fascia of the mesentery and is the end of the avascular plane. In patients with rectal cancer, this plane is the "holy plane." The avascular plane is also present below Waldeyer's fascia and requires incision to release the rectum from the pelvic floor musculature. A total mesorectal excision with complete intact mesenteric envelope is essential to decrease local recurrence of the cancer in the pelvis.

The laparoscopic retraction of the rectum should be performed bluntly without grasping of the bowel or mesorectum. The retraction of the bladder and the uterus or prostate can be made safe with blunt retraction by an open grasper to lift the anterior tissues away from the rectum. Long (45-cm) instruments are essential. During the anterior dissection at the level of the cul-de-sac, the rectum is then gently pushed posteriorly to provide downward countertraction. The dissection plane in the anterior pelvis is critical to the protection of nerves behind the prostate or vagina that control sexual function. Denonvilliers's fascia is the plane that marks the anterior extent of the mesenteric envelope of the rectum below the cul-de-sac. A cancer in the anterior rectum should be treated with removal of Denonvilliers's fascia. This places the nerves at risk for damage along the anterior surface of Denonvilliers's fascia, behind the seminal vesicles and the prostate. The rectovaginal septum in female patients is also very close to the anterior surface of the rectum, and Denonvilliers's fascia is a landmark for protecting the rectum and maintaining an intact mesorectal excision. The avascular tissue plane outside Denonvilliers's fascia provides a guide to safe appropriate pinpoint dissection in the low anterior pelvis caudal to the cul-de-sac.

The middle hemorrhoidal vessels cross from the internal iliac vessels in the lateral pelvic side wall to enter the mesentery of the rectum at the lower portion of the pelvis in the anterolateral position. The splanchnic nerves run just outside the mesentery along this pelvic side wall, and the crossing fibers of the nerves carrying motor and sensory impulses to the rectum extend along the sides of the blood vessels through the anterolateral ligaments. A dissection plane in the middle of these ligaments provides protection to the laterally placed splanchnic nerve trunks and avoids damage to the mesenteric envelope and lymphatic vessels along the side of the rectal wall. The division of these vessels can be accomplished with the electrocautery or with sealing devices, deep in the pelvis to control blood loss. Precise use of electrocautery is important to protect the lateral nerves. A hook cautery or "paddle" tip can be used to reduce spread of damage. Division of the anterior lateral ligaments releases the rectum from the attachments in the low pelvis. Upward traction on the rectum then provides exposure to the deep pelvis posteriorly. Low rectal transection may not be accomplished adequately with laparoscopic stapling instruments. The author's preference is to place a double staple line with cutting transverse stapler through Pfannenstiel's incision in the suprapubic site. A wound protection or hand access port provides radial retraction of the edges of the incision (Figure 7). Control of the transverse staple line with adequate distal margin below the tumor is essential in cases of malignancy. Multiple staple firings with endoscopic GIA-type staplers may actually increase the risk of anastomotic leak in patients undergoing laparoscopic low anterior resection.

Results of numerous studies available suggest that a robotic approach may facilitate dissection of the pelvis. The parallel alignment of the three instrument arms in the pelvis and the three-dimensional camera, all controlled by the surgeon, gives better control of traction-countertraction and sharp dissection with depth perception. The Robotic versus Laparoscopic Resection for Rectal Cancer (ROLARR) study is underway to compare the surgical outcomes and conversion rate between robotic and laparoscopic anterior resection of the rectum. The University of Leeds in the United Kingdom is the lead institution, and the study includes international investigational sites.

When rectal resection is performed and a low anastomosis may be needed, splenic flexure mobilization should be performed and the inferior mesenteric artery and vein should be divided at their origins to allow the left colon to reach all the way into the pelvis. Because of the sigmoid colon's poor blood supply and noncompliant wall of thick muscle, it should not be used as the anastomotic or preanastomotic segment. The sigmoid is almost inevitably affected by the neoadjuvant radiation in cases in which pretreatment is indicated. The functional outcome is compromised in an end-to-end anastomosis with the sigmoid. Some surgeons always use a pouch made from the last 5 cm of the bowel if the sigmoid is used as the proximal component. If the splenic flexure is freed to allow the left colon to act as the proximal component, the more compliant portion of colon is able to function as a reservoir without a pouch.

Crohn's Disease

Laparoscopy is well recognized as a minimally invasive approach in patients with Crohn's disease and is beneficial to their early recovery and quality of life. The reduction in postoperative adhesions allows an easier second operation in patients who are at high risk for needing a repeat surgical treatment. The lower risk of surgical site infection is a true benefit in patients who are usually immunocompromised. In fact, a review of the National Surgical Quality Improvement Projects showed that ileocolic resection for Crohn's disease results in lower rates of sepsis or pneumonia, shorter length of hospital stay, and overall improved outcome.

The recurrence after resection with laparoscopic approaches is unchanged from that after open surgical approaches. The use of HALS facilitates the minimally invasive approach to complicated cases of Crohn's disease. For example, a patient with a phlegmon and a fistula might be amenable to a laparoscopic approach with a hand-assisted technique. The use of the surgeon's hand clarifies anatomy and prevents converting to an open operation. Fracture of inflammatory adhesions by the finger facilitates identification of individual loops of secondarily involved intestine and limits the amount of intestine that otherwise might have been resected. As a result, short bowel syndrome is avoided. The principle of starting with a laparoscopic approach and converting to a hand-assisted approach early on can usually avoid an open conversion and all the associated problems such as a longer hospital stay, high infection rate, and more adhesions. Therefore, the recommendation should be to attempt a minimally invasive approach in most circumstances.

Ulcerative Colitis

Numerous researchers have investigated the use of a laparoscopic approach to a total proctocolectomy, ileal pouch, and anal anastomosis for ulcerative colitis. The results of their retrospective studies show that there is a decrease in fistula formation if a laparoscopic approach is utilized and a stoma is in place for protection. A three-stage procedure for patients who have severe fulminant colitis may be an improvement in the management of these patients because of the avoidance of pouch leak and abscess. Decreases in overall complications have been documented in patients undergoing three-stage procedures, in comparison with two-stage procedures. The three-stage procedure incorporates a laparoscopic total abdominal colectomy, ileostomy, and construction of Hartmann's pouch of the rectum, followed by a laparoscopic completion proctectomy and pouch construction with a diverting loop ileostomy. The third stage is closure of the ileostomy. The laparoscopic approach has been shown to result in ileostomy closure 20 days sooner for the laparoscopic two-stage ileal pouch anal anastomosis than for the open version. In comparison with the open procedure, the three-stage laparoscopic procedure results in accomplishment of the ileoanal pouch anastomosis 49 days sooner and ileostomy closure for the third stage 17 days sooner.

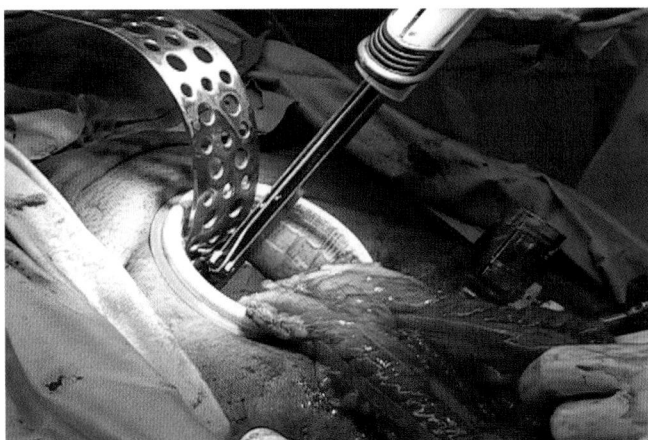

FIGURE 7   Laparoscopic low anterior resection. The rectum and sigmoid are pulled through the incision. *(From Fleshman JW, Birnbaum EH, Hunt SR, et al [eds]: Atlas of surgical techniques for colon, rectum, and anus, Philadelphia, 2012, WB Saunders.)*

Selecting criteria of patients for the three-stage approach include high dose of immunosuppressants in the presence of fulminant colitis and malnutrition. All other patients are well served by a two-stage approach.

The National Inpatient Sample data show that 29% of patients with ulcerative colitis have been treated laparoscopically since 2004. In the single year 2008, that number increased to 41%. A database review also showed a decrease in complications—specifically, surgical site infection, pneumonia, blood loss, and sepsis—for the laparoscopic components of total abdominal colectomy and ileoanal pouch anastomosis.

A retrospective review from the Cleveland Clinic showed that laparoscopic total proctocolectomy and ileoanal pouch anastomosis resulted in fewer complications than did open surgery. This has the "downstream" effect of improving fertility in female patients, with a 50% conception rate in such women who tried to become pregnant (in compared with <30% of those who underwent open operation).

The literature now has several small series of SILS approaches to ulcerative colitis. There seems to be no increase in complications, even though the operative approach is lengthier and is more of a struggle than the laparoscopic approach. Patients should be selected carefully for undergoing this technically demanding procedure. One might add that the patient should carefully select the surgeon as well. Robotic-assisted SILS may make this procedure more feasible when wristed instruments become available for SILS robotic instrumentation.

Diverticulitis

Diverticulitis can be one of the most complicated and difficult disease processes that a colorectal surgeon or general surgeon encounters in the operating room. For this reason, the laparoscopic approach for diverticulitis was slow to be accepted within the surgical community. Numerous studies in the 1990s elucidated the limitations of laparoscopic surgery for the treatment of diverticulitis. Surgeons feared an increase in anastomotic leak rate and bowel injury beyond the area of disease. Although these fears have not been supported and the potential complications have not appeared, the use of the laparoscopic approach to diverticulitis is still under a fair amount of scrutiny. A systematic review of diverticulitis and laparoscopy included 21 studies that are currently in the literature. The review concluded that laparoscopy provided a shorter length of hospital stay and a slightly increased operating time. Complication rates in patients with complicated diverticulitis were decreased in the laparoscopic cases, even though there was wide variability in conversion rates (between 30% and 70%). Hand-assisted laparoscopic sigmoid resection, however, may actually decrease the operating time and decrease the conversion rate by adding an additional safety factor of having a hand through a small incision present in the abdomen during the dissection, as mentioned in the section on Crohn's disease. Several reports suggest that laparoscopic lavage for treatment of diverticular perforation is safe and may be a treatment for the future. The majority of these reports concern patients with abscess perforations (Hinchey class III) and very few suggest this is appropriate for feculent peritonitis (Hinchey class IV). Oversewing of the perforation and placement of drains may be the only treatment needed. With laparoscopic and hand-assisted techniques for sigmoid resection, the rate of complications was decreased, and the numbers of complications of these two techniques were equal. The complication rate was improved over the open procedures. Regardless of the chosen technique, a complete resection of the sigmoid colon down onto soft normal rectum is necessary to prevent recurrent diverticulitis. A simple technique to guarantee resection at the normal rectum is to pass a 29-mm circular stapler to the level of planned resection. If the bowel easily accepts this large diameter, the surgeon can be confident the resection line is on the soft rectum.

Enthusiasm for transanal extraction of the diverticular segment at the end of the procedure is limited. This step may reduce infection in the abdominal wall by eliminating an extraction site. Even when the patient has a positive culture from the pelvis after the rectal stump is opened to remove the specimen, there is no increase in infection. A report from Argentina showed that there was no decrease in sexual function 34 months after the transvaginal specimen extraction that followed laparoscopic sigmoid colectomy in middle-aged women. Transanal extraction would not be expected to affect sexual function, but it might result in a pelvic inflammatory process that would affect fertility negatively.

The National Inpatient Sample Database has provided data that confirm laparoscopic sigmoid colectomy increased to 39% of elective cases being performed for diverticulitis. Overall, laparoscopic sigmoid colectomy was being performed in 32% of patients with diverticulitis, and 94% of all patients undergoing elective surgery received a primary anastomosis. The urgent procedures performed laparoscopically still had a fairly high rate of stoma formation (54%). A review from the Mayo Clinic showed that a leak rate of 1.5% could be expected, even when complicated and uncomplicated cases were compared. A hand-assisted approach was utilized in the majority of these patients and may explain the lack of difference between the leak rates in complicated and uncomplicated cases. In the setting of extreme fibrosis and inflammation, early conversion to an open operation is the best approach for the patient and the surgeon. It reduces the chance of intraoperative complication and shortens operative time to reasonable length.

Colon Cancer

Numerous international and national trials in which laparoscopic and open resection of colon cancer were compared have shown that the laparoscopic approach is safe and results in equivalent, if not slightly improved, oncologic outcomes for colon cancer. The most recent report of laparoscopic treatment of colon cancer documented that laparoscopy may actually reduce the circulating levels of cancer-supporting growth factors, in comparison with open resection. This may have some implications for distant recurrence and may be an indicator that a less invasive approach is important for long-term treatment of cancer.

Conversion to an open operation during a laparoscopic approach does not seem to affect cancer outcomes. The original fear that laparoscopy would cause an increase in intraabdominal carcinomatosis and seeding of tumor in the trocar sites has been unfounded. Good oncologic technique has prevented both of these possibilities.

The experience of the surgeon and willingness to convert early may be important with regard to the fact that conversion does not result in higher local tumor recurrence rates. The most common reasons for converting to an open operation are large tumor size with local invasion and adhesions. These can be identified early in the procedure, and the operation can be switched to either a hand-assisted approach or an open approach to avoid untoward oncologic outcomes. The SILS approach to colon cancer has been shown to be almost equal to a laparoscopic procedure with regard to lymph node harvest, negative margins, and recurrence. The case-matched controlled, retrospective study from Scott and White Clinic revealed that the patients who underwent laparoscopy had a higher rate of conversion to an open procedure than those who underwent the SILS approach (15.4% vs 11.5%). It is important to remember that a conversion to a multiport technique or a HALS approach preserves the majority of benefits of a minimally invasive approach.

Rectal Cancer

Rectal cancer is being considered an opportunity for laparoscopic treatment. There are numerous reports of rectal resection. The

Colorectal Cancer Laparoscopic or Open Resection (COLOR II) trial showed that laparoscopic treatment of rectal cancer is safe and feasible and results in similar complication rates and early oncologic outcomes as an open procedure. The Alliance Z6051 trial has closed to accrual after entering the required 480 patients. The endpoint of this trial is the surgical specimen, as a surrogate for oncologic outcome. Negative radial and distal margins and a good quality total mesorectal excision (TME) specimen are the primary outcomes for this trial. For the first time in a trial, photodocumentation of the rectal specimen has been utilized for quality control of the surgical technique. The quality of the TME specimen (complete, nearly complete, incomplete) is being incorporated into the pathology reports for these patients to document the quality of the surgery that was performed. A report from the COREAN (from Korea) trial showed that a randomization of laparoscopic versus open technique resulted in equivalent outcomes for stage II and III rectal cancer. Patients who underwent the laparoscopic procedure showed less blood loss, shorter length of hospital stay, less requirement for pain medicine, and a 91% of complete to near-complete TME in the rectal specimen, in comparison with 88% of patients who underwent the open procedure. There was only a 1.2% conversion rate for the patients who underwent laparoscopy.

Innovations are ongoing in the surgical treatment of rectal cancer. Transanal endoscopic proctectomy for rectal cancer has been reported in a small group of men treated in France, with a 6% conversion rate, and 80% to 87% specimens were of good quality. However, there was 30% incidence of local recurrence in 30 patients reported (12% at 21 months) with this technique. This technique needs further study.

Robotic proctectomy has been compared retrospectively with laparoscopy in a large group of patients treated in Melbourne, Australia. The oncologic outcomes have been shown to be equivalent. A decreased conversion rate was noted in patients who underwent robotic proctectomy.

In another study from Brisbane, Australia, the laparoscopic approach to a proctectomy was compared with the hybrid laparoscopic approach, in which the rectal dissection is performed with open technique through a small open incision above the pubis. The incidence of pelvic abscess and complications was much higher in the patients who underwent the hybrid procedure, but there was no change in local recurrence or survival. Transanal endoscopic total mesorectal excision and SILS left colectomy and transanal/transabdominal laparoscopic and endoscopic proctectomy have been shown to be feasible in both cadavers and living humans. No long-term data are available.

COMPLICATIONS AND LEARNING CURVE OF LAPAROSCOPIC COLECTOMY

Even though laparoscopy provides a minimally invasive approach with smaller incisions, there is a minimal change (1 to 2 days) in the length of hospital stay and recovery of the patient in comparison with the open approach. Much of the improvement in recovery was noted after the discharge time frame; laparoscopically treated patients tend to return to activities of daily living faster. There is an emphasis on the early recovery program in combination with laparoscopic colectomy. The early recovery program seems to improve recovery, beyond the improvements contributed by the laparoscopic approach, by shortening the length of hospital stay to as little as 2 days after a laparoscopic colectomy. The early recovery program is a hospital wide, multidisciplinary approach that focuses on the patient to "improve" recovery by limiting complications, reducing iatrogenic effects on

postoperative bowel functioning, and controlling pain. Fluid restriction, limits on narcotics, early ambulation, and feeding all contribute.

The learning curve for a laparoscopic colectomy has been shown to be variable. A study from Osaka, Japan, showed that the time needed for a surgeon to perform laparoscopic colectomy stabilizes after 50 cases. Conversion rates greatly diminish after 150 cases, and the complications decrease after 200 cases. The leak rate was 14% at the beginning and decreased to 4% after 200 cases. Other studies have shown that HALS can reduce the number of cases needed to decrease conversion and operating room time to approximately 100 cases. The operating time is decreased with HALS without compromising length of hospital stay or complication.

The American College of Surgeons' National Surgical Quality Improvement Program (NSQIP) database has shown that the likelihood for high-level complications is lower for laparoscopic than for open cases, even after risk adjustment. The National Inpatient Sample Database showed that thromboembolic complications after colectomy in 149,000 patients was decreased by almost half in the patients who underwent the laparoscopic procedure, in comparison with patients who underwent the open procedure, and seemed to be related to the presence of inflammatory bowel disease, rectal operation, malignancy, obesity, and congestive heart failure as risk factors.

In conclusion, laparoscopic colectomy and proctectomy are feasible techniques in the treatment of colorectal disease. The studied approach to adopting these techniques is based on surgical research that provides data for evidence-based care in colorectal disease. The use of new technology is sometimes enticing for marketing purposes or for the pleasure of performing a new operation. Early adoption of these procedures must be balanced against the realities that on occasion, new technology is not of benefit to the patient or the medical system. An example in which enthusiasm has outdistanced evidence-based evaluation is the case of robotic colectomy and proctectomy. As time goes forward, cost effectiveness will need to be evaluated as resources become more limited. Patient care must always be at the forefront of concern when surgeons adopt new techniques in the technology.

SUGGESTED READINGS

Ahmed Ali U, Keus F, Heikens JT, et al: Open versus laparoscopic (assisted) ileo pouch anal anastomosis for ulcerative colitis and familial adenomatous polyposis [Review], *Cochrane Database Syst Rev* (1):CD006267, 2009.

Gaertner WB, Kwaan MR, Madoff RD, et al: The evolving role of laparoscopy in colonic diverticular disease: a systematic review, *World Journal of Surgery* 37(3):629–638, 2013.

Greenblatt DY, Rajamanickam V, Pugely AJ, et al: Short-term outcomes after laparoscopic-assisted proctectomy for rectal cancer: results from the ACS NSQIP, *J Am Coll Surg* 212(5):844–854, 2011.

Jayne DG, Thorpe HC, Copeland J, et al: Five-year follow-up of the Medical Research Council CLASICC trial of laparoscopically assisted versus open surgery for colorectal cancer, *Br J Surg* 97(11):1638–1645, 2010.

Kang SB, Park JW, Jeong SY, et al: Open versus laparoscopic surgery for mid or low rectal cancer after neoadjuvant chemoradiotherapy (COREAN trial): short-term outcomes of an open-label randomized controlled trial, *Lancet Oncol* 11(7):637–645 2010.

Masoomi H, Kang CY, Chaudhry O, et al: Predictive factors of early bowel obstruction in colon and rectal surgery: data from the Nationwide Inpatient Sample, 2006–2008, *J Am Coll Surg* 214(5):831–837, 2012.

Pendlimari R, Holubar SD, Dozois EJ, et al: Technical proficiency in hand-assisted laparoscopic colon and rectal surgery: determining how many cases are required to achieve mastery, *Arch Surg* 147(4):317–322, 2012.

Surgical Care and Outcomes Assessment Program (SCOAP) Collaborative, Kwon S, Billingham R, et al: Adoption of laparoscopy for elective colorectal resection: A report from the Surgical Care and Outcomes Assessment Program, *J Am Coll Surg* 214(6):909–918.e1, 2012.

MINIMALLY INVASIVE ESOPHAGECTOMY

Luis F. Tapias, MD, and Christopher R. Morse, MD

OVERVIEW

Transhiatal esophagectomy and Ivor Lewis esophagectomy are the two most commonly performed operations for esophageal pathology. Both are complex procedures that are often associated with high morbidity and mortality. Because esophagectomy is frequently performed in elderly patients with many coexisting medical comorbidities, increasing interest has been found in minimally invasive approaches in an attempt to improve early postoperative outcomes. Minimally invasive esophagectomy (MIE) has the potential for an easier postoperative recovery with fewer cardiopulmonary and infectious complications. In addition, enhanced visualization of abdominal and mediastinal structures by means of a minimally invasive approach may facilitate intraoperative steps, reduce injury to neighboring structures, improve lymph node harvest, and decrease blood loss.

In 1992, Cuschieri and colleagues described a technique of esophagectomy with a staged procedure that combined a right thoracoscopic approach in the prone position with a midline laparotomy and cervical anastomosis. In 1995, DePaula and colleagues reported a small series of laparoscopic transhiatal esophagectomies. Subsequently, in 1998, Luketich and colleagues reported a combined thoracoscopic and laparoscopic approach to esophagectomy that consisted of a thoracoscopic mobilization of the esophagus, the laparoscopic creation of the gastric conduit, and a neck anastomosis. Watson and colleagues later reported a minimally invasive Ivor Lewis technique in 1999 and described a laparoscopic construction of the gastric conduit followed by thoracoscopic intrathoracic anastomosis.

INDICATIONS

The most common indication for MIE is esophageal cancer (stages I to IIIA), although esophagectomy may be used in rare, end-stage, benign esophageal disorders such as achalasia. At present, no absolute contraindications exist, although advanced training in minimally invasive esophageal surgery is encouraged. Minimally invasive esophagectomy as performed for cancer can be performed in patients who have or have not received neoadjuvant chemoradiation. Obesity and previous abdominal or thoracic surgery can lead to more technically demanding MIE, but they are not contraindications. In any case, safety should be foremost, and the surgeon must maintain a low threshold to convert the operation to an open procedure, either in the abdominal or thoracic stages of the operation, if needed. The most common esophageal cancer in the United States is adenocarcinoma, often associated with Barrett's esophagus, which leads to a preference for a minimally invasive Ivor Lewis approach, although the steps are easily modified to a laparoscopic transhiatal or a modified McKeown's technique. The steps to an Ivor Lewis approach and the additional modifications to include a cervical anastomosis are described.

PREOPERATIVE PREPARATION

The preoperative evaluation for a minimally invasive esophagectomy is no different than that for a patient undergoing an open procedure.

The two primary issues are whether a patient is resectable and whether the patient has sufficient cardiopulmonary reserve to tolerate the operation. Staging of esophageal cancer includes an upper endoscopy, endoscopic ultrasound scan (EUS), computed tomographic (CT) scanning, and positron emission tomographic (PET) imaging. Upper endoscopy is performed to identify the proximal and distal extent of the tumor, which may impact on the type of procedure; this is often done in the operating room at the time of the operation. The primary benefit of EUS is to determine the degree of invasion of the esophageal wall by tumor and adjacent lymph node status. Patients with T3 or N1 disease are typically treated with induction chemoradiotherapy before esophagectomy. CT imaging is useful to determine the presence of bulky nodal disease within the abdomen. Bulky disease limited to the celiac nodal basin does not preclude esophagectomy, provided significant response to induction therapy is seen. The addition of PET imaging, often in conjunction with CT scan, increases the sensitivity in detection of distant metastatic disease. PET is not particularly helpful in identification of periesophageal nodal disease because activity within these nodes often is obscured by the primary tumor.

Patients should undergo a thorough evaluation to determine medical suitability for operation. This includes a cardiac stress test and, if indicated, coronary angiography. Patients with a significant tobacco history also should undergo pulmonary function testing. In addition, most patients with locally advanced cancer have some degree of dysphagia and weight loss before diagnosis. Dysphagia often improves with induction therapy. The placement of either an esophageal stent or a percutaneous gastrostomy tube is strongly discouraged for any patient who may be an operative candidate. Esophagectomy may still be performed in these situations, although it is technically more challenging.

MINIMALLY INVASIVE IVOR LEWIS ESOPHAGECTOMY

A minimally invasive Ivor Lewis esophagectomy is preferred because it allows excellent visualization of mediastinal structures and a complete thoracic lymph node harvest and minimizes recurrent laryngeal nerve injuries and the creation of a tension-free anastomosis. A minimally invasive Ivor Lewis esophagectomy is performed in two stages. In the first stage, laparoscopic mobilization of the stomach and construction of the gastric conduit is performed with the patient in a supine position. In the second stage, the patient is repositioned to a left lateral decubitus position for mobilization of the thoracic esophagus, mediastinal lymph node dissection, removal of the surgical specimen, gastric pull-up, and construction of an intrathoracic esophagogastric anastomosis. Narrowing of the gastric tube too much is discouraged, and an attempt should be made to preserve the width at approximately 5 to 6 cm. A pyloroplasty or pyloromyotomy is not routinely performed. A jejunostomy is routinely performed in all patients.

Surgical Technique

The patient is placed supine, and the surgeon stands to the patient's right and the assistant to the left. The initial step is to perform an on-table esophagogastroduodenoscopy (EGD) to confirm tumor location, the presence of Barrett's esophagus, and the suitability of the stomach as a conduit for reconstruction. Five initial laparoscopic ports are placed in the upper abdomen in a paramedian fashion (Figure 1). A 10-mm, 30-degree laparoscope is used. The abdomen is examined for metastatic disease, and a liver retractor is placed through the most lateral port on the right side. Dissection is begun

The gastric conduit is created with endoscopic staplers, starting at the incisura; a sixth laparoscopic port is placed in the right lower quadrant for this purpose. The right gastric artery is often preserved. Remember to withdraw or remove the nasogastric tube before conduit creation. The stomach is divided up to the cardia with multiple fires of an endoscopic stapler, keeping a 5-cm to 6-cm width to the conduit along the greater curvature (Figure 3). The first staple firing along the lesser curve is typically a vascular load to control vessels in this area. To set up conduit creation, the assistant grasps the fundus along the greater curvature and gently stretches it towards the spleen; a second grasper is placed on the antrum, and a slight downward retraction is applied. Light tension superiorly and inferiorly on the stomach can extend the length of the conduit and allow the creation of a straight staple line. Prevention of spiraling of the stomach is critical as the staple line is advanced proximally.

A jejunostomy is placed (Flexiflo Laparoscopic Jejunostomy Kit, Abbott Laboratories, Abbott Park, Ill) in the left lower quadrant. Rotating the transverse colon up towards the hiatus, the ligament of Treitz is identified. Moving 30 to 40 cm down the jejunum, a loop of small bowel is tacked to the abdominal wall with an endostitch device. Facilitating this step is the additional 12-mm port initially placed in the lower right quadrant during creation of the gastric conduit. A needle and then a guidewire are passed into the jejunum with laparoscopic vision. Proper placement of the catheter is confirmed by observing distension of the jejunum as air is insufflated into the needle catheter. The jejunum surrounding the feeding tube is then tacked to the abdominal wall with several additional endostitches.

Finally, with an endostitch, the most superior portion of the gastric tube is then stitched to the specimen (Figure 4). The stitch maintains correct orientation of the gastric conduit as it is delivered into the chest. The laparoscopic portion of the procedure is completed by dividing the phrenoesophageal membrane. The crura are also assessed to determine whether a stitch should be placed to avoid herniation of the conduit into the chest.

The patient is turned to the left lateral decubitus position for the thoracoscopic mobilization of the esophagus and creation of an intrathoracic anastomosis. The surgeon stands to the back of the patient, and the assistant stands to the front. After lung isolation is achieved, five thoracoscopic ports are placed (Figure 5). A 10-mm camera port is placed in the 7th or 8th intercostal space, anterior to the midaxillary line. A 10-mm port is placed at the 8th or 9th intercostal space, posterior to the posterior axillary line, for the ultrasonic coagulating shears. A 10-mm port is placed in the anterior axillary line at the 4th intercostal space, through which a fan-shaped retractor retracts the lung anteriorly to expose the esophagus. A 5-mm port is placed just anterior to the tip of the scapula and is used for retraction by the surgeon. A final port is placed at the sixth rib, at the anterior axillary line for suction, and is critical in the creation of the anastomosis.

The initial step is to place a stitch in the central tendon of the diaphragm to facilitate visualization of the gastroesophageal junction; this suture is brought out through a 1-mm incision in the anterior chest wall, retracting the diaphragm inferiorly and anteriorly. Dissection in the chest begins by dividing the inferior pulmonary ligament. In taking down the inferior pulmonary ligament, dissection onto the pericardium is important because it is the medial aspect of the dissection. The inferior pulmonary vein is retracted anteriorly, and the dissection is carried along the pericardium, mobilizing the subcarinal lymph packet. At risk during the mobilization the subcarinal nodes is the posterior, membranous wall of the right mainstem bronchus, which should be clearly identified. With complete dissection of the subcarinal space, the left mainstem bronchus should be identified. The subcarinal nodal package is removed with the specimen. The mediastinal pleura is then opened along the hilum to the level of the azygos vein. The mediastinal pleura is opened above the azygos vein, and with complete dissection around the azygos vein, it is divided with a vascular load of an endoscopic stapler.

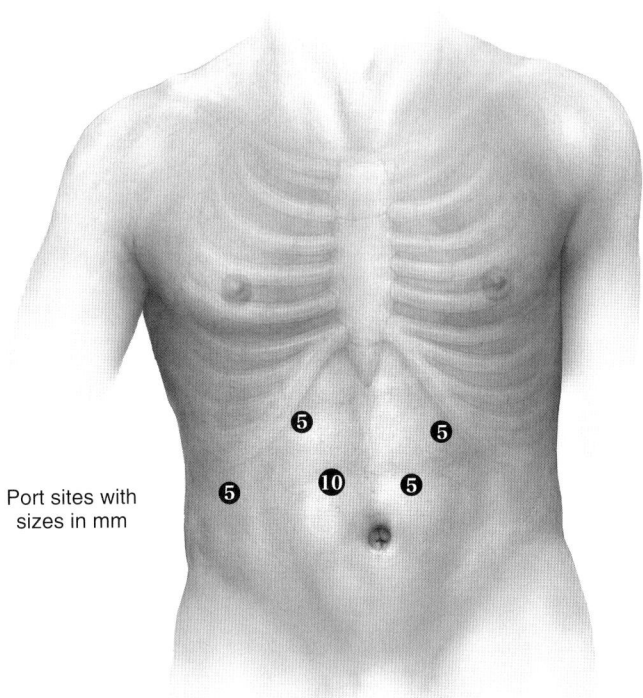

Port sites with sizes in mm

FIGURE 1 The patient is initially positioned in the supine position, and a double lumen endotracheal tube is placed in preparation for the thoracoscopic mobilization of the esophagus. Five abdominal ports are used for the gastric mobilization. A marking pen is used to trace the midline from the xiphoid to the umbilicus, and this line is further divided into thirds. To avoid potential injury to any abdominal viscera or organs, the initial port is placed via an open technique. The two midclavicular ports are placed on the lower third of the marked line to assist with gastric mobilization. *(From Tsai WS, Levy RM, Luketich JD: Technique of minimally invasive Ivor Lewis esophagectomy,* Op Tech Thorac Cardiovasc Surg *14(3):177, 2009; Fig. 1.)*

by taking down the gastrohepatic ligament and exposing the right crus. The phrenoesophageal ligament is divided, and the distal esophagus is mobilized, with care taken to keep all of the surrounding tissue with the specimen. The gastrocolic omentum is divided, and careful attention is paid to preserving the right gastroepiploic artery (Figure 2). Dissection is carried up the greater curve, further mobilizing the stomach by dividing the short gastric arteries where the dissection moves close to the greater curvature. The left crus is exposed, and the esophagus is mobilized into the mediastinum. All attachments between the posterior aspect of the stomach and the anterior surface of the pancreas are divided to the level of the pylorus. From the lesser curve side of the stomach, the left gastric artery is dissected to its base with all nodal tissue included in the specimen. A stapler is placed at the base of the artery and vein, and they are divided.

The authors do not routinely perform a pyloroplasty because they have observed at their institution a low incidence of gastric outlet obstruction after esophagectomy among patients who did not undergo a pyloric drainage procedure. Furthermore, should delayed gastric emptying present in the postoperative period, it can be managed conservatively or with endoscopic balloon dilation of the pylorus in most patients. If a pyloroplasty is to be performed, the pylorus is opened with ultrasonic shears and the pylorus closed transversely in an interrupted fashion with an Endostitch device (Covidien, Mansfield, Mass) with nonabsorbable suture. Alternatives to pyloroplasty include pyloromyotomy or botulinum toxin injection of the pylorus.

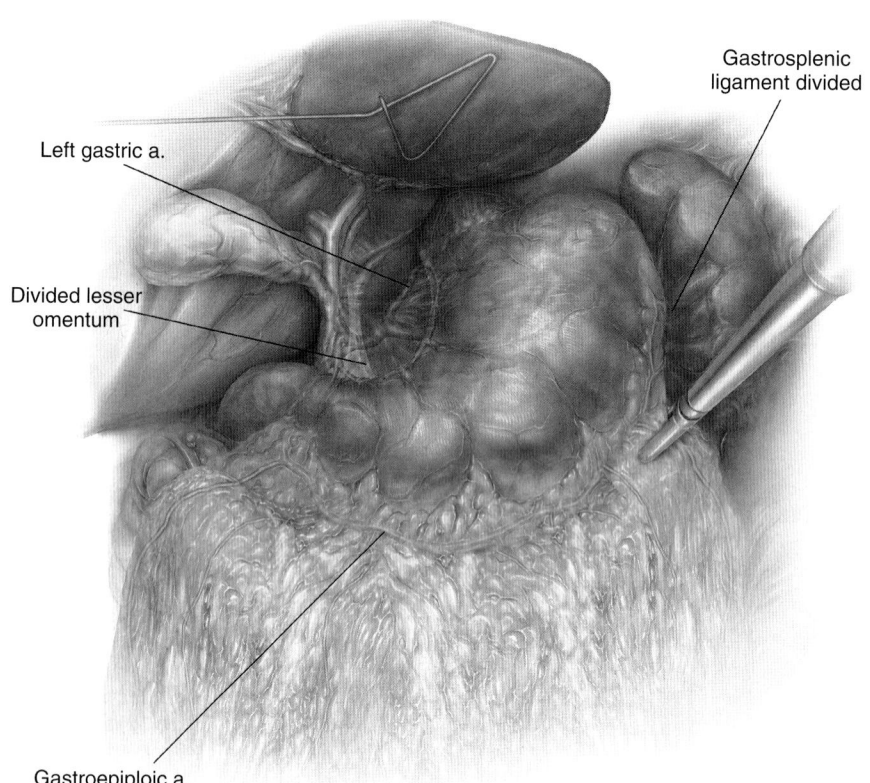

Gastrosplenic ligament divided

Left gastric a.

Divided lesser omentum

Gastroepiploic a.

FIGURE 2 After an initial inspection of the peritoneal surfaces and the liver to rule out any metastatic disease, the gastrohepatic omentum is opened. The left gastric artery/vein pedicle is identified, and by tracing its course proximally, the celiac lymph nodes are then examined. A complete lymph node dissection is performed to include the celiac nodes, sweeping all nodal and fatty tissue with the specimen; the nodal dissection is continued along the splenic artery and the superior border of the pancreas. This plane continues cephalad toward the right and left crus, continuous with the preaortic dissection plane into the lower thoracic cavity. If any lymph nodes appear suspicious for metastatic involvement, they are dissected and sent for frozen-section analysis. If the nodes do not appear malignant or are pathologically free of cancer on analysis, dissection of the right crus is initiated to mobilize the lateral aspect of the esophagus. *(From Tsai WS, Levy RM, Luketich JD: Technique of minimally invasive Ivor Lewis esophagectomy,* Op Tech Thorac Cardiovasc Surg *14(3):178, 2009; Fig. 2.)*

Posteriorly, the pleura is divided and the esophagus dissected away from the chest wall and aorta. All aortoesophageal vessels encountered during this portion of the procedure should be clipped before division. Any tissue suspicious for lymphatic branches arising from the thoracic duct is meticulously clipped and divided to prevent chylothorax. If injury to the thoracic duct is a concern, this structure can be ligated en masse at the level of the diaphragm. With the esophagus mobilized medially and laterally, the specimen is pulled into the chest with the attached gastric conduit. Care should be taken to only bring in enough gastric tube to reach the proximal esophageal remnant because redundant gastric conduit above the diaphragm is a source of delayed poor gastric emptying as a result of the S loop of gastric conduit this may create. The gastric tube must remain properly oriented with the staple line, continuing to face the lateral chest wall with this avoiding spiraling or 360-degree twisting of the conduit. The stitch is cut between the specimen and the conduit, and the specimen is retracted anteriorly and superiorly. The dissection continues posteriorly to mobilize the esophagus completely off the contralateral pleura. When dissecting the esophagus above the level of the azygos vein, the dissection plane moves to the wall of the esophagus. This avoids injury to the recurrent laryngeal nerve. Lymph nodes above the azygos vein are not routinely harvested.

The posterior incision is increased to a total of 4 cm; a wound protector is placed. The esophagus is transected with Endo Shears (Covidien, Mansfield, Mass) at a level appropriate for the tumor. The specimen is removed through the wound protector and sent for pathologic analysis of the margins. The anvil of a 28-mm end-to-end anastomosis (EEA) stapler is placed in the proximal esophagus, and a purse-string suture is placed and tied to secure the anvil in position (Figure 6). A second purse-string suture is placed to further secure the anvil and pull in any mucosal defects. The gastric conduit is then pulled to the apex of the chest, and the ultrasonic shears are used to open up the tip of the gastric conduit along the staple line. The EEA stapler is placed through the posterior- inferior port, which had been enlarged and positioned in the conduit. The stapler

tip is brought out along the greater curve of the gastric conduit to join the anvil. Before the anastomosis is created, the amount of conduit that will lie in the chest is carefully ascertained. A common mistake is to bring an excess amount of stomach into the chest in an effort to minimize tension on the anastomosis. This excess conduit often assumes a sigmoid curve above the diaphragm and may lead to significant problems with gastric emptying. In addition, ensuring proper orientation of the stomach is critical to prevent twisting. The tip of the stapler and the anvil are docked, and the stapler is fired, creating a circular esophagogastric anastomosis (side of gastric conduit to end of esophagus) at approximately the level of the azygos vein. The excess stomach (the gastrostomy through which the stapler was placed) is trimmed with several loads of an articulating linear endoscopic stapler, and a 28F chest tube and a Blake drain (Ethicon Inc., Somerville, NJ) are placed adjacent to the anastomosis (Figure 7).

LAPAROSCOPIC TRANSHIATAL ESOPHAGECTOMY

Laparoscopic transhiatal esophagectomy is a two-stage operation. The patient is initially positioned supine for the laparoscopic construction of the gastric conduit and transhiatal mobilization of the esophagus. In a second stage, the cervical esophagus is mobilized through a neck incision with removal of the esophageal specimen and gastric pull-up. An esophagogastric anastomosis is performed in the neck. The initial port placement and mobilization of the stomach are similar to the Ivor Lewis approach. The esophagus at the hiatus is initially mobilized, the greater curve of the stomach dissected from the greater omentum to preserve the gastroepiploic artery, the lesser curve of the stomach is mobilized dividing the left gastric artery and vein, and the gastric conduit is created. A jejunostomy is placed. In the last step of the abdominal phase of this procedure, the esophagus

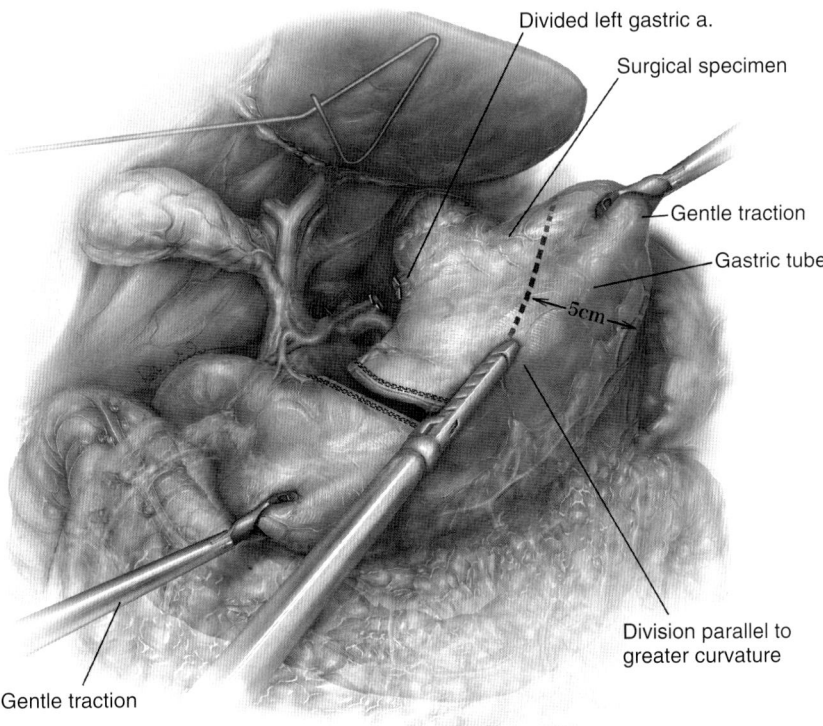

Divided left gastric a.

Surgical specimen

Gentle traction

Gastric tube

5cm

Division parallel to
greater curvature

Gentle traction

FIGURE 3 Once the stomach and celiac lymph nodes are completely mobilized, the left gastric artery and vein are divided with a vascular load on the Endo GIA (Covidien, Mansfield, Mass) stapler. This is done by approaching the pedicle from the lesser curve. The pedicle must be dissected completely clean with all celiac nodes swept up into the specimen. Once the pedicle is divided, the distal esophagus, gastric fundus, and antrum should be completely mobilized. The gastric tube is usually created before the completion of the pyloroplasty and placement of the feeding jejunostomy tube because this provides time to assess the viability of the gastric tube as a conduit before bringing it into the chest. The first stapler used for creating the gastric conduit contains a vascular load to control bleeding from the adipose tissue and vessels along the lesser curve. The stapler is placed just up to, but not onto, the gastric antrum, which is usually thick and requires staples appropriate for thick tissue. The initial 5/12-mm right midclavicular port is changed to a 15-mm port to allow for the placement of a 4.8-mm Endo GIA stapler (Autosuture, Covidien). An additional 12-mm port is placed in the right lower quadrant to assist with the creation of the gastric tube. *(From Tsai WS, Levy RM, Luketich JD: Technique of minimally invasive Ivor Lewis esophagectomy, Op Tech Thorac Cardiovasc Surg 14(3):181, 2009; Fig. 5.)*

is mobilized through the esophageal hiatus circumferentially as high as possible in an effort to reach the cervical esophageal dissection plane. If needed, a portion of the crus of the diaphragm is divided to enlarge the esophageal hiatus to facilitate exposure and transhiatal delivery of the surgical specimen. The tip of the gastric conduit is sutured to the surgical specimen. The abdominal operation is now halted, and the neck procedure is started. Through a horizontal left neck incision, the platysma is divided and the sternocleidomastoid muscle is retracted laterally. The inferior thyroidal vessels and the omohyoid muscle are divided. Blunt dissection of the esophagus is carried inferiorly to join the laparoscopic mediastinal dissection plane. Once the entire esophagus is mobilized, the specimen is removed through the cervical incision, pulling along with it the gastric conduit. The laparoscope is now placed back into the abdomen to allow direct visualization of the gastric tube and avoid trauma or spiraling of the conduit. The esophagus is divided 4 cm distal to the upper esophageal sphincter. On confirmation of a negative margin for carcinoma or Barrett's esophagus, an esophagogastric anastomosis is performed in the neck with either a two-layer hand-sewn or a stapled technique.

THORACOSCOPIC AND LAPAROSCOPIC ESOPHAGECTOMY WITH CERVICAL ANASTOMOSIS

A combined thoracoscopic and laparoscopic esophagectomy with cervical anastomosis is a three-stage operation. Initially, the patient is placed in the left lateral decubitus position, and the thoracic esophagus is mobilized in a similar fashion to a minimally invasive Ivor Lewis esophagectomy. However, above the azygos vein, the parietal pleura is left intact to limit mediastinal contamination in the event of a cervical anastomotic leak. Dissection is carried up to the thoracic inlet with circumferential mobilization of the esophagus. Once the esophagus is completely mobilized, the patient is placed supine, and the abdominal portion of the operation begins. Again, this portion of the procedure is similar to the previously described gastric mobilizations. At the conclusion of the gastric mobilization, the neck dissection is completed in a similar fashion as that described for a minimally invasive transhiatal approach. Once the cervical anastomosis is complete, the surgeon returns to the laparoscopic view and

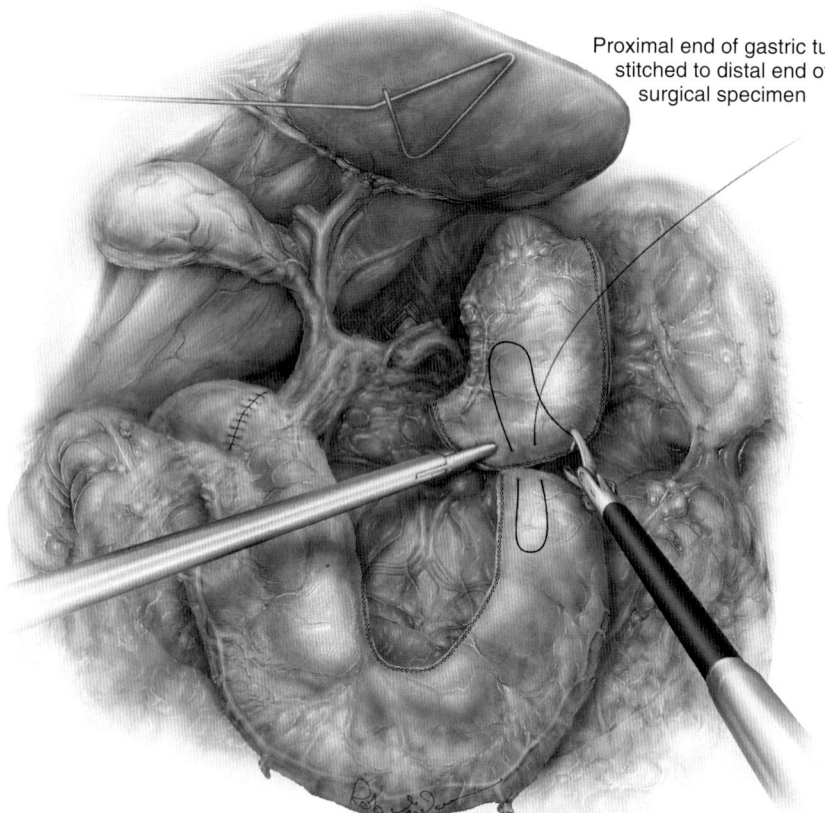

Proximal end of gastric tube stitched to distal end of surgical specimen

FIGURE 4 The most superior portion of the gastric tube is stitched to the specimen. The stomach must be kept aligned correctly so that, during the mobilization of the conduit into the chest, it does not twist in the abdomen. This is ensured by suturing the greater curvature along the short gastric vessels to the staple line of the proximal gastric remnant. *(From Tsai WS, Levy RM, Luketich JD: Technique of minimally invasive Ivor Lewis esophagectomy, Op Tech Thorac Cardiovasc Surg 14(3):185, 2009; Fig. 9.)*

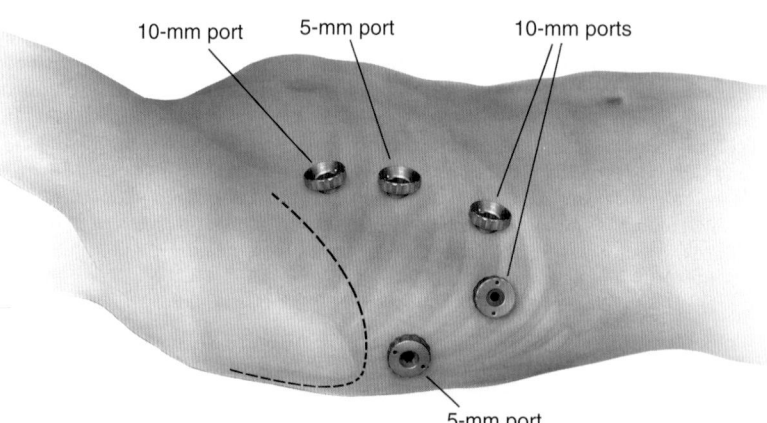

10-mm port   5-mm port   10-mm ports

5-mm port

FIGURE 5 The patient is then turned to the left lateral decubitus position for the thoracoscopic mobilization of the esophagus and creation of the intrathoracic anastomosis. Five thoracoscopic ports are used. A 10-mm camera port is placed in the 7th or 8th intercostal space, just anterior to the midaxillary line. The working port is a 10-mm port that is placed at the 8th or 9th intercostal space, posterior to the posterior axillary line. Another 10-mm port is placed in the anterior axillary line at the 4th intercostal space, through which a fan-shaped retractor aids in retracting the lung to expose the esophagus. A 5-mm port is placed just inferior to the tip of the scapula, and this is used by the surgeon's left hand for countertraction. A final port is placed at the sixth rib, at the anterior axillary line for suction, and is important in the creation of the anastomosis. *(From Tsai WS, Levy RM, Luketich JD: Technique of minimally invasive Ivor Lewis esophagectomy, Op Tech Thorac Cardiovasc Surg 14(3):187, 2009; Fig. 11.)*

Gastroesophageal anastomosis with EEA stapler

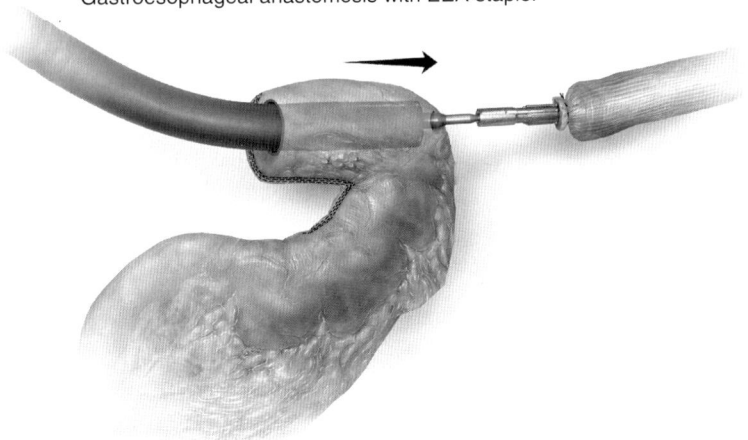

FIGURE 6   The anvil of a 28-mm end-to-end anastomosis *(EEA)* stapler is placed in the proximal esophagus and a 2.0 endo stitch purse-string suture is placed and tied (intracorporeal technique) to secure the anvil in position. It is technically challenging to make this first stitch perfect because the anvil has a tendency to migrate out of the open end of the proximal esophagus. For this reason, a second purse-string suture is placed to further secure the anvil and pull in any mucosal defects, thereby ensuring complete rings after EEA firing. Ordinarily, a 28-mm EEA stapler is used in an attempt to minimize the risk of stricture and decrease need for postoperative dilations. In most cases, the 28-mm anvil is secured without difficulty. On rare occasion, a Foley balloon catheter must be used to dilate the proximal esophagus. Should the Foley balloon catheter fail, a 25-mm stapler is then used. The gastric conduit is then pulled to the apex of the chest, and the ultrasonic shears are used to open up the tip of the gastric conduit along the staple line. The EEA stapler is placed through the posterior-inferior port, which had been enlarged, and positioned in the conduit. The stapler tip is brought out along the greater curve of the gastric conduit to join the anvil. Before creating the anastomosis, the amount of conduit that will lie in the chest is carefully estimated. A common mistake is to bring an excess amount of stomach into the chest in an effort to minimize tension on the anastomosis. This excess conduit often assumes a sigmoid conformation above the diaphragm and may lead to significant problems with gastric emptying. In addition, ensuring proper orientation of the stomach is critical to prevent twisting. *(From Tsai WS, Levy RM, Luketich JD: Technique of minimally invasive Ivor Lewis esophagectomy, Op Tech Thorac Cardiovasc Surg 14(3):189, 2009; Fig. 13.)*

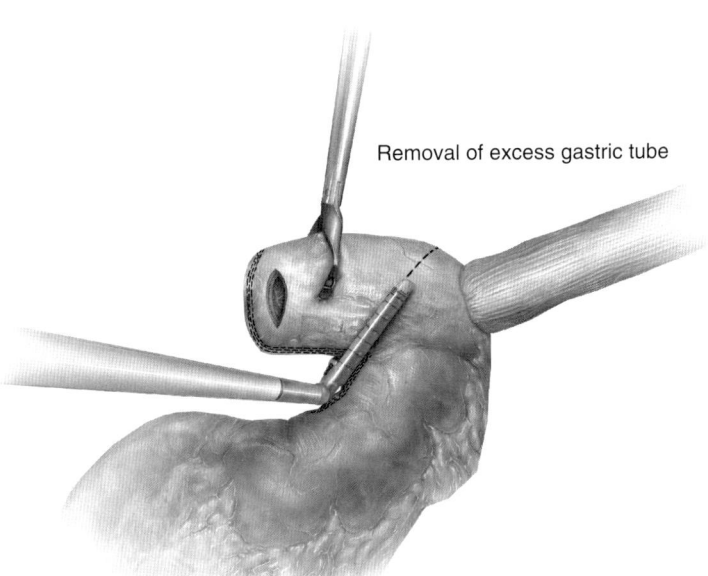

Removal of excess gastric tube

FIGURE 7   The tip of the stapler and the anvil are docked, and the stapler is fired, creating a circular esophagogastric anastomosis, joining the side of the gastric conduit to the end of esophagus, at approximately the level of the azygos vein. The excess gastric tip (the gastrostomy through which the stapler was placed) is trimmed with several loads of an articulating linear stapler, with care taken not to injure the omental pedical wrap that was mobilized along the greater curvature. Endoscopy is not routinely performed to evaluate the anastomosis. *(From Tsai WS, Levy RM, Luketich JD: Technique of minimally invasive Ivor Lewis esophagectomy. Op Tech Thorac Cardiovasc Surg 14(3):190, 2009; Fig. 14.)*

gently pulls downward on the pyloroantral area to retrieve any excess gastric tube that may have been pulled up into the chest during the neck anastomosis and mobilization. The gastric conduit is then tacked to the hiatus.

POSTOPERATIVE CARE

Patients undergo extubation in the operating room. Epidural analgesia is not routinely used after MIE Ivor Lewis at the authors' institution, and pain is managed with rib blocks, patient-controlled analgesics, and ketorolac. Postoperative management includes the initiation of tube feeds on postoperative day 2. The nasogastric tube is typically removed on postoperative day 5, and a barium swallow is performed to assess gastric emptying and anastomotic integrity. If results are normal, this is followed by the initiation of a clear liquid diet, advanced over 3 weeks. Tube feedings are cycled to the evenings, and the jejunostomy is removed at the first office visit.

RESULTS

Luketich and colleagues published in 2012 the largest series to date on MIE with 1011 patients, including 481 patients who received a minimally invasive three-field McKeown's-type esophagectomy and 530 patients who received a minimally invasive Ivor Lewis esophagectomy. Among the patients who underwent an Ivor Lewis MIE, they reported a median intensive care unit (ICU) length of stay of 2 days and a median hospital length of stay of 7 days. Conversion to open rate was 4%. Major morbidity included empyema in 5% of the cases, anastomotic leak requiring reoperation in 5%, gastric tube necrosis in 2%, and vocal fold paresis or paralysis in 1%. In addition, in the authors' experience, chylothorax occurred in 5% of patients, with only 2.5% needing ligation of the thoracic duct. Furthermore, Luketich and colleagues reported an operative mortality rate of 1.68%. Adequacy of resection was reported in terms of a negative margin, achieved in 98% of patients, and the median number of lymph nodes examined was 21.

When compared with open esophagectomy, the authors found at their institution that minimally invasive Ivor Lewis esophagectomy is associated with decreased intraoperative blood loss, less intraoperative intravenous fluid administration, shorter duration of nasogastric tube drainage, faster initiation of oral intake, and decreased ICU and hospital length of stay. Oncologic outcomes were comparable when examining the number of lymph nodes retrieved and compromise of resection margins. Importantly, MIE was associated with a significantly lower incidence of pulmonary complications when compared with open procedures.

SUMMARY

Minimally invasive esophagectomy can be performed safely with reasonable operative times, markedly less morbidity and mortality, excellent anastomotic integrity, and consistent initial oncologic outcomes. Because pulmonary complications carry a poor prognosis, the ability to decrease and eliminate them is critical, which seems to be achieved with a minimally invasive esophagectomy in several studies. Although long-term oncologic outcomes are being evaluated, initial short-term results indicate that a minimally invasive esophagectomy is at least equivalent to its open counterpart. MIE should be performed in centers with experience in advanced minimally invasive esophageal surgery. Certainly, further prospective studies are needed to confirm these results, such a large multicentered, randomized, controlled trial.

SUGGESTED READINGS

Bizekis C, Kent MS, Luketich JD, et al: Initial experience with minimally invasive Ivor Lewis esophagectomy, *Ann Thorac Surg* 82:402–407, 2006.

Luketich JD, Pennathur A, Awais O, et al: Outcomes after minimally invasive esophagectomy: review of over 1000 patients, *Ann Surg* 256(1):95–103, 2012.

Sihag S, Wright CD, Wain JC, et al: Comparison of perioperative outcomes following open versus minimally invasive Ivor Lewis oesophagectomy at a single, high-volume centre, *Eur J Cardiothorac Surg* 42(3):430–437, 2012.

Tapias LF, Morse CR: Minimally invasive Ivor Lewis esophagectomy after induction therapy yields similar early outcomes to surgery alone, *Innovations (Phila)* 6(5):331–336, 2011.

Tapias LF, Morse CR: A preliminary experience with minimally invasive Ivor Lewis esophagectomy, *Dis Esophagus* 25(5):449–455, 2012.

Laparoscopic Treatment of Esophageal Motility Disorders

Edward D. Auyang, MD, MS, and
Carlos A. Pellegrini, MD, FACS, FRCSI (Hon)

INTRODUCTION

Esophageal motility disorders are the result of disruption of the complex swallowing mechanism that simultaneously propels food boluses through the esophagus and prevents aspiration. The etiology of these disorders is not clearly understood, although the several proposed theories have included genetic, immunologic, and infectious mechanisms. These disorders usually manifest themselves in one of the two ends of the spectrum: hypercontractility in the form of "nutcracker" esophagus or diffuse esophageal spasm or hypocontractility, as with the complete aperistalsis of achalasia. Most of these disorders have no effective cure and are only treatable symptomatically with medications and endoscopic or surgical therapy. Achalasia is the most common esophageal motility disorder. Etiology is not known and cure is not possible, but surgery is extremely effective to resolve dysphagia, which is its main symptom. Patients present clinically with dysphagia and regurgitation. The gold standard for diagnosis is manometry, and the hallmark of the disease is the absence of peristalsis combined with impaired relaxation of the lower esophageal sphincter (LES). In 60% of patients, LES pressure is elevated. Barium esophagram, a useful study, typically has the pathognomonic appearance of a dilated esophagus with a distal esophageal "bird's beak" tapering. Upper gastrointestinal (GI) endoscopy further confirms the radiographic finding and is used to rule out other disease processes that may mimic achalasia, such as peptic strictures or neoplasms. In addition to achalasia, patients with esophageal dysmotility may present with the rare entity of epiphrenic diverticula.

These diverticula, found in the distal 10 cm of esophagus, are formed when weakness of the esophageal muscularis in the setting of esophageal dysmotility results in a functional obstruction. Symptoms and diagnostic evaluation are identical to those for achalasia.

In this chapter, the authors describe the technique for laparoscopic Heller myotomy for the treatment of achalasia, address the challenges of revisional surgery after previous surgical myotomy and treatment of end-stage achalasia, and describe the technique for the laparoscopic treatment of epiphrenic diverticula.

LAPAROSCOPIC HELLER MYOTOMY AND PARTIAL FUNDOPLICATION FOR ACHALASIA

Before elective surgery, patients who have a dilated esophagus as identified on preoperative studies are instructed to be on a liquid-only diet for 4 to 5 days in advance of the operation to help reduce the risk of aspiration of esophageal contents during induction of anesthesia. Preoperative subcutaneous heparin for deep vein thrombosis (DVT) prophylaxis and a first-generation cephalosporin for antibiotic prophylaxis are routinely administered before incision. The patient is positioned on the operating table on top of a bean bag. An upper-body warming device and bilateral lower extremity sequential compression devices (SCDs) are applied. A Foley catheter is placed given the anticipated duration of the operation. General anesthesia is induced, and the patient is placed in a low-lithotomy position. The bean bag is evacuated to form a "seat," thus preventing slipping when the patient is in reverse Trendelenburg's position. Both arms are tucked to allow for placement of a self-retaining retractor by the patient's right arm. The surgeon stands between the patient's legs, and the laparoscopic monitor is placed in the midline directly over the patient's upper chest for direct viewing.

Pneumoperitoneum is obtained with a Veress needle technique at the left subcostal margin. Preference, for safety reasons, is placement of the first trocar with direct vision with an 11-mm bladless optical trocar. A 10-mm trocar is placed at a left supraumbilical location approximately 1 hand width below and medial to the left subcostal port. A 10-mm left flank assistant port and a 5-mm right subcostal working port are then placed. Finally, a Nathanson's liver retractor is placed at a subxiphoid location without a port, or for patients with a large liver, a paddle liver retractor is placed through a right flank 11-mm port. The patient is then placed in steep reverse Trendelenburg's position (Figure 1).

A point approximately one third of the way distal to the gastroesophageal junction (GEJ) along the greater curve is chosen, and the short gastric vessels are divided proximally with an energy device. The hiatus is then dissected starting along the left crus and proceeds counter-clockwise anteriorly. The gastrohepatic ligament is then divided, and the right crus is dissected in a clockwise fashion to meet the left-sided dissection (Figure 2). The posterior window of the GEJ is opened so that a ½-inch Penrose drain can be placed around the GEJ to facilitate inferior retraction of the esophagus. This allows for a high mediastinal dissection to be performed to lengthen the esophagus and create the distance for an anterior esophagomyotomy 8 cm proximal to the GEJ. In addition, this window is used for creation of the Toupet fundoplication after the myotomy is completed (Figure 3).The anterior vagus nerve is identified and preserved during this dissection (Figure 4). The gastroesophageal fat pad is dissected away from the GEJ and resected to facilitate identification of the exact place in which the esophagus becomes stomach so that the distal extent of the myotomy on the anterior cardia of the stomach can be appropriately identified.

Once the anterior surface of the esophagus, GEJ, and cardia are free and the anterior vagus nerve is mobilized, the myotomy can be performed. A 52F lighted esophageal bougie is passed transorally by the anesthesiologist or the surgeon with the tip positioned in the

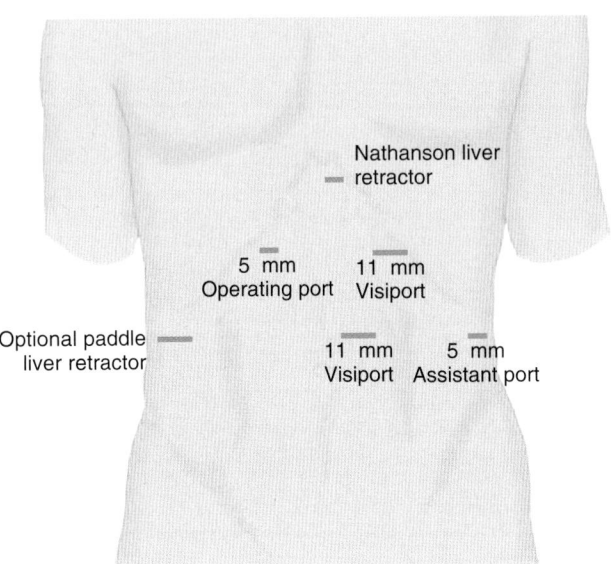

FIGURE 1   Port placement.

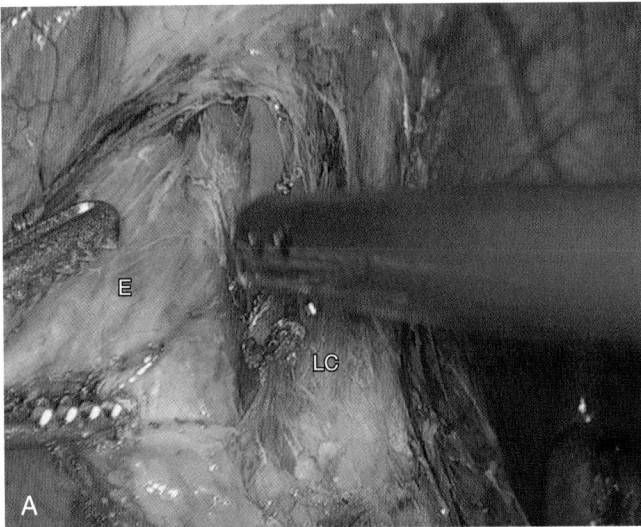

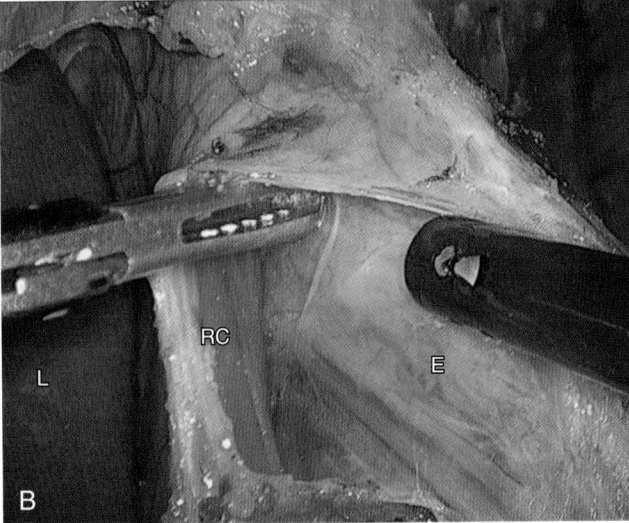

FIGURE 2   A, Left and **(B)** right crural dissection. *E,* Esophagus; *L,* liver; *LC,* left crus; *RC,* right crus.

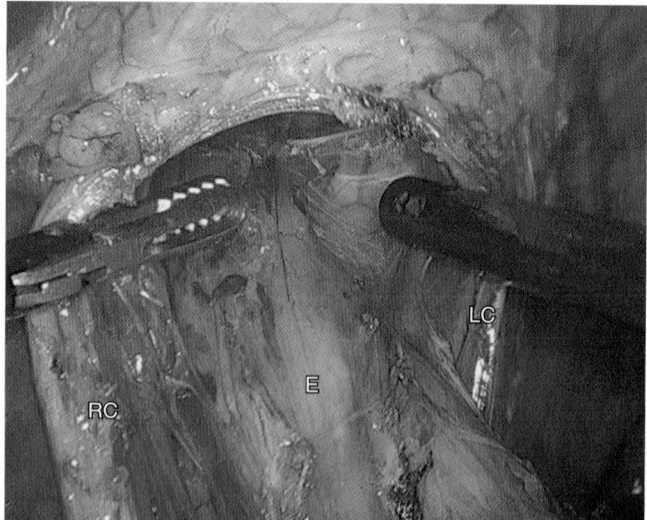

FIGURE 3   Mediastinal dissection. *E*, Esophagus; *LC*, left crus; *RC*, right crus.

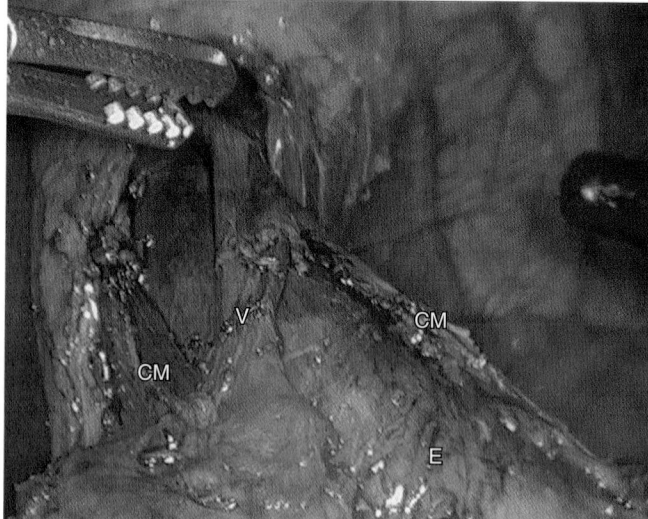

FIGURE 5   Complete myotomy. *CM*, Esophageal circular muscle; *E*, esophagus; *V*, vagus nerve.

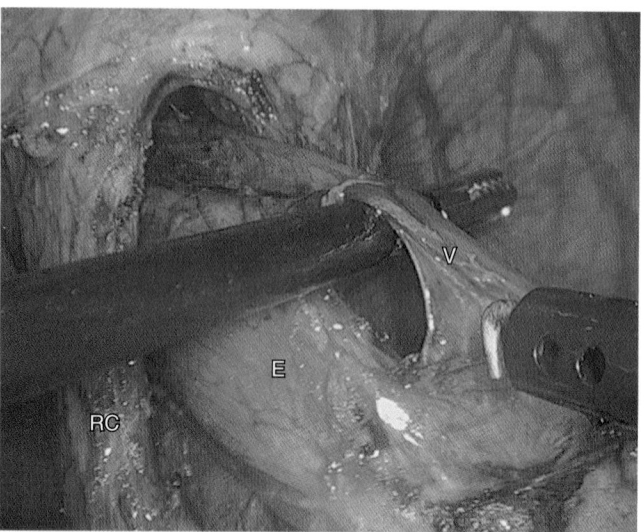

FIGURE 4   Identification of anterior vagus nerve during dissection. *E*, Esophagus; *RC*, right crus; *V*, vagus nerve.

body of the stomach. A clamp is placed through the left lateral assistant port to spread the anterior esophagus and stomach over the Bougie to provide tension on the muscle fibers, facilitating the division of the muscle. The myotomy is started distally on the cardia of the stomach from a distance at least 3 cm distal from the previously identified GEJ. This is absolutely critical to ensure a complete myotomy and adequate division of the fibers of the GEJ. The superficial muscle is carefully scored with an L-hook monopolar cautery, with extreme care taken not to cauterize too deeply and cause a mucosal perforation. The L hook is then used to divide the longitudinal and oblique muscle fibers of the stomach without the use of energy. This is the most difficult portion of the myotomy as the fibers cross in multiple directions and do not separate easily from the underlying mucosa. The dissection progresses proximally to the GEJ and further along the distal esophagus to a point at least 8 cm proximal to the GEJ. In the vicinity of the GEJ, the anterior vagus needs to be retracted from the right lateral position to the left lateral position to facilitate the proximal progression of the myotomy (under the vagus nerve). The esophageal longitudinal and circular muscle fibers are also divided without the use of energy because the

underlying mucosa is very thin. The lighted Bougie helps for identification of undivided esophageal circular muscle fibers as the myotomy is completed (Figure 5). If bleeding is encountered during the myotomy, it can usually be controlled with direct pressure. Electrocautery is not recommended on the mucosa because thermal injury is very likely. Perforations can occur during the creation of the myotomy and should not be regarded as a complication. If a perforation of the mucosa occurs, it is usually easily identified and can be repaired primarily with 4-0 absorbable interrupted stitches.

Once a myotomy of adequate length is completed (6 to 8 cm proximal to the GEJ on the esophagus and 3 cm onto cardia of stomach), the antireflux procedure is performed. A fundoplication is routinely performed because the incidence rate of reflux after Heller myotomy is more than 50%. A partial fundoplication is chosen over a complete fundoplication as to avoid persistent dysphagia. The authors' preference is for the Toupet partial posterior fundoplication because of the lower rate of postoperative dysphagia compared with an anterior Dor fundoplication. The first step in creation of the Toupet fundoplication is passage of the tip of the gastric fundus posterior to the GEJ and securing it to the right crus with 2-0 silk at two locations, anterior and posterior. Next, the fundic tip is sutured to the right edge of the myotomy with three 2-0 sutures. The proximal fundus is then sutured to the left edge of the myotomy with three 2-0 silk sutures and finally to the left crus. This configuration not only helps reduce reflux but also "tents" the myotomy apart, in theory reducing the chance of scarring and reformation of anterior muscular fibers (Figure 6). An anterior Dor fundoplication is used when one of the following two scenarios is encountered: (1) a mucosal perforation has occurred, and the fundoplication is used as a buttress for the mucosal repair; and (2) the Toupet fundoplication when fashioned creates too much bulk and posterior angulation of the GEJ. Experience reported by Duranceau's group at the University of Montreal with the use of the Nissen fundoplication has shown that although this operation is more effective in preventing reflux, a larger number of patients have recurrent dysphagia compared with a partial (posterior or anterior) fundoplication. On very rare occasion when a patient is older, has near end-stage achalasia, and has a severely dilated esophagus, a fundoplication is not performed at all for concern of causing dysphagia. The risk of reflux is accepted, and the patient is placed on life-long proton pump inhibitor therapy.

At the completion of the operation, an intraoperative upper endoscopy is performed to evaluate for adequate length of the myotomy and appropriate anatomic configuration of the fundoplication and to look for evidence of mucosal perforation. The abdomen

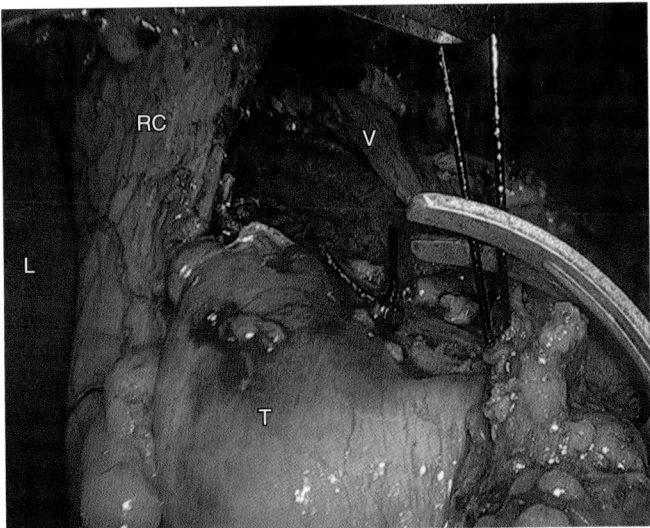

FIGURE 6 Toupet fundoplication. *L*, Liver; *RC*, right crus; *T*, Toupet fundoplication; *V*, vagus nerve.

is finally desufflated, and the incisions are closed with 4-0 dissolvable suture. After surgery, patients are started on a clear liquid diet the day of the operation and advanced to a soft diet the following day. Patients are typically discharged on the first postoperative day. For the subsequent 6 weeks, while inflammation and edema from the operation are resolving, patients are on a modified diet and instructed to specifically avoid eating breads, raw vegetables, and pieces of meat to avoid food impaction.

REVISIONAL SURGERY AFTER HELLER MYOTOMY

Treatment of recurrent or persistent dysphagia after previous Heller myotomy can be very challenging. The most important element is to define the anatomy and its relationship to the patient's recurring or returning symptoms (overwhelmingly dysphagia). A thorough evaluation is necessary to determine the etiology of dysphagia and whether it is amenable to surgical revision. The first step involves obtaining all possible records before the patient's initial myotomy, in particular finding confirmatory testing that the patient had an accurate diagnosis of achalasia to begin with. The patient's operative report is critical to determine whether an adequate length myotomy was performed initially and what type of, if any, fundoplication was performed. A thorough history from the patient can provide further information. Whether or not symptoms improved after initial myotomy and how soon they recurred can suggest whether the operation performed was initially effective. Specifically, whether a patient had moderate or substantial weight gain after an operation is a key determinant of prior surgical success.

After a thorough history and review of records, multiple tests are used to determine the cause of dysphagia. To use each test, the etiologies for dysphagia need to be recognized. The three most common etiologies for persistent or early dysphagia are: (1) inaccurate diagnosis of achalasia; (2) incomplete myotomy (or excessive scarring of a well-done myotomy); and (3) excessively tight fundoplication or crural closure. Recurrent or late dysphagia is most likely the result of late scarring and fibrosis at the site of previous myotomy, although peptic strictures, herniated fundoplication, and esophageal neoplasms also should be considered. On the basis of this understanding, the information that each test provides can be interpreted. Upper GI barium swallow provides anatomic and functional information about the esophagus. If there is a specific point of obstruction or if there is a problem with the fundoplication, such

as wrap herniation, this can be identified on the upper GI examination. Upper endoscopy can identify additional causes of dysphagia, such as esophagitis, esophageal diverticuli, strictures, and neoplasms. In the absence of anatomic causes for dysphagia, esophageal manometry is used to confirm the diagnosis of achalasia and for assessment of the LES. With a diagnosis of achalasia and persistent incomplete LES relaxation, a patient with these findings may be a candidate for a redo myotomy. Finally, 24-hour pH testing can assess whether the patient has quantitative acid reflux that may be responsible for dysphagia.

Initial treatments for patients with post-Heller dysphagia from incomplete myotomy or recurrent scarring may include endoscopic therapies such as pneumatic dilation. However, for patients who have a clearly identifiable stricture or area of narrowing and are fit for surgery, a redo myotomy, or a laparoscopic revision, may provide a benefit. The redo operation is approached laparoscopically with ports placed in an identical fashion to a laparoscopic Heller myotomy. If a fundoplication was previously performed, this is taken down and all adhesions are lysed to restore the original anatomy as best as possible. The myotomy is then made lateral to the original myotomy and extended at least 4 cm onto the gastric cardiac and as far proximally up the esophagus as is possible with a minimal distance of 6 to 8 cm. Extreme care must be taken for this dissection to avoid making a myotomy over the previous location and perforating the stomach or esophagus because the contour of the muscular fibers may be altered from fibrosis. After completion of this new myotomy, a Toupet fundoplication is typically performed that is constructed in a similar fashion as described previously. Criteria for choosing to perform a Dor fundoplication or no fundoplication are identical for the revisional operation as they are for a first-time operation.

Revisional surgery after previous Heller myotomy for achalasia is an operation that should only be undertaken by surgeons who have a large amount of experience with Heller myotomy and revisional foregut operations. Distortion of original anatomy from adhesions and scar can make a redo operation particularly challenging and can result in a higher complication rate when performed by the less experienced surgeon. Furthermore, an injury to the mucosa, most often a laceration during the dissection, may require an esophagectomy, and the surgeon should be prepared to do so. It is, therefore, important for the surgeon to understand the etiologies of recurrent or persistent dysphagia and recognize when a referral should be made to a more specialized center for a redo operation.

LAPAROSCOPIC TREATMENT OF END-STAGE ACHALASIA

Although laparoscopic Heller myotomy with partial fundoplication is a successful treatment for most patients diagnosed with achalasia, there is a subset of patients who have end-stage achalasia and a severely dilated and tortuous esophagus in which a myotomy will not improve symptoms. It is in this patient population that esophagectomy is considered. Critical decision-making points for offering an esophagectomy are focused around a patient's age, comorbidities, and ability to tolerate the operation. Unfortunately, end-stage achalasia is usually diagnosed in elderly, severely malnourished patients. These are also the patients who are less likely to tolerate an esophagectomy and in whom endoscopic therapies such as botulinum toxin or pneumatic dilation should be strongly considered (Figure 7).

LAPAROSCOPIC TREATMENT OF EPIPHRENIC DIVERTICULA

Surgical treatment of epiphrenic diverticula is composed of three components: resection of the diverticulum, esophagomyotomy, and fundoplication. Historically, this procedure has been performed with a thoracic approach, either with video-assisted thoracoscopic

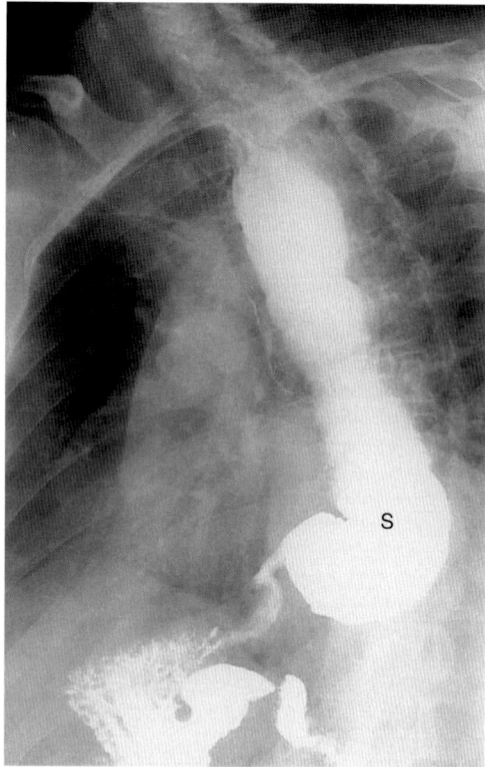

FIGURE 7 Sigmoid esophagus. *S,* Dilated, sigmoid esophagus.

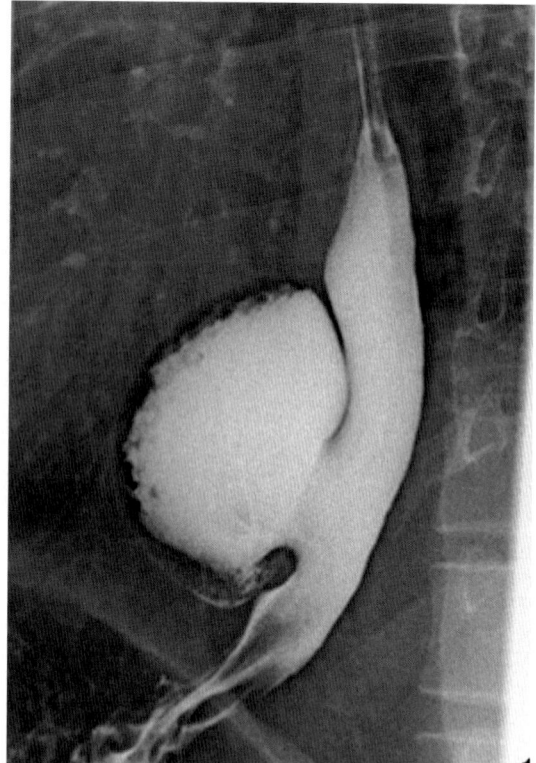

FIGURE 8 Epiphrenic diverticulum.

surgery (VATS) or open thoracotomy. In fact, many institutions still prefer the thoracic approach. With the development of laparoscopy, the transabdominal approach has been shown to provide good visualization and access to the distal esophagus. In addition, there may be less pain and morbidity compared with a thoracic approach (Figure 8).

The operative approach to the epiphrenic diverticulum is identical to the approach for laparoscopic Heller myotomy. Five ports are placed as described previously. The short gastric vessels are divided, the left and right crus are dissected free from the esophagus, and the esophageal attachments to the mediastinum are dissected as superiorly as possible. Any adhesions between the diverticulum and esophagus are also freed to show the neck of the diverticulum. The vagus nerve, which often is overlying the diverticulum, is protected and retracted. The diverticulum is then resected with an endoscopic linear stapler (3.5-mm staple width) over a 50F lighted bougie to prevent esophageal narrowing. The Heller myotomy and fundoplication are then performed with the technique described previously. The fundoplication may be a Dor or a Toupet. It usually does not reach the area of the diverticulum, and thus, the choice has to do with the myotomy, not with the diverticulectomy. With that in mind, the principles and rationale described previously for patients with achalasia are applied. An esophagram is obtained 2 days after the operation to evaluate for esophageal leak and narrowing. If the esophagram does not show any residual diverticulum or leak, the patient is started on a liquid diet and is discharged the following day on the modified diet described previously.

SUMMARY

Esophageal motility disorders are rare and complex diseases that can manifest themselves in a variety of clinical forms. Achalasia is a disorder in which aperistalsis leads to severe dysphagia, regurgitation,

and weight loss. Laparoscopic Heller myotomy with Toupet fundoplication is the preferred approach to patients who have achalasia. Revisional surgery for persistent or recurrent dysphagia is a feasible option in patients who have a clear surgically correctable problem but should be performed by experienced foregut surgeons. In addition, esophagectomy may provide an option for patients with severe end-stage achalasia who can tolerate the operation and in whom Heller myotomy will not provide a benefit. Epiphrenic diverticula are rarer entities that may be the result of esophageal dysmotility. A laparoscopic diverticulectomy in combination with Heller myotomy with Toupet fundoplication can provide a successful result and may have less pain or morbidity compared with thoracic and thoracoscopic approaches.

SUGGESTED READINGS

Oelschlager BK, Chang L, Pellegrini CA: Improved outcome after extended gastric myotomy for achalasia, *Arch Surg* 138(5):490–495, 2003.

Petersen RP, Pellegrini CA: Revisional surgery after Heller myotomy for esophageal achalasia, *Surg Laparosc Endosc Percutan Tech* 20:321–325, 2010.

Rawlings A, Soper NJ, Oelschlager BK, et al: Laparoscopic Dor versus Toupet fundoplication following Heller myotomy for achalasia: results of a multicenter, prospective, randomized-controlled trial, *Surg Endosc* 26(1):18–26, 2012.

Soares RV, Montenovo M, Pellegrini CA, et al: Laparoscopy as the initial approach for epiphrenic diverticula, *Surg Endosc* 25(12):3740–3746, 2011.

Woltman TA, Oelschlager BK, Pellegrini CA: Surgical management of esophageal motility disorders, *J Surg Res* 117:34–43, 2004.

Wright AS, Williams CW, Pellegrini CA, et al: Long-term outcomes confirm the superior efficacy of extended Heller myotomy with Toupet fundoplication for achalasia, *Surg Endosc* 21(5):713–718, 2007.

Zhu ZJ, Chen LQ, Duranceau A: Long-term result of total versus partial fundoplication after esophagomyotomy for primary esophageal motor disorders, *World J Surg* 32(3):401–407, 2008.

Laparoscopic Adrenalectomy

Lee L. Swanstrom, MD, FACS

INTRODUCTION

Since laparoscopic access to the adrenal gland was first introduced in the early 1990s by Gagner, Park, and others, it has become the standard approach for almost all indications. This includes both benign and malignant indications, with the sole exceptions being more advanced cancers and when it is part of a secondary resection such as a radical nephrectomy. The techniques of laparoscopic adrenalectomy have mostly reproduced the approaches of open approaches with some important exceptions: the first being the lateral decubitus approach, which is now the standard technique. Other variations have paralleled the evolutions of laparoscopic surgery in general: single port approaches, mini-laparoscopy, and robot-assisted laparoscopy. Finally, there have been some animal studies of flexible endoscopic adrenalectomy by natural orifice transluminal endoscopic surgery (NOTES) approaches.

INDICATIONS

Indications for adrenalectomy can be either benign or malignant. By far the most common indications for adrenalectomy are benign endocrine tumors or lesions suspected of being endocrine tumors. Endocrinologically active tumors can secrete cortical steroids (cortisol, adrenal androgens, and aldosterone) or medullary hormones (epinephrine or norepinephrine) and therefore be detected by various hormone-related systemic symptoms. They can also be nonsecreting and picked up as incidental findings on computed tomographic (CT) scans or magnetic resonance imaging (MRI)—hence the term *incidentalomas*. In general, any patient documented to have an adrenal lesion and symptoms related to hormone secretion—and even those who have an asymptomatic lesion but elevated adrenal hormones—should have an adrenalectomy. Particularly problematic are symptomatic patients with elevated hormones and no lesion seen on imaging studies. For these patients, more sophisticated methods such as radionuclide scans or radiologically performed direct venous sampling may be helpful to localize the tumor. Finally, one or both normal glands may be removed in patients with medically uncontrollable Cushing's syndrome caused by pituitary tumors.

Primary adrenal malignancies are relatively rare. They include the malignant transformation of the usual endocrine tumors as well as some others, such as adrenal cortical cancer, lymphomas, leiomyosarcomas, pheochromocytomas, and metastatic cancers. Early and incidentally discovered cancers are treated effectively by laparoscopic approaches, but more advanced tumors requiring nodal field or adjacent organ resection are most commonly approached through open surgery or at least undergo a high conversion rate. Finally, the adrenal is a not infrequent site of metastases from a variety of tumor types (lung and ovarian being perhaps the most common). Indications for laparoscopic adrenalectomy are summarized in Table 1.

TECHNIQUES

Patient preparation is generally as it would be for any patient undergoing laparoscopic surgery: preoperative single shot of a first-generation cephalosporin, antithrombosis measures (aggressive ones in the case of adrenal malignancy), as well as addressing electrolyte imbalance frequently seen in hormonally active tumors. The exception is active pheochromocytomas, where surgical manipulation of the tumor can lead to wild swings of blood pressure, although less so with laparoscopic resection. It is recommended that these patients have 3 weeks of preoperative beta and alpha blockade managed by an endocrinologist.

Patient Position

Patients undergoing an adrenalectomy will be placed in one of three basic positions: anterior (supine), lateral (lateral decubitus), or prone. Anterior is seldom used unless an additional procedure is indicated, as retraction and exposure of this most deeply placed organ is difficult and requires additional ports. A suspected cancer might be one such indication, as wide nodal resection is indicated as well as an abdominal exploration. Either the lateral or the posterior approach can be used routinely, although a relative indication for the posterior approach is the need for bilateral adrenalectomy, and a relative contraindication for the posterior approach is a large tumor.

Lateral Approach

The lateral approach works because the position allows the multitude of organs overlying the adrenal gland to fall away. A beanbag support should be placed on the table and the patient positioned with the umbilicus over the break in the table. After anesthesia, the patient is rolled to almost a full lateral decubitus position (lesion facing up) with an axillary roll for nerve protection and the arms appropriately positioned. The table is "broken" enough that the flank is even with the iliac crest and the lower rib margin. The beanbag is deflated and the patient taped well to the operating table and checked carefully for pressure points (Figure 1). After draping, the table is rolled dorsally, and initial access is obtained by either the Veress or the Hasson technique. The initial port is placed in the lateral rectus margin 10 cm below the costal margin. Two or three additional ports (2.5-5 mm) are placed along the costal margin, as illustrated in Figure 2. The surgeon and assistant stand on the same side of the table facing the patient's belly.

On the left, the native attachments of the colon splenic flexure are taken down if needed to place the posterior-most port. Because the adrenal gland lies behind the spleen, the lateral splenic peritoneal attachments are divided to let the spleen roll forward by gravity. The upper margin of the left kidney is identified by palpation and a small window in Gerota's fascia. Alternatively, particularly in very obese patients, laparoscopic ultrasound can identify the key landmarks of the superior kidney and left renal vessels, which is the angle that contains the left adrenal gland. In most cases, the lateral and inferior margin of the gland is first identified. This is done by carefully dividing the retroperitoneal fat to visually identify the unique greenish/yellow color of the adrenal (Figure 3). Dissection is performed using an energy device like an ultrasonic scissor and a "no touch" technique in which the surgeon concentrates on retracting the adrenal gland without grasping it directly but rather grasping peri-adrenal fat or simply pushing it or levering it with a grasper or suction. The gland is progressively dissected free, heading toward the deepest portion, which lies next to the renal vasculature. It should be noted that every millimeter of the dissection should be done with hemostatic instruments. This is because small vessels enter the gland in unpredictable patterns and energy prevents blood staining the tissues, which can make identification of the tissue planes difficult. The adrenal vein on the left is usually the last attachment to be divided, and division is usually safely done with bipolar or harmonic energy.

TABLE 1: Current indications for surgical intervention in adrenal pathology

Indication	Benign	Malignant
Incidentaloma	Growing	>5 cm
Aldosteronoma	Symptomatic	Evidence of invasion
Cortisolinoma	Hypertension	Adjacent invasion, large size
Pheochromocytoma	Blood pressure problems	Invasion or metastasis on imaging
Adrenal metastasis	Lesions on imaging	Associated lung, kidney, ovarian, and other lesions

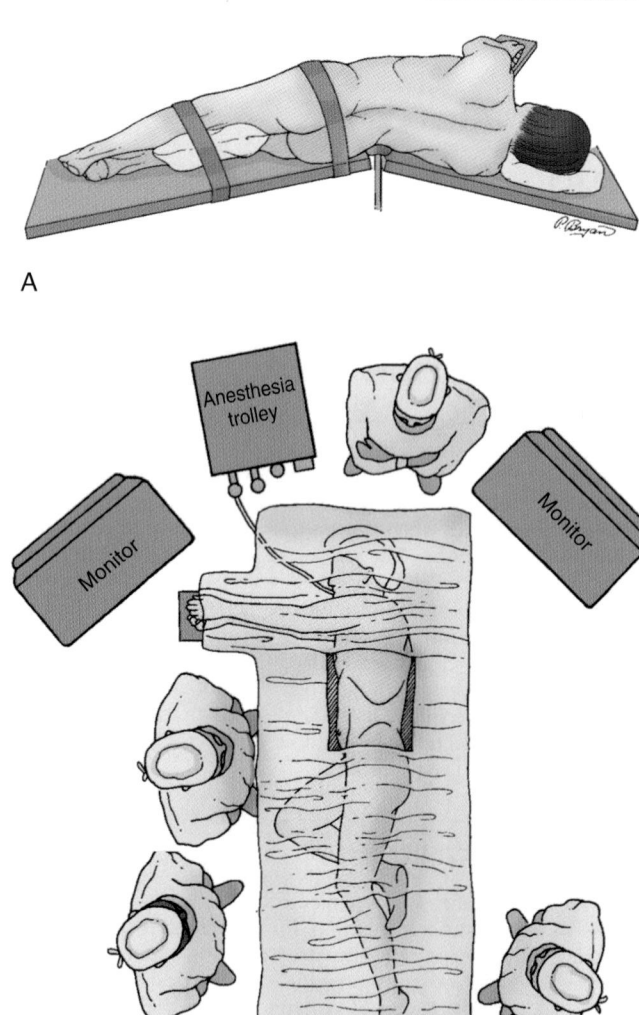

FIGURE 1   **A,** Patient positioning for lateral approach to left laparoscopic adrenalectomy (kidney rest and table break are positioned at the iliac crest). **B,** Operating room setup and patient positioning for laparoscopic adrenalectomy. *(Modified from Smith CD, Weber CJ, Amerson JR: Laparoscopic adrenalectomy: new gold standard, World J Surg 23:389-396, 1999.)*

The resected gland is placed in an impervious specimen bag and retrieved by slightly increasing the largest port site. After carefully inspecting the resection bed for hemostasis, this widened port site is closed with a suture passer and full-thickness absorbable sutures.

For the right adrenal gland, port placement is the same. The triangular ligament of the right liver lobe is completely divided to free the bare area and let the right lobe roll forward. There is typically little fat in the retroperitoneum of the right side, due to the compression of the liver. The adrenal, in fact, is often visible through the peritoneum. The peritoneum is opened vertically over the gland and once again with a "no touch" technique and energy the whole way. Dissection progresses from lateral to medial until the lateral margin of the vena cava is visualized. Precise and gentle dissection is performed to separate the medial gland from the vena cava until the right adrenal vein is well visualized. It should be controlled by clips, at least on the vena cava side, before being divided. Once again, the gland is placed in a bag and the bag withdrawn to the incision to allow the gland to be extracted.

Posterior Approach

For the posterior approach, the patient is positioned in the prone position. An orthopedic spine bed is best, but a standard bed is possible with specialized pads and bolsters. Before prepping and draping the bed or table, all possible points of pressure to the patient are addressed (Figure 4).

As the "landscape" for posterior port placement is quite limited, being confined in the angle between the posterior costal margin and the lateral edge of the paraspinous muscle, it is critical that small ports be used and placed very precisely (Figure 5). There is typically only room for three ports on each side, but if well placed, this is all that is needed, as there are no adjacent organs to retract with this approach. External ultrasound can be used to map out the position of the kidney and adrenal gland and mark the position on the skin. This allows for the most accurate placement of two 5-mm ports. The central port is 10 mm. Either an "optically directed" port or a direct cutdown technique is used to access the retroperitoneal space. A hernia-dissecting balloon is inflated to create the retroperitoneal space. Relatively high pressure carbon dioxide (CO_2) is used for insufflations (15-16 mm Hg). Often the adrenal gland can be seen at the base of this dissection (Figure 6). The additional 3-mm or 5-mm ports are placed under vision. Dissection of the gland is performed as previously described, using a "no touch" technique as much as possible and a sealing energy technology. As the dissection starts on the posterior aspect of the gland, it is not unusual for the main vascular supply to be encountered early in the dissection, requiring its control with energy or clips, depending on its size. Care must be

taken to avoid injury to the peritoneum, as this can result in the collapse of the retroperitoneal space and loss of exposure. The specimen is bagged and removed through a widened port site. The port site fascia is usually not closed.

COMPLICATIONS

Laparoscopic adrenalectomy is not a particularly risky surgery; mortality due to the surgery is essentially unknown, although certain disease states, such as adrenal cortical cancer and Cushing's syndrome, have high associated morbidity and mortality rates. Intraoperative morbidity is primarily related to organ injury during surgery, for example, injury to proximal organs (spleen, liver, colon, etc.). Although this happens less than 5% of the time, it often occasions

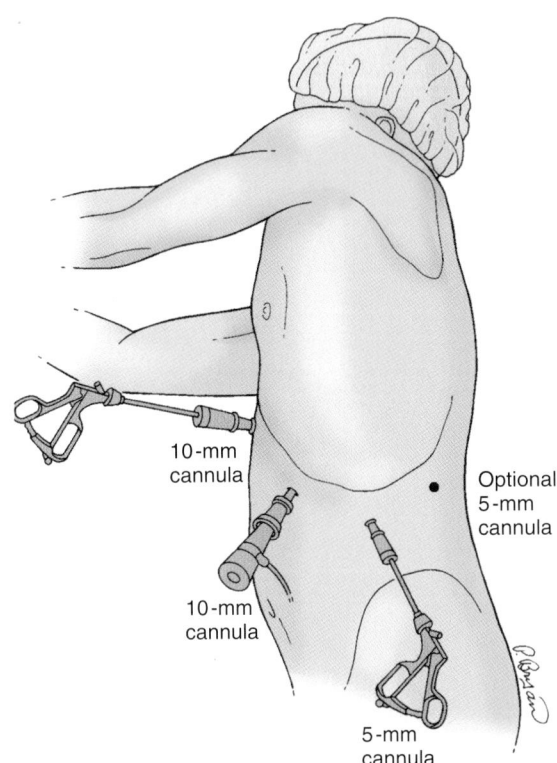

FIGURE 2 Trocar placement and instrument placement for left laparoscopic adrenalectomy. *(Modified from Smith CD, Weber CJ, Amerson JR: Laparoscopic adrenalectomy: new gold standard,* World J Surg *23:389-396, 1999.)*

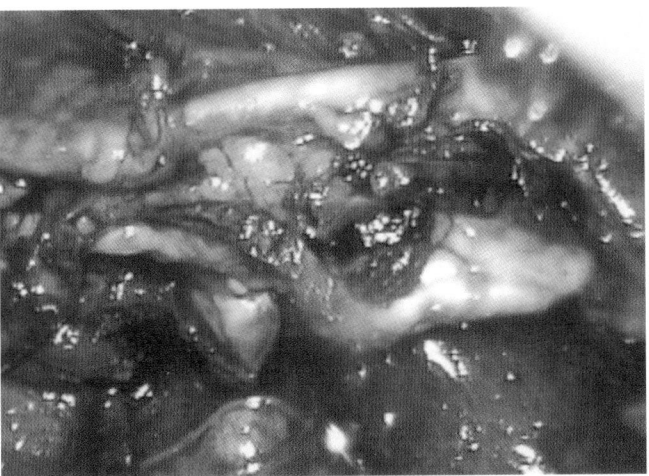

FIGURE 3 Division of the retroperitoneal fat reveals the distinctive green/yellow color of the adrenal gland.

conversion to open surgery. Injury or disruption of the gland may not be strictly a "complication," but it represents a technical error that may compromise patient treatment and therefore should be avoided. The major dramatic complication associated with laparoscopic adrenalectomy is the same as for open adrenals, that is, bleeding. This can be intraoperative bleeding due to adjacent organ injury (spleen, liver), an escaped blood vessel (arterial or venous), or, most dramatically, an injury to one of the major vessels that lie close to the adrenal gland. It can also be delayed bleeding happening typically hours to days following the procedure and primarily due to the vascular nature of the paraadrenal environment.

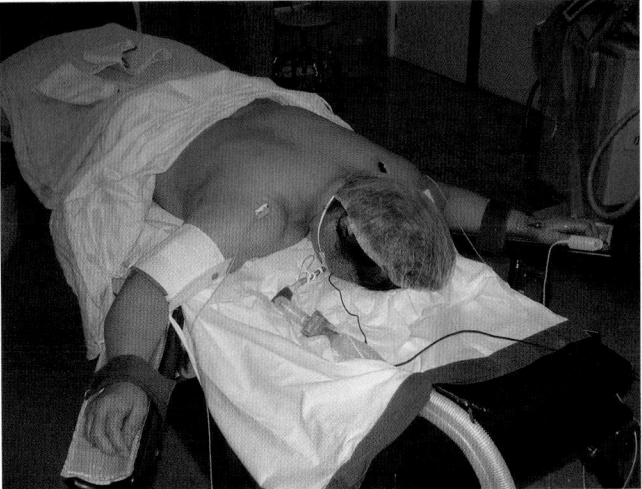

FIGURE 4 The posterior approach requires the patient to be placed in the prone position.

The dreaded complication of an injury to a major vascular structure during dissection justifies its concern, as conversion to control is difficult to impossible depending on the patient position (lateral decubitus vs posterior). Fortunately, structures most at risk are the vena cava or renal vein, and positive pressure CO_2 insufflation tamponades the bleeding and can permit a careful clip application or suture repair if the surgeon does not panic and lose control of the situation.

Other complications might include wound problems or hernias but more commonly would be associated with underlying endocrine disorders associated with the primary disease states, such as electrolyte disturbance or endocrine insufficiency. These potentialities may be a good opportunity for surgeons to establish a close working relationship with endocrinology specialists.

POSTOPERATIVE CARE

Patients can be expected to have a moderate amount of pain following laparoscopic adrenalectomy. Typically they would stay in the hospital for approximately 24 hours with at least a hematocrit/hemoglobin check before discharge. Patients with more complex problems such as extreme hypertension, profound electrolyte problems, or need for replacement steroid therapy, may need longer hospital stays as well as more frequent blood work. For most patients, no physical restrictions are placed, and most return to full work activities in 2 weeks.

OUTCOMES

Laparoscopic approaches to adrenal pathologies are highly successful. Conversion to an open procedure is needed less than 5% of the time for benign disease and 20% for malignancies. Otherwise, success rates for disease cure or palliation closely mimic results from open surgery with documented advantages of less pain, shorter hospital stays, and a quicker return to normal activity.

THE FUTURE: EVEN LESS INVASIVE SURGERY

There is movement afoot to further reduce the physiologic impact of laparoscopic surgery. Single-incision surgery (e.g., single-incision laparoscopic surgery [SILS], laparoendoscopic single-site surgery

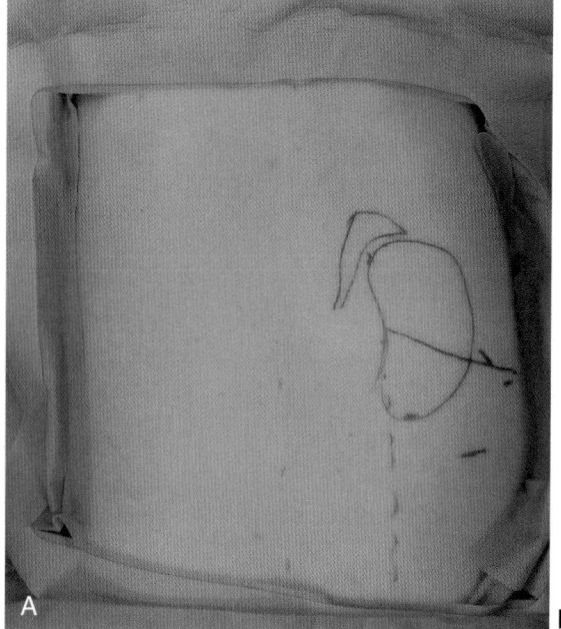
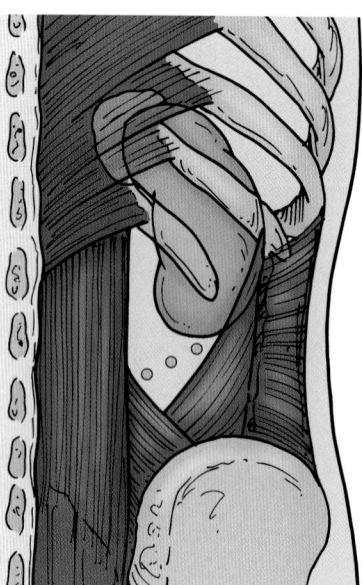

FIGURE 5 Posterior port placement has to be done carefully as there is limited space for placement.

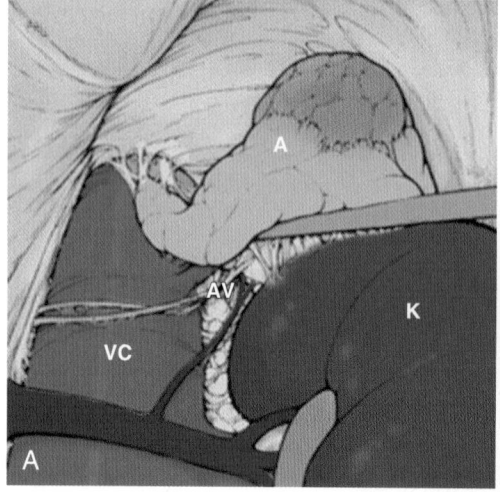
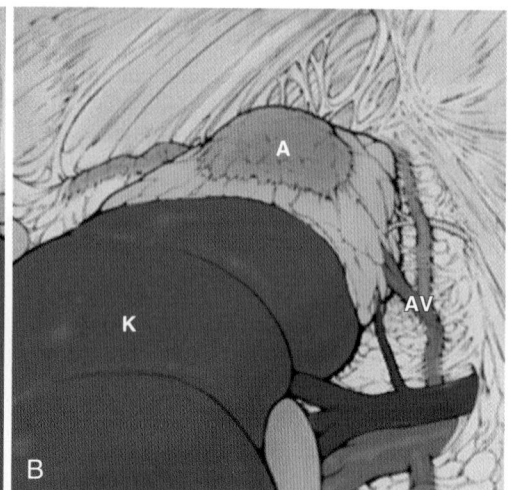

FIGURE 6 Posterior retroperitoneal endoscopic adrenalectomy. **A,** Right. **B,** Left. A, Adrenal; AV, adrenal vein; K, kidney; VC, vena cava. (Modified from Walz MK: Minimally invasive adrenal gland surgery [in German], Chirurg 69:613-620, 1998.)

[LESS], trans umbilical surgery [TUS]), mini-laparoscopy, and NOTES are being explored in hopes of improving cosmesis, decreasing postoperative pain, and speeding recovery. These less invasive approaches are either just in the process of being adopted (SILS) or are in the exploratory stage, and there are no definitive outcomes data to define their exact place in adrenal surgery.

Single-incision Laparoscopic Surgery Approach

Accessing the adrenal laparoscopically through a single incision (the SILS approach) has the best comparative outcomes data to support its use. Several prospective studies have been published showing feasibility and some patient advantages: decreased pain and better cosmetics primarily. Single-incision adrenalectomy is performed either with a specially designed multiple-port device, placed through a 1.5-cm to 2.5-cm incision, or by making a single skin incision and placing several small laparoscopic ports through the fascia (Figure 7). Drawbacks of such an approach include the ergonomic difficulties of multiple parallel instruments and the laparoscope, which make

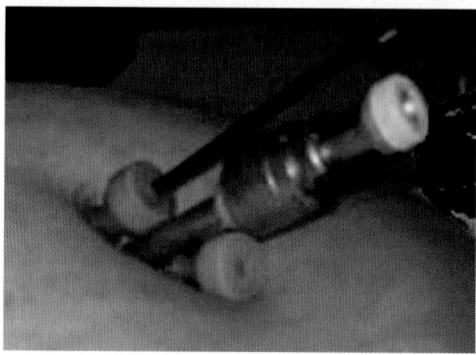

FIGURE 7 One technique of single-port surgery involves a single 2.5-cm skin incision with three 5-mm ports placed through the fascia. The fascial incisions can be connected at the end of the case to remove the specimen.

such approaches more technically demanding, and theoretic concerns about increased wound problems. Still, most would recognize that adrenalectomy is almost the perfect procedure for this approach, as it involves a small organ, in a tight space, with a limited number of instruments needed, and requiring no suturing.

Mini-Laparoscopy

Laparoscopy using 2-mm to 3-mm instruments, so-called mini-laparoscopy, is enjoying somewhat of a renaissance as surgeons and patients aim to further reduce the morbidity rate of standard laparoscopy. It has also been facilitated by the availability of new alloys and materials that make very rigid, small instruments possible. Adrenalectomy certainly makes sense for this approach, as the adrenal gland is a small lightweight organ and is usually located in a tight constrained space. Perhaps because it is so close to the, now standard, 5-mm port approach, there has been little in the literature documenting benefits or problems with mini-lap adrenalectomy.

Robot-Assisted Laparoscopic Adrenalectomy

As with all laparoscopic surgery, robots have invaded the field. There are several reports describing the use of the da Vinci telemanipulator (Intuitive Surgical, Sunnyvale, Calif) to perform adrenalectomy. Users report great benefits in surgeon ergonomics but no documented clinical outcomes benefit to the patient. Also, the use of the da Vinci is expensive, takes longer, and requires the use of larger ports than standard laparoscopy. It would seem that, until a surgeon/computer interface is fully realized (e.g., image registration for the localization of the gland and its vasculature), the "robot," as it currently exists, is little else than a marketing deception.

NOTES Adrenalectomy

NOTES is perhaps the ultimate expression of minimally invasive surgery. This postulates the fusion of the low-impact nature of even fairly aggressive endoscopic interventions, such as endoscopic retrograde cholangiopancreatography (ERCP), pancreatic pseudocyst drainage, and endoscopic submucosal dissection (ESD), which typically resulted in patients being pain free and back to work in a day or two, with true surgical procedures such as adrenalectomy. Although laparoscopic adrenalectomy is a true advance over open surgery in terms of patient impact, it still entails an operating room, a hospital stay, weeks off work, scars, and pain. The possibility of doing this as an outpatient procedure under sedation, with full activity the next day (as after polypectomy or ERCP), has been the driving force behind the push for an endoscopic surgical approach. Because of its small size, extraabdominal location, and distinctive anatomy, the adrenal gland was an early target of the NOTES investigations. Initial animal and cadaver studies documented its accessibility either transvaginally or transrectally using flexible retroperitoneoscopy. Whether these approaches are the future of treatment of adrenal disease is conjectural, but it does open the door to thinking beyond the traditional surgical approaches to the gland and its diseases.

SELECTED READINGS

Liao CH, Chueh SC, Wu KD, et al: Laparoscopic partial adrenalectomy for aldosterone-producing adenomas with needlescopic instruments, *Urology* 68(3):663–667, 2006.

Nigri G, Rosman AS, Petrucciani N, et al: Meta-analysis of trials comparing laparoscopic transperitoneal and retroperitoneal adrenalectomy, *Surgery* 153(1):111–119, 2013.

Pineda-Solís K, Medina-Franco H, Heslin MJ: Robotic versus laparoscopic adrenalectomy: a comparative study in a high-volume center, *Surg Endosc* 2012 [Epub ahead of print].

Sroka G, Slijper N, Shteinberg D, et al: Laparoscopic adrenalectomy for malignant lesions: surgical principles to improve oncologic outcomes, *Surg Endosc* 2013 [Epub ahead of print].

Walz MK, Groeben H, Alesina PF: Single-access retroperitoneoscopic adrenalectomy (SARA) versus conventional retroperitoneoscopic adrenalectomy (CORA): a case-control study, *World J Surg* 34(6):1386–1390, 2010.

Zou X, Zhang G, Xiao R, et al: Transvaginal natural orifice transluminal endoscopic surgery (NOTES)-assisted laparoscopic adrenalectomy: first clinical experience, *Surg Endosc* 25(12):3767–3772, 2011.

MINIMALLY INVASIVE PARATHYROIDECTOMY

Tracy S. Wang, MD, MPH, and
Julie Ann Sosa, MD, MA, FACS

Primary hyperparathyroidism (pHPT) is defined as the presence of elevated serum calcium levels in the setting of elevated or inappropriately high normal serum parathyroid hormone (PTH) levels. Recent studies have shown that a small subset of patients with normal serum and ionized calcium levels but elevated PTH levels may also have the disease, termed normocalcemic pHPT. Overt manifestations of pHPT include nephrolithiasis, pancreatitis, peptic ulcer disease, pathologic bone fractures, and neuropsychiatric disorders; more subtle symptoms, such as fatigue, weakness, forgetfulness, depression, and bone and joint pain, are subjective and more difficult to attribute solely to parathyroid disease. The overwhelming majority of patients today presents with asymptomatic disease that is identified serendipitously on the basis of automated serum screening.

Surgery remains the sole curative treatment for pHPT and is recommended for all patients with symptomatic disease and for patients with asymptomatic disease who meet current consensus guidelines for parathyroidectomy. These guidelines include age less than 50 years, serum calcium 1.0 mg/dL or more above the upper limit of normal, osteoporosis (T score, ≤−2.5), history of a pathologic bone fracture, and reduced renal function (glomerular filtration rate [GFR], <60). However, given recent evidence that shows improved neurocognitive performance and quality of life in patients after curative parathyroidectomy, the authors believe that parathyroidectomy by experienced parathyroid surgeons should be considered as a treatment option for all patients with pHPT who are amenable to surgical consultation and who are deemed to be reasonable surgical candidates.

The most common etiology of pHPT is a single parathyroid adenoma (80% to 85%); other causes are multigland hyperplasia, including double adenomas (10% to 15%), and rarely, parathyroid cancer (<1%). Given that most cases result from a single abnormal parathyroid, the development of improved imaging techniques for preoperative localization and the introduction of intraoperative parathyroid hormone (IOPTH) monitoring have allowed minimally invasive parathyroidectomy (MIP) to become the new gold standard for patients undergoing parathyroidectomy for sporadic pHPT, with equivalent cure rates and lower complication rates (recurrent laryngeal nerve injury and hypoparathyroidism) than with conventional bilateral neck exploration. Another benefit of a focused approach is the ability to perform parathyroidectomy with local anesthesia with an ipsilateral cervical block and sedation in the ambulatory setting.

Considerable debate exists, however, regarding the definition of a minimally invasive parathyroidectomy, with respect to extent of surgical exploration, length of incision, and use of intraoperative adjuncts, such as IOPTH monitoring. The authors believe that the appropriate definition of a minimally invasive parathyroidectomy is a focused, uniglandular exploration based on accurate preoperative localization, with use of IOPTH measurements as a guide for determination of intraoperative biochemical cure and with use of the radio-guided gamma probe or ex vivo parathyroid aspiration as intraoperative confirmation of the culprit lesion.

PREOPERATIVE PARATHYROID LOCALIZATION

Minimally invasive parathyroidectomy is dependent on accurate preoperative localization; failure of preoperative localization may necessitate conversion to bilateral exploration with attendant increases in operative time, increased hospital stay, and risk of complications. Common imaging studies include cervical ultrasound scan, technetium Tc 99m sestamibi with single-photon emission computed tomography (SPECT), and four-dimensional computed tomographic (4D-CT) scan. The preoperative imaging algorithm is highly surgeon and institution dependent, although patient characteristics such as renal function, contrast allergies, and body habitus also must be taken into consideration.

Cervical ultrasound scan is inexpensive and noninvasive and provides detailed anatomic information regarding both thyroid and parathyroid pathology (Figure 1). The sensitivity of ultrasound scan in detection of abnormal parathyroid glands ranges from 48% to 93%, with a recent meta-analysis finding a pooled sensitivity of 76% and a positive predictive value (PPV) of 93%, whether performed by surgeons or radiologists. Ultrasound scan has the advantage of being able to detect any thyroid pathology that may require further

evaluation with fine-needle aspiration biopsy before surgery. Ultrasound scan is limited by the inability to accurately identify ectopic parathyroid adenomas in the mediastinum and retroesophageal locations.

Sestamibi scans use the metabolic activity of hyperfunctional parathyroid glands to identify abnormal parathyroid tissue, and the addition of SPECT provides three-dimensional information, rather than a planar view alone (Figure 2). Pooled sensitivity of sestamibi-SPECT is 79%, with a PPV of 91%; factors that influence accuracy of sestamibi-SPECT include the severity of pHPT, serum calcium, PTH, 25-OH vitamin D levels, and oxyphil cell content in the parathyroid adenoma. Adenoma location, size, and presence of multiglandular disease or thyroid nodules further limit the sensitivity of both sestamibi-SPECT and ultrasound scan.

Because of the limitations of both ultrasound scan and sestamibi-SPECT, 4D-CT scan has emerged as an additional modality for preoperative imaging; it uses the three-dimensional aspect of CT scans with the added dimension of changes in perfusion of intravenous contrast over time. Visualization of differences in perfusion (rapid uptake and washout) allow for identification of hyperfunctional parathyroid glands (Figure 3). The sensitivity and PPV of 4D-CT scan in detection of abnormal parathyroid tissue are 89% and 94%, respectively, but decrease to 72% and 75% when performed in patients with previously negative or inconclusive ultrasound scan and sestamibi-SPECT. Limitations of 4D-CT scan include the use of intravenous contrast and exposure to ionizing radiation.

The diagnosis of pHPT is not influenced by the results of imaging because the diagnosis is biochemical. However, imaging studies are crucial because accurate preoperative localization allows surgeons to maximize opportunities for a minimally invasive approach. A recent cost analysis suggests that the combination of ultrasound scan, sestamibi-SPECT, and if necessary, 4D-CT scan was the most cost-effective approach to preoperative imaging, followed by a combination of ultrasound scan and 4D-CT scan. The use of sestamibi-SPECT alone and bilateral exploration with no preoperative imaging were the least cost-effective modalities. The cost effectiveness is dependent on the accuracy of each study, which is highly dependent on institutional idiosyncrasies in technique and interpretation. Therefore, surgeons must know their institutional data to determine the optimal algorithm for preoperative imaging.

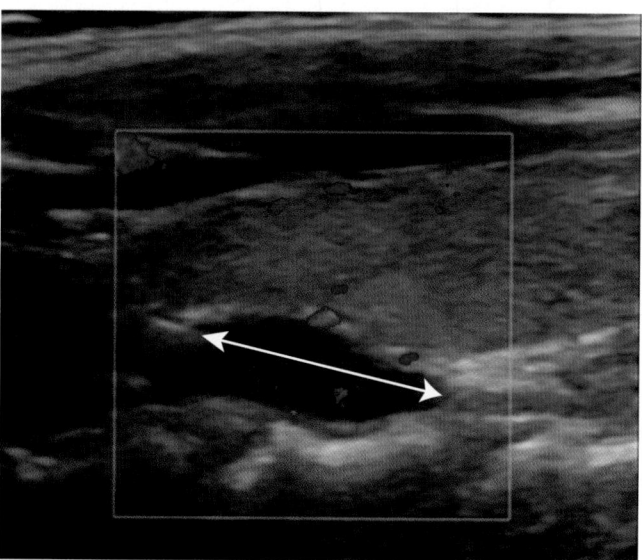

FIGURE 1   Ultrasound scan, depicting parathyroid adenoma.

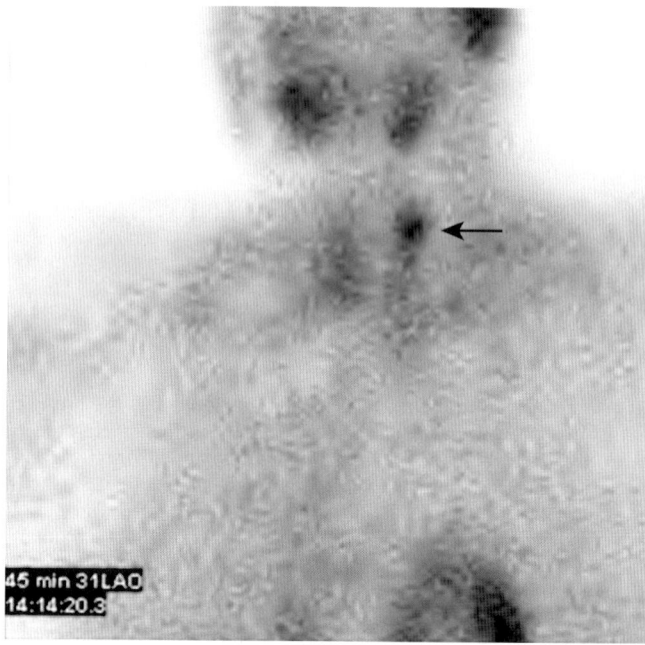

FIGURE 2   Sestamibi scan, depicting left-sided parathyroid adenoma.

Given all of the previous considerations, the authors favor the use of cervical ultrasound scan and sestamibi-SPECT in all patients with pHPT before parathyroidectomy. If these imaging study results are negative or discordant, 4D-CT scan is then used. For patients undergoing reoperative parathyroidectomy for persistent or recurrent pHPT, concordant preoperative localization studies are crucial to facilitating minimally invasive parathyroidectomy, and consideration should be given to obtaining a 4D-CT a priori. Additional invasive localization techniques may include ultrasound scan with aspiration and PTH sampling of nodules presumed to be abnormal parathyroid tissue or arteriography with venous sampling. Any patient with thyroid nodules that meet criteria for fine-needle aspiration (FNA) based on size or appearance should undergo further evaluation so that concomitant thyroidectomy can be performed, if necessary (Figure 4).

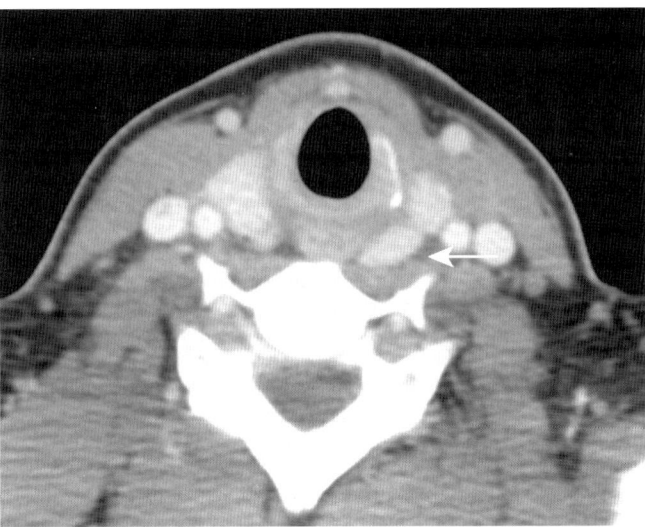

FIGURE 3 Four-dimensional computed tomographic scan, depicting left-sided parathyroid adenoma.

INTRAOPERATIVE ADJUNCTS

A major advance in the surgical management of pHPT was the development of a rapid immunoassay, predicated on the short half-life of PTH (approximately 3 to 5 minutes), that allowed for intraoperative PTH testing. IOPTH monitoring is a crucial adjunct for parathyroid surgery, and minimally invasive parathyroidectomy should not be performed without it. In brief, PTH levels are obtained before incision (baseline), at the time of excision of the parathyroid gland (time zero, when a spike in the PTH level can occur as a result of manipulation of the culprit gland during resection), and at 5-minute to 10-minute intervals after excision until the PTH level has fallen by an appropriate decrement. PTH levels can be obtained from either a peripheral intravenous catheter (preferred) or an arterial line.

Several valid criteria are used for interpretation of IOPTH testing. The Miami criterion consists of a drop of 50% or more from the baseline or time-zero level, whichever is higher, 10 minutes after removal of all abnormal glands; with this criterion, the reported cure rate (eucalcemia and normal PTH levels at 6 months after surgery) is 97%. The authors favor a more stringent criterion, which requires a decrease of 50% or more from the baseline or time-zero level, whichever is higher, *and* a decrease into normal range 10 minutes after removal of all abnormal glands. Failure to meet criteria, whichever is used, mandates further operative exploration and is highly suggestive of the presence of multigland disease. Overall success rates for parathyroidectomy are equivalent (95% to 98%), irrespective of the criterion used.

Radio-guided parathyroidectomy with the handheld gamma probe is a less frequently used intraoperative adjunct. The principle behind use of the gamma probe is that hyperfunctional parathyroid tissue retains technetium 99m sestamibi longer than surrounding tissues; therefore, a handheld gamma probe is used to localize the abnormal parathyroid gland during surgery. The patient receives an injection of sestamibi approximately 1 hour before surgery. In the operating room, a background count is determined with scanning of normal thyroid tissue; after incision, the gamma probe is used to scan for in vivo counts that are higher than background. After identification and resection of the parathyroid gland, an ex vivo count of the resected gland is obtained; parathyroid tissue is confirmed if the ex

FIGURE 4 Parathyroid imaging algorithm. *4DCT,* Four-dimensional computed tomographic scan; *FNA,* fine-needle aspiration; *MIP,* minimally invasive parathyroidectomy; *pHPT,* primary hyperparathyroidism; *SPECT,* single-photon emission computed tomography.

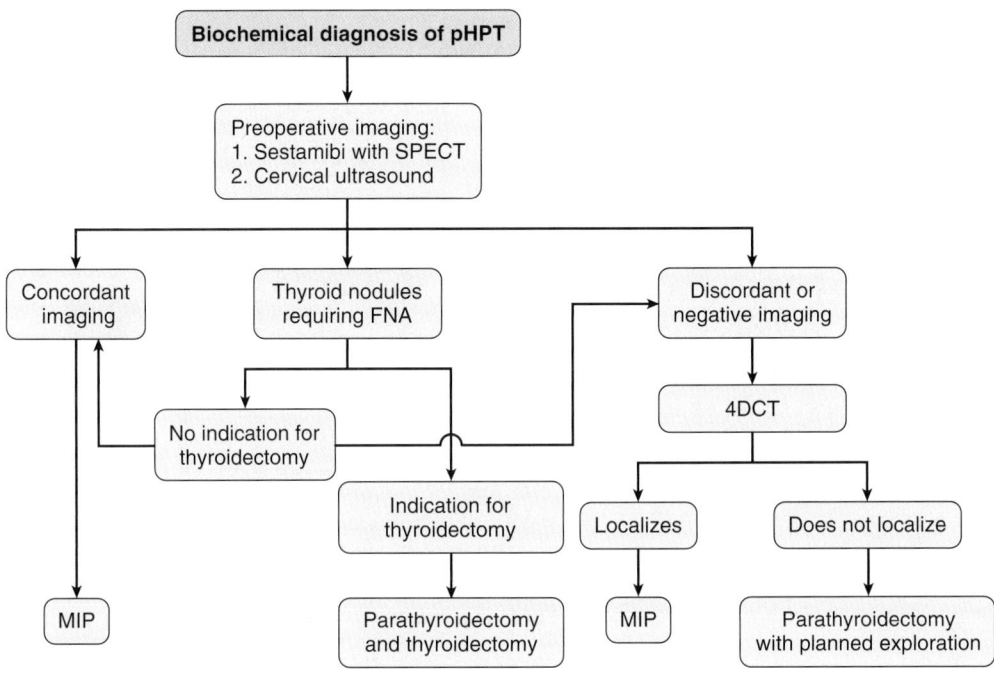

vivo–to-background ratio is 20% or more. Although radio-guided parathyroidectomy can facilitate dissection in reoperative cases, use of the gamma probe has not been shown to have improved success rates compared with IOPTH monitoring and does not confirm that all hyperfunctional tissue has been removed; therefore, the authors do not use radio-guided parathyroidectomy in their practices.

SURGICAL APPROACH

All patients undergoing consideration for parathyroidectomy should undergo a thorough history and physical examination, with careful review of biochemical results to confirm the diagnosis. Patients who report voice hoarseness or who have had prior anterior neck surgery, including previous thyroidectomy, parathyroidectomy, carotid endarterectomy, or cervical spine surgery, should undergo laryngoscopy for documentation of recurrent laryngeal nerve function. All localization studies should be reviewed by the operating surgeon. In addition, sequential compression devices are used in all patients; perioperative antibiotics are not routinely used.

The surgical approach for minimally invasive parathyroidectomy requires consideration of several factors, including appropriate venous/arterial access to obtain IOPTH samples, type of anesthesia (general or locoregional), placement of the incision, and extent of exploration based on the results of IOPTH testing. Patients should have a peripheral, large-bore intravenous catheter placed, preferably in the antecubital position, for administration of medications and fluids and for IOPTH sampling. In patients with difficult venous access, a second intravenous catheter or radial arterial line is sometimes necessary.

The two options in the anesthetic management of patients undergoing parathyroidectomy are general anesthesia and monitored anesthesia care with a surgeon-administered cervical block. General anesthesia is the mainstay of parathyroidectomy and is appropriate for patients with known multigland, familial, or secondary hyperparathyroidism; nonlocalized parathyroid disease on patient imaging; patient anxiety or claustrophobia; and patient preference. However, for patients with well-localized disease, cervical block anesthesia can be considered. Patients are given intravenous sedation by the anesthesia team; propofol has been shown to distort the results of the IOPTH assay and should be avoided, particularly if there is not a dedicated catheter for IOPTH measurements. A superficial cervical block with a 1:1 mixture of 1% lidocaine and 0.25% bupivacaine is administered posterior and deep to the sternocleidomastoid muscle; local infiltration also is performed at the incision (Figure 5). This approach is generally well tolerated; in one recent study, reasons for conversion to general anesthesia included unrecognized thyroid pathology requiring thyroidectomy, technical difficulties related to adequate protection of the recurrent laryngeal nerve, and patient discomfort. Potential advantages of cervical block anesthesia include decreased operating time, costs, reduced postoperative nausea and vomiting and more rapid discharge, and decreased need for oral pain medication. Importantly, it allows the surgical team to test the patient's phonation during the operation to ensure the continued integrity of the recurrent laryngeal nerve during the dissection. If a bilateral exploration is needed, a contralateral cervical block can be performed safely as long as the patient is comfortable and the surgeon deems that it is safe to proceed. Confirmation of intact patient phonation must be ensured because inadvertent block of bilateral recurrent laryngeal nerves can result in an airway emergency.

Irrespective of choice of anesthesia, patients should be placed in a beach-chair position, with arms tucked and adequate protection afforded to pressure points, and a shoulder roll (the authors use an inflatable intravenous [IV] bag) is inserted under the upper back to facilitate slight extension of the neck (Figure 6). A traditional Kocher's incision used for thyroidectomy is a transverse, slightly curved incision approximately two fingerbreadths above the sternoclavicular joint. A similar incision of approximately 2 to 4 cm in length is preferred for parathyroidectomy. In patients with good preoperative localization, some surgeons favor placing the incision to the right or left of midline. However, should bilateral exploration be necessary, the incision needs to be substantially extended; therefore, a symmetrical, midline incision is preferred. The subcutaneous tissues and platysma are divided transversely; subplatysmal skin flaps can be raised with electrocautery. The median raphe should be identified, and the strap muscles divided vertically in the midline and separated from the thyroid gland.

FIGURE 5   Cervical block anesthesia. *(From Udelsman R: Unilateral neck exploration under local or regional anesthesia. In Gagner M, Inabnet W III, editors:* Minimally invasive endocrine surgery, vol 1, *Philadelphia, 2002, Lippincott Williams & Wilkins.)*

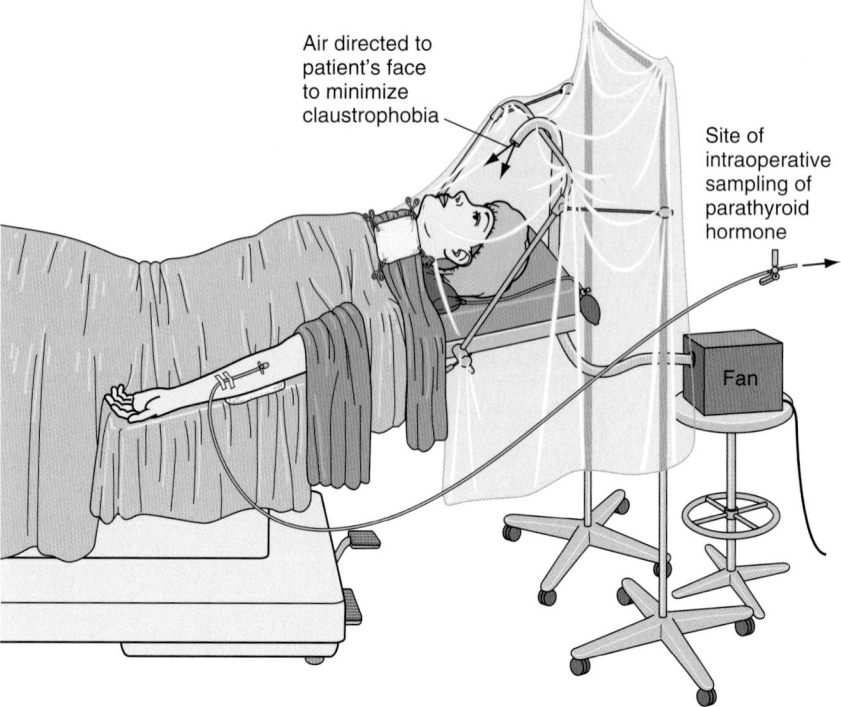

Air directed to patient's face to minimize claustrophobia

Site of intraoperative sampling of parathyroid hormone

Fan

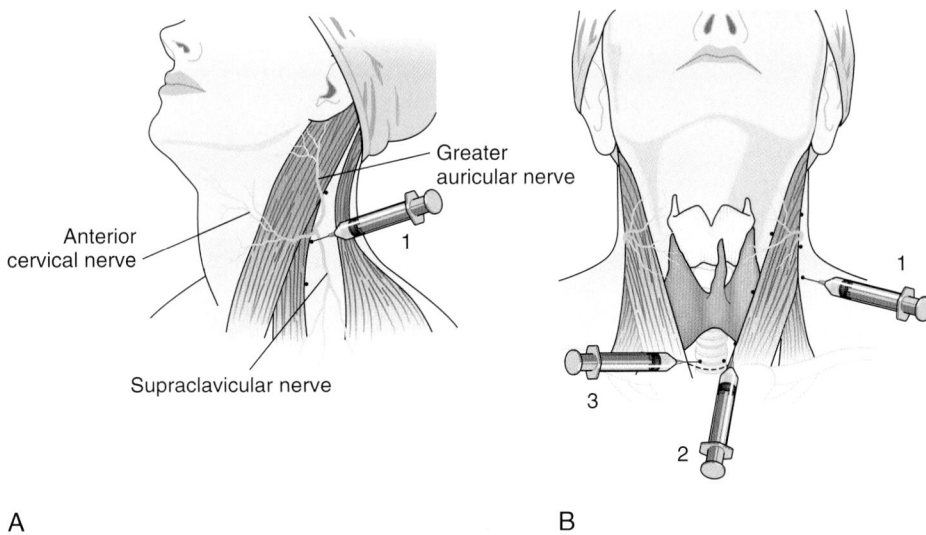

FIGURE 6 Patient positioning in the operating room, when cervical block anesthesia is used. **A,** A superficial cervical block is administered posterior and deep to the sternocleidomastoid muscle. **B,** A local field block also is performed. *(From Udelsman R: Unilateral neck exploration under local or regional anesthesia. In Gagner M, Inabnet W III, editors: Minimally invasive endocrine surgery, vol 1, Philadelphia, 2002, Lippincott Williams & Wilkins.)*

Surgical exploration should begin on the side suggested by preoperative imaging. Understanding of parathyroid gland embryology is essential for surgeons performing parathyroidectomy. Most patients have four parathyroid glands: two superior glands (derived from the fourth pharyngeal pouch) and two inferior glands (derived from the third pharyngeal pouch). The superior glands typically are located posterior to the recurrent laryngeal nerve and posteromedial to the superior thyroid lobe; ectopic glands may be located in a retroesophageal location. The inferior glands are more variable but typically are anterior to the recurrent laryngeal nerve and inferior and lateral to the inferior portion of the thyroid lobe. Ectopic inferior parathyroid glands may be located in the thymus, thyrothymic tissue, anterior mediastinum, or carotid sheath.

Several technical considerations are to be noted during exploration. First, depending on location of the adenoma, the thyroid may need to be mobilized; however, if possible, ligation of arteries and veins to the thyroid should be minimized, for risk of postoperative hypothyroidism. Second, care must be taken at all times to protect the recurrent laryngeal nerve, particularly for superior, retroesophageal parathyroid glands. Once the nerve is identified, electrocautery and suction irrigation should be used with caution. Third, the parathyroid adenoma should be manipulated as little as possible, so that the gland does not secrete PTH and cause a spike in IOPTH levels and to avoid rupture of the parathyroid capsule, leading to potential seeding of parathyroid cells and future parathyromatosis. If the parathyroid capsule is ruptured, the parathyroid bed should be copiously irrigated with hypotonic solution (water) before closure. A small amount of an absorbable hemostatic agent may be placed in the area of dissection before closure. The strap muscles and platysma are closed with running or interrupted 3-0 vicryl sutures, and the skin is closed with a 5-0 polypropylene suture, which is removed before patient discharge, or an absorbable subcutaneous stitch or skin adhesive alternative.

Assuming an abnormal parathyroid gland is identified and resected (Figure 7), IOPTH results should be obtained before leaving the operating room. If IOPTH levels fail to decrease appropriately, further exploration is mandatory. The authors prefer to identify all remaining parathyroid glands before resection, beginning with the ipsilateral parathyroid gland. Once all glands have been identified, the decision can be made as to the extent of surgical resection. If all four parathyroid glands are clearly abnormal, a subtotal parathyroidectomy should be performed, with the remnant parathyroid gland chosen being the gland that might easiest be accessed (usually an inferior gland) should the patient have recurrent pHPT develop and need a reoperative procedure. The subtotal parathyroidectomy

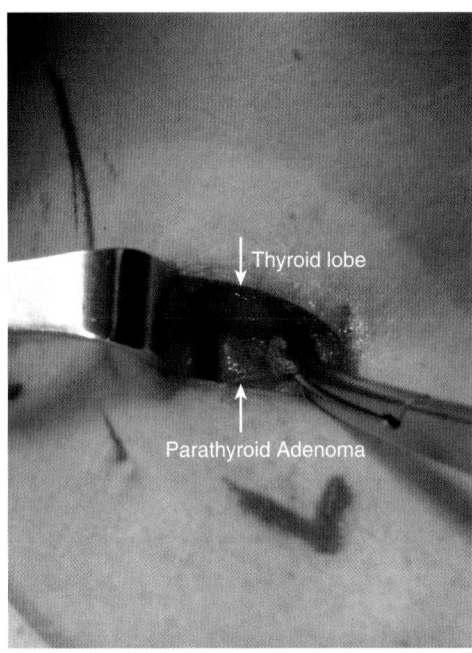

FIGURE 7 Identification of an inferior parathyroid adenoma.

should be performed first to ensure viability of the remnant parathyroid gland, followed by resection of remaining abnormal glands and repeat IOPTH monitoring. A titanium clip can be left on the subtotal parathyroid gland to facilitate future identification of the remnant if there is a recurrence of pHPT. The authors do not routinely biopsy glands that appear to be normal to avoid potential devascularization of that gland. Rarely, because of manipulation of the parathyroid gland during exploration and a spike in preexcision PTH levels, IOPTH levels may fail to normalize at 10 minutes after excision. If, based on the judgment of an experienced parathyroid surgeon, preoperative imaging results and adenoma size suggest that multigland disease is unlikely, the operation can be terminated and a PTH result obtained in the recovery room, with return to the operating room should the appropriate decrease in PTH levels fail to occur there. If a suspected parathyroid carcinoma is encountered based on disease presentation, imaging, and intraoperative findings, conversion to general anesthesia should occur, followed by ipsilateral thyroid

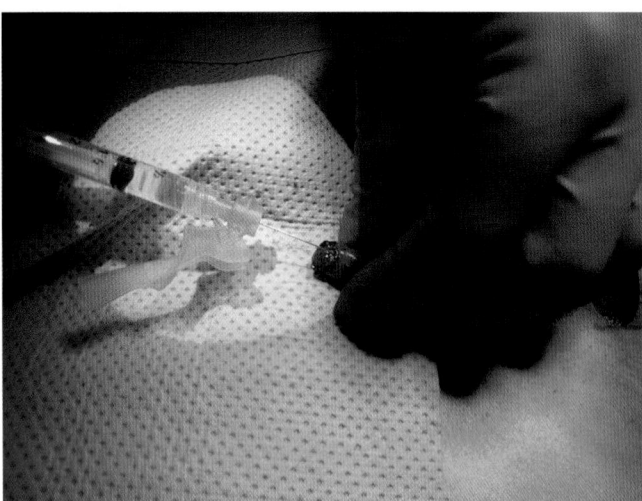

FIGURE 8   Ex vivo parathyroid aspiration.

lobectomy en bloc with the involved parathyroid gland and central lymph node dissection. Frozen section biopsy of the involved parathyroid gland should not be performed.

In addition to IOPTH monitoring, confirmation that parathyroid tissue has been resected is helpful, either with a frozen section or with ex vivo parathyroid aspiration (Figure 8). After resection of the parathyroid, a 25-gauge needle is used to aspirate tissue from the parathyroid gland; the syringe should contain a small amount of saline solution. This sample can then be run with the IOPTH samples; PTH levels that are significantly above serum PTH or above the upper limit of detection on the laboratory machine are considered to be positive confirmation that the resected tissue is parathyroid.

POSTOPERATIVE MANAGEMENT

Minimally invasive parathyroidectomy may be performed as an outpatient procedure; considerations for overnight observation include conversion to bilateral exploration, resection of more than one parathyroid gland, patient comorbidities, distance travelled, and patient preference. Inpatients should have a serum calcium and PTH level obtained on the morning after surgery. Patients should be discharged on calcium supplementation and instructed on recognition and management of symptoms of postoperative hypocalcemia, including perioral and extremity tingling or numbness. Vitamin D

supplementation with calcitriol is used in patients who experience hypocalcemic symptoms overnight that is refractory to calcium supplementation alone and in those who have undetectable PTH levels on postoperative day 1.

Patients are seen in the clinic approximately 1 week after surgery; serum calcium, PTH, and 25-OH vitamin D levels are obtained at that time and supplementation adjusted accordingly. Daily calcium supplementation is recommended for at least 6 months after surgery. Patients are seen in follow-up, in conjunction with their endocrinologist or primary care physician, with serum calcium and PTH levels at 6 months, 12 months, and annually, because 2% to 3% of patients have recurrent pHPT develop. Cure from primary hyperparathyroidism is defined as normalization of serum calcium level 6 months after parathyroidectomy. Studies have shown that up to 44% of patients have elevated PTH levels in the setting of normal calcium levels after curative parathyroidectomy, possibly from vitamin D deficiency, chronic renal disease, or bone remineralization.

Postoperative complications include recurrent laryngeal nerve injury that leads to transient or permanent voice changes and permanent hypoparathyroidism that necessitates chronic calcium and vitamin D supplementation. In the hands of experienced parathyroid surgeons, rates of these complications should be 1% to 2%, in conjunction with cure rates of more than 95%. Recent studies have shown the importance of surgeon volume in parathyroid surgery and suggest that surgeons who perform 30 to 50 or more parathyroidectomies per year are most likely to achieve appropriate cure rates with acceptable rates of morbidity.

SUGGESTED READINGS

Bilezikian JP, Khan AA, Potts JT: Guidelines for the management of asymptomatic primary hyperparathyroidism: summary statement from the Third International Workshop, *J Clin Endocrinol Metab* 94:335–339, 2009.

Cheung K, Wang TS, Farrokhyar F, et al: A meta-analysis of preoperative localization techniques for patients with primary hyperparathyroidism, *Ann Surg Oncol* 19:577–583, 2011.

Richards ML, Thompson GB, Farley DR, et al: An optimal algorithm for intraoperative parathyroid hormone monitoring, *Arch Surg* 146:280–285, 2011.

Roman SA, Sosa JA, Pietrzak RH, et al: The effects of serum calcium and parathyroid hormone on psychological and cognitive function in patients undergoing parathyroidectomy for primary hyperparathyroidism, *Ann Surg* 253:131–137, 2011.

Wang TS, Cheung K, Farrokhyar F, et al: Would scan, but which scan? A cost-utility analysis to optimize preoperative imaging for primary hyperparathyroidism, *Surgery* 150:1286–1295, 2011.

Wang TS, Roman SA, Cox H, et al: The management of thyroid nodules in patients with primary hyperparathyroidism, *J Surg Res* 154:317–323, 2009.

LAPAROSCOPIC LIVER RESECTION

Jay A. Graham, MD, and
Lynt B. Johnson, MD, MBA, FACS

OVERVIEW

Laparoscopy has forever changed the landscape of surgery. Although hepatobiliary surgery remained the last bastion of "maximal

invasiveness," recently there has been a rise in the implementation of laparoscopy for complex liver operations. The inherent high risks associated with hepatic resection initially tempered enthusiasm for these laparoscopic pursuits, but in recent years, techniques to safely perform hepatic resections have evolved.

Concerns about the perceived lack of control of hemorrhage from hepatic vasculature during laparoscopic procedures gave pause to even the heartiest surgeons. As a result, early experience with laparoscopic liver surgery began with nonanatomic wedge resection for lesions located on the anterior surface. While some attempted the relatively straightforward left lateral segmentectomy laparoscopically, it was not until the advent of the hand-assisted technique that formal liver resection became feasible for many hepatobiliary surgeons.

This divergence from the purely laparoscopic instrumentation of the liver had many distinct advantages. Practically, the hand is the most useful retractor, offering expedient conformational change and unmatched haptic feedback. As such, intracorporeal hand insertion during laparoscopic resection gives the surgeon enhanced tactile stabilization of the liver, allowing for more precise mobilization and dissection of the target lobe. In addition, the hand port serves as a retrieval site for the surgical specimen.

This new approach has offered the patient an alternative to the traditional bilateral subcostal incision and thereby tendered the marked benefits of limited incisions inherent to minimally invasive surgery. This laparoscopic advance has extended into all forays of surgery with an ensuing decrease in incision size, which translates into less pain for the patient. With less pain comes earlier mobility, which results in decreased morbidity and reduced length of stay. Secondarily, direct costs may be reduced with the use of laparoscopic techniques as a result of the earlier hospital discharge.

Heretofore laparoscopic hepatic resection has seemed far afield, but the subsequent innovation has shifted the paradigm. To this end, laparoscopy as applied to hepatic surgery is germane to discussions of "best practices" and offers a technical approach that should be considered for many patients with liver pathology.

PREOPERATIVE EVALUATION

Evaluation of patients suitable for laparoscopic hepatic resection begins in the clinic. Patients often have preconceived notions, so it is important to balance heightened expectations with the reality of the situation. As such, preoperative evaluation generally begins with a comprehensive assessment of all organ systems. Although this approach is no different for any surgical candidate, particular attention should be paid to the cardiac and pulmonary physiology of the patient. These systems, more so than others, can be severely impacted during insufflation of the abdomen.

Systems-Based Clinical Evaluation

At a minimum, a complete blood count, chemistry, and coagulation panel should be obtained. In addition, a chest x-ray and an electrocardiogram (EKG) should be acquired if the patient is older than 50 years or has a history of heart disease. Cardiac risk stratification is of upmost importance, and every effort should be made to follow the American Heart Association (AHA) guidelines for cardiovascular evaluation for noncardiac surgery. Surgeons should also familiarize themselves with the assessment of metabolic equivalents (METs), as this is a reflection of estimated functional capacity and is paramount to guiding the appropriate preoperative testing. Generally, patients with good or borderline functional status may not have pulmonary issues that preclude surgery. However, patients with chronic respiratory disease should be optimized with bronchodilators, steroids, antiinflammatory agents, breathing exercises, and/or chest physiotherapy (Box 1).

Physical examination of the patient's heart and lungs may clue the clinician into possible cardiopulmonary disease and prompt further testing. Examination of the abdomen is also crucial to the preoperative evaluation. A larger body habitus will make the target lobe mobilization more difficult. Visual inspection and the finding of scars can often hint at the difficulty and improbability of pursuing laparoscopic resection due to suspected adhesive disease. Additionally, physical examination may promote a dialogue with the patient regarding the likelihood of conversion to an open approach. Axial imaging also plays an important role in operative planning.

Axial Imaging Preoperative Planning

Patients generally seek clinical evaluation with a computed tomographic (CT) or magnetic resonance imaging (MRI) scan in hand. It is important to assess lesion location and morphology with an understanding of segmental liver anatomy. As such, the location of the lesion and its relationship to the hepatic vasculature can predicate a partial, formal right, left, or extended hepatectomy.

This preoperative method of evaluation is not consigned solely to laparoscopic liver surgery, and the tumor growth pattern, prior foregut surgery, or liver morphology may contraindicate for minimally invasive surgery. Evidence of extrahepatic tumoral extension or hepatomegaly can make intracorporeal mobilization difficult and therefore preclude laparoscopic resection. Although these findings are relative contraindications, they are not binding, and some espouse the notion that one can always begin laparoscopically and convert if necessary. In our experience, the conversion rate is approximately 5%.

Relative Contraindications to Laparoscopy

Although refractory hypotension is the only absolute contraindication to laparoscopy, there are many situations that make its use ill advised. In general, patients with an American Society of Anesthesiologists (ASA) classification of 4 or higher should not undergo laparoscopic procedures because hemodynamic instability is likely to arise in the setting of a pneumoperitoneum. As such, patients with poor cardiopulmonary reserve should temper the surgeon's enthusiasm for laparoscopic pursuits. However, rarely is the surgeon confronted with such obvious and straightforward clinical decisions.

The assessment of the risks and benefits of alternative operative approaches underscores the relative contraindications for laparoscopic liver resection. In our experience, patients who have had prior open foregut surgery are generally poor candidates for a laparoscopic approach, given the likely adhesive disease. Moreover, bulky pathology or hepatomegaly usually predicates open surgery, as hepatic mobilization can be problematic (Box 2). In contrast, laparoscopic resection for malignancy has been shown to be safe, which parallels the findings for treatment of other intraabdominal organ cancers.

BOX 1: Preoperative evaluation

Complete blood count
Basic metabolic panel
Coagulation panel
Chest x-ray
Electrocardiogram
Cardiac risk stratification (AHA)
Pulmonary function optimization
Physical examination
Axial imaging

AHA, American Heart Association.

BOX 2: Relative contraindications to laparoscopic hepatic resection

ASA classification ≥ 4
Poor cardiopulmonary reserve
Prior open foregut surgery
Large (>10 cm) posterior lesions
Hepatomegaly

ASA, American Society of Anesthesiologists.

ANESTHESIA AND INTRAOPERATIVE MONITORING

Surgeons must be intimately aware of the physiologic consequences of laparoscopy. Open communication with the anesthesiologist is crucial to anticipating and correcting the various problems that may arise. Patients with significant comorbidities need to be mindfully approached because profound changes in cardiopulmonary regulation may result from relatively minor alterations in abdominal pressure.

Hemodynamic complications due to insufflation are well documented, some of which may be deleterious and even result in death. Cardiac filling is often reduced, as manifested by lower left ventricular end-diastolic volumes due to increased abdominal pressure and abridged venous forward flow. A decrease in cardiac output is the primary indicator of the decline in right heart filling with the establishment of a pneumoperitoneum, especially in the context of patient positioning with reverse Trendelenburg. Both entities can severely limit venous return and ultimately result in a 20% to 60% reduction in cardiac index. Patients with ventricular systolic dysfunction are especially at risk. Hypotension should prompt pneumoperitoneum reduction and intravenous fluid resuscitation to counter these effects.

The occurrence of cardiac arrhythmias during laparoscopy is well chronicled. The rapid stretching of the peritoneum during initial insufflation often elicits a vagal response that can cause profound bradycardia and decreased inotropy. Prompt release of the pneumoperitoneum usually results in return of a normal rhythm. Likewise, carbon dioxide (CO_2) can be absorbed during laparoscopy and decrease the threshold for arrhythmias by irritating the myocytes and altering the conduction pathways.

The respiratory effects of laparoscopy are also notable, as they are both mechanical and due to the aforementioned gas exchange issues. Specifically, there is a reduction in functional reserve capacity (FRC) and lung compliance during abdominal insufflation. While there is a transient decrease in pulmonary shunt on initial insufflation with a concomitant rise in PaO_2, ultimately the elevated diaphragm and resultant decrease in FRC can cause hypoxemia, especially in obese patients or in patients with preexisting pulmonary disease. Therefore, patients with a larger body habitus, and also those with preexisting pulmonary disease, should be managed with higher positive-pressure ventilation and minute ventilation.

Surgical dissection during laparoscopy can also result in noticeable changes in ventilatory physiology and increase the chance of vascular embolic phenomenon. While the resultant hypercapnia is manageable by increasing the minute ventilation, the potential for symptomatic CO_2 gas embolism must be recognized. CO_2 gas embolism is likely an underrecognized occurrence due to its high solubility and diffusion. However, this risk may be heightened, especially with laparoscopic hepatic parenchymal transection due to exposure of the vast network of cut vessels to the pneumoperitoneum. As such, in the event of a rapidly dropping end-tidal CO_2 (E_TCO_2) and cardiopulmonary instability, evacuation of the pneumoperitoneum, volume resuscitation, and maneuvers to place the patient in left lateral decubitus position should commence.

To guard against such mishaps, it is critical that the patient is monitored with more than the usual array of instruments for general anesthesia. Given the potential for rapidly progressing and deleterious events, the patient should have, at a minimum, a radial or femoral arterial line placed. More often than not, it is also recommended to have central venous access should the patient need emergent blood volume replacement. Central venous pressure (CVP) monitoring is also of utmost importance. Blood loss is markedly limited if the liver transection is performed with a low CVP (<5 mm Hg). Secondarily, a central line allows the anesthesiologist to perform an acute normovolemic hemodilution (ANH). In our institution, routine use of a low CVP and ANH for hepatic resection has limited blood loss and reduced the need for allogeneic blood transfusion in patients undergoing major hepatic resections.

OPERATIVE TECHNIQUES

Numerous methods of laparoscopic resection have gained popularity with increased sharing and collaboration in the surgical community. Recognizing the diversity of these laparoscopic techniques used for liver resection, a panel of 45 well-known hepatobiliary surgeons worked to establish a standard classification system and summarize a unified position statement on safety and efficacy of laparoscopic liver resection. This panel of experts agreed on the terms *pure laparoscopy*, *hand-assisted*, and *hybrid technique* to describe the various approaches.

Pure Laparoscopy

Pure laparoscopy is usually used for wedge resections of anterior lesions of the liver or masses located in the left lateral segment, but it has been used for major lobe resections as well. Access is gained into the abdomen, depending on the surgeon's preference, and an umbilical 10-mm trocar is placed. Safe trocar insertion is of paramount importance. Viscus perforation and vasculature laceration can occur as a result of unintended and uncontrolled insertion. Although these injuries happen infrequently, significant morbidity, including death, can result. As such, the most reliable way of preventing trocar placement injury is macrobracing. This technique involves the use of the nondominant hand to counter the loss of resistance as the trocar tip penetrates the fascia and peritoneum.

After insufflation, the patient is moved into the reverse Trendelenburg position to enable sighting of the hilar structure and to position the small bowel in the lower abdomen and pelvis. Two to three trocars are placed under direct visualization to facilitate triangulation of the intended surgery site. Here, laparoscopic ultrasound is of great use to determine the depth of the mass and its juxtaposition to vasculature. Lesions on the liver surface may be wedged out with the use of laparoscopic adaptations of the Harmonic scalpel (Ethicon Endo-Surgery, Blue Ash, Ohio), LigaSure (Covidien, Boulder, Colo), Enseal (Ethicon Endo-Surgery, Blue Ash, Ohio), or any other bipolar energy device.

More formal laparoscopic liver resection requires far more expertise and level of comfort when dissecting the liver. Although bleeding is not unusual during hepatic parenchymal division, the potential lack of expedient vascular control during life-threatening hemorrhage with minimal access is worrisome. As such, we take a far more conservative approach with anatomic liver resection, opting for use of the hybrid technique. Nevertheless, the literature is replete with examples of pure laparoscopic liver formal resection.

Generally, the hilum is dissected and the respective hepatic artery ligated and divided. The portal vein to the affected side is then clamped. Transection then begins in the usual fashion, and major vasculature is controlled with laparoscopic stapling devices. The major bile ducts are also stapled, and the specimen is extirpated through an extended umbilical incision. For this reason, it is more prudent to attempt larger resections with the alternative hand-assisted and hybrid techniques, given the similarity in the incision size.

Hand-Assisted Technique and the Hybrid Technique

Whereas the incision that accommodates the hand port is the same for the hand-assisted and the hybrid techniques, there are some definitive differences. Both operative procedures employ the hand as a retractor, but hand-assisted liver resection implies that the resection is performed entirely intracorporeally. Conversely, the hybrid technique is a practice of using the hand to mobilize the liver with subsequent removal of the hand port so as to perform the liver transection in an open fashion without extending the incision. Our institution favors the hybrid approach because we intuitively feel that this technique provides a more expeditious and practical manner for mobilization, parenchymal dissection, and removal of the liver specimen. Nevertheless, because surgeons of great skill have been trained in both methods, the optimum procedure is the one that favors the comfort level of the practitioner. Here we will describe the hybrid approach to liver resection, but the details are applicable to any system of laparoscopy using the hand.

A 7.5-cm subxiphoid incision is made, and a hand port (GelPort Laparoscopic System, Applied Medical, Rancho Santa Margarita, Calif) is inserted for hand assistance (Figure 1). A pneumoperitoneum is established after a standard Hassan trocar insertion periumbilically, and a 5-mm trocar is placed obliquely in the right or left subcostal margin depending on the location of the target lobe. As described earlier, great care must be taken when inserting trocars intraabdominally because of the inherent potential for vascular or viscus injury. The periumbilical trocar placement can be particularly risky because of its larger size and the relatively blind nature of insertion. This possibility can be minimized by introducing the trocar using the Hassan cut-down technique. One hand should be placed into the abdomen through the subxiphoid incision to receive the trocar as the other is used to gently advance the port-system through the fascia. Alternatively, a malleable retractor can be used to displace the bowel and to minimize the consequences of inadvertent and uncontrolled thrusting.

After safe insufflation of the abdomen, the operation begins with mobilization of the liver after positioning the patient in reverse Trendelenburg. Laparoscopic diathermic energy-based devices are used to divide the visceral attachments and triangular and coronary ligaments. The side of hepatic pathology dictates right or left hand insertion for hepatic lobe retraction.

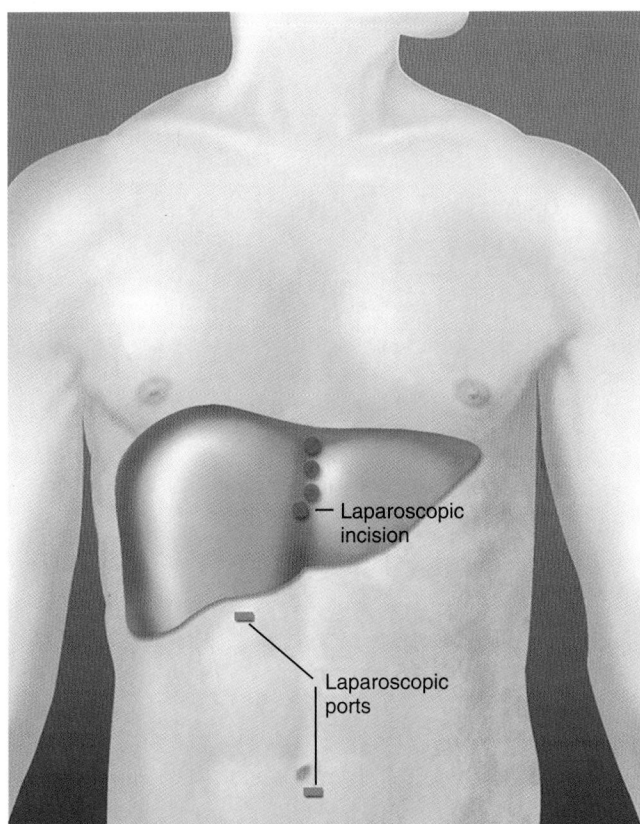

FIGURE 1   A 7.5-cm subxiphoid incision is made, and a hand port (GelPort Laparoscopic System, Applied Medical, Rancho Santa Margarita, Calif) is inserted for hand assistance.

The hand is an optimal retractor because of its ability to conform to the contours of the liver and displace pressure to the entire organ, preventing possible parenchymal injury. Moreover, intracorporeal hand insertion during laparoscopic assisted resection gives the surgeon enhanced tactile stabilization of the liver; this allows for more precise mobilization and dissection of the target lobe. Hand assistance also promotes safety in affording the surgeon with an expedient method of manual control of hemorrhage during a potential vascular mishap.

Furthermore, the laparoscopic camera aids in the operative procedure by enhancing acuity and magnification. Optic capture offered by laparoscopy can secondarily facilitate the identification and division of tangential structures. Angled lenses can offer an even greater advantage through visualization and ligation of the posterior medial vessels such as the retrocaval short hepatic veins during a right hepatectomy. These retroperitoneal short vessels can be divided in the aforementioned fashion or through the hand port after exsufflation.

Once the target liver lobe has been mobilized by division of all peritoneal reflections, the abdomen is exsufflated and the hand port is removed. Because exposure is of paramount importance, we recommend the use of a retractor system. We prefer the BOOKWALTER retractor system (Codman and Shurtleff, Raynham, Mass), but any variation will do. With adequate and uncompromised retraction, extrahepatic hilar vasculature ligation and division then ensue to lessen blood loss during liver transection. Of note, vascular anomalies are far from unusual, and the surgeon must be mindful to assess for aberrant right and left hepatic arteries. Next, the parenchymal dissection through the hard port incision is accomplished with the aid of ultrasonography and ultrasonic surgical aspirators (CUSA, Integra Lifesciences Corp, Plainsboro, NJ) to identify the venous entities. During cases of major resection, the hanging maneuver as described by Dr. Belghiti is used, with an umbilical tape passed anterior to the vena cava. We ardently believe the biliary ductal system should be managed during intrahepatic dissection to prevent injury to the contralateral duct.

For living donor hepatectomies, the hepatic artery, portal vein, and hepatic vein branches are kept intact as the parenchymal division is completed. The patient is then heparinized prior to the dissection of the target vascular structures and ultimate division. Subsequently, the specimen is removed through the hand port site.

Right Hepatectomy Using the Hybrid Technique

After mobilization of the right hepatic lobe by division of the falciform and triangular ligaments, we exsufflate the abdomen, remove the hand port, and secure the retractor system to expose the liver through the midline abdominal incision. Next, we place lap pads behind the liver to bring the hilum into better view.

Prior to dissection, we methodically palpate for a replaced right hepatic artery. Hepatic arterial anomalies are so frequent that they are almost the norm; therefore, a clear distinction of lobar inflow should be made prior to ligation. The middle hepatic artery can be easily mistaken for a right hepatic artery, especially in the setting of a replaced artery, and division can have severe implications for segments 4A and 4B. While we do not routinely use a Doppler to map the arterial routes, we completely dissect out the right hepatic artery. Here we ligate and divide the right hepatic artery and dissect posteriorly to delineate the portal vein. The right portal vein is circumferentially mobilized superiorly and divided. This devascularizes the right lobe inflow and results in demarcation of the liver. The right hepatic vein is then identified on the superior aspect of the liver and is divided using an articulating laparoscopic stapling device (EndoPath ETS, Ethicon Endo-Surgery, Blue Ash, Ohio) to ensure safe control of this very large vessel off of the inferior vena cava.

We routinely use intraoperative ultrasound to characterize and mark the course of the middle hepatic vein, as relying on ischemic demarcation can result in injury to a slightly laterally positioned vessel. Using the aforementioned hanging maneuver, we proceed with liver division, being mindful to stay to the right of the middle hepatic vein. We opt to ligate the right hepatic duct during intraparenchymal division because contralateral bile duct ischemia can occur if extrahepatic dissection is attempted. The specimen is then removed through this incision.

Left Hepatectomy Using the Hybrid Technique

A left hepatectomy using the hybrid technique follows many of the same steps that were previously discussed. Again, one should be mindful of arterial variances, especially a replaced left hepatic artery coming from the left gastric artery. After correct identification and division of the middle and left hepatic arteries, dissection of the left portal vein begins by working posteriorly to the ligated arterial vasculature. Traditionally, the caudate lobe is spared in formal left hepatic lobe resections, and therefore the surgeon should preserve the portal venous branches from the left portal vein into this segment.

Next, the middle hepatic vein is characterized using intraoperative ultrasound, and its course is marked on the surface of the liver using electrocautery. The middle and left hepatic veins are then divided with a laparoscopic stapling device, and parenchymal transection begins in the standard fashion.

OPERATIVE METRICS

In a recent study, we compared our experience of conventional open liver resection to laparoscopic liver resection. As expectant, the laparoscopic approach with hand assistance and parenchymal dissection through the hand port incision had equivalent operative metrics with shortened length of stay. Reports like those issued by Koffron et al have shown that laparoscopic resection is less expensive because of the shortened hospital stay. This finding reflects what has already been conclusively shown with laparoscopic cholecystectomy, fundoplication, and gastric bypass surgery.

As efficiency pressures continue to rise, the laparoscopic approach for liver resection will likely be further embraced. To this end, we surmise that the hybrid technique will gain favor, as it more closely assimilates the skills that hepatobiliary surgeons already possess. Moreover, this technique offers the most palatable setting of safety with the use of the hand for liver mobilization and prompt control of bleeding vasculature.

Practically, the hand is the best-known liver retractor, as it is atraumatic and offers varying degrees of facile mobility. Moreover, with this approach, we are able to substantially minimize the incision for an open liver resection as the standard subcostal incision can approach 35 cm. Accordingly, we believe that the potential long-term sequelae of the traditional bilateral subcostal incision with midline extension, which include abdominal wall hernias and paresthesias, may be lessened.

CONCLUSION

Since Dr. Jean Louis Lortat Jacob detailed the first published hepatectomy using the roadmap map laid out by Claude Couinaud, the field of liver surgery has seen a celebrated rise in the capability to offer resection with lower rates of morbidity and mortality. It is evident that with the arrival of the twenty-first century, the emergence of laparoscopy embodies a marriage of uncompromised surgical technique and better outcomes for our patients.

Newer approaches have allowed surgeons to bridge the gap between operative technique and improved outcomes. This occurrence has been largely device-driven, and industry has taken a lead role in these advancements. Laparoscopy has emerged as an advancement that embodies these efforts to improve medical care and represents a significant change to the landscape of surgery. As such, we are in the renaissance of minimally invasive surgery with innovation guiding a renewed operative approach to intraabdominal pathology. Liver surgery, although initially late to embrace laparoscopy, is now gaining momentum in this paradigm shift. The advent of innovative laparoscopic tools that mirror what is used conventionally have facilitated this transition.

SUGGESTED READINGS

Belghiti J, Guevara OA, Noun R, et al: Liver hanging maneuver: a safe approach to right hepatectomy without liver mobilization, *J Am Coll Surg* 193(1):109–111, 2001.

Bhojani FD, Fox A, Pitzul K, et al: Clinical and economic comparison of laparoscopic to open liver resections using a 2-to-1 matched pair analysis: an institutional experience, *J Am Coll Surg* 214(2):184–195, 2012.

Buell JF, Cherqui D, Geller DA, et al: The international position on laparoscopic liver surgery: The Louisville Statement, 2008, *Ann Surg* 250(5):825–830, 2009.

Fong Y, Jarnagin W, Conlon KC, et al: Hand-assisted laparoscopic liver resection: lessons from an initial experience, *Arch Surg* 135(7):854–859, 2000.

Johnson LB, Graham JA, Weiner DA: Smirniotopoulos J. How does laparoscopic-assisted hepatic resection compare with the conventional open surgical approach? *J Am Coll Surg* 214(4):717–723, 2012.

Koffron AJ, Auffenberg G, Kung R, et al: Evaluation of 300 minimally invasive liver resections at a single institution: less is more, *Ann Surg* 246(3):385–392; discussion 92–94, 2007a.

Koffron AJ, Kung RD, Auffenberg GB, et al: Laparoscopic liver surgery for everyone: the hybrid method, *Surgery* 142(4):463–468; discussion 468.e1–468.e2, 2007b. Erratum in: *Surgery* 143(2):301, 2008.

Lortat-Jacob JL, Robert HG, Henry C: [Excision of the right lobe of the liver for a malignant secondary tumor], *Archives des maladies de l'appareil digestif et des maladies de la nutrition* 41(6):662–667, 1952.

Thenappan A, Jha RC, Fishbein T, et al: Liver allograft outcomes after laparoscopic-assisted and minimal access live donor hepatectomy for transplantation, *Am J Surg* 201(4):450–455, 2011.

Staging Laparoscopy for Gastrointestinal Cancer

Steven D. Wexner, MD, PhD (Hon), FACS, FASCRS, FRCS (Ed), and Elisabeth C. McLemore, MD, FACS, FASCRS

OVERVIEW

Staging laparoscopy can detect radiographically occult metastases and lead to changes in the therapeutic plan for a significant number of patients. Compared with staging laparotomy, staging laparoscopy is associated with a shorter hospital length of stay, reduced pain, lower morbidity, shorter recovery time, and reduced cost. In addition, staging laparoscopy can minimize potential delays in patient access to chemotherapy and radiation therapy and facilitates appropriate selection of patients for palliative therapy.

The improvement in laparoscopic instrumentation and technical ability over the past few decades has resulted in a sensitivity of laparoscopic metastatic detection equivalent to that achieved during open exploration. Intraoperative laparoscopic ultrasound scan can be more sensitive than either preoperative computed tomographic (CT) scan or magnetic resonance imaging (MRI). The concern for the risk of port-site metastasis and peritoneal carcinomatosis as a result of laparoscopic assessment of an abdominal malignant process has abated. However, controversy regarding selective versus routine use of staging laparoscopy has yet to be settled for a subset of patients with cancer.

GENERAL TECHNIQUE

A proposed assessment of the indications and contraindications for staging laparoscopy for specific tumor types is listed in Table 1. Contraindications include severe adhesive disease, intolerance to the establishment of pneumoperitoneum, poor cardiovascular or pulmonary reserve that precludes operative intervention, and uncorrectable coagulopathy. Before a diagnostic or staging laparoscopic procedure is started for a gastrointestinal malignancy, the surgeon must ensure that adequate pathologic expertise is available. Most operations require several frozen-section analyses of biopsy specimens. A phone call from the operating room to the pathologist at the beginning of the case frequently facilitates and hastens the diagnosis, thereby shortening the overall operative time.

With a 30-degree or 45-degree laparoscope, a thorough inspection of the suprahepatic and infrahepatic spaces, diaphragm, surface of the bowel, lesser sac, root of the transverse mesocolon and small bowel, ligament of Treitz, paracolic gutters, and pelvis should be performed. In the case of pancreatic cancer, the lesser sac is opened, and the pancreas and posterior aspect of the stomach are examined. During the inspection, any intraperitoneal fluid or ascites should be aspirated for cytology if suspicious, or as directed per institutional protocol. A biopsy of the abdominal wall, diaphragm, mesentery, or other implants should be taken and assessed with fresh frozen techniques. Peritoneal lavage is performed according to protocol or surgeon preference. Subsequently, the primary tumor can be assessed for possible node involvement that may preclude surgical resection, extraserosal invasion, and infiltration into surrounding structures.

Laparoscopic ultrasound scan is often performed if inspection is uninformative, or if a significant chance of a liver metastasis is present. Intraoperative ultrasound scan has an obvious and important role in surgical decision making for hepatobiliary and pancreatic malignancies. With use of a multifrequency laparoscopic ultrasound probe with a flexible transducer tip, sonographic evaluation should include the deep hepatic parenchyma, portal vein, and mesenteric vessels, and assessment of the involved organ with the primary tumor and its associated nodes. In general, with the probe frequency set to 5 MHz, the liver parenchyma can be systematically assessed, starting from right to left anteriorly then posteriorly. Increasing the probe frequency to 7 MHz allows for further evaluation of the extrahepatic bile ducts and associated nodes, and the long axis in a relatively transverse plane, either directly or through the overlying omentum. For metastatic and primary liver malignancies, an ultrasound scan–guided core biopsy should be taken for suspicious lesions that preclude curative resection. Color-flow Doppler imaging can be used to assess portal and hepatic vasculature and the relationship of these structures to any tumors visualized. For visualization and inspection of the areas listed previously, the patient should be securely positioned with appropriate padding to prevent intraoperative patient position migration or soft tissue damage during liberal adjustment of the operating room table position.

ESOPHAGEAL CANCER

Combined thoracoscopy and laparoscopy for esophageal cancer has been reported to achieve nearly 90% accuracy in documentation of locally advanced disease with nodal involvement. The addition of laparoscopic ultrasound scan during staging has been reported to increase the detection rate for metastasis by 8% with little impact on the false-negative rate. Laparoscopic evaluation allows for assessment of liver and peritoneal metastasis and celiac nodal involvement. Staging laparoscopy results in more significant changes to the treatment plan for patients with lower esophageal and proximal gastric tumors when compared with patients with mid to upper esophageal lesions. At the time of diagnostic laparoscopy, enteral feeding access can be established as necessary to proceed with palliative or neoadjuvant therapy. Thoracoscopic evaluation is performed in the right chest cavity with the patient in left lateral decubitus position with table splitting. Mobilization of the inferior pulmonary ligament allows for assessment of the intrathoracic esophagus, paraesophageal tissues, and subcarinal lymph nodes. Major complications related to laparoscopic staging for esophageal cancer are rare.

GASTRIC ADENOCARCINOMA

Currently, routine preoperative staging for gastric adenocarcinoma in the United States includes esophagogastroduodenoscopy (EGD) with endoscopic ultrasound scan, high-quality cross-sectional imaging, positron emission tomography (PET), and staging laparoscopy. Multiple studies have documented the value of staging laparoscopy. When lymph node–positive disease is discovered at the time of diagnostic laparoscopy in patients without obstructive symptoms, most patients can proceed with systemic chemotherapy without obstruction or bleeding developing. Multidisciplinary clinical staging and medical therapy at high-volume medical centers has been associated with improved oncologic outcomes.

In an attempt to better define those patients who may benefit from staging laparoscopy, Sarela and colleagues from Memorial Sloan Kettering Cancer Center reviewed 657 gastric cancer patients with minimal symptoms and no clinical evidence of metastatic disease on clinical staging spiral CT cross-sectional imaging. Metastatic disease was detected in 31% of patients. Multivariate analysis revealed that radiographically occult metastatic disease was more prevalent in patients with gastroesophageal junction lesions, diffuse gastric

TABLE 1: Indications and contradictions for staging laparoscopy for specific tumor types

Tumor type	Indications	Contradictions
Pancreatic adenocarcinoma	Detection of unsuspected locally advanced disease in patients with resectable disease based on preoperative imaging Consideration of peritoneal lavage before definitive surgery per individual protocol Selection of palliative treatment with locally advanced disease without evidence of metastatic disease Assessment before planned neoadjuvant chemoradiation	Metastatic disease that is evident on CT scan
Gastric adenocarcinoma	T3 or T4 disease without evidence of nodal and distal metastasis Gastroesophageal junction tumors Questionable lymph nodes on imaging	Need for palliative procedures for obstruction, hemorrhage, or perforation; proceed with surgery T1 or T2 disease can proceed with resection without diagnostic laparoscopy
Esophageal tumors	Candidates for neoadjuvant chemotherapy Candidates for curative resection and negative preoperative imaging	
Colorectal cancer	Patients with resectable liver metastases without evidence of extrahepatic metastasis	Unresectable, nonablatable hepatic disease
Primary hepatic tumors	Candidates for curative resection based on size and location with adequate hepatic reserve	Tumors with major vessel or organ invasion
Biliary tract tumors	Known or suspected gallbladder cancer without unresectable or metastatic disease T2 or T3 hilar cholangiocarcinoma	T1 gallbladder cancer incidentally found during cholecystectomy
Lymphoma	Need for tissue diagnosis in the absence of peripheral lymphadenopathy	

CT, Computed tomographic.
Modified from Hori Y: Restaging after treatment or when recurrence is suspected: SAGES Guidelines Committee: diagnostic laparoscopy guidelines, Surg Endosc 22(5):1353-1382, 2008.

tumors, poor differentiation, and age less than 70 years. In patients with preoperative imaging that revealed lymphadenopathy greater than 1 cm (49%) in diameter and T3 or T4 tumors (63%), a higher incidence of radiographically occult metastatic disease was found.

COLORECTAL LIVER METASTASIS AND HEPATOBILIARY PRIMARY TUMORS

Staging laparoscopy is seldom used in the primary treatment of colorectal cancer. Furthermore, the combination of PET, CT scan, and MRI has decreased the need for diagnostic laparoscopy for colorectal liver metastasis. However, diagnostic laparoscopy used in conjunction with laparoscopic ultrasound scan as a prelude to liver resection can identify factors that preclude curative resection in up to 25% of cases. The overall benefit of diagnostic laparoscopy for the determination of a nonresection candidate is nearly 40% for primary liver tumors and 12% for colorectal liver metastasis. The largest study of staging laparoscopy for hepatocellular carcinoma was notable for avoidance of a nontherapeutic laparotomy in 16% of patients. Routine staging laparoscopy for intrahepatic cholangiocarcinomas has resulted in avoidance of unnecessary operative intervention in 27% of patients treated at Memorial Sloan-Kettering Cancer Center.

In patients with hilar cholangiocarcinomas, the addition of intraoperative ultrasound scan increased the yield for detection of tumors not amenable to surgical resection by nearly 20%.

Many patients undergo percutaneous ablative procedures for malignant hepatic lesions. Although these procedures can sometimes be performed in radiology suites, most surgeons believe strongly that these patients are best served in a setting in which staging laparoscopy and laparoscopic ultrasound scan–guided ablation can also be performed. Nearly 40% of patients with unresectable disease have either extrahepatic disease or additional, small-volume disease in the liver that is not detected on preablative imaging. Therefore, patients undergoing percutaneous liver ablative procedures are at risk for undertreatment or overtreatment of the true disease burden.

PANCREATIC AND PERIAMPULLARY ADENOCARCINOMAS

Although the first case series of staging laparoscopy for pancreatic cancer was described by Cushchieri in 1978, minimally invasive techniques for the management of pancreatic cancer have been slow to progress and gain national participation. With the evolution of staging to include pancreatic helical CT imaging with fine cuts, the diagnostic yield of staging laparoscopy over the past few decades has decreased from 35% to approximately 13%. Therefore, some surgeons have argued for the selective use of staging laparoscopy. Evidence suggests that laparoscopy should be reserved for tumors in the body or tail of the pancreas and tumors larger than 3 cm and for cases with preoperative CA 19-9 levels greater than 100 U/mL. With regard to ampullary, duodenal, and distal bile duct tumors, the addition of diagnostic laparoscopy to dynamic CT scanning appears to identify an additional 10% of patients with unresectable disease.

LYMPHOPROLIFERATIVE DISEASES

Staging laparoscopy for lymphoproliferative disorders is similar to traditional staging laparotomy and can include liver biopsy, splenectomy, and lymph node sampling of iliac, celiac, portal, mesenteric, and periaortic nodes and excision of abnormal nodes identified before surgery with marking of the area of excision with clips. Surgeons may elect to perform oophoropexy posterior to the uterus to improve the patient's fertility. The positive diagnostic yield is related to degree of tissue sampling, experience with laparoscopy, and complete mobilization of the colon, duodenum, and pancreas. Surgeons are most often requested to biopsy abnormal-appearing lymph nodes in the mesentery detected on cross-sectional imaging. The entire node does not need to be removed in some cases; simply obtaining large biopsies with a cupped biopsy instrument may be adequate. Before leaving the operating room, it is important to receive confirmation from the pathologist regarding the diagnosis and ensure that the amount of tissue collected is adequate for flow cytometry or other pathologic evaluation.

A core needle biopsy obtained by a radiologist is an option in some cases. For example, image-guided core needle biopsy may be preferred in those patients with lymphadenopathy that is difficult to reach surgically, such as enlarged lymph nodes posterior to the renal vessels. In addition, image-guided lymph node biopsy is also an attractive alternative in patients who are at high risk or cannot tolerate anesthesia. Although percutaneous biopsy is less invasive, percutaneous biopsy remains inferior to the diagnostic accuracy of laparoscopic biopsy, which has been shown to be greater than 90%.

NATURAL ORIFICE TRANSLUMINAL ENDOSCOPIC SURGERY

Staging peritoneoscopy with natural orifice transluminal endoscopic surgery (NOTES) is a novel diagnostic approach that is currently undergoing evaluation. The methodology of NOTES has been validated in human and animal models. Transvaginal, transgastric, and transcolonic techniques have been described in the literature. In the Netherlands, Voermans and colleagues showed that transcolonic peritoneoscopy was inferior to standard laparoscopy in detection of peritoneal metastases in an animal model (53% vs 95%). Conversely, diagnostic transgastric endoscopic peritoneoscopy was found to have a 95% concordance with laparoscopic exploration for assessment of peritoneal metastasis with no infectious complications at The Ohio State University. Further research and development continue to evolve the means to endoscopically close the natural orifice entry site. At this time, diagnostic natural orifice endoscopic peritoneoscopy is considered an investigative technique and should only be performed with Institutional Review Board (IRB) approval and participation in Natural Orifice Surgery Consortium for Assessment and Research (NOSCAR).

SUMMARY

Advances in preoperative CT scan, endoscopic ultrasound scan, MRI, and PET cross-sectional imaging, and staging laparoscopy, have given physicians more detailed information with which to tailor oncologic therapies within standard national guidelines. By eliminating the need for laparotomy to assess tumor location and surgical resection candidacy, staging laparoscopy continues to play an important role in defining the next appropriate steps in the management of patients with gastrointestinal, hepatobiliary, pancreatic, and lymphoproliferative malignancies. Although routine use of staging laparoscopy continues for esophageal and bile duct malignancies, some investigators have argued for selective utilization of staging laparoscopy for gastric and pancreatic malignancies. As radiographic imaging, endoscopic ultrasound scan, and other staging modalities evolve, clinical trials will continue to further specify the role of laparoscopic investigation of patients with gastrointestinal malignancies.

SUGGESTED READINGS

Karanicolas PJ, Elkin EB, Jacks LM, et al: Staging laparoscopy in the management of gastric cancer: a population-based analysis, *J Am Coll Surg* 213(5):644–651, 2011.

Muntean V, Oniu T, Lungoci C, et al: Staging laparoscopy in digestive cancers, *J Gastrointestin Liver Dis* 18(4):461–467, 2009.

Rieder E, Swanstrom LL: Advances in cancer surgery: natural orifice surgery (NOTES) for oncological diseases, *Surg Oncol* 20(3):211–218, 2011.

Society of American Gastrointestinal and Endoscopic Surgeons: Diagnostic laparoscopy guidelines, *Surg Endosc* 22:1353–1383, 2008.

Winner M, Allendorf JD, Saif MW: An update on surgical staging of patients with pancreatic cancer, *JOP* 13(2):143–146, 2012.

LAPAROSCOPIC PANCREAS SURGERY

Martin A. Makary, MD, MPH

Laparoscopic pancreas surgery can be difficult to learn, but once mastered and applied appropriately, the approach yields clinical benefits for patients: namely, reduced wound complications and decreased postoperative pain. In the author's experience in performing 270 laparoscopic pancreas operations at Johns Hopkins Hospital, the wound infection rate is 1%, in comparison with 11% for open pancreas surgery. In addition, the laparoscopic approach is associated with decreased postoperative narcotic utilization, decreased time to ambulation, and increased activity level at discharge: patient-centered outcomes that are improved over those of open surgery. These benefits have implications for other outcomes because wound complications and decreased activity are risk factors for secondary complications and increased costs. Infection is an independent predictor of hospital readmission, and the presence of a wound complication often delays postoperative adjuvant therapy. Furthermore, the decrease in pain is of value, in view of the goal of a good quality of life for many patients with cancer and a poor prognosis. Kendrick and Cusati (2010), in one series, reported that laparoscopic pancreas surgery was associated with no superficial surgical site infections and a reduced length of stay. Other authors have also reported significantly decreased rates of incisional hernia and postoperative bowel obstruction, complications that occur in as many as 20% of patients after open surgery. Another benefit of laparoscopy may be improved cosmesis, an outcome of particular value in young patients who classically present with a pancreas cyst or neuroendocrine tumor. Many of the outcomes favorably influenced by laparoscopy (surgical infection, pain level, and patient satisfaction) are metrics increasingly being used by both surgical registries and payers to measure quality in surgery. In addition, the author has found that the 12-times magnification of new laparoscopic high-definition cameras allows the surgeon to visualize the anatomy better than does open surgery.

LAPAROSCOPIC WHIPPLE

The percentage of Whipple procedures performed laparoscopically at Johns Hopkins Hospital is increasing, and it is expected that the majority of Whipple operations will be performed laparoscopically by 2025. The laparoscopic approach is offered as the procedure of choice for patients who require a Whipple operation and do not have large (>5 cm) tumors or in whom tumors do not involve the large segment of the portal vein. Although other authorities have described laparoscopic resection of a long segment of the portal vein, the author's experience has been limited to partial vein resections managed with a laparoscopic side-biting vascular clamp.

The steps of a laparoscopic Whipple procedure (in order) are listed here and described afterwards:

1. Perform staging laparoscopy
2. Open the lesser sac
3. Resect a common hepatic artery lymph node
4. Divide the gastroduodenal artery
5. Divide the distal stomach
6. Dissect the portal structures
7. Perform cholecystectomy, and divide common bile duct
8. Divide the pancreas after separation from superior mesenteric vein
9. Perform Kocher maneuver
10. Divide jejunum
11. Mobilize the ligament of Treitz
12. Identify the superior mesenteric artery
13. Divide the uncinate/retroperitoneal attachments, and extract specimen
14. Extract jejunum through ligament of Treitz defect
15. Perform retrocolic pancreaticojejunostomy and hepaticojejunostomy
16. Perform antecolic (retrogastric) gastrojejunostomy
17. Drain placement

Technique

Peritoneal access is achieved through the caudal aspect of the umbilicus in a Hassan technique. Once the abdomen is distended, a left subcostal 12-mm bladeless VersaStep port (Covidien, Mansfield, Mass) is placed followed by a 5-mm bladeless VersaStep port left of the umbilicus so that there are two working ports on the patient's left side. The right-sided abdominal ports are then placed by insertion of a 5-mm port at the right subcostal region along the midclavicular line. Caudal to this port, two additional 12-mm ports are inserted so that there are two working ports on each side of the patient, as well as a port for a fan retractor to retract the duodenum and pylorus. A 10-mm, 45-degree laparoscope is used for visualization. The abdomen is explored for metastatic disease.

The lesser sac is accessed through the gastrocolic ligament to the second part of the duodenum. The right colon, including hepatic flexure, is sometimes mobilized. The gastroduodenal artery is then skeletonized, and a silk suture and one or two 10-mm clips are used on the proximal side. The artery is divided with a sealant device. The stomach is then divided just proximal to the pylorus with an Endo GIA stapling device (Covidien) with green or black loads (at least 4.8-mm size) for a classic-type Whipple procedure. A cholecystectomy is then performed, and the common bile duct is divided proximal to the entry site of the cystic duct, which enables the gallbladder to remain with the specimen for subsequent extraction.

The portal vein is then dissected from above the pancreas, and the superior mesenteric vein is dissected from below. A tunnel behind the pancreatic neck is created.

The transverse mesocolon is then raised cephalad to identify the ligament of Treitz. At approximately 15 cm distal to the ligament of Treitz, the small bowel is divided with an Endo GIA stapling device (Covidien) with a white load (2.5 mm). Each stapled end of the jejunum is sewn together with a 10-cm air knot so that the distal segment can later be pulled through the ligament of Treitz defect for the eventual reconstruction. The small bowel mesentery is also divided proximally to the ligament of Treitz, which is mobilized. Turning attention to the patient's right side, the surgeon then identifies the superior mesenteric artery, and the branches of the artery and vein going into the Whipple specimen are divided with the LigaSure (Figure 1) (Covidien); clips are used as needed on larger branches. The Whipple specimen is then extracted out in a 15-mm bag through the umbilicus. The jejunum is extracted intact initially. The fascia and skin defects are extended to approximately 3 to 4 cm for the extraction.

The small bowel is passed through the ligament of Treitz in order to perform an end-to-side pancreaticojejunostomy. This is performed in a handsewn manner over a pancreatic duct stent with the use of a 3F, 5F, or 8F pediatric feeding tube placed into the duct (Figure 2) and into a 2-mm to 3-mm opening in the side of the jejunum. Two running 3-0 barbed stitches (V-Loc sutures; Covidien) are used for the front and back side of the pancreaticojejunostomy. The hepaticojejunostomy is then performed with placement of a single layer of 4-0 Vicryl stitches handsewn in an interrupted manner. The gastrojejunostomy is then performed in an antecolic retrogastric manner along the posterior wall of the stomach in a stapled side-to-side technique with an Endo GIA 60 stapler. The resulting defect is then closed with interrupted stitches.

In patients in whom the pancreas is soft, a surgical drain is then placed near the anastomoses. All 12-mm port sites are closed at the level of the fascia.

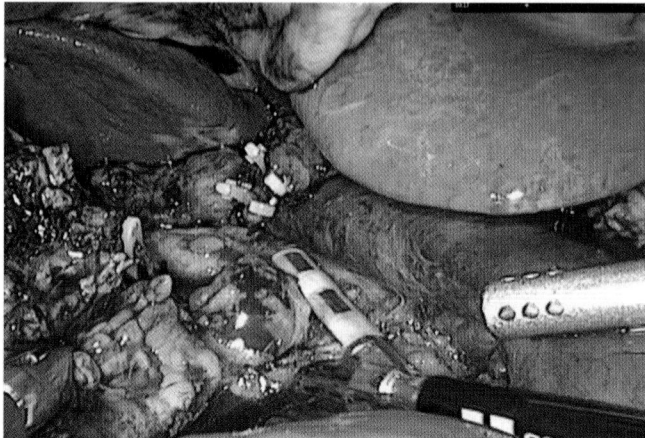

FIGURE 1 Uncinate dissection: division of the pancreas along the portal vein and superior mesenteric artery. (Gastroduodenal artery is clipped with the white clips above.)

Of note, for all of the author's advanced laparoscopic pancreas procedures, a No. 10 blade scalpel and Mayo scissors are always kept on the Mayo stand in case a rapid conversion to open procedure is necessary. Unlike other laparoscopic procedures, laparoscopic pancreas surgery may have to be converted expeditiously to an open approach because of the intimate proximity of the large vessels in the region. The author also makes sure that no pop-off stitches are used

because these can easily pop off inadvertently while in the insufflated field. Care is taken to make sure hypercarbia is managed appropriately if it is noted from an elevated end-tidal CO_2 level.

The author does not use the robot for the laparoscopic Whipple procedure because of the longer operative time currently associated with robotic surgery; however, it may be a useful tool for performing the reconstruction, and future generations of robotic devices may yield advantages not yet realized. In the author's most recent 50 laparoscopic Whipple procedures, mean operative time was 5 hours, 25 minutes. Postoperative management follows a similar pathway as for the open Whipple procedure, although narcotic utilization and activity level during the inpatient recovery are noticeably improved with the laparoscopic approach.

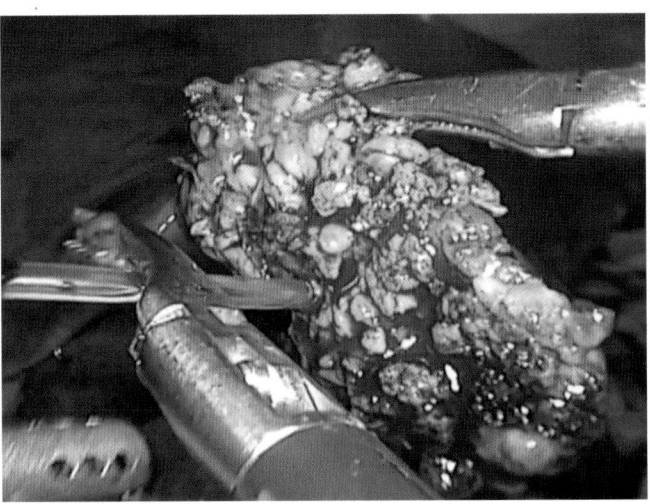

FIGURE 2 Placing a pancreatic duct stent into the divided pancreas.

LAPAROSCOPIC DISTAL PANCREATECTOMY

Most distal pancreas tumors are ideal candidates for laparoscopic resection. The author offers a laparoscopic distal pancreatectomy to patients who have lesions that do not involve the celiac or mesenteric vessels and are less than 6 or 7 cm in size. The author routinely attempts spleen preservation when there is no suspicion of malignancy, and the spleen can be spared in 70% of distal pancreatectomies in this setting (Figure 3 and 4). Of importance is that in cases in which malignancy is suspected on the basis of imaging studies or a family history of pancreas cancer, the author removes the spleen with the tail of the pancreas en bloc to achieve a wide resection of

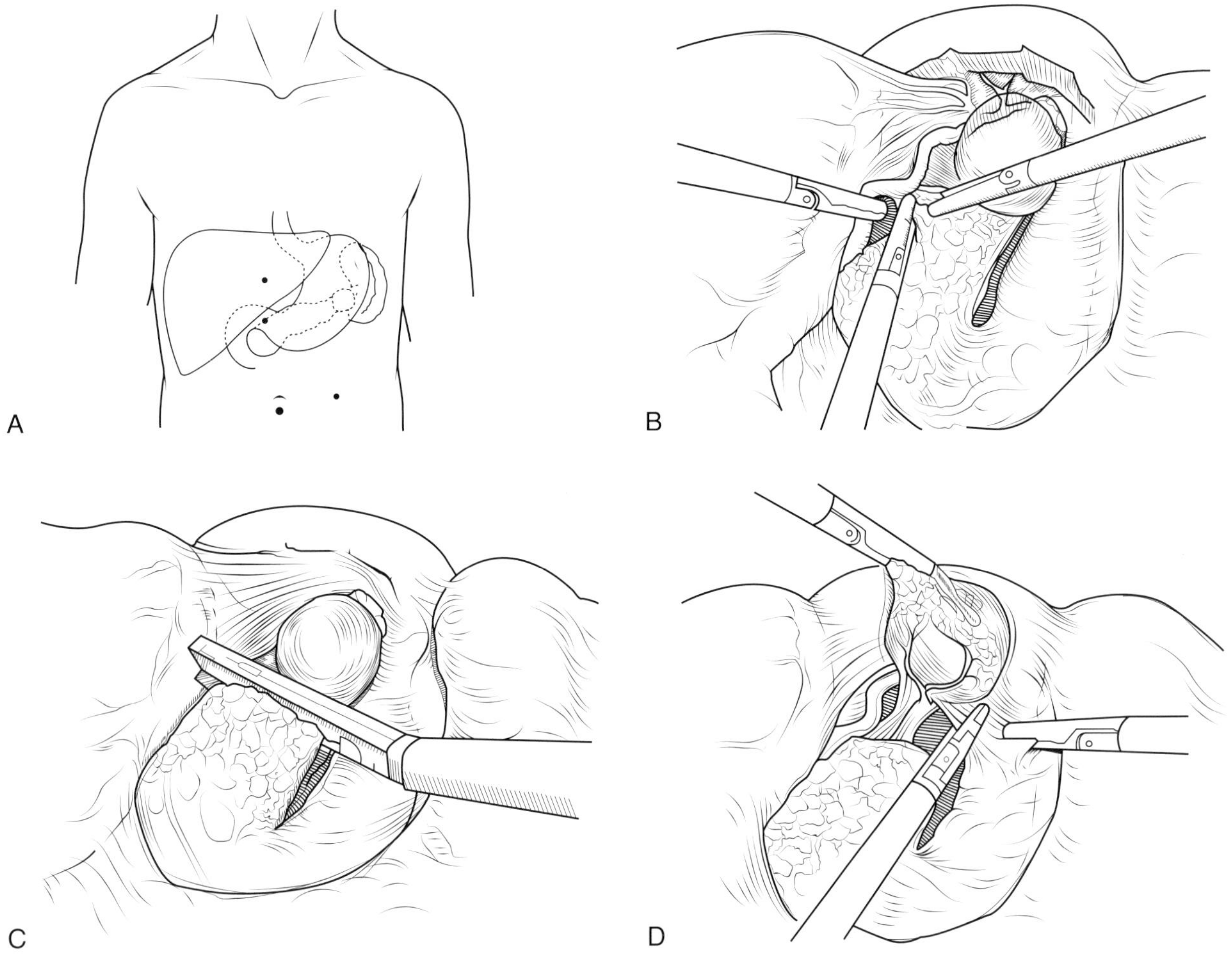

A

B

C

D

FIGURE 3 Spleen preserving distal pancreactomy: port site placement and vessel-preserving technique.

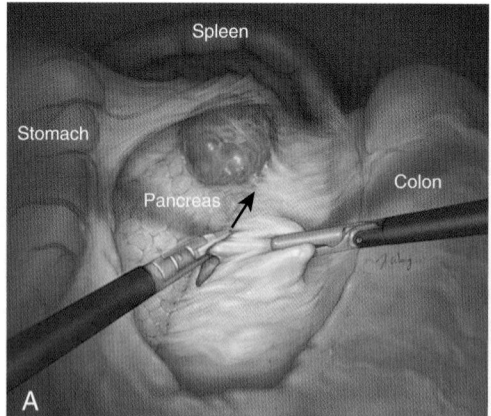
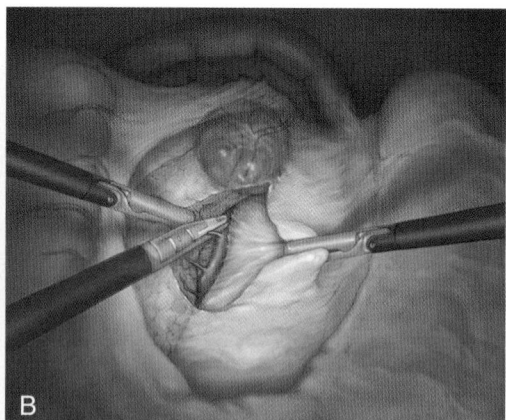

FIGURE 4 **A** and **B,** Laparoscopic distal pancreatectomy. (© Jenny Wang, 2008.)

the lymph node basin in the area of the splenic vessels and splenic hilum. In the author's experience, laparoscopic distal pancreatectomy can result in improved patient outcomes and an increased likelihood for splenic preservation in appropriate situations.

Preoperative Tattooing

For small lesions of the pancreatic neck, body, and tail, particularly those that are posterior, the author uses a novel technique to tattoo pancreatic lesions to facilitate identification at the time of laparoscopic surgery. In each patient scheduled for a laparoscopic distal pancreatectomy, the pancreatic lesion is tattooed via an endoscopic transgastric technique under endoscopic ultrasound guidance before surgery (Figure 5). Using an endoscopic 22-gauge needle, the surgeon injects a total of 5 mL of concentrated purified carbon particles (GI Spot dye; GI Supply, Camp Hill, Pa) are injected into the pancreatic parenchyma immediately proximal to the tumor. The dye is injected to create a vertical line deep in the pancreas parenchyma because the dye may need to be identified from the posterior aspect of the gland during the dissection.

Preoperative marking enables the surgeon to quickly identify the location of the tumor at the time of laparoscopy and guides the decision of where to divide the gland. The author has found that tattooing significantly decreases the author's operative time for distal pancreatectomy. Furthermore, it helps avoid the awkward situation of missing a subtle tumor in the resected specimen—a hazard of the decreased tactile sense in laparoscopic palpation with long instruments. Even large tumors detected on computed tomography, which a surgeon can anticipate identifying easily, can be surprisingly difficult to find because of the homogeneous color of the pancreas and its retroperitoneal bed.

Technique

The laparoscopic distal pancreatectomy steps (in order) are listed as follows and described afterwards:

- Perform staging laparoscopy
- Open the lesser sac
- Perform takedown of the splenic flexure of the colon
- Distinguish the splenic vessels from the hepatic vessels
- Divide splenic artery unless the spleen is preserved
- Mobilize the distal pancreas, and divide splenic vein if splenectomy is performed
- Extract specimen
- Place a drain in the divided stapled pancreas

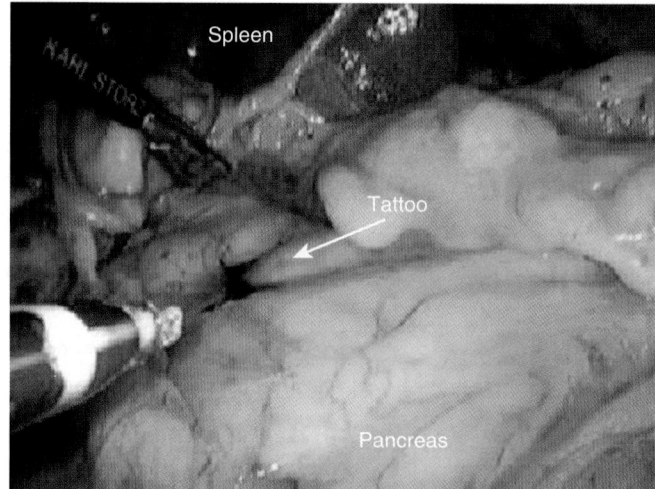

FIGURE 5 **A** and **B,** Tail of pancreas with tattoo and spleen in background. (© Jenny Wang, 2008.)

The author places an infraumbilical port with a Hassan method. Two ports placed in the upper midline (or right of midline) and one port in the left lower quadrant are inserted under direct visualization (see Figure 4). The precise locations of these ports depend on the location of the tumor, the intention to preserve the spleen, and the patient's body habitus. Once local landmarks are identified, the gastrocolic omentum and short gastric vessels are divided, followed by takedown of the splenic flexure of the colon to achieve wide visualization of the lesser sac. Mobilization of the gland is easiest from the inferior border of the gland (see Figure 5). Thus, beginning with the inferior approach facilitates dissection of the posterior aspect of the gland from the retroperitoneal bed. The splenic artery and vein branches can be visualized from underneath the pancreas, and the author alternates dissection of the splenic vessels from above and below the gland according to which exposure best offers visualization.

Once the pancreas is clear from the splenic vessels to allow for division of the gland, the author attempts to dissect as much of the tail as possible, freeing the entire tail when feasible. The gland is divided with a stapler with a size chosen on the basis of the pancreas thickness. On occasion, the author has used a reticulating stapler reinforced with a bioabsorbable staple line material (GORE SEAM-GUARD, Gore Medical, Newark, Del). The specimen is removed with an Endo Catch bag (Covidien), and a surgical drain is place at the cut end of the pancreas.

Laparoscopic Distal Pancreatectomy With Splenectomy

When a malignancy is suspected or a technical reason necessitates removal of the spleen, the author chooses to mobilize the spleen after individual division of the splenic artery, splenic vein, and gland. Care is taken to ensure that the splenic artery is not confused with the hepatic artery. Dissection of the splenic artery toward the spleen is sometimes necessary to ensure that the splenic artery is not mistaken for the hepatic artery. The splenic artery and the vein, respectively, are each ligated in turn with a vascular stapler; sometimes these vessels are approached from the posterior aspect of the gland. The spleen is mobilized from its attachments as the last step of the operation.

When the spleen is removed for technical or anatomic (nononcologic) reasons, the author divides the pancreas from the spleen to morcellate (liquefy) the spleen for easy extraction from the peritoneum. The intact specimen is freely suspended in the insufflated abdomen, and then the spleen is divided from the tail of the pancreas with a series of GIA staplers fired close to the spleen to avoid leaving residual pancreatic tissue or lymph nodes on the spleen side. This intracorporeal separation allows for removal of the pancreas intact and the spleen by the morcellation technique. However, a stitch or orientation via the tattoo is needed to identify the true pancreatic margin. This piecemeal extraction method is not applicable when an oncologic margin could be threatened by the intracorporeal separation of the pancreas and spleen. In this case, the specimen is removed en bloc in an Endo Catch bag, which necessitates a small extension of the midline 12-mm port sites. A frozen-section analysis is performed intraoperatively to confirm a negative and adequate margin of resection before the operation is completed.

At all times, an Endo GIA 2.5-mm (white vascular load) stapler is open, loaded, and ready to use in case of injury to the splenic vessels. Clips are avoided because stapling devices cannot engage on a clip. As a precaution, the author always keeps a fresh 10-blade scalpel and curved heavy Mayo scissors ready at all times in case a rapid conversion to an open operation is needed to control bleeding.

Patient Outcomes

Patients are admitted to the surgical floor for a typical hospital stay of 2 to 4 days after surgery. The author has observed that these patients behave clinically similar to patients who have undergone laparoscopic cholecystectomy and adrenalectomy: they often require little or no narcotic pain medication. Wound complications are rare after the laparoscopic technique; however, the pancreatic leak rate for all types of laparoscopic pancreas surgery is identical to that for the open operation.

LAPAROSCOPIC CENTRAL PANCREATECTOMY

Less common procedures such as a central pancreatectomy entail the same principles and indications as the open procedure. The author has found that these procedures are ideal in patients who are at risk for developing diabetes or worsening insulin dependence after pancreas surgery. To perform central pancreatectomy, central masses are approached in the same way as in a laparoscopic Whipple procedure, whereby the surgeon delineates the vascular anatomy and creates a tunnel behind the neck of the pancreas.

LAPAROSCOPIC TOTAL PANCREATECTOMY WITH ISLET AUTOTRANSPLANTATION

The author has found laparoscopy to be ideal for patients who require a pancreatectomy for chronic pancreatitis because of the decreased pain benefits, inasmuch as the pain is often challenging to manage. During the procedure, after the pancreas is resected with the techniques described previously, the author performs the hepaticojejunostomy and gastrojejunostomy while the islets are being prepared in the laboratory in the operating room. Once the islet solution is ready for autotransplantation into the liver, the author places a metal hollow-bore 16-gauge needle with intravenous tubing attached through a 12-mm port site. From within the peritoneal cavity, the author uses laparoscopic instruments to place the needle into the splenic or portal vein. The islet infusion is then delivered, the needle is subsequently removed, and direct pressure is applied to the puncture site of the vein to achieve hemostasis (Figure 6).

OLDER AND HIGH-RISK PATIENTS

The author has found that frail older patients and other high-risk patients are ideal candidates for the minimally invasive approach. For such patients, the author uses the lowest insufflation pressures (usually 9 to 11 mm Hg), which allows good visualization. Using appropriate monitoring, the author has observed that the recovery benefits of a laparoscopic resection are magnified in octogenarian patients who have undergone the procedure. As is true for young patients, laparoscopic distal pancreatectomy in frail older patients is a shorter procedure and is associated with less physiologic stress to the patient. Moreover, the decreased postoperative pain associated with laparoscopy allows patients to ambulate earlier and more frequently than patients who undergo open surgery, which decreases the risk of thrombosis.

CONCLUSION

The author's technique and experience with laparoscopic pancreas surgery have been described. A strong foundation with open pancreas surgery is an important prerequisite for developing skills in laparoscopic pancreas surgery. In summary, when applied appropriately, laparoscopy is associated with decreased wound complications

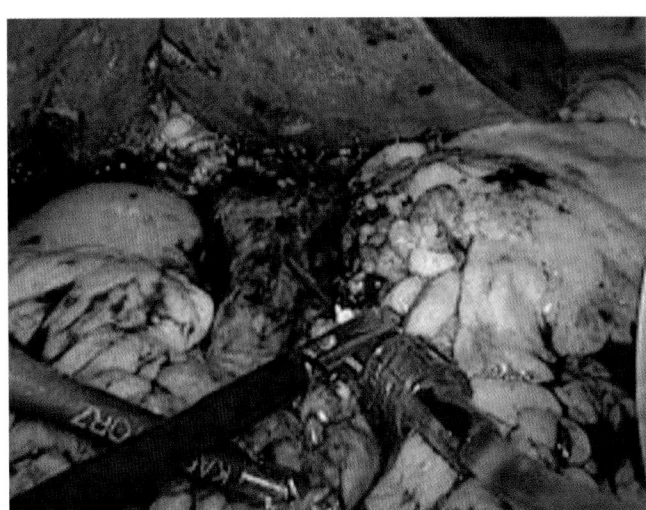

FIGURE 6 Laparoscopic islet autotransplantation infusion into portal vein.

and less pain for patients, and it minimizes the risk for long-term complications such as incisional hernia and small bowel obstruction. In the setting of cancer, an adequate lymphadenectomy with an en bloc resection can be accomplished with a wide resection of the regional lymph nodes. Furthermore, in the absence of a large wound, laparoscopic distal pancreatectomy for cancer allows for a shorter interval to adjuvant therapy when indicated. Laparoscopy is particularly ideal for candidate patients with decreased physiologic reserve or cardiopulmonary risk factors. In the future, improved surgical techniques may decrease the learning curve and enable more patients to benefit from the decreased complications observed.

ACKNOWLEDGMENTS

The author thanks Ms. Jenny Y. Wang of the Johns Hopkins University Graduate School for Art Applied to Medicine, who has demonstrated the procedure through the drawings presented in this chapter. The illustrations are copyrighted to Jenny Wang, 2008.

SUGGESTED READINGS

Boutros C, Ryan K, Katz S, et al: Total laparoscopic distal pancreatectomy: beyond selected patients, Am Surg 77(11):1526–1530, 2011.
Bruzoni M, Sasson AR: Open and laparoscopic spleen-preserving, splenic vessel-preserving distal pancreatectomy: indications and outcomes, J Gastrointest Surg 12:1202–1206, 2008.
Kendrick ML, Cusati D: Total laparoscopic pancreaticoduodenectomy: feasibility and outcome in an early experience, Arch Surg 145(1):19–23, 2010.
Kooby DA, Gillespie T, Bentrem D, et al: Left-sided pancreatectomy: a multicenter comparison of laparoscopic and open approaches, Ann Surg 248:438–446, 2008.
Makary MA, Warshaw AL, Centeno BA, et al: Implications of periotoneal cytology for pancreatic cancer management, Arch Surg 133:361–365, 1998.
Newman NA, Lennon AM, Edil BH, et al: Preoperative endoscopic tattooing of pancreatic body and tail lesions decreases operative time for laparoscopic distal pancreatectomy, Surgery 148(2):371–377, 2010.
Venkat R, Edil BH, Schulick RD, et al: Laparoscopic distal pancreatectomy is associated with significantly less overall morbidity compared to the open technique: a systematic review and meta-analysis, Ann Surg 255(6):1048–1059, 2012.

LAPAROSCOPIC BYPASS FOR PANCREATIC CANCER

Peter Nau, MD, MS, and Peter Muscarella, MD

BACKGROUND

Pancreatic cancer is the ninth most common cancer in the United States, with approximately 44,030 cases in 2011. Of those, 37,660 will succumb to the disease, making pancreatic cancer the fourth most common cancer causing death. Five-year survival for all stages remains low at 6%. To date, adjuncts to surgical therapy remain inadequate. An R0 resection offers the best chance for cure, but only 10% to 20% of patients will have resectable disease at time of presentation. Consequently, surgical management of pancreatic cancer is often performed for palliation rather than with a curative intent.

Given the high rates of locally invasive and metastatic disease at presentation, many patients are found to have unresectable tumors prior to surgical intervention by evaluation with radiographic and endoscopic staging modalities. With the sensitivity of high-resolution multidetector computed tomography for predicting resectability as high as 96%, this has become increasingly common. In these clinical scenarios there is an opportunity to palliate the patient outside of the operating suite.

The use of endoscopically placed stents for palliation of biliary obstruction has been shown to be a successful modality for patients who are not surgical candidates. The use of metallic stents in these cases is preferred because they are associated with a lower risk of recurrent biliary obstructions. Endoscopic palliation of gastric outlet obstruction (GOO) is also well described. In the multicenter, randomized SUSTENT trial, endoscopic palliation was compared to surgical bypass for the treatment of malignant GOO. In this study, stent placement proved to be a superior treatment for patients with a life expectancy of 2 months or less. However, in those with increased predicted survival, endoscopic palliation was associated with more major complications at a higher mean hospital cost. Furthermore, in the patients who had a longer anticipated life expectancy there were statistically significant increases in food intake, fewer recurrent obstructive symptoms, and a decreased necessity for reinterventions in those who underwent a surgical gastrojejunostomy. It should not go unnoticed that this study was limited by a low patient accrual. This is not unexpected given patient preference for a minimally invasive procedure, thus complicating the extrapolation of the data to a wider population. That being said, current literature supports the use of metallic stents for the endoscopic palliation of biliary obstruction. Additionally, in those with GOO and an estimated life expectancy of 2 months or less, an endoscopic approach is reasonable. Outside of that time frame, the procedure is fraught with complications and increased costs, and it should not be included in the physician's therapeutic armamentarium.

There is little debate that the palliation of GOO secondary to locally invasive disease is associated with an improved quality of life. However, given that as few as 10% of patients with unresectable periampullary malignancies progress to a GOO, the concept of addressing gastric drainage prophylactically is more controversial. In an effort to address this issue, the group at Johns Hopkins Medical Institution completed a prospective, randomized study for prophylactic retrocolic gastrojejunostomy versus no intervention in patients found intraoperatively to have unresectable periampullary carcinomas. They noted that the addition of the prophylactic procedure decreased the incidence of late GOO without a concomitant increase in morbidity or length of stay. A review of the Cochrane Database further clarified the issue, confirming that a prophylactic gastrojejunostomy is indicated in all patients with unresectable periampullary carcinoma already undergoing surgical exploration. Whether the prophylactic procedure should be completed outside of the situation where the abdomen is already open remains controversial.

GASTRIC OUTLET OBSTRUCTION

Laparoscopic Gastrojejunostomy

Technical considerations for laparoscopic gastrojejunostomy begin with appropriate thrombotic and antibiotic prophylaxis. Following placement of an indwelling Foley catheter and temporary orogastric tube, positioning of the patient is completed. At our institution we prefer the split leg position with the arms abducted and foot boards in place. All pressure points are protected, and the patient is secured to the bed to allow for deep Trendelenberg positioning. This positioning places the operative surgeon on the patient's right with the assistant on the left and a camera holder between the patient's legs.

Accessing the abdomen can be accomplished via an open, cutdown or closed technique. It is our preference to use a veress needle placed in the left upper quadrant to establish pneumoperitoneum. We find that placement of the camera port in the periumbilical position is more consistent when performed following distention of the abdominal wall. Generally, the periumbilical port is placed cephalad to the umbilicus, approximately 15 to 17 cm caudal to the xyphoid process. For this operation, a 10-mm, 30-degree scope is used due to the associated increased illumination and better optics, necessitating a 10-mm supraumbilical port. In total, three additional ports are placed. These are placed with a gentle curve or U-shape conformation with the apex at the midline port. Two ports are placed in the left abdomen. These are placed no less than 1 handbreadth apart to optimize ergonomics and minimize crossing of instruments. The trocars can be 5 mm in size to minimize pain and potential postoperative morbidity. The right-sided trocar should be placed to mirror the medial port on the left, with an option for a fifth port placed more laterally if necessary for bowel manipulation or when it is elected to close the common defect in the gastrojejunostomy via intracorporal suturing techniques. A 12-mm trocar is placed at the more medial right sided port to facilitate stapling and/or intracorporal suturing. In the event that a robotic-assisted procedure is chosen, trocar placement must be more spread out to prevent the arms from colliding with one another.

The operation is begun by examining the small bowel mesentery and the omentum. A foreshortened mesentery or one that is infiltrated with tumor is not amenable to a bypass procedure. Further, the inability to reflect the omentum cephalad may make a laparoscopic procedure prohibitively difficult. In these situations the minimally invasive approach may not be feasible and an open technique should be considered.

Next, the transverse colon is elevated using atraumatic bowel graspers, and the ligament of Treitz is identified. The small intestine is elevated and oriented in an antecolic, isoperistaltic position adjacent to the greater curvature of the stomach. Having verified that the small intestine reaches without undue tension, the lesser sac is entered and the short gastric vessels are ligated with a laparoscopic energy device. It may be unnecessary to ligate all vessels high up on the greater curvature. The goal of this maneuver is to mobilize and expose the greater curvature of the stomach to allow for the creation of a retrogastric anastomosis. This does necessitate the division of any retrogastric attachments to the retroperitoneum. For the most part, this is an avascular dissection. However, it is best completed with a laparoscopic energy device to secure hemostasis. Pancreatitis related to the underlying disease process and associated obstruction may complicate this task. Attention should be paid to the transverse colon and its associated mesentery because injury to these structures can complicate the operation and postoperative hospital course. Placing the patient in reverse Trendelenburg position following mobilization of the stomach will facilitate visualization by allowing the colon to fall out of the operative field. Prior to creation of the anastomosis, a single proximal tacking stitch between the jejunum and stomach is placed to orient the specimens. Next, using electrocautery, enterotomies are made in the antimesenteric border of the jejunum and the posterior wall of the stomach adjacent to the greater curvature. The anastomosis is created using a laparoscopic stapling device (Figure 1). We use staplers with a 60-mm staple length and a depth of no less than 3.5 mm. Staple depth may be increased at the discretion of the operative surgeon based on the thickness of the stomach wall.

Closure of the common enterotomy can be accomplished with intracorporal suturing or an additional firing of the laparoscopic

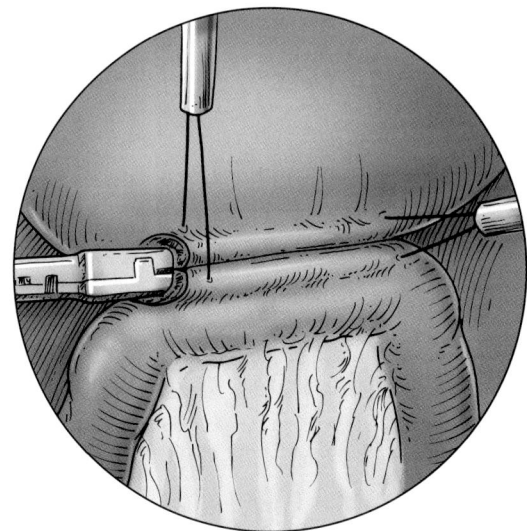

FIGURE 1   Sketch of the gastrojejunostomy, orienting of the antimesenteric border of the jejunum, and the greater curvature of the stomach prior to staple line creation. *(From Tsiaosssis J, Tsiotos GG: Gastroenterostomy. In Calvien PA, Sarr MG, Fong Y, editors:* Atlas of upper gastrointestinal and hepato-pancreato-biliary surgery, *Heidelberg, 2007, Springer-Verlag.)*

stapling device. A hand-sewn closure is completed in two layers. The inner layer is comprised of a running 3-0 absorbable suture, with an outer layer of interrupted 3-0 nonabsorbable suture to imbricate the edges of the anastomosis. We have found that using two running sutures starting at both ends and then tying them together in the middle is preferable for the inner layer and may decrease the risk of leaks at the ends of the closure. In some hands this procedure may be more reliably completed with the use of a laparoscopic suturing device such as the EndoStitch (Covidien, Norwalk, Conn). In the event that a stapled closure is chosen, attention should be paid to the efferent limb, as this lumen can be easily narrowed. Alternatively, a robotically assisted anastomosis can be fashioned (Figure 2). This technology is particularly suited for suturing and can facilitate creation of a hand-sewn gastrojejunostomy. Assessment of the anastomosis is accomplished via endoscopic insufflation of the stomach while submerging under saline to evaluate for air bubbles. All 10-mm fascial defects are closed at our institution. This is accomplished with a standard figure-of-eight stitch of a large-caliber absorbable suture (0-0 or 1-0) after desufflation of the abdomen or with a suture passer under laparoscopic guidance.

Postoperatively, the patients are kept nil per os (NPO) overnight. On the morning of postoperative day 1, the Foley catheter is removed, and a clear liquid diet is initiated. The diet is advanced as tolerated. In the event that postprandial nausea and delayed gastric emptying are encountered, metoclopramide or erythromycin and antiemetics can be administered. Patients are discharged once they are able to tolerate a diet, with return of gastrointestinal tract function.

LAPAROSCOPIC BILIARY BYPASS PROCEDURES

While feasible, a minimally invasive approach to the palliation of a biliary obstruction is more technically demanding. Moreover, given the complexity of the procedure and decreased morbidity of an endoscopically placed stent, it is easy to see why the majority of malignant biliary obstructions are addressed with biliary stenting rather than by surgical bypass. However, in the event that endoscopic

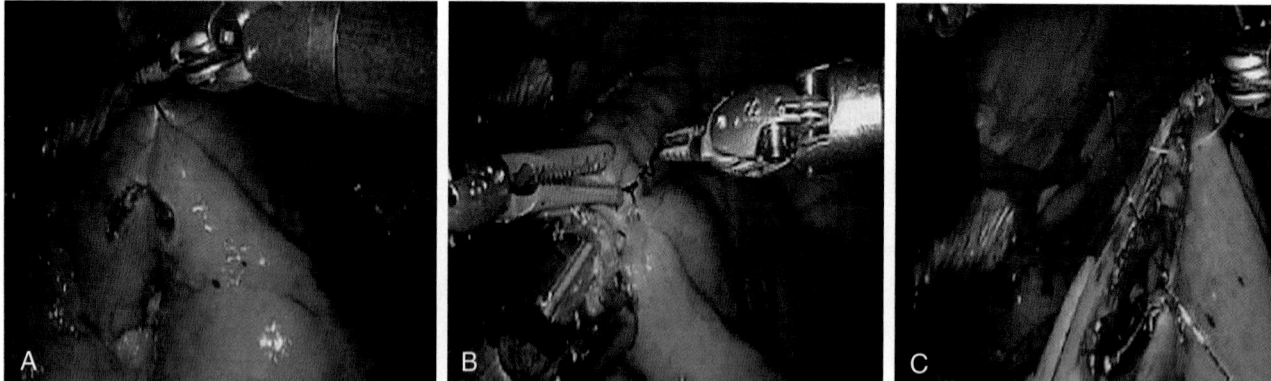

FIGURE 2 Sequential steps illustrating the robotic-assisted gastrojejunostomy. **A,** Tacking the jejunum to the posterior gastric wall, with subsequent creation of enterotomies for staple firing. **B,** Creation of the gastrojejunostomy with a laparoscopic stapling device. **C,** Suture closure of the common enterotomy.

means are not feasible or have failed, the incorporation of this procedure with a gastrojejunostomy to palliate the obstructive symptoms may be necessary.

Laparoscopic Cholecystojejunostomy

Laparoscopic cholecystojejunostomy is well described in the literature. In this procedure the technical demands of a hand-sewn anastomosis are circumvented with the creation of a stapled anastomosis between a distended gallbladder and the jejunum. This is appealing in that it mirrors the procedure performed with an open approach. Further, it requires only token dissection, minimizing the procedure-related morbidity to which the patient is exposed. It has been recommended that this procedure only be considered in those with a radiographically proven patent hepatocystic junction that is well removed from the malignant obstruction. With that said, this operation has fallen out of favor due to a documented 4.4-fold increase in the necessity for reintervention in the population when compared to those that are palliated with a hepaticojejunostomy. In the setting of a palliative operation, we believe this is prohibitively high, making the cholecystojejunostomy a procedure of historic interest only.

Laparoscopic Choledochoduodenostomy

Given the proximity of the duodenum and the common practice of creating a choledochoduodenostomy for refractory calculous disease, it has been proposed to adopt this technique for the treatment of malignant obstructions. Given the nature of the underlying pathology and the propensity for extension of the malignant process, this may be an inadequate or difficult operation in this patient population. The decision to incorporate this methodology for a biliary bypass should only be made when a thorough inspection of the right upper quadrant has convinced the surgeon that extension of the tumor will not cause a recurrent obstruction. Given the propensity for the development of a GOO, it has been suggested that this procedure should be performed with a concomitant palliative gastrojejunostomy.

Technical considerations that arise with the addition of a biliary anastomosis include the necessity of the fifth, right-sided trocar and the need for effective liver retraction. We prefer to use a self-retaining Nathanson liver retractor placed through a subxiphoid stab incision for hands-free exposure of the hepatoduodenal ligament. Using the aforementioned port configuration, a Cattell-Braasch maneuver is performed so as to obtain enough mobility that a tension-free anastomosis can be created. Next, the common bile duct is dissected out from its lateral position in the hepatoduodenal ligament. This is

easiest with laparoscopic Maryland forceps and intermittent application of the cautery using the hook dissector. Finally, prior to completion of the anastomosis, a cholecystectomy is completed using standard surgical techniques.

We use a diamond-shaped anastomosis, employing a 1-cm to 2-cm longitudinal duodenotomy and a 1-cm to 2-cm choledochotomy. The apices of the choledochotomy are secured to the midpoints of the duodenotomy (Figure 3). This is completed with a hand-sewn technique using interrupted stitches of 5-0 or 6-0 absorbable, monofilament suture. Alternatively, the back row of the anastomosis can be created using a running suture. Creation of the anastomosis is a complex procedure, but it may be facilitated by placement of the most lateral stitches first. In this way, the anastomosis is orientated and anchored in place for further stitch placement. It is the standard practice at this institution to leave a single 19F Jackson-Pratt (JP) drain in the dependent portion of the right upper quadrant to drain any potential anastomotic leaks. A nasogastric tube is placed in all cases that involve a biliary anastomosis. Postoperative care includes maintenance of a nasogastric tube to low intermittent suction and NPO status while awaiting return of bowel function. Typically, in the absence of any bilious drainage, the JP drain is removed prior to discharge.

Laparoscopic Choledochojejunostomy

Choledochojejunostomy maximizes symptom resolution while minimizing potential morbidity. This operation is set up similarly to the aforementioned choledochoduodenostomy with a five-port technique. A prophylactic gastrojejunostomy may be created proximal to the choledochojejunostomy, but it requires a diverting entero-enterostomy. This procedure is technically challenging when performed laparoscopically, and the risks may outweigh any potential benefits. We prefer an antecolic, loop choledochojejunostomy to the creation of a Roux-en-Y because it eliminates the potential morbidities of small bowel division and the additional anastomosis. Having completely mobilized the stomach and reflected the colon in a caudal direction, the jejunum is approximated to the hepatoduodenal ligament and stomach to ensure that tension-free anastomoses can be created. The choledochojejunostomy is then fashioned in a manner mirroring the choledochoduodenostomy.

It should be noted that robotic-assisted techniques are uniquely suited for the creation of these difficult biliary anastomoses. The three-dimensional optics and increased degrees of freedom provided by the DaVinci Surgical System (Intuitive Surgical, Inc., Sunnyvale, Calif) facilitate what is otherwise a prohibitively difficult procedure in most surgeons' hands. To incorporate the robot in this operation, complete mobilization of the duodenum and stomach is completed.

of patients in whom cure is not possible due to metastatic or locally advanced disease. Endoscopic stenting may be useful in many patients, but surgery continues to play a role in patients who are found to have unresectable disease at the time of surgical exploration or who have failed or are not candidates for endoscopic therapy. In addition, surgical palliation may have better results for patients whose life expectancies are more than several weeks. The role for palliative gastric bypass is unclear, but the procedure appears to offer benefit for patients who are already undergoing surgery for exploration and/or biliary bypass procedures. Minimally invasive techniques offer the potential benefits of decreased morbidity, pain, and hospital length of stay when performed by experienced surgeons. Robotic-assistance with these procedures may improve outcomes for many surgeons, offering improved visualization and suturing capability for these sometimes difficult anastomoses.

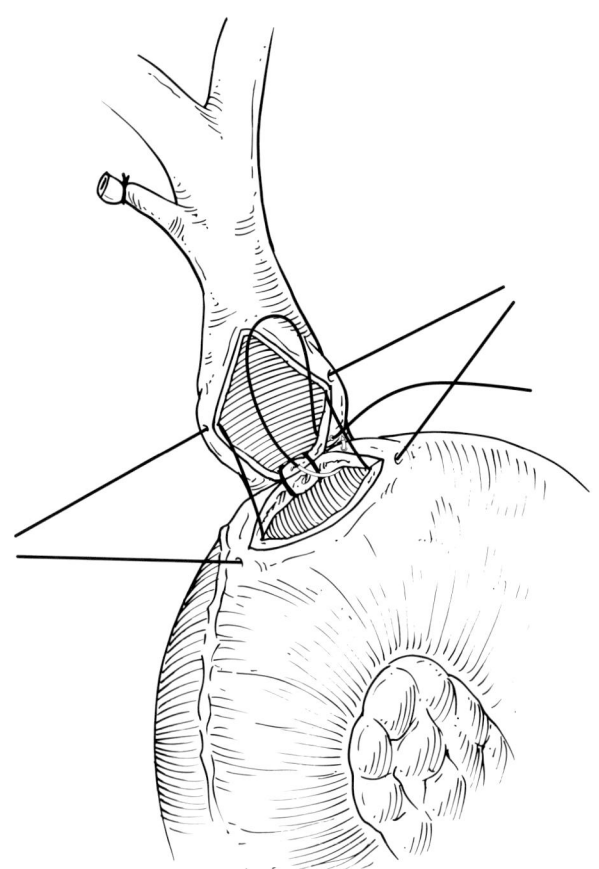

FIGURE 3 Creation of a side-to-side choledochoduodenostomy. Stay sutures aid in orienting the bowel. *(From Riall TS: Choledochoduodenostomy and Hepaticojejunostomy. In Townsend CM, Evers BM, editors: Atlas of general surgical techniques, St. Louis, 2010, Saunders.)*

After having oriented the jejunum in position, the robot is docked and the anastomosis completed. The means for completion of the concomitant gastrojejunostomy is left at the discretion of the surgeon. Postoperative care mirrors that for the choledochoduodenostomy.

CONCLUSIONS

Pancreatic cancer is a common cause of cancer death, and most patients present with advanced disease. Palliation of biliary and gastric outlet obstruction is necessary for many of the 80% to 90%

SUGGESTED READINGS

Contreras CM, Stanelle EJ, Mansour J, et al: Staging laparoscopy enhances the detection of occult metastases in patients with pancreatic adenocarcinoma, *J Surg Oncol* 100(8):663–669, 2009.

Espat NJ, Brennan MF, Conlon KC: Patients with laparoscopically staged unresectable pancreatic adenocarcinoma do not require subsequent surgical biliary or gastric bypass, *J Am Coll Surg* 188(6):649–655; discussion 655–657, 1999.

Gurusamy KS, Kumar S, Davidson BR: Prophylactic gastrojejunostomy for unresectable periampullary carcinoma, *Cochrane Database Syst Rev* (10):CD008533, 2010.

Jeurnink SM, Steyerberg EW, van Hooft JE, et al: Surgical gastrojejunostomy or endoscopic stent placement for the palliation of malignant gastric outlet obstruction (SUSTENT study): a multicenter randomized trial, *Gastrointest Endosc* 71(3):490–499, 2010.

Kazanjian KK, Reber HA, Hines OJ: Laparoscopic gastrojejunostomy for gastric outlet obstruction in pancreatic cancer, *Am Surg* 70(10):910–913, 2004.

Lillemoe KD, Cameron JL, Hardacre JM, et al: Is prophylactic gastrojejunostomy indicated for unresectable periampullary cancer? A prospective randomized trial, *Ann Surg* 230(3):322–328; discussion 328–330, 1999.

Moss AC, Morris E, Mac Mathuna P: Palliative biliary stents for obstructing pancreatic carcinoma, *Cochrane Database Syst Rev* (1):CD004200, 2006.

Navarra G, Musolino C, Venneri A, et al: Palliative antecolic isoperistaltic gastrojejunostomy: a randomized controlled trial comparing open and laparoscopic approaches, *Surg Endosc* 20(12):1831–1834, 2006.

Sarr MG, Cameron JL: Surgical management of unresectable carcinoma of the pancreas, *Surgery* 91(2):123–133, 1982.

Urbach DR, Bell CM, Swanstrom LL, et al: Cohort study of surgical bypass to the gallbladder or bile duct for the palliation of jaundice due to pancreatic cancer, *Ann Surg* 237(1):86–93, 2003.

Laparoscopic Management of Pancreatic Pseudocyst

Andre Ilbawi, MD, and
Karen D. Horvath, MD, FACS

OVERVIEW

With the improved understanding of the complications of acute pancreatitis in the last half century, more precise morphologic terms have evolved. The most recent revision of the 1992 Atlanta Symposium terms should be used for all clinical and research communications (Table 1). With use of these descriptors, a pancreatic pseudocyst is a fluid-filled collection with minimal or no necrosis. It forms after disruption of the pancreatic duct leaking activated pancreatic enzymes into the peripancreatic tissues. The resultant inflammatory reaction stimulates a fibrous pseudocapsule to form after about 4 weeks. Pseudocysts can form after an episode of acute pancreatitis (2% to 10%) or after an acute exacerbation of chronic pancreatitis (20% to 40%). In contrast, patients who have development of necrotizing pancreatitis, with resulting necrosis of the pancreatic gland or peripancreatic tissues, do not present with a pseudocyst but instead with a walled-off necrosis (WON). These two entities are often confused in clinical and research communications, and each carries a different management algorithm and prognosis. At its most fundamental level, appropriate management depends first on accurate diagnosis: does this patient have a pancreatic pseudocyst or WON? This is followed by the characterization of the process as sterile or infected, which also informs decision making.

Once the diagnosis of a pseudocyst is established, the next step is to decide if, when, and how to intervene. Minimally invasive approaches are now considered standard of care, so optimal management necessitates a multidisciplinary approach.

CLINICAL FEATURES

Pseudocysts develop from acute fluid collections that persist for more than 4 weeks after an episode of acute interstitial edematous pancreatitis. Spontaneous resolution may occur after sealing of the ductal leak with reabsorption of the fluid. The most common symptom is abdominal pain, which is present in 80% to 90% of patients. Nausea, emesis, early satiety, or weight loss can also be presenting symptoms. On examination, an epigastric mass is found in 50% of patients. General tenderness may be present on physical examination. Rarely, patients may also have signs that result from an obstructive process such as jaundice. A mildly elevated amylase may be present in up to 76% of patients.

PREOPERATIVE WORKUP

Preoperative radiographic studies establish the diagnosis and help guide therapy. A contrast-enhanced computed tomographic (CT) scan (CECT) should be performed in all patients. Radiographically, pseudocysts are surrounded by a well-defined wall with few to no nonliquid components. High-density material within the fluid collection on CECT of more than 20 Hounsfield units should be suspicious for the presence of WON. The CECT should be reviewed with an eye towards establishing the proximity to adjacent structures and cyst wall thickness; identifying any sequelae of portal hypertension or venous thrombosis, such gastric varices lying in the path of the planned operation; and revealing an infectious process (i.e., presence of gas) or a pseudoaneurysm.

An ultrasound scan of the gallbladder should be performed in all patients, and a cholecystectomy should be planned if gallstones or sludge are present. The utility of preoperative endoscopic retrograde cholangiopancreatography (ERCP) in patients with a pseudocyst is debated, but the procedure does offer information regarding ductal anatomy, undetected multiplicity, and areas of disruption or stenosis of the duct that should lead away from percutaneous or endoscopic management. Definitive intervention should be done 24 to 48 hours after ERCP because manipulation carries a high incidence of introducing infection. Other imaging modalities such as transabdominal ultrasound scan, magnetic resonance cholangiopancreatography (MRCP), and endoscopic ultrasound scan are useful adjuncts in select patients.

A cystic neoplasm of the pancreas must be distinguished from a pseudocyst. Approximately 20% of lesions originally thought to be pseudocysts are estimated to eventually be found to be cystic neoplasms. Suspicion for a cystic neoplasm should be heightened in patients with no history of acute pancreatitis and no risk factors for chronic pancreatitis. Prior imaging should be obtained, with a focus on interval changes and associated radiographic findings that would indicate a recent history of acute pancreatitis, such as peripancreatic inflammation, pancreatic ascites, pleural effusions, and absence of septa within the pseudocyst. Aspiration with evaluation of fluid content can be helpful. Pseudocysts usually contain an elevated amylase value of more than 5000 IU/mL, whereas elevated carbohydrate antigen 19-9 (CA19-9) and carcinoembryonic antigen (CEA) values are concerning for a cystic neoplasm.

A related pathologic entity in the differential diagnosis is a delayed postnecronectomy pseudocyst that occurs after endoscopic drainage or necronectomy of a WON. This unusual pseudocyst occurs in the recovery phase of a patient with necrotizing pancreatitis and is the result of disconnected pancreatic tail syndrome that occurs when a viable but orphaned portion of distal pancreas secretes pancreatic fluid into a cavity forming a pseudocyst.

OPERATIVE INDICATIONS

Pseudocyst drainage is indicated with symptomatic or enlarging conditions or with development of complications, such as infection, bleeding, or rupture. Surgical convention also supports intervention for a pseudocyst size of more than 6 cm that persists beyond 4 to 6 weeks because larger cysts are associated with a higher complication rate. Intrasplenic or perisplenic pseudocysts are thought to have a higher incidence of hemorrhage and are thus also managed operatively.

Relative contraindications to an internal surgical drainage procedure include acute fluid collections with an immature capsule and those that are grossly infected.

PROCEDURE SELECTION

Selection of the best approach for definitive management is complex and depends on many factors. Decisions can be influenced by the local anatomy, presence of sinistral hypertension, and communication with the pancreatic duct; presence of infection; suspicion of a cystic neoplasm; the size, number, and location of pseudocysts; the presence of chronic pancreatitis; and the medical status of the patient. Management of a pancreatic pseudocyst should be customized for each patient and is best decided in consultation with a

TABLE 1: Revised Atlanta classification terms

	Interstitial edematous pancreatitis Acute inflammation of the pancreatic parenchyma and peripancreatic tissues, but without recognizable necrosis of pancreatic parenchyma or peripancreatic tissues.	Necrotizing pancreatitis Inflammation associated with pancreatic parenchymal necrosis or peripancreatic necrosis.
Early (1st 4 wk after onset of pancreatitis)	Acute fluid collection Peripancreatic fluid associated with IEP with no associated peripancreatic necrosis. This term applies only to areas of peripancreatic fluid seen within the first 4 wk after onset of IEP.	Acute necrotic collection A collection containing variable amounts of both fluid and necrosis associated with necrotizing pancreatitis; the necrosis can involve the pancreatic parenchyma or the peripancreatic tissues.
Late (≥4 wk after onset of pancreatitis)	Pancreatic pseudocyst A complete encapsulated collection of fluid outside the pancreas with minimal (<5%) or no necrosis usually requires more than 4 wk after onset of IEP to mature and has a well-defined inflammatory wall; rarely, a pancreatic pseudocyst may develop in a patient with necrotizing pancreatitis after treatment with necronectomy, usually related to disconnected duct syndrome.	Walled-off necrosis An encapsulated collection of pancreatic or peripancreatic necrosis that persists for >4 wk after onset of necrotizing pancreatitis and has a well-defined inflammatory wall.

IEP, Interstitial edematous pancreatitis.

multidisciplinary team composed of an interventional radiologist, an endoscopist, and a surgeon.

Pseudocysts are treated most effectively with internal drainage, which is done through the surgical or endoscopic creation of a cystenterostomy. Endoscopic transmural cystenterostomy with the use of endoscopic ultrasound scan (EUS) and color Doppler offers a less invasive option when the pseudocyst is mature and has a favorable anatomy and location. However, accumulating evidence suggests that endoscopic drainage may have higher rates of failure, sepsis, and bleeding. Still, it is the most common form of drainage procedure used in the United States, which leaves the surgeon for the most difficult cases.

Surgical intervention is the standard when endoscopy is not a viable option, when concern exists for a cystic neoplasm, and when complications related to chronic pancreatitis are present, such as pancreatic duct strictures and stones. Operative internal drainage can be accomplished with cystenterostomy, usually cystgastrostomy or cystjejunostomy. In general, cystgastrostomy has a decreased operative time and faster recovery. The two laparoscopic cystgastrostomy approaches are the anterior approach and the posterior approach. The anterior approach is technically less demanding but requires that the stomach be widely adherent to the cyst. The posterior approach avoids an additional gastrotomy and is thought to allow more precise cyst visualization and dissection. It also provides a greater tissue yield for histopathology and is associated with a lower risk of recurrence from occlusion. A transgastric approach has also been described but requires specialized equipment (e.g., intraluminal trocars) and can be technically challenging. Multiple pseudocysts and giant pseudocysts (>10 cm) are best managed with cystjejunostomy. This approach minimizes the formation of dependent residual pockets, which are prone to infection. Finally, the presence of common duct stenosis or pancreatic duct dilation favors cystjejunostomy that can drain both the pseudocyst and the dilated ductal system. Cystduodenostomy has very few indications.

Pseudocyst resection is an alternative to surgical cystenterostomy for moderately sized chronic pseudocysts and for a pseudoaneurysm in close association with the pseudocyst. Most resections for pseudocysts involve a distal pancreatectomy with or without concomitant splenectomy. Roux-en-Y pancreaticojejunostomy can be used if a distal pancreatic stump remains in situ.

Percutaneous catheter drainage should be reserved for either poor operative candidates or infected pseudocysts because of the risk of persistent pancreaticocutaneous fistula. Early recurrence is high, approaching 80%. Transpapillary stenting is effective when used with a communicating pseudocyst, particularly if it is solitary, smaller than 6 cm, and remote from the gastric or duodenal wall.

PREOPERATIVE PLANNING

Preoperative planning should include a gastroduodenoscopy to exclude gastric or duodenal pathology. It is also important to ensure that surgical pathology is available for frozen-section analysis of the pseudocyst wall before cystenteric drainage. The patient is placed in the supine position with the surgeon to the patient's left. A nasogastric tube and Foley catheter should be placed. A first generation cephalosporin is administered before surgery. Port placement may be modified if laparoscopic cholecystectomy is also planned. Critical surgical principles for laparoscopic cystenterostomy are listed in Box 1.

LAPAROSCOPIC CYSTGASTROSTOMY

Anterior Approach

Hasson's technique is used to gain access to the peritoneal cavity at the umbilicus. Three additional ports are placed (Figure 1). The left lobe of the liver is retracted cephalad, exposing the entire anterior gastric wall. An anterior gastrotomy (extending 4 to 5 cm) is made with ultrasonic shears or Harmonic scalpel (Ethicon Endosurgery, Cincinnati, Ohio) to expose the posterior gastric wall.

The pseudocyst is identified by visualizing a bulge on the posterior wall of the stomach. Laparoscopic ultrasound scan should be used to verify the location, map out the planned cystogastrostomy, and define the presence of large interposing blood vessels. The pseudocyst should be aspirated to assist in localization, obtain sample for

gram stain, and establish the thickness of the common wall. The pseudocyst is then entered with an incision on the posterior wall of the stomach with a Ligasure device (Covidien, Boulder, Colo) or ultrasonic shears for an incision length of 4 to 6 cm (Figure 2). Simple electrocautery alone is insufficient because of concern for postoperative hemorrhage. A biopsy of the pseudocyst wall is sent. The interior of the pseudocyst is examined with the laparoscope, then the cavity is aggressively irrigated and debris removed with a blunt grasper. The cavity is inspected for hemostasis.

The cystgastrostomy can be created with an endoscopic linear 45-mm stapler, and a wedge or diamond-shaped cystgastrostomy is made (Figure 3). An alternate approach to ensure apposition and control hemostasis is to create the cystgastrostomy with running, locked full-thickness sutures. The anterior gastrotomy is closed with a running, continuous suture or linear stapler (Figure 4).

BOX 1: Critical surgical principles

1. Place the patient on a padded bean bag if patient position is to be changed during the procedure.

2. Be prepared to perform a splenectomy if a distal pancreatectomy is planned.

3. Use of intraoperative ultrasound scan is a critical adjunct in defining anatomic relationships, the presence of multiple cysts, and the location of the common bile duct and pancreatic duct.

4. Rule out pseudoaneurysm with Doppler-guided ultrasound scan.

5. Consider use of a hand-assist device if the dissection is difficult.

6. Access the cyst in a dependent location to optimize pseudocyst drainage. Aspirate first, then create cystotomy with electrocautery alongside the needle.

7. Biopsy cyst wall to rule out cystic neoplasm.

8. Débride content of the pseudocyst thoroughly but with caution to avoid bleeding.

9. Cystenteric anastomosis should be 3 to 5 cm to prevent premature closure and recurrence.

10. Ensure hemostasis of friable pseudocyst wall with either an endoscopic stapler or a suture ligation with a continuous, locking closure.

11. Interrogate the cystgastrostomy with submersion in saline solution as the stomach is insufflated via the nasogastric tube.

12. Consider placing omentum over cystenterostomy.

13. Place a closed suction drain to identify and control potential postoperative fistulae.

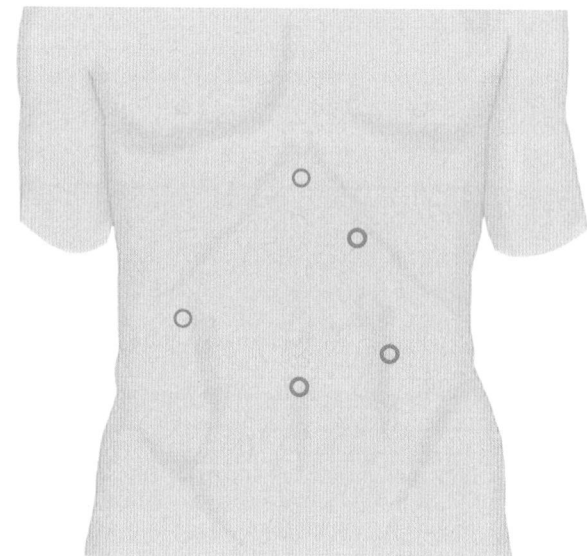

FIGURE 1   General port placement for cystenterostomy. For anterior cystgastrostomy, the epigastric port is often not needed. *(From Kaban GK, Perugini RA, Czerniach DR, et al: Pancreatic pseudocyst drainage, Op Tech Gen Surg 6(1):55-62, 2004.)*

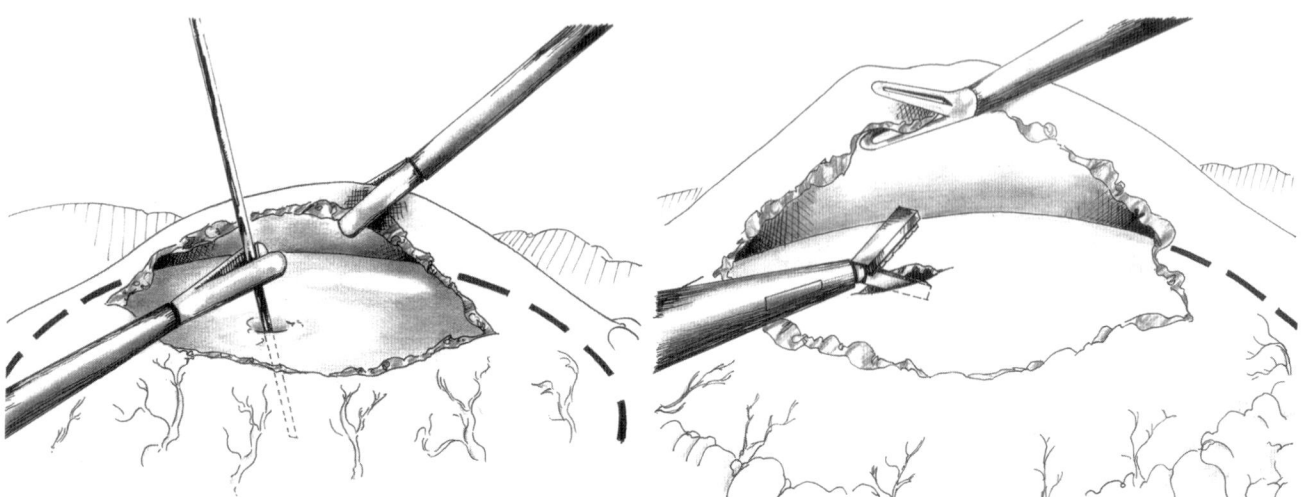

FIGURE 2   Anterior approach. After anterior gastrotomy, the cyst is aspirated in a dependent position to confirm its location and to prepare for a cystotomy to be made transversely along the access site. *(From Kaban GK, Perugini RA, Czerniach DR, et al: Pancreatic pseudocyst drainage, Op Tech Gen Surg 6(1):55-62, 2004.)*

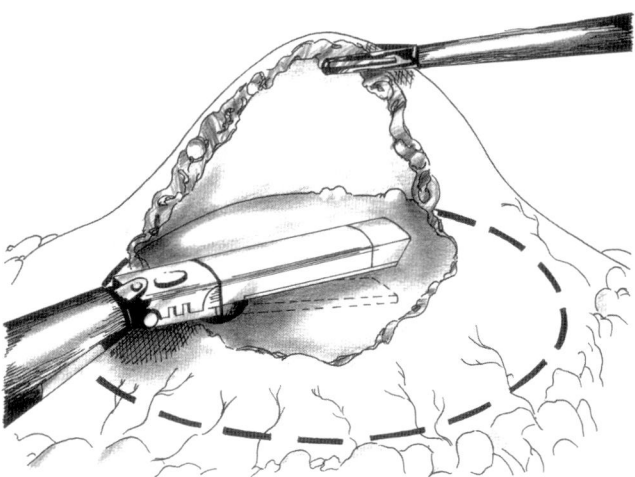

FIGURE 3   Anterior approach. A stapling device can be used to extend the cystgastrostomy, usually with 2.5-mm staples. Thicker walled pseudocysts require staples of 3.5 mm of larger. Intracorporeal suturing may be necessary. *(From Kaban GK, Perugini RA, Czerniach DR, et al: Pancreatic pseudocyst drainage,* Op Tech Gen Surg *6(1):55-62, 2004.)*

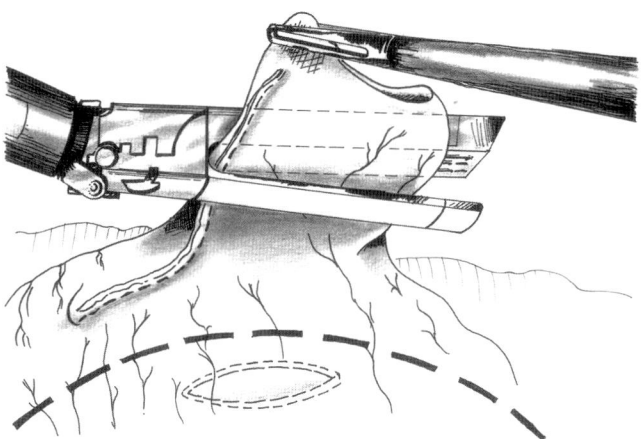

FIGURE 4   Anterior approach. The anterior gastrotomy is closed with an endoscopic linear stapler or running suture. *(From Kaban GK, Perugini RA, Czerniach DR, et al: Pancreatic pseudocyst drainage,* Op Tech Gen Surg *6(1):55-62, 2004.)*

Posterior Approach

The posterior, or lesser sac, approach can be used when the pseudocyst resides close to the inferior edge of the stomach. The posterior gastric wall is directly accessed for the cystgastrostomy through one gastrotomy.

Standard laparoscopic access is obtained, and the left lobe of the liver retracted as described previously. The lesser sac is entered by dividing the gastrocolic ligament; this is often tedious and challenging given the prior inflammatory process, distorted anatomy, and adhesions. The anterior gastric wall is retracted cephalad. The pseudocyst is exposed and skeletonized to the area where it is closely adherent to the posterior gastric wall. A needle is passed to aspirate the cyst fluid for analysis as described previously. A biopsy of the cyst wall is sent. A cystotomy is made to accommodate the linear stapler. The optimal position of the gastrotomy can be confirmed with simultaneous introduction of a gastric endoscope. A gastrotomy is created about 3 to 5 cm along the posterior gastric wall directly opposite the cystotomy. A linear staple is used to create the

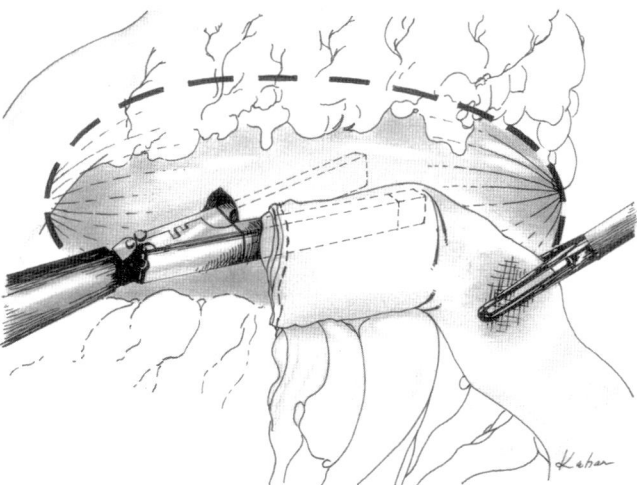

FIGURE 5   Laparoscopic cystjejunostomy. The cystjejunostomy is created in the most dependent portion of the cyst, oriented in an antimesenteric fashion. *(From Kaban GK, Perugini RA, Czerniach DR, et al: Pancreatic pseudocyst drainage,* Op Tech Gen Surg *6(1):55-62, 2004.)*

cystogastrostomy. The common defect is closed with interrupted or running sutures or an additional laparoscopic stapler.

LAPAROSCOPIC CYSTJEJUNOSTOMY

Access to the peritoneal cavity is achieved through an initial 10-mm periumbilical port, and pneumoperitoneum is established. Three additional ports are placed in the bilateral upper abdomen. If a linear stapler will be used, a 12-mm port is also placed in the left lower quadrant. The transverse colon and omentum are retracted cephalad. The pseudocyst often bulges through the transverse mesocolon just to the left of the middle colic vessels. If not, it can be accessed through the lesser sac. Careful attention must be paid to the central middle colic pedicle, which can be obscured by thickened overlying peritoneum and saponified adipose tissue from prior inflammation. The preferred site of access is just superior and lateral to the ligament of Treitz. The most dependent portion of the pseudocyst is identified with ultrasound scan assistance and aspirated as described previously. The cystotomy is created with the Ligasure or Harmonic scalpel, and a biopsy of the cyst wall is performed. Inspection and débridement of the pseudocyst are performed before proceeding with the Roux-en-Y reconstruction.

The ligament of Treitz is identified, and the jejunum is transected 20 cm distal to this point with a linear stapler. The mesentery is divided in the direction of the root of the mesentery in a way to ensure adequate blood flow to the Roux limb. The jejunojejunostomy is created approximately 40 cm distal to the transection site. The mesenteric defect should be closed. The Roux limb is brought up to the pseudocyst either directly opposed to the mesocolon or through a window in the transverse mesocolon to which it is later secured. It is then tacked to the pseudocyst to achieve optimal orientation for linear stapling, ensuring the distal loop of bowel is approximated to the pseudocyst in the longitudinal plane and is antimesenteric (Figure 5). A small incision is made in the jejunum opposite to the one previously made in the pseudocyst. Hemostasis is ensured through direct inspection. The cystjejunostomy is fashioned to a total length of 5 cm or greater. This is done either with a laparoscopic linear stapler or a running or interrupted suture. The cystenterotomy is closed with a single layer of interrupted suture. A closed suction drain should be left. The abdomen is inspected and irrigated followed by fascial closure of any port 10 mm or more.

A lateral, side-to-side pancreaticojejunostomy may be necessary in patients with chronic pancreatitis and a dilated pancreatic duct. Additional pseudocysts can be incorporated into the laterally positioned Roux limb.

POSTOPERATIVE CARE

Enteral feeding can begin usually at about 48 hours after laparoscopic cystenterostomy. This is the case even with Roux-en-Y reconstruction as reflux into the cyst is minimal and prolonged ileus is rare. Postoperative bleeding from the pseudocyst capsule or anastomosis should be managed with endoscopic electrocoagulation, laparoscopy, or laparotomy. Bleeding may also arise from avulsion or laceration of peripancreatic arteries or veins during cyst débridement and may require emergent coil embolization. Drain fluid may be assayed for amylase if there is a concern for anastomotic dehiscence. Persistent postoperative fever of unclear etiology should be worked up with an abdominal CT scan with oral contrast to rule out premature closure of the cystenterostomy or formation of an abscess.

OUTCOMES AND COMPLICATIONS

Limited reports exist that compare laparoscopic and open cystenterostomy, and no comparative studies are found for the different laparoscopic approaches to cystgastrostomy or cystjejunostomy. Given the low prevalence of true pseudocysts, these studies are unlikely to become available. The proposed advantages of a laparoscopic approach are less postoperative pain, smaller scar, shortened stay, and more rapid return to activities. Recurrence rates on published series of laparoscopic management of pseudocysts range from 0 to 2%, with a morbidity rate of 3% to 33%. Use of a laparoscopic stapler is thought to possibly carry a lower bleeding risk.

BRIEF COMMENT ON WALLED-OFF NECROSIS

WON occurs at a much greater frequency than pseudocyst formation. If a patient is determined to have WON and not a pancreatic pseudocyst, the options for effective drainage are different. There now exist prospective safety and efficacy and randomized controlled trial data to support superior short-term and long-term clinical outcomes and cost benefits with a step-up approach to WON. The step-up approach involves initial percutaneous drainage of a symptomatic WON followed by a more invasive drainage procedure when necessary. Classically, the step-up approach was described with the videoscopic-assisted retroperitoneal débridement technique, although any endoscopic, laparoscopic, or open approach can be substituted.

SUGGESTED READINGS

Banks PA, Bollen TL, Dervenis C, et al: Acute Pancreatitis Classification Working Group: classification of acute pancreatitis: 2012: revision of the Atlanta classification and definitions by international consensus, *Gut* 62(1):102–111, 2013.
Cannon JW, Callery MP, Vollmer CM Jr: Diagnosis and management of pancreatic pseudocysts: what is the evidence? *J Am Coll Surg* 209:385–393, 2009.
Davila-Cervantes A, Gomez F, Chan C: Laparoscopic drainage of pancreatic pseudocysts, *Surg Endosc* 18(10):1420, 2004.
Kaban GK, Perungini RA, Czerniach DR, et al: Pancreatic pseudocyst drainage, *Op Tech Gen Surg* 6(1):55–62, 2004.
van Santvoort HC, Besselink MG, Bakker OJ, et al, for the Dutch Pancreatitis Study Group: A step-up approach or open necrosectomy for necrotizing pancreatitis, *N Engl J Med* 362(16):1491, 2010.

VIDEO-ASSISTED THORACIC SURGERY

Christopher M. Sciortino, MD, PhD,
Benedetto Mungo, MD, and Daniela Molena, MD

INTRODUCTION

Video-assisted thoracic surgery (VATS) is the minimally invasive alternative to open thoracotomy for thoracic procedures. It has become an invaluable technique for the diagnosis and treatment of thoracic disease. Thoracoscopy was first described in 1910 by a Swedish internist, Hans Christian Jacobaeus, who used a rigid cystoscope to perform pleural inspection and adhesiolysis for tuberculosis. Today, VATS is used for a wide spectrum of diseases by both thoracic and general surgeons. This chapter outlines the indications and the general technique of VATS.

INDICATIONS FOR VIDEO-ASSISTED THORACIC SURGERY AND PATIENT SELECTION

The indications for the VATS approach are nearly identical to those for open thoracotomy. Box 1 lists the surgical applications for VATS. Relative contraindications to VATS are listed in Box 2. The contraindications would be similar to the relative contraindications to open thoracotomy with the possible exception of fused pleural space and tumor involvement of the chest wall.

Advantages of VATS over the open thoracotomy approach include less pain, lower rates of postoperative pneumonia, and shorter hospital stays. Disadvantages of VATS include limited exposure, inability to palpate all but superficial structures, the need for specialty equipment, two-dimensional view of the operative field, and the potential need for emergency conversion to open thoracotomy if major airway or vascular disruption should occur.

No matter which technique is utilized, careful preoperative workup must be performed to ensure that the patient is a suitable candidate for the planned thoracic procedure. The workup includes a general medical evaluation, preoperative imaging, laboratory tests, pulmonary function testing, and cardiac evaluation if applicable.

BOX 1: Common applications for video-assisted thoracic surgery approach to the thorax

Diagnostic thoracoscopy
Pleural biopsy
Lymph node biopsy
Decortication
Pleurodesis
Wedge resection
Lobectomy
Pneumonectomy
Mediastinal tumor excision
Thymectomy
Pericardial window
Resection of benign esophageal tumors
Esophageal diverticulectomy
Esophageal myotomy
Paraesophageal hernia repair
Minimally invasive esophagectomy
Sympathectomy
Pulmonary vein isolation
Lung volume reduction surgery
Diaphragm plication

BOX 2: Relative contraindications to VATS

Dense pleural adhesion (obliterated pleural space)*
Pulmonary hilar lesion*
Superior sulcus tumor*
Small (<1 cm), deeply located pulmonary nodule*
Extensive tumor involvement of the chest wall*
Severe hemorrhage*
Inability to achieve ipsilateral lung isolation
Hemodynamic instability
Ventilator dependency
Coagulopathy
Inadequate visualization
Severe thoracic or spinal deformities (e.g., scoliosis or pectus excavatum)
Inability to tolerate single lung ventilation
Noncompliant lung
Severe emphysema

*Specific to video-assisted thoracic surgery (VATS) in comparison with open thoracotomy.

Pulmonary function tests are used to help predict (1) whether the patient can tolerate one lung ventilation for the proposed procedure and (2) whether the patient has the physiologic reserve to tolerate any planned pulmonary resection. Figure 1 is a useful algorithm to assess patient's eligibility for lung resection on the basis of preoperative lung function.

SURGICAL SETUP AND EQUIPMENT

Anesthesia

Thoracic surgical procedures require an experienced anesthesia team familiar with single-lung ventilation. The expertise includes the ability to place and troubleshoot double-lumen tubes or bronchial blockers, as well as the ability to manage hemodynamic shifts that result from single-lung ventilation (e.g., shunt physiology).

The majority of patients who undergo a thoracic surgical procedure have an epidural catheter placed before the procedure for intraoperative and postoperative analgesia management. Routine use of epidural analgesia significantly decreases postoperative pain and respiratory complications. All patients undergoing major lung resection should have an arterial cannula placed for hemodynamic monitoring and frequent blood gas analysis. Central venous access is utilized on a case-by-case basis.

Patient Positioning

Figure 2 illustrates the basic positioning for most VATS procedures. The patient is placed in the lateral decubitus position, with an axillary roll. The bed is flexed all the way to help separate the ribs and open the intercostal spaces, but, of most importance, to allow the hip to descend below the line of the chest wall to avoid interference with instruments manipulation. The neck is supported to keep the spine straight. The lower arm is placed on an arm board with copious padding to minimize the risk of neuropraxia, and the upper arm is either rested on pillows or preferably supported by commercially available arm holders or retractors in a manner that gives access to the entire chest and axilla. The patient is supported on each side either with a bean bag or rolled sheets. Broad silk tape is used to stabilize the hips. The legs are well padded, especially on the knees and ankles; the inferior leg is bent to approximately 90 degrees; and the superior leg is straight.

Equipment

The basic VATS imaging equipment is similar to that for laparoscopy and consists of a fiber optic light source and an imaging system linked to the operative camera. For most adult procedures, the authors use a 10-mm scope (30 or 45 degrees) attached to the camera head. The current generation of cameras offers high-definition resolution with the capacity for continuous recording of procedures. Carbon dioxide insufflation is not routinely used in VATS; however, it is occasionally used to help compress the isolated lung when endoluminal suction is insufficient, to increase the intrathoracic volume by pushing the diaphragm down, and to stabilize the mediastinum by decreasing contralateral respiratory excursions. The insufflation pressure should be kept low (the authors recommend not exceeding 8 mm Hg), and attention to hemodynamic changes is imperative because the lack of compliance of the chest wall (in relation to the abdomen) can result in a rapid decrease in venous return or mediastinal shift, both of which could cause a profound drop in blood pressure.

Surgical instruments for VATS procedures are also similar to those for laparoscopy. Long channel graspers, dissectors, and scissors are utilized for their designed purpose. Instruments unique to VATS include specially designed lung graspers (Figure 3) with a broad-based shape to minimize tissue trauma and tearing during lung manipulation. Monopolar electrocautery is used for dissection and hemostasis and can be engaged either through the connection on endothoracic instruments or through the use of an extended-length electrocautery pen. Ultrasonic dissector–coagulator (Harmonic scalpel; Ethicon, Bridgewater, NJ) systems are often utilized in VATS procedures and have less heat dispersion and a protected jaw arm, which can be important during dissection in the region of delicate structures such as nerves and thin vessels. A bendable argon beam (Bend-A-Beam; ConMed, Utica, NY) can be useful for overcoming the limitations of a rigid chest cavity and allows reaching around the lungs or the convexity of the chest wall.

Endoscopic staplers are the modern mainstay of resections by VATS (Figure 4). Most staplers used in VATS are capable of simultaneously stapling and cutting. Characteristics of currently available staplers include a variety of lengths (from 30 to 60 mm), varying staple heights, and the ability to roticulate. The length of stapler should be carefully chosen according to amount of tissue that must

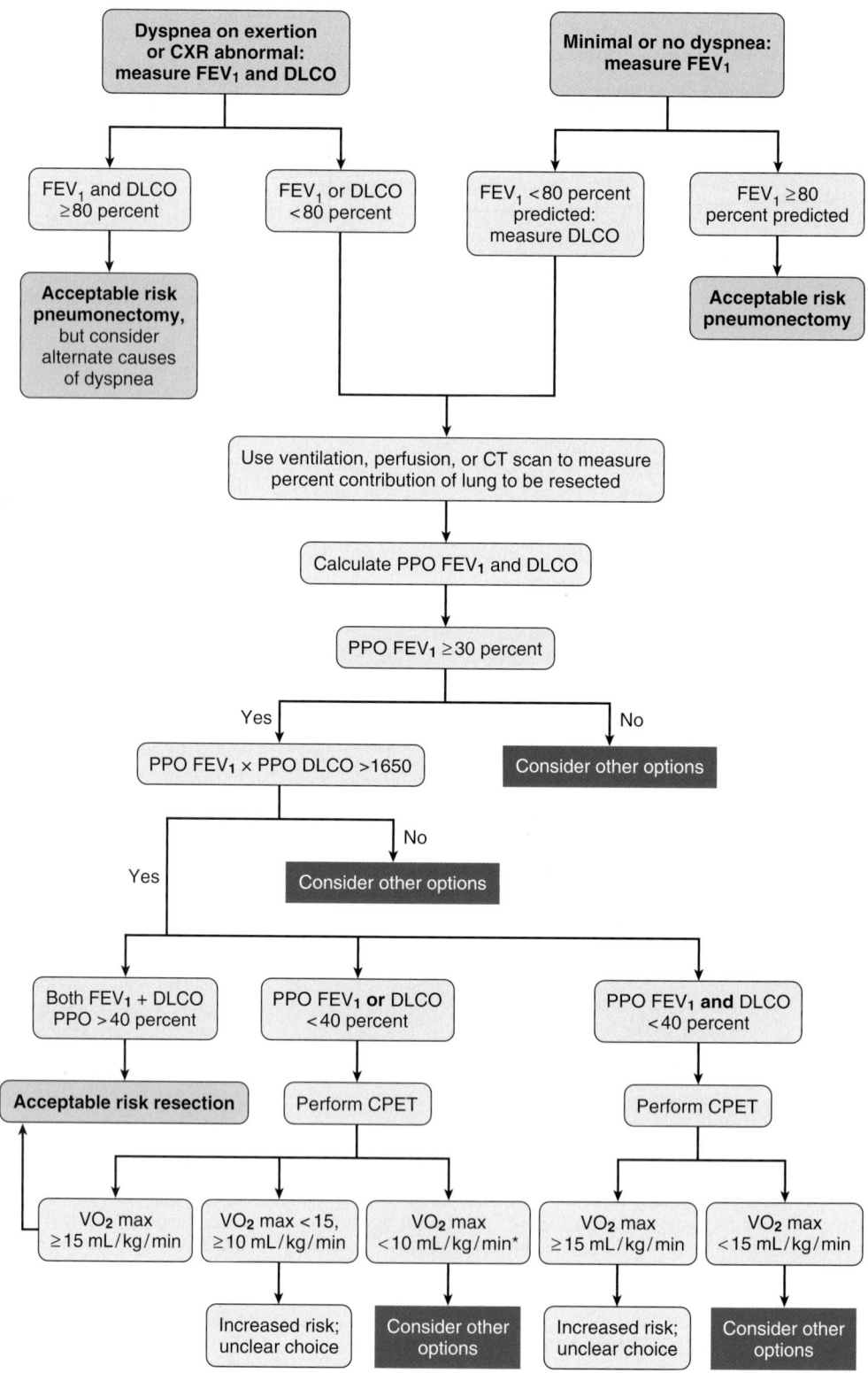

FIGURE 1 Evaluation for lung resection. *VO_2 max <10 mL/kg/min is approximately equivalent to walking less than 25 shuttles on two shuttle walks or less than 1 flight of stairs. *CPET,* Cardiopulmonary exercise test; *CT,* computed tomographic; *CXR,* chest radiograph; *DLCO,* diffusion capacity of carbon monoxide; FEV_1, forced expiratory volume in 1 second; *PPO,* predicted postoperative; VO_2, oxygen consumption. *(Data from Colice GL, Shafazand S, Griffin JP, et al: Physiologic evaluation of the patient with lung cancer being considered for resectional surgery, Chest 132:161S, 2007.)*

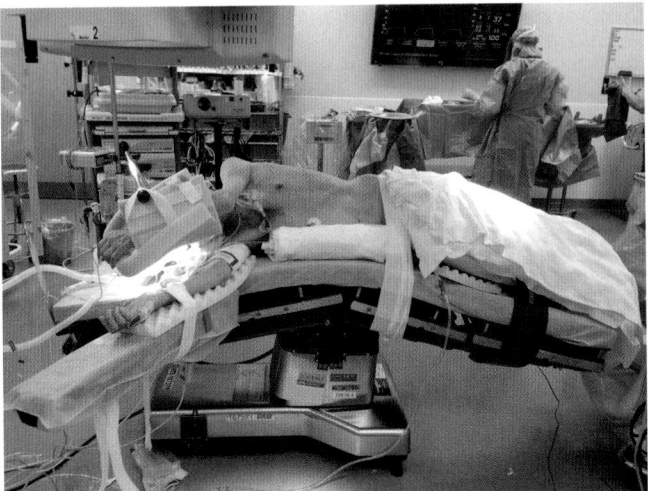

FIGURE 2 Patient positioning for video-assisted thoracic surgery (VATS). The patient is placed in the lateral decubitus position with axillary roll. Padding is placed under the neck to ensure alignment of cervical spine. Rolls are placed on either side of the patient to stabilize the torso. Silk tape is used to secure the position of the hips. Padding is placed around arms and between legs to minimize the risk of neuropraxia.

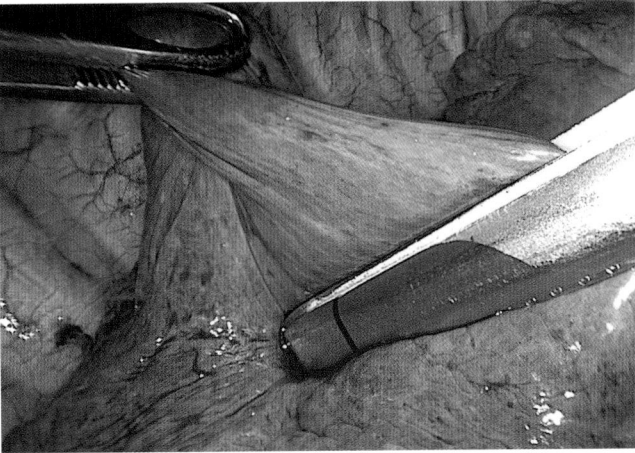

FIGURE 4 Intraoperative view of a video-assisted thoracic surgery (VATS) procedure. In a pulmonary resection, the surgeon uses an endoscopic stapling device to quickly divide both pulmonary parenchyma and vessels, while excellent pneumostasis and hemostasis is maintained.

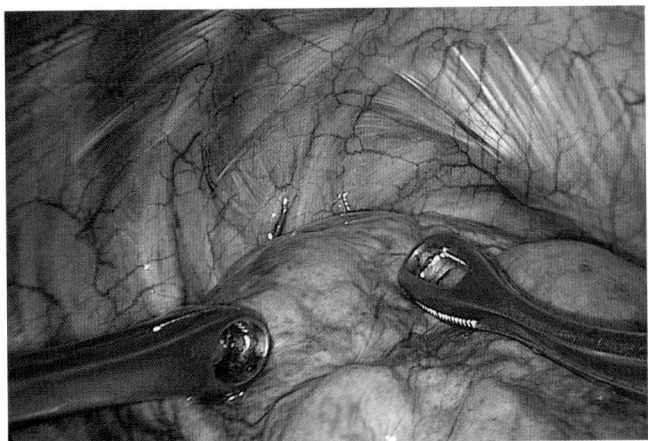

FIGURE 3 Intraoperative view of a video-assisted thoracic surgery (VATS) procedure. Note the peculiar shape of the atraumatic tissue graspers, specifically designed for the lung parenchyma.

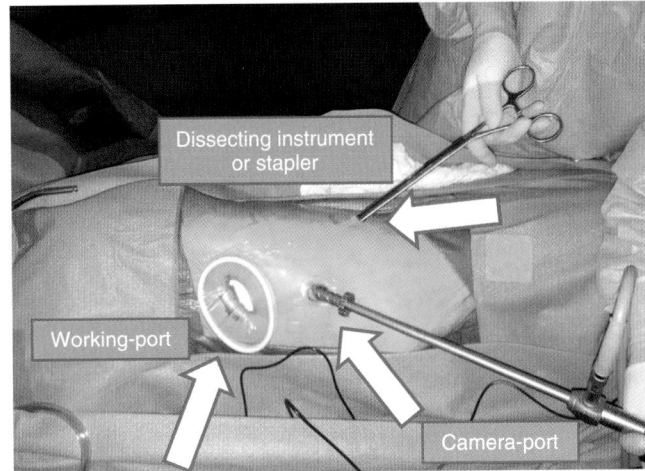

FIGURE 5 The triangulation principle of thoracoscopic port placement. The optic channel is often placed centrally and should maintain an angle of 30 to 60 degrees between it and any other instruments. A wound retractor is useful to separate the soft tissues and allow easy introduction of instruments through the working port.

be resected, the location in relation to the chest wall and mediastinum, and the patient's chest cavity volume. Because of the closed and fixed confines of the chest cavity, longer staplers are difficult to manipulate in small patients or for lung resections close to the chest wall. The staples' height is chosen on the basis of the thickness of the tissue that needs to be sealed; for example, 2-mm to 2.5-mm staples are used for blood vessels and very thin lung parenchyma, whereas 4.8-mm staples are used for thick lung parenchyma or a lobar bronchus.

Several products exist to reinforce staple lines and are compatible with most staplers. They are marketed as a means to decrease air leaks at staple lines, decrease the duration of chest tube drainage, and potentially decrease the length of hospital stay. Only one biologic glue (Progel; Neomend, Irvine, Calif) has been approved by the U.S. Food and Drug Administration for application to the lung, and it is specifically designed for sealing small tears on the surface of the lung and at staple sites to decrease air leaks. The added cost of these materials

limits their routine use; therefore, the authors utilize them selectively in patients at high risk for prolonged air leaks.

Port Site Placement

Port site placement is the most important factor for the successful performance of thoracic procedure by VATS. Triangulation to the desired intrathoracic target is hindered by the rigidity of the chest wall, limited intercostal space, the diaphragm, the heart, and the scapula. Typically, for a three-port technique, one port is placed in the seventh or eight intercostal space along the posterior axillary line, and it is used to introduce the camera. The second port site is usually placed in the eight intercostal space in line with the tip of the scapula, and it is used for retraction or stapling, or both. A third port is positioned in the fourth or fifth intercostal space in the midaxillary line (Figure 5). This affords enough port separation at the skin level to allow for adequate instrument spacing in the chest to work without crossing instruments. However, the placements of these ports can be modified after initial thoracoscopy to optimize instruments' position. Minor procedures such as pleural inspection and biopsy can be performed with a single port. In most procedures, two to four ports are used, and in some instances, the more proximal port may be lengthened to allow multiple instruments to be placed through it ("working port").

BASIC TECHNIQUE AND EMERGENCY CONVERSION TO THORACOTOMY

Basic Technique of Video-Assisted Thoracic Surgery

After induction of anesthesia and endotracheal intubation, a diagnostic bronchoscopy is performed to evaluate the airways, clear any secretions, and ensure proper position of the double-lumen endotracheal tube. The patient is then carefully positioned, prepared, and draped. The desired lung is isolated to allow adequate time for collapse. The port sites are marked and, after the skin is incised, electrocautery is used to dissect to the level of the rib space. The chest is entered by electrocautery dissection on the superior aspect of the rib to avoid the intercostal bundle. The authors utilize short metal bullet-tipped trocars for the camera port to keep the track open and protect the camera during entry. If insufflation is used, thoracoscopic trocars with a unidirectional valve should be placed through each incision, to avoid air leakage. The camera is coated with antifog solution and carefully placed in to the thoracic cavity for initial inspection and evaluation of lung isolation. Adhesions are taken down either with the Harmonic scalpel or with electrocautery. Excessive torque should be avoided while the VATS instrument is manipulated to avoid postoperative intercostal neuritis. Vascular structures are circumferentially dissected before stapler engagement to ensure that the stapler can be placed with minimal tension on the vessel. Once the desired specimen is dissected free, it is retrieved from the chest via a specimen bag to prevent chest wall seeding. After the specimen is removed, the surgical site is inspected and then irrigated and cleared of any fluid and clot. Chest tubes are placed under direct vision through port sites before lung reexpansion. The lung is reinflated under direct vision to assess for areas of persistent atelectasis, to ensure adequate filling of the chest cavity, and to evaluate all staple lines for leaks. The chest wall muscles are approximated with absorbable suture to avoid lung herniation, and a subcuticular suture is used to close the skin.

Conversion to Thoracotomy

The need for conversion from VATS to open thoracotomy is always a possibility, and the operating room should be prepared for this event. This typically occurs in the situation in which there is unexpected bleeding or airway disruption or if it is unsafe or impractical to proceed by VATS (e.g., tumor extends to the hilum). In the nonemergency setting, a muscle-sparing thoracotomy can be considered. However, in the urgent/emergency conversion, a non–muscle-sparing thoracotomy can be performed. Bleeding can occasionally be controlled by compression with a sponge stick while the thoracotomy is opened. It is important to have proper retractors and other equipment readily available when VATS is performed, in case there is a need to quickly convert to thoracotomy.

SUMMARY

VATS represents a safe and feasible alternative to thoracotomy for a wide range of surgical procedures. It offers surgical and oncologic outcomes comparable with those of traditional surgery and, moreover, provides some adjunctive benefits, such as less postoperative pain and faster recovery. Future technologic achievements, targeted to overcome the known limitations of this technique, will contribute to further extension of its indications and use.

SUGGESTED READINGS

Acuff TE, Mack MJ, Landreneau RJ, et al: Role of mechanical stapling devices in thoracoscopic pulmonary resection, *Ann Thoracic Surg* 56(3):749–751, 1993.

McKenna RJ Jr, Houck W, Fuller CB: Video-assisted thoracic surgery lobectomy: experience with 1100 cases, *Ann Thoracic Surg* 81:421–426, 2006.

Sedrakyan A, van der Meulen J, Lewsey J, et al: Video assisted thoracic surgery for treatment of pneumothorax and lung resections: systematic review of randomised clinical trials, *BMJ* 329(7473):1008, 2004.

Shaw JP, Dembitzer FR, Wisnivesky JP, et al: Video-assisted thoracoscopic lobectomy: state of the art and future directions, *Ann Thorac Surg* 85(2):S705–S709, 2008.

Swanson SJ, Meyers BF, Gunnarsson CL, et al: Video-assisted thoracoscopic lobectomy is less costly and morbid than open lobectomy: a retrospective multiinstitutional database analysis, *Ann Thorac Surg* 93(4):1027–1032, 2012.

LAPAROSCOPIC SURGERY FOR MORBID OBESITY

Kashif A. Zuberi, MD, Thomas Magnuson, MD, and Michael A. Schweitzer, MD

The morbid obesity epidemic continues to spread throughout industrialized nations. It is a condition with a heterogeneous etiology, including genetic, psychosocial, and environmental factors.

Prevention methods have currently been unable to halt the further spread of this disease. Obesity has been linked to increased healthcare costs, common physiologic derangements, reduced quality of life, and increased overall mortality. More than one third of adults and almost 17% of children in the United States are obese.

Medical therapy that can cause sustained significant weight loss may be years away. Bariatric surgery, when combined with a multidisciplinary team, continues to be the only proven method to achieve sustained weight loss in most patients. Bariatric procedures modify gastrointestinal anatomy and, in some cases, enteric hormone release to reduce caloric intake, reduce absorption, and alter metabolism to achieve weight loss. Currently, the three most common bariatric operations in the United States are Roux-en-Y gastric bypass, adjustable gastric band, and the vertical sleeve gastrectomy (Boxes 1, 2, and 3). The sleeve gastrectomy is part of a duodenal switch with biliopancreatic diversion. It has been used in patients at higher risk as a first-staged weight loss procedure, where the plan is to induce a significant weight loss and then offer patients a revision to a gastric bypass or duodenal switch with biliopancreatic diversion when they have achieved a safer weight. It is also now used as a primary bariatric operation with weight loss results that are better than adjustable gastric band but without the intestinal malabsorption issues seen after gastric bypass. Duodenal switch with biliopancreatic diversion has never been a popular weight loss surgery because of the significant malnutrition that accompanies this procedure (Box 4). All four of these operations can be performed laparoscopically in most patients.

PREOPERATIVE EVALUATION

The National Institutes of Health Consensus Development Conference Statement for Gastrointestinal Surgery for Severe Obesity was issued in 1991 and is still regarded as the starting point for criteria to accept patients in a surgical weight loss program. Patients are considered morbidly obese and candidates for surgery if they have a body mass index (BMI) of at least 35 kg/m², with an obesity-related comorbidity or greater than 40 kg/m². Recommendations are that patients should have tried dieting in the past before surgical therapy is considered as a treatment option (Box 5).

In evaluation of a potential patient for bariatric surgery, a multi-disciplinary team should be used. This team should include a dietitian and mental health professional, whose purpose is to obtain dietary and behavioral eating history, discuss postoperative dietary expectations, and decide whether the patient is appropriate for bariatric surgery. Support for the surgery from family members and friends is helpful. If the team believes that the patient is not appropriate for surgery, then consideration should be given to nonoperative medical management with appropriate counseling and surgery should be reconsidered or denied indefinitely.

Patients with severe end organ disease, such as end-stage heart failure or respiratory failure, are at higher risk for morbidity and mortality. Surgery is not necessarily contraindicated for these patients, but weight loss alone may not significantly correct end-stage heart or lung disease. Patients with cirrhosis may be at higher risk

---

BOX 1: Gastric bypass

Advantages
- Proven weight loss over 5 years
- Better weight loss than restrictive-only operations
- Proven improvement in medical comorbidities
- Mortality rate less than 1% at most centers

Disadvantages
- Malabsorption
- Marginal ulcer
- Stomal stenosis
- Inability to easily access distal stomach
- Internal hernia
- Small bowel obstruction
- Iron deficiency anemia
- Calcium and vitamin B_{12} deficiency

BOX 2: Adjustable gastric band

Advantages
- Reversible
- Least invasive (no stapling of the stomach)
- Lowest risk of death
- No malabsorption

Disadvantages
- Erosion
- Esophageal dilation
- Breakage
- Port problems
- Slippage or prolapse
- May worsen GERD
- Failure to lose weight
- Lower average weight loss

GERD, Gastroesophageal reflux disease.

BOX 3: Sleeve gastrectomy

Advantages
- Better weight loss than with adjustable gastric band
- Proven improvement in medical comorbidities
- Easier to perform than gastric bypass, especially if BMI is high
- No intestinal malabsorption
- No risk of marginal ulcers
- Preserved pylorus means less risk of dumping
- Ability to convert to gastric bypass or DS-BPD
- Mortality rate less than 1% at most centers

Disadvantages
- Not reversible
- Large portion of stomach removed
- A proximal leak is difficult to treat
- Stricture (incisura angularis)

BMI, Body mass index; DS-BPD, duodenal switch with biliopancreatic diversion.

BOX 4: Duodenal switch with biliopancreatic diversion

Advantages
- Excellent weight loss
- Proven improvement in medical comorbidities
- Preserved pylorus means less risk of dumping
- Less risk of marginal ulcers

Disadvantages
- Increased risk of protein malabsorption
- Increased risk of fat-soluble vitamin malabsorption (A, D, E, and K)
- Iron deficiency anemia
- Diarrhea and excess gas more common
- Internal hernia
- Higher complication rate
- Higher risk of osteoporosis

BOX 5: Patient requirements for bariatric surgery

1. Patients with a BMI of 40 kg/m² or greater are potential candidates for bariatric surgery.
2. Patients with a BMI of 35 to 40 kg/m² with significant obesity-related comorbidity are also potential candidates for bariatric surgery.
3. Patients with a history of dieting.
4. Patients with no recent substance abuse.
5. Patients should be evaluated by a multidisciplinary team that includes a dietitian and psychologic evaluation before surgery.

BMI, Body mass index.

for surgery but certainly may benefit from weight loss. Patients who are morbidly obese may be rejected for heart, lung, liver, or kidney transplant and, therefore, may benefit from bariatric surgery-induced weight loss. Patients who are nonambulating or bedridden should also be considered at high risk for postoperative complications.

Currently, patients with type 2 diabetes with a BMI of 30 to 35 kg/m² are being studied for whether they would benefit from bariatric surgery. The U.S. Food and Drug Administration (FDA) has approved the adjustable gastric band for this subgroup of patients.

PREPARING THE PATIENT IN THE OPERATING ROOM

On the morning of surgery, the patient is injected subcutaneously with low molecular-weight heparin to prevent venous thromboembolic complications. A peripheral intravenous (IV) line is placed, and an appropriate antibiotic is administered intravenously. The patient is placed on the operating room table in the supine position with a footboard. Appropriate padding of the patient is important because these particular patients are at increased risk for compression-related injuries. Sequential compression devices are placed on the lower extremities if they fit. General anesthesia is performed, and then a urinary catheter is inserted. The anesthetist inserts, applies suction to, and then immediately removes the oral-gastric tube before starting the operation. Esophageal temperature probes are not recommended because these can migrate into the stomach during stapling. The operating surgeon stands on the patient's right side, and the assistant on the left (Figure 1). Entering the abdomen in morbidly obese patients is safe with direct vision with a device that allows visualization of the abdominal wall layers sequentially with a 0-degree laparoscope inserted inside of it. Initial access in each procedure is through a left upper quadrant 12-mm incision.

TECHNIQUES

Laparoscopic Antecolic Antegastric Roux-en-Y Gastric Bypass Operative Technique

The abdomen is then insufflated with carbon dioxide to a pressure of 15 mm Hg, a 45-degree angled laparoscope is inserted, and an additional four ports are placed (a 5-mm trocar at the right subcostal margin, a 5-mm inferior to the left upper quadrant 12-mm trocar, a 12-mm trocar in the right upper quadrant, and a 12-mm trocar in the upper abdominal midline). The omentum and transverse colon are retracted cephalad until the transverse colon mesentery is visualized. Anterior retraction of the mesentery allows visualization of the jejunum at the ligament of Trietz. The jejunum is then transected with a linear stapler loaded with a 60-mm–length cartridge containing variable staple sizes from 2.0 to 3.0 mm for medium-thickness

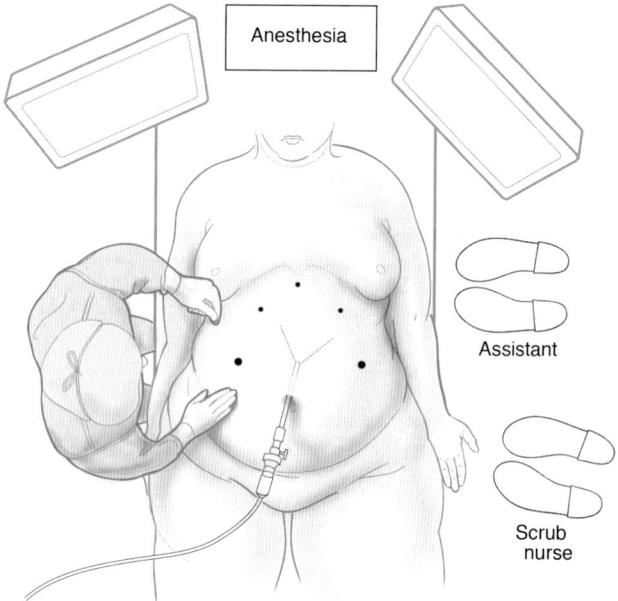

FIGURE I Positioning for laparoscopic gastric bypass. *(Illustration used with permission from Cameron JL, Sandone C:* Atlas of gastrointestinal surgery, *ed 2, vol II, Shelton, CT, in press, PMPH-USA.)*

tissue, approximately 40 cm to 75 cm distal to the ligament of Trietz. A long enough section of mesentery is usually found here so that the Roux limb can be placed in the antecolic antegastric position and safely reach the gastric pouch without any significant tension. The mesentery is divided with a linear stapler loaded with a 2.0-mm staple cartridge, and then the ultrasonic shears are used to extend this division as much as necessary so that the proximal Roux limb is able to safely reach the gastric pouch. A stay suture is placed on the proximal Roux limb, and then the bowel is run approximately 60 to 100 cm distal to the stapled off end. A stay suture is placed here to mark where the stapled side-to-side jejunojejunostomy will be constructed with the end of the biliopancreatic limb. The anastomosis is performed with a linear stapler loaded with a 60-mm–length cartridge containing variable staple sizes from 2.0 to 3.0 mm that is inserted through small enterotomies made with the ultrasonic shears below the stay suture (Figure 2). The enterotomy opening is then closed with firing of a similar linear stapler that has been placed under two stay sutures at each end of the opening (Figure 3). An unzipping stitch is placed in the crotch of the stapled anastomosis, and an antiobstruction stitch is placed to keep the Roux limb from kinking at the jejunojejunostomy. The mesenteric defect is then closed with a running suture. Clips or sutures are placed on the staple line if there is any bleeding. The greater omentum is divided in half with an ultrasonic dissector or vessel-sealing device along its entire length up to the border of the transverse colon.

Next, the patient is placed into steep reverse Trendelenburg's position. The legs and feet are then checked to ensure they are still straight and on the footboard. The left lateral segment of the liver is retracted with a Nathanson's retractor through a subxiphoid 4-mm puncture, which is then held in position with a movable arm that attaches to the operating room table (Iron Intern with Nathanson's liver retractors, Automated Medical Products Corp., Edison, NJ). The procedure then begins with dissecting the peritoneal attachments at the angle of His to expose the left crus, followed by the bare area of the gastrohepatic omentum to enter the lesser sac. Division of the neurovascular bundle on the lesser curvature side of the stomach just distal to the left gastric vein is done with a linear stapler with a

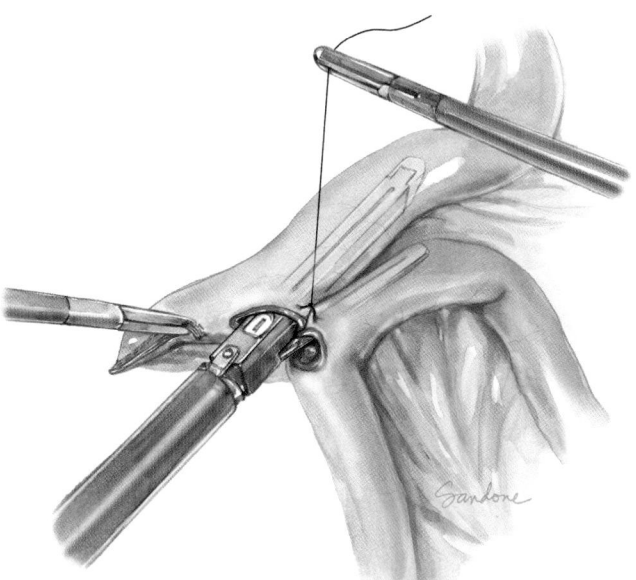

FIGURE 2 A linear stapler is used to create the jejunojejunostomy. *(Illustration used with permission from Cameron JL, Sandone C: Atlas of gastrointestinal surgery, ed 2, vol II, Shelton, CT, in press, PMPH-USA.)*

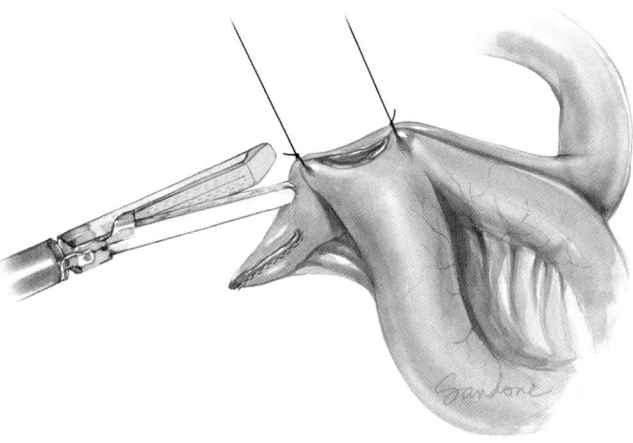

FIGURE 3 Closure of jejunojejunostomy opening. *(Illustration used with permission from Cameron JL, Sandone C: Atlas of gastrointestinal surgery, ed 2, vol II, Shelton, CT, in press, PMPH-USA.)*

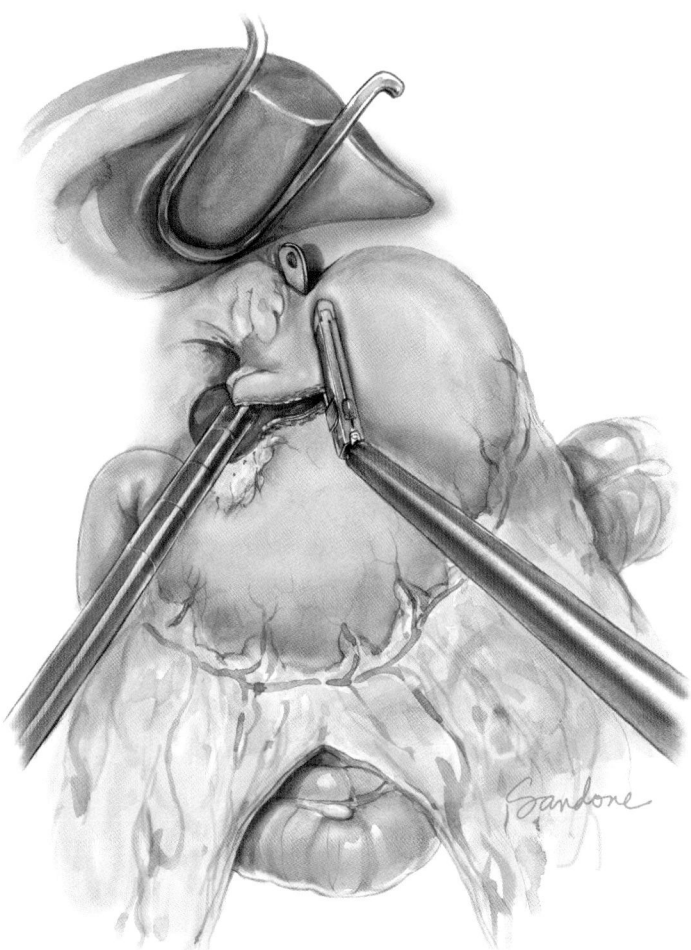

FIGURE 4 Stapled division of stomach. *(Illustration used with permission from Cameron JL, Sandone C: Atlas of gastrointestinal surgery, ed 2, vol II, Shelton, CT, in press, PMPH-USA.)*

2.0-mm staple cartridge. Next, a linear stapler loaded with a 60-mm–length cartridge containing variable staple sizes from 3.0 to 4.0 mm is first used to divide the stomach, followed by successive firings of a linear stapler containing 60-mm–length cartridges with variable staple sizes from 2.0 to 3.0 mm. The first gastric staple transection is started on the lesser curve side just below the left gastric vein and is then followed by sequential stapling until completion at the angle of His so that the proximal gastric pouch created is 15 to 20 mL in size (Figure 4). It is important to retract the posterior fundus downward and bring the stapler around the tissue at the angle of His to avoid making a large fundal pouch. This is prevented by entering the open space of the lesser sac after the first stapled division of the stomach and then dissecting through to the angle of His with an articulating dissector instrument that can then lock in place after forming a right angle. The articulating dissector can then be used to retract the fundus inferiorly while stapling sequentially to the angle of His. The stomach staple lines on both sides should be inspected for adequate

staple formation, bleeding, and ischemia. Bleeding staple lines are usually easily taken care of with a clip or direct suture ligation.

The Roux limb is brought up antecolic antegastric with care to avoid a twist in the mesentery. The Roux limb is then sutured to the gastric pouch staple line approximately where the first and second gastric staple lines intersect. A small enterotomy is made below the stay suture in the Roux limb and a similar size gastrotomy in the pouch to place the linear stapler loaded with a 45-mm–length cartridge containing variable staple sizes from 3.0 to 4.0 mm to create the gastrojejunostomy where only the first 30-mm of the staple cartridge are used (Figure 5). A stay suture is placed on the lesser curve (right) side of the opening; it is then used to retract the posterior part of the anastomosis to the left and anterior, thereby exposing the entire posterior side. A running 2-0 suture is then placed starting posterior on the left side and continuously run to the stay suture on the right side, which it is tied too (Figure 6). The anesthesia team carefully passes a 32F blunt round-end bougie from the mouth and then through the gastrojejunal anastomosis and into the Roux limb. A stay suture is placed at the halfway point of the opening between the end stay sutures. This stay suture and the stay suture on the left (angle of His side) are used to elevate the tissue so that the linear stapler loaded with a 60-mm–length cartridge containing variable staple sizes from 3.0 to 4.0 mm can be used to close the openings. The stapler is brought down on top of the bougie while retracting the tissue to be transected. This firing then closes most of the opening,

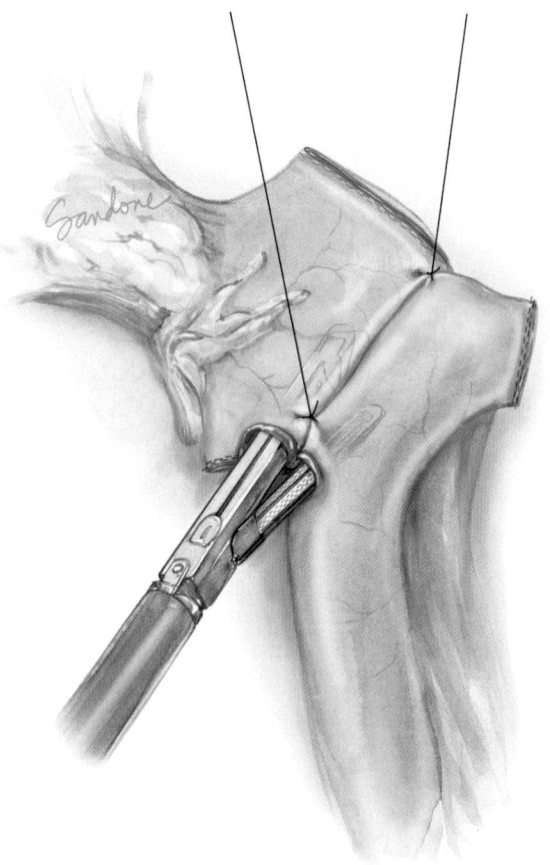

FIGURE 5   A linear stapler is used to create the gastrojejunostomy. *(Illustration used with permission from Cameron JL, Sandone C: Atlas of gastrointestinal surgery, ed 2, vol II, Shelton, CT, in press, PMPH-USA.)*

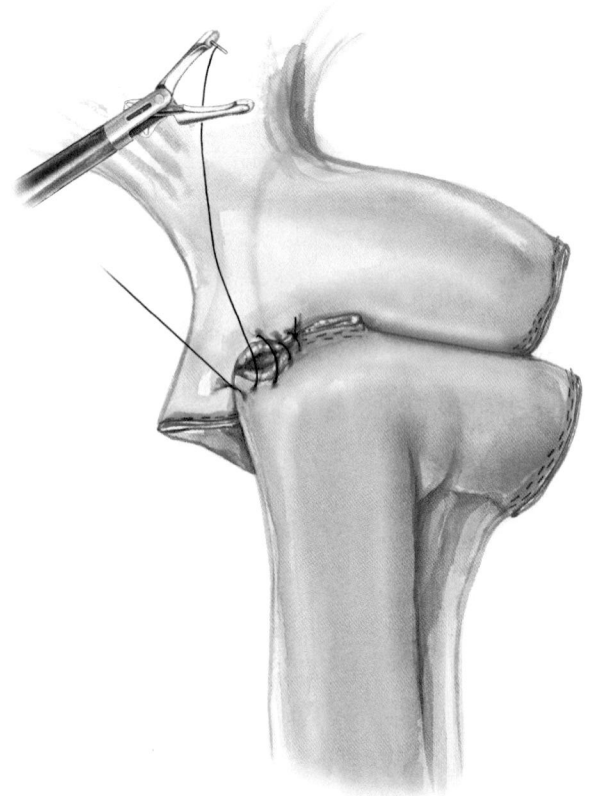

FIGURE 7   The opening used for the linear stapler is then closed with a running suture. *(Illustration used with permission from Cameron JL, Sandone C: Atlas of gastrointestinal surgery, ed 2, vol II, Shelton, CT, in press, PMPH-USA.)*

and the small remaining defect on the right side is easily closed with a 2-0 suture (Figure 7). Alternatively, the entire opening could be closed with a running 2-0 suture. The gastrojejunal anastomosis is then completed by running a 2-0 suture to cover the entire anterior and lateral sides in a second layer. The resultant anastomosis is approximately 12 mm in diameter and has been completely encircled by multiple continuous running 2-0 suture. An air leak test can be performed if desired to test the gastrojejunal anastomosis.

The operating room table is taken out of steep reverse Trendelenburg's position, and the mesenteric defect is then closed between the Roux limb mesentery and the transverse mesocolon, up to the transverse colon with running 2-0 suture. This is to help prevent an internal hernia through Peterson's defect. The remaining jejunojejunostomy mesenteric defect is then closed with a running suture. A drain is placed in the left upper quadrant by the anastomosis, and the trocars are removed with direct vision. Long-acting local anesthetic is placed in the wound, and the sites are closed with an absorbable subcuticular suture and glue (Figure 8).

Laparoscopic Adjustable Gastric Band

The 45-degree angled viewing laparoscope is inserted, and an additional three trocars (a 12-mm trocar in the upper abdominal midline and two right upper quadrant 5-mm trocars) are placed with direct vision. The angle of His attachments are taken down with blunt dissection, and the gastrohepatic omentum in the bare area is divided with a hook electrocautery. The right crus is identified. After the hook cautery is used to divide peritoneal tissue, an articulating dissector is then placed from the right crus side to the angle of His, with gentle rotating side-to-side motion as it is advanced forward; it is then

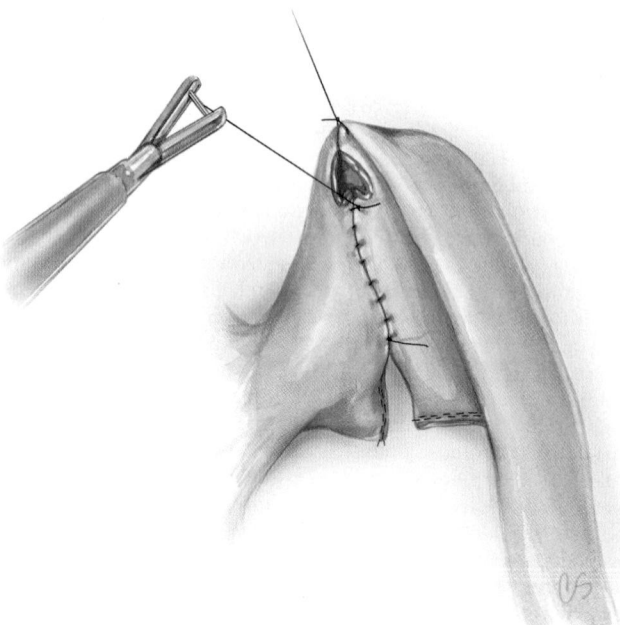

FIGURE 6   Reinforcing the posterior staple line of the gastrojejunostomy. *(Illustration used with permission from Cameron JL, Sandone C: Atlas of gastrointestinal surgery, ed 2, vol II, Shelton, CT, in press, PMPH-USA.)*

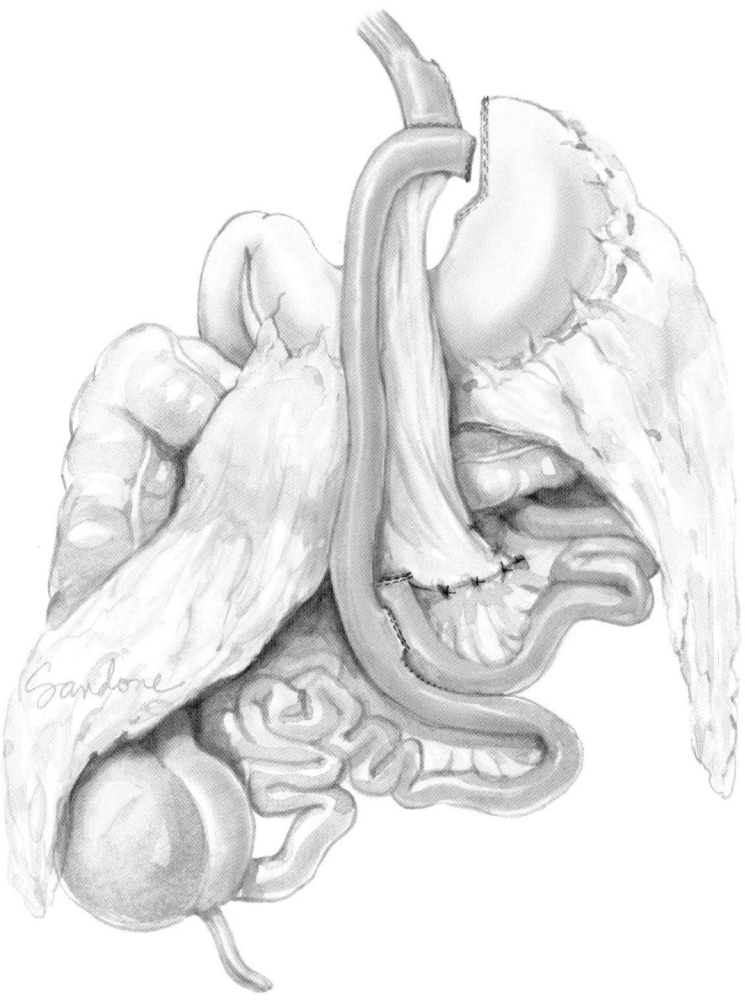

FIGURE 8 Antecolic antegastric Roux-en-Y gastric bypass. *(Illustration used with permission from Cameron JL, Sandone C: Atlas of gastrointestinal surgery, ed 2, vol II, Shelton, CT, in press, PMPH-USA.)*

flexed into a right angle and locked. The 12-mm left upper quadrant trocar is removed, and a 15-mm trocar is placed. The adjustable band is placed into the abdomen through the 15-mm trocar. The band tubing is then placed through the opening in the articulating dissector and then brought over to the right crus side (Figure 9). The tubing is removed from the dissector and then placed through the buckle of the band. The buckle is then locked. Next, one to four interrupted 2-0 nonabsorble sutures are placed from the fundus to the proximal stomach (superior to the band). It is easier to work closer to the angle of His side of the stomach and then sew towards the patient's right side (Figure 10). The buckle of the band should not be covered because of increased risk of erosion. The anterior fundal wrap over the band should be without tension. The tubing of the band is grasped and removed through the left upper quadrant trocar site. The trocars are then removed. A subcutaneous pocket is formed on the anterior side of the fascia, and the port is connected to the band tubing and then secured to the fascia. It is important to check the tubing and ensure it has no kinks as it enters the fascia. The site is irrigated, and then all the trocar sites are closed with subcuticular suture and glue (Figure 11).

Laparoscopic Vertical Sleeve Gastrectomy

Laparoscopic vertical sleeve gastrectomy was initially used as a first-stage operation in patients at high risk or in patients whose super

morbid obesity made a laparoscopic-only approach difficult. After 12 to 24 months of weight loss, a second-stage operation could be used in those who were still at a high BMI and wanted to be revised to a laparoscopic Roux-en-Y gastric bypass or a laparoscopic duodenal switch with biliopancreatic diversion. This staged approach is designed to reduce operative risk by improving comorbidities and reducing the technical challenges associated with super morbidly obese patients. Recent data has shown that sleeve gastrectomy is an effective operation for weight loss, resulting in 40% to 60% excess body weight loss as the primary treatment alone. It is easier to perform and has less complications then a Roux-en-Y gastric bypass or duodenal switch with biliopancreatic diversion. It does not involve a large foreign body that can be at risk to erode or slip as with an adjustable gastric band. It also avoids the intestinal malabsorption and small bowel obstruction risks seen with gastric bypass or duodenal switch with biliopancreatic diversion.

As previously described, entry to the abdominal cavity starts with a 12-mm trocar placed with direct vision through a left upper quadrant incision. The abdomen is then insufflated with carbon dioxide to a pressure of 15 mm Hg, a 45-degree angled laparoscope is inserted and an additional three ports (a 5-mm trocar at the right subcostal margin, a 15-mm trocar in the right upper quadrant, and a 12-mm trocar just to the left of the upper abdominal midline) and a subxiphoid liver retractor are placed with direct vision. The operation starts with division of the stomach's greater curvature blood supply with a vessel-sealing device to divide the gastrocolic and gastrosplenic

FIGURE 9   The band tubing attached to the articulating dissector is then brought around the posterior stomach, from patient's left to right side. *(Illustration used with permission from Cameron JL, Sandone C: Atlas of gastrointestinal surgery, ed 2, vol II, Shelton, CT, in press, PMPH-USA.)*

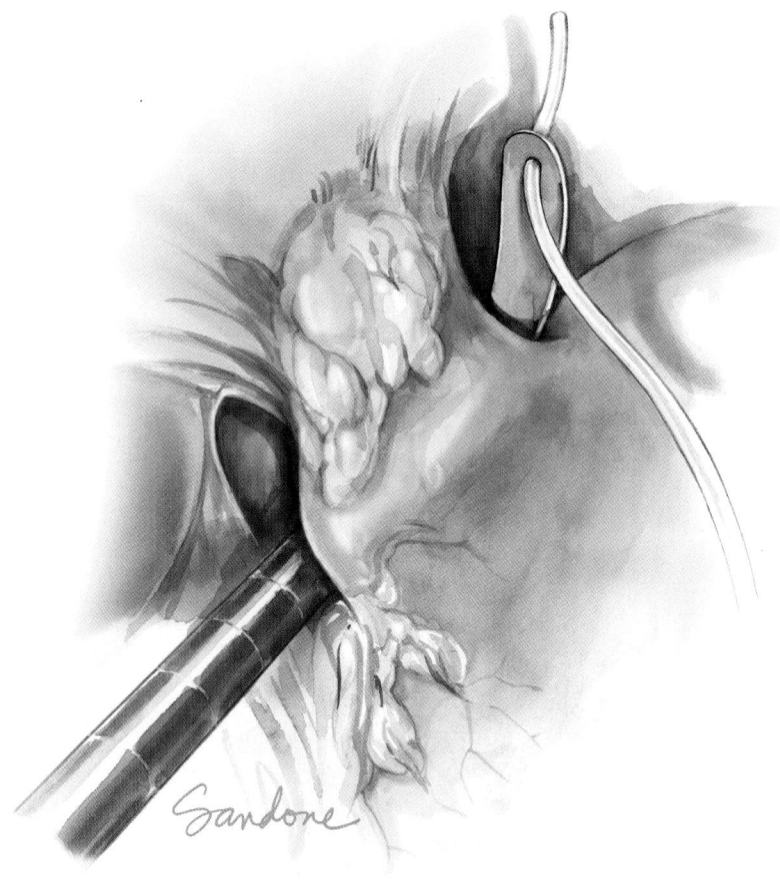

FIGURE 10   An anterior gastric wrap is performed with interrupted nonabsorbable sutures. *(Illustration used with permission from Cameron JL, Sandone C: Atlas of gastrointestinal surgery, ed 2, vol II, Shelton, CT, in press, PMPH-USA.)*

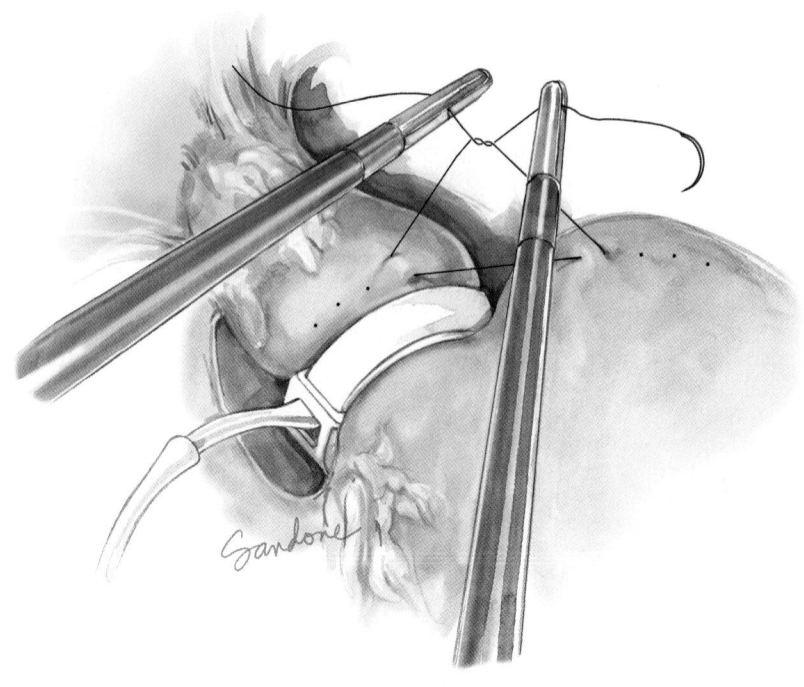

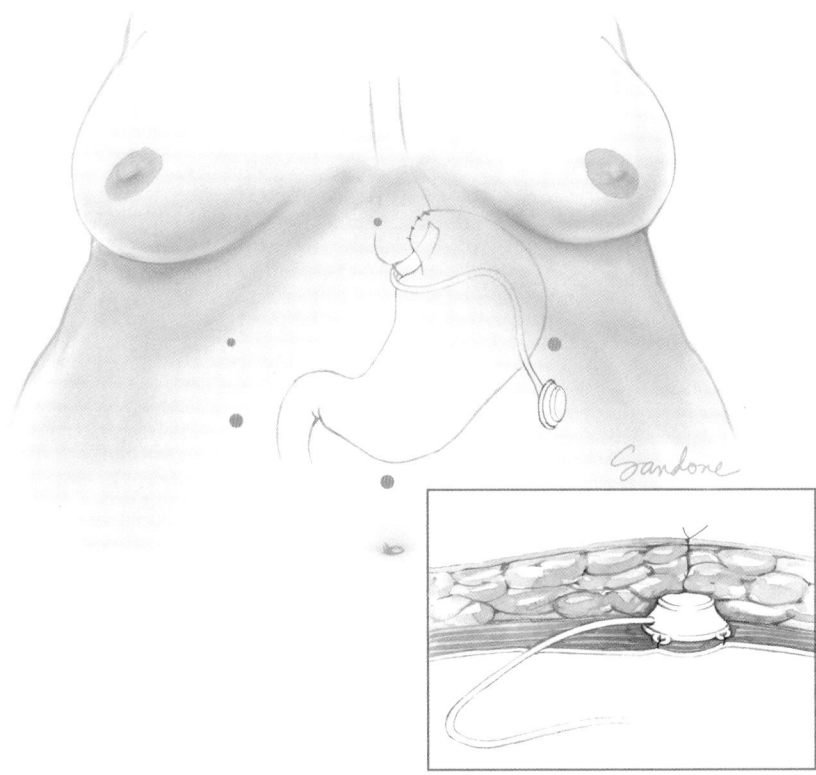

FIGURE 11   Adjustable gastric band with port placement in the left upper quadrant. *(Illustration used with permission from Cameron JL, Sandone C: Atlas of gastrointestinal surgery, ed 2, vol II, Shelton, CT, in press, PMPH-USA.)*

ligaments close to the stomach (Figure 12). A stay suture is placed 6 to 7 cm from the pylorus-duodenal junction. A 40F bougie is inserted transorally and brought down alongside the lesser curve until it lays against the stomach wall to the patient's right of the stay suture. Next, a narrow gastric tube is created with a linear cutting stapler starting on the patient's right side of the stay suture and sequentially stapling towards the angle of His alongside a 40F bougie. The surgeons should confirm that the bougie is on the lesser curve side of the stapler.

The stomach is first divided with two firings of the linear stapler loaded with 60-mm–length cartridges containing variable staple sizes from 4.0 to 5.0 mm for extra thick tissue. The stomach is continued to be divided with a linear stapler loaded with 60-mm–length cartridges containing variable staple sizes from 3.0 to 4.0 mm. The stomach is divided next to the bougie all the way up to the angle of His where the lateral stomach is separated (Figure 13). Care is taken not to leave any fundus behind and not to apply the stapler too close to the gastroesophageal junction. Hemostasis of the gastric staple line can be secured with running sutures or clips. The resected stomach is extracted intact through the 15-mm trocar site, after widening the fascial opening with a clamp device. If the surgeon desires, the staple line can be evaluated with an underwater leak test either with an orogastric tube or an endoscope. A drain is placed in the left upper quadrant and brought out through the 5-mm trocar site. The ports are removed with direct vision after first closing the 15-mm port site suture passing device. Long-acting local anesthetic is placed in the wounds, and the sites are closed with subcuticular sutures (Figure 14).

Laparoscopic Biliopancreatic Diversion With Duodenal Switch

The laparoscopic duodenal switch with biliopancreatic diversion (DS-BPD) is primarily a malabsorptive operation that involves preservation of the gastric pylorus and creation of a short, 100-cm ileal

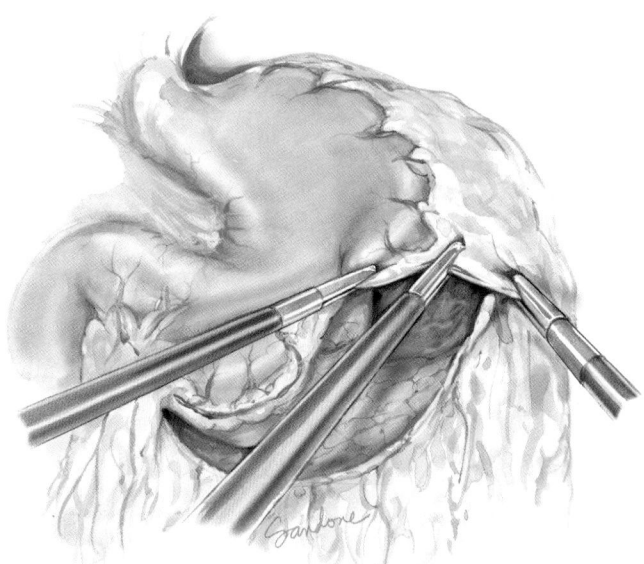

FIGURE 12   Division of the vascular supply next to the greater curvature of the stomach. *(Illustration used with permission from Cameron JL, Sandone C: Atlas of gastrointestinal surgery, ed 2, vol II, Shelton, CT, in press, PMPH-USA.)*

"common channel," where food and biliopancreatic enzymes are allowed to mix. Because of the potential for malabsorption-related nutritional deficiencies and the complexity of the operation, DS-BPD is the least common bariatric operation performed in the United States when compared with gastric bypass, sleeve gastrectomy, and adjustable gastric banding.

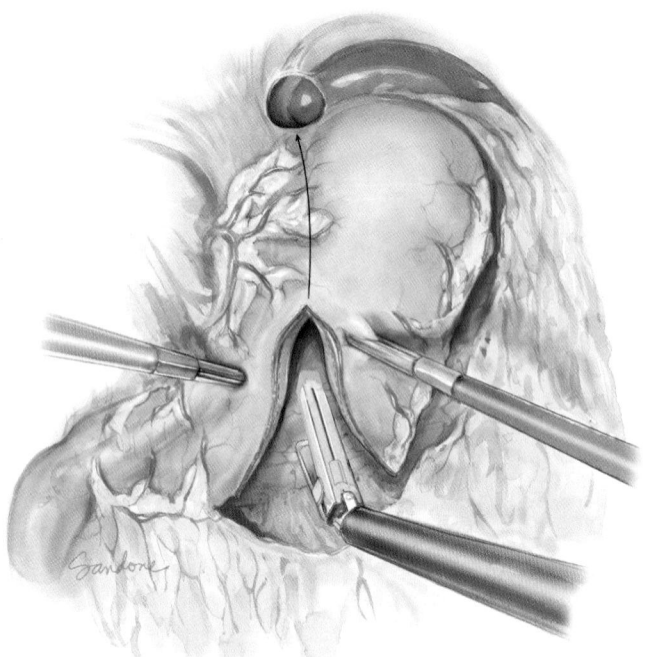

FIGURE 13 Linear stapler used to vertically divide the stomach close to the lesser curve. A 40F bougie is used to calibrate the size of the remaining stomach. *(Illustration used with permission from Cameron JL, Sandone C: Atlas of gastrointestinal surgery, ed 2, vol II, Shelton, CT, in press, PMPH-USA.)*

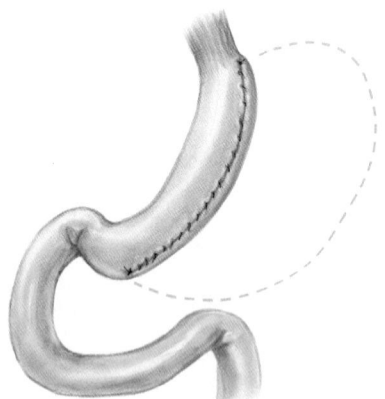

FIGURE 14 Vertical sleeve gastrectomy. *(Illustration used with permission from Cameron JL, Sandone C: Atlas of gastrointestinal surgery, ed 2, vol II, Shelton, CT, in press, PMPH-USA.)*

As previously described, entry to the abdominal cavity starts with a 12-mm trocar placed with direct vision through a left upper quadrant incision. The abdomen is then insufflated with carbon dioxide to a pressure of 15 mm Hg, a 45-degree angled laparoscope is inserted, and an additional four ports (a 5-mm trocar at the right subcostal margin, a 5-mm inferior to the left upper quadrant 12-mm trocar, a 15-mm trocar in the right upper quadrant, and a 12-mm trocar in the upper abdominal) and a subxiphoid liver retractor are placed with direct vision. The operating surgeon stands on the patient's left side for the small intestinal part of the operation, and the assistant on the right. The left-sided ports are the surgeon's operating ports for the ileoileostomy part of the procedure. The operating room table is then placed flat, and the omentum and transverse colon

are retracted cephalad. The cecum and ileocecal valve are then identified, and the ileum is measured back 100 cm proximal to the cecum. A stay suture is placed, and then another 150 cm of ileum is measured proximal from the suture. This is where the ileum is transected with a linear stapler loaded with a 60-mm–length cartridge containing variable staple sizes from 2.0 to 3.0 mm. The mesentery is divided with the ultrasonic shears, and a stay suture is placed on the distal transected bowel to mark the Roux end that will connect to the duodenum. The proximal divided bowel is the biliopancreatic limb, which is brought down to the previous stay suture marking the ileum at 100 cm from the cecum. A stapled side-to-side ileoileostomy is then constructed. Care should be taken to avoid a twist or misalignment of the bowel at this point. The anastomosis is performed as the previously described enteroenterostomy in the gastric bypass section.

Next, the patient is placed in steep reverse Trendelenburg's position, and a liver retractor is placed in the subxiphoid position to retract the left lateral segment of the liver. As previously described, a sleeve gastrectomy is then performed, with a 48F instead of a 40F bougie, and then it is removed after completion. Attention is then turned toward the duodenum, which is freed from its lateral attachments, with great care taken to not injure any of the structures in the hepatoduodenal ligament. The duodenum is divided approximately 2 to 4 cm distal to the pylorus with a linear stapler loaded with a 60-mm–length cartridge containing variable staple sizes from 3.0 to 4.0 mm (Figure 15). The omentum is split, and the Roux limb is brought antecolic up to the proximal duodenal end. Two stay sutures are placed for a side-to-side anastomosis. Under the inferior stay suture, both ends are opened and a linear stapler loaded with a 45-mm–length cartridge containing variable staple sizes from 3.0 to 4.0 mm is placed for 2.5 to 3 cm and fired (Figure 16). A 40F bougie is placed through the anastomosis. The opening is now closed with a running suture. Multiple seromuscular interrupted sutures are placed circumferentially. The mesenteric defect is then closed between the Roux limb mesentery and the transverse mesocolon, up to the transverse colon. A drain is left by the stomach, and another drain is left by the ileoduodenal anastomosis. The trocars are removed, and local anesthetic is injected, followed by a subcuticular closure of the trocar sites (Figure 17).

Laparoscopic Gastric Plication

Laparoscopic gastric greater curvature plication is an emerging restrictive bariatric procedure that successfully reduces the gastric volume with plication of the gastric greater curvature. Its main advantages are the reversibility of the technique, no staple line needed, and no foreign body. Currently, it is under investigational protocol at several institutions in the United States. The procedure consists of separating the greater omentum and attachments of the spleen from the greater curvature of the stomach. The anesthesiologist places a bougie into the stomach or a flexible endoscope may be used in its place. The surgeon then starts inverting the stomach 2 cm from the angle of His on the greater curvature side with either running or interrupted sutures to approximately 5 to 6 cm from the pylorus. A second row of sutures are usually placed to further fold the stomach inward and create more restriction. Current studies have shown short-term efficacy in weight reduction. However, further studies are needed to determine long-term efficacy and safety because the rates of complications may increase over time along with weight regain. Acute gastric perforation, leak at the suture line, obstruction, and intussusception are all possible complications.

POSTOPERATIVE MANAGEMENT

Most patients are transferred after routine monitoring in the recovery room. Patients with moderate to severe obstructive sleep apnea are prescribed (CPAP [continuous positive airway pressure]) during

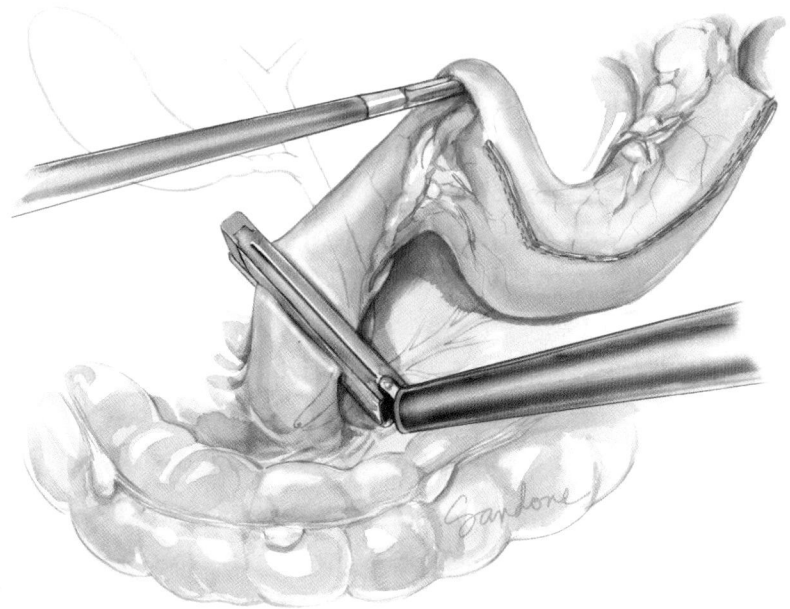

FIGURE 15   The duodenum is divided with a linear stapler. *(Illustration used with permission from Cameron JL, Sandone C: Atlas of gastrointestinal surgery, ed 2, vol II, Shelton, CT, in press, PMPH-USA.)*

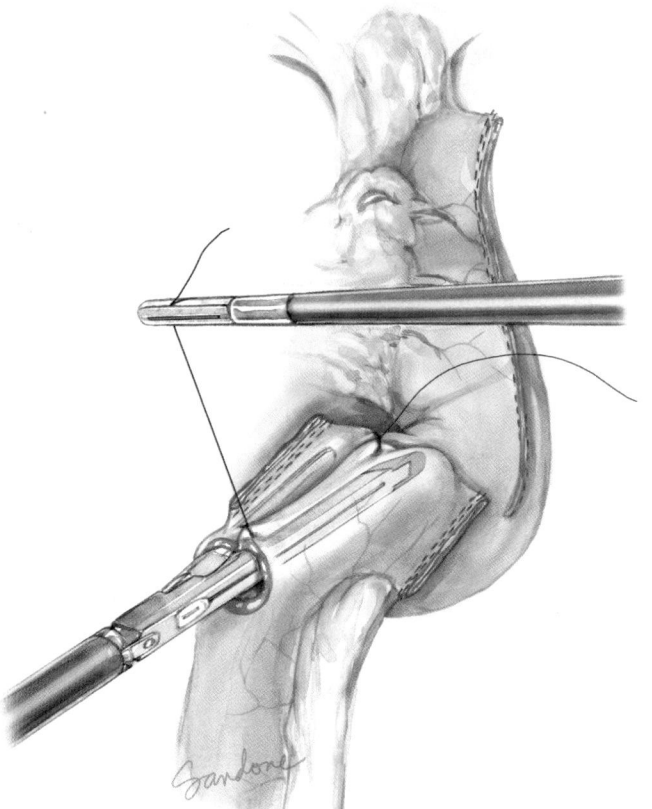

FIGURE 16   The duodenoileostomy is created with a linear stapler. *(Illustration used with permission from Cameron JL, Sandone C: Atlas of gastrointestinal surgery, ed 2, vol II, Shelton, CT, in press, PMPH-USA.)*

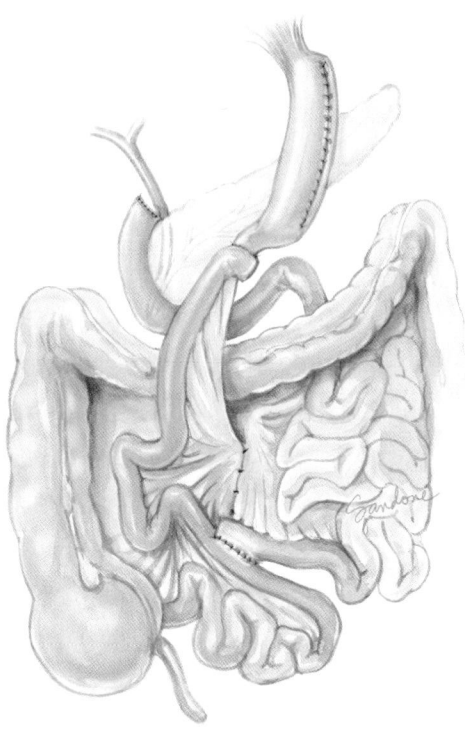

FIGURE 17   Antecolic duodenal switch with biliopancreatic diversion. *(Illustration used with permission from Cameron JL, Sandone C: Atlas of gastrointestinal surgery, ed 2, vol II, Shelton, CT, in press, PMPH-USA.)*

sleep, if they are able to tolerate it or use it routinely at home. Low molecular-weight heparin is continued during hospitalization for most patients, and some patients who are at higher risk for venous thromboembolism may be treated at home for an entire month after surgery. The patient is usually in a chair or ambulating within the first 12 hours. Pain is managed with a patient-controlled analgesia delivery device for the first evening, and the patient is encouraged to use the incentive spirometer while awake.

Patients for adjustable gastric band are given a liquid diet the following morning and then discharged to home. Patients for gastric bypass and duodenal switch are started on a limited liquid diet on postoperative day 1, and then the quantity of liquids is advanced as tolerated on day 2 with discharge planned that day. Patients for sleeve gastrectomy are given a nonsugar liquid diet on postoperative day 1 and usually advanced over the course of the day, with an aim to discharge that day or the following morning. Patients after all four operations remain on a nonsugar noncarbonated liquid diet that includes protein drinks for the first week after surgery. They are then advanced to a puree diet that still includes protein drinks for the following 3 weeks, at which time they start to introduce solid foods. Selective upper gastrointestinal series radiography is used in patients who have a sustained heart rate over 120 bpm, respiratory distress, fever, increasing abdominal pain or chest pain. The drain is removed before discharge.

Follow-up is in 2 weeks for all patients. Patients are highly encouraged to go to monthly support group meeting and see the dietitian on a routine basis, along with a mental health professional if needed or requested.

Patients for adjustable gastric band are evaluated for their first fill at the 6-week postoperative appointment. Patients who, despite making healthy food choices, have stopped losing weight, who report no "restriction" with solid foods, and who are consistently hungry in between meals get a fill. Patients are then asked to follow-up in 2 months. Band position and tightness can be assessed with fluoroscopy if necessary in patients who, despite repeated fills, continue to have no restriction. Patients who report continued vomiting, abdominal pain, or severe gastroesophageal reflux disease (GERD)–like symptoms should also be evaluated with an upper gastrointestinal fluoroscopic study.

All patients are placed on a multivitamin and calcium after surgery. Menstruating women are placed on iron to prevent anemia. Patients for gastric bypass are recommended to take vitamin B_{12}, and patients for duodenal switch with biliopancreatic diversion are advised to take supplements that include the fat-soluble vitamins A, D, E, and K. Patients who have not had their gallbladder previously removed are placed on ursodiol 300 mg twice a day for 6 months to reduce the risk of symptomatic cholelithiasis during the rapid weight loss phase after gastric bypass, sleeve gastrectomy, or DS-BPD surgery. Follow-up is usually around 3, 6, 12, 18, and 24 months, followed by every year thereafter. An iron panel and hematologic, electrolyte, and liver function laboratory tests are obtained at 3 months, and vitamin B_{12} 25-hydroxy vitamin D and PTH levels, are added at 1-year visits. Patients who are not taking in enough protein by diet history may need prealbumin checked along with nutritional counseling. Patients for DS-BPD may also need the additional vitamins A, E, and K tested for after surgery.

OUTCOMES AND COMPLICATIONS

Buchwald and colleagues conducted a meta-analysis of the bariatric literature in 2003. They found that mean excess weight losses for adjustable gastric band, Roux-en-Y gastric bypass, and biliopancreatic diversion with or without duodenal switch were 48%, 62%, and 70%, respectively. Mortality rates were 0.1%, 0.5%, and 1.1%, respectively, for the three operations. Type II diabetes was found overall to be completely resolved in 77% of patients and improved in an additional 9% of patients. Hyperlipidemia, hypertension, and obstructive sleep apnea were improved in 70%, 79%, and 84%, respectively. Schauer and associates showed in a randomized prospective trial that obese patients with uncontrolled type II diabetes had significant improvement in glycemic control after both Roux-en-Y gastric bypass and sleeve gastrectomy compared with medical therapy alone. The mean glycated hemoglobin was 9.2% before the study; after 12 months, the mean decreased to 7.5% in the medical therapy alone group, 6.4% in the gastric bypass group $(P < 0.001)$, and 6.6% in the sleeve gastrectomy group $(P = 0.003)$. Patient weight loss was only −5.4 kg in the medical therapy group as compared with the gastric bypass and sleeve gastrectomy groups (−29.4 kg and −25.1 kg, respectively; $P < 0.001$) at 12 months follow-up. In a large retrospective cohort study comparing bariatric surgery patients matched with morbidly obese patients who did not undergo surgery, Adams and

colleagues found a 40% reduction in mortality rate after 7.1 years with the surgery group. The significant decrease in the long-term mortality rate was attributed to a decrease in coronary artery disease, type II diabetes, and cancer-related deaths.

Pulmonary embolism and sepsis from an anastomotic leak are the two leading causes of death in the postoperative period after bariatric surgery. Both complications are less than 1% at most bariatric surgery centers that are part of the American College of Surgeons Bariatric Surgery Center Network Accreditation program. Perioperative measures to reduce the risk include: chemoprophylaxis, sequential compression devices (if they can safely fit the patient's lower extremity), and early ambulation. Some centers go beyond the routine in-hospital prophylaxis by placing patients who may be at higher risk for venous thromboembolism on low molecular-weight heparin anywhere from 10 days to a month after discharge from the hospital. These patients may include those who have a history of pulmonary embolism or deep venous thrombosis, poor ambulation, severe venous stasis disease, and possibly a BMI of more than 70 kg/m². Inferior vena cava filters are also used in some select patients who may be at higher risk for death from pulmonary embolism. It is unclear to date whether these extra measures used to prevent venous thromboembolism (VTE) are helpful because no randomized trials specifically address the morbid obese patient population that undergoes bariatric surgery.

Prevention of a leak is one of the primary ways to decrease mortality after bariatric surgery. The most common area for a leak to occur after gastric bypass is at the gastrojejunostomy. However, a leak may also occur at the distal stomach staple line or the jejunojejunostomy. There are several ways of performing the upper anastomosis of a GBP or DS-BPD that include circular stapler, linear stapler, hand-sewn, and a combination of stapling with an outer layer of suturing. This may account for variation in the reported rates of a leak, stomal stenosis, and marginal ulcer. At Johns Hopkins, the laparoscopic Roux-en-Y gastric bypass leak rate is less than 0.3% with the previously described technique that has an inner stapled layer and essentially an outer layer consisting of multiple running sutures.

Box 6 shows the published complication rate after laparoscopic gastric bypass. The authors have used an antecolic antegastric technique for more than 7 years, which has reduced the internal hernia rates to less than 2%. The authors continue to close the defect between the transverse mesocolon and the Roux limb mesentery up to the transverse colon along with the enteroenterostomy defect in both the gastric bypass and the DS-BPD operations. Stomal stenosis after gastric bypass most commonly occurs between 2 to 6 weeks after surgery but occasionally may be seen later in conjunction with a marginal ulcer. Greater than 90% of these patients respond to balloon dilation; however, late-occurring strictures are less likely to heal and may require revision of the gastrojejunostomy with or without a truncal vagotomy. A marginal ulcer after gastric bypass can occur on the jejunal side of the gastrojejunal anastomosis, and again, greater than 90% heal with proton pump inhibitor therapy. Patients should

---

BOX 6: Complications for 251 cases

Stomal stenosis: 10 (4%)
Marginal ulcer: 11 (4%)
Symptomatic gallstones: 8 (3%)
Internal hernia: 4 (2%)
Postoperative bleeding: 5 (2%)
Stroke (minor): 1 (0.4%)
Trocar hernia: 0 (0)
Deep venous thrombosis: 0 (0)
Pulmonary emboli: 0(0)
Wound infection: 0 (0)
Leaks: 0 (0%)
Death: 1 (0.4%)

be asked if they are smoking, using nonsteroidal antiinflammatory drugs (NSAIDs), or drinking large quantities of caffeinated drinks (coffee, tea, etc.) because these have all been attributed with marginal ulceration. The most common location of a stricture seen after sleeve gastrectomy is at the incisura angularis. These strictures may respond to balloon dilation, otherwise a revision to a gastrojejunostomy proximal to the stricture may be needed.

The laparoscopic adjustable gastric band (LAGB) operation has a lower 30-day major complication rate when compared with gastric bypass, sleeve gastrectomy, and DS-BPD. However, long-term complications after LAGB appear to be higher, with rates above 20%. Cottam and colleagues in a case-controlled matched-pair cohort study showed excess weight loss is greater after gastric bypass when compared with LAGB (74% vs 51%, respectively; $P < 0.001$) at 3 years. Type II diabetes resolved more frequently after gastric bypass (78% vs 50%, respectively; $P = 0.01$). The most common complications after LAGB are port/tubing breakage, flipped port, gastric prolapse or band slippage, and GERD. Gastric prolapse or band slippage entails cephalad herniation of the stomach through the band, resulting in a larger pouch and, in some cases, near or total gastric outlet obstruction. Erosion of the band into the stomach lumen is a complication reported in ~1% of cases and requires removal of the band. Infection of the band system is also seen in ~1% of cases and again requires removal. GERD symptoms that develop when inflating the band with saline solution to increase restriction may require removal of the some or all of the fluid. Patients who have an obvious hiatal hernia at the time of surgery may benefit from a crural repair at the time of gastric band placement.

ENDOSCOPIC APPROACHES TO THE MANAGEMENT OF OBESITY

Transoral endoluminal interventions performed entirely through the gastrointestinal tract with flexible endoscopy offer the potential for an ambulatory weight loss procedure without any incisions on the abdominal wall. The restrictive procedures include intragastric balloon treatment, endoluminal sutured gastroplasty, and transoral stapled gastroplasty. The malabsorptive procedures include duodenojejunal bypass sleeve and gastroduodenojejunal bypass sleeve. Other procedures that have been performed with varying degrees of short-term success include intragastric injection of botulinum toxin type A and gastric electrical stimulation.

The most widely studied of these therapies is the intragastric balloon. Although this device is currently not FDA approved for use in the United States, it has been used in Europe, Canada, Mexico, India, and South America with adequate short-term results. The most common complication is nausea and vomiting, but more serious complications, such as gastric erosions, ulcerations, and bowel obstructions, have been noted. There are ongoing trials looking at the use of flexible endoscopically guided staplers or suture devices to create a gastric sleeve along the lesser curvature of the stomach. Flexible endoscopic suturing devices have also been used to reduce

the size of the stoma and gastric pouch in patients who have had weight regain after gastric bypass. Unfortunately, long-term weight loss has not been proven with these devices.

Malabsorptive procedures, such as the duodenojejunal bypass sleeve, use a prosthetic barrier device that intraluminally bypasses the necessary areas of absorption in the duodenum and the upper part of the jejunum. A gastroduodenojejunal bypass sleeve has also shown promise in very short-term results with regards to weight loss and glycemic control. Long-term results and safety profile studies are needed with these devices.

Endoscopic therapy for weight loss is in its infancy; newer therapies are constantly being introduced and tested. If appropriate efficacy and safety profiles can be established, these products may be introduced into the clinical mainstream practice.

COMMENTS

Bariatric surgery continues to be the only effective means of producing weight loss in most patients. It has been shown to reduce or even eliminate comorbidities associated with a high BMI. Mortality and leak rates less than 1% have been published by several leading surgical centers committed to bariatric surgery. Laparoscopic techniques have been shown in randomized prospective studies over open approaches to significantly reduce perioperative wound complications and incisional hernias. Appropriate attention to the risks and benefits of the procedure along with the individual patient's medical risks requires consultation and joint decision making between the physician and the patient. Center of excellence certification programs are collecting outcome data that will not only help to document in the future the beneficial long-term effects of bariatric surgery but will also define acceptable outcomes and complication rates.

SUGGESTED READINGS

Adams TD, Gress RE, Smith SC, et al: Long-term mortality after gastric bypass surgery, *N Engl J Med* 357:753–761, 2007.

Buchwald H, Avidor Y, Braunwald E, et al: Bariatric surgery: a systemic review and meta-analysis, *JAMA* 292:1724–1728, 2004.

Cottam DR, Atkinson J, Anderson A, et al: A case-controlled matched pair cohort study of laparoscopic Roux-en-Y gastric bypass and Lap-Band patients in a single US center with three-year follow-up, *Obes Surg* 16:534–540, 2006.

Schauer PR, Kashyap SR, Wolski K, et al: Bariatric surgery versus intensive medical therapy in obese patients with diabetes, *N Engl J Med* 366:1567–1576, 2012.

Schweitzer MA, Lidor A, Magnuson TH: 251 consecutive laparoscopic gastric bypass operations using a 2 layer gastrojejunostomy technique with a zero leak rate, *J Laparoendosc Adv Surg Tech A* 16:83–87, 2006.

Steele KE, Prokopowicz GP, Magnuson T, et al: Laparoscopic antecolic Roux-en-Y gastric bypass with closure of internal defects leads to fewer internal hernias than the retrocolic approach, *Surg Endosc* 22:2056–2061, 2008.

Wittgrove AC, Clark WG: Laparoscopic gastric bypass Roux-en-Y: 500 patients: technique and results, with 3–60 month follow-up, *Obes Surg* 10:233–238, 2000.

Laparoscopic Donor Nephrectomy

Dorry Segev, MD, PhD

Once the patients and the team decided to proceed with the transplant, an extra professional burden falls on the surgeon performing the donor nephrectomy because his patient is expected to survive normally.

Joseph Murray, MD, Nobel Lecture, December 8, 1990

OVERVIEW

Every year since 2000, approximately 6000 healthy individuals in the United States undergo uninephrectomy for the purposes of kidney donation to a family member, a friend, or even a stranger. This rate has doubled since 1995 (Figure 1), the year the laparoscopic donor nephrectomy was developed and first described by Ratner and colleagues (1995) at Johns Hopkins Medical Center. At this point, nearly all donor nephrectomies in this country are performed laparoscopically, either through traditional (pure) laparoscopy or hand-assisted techniques (Figure 2). Although the significant increase in live donor kidney transplantation between 1995 and 2000 was probably inspired by the decrease in the problems of a minimally invasive approach (pain, scar, duration of convalescence), risks are still associated with this operation, and minimizing and understanding these risks remain high priorities for the transplant community.

To help clinicians better understand the laparoscopic donor nephrectomy, this chapter explores the evaluation of the live kidney donor, contraindications to donation, the intraoperative approach, and postoperative management. Short-term risks are discussed, as are what are known and unknown about long-term risk.

EVALUATION OF THE LIVE KIDNEY DONOR

In general, live kidney donors should be both physically and mentally well, with adequate social and financial support. A thorough, careful medical history is obtained, and donors undergo physical examination, laboratory screening, and radiographic assessment. Creatinine clearance is determined, urinalysis and culture are examined, complete blood cell count and chemistry profiles are obtained, and screening for infectious diseases (including cytomegalovirus [CMV], Epstein-Barr virus [EBV], varicella-zoster virus [VZV], human immunodeficiency virus [HIV], syphilis, hepatitis, and tuberculosis) is performed.

Transplantation centers often conduct the evaluation in various phases to save donor candidates the cost and burden of additional testing if they are excluded in an earlier phase. Donors who pass early screening tests eventually undergo in-person consultation by a nephrologist, a surgeon, a psychologist or psychiatrist, a nurse coordinator, a social worker, and an independent living donor advocate. Later phase screening might include mammography, cardiac evaluation such as echocardiography or stress testing, pulmonary testing, colonoscopy, Papanicolaou smear, or prostate-specific antigen measurement (PSA).

All donors undergo abdominal imaging to confirm the presence of two kidneys and map the hilar anatomy; although it is unusual for a donor to be excluded on the basis of vascular abnormalities, this does occur on occasion, but of more importance is that a preoperative understanding of the vascular anatomy can assist with choice of kidney, as well as of the intraoperative approach. The left kidney is commonly the kidney of choice, because of its longer renal vein and lack of proximity to the liver, unless abnormalities or other inequalities between the kidneys exist.

CONTRAINDICATIONS

Age of younger than 18 years is considered a contraindication to donation in almost all cases. Diabetes mellitus, significant cardiac disease, and vascular disease are also considered absolute contraindications, as are most active malignancies. HIV infection is an exclusion criterion currently dictated by congressional law, in addition to the potential risk of HIV-related renal disease. Active infection is generally a contraindication, particularly if systemic. Untreatable psychiatric illness, active substance abuse, and severe neurologic deficits are also contraindications. Debated contraindications include decreased creatinine clearance, insulin resistance, obesity, and hypertension; the level for exclusion varies among transplantation centers, and some centers have written extensive protocols for evaluating, approving, and monitoring donors with these conditions.

OPERATIVE APPROACH

The patient is positioned in a modified lateral decubitus position, with the ipsilateral side (the side of the kidney intended for donation) upward. A periumbilical camera port, a subxyphoid operating port, and a left lateral operating port are placed. Pfannenstiel's incision, 6 to 8 cm long, is also made for eventual extraction; until then, the fascial incision is limited to a single port, and a retractor is placed through this site for medial retraction of the colon throughout the operation. A left nephrectomy is usually performed inasmuch as the left kidney is preferred (all other things equal) because of its longer vein. The right nephrectomy is performed in a very similar manner, in mirror image; an additional upper-abdominal port is often needed for liver retraction.

Dissection begins with medial reflection of the descending colon to the left margin of the aorta. As this reflection progresses, the elements of the hilum are visualized, including the renal vein, the gonadal vein, and the ureter. Keeping the mesoureter intact, so as to avoid devascularizing the ureter, the surgeon creates a plane between the ureteral pedicle (including the ureter, the mesoureter, and the gonadal vein) and the psoas muscle. This plane proceeds along the lateral margin of the aorta from the caudalmost extent of the dissection, usually where the ureter crosses the psoas muscle, in a cephalad manner towards the hilum; the ureteral pedicle is elevated during this process to assist in defining this plane. As the dissection approaches the renal vessels, small lumbar tributaries to the renal vein are occasionally encountered and must be ligated carefully.

Hilar dissection includes definition of the renal vein, ligation of the adrenal vein, definition of the renal artery to its base, and division of the periaortic tissue between the renal vein and artery (Figure 3). This is usually accomplished as listed, although anatomic variations are common and may require a different order of operations; gentle anterior retraction of the vein is often required to visualize the artery. Once the hilum is carefully dissected, the upper pole of the kidney is separated from the adrenal gland; it is important to carefully define the extrarenal route of the artery to protect it from injury during this upper pole dissection. Continuing cephalad, the surgeon divides the splenorenal ligament, following the plane along the upper pole of the

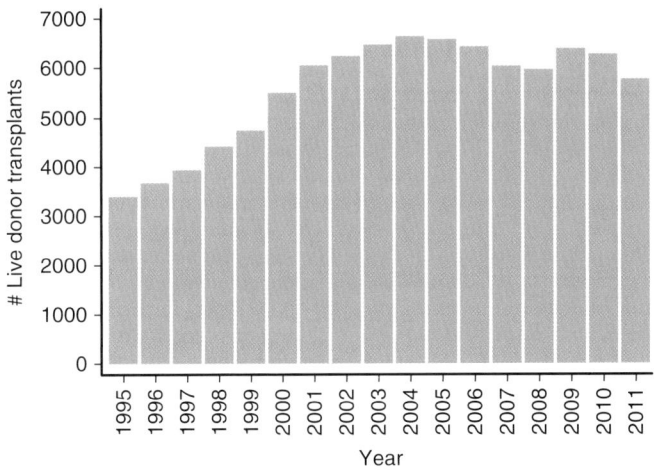

FIGURE 1   Number of live donor kidney transplantations in the United States, by year. *(Data from the Organ Procurement and Transplantation Network.)*

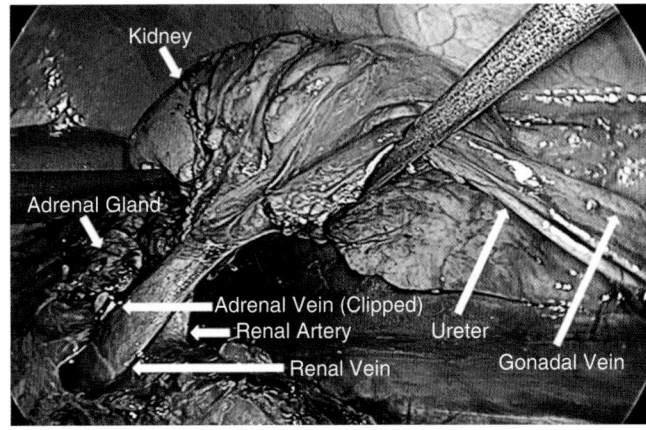

FIGURE 3   Hilar anatomy of the left kidney during a laparoscopic donor nephrectomy.

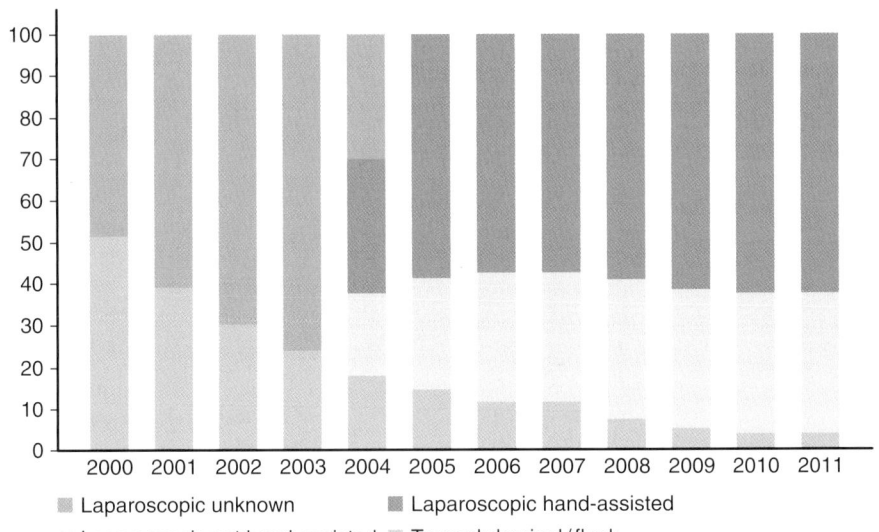

Laparoscopic unknown   **Laparoscopic hand-assisted**
Laparoscopic not hand-assisted   **Transabdominal/flank**

FIGURE 2   Percentage of donor nephrectomies in the United States performed laparoscopically, by year. *(Data from the Organ Procurement and Transplantation Network.)*

kidney to avoid injury to nearby structures such as the pancreas and spleen.

If the donor operation is coordinated with a recipient room, the donor operation typically does not proceed beyond this point until there is confirmation of safe induction of anesthesia in the recipient or identification of appropriate arterial and venous conduits for the allograft. Furosemide and mannitol are administered to the donor, the ureter and gonadal vein are divided distally, and the kidney is separated from its posterolateral attachments. After the surgeon verifies that the kidney remains attached by only the renal artery and vein, heparin is administered to the donor. The Endo Catch bag is placed through Pfannenstiel's incision, and the camera is moved from the periumbilical port to the lateral port to facilitate the appropriate angle for the endovascular stapler. To remove the kidney through Pfannenstiel's incision, the fascia are further opened to accommodate the kidney in the Endo Catch bag. Protamine is administered, and the kidney is removed for backtable flushing. After the fascia are closed, the abdomen is reinsufflated to confirm hemostasis and integrity of nearby structures, including the spleen and mesocolon.

An alternative approach, the Hopkins group has reported vaginal extraction of the kidney for donation. In lieu of extraction through Pfannenstiel's incision, a transverse posterior colpotomy at the apex of the posterior fornix is used, leaving the donor with only port sites.

It is absolutely imperative to control the renal artery by using a tissue transfixion technique such as suture ligation or staples anchored within the vessel wall. The use of nontransfixing devices (such as the Hem-o-lok clip) has been associated with fatal hemorrhagic complications because these devices, not anchored to the vessel wall, can dislodge. In spite of a class II recall by the U.S. Food and Drug Administration, there is evidence that these clips are still in use, which puts live kidney donors, and the entire practice of live donor kidney transplantation, at avoidable and unnecessary risk.

POSTOPERATIVE MANAGEMENT

The usual length of a hospital stay after live donor nephrectomy is approximately 2 days. Most postoperative management is relatively self-evident and consistent with management of other abdominal operations that do not involve entry into a hollow viscus. It is prudent to measure the donor's hemoglobin on the first postoperative day, in view of the location of the dissection and the intraoperative heparinization, as well as the creatinine level, which is expected to rise about 50%. In general, donors who do not experience complications are seen for one in-person postoperative outpatient visit and are otherwise monitored by phone unless otherwise necessary. Interval reporting of donor follow-up to the Organ Procurement and Transplantation Network is required throughout the first 2 years after donation.

RISKS

The main operative risks arise from the transabdominal nature of the operation, including damage to abdominal viscera, particularly those near the kidney. Because major tributaries of the venae cavae and aorta are dissected and ligated, bleeding can be profuse on rare occasion. In a study of more than 80,000 living kidney donors, (Segev et al., 2010) the risk of perioperative death was estimated to be 3.1 per 10,000 donors (95% confidence interval: 2.0 to 4.6); although this incidence is extremely low, the potential of death from this operation is not treated lightly, inasmuch as the donor undergoing the operation gains no direct medical benefit from doing so.

The greater worry is the long-term risk after kidney donation. The risk of death over the long term does not seem to be higher in persons who donated a kidney than in healthy nondonor controls, regardless of age; however, many questions remain regarding risk of long-term medical sequelae attributable to donation. Unfortunately, most studies lack an appropriate nondonor comparison group, and so most of the available evidence is limited to studies of donors versus other donors. For example, there is strong evidence that African American donors have a higher incidence of postdonation hypertension, diabetes, and kidney disease.

CONCLUSION

On the basis of currently available data, it seems reasonable for a healthy individual to undergo nephrectomy for the purposes of kidney donation, if the individual is carefully screened and approved by a transplantation center. Most donor operations are performed laparoscopically, either with hand assistance or, as described in this chapter, with pure laparoscopic techniques. Risk remains low, although it is not fully quantified because of limitations in research and follow-up of donors, as well as the relatively short history of this operation. Efforts to increase live donation in response to the worsening organ shortage are ongoing, in parallel with efforts to understand and minimize postdonation risk.

SELECTED READINGS

Allaf ME, Singer AL, Shen W, et al. Laparoscopic live donor nephrectomy with vaginal extraction: initial report, *Am J Transplant* 10(6):1473–1477, 2010.

Berger JC, Hoque M, Garonzik-Wang JM, et al: Living kidney donors over the age of 70: donor and recipient outcomes, *Clin J Am Soc Nephrol* 6(12):2887–2893, 2011.

Friedman AL, Peters TG, Jones KW, et al: Fatal and nonfatal hemorrhagic complications of living kidney donation, *Ann Surg* 243(1):126–130, 2006.

Ratner LE, Ciseck LJ, Moore RG, et al: Laparoscopic live donor nephrectomy, *Transplantation* 60(9):1047–1049, 1995.

Segev DL, Muzaale AD, Caffo B, et al: Short-term and long-term survival in a 15-year cohort of all live kidney donors in the United States, *JAMA* 303(10):959–966, 2010.

LAPAROENDOSCOPIC SINGLE-SITE SURGERY AS AN EVOLVING SURGICAL APPROACH

John C. LaMattina, MD and Rolf N. Barth, MD

The ability to consolidate multiple laparoscopic port and specimen extraction sites within one incision hidden within the umbilicus provides the impetus for utilizing a single-port approach in surgery. The benefits of improved cosmetic outcomes have been tempered by the learning curve and potential risks associated with adopting a new and potentially more difficult technique. Nonetheless, the availability of multiple single-port devices has allowed for application and progressive experience in general surgery, urology, and gynecology (Table 1).

Single-port laparoscopy has been referred to by a number of terms, some of which are proprietary. Current consensus statements have supported preference for the term laparoendoscopic single-site (LESS) surgery. However, other terms are utilized in both academic literature and commercial marketing. These include single-site laparoscopy (SSL), single-port laparoscopy (SPL), single-incision laparoscopic surgery (SILS), and embryonic natural-orifice transumbilical endoscopic surgery (e-NOTES). It is important to recognize that these descriptors refer to a common technical approach. Most single-port procedures are performed through a transumbilical approach.

TRAINING AND LEARNING CURVE

A multidisciplinary international consortium met in 2008 to create recommendations for the emerging technology of single-port laparoscopy. The consortium's statement supported stepwise training for LESS surgery, including inanimate trainers, training on animals, observation, and mentoring/proctoring. The importance of patient safety in applying this technology was highlighted, and a specific statement was included to encourage the use of accessory 2-mm needlescopic ports to assist with the surgical procedure. The accessory needlescopic site is most beneficial during the learning curve in utilizing single-port surgery.

The authors' experience introducing this technique for donor nephrectomy in 2009 followed a similar approach of observation and mentorship, use of animal models, and proctoring. Of importance is that they maintained an extremely low threshold for additional port placement if progress slowed or technical difficulties were encountered. One reasonable approach for learning the single-port technique is progressive port minimization during the learning curve, with decreased use and number of additional ports as expertise with the LESS technique is obtained. The authors utilized the needlescopic ports in the majority of early cases (first 50) and required needlescopic or additional ports in fewer than 10% of subsequent cases. After the initial 25 cases, there was no statistical difference between LESS donor nephrectomy times and the times of historic controls.

TABLE 1: Identified current laparoendoscopic single-site (LESS) procedures in various surgical specialties*

High-volume procedures	Intermediate-volume procedures	Low-volume procedures
Cholecystectomy	Adrenalectomy	Bariatric procedures
Appendectomy	Splenectomy	Myomectomy
Inguinal hernia repair	Hysterectomy	Prostate resection
Oophorectomy	Pelvic organ prolapse	Cystectomy
Salpingectomy	Donor nephrectomy	Partial nephrectomy
Endometriosis surgery	Ureteral reimplantation	Retroperitoneal lymph node dissection
Tubal ligation	Ileal interposition	Esophageal myotomy
Pyeloplasty	Small bowel resection	Distal pancreatectomy
Simple nephrectomy	Fundoplication	
Renal cyst decortication		
Ablative renal surgery		
Pelvic lymphadenectomy		
Nephrectomy		
Gastric banding		
Colon resection		

*Tabulated according to anticipated surgical volumes.
From Gill IS, Advincula AP, Aron M, et al: Consensus statement of the consortium for laparoendoscopic single-site surgery, Surg Endosc 24(4):762–768, 2010.

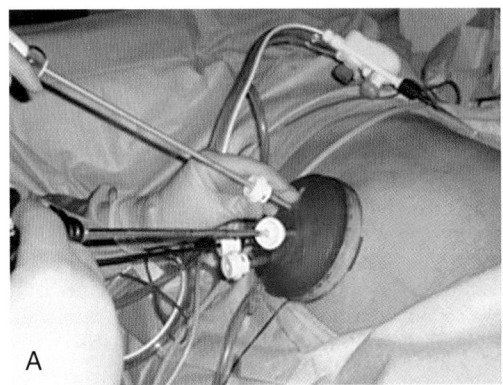
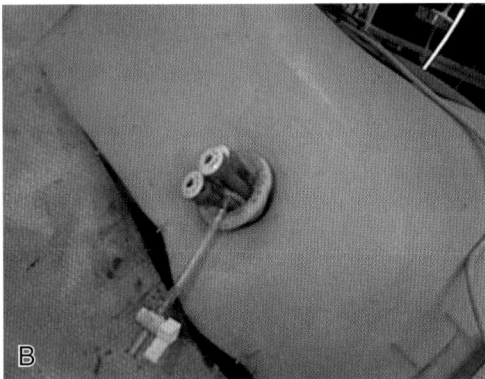

FIGURE 1 Single-port devices available are either **(A)** gel-based devices (Gelpoint, Applied Medical, Rancho Santa Margarita, Calif) or **(B)** more compact solid port designs (SILS Port, Covidien, Mansfield, Mass).

DEVICES AND INSTRUMENTS

Multiple commercial port devices are available for LESS surgery. The predominant difference is between gel-based devices (GelPOINT Advanced Access System and GelPort Laparoscopic System, Applied Medical, Rancho Santa Margarita, Calif), and more compact solid port designs (SILS Port, Covidien, Mansfield, Mass; Quadport, Olympus, Center Valley, Pa; Single Port Access Device, Ethicon, New Brunswick, NJ) (Figure 1). Single-port systems include the required insufflation port and accommodate three, four, or five ports sized between 5 and 15 mm. Ports are placed via open techniques under direct visualization and are either placed directly through the fascia or attached to wound retractor components. The incisions required to accommodate the ports vary from 22 mm to more than 70 mm. Most single-port systems also include a ventilation valve because the accumulation of vapor and aerosolized materials can significantly impair visualization.

Optical laparoscopic equipment need not be specifically modified for single-port surgery. Both 5-mm and 10-mm standard laparoscopic cameras can be utilized. Because of the umbilical port placement and the close proximity of operative instruments, some benefit is obtained from the use of bariatric-length cameras and right-angle light cord adaptors. The 5-mm cameras provide less illumination than do 10-mm systems. Articulating cameras are available and, with experience, provide some benefit in reducing interference with operative instruments (Figure 2, *A*). Depending on the application, experience in using both articulating and standard cameras in a single-port device can be helpful, inasmuch as one or the other could result in less interference between operative instruments and contamination of the camera lens, which would provide a more optimal visualization of the operative field. The ability to navigate the camera to reduce interference with operative instruments is a key component of success with single-port techniques.

No specialized instruments are needed to perform single-port procedures. The use of standard energy devices, clip appliers, and staplers is enabled by all available port devices. Articulating instruments are available for dissection, grasping, and cutting (see Figure 2, *B*). With progressive experience in using articulating instruments, some benefits can be realized with improved mobility that is inherently limited by a single-site approach. Nonetheless, none of the articulating instruments are needed to successfully accomplish the variety of surgical procedures currently being performed. One important concept is the use of instruments of different lengths to separate the surgeon's hands at different distances externally. For instance, combining bariatric-length suction-irrigator devices and Maryland dissectors with standard-length instruments can allow for separation of the surgeon's hands in different planes and reduce external hand conflicts.

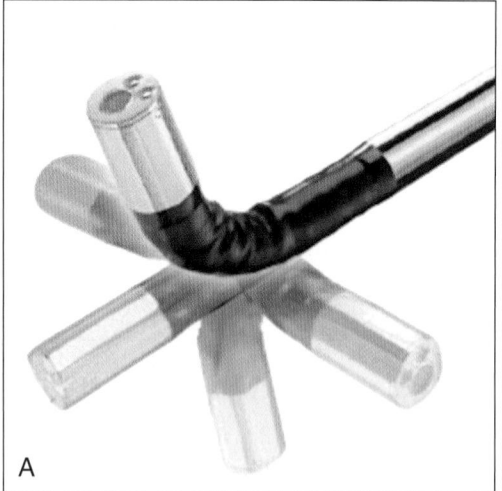 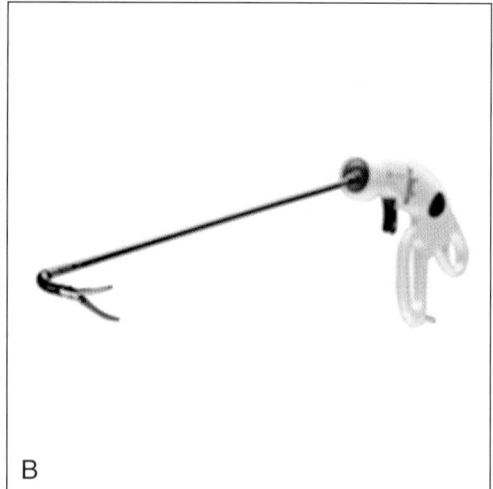

FIGURE 2 Articulating camera and instruments are available for single-port systems. **A,** Articulating 5-mm camera (Olympus LTF-VP Deflectable Tip Video Laparoscope, Center Valley, Pa); **B,** Articulating 5-mm dissecting device (SILSDISSECT36 Single Use Articulating Dissector with Monopolar Cautery, Covidien, Mansfield, Mass).

TRANSUMBILICAL APPROACH

The primary benefit of LESS surgery is improved cosmesis, which is best achieved when the port is inserted transumbilically. Although transumbilical port placement is most common, alternative port site placements have been utilized for other procedures, such as bariatric surgery. Depending on the device utilized and the required length of extraction incision, total incision lengths can vary from 2 to 7 cm (or longer). The invagination of the umbilicus allows for the majority of the incision length to be camouflaged, which results in apparent incision lengths of 3 to 4 cm. Healing and contraction of the umbilical incision over time further minimizes the postoperative scar so that it becomes barely visible (Figure 3). The rationale supporting LESS surgery may be poorer for procedures in which larger incisions are needed for specimen extraction.

One weakness of the transumbilical approach is the potential for umbilical incisional hernias. The presence of incidental umbilical defects has been noted in approximately 25% of potential kidney donors. The fascia incision can be closed by a variety of techniques, and the authors generally perform interrupted closures with No. 1 polydioxanone suture. The authors have observed umbilical hernias in 2% of kidney donors, and although this surgical complication rate is comparable with that in other approaches, the authors do specify this risk in the consent process. For procedures that do not necessitate significant extraction incisions (e.g., gastric bypass), port site hernia rates of less than 1% (similar between single- and multiple-port approaches when a 15-mm port was utilized) have been described. The authors' center experience also suggests that obese patients or patients who engage in extreme physical exertion within months of donation are more susceptible to hernia development. In addition, target operative anatomy may be displaced significantly from the umbilicus in obese patients, in comparison with nonobese patients (Figure 4). Achieving instrument reach may require modification of port placement from the transumbilical site in these patient populations.

NEPHRECTOMY

The availability of kidney transplantation is dependent on substantial numbers of living donors to address the nearly 100,000 patients currently awaiting renal transplantation. Of the approximately 18,000 kidney transplantations performed annually in the United States, approximately 33% involve kidneys from living donors. Nearly all renal donations in the United States are currently performed via laparoscopy (hand-assisted or total laparoscopic approaches).

Extensive preoperative imaging is performed to ensure knowledge of vascular anatomy to allow for optimal surgical planning. Kidney donors are typically otherwise in excellent health without comorbid conditions. Thus improved cosmesis could be viewed as one advantage of LESS donor nephrectomy. The potential to attract kidney donors or encourage recipients to ask possible donors is one rationale for this surgical procedure.

The use of LESS approaches in renal surgery and living-donor kidney donation was first reported by Gill and colleagues (2008) at the Cleveland Clinic Foundation. In this initial series, they described technical feasibility, safety, and good outcomes for renal donation. The authors' experience with more than 250 LESS donor nephrectomies has provided evidence of the safe and routine application of this technique. The authors have found equivalent safety, complication rates, and transplantation outcomes in their patients in comparison with historic laparoscopic controls. The authors have additionally noted that kidney donors who donated via LESS donor nephrectomy approaches reported higher satisfaction with the donation process than did donors who donated via a totally laparoscopic multiport approach. Whether this will translate into increased interest and higher numbers of kidney donors has yet to be revealed.

The technical learning curve was overcome after the first 25 cases, with subsequent operative times that were not significantly different from those of totally laparoscopic approaches. Four surgeons at the authors' center have been able to achieve proficiency in the LESS approach and can perform LESS donor nephrectomy independently. In addition, the authors have participated in training surgeons from other centers who have then applied the technique successfully. Two important principles are (1) the addition of laparoscopic ports if the procedure appears to stop making progress and before complications arise and (2) the presence of an additional trained surgeon to help in decision making and expedient extraction of the renal allograft after vascular division. The few other centers in which this approach has been used have reported similar results in regard to donor safety and transplantation outcomes.

CHOLECYSTECTOMY

Cholecystectomy is one of the most common general surgery procedures, and laparoscopy has one of the most extensive applications in this procedure. The moderately sized tissue specimen can be removed through the single-port incision without extension, whereas removal through a 12-mm laparoscopic trocar site occasionally requires extending the incision length. In contrast to donor nephrectomy, inasmuch as cholecystectomy is often performed urgently, the target

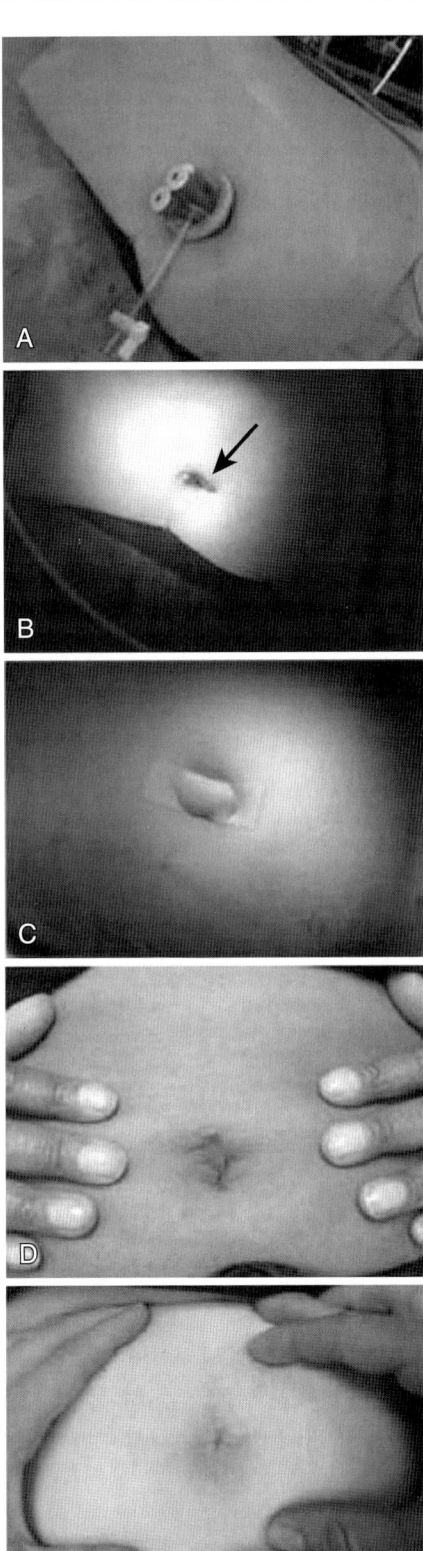

FIGURE 3 Single-port placement and cosmetic outcomes of nephrectomy. **A,** Transumbilical placement of SILS Port (Covidien). **B,** Immediate postoperative appearance after subcuticular closure. **C,** Bandage placement. **D,** Cosmetic outcome at 6 months. **E,** Cosmetic outcome at 2 years. *(From Barth RN, Phelan MW, Goldschen L, et al: Single-port donor nephrectomy provides improved patient satisfaction and equivalent outcomes, Ann Surg 257(3):527–533, 2013.)*

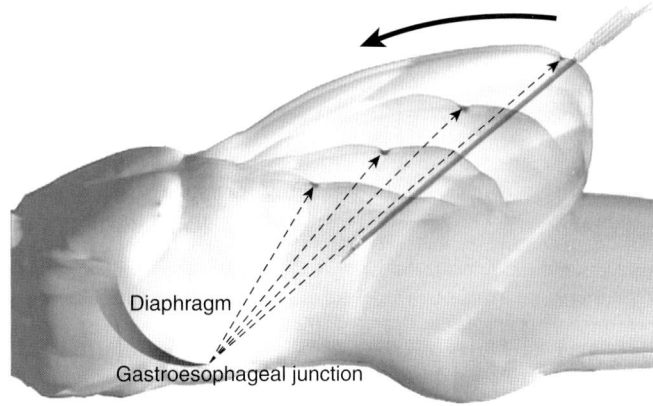

FIGURE 4 Umbilical recession in obese patients. *(Reproduced, with permission, from El-Ghazaly TH, Saber AA: Single incision laparoscopic surgery [SILS™] and trocar reduction strategies for bariatric procedures. In Deitel M, Gagner M, Dixon JB, et al [eds]: Handbook of obesity surgery, Toronto, 2010, FD-Communications, pp. 190–197. From Saber AA, El-Ghazaly TH, Dewoolkar AV, et al: Single-incision laparoscopic sleeve gastrectomy versus conventional multiport laparoscopic sleeve gastrectomy: technical considerations and strategic modifications, Surg Obes Relat Dis 6[6]:658–664, 2010.)*

anatomy has associated inflammation, and extensive imaging cannot be performed before surgery. Despite these differences, general surgeons have applied LESS cholecystectomy with good outcomes.

Studies performed to address concerns that the single-port approach could result in higher complication rates have yielded conflicting data. It is more technically challenging to demonstrate the "critical view" that can typically be readily achieved with triangulated instrument placement and gallbladder retraction. Multiple approaches to gallbladder retraction via the single-port have been utilized, including accessory needlescopic ports or transabdominal retaining sutures. One randomized study of only 21 patients who underwent LESS cholecystectomy did reveal increased rates of complications, including hernia, bleeding, and a retained stone. Larger series have demonstrated results similar to those of standard multiport approaches without any increase in biliary or other complications. Operative times also appear to normalize to multiport techniques with progressive experience; some centers have reported a learning curve of as few as five patients. One randomized trial of 150 patients assigned to undergo either LESS or conventional laparoscopic cholecystectomy demonstrated (1) that patients who underwent LESS procedures had improved pain scores, decreased analgesic use, and better survey responses for cosmesis and quality of life, and (2) no increase in reported complications. Other trials have confirmed the improved cosmetic appearances but have not demonstrated significant differences with pain or convalescence. Another randomized study determined that although initial pain scores are the same between LESS and multiport approaches, pain scores decreased to a greater degree in the patients who underwent LESS procedures after the first 6 to 12 hours.

The concern for hernia formation has been highlighted by other data. One multicenter randomized trial of 200 patients undergoing either LESS or multiport cholecystectomy revealed a significant difference in rates of hernia formation (8.4% vs 1.2%, $P = 0.03$) after 1 year of follow-up. These results differ from those of other large reviews of LESS cholecystectomy, in which incisional hernia rates were reported to be between 1% and 2%. Unlike extraction incisions for other surgical resections via single-port approaches, the required extraction incision for cholecystectomy does not generally require extension. Longer term follow-up of hernia rates are of significant importance in more accurately defining whether risk is increased with LESS approaches.

BARIATRIC SURGERY

The successful application of single-site approaches in bariatric surgery has been reported for gastric banding, sleeve gastrectomy, and Roux-en-Y gastric bypass procedures. Because gastric banding necessitates an adequate incision length for the implantable band device, this provides a good indication for the LESS approach. The technical feasibility and safety of the LESS approach for gastric banding were first reported in 2010 and confirmed in a larger series in 2012. In one series, additional port placement was required in 6% of patients, and no open conversions or blood transfusions were required. Recommendations were made for additional port placement after increased operative times (>60 minutes) with the single-port device.

Sleeve gastrectomy requires extraction of the resected gastric remnant, which necessitates extension of individual port sites when performed via a multiport approach. On the other hand, the longer incision length required for the single-port device is typically sufficient for specimen extraction. In one small series, sleeve gastrectomy entailed increased operative times with LESS surgery but resulted in decreased pain and analgesic requirements.

Roux-en-Y gastric bypass has also been performed via a single-port technique, with success rates equivalent to those of multiport approaches and with better patient satisfaction scores. The LESS procedures were performed by experienced bariatric surgeons (>400 procedures), but still resulted in longer operative times, with subjective appreciation of increased technical difficulty. Because gastric bypass does not involve specimen extraction or device implantation, the use of a single-port approach is based on the potential for improved cosmesis and decreased pain.

COLECTOMY

Single-port approaches have also been increasingly utilized and explored for both benign and oncologic colonic resections. Although technical considerations in the transition from multiport to single-port approaches in performing a colectomy are similar with regard to triangulation as for other procedures, laparoendoscopic single-site colectomy introduces the additional variable of an increased specimen size.

A meta-analysis of more than 500 patients who underwent LESS colorectal surgical procedures demonstrated equivalent outcomes, with decreased blood loss, hospital stay, and incision size in comparison to an equal cohort of patients undergoing standard laparoscopic procedures. No differences were reported with overall outcomes, rates of conversion to open surgery, or oncologic outcomes for tumor resection. In another large single-center report, researchers described their experience with more than 200 LESS colectomies for predominantly diverticular disease. Patients underwent sigmoid/left colectomy or high anterior resection. Open conversion rates were 6% and were generally attributed to difficulty with laparoscopic dissection in diverticular disease. Right-sided colectomies appear equally feasible. A report in which more than 40 LESS right hemicolectomies were compared with 100 conventional laparoscopic right hemicolectomies performed mostly for oncologic indications revealed equivalent oncologic outcomes and complication rates. LESS approaches resulted in an equal rate of conversion to open surgery (5%) as conventional surgery. Of the patients who underwent LESS surgery, 7.5% required additional port placement.

URGENT INDICATIONS

New technical approaches in laparoscopy may be difficult to use for urgent surgical indications; such cases may occur on nights and weekends when the surgeon is likely to encounter surgical staff who are less familiar with instrumentation and devices. Nonetheless, LESS surgery does not require unique laparoscopic instrumentation outside of the single-port device. Predicted differences in operative time, especially during the learning curve for single-port approaches, may be a driving consideration of which patients are candidates for LESS surgery for more urgent indications. Despite these challenges, LESS surgery is possible for urgent procedures. A trial of nearly 200 patients undergoing urgent appendectomy via either multiport or LESS approaches demonstrated slightly increased operative times (6 minutes) and decreased pain levels postoperatively in the patients who underwent LESS surgery. Appendix extraction was possible via the 12-mm port site in the patients who underwent multiport surgery and via the 2-cm single-port site in those who underwent LESS surgery. In this study, both groups included pediatric patients.

UROLOGIC SURGERY

LESS surgery has been reported for numerous urologic procedures, including pyeloplasty, nephrectomy, adrenalectomy, and prostatectomy. Much of the early experience with LESS procedures and the translation from animal models to human procedures focused on laparoscopic nephrectomy. The technical modifications required for LESS surgery were investigated and evaluated in urologic applications before more widespread marketing and availability of single-port devices. Initial descriptions focused on the feasibility and limitations of the approaches. In later randomized studies, outcomes were compared with those of multiport approaches; patient satisfaction with cosmesis was improved, return to activity was quicker, and postoperative pain was decreased.

A review of more than 1000 LESS urologic procedures from 18 academic institutions around the world demonstrated that nearly 50% of single-port procedures were directed toward renal tumors or cysts. Overall, a 3.3% complication rate was reported (the majority of these were minor), 23% of cases required additional port placement, and fewer than 1% of cases required conversion to open surgery. Of interest is that 13% of cases involved the use of robotic assistance through the existing GelPort platform (Applied Medical, Rancho Santa Margarita, Calif). Robotic-assisted LESS surgery has demonstrated its feasibility but, conversely, also has limitations, which illustrates the continued demand for technical advancements in the available instrumentation and compatible robotic platforms. Robotic surgery has a strong place in the current repertoire of urologic surgery, and thus the combination of single-site approaches and robotic surgery has the potential to drive further innovation in surgery that will enable broader application.

GYNECOLOGIC SURGERY

Gynecologic surgeons have likewise introduced LESS approaches. In an initial report, applications of both manual and robotic single-site approaches were described for such indications as pelvic staging, oophorectomy, hysterectomy, and ovarian cystectomy. As noted in urologic applications, the hybrid approach of utilizing robot-assisted laparoscopy may represent one technique that enables single-site surgery.

ROBOTIC SINGLE-PORT APPROACH

The U.S. Food and Drug Administration (FDA) approved a single-port platform for the robotic da Vinci Surgical System (Intuitive Surgical, Sunnyvale, Calif; Figure 5). In the United States, this device is approved for only cholecystectomy; however, European investigators have used these devices for urologic and gynecologic procedures. Initial reports demonstrate the safety of this platform in robotic

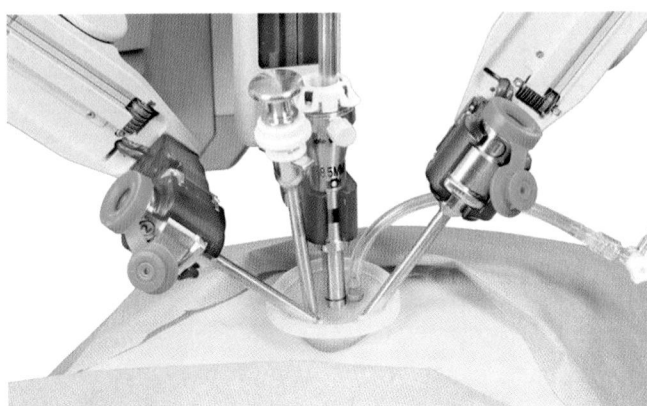

FIGURE 5 Single-port platform for the robotic da Vinci Surgical System (Intuitive Medical, Sunnyvale, Calif).

single-port cholecystectomy procedures. The robotic platform offers specific advantages in terms of improved ergonomics, reduced "sword-fighting" between instruments, and improved optical systems. However, the robotic single-port platform does not yet allow for the use of articulating robotic instruments, which are one of the most compelling technical advantages of using the robotic approach in surgery. The development of similarly articulating instrumentation for the single-port robotic platform will be a significant step in improving the current limitations of manual single-site laparoscopic approaches. Once developed, fully articulating robotic single-port platforms may eliminate many of the limitations that exist with current single-port laparoscopic surgery.

As previously described, urologic and gynecologic surgeons with experience in robotic surgery have been utilizing standard robotic instruments through a single incision via a GelPort device with success. This approach allows for the substantial benefits that robotic surgery incorporates in terms of articulating instruments, three-dimensional optical systems, and improved ergonomics for the surgeon. These specialties have embraced training in and clinical applications for robotic surgery and are well positioned to make advances in robot-assisted single-port surgery.

Future combinations of image-guided surgery involving computed tomographic (CT) scans and fluorescent dye may enable robotics to improve many surgical approaches. Image-guided robotic surgery with the use of three-dimensional CT scan overlays has been described for renal tumors, and real-time ultrasound guidance for robotic navigation has been reported for prostatectomy. Combination with indocyanine green that can be detected with fluorescence imaging can also allow for real-time imaging of biliary anatomy. These technical advances, in combination with robot-assisted single-port approaches, have the potential to improve safety through real-time anatomic imaging.

COST CONSIDERATIONS

The application of new technology has associated costs dependent on instrumentation and port devices. The incremental benefits of new technologic approaches should thus be weighed against the potential for substantially increased costs. Limited cost analyses have been performed for single-port surgery; however, a few researchers have described an increased incremental cost of $200 to $800 per case.

One favorable factor for single-port surgery is a comparable equipment platform used in standard laparoscopy. The cost of individual ports required for multiport surgery (usually three or four ports of various sizes) is consolidated into the cost of a single-port access system that includes all necessary ports. The surgery can be performed with existing reusable and disposable laparoscopic instruments, which eliminates a potential cascade of new instrument charges. Existing stapling devices, energy devices, clip appliers, retrieval bags, and other equipment can all be used through the available single-port devices. In addition, the optic systems utilized for standard laparoscopy can be applied to single-port laparoscopy (5-mm or 10-mm camera systems, or both, depending on the single-port system utilized).

Most authorities describe normalization of operative times after appropriate learning curves, which thus eliminates longer surgical or anesthetic times from any cost differential. Furthermore, the single-port approach does not require any unique operating room setup that could affect setup times and personnel requirements.

Cost can be increased in association with a small number of flexible and articulating laparoscopic instruments designed for single-port use. However, these instruments have not proved to be essential for any of the currently applied surgical procedures. Further refinements and experience may allow single-port surgery to proceed with fewer limitations in the future. One item that the authors and others have found beneficial is a flexible camera. The ability to improve visualization and navigate the camera away from any interference with other instruments has improved surgeons' capacity to perform the procedure safely with decreased operative times. These cameras can also provide high-definition digital images (in contrast to older analog systems) that further facilitate the operation.

On the other hand, significant cost is associated with developing a robotic assist approach. Robotic surgery requires a specialized operating room setup, and personnel must be familiarized with the equipment, the actual robotic device and all associated instruments, camera systems, and comparatively longer operative times. The single-port approach is relatively simple and inexpensive in comparison.

CONSENT ISSUES

Although the use of LESS surgical approaches does not require any new consent process, adequate informed consent does take on additional requirements. The devices utilized are FDA approved and have been employed in a wide variety of applications. Nonetheless, the ability to demonstrate individual proficiency with LESS approaches is important, and the authors recommend discussing the novel approach with patients in the consent process. A published consensus statement from the Society of University Surgeons supported an informed consent process that includes a specific discussion of the innovative aspects of the surgical procedure. In addition, survey data revealed that patients believe that information for consent must include knowledge of whether their operation was the surgeon's first case with the innovative procedure, clarification of the novelty of the technique in comparison with standard approaches, and potential risks of the novel approach. Informed consent will be strengthened by presentation of the individual surgeon's experience and complications with LESS surgery. Because the primary benefit is cosmetic, this must be weighed against any potential risks to the patient and put in the context of each surgeon's experience.

The authors also discuss the placement of additional ports in approximately 10% of donor nephrectomy cases. Similarly, conversion from laparoscopic to open approaches is always discussed, and the authors provide conversion rates for the specific procedure. The authors believe that for surgeons proficient in LESS surgery, the hierarchy of preferred approaches for certain procedures should be LESS surgery, multiport laparoscopy, hand-assisted laparoscopy, and finally open surgery.

STRATEGIES FOR SUCCESSFUL INCORPORATION OF THE SINGLE-PORT TECHNIQUE

Operative room setup is quite similar to standard laparoscopic procedures, except that both the surgeon and assistant operate through a single access point, which results in crowding (Figure 6). The primary difficulty that most surgeons encounter when transitioning to a single-port technique is the proximity of the surgical instruments that they pass through the single-port device. In addition to placing the instruments in very close proximity, the surgeon's and assistant's hands also tend to interfere with each other (Figure 7). This creates both "sword-fighting" between instruments and physical discomfort for the surgeon. A number of strategies have been developed to address these "steric hindrances." Although it is contrary to standard laparoscopic teaching, the authors find it easiest to cross the instruments inside the abdomen. This enables the surgeon's hands to obtain space between them. The surgeon can increase the space by using instruments of different length, which positions the hands at different distances from the patient. The surgeon can further enhance positioning by holding the instruments with the palms downward, placing the instrument handles outward. Larger devices, such as the GelPort device, are easier for those first becoming familiar with the technique because the distances between ports is much larger. The disadvantage of these ports, however, is that they require larger skin and fascial incisions. Some surgeons have found articulating instruments to be of assistance as well.

The authors have been able to minimize interference by having the assistant operate a 5-mm flexible camera. The assistant is able to angulate the camera downward, providing a bird's-eye view of the region of interest. A right-angle camera cord adapter creates more space for the operator.

Newer ports have incorporated a venting system, which eliminates the troublesome fogging and visual disruptions associated with earlier designs. Such ports tend to require higher CO_2 flow rates, but they vastly improve visualization.

The authors emphasize the importance of early placement of additional ports in the event of difficulty visualizing or mobilizing

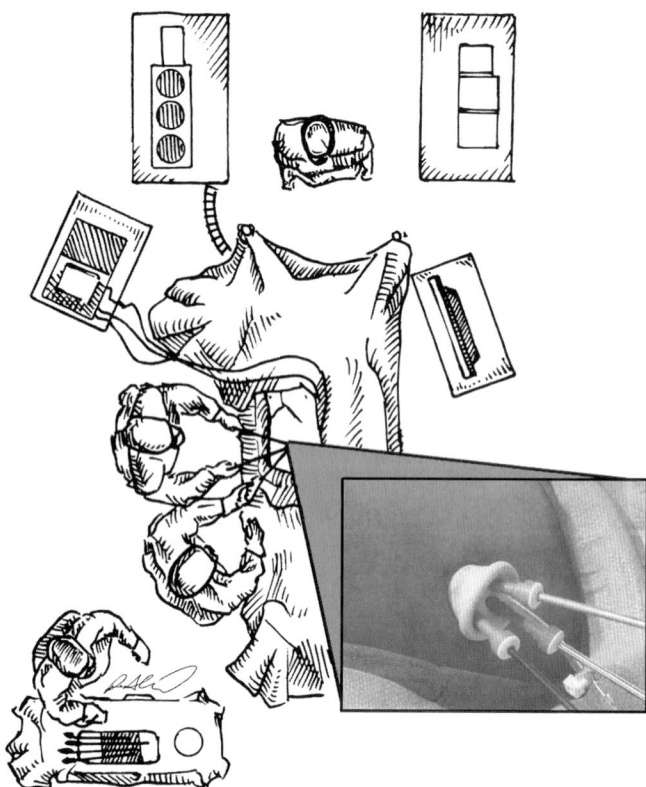

FIGURE 6 Operating room setup for single-port donor nephrectomy. Patient position and operating room setup are similar to those for standard laparoscopic nephrectomy. Surgeon and assistant are in close proximity as multiple instruments and camera are inserted through the umbilical port. The assistant operating the camera or additional instrument must pay attention to avoiding interference with the primary surgeon's instruments. *(From Morris PJ, Knechtle SJ:* Kidney transplantation—principles and practices, *Philadelphia, 2008, Elsevier.)*

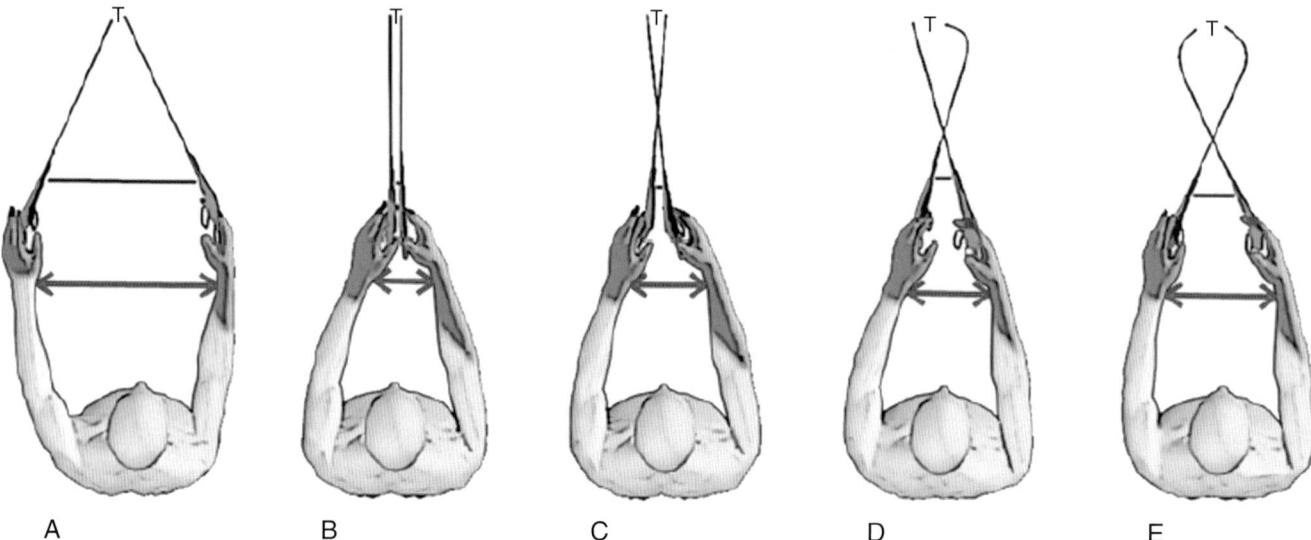

FIGURE 7 Multiport laparoscopy **(A)** versus single-incision laparoscopic surgery hand-instrument **(B** to **E)** orientations. *T*, Target. *(Reproduced, with permission, from El-Ghazaly TH, Saber AA: Single incision laparoscopic surgery [SILS™] and trocar reduction strategies for bariatric procedures. In Deitel M, Gagner M, Dixon JB, et al [eds]:* Handbook of obesity surgery, *Toronto, 2010, FD-Communications, pp 190–197. From Saber AA, El-Ghazaly TH, Dewoolkar AV, et al: Single-incision laparoscopic sleeve gastrectomy versus conventional multiport laparoscopic sleeve gastrectomy: technical considerations and strategic modifications,* Surg Obes Relat Dis *6[6]:658–664, 2010.)*

the target anatomy. They have found that the presence of two surgeons comfortable in LESS surgery to assist in decision-making and surgical exposure is crucial for success in challenging cases.

CONCLUSIONS

The primary benefit of LESS surgery is improved cosmesis for the patient. This benefit is most pronounced when the port is placed in a transumbilical location and the entire incision can be contained within the umbilicus. Applications in general surgery, urology, gynecology, and living donor nephrectomy have been reported, and growing experience supports application of LESS techniques. A learning curve to obtain experience with these new devices does exist, and not all surgeons may be able to safely master use of a single-port approach. Commitment to adding additional ports when technical challenges arise is paramount to avoid complications.

SUGGESTED READINGS

Barth RN, Phelan MW, Goldschen L, et al: Single-port donor nephrectomy provides improved patient satisfaction and equivalent outcomes, *Ann Surg* 257(3):527–533, 2013.

Biffl WL, Spain DA, Reitsma AM, et al: Responsible development and application of surgical innovations: a position statement of the Society of University Surgeons, *J Am Coll Surg* 206(3):1204–1209, 2008.

Bucher P, Pugin F, Buchs NC, et al: Randomized clinical trial of laparoendoscopic single-site versus conventional laparoscopic cholecystectomy, *Br J Surg* 98(12):1695–1702, 2011.

Gill IS, Advincula AP, Aron M, et al: Consensus statement of the consortium for laparoendoscopic single-site surgery, *Surg Endosc* 24(4):762–768, 2010.

Gill IS, Canes D, Aron M, et al: Single port transumbilical (E-NOTES) donor nephrectomy, *J Urol* 180(2):637–641, 2008; discussion, *J Urol* 180(2):641, 2008.

NOTES: WHAT IS CURRENTLY POSSIBLE?

Faming Zhang, MD, PhD, and
Anthony N. Kalloo, MD

OVERVIEW

Natural orifice transluminal endoscopic surgery (NOTES) has gained a great deal of attention from gastroenterologists and surgeons all over the world since its introduction in 2000. More than 1000 reports describing various applications of NOTES in both animal and human experiments (Table 1) have been published since that time. More than 110 reports associated with NOTES were published in 2011. More than 30 currently open clinical trials in humans are officially registered in the U.S. government Web-based registry (http://www.clinicaltrials.gov). NOTES-associated procedures have been performed in several thousand patients. The concept is continuously expanding as industry develops new enabling technologies for NOTES.

The basic aim of scarless surgery through a natural orifice such as the mouth, vagina, and anus is to dramatically reduce the surgical effect on the patient and to improve surgical outcomes. At a minimum, this concept has introduced a new era in minimally invasive surgery: the avoidance of skin incisions, with a resulting decrease in physical and psychologic disability; direct patient benefits, such as less pain; and allowing the conversion of standard inpatient surgical interventions into outpatient clinic procedures.

The acronym *NOTES* has become a mark of innovative, minimally invasive surgery. In 2004, Rao and Reddy brought attention to NOTES with their description of the first human NOTES procedure (transgastric appendectomy). In 2005, the American Society of Gastrointestinal Endoscopy (ASGE) and the Society of American Gastrointestinal and Endoscopic Surgeons (SAGES) formed a NOTES working group, the Natural Orifice Surgery Consortium for Assessment and Research (NOSCAR). This committee subsequently identified the fundamental challenges to be addressed and outlined a pathway for the responsible development and evolution of NOTES.

Under the auspices of NOSCAR, the field of NOTES has advanced tremendously since its inception, and exciting and well-designed research has been published. Both randomized controlled trials and results from large national and international registries have been published. NOTES should no longer be viewed as merely a more cosmetic way to perform surgery. NOTES has the potential to decrease postoperative pain and anesthesia requirements, better preserve immune function, and accelerate patient recovery.

It is not surprising that some medical practitioners still doubt the potential and clinical relevance of NOTES. NOTES was initially criticized as unrealistic, dangerous, and unnecessary. This situation is similar to that of the early era of laparoscopic surgery, when the first laparoscopic cholecystectomy was performed in a human in 1985. However, the substantial number of published laboratory studies and clinical trials are a reflection of the significant interest and application by endoscopists and surgeons. Novel interventions for NOTES (see Table 1) have been developed, such as endoscopic ultrasonography (EUS)-guided approach to NOTES interventions, endoscopic local full-thickness resection for gastrointestinal stromal tumors, (GIST) and per-oral endoscopic myotomy (POEM). Many diseases formerly treated only by conventional surgical interventions are now more often treated by endoluminal procedures at many centers worldwide.

TREATMENT AND METHODS

The adoption of NOTES into clinical practice is strongly dependent on device development. NOTES procedures involving available or "standard" instruments are highly demanding, even for experienced endoscopists or laparoscopists. The sophisticated systems enabling pure NOTES procedures are still limited, and most remain in prototype. However, many creative, flexible endoscopists and laparoscopists have overcome these technical challenges, making some pure NOTES procedures a clinical reality with the use of conventional endoscopes and accessory devices. Advanced NOTES platforms and devices (Figure 1), such as the EndoSAMURAI with two arms (Olympus Corp.), the new flexible endoscope for NOTES (Boston Scientific), or the ANUBIScope (Karl Storz), all enable laparoscopic-like trangulation. The ability to perform intracorporeal suturing is still in the prototype phase, but the launching of such devices will prompt a huge step forward. A new closure device by OVESCO (Tübingen, Germany) is capable of providing full-thickness closure

TABLE 1: The expanding spectrum of NOTES procedures in animals and humans

Orifice routes	Procedure	Animal	Human
Transvaginal	Cholecystectomy	X	X
	Appendectomy	X	X
	Nephrectomy	X	X
	Partial gastrectomy	X	X
	Liver biopsy	X	X
	Pancreatectomy	X	
	Descending colon resection	X	X
	Splenectomy		X
	Liver resection		X
	Renal cyst resection		X
	Salpingectomy		X
	Hernia repair		X
	Adjustable gastric banding		X
	Retroperitoneoscopy		X
Transgastric/ duodenal	Cholecystectomy	X	X
	Appendectomy	X	X
	Full-thickness resection	X	X
	Peritoneoscopy	X	X
	Liver biopsy	X	X
	EUS-guided NOTES	X	X
	Omental patch repair perforation	X	X
	Gastrojejunostomy	X	
	Pancreatectomy	X	
	Omentectomy	X	
	PEG tube salvage		X
	Retroperitoneal access		Cadavers
Transesophageal	Tunneling/Heller myotomy	X	X
	Vagotomy	X	
	Antireflux therapy	X	
	Lymphadenectomy	X	
	Pleural biopsy	X	
	Pericardial/cardial interventions	X	
Transrectal	Proctosigmoidectomy	X	X
	Full-thickness colon resection	X	Cadavers
	Transanal pull-through		X
Transvesical	Peritoneoscopy	X	
	Varicocelectomy	X	
Transpharyngeal	Mediastinal exploratory	X	
Transtracheal	Thoracic exploration	X	
Transoral	Thyroidectomy	X	Cadavers

EUS, Endoscopic ultrasonography; *NOTES,* natural orifice transluminal endoscopic surgery; *PEG,* percutaneous endoscopic gastrostomy.

of the intestinal wall. The ability to provide secure closure is one of key potential barriers to clinical NOTES (Figure 2).

Pure NOTES involves introduction of instruments through a natural orifice route only, without any transluminal assistance. The term *hybrid* is used to describe procedures that involve any type of transabdominal assistance. Hybrid NOTES can be categorized into two types: NOTES-assisted laparoscopy and laparoscopy-assisted NOTES. The critical methods are analyzed according to transluminal access routes in clinical trials.

Transvaginal access is the most frequently reported NOTES access route in clinical trials. In most cases of transvaginal NOTES procedures reported so far, surgeons have utilized a hybrid NOTES approach, in which at least one laparoscopic port has been used for insufflations, visualization, retraction, or initial dissection. This is important, at least at the initial research stage, to prevent complications. Zornig and colleagues published the first comparative study of hybrid NOTES procedures with laparoscopy in a series of 216 patients. The transvaginal technique starts with a 5-mm incision deep in the umbilicus, insufflation of the abdomen, and diagnostic laparoscopy. The average time was 52 minutes for transvaginal NOTES and 35 minutes for laparoscopy. The postoperative frequencies of sexual intercourse were the same in both patient groups. The matched-pair study further showed that transvaginal NOTES is safe, did not lead to any serious complications, and was followed by only one infection. In comparison with laparoscopy, transvaginal NOTES obviously has a better cosmetic result; produces less pain, fewer wound infections, and fewer trocar hernias; and is associated with shorter hospital stays and sick leave. The first pure transvaginal NOTES right nephrectomy—in a 58-year-old woman suffering from recurrent urinary tract infection and an atrophic right kidney—was reported by Kaouk and colleagues in 2010 (Figure 3). Other transvaginal procedures performed include appendectomy, colectomy, partial/sleeve gastrectomy, retroperitoneoscopy, liver resection, splenectomy, and renal cyst resection. The shortcomings of a transvaginal NOTES approach include applicability only to women; reported risk of injury to bladder, urethral, vulva, small bowel, colon, and rectum; and the potential risk of infertility.

Transgastric NOTES is the second most common NOTES access method. Most transgastric NOTES procedures were performed as a hybrid procedure that included the use of laparoscopic port guidance and insufflations. Pure NOTES gastrostomies are typically performed in the anterior stomach with needle knife puncture and balloon dilation. Nau and colleagues reported transgastric NOTES peritoneoscopy in a series of 130 patients. Eighty patients were enrolled for evaluation of diagnostic accuracy and utility. The diagnostic transgastric peritoneoscopy was completed in 20 patients with pancreatic head masses and found to have a 95% concordance with laparoscopic findings for assessment of peritoneal metastasis. There was no significant difference in the ability to adequately explore the four quadrants between patients with preinsufflation of the abdomen and in those without, no difference between the endoscopic and laparoscopic pressure readings of the peritoneal cavity, and no difference in pressure readings of the peritoneal cavity between patients with and without a surgical history. In the evaluation of 100 consecutive patients, the risk of bacterial contamination secondary to per-oral and transgastric entry was clinically insignificant. The use of proton pump inhibitors did not result in a higher bacterial load in the peritoneal cavity. Bingener and colleagues showed the clinical efficacy of endoscopic transluminal omental patch repair for perforated peptic ulcer. In their study, 49 patients with a perforated peptic ulcer in the gastric, duodenal, or other region of intestine underwent transluminal omental patch repair. Bingener and colleagues showed that a 10-mm-diameter ulcer opening is required for performing transluminal inspection, irrigation, and drainage and for endoscopic luminal omental patch closure. Most patients with a peptic ulcer would be theoretically eligible for a pure transluminal endoscopic or hybrid procedure. Other transgastric NOTES procedures performed, including cholecystectomy, appendectomy, full-thickness resection with

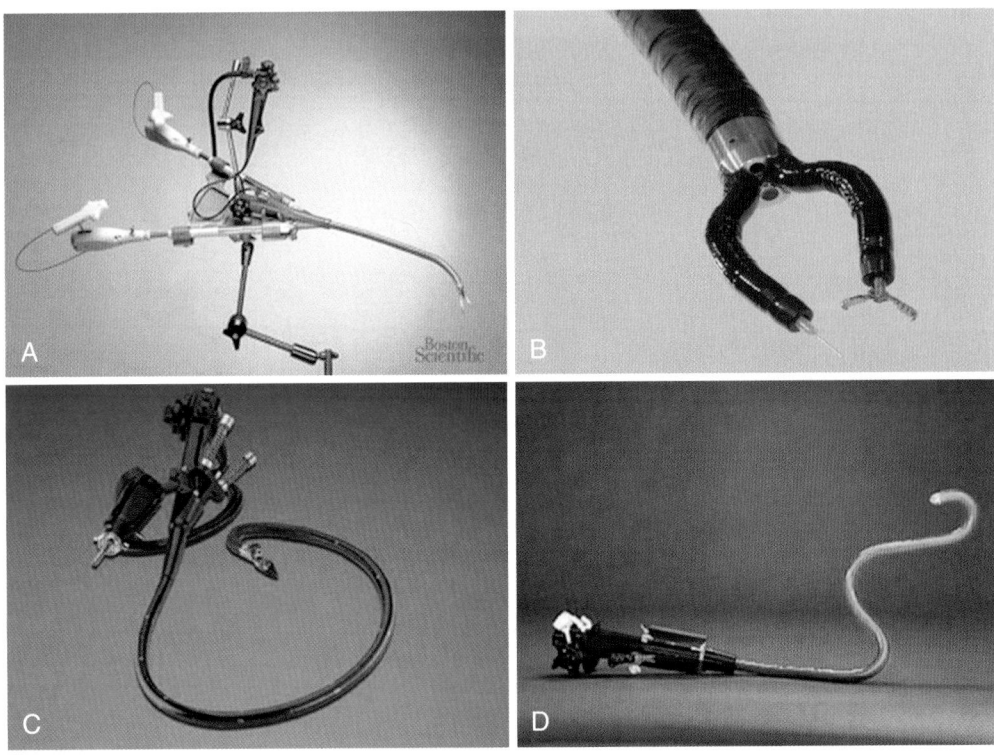

FIGURE 1 Devices for natural orifice transluminal endoscopic surgery (NOTES). **A,** New flexible endoscope for NOTES (Boston Scientific). **B,** EndoSAMURAI with two arms (Olympus Corp.). **C,** ANUBIScope (Karl Storz). **D,** TransPort (USGI Medical).

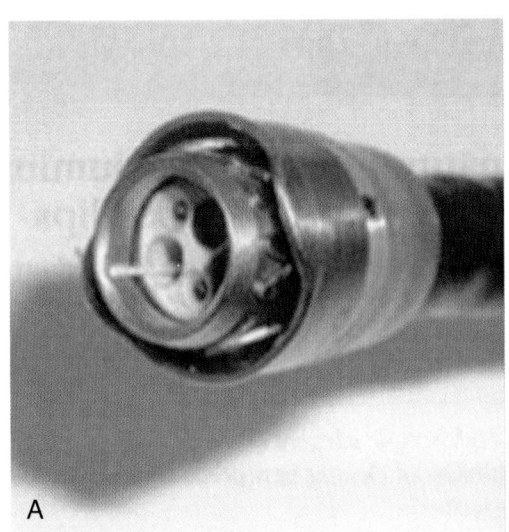

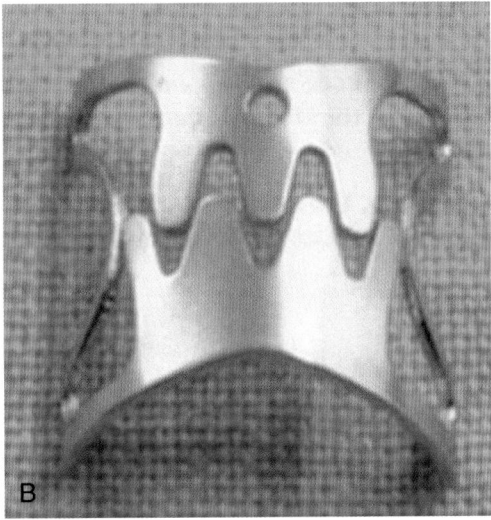

FIGURE 2 Closure devices (OVESCO, Tübingen, Germany). **A,** OTSC (Over-The-Scope Clip) Twin Grasper. **B,** OTSC Clip.

or without submucosal tunneling, liver biopsy, and endoscopic ultrasonography–guided NOTES. The lack of a foolproof device for the facile and safe closure of the gastric defect is the sole factor limiting a transgastric NOTES approach.

The first transesophageal NOTES procedures in humans was POEM, for treatment of achalasia, as reported by Inoue and colleagues in 2009. POEM is based on the esophageal submucosal tunneling technique. A long submucosal tunnel is created (mean length, 12.4 cm), followed by endoscopic myotomy of circular muscle bundles for a total length of 8.1 cm (2.0 cm in cardia). The flaps act as a seal that prevents mediastinal contamination and can be closed with various tissue-approximating devices at the conclusion of the procedure (Figure 4).

Transrectal NOTES access is increasingly being facilitated by transanal endoscopic microsurgery (TEM) platform or performed through direct transrectal trocar insertion. New developments in flexible endoscopic platforms and instruments such as flexible staplers with TEM–like platforms could enable pure NOTES colorectal surgery via the transanal route in the near future.

NOTES: WHAT WILL BE POSSIBLE IN THE NEAR FUTURE?

It should be acknowledged that NOTES is not about adapting laparoscopic concepts with its focus on triangulation; instead, it entails performing inline procedures along a single axis, as with standard flexible endoscopy. The ability to resect large portions of the gastric mucosa successfully with the endoscopic techniques has demonstrated that triangulation is not necessary for dissection. The future of NOTES will hinge on techniques and devices that facilitate inline complex procedures.

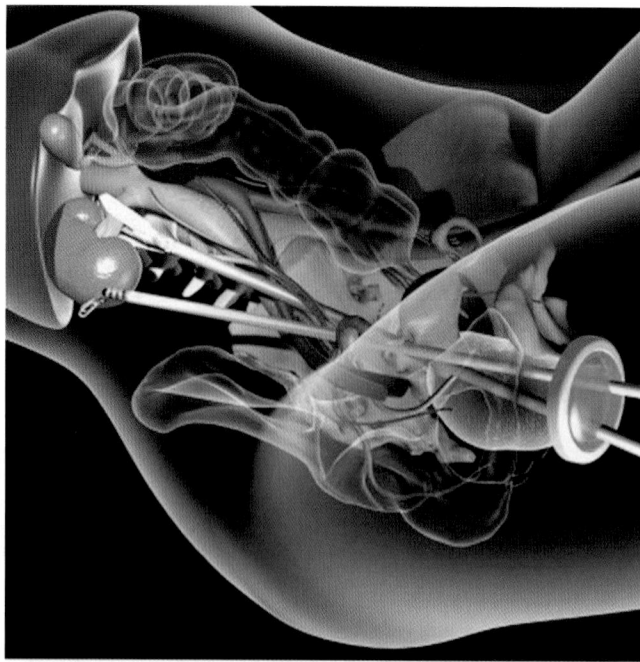

FIGURE 3   Operative illustration of transvaginal nephrectomy.

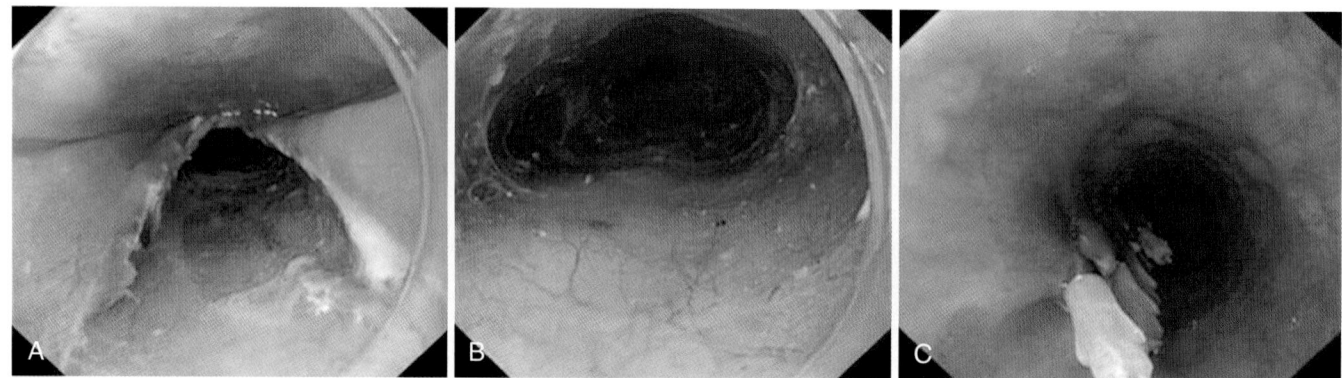

FIGURE 4   A-C, Transluminal submucosal tunneling and closure.

The spectrum of therapeutic flexible endoscopy performed by gastroenterologists inside the lumen has widened since the introduction of NOTES. However, it remains unclear who should be trained for performing NOTES and which discipline is primarily involved with NOTES. The fourth Euro-NOTES workshop yielded the consensus statements of NOTES in 2011. According to the consensus, it appears reasonable for a diagnostic approach to be performed by a gastroenterologist; a therapeutic NOTES procedure will probably be performed by a surgeon. The current situation of training surgeons in flexible endoscopy and training gastroenterologists in laparoscopic surgery cannot be regarded as an ideal solution. An ideal goal would be to achieve combined endoscopic/laparoscopic operating room suites with common wards and staff, common conferences, and a substantial volume of "crossover cases" between surgery and endoscopy.

NOTES is one of the most exciting current developments in minimally invasive endoscopic surgery. Since its theoretical conception in 2000, transluminal procedures without visible scars have been performed via natural orifices by creative endoscopists and surgeons conducting minimally invasive operations worldwide. Some NOTES procedures have become regular minimally invasive therapies at many clinical centers in some areas or countries, such as those in Europe and South America, Japan, and China. NOTES is continuing to evolve and is here to stay.

SUGGESTED READINGS

American Society of Gastrointestinal Endoscopy, Society of American Gastrointestinal and Endoscopic Surgeons: ASGE/SAGES Working Group on Natural Orifice Translumenal Endoscopic Surgery White Paper October 2005, *Gastrointest Endosc* 63:199–203, 2006.

Inoue H, Minami H, Kobayashi Y, et al: Peroral endoscopic myotomy (POEM) for esophageal achalasia, *Endoscopy* 42:265–271, 2010.

Khashab MA, Kalloo AN: NOTES: current status and new horizons, *Gastroenterology* 142(4):704–710, 2012.

Meining A, Feussner H, Swain P, et al: Natural-orifice transluminal endoscopic surgery (NOTES) in Europe: summary of the working group reports of the Euro-NOTES meeting 2010. *Endoscopy* 43:140–143, 2011.

Nau P, Ellison EC, Muscarella P Jr, et al: A review of 130 humans enrolled in transgastric NOTES protocols at a single institution, *Surg Endosc* 25:1004–1011, 2011.

Zornig C, Siemssen L, Emmermann A, et al: NOTES cholecystectomy: matched-pair analysis comparing the transvaginal hybrid and conventional laparoscopic techniques in a series of 216 patients, *Surg Endosc* 25:1822–1826, 2011.

INDEX

Page numbers followed by *f* indicate figures; *t*, tables; and *b*, boxes.